Primary Pediatric Care

PRIMARY PEDIATRIC CARE

EDITOR-IN-CHIEF

ROBERT A. HOEKELMAN, M.D.
Professor of Pediatrics
University of Rochester School of Medicine and Dentistry
Rochester, New York

CO-EDITORS

STANFORD B. FRIEDMAN, M.D.
Professor of Pediatrics
Division of Adolescent Medicine, Department of Pediatrics
Albert Einstein College of Medicine/Montefiore Medical Center
Bronx, New York

NICHOLAS M. NELSON, M.D.
Professor of Pediatrics
The Pennsylvania State University College of Medicine
The Milton S. Hershey Medical Center
Hershey, Pennsylvania

HENRY M. SEIDEL, M.D.
Professor of Pediatrics
The Johns Hopkins University School of Medicine
Baltimore, Maryland

MICHAEL L. WEITZMAN, M.D.
Edward H. Townsend Professor of Pediatrics
University of Rochester School of Medicine and Dentistry
Rochester, New York

ASSOCIATE EDITOR

MODENA E. H. WILSON, M.D., M.P.H.
Professor of Pediatrics and Health Policy Management
The Johns Hopkins University School of Medicine
Baltimore, Maryland

THIRD EDITION

with **431** *illustrations*

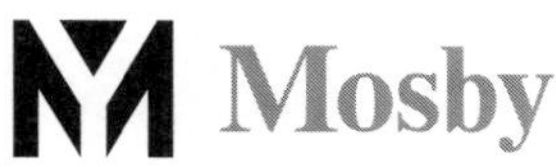

St. Louis Baltimore Boston Carlsbad Chicago Naples New York Philadelphia Portland
London Madrid Mexico City Singapore Sydney Tokyo Toronto Wiesbaden

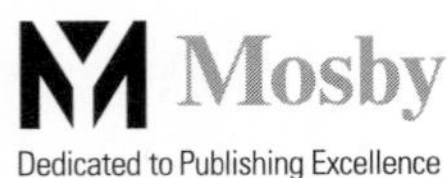

Dedicated to Publishing Excellence

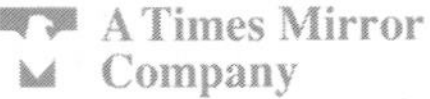

Vice President and Publisher: Anne S. Patterson
Editor: Laurel Craven
Managing Editor: Kathryn H. Falk
Developmental Editor: Carolyn M. Kruse
Project Manager: Patricia Tannian
Project Specialist: John Casey
Book Design Manager: Gail Morey Hudson
Manufacturing Manager: Dave Graybill
Cover Design: Teresa Breckwoldt

THIRD EDITION

NOTE: The indications for and dosages of medications recommended conform to practices at the present time. References to specific products are incorporated to serve only as guidelines and are not meant to exclude a practitioner's choice of other, comparable drugs. Many oral medications may be given with more scheduling flexibility than implied by the specific time intervals noted. Individual drug sensitivity and allergies must be considered in drug selection.

Every attempt has been made to ensure accuracy and appropriateness. New investigations and broader experience may alter present dosages schedules, and it is recommended that the package insert of each drug be consulted before administration. Often there is limited experience with established drugs for neonates and young children. Furthermore, new drugs may be introduced, and indications for use may change. This rapid evolution is particularly noticeable in the use of antibiotics and cardiopulmonary resuscitation. The clinician is encouraged to maintain expertise concerning appropriate medications for specific conditions.

Printed in the United States of America
Composition by The Clarinda Company
Printing/binding by Rand-McNally

Mosby–Year Book, Inc.
11830 Westline Industrial Drive
St. Louis, Missouri 63146

Library of Congress Cataloging in Publication Data

Primary pediatric care / editor-in-chief, Robert A. Hoekelman; co-editors, Stanford B. Friedman . . . [et al.]; associate editor,
Modena E.H. Wilson.—3rd ed.
p. cm.
Includes bibliographical references and index.
ISBN 0-8151-4547-0
1. Pediatrics. I. Hoekelman, Robert A.
[DNLM: 1. Pediatrics. 2. Primary Health Care. WS 100 P9526 1997]
RJ45.P673 1997
618.92—dc20
DNLM/DLC
for Library of Congress 96-28962
CIP

96 97 98 99 00 / 9 8 7 6 5 4 3 2 1

Contributors

ALICE D. ACKERMAN, M.D.

Associate Professor of Pediatrics and Anesthesiology
Vice Chair for Clinical Practice
Chief, Division of Pediatric Critical Care Medicine
Department of Pediatrics
University of Maryland School of Medicine
Baltimore, Maryland
28: Fluid Therapy

HENRY M. ADAM, M.D.

Associate Professor of Pediatrics
Albert Einstein College of Medicine
Montefiore Medical Center
Bronx, New York
25: Management of Fever

GERALD R. ADAMS, Ph.D.

Professor, Department of Family Studies
University of Guelph
Guelph, Ontario, Canada
105: Runaway Youth

ELIZABETH MELLER ALDERMAN, M.D.

Assistant Professor of Pediatrics
Division of Adolescent Medicine
Albert Einstein College of Medicine
Montefiore Medical Center
Bronx, New York
57: Child Custody

THOMAS F. ANDERS, M.D.

Professor of Psychiatry
University of California, Davis
Davis, California
85: Nightmares and Other Sleep Disturbances

JOEL M. ANDRES, M.D.

Professor and Chief
Department of Pediatric Gastroenterology
University of Florida College of Medicine
Gainesville, Florida
148: Jaundice

TRINA M. ANGLIN, M.D. Ph.D.

Section of Adolescent Medicine
Department of Pediatrics
University of Colorado
Denver, Colorado
108: Violent and Aggressive Behavior

SUSAN S. ARONSON, M.D.

Clinical Professor of Pediatrics
Medical College of Pennsylvania and Hahnemann University
Philadelphia, Pennsylvania
59: Child Care and Early Education Programs

BARABARA L. ASSELIN, M.D.

Assistant Professor of Pediatrics
Division of Pediatric Hematology/Oncology
University of Rochester School of Medicine and Dentistry
Rochester, New York
227: Leukemias

LEWIS A. BARNESS, M.D.

Professor of Pediatrics
University of South Florida College of Medicine
Tampa, Florida
130: Failure To Thrive

NANCY K. BARNETT, M.D.

Associate Professor
Departments of Pediatrics and Dermatology
The Johns Hopkins University School of Medicine
Baltimore, Maryland
111: Alopecia and Hair Shaft Anomalies
145: Hyperhidrosis
160: Pruritus
161: Rash
196: Contact Dermatitis
222: Insect Bites and Infestations

STEPHEN R. BARONE, M.D.

Instructor, Pediatrics
New York University School of Medicine
North Shore University Hospital
Manhasset, New York
221: Infectious Mononucleosis and Epstein-Barr Virus Infections

TODD F. BARRON, M.D.

Assistant Professor of Pediatrics
The Pennsylvania State University College of Medicine
The Milton S. Hershey Medical Center
Hershey, Pennsylvania
286: Increased Intracranial Pressure

JOHN BAUM, M.D.

Professor Emeritus of Medicine
University of Rochester School of Medicine and Dentistry
Rochester, New York
149: Joint Pain

WILLIAM R. BEARDSLEE, M.D.

Chairman, Department of Psychiatry
Judge Baker Children's Center;
George P. Gardner/Olga M. Monks Professor of Child Psychiatry
Harvard Medical School
Boston, Massachusetts
52: Mental Health of the Young: An Overview

MARK F. BELLINGER, M.D.

Professor of Surgery
University of Pittsburgh School of Medicine;
Chief of Pediatric Urology
Children's Hospital of Pittsburgh
Pittsburgh, Pennsylvania
164: Scrotal Swelling
229: Meatal Ulceration

ROBERT J. BERKOWITZ, D.D.S.

Associate Professor
Departments of Clinical Dentistry and Pediatrics
Chief, Division of Pediatric Dentistry
University of Rochester School of Medicine and Dentistry;
Director, Pediatric Dentistry Program
Eastman Dental Center
Rochester, New York
22: Prevention of Dental Caries

CHESTON M. BERLIN, Jr., M.D.

University Professor of Pediatrics
Professor of Pharmacology
The Pennsylvania State University College of Medicine
The Milton S. Hershey Medical Center
Hershey, Pennsylvania
219: Iatrogenic Disease
278: Drug Overdose

WALLACE F. BERMAN, M.D.

Associate Professor of Pediatrics
Chief, Pediatric Gastroenterology
Medical College of Virginia
Richmond, Virginia
135: Gastrointestinal Hemorrhage

ANDREW S. BERNSTEIN, M.D.

Medical Director
The Young People's Health Connection
Public Health Department of Baltimore City
Baltimore, Maryland
290: Rape

ROBERT J. BIDWELL, M.D.

Associate Professor of Pediatrics
Director of Adolescent Medicine
John A. Burns School of Medicine
University of Hawaii
Honolulu, Hawaii
100: Homosexuality: Challenges of Treating Lesbian and Gay Adolescents

GLENN H. BOCK, M.D.

Associate Professor of Pediatrics
Uniformed Services of the Health Sciences
Bethesda, Maryland;
Medical Co-Director
Pediatric Kidney Center
Fairfax Hospital for Children
Falls Church, Virginia
210: Hemolytic-Uremic Syndrome
212: Henoch-Schönlein Purpura
269: Urinary Tract Infections
284: Hypertensive Emergencies
291: Acute Renal Failure

JOSEPH E. BOGGS, Ph.D.

Assistant Professor
Department of Psychology
DePauw University
Greencastle, Indiana
93: Consultation and Referral for Behavioral and Developmental Problems

WILLIAM E. BOYLE, Jr., M.D.

Professor of Pediatrics and Community and Family Medicine
Dartmouth Medical School
Hanover, New Hampshire
6: The Pediatric History

NANCY E. BRAVERMAN, M.D.

Postdoctoral Fellow, Department of Pediatrics
The Johns Hopkins University School of Medicine
Baltimore, Maryland
20:3: Screening—Recognition of Genetic-Metabolic Diseases by Clinical Diagnosis and Screening

T. BERRY BRAZELTON, M.D.

Professor Emeritus of Pediatrics
Harvard Medical School
Boston, Massachusetts
74: Developmental Approach to Behavioral Problems

DAVID I. BROMBERG, M.D.

Assistant Professor of Pediatrics and Psychiatry
University of Maryland School of Medicine
Baltimore, Maryland
75: Interviewing Children
78: Colic
288: Pneumothorax and Pneumomediastinum

JOHN G. BROOKS, M.D.

Professor and Chairman
Department of Pediatrics
Dartmouth Medical School
Hanover, New Hampshire
265: Sudden Infant Death Syndrome

MICHAEL G. BURKE, M.D.

Assistant Professor, Department of Pediatrics
The Johns Hopkins University School of Medicine;
Chairman, Department of Pediatrics
St. Agnes Hospital
Baltimore, Maryland
128: Extremity Pain

DEBORAH E. CAMPBELL, M.D.

Associate Professor of Pediatrics
Albert Einstein College of Medicine;
Acting Director, Division of Neonatology
Montefiore Medical Center
Bronx, New York
20:7: Screening—Screening for Drugs

PRESTON W. CAMPBELL, M.D.

Department of Pediatrics
Division of Pulmonary Medicine
Vanderbilt University School of Medicine
Nashville, Tennessee
247: Pneumonia

MARY T. CASERTA, M.D.

Assistant Professor
Department of Pediatrics
University of Rochester School of Medicine and Dentistry
Rochester, New York
287: Meningococcemia

ROBERT W. CHAMBERLIN, M.D., M.P.H.

Adjunct Professor
School of Health and Human Services
University of New Hampshire
Durham, New Hampshire;
Adjunct Professor of Pediatrics
Dartmouth Medical School
Hanover, New Hampshire
5: Community-wide Approaches to Promoting the Health and Development of Families and Children

PATRICIA M. CHUTE, Ed.D.

Director, Cochlear Implant Center
Manhattan Eye, Ear, and Throat Hospital
New York, New York
137: Hearing Loss

EDWARD B. CLARK, M.D.

Professor and Chair
Department of Pediatrics
University of Utah School of Medicine
Salt Lake City, Utah
115: Cardiac Arrhythmias
138: Heart Murmurs
142: High Blood Pressure in Infants, Children, and Adolescents
195: Congenital Heart Disease

HARVEY J. COHEN, M.D., Ph.D.

Professor and Chair
Department of Pediatrics
Stanford University School of Medicine;
Chief of Staff
Lucile Salter Packard Children's Hospital at Stanford
Palo Alto, California
113: Anemia and Pallor

MICHAEL I. COHEN, M.D.

Professor and Chairman
Department of Pediatrics
Albert Einstein College of Medicine
Montefiore Medical Center
Bronx, New York
95: Challenges of Delivering Health Care to Adolescents

MICHAEL W. COHEN, M.D.

Clinical Professor
Director, Attention Disorders Center
Department of Pediatrics
University of Arizona College of Medicine
Tucson, Arizona
82: Enuresis

CYNTHIA H. COLE, M.D.

Assistant Professor of Pediatrics
Tufts University Medical School
Boston, Massachusetts
143: Hirsutism, Hypertrichosis, and Precocious Sexual Hair Development
146: Hypotonia

ARNOLD H. COLODNY, M.D.

Clinical Professor of Surgery
Harvard Medical School;
Senior Surgeon
Children's Hospital
Boston, Massachusetts
250: Pyloric Stenosis

COLLEEN L. COOK, M.D.

Assistant Professor of Pediatrics
The Pennsylvania State University College of Medicine
The Milton S. Hershey Medical Center
Hershey, Pennsylvania
293: Status Asthmaticus

W. CARL COOLEY, M.D.

Associate Professor of Pediatrics
Director, Center for Genetics and Child Development
Dartmouth Medical School
Hanover, New Hampshire
61: Family-Centered Care in Pediatric Practice

R. STEVEN COUCH, M.D.

Assistant Professor of Pediatrics
Vanderbilt University School of Medicine;
Assistant Medical Director for Pediatrics
Vanderbilt Stallworth Rehabilitation Hospital
Nashville, Tennessee
38: Cerebral Palsy

SUSAN M. COUPEY, M.D.

Professor of Pediatrics
Albert Einstein College of Medicine;
Associate Director, Division of Adolescent Medicine
Montefiore Medical Center
Bronx, New York
99: Drug, Alcohol, and Tobacco Abuse
106: Adolescent Sexuality

DAVID R. CUNNINGHAM, Ph.D.

Professor of Surgery (Audiology)
Director, Division of Communicative Disorders
University of Louisville School of Medicine
Louisville, Kentucky
20:9: Screening—Auditory Screening

JOSEPH R. CUSTER, M.D.

Associate Professor of Pediatrics
Director, Pediatric Critical Care Medicine
University of Michigan School of Medicine
Ann Arbor, Michigan
292: Shock
Appendix B: Special Procedures

PHILIP W. DAVIDSON, Ph.D.

Professor of Pediatrics and Psychiatry (Psychology)
University of Rochester School of Medicine and Dentistry;
Director, Strong Center for Developmental Disabilities
Rochester, New York
10: Communication with Parents and Patients
Appendix D: Common Psychological and Educational Tests

PAMELA K. DEN BESTEN, D.D.S.

Associate Professor
Department of Growth and Development
Chair, Division of Pediatric Dentistry
University of California
San Francisco, California
22: Prevention of Dental Caries

MICHAEL D. DETTORE, D.O.

Assistant Professor of Pediatrics
The Pennsylvania State University College of Medicine
The Milton S. Hershey Medical Center
Hershey, Pennsylvania
293: Status Asthmaticus

JOHN M. DIAMOND, M.D.

Associate Professor of Psychiatry
East Carolina University School of Medicine
Greenville, North Carolina
103: Mood Disorders in Children and Adolescents

CYNTHIA A. DOERR, M.D.

Children's Hospital and Health Center
Division of Infectious Diseases
San Diego, California
267: Tuberculosis

JAY N. DOLITSKY, M.D.

Assistant Professor of Otolaryngology
New York Medical College;
Director of Medical Student Education
New York Eye and Ear Infirmary
New York, New York
204: Foreign Bodies of the Ear, Nose, Airway, and Esophagus

JOHN H. DOSSETT, M.D.

Professor of Pediatrics
The Pennsylvania State University College of Medicine
The Milton S. Hershey Medical Center
Hershey, Pennsylvania
17: Immunizations
162: Recurrent Infections
180: Acquired Immunodeficiency Syndrome (AIDS) and Human Immunodeficiency Virus (HIV) Infection
197: Contagious Exanthematous Diseases

ANA M. DUARTE, M.D.

Director, Division of Dermatology
Children's Skin Center
Miami Children's Hospital
Miami, Florida
186: Atopic Dermatitis
255: Seborrheic Dermatitis

HOWARD DUBOWITZ, M.D.

Associate Professor of Pediatrics
University of Maryland School of Medicine
Baltimore, Maryland
56: Child Abuse and Neglect

DAVID L. DUDGEON, M.D.

Professor of Surgery and Pediatrics
Case Western Reserve University
Cleveland, Ohio
207: Gastrointestinal Obstruction

REGGIE E. DUERST, M.D.

Associate Professor of Pediatrics
University of Rochester School of Medicine and Dentistry
Rochester, New York
157: Petechiae and Purpura

WILLIAM A. DURBIN, Jr., M.D.

Professor of Pediatrics and Medicine
University of Massachusetts Medical School
Worcester, Massachusetts
118: Cough

PAUL H. DWORKIN, M.D.

Professor and Associate Chairman of Pediatrics
Head, Division of General Pediatrics
University of Connecticut School of Medicine
Farmington, Connecticut;
Director/Chairman of Pediatrics
Saint Francis Hospital and Medical Center
Hartford, Connecticut
20:1: Screening—General Considerations
72: School Learning Problems and Developmental Differences

DAVID R. EDELSTEIN, M.D.

Clinical Associate Professor
Department of Otorhinolaryngology
Cornell University Medical College;
Chief, Nasal and Sinus Service
Department of Otolaryngology
Manhattan Eye, Ear, and Throat Hospital
New York, New York
127: Epistaxis

WENDI G. EHRMAN, M.D.

Assistant Professor of Pediatrics
Medical College of Wisconsin
Milwaukee, Wisconsin
234: Obesity

MARVIN S. EIGER, M.D.

Associate Clinical Professor of Pediatrics
The Mount Sinai School of Medicine;
Attending Pediatrician
The Beth Israel Medical Center
New York, New York
16:2: Nutrition—Feeding of Infants and Children

ROBERT E. EMERY, Ph.D.

Professor and Director of Clinical Training
Department of Psychology
University of Virginia
Charlottesville, Virginia
58: Children and Divorce

NORBERT B. ENZER, M.D.

Professor and Chairman, Department of Psychiatry
Michigan State University
East Lansing, Michigan
87: Phobias

LEONARD D. ERON, Ph.D.

Professor of Psychology
University of Michigan;
Research Scientist
Institute for Social Research
Ann Arbor, Michigan
66: Violence in Television and Video Games: Influence on Children and Adolescents

ALLEN ESKENAZI, M.D.

Assistant Professor of Pediatrics
Division of Hematology/Oncology
University of Maryland School of Medicine
Baltimore, Maryland
166: Splenomegaly
220: Idiopathic Thrombocytopenia

JEFFREY M. EWIG, M.D.

Assistant Professor of Pediatrics
Albert Einstein College of Medicine
Montefiore Medical Center
Bronx, New York
36: Cystic Fibrosis

†MARY FARREN, R.N., M.S.

Senior Nursing Educator
Department of Community Health Nursing
University of Rochester School of Nursing
Rochester, New York
73: Nursing Roles in School Health

MARIANNE E. FELICE, M.D.

Professor and Vice Chair, Department of Pediatrics
Director, Division of Adolescent Medicine
University of Maryland Medical Systems
Baltimore, Maryland
24: The Ill Child
290: Rape

MARTIN A. FINKEL, D.O.

Professor of Clinical Pediatrics
Acting Chairman, Department of Pediatrics
University of Medicine and Dentistry of New Jersey
School of Osteopathic Medicine
Medical Director, Center for Children's Support
Stratford, New Jersey
56: Child Abuse and Neglect

PHILIP FIREMAN, M.D.

Professor of Pediatrics
University of Pittsburgh School of Medicine;
Director, Department of Allergy, Immunology, and Rheumatology
Children's Hospital of Pittsburgh
Pittsburgh, Pennsylvania
185: Asthma

MARTIN FISHER, M.D.

Associate Professor of Pediatrics
New York University School of Medicine;
Chief, Division of Adolescent Medicine
North Shore University Hospital
Manhasset, New York
98: Anorexia and Bulimia Nervosa

LOIS T. FLAHERTY, M.D.

Adjunct Associate Professor
Department of Psychiatry
Division of Child and Adolescent Psychiatry
University of Maryland School of Medicine
Baltimore, Maryland
168: Strange Behavior

THOMAS P. FOLEY, Jr. M.D.

Professor of Pediatrics
Director, Division of Endocrinology, Metabolism, and Diabetes Mellitus
University of Pittsburgh School of Medicine
Pittsburgh, Pennsylvania
218: Hypothyroidism

†Deceased.

GILBERT B. FORBES, M.D.

Professor Emeritus of Pediatrics
University of Rochester School of Medicine and Dentistry
Rochester, New York
16:1 Nutrition—Nutritional Requirements

LINDA M. FORSYTHE, M.D.

Instructor in Pediatrics
Harvard Medical School;
Clinical Assistant, Child Psychiatry
Massachusetts General Hospital
Boston, Massachusetts
79: Conduct Disorders

SHARON L. FOSTER, Ph.D.

Professor of Psychology
California School of Professional Psychology
San Diego, California
86: Peer Relationship Problems

HOWARD R. FOYE, Jr., M.D.

Clinical Associate Professor of Pediatrics
University of Rochester School of Medicine and Dentistry
Rochester, New York
15: Anticipatory Guidance

MARY PAT FRANCISCO, M.D.

Fellow in Pediatric Gastroenterology
Department of Pediatrics
University of Florida College of Medicine
Gainesville, Florida
148: Jaundice

T. EMMETT FRANCOEUR, M.D., C.M. F.R.C.P. (C)

Associate Professor of Pediatrics
McGill University School of Medicine
Montreal, Quebec, Canada
117: Constipation

ELAINE M. FRANK, Ph.D.

Assistant Professor
Speech-Language Pathology and Audiology
University of South Carolina
School of Public Health
Columbia, South Carolina
19: Language and Speech Assessment

CARL A. FRANKEL, M.D., F.A.C.S.

Pediatric Ophthalmologist
Harrisburg, Pennsylvania
163: The Red Eye
167: Strabismus
236: Ocular Foreign Bodies
237: Ocular Trauma
249: Preseptal and Orbital Cellulitis

CHRISTOPHER N. FRANTZ, M.D.

Professor of Pediatrics
Chief, Pediatric Hematology/Oncology
University of Maryland School of Medicine
Baltimore, Maryland
220: Idiopathic Thrombocytopenia

STANFORD B. FRIEDMAN, M.D.

Professor of Pediatrics
Albert Einstein College of Medicine
Montefiore Medical Center
Bronx, New York
24: The Ill Child
76: Concepts of Psychosomatic Illness
93: Consultation and Referral for Behavioral and Developmental Problems
96: Conversion Reactions in Adolescents

JOHN H. FUGATE, M.D.

Pediatric Intensivist
Children's Healthcare-Minneapolis and North Memorial Medical Center
Minneapolis, Minnesota
292: Shock

KEITH J. GALLAHER, M.D.

Clinical Assistant Professor of Pediatrics
University of North Carolina
Chapel Hill, North Carolina;
Attending Neonatologist
Cape Fear Valley Medical Center
Fayetteville, North Carolina
46: Signs and Symptoms of Neonatal Illness

DAISY CAPISTRANO GARCIA, M.D.

Attending Neonatologist
Hutzel Hospital
Detroit, Michigan
49: Neonatal Drug Abstinence Syndrome

JOHN P. GEARHART, M.D.

Professor of Urology
The Johns Hopkins University School of Medicine;
Director of Pediatric Urology
The Brady Urological Institute
Baltimore, Maryland
217: Hypospadias, Epispadias, and Cryptorchism

HARRY L. GEWANTER, M.D.

Assistant Medical Director
Director of Pediatric Rheumatology
Children's Hospital
Richmond, Virginia
224: Juvenile Arthritis

KATHLEEN L. GIFFORD, R.N.

Neonatal Research Nurse
Department of Pediatrics
The Pennsylvania State University College of Medicine
The Milton S. Hershey Medical Center
Hershey, Pennsylvania
44:4: Neonatal Adaptations—Adjustment Period

JULIUS G. GOEPP, M.D.

Assistant Director, Pediatric Emergency Medicine
Department of Pediatrics
The Johns Hopkins University School of Medicine
Baltimore, Maryland
264: Stomatitis
274: Dehydration

MELANIE A. GOLD, D.O.

Assistant Professor
Department of Pediatrics
University of Pittsburgh Medical School
Pittsburgh, Pennsylvania
55: Gay- and Lesbian-Parented Families

ARCHIE S. GOLDEN, M.D., M.P.H.

Associate Professor of Pediatrics
The Johns Hopkins University School of Medicine;
Chairman, Department of Pediatrics
The Johns Hopkins Bayview Medical Center
Baltimore, Maryland
193: Cleft Lip and Cleft Palate

DONALD A. GOLDMANN, M.D.

Professor of Pediatrics
Division of Infectious Diseases
Children's Hospital Medical Center
Harvard Medical School
Boston, Massachusetts
208: Giardiasis
246: Pinworm Infestations

ROBERT E. GREENBERG, M.D.

Professor, Department of Pediatrics
University of New Mexico School of Medicine
Albuquerque, New Mexico
199: Diabetes Mellitus
275: Diabetic Ketoacidosis

JOSEPH GREENSHER, M.D.

Professor of Pediatrics
State University of New York Health Science Center
Stony Brook, New York;
Medical Director and Associate Chairman
Department of Pediatrics
Winthrop-University Hospital
Mineola, New York
23: Injury Prevention
Appendix A: Pediatric Basic and Advanced Life Support

SYLVIA P. GRIFFITHS, M.D.

Professor Emeritus of Clinical Pediatrics
Columbia University College of Physicians and Surgeons
New York, New York
252: Rheumatic Fever

LINDSEY K. GROSSMAN, M.D.

Associate Professor and Chief
Ambulatory Pediatrics
The Ohio State University;
Associate Medical Director, Ambulatory Services
Children's Hospital
Columbus, Ohio
119: Dental Stains
153: Malocclusion
214: Herpes Infections

JOHN H. GUNDY, M.D.

Associate Clinical Professor of Pediatrics
Yale University School of Medicine
New Haven, Connecticut
7: The Pediatric Physical Examination

CAROLINE BREESE HALL, M.D.

Professor of Pediatrics and Medicine
University of Rochester School of Medicine and Dentistry
Rochester, New York
152: Lymphadenopathy
189: Bronchiolitis
273: Croup (Acute Laryngotracheobronchitis)
280: Epiglottitis

DAVID E. HALL, M.D.

Consulting Pediatrician
Scottish Rite Children's Medical Center
Atlanta, Georgia
262: Sports Injuries
282: Head Injuries

WILLIAM J. HALL, M.D.

Professor of Medicine and Pediatrics
Vice Chair, Department of Medicine
University of Rochester School of Medicine and Dentistry;
Chief, Department of Medicine
Rochester General Hospital
Rochester, New York
189: Bronchiolitis
273: Croup (Acute Laryngotracheobronchitis)
280: Epiglottitis

J. ALEX HALLER, Jr., M.D.

Professor of Surgery
Pediatrics and Emergency Medicine
The Johns Hopkins University School of Medicine
Baltimore, Maryland
242: Pectus Excavatum and Pectus Carinatum
281: Esophageal Burns

MARILYNN HAYNIE, M.D.

Harvard Medical School
Boston, Massachusetts
35: Children Assisted by Medical Technology

THOMAS A. HAZINSKI, M.D.

Professor and Vice-Chairman
Department of Pediatrics
Vanderbilt University School of Medicine
Nashville, Tennessee
178: Wheezing
247: Pneumonia

ALICE B. HEISLER, M.D.

Assistant Professor of Pediatrics and Child Psychiatry
Walter P. Carter Center
University of Maryland School of Medicine
Baltimore, Maryland
89: Self-Stimulating Behaviors

FRED J. HELDRICH, M.D.

Associate Professor of Pediatrics
The Johns Hopkins University of School of Medicine
Director, Pediatric Residency Training Program
St. Agnes Hospital
Baltimore, Maryland
125: Dysuria
243: Pertussis (Whooping Cough)
253: Rocky Mountain Spotted Fever

NEIL E. HERENDEEN, M.D.

Assistant Professor of Pediatrics
University of Rochester School of Medicine and Dentistry
Rochester, New York
182: Animal Bites
198: Cystic and Solid Masses of the Face and Neck

DONNA M. HILL, Ph.D., R.N., C.S.

Associate Professor of Clinical Nursing
University of Rochester School of Nursing
Rochester, New York
73: Nursing Roles in School Health

ROBERT A. HOEKELMAN, M.D.

Professor of Pediatrics
University of Rochester School of Medicine and Dentistry
Rochester, New York
3: Child Health Supervision
6: The Pediatric History
10: Communication with Parents and Patients
20:2: Screening—The Physical Examination As a Screening Test
134: Foot and Leg Problems
266: Tonsillectomy and Adenoidectomy

GEORGE W. HOLCOMB III, M.D.

Assistant Professor
Departments of Surgery and Pediatrics
Vanderbilt University Medical Center
Nashville, Tennessee
32: Minimally Invasive Surgery

NEIL A. HOLTZMAN, M.D., M.P.H.

Professor of Pediatrics
The Johns Hopkins University School of Medicine
Baltimore, Maryland
20:3: Screening—Recognition of Genetic-Metabolic Diseases by Clinical Diagnosis and Screening

KYLE D. HOUSER, M.Ed., M.A.

Department of Pediatrics
Strong Center for Developmental Disabilities
University of Rochester School of Medicine and Dentistry
Rochester, New York
Appendix D: Common Psychological and Educational Tests

BARBARA J. HOWARD, M.D.

Assistant Professor of Pediatrics
The Johns Hopkins University School of Medicine
Baltimore, Maryland
226: Labial Adhesions

SHARON GENEVIEVE HUMISTON, M.D., M.P.H.

Assistant Professor
Departments of Emergency Medicine, Pediatrics, and Community and Preventive Medicine
University of Rochester School of Medicine and Dentistry
Rochester, New York
279: Envenomations

HEIDI M. INDERBITZEN, Ph.D.

Assistant Professor of Psychology
University of Nebraska at Lincoln
Lincoln, Nebraska
86: Peer Relationship Problems

MICHAEL JELLINEK, M.D.

Harvard Medical School
Boston, Massachusetts
79: Conduct Disorders

JERRI ANN JENISTA, M.D.

Attending Pediatrician
Department of Pediatrics and Emergency Medicine
St. Joseph Mercy Hospital
Ann Arbor, Michigan
203: Enterovirus Infections
254: Roseola and Related Diseases: HHV-6 and HHV-7 Infections

ALAIN JOFFE, M.D., M.P.H.

Associate Professor and Director of Adolescent Medicine
The Johns Hopkins University School of Medicine
Baltimore, Maryland
112: Amenorrhea
122: Dysmenorrhea
150: Limp
173: Vaginal Bleeding
174: Vaginal Discharge
258: Sexually Transmitted Diseases

DENNIS L. JOHNSON, M.D.

Professor of Surgery and Pediatrics
Director of Pediatric Neurosurgery
The Pennsylvania State University College of Medicine
The Milton S. Hershey Medical Center
Hershey, Pennsylvania
215: Hydrocephalus

R. JOSEPH JOPLING, M.D.

Pediatric Practitioner
Willow Creek Pediatrics
Salt Lake City, Utah
21: Counseling Families on a Healthy Life-style

NICHOLAS JOSPE, M.D.

Associate Professor
Division of Pediatric Endocrinology
Strong Memorial Hospital
University of Rochester School of Medicine and Dentistry
Rochester, New York
216: Hyperthyroidism

LINDA J. JUSZCZAK, R.N., M.S., M.P.H.

Senior Teaching Associate in Pediatrics
Project Director, School-based Health Centers
North Shore University Hospital
Cornell University Medical College
Manhasset, New York
39: The Chronically Ill and Disabled Child in School

RUTH K. KAMINER, M.D.

Professor of Pediatrics
Albert Einstein College of Medicine;
Associate Director for Medical Services
Children's Evaluation and Rehabilitation Center
Rose F. Kennedy Center
Bronx, New York
18: Identification of Developmental Delays and the Early Intervention System

AUBREY J. KATZ, M.D.

Chief, Pediatric Gastroenterology
Newton-Wellesley Hospital
Center for Pediatric Gastroenterology
Waltham, Massachusetts
206: Gastrointestinal Allergy
209: Gluten-Sensitive Enteropathy (Celiac Sprue)

BRADLEY B. KELLER, M.D.

Assistant Professor of Pediatrics and Physiology
University of Rochester School of Medicine and Dentistry
Rochester, New York
283: Heart Failure

KENNETH KENIGSBERG, M.D.

Assistant Clinical Professor of Surgery
Cornell University Medical College;
Chief, Division of Pediatric Surgery
North Shore University Hospital
Manhasset, New York
109: Abdominal Distention
141: Hepatomegaly

JOHN H. KENNELL, M.D.

Professor of Pediatrics
Case Western Reserve University School of Medicine;
Chief, Division of Child Development
Rainbow Babies and Children's Hospital
Cleveland, Ohio
44:6: Neonatal Adaptations—Pediatric Support for Parents

THOMAS J. KENNY, Ph.D.

Professor of Pediatrics
University of Maryland School of Medicine
Baltimore, Maryland
34: Mental Retardation

MARK D. KILGUS, M.D., Ph.D.

Assistant Professor
Department of Neuropsychiatry and Behavior Sciences
University of South Carolina School of Medicine
Columbia, South Carolina
80: Cross-Sex Behavior

MARSHALL H. KLAUS, M.D.

Adjunct Professor of Pediatrics
University of California
San Francisco, California
44:6: Neonatal Adaptations—Pediatric Support for Parents

MAURICE D. KOGUT, M.D.

Professor and Chair
Department of Pediatrics
Wright State University School of Medicine
Dayton, Ohio
285: Hypoglycemia

DAVID N. KORONES, M.D.

Assistant Professor of Pediatrics
University of Rochester School of Medicine and Dentistry
Rochester, New York
113: Anemia and Pallor

SABINE KOST-BYERLY, M.D.

Assistant Professor
Department of Anesthesiology and Critical Care Medicine
The Johns Hopkins University School of Medicine
Baltimore, Maryland
26: Management of Acute Pain in Children

LEONARD R. KRILOV, M.D.

Associate Professor of Pediatrics
Cornell University Medical College;
Chief, Pediatric Infectious Diseases
North Shore University Hospital
Manhasset, New York
192: Chronic Fatigue Syndrome
221: Infectious Mononucleosis and Epstein-Barr Virus Infections

ROBERT K. KRITZLER, M.D.

Clinical Assistant Professor of Pediatrics
University of Maryland School of Medicine;
Physician-in-Chief
Kaiser Permanente Medical Group
Baltimore, Maryland
165: Sexual Developmental Alterations

MICHAEL A. LACORTE, M.D.

Professor of Clinical Pediatrics
New York University School of Medicine;
Chairman, Department of Pediatrics
The Brooklyn Hospital Center
Brooklyn, New York
20:4: Screening—Cardiac Screening

JOHN M. LEVENTHAL, M.D.

Professor of Pediatrics and Child Study Center
Yale University School of Medicine
New Haven, Connecticut
65: Sexual Abuse of Children

SUSAN E. LEVITZKY, M.D.

Assistant Clinical Professor of Pediatrics
Albert Einstein College of Medicine
New York, New York
144: Hoarseness

SAMUEL M. LIBBER, M.D.

Assistant Professor of Pediatrics
The Johns Hopkins University School of Medicine
Baltimore, Maryland
158: Polyuria

GREGORY S. LIPTAK, M.D., M.P.H.

Associate Professor of Pediatrics
University of Rochester School of Medicine and Dentistry
Rochester, New York
33: Physical Disability and Chronic Illness
38: Cerebral Palsy
200: Diaper Rash
260: Spina Bifida

GEORGE A. LITTLE, M.D.

Professor of Pediatrics and Obstetrics/Gynecology
Dartmouth-Hitchcock Medical Center
Hanover, New Hampshire
42: The Fetus at Risk
43:2: Perinatal Medicine—Perinatal Transport

DONALD LONDORF, M.D., C.M., F.R.C.P. (C), F.A.C.E.P.

Assistant Professor of Emergency Medicine
University of Rochester School of Medicine and Dentistry
Rochester, New York
279: Envenomations

DONALD P. LOOKINGBILL, M.D.

Professor, Department of Medicine
Chief, Division of Dermatology
The Pennsylvania State University College of Medicine
The Milton S. Hershey Medical Center
Hershey, Pennsylvania
179: Acne
187: Bacterial Skin Infections
202: Drug Eruptions
270: Verrucae (Warts)

STEVEN E. LUCKING, M.D.

Associate Professor of Pediatrics
Chief, Division of Pediatric Critical Care
The Pennsylvania State University College of Medicine
The Milton S. Hershey Medical Center
Hershey, Pennsylvania
271: Airway Obstruction
277: Drowning and Near-Drowning

HAROLD L. LUPER, Ph.D.

Professor, Department of Audiology and Speech Pathology
University of Tennessee
Knoxville, Tennessee
90: Stuttering

JED G. MAGEN, D.O.

Assistant Professor and Director
Psychiatry Residency Training Program
Michigan State University
East Lansing, Michigan
87: Phobias

LOIS A. MAIMAN, Ph.D.

Chief, Prevention Research Branch
Division of Epidemiology, Statistics, and Prevention Research
National Institute of Child Health and Human Development
National Institutes of Health
Bethesda, Maryland
12: Compliance with Pediatric Health Care Recommendations

M. JEFFREY MAISELS, M.B., B.Ch.

Clinical Professor of Pediatrics
Wayne State University School of Medicine and
University of Michigan Medical School;
Chairman, Department of Pediatrics
William Beaumont Hospital
Royal Oak, Michigan
44:1: Neonatal Adaptations—Peripartum Considerations
44:4: Neonatal Adaptations—Adjustment Period
48: Critical Neonatal Illnesses

MARILYN J. MANCO-JOHNSON, M.D.

Professor, Department of Pediatrics
University of Colorado Health Sciences Center;
Director, Mountain States Regional Hemophilia Center
Denver, Colorado
276: Disseminated Intravascular Coagulation

RONALD V. MARINO, D.O., M.P.H.

Associate Professor of Clinical Pediatrics
State University of New York College of Medicine
at Stony Brook;
Director, General Pediatrics
Winthrop University Hospital
Mineola, New York
71: School Absenteeism and School Refusal

ROBERT W. MARION, M.D.

Associate Professor of Pediatrics
Director, Division of Genetics
Albert Einstein College of Medicine
Montefiore Medical Center
Bronx, New York
268: Umbilical Anomalies

KEITH H. MARKS, M.D., Ph.D.

Professor of Pediatrics
Division of Newborn Medicine
The Pennsylvania State University College of Medicine
The Milton S. Hershey Medical Center
Hershey, Pennsylvania
48: Critical Neonatal Illnesses

THOMAS A. MASSARO, M.D., Ph.D.

Harrison Foundation Professor of Medicine and Law
Department of Pediatrics
University of Virginia
Charlottesville, Virginia
4: Legal and Ethical Issues for the Pediatrician

REBECCA RIBOVICH MATSAKIS, M.D.

Assistant Professor of Pediatrics
The Johns Hopkins University School of Medicine
Baltimore, Maryland
251: Reye Syndrome

ÅKE MATTSSON, M.D.

Professor of Psychiatry
East Carolina University School of Medicine
Greenville, North Carolina
103: Mood Disorders in Children and Adolescents
104: Suicidal Behavior in Children and Adolescents

LYNNE G. MAXWELL, M.D.

Associate Professor of Anesthesiology, Critical Care Medicine, and Pediatrics
The Johns Hopkins University School of Medicine
Baltimore, Maryland
8: Preoperative Assessment
26: Management of Acute Pain in Children
248: Postoperative Management of the Pediatric Outpatient: Surgical and Anesthetic Aspects

JAY H. MAYEFSKY, M.D., M.P.H.

Associate Professor of Pediatrics
Finch University of Health Sciences
The Chicago Medical School;
Senior Attending Physician
Division of Ambulatory Pediatrics
Cook County Children's Hospital
Chicago, Illinois
124: Dyspnea

ELIZABETH R. McANARNEY, M.D.

Professor and Chair
Department of Pediatrics
University of Rochester School of Medicine and Dentistry
Rochester, New York
107: Adolescent Pregnancy and Parenthood

MARGARET C. McBRIDE, M.D.

Associate Professor of Neurology and Pediatrics
University of Rochester School of Medicine and Dentistry
Rochester, New York
256: Seizure Disorders
294: Status Epilepticus

LAURA K. McCORMICK, Dr. P.H.

Assistant Professor of Behavioral Sciences
University of Texas Health Science Center—Houston
School of Public Health
Houston, Texas
68: School Health Education

HIRAM L. McDADE, Ph.D.

Associate Professor of Speech-Language and Audiology
University of South Carolina
School of Public Health
Columbia, South Carolina
19: Language and Speech Assessment

DIANE L. McDONALD, M.D.

Instructor, Department of Pediatrics
The Johns Hopkins University School of Medicine
Baltimore, Maryland
121: Dizziness and Vertigo
170: Syncope

ROBERT H. McLEAN, M.D.

Professor of Pediatrics
University of Maryland School of Medicine
Baltimore, Maryland
126: Edema

JAMES W. McMANAWAY III, M.D.

Associate Professor of Ophthalmology and Pediatrics
The Pennsylvania State University College of Medicine
The Milton S. Hershey Medical Center
Hershey, Pennsylvania
163: The Red Eye
167: Strabismus
175: Visual Problems
236: Ocular Foreign Bodies
237: Ocular Trauma
249: Preseptal and Orbital Cellulitis

RAKESH MENON, M.D.

Clinical Instructor in Pediatrics
State University of New York Health Science Center at Brooklyn
Brooklyn, New York
20:4: Screening—Cardiac Screening

RUTH J. MESSINGER, M.S.W.

Coordinator, Social Work Services
Department of Pediatrics
University of Rochester School of Medicine and Dentistry
Rochester, New York
10: Communication with Parents and Patients

GEOFFREY MILLER, M.D., M.R.C.P., F.R.A.C.P.

Professor of Pediatrics and Neurology
Baylor College of Medicine
Houston, Texas
38: Cerebral Palsy

MARVIN E. MILLER, M.D.

Professor of Pediatrics and Obstetrics/Gynecology
Wright State University School of Medicine;
Director of Medical Genetics and Birth Defects
Children's Medical Center
Dayton, Ohio
40: Approaches to Genetic Diseases
45: Skin Lesions of the Neonate
129: Facial Dysmorphism

HOWARD C. MOFENSON, M.D.

Professor of Pediatrics and Emergency Medicine
State University of New York Health Science Center
Stony Brook, New York;
Director, Long Island Regional Poison Control Center
Winthrop-University Hospital
Mineola, New York
23: Injury Prevention
Appendix A: Pediatric Basic and Advanced Life Support

RICHARD T. MOXLEY III, M.D.

Professor of Neurology and Pediatrics
University of Rochester School of Medicine and Dentistry;
Director of Neuromuscular Disease Center
Strong Memorial Hospital Medical Center
Rochester, New York
37: Muscular Dystrophy

DENNIS J. MUJSCE, M.D.

Associate Professor of Pediatrics
Division of Newborn Medicine
The Pennsylvania State University College of Medicine
The Milton S. Hershey Medical Center
Hershey, Pennsylvania
50: High-Risk Follow-up

PHILIP R. NADER, M.D.

Professor and Director
Community Pediatrics
University of California at San Diego
San Diego, California
67: Overview of School Health and School Health Program Goals

NICHOLAS M. NELSON, M.D.

Professor of Pediatrics
The Pennsylvania State University College of Medicine
The Milton S. Hershey Medical Center
Hershey, Pennsylvania
9: Structural and Functional Analysis of Body Systems
43:1: Perinatal Medicine—Overview
44:1: Neonatal Adaptations—Peripartum Considerations
44:2: Neonatal Adaptations—Physiological Status of the Healthy Infant
44:3: Neonatal Adaptations—Recovery Period
44:4: Neonatal Adaptations—Adjustment Period
44:5: Neonatal Adaptations—Establishment of Equilibrium
50: High-Risk Follow-up

KATHERINE NITZ, Ph.D.

Assistant Professor, Department of Pediatrics
University of Maryland School of Medicine
Baltimore, Maryland
34: Mental Retardation

ROBERT J. NOLAN, Jr., M.D.

Assistant Professor of Pediatrics
Deputy Chairman for Education and Training
The University of Texas Health Science Center at San Antonio
San Antonio, Texas
289: Poisoning

C. JEAN OGBORN, M.D.

Assistant Professor, Department of Pediatrics
Subdepartment of Pediatric Emergency Medicine
The Johns Hopkins University School of Medicine
Baltimore, Maryland
147: Irritability

KAREN OLNESS, M.D.

Professor of Pediatrics, Family Medicine and International Health
Division of General Academic Pediatrics
Case Western Reserve University School of Medicine
Cleveland, Ohio
11: Cultural Issues in Primary Pediatric Care

ENRIQUE M. OSTREA, Jr., M.D.

Professor of Pediatrics
Wayne State University School of Medicine
Detroit, Michigan
49: Neonatal Drug Abstinence Syndrome

CHARLES N. PAIDAS, M.D., F.A.C.S., F.A.A.P.

Assistant Professor
Departments of Surgery, Pediatrics, Oncology, and Anesthesia and Critical Care Medicine
The Johns Hopkins University School of Medicine
Baltimore, Maryland
248: Postoperative Management of the Pediatric Outpatient: Surgical and Anesthetic Aspects

JUDITH S. PALFREY, M.D.

Chief, Division of General Pediatrics
Children's Hospital
Boston, Massachusetts
35: Children Assisted by Technology

JAMES PALIS, M.D.

Assistant Professor of Pediatrics
University of Rochester School of Medicine and Dentistry
Rochester, New York
223: Iron Deficiency Anemia

CHARLES PALMER, M.B., Ch.B.

Associate Professor of Pediatrics
The Pennsylvania State University College of Medicine
The Milton S. Hershey Medical Center
Hershey, Pennsylvania
47: Common Neonatal Illnesses

FRANCES C. PAOLINI-MASUCCI, M.S.W.

Assistant Director for Social Work Services
Department of Pediatrics
Montefiore Medical Center
Bronx, New York
97: Counseling Parents of Adolescents

GUY S. PARCEL, Ph.D.

Professor and Director
Center for Health Promotion Research and Development
University of Texas Health Science Center
Houston, Texas
68: School Health Education

SIMON C. PARISIER, M.D.

Professor and Chairman, Department of Otolaryngology
Manhattan Eye, Ear, and Throat Hospital
New York, New York
137: Hearing Loss

MARGARETE PARRISH, Ph.D., M.S.W., L.C.S.W.(C)

Assistant Professor of Pediatrics and Social Work
University of Maryland School of Medicine
Baltimore, Maryland
290: Rape

EVAN G. PATTISHALL III, M.D.

Associate Professor of Pediatrics
The Pennsylvania State University College of Medicine
The Milton S. Hershey Medical Center
Hershey, Pennsylvania
191: Chickenpox

DAVID S. PELLEGRINI, Ph.D.

Practicing Psychologist
Washington, D.C.
77: Prediction of Adult Behavior from Childhood

ROBERT A. PENDERGRAST, Jr., M.D., M.P.D.

Assistant Professor of Pediatrics
The Johns Hopkins University School of Medicine
Baltimore, Maryland;
Pediatrics and Adolescent Medicine Practitioner
Patuxent Medical Group
Columbia, Maryland
114: Back Pain

JAY A. PERMAN, M.D.

Professor and Chair
Department of Pediatrics
Medical College of Virginia
Richmond, Virginia
213: Hepatitis

ELLEN C. PERRIN, M.D.

Department of Pediatrics
University of Massachusetts School of Medicine
Worcester, Massachusetts
55: Gay- and Lesbian-Parented Families
64: Teaching Parents about Effective Discipline

SHERIDAN PHILLIPS, Ph.D.

Associate Professor of Psychiatry
University of Maryland School of Medicine
Baltimore, Maryland
92: Options for Psychosocial Intervention with Children and Adolescents
93: Consultation and Referral for Behavioral and Developmental Problems

MICHAEL E. PICHICHERO, M.D.

Professor of Microbiology and Immunology, Pediatrics, and Medicine
University of Rochester School of Medicine and Dentistry
Rochester, New York
225: Kawasaki Disease
263: Staphylococcal Toxic Shock Syndrome

SERGIO PIOMELLI, M.D.

Professor of Pediatrics
Columbia University College of Physicians and Surgeons
New York, New York
20:6: Screening—Screening for Lead Poisoning

S. MICHAEL PLAUT, Ph.D.

Associate Professor of Psychiatry
University of Maryland School of Medicine
Baltimore, Maryland
14: Assessing the Medical Literature

CHARLES E. PLESS, M.D.

Montreal Children's Hospital
Montreal, Quebec, Canada
2: Morbidity and Mortality among the Young

IVAN B. PLESS, M.D.

Professor of Pediatrics, Epidemiology, and Biostatistics
McGill University School of Medicine;
Director, Community Pediatric Research
Montreal Children's Hospital
Montreal, Quebec, Canada
2: Morbidity and Mortality among the Young

LESLIE P. PLOTNICK, M.D.

Associate Professor of Pediatrics
The Johns Hopkins University School of Medicine
Baltimore, Maryland
158: Polyuria
165: Sexual Developmental Alterations

KEITH R. POWELL, M.D.

Professor and Associate Chair for Clinical Affairs
Department of Pediatrics
University of Rochester School of Medicine and Dentistry
Rochester, New York
31: Antimicrobial Therapy
230: Meningitis

GREGORY E. PRAZAR, M.D.

Pediatric Practitioner
Exeter Pediatric Associates
Exeter, New Hampshire
84: Lying and Stealing
91: Temper Tantrums and Breath-Holding Spells
96: Conversion Reactions in Adolescents

RICHARD OWEN PROCTOR, M.D., M.P.H.&T.M. (Tropical Medicine)

Regional Director, Region 6/5S
Texas Department of Health
Houston, Texas
241: Parasitic Infestations

EVA G. RADEL, M.D.

Director, Division of Pediatric Hematology/Oncology
Albert Einstein College of Medicine
Montefiore Medical Center
Bronx, New York
29: Blood Products and Their Uses
211: Hemophilia and Other Hereditary Bleeding Disorders

ROBERT F. REISS, M.D.

Division of Laboratory Hematology and Transfusion Medicine
Columbia University College of Physicians and Surgeons
New York, New York
20:5: Screening—Screening for Anemia

GEORGE A. REKERS, Ph.D.

Professor of Neuropsychiatry and Behavioral Science
University of South Carolina School of Medicine
Columbia, South Carolina
80: Cross-Sex Behavior

JULIUS B. RICHMOND, M.D.

John D. McArthur Professor Emeritus of Health Policy
Harvard Medical School
Boston, Massachusetts
52: Mental Health of the Young: An Overview

SARAH M. RODDY, M.D.

Associate Professor of Pediatrics and Neurology
Loma Linda University School of Medicine
Loma Linda, California
155: Nonconvulsive Periodic Disorders
256: Seizure Disorders
294: Status Epilepticus

LANCE E. RODEWALD, M.D.

Associate Professor of Emergency Medicine and Pediatrics
Chief, Division of Pediatric Emergency Medicine
University of Rochester School of Medicine and Dentistry
Rochester, New York
12: Compliance with Pediatric Health Care Recommendations

PAUL T. ROGERS, M.D.

Instructor, Department of Pediatrics
The Johns Hopkins University School of Medicine
Baltimore, Maryland
201: Down Syndrome: Managing the Child and Family

BERYL J. ROSENSTEIN, M.D.

Professor of Pediatrics
Director, Cystic Fibrosis Center
The Johns Hopkins University School of Medicine
Baltimore, Maryland
116: Chest Pain
140: Hemoptysis
172: Torticollis

EDWARD J. RULEY, M.D.

Professor of Pediatrics
Uniformed Services of the Health Sciences
Bethesda, Maryland;
Medical Co-Director, Pediatric Kidney Center
Fairfax Hospital for Children
Falls Church, Virginia
20:8: Screening—Use of Urinalysis and the Urine Culture in Screening
139: Hematuria
159: Proteinuria
183: Anuria/Oliguria
233: Nephrotic Syndrome
235: Obstructive Uropathy and the Vesicoureteral Reflux

OLLE JANE Z. SAHLER, M.D.

Adjunct Professor of Pediatrics
University of Rochester School of Medicine and Dentistry
Rochester, New York
51: Theories and Concepts of Development As They Relate to Pediatric Practice
Appendix D: Common Psychological and Educational Tests

MORTON E. SALOMON, M.D.

Associate Professor of Pediatrics and Emergency Medicine
Albert Einstein College of Medicine;
Director of Adult and Pediatric Emergency Services
Montefiore Medical Center and North Central Bronx Hospital
Bronx, New York
169: Stridor

EDWARD J. SALTZMAN, M.D.

Clinical Professor of Pediatrics
University of Miami School of Medicine
Miami, Florida
1: The Health Care Delivery System

JOHN SARGENT, M.D.

Associate Professor of Psychiatry and Pediatrics
Director, General and Child and Adolescent Psychiatry Training
University of Pennsylvania School of Medicine
Philadelphia, Pennsylvania
60: Family Interactions: Children Who Have Unexplained Physical Symptoms

RICHARD M. SARLES, M.D.

Professor and Director, Division of Child and Adolescent Psychiatry
University of Maryland School of Medicine
Baltimore, Maryland
89: Self-Stimulating Behaviors
93: Consultation and Referral for Behavioral and Developmental Problems
154: Nervousness

LAWRENCE A. SCHACHNER, M.D.

Professor of Pediatrics and Dermatology
Director, Division of Pediatric Dermatology
University of Miami School of Medicine
Miami, Florida
186: Atopic Dermatitis
255: Seborrheic Dermatitis

ERIC A. SCHAFF, M.D.

Associate Professor of Family Medicine and Pediatrics
University of Rochester School of Medicine and Dentistry
Rochester, New York
41: Contraception and Abortion

L.R. SCHERER III, M.D.

Clinical Associate Professor of Pediatric Surgery
Director of Kiwanis-Riley Trauma Life Center
Indiana University School of Medicine
Indianapolis, Indiana
295: Thermal Injuries

THERESE K. SCHMALBACH, M.D.

Director of Clinical Research
Vertex Pharmaceuticals
Cambridge, Massachusetts
30: Clinical Pharmacology

BARTON D. SCHMITT, M.D.

Professor of Pediatrics
University of Colorado School of Medicine;
Director, General Pediatrics Consultations
The Children's Hospital
Denver, Colorado
81: Encopresis

MARCIE B. SCHNEIDER, M.D.

Assistant Professor of Pediatrics
Cornell University Medical College;
Associate Chief, Division of Adolescent Medicine
North Shore University Hospital
Manhasset, New York
39: The Chronically Ill and Disabled Child in School

S. KENNETH SCHONBERG, M.D.

Professor of Pediatrics
Albert Einstein College of Medicine
Montefiore Medical Center
Bronx, New York
20:7: Screening—Screening for Drugs
99: Drug, Alcohol, and Tobacco Abuse

KENNETH C. SCHUBERTH, M.D.

Associate Professor of Pediatrics
The Johns Hopkins University School of Medicine
Baltimore, Maryland
181: Allergic Rhinitis

CINDY L. SCHWARTZ, M.D.

Associate Professor of Oncology and Pediatrics
Associate Director of Pediatric Oncology for Clinical Programs
The Johns Hopkins University School of Medicine
Baltimore, Maryland
190: Cancers in Childhood

KATHLEEN B. SCHWARZ, M.D.

Associate Professor of Pediatrics
The Johns Hopkins University School of Medicine
Baltimore, Maryland
213: Hepatitis

EDWARDS P. SCHWENTKER, M.D.

Associate Professor of Orthopaedics and Rehabilitation
The Pennsylvania State University College of Medicine;
Medical Director of Rehabilitation
The Milton S. Hershey Medical Center
Hershey, Pennsylvania
239: Osteomyelitis
257: Septic Arthritis

GEORGE B. SEGEL, M.D.

Professor of Pediatrics, Medicine, and Genetics
Associate Chair for Academic Affairs
Department of Pediatrics
Chief, Division of Pediatric Genetics
University of Rochester School of Medicine and Dentistry
Rochester, New York
152: Lymphadenopathy

HENRY M. SEIDEL, M.D.

Professor of Pediatrics
The Johns Hopkins University School of Medicine
Baltimore, Maryland
13: The Art of Consultation
62: Health Needs of Parents
136: Headache
154: Nervousness
217: Hypospadias, Epispadias, and Cryptorchism

WILLIAM A. SHINE, Ed.D.

Superintendent of Schools
Great Neck, New York
70: School Behavior Problems

DAVID M. SIEGEL, M.D., M.P.H.

Associate Professor of Pediatrics and Medicine
University of Rochester School of Medicine and Dentistry
Rochester, New York
149: Joint Pain
228: Lyme Disease

ARNOLD T. SIGLER, M.D.

Associate Professor of Pediatrics
The Johns Hopkins University School of Medicine
Baltimore, Maryland
131: Fatigue and Weakness

EDWARD M. SILLS, M.D.

Associate Professor of Pediatrics
The Johns Hopkins University School of Medicine;
Director, Pediatric Rheumatology
The Johns Hopkins Hospital
Baltimore, Maryland
238: Osteochondroses
261: Spinal Deformities

NANCY E. SIMEONSSON, R.N., M.P.H.

Director of Nursing Services
Frank Porter Graham Child Development Center
Chapel Hill, North Carolina
20:12: Screening—Developmental Surveillance and Intervention

RUNE J. SIMEONSSON, Ph.D., M.S.P.H.

Professor of Education, Research Professor of Psychology
University of North Carolina
School of Education
Chapel Hill, North Carolina
20:12: Screening—Developmental Surveillance and Intervention

MARK D. SIMMS, M.D.

Associate Professor of Pediatrics
Medical College of Wisconsin
Milwaukee, Wisconsin
53: Foster Care and Adoption

JEAN C. SMITH, M.D.

Clinical Associate Professor of Pediatrics
University of North Carolina
Chapel Hill, North Carolina
110: Abdominal Pain

SHIRLEY A. SMOYAK, Ph.D., R.N.

Professor of Planning and Public Policy
Rutgers—The State University of New Jersey;
Director, Public Health Program
The Bloustein School of Planning and Public Policy
Senior Researcher, Institute for Health, Health Care Policy and Aging Research
New Brunswick, New Jersey
54: Changing American Families

DAVID M. SNYDER, M.D.

Associate Clinical Professor of Pediatrics
University of California at San Francisco School of Medicine
San Francisco, California;
Medical Director, Developmental and Behavioral Pediatrics
Valley Children's Hospital
Fresno, California
74: Developmental Approach to Behavioral Problems

MARY V. SOLANTO, Ph.D.

Associate Professor of Pediatrics
Albert Einstein College of Medicine
Bronx, New York;
Senior Psychologist
Schneider Children's Hospital
Long Island Jewish Medical Center
New Hyde Park, New York
69: Attention Deficit/Hyperactivity Disorder

BARBARA STARFIELD, M.D.

University Distinguished Professor of Pediatrics
The Johns Hopkins University School of Medicine;
Head, Division of Health Policy
The Johns Hopkins University School of Hygiene and Public Health
Baltimore, Maryland
1: The Health Care Delivery System

JEFFREY R. STARKE, M.D.

Associate Professor of Pediatrics
Baylor College of Medicine
Houston, Texas
267: Tuberculosis

CAROLE A. STASHWICK, M.D., Ph.D.

Assistant Professor of Pediatrics
Dartmouth Medical School
Hanover, New Hampshire
177: Weight Loss

DAVID M. STEINHORN, M.D.

Assistant Professor of Pediatrics and Anesthesiology
SUNY at Buffalo
Buffalo, New York
135: Gastrointestinal Hemorrhage

CATHERINE STEVENS-SIMON, M.D.

Assistant Professor of Pediatrics
University of Colorado Health School of Medicine
Denver, Colorado
107: Adolescent Pregnancy and Parenthood

R. SCOTT STRAHLMAN, M.D.

Instructor, Department of Pediatrics
The Johns Hopkins University School of Medicine
Baltimore, Maryland;
Clinical Director of Pediatrics
Columbia Medical Plan
Columbia and Frederick, Maryland
184: Appendicitis
205: Fractures and Dislocations

LAURENCE I. SUGARMAN, M.D.

Clinical Assistant Professor, Department of Pediatrics
University of Rochester School of Medicine and Dentistry
Rochester, New York
27: Hypnosis and Biofeedback Therapy

CIRO V. SUMAYA, M.D.

Professor of Pediatrics and Pathology
The University of Texas Health Science Center;
San Antonio, Texas
221: Infectious Mononucleosis and Epstein-Barr Virus Infections

DENNIS M. SUPER, M.D., M.P.H.

Associate Professor of Pediatrics
Case Western Reserve University
Cleveland, Ohio
44:5: Neonatal Adaptations—Establishment of Equilibrium
245: Phimosis

AMY L. SUSS, M.D.

Assistant Professor of Pediatrics
State University of New York Health Science Center at Brooklyn;
Director, Division of Adolescent Medicine
Children's Medical Center
Brooklyn, New York
83: Fire-setting

PETER G. SZILAGYI, M.D., M.P.H.

Associate Professor of Pediatrics
University of Rochester School of Medicine and Dentistry;
Chief, Ambulatory Pediatrics
Children's Hospital at Strong
Rochester, New York
182: Animal Bites
198: Cystic and Solid Masses of the Face and Neck

PHILIP E. THUMA, M.D.

Associate Professor of Pediatrics
The Pennsylvania State University College of Medicine
The Milton S. Hershey Medical Center
Hershey, Pennsylvania
194: The Common Cold
244: Pharyngitis and Tonsillitis

MARTIN H. ULSHEN, M.D.

Professor of Pediatrics and Nutrition
Chief, Division of Gastroenterology
University of North Carolina School of Medicine
Chapel Hill, North Carolina
120: Diarrhea and Steatorrhea
151: Loss of Appetite
176: Vomiting

ÉLISE W. VAN DER JAGT, M.D., M.P.H.

Associate Professor of Pediatrics and Critical Care
University of Rochester School of Medicine and Dentistry
Rochester, New York
132: Fever
133: Fever of Unknown Origin

ROBERT C. VANNUCCI, M.D.

Professor of Pediatrics
The Pennsylvania State University College of Medicine
The Milton S. Hershey Medical Center
Hershey, Pennsylvania
188: Brain Tumors

SUSAN VIG, Ph.D.

Assistant Professor of Pediatrics
Albert Einstein College of Medicine;
Senior Psychologist
Children's Evaluation and Rehabilitation Center
Rose F. Kennedy Center
Bronx, New York
18: Identification of Developmental Delays and the Early Intervention System

WALTER J. WADLINGTON, LL.B.

James Madison Professor of Law
University of Virginia School of Law
Charlottesville, Virginia
4: Legal and Ethical Issues of Pediatric Medicine

ALLEN R. WALKER, M.D.

Assistant Professor of Pediatrics
Director, Pediatric Emergency Medicine
The Johns Hopkins University School of Medicine
Baltimore, Maryland
272: Coma

ROBERT F. WARD, M.D.

Assistant Professor of Otolaryngology
Cornell University Medical College;
Attending Physician
Department of Otolaryngology
The New York Hospital;
Assistant Attending Physician
Manhattan Eye, Ear, and Throat Hospital
New York, New York
204: Foreign Bodies of the Ear, Nose, Airway, and Esophagus

RICHARD C. WASSERMAN, M.D., M.P.H.

Associate Professor of Pediatrics
University of Vermont College of Medicine
Burlington, Vermont
20:10: Screening—Vision Screening

KRISTI WATTERBERG, M.D.

Associate Professor of Pediatrics
The Pennsylvania State University College of Medicine
The Milton S. Hershey Medical Center
Hershey, Pennsylvania
46: Signs and Symptoms of Neonatal Illness

IRVING B. WEINER, Ph.D.

Professor of Psychiatry and Behavioral Medicine
University of South Florida College of Medicine
Tampa, Florida
88: Psychosis
102: Juvenile Delinquency

MICHAEL H. WEISS, M.D.

Clinical Associate Professor of Otolaryngology
State University of New York Health Science Center at Brooklyn;
Director, Division of Otolaryngology
Maimonides Medical Center
Brooklyn, New York
137: Hearing Loss

MARK D. WEIST, Ph.D.

Assistant Professor of Psychiatry
University of Maryland at Baltimore
Baltimore, Maryland
92: Options for Psychosocial Intervention with Children and Adolescents

ESTHER H. WENDER, M.D.

Clinical Professor of Pediatrics
Albert Einstein College of Medicine
Bronx, New York;
Director, Child Health Services
Westchester County Department of Health
Hawthorne, New York
69: Attention Deficit/Hyperactivity Disorder
101: Interviewing Adolescents

STEVEN L. WERLIN, M.D.

Professor of Pediatrics
Director of Pediatric Gastroenterology
Medical College of Wisconsin
Milwaukee, Wisconsin
123: Dysphagia

JOHN SCOTT WERRY, M.D.

Professor Emeritus of Psychiatry
University of Auckland
Auckland, New Zealand
171: Tics

CHARLES F. WHITTEN, M.D.

Distinguished Professor Emeritus of Pediatrics
Associate Dean for Special Programs
Director, Comprehensive Sickle Cell Center
The Wayne State University School of Medicine
Detroit, Michigan
20:11: Screening—Sickle Cell Conditions

DONNA E. WIENER, M.D.

Assistant Professor of Pediatrics
Division of Pediatric Education
Montefiore Medical Center
Albert Einstein College of Medicine
Bronx, New York
95: Challenges of Delivering Health Care to Adolescents

RICKEY L. WILLIAMS, M.D., M.P.H.

Clinical Lecturer in Pediatrics
University of Arizona
Tucson, Arizona
63: Latchkey Children: Children in Self-Care
240: Otitis Media and Otitis Externa
259: Sinusitis

CRAIG M. WILSON, M.D.

Assistant Professor in Pediatrics, Geographic Medicine, and Microbiology
University of Alabama at Birmingham
Birmingham, Alabama
208: Giardiasis
246: Pinworm Infestations

MODENA E.H. WILSON, M.D., M.P.H.

Professor of Pediatrics and Health Policy and Management
The Johns Hopkins University School of Medicine
Baltimore, Maryland
156: Odor (Unusual Urine and Body)

BEATRICE L. WOOD, Ph.D.

Assistant Professor in Psychiatry and Pediatrics
State University of New York at Buffalo
Buffalo, New York
51: Theories and Concepts of Development As They Relate to Pediatric Practice

KATHLEEN A. WOODIN, M.D.

Assistant Professor of Pediatrics
University of Rochester School of Medicine and Dentistry
Rochester, New York
Appendix C: Miscellaneous Values

JEROME Y. YAGER, M.D.

Associate Professor of Pediatrics
Royal University Hospital
Saskatoon, Saskatchewan, Canada
188: Brain Tumors

W. SAM YANCY, M.D.

Clinical Professor of Pediatrics
Associate Clinical Professor of Psychiatry
Duke University Medical Center
Durham, North Carolina
94: Adolescence

MYRON YASTER, M.D.

Associate Professor of Anesthesia/Critical Care Medicine and Pediatrics
The Johns Hopkins University School of Medicine;
Director, Pediatric Pain Service
Children's Center, The Johns Hopkins Hospital
Baltimore, Maryland
8: Preoperative Assessment
26: Management of Acute Pain in Children
248: Postoperative Management of the Pediatric Outpatient: Surgical and Anesthetic Aspects

MICHAEL W. YOGMAN, M.D.

Assistant Professor of Pediatrics
Tufts University Medical School
Boston, Massachusetts
74: Developmental Approach to Behavioral Problems

RICHARD S.K. YOUNG, M.D., M.P.H.

Associate Clinical Professor of Pediatrics and Neurology
Yale University;
Chair, Department of Pediatrics
Hospital of Saint Raphael
New Haven, Connecticut
231: Meningoencephalitis

Foreword

Primary care has become the recognized term for the field of general medicine practiced largely in the office and community. The term now is highly visible, whereas 2 decades ago it was scarcely known. Our nation's need for more primary care doctors is the subject of great debate, as is how to accomplish this. In contrast to 2 decades ago, primary care has achieved academic respectability; both faculty and practitioners are in demand. It is a field whose time in the sun is now. This textbook, *Primary Pediatric Care,* now in its third edition, has been one of the major forces leading to acceptance of the field because of its contribution to the knowledge base necessary to educate students, residents, fellows, and practitioners in the field. It recognizes that the care of children is broad and complex and requires the ability to synthesize biological and psychosocial data, to have skills of communication, and to understand, as the editors state, "the determinants and reflections of health and disease."

This text also provides essential information about the health care system, as well as knowledge about promotion of health and prevention of disease, aspects of pediatric practice that account for nearly half of pediatric visits. It deals with complex medical-social issues such as substance abuse, contraception and abortion, adoption, children of gay or lesbian parents, school problems, child abuse, and delinquency—topics difficult to find in traditional pediatric texts—but does not neglect presentation of the traditional clinical problems. Its focus is always on prevention and on diagnosis and treatment of disease presenting in the office or primary care setting rather than in the hospital, although some of these conditions, especially if not diagnosed and treated early, require hospitalization. This ability to deal broadly and comprehensively with child health distinguishes the primary care pediatrician. This text provides the knowledge to allow pediatricians to fulfill this role effectively.

In the past, much of this typical information was gained after starting in practice, if ever. Today there is a research-based knowledge of many of these complex issues. This up-to-date text documents this research base, essential for anyone providing continuing health care for children.

Textbooks, similar to all species, have a primary task—survival in a changing world. To have reached a third edition, *Primary Pediatric Care* demonstrates survival skills in today's rapidly changing world. It provides the primary care pediatrician, as well as the student, resident, fellow, and other practitioners, with the knowledge to survive and to thrive, and more important, to provide health care of high quality to children—the hope for the future of our human species.

Robert J. Haggerty, M.D.

Professor and Chair Emeritus
Department of Pediatrics
University of Rochester
School of Medicine and Dentistry

Preface

The practice of pediatrics has become increasingly complicated over the years, as knowledge of the etiology, pathophysiology, and management of physical, emotional, behavioral, and social ills has developed more rapidly and fully.

Although the dimensions of pediatrics have grown, the education of the pediatrician has remained, for the most part, disease-oriented and pathophysiological in substance. Educators, despite the recommendations made by the Task Force on Pediatric Education in 1978, have demonstrated minimal awareness of the gap between this disease orientation and the actual practice of primary health care, and they have made only token efforts to adjust teaching programs to reflect the actual practice of the majority of pediatricians. In fact, the pathophysiological priority has been maintained in the belief that, given a sound disease-oriented experience, the primary care provider can acquire the other, softer, "easier" knowledge of health care "on the job." This belief is unjustified.

Knowledge of pathophysiology is essential to the understanding of disease and of normalcy; however, it is not sufficient in itself to ensure success in the management of illness. An understanding of illness requires both an understanding of health per se and of the greater complexities of health.

The purpose of this text is to provide much of the pertinent information concerning the *determinants and reflections of health and of disease*. The primary provider of health care to the young should be in command of this information, which constitutes a body of knowledge not now conveniently available to the student and practitioner in one repository. It may seem more subjective than the "harder" pathophysiological knowledge base and, therefore, less scientific. It is not. Indeed, its variables are infinite and its experiments more difficult to control. Although pathophysiological knowledge is treated throughout this text, the book focuses on the *determinants* of health and disease; it attempts to be comprehensive only in regard to this body of knowledge. The reader is referred to other sources when information in greater depth in other areas is required. Cited references to scientific publications are used, and contributors have been asked to identify and clarify controversial issues.

The scope of this text, then, is different from that of traditional pediatric texts in that *all* aspects of *health* care are considered. The breadth and depth of the discussion of *illness,* however, are limited to that information which the primary care provider needs to function effectively in his or her role. The rarer diseases and the esoteric points in etiological pathophysiological and therapeutic considerations of the more common disease are not included here. The message is that the physical and emotional health of the child can be adequately maintained by the primary care provider (1) through well-child visits, which focus on prevention and early detection of disease and of psychosocial dysfunction, and (2) through competent management of acute and chronic illness with or without the help of other professionals.

In using this text, our readers are asked to keep in mind the following five questions: (1) What does the primary care provider need to know about the condition or disease being described to recognize it? (2) How should the condition be managed? (3) When should consultation be sought or referral to a specialist be made? (4) What can the primary care provider expect the consultant to do for the patient? and (5) What role should the primary care provider play in the management of care after a referral has been made? Certain general considerations to guide one's thinking include prevention, screening, and emergency management, as well as collaborative care, follow-up care, and costs. Family, community, environmental, and political influences on the presentation and outcome of the condition also must be considered.

We hope that this book will provide *all* primary health care practitioners much of the information required to understand and manage the various problems they encounter in caring for the young. It would be extremely difficult, if not impossible, for any one text to provide all the information such practitioners require. We do not pretend to do so but urge the reader (student or practitioner) to seek that information not found herein from references we have provided or from other comprehensive pediatric textbooks that emphasize different elements of the health care of the young.

This textbook would not have been published without the help and support of many persons. The names and affiliations of the 281 contributing authors are given in the list of contributors.

Our publishers provided us with the essentials editors need: opportunity, direction, proficiency, provocation, criticism, and, above all, reassurance and patience. Laurel Craven, Kathryn H. Falk, Carolyn M. Kruse, Robin Sutter, Jennifer Byington, and John Casey gave us these and more.

Extensive editorial comment and direction were given by Sydney A. Sutherland. Her assistance in ensuring the seemingly impossible—the smooth and continual communication among authors, editors, and publishers—has been especially appreciated. A special thanks also goes to Mrs. Francine Cheese for editorial support and to Mary Sharkey for her diligent editorial help.

We thank all of these good people for their interest, expertise, and understanding.

Robert A. Hoekelman
Stanford B. Friedman
Nicholas M. Nelson
Henry M. Seidel
Michael Weitzman

Introduction

Robert A. Hoekelman

There is no doubt that those who are concerned with the delivery of child health care face serious difficulties in finding the resources and mechanisms to ensure that all children in need of preventive, maintenance, and curative services receive them. No matter how the pediatric health care pie is sliced, as it currently exists, all the appetites will not be satisfied. This is true for those who seek these services and even more so for the greater numbers who are in need yet do not recognize that need or do not have the resources to seek the appropriate care.

Any review of health care needs and prospects for meeting them demands an assessment of the services that are required, how these can be organized and delivered effectively and efficiently, who will deliver these services, and how these persons can be prepared to do so.

Traditionally, primary care pediatricians have conducted high-volume practices in solo or partnership arrangements. They have provided preventive services and health maintenance supervision and have managed acute minor illnesses on an ambulatory basis. Only a small part of their efforts, however, have been spent in the diagnosis and treatment of serious illness in the hospital, for which most of their postgraduate training prepared them. These problems have increasingly been referred to subspecialty pediatricians located in large medical centers, either because primary care pediatricians have not had the time to deal with them or because their knowledge and skills in the management of severe illness have atrophied from disuse.

Most pediatricians have learned to do what they do through on-the-job experience rather than through formal training, albeit this has changed to some extent in recent years with increasing emphasis being placed on ambulatory care training. To many, the content of private practice comes somewhat as a surprise. Some pediatricians are not satisfied with this role and turn to subspecialty training and practice, but most adjust quickly and find primary care practice extremely rewarding.

There are, however, forces coming to bear on the future of primary pediatric practice over which the individual physician has little or no control. These forces are as follows:

1. The incidence of serious disease in childhood is decreasing because of public and individual preventive health measures: therefore the number of these illnesses occurring in a single practice is diminishing.
2. The reproductive behavior of the population is changing. The use of contraceptive devices and the liberalization of abortion laws have decreased the birth rate significantly, particularly in the populations served by most pediatricians. Infant mortality, prematurity, and morbidity have diminished as well, and the regionalization of perinatal care has transferred the management of most high-risk newborn infants from the primary care pediatrician to neonatologists in regional centers.
3. The rapid increase in medical knowledge and technology has produced methods of treatment for many childhood diseases that can be provided only in large institutions by specialists who devote most of their efforts to these problems. The primary care physician, therefore, cannot morally or ethically elect to continue to care for these patients.
4. Other professionals have demonstrated their ability to provide competently much of the care currently undertaken by the practicing pediatrician. Family practitioners, pediatric nurse practitioners, and physicians' assistants are capable of providing those services, working with or independent of the pediatrician.
5. Private practice is moving toward consumer control. Demands are being made on the practitioner to institute new organizational and financial arrangements in the provision of primary care. Issues of cost, availability, acceptability, accountability, and efficacy of care provided must be dealt with by each practitioner.

These forces need not be viewed negatively; rather, they can be used by pediatric practitioners to improve the health care available to children. Pediatric practice will need to be reorganized to meet the needs of all children, not just those for whom care is sought. Care must also become more continuous and comprehensive and must be coordinated with the health-related needs of children that are met by others. Pediatricians will have to relate to the broader issues that affect the health of children within the family structure, within the community, and within the greater environment.

The list of these issues, long neglected, is extensive and includes specific problems within the areas of education (attaining full intellectual potential), communication (understanding and being understood), socialization (behaving appropriately with others), and normalization (functioning within acceptable limits) for both well and ill children. Efforts to deal with these issues effectively will need to be directed through the community. The prospect for success in effecting improvement in the health of children is probably greater along this avenue than in the provision of individual health care. It is clear that practicing pediatricians cannot accomplish these goals without working collaboratively with other professionals within and outside the practice setting.

This change in the complexion of primary care practice requires changes in our system of undergraduate and graduate medical education. The curriculum must be altered to include educational objectives commensurate with the activities of primary care physicians and to exclude objectives that are no longer pertinent to practice. Early identification of students who plan to enter primary care versus those who plan on subspecialty practice within academia or outside is needed, and interdisciplinary education with other professionals who will be working collaboratively with physicians in team-oriented care needs to be instituted. In addition, the milieu in which medical education takes place must be supportive of the broader concept of the practice of primary care.

Primary care has been defined to the satisfaction of almost everyone, and educational programs to prepare physicians to provide such care to children have emerged in response to reason, demand, and dictum. Questions now arise as to who should provide the bulk of that care and how it can best be organized to ensure that the health care needs of all our children are met. The politics of primary pediatric care begin to occupy more of our thoughts and discussion.

Part One of this book, Overview of Pediatric Care, presents an analysis of pediatric care in the United States including how it is delivered, the morbidity and mortality that occur, the application of child health supervision designed to promote health and reduce morbidity and mortality, the legal issues that affect the way pediatrics is practiced, and the methods used in delivering pediatric care within the community.

Part Two, Evaluation and Communication, addresses the diagnostic process, which begins with construction of a data base through the gathering of historical information concerning the patient's illness, the conducting of a complete examination to detect deviations from the normal physical status, and the performing of specific tests to analyze the structure and function of the body systems that may be involved. The process continues with assimilation of the information gathered to reach a provisional or definitive diagnosis, with or without assistance from consulting specialists and the medical literature. It moves to communication of the diagnosis to the patient and parents so that they understand what the problem is, what can be done to solve it, and what their role is in its management.

Pediatric patients must be managed with the understanding that they are dependent on others to ensure their optimum growth and development, their protection from the acquisition of disease, and their recovery from illness. Those responsible for these assurances are, in turn, dependent on health professionals to guide them in the use of the means by which those assurances can best be realized.

Part Two continues with a discussion of how practitioners perceive and respond to the cultural issues that affect how medicine is practiced among selected ethnic populations and how compliance with pediatric health care recommendations can be enhanced in general, both at the primary care level and at the level of consultation with subspecialists. It ends with how physicians communicate with each other through the medical literature.

Part Three, Principles of Patient Care, explores the general principles of prevention and treatment that are applicable to the comprehensive care of the young. It deals with the maintenance of health in well children and with therapies directed to acutely and chronically ill children, stressing aspects of illness care that are unique to the pediatric patient.

Practitioners of medicine in the United States and other highly developed nations often approach health care of children as though it were separate from that of the rest of the family. Yet common sense tells us that attention to the mother, her pregnancy, the fetus, and the birth process is mandatory for optimal care of the child. These are addressed in Part Four, The Reproductive Process.

Understanding the mother's genetic makeup is essential for the physician who is in the position of giving advice about continuing a pregnancy or undertaking another one. Similarly, an understanding of conception control methods and abortion issues is necessary.

The environment of the developing baby likewise influences the outcome of pregnancy; therefore knowledge of the transfer of noxious substances across the placenta is valuable, as is familiarity with diagnostic methods such as amniocentesis, ultrasound, and fetoscopy.

As the identification of risk during pregnancy becomes better understood, the developing fetus can be made safe from adverse intrauterine influences. Nutritional requirements of the fetus are now better understood, one consequence being that most physicians no longer starve the mother to keep her weight down during pregnancy.

Personal adaptation (both emotional and physical) of women to pregnancy has been given new emphasis in an attempt to provide caring, individual prenatal services. The involvement of physicians, nurse practitioners, other health workers, and laypersons in educational programs for pregnant women has led to improved services for women and children.

Development of regional facilities and programs for high-risk perinatal patients has promoted successful pregnancies, just as tertiary care obstetric and newborn services have improved the outcome for newborns and older infants who have serious medical problems.

Part Five, The Newborn, addresses the specifics of the care of the newborn baby from the primary care practitioner's perspective. Even though much of the technology described is applied by neonatologists, the practitioner must be able to recognize those situations in which neonatologists should be consulted and must be able to apply initial therapeutic measures to stabilize the condition of the sick infant until help can be obtained.

Children are the center of a "universe"; they are surrounded in successive rings by the family and the community. In Part Six, Psychosocial Issues in Child Health Care, we address not only specific diagnoses and problems, but also the theories of psychological development and the influences of the family, the school, and society on the psychological and physical well-being of infants, children, and adolescents.

Although the pediatric patient's demographic characteristics (age, sex, race, socioeconomic status), ethical influences, and geographic and seasonal environments direct a practitioner's thoughts to specific diagnoses, the presenting signs and symptoms are more persuasive. They immediately bring to mind many diagnostic possibilities and rule out many others. Differential diagnosis begins with consideration of the potential cause of each sign observed by the examiner and each symptom experienced by the patient. It ends when only one cause remains to explain all of the patient's signs and symptoms—at least this usually is the case.

Seventy signs and symptoms commonly encountered in pediatric practice are discussed in Part Seven, Presenting Signs and Symptoms. Most also are mentioned in other parts of the book in discussions of specific diseases.

Pediatric practice surveys, among other things, catalog the diagnoses made by pediatricians for patients they care for in their offices. The 92 diagnoses discussed in Part Eight, Specific Clinical Problems, along with well-child care, constitute the reasons for most office visits made to pediatricians. Almost all the rest of the visits are related to various psychosocial issues discussed in Part Six. These 92 diagnoses also include most of the reasons for hospitalization of pediatric patients beyond the newborn period. The 25 remaining reasons for hospitalization in this age group (except for those due to a small number of rare diseases) are discussed in Part Nine, Critical Situations.

The primary care pediatric practitioner is seldom called on to intervene in critical situations that threaten the life of an infant, child, or adolescent. However, regardless of the practice location and the availability of subspecialists who assist in such instances, each practitioner should be prepared to make appropriate decisions or to take immediate actions that will lead to positive outcomes in such situations. To this end, the methods for management of emergency life-threatening conditions are presented. Appendix A details the methods required for Pediatric Basic and Advanced Life Support. Appendix B, Special Procedures, provides detailed instructions for performing the procedures that may be required in the management of the critical situations described.

Appendix C, Miscellaneous Values, and Appendix D, Common Psychological and Educational Tests, provide the balance of the information pediatric practitioners need to aid themselves in the interpretation of data gathered for the assessment and management of their patients.

Contents

Primary Pediatric Care

PART ONE

Overview of Pediatric Care

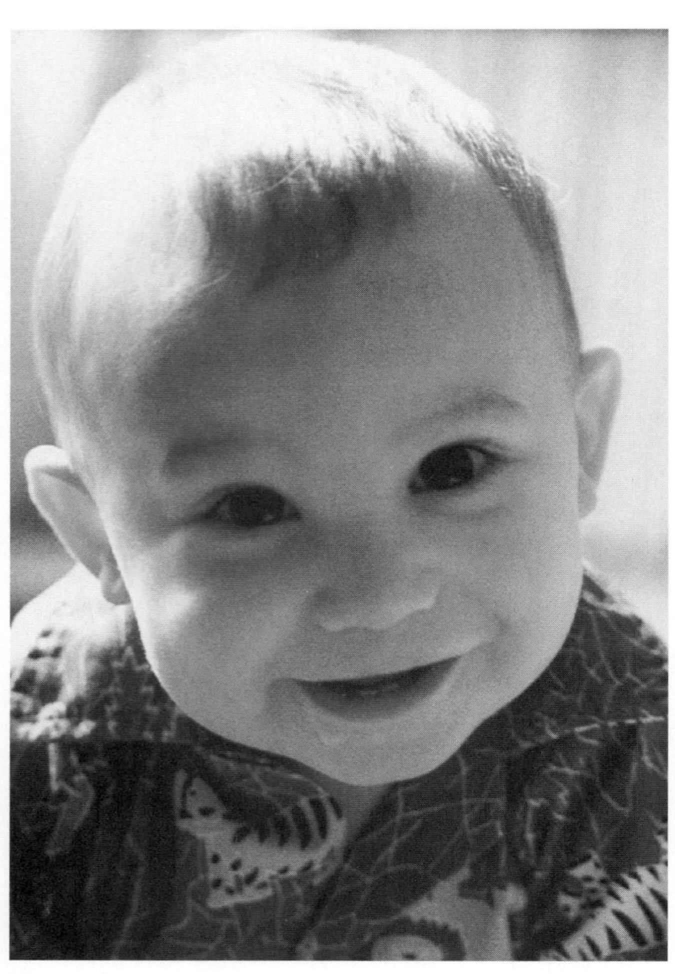

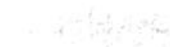

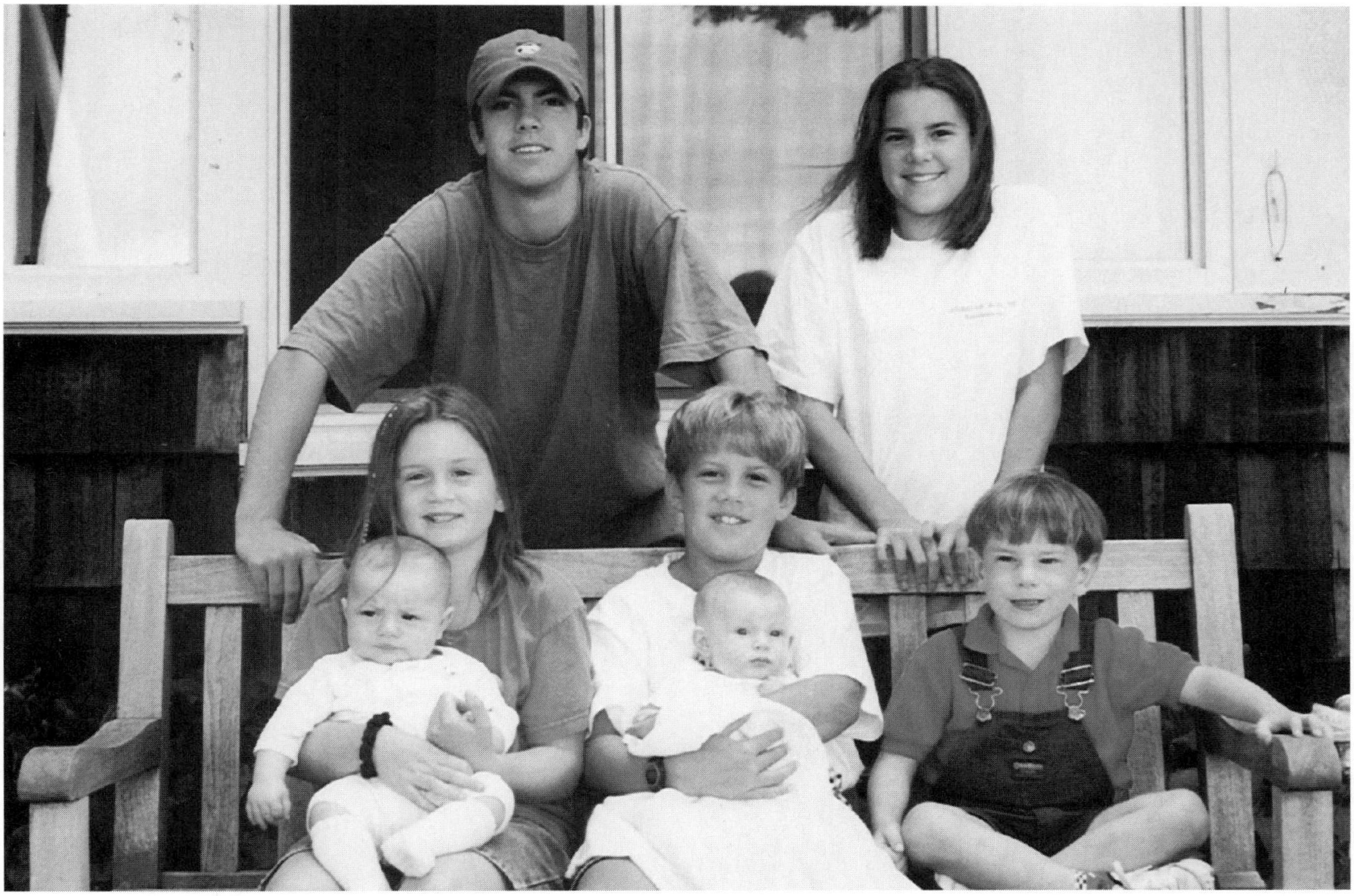

1 The Health Care Delivery System

Edward J. Saltzman and Barbara Starfield

As the medical specialty devoted to the health of infants, children, adolescents, and young adults, pediatrics plays an important role in the U.S. health care system. Over the past 50 years, the number of pediatricians, their characteristics, and the characteristics of pediatric practice have changed dramatically, all in concert with the vast increase in medical knowledge, technical advances, and social change.

In 1992 the United States had 45,881 pediatricians, a significant share (7%) of the total number of physicians.[9] Women are increasingly represented in pediatrics; in 1993, 40% of all U.S. pediatricians were women, a higher percentage than in all other fields of medicine (18% of women physicians are pediatricians).

The 1993 female-male ratio of 40/60 in pediatrics will continue to change; in 1993, for example, 59.5% of pediatric residents were women.[4] A large proportion of pediatricians are young (Table 1-1), and women are the majority at younger ages.

In 1992 there were 7225 pediatric residents.[4] The 1994 National Residency Matching Program resulted in 10.9% of U.S. medical school graduates undertaking pediatric programs,[8] up slightly from 10.5% in 1993.[7] Of the 2073 positions offered for 1994, 1900 were filled (91.7%), 1435 by U.S. graduates (69.2% of all positions offered, and 75.5% of all positions filled). Also in 1994, 88 residency programs in combined internal medicine–pediatrics matched 332 first-year residents, an increase of 200% over the number in 1988.[7,8,12]

International medical graduates constitute a significant number of America's pediatricians. In 1992, of the 144,000 international medical graduate physicians in the United States (22% of all physicians), 13,056 (9.1%) were pediatricians.[9] They represented 28.9% of all pediatricians that year.

Currently, 60% of pediatric residency graduates enter primary care practice directly, a figure that has remained stable over the past decade.[6] Although 40% of pediatricians enter subspecialty training, fewer than 20% of certified pediatricians are also certified in subspecialties, and even fewer practice subspecialties exclusively. However, in 1993, 86.5% of practicing pediatricians were in primary care exclusively or in part, compared to 95% in 1970. Table 1-2 shows the number of practitioners in each of the pediatric subspecialties certified by the American Board of Pediatrics through 1994.

A 1992 survey of members of the American Academy of Pediatrics who practice direct patient care revealed that the most common practice organization was single or multiple partnership. As managed care arrangements increase, group practice, either in single-specialty or multispecialty form, is expected to continue to flourish.[5]

Pediatricians engaged in direct patient care practice an average of 47.2 weeks a year, a figure that has gone unchanged since 1980. On the average, pediatricians in a group practice spend almost 2 weeks less per year at work than those in practice alone.[13] Practicing pediatricians average 49.2 hours a week in direct patient contact, 3.2 hours in activities related to patient care (performing and interpreting diagnostic studies, consulting with other physicians, and talking with patients or parents by telephone), and 5.2 hours in administrative, teaching, or research activities. Thus the average practicing pediatrician has a 57.6-hour workweek.[13]

The number of hours pediatricians spent in the office each week increased slightly between 1984 and 1994 (from 29 to 32), with a corresponding decrease in hospital hours (from 9 to 7.6 hours).[13]

According to the most recent National Ambulatory Medical Care Survey (NAMCS), in 1992, 96.1 million visits were made to pediatricians, accounting for 12.6% of the 762 million ambulatory care office visits made to all physicians in the United States.[11] For pediatricians, this was an increase of more than 20 million visits over the previous year, when 76.4 million visits (11.1%) were made to pediatricians.[10] The reason for this striking increase is unclear, given that it is disproportionate to the rise in the number of visits by patients of all ages and that the age groups that visit pediatricians make fewer visits per 100 individuals than any other age groups. For example, in 1991, those under 15 years of age made 224.8 visits per 100 persons, and 15- to 24-year-olds made 178.2 visits; the average for all ages, including these two groups, was 269.3.[10]

Many patients in the two primary pediatric age groups (commonly, birth to 14 years of age, and 15 to 24 years of age) receive regular care from family practice physicians and internists. NAMCS data for 1991 showed that children under 15 years of age made 100.6 million visits to pediatricians, family practice physicians, and internists; adolescents and young adults (ages 15 to 24) made 27.4 million such visits. In the younger group, pediatricians accounted for 69% of those visits, family medicine practitioners, 29%, and internists, about 2%. In the older age group, however, pediatricians accounted for only 12.3% of visits, whereas family medicine practitioners accounted for 65.3% and internists, 22.4%.[10] Clearly, pediatricians provide a medical home formost preschoolers and grammar and junior high school children. Their influence on the health care of adolescents and young adults wanes appreciably, despite the efforts of many pediatricians to attract them to their practices.

A major study by the Graduate Medical Education National Advisory Committee (GMENAC) in 1981 concluded that a surplus of pediatricians would exist by the 1990s. However, this may not prove true because the number of pediatricians needed to care for the child population in fact, has increased. Women pediatricians, as a group, work fewer hours than their male counterparts; thus more pediatricians will be needed in the work force to care for the same number of children.

Table 1-1 Distribution of Nonfederal U.S. Pediatricians by Age and Sex (1993)*

		Age groups				
Sex		<35	35-44	45-54	55-64	≥65
Male	58.8	19.3	32.6	24.2	15.0	8.9
Female	41.2	37.2	37.7	17.0	5.3	2.8

*Percentages for 46,059 pediatricians.
Modified from Roback G et al: *Physician characteristics and distribution in the US*, Chicago, 1994, The American Medical Association.

Table 1-2 Number of Board-Certified Pediatric Subspecialists* through 1994

Adolescent medicine (1994)†	209
Cardiology (1961)	1185
Critical care (1987)	567
Emergency medicine (1992)	491
Endocrinology (1978)	642
Gastroenterology (1990)	387
Hematology/oncology (1974)	1207
Infectious diseases (1994)	501
Neonatology/perinatology (1975)	2787
Nephrology (1974)	452
Pulmonology (1986)	462
Rheumatology (1992)	125
Total	9015

Data obtained from the American Board of Pediatrics.
*Certified by the American Board of Pediatrics as of Dec. 31, 1994.
†Year in parentheses indicates when subspecialty board was established.

Also, pediatricians' workload could increase dramatically if changes in our political system bring about universal health insurance, which would cover the approximate 12 million children now uninsured. Other pediatrician-demand factors could be inclusion of Medicaid in the "covered" system, the expected increased coverage of well-child care by third-party payers, and recently recommended increases in the number of health supervision visits, especially in the adolescent years. Current health-related school, behavioral, and social problems, (e.g., substance abuse, eating disorders, mental illness, sexually transmitted disease, consequences of adolescent sexual behavior, learning disabilities, and the school drop-out rate) increasingly generate a need for more pediatricians.

Part of the increased demand might be met by nurse practitioners and other child health associates working with pediatricians in their practices, in the schools, and in the community. In 1994, approximately 4000 pediatric nurse practitioners worked in such ways with an estimated 6000 to 9000 pediatricians.

ORGANIZATION OF PRACTICE

Almost 60% of pediatricians practice in urban areas (about half in inner city locations); 30% practice in suburbia, and the remainder are found in small rural towns.[5] Except for those practicing in sparsely populated areas, which have limited hospital and technical support services and few pediatric specialists, pediatricians generally practice in a similar manner throughout the United States.

Traditionally, pediatrics has been an office-based specialty; more than 85% of pediatricians who see patients (excluding resident physicians) are office based. Pediatricians practice mostly in small groups or in individual private offices, where they make their own decisions about the focus and scope of their practice, their office equipment and arrangements, and their method of charging for services rendered. Most payment systems involve a fee for service arrangement. According to a 1993 survey by the American Academy of Pediatrics, most pediatricians are self-employed.[4]

However, this type of organization rapidly is being replaced by "managed care," in which various aspects of providing services, as well as paying for them, are controlled. Patient care is managed through a variety of approaches, including utilization reviews and controls, and nontraditional forms of financial arrangements, such as capitation and incentive payments.

Utilization review may take three forms. *Prospective utilization review* requires approval before hospitalization, consultation, or use of certain ambulatory diagnostic services. *Concurrent utilization review* involves scrutiny of hospitalized patients to ensure the earliest discharge possible, often through arrangements for home health care and ambulatory center–based services. This may be done by third-party payers for hospitalization if payment involves a per diem rate or by the hospital if the payment system calls for a fixed amount based on the patient's DRG (diagnosis-related group). *Retrospective utilization review* allows payment to be denied if distortion of facts led to approval for hospitalization, consultation, or ambulatory diagnostic studies.

The trend toward group practice likely will continue, given the explosive growth of managed care and the advantage to third-party payers, who seek "larger offices" so as to provide more complete medical coverage and greater concentration of patients in fewer offices. The "on-call" schedules, cost savings, and medical camaraderie also are appealing features of group practice. Other means of organizing services have existed for many decades, but only recently have the alternative health care delivery systems begun to increase in importance and number. These systems, which attempt to manage and finance the delivery of health care, constitute the "alphabetizing" of medical care: HMOs, IPAs, PPOs, and the newer form of managed care, EPOs.

Health Maintenance Organizations (HMOs)

In 1932 the Committee on the Costs of Medical Care (a self-created, voluntary committee of government and public health groups) recommended that health care be furnished by organized groups of health professionals, preferably in a hospital, on a group prepayment basis. The idea drew little interest in the medical profession, which devoted its energies to an alternative mechanism for improving access to care—private insurance, under which physicians were to be reimbursed on a fee for service basis for covered services. The prepayment idea grew very slowly; by the early 1980s, only 2% of physicians and less than 5% of the U.S. population were involved. However, in the 1980s, rapidly exploding medical care costs under the fee for service insurance system provided the impetus for new thinking about prepayment. In 1981 there were 260 HMOs; by 1990 615 had been established. By 1993 an estimated 43 million Americans were enrolled in such organizations. By 1994, there were fewer HMO plans than in 1990 (540), but more enrollees—49 million.[15]

Five characteristics distinguish HMOs: (1) a defined population of enrolled members, (2) payments determined in advance for a specific period of time, (3) a contractual responsibility on the part of the organization to provide or ensure medical services, (4) voluntary enrollment, and (5) direct provision of medical services, with the HMO and its physician members assuming at least part of the financial risk of loss in providing services.

There are four major types of HMOs:

- *Staff Model:* In this type of HMO, a group of physicians either are salaried employees of a specially formed group practice that is an integral part of the HMO plan, or are salaried employees of the HMO. Under this model, medical services are provided at HMO-owned health centers.
- *Group Model:* Group models are divided into two kinds: (1) the closed panel type, under which medical services are provided in HMO-owned health centers or in satellite clinics by physicians who belong to a specially formed but legally separate medical group that serves only the HMO; and (2) a system under which the HMO contracts with an existing, independent group of physicians to deliver medical care. In the latter case, the group receives a capitation for each enrollee plus a share of the group's net income, if any; individual physicians may receive a salary, may share the income equally, or may be paid according to their productivity.
- *Network Model:* A network HMO is an organizational form in which the HMO contracts for medical services within a network of medical groups, usually of different types.
- *Individual Practice Association (IPA) model:* The IPA model is a form of HMO in which physicians practice in their own offices and participate in a prepaid health care plan. The physicians charge enrolled patients agreed-upon rates and bill the IPA on a discounted fee for service or a capitated basis. The physicians often continue to see their own patients (non-HMO patients) along with HMO patients. IPAs currently are the dominant HMO model; they accounted for 65% of all plans by the end of 1993. Network models accounted for 13%, group models, 13%, and staff models, 10%.[4]

In the typical HMO, patient care can be given only by providers (doctors, hospitals, special laboratories, and roentgenographic facilities) who either are employees of the HMO or have contracted with the HMO to provide specific services for a specific fee. Under this system patients cannot choose to receive their care from a physician unless the physician or facility is on the HMO roster (network). In return for this limitation of freedom, the payers (usually employers but sometimes enrollees directly) are guaranteed that their costs for medical care will not exceed a predetermined value. It is the HMO and, through it, the physicians and hospitals who are at risk for excessive expenses.

The predetermined cap on cost to the medical consumer is the most appealing aspect of this type of medical system. HMOs (and other managed care systems) emphasize such cost-control methods as preadmission authorization, preadmission diagnostic testing, early hospital discharge, outpatient surgery, preauthorization for consultations, and restricted drug formulary policies. All these measures are designed to reduce medical costs and, thereby, medical insurance premiums.

The results of a poll conducted by the American Medical Association (AMA) indicated that HMO members were as satisfied with the medical care they received as were patients treated under traditional indemnity plans.[1] The HMO loss experience with malpractice claims also closely parallels that of fee for service care.

Despite HMOs' proven ability to hold down costs while ensuring quality, many people who are given a choice prefer a plan that has some elements of traditional medical practice, even if it costs more. For example, under "point of service" (POS) plans, enrollees may receive services outside the provider network without special referral authorization, but with the expense of additional deductible costs and/or extra copayments. Generally, this kind of coverage carries a limitation much like that for indemnity insurance; namely, a ceiling on reimbursement.

Preferred Provider Organizations (PPOs)

The increase in HMOs between 1981 and 1994 was remarkable. But another form of organization, the PPO, grew even faster—from about 20 plans serving just a few members in 1981 to 802 plans with approximately 79 million enrollees in 1994.

The PPO is an association of physicians or hospitals that contracts with employers or insurers to provide services on a discounted fee for service or capitated basis. Pediatricians are popular with PPO insurers. The population pediatricians serve generally is not costly, and PPO insurers like to have young families (who make relatively few demands on the health care system) in their plans. PPOs differ from the traditional insured, fee for service arrangements by contracting to provide services to specific populations and by agreeing to a review of use and claims experiences to control an overuse of services (visits and procedures). In contrast to HMO physicians, PPO physicians incur no financial risk from overuse of services.

PPOs also maintain their own network of providers and facilities and encourage their enrollees to stay in the network by increasing their costs if they go elsewhere. Other cost-containment mechanisms are utilization review and use of a "gatekeeper."

The "gatekeeper" concept helps to control costs by creating a system under which all patients first are seen by the primary care physician, who is the only person who can refer the patient for consultations, ambulatory diagnostic tests, or nonemergency services. Gatekeepers are likely to avoid excess referrals because the PPOs regularly monitor each physician's referral patterns. If the referrals seem excessive to the plan's administrators, attempts are made to reeducate the physician to PPO protocols. If this does not work, the physician may be dismissed from the PPO. Patients who bypass the gatekeeper are penalized financially.

The major factor stimulating the growth of PPOs is the belief that they offer a greater choice of providers that do HMOs. However, with the current abundance of hybrid HMO plans, the differences between many of these plans in terms of choice of physician are marginal.

Exclusive Provider Organizations (EPOs)

In an effort to offer features like an HMO's, the PPOs have developed the EPO, or exclusive provider organization. This system combines the restrictive structure of the HMO provider panel (no out-of-network usage) with the payment structure and flexibility (multiple network providers) of a PPO. In their purest form, EPOs offer members an all-or-nothing approach to coverage. Unlike PPOs, which require patients to pay part of the cost of care, EPOs usually do not require copayments; however, they also do not pay any bills arising from the use of unapproved providers (PPOs pay a portion of the cost of out-of-network care). Generally, the choice of physicians in an EPO is more limited than in a PPO; physicians are selected on the basis of their reputation in the community, cost, and popularity with patients. EPOs also offer companies larger discounts and have tighter utilization review than other managed care models. The exclusive provider generally is paid on a discounted fee for service basis, as with PPOs and IPAs, rather than by capitation (as in staff or group model HMOs). Many physicians find the EPOs' fee for service reimbursement attractive.

By 1995 about 85% of insured Americans were enrolled in some type of managed care plan. About 25% of these were in HMOs (8% in staff or group models, 13% in IPAs, and 4% in POS plans), another 25% were in PPOs or other systems involving incentives or mandates to increase use of specific network providers, about 35% were in managed indemnity plans, and about 15% (largely Medicare and Medicaid patients) were in some form of managed care (Weiner J: Personal communication, 1995).

Tax-supported Programs

Although government agencies always have assumed at least some responsibility for health services of those unable to provide for their own, the need for a more concerted effort became evident as the Depression of the 1930s deepened and access to medical care failed to spread to the entire population. Title V of the Social Security Act of 1935 was responsible for the substantial involvement of local health departments in certain aspects of health care delivery.

Health Department Programs. Local health departments provide a sizable proportion of preventive and case-finding services, particularly in rural and central city areas. But as a result of the wave of "privatization" in the 1980s, their involvement in direct delivery of services has been reduced markedly. Health department efforts now are concentrated largely on environmental health and communicable disease control. In many cities, health departments operate a municipal hospital, but even this role has declined. Where such hospitals exist, they often are overwhelmed by the challenges of AIDS (acquired immune deficiency syndrome) and related problems and the difficulty in finding adequate reimbursement for services provided to those lacking insurance.

Some services are provided in schools, particularly in areas where children otherwise would not receive them. These services often are supported by general tax revenues or by direct grants from federal agencies and are administered by local departments of education or health. Preeminent among such services are those related to essential preventive services. For example, all states have established some immunization as a prerequisite for school attendance. Many also require a physical examination, which may be repeated periodically during the years the child is in school.

Community Health Centers. Started in the mid-1960s as an effort to provide comprehensive health care for groups with little access to medical care, community health centers have grown into a network of facilities that by 1995 were providing care for almost 7 million poor and underserved individuals in the 50 states, Puerto Rico, and the District of Columbia. The centers are funded primarily by grants from the federal government through programs for community health centers and migrant health centers, the National Health Services Corp., Maternal and Child Health (MCH) block grants to states, and the Urban Indian Health Program. Many centers also try to attract patients with private insurance or Medicaid, which contributes 30% to 50% of the operating budgets of most community health centers. Yet these facilities reach less than 25% of the country's medically underserved.

Social Security Programs. Two of the Social Security amendments of the mid-1960s had a significant impact on health care delivery for children. Medicaid, authorized by Title XIX of the Social Security Act, provides a means of paying for medical care, through tax dollars, for those who cannot afford it. Originally it was intended that medical care be provided through existing systems, primarily independent office practices.

Medicaid is a joint federal/state program, supported by both federal and state contributions. The federal government sets a minimum of services to be provided, although states may limit the duration of the these services. Eligibility is based primarily on low family income. Medicaid accounts for a greater proportion of all expenditures of health services for children than for adults, but the share of Medicaid payments for children is low despite the large proportion of children among the eligible.

States vary widely in their eligibility requirements for Medicaid. Nationally, fewer than 50% of families with an income below the national poverty level are covered. States often do not cover even those children eligible for Medicaid; the proportion covered varies from a small minority in some jurisdictions to a substantial majority in others. In response to this situation, Congress has encouraged (and in some cases mandated) incremental additions, starting with infants and young children. States must cover children under age 6 in families with incomes up to 133% of the poverty level. Effective July 1, 1991, coverage of poor children ages 6 to 19 has been required and is to be phased in over the following 10 years. If universal health coverage is ever attained in the United States, it is expected that the Medicaid program will be phased out because everyone automatically should be eligible for any national plan.

Title V Amendments. The original Social Security Title V program, enacted in 1935, supported a variety of programs designed to deliver health services to mothers and children; these were administered predominantly by the states. The law was amended significantly between 1963 and 1967 to provide funds to support services in low-income and rural areas for maternal and child health clinics, family planning, regionalized infant care, and dental care. In the 1980s these were replaced by the "new federalism," which provided "block" grants to the states for maternal and child health services, to cover Supplemental Security Income for disabled children (i.e., children with chronic health problems), to fund programs for preventing lead-based paint poisoning and sudden infant death syndrome (SIDS), and to support hemophilia treatment centers, and adolescent pregnancy and genetics services.

However, the concern of Congress and children's advocates about the diminished reporting and accountability mechanisms for block grants in general, the extension of health services financing through Medicaid, and the evolution of new principles of care promoted a series of amendments to Title V, beginning in the mid-1950s and culminating in the Omnibus Budget Reconciliation Act of 1989 (OBRA '89). Under these amendments, new requirements were established for state MCH programs for (1) planning and supporting community-based systems of coordinated, family-centered care for all mothers and children, (2) strengthening linkages with Medicaid to assure enrollment of eligible pregnant women and children, and (3) adopting appropriate quality standards. OBRA '89 also extensively codified block grant reporting requirements.

In most southern, midwestern, and western states, which have large networks of county and local health departments, services (including well-child care, antenatal care, health screening, and immunizations) traditionally have been provided directly through government agencies in local health clinics and schools. In other areas, particularly the Northeast, the more common approach has been for state maternal and child health agencies to contract with an array of private providers and community health centers for provision of public MCH services. With respect to Title V–mandated care for children with chronic illnesses or other disabling health conditions, services have been provided through a combination of contractual arrangements with tertiary medical centers and state-operated itinerant clinics in rural areas.

These welcome expansions in Medicaid and the new responsibilities in planning and oversight enacted in the late 1980s, coupled with the emergence of managed care organizations in the 1990s, continue to change the nature and scope of public maternal and child health services in accommodating the contemporary needs of women and children.

Hospital-based Services

In 1993, 1 in 8 physician encounters with individuals under age 18 occurred in a hospital.[5] That number is increasing, particularly among very young children and the poor. Although numerous studies have been done in individual outpatient departments of teaching hospitals, little is known about the amount, scope, and type of care provided nationwide. Most medical services in these facilities are provided by physicians in training, who rotate through outpatient departments as part of their postgraduate education. This hospital-based sector of care is particularly prevalent in central city areas near teaching hospitals, through which many children receive most of their health care.

The 1990s have seen the emergence and growth in numbers of the pediatric hospital-based subspecialties of critical care medicine (intensivists) and emergency medicine. These physicians offer in-hospital care through direct access to hospitalized patients or referrals from pediatric generalists. Aside from having special expertise in their respective fields, these physicians offer 24-hour availability on site in pediatric intensive care units and emergency rooms.

PRACTICE CHARACTERISTICS

Style and Content

Through much of the early and middle twentieth century, the practicing general pediatrician was the daily expert, always on call in the office for families in need, or making frequent house calls or hospital rounds. The practitioner worried about, comforted, and ministered to both well and sick newborns, premature infants, sick children out of the hospital, and especially children who were hospitalized. General pediatricians diagnosed and treated rheumatic fever, glomerulonephritis, all forms of contagious disease, and most forms of cardiac, neurologic, and allergic diseases. In short, they dealt with all "minor" and most major illnesses. Subspecialists were few and far between, found only in academic medical centers. Concepts such as "primary," "secondary," and "tertiary" care were unknown, and the hospital-based pediatric intensivist, neonatologist, as well as other subspecialists, did not exist. There was little time for health education because the pediatrician had to provide definitive care for all childhood diseases.

Today, the office-based (or primary care) pediatrician deals with illnesses that are only potentially serious. The patient almost always is seen in the office, rarely in the hospital, and almost never in the home. The variety of illnesses treated today does not even remotely resemble that of the past. Upper respiratory disease (including ear infections), moderate lower respiratory problems, feeding problems, gastrointestinal upsets, and minor trauma account for 75% to 85% of illness care. But the health care needs of children are changing; a large portion of practice time now is spent on wellness care, dealing with family dynamics, and managing the "new morbidities." Most primary care pediatricians devote much of their effort to the following:

- Providing prenatal counseling
- Preventing accidents by giving advice about seat belts, smoke alarms, water safety, home safety, poison control, and bicycle helmets
- Discussing the child's education with the family and supporting the achievement of educational goals from infancy through adolescence
- Becoming an expert in abuse avoidance, whether it be drug abuse, child abuse, or parental abuse
- Providing advice and support during divorce or other marital crises
- Advising families on life-style goals, such as the need for family time and for an understanding of work-related time constraints and stresses and how the family copes with them
- Promoting good health through advice on a prudent diet and nutrition, exercise, and avoidance of bad health habits, such as smoking
- Encouraging community activism through knowledge and use of common resources and involvement with

school boards, religious groups, school athletic programs, and community facilities

- Devoting time to the care of adolescents and young adults, with the twin goals of being able to provide guidance and anticipate problems and to be helpful in solving such problems; areas of special attention include sex education, understanding one's sexuality, avoiding sexually transmitted diseases, preventing drug and alcohol abuse and teenage pregnancy, and advising about education and career goals

The time a pediatrician spends in office practice remains challenging and interesting, although it is channeled differently than in the past.

Because the typical practitioner wants to be (and is becoming) less involved with illnesses that require time-consuming workups or acute care management, either on an outpatient or an inpatient basis, care increasingly is becoming limited to the office. Office-based pediatricians are spending less time in the hospital than in the past; in 1991, practicing pediatricians spent only 15% of their time on hospital rounds, a 9% decrease from 1984.[13]

Referrals to hospital-based neonatologists have become commonplace, even for normal newborn care. This "in-house, always available" service saves time for the office-based pediatricians by reducing the need to visit the hospital. It also ensures that patient care is supervised on site. The success of this delegation of care, even when subspecialty care may not be needed, may be giving rise to a new type of pediatrician—the hospital-based pediatric generalist, who is located in community and teaching hospitals and who provides both consultations and total inpatient care for referred patients.

One third of all patients of primary care pediatricians are under 1 year of age, and one fourth are between 1 and 4 years of age. The proportion of patients 19 years or older is very small; however, nearly 43% of pediatricians see patients 19 to 21 years old, and 1 in 5 see patients over 21 years of age.[3]

In 1993 pediatricians reported that 29% of their patients were eligible for Medicaid, and 9% reported that 75% or more of their patients were on Medicaid[5]; 14% reported that none of their patients were on Medicaid, but some of these physicians were in military practices, where such coverage is unnecessary. Pediatricians averaged 5.2 hours a month in volunteer activities, although 51% of the respondents spent no time in volunteer activities.[3] Volunteer activities included providing free health care, consulting for schools and government agencies, and providing health education to community and church organizations.

Recently, pediatric residency programs have begun to emphasize involvement in community health care and other community-related activities, but the extent to which this will change the health care outcomes of children in need is unknown.

Extended Hours and Satellite Offices

Families in which both parents work and one-parent families now make up the majority of families in the United States. As a result, group or solo practices in which physicians share coverage have been forced to extend their office hours to provide coverage during evenings and on weekends, in addition to the traditional on-call coverage at night. This is a radical departure from the office hours that pediatricians traditionally provide.

After-hours coverage is provided in settings the group finds convenient, such as using their own office or arranging for an examination suite provided by the local hospital. In these settings, many pediatricians join forces for after-hours or weekend coverage. They take turns covering the telephone and meeting patients' needs, with prompt referral back to the patient's designated doctor. This provides efficient off-hours medical care and affords each practitioner more time for rest, relaxation, and pursuing personal interests.

Pediatricians also have embraced the concept of the satellite office as a response to the movement of young families to the suburbs. These offices offer the same complete pediatric care available in the "main" office but are more accessible to suburban dwellers. Satellite offices often outgrow the main office as communities change in character or demographics and establish an identity of their own.

Professional Liability

Pediatricians are part of a socioeconomic medical environment marked by skyrocketing professional liability claims and, concomitantly, very high professional liability insurance premiums. Some pediatricians pay premiums as high as $20,000 to $25,000 a year, which constitutes a significant percent of gross revenue. In earlier times, litigation involved surgeons and surgical procedures almost exclusively. Today, failure to diagnose illness and anticipate drug reactions is high on the list of causes of lawsuits against pediatricians. Pediatricians who fail to diagnose meningitis or sepsis, who delay in diagnosing congenital dislocation of the hip or congenital hypothyroidism, or who experience problems with managing croup versus epiglottitis, for example, are at high risk for malpractice suits. Because of the variability among states in statutes of limitation for filing malpractice claims on behalf of minors or because of failure to set limits ("caps") for malpractice awards, pediatricians are at risk not only for high awards but for settlement many years after the alleged malpractice occurred. Many legal remedies have been proposed to adjust these claims reasonably; so far, these remedies have had little fiscal impact except in a few states.

In the 1993 survey of its members, the American Academy of Pediatrics (AAP) found that there had been no significant pattern of change in medical liability experience for pediatricians in the past 6 years.[4]

- The percentage of pediatricians reporting a suit for malpractice in 1992 was 29.9, up from 26.9 in 1987 and 27.9 in 1990.
- The percentage of pediatricians who reported being a party to a claim or suit for malpractice while a resident in 1992 was 8.4%.
- The average number of years in practice among pediatricians who have been sued is nearly the same for all 3 years (18.6 years in 1992, 18 in 1990, and 18.6 in 1987).
- In 1992, 62.5% of the pediatricians sued reported the hospital as the site of the alleged malpractice and 32.1% the office as the alleged site.
- Just over 29% of cases were settled out of court in 1992; in 35.1% of cases, the plaintiff dropped the suit.

WAYS TO AVOID MALPRACTICE SUITS

Standards

- Meet normative standards of health care delivery (i.e., according to expert opinion as found in medical textbooks and articles in scientific journals) and/or empiric standards (i.e., according to local medical practice).

Communication

- Use positive methods in communicating with patients and parents, showing respect, understanding, concern, and compassion.
- Train staff to be sensitive to a patient's needs at all times.
- Train staff to manage patient telephone calls properly and to log all incoming and outgoing telephone calls, including patient problems and instructions given.

Documentation

- Record on the first page of a patient's chart his or her drug allergies and problem list.
- Record for each visit the history, findings on physical examination (including pertinent negative findings), diagnostic tests ordered (including their results), and treatment prescribed in sufficient detail for purposes of recall.
- Record all immunizations given and all screening test results.
- Record all telephone calls during which medical information about the patient was received or advice was given; include date and time.
- Place in the patient's chart discharge summaries of hospitalizations, and referral letters to and responses from consultants.

- In 1992 most pediatricians who had been sued (54.8%) reported that the plaintiff was a patient who was not seen regularly by them. Among pediatricians reporting that the plaintiff was not a regular patient, about one third said the claim involved on-call coverage.
- In the 1990 and 1992 AAP surveys, 11.4% of pediatricians responding stated that fear of a malpractice suit prevented them from participating in community-based activities.
- Claims against pediatricians in 1993 had the highest average indemnity payment of the 24 medical specialties studied in the Data Sharing Project of the Professional Insurance Association of America. The average indemnity payment of $206,230 per claim for pediatricians compares with the average of about $133,000 for all medical specialties included in the study. Claims involving errors or delays in diagnosing meningitis accounted for more than 15% of the claims paid; 10% of the claims paid involved prescribed drugs.

In an attempt to cope with a litigious environment, pediatricians continue to make prudent referrals, test appropriately, maintain better records, spend adequate time with patients, and use other techniques to avoid risk (see the box above). However, there is no evidence that either these approaches or the annual risk-management educational programs on reducing medical malpractice suits are effective. Defensive medicine has had an economic impact by increasing expenditures for medical care. Some of these practice changes may constitute improvements in medical care; others may be unnecessary or even harmful. Because of a perceived change in physician-patient relationships resulting from the threat of liability, the pleasure of practice lessens. Hope for a change that is both fair and equitable to the public and the medical profession depends on societal attention to this difficult problem.

SCOPE OF PEDIATRIC PRACTICE

Until recently, the types of services provided by the nation's pediatric practitioners were unknown. Because of the rising cost of health care, practitioners increasingly are being required to document services rendered to determine how money is being spent and whether increased costs have resulted in improved health. Although sporadic studies of individual practices have appeared since the 1930s, nothing in the way of national practice data existed until the development of the National Ambulatory Medical Care Survey (NAMCS) by the National Center for Health Statistics in the early 1970s. NAMCS is a periodic survey of office-based practices; in 1992 the survey was expanded to include hospital outpatient departments and emergency rooms. These surveys do not include care provided in tax-supported service programs.

Tables 1-3 through 1-6 provide statistics gathered by NAMCS in 1991 regarding U.S. office-based practices, including the most common diagnoses, the disposition and duration of visits, the therapeutic services rendered, and the drugs prescribed, by therapeutic classification.[10] A relatively large proportion of children require a repeat visit to the same physician, and some require a visit to another physician (Table 1-4); this indicates the need to integrate care over several visits, both to the original physician and to consultants. Ensuring continuity is a major challenge to physicians in primary care.

All children are supposed to have a "medical home" that provides continued, integrated care over time. Even for children who have a regular source of care, this source does not always provide all the required services, nor does it always integrate the services that the child has received elsewhere. Many children who have a physician whom they identify as their regular source of care actually go to another physician when they need medical services. Moreover, physicians in primary care facilities may not be aware of these visits elsewhere or of what occurred, even though this may influence significantly the patient's response to subsequent care.

This fragmented, uncoordinated care presents a major challenge to our health care system. If practitioners, health programs, and health institutions continue to function as separate and uncoordinated agencies, and if individuals continue to seek care from so many sources, duplication of services probably will result in an ever-increasing cost of care without commensurate gains. In fact, effectiveness is likely to diminish because patients are given conflicting advice and treatment by different practitioners. The extent to which man-

Table 1-3 Ten Most Common Diagnoses in Pediatric Office Visits (1991)

Rank	Diagnosis	Number of visits (thousands)	Percentage of visits	Cumulative percentage
	All Visits	74,646	100.0	
1	Health supervision of infant or child	13,854	18.6	18.6
2	Suppurative and unspecified otitis media	8099	10.8	29.4
3	Acute upper respiratory infections of multiple or unspecified sites	6673	8.9	38.4
4	General medical examination	3776	5.1	43.5
5	Acute pharyngitis	3255	4.4	47.8
6	Chronic sinusitis	2723	3.6	51.5
7	Bronchitis, not specified as acute or chronic	1865	2.5	54.0
8	Asthma	1718	2.3	56.3
9	Personal history of certain other diseases	1624	2.2	58.4
10	Viral infection in conditions classified elsewhere	1528	2.0	60.5

Modified from Shappert SM: National Ambulatory Medical Care Survey: 1992 summary: advance data for vital and health statistics: no 253, Hyattsville, Md, 1994, The National Center for Health Statistics.

Table 1-4 Disposition and Duration of 74.6 Million Pediatric Office Visits (1991)

Disposition of visit	Percentage of visits
No follow-up planned	13.3
Return at specified time	49.9
Return if needed	37.0
Telephone follow-up planned	3.5
Refer to other physician	1.8
Return to referring physician	0.1
Admit to hospital	0.2
Other	0.6
Duration of visit	
<1 min	0.5
1-5 min	7.3
6-10 min	33.0
11-15 min	38.4
16-30 min	18.9
>30 min	1.9

Modified from Shappert SM: National Ambulatory Medical Care Survey: 1992 summary: advance data for vital and health statistics: no 253, Hyattsville, Md, 1994, The National Center for Health Statistics.

Table 1-5 Therapeutic Interventions in 74.6 Million Pediatric Office Visits (1991)

Medication therapy	Percentage distribution
Drug visits*	69.5
One drug	42.5
Two drugs	17.3
Three drugs	7.0
Four drugs	2.0
Five drugs	0.7
Visits without mention of medication	30.5
Counseling/education and other therapy†	
None	61.7
Growth/development	20.8
Diet	17.2
Other counseling	12.3
Family/social	6.4
Exercise	4.0
Cholesterol reduction	0.6
Weight reduction	0.6
Family planning	0.4
Alcohol abuse	0.4
Drug abuse	0.3
Smoking cessation	0.3
Psychotherapy	0.3
Physiotherapy	0.2
Other therapy	1.2

Modified from Shappert SM: National Ambulatory Medical Care Survey: 1992 summary: advance data for vital and health statistics: no 253, Hyattsville, Md, 1994, The National Center for Health Statistics.
*Drug visits are visits at which one or more medications are ordered or provided by the physician; includes new and continuing medications.
†More than one therapy may have been involved in a single visit.

aged care systems actually reduce the fragmentation of care still is unknown.

In most other industrialized nations, health services are regionalized; services are organized according to the degree to which they are needed. Services required frequently or by by large portions of the population are provided on the local or community level and thus are very accessible. These systems are called primary health services.

The experience of prepaid group practices, which by definition provide care for a specific population, is useful in determining how many physicians may be needed to ensure accessibility to primary care services. A ratio of 1 child health physician per 2000 children has proved generally satisfactory, but the ratio of 1:2500 may be more realistic, considering the mobility of our population and the number of people who count themselves as patients, even though they rarely are seen.

Physicians in primary care (all family practice physicians and most pediatricians and internists) should assume responsibility for providing a broad spectrum of care (both preventive and curative) over time and for coordinating all the care their patients receive, including that from specialists. When primary care physicians need advice on difficult cases, they should refer patients for consultation to secondary health facilities, which are more centralized than the primary care facilities and usually are located in community hospitals. Patients who require care for complicated and unusual illnesses should be referred to tertiary care facilities, usually university medical centers, which are even more centralized and

Table 1-6 Drugs Prescribed in 74.6 Million Pediatric Office Visits (1991)

Therapeutic classification	Number of drugs prescribed (thousands)	Percentage distribution
All drugs prescribed	81,746	100.0
Antimicrobial agents	25,825	31.6
Immunologic agents	17,196	21.0
Respiratory tract drugs	15,842	19.4
Skin/mucous membrane agents	4661	5.7
Drugs used for pain relief	4254	5.2
Hormones and related agents	2066	2.5
Metabolic and nutrient agents	1637	2.0
Gastrointestinal agents	1563	1.9
Ophthalmic agents	1452	1.8
Psychopharmacologic drugs	641	0.8
Cardiovascular-renal drugs	525	0.6
Neurologic drugs	249	0.3
Hematologic agents	228	0.3
Other and unclassified drugs	5609	6.9

Modified from Shappert SM: National Ambulatory Medical Care Survey: 1992 summary: advance data for vital and health statistics: no 253, Hyattsville, MD, 1994, The National Center for Health Statistics.

carry out training and research functions as well. The tertiary care centers provide services that require a high degree of technical expertise. The expensive equipment needed for these specialties should be located only in tertiary centers and not in every health center that desires it and can get the money to buy it (as is often the case). To date, however, no national priority has been established to develop such a regional system of health services for children.

Reimbursement Issues

The net income for pediatricians averaged $119,300 in 1993, up from $111,800 in 1991.[2] This placed their income fourth from the bottom among disciplines (above family medicine and general practitioners and psychiatrists). Despite this increase, pediatricians typically earn 15% less than the median for all nonsurgical specialists and 21% less than office-based MDs and DOs in private practice in all fields combined.

One reason for this income lag is the high proportion of women pediatricians, whose fees are the same as their male colleagues, but whose income is lower because many women pediatricians work shorter hours in order to meet family obligations. This factor also may be reflected in the decline in the average number of visits made to pediatricians per week, from 153 in 1988 to 142 in 1992.[3] Another factor limiting pediatricians' income may be their heavy reliance on managed care—36% of all patient visits in 1992, a much higher percentage than in other fields of primary care. Also, pediatrics is a specialty that requires counseling and listening more than performing procedures, and reimbursement favors performing procedures.

In a 1994 survey by the American Academy of Pediatrics,[5] pediatrician members reported the following distribution of payment methods used by their patients: Blue Cross/Blue Shield, 17.1%; other private insurance (indemnity, HMO, PPO, and the like) 38.7%; Medicaid, 29%; Medicare, 2.6%; and uninsured/self-pay, 12.4%. Overall, of insured patients (both public and private), approximately 60% were in nontraditional, managed care systems: HMOs, 28.2%; PPOs, 14.9%; IPAs, 5.1%; and other plans, 11.8%. The remaining 30% were in a traditional fee for service system.

In 1992 Congress adopted a new relative value system of reimbursement to pay physicians for care of the elderly under the Medicare program. This system, called the Resource-Based Relative Value Scale (RBRVS), measures work in four dimensions: (1) time, (2) mental effort and judgment, (3) technical skill and physical effort, and (4) psychological stress. The RBRVS tends to equalize reimbursement by lowering fees for technical procedures and raising fees for "cognitive services." By late 1994, a pediatric RBRVS was under development, to ensure that pediatricians would be reimbursed according to the same principles as those underlying the RBRVS fee schedule that the Health Care Financing Administration (HCFA) uses to reimburse Medicare providers.

Impact of Reimbursement on the Scope of Services

The proportion of the U.S. population covered by health insurance increased from 47% in 1950 to 82% in 1994. Coverage varies with each plan and its benefit package, and the nature of the benefits determines both the physician's and the patient's choices in treatments and services.

Children with no health insurance are significantly less likely to see a physician for necessary health care than are children with insurance. According to the 1987 National Medical Expenditure Survey, of children with sore throats, 40% of those insured were taken to a physician, but more than 60% of those uninsured were not. The figures were comparable for acute ear pain (32.1% versus 49.1%), recurrent ear infections (14.9% versus 33.2%), and asthma (35.4% versus 50.6%).[14]

The proportion of the population covered by private insurance varies markedly according to family income. Fewer than 15% of children in poor families have private health insurance, compared with more than 90% of those in higher income families.

Some of the cost of care for indigent children is paid directly by the government. This tax-supported contribution comprises two parts: direct services to mothers and children provided by local, state, and federally supported health care agencies and payment systems (largely Medicaid) channeled through the "private" health care system.

Data from the National Center for Health Statistics, gathered over the past decade, show that children are less likely than the population as a whole to be covered by private health insurance; preschoolers are much less likely than other children to have private insurance. Poor and especially near-poor children are much less likely than children who are not poor to have any coverage for medical care, regardless of whether they have a disability as a result of medical problems. Children in low-income families are more compromised if they have no insurance coverage than are adults. Meager family funds must be rationed; illness in low-income adults, particularly if they work, has greater immediate economic consequences than does illness in children. This explains why children in the "gray" area, whose families neither qualify for government help nor can afford insurance, are less likely than other children to see a health care practitioner when they are ill.

Only a minority of traditional indemnity insurance plans pay providers for any preventive services, but the newer managed care plans that are becoming so popular with both the payer and the consumer almost always cover such services. These plans not only pay the provider fees but also energetically market health information and patient reminder notices to make sure their enrollees avail themselves of this preventive care.

In 1986, Florida, with the help of the American Academy of Pediatrics, became the first state to mandate private health insurance coverage for health supervision. Under the Child Health Incentive Reform Plan (CHIRP), a certain number of visits are covered without a deductible payment by the parents. To the extent that other states follow this lead in mandating coverage for preventive services, such legislation will enhance the role of the pediatrician in furthering child health.

As of 1994, California, Connecticut, the District of Columbia, Hawaii, Iowa, Massachusetts, Maryland, Minnesota, Montana, New York, Ohio, and Rhode Island also had CHIRP-type legislation, although all had different ages and care mandates. Of concern, however, is the growth in industry's attempts to provide employee "self-insurance" health care programs, which are exempted from state laws mandating coverage of certain services. Because the cost of health insurance continues to escalate, small and large businesses are looking for a less costly method of providing health services for their employees. By using self-insurance plans, the employer can save money by eliminating some of the benefits currently required by law (e.g., coverage of children and other dependents) and can establish higher deductibles and copayments. Eliminating coverage for dependents in this way could affect children and their pediatricians adversely.

The sustained rise in medical care costs is responsible for much congressional interest in controlling certain aspects of medical practice. However, the debate over whether this control should reside with government agencies or be delegated to insurance companies, professional organizations, or hospitals, as well as over the scope of activities to include under those controls, to date have impeded implementation of any serious federal cost-control proposal.

A major attack on the escalation of medical care costs was instituted by the Department of Health and Human Services through the Social Security Act Amendments of 1983, which mandated the use of diagnosis-related groups (DRGs) as the basis for reimbursing hospitals for patient care. Until then, hospitals were reimbursed according to per diem rates and the diagnostic and therapeutic procedures performed. Under the DRG system, care for Medicare recipients (mostly those over age 65) is reimbursed according to the diagnosis established on admission. All diagnoses have been grouped into 467 categories, each of which is relatively homogeneous with respect to length of hospital stay and costs. Hospitals receive a specific sum for each DRG, regardless of the patient's actual length of stay or the number of procedures performed.

The National Association of Children's Hospitals and Related Institutions (NACHRI) developed pediatric DRGs for use in children's hospitals in 1988 and updated them in 1990. If a DRG-like system (for fee for service payments) or a "case-mix" system (for capitated payment) is ever developed, and if preventive care, including counseling and guidance coverage, is provided, pediatric practice should be improved substantially.

QUALITY OF CARE

The medical profession has always claimed responsibility for regulating entry into its ranks and for assessing the quality of care provided. Although state boards have the legal authority to dispense licenses to practice, all states delegate this authority to the profession, which nominates candidates, whom the state then licenses. Individuals merely must demonstrate that they graduated from medical school and can achieve a passing grade on a cognitive examination developed by the profession itself, either in the state (state licensing examinations) or nationally (the National Board of Medical Examiners or the Federation of State Licensing Boards, i.e., "Flex" examinations).

Many specialties have their own certifying examinations. By the end of 1994, the American Board of Pediatrics had certified 55,130 pediatricians in general pediatrics. Of these, 9015 had been certified as subspecialists (see Table 1-2). Approximately 85% of those practicing pediatrics as generalists or subspecialists are board certified (Oliver TK, senior vice president, American Board of Pediatrics: personal communication, 1995.)

The American Board of Pediatrics requires certification renewal every 7 years for pediatricians certified in 1988 or thereafter. This requires successful completion of the Program for Renewal of Certification in Pediatrics (PRCP), which includes a structured home study curriculum and a supervised, open-book written examination. Diplomates certified before 1988 may choose to renew their certification by voluntarily completing the PRCP.

Most health provider organizations use certification and recertification data as one means of ensuring quality of care, requiring their pediatricians to be either board certified (having passed the written examination) or board eligible (having completed 3 years of pediatric residency training in an accredited program) with certification within 5 years of completion of residency training. Whether recertification will be required by these organizations is unclear as yet. Up to this point, there is no requirement that pediatricians demonstrate competence under the conditions of actual practice, either when they enter practice or at any time afterward. However, a few managed care organizations regularly assess some aspects of quality of care for both adults and children; these efforts may expand in the future.

Medical School Accreditation

Medical schools are accredited by the Liaison Committee on Medical Education, which is composed of representatives of the American Medical Association (AMA) and the Association of American Medical Colleges.

Medical schools qualify for accreditation by demonstrating to the Liaison Committee that they offer (1) a "sound educational program," which provides students the opportunity to acquire a solid basis of education in medicine and fosters the development of lifelong habits of scholarship and service; (2) scientific research; (3) graduate education through both clinical residency programs and advanced degree programs in the basic medical sciences; and (4) continuing education aimed at maintaining and improving the competence of professionals engaged in caring for patients.

Hospital Accreditation

To be accredited, hospitals must receive approval from the Joint Commission on Accreditation of Health Care Organizations, a council composed of representatives of the American Medical Association, the American Hospital Association, the American College of Surgeons, and the American College of Physicians. Accreditation, both of hospitals and medical schools, is essential to the financial viability of those institutions. Most third-party payers (the government and insurance companies) that reimburse hospitals or contribute to the support of medical schools require them to be accredited as a condition for payment.

Assurance of Quality Care

The passage of federal legislation stimulated the profession to demonstrate its involvement in assuring quality of care. Review of medical activities in hospitals was the first step proposed, largely because hospital costs assume a disproportionate share of the health care dollar. The Professional Standards Review Organization (PSRO) Act, passed in 1972, required that hospital admission of patients covered by government payments be reviewed for justifiability and that hospitals periodically designate individual diagnoses for which all medical records of patients with those diagnoses would be audited to determine the adequacy of care. Although opposed by many physicians, these requirements stimulated the profession to specify standards of care for common problems requiring hospitalization. However, continued opposition by the profession, inability to demonstrate unequivocally that costs were reduced as a result of quality assurance activities, and general government policy to reduce government regulation led to severe restrictions in the program and eventually to its demise.

A new program, professional review organizations (PROs), was established by the Tax Equity and Fiscal Responsibility Act (TEFRA) of 1982 as a means of reviewing the completeness, adequacy, and quality of care, primarily in hospitals. In contrast to the PSROs, which were nonprofit physician organizations, PROs could be for-profit groups and fiscal intermediaries that won the contracts from the federal government for monitoring health care use. Although these PROs currently review diagnostic information and completeness and adequacy of care, as well as appropriateness of admissions, for the elderly (patients covered by Medicare), this type of monitoring probably will spread to other groups of patients covered by government and even private insurers.

Studies have shown that the organization in which a physician practices has a greater influence on the quality of practice than the physician's individual characteristics. Team practice, in which nurses and community health workers share responsibility with the physician for certain aspects of care, is likely to result in both greater recognition of patients' problems and greater likelihood that they will be addressed by the physician. Prepaid group practices in which several physicians share fiscal accountability also is likely to result in greater consideration of the necessity and justifiability of professional actions.

In a health system that allows patients to seek care anywhere they choose, those who fail to obtain relief of their complaints often seek subsequent care elsewhere. Thus physicians may not be in a position to observe the impact of their services. Conversely, no mechanism exists by which patients who are cured can apprise their physician of this. Most physicians are unable to assume responsibility for follow-up care of a patient if the patient does not voluntarily return for care. As the costs of care become an increasing concern of third-party payers (government, insurance companies, and employers), duplication of services, as reflected in visits to different care providers for the same problem, will become evident. As a result, physicians may be encouraged to assume greater responsibility for episodes of illness rather than just for individual visits made by patients; managed care systems will encourage such assumption of responsibility. This is likely to make physicians more aware of deficiencies that may exist in current medical practice.

The historical prerogative by which physicians decide what practices constitute "good quality" is being altered by a movement toward greater public accountability. "Good quality" is an issue for the present, in that it responds to the clamor from the public, government, and insurance carriers to hold physicians accountable for costs of health care and the quality of the medical care they render.

It appears likely, however, that certain aspects of practice will remain under physicians' control. The first such aspect is the selection of students for entrance into medical school. Ever since the Flexner Report (1910), the upper social classes have been overrepresented in the profession of medicine compared with their proportion in the general population. The high and continually rising cost of medical education without substantial government subsidy of those who cannot afford it is a powerful deterrent to applications from such students.

The second aspect is practice location. In many countries with national health insurance, physicians are not reimbursed for their services if they locate their practices in areas that already have a sufficient number of physicians. In the United States, there are no deterrents to physicians locating wherever they please and wherever they can obtain a license.

The third aspect likely to remain in the professional domain is the disciplining of physicians. In some countries patients' dissatisfaction and complaints can be addressed to government agencies, which consider them and then exonerate or recommend sanctions (usually financial) against the physician. The medical profession in the United States has been rather impotent in disciplining its members in any meaningful way because there is no way to impose sanctions short of revoking a license, which is hardly ever done. To date, both professional and legislative bodies have failed to come to grips with this issue.

The fourth aspect likely to remain in the hands of the profession is control over the technical areas of medical care. As new technology is developed, it often is used without adequate prior assessment of its costs and benefits. Although pressure to reduce the rate of growth in medical care costs (which largely are a result of increased use of technology) undoubtedly will lead to attempts to restrain some of physicians' practices, actual control over these practices is likely to be assumed by the organizations that employ or pay physicians. The profession itself, however, may retain development of policies concerning these controls.

There is a natural concern about possible limitations and reductions in the use and availability of care. Patterns of care in the United States, including the rate of use of tests, procedures, and hospital beds, vary from region to region and from physician to physician by as much as tenfold. What is appropriate usage? The purchasers of care, industry and consumers alike, want answers. Demands are being made for health care outcome data that use various clinical practice guidelines (CPGs) to determine the best medical management strategies. Once these strategies have been agreed upon by the insurer's panel of physician experts, payment for implementing other strategies will be denied, particularly if the other strategies are more costly or less effective than the approved ones. Malpractice liability also has created a need for review of these data in an effort to reduce liability somewhat.

An array of initiatives designed to define and improve the quality of health care has been developed over the past decade. One of these stands out and can be attributed to the writings of W. Edwards Deming, whose work gained wide acceptance in Japan after World War II. Deming and others promoted a specific process for improving quality in manufacturing and other industries. The goal of the process, called continuous quality improvement (CQI) or total quality management (TQM), is to set into motion a permanent method of evaluating production quality by setting standards, improving performance, determining where standards are not being met, changing performance to meet the new standards and, when necessary, redefining the standards on the basis of what was learned throughout the cycle. The goal is a continuous spiral of improved quality in the final product. Some CPGs have been developed by the American Academy of Pediatrics in concert with the American Academy of Family Practice, the federal Agency for Health Care Policy and Research, and other organizations. Many hospitals and managed care organizations already are applying these principles of quality assurance; the development of CPGs is one example.

EFFECTIVENESS OF CARE

Although all practitioners must demonstrate at least a minimal amount of theoretical knowledge as a condition of licensure before they enter practice, the relationship between performance in tests and subsequent quality of practice has never been demonstrated. Even the procedure by which physicians become certified as "specialists" provides dubious assurance of high quality. As noted above, practice organization (e.g., group practice, teaching hospital practice) is more important as a determinant of quality than are individual physician characteristics. Board certification, apart from its relationship to longer lengths of postgraduate training, appears to have no relationship to practice quality. Continuing education requirements and periodic recertification procedures imposed by professional organizations are unlikely to improve the situation unless the model of quality of care on which the original educational and certification procedures are based is broadened to encompass assessment of the impact of services on health status.

Up to this point, this chapter has examined issues relating to the structure and process of medical care. Manpower, the organization of care, accessibility, and costs reflect the structure, or form, of health services. The process of care has been addressed in the discussion of quality, which involves recognizing patients' problems, further gathering of data to arrive at medical diagnoses, instituting therapy, and reassessing to ensure optimal response to therapy. As has been shown, patients contribute to the process of care by deciding whether to seek it (utilization), accept it, and understand it and comply with recommendations. The third means by which care may be evaluated is based on the attainment of goals, or outcomes. Outcomes may be divided into four categories: deaths, illness and injury, disability, and others.

Improving Health and Well-Being: Outcomes of Care

The significant declines in mortality over the past century can be attributed more to improvements in public health than to specific technologic advances applied to individual patients. The discovery of antibiotics is the only scientific advance applied to individual patients who are ill that has had a major impact in improving length of life; even here, the predominant, albeit not the only, effect seems to have been to reduce deaths in the elderly from acute infectious complications of chronic illness. The marked improvement in life expectancy over the past century has resulted primarily from lowered infant mortality. Infant mortality began to decline long before specific medical interventions were imposed, and the decline resulted from general improvements in sanitation, maternal nutrition, hygiene, and infant feeding.

Deaths are registered uniformly and therefore are available and easily tabulated. But after infancy, deaths in childhood are so relatively infrequent that they are an insensitive indicator of the value of medical interventions.

Perhaps measuring the value of personal health services delivery in terms of a reduction in mortality is too great an expectation. Rather, some say that the measure of the system should be a reduction in the occurrence of disease and its manifestations—morbidity. But even here, it is unclear that physicians make a critical difference. Certainly the introduction of immunization has been responsible for large declines in the incidence of diphtheria, tetanus, pertussis, poliomyelitis, rubeola, rubella, and *Haemophilus influenzae* type b and hepatitis B infections and for the eradication of smallpox. But once again, it is the public health sector rather than the practice of individual physicians that has been most responsible. Federal funds to support immunizations have been crucial to the effectiveness of these programs; attempts to reduce or eliminate federal support have led to reduced immunization and to disease epidemics among children, particularly the poor.

Illness and injury data are obtainable only for those few conditions for which reporting is mandated by law because of their potential public health impact (contagiousness), such as rubella, rubeola, and hepatitis; however, these causes of morbidity constitute a small proportion of the health problems of children. National health surveys, including household surveys and surveys of practitioners' offices, are an important source of information about the prevalence of other child health conditions.

The ongoing household survey administered by the Department of Health and Human Services' National Center for

Health Statistics obtains information about disability from a sample of the population. Disability is ascertained by asking questions about limitations on activity resulting from chronic conditions and about restrictions on usual daily activity or confinement to bed as a result of acute conditions.

Increasingly, the impact of medical care is being measured; evidence exists that individuals are more or less comfortable, more or less satisfied with their health, more or less able to achieve their physical and intellectual potential, and more or less able to control physical, emotional, and social threats to their health. The pediatric practitioner of the future will be confronted more with these new concepts of disease and health than with the acute illnesses that have preoccupied the child health practitioner of the past.

The impact that health services can be expected to have, even under the best of circumstances, is limited by the role of other forces. At least four factors determine an individual's state of health (Fig. 1-1). Genetic constitution is the basic determinant. People differ in predisposition to specific illnesses and in response to their treatment largely because of differences in their genotypes. Probably the second most important determinant of an individual's state of health is his or her social and physical environment. Where individuals live, how they work, the food available to them, and the stresses imposed upon them by the social system all affect how healthy they are and how well they resist insults to their health. Children particularly are vulnerable to the effects of the physical and social environment, because they are even less able than adults to select their surroundings and exposures. The third most important ingredient is the role that individuals themselves play in their behavior. Although young children are less likely to determine their life patterns than are adults (whose smoking, drinking, eating, and driving behaviors are major underlying causes of death), the patterns set for them by their parents influence not only how ill health is dealt with in childhood, but also how well they are taught behavior destined to affect their health in later life. The final and probably least critical determinant of health, except in unusual situations, is the provision of medical services.

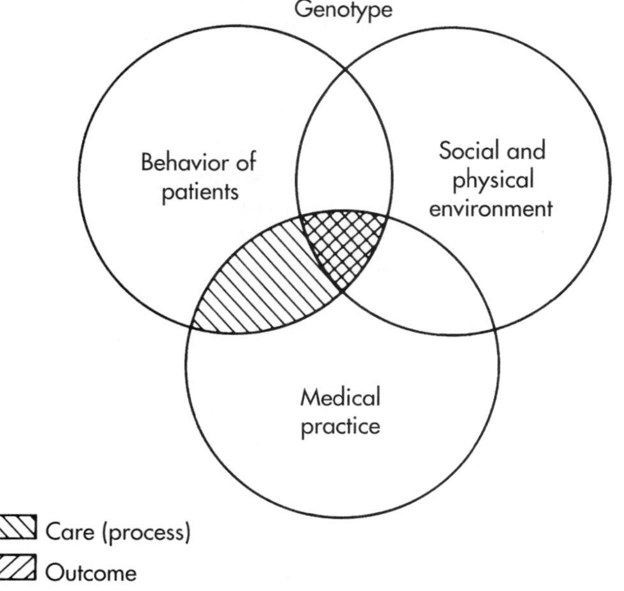

FIG. 1-1 Determinants of health status.

Who Defines "Good Care"?

Consumers and providers of health services differ in the priorities they place on the three main elements of care: access, cost, and quality. Costs of and access to medical care are of prime importance to consumers. In contrast, neither access nor cost is an important component of medical school training, which focuses almost exclusively on how to make a diagnosis, how to support this diagnosis with appropriate information from the history, physical examination, and laboratory findings, and how to institute treatment appropriate to the diagnosis. The nature of most educational settings (university-based, research-oriented, with generally a highly specialized faculty) is responsible for the following important limitations in medical training:

1. The educational process focuses largely on the biochemical and biophysical bases of disease processes. In contrast, relatively little attention is devoted to understanding the social, occupational, and environmental causes of ill health, although these are major determinants of disease.
2. The diagnostic process emphasizes assigning single causes for disease and arriving at a single diagnosis. It is more appropriate today to consider multiple causes of a disease. Moreover, one disease often is complicated and modified by the presence of another disease or a genetic, environmental, or psychosocial factor.
3. Insufficient attention is paid to the concept of human variability. In medical education, little attention is paid to the reasons why some individuals who are predisposed to disease stay well whereas others succumb, and why some respond to therapy and others do not.
4. Students' exposure to patients' illnesses are short term. Education, composed of blocks of time in various specialties, does not prepare students to assume long-term responsibility for patients, as will be required in the subsequent practice of medicine.
5. Students learn about illnesses either through reading about them or by participating in the care of ill patients. In both instances, their knowledge is derived primarily from experiences with patients at university-affiliated hospitals. Patients appearing for care at such institutions are not representative of the population as a whole or even of the patients whom the students will subsequently meet as practitioners.

In the education of physicians, "quality" of care, characterized by the use of optimal techniques in arriving at diagnostic and therapeutic decisions, is virtually the only dictum emphasized. With this limited concept of "quality," it might be expected that at least diagnosis and therapy would be optimum in clinical practice. Unfortunately, this is not the case, as the following situations indicate.

Many well-accepted diagnostic strategies are of unproven usefulness, and some are actually harmful. For example, studies have shown that patterns of laboratory use may bear little or no relation to patients' needs. The extent of error, both in clinical observations and in laboratory findings, appears largely unrecognized by physicians. Outcome data will help to define these errors.

Many commonly applied therapeutic maneuvers are of unproven usefulness and may be dangerous. For example, several studies demonstrate that surgical rates in the United States are much higher than in other developed countries, without any demonstrable difference in the need for surgery as defined by prevalence of disease or illness. Even within the United States, the number of hospital admissions, the length of stay in the hospital, and the rate of surgical procedures vary markedly from area to area, unrelated to differences in medical need. Outcome data will help determine the usefulness of various therapeutic maneuvers.

Another problem is the misuse of drug therapy. For many physicians, drug manufacturers' representatives and advertisements are the primary sources of information on new drugs. Several surveys have shown a widespread lack of appreciation of the dangers of many drugs and much unwarranted use of drugs. Outcome data will be helpful in determining the usefulness of drugs by helping physicians prescribe them more appropriately.

Even when diagnostic and therapeutic interventions can be shown to be appropriate and efficacious, applying them does not necessarily produce the desired outcome. This is because adequate diagnosis and therapy, although necessary for high-quality care, are by themselves insufficient. The treatment of illness and the maintenance of health also require the participation of patients and potential patients and a supportive social and physical environment, as Fig. 1-1 shows. The very best quality of care, defined as efficacious diagnosis and treatment, will fail to achieve its effect if those who require it and can benefit from it do not appear for care, if they fail to understand and accept it, or if they are unwilling to comply with the prescribed therapy (Fig. 1-2).

For these reasons, the traditional definition of quality of care should be broadened from its concentration on diagnostic and therapeutic strategies to include two additional facets of medical practice: problem recognition and follow-up with reassessment.

Problem Recognition

The application of diagnostic or therapeutic strategies requires first that problems, or potential problems, be recognized. Evidence indicates that the existence of many types of health problems often is overlooked.

Physicians are consistently poorer at recognizing the existence of significant behavior problems and social factors related to illness than they are at recognizing problems with obvious biophysiologic or anatomic manifestations. But even organic problems may be neglected. Many children, and adults, too, have health conditions that their physicians fail to follow, even when information about these conditions is available. Failure to recognize the problems that patients bring to physicians is a serious shortcoming in the provision of health services, because it has been shown that this failure is associated both with decreased patient satisfaction and failure to follow medical advice. Without recognizing the full range of patients' problems, no diagnostic strategy or therapeutic intervention can be fully effective.

Problem recognition also extends to prevention of disease. One type of prevention, primary prevention, is traditional to pediatricians. It consists of recognizing susceptibility to disease and applying measures to prevent it from occurring. Immunizations are the most obvious example of primary prevention, but prevention goes far beyond this. Sometimes only certain people are at risk of acquiring disease later in life; pediatricians must direct efforts at discovering who these people are, at keeping them under surveillance, and at trying to eliminate the situations that allow the illness to develop. This is known as secondary prevention. As social, occupational, environmental, and behavioral factors become recognized as important antecedents of many chronic illnesses, pediatricians will become more involved in activities directed toward preventing them.

Up to now, secondary prevention has not been a common feature of pediatric practice, and when children at risk have been identified, it generally has been at the initiative of government and social agencies. Examples of such efforts include hearing and vision screening in schools, special screening programs for specific disease in special populations (sickle cell anemia, Tay-Sachs disease), and state-mandated neonatal screening for inherited metabolic disorders (e.g., phenylketonuria). A major challenge for pediatricians is recognizing and dealing with occupational hazards that result in

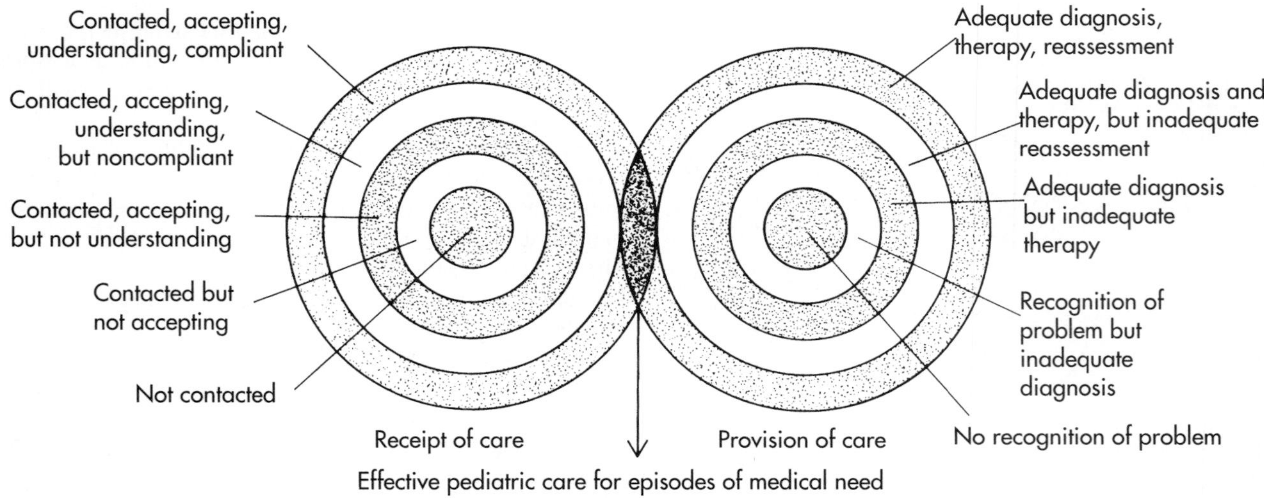

FIG. 1-2 The process of pediatric care.

parents unknowingly exposing their children to toxic materials invisibly carried home from the workplace. Ultimately, pediatricians must assume responsibility for coordinating all the care of children, including primary and secondary prevention, as well as treating manifest illness.

Follow-up and Reassessment

To ensure that diagnostic procedures and instituted therapy are adequate and that problems are being resolved as expected, patients must be monitored; this is known as outcomes assessment.

Medical textbooks and teaching rarely include information that would help the practitioner define appropriate intervals for reassessing particular health problems. Such information would have to come from careful studies of the natural history of patients' problems, with and without intervention, and such studies are rare. Moreover, little is known about the extent to which practitioners follow up problems they treat. When the issue has been examined, it has been found that failure to follow up on treated patients results in unresolved health problems. At the very least, it produces a highly inefficient health care system; care is paid for, but no benefit is gained. At the most, it will ultimately lead to societal demands for greater accountability of the profession.

It seems likely that future physicians will be encouraged, and perhaps even required, to keep certain types of data about the children in their practices. A data set for hospitals to use for each patient admitted and a similar set for ambulatory care have been accepted by the National Committee for Health Statistics and recommended for wide use. These include registration data (patient identification number, name, address, birth date, sex, race, and marital status) and encounter data (facility identification number, provider identification number, patient identification number, source of payment, date of encounter, patient's purpose for visit, physician's diagnosis, diagnostic and management procedures, and disposition). Adoption of this or a similar system for collecting information in a standardized way will facilitate the understanding of health and disease processes and the role medical care plays in influencing them.

A national collaborative research network, under the aegis of the American Academy of Pediatrics, has been developed that involves hundreds of office-based pediatricians in scientific inquiry about child health problems and their care. Participation in such networks can provide a stimulating experience for pediatricians and engage them in a lifelong process of continuing education and intellectual renewal. Pediatric practitioners who are involved contribute in a major way to improving knowledge about the distribution and nature of child health problems and their responsiveness to medical therapy.

REFERENCES

1. *AMA News,* Aug. 17, 1992.
2. *AMA News,* March 7, 1994.
3. American Academy of Pediatrics, Department of Research: Career characteristics of pediatricians: working paper no 17, Elk Grove, Ill, 1992, The Academy.
4. American Academy of Pediatrics, Department of Research: Periodic survey: no 21, Elk Grove, Ill, 1993, The Academy.
5. American Academy of Pediatrics, Department of Research: Periodic survey of fellows: no 25, Elk Grove, Ill, 1994, The Academy.
6. Federation of Pediatric Organizations: Graduate medical education and pediatric work force issues and principles, *Pediatrics* 93:1018, 1994.
7. Randlett R: Report of the National Resident Matching Program, *Acad Med* 68:502, 1993.
8. Randlett R: Report of the National Resident Matching Program, *Acad Med* 69:508, 1994.
9. Roback G et al: *Physician characteristics and distribution in the US,* Chicago, 1994, The American Medical Association.
10. Shappert SM: National Ambulatory Medical Care Survey: 1991 summary, Vital and Health Statistics, Series 13, no 116, 1994.
11. Shappert SM: National Ambulatory Medical Care Survey: 1992 summary: advance data from Vital and Health Statistics, no 253, Hyattsville, Md, 1994, The National Center for Health Statistics.
12. Shubiner H et al: Perspectives of current trainees in combined internal medicine-pediatrics, *Am J Dis Child* 147:885, 1993.
13. *Socioeconomic characteristics of medical practice,* Chicago, 1992, The American Medical Association.
14. Staddard JJ et al: Health insurance status and ambulatory care for children, *N Engl J Med* 330:1420, 1994.
15. Stout N: *Managed care digest: HMO edition,* Kansas City, Mo, 1994, Marion Merrill Dow.

2 Morbidity and Mortality Among the Young

Ivan B. Pless and Charles E. Pless

Understanding the major causes of death, disease, and disability in children and adolescents is central to the efforts of all who serve the young. The goal must be to prevent the preventable with respect to disease and its consequences and to limit disability resulting from the unpreventable. Moreover, the patterns of mortality and morbidity over time provide a basis for predicting future child health needs. The *mortality* rate is the proportion of children who die in a given time period; it may be age, sex, or disease specific. *Morbidity* rates describe the proportion of children who are affected by any illness or impairment at a given time or over a specified period of time.[28]

Variations in these statistics often are attributable to socioeconomic differences, but they also may reflect differences in medical care. For example, much of the variation in infant mortality from state to state follows a pattern of aggregate economic well-being. But this is inevitably confounded by the amount and sophistication of health care available in these areas. Thus rates generally are lower in the wealthier Northeast than in the poorer Southeast. Likewise, important differences between the races persist that undoubtedly reflect both socioeconomic and medical care factors (Fig. 2-1).

International comparisons add another perspective to mortality statistics. The outstanding causes of death vary greatly between the United States and countries in Latin America, where infant mortality ranges from 20 to 105 per 1000 live births.[36] However, in 1991, the United States ranked twenty-first among the 25 countries with the lowest infant death rates. The rate in 1992 was 8.5 per 1000—only a 5% improvement over the previous year.[40] For some, this disappointing performance is a reflection on the serious shortcomings in the availability of antenatal and postnatal care for many U.S. citizens.

HEALTH STATISTICS

Health statistics comprise births, deaths, and other measures of the occurrence of disease and may be expressed as prevalence or incidence. *Prevalence* is the proportion of individuals in a population who have a specific disease at any particular time; *incidence* is the proportion who develop new cases of a disease over any given period of time.[28] Both rates are expressed only in relation to those who are potentially at risk for a particular disorder (e.g., both sexes are not included in the denominator when figures on circumcisions or teenage pregnancies are presented). Most of the morbidity rates described in this chapter are prevalence rates per 1000 children under 18 years of age. Mortality statistics, however, usually are given as rates per 100,000. As a rule, crude rates alone are of little use when comparing different populations or groups. They must be standardized using statistical procedures to allow for differences, such as age and sex distribution, among the populations being compared.

National statistics can be used to estimate roughly what will be seen in an individual pediatric practice. For example, in a typical practice of 2500 to 3000 patients, given a prevalence of asthma of nearly 40 per 1000, a pediatrician may expect to be providing care for about 120 asthmatic children at any given time. However, even over a 10-year period and allowing for patient turnover of 10% per year, the same physician will see only a few cases of any less common disorder. Because the applicability of national estimates varies considerably from region to region, this variability should be taken into account when applying such estimates to specific settings.

Birth Rates

Around 1955, when the birth rate was approximately 24 per 1000, a striking decline in the rate began in the United States. By 1974 it had fallen to 15 per 1000. However, between 1986 and 1990, it increased 11%, so that in 1991, the rate was 16.3 per 1000.[23] The implications of this trend are important in relation to the absolute size of the child population and its size relative to the elderly. Both factors influence the number of health professionals and hospital beds needed to care for children properly.

The fertility rate (the birth rate among women of childbearing age) fell 35% between 1950 and 1992 with the rate in 1992 being 69.6 per 1000.[23] The effect of this fall on the actual number of children born was countered to some degree by the larger number of women of childbearing age, who were born during the postwar baby boom. Numerous factors are involved in the decline in fertility. It is widely believed that the state of the economy during this time played a large role, as did the growing desire to limit family size for other reasons. Certainly the widespread availability of more effective methods of contraception, such as contraceptive pills, and the growing number of legal abortions also were important factors.[31]

Unmarried teenage pregnancies are a cause of morbidity and mortality for both mother and child, especially for mothers under 15 years of age. Preterm deliveries are much more common for African-American teenage mothers than for Caucasians.[4] Of the babies born in 1991 to young women in this age group, 13.7% weighed less than 2500 grams.[23] The birth rate for unmarried teenagers 15 to 19 years old doubled between 1970 and 1991, from 22.4 to 44.8, and the pregnancy rate increased even more. The availability of legal abortions, one third of which were performed on women in this age group, has prevented the teenage birth rate from rising even faster.

Leading Causes of Death

Although preventing premature death is a priority for all pediatricians, the amount of attention given to any specific cause is not always commensurate with its importance. For

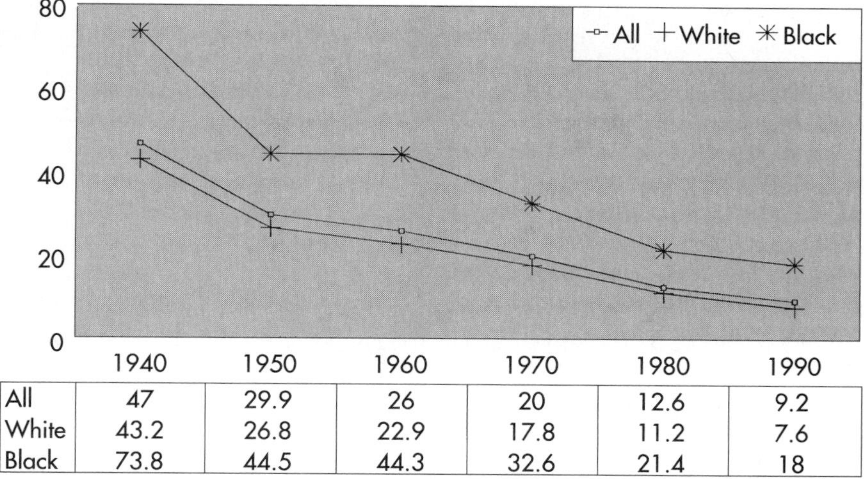

	1940	1950	1960	1970	1980	1990
All	47	29.9	26	20	12.6	9.2
White	43.2	26.8	22.9	17.8	11.2	7.6
Black	73.8	44.5	44.3	32.6	21.4	18

FIG. 2-1 U.S. infant mortality rates, 1940-1990. Deaths per 1000 live births during the first year of life. The 1992 U.S. infant mortality rates (those most recently available at this writing) were 8.5 for all infants, 6.9 for Caucasian infants, and 16.8 for African-American infants.

(Data from United States Center for Health Statistics: Annual summaries of vital statistics.)

example, as Table 2-1 shows, accidents are the most common cause of death after the first year of life, but much less time is devoted to preventing them than to the care of minor illnesses or of major illnesses with lower mortality rates than accidents.

Main Causes of Death by Age Group

In 1992 the infant mortality rate reached an all-time low of 8.5 per 1000 live births, a drop of 82% since 1940.[40] This is due to improvements in the treatment of perinatal disorders (particularly asphyxia and other respiratory conditions), immaturity, and gastrointestinal problems. Despite this remarkable record, almost 50% of all deaths up to 18 years of age still occur during the first year of life; as stated earlier, this key statistic is still not as good in the United States as it is in many other, less wealthy countries.

Moreover, in 1960 the infant mortality rate for African-Americans was 44.3 per 1000 live births, compared with 22.9 per 1000 for Caucasians; in 1992 the respective rates were 16.6 and 6.9 per 1000. Thus, although rates for both races have improved, they have begun to level off, and the gap has ceased to narrow since 1980 (see Fig. 2-1).

The causes of death in children over 1 year of age have changed remarkably little over time, although the trend generally is one of consistent improvement. In the 1 to 14 age group, accidents (unintentional injuries) followed by malignancies and congenital anomalies are the main causes. A particularly disturbing change, however, is the rise in homicides. Between 1968 and 1992 the rate increased from 1.5 to 2.8 per 100,000 for those 1 to 4 years of age, and from 0.6 to 1.6 for those 5 to 14 years of age. On average, these trends represent a worsening of about 60% in just over 3 decades.

Of particular concern is the alarming increase in firearm deaths among teenage African-American boys ages 15 to 19 between 1984 and 1988—an increase that almost certainly has continued.[8] For African-American girls ages 10 to 14, the firearm death rate more than doubled in a single year, from 1987 to 1988.

In 1992 the death rate in the age group 15 to 24 years was 95.6 per 100,000; 76% of the almost 35,000 deaths in that age group were caused by accidents, homicide, and suicide, in that order (see Table 2-1). Hence, in this age group, and across all ages, the most promising opportunities for further reducing death rates lie with preventing serious injuries and with gaining greater understanding of the social and psychological factors that lead to suicide and homicide (see Chapters 104, Suicidal Behavior in Children and Adolescents, and 108, Violent and Aggressive Behavior).

Temporal Trends by Specific Cause of Death

The rates of infant deaths resulting from pneumonia, bronchitis, and meningitis have remained almost stable since 1952, and deaths from most congenital abnormalities are virtually unchanged since 1932. For example, the death rate for congenital heart disease still is approximately 20 per 100,000, probably because improved technology (e.g., open heart surgery) has resulted only in the postponement of death.

Sudden infant death syndrome (SIDS), which long has been of great interest to epidemiologists, now receives more attention from clinicians. Several studies suggest a fairly consistent incidence over time of about 2 to 3 in 1000 live births, but little is known about the causes or the prevention of the syndrome. (SIDS is discussed in greater detail in Chapter 265.)

Another area of concern is the number of injuries and deaths resulting from child abuse and neglect, but accurate estimates are difficult to obtain. The incidence ranges from 6.3 per 1000 for newborns to 2-year-olds to 22.6 per 1000 for those 12 to 14 years of age.[6] Most of the deaths occur in infants and young children. Injuries are more common in older children but are less severe and thus less likely to be reported as abuse.

An illuminating report produced by the National Center for Health Statistics (NCHS) highlights the large decline in death rates during the last half of the twentieth century and the increasing proportion of deaths caused by injuries and vio-

Table 2-1 Major Causes of Death by Age: Birth Through 24 Years, United States, 1992*

Cause of death	Age (yr) <1	1-4	5-14	15-24	1-14	0-24	Total no. of deaths
Accidents (E800-E949)	20.5 [4]	9.3 [1]	9.3 [1]	37.8 [1]	11.3 [1]	22.1 [1]	20,336
Perinatal conditions (760-779)	389 [1]	0.7	0.1	—	0.8	17.4 [2]	15,708
Homicide (E960-978)	8.1	2.8 [5]	1.6 [3]	22.2 [2]	2.0 [4]	10.2 [3]	9362
Congenital anomalies (740-759)	186.2 [2]	5.5 [2]	1.2 [4]	1.2	2.5 [3]	10 [4]	9203
Suicide (E950-959)	—	—	0.9	13.0 [3]	0.6	5.6 [5]	5007
Neoplasms (140-239)	3.9	3.5 [3]	3.3 [2]	5.3 [4]	3.4 [2]	4.1	3809
Infections (001-139; 320-322; 466; 480-487; 590)	29.4 [3]	3.0 [4]	1.0 [5]	2.7 [5]	1.6 [5]	3.3	3000
Cardiovascular (390-398; 402; 404-429)	17.9 [5]	1.8	0.8	2.7 [5]	1.1	2.4	2254
Cerebrovascular (430-438)	4.1	0.3	0.2	0.5	0.2	0.5	477
Pulmonary (490-496)	1.1	0.4	0.3	0.5	0.3	0.4	397
Renal (580-589)	4.7	<0.1	0.1	0.2	0.1	0.3	282
Gastrointestinal (531-33; 540-543; 550-553; 560; 571; 574-575)	2.5	0.1	0.1	0.2	0.1	0.3	278
Anemias (280-285)	1.2	0.4	0.3	0.3	0.3	0.3	302
Diabetes (250)	0.0	0.0	0.2	0.4	0.1	0.2	167
Pregnancy complications (630-676)	0.0	0.0	0.0	0.3	0.0	0.1	111
Nutritional deficiencies (260-269)	0.5	0.0	0.0	0.0	0.0	0.0	40
All other external causes (E980-E999)	1.0	0.2	0.1	0.9	0.1	0.5	461
All other diseases	194.7	8.5	3.3	7.2	4.9	14	12,939
Total (rate)	865.7	43.6	22.5	95.6	28.8	91.3	
Estimated population (thousands)	4000	15,512	36,542	36,147	51,964	92,111	
Number of deaths	34,628	6764	8193	34,548	14,957	84,133	84,133

Adapted from the National Center for Health Statistics: Advance report of final mortality statistics: 1992, Monthly vital statistics report, vol 43, no 6, suppl, Hyattsville, Md, 1994, Public Health Service.
Figures in parentheses indicate International Classification of Disease, 9th revision, 1975 categories. Figures in brackets indicated ranking (1-5).
*Deaths per 100,000.

lence.[9] It also calls attention to the sizable race, sex, and geographic differences in many causes of death, especially injuries.

As well as the wealth of specific statistical information provided, the report by Fingerhut and Kleinman[9] makes an important conceptual distinction. The authors introduce the terms "natural" to refer to "medical" (i.e., noninjury) disease categories and "external" to refer to all others (i.e., accidents, homicide, and suicide). The distinction is important because physicians traditionally concern themselves primarily with medical disorders, even though the external category encompasses the most important causes of death at all ages after the first year of life. Deaths in both categories follow a U-shaped pattern by age; children ages 4 to 12 years have the lowest rate, and those younger and older have higher rates. Among younger children the rates are largest for natural causes; in adolescence, external causes dominate.

As stated, most trends over time are encouraging. Although most of the dramatic improvements in all age groups occurred during the first half of the century, mortality rates continued to fall, except among those 15 to 19 years of age. Since 1970 these rates have declined still further, between 37% and 50% in those under 9 years of age, but much less (about 25%) among older children and adolescents. However, the patterns are quite different for the two major categories; natural causes fell by about 70% in all age groups since the early 1930s, and external causes declined by only about 30%.

But the trends for some natural causes are considerably less impressive. For example, among 5- to 14-year-olds, deaths from infectious illnesses fell by only 20%; much the same is true for deaths from neoplasms over this period.

Of special interest is the shift in relative importance between the two categories. Between 1900 and 1950, the proportion of deaths among 5- to 9-year-olds resulting from external causes rose from 9% to nearly 40%; the same general pattern is seen for the other age groups as well. This reflects both growing success in combating natural causes and absolute increases in deaths from injuries. The data also show that the more recent improvements, although widespread, are distributed unequally within the population; for example, the decline in death rates since 1979 has been more rapid among Caucasian children than among African-American children.

The importance of injuries as a cause of death in the 1980s and 1990s is underscored both by the NCHS report and by other such data.[14,16] Although injuries remain the leading cause of death in all age groups over 1 year, their decline since 1975 has been impressive but uneven. In the age group 1 to 14 years, the rate has fallen by nearly 30%, whereas among those 15 to 24 years, the decline has been only about half as great, approximately 18%.[41]

Hoekelman and Pless[16] suggest that the trends described above are unlikely to be the result of any methodologic artifacts and that in the case of natural or "medical" causes, much of the credit for the improvement must be given to advances in medical technology such as vaccines, antibiotics, and surgical techniques. In comparison, the external causes reflect societal phenomena, only some of which have been identified: counseling, health education, seat belt legislation, and reductions in motor vehicle speed limits. However, it must be noted that in some age groups, the death rate actually has increased in certain categories since 1975; these categories include cardiovascular and renal diseases, perinatal conditions, homicides, and suicides. In the case of the first two conditions, part of the explanation may be greater diagnostic accuracy and measures that prolonged survival, so, in effect, deaths that would have occurred in one age group have been postponed to another. Explanations for the rise in homicides and suicides are, sadly, all too apparent: an increase in societal violence generally, the popularity of firearms, and widespread pessimism among many young people.

International Comparisons

Apart from the disappointing infant mortality statistics described earlier, at the international level, the United States in 1985 had the highest injury death rate compared with those of eight other developed countries; this is true for all age groups, with few exceptions.[41] The rates for homicide and suicide among teenagers (ages 15 to 19) also are the highest, except for suicide among Canadian teenage boys. In contrast, the differences are much less pronounced for deaths resulting from natural causes, and generally the rankings for the United States are in the midrange for all age groups.

MORBIDITY AND DISABILITY

Clinicians need to distinguish morbidity from disability. "Disability" is defined by the National Center for Health Statistics as "a general term used to describe any temporary or long-term reduction of a person's activity as a result of an acute or chronic condition." For practical purposes, days in bed, days off from school, and days of limited activity are the measures most commonly used for disability. However, children frequently experience an illness (or an episode of morbidity) that is not accompanied by any notable disability. Those with colds, for example, may attend school and play actively, and even children with a limb in a plaster cast often participate in vigorous athletics.

Disability

The most important aspect of morbidity is the extent of disability that it produces. Because there is no universally accepted way to assess disability, several indicators are used to describe the extent and manner in which illnesses are manifested. A common factor in most indicators is an estimate of functional impairment, as reflected in alterations of usual activities. However, "usual activities" depend on age. Moreover, many childhood illnesses, such as asthma and epilepsy, are episodic. Thus even with a chronic disorder, levels of disability may vary greatly from one day to the next. It is particularly difficult, therefore, to judge the overall disability of children who have chronic disorders. To confuse matters further, parents of handicapped children may fail to distinguish between what is "usual" for their child and what is usual for the child's healthy peers.

Many observers have been troubled by the possibility that efforts to save sick newborns might result in an increasing societal burden to care for more disabled or handicapped individuals. In fact, however, some reports suggest that the incidence of cerebral palsy is decreasing among infants who have received good neonatal care. Furthermore, several studies have noted a falling number of low-birth-weight and premature babies. This trend, combined with improved care for such babies in neonatal intensive care nurseries, may have had a significant impact on both infant mortality and the quality of survival.[1] The net effect may be an appreciable reduction of handicaps that are secondary to birth factors. But in Sweden the decrease in the incidence of cerebral palsy, first noted in the early 1960s, appears to have reversed. Hagberg and colleagues[12] reported that the rate for the years 1967 to 1970 (about 1.4 per 1000 live births) has risen sharply. Between 1979 and 1982 the average crude prevalence was 2.17 per 1000. Although more recent figures are not available, the fear that improved technology might have adverse effects is not without substance and reflects in particular the impact of this technology on ever-smaller and younger preterm infants, who are surviving in increased numbers.[34]

An average child misses 5.3 days of school per year because of illness or injury. Most such absences (58%) are caused by respiratory disorders. Infective and parasitic diseases account for 20%, injuries for 8.2%, digestive system conditions for 4.5%, and all other acute conditions for 9.5%. On average, girls miss considerably more school than boys; however, boys are almost twice as likely to be absent because of injuries.

An analysis of trends in disability, based on parental reports of the proportion of children whose activity is limited due to chronic illness, indicates a near doubling of rates since 1960.[24] In 1960 1.8% of children under 17 years of age had activity limitations of some degree; 0.9% were limited in their major activity. By 1981 these figures had risen to 3.8% and 2%, respectively. The percent change between 1964 and 1978 was much greater among children who were not poor than among the poor. Although a number of methodological factors may account for some of these findings, it is likely that these factors account for only a small part of the trend.

International Comparisons. Three commonly used indicators—disability days, bed days, and the percentage of those whose activities were limited during the preceding 2 weeks—based on parents reports, were compared for Canada and the United States.[17] Distinctions depended on whether an illness or injury prevented a child from carrying on the major activity typical of his or her age group (e.g., ordinary play with other children or school attendance), whether it only limited the amount or kind of major activity performed, or whether it restricted only strenuous activities such as athletics.

In 1978-79 children under age 15 in the United States had more disability days per person per year than their peers in Canada (11.1 versus 8.7) and also had more bed days per person per year (5.2 versus 3.6); the percentage with limitations of activities was higher for U.S. children than for Canadian children (3.7 versus 2.8). During the same period the death rates were comparably greater in the United States: for those under age 15, 128 in the United States compared with 116 in Canada; the difference was especially marked for those under age 1 year and reversed somewhat for those between 10 and 14 years of age.[17]

Population-based Morbidity and Disability. Ogden Nash defined the family as "a unit composed not only of children, but of men, women, the occasional animal, and the common cold." The cold remains the dominant illness of childhood and one that occupies a disproportionate share of the physician's time and skill in view of its usually self-limiting nature. Together, upper respiratory and gastrointestinal tract infections account for more than 60% of all acute childhood illnesses. In addition, about one third of all children have at least one accident each year, and 3% of these require hospitalization. Approximately 1 child in 10 has a chronic physical illness by age 15, at least 5% of all children have emotional problems, and roughly 3% are handicapped because of low intelligence. A precise figure for the constellation of problems encompassed by the rubric "learning disorder" is impossible to determine; the reported range is 3% to 23%.

Acute Illness

Over the past 25 years the incidence of infectious diseases has declined impressively in the United States because of the development of effective vaccines.[21] The elimination of smallpox and the virtual extinction of poliomyelitis and the serious sequelae of mumps and measles are excellent examples of the success of vaccine technology. An important role in these advances was played by the development of improved, more stringent methods of field-testing procedures, which is essential to ensure the safety and effectiveness of the vaccines. The immunization story is one of the major triumphs of public health, and it is one in which the practicing community has played a key role.

However, the development of effective vaccines illustrates an age-old and continuing problem: how to ensure that good technology is implemented fully, promptly, and appropriately. Currently it is estimated that nearly 40% of 2-year-olds have not received recommended immunizations.[10] In most parts of the country immunizations are provided by private practitioners, but in some areas public health departments also are involved. As a result, adequate immunization records are difficult to maintain. Perhaps partly because of poor tracking, on several occasions since the mid-1970s there have been alarming increases in measles, often with serious sequelae. With the help of well-directed government funding, the number of cases fell from 57,000 in 1977 to 3211 between 1982 and 1983. However, from this nadir in 1983, "the number of reported cases approximately doubled in the next 5 years, and in 1989 to 1990 the United States experienced the worst epidemic of measles in nearly 2 decades, with nearly 46,000 cases and 130 deaths."[21] It appears that this reflects at least partly the withdrawal of government funding for immunizations and the failure of many funded programs to reach preschool, lower-income children. This should be overcome by the Comprehensive Childhood Immunization Act of 1993, enacted by Congress, which provided what is, in effect, free vaccine for children insured by Medicaid and others who lack insurance that covers immunizations.[10] Obviously, still greater success in this area depends heavily on continued federal involvement.

Apart from infectious diseases and the acute, usually viral illnesses normally seen in physicians' offices, the remaining acute disorders are those treated in emergency departments (ED) or outpatient departments (OPD). The National Hospital Ambulatory Medical Care Survey, initiated in 1991, found that children under age 15 accounted for 25% of all ED visits, making on average nearly 40 visits per 100 persons per year. For visits classified as "urgent," the rate was 15.7; for those classified as "nonurgent," the rate was 24.2.[18] Nearly the same proportion (22.5%) of all OPD visits were made by children (22.5 visits per 100 persons per year), although only 13.5 of all OPD visits were to pediatric departments.[19]

Chronic Disorders

Chronic conditions affect children less often than acute disorders, so the rate of occurrence for a chronic condition usually is expressed as the prevalence in 1000 persons under 18 years of age. The rates per 1000 based on the 1988 National Health Interview Survey are shown in Table 2-2.[25] Respiratory (96.8) and skin allergies (32.9) have the highest rates, followed by asthma (42.5). Disorders of speech, hearing, and vision combined affect 54.2 children per 1000. An interesting feature in this table are the sharp and as yet unexplained differences in the rates in the ethnocultural groups listed, as

Table 2-2 Prevalence of Specific Chronic Conditions Among Children Under Age 18*

Condition	All	White	Black	Hispanic
Respiratory allergies	96.8	114.7	53.6	47.4
Asthma	42.5	42.0	51.3	35.1
Eczema and skin allergies	32.9	36.7	21.7	19.2
Speech defects	26.2	24.0	34.5	35.4
Digestive allergies	22.3	27.0	9.9	8.4†
Deafness and hearing loss	15.3	18	6.0†	15.2
Heart disease	15.2	18.3	7.7†	10.0
Musculoskeletal impairments	15.2	15.8	10.6	15.2
Blindness and vision loss	12.7	13.8	8.7†	13.3
Anemia	8.8	8.9	9.2†	7.5†
Arthritis	4.6	4.8	5.4†	2.0†
Epilepsy and seizures	2.4	1.9	2.4†	6.2†
Sickle cell disease	1.2†	<0.1†	7.1†	0.3†
Diabetes	1.0†	1.3†	<0.1†	0.3†
Other	19.8	23.6	10.2	9.2†

Adapted from Newacheck P, Stoddard J, McManus M: *Pediatrics* 91:1031, 1993.

*United States, 1988; cases per 1000.

†Prevalence estimate has a relative SE >30.

seen, for example, for asthma, where the rate among African-Americans is one third greater than among Hispanics. These national figures may or may not be consistent with those found at the level of the community; hence, as stated earlier, they can be used only as a rough guide to what may be expected in a typical practice.

Hospital Morbidity

Another important measure of morbidity is hospitalization. The advantage of this measure is that in many countries statistics based on discharge diagnoses are collected routinely, making comparisons possible.

The 1992 Summary of the National Hospital Discharge Survey reported that just under 2.5 million children under 15 years of age were discharged from short-stay hospitals that year.[11] Expressed as a rate, this is 45.3 per 1000 population (50.8 for boys and 40.8 for girls). The average length of stay was 4.9 days for both sexes; there were no significant differences between boys and girls.

As shown in Table 2-3, for all children under age 15, the hospitalization rates per 10,000 population in 1992 for the three leading diagnostic categories were: respiratory, 131.3; injury and poisoning, 53.3; and digestive system, 44.5. The conditions responsible for the longest lengths of stay, however, were different: mental disorders required, on average, 16.4 days; perinatal conditions, 12.3 days; and diseases of the circulatory system, 7.4 days. As in most previous years, the procedures performed most often for those under age 15 were operations on the digestive system (389 per 100,000; e.g., appendectomy), operations on the musculoskeletal system (306; e.g., open reduction of fractures), and heart surgery (272). ENT procedures were performed on 212 per 100,000 children; of these, nearly half (90.8) were tonsillectomies.[11]

The previously cited NCHS report also compares hospitalization rates for children in the United States and Canada.[17] Although Canada has a system of comprehensive health insurance that covers all hospital costs, in many other respects the populations and systems of care are similar. The study was prompted by the finding that the hospital discharge rate for children in the United States during 1980 was among the lowest of the seven Western countries examined, whereas the rate in Canada was 42% higher (67 per 1000 versus 95 per 1000 population, respectively). It also was found that children in Canada had a longer average length of stay in the hospital (5.3 versus 4.4 days) but that the proportion of sick newborns was considerably higher in the United States.

A more recent study[14] shows that in the United States, the rate of discharges remained unchanged between 1971 and 1983 (approximately 70 per 1,000), whereas the rate in Canada fell from 112 to 89 during the same period. However, between 1983 and 1987, there was a 27% decline in hospitalizations in the United States compared with a fall of only 6% in Canada.

In the NCHS report, even larger variations between the two countries were found for specific diagnostic groups (e.g., tonsillectomy and adenoidectomy, upper respiratory infections—each showing much lower rates for children in the United States); these, in turn, varied by age. It is not clear what accounts for these differences. On the surface they may suggest that children in the United States are healthier than those in Canada. However, this explanation seems unlikely because, as has been stated, disability rates are higher in the United States. In particular, hospitalization data do not tell whether the differences represent the greater emphasis placed on ambulatory care or the existence of financial barriers to hospital care in the United States.

Substantial differences in hospitalization patterns also have been found within the United States. A report by Perrin and colleagues[27] covering a wide range of conditions shows that the rate of admissions in Boston was more than twice that in Rochester, New York, whereas that for New Haven, Connecticut, fell between the two. Although, again, socioeconomic differences may partly explain these variations, it seems likely that differential access to primary care also plays a significant role.

Table 2-3 Hospital Morbidity: Inpatient Discharge Rate at Short-Stay Hospitals by Diagnosis and Average Stay (Children Under Age 15)*

Condition	Rate	Average stay (days)
Respiratory (460-519)†	131.3	3.5
Injury and poisoning (800-999)	53.3	3.7
Digestive system (520-579)	44.5	3.7
Infectious and parasitic (001-139)	36.3	4.0
Nervous system (320-389)	24.7	3.7
Congenital anomalies (740-759)	24.5	6.9
Endocrine, nutritional, and metabolic (240-279)	20.2	5.2
Genitourinary (580-629)	13.4	4.0
Mental (290-319)	13.1	16.4
All	329.4	4.9

Adapted from: Graves EJ: 1992 Summary: National Hospital Discharge Survey: advance data from Vital and Health Statistics, no 249, Hyattsville, Md, 1994, National Center for Health Statistics.

*United States, 1992; rates per 10,000.

†Figures in parentheses indicate International Classification of Disease, 9th revision, 1975 categories.

Practice-based Morbidity

In Britain and most of Europe, pediatricians serve almost exclusively as consultants to general practitioners and, accordingly, are only involved in a small proportion of all child-physician encounters. More than half of their work involves the diagnosis and treatment of serious, complex chronic illnesses, toward which their training is heavily oriented. In contrast, most pediatricians in the United States and Canada concentrate on primary care; consequently, the spectrum of illness they see is quite different from that seen by their European counterparts and also differs greatly from the case mix encountered during residency training.

Although few data are available, it appears that office practice in most communities in the United States increasingly has become focused on well-child care and the care of children who have minor infectious illnesses. One reason may be the growth of pediatric subspecialties and the inclination of primary care physicians to refer many complex disorders to specialists. Another reason may be the loss of many older children to physicians in internal medicine. Starfield and colleagues[35] reported that in 1983, pediatricians were involved in 6% of all medical encounters involving those 15 to 19 years of age; even in the 10 to 14 age group, the proportion was only 25.5%. In both these older age groups, general practitioners and other physician specialists saw far more patients than did pediatricians. Nonetheless, most of the common infectious illnesses (e.g., otitis media, throat infections, pneumonia, diarrhea) are managed by pediatricians. Nationally, however, general practitioners provide almost as much preventive and psychosocial care (35.8% and 19.5%, respectively) as do pediatricians (44.2% and 16.5%), and considerably more surgical care.

In the 1990 National Ambulatory Medical Care Survey (NAMCS), it was reported that 19.6% of all office visits were made by children under age 15—an average of 2.5 visits per year.[33] Interestingly, Caucasian children made an average of 2.6 visits per year, whereas African-American children made only 1.5 visits per year. Of all office visits, 13.7% were to pediatricians; this represents an average of 33 visits per 100 persons per year.

Although practices vary, the general pattern is that the more complex and challenging chronic disorders rarely are seen in everyday practice.[29] On the whole, NAMCS, which is conducted periodically by the National Center for Health Statistics, shows that only 10% of all visits to pediatricians are for serious problems. Based on information obtained through NAMCS, Woodwell[42] reports that nearly 25% of all visits to pediatricians (generalists and subspecialists combined) are for well-baby examinations, general medical examinations, or inoculations. Cough and ENT complaints account for a further 32% of all visits. Noteworthy at the opposite extreme is the small proportion of visits for emotional or behavioral reasons—1% overall. But this figure rises progressively through the age groups; among those 15 to 19 years old, the proportion is 3.3%.

Use of Health Services

The development of a rational health care system should be based on the results of studies about how health services are used by children.

Patients who have symptoms of equal severity seek medical attention, if at all, at different times. The explanation for this takes into account both what the symptom is and how disruptive it is to the individual and the family. Convenience and finances, as well as a broad range of sociocultural factors, influence the decision to seek care.[3] For example, the belief that a perceived symptom is serious or that medical care is appropriate varies considerably among cultural, ethnic, and religious groups. Although little can be done to influence such beliefs, much can be done to affect some of the cost factors involved. It is estimated that the proportion of children in the United States who have no private or public health insurance increased roughly from 13% to 18% between 1977 and 1987; among poor and low-income families, the increase was from 21% to 31%.[7] A recent report concludes, "As compared with children with health insurance, children who lack health insurance are less likely to receive medical care from a physician when it seems reasonably indicated and are therefore at risk for substantial avoidable morbidity."[37]

Several studies of the use of medical care[32,38] also report correlations between the child's age, the mother's marital status and education, race, parental occupation, number of children, access to care, and use of medical services. However, different patterns are found for short-term (2 weeks or less) and long-term use of health care, as well as for the use of preventive and curative services.

Stress resulting from causes other than illness frequently determines the tolerance a parent may have for a child's symptom. Roghmann and Haggerty[30] distinguish between acute and chronic stress because each influences the use of medical services differently. For example, poor families live with stress every day, and it has been suggested that they are "crisis oriented"; that is, only when a symptom becomes extremely severe is the decision made to seek medical advice.

Many epidemiologists suggest that medical care itself may be less important in determining health than is social class. The pervasiveness of the influence of social factors on health is evident in countries such as Great Britain, where there is no barrier to care based on income. Although Great Britain has had universal health care since 1945, several studies show that social class continues to be correlated significantly with many measures of child health. However, other reports have shown that income-related problems may be ameliorated by reducing barriers to accessibility.[20] In an experiment,[2] low-income families were provided with a model of care similar to that provided in a middle-class group practice. Compared with a control group that received episodic care, the experimental group had fewer hospitalizations, operations, and illness visits, obtained more preventive services and more health supervision visits, and reported greater satisfaction—all at a relatively low cost.

Changes in health care delivery in other countries show similar results. After the introduction of universal health insurance in Canada, for instance, increases were reported in the number of lower-income families seeking early prenatal care, postpartum checkups, and postnatal examinations of infants. Increases in the percentage of individuals consulting physicians for symptoms related to measles, tonsillitis, diarrhea, and vomiting also were noted.[39]

Current Public Health Issues: Prevention and the New Morbidity

The term *new morbidity* has been used to draw attention to a group of child health problems that assumed growing importance during the 1960s.[13] Although none of the problems, strictly speaking, were "new," they had gained in prominence as many of the causes of the old, traditional morbidity declined. Thus, in place of nutritional and vitamin deficiencies, for example, more attention now is being paid to school and behavioral problems, accidents, and problems of adolescence, and the demand is growing for a more comprehensive approach to the care of children who have chronic disorders.

The argument for adopting community strategies to deal with these problems is strengthened by the complex, interacting factors that characterize much of the new morbidity. No single etiologic factor predominates, nor are these problems amenable to single or simple forms of treatment. Many involve, simultaneously and equally, dysfunction in the child, in the family, and in the community. For example, biological, psychological, and sociological forces are at work in most school and behavioral problems.

The greatest challenge presented by the new morbidity is the oldest of all—prevention. A group of scientists led by Breslow[5] systematically assessed many preventive measures aimed at children. Much the same sort of exercise was conducted in Canada by a task force responsible for evaluating periodic health examinations (e.g., routine checkups or, in the case of infants, well-baby care).[26] Further assessments of how much and what kind of preventive care is scientifically supportable[15,39] conclude that it is not yet possible to prove the value of many procedures listed in the American Academy of Pediatrics' Guidelines for Childhood Health Supervision. Nonetheless, there is some basis for recommending that primary and secondary prevention of conditions such as maladjustment, smoking, dental caries, malnutrition, accidents, communicable diseases, and unwanted pregnancies is warranted, but only at specified intervals or ages. In some cases, screening for prevention is justified only for well-defined, high-risk subgroups. How these procedures can be implemented most effectively, whether some of these can be done efficiently and properly in private practice, and how the effects are to be evaluated still must be determined. Also to be resolved are questions about how such preventive services are best organized and financed. This is especially challenging in the context of the health care reforms recently attempted in the United States.

REFERENCES

1. Alberman E: Low birthweight and prematurity. In Pless IB, editor: *The epidemiology of childhood disorders,* New York, 1994, Oxford University Press.
2. Alpert JJ et al: Delivery of health care for children: report of an experiment, *Pediatrics* 57:917, 1976.
3. Andersen RA: Behavioral model of families' use of health services, Center for Health Administration Studies, Research Series, Chicago, 1968.
4. Blankson SP et al: Health behavior and outcomes in sequential pregnancies of black and white adolescents, *JAMA* 269:1401, 1993.
5. Breslow L et al: *Preventive medicine USA: theory, practice, and application of prevention in personal health services,* Canton, Mass, 1976, Watson.
6. Christoffel KK: Intentional injuries: homicide and violence. In Pless IB, editor: *The epidemiology of childhood disorders,* New York, 1994, Oxford University Press.
7. Cunningham PJ, Monheit AC: Insuring the children: a decade of change, *Health Affairs* 9:76, 1990.
8. Fingerhut LA et al: Firearm mortality among children, youth, and young adults 1-34 years of age: trends and current status: United States, 1979, Monthly vital statistics report, vol 39, no 11, suppl, Hyattsville, Md, 1991, National Center for Health Statistics.
9. Fingerhut LA, Kleinman JC: Trends and current status in childhood mortality: United States, 1900-85, DHHS Pub No (PHS) 89-1410, Washington, DC, 1989, Public Health Service, US Department of Health and Human Services.
10. Freed GL, Katz SL: The Comprehensive Childhood Immunization Act of 1993, *N Engl J Med* 329:1957, 1993.
11. Graves EJ: 1992 Summary: National Hospital Discharge Survey: advance data from Vital and Health Statistics, no 249, Hyattsville, Md, 1994, National Center for Health Statistics.
12. Hagberg B et al: The changing panorama of cerebral palsy in Sweden. V. The birth year period 1979-82, *Acta Paediatr Scand* 78:283, 1989.
13. Haggerty RJ: The boundaries of health care, *Pharos* 35:106, 1972.
14. Hodge M, Dougherty G, Pless IB: Pediatric mortality and hospital use: a comparison of Canada and the United States, 1971-1987, *Am J Public Health* (in press).
15. Hoekelman RA: An appraisal of the effectiveness of child health supervision, *Curr Opin Pediatr* 1:146, 1989.
16. Hoekelman RA, Pless IB: Decline in mortality among young Americans during the twentieth century: prospects for reaching national mortality-reduction goals for 1990, *Pediatrics* 82:582, 1988.
17. Kozak LJ, McCarthy E: Hospital use by children in the United States and Canada, National Center for Health Statistics, Vital and Health Statistics Series 5, no 1, DHHS Pub No (PHS) 84-1477, Washington, DC, 1984, US Government Printing Office.
18. McCaig LF: National Hospital Ambulatory Medical Care Survey: 1992 emergency department summary: advance data from Vital and Health Statistics, no 245, Hyattsville, Md, 1994, National Center for Health Statistics.
19. McCaig LF: Outpatient department summary: National Hospital Ambulatory Medical Care Survey, 1992: advance data from Vital and Health Statistics, no 248, Hyattsville, Md, 1994, National Center for Health Statistics.
20. McDonald AD et al: Effects of Quebec Medicare on physician consultations for selected symptoms, *N Engl J Med* 289:1174, 1974.
21. Mortimer EA: Communicable diseases. In Pless IB, editor: *The epidemiology of childhood disorders,* New York, 1994, Oxford University Press.
22. National Center for Health Statistics: Advance report of final mortality statistics: 1992. Monthly vital statistics report, vol 43, no 6, suppl, Hyattsville, Md, 1994, Public Health Service.
23. National Center for Health Statistics: Advance report of final natality statistics: 1991, Monthly vital statistics report, vol 42, no 2, suppl, Hyattsville, Md, 1993, Public Health Service.
24. Newacheck P, Budetti PP, McManus P: Trends in childhood disability, *Am J Public Health* 74:232, 1984.
25. Newacheck P, Stoddard J, McManus M: Ethnocultural variations in the prevalence and impact of childhood chronic conditions, *Pediatrics* 91:1031, 1993.
26. The periodic health examination, *Can Med Assoc J* 121:1193, 1979.
27. Perrin JM et al: Variations in rates of hospitalization of children in three urban communities, *N Engl J Med* 320:1183, 1989.
28. Pless IB: Concepts, terms, and methods. In Pless IB, editor: *The epidemiology of childhood disorders,* New York, 1994, Oxford University Press.
29. Pless IB, Satterwhite B, Van Vechten D: Chronic illness in childhood: a regional survey of care, *Pediatrics* 58:37, 1976.
30. Roghmann KJ, Haggerty RJ: Daily stress, illness, and use of health services, *Pediatr Res* 7:520, 1973.
31. Roghmann KJ: The impact of the New York state abortion law. In Haggerty RJ, Roghmann KJ, Pless IB, editors: *Child health and the community,* ed 2, New Brunswick, NJ, 1993, Transaction.
32. Rosenstock IM: Why people use health services. II, *Milbank Mem Fund Q* 44:94, 1966.
33. Schappert SM: National Ambulatory Medical Care Survey: 1990 summary: advance data from vital and health statistics: no 213, Hyattsville, Md, 1992, National Center for Health Statistics.
34. Stanley FJ, Blair E: Cerebral palsy. In Pless IB, editor: *The epidemiology of childhood disorders,* New York, 1994, Oxford University Press.
35. Starfield B et al: Who provides health care to children and adolescents in the United States? *Pediatrics* 74:991, 1984.
36. *The state of the world's children: 1991,* New York, 1992, Oxford University Press for UNICEF.
37. Stoddard JJ, St. Peter RF, Newacheck PW: Health insurance status and ambulatory care for children, *N Engl J Med* 330:1421, 1994.
38. Suchman EA: Social patterns of illness and medical care, *J Health Hum Behav* 6:2, 1965.
39. US Congress, Office of Technology Assessment: Healthy children: investing in the future, Pub No OTA-H-345, Washington, DC, 1988, US Government Printing Office.
40. Wegman ME: Annual summary of vital statistics: 1993, *Pediatrics* 93:743, 1993.
41. Williams BC, Kotch JB: Excess injury mortality among children in the United States: comparison of recent international statistics, *Pediatrics* 86 (suppl):1067, 1990.
42. Woodwell D: Office visits to pediatric specialists: 1989: advance data from vital and health statistics: no 208, Hyattsville, Md, 1992, National Center for Health Statistics.

SUGGESTED READING

Pless IB, editor: *The epidemiology of childhood disorders,* New York, 1994, Oxford University Press.

3 Child Health Supervision

Robert A. Hoekelman

We credit George Armstrong as the father of ambulatory pediatrics and the champion of health maintenance and disease prevention in the individual child—this at a time in nineteenth century England when most of his colleagues were concerned only with the treatment of illness. In the United States child health supervision had its beginnings in the milk stations and child health conferences of our large cities, where babies were brought to be fed, weighed, examined, and immunized against contagious diseases. It was the conviction that child health supervision is vital that provided the fundamental impetus for establishment of the American Academy of Pediatrics (AAP) and that continues to be the principle upon which pediatrics as a special discipline is based. At the American Public Health Association's 1955 conference on health supervision of young children, health was defined as "a state of physical, mental, and social well-being, not merely the absence of disease or infirmity"; the objective of health supervision for children was deemed to be "to keep the well child well and promote the highest possible level of his complete well-being."[4]

It has not been documented how the frequency and content of well-child visits evolved. However, in 1967, the AAP established guidelines (later called recommendations) for child health supervision based on observed practices and expert opinion. These were revised twice during the 1970s, three times during the 1980s, again in 1991 and, most recently in 1995.[1] These revisions, also based on observations and opinions, in most instances called for an increase in the number of visits and procedures to be conducted during each scheduled visit. Table 3-1 shows the general growth in the number of child health supervision visits recommended by the AAP between 1967 and 1995. The 1995 recommendations call for 27 health supervision visits during the first 21 years of life (Fig. 3-1), in addition to a prenatal visit and at least one visit in the hospital after birth. The recommendations are designed for children who receive competent parenting, who have no manifestations of any important health problems, and who are growing and developing satisfactorily. Additional visits may be necessary if circumstances suggest variations from normal.[1]

Now, 28 years after the first guidelines were introduced, many pediatric practitioners and investigators have begun to reexamine the objectives of child health supervision and the methods by which those objectives can be met realistically in terms of needs, costs, and benefits.

OBJECTIVES

The goals of child health supervision have been categorized in several ways. However, there are three basic objectives:

1. Prevention of disease
   a. Immunization
   b. Health education
2. Early detection and treatment of disease
   a. History
   b. Physical examination
   c. Screening
3. Guidance in psychosocial aspects of child rearing

Prevention of Disease

The first objective is accomplished mostly through immunization against specific communicable diseases and through health education, initially directed to the parents and later to the child when he or she reaches the age of understanding. These educational efforts concern nutrition, dental hygiene, leading healthy life-styles, and injury prevention. The aim of this approach is to improve individual and public health. These elements of disease prevention are discussed in detail in Chapter 16, Nutrition, Chapter 21, Counseling Families on Healthy Life-styles, Chapter 22, Prevention of Dental Caries, and Chapter 23, Injury Prevention.

Early Detection and Treatment of Disease

The second objective is based on the presumption that early intervention in identified illnesses results in increased cure rates and decreased disability.

Through history-taking and physical assessment of how well or poorly an infant or child is growing and developing compared with suggested norms, invaluable criteria are developed for identifying either wellness or underlying disease. In this sense, these activities are screening tests as much as are the specific tests pediatricians use routinely to detect anemia, urinary tract infections, tuberculosis, phenylketonuria, sickle cell disease, lead intoxication, and other illnesses in asymptomatic, seemingly normal infants and children.

The principles and techniques of history-taking and the physical examination of infants, young children, and adolescents are detailed in Chapters 6, The Pediatric History, and 7, The Pediatric Physical Examination. The use of the physical examination for early detection of disease is discussed in Chapter 20, Screening, as are the specific screening tests used. The methods by which motor, intellectual, social, and emotional development are assessed and monitored in well children are discussed in Chapter 18, Identification of Developmental Delays and the Early Intervention System, Chapter 19, Language and Speech Assessment, and Chapter 74, Developmental Approach to Behavioral Problems.

Guidance in Psychosocial Aspects of Child Rearing

The psychosocial aspect of child health supervision often is placed under the rubrics of advice, anticipatory guidance, counseling, and reassuring the parents about their concerns and that they are doing a good job. Well-child visits offer an opportunity to identify potential and real problems in psychosocial adjustment, to prevent potential disorders, to treat

RECOMMENDATIONS FOR PREVENTIVE PEDIATRIC HEALTH CARE

Committee on Practice and Ambulatory Medicine

Each child and family is unique; therefore, these **Recommendations for Preventive Pediatric Health Care** are designed for the care of children who are receiving competent parenting, have no manifestations of any important health problems, and are growing and developing in satisfactory fashion. **Additional visits may become necessary** if circumstances suggest variations from normal.

These guidelines represent a consensus by the Committee on Practice and Ambulatory Medicine in consultation with national committees and sections of the American Academy of Pediatrics. The Committee emphasizes the great importance of **continuity of care** in comprehensive health supervision and the need to avoid **fragmentation of care.**

A **prenatal visit** is recommended for parents who are at high risk, for first-time parents, and for those who request a conference. The prenatal visit should include anticipatory guidance and pertinent medical history. Every infant should have a newborn evaluation after birth.

	INFANCY[3]								EARLY CHILDHOOD[3]					MIDDLE CHILDHOOD[3]				ADOLESCENCE[3]											
AGE[4]	NEWBORN[1]	2-4d[2]	By 1mo	2mo	4mo	6mo	9mo	12mo	15mo	18mo	24mo	3y	4y	5y	6y	8y	10y	11y	12y	13y	14y	15y	16y	17y	18y	19y	20y	21y
HISTORY																												
Initial/Interval	•	•	•	•	•	•	•	•	•	•	•	•	•	•	•	•	•	•	•	•	•	•	•	•	•	•	•	•
MEASUREMENTS																												
Height and Weight	•	•	•	•	•	•	•	•	•	•	•	•	•	•	•	•	•	•	•	•	•	•	•	•	•	•	•	•
Head Circumference	•	•	•	•	•	•	•	•	•	•	•																	
Blood Pressure												•	•	•	•	•	•	•	•	•	•	•	•	•	•	•	•	•
SENSORY SCREENING																												
Vision	S	S	S	S	S	S	S	S	S	S	S	O[5]	O	O	S	S	O	S	O	S	S	O	S	S	O	S	S	S
Hearing[6]	S/O	S	S	S	S	S	S	S	S	S	S	O	O	O	S	S	O	S	O	S	S	O	S	S	O	S	S	S
DEVELOPMENTAL/ BEHAVIORAL ASSESSMENT[7]	•	•	•	•	•	•	•	•	•	•	•	•	•	•	•	•	•	•	•	•	•	•	•	•	•	•	•	•
PHYSICAL EXAMINATION[8]	•	•	•	•	•	•	•	•	•	•	•	•	•	•	•	•	•	•	•	•	•	•	•	•	•	•	•	•
PROCEDURES – GENERAL[9]																												
Hereditary/Metabolic Screening[10]	←	—	•																									
Immunization[11]	•	—	→	•	•	•		←	•	→			←	•	→			•	—	—	—	—	→					
Lead Screening[12]							•	→			•																	
Hematocrit or Hemoglobin			←	—	—	—	•											←	—	—	—	•[13]	—	—	—	—	—	→
Urinalysis														•				←	—	—	—	•[14]	—	—	—	—	—	→
PROCEDURES – PATIENTS AT RISK																												
Tuberculin Test[15]								*	*	*	*	*	*	*	*	*	*	*	*	*	*	*	*	*	*	*	*	*
Cholesterol Screening[16]											*	*	*	*	*	*	*	*	*	*	*	*	*	*	*	*	*	*
STD Screening[17]																		*	*	*	*	*	*	*	*	*	*	*
Pelvic Exam[18]																		*	*	*	*	*	*	← *	*	* [18]	*	* →
ANTICIPATORY GUIDANCE[19]	•	•	•	•	•	•	•	•	•	•	•	•	•	•	•	•	•	•	•	•	•	•	•	•	•	•	•	•
Injury Prevention[20]	•	•	•	•	•	•	•	•	•	•	•	•	•	•	•	•	•	•	•	•	•	•	•	•	•	•	•	•
INITIAL DENTAL REFERRAL[21]								←	—	—	—	•																

1. Breastfeeding encouraged and instruction and support offered.
2. For newborns discharged in less than 48 hours after delivery.
3. Developmental, psychosocial, and chronic disease issues for children and adolescents may require frequent counseling and treatment visits separate from preventive care visits.
4. If a child comes under care for the first time at any point on the schedule, or if any items are not accomplished at the suggested age, the schedule should be brought up to date at the earliest possible time.
5. If the patient is uncooperative, rescreen within six months.
6. Some experts recommend objective appraisal of hearing in the newborn period. The Joint Committee on Infant Hearing has identified patients at significant risk for hearing loss. All children meeting these criteria should be objectively screened. See the Joint Committee on Infant Hearing 1994 Position Statement.
7. By history and appropriate physical examination: if suspicious, by specific objective developmental testing.
8. At each visit, a complete physical examination is essential, with infant totally unclothed, older child undressed and suitably draped.
9. These may be modified, depending upon entry point into schedule and individual need.
10. Metabolic screening (eg, thyroid, hemoglobinopathies, PKU, galactosemia) should be done according to state law.
11. Schedule(s) per the Committee on Infectious Diseases, published periodically in *Pediatrics.* Every visit should be an opportunity to update and complete a child's immunizations.
12. Blood lead screen per AAP statement "Lead Poisoning: From Screening to Primary Prevention" (1993).
13. All menstruating adolescents should be screened.
14. Conduct dipstick urinalysis for leukocytes for male and female adolescents.
15. TB testing per AAP statement "Screening for Tuberculosis in Infants and Children" (1994). Testing should be done upon recognition of high risk factors. If results are negative but high risk situation continues, testing should be repeated on an annual basis.
16. Cholesterol screening for high risk patients per AAP "Statement on Cholesterol" (1992). If family history cannot be ascertained and other risk factors are present, screening should be at the discretion of the physician.
17. All sexually active patients should be screened for sexually transmitted diseases (STDs).
18. All sexually active females should have a pelvic examination. A pelvic examination and routine pap smear should be offered as part of preventive health maintenance between the ages of 18 and 21 years.
19. Appropriate discussion and counseling should be an integral part of each visit for care.
20. From birth to age 12, refer to AAP's injury prevention program (TIPP®) as described in "A Guide to Safety Counseling in Office Practice" (1994).
21. Earlier initial dental evaluations may be appropriate for some children. Subsequent examinations as prescribed by dentist.

Key: • = to be performed * = to be performed for patients at risk S = subjective, by history O = objective, by a standard testing method ←•→ = the range during which a service may be provided, with the dot indicating the preferred age.

NB: Special chemical, immunologic, and endocrine testing is usually carried out upon specific indications. Testing other than newborn (eg, inborn errors of metabolism, sickle disease, etc.) is discretionary with the physician.

The recommendations in this publication do not indicate an exclusive course of treatment or serve as a standard of medical care. Variations, taking into account individual circumstances, may be appropriate.

FIG. 3-1

Table 3-1 American Academy of Pediatrics Recommendations for Child Health Supervision

Number of visits	Infancy (birth-1 yr)	Early childhood (1-4 yr)	Late childhood (5-12 yr)	Adolescence/ young adulthood (13-21 yr)	Total
1967	5	4	3	2	14
1982	6	5	5	4	20
1991	7	5	5	4	21
1995	7	5	6	9	27

actual disorders early in their course, and to make referrals for children and their families with gross interpersonal relationship problems that are beyond the therapeutic scope of the primary care practitioner. Anticipatory guidance in these areas is discussed in Chapter 15, Anticipatory Guidance.

Continuity of Care

Some feel that there is a fourth objective of well-child care: continuity of care. This actually can be considered more an outcome of well-child care than an objective, since it speaks to the establishment of a meaningful relationship between the pediatrician and the parents and child. It implies that regular visits produce familiarity, trust, and respect and that these enable the physician to be more effective in managing all aspects of health and illness care.

That continuity of care makes a difference in these respects, however, has not been proven, and although it seems a logical assumption, a physician who demonstrates interest in and concern for the child and family can establish a meaningful relationship instantly without that prior experience of continuity. Conversely, meaningful relationships can dissolve just as quickly if interest and concern are not sustained, regardless of past performance.

EVALUATION OF THE EFFECTIVENESS OF CHILD HEALTH SUPERVISION

The basis of the effectiveness of child health supervision (and of illness care also) lies in the pediatrician's ability to influence the parents to follow the advice and prescriptions given them. Professional competence is of little use if parental compliance is not obtained. The level of compliance is positively correlated with satisfaction, and satisfaction with effective communication between the parent and the physician, nurse, or other health professional. These interactions are extremely complex and, in part, relate to addressing the parent's concerns and expectations and the need to understand the rationale for recommendations made. The degree of satisfaction and compliance achieved depends on the extent to which these needs are acknowledged and met and on the parent's perception of the physician's empathy and view of him or her as a person (reflexive self-concept). These perceptions are formed very rapidly, often in the first moments of communication. The means by which communication and maternal compliance are enhanced are discussed in detail in Chapters 12, Compliance with Pediatric Health Care Recommendations, and 13, The Art of Consultation.

On the basis of observation of individual practitioners, there is reason to believe that health professionals are doing a good job in meeting the objectives of child health supervision for *some* of their patients and their families. However, this is not the case for most of our children nationwide. Studies of the levels of child health care achieved for specific population groups demonstrate that, for most children, practitioners fall far short of their goals. These data show that in poor urban and rural areas, fewer than 5% of children receive a level of well-child care consistent with the AAP's recommendations, and even in relatively affluent suburban and rural communities, only one third to two fifths of children receive care at that level.[15]

There are indications that practitioners are not meeting the objectives of well-child care for the vast majority of children whose parents seek such care for them. Time-motion studies of pediatricians conducting well-child care have shown that very little time is spent on individual well-child visits—12 minutes on average. This has been true for private as well as clinic patients. One must question whether the objectives of well-child care can be reached in such a short time. These studies show that pediatric nurse practitioners working in the same practices spend considerably more time on well-child care (20 to 30 minutes per visit) than do their physician colleagues.

Very few studies have assessed the content of well-child visits in terms of the amount of time pediatricians and parents spend discussing psychosocial issues and concerns. Reisinger and Bires[14] demonstrated that anticipatory guidance constituted only about 8.4% of the total time pediatricians spent in well-child visits. The practitioners studied averaged 52 seconds in providing such guidance, with a high of 97 seconds for visits involving infants 5 months of age or younger and a low of 7 seconds for patients 13 to 18 years of age.

The AAP's guidelines for health supervision are controversial because of concerns that (1) there have been no data to indicate the need for so many visits or the value of what is done during them, save administering immunizations; and (2) there are not nor will there ever be enough health care professionals (pediatricians, family medicine practitioners, nurse practitioners, or physician's assistants) to deliver such care to all or even a significant portion of our children.[3,11] Others are concerned that adhering to these guidelines ensures that the maldistribution of pediatricians (too many in suburban areas and not enough in inner city, urban, and rural areas) will continue, denying underserved children access to all facets of child health care.[6]

During the past 30 years many investigators have reviewed the overall effectiveness of child health supervision; these reviews were incorporated into a 1988 report by a study group of the Office of Technology Assessment (OTA) of the U.S. Congress. The report was an in-depth study of preventive child health services, including well-child care.[16] The study group's conclusions ranged from strongly negative to strongly positive, based on its opinion regarding intervening or process outcomes the group viewed as bad (high costs, uneven personnel distribution, overdependence of parents on health care providers) or good (parent and provider satisfaction, improved parental compliance with provider instructions, better acute care through establishment of an informed and trusting relationship). However, the study group was unable to base its conclusions on any studies that meet Elinson's accepted criteria for determining the worth of health care intervention.[5] These criteria require that studies be prospective, involve some planned intervention (e.g., child health supervision as recommended by the AAP) designed to achieve specific end points (e.g., improved child health in terms of decreased mortality and morbidity), and include control as well as experimental groups. Meeting Elinson's criteria presents some difficulties in evaluating the effectiveness of child health supervision.

In its 1977 report, the AAP's Ad Hoc Committee on the Value of Preventive Child Health Care[10] stated, in applying Elinson's criteria to child health supervision, that preventive child health care is a process applied throughout infancy and childhood and that it would require study over many years if its overall value were to be proven. This creates problems in maintaining sample and investigator continuity, because patient mobility and academic permanency (a condition affecting potential researchers) often is short-lived. Patient mobility could be counteracted by appropriately increasing the size of the initial experimental and control groups to allow for losses. Maintaining investigator continuity would require personal commitment and good health over time; these requisites, particularly that of continuity, are not always assured for academicians, who are most likely to be chosen for principal investigator positions in studies of this type.

The end points chosen could include indices of health and illness, school performance, or psychosocial adjustment. However, new instruments for measuring indices in any of these areas would have to be developed, particularly to maintain uniformity throughout the samples. Large samples would be required, because there would be multiple intervening independent variables, and the differences in the end points most likely would be small. A multicenter study design would be required to overcome geographic, economic, and cultural population variables; this would compound the investigator-continuity problems and create difficulties in standardization.

Any long-range study carries the risk of process and measurement obsolescence. For example, new preventive care procedures could become operative at midpoint and distort planned end point measures; or end points considered significant at the beginning of the study may no longer be significant at the end of the study because of social, political, educational, or medical changes.

The cost of conducting a study of this type would be extremely high, and the prospects for assured, continued funding, even with sanction and direction from the AAP, might not be bright.

Another consideration is the ethical issue of withholding from children in the control group methods of medical management considered valuable. This could be addressed through a passive relationship with the control group and an aggressive promotion of the AAP's preventive care recommendations with the experimental group. A retrospective approach could be used with the control group consisting of children who had received no or few preventive health care services, but this would not meet Ellison's prospective criterion.

The Ad Hoc Committee on the Value of Preventive Child Health Care recognized that the task it recommended is complex and will require considerable time and effort to complete. Nevertheless, it is the only way to determine the overall effectiveness of the child health supervision schedules recommended by the AAP.

To these limitations on studying the overall effectiveness of child health supervision, the OTA study group[16] added the observation that, "The health status of children in particular (and the population in general) is far more strongly determined by social and economic factors than by the nature of medical care; hence, the contribution that well-child care can make to health outcomes is likely to be modest, and studies to detect these modest contributions must be based on very large samples. Few available studies of the effectiveness of child health care have had very large samples. None of them directly address the question of the overall effectiveness of well-child care."

The OTA study group's review of the literature evaluating the effectiveness of well-child care as a whole concludes that well-child care as now performed (other than immunization) has no overall effect on childhood mortality or morbidity and exerts little influence on developmental and social functioning outcomes. In 1990 the Canadian Task Force on Periodic Health Examination reached the same conclusion.[2] Despite this, child health supervision will remain the basis upon which most pediatric practices are built, because it provides parental and physician satisfaction and reassurance (in some cases conviction) that well-child visits keep children well and prevent serious illnesses.

ALTERATION OF STANDARDS

If society accepts the premises that large segments of the child population are not receiving what practitioners feel to be optimal health care and that good health care is an inherent right of all citizens and not simply a privilege available to those who can afford it, it becomes obvious that practitioners must compromise their standards of adequate well-child care, the methods of delivering that care, or both.

In regard to changing the standards of child health supervision, practitioners must consider the fact that there is some substantiation that reducing the frequency of visits, at least for infants identified as low risk, does not alter the outcomes in terms of their physical health.[7,9] Thus the number of visits could be reduced by half without compromising one aspect of the quality of care. Practitioners must consider that some children may require only minimal health supervision other than completion of immunization schedules, whereas others will require much, much more.

Another alternative would be to use health care providers other than physicians for child health care. For the most part, pediatricians have been reluctant to do this for a variety of reasons, not the least of which is their concern that the quality of child health supervision would diminish under these circumstances. However, there is good evidence that using nonphysicians, particularly pediatric nurse practitioners, for most elements of well-child care does not reduce the quality of that care. Studies performed in private practices, prepaid group practices, and university hospital clinics have demonstrated that pediatric nurse practitioners are entirely competent to provide well-child care and that the care they render does not result in altered health outcomes, increased utilization, decreased compliance, or decreased parental satisfaction. Equally important, this model is less expensive than that in which the physician provides all elements of well-child care.

Providing health education and guidance in the psychosocial aspects of child rearing to groups of parents also is a means of reducing professional time expended on child health supervision visits, and this method has proved satisfactory to some practitioners and parents.[13]

Consideration of the costs of care must include (1) use of physician time that might be more effectively applied to other health problems; (2) the extent to which taxes should be used to support activities that have so few proven beneficial outcomes; and (3) a family's ability to afford the fees charged, the expenditures for transportation and baby-sitting services while the parent is away from home, and the loss of income for working parents who must comply with the daytime visit schedules of private practices, clinics, and health centers. Having public health nurses provide all aspects of child health supervision in the homes of underprivileged women and children has proved to be a cost-effective method of delivering such services to a population at high risk that would not receive them otherwise.[12]

DISCUSSION

From the early 1930s through the late 1980s, numerous practice-based studies and those conducted by the National Center for Health Statistics (the National Ambulatory Medical Care Survey) have shown that 30% to 45% of primary care pediatric office visits are for child health supervision and that more than 50% of some primary care pediatricians' office time is spent in this activity. These percentages have risen over time as visits and procedures have been added to the AAP recommendations, and they most surely will rise again with the 1995 increase in recommended visits, from 20 to 27 between birth and age 21.*

*This increase was based on the Bright Futures Project, which was sponsored by the U.S. Public Health Service's Maternal and Child Health Bureau and by the Medicaid Bureau of the Health Care Financing Administration. The project's findings were published in 1994[8] and were approved by 16 national medical, nursing, and child advocacy organizations, including the AAP, the AMA, and the American Nurses Association (ANA). They were officially adopted by the AAP in 1995.[1]

In adhering to the AAP's guidelines, pediatricians would limit the number of children they can care for who have other health and illness care needs that currently are unmet. It seems that practitioners either must explore further the evidence at hand to determine if they can reduce the frequency of well-child visits or employ others to conduct such visits. Practitioners need to change their perspective on traditional professional roles and methods and focus on the goal of meeting the health supervision and illness care needs of all children.

REFERENCES

1. American Academy of Pediatrics, Committee on Practice and Ambulatory Medicine: Recommendations for preventive pediatric health care, *Pediatrics* 96:373, 1995.
2. Canadian Task Force on Periodic Health Examination: Periodic health examination: 1990 update, *Can Med Assoc J* 143:867, 1990.
3. Chamberlin RW, Schiff DW, Rogers KD: Are routine periodic child health visits beneficial? In Smith DH, Hoekelman RA, editors: *Controversies in child health and pediatric practice,* New York, 1981, McGraw-Hill.
4. Committee on Child Health: Health supervision of young children, New York, 1955, American Public Health Association.
5. Elinson J: Effectiveness of social action programs in health and welfare; from Assessing the Effectiveness of Children's Health Services, Report of the Fifty-Sixth Ross Conference on Pediatric Research, Columbus, Ohio, 1967, Ross Laboratories.
6. Fossett JW, Peterson JA: Physician supply and Medicaid participation, *Med Care* 27:386, 1989.
7. Gilbert JR et al: How many well-baby visits are necessary in the first 2 years of life? *Can Med Assoc J* 130:857, 1984.
8. Green M, editor: *Bright futures: guidelines for health supervision of infants, children, and adolescents,* Arlington, Va, 1994, National Center for Education in Maternal and Child Health.
9. Hoekelman RA: What constitutes adequate well-baby care? *Pediatrics* 55:313, 1975.
10. Hoekelman RA, Thompson HC: Value of preventive child health care, Evanston, Ill, 1977, American Academy of Pediatrics.
11. Hoekelman RA: Well-child visits revisited, *Am J Dis Child* 137:17, 1983.
12. Olds DL, Kitzman H: Can home visitation improve the health of women and children at environmental risk? *Pediatrics* 86:108, 1990.
13. Osborn LM, Woolley FR: Use of groups in well-child care, *Pediatrics* 67:701, 1981.
14. Reisinger KS, Bires JA: Anticipatory guidance in pediatric practice, *Pediatrics* 66:889, 1980.
15. Staub HP et al: Health supervision of infants on the Cattaragus Indian Reservation, New York, *Clin Pediatr* 15:44, 1976.
16. US Congress, Office of Technology Assessment: Healthy children: investing in the future, Pub No OTA-H-345, Washington, DC, 1988, US Government Printing Office.

SUGGESTED READING

Hoekelman RA: An appraisal of the effectiveness of child health supervision, *Curr Opin Pediatr* 1:146, 1989.

4 Legal and Ethical Issues for the Pediatrician

Thomas A. Massaro and Walter J. Wadlington

In today's complex society, primary pediatric care often extends beyond traditional medical boundaries; those who care for children are involved increasingly with the broader social issues that confront our society. To serve as effective advocates for children in this environment, pediatricians must understand not only the contemporary political and social milieu, but also the legal and ethical structures that operate within it. This chapter examines some common ethical and legal problems encountered in everyday pediatric practice.

LEGAL AND ETHICAL REASONING—SIMILAR METHODOLOGIES

Ethical and legal systems both seek to guide human conduct. Ethics concentrates on the values on which behaviors are based, whereas the law attempts to define basic behaviors that support the smooth functioning of society. In pediatrics, the distinction between the ethical and the legal sometimes is blurred (especially if issues of medical malpractice are treated separately). There are many similarities in process between the two disciplines. Both tend to be case driven, and both require careful interpretation of specific facts. Both seek to apply historical precedents to current deliberations. Conceptual frameworks such as the algorithm describing the different levels of analysis (from theory to principle to rule to recommendation for particular actions) originally developed for bioethical deliberations[1] can be applied equally well to legal thought.

THE LEGAL SYSTEM

For many of us, it would be simpler if "the law" were a single logical structure—a geometry that develops in an orderly fashion from a set of basic assumptions. In reality, at least three independent constructs constitute the legal system that affects children: (1) common law or case law based on judicial decisions; (2) statutory law generated through legislative action; and (3) administrative law shaped by the growing governmental regulatory process that exists simultaneously in separate federal and state systems. And because most issues affecting children are based on state rather than federal law, the rulings and interpretations may differ significantly from one jurisdiction to another.

DECISION MAKING BY AND FOR CHILDREN

Decisions Regarding Medical Care

Historically, under common law, minors were presumed to be incompetent; that is, unable to make decisions on their own behalf until they reached "majority." In most states today, majority arrives on the eighteenth birthday (although special restrictions may apply for certain situations such as purchasing alcoholic beverages). Pediatricians will argue that a single chronological milestone defining "competency" runs counter to what we know about human development and that the attainment of competency is an incremental maturation process that brings increased capacity and responsibility along the way. For example, children of 11 or 12 years of age who can begin to handle conflicting viewpoints may be in a position to understand treatment alternatives, but the law historically draws a more rigid line between competency and incompetency. Fortunately, however, this strict interpretation is gradually being modified in both case law and legislation. A more flexible definition of competency is emerging, and pediatricians should be prepared to endorse those changes whenever possible. As part of this trend, most states have defined *emancipated minors,* and many have accepted *mature minor doctrines* through case law or formally through the development of legislation.

The Emancipated Minor

Emancipation is a means for declaring that a minor can conduct legal affairs as an adult. Once an amorphous, common law theory that forced determination of the details of each specific case,[2] the concept increasingly has been codified to provide certainty through judicial decree sought after a child reaches a certain age, usually 16.[3] Emancipation also may be effected by a minor's marriage, but parental consent generally is required in jurisdictions allowing marriage at an age below majority. Many jurisdictions have enacted statutes for such purposes as permitting a minor parent to relinquish a child for adoption or to donate blood.

The Mature Minor

In recent years there has been progress toward empowering minors to make decisions relating to medical care for themselves, even when general emancipation doctrines do not apply. Although in most cases the principle still applies that someone who has legal authority (usually a parent) must consent to nonemergency medical care to avoid a possible action for battery (the unauthorized invasion of a person's protected bodily interest), exceptions have been created through special "minor consent" doctrines in most states; these typically allow a minor to consent to treatment (without additional parental approval) for certain conditions or procedures such as crisis counseling, communicable disease, family planning (not including abortion), or substance abuse. Some states have gone farther by enacting statutes allowing a mature minor to consent to health care procedures in general.[4]

Although it might be assumed that the special laws dealing with medical consent reflect increasing concern about expanding the general decision making autonomy of minors, they actually were based largely on medical expediency. If children in the specified circumstances would be unwilling to consult with their parents, they might not seek care. The laws also may be regarded as an acknowledgment of change, or a breakdown, in traditional family relationships. Legally, many of these laws leave some perplexing, unresolved issues for pediatricians. In many jurisdictions, important legal concerns remain unanswered, such as patient confidentiality (when is it appropriate to inform the parents of a sexually active consenting minor of an IUD placement?), financial responsibility (can an insurance claim be filed under a family policy without notifying the parent?), and informed consent (at what point is the patient intellectually capable of making a decision that rationally considers the alternatives?). The new laws also pose ethical dilemmas regarding whether or how to protect the privacy and decision making autonomy of the minor, even when this may delay or preclude parental involvement.

The question of what information must be disclosed to a child is the reverse of the confidentiality issue; that is, what we are obliged to tell a child despite parental objections. Sigman, Kraut, and La Puma[5] describe an interesting ethical dilemma regarding disclosure of the diagnosis of cystic fibrosis against the wishes of the parents. Accepting that while the patient was young, withholding information was ethical behavior as long as the physician's personal and professional value system was not violated, the authors conclude that with increasing maturity, the nondisclosure is less defensible.

Terminal Illness

An especially difficult and often controversial issue is whether a minor patient can authorize life support measures to be withdrawn. Many states have natural death acts that allow a competent individual to declare a treatment pattern to be followed in the event of subsequent incompetence and terminal illness, but most of these laws directly or indirectly exclude children. Texas is one of a few states that include children in their natural death provisions. A review of the Texas experience over a 3-year period indicated that this inclusion creates no extraordinary legal or ethical problems. Seventeen patients ranging in age from 2 days to 15 years were involved. Thirteen declarations actually were implemented, and bioethics committee consultation was required in only two cases.[6]

In the absence of applicable legislation, the issues surrounding withdrawal of support can be very complex and often are channeled through the courts. (Four states address the issue of a child's right to die directly; three others provide some direction for caregivers.) A case study in the medical literature in 1973 explained the process by which a 16-year-old was allowed to withdraw from dialysis after she had rejected a kidney transplant.[7] There was no legal intervention, and the discussion focused largely on ethical issues.

Case law in this area varies significantly across jurisdictions. In late 1989 the Supreme Court of Illinois held that a 17-year-old who had leukemia and who needed blood transfusions was a "mature minor" who could refuse transfusion because of her right to the free exercise of her religion.[8] Reasoning that Illinois law allows individuals over age 12 to seek medical attention for certain conditions, permits pregnant or unmarried women under 18 to consent to treatment, and has accepted the "mature minor" concept in other contexts, the court concluded that the common law right to control one's health care with regard to decisions of terminal illness also should extend to mature minors, especially as the child approaches the age of majority.[9] A Maine court allowed premajority statements of a terminally ill patient who later entered a vegetative state to be used as evidence of his wish not to be kept alive in such a condition.[10] But a Texas court would not apply the rationale of the Illinois decision in the case of a 16-year-old who refused consent to a transfusion and executed a document releasing his physician from any liability,[11] explaining that Texas had no equivalent mature minor doctrine.

Minors as Organ Donors

The issue of whether a parent can authorize inter vivos (close to death) donation of an organ (usually a kidney) from one of his or her minor children to another has reached several different courts. Ordinarily a guardian is charged with acting to further the interests of the ward, and one line of reasoning would question whether such a donation is of any benefit to the ward. At least two courts have held that it is not,[12] although others have been willing to permit such a donation by rationalizing a benefit to the donor who otherwise might suffer guilt or other psychological reactions on later learning that she might have saved her sibling but did not.[13] Developments in immunosuppression have obviated some of the previous pressures, particularly in cases involving identical siblings. Procedures for using cadaver tissue usually are governed by the same rules applicable to adult decedents, though minors typically are not permitted to make donations to be effective on their death.[14]

Minors as Research Subjects

The issue of children as research subjects is derived from the notion that children are incompetent and therefore unable by definition to make informed decisions about alternatives. Although research data suggest that older children are no less likely than adults to appreciate the implications of the research process fully, the concept that majority is required for informed consent has been supported. As a result, we do not allow children to participate in experimentation that poses a serious threat to them, even if it benefits others. Federal regulations support the ethical position that a parent or guardian may consent to participation in a study benefiting others only if it imposes "minimal risk" to the child. Of course, in one sense this merely shifts the debate to the interpretation of "minimal risk." If a study involves more than minimal risk, as appropriately defined, *and* offers the potential of direct benefit to the child, an institutional review board (IRB) must determine if (1) the risk is justified by the potential benefit; (2) the risk is no greater than that posed by existing available treatments; and (3) the assent of the child and the permission of one parent has been obtained.

Civil Commitment

In *Parham v. J.R.*,[15] the U.S. Supreme Court ruled in 1979 that the due process clause of the Constitution did not require Georgia to provide an initial adversary hearing when a minor was committed involuntarily by the parents to a mental institution because "natural bonds of affection lead parents to act in the best interests of their children." However, some states do provide for an administrative hearing for minors over a certain age (e.g., 14 years) if they object to being institutionalized for mental illness or psychiatric problems.[16]

Brain Death

The success of solid organ transplantation in children has brought considerable attention to the diagnosis of brain death in young patients. Over the past several years, a consensus has developed that the criteria for brain death in adults can be applied to children, including full-term newborns over 7 days old. Premature newborns and all infants under 1 week old are excluded because of the difficulty in establishing appropriate criteria and because some brainstem functions may not be developed fully and therefore cannot be determined reliably.[17]

THE RELATIONSHIP BETWEEN PARENT AND CHILD

Background

Common law once regarded children as tantamount to property of their parents, who were entitled to their earnings but required to provide for their basic needs. The concept of "child as chattel" has changed, but parents retain decision making authority on behalf of the child, and their duties of support have expanded. However, courts have begun to recognize that a child's interests may not always coincide with those of the parents, who do not always act in the best interests of their offspring. And child protection initiatives emanating from the *parens patriae* doctrine (literally the state as parent or protector) now permit much broader state intervention in response to detrimental action or inaction by a parent.

Legal Status

Determining the legal and biological parents is an important part of the history-taking and care-planning process. Developments in assisted conception may well provide the ultimate catalyst for revision of the outmoded rules that still characterize much of our law regarding establishment of parentage,[18] but until that time, pediatricians must work within an inefficient and often confusing structure. It was long presumed legally that a child born to a married woman cohabiting with her husband was the latter's legitimate offspring.[19] With current laboratory techniques that can not only exclude a possible father, but also establish a high degree of probability of paternity in many cases, challenges increasingly are being registered. When paternity claims have been substantiated by these techniques, courts generally have responded by giving additional rights and responsibilities to the claimant.

A recent series of constitutional decisions has recognized greater rights for fathers of children born out of wedlock when these fathers come forward or are identified in a timely fashion and when they wish to develop parental relationships with their children.[20] Those rights may include visitation or custody or the need for paternal consent to an adoption. An unwed father who has established a good working relationship with his child usually can preclude adoption by someone else without his consent.[21] States have established specific procedures, sometimes including a "putative father registry," to deal with legal problems of the father who does not come forward to establish such a relationship. Failure to meet the requirements of such schemes can effectively preclude the assertion of parental rights by a biological father.[22]

A state also can choose to fix legal parentage in a person not the biological parent. This was made clear when the U.S. Supreme Court upheld application of a California law that effectively blocked a putative biological father's attempt to establish his paternity of a child born to a woman married to someone else, even though the plaintiff had once lived with the mother and child.[23]

Although these issues previously were more a matter of paternity, gestational surrogacy has begun to raise them on the maternal side as well. Already one court has determined that in some instances a gestational mother can be regarded as the legal mother in preference to the oocyte donor seeking maternal rights after a child's birth,[24] although a proposed legislative model would hold to the contrary.[25]

Limits on the Parental Role in Medical Decision Making

Questions about the scope and correctness of parental decisions and the degree to which they may be overridden by the state continue to arise. At one time parental authority to authorize or decline medical treatment for a child was very broad.[26] But more recently, legislative and judicial action have combined to permit courts to review and overrule parental decisions in life-threatening situations. Typical among these were cases in which a parent refused to authorize a blood transfusion for an operation that held promise for a cure, with almost certain death the alternative.[27] Because such parental objections often were motivated by sincerely held religious beliefs, federal constitutional issues of freedom of religion were posed. In appointing a guardian to make the medical decision, many courts echoed a pithy statement from an earlier constitutional case that did not involve medical intervention:

> Parents may be free to become martyrs themselves. But it does not follow that they are free, in identical circumstances, to make martyrs of their children before they have reached the age of full and legal discretion where they can make that choice for themselves.[28]

In a more recent series of cases, courts have shown willingness to intervene in the parental decision making process in other than life-threatening cases. A major turning point was a New York case in which the parent of a child who had neurofibromatosis with significant unilateral facial hypertrophy would not consent to blood transfusions necessary for ameliorative, cosmetic surgery. The Family Court determined:

> [T]his court's authority to deal with the abused, neglected or physically handicapped child is not limited to "drastic situations" or to those which constitute a "present emergency," . . . the Court has a "wide discretion" to order medical and surgical care and treatment for an infant even over parental objection, if in the Court's judgment the child's health, safety or welfare requires it.[29]

The judge added that:

> If this court is to meet its responsibilities to this boy, it can neither shift the responsibility onto his shoulders nor can it permit his mother's religious beliefs to stand in the way of obtaining through

corrective surgery whatever chance he may have for a normal, happy existence, which . . . is difficult of attainment under the most propitious circumstances, but will unquestionably be impossible if the disfigurement is not corrected.[30]

Recently the issues have resurfaced in the form of criminal prosecution against parents whose children died after they were treated through prayer rather than medicine. The results have varied, depending on matters of individual statutory interpretation[31] and whether laws allowing religious exceptions to medical treatment in some instances but not in others provide adequate notice for parents as to when their conduct is punishable.[32] Other cases are arising regarding cultural rather than religious differences in medical treatment, and courts continue to grapple with establishment of standards for determining when intervention is appropriate, trying to include factors such as probability of success and quality of life (or what can be regarded as medical success).[33]

Do Not Resuscitate (DNR) Decisions by Parents

In 1984 the Georgia Supreme Court confronted the issue of whether parents could permit removal of life support from a terminally ill minor in a persistent vegetative state.[34] The court held that once the diagnosis had been made and confirmed by two uninvolved physicians, the parents could decide in the exercise of the minor's right to refuse treatment. Subsequently, in *In re Doe,*[35] the same court faced the situation of two parents disagreeing over the proper medical course for their 13-year-old terminally ill child. The court held that the two parents shared equally in decision making and if one disagreed with the decision to forego CPR, the hospital must follow the Georgia statute's presumption that every patient is presumed to consent to resuscitation. Illinois has codified authority in surrogate decision making and has specifically included decisions for children in that priority setting.

Parental Duties

Parents are required not only to support their children, but also to provide necessary medical and other care. The state, acting through its courts, can exercise considerable child protection authority under the common law doctrine of *parens patriae*. But the scope of these parental duties and the legal response to failure to perform them today are widely defined by statute as well. In addition, overriding parental decisions on medical care, courts may remove the child from parental custody and, in the most severe cases, terminate parental rights. Criminal sanctions also may be imposed for neglect or abuse.

Termination of Parental Rights

To involuntarily terminate parental rights, the state must support its allegations by clear and convincing evidence, a fairly high standard of proof.[36] At one time the underlying basis for such termination typically was couched in general language, such as "unfitness." Today statutes more often set forth specific circumstances under which termination can be justified, such as continual danger in returning a child to a home after removal for severe abuse or neglect. Generally the state must take steps to try to remedy the conditions that led to separation and to reunite parents with their children, but the statutes typically fix a time after which termination proceedings can proceed if such attempts are unsuccessful. A major effect of terminating parental rights is to make a child eligible for adoption rather than foster care.

Although many of the cases in which termination takes place involve clear cases of abandonment or physical abuse, termination also may be effected when parents are physically or mentally incapable of meeting their child's special medical needs.[37]

Reporting Statutes

Child abuse reporting statutes require or seek to promote notification of a public official or agency of cases involving children who are abused or neglected by their families.[38] Although initially regarded by many as focusing principally on physical abuse, the definitions of the conduct or conditions that must be reported now often are tied into those contained in child abuse, neglect, and endangerment statutes generally. Most of the latter are broad enough to include failure to provide necessary medical care, known increasingly as "medical neglect"; therefore this may be a condition that must be reported.

Most reporting statutes require physicians and other health care providers to report suspicious events or circumstances that become known to them in their professional capacity. Almost all provide some specific sanction for not reporting, and there also is the possibility of a civil action for damages against one who willfully fails to report as required by the statute, although for such an action to be successful, it must be established that the failure to report contributed significantly to a subsequent injury that might have been averted.[39] The statutes usually immunize good faith reporters from damage awards based on their action. Many also render the physician-patient privilege inapplicable in cases subject to required reporting and authorize physicians to take photographs of a child's injuries (see Chapter 56, Child Abuse and Neglect).

Custody and Visitation after Separation or Divorce

The basic duty of both parents to support their children continues after divorce. The father's obligation once was considered primary, but today the amount of support ordinarily is based on the ability of the respective parties to contribute.

When one parent is awarded primary custody of a child upon the separation or divorce of a couple, the noncustodial parent usually is entitled to visitation privileges unless it is determined that such contact would be harmful or detrimental to the child. In an increasing number of cases, courts are making "joint" or "shared" custody awards. The terminology often is used loosely; such an award may provide for joint physical custody, in which the child spends a substantial amount of time with each parent, or for joint legal custody, in which one parent may be the primary physical custodian, with the other sharing in decisions about matters such as medical care and education. Joint custody generally is explained as reflecting the state's desire to assure maximum involvement by both parents in the rearing of their child. Usually, courts will not make a joint custody award if the parents strongly oppose it or if their personal relationship would make it difficult or impossible for them to carry it out successfully[40] (see Chapter 58, Children of Divorce).

ADOPTION

Adoption establishes a parent-child relationship between individuals not so related by blood kinship, substituting adoptive parents for the birth (or previously adopting) parents. The consent of the child's parents is required unless their rights have been terminated, although some states provide a method through which courts can override a parental objection when consent is withheld contrary to the child's best interests.[41] Notification of the parents is required, in any event, to ensure due process of law,[42] and the courts have shown reluctance to permit adoption over parental objection if parental rights have not been terminated and if there is no basis for such termination, such as unfitness.[43]

Placement Issues

Placement can be classified as "agency" or "private" according to whether a state or state-licensed agency serves as an intermediary between birth and adoptive parents. Although physicians (particularly obstetricians) at times have become directly involved in the private placement process, some jurisdictions now hold that any "placing" activity is unlawful for professionals such as physicians and lawyers unless they formally qualify as child welfare agencies.[44] A few jurisdictions even make it difficult or impossible to process adoptions for children not placed through an agency. However, nonagency placements with close relatives and stepparents are not only permitted widely but often can proceed under streamlined procedures facilitating them.

Confidentiality of Adoptions

States generally have provisions allowing anonymous placement through an agency shortly after a child's birth. A new birth certificate is entered, and information about the birth parents is sealed, to be opened only on court order. In what can be described as a "search for roots," some adopted children later seek to determine their birth identity.[45] One strategy is to seek out records or information from obstetricians or pediatricians who had medical contact with the child before placement. Physicians should be aware that such information usually is legally confidential. In a case in which a physician gave an adopted child a letter incorrectly stating that the child needed to know her birth mother's identity because the latter had been given diethylstilbestrol (DES) during pregnancy, it was determined that the birth mother had a legal cause of action against the physician for breach of a confidential relationship.[46]

In some instances it may be important to construct a genetic history for an adopted child when neither the adoptive parents nor the child know the identity of the birth parents. The courts have been reluctant to fully open the files to the parties[47]; rather, they have sought to obtain such information through confidential means when feasible. It now is common for adoption agencies to try to obtain and keep genetic information so that it can be made available, if needed, without having to reveal the birth parents' identities.

Subsidized Adoption

Subsidized adoption is a method through which the state can provide financial assistance to adoptive parents of "special needs" children. It was given considerable impetus by amendments to the Social Security Act in 1982,[48] and today such programs, operated by the states with joint federal and state funding, have succeeded in integrating many "hard to place" children with adoptive families rather than relegating them to the uncertain world of long-term foster care.[49] Typically, the state negotiates a contract with the individual adopters based on the child's special needs and the adopters' ability to support them. Medical care can be assured by extending Medicaid eligibility to the child regardless of whether the adopting parents would qualify for it. This has produced occasional problems of adjusting payments guaranteed by the adopting state if the child moves to another state that has different Medicaid coverage.

Open Adoption

Today advocacy is increasing for "open" adoption, under which a natural parent could retain some rights, such as visitation, after adoption. Many if not most state statutes seem to preclude such an approach without amendment.[50] However, several courts have allowed at least limited enforcement of a contract between a birth parent and adoptive parents for what would be tantamount to an open adoption.[51] In one such case, the natural parent was a mother who executed a divorce settlement agreement providing that she would maintain visitation rights, although she agreed that her ex-husband's new wife could adopt the child.[52]

Revocation and Actions for Fraud or "Wrongful Adoption"

Some states once allowed adoptive parents to rescind the adoption of a child who manifested serious congenital difficulties within a specified time. The strong majority approach today is to provide no avenue for revocation for such a reason once an adoption decree has become final. However, some courts now recognize actions for monetary damage based on fraud or "wrongful adoption" against placing agencies who negligently or fraudulently fail to reveal to adopters such known problems as a background of incest[53] or hereditary conditions such as Huntington disease.[54]

THE "BABY DOE" REGULATIONS AND THEIR LEGACY

After several widely publicized cases addressing parental authority to decline treatment for severely defective neonates, in 1983 the secretary of the Department of Health and Human Services (DHHS) announced an "interim final regulation" dealing with neonates in hospitals receiving federal funds. Based on section 504 of the Rehabilitation Act of 1972, which focuses on discrimination against "otherwise qualified handicapped individuals," the regulation required conspicuous posting of signs in pediatric and neonatal wards urging anyone knowing of denial of food or customary medical care to a defective infant to notify DHHS, which was authorized to intervene immediately through a special investigative squad. The regulation was soon judicially invalidated[55] because of the agency's procedural failure to comply with rule making requirements, although the court also indicated that the rule was arbitrary and capricious. A subsequent regulation, which also encouraged establishing "infant care review committees," was set aside as exceeding the agency's authority under the Rehabilitation Act.[56] By then, Congress had conditioned state participation in a federal program for prevention and treatment of child neglect and abuse on providing a mechanism for responding to reports of medical neglect, including "withholding of medically indicated treatment from disabled infants with life-threatening conditions."[57] As a result of this process, protecting defective neonates from discrimination based on disability now rests largely in the hands of the states, whose provisions may vary significantly. The ethical issues of how to balance the interests of a defective neonate, the parents, and the state continue to confront the pediatrician/neonatologist, who probably has greater discretion now than during the *Baby Doe* era.

FETAL ALCOHOL SYNDROME AND "CRACK" BABIES

Workable legal responses to problems of newborn infants who have fetal alcohol syndrome (FAS) or problems relating to maternal drug use during pregnancy have been particularly elusive. The problem is that many legal tools used for child protection, such as removal from parental custody and placement in foster care, termination of parental rights, or subsidized adoption, are not feasible in most cases.

Several jurisdictions have sought to prosecute mothers under criminal statutes forbidding delivery of controlled substances to minors, even though this was not envisioned by the drafters of such penal provisions. The attempts have been largely unsuccessful, although some have required litigation to the appellate court level before favorable resolution on the mother's behalf.[58]

Some states have added special provisions in their child protection or other statutes that focus specifically on neonates affected by maternal substance abuse. Florida's abuse and neglect statute, for example, provides that harm to a child's welfare can occur when a parent inflicts physical or mental injury. Such injury specifically includes physical dependency of a newborn infant upon a controlled drug except for drugs administered in conjunction with a detoxification program or drugs administered in conjunction with medically approved treatment procedures. However, the statute also provides that "no parent of such a newborn infant shall be subject to criminal investigation solely on the basis of such infant's drug dependency . . ."[59]

TORT ACTIONS BY AND AGAINST MINORS

The law of torts deals with compensation in money damages for injury to person or property. An intentional tort involves an unauthorized invasion of some legally protected interest such as the right to bodily integrity,[60] mentioned earlier in the context of obtaining a patient's consent to a medical procedure in order to preclude a battery action. The more usual action to recover for medical injury is based on negligence, which extends to cases of actual harm caused by unreasonable departure from a normative standard with regard to someone who is owed such a duty of care.[61] Punitive damages, designed more for deterrence than compensation, sometimes may be awarded in intentional tort actions; they are likely to be awarded in negligence actions only in cases of recklessness or grossly negligent conduct, if at all.

A minor must bring a legal action through a legal representative, such as a parent. In many states the statute of limitations, which determines how long an injured person has in which to sue after the event causing an injury, does not begin to "toll" for a minor until the age of majority. This can produce what actuaries refer to as a "long tail," which means that one injured as an infant may still bring an action at age 19 or even later. Some states have enacted legislation shortening the statute of limitations for medical malpractice actions of minors,[62] although several such statutes have been determined unconstitutional because of their unequal application to other types of injuries. The statute of limitations can be especially important for a physician whose insurance is based on coverage of "claims made" during the insurance year rather than by "occurrence," which would include claims whenever filed if they were based on conduct during the year of coverage.

Two states, Virginia[63] and Florida,[64] have enacted special "no fault" compensation systems to deal with the problems of infants who sustain severe, permanently disabling injuries during the birth process.

Liability of Minors

In most states minors are liable for their own torts, whether negligent or intentional.[65] Although parents historically were not vicariously liable for the damage caused by their children, many jurisdictions have adopted statutes imposing such liability on them up to a specified (usually fairly low) ceiling for certain willful or malicious acts.[66]

The doctrine of intrafamily immunity once precluded actions by children against their parents, but this has been widely abrogated to permit children to sue their parents for injury except when it is based on discretion in the exercise of parental control and authority.[67]

CONCLUSIONS

Our society is changing rapidly, and children are greatly influenced by those changes. The environments in which they live and the issues they face are more complex. Older children are being given more responsibility to participate in decisions that affect them. Pediatricians must understand the changing social climate and, wherever possible, be prepared to help direct these changes. Although no busy practitioner can completely grasp all the legal and ethical issues involved, primary care pediatricians serve their patients well by having some understanding of the basic trends and by being able to offer some direction to the children and families who look to them for advice.

REFERENCES

1. Beauchamp TL, Childress JF: *Principles of biomedical ethics,* ed 3, New York, 1989, Oxford University Press.
2. See Gottesfeld: The uncertain status of the emancipated minor: why we need a uniform statutory emancipation of minors act (USEMA), *USF L Rev* 15:473, 1981.
3. See, e.g., Va. Code §§ 16.1-33, -334 et seq. (Cum. Supp. 1993).
4. See, e.g., Ark. Code § 20-9-602(7); Miss. Code § 41-41-3(h) (Rev. 1993).
5. Sigman GS, Kraut J, La Puma J: Disclosure of a diagnosis to children and adolescents when parents object, *Am J Dis Child* 147:764, 1993.

6. Jefferson LS et al: Use of the Natural Death Act in pediatric patients, *Crit Care Med* 19:901, 1991.
7. Schowalter, Fernholt, Mann: The adolescent's decision to die, *Pediatrics* 51:91, 1973.
8. *In re E.G.*, 549 N.E.2d 322 (Ill. 1990).
9. 549 N.E.2d at 327.
10. *In re Swan*, 569 A.2d 1202 (Me. 1990).
11. *O. G. v. Baum*, 790 S.W.2d 840 (Tex. App. 1990).
12. See *Lausier v. Pescinski*, 226 N.W.2d 180 (Wis. 1975); *In re Richardson*, 284 So.2d 185 (La. App. 1973).
13. See *Hart v. Brown*, 289 A.2d 386 (Superior Ct., Conn. 1972); *Little v. Little*, 576 S.W.2d 493 (Tex. Civ. App. 1979).
14. See Uniform Anatomical Gifts Act §§ 2,3 (1987).
15. 442 U.S. 854 (1979).
16. See *In re Roger S.*, 569 P.2d 1286 (Cal. 1977); Dillon et al: In re Roger S: The impact of a child's due process victory on the California mental health System, 70 *Calif L Rev* 70:373, 1982.
17. Kohrman MH: Brain death in neonates, *Semin Neurol* 13:116, 1993.
18. For discussion, see Wadlington: Baby M: catalyst for family law reform? *J Contemp Health Law and Policy* 5:1, 1989; Wadlington: Contracts to bear a child: the mixed legislative signals, *Idaho L Rev* 29:383, 1992-1993.
19. Clark H: The law of domestic relations in the United States, 190 (1988).
20. See *Stanley v. Illinois*, 405 U.S. 645 (1972).
21. *Caban v. Mohammed*, 441 U.S. 380 (1979).
22. *Lehr v. Robertson*, 463 U.S. 248 (1983).
23. *Michael H. and Victoria D. v. Gerald D.*, 491 U.S. 110 (1989).
24. *Johnson v. Calvert*, 851 P.2d 776 (Cal. 1993).
25. Uniform Status of Children of Conception Act, § 2. 9 U.L.A. 50.
26. See *In re Tuttendario*, 21 Pa. Dist. 561 (Q.S. Phila. 1912); Wadlington W: Minors and health care: the age of consent, *Osgoode Hall L J* 11:115, 1973.
27. See, e.g., *People ex rel. Wallace v. Labrenz*, 104 N.E.2d 769 (Ill. 1952); *State v. Perricone*, 181 A.2d 751 (N.J. 1962).
28. See *Prince v. Massachusetts*, 321 U.S. 159 (1944).
29. *In re Sampson*, 317 N.Y.S.2d at 641, 654 (1970).
30. Id. at 657.
31. *Walker v. Superior Court*, 763 P.2d 852 (Cal. 1988).
32. *Hermanson v. State*, 604 So.2d 775 (Fla. 1992).
33. See Wadlington W: Medical decision making for and by children: tensions between parent, child, and state, *Illinois Law Review* :301, 1994.
34. *In re L. H. R.*, 321 S.E 2d 716 (Ga. 1984).
35. 418 S.E.2d 3 (Ga. 1992.)
36. *Santosky v. Kramer*, 455 U.S. 745 (1982).
37. *In Re M.L.G.*, 317 S.E.2d 881 (Ga. App. 1984).
38. See Kempe et al: The battered child syndrome, 181 JAMA 181:17, 1962; Paulsen, Parker, Adelman: Child abuse reporting laws: some legislative history, *Geo Wash L Rev* 34:482, 1966. [Add citation to 4th Ed. of Kempe, Helfer and Krugman.]
39. *Landeros v. Flood*, 551 P.2d 389 (Cal. 1976).
40. See *In re Marriage of Weidner*, 338 N.W.2d 351 (Iowa 1983).
41. See, e.g., Va. Code § 63.1-225 (Cum. Supp. 1993).
42. *Armstrong v. Manzo*, 380 U.S. 545 (1965).
43. See, e.g., *Malpass v. Morgan*, 192 S.E.2d 794 (1972); *Joliff v. Crabtree*, 299 S.E.2d 358 (1983).
44. See, e.g., Va. Code §§ 63.1-220.1, 63.1-238.1.
45. *In Re Roger B.*, 418 N.E.2d 751, appeal dismissed 454 U.S. 806 (1981).
46. *Humphers v. First Interstate Bank*, 696 P.2d 581 (Or. 1984).
47. See *In re Roger B.*, 418 N.E.2d 751 (Ill. 1981), appeal dismissed 454 U.S. 806.
48. 42 U.S.C.A. § 602(1) (20).
49. See Bussiere: Federal adoption assistance for children with special needs, *Clearinghouse Review* 587, 1985; Rosenthal: Outcomes of adoptions of children with special needs, 3 *The Future of Children*, No.1, at 77 (Spring 1993).
50. See the discussion of the New York Court of Appeals in *Matter of Gregory B.*, 542 N.E.2d 1052 (N.Y. 1989).
51. See, e.g., *Michaud v. Wawruck*, 551 A.2d 738 (Conn. 1988).
52. *Weinschel v. Strople*, 466 A.2d 1301 (Md. 1983).
53. *M.H. and J.L.H. v. Caritas Family Services*, 488 N.W.2d 282 (Minn. 1992).
54. *Meracle v. Children's Service Society of Wisconsin*, 439 N.W.2d 532 (Wis. 1989).
55. *American Academy of Pediatrics v. Heckler*, 561 F. Supp. 395 (D. D.C. 1993).
56. *Bowen v. American Hospital Ass'n*, 476 U.S. 610 (1986).
57. 42 U.S.C.A. §§ 5102, 5103 (b) (2).
58. See, e.g., *Johnson v. State*, 602 So.2d 1288 (Fla. 1992)
59. Fla. Stat. Ann. 415.503 (9) (a) 2.
60. ALI (American Law Institute), Restatement (Second) of Torts Chapter 1 (1977).
61. ALI (American Law Institute), Restatement (Second) of Torts Chapter 2 (1977).
62. See, e.g., Va. Code § 8.01-243.1 (1992 Repl. Vol.).
63. Va. Code §§ 38.2-5001 et seq. (1990 Repl. Vol.)
64. Fla. Stat. Ann. 766.301 et seq.
65. See Prosser, Keeton: The law of torts 1071, St Paul, 1984, Foundation.
66. See, e.g., Va. Code §§ 8.01-43, -44 (Cum. Supp. 1992).
67. *Burnette v. Wahl*, 588 P.2d 1105 (1978).

5 Community-wide Approaches to Promoting the Health and Development of Families and Children

Robert W. Chamberlin

Many of our major child health and developmental problems, such as low-birth-weight babies, infant deaths, child abuse and neglect, and school failure, are related to poor family functioning.[5,6] Before the child is born, family dysfunction manifests itself in the physician's office as poor health habits that affect the outcome of the pregnancy, such as inadequate prenatal care, poor nutrition, too closely spaced pregnancies, and use of cigarettes, alcohol, and drugs. After the child is born, family dysfunction shows up as poor parenting skills, such as lack of or inappropriate developmental stimulation, abuse and neglect, exposure to hazardous environments, and inadequate use of preventive services.

Currently, American families are trying to function under increasingly heavy stress at a time when traditional family and community support systems have eroded.[10,12] Common risk factors for family dysfunction include: being a single parent; working for companies that do not have paid pregnancy and child care leave or flexible hours; lacking access to affordable, high-quality day care; not having enough money to meet the basic expenses of food, clothing, medical care, and housing; being young and inexperienced in child rearing without grandparents available and willing to help out; living in isolated circumstances because of lack of transportation or unsafe neighborhoods; or having a child who is difficult to care for or too many children for one's coping capacity.

Families that face these risk factors are in all of our communities as a result of high divorce rates and out-of-wedlock births; teenage pregnancies; geographic mobility and residence in "mega" suburbs or inner city ghettoes that have lost their sense of cohesiveness; a shifting economy that has replaced high-paying manufacturing jobs with lower-paying service jobs; and the increasing cost of housing, medical care, food, and transportation.

Although the physician can provide some education and support during individual office visits, he or she must combine forces with other community providers and leaders to see that basic community support systems are in place for all parents and children.

Most state government and local community responses to these changes are latent and come into play only after some crisis has affected a family or child, such as a low-birth-weight baby who needs intensive care, abuse or neglect, failure in school, or becoming homeless.[4,13] However, public health experience has taught us that when risk factors are widespread throughout all levels of the population and risk scores assume a bell-shaped distribution curve with most of the population falling in the medium-risk range, a community-wide approach is more effective because primary prevention works best by preventing low- and medium-risk families from becoming high-risk families. This is because there are many more medium-risk families that will become high risk as their life circumstances change than there are high-risk families that will be rehabilitated by some kind of intensive intervention[15] (Fig. 5-1).

For example, we no longer try to prevent heart disease by paying attention only to those who have had heart attacks. Instead, we try to reduce the risk of the population at large by helping people change habits they have that are related to heart disease such as avoiding exercise, becoming obese, and smoking cigarettes. A similar argument can be made for families. In the long run, reducing family stress and helping families cope are more effective in preventing all the above-mentioned problems than trying to rescue families after they have become severely dysfunctional. The problem with this approach, however, is that community-wide efforts are difficult to carry out and take time to become effective. They require interagency collaboration at the state and local levels; development of an array of parent education and support programs; social marketing, advocacy, and fund raising; and training of community leaders in primary prevention. Fortunately, we have examples from this country and abroad of how this can be done.

IMPLEMENTING COMMUNITY-WIDE APPROACHES

At a 1987 conference funded by the Ford Foundation and the Division of Maternal and Child Health, an agency of the federal Health Resources and Services Administration (HRSA), a number of successful community-wide preventive and promotive programs used in the United States and abroad were studied; the following basic elements common to all were identified[5,6]:

1. A geographic catchment area to be covered was defined.
2. A broad-based constituency of area leaders was developed to (1) establish a data base for needs and for assessing and monitoring program effects over time, (2) develop a framework to guide program development and coordination, and (3) identify priorities for filling in missing pieces.
3. A comprehensive, coordinated array of programs was created to meet the needs of different families at different times in their lives. These programs would be those of proven value, such as home visits to new mothers and families having special needs; parent-child drop-in

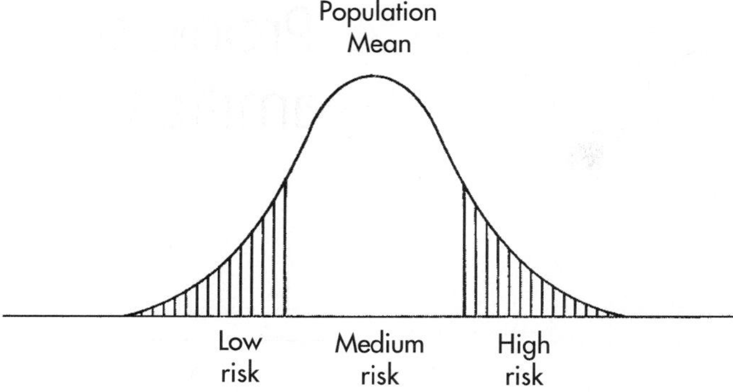

FIG. 5-1 Distribution of risk scores for family dysfunction.

centers to promote parental competence and self-esteem and provide peer support; early childhood programs to promote the social, emotional, and cognitive skills of young children; work site and school site parenting programs; and wellness programs for prenatal and well-child care.

4. Social marketing techniques were used to educate the public about the need for parent education and support and early childhood programs.
5. Stable, long-term funding was established, a task often accomplished through local and statewide advocacy groups created to promote partial funding through legislation and private and public collaboration.

The consensus at the conference was that communities must have local control over priorities and the daily running of the programs, but the state or some other regional body can help by providing start-up money and technical assistance and by developing standards to ensure the quality of the programs.

These basic elements are similar to those that emerged from the World Health Organization (WHO) Healthy Cities experience and other community-based interventions.[1,3]

Stanford Heart Disease Prevention Project

One of the best examples of how to implement a community-wide preventive and promotive program is the Stanford Heart Disease Prevention Project, which developed a three-part ecologic framework to guide program development and coordination[11] (see the box on p. 40.) The column on the right shows the status indicators followed to monitor the success of the project, in this case the frequency of various types of cardiovascular disease. For families, the status indicators might be the rates for low-weight births, child abuse, school readiness, and dropping out of school. The middle column shows factors that influence individual risk factors related to the occurrence of the condition or disease. These influencing factors include knowledge about risk factors and what to do to reduce one's susceptibility to them, attitudes and beliefs about one's susceptibility to the condition in question, and the effectiveness of the proposed preventive strategies. This column also identifies specific individual habits and skills related to the occurrence of preventable problems. For heart disease, these include diet and exercise and how to resist peer pressure to smoke. For child health and developmental outcomes, examples would be health habits of the mother related to pregnancy outcome and parenting skills related to promoting the health and development of the child at various times.

The column on the left identifies all those social context factors that influence individual knowledge and behavior. Among these are immediate social level variables such as family traditions and the local peer culture. Next come organizational level variables such as school health curricula, practices of health care providers, and work site programs and policies. At the community level are variables such as what is reflected in the mass media, local and state policies and regulations affecting individual behavior and attitudes, and residents feeling a sense of community where they live. By using this overall framework, one can identify where a particular community is on any one of these variables and set priorities for adding, altering, or coordinating programs and services. The Stanford group also has worked out a sophisticated approach to social marketing, including how to identify different segments of the population to reach, how to develop messages and activities that will be understood and followed, and how often and by what method to deliver this information.[7] Finally, the group has developed a number of skills for building a broad-based constituency to support preventive programs. Much of this technology can be adopted to promote healthy families and children.

Brookline Early Education Program

An example of a successful neighborhood-based, community-wide preventive program for families and children is the Brookline Early Education Program, implemented as a demonstration project in Brookline, Massachusetts, in the 1970s.[9] This project, based in a school district, consisted of four components: a home visitor program, a parent drop-in center, a center-based early childhood program, and periodic health and development screening. The home visits and parent groups focused on "understanding normal child development, developing networks of people who cared about and assisted each other, and developing a sense of community, a sense of belonging to the town." Any new parent living in the area was eligible to participate. The outcome measures were the effects of the program on parents and on the children's functioning in school.

The Brookline program found no one component to be crucial for all families. Rather, validation of the parent's role was found to be the essence of any component, and different parents found this in different ways, such as from their child's teacher, from the pediatrician or nurse, from the psychologist after the examinations, from the home visitor, or from "networking" with other parents. The program also taught parents the importance of understanding and appreciating their child as a unique and important individual, of understanding the rate of their child's development, including the wide range of normal development, and of realizing that no child is perfect. The program also fostered friendships among the parents of the children. Parents whose children are now in the eight or ninth grade have said that they still maintain those friendships, even with some families who have moved.

The children who participated in the program were found to be more socially competent on entering school and to have significantly fewer reading problems at the end of second grade. One of the most important findings of the study was that families under the heaviest stress needed more intensive outreach services such as home visits for their children to achieve significantly in reading. The need for more intensive services for families at higher risk of family dysfunction also

STANFORD MODEL FOR PREVENTION OF HEART DISEASE

Community health education program	Factors that influence individual risk of disease	Rates of coronary heart disease
Social level variables	**Awareness and knowledge about**	**Chronic disease**
Parental behaviors	Cardiovascular risk factors	Angina pectoris
Peer pressure	Community resources	Myocardial infarction
Social-cultural norms		
	Attitudes and beliefs about	**Premature death**
Organizaitonal level variables	One's probability of developing heart disease	Heart attack
School health curricula		Stroke
Work site facilities and policies	**Skills**	
Grocery store labeling	Resisting peer pressure	
	Reading labels	
Community level variables		
Mass media	**Behaviors**	
Labeling laws	Diet and nutrition	
Social trends for smoking, exercise, and diet	Physical activity	
	Demography	
	Socioeconomic status	
	Age	
	Gender	

From Stanford Heart Disease Prevention Project.

was a central finding in the review of successful health, education, and support programs described by Schorr.[16] The Brookline program has provided a model for the implementation of statewide, school-based parent education and support programs in Minnesota and Missouri.[9]

Addison County Parent/Child Center

An example of a community-wide approach to promoting the health and development of families and children in a more rural setting comes from Addison County, Vermont.[14] The Addison County Parent/Child Center, located in Middlebury, the county's largest town, has programs involving 1500 families in 23 towns in a county having a total population of about 32,000. This program has evolved over 10 years. The basic principles of the program are building the self-esteem of parents and children, developing communication skills, and building a sense of community where people live. Center-based activities include providing affordable child care of high quality, training child care workers, providing an early intervention program for children who have disabilities, and providing support groups for individuals undergoing a variety of life crises and transitions. Parental self-esteem is promoted through a variety of opportunities for learning and skill building, including learning to drive and repair cars, to cook and sew, and to read and get a high school equivalency diploma, and also to learn about child care and parenting and to develop skills such as typing and word processing. Outreach activities include holding toddler play groups weekly in nine towns throughout the county. There is a home visitor program for first-time parents and for families who have special needs. Programs are held in schools on such topics as family life, teenage parents, and how to develop communication skills and resist peer pressure for participation in sex or use of cigarettes, drugs, and alcohol. Community building is fostered by holding spaghetti dinners and promoting events such as family fairs and toddler Olympics. Transportation is provided to all activities. A recent evaluation of the program by the University of Vermont has shown a considerable decrease in teenage pregnancy, as well as in births of low-weight babies, infant mortality, child abuse, and school dropout in the county.

This program has been so successful that parent-child centers have been started in all Vermont counties, and the legislature funds about 25% of each center's budget through an annual line item appropriation. Vermont also has developed a strong statewide advocacy group called the Children's Forum, which has successfully turned out a large number of parents to lobby on its behalf when funding decisions are being made by the legislature. Other states, such as Connecticut and Maryland, also are starting networks of parent-child centers.[17]

ROLE OF THE PRIMARY HEALTH CARE PROVIDER

Some physicians have responded to altered family conditions by employing a social worker or psychologist to work directly with families in the practice and by holding group meetings for parents. A partnership in Norway, Maine, has combined a traditional fee for service practice with a variety of programs serving a greater geographic catchment area of about 10,000 residents.[2] These additional programs include an early intervention program for children who are developmentally delayed and an associated nursery school that provides "mainstreaming" experiences. A parent drop-in center was added later that offers information, referral services, and exercise classes, as well as other informal activities for parents and children. To qualify for funds from state agencies and other sources, the practice has been established as a nonprofit health and service agency called the Child Health Center of Norway, Maine. This broader orientation has resulted in a close relationship with other community services that refer families to the center, such as the area public health nurses, the local child abuse prevention councils, and the local school systems. The Academy of Pediatrics' Healthy Tomorrows Program is helping to fund innovative programs such as this. Pediatric departments in hospitals and medical schools also have become more community oriented. The University of Rochester in Rochester, New York, has a program that pioneered in this direction.[8] The Martin Luther King–Drew Medical Center's Department of Pediatrics serves the Watts area in inner city Los Angeles.[16] This group operates on the principle that the health care of children can be addressed only in the context of their surroundings. Thus the department has been instrumental in establishing a model child care center, a family day care network, a Head Start program, a training program for child care workers, and a consortium of community early childhood centers. Members of the department also have become involved in a program for teenage mothers at the local high school and have helped develop a magnet high school for the health professions, in which students from all over Los Angeles combine high school classes with apprenticeships in the King-Drew Medical Center laboratories.

SUMMARY

Primary prevention works by preventing low- and medium-risk families from becoming high-risk families. Because of the widespread distribution of risk factors for family dysfunction in all segments of our communities and the bell-shaped distribution curve of family risk scores, it is necessary to develop comprehensive, coordinated, nondeficit-oriented community-wide approaches to promoting healthy families and children if we hope to reduce significantly the incidence of such problems as low-birth-weight babies, child abuse, and failure in school.

We know what basic programs are needed, and most of the technology for developing community-wide approaches has been worked out and is available. However, to get these basic programs, pediatricians and other primary health care providers must become advocates for families and children and must educate legislators and public officials on the penny-wise, pound-foolish nature of the current practices, which tend to wait until a family or child is severely dysfunctional before providing services.

REFERENCES

1. Ashton J, editor: *Healthy cities,* Philadelphia, Pa, 1992, Open University Press.
2. Bauer S: Report of the Maine Delegation: the Norway, Maine, Child Health Center. In Chamberlin RW, editor: *Beyond individual risk assessment: community-wide approaches to promoting the health and development of families and children,* Washington, DC, 1988, National Center for Education in Maternal and Child Health.
3. Bracht N, editor: *Health promotion at the community level,* Newbury Park, Calif, 1990, Sage.
4. Bronfenbrenner U, Weiss HB: Beyond policies without people: an ecologic perspective on child and family policy. In Zigler E, Kagan SL, Klugman E, editors: *Children, families, and government,* Cambridge, England, 1983, Cambridge University Press.
5. Chamberlin RW, editor: *Beyond individual risk assessment: community-wide approaches to promoting the health and development of families and children,* Washington, DC, 1988, National Center for Education in Maternal and Child Health.
6. Chamberlin RW: Preventing low birth weight, child abuse, and school failure: the need for comprehensive, community-wide approaches, *Pediatr Rev* 13:64, 1992.
7. Farquhar J, Maccoby N, Wood P: Education and communication studies. In Holland W, Deters R, Knox G, editors: *Oxford textbook of public health,* vol 3, Oxford, England, 1985, Oxford University Press.
8. Haggerty R, Roghmann K, Pless I, editors: *Child health and the community,* ed 2, New York, 1993, New Brunswick, NJ, Transaction.
9. Hauser-Cram P et al: *Early education in the public schools: lessons from a comprehensive birth-to-kindergarten program,* San Francisco, Calif, 1991, Jossey-Bass.
10. Hobbs N et al: *Strengthening families,* San Francisco, Calif, 1984, Jossey-Bass.
11. Jackson C: A community-based approach to preventing heart disease: the Stanford experience. In Chamberlin RW, editor: *Beyond individual risk assessment: community-wide approaches to promoting the health and development of families and children,* Washington, DC, 1988, National Center for Education in Maternal and Child Health.
12. Kagan S et al, editors: *Family support programs,* New Haven, Conn, 1987, Yale University Press.
13. Kozol J: *Rachel and her children: homeless families in America,* New York, 1988, Fawcett.
14. Mitchell C: Report of the Vermont Delegation: the Addison County Parent/Child Center. In Chamberlin RW, editor: *Beyond individual risk assessment: community-wide approaches to promoting the health and development of families and children,* Washington, DC, 1988, National Center for Education in Maternal and Child Health.
15. Rose G: Sick individuals and sick populations, *Int J Epidemiol* 114:32, 1985.
16. Schorr L: *Within our reach: breaking the cycle of disadvantage,* New York, 1988, Anchor Doubleday.
17. Weiss H: State family support and education programs: lessons from the pioneers, *Am J Orthopsychiatry* 59:32, 1989.

SUGGESTED READINGS

Chamberlin RW: Home visiting: a necessary but not in itself sufficient program component for promoting the health and development of families and children, *Pediatrics* 84:178, 1989.

Olds D et al: Improving the life course development of socially disadvantaged mothers: a randomized trial of nurse-home visitation, *Am J Public Health* 78:1436, 1988.

PART TWO

Evaluation and Communication

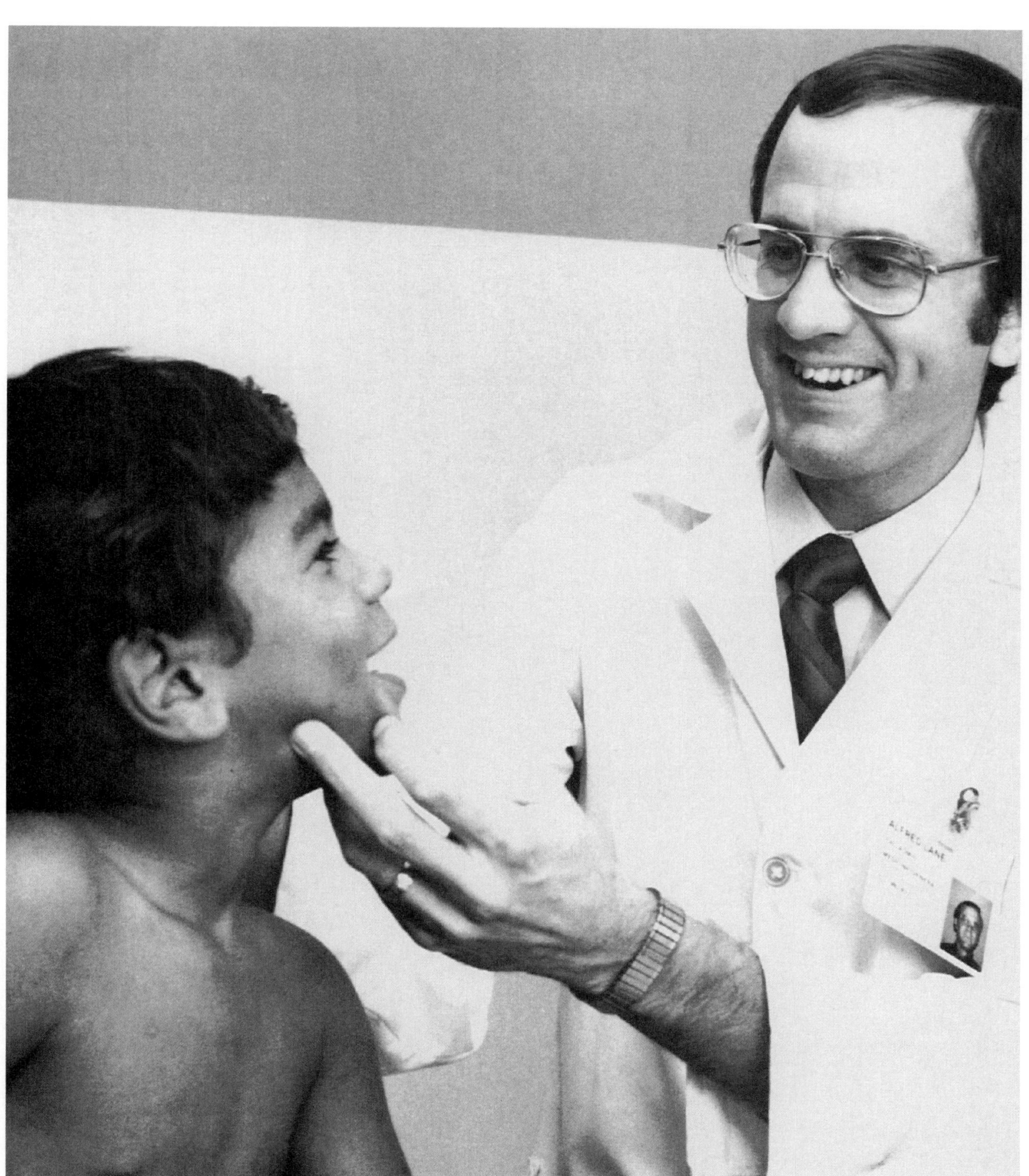
ALFRED LANE

6 The Pediatric History

William E. Boyle, Jr., and Robert A. Hoekelman

A good history carefully obtained from an intelligent mother . . . puts the physician in possession of a fund of information about the patient which is of greatest value, not only in arriving at a diagnosis in the illness for which he is consulted, but is exceedingly helpful in the future management of the child.

L. Emmett Holt, 1908[1]

Perhaps in no other medical field is a history as important as it is in pediatrics. For early detection of problems related to health (including growth, development, and nutrition) and for prevention of future difficulties, the practitioner must have a thorough knowledge of the child and the family, their lifestyle, and their environment. Unlike in most other areas of medicine, the pediatric history usually is given by someone other than the patient. Thus a certain amount of subjectivity and objectivity is lost. Signs and symptoms are filtered through parental perspectives before emerging as historical data and therefore are influenced by parental hopes and fears. A pediatric history is a compilation of information gathered in a variety of ways—through interviews, direct observations, questionnaires, and medical records—that usually provides a concise record of the child and the family.

In the past, training in interviewing and history-taking took place in an acute illness situation in which the concern or complaint was readily stated or easily seen. Today, however, children are treated for an increasing number of psychosocial problems, usually in an outpatient setting. These problems may include learning difficulties, chronic or handicapping conditions, or behavioral or developmental problems—all of which require sensitive, insightful listening. Thus the pediatrician must have a thorough knowledge of the child's health status, developmental stage, and cognitive level, as well as the family's functional characteristics, belief systems, and socioeconomic circumstances.

Much of pediatrics has to do with vague questions or concerns, such as "Why does she cry so much?" "Why is he so thin?" or "Is that cough serious?" These concerns must be answered and expectations dealt with if the encounter is to be fruitful. If the physician and parent or patient have different perceptions of the problem, the physician must attempt to "tease out" and understand the patient's or parents' concerns.

Much transpires during the initial interview between a practitioner and a family other than the gathering of a history. The tone of all future encounters is established, and ideally the family begins to develop a trusting, confident relationship with the practitioner. Just as the practitioner is trying to assess the problem at hand, so, too, are the parents (and child) "sizing up" the practitioner and trying to feel comfortable with him or her. A warm, friendly, nonjudgmental, courteous manner certainly facilitates this.

History-taking requires some degree of decision making on the part of the interviewer as to what is relevant. It is not merely the gathering of a list of all symptoms and pertinent historical "negatives"; it also involves the synthesis of various facts, attitudes, and observations. To do this well requires experience, tact, and some degree of intuition. It is a difficult task. Compiling a history is accomplished best if, for each visit, the practitioner can obtain the answers to three questions: "Why did you come today?"; "What are you worried about most?"; and "Why does that worry you?" The answers not only direct further inquiry, but also provide clues to parent and patient concerns that need to be allayed or dealt with directly during the visit and perhaps thereafter. For example, a parent who brings a child to a physician because of swollen cervical lymph nodes may be worried that they represent the first signs of malignancy, because an aunt who died of Hodgkin disease had the same problem. Parents, older children, and adolescents need to be told what symptoms and signs do *not* represent, as well as what they do represent, especially if the parents and patient are worried that the symptoms and signs indicate a serious or fatal illness.

SETTING AND AMBIENCE

Although pediatric histories are taken in a variety of locations, a comfortable environment should be used to enhance communication. If the practitioner projects courtesy, interest, and a desire to help, a trusting, positive relationship is likely to develop. Patients and parents are acutely aware of *what the physician thinks of them* or what they perceive the physician's opinion to be—the *reflexive self-concept.* ("The doctor thinks I'm a good parent.") If the reflexive self-concept is high, parent (or patient) satisfaction and compliance with management recommendations are more likely to be high. Some questions to consider are: Does the practitioner imply disinterest in the patient by allowing constant interruptions by others during the history-taking? Is privacy ensured? Are children made comfortable? Is there a place for clothing and belongings (other than a lap)? Obviously, seating should be available for all, and the history-taker should remain seated for the session. Parents or guardians should be called by their formal names (Mrs. Williams, Mr. Adams), unless a personal relationship has been established that enables the use of first names, rather than "Mother," "Dad," or "Grandma." Children should be referred to by their first names, for example, "Chris" or "Jane," rather than "he," "she," or "the baby." Notes can be taken as long as this does not distract from the continuity or spontaneity of the interview. Most parents find coping with more than one child disruptive and distracting, so seeing more than one child at a time or having others in the room should be discouraged. Formula and toys should be available to help quiet infants and toddlers if necessary.

Clothing and appearance may affect the ease with which a relationship is established. Parents and children view a visit to the pediatrician as a special occasion and frequently dress accordingly. They hope their practitioner will view the visit in the same manner. The practitioner's dress should be appropriate to the population served and consistent with local values. Most pediatricians do not wear a white coat because it may evoke fearful memories for the child, although this has never been substantiated.

TYPES OF INTERVIEWS

The pediatric history is obtained in a variety of settings and for a variety of reasons. The initial history may be taken during an interview with the parents before their baby's birth, in the hospital after the birth, in the physician's office during the first visit for whatever reason, in an emergency room at the time of an acute illness, or in a hospital room after admission for a specific illness or elective surgery. The time devoted to the initial interview and the amount of information gathered depends on the circumstances. Likewise, subsequent history-taking will vary in depth and breadth, depending on the reason for the visit and the amount of time that has elapsed since the last visit.

This chapter focuses on the information to be gathered and the techniques used in obtaining the comprehensive pediatric history, which usually is accomplished in a single sitting. Circumstances may preclude completion of this exercise during the initial visit, however, and much of the information will have to be gathered at subsequent visits. For example, the initial history obtained for a child who has acute otitis media and who is "squeezed in" during fully scheduled office hours will be brief and related primarily to the chief complaint. The rest of the history can be obtained during a scheduled follow-up visit when adequate time is allotted for this purpose.

Prenatal Interview

Ideally, the parents should have their first encounter with a pediatrician before their baby is born. To many, the idea of bringing a baby in utero to the pediatrician seems strange, but much information can be gathered at this time, and a strong, understanding relationship between the parents and the pediatrician can be fostered. In addition, problems can be identified and intervention instituted then, rather than waiting until the frantic, unsettled postpartum period. An example is the isolated, deprived, pregnant woman who should be identified before she delivers so that appropriate social and psychological support can be provided.

Pregnancy is much more than a period of gestation, growth, and development of a fetus. During this time the mother must adapt to profound psychobiological changes. A life grows within her, distorting her self-image and causing nausea and then fatigue and disequilibrium. She feels obese and uncomfortable. After quickening, she begins to identify this life within her as a separate individual and to fantasize about its sex, size, and soundness. Frequently she becomes introspective and withdrawn, which may stress her marital relationship. Spousal physical abuse is not uncommon during pregnancy. As her term approaches, the mother wants the discomfort of pregnancy to end, yet she views the work of labor and delivery with some trepidation. All this is hard work for both her body and her psyche. Many women have spent high school or college years preparing for careers, and approaching motherhood frequently means temporarily relinquishing a rewarding position or prestigious job. It means embarking on a new "career" without much training and often without much status. In addition, our society is mobile. There are fewer extended families and thus fewer experiences and less advice such families can bring to the task of child rearing. Most young couples live alone and often are far removed from parents and siblings. These couples seldom have a wide range of friends on whom they can rely for help and support. Because of these societal changes, young couples usually find coping with the stresses of parenthood difficult and often turn to professionals for support and assistance.

Ideally, the person who has cared for the woman throughout her pregnancy and delivery and who understands her needs should be the person who will help her understand her new role as a mother. In many communities this is not done. Obstetricians traditionally care for women only throughout pregnancy and the immediate postpartum period. Pediatricians traditionally assume care of the infant at birth. Many women find it difficult to leave someone who has supported them through a difficult psychobiological change and to develop a new relationship while they learn the new role of motherhood. Thus a prenatal interview can greatly assist in this transition.

Prenatal interviews do not need to be long or detailed; 20 to 30 minutes should suffice. In addition to gathering facts, the pediatrician should set a tone for future encounters. Husband and wife should be interviewed together, if possible, both to air parental concerns and to help them support each other. All parents are anxious about their adequacy and the health of their unborn infant, and a supportive attitude and tacit acknowledgment that these fears are understandable can be most helpful.

Taking a thorough family history is *one* way of evidencing concern, not just for the child but for the entire family. Parents should understand the physician's interest in them as individuals and not merely as Bob's or Ann's mother and father.

During a typical prenatal interview, plans for labor and delivery should be discussed, as well as a program of childbirth education and the type of infant feeding that is contemplated. It is wise at this time to point out certain safety issues that the parents should attend to before their baby comes home, such as obtaining a child safety seat and a smoke detector and setting the hot water heater at a safe temperature (see Chapter 23, Injury Prevention). Circumcision should be discussed, unless the couple has learned through tests that their baby is a girl. It also is helpful to point out to the parents that they obviously have imagined a variety of circumstances for their child, which the practitioner can understand and will help with if they arise. It should be noted whether one or both parents desire a child of a particular sex, which may affect their abilities as parents.

The mother's blood type, medications taken, and rubella status (if known) should be elicited. Genetic information should be gathered about both sets of grandparents. In addition to inherited disorders and birth defects, familial tendencies such as obesity, hypertension, and short stature should be investigated. It also is wise to ask what the couple's own parents were like, because parenting techniques and styles frequently are passed from one generation to the next.

After dealing with the family history, the practitioner needs to gather some information about other supportive individuals. Who will help out when the baby comes home? Will the husband have a paternity leave of some sort? Grandparents traditionally visit shortly after delivery, and the pediatrician should point this out and ask if they will be helpful or another burden. He or she also should inquire if transportation and a telephone are readily available. The physician should be alert at all times for evidence of undue stress, isolation, and prior deprivation, since these factors are known to be predictors of poor parenting. The parents will want to know when the pediatrician will see the baby in the hospital, what the appointment schedule will be, and how the pediatrician can be reached. Fees for visits also can be discussed at this time.

The parents should be allowed to ask questions about their concerns. It is best to support their instincts rather than to direct and show one's own personal bias. The pediatrician should anticipate certain normal variations such as sleepy babies, the postpartum "blues," and the physiological slump that lasts from 6 to 8 weeks after birth. Parental questions may seem trivial (skin care, type of diapers), but all evolve around the question "Will we be good parents?" Strong reassurance that their instincts are good serves to reinforce and strengthen the couple's tendencies toward good parenting and leads to a confident beginning as parents.

At the conclusion of the interview the practitioner should have an idea of the parents' life-style and coping mechanisms, and they should feel reassured that they have a supportive person who will help them enter parenthood.

As prenatal interviewing has become more widespread, interview requests for second or subsequent pregnancies have become more common. These generally are not quite so formal and can take place during the routine health maintenance visits of an older child. Parental concerns deal not only with the health and soundness of the unborn, but also with coping with another child. "Will I be able to divide myself and still survive?" The mother finds herself torn between her baby in utero and her baby at home, and this issue must be addressed. Inappropriately, she may have her child attempt new developmental tasks such as toilet-training so that in essence she will have only one baby. She also may force a child to "grow up" and relinquish a crib, stroller, or high chair. All these efforts should be discouraged. Separation at the time of delivery can be a problem for a child, who must be told that mommy will leave for a while and then return. This should be done shortly before the expected confinement. The mother's departure can be made easier by having the child help the mother pack for her hospital stay. The separation also will stress the supports the family has developed, and the practitioner should review these at this time. It likewise is important to recount the previous birth experience, to identify conflicts or problems and thus avoid them a second time. The mother should be reassured that she will be able to cope and that support will be available.

Comprehensive Pediatric History Interview

Traditionally, history-taking has been a stepwise delineation of the events that led to the practitioner-patient encounter. Most practitioners learned this technique while dealing with hospitalized or acutely ill children, where the problem frequently was visible or obvious. Fortunately, a great deal of history-taking now takes place in settings other than the hospital and frequently does not involve illness. Therefore, this discussion will focus on the *pediatric interview,* of which historical data are merely a part. The interview should include observation of behavior and family interactions. Essentially, a history is a narrative about an encounter between practitioner and parent and child that includes subjective and objective data and omits some details considered irrelevant.

The box on pp. 49 to 51 is a suggested outline for components of a *comprehensive pediatric history.* In certain settings some of the data already will have been gathered, but a thorough knowledge of each component of the history is essential. Obviously, under certain circumstances it may be necessary to gather other information; the boxed material merely suggests a general format.

Usually the interview begins with the parents stating the concerns that led to the present encounter—the *chief complaint.* The parents should then be allowed, with as little interruption as possible, to relate the history as they recall it. Certain areas may be amplified and clarified, but direct or challenging questions should be avoided. After eliciting the chief complaint, the practitioner should enumerate the events associated with it in an orderly sequence *(present illness).* In addition to facts, parental concerns and feelings about these symptoms should be elicited. The parents should be asked to speculate on what they think is causing the complaint or symptom. This information can be valuable in several respects. First, it demonstrates the level of parental concern, which may influence subsequent care and treatment. Thus, parents who equate nosebleeds with leukemia will need more than simple reassurance. Second, parental concerns about causation may color the history a great deal; for example, their concern about developmental delay can influence the information they supply about achievement of early milestones. It always is important to discover how the present illness affects the rest of the family. This information will help the physician better understand the family's concerns about and responses to a given symptom or illness and what, if any, secondary gain exists for the child.

Although the chief complaint must remain the central focus of the interview, it frequently is obvious that it is not the main problem. This especially is true when dealing with very young children. Tired, anxious, or frightened parents often perceive their reactions to an infant as being abnormal in some way; they then project this as something being wrong with the baby. This makes seeking help acceptable. Once the practitioner recognizes this, he or she should try to create an atmosphere that allows the parents to express all their concerns. Questions such as, "Are there any other problems with Kathy you would like to discuss?" or "Is there anything else bothering you about Teddy?" might facilitate communication.

After the present illness has been defined and elaborated upon, certain significant events should be enumerated *(past* medical history). Much of this material is factual and can be obtained by using a direct question and answer format. Significant events such as operations, serious injuries, and hospitalizations should be verified by obtaining and reviewing appropriate hospital records.

When obtaining the patient's early history, the practitioner should elicit medically significant facts from conception to the onset of the present illness. All areas delineated in the box on pp. 49 to 51 should be touched on to some degree. The amount of information obtained may vary, but prenatal problems such as bleeding, eclampsia, or infection should be noted, and birth weight, type of delivery, and neonatal problems, if any, must be described. Information about nutrition can reveal a great deal about family dynamics and parental perceptions and expectations. "Tell me how Jennifer eats" frequently brings forth a torrent of information, but its value, nutritionally speaking, may be limited. "Good eaters" and "picky eaters" frequently weigh the same, and those who "hardly eat a thing" often are overweight.

In dealing with issues of development, it frequently is best to ask an indirect question, such as "Tell me what Connor did during his first (or second) year." This usually elicits much more information than do direct questions about motor milestones. The practitioner should seek information concerning the level of skill rather than the age of achievement; for example, it is more important to know that the child could make simple wants known at age 2 than the age when the first word was uttered. Some information about social adaptability and temperament should be obtained (see Chapters 75, Interviewing Children, and 101, Interviewing Adolescents).

Previous health care is important, and the child's immunization status is a significant part of the early history. The practitioner should record all immunizations, skin tests, and pertinent screening information on a separate sheet that is readily accessible and retrievable. Filling out a few history forms later for camp or entry into preschool will prove the value of this record.

Allergies and allergic reactions also are an important part of the early history. Specific allergic reactions should be described in as much detail as possible to clarify the reaction. For example, ampicillin can cause a variety of cutaneous and gastrointestinal reactions, but only urticaria is a true allergic response to the medication. Idiosyncratic reactions to drugs such as phenothiazides also should be described.

The *family history* contains variable information but often is difficult to construct. An attempt should be made to trace back at least two generations on each side of the family, and any data obtained should be recorded appropriately. Fig. 6-1 shows one method of recording such data. The names, birth dates, and health of the three generations concerned usually are listed below the pedigree (although not shown here), using a number indicating each person. As more data such as births, deaths, and disease become available, they can be added easily.

Consanguinity of parents should be investigated specifically by asking if the parents are related by blood. In addition to seeking known inherited diseases such as diabetes, hemophilia, or neuromuscular disorders, the practitioner should note familial tendencies such as obesity, short stature, early heart disease, and hypertension. Sometimes it is appropriate to inquire about the parenting techniques of forebears. It has been shown that abusive parents frequently were deprived or abused as children. It also is important to ask specifically about the health of the parents' brothers or sisters, since they often are overlooked during an interview.

The *psychosocial history* describes the child in his or her present milieu and relationships with family, peers, school, and community. This should include information about the physical setting (e.g., housing), environment, and degree of isolation. Determining how children spend the day, who cares for them, what they like to do, and what their hobbies are is important. Inquiry should be made about the support system within the family; for example, the nature of an extended family, supportive or conflicting roles, the elements of stress that exist for this child, and how the child and family cope with them.

The psychosocial history also should touch on the parents' attitudes toward discipline and expectations about achievement. When appropriate, the practitioner should determine how the parents compare this child to his or her siblings or to other children. It also is appropriate at this time to ask the parents to describe the child's temperament (e.g., "mellow," "fiesty," "lazy"), as well as what they see as his or her strengths.

The *review of systems* should be detailed completely to obtain a baseline evaluation of all systems and their level of function. Children change over time, and various systems may be the target of stress or disease processes. Therefore, the practitioner should reassess all organ systems periodically and record their apparent level of function.

INTERVIEWING TECHNIQUES

Although most interviews are direct and straightforward, difficulties occasionally are encountered. Certain pitfalls can be avoided by changing the interview format or adapting particular strategies. Clarification of certain terms always is essential. For example, *diarrhea* and *flu* mean different things to different people, and no true communication can occur until such terms are defined. The temporal nature of complaints also must be assessed carefully. Children who are "always sick" may have recurrent infections that clear in 5 to 7 days, or they may have a perpetually runny nose, which is seen in some children who have allergies.

If the patient has been seen before, the practitioner should review the child's medical record before the visit to refresh his or her memory on past health and illnesses that may relate to the reason for the current visit. Consultants should review the letter of referral and the reason for and goals of the visit before interviewing the parents and patient.

Many parents see their skills as parents being challenged during the pediatric interview: "After all, if we did things right, we wouldn't need to see the doctor." They become defensive and may answer questions "ideally." At the same time, they want to share fears and worries with a caring, empathetic practitioner. The pediatrician must strive to develop this trusting relationship. By being facilitative, he or she enables the parents to ventilate fears and frustrations and sort out thoughts. Statements such as "That must have worried you" or "I bet that's upsetting" let parents know that the practitioner is concerned with much more than the facts in the interview. On the other hand, statements or questions sug-

COMPREHENSIVE PEDIATRIC HISTORY

The following comprehensive pediatric history is exhaustive and obviously not meant to be used in its entirety with all patients. However, depending on the patient's age and sex and the nature of the chief complaint and the present illness, the interviewer will need to explore in depth some or all of the subjects listed. In most instances common sense must be used in deciding how much information should be gathered.

Date of interview

Identifying data

Record the date and place of birth, sex, race, religious preference, nickname (particularly for children 2 to 10 years of age), parents' first names (and last names, if different), and where the parents can be reached during work hours.

Source of and reason for referral

Source of the history

This may be the parents, the patient, or sometimes a relative or friend. As a practitioner, you should record your judgment of the validity of the source's reporting. Other possible sources of the history are the patient's medical record, or a letter from a referring physician or the school nurse.

Chief complaints

When possible, quote the parents or the patient. Clarify whether these complaints are the concerns of the parents, the patient, or both. In some instances they are the concerns of a third party, such as a teacher.

Present illness

This should be a clear, chronological narrative of the problems for which the patient is seeking care. Include the onset of the problem, the setting in which it developed, its manifestations and treatments, its impact on the patient's life, and its meaning to the patient or the parents, or both. Describe the principal symptoms in terms of (1) location, (2) quality, (3) quantity or severity, (4) timing (i.e., onset, duration, and frequency), (5) setting, (6) factors that have aggravated or relieved these symptoms, and (7) associated manifestations. Relevant data from the patient's chart, such as laboratory reports, also belong in the Present Illness section, as do significant negatives (i.e., the absence of certain symptoms that will aid in differential diagnosis). Include how each member of the family responds to the patient's symptoms, their concerns about them, and whether the patient achieves any secondary gains from them.

Past medical history

General state of health as the parents or patient perceives it

Birth history

This is particularly important during the first 2 years of life and when dealing with neurological and developmental problems. Review the hospital records if preliminary information from the parents indicates significant difficulties before, during, or after delivery.

Prenatal history

Determine the mother's health before and during the pregnancy, including nutritional patterns and specific illnesses related to or complicated by the pregnancy; doses and duration of all legal and illegal drugs taken during the pregnancy (including alcohol ingestion and cigarette smoking); weight gain; vaginal bleeding; duration of the pregnancy; and the parents' attitudes toward the pregnancy and parenthood in general, and toward this child in particular.

Natal history

Determine the nature of the mother's labor and delivery, including degree of difficulty, analgesia used, and complications encountered; birth order, if a multiple birth; and birth weight.

Neonatal history

Determine the onset of respirations; resuscitation efforts; Apgar scores and estimation of gestational age; specific problems with feeding, respiratory distress, cyanosis, jaundice, anemia, convulsions, congenital anomalies, or infection; the mother's health after delivery; separation of the mother and infant and the reasons for this; the mother's initial reactions to her baby and the nature of bonding; and patterns of crying and sleeping and of urination and defecation.

Feeding history

This is particularly important during the first 2 years of life and in dealing with problems of undernutrition and overnutrition.

Infancy

Breast-feeding—frequency and duration of feeds, use of complementary or supplementary artificial (formula) feedings, difficulties encountered, time and method of weaning. *Artificial (formula) feeding*—type, concentration, amount, and frequency of feeds; difficulties encountered (regurgitation, colic, diarrhea); timing and method of weaning. *Vitamin and iron supplements*—type, amount given, frequency, and duration. *Solid foods*—types and amounts of baby foods given; when introduced, and infant's response; introduction of junior and table foods; start of self-foods; start of self-feeding; and the mother's and child's responses to the feeding process.

Childhood

Eating habits—likes and dislikes, specific types and amounts of food eaten, parents' attitudes toward eating in general and toward this child's undereating or overeating, and parents' response to any feeding problems. With childhood feeding problems, the parents may need to keep a diet diary for 7 to 14 days to allow accurate assessment of the child's food intake.

Growth and development history

This is particularly important during infancy and childhood and in dealing with problems such as delayed physical growth, psychomotor and intellectual retardation, and behavior disturbances.

Physical growth

Determine the actual (or approximate) weight and height at birth and at 1, 2, 5, and 10 years; record any history of slow or rapid gains or losses; and note the tooth eruption and loss pattern.

Modified from Bates B, Hoekelman RA: Interviewing and the health history. In Bates B, editor: *A guide to physical examination and history taking,* ed 6, Philadelphia, 1995, JB Lippincott.

COMPREHENSIVE PEDIATRIC HISTORY—cont'd

Developmental milestones

Determine the ages at which the patient: held head up while prone; rolled over from front to back and back to front; sat with support and alone; stood with support and alone; walked with support and alone; said first word, combinations of words, and sentences; tied own shoes; and dressed without help.

Social development

Sleep—amount and patterns during the day and at night; bedtime routines; type and location of bed; nightmares, terrors, and somnambulation. *Toileting*—methods of training used; when bladder and bowel control were attained; occurrence of accidents or of enuresis or encopresis; parents' attitudes; terms used in the family for urination and defecation (important to know when a young child is admitted to the hospital). *Speech*—hesitation; stuttering; baby talk; lisping; estimate of the number of words in the child's vocabulary. *Habits*—bed-rocking; head-banging; tics; thumb-sucking; nail-biting; pica; ritualistic behavior; use of tobacco, alcohol, or drugs. *Discipline*—parents' assessment of child's temperament and response to discipline; methods used and their success or failure; negativism; temper tantrums; withdrawal, aggressive behavior. *Schooling*—experience with day care, nursery school and kindergarten; age and adjustment on entry; current level of parents' and child's satisfaction; academic achievement; school's concerns. *Sexuality*—relationships with members of the opposite sex; inquisitiveness about conception, pregnancy, and girl-boy differences; parents' responses to child's questions, and what they have taught him or her about masturbation, menstruation, nocturnal emissions, the development of secondary sexual characteristics, and sexual urges; dating patterns. *Personality*—degree of independence; relationships with parents, siblings, and peers; group and independent activities and interests; congeniality; special friends (real or imaginary); major assets and skills; self-image.

Childhood illness

Determine the specific illnesses the child has had, such as rubeola, rubella, chickenpox, or mumps, as well as any recent exposures to communicable childhood diseases.

Immunizations

Record the specific dates of administration of each vaccine so that a booster program can be maintained throughout childhood and adolescence; also record any untoward reactions to a vaccine. The parents should have their own written record of the child's immunizations.

Screening procedures

Record the dates and results of any screening tests. For all children, these tests should include vision, hearing, tuberculin tests, urinalysis, and hematocrit, as well as phenylketonuria, galactosemia, and other genetic-metabolic disorders. For certain high-risk children, additional tests may include sickle cell, the human immune deficiency virus (HIV), blood lead, cholesterol, alpha-1-antitrypsin deficiency, and any other screening that may be indicated.

Operations, injuries, and hospitalizations

Elicit the details of these events and the child's and parents' reactions. If the child is old enough, ask age-appropriate questions about safety and about preventing injuries.

Allergies

Pay particular attention to the allergies that are more prevalent during infancy and childhood—eczema, urticaria, perennial allergic rhinitis, asthma, food intolerance, and insect venom hypersensitivity.

Current medications

Include home remedies, nonprescription drugs, and medicines borrowed from family members or friends. If it seems that the patient might be taking one or more medications, survey one 24-hour period in detail: "Take yesterday, for example. Starting from when he woke up, what was the first medicine Thomas took? How much? How often during the day did he take it? What is he taking it for? What other medications . . .?"

Family history

Record the education attained, job history, emotional health, and family background of each parent or parent substitute; the family's socioeconomic circumstances, including income, type of dwelling, and neighborhood; parents' work schedules; family cohesiveness and interdependence; support available from relatives, friends, and neighbors; ethnic and cultural milieu in which the family lives; parents' expectations of the patient and attitudes toward him or her in relation to siblings. (All or part of this information can be recorded in the Present Illness section, if pertinent to it, or under Psychosocial History.)

Also record the age and health or age and cause of death of each immediate family member, including the parents (see Fig. 6-1). Ascertain consanguinity of the parents by inquiring if they are "related by blood."

Note the occurrence in the family of any of the following conditions: diabetes, tuberculosis, heart disease, high blood pressure, stroke, kidney disease, cancer, arthritis, anemia, headaches, mental illness, or symptoms resembling those of the patient.

Psychosocial history

This is an outline or narrative description that captures the important and relevant information about the patient as a person:

The patient's life-style, home situation, and "significant others"

A typical day—how the patient spends his or her time between arising and going to bed

Religious and health beliefs of the family that are relevant to perceptions of wellness, illness, and treatment

The patient's outlook on the future

Review of systems

General. Usual weight, recent weight change, weakness, fatigue, fever, pallor.

Skin. Rashes, lumps, itching, dryness, color change, changes in hair or nails.

Head. Headache, head injury.

Eyes. Vision, glasses or contact lenses, last eye examination, pain, redness, excessive tearing, double vision.

Ears. Hearing tinnitus, vertigo, earaches, infection, discharge.

Continued.

COMPREHENSIVE PEDIATRIC HISTORY—cont'd

Nose and Sinuses. Frequent colds, nasal stuffiness, hay fever, nosebleeds, sinus trouble.

Mouth and Throat. Condition of teeth and gums, bleeding gums, last dental examination, frequent sore throats, hoarseness.

Neck. Lumps in the neck, swollen glands, goiter, pain in the neck.

Breasts. Lumps, pain, nipple discharge.

Respiratory. Cough, sputum (color, quantity), hemoptysis, wheezing, asthma, bronchitis, pneumonia, tuberculosis, pleurisy; results of last chest roentgenogram.

Cardiac. High blood pressure, rheumatic fever, heart murmurs; dyspnea, cyanosis, edema; chest pain, palpitations; results of past electrocardiograms or other heart tests.

Gastrointestinal. Trouble swallowing, loss of appetite, nausea, vomiting, vomiting of blood, indigestion; frequency of bowel movements, change in bowel habits, rectal bleeding or black, tarry stools, constipation, diarrhea; abdominal pain, food intolerance, excessive passing of gas; jaundice, hepatitis.

Urinary. Frequency of urination; polyuria; nocturia; dysuria; hematuria; urgency; hesitancy; incontinence; urinary tract infections.

Genitoreproductive. *Male*—discharge from or sore on penis; history of venereal disease and its treatment; hernias; testicular pain or masses; frequency of intercourse; libido; sexual difficulties; sexual preference.

Female—age at menarche; regularity, frequency, and duration of periods; amount of bleeding, bleeding between periods, last menstrual period; dysmenorrhea; discharge, itching, venereal disease and its treatment; number of pregnancies, number of deliveries, number of abortions (spontaneous and induced); complications of pregnancy; birth control methods; frequency of intercourse; libido; sexual difficulties; sexual preference.

Musculoskeletal. Joint pains or stiffness, arthritis, backache; if these are present, describe location and symptoms (e.g., swelling, redness, pain, stiffness, weakness, limitation of motion or activity); muscle pains or cramps.

Neurological. Fainting, blackouts, seizures, paralysis, local weakness, numbness, tingling, tremors, memory loss.

Psychiatric. Nervousness, tension, moodiness, depression.

Endocrine. Thyroid trouble, heat or cold intolerance, excessive sweating, diabetes, and excessive thirst, hunger, or urination.

Hematological. Anemia, easy bruising or bleeding, past transfusions and possible reactions to them.

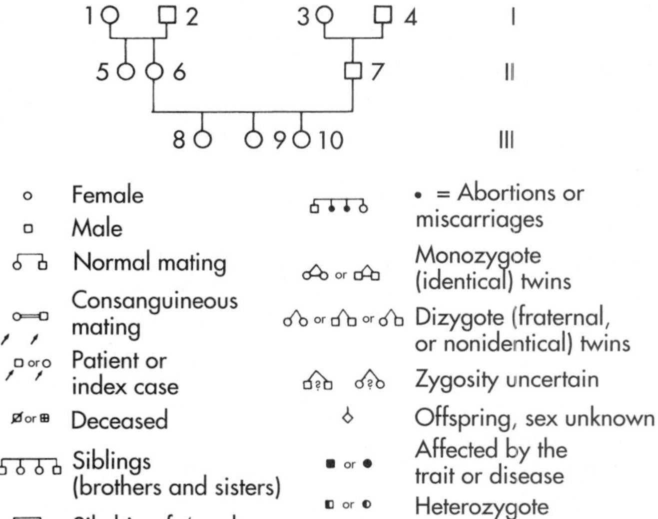

FIG. 6-1 Chart and symbols used to construct a family history, or family pedigree. The Roman numerals indicate generations.

gesting that the parents have not managed their child's illness properly, such as "You should have brought Gretchen in sooner," or "It would have been better not to have fed Stephanie," or "Why did you do *that?*" always should be avoided.

The techniques used to obtain a complete and accurate history vary with the situation and the person being interviewed.

Types of Questions

In emergencies, the practitioner should ask only direct questions (non-open-ended) that quickly elicit the important facts needed to make treatment decisions. In nonemergencies, where time is not a factor, direct questions should be used to obtain identifying data and information about pregnancy, birth, growth and development, feeding, immunizations, screening tests, previous illnesses, injuries and hospitalizations, family history, and review of systems.

Direct questions should be asked one at a time. Rapid-order direct questions, such as "Has Karl ever had eczema, hay fever, asthma, or allergic reactions to drugs?" are logical to the questioner but are likely to confuse the respondent and lead to an overall "no" answer when a "yes" would be appropriate for one or more of the elements of the question.

Indirect (open-ended) questions are extremely useful in eliciting the present illness and psychosocial history. The extreme type of open-ended question—"How does Bonnie spend a typical day?"—is discussed below. The answers to open-ended questions often provide clues to underlying, unstated problems and cues for pursuing specific elements of the patient's illness. However, use of open-ended questions may have to be curtailed because of time limitations, parental verbosity, or the parents' inability to focus on the information sought.

Direct questions also are important in eliciting the details of the present illness and the psychosocial history. For example, if a cough is mentioned as a symptom in the patient's illness, the following sequence of direct questions is appropriate: "How long has Bobbie had the cough?"; "When does he have it?"; "Does it wake him up at night?"; "What does it sound like?"; "Does he cough up any phlegm?"; "How much?"; "What does it look like?" Thus, open-ended questions identify the direction for further inquiry, and direct questions help to determine the importance of the symptoms or signs identified.

Leading direct questions—for example, "Does Sarah Jane do well in school?"—should be avoided because they are more likely to result in "expected," affirmative answers than are nonleading, direct questions, such as "What kinds of grades does Sarah Jane get in school?"

Helping the Parent or Patient Communicate

Throughout the interview the parents or patient should be assisted in several ways to relate all necessary information fully. The practitioner should use medical terminology understood by the parents or patient. Words such as *tinnitus, palpitation,* and *incontinence* may have little meaning to the parents or patient, who often will be too embarrassed to ask for a definition and may simply answer "no" when asked if those signs and symptoms are present.

The interview process is one of interaction between the practitioner and the parents or patient. The person providing information should do most of the talking and the practitioner most of the listening. However, the practitioner can encourage the parents or patient to communicate their story by using the following seven techniques.

1. *Facilitation.* This is designed to convey interest in what the parent or patient is saying. Maintaining eye contact, leaning forward, nodding in affirmation, and saying "yes," "uh huh," "I see," and the like, all convey interest and encourage the parent or patient to continue.
2. *Reflection.* Repetition of words the parent or patient has said encourages him or her to provide more detail, as is demonstrated in the following example:

Parent: Kara woke up in the middle of the night breathing hard.
Interviewer: Breathing hard?
Parent: Yes, she seemed to be breathing fast and making a wheezing noise.
Interviewer: A wheezing noise?
Parent: Yes, in and out—a musical wheezing sound.

By using reflection, the interviewer was able to elicit the nature of the child's breathing difficulty without influencing its description or diverting the parent's thoughts.

3. *Clarification.* The interviewer often must clarify what the parent or patient has said; for example, "What do you mean by 'Rob wasn't acting right'?"
4. *Empathy.* Recognizing and responding to a parent's or patient's feelings of concern, fear, or embarrassment show understanding and acceptance and encourage continued expression of the emotion. "I can understand why that upset you" or "That must have been difficult to deal with" is an empathetic expression that tells the parent or patient that the practitioner appreciates what he or she has been experiencing and is sympathetic. The practitioner also can ask the parent or patient how he or she feels or felt about a particular situation that has been related. This displays an interest in the parent's or patient's feelings as well as in the medical facts.
5. *Confrontation.* This technique is used to clarify what seems to be a contradiction between the parent's or patient's feelings and actions: "You say Sally loves school but misses a lot because she has an upset stomach most mornings." Although confrontation is used to seek clarification, it also may lead to interpretation of the meaning of the contradiction.
6. *Interpretation.* This technique is used to move beyond clarification to an inference to be made from the circumstances presented. Thus the above example might lead to the following statement and questions by the practitioner: "Maybe there is some relationship between Sally's upset stomach and her wanting or not wanting to go to school. Do you think that's possible?"
7. *Recapitulation.* This technique is especially useful when a long and complicated or an unusual history is presented. The practitioner summarizes to the parent or patient the history as the practitioner understands it. This may be done at more than one point during the interview and serves to confirm the validity of the history. It also allows for possible changes.

Hindrances to Communication. Although a calm, reserved, interested demeanor is important to enhance communication, the practitioner must guard against appearing casual. Constant eye contact with the parent, interrupted by glances at the child (if present), should be maintained. Evidence of boredom or impatience—looking away from the parents or patient, tapping the fingers or a pencil on a tabletop, or rushing through the interview—must be avoided. Inappropriate smiling or laughter also hinders good communication. The parents or patient always should feel that they have the practitioner's undivided attention. If time is short, the parents or patient should be informed and another appointment made for completing the interview.

Interviewing the Child

A great deal of information can be gained by interviewing the child directly (see Chapter 75, Interviewing Children). Many children interact spontaneously with the pediatrician and readily answer direct questions. Often only the child can reveal the severity of the pain or the extent of the symptoms. Sometimes it is better to approach children indirectly, such as encouraging them to talk about their symptoms, than to seek direct answers. For example, "Tell me about your cold, Gordon" is preferable to "Do you cough?" The pediatrician should always support the child's "own story." It should be taken seriously, and confidences should not be violated except in unusual circumstances.

With chronic problems, such as constipation or enuresis, it is helpful to review with patients their knowledge of the complaint. Patients can be asked what they were told before coming to the physician's office, how they feel about the visit, how their symptoms affect them and alter their lifestyle, and whether they are able to attend school and carry out all their regular activities. It also is important to ask children what they think is causing their symptoms, what they are worried about, and why it worries them.

Interviewing the child provides another opportunity to assess parent-child interaction. Many parents cannot let their child speak without addition, interruption, or correction. A school-age child who clings to a parent and cannot be coaxed to make eye contact with the practitioner or interact in any way probably is overly shy and dependent. As adolescence approaches, parent-child conflicts become more intense. Given the chance, many adolescents will make this obvious.

Under these circumstances, separate interviews probably are preferable (see Chapter 101, Interviewing Adolescents).

"Typical Day" Technique. In many situations information about a child's typical day can be very helpful and informative, and most parents can relate this information readily. In addition to concrete material (e.g., sleep patterns and feeding activities), much can be learned about areas of stress and harmony within a family. As with other aspects of the history, such information should be obtained as objectively as possible. Parents frequently find it difficult to discuss situations without seeking approval, even if tacit, of their own actions. Mothers who are confused or unsure of themselves frequently may ask advice on a particular aspect of their child's behavior as it is presented in the description of the child's typical day; however, it is best to defer answers until the entire day has been described.

Discussion can begin with an introduction, such as "To find out more about Kim, I am going to ask you to tell me how she spends a typical day." The practitioner should then begin by asking what time the patient arises and what happens. Some parents will launch into vivid descriptions and will require little direction, whereas others must be encouraged. Details can be elicited by asking some simple questions, such as "What is her mood on awakening?", "Who takes care of her?", and "What does she usually eat for breakfast?" Discussion can include food likes and dislikes, skill in eating, and conduct at the table. The practitioner also can learn about the child's activities, habits, and television viewing practices. The subject of discipline might come up during this discussion, and the parents' beliefs about prohibitions and punishments can be ascertained.

Lunchtime, afternoon rest periods, and activities are reviewed in much the same way. Descriptions of trips to the market or to other stores can provide information about behavior with others and reactions to new experiences.

The evening meal often is stressful in many families, and how it proceeds can provide many clues to family dynamics. For example, the practitioner should find out when the parents arrive home, whether the child eats with the parents, and if so, the types of interactions that occur. Information about the events surrounding preparation for sleep, bedtime rituals, and sleeping patterns also is important.

At the end of such an interview, it should be possible to assess not only the child's style and temperament but also the family's strengths and weaknesses. This information is essential for advising parents of children who are having developmental and maturational problems.

QUESTIONNAIRES

In certain instances, parental questionnaires may be used to supplement the history. Some may be used as part of a general health appraisal, whereas others are more applicable to a specific problem. The Framingham Safety Survey is part of The Injury Prevention Program (TIPP) of the American Academy of Pediatrics. It is the basis of office counseling on injury prevention in child health supervision. Questionnaires are especially helpful for assessing school problems and developmental issues. The Denver Prescreening Developmental Questionnaire–Revised (R-PDQ), and the Achenbach Child Behavior Checklist (CBC) are but two examples (see Appendix D for more information about these questionnaires and others). The practitioner will be wise to be thoroughly familiar with the questionnaire format and its pitfalls before using it; all may supply additional information, but all also may be subject to observer bias and should be interpreted accordingly.

RECORDING HISTORICAL INFORMATION

There are two main goals in recording the historical data gained in an interview. First, the patient's symptoms and medical history, which will help in formulating a diagnosis and therapeutic plan, are documented. This serves as a legal record of the practitioner-patient encounter. Second, a reasonable account of the patient's medical status is made available to others who also are involved in the patient's care and to the person who initially gathered the information.

The historical data base should contain all the medically significant facts of the child's life. The recorded history is a synthesis of material and observations gained during the interview, compiled in a legible, retrievable form.

The present illness must be recorded clearly and concisely. Consistency is paramount, especially when dealing with events in time. Events must be recorded by using either of these methods: "Dick developed a cough on March 17" or "Dick developed a cough 5 days before our interview on March 23." "Tuesdays" and "Fridays" are difficult to identify 2 weeks after an interview.

Data obtained during an interview can be recorded in a variety of ways, ranging from tape-recording the entire session, a method often used by psychiatrists, to merely noting "Dx—acute otitis media; Rx—amoxicillin × 10 days" on an index card. Records should be legible, and much of the data should be retrievable without having to pore over volumes of paper. This requires some foresight and planning so that different parts of the history can be separated for later use. Ideally the historical data base should be standard and uniform. However, certain problems (hip clicks, birthmarks) change with time and vary by age and sex (menstrual irregularities), by type of population served, and by geographic locale.

A variety of questionnaires have been developed to facilitate development of the data base. These are designed to be age appropriate and can be filled out by the parent or by a nurse, physician's assistant, or other office personnel. Such questionnaires can be used to gather a large amount of data quickly, thoroughly, and concisely. However, they also present several drawbacks. First, questions tend to be answered in an idealized way because parents usually have a skewed opinion of their children. Second, all logical sequencing of information gathering is lost, and degrees of concern are not readily expressed. Third, unless the data base is updated frequently by subsequent questionnaires, much of the information soon becomes irrelevant.

Gathering and recording a history and communicating compassionately and courteously with patients and their families are difficult tasks. These are not innate skills, but rather require work, insight, perseverance, and practice. The work is hard, but the rewards are great.

REFERENCE

1. Holt LE: *The diseases of infancy and childhood,* New York, 1908, Appleton-Century-Crofts.

SUGGESTED READINGS

Bates B, Hoekelman RA: Interviewing and the health history. In Bates B, editor: *A guide to physical examination and history taking,* ed 6, Philadelphia, 1995, JB Lippincott.

Cassell EJ: *Talking with patients,* vol 2, *Clinical technique,* Cambridge, Mass, 1985, MIT Press.

Feinstein AR: *Clinical judgment,* Baltimore, 1967, Williams & Wilkins.

Klaus MH, Kennell JH: *Parent-infant bonding,* ed 2, St Louis, 1982, Mosby.

Thornton SM, Frankenburg WK, editors: Child health care communications, Johnson & Johnson Pediatric Round Table No 8, 1983.

Wessel MA: The prenatal pediatric visit, *Pediatrics* 32:826, 1963.

7 The Pediatric Physical Examination

John H. Gundy

The examination of an infant or child by a physician or nurse practitioner can accomplish several goals simultaneously. With children, as opposed to adults, the physical examination often is the first direct contact between the examiner and the patient, the history having been obtained primarily from a parent. Therefore one of the crucial outcomes of the examination is the relationship that will be initiated and continued between the physician and the child. The quality and quantity of care plans and the child's future attitude in medical settings will depend in part on this relationship. This chapter emphasizes approaches to examining children of different ages that will enhance the physician-child relationship.

The physician-*parent* relationship, which is initiated when the history is taken, can be enhanced further during the physical examination if the practitioner takes a relaxed, gentle approach toward the child and, no less important, performs a thorough examination appropriate to the setting and the chief complaint. Parents develop trust in physicians in a number of ways, not the least of which is the consideration the practitioner shows for the child's fears and the parents' concern about a particular symptom or sign. For each organ system discussed in this chapter, the common symptoms for which physicians are consulted are linked to a suggested level of "completeness" in performing a physical examination.

The physician must be sensitive to the potential for iatrogenic concerns initiated by his or her comments during the examination and should anticipate the child's wondering, "What's wrong with me?" and the parent's worrying, "What did I do wrong?" Reactions such as these are very common. A thorough grounding in the normal stages of growth and development of the organ systems and the body as a whole allows the examining physician to respond to such questions by emphasizing the normal physical findings, as well as by interpreting abnormal findings in the context of normal developmental patterns. The description of each organ system in this chapter begins with important stages of growth and development, particularly those steps that can be monitored by serial physical examinations. The characteristics of common physical abnormalities will be linked whenever possible to the child's age and stage of growth.

The physical examination has limited value as a screening mechanism for occult disease (see Chapter 20, Two, The Physical Examination as a Screening Test) and has proved to be much less productive in detecting problems in school children, for instance, than is a comprehensive history. In general, the physical examination of children confirms abnormalities suggested by the history, as well as normal growth and development. When the child is examined in the presence of one or both parents, the physical examination can provide strong clues about the strength and characteristics of the parent-child relationship.

Each portion of the physical examination is discussed according to the special characteristics of each of five age groups: newborn period, infancy (1 week to 12 months), early childhood (1 to 5 years), late childhood (6 to 12 years), and adolescence (12 to 18 years).

APPROACH TO THE PATIENT

Newborn Period

At least one examination of the newborn infant should be performed in the presence of one or both parents, to facilitate both evaluation of the parent-infant relationship and to address the parents' questions about their baby. A newborn infant is examined immediately after birth to assess the adequacy of pulmonary ventilation and the integrity of the cardiovascular system and the central nervous system (CNS). While assessing the need for resuscitation, the examiner should minimize exposure of the wet infant to cool ambient air by drying the infant with a towel and conducting the examination under a warming device.

Recovery from the birth process is measured by using the Apgar scale, with scores of 0, 1, or 2 given for degree of cyanosis, respiratory rate, heart rate, reflex irritability (reaction to a soft catheter introduced into the external nares), and muscle tone (Table 7-1). The infant is rated at 1 and 5 minutes after birth; total scores below 7 or 8 at 1 minute usually indicate some degree of CNS depression, and scores below 3 or 4 indicate severe depression requiring resuscitation. If the Apgar score is 8 or higher at 5 minutes and the baby's airway is clear, the rest of the body is surveyed briefly to identify gross congenital abnormalities and to estimate gestational age. After the baby is weighed, the weight–gestational age category is determined by using a standard gestational age growth chart (see Fig. 35-4), with certain risks predictable for each group (hypoglycemia and congenital anomalies in babies small for gestational age, hypoglycemia and infant of a diabetic mother in babies large for gestational age). The neuromuscular part of the gestational age determination ideally is postponed until the infant is fully stabilized (12 to 48 hours after birth), as shown in Fig. 36-8.

In many hospitals a second, more thorough examination is performed within 12 hours of birth to assess the degree of recovery from the birth process and to determine the presence or absence of signs of respiratory distress and the ability to feed. This examination can serve as a safety check before transferral of the baby from the "transition" nursery to the "routine" nursery. It should take place in a warmed environment with the baby undressed to allow careful observation of the respiratory rate, the degree of respiratory effort, as evidenced by intercostal retractions, the color, and spontaneous activity. Often quiet babies can arouse themselves with a "startle," or Moro, response that can interfere with the examination. Giving the baby something to suck on (rubber

Table 7-1 The Apgar Score

Sign	Score 0	Score 1	Score 2
Heart rate	Absent	<100	>100
Respiratory effort	Absent	Weak, irregular	Good, crying
Muscle tone	Flaccid	Some flexion of extremities	Well flexed
Reflex irritability (catheter in nose)	No response	Grimace	Cough or sneeze
Color	Blue, pale	Body pink; extremities blue	Completely pink

From Klaus MH, Fanaroff AA: *Care of the high-risk neonate,* ed 4, Philadelphia, 1993, WB Saunders.

nipple, examiner's finger, or baby's fist), and holding the baby's arms against the sides will help keep the infant as relaxed as possible; performing the examination several hours after a feeding is ideal. Although it is important to assess the intensity and pitch of the cry, as many of the painless parts of the examination as possible should be performed before fully arousing the baby. Therefore, with the baby supine and after making general observations, many examiners begin by listening to the heart and lungs, then palpating the abdomen before examining the remaining systems, leaving the usually uncomfortable abduction of the hips until last.

Examination of the undressed baby with the parents present just before discharge affords the opportunity to point out normal findings, answer questions about perceived imperfections (and sometimes allow both parents a first look at their baby's entire body), discuss care of the circumcision and umbilicus, and observe the quality of the parent-infant attachment while the baby is held or fed. Holding the baby en face (the mother's face is rotated so that her eyes and those of the infant meet fully in the same vertical plane of rotation, as shown in Fig. 7-1), smiling at the baby, responding to signs of hunger or satiation, and talking about the baby positively and confidently all are signs that strong parent-infant bonds are being formed and have been enhanced by the hospital experience.

Infancy

Infants between the ages of 1 and 6 months almost always are a pleasure to examine because of their responsiveness to the examiner's face and their increasing interest in environmental objects such as tongue depressors and penlights. At this age infants can be examined successfully on the examination table, with the parent usually standing close beside the table. With the infant unclothed except for the diaper, the practitioner should observe for spontaneous activity, state of alertness, and responsiveness to both the examiner and the parent. The order of the examination varies. If the infant is asleep in the parent's lap or held upright at the breast or shoulder, the heart and respiratory rates can be obtained, and the heart, lungs, and even the abdomen can be examined without waking the baby. Again, the relatively uncomfortable abducting of the hips and speculum examination of the tympanic membranes are best left until last. Prolonged or painful procedures, such as deep palpation of the abdomen or a rectal examination, are best done while the baby is being fed. The infant should be examined as if physically attached to the parent, and the parent's response, especially to painful procedures, should be noted. Sometimes the parent may appropriately thank the examiner for removing an irritable, crying baby to the examining table (or to another room if on a house call), but the physician must never be lulled into thinking that the isolated examination of the infant is a complete examination. With a chronically hospitalized baby, a continuous care nurse may substitute for an absent parent during the examination.

Infants 6 to 12 months of age are increasingly difficult to examine because of their normally developing anxiety about faces other than their parents' and the perceived separation from the parent. Offering interesting objects or allowing infants to sit and reach for objects or to walk or crawl around the office can help distract them. Direct eye contact with the strange face of the examiner can be especially frightening to the baby. Examination at these ages usually is easier if the baby is held in the parent's arms or on the parent's lap. In many clinical situations, direct observation of a breast-feeding or bottle-feeding is extremely useful and can help in identifying problems such as improper feeding techniques, weak sucking movements, and dysfunctional swallowing.

Early Childhood

With children 1 to 5 years old, the most effective initial approach is to form a supportive relationship with the parent or an older sibling, who, it is hoped, will become the physician's ally in the examination of the child. This alliance is aided by identifying the parent's emotional state and anxiety level during the history and then "tuning in" nonjudgmentally. For instance, if the parent appears both anxious about the child's symptoms and guilty about having had to bother the physician, the physician might say, "I know it can be frightening to hear a baby cough like that, and I'm glad you brought him in to be examined." A parent who appears angry sometimes can be "defused" by a remark such as, "I know how aggravating it must be to have to bring your child in for so many ear infections." Tired, worn-out parents will work with a physician who is sympathetic, but they can be distracting and even disruptive if they receive nonverbal and verbal messages that they are dressed improperly, somewhat less than adequate as parents, or a general nuisance to those who practice medicine.

In most situations, children in this age group are easiest to examine while being held by the parent, a position that also is comforting to the child when the history is initiated. A few toys and books on a low table, colorful photographs and children's drawings on the walls, and the absence of a white coat on the examiner often leads children to relax and encourages them to leave the parent and explore the office. It can be helpful to offer the child a piece of examining equipment such as a stethoscope or percussion hammer to handle while the

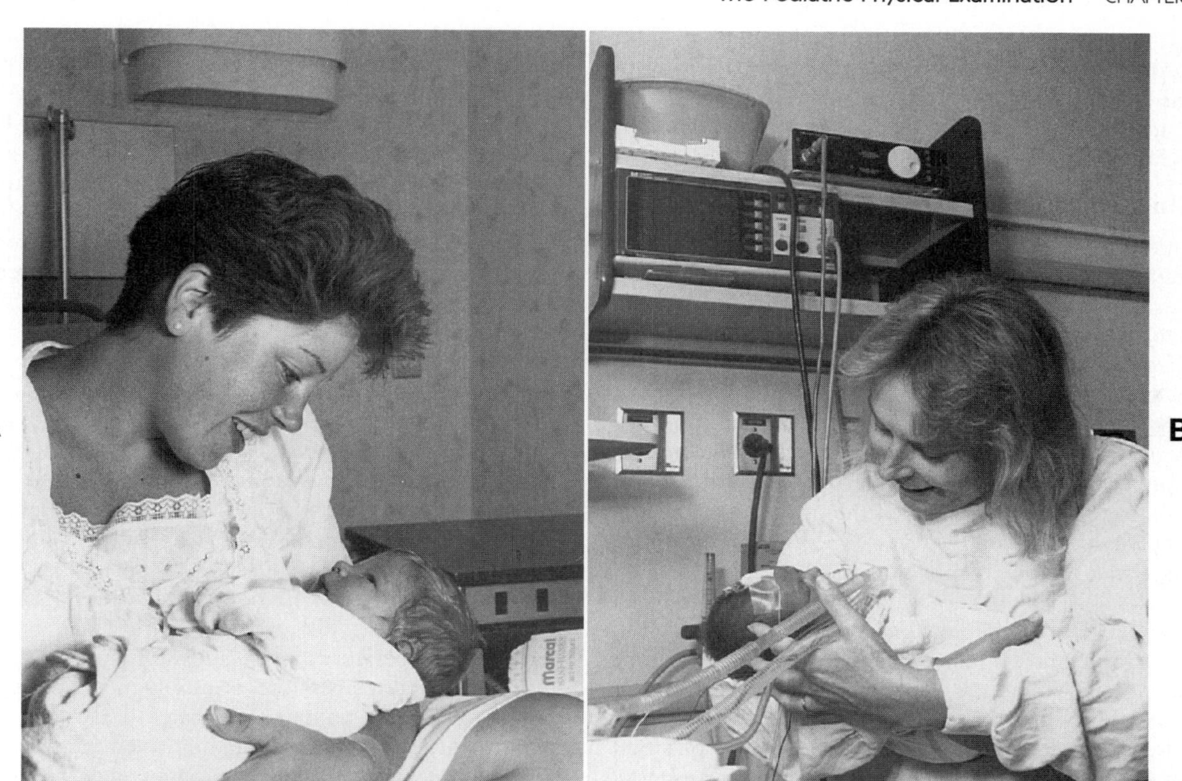

FIG. 7-1 **A,** Full-term 1-day-old infant looking "en face" eye to eye with his mother. **B,** The mother of a 2-day-old, 31-week, 1400 g premature infant on a ventilator positions herself so that she can look eye to eye with her son.

(Courtesy Ruth A. Lawrence, M.D.)

history is being taken. The examiner often can alleviate fear by showing the child what an otoscope is and demonstrating its use before using it on the child. Observing the child's handling of objects and interest and confidence in exploring a new environment, as well as the parent's reaction to the child's curiosity or fear, gives the examiner information important to understanding the child's developmental status and anticipating the parent's ability to cope with any problems the child may have.

In general, older children in this age group are increasingly able to communicate verbally with the examiner. A conversation that starts about the child's cat or siblings can lead to a description of what is about to be done. Continuing to describe what is being done ("I am now listening to your heart beating") can soothe even the child who starts off by screaming and kicking. With a frightened child, the parent may interpret prolonged silence on the examiner's part as disgust or anger with the child or parent. Also, a continuing conversation with the parent and the child during the examination signals to the child that the examiner is on the parent's side, and this may increase the child's confidence that nothing too drastic will be done.

It is best to have the child remain dressed until just before the examination, some of which can be accomplished by only partly removing pieces of clothing. Even before having the parent undress the child, important general observations about the child can be made, such as the activity level, gross and fine motor coordination, receptive and expressive language function, skin color, respiratory rate, and ability to cope with a foreign environment. Some specific portions of a developmental assessment, such as throwing and catching a ball or drawing a circle, often can break the ice and help the child into a gamelike atmosphere that can be continued throughout the examination.

Again, the order of the examination should be flexible; painful procedures (ears, throat) and frightening ones (anything that requires lying down) should be postponed until last. A steady pace, coupled with gentle but firm anticipatory statements ("Now I'm going to have you lie down so I can listen to your tummy"), enhances a relatively brief encounter, which in turn keeps the parent on the practitioner's side.

It often is necessary to restrain the child, for instance, to accomplish an adequate examination of the tympanic membranes. This can be done in a number of ways, all enhanced by continuing the descriptions and discussions calmly. The parent usually is the best assistant. The child can be restrained by holding the outstretched arms against the child's head or against the child's abdomen while the examiner's body and one elbow immobilize the lower half of the child's body. The parents should be reassured that struggling is a normal response to an examination in this age group, but that it can be aggravated if the parents berate or threaten the child. The examiner's goal should be to evaluate the child's health and illness while maintaining the trust and confidence of both the child and parent. Achieving this goal requires long hours of practice, the flexibility to ask other professionals for help when the examiner's (or the parent's) patience is about to run out, and, most important, an enjoyment of the diversity, unpredictability, and spontaneity of children.

Late Childhood

Children 6 to 12 years old usually are a pleasure to examine and rarely present any problems. A key ingredient for a successful examination is a relaxed conversation with the child about subjects such as school, hobbies, or favorite friends, interspersed with brief comments about the examination itself. Occasionally, a child who had an unpleasant experience with a physician as an infant will need more time for the preparatory description of the examination. School-age children usually prefer to wear a simple drape over their underpants, and they also prefer that siblings of the opposite sex be kept out of the room, particularly when the genitalia are examined. The order of the examination can be the same as for adults (vital signs, then head to foot), with care taken to anticipate any painful manipulations or procedures. As with younger children, the examiner can make the following critical observations without the actual "laying on of hands": activity level, ability to follow simple directions, ability to read passages of varying difficulty and to write, clarity of articulation, mood, level of neuromaturational functioning as tested by tasks such as hopping on one foot and rapidly alternating hand movements, and the relationship with the parent.

Adolescence

Most adolescents (12 to 18 years) prefer being examined without their parents in the room. They respect a straightforward, uncondescending approach, and parents respect the examiner who approaches adolescents as though they were adults. Decisions about who will be present should be discussed before the examination. With the parent out of the room, the examiner can review pertinent history or concerns directly with the adolescent. Most pubertal boys and girls have concerns about what is happening to their body, and a physical examination allows the examiner to explain and try to alleviate these concerns. Some special clinics for adolescents use brief, self-administered questionnaires so that the examiner can tune in to the adolescent's present concerns more quickly. While performing the examination, the examiner can reassure the pubertal child about normal developmental stages such as unilateral gynecomastia in boys, rapidly enlarging feet, the beginning of acne, and the interrelationships of the adolescent growth spurt and sexual development. The examiner's ability to approach the child's emerging sexuality factually or nonanxiously will help adolescents view themselves, at least briefly, with objectivity. Instruction in breast and testicular self-examination can help in this regard.

VITAL SIGNS AND EVALUATION OF SOMATIC GROWTH

Just as general observation of a child's behavior can give important clues about the child's general level of functioning, measuring vital signs and the characteristics of somatic growth often provides the basis for decisions about the child's overall health or illness. An abnormal vital sign or physical measurement often is the only outward indication of a problem in a child. Interpretation of vital signs and physical measurements depends on a knowledge of the normal biological changes of the growing infant, child, and adolescent. One principal characteristic of human growth is that different organ systems mature at different rates and times throughout fetal life, infancy, and childhood. Fig. 7-2 compares the longitudinal growth of the body as a whole with three component tissues: lymphoid, neural, and genital.

Temperature

Body temperature usually is measured rectally in infants and in children up to 6 or 7 years of age, and orally in older children who can understand directions about retaining the thermometer. A device that measures the temperature in the external ear canal can give readings that are roughly comparable to the infant's rectal temperature or the child's oral temperature. The axillary temperature sometimes is measured, especially in infants whose bottoms are excoriated or in small premature infants. This reading generally is 2° F lower than the rectal temperature and 1° F lower than the oral temperature. The rectal temperature usually is measured with the infant or child held prone on the parent's lap (Fig. 7-3). The buttocks are separated, and the lubricated thermometer is inserted through the anal sphincter at an angle of about 20 degrees above the horizontal for a distance of 1½ inches. The thermometer is held in place for approximately 1 minute, either by the examiner or by the parent. Because of the relative thermal instability of newborns, especially prematurely born babies, the ambient temperature often is measured and recorded at the same time and sometimes can explain an abnormally elevated or depressed rectal temperature. Newborns' temperatures normally are higher than those of older children, averaging approximately 99.5° F (37.5° C) during the first 6 months of life. The temperature falls below 99° F (37.2° C) after age 3 and reaches 98° F (36.7° C) by age 11. A circadian rhythm of body temperature is observable by age 2 and is well developed by age 5, with increasingly higher temperatures during the daylight hours and a fall in temperature during the night (Fig. 7-4). In infants and children there often is little relationship between the degree of temperature elevation and the severity of illness. In fact, hypothermia sometimes develops in infants who have profound infection, and children can have rectal temperatures as high as 101° F (38.3° C) after vigorous activity. It is not uncommon for children admitted to the hospital for elective procedures to have elevated temperatures initially, probably because of transient anxiety.

Pulse

The heart rate is measured by palpating the peripheral pulse (femoral, radial, or carotid arteries), by observing the pulsating anterior fontanelle, or by palpating or auscultating the heart directly. The pulse can be increased significantly in normal infants and children by anxiety, fever, and exercise before or during the examination, as well as by inflammatory illnesses, shock, and congestive heart failure. Major changes occur in the resting heart rate with increasing age, probably reflecting increasing functional control by the vagus nerve (Table 7-2). A circadian rhythm in the heart rate is observed

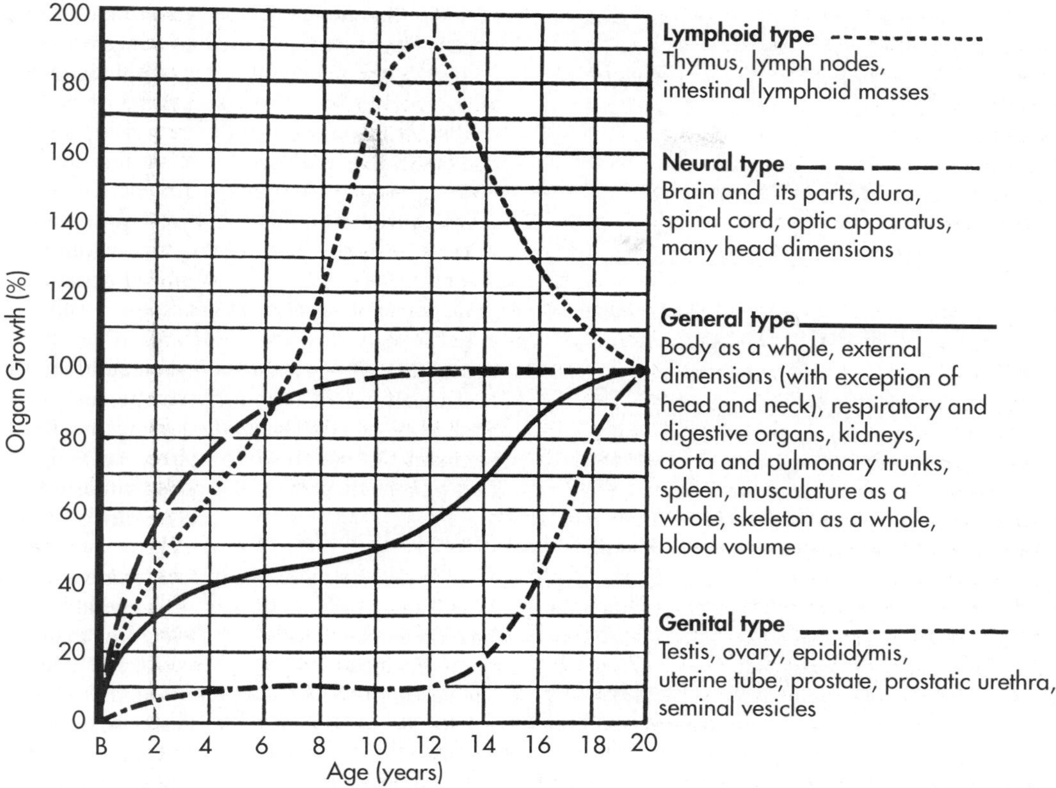

FIG. 7-2 Differential organ growth curves.
(From Harris JA et al: *The measurement of man,* Minneapolis, 1930, University of Minnesota Press.)

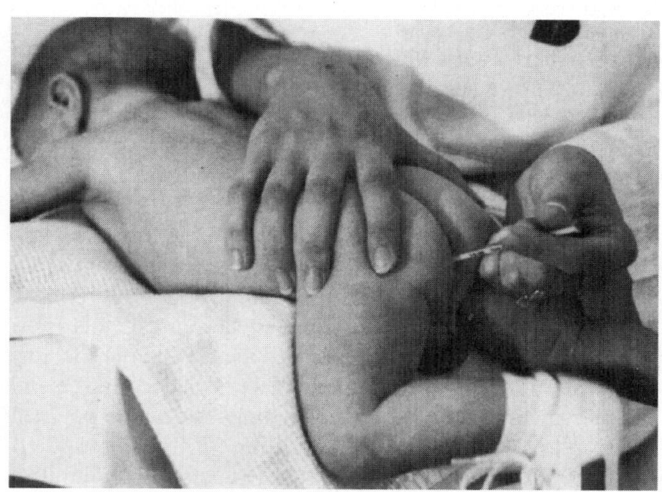

FIG. 7-3 Temperature measurement in infants.
(Photograph by P. Ruben.)

Table 7-2 Average Heart Rate for Infants and Children at Rest

Age	Average rate	Two standard deviations
Birth	140	50
First month	130	45
1-6 mo	130	45
6-12 mo	115	40
1-2 yr	110	40
2-4 yr	105	35
6-10 yr	95	30
10-14 yr	85	30
14-18 yr	82	25

From Lowrey GH: *Growth and development of children,* ed 8, Chicago, 1986, Mosby.

by age 2, with a fall of 10 to 20 beats/min during sleep; an absence of this rate slowing with sleep can be helpful in diagnosing acute rheumatic fever or thyrotoxicosis.

The examiner also should assess the rhythm of the heartbeat; equal spacing between consecutive beats is recorded as regular sinus rhythm (RSR). The cardiac rhythm more commonly is irregular than regular, especially in early and late childhood, reflecting sinus arrhythmia and increasing vagal control. Extrasystoles, appearing as irregularly spaced beats with or without a compensatory pause, are common in healthy children, usually can be abolished by exercise, and rarely occur as the only physical finding of underlying heart disease. Heart rates above 180 beats/min (especially if rigidly regular) in infants beyond the neonatal period may indicate atrial *tachycardia.* Other arrhythmias in children are rare and occur mostly in those who have underlying heart disease (e.g., congenital heart disease, rheumatic fever, and Kawasaki disease). Tachycardia with shock in infants and children usually is associated with a weak pulse and cold, sweaty extremities. Tachycardia caused by congestive heart failure usually coexists with significant tachypnea, with or without hepatic enlargement. Heart block can occur in children who have Lyme disease with myocardial involvement.

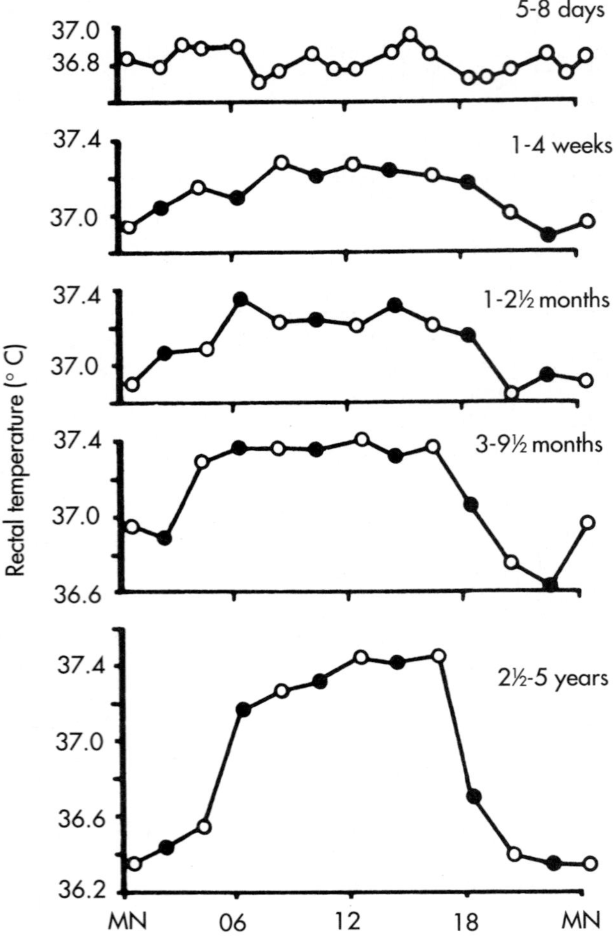

FIG. 7-4 Mean rectal temperature at different hours in groups of infants at different ages. Except in the youngest group, measurements were made every 4 hours. The hollow and solid circles represent different groups of 3 to 18 infants observed over 2 to 11 days. *MN,* Midnight.

(From Davis JA, Dobbing J: *Scientific foundations of pediatrics,* ed 2, Baltimore, Md, 1981, University Park Press.)

Respirations

Observations of the rate, depth, and ease of respiration begin at the first encounter with the child. The rate of respiration, like the heart rate, is influenced significantly by emotion and exercise, making it necessary to wait in some instances until a resting state is reached or to count the rate immediately if the infant or child is first encountered asleep. The rate may be counted by observing abdominal excursion in infants and thoracic excursion in children, ideally at a moment when the child is not paying attention to the examiner. In a sleeping infant the respiratory sounds may be counted with the bell of the stethoscope held just in front of the nose.

The respiratory rate varies with age, reflecting variables such as aspirated amniotic fluid in the newborn and increasing numbers of alveoli and increasing lung compliance with postnatal growth. The rate varies between 30 and 80 breaths/min in a newborn, 20 and 40 breaths/min in infancy and early childhood, and 15 and 25 breaths/min in late childhood; the adult level of 15 to 20 breaths/min is reached by age 15. Because changes in the respiratory rate are common over short periods, the rate should be counted for at least 1 minute, especially in crying or excited infants. The respiratory rate must be observed for several minutes in newborns, especially premature babies less than 2 kg and 36 weeks of gestational age, to discover apneic episodes (absent respirations for 20 seconds or more) and periodic breathing (apneic periods lasting between 5 and 10 seconds). In early and late childhood, irregular respirations such as Cheyne-Stokes breathing are seen only in severely ill children, such as those who have overwhelming infection or severe head trauma.

Depth of respiration is determined subjectively and compared with norms observed for that age group; deep breathing may be observed in states of metabolic acidosis, and shallow breathing in severe obstructive states such as asthma. Ease of respiration is partly a subjective determination, as in estimating the degree of dyspnea, and is discussed in the section of this chapter on the chest and lungs.

Blood Pressure

In recent years there has been an interest in the possibility of identifying individuals who have essential hypertension before they reach adulthood. In addition, due to the improvements in intensive care technology, blood pressure is determined in hospitalized infants and children more regularly. It is essential to measure the blood pressure when evaluating a child who is suspected of having congenital heart disease or chronic renal disease or who is unconscious. Blood pressure measurements in healthy ambulatory patients are compared with standard norms. The auscultatory method of determining blood pressure is useful and is practiced in children over age 5 or 6; between ages 2 and 5, some children are cooperative, but others become agitated and anxious. It is helpful to remember that the blood pressure of hospitalized children, especially those admitted for elective reasons, is higher during the first 1 or 2 days and then tends to plateau at lower levels; the blood pressure of sick hospitalized children tends to remain constant throughout the hospitalization. Several determinations may be needed to obtain values unaffected by anxiety. Having children "watch the silver column rise" and explaining that the cuff will gently squeeze their arm usually reduces anxiety.

The size of the cuff is important because a cuff that is too small will produce falsely elevated values. The optimal cuff size is one that covers two thirds of the distance between the antecubital fossa and the shoulder or between the popliteal fossa and the hip. The rubber bag inside the cuff should encircle the extremity. Every site where infants and children are examined should have cuffs ranging from 1 to 4 inches in width.

With the auscultation method, the point where the sounds are first heard is recorded as the systolic pressure, and the point where the sounds disappear is recorded as the diastolic pressure. When the pulse sounds cannot be auscultated, a distal artery (radial, popliteal, or dorsalis pedis) can be palpated; the point where the first pulsation is felt is about 10 mm Hg lower than the auscultated systolic pressure. The flush method can be used in infants and young children. The elevated extremity, with the uninflated cuff in place, is stroked and "milked" from the hand to the elbow. The cuff then is inflated to a point above the estimated systolic pressure, and the pressure is slowly released. A sudden flush or reddening of the extremity, compared with the color of the opposite extremity, will occur at a point approximately halfway between the systolic and diastolic pressures. Normally, the systolic pressure is higher in the lower extremities, and the diastolic pressure is the same in the arms and legs.

Somatic Growth

Assessing somatic growth is crucial in every evaluation of an infant or a child because growth is the central characteristic of normal children and deviations from the child's norm provide an early warning of pathological processes. Several tools are available to aid in this evaluation; the most important, however, are growth charts, constructed either by longitudinal, serial measurements of a single cohort of children or by measurements of large numbers of children of different ages over a brief period. Although physical measurements of a child at a single point in time will give some useful clinical information, serial measurements over months or years provide an accurate record of the infant's or child's overall general pattern of growth, with deviations from the subject's norm indicating some intrinsic defect or environmental insult. The physical measurements used most often in assessing children are height and weight and, in infants and young children, the head circumference as well. To be clinically useful, all these measurements should be made with care and using a consistent technique.

Of the different growth charts currently available, the most recent were published by the National Center for Health Statistics. These include length for age or stature for age, weight for age, head circumference for age (to 36 months), and weight for length or weight for stature from birth to puberty. Separate charts are available for boys and girls of two age groups: birth to 36 months and 2 to 18 years (Figs. 7-5 to 7-16). The percentile lines on these charts indicate the number of normal children expected to fall above and below the index child's measurement. For instance, a 2-year-old girl whose length is 34 inches is in the 50th percentile for length; 50% of all normal 2-year-old girls will be expected to be taller, and 50% shorter.

Other growth charts indicate the mean and standard deviations from the mean by chronological age. Standard deviations (SD) are defined mathematically; for example, 1 SD above and below the mean includes about 67% of the measurements, and 2 SD above and below the mean includes about 95% of the measurements.

Velocity growth curves (Fig. 7-17) are used to measure differential rates of growth at different ages, especially among adolescents and children suspected of having endocrine disorders. These charts illustrate the two periods of rapid growth—infancy and puberty—and the differences by sex at puberty.

Height. Standing height can be measured fairly accurately in children over age 2 or 3. Some growth charts, such as Stuart's, use standing height measurements beginning at age 6; others, such as the new National Center for Health Statistics charts, plot standing heights beginning at age 2. Stand-up scales with attachments for measuring height generally are inaccurate. Short of buying an expensive wall-mounted apparatus (Stadiometer), accurate measurements can be made by attaching a graduated tape or ruler to a wall and placing a flat surface on top of the head to determine the height (Fig. 7-18). This measurement should be made with the child standing in stockings or bare feet, with his or her heels back and shoulders just touching the wall.

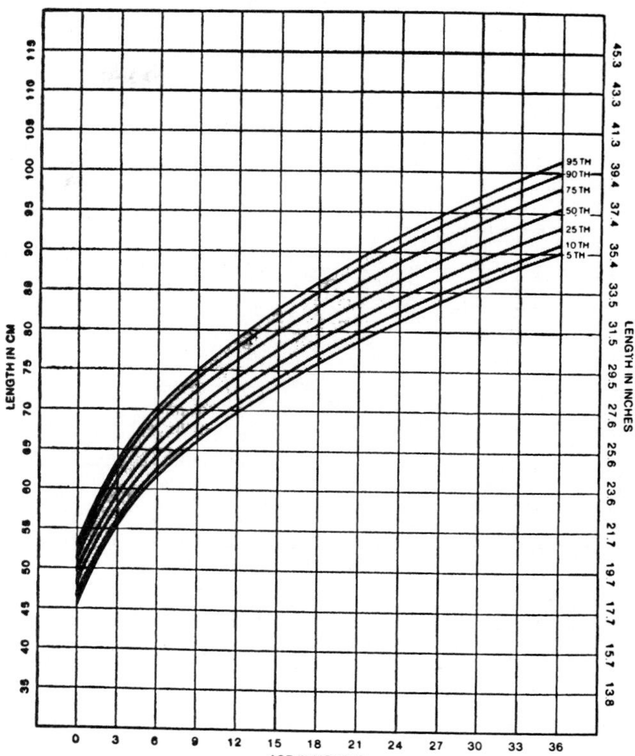

FIG. 7-5 Girls from birth to 36 months: length by age.
(Modified from Hamill VV, Drizd TA, Johnson CL et al: *Am J Clin Nutr* 32:607, 1979.)

Length of Infants. This is measured most accurately by using flat boards placed across and perpendicular to the examining table in contact with the vertex of the head and the soles of the feet and reading the measurement from a scale attached to the surface of the table (Fig. 7-19); care must be taken, in newborns particularly, to extend the hips and knees fully.

Weight. Infants are weighed on "infant" scales, with the baby clothed only in a diaper. Children old enough to stand are weighed in their underpants on stand-up scales. Stand-up scales, because of their usually wobbly base, may be frightening to children 1 to 3 years old, and sometimes the child must be weighed by subtracting the parent's weight from the combined parent-child weight. Ideally, serial measurements are made by using the same scale. In most normally growing children the height and weight measurements, when plotted on growth charts, fall within two standard percentile lines of each other (e.g., the 3rd, 10th, 25th, 50th, 75th, 90th, and 97th percentiles). Children whose measurements are either above the 97th or below the 3rd percentile require further evaluation, as do children whose height and weight differ by more than two percentile lines or categories.

Head Circumference. The head circumference is measured and plotted on a standard growth chart during each health maintenance examination from birth to age 2, the period of maximum rate of brain growth. With children over age 2, head circumference measurements are obtained at the initial examination of any child and when any component of the growth curve has been abnormal.

The measurement is made by placing a cloth tape mea-

GIRLS WEIGHT BY AGE PERCENTILES
AGES BIRTH-36 MONTHS

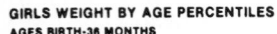

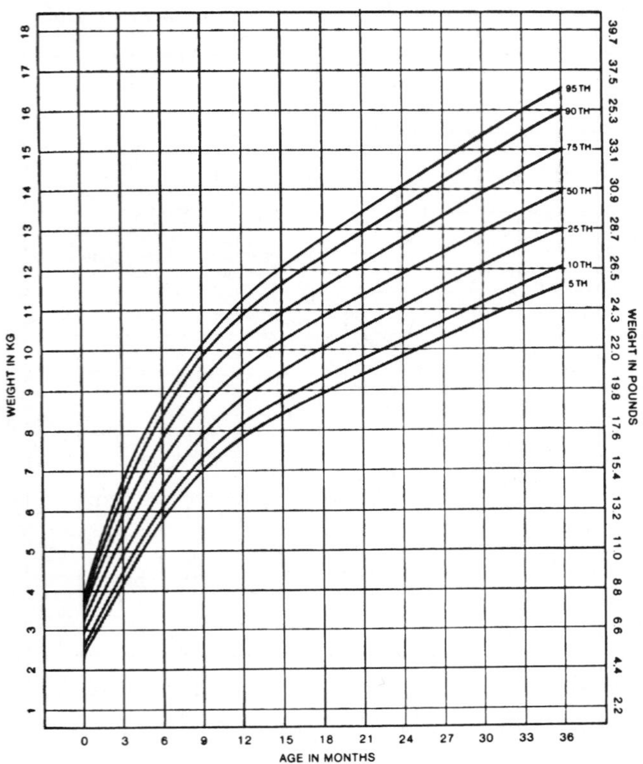

FIG. 7-6 Girls from birth to 36 months: weight by age.

(Modified from Hamill VV, Drizd TA, Johnson CL et al: *Am J Clin Nutr* 32:607, 1979.)

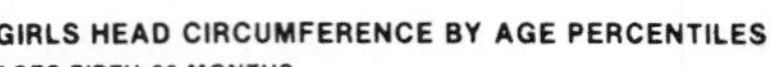

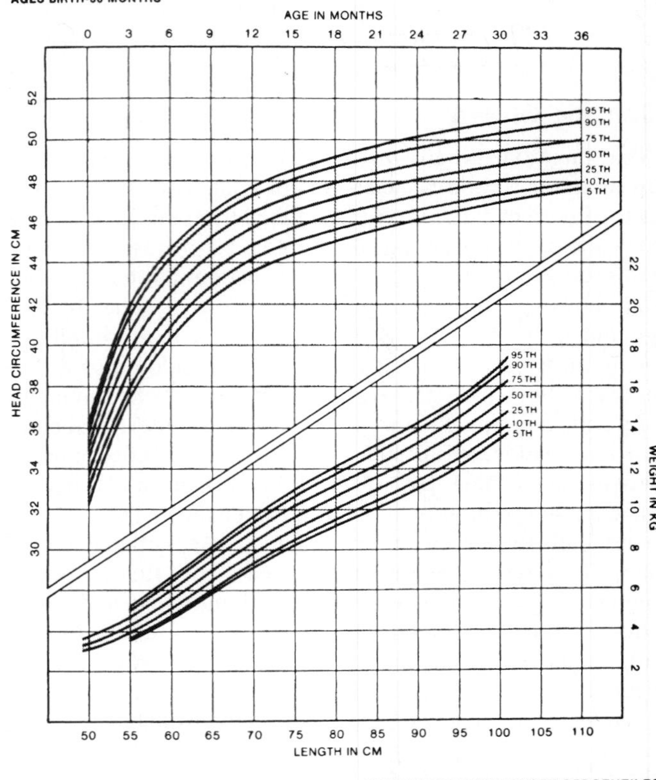

GIRLS WEIGHT BY LENGTH PERCENTILES
AGES BIRTH-36 MONTHS

FIG. 7-7 Girls from birth to 36 months: head circumference by age and weight by length.

(Modified from Hamill VV, Drizd TA, Johnson CL et al: *Am J Clin Nutr* 32:607, 1979.)

sure around the maximum occipitofrontal circumference, taking three separate readings and selecting the largest value. When measuring the heads of infants, it usually is necessary to have the infant supine with the arms held firmly against the body by the parent or a nurse; with children, the examiner can improve cooperation by first demonstrating the use of the measuring tape on himself or herself.

Chest and Other Measurements. In newborns the chest circumference is compared with the head circumference, the head having a larger circumference. The chest circumference normally equals and then exceeds the head circumference during the first year of life. Chest circumference is measured at the level of the nipples midway between expiration and inspiration. Another chest measurement sometimes used in following up children who have chronic pulmonary disease is the thoracic index, obtained by dividing the anteroposterior diameter by the transverse chest diameter. This index normally decreases from 0.85 at birth to 0.74 at age 6 because of the more rapid growth of the transverse diameter. The transverse (side-to-side) diameter and anteroposterior (sternum-to-vertebrae spinous process) diameter are measured most accurately with special calipers at the level of the nipples. Additional somatic measurements can help in the evaluation of children whose somatic growth is abnormal. The ratio of the upper half of the body to the lower half is obtained by measuring the distance from the crown to the symphysis pubis and then from the symphysis pubis to the floor (or, with an infant, to the heel) while the child is standing. This ratio changes from 1.7:1 in the newborn to 1:1 in the adult. The arm span, normally equal to the standing height, is measured from fingertip to fingertip of the third fingers with the arms outstretched. Norms for these measurements by age and by height are available in pediatric endocrinology textbooks.

ORGAN SYSTEMS

Skin

During the development of the fetus, neural crest cells, or melanoblasts, which have the potential for producing melanin, migrate from the dorsal region of the developing embryo. Under genetic control and mediated by tyrosinase, the melanoblasts produce varying amounts and shades of melanin, which make up the pigment of the skin, hair, and irides. Midline, ventral areas of defective pigmentation, such as piebaldism, can result from several developmental causes and sometimes are associated with defects in the development of the neural crest cells that give rise to the bipolar cells of the auditory nerve. Individuals in whom tyrosinase is absent lack pigmentation and have albinism. Localized areas of depigmentation shaped like a leaf are seen in tuberous sclerosis.

The periderm is a superficial layer of epidermis with absorption properties that normally is shed before birth; persistence of the periderm is seen in the "collodion baby" and in

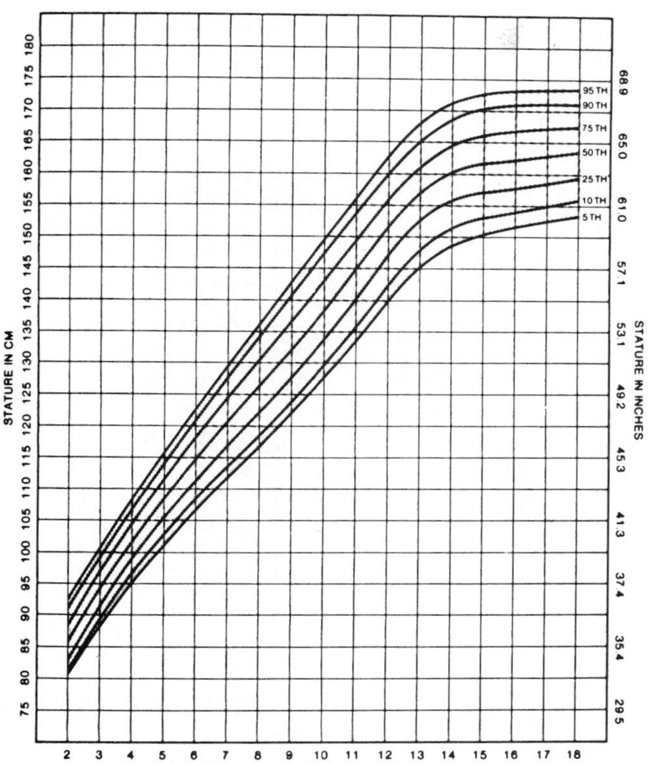

FIG. 7-8 Girls from 2 to 18 years: stature by age.

(Modified from Hamill VV, Drizd TA, Johnson CL et al: *Am J Clin Nutr* 32:607, 1979.)

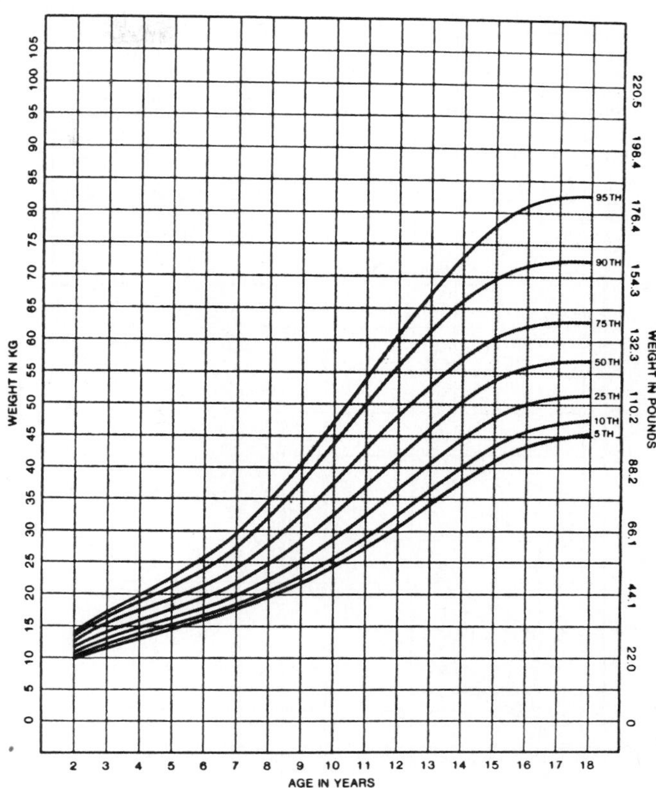

FIG. 7-9 Girls from 2 to 18 years: weight by age.

(Modified from Hamill VV, Drizd TA, Johnson CL et al: *Am J Clin Nutr* 32:607, 1979.)

forms of congenital ichthyosis. Hair follicles begin developing during the third fetal month, and skin keratinization first occurs at their openings. Sebaceous glands, whose secretions contribute to the formation of vernix caseosa, are active starting in the latter months of pregnancy; after birth, they are relatively inactive until puberty. Apocrine glands are formed in the fetus but are not developed fully until puberty. Sweat glands, which grow most rapidly between the twenty-second and twenty-fourth fetal weeks, are inactive in the fetus. They become active in the newborn after several weeks and reach a maximal rate of activity by age 2. Sweat gland secretion may be under some degree of cortical control, which may explain children's tendency to sweat at all times and adults' tendency to sweat more while asleep.

Adipose tissue begins to develop during fetal life and constitutes 28% of the body weight at term. The number of fat cells increases especially rapidly during the first year of life, with adipose tissue constituting 40% to 70% of the body weight at 4 months of age. Cell numbers increase at a slower rate until puberty, when a second growth spurt occurs. In adults, adipose tissue constitutes 15% to 40% of body weight in men and 25% to 50% in women. The fat content of adipose tissue in a nonobese individual increases from 40% at birth to 80% in the adult.

Examination of the skin often yields important clues to both normal and pathological systemic processes. For instance, the characteristics of the newborn's skin reflect, in part, the length of gestation, and such observations as the opacity of the skin and the distribution of body hair can help determine the gestational age. The onset, distribution, and characteristics of some exanthems are specific for certain infectious diseases of children, and a few lesions are associated with abnormalities of other organ systems, especially the central nervous system (the phakomatoses). The skin, therefore, should be thoroughly examined in each newborn, each acutely ill or febrile child, and each child in whom congenital anomalies are suspected. A thorough examination of the skin involves noting the skin's color, consistency, and turgor; the distribution and type of lesions; and the characteristics of the sweat and sebaceous glands, the body and scalp hair, and the nails.

Newborn Period. During the first minutes after birth, the newborn's Apgar score is determined partly by assessment for the presence and distribution of cyanosis. A normal, nonchilled newborn usually progresses from generalized cyanosis to generalized pinkness while normal respirations are established during the first 5 to 10 minutes of extrauterine life. Acrocyanosis, especially on exposure to a cool environment, is common in newborns for several weeks after birth, as is mottling of the skin, a latticelike pattern of pale and dark areas that appear especially on the extremities. Severe cold stress can cause generalized cyanosis. Occasionally, in newborns, transient cyanosis of an entire half of the baby (harlequin color change) or of one or more extremities is noted, presumably as the result of temporary vascular instability.

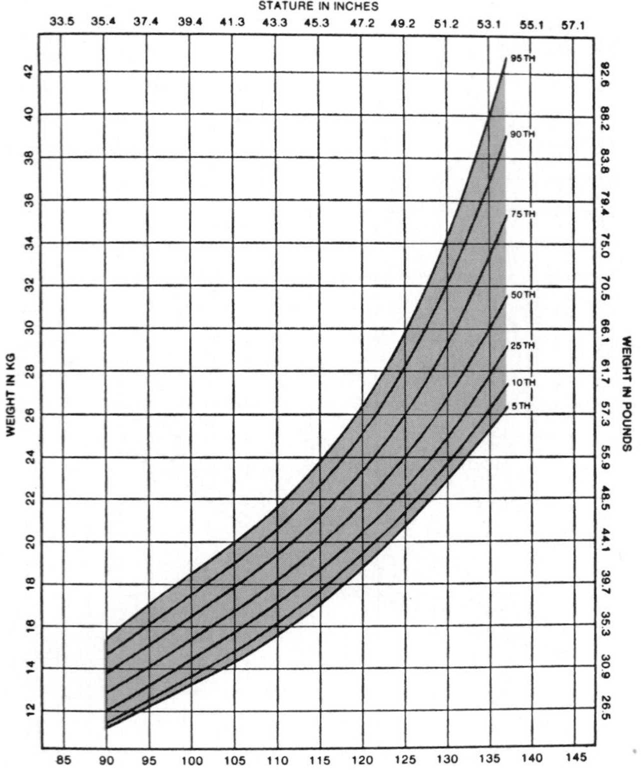

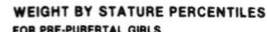

FIG. 7-10 Prepubertal girls: weight by stature.

(Modified from Hamill VV, Drizd TA, Johnson CL et al: *Am J Clin Nutr* 32:607, 1979.)

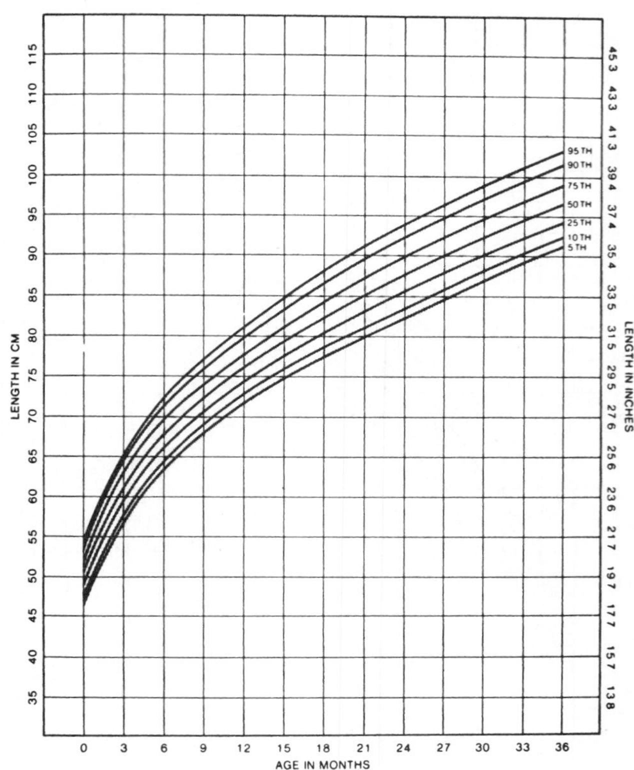

FIG. 7-11 Boys from birth to 36 months: length by age.

(Modified from Hamill VV, Drizd TA, Johnson CL et al: *Am J Clin Nutr* 32:607, 1979.)

Persistent generalized cyanosis usually is a sign of depression caused by maternal drugs or anesthesia, primary pulmonary disease, congenital heart disease, overwhelming infection, or hypoglycemia. Plethora in newborns may indicate high levels of hemoglobin (seen, for instance, in the twin-to-twin transfusion syndrome), and pallor in newborns may be a sign of anemia or cold stress or, less commonly, of congestive heart failure or shock.

A newborn's skin is covered by varying amounts of white, greasy, vernix caseosa, with larger amounts present in preterm babies. The newborn's skin color is determined partly by the amount of subcutaneous fat present. Premature babies have a smaller amount of subcutaneous fat and generally appear redder than full-term babies; their skin also is more transparent, and therefore subcutaneous blood vessels are more visible. Yellow staining of the vernix by meconium suggests that birth was preceded by acute fetal distress; with more prolonged fetal distress, as in the postmature baby who has placental insufficiency, the yellow (or yellow-green) staining can involve the umbilicus and nails. The skin tends to progress from being smooth to scaly, with varying amounts of desquamation and fissuring as the gestation progresses from preterm to postterm. This latter condition usually changes to normal, smooth skin without specific treatment within 1 to 2 weeks. Nonspecific edema, especially of the hands and feet, is less prominent as the gestational age approaches term. Generalized or localized petechiae, ecchymoses of the scalp or face, lacerations of the external ears, and diffuse or localized scalp edema all can be caused by physical trauma sustained during birth.

Jaundice can be expected to appear in at least 50% of normal term babies and in a higher percentage of preterm babies in the third or fourth day of life, usually indicating the presence of physiological jaundice. However, jaundice appearing at any time during the neonatal period may be an early sign of infection or of metabolic or primary hepatic disease. The early onset of jaundice also raises the question of blood group incompatibility and erythroblastosis. Clinically apparent jaundice usually indicates a serum bilirubin of at least 6 mg/dl, although the lack of subcutaneous fat in premature infants may delay its detection. Because of the variable lighting in many newborn nurseries and maternity units, clinical estimation of the bilirubin level is notoriously inaccurate, although some experienced neonatologists find that jaundice tends to progress from the head to the proximal and then distal extremities with increasing serum concentrations of bilirubin. The most consistent observations can be made by examining the skin in direct daylight. The presence of jaundice is best appreciated after pressure is applied to an area of skin over the forehead or sternum with the flat surface of a glass slide to empty the capillary bed.

The amount of melanin in the skin varies at birth. Babies of African-American parents may demonstrate very little as neonates. Pigmented areas over the lumbar region and buttocks, known as mongolian spots, commonly are present in

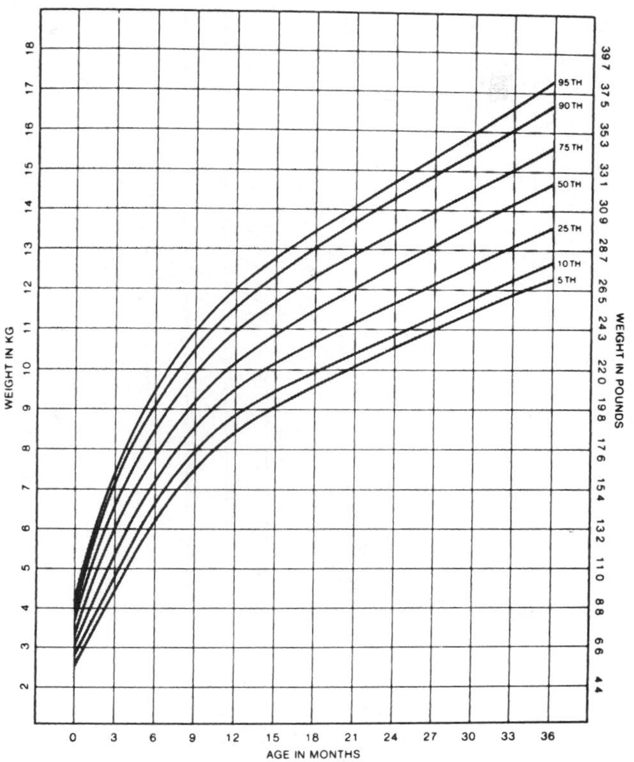

FIG. 7-12 Boys from birth to 36 months: weight by age.

(Modified from Hamill W, Drizd TA, Johnson CL et al: *Am J Clin Nutr* 32:607, 1979.)

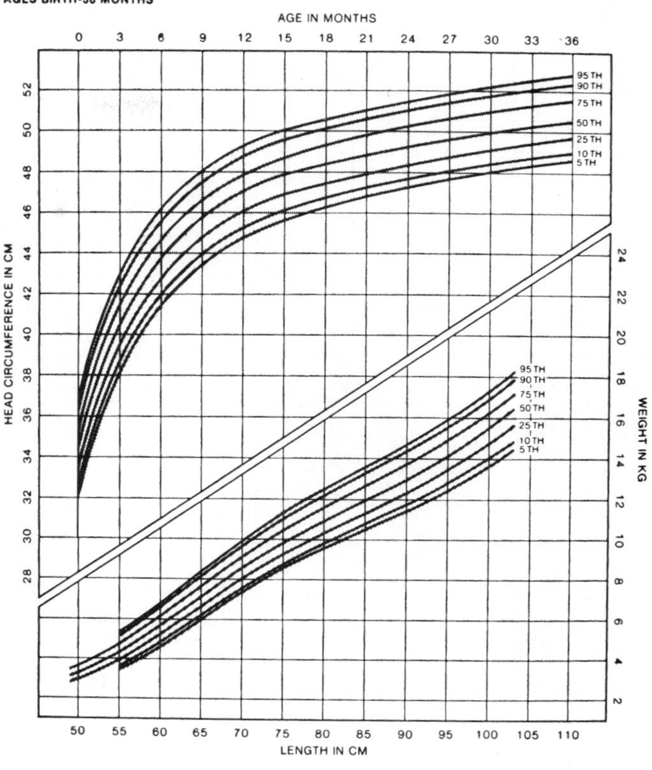

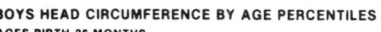

FIG. 7-13 Boys from birth to 36 months: head circumference by age and weight by length.

(Modified from Hamill W, Drizd TA, Johnson CL et al: *Am J Clin Nutr* 32:607, 1979.)

black, darker-complexioned white, and Asian babies at birth. They become less prominent and eventually disappear during childhood. A number of other spots can be seen on a healthy newborn's skin, including the common telangiectasias (nevus flammeus) on the eyelids, bridge of the nose, upper lip, and nape of the neck, which usually disappear during infancy; red or purple strawberry hemangiomas or more deep-seated, cavernous hemangiomas; tiny white papules on the nose, cheeks, forehead, and occasionally the trunk caused by plugging of the sebaceous glands (milia); pinpoint vesicles with or without surrounding erythema caused by plugging of the sweat glands (miliaria); erythematous flares with central pinpoint white vesicles or papules, known as erythema toxicum, which may appear and disappear over several hours during the first week of life; and areas of either decreased or increased pigmentation, café-au-lait spots being one example, which may occur in isolation or may be associated with generalized disease, such as neurofibromatosis.

The newborn's skin often is covered with fine lanugo hair, more prominently seen in premature infants, which is lost after several weeks of life. Scalp hair at birth, which varies in amount, commonly is shed and replaced by permanent hair of a different degree of pigmentation. The fingernails may be long in postmature babies, and their color can be influenced by amniotic fluid staining and melanin pigmentation of the nail beds. Incurving of the lateral margins of the toenails is common and can be associated with local inflammation. Examination of the fingerprint and palmar crease patterns in newborns sometimes is useful because of the association of abnormal dermatoglyphics with certain chromosomal abnormalities and intrauterine infections.[7] Magnification is essential in determining the fingerprint pattern on the distal phalanges and the position of the axial triradius of the palm. A single transverse palmar crease (simian line) can occur in normal individuals but more commonly is associated with chromosomal abnormalities such as Down syndrome.

The newborn's skin should be checked carefully for defects and sinus tracts, especially over the entire length of the spine and the midline of the head from the nape of the neck to the bridge of the nose. Sinus tracts sometimes communicate with intracranial and intraspinal spaces or masses, as with dermoid cysts and encephaloceles. Preauricular sinuses may or may not communicate with a persistent brachial cleft space. A more common minor abnormality of the preauricular area is the skin tag, which usually has a cartilaginous core.

Infancy. Careful inspection of a completely undressed infant during health maintenance checks often will reveal minor abnormalities such as cradle cap and diaper dermatitis, the sometimes chronic lesions of infantile acne that first appear at 3 to 4 months of age, and less commonly, scattered ecchymoses of varying ages that can signal child abuse. Palpation of the skin, preferably over the lateral abdominal wall, allows qualitative measurement of subcutaneous adipose tis-

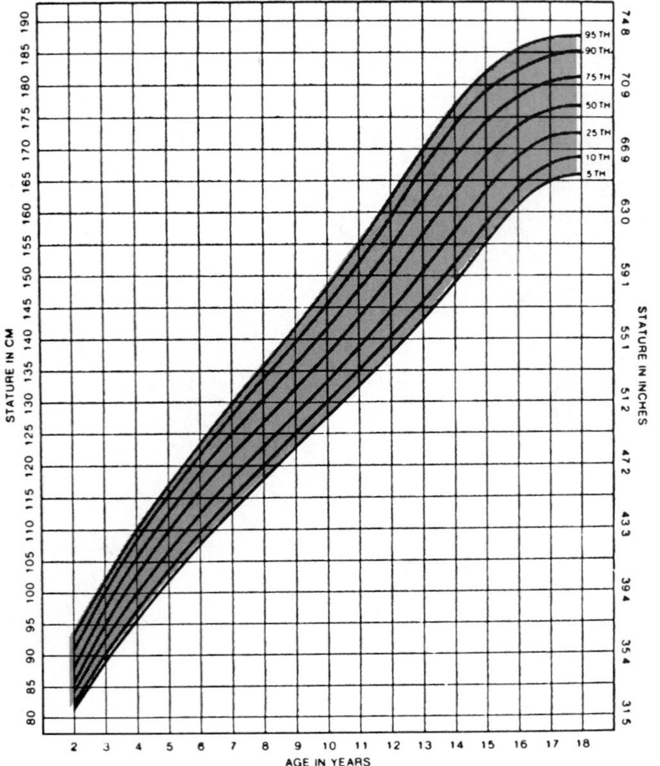

FIG. 7-14 Boys from 2 to 18 years: stature by age.

(Modified from Hamill VV, Drizd TA, Johnson CL et al: *Am J Clin Nutr* 32:607, 1979.)

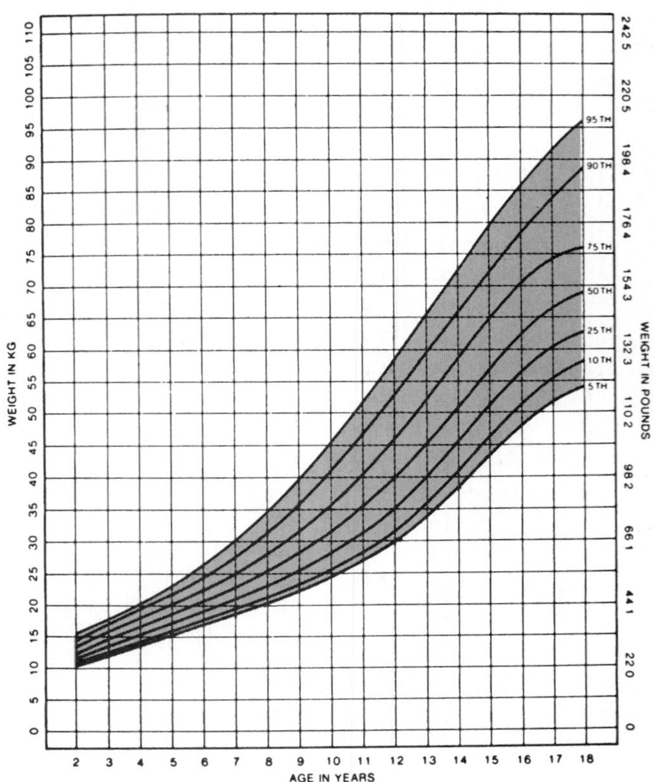

FIG. 7-15 Boys from 2 to 18 years: weight by age.

(Modified from Hamill VV, Drizd TA, Johnson CL et al: *Am J Clin Nutr* 32:607, 1979.)

sue during infancy and also observation of skin turgor (the rate of return to resting position after the skin is lifted and released), which is decreased with dehydration.

Early and Late Childhood. For all children, evaluation of acute or chronic rashes is helped greatly by a careful description of the rash's major characteristics (macular, papular, pustular, vesicular, petechial, ecchymotic, oozing, scaly, exfoliative, abraded, erythematous, or pigmented), location (trunk, face, extremities, or intertriginous or hairy areas), developmental history, and temporal association with other signs and symptoms. In fact, most infectious exanthems of children are diagnosed by certain constellations of these factors. One recently described infectious disease, Lyme disease, is diagnosed in its early stages solely by a rash (expanding, red, macular rash with or without a central mark from a tick bite) (see Chapter 228).

Adolescence. Examination of the skin of adolescents allows monitoring of important pubertal changes such as areolar pigmentation, pigmentation of the external genitalia, development of pubic and axillary hair, increased functioning of sweat and apocrine glands, and an increase in subcutaneous fat. The prominent signs of acne vulgaris on the face and trunk can be anticipated in many adolescents.

Head and Face

The rapid rate of brain growth during infancy and childhood explains the increased size of the head relative to body length in newborns and infants as contrasted with that of adults. The facial contours and dimensions change considerably during the first 10 years of life, reflecting the downward and forward growth of the mandible and vertical growth of the maxilla and nasal bones. These changing proportions are best summarized by the proportion of cranium to face volumes at different ages: 8:1 at birth, 5:1 at age 2, and 2:1 by age 18. A thorough examination of the head includes measuring the head circumference and plotting the value on a standard growth chart, observing the shape and symmetry, and palpating the sutures and fontanelles; occasionally percussion, auscultation, and transillumination are needed. The head should be examined thoroughly in clinical situations involving growth or developmental failure, suspected trauma, a seizure disorder, or fever in an infant and as part of every health maintenance examination from birth to age 2.

Newborn Period. The newborn's skull is composed of partly calcified, bony plates that interface with each other at predictably located suture lines. The major sutures palpable at birth are the coronal, lambdoid, sagittal, and metopic sutures (Fig. 7-20). Because of overriding of one cranial bone on another after molding of the skull during the descent through the birth canal, the newborn's sutures often feel like ridges. The anterior fontanelle is located at the junction of the sagittal and coronal sutures and varies considerably in size in normal infants; it usually measures about 1 inch at its greatest diameter and is diamond shaped. The posterior fon-

WEIGHT BY STATURE PERCENTILES
FOR PRE-PUBERTAL BOYS

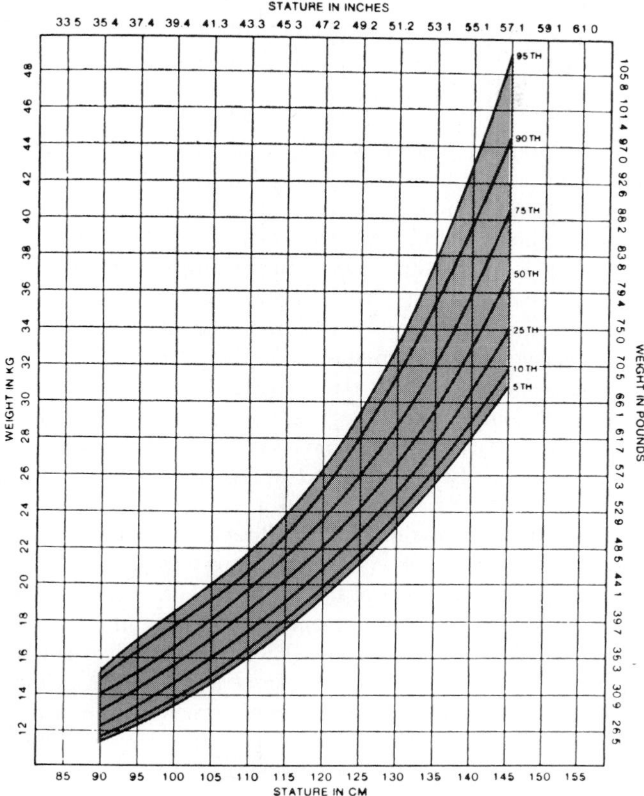

FIG. 7-16 Prepubertal boys: weight by stature.

(Modified from Hamill VV, Drizd TA, Johnson CL et al: *Am J Clin Nutr* 32:607, 1979.)

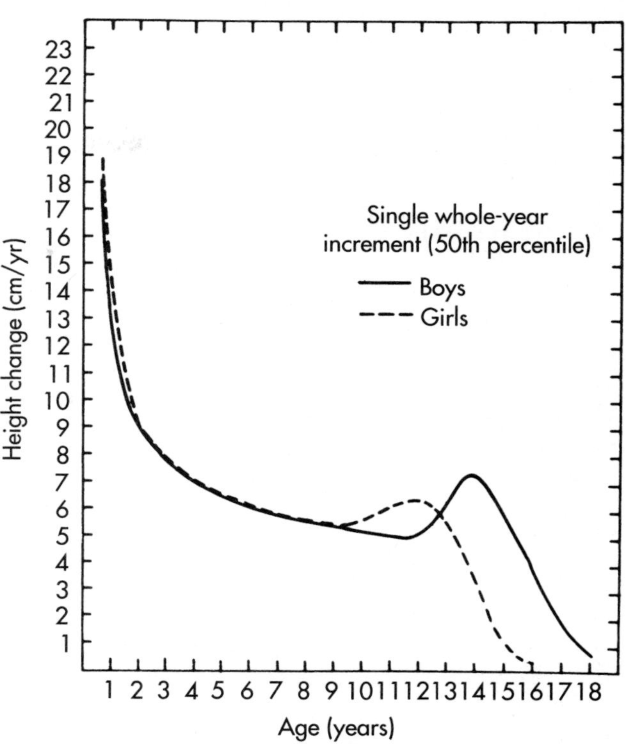

FIG. 7-17 Velocity curves for length and height for boys and girls based on intervals of 1 year.

(From Lowrey GH: *Growth and development of children*, ed 8, Chicago, 1986, Mosby.)

tanelle, found at the junction of the sagittal and lambdoid sutures, only occasionally is palpable at birth. Vascular pulsations, transmitted by the cerebrospinal fluid (CSF), normally can be seen over the anterior fontanelle. With normal CSF pressure and with the infant in an upright position and not crying, the anterior fontanelle is soft and flat upon palpation. A bulging fontanelle is a sign of increased intracranial pressure; a depressed fontanelle is a sign of decreased intravascular volume, as in dehydration.

At birth it is common to palpate localized edema over one or more areas of the head. A palpable swelling, particularly over the vertex, that recedes after 1 or 2 days represents subcutaneous edema and is called *caput succedaneum*. Swollen areas whose margins are limited to suture lines and that often require weeks to recede represent subperiosteal hemorrhage and are called *cephalhematomas*. These resolve partly by calcification, which initially may feel like a mass with a heaped-up bony rim and a soft center. Other commonly seen effects of the birth process include linear or curved abraded or lacerated areas, especially over the zygomatic arches and preauricular areas, resulting from use of obstetric forceps. The infant's face may be asymmetrical at birth because of intrauterine positioning with the chin touching one shoulder. Facial palsy, manifested by a drooping corner of the mouth during crying, usually is caused by obstetric forceps exerting pressure over the facial nerve in the preauricular area.

The cranial bones normally become firmer upon palpation

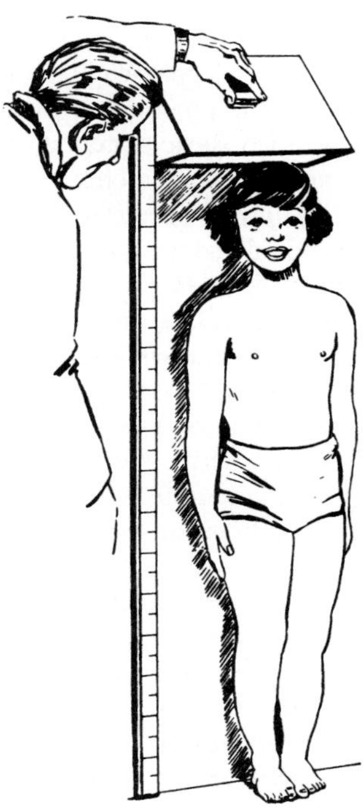

FIG. 7-18 Measurement of height.

(From Evaluation of body size and physical growth of children, 1976, Rockville, Md, the Maternal and Child Health Program, US Department of Health, Education, and Welfare.)

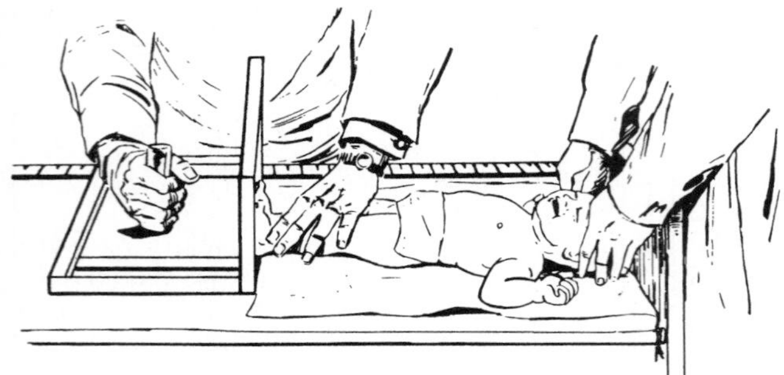

FIG. 7-19 Measurement of length in the infant.
(From Evaluation of body size and physical growth of children, 1976, Rockville, Md, the Maternal and Child Health Program, US Department of Health, Education, and Welfare.)

with increasing gestational age. One exception occurs when the sutural edges of the cranial bones are pliable and "springy," a condition known as *craniotabes,* which is found in many normal infants and in rare cases is a sign of rickets. A disproportionately large head at birth may indicate hydrocephalus or intrauterine growth retardation in which overall brain growth often is relatively normal.

Transillumination of the newborn and infant head is useful in evaluating asymmetrical or disproportionately large heads as well as unexplained neurological signs and symptoms. The procedure is accomplished in a completely darkened room by use of a bright light source, such as a three-battery flashlight or a special high-intensity light. If a flashlight is used, it should be fitted with a soft foam rubber collar and held against the head tangentially in such a way as to allow uniform intensity of illumination of the head around the full circumference of the light. Localized bright spots may indicate acquired problems, such as subdural effusions, or congenital defects, such as porencephalic cysts. The entire head will "light up" in the presence of hydranencephaly.

Infancy, Childhood, and Adolescence. By measuring and plotting serial occipitofrontal head circumferences, the examiner can monitor the normal growth of the brain within the normally yielding cranial bones, which are separated from each other by suture lines that remain patent until brain growth is complete. A head circumference that is increasing at an abnormally slow rate may indicate either a slowly growing brain (intrinsic or acquired defect) or cranial sutures that have closed too soon (craniosynostosis). The normally proportioned small head is called *microcephaly,* and a small head associated with premature suture closure is labeled according to the shape distortion caused by the suture involved (scaphocephaly, plagiocephaly, acrocephaly).

Craniosynostosis, a diagnosis that requires confirmation by roentgenography, often is associated with prominence or ridging of the involved suture line. A head that is growing too rapidly when compared with the rate of height and weight gain always should be evaluated for hydrocephalus and subdural effusions. Sometimes the head is just asymmetrical, with a normally increasing head circumference; this suggests either intrauterine or extrauterine positional effects, such as the flat occiput seen in babies who are left to lie for long periods and the flattening of one occipital bone and the opposite frontal bone sometimes associated with torticollis (cranioscoliosis). Prominent frontal bone bossing, with or without associated saddle-nose deformity, may be a sign of the developing osteomyelitis associated with congenital syphilis. The anterior fontanelle normally is not palpable after 18 months of age and may disappear as early as 3 months of age.

Percussion of the head by directly tapping with the middle finger normally elicits a flat sound. A "cracked pot" sound may be heard in infants whose fontanelle is open or in infants with increased intracranial pressure whose fontanelle is closed, as is seen with hydrocephalus. Auscultation of the head for localized bruits, indicating vascular anomalies, is included in the evaluation of children who have seizures or other neurological abnormalities. Up to age 5, however, systolic or continuous bruits may be heard over the temporal areas in normal children.

Examination of the face begins with an overall impression, which occasionally yields important diagnostic clues, such as the dull, immobile face associated with hypothyroidism; the open-mouthed expression of the child who has chronic nasopharyngeal obstruction caused by hypertrophied adenoids; the multiply bruised face of the battered child; and the small nose, open mouth, and prominent epicanthal skinfolds of the child who has Down syndrome. Facial puffiness, or edema, especially involving the eyelids, can be an early sign of fluid retention secondary to acute or chronic renal disease or congestive heart failure. The distance between the eyes, usually measured as the interpupillary distance, can be increased as well as decreased in a number of syndromes of chromosomal origin and with other developmental anomalies.

The Chvostek sign, elicited by tapping the cheek just under the zygoma and causing unilateral facial grimacing, sometimes is a sign of hypocalcemia or hyperventilation tetany in older children; it also can be present in normal infants and young children.

Parotid gland swelling often is difficult to distinguish from cervical adenitis. The swollen parotid gland lies mainly anterior to the angle of the mandible and often pushes the ear pinna away from the side of the head, which can be seen when the patient is viewed from behind. Swelling and tenderness below a line drawn from the angle of the mandible to the mastoid process is caused by cervical adenitis. Nonobstructive parotitis usually is viral: when acute, it usually is caused by the mumps; when recurrent or chronic, human immunodeficiency virus (HIV) should be considered (see Chapters 180, Acquired Human Immunodeficiency Syndrome (AIDS) and Human Immunodeficiency Virus (HIV) Infection, and 196, Contact Dermatitis).

Eyes

Studies of the process of mother-infant bonding during the neonatal period highlight the functional importance of an intact visual system in babies from the first minutes after birth.[4] Although examination of the eye is important in picking up clues to congenital and acquired systemic abnormalities, the overriding goal of examining the eyes of infants and children is to ascertain that normal functioning is taking place and that potentially remediable processes affecting visual acuity are detected early.

At birth the eye is almost full grown compared with the other organs and the body. By this time the retina is com-

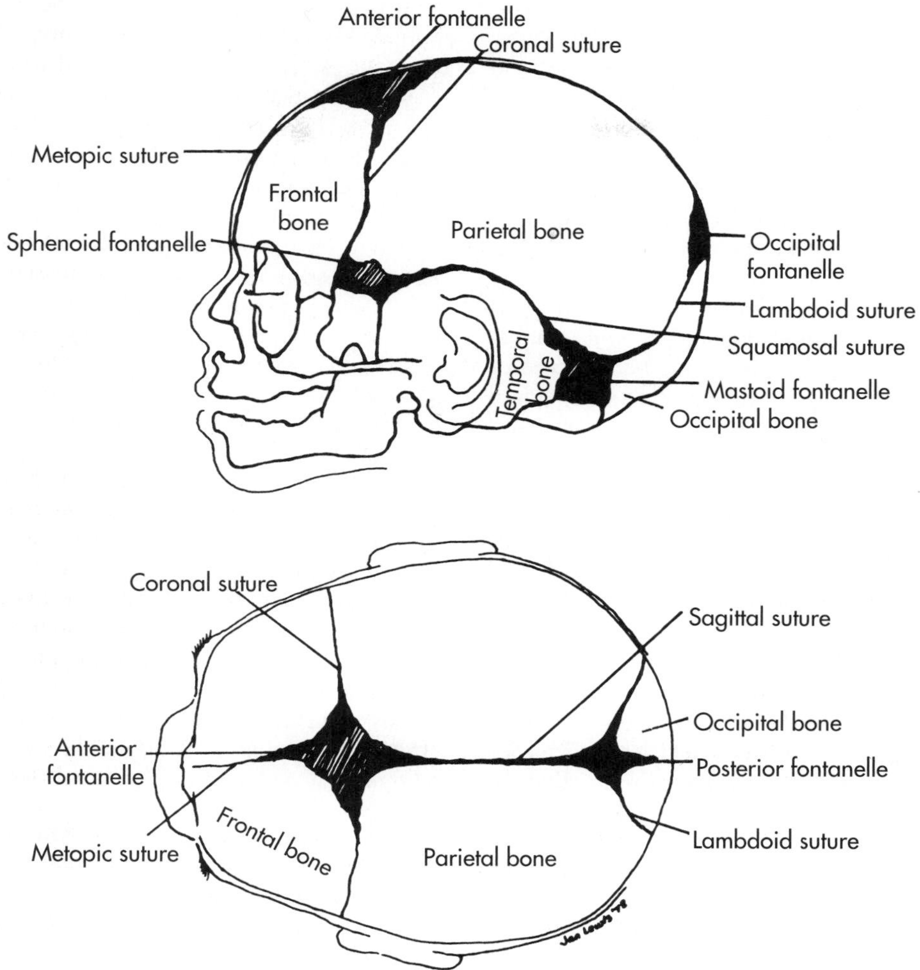

FIG. 7-20 Two views of the neonatal skull, showing clinically important fontanelles and sutures. (From Scanlon JW et al: *A system of newborn physical examination,* Baltimore, 1979, University Park Press.)

pletely developed except for the central foveal region, which is fully developed by 4 months of age, as is myelination of the central optic radiations and differentiation of the optic cortex. The cornea increases in diameter from 10 mm at birth to the final adult size of 11.5 mm. The lens doubles in weight between birth and age 20 and then increases another 50% by age 80. The pupillary reflex to light is functioning by 29 to 31 weeks of gestation. At birth the globe tends to be short in relation to the focusing ability of the lens and cornea (hypermetropia), and up to age 12 to 14 the globe gradually lengthens with a resulting tendency for visual images to be focused in front of the retina (myopia).[9] At birth babies can respond to faces and to colored as well as black and white objects. The fixed focal length of the newborn's eyes (20 cm), along with the aforementioned factors and distracting influences (startle reflex, hunger, temperature changes), limit the newborn's ability to respond visually for more than brief moments.

The ability to accommodate is present by 4 months of age, and the ability to follow a moving light through different planes at various angles from the face is developed fully by 6 months of age.

Examination of the eye is an important part of every examination of an infant or child. The completeness of the examination may vary according to the reason for the visit (health maintenance versus emergency head trauma) and the chief complaint (headaches versus a sprained knee). A thorough examination of the eye includes observation of the lids, including eyelashes, tear ducts, and glands; the conjunctiva; the sclera and cornea; the pupils, including reaction to light and accommodation; and the lens. Globe size and intraocular pressure should be estimated, and the extraocular movements should be tested to note any presence of nystagmus or strabismus. Examination of the fundus includes assessment of the optic disk, macula, retina, and central vessels; this should be done in every child who is examined because of headache, head trauma, or other suspected intracranial lesion. Assessment of visual acuity should be part of every health maintenance examination.

Newborn Period. Several attempts may be required to examine a newborn's eyes completely because of transient edema of the eyelids caused by the birth process or by the conjunctivitis induced by silver nitrate instillation soon after birth. The upper eyelid may have a midline notch from incomplete fusion of its embryonic medial and lateral portions. The eyelids normally are fused until the eighth month of gestation. The lids often are slippery with vernix caseosa and conjunctival exudate, which should be removed gently with a dry cloth, allowing separation of the lids with a finger placed on each lid. Occasionally, one or both eyelids will be everted after birth. Episcleral and subconjunctival hemorrhages, either focal or diffuse, commonly are present after birth and can be expected to recede spontaneously. Less commonly, hyphema (blood in the anterior chamber) may be present. Cloudiness of the cornea can be caused by congenital glaucoma and requires ophthalmological consultation. Opaque particles or strands in the lens may be cataracts or remnants of the artery that supplies the lens in its early stages of development (hyaloid artery). This iris often is less pigmented at birth; its final color develops during the first year of life. Although a ring of white specks around the periphery of the iris (Brushfield spots) is present in some normal infants, it is more prominent and common in children who have Down syndrome. Defects in the iris, particularly in the ventral aspect, can be associated with parallel defects in the lens and retina (colobomas) and represent incomplete closure of the embryonic optic fissure.

Careful examination of the newborn's retina is difficult without the use of mydriatics. The appearance of a "red reflex," seen when the ophthalmoscope is held 10 to 12 inches in front of the eye, ascertains that no major obstructions in light are present between the cornea and the retina, such as corneal opacities, cataracts, and retinal tumors. Funduscopic examination of the newborn is indicated in babies in whom the red reflex is absent, in babies who have been given supplemental oxygen, and in babies in whom CNS trauma or septicemia is suspected. In some newborn nurseries every newborn is given a funduscopic examination. With the ophthalmoscope, the cornea usually can be seen at +20 diopters, the lens at +15 diopters, and the fundus at 0 diopters. The fundus is examined 30 minutes after instillation of a drop of 2.5% phenylephrine (Neo-Synephrine) ophthalmic solution in each eye, optimally with the assistance of another person who can offer the baby a sugar nipple. The physician notes the size and color of the optic disk and macula and any areas of hemorrhage or increased or decreased pigmentation of the retina. In newborns and infants the optic disk is paler than in older children, the peripheral retina vessels are not well developed, and the foveal light reflection is absent. Papilledema rarely occurs before age 3 because of the ability of the fontanelles and open sutures to absorb increases in intracranial pressure.

Perhaps the most productive method for observing both the structure and function of the newborn's eyes is for the examiner to hold the infant upright, in which position the infant often opens his or her eyes spontaneously. Abnormalities in the size of the eyes should be noted, inasmuch as microphthalmia is a part of several rare congenital defect syndromes. Any upward or downward slanting of the axis of the eyelids (palpebral fissures) also should be noted; upward slanting is characteristic of children who have Down syndrome. Although inner epicanthal folds can occur in normal infants, they are common in children who have Down syndrome and in those with other chromosomal abnormalities. The setting-sun sign (a portion of the white sclera is seen between the upper lid margin and the iris) occurs in some normal premature and full-term infants, but persistence suggests the possibility of hydrocephalus.

When the baby is held at arm's length and turned slowly in one direction (Fig. 7-21), the eyes turn toward that direction. When rotation stops, the eyes turn toward the opposite direction after a few quick, unsustained, nystagmoid movements. More sustained nystagmus with this maneuver or at rest may indicate blindness or other CNS problems. When just the head is moved slowly through its full range of motion, the eyes do not move but remain in their original position (doll's eye reflex). This maneuver can demonstrate paresis of the lateral rectus muscle. Strabismus, the condition in which the visual axes of both eyes in fixing a distal point are not parallel, commonly is seen as an intermittent phenomenon in normal newborns and may persist up to 6 months of age. The infant should be examined carefully for inward deviation of the eye, or esotropia, and outward deviation, or exotropia—whether alternating, fixed, or transient. Prominent epicanthal folds sometimes can give the erroneous impression of strabismus. Any fixed divergence of the eyes and any transient outward divergence in the newborn require immediate neurological and ophthalmological consultation.

Visual acuity in the newborn is assessed indirectly by means of visual reflexes such as consensual pupillary constriction in response to a bright light; blinking in response to a bright light and to an object moved quickly toward the eyes; and opticokinetic nystagmus, which the normal infant demonstrates when a cylinder that has alternating vertical black and white lines is rotated at specified distances from the eyes.

Infancy. In addition to the findings on the examination described for the newborn, a few common problems particularly affect young infants. Tears often are not present at birth but are produced by 4 months of age. The nasolacrimal duct, however, sometimes is not patent until 1 year of age, leading to a chronically tearing eye with or without purulent discharge. Pressure over the nasolacrimal sac on the medial edge of the lower eyelid will confirm the diagnosis of nasolacrimal duct obstruction by yielding mucoid or purulent fluid. Usually there is minimal or no conjunctival inflammation,

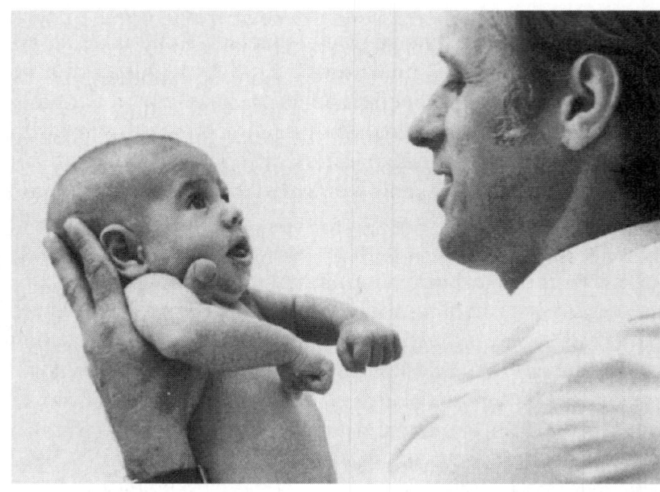

FIG. 7-21 Vestibular function testing in the infant. (Photograph by P. Ruben.)

and ophthalmological consultation is not indicated unless the tearing and discharge persist beyond 12 months of age.

Although acute conjunctival inflammation with purulent exudate sometimes occurs in neonates in reaction to the routine instillation of silver nitrate drops, another cause that must be considered is infection by *Neisseria gonorrhoeae, Staphylococcus aureus,* or *Chlamydia trachomatis. C. trachomatis* can be diagnosed by the presence of cytoplasmic material in the epithelial cells of conjunctival scrapings. An acutely red, tearing eye in infants often is caused by corneal abrasions inflicted by the infant's own fingernails; this diagnosis can be confirmed by placing a damp fluorescein strip in the corner of the eye and observing the green staining of the abraded corneal epithelium.

Unilateral or bilateral ptosis of the lids may be appreciated better after the immediate postbirth period; it may be a familial trait, part of a syndrome of congenital anomalies, or the result of oculomotor nerve palsy. Unilateral exophthalmos, or protrusion of the eye, can result from a retroorbital tumor or abscess.

Childhood and Adolescence. After the neonatal period and up to 3 to 5 years of age, visual acuity continues to be determined by the observations of the parents and the examiner. By 4 weeks of age the infant can fixate on an object; by 6 weeks, coordinated movements in following an object are seen. By 3 months the infant can follow an object moving across his or her midline, and convergence of the eyes is present. Beginning at 4 to 5 months the infant can reach for and grasp objects. Increasing recognition of familiar objects and faces by 5 to 6 months of age confirms normally developing cortical as well as visual systems. Between 1 and 3 years of age the infant responds to and uses brightly colored toys and children's books and can circumnavigate the examiner's office. Standardized tests of visual acuity for children under age 3 have been developed. These tests require the child to "match" a toy or ball with small "test" objects that the examiner holds. These tests, which are not widely known or used, may offer the child health worker a useful screening tool.

Infants and children who fail to perform according to the tests outlined here should be examined further for blindness or mental retardation. Besides instances of blindness that are genetically determined or caused by perinatal insults, amblyopia (or reduced visual acuity) results from suppression of one or two unequal images in the visual cortex. Its importance is that it can be reversed only if diagnosed early enough (by age 6 at the latest) to allow treatment of the underlying cause. There are two major categories of causes of *amblyopia:* obstructive amblyopia secondary to a cataract, corneal opacity, or severe ptosis and amblyopia ex anopsia secondary to uniocular squint (strabismus) or refractive (anisometropia) error. *Strabismus* is detected by using the pupillary light reflex and the cover tests. The symmetry of the pupillary light reflex is observed while the child focuses on a penlight 12 inches from the eyes; asymmetry indicates esotropia or exotropia. In the cover test, with the child focusing on the penlight, the visual axis of one eye is interrupted by the examiner's hand; any movement of the uncovered eye indicates strabismus.

Loss of visual acuity in one eye detected during a screening evaluation often is the first indication of amblyopia. Vision is screened by using the Snellen illiterate E chart for children between the ages of 3 and 5 and the Snellen E chart for children 5 years of age and older (see Chapter 20, Ten, Vision Screening).

The most common abnormalities of children's eyes seen in an ambulatory setting are swelling and redness of the eyelids and a red, tearing eye. Swelling and redness of the eyelids occur with obstruction of the nasolacrimal duct, blepharitis, hordeolum, and chalazion. Edema, tenderness, and warmth of the eyelid, usually indicative of periorbital cellulitis, can be caused by infection resulting from local trauma or insect bites, or they can be associated with upper respiratory tract infections and otitis media. Orbital cellulitis is characterized by marked lid edema, proptosis, chemosis, reduced vision, and decreased motility with pain on movement of the globe (see Chapter 249, Preseptal and Orbital Cellulitis). A red, tearing eye can be caused by acute conjunctivitis, subconjunctival hemorrhage, keratitis, acute iridocyclitis, and acute glaucoma. Conjunctivitis characterized by prominence of the conjunctival blood vessels is one of the signs of Kawasaki disease. Evaluation of children who have sustained head trauma or who are suspected of having an overwhelming infection requires careful, repeated testing of the extraocular movements in the six cardinal fields of gaze and of the pupillary light reflex and observation of the conjunctivae and fundi, looking for unilateral abnormalities, hemorrhage, and papilledema. For example, lateral rectus muscle palsy often is the earliest sign of increased intracranial pressure (see Chapter 286, Increased Intracranial Pressure).

Ears

The inner ear develops early in the first trimester of pregnancy, and response to sound can be shown in the twenty-sixth fetal week. At birth the cochlea and vestibule are anatomically mature.

Successful examination of the ears in infants and children, a skill that requires years of practice to develop, is extremely important because of the high incidence of middle ear abnormalities in children. The student should approach the use of the otoscope and the almost universal presence of ceruminous impediments to visualization of the external auditory canal in children with patience and a willingness to ask for confirmation of findings as often as needed. The practitioner should include a thorough examination of the ears in every physical examination, noting the characteristics of the external ear, external canal, and tympanic membrane and assessing hearing acuity.

Newborn Period. The external ear is flat and shapeless until 34 weeks of gestation; once folded, it may remain so unless placed back in the flat position. Between 34 and 40 weeks of gestation, an incurving of the periphery of the pinna develops, along with an increasing ability to return spontaneously from the folded to the flat position. Minor anomalies in the shape of the external ear should be noted, including the occasional preauricular skin tags or preauricular sinuses. The position of the upper attachment of the external ears should be noted in relation to a line connecting the inner and outer canthus of the eye. Attachments that fall below this line sometimes are associated with other congenital abnormalities, particularly renal agenesis. The patency of the external auditory canals can be determined by direct observation after pulling the pinna away from the side of the head. The tympanic membrane is coated with vernix caseosa for several days after birth and usually cannot be visualized.

Auditory screening in neonates begins with identifying those at risk for hearing loss because of a familial hearing disorder, intrauterine viral infection, hyperbilirubinemia, with bilirubin levels above 20 mg/dl, previous treatment with an ototoxic drug (e.g., gentamycin), or defects of the ear, nose, or throat. Neonates with any of these factors should be screened for hearing loss. Their subsequent language development should be monitored closely, and they should be referred to an audiologist for any signs suggesting hearing loss (see Chapter 20, Nine, Auditory and Speech Screening).

Infancy and Childhood. Several techniques can help the practitioner visualize the tympanic membrane. The infant's head should be stabilized to prevent painful jamming of the speculum into the ear canal. This sometimes can be accomplished by having the parent or a nurse hold the infant against his or her chest with the infant's head on one and then the opposite shoulder. The head usually is stabilized best by laying the infant supine on the examining table and having the parent or a nurse hold the baby's arms against the body or extended on either side of the head. Providing some type of visual distraction, as well as verbal reassurances, while positioning the infant usually affords the examiner a brief, struggle-free period for performing the otoscopic examination. Varying amounts of resistance are almost universal, however, and a rapid examination is desirable for the infant, the parents, and the examiner. One hand is used to grasp the ear pinna and gently pull it laterally and posteriorly to straighten the lumen of the external canal. In infants, the external canal tends to be perpendicular to the temporal bone, with a slight upward angle (further growth of the skull will give the canal a slightly anterior and downward direction). If the otoscope is held upside down, the infant's head can be stabilized further by the hand holding the ear pinna and the ulnar surface of the hand holding the otoscope (Fig. 7-22).

The examiner can further stabilize the infant's body by leaning across the chest and abdomen. The ear speculum then is introduced into the external canal and gently advanced to the point where the bony portion of the canal prevents further entry. Cerumen, which can be soft, firm, or flaky and varies from white to dark brown, may have to be removed. A flexible, wire-loop ear curette can remove small to moderate amounts of soft cerumen and poses less risk of abrading the canal wall or tympanic membrane than does a rigid curette. Curetting is done most safely through the otoscopic head. Larger amounts of hard, inspissated cerumen may require irrigation with warm water and sometimes prior treatment with softening agents such as hydrogen peroxide. An ear canal filled with purulent exudate usually indicates acute otitis media with perforation or otitis externa (the latter is accompanied by pain when the pinna is moved); irrigation usually is unsuccessful and may be dangerous, especially with perforation of the tympanic membrane. Several sizes of specula should be tried to find the largest size that fits into the ear canal, thus allowing visualization of the largest area of tympanic membrane. The otoscope usually must be rotated to view all the important landmarks.

A normal tympanic membrane (Fig. 7-23) is semitransparent, roughly cone shaped, and inclined away from the examiner. The light reflex in the anteroinferior quadrant often is the first landmark seen, with its origin at the central umbo. The examiner, moving the light superiorly from the umbo, can see the long process of the malleus through the membrane, which ends in a bony protuberance that marks the junction of the pars tensa inferiorly and the pars flaccida superiorly. Vague outlines of the incus sometimes can be seen in the posterosuperior quadrant. Air insufflation, by means of a diagnostic otoscopic head fitted with a mouth tube or small bulb, permits direct observation of the eardrum's movement as positive and then negative pressure gently is applied (pneumatoscopy).

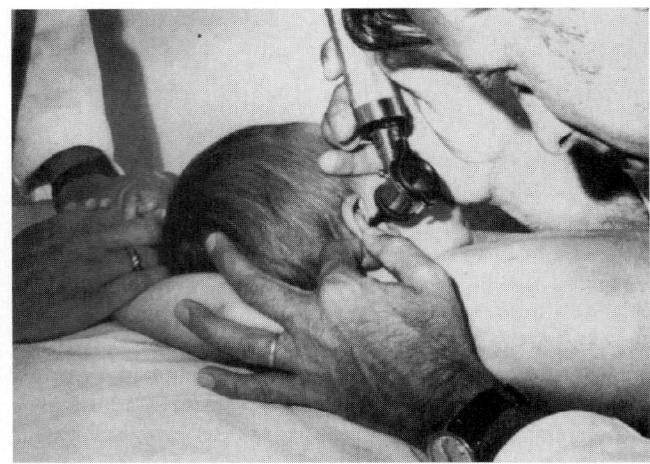

FIG. 7-22 Otoscopic examination of the child. (Photograph by P. Ruben.)

As acute otitis media develops, the tympanic membrane becomes increasingly opaque and erythematous, usually progressing superiorly to inferiorly, with progressive outward bulging and eventual loss of the outlines of the malleus and of the light reflex. Air insufflation will demonstrate decreasing mobility and sometimes the changing menisci of fluid levels within the middle ear. As the condition heals, these changes resolve inferiorly to superiorly; final resolution of opacity, limited motion, and fluid levels sometimes requires several months.

Bullous myringitis appears as a bubblelike swelling that can almost fill the bony portion of the external ear canal. Blood behind the eardrum, either red or purple, is a sign of basilar skull fracture and should be looked for in children who have suffered head trauma. White plaques on the eardrum are scars from old infections. A white mass in the posterosuperior quadrant may be a cholesteatoma, which is present with chronic obstructive middle ear disease. When examining acutely ill children suspected of having a middle ear infection, the mastoid process should be inspected for overlying swelling and erythema and palpated for tenderness—signs of acute mastoiditis.

In infants, auditory acuity is screened directly and indirectly. The indirect method is based on the effect of normal hearing on language development. Normal infants make cooing sounds (semipurposeful vocalization of vowel sounds) by 6 weeks of age, laugh out loud by 3 months, babble (repetitive sounds, such as "baabaa") by 6 months, echo sounds made in their presence by 9 months, and say their first mean-

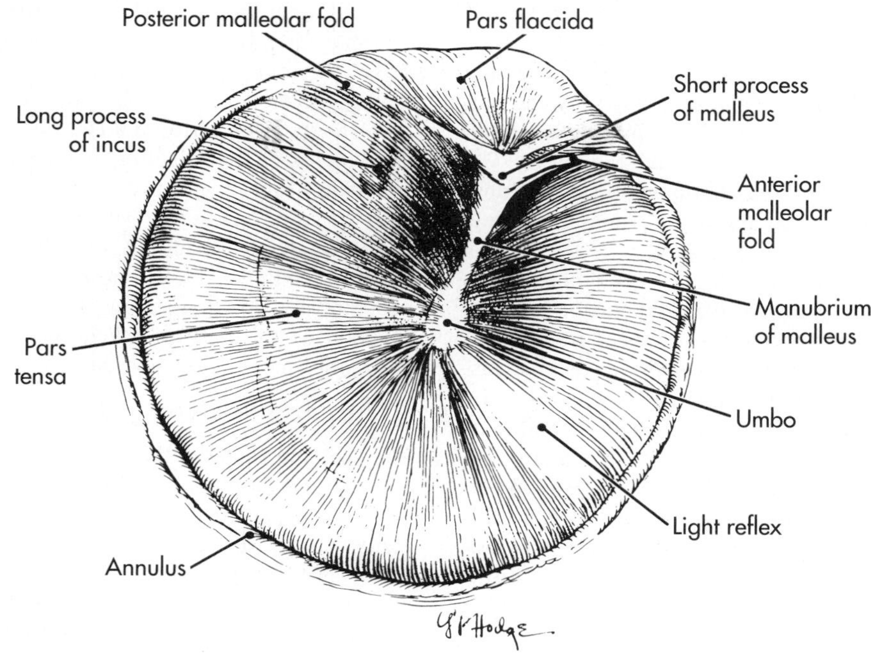

FIG. 7-23 Anatomy of the tympanic membrane.
(From Strome M, editor: *Differential diagnosis in pediatric otolaryngology,* Boston, 1975, Little, Brown.)

ingful word between 12 and 15 months. An infant who fails to progress beyond any of these developmental stages or who regresses should be examined further for hearing loss, as well as for mental retardation.

Hearing can be assessed qualitatively by noting the infant's response to a nearby sound, which is made without visually distracting the infant and without producing vibrations of the air or the surface on which the infant is lying. Responses often are difficult to interpret but include blinking the eyes in a neonate, momentarily ceasing body movements at 1 to 2 months, and turning the head toward the sound by 3 to 4 months. The test sounds can be made by snapping the fingers or ringing a bell. With older infants, tongue clucking produces a test sound with the frequencies of normal speech (500 to 2000 Hz). Asking the parents about the infant's responses to sounds may be as reliable as simple office screening.

In children 1 to 5 years of age, normal hearing is necessary for language development beyond the one-word stage. Hearing can be screened by whispering, as softly as possible, a number into the child's ear and asking the child to repeat it or by asking the child if he or she can hear a ticking watch held a few inches from either ear.

Audiometric testing is indicated for any infant or child who fails any of these qualitative tests, and formal testing should be a routine procedure for children before they start school. Because of the high incidence of middle ear infections among infants and preschool children, hearing screening is routine in many offices and well-child clinics, both in following up known infections and as an annual procedure (see Chapter 20, Screening).

Late Childhood and Adolescence. The tympanic membrane in this age group usually can be examined without resistance, with the child sitting. If the child has ear pain or has had a previous painful examination, the supine position will make head stabilization easier. A qualitative hearing test for children in this age group can be accomplished by using tuning forks, particularly those with frequencies in the human voice range of 500 to 2000 Hz. The examiner's own acuity, presuming that it is normal, can be compared with the child's. Comparing bone and air conduction (Rinne test) and testing for lateralization of bone conduction with the handle of the tuning fork held against the midforehead (Weber test) can distinguish qualitatively between conductive and nerve hearing loss; with conductive loss, air conduction is less than bone conduction, and there is lateralization to the affected ear. Audiometric screening for this age group is routine in many schools. Some children who have chronic middle ear disease have fluctuating hearing loss that can be missed on a single puretone screening. In such cases, pneumatoscopy and impedance audiometry can provide the definitive diagnosis.

Nose

The relative size and shape of the nose normally are influenced by the downward and forward growth of the maxillary bones and, to a lesser extent, by the increase in the bizygomatic width during childhood. The bony orbits are nearer adult size in the newborn than are the other facial bones, and the palate grows most rapidly during the first year of postnatal life. The paranasal sinuses are represented only by the centrally placed ethmoid sinuses at birth; the maxillary sinuses develop from birth and usually are apparent on roentgenograms by age 4 and the sphenoid sinuses by age 6. The frontal sinuses usually have reached the level of the roof of the orbits by age 6 to 7. The nose humidifies incoming air and traps bacteria and noxious materials in its continuous mucous blanket, moving them toward the pharynx by ciliary action. Olfactory function appears to be present at birth and to increase with age.

A thorough examination of the nose involves inspecting the external form, the condition of the external nares, the mucous membranes of the septum, and the turbinates and floor of the nose, as well as describing any exudate present. The nose should be examined in all newborns and in all children who have upper respiratory tract symptoms, noisy breathing, epistaxis, head trauma, headache, and fever.

Newborn Period. In examining the newborn's nose, it is important to rule out the presence of unilateral or bilateral choanal atresia, which can produce severe respiratory distress, inasmuch as most newborns are unable to breathe easily through their mouths. This examination is performed by introducing a soft No. 8 feeding tube into each external naris and advancing the catheter to the pharynx. Advancing the feeding tube farther into the stomach rules out esophageal obstructions such as atresia and allows aspiration of the amniotic fluid from the stomach. A simpler technique for testing choanal patency is to close one and then the other nostril while holding the mouth closed. Obstructed nasal breathing sometimes is seen briefly after birth because of inhaled blood and amniotic debris, which can cause moderate to severe distress, especially in those few infants who have congenitally narrow nasal cavities. A profuse, purulent nasal discharge in the neonatal period could suggest the presence of congenital syphilis.

Infancy, Childhood, and Adolescence. By elevating the tip of the child's nose and using a nasal speculum, the practitioner can inspect the membranes covering the nasal septum, floor of the nose, and inferior, middle, and superior turbinates in the lateral nasal wall for signs of inflammation and bleeding points. The nasal septum occasionally is deviated to one side, sometimes obstructing breathing on that side. The fairly common occurrence of intranasal foreign bodies should be anticipated when examining any child who has chronic nasal discharge, with or without associated bleeding. Epithelial polyps of the nasal mucosa are rare in children and usually indicate underlying cystic fibrosis or chronic allergic rhinitis. A pale, swollen, boggy nasal mucosa indicates allergic rhinitis, whereas with viral rhinitis the nasal membranes are red and bleed easily. Sinusitis should be suspected whenever purulent exudate appears from beneath any of the three nasal turbinates, especially in a child who has a history of chronic nasal congestion, chronic tracheobronchitis, recurrent otitis media, and fever. Transillumination of the paranasal sinuses in younger children is of limited value to physicians other than otorhinolaryngologists because of the variable development of the sinuses before ages 8 and 10. After 10 years of age the frontal sinuses can be transilluminated in a darkened room by holding a bright light source (transilluminator attachment for an otoscope-ophthalmoscope handle) against the superomedial aspect of the orbit; the maxillary sinuses can be transilluminated by holding the light against the lateral aspects of the hard palate within the closed mouth.

Clear fluid draining from the nose after head trauma should be tested for sugar, which is present with a CSF leak. In a child who has a history of epistaxis, the anteroinferior portion of the septum is a common location of prominent blood vessels that bleed easily, especially when aggravated by local inflammation and self-inflicted abrasions.

Swelling around the bridge of the nose can be caused by a cavernous hemangioma or, less commonly, a nasal encephalocele. Erythematous swelling that involves the lateral portion of the bridge of the nose and adjacent eyelids can be a sign of orbital or periorbital cellulitis, which requires immediate intensive investigation and treatment.

Primary care physicians often are asked to examine a child who has suffered trauma to the nose. Consultation with a subspecialist should be sought immediately if the child has prolonged bleeding from the nose after an injury, there is evidence of a septal hematoma, or there is any question of depression of the base of the nose or of deviation from the nose's normal straight-line vertical axis.

Mouth and Pharynx

The size and shape of the mouth and pharynx change during infancy and childhood, with further growth during the first year of the hard palate and also of the mandible, which expands on all surfaces through the second year, extending downward and forward as a result of mandibular condylar growth. The most useful clinical evidence of growth about the mouth is the eruption, further growth, and shedding of the 20 primary (deciduous) teeth, with subsequent eruption of the 32 secondary (permanent) teeth. Intrauterine tooth growth begins during the second fetal month. The deciduous teeth usually begin to erupt by the sixth month of extrauterine life; roughly one new tooth erupts for each month after 6 months of age, with eruption of all deciduous teeth by 28 to 36 months of age. Table 7-3 summarizes the chronology of eruption and shedding of teeth in the growing human. Shedding of the deciduous teeth and eruption of the permanent teeth normally begin at age 5 in boys and age 5½ in girls and continue through age 14, with eruption of the permanent teeth completed by age 20.

The pharyngeal tonsils steadily increase in size during childhood and then begin to recede during puberty, a pattern of growth shared with adenoidal lymphoid tissue and peripheral lymph nodes.

The mouth and pharynx should be examined carefully during all health maintenance visits and in all children who have respiratory symptoms, fever of unknown origin, and ear or facial pain. A complete examination involves inspecting and palpating the lips, buccal mucosa, gingiva, hard palate, and mandible, as well as inspecting the teeth, tongue, soft palate, tonsillar pillars, tonsils, and posterior pharyngeal wall.

Newborn Period. The newborn's mouth often is examined initially by means of the sucking reflex, with the examiner's finger inside the baby's mouth; this can quiet the baby and expedite other parts of the examination. The relative size of the mandible is noted (small mandibles sometimes are associated with underdevelopment of other facial bones as a result of a generalized or genetic disorder). Clefts of the upper lip may be unilateral, bilateral, or midline and may be associated with palatal clefts. A common normal variant is a prominent mucosal fold connecting the inner midline of the upper lip to the posterior portion of the upper gum, leaving a deep notch in the midline of the gum. The upper and lower gums have finely serrated borders. Occasionally, small white mucus-retention cysts, which may be mistaken for teeth, are present. White retention cysts at the midline of the posterior border of the hard palate are known as Epstein pearls. Both

Table 7-3 Most Common Pattern of Dental Development

Dental age (yr)	Erupting*		Exfoliating	
0-1	b a	a b		
	b a	a b		
1-2	c	c d		
	d c	c d		
2-3	e	e		
	e	e		
3-4				
4-5				
5-6	6	6		
	6 1	1 6	a	a
6-7	1	1	a	a
	2	2	b	b
7-8	2	2	b	b
8-9				
9-10				
10-11	4	4	d	d
	4 3	3 4	d c	c d
11-12	5 3	3 5	e c	c e
	5	5	e	e
12-13	7	7		
	7	7		
16-24	8	8		
	8	8		

From Barkin RM, Rosen P: *Emergency pediatrics,* ed 4, St Louis, 1994, Mosby.
**a-e,* Primary teeth; *1-8,* secondary teeth.

types of mucus-retention cysts disappear spontaneously within a few months. Filmy, patchy white membranes over the gingiva, inner lips, and buccal mucosa that cannot be removed by scraping and that sometimes overlie an erythematous base can be seen in some healthy newborns; these are characteristics of monilial stomatitis, or thrush.

A prominent tongue, which may protrude from the mouth, is seen in congenital hypothyroidism and in Down syndrome. A frenulum attaches to the tongue's inferior surface and may extend almost to the tip. When this is thickened and shortened, protrusion of the tongue is limited. Although a source of concern to parents, this "tongue tie" rarely interferes with speech and requires no treatment. Salivation is relatively scanty in a normal newborn; therefore, excessive collection of saliva and mucus in the mouth should prompt investigation for esophageal atresia.

A newborn's pharynx is difficult to visualize except during crying because of the strong gag reflex induced by the tongue blade, which may cause the pharynx to fill with stomach contents. Tonsillar tissue is not visible in newborns.

The quality of the infant's cry should be noted. A strong, lusty cry indicates a healthy baby whose airways and lungs are functioning normally; expiratory grunting is associated with respiratory distress; inspiratory stridor is caused by a number of lesions obstructing internal and external airways; a high-pitched cry suggests intracranial diseases, either congenital or acquired; a hoarse cry suggests hypocalcemic tetany or cretinism; and absence of a cry suggests severe illness or mental retardation.

Infancy, Childhood, and Adolescence. Because it usually is difficult to examine the mouth and pharynx of preschool children, these attempts are best saved until the end of the examination. Some manner of restraint usually is required; one of the most effective methods is to have the child seated on the mother's lap with the child's head held stationary by the mother's hand (Fig. 7-24). Some infants and toddlers will permit a brief period of "looking at the teeth," with the tongue depressor used gently to retract the lips and buccal mucosa. A crying infant usually gives the examiner struggle-free glimpses of the mouth and pharynx without the need for manipulation. While adequately restrained, a closed-mouthed, frightened infant or child can be examined by slipping the tongue depressor between the teeth and onto the tongue. In older children, firm pressure on the anterior half of the tongue, with the tongue not protruded, will suffice; in infants the gag reflex usually must be induced by slipping the tongue depressor onto the posterior half of the tongue. In general, sick children including those who have respiratory tract infections are the most reluctant to have the physician peer into their mouth. Healthy children, on the other hand, sometimes can be persuaded to say "aaah" if the practitioner describes and even demonstrates on a favorite doll or toy animal.

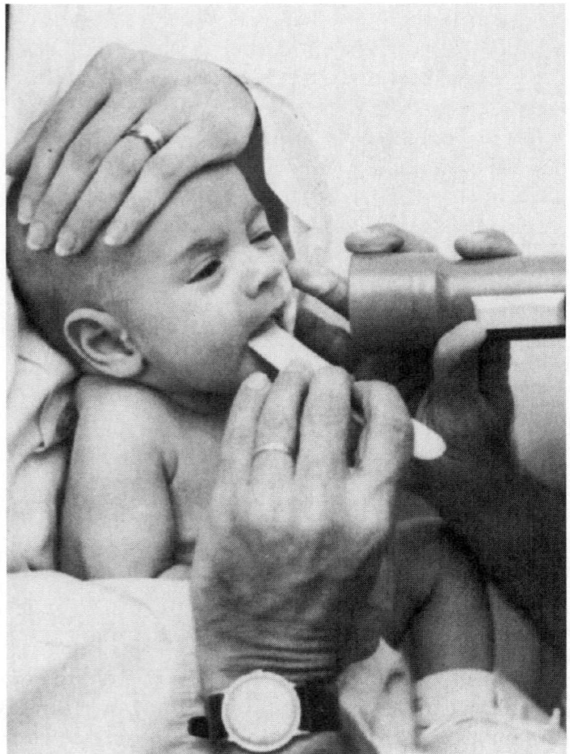

FIG. 7-24 Examination of the pharynx in the infant. (Photograph by P. Ruben.)

Salivation normally increases to full capacity during the third month of life, the age when salivary drooling first is observed because of the infant's limited ability to swallow and the lack of lower front teeth to serve as a dam. Increased salivation associated with respiratory distress and fever usually suggests herpes simplex stomatitis or epiglottitis. Salivation also may increase temporarily with the eruption of new teeth. During the winter months the lips can be dry and cracked, especially at the corners of the mouth. Deeper fissures at the corner of the mouth, cheilosis, occur in several states of nutritional deficiency and when infected by *Monilia albicans*.

The gingivae should be inspected for localized as well as diffuse inflammatory lesions. Shallow, white-based ulcers with surrounding erythema can be seen, usually singly, on the gingivae in association with upper respiratory tract infections. Numerous gingival ulcers with concomitant involvement of the tongue and lips associated with increased salivation, fever, and pain usually result from primary herpes simplex infection, which is most common during the first years of life. Recurrent herpes simplex stomatitis, or "cold sores," involving the lips can occur after the primary bout of stomatitis. Localized or diffuse gingival inflammation most often is associated with dental disease, particularly plaque buildup at the gingival borders because of inadequate tooth brushing. Dental abscesses sometimes exhibit an erythematous soft tissue mass that exudes pus opposite the root of the involved tooth. Gingivae that bleed easily most often reflect poor mouth hygiene and irritation by bacterial plaque, but the condition can signal, albeit rarely, blood dyscrasia, a clotting deficit, or vitamin C deficiency (scurvy).

The buccal mucosa can be involved with nonspecific ulcerative processes, but occasionally it is the site of important signs of specific infectious diseases. In measles, on the second or third day of the illness, before the onset of the generalized rash, Koplik spots can be seen on the buccal mucosa; these are white pinpoint spots that appear at the level of the lower teeth. In parotitis, usually caused by the mumps virus but occasionally by other organisms, Stensen duct openings, found at the level of the upper molars, are red, swollen, and tender. Scattered white ulcers of varying size can appear on the buccal mucosa in chickenpox. In Kawasaki disease several abnormalities can be seen, including cracked, fissured lips and diffuse redness of the pharynx. Chronic thrush may be an early sign of HIV infection in infants and children.

The teeth are counted with the expectation that the infant will have, on the average, one tooth for each month of age past 6 months up to 28 to 36 months of age, when the full complement of primary teeth will have erupted. Delayed tooth eruption can accompany either serious chronic disease or generalized developmental delay. In infants, the individual teeth are examined for localized or generalized enamel hypoplasia, which can reflect a variety of causes, including hereditary enamel hypoplasia, intrauterine insults such as infections, and prematurity (Fig. 7-25). The infant's teeth may have a permanent yellow, gray, or brown discoloration if the mother took tetracycline during her pregnancy or if the baby was treated with the drug; mottled, pitted teeth with a lusterless, opaque enamel may be the result of an excessive fluoride intake. Oral iron preparations can stain the teeth green, as can an elevated bilirubin level during the neonatal period.

The spacing of the teeth should be observed, giving special attention to teeth that are too close together or too far apart, both of which may cause spacing problems later on. Dental occlusion can be checked by having the child bite down and then observing for maxillary protrusion (overbite) or mandibular protrusion (underbite). Malocclusion has numerous causes, including chronic mouth breathing caused by nasal or nasopharyngeal obstruction, the rare instances of mandibular overgrowth secondary to temporomandibular arthritis in juvenile rheumatoid arthritis, and maxillary overgrowth in untreated hereditary hemolytic anemias, such as Cooley anemia.

The texture and appearance of the tongue may indicate specific diseases. Dryness, with or without coating, may be seen in chronic mouth breathing or in states of dehydration. Strawberry tongue, a result of the prominence of the papillae, is seen during the course of scarlet fever and in Kawasaki disease. Thrush and herpes simplex, previously described, can involve the tongue. Geographic tongue, in which the surface has the appearance of a relief map, may be nonspecific or may be associated with underlying allergic disease. Deep furrows in the tongue (scrotal tongue) have no significance. Fine and gross tremor of the tongue, including fasciculations and fibrillations, can be seen in both CNS disease (e.g., Sydenham chorea) and peripheral nerve and neuromuscular junction diseases (Werdnig-Hoffmann disease).

Petechiae sometimes are present on the hard and soft palates in association with pharyngitis, especially streptococcal pharyngitis. The upward motion of the uvula and soft palate should be confirmed during phonation and with the gag reflex to rule out paralysis. A bifid uvula (Fig. 7-26) should be recognized because it can be associated with a submucous cleft of the soft palate. In this condition the soft palate is relatively short and does not reach the posterior pharyngeal wall. Palatal closure against the posterior pharyngeal wall, essential for normal articulation and voice resonance, can be aided in this condition by the presence of hypertrophied nasopharyngeal lymphoid tissue. Therefore during the preoperative examination of a child scheduled for adenoidectomy, the practitioner should check for submucous cleft of the palate because it may affect the decision to operate (see Chapter 266, Tonsillectomy and Adenoidectomy).

The anterior and posterior pillars that border the tonsils are difficult to distinguish in most infants. The tonsils (palatal tonsils) are proportionately larger in preschool and school-age children than in adults. Tonsillar size is estimated arbitrarily on a scale of 1 to 4+, 1+ indicating easy visibility and 4+ indicating that the tonsils meet in the midline. The tonsils normally appear more prominent during gagging or crying, and their relative size can be assessed accurately only while the infant or child is at rest. The tonsillar crypts normally contain varying amounts of desquamated cells, which appear as white spots on the surface. However, true tonsillar exudate usually is less localized to the crypts and extends over a greater portion of the surface. Some examiners try to distinguish the color of the exudate—yellow being more common with streptococcal infection, white with viral infections, and gray with diphtheria. The only reliable way to determine cause, at least for the presence or absence of group A beta-hemolytic streptococci, is to obtain a throat culture, especially of the tonsillar exudate in children over 2 to 3 years of age. Tonsillar erythema and edema, which also should be noted, are particularly conspicuous with streptococcal infection.

Shallow, white-based ulcers that have erythematous edges, which may involve the adjacent pillars and posterior pharynx, suggest herpangina, caused by coxsackievirus A, and can be distinguished from the more anterior location of the herpes simplex ulcers. The diphtheritic membrane may be confluent over the tonsils, pharynx, and uvula, and bleeding ensues when the membrane is pulled away. In infants a diffusely red pharynx and tonsillar area, with or without exudate, most likely has a viral origin. A peritonsillar abscess is suggested by asymmetrical enlargement of the tonsils, often associated with lateral displacement of the uvula.

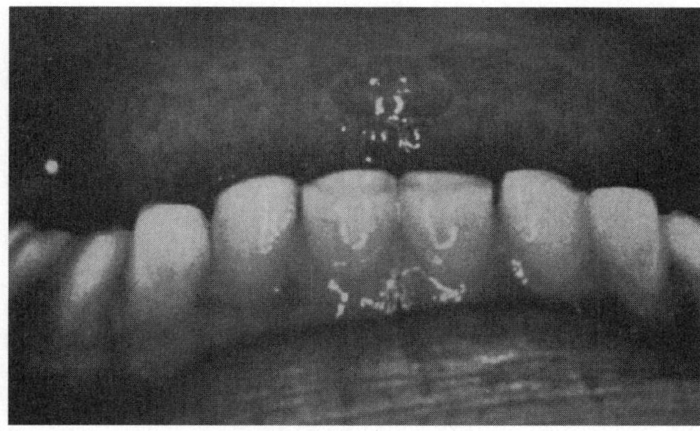

FIG. 7-25 Enamel hypoplasia in a premature child.

(From McDonald RE, Avery DR: *Dentistry for the child and adolescent,* ed 5, St Louis, 1987, Mosby.)

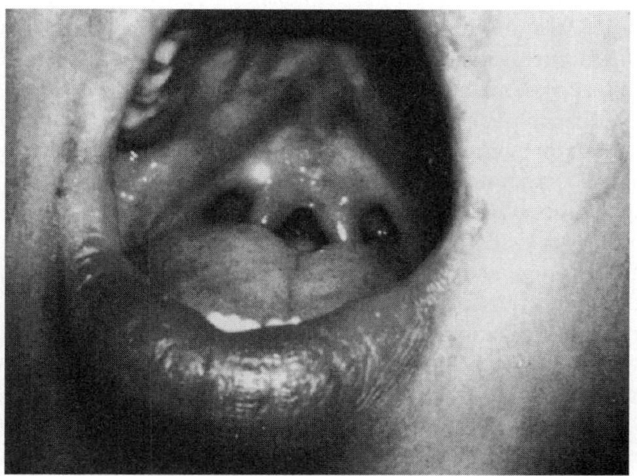

FIG. 7-26 Submucosal cleft palate with bifid uvula.

The posterior pharyngeal wall should be inspected for evidence of lymphoid hyperplasia, which has a "cobblestone" appearance and indicates chronic postnasal drainage, as seen in chronic allergic rhinitis or bacterial sinusitis. Postnasal drainage into the pharynx is to be expected in infants and children who have upper respiratory tract infections, and the characteristics of the mucus suggest various causes. Clear mucus is present in allergic rhinitis or in the early stages of acute rhinitis, whereas purulent mucus appears in the late stages of a viral rhinitis or with chronic bacterial sinusitis.

The presence and size of the adenoidal lymphoid tissue can be estimated indirectly by noting the amount of mouth breathing at rest, by observing the ease of breathing through the nostrils, and by noting any nasality to the voice. Direct palpation of the adenoids with a finger introduced through the mouth and around the soft palate is uncomfortable and difficult for all involved. Using the nasopharyngeal mirror for this purpose is most helpful to those who use it every day, such as otolaryngologists.

The epiglottis sometimes is visualized by chance when the throat of a child who has an upper respiratory tract infection is examined. In children who have croupy cough, especially if of sudden onset and associated with high fever, drooling, and signs of upper airway obstruction, the epiglottis must be visualized to rule out acute bacteral epiglottitis, a true emergency in children (see Chapter 280, Epiglottis). The epiglottis may be swollen several times its usual size and is cherry red. Because of the danger of complete airway obstruction and of cardiac arrest during this examination, endotracheal tubes, a tracheotomy set, and an oxygen source should be at hand. Some primary care physicians choose to rely on a lateral neck roentgenogram initially to evaluate the size of the epiglottis and postpone direct visualization until a surgeon is present.

Neck

The neck is relatively short in infants and lengthens during childhood as a result of vertebral growth. Consequently the epiglottis descends from the level of the first cervical vertebral body at birth to the lower third of the third cervical vertebral body by adulthood. The larynx is one third the adult size at birth. It grows rapidly until age 3, becoming wider as well as longer, and then grows slowly until puberty, when another rapid increase in all dimensions occurs, especially in boys. The trachea at birth is approximately one third the adult length, and both the anteroposterior and lateral diameters of the trachea increase by nearly 300% from birth to puberty. The thyroid gland increases approximately 10 times in weight from birth through puberty, with most growth occurring during puberty. Cervical lymph nodes, a few of which may be palpable at birth, increase in size, following the growth curve for the body's lymphatic tissues in general; those in most normal children are less than 1 cm in diameter. The neck should be examined thoroughly from time to time in healthy infants and children and always in children who have a respiratory or febrile illness. This examination has two parts: (1) noting the overall neck dimensions; the resistance to passive motion; the size and location of the lymph nodes, thyroid gland, and other masses; and the status of neck vessels; and (2) palpating the trachea.

Newborn Period. The newborn's relatively short neck should be inspected for position and overall size. Torticollis, a condition in which the head is tilted to one side with the chin rotated toward the opposite shoulder, usually is associated with a palpable hematoma of the involved sternocleidomastoid muscle. It is believed to arise from a birth injury and may require physical therapy. Opisthotonos, in which the neck and back are held in extreme extension, is an ominous sign that indicates either meningeal irritation or, in an infant who has jaundice, kernicterus. In infants, frequent opisthotonic positioning associated with a relative paucity of trunk flexion movements may be an early sign of the spasticity of cerebral palsy. An unusually short neck may indicate cervical spine anomalies (Klippel-Feil syndrome), and a webbed neck is seen in Turner syndrome. The newborn clavicles should be palpated routinely to rule out clavicular fractures, which usually occur at the junction of the middle and outer thirds of the bone and can occur during birth. Palpable neck masses in the newborn include the midline thyroglossal duct cyst, the supraclavicular cystic hygroma, which transilluminates, and brachial cleft cysts with or without associated skin tags and fistulas along the anterior border of the sternocleidomastoid muscle. Palpable cervical lymph nodes in normal newborns usually are less than 5 mm in diameter. A crackly sensation upon palpation in the supraclavicular areas usually indicates pneumomediastinum.

Infancy, Childhood, and Adolescence. When palpably enlarged lymph nodes are found, the examiner should note their location, size and number, consistency, tenderness, mobility, and attachment to other structures. Anterior cervical lymph nodes commonly enlarge in association with upper respiratory tract infections, dental infections, and stomatitis and less commonly with mycobacterial infection. Enlargement of the posterior cervical nodes is common secondary to insect bites or inflammatory lesions of the scalp. Cervical lymph nodes are enlarged generally with many viral syndromes, especially rubella, measles, and infectious mononucleosis. Lymph nodes enlarged because of an inflammation usually return to normal size days or weeks after the primary infection has subsided. One or more enlarged cervical lymph nodes, combined with other signs, are seen in Kawasaki disease. Lymph nodes that are enlarging without any signs of infection suggest Hodgkin disease and other lymphomas. Chronically enlarged lymph nodes can be seen throughout the body in HIV infection (see Chapter 180, Acquired Immunodeficiency Syndrome (AIDS) and Human Immunodeficiency Virus (HIV) Infection).

Every infant and child who has an acute illness should be checked for nuchal rigidity, an important sign of meningeal irritation from meningitis. Ideally the infant or child should be quiet and relaxed, lying supine as the examiner gently lifts the head from the examining table with a hand at either side of the infant's head and notes the degree of suppleness and any resistance to flexion. Flexion of the thighs associated with neck flexion (Brudzinski sign) and flexion of the extended lower extremity while its opposite is fully extended and flexed 90 degrees at the hip (Kernig sign) are present less often in infants who have meningitis than in older children and adolescents. A child who has nuchal rigidity is unable to touch the chin to the chest and assumes a tripod position when asked to sit up, that is, rests backward on extended arms while the legs are extended on the examining table.

The thyroid gland normally is difficult to palpate, if palpable at all, before puberty; it should be palpated, as should the trachea, from in front of and from behind the child. An enlarged thyroid can occur in children who have euthyroid, hypothyroid, or hyperthyroid states, and it can be caused by iodine deficiency as well as iodine excess (from cough medicines containing iodine), congenital or familial blockage of thyroxine synthesis, thyroiditis, diffuse or nodular hyperplasia, and, in rare cases, carcinoma. Normally the trachea is slightly deviated to the right; deviation from this norm indicates mediastinal shift, as may occur with foreign body–induced atelectasis and pneumothorax. Neck venous pulsations and distention, usually difficult to determine in infants because of their relatively short necks, can give clues to heart disease and congestive heart failure in older children.

Children who have painful or limited neck motion should be checked for a full range of flexion, extension, lateral rotation, and lateral flexion. A fairly common cause of limited head motion is wryneck, or torticollis, which can occur after a play injury or sometimes a respiratory tract infection. The head is tilted to one side, with sternocleidomastoid tenderness on the long or stretched side (as distinguished from neonatal torticollis, in which the involved sternocleidomastoid muscle is on the short side); the underlying cause of wryneck is a rotary subluxation of the first two cervical vertebrae.

Chest and Lungs

The chest wall in the fetus and newborn is round; with further growth it gradually flattens, with the lateral diameter exceeding the anteroposterior diameter. The thoracic index (transverse/anteroposterior diameter) is measured serially in some clinics that treat children who have chronic obstructive lung disease, such as cystic fibrosis, as a means of monitoring the degree of formation of a "barrel chest." The infant's chest wall is relatively thin compared with an adult's; therefore heart and lung sounds are transmitted more clearly. Respirations are predominantly abdominal in infants, reflecting the greater role of the diaphragm; by age 6 they are predominantly thoracic, reflecting the increased role of the thoracic musculature in normal breathing.

By 16 weeks of gestation the bronchial tree is fully developed, with the adult number of segments and subsegments. Alveoli, in comparison, are just forming by the time of birth, with only 8% of the average adult number present. The number of alveoli increases until age 8, after which they primarily increase in size rather than in number until adulthood. Pulmonary blood vessels develop parallel to the developing bronchial tree and alveoli, and increasing amounts of muscle appear in the walls of the more distal arterioles over time. By 28 weeks of gestation, airway and blood vessel development usually is adequate for gas transfer. By 34 to 36 weeks of gestation, sufficient amounts of a surface-active lipid are present within the alveoli to maintain them in a partly expanded position, rather than remaining collapsed at the end of each expiration. As noted previously, the respiratory rate declines with age, partly because of further postnatal development of the alveoli, with a resulting increase in lung volume.

The breasts of many normal male and female infants, are transiently hypertrophied at birth, sometimes producing small amounts of clear or white fluid, called *witch's milk.* This hypertrophy normally disappears by 2 to 3 months of age. Many pubertal boys have transient unilateral or bilateral firm, sometimes painful, subareolar masses that disappear within a year of onset. A girl's pubertal breast development often is asymmetrical and proceeds through several stages, starting with an increase in the areolar diameter between ages 8 and 13, and is completed between ages 12 and 19 (Fig. 7-27).

The chest and lungs should be examined thoroughly in every child who has any respiratory symptoms, fever, abdominal pain, or chest pain. The examiner should note size, symmetry, movement with respirations, localized tenderness or masses, and breast characteristics. The three goals of an examination of the lungs using observation, percussion, and auscultation are (1) to determine the nature of respiration, including rate, depth, and ease, (2) to establish the adequacy of gas exchange, as indicated by signs of hypoxia or hypercapnia, and (3) to localize disease. The examiner should use and become familiar with the sound characteristics of one stethoscope. Except when auscultating the chest of a small premature baby, an adult-sized stethoscope with both a bell and a diaphragm generally is effective for examining infants and children of all ages.

Newborn Period. During the few moments after birth, the adequacy of the developing lungs for gas exchange (which is influenced by factors such as maternal anesthesia, birth trauma, and the normality of the infant's central nervous and cardiovascular systems) is grossly assessed by the Apgar score, which includes observations about the color and initiation of respirations. Once normal respirations have been established, the baby's chest is inspected for deformities, such as a markedly bulging or markedly concave sternum (pectus carinatum or excavatum); asymmetry caused by uneven chest expansion, absence of or deformed ribs, or absence of the pectoral muscle; and overall size, inasmuch as small thoracic cages are a feature of several congenital anomalies. The respiratory rate normally falls from as high as 60/min immediately after birth to 30 to 40/min by several hours of age. In a normal newborn the auscultated breath sounds are heard easily and have a higher pitch than those in the older child and adult.

A newborn in respiratory distress from any cause exhibits some or all of the following signs: tachypnea, cyanosis, expiratory grunting, intercostal retractions (subcostal, substernal, and supraclavicular retractions are also possible), and decreased air entry, as measured by decreased breath sounds. If a pulse oximeter is not available, the Downes score (Table 7-4) is a useful clinical tool for serially monitoring the severity of newborn respiratory distress, particularly that caused by hyaline membrane disease. Persistent scores of 5 or higher usually indicate that respiratory assistance is needed. Simple auscultation of a newborn in respiratory distress should aid in the diagnosis of (1) unilateral lesions, such as aspiration pneumonia, congenital diaphragmatic hernia, congenital hypoplastic segments or emphysema, and unilateral pneumothorax and (2) congenital heart disease and heart murmurs.

The respiratory rate of newborns, particularly premature newborns, can be quite irregular during the first few days of life and sometimes can slow to the point of apnea. Two patterns should be differentiated in premature infants. *Periodic breathing* is associated with relatively brief periods of apnea lasting 5 to 10 seconds, usually without secondary bradycardia. It occurs more commonly when the baby is awake and

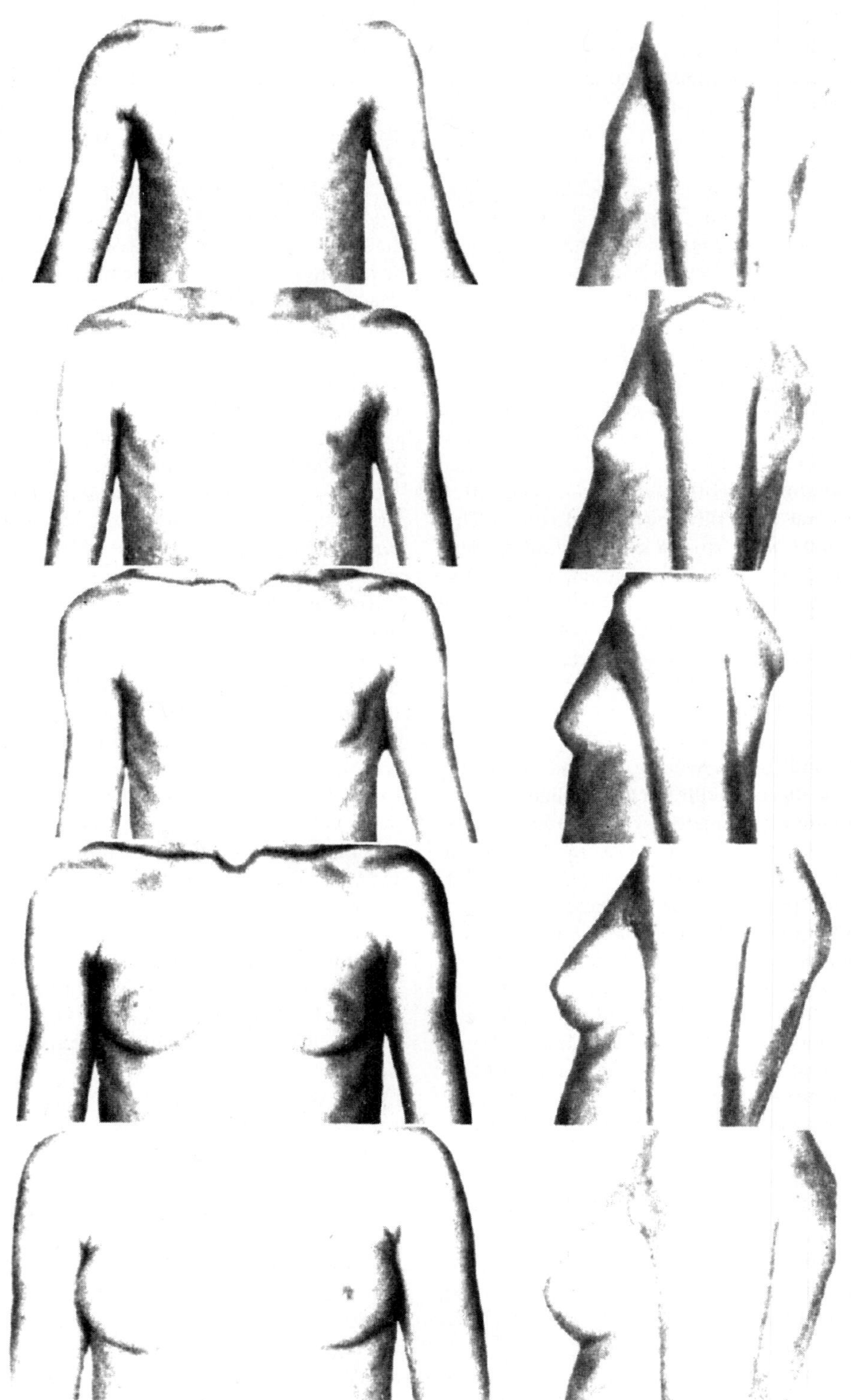

FIG. 7-27 Stages of development of the female breast.
(From Tanner JM: *Growth at adolescence,* ed 2, Oxford, 1962, Blackwell.)

is uncommon before 5 days of age. True apneic spells, on the other hand, last longer than 20 seconds, are associated with bradycardia, can be associated with pulmonary disease, and are more common in infants who weigh less than 1250 g.

Infancy, Childhood, and Adolescence. In these children, auscultation and percussion, along with observation of breathing patterns, are particularly useful techniques for evaluating the chest and lungs. Auscultation often is accomplished most successfully when the infant or child is only minimally aware of being examined—for example, while asleep, being fed, or being held up to the parent's shoulder. When preschool children are asked to "take a deep breath,"

Table 7-4 Downes Score: A Method for Monitoring Respiratory Distress

Score	0	1	2
Respiratory rate (breaths/min)	60	60-80	>80 or apneic episode
Cyanosis	None	In air	In 40% oxygen
Retractions	None	Mild	Moderate to severe
Grunting	None	Audible with stethoscope	Audible without stethoscope
Air entry (crying)	Clear	Delayed or decreased	Barely audible

From Downes JJ: *Clin Pediatr* 9:326, 1970.

they often hold their breath. It is easier to start by auscultating while the child breathes at a resting level. If the child is crying, the inspiratory phase can be thoroughly auscultated, but predominantly expiratory adventitious sounds, such as wheezes, can be missed. After the examiner listens to breath sounds at rest or during crying, a useful technique for accentuating adventitious sounds, particularly during the expiratory phase, is inducing forced expiration. The examiner may do this by holding the hands on opposing anterior and posterior sides of the chest, with the stethoscope in one hand held against the chest, and gently squeezing the hands together as expiration is ending.

Breath sounds in infants and children tend to be audible during both inspiration and expiration (i.e., bronchovesicular) and are heard more clearly than in adults. Secretions in any part of the respiratory tree usually are loudly audible throughout the chest, and the examiner should repeat his or her observations to rule out transmitted sounds from the nose or pharynx. It is tempting for inexperienced examiners to suspect pneumonia in most children evaluated for acute respiratory illnesses because of the fairly usual occurrence of tracheal and bronchial inflammation with common viral infections. The more or less generalized coarse rhonchi (continuous, low-pitched sounds) from bronchial secretions and the wheezes (higher pitched, predominantly expiratory) from bronchiolar secretions should be distinguished from the much less common, usually localized, crackling rales caused by alveolar fluid or exudate and heard best at the end of inspiration. Pneumonia in infants and young children almost always is accompanied by fever and tachypnea, whereas rales, bronchial breath sounds, dullness to percussion, and a productive cough are less common findings than in adults.

Several objective signs of respiratory distress can be seen in infants and children. Orthopnea occurs in children who have asthma or congestive heart failure. Maximal use of accessory muscles of respiration produces several useful physical signs, including head bobbing, seen especially in infants, with the head bobbing forward in synchrony with each inspiration, and flaring of the nasal alae, resulting from contraction of the anterior and posterior dilator naris muscles. These signs indicate increased work of breathing, or inspiratory efforts shortened by pain, as occurs in pleuritis or thoracic trauma. Intercostal retractions, an exaggerated inspiratory sinking in of intercostal and sometimes supraclavicular soft tissue, indicate increased inspiratory effort and reflect airway obstruction and lung stiffness. Bulging of the intercostal space during expiration occurs with increased expiratory effort, such as in asthma, bronchiolitis, and cystic fibrosis. Subcostal retractions, seen anteriorly at the lower costal margins, reflect flattening of the diaphragm and occur in conditions with diffuse lower airway obstruction. Substernal retractions can be seen in children who have severe upper airway obstruction and in newborns, especially premature infants, who have various pulmonary diseases. Audible wheezes usually indicate obstruction of the larger airways, and grunting can be associated with pneumonia, chest pain, and respiratory distress syndrome in neonates. A "thud" may be heard on inspiration in children who have a tracheal foreign body as the object moves in response to airflow.

The adequacy of gas exchange is judged primarily by seeking signs of hypoxia. Cyanosis, which results when the amount of reduced hemoglobin in the capillaries exceeds 5 g, is either peripheral (as with exposure to a cold environment) or central (seen as blue mucous membranes), the latter being of pulmonary or cardiac origin. Tachycardia, dyspnea on exertion, and CNS depression are additional signs of hypoxia that can be critical in following up a child who has marginally adequate gas exchange, as in severe croup. Progressive signs of hypercapnia in acute respiratory illnesses include hot hands, small pupils, engorged fundal veins, muscular twitching, coma, and papilledema.

Localization of intrathoracic lesions in children is aided by palpating for tracheal deviation and observing for unequal respiratory movements of one half of the chest, localized areas of dull or flat percussion notes, and the presence of tactile fremitus. Percussion also can be used to delineate the lung boundaries in inspiration and expiration.

Heart

The major anatomical characteristics of the heart form long before birth, as do most congenital heart defects. In a normal newborn's heart the right ventricle has a muscle mass equal to that of the left ventricle, reflecting the fetal circulation in which both ventricles pump blood into the systemic circulation, the right through the ductus arteriosus. After birth the left ventricle gains weight relative to the right ventricle, reaching the adult weight ratio of approximately 2:1 by age 1, reflecting the major changes in postnatal circulation. At birth, or shortly thereafter, the ductus arteriosus normally closes, and the flap of the foramen ovale is held closed by the rise in pressure in the left atrium. As many as half of all newborns have transient murmurs during the first 24 to 48 hours of life, some of which are caused by a late-closing ductus arteriosus.

Congenital heart defects can be classified according to the embryonic stages of development during which an abnormality arises: position anomalies (dextrocardia with or without situs inversus), anomalous growth of the atrial chambers (atrioventricular canal, ostium primum defect, persistent foramen ovale), anomalous bulboventricular growth and septation (ventricular septal defect, tetralogy of Fallot, double outlet right ventricle, transposition of the great vessels), and maldevelopment of the truncus (truncus arteriosus, patent ductus arteriosus, coarctation of the aorta).

The significant and normal changes in pulse and blood pressure that occur with age in infants and children have been described earlier in this chapter. It is important to remember that optimal auscultation of the heart requires use of a stethoscope with both a bell and a diaphragm, the bell picking up lower-pitched sounds and the diaphragm picking up higher-pitched ones. Proper use of the bell involves holding it lightly against the chest while the diaphragm is pressed firmly to the chest. Stethoscope tubing should be no more than 10 to 12 inches long. During auscultation, gentle traction on the earpiece end of the stethoscope enhances the audibility of heart sounds by making a tighter seal between the earpiece and the examiner's external auditory canal. Because infants have relatively rapid heart rates, detecting abnormalities in their heart sounds demands that each of the two major heart sounds be listened to in isolation, giving attention to each interval between these sounds. As in adults, the heart is auscultated initially over the four cardinal areas (apex, or *mitral area;* lower left sternal border, or *tricuspid area;* second left intercostal space at the sternal margin, or *pulmonary area;* and second right intercostal space, or *aortic area*). Auscultation then proceeds to the remainder of the precordium and chest, including the infraclavicular and supraclavicular area, the axillae, the back, and the neck.

A thorough examination of the heart should be part of all physical examinations of infants and children; it involves noting the heart rate and rhythm, heart size, and characteristics of the first and second heart sounds, especially in the second left interspace. With murmurs, the following information should be recorded: timing in the cardiac cycle (early, late, or pansystolic; protodiastolic, middiastolic, or presystolic), quality (blowing, harsh, rumbling, musical, or other), grade of maximal intensity (on a scale of I to VI, with V and VI being associated with a palpable thrill), duration, point of maximal intensity, and transmission. In all infants and children whose findings suggest congenital heart disease, palpation of peripheral pulses is especially important to determine if the pulses in the lower extremities are diminished and those in the upper extremities increased, as occurs with coarctation of the aorta. Blood pressure is measured as described earlier in this chapter.

Newborn Period and Infancy. An infant's general appearance can provide clues to underlying heart disease and may mandate a more sophisticated cardiac examination. Examples of conditions frequently associated with congenital heart disease are Down syndrome (endocardial cushion defect), Turner syndrome (coarctation of the aorta), trisomy 13, trisomy 18, and congenital rubella syndrome (patent ductus arteriosus, pulmonary stenosis). Important clinical signs of significant heart disease include cyanosis, growth failure, and lethargy. The most prominent signs of congestive heart failure in infants are tachypnea, tachycardia, and liver enlargement. Peripheral edema and pulmonary rales are late findings and therefore not as helpful as in adults. Visible chest pulsations can indicate a hyperdynamic state caused by an increased metabolic rate or an inefficient pumping action from valvular or septal incompetency or other defect. Dextrocardia is suggested by a right-sided cardiac impulse and may be associated with abdominal situs inversus (reversal of the position of the liver, spleen, and intestines).

The apical impulse in infants normally is palpated in the fourth left interspace just outside the midclavicular line; after age 7 it is in the adult position of the fifth left interspace in the midclavicular line. The point of maximal impulse of the heart can suggest individual ventricular enlargement. An impulse at the xiphoid process or lower left sternal border suggests right ventricular hypertrophy, whereas an impulse maximal at the apex suggests left ventricular hypertrophy.

Infants' heart sounds often are difficult to differentiate from their breath sounds because the pitches and rates of each can be similar. Watching the abdominal excursions with respiration and palpating a peripheral pulse while auscultating the chest can aid in this differentiation. The examiner should be prepared to spend at least several minutes listening to the precordial area, at which time the heart and respiratory rates and rhythms can be determined. For each heart sound, the intensity, point of maximal intensity, and degrees of splitting should be noted. Normally the second heart sound is louder than the first in the second left interspace and often is split (reflecting the pulmonary valve closing after the aortic valve); the split often widens with inspiration. Examples of abnormalities of the heart sounds are the loud first sound heard at the apex in mitral stenosis; the loud second sound in the pulmonary area, indicating pulmonary hypertension; and the fixed, split-second sound in the pulmonary area with atrial septal defect. A third heart sound can be heard at the apex of normal children and should be distinguished from the higher intensity, third-sound gallop that occurs with tachycardia and indicates congestive heart failure.

Heart murmurs are more difficult to localize in infants than in children and adolescents because in infants they often are so well transmitted and heard throughout the chest. Gross anatomical localization can be helpful, however, as illustrated by (1) the prominence over the back of the murmurs of coarctation of the aorta and some cases of patent ductus arteriosus, (2) the precordial systolic murmur of ventricular septal defect growing louder as the examiner descends the left sternal border to the xiphoid, and (3) the murmur or murmurs of peripheral pulmonary artery stenosis becoming louder as the examiner moves the stethoscope laterally from the precordium. On the other hand, the typical to-and-fro continuous murmur of patent ductus arteriosus described in older children may be absent in affected infants and represented only by a precordial systolic murmur.

Childhood and Adolescence. A cardiac examination in children and adolescents follows the outline already given and is different from the examination of infants largely because of the need to distinguish organic murmurs from the "innocent" murmur, which occurs in as many as 50% of normal children. Innocent murmurs are unassociated with any symptomatic, roentgenographic, or electrocardiographic evidence of heart disease, and the three types have several characteristics in common. They usually are low pitched and therefore heard best with the bell. They are musical or vibratory (see Fig. 7-28), as distinguished from the more complex range of frequencies of "significant" murmurs. Their intensity usually is no greater than I or II/VI, and both their presence and intensity vary with change in the child's position

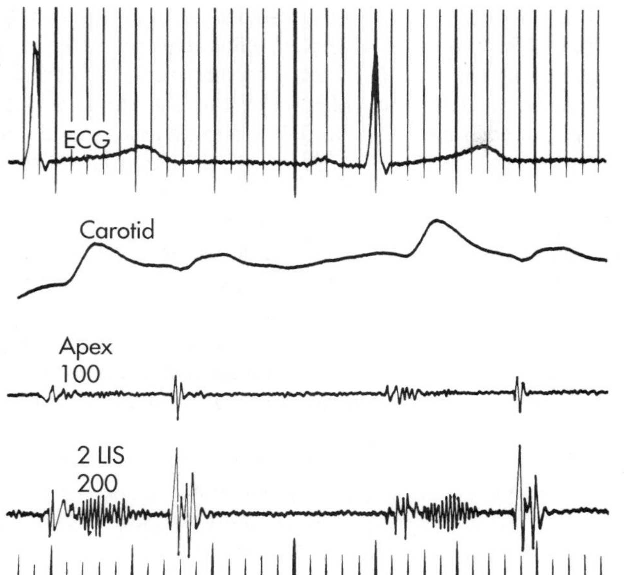

FIG. 7-28 An innocent murmur: phonocardiogram. Note the even harmonic quality of a stringlike murmur. *2 LIS,* Second left interspace.

(From Nadas AS, Fyler DC: *Pediatric cardiology,* ed 3, Philadelphia, 1972, WB Saunders.)

or respiratory phase. Innocent murmurs are heard most commonly either at the second left interspace or halfway between the lower left sternal border and the apex. At these sites the murmurs are of short duration and occur early in systole. A third common location is above or below either clavicle, where the murmur is called a *venous hum.* This is an impressive sounding murmur, often continuous throughout systole; it is heard best with the child sitting and does not occur in the supine position.

In contrast to innocent murmurs, significant murmurs usually, but not always, are of greater intensity, are less localized, and are more likely to radiate over parts of the chest; they also usually do not change in loudness with a change in the child's position or respiratory phase. Systolic murmurs can be classified as *stenotic, regurgitant,* or *uneven.* Stenotic systolic murmurs are associated with a pressure gradient across the aortic or pulmonary valve and are of high frequency, are diamond shaped, and are transmitted to the neck. Soft systolic murmurs heard in the pulmonary area and associated not with a valvular pressure gradient but with increased flow are present with an atrial septal defect. Atrioventricular valve regurgitant murmurs begin immediately with the first sound, are either decreased or pansystolic, are blowing in character, and are best heard at the lower left sternal border or at the apex, radiating to the axilla and back. The murmur of mitral insufficiency, which is heard at the apex in a large percentage of children who have acute rheumatic fever, can be transient and soft; its discovery can be aided by auscultating over the apex with the child supine and rotated partly onto the left side. The systolic murmur along the left sternal border heard with a ventricular septal defect usually is pansystolic but has a harsher quality than the atrioventricular valve regurgitant murmurs and is transmitted less well to the axilla, neck, and back. An uneven systolic murmur is heard with patent ductus arteriosus along the upper left sternal border. Although pansystolic with or without a diastolic component, the sound of the murmur varies in pitch and intensity from beat to beat.

Most diastolic murmurs are caused by three types of cardiac abnormalities. Protodiastolic murmurs of high pitch with a crescendo-decrescendo pattern are heard with aortic or pulmonary valve regurgitation. Middiastolic murmurs, which are low pitched, rumbling, often crescendo in pattern, preceded by an opening snap and followed by an accentuated first sound, are heard with mitral (and, in rare cases, tricuspid) stenosis. Diastolic flow murmurs, occurring with all large left-to-right shunts and with acute rheumatic fever in association with mitral regurgitation, are caused by increased flow through a normal-sized atrioventricular orifice and are of low frequency, are early or middiastolic in timing, and are associated with a loud third heart sound.

Continuous murmurs (i.e., murmurs that extend through systole into diastole) are heard most commonly with patent ductus arteriosus and sometimes are called "machinery" murmurs. These murmurs usually are loud, high pitched, and heard along the left upper sternal border, radiating to the neck and back.

The most common presenting signs of congestive heart failure in children, as in infants, are tachypnea, orthopnea, liver enlargement, and sometimes increased sweating. Peripheral edema and pulmonary rales tend to be late findings. In children, the appearance of facial edema more commonly indicates either an allergic reaction or renal disease, such as acute glomerulonephritis. Swelling and redness of the hands and feet are features of Kawasaki disease, as is congestive heart failure (and in a small number, myocardial infarction). Heart failure in children most often occurs with acute or chronic myocarditis (especially acute rheumatic fever), in some children with congenital heart disease, in overwhelming infections, and in hypovolemic states.

Hypertension in children usually is of renal origin, once anxiety has been ruled out. The types of underlying renal disease include acute illnesses such as acute poststreptococcal glomerulonephritis and acute pyelonephritis, end stages of various chronic renal diseases (glomerulonephropathies, chronic obstruction or infection, developmental renal anomalies), kidney tumors such as Wilms tumor, and renal vessel thrombosis and anomalies. Other causes of hypertension include those related to the central nervous system (poliomyelitis, encephalitis, increasing intracranial pressure of many causes), cardiovascular disease (coarctation of the aorta and aortic run-offs, as with patent ductus arteriosus, anemia, and thyrotoxicosis), endocrine-metabolic disturbances (cortisone therapy, pheochromocytoma, Cushing disease, congenital adrenal hyperplasia, primary aldosteronism, and porphyria), lead and mercury poisoning, and essential hypertension, in which none of these conditions exists. Increasing experience in the routine measurement of blood pressure in children and adolescents suggests that essential hypertension may be more prevalent among adolescents than was previously believed, especially among those who have a family history of hypertension.

The physical findings of heart disease in infants and children only begin to define the nature of the etiology of the disease. Chest roentgenography and electrocardiography, as well as echocardiography, phonocardiography, and cardiac catheterization, are used to define the basic lesion further. Thus physical examination of the heart is an important step in cardiac diagnosis but is only the first of many steps that require interpretation by a qualified cardiologist.

Abdomen

The size and shape of the abdomen change with age, reflecting, in part, changes in the intraabdominal and intrathoracic organs. During the neonatal period the abdomen is relatively protuberant because of (1) the intrathoracic expansion of the lungs with downward movement of the diaphragm and (2) the relatively large liver caused by intrauterine extramedullary hematopoiesis. The first meconium stool usually is passed within 24 hours of birth, and intestinal gas is visible by roentgenogram throughout the normal bowel by 48 hours of age. The horizontal position of the stomach within the abdomen in infancy accounts for the increased postprandial protuberance of the epigastric area. The more vertical, adult position of the stomach is developed slowly throughout childhood. The stomach's capacity increases rapidly during the first years of life, from an average of 30 to 90 ml at birth to 210 to 360 ml at age 1 and 500 ml at age 2; it then increases slowly to the adult capacity of 750 to 900 ml. Abdominal protuberance in preschool children is caused by a transient, normal lumbar lordosis. The abdominal musculature is relatively hypotonic at birth, allowing deep palpation. Midline defects include the relatively common and usually transient diastasis recti, the fairly common umbilical hernia, and the rare omphalocele.

The abdomen should be examined thoroughly during all health maintenance examinations and in children who have gastrointestinal symptoms, fever, cough, and any other evidence of acute illness. This examination involves inspection of the abdominal contour and size; palpation for tenderness and an enlarged liver, spleen, kidneys, or masses; percussion; and auscultation of bowel sounds. Examination of the rectum is indicated in all children who show evidence of an intraabdominal or a pelvic disorder or who have fecal elimination problems or rectal bleeding.

Newborn Period and Infancy. Absence of the normal prominence of the abdomen in a newborn should lead to further investigation for diaphragmatic hernia or high intestinal atresia. Subcutaneous abdominal wall blood vessels are easily visible in most infants because of their relatively small amount of subcutaneous fat. Abdominal movement is due to the prominent role of the diaphragm in breathing and, in addition, to intestinal peristalsis. Visible peristaltic waves can be observed over any quadrant of the abdomen, especially in premature babies, who have relatively thin abdominal walls. Prominent gastric peristaltic waves moving from left to right across the upper portion of the abdomen are present with congenital pyloric stenosis, which usually manifests by 4 to 6 weeks of age.

The umbilical stump is inspected at birth for meconium (yellow) staining, a sign associated with chronic fetal distress. The normal umbilicus contains two ventrally placed, thick-walled, smaller arteries and one dorsally placed, thin-walled, larger vein. In the past, infants who had a single umbilical artery were believed to have a higher than normal incidence of congenital malformations, but this finding recently has been shown to have no significance if it is an isolated anomaly. The umbilical stump, if left uncovered after birth, shrinks to a relatively hard, dark brown eschar, which normally separates from the abdomen by 1 to 2 weeks after birth. The central core area of the umbilicus usually is covered with skin no later than 3 to 4 weeks of age, a process that sometimes is delayed by growth of pink granulation tissue (umbilical granuloma). Transient spotty bleeding of the umbilical area after separation of the umbilical eschar is common and usually lasts no longer than a few days. Chronic drainage of clear fluid from the umbilicus suggests the presence of persistently patent urachus, a urachal cyst, or a communicating Meckel diverticulum or omphalomesenteric duct. Erythema of the periumbilical skin with or without purulent or foul-smelling discharge suggests omphalitis, a local infection that can spread rapidly to the bloodstream and meninges. Umbilical hernias may be associated with palpable abdominal wall defects that vary from 0.5 to 5 or 6 cm in diameter and that protrude equally as far, especially when the infant is crying or straining.

A light touch of the examining fingers against the infant's abdominal wall usually contacts the liver edge, 1 to 2 cm below the right costal margin. A spleen tip may be palpated in normal infants at the left costal margin. Midline structures such as the enlarged pylorus of infants who have pyloric stenosis sometimes are difficult to palpate because of the contraction of the rectus muscles. Holding the infant's thighs in a flexed position and palpating while the infant is sucking usually will permit deep, midline palpation. The kidneys are accessible to palpation, especially at birth, by the technique of ballottement. One hand is held with the fingers in the costovertebral angle while the other hand presses downward from the anterior costal margin. The posterior hand then "flips" the kidney toward the anterior hand, which usually can "catch" the lower pole of the kidney. It also can be felt as it drops back against the posterior hand. In this manner, symmetry of kidney size can be determined. A unilaterally large kidney occurs with a multicystic kidney, unilateral hydronephrosis, Wilms tumor, invasive neuroblastoma, or renal vein thrombosis. Other palpable abdominal masses include the dilated bladder secondary to urethral obstruction, the bilateral flank masses of hydronephrosis and polycystic kidney disease, duplications of the bowel, and rare primary hepatic tumors. Palpable masses associated with signs of intestinal obstruction (vomiting, abdominal distention, and failure to pass stool) include the meconium masses associated with imperforate anus, Hirschsprung disease, meconium plug syndrome, and meconium ileus; midgut volvulus associated with intestinal malrotation; and the sausage-shaped, usually right lower quadrant abdominal mass of intussusception associated with bloody or currant jelly stools. Infants who have signs of intestinal obstruction and no palpable mass require immediate further evaluation for congenital atresia or stenosis of any portion of the bowel, peritonitis, and, in premature infants, necrotizing enterocolitis.

Percussion of an infant's abdomen can be helpful in determining the size of organs or masses and also outlines the relatively large area of the upper portion of the abdomen filled by the stomach. Ascites may accompany peritonitis, liver or kidney disease, and lymphangiomas of the small bowel mesentery. Bowel sounds (peristaltic sounds) are metallic tinkling sounds heard normally every 10 to 30 seconds. They occur more frequently with intestinal obstruction or gastroenteritis and are diminished with ileus, which can accompany almost any infectious process in infants, especially pneumonitis or gastroenteritis.

A rectal examination, performed with the fifth finger, can be useful in differentiating bladder from sacral masses, in palpating the uterus, and in detecting the absence of rectal feces in some infants who have Hirschsprung disease. Some practitioners prefer to use the index finger for this examination because of its greater length, flexibility, sensitivity, and mobility.

Childhood and Adolescence. The shape of the abdomen becomes increasingly scaphoid in school-age children, with the exception of children who have exogenous obesity. Frightened, uncomfortable, or ticklish children can be examined successfully if the thighs are held in partial flexion and the abdomen is approached first with the stethoscope. While listening for bowel sounds, the stethoscope can be pushed gently into the abdomen, and areas of rigidity or tenderness can be noted. The examiner's hands should be warm, and in older children, deep breathing will enhance abdominal palpation. Another useful technique is placing the child's hand between the abdominal wall and the examiner's hand. It can be especially difficult to detect rigidity or tenderness in a crying or nonverbal child. The examiner can watch for facial grimacing and can attempt to "catch" the brief instant of relative relaxation of the abdomen at the end of expiration. The protuberant abdomen of a child whose lungs are hyperexpanded and who experiences forceful abdominal muscle contractions on expiration and sore abdominal muscles (present, for instance, in status asthmaticus) can be especially difficult to examine for intraabdominal abnormalities. Having such a child raise his or her head from the supine position usually lessens intraabdominal pain but increases abdominal muscle soreness.

Abdominal tenderness in children can be localized by the responses to direct palpation, by referred pain on rebound tenderness, by "shake" tenderness in which the child's pelvis is lifted gently off the examining table and gently shaken, by pain accompanying hyperextension of the hips (psoas sign) or flexion and external rotation of the hip with the knee held in flexion (obturator sign), and by palpating a finger in the rectum against the posterior pelvic wall. Tenderness from an inflamed appendix usually is maximal in the right lower quadrant. Diffuse tenderness can accompany paralytic ileus secondary to extraabdominal or intraabdominal infection, as well as the more serious peritonitis or perforated abdominal organ or viscus. Midline tenderness, especially in the lower portion of the abdomen, can be elicited by palpating the abdominal aorta or a full bladder.

If the abdomen is soft, the cecum and sigmoid colon often can be rolled between the examining fingers and the adjacent iliac crest. The entire colon sometimes is palpable when filled with feces in association with functional fecal retention. In normal children, the tip of the spleen and the edge of the liver may be palpable, especially on deep inspiration. The spleen commonly enlarges in association with a number of acute infectious diseases and with a number of blood dyscrasias. The liver can enlarge as a result of heart failure, hepatitis, septicemia, metastatic tumor, blood dyscrasia, and various storage diseases. Upper quadrant direct tenderness or shock tenderness (elicited by gently pounding the lower anterior rib cage), which may be signs of liver or splenic bleeding or rupture, should be investigated in all children who have sustained trauma to the abdomen.

Genitalia

By the end of the third fetal month the undifferentiated fetal gonad has developed into an ovary or, under the influence of the XY chromosome, into a testis. With production of testosterone by the fetal testis (the medulla of the fetal gonad), the wolffian duct system further develops into the epididymis, ductus deferens, and seminal vesicles; development of the müllerian duct system is inhibited by an as yet unidentified factor. The testes descend into the scrotum between the seventh and eighth months of gestation, followed by a sleeve of parietal peritoneum, the processus vaginalis, which closes off in most babies by the time of birth. At the time of birth one or more testes are undescended in 3% to 4% of male babies. Most of these descend by 3 months of age, leaving 1% of babies by age 1 year with unilateral or bilateral undescended testes. The processus vaginalis can remain patent and retain its connection with the peritoneal cavity, causing an inguinal hernia that usually is apparent within a few months after birth. A fluid-filled segment of the processus vaginalis within the scrotum, a hydrocele, is present in 10% of male babies and can be associated with an inguinal hernia. Many hydroceles apparent at birth disappear spontaneously within the first few months of life.

In the absence of fetal testosterone and another undetermined factor, the müllerian duct system develops into the fallopian tubes, uterus, and upper vagina. After birth, as a result of withdrawal of maternal estrogen, the uterus decreases in size and then grows slowly back to its birth size by age 5. By age 10 the corpus of the uterus has grown to a size equal to that of the uterine cervix. The cervix grows rapidly again in the premenarcheal years, followed by further growth of the uterine corpus.

The development of secondary sex characteristics during puberty varies considerably as to time of onset, duration, and sequential timing in both boys and girls (Figs. 7-29 and 7-30). In girls, breast development begins between the ages of 8 and 13 and is completed between the ages of 12 and 19. The development of pubic hair roughly parallels breast development. The peak velocity of growth in height occurs, on the average, 1 year after the onset of breast development, whereas menarche occurs approximately 2 years after the onset of breast development. In girls, puberty lasts between 1½ and 6 years.

In boys, testicular enlargement precedes the development of pubic hair, processes that begin between the ages of 9½ and 13½. An increase in the size of the penis parallels an increase in testicular size, following an initial lag phase. The peak velocity of growth in height occurs later in boys than in girls, commencing at an average age of 14 years. Puberty in boys lasts between 1.8 and 4.7 years.

The stages of development during puberty in boys and girls are illustrated in Figs. 7-31 and 7-32. Sequential recording of a given child's progress can be used both to diagnose abnormal development and to reassure a worried normal adolescent.

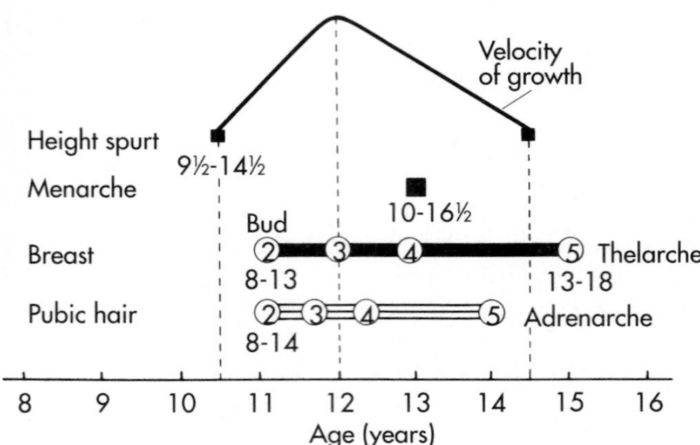

FIG. 7-29 Sequence of events in adolescent girls. An average girl is represented; the range of ages within which some of the events may occur is given by the figures placed directly below the bars.

(From Marshall WA, Tanner JM: *Arch Dis Child* 45:13, 1970.)

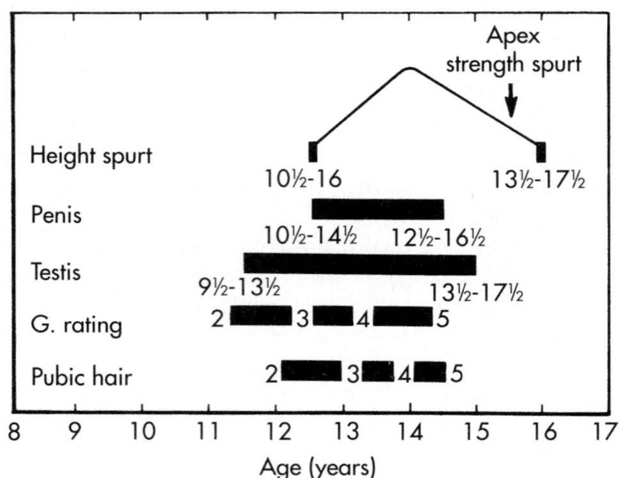

FIG. 7-30 Sequence of events in adolescent boys. An average boy is represented; the range of ages within which some of the events may occur is given by the figures placed directly below the bars.

(From Marshall WA, Tanner JM: *Arch Dis Child* 45:13, 1970.)

Thorough examination of the external genitalia is mandatory immediately after birth to allow rapid evaluation of babies whose genitalia are ambiguous. The external genitalia are examined during all health maintenance examinations and in all children seeking medical attention for abdominal pain. The penis, testes, and external inguinal rings should be examined in boys, the clitoris, labia majora and minora, vaginal orifice, urethral orifice, and external inguinal rings in girls. Internal inspection of the vagina and cervix and bimanual palpation of the internal genitalia are not part of the routine examination of children; they are, however, performed in the evaluation of problems such as vaginal discharge or bleeding (see the following discussion).

When the primary care physician evaluates an infant, a child, or an adolescent for suspected sexual abuse, the child and parent must be prepared with patience and with attention to their fears and concerns. The child must have some control over the position, draping, and pace of the examination and should not be restrained. The examination can proceed with the child supine in the mother's lap, supine on the examining table in a frog-leg position, in a lateral decubitus position with the knees drawn up to the chest, or in a knee-chest position. The examiner should explain and answer questions both before and during each step. After the body as a whole is inspected for signs of trauma, the external genitalia and anus are observed for old or new abrasions or lacerations (facilitated by prior application of toluidine blue dye), scars, hyperpigmentation, verrucae, and enlarged orifices. The hymen is inspected for shape, stretching, injury, or thickening; a vaginal orifice larger than 4 mm in prepubertal children is thought by some to be associated with prior vaginal penetration.[2,3,5] All findings should be recorded clearly, with diagrams, if necessary, for possible use in future child protective custody hearings. Culture specimens of perineal tissue or exudate, or both, are obtained routinely to detect *Neisseria gonorrhoeae,* if present, and, when suspected, *Chlamydia trachomatis,* herpes simplex virus, and *Trichomonas* and *Gardnerella* organisms. Venereal warts (condyloma acuminatum) can be seen in their earliest stages after application of 3% to 5% acetic acid solution to perineal tissues; their presence suggests sexual molestation.

Newborn Period. The appearance of the external genitalia at birth provides information that is useful in assessing gestational age. In boys, the testes are undescended before the thirtieth week of gestation, are high in the inguinal canal between the thirtieth and thirty-sixth weeks, and normally have completely descended into the scrotum by 40 weeks. The scrotal rugae appear, progressing inferiorly to superiorly, between the thirtieth and fortieth weeks. In girls, the labia majora are widely separated and the clitoris is prominent up to the thirty-sixth week; by 40 weeks the labia majora completely cover the labia minora and clitoris.

A white vaginal discharge, occasionally mixed with blood, can be seen for several days after birth, the result of withdrawal from the relatively high levels of maternally derived estrogen. Maternal estrogen also can cause a transient hypertrophy of the labia majora, as seen at birth. The urethral and vaginal orifices can be visualized by downward and lateral traction on each side of the perineum (Fig. 7-33). The hymen varies in thickness and size, the central orifice usually measuring up to 4 mm in diameter in infants. Rarely is the hymen imperforate at birth.

The foreskin of the penis usually is nonretractable at birth, a condition that can persist for years. Ordinarily, sufficient retraction is possible to allow visualization of the external urethral meatus at the tip of the glans penis. The ventral surface of the penis should be inspected at birth for hypospadias (an abnormal position of the external urethral meatus located anywhere between the midline scrotum to the tip of the glans), because its presence is a contraindication to circumcision. Hypospadias may be accompanied by chordee, a fixed, downward bowing of the penis. In rare cases the urethral meatus is located on the dorsal surface of the penis, a condition known as epispadias. After circumcision the glans penis and the remaining lip of foreskin are swollen and erythematous for several days.

Palpation of the testes should proceed downward from the

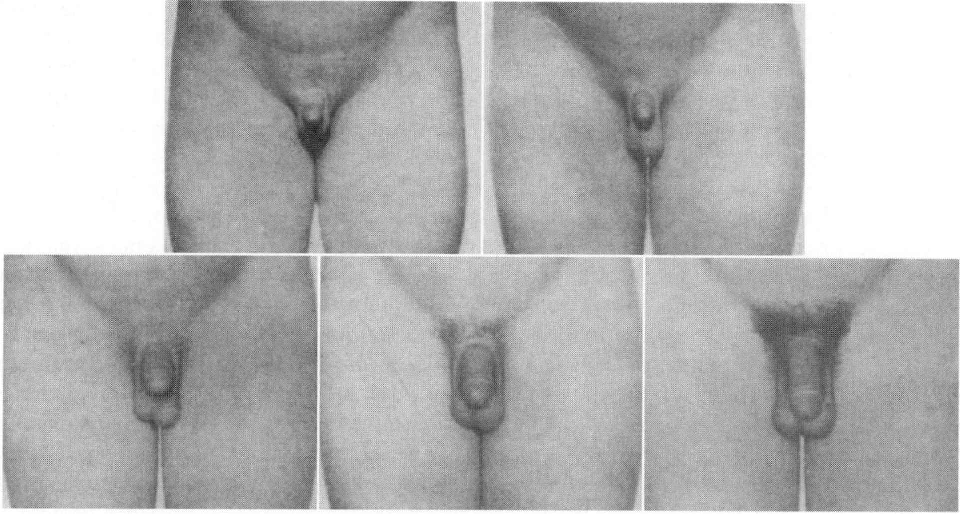

FIG. 7-31 Standards for genitalia maturity ratings in boys.
(From Tanner JM: *Growth at adolescence,* ed 2, Oxford, 1962, Blackwell.)

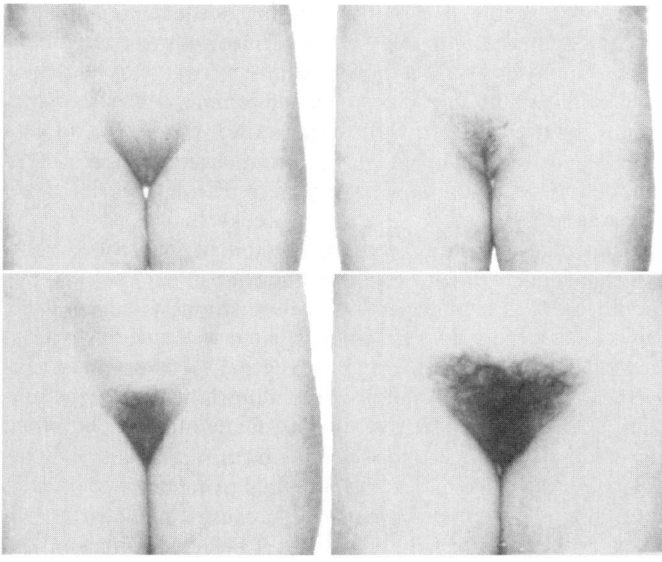

FIG. 7-32 Stages of development of pubic hair in girls. Stage 1 is not shown, since there is no pubic hair in this stage.
(From Tanner JM: *Growth at adolescence,* ed 2, Oxford, 1962, Blackwell.)

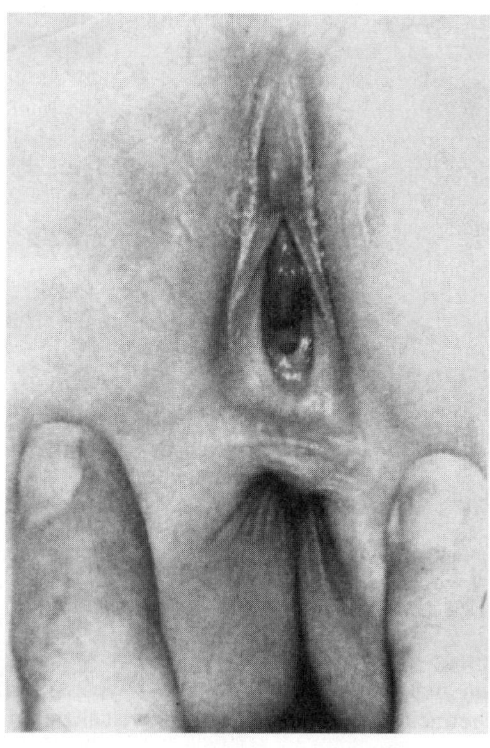

FIG. 7-33 Inspection of the infant vulva.

external inguinal ring to the scrotum to counteract the active cremasteric reflex in infants. This technique is important in diagnosing the undescended testis accurately. Inguinal hernias in infants occur as unilateral or bilateral inguinal and scrotal bulges that usually are reducible and may appear only with crying or straining. Hydroceles are scrotal and sometimes inguinal masses that often are attached to the testes and are nonreducible and nontender and that transilluminate.

In rare cases the appearance of the external genitalia may make it difficult to determine gender. For instance, there may be a midline phallus with apparent scrotal hypospadias and partly fused scrotal-appearing skin with no palpable scrotal masses. In this situation, careful inspection and in some cases probing of the midline of the perineum for a vaginal orifice is an important first step in diagnosing ambiguous external genitalia in a female baby, as is rectal examination to palpate for the presence of a uterus.

Infancy and Early Childhood. Several minor physical abnormalities are common during the first years of life. In boys, ammoniacal dermatitis involving the perineum (diaper rash) in either a circumcised or an uncircumcised infant can cause balanitis, an acute inflammation of the glans penis, which sometimes is associated with purulent exudate. After an episode of balanitis, the external urethral meatus may become stenotic, causing a narrow urinary stream and prolonged emptying of the bladder. Balanitis in an uncircumcised boy can leave adhesions between the glans penis and the foreskin, preventing retraction of the foreskin.

It is important to diagnose an undescended testis accurately because corrective surgery can protect the functioning of a normal, undescended testis only if performed during the first few years of life. An acutely tender testis may indicate torsion of the testis, orchitis, a complication of mumps that commonly occurs in young men, or epididymitis.

In female infants, paper-thin adhesions between the labia minora are common during the first few years of life, sometimes completely covering the vulvar vestibule, with a small opening through which urine escapes. These vulvar adhesions sometimes can be parted by applying gentle pressure laterally on the labia majora. They also will disappear if a cream containing estrogen is applied for several weeks.

Vulvovaginal discharge in preschool-age girls most often is caused by vaginal foreign bodies, usually bits of toilet paper; occasionally a specific bacterial organism can be cultured, or pinworms may be discovered. Cultures that are positive for *N. gonorrhoeae* and *C. trachomatis* almost always indicate sexual abuse. Making these diagnoses occasionally requires vaginoscopy with a special instrument, such as the Huffman vaginoscope or a nasal speculum (Fig. 7-34). Vaginal specimens for smears and cultures can be obtained with the least pain by first instilling a small amount of sterile nutrient broth into the vagina with a medicine dropper.

Although digital examination of the vagina usually is not possible in prepubertal girls, the uterus can be palpated for size, shape, and tenderness with one hand placed over the lower portion of the abdomen and a finger of the other hand inserted into the rectum.

During a rectal examination in a girl, the cervix is the predominant part of the uterus that is palpable; the ovaries normally are not felt. Examination of the rectum in both boys and girls usually is helped by telling the child that "this will be just like having your temperature taken" and by talking with the child in a relaxed manner while performing the examination.

Late Childhood. Children usually begin to have uncomfortable feelings about being undressed in front of adults by the time they reach the age of 5 or 6. Soliciting reassurance from the parent and using drapes or gowns may make the examination of school-age children easier.

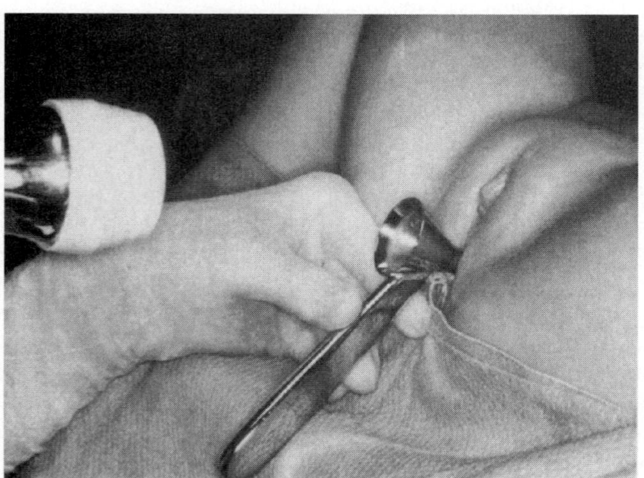

FIG. 7-34 Inspection of the vagina, using a children's vaginoscope and simple illumination with a flashlight.

Occasionally, secondary sex characteristics begin to develop in children in this age group. Evaluation of such children must distinguish among premature thelarche, premature menarche, and precocious puberty.

One method for examining normally retractile testes is to palpate the scrotum with the boy squatting; the examiner begins to palpate over the inguinal areas and works downward onto the scrotum. This technique is especially helpful when examining boys with exogenous obesity, whose external genitalia may be "engulfed" in excess peripubic and perineal adipose tissue. By age 4 it usually is possible to palpate for an inguinal hernia over the external inguinal ring while the boy coughs, with the examining finger inserted into the scrotal tissue and slid upward into the inguinal canal. Tender, acute swelling of the scrotum can be caused by torsion of the testes, epididymitis, orchitis (often caused by mumps), or an incarcerated inguinal hernia.

Adolescence. Examination of an adolescent's genitalia presents the practitioner with an opportunity to reassure the adolescent about the normal progression of the stages of puberty. The examiner should remember that adolescents have an excellent ability to deny real concerns and worries; therefore, the physician should be especially sensitive to questions that might relate to a concern about venereal disease, pregnancy, or even cancer. Honest, direct answers to the adolescent's questions, coupled with a careful description of the examination before it is performed, will help to establish a trusting relationship.

Bimanual palpation of the uterus, as just described, usually is adequate when examining prepubertal and virginal pubertal girls. A complete pelvic examination is indicated for any adolescent who has vaginal discharge, dysuria, pyuria, lower abdominal pain, irregular vaginal bleeding, or amenorrhea, and for a sexually active adolescent. This examination is aided by proper instruments, including a vaginoscope or small speculum, culture media, glass slides, and a cytology fixative. The physician should be patient and gentle, minimizing painful procedures and embarrassment for the patient. After the external genitalia have been inspected and the internal organs have been examined with a speculum or vaginoscope, the uterus and ovaries are palpated using the bimanual technique; normally the ovaries are not palpable. Specimens should be obtained periodically in sexually active adolescents to culture for *N. gonorrhoeae* and *C. trachomatis* and to evaluate cervical cytology for herpes virus effects.

Musculoskeletal System

The changes in the musculoskeletal system of infants, children, and adolescents over time give the examiner the most visible evidence of human growth. If a child's sequential measurements of height fall within the norms of a standard growth curve, this is strong evidence not only that bone growth is normal, but also that the numerous factors necessary for normal growth are operating appropriately. In addition, because of its visibility, the musculoskeletal system most often is the source of questions from parents concerning possible deviations from normal, including the possible effects of trauma, a leading cause of morbidity and mortality in children.

The outward manifestations of growth of the trunk and extremities reflect primarily growth of bone, muscle, and adipose tissue. Bone grows in the fetus starting with cartilage, then from the primary centers of ossification, primarily in the long bones. Postnatally, new bone formation occurs in secondary centers of ossification at the ends of long bones and the vertebral bodies and in the membranes of the flat bones of the cranium and clavicle. In addition to longitudinal growth of long bones and vertebral bodies, internal remodeling takes place throughout infancy and childhood, resulting in less dense bone, a changing thickness of the bone cortex, and changing amounts of red marrow and fat within the diaphyses of bone. In addition to hormonal factors, bone remodeling is influenced by mechanical forces caused by muscle attachments and gravity. Bone growth is completed with ossification of the growth cartilage and union of the epiphyses and diaphyses of long bones by age 25. The roentgenographic appearance of the onset, size, and shape of secondary ossification centers can be compared with established norms in determining the bone age, a measurement that despite its variability can be helpful in assessing children who are suspected of having abnormal growth.

Growth in stature predominates in the lower extremities before puberty and in the trunk during puberty. The distal extremities reach adult size before the proximal extremities—thus the common complaint of preadolescent children that their feet are too big.

Muscle growth, which results from increases in the number, size, and length of cells, proceeds throughout childhood according to the following increasing proportions of muscle mass to body weight: 1:5 to 1:4 at birth, 1:3 in early adolescence, and 2:5 in early maturity. A spurt in the increase in muscle cell numbers occurs at age 2, and maximal increase occurs between the ages of 10 and 16. Muscle cell size increases faster in girls than in boys between the ages of 3 and 10, but after age 14, boys surpass girls in both the number and size of muscle cells. The number of muscle fibers increases slowly until the fifth decade of life.

A thorough evaluation of the musculoskeletal system should be part of every newborn examination, every child health maintenance examination, and the examination of any child who has an abnormality of growth, stature, or gait. It includes an appraisal of (1) posture, position, and gross deformities, (2) skin color, temperature, and tenderness, (3) bone or joint tenderness, (4) range of joint motion, (5) muscle size, symmetry, and strength, and (6) the configuration and motility of the back.

Newborn Period. The position and appearance of the extremities at birth can reflect intrauterine position. The folded position of the lower extremities on the abdomen in the fetus results in the common appearance in newborns of externally rotated, somewhat bowed, lower extremities and everted feet. A baby born after a breech presentation often has markedly flexed hips and extended knees. Traction on the brachial plexus during delivery can cause what usually is a temporary paresis of the proximal upper extremity muscles (Erb palsy), most often appearing as an asymmetrical Moro reflex (see p. 95). Another common cause of an asymmetrical Moro reflex resulting from a birth injury is a fractured clavicle, which can be confirmed by palpating an area of crepitance, usually over the distal third of the clavicle.

Gross deformities should be recognized at birth, both for early treatment and for possible clues to generalized genetic or metabolic diseases. Relatively common deformities include short or absent extremities, absence of one bone in an extremity, hypertrophy of one bone in an extremity or of an entire half of the body (hemihypertrophy), extra fingers or toes (polydactyly), webbed or fused fingers or toes (syndactyly), and annular constricting bands around a portion of an extremity with or without distal amputation or lack of development. The ratio of extremity length to body length should be noted. In a normal newborn the ratio of the upper segment of the body to the lower segment (above and below the symphysis pubis) is approximately 1.7:1. In various types of dwarfism the extremities alone may be short, as in achondroplasia, or both extremities and trunk may be shortened, as in Morquio disease. The entire length of the vertebral column should be examined and palpated for bony defects with or without overlying skin defects.

The joints should be tested for range of motion, noting any asymmetry, undue tightness, or contractures, as well as the muscle tone. A floppy or hypotonic baby may have CNS disease, a metabolic disturbance, primary muscle disease, or anterior horn cell disease. Limited unilateral joint motion with or without associated bone or joint tenderness and fever should be investigated extensively as a possible sign of osteomyelitis.

Perhaps the most important part of the examination of a newborn's extremities is the examination of the lower extremities, giving special attention to the hips and feet. The hips are examined particularly to rule out congenital dislocation, a condition that is relatively easy to treat, with good results, *if* treatment is started early. The examiner tests for an unstable or actually dislocated femoral head by abducting one hip at a time and feeling for a click when the femoral head passes back into the acetabulum. This maneuver usually requires 70 to 80 degrees of hip abduction. Downward pressure over the hips transmitted through the flexed knee can be used to attempt to produce posterior dislocation of the femoral head (Fig. 7-35). The click or clunk of the reducing femoral head should be distinguished from the clicks felt with rotation of the hip and the click felt with simultaneous movement of the knee. After the newborn period, the hip click (Ortolani sign) heard with congenitally dislocated hips disappears, and other signs become helpful in making this diagnosis. The thigh may appear shorter on the affected side, the thigh skinfolds may be asymmetrical (although this occurs in some normal babies), and the hip will have limited abduction on the affected side. Tight hip abductors in the neonatal period are not a sign of congenital hip dislocation.

A newborn's and an infant's feet often appear flat because of a plantar fat pad that gradually disappears during the first 1 to 2 years of life. The most severe foot deformity at birth is the equinovarus deformity, or clubfoot. True clubfoot deformities cannot be corrected passively, nor do they correct with stroking of the foot's lateral side. This deformity comprises fixed forefoot adduction, fixed inversion especially of the hindfoot, equinus position, internal tibial torsion, and small calf muscles.

Viewing the sole of the resting foot (not spontaneously inverted or everted) allows observation for the normal single anteroposterior plantar axis. In metatarsus varus deformity

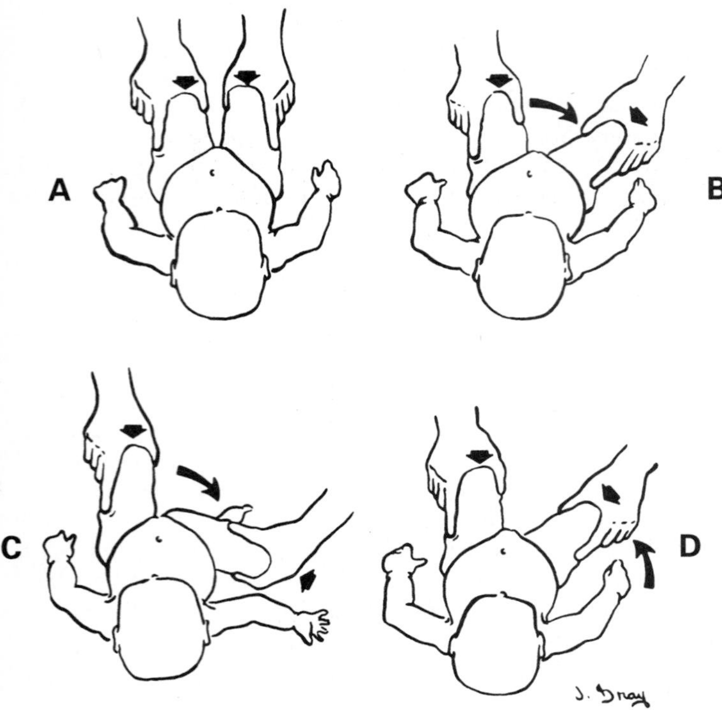

FIG. 7-35 Examination for congenital dislocation of the hip. **A,** Downward pressure is exerted on the hips to produce posterior dislocation. **B,** The hip to be examined is then abducted. **C** and **D,** A positive Ortolani sign is elicited by feeling the head reenter the acetabulum with a click. The examiner's finger is on the baby's greater trochanter during all phases of the examination.

(From Stanisavljevic S: *Diagnosis and treatment of congenital hip pathology in the newborn,* Baltimore, 1964, Williams & Wilkins.)

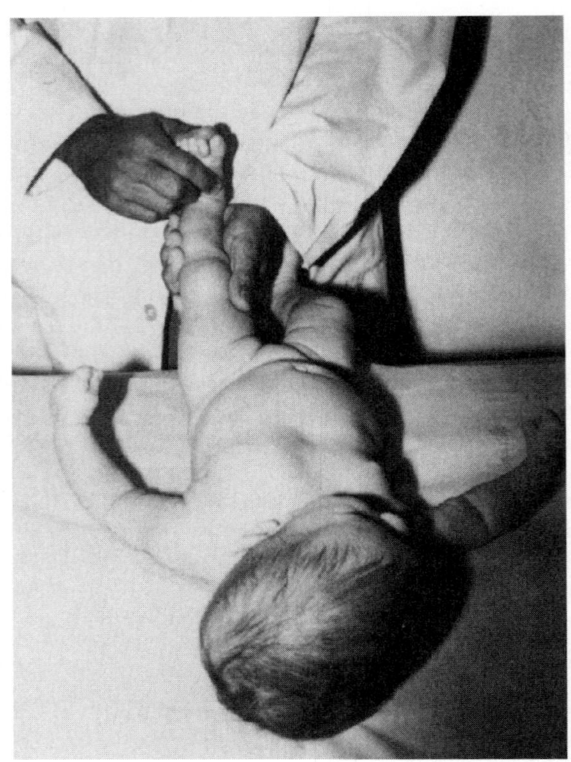

FIG. 7-36 Examination of the lower extremities.

(Photograph by P. Ruben.)

the forefoot is adducted in relation to the hindfoot, thus describing two anteroposterior axes, and this position is not correctable by stroking the foot's lateral border. In calcaneovalgus deformity the foot is dorsiflexed and everted.

One way to examine the alignment of a lower extremity is shown in Fig. 7-36. With the infant supine, an imaginary line is drawn that connects the anterior superior "iliac" spine with the midpatella and continues down to the foot; if the line falls medial to the first toe, external tibial torsion is present; if it falls lateral to the second toe, internal tibial torsion is present. See Chapter 134 for a complete discussion of developmental orthopedic variations of the lower extremities.

Infancy and Early Childhood. An infant's lower extremities often remain bowlegged with externally rotated feet for the first 1 to 2 years of life. With ambulation, the feet gradually assume the straight-ahead position, and the knockknee, or genu valgum, position normally is seen between the ages of 2 and 6 or longer.

Severe bowing of the legs raises the question of rickets or epiphyseal damage from inflammation or trauma (Blount disease). The infant who toes in should be examined for metatarsus varus, internal tibial torsion, or femoral anteversion. Flatfeet, or feet without a longitudinal arch, are common, especially in children who have generalized ligamentous laxity.

A toddler's lower extremities are examined best by first observing the spontaneous gait with the infant undressed. The normal gait usually is wide based and somewhat unstable, with prominent lumbar lordosis. Then, especially if positional deformities are noted, a careful examination of the hips, knees, legs, ankles, and feet with the child in the supine position can confirm the presence of any fixed deformity. A child who has a limp should be examined carefully for signs of trauma; localized bone or joint tenderness from fracture or infection; joint effusions with limited range of motion from trauma, infection, or noninfectious arthritis; peripheral muscle weakness; unilateral or bilateral spasticity, especially manifested by a tight Achilles tendon; and proximal muscle weakness, particularly weakness resulting from unrecognized hip disease such as congenital dislocated hip or coxa vara. Testing for the last-named condition can be done by having the child raise one foot while standing. This normally produces an elevation in the contralateral hip. Inability of the hip abductors to elevate the contralateral hip is considered a positive Trendelenburg sign (Fig. 7-37).

Child abuse should be suspected in all cases of trauma if (1) the history of the injury is inconsistent with its severity; (2) there are signs of multiple blunt trauma to the extremities, trunk (especially the buttocks), and face; (3) trauma is recurrent; and (4) significant delay occurs between the episode of injury and the request for medical attention.

The infant who has a tender elbow held in pronation, usually after a pulling episode (nursemaid elbow), suffers from subluxation of the radial head, which can be reduced easily by supinating the arm while applying pressure to the radial head.

Late Childhood and Adolescence. A limp in a child between the ages of 4 and 8, especially if accompanied by knee

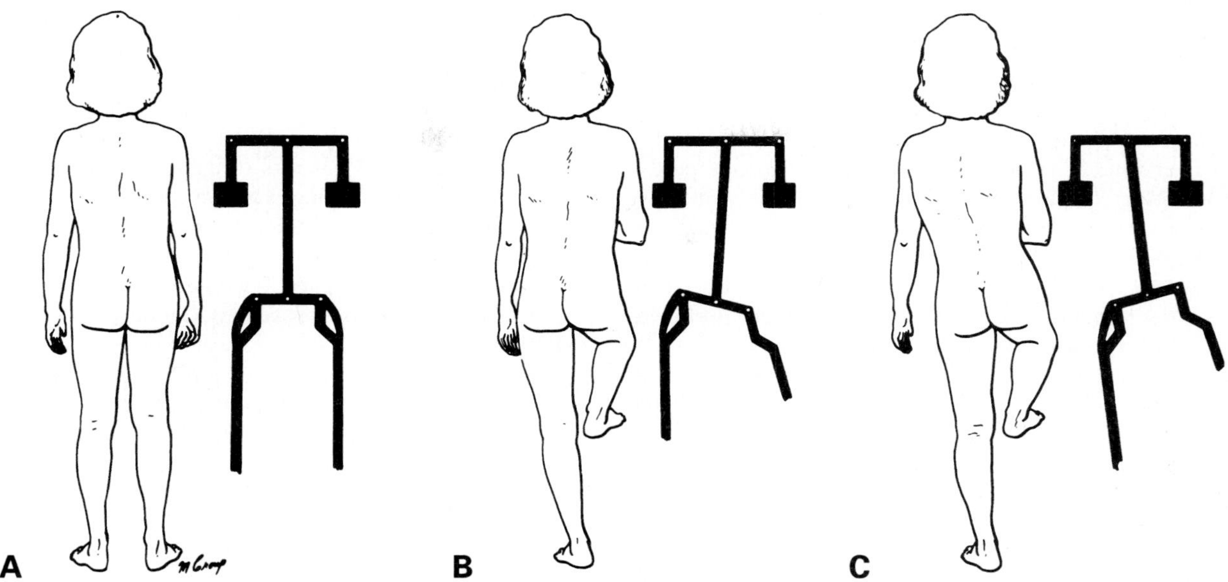

FIG. 7-37 Trendelenburg sign, showing weakness of the gluteus medius muscle. **A,** Normal standing. **B,** Dropping of the pelvis of the contralateral side when standing on the affected leg. **C,** Compensation for weakness when walking by shifting the center of gravity of the trunk to elevate the pelvis on the opposite side.

(From Ferguson Am Jr: ***Orthopaedic surgery in infancy and childhood,*** ed 5, Baltimore, 1981, Williams & Wilkins.)

pain, suggests Legg-Calvé-Perthes disease, as well as the conditions previously mentioned. The same symptoms in a child between the ages of 9 and 12 may be caused by a slipped femoral capital epiphysis. Tenderness over the tibial tubercle may be a sign of Osgood-Schlatter disease. Painful heels can be caused by partial evulsion of the Achilles tendon, retrocalcaneal bursitis, or plantar fasciitis.

In the examination of an injured knee, the following elements should be tested: the medial and lateral collateral ligaments, by abducting and adducting the tibia on the femur; the cruciate ligaments, by pulling the tibia forward, then pushing it backward with the knee flexed; the medial and lateral menisci, by extending the knee with the foot held in eversion and then inversion; the patella, by pushing it posteriorly against the femur; and the joint space for effusion, by pressing over the suprapatellar bursa and then attempting ballottement of the patella.

School-age children and adolescents should be examined for scoliosis, or lateral curvature of the vertebral column. Significant spinal curvature can be seen with the child standing erect; lesser degrees of curvature can be observed by having the child bend forward approximately 50 degrees, letting the shoulders droop forward and the arms hang freely. The examiner then looks for a unilateral elevation of the lower thoracic ribs and flank, which accompanies the rotational deformity of scoliosis (Fig. 7-38).

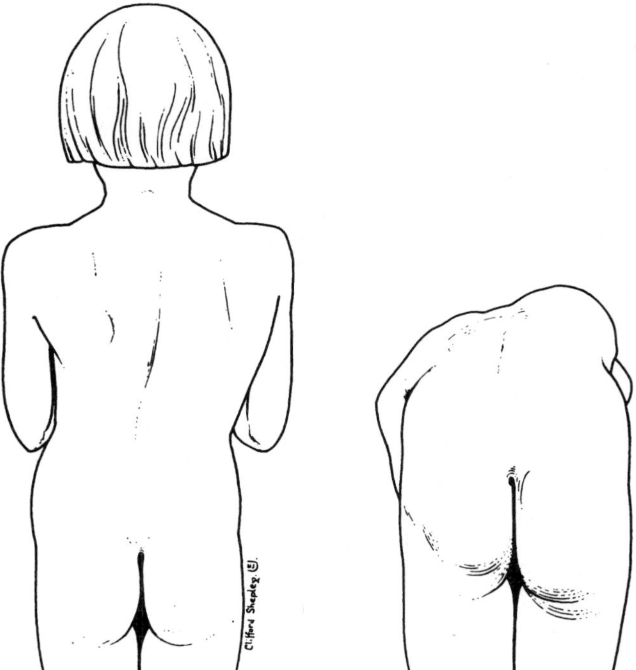

FIG. 7-38 Examination for scoliosis.

(From James JIP: ***Scoliosis,*** Edinburgh, 1976, E&S Livingstone.)

Nervous System

Compared with other organ systems, the manifestations of nervous system growth in infants and children are the most dynamic. Therefore the definitions of normal for any sign that reflects the state of the nervous system or one of its parts are critically age dependent. These norms also demonstrate wide variation among individuals, as well as within a single individual on different days and under variable conditions. The growth and integrity of the growing nervous system can be assessed in two ways. One way is to describe the changes in a child's abilities in various behavioral areas over time, in reference to established norms; this "developmental assessment" is discussed in Chapter 20, Twelve, Developmental Surveillance and Intervention. The other method is neurological assessment, in which often-changing physical signs that reflect the state of subsystems of the nervous system are described over time. The developmental stage depends partly on the neurological stage, but it also is influenced greatly by the child's environmental experiences. The major goal of neurological assessment in children is to monitor the maturation of the nervous system, although the methods described for localizing nervous system lesions in adults are useful in evaluating certain problems in children.

The nervous system grows most rapidly during fetal and early postnatal life, reaching approximately one fourth the adult size at birth, one half by age 1, four fifths by age 3, and nine tenths by age 7. At the cellular level there are two distinct peaks of growth rate. The first involves neuroblasts, which multiply between 10 and 18 weeks of fetal life; after this time, the number of neuronal cells probably increases very little. The second and more striking spurt of brain growth occurs between midgestation and approximately 18 months of age and reflects multiplication of glial cells, production of myelin by the glial cells, and development of dendrites and synaptic connections. Myelination continues relatively rapidly until age 4, after which it gradually increases to adult levels.

The growth of the spinal cord, after fusion of the neural folds cranially and caudally, initially is most rapid in the lumbar and cervical regions, with the thoracic region developing most rapidly during the third trimester of pregnancy. During the third fetal month the developing vertebral column grows more rapidly than the spinal cord, and as a result, the cordal end of the spinal cord moves cranially from the level of the fourth lumbar vertebra in the fifth month to the adult level of the first or second lumbar vertebra by the second postnatal month. Myelination of the cord proceeds cephalocaudad.

Spontaneous and reflexive motor activity, reflecting developing muscular innervation and spinal reflex arcs, begins during the tenth week of fetal life. At 12 weeks of fetal age a primitive rooting and grasp response can be seen; withdrawal of the lower extremities in response to stimulation of the feet and the gastrocnemius stretch reflex are seen at 16 weeks; by 19 weeks, regular respiratory movements are seen in response to hypoxia. Tonic myotactic reflexes, responsible for the recoil of an extended extremity, are well developed in the term infant. The rhythmicity of rhythmic motor neuron activity, which is responsible for jerky repetitive movements during activity (e.g., the jerking jaw movements that accompany crying), increases with increasing gestational age. At term, stretch reflexes, such as the knee jerk, are diminished by sleep, whereas exteroceptive reflexes (superficial abdominal and Babinski reflexes) are not.

The normal sequence of changes in an infant's posture, muscle tone, and reflexes that occurs with increasing gestational age from 28 to 40 weeks has been described by several observers and, despite their differences, can be used in assessing a neonate's gestational age (Fig. 7-39). Similarly, the persistence and eventual cessation of certain characteristics of the infant's posture, tone, and reflexes follow a defined pattern with age. Changes in the infant's and child's developmental abilities (see Chapter 20, Twelve, Developmental Surveillance and Intervention) also are based on the continuing maturation of the nervous system.

An additional behavioral characteristic of the maturing nervous system is the change in sleep-wake cycles with age. The neonate's sleep-wake cycle usually is quite irregular, but it becomes regular by 15 weeks of age. Rapid eye movement (REM) sleep occurs during a greater proportion of sleeping time in infants than in adults. A small number of neonates are found to have irregular respirations during sleep, sometimes to the point of apnea, a condition that has been discarded as a precursor of sudden infant death syndrome (SIDS).

A neurological examination should be performed on every neonate and on infants and preschool children during health maintenance visits. Other indications for a careful neurological assessment include developmental delay, failure in school, abnormal social behavior, headache, head trauma, seizures, sensory disturbances, changes in states of consciousness, abnormal gait, recent personality change, and fever of unknown origin. Structural and functional abnormalities of the nervous system of infants and children can produce delays in the normal maturational sequences and localizing signs. Therefore the neurological assessment must include observation of spontaneous and elicited activity that reflects brain maturation, as well as the ordered sequence of the neurological examination as described for adults.

Several authors have suggested ways to organize the neurological examination in the younger age groups. Prechtel and Beintema[6] have described a system for neonates; Amiel-Tison,[1] one for infants during the first year of life; and Touwen and Prechtl,[8] one for children who have behavioral or learning disabilities. The box on p. 95 presents a method of organizing the data of a neurological examination; this scheme combines parts of the age-specific evaluations with the standard adult neurological examination.

Various components of this summary are discussed in other chapters in this text. The following sections highlight the approach to the neurological examination of children of different age groups, including major areas of emphasis for each group.

Newborn Period and Infancy. Careful observation is the most important tool in the neurological examination of the newborn and infant, taking into account the optimal environmental conditions previously described. Even when an infant is asleep and dressed, the examiner can note the posture, especially the degree of flexion of the extremities; any hyperextension of the neck, including overt opisthotonos; the symmetry of the position of the extremities; and the amount, quality, and symmetry of spontaneous movements, including tonic or clonic convulsions. Holding the thumb curled under the flexed fingers is a sign present with many brain abnormalities (cerebral thumb). In normal premature infants, continuous athetoid movements are common (e.g., simultaneous flexion of the elbow and rotation of the upper portion of the arm). Athetoid postures also are common in term infants. Tremor with or without crying is seen in many healthy newborns during the first days of life. Spontaneous assumption of the tonic neck position (extension of the ipsilateral extremities after rotation of the head to one side) may occur in normal infants, but an obligatory tonic neck reflex (one that always is present) is abnormal. The face is observed for ex-

Menstrual age (weeks)

28 29 30 31 32 33 34 35 36 37 38 39 40 41 42

Withdrawal reflex
Pupil reaction to light
Palmar grasp reflex
Moro reflex (abduction and exten.)
Crossed extensor reflex
Recoil of legs, prone position
Glabella tap reflex
Cremasteric reflex
Rooting reflex
Recoil of legs, supine position
Standing response
Recoil of arms, supine position
Traction response (flexion of elbows)
Moro reflex (adduction and flexion)
Traction response (head control)
Stepping movements
Neck righting reflex
Head rising in prone position
Crossed extensor reflex (adduction)

28 29 30 31 32 33 34 35 36 37 38 39 40 41 42

Menstrual age (weeks)

· · · · · · · Not yet present in all cases
– – – – Developing from immature to mature pattern
——— Fully developed

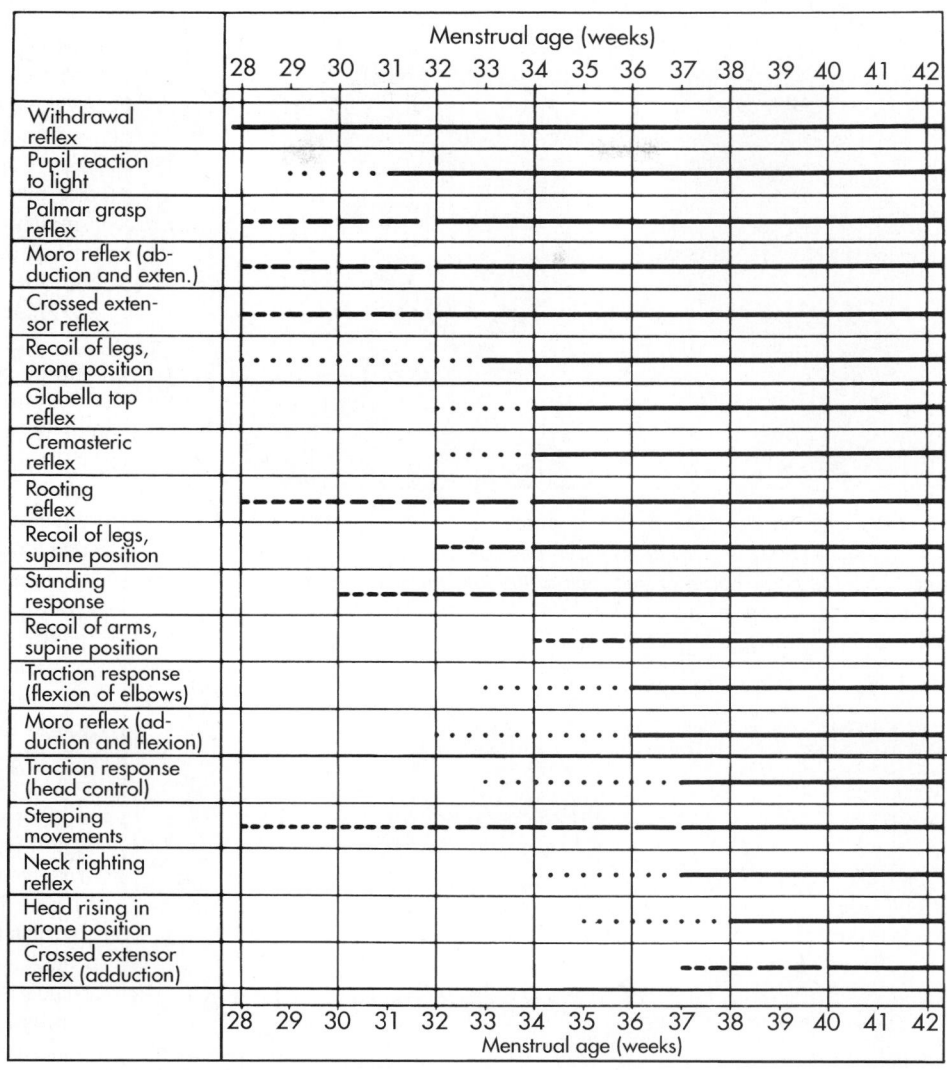

FIG. 7-39 Developmental sequence of various reflexes and motor automatisms.

(From Davis JA, Dobbing J, editors: *Scientific foundations of paediatrics*, ed 2, Baltimore, Md, 1981, University Park Press.)

pression (alert, bland, fussing, crying); symmetry of eye closure after a tap on the glabella (glabella reflex); and symmetry of position and movement of the eyes, including presence of symmetry and pupillary constriction and blinking of the eyelids in response to a hand clap approximately 12 inches from the infant's face.

With the baby undressed, resistance to passive stretch is tested in the extremities, trunk, and neck, noting particularly any symmetrical and asymmetrical increase or decrease. Many infants in whom spasticity develops later are hypotonic during the neonatal period. Symmetry of the biceps, patellar, superficial abdominal, cremasteric, and anal reflexes is noted, and eliciting ankle clonus (recording the number of beats obtained) is attempted. The palmar and plantar grasps are tested (Fig. 7-40) for differences of intensity between the two sides (unilaterally decreased in Erb palsy, for instance) or bilateral absence, as with cord lesions. As Fig. 7-40 shows, it is important to press the infant's palm from the ulnar side, with the infant's head in the midline position. The Babinski reflex (with a flexor response and fanning of the toes), which is expected in normal newborns, is tested for symmetry, as is the withdrawal reflex of the lower extremities.

The rooting response is elicited while the baby's hands are held against the chest (Fig. 7-41). In addition to the response shown, with stimulation of the upper lip, the mouth is opened and the head is retroflexed; with stimulation of the lower lip, the mouth opens and the jaw drops. This reflex is absent in depressed infants; when the examiner's fingers are placed into the infant's mouth, the sucking response is decreased in strength, frequency of sucks, and duration.

In the traction response test (Fig. 7-42), the examiner pulls the supine infant into a sitting position and notes the degree of resistance to extension of the arms at the elbow and the degree to which the head is held upright. In a term infant

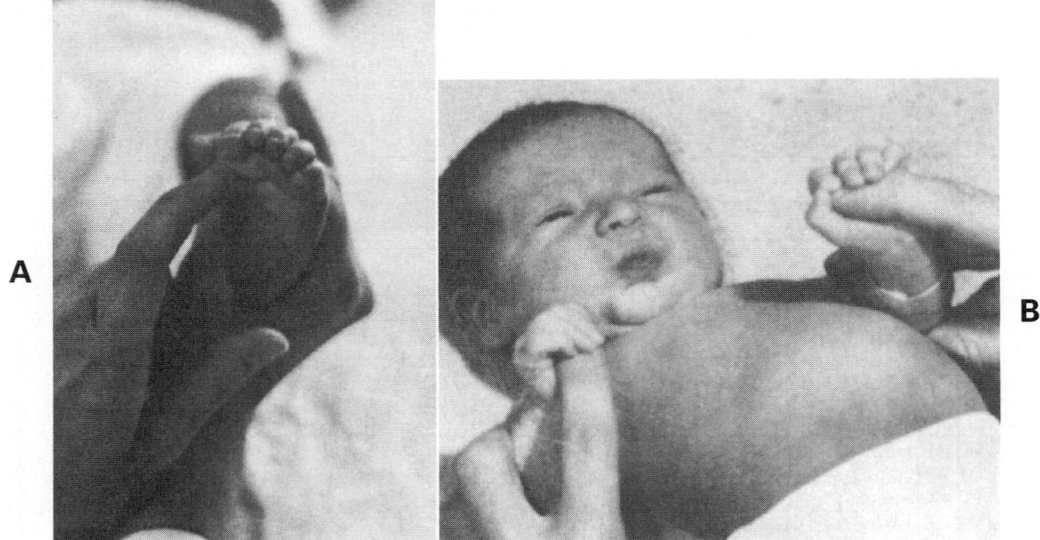

FIG. 7-40 **A,** Plantar grasp. **B,** Palmar grasp.

(**A** From Whaley LF, Wong DL: *Nursing care of infants and children,* ed 4, St Louis, 1991, Mosby; **B** From Prechtl HFR: *The neurological examination of the full-term newborn infant,* ed 2, London, 1977, Heinemann.)

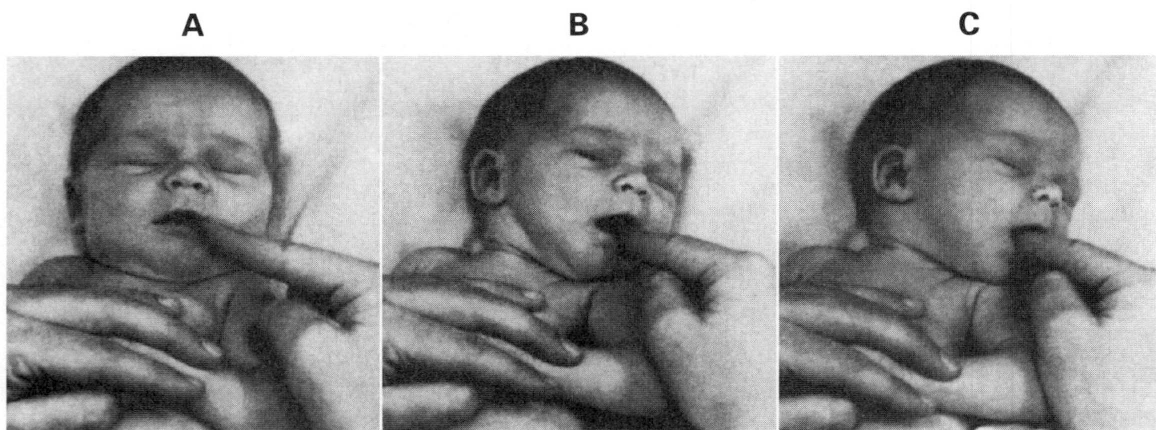

FIG. 7-41 Rooting response. **A,** Stimulation. **B,** Head turning. **C,** Grasping with the mouth.

(From Prechtl HFR: *The neurological examination of the full-term newborn infant,* ed 2, London, 1977, Heinemann.)

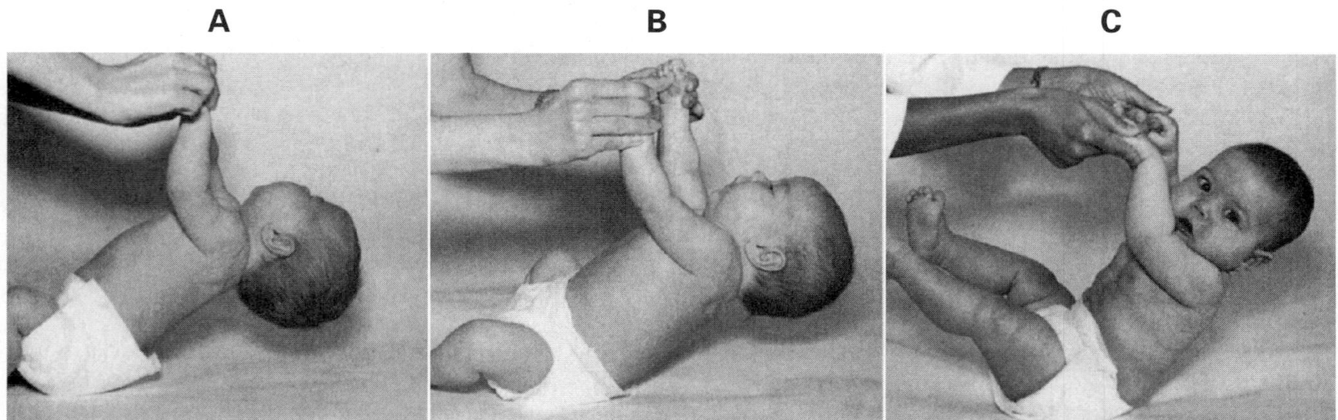

FIG. 7-42 Sitting development. **A,** First 4 weeks or so: complete head lag when being pulled into sitting position. **B,** About 2 months: considerable, but not complete, head lag when being pulled into sitting position. **C,** 4 months: no head lag when being pulled into sitting position.

(From Whaley LF, Wong DL: *Nursing care of infants and children,* ed 2, St Louis, 1983, Mosby.)

ORGANIZATION OF THE PEDIATRIC NEUROLOGICAL EXAMINATION

Conditions under which the examination is conducted
- Child's behavioral state
- Environmental conditions

Mental status
- State of consciousness
- Language (receptive and expressive)
- Cognitive functioning
- Mood
- Social and self-awareness

Station and gait

Head
- Skull
- Cranial nerves I to XII

Motor
- Muscle size, symmetry, contractures, tone, and strength
- Spontaneous activity when prone, supine, sitting, standing, and walking, including fine and gross motor abilities
- Resistance to passive stretch
- Coordination
- Involuntary movements, including fasciculations, tremor, chorea, athetosis, dystonia, and myotonic jerks

Sensory

Reflexes
- Neonatal
- Deep tendon reflexes, including plantar response
- Abdominal, cremasteric, and anal reflexes
- Clonus

Autonomic nervous system
- Cardiac and respiratory rate, bladder functioning, temperature control

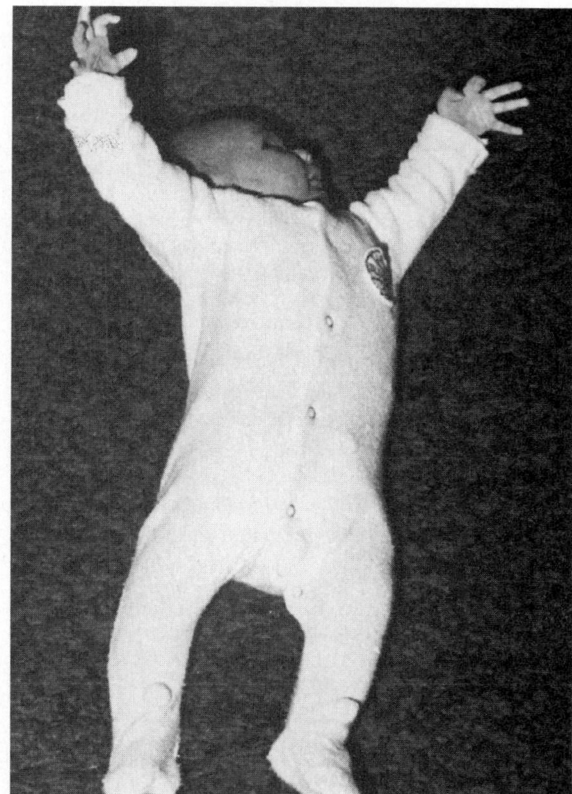

FIG. 7-43 Moro response.

(From Whaley LF, Wong DL: *Nursing care of infants and children,* ed 4, St Louis, 1991, Mosby.)

some degree of flexion of the elbow is maintained, and head control is relatively weak, with neither head flexors nor extensors predominating.

The Moro response is a critically important sign of an intact nervous system, particularly during the neonatal period. It is best elicited, as shown in Fig. 7-43, by supporting the infant's body in one hand, then suddenly allowing the head to drop a few centimeters with the other hand during a moment when the head is midline and the neck muscles are relaxed. A complete Moro response consists of symmetrical abduction of the upper extremity at the shoulder, extension of the forearm at the elbow, and extension of the fingers, all followed by abduction of the arm at the shoulder. The Moro response also can be elicited by holding the baby supine and then suddenly lowering the entire body about 12 inches and by producing a sudden loud noise.

The prone infant is observed for spontaneous head movements (brief lifting or turning from side to side), spontaneous crawling movements, and the incurvation, or Galant, reflex (lateral curvation of the trunk after stimulation with a finger or pin along a paravertebral line from the shoulder to the buttocks about 3 cm from the midline). The infant then is held prone in the air with the examiner's hands around the chest. The normal newborn is somewhat flaccid during this maneuver, but the hypertonic or opisthotonic baby will lift the head and extend the lower extremities to varying degrees. With the infant still upright, the placing and stepping responses are noted. In the placing response, the dorsum of one foot is allowed to brush against the undersurface of a tabletop edge and is followed normally by simultaneous flexion of the knees and hips and placement of the stimulated foot on the table. In the stepping response, the soles of the feet are allowed to touch the surface of the table, which elicits alternating stepping movements with both legs.

Throughout the neurological examination, the practitioner should note the quality and duration of the infant's cry, and he or she should listen for the high-pitched, excessive, or weak cries that can accompany brain lesions. Cranial nerve testing is completed by testing the corneal and jaw jerk reflexes (cranial nerve V); the response during rotation of the upright infant's eyes to turning in the same direction he or she is moved (vestibular cranial nerve VIII); the gag reflex, symmetrical elevation of the palate and swallowing movements (cranial nerves IX and X); and by observing for torticollis (cranial nerve XI) and the symmetry of the tongue, including observation for fasciculations (cranial nerve XII).

The results of all these maneuvers occasionally indicate a localized brain lesion, such as hemiparesis secondary to intracranial bleeding. More often, however, the general state of the infant's nervous system is determined to be normal, hyperexcitable, apathetic, or comatose. The physician must

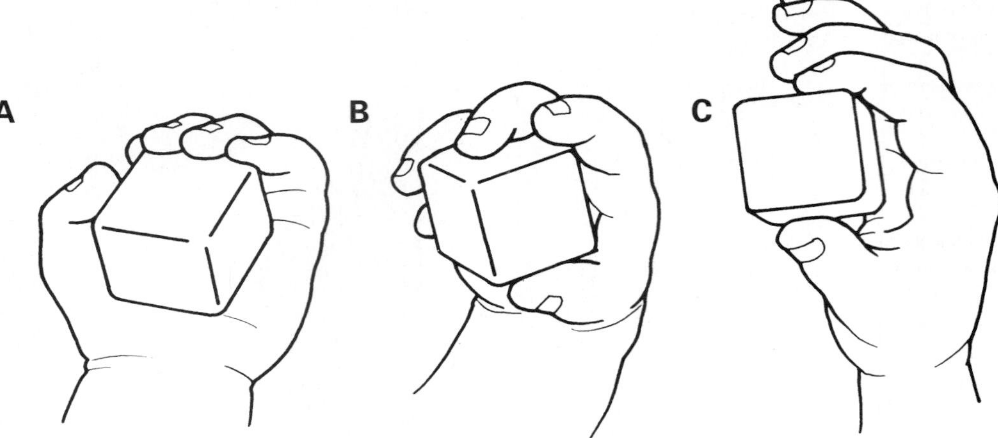

FIG. 7-44 Manipulation. **A,** 6 months: immature palmar grasp of a cube. **B,** 8 months: grasp at the intermediate stage. **C,** 1 year: mature grasp of a cube.

then decide what further diagnostic tests are indicated and the frequency of follow-up examinations.

As the infant matures, the neonatal reflexes (automatisms) disappear. Persistence of neonatal reflexes beyond age appropriate norms for their disappearance usually indicates nervous system abnormality. Some of the techniques for examining neonates are continued during the first year to ascertain whether strength and coordination have developed further. For instance, a normal 3-month-old infant no longer demonstrates head lag when pulled to a sitting position; a 5-month-old infant lifts its head from the supine position when about to be pulled up; and he or she sits without support between 5 and 8 months of age. The infant usually walks without support between 12 and 18 months of age.

It is important to monitor the development of hand coordination. A normal infant can reach and grasp objects by 5 months of age, transfer objects from hand to hand by 7 months, and pick up a raisin using a pincer grasp by 10 months (Fig. 7-44). After 8 months of age, a normal infant demonstrates symmetrical parachute and lateral propping reactions. The parachute reflex can be assessed using a flinging motion of the ventrally suspended infant toward the examination table, which should elicit extension of the arms. In the lateral propping reaction, the sitting infant is pushed to one side, and the arms should extend to prevent falling. During these maneuvers the examiner looks for asymmetrical movement.

Early and Late Childhood. Further growth of the nervous system in infants and children is monitored by observing walking, the development of speech and language abilities, interaction with parents, and the ability to manipulate small objects, use pencils and crayons, climb and run, throw and catch a ball, and follow simple directions. Muscle strength in the lower extremities is best tested by observing gait, heel and toe walking, standing and hopping on one leg, and the ability to rise from the floor from a supine position. Coordination can be observed in all these maneuvers, as well as in heel-to-shin, finger-to-nose pointing, and tandem walking. If the child's development is delayed or if the child has a history of school failure, further testing of neurophysiological maturation (described in Chapter 20, Twelve, Developmental Surveillance and Intervention) can help define both abilities and areas that need special attention.

As with infants, the neurological examination of school-age children who have nervous system abnormalities usually defines some degree of maturational delay. Localizing neurological signs are less common, occurring in children most often as a result of traumatic intracranial bleeding or brain tumors or after CNS infection.

Adolescence. Although reading ability and comprehension, improved coordination, and increased strength all can be used to monitor further neuromuscular maturation in adolescents, the neurological examination in this age group is similar to the adult examination. When evaluating a young person's mental status, the examiner should remember that many normal adolescents display variable mood swings, confused thinking, and resistance to authority.

REFERENCES

1. Amiel-Tison C: A method for neurological evaluation within the first year of life, *Curr Probl Pediatr* 8, 1976.
2. Berenson AB et al: Appearance of the hymen in prepubertal girls, *Pediatrics* 89:387, 1992.
3. Chadwick DL et al: *Color atlas of child sexual abuse,* Chicago, 1989, Mosby.
4. Klaus MH, Kennell JH: *Bonding: the beginnings of parent-infant attachment,* St Louis, 1983, Mosby.
5. McCann J et al: Genital injuries resulting from sexual abuse: a longitudinal study, *Pediatrics* 89:307, 1992.
6. Prechtl H, Beintema D: *The neurological examination of the full term newborn infant,* London, 1964, Heinemann.
7. Smith DW: *Recognizable patterns of human malformation,* Philadelphia, 1976, WB Saunders.
8. Touwen BCL, Prechtl H: *The neurological examination of the child with minor dysfunction,* London, 1970, Heinemann.
9. Zadnik K et al: The effect of parental history of myopia in children's eye size, *JAMA* 271:1823, 1994.

SUGGESTED READINGS

American Academy of Pediatrics, Joint Committee on Infant Hearing: Position statement 1982, *Pediatrics* 70:496, 1982.

Davis JA, Dobbing J: *Scientific foundations of paediatrics,* ed 2, Baltimore, Md, 1981, University Park Press.

Ferguson AB: *Orthopaedic surgery in infancy and childhood,* ed 4, Baltimore, 1975, Williams & Wilkins.

Gammon JA: Visual system screening in infants and young children, *Pediatr Rev* 4:71, 1982.

Hoekelman RA: The pediatric physical examination. In Bates B, editor: *A guide to physical examination and history taking,* ed 6, Philadelphia, 1995, JB Lippincott.

James JIP: *Scoliosis,* Edinburgh, 1976, E&S Livingstone.

Lowrey GH: *Growth and development of children,* ed 8, Chicago, 1986, Mosby.

Lynch A: Use of health history in upgrading school health care. Paper presented at the annual meeting of the New Orleans American Public Health Association, New Orleans, September 1974.

McDowell F, Wolff HG: *Handbook of neurological diagnostic methods,* Baltimore, 1960, Williams & Wilkins.

Nadas AS, Fyler DC: *Pediatric cardiology,* ed 3, Philadelphia, 1972, WB Saunders.

Smith TF, O'Day D, Wright PF: Clinical implications of preseptal (periorbital) cellulitis in childhood, *Pediatrics* 62:1006, 1978.

Stanisavljevic S: *Diagnosis and treatment of congenital hip pathology in the newborn,* Baltimore, 1964, Williams & Wilkins.

Wilkin L: *The diagnosis and treatment of endocrine disorders in childhood and adolescence,* ed 3, Springfield, Ill, 1965, Charles C Thomas.

8 Preoperative Assessment

Lynne G. Maxwell and Myron Yaster

Ambulatory or same-day surgery provides significant medical, psychological, and economic benefits to children and their families.[17,18,32] Indeed, it now constitutes more than 50% of all surgery performed in children. Much of the preoperative and postoperative patient care that in the past was provided in the hospital by the surgeon and anesthesiologist now is being performed by the child's pediatrician. Indeed, the pediatrician often is asked "to clear" children for surgery, with little, if any, guidance as to what this means. This chapter reviews the effects of anesthesia on children and highlights those aspects of the child's history and physical examination of particular importance to the anesthesiologist and surgeon.

EFFECTS OF GENERAL ANESTHESIA

General anesthesia abolishes the sensation of pain (analgesia), produces muscle paralysis, amnesia, and a loss of consciousness, and inhibits the adrenal-stress response to pain and surgery. Although the drugs that produce general anesthesia have very narrow therapeutic indices, modern anesthetic practice produces few, if any, perioperative complications. Nevertheless, children and their parents dread the entire experience of surgery. Young children are afraid of separation from their parents, older children fear potential mutilation and death, and teenagers fear all of this plus loss of control.[33] Young children often will struggle, scream, and cry when either separated from their parent(s) or when anesthesia is being induced, particularly if the induction technique is a "mask breathe down." This struggle (sometimes referred to as "brutane" anesthesia) often leads to a stormy induction of anesthesia and significantly increases the risks of airway compromise (laryngospasm, coughing, breath holding, and so forth), anesthetic overdose (hypotension), and arrhythmias, particularly when halothane is used as the induction agent. Furthermore, memories of this struggle or of the separation from one's parents may be long lasting, indeed, even longer lasting than the experience of surgery itself.

Parents fear for their child's life and safety as well. This sense of terror and foreboding is compounded by a sense of inadequacy and guilt. Rather than protecting their child from pain and suffering, they feel responsible for "causing" it or "allowing" it to happen.

Is this fear and foreboding necessary, and can it be allayed? Ultimately, this depends on how safe anesthesia actually is. Between 1978 and 1982, anesthesia *mortality* for French children less than 15 years of age was 1 in 40,000.[28] The incidence of anesthetic complications was 0.7/1000; cardiac arrest occurred in 12 of 40,000 patients but resulted in only one death. The incidence of complications was much higher in infants less than 1 year (4.3/1000). In a study reviewing the experience in an American hospital from 1969 to 1983, the overall mortality rate was 0.9/10,000 anesthetics with an incidence of cardiac arrest of 1.7/10,000.[11] In this study, children less than 12 years of age had a threefold higher incidence of cardiac arrest (4.7/10,000) when compared with adult patients (1.4/10,000).[11] Complications leading to cardiac arrest in these studies were due largely to complications of airway management (laryngospasm, difficult intubation, and pulmonary aspiration of gastric contents) or were secondary to halothane overdosage (hypotension, arrhythmia, or both). Infants less than 1 month have the greatest risk of serious intraoperative complications (cardiac arrest) and the highest perioperative death rates because they are more likely to be having major surgery (intrathoracic or intraabdominal) than are older children and are "sicker" (a greater percentage are ASA physical status 3 to 5) (see below). A recent review of closed anesthesia malpractice claims revealed that pediatric cases were related to respiratory events with a greater frequency than adult cases (43% vs. 30%), and the mortality rate was greater in the affected children (50% vs. 35%).

The American Society of Anesthesiologists (ASA) Physical Status classification (Table 8-1) provides a convenient method of summarizing the patient's physical condition and also may provide a means of assessing the relative risk of anesthesia. ASA physical status (PS) 1 patients are healthy and have no underlying disease, whereas ASA PS 4 patients are significantly incapacitated by their underlying disease. Other factors associated with increased preoperative risk are multiple coexistent diseases and the need for emergent surgery. The anesthetic mortality rate in healthy ASA PS 1 children requiring elective surgery is probably less than 1 in 50,000.

Children who are candidates for outpatient surgery generally are in the ASA PS 1 and 2 groups. Therefore, among ASA PS 1 and 2 children who require elective surgery, factors that could impose any additional perioperative risk (e.g., upper respiratory infection, recent meal) are considered unacceptable. ASA PS 3 and even 4 patients increasingly are undergoing outpatient surgery because insurance companies are refusing to pay for inpatient care. Unfortunately, whether this is safe or desirable is irrelevant. Because of the increased risk to these children, direct communication between the pediatrician and anesthesiologist is advised well in advance of the planned surgical procedure.

ANESTHETIC RELEVANCE OF THE HISTORY AND PHYSICAL EXAMINATION

The preoperative evaluation is concerned directly with the aspects of the child's history and physical examination that can affect the course of the anesthetic and perioperative management. This evaluation of children for anesthesia depends on

Table 8-1 ASA Physical Status Classification for Preoperative Assessment of Patients

PS 1	A normal healthy patient
PS 2	A patient with mild systemic disease
PS 3	A patient with severe systemic disease
PS 4	A patient with a severe systemic disease that is a constant threat to life
PS 5	A moribund patient who is not expected to survive without the operation

American Society of Anesthesiologists, Inc: ASA Relative Value Guide, Park Ridge, Ill, 1996.
PS, Physical Status.

an understanding of how anesthesia affects their normal physiology. The areas of primary concern in the history are related to neuromuscular, cardiovascular, respiratory, endocrine, and hematological or oncological diseases. The areas of key interest to the anesthesiologist in the physical examination are related to airway anatomy, the presence of stridor, wheezing, or murmurs, and evidence of preexisting neurological deficit. Many departments of anesthesiology will provide the pediatrician with a history and physical form for the purpose of reporting the preoperative evaluation (Fig. 8-1).

AIRWAY AND PULMONARY FUNCTION

General anesthesia alters respiratory function significantly at virtually every level. Early effects result from excitation of airway reflexes (laryngospasm, increased secretions, and bronchospasm) before the achievement of a depth of anesthesia appropriate for surgery during the inhalational induction of general anesthesia. The effects of anesthesia include decreased contractility of respiratory muscles, depressed ciliary clearance, depression of the central respiratory response to hypoxia and hypercarbia, decreased lung volume, and increased intrapulmonary shunting. These effects can result in serious and potentially life-threatening consequences, including upper airway obstruction, hypoventilation or apnea, and hypoxemia. The presence of underlying conditions (e.g., prematurity) or respiratory or airway diseases (e.g., asthma or bronchopulmonary dysplasia) compounds the risks of anesthesia greatly for the child. Therefore detailed information about preexisting respiratory disease should be available for the anesthesiologist.

Upper Respiratory Tract Infections

Children who have acute or recent viral or bacterial upper respiratory infections (URI) are at increased risk for airway and pulmonary complications during anesthesia.[3,16] This risk exists during the acute infection and persists for up to 6 weeks after the infection has run its course.[10] Anesthetic complications that occur commonly in children who have an acute URI or during their convalescence include bronchospasm, laryngospasm, acute subglottic edema with stridor, intraoperative and postoperative hypoxia, atelectasis, and postextubation croup. Endotracheal intubation increases the risk of respiratory complications significantly. Unfortunately, avoiding intubation often is impossible.

Interestingly, several studies have found no significant increase in respiratory complications among children anesthetized with an acute URI.[22] This has led some to advocate *not* canceling surgery for these children. It is our belief that the physiological, psychological, and financial implications of delays in surgery must be weighed against the risks of increased perioperative complications of anesthetizing a child who has a URI. Patients who have systemic manifestations, such as fever greater than 38.5° C, purulent nasal discharge, and lower respiratory symptoms such as productive cough, crackles, wheezes, or positive chest radiograph findings should have the surgical procedure delayed for 4 to 6 weeks after the resolution of symptoms.[10] Surgery and anesthesia usually can proceed safely in children who have none of these symptoms, particularly if they do not require endotracheal intubation (Fig. 8-2).

Asthma

Asthma is one of the most common and most serious underlying medical conditions that can affect patients undergoing general anesthesia.[9,12] Many procedures performed routinely during anesthetic management, most notably laryngoscopy and intubation, are potent and intense stimuli that produce bronchospasm. Intraoperative bronchospasm can be catastrophic; it may make ventilation difficult, if not impossible, and may result in hypercarbia, acidosis, hypoxia, cardiovascular collapse, and death. Fortunately, this need not and should not happen. Maximal preoperative optimization of a patient's medical management may prevent or, at the very least, limit all of the perioperative complications of asthma ("the best defense is a good offense"). In general, asthma medical therapy must be escalated preoperatively even in well-controlled or asymptomatic patients to limit or prevent intraoperative bronchospasm. Thus the child who takes asthma medications only on an as-needed ("prn") basis should begin his or her inhaled beta-agonists or oral medications 3 to 5 days preoperatively.[19,24] The child taking medications on a chronic basis (oral or inhaled) should have steroids added in doses that would be used for an acute exacerbation of this disease. Finally, the "difficult" asthmatic child who takes bronchodilators and steroids regularly requires either intensification in the frequency of nebulizer treatments, added bronchodilators, increased steroids, or on occasion, all of these.[19]

The child taking theophylline requires special attention. Serum levels (therapeutic range, 10 to 20 μg/ml) should be measured to optimize drug dosing and guide intraoperative bronchodilator therapy. Intraoperatively, the acute administration of intravenous doses of aminophylline is dangerous, even in the setting of low blood levels, because the interaction of high levels of aminophylline and inhalation general anesthetic agents often produces cardiac dysrhythmias, and wheezing may be treated adequately intraoperatively by the use of beta-agonists, steroids, and intravenous lidocaine (which also suppresses airway reflexes).

Elective surgery should never be performed in children who are wheezing actively or who have had a recent asthma attack. Decreased peak expiratory flow and FEV_1 occur in adults and children for up to 6 weeks following an acute asthma attack, and airways are more responsive and prone to bronchospasm in this period (see Upper Respiratory Tract Infections). Therefore a recent asthma exacerbation requiring hospital admission or emergency therapy within 6 weeks of

PREOPERATIVE EVALUATION/HISTORY AND PHYSICAL

DATE: ____________ TIME ______ AGE _____ SEX ____ RACE ____

PROCEDURE ____________________

DIAGNOSIS ____________________

MEDICATIONS ____________________

ALLERGIES ____________________

STAMP PATIENT'S IDENTIFICATION OR PRINT CLEARLY

NURSING UNIT / CLINIC

JHH HISTORY NUMBER

PATIENT'S NAME (LAST, FIRST, M.I.)

USE BALLPOINT PEN

PAST MEDICAL HISTORY AND REVIEW OF SYSTEMS

YES	NO	CARDIOVASCULAR
□	□	MI
□	□	HYPERTENSION
□	□	ARRHYTHMIA
□	□	ANGINA
□	□	CHF
□	□	VALVULAR DISEASE
□	□	PERIPHERAL VASC. DISEASE
□	□	PAST CARDIAC SURGERY
□	□	OTHER
		PULMONARY
□	□	SMOKING Hx
□	□	ASTHMA
□	□	COPD/EMPHYSEMA/BPD
□	□	OTHER
		RENAL
□	□	RENAL FAILURE
□	□	OTHER

YES	NO	HEPATIC
□	□	HEPATITIS
□	□	OTHER
		ENDOCRINE
□	□	DIABETES
□	□	OTHER
		INFECTIOUS
□	□	SEPSIS
□	□	OTHER
		NEUROLOGIC
□	□	SEIZURE
□	□	ELEVATED ICP
□	□	CEREBROVASC. DISEASE
□	□	NEUROMUSCULAR DISORDER
□	□	OTHER
		GASTROINTESTINAL
□	□	G.E. REFLUX/HIATAL HERNIA
□	□	BOWEL OBSTRUCTION
□	□	OTHER

YES	NO	HEMATOLOGIC
□	□	SICKLE CELL
□	□	COAGULOPATHY
□	□	PREGNANCY/TRANSFUSION WITHIN LAST 3 MONTHS Y/N
□	□	OTHER
		PEDIATRICS
□	□	PREMATURITY
□	□	CONGENITAL ABN.
□	□	APNEA
□	□	OTHER
		OBSTETRICS
□	□	PREECLAMPSIA/ECLAMPSIA
□	□	PREMATURITY
□	□	PLACENTA PREVIA/ABRUPTIO
□	□	LMP______
□	□	OTHER
		ANESTHETIC DIFFICULTIES
□	□	DIFFICULT INTUBATION
□	□	FAMILY HISTORY
□	□	OTHER
		DRUG USE
□	□	ETOH
□	□	OTHER

□ HISTORY UNKNOWN EXCEPT AS NOTED ABOVE

EXPLANATION OF POSITIVE DATA ____________________

PHYSICAL EXAMINATION BP (RANGE): __________ P ______ R ______ T _____ WT ______ (lbs.) (Kg.)

LABS:

H&P PERFORMED BY ____________

ECG FINDINGS: ____________

RISK FACTORS:

HEMODYNAMIC COMPROMISE ________ OTHER ________

CRITICAL AIRWAY ________

FULL STOMACH ________ LAST PO ________

IMPRESSION: ASA STATUS | 1 | 2 | 3 | 4 | 5 | E | ____________

REVIEWED BY: M.D. | DATE TIME

CHART COPY

FIG. 8-1 Example of preoperative evaluation/history and physical examination form. (From the Johns Hopkins Hospital, Department of Anesthesiology and Critical Care Medicine, 1988.)

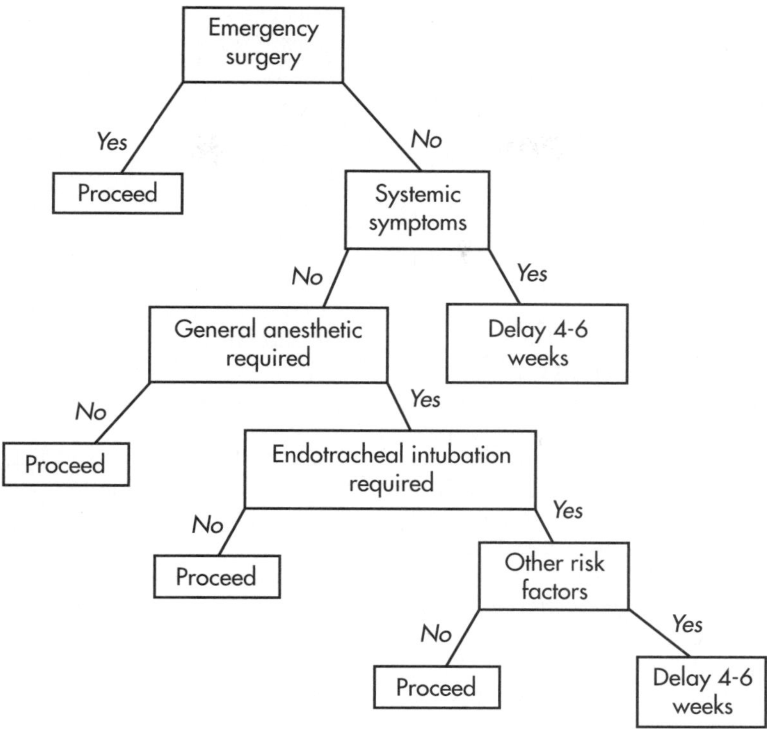

FIG. 8-2 Suggested clinical decision tree for patients who have a recent history of upper respiratory infection being evaluated for surgery.
(From Martin LD: *Pediatr Clin North Am* 41:121, 1994.)

surgery precludes elective surgery. *Elective* surgery in asthmatic children who have an upper respiratory tract infection should be delayed 6 weeks, even if they have no wheezing on ausculation, because the incidence of bronchospasm is likely to be increased greatly beyond that seen in nonasthmatic children—an elevenfold increase in respiratory complications when children require endotracheal intubation as part of anesthetic management.

Corticosteroids are extremely effective in preventing perioperative wheezing, even in patients who have severe asthma.[19] Patients should receive 1 mg/kg of prednisone orally once daily for 3 days before surgery and on the morning of surgery. Although the chronic administration of high-dose corticosteroids for the treatment of asthma can be associated with severe systemic side effects, the short-term perioperative administration just described is safe and most effective in decreasing the incidence of perioperative bronchospasm. All oral medications may be taken with small amounts of water on the morning of surgery.

Pulmonary Function Tests

Pulmonary function tests often are used to assess the response to bronchodilator therapy in patients whose bronchospasm is reversible. Although they rarely are necessary preoperatively in patients who have uncomplicated asthma, these tests may be useful in predicting whether children who have pulmonary or thoracic cage abnormalities are at increased risk for anesthetic complications. The studies used most commonly are pulse oximetry, forced vital capacity (FVC), and forced expired volume in the first second of expiration (FEV_1). The absolute values obtained and the ratio of the two measurements (FEV_1/FVC) are useful predictors of the need for postoperative mechanical ventilation among patients at risk (e.g., kyphoscoliosis). In adults, an FEV_1/FVC <50%, an FEV_1 <35% predicted, or an absolute FVC <25 ml/kg is associated with inadequate postoperative ventilation and usually results in prolonged mechanical ventilation. However, the accurate measurement of FEV_1 and FVC requires patient cooperation; therefore it usually is not possible to obtain reliable results in children younger than 6 years.

PREMATURITY AND APNEA

Infants born prematurely (<37 weeks) have a significantly increased risk of developing postoperative apnea (>15 seconds).[29] Former preterm infants who undergo general anesthesia have an increased incidence of apnea, periodic breathing, and bradycardia for up to 24 hours after surgery when compared with full-term infants. Regardless of a patient's age, all general anesthetics, sedatives, hypnotics, and opioids produce dose-dependent and drug-specific alterations in the mechanics and central control of the respiratory system. This places the prematurely born infant at particular risk for developing apnea because the central and peripheral chemoreceptors are immature and limit effective responses to hypoxia and hypercarbia, even without the additional burden of drug-induced depression. Furthermore, the general anesthetics decrease muscle tone in the airways, chest wall, and diaphragm and thereby depress the ventilatory response to hypoxia and hypercarbia further.

Several studies have demonstrated an increased risk for apnea to develop postoperatively in former preterm infants undergoing minor and major surgical procedures.[15] This risk can be minimized by the perioperative administration of caffeine (or theophylline), the use of spinal anesthesia instead of general anesthesia, and the delaying of surgery until the child is older than 48 to 60 postconceptual weeks.[30,31] Welborn et al. in a double-blind study demonstrated that 10 mg/kg of caffeine base (which is equivalent to 20 mg/kg of caffeine citrate or benzoate) given intravenously after the induction of general anesthesia virtually eliminated postoperative apnea.[30] These same investigators and others also have demonstrated that spinal anesthesia (particularly in inguinal hernia surgery) decreased the risk of postoperative apnea significantly.[31] Nevertheless, it is our belief, albeit conservative, that the risk of postanesthesia apnea has been defined clearly and that the use of caffeine and spinal anesthesia as prophylaxis has been studied only in very small patient populations. Therefore, it is our practice to admit all at-risk patients, regardless of the anesthetic technique used, to monitored, high-surveillance in-patient units for 24 hours after anesthesia and surgery.

In addition, former premature infants who were intubated and ventilated as neonates are at increased risk for subglottic stenosis. While a negative history does not exclude the diagnosis, a history of croup or stridor is a very important warning sign of possible subglottic narrowing.

BRONCHOPULMONARY DYSPLASIA

Bronchopulmonary dysplasia (BPD) significantly complicates the anesthetic management of children. Several effects of anesthesia, together or separately, produce life-threatening consequences. Pulmonary vasoconstriction following anesthetic induction can aggravate ventilation-perfusion mismatch and lead to profound hypoxemia. Anesthetic effects on myocardial contractility can result in impaired right ventricular function, reduced cardiac output, pulmonary hypoperfusion, and profound cardiovascular compromise with hypoxemia resembling acute cor pulmonale. Increased airway reactivity during induction of or emergence from anesthesia can result in a severe exacerbation of BPD with an increased ventilation-perfusion mismatch. Increased oral and bronchial secretions induced by the anesthetic can compromise airflow and lead to airway or endotracheal tube plugging. Because of diminished respiratory reserves in these patients, such plugging can cause death quickly. These children also may have a degree of increased airway reactivity and tracheomalacia. Intraoperative bronchospasm or airway collapse poses a serious intraoperative risk. Finally, infections of the respiratory tract occur frequently in children who have BPD, and the presence of pneumonia can complicate the perioperative course significantly.

It is essential that the pulmonary status of these children be optimized before surgery and anesthesia. Bronchodilators, antibiotics, diuretics, and corticosteroid therapy all may benefit these children. Respiratory infections or bronchospasm in children who have BPD must be treated thoroughly before elective surgery. In children who have severe BPD and bronchospasm, preoperative treatment with increased inspired oxygen tension may decrease pulmonary vasoreactivity and improve cardiovascular function. The possibility of associated right ventricular dysfunction always should be considered and, where indicated, evaluated with ECG and echocardiography. Because these children are at major risk for perioperative mortality and morbidity, the situation should be explained to parents before surgery. In addition, these children may require continuous postoperative monitoring and ventilation for an extended period (24 to 48 hours). Risks of general anesthesia and intubation in these children sometimes can be avoided with the judicious use of regional anesthesia (caudal or spinal) for operations such as hernia repair in infants under 6 months. Parents must be cautioned, however, that regional anesthesia may not be 100% successful and that intubation might still be required.

OBSTRUCTIVE SLEEP APNEA

Children who have long-standing obstructive sleep apnea secondary to adenotonsillar hypertrophy, obesity, or other cause also can develop significant pulmonary hypertension and cor pulmonale.[8] Like children who have BPD, these youngsters also are at risk for perioperative hypoxemia and acute right heart failure. Patients at greatest risk are those who demonstrate daytime somnolence, complete or frequent obstructive apnea events, cyanosis during sleep, or signs of cardiopulmonary dysfunction.[8] Preoperatively, these children should undergo a hematocrit, chest radiograph, ECG, and echocardiogram. Postoperatively, they should be admitted to the pediatric intensive care unit because the incidence of obstructive events actually may increase during the first 24 hours after surgery.

CARDIOVASCULAR

All anesthetic agents can affect the normal cardiovascular system profoundly and adversely. The sinus node, conduction system, and myocardial contractility all can be depressed by general anesthetics. Moreover, general anesthesia alters both preload and afterload by relaxing vascular smooth muscle tone. General anesthetics also attenuate hypoxic pulmonary vasoconstriction and thereby impair ventilation perfusion matching. Finally, halothane, the potent vapor anesthetic used most commonly in pediatric patients, may produce arrhythmias, even in patients who have no underlying conduction defects. Although severe arrhythmias are possible in normal children theoretically, they are more common in those receiving other drugs that are arrhythmogenic, such as epinephrine (often injected by surgeons to cause vasoconstriction and decrease surgical bleeding) or aminophylline. Other patients at increased risk are those who have underlying conduction abnormalities, especially syndromes associated with a prolonged QT interval. More commonly, however, the only manifestations of halothane's effects on the conducting system are occasional PVCs or bigeminy, both of which are seen frequently in association with hypercarbia due to hypoventilation or with "light" or inadequate anesthesia. These mild dysrhythmias are treated easily by increasing the minute ventilation or the depth of anesthesia.

Important, common effects of inhalation agents on the cardiovascular system include vasodilation and depression of myocardial contractility. These actions often combine to cause some degree of hypotension, which may be severe in patients who are relatively hypovolemic because of prolonged fasting or extraordinary fluid losses (diarrhea, vomiting, hemorrhage). The presence of underlying heart disease (e.g., congestive heart failure, dysrhythmias, and intracardiac shunts) magnifies the inherent risks of anesthesia. Accordingly, thorough cardiovascular assessment is a critical part of preoperative preparation.

Intracardiac Shunts

Most anesthetic agents decrease vascular tone and thus decrease both pulmonary and systemic vascular resistance. The relative changes in these resistances can alter the dynamics of intracardiac shunts. Thus, during general anesthesia a left-to-right intracardiac shunt (e.g., ventricular septal defect) may produce pulmonary over-circulation and failure. In contrast, during anesthesia pulmonary vascular resistance may increase acutely as a consequence of hypoxia, hypercarbia, acidosis, and hypotension. Thus a predominantly left-to-right shunt can be converted to a right-to-left shunt, which can have catastrophic consequences (e.g., hypoxemia, or acute cor pulmonale). Children who have intracardiac shunts also can have "paradoxical embolism" produced by air or a thrombus traveling from the venous circulation into the systemic circulation (e.g., cerebral arteries). For these reasons, intracardiac shunts must be identified preoperatively.

Murmurs

Cardiac murmurs are common in children (see Chapter 138). Murmurs are either "functional" or pathological. It is imperative that patients who have congenital anomalies of the heart or great vessels be identified before anesthesia. In general, the child who has a murmur but who has a normal S_1 and S_2, normal exercise tolerance, is acyanotic, and is growing well will tolerate a general anesthetic without complication. However, even asymptomatic patients who have a previously unrecognized pathological murmur should be assessed appropriately and may require antibiotic prophylaxis. Appropriate preoperative evaluation reasonably includes a thorough physical examination and electrocardiogram. If there is any question of a cardiac abnormality, preoperative echocardiography and evaluation by a pediatric cardiologist are necessary.

The presence of an abnormal murmur, cyanosis, decreased exercise tolerance, poor weight gain, sweating, decreased femoral pulses, or a precordial heave necessitates a more complete preoperative evaluation (hematocrit, ECG, chest radiograph, oxygen saturation, and cardiology consultation). If a child who has known congenital heart disease presents for preoperative evaluation, the precise details of any previous surgery, current intracardiac anatomy, cardiac conduction defects, and myocardial function should be documented and the anesthesiologist informed of the findings before surgery. Any anatomical defects should be described and the amount of intracardiac shunting and resting arterial saturation quantified. The pediatrician or cardiologist also should note the cardiac medications the child is taking and any recent changes in the child's status.

Subacute Bacterial Endocarditis Prophylaxis

Antibiotic prophylaxis to prevent bacterial endocarditis is indicated for children who have congenital heart disease and are undergoing any procedure in which the patient is at risk for transient bacteremia (e.g., dental, sinus, airway, genitourinary, gastrointestinal) or when the surgical site, though normally sterile, is contaminated. In addition to patients who have shunts, patients who have hemodynamically insignificant lesions (bicuspid aortic valve, mitral valve prolapse, or a history of infective carditis) also require perioperative prophylaxis. All patients who have undergone palliative or corrective cardiac operations require prophylaxis for the rest of their lives. The only exceptions are those children who have had a patent ductus arteriosus ligated or who have had a primary closure of a secundum atrial septal defect without a prosthetic patch; these two groups of patients require prophylaxis for only the first 6 months postoperatively. Oral endotracheal intubation by itself is not an indication for SBE prophylaxis, but nasotracheal intubation does require prophylaxis. The antibiotic regimen recommended by the American Heart Association[2] should be followed (see the box on p. 104). It usually is acceptable for the antibiotic to be given when the IV is started after induction of anesthesia because the interval between start of the IV and the incision generally is long enough (5 minutes) to achieve adequate blood levels. It is unnecessary to start an IV in a child who is awake solely to administer antibiotics for SBE prophylaxis. The necessity for continuing the antibiotic therapy postoperatively should be emphasized to the family because the child may be discharged as soon as 1 to 2 hours after surgery.

NEUROMUSCULAR DISEASES

Anesthetic agents affect the CNS globally in addition to providing anesthesia. Although suppression of awareness and central responses to pain are desirable, anesthetics also inhibit vital central nervous system functions. Thus respiratory depression, inhibition of autonomic tone, and impaired reflex regulation all occur during general anesthesia. Anesthetics also alter cerebrovascular tone, autoregulation, and intracranial fluid dynamics. Thus anesthetic agents that cause cerebrovascular dilation can alter intracranial space compliance and cerebral perfusion pressure. The potent inhalational agents (halothane, enflurane, isoflurane, desflurane, and sevoflurane) produce sluggish motor reflex responses and impair coordination, effects that may persist for hours after cessation of anesthetic administration. Preexisting neuromuscular weakness may be exacerbated significantly. The normal child may manifest long tract signs transiently, including hyperextension and hypertonicity associated with extensor plantar reflexes. There may be anisocoria or exacerbation of underlying hemiparesis. Although most general anesthetics are anticonvulsants, patients may have seizures after clinically appropriate doses of enflurane and methohexital; thus these agents usually are avoided in patients who have a known seizure disorder. Finally, chronic or acute preoperative ingestion of CNS stimulants (e.g., methylphenidate, cocaine, and amphetamines) may increase anesthetic requirements significantly.[4]

For these reasons the presence of central neurological or peripheral neuromuscular abnormalities must be documented preoperatively. Because virtually all anesthetics produce cerebral vasodilation and thereby may increase intracranial pressure, children at risk for intracranial hypertension (e.g., hydrocephalus, brain tumor, and blocked ventriculoperitoneal

ANTIBIOTIC REGIMENS FOR INFECTIVE ENDOCARDITIS PROPHYLAXIS

Upper respiratory tract surgical procedures (including oral surgery and dental procedures causing gingival bleeding)

1. Standard regimens
   a. Amoxicillin 50 mg/kg (up to 3 g) po 1 hr before the procedure and ½ the initial dose 6 hr later.
   b. For children unable to take oral medications, parenteral ampicillin 50 mg/kg (up to 2 g) 30 min before the procedure and ½ the initial dose 6 hr later.
2. Regimen for those who have intracardiac prosthetic valves or systemic-pulmonary shunts
   Parenteral ampicillin 50 mg/kg (up to 2 g) plus parenteral gentamicin 2.0 mg/kg (up to 80 mg), given 30 min before the procedure. Oral amoxicillin 25 mg/kg (up to 1.5 g) is given 6 hr after the initial antibiotics, or the parenteral regimen can be repeated 8 hr after the first dose. Many authorities recommend one of the above standard regimens for this high-risk group.
3. Regimen for penicillin-allergic patients
   a. Oral: Erythromycin ethylsuccinate or stearate 20 mg/kg (up to 800 mg of erythromycin ethylsuccinate or ≤1 g of erythromycin stearate) 2 hr before the procedure, followed by ½ the initial dose 6 hr later. Alternative regimen: Clindamycin 10 mg/kg (up to 300 mg) po 1 hr before the procedure, followed by ½ the initial dose 6 hr later.
   b. Parenteral: Clindamycin 10 mg/kg IV (up to 300 mg) 30 min before the procedure, followed by ½ the initial dose 6 hr later.
   c. Parenteral for patients who have intracardiac prosthetic material or systemic-pulmonary shunts: Vancomycin 20 mg/kg IV (up to 1g) given over 1 hr, starting 1 hr before the procedure.

For GI/GU surgical procedures

1. Standard regimen: Parenteral ampicillin and gentamicin 30 to 60 min before the procedure and again 8 hr later. Alternatively, oral amoxicillin may be given 6 hr after the initial antibiotics. Dosages are the same as for upper respiratory tract surgery.
2. Oral regimen for minor procedures in a low-risk patient: Amoxicillin 50 mg/kg (up to 3 g) 1 hr before the procedure and ½ the initial dose 6 hr later.
3. Regimen for penicillin-allergic patients: IV vancomycin and gentamicin 1 hr before the procedure, with a repeat dose 8 hr later. Dosages are the same as given for upper respiratory tract surgical procedures.

shunts) must be identified before surgery. Any existing CSF shunt must be evaluated appropriately for patency and proper functioning before surgery. In addition, because residual anesthetic effects may impair airway reflexes in the immediate postoperative period, any evidence of brainstem dysfunction (vocal cord paralysis, swallowing dysfunction, and/or aspiration) should be noted in the preoperative evaluation.

Patients who have neuromuscular and degenerative diseases are at increased risk of postoperative weakness. This may require postoperative respiratory care and even prolonged mechanical ventilation. In children who have progressive diseases of nerve or muscle, hyperkalemia or malignant hyperthermia occur more commonly after succinylcholine administration. Indeed, the fear of fatal hyperkalemia following succinylcholine administration in patients who have undiagnosed muscular dystrophy has led the Food and Drug Administration recently to contraindicate the use of succinylcholine in routine intubations in all children.

Patients receiving anticonvulsant medication should have blood concentrations measured to ensure therapeutic levels perioperatively. These children may require perioperative IV administration of anticonvulsants because postoperative fasting or vomiting may not allow maintenance of therapeutic blood levels with orally administered drugs. However, most anticonvulsants have very long half-lives, and the omission of one dose will not decrease the blood level significantly. Patients who have been seizure-free for 2 years and have had no adjustment of their anticonvulsant dose probably do not require the determination of anticonvulsant levels, but the anesthesiologist should be informed to make sure that he or she agrees with this plan.

ENDOCRINE

Anesthesia and surgery subject the child to significant stresses. Children have greatly increased circulating levels of epinephrine, norepinephrine, and cortisol during surgery. The insulin/glucagon relationship is altered dramatically. Moreover, a stress-related catabolic state persists long after the day of surgery. Therefore the child undergoing surgery should be in the best nutritional state possible before elective surgery is contemplated.

The stress associated with surgery produces a hyperglycemic response because of increased levels of circulating corticosteroids and catecholamines, even with prolonged preoperative fasting. However, in infants and small children, even mild fasting can be associated with perioperative hypoglycemia, especially in infants less than 1 year or who have a history of premature birth.

Diabetes Mellitus

The most common endocrinological problem in the perioperative period is diabetes mellitus. Insulin-dependent diabetic children experience significant perioperative difficulties, even when their control is good. Brittle or noncompliant diabetic patients have additional problems, including an increased risk of perioperative hypoglycemia or hyperglycemia, osmotic diuresis, intravascular hypovolemia, and altered mental status. It is essential to document the child's insulin regimen, the degree of compliance, how well the blood glucose concentration is controlled, and whether the child has any adverse effects of a short to moderate fast. A recent growth history also is useful to indicate how well controlled the child's diabetes may be. Various techniques for managing preoperative insulin therapy have been proposed (Table 8-2). We generally recommend that the child follow routine preoperative fasting guidelines for surgery—namely, that children do not eat solids foods (including breast milk) for at least 6 hours before surgery.[25,26] Patients are allowed to drink clear liquids for up to 2 to 3 hours before surgery.[25,26]

The insulin dose should be decreased to half of the child's usual morning dose on the day of surgery and given as

Table 8-2 Protocols for Perioperative Insulin Therapy

Classic regimen (morning of surgery)	Start IV infusion 5% dextrose in 0.45% saline at 1500 ml/m²/day Administer ½ usual morning insulin dose Check blood glucose before induction and during anesthesia
Continuous insulin infusion (morning of surgery)	Start IV infusion 5% dextrose in 0.45% saline at 1500 ml/m²/day Add 1-2 units of insulin per ml of 5% dextrose Check blood glucose before induction and during anesthesia
Insulin- and glucose-free regimen (for operative procedures of short duration on the morning of surgery)	Withhold morning insulin dose If indicated for the procedure: glucose-free solution (e.g., lactated Ringer) at maintenance rate Check blood glucose before induction and during anesthesia

soluble insulin. This seems reasonable because mild to moderate hyperglycemia (without ketosis) usually does not present a serious problem to the child, whereas hypoglycemia has devastating consequences. In the anesthetized child, the usual signs of hypoglycemia (tachycardia, diaphoresis, lethargy progressing to obtunded mental status) are masked and a significant hypoglycemic insult can occur intraoperatively with little evidence of it until attempts are made to awaken the child. Heavy preoperative sedation also is avoided in diabetic children so that their level of consciousness can be assessed readily during the perioperative period.

Patients on long-term corticosteroid therapy and those who have congenital adrenal insufficiency have suppression of the hypothalmic-pituitary-adrenal axis; therefore they cannot manifest an appropriate stress response and are at risk for severe hemodynamic compromise (Addisonian crisis). Long-term corticosteroid therapy is used commonly for a variety of illnesses. The severity of the underlying disease state and any associated complications must be noted appropriately, as should side effects of steroid therapy, including Cushingoid facies, vascular and bleeding abnormalities, myopathy, and cardiomyopathy. For these reasons, children who are receiving long-term or intermittent corticosteroid therapy should be treated with corticosteroids for 24 hours before surgery. "Stress doses" of steroids are administered commonly to patients on chronic steroid therapy. Although this is of theoretical benefit, the necessity of this regimen has not been substantiated in human studies. In fact, studies in patients undergoing surgery suggest that such stress doses are unnecessary. Even so, until this issue is resolved, we recommend the administration of 2.5 to 5 mg/m^2 of prednisone orally the night before and 25 to 50 mg/m^2 of hydrocortisone after the IV is started before or after anesthetic induction.

HEMATOLOGICAL

Hematological conditions that may complicate perioperative management include anemia, sickle cell disease, and the presence of a bleeding diathesis (e.g., factor deficiency syndromes and chronic aspirin therapy). Anemia is associated with a reduction in the oxygen-carrying capacity and a secondary increase in cardiac output. Anemia often is tolerated well; unfortunately, many perioperative events (e.g., blood loss or anesthesia-induced myocardial depression) can subject the child with intact and compensated cardiac function to cellular hypoxia and cardiovascular collapse when the stresses of anesthesia and surgery overwhelm the anemic patient's delicate balance of oxygen supply and demand. Furthermore, an anemic child is more likely to need blood transfusions perioperatively if significant bleeding occurs, whereas even in the face of moderate amounts of blood loss, it is common to avoid administration of blood products in children who have normal preoperative hemoglobin. Although the hemoglobin value at which individual anesthesiologists choose to transfuse varies greatly, most anesthesiologists allow a normal child's hemoglobin to decline to 7 to 8 g/dl before he or she transfuses blood.

A child who has a previously undiagnosed anemia may have a serious underlying disorder such as sickle cell anemia or blood dyscrasia that requires additional evaluation before surgery. Thus the cause of any significant anemia (hemoglobin <9) should be determined preoperatively. Nutritional causes (e.g., iron deficiency) often require relatively brief periods of therapy to improve the child's anemia. The presence of a mild anemia should not delay urgent surgery. For elective surgery, consultation with the anesthesia and surgical team may be required. Nevertheless, the incidence of previously undetected anemia in children presenting for elective surgery is extremely low. Therefore, *we do not advocate routine determination of hematocrit and hemoglobin* if studies performed previously as part of well child care have been normal (see Preoperative Laboratory Testing below).

Sickle Cell Anemia

Patients who have sickle cell anemia (SSA) have an increased risk of complications from general anesthesia and surgery. Sickling readily occurs with hypoxia, hypercarbia, acidosis, hypothermia, hypovolemia, and hypoperfusion states, all of which can occur perioperatively. Decreased functional residual capacity and altered ventilation-perfusion ratios, which occur commonly during general anesthesia, may give rise to transient hypoxemia, which may precipitate sickling and contribute to postoperative acute chest syndrome. Immobility, vasoconstriction, increased insensible fluid loss, and position on the operating table may produce regional hypoperfusion and stasis. Children who have SSA and who are significantly anemic may benefit from simple red cell transfusions preoperatively. For prolonged or extensive operations, multiple simple or exchange transfusions to achieve hemoglobin S levels less than 30% are recommended.[13] Measures should be taken to ensure adequate perioperative hydration, especially because patients who have SSA and, to a lesser extent, children who have sickle trait have hyposthenuria, and the urine will remain inappropriately dilute, even in the face of significant intravascular volume depletion.

Sickle cell anemia frequently is associated with cardiomyopathy, nephropathy, central and peripheral neuropathy, or chronic respiratory dysfunction—all of which may complicate general anesthesia or the perioperative course. Because of the potential for further impairment during general anesthesia, it is necessary to document the degree of involvement of these organ systems. The preoperative assessment also should describe the type of sickle crises the child usually experiences and the date of the most recent crisis. The pediatrician should note the extent of preexisting disease and consult with the anesthesiologist regarding the need for special preoperative preparation, including transfusion therapy. Other forms of hemoglobinopathies such as Cooley anemia, sickle-C, and thalassemia have important anesthetic implications, and such diagnoses should be communicated to the anesthesiologist.

An underlying bleeding diathesis may create serious problems in the perioperative period because of increased intraoperative and perioperative blood loss, CNS and other organ damage from hemorrhage, and hematoma formation. Children who have factor deficiencies are at greatly increased risk for perioperative bleeding unless they receive factor replacement before, during, and after surgery. For minor operations the goal is 25% to 40% of normal factor levels preoperatively; for major procedures the target is 50% of normal with repeat doses administered intraoperatively to maintain that level. Children receiving aspirin therapy may have a higher risk for bleeding because of platelet dysfunction. This usually presents no problems for minor procedures, but such patients may benefit from discontinuation of aspirin therapy 1 week before a major procedure.

Transfusions

Questions frequently are raised by parents regarding transfusion practices. Parents are anxious about the infectious risks of transfusion, and some may have religious objections. Parents should be informed realistically about the risks of excessive blood loss in the operation their child faces. Children as small as 30 kg who have normal hematocrits may donate autologous blood in advance of elective procedures. This possibility should be discussed with the surgeon and arranged through the hospital blood bank. Some blood banks will allow "directed" donation (allogenic or homologous blood), in which a family member who has the same blood type as the patient donates blood for a specific family member. It must be remembered that some blood banks do not screen directed donor units for HIV or hepatitis and that these units may represent a greater risk of infection than the regular blood supply.

SPECIAL PROBLEMS

Malignant Hyperthermia

Malignant hyperthermia is a rare (1:15,000 children; 1:40,000 adults), potentially lethal disorder of acute hypermetabolism induced almost exclusively by exposure to volatile anesthetics (halothane, enflurane, and isoflurane) and succinylcholine.[14,27] It is an inherited disorder of intracellular calcium regulation and is a widespread membrane defect that exists in many cell types, particularly skeletal muscle. Fortunately, it can be prevented by avoiding triggering agents if the diagnosis is known or suspected. Because of the high risk of mortality, the pediatrician should note any history of anesthetic problems in the patient and family, especially if high fevers were involved. Preoperative preparation for such children includes consultation with the surgeon and anesthesiologist and avoidance of triggering agents. Dantrolene sodium, a direct-acting muscle relaxant, has been used with great success in treating the full-blown disease and may be used prophylactically.

Oncology

Children who have received certain chemotherapeutic agents may be at increased risk during the perioperative period because of the adverse effects of therapy. Bleomycin, BCNU, busulfan, cyclophosphamide, and methotrexate all have been associated with pulmonary fibrosis.[1] Exposure to even the modest levels of supplemental oxygen required for all patients who receive general anesthesia may aggravate the underlying lung disease greatly. Myocardial damage has been reported with cyclophosphamide, doxorubicin, adriamycin, m-AMSA, and radiation therapy. Inhalational anesthetics are arrhythmogenic and depress myocardial contractility. Patients who have myocardial damage may develop hypotension, even at low concentrations of inhaled anesthetics. Perioperative hypercarbia and stress can increase the risks of arrhythmia further. Consequently, the preoperative history should include the type and amount of chemotherapy and the extent of any associated complications. In addition to the physical examination, evaluation may include, depending on the history, chest radiographs, arterial blood gas measurements, an electrocardiogram, and echocardiography to document the extent of cardiorespiratory involvement. A patient who is asymptomatic and whose activity is unrestricted may need no additional laboratory tests. Preoperative communication of this information to the anesthesiologist will help identify children who require further evaluation.

Connective Tissue Disorders

Children who have connective tissue disorders may have multiple organ system involvement. These patients often are treated with aspirin or other nonsteroidal antiinflammatory drugs (NSAIDs), which may complicate their perioperative management further by causing a bleeding diathesis due to platelet dysfunction. The effect of aspirin and NSAIDs on platelet function is long-lived, and aspirin or other nonsteroidal antiinflammatory drugs should be stopped 1 week preoperatively. If these drugs cannot be stopped, a bleeding time may be performed to evaluate the extent of platelet impairment. Determination of prothrombin and partial thromboplastin times will not reflect this abnormality.

Patients who have connective tissue disorders may have associated dysphagia and esophageal dysmotility, which can predispose patients to pulmonary aspiration of gastric and esophageal contents. Extensive fibrosis of the temporomandibular or cricoarytenoid joint can complicate airway management and endotracheal intubation. Pulmonary infiltration and fibrosis may complicate intraoperative care by causing hypoxemia. Hematological abnormalities, including anemia of chronic disease, may complicate management even further. Again, the history should focus on the extent of disease, the type of treatment, and the child's response to therapy. Laboratory assessment may include an ECG, a chest radiograph, electrolytes, blood urea nitrogen, creatinine, hemoglobin, hematocrit, and platelet levels, as well as evaluation of the peripheral blood smear. A patient who has quiescent disease and who has regular follow-up may need nothing other than his or her hematocrit determined.

MEDICATIONS

Children receive medications regularly for many illnesses. The dosage should be adjusted to ensure adequate therapeutic levels perioperatively. The medications ordinarily are continued at usual doses up to and including the day of surgery. The two current exceptions to this practice are the use of monoamine oxidase (MAO) inhibitors and tricyclic antidepressants (TCA). The MAO inhibitors infrequently are encountered in younger children and adolescents; however, TCAs, such as imipramine and its analogs, are used commonly in the treatment of enuresis. In children receiving MAO inhibitors, the administration of meperidine (Demerol) or pancuronium (Pavulon) can have profound, catastrophic consequences (malignant hypertension and tachycardia, the neuroleptic malignant syndrome).[5] The TCAs can produce significant conduction abnormalities undetected by electrocardiography; moreover, when combined with the volatile anesthetic halothane, TCAs have resulted in life-threatening arrhythmias in the perioperative period. Therefore it is best to discontinue these agents 2 to 3 weeks before the scheduled operation. If this cannot be done without risk to the patient, preoperative consultation with the anesthesiologist is necessary.

RELEVANT ASPECTS OF THE PHYSICAL EXAMINATION

The physical examination is directed at the general state of health and specifically to discover conditions that could complicate anesthesia. The cardiovascular and respiratory systems demand close attention and documentation. Neurological status should be evaluated and preexisting deficits specifically documented. Recording of all abnormalities will assist the anesthesiologist in developing an appropriate plan.

The pediatrician should note the general body habitus, height, weight (in kg), and percentiles. An obese or Cushingoid child can have significant hypoventilation or airway obstruction in the supine position and under anesthesia and is at increased risk for aspiration pneumonitis. A careful examination of the head and neck is essential. A short neck, large tongue, and a small mandible all constitute sources of airway obstruction and may lead to delay or impossibility in intubating the trachea because of the difficulty in seeing the glottic opening. Midfacial or maxillary hypoplasia may present similar problems. In addition to difficulty with intubation, such patients may have airway obstruction on induction of anesthesia and difficulty with ventilation.

In addition to having the above airway concerns because of large tongues and relatively hypoplastic midface, patients who have Down syndrome may have atlantoaxial instability. This may manifest only under general anesthesia and neuromuscular blockade and can result in damage to the cervical spinal cord.[20,21] Parents should be questioned regarding any neurological symptoms such as long-track signs (hyperreflexia, Babinski, and clonus), hand weakness, or bladder and bowel dysfunction. History of torticollis or neck pain should be elicited. Even in the absence of symptoms, we recommend that children who have Down syndrome and are 2 years or older have lateral flexion and extension radiographs of the cervical spine before anesthesia in order that patients at risk for subluxation be identified. Some children over 5 years will have had these films as a requirement for their participation in Special Olympics. If radiographs reveal an atlantodens interval of greater than 5 mm (usually maximal in the flexion view), the child should be referred for orthopedic or neurosurgical consultation before elective surgery.

Some "dwarfing" syndromes can be associated with airway and cardiorespiratory abnormalities that can present significant problems perioperatively. In all children, the presence of loose or fractured teeth must be documented to guard against potential aspiration, because the teeth and oral mucosa may be subject to trauma during airway manipulation.

Preoperative vital signs, including weight in kg, temperature, respiratory rate, heart rate, and blood pressure should be noted. Preoperative recognition of any cardiovascular compromise may prevent significant perioperative problems. For example, patients who have significant chest wall or thoracic deformities (e.g., severe scoliosis and dwarfism) can have marked cardiorespiratory compromise manifested as decreased lung volumes and pulmonary function and have myocardial strain evident on ECG or echocardiogram. Such patients are at risk for intraoperative complications and prolonged postoperative mechanical ventilation. Therefore they need preoperative pulmonary function studies and evaluation of their myocardial function to enable the anesthesiologist to design the optimal anesthetic plan.

LABORATORY EXAMINATION

Laboratory studies are performed to detect significant physiological abnormalities that may prove hazardous to the child perioperatively. In an otherwise healthy child scheduled for outpatient surgery, routine laboratory tests rarely are indicated. Routine preoperative chest radiographs in well children have failed to detect abnormalities of major anesthetic or surgical consequence.[6] Screening tests for hemoglobin and hematocrit values commonly are obtained in the hope of identifying and treating those who have significant anemia. However, recent studies indicate that the incidence of previously undetected anemia in children presenting for elective surgery is extremely low (0.29%).[7,23] Furthermore, outpatient procedures can be performed safely, even in the presence of mild (hematocrit 27% to 35%) anemia. Therefore we do not advocate routine determination of hematocrit and hemoglobin if previous studies performed as part of well-child care have been normal. However, African-American children who have not had a hemoglobin/hematocrit determination after 6 months of age should have a hemoglobin or hematocrit and a sickle cell screening test. Electrolyte abnormalities of any consequence are extremely rare in healthy children; preoperative screening for such deviations usually is unhelpful and does not alter the anesthetic management. Even in hospitalized patients who might be expected to have an incidence of laboratory abnormalities higher than that found in "healthy outpatients," routine testing is not indicated. Screening preoperative urinalysis also failed to discover serious underlying problems in the vast majority of children studied (99.5% of 1859 patients <19 years of age).[6] Therefore we do not obtain these tests in healthy children scheduled for elective surgery.

Performing routine preoperative pregnancy tests in adolescent females remains controversial. Because of the high rate of sexual activity among increasingly younger teenagers and because all anesthetic medications increase the incidence of abortion and are potential teratogens at various doses, it seems prudent to ask whether the patient is sexually active. If so, the date of the last menstrual period should be documented, and the pediatrician should consider obtaining a screening test for pregnancy and informing the family of potential risks if the test is positive. Some anesthesiologists are reluctant to involve themselves in this aspect of their patient's lives, citing privacy issues, and are uncomfortable communicating with families about unexpectedly positive results. The pediatrician, having a longstanding relationship with the teenager and family, may be more comfortable dealing with this issue.

While the healthy child needs almost no preoperative laboratory tests, the situation is entirely different for children who have a history of or the presence of an abnormality. For example, it is helpful to obtain a chest radiograph in a patient who has a history of chronic aspiration or lower airway disease. Knowing the hemoglobin level is important in the child who has sickle cell disease or cardiac disease. A child who has cardiovascular disease on digoxin therapy should have his or her serum sodium, potassium, and digoxin levels measured. An ECG is warranted in a child who has obstructive sleep apnea, BPD, congenital heart disease, or severe scoliosis. In these and similar circumstances, preoperative testing is aimed at detecting and quantifying underlying abnormalities associated with known disease that can lead to life-threatening complications during anesthesia.

SUMMARY

Preoperative evaluation and preparation is directed toward minimizing the intrinsic risks of anesthesia and surgery by having the child in the healthiest possible condition before surgery. The pediatrician can contribute to this goal by understanding the effects of general anesthesia on the physiology of children. This allows an appreciation of the anesthesiologist's concerns regarding underlying diseases, which may appear "stable" (and, therefore, of little present concern to the pediatrician) but which may have grave consequences during anesthesia. The preoperative evaluation is designed to ensure that the child's preoperative needs can be met by providing the anesthesiologist both qualitative and quantitative information regarding the child's state of health and disease. The relationship between the child, parents, and pediatrician places the latter in an ideal position to prepare families for their children's surgical experience.

REFERENCES

1. Burrows FA, Hickey PR, Colan S: Perioperative complications in patients with anthracycline chemotherapeutic agents, *Can Anaesth Soc J* 32:149, 1985.
2. Dajani AS et al: Prevention of bacterial endocarditis. Recommendations by the American Heart Association, *JAMA* 264:2919, 1990.
3. DeSoto H et al: Changes in oxygen saturation following general anesthesia in children with upper respiratory infection signs and symptoms undergoing otolaryngological procedures, *Anesthesiology* 68:276, 1988.
4. Eger EI: MAC. In Eger EI, editor: *Anesthetic uptake and action,* Baltimore, 1974, Williams & Wilkins.
5. Evans-Prosser CD: The use of pethidine and morphine in the presence of monoamine oxidase inhibitors, *Br J Anaesth* 40:279, 1968.
6. Farnsworth PB et al: The value of routine preoperative chest roentgenograms in infants and children, *JAMA* 244:582, 1980.
7. Hackmann T, Steward DJ, Sheps SB: Anemia in pediatric day-surgery patients: prevalence and detection, *Anesthesiology* 75:27, 1991.
8. Helfaer MA, Wilson MD: Obstructive sleep apnea, control of ventilation, and anesthesia in children, *Pediatr Clin North Am* 41:131, 1994.
9. Hirshman CA: Airway reactivity in humans: anesthetic implications, *Anesthesiology* 58:170, 1983.
10. Jacoby DB, Hirshman CA: General anesthesia in patients with viral respiratory infections: an unsound sleep? *Anesthesiology* 74:969, 1991.
11. Keenan RL, Boyan CP: Cardiac arrest due to anesthesia: a study of incidence and causes, *JAMA* 253:2373, 1985.
12. Kingston HG, Hirshman CA: Perioperative management of the patient with asthma, *Anesth Analg* 63:844, 1984.
13. Lanzkowsky P et al: Partial exchange transfusion in sickle cell anemia: use in children with serious complications, *Am J Dis Child* 132:1206, 1978.
14. Larach MG et al: Prediction of malignant hyperthermia susceptibility by clinical signs, *Anesthesiology* 66:547, 1987.
15. Liu LM et al: Life-threatening apnea in infants recovering from anesthesia, *Anesthesiology* 59:506, 1983.
16. Martin LD: Anesthetic implications of an upper respiratory infection in children, *Pediatr Clin North Am* 41:121, 1994.
17. Maxwell LG, Deshpande JK, Wetzel RC: Preoperative evaluation of children, *Pediatr Clin North Am* 41:93, 1994.
18. Pasternak LR: Outpatient anesthesia. In Rogers MC et al, editors: *Principles and practice of anesthesiology,* St Louis, 1993, Mosby.
19. Pien LC, Grammer LC, Patterson R: Minimal complications in a surgical population with severe asthma receiving prophylactic corticosteroids, *J Allergy Clin Immunol* 82:696, 1988.
20. Pueschel SM: Atlantoaxial instability and Down syndrome, *Pediatrics* 81:879, 1988.
21. Pueschel SM, Scola FH: Atlantoaxial instability in individuals with Down syndrome: epidemiologic, radiographic, and clinical studies, *Pediatrics* 80:555, 1987.
22. Rolf N, Cote CJ: Frequency and severity of desaturation events during general anesthesia in children with and without upper respiratory infections, *J Clin Anesth* 4:200, 1992.
23. Roy WL, Lerman J, McIntyre BG: Is preoperative haemoglobin testing justified in children undergoing minor elective surgery? *Can J Anaesth* 38:700, 1991.
24. Sauder RA et al: Methylprednisolone increases sensitivity to beta-adrenergic agonists within 48 hours in Basenji greyhounds, *Anesthesiology* 79:1278, 1993.
25. Schreiner MS: Preoperative and postoperative fasting in children, *Pediatr Clin North Am* 41:111, 1994.
26. Schreiner MS, Triebwasser A, Keon TP: Ingestion of liquids compared with preoperative fasting in pediatric outpatients, *Anesthesiology* 72:593, 1990.
27. Schwartz L, Rockoff MA, Koka BV: Masseter spasm with anesthesia: incidence and implications, *Anesthesiology* 61:772, 1984.
28. Tiret L et al: Complications related to anaesthesia in infants and children: a prospective survey of 40,240 anaesthetics, *Br J Anaesth* 61:263, 1988.
29. Welborn LG, Greenspun JC: Anesthesia and apnea: perioperative considerations in the former preterm infant, *Pediatr Clin North Am* 41:181, 1994.
30. Welborn LG et al: High-dose caffeine suppresses postoperative apnea in former preterm infants, *Anesthesiology* 71:347, 1989.
31. Welborn LG et al: Postoperative apnea in former preterm infants: prospective comparison of spinal and general anesthesia, *Anesthesiology* 72:838, 1990.
32. Yaster M et al: The night after surgery: postoperative management of the pediatric outpatient—surgical and anesthetic aspects, *Pediatr Clin North Am* 41:199, 1994.
33. Zuckerberg AL: Perioperative approach to children, *Pediatr Clin North Am* 41:15, 1994.

9 Structural and Functional Analysis of Body Systems

Nicholas M. Nelson

The essential task of the physician, perhaps more than that of the surgeon, is problem delineation. To be sure, the medical practitioner is involved in the solution of problems, once defined, but these solutions tend to emphasize the enhancement of normal and the suppression of abnormal physiological responses, often by pharmacological means, rather than by the surgeon's direct attack on an anatomical structure that has been altered by disease or development.

The symptoms of which the patient complains and the signs that the physician elicits serve to suggest involvement of one or more organ systems, so the patient's history and physical examination together may be viewed as what applied mathematicians and statisticians call exploratory data analysis. In this earliest phase of clinical problem-solving, the physician assembles the differential diagnosis and then orders that list in descending likelihood, based on his or her knowledge of the epidemiology and, particularly, the natural history of the diseases in question.

This chapter is concerned with a succeeding phase of clinical investigation—the "workup," or confirmatory data analysis, wherein the physician's suspicions, intuitions, and knowledge of the location and extent of the patient's condition are confirmed or denied. Of course, many of the problems encountered in primary care are self-evident or otherwise sufficiently familiar as not to require investigation beyond the history or physical examination; yet, no primary care practitioner is likely to see many patients without recourse to the clinical laboratory and radiological or other consultative support of his or her effort to define the patient's problem. During this effort the practitioner increasingly must bear in mind the cost-benefit ratio of the investigations proposed—"cost" to include not only the fiscal but also the morbid and even mortal risks of the procedures under consideration, as constantly displayed against the benefits likely to be returned in the form of useful or definitive diagnostic information. A sequence of investigations should be planned that is pertinent to the organ system indicated by exploratory analysis of the clinical data gathered and that is coordinated with the current differential diagnosis. This list should begin with those procedures that are inexpensive, noninvasive, and of high sensitivity to many diseases ("coarse focus") but of low specificity for any single disease ("fine focus").

GENERAL ASSESSMENT

The quintessence of pediatrics, in contrast to other clinical disciplines, is its constant concern with the changes that accompany the growth and development of its patients. The child seriously involved with disease usually announces the intensity of that involvement by primary or secondary disruptions of somatic growth and psychomotor development, almost regardless of precise etiology. These aspects are treated in much greater depth elsewhere in this volume, but Tables 9-1 and 9-2 set out some of the more important benchmarks against which the pediatrician measures the patient's progress in these areas.

The Lubchenco, Wright, and Babson charts help the neonatologist assess the growth of premature infants, just as the National Center for Health Statistics charts (which largely have displaced the "Harvard" or "Iowa" or "Wetzel grid" standards of an earlier era) serve those who are concerned with the growth of children from term birth through adolescence. The Dubowitz examination inverts the usual approach to developmental assessment by using established age norms of physical and neuromotor characteristics to estimate gestational age; it assumes that the child being assessed is developed normally for his or her gestational age (which is to be estimated), in contrast to the more typical process of referring the assessed stage of growth and development to the child's (known) age.

The available tools for developmental assessment of the young infant necessarily emphasize motor over cognitive phenomena, and many feel that true cognition is best estimated by the adaptive and language components of the various screening instruments. The alleged cultural "loading" of most of the formal psychometric estimators of intelligence (Table 9-2) has brought them under political and popular critical fire; yet, whatever their "fairness," their position as valid predictors of school performance has not been challenged.

The screening tests noted in Table 9-2 are sufficiently simple and brief to administer, after reasonable practice, as to merit consideration for inclusion in a primary care practice, either as a routine assessment or as a preliminary to formal psychometric testing upon symptomatic indication. (See Appendix D, Table D-1 for a description of the tests listed in Table 9-2.)

ORGAN IMAGING

The past 2 decades have witnessed such rapid and fundamental changes in organ imaging, as scintigraphic, sonographic, magnetic, and computer technologies have intermarried with that of radiation, that some departments of radiology have seriously considered changing their names to departments of "medical imaging." In some areas the field also is shifting from one in which the technician occupies the major portion of the patient's experience to one in which the radiologist (imagist?) dominates, especially in the techniques of angiointervention and ultrasound. Throughout the development

Table 9-1 Assessment of Growth

Examination	
Basic	**Specialized**
General	
Growth charts	
Cross sectional	Cell size (RNA)
Premature infant	Cell number (DNA)
Lubchenco, Usher (weight, length, head)[3,5,9]	
Infant and child	
NCHS (weight, length, head)[4]	
Nellhaus (head)[7]	
Longitudinal	
Premature infant	
Wright (weight)[10]	
Babson, Marks (weight, length, head)[1,6]	
Infant and child	
Tanner (weight, length)[8]	
Chemical	
Alkaline phosphatase	N2-balance K-balance
Bone age	
Knee (newborn)	
Hand, wrist (child)	
Body fat	
Skinfold thickness	Underwater weight
Harpenden calipers	Total body water ^{40}K distribution

of the field, the goals of optimum resolution of the tissue of interest and its optimum differentiation from neighboring tissues of noninterest have come into constant conflict with the restraints of cumulative radiation dosage and the desire to minimize invasiveness. Great strides recently have been made in diminishing risk while increasing definition but at such an increase in the cost of technology as to question seriously the relative contribution of these techniques toward establishing and maintaining the public health. Before dismissing technological advance in medicine on grounds of cost alone, however, physicians, if not politicians, might well reflect upon the "costs" of the modern computed tomographic or magnetic resonance documentation of a posterior fossa tumor in a 4-year-old (and in *40 minutes*) versus the "lesser costs" of an obsolete evaluation extracted through the pain and risk of a pneumoencephalogram, a ventriculogram, or cerebral angiography (with luck, in *5 days*).

Table 9-3 offers a survey of current imaging techniques and their ability to contribute to our understanding of the patient.

Roentgenography

Still the gold standard against which to measure the resolving power of any imaging technique, classic roentgenography, nevertheless, rarely has been able to differentiate the soft tissues of interest within a body region unless abetted by natural (air) or artificial (barium, iodine, or other radiopaque compound) increases in contrast. This is because the transmission of roentgen rays through body tissues is a function of their radioabsorption—mineral and bone being the most opaque, water and air being the least. Water, blood, and muscle, unfortunately, are so similar in radiopacity as to render most difficult the precise appreciation of anything more than gross organ dimension within the abdomen, for instance. Angiography, urography, bronchography, and other techniques for instilling contrast agents are very valuable, but all require some level of invasiveness, and many require local or general anesthesia. Moreover, the contrast agents themselves are not benign—for example, they may produce anaphylaxis or hemiplegia after cerebral angiography or myocardial ischemia after coronary angiography. Digital subtraction techniques in venous or arterial angiography can improve differentiation from confusing background structures and even diminish the dose of contrast agent required but not the necessity for invading the vascular tree.

Radionuclide Imaging

One of the happier aspects of the nuclear age has been the discovery or development of a vast array of radioactive and nonradioactive isotopic tracer elements without which most of modern biochemistry and even archaeology and paleontology could not have proceeded. Nuclear medicine has emphasized the attachment of a radioactive label with requisite physical characteristics to a biologically active carrier molecule, concentrated by natural body processes into the target area or organ, there to emit gamma radiation, which is then recorded, typically by a scintillation camera. This concentration in normal tissues means that diseased areas usually are revealed as areas of altered accumulation of radioactivity, because of loss of microvasculature and replacement of normal tissue. Occasionally, areas of abnormal increases in blood flow are displayed by inflamed tissues or tumors.

Because these synthetic radiopharmaceuticals reside and radiate within the body, they must have either a short half-life ($t_{1/2}$) for radiation or be rapidly excreted or both. On the other hand, the $t_{1/2}$ must be long enough to allow for transport from the site of preparation to that of instillation into the patient. Technetium (Tc) is an element that naturally (without carrier) concentrates especially well in the choroid plexus, the salivary and thyroid glands, and the stomach, but the basic reasons for its prominence as a label in Table 9-4 are its relative ease of preparation, its $t_{1/2}$ of 6 hours, and its gamma emission at energy levels (140 Kv) that prevent absorption by the body (up to 20 Kv), yet are below those levels (above 600 Kv) where radiation scatter becomes so gross as to render organ delineation hopeless. Indeed, the poor resolving power of most radionuclide techniques has in many instances led to their gradual displacement by equally noninvasive ultrasound or computed tomography (CT), wherever the issue has been only that of delineating organ structure. SPECT (single photon emission computed tomography) scans, in particular, have improved resolution significantly.

The carrier molecules for certain radionuclide techniques, however, are specific examiners of an organ's function (e.g., ^{99m}Tc DTPA in the assessment of glomerular filtration, or ^{99m}Tc sulfur colloid, which is phagocytosed by Kuppfer cells) and therefore can challenge nuclear magnetic resonance imaging (MRI) and positron emission tomography (PET) on the

Table 9-2 Assessment of Development

	Social adaptation	Language	Cognition and intellect	Perception and motion	Emotion and projection	Academic achievement
Screening tests						
Premature newborn						
Ballard Gestational Aging—expanded				X		
Term newborn						
Brazelton Behavioral Assessment Scale	X					
Infant and child						
Denver Developmental Screening Test	X	X		X		
Developmental Profile II*	X	X	X	X		
Vineland Adaptive Behavior Scales*	X	X		X		
Psychometric tests						
Bayley Scales of Infant Development II	X	X	X	X		
Developmental Test Visual-Motor Integration				X		
Stanford-Binet Intelligence Scale IV			X			
Test of Language Development		X				
Wechsler Individual Achievement Test						X
Wechsler Intelligence Scale for Children III			X			
Child Behavior Checklist*					X	
Pediatric Behavior Scale*					X	

*Parental observation.

Table 9-3 Imaging Techniques*

	Usefulness for delineation of			
Modality	**Static structure**	**Dynamic motion**	**Metabolic function**	**Imaging criterion**
Ultrasound	++	+++	0	Acoustic impedance
Magnetic resonance imaging (MRI)				
Hydrogen	++	+	0	Water content
Phosphorus	+	0	++	Energy metabolism
Radionuclide nuclear scintigraphy	+	+	++	Gamma emission
Single photon emission computed tomography (SPECT)	++	++	0	
Positron emission tomography (PET)	+	0	++	Positron emission (metabolic activity)
Roentgenography				
Standard roentgenogram	+++	0	0	Roentgen ray density (enhanced spectrum)
Computed tomography (CT)	++	+	0	
Angiography				
Standard	+++	0	0	
Cine/video	++	+++	0	
Digital subtraction	++	0	0	(reduced background)
Fluoroscopy	++	+++	0	

*In approximate ascending order of energizing radiation sustained by the patient.

grounds of informed functional analysis of certain organs. Few sights, for instance, are more rewarding to the pediatric surgeon, faced with a child who has massive rectal bleeding, than a positive "Meckel diverticulum scan," where the pertechnetate label has concentrated in the parietal cells of ectopic gastric tissue and thus narrowed the surgeon's otherwise unguided search throughout the intestine for an attackable bleeding site.

Ultrasonography

The precocious infancy of ultrasonography is just now maturing into an adolescence in which it already has become the fundamental means for assessment of fetal growth and development, as well as for neonatal and infant intracranial examination, not to mention its earlier and continuing contributions in cardiology (echocardiography) and in the examination of the abdominal viscera, the orbit, and the hip. Although to the untrained eye the current interpretation of ultrasonic scans may seem to approach the mystic, image quality nonetheless is vastly superior to that of radionuclide imaging. There is no ionizing radiation, and the sound energy levels used are believed to be far below the threshold for tissue damage.

The critical factor for tissue differentiation is acoustic im-

Table 9-4 Radionuclide Scans

Organ	Label	Carrier	Concentration mechanism
Liver	^{99m}Tc	Sulfur colloid	Phagocytosis (Kuppfer cells)
	^{99m}Tc	HIDA	Active transport (extrahepatic cells)
	^{99m}Tc	PIPIDA	Active transport (biliary cells)
Kidneys	$^{99m}TcO_4$	None	Flow diffusion
	^{99m}Tc	DTPA	Active transport (glomerulus)
	^{125}I	Thalamate	Active transport (glomerulus)
	^{131}I	Hippuran	Active transport (tubule)
Lungs	^{133}Xe	None	Active transport (alveolar gas)
	^{99m}Tc	HSA (macroaggregated)	Capillary blockade
Heart	$^{99m}TcO_4$	None	Flow diffusion
Blood pool	^{99m}Tc	HSA	Compartmentation
	^{99m}Tc	RBC	Compartmentation
Spleen	^{99m}Tc	Sulfur colloid	Phagocytosis (Kuppfer cells)
RE system	^{99m}Tc	RBC	Sequestration
Gut	$^{99m}TcO_4$	None	Active transport (parietal cells)
Abscess, tumor	^{67}Gallium	None	? Transport (inflammatory cells)
			? Diffusion (tumor cells)
Bone	^{99m}Tc	Diphosphonate	Active transport
Thyroid	$^{99m}TcO_4$	None	Flow diffusion
	^{131}I	None	Active transport (thyroid cells)
Adrenal	^{131}I	Cholesterol	Active transport (cortical cells)
	^{125}I		
CSF	^{99m}Tc	HSA	Compartmentation
Brain	$^{99m}TcO_4$	None	Active transport (choroid plexus)

HIDA, Hepatoimidodiacetic acid; *PIPIDA*, paraisopropylimidodiacetic acid; *DTPA*, diethylenetriamine pentaacetic acid; *HSA*, human serum albumin; *RBC*, red blood cells; *RE*, reticuloendothelial; *CSF*, cerebrospinal fluid

pedance (analogous to radiodensity), but the range of values displayed by various tissues is much wider than that for radiation. Hence, blood or water in the ultrasonogram (in contrast to the unenhanced roentgenogram) is distinguished easily from connective tissue and muscle; on this fact rests modern echocardiography. Bone, however, is nearly opaque to ultrasound, so the cranial and thoracic contents can be examined only through the sonic "windows" offered by the open anterior fontanelle, an intercostal space, the subxiphoid region, or the suprasternal notch.

M (for motion) -mode ultrasonography, videorecorded in "real time," two-dimensional sector or linear array scanning, and Doppler scans form the sonic dynamic equivalents of classic fluoroscopy or cineangiography. By these techniques the motions of the heart and its valves, the fetus, the lungs, and the flow of blood can be viewed, reviewed, and analyzed, often by the same analytical formulas developed and substantiated through the more invasive techniques of angiography.

To the advantages of relative safety, high image quality, and the dynamic, as well as static, recording afforded by ultrasonography can be added the highest degree of portability of all the imaging techniques—the equipment is brought to the bedside easily on vehicles substantially smaller and lighter than the usual "portable" roentgenography machine. However, imaging still requires a high degree of patience, experience, and artistry on the part of the examiner wielding the sonic transducer, so interpretability of recordings is much more in direct proportion to the expertise of the physician or technician at the bedside than is the case in, say, roentgenography.

Computed Tomography (CT)

Computed tomography is derived from the earlier methods of plain tomography, wherein either the roentgen ray tube or the film cassette (or both) are rotated during exposure so as to blur all tissues except those at the axis of rotation. With CT, a computer enhancement of the digitally analyzed "gray scale" of received roentgen ray transmission vastly widens the scale of appreciable radiodensity differences between tissues beyond that of the "mineral-bone-water-air" scale of classic roentgenography. The body, thus, is viewable as a sequence of axial planar "cuts," reminiscent of the frozen whole-body sections of gross anatomy. However, the technique is relatively slow to complete a cut and usually requires contrast enhancement. Moreover, it is distinctly static, quite expensive, and most certainly nonportable. Nonetheless, it has revolutionized clinical neurology and essentially has made pneumoencephalography and ventriculography obsolete, while relegating cerebral angiography to the status of a strictly preoperative procedure. The diagnostic acumen and therapeutic capabilities of virtually all the surgical subspecialties have been enhanced similarly by CT cuts through the body part of their interest, from orbit to ankle.

Positron Emission Tomography (PET)

Related to CT scanning in that tomography is used to produce a tissue "slice," PET scans view the positrons emitted by appropriately excited body tissues rather than roentgen rays. If the excitation is produced by isotopes of metabolically active molecules and compounds (e.g., oxygen and glucose), it becomes possible to examine sites of metabolic activity (and blood flow to them). The concept is similar to, but much more rapidly and accurately defined than, radionuclide scans. However, the equipment is expensive, nonportable, and must be close to the cyclotron or other heavy nuclear gear required to produce the short-lived isotopes. PET scanning, thus, is much more a research tool than a practical one for clinical management.

Magnetic Resonance Imaging (MRI)

MRI is the newest, and in some ways the most promising (but hardly the least expensive), imaging technique for general use. It is beginning just now to blossom and assume its place in the diagnostic imaging armamentarium. It also is noninvasive (and nonportable) and is based on the phenomenon of the magnetic resonance of uniform spin, induced in the atomic particles of all tissues placed in a strong magnetic field and then struck by a radiofrequency pulse delivered at the natural vibrational frequency of the atom in question (e.g., hydrogen). As the imposed radiofrequency pulse subsides, the atomic particles "relax" into their natural random spin orientation and emit a recordable electromagnetic pulse, the density scale of which is a function of the density of that atom in the tissue so bombarded.

If the imposed radiofrequency pulse is "tuned" (like a radio or TV receiver) to resonate in hydrogen nuclei (protons), then the emitted electromagnetic pulse reflects the varying water (i.e., hydrogen proton) content of those tissues. If, on the other hand, the pulse is tuned to the phosphorus atom, intimately involved in most of the body's energy-transforming biochemical reactions, then the recorded image (as in PET scanning) tends to reflect metabolic activity within the tissues examined. Although the image quality of MRI hydrogen scanning already compares favorably with or exceeds that of CT and PET scanning, it is too early to specify whether the promise of bloodless biochemical biopsy through MRI (phosphorus or other atom) can be realized.

SYSTEMIC EVALUATION

The assessment of structure and function of the organ systems within the body involves both biochemical and biophysical means for tracing the effectiveness with which an organ performs its tasks. Disruptions of gross structure need not impair function (e.g., hepatic metastases), and disruptions of function need not impair gross structure (e.g., renal tubular acidosis); thus evaluation of both often is necessary to rule out disease, especially in those organs that have multiple functions, such as the liver and kidneys.

The functional evaluation of the heart and circulation, the respiratory tract, the neuromotor system, the skin, the eyes, and the ears is accomplished largely by the physician during the physical examination. In contrast, physiological assessment of the hematopoietic, immune, and endocrine systems, the kidneys and the urinary tract, and the liver and intestinal tract, depends heavily on laboratory tests. In all, however, a careful medical history designed to test, by system-oriented symptomatic questioning, the presence or absence of normal organ function should direct the exploration of the patient's problem and contribute most to its solution.

Table 9-5 Heart and Circulation

	Examination	
	Basic	**Specialized**
Structure	Chest roentgenogram	Radionuclide scan Echocardiogram Angiography
Function		
Hemodynamics		
Preload	Auscultation	Echocardiogram
Contractility	Sphygmomanometry	Echocardiogram
Afterload	Electrocardiogram	Echocardiogram
Distribution of flow	Oximetry Blood gases	Radionuclide scan Cardiac catheterization Thermodilution Dye dilution Angiography
Microcirculation	Stress exercise testing Maximum O_2 consumption	

Heart and Circulation

Appropriate indicators for investigation of this system (Table 9-5) may range from a presumably innocent cardiac murmur to cyanosis and frank heart failure. The increasing sophistication of echocardiography has relegated formal catheterization largely to the category of a preoperative and postoperative intervention to be undertaken when accurate measurement of chamber pressures and pulmonary and systemic flow ratios is necessary. Stress (exercise) testing is used to evaluate the cardiovascular response to the aerobic demands of physical activity.

The hemodynamic stress placed on the heart by excessive venous return (preload) or excessive outflow resistance (afterload) tends to produce dilation or hypertrophy, respectively, of the chamber so loaded. Preload may be estimated clinically by measurement of venous pressure, detection of "flow" murmurs, and roentgenographic assessment of pulmonary vasculature and the like, whereas the more difficult judgment of afterload depends on the site or sites of vascular resistance—at the outflow tract (stenotic semilunar valves), in the great vessels (coarctation), or at the level of the resistance vessels themselves (diastolic hypertension). A sense of chamber wall thickness may be derived from electrocardiography (in the amplitude of QRS deflections), but the echocardiogram has become the modern gold standard for measuring chamber diameters and wall and valve dimensions. Moreover, cardiovascular shunts may be traced during the echocardiogram by simple saline injections or (color) Doppler echocardiography, whereas chamber hemodynamics (ejection fraction, circumferential shortening velocity, and fractional shortening) may be measured accurately and repeatedly as clinical indices of myocardial contractility.

The invasive procedures (cardiac catheterization, angiography, venography) now are generally reserved for those situations requiring precise anatomical detail (pulmonary artery)

Table 9-6 Lungs and Respiratory Tract

	Examination	
	Basic	**Specialized**
Structure		

Overall	Chest roentgenogram
	Fluoroscopy
	Sinus roentgenograms, CT scan
	Barium swallow
	Sputum
	  Analysis
	  Culture
		Nasopharyngoscopy
		Bronchoscopy (flexible, rigid)
		Laryngoscopy

Lung volumes	Spirometry Pneumotachometry Tomograms	Gas dilution (N_2, H_2) Body plethysmography Bronchography Angiography Puncture Biopsy
Function		
Ventilation	Spirometry Flow rates	Gas washout (N_2, H_2) Flow-volume loops Occluded breath-mouth pressure Radionuclide scan Body plethysmography
Perfusion		Radionuclide scan Gas absorption (N_2O, acetylene)
Diffusion		Diffusing capacity (CO, O_2)
Gas exchange	Oximetry Transcutaneous blood gases Arterial blood gases	Alveolar-arterial (O_2, CO_2, N_2) gas gradients

Mechanics		Body plethysmography
		  Compliance
		  Resistance

Stress	Exercise Cold air breathing	

or pressure/flow data, generally in anticipation or documentation of surgical repair, or for frank vascular intervention.

Lungs and Respiratory Tract

The patient who has symptoms referable to the respiratory tract (e.g., cough and hyperpnea) may be suffering from more global disease (allergy or diabetic ketoacidosis), but those children who have signs of impending or actual respiratory failure (dyspnea or cyanosis) usually are found to have significant disruption of lung tissue, most often the airways.

The overall aim and usual result of pulmonary function testing (Table 9-6) is the classification of the child's problem as either "obstructive" or "restrictive." Obstructive disease of the airways (asthma or other bronchospastic disease and cystic fibrosis) slows flow rates and alters gaseous outflow curves and flow-volume loops, often producing secondary increases in residual lung volume and functional residual capacity. Restrictive lung disease (pneumonia, hyaline membrane disease, neurological disease, or other conditions that impair the thoracic "bellows") encompasses those processes that restrict or replace alveolar volume and ventilation.

Unfortunately, most of the apparatus and maneuvers developed to assess pulmonary function require a level of understanding and cooperation on the part of the patient that is beyond the capabilities of most children under about 5 to 7 years of age unless they are swaddled and satiated (i.e., essentially "thalamic") newborn infants. Hence in practical terms the clinical assessment of pulmonary function in most cases is reduced to simple flow studies (e.g., Wright peak flowmeter) and estimates of gas exchange (oximetry and transcutaneous or arterial blood gases).

Kidneys and Urinary Tract

Critical disruption of renal function (Table 9-7) can be notoriously subtle and insidious, evoking no detectable symptoms until far advanced. Hence the cautious physician usually includes a urinalysis and determinations of blood urea nitrogen (BUN) and creatinine in the evaluation of any child whose growth or general health is at all in question, even in the presence of a normal urinalysis. Manifestation of renal disease in a younger child often is in the form of an abdominal mass (hydronephrosis, Wilms tumor, or cystic disease),

Table 9-7 Kidneys and Urinary Tract

	Examination	
	Basic	**Specialized**
Structure	Ultrasound Intravenous urography CT scan ^{99m}Tc DTPA scan	^{131}I hippuran scan Angiography Retrograde cystourethrography Cystoscopy Biopsy
Function		
Urinary tract	Urinalysis	Voiding cystourethrogram Cystometrics
	BUN Creatinine	Lasix-stimulated diethylene triamine pentacetic acid (DTPA) scan
Glomerulus	Urine flow Creatinine clearance	^{125}I thalamate scan (captopril-stimulated) Inulin clearance
Tubule	Fluid restriction test Phosphate clearance Urine and serum electrolytes	Vasopressin test Paraamino hippurate (PAH) clearance NH_4Cl loading test

the delineation of which is the special and spectacular province of the ultrasonogram; indeed, these renal lesions currently are being detected during careful *fetal* ultrasound examination. Hence urography is now used only rarely to assess extrarenal retroperitoneal disease and is limited to evaluation of the renal pelvis and ureter per se, complementary to the ultrasound examination and CT scan.

Intestinal Tract

The modes for investigation of the gastrointestinal tract (endoscopy excepted) have changed less in the last generation, perhaps, than those of any other organ system (Table 9-8); the development of flexible fiberoptic instrumentation has placed nearly the entire alimentary canal under direct scrutiny by endoscopic procedures that, if unpleasant and requiring sedation or anesthesia, are nonetheless accurate and repeatable. In contrast to the older child and adult, fundamental gastrointestinal disease in the younger child involves malformations more frequently than chronic inflammation (e.g., enteritis and colitis), despite the prominence of acute gastrointestinal intercurrent infectious illness in any primary pediatric practice.

Liver

Beyond the newborn period, in which hyperbilirubinemia is a daily concern, primary liver disease other than hepatitis is relatively rare among children. However, the liver is frequently yet secondarily involved in multisystemic disease (vascular congestion and obstructions, abscess, storage disease) because of its strategic vascular location and global metabolic activity. The omnipresent, multimembered "liver panels" much beloved by younger house officers often produce information redundant to the usually sufficient items shown in Table 9-9. The assessment of bile flow in the jaundiced but acholic young infant continues to frustrate the pediatrician attempting to distinguish biliary atresia from "neonatal hepatitis" by such fallible means as ^{131}I rose bengal liver excretion or red cell peroxidation (as an index of gastrointestinal bile-assisted vitamin E absorption), but improvements in the safety of direct (endoscopic or transhepatic) cholangiography have served to diminish delay in selecting candidates for hepatic portoenterostomy (Kasai procedure) or, more recently, liver transplantation.

Table 9-8 Intestinal Tract

	Examination	
	Basic	**Specialized**
Structure	Abdominal plain roentgenogram Flat Upright Contrast/fluoroscopy Barium esophagogram Upper GI series Barium enema Ultrasound scan	Computed tomography Radionuclide scan Endoscopy Esophagoscopy Gastroduodenoscopy Cholangio-pancreatography Colonoscopy Biopsy
Function		
Peristalsis	Contrast fluoroscopy	Manometry
Secretion	Gastric pH	Duodenal aspiration Enzymes Bile
Absorption	Fecal analysis Reducing sugar Fat Trypsin Alpha-1-antitrypsin Loading (tolerance) tests Oral glucose D-xylose Serum carotene	Hydrogen breath test ^{51}CrCl excretion Mucosal enzymes (biopsy)

Table 9-9 Liver

	Examination	
	Basic	**Specialized**
Structure	Ultrasound	Computed tomography
	Radionuclide scan	
	^{131}I rose bengal	
	^{99m}Tc PIPIDA	Endoscopy
		Cholangio-pancreatography
		Transhepatic/operative cholangiography
		Biopsy
		Splenoportography
Function		
Protein synthesis	Serum albumin	
	Prothrombin time	
	Gamma globulin	Electrophoresis
Biotrans-formation	SGOT	5′-Nucleotidase
	SGPT	Gamma-glutamyltransferase
		Leucine aminopeptidase
Conjugation	Bilirubin (direct/total)	
Excretion	Alkaline phosphatase	
Bile flow	Duodenal intubation	^{131}I rose bengal
		Red cell peroxidation
		^{99m}Tc IDA
Special		NH_3
		Alpha-1-antitrypsin
		Ceruloplasmin

PIPIDA, Paraisopropylimidodiacetic acid; *IDA,* imidodiacetic acid; *SGOT,* serum glutamic-oxaloacetic transaminase; *SGPT,* serum glutamic-pyruvic transaminase.

Table 9-10 Neuromuscular and Central Nervous Systems

	Examination	
	Basic	**Specialized**
Structure	Plain skull roentgenograms	
	Ultrasound	
		CT, MRI scans
		Radionuclide (^{99m}Tm) scan
		PET scan
		Myelography
		Cerebral angiography
		Biopsy
		Muscle
		Nerve
		Brain
Function		
Sensory	Neurological exam	
Vision	Vision testing	VER, ERG, EOG, FPL
Hearing	Perimetry	BAER
Cutaneous	Audiometry	SER
	EEG	
Motor	Neurological exam	EMG, MEP
	EEG	EOG
	CPK	Nerve conduction study
Integrated	Developmental testing	Psychometric evaluation
Global	CSF	Subdural tap
		Ventricular tap

PET, Positron emission tomography; *VER,* visual evoked responses; *ERG,* electroretinography; *EOG,* electrooculogram; *FPL,* forced preferential looking; *BAER,* brainstem auditory evoked responses; *SER,* somatosensory evoked responses; *EEG,* electroencephalogram; *EMG,* electromyogram; *MEP,* motor evoked potential; *CPK,* creatine phosphokinase; *CSF,* cerebrospinal fluid.

Nervous and Neuromuscular Systems

Perhaps more than in any other organ system, functional assessment of the nervous and neuromuscular systems is accomplished principally during the performance of a careful neurological examination, especially of the older child, for whom communication is not a barrier. The evaluation of no other system, however, has been as revolutionized by the development of ultrasound, CT, and MRI (Table 9-10), which has all but obliterated the need for invasive studies (pneumoencephalography, myelography, ventriculography). Moreover, evoked response testing has placed the assessment of the visual and auditory apparatus of the young infant on more secure ground than did the traditional bedside maneuvers. Yet, true vision and hearing require integrated processing of the signals documented (by evoked potentials, say) as being received and sent along the optic and acoustic nerves, so the possibility of "cortical" blindness or deafness still is investigated best by the behavioral responses of an alert and cooperative patient.

Eye and Ear

The primary care pediatrician's involvement with eyes and ears is properly limited to first aid and functional screening, despite the prominence of conjunctivitis and otitis media and externa in any such practice. His or her role, then, is largely that of prevention and limitation of disease by referral of those patients whose response to relatively straightforward treatment of upper respiratory and ocular problems is unsatisfactory. The development of practical impedance tympanometry has served to sharpen the indications for such referral. Tables 9-11 and 9-12 set out some of those procedures by which the ophthalmologist and otolaryngologist seek to define the finer aspects of structure and function. Both disciplines have developed a number of individuals who confine their practice to children.

Skeleton

Pertinent modalities for assessing the body's bony support are set out in Table 9-13, the radionuclide scans being particularly valuable in the investigation of infectious or metastatic involvement of bone. Radioimmunoassay procedures have brought measurement of the hormones pertinent to bone metabolism (parathyroid hormone, calcitonin, and the vitamin D system) out of the research laboratory and into clinical medicine.

Skin and Appendages

Functional disruptions of cutaneous function are much less frequent causes for presenting complaint than are the itches,

Table 9-11 Eye

	Examination	
	Basic	**Specialized**
Structure	Ultrasound	CT scan
Media	Direct ophthalmoscopy	Indirect ophthalmoscopy
Retina	Fluorescein dye (conjunctivae)	Slit-lamp biomicroscopy Ophthalmic ultrasound Fluorescein angiography
Function		
Intraocular pressure		Indentation (Schiøtz) tonometry Applanation tonometry (Perkins)
Visual response	Startle reflex Fixation	Optokinetic nystagmus Electrooculogram Electroretinogram Visual evoked responses
Ocular alignment	Corneal light reflex (Hirschberg's method) Alternate cover tests	
Ocular motility	Conjugate eye movements	
Visual acuity	Snellen charts Illiterate "E" charts	Refraction Retinoscopy Forced preferential looking
Visual fields	Confrontation Attraction	Perimetry Scotometry
Color vision	Pseudoisochromatic test (Ishihara test)	Farnsworth-Munsell D-100 color test

Table 9-12 Ear

	Examination	
	Basic	**Specialized**
Structure	Head light and mirror Pneumatic otoscopy	Microscopic otoscopy Computed tomography Magnetic resonance imaging
Function		
Hearing	Visual response Play response Speech response Impedance audiometry Conventional audiometry	BAER* Central auditory processing Cochleography
Vestibular	Bárány chair (or equivalent) Caloric stimulation	Electronystamography Posturography
Eustachian tube		Pressure-flow study
Sound conduction	Impedance tympanometry	

*Brainstem auditory evoked responses.

Table 9-13 Bone

	Examination	
	Basic	**Specialized**
Structure	Physical examination Plain roentgenograms Ultrasound (joints) CT scan MRI	Radionuclide scan ^{99m}Tc polyphosphate ^{67}Gallium citrate Roentgen-ray absorptiometry Arthrocentesis Bone biopsy
Function	Alkaline phosphatase Ca, P	Parathyroid hormone Calcitonin Vitamin D_3 25-OH-D_3 1,25-$(OH)_2$-D_3

rashes, and eruptions that consume much of the pediatrician's day; such disruptions most often reflect general systemic disease, usually of infectious or iatrogenic origin. The hand lens is the technological support used most frequently by the inspecting dermatologist, yet exudates, scrapings, and cuttings occasionally require detailed analysis, as indicated in Table 9-14.

Endocrine System

Confirmatory data analysis in this system almost exclusively is functional in nature and dependent on the radioimmunoassay laboratory (Table 9-15), whether the fluid examined be blood or urine, the latter being viewed as an "integrating averager" of hormone secretion (which in blood often displays pulsatile or diurnal rhythms). To be sure, roentgenographic, ultrasound, angiographic, MRI, and radionuclide techniques often are used for a rather gross overview of endocrine organ outlines (sella turcica, adrenal cortex, and thyroid), but picogram quantities of hormones and small clusters of specialized cells are beyond the powers even of histological techniques for resolution of structure. In most cases in Table 9-15,

Table 9-14 Skin and Appendages

	Examination	
	Basic	**Specialized**
Structure	Inspection	
	Direct (hand lens)	Dark field
	Wood's lamp	Biopsy
		Immunofluorescent studies
	Exudates (bacteria)	
	Smear	
	Culture	
	Scrapings	
	Direct oil (scabies)	
	KOH (fungi)	
	Tzanck smear (herpes)	Cuttings (chemical analyses)
		Hair
		Nails
Function		
Vasoreactivity		Catechol iontophoresis
		Skin blood flow
Sweating	Starch-iodine examination	
	Pilocarpine iontophoresis	

a "negative feedback axis" is involved that shuts down the hypothalamic activation of the pituitary gland's stimulation of end-organ hormone production. An increased end-organ hormonal level in the blood is the (negative) signal that impedes further trophic hormone release—analagous to the increased heat that shuts off the living room thermostat.

The suspicion of end-organ malfunction and even the measurement of some of the pertinent hormones (especially adrenal and thyroid) are in the province of the primary pediatrician, but detailed assessment of the pituitary and hypothalamic feedback loops by various evocative tests (see Table 9-15) normally is under the proper jurisdiction of the pediatric endocrinologist.

Blood

Although structural assessment of at least the circulating elements in the hematopoietic system is part of the armamentarium of any physician, the hematologist should be called on to examine the disruption of hemostasis, which may be suggested by the various screening tests of clotting function (Table 9-16). Yet the pediatrician's most frequent contact with this system probably is in tracing its involvement with disease of nutritional, infectious, or cancerous origin.

Immune System

The body's immunological defenses constitute an elaborate system that has evolved over eons of assault by "nonself"

Table 9-15 Endocrine System

End-organ hormones	Intermediaries	Releasers
Adrenal cortex	ACTH (corticotropin)	CRH (corticotropin-releasing hormone)
Cortisol		
Aldosterone	Angiotensin II (kidneys)	
Dehydroepiandrosterone		
Adrenal medulla		
Epinephrine		
Norepinephrine		
Dopamine		
Gonads		
Testosterone	FSH (follicle-stimulating hormone)	LH-RH (luteinizing hormone–releasing hormone)
Estradiol	LH (luteinizing hormone)	
Progesterone		
Thyroid		
Triiodothyronine (T_3)	TSH (thyroid-stimulating hormone [thyrotropin])	TRH (thyroid-releasing hormone)
Thyroxine (T_4)		
Parafollicular cells		
Calcitonin		
Parathyroid		
Parathyroid hormone	Vitamin D	
Growth		
Somatomedin action	GH (growth hormone, somatotropin)	GHRH (growth hormone–releasing hormone)
		Somatostatin (inhibits release)
Lactation		
Direct action	PRL (prolactin)	PRH (prolactin-inhibiting hormone)
Melanocyte	MSH (melanocyte-stimulating hormone)	MRF (melanocyte-releasing factor)
Direct action		
Distal renal tubule		
Direct action	ADH (arginine vasopressin)	
Uterus		
Direct action	Oxytocin	

Table 9-16 Blood and Hematopoietic System

	Examination	
	Basic	**Specialized**
Structure	Hemoglobin	Marrow biopsy
	Hematocrit	Marrow culture
	Reticulocyte count	
	Cell counts	
	Red cell	
	White cell	
	Platelet	
	Peripheral smear	
	Marrow aspiration	
Function		
Neutrophil		
Chemotaxis	Rebuck skin window technique	Boyden chamber
Phagocytosis		Vital staining (myeloperoxidase)
Bacterial killing	Nitroblue tetrazolium test	Chemiluminescence
Red cell		
Gas transport	Hemoglobin electrophoresis	Po_2 at 50% saturation; 2,3-diphosphoglycerate
Membrane stability	Osmotic fragility	Peroxidation
		NADPH* generation
Glycolysis		
Hemostasis		
Total	Clotting time	
Vascular phase	Tourniquet test	
Platelet phase	Bleeding time	Platelet aggregation
	Clot retraction	
Phase III	Thrombin time	Fibrinogen, factor XIII
Phase II	Prothrombin time (PT)	Prothrombin, factors V, VII, and X
Phase I	Partial thromboplastin time (PTT)	Thromboplastin generation
	Prothrombin consumption	Factors VII, VIII, IX, XI, and XII

**NADPH,* Nicotinamide adenine dinucleotide phosphate.

Table 9-17 Immune System

	Examination	
	Basic	**Specialized**
Structure		
Lymphocytes		
Overall	Lymphocyte count	Biopsy (node, thymus, spleen, gut)
T cells	Lateral chest roentgenogram	
	Rosette formation (sheep RBC)	Monoclonal markers (helper, suppressor)
B cells	Serum IgG, IgM levels	IgM cell markers
	Serum isohemagglutin levels	
Complement system	Total hemolytic complement level	Specific complement protein levels (C3,C4)
Allergen system	Total IgE (radioimmunoassay)	
Function		
T cell	Skin tests (tuberculin, *Candida*)	Stimulated lymphocyte culture
B cell	Skin tests (Schick test)	Stimulated lymphocyte culture
Allergen	Eosinophils	Provocative testing (airways)
	Skin testing	Prausnitz-Küstner passive transfer
	Specific radioallergosorbent tests (RAST)	Leukocyte histamine release

invaders, potential or real. The developmental costs of this system to the species have been the very common occurrence of those atopic individuals who overreact to the antigens in their environment (with reactions of eczema, asthma, or rhinitis), the much rarer occurrence of individuals who, by confusing self with nonself, develop "autoimmune" disease (e.g., myasthenia gravis, rheumatic fever, glomerulonephritis, and possibly diabetes), and those unfortunates whose normal immune defenses have been impaired naturally (through infection with the human immune deficiency virus [HIV]) or

ETIOLOGICAL CLASSIFICATION OF DISEASE ORIGIN

Genetic and developmental
Nutritional
Infectious
Neoplastic
Traumatic and physical agents
Hypersensitivity
Psychogenic
Unknown or unclassified

MECHANISMS OF BIRTH DEFECTS

Single mutant gene

Autosomal dominant (e.g., achondroplasia, neurofibromatosis, polycystic kidney)
Autosomal recessive (e.g., adrenogenital syndrome, cystic fibrosis, sickle cell disease)
X-linked (e.g., chronic granulomatous disease, glucose 6-phosphate dehydrogenase [G6PD] deficiency, hemophilia A)

Chromosomal disorders
Aneuploidy
Monosomy
XO: Turner's syndrome
Trisomies
13: Patau's syndrome
18: Edwards' syndrome
21: Down syndrome
XXY: Klinefelter's syndrome
XYY
XXX

Structural changes
Translocations (balanced, unbalanced)
Robertsonian
Reciprocal
Deletions
Chromosome 5: cri-du-chat syndrome
Breakage

Multifactorial (gene-environment interaction)
Single congenital
Cardiac defects
Cleft lip or palate
Meningomyelocele
Age related
Diabetes
Schizophrenia

whose immune defenses must be artificially crippled to improve the likelihood of successful transplantation of foreign tissues and organs.

The frustrating frequency with which parents and pediatricians deal with infections contracted by the "immunological virgins" who are their children often has led to fruitless attempts to document immunological incompetence. Most often, however, quiet epidemiological reflection will indicate that recurrent infections among otherwise healthy young American children usually are caused by a plethora of microbial invaders (particularly well-concentrated in day care centers) rather than by any paucity of defenses. Relatively simple screening tests of immediate and delayed hypersensitivity, and of antibody level usually are sufficient to dispel doubt.

The availability of radioallergosorbent tests (RAST) (Table 9-17) for specific antigen-associated IgE has considerably simplified, not to mention humanized, the allergic evaluation of the symptomatic child under consideration for desensitization therapy; however, it should never replace a careful historical review of the onset and offset of those symptoms.

PRENATAL DIAGNOSTIC SCREENING FOR BIRTH DEFECTS

Indications

Advanced maternal age
Known "carrier"
 Balanced translocation
 X-linked
Previous affected child
 Trisomy
 Neural tube defect

Procedures

Radiography
Ultrasound
Chorionic villus sampling
Amniocentesis
Amniography
Fetoscopy

Amniotic fluid analysis

Fluid (secretory products)
 Alpha-fetoprotein
Cultured cells
 Karyotype
 Enzymatic analysis
 Genome (DNA)
  Molecular hybridization
  Restriction endonucleases

ETIOLOGICAL DELINEATION

It is a sweet irony that a textbook of pediatrics, such as this volume, can now afford a relative neglect of nutritional and infectious disease on the ground that, at least in developed countries, social, sanitary, economic, and medical advances have diminished the prominence of the serious nutritional and infectious diseases that brought pediatrics into being. A concurrent and corollary emphasis on problems of early development (perinatology, neonatology, and congenital anomalies) and behavior (a principal focus of this volume) likely will characterize the pediatrics of the next 100 years. Hence, within the usual etiological classification of disease (see the

Table 9-18 Genetic Screening

Examinations	
Basic	**Specialized**
Newborn (nonselective mass screening)	
Blood bacterial inhibition assay (Guthrie test)	
Phenylalanine (phenylketonuria)	
Leucine (maple syrup urine disease)	
Methionine (homocystinuria)	
Tyrosine (tyrosinemia)	
Fluorescent spot test (Beutler)	
Galactose (galactosemia)	
Radioimmunoassay	
Thyroxine (hypothyroidism)	
Infant (symptomatic)	
Blood	
Ca, Mg, electrolytes	
pH, sugar, ketone, NH_3	
Urine	
Odor	
Sugar	
Ketones	
Amino acids	
Direct reagent spot test	Amino acids
$FeCl_3$	High-pressure liquid chromatography
Dinitrophenylhydrazine	
Ketoacids	Organic acids
Nitrosonaphthol	Gas chromatographic mass spectroscopy
Tyrosine	
Cyanide/nitroprusside	
Cystine	
Homocystine	
Paper or thin-layer chromatography	
Carbohydrates	
Benedict solution (Clinitest)	
Reducing sugar	
Glucose oxidase (Labstix)	
Glucose	
Toluidine blue	
Mucopolysaccharides	

Table 9-19 Assessment of Genetic Disease

Examinations	
Basic	**Specialized**
Pedigree	Genotype
	Karyotype
	(cultured)
Proband	Amniotic cells
Phenotype	Leukocytes
Dysmorphological	Bone marrow
Dermatoglyphic	Genome mapping
	Specific protein product
	Enzyme
	Skin fibroblast culture
	Red cells
	Substrate/metabolic product
	Urine
	Blood
	Tissue culture

Table 9-20 Assessment of Infectious Diseases

Examinations	
Basic	**Specialized**
Epidemiology	
Body fluids/exudates/tissues	
Direct examination	
Method	
Saline suspension	Special stains
Potassium hydroxide preparation	Dyes
	Fluorescent antibodies
Gram stain	Electron microscopy
Tzanck preparation	
Light microscopy	
Laboratory culture	
Appropriate selective media	
Typing	
Antibiotic sensitivity	Typing
Enzymatic screening	Phage
	Serologic
	Specific antibody responses
	Complement fixing
	Neutralizing
	Hemagglutination inhibiting
	Precipitating
	Special serologic assays
	Monospot, Epstein-Barr titer
	Venereal Disease Research Laboratory (VDRL)
	Fluorescent antibodies
	Radioimmunoassay (RIA)
	Enzyme-linked immunosorbent assay (ELISA)

box on p. 120), we here will consider only briefly and broadly those of genetic or infectious origin. Discussions of psychogenic disease are found throughout this volume, whereas the possibility of iatrogenic disease lurks in every contact between child and primary pediatrician, particularly when the latter is oriented to treatment rather than to *thinking* and reflecting on the fact that the vast majority of his or her sick patients are dealing with self-limited, intercurrent illnesses that usually require only sympathetic support and symptomatic treatment. The pediatrician's therapeutic zeal is better reserved for those few life-threatening emergencies discussed elsewhere in this book.

Genetic Disease

It could be argued that hemolytic disease of the newborn and the prevention of those cases caused by the D-antigen represent a model approach to genetic disease. Few, if any, other known genetic diseases, however, result in an individual who is phenotypically normal but thrust into the genetically inhospitable environment of a "foreign" amniotic sac (although who now could stipulate that such is not the mechanism for production of some "multifactorial" congenital anomalies?).

Table 9-21 Perinatal Infections (Relative North American Incidence)

Common	Rare	"Retired"
Viral		
Cytomegalovirus		Rubella
Hepatitis B	Varicella	
Herpes	Coxsackievirus	
Bacterial		
Streptococcus B	*Staphylococcus aureus*	Streptococcus A
Escherichia coli	*Pseudomonas*	Syphilis
(especially K1)	*Klebsiella-Enterobacter*	Gonorrhea
Listeria	*Proteus*	
	Pneumococcus	
	Pertussis	
	Haemophilus influenzae	
Other		
Chlamydia		
Mycoplasma		
Toxoplasma		

Table 9-22 Respiratory and Pharyngeal Infections (Relative North American Incidence)

Common	Rare	"Retired"
Viral		
Respiratory syncytial virus	Coxsackievirus	Measles
Parainfluenza	Epstein-Barr virus	
Influenza	Herpesvirus	
Rhinovirus	Coronavirus	
Adenovirus		
Bacterial		
Streptococcus A	*Staphylococcus*	Tuberculosis
Pneumococcus	*aureus*	Diphtheria
Haemophilus influenzae	*Legionella*	Pertussis
Other		
Mycoplasma		
Chlamydia		

A classification of the mechanisms of birth defects is offered in the box on p. 120 along with some pertinent examples. Current prenatal diagnostic screening approaches to the prevention of birth defects (actually preventing the birth of those who are defective) are shown in the box on p. 120. Although crude, this scheme can be effective—yet, apart from advanced maternal age (as an index of risk for nondisjunction during meiosis), entry into such a system is by definition purchased at the price of a previous genetic disaster. Genetic engineering for gene replacement or alteration of established genetic disease is yet, analagously speaking, somewhere between Isaac Newton's discovery of the law of universal gravitation and human arrival on the surface of the moon—that is, much engineering remains to be done.

The pediatrician, however, is called on now to be aware of and to deal with the genetic disease already established in the patient. He or she must attempt to clarify the clinical presentation, always suspicious of the possibility of an inborn error of metabolism, particularly among those infants who are phenotypically normal, yet give a history of vomiting, dysphagia, and neurological catastrophe (severe alterations in muscle tone, seizures, or coma) after exposure to ingested sugars or protein. A scheme for screening infants with regard

Table 9-23 Gastrointestinal and Diarrheal Infections (Relative North American Incidence)

Common	Rare	"Retired"
Viral		
Rotavirus	Norwalk virus	Poliovirus
Echovirus		
Coxsackievirus		
Adenovirus		
Bacterial		
Escherichia coli	*Yersinia*	Cholera
Enteropathogenic	*Salmonella*	Typhoid
Enterovirulent	*Shigella*	
Enteroinvasive	*Campylobacter*	
Other		
Giardia	Tapeworm	
	Amebiasis	

Table 9-24 Other Significant Infectious-Disease Agents (Relative North American Incidence)

Common	Rare	"Retired"
Bacteria		
Staphylococcus	*Yersinia*	Tetanus
aureus	*Campylobacter*	*Haemophilus*
	Brucella	*influenzae* B
	Meningococcus	
	Clostridium difficile	
	Leptospira	
	Actinomycosis	
	Nocardiosis	
Viruses		
Hepatitis A	Arthropod borne	Mumps
	(arbovirus)	Rabies
		Smallpox
		Rubella
		Hepatitis B
		Varicella
Rickettsiae	Spotted fever	Typhus
Fungi/yeast		
Tinea	Coccidioidomycosis	
Candida	*Cryptococcus*	
	Aspergillosis	
	Histoplasmosis	
Protozoa	Amebiasis	Malaria
	Sporozoea	
	Pneumocystis carinii	
Helminths		
Ascaris	*Toxocara caris*	Hookworm
Enterobius		*Trichinella*

Table 9-25 Opportunistic Infections

Agents

Many
- Low virulence
- Unusual pathogens

Opportunities

Natural

Development
- Anatomical defects of the skin
- Premature infant (small inoculum)
- Term infant (large inoculum)
- Immune defect

Disease
- Cystic fibrosis
- Diabetes
- Malignancy
- Nephrotic syndrome
- Sickle cell disease

Acquired

- Acquired immune deficiency syndrome (AIDS)
- Burns
- Malnutrition
- Trauma

Iatrogenic

Anatomical invasion
- Surgical procedures
- Dental procedures
- Indwelling catheters and shunts
  - Urinary
  - Vascular
  - Peritoneal
  - Ventricular

Ecological disruption
- Antibiotics
- Inhalation therapy

Immune interference
- Suppression
  - Malignancy
  - Transplantation
- Splenectomy

to the more common (although all are relatively rare) inborn errors of metabolism is displayed in Table 9-18.

In those infants who are abnormal phenotypically, the pediatrician must strive to identify the dysmorphological pattern presented, often in consultation with an appropriate atlas of known defects or a clinical geneticist. The painstaking work of establishing the family pedigree (often a severe challenge in this nation of mobile immigrants) must be undertaken to provide the essential groundwork for genetic counseling. The genotype must be established, where possible (Table 9-19), and biochemical efforts to assay the putative missing enzyme, abnormal substrate (e.g., the glucocerebroside in Gaucher disease), or deficient protein product (e.g., factor VIII in hemophilia) undertaken to identify the affected biochemical pathway.

Prompt detection of some inborn errors (phenylketonuria and maple syrup urine disease) can lead to a rewarding plan for prevention of mental retardation. Some families (those who have a child who has trisomy 21 syndrome) will require consistent, sympathetic support over a long period of time; others (those who have a child who has trisomy 13 or 18) may require more intensive support over a shorter period of time. It is the pediatrician's duty early to decide which type of problem the patient represents.

Infectious Disease

The prior claims to possession of the planet anciently established by the one-celled organisms, the evolution of host defenses by "higher forms" to combat the threat of those microbes, and the genetic ingenuity regularly displayed by such organisms in rapidly developing resistance to human antimicrobials all suggest that infectious diseases will forever remain a fundamental concern for all primary care practitioners, most especially pediatricians. Although most of the great scourges have subsided (for now) in developed countries (e.g., "summer diarrhea," polio, and smallpox), good fortune in genetically driven "antigenic shifts" (e.g., influenza and staphylococcal and streptococcal diseases) apparently has played at least as important a role as clean water, good housing, antimicrobials, and vaccines. Yet every young child who has intact host defenses can, in any society, be overwhelmed by too large an inoculum in the process of developing immunity first-hand.

The basic diagnostic approaches to the infected child are outlined in Table 9-20, the most powerful tool being the practitioner's constant epidemiological awareness of the endemic or invasive infectious disease currently prevalent in his or her community ("what's going around"). A selected microbial demography of common pediatric infectious diseases is set out in Tables 9-21 to 9-24. Of increasing concern are the many opportunistic infections (Table 9-25) that complicate the course of those patients already suffering from serious primary disease, whose host defenses have been assaulted and diminished by human or natural intervention.

REFERENCES

1. Babson SG: Growth of low-birth-weight infants, *J Pediatr* 77:11, 1970.
2. Ballard JL et al: New Ballard Score, expanded to include extremely premature infants, *J Pediatr* 119:417, 1991.

3. Battaglia FC, Lubchenco LO: A practical classification of newborn infants by weight and gestational age, *J Pediatr* 71:161, 1967.
4. Hamill PC et al: Physical growth: National Center for Health Statistics Percentiles, *Am J Clin Nutr* 32:607, 1979.
5. Lubchenco LO, Hansman C, Boyd E: Intrauterine growth in length and head circumference as estimated from live birth at gestational ages from 26 to 42 weeks, *Pediatrics* 37:403, 1966.
6. Marks KH et al: Head growth in sick premature infants: a longitudinal study, *J Pediatr* 94:282, 1979.
7. Nellhaus G: Head circumference from birth to eighteen years: practical composite international and interracial graphs, *Pediatrics* 41:106, 1968.
8. Tanner JM, Whitehouse RH: Clinical longitudinal standards for height, weight, height velocity, weight velocity, and stages of puberty, *Arch Dis Child* 51:170, 1976.
9. Usher R, McLean F: Intrauterine growth of live-born Caucasian infants at sea level: standards obtained from measurements in 7 dimensions of infants born between 25 and 44 weeks of gestation, *J Pediatr* 74:901, 1969.
10. Wright K et al: New postnatal growth grids for very low birthweight infants, *Pediatrics* 91:922, 1993.

SUGGESTED READINGS

Frankenburg WK, Camp BW: *Pediatric screening test*, Springfield, Ill, 1975, Charles C Thomas.

Thorpe HS, Werner EE: Developmental screening of preschool children, *Pediatrics* 53:362, 1974.

10 Communication with Parents and Patients

Ruth J. Messinger, Philip W. Davidson, and Robert A. Hoekelman

One important goal of any diagnostic procedure is to simplify the choice of treatment and clarify the prognosis. An extremely important component of this goal is conveying pertinent information to the child or to his or her parents or advocates. In most clinical circumstances in which the illness is minor or carries an excellent prognosis, such information is presented straightforwardly by the diagnostician to the patient or the parents. In those cases that involve children who are gravely ill, severely handicapped, mentally retarded, learning disabled, or emotionally disturbed, however, the situation becomes far more complex for clinicians, patients, and parents. Parents, years after the fact, vividly remember how and when the "bad news" was told. The interpretive presentation therefore must become part of a broader counseling session that deals with feelings and emotions, as well as facts, to ensure understanding of the information being shared.

This chapter focuses on the process of information sharing with parents or patient as an extension of the diagnostic process itself. The goal of interpreting diagnostic findings is more than merely announcing technical information. The real objective in providing that information is to establish a partnership between the provider and parents that will enhance the parents' capacity to respond appropriately to their child's illness and to comply with the recommended treatment.

Recent legislative changes that mandate participation by parents in decisions about their children who have special needs and that emphasize family-centered, coordinated, case-managed care make this partnership even more crucial. Part H of the Individuals with Disabilities Education Act (Public Law #100-476), for example, specifically mandates parent-driven planning of service provision to their offspring ages 0 to 2 who have disabilities.

There is no one blueprint for building the very important relationship between clinician and parents; however, interpretation of the physician's findings to parents, without unnecessary delay, is essential in case management, as is the need to attend to the family's expectations and questions initially and over time. Klein[4] provides an in-depth analysis of how professionals' negative attitudes toward and absence of respect for parents can interfere with constructive communication about a child's diagnosis and treatment. This dialogue may be complicated further when clinicians become frustrated by their inability to cure or "save" the child, when they know that there are no local resources to deal with the child's problem, or when the parents ask questions that the clinician cannot answer.

A professional-parent relationship based on the posture, "I have the information, and I know what's best for your child," represents a basic misinterpretation of the kind of relationship between parent and clinician that is necessary when information about a complex and threatening illness has to be shared. Diagnosis and treatment are biomedical, but psychosocial and educational matters and their presentation to parents are decidedly nonmedical; such presentation is itself a psychosocial process of interpersonal communication. It is inappropriate to assume that simply "having the information" or knowledge about "what's best" for the child is sufficient for communicating diagnostic, therapeutic, and prognostic information to the parents. Parents usually know their child better than anyone else and are central as nurturers, caretakers, and guardians of their children.

Myers[7] cautions that to communicate effectively, clinicians must maintain a flow of information between parents and themselves; simply telling parents the facts of an evaluation does not guarantee that they will hear or understand. Fuller and Geis,[2] Lynch and Staloch,[6] and Triggs and Perrin[8] agree that clinicians must communicate with the parents, and the parents with them, for an understanding to be achieved. Such communication can be described in general terms, but its effective implementation depends on careful individual planning and a reasonable investment of time.

The box on p. 126 outlines a method for conducting an "interpretive" conference. The format outlines four major steps, each equally important, that are essential for an effective outcome. It is applicable when the child is evaluated by the clinician (physician, nurse, psychologist, social worker, or educational specialist) alone or when several professionals have been involved as members of an interdisciplinary team in the diagnostic evaluation.

PREPARATION FOR AN INTERPRETIVE CONFERENCE

The interpretive conference must be planned beforehand to ensure that the conference will achieve its purpose. The conference should occur as soon as possible after the examination and testing of the patient. The clinician who conducts the conference is best prepared, both emotionally and cognitively, immediately after the last visit or staffing conference, and parents are anxious to hear about the outcome of the evaluation as soon as possible.

If more than one professional is involved in the conference, the basic aim should be to establish maximum communication between parents and professionals while this expertise is available to ensure that most parental questions can be answered effectively. With certain conditions, such as mental retardation and learning or emotional disorders, the physician may not be included in the conference or may not be the primary spokesperson. In these circumstances the psychologist, special educator, or social work clinician might serve that role.

Sometimes the parents view the physician as an authority figure. The implication of this perception is that the credibil-

INTERPRETIVE CONFERENCE FORMAT OUTLINE

- I. Entry pattern
  - A. Review of evaluation procedures conducted
  - B. Parents' and child's perceptions
  - C. Restatement of parental concerns
    - 1. Main worry
    - 2. Additional concerns
- II. Presentation of findings
  - A. Encapsulation: brief overview
  - B. Reaction by parents and patient
  - C. Detailed findings
    - 1. Reactions to normal test results
    - 2. Reactions to abnormal test results
- III. Recommendations—only after time has been allowed for reactions
  - A. Restatement of concerns with both parents
  - B. Recommendations—one at a time
  - C. Reactions after each recommendation
  - D. Sharing with the child
- IV. Summary
  - A. Repetition of findings, in varied wording if possible
  - B. Restatement by parents or patient
  - C. Planning for future contacts

ity of a team that does not include the physician may be impaired. On the other hand, the physician need not automatically be cast in the role of leader at an interpretive conference unless the bulk of the information to be discussed is biomedical. In no case should the interpretation of technical material to parents be left in the hands of nonprofessionals or professionals whose lack of expertise could lead to parental misunderstanding. Also, the information should not be revealed by someone who did not participate in the diagnostic workup.

Once the team members have been selected, they should meet long enough to organize the conference, following the outline in the box above. This planning session should allow enough time to ensure that all the team members agree on the major information to be shared with the parents and that all terminology is understood. Team members also should select a leader who will structure the conference. This is of paramount importance because organization of the conference is the key to satisfactory communication. The leader's responsibility is to control the flow of information from professionals to parents and vice versa to ensure two-way communication. *Control* implies not only organization but also a certain empathic sensitivity for the parents' feelings and reactions so that emotional highs and lows can be adequately recognized, permitted, and dealt with respecting families' cultural proscriptions and without the purpose of the conference being disrupted.

The clinician who is to present the information alone also should plan the presentation, following the same procedures recommended for the team. Preparation especially is important for individual presentations because the individual has a more difficult task of control than does the group once the conference has begun. In this circumstance the clinician continuously must be the spokesperson, without having the chance to listen to another professional present information while organizing his or her own thoughts or "picking up" on points that others have not made clear or have not made at all.

CONDUCTING THE CONFERENCE

Entry Pattern

The beginning of the interview often sets the tone for what follows. It is assumed that planning has included those physical requirements that create an empathic climate, privacy, and freedom from interruption.

A review of what has been done diagnostically should be shared with a minimum of technical jargon so that parents will not be intimidated when asked to discuss their "main worry." During such a discussion a "hidden agenda" often surfaces, related either to the cause of the problem or to the problem itself. Therefore, before the information is presented to the parents, the parents' perception of the child and the child's current situation should be sought. For example, the practitioner might ask both parents, "How do you see Mary's problems and strengths today?" Even if both parents have accompanied their child throughout the evaluation, each may have different knowledge about and reactions to what is happening.[1] This also is an appropriate time to ask what others have told them of their child's condition.

Presentation of Findings

Dwelling on technical data that do little to enhance the parents' understanding of their child's disorder accomplishes nothing and may interfere with establishing good professional-parent communication. Such data only serve to confuse, rather than clarify, the parents' concerns. When several different tests have been done in a lengthy, technical evaluation, it is especially helpful for parents to understand that the data presented summarize the results of all those tests.

Some parents need a name for their child's illness or problem. If labels have not already been used by others, they may well be in the future. Most parents want honest appraisals and will resent ambiguous assurances that border on deception. For example, if an infant has been born having fetal alcohol syndrome, the parents should be told that that is the diagnosis rather than given vague or technical terms such as "multiple craniofacial and other anomalies" to explain their child's condition.

The practitioner(s) should focus on the parents' own perceptions of their child when explaining findings, particularly as these may relate to the parent's experiences with other children. Age or grade equivalents rather than ratio scores are useful when it is necessary to convey the presence of developmental delay or immaturity. For example, the clinician might say, "Your daughter seems in many ways to behave more like a 10-year-old than a 15-year-old. That is what the psychological testing indicates when it finds your daughter has an IQ of 55." It is clearer to say, "Joey reads and understands written information more like a third grader than a ninth grader" than to say, "Your son's test scores show 'scatter,' and he has a learning disability." It often is said that after the parents hear the bad news, they hear very little else. Krahn et al[5] reiterate parents' need to hear something positive in the "informing" interview. For this reason the actual presentation should begin with areas of strength or normality. Abnormal findings, stated honestly but gently, should be restated more than once and by using different words to convey the same findings. Indeed, Kaminer and Cohen[3] emphasize the relationship between empathy and honesty: "The literature documents that communication skills can be taught or at least improved. Acquiring an understanding heart seems to be more difficult." Parents should be encouraged to react to the diagnosis of the problem and to accept their feelings, including the anger that is often directed at the clinician. Responses that reflect shock, guilt, bereavement, and inadequacy frequently are seen in various intensities and combinations. Communication at this level also is influenced by any sociocultural and educational differences between the professionals and the parents.

Recommendations

Specific information should be shared at a pace that can be handled emotionally and cognitively. Parents seldom feel comfortable asking for clarification, but if they are asked to restate their "main worry" and other worries, the practitioner's recommendations can become meaningful and relevant. Parents usually find it helpful to receive recommendations that include, among other things, communication with other parents who have a child with a similar problem and referral elsewhere for help.

Recommendations are not complete until the interpreter and both parents are able to decide what will be communicated to the child and who will do it. Parents' wishes and the cognitive and emotional development of the child are important considerations in this very important issue.

SUMMARY

After recommendations have been shared and before the session is terminated, findings once again should be highlighted. One successful method for obtaining feedback is to ask parents to restate what they heard and what decisions were made. This provides the professional with the parents' perception and understanding of the problem and allows for further clarification, if necessary.

Often, more than one "interpretive" session is indicated. This can be planned by arranging for parents to contact the clinician by telephone (at a definite time) after they have had time to think about and react to the information that was shared or when further questions and concerns arise. The session should be terminated only after the clinician has stated a willingness and an ability to participate in a therapeutic alliance with the parents.

Discussion of diagnostic findings is a dynamic process that is an initial step in building a therapeutic milieu. The model presented here organizes a typically complex, often unwieldy, process between the professional and the parents that easily can end disastrously and decrease chances for successful therapeutic intervention with the patient. If the clinical findings, diagnosis, and prognosis are presented clearly during the conference, two-way communication will be fostered because both the professional and the parents can identify the limits of the situation and focus on the problems that can be dealt with successfully. This method of imparting information enhances the professional-parent relationship and encourages immediate and future communication and compliance with recommendations.

REFERENCES

1. Bailey D, Blasco P, Simeonsson R: Needs expressed by mothers and fathers of young children with disabilities, *Am J Ment Retard* 97:1, 1992.
2. Fuller R, Geis S: Communicating with the grieving family, *J Fam Pract* 21:139, 1985.
3. Kaminer R, Cohen H: How do you say, "Your child is retarded"? *Contemp Pediatr* 5:36, 1988.
4. Klein S: The challenge of communicating with parents, *Dev Behav Pediatr* 14:3, 1993.
5. Krahn G, Hallum A, Kime C: Are there good ways to give 'Bad News'? *Pediatrics* 91:3, 1993.
6. Lynch EG, Staloch NH: Parental perceptions of physicians' communication in the informing process, *Ment Retard* 26:77, 1988.
7. Myers B: The informing interview, *Am J Dis Child* 137:572, 1983.
8. Triggs EG, Perrin E: Improving communication about behavior and development, *Clin Pediatr* 28:185, 1989.

SUGGESTED READINGS

Able-Boone H, Dopecki PR, Smith MS: Parent and health care provider communication and decision making in the intensive care nursery, *Child Health Care* 18:133, 1989.

Fletcher AB, Saren AV: Communicating with parents of high-risk infants, *Pediatr Ann* 17:477, 1988.

Greenberg LW et al: Giving information for a life-threatening diagnosis, *Am J Dis Child* 138:649, 1984.

Johnson SH: Ten ways to help the families of a critically ill patient, *Nursing* 1:50, 1986.

Sharp MC, Strauss RP, Horch SC: Communicating medical bad news: parents' experiences and preferences, *J Pediatr* 121:539, 1992.

Stone D: A parent speaks: Professional perceptions of parental adaptation to a child with special needs, *Child Health Care* 18:174, 1989.

Turnbull AP, Turnbull HR, editors: *Parents speak out: then and now,* Columbus, Ohio, 1985, Merrill.

11 Cultural Issues in Primary Pediatric Care

Karen Olness

You are working in a pediatric emergency room, and you evaluate an 11-month-old child who was born in the Middle East. He has had a fever and cold for a week. On examination you find signs of otitis media and round ulcerated areas on both wrists. The family explains that they were treating the child with crushed garlic cloves taped onto the child's wrists.

You are a middle-aged pediatrician working in the outpatient department of a large county hospital. A Hmong child is brought in with a cold and fever. You conduct a thorough examination, including otoscopy, and diagnose otitis media. Through the interpreter you prescribe amoxicillin and arrange for a follow-up appointment. Two days later the child, who is still febrile, returns in the company of 10 adult relatives and the interpreter. You begin an examination. However, when you reach for the otoscope, the interpreter says that the family requests that you not use it.

You are working in a small group practice and have many Mexican-American families as clients. One of the nurse assistants is Mexican-American, and she brings her children to the practice for well-child care. She is well liked by families and colleagues within the practice. One day she mentions that her 4-year-old son is ill and asks to leave early. You offer to see him, and she replies that he has *empacho,* a gastrointestinal illness and that she is taking him to see a healer in the family. She says that *empacho* cannot be cured by conventional medical treatment.

The above examples represent the types of cross-cultural situations encountered by pediatricians. As they become familiar with the particular belief guiding the use of garlic plasters or the use of an otoscope or the diagnosis of *empacho,* pediatricians learn how to cope with these situations. More complex cross-cultural issues are those never manifested overtly by clients; they can result in noncompliance, the seeking of another physician, or misinterpretation of the diagnosis and treatment. The goal of transcultural medicine, now taught in many medical schools, is not to familiarize physicians with all cultural issues related to medicine but rather to sensitize physicians to different cultural beliefs (see the box on p. 129). It is hoped that they may take into account different expectations regarding their roles and different explanations for disease that evolve from varying cultural beliefs.

American child health professionals have more cross-cultural issues to consider than do child health professionals in any other country, and they receive little guidance and preparation for these issues. American child health providers encounter cross-cultural issues when diagnosing and treating families who are newcomers to the United States[13] or those whose cultural heritages relate to parents or grandparents who immigrated to the United States. Furthermore, American child health providers are mobile and may themselves work in several different cultural environments during a lifetime. In the future it is likely that the services of American child health experts will be required increasingly in Third World areas,[10,34] where 90% of the world's babies are born.

DEFINITIONS

Americans living in urban areas encounter cultural differences every day and may be unaware of them as they work, shop, and play. Culture, cultural norms, and one's perception of social self all play a part in the way reality is defined. *Social self* refers to the way individuals perceive or present themselves to others. It includes the degree of acceptance of the culture or subculture the individuals are in and how they project that acceptance or rejection to those around them. *Culture* is defined as a way of life for a group of people: how they work; how they relax; their values, prejudices, and biases; and the way they interact with one another. This involves *cultural norms,* which are ethical and moral or traditional principles of a given society. Cultural norms usually are unwritten but, nevertheless, are understood as the rules and values by which a culture functions. People are expected to abide by these unwritten rules or norms. When they violate these, they may be criticized or ostracized by others within the culture. Cultural norms include unwritten definitions of health, sickness, and abnormality.

A popular current phrase is "the culture of the workplace." Managers use this phrase often; yet those within a work environment are not provided guidelines for assessing their own cultural norms and how they may fit or conflict with the culture of a workplace. It is possible for a pediatrician to feel comfortable in a children's hospital (i.e., workplace), whether that pediatrician is American or French or Ethiopian, but to feel distinctly out of place in social, recreational, or political aspects of that society. The workplace culture often becomes the principal and most comfortable culture for health professionals, regardless of their own ethnic background, age, sex, or linguistic abilities.

Cross-cultural discomforts in the pediatric workplace may arise from efforts to communicate with families who have different cultural norms.[15,20] The child health professional may feel uncomfortable in spite of efforts to be nonjudgmental, because cultural norms are powerful determinants of a person's perceptions. Furthermore, medical training itself is an enculturating process leading one to hold the same values as one's medical peers.

Explanations of Disease: Cultural Variations

Namboze[25] noted that cultural beliefs about disease causation in Ganda society fall under the following categories: magical, supernatural, infectious, and hereditary. She notes

WAYS TO DEVELOP CULTURAL SENSITIVITY

1. Recognize that cultural diversity exists.
2. Demonstrate respect for people as unique individuals, with culture as one factor that contributes to their uniqueness.
3. Respect the unfamiliar.
4. Identify and examine your own cultural beliefs.
5. Recognize that some cultural groups have definitions of health and illness as well as practices that attempt to promote health and cure illness, which may differ from the provider's.
6. Be willing to modify health care delivery in keeping with the patient's cultural background.
7. Do not expect all members of one cultural group to behave in exactly the same way.
8. Appreciate that each person's cultural values are ingrained and therefore very difficult to change.

From Stulc DM: The family as a bearer of culture. In Cookfair JM: *Nursing process and practice in the community,* St Louis, 1990, Mosby.

that some of these beliefs are beneficial and can be included in health teaching. Others are harmless and best left alone by child health professionals; some cultural practices, however, are harmful.

Garlic, mentioned in the first vignette, has been part of healing folklore in many cultures. Like many herbal treatments, it may cause multiple adverse effects in addition to local burns.[8]

Bill Moyers' book, *Healing and the Mind,*[24] following his PBS television series, was on the *New York Times* bestseller list for months. The National Institutes of Health, responding to congressional demand, has developed an Office of Alternative Medicine.

Empacho, mentioned in the earlier vignette, is a gastrointestinal disorder attributed to food or saliva getting "stuck." It is believed to be caused by ingesting too much or by eating either the wrong food or at the wrong time. Infants can get *empacho* by swallowing too much saliva during teething, and adults may get it as a result of anxiety.[19,27] Folk healers treat *empacho* with diet change, laxatives, herbal teas, and massage. A study of 67 Puerto Rican parents in Connecticut found that 64% said a child had had *empacho.*[27]

Many ethnic groups within the United States bring their ill children to both pediatricians and traditional healers within the community.[5,16,17,26] Special ceremonies, herbal remedies, chanting, and prayer often are prescribed by the latter. It is unusual for the family to share this information with their pediatricians unless the pediatrician is of the same ethnic group, speaks the same language, or has a long-standing, trusting relationship with the family.

It should be noted that well-educated American parents may purchase vitamins, minerals, and food supplements at health food stores or consult chiropractors for their children and also may not inform their pediatricians about all treatments being used.

A recent survey of American adults found that 34% reported using at least one unconventional therapy in the past year. A third of these saw providers for unconventional therapy, making an average of 19 visits in 1 year. The type of therapy included relaxation and imagery techniques, chiropractic and spiritual healing, commercial weight-loss programs, megavitamin therapy, homeopathy, acupuncture, and massage.[6]

A Minnesota physician who works at St. Paul–Ramsey Medical Center International Clinic was infertile and decided to consult an herbalist and a shaman while she was visiting a Hmong village in Thailand. Treatment included drinking a mixture of dried bugs, alcohol, and mucus. A year later her daughter was born.[11] She believes that patients should be encouraged to use both their traditional and our medical systems.

CULTURAL ASSESSMENT

Appraising a patient's or parent's cultural beliefs, values, and customs is an essential part of health assessment[30] (Table 11-1). In Leininger's opinion, a cultural assessment is as important as a physical or psychological assessment.[18] Cultural assessments can be used to understand behavior that otherwise could be interpreted as negative or noncompliant.

It is important to remain sensitive to individual differences within the cultural groups while gathering information concerning a particular family; it is important not to make stereotypical assumptions. Problems arise when a negative attitude comes from these erroneous assumptions. For example, although alcoholism is prevalent in many Native American tribes, it would be erroneous to assume that any Native American treated is an alcoholic. Developing a false sense of cultural knowledge can impede the practitioner from learning specific aspects about a particular culture. An accurate understanding of several cultures would certainly take an anthropologist years of study. The best recommendation is to review the available literature and interview colleagues who are members of a specific cultural group. Observation and interview are two useful tools when assessing cultural background.[3,30] Tripp-Reimer, Brink, and Saunders present several aspects to the cultural assessment that involve the following[33]:

- Ethnic group affiliation and racial background
- Major values and beliefs
- Health beliefs and practices
- Religious influences or special rituals
- Language barriers and communication styles
- Parenting styles and role of the family
- Dietary practices

The American Medical Association distributes a manual on providing culturally competent care for adolescents.[1] This guide lists open-ended questions to facilitate understanding of how an adolescent from another culture perceives his or her health problem; for example, "Apart from me, who do you think can help you get better?"

Ethnic Group Affiliation and Racial Background

Racial background refers to specific physical and structural characteristics. These characteristics are transmitted genetically and distinguish one group from another. Some diseases are more prevalent for genetic reasons in certain racial or ethnic groups, such as sickle cell anemia in African Americans

Table 11-1 Characteristics of Culturally Diverse Families*†

	Origin	
	Eastern Asian	**Hispanic**
Ethnic affiliation/racial background	Pacific Islands, Japan, China, Phillipines, Korea, Vietnam, Laos Characteristics include Mongolian spots or irregular areas of deep-blue pigmentation, commonly seen in sacral/gluteal regions. Lactase deficiency is common.[4] Sensitive to alcohol, characterized by hypotension, tachycardia, and bronchial constriction in Japanese.[8]	Puerto Rican, Cuban, Mexican, and South and Central American. Ancestry can be Aztec and Mayan, Spanish, and African blacks. *Although some pride themselves on "mixed" descent, others do not.*
Major values/beliefs	Dignity paramount; important to "save face." Emotions should be controlled to think logically and to judge objectively. *Tendency to keep problems to themselves.*	Loyalty to family is more important than individual needs. Belief: humans have very little control over their future; they stress the "will of God."
Health beliefs/practices	Disease is caused by imbalance between opposing forces of yin and yang. Disharmony results from improper care of body or unhappiness with oneself or society; can result in disease. *Balance is disrupted by blood being drawn for tests. Therefore, there is a reluctance to cooperate. Problem: when herbal medicines are taken along with prescribed medications, effects are unknown but patients should be warned that one might weaken the other.*	Health is considered a gift from God; illness is punishment for wrongdoing. Cure is sought from *curanderos* (folk healers) who use prayer, ritual, and laying on of the hands. Less common disorders are will of God. *Health is considered a balance among the four humors of the body* (blood, phlegm, black bile, and yellow bile). "Hot" diseases require "cold" treatment and vice versa. For example: Penicillin is considered "hot" and may not be taken if patient has fever. *Noncompliance* results.
Religious influences	Families may practice Buddhism, Confucianism, Taoism, or "Western" religions (Judaism or Christianity). Confucianism stresses duty toward others; Taoism, self-realization through harmony, which influences followers to avoid conflict. Buddists believe their present lives predetermine their destiny. Death is accepted as a natural part of the life cycle. Many prefer to die in their own home. Belief: a person who dies outside of the home will become a wandering soul with no place to rest.	Approximately 85% to 90% are Catholic.[18] Priest plays important role as spiritual leader and adviser.
Language barriers/ communication styles	May smile or laugh to mask emotions or nod "yes" even when they disagree. To question authority figures or to look directly into eyes is considered sign of disrespect. Eastern Asians may wait silently rather than ask questions because they believe the health care provider will know best. *Use of touch through handshaking is uncomfortable;* should be avoided unless the patient offers first. Needs permission before touching head. (Belief: head is sacred part of body.) Disrespectful to point toe in someone's direction or show bottom of shoes while crossing legs. (Belief: foot is the lowliest part of the body.) Many Eastern Asians will offer food or drink; it is disrespectful not to accept. Wait until patient partakes first.	Spanish is the predominant language. *Translators should be same sex as patient because modesty is valued and may make sexual discussion uncomfortable.* Touch is an acceptable form of expression and may be used among friends and family through hugging, kissing, and holding hands.

*It is very important to use this chart as a guideline for information concerning culturally diversified families rather than as a set of restrictions and rules. Suggested readings and references along with patient/family interviews will be helpful in obtaining more information about a particular group of people. Potential problems are set in italics.

Data from Stulc DM: The family as a bearer of culture. In Cookfair JM: *Nursing process and practice in the community,* St Louis, 1991, Mosby.

†Readers should be aware that these categories (e.g., Native American, Eastern Asian, and so on) are *general categories* only and that, for instance, not all Eastern Asian people have rice as their main starch. Nonetheless, we find the categories useful as an example of how cultures can differ *in general.*

Table 11-1 Characteristics of Culturally Diverse Families*†—cont'd

	Origin	
	Eastern Asian	**Hispanic**
Parenting styles/role of the family	Extended family may live together. In more traditional families, the father is the authority figure. Early childhood parenting is permissive. Infants seldom cry. Feed on demand. Weaning takes place later than in Anglo-American infants. Parents may allow children to sleep with them. At age 5 or 6, sterner discipline in which obedience is stressed begins. Physical and nonphysical (scolding and shaming) disciplinary techniques are implemented. Aggression (fighting) is disapproved of and admonished. The mother is the primary disciplinarian and plays the major role in child rearing.[26]	Strong sense of family exists. Many live in extended families. Communities are paternalistic, so men must be considered in all decisions; however, they are minimally involved in child care. Children are highly valued. Parents provide much physical attention. Independence is encouraged in boys; girls are protected. *Respect for authority figures may cause adults to feign agreement or understanding.* Attitude that "problems" should stay within family.
Dietary practices	Rice is the main starch. Milk is not readily consumed because a taste for it has not been acquired. *Possible lactose intolerance. Calcium acquired through soybeans, small bony fish, sesame seeds, and tofu.*	Basic staples: rice and beans, along with corn, fruits such as green bananas, and chilis. Diet is high in vegetable protein, carbohydrates, smaller amounts of animal protein and calcium.[18] *Hispanics see fat babies as a sign of good health.* Putting additional cereal in bottle is a common practice. *Consider "hot" and "cold" foods in diet as a part of treatment.* Believe that "hot" foods, (chili peppers, grains, kidney beans, alcoholic beverages, beef, lamb) are more easily digested than "cold."[7]

	Origin	
	Native American	**African American**
Ethnic affiliation/racial background	400 Indian tribes in United States and Canada; more than 280 reservations. No one language or style of dress.	Heterogeneous group, the majority of whom are descendents of people from West Africa (formerly Ivory Coast). *Sickle cell anemia is common in blacks, along with glucose-6-phosphate dehydrogenase (G6PD) deficiency.*
Major values/beliefs	Respect for harmony between humans and nature, generosity, sharing of possessions, personal integrity and bravery, brotherhood, compassion for others. Competitive behavior discouraged.	Orientation toward the present rather than the future, *implications for preventive health maintenance.* Orientation to time is flexible in terms of schedules and appointments. Needs of family are valued over punctuality.
Health beliefs/practices	Health is a state of harmony between humans and nature. Illness is caused by witchcraft, violation of taboos, possession by spirits, loss of soul, disease or object intrusion into the body.[31] Prevention may involve wearing a talisman or carrying a special sack of herbs.	Health beliefs for low-income black Americans are described as a blend of elements from Africa, folk medicine, selected aspects of modern scientific medicine, with others of Christianity, voodoo, and magic. Southern communities use roots, herb potions, oils, powders, tokens, rituals, and ceremonies. Prayer is used as a method of treatment because illness is a punishment for failure to abide by God's rules.
Religious influences	Religion plays an integral part. Mountains, rivers, and all geographical features considered sacred.	After the Civil War, religion provided support for struggle with poverty, unemployment, and overcrowded living. Leadership often attained through church roles. Ministers play an important role in community and provide support during stress.
Language barriers/ communication styles	Many different languages exist. Many tribes value nonverbal language. Periods of silence might mean one is becoming sensitive to environment or gathering thoughts for greater impact when speaking. Do not value individuals who hurry speech, interrupt, and interject. Sensitive to nervous mannerisms. Appreciate hand shake and eye contact. Unwavering eye gaze should be avoided because it is viewed as insulting.	Health care providers from dominant white cultures create barriers and prevent effective communication. Attempts to imitate stereotypical and stylized "black English" may be perceived as mockery and should be avoided.

Table 11-1 Characteristics of Culturally Diverse Families*†—cont'd

	Origin	
	Native American	African American
Parenting styles/role of the family	Clan membership is inherited through the mother. Elders are respected. Parents value children highly. Children are seldom disciplined by raising of the voice or by use of physical force. Parents instill respect not only for elders but also for worthy objects within nature.	Close-knit circle of relatives and family is the norm; all participate in child rearing. Thus structure is seen as buffer from stress.[28] Socialization of black children can pose special challenges.[1,34] "To raise a black child without any notion that he is viewed differently because of race would be disastrous."[34] The child's individuality is highly valued. First-born children tend to receive more mothering. Adolescent girls are encouraged to accept more responsibilities; teenage boys are given freedom from responsibility.
Dietary practices	Foods may be used in ceremonies to ward off illness or to regain health. Delaware Indians prohibit eating meat during a febrile illness. One restriction, such as cow's milk, is based on prevalent lactose intolerance.[35] Corn, squash, and beans are typical staples.	Salt pork as a seasoning is common and greens such as collard, mustard, chard, and kale are common. Vinegar and hot peppers are condiments. Boiling and frying are the main method of preparation. *Hypertension and strokes cause high mortality among black Americans, with men 15.5 times more affected than their white counterparts.*[29]

and Tay-Sachs disease in families of Ashkenazi Jewish origin.

Within the boundaries of one country, such as Uganda or Laos, there may be scores of different tribes who vary with respect to physical characteristics, genetically transmitted diseases, and health beliefs. On the other hand, some beliefs and life-styles that affect health are common to ethnic groups that could not have had communication with one another. An example of this is the child rearing habit that leads to toddler malnutrition. After giving birth, the mother is isolated with the new baby for several weeks. The older toddler, who has been with the mother continually before the sibling's birth, is now rejected. He is depressed, eats poorly, and develops malnutrition. The word *kwashiorkor,* an African tribal word, means "disease of the deposed or separated child."

Health Beliefs and Practices

Viewpoints on health and healing vary from group to group. The basic definition of illness stems from a dominant American culture and is based on Western scientific thought, which views illness as a breakdown in a body part because of invasion by an organism.[24,30] Extreme effort is necessary to see illness and healing from a different perspective. Sensitivity is important because a lack of it can affect patient safety. The issue of pain is dealt with in Zborowski's classic study.[37] While the dominant American culture values stoicism and nonemotional expressions of pain, other cultures may express pain through screaming, moaning, and verbal complaining. An understanding of these differences is essential in assessing and treating pain in children.[2]

Beliefs and perceptions regarding disabilities relate to culture. Many Asian societies are concerned about the spiritual cause of a disability, for example, failure to follow a tradition. A child born with a disability may be the recipient of punishment assigned to a parent or relative.[7] These beliefs are present among Americans from Asian cultures and may affect whether rehabilitation treatment is perceived as important.

Religious Influences or Special Rituals

The dominant culture has separated "church and state" for so many years that it is quite common to separate those entities in health care as well. However, for many cultures, religion still influences beliefs strongly concerning health and illness, death, and treatment. It is important to assess the role of significant religious leaders, especially during times of life-threatening illness. Special religious ceremonies may be comforting to the ill child and to family members. These should be integrated into the treatment.

Language Barriers and Communication Styles

Determining which language is spoken at home is essential in assessing the culture.[30] Although the family and child may speak English, their words and understanding, especially of cognitive expression, may be limited. It is recommended that an interpreter accompany the primary caregiver when explaining potentially complex topics. Assessing a family's ability to read and write in English also is important.

Nonverbal communication may have different meanings in different cultures. Many Eastern Asian–Americans nod out of respect, not necessarily out of understanding. Some behaviors can lead to alienation and eventually withdrawal; thus their meanings are essential in keeping communication open. In Bulgaria, one nods the head to mean "no" and moves the head back and forth to denote "yes."

Parenting Styles and Role of Family

Understanding that "parenting is neither good nor bad in any culture, simply different," is the basis of acknowledging differing cultures' attitudes toward the family.[4] It is inaccurate to assume that the dominant American culture has all the answers when it comes to parenting. While the dominant

American culture may value independence in children, another culture may value submissiveness.[30] Attitudes toward family members vary with each culture. Culture will address how different members' advice is regarded and whether those members are involved in decisions. Culture also will affect the values held about children, family structure, and gender.[9] Parental attitudes regarding infant development and sleeping arrangements often reflect cultural values.[22]

Dietary Practices

Diet is an integral part of a person's culture. Dietary practices can include not only preferences and dislikes of particular foods but also food preparation, consumption, frequency, time of eating, and utensils used. When a prescribed diet is part of a patient's treatment, it is essential to assess the cultural influences involved. Consulting a nutritionist, a cultural informant, or colleagues of various ethnic backgrounds can be helpful.

In Table 11-1, four different cultures are outlined according to seven points of assessment. There is a tendency to assume that all members of a similar cultural background share commonalities, such as language, religion, and viewpoints.[32] Knowing the differences of the backgrounds within the different cultures is essential to becoming sensitive to cultural assessments.

HOW PEOPLE INTERACT: EXPECTATIONS FOR APPROPRIATE BEHAVIOR

Perhaps in a century, all people of the world will share a common culture with respect to appropriate interactions. The U.S. population has scores of views regarding appropriate interpersonal interactions.[21] More than a common language is required to develop a consensus regarding, for example, eye contact, touching, personal space or territory, appearance, gestures, use of the voice, greetings, partings, and facial expressions. Even responses to pain vary among cultural groups, including subcultures in the United States.[2,14] Most humans tend to use the rules regarding these interactions developed from childhood cultural experiences. Complicating this within the United States is that chaotic living situations for children may not provide models for appropriate interpersonal interactions. Young children who watch television a great deal and who are unable to distinguish what is real from what is not (acting) often imitate unusual or inappropriate interpersonal interactions.

In diplomatic circles there are norms, some of them written, with respect to communication. Diplomats are encouraged to learn about cultural norms within their host country, for example, who can shake hands, how close to another one stands at a reception, and how much eye contact is allowed. Yet diplomats make mistakes and therefore are misinterpreted. American child health professionals who interact with peers from other cultures should study cultural norms before working with foreign colleagues, whether in this country or their own. Visitors from East Africa and Southeast Asia often complain that they find American friendliness superficial. The immediate pleasant friendliness of Americans would represent a more advanced stage of personal intimacy and friendship in their cultures, and they are offended when they discover that it does not necessarily reflect depth. They also find it difficult to accept gifts from Americans because, in many cultures, gifts are only in exchange for something or to acquire an advantage. Direct expression of feelings is inappropriate and considered bizarre in many cultures. In Thailand, for example, one turns anger toward another object, either animate or inanimate, called "prachot."[12] This is done consciously to alert the person (who is the object of one's displeasure and annoyance) to how the injured party feels. In Southeast Asia, avoiding confrontation is considered positive and expressing anger, hatred, and annoyance overtly is considered negative.

There are a number of training programs to increase sensitivity among people toward varying cultural norms and values. Pediatricians who plan to work in other cultures may benefit from a game ("Bafa-bafa") in which participants are divided into two groups and provided with values, expectations, and customs of a new culture.[29]

PERCEPTUAL DIFFERENCES AMONG CULTURES

Perceptual differences among various groups of humans relate not only to group beliefs, customs, and experiences but also to differences in sensory systems that may have evolved in response to the need for individual survival or to society's needs. These are well-documented differences in auditory, visual, musical, and tactile skills and may relate to differences in eye-hand coordination, information processing, and language and spatial perceptions.

Some of the differences may be genetic, but others reflect the emphasis, focus, and practice of a skill within a culture. For example, an infant's perceptual abilities are modified by listening to a particular language. Syllables, words, and sentences used in all human languages are formed from a set of speech sounds called *phones*. Only part of the phones are used in any particular language. Young infants can discriminate nearly every phonetic contrast, but this broad-based sensitivity declines by 1 year of age.[35] Adults have difficulty discriminating phones that do not connote meaning in their own native language and thus are handicapped when learning a new language. English-speaking natives have difficulty in perceiving the difference between two "k" phonemes (sounds) used in Thai. Japanese-speaking adults have difficulty distinguishing between the English */ra/* and */la/*. Adults who learn another language early but who do not practice the language as they mature may lose their ability to differentiate among its sounds.

Learning the language of another culture is essential to understanding that culture. Dependency on bilingual translators or interpreters is fraught with the likelihood of misunderstanding, especially in medicine. In some cultures, the status of the interpreter affects what information is provided by the patient and how it is prepared for the ears of the foreign health professional. If the patient is of "higher" status than the interpreter, an awkward situation can result for the interpreter. If the interpreter has little specific knowledge regarding health and medical matters, translation is less than ideal. Furthermore, abstract concepts may not translate well from English to other languages. For example, it is much more difficult to express abstract concepts in Norwegian or in Russian than in English. Many words from Western languages do not exist in Asian languages; therefore the concepts do not exist. Similarly, some Asian concepts cannot be expressed in English. The Lao language, for example, is richer in terms of words related to family relationships than is the English language.

Many studies have demonstrated that information processing differs among cultures. For example, a study of university students from four cultures demonstrated culturally dependent differences in processing information that affected choices of color dominance.[28] Numerous studies have demonstrated cultural differences in children's preferences for colors and shapes. For example, one study demonstrated that African children clearly prefer color to form into their adolescence.[31] Euro-American children, however, selected form over color from kindergarten age into adulthood. Language structure may determine perceptual preference with respect to form or color. For example, Navajo children demonstrate form preferences, and the Navajo language uses different labels for the same objects in different tenses. How often do child health professionals consider how information processing or preferences by a child or his or her parent may depend on the original language or cultural background? Morely[23] has noted that information processing styles, preferences for forms and colors, and educational background must be considered in preparing health education materials for use in developing countries. This also should be an important consideration in planning health education in the United States.

ETHICAL ISSUES IN CROSS-CULTURAL MEDICINE

Many ethical issues operate in making transcultural diagnostic and treatment decisions. These relate to communication barriers, varying explanations for disease, and different expectations regarding what is honest or valuable.

Can an American pediatrician truly explain a surgical consent form to newly arrived parents of a Southeast Asian baby? When newly arrived refugees fear they will be returned and therefore sign anything or do anything to gain favor, is it ethical to ask them to sign a consent form to have blood drawn for clinical research?

Mental illness is defined very differently among cultures.[17,36] Is it ethical to use psychotherapy when therapist and patient are unmatched ethnically?

REVERSE CULTURE SHOCK

Child health professionals who spend substantial time working in different cultures may find the culture shock when returning to the United States to be as noticeable as the shock when arriving in the new culture. In fact, a benefit of cross-cultural travel (if it goes beyond Western hotels and into indigenous communities) is that one becomes sensitized to cultural norms. We may recognize idiosyncracies of our own cultures, such as loud voices, frenetic days, instant breakfasts, direct expression of feelings, pampered pets, or written invitations to social events. We may be uncomfortable in our forays to department stores that provide too many choices.

SUMMARY

Cross-cultural issues in pediatrics affect communication, expectations, and medical explanations. Pediatricians, while enculturated by their specialty training, also have individual ethnic norms that affect their beliefs and values. It is therefore helpful for child health professionals to learn about beliefs of their colleagues and patients. Wherever there may be a strong belief in a folk explanation for the cause of an illness, pediatricians are likely to be most successful if they acknowledge the belief and attempt to work with it. When simultaneous use of a traditional and Western medical regimen is possible and will do no harm, it is likely to enhance long-term, trusting relationships. Awareness of cultural evolution, perceptual differences related to cultural background, and implications for decision making with respect to children is essential for child health professionals throughout the world.

REFERENCES

1. American Medical Association: *Culturally competent health care for adolescents: a guide for primary care providers,* Chicago, 1994, Department of Adolescent Health, AMA.
2. Bernstein B, Pachter LM: Cultural considerations in children's pain. In Schecter NL, Berde C, Yaster M, editors: *Pain in infants, children, and adolescents,* Baltimore, 1993, Williams & Wilkins.
3. Bloch B: Bloch's assessment guide for ethnic/cultural variations. In Orque M, Bloch B, Monrroy I, editors: *Ethnic nursing care: a multicultural approach,* St Louis, 1983, Mosby.
4. Brink P: An anthropological perspective on parenting. In Horowitz J, Hughes C, Perdue B, editors: *Parenting reassessed: a nursing perspective,* Englewood Cliffs, NJ, 1982, Prentice-Hall.
5. Colehan JL: Navajo Indian medicine: implications for healing, *J Fam Pract* 10:55, 1980.
6. Eisenberg DM et al: Unconventional medicine in the United States, *N Engl J Med* 328:246, 1993.
7. Fitzgerald M, Armstrong J: Culture and disability in the Pacific, *International Exchange of Experts and Information in Rehabilitation Newsletter,* Jan 1993.
8. Garty BZ: Garlic burns, *Pediatrics* 91:658, 1993.
9. Harwood RLK: The influence of culturally derived values on Anglo and Puerto Rican mothers' perception of attachment behavior, *Child Dev* 63:822, 1992.
10. Jelliffe DB, Bennett FJ: Indigenous medical systems and child health, *J Pediatr* 57:248, 1960.
11. Kelly M: Healing the transcultural medicine gap, *Health Sciences,* University of Minnesota, Fall 1993.
12. Klausner W: *Conflict or communication,* Bangkok, 1978, Business in Thailand Publications.
13. Knoll T: *Becoming Americans, Asian sojourners, immigrants, and refugees in the Western United States,* Portland, Ore., 1982, Coast to Coast Books.
14. Konner M: Minding the pain, *The Sciences* 30:6, 1990.
15. Korbin JE, Johnston M: Steps toward resolving cultural conflict in a pediatric hospital, *Clin Pediatr* 21:259, 1982.
16. Krajewski J: Folk-healing among Mexican American families as a consideration in the delivery of child welfare and child health care services, *Child Welfare* 70:157, 1991.
17. Krener PG, Sabin C: Indochinese immigrant children problems in psychiatric diagnosis, *J Am Acad Child Psychiatry* 24:453, 1985.
18. Leininger M: *Transcultural nursing: concepts, theories, and practices,* New York, 1978, John Wiley & Sons.
19. Lozoff B, Kamath KR, Feldman RA: Infection and disease in South Indian families: beliefs about childhood diarrhea, *Human Organization* 34:353, 1975.
20. Lynch EW, Hanson MJ, editors: *Developing cross-cultural competence: a guide for working with young children and their families,* Baltimore, 1992, Paul H. Brooks.
21. Marsh P: *Eye to eye: how people interact,* Topsfield, Mass., 1988, Salem House.
22. Morelli GA et al: Cultural variation in infants' sleeping arrangements: questions of independence, *Developmental Psychology* 28:604, 1992.

23. Morley D: Beliefs and attitudes to child-rearing and disease. In Morley D, editor: *Paediatric priorities in the developing world,* London, 1973, Butterworths.
24. Moyers W: *Healing and the mind,* New York, 1993, Doubleday.
25. Namboze JM: Health and culture in an African society, *Soc Sci Med* 17:2041, 1983.
26. Olness KN: Cultural aspects in working in Lao refugees, *Minn Med* 62:871, 1979.
27. Pachter LM, Bernstein B, Osorio A: Clinical implications of a folk illness: empacho in mainland Puerto Ricans, *Med Anthropol* 13:285, 1992.
28. Schkade LL, Ramani S, Masakazu J: Human information processing and environmental complexity: an experiment in four cultures, *ASCI J Management* 8:56, 1978.
29. Shirts RG: *Bafa'Bafa': a cross-cultural simulation,* Del Mar, Calif, 1977, Simile.
30. Stulc DM: The family as a bearer of culture. In Cookfair JM: *Nursing process and practice in the community,* St Louis, 1991, Mosby.
31. Suchman RG: Cultural differences in children's color and form preferences, *J Soc Psychol* 70:3, 1966.
32. Theirderman S: Workshops in cross-cultural health care: the challenge of "ethnographic dynamite," *Journal of Continuing Education in Nursing* 19:25, 1988.
33. Tripp-Reimer T, Brink P, Saunders J: Cultural assessment: content and process, *Nurs Outlook* 32:78, 1984.
34. *UNICEF: the state of the world's children,* New York, 1994, UNICEF.
35. Werker JF: Becoming a native listener, *Am Scientist* 77:54, 1989.
36. Westermeyer J: *Poppies, pipes, and people: opium and its use in Laos,* Berkeley, Calif, 1982, University of California.
37. Zborowski M: Cultural components in response to pain, *Journal of Social Issues* 8:16, 1952.

SUGGESTED READINGS

Chesney AP et al: Mexican-American folk medicine: implications for the family physician, *J Fam Pract* 11:567, 1980.

Fabrega H, Tyma S: Language and cultural influences in the description of pain, *Br J Med Psychol* 49:349, 1976.

Grouse LD: The far-away look, *JAMA* 244:2053, 1980.

Henderson G, Primeaux M: *Transcultural health care,* Menlo Park, Calif, 1981, Addison-Wesley.

Lin TV: Psychiatry and Chinese culture, *West J Med* 139:58, 1983.

Logan B, Semmes C: Culture and ethnicity. In Logan B, Dawkin C, editors: *Family-centered nursing in the community,* Menlo Park, Calif, 1986, Addison-Wesley.

Mattson S: The need for cultural concepts in nursing curriculum, *J Nurs Educ* 26:206, 1987.

Olness KN: On "Reflections on caring for Indochinese children and youths" *J Dev Behav Pediatr* 7:129, 1986 (commentary).

Vogel V: American Indian medicine. In Henderson G, Primeaux M, editors: *Transcultural health care,* Menlo Park, Calif, 1981, Addison-Wesley.

12 Compliance with Pediatric Health Care Recommendations

Lois A. Maiman and Lance E. Rodewald

The success of outpatient therapy depends on (1) the physician's ability to diagnose the illness correctly and to offer efficacious treatment and (2) the patient's compliance with the therapeutic plan. Although the physician's role in successful therapy has been emphasized in theory, factors that influence patient cooperation are not an integral aspect of medical education. The consequences of noncompliance are seen in everyday pediatric practice, for example, wheezing children who have asthma whose blood shows no detectable theophylline and children who have diabetes who have repeated episodes of ketoacidosis and highly elevated hemoglobin A_{1c} levels. Although not all therapeutic failures are due to noncompliance, the differential diagnosis in a child unresponsive to therapy should include a compliance-oriented history that indicates whether the child has taken the medication. This chapter addresses practical steps the pediatrician can take to enhance patient compliance.

Many studies have documented low rates of parental compliance concerning prescribed regimens for their children. Although the rates of noncompliance vary with the characteristics of the condition, treatment, and patient, a recent review of the literature by Dunbar-Jacobs et al.[17] reveals that at least 33% of the subjects in most studies fail to follow the practitioner's advice. Moreover, when the recommended action is for prevention or requires sustained behavior, as in chronic illnesses, only about 50% of patients are compliant. As Haynes[24] notes, "In an era when efficacious therapies exist or are being developed at a rapid rate, it is truly discouraging that one half of the patients for whom appropriate therapy is prescribed fail to receive full benefits through inadequate adherence to treatment."

Dramatic evidence of noncompliance exists with regard to 10-day antibiotic regimens for otitis media and streptococcal pharyngitis. Studies[6,19,21,23] show that 40% to 80% of children do not receive the entire course of treatment; moreover, compliance is less than 50% by the fifth day of treatment.[2] Similar low rates of compliance are found in the self-management of chronic conditions such as diabetes. The importance of participation by the patient and family in the management of juvenile diabetes is widely recognized; the therapeutic regimen necessitates a continuous process of both prescriptive (e.g., administration of insulin or urine testing) and proscriptive (e.g., management of diet or exercise) behaviors. Complex regimens of long duration that require the alteration of existing behavior patterns usually are associated with inadequate levels of patient compliance, which is certainly the case with juvenile diabetes.

In reviewing the determinants of compliance, Becker and Maiman[5] describe how poor compliance creates significant barriers to effective delivery of medical care. Noncompliance weakens or invalidates the potential benefits of the prescribed regimen, and it frequently exposes the patient to additional medical tests or alternative therapies that may be duplicative or unnecessary (and that may result in iatrogenically poor outcomes). It also interferes with the pediatrician-parent relationship (e.g., dissatisfaction about poor medical outcomes resulting from noncompliance; negative reactions by pediatricians to "problem" patients), and it prevents accurate evaluations of the treatment's efficacy.

Unfortunately, research (much of which has focused on pediatric patients)[25] shows that there are no readily observable characteristics of poorly compliant patients that might permit easy identification, nor do individuals reveal their noncompliance without specific efforts by the pediatrician to assess levels of adherence. Moreover, physicians appear unable to predict their patients' likely compliance any more accurately than one could by chance.[10,16]

Practitioners overestimate the compliance rates of their own patients and underestimate the compliance rates of their colleagues' patients. Furthermore, practitioners are inclined to blame noncompliance on the patient's personality, and in general they express little desire to understand the problem and little sympathy for the uncooperative patient. Studies of medical students show that their compliance-related attitudes and behaviors resemble those of patients in general.[7]

Numerous studies have shown that sociodemographic characteristics (mother's age, race, education, income, marital status) do not predict compliance. One consistent exception is the association of noncompliance with the extremes of age, possibly because young children are more resistant to taking bad-tasting medicine and elderly persons may be forgetful. Research on personality traits of the patient (e.g., illness dependency, authoritarianism, and frustration tolerance) has not found significant associations between these factors and compliance. Therefore the pediatrician must view every child caretaker as a potential noncomplier.

STRATEGIES FOR IMPROVING PATIENT COMPLIANCE

Given the dramatic rates of noncompliance and the difficulty it causes, pediatricians need to learn about the causes of noncompliance and its cure. Although no solution has been discovered, research during the past 2 decades, including systematic study of adherence in pediatric populations, has yielded substantial practical knowledge and techniques for increasing treatment compliance in pediatric practice. This chapter discusses some major factors that contribute to noncompliance and describes steps pediatricians can take to reduce the problem.

Providing Information

A logical starting point for influencing the likelihood of adherence to therapy is the pediatrician's instructions. Some parents will not really understand (i.e., know) what is expected of them after the visit.

Knowledge affects compliance in several ways: (1) knowledge about certain details of prescribed therapy (e.g., the duration of the regimen, dosage, and frequency of administration) is essential for correct compliance; (2) parents frequently do not possess all the information they need to follow the regimen; and (3) provision of the necessary information rarely is sufficient to produce adequate patient cooperation because of the other variables, such as poor recall or insufficient motivation on the part of the caretaker.

Studies by Ley and co-workers[34,35] show that patient recall declines rapidly; about 50% of the information given to patients is forgotten 15 minutes after meeting with the physician. Patients remember best what occurred during the first one third of the visit and remember more about the diagnosis than about the details of the prescribed therapy. In a study of communication between pediatricians and mothers, Korsch and co-workers[32] demonstrated inadequate maternal comprehension of terms such as "incubation period" (interpreted as instructions to stay in bed) and "lumbar puncture" (identified as draining of the lungs). Considerable variation in understanding has even been shown for terms such as "evening" and "with meals" applied to directions for administering medications. This confusion suggests the need either to explain many of the most common medical terms or to provide substitute terms.

These findings point to several strategies for modifying features of physician-parent communication. The pediatrician should provide the parent with individualized, written instructions (preferably written in the parent's presence). The best results are obtained when the pediatrician describes the details of the regimen orally, writes them down, and reviews the written instructions. Second, the physician should emphasize the important details of the regimen and avoid causing "information overload"; general information about the disease and about the specific action of the medication is unlikely to increase compliance. Finally, detailed therapeutic instructions should be presented early in the discussion about treatment.

Changing Characteristics of the Regimen

Compliance is reduced when the regimen is complex, inconvenient, or expensive, is of long duration, or requires an alteration of the patient's life-style.[26,31,33,42] Although a particular regimen may not be modifiable, the pediatrician should consider several methods to improve compliance. The regimen can be simplified by reducing the number of medications prescribed and the number of doses given per day (if clinically appropriate) and by administering doses simultaneously when more than one medication is required. Other effective approaches include avoiding the prescription of medications that are not essential to the treatment (such as use of a decongestant with the antibiotic prescribed for otitis media) and minimizing both inconvenience and forgetfulness by matching the regimen to the parent's and child's regular daily activities.

The duration of the regimen may not be modifiable, but we suggest using the shortest regimen consistent with good medical practice. In long-term therapy, strategies for inducing a feeling of "shorter regimen duration" include scheduling follow-up visits in quick succession to demonstrate progress and telephoning the parent 3 to 4 days after the visit to check on progress or problems with the regimen. If life-style (e.g., diet and exercise) must be modified, Dunbar and Stunkard[18] suggest that changes be introduced one at a time, that whatever compliance is achieved be reinforced, and that the next therapeutic task be added. Finally, the physician may be able to reduce the cost of the treatment by prescribing generic drugs, refraining from prescribing unnecessary drugs, and encouraging shopping for the most economical prescription rates.

Altering Health-related Beliefs

Current medical training does not emphasize ways to encourage patient education and motivation. Few schools attempt to teach the medical student how to identify conditions under which patients will follow advice, the methods most likely to generate effective communication with patients, or interviewing skills that will determine what the patient knows, believes, or is concerned about.

Patients' beliefs about their health, illness, and its treatment strongly influence the probability of compliance. Evidence[28] supports a health belief model, which hypothesizes that whether an individual will follow a practitioner's advice often depends on four factors: (1) *health motivation*—degree of interest in and concern about health matters in general, (2) *susceptibility*—perceptions of vulnerability to the particular illness (or to its sequelae), including acceptance of the practitioner's diagnosis, (3) *severity*—perceptions concerning the probable seriousness of the consequences, on both bodily and social dimensions, of contracting the illness or of leaving it untreated, and (4) *benefits and costs*—an evaluation of the advocated health behavior concerning its probable effectiveness in preventing or treating the condition, weighed against estimates of various barriers that might be involved in undertaking the recommended action (e.g., financial expense, physical or emotional discomfort, inconvenience, or possibility of adverse side effects).

Data emphasizing the importance of these health benefits in pediatric settings are available from studies[12,22,29] of cooperation with many different types of recommended therapies. These studies ranged from participation in screening programs to compliance with various short- and long-term medication regimens. A study by Becker and co-workers[4] indicates that mothers who are concerned about their child's illness, feel that their child is vulnerable to otitis media and perceive it as a threat to the child, and who believe in the accuracy of the diagnosis and have confidence in the benefits of the medication are more likely to comply with a 10-day antibiotic regimen for otitis media than mothers who do not have these beliefs.

These findings, including the successful role of health beliefs in compliance by adults with their own regimens, together with research[31] demonstrating that health attitudes and perceptions can be altered, support the recommendation by Podell[41] that more attention be paid to monitoring and motivating the patient or parents regarding health beliefs. Mathews and Hingson[39] suggest that a compliance-oriented history of health beliefs be a routine part of the patient or parent interview. For example, the practitioner should determine whether the mother shows appropriate concern about the child's health problem, agrees with the diagnosis, perceives the child's illness as serious, believes the recommended therapy will work, fears medication side effects, or feels the regimen will be too hard to follow.

Giving attention to health beliefs during the diagnostic phase of the visit helps the practitioner determine what beliefs might cause noncompliance and what content should be emphasized in teaching. In developing a strategy for effective persuasion, the practitioner should know that simply providing the correct facts sometimes is sufficient; at other times more extensive discussion or motivating appeals, such as fear, parental or family responsibility, or pride, may be required. In other instances recommendations by sources of information viewed as being credible, such as other patients (or their parents) for whom the same treatment was successful, may be beneficial. The pediatrician should encourage parents to discuss their concerns about the diagnosis or the treatment and to disclose *all* their worries about their child's illness and treatment.

The positive effects of practitioner awareness on patient compliance have been illustrated in controlled trials.[27,37] A recent study directed the intervention to the pediatrician to increase his or her knowledge and use of compliance-enhancing strategies, and subsequently to improve mothers' compliance with an antibiotic regimen for their child's otitis media.[37] One of three groups of randomly assigned pediatricians was given special 5-hour tutorials, with accompanying printed materials that emphasized the difficulties experienced by parents in complying with their child's treatment plans and possible strategies for enhancing compliance (including modifying parents' health beliefs). The second group received only the printed materials; the third, the control group, received nothing. Both educational formats produced increases in pediatrician knowledge about compliance-enhancing techniques. Mothers of children whose pediatricians were in the study group used the prescribed antibiotic regimen more correctly and consistently than did mothers of control-group pediatricians. The positive influence of physician education on patient compliance suggests that health care organizations should provide training for all staff members in compliance-oriented history taking and other compliance-related techniques.

Improving Practitioner-Patient Interaction

Numerous aspects of practitioner-patient interaction, such as impersonality and brevity of encounter,[11,30] negatively affect patient behavior. Lack of communication, particularly communication of an emotional nature, usually is the problem. According to Davis,[16] patterns of communication that deviate from the patient's expectations of the practitioner-patient relationship are associated with a patient's failure to comply with a practitioner's advice. Such deviations include interactions in which tension is not released and in which the practitioner is formal, rejecting, or controlling, in addition to interactions in which the practitioner disagrees completely with the patient or interviews the patient at length without giving subsequent feedback.

Many investigations[3,20,32,45,46] have shown that good pediatrician-mother interaction is associated with positive outcomes for children, including appointment keeping, problem resolution, and compliance. Frances and co-workers[22] report that a mother's compliance with a regimen prescribed for her child and her own satisfaction are increased when the affective elements of the communication are enhanced (e.g., when she feels the practitioner is friendly and understands the complaint, when her expectations from the medical visit are met, and when she receives an explanation of the diagnosis and cause of the child's illness). In another study of pediatrician-mother interaction, by Liptak and co-workers,[36] the extent of a pediatrician's awareness of maternal concerns and the adequacy of communication were directly related to two outcomes in well-child care: mother-child adaptation and maternal satisfaction with medical care.

How this interaction may affect compliance and parental concerns is suggested by studies of otitis media and asthma. When communication between the practitioner and parents includes agreement on the child's diagnosis and the need for follow-up visits and an explanation of the details of the regimen, compliance with administering a 10-day antibiotic regimen for otitis media and keeping the follow-up appointments was increased.[3] Further, a descriptive study by Clark and co-workers[13] of problems confronting parents of children who have asthma showed that practitioner-patient communication often is inadequate. Major concerns of almost 50% of the parents were lack of information from the child's physician, difficulty in comprehending responses to questions, and lack of discussion on preventive measures.

Increasing Patient Supervision

Another important dimension of the practitioner-patient interaction concerns the amount of supervision. A variety of "before-and-after" studies[24,43] have shown increased patient cooperation when outpatient visits are increased, home visits are added, patients receive negative feedback concerning their noncompliance, and patients receive continuity of care. Methods of continually monitoring compliance include calling the parents to remind them of the regimen or the follow-up visit, requesting that empty bottles or those containing unused pills be brought to the next visit, and instructing the parents or patient to keep a record of the time and dose of daily medication administration. Monitoring blood levels of medications taken on a continuing basis, such as anticonvulsants and theophylline, also helps detect noncompliance. When techniques to measure blood levels are unavailable for a specific medication, indirect measures can be used (e.g., ascertaining appropriate suppression as a result of the prednisone regimen by obtaining a cortisol level in a steroid-dependent child who has asthma).

A development that attempts to capitalize on and in some ways improve the relationship between practitioner and patient is the *therapeutic contract*. Lewis and Michnich[33] describe the technique by which both parties set forth a treatment goal, decide the specific obligations of each party in attempting to achieve that goal, and then set a time limit for its achievement. Support for the practitioner-patient contract as a tool for increasing patient compliance is reported for pediatric weight reduction, dietary management, and exercise recommendations.

Enlisting Family Support

Members of the patient's family can remind, assist, encourage, and reinforce the patient or parent in following medical advice. Supportive and successful helping efforts are associated with greater compliance and are especially important in the motivation and compliance of a chronically ill child.

For example, in studies[8,44] of weight control, investigators found that persons who were assisted by another family member in the reinforcement of proper eating behavior were more likely to lose weight and to maintain that weight loss. Similar outcomes have been noted concerning the family's influence on compliance with recommendations for obtaining immunizations and other preventive measures and for taking medications. Several studies[2,5,40,41] of family-level variables have documented relationships between the extent of patient compliance and a family's own health beliefs and the family's evaluation of the patient's illness and recommended treatment. Compliance is enhanced when the normal roles and routines of the family are compatible with the patient's illness or when family members are willing to incorporate changes in their daily lives and environment to accommodate the demands of the illness.

However, the family also can have a negative effect on a child's willingness to cooperate with care. Parents who have chronically ill children are faced with tasks often in conflict: first, implementing the regimen at home and removing the immediate threat of medical crisis; and second, enabling the child to take developmentally appropriate steps in assuming responsibility for compliance with treatment.[1] Therefore the practitioner should carefully evaluate the role of family members in the patient's therapy and attempt to maximize their potential constructive contributions and minimize their possible destructive influences.

Using Other Health Care Providers

The physician can benefit from the compliance-oriented interventions of other health care practitioners, who can provide additional assessment, instruction, clarification, and reinforcement. Marston[38] contends that nurses, by virtue of their numbers and amount of patient contact, have the greatest potential of any group of health professionals for affecting patient health behavior. Important nursing compliance-related activities include developing patient contracts, instituting behavior modification, diagnosing or monitoring adherence levels, using health education to clarify the regimen, developing strategies to change health attitudes, and enlisting support of the patient's family and other significant persons.

A review of investigations by Canada[9] emphasizes the potential role of the pharmacist in enhancing patient compliance. Consultation with the pharmacist before hospital discharge led to a 75% reduction in a high baseline rate of deviation from prescribed drug regimens. In the case of outpatients, counseling by pharmacists (including written reinforcement of counseling information and telephone or mailed reminders of when the patient's supply of medication was scheduled to run out) increased the percentage of prescriptions refilled on time and decreased the proportion of nonrefills. Suggestions for pharmacist involvement include actions to be taken if the patient fails to pick up the original prescription, written instructions on special precautions to be taken with various types of drugs, and maintenance of a patient medication profile. Implementation of these suggestions could aid in preventing overdose, allergic reactions, and adverse drug interactions, and they also could serve to monitor compliance.

SUMMARY

This chapter summarizes the results of a variety of studies about the problem and determinants of patient compliance. Despite Osler's observation[15] that "the desire to take medicine is perhaps the greatest feature which distinguishes man from animals," the practitioner's problem in delivering efficacious care often is not selecting a treatment regimen but rather obtaining patient—and with the child patient, *parent*—cooperation with the recommended therapy. Desired outcomes, such as improved communication, greater satisfaction of the parent with the visit, and willingness to follow the therapeutic plan, are more likely when the physician employs communication and regimen management strategies.[14]

We suggest a multifactorial approach to understanding and increasing compliance, and we encourage the practitioner concerned with increasing cooperation with therapies to try to (1) improve the patient's or parents' knowledge of the specifics of the regimen, reinforce essential points with review, discussion, and clearly written instructions, and to emphasize the importance of the therapeutic plan; (2) take appropriate steps to reduce the cost, complexity, duration, and amount of behavioral change required by the regimen and to increase the convenience of the regimen; (3) obtain a compliance-oriented history of previous experiences and present health beliefs and, when necessary, employ strategies to modify the patient's or parents' perceptions that might inhibit compliance; (4) improve levels of satisfaction, particularly with the practitioner-patient relationship, and encourage questions concerning the diagnosis and proposed therapy; (5) arrange for continued monitoring of subsequent compliance to treatment (e.g., establish specific follow-up appointments and telephone reminders); (6) enlist family support for the therapeutic regimen; and (7) use other members of the health care team.

REFERENCES

1. Anderson BJ, Coyne CC: Family context and compliance behavior in chronically ill children. In Krasnegor NA et al, editors: *Developmental aspects of health compliance behavior,* Hillsdale, NJ, 1993, Lawrence Erlbaum Associates.
2. Baric L: Conjugal roles as indicators of family influence on health-directed action, *Int J Health Educ* 13:58, 1970.
3. Becker MH, Drachman RH, Kirscht JP: Predicting mothers' compliance with pediatric medical regimens, *J Pediatr* 81:843, 1972.
4. Becker MH, Drachman RH, Kirscht JP: A new approach to explaining sick-role behavior in low-income populations, *Am J Public Health* 64:205, 1974.
5. Becker MH, Green LW: A family approach to compliance with medical treatment: a selective review of the literature, *Int J Health Educ* 18:173, 1975.
6. Bergman AB, Werner RJ: Failure of children to receive penicillin by mouth, *N Engl J Med* 268:1334, 1963.
7. Blackwell B et al: Teaching medical students about treatment compliance, *J Med Educ* 53:672, 1978.

8. Brownell KD et al: The effect of couples training and partner cooperativeness in the behavioral treatment of obesity, *Behav Res Ther* 16:323, 1978.
9. Canada AT: *The pharmacist and drug compliance.* In Sackett DL, Haynes RB, editors: *Compliance with therapeutic regimens,* Baltimore, 1976, Johns Hopkins University.
10. Caron HS, Roth HP: Patients' cooperation with a medical regimen, *JAMA* 203:922, 1968.
11. Charney E: Patient-doctor communication, *Pediatr Clin North Am* 19:263, 1972.
12. Charney E et al: How well do patients take oral penicillin? A collaborative study in private practice, *Pediatrics* 40:188, 1967.
13. Clark NM et al: Developing education for children with asthma through study of self-management behavior, *Health Educ Q* 7:278, 1980.
14. Clark NM et al: Physician-patient partnership in managing chronic illness, *Acad Med* 70:957, 1995.
15. Cushing H: *The life of Sir William Osler,* vol 1, New York, 1925, Oxford University.
16. Davis MA: Variations in patients' compliance with doctors' orders: analysis of congruence between survey responses and results of empirical investigation, *J Med Educ* 41:1037, 1966.
17. Dunbar-Jacob JM, Dunning EJ, Dwyer K: Compliance research in pediatric and adolescent population: two decades of research. In Krasnegor NA et al, editors: *Developmental aspects of health compliance behavior,* Hillsdale, NJ, 1993, Lawrence Erlbaum Associates.
18. Dunbar JM, Stunkard AJ: Adherence to diet and drug regimen. In Levy R et al, editors: *Nutrition, lipids, and coronary heart disease,* New York, 1979, Raven Press.
19. Elling R, Whittemore R, Green M: Patient participation in a pediatric program, *J Health Hum Behav* 1:183, 1960.
20. Falvo D, Woehlke P, Deichmann J: Relationship of physician behavior to patient compliance, *Patient Counsel Health Educ* 2:185, 1980.
21. Feinstein AR et al: A controlled study of three methods of prophylaxis against streptococcal infection in a population of rheumatic children, *N Engl J Med* 260:697, 1959.
22. Frances V, Korsch BM, Morris MJ: Gaps in doctor-patient communication: patients' response to medical advice, *N Engl J Med* 280:535, 1969.
23. Gordis L, Markowitz M, Lilienfeld AM: Studies in the epidemiology and preventability of rheumatic fever. IV. A quantitative determination of compliance in children on oral penicillin prophylaxis, *Pediatrics* 43:173, 1969.
24. Haynes RB: A critical review of the "determinants" of patient compliance with therapeutic regimens. In Sackett DL, Haynes RB, editors: *Compliance with therapeutic regimens,* Baltimore, 1976, Johns Hopkins University Press.
25. Haynes RB, Taylor DW, Sackett DL: *Compliance in health care,* Baltimore, 1979, Johns Hopkins University Press.
26. Hellmuth GA, Johannsen WJ, Sorauf T: Psychological factors in cardiac patients, *Arch Environ Health* 12:771, 1966.
27. Inui TS, Yourtee EL, Williamson JW: Improved outcomes in hypertension after physician tutorials: a controlled trial, *Ann Intern Med* 84:646, 1976.
28. Janz NK, Becker MH: The health belief model: a decade later, *Health Educ Q* 11:1, 1984.
29. Johnson AJ et al: *Epidemiology of polio vaccine acceptance: a social and psychological analysis,* monograph series no. 3, Jacksonville, Fla, 1962, Florida State Board of Health.
30. Joyce CRB et al: Quantitative study of doctor-patient communication, *Q J Med* 38:183, 1969.
31. Kirscht JP: Research related to modification of health beliefs, *Health Educ Monogr* 2:455, 1974.
32. Korsch BM, Gozzi EK, Francis V: Gaps in doctor-patient communication. I. Doctor-patient interaction and patient satisfaction, *Pediatrics* 42:855, 1968.
33. Lewis CE, Michnich M: Contracts as a means of improving patient compliance. In Barofsky I, editor: *Medication compliance: a behavioral management approach,* Thorofare, NJ, 1977, Charles B Slack.
34. Ley P: Primacy, rated importance, and the recall of medical statements, *J Health Soc Behav* 13:311, 1972.
35. Ley P et al: A method for increasing patients' recall of information presented by doctors, *Psychol Med* 3:217, 1973.
36. Liptak GS, Hulka BS, Cassel JC: Effectiveness of physician-mother interaction during infancy, *Pediatrics* 60:186, 1977.
37. Maiman LA et al: Improving pediatricians' compliance-enhancing practices: a randomized trial, *Am J Dis Child* 142:773, 1988.
38. Marston M: Compliance with medical regimens: a review of the literature, *Nurs Res* 19:312, 1970.
39. Matthews D, Hingson R: Improving patient compliance: a guide for physicians, *Med Clin North Am* 61:879, 1977.
40. Oakes TW et al: Family expectations and arthritis patient compliance to a hand-resting splint regimen, *J Chronic Dis* 22:757, 1970.
41. Picken B, Ireland G: Family patterns of medical care utilization: possible influences of family size, role and social class on illness behavior, *J Chronic Dis* 22:181, 1969.
42. Podell RN: *Physician's guide to compliance in hypertension,* West Point, Penn, 1975, Merck.
43. Rokart JF, Hofmann PB: Physician and patient behavior under different scheduling systems in a hospital outpatient department, *Med Care* 7:463, 1969.
44. Saccone AJ, Israel AC: Effects of experimenter versus significant other controlled reinforcement and choice of target behavior on weight loss, *Behav Ther* 9:271, 1978.
45. Starfield B et al: Patient-doctor agreement about problems needing follow-up visit, *JAMA* 242:344, 1979.
46. Starfield B et al: The influence of patient-practitioner agreement on outcome of care, *Am J Public Health* 71:127, 1981.

13 The Art of Consultation

Henry M. Seidel

The major purpose of consultation is to gain assistance in the diagnosis, treatment, or management of a patient's problem, as well as to reassure the patient and family. A practitioner often wants similar reassurance, sometimes for legal reasons. Unfortunately, an insecure practitioner may hesitate to ask for consultation for fear of being thought incompetent. "Going it alone" is not always in the patient's best interest. That interest cannot be compromised by someone who does not recognize the limits of individual knowledge and competence in a time when omniscience is beyond anyone's capacity. Trust in the relationship between the practitioner and patient and family is essential; it usually is reinforced, not undermined, by appropriate consultation. Patients and parents appreciate and respond to a practitioner's candor in defining the areas of his or her expertise and in stating limitations. Sound communication maintains trust, whatever the consultant contributes, and requires the role of each participant in the process to be clearly defined. These fundamental principles apply, whether the practice arrangement of the referring physician and the consultant is a health maintenance organization, a large group practice, or a fee-for-service setting.

A consultation is not a referral. The physician who requests a consultation is not intending to transfer care to another physician or even, necessarily, to share care with another physician. In some circumstances, a referral or a transfer of care may be appropriate. More often, a sharing of care serves the best interests of the patient.

PRIMARY CARE PROVIDERS

The primary care provider is responsible for arranging a consultation. Its ultimate value depends in large part on how skillfully it is managed by that practitioner. The need for consultation often arises during the stress of an acute illness, a time when the family and patient may react to the suggestion with increased anxiety about the gravity of the illness. This anxiety can be tempered by acknowledging it and by putting any underlying fears in appropriate and honest context. In addition, problems in choosing a consultant can be anticipated if there is frank discussion of skills, personalities, and cost.

The information given to the consultant by the referring physician provides the basis for a successful response. Any behavioral, emotional, social, and economic factors that can influence decision making should be made clear. Problems must be stated concisely, and individual responsibilities for the patient's continuing care should be arranged according to the competence, knowledge, and particular skills of the physicians involved. The primary care provider orchestrates the entire process and must be available to keep all participants fully informed to maintain their optimal contributions. The consultant must clearly understand the goals of the interaction and that the primary care provider's role in the decision-making process is not abdicated. The time at which the patient returns to the primary care physician must be clearly defined. The consultant may need to continue contact with the patient, however, and these visits often may parallel primary care visits. When the relationship with the consultant ends, the primary care physician must ensure follow-up care.

NONPHYSICIAN HEALTH PROFESSIONALS

Over the past several decades the work of the primary pediatrician has been increasingly complemented by that of nonphysician health professionals. The team of health workers may include nurses, nurse practitioners, and physician assistants; physical, occupational, and speech therapists; educational, developmental, and clinical psychologists; audiologists; social workers; and nutritionists. The pediatrician is responsible for understanding the resources provided by these professionals, referring patients to them when indicated, and maintaining effective communication among all involved.

The rules for communication are the same as those that govern consultation with another physician. Three-way interaction is essential when the patient requires care that is not within the competence of the pediatrician or that demands time that the pediatrician does not have. The nonphysician health professional takes on all the responsibilities of any consultant, including that of maintaining open and respectful communication.

CONSULTANTS

The patient and family often are understandably anxious about the unresolved problem presented to the consultant. Concerns about illness and practical considerations of cost must be understood. The consultant should avoid demeaning the primary practitioner because any hint of incompetence or error, verbal or nonverbal, can destroy trust among all participants. Sometimes hindsight, new information, or superior knowledge might prompt a criticism of past management. This must be constructive and must be discussed without hesitancy with the referring physician in private. Health care decision making should, however, tolerate disagreement; many times two or more valid approaches to a problem are possible. Nevertheless, when there is evidence of possible incompetence, the needs of the patient always come first. This is a circumstance that demands honesty and delicacy and, at times, a difficult step—the provision of information to responsible authorities in hospitals, medical societies, and licensing boards. Indeed, once the consultant agrees to consultation, legal responsibility in all its dimensions is assumed.

The consultant cannot rely solely on the observations of others. Information should be obtained independently because the answer to a puzzle may lie in a retaken history, a discriminating observation during the physical examination, or a reevaluation of laboratory data. Reconstruction, reinterpretation, and careful attention to detail are critical.

The consultant must make recommendations promptly, either in person or by telephone. Findings and recommendations must be documented on the hospital chart or in the consultant's office file and also in a letter to the referring practitioner. All information shared with the patient and family must also be made available to the primary physician in timely fashion. If the patient and family circumvent the primary physician and seek additional advice without his or her knowledge, an awkward or threatening situation for the primary care provider could result. The consultant must be sensitive to this while still holding the patient's needs paramount.

The pediatrician who is asked to consult should be aware that many physicians who ask for consultation may not have the necessary education and training for continuing management of a given child's problem. One should be sensitive to this possibility and to the delicate issue that arises from a perception of competition between pediatricians and family practitioners. The reality here is far less than the supposition; nevertheless, it cannot be ignored. Again, the patient's needs must remain paramount, and the consulting pediatrician must be prepared to share care and to accept a transfer of responsibility without usurping that responsibility inappropriately.

Cost Containment

Second opinions have been suggested, particularly when surgery is being considered, as a means of ensuring an appropriate and perhaps cost-saving decision. Ideally, only necessary surgery is performed, and the expectation is that a second opinion will ensure this. There is no certainty, however, that the second opinion is more valid if it contradicts the first. An obvious absurdity can result if the patient is subjected to the opinion of a third expert to overcome a tie vote. This can be avoided if the rules of consultation are scrupulously observed and if the consultant is objective. Referring physicians should take care that no conflict of interest exists between them and the clinicians they consult. Further opinions rarely are necessary when a primary physician and a consultant communicate well with each other and, above all, keep the patient fully and appropriately informed.

Recommendations made by the consultant are not binding and may be rejected by the patient and family and referring physician. They all retain the privilege of being involved in the final decision. The consultation process does lose value if it is diluted by too many opinions, so the referring physician must see that balance is maintained. Thus optimal patient care requires the orchestrating hand of the primary pediatrician while a variety of individuals contribute their special skills to understanding and solving the patient's problems. Certainly, should the consultant's advice be rejected after clear and open discussion with everyone concerned, the reasoning underlying the entire process from the beginning to end must be clearly documented. Unhappily, the courts, often wrongly, give greater weight to the consultant in a legal proceeding.

A CAVEAT

The consultative process can be abused. Used in excess and without clear need, it can confuse the patient, add to cost, and depersonalize individual care. What Peter Berczeller has characterized as "management by committee" underlies much of a resident's experience in recent years, as more and more people are involved in the continuing management of one person's problems. Judicious self-reliance is no longer as often the tempering factor it must be if a mature clinician is to develop. *Judicious* is an important word. One must respect one's limits. That is achievable without surrendering the responsibility to orchestrate and to keep the consideration of the patient "whole."

REASONS FOR CONSULTATION WITH PHYSICIANS AND NONPHYSICIANS IN A VARIETY OF HEALTH AND MEDICAL DISCIPLINES

1. Uncertainty in diagnosis
2. Confirmation of diagnosis
3. Specific skill required for diagnostic process, for example:
   a. Pediatric subspecialist—to perform a variety of diagnostic techniques
   b. Radiologist—to consider all the "imaging" modalities and to select them appropriately
   c. Endoscopist—to see a lesion and perform a biopsy
   d. Surgeon—to explore and remove a lesion, to obtain a biopsy specimen, or to correct a problem
   e. Pathologist—to interpret the nature of the tissue removed
   f. Psychologist, psychiatrist, and mental health counselor—to search for more subjective insights
   g. Teacher and social worker—to discover aspects of patient and family life unknown to the referring physician
4. Uncertainty as to appropriate management or therapy, or both
5. Specific skill required for therapy or management, or both, for example, the variety of surgical disciplines
6. Reassurance for the patient and family or the primary pediatrician, for example:
   a. Reassurance as to the diagnosis (even in the face of certainty)
   b. Reassurance as to a suggested course of action
7. Assistance in long-term follow-up and management of chronic illness, for example:
   a. Physical therapist
   b. Occupational therapist
   c. Rehabilitationist
   d. Schoolteacher

GUIDELINES FOR REQUESTING A CONSULTATION

- Be precise in stating your goals for the consultation and the information you need.
- Be aware of uncertainty in the patient and family and in yourself, and be prepared to take every step necessary to resolve it.
- Keep the needs of the patient and family sharply in mind, and keep them well-informed and active in the decision-making process.
- Clarify the extent to which you want only to consult or to which you want to refer and share in the care of the patient; do not abdicate your role in decision making.
- Do not abdicate your responsibilities for keeping informed, coordinating information, and maintaining continuity and communication with all the persons involved; this, of course, requires precise and detailed record keeping.

GUIDELINES FOR PROVIDING A CONSULTATION

- Be precise and prompt in providing information, using language appropriate to each of the persons involved; different professionals have different jargon, but patients have variable understanding of jargon, most often none at all.
- Keep the patient and family informed but not without parallel or prior information to the referring physician.
- Be available for sharing, but not usurping, the privilege of care for a child who is referred by someone more specifically experienced in the care of adults.
- Keep thorough records and always provide the referring physician with a detailed consultation note; do not rely solely on spoken communication, whether in person or on the telephone.
- Define information with your own observations; accept the word of others only in rare circumstances.
- Be wary of "off-the-cuff" corridor or telephone consultation; when there is the least uncertainty, see the patient.

The accompanying boxes outline situations in which a practitioner may decide that a consultation would be in the best interests of the patient and family.

SUGGESTED READINGS

Balint M: *The doctor, his patient, and the illness,* New York, 1972, International Universities Press.

Bursztajn H et al: *Medical chances: how patients' families and physicians can cope with uncertainty,* New York, 1981, Delacorte Press/Seymour Lawrence.

Committee on Standards of Child Health Care: *Communication with nonphysician health personnel,* Evanston, Ill, April 1979, American Academy of Pediatrics.

Berczeller PH: The malignant consultation syndrome. *Hosp Pract* September 15:33, 1991.

Nazarian LF: On consulting and being consulted, *Pediatr Rev* 13:124, 1992.

Wilde JA, Pedroni AT Jr: The do's and don'ts of consultations, *Contemp Pediatr,* May 1991, p 23.

Editorial note: Contrasts in academic consultation, *Ann Intern Med* 94:537, 1981.

Stickler GB: The pediatrician as a consultant, *Am J Dis Child* 143:73, 1989.

Stickler GB: Telephone etiquette, *Am J Dis Child* 143:520, 1989.

Symposium: When the pediatrician is the consultant, *Contemp Pediatr* 5:96, 1988.

Tumulty PA: *The effective clinician,* Philadelphia, 1973, WB Saunders.

14 Assessing the Medical Literature

S. Michael Plaut

Two studies published the same year in the same journal reported on the relationship between marijuana smoking and testosterone levels in young adult men.[4,5] One study reported a statistically significant dose-related relationship between these two variables; the other could find no relationship. What is a practitioner to make of this discrepancy in results? Perhaps the answer lies in the methods used in the two studies. The first study used retrospective self-reports of marijuana smoking in the subjects' normal environment. In the second study testosterone levels were measured before, during, and after the smoking of standardized, government-issued "joints" in a controlled institutional environment. Can either of these methods be considered inherently better than the other? Both studies used certain screening devices to minimize suspected extraneous factors that might affect the results. But were all such factors accounted for? In dealing with a value-laden topic about which the reader might have some prejudices, the interpreter must ask whether personal feelings color his or her interpretation of the data. Thus a number of factors, including logistic and methodological limitations, the possibility of human bias, and a practitioner's knowledge of the field and its technology, are involved in the appropriate interpretation of a scientific study.

IMPORTANCE OF CRITICAL EVALUATION

"The physician," writes Dykes,[3] "will be equipped to allow the public access to high quality medical care only to the extent that he has been able to keep up with and to grasp the import of advances in the science of medicine." To maintain currency in his or her field, the practitioner must maintain a level of dissatisfaction with the status quo in clinical medicine and a commitment to the idea that science itself "depends for its vitality on a milieu that fosters vigorous, open dissent."[3] Beveridge wrote, "Nothing could be more damaging to science than abandonment of the critical attitude and its replacement by too ready acceptance of hypotheses put forward on slender evidence."[1] This chapter discusses factors important to the critical evaluation of research data, as well as guidelines useful for interpreting that data.

Limitations of Individual Studies

No matter how well conceived and designed a study is, and regardless of how effectively its results are communicated, certain necessary limitations must be taken into account in interpreting its value.

Scope and Feasibility. As implied by the discussion of the previous two studies, certain decisions must be made in designing a study—decisions that eventually define the nature and extent of the study's usefulness. The investigator may opt for the natural conditions of a field study or for the higher level of control afforded by a laboratory or institution. Although a heterogeneous subject population allows greater generalization from the results, a homogeneous sample tends to reduce variability in the data, and thus fewer subjects are required to obtain conclusive results. Although an investigator may wish to observe many aspects of a phenomenon, the number of variables that can be accounted for will be limited by factors such as the investigator's breadth of expertise, the amount of blood or tissue that can be collected, a subject's ability to concentrate for long periods in completing questionnaires, or the possibility that measurement of one variable might influence the reliability of another.

Relevance and Application. Because an investigator must set limits when designing a study, these limits must extend to the interpretation and applicability of the data. For example, although human studies may be considered more relevant than animal studies for clinical purposes, animal studies have the advantage of allowing a measure of manipulation and control that only rarely is possible with human subjects. Any one study can investigate only a relatively small facet of the larger conceptual problem it attempts to address. Thus the ultimate value of any study depends on replication of the findings in different research settings and synthesis of these findings into a comprehensive picture of the field of study.

Medium of Presentation. Review papers and books are the best sources of comprehensive summaries of research findings. However, although such sources have the advantage of a longer perspective on a field of study, they do not have the currency of the journal article or meeting presentation. Besides being current, a journal article has the additional advantages of procedural detail and peer review before publication. Although information presented at a scientific meeting or in a professional "throwaway" publication has a shorter time lag, it often has not undergone thorough peer review. Thus a practitioner must consider the source of the information in evaluating its scientific merit or practical relevance.

Human Element in Research

A second major consideration when assessing scientific literature is the individual contribution each participant makes to the research process. As suggested in the aforementioned marijuana studies, cultural or personal values probably color an individual's approach to a research area. In addition, researchers may respond to real or implied institutional pressures to produce a certain quantity of research output. Such pressures may affect many aspects of the research process, from the choice of a research question based on expediency, to excessive haste in publishing the results. An investigator's emotional investment in his or her research may be especially high in areas that might be considered "faddish" or controversial or that reflect a strong theoretical or cultural bias. Examples in developmental research include the areas of mother-infant bonding, hyperactivity, and intelligence testing. Even at best, the knowledge of a researcher, reviewer, or reader is finite, and this limitation may become most apparent in dealing with multidisciplinary issues. As Dykes has written, "Physicians must recognize the fallibility of even our species' greatest intellects. . . . The biases of eminent men are still biases."[3]

Subjective factors may influence the evaluation of research in many ways; a few common examples are given here.

Dichotomous Thinking. Practitioners often tend to oversimplify their thinking about natural phenomena by placing the phenomena in categories rather than on continua. Thus mental illness has either a behavioral or a biological origin, adult traits are determined either genetically or environmentally, and diseases are either physical or psychosomatic. A practitioner may be inclined to think of research subjects as being either normal or abnormal, depending on the issue in question. Although such categorization often is useful or even necessary, few biological questions have a simplistic, all-or-nothing answer. It usually is more fruitful to think in terms of the degree to which each of several factors may interact to influence a phenomenon, rather than attempting to attribute the cause exclusively to one factor or another.

Overemphasis on Results and Applications. An author's interest in publication or a reader's interest in application often may lead him or her to be "data oriented" in conducting or evaluating research. The value of a study, however, can be determined only by examining the methods used to gather the data. Factors such as the validity of operational definitions, the proper use of controls, the choice of subject population, and the use of suitable methods and procedures for collecting and analyzing data are critical to appropriate interpretation of results.

Conformance to Expectations. Claude Bernard once said that "men who have excessive faith in their theories or ideas are not only ill-prepared for making discoveries; they also make poor observations."[1] Although research papers often are written as though the results obtained were exactly as predicted in the introduction, this rarely is the case. Many scientific discoveries are made by the alert, open-minded observer of an unexpected finding. Bernard further admonishes the scientist to forget his or her hypothesis once the study begins, and the reader of a paper should do the same. As mentioned earlier, it is only by challenging one's expectations and assumptions that any scientific field can be advanced.

Assumed Attributes of Design. Readers of research papers sometimes assume that certain attributes of scientific studies are universally desirable, such as using control or comparison groups of subjects, randomizing procedures, and using large numbers of subjects. However, none of these procedures is necessarily of service to the research question being asked. For example, a hypothesis about the relationship between two characteristics (e.g., nutritional status and school performance) of a given subject population does not need a control group to be tested adequately, *unless* the prediction is that the relationship between those characteristics is not of the same magnitude in another subpopulation, as defined by age, race, sex, or other relevant qualities. However, the absence of a control group also means that the group studied cannot necessarily be considered *distinctive* on the basis of a single study. Nutritional status may be found to be related to school performance in a group of diabetic children, but this cannot be considered uniquely characteristic of such children unless nondiabetic children are studied similarly.

Belief in Technical Complexity. Studies often appear more credible when highly technical procedures are described in detail. However, simply because a study employs a standardized questionnaire or test to measure some aspect of social interaction or because a computer is used to analyze data does not necessarily mean that the methods used were appropriate to the research question or that the data derived from these procedures led to valid conclusions.

Excessive Skepticism toward the Research Process. Because they are aware that human frailties and technical limitations are real elements of the research process, some practitioners may become *hypercritical* of all research results. It should be apparent, however, that the cause of biomedical science would not be served either by total acceptance or total rejection of all scientific endeavor. A spirit of openness and curiosity and a healthy skepticism toward scientific thinking are necessary no matter whose work the practitioner evaluates. This kind of attitude can make science both exciting and productive.

Influence of Socially Validated Standards. It also is important to realize that many of the practices of science are determined, at least in part, by social standards within the broad community of scientists or within society itself. Thus what is now considered unethical scientific practice might not have been so 30 or 40 years ago. Other socially validated standards include authorship practices, expectations for frequency of publication, levels of statistical significance that define the reliability of data, and even the use of statistical criteria for interpreting data. These practices not only vary with the passage of time and social events but also differ among various scientific specialities.

USEFUL KNOWLEDGE AND SKILLS

The preceding section emphasized the attitudinal aspects of effective research critique. Certain knowledge and skills also are extremely useful for competently evaluating research results.

Content and Methods

An important characteristic of research is that it builds on the thinking and findings of the past. Therefore some knowledge of the literature of the field in question will help the reader determine whether the rationale for a given study and the techniques and procedures used are based on current practices, controversies, or interpretations.

Minimizing Bias and "Confounds." Probably the greatest number of errors made in interpreting data derive from a poor understanding of the importance of instituting good operational definitions and control procedures and accounting for confounded variables in conducting any research. For example, in the study by Kolodny and coworkers[4] mentioned earlier, any statement made about differences in testosterone levels between users and nonusers of marijuana had to account for the possibility that users and nonusers of marijuana may have used other substances to a different extent than did nonusers of marijuana, inasmuch as such substances also might alter levels of testosterone. Without accounting for this possible *confound,* it would be difficult to attribute any difference between the groups to marijuana use per se. Thus, by taking a good history, the investigator can control for the possible effect of substances other than that under study. In addition, because this study was based on reported use of "street variety" marijuana, the *operational definition* of marijuana necessarily included any impurities that might be contained in the joints smoked by the study subjects.

Data Presentation and Analysis. Another frequent impediment to interpretation of scientific findings is difficulty understanding and interpreting statistical terms and test results. For example, the concept of *variance* is basic to an understanding of the quantitative expression of data, yet it often is overlooked in their interpretation. Nonetheless, as illustrated in Fig. 14-1, a practitioner's interpretation of the difference between two means must depend on the spread of individual data points around those means. The more dispersed the data are around the mean, the less certain the practitioner can be about the distinction between groups of subjects. Beveridge[1] has suggested that practitioners try to learn at least enough about statistical methods to maintain some respect for them and to know when to consult someone else. A course in basic statistics, coupled with hands-on problem solving, will help the practitioner feel more at ease with these concepts and methods.

Literature Search Techniques. For some clinicians, reviewing scientific literature involves reading the journals to which they subscribe and attending professional meetings. However, if a clinician wishes to pursue any area of research in greater depth, he or she should have some knowledge of the most advanced techniques for keeping up with and researching specialized literature. In addition to a number of publications that can be found in medical libraries or obtained by subscription (e.g., *Current Contents, Index Medicus,* and *Science Citation Index),* an increasing number of computer search services are available that can be invaluable for gaining a historical perspective or maintaining a current awareness in any field. Such services are accessible not only through libraries, but also through personal computer–based programs such as *Grateful Med,* from which one can search a number of data bases from any computer that has a modem. With such programs it is possible not only to search the literature, but also to obtain abstracts and authors' addresses and to order reprints of articles.

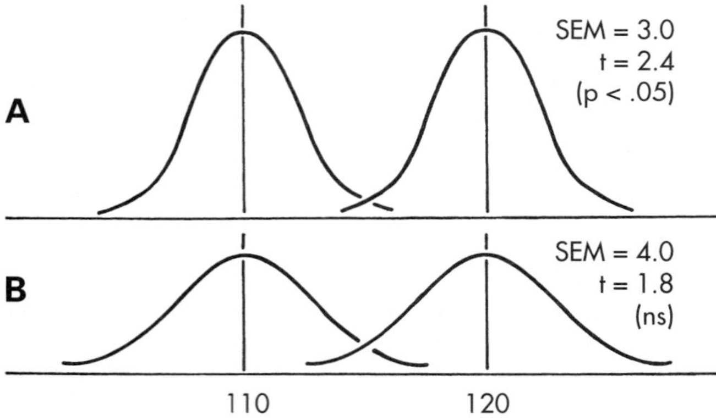

FIG. 14-1 The importance of variance in determining the significance of a difference between means using the *t* test. Once *t* is computed, a table is consulted to determine whether it meets the criterion for significance. **A,** The smaller variance, or standard error of the mean (SEM), leads to a larger *t* value and thus to the conclusion that a difference between means of that magnitude could have occurred by chance less than once in 20 times ($p < 0.05$). This is not the case in **B,** even though the means are the same, because the variances (SEMs) are too large. Thus the difference is considered not significant *(ns).*

(From Plaut SM: Psychosocial aspects of scientific investigation. In Balis GU et al, editors: ***The psychiatric foundations of medicine: dimensions of behavior,*** London, 1978, Butterworth.)

Scientific Communication. It is easier to assess the value of a paper or presentation realistically if the practitioner has some appreciation for the processes by which scientific data are disseminated. Learning how to prepare a good paper or presentation can help a clinician in assessing the quality of others' work. Some knowledge of the screening processes involved in selecting research reports for presentation or publication also is useful. For example, journals typically submit their papers to a more rigorous peer review process than do meeting program committees, and the extent of peer review a report undergoes varies somewhat even within those two spheres.

Nature of the Research Process. Finally, intensive involvement with a research project can go a long way toward acquainting the clinician with both the technical and the human aspects of the research process. The value of supervised research training early in a career cannot be overemphasized. If such an experience is not possible, participation in a research methodology course or journal club can provide some guided experience in critical evaluation of research reports. A third but less effective alternative is reading in some of the aforementioned areas.

EVALUATION GUIDELINES

A research study should be timely, reflecting a knowledge of current developments in its field of interest and using current methodology. Usually the author need not provide a comprehensive review of the literature. Rather, he or she should demonstrate that the study accounts for relevant knowledge, issues, and controversies related to the topic of interest.

Method

The study's stated purpose, the definitions of variables and terms, the methods and procedures used, the reporting of data, and the interpretation of results all should show a logical consistency. Returning to the marijuana studies, one was based on the use of street marijuana, which could have contained impurities, preventing the investigator from conclusively attributing any effects to marijuana per se. The other used joints manufactured and standardized specifically for the study, resulting in a more specific operational definition of the independent variable *marijuana.* If a practitioner wishes to apply the results of these studies, he or she must consider which of the two operational definitions is more relevant to his or her purpose. Which is relevant: whether smoking marijuana itself affects testosterone levels in a controlled, institutional setting, or whether the experience of using marijuana in more customary situations is related to levels of this hormone? Each of these questions is more relevant for certain readers and for certain purposes of application or further investigation.

An important and oft-stated rule of thumb for writing the methods section of a paper is that it should, according to Day,[2] "provide enough detail that a competent worker can repeat the experiments. . . . The cornerstone of the scientific method *requires* that your results, to be of scientific merit, must be reproducible; and, for the results to be adjudged reproducible, you must provide the basis for repetition of the experiments by others." A complete presentation also makes it easier to evaluate the timeliness, relevance, and effectiveness of the methods and procedures used.

Results

Authors sometimes tend to present only the results of statistical tests, as though the only intent of the study were to report the difference between two groups of subjects or a relationship between two variables. It is important that sufficient descriptive data be presented so that the reader can see the data on which these statistical tests were performed. However, journals' space limitations require that authors make some judgments as to which data are best presented in graphs, tables, or text, or not at all. The practitioner's primary concern should be that the questions addressed by the study are reflected appropriately in the data presented and that any interpretation of results is supported by the actual presentation of relevant data. At times there may be relatively subtle aspects of data presentation that the reader should consider. For example, if an author reports relative changes in the scores of two groups of subjects over time as the percentage of an initial value, the practitioner should expect that the author also will provide some information about the initial values themselves. If a group of children performed extremely well on an achievement test, it might not be appropriate to expect that an experimental training program would improve their scores on that particular test.

Statistical Analysis

The following three factors should be considered in evaluating the use of statistical methods.

Relevance to the Research Question. The statistical methods used should reflect the nature of the question asked by the study. For example, if an author were to predict a systematic relationship between body weight and blood pressure in a group of young adolescents, dividing the children into two discrete groups of body weight and comparing the mean blood pressures by use of a t test would not provide the most sensitive method for exploring this question. A correlational technique that takes into account the individual weights of the children would be a more sensitive and appropriate way to proceed.

Conformance to Underlying Assumptions. Appropriate use of any statistical test is based on certain assumptions about the data. For example, certain tests require that the data approximate a normal, or gaussian, distribution, that the number of observations exceeds a certain level, or that two groups of data being compared be independently acquired. If a test that is used to analyze a body of data does not meet its underlying assumptions adequately, inappropriate conclusions may result.

Use of Appropriate Documentation. If the statistical tests used are not as widely known as, for example, the chi-square, t test, or Pearson correlation, the author should provide a reference to the source of the test used. Noting that a particular computer was used to analyze the data is not acceptable documentation. The work of a computer is no more effective than the program it is asked to follow, and the program itself must reflect an appropriate statistical method. Finally, the reader should expect the author to identify all tests used and, in most cases, to report actual results. The simple assertion that "the difference was significant ($p < 0.05$)" does not allow the reader to address the statistical issues outlined here.

Discussion

The reader should determine whether the interpretation of results is consistent with and limited to the data presented. Were conclusions based on data that were either not presented or ambiguous? Does the author generalize inappropriately to populations that have different characteristics from those of the one observed? Sound data and clear thinking usually result in a logical, concise interpretation. As mentioned previously, a scientist's effectiveness often is related to alertness to the unexpected finding and a willingness to consider various alternative explanations for a phenomenon. Regardless of whether the author of a paper considers such alternatives, the reader should be as alert to what is not included in the discussion section as to what is. As Beveridge[1] has said, "The most difficult mental act of all is to rearrange a familiar bundle of data, to look at it differently and escape from the prevailing doctrine."

SUMMARY

In assessing medical literature, the practitioner must remember that any study's value is limited by certain technical considerations and that every aspect of research is affected somewhat by the psychosocial milieu of both researcher and audience. Good scientific pursuit and effective critique require an understanding these facts, a conscious effort to look at relationships in new and unexpected ways, and a certain level of technical knowledge in the area of research methodology. Conscientious, competent evaluation of research does not simply serve the clinician and his or her patients; ultimately, it enhances the quality of published research.

REFERENCES

1. Beveridge WIB: *The art of scientific investigation,* ed 3, New York, 1957, Vintage.
2. Day RA: *How to write and publish a scientific paper,* ed 3, Phoenix, 1988, Oryx.
3. Dykes MHM: The physician: the key to the clinical application of scientific information, *JAMA* 237:239, 1977.
4. Kolodny RC et al: Depression of plasma testosterone levels after chronic intensive marihuana use, *N Engl J Med* 290:872, 1974.
5. Mendelson JH: Plasma testosterone levels before, during and after chronic marihuana smoking, *N Engl J Med* 291:1051, 1974.

SUGGESTED READINGS

Feinstein AR: *Clinical epidemiology: the architecture of clinical research,* Philadelphia, 1985, WB Saunders.

Fletcher RW, Fletcher SW, Wagner EH: *Clinical epidemiology—the essentials,* Baltimore, 1982, Williams & Wilkins.

Kilby SA, McAlindon MN: Searching the literature yourself: why, how and what to search. In Arnold JM, Pearson GA, editors: *Computer applications in nursing education and practice,* New York, 1992, National League for Nursing.

Shockley JS: *Information sources for nursing: a guide,* New York, 1988, National League for Nursing.

PART THREE
Principles of Patient Care

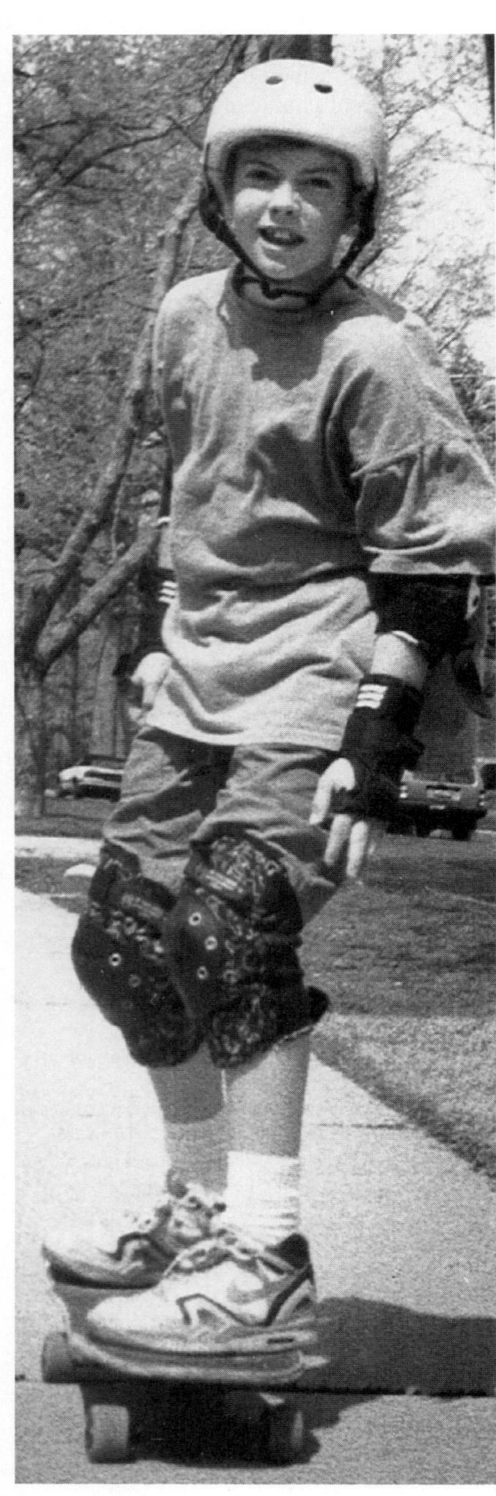

SECTION ONE

PREVENTION OF DISEASE

SECTION TWO

TREATMENT OF DISEASE

SECTION THREE

MANAGEMENT OF CHRONIC ILLNESS

15 Anticipatory Guidance

Howard R. Foye, Jr.

Anticipatory guidance is the key to achieving the primary goals of pediatric care of promoting health and preventing disease. Providing anticipatory guidance in primary care is challenging because of the range and complexity of appropriate issues, the enormous individual differences among normal children and their families, and the limited time available in health supervision visits. Other than the time constraints involved, these challenges can be the greatest source of interesting variety and rewarding physician-patient interactions in the practice of primary pediatric care.

Three major activities are involved in anticipatory guidance: (1) gathering information, (2) establishing a therapeutic alliance, and (3) providing education and guidance. Many discussions of anticipatory guidance focus only on the third element. Without the first two, however, education and guidance often is misguided or ineffective.

GATHERING INFORMATION AND ESTABLISHING A THERAPEUTIC ALLIANCE

Gathering information through careful history-taking and observation is a prerequisite if the pediatrician is to understand and respect the unique qualities of the child and family. Effective anticipatory guidance, like any teaching, should begin with an understanding of the student's knowledge base, preconceptions, and motivation; guidance is effective to the extent that it is targeted to the individual. A therapeutic alliance between the parents and the physician, based on mutual trust and respect, is another prerequisite for effective anticipatory guidance. Besides enhancing the effectiveness of teaching, this alliance can be a powerful source of emotional support. By listening respectfully, sympathizing with the parents' frustrations, and reinforcing effective parenting positively, the pediatrician can help the parents gain a sense of competence and confidence in their parenting. As the child develops, it becomes increasingly important to establish a therapeutic alliance directly with the child. This relationship is crucial to support and anticipatory guidance as the child becomes more independent.

The box on p. 152 outlines information that should be gathered before anticipatory guidance is provided. The two major categories are information about the *child* and information about the *child's environment.* Traditional pediatric health care focuses on the child, particularly on issues of promoting physical health, preventing disease, detecting and treating disorders, and monitoring for developmental milestones. More recently, pediatric health care has broadened its focus to include issues of behavior and the environment in which the child is developing. The list is imposing, particularly with the time limitations of primary care visits, but at least brief attention must be given to these areas to target anticipatory guidance appropriately. Prior knowledge of the child and family obviates the need to survey all these topics at each visit, although frequent updates are important.

Some fundamental principles about the prerequisites for anticipatory guidance need to be highlighted:

1. The parents and child must be given the opportunity to express their concerns at the beginning of every visit; the pediatrician's agenda for the visit will not get their attention until the physician has addressed *their* agenda.
2. Because it is important to develop a good relationship with the child as well as the parents, the pediatrician should interact warmly with the child at each visit. Even if only briefly, the physician should greet, talk, and play with the child before proceeding to more threatening procedures such as a physical examination and immunizations.
3. The pediatrician always should inquire about how things are going for the parents. Particularly in today's society of fragmented families, parenting can be lonely and demanding. To be a good nurturer, a person needs to be nurtured. The physician should take advantage of every opportunity to compliment the parents and encourage them to save time for themselves and each other. By supporting the parents and helping them support each other, the pediatrician indirectly can help the parents nurture their child.

Two questions that bear frequent repeating are:

—What do you and your child enjoy doing together?

—Is there enough time for spontaneity—for listening to your child and for doing what the child wants to do with you?

PROVIDING EDUCATION AND GUIDANCE

With the information outlined in the box, the pediatrician is in a position to provide anticipatory guidance. This is particularly important because time does not permit guidance on all potentially important topics. Table 15-1 suggests topics for anticipatory guidance by age. For general categories, some discussion, education, or guidance is warranted at each health supervision visit. Examples of more specific topics likely to be relevant at specific ages are listed under the headings.

Many potentially important topics may be overlooked if anticipatory guidance is limited to topics linked to specific ages. Topics that may be among the most important at any age and therefore always worthy of consideration include:

1. *Family stresses* (e.g., single parenthood, divorce, separation, moving, illness, death, unemployment)

PERTINENT INFORMATION FOR ANTICIPATORY GUIDANCE

A. Information about the *child*
   1. *Concerns:* expressed by parent or child
   2. *Health:* current status and follow-up of past problems
   3. *Routine care:* feeding, sleep, and elimination
   4. *Development:* evaluated by school performance or with standardized tests (e.g., Denver Developmental Screening Test,[6] Early Language Milestone Scale[3])
   5. *Behavior:* temperament and interaction with family, peers, and others

B. Information about the child's *environment*
   1. *Family composition* (at home)
   2. *Caregiving schedule:* who and when
   3. *Family stresses:* (e.g., work, finances, illness, death, moving, marital and other relationships)
   4. *Family supports:* relatives, friends, organizations, material resources
   5. *Stimulation* in the home
   6. *Stimulation/activities* outside the home, (e.g., preschool/school, peers, organizations)
   7. *Safety*

2. *Temperament*[8]
3. *Hurried children*[4]—tight schedules and pressure to achieve and grow up fast
4. *Self-esteem*—development of a sense of competence[9]

The lists in Table 15-1 should not limit the pediatrician's scope but merely serve as examples and reminders. Much anticipatory guidance will follow from information gathered at the beginning of the visit, including new concerns of the parent or child and follow-up of old problems. The following sections supplement information in Table 15-1 by listing the major developmental tasks of each period and discussing related anticipatory guidance issues briefly.

Prenatal Visit

The family's developmental tasks in the period before delivery involve planning and preparing for the birth and early care of the infant. The main goal of the prenatal visit is to begin the development of a therapeutic alliance with the family. Specific objectives include learning about the family's health and social history and discussing their plans and concerns about the remainder of the pregnancy, labor, delivery, and early child care. Other objectives include a discussion of the nature of the pediatrician's working relationship with the family and details about how the practice functions.

Newborn Visits

During the newborn period, the major developmental tasks for infants involve the transition to the extrauterine environment. The major tasks for parents include bonding and learning to respond appropriately to the emotional and physical needs of their infant. The objectives of newborn pediatric care include assessing the infant's physical status, behavioral individuality, and caregiving environment at home; managing health problems; and promoting bonding and parenting competence and confidence.

Up to 6 Months

The major developmental tasks in the first 6 months include socioemotional development (caregiver-infant reciprocity[2]), cognitive development (attention to events in the external environment), and physical development (rapid growth and visually guided manipulation with the hands).

Reciprocity is a term used to describe the achievement of mutually satisfying and predictable interactions between an infant and a caregiver. The development of reciprocity is influenced both by the clarity and predictability of the cues provided by the infant and by the caregiver's sensitivity, responsiveness, and predictability. This is an important period of learning for all participants in these interactions. Learning is more difficult when the infant is irritable or unpredictable or when the caregiver's responsiveness is hindered by fatigue, depression, or distractions caused by family stress. The following anticipatory guidance may be helpful: (1) anticipatory teaching about the normal unpredictability of feeding and sleeping schedules and the frequency of unexplained episodes of crying in the first few months, (2) discussion of the parenting of infants with various temperaments, and (3) discussion and counseling about issues that may be interfering with the caregiver's ability to provide a responsive environment for the infant.

The major cognitive developmental task for the infant in this period involves a shift from activities centered on the body (e.g., sucking) to a greater interest in the external environment. At first this is manifested by increasing visual and auditory attention to external events. Then, from 4 to 6 months of age, the infant's ability to visually guide the grasp and manipulate objects progresses rapidly.

6 to 12 Months

The major developmental tasks of the infant 6 to 12 months old include socioemotional development (attachment,[1] basic trust versus mistrust[5]), cognitive development (object permanence, early means-end relationships[7]), and physical development (mobility).

The concepts of attachment and basic trust are similar. Basic trust develops in the first year to the extent that an infant learns that the caregiver is a predictable and reliable provider of essential physical and emotional needs. Trust in this most important aspect of the external environment, the primary caregiver, is believed to result in more confident exploration of the wider environment during the second year, when autonomy becomes the major socioemotional issue. Attachment theorists refer to this as *exploration from a secure base.* An infant who is insecurely attached (who mistrusts more than trusts) because of unpredictable or unreliable caregiving in the first year will more likely be inhibited in exploring the environment. The insecurely attached infant also is more likely to be clinging and demanding as a result of insecurity about the caregiver's availability. These behaviors may lead to the erroneous conclusion that the infant is too "attached" to the caregiver. It is important to remember, however, that most infants go through a period of separation anxiety toward the end of the first year, when clinging behavior increases. Also, some infants who temperamentally are more

Table 15-1 Topics of Anticipatory Guidance

Prenatal and newborn

Prenatal visit

1. *Health:* pregnancy course; worries; tobacco, alcohol, drug use; hospital and pediatric office procedures
2. *Safety:* infant car seat, crib safety
3. *Nutrition:* planned feeding method
4. *Child care:* help after birth, later arrangements
5. *Family:* changes in relationships (spouse, siblings), supports, stresses, return to work

Newborn visits

1. *Health:* jaundice, umbilical cord care, circumcision, other common problems, when to call pediatrician's office
2. *Safety:* infant car seat, smoke detector, choking, keeping tap water temperature below 120° F
3. *Nutrition:* feeding, normal weight loss, spitting, vitamin and fluoride supplements
4. *Development/behavior:* individuality, "consolability," visual and auditory responsiveness
5. *Child care:* importance of interaction, parenting books, support for primary caregiver
6. *Family:* postpartum adjustments, fatigue, "blues," special time for siblings

First year

Up to 6 months

1. *Health:* immunizations, exposure to infections
2. *Safety:* falls, aspiration of small objects or powder, entanglement in mobiles that have long strings
3. *Nutrition:* supplementing breast milk or formula, introducing solids, iron
4. *Development/behavior:* crying/colic, irregular schedules (eating, sleeping, eliminating), response to infant cues, reciprocity, interactive games, beginning eye-hand coordination
5. *Child care:* responsive and affectionate care, caregiving schedule
6. *Family:* return to work, nurturing of all family relationships (spouse and siblings)

6-12 months

1. *Safety:* locks for household poisons and medications; gates for stairs; ipecac; poison center telephone number; outlet safety covers; avoiding dangling cords or tablecloths; safety devices for windows/screens; toddler car seat when infant reaches 20 pounds; avoiding toys that have small detachable pieces; supervise child in tub or near water
2. *Nutrition:* discouraging use of bottle as a pacifier or while in bed; offering cup and soft finger foods (with supervision); introducing new foods one at a time
3. *Development/behavior:* attachment, basic trust versus mistrust, stranger awareness, night waking, separation anxiety, bedtime routine, transitional object
4. *Child care:* prohibitions few but firm and consistent across caregiving settings; defining discipline as "learning" (not punishment)
5. *Family:* spacing of children

Second year

1-2 years

1. *Health:* immunizations
2. *Safety:* climbing and falls common; supervising outdoor play; ensuring safety caps on medicine bottles; noting dangers of plastic bags, pan handles hanging over stove, and space heaters
3. *Nutrition:* avoiding feeding conflicts (decreased appetite is common); period of self-feeding, weaning from breast or bottle; avoiding sweet or salty snacks
4. *Development/behavior:* autonomy versus shame/doubt, ambivalence (independence/dependence), tantrums, negativism, getting into everything, night fears, readiness for toilet training, self-comforting behaviors (thumb sucking, masturbation), speech, imaginative play, no sharing in play, positive reinforcement for desired behavior
5. *Child care:* freedom to explore in safe place; day care; home a safer place to vent frustrations; needs show of affection, language stimulation through reading and conversation
6. *Family:* sibling relationships, parents modeling of nonaggressive responses to conflict (including their own conflict with their toddler)

Preschool

2 to 5 years

1. *Health:* tooth brushing, first dental visit
2. *Safety:* needs close supervision near water or street; home safety factors include padding of sharp furniture corners, fire escape plan for home, and locking up power tools; should have car lap belt at 40 pounds and bike helmet; should know (a) name, address and telephone number, (b) not to provoke dogs, and (c) to say "no" to strangers
3. *Nutrition:* balanced diet; avoiding sweet or salty snacks; participating in conversation at meals

Continued.

Table 15-1 Topics of Anticipatory Guidance—cont'd

2 to 5 years—cont'd

4. *Development/behavior:* initiative versus guilt; difficulty with impulse control and sharing; developing interest in peers, high activity level; speaking in sentences by age 3; speech mostly intelligible to stranger by age 3, reading books; curiosity about body parts; magical thinking, egocentrism
5. *Child care/preschool:* needs daily special time with parents, bedtime routine; talking about day in day care; limiting TV watching with child, reprimanding privately, answering questions factually and simply; adjusting to preschool, kindergarten readiness
6. *Family:* chores, responsibilities

Middle childhood
5 to 10 years

1. *Health:* appropriate weight; regular exercise; somatic complaints (limb and abdominal pain, headaches); alcohol, tobacco, and drug use; sexual development; physician and child dealings (more direct)
2. *Safety:* bike helmets and street safety; car seat belts; swimming lessons; use of matches, firearms, and power tools; fire escape plan for home; saying "no" to strangers
3. *Nutrition:* balanced diet, daily breakfast, limiting sweet and salty snacks, moderate intake of fatty foods
4. *Development/behavior:* industry versus inferiority, need for successes, peer interactions, adequate sleep
5. *School:* school performance, homework, parent interest
6. *Family:* more time away but continuing need for family support, approval, affection, time together, and communication; family rules about bedtime, chores, and responsibilities; guidance in using money; parents should encourage reading; limiting TV watching and discussing programs seen together; teaching and modeling nonviolent responses to conflict
7. *Other activities:* organized sports, religious groups, other organizations, use of spare time

Adolescence
Discuss with adolescent

1. *Health:* alcohol, tobacco, and drug use, health consequences of violence, dental care, physical activity, immunizations
2. *Safety:* bike and skateboard helmet and safety, car seat belts, driving while intoxicated, water safety, hitchhiking, risk taking
3. *Nutrition:* balanced diet, appropriate weight, avoiding junk foods
4. *Sexuality:* physical changes, sex education, peer pressure for sexual activity, sense of responsibility for self and partner, OK to say no, preventing pregnancy and sexually transmitted diseases, breast and testes self-examination
5. *Development/relationships:* identity versus role confusion, family, peers, dating, independence, trying different roles, managing anger other than with verbal and physical attacks
6. *School:* academics, homework
7. *Other activities:* sports, hobbies, organizations, jobs
8. *Future plans:* school, work, relationships with others

Discuss with parents

1. *Communication:* allowing adolescents to participate in discussion and development of family rules; needs frequent praise and affection, time together, interest in adolescent's activities
2. *Independence:* parent and child ambivalence about independence; expecting periods of estrangement; promoting self-responsibility and independence; still needs supervision
3. *Role model:* actions speak louder than words—parents provide model of responsible, reasonable, nonviolent, and compassionate behavior

timid or socially withdrawn may have an extended period of "clinginess."

Object permanence means that the infant now understands that objects continue to exist even when they are not present in the immediate physical environment. Calls for an absent primary caregiver often are the earliest evidence that the infant has developed this cognitive ability. Separation anxiety and night waking also may be manifestations of this new achievement. A budding understanding of means-end relationships is apparent in the infant's ability to remove a barrier or to use a second object to retrieve a toy that is out of reach. Another manifestation may be the infant's association of the coat closet with Mommy's departure and therefore the bitter protests that occur when the mother approaches the closet.

Increasing mobility has many implications for anticipatory guidance, particularly regarding issues of safety.

1 to 2 Years

The major developmental tasks of the 1- to 2-year-old include socioemotional development (autonomy versus shame and doubt[5] and ambivalence regarding dependence and independence), cognitive development (exploration, early language, "pretend" play), and physical development (ambulation and slower growth).

The issue of autonomy is at the heart of "the terrible twos," which actually start during the second year of life. This period is characterized by frustrating, dramatic behavioral shifts from stubborn independence ("I want to do it myself" and "no" to most parental requests) to infantile clinging and dependence. Parents often wish that their child were both more independent and less independent at the same time. The wild fluctuations are related to the child's newly acquired walking and climbing skills, as well as his or her eagerness to explore, which often outstrips the cognitive ability to anticipate danger or surprise. The brazen explorer quickly can be reduced to a tearful clinger to mommy's skirt.

The second year is a very exciting time for cognitive development. The developing ability to understand and to use language is a manifestation of the child's cognitive ability to use symbols for objects. By age 2, the child's play becomes a theater for imitating past events and demonstrating a budding ability to think symbolically and creatively.

A decline in the growth rate in the second year is the cause of one of the most frequent parental concerns in this period: "He eats like a bird." Explaining normal growth and intake usually reassures the parents.

Preschool: 2 to 5 Years

The major developmental tasks of the preschool period include socioemotional development (initiative versus guilt,[5] mastery [e.g., toilet training], and peer interactions with true sharing), cognitive development (speech, deferred imitation, and imagination), and physical development (steady growth and increasing coordination).

The initiative that characterizes this period is demonstrated in widening interactions with the physical environment and with people outside the family. Good parenting involves giving the child opportunities to exercise initiative and to experience mastery over new challenges, while ensuring close supervision to provide necessary support and encouragement and to prevent harm. An overprotective or restrictive caregiving environment may result in fear or guilt and may inhibit initiative and the developing sense of self-mastery. A caregiving environment that pushes the child too hard toward "independence" may not provide enough supervision and support to allow the child to master the developmental tasks of this period.

During the preschool period, language develops so remarkably that it is easy to forget that the preschooler's thinking often is still illogical. It is characterized by an egocentrism that cannot comprehend a perspective other than the child's own and assumes that other people have seen and experienced exactly what the child has. It also is characterized by magical thinking—the blurring of fantasy and reality; wishes, dreams, and actual events are not clearly distinguished. These logical limitations may help explain the common occurrence of irrational fears and exasperating misunderstandings between parent and child. A wish that a new sibling would go away may be a frightening source of guilt and self-blame when the new infant is hospitalized. The child may think that wishing made it happen. Careless comments by a parent also may be a source of anxiety for a child who cannot distinguish a threat from reality.

Middle Childhood: 5 to 10 Years

The major developmental tasks of middle childhood include socioemotional development (industry versus inferiority[5]), cognitive development (concrete logical thinking,[7] basic functions of mathematics, and classification of objects), and physical development (preadolescence).

This is the period when the pediatrician should increasingly engage the child directly in discussions and anticipatory guidance. By the end of this period, some physicians already are spending part of each visit alone with the child.

Middle childhood is the period when critical appraisal of a child's abilities begins in earnest. Although preschool children (and their parents) frequently compare themselves with their age mates, comparisons become much more quantitative and official in middle childhood. Tests and opportunities for public humiliation in school are unending. Even when teachers are careful to avoid overt comparisons, the children know how they measure up. After-school activities, particularly sports, often are highly competitive. It is easy to understand how a child may develop a sense of inferiority, particularly in a culture that so emphasizes being number one, as if anything else is not good enough.

The socioemotional task of industry (i.e., motivation to succeed through work) requires that the child experience success. Lack of success in tasks leads to a feeling of inferiority, discouragement, and giving up. This is an important issue for anticipatory guidance, because parents also may have accepted the notion that the child is not good at anything. Some creative thinking must be done to provide successful experiences for each child so that lack of motivation does not rob the child of his or her potential.

Adolescence

The major developmental tasks of adolescence include socioemotional development (identity versus role confusion[4]), cognitive development (abstract and hypothetical thinking[5]), and physical development (puberty).

Adolescence frequently is described as comprising three stages. Early adolescence (roughly 10 to 13 years of age) is the period of most rapid physical growth and sexual development. Because of the rapid changes, many children are preoccupied with their bodies and with comparing themselves with their peers. In addition, they begin to separate from their parents, frequently challenging parental authority. During middle adolescence (roughly 14 to 17 years of age), preoccupation with physical changes lessens. This period is characterized by intense involvement with peers, conflicts over independence with parents and, often, sexual exploration. Late adolescence (roughly 18 years of age to 21) is characterized by increased concern over future plans, including college studies and career plans. Social skills are more advanced, and many adolescents are involved in committed, intimate relationships.

LITERATURE FOR PARENTS AND CHILDREN

Literature for parents and children's books frequently are valuable supplements to discussions with the pediatrician about topics of anticipatory guidance. Often practitioners lack sufficient time to discuss an issue in depth in the office. One alternative is to begin a discussion in the time available and then suggest a pertinent reference. Literature references for the parents and child are listed at the end of the chapter; however, follow-up is crucial. Perhaps the next regular visit is soon enough, but it always is appropriate to invite the family to call or to make an appointment if family members wish to discuss further questions sooner. Of course, sometimes a definite follow-up visit or referral should be scheduled immediately.

A note of caution is warranted about recommending books. Some parents have a tendency to overintellectualize parenting—to place too much reliance on specific "expert" advice that is not individualized to their family. Good literature for parents points out that specific advice needs to be tailored to the unique qualities of the child and the parents and to the environment in which they live. Good parenting involves more than general knowledge about children and behavior management; it also involves sensitivity and responsiveness to the special qualities of each child and self-awareness about how the parent's feelings and events in the environment influence interactions with the child. Written advice alone, therefore, is not sufficient. The parents must interpret and modify the advice to fit their situation. Some can do this themselves; many will benefit from anticipatory guidance by the pediatrician.

Most parents will want to have at least one of the following books:

Brazelton TB: *Working and Caring,* Reading, Mass., 1984, Addison-Wesley Publishing Co., Inc. A wonderful book for parents trying to balance working and child care—honest and positive.

Hoekelman R, MacDonald N, and Baum D: *The New American Encyclopedia of Children's Health,* New York, 1989, New American Library Publishing Co., Inc. A handy A to Z guide written especially for parents; this book addresses their common concerns.

Leach P: *Your Baby and Child from Birth to Age Five,* New York, 1986, Alfred A. Knopf, Inc. Another superb, wide-ranging reference with an emphasis on child development.

Spock B, Rothenberg M: *Dr. Spock's Baby and Child Care,* New York, 1985, Pocket Books. This updated classic is still an invaluable, enjoyable, wide-ranging book for parents.

The following professional texts contain extensive, annotated bibliographies of parent and child literature on a wide variety of topics (health and development):

Dixon S, Stein M: *Encounters with Children: Pediatric Behavior and Development,* Chicago, 1987, Mosby.

Sahler OJ, McAnarney E: *The Child from Three to Eighteen,* St. Louis, 1981, Mosby.

REFERENCES

1. Bowlby J: *Attachment,* ed 2, New York, 1983, Basic Books.
2. Brazelton TB, Koslowski B, Main M: The origins of reciprocity: the early mother-infant interaction. In Lewis M, Rosenblum L, editors: *The effect of the infant on its caregiver,* New York, 1974, John Wiley & Sons.
3. Coplan J: Evaluation of the child with delayed speech or language, *Pediatr Ann* 14:203, 1985.
4. Elkind D: The hurried child: growing up too fast too soon, Reading, Mass, 1981, Addison-Wesley.
5. Erikson E: *Childhood and society,* thirty-fifth anniversary edition, New York, 1986, WW Norton.
6. Frankenburg W, Sciarillo W, Burgess D: The newly abbreviated and revised Denver Developmental Screening Test, *J Pediatr* 99:995, 1981.
7. Ginsburg H, Opper S: *Piaget's theory of intellectual development,* ed 3, Englewood Cliffs, NJ, 1988, Prentice-Hall.
8. Thomas A, Chess S, Birch H: *Temperament and behavior disorders in children,* New York, 1968, New York University Press.
9. White R: Motivation reconsidered: the concept of competence, *Psychol Rev* 66:297, 1959.

SUGGESTED READINGS

Brazelton TB: Anticipatory guidance, *Pediatr Clin North Am* 22:533, 1975.

Casey P, Sharp M, Loda F: Child-health supervision for children under 2 years of age: a review of its content and effectiveness, *J Pediatr* 95:1, 1979.

Chamberlin R, Szumowski E, Zastowny T: An evaluation of efforts to educate mothers about child development in pediatric office practices, *Am J Public Health* 69:875, 1979.

Committee on Psychosocial Aspects of Child and Family Health, American Academy of Pediatrics: Guidelines for health supervision. II, Elk Grove Village, Ill, 1988, The Academy.

Prothow-Stith D: *Deadly consequences,* New York, 1991, Harper Collins.

16 Nutrition

ONE

Nutritional Requirements

Gilbert B. Forbes

To live, to grow, and to thrive, human beings must take in nutrients from their environment. Before birth these are supplied by the mother; thereafter, they must be ingested. If too little is provided, the infant or child will not grow and may become ill; too much may lead to toxicity or obesity. Nutritionists have tried for decades to define the optimum intakes for various nutrients; a few are known, yet for most the only data available are in the form of educated guesses. In an attempt to cover the maximum conceivable need (because individuals vary in size, there may be individual differences in requirements), quasiofficial bodies such as the National Academy of Sciences have recommended generous allowances of most nutrients. Although this would provide for the upper extremes of need, in effect it advises most of the population to eat more than they need. Dietary surveys among healthy individuals thus show that the diets of many people do not satisfy the listed recommended dietary allowances. Perhaps this is just as well, inasmuch as overnutrition now is a greater problem in this country than undernutrition, and there is concern over the possibility that the former may shorten the life span.

Nutritional requirements can be considered on the basis of age, body size, growth rate, physiological losses (as in menstruation and lactation), and caloric intake. The following discussion deals primarily with the normal child; for the most part, situations that call for special nutritional advice are dealt with in other chapters.

Note should be taken of the contribution of food technology to the modern nutritional scene: the pasteurization of milk, the addition of certain vitamins and minerals to some foods, alterations in milk composition to serve the needs of young infants better, hypoallergenic formulas, and the special formulas for infants who have certain inborn errors of metabolism (e.g., phenylketonuria). All this has made it possible to feed the majority of infants most satisfactorily. The only undesirable consequence has been a decline in breast-feeding; although of minor nutritional importance in Western society, this decline may be disadvantageous in poor countries and in depressed areas where sanitation is inadequate and the supply of animal protein is meager. However, interest in breast-feeding has revived in recent years in all societies.

ENERGY

Energy Metabolism

The body continuously expends energy, in the form of heat and work. Body temperature must be maintained, physical activity provided for, and the processes of digestion, cellular transport, and tissue synthesis supported. The unit of energy generally employed in metabolism is the kilocalorie (kcal),* usually designated simply as a *calorie* (Cal). Foods have approximately the following energy equivalents when burned in the body:

1 g protein = 4 calories (protein is 16% nitrogen)
1 g carbohydrate = 4 calories
1 g fat = 9 calories

It is axiomatic that the body cannot exist on only one or even two of these sources of energy, so it is fortunate that nature has provided a mixture of the three in many foods. Satisfactory, palatable diets for infants and children (and adults, too) provide 8% to 15% of total calories from protein and 30% to 50% each from fat and carbohydrate.

Energy intake is put to five broad uses:

1. *Basal metabolism.* This term refers to energy expenditure at rest in the fasting state. On a body weight basis, the basal metabolic rate (BMR) is higher in infants than in adults, primarily because (1) infants' surface area to weight ratio is higher, (2) a certain amount of infants' "basal" energy is used for growth, and (3) the relative size of the viscera and brain (the most metabolically active organs in the body) is considerably greater in infants. During the first year of life the BMR is about 55 Cal/kg/day; thereafter this value diminishes gradually to the adult level of about 25 to 30 Cal/kg/day. Because adipose tissue has a low metabolic rate, the BMR *per kilogram of body weight* is lower in obese individuals than in thin ones and in women compared with men. However, the BMR bears a linear relationship to *lean weight* in adolescents and adults.
2. *Requirement for growth.* The synthesis of tissue obviously requires energy. The exact amount is not known, but studies of young children recovering from malnutrition and studies of intentionally overfed adults show that 4 to 8 extra calories are required for each gram of weight gain. During the first 4 months of life, one third of the total caloric intake is used for growth. By the end of the second year of life, this has dropped to 1% to 2% of calories.
3. *Energy lost in excreta.* Some nitrogen is excreted in the urine, and feces contain both protein and fat. It is estimated that such losses constitute about 10% of the energy intake of the normal diet.
4. *Specific dynamic action.* Resting metabolism rises somewhat after a meal, especially after a generous protein intake, and may not return to the baseline for several hours. The amount of energy dissipated in this manner is estimated to be 5% to 10% of total calories ingested.

*A kilocalorie is the amount of heat required to raise the temperature of 1 kg of water by 1° C (from 14.5° to 15.5° C); it equals 1000 small calories. Some would like to replace this with another unit of energy, the *joule* (equivalent to 10^7 ergs), which physical scientists commonly use. One kilojoule (kJ) equals 0.239 kcal; to convert kilocalories to kilojoules, multiply by 4.18.

5. *Requirement for physical activity.* Studies of adults show that sedentary men require about 2700 Cal/day and very active men, 4000; for women, these values are 2000 and 3000 Cal/day, respectively. Thus, very active people need 1½ times more food. Although estimates of this sort are not available for infants and children, casual observation confirms that physical activity varies from person to person. Some infants are more restless than others, and, obviously, the energy expenditure of high school athletes is different from that of their spectator friends. Because a major portion of the total energy expenditure is directly proportional to body weight, large persons expend more energy in a given task and at rest.

Table 16-1 lists energy expenditures for adults (these values would apply to late adolescents, as well) for various activities. The total daily energy requirement as a function of age and sex is depicted in Fig. 16-1. These data are based on reports by the Food and Nutrition Board of the National Academy of Sciences and the World Health Organization. The diagram shows the estimated average requirement. Note the sex difference both in total calories and calories per kilogram during adolescence. This is due to (1) boys' greater lean weight and (2) their greater physical activity. The values for individuals 19 to 20 years of age equal those for young adults.

In this context, it is instructive to consider the growth of the lean body mass (LBM) inasmuch as this represents the bulk of the body's metabolically active tissue, whereas the adipose tissue component is relatively inert. The data shown in Fig. 16-2 are based on total body potassium measurements.* Note that the LBM growth curve differs from that of total body weight, because the latter includes a variable proportion of fat. The adolescent growth spurt in LBM is considerably greater for boys than for girls. It should be obvious that an adolescent boy has a greater need for calories and for many nutrients, particularly calcium and nitrogen. Indeed, in the midst of his adolescent growth spurt, a boy's need for iron to provide growth of blood volume and muscle mass may equal that of a postmenarcheal girl.

*One of the naturally occurring isotopes of potassium (^{40}K) is radioactive, and the body contains enough of this isotope to allow its measurement by specially designed scintillation counters. Because potassium is found only in lean tissue, LBM can be estimated.

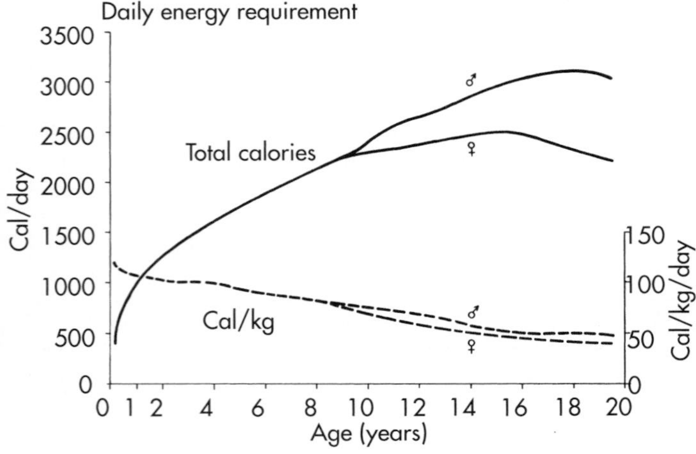

FIG. 16-1 Daily energy requirement as a function of age and sex.

Fig. 16-1 shows the *average* energy requirement. Larger individuals need more calories, both for maintenance and for a given degree of physical activity; smaller people need less. This amounts to 18 to 20 calories a day for each kilogram of weight difference. Under normal circumstances, appetite is a good indicator of energy need. In situations of abnormal growth, either too little or too much, this chart can help the pediatrician determine whether the stated intake of food is appropriate and thus whether food intake could be a contributing factor.

Low-birth-weight neonates need a generous intake of calories (i.e., 130 to 150 Cal/kg/day) to provide for "catch-up" growth, and their inadequate fat stores demand that feeding be started as soon after birth as possible.

One additional point is worth noting: if calories are obtained from a variety of foods, an adequate intake of calories usually ensures an adequate intake of essential nutrients. Therefore calories should be the first item evaluated in assessing a dietary history.

Pregnancy and Lactation

The recent increase in the number of teenage pregnancies demands that pediatricians and child health personnel be aware of the extra energy requirements for pregnancy and lactation. Studies of chronically undernourished poverty groups have shown that birth weight and the chances of infant survival can be improved by providing additional calories during pregnancy; it now generally is admitted that a weight gain of 10 to 13 kg is desirable. Weight gain during pregnancy, as well as the prepregnancy weight, influences birth weight. The extra energy cost to the mother is estimated at 150 to 300 Cal/day throughout pregnancy, depending on how much she curtails her physical activity. Although based on adults, these figures should pertain equally well to the pregnant teenager.

Lactation requires even more energy. Each deciliter of milk produced contains 72 calories, and milk production is said to be 80% efficient; thus 90 extra calories must be ingested by the mother for each deciliter of milk produced. The total milk production of 850 ml/day, therefore, requires an extra 760 calories. An underweight mother should be urged to get more than this, whereas the well-nourished mother needs less—perhaps only an extra 500 Cal/day—because she can draw on her generous fat stores.

PROTEIN

Proteins are high-molecular-weight polypeptides that serve many functions in the body. Enzymes are proteins, as are antibodies and some hormones; hemoglobin, plasma albumin, and the contractile elements of muscle also are proteins. All proteins are composed of some 20 amino acids, in varying

Table 16-1 Calories (kcal) Expended per Hour by Adults

	Calories	
Activity	**Men**	**Women**
Sleeping	65	54
Sitting quietly	83	69
Walking (3 miles/hr)	220	180
Swimming, tennis	400	300
Rowing	450+	360+

proportions; the function of a particular protein is governed by the sequence of amino acids within the molecule. Of these amino acids, nine cannot be synthesized by the body; therefore they are known as *essential amino acids*—histidine, isoleucine, leucine, lysine, methionine, phenylalanine, threonine, tryptophan, and valine. There are indications that cystine and taurine may be essential for low-birth-weight infants; these essential amino acids must be supplied in food.

As with energy, the body needs a constant supply of protein; during growth, new tissue must be synthesized because *all* tissues (even bone and adipose tissue) contain protein. Even during adult life there is a constant turnover of protein, with some nitrogen being lost in the urine even on a protein-free diet and during fasting. There is a protein requirement for growth and maintenance, and this is an unremitting requirement because the body has no storage site for protein. An inadequate supply results in a slowing of growth, a compromise of many body functions, and the wasting of muscle; in severe deprivation, impaired resistance to infection, reduced mentality, and even death may result.

Ingested protein first must undergo hydrolysis, a process begun in the stomach and carried to partial completion in the upper small intestine, mainly by pancreatic enzymes. The resultant amino acids and small peptides then are transported by specific metabolic processes (which themselves involve special proteins) into the interior of the intestinal mucosal cells (the peptide bonds having been split at the brush border), and the amino acids are absorbed into the portal blood.

The end products of protein metabolism appear in the urine mainly as urea, the deaminated amino acids being either converted to carbohydrate and fat or burned to carbon dioxide and water.

Biological Quality

The variable amino acid composition of food proteins leads to variations in the efficiency with which they supply the body's needs. The methods for estimating the biological quality of a given protein include tests on animals, observation of the growth of children on differing diets, nitrogen balance studies on adult volunteers, and a chemical score based on the amino acid content. Although these do not always yield the same result, the biological quality of the proteins in various food groups generally is agreed upon. In Table 16-2, the two sources with the highest quality protein are arbitrarily assigned a score of 100. Simply stated, a child must ingest more of a low-quality protein to achieve proper nutrition and the desired growth rate. The low quality of vegetable proteins is due to relative deficiencies of one or more essential amino acids. For example, wheat is low in lysine, corn is low in lysine and tryptophan, rice is low in lysine and threonine, and beans are low in methionine. Commercial formulas based on processed soy flour have proved satisfactory for infants. Some vegetables are so low in protein (e.g., cassava has only 0.35 g of protein per 100 Cal) that it becomes impossible to eat enough to meet the protein need. However, a judicious mixture of vegetables can yield a most satisfactory result. Strict vegetarians have survived in apparent health for many years, and tests of suitable vegetable mixtures have shown good results in the treatment of protein malnutrition.

Generally speaking, it is wise to include some animal protein in the diet; even if only a third of the total protein in-

Table 16-2 Relative Biological Quality of Food Protein

Food	Score
Human milk	100
Whole egg	100
Cow milk	95+
Meat	80+
Processed soy flour	80+
Vegetable proteins	50-70

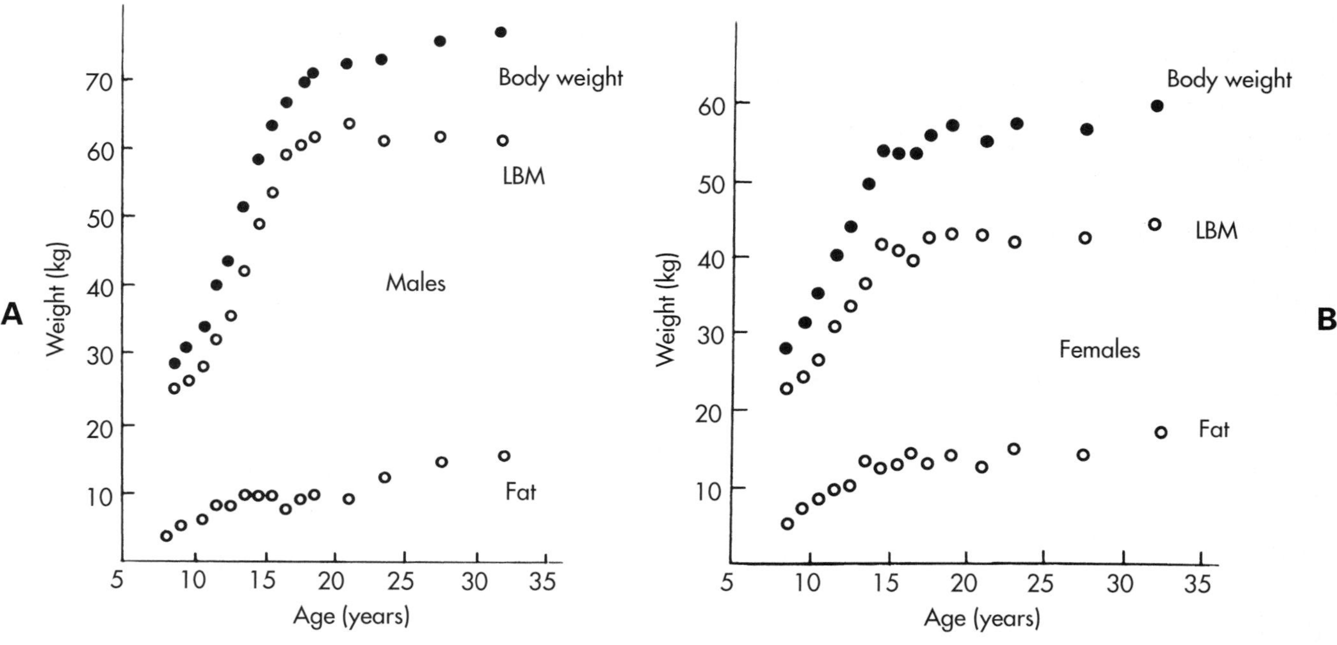

FIG. 16-2 Mean body weight and estimated lean body mass *(LBM)* and fat by ^{40}K counting for 604 males **(A)** and 467 females **(B)** ages 8 to 35 years.

take comes from this source, the risk of a specific amino acid deficit becomes negligible.

Requirement

There are many problems in estimating the precise protein requirement for any age; these include variations in growth rate, the size of the lean body mass, protein quality, and finally and most important, the technical and ethical difficulties in carrying out the necessary experiments on human beings. Indeed, estimates for the early months of life are based on the average intake of human milk by infants who appear to be thriving. Fig. 16-3 represents a composite of estimates by the National Academy of Sciences (NAS) and the World Health Organization (WHO). It should be noted that the usual American diet, which derives 12% to 15% of calories from protein (human milk is an exception: 8%) and an average per capita consumption of 100 g, provides protein well in excess of actual need.

It is important to note that the protein requirements (per kilogram of weight) of a young infant are relatively high compared with those of the older child or adult. High-quality protein is important for young infants, and a reasonable intake of milk ensures that is achieved. However, there is no particular advantage to providing protein in excess of actual need, inasmuch as the excess cannot be stored and therefore is metabolized as an energy source and appears in the urine as urea and amino acids. Studies of infants recovering from severe malnutrition have shown that satisfactory recovery can be achieved at protein intakes as low as 2.5 g/kg. In fact, there is serious doubt that diets really high in protein are needed under any circumstances save those associated with abnormal protein losses (e.g., as with extensive burns or gastrointestinal disease).

Several groups require special consideration. The rapid growth rate of low-birth-weight newborns demands a protein intake of 3 to 4 g/kg during the early months of life. Lactating women need an extra supply: 850 ml of human milk contains 10 g of protein; under the assumption that protein utilization is only 60% efficient, the mother should receive an extra 17 g of protein daily. The extra demand for protein during pregnancy is appreciable but not great; the body of the term newborn contains about 400 g of protein, to which should be added the 500 g contained in the placenta, gravid uterus, and breasts and in the expanded blood volume. Most of this increased need for protein occurs during the latter half of pregnancy, when it averages 6 g/day.

Excessive amounts of protein (5 g/kg or more) can lead to toxicity. The concentration of blood urea nitrogen rises, the urine may contain albumin and casts and, if water intake is low, the excessive renal solute load leads to an increase in obligatory renal water excretion and to dehydration; that plus the increased specific dynamic action can result in fever, the so-called protein fever.

FAT

Fat is a constituent of all body tissues. The term *fat* is applied to a heterogeneous group of low-molecular-weight compounds that contain fatty acids and that have in common the property of being soluble in solvents such as chloroform and ether. Neutral fats, or triglycerides, are fatty acid esters of glycerol. They serve the functions of energy storage and insulation against the cold and provide a cushion for internal organs. This depot fat accounts for about 14% of body weight in term newborns and 10% to 30% in adults. Fig. 16-2 shows that body fat content varies with age and sex. Obese individuals may have as much as 50% fat.

The high energy content of adipose tissue (composed of fat-laden adipocytes and a connective tissue stroma) is due to two factors: the high caloric value of fat itself (which has the energy equivalent of gasoline), and the fact that, unlike with protein and carbohydrate, fat deposition is not accompanied by an increase in tissue water. This makes for efficient energy storage; indeed, a moderately thin adult can survive fasting for at least a month, and the very obese have survived for as long as 250 days. Newborn animals (including humans) and adult hibernators have a special adipose organ—brown fat—that supplies energy quickly in response to cold.

Fatty acids are classified according to the number of

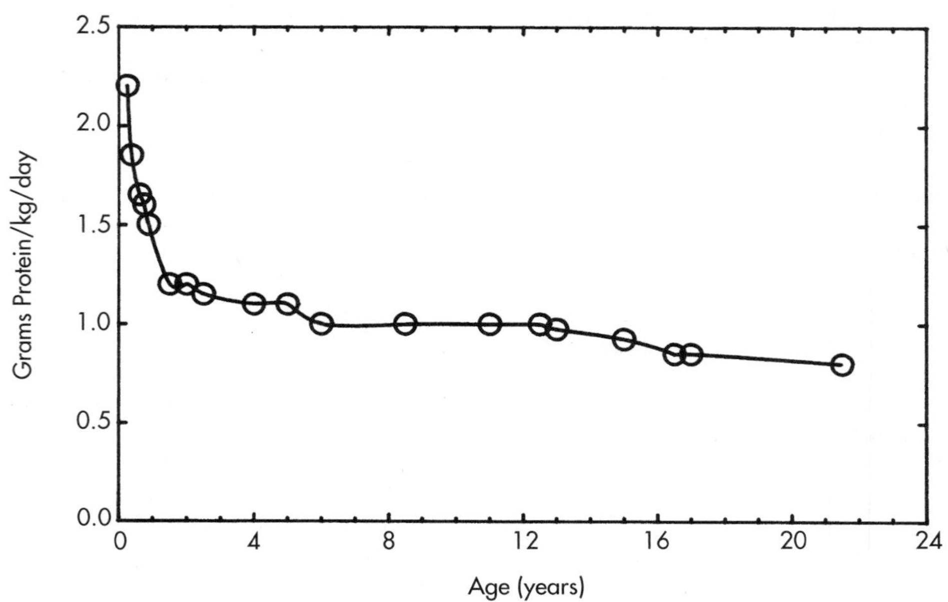

FIG. 16-3 Estimates of protein requirements as a function of age.

double bonds in the hydrocarbon chain. *Saturated fat* contains a relatively small percentage of fatty acids having double bonds, and *polyunsaturated fat* contains a high percentage of fatty acids having such bonds. Generally, the former have higher melting points and thus a firmer consistency at room temperature (compare lard and corn oil). Fats of vegetable origin tend to be more unsaturated than those of animal origin; human milk fat is less saturated than cow milk fat. In addition to neutral fats, there are other fats. Some contain phosphorus or galactose, which are essential components of tissue. Some—the lipoproteins—are linked to protein; these contribute to the stability of cell membranes and serve in combination with proteins and polysaccharides as structural components of cells (lysozymes and myelin sheaths are examples).

With the exception of linoleic, linolenic, and arachidonic acids, the multitude of fats found in the body can be formed from protein or carbohydrate precursors. Although symptoms and signs of essential fatty acid deficiency (dermatitis and impaired growth and lipid transport) have been observed under experimental conditions and in patients fed parenterally for long periods, the requirement is low—only 1% to 2% of total calories—thus such deficiencies have not been described under natural circumstances. Essential fatty acids are precursors of an important series of compounds, the prostaglandins. Cholesterol, which is a sterol and not a fat in the true sense, plays an important role in metabolism. It is a precursor of bile acids, vitamin D, adrenocortical steroids, and sex hormones. It is synthesized in the body and thus is present in foods of animal origin, and its absorption by the intestine is facilitated by a high-fat diet. Diets high in fat and cholesterol are thought to accelerate the process of atherosclerosis.

Fat digestion occurs in the upper small intestine by the action of pancreatic and intestinal lipases, which split off two fatty acids from glycerol. The 2-monoacyl glycerol residue combines with bile salts to form micelles (which, incidentally, incorporate fat-soluble vitamins and cholesterol), which act to dissolve the free fatty acids and are taken up by the mucosal cells. Here the triglycerides are reconstituted and released into the lymph as chylomicrons. Short- and medium-chain fats (12-carbon chains or less) are handled differently; these are hydrolyzed by the brush border of mucosal cells, and the resultant fatty acids are released into the portal vein.

Fat exists in several forms in plasma: as triglycerides, free fatty acids, lipoproteins, and phospholipids. Fatty acids are a source of energy for muscle, and they can be esterified by adipocytes to form depot fat; they also can be synthesized in liver and adipose tissue from dietary carbohydrate precursors.

Unsaturated fatty acids that have a double bond at the third carbon from the methyl terminal (alpha-linolenic acid is one such omega-3 fatty acid) are present in significant amounts in marine fish oils. These fatty acids and their derivatives reduce platelet aggregation and appear to retard the progress of atherosclerosis. Fish-eating populations have less atherosclerotic disease and also have slightly longer bleeding times.

CARBOHYDRATES

As the name implies, carbohydrates are a series of compounds composed of carbon, hydrogen, and oxygen. They generally are classified into three groups: monosaccharides, which contain five or six carbon atoms (e.g., glucose and fructose); disaccharides, which have 12 carbon atoms (e.g., sucrose and lactose); and polysaccharides, which are high-molecular-weight polymers (e.g., glycogen and starch are examples). Their main function is to supply energy, although certain specialized forms are involved in antigen-antibody reactions. Deoxyribonucleic acid (DNA) and ribonucleic acid (RNA) both contain a five-carbon sugar (deoxyribose and ribose, respectively); glucose and galactose are essential constituents of tissues such as collagen and cerebrosides; and the various glycoproteins have specialized functions.

Some tissues, such as muscle, can use fatty acids as a prime source of energy, but the brain derives most of its energy from glucose. In theory, the body can exist without dietary carbohydrate (CHO) because it can be formed from protein and fat; however, diets that are very low in CHO (less than 5% of calories) quickly lead to excessive combustion of fat and a rise in fatty acid and ketone body levels in the blood, and thus to acidosis. This is what occurs when a ketogenic diet is used to treat epilepsy.

Monosaccharides require no digestion. Disaccharides are hydrolyzed in the upper small intestine by specific enzymes. Digestion of starch begins in the mouth (salivary amylase) and is carried to completion in the intestine by the action of pancreatic amylase and specific disaccharidases in the brush border of the jejunal epithelial cells. The resultant mixture of simple sugars, principally glucose, is taken into the mucosal cells and then into the portal circulation. In the liver, fructose and galactose are converted to glucose; some glucose is released to the general circulation, and some is stored as glycogen. The entry of glucose into cells of all types, save brain cells, is facilitated by the action of insulin. The level of blood glucose is maintained by the combined action of pituitary and adrenal, as well as pancreatic, hormones.

Diets very high in monosaccharides or disaccharides may cause diarrhea, and consuming these sugars (particularly sucrose) in a physical form that adheres to the teeth promotes dental caries. Generally, the proportions of protein, CHO, and fat in the diet can vary considerably without metabolic or nutritional risk. The limits are rather wide: protein, 8% to 20% of calories; CHO, 15% to 60% of calories; and fat, 25% to 60% of calories. Contrary to widespread belief, obesity is *not* the result of an abnormal distribution of calories among these three dietary components (e.g., starches are no more "fattening" than fat); rather, it is the *total* caloric intake that is at fault. There is evidence that high-fat diets, particularly those that provide large amounts of saturated fats and cholesterol, can be detrimental to health; however, an excess of total calories and a sedentary life-style also are important in this regard.

WATER

All tissues contain water (dental enamel has 1% to 2%), and for most tissues this is the principal constituent. Most chemical reactions take place only in an aqueous medium, and the rate of water turnover in the body is relatively high. Thus it is no accident that most edible foods contain large amounts of this dietary essential.

Water is continuously lost from the body by a number of routes. There is an obligatory loss in urine because the kidney has a limited capacity to produce a concentrated urine.

In children and adults this limit is about 1400 mOsm/L,* corresponding to a specific gravity of about 1.040. Thus diets high in solutes, which are largely excreted in the urine (nitrogen, sodium, phosphorus), call for a large urine volume. It should be noted that very young infants are able to achieve a urine concentration of only 700 mOsm/L. Water also is lost continuously from the lungs and skin in the absence of sweating, the so-called insensible water loss, the amount of which is roughly proportional to the BMR. Such losses amount to about 10 ml/kg/day in an adult and 30 ml/kg/day in an infant. Water loss through sweating varies with the environmental temperature and humidity and with physical activity. Under extreme conditions an adult can lose 500 ml/hr through sweating.

Daily fecal water loss amounts to about 150 ml in an adult and 10 ml/kg in an infant.

Besides food and drink, the body has its own source of water. The burning of fat and CHO produces carbon dioxide and water (H_2O), the so-called water of oxidation (100 g of fat yields 107 ml H_2O, 100 g of glucose yields 60 ml H_2O). For an adult, this amounts to about 300 ml/day and for an infant, about 90 ml/day. Fig. 16-4 depicts the overall water economy for the average infant and the average adult. It is apparent that the infant is at greater risk from water deprivation inasmuch as infants' water turnover is much larger—about 16% of total body water each day, compared with about 6% per day in adults. Likewise, infants are at greater risk from conditions that accelerate water loss (e.g., vomiting and diarrhea), from heat stress, and from diets that provide excessive amounts of solute for urinary excretion (high protein, high salt). It is no accident that human milk has a high ratio of water to solute.

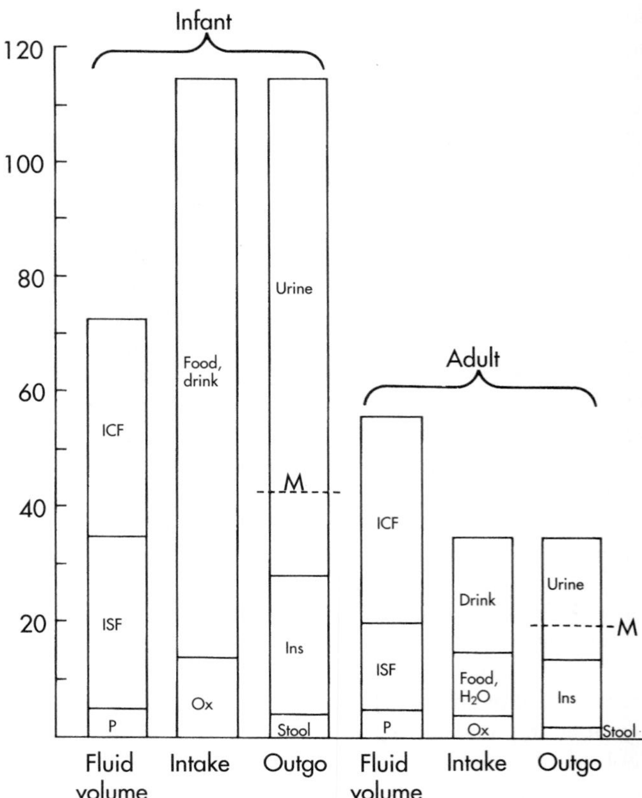

FIG. 16-4 Comparisons of body fluid volumes (percentage of body weight) and daily intake and outgo of water (ml/kg) for an infant and an adult. The values shown are averages and vary somewhat with the method used and the subject's fat content. *Dashed line (M),* Value for minimal water expenditure; *P,* plasma volume; *ISF,* interstitial fluid volume; *ICF,* intracellular fluid volume; *Ox,* water of oxidation; *Ins,* insensible water loss.

(From Farmer T, editor: *Pediatric neurology,* ed 3, New York, 1983, Harper & Row.)

MINERALS

The diet must provide the minerals that are essential components of body tissues. A deficiency of these minerals leads to diminished growth and to disease, and excessive intakes may result in toxicity. Table 16-3 provides information on the functions, dietary sources, and requirements for minerals for which requirements have been estimated. Except for iron and fluoride, a well-balanced diet provides a satisfactory intake of minerals. Iron deficiency now is the most common nutritional deficiency in this country. Attempts to improve this situation have been made through iron fortification of cereal products and infant formulas. Fluoride is added to the drinking water in many communities, as well as to toothpastes.

It should be mentioned here that the average American diet provides a generous amount of salt, to the point that some nutritionists are concerned about this as a possible factor in the pathogenesis of hypertension.

Besides those listed in Table 16-3, a number of minerals are known to be essential for animals and presumably for humans. These are chloride, chromium, manganese, molybdenum, nickel, silicon, tin, and vanadium. Deficiencies of these minerals are unlikely except with protracted parenteral feeding or, in the case of chloride, with excessive vomiting.

VITAMINS

As the word itself implies, vitamins are necessary for proper tissue function and thus for growth. These compounds act as cofactors for a number of enzymes. Most cannot be synthesized in the body and so must be supplied in the diet. Exceptions to this rule include vitamin D (activation of skin sterols by sunlight) and vitamin K (synthesized by intestinal bacteria). Small amounts of vitamin B_{12} are manufactured by intestinal bacteria, and some niacin is produced by conversion from tryptophan, but not in quantities sufficient to meet requirements. Vitamin deficiencies result in disease, and excessive intakes may lead to toxicity. The story of the discovery of the relationship of certain diseases to dietary inadequacies, of the presence of certain "vital amines" in trace amounts of food, and of the elucidation of their chemical structures and metabolic functions is fascinating, as well as intimately associated with the development of modern nutritional science.

Table 16-4 lists the vitamins known to be important for

*An osmole is the molecular weight in grams of an osmotically active particle, whether it be a nonionized compound such as glucose or urea or an ion such as Na^+ or Cl^-. A milliosmole (mOsm) is one thousandth of an osmole.

Table 16-3 Nutritionally Important Minerals

Mineral	Function	Physiology	Effects of deficiency	Effects of excess	Daily requirement	Sources
Calcium	Structure of bone, ion transport across cell membranes, neuromuscular excitability, blood coagulation	Absorption aided by vitamin D and parathyroid hormone (PTH), hindered by phosphate; PTH facilitates release from bone, thyrocalcitonin inhibits; gravity and muscle tension needed for skeletal stability	Osteoporosis only with severe deficiency, muscle paralysis, or malabsorption	Hypercalcuria with excessive vitamin D, and immobilization	Infants—400-600 mg Adolescents—600-700 mg Pregnancy (latter half), lactation—1000-1200 mg	Milk, cheese, green leafy vegetables, beans, canned salmon
Copper	Cofactor for certain enzymes, cross-linking of collagen	Plasma level 110 μg/dl, mostly as ceruloplasmin; intestinal absorption hindered by excessive zinc	Anemia, osteoporosis, defective myelination	None, except with massive ingestion	0.5-2 mg	Liver, meats, grains
Fluoride	Bone and tooth structure, resistance to caries	Deposited in bone as fluorapatite	Tendency for dental caries	4-8 mg/day—mottled teeth 20+ mg/day for long periods—osteosclerosis Large doses—acute poisoning	1 mg/L in drinking water	Seafoods, many municipal water supplies
Iodine	Constituent of thyroid hormone	Concentrated in thyroid gland	Simple goiter, endemic cretinism	Iodism	40-150 μg	Seafoods, iodized salt
Iron	Constituent of hemoglobin, myoglobulin, enzymes	Absorption regulated by gastrointestinal mucosa, level of blood hemoglobin; menstrual loss averages 0.7 mg/day	Anemia; if severe, cardiac failure, poor growth, lethargy	Hemosiderosis, poisoning by medicinal iron	Infants—1 mg/kg Adolescents—10-18 mg	Liver, whole grains, eggs, legumes, meat
Magnesium	Cofactor for enzymes, neuromuscular excitability	Principal cation of intracellular fluid	Tetany, hypocalcemia	Poisoning from medicinal magnesium (intravenous or intramuscular)	Infants—4 mg/kg	Meat, cereals, milk
Phosphorus	Constituent of phospholipids, ATP, nucleic acids; intermediary metabolism	Absorption regulated by vitamin D, dietary calcium, PTH; latter affects renal excretion	Muscle weakness; dysethesia; rickets in premature infants	In newborn, hypocalcemia	Infants—two thirds of calcium requirement All others—same as calcium requirement	Most foods
Potassium	Cellular transport, CHO and protein metabolism, membrane potential in muscle and nerve	Principal cation of intracellular fluid; regulation by adrenocortical steroids	Muscle weakness, abdominal distention, cardiac failure, alkalosis	Cardiac failure	1.5-2 mEq/kg	All foods
Selenium	Constituent of glutathione peroxidase	Interaction with vitamin E, heavy metals	Cardiomyopathy; muscle degeneration (animals)	Animals—"blind staggers"	Adults—50-200 μg	Seafood, liver, meat
Sodium	Osmotic pressure, cellular transport, extracellular fluid volume	Principal cation of extracellular fluid; regulation by adrenocortical hormones	Weakness, dehydration	Edema; CNS irritability if severe	2 mEq/kg	Most foods
Zinc	Constituent of enzymes	Absorption impaired by diet high in calcium, fiber	Growth failure, hypogonadism, reduced taste acuity	None except with massive ingestion	Children—6 mg Adults—15 mg	Meat, especially pork, whole grains, nuts, cheese

Table 16-4 Nutritionally Important Vitamins

Vitamin	Characteristics	Biochemical action	Effects of deficiency	Effects of excess	Daily requirement	Food sources
Vitamin A (retinol); 1 IU = 0.3 μg retinol	Fat soluble, heat stable; bile necessary for absorption, specific binding protein in plasma; stored in liver	Component of visual purple; integrity of epithelial tissues, bone cell function	Night blindness, xerophthalmia, keratomalacia, poor growth, impaired resistance to infection	Hyperostosis, hepatomegaly, alopecia, increased cerebrospinal fluid pressure	Infants—300 μg Adolescents—750 μg Lactation—1200 μg	Milk fat, eggs, liver
Provitamin A (beta-carotene); one sixth the activity of retinol	Converted to retinol in liver, intestinal mucosa			Carotenemia		Dark green vegetables, yellow fruits and vegetables, tomatoes
Biotin	Water soluble; synthesized by intestinal bacteria; deficiency with large intake of egg *white*, total parenteral nutrition	Coenzyme	Dermatitis, anorexia, muscle pain, pallor	Unknown	Unknown	Liver, egg yolk, peanuts
Cobalamin (vitamin B_{12})	Slightly soluble in water, heat stable only at neutral pH, light sensitive; absorption (ileum) dependent on gastric intrinsic factor; cobalt a part of the molecule	Coenzyme component; red blood cell maturation; CNS metabolism	Pernicious anemia, neurological deterioration	Unknown	1-2 μg	Animal foods only; meat, milk, eggs
Folacin (group of compounds containing pteridine ring, *p*-aminobenzoic and glutamic acids)	Slightly soluble in water, light sensitive, heat stable; some production by intestinal bacteria; ascorbic acid involved in interconversions; interference from oral contraceptives, anticonvulsants	Tetrahydrofolic acid (the active form): synthesis of purines and pyrimidines, and methylation reactions	Megaloblastic anemia	Only in patients with pernicious anemia not receiving cobalamin	Infants—60 μg Adolescents—200 μg Pregnancy—400 μg	Liver, green vegetables, cereals, oranges
Niacin (nicotinic acid, nicotinamide)	Water soluble, heat and light stable; availability from corn enhanced by alkali; synthesized in the body from tryptophan (60:1), some by intestinal bacteria	Component of coenzymes I and II (NAD, NADP); many enzymatic reactions	Pellagra: dermatitis, diarrhea, dementia	Nicotinic acid (not the amide): flushing, pruritus	6.6 mg/1000 Cal	Meat, fish, whole grains, green vegetables
Pantothenic acid	Water soluble, heat stable	Component of coenzyme A; many enzymatic reactions	Observed only with use of antagonists; depression, hypotension, muscle weakness, abdominal pain	Unknown	Unknown—estimated at 5-10 mg	Most foods

Vitamin B_6 (pyridoxine, pyridoxal, pyridoxamine)	Water soluble, heat and light labile; interference from isoniazid; pyridoxal is the active form	Cofactor for many enzymes	Dermatitis, glossitis, cheilosis, peripheral neuritis; infants—irritability, convulsions, anemia	Polyneuropathy	Infants—0.2-0.3 mg Adults—1-2 mg	Liver, meat, whole grains, corn, soybeans
Riboflavin	Water soluble, light labile, heat stable; synthesis by intestinal bacteria (?)	Cofactor for many enzymes	Photophobia, cheilosis, glossitis, corneal vascularization, poor growth	Unknown	0.6 mg/1000 Cal	Meat, milk, eggs, green vegetables, whole grains
Thiamine (vitamin B_1)	Heat labile; absorption impaired by alcohol; requirement a function of CHO intake; synthesis by intestinal bacteria	Coenzyme for decarboxylation, other reactions	Beriberi; neuritis, edema, cardiac failure; hoarseness, anorexia, restlessness, aphonia	Unknown	0.4 mg/1000 Cal	Liver, meat, milk, whole grains, legumes
Ascorbic acid (vitamin C)	Easily oxidized, especially in presence of copper, iron, high pH; absorption by simple diffusion	Exact mechanism unknown; functions in folacin metabolism, collagen biosynthesis, iron absorption and transport, tyrosine metabolism	Scurvy	Massive doses may lead to temporary increase in requirement	Infants—10-20 mg Adolescents—30 mg	Citrus fruits, tomatoes, cabbage, potatoes, human milk
Vitamin D (D_2—activated calciferol; D_3—activated dehydrocholesterol); 1 IU = 0.025 μg	D_2 from diet, D_3 from action of ultraviolet light on skin; hydroxylated sequentially in liver and kidney to form 1,25-dihydroxycholecalciferol, the active compound; regulated by dietary calcium and PTH; now called a hormone; anticonvulsant drugs interfere with metabolism	Formation of calcium transport protein in duodenal mucosa; facilitates bone resorption and phosphorus absorption	Rickets, osteomalacia	Hypercalcemia, azotemia, poor growth, vomiting, nephrocalcinosis	Infants—10 μg (400 IU) Others—2.5-10 μg (100-400 IU)	Fortified milk, fish liver, salmon, sardines, mackerel, egg yolk, sunlight; human milk not an adequate source
Vitamin E; 1 IU = 1 mg alpha-tocopherol acetate	Stored in adipose tissue, transported with beta-lipoproteins; absorption dependent on pancreatic juice and bile (iron may interfere); requirement increased by large amounts of polyunsaturated fats	Antioxidant; role in red blood cell fragility	Hemolytic anemia in premature infants; otherwise, no clear-cut deficiency syndrome in humans	Unknown	Infants—4 mg Adolescents—15 mg	Cereal seed oils, peanuts, soybeans, milk fat, turnip greens
Vitamin K (naphthoquinones)	Fat soluble, bile necessary for absorption, synthesis by intestinal bacteria	Blood coagulation: factors II, VII, IX, X	Hemorrhagic manifestations	Water soluble analogs only: hyperbilirubinemia	Newborn—single dose of 1 mg; thereafter 5 μg/day Older infants and children—unknown	Cow milk, green leafy vegetables, pork liver

humans, including the chemical name, function, estimated dietary requirement, dietary sources, and toxicity level.

It should be noted that certain foods are fortified with vitamins. By law, vitamin D must be added to milk, and vitamins now are added to many commercial infant formulas, to certain cereal products, to some breads, to fruit substitute drinks, and to other foods. Vitamin products are sold widely. As a result, overt vitamin deficiencies now are rare in the United States. Nevertheless, infants and children are at greater risk than adults because their requirements are proportionally greater, and thus dietary deficiency results in disease more quickly.

Recent claims have been made that massive intakes of vitamin C and the B complex will protect against respiratory tract infection and atherosclerosis and will ameliorate abnormal behavior and poor school performance. Such claims for *megavitamin therapy* and *orthomolecular treatment* are without merit.

A daily intake of 400 μg of folic acid, started before conception and continued during pregnancy, has been associated with a significant decrease in the incidence of neural tube defects (see Table 16-4). For women who have borne an infant who has such a defect, a daily intake 10 times greater (i.e., 4 mg), begun before conception, is recommended.[3]

NUTRITION IN THE UNITED STATES TODAY

Of the many factors that bear on today's nutritional scene, none has had a greater impact than *food technology* and *sanitation*. These modern developments have resulted from combined action by the government, industry, nutritional scientists, and physicians.

Before the turn of the century, the greatest hazards to infant health were infection and improper food. The whole history of infant nutrition is one of attempts to devise a satisfactory milk for babies who could not be fed at the breast. It was the realization in the past that raw cow milk was not a satisfactory food for young infants that led the fortunate few to employ wet nurses for their young.

The following features of raw cow milk render it less than suitable for young infants. *Bacterial contamination* arises from several sources: the cow herself (tubercle bacilli, streptococci [mastitis is common in high-producing herds], and *Brucella* organisms) and the various humans who handle the milk, any one of whom may add bacteria to the milk from respiratory or cutaneous foci. Lack of suitable refrigeration in former days (or in some areas still) accentuated the problem.

Cow milk contains about three times as much protein as human milk, and it is this high protein content (a large fraction of which is casein) that accounts for the formation of tough, voluminous curds on gastric acidification and thus leads to *impaired digestibility*. According to casual observation, formula-fed infants have larger stool volumes than do breast-fed babies.

The sum total of solutes available for renal excretion is 2½ times higher in cow milk than in human milk, and this *high solute load* calls for a higher obligatory urine volume; thus the infant is at greater risk from hot weather. For the newborn, the high phosphorus content of cow milk is one factor in the pathogenesis of neonatal hypocalcemia. Raw cow milk supplies barely enough *ascorbic acid* (21 mg/L) to prevent scurvy, and unfortunately, the process of pasteurization destroys about half the vitamin present. A few infants are *allergic* to cow milk protein and suffer gastrointestinal disturbances or eczema as a result.

Modern technology has overcome these difficulties. Pasteurization, combined with mandated refrigeration, has virtually eliminated bacterial contamination; evaporated milk and commercial infant formulas are sterile and keep well without refrigeration. Heat treatment also improves digestibility, and diluting the milk with water and adding carbohydrate to restore the caloric content reduces the solute load.

Industry also has modified modern cow milk formulas by adding ascorbic acid, vitamin D, and iron, reducing the phosphorus content, developing hypoallergenic milks based on soybean and hydrolyzed casein, reducing the sodium and protein content, and substituting vegetable fat for milk fat. Some commercial infant formulas contain added vitamin E and B complex, some are free of lactose (this sugar might not be tolerated by babies who have gastrointestinal disorders), and others contain hydrolyzed protein as a source of nitrogen. This wide variety of infant formulas makes it possible to feed every baby satisfactorily by formula from nonhuman sources. Modern technology has wrought a change of unprecedented magnitude in infant welfare.

However, these technological advances have two disadvantages: cost and the decline in breast-feeding. Cost is a problem for poor Americans and a major stumbling block to the exportation of food technology to poverty-stricken nations. Moreover, the more advanced the technology, the higher the cost. For example, a mother who nurses her 2- to 3-month-old infant needs only an extra pint of pasteurized milk each day to satisfy the additional calcium and protein requirements, plus an extra two slices of bread and one potato (or 10 g of butter) to complete the caloric need, together with vitamin D drops for the baby. Using an evaporated milk–water–Karo syrup formula also is inexpensive (additional vitamin C is needed), whereas the cost of a commercial ready-to-feed formula complete with added vitamins is considerably greater.

The ease and convenience of formula feeding have led inevitably to a decline in breast-feeding in our society and even in some developing countries. There is some evidence of an immunological advantage in human milk and for better absorption of iron, zinc, and fat; furthermore, the lack of contamination and the psychological benefit that may accrue with nursing are clear advantages. It is appropriate, therefore, to encourage breast-feeding in situations in which sanitation is poor, refrigeration is lacking, and cost is critical. It is encouraging to note that many more mothers have chosen to nurse their babies in recent years. However, it should be remembered that human milk contains very little vitamin D; thus nurslings must be given this vitamin, and mothers should be advised to eat a well-balanced diet.

Governmental regulations, public health activities, and governmental assistance are of the utmost importance to the modern nutritional scene. Municipal water supplies are now pure, and pasteurization is a uniform requirement for the sale of cow milk commercially. Dairy cattle are tested for tuberculosis and brucellosis, and those that have mastitis are removed from milk production. Other measures include inspection of food handlers and meats, inspection of restaurant kitchens, codes for infant formulas shipped from one state to another, and codes for canned foods. The result is that diseases such as typhoid fever, bovine tuberculosis, trichinosis, botulism, and staphylococcal food poisoning now are rare.

Many studies have shown the deleterious effects of severe infection, particularly gastroenteritis, on nutrition (vitamin turnover increases, and nitrogen balance becomes negative). The high prevalence of infantile malnutrition in developing countries is due in part to the occurrence of repeated infections. The Food and Drug Administration (FDA) was formed in 1938; this agency has the authority to regulate, among other things, food quality, food labeling, use of food additives, and vitamin fortification. The Federal Trade Commission (FTC) monitors advertising claims. These measures have resulted in better, cleaner, and more wholesome food. One of the most dramatic improvements was effected by the mandatory addition of vitamin D to milk, which has led to virtual elimination of dietary deficiency rickets in this country.

Food assistance programs are now fairly widespread. These include school lunch programs, the food stamp program, the program for women, infants, and children (WIC) and, in reality, the farm subsidy program. As a result, families that have limited financial means can augment their otherwise meager food supply. Millions of people are receiving food stamps, and 600,000 are enrolled in the WIC program.

Finally, local, state, and federal governments play an important role in providing free or low-cost health care for poor people and salaries for school and public health nutritionists and for helping to defray the cost of special foods for children who have certain diseases, such as phenylketonuria.

The result of these efforts, both industrial and governmental, is that with but one exception (iron deficiency anemia), overt nutritional deficiency now is uncommon in the United States, and obesity and dental caries have become the most prevalent "nutritional" conditions.

Two quasiofficial organizations have published recommendations for nutritional allowances (*not* requirements): the Food and Nutrition Board of the National Academy of Sciences–National Research Council and the Food and Agricultural Organization (FAO) of the United Nations. The former organization publishes a series of pamphlets at roughly 5-year intervals (the most recent one in 1989) that include a listing of recommended dietary allowances (RDAs) for people of all ages. These are based on knowledge of actual requirements, to which is added a generous "safety factor" to account for supposed individual variation in requirements and for variations in food quality. Except for calories, the "recommended" amounts all are in excess of actual need for the average individual; therefore it is not surprising that dietary surveys reveal that a sizable proportion of the population consumes less of many nutrients than the NAS recommends. The FAO recommendations are closer to actual requirements for protein, calcium, and a number of vitamins (see WHO *Handbook*); unfortunately this list of nutrients is not as complete as the one published by the NAS.

POSSIBLE ROLE OF INFANT AND CHILD NUTRITION IN ADULT HEALTH

Generally, the nutritional status of infants and children today is reasonably good. Some experts say our biggest challenge is the adult—that is, whether current infant feeding practices are compromising their health and longevity.

Several facts have been established. An intake of fluoride in early life, at a time when dental enamel is forming, results in a long-term diminution of the dental caries rate. It is known that a high intake of sucrose, particularly in solid, sticky foods, predisposes a person to dental caries; thus early learning of food habits that minimize the consumption of such foods should be beneficial.* Childhood obesity tends to persist into adult life, and this obesity shortens life span; therefore, attempts to prevent childhood obesity are important. Severe malnutrition in *early life* may impair intellectual performance† and should be avoided through procedures such as early feeding of premature infants, use of intravenous alimentation in certain critical situations, and early requests for medical advice and treatment of diseases that compromise nutrition during infancy.

The most challenging question relates to atherosclerosis and its cardiac and cerebral consequences. (This discussion forgoes consideration of the inherited abnormalities of lipoprotein metabolism associated with early onset arterial disease.) Arterial changes (the fatty streaks) appear in childhood, and by age 20 an appreciable percentage of men already have atherosclerotic plaques. The dietary components that have been considered as possible factors in initiating or intensifying this aging process are total calories, animal protein, saturated fats, and cholesterol. Cross-cultural surveys of adult autopsies reveal that any or all of these factors may be at fault; there also is some evidence that "postcoronary" adults who limit their intake of calories, saturated fat, and cholesterol have a better prognosis. The possible preventive role of fish has been mentioned earlier; however, certain species now are contaminated with mercury and polychlorinated hydrocarbons and therefore should not be eaten.

Experiments conducted many years ago showed that rats fed (from weaning) an amount of food equal to about two thirds of their usual intake lived much longer and had less arterial disease and fewer tumors that those fed ad libitum. These results have been confirmed by Ross,[2] who states, "The effects of chronic restriction in food intake on laboratory animals have been so apparent that it is difficult to avoid concluding that no environmental factor so decisively reduces the rate or expression of the aging process," and, "The mechanisms through which nutrition influences the aging processes are already operative during the *youthful stage* of life [italics mine]." If dietary restriction is postponed until maturity, the benefits are not as great.

Recent surveys show that Americans' average protein intake is at least twice the estimated requirement, that average milk consumption is about a pint a day, that solid food supplements are offered to infants at a very early age, and that obesity is prevalent; thus the results of the animal experiments are worth serious consideration. Berry[1] makes this cogent

*Statements by manufacturers reveal a generous consumption of sucrose. For the United States, this amounts to about 50 kg per capita per year, equivalent to 125 g, or 500 calories, per day. Furthermore, this figure has remained fairly constant over the past 50 years.

†There is reasonable evidence of such an effect when malnutrition occurs in the early months of life, and particularly when it is prolonged. In late infancy and childhood the effect has not been demonstrated clearly, probably because brain maturation is well on its way to completion. Nor has nutritional deprivation during pregnancy been shown to impair intellectual performance of the offspring. The effect of malnutrition per se is very difficult to study because it is almost always accompanied by cultural or emotional disadvantages.

comment: "Throughout the world the State does not accept the responsibility to protect its individuals from overnutrition." It is of interest that strict vegetarians are leaner and have lower levels of serum lipids and lower blood pressures than do nonvegetarians.

Some students of nutrition claim that there is evidence that modern refined foods have a deleterious effect, in that their consumption favors the incidence of diverticulosis and colonic tumors. These individuals advocate a diet that is higher in fiber, such as whole grain cereals, bran, and raw vegetables. Others caution against an excess of dietary fiber because this may interfere with the absorption of certain minerals.

Committees of the U.S. Senate and of the American Heart Association suggest that it would be advantageous for everyone to reduce his or her intake of saturated fats, refined sugar, salt, and cholesterol while proportionally increasing the amount of complex carbohydrates, and to balance energy intake with energy expenditure. These "dietary goals" should apply to children (but *not* infants) as well as to adults.

"WELL-BALANCED" DIET

Consuming a variety of foods is the best protection against nutritional deficiency. Except for the first few months of life, when milk is the principal if not the sole food, the daily diet should include items from each of the following general food groups, known in nutritional circles as "the basic four": (1) meat, fish, poultry, eggs, (2) dairy products (milk, cheese, milk products), (3) fruits and vegetables, and (4) cereals. The U.S. Department of Agriculture has depicted these as a food "pyramid," with high-frequency foods placed at the bottom. Today, the term *junk food* often is heard in reference to prepared foods high in refined carbohydrate and low in protein and vitamins, full of so-called empty calories. These foods do supply energy, and one cannot help thinking of the simpler life of previous generations, when foods of similar composition (e.g., apple pie, cake with thick frosting, jellied preserves, and home-canned fruits) were consumed freely, without opprobrium, their production considered the hallmark of a successful housewife.

Vegans, the colloquial term for strict vegetarians, should be counseled by a nutritionist because their diet is devoid of vitamin B_{12} and is likely to be low in calcium. Grains and vegetables must be chosen so as to include all the essential amino acids.

All those who follow "fad diets" of one sort or another and those who limit their food intake voluntarily in an effort to lose weight also should receive nutritional guidance, inasmuch as such diets may lack one or more essential nutrients. There are now reports of growth failure in adolescents who consume low-fat diets, for such diets usually are too low in calories.

TWO
Feeding of Infants and Children

Marvin S. Eiger

Infant nutrition should be considered a holistic enterprise. After the initial physical examination and the pronouncement that the baby is normal, the mother's primary concern becomes how she will nourish her infant. During pregnancy, maternal good health, a carefully supervised dietary intake, and adequate rest ensure proper nutrition of the fetus. This symbiotic union persists once infant and mother become two separate beings, and adequate nutrition for the infant becomes a more purposeful procedure, the details of which absorb much of the mother's time and energy during the first 6 to 12 months of the infant's life. This is the period of most rapid extrauterine growth, during which infants double their birth weight in the first 5 months and triple it by the twelfth month. Food during this period satisfies both physical and emotional growth, and the setting in which it is provided is of paramount importance to the infant, whose oral orientation translates food into ego satisfaction. Thus the practice of infant feeding cannot be based solely on *what type of milk* the infant should receive. Numerous other factors must be considered.

Most infants appear to grow normally and maintain a satisfactory state of health despite variations in nutritional management. The goal of infant nutrition is to produce an adequately (but not overly) nourished child whose diet is readily digestible, with all the essential nutrients provided through a reasonable distribution of calories derived from protein, fat, and carbohydrate. Because the pattern and content of feeding in infancy strongly affects dietary habits later in life, considerable care must be given to constructing the early dietary milieu.

Based on studies of nutritional requirements in infancy, reasonable dietary recommendations for full-term infants are 7% to 16% of calories from protein, 30% to 55% from fat, and the remainder from carbohydrate.[4] Human milk provides approximately 7% of calories from protein, 55% from fat, and 38% from lactose. Most commercially prepared formulas in the United States are modeled after human milk and provide 9% to 15% of calories from protein, 45% to 50% from fat, and the remainder from carbohydrate, usually lactose.

With the possible exceptions of vitamin D, iron, and fluoride, the infant fed breast milk from a healthy mother apparently receives more than adequate nutrition without further supplementation for at least the first 6 months of life. Thus, from a physiological and teleological point of view, the maxims "breast is best" and "human milk is for humans, cow milk is for cows" are unchallengeable. Only in the past 50 years or so has there been any question as to whether a mother would breast-feed her baby. With the advent of pasteurization, dependable refrigeration, and production of formulas from cow milk, alternatives have been provided. Thus the decision to breast-feed depends on several factors: the customs of the community, life-style, the mother's personality, and the attitudes of the obstetrician, pediatrician, and family. In 1980 the American Academy of Pediatrics, in its strongest statement ever, advised pediatricians and other health providers for children of the importance of and the need to recommend breast-feeding over formula feeding. The pediatrician must be aware of the advantages of human milk over cow milk for infant feeding and encourage mothers to breast-feed. However, the pediatrician must remain sensitive to the mother's own feelings and needs.

COMPARISON OF HUMAN MILK AND COW MILK

Milk is the primary source for satisfying nutritional needs during the entire first year of life. Solid foods are unnecessary for most infants until at least 4 to 6 months of age. Therefore it is essential that the physician be knowledgeable about the composition of human milk and cow milk. The manufacturers of infant formulas constantly attempt to modify cow milk to produce a product comparable to human milk. It is of interest that the growth rates of the human infant and the calf are different. An infant takes two to three times longer than a calf to double its birth weight. Inasmuch as cow milk contains 3.5 g of protein per deciliter to human milk's 1.1 g, a ratio of 3 : 1, the symmetry of nature is satisfied. (See Table 16-5 and Appendix C, Tables C-11 and C-12, for comparisons of human milk and various cow milk formulas.)

Besides the larger amount of protein in cow milk than in human milk, the proteins in the two milks have qualitative differences. The percentage of casein, as compared with whey proteins (lactalbumin and lactoglobulins), is higher in cow milk. Both proteins have high biological value, but casein causes higher curd tension in the infant's stomach and thus must be treated by homogenization, heating, and acidification for better digestion.

The fat of cow milk (butterfat) contains predominantly saturated fatty acids and is less well digested by infants than is the fat of human milk, which contains predominantly monounsaturated fatty acids such as oleic acid and adequate amounts of polyunsaturated fatty acids such as essential linoleic acid. The fat composition in human milk allows for excellent fat and calcium absorption and ensures that all essential fatty acids are provided. Human milk, in contrast to cow milk, is rich in lipase which when added to intestinal lipase, aids in the rapid splitting of free fatty acids from triglycerides to ensure quick absorption. It has been shown that free fatty acids are the most important sources of energy for the young infant, and the lipase in human milk makes these free fatty acids available rapidly, even before digestion with intestinal lipase begins.

Lactose is present in higher concentrations in human milk than in the milk of any other mammal. Lactose is split into glucose and galactose. Galactose is synthesized into galactolipid, which is an essential component of the central nervous system in mammals. In most commercial formulas, lactose is provided as the carbohydrate in a percentage similar to that found in human milk.

The total ash content of human milk (0.2%) is less than one third that of cow milk (0.7%); this provides a greater margin of safety for renal excretion during illness in early infancy.

BREAST-FEEDING VERSUS ARTIFICIAL FEEDING*

Many studies indicate that breast-fed infants develop fewer gastrointestinal infections, respiratory illnesses, and allergic reactions than do artificially fed infants.[6,7,10] These differences are most striking in the developing countries, where poor sanitary practices prevail. However, breast-feeding affords a large degree of protection against illness to infants in the developed countries as well. This protection is based on the presence of secretory antibodies in colostrum; the bifidus factor in human milk, which promotes the development of the characteristic intestinal microflora of *Lactobacillus bifidus;* and other host factors (Table 16-6). Each year researchers add more defensive factors found in breast milk to this list of properties. The infant acquires maximum protection against infection if breast milk alone, without solid foods, is offered until 6 months of life.

The immunological advantages of breast milk are most evident during the infant's first half year, but protection against many pathogens does endure through the toddler period. Breast-feeding offers greatest protection against diarrheal disease and against serious respiratory disease (wheezing, bronchitis, bronchiolitis, pneumonia) rather than uncomplicated respiratory tract infections. Bottle-feeding increases the risk of otitis media and of hospitalization for bacterial infections, septicemia, and meningitis.[3]

Breast-fed infants have been shown to have a lower incidence of allergic diseases when foreign food antigens are avoided for the first 6 months of life.[4] In one study of more than 20,000 infants, those who were fed artificially were seven times as likely to develop eczema as those who were completely breast-fed.[8] The first 6 months is the period in which infants' passively acquired transplacental antibodies are being replaced with their own; thus lack of exposure to foreign food antigens in the breast-fed infant presumably results in a reduced frequency of allergic reactions. Infants are never allergic to their mother's milk, whereas allergy to cow milk does occur.

An infant can digest human milk much more easily than the milk of other mammalian species. Breast milk forms softer curds in the infant's stomach than does cow milk and is assimilated more rapidly. Although it contains less protein than cow milk, virtually all the protein in breast milk is used by the infant, whereas about half the protein in cow milk is passed in the stool. A breast-fed infant rarely gets diarrhea and rarely becomes constipated because breast milk does not form hard stools in the intestinal tract.

Breast milk has no synthetic compounds, no preservatives, and no artificial ingredients. It is always available at the right temperature and the right consistency. Suckling at the breast is good for the infant's tooth and jaw development. Nursing is technically different from artificial feeding in that the bottle-fed infant does not have to exercise the jaws so energetically, inasmuch as light sucking alone produces a rapid flow of milk. Bottle-fed infants use their tongue in a manner quite opposite that of the breast-fed baby; the flow of milk through the rubber nipple is produced by a tongue-thrusting motion with each suck while the infant's lips create a negative pressure in the oral cavity, thus suctioning milk from the bottle.

The breast-fed baby places the tongue over the lower jaw, where it remains throughout the nursing session, and draws the nipple by suction well into the mouth, elongating it to three times its normal length and extending it to the junction between the hard and soft palates. The elongated nipple rests in a trough formed by the U-shaped tongue. As each suckling cycle is initiated, the infant's jaws compress the milk sinuses just under and proximal to the areola, pinching off a bolus of milk and propelling it toward the posterior pharynx by a peristaltic, wavelike motion. This rollerlike movement, which begins at the anterior tip of the tongue and progresses toward its base, effectively strips the milk bolus from the base of the nipple out toward its tip, where it exits into the infant's mouth and is swallowed (Fig. 16-5). The jaw muscles

*See Chapter 44, Four, Adjustment Period, for additional discussion of breast-feeding.

Table 16-5 Comparison of Nutrients in Formulas and Mature Human Milk

Component (per dl)	Recommended daily dietary allowances (0-6 months)	Human milk—values variable	"Humanized" formulas: Enfamil with iron	Similac with iron	SMA	Evaporated milk, 1:1 dilution	Evaporated milk 13 oz, water 19 oz, carbohydrate 1 oz	Whole milk 3.5% fat
Calories (kcal)	117 kcal/kg	67-75	67	68	67	69	67	66
Protein (g)	2.2 g/kg	1.1	1.5	1.6	1.5	3.5	2.8	3.5
Fat, total (g)	Not listed	4.5	3.7	3.6	3.6	3.8	3.0	3.5-3.7
Saturated		2.2	1.2	1.4	1.6	2.4	1.9	2.2
Unsaturated		2.3	2.5	2.2	2.0	1.4	1.1	1.3
Cholesterol (mg)	Not listed	7-47	1.4	1.6	3.3	10-34	8-28	10-35
Carbohydrate (g)	Not listed	6.8 lactose	7 lactose	7.1 lactose	7.2 lactose	4.8 lactose	7.0 lactose sucrose	4.9 lactose
Calcium (mg)	360	34	55	58	44	126	100	118
Phosphorus (mg)	240	14	46	43	33	102	81	92
Sodium (mg)	Not listed	16	28	25	16	60	48	50
Potassium (mg)	Not listed	51	69	75	56	152	122	137
Magnesium (mg)	60	4	4	4	5	12	10	12
Iron (mg)	10	0.05	1.2	1.2	1.3	0.05	0.04	0.05
Copper (μg)	Not listed	40	60	40	50	Estimate 30	Estimate 20	30
Zinc (mg)	3	0.3-0.5	0.4	0.5	0.4	0.3-0.5	0.2-0.4	0.3-0.5
Iodine (μg)	35	3	7	10	7	5	4	5
Vitamin A (IU)	1400	200	170	250	264	185	150	140
Thiamine (mg)	0.3	0.016	0.05	0.07	0.07	0.03	0.02	0.17
Riboflavin (mg)	0.4	0.036	0.06	0.1	0.1	0.19	0.16	0.17
Niacin (mg)	5	0.1	0.8	0.7	0.7	0.1	0.1	0.1
Pyridoxine (mg)	0.3	0.01	0.04	0.04	0.04	0.04	0.03	0.06
Folacin (mg)	0.05	0.005	0.01	0.005	0.005	0.005	0.004	0.005
Vitamin B_{12} (μg)	0.3	0.03	0.2	0.2	0.1	0.08	0.06	0.4
Vitamin C (mg)	35	4	5	6	6	0.5	0.4	1
Vitamin D (IU)	400	2	42	40	42	Fortified 40	Fortified 32	Fortified 42
Vitamin E (IU)	4	0.2	1.3	1.5	1	0.04	0.03	0.04
Vitamin K (μg)	Not listed	1.5	6	9	5.8	Estimate 6	Estimate 5	6

Data from Fomon SJ: *Infant nutrition,* ed 2, Philadelphia, 1980, WB Saunders; and the Committee on Dietary Allowances: *Recommended dietary allowance,* ed 9, rev ed, Washington, DC, 1980, National Academy of Sciences.

Table 16-6 Host Resistance Factors in Human Milk

Components	Proposed mode of action
Growth factor of *L. bifidus*	*L. bifidus* interferes with intestinal colonization of enteric pathogens
Antistaphylococcal factor	Inhibits staphylococci
Secretory IgA and other immunoglobulins	Protective antibodies for the gut and respiratory tract
C4 and C3	C3 fragments have opsonic, chemotactic, and anaphylatoxic activities
Lysozyme	Lysis of bacterial cell wall
Lactoperoxidase-H_2O_2-thiocyanate	Killing of streptococci
Lactoferrin	Kills microorganisms by chelating iron
Leukocytes	Phagocytosis
	Cell-mediated immunity—production of IgA, C4, C3, lysozyme, and lactoferrin

are thus strenuously exercised, encouraging the development of well-formed jaws and straight, healthy teeth.[17]

Because of this fundamental difference between *suckling* at the breast and *sucking* on a bottle or pacifier, a very young infant (under 6 weeks of age) should be fed exclusively on the breast lest "nipple confusion" occur. This is a development that may ensue in *some* young infants, full-term as well as preterm, whereby too early introduction of a rubber nipple, and the tongue-thrusting that it requires to control rapid milk flow, prevents the necessary conditioning mechanism essential to the development of proper suckling technique. Suckling at the breast is not instinctual in humans, as it is in other mammals; rather, it is a learned response for both mother and baby, and in the early weeks much time, attention, and support must be devoted to this educational process.

Perhaps most important, although most nebulous, are the psychological benefits the infant derives from breast-feeding.[1] Factors such as the more intimate interaction between the breast-feeding mother and child and the more immediate satisfaction of the nursing baby's hunger seem to augur healthier mental development. The infant also gains a sense of security from the warmth and closeness of the mother's body. Breast-feeding eliminates the practice of bottle propping; the infant, of necessity, must be drawn close at each feeding. Although the bottle-feeding mother also can show her love for her baby by holding and cuddling the baby at feeding times, in actual practice she may do less of this, and of course she cannot duplicate the *unique* skin-to-skin contact between the nursing mother and her infant. Montagu[13] states, "The breast-feeding relationship constitutes the foundation for the development of all human social relationships, and the communications the infant receives through the warmth of the mother's skin constitute the first of the socializing experiences of his life." Babies gain a sense of well-being from secure handling, and mothers who nurse their infants successfully often seem more confident in managing them. Whether the woman who is sure of her maternal abilities is more likely to breast-feed—or whether the experience itself infuses her with self-confidence—is difficult to determine. Mothers who nurse may be better able to soothe their babies when they are upset, perhaps because the very act of putting them to the breast is such a comfort to them that the mother does not have to search for other methods of reassurance.

The mother, also, gains distinct benefits from breast-feeding. These include (1) stimulation, by suckling, of oxytocin secretion, which fosters uterine contractions, hastens postpartum uterine involution, and inhibits postpartum hemorrhaging, (2) convenience, obviating the need to prepare formula, sterilize nipples and bottles, and refrigerate formula when traveling, (3) economy, (4) esthetics—breast-fed infants smell better because the odor of both bowel movements and spit-up milk is less offensive than that of bottle-fed infants, (5) decreased risk of postpartum thromboembolism and premenopousal breast cancer[14] and (6) emotional satisfaction and a sense of fulfillment.

The "nursing couple," mother and baby, forge an especially close and interdependent relationship. The baby depends on the mother for sustenance and comfort, and the mother looks forward to feeding times to gain a pleasurable sense of comfort with her infant and a period of rest and relaxation during her busy day. Because of this unique relationship, many women consider the nursing months among the most fulfilling times of their lives.

A mother should not breast-feed unless she is fully convinced that she wants to. In most instances the wishes of the baby's father affect the decision to breast-feed inasmuch as he, because the extended family has been replaced by the nuclear family, has become the nursing mother's chief support system. For most women, nursing is accomplished easily; however, if for any reason the desire to breast-feed is lacking or poorly supported, initiating or continuing nursing may be difficult and may produce emotional strains that could disrupt the mother-child-father relationships. Physicians should support the mother completely whether her decision is to nurse, not to nurse, or to discontinue nursing, regardless of their personal opinions on the matter.

For a working mother, breast-feeding requires a great deal of patience, development of time-saving routines, and cooperation at the workplace, where privacy for expressing milk and storage facilities should be available. Many large corporations are recognizing this need and realizing the economic and psychological advantages of enabling nursing mothers to return to work early. Lightweight, efficient, easy-to-use electric pumps can be rented inexpensively over the long term and can be left at the workplace so that milk can be expressed, refrigerated, and taken home for the infant's next-day feeding. If expressed milk is to be used within 48 hours, it may be placed in the refrigerator; if frozen immediately after collection and kept in the freezer, it should be used within 6 months. A sympathetic family and physician and access to various support systems will help the working mother to continue nursing.[15]

BREAST-FEEDING

Basis of Lactation

Successful breast-feeding depends on a strongly motivated mother, a healthy infant who has a strong sucking impulse, and a physician who is confident and competent in his or her knowledge of the anatomy of the mammary gland, the com-

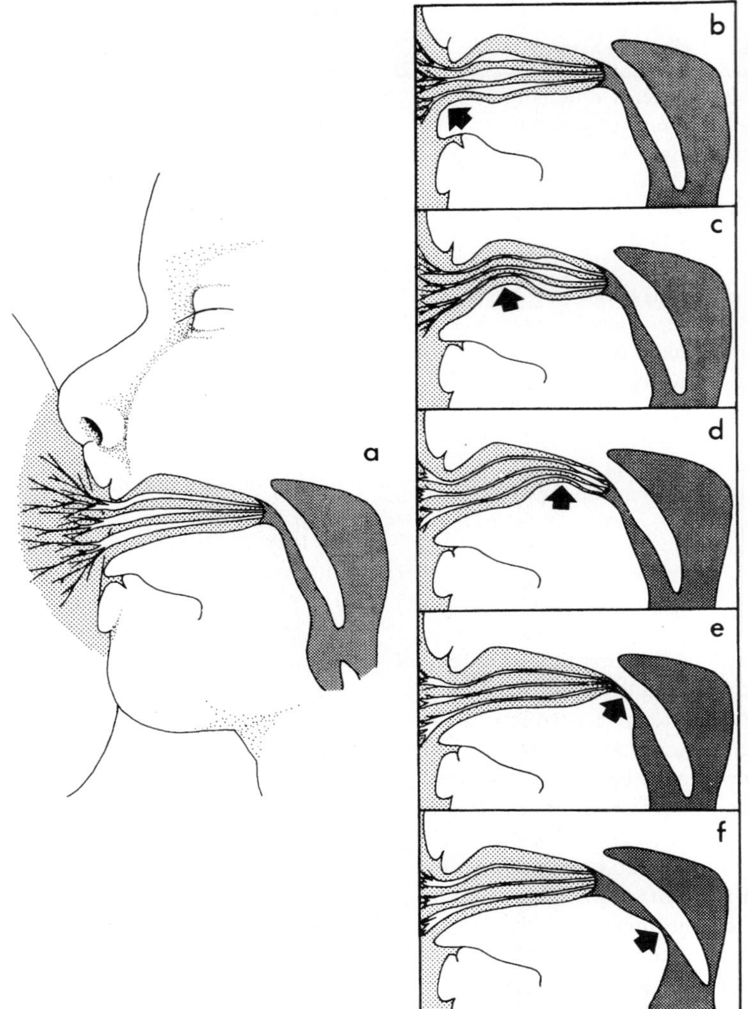

FIG. 16-5 Complete "suck" cycle. **a,** The infant's jaws compress the sinuses, and the nipple is drawn into the mouth with the tip at the junction of the hard and soft palates; the tongue is cradling the nipple. **b,** The lower jaw constricts the nipple base, pinching off the milk bolus, and the anterior tip of the tongue begins a wavelike motion. **c,** The rollerlike tongue action moves milk posteriorly. **d** and **e,** A wave of compression pushes the milk into the oropharynx, where it is swallowed. **f,** The jaw lowers, allowing the milk to flow into the nipple base again as the next "suck" cycle begins.

(From Woolridge MW: *Midwifery* 2:166, 1986.)

position of human milk (see Table 16-5), and the neurohormonal control of lactation.

Directly beneath and behind the areola is a group of milk pools, or lactiferous sinuses, that with proper "latch-on," the nursing infant's jaws compress, squeezing milk into and along the pores of the nipple. The nipple itself is merely a spout through which the milk is conducted into the infant's mouth and should not itself be traumatized by the infant's jaws. The sinuses are widened parts of the lactiferous ducts, of which there are 15 to 20, each emptying into the nipple. At their proximal ends within the breast, the ducts branch off into smaller canals, called *ductules*. At the end of each ductule is a grapelike structure composed of a cluster of tiny, rounded saclike alveoli, in which the milk is made. The ducts and the alveoli are surrounded with myoepithelial cells that contract (in response to oxytocin), squeezing the milk into and through the entire duct system, finally ending up in the sinuses. Clusters of alveoli compose the lobules, which are bound together by connective tissue, richly interwoven with blood vessels and lymphatics into the 15 to 20 lobes in each breast. Each lobe is connected to one duct, and each duct empties into one opening on the nipple (Fig. 16-6).

Physiology of Lactation

Successful lactation is a simple process, the result of reflex interactions between the nursing couple; it is based on the superimposition of two reflex triangles, the *prolactin* (or milk secretion) *reflex* and the *letdown* (or milk ejection) *reflex*.

Prolactin Reflex. When the infant suckles at the breast, the maternal anterior pituitary gland is stimulated, via the vagus nerve and the hypothalamus, to secrete the hormone prolactin, which acts on the breast alveoli to produce milk. Prolactin secretion is determined by how often the infant stimulates the nipple and areola. Until the milk supply is well es-

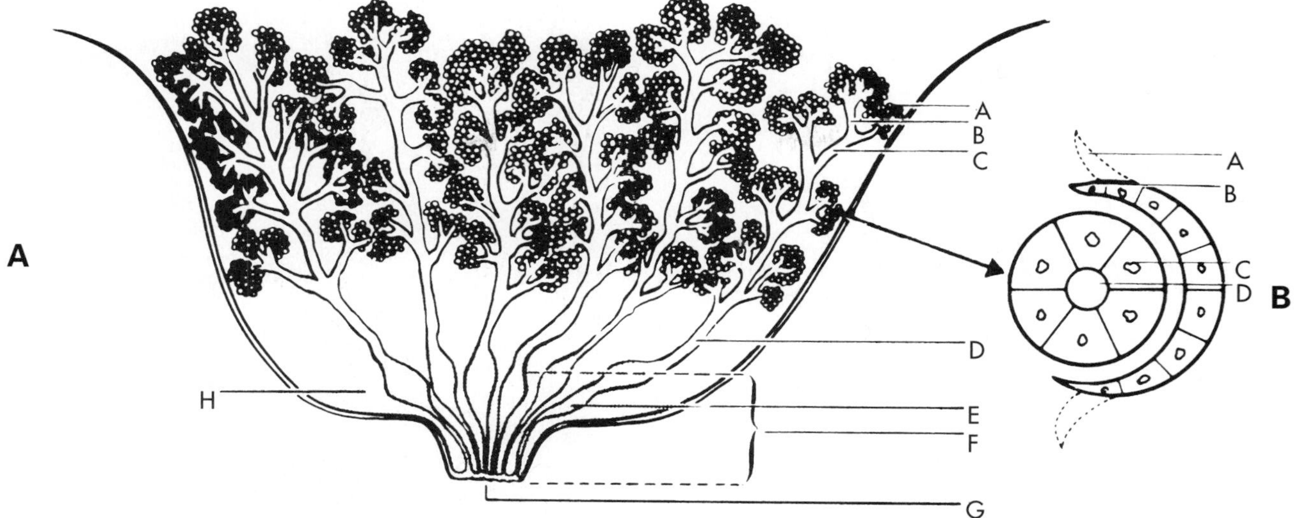

FIG. 16-6 **A,** Diagram of the breast as a "forest of trees." With full development of the uterine-menstrual cycle, groups of gland-secreting cells (alveoli) bud from the small ducts (ductules). The alveoli secrete milk under the influence of prolactin, a hormone of the pituitary gland. *A,* Alveolus; *B,* ductule; *C,* duct; *D,* lactiferous duct; *E,* lactiferous sinus; *F,* ampulla; *G,* nipple pore; *H,* areolar margin. **B,** Diagram of an alveolus. Gland-secreting cells are arranged in a circle around the ductule opening. The alveolus is surrounded by a contractile cell. When sucking begins, this cell, under the influence of oxytocin from the pituitary gland, contracts and squeezes the milk into the duct system; this reflex is called *letdown. A,* Uncontracted myoepithelial cell; *B,* contracted myoepithelial cell; *C,* gland-secreting cell; *D,* ductule opening.

(From Applebaum RM: *Pediatr Clin North Am* 17:205, 1970.)

tablished, which normally takes 3 to 6 weeks of total breast-feeding without supplementation with either water or formula, the breasts require stimulation on an average of 8 to 12 times each 24-hour period.

Letdown Reflex. This originally was a dairy term, referring to the cow's ability to "let down" her milk. It is essential for getting the milk to the baby and can be inhibited by anxiety, illness, breast engorgement, pain, emotional tension, and fatigue. *Maternal confidence* and reassurance are required for this reflex to work efficiently. After the infant has been nursing for 2 to 3 minutes, the posterior pituitary gland releases oxytocin, another hormone that, traveling through the bloodstream to the breast, contracts the myoepithelial cells surrounding the alveoli and milk ducts, causing the milk to be ejected toward the lactiferous sinuses (Fig. 16-7). The cell membranes of the secretory cells rupture during this process, so larger and more concentrated fatty globules and protein particles are added to the milk. This high-calorie fatty milk is called "hindmilk"; it constitutes the final two thirds of the volume of milk during each individual nursing session and is added to the previous one third of "foremilk" produced during the height of the earlier prolactin secretion phase. A vigorous letdown reflex thus increases the caloric content of the milk and, by forceful ejection, refills the milk sinuses with the rich, creamy "hindmilk" that ensures rapid weight gain when the infant obtains it regularly. Ensuring adequate drainage of milk through an effective letdown reflex prevents engorgement and is essential for successful lactation.

Technique of Nursing

Stimulation of the breasts by frequent nursing very early in the postpartum hours encourages milk flow and provides an adequate milk supply rapidly. The infant should be placed on the mother's abdomen and put to the breast in the delivery room or, if this is not possible, soon after the initial newborn physical examination. In many hospitals one or two feedings of sterile water precede the first milk feeding to rule out esophageal anomalies. In most normal-appearing, full-term infants, this is not necessary; also, it may lead to nipple confusion and may delay initiation of breast-feeding.

In the first few days after delivery, the breast produces colostrum, a low-fat, high-protein milky fluid rich in fat-soluble vitamins and antibodies. Colostrum sustains the newborn until the "real" milk comes in, on approximately the sixth day. The breast-fed baby is a hungry baby who cries often to be fed; this is a normal response that occurs at 1- to 3-hour intervals in the first 4 to 6 weeks of life. Because breast milk is more digestible than cow milk, a breast-fed infant's stomach empties more rapidly. Therefore breast-fed babies require feeding more often than bottle-fed babies (8 to 12 feedings in 24 hours versus 6 for a bottle-fed baby).

Optimal breast-feeding is "demand" feeding. Maximal milk production occurs when engorgement is reduced and the breast is emptied frequently by the infant. A breast emptied of milk quickly produces more, and a natural state of equilibrium is established between the mother and the infant.

Successful breast-feeding can be thwarted by overrigid hospital administrators' concern for a germ-free environment and tight nursing and medical staff regulations, which can be extremely inconvenient for the nursing couple. The optimal physical and emotional health of mothers and infants sometimes demands certain changes in many traditional hospital procedures. Demand feeding of the breast-fed infant ideally is effected by a complete rooming-in program. The in-

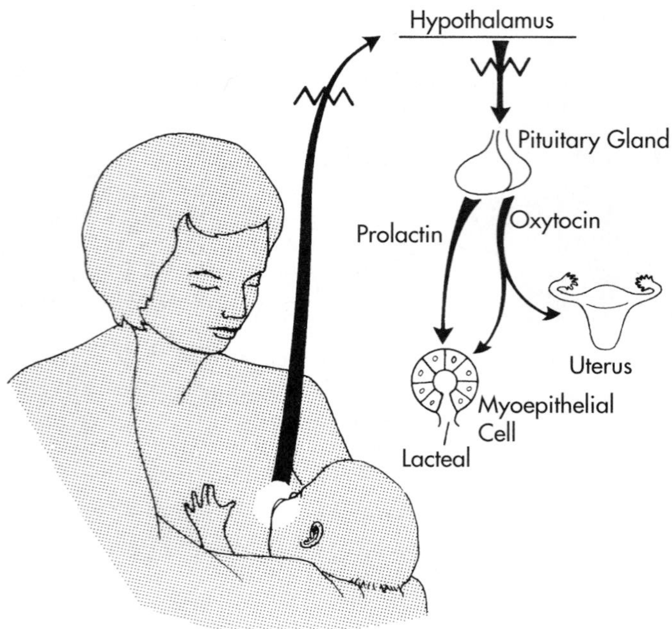

FIG. 16-7 Diagrammatic outline of the ejection reflex arc. The infant's suckling stimulates mechanoreceptors in the nipple and areola that send stimuli along nerve pathways to the hypothalamus, which, in turn, stimulates the posterior pituitary to release oxytocin. The bloodstream carries the oxytocin to the breast and the uterus. In the breast, oxytocin stimulates the myoepithelial cell to contract and eject milk from the alveolus. Prolactin, which is secreted by the anterior pituitary gland in response to the infant's suckling, effects milk production in the alveolus. Stress, such as pain or anxiety, can inhibit letdown, whereas the sight or cry of an infant can stimulate it.

(From Lawrence RA: *Breastfeeding: a guide for the medical profession,* ed 4, St Louis, 1994, Mosby.)

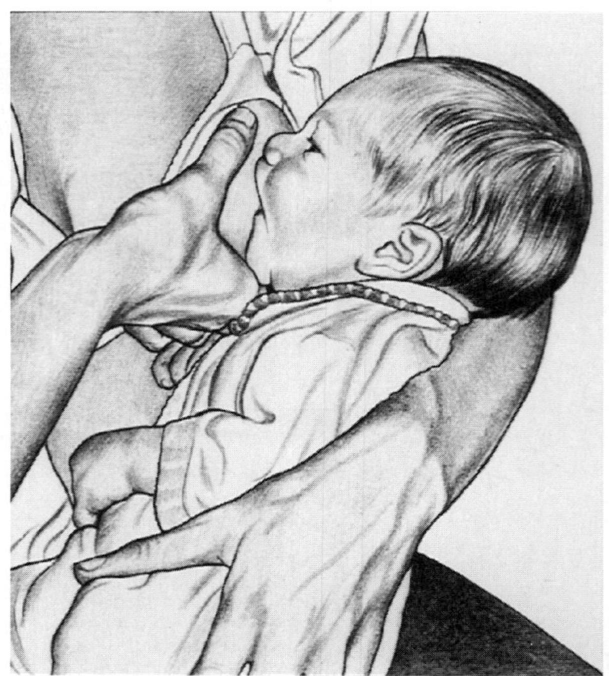

FIG. 16-8 Correct latch-on position: The baby faces the mother directly, his stomach against hers, his head, which is kept in line with his body, resting in the crook of his mother's arm. The mother uses the C-hold to support her breast.

(From Eiger MS, Olds SW: *The complete book of breastfeeding,* New York, 1987, Workman, Bantam.)

fant should be allowed to be with the mother for as long as possible to allow the mother to become acquainted with her new infant and to accustom herself to the baby's natural eating and sleeping rhythms.

A comfortable position, either sitting or lying, is essential for successful nursing. The *cradle* position, the most commonly used hold, is best accomplished with the mother sitting in an armless chair, the leg on the side on which she is nursing resting on a footstool, and a pillow on her lap supporting the forearm on which her baby is resting. Her infant should be facing her directly, his stomach against hers, his head in line with his body, his neck in the bend of her elbow, with her hand on his buttocks so that he is pulled up close, with his face almost touching the breast. The mother's free hand then grasps her breast in the C-hold: thumb on top and well behind the areola, index finger opposite, below, and again well behind the areola, with the other three fingers supporting the breast from underneath. In this position the infant's mouth directly opposes the nipple, which the mother should stroke patiently against the infant's lower lip (rooting reflex) until the baby's mouth opens quite wide to accept the nipple; at this point the mother pulls the baby's head firmly onto the breast, inserting the nipple deep into his mouth and allowing him to close his jaws over the base of the nipple for proper and effective *latch-on* (Fig. 16-8). When feeding on the first side is complete, the mother breaks the suction by placing her fifth finger into the corner of the infant's mouth before transferring him to the other breast.

An effective latch-on, or attachment of the baby to the breast, is essential for efficient and painless initiation of lactation. Although breast-feeding is a natural process, it is the result of the transmission to the new mother of a generationally accumulated experience that is to a great extent lacking in our modern, technologically oriented Western society, in which the extended family has been replaced by its inadequate nuclear counterpart and wherein the central hospital nursery severely interferes with the necessary interaction between mother and infant.[12] The latch-on is not instinctual, and the new mother must be taught by trained, knowledgeable personnel in the immediate postpartum hours how to perform it properly. Breast-feeding should not be painful, even at the beginning, and with the correct latch-on technique it will be comfortable for the mother, allowing an effective letdown and early, rapid establishment of a rhythm of frequent draining and filling of the breasts, which is essential to building a dependable milk supply.

No time limit should be imposed on nursing on each breast, even in the early days, because the infant's jaws will not traumatize the nipple if the mother uses the correct latch-on technique.[11] In the first few weeks, however, the baby should be encouraged to stimulate both breasts at each nursing session, and the breast used last at the previous feeding should be used first at the next feeding. The mother should be taught to listen for her infant's swallowing sounds (short, sighinglike noises), rather than observing the suckling, as an indication that her baby is removing milk from her breast. The ideal ratio is no more than one to two sucks per swallow. After the first few weeks, when the milk supply is adequate, an older, thriving infant may desire to remain on one breast throughout the entire feeding to obtain the benefits of the rich, satiety-producing hindmilk, and the mother should be told that this is acceptable so long as the breasts are alternated at ensuing feeding sessions.[16]

Breast-fed babies may lose up to 10% of their birth weight, but the initial weight loss can be decreased markedly by immediately initiating nursing in the delivery suite, by allowing frequent, unrestricted demand feeding sessions with mother and baby rooming-in together, by avoiding supplementation with either water or formula, and with the constant support of trained medical and nursing personnel. Attention must be given in the early weeks to the adequacy of the buildup of the maternal milk supply. The infant *under 1 month of age* who is ingesting sufficient mother's milk is never constipated and should be having at least four or more stools per 24-hour day. Fewer than that number, even if the infant is wetting frequently, is a danger sign, and intervention is needed. Close follow-up is in order for breast-fed infants who lose more than 5% to 7% of their weight or who have other risk factors (e.g., early hospital discharge, feeding-related jaundice, or birth by cesarean section). In the early weeks bottle supplementation should be used rarely because of the physiological differences between *suckling* (breast) and *sucking* (bottle), and the consequent risk of nipple confusion. Many new and exciting techniques have been developed to increase an insufficient milk supply, and formula supplementation at the breast with nursing supplementers is available to tide the infant over, without undermining the development of the suckling mechanism, until the mother's milk supply increases.

Drugs in Breast Milk

All drugs that a lactating woman ingests appear in the breast milk, usually in amounts that do not approximate the concentration in the mother's plasma. The total amount excreted into the milk after a single maternal dose is a function of time and nursing frequency; for most drugs, the amount is less than 1% to 2% of the amount the mother takes.[1] Reasonable concern exists about the effect on the nursing infant of substances the mother ingests. The effect on the infant is determined by the volume of milk ingested, the amount absorbed from the intestine, the activity of the drug, the infant's sensitivity to and tolerance of the specific substance, the cumulative effect of chronicity of therapy with the particular drug, and the infant's size and maturity. Maternal dosing immediately after a nursing session minimizes the entry of the substance into the milk at the next feeding, inasmuch as the peak maternal plasma level follows the curve of peak milk production. Short-acting preparations should be prescribed, if possible, rather than long-acting forms. Data rapidly are becoming available to guide practitioners' recommendations to mothers regarding the drugs they can take without fear of affecting their babies adversely.[2]

The factors that affect the appearance of a drug in breast milk are its lipid solubility, its pK_a, its protein-binding ability, and the pH of the milk. Un-ionized drugs that have a high lipid solubility are transported better than ionized ones. The concentration of a drug in breast milk depends on the volume of mammary alveolar cells and the concentration of unbound drug in the mother's plasma. Drugs usually diffuse through membranes passively, depending on the concentration gradient and their lipid solubility. The pH of breast milk is approximately 7.0 and that of plasma is approximately 7.4; therefore weak acids usually have low milk/plasma ratios, whereas weak bases are likely to have high ratios. Most drugs for which specific information is available can be grouped into categories relating to their potential effect on the nursing infant (Tables 16-7 through 16-11). Steroids, when taken in large doses over time by the mother, can suppress growth and interfere with endogenous steroid production in the infant. Infants who have a glucose-6-phosphate dehydrogenase (G6PD) deficiency may suffer hemolysis from ingesting nalidixic acid, sulfonamides, and other oxidant drugs in breast milk. Chronic salicylate ingestion by the mother can produce hemorrhagic problems in her breast-feeding infant.

Table 16-7 Drugs Contraindicated during Breast-Feeding

Drug	Reason for concern
Bromocriptine	Suppresses lactation; may be hazardous to the mother
Cocaine	Cocaine intoxication
Cyclophosphamide	Possible immune suppression; unknown effect on growth or association with carcinogenesis; neutropenia
Cyclosporine	Possible immune suppression; unknown effect on growth or association with carcinogenesis
Doxorubicin*	Possible immune suppression; unknown effect on growth or association with carcinogenesis
Ergotamine	Vomiting, diarrhea, convulsions (doses used in migraine medications)
Lithium	One-third to one-half therapeutic blood concentration in infants
Methotrexate	Possible immune suppression; unknown effect on growth or association with carcinogenesis; neutropenia
Phencyclidine (PCP)	Potent hallucinogen
Phenindione	Anticoagulant; increased prothrombin and partial thromboplastin time in one infant; not used in the United States

From the Committee on Drugs, American Academy of Pediatrics: *Pediatrics* 93:137, 1994.
*Drug is concentrated in human milk.

Antibiotics usually do not produce acute adverse effects in breast-fed infants (see Chapter 31, Antimicrobial Therapy). However, continuous ingestion of the aminoglycosides may alter an infant's intestinal flora, may affect some immune mechanisms adversely, and may predispose him or her to hypersensitivity. Tetracycline ingestion through breast milk has not been reported to cause mottled teeth in breast-fed infants, even when tetracyclines are found in high concentrations in breast milk, probably because the calcium complexing of tetracyclines in milk interferes with their absorption by the infant.

Lactating mothers must always be aware that anything they ingest may pass into their milk and have an undesirable effect on the infant. Physicians, dentists, and paramedical personnel responsible for prescribing drugs should be informed

Table 16-8 Drugs of Abuse: Contraindicated during Breast-Feeding*

Drug	Reason for concern
Amphetamine†	Irritability, poor sleeping pattern
Cocaine	Cocaine intoxication
Heroin	Tremors, restlessness, vomiting, poor feeding
Marijuana	Only one report in the literature; no effect mentioned
Nicotine (smoking)	Shock, vomiting, diarrhea, rapid heart rate, restlessness; decreased milk production
Phencyclidine	Potent hallucinogen

From the Committee on Drugs, American Academy of Pediatrics: *Pediatrics* 93:137, 1994.

*The AAP's Committee on Drugs strongly believes that nursing mothers should not ingest any of the compounds listed in this table. Not only are they hazardous to the nursing infant, they also are detrimental to the mother's physical and emotional health. Obviously, this list is not complete; nursing mothers should not ingest *any* drug of abuse, even if no adverse reports are found in the literature.

†Drug is concentrated in human milk.

Table 16-9 Radioactive Compounds Requiring Temporary Cessation of Breast-Feeding*

Drug	Recommended period of no breast-feeding
Copper 64 (^{64}Cu)	Radioactivity in milk present at 50 hr
Gallium 67 (^{67}Ga)	Radioactivity in milk present for 2 wk
Indium 111 (^{111}In)	Very small amount present at 20 hr
Iodine 123 (^{123}I)	Radioactivity in milk present up to 36 hr
Iodine 125 (^{125}I)	Radioactivity in milk present for 12 d
Iodine 131 (^{131}I)	Radioactivity in milk present for 2-14 d, depending on study
Radioactive sodium	Radioactivity in milk present for 96 hr
Technetium-99m (^{99m}Tc), ^{99m}Rc macroaggregates, ^{99m}Tc O4	Radioactivity in milk present for 15 hr to 3 d

From the Committee on Drugs, American Academy of Pediatrics: *Pediatrics* 93:137, 1994.

*A nuclear medicine physician should be consulted before a diagnostic study is performed so that the radionuclide with the shortest excretion time in breast milk can be used. Before the study the mother should pump her breasts and store enough milk in the freezer for feeding the infant; after the study she should pump her breasts to maintain milk production but should discard all milk pumped for the time that radioactivity is present in the milk. A radiology department can screen milk samples for radioactivity before the mother resumes nursing.

Table 16-10 Drugs Whose Effect in Nursing Infants Is Unknown but May Be of Concern

Psychotropic drugs (those listed in the Antianxiety, Antidepressant, and Antipsychotic categories) are of special concern when given to nursing mothers for long periods. Although there are no case reports of adverse effects in breast-feeding infants, these drugs appear in human milk and thus conceivably could affect short-term and long-term functioning of the central nervous system.

Drug	Reported or possible effect
Antianxiety	
Diazepam	None
Lorazepam	None
Midazolam	—
Perphenazine	None
Prazepam*	None
Quazepam	None
Temazepam	—
Antidepressants	
Amitriptyline	None
Amoxapine	None
Desipramine	None
Duthiepin	None
Doxepin	None
Fluoxetine	—
Fluvoxamine	—
Imipramine	None
Trazodone	None
Antipsychotic	
Chlorpromazine	Galactorrhea in the mother; drowsiness and lethargy in the infant
Chlorprothixene	None
Haloperidol	None
Mesoridazine	None
Chloramphenicol	Possible idiosyncratic bone marrow suppression
Metoclopramide*	None described; dopaminergic blocking agent
Metronidazole	In vitro mutagen; may discontinue breast-feeding 12-24 hr to allow excretion of dose when the mother is given single-dose therapy
Tinidazole	See metronidazole

From the Committee on Drugs, American Academy of Pediatrics: *Pediatrics* 93:137, 1994.

*Drug is concentrated in human milk.

that the mother is breast-feeding so that care can be taken in prescribing a drug compatible with the nursing baby. Should it be necessary to prescribe a medication that is incompatible with breast-feeding, a reasonable, safe alternative almost always can be substituted. Nursing should never be terminated arbitrarily because of the need for maternal therapy. If breast-feeding must be stopped temporarily, a breast-pumping regimen to maintain the mother's milk supply and the continuous support of the family and sympathetic medical personnel will allow it to be resumed successfully. Over-the-counter (OTC) medications taken for a short time rarely present problems for the nursing baby, but caution should be used with them as well.

Complications of Breast-Feeding

The complications of nursing usually pertain to difficulties the mother experiences, but occasionally an infant will become seriously ill for a prolonged period and will be unable to nurse adequately. During brief illnesses in which feeding at the breast is not possible, the breast can be emptied peri-

Table 16-11 Drugs Associated with Significant Effects on Some Nursing Infants (Should Be Given with Caution to Nursing Mothers)

Drug	Reported effect
5-Aminosalicylic acid	Diarrhea (one case)
Aspirin (salicylates)	Metabolic acidosis (one case)
Clemastine	Drowsiness, irritability, refusal to feed, high-pitched cry, neck stiffness (one case)
Phenobarbital	Sedation; infantile spasms after weaning from milk containing phenobarbital, methemoglobinemia (one case)
Primidone	Sedation, feeding problems
Sulfasalazine (salicylazosulfapyridine)	Bloody diarrhea (one case)

From the Committee on Drugs, American Academy of Pediatrics: *Pediatrics* 93:137, 1994.
When possible, the blood concentration in the infant should be measured.

odically during maternal-infant separation with an electric breast pump and the infant fed the expressed breast milk through a nursing supplementer or a bottle, depending on the baby's age and maturity.

Nipples will not become sore and cracked if careful attention is paid to the correct latch-on technique, proper positioning, and preventing engorgement. Pain on latch-on is a signal that the baby must be removed from the breast and the positioning corrected immediately. Mothers should be aware that breast-feeding is pleasurable, and the adage that "if it hurts, then it is wrong" is valid. If the nipple is traumatized, treatment consists of exposing the nipple to the air, relieving engorgement by frequent feeding or mechanical pumping, *avoiding* use of creams or ointments because the nipple pores are easily blocked and the areolar tissue easily macerated, and applying the mother's own expressed breast milk to the nipples. These measures, of course, are coupled with instruction in proper positioning and latch-on.

Incomplete emptying of part of the breast easily can lead to a plugged duct in that area. Nursing mothers should palpate their breasts regularly to become aware of full areas, which when found should be treated with breast massage and specific positioning of the infant on that breast in order to empty, frequently and effectively, the area under suspicion.

Breast engorgement and plugged ducts, when unattended to, can quickly lead to mastitis, which is *not* a contraindication to continued nursing. Even if fever, breast tenderness, and erythema develop, there is ample evidence that administering antibiotics and continuing nursing—because it relieves engorgement and thus ensures drainage of the affected areas—will prevent many cases of mastitis from progressing to breast abscesses, which may require surgical incision. The infant who nurses on the infected breast does *not* become ill and is in *no* danger. Feeding from the affected breast may be temporarily discontinued just after surgical drainage, but breast-feeding may be resumed from that breast after the wound has healed.

Concomitant with the resurgence of breast-feeding in the 1980s has been a rapid expansion of knowledge in the field of lactation; a new specialist, the lactation consultant, armed with innovative intervention techniques, has emerged to aid the physician in diagnosing and treating problems of the nursing couple. Lactation consultants certified by the International Board of Lactation Consultant Examiners are identified by the degree IBCLC (International Board-Certified Lactation Consultant) as individuals who have acquired in-depth knowledge and special skills to help mothers with breast-feeding problems. A busy pediatrician who may be unable to devote the required amount of attention to these time-consuming, common, and often urgent problem solving needs of nursing mothers benefits his or her patients by referring them to a certified lactation consultant. The lactation consultant has clarified the concept of "insufficient milk syndrome," which actually is a composite of maternal and infant etiological factors that usually are correctable with supportive professional management.

ARTIFICIAL FEEDING

If bottle-feeding is chosen, or if breast-feeding is not feasible or successful, the infant will still thrive on an artificially prepared formula. Commercially prepared formulas for normal infants are modifications of whole cow milk that approximate the composition of human milk. Thus the "humanized" formulas compare favorably with breast milk in their content of protein, carbohydrate (lactose), and saturated and unsaturated fats. Special formulas are available for milk-intolerant infants and for those who have specific malabsorptive problems (see Appendix C).

Feeding Schedule

When bottle-feeding is used, a demand schedule should be encouraged, as with the breast-fed infant. Bottle-fed babies should be fed only as much as they desire, although maternal pressure may subtly urge them to empty the bottle. This should be discouraged inasmuch as overfeeding at this age may establish a pattern of eating that eventually will result in obesity. Because the gastric emptying time of bottle-fed babies is longer, they require less frequent feedings than do breast-fed babies. An artificially fed infant usually shows a greater weight gain than a breast-fed infant. There is no evidence that this increased weight gain is desirable; indeed, it probably is not.

Whether breast- or bottle-fed, an infant who is fed on demand will adjust intake to needs for growth. The following patterns, with some variation, usually are established:

Age (mo)	Number of feedings per 24 hours
Birth-1	6-8
2-6	4-5
7-10	3-4
11-12	3

Age (mo)	Ounces per feeding
1	2-4
2	5
3	5-6
4	6-7
5-12	8

It should be noted that during the second or third month of life, most infants eliminate the night feeding.

PREPARATION AND TERMINAL STERILIZATION OF INFANT FORMULA

Preparation

1. Measure the prescribed number of ounces of hot water into a clean quart pitcher.
2. Stir in the carbohydrate. Measure powdered sugar with a standard-size tablespoon and level each spoonful with a table knife.
3. Add the prescribed number of ounces of milk to the formula and stir to mix well.
4. Pour the formula into clean nursing bottles.
5. Put nipples and caps on the bottles, leaving the caps loose.

Sterilization

1. Put the bottles of formula on a rack in the sterilizer or deep kettle. Caps should be loose, not screwed on tightly. Put about 3 inches of water in the sterilizer, and cover.
2. Bring the water to a boil over moderate heat, then allow to boil gently (with the sterilizer still covered) for 25 minutes.
3. Remove the sterilizer from the heat. Leave it closed (do not even lift the lid) until the side of the sterilizer has cooled enough so that you can touch it with the palm of your hand.
4. Open the sterilizer. Then cool the bottles gradually, adding a small amount of cool water to the hot water in the sterilizer. (Gradual cooling prevents "skimming," which frequently causes nipple clogging.)
5. Remove the cooled bottles and screw the caps tight.
6. Store the bottles of formula in the refrigerator.

Preparation of Formula

In the United States, most artificial feeding with cow milk is accomplished with proprietary formulas prepared commercially and supplied as "ready to feed" or "easy to mix" in presterilized bottles and cans. The ready-to-feed formulas are supplied with attached nipples in 4-, 6-, and 8-ounce disposable bottles and in 1-quart cans. Ready-to-feed formulas offer convenience to mothers who must travel with their infants and often are used as complementary and supplementary feedings for breast-fed babies, but they are too expensive for most families to use everyday. Easy-to-mix, concentrated formulas are supplied in 13-ounce cans of liquid, which is mixed with equal amounts of water, and in 6-ounce cans of powder, which is mixed with appropriate amounts of water, usually in a 1:2 ratio.

In some parts of the United States and the rest of the world, the cost of commercially prepared formula is too high for mothers who cannot or choose not to breast-feed, and a home-prepared formula is used.

Calculation of the ingredients needed for a home-prepared infant formula made from whole cow milk (20 Cal/oz) or evaporated milk (44 Cal/oz) is based on four principles: (1) All formulas should contain milk, water, and carbohydrate and have an energy content of approximately 20 Cal/oz; (2) full-term infants require 110 to 120 Cal/kg and 150 to 180 ml of fluid per kilogram each day; (3) 2 ounces of evaporated milk (EM) or 4 ounces of whole milk (WM) per kilogram are required each day; and (4) most infants require feeding five or six times every 24 hours. According to these principles, a 24-hour supply of formula for a 10-pound (4.5 kg) baby would consist of approximately 500 calories and 750 ml. The amount of EM required would be 10 ounces (300 ml),* which would provide 440 calories. The balance of fluid required (450 ml) would be made up with water, and the balance of 60 calories would be supplied with carbohydrates (e.g., table sugar, 60 Cal/tbsp; Karo, 60 Cal/tbsp; and Dextri-Maltose, 30 Cal/tbsp). The formula, then, would consist of 10 ounces of evaporated milk, 15 ounces of water, and 1 to 2 tablespoons of carbohydrate (depending on the kind used). The 25 ounces of formula would contain 500 calories, or 20 Cal/oz, and would be divided into five or six bottles, each containing 4 to 5 ounces. When larger amounts of formula are needed or when whole milk is used, the four formula principles can be met by either of the following mixtures: 13 ounces of EM, 19 ounces of water, and 120 calories (2 to 4 tablespoons) of carbohydrates; 23 ounces of WM, 9 ounces of water, and 180 calories (3 to 6 tablespoons) of carbohydrates. These formulas would meet the needs of a baby weighing 6 kg or more. A fifth principle of artificial feeding is that babies rarely require more than 1 quart of formula per 24 hours.

The method of mixing formulas described previously assumes that a full 24-hour supply will be prepared. Single 8-ounce feedings (3 ounces of EM, 5 ounces of water, and 30 calories of carbohydrate) or fractions thereof can be mixed, based on the amount the baby usually takes.

Depending on where the family lives, the mother may need to be instructed to prepare her infant's formula under aseptic conditions or to use terminal sterilization; milk is a rich culture medium, and significant contamination may result if neither of these methods is used in areas where the purity of the water supply is sometimes questionable. However, in most urban areas with safe water systems, sterilization is unnecessary. The box above presents, in instructional form, a step-by-step method of preparing and sterilizing infant formulas. This process should be followed when well water is used and when organism counts in tapwater are too high. Aseptic methods of preparing single feedings or 24-hour supplies of formula also can be used under these circumstances. With these methods, the water, bottles, nipples, and utensils must be boiled beforehand. Refrigerating prepared formula reduces the number of bacteria found in contaminated bottles. Realistically, as Kendall and colleagues[9] and others have shown, fewer than half of mothers can prepare a sterile formula using either method. If a pediatrician suspects that a mother is unlikely to use aseptic or terminal sterilization tech-

*For ease of calculation, 1 ounce is considered to contain 30 ml.

niques, a presterilized proprietary formula or single-feeding mixture should be used. It probably is wise to use some form of sterile formula preparation during the first 4 months of life.

Although most mothers warm their infant's bottle before feeding, there is no evidence that babies prefer their milk warmed. Parents should be cautioned to avoid warming baby bottles in microwave ovens, which can result in overheating of the formula and can cause esophageal burns on ingestion. In addition, steam can form inside the bottle, causing an explosion.

VITAMIN SUPPLEMENTS

Except for vitamin K, most infants have adequate vitamin stores from birth until rapid postnatal growth ensues at 10 to 14 days of life; vitamin supplementation should begin by that time. Most commercially prepared formulas have an adequate vitamin content; therefore, except for babies with special needs, infants given these formulas do not need additional vitamins. Although human milk can be expected to satisfy the recommended requirements for vitamins A, C, and E and the B vitamins, it may be advisable to provide breast-fed infants with a preparation containing the minimum daily requirement of vitamin D if the mother's vitamin D intake is inadequate or if the mother's or infant's exposure to sunlight is limited.

Infants fed home-prepared formulas should receive supplemental vitamins (A, C, and D) as well as iron and fluoride. These are available commercially in a combination liquid (TRI-VI-FLOR with Iron) of which 1 ml is given orally by dropper daily.

FLUORIDE SUPPLEMENTS

All children over 6 months of age living in areas that lack adequate fluoridation of the water supply should receive daily fluoride supplements because flourides have been demonstrated to inhibit the development of dental caries (see Table 22-1 for flouride supplemental dosage schedule).

IRON SUPPLEMENTATION IN INFANCY

The AAP's Committee on Nutrition recommends that during the first year of life, infants should have an iron intake of 1 mg/kg/day, to a maximum of 15 mg/day, to prevent the development of iron deficiency anemia. Milk, both human and cow, is deficient in iron. Commercial formulas are supplemented with 8 to 12 mg of iron/liter. Breast-fed infants need not receive this amount of iron with their vitamin supplements because the small amount of iron in breast milk is almost completely bioavailable to the nursing infant; thus breast milk provides sufficient iron until the sixth month of life.

WEANING

Weaning customs vary considerably around the world. In many countries, babies routinely are nursed well into the second and sometimes the third year of life. In the United States and some other Western countries, mothers plan to wean their babies from the breast sometime between 6 and 15 months of age. By 6 months of age, babies in an industrialized society can meet their nutritional needs through cow milk formula and a wide variety of solid foods because their gastrointestinal tract has matured and they have developed the digestive ability to handle foreign proteins. Breast milk no longer is as important to them as when it provided their only source of nourishment. After 9 months a nursing mother usually produces less milk, and her letdown reflex becomes sluggish. However, the emotional benefits that a mother and baby derive from breast-feeding are just as great at 9 months or at 1 year or even later. The age at which the infant is weaned from the breast should be based on a mutual decision between mother and infant. Child-led weaning is commonly practiced throughout the world; however, in the United States, various social and cultural factors tend to dictate earlier weaning than in other countries. Mothers who are having a gratifying breast-feeding experience and who are made aware of the nutritional, immunological, and emotional benefits their nursing infants enjoy throughout and even beyond the breast-feeding period will want to continue as long as possible, and it behooves the pediatrician to urge them to do so. If weaning occurs when the infant is under 12 months of age, cow milk formula should be provided in a bottle or cup. The older infant may be weaned directly to whole milk from a bottle or cup.

The process of weaning should be gradual and should begin with substitution of one breast-feeding with a bottle or cup feeding, usually at the midday meal. Once the bottle or cup is accepted, other breast-feedings are similarly eliminated and replaced gradually over a period of 1 to 4 weeks. The mother's milk supply will diminish during this time because the stimulus of regular emptying of the breast is removed. However, some mothers can continue one or two breast-feedings over several months should they so choose.

Occasionally, because the mother or infant becomes ill or because a complication of nursing arises, breast-feeding must be discontinued abruptly. To reduce her discomfort, the mother should wear a tight breast binder, reduce her fluid intake, and apply ice packs to her breasts. Taking 20 mg of stilbestrol orally each day for 3 days also is effective in reducing her discomfort and in "drying up" her milk supply; however, this seldom is necessary. Whenever possible, weaning should not be instituted during very warm weather because some babies initially will refuse any feeding other than breast milk for as long as 24 to 48 hours. A formula-fed infant can be weaned from a bottle to whole cow milk from a cup by 9 to 12 months of age.

Skim milk should not be given to infants until they reach at least 2 years of age because up to that point milk serves as the major source of food, and skim milk would provide too few calories, an excess of protein, and an inadequate amount of essential fatty acids.

FEEDING SOLID FOODS

Introduction to Solid Foods

From a developmental point of view, there are cogent reasons why solids should not be added to the infant's diet before 4 to 6 months of age. When a solid object such as a spoon or a tongue depressor is introduced between the lips of a young baby, she purses her lips, raises her tongue, and pushes against the object vigorously (extrusion reflex). By 4 to 6 months the behavior changes so that when a spoon is inserted between the lips, they part, the tongue depresses, and food placed in the mouth is drawn to the back of the pharynx and swallowed. Thus the physiologically appropriate time to begin feeding solids is somewhere between 4 and 6 months. Somewhat later, at about 7 to 9 months of age, rhythmic biting movements begin even in the absence of teeth; foods requiring some chewing may be added to the diet at this time.

Schedule for Solid Foods

An appropriate regimen for introducing solid foods begins with grains and fruits. Rice cereal appears to be the least allergenic of the cereals and thus should be offered first. Progression through vegetables, meats, and eggs can be accomplished in the following manner:

5-6 mo	Cereals and fruits
6-7 mo	Meats and vegetables
7-8 mo	Egg yolk
8-9 mo	Egg white

To ensure an adequate amount of protein, fat, and carbohydrate during the sixth to twelfth months, infants should be offered and should consume no more than an average of 28 ounces of milk each day in addition to their quota of solids. An example of an infant diet in this age group follows:

Breakfast	Cereal and milk
Midmorning snack	Cup of orange juice
Lunch	Meat, yellow or green vegetables, fruit, milk
Midafternoon snack	Cup of orange juice or milk
Dinner	Cottage cheese or yogurt, egg, vegetable, fruit, and milk
Bedtime	Milk

Solid foods can be prepared easily from fresh ingredients that are pureed in a food grinder or blender, or commercially prepared baby foods may be used.

In late infancy and particularly during the toddler period (12 to 30 months of age), a normal physiological decline in appetite occurs, paralleling the decrease in growth rate. The parents should be made aware both of this normal decline in interest in food, particularly at meal times, and also of the concomitant reduction in milk intake, which may drop to 16 ounces a day by 24 to 36 months of age. By 4 to 7 years of age the appetite normally increases, as does the growth rate. The intake of *total* calories increases rapidly during the first year of life, then less rapidly to about age 4, and then increases rapidly again. The average full-term infant, by 7 to 10 days of life, will consume approximately 300 calories; thereafter, the first-year increment is nearly 600 Cal/day, the second-year increment nearly 275 Cal/day, the third- and fourth-year increments nearly 100 Cal/day, and the fifth- to seventh-year increments nearly 130 to 140 Cal/day. Thus, despite a decrease in appetite, the actual *intake of calories* does not decrease during the preschool period and growth patterns remain satisfactory.

PRUDENT DIET FOR THE SCHOOL-AGE CHILD AND THE ADOLESCENT

The diet of a school-age child and an adolescent should be similar to that of an active adult; however, the extra caloric needs created by the period of rapid growth should be taken into account. Dietary habits and food preferences are closely linked with early associations and family influences. *Children will eat what they see their families eat.* Parents must be told that their infants and young toddlers will crave salt and sugar in their foods as older children and adults *if that is what they have been accustomed to in early life.* Basically, preparing foods without additives for infants and young children will ensure adequate nutrition and lay the groundwork for sound eating habits in later life.

The pediatrician is in a position to educate entire families in ways to eat more healthful foods in an attempt to prevent obesity and atherosclerosis. Physicians need to know the facts about good nutrition if they are to effect changes in the lifetime habits of families that involve consuming fewer calories and less fat, salt, and refined sugars.

The American Health Association has endorsed a prudent diet for the child and adolescent, which in simplified form has the following requirements:

- A high-quality protein with every meal
- Milk (preferably skimmed) and other low-fat dairy products
- Vegetables high in vitamin A
- Fruits for vitamin C
- Whole grain or enriched breads or cereals
- Vegetable oils high in polyunsaturated fats
- Meat—four servings per week of 4 ounces each
- Fish (a good source of polyunsaturated fats)—one to two times a week
- Poultry (low fat)—one to two times a week
- Dark green, leafy, or deep yellow vegetables—at least four times a week, preferably once a day
- Eggs—a maximum of four a week

A prudent diet thus limits the use of fatty meats, high-fat dairy products, eggs, and hydrogenated shortenings and promotes the consumption of fish and the substitution of polyunsaturated vegetable oils and margarines for butter, lard, and other saturated fats.

REFERENCES

Nutritional Requirements

1. Berry WTC: Nutrition in a health service. In McLaren DS, Burman D, editors: *Textbook of paediatric nutrition,* New York, 1976, Churchill Livingstone.
2. Ross MH: Nutrition and longevity in experimental animals. In Winick M, editor: *Nutrition and aging,* New York, 1976, John Wiley & Sons.
3. Rosenberg IH: Folic acid and neural-tube defects: time for action? *N Engl J Med* 327:1875, 1992.

Feeding of Infants and Children

1. Berlin CM: Drugs and chemicals in breast milk, personal communication, June 26, 1989.
2. Committee on Drugs, American Academy of Pediatrics: The transfer of drugs and other chemicals into human milk, *Pediatrics* 93:137, 1994.
3. Cunningham AS, Jelliffe DB, Jellife EFP: Breast-feeding and health in the 1980s: a global epidemiological review, *J Pediatr* 118:659, 1991.
4. Eiger MS, Olds SW: *The complete book of breastfeeding,* New York, 1987, Workman, Bantam.
5. Fomon SJ: *Infant nutrition,* ed 2, Philadelphia, 1974, WB Saunders.
6. Goldman AS, Smith CW: Host resistance factors in human milk, *J Pediatr* 82:1082, 1973.
7. Goldman AS: The immune system of human milk: antimicrobial, anti-

inflammatory, and immunomodulating properties, *Pediatr Infect Dis J* 12:664, 1993.
8. Grules CG, Sanford HN: The influence of breast and artificial feeding on infantile eczema, *J Pediatr* 9:223, 1936.
9. Kendall N, Vaughn VC, Kusakcioglu A: Study of preparation of infant formulas, *Am J Dis Child* 122:215, 1936.
10. Lawrence RA: *Breastfeeding: a guide for the medical profession,* ed 3, St Louis, 1989, Mosby.
11. L'Esperance C, Frantz K: Time limitation for early breastfeeding, *J Obstet Gynecol Neonatal Nurs* 14(2):114, 1985.
12. Lozoff B et al: The mother-newborn relationship: limits of adaptability, *J Pediatr* 91:1, 1977.
13. Montagu A: *Touching: the human significance of the skin,* New York, 1971, Harper & Row.
14. Newcomb PA et al: Lactation and reduced risk of premenopausal breast cancer, *N Engl J Med* 330:82, 1994.
15. Olds SW: *The working parents' survival guide,* New York, 1983, Bantam.
16. Woolridge MW: Colic, "overfeeding," and symptoms of lactose malabsorption in the breast-fed baby: a possible artifact of feed management? *Lancet* 2:382, 1988.
17. Woolridge MW: The anatomy of infant sucking, *Midwifery* 2:164, 1986.

SUGGESTED READINGS

Nutritional Requirements

American Psychiatric Association Task Force: *Megavitamins and orthomolecular therapy in psychiatry,* Washington, DC, 1973, The Association.

Burkitt DP, Walker ARP, Painter NS: Dietary fiber and disease, *JAMA* 229:1068, 1974.

Fomon SJ: *Infant nutrition,* ed 2, Philadelphia, 1974, Saunders.

Food and Nutrition Board, National Academy of Sciences: *Recommended dietary allowances,* ed 10, Washington, DC, 1989, The Academy.

Forbes GB: Food fads: safe feeding of children, *Pediatr Rev* 1:207, 1980.

Forbes GB: *Human body composition: growth, aging, nutrition, and activity,* New York, 1987, Springer-Verlag.

Forbes GB, Woodruff CW, editors: *Pediatric nutrition handbook,* ed 2, Elk Grove Village, Ill, 1985, American Academy of Pediatrics.

Grand RJ, Sutphen JL, Dietz WH, editors: *Pediatric nutrition,* Boston, 1987, Butterworth.

Hytten FE, Leitch I: *Physiology of human pregnancy,* ed 2, Oxford, 1971, Blackwell Scientific.

Klein PS, Forbes GB, Nader PR: Effects of starvation in infancy (pyloric stenosis) on subsequent learning abilities, *J Pediatr* 87:8, 1975.

Leaf A, Weber PC: Cardiovascular effects of n-3 fatty acids, *N Engl J Med* 318:549, 1988.

Lechtig A et al: Maternal nutrition and fetal growth in developing countries, *Am J Dis Child* 129:553, 1975.

McCann ML, Schwartz R: The effects of milk solute on urinary cast excretion in premature infants, *Pediatrics* 38:555, 1966.

McKigney JI, Munro HN, editors: *Nutrient requirements in adolescence,* Cambridge, Mass, 1976, MIT Press.

Mertz W: The essential trace elements, *Science* 213:1332, 1981.

Pike RL, Brown ML: *Nutrition: an integrated approach,* ed 2, New York, 1975, John Wiley & Sons.

Rush D, Davis H, Susser M: Antecedents of low birth weight in Harlem, New York City, *Int J Epidemiol* 1:393, 1972.

Sacks FM et al: Plasma lipids and lipoproteins in vegetarians and controls, *N Engl J Med* 292:1148, 1975.

Stein Z et al: *Famine and human development,* New York, 1975, Oxford University Press.

Tsang RC, Nichols BL, editors: *Nutrition during infancy,* Philadelphia, 1988, Hanley & Belfus.

Walker WA, Watkins JB, editors: *Nutrition in pediatrics,* Boston, 1985, Little, Brown.

Waterlow JC, Alleyne GAO: Protein malnutrition in children. In Anfinsen CB Jr, Edsall JT, Richards FM, editors: *Advances in protein chemistry,* vol 25, New York, 1971, Academic Press.

World Health Organization: Energy and protein requirements. Report of a Joint FAO/WHO/UNU expert consultation, Tech Rep Series 724, Geneva, 1985, WHO.

Feeding of Infants and Children

Applebaum RM: The modern management of successful breast feeding, *Pediatr Clin North Am* 17:1, 1970.

Auerbach KG, Riordan J: *Breastfeeding and human lactation,* Boston, 1993, Jones & Bartlett.

Bakwin H: Feeding program for infants. I, *Fed Proc* 23:1, 1964.

Beal VA: On the acceptance of solid foods and other food patterns of infants and children, *Pediatrics* 20:448, 1957.

Bennett I, Simon M: *The prudent diet,* Port Washington, NY, 1973, David White.

Briggs G, Freeman R, Yaffe S: *Drugs in pregnancy and lactation,* ed 2, Baltimore, 1986, Williams & Wilkins.

Eiger MS, Rausen AR, Silverio J: Morbidity of breast-fed vs bottle-fed infants, *Clin Pediatr* 23:9, 1984.

Gerard JW: Breastfeeding: second thoughts, *Pediatrics* 54:6, 1974.

Grules CG, Sanford HN: The influence of breast and artificial feeding on infantile eczema, *J Pediatr* 9:223, 1936.

Kendall N, Vaughn VC, Kusakcioglu A: Study of preparation of infant formulas, *Am J Dis Child* 122:215, 1971.

Lawson D, Conlon J: *Superbaby cookbook,* New York, 1974, Macmillan.

Minchin M: *Breastfeeding matters,* Australia, 1985, Alma.

Oseid BJ: Breastfeeding and infant health, *Clin Obstet Gynecol* 18:149, 1975.

Reina D: Infant nutrition, *Clin Perinatal* 2:373, 1975.

Winikoff B, Baer EC: The obstetrician's opportunity: translating "breast is best" from theory to practice, *Am J Obstet Gynecol* 138:105, 1980.

17 Immunizations

John H. Dossett

BASIC CONCEPTS

General Immunity

General immunity, sometimes called *natural immunity*, refers to a general and immunologically mediated resistance to infection caused by microbial organisms of low virulence. Infection with such organisms may be inhibited by (1) broadly cross-reacting or nonspecific antibodies, (2) antibodies plus complement, (3) complement alone, or (4) phagocytosis, which is mediated by general rather than specific opsonins. Because most microbes are in this category, human beings who have normal host resistance can live and grow in a physical environment teeming with microbes. Water, food, soil, and air all are alive with microbial organisms, yet humans are not constantly being infected.

Specific Immunity

In contrast to low-virulence organisms, which can be repressed through general immunity, hundreds of highly virulent microbes possess specific characteristics that allow them to produce human disease. Moreover, the body must produce specific immunologically mediated responses to rid itself of such organisms or to protect itself from them. This specific immunity is called *acquired immunity*, which may be acquired either actively or passively.

Active Immunity. "Active" immunity refers to endogenous development of specific immunity in response to contact with microbial antigens. This immunity occurs within the host; it may be either humoral or cellular immunity but usually is both. The microbial antigens responsible for active immunity can be derived either from intact living microbial organisms or from nonliving microbial antigens.

Living Microbial Antigens. Most active immunity is acquired spontaneously, in that it results from random community-acquired infections. These usually are infections that have wild-strain microbes, and they may or may not be associated with a clinical illness. An example of such immunity would be the protection against subsequent episodes of chickenpox, mumps, and polio conferred by having contracted the natural disease. Some individuals are protected against such diseases as the result of an unrecognized infection.

In contrast to such spontaneously acquired immunity, which may be associated with significant morbidity and mortality, is the notion of *electively induced immunity*, or immunoprophylaxis, the principal subject of this discussion. Intrinsically associated with electively induced immunity is the ideal of preventing illness, both the kind caused by community-acquired infections and that caused by the actual immunizing agent. Fortunately, this two-part goal largely has been achieved for many infectious diseases, and the scientific and human interest stories of the research, development, and implementation of these triumphs constitute some of the greatest dramas of the twentieth century.

Immunoprophylaxis. Immunoprophylaxis may be accomplished with the antigens of either living or nonliving microbes. Each has advantages and disadvantages (see the box on p. 183). A live vaccine induces a "controlled infection"; the objective is to effect protective immunity without causing significant clinical illness. This control is sought by managing (1) the virulence of the infectious agent, (2) the size of the inoculum, and (3) the site of infection. Examples of *attenuated live vaccines* (those having diminished virulence) are the measles, rubella, mumps, and Sabin polio vaccines.

Immunity also may be induced by giving controlled amounts of *killed microbial antigens*. Under this principle, specific microbial components or killed whole microbes are administered to stimulate endogenous production of protective immunity. Examples of killed whole microbe vaccines are the pertussis, influenza, and Salk polio vaccines. Examples of specific microbial component vaccines are the tetanus, diphtheria, pneumococcal, meningococcal, and hepatitis B vaccines.

Passive Immunity. The major remaining method of acquiring protective immunity is through acquisition by the host of *preformed host defense factors* (humoral antibodies, transfer factor, or competent cells) from an exogenous source. Examples of such passive immunity are (1) placental transfer of maternal IgG to newborn infants, (2) administration of immune serum globulin to protect against hepatitis A and measles, and (3) administration of varicella-zoster immunoglobulin (VZIG) or hepatitis B immunoglobulin (HBIG) to protect against chickenpox or hepatitis B. In general, passive immunity is used to supply a measure of protection to individuals who already have been exposed to a virulent infectious agent or to those at high risk of being exposed to such an agent to which they have no active immunity. The relative advantages and disadvantages of active and passive immunoprophylaxis are shown in the box on p. 183.

Epidemic Control and Prevention

Three major control strategies guide the use of immunoprophylaxis to prevent the epidemic spread of infections: spot control, herd control, and selective control.

Spot Control. Spot control involves immunization of known and potential contacts of infected individuals to prevent the disease from spreading. To apply this principle, infected individuals must be readily identifiable so that they can be isolated and their contacts immunized. Clearly, communicable diseases characterized by significant subclinical infection do not lend themselves to this method. Smallpox is a good example of a disease against which this method has been successful. Conversely, the high incidence of subclini-

ADVANTAGES AND DISADVANTAGES OF LIVE ATTENUATED AND KILLED VACCINES

Live attenuated vaccines
Advantages

- Produce controlled infections that emulate natural immunity
- More likely to provide long-lasting or permanent immunity than are killed vaccines

Disadvantages

- Risk of vaccine-induced disease in recipient
- Risk of vaccine strain spreading to another person

Killed vaccines
Advantages

- No risk of vaccine-induced infection
- May use purified antigens
- Safe for immunocompromised individuals
- Safe for pregnant women

Disadvantages

- Immunity less likely to be prolonged or permanent

ADVANTAGES AND DISADVANTAGES OF ACTIVE AND PASSIVE IMMUNOPROPHYLAXIS

Active immunity
Advantage

- Prolonged or permanent protection

Disadvantages

- Protection delayed
- Risks related to the use of live organisms
- Difficulty getting vaccine to at-risk populations
- Only weak immune response in some young hosts

Passive immunity
Advantage

- Immediate protection

Disadvantages

- Brief term of protection
- Risk of serum sickness
- Active immune response to some vaccines inhibited
- Protection frequently given too late

cal infection in poliomyelitis (polio) makes it unsuitable for the spot control strategy.

Herd Control. Herd control involves reducing the number of people susceptible to a given communicable disease to the point where it becomes impossible for the disease to spread in epidemic proportions. Being able to keep polio under control is a good example of how this strategy is applied; even though isolated clinical and subclinical cases occur, they cannot reach epidemic proportions because most of the population has been immunized and therefore is not at risk. This strategy also has been remarkably successful in preventing rubella and rubeola epidemics; it will be even more successful when a larger majority of the population is removed from the at-risk category through effective immunization.

Selective Control. The selective control strategy is based on the assumptions that specific groups of people are at significant epidemiological risk for certain communicable diseases and that the rest of the population is at low risk for such infection. Thus only the specific groups at risk are selected for immunization. For example, hemodialysis patients and male homosexuals are at great risk for infection with the hepatitis B virus; therefore they are selectively chosen as groups for whom the hepatitis B vaccine is recommended.

Limitations of Vaccines

Clearly, the goal of public health agencies and infectious disease specialists is to develop methods to prevent all infectious diseases. However, some important communicable diseases have not succumbed either to environmental or to immunological control with vaccines. For instance, a vaccine made from group A streptococci theoretically could cause rheumatic fever, although there is no evidence of this. A number of vaccines induce an excellent immune response in older children and adults but a poor one in young children. For example, the pneumococcal vaccine is ineffective in children under age 2, its major target population, because although *Streptococcus pneumoniae* strains cause frequent, severe diseases in young children, those under 2 years of age do not make protective antibodies on being vaccinated. Similarly, *Haemophilus influenzae* type b until recently was the leading cause of childhood meningitis, but the first vaccines produced from these bacteria induced only a poor antibody response in the target population (again, children under age 2). Fortunately, the *H. influenzae* type b polysaccharides now have been linked successfully with proteins that render these conjugate vaccines immunogenic in young infants.

The ultimate criterion for any vaccine's effectiveness is whether it protects the vaccinated person against the target disease. Unfortunately, no reliable, inexpensive laboratory tests are available for determining the level of protection a given person has acquired. Specifically, it would be prohibitively expensive to test every person after each vaccination to determine antibody titers. Field studies, however, have determined the dosage of vaccine and the number of doses that render a vaccine 90% to 95% protective. For example, a single dose of measles vaccine given after age 1 protects more than 95% of infants. In contrast, no more than 70% of infants are protected after a single dose of pertussis vaccine; only after three doses is 85% protection approached.

The laboratory criteria for protection have been rather arbitrarily established for some diseases. With rubella, for example, it is recommended that any woman in her childbearing years whose rubella antibody titer is below 10 be vaccinated, regardless of whether she had been vaccinated previously. Certainly some women whose titers are below 10 are protected, but the consequences of gestational rubella justify this arbitrary recommendation.

PRACTICE OF IMMUNIZATION

With a few exceptions, it is clear that all children should be immunized. However, *no vaccine is perfectly safe and always effective.* Consequently, the risk of infection—morbidity and mortality—must be weighed against the risks and benefits of the corresponding vaccination.

It is good practice to discuss these issues with parents and guardians; they are entitled to know the risks of infection (incidence, morbidity, and mortality) and the benefits and risks of the corresponding vaccinations. Although the law requires vaccination for several of the common childhood infections as a condition for attending school, parents need accurate information so that they are informed participants in decisions about the immunization of their children.

Many of the current practices in immunization have evolved from attempts to minimize the cost, inconvenience, and discomfort of administering the vaccine without compromising its efficacy or safety. Consequently, many vaccines have been combined to meet these goals, such as diphtheria, tetanus, pertussis, and *H. influenzae* (DTP-Hib), and measles-mumps-rubella (MMR).

Also, the recommended schedule for administering vaccines is selected rather arbitrarily to synchronize with a reasonable schedule for health supervision during infancy. There is certainly nothing sacred about a primary schedule for immunization at 2, 4, and 6 months of age. It is important, however, to monitor a child's growth and development in the first year of life at these intervals, and such a schedule conveniently meshes with effective immunization.

The schedule generally recommended has been endorsed by the Advisory Committee on Immunization Practices (ACIP) of the U.S. Public Health Service, the AAP's Committee on Infectious Diseases, and by the American Academy of Family Physicians (Table 17-1).

Table 17-1 Recommended Childhood Immunization Schedule—United States, January 1996*

Vaccine	Birth	1 mo	2 mo	4 mo	6 mo	12 mo	15 mo	18 mo	4-6 yr	11-12 yr	14-16 yr
Hepatitis B†‡	Hep B-1										
			Hep B-2		Hep B-3					Hep B‡	
Diphtheria, tetanus, pertussis§			DTP	DTP	DTP	DTP§ (DTaP at 15 + m)			DTP or DTaP	Td	
H. influenzae type b‖			Hib	Hib	Hib‖	Hib‖					
Polio¶			OPV¶	OPV	OPV				OPV		
Measles, mumps, rubella#						MMR			MMR# or	MMR#	
Varicella-zoster virus vaccine**							Var			Var**	

From American Academy of Pediatric Committee on Infectious Diseases: *Pediatrics* 97:143, 1996.

*Approved by the Advisory Committee on Immunization Practices (ACIP), the American Academy of Pediatrics (AAP), and the American Academy of Family Physicians (AAFP). Vaccines are listed under the routinely recommended ages. Bars indicate range of acceptable ages for vaccination. Shaded bars indicate *catch-up vaccination:* at 11-12 years of age, hepatitis B vaccine should be administered to children not previously vaccinated, and varicella-zoster virus vaccine should be administered to children not previously vaccinated who lack a reliable history of chickenpox.

†*Infants born to HBsAg-negative mothers* should receive 2.5 μg of Merck vaccine (Recombivax HB) or 10 μg of SmithKline Beecham (SB) vaccine (Engerix-B). The second dose should be administered ≥1 month after the first dose. *Infants born to HBsAg-positive mothers* should receive 0.5 mL hepatitis B immune globulin (HBIG) within 12 hours of birth and either 5 μg of Merck vaccine (Recombivax HB) or 10 μg of SB vaccine (Engerix-B) at a separate site. The second dose is recommended at 1 to 2 months of age and the third dose at 6 months of age. *Infants born to mothers whose HBsAg status is unknown* should receive either 5 μg of Merck vaccine (Recombivax HB) or 10 μg of SB vaccine (Engerix-B) within 12 hours of birth. The second dose of vaccine is recommended at 1 month of age and the third dose at 6 months of age

‡Adolescents who have not previously received three doses of hepatitis B vaccine should initiate or complete the series at the 11- to 12-year-old visit. The second dose should be administered at least 1 month after the first dose, and the third dose should be administered at least 4 months after the first dose and at least 2 months after the second dose.

§DTP4 may be administered at 12 months of age, provided at least 6 months have elapsed since DTP3. DTaP (diphtheria and tetanus toxoids and acellular pertussis vaccine) is licensed for the fourth and/or fifth vaccine dose(s) for children 15 months of age or older and may be preferred for these doses in this age group. Td (tetanus and diphtheria toxoids, adsorbed, for adult use) is recommended at 11 to 12 years of age if at least 5 years have elapsed since the last dose of DTP, DTaP, or DT.

‖Three *H. influenzae* type b (Hib) conjugate vaccines are licensed for use in infants. If PRP-OMP (PedvaxHIB [Merck]) is administered at 2 and 4 months of age, a dose a 6 months is not required. After completing the primary series, any Hib conjugate vaccine may be used as a booster.

¶Oral poliovirus vaccine (OPV) is recommended for routine infant vaccination. Inactivated poliovirus vaccine (IPV) is recommended for persons with a congenital or acquired immune deficiency disease or an altered immune status as a result of disease or immunosuppressive therapy, as well as their household contacts, and is an acceptable alternative for other persons. The primary three-dose series for IPV should be given with a minimum interval of 4 weeks between the first and second doses and 6 months between the second and third doses.

#The second dose of MMR is routinely recommended at 4 to 6 years of age or at 11 to 12 years of age but may be administered at any visit, provided at least 1 month has elapsed since receipt of the first dose.

**Varicella-zoster virus vaccine (Var) can be administered to susceptible children any time after 12 months of age. Unvaccinated children who lack a reliable history of chickenpox should be vaccinated at the 11- to 12-year-old visit.

Interrupted Schedule

Contrary to common belief, interruption of the recommended schedule does not require restarting the entire immunization program. *Immunization of preschool children should proceed from the point at which it was interrupted, regardless of the interval since the last dose was given* (Table 17-2).

Unimmunized Children

Children who were not immunized in the first year of life may be started on a course of primary immunization any time before age 7. The schedule should be modified for these children so that they are protected against as many of the communicable diseases as possible. Therefore it is recommended that they initially receive MMR, DTP, Hib, HBV, and oral polio vaccine (OPV), followed by subsequent DTP, Hib, and OPV doses at 4-week intervals. This should be continued until the child has received three doses each of DTP and OPV and no more than three more of Hib, depending on the child's age. Except in measles epidemics, MMR should not be given until the child is 12 months old. Children who start or resume vaccinations after age 5 do not need the Hib vaccine, and those 7 and older should not be given the pertussis vaccine (Table 17-2).

Vaccine Interference

Some physicians believe that active response to one vaccine may interfere with the host response to another vaccine, but large field studies have demonstrated that this is not true. For instance, DTP and MMR give good responses to each of the components in these combined vaccines. Moreover, all these combinations (DTP, Hib, OPV, and MMR) may be given simultaneously without interfering with each other.

Intercurrent Illnesses and Vaccination

A mild upper respiratory tract infection or a mild episode of diarrhea should not preclude routine vaccination. Fever per se should not be considered a contraindication to immunization. This practice has resulted in too many unimmunized children. The decision to defer immunization should be based on the physician's assessment of the severity of the illness and not on the degree of temperature elevation. Immunization should be deferred in children who have moderate or severe medical illnesses.

Table 17-2 Recommended Immunization Schedules for Children Not Immunized in the First Year of Life

Recommended time/age	Immunization(s)*†	Comments
	Younger than 7 years	
First visit	DTP, Hib, HBV, MMR, OPV	If indicated, tuberculin testing may be done at same visit. If child is 5 yr of age or older, Hib is not indicated.
Interval after first visit:		
1 mo	DTP, HBV	OPV may be given if accelerated poliomyelitis vaccination is necessary, such as for travelers to areas where polio is endemic.
2 mo	DTP, Hib, OPV	Second dose of Hib is indicated only in children whose first dose was received when younger than 15 mo.
≥8 mo	DTP or DTaP,‡ HBV, OPV	OPV is not given if the third dose was given earlier.
4-6 yr (at or before school entry)	DTP or DTaP,‡ OPV	DTP or DTaP is not necessary if the fourth dose was given after the fourth birthday; OPV is not necessary if the third dose was given after the fourth birthday.
11-12 yr	MMR	At entry to middle school or junior high school.
10 yr later	Td	Repeat every 10 yr throughout life.
	7 Years and older§‖	
First visit	HBV,¶ OPV, MMR, Td	
Interval after first visit:		
2 mo	HBV,¶ OPV, Td	OPV may also be given 1 mo after the first visit if accelerated poliomyelitis vaccination is necessary.
8-14 mo	HBV,¶ OPV, Td	OPV is not given if the third dose was given earlier.
11-12 yr	MMR	At entry to middle school or junior high.
10 yr later	Td	Repeat every 10 yr throughout life.

From Peter G, editor: *1994 Red Book: Report of the Committee on Infectious Diseases,* ed 23, Elk Grove Village, Ill, 1994, American Academy of Pediatrics.

*If all needed vaccines cannot be administered simultaneously, priority should be given to protecting the child against those diseases that pose the greatest immediate risk. In the United States, these diseases for children younger than 2 years usually are measles and *Haemophilus influenzae* type b infection; for children older than 7 years, they are measles, mumps, and rubella (MMR).

†DTP or DTaP, HBV, Hib, MMR, and OPV can be given simultaneously at separate sites if failure of the patient to return for future immunizations is a concern.

‡DTaP is not currently licensed for use in children younger than 15 mo of age and is not recommended for primary immunization (i.e., first three doses) at any age.

§If person is 18 yr or older, routine poliovirus vaccination is not indicated in the United States.

‖Minimal interval between doses of MMR is 1 month.

¶Priority shold be given to hepatitis B immunization of adolescents.

Note: For varicella-zoster virus vaccine, see Table 17-1.

Barriers to Use of Immunoprophylaxis

Despite the established vaccines' long record of safety and success, many people in the United States still are susceptible to preventable infectious illnesses. Unfortunately, this is not because the vaccines have failed, but because vaccination has been neglected for a significant number of children and adolescents. This neglect is the result of general ignorance of the target diseases and fear of or hostility toward the vaccines. The current (and subsequent) generation of young parents has had no experience with the ravages of polio, measles, diphtheria, pertussis, or tetanus; consequently, they have no experiential reason to fear these diseases, as did previous generations. Often even young physicians have never seen these diseases, which makes it difficult for them to convince parents of the urgency of immunization.

The general lack of knowledge about these once common and devastating diseases is so widespread that formal instruction in their history and control might profitably become part of the core curriculum in high school. Surely such information is as important to young people and to society as are driver's education and sex education.

Efficacy of Vaccines

A vaccine's efficacy is the efficiency with which it protects vaccinated individuals against disease in settings in which virtually everyone is exposed uniformly to the infectious agent. Vaccine efficacy (VE) is calculated as follows:

$$VE\ (\%) = \frac{ARU - ARV}{ARU} \times 100$$

where *ARU* and *ARV* represent the attack rates in unvaccinated *(ARU)* and vaccinated *(ARV)* subjects.

International Travel

Several communicable diseases that no longer are a threat in North America remain endemic to other parts of the world. For specific information on the risks of infection in the various countries, the Centers for Disease Control and Prevention (CDC) annually publishes *Health Information for International Travel.* This always current resource provides appropriate recommendations to avoid infection with yellow fever, typhus, cholera, plague, malaria, typhoid fever, hepatitis A, and hepatitis B.

SPECIFIC IMMUNIZATIONS

Diphtheria Immunization

Fifty years ago diphtheria was a common respiratory illness with a fatality rate that ranged from 5% to 10%. In the past 5 to 6 years, fewer than 100 cases have been reported annually, but some deaths occur each year.

Vaccine. Diphtheria vaccine is a toxoid produced from virulent bacterial toxin in toxigenic strains of *Corynebacterium diphtheriae*. It is a good antigen that induces excellent antitoxin titers.

Administration. Diphtheria toxoid generally is given to infants in combination with the tetanus, pertussis, and *Haemophilus influenzae* type b vaccines (DTP-Hib); in children, over age 7, the diphtheria vaccine may be combined with just tetanus toxoid. Because diphtheria toxoid is more likely to cause adverse reactions (e.g., fever, local tenderness), an adult vaccine (Td) is recommended for those older than 7 years of age. Td contains the standard amount of tetanus toxoid but only 20% of the diphtheria toxoid supplied by DTP or DT.

Adverse Reactions. Diphtheria toxoid is a safe vaccine; its only proven side effects are a low incidence of fever and mild pain at the injection site.

Efficacy. The primary series of DTP is more than 90% effective in preventing serious diphtheritic infections. However, it does not prevent the individual from carrying *C. diphtheriae* on the skin or in the nasopharynx. The vaccine is believed to be protective for at least 10 years and perhaps for much longer.

Target Population. Young children particularly are susceptible to the myocarditis and neuritis of *C. diphtheriae* infection. Most cases occur among unimmunized children and adults.

Tetanus Immunization

The general use of tetanus toxoid has produced a dramatic decline in the number of tetanus cases seen in the United States. However, approximately 100 cases per year continue to be reported. In recent years more than half of these cases have occurred in individuals over age 50 who had not been immunized or were only partly immunized or whose immunization status was unknown.

Vaccine. The tetanus vaccine is a toxoid made from the virulent neurotoxin of *Clostridium tetani.*

Administration. In preschool children, tetanus toxoid usually is administered in combination with the diphtheria, pertussis, and *Haemophilus influenzae* type b vaccines (DTP-Hib). In children age 7 or older and adults, a diphtheria-tetanus preparation with a smaller amount of diphtheria toxoid (Td) is used (see Diptheria Immunization, above).

Adverse Reactions. The only proven side effects of tetanus toxoid are a low incidence of mild fever and mild tenderness at the injection site.

Efficacy. Tetanus toxoid is remarkably effective and generally induces protective antitoxin levels that persist at least 10 years after full immunization.

Target Population. Because the human body has little natural immunity to tetanus toxin and because strains of *C. tetani* are found everywhere, everyone, no matter what age, should be immunized with tetanus toxoid.

Wound Type and Risk of Tetanus. The risk of tetanus can be categorized as follows:

1. Wounds are particularly prone to tetanus contamination if they are more than 24 hours old, contain devitalized tissue, or are heavily contaminated with bacteria. Some examples of these types of wounds are injuries involving farm machinery, abdominal gunshot wounds, and some crush injuries caused by automobile and motorcycle accidents.
2. Wounds are moderately prone to tetanus if the injury involves moderate bacterial contamination, extension into muscle, crushing of tissue, or a tissue puncture.
3. Wounds are not prone to tetanus if they are clean, usually less than 24 hours old, not associated with tissue crushing or puncture, and do not extend into muscle (Table 17-3).

Table 17-3 Guide to Tetanus Prophylaxis in Wound Management*

History of tetanus immunization	Type of wound and type of vaccine given		
	Clean minor wound	Moderately tetanus prone	Very tetanus prone
Incomplete or uncertain	Td	Td + TIG-H (250 U)	Td + TIG-H (250-500 U)
Fully immunized but >10 yr since last dose of Td	Td	Td	Td
Fully immunized but 5-10 yr since last dose of Td	None	Td	Td
Fully immunized but <5 yr since last dose of Td	None	None	None

*Schedule recommended by the U.S. Public Health Service's Advisory Committee on Immunization Practices.

Td, Tetanus and diphtheria toxoids (adult type); *TIG-H,* Tetanus immunoglobulin–human, a specific tetanus antitoxin collected from human volunteers.

NOTE: 1. Children under age 7 should be given DTP rather than Td.

2. A full primary series comprises two doses of tetanus toxoid 2 months apart, plus a booster dose at least 6 months after the second dose.

Pertussis Immunization

During the 1930s and 1940s pertussis was a leading cause of infectious mortality and morbidity among children. The general use of pertussis vaccine has remarkably reduced the number of deaths from pertussis. However, the incidence of pertussis is still unacceptably high—approximately 2500 cases a year. This includes a mortality rate of 0.4% and an encephalopathy rate of 0.9%. Since the 1950s all deaths and serious complications have occurred in children under 1 year of age.

Vaccine. Pertussis vaccine is a crude vaccine prepared from killed whole organisms. Two new acellular pertussis vaccines have been licensed for use in children 18 months and older. These vaccines are as protective as the whole cell vaccine and have significantly fewer adverse effects.

Administration. The vaccine usually is given in combination with the tetanus and diphtheria toxoids (DTP). Because the greatest mortality and morbidity of pertussis occur in young children, the vaccine should be started at 2 months of age; however, it is not indicated for children over age 7.

Adverse Reactions. Pertussis vaccine is associated with a higher incidence of reactions and complications than are most other vaccines. More than half of children immunized have temporary tenderness at the DTP injection site, and approximately half have mild, brief systemic signs such as fever, irritability, or lethargy. More serious reactions, such as convulsions and hypotonic hyporesponsiveness, occur in approximately 1 in 2000 cases. Virtually all these children recover quickly and without sequelae.

Grave complications are much less common. Encephalopathy occurs in approximately 1 in 100,000 cases, and permanent neurological sequelae occur in approximately 1 in 300,000. However, recent data indicate quite clearly that pertussis immunization cannot be linked statistically to encephalopathy, neurological damage, or death. The risk of a repeat reaction should be weighed against the potential benefit of immunization. For example, a high fever or febrile seizure may well be controlled by a prophylactic antipyretic administered before and after subsequent immunization. Thus each case should be analyzed on an individual basis.

Efficacy. Pertussis is a highly communicable disease, with an attack rate as high as 90% in unimmunized household contacts. However, the vaccine, which has a calculated efficacy of 80% to 85%, is highly effective in preventing or attenuating the disease and thus preventing serious complications.

Target Population. All children except those who have an evolving neurological illness should be immunized. Children who have stable neurological deficits should be immunized, just as any other child.

Risk/Benefit. In recent years great popular concern has arisen about the safety of the pertussis vaccine. Much of this concern has been fueled by erroneous information about the incidence of encephalopathy and permanent neurological sequelae. Because of this misinformation, many parents have chosen not to have their infants vaccinated for pertussis.

Although the vaccine does have risks, the risk of death or encephalopathy from pertussis infection in an unimmunized child is much greater. Recently, when pertussis immunization in Great Britain and Japan dropped from 80% to 30%, large epidemics of pertussis followed in both countries. Projections from these recent epidemics indicate that *the risk of pertussis-related death is 10 times greater in an unimmunized population than in an immunized population of children.* With a cohort of 3.5 million births per year, the projected number of deaths from pertussis and pertussis vaccination is 44 per year; the same group without vaccination is projected to have 457 deaths. A similar tenfold greater incidence is projected for frequency of hospitalization, episodes of encephalitis, and cost in an unimmunized cohort of children.[2] The new acellular pertussis vaccines are licensed and used in children 18 months of age or older. These vaccines are remarkably effective and have few side effects. The FDA likely will license acellular vaccines for primary immunizations in infants during 1996 and 1997.

Polio Immunization

Before the Salk inactivated polio vaccine (IPV) was introduced in 1955, more than 18,000 cases of paralytic polio were reported in epidemic years. However, in one of the most dramatic public health success stories, the general use of polio vaccine has almost eradicated paralytic polio in highly developed countries. Even so, 5 to 15 cases are reported in the United States each year, usually among unimmunized individuals such as illegal aliens or those who for various reasons refused or did not seek immunization.

Vaccine. The first polio vaccine licensed (1955) was the IPV. After a primary series of immunizations, it protected the child against paralytic disease but not against polio *infection.* In 1963 the Sabin oral polio vaccine (OPV), a live, attenuated poliovirus, was licensed. All three serotypes of poliovirus have been combined into a highly effective, trivalent vaccine that provides gastrointestinal mucosal immunity to infection. Moreover, the vaccine virus may spread through the fecal-oral route, much like the spread of wild virus; this has the added advantage of immunizing secondary and tertiary contacts.

Administration. OPV is given by mouth and should be started at the 2- or 4-month visit. Second and third doses of OPV are recommended at 2-month intervals thereafter. Booster doses are recommended at approximately 18 months of age and again when the child starts school. OPV may be given at the same time as DTP-Hib and MMR if the primary immunizations have been delayed beyond the first birthday. It has been shown that *breast milk with antibodies to polio is capable of neutralizing the vaccine but does not interfere with the development of immunity;* therefore breast-fed babies also should be immunized according to the routine recommended schedule.

Adverse Reactions. OPV is remarkably safe, producing virtually no minor reactions. A few cases of vaccine-associated paralytic disease have been reported—the risk in primary vaccinees is approximately 1 in 19 million cases. If paralytic disease in close contacts of vaccinees also is counted, the risk is approximately 1 in 4 million. Whichever is the case, the benefit of polio vaccination is overwhelming.

Efficacy. Polio is a highly communicable disease that spreads rapidly through unimmunized populations, as witnessed in a recent epidemic in Taiwan. Calculations from recent experiences have estimated the vaccine's efficacy as 82% after one dose, 96% after two doses, and 98% after three doses.

Target Population. All children should be given the trivalent oral polio vaccine except for those with immune deficiency syndromes and their household contacts.

Measles Immunization

Until the 1960s approximately 500,000 cases of measles were reported in the United States each year. Because of underreporting, the actual number may have been five times that figure or more. The major complications of measles are encephalitis and bronchopneumonia; approximately one case of encephalitis or pneumonia occurs in every 1000 cases of measles, often resulting in death or neurological sequelae of varying severity. In the large measles epidemics that occurred before the 1960s, as many as 1 in 15 of the affected children died.

Vaccine. Live measles virus vaccine is prepared in chick embryo cells from the Edmonston-B strain, which has been attenuated further. The vaccine is used primarily in combination with the mumps and rubella vaccines (MMR). However, the measles vaccine is available in a monovalent form or in combination with rubella only (MR).

Administration. It is recommended that the measles vaccine be given at 15 months of age, along with rubella and mumps (MMR), inasmuch as *children immunized before 1 year of age are less likely to make protective antibodies because of neutralization of the vaccine by maternal antibodies.* The measles vaccine may be given at the same time as other vaccines if the child has not been immunized according to the recommended schedule. A second dose of MMR should be given when the child starts school. It is most important that the vaccine be handled properly; to prevent inactivation, it should be transported and stored at 35.5° to 50° F (2° to 10° C) and protected from light.

Adverse Reactions. The measles vaccine has an outstanding safety record. Fever that may last up to 5 days develops in approximately 5% of vaccinees between the sixth and tenth day after vaccination. Usually no other symptoms occur, although transient rashes have been reported in 3% to 5% of vaccinees.

People who have received the killed measles vaccine are more likely to have fever and local tenderness when revaccinated with live measles vaccine. However, this risk is far less than their risk of severe atypical measles on exposure to wild measles virus.

Efficacy. The development of measles antibodies protects at least 95% of measles vaccinees from clinical measles. A single dose at approximately 15 months of age protects for at least 15 years and usually for a lifetime. General use of the vaccine has resulted in a 99% reduction in the number of reported measles cases.

Target Population. Anyone who has not had measles infection or measles immunization is at risk for infection. Individuals born before 1957 are likely to have had measles; those born after 1957 should be immunized unless they have had (1) physician-diagnosed measles, (2) serological evidence of measles immunity, or (3) measles immunization subsequent to the person's first birthday. In the 1980s, more than half of measles cases occurred in adolescents and young adults. Clearly, greater emphasis must be placed on immunizing young people of high school and college age. Most states have passed legislation requiring evidence of measles immunity for a child to attend school, and many colleges require measles revaccination before matriculation. Preschool children remain at risk and should be immunized promptly at 15 months of age.

Revaccination. Through the 1980s many epidemics of measles occurred in teenagers and young adults. This appeared to be partly the result of waning immunity in those who had been vaccinated at 15 months of age. Consequently, it is now recommended that all children and young adults (ages 5 to 21 years) have a second measles vaccination. This second dose preferably is given when the child starts school; however, those who have not received a second dose should receive it at whatever age they are identified. In the 1990s, young people in middle school, high school, and college should be targeted for revaccination.

Contraindications. As with all live virus vaccines, there is a theoretical risk of fetal infection if pregnant women are vaccinated. However, no direct experiences with any of the common vaccines (MMR and OPV) have confirmed this fear. MMR vaccination should not be postponed because of a mild upper respiratory tract infection. Again, fever per se should not be considered a contraindication to MMR vaccination.

Children who have had anaphylactic reactions to eggs should not be immunized; such children are so rare, however, that this risk hardly ever precludes measles immunization.

If a child is immunocompromised (e.g., has leukemia, lymphoma, or disseminated malignancy) or is undergoing steroid therapy, a specialist in the field should be consulted before the child is given a live virus vaccine. It generally is agreed that children infected with the human immunodeficiency virus (HIV) should be given the MMR vaccine, but that the enhanced inactivated poliovirus vaccine (EIPV), rather than the live poliovirus vaccine, should be used.

Mumps Immunization

Mumps generally is a benign infection commonly characterized by fever and parotitis. At least 30% of cases are subclinical, and about 15% of affected patients have meningeal signs but recover without sequelae. Rare nerve deafness is the primary serious permanent sequel. Since the mumps vaccine was introduced in 1967, its general use has resulted in a 98% reduction in the number of cases of mumps reported annually.

Vaccine. The mumps vaccine is an attenuated live virus prepared in chick embryo cultures. It produces a subclinical infection that has virtually no side effects. It most often is combined with measles and rubella vaccines to reduce the cost and discomfort of injections.

Administration. The mumps vaccine should be given to all generally healthy children at 15 months of age, and it should be given with the measles and rubella vaccines (MMR). As with the measles vaccine, mumps vaccine should be transported and stored at 35.5° to 50° F (2° to 10° C) and protected from light. A single dose of the mumps vaccine can be expected to provide durable, probably lifelong immunity.

Adverse Reactions. There are rare reports of fever and rash temporally related to mumps vaccination. Reports of seizures and encephalitis are rare; the incidence of these is even lower than the incidence of central nervous system dysfunction expected in the general population.

Efficacy. The efficacy of the mumps vaccine, calculated in several studies, ranges from 80% to 90%. Measurable antibodies develop in more than 90% of those vaccinated.

Target Population. Because of interference from maternally transported antibodies, protective antibodies are less likely to develop in children immunized before 1 year of age. However, all children and young adults who have not been immunized or have not had clinical mumps would benefit from the vaccine. Vaccination poses no additional risk to individuals who actually may have had preceding subclinical mumps or to those whose immunization status is uncertain. The cost/benefit ratio of the mumps vaccine has been clearly documented. Because adolescents and young adults born after 1967 are less likely to have been immunized by natural infection, special emphasis should be placed on immunizing this group.

Rubella Immunization

Rubella is one of the common childhood exanthems usually manifested by a brief, low-grade fever, suboccipital and postauricular lymphadenopathy, and mild arthralgia. It produces transient arthritis in infected adolescents and young adult women. Before the rubella vaccine came into general use, the disease occurred in epidemic form approximately every 7 years. Infection of pregnant women is complicated by a high incidence of fetal infection, which results in a high incidence of fetal death, malformation, and neurological sequelae—the major public health problem posed by rubella. Since 1980 more than 75% of rubella cases have occurred in young adults over age 15.

Vaccine. The live rubella vaccine is an attenuated rubella virus prepared in a human diploid cell culture. It is produced as a monovalent vaccine and also in combination with the measles vaccine (MR) or the mumps and measles vaccines (MMR). The vaccine produces subclinical infection in those vaccinated but does not spread to susceptible contacts.

Administration and Target Population. All children, adolescents, and young adults who do not have serological evidence of rubella immunity should be vaccinated. It is recommended that infants receive the vaccine in combination with the measles and mumps vaccines at 15 months of age. Because most adolescents and young adults who have not been vaccinated against rubella also have not been vaccinated against measles or mumps, they, too, should receive the MMR vaccine.

Although general immunization of young children has prevented large, statewide epidemics, small epidemics still occur regularly in high schools and colleges, on military bases, and in businesses that employ many young people. These young people constitute a major targeting priority because they are in their peak childbearing years. *All women who attend prenatal clinics should be screened for rubella immunity* so that those who are susceptible can be immunized immediately after giving birth. *A history of rubella is not reliable and should not be accepted in lieu of vaccination.*

Adverse Reactions. A significant number of vaccinees (30%) may have a transient rash, lymphadenopathy, or arthralgia. Approximately 1% have self-limited arthritis; this reaction occurs more often in women than in children.

The primary concerns with the rubella vaccine have been that (1) young women in their first trimester of pregnancy might be vaccinated inadvertently, and (2) the vaccine virus might be as teratogenic as the wild virus. The first concern has been confirmed in that at least 1000 pregnant women have received the rubella vaccine inadvertently. However, in none of these women has congenital rubella syndrome been diagnosed. A few of the infants also were infected, but they had no illness attributable to the vaccine virus. Even so, *it is recommended that women known to be pregnant not be vaccinated with rubella vaccine or with any other live virus vaccine.* If, however, such vaccination occurs inadvertently, there is no reason to recommend termination of the pregnancy.

Efficacy. Protective antibodies develop in approximately 95% of susceptible individuals over 1 year of age who receive a single dose of rubella vaccine. This immunity is long term and confers probably lifelong protection against viremia and clinical illness.

Hepatitis B Immunization

The hepatitis B virus infects approximately 200,000 people a year in the United States, resulting in about 10,000 hospitalizations and 250 acute deaths. Many more deaths occur from later complications, such as cirrhosis or hepatoma. The risk of infection is concentrated in certain groups, such as male homosexuals, institutionalized developmentally disabled children, certain health care personnel, and household contacts of infected individuals.

Vaccine. The hepatitis B vaccine is a recombinant gene product in which hepatitis B surface antigen (HB_SAg) is harvested from yeast that has the gene coding for HB_SAg incorporated into its DNA. This vaccine has no connection to blood or other mammalian tissue.

Administration. The dose for adults is 10 μg (1 ml); for children under age 9, the dose is reduced to 5 μg (0.5 ml). Three doses are needed to raise protective antibodies. These doses apply only to Recombivax. Engerix-B has a different content of antigen that results in a two to four times higher antigen dose, depending on age. Physicians should consult the package insert for the appropriate dose. The first two doses are given 1 month apart; the third dose is given 6 months after the first. These are all given intramuscularly (see the box below).

Adverse Reactions. Approximately 15% of vaccine recipients have mild tenderness at the injection site.

Efficacy. Protective antibodies develop in more than 90% of healthy adults after three intramuscular doses of HBV vaccine. Up to 95% of susceptible vaccinees in field trials have been protected against hepatitis B infection.

Target Population. Because of the increasing incidence of hepatitis B disease, the availability of safe, effective vaccines, and the declining cost of these vaccines *the general recommendation is that all children be immunized with hepatitis B vaccine.*

Pediatricians encounter infants born to mothers who test positive for HB_SAg, as well as children who live in households with chronic HBV carriers. Babies born to mothers who have HB_SAg positivity are particularly vulnerable; they should receive hepatitis B immunoglobulin (HBIG) *and* the HBV vaccine. Follow-up serological testing (anti-HB_SAg) should be done when the infant is 12 to 15 months of age to determine the vaccine response. It is recommended that children older than 12 months from households that have chronic carriers receive the vaccine only. Children younger than 12 months of age should receive both HBIG and HBV vaccine (see the box below, left). Perinatal transmission of HBV can be prevented by screening all pregnant women for HB_SAg and by administering HBIG and the HBV vaccine to the newborn infants of mothers who are HBV carriers. Some states require universal prenatal screening for HB_SAg.

HEPATITIS B PROPHYLAXIS FOR PERINATAL AND HOUSEHOLD EXPOSURE

1. Infants born to mothers who test positive for hepatitis B antigens have a great probability of being infected (HB_SAg positive, 25% probability; HB_eAg positive, 85% probability). Infection may occur anytime in the first year after birth.
2. Infants infected with HBV have a 90% probability of becoming chronic HBV carriers.
3. Perinatal administration of HBIG is 75% effective in preventing chronic infection.
4. Perinatal administration of HBIG and the HBV vaccine is 90% effective in preventing chronic infection.
5. Both HBIG and the HBV vaccine are recommended.

		Perinatal exposure	Household contact
HBIG			
	Dose	0.5 ml IM	For infants <12 months of age only
	Timing	Within 12 hr of birth	
HBV vaccine			
	Dose	0.5 ml IM	0.5 ml IM
	Timing	Within 2 mo of birth, repeated at 1 mo and 6 mo after the initial dose (may be given at the same time as HBIG and other childhood immunizations)	When contact is identified; repeat after 1 mo and 6 mo

Influenza Immunization

Infection with the influenza virus produces an illness generally manifested by fever, cough, paratracheal pain, and myalgia. Its primary morbidity and mortality occur among older adults and the chronically ill.

Influenza infections arise every winter, but large epidemics develop when major shifts occur in the antigenic structure of the prevalent strains. Influenza A viruses are classified on the basis of their hemagglutinin and neuraminidase antigens. Three subtypes of hemagglutinin (H_1, H_2, and H_3) and two subtypes of neuraminidase (N_1 and N_2) have been recognized in the strains that cause human disease. Immunity to a specific hemagglutinin protects against infections and serious disease. *Because influenza A virus antigens are always changing, a reliable vaccine for protecting susceptible populations is particularly difficult to develop.*

Immunization Strategy. Each summer the ACIP attempts to predict the subtypes of influenza virus likely to be prevalent in the coming respiratory virus season. This prediction is based on analysis of the strains most prevalent at the end of the previous season. On the basis of these predictions, vaccine is prepared and distributed in the late summer and fall of each year.

Vaccine. The vaccines are either whole virus or split virus preparations that have been grown on chick embryo cells. In recent years the vaccines have been purified of virtually all egg protein, and the antigen concentration has been stabilized.

Administration and Target Population. Recommendations on the number of doses and the target population vary from year to year, but current CDC recommendations are published in a number of readily available sources each summer; *Morbidity and Mortality Weekly Reports* is a good source. *Children who have a chronic illness are at greater risk for serious complications and are the only children who should be vaccinated.* The following conditions warrant administration of the influenza vaccine:

1. Chronic pulmonary disease (e.g., cystic fibrosis, asthma, severe scoliosis, bronchopulmonary dysplasia, and neuromotor diseases that compromise ventilation)
2. Heart disease with altered circulatory dynamics
3. Chronic renal disease with azotemia
4. Diabetes mellitus and other metabolic diseases
5. Immunocompromised conditions
6. Severe chronic anemias

Adverse Reactions. A mild induration at the injection site develops in approximately one third of vaccine recipients. Systemic reactions of fever, malaise, or myalgia occur infrequently. In 1976 a temporal association was noted between administration of the "swine" influenza vaccine and the development of Guillain-Barré syndrome (GBS) in adults. No increase in GBS has been seen after influenza vaccinations since 1978.

Rabies Prevention

Rabies almost has been eliminated from humans in the United States, largely because of compulsory rabies vaccination of dogs. Even so, thousands of people are injured annually by rabid or potentially rabid animals. Now that rabies for the most part has been controlled among domestic animals, *wild animals (especially skunks, foxes, raccoons, and bats) account for approximately 75% of animal rabies.* Because rabies is such a lethal disease, anyone exposed to the risk of rabies infection needs to be immunized.

Vaccine. The currently recommended vaccine is a human diploid cell (rabies) vaccine (HDCV). It is an inactivated virus vaccine that produces good antibody responses with only mild side effects. This vaccine has replaced the duck embryo vaccine (DEV), which requires four times as many injections, has more side effects, and produces much lower antibody titers.

Human rabies immune globulin (RIG) is prepared from the plasma of hyperimmunized human donors. It is standardized to contain 150 IU of rabies-neutralizing antibodies per milliliter.

Administration and Target Population. Children who are bitten or scratched by animals known to be able to carry rabies should be regarded as having been exposed to rabies. Decisions about rabies prophylaxis should be based on information about (1) the circumstances of the bite or nonbite injury, (2) the species of animal, (3) the animal's health (when possible), and (4) the type of exposure.

Circumstances of the Bite or Nonbite Injury (Provoked or Unprovoked). An unprovoked attack is more likely to indicate that the animal is rabid. Bites or scratch injuries incurred while attempting to feed, pet, or handle an apparently healthy animal generally should be regarded as provoked injuries.

Species of Animal. A few species are more likely than others to be infected with the rabies virus. In the United States, since 1960 these animals have included skunks, raccoons, foxes, bats, coyotes, and bobcats. Any possible rabies exposure (bite or nonbite) to these animals requires postexposure prophylaxis unless the animal is tested and shown to be free of rabies.

Rodents such as squirrels, chipmunks, rats, mice, hamsters, guinea pigs, and gerbils, as well as rabbits, are only rarely infected and have not been known to cause human rabies in the United States. Consequently, bites by such animals are almost never an indication for rabies prophylaxis.

Health of the Implicated Animal. *Any healthy domestic dog or cat that bites a child should be confined and observed for 10 days.* If the animal shows any signs of illness during this time, it should be evaluated by a veterinarian. If signs suggesting rabies develop, the animal should be humanely killed and the head submitted to a qualified laboratory for rabies examination. Any stray domestic dog or cat that bites a person should also be confined and observed for clinical signs of rabies.

Signs of rabies in wild animals cannot be interpreted reliably; therefore any wild animal that bites or scratches a person should be killed, if possible, and submitted for examination. If fluorescent antibody examination of the brain tissue of any animal (domestic or wild) is shown to be negative for rabies, the injured person does not need to be treated.

Type of Exposure (Bite and Nonbite). Rabies is transmitted by introduction of the virus into cuts and wounds or through contamination of mucous membranes. A *bite* is defined as any penetration of the skin by the animal's teeth. Nonbite exposure includes scratches, cuts, open wounds, or mucous membranes contaminated by an animal's saliva or other potentially infected materials.

Postexposure Prophylaxis. Immediately and thoroughly washing all bite and nonbite wounds with soap and water is as important as immunization in preventing rabies. The decision to administer rabies prophylaxis should never be made lightly, because it requires multiple injections, considerable expense, and some risk of side effects (see Table 17-4 for guidelines for postexposure antirabies treatment). Rabies prophylaxis always should include HDCV and RIG. RIG is given only once, at the beginning of treatment. The dose is 20 IU/kg. If possible, half the dose should be infiltrated around the site of exposure and the rest given intramuscularly. Five 1 ml doses of HDCV are given intramuscularly on days 1, 3, 7, 14, and 28. A serum specimen for rabies antibody testing should be collected 2 to 3 weeks after the last injection. Testing for rabies antibodies can be arranged through a state health department laboratory. If antibody response is not confirmed, the patient should receive a booster dose of the vaccine.

Adverse Reactions. Approximately 25% of those given HDCV report local reactions such as pain or swelling at the

Table 17-4 Postexposure Antirabies Treatment Guide*

Species of animal	Animal's condition at time of attack	Treatment of exposed person
Wild skunk, fox, coyote, raccoon, or bat	Regard as rabid	HDCV† and RIG
Domestic dog or cat	Healthy	None‡
	Unknown (escaped)	Call public health official
	Rabid or suspected of being rabid	HDCV and RIG‡
Other	Consider individually	

Modified from the Report of the Committee on Infectious Disease: *Red book,* ed 19, Evanston, Ill, 1982, American Academy of Pediatrics.
HDCV, Human diploid cell (rabies) vaccine; *RIG,* (Human) rabies immune globulin.
*These recommendations are only guidelines; they should be applied in conjunction with information about the species of animal involved, the circumstances of the bite or nonbite exposure, the animal's vaccination status, and whether rabies is present in the region.
†The vaccine is discontinued if the animal is killed at the time of the attack and subsequent fluorescent antibody tests are negative for rabies.
‡HDCV and RIG are begun at the first sign of rabies in a biting dog or cat during the 10-day holding period.

injection site. Mild systemic reactions (e.g., headache, dizziness, and muscle aches) occur in 20% of recipients. Rabies prophylaxis should not be discontinued because of these mild adverse reactions, which usually can be managed with aspirin or other antiinflammatory agents.

Efficacy. The regimen described previously has been used in more than 150 people who were bitten by animals known to be rabid. No cases of rabies developed.

Smallpox Immunization

Not one case of smallpox has been seen in the United States since 1947. The last community-acquired cases of smallpox in the world occurred in the fall of 1979. Consequently, the risk of complications from the vaccine far outweighs any risk of acquiring smallpox. For this reason, routine smallpox immunization no longer is recommended. Vaccination now is indicated only for laboratory workers directly involved with smallpox or closely related viruses. Vaccination is not indicated for international travel.

Pneumococcal Vaccination

Virulent strains of *Streptococcus pneumoniae* are a major cause of morbidity and mortality in the very young, in older adults, and in certain patients who have host defense deficiencies. Several controlled trials over 3 decades have demonstrated that polyvalent pneumococcal vaccines can reduce significantly the incidence and mortality of pneumococcal disease caused by the specific strains incorporated into the vaccine. In the first 2 years of life, about 20% of all children develop otitis media caused by pneumococci; half the cases of pneumococcal meningitis occur in young children. Unfortunately, however, this major pediatric target population does not respond to pneumococcal vaccination by developing protective antibody titers. The recent, highly successful development of *H. influenzae* type b polysaccharide/protein conjugate, which is immunogenic in young children, gives encouragement that similar techniques can be applied to pneumococcal vaccines.

Vaccine. The current pneumococcal vaccine is polyvalent and contains the polysaccharides of 23 common pneumococcal strains, which account for 85% of the *S. pneumoniae* isolates. Each 0.5 ml dose of vaccine contains 25 mg of purified polysaccharide from each of the 23 strains.

Administration. The vaccine (0.5 ml) should be given intramuscularly or subcutaneously in the thigh or deltoid muscle. Intradermal injections have been associated with severe local reactions.

Adverse Reactions. Local erythema and mild soreness occur in approximately half of vaccine recipients. Severe adverse reactions have been rare. However, because more severe local and systemic reactions are common in adults given a second immunization, booster doses or repeat immunizations are contraindicated for adults. The safety of second doses in children has yet to be determined.

Efficacy. In vaccine recipients over age 2, immunization has demonstrated variable efficacy, from little protection up to an 80% reduction in the incidence of type-specific pneumococcal diseases, including pneumococcal bacteremia, pneumonia, and otitis media.

Target Population. The pneumococcal vaccine is recommended for everyone over age 50. Younger people at increased risk of acquiring pneumococcal disease and of death also should be immunized, such as those with congenital and traumatic asplenia, sickle cell disease, nephrotic syndrome, or other immune deficiency syndromes. Individuals who have Hodgkin disease should be immunized before beginning therapy. It is recommended that the pneumococcal vaccine be given *in addition to* penicillin prophylaxis when there is a valid indication for chronic penicillin prophylaxis.

Haemophilus Influenzae Type B Immunization

Before the conjugated *Haemophilus influenzae* type b (Hib) vaccines were introduced, *H. influenzae* type b meningitis affected 15,000 to 20,000 children a year in the United States, making it the leading cause of acquired mental retardation. Besides posing this threat, Hib diseases caused many other serious infections, such as epiglottitis, pericarditis, pneumonia, orbital cellulitis, and bone and joint infections. More than 75% of these infections occurred in children under age 2.

Vaccine. In the late 1980s, several vaccines were developed that linked *H. influenzae* type b polyribosyl ribitol phosphate (PRP) to various protein antigens, such as diphtheria toxoid (PRP-D), tetanus toxoid (PRP-T), and the outer membrane protein complex (PRP-OMP) of *Neisseria meningitidis*. Another vaccine with exciting potential was produced when *H. influenzae* type b oligosaccharide was conjugated to cross-reacting material (^{197}CRM), a nontoxic mutant diphtheria toxin (HbOC). Three of these conjugate vaccines have induced excellent anti-PRP titers in young infants.

In October 1990, the U.S. Food and Drug Administration (FDA) approved the HbOC vaccine (HibTITER, from Lederle-Praxis Biologicals) for administration to infants beginning at 2 months of age. Within months the incidence of Hib diseases had been reduced dramatically. Since then, these devastating and formerly common infections have become uncommon. This clearly is a public health triumph comparable to the success of the pertussis and polio vaccines.

Administration and Target Population. It is recommended that all infants receive four doses of a conjugated Hib vaccine, which should be given at 2, 4, and 6 months of age, plus a booster dose given at 12 to 15 months of age (see Table 17-1). Only two initial doses, at 2 and 4 months, are needed when using PRP-OMP (Pedvax HIB, Merck, Sharp & Dohme).

Adverse Reactions. Approximately half of all vaccine recipients have mild fever and a mild reaction at the injection site. A significant fever develops in only 1% of those immunized. When this vaccine is given simultaneously with DTP, the incidence of reactions is no greater than with DTP alone.

Efficacy. Several controlled trials and postmarketing experience indicate that the efficacy of these vaccines in preventing invasive disease due to Hib is greater than 90%. In fact, invasive disease in a fully immunized child should raise the question of an unrecognized immunodeficiency.

Meningococcal Immunization

Meningitis and bacteremia caused by *Neisseria meningitidis* continue to cause significant morbidity and mortality among children. The secondary attack rate among household contacts is about 0.3%. However, in epidemics this secondary attack rate can increase at least tenfold (3% to 10%), and these epidemics have dictated the need for an effective vaccine. Purified polysaccharide vaccines to serotypes A, B, and C have been tested. The A and C vaccines are safe and effective, but the type B vaccine is a weak antigen that results in poor antibody responses. This is particularly important because most cases of meningococcal disease in the United States during the past decade have been caused by group B strains.

Vaccine. Currently four vaccine preparations are available: monovalent group A and group C vaccines, a bivalent vaccine that contains both group A and group C polysaccharides, and a quadrivalent vaccine that includes group A, group C, group Y, and group W135 polysaccharides.

Administration. Vaccinees receive 50 μg of the component antigens, which are given subcutaneously.

Adverse Reactions. Adverse reactions are rare. Approximately 5% of vaccinated children have transient erythema; local tenderness is rare.

Efficacy. Under epidemic conditions, the group A vaccine has proved effective in children over 6 months of age. Under the same conditions the group C vaccine was highly effective in children over age 2 but less protective for younger children. In its failure to protect very young children, the group C vaccine is similar to the pneumococcal vaccine.

Target Population. The meningococcal vaccine currently is recommended for use in epidemic outbreaks of group A or group C disease. Clearly, travelers should be immunized if they plan to visit a city or country undergoing such an epidemic. Local epidemics should be defined in conjunction with state health departments and the CDC before large-scale vaccination is implemented.

Vaccination should be considered, along with chemoprophylaxis, for household contacts, day care contacts, and selected hospital contacts when the index case is found to be infected with a group A or group C strain of *N. meningitidis.*

Varicella Immunization

Varicella (chickenpox) generally is a self-limited infection with only moderate morbidity (and in rare cases long-term sequelae) among healthy individuals. However, recent advances in intensive care and chemotherapy have greatly increased the number of immunocompromised children, for whom varicella infection can mean serious disease and death. The addition of Reye syndrome and neonatal varicella to the list of established varicella complications has sparked interest in developing appropriate vaccines.

Vaccine. The OKA and KMcC strains have been tested and have proved safe and immunogenic in children. Moreover, significant antibody titers have persisted for longer than 5 years, and vaccinated children have been protected when exposed to active chickenpox.

Administration and Target Population. The OKA vaccine was licensed by the FDA in the spring of 1995. A single dose is recommended for all healthy children over 1 year through 12 years of age who do not have a reliable history of varicella infection. Adolescents and adults should receive two doses 4 to 8 weeks apart. Although varicella usually is a self-limited infection, the risk of unpleasant and sometimes life-threatening complications is such that this vaccine can be recommended for all children. Vaccination is especially important for individuals who reach adolescence (beyond 12 years of age) or adulthood without having had chickenpox because the disease and its complications (including death) are much more severe in these older groups than in children.

Adverse Reactions. Approximately 5% of vaccinees develop a rash between the sixth and tenth day after vaccination. The rash consists of erythematous papules rather than the vesicles seen in naturally occurring chickenpox. The risk of vaccine-associated varicella-zoster and demyelination syndromes is not known. Careful postlicensing follow-up will answer these questions.

Persons who are immunocompromised for any reason should not be given varicella vaccine. However, an immunocompromised person in the same household as a varicella vaccinee is not at risk unless the vaccinee develops a rash, in which case contact with the immunocompromised person should be avoided until the rash disappears.

Persons allergic to neomycin should not be given varicella vaccine because it contains trace amounts of neomycin.

Pregnant women should not be given varicella vaccine because the vaccine's effects on fetal development are unknown. Pregnancy should be avoided for at least 1 month after vaccination. A pregnant woman living in the household of a potential vaccinee is not a contraindication to vaccination.

Varicella vaccine should not be given to persons with moderate or severe illness, since it is not yet known whether such illness will interfere with the development of immunity.

It is recommended that salicylates not be administered for 6 weeks after the varicella vaccine is given because of the association between Reye syndrome, natural varicella, and salicylates. To date, no cases of Reye syndrome have been reported in varicella vaccinees.

Efficacy. Accurate information about varicella vaccine efficacy is as yet not available. However, preliminary data indicate that the vaccine protects to a limited extent (if at all) against infection, to a greater extent against varicella disease, and very well against severe complications of the disease.

Tuberculosis Immunization

After a long decline in the incidence of tuberculosis in the United States, recent years have seen a dramatic increase in the number of people contracting tuberculosis. From 1985 to 1992 there was approximately a 35% increase in cases of tuberculosis in children 0 to 14 years of age and a 55% increase in adults 25 to 44 years of age.[1] For this reason, the strategy for controlling tuberculosis in the United States has been to identify and treat cases that arise and to follow up patients' contacts with close surveillance. Vaccination has been reserved for selected groups.

Vaccine. Bacille Calmette-Guérin (BCG) is an attenuated strain of *Mycobacterium bovis.* All current vaccines are derived from the original strain.

Administration. BCG is given intradermally. Newborn infants receive 0.05 ml; older infants and children receive 0.1 ml. The vaccine should be given 2 to 3 months before the anticipated exposure, and the tuberculin skin test is repeated 2 to 3 months after vaccination. If the skin test shows a negative reaction, the BCG vaccination should be repeated.

Adverse Reactions. Adverse reactions vary according to the vaccine strain. The product licensed for use in the United States has a 1% to 10% rate of adverse effects, the most common being ulceration at the vaccination site and regional lymphadenitis.

Efficacy. *BCG has proved effective in preventing clinical tuberculosis among selected infants at great risk for becoming infected with the tubercle bacillus.* It also is protective for the general population in developing countries where tuberculosis is still prevalent.

Target Population. Infants born to mothers who have active (sputum-positive) tuberculosis are at significant risk of developing disseminated tuberculosis. BCG should be given to any such infant, who should be separated from the mother until she has had adequate treatment. Infants and children who have repeated exposure to individuals who have multidrug-resistant tuberculosis also should be considered for immunization. A diligent effort should be made to identify any other infected persons in the infant's environment so that they also can be "separated" and treated. The vaccinated infant should remain separated from any infected person until the patient's sputum is negative for the tubercle bacillus or until the infant's tuberculin skin test (PPD) shows an antibody response to BCG vaccination.

Individuals whose PPD test results are negative and people likely to enter areas where repeated exposure to untreated tuberculosis is probable are candidates for BCG vaccine. The latter category would include Peace Corps families, some military families, some missionary families, and health care professionals working in certain areas of the world.

Contraindications. BCG should not be given to immunocompromised individuals. Pregnancy, burns, and skin infections also are specific contraindications to BCG immunization.

The duration of tuberculin skin test positivity after BCG vaccination is unknown. Consequently, a positive reaction to PPD after BCG vaccination may be confusing. If a person vaccinated with BCG has a large skin reaction that is compatible with exposure to tuberculosis, the reaction should be interpreted as being disease related and should not be attributed to the BCG vaccination.

Typhoid Immunization

The remarkable decline in the incidence of typhoid fever in the United States is the result of general public health measures such as good plumbing and a clean water supply and is not attributable to the typhoid vaccine.

Vaccine. Killed typhoid vaccines produce significant antibody titers in 70% to 80% of those immunized. These antibody titers are protective against a small inoculum of *Salmonella typhi,* but a large inoculum can easily overcome the resistance of immunized individuals. Moreover, the vaccines regularly produce local pain, regional adenopathy, and systemic reactions of significant fever and malaise.

Target Population. *Because of its limited protection and frequent untoward side effects, typhoid vaccine rarely is recommended.* It may be used in community or institutional outbreaks of typhoid fever and in individuals who have intimate exposure to typhoid carriers.

Cholera Immunization

The risk of cholera to those who travel to endemic areas is small. Even so, the best protection is to avoid any potentially contaminated water or food; the *currently available vaccines are not very effective.*

Target Population. The cholera vaccine is recommended only for individuals required to show evidence of cholera vaccination to gain entrance to a specific country. A single primary immunization (0.2 ml for children 1 to 5 years of age, 0.3 ml for those 5 to 10 years of age, and 0.5 ml for those over age 10) is sufficient to satisfy regulations.

FUTURE VACCINE DEVELOPMENT

The conjugation technology so successfully used in *Haemophilus influenzae* type b (Hib) vaccines is being applied to other bacteria that have polysaccharide capsules such as *Streptococcus pneumoniae* and *Neisseria meningitidis.* A conjugated pneumococcal vaccine very likely will be licensed soon. Its public health implications are as dramatic as the recent Hib vaccine experience.

Other new and improved vaccines on the short-term and long-term horizons include those for hepatitis A, typhoid, cholera, shigella, enterotoxigenic *Escherichia coli,* tetravalent rotavirus, respiratory syncytial virus, influenza and parainfluenza viruses, group B streptococcus, herpes virus types 1 and 2, *Borrelia borgdorferi* (Lyme disease), maleria, and *Mycobacterium tuberculosis.*[3] A vaccine to prevent HIV infection will take longer to develop than most of these, despite our tremendous investment in it.

We can look forward to new combinations of live vaccines (MMR + varicella + OPV + tetravalent rotaviruses) and of attenuated vaccines (DPT + Hib + IPV + HBV + selected pneumococcal and meningococcal conjugates).[3]

The Children's Vaccine Initiative (CVI) presented at the 1990 Summit of World Leaders on Children defines a goal of developing a single supervaccine that "could be given orally once at or near birth, provide immunity for life, require no boosters, permit storage without refrigeration, obviate the need for needles and syringes, and protect against as many as 20 diseases at once."[4] CVI, with backing from UNICEF, the World Health Organization, the United Nations Development Program, the World Bank, and the Rockefeller Foundation, plans to effect collaboration in and integration of new vaccine research and development among private manufacturers and national vaccine institutes in developed countries to reach this goal.

REFERENCES

1. Center for Disease Control and Prevention: Tuberculosis morbidity: United States, 1992, *MMWR* 42:696, 1993.
2. Cherry JD et al: Report of the Task Force on Pertussis and Pertussis Immunization, 1988, *Pediatrics* 81 (suppl):939, 1988.
3. Katz SL: Prospects for childhood immunization in the next decade, *Pediatr Ann* 22:733, 1993.
4. Robbins A, Freeman P, Powell KR: International childhood vaccine initiative, *Pediatr Infect Dis J* 12:523, 1993.

SUGGESTED READINGS

Advisory Committee on Immunization Practices (ACIP) U.S. Public Health Service. Recommendations published annually in *Morbidity and Mortality Weekly Report (MMWR).*

Peter G, editor: *1994 Redbook: Report of the Committee on Infectious Diseases,* ed 23, Elk Grove Village, Ill, 1994, American Academy of Pediatrics.

18 Identification of Developmental Delays and the Early Intervention System

Ruth K. Kaminer and Susan Vig

A fundamental screening principle states that positive findings must be followed by appropriate evaluations and treatment. Therefore, when a pediatrician identifies a child who has delayed development, that child needs to be connected to the newly available early intervention system. The importance of early intervention as a national concern has been reflected in recent federal legislation. The Amendments to the Education of the Handicapped Act (Part H of PL 99-457), enacted by Congress in 1986 and subsequently incorporated into the Individuals with Disabilities Education Act (IDEA) of 1989, gave the states the option of participating in the early intervention system, and all 50 states chose to do so. The legislation requires participating states to develop a coordinated, comprehensive, multidisciplinary system of early intervention services for young children (birth to 3 years) and their families.

Key components of the legislation include a definition of developmental delay, a comprehensive child find and referral system, a public awareness program, policy regarding personnel standards, and procedural safeguards to ensure protection of confidentiality and the rights of families to due process. In each state a lead agency is designated to administer, supervise, and monitor early intervention programs and activities; most states have assigned these roles to the Department of Education or the Department of Health. Early intervention legislation requires a comprehensive, multidisciplinary evaluation to determine the needs of children and families. After evaluation, family members and professionals work together to develop an Individualized Family Service Plan (IFSP) that describes services, supports, and coordination of services to be provided for the child and family.

Pediatricians play an important role in this process by identifying and serving children who are developmentally delayed. Good pediatric practice embodies the principles on which the IDEA legislation is based—a family orientation and an awareness of the need to support a child's future independent functioning. Pediatricians have learned that any factor affecting a child's functioning impacts the parents and family, regardless of whether the cause of such limitations is known.

The pediatrician's role in identifying and serving children who are developmentally delayed may be interpreted narrowly or broadly, depending to some extent on the physician's training, interest, and level of comfort (see Chapter 20, Twelve, Developmental Surveillance and Intervention). However, minimal expectations include screening for developmental delays by routinely asking the parents about their concerns during health maintenance visits, judiciously using appropriate, validated screening instruments, and referring children whose development is questionable or delayed for evaluation and services. Routine screening of vision and hearing in preschoolers is an accepted part of health maintenance.

For those pediatricians who have a greater interest in developmental disabilities, other roles include participating with other professionals in multidisciplinary evaluations of the child's delay, helping the parents understand the child's strengths and weaknesses, interpreting medical information for early intervention providers, and monitoring the progress of any interventions. Parents need and value the support of their pediatrician in dealing with the possibility or reality of developmental delay in their child.[2]

Although many pediatricians are actively involved in identifying, evaluating, referring, and managing children who are developmentally delayed, the following barriers, which may prevent some pediatricians from getting involved in these roles, have been noted.

1. *Reluctance to identify developmental delays because the physician has to confront the parents with the possibility of these delays.*

Just as pediatricians share the parents' enjoyment of their children's developmental progress, they share their distress when it becomes necessary to question the adequacy of that progress. Some parents wait for the pediatrician to voice the concerns they have begun to feel, and they interpret the physician's silence as an indication that no problem exists. By routinely questioning parents about development and behavior at all contacts and observing the child's development along with the parent, the pediatrician creates a comfortable atmosphere for discussing concerns identified either by the parents or the pediatrician.

2. *Questioning the efficacy of early intervention.*

A pediatrician who is convinced that early intervention will help a child and family is more likely to try to identify a child who needs this service. Current literature contains well-designed studies documenting the efficacy of early intervention in improving children's developmental outcomes. The Infant Health and Development Program, an extensive eight-site clinical trial for low-birth-weight infants, demonstrated such an impact. Children who had participated for 3 years with their families in this comprehensive early intervention program, which provided health, developmental, and family services, had higher mean IQs and fewer maternally reported behavior problems at corrected age 36 months than controls.[3] Follow-up studies of economically disadvantaged children have shown that daily participation in intensive, center-based early intervention is associated with higher IQ, stronger school achievement, and fewer failing grades at age 12.[4] In general, the best developmental outcomes have been associated with early intervention programs that are comprehensive, involve the family as well as the child, and focus on strengthening the parent-child relationship.[1] The two groups that appear to benefit most are children who have biological risk factors and are growing up in adverse circumstances, and all children who have mild degrees of developmental delay.

3. *Concerns about overidentifying delays, upsetting the family, and subjecting the child to unnecessary evaluations.*

Sensitive exploration of possible delays harms neither the parents nor the child, whereas avoiding the issue may be detrimental. Evaluation is a way of gaining a better understanding of the child and, when necessary, may serve as a ticket into the system of developmental services.

4. *Lack of familiarity with resources and service systems.*

Pediatricians may not have the time to be actively involved in the early intervention system; however, they must inform themselves on how to connect their patients and families to this system so that the children may obtain services to which they are entitled. Literature for patients can be obtained from the state's Part H lead agency and should be available in the pediatrician's office. Most medical school–affiliated pediatrics departments have specialists in developmental disabilities who are a useful resource for evaluation and referral to publicly funded services.

It is painfully common for clinicians evaluating children who have developmental disabilities to hear from parents that the pediatrician reassured them about the child's delay by saying "he'll outgrow it." Although children may outgrow various problems, a physician should always investigate the parents' concerns before reassuring them. Without careful screening and monitoring of the development of all children, only those who have more severe delays are likely to be identified. There is evidence that intervention may make the most critical difference in the development, behavior, and success of children whose delays are mild.

REFERENCES

1. Bennett FC, Guralnick MJ: Effectiveness of developmental intervention in the first five years of life, *Pediatr Clin North Am* 38:1513, 1991.
2. Committee on Children with Disabilities, American Academy of Pediatrics: Pediatrician's role in the development and implementation of an Individualized Education Plan (IEP) and/or an Individualized Family Service Plan (IFSP), *Pediatrics* 89:340, 1992.
3. The Infant Health and Development Program: Enhancing the outcomes of low-birth-weight, premature infants, a multisite, randomized trial, *JAMA* 263:3035, 1990.
4. Ramey CT, Ramey SL: Effective early intervention, *Ment Retard* 30:337, 1992.

19 Language and Speech Assessment

Hiram L. McDade and Elaine M. Frank

Each child who enters school is assumed to possess a fully developed system of spoken language skills, and this system is the foundation for teaching higher levels of communication. The late talker, the 3-year-old whose speech is unintelligible, or the child who has a limited vocabulary or word-finding difficulties invariably becomes conspicuous again when he or she needs special assistance in reading, spelling, writing, and mathematics. Often, early remedial services are not provided for these children because of a "wait and see" attitude among health professionals. Actually, Johnny, who didn't begin talking until he was 2 years old and whose speech could not be understood until he was 4 years old, never outgrew his problem. It simply was manifested in other channels of language learning. The literature is compelling regarding the relationship between failure in reading and writing in the primary grades and a history of earlier communication difficulties.[1,7] In fact, of the various skills assessed on standardized intelligence tests, the items most predictive of later academic performance are language based. For this very reason, assessment of any child's readiness for school must give primary consideration to the adequacy of his or her general communicative abilities.

HEARING ASSESSMENT

Because normal speech and language development require an intact auditory system, a hearing assessment is an integral part of any developmental screening. It should be noted, however, that children who have recurrent otitis media frequently pass pure-tone screenings for two reasons: (1) the resultant hearing loss usually is intermittent, and (2) the test signals often are presented at increased levels to compensate for the noise level of the examination room. Thus, hearing screenings are inadequate follow-up procedures for children who have been diagnosed as having persistent or serious otitis media. Such children require full audiological testing.[3] More recently, tympanometry has become a routine component of hearing assessments.[4] Coupled with the results of a pure-tone screening, tympanograms help identify a potential conductive component (middle ear problems) that otherwise might be missed.

SPEECH AND LANGUAGE DEVELOPMENT

As in other developmental areas, obtaining a thorough history is an important step in assessing a child's oral communication skills. Because the emergence of certain critical speech and language abilities follows a relatively stable timetable, a child's competency may be compared with these norms, either by history or by direct observation. The purpose of such "screenings" (formal or informal) is not to diagnose but to identify those in need of further testing. Consequently, children who fail to measure up to normative data should be referred to a speech-language pathologist. Such a referral provides two benefits: (1) children found to be deficient in speech and language abilities are assured early intervention, and (2) children whose developmental status remains uncertain may be reassessed at appropriate intervals. For the latter group, the evaluation provides objective baseline data that allow the examiner to measure the child's rates of progress over time.

The acquisition of first words (at approximately 12 months of age) is the initial evidence of a child's language development. In general, children who are still nonverbal at 18 months of age should be referred for further testing.[2] However, a word of caution about the achievement of this developmental milestone: in their eagerness for and anticipation of the child's development of speech, parents frequently interpret the utterances "mama" and "dada" as meaningful words. These vocalizations usually are merely a function of the child's advanced babbling stage, and if the examiner accepts them as words, a spuriously low age level will be assigned to the acquisition of first words (e.g., 6 or 8 months). For this reason, more detailed information should be obtained by asking the parents how old their child was when he or she spoke first words other than "mama" or "dada."

The emergence of two-word phrases is a significant milestone in language learning. It is at this stage that the rudimentary rules of grammar are first evidenced. The term *grammar* here refers to (1) syntax, or the rules that govern how words may be combined to form phrases and sentences, and (2) morphology, which determines how the sounds that make up a word may be altered to modify its meaning, such as plural, possession, and verb tense.[2] As a child develops the ability to combine words (through the acquisition of syntax), the meaning of each utterance becomes more apparent, making the child a better communicator. Normal children as young as 18 months of age begin producing two-word combinations. A child who has failed to achieve this milestone by 24 months of age should be referred for further testing.

By age 3, most children have a spoken vocabulary of more than 500 words. In addition, their grammatical skills have developed to the point where they routinely speak in three- and four-word sentences. At this age the basic rules of morphology are fine tuned. Plural, possessive, and past tense forms of words are beginning to be mastered, and use of pronouns such as I, me, you, and mine is common. Three-year-olds demonstrate an appropriate understanding of *why* questions, indicating an appreciation of cause and effect. The speech of a 3-year-old is highly intelligible, and despite frequent mispronunciations, a stranger has no difficulty understanding the child. In short, 3-year-olds have the capacity to carry on a reasonable conversation with an adult.[6]

The language of 4-year-olds approaches adult competency

with respect to grammatical skills. Unlike 2- and 3-year-olds, 4-year-olds speak in complete sentences. Rarely are words omitted from the four- and five-word sentences that these children typically produce. Although 4-year-olds do not have as many different ways to say the same things as do older children, they usually have at least one way to express all thoughts and desires. The vocabulary of a 4-year-old also is quite extensive. By this age most children can recognize and name several colors, count to 10 by rote, understand the prepositions in, on, under, beside, in front, and in back (but not behind until age 5), and answer complex questions, such as "How much?" "How long?" and "What if . . . ?"

By age 5, children have developed most of the language-based concepts that are important for schooling. They can sort and classify objects by category, name all the basic colors, and understand the concept of time (which allows them to answer *when* questions) and the concept of numbers up to 10 integers. Their articulation skills also are developed fully by age 5. Any residual mispronunciations at this point represent disordered speech and should prompt immediate referral to a speech-language pathologist (see Chapter 90).

INTELLIGIBILITY OF SPEECH

In the course of normal development, it is common for children to mispronounce certain sounds or to have difficulty producing particular words. The mastery of sounds in the language is a gradual process that takes place over a period of 3 to 4 years. Unfortunately, many children whose speech is disordered are not identified as such until later years because their deviant articulation patterns occur during a time when adults expect a certain amount of mispronunciation. There are differences, however, between normal and disordered speech, even as early as 2 to 3 years of age. Our tolerance for mispronunciations during this developmental period often prevents us from discerning these differences. The speech-language pathologist is trained specifically to determine if the pattern of misarticulation exhibited by a particular patient is common for normal children or indicates disordered speech and, thus, is not likely to be self-corrected.

One important factor the health professional must consider is the child's intelligibility. Young children who are acquiring a sound system normally are understood easily, despite their frequent misarticulations.[6] That is, regardless of the conspicuousness of their speech errors, normal children have little trouble communicating, even with unfamiliar listeners. In contrast, a child who is unintelligible, or whose parents report difficulty understanding his or her speech, is exhibiting a pattern of misarticulation that is not part of normal development.[2] Such a child is less likely to outgrow the problem and thus requires thorough evaluation to determine the need for speech therapy.

ACQUIRED SPEECH AND LANGUAGE DISORDERS IN CHILDREN

Acquired brain injury in children and adolescents may result in significant speech or language dysfunction. Acquired communication disorders frequently occur secondary to an open or closed traumatic brain injury (TBI), anoxia, or cerebral infection. TBI is by far the leading cause of brain injury among children; each year, 150,000 to 200,000 children are hospitalized for this condition. Falls are the most common cause of injury, followed by bicycle accidents, motor vehicle accidents, and child abuse. Open head injuries from gunshot wounds have increased among children and adolescents.[5] Among children who have a TBI, studies have reported a high rate of risk taking, limited judgment, and learning problems. Contrary to previous thought, young children (birth to age 4) who experience a brain injury have a poorer prognosis for normal communicative function than school-age children or adolescents. A brain injury often interferes with acquisition of new knowledge and skills. Older children have the advantage of knowledge acquired before the brain injury.[8]

TBI can result in a focal or, more often, diffuse brain injury (see Chapter 282). TBI often results in sequelae involving language problems, which may include disorganized, tangential, wandering discourse, imprecise language, word retrieval difficulties, disinhibited, socially inappropriate language, ineffective use of contextual cues, restricted output and lack of initiation, difficulty comprehending extended language in spoken or written form, difficulty detecting main ideas, difficulty following rapidly spoken language, difficulty understanding abstract language, including indirect or implied meaning, and inefficient verbal learning due to reduced memory ability.[8] Because these problems are different from the grammatical difficulties typical of children who have developmental problems, they frequently are misunderstood and not seen as being symptomatic of a language disorder. Speech disturbances can include apraxic speech, characterized by difficulty initiating and programming speech, or dysarthric speech due to paralysis or paresis of oral or pharyngeal musculature.

Standardized testing may not be sensitive to the communicative-intellectual effects of TBI. Insightful clinical evaluation of speech and language function is essential in determining the need for rehabilitative or specialized educational intervention. Although a positive correlation between initial indices of severity (including the Glasgow coma scale and the length of coma) and the long-term outcome is relatively strong, individual outcomes may vary. Children who have a mild head injury and only a short-term loss of consciousness may require minimal medical intervention but still may experience interruption in normal cognitive functioning. Behavioral changes, including easy fatigability, inconsistent performance, and slow processing, often are evident. Children who have a more severe head injury may require intensive speech and language inpatient rehabilitation and outpatient follow-up.

Therapeutic intervention goals may be rehabilitative or compensatory. Rehabilitation of attention, awareness, perception, memory, learning, organization, social cognition, problem solving, and general executive system functioning are necessary for cognitive processing and language functioning. Compensatory techniques may include memory devices, organizational patterning, or referent cues. Stimulating speech programming and muscular strengthening may improve oral communication, or compensatory techniques may be required in the form of augmentative communicative devices (e.g., communication boards or computerized speech). Successful educational reentry for children who have a TBI should include assistance in school programming and inservice for family, teachers, other school personnel, and the child's peers. Children whose TBI is significant will need continued monitoring through successive developmental stages to achieve maximum functional ability and academic success.

REFERENCES

1. Aram D, Ekelman B, Nation J: Preschoolers with language disorders: 10 years later, *J Speech Hear Res* 27:232, 1984.
2. Berko Gleason J: *The development of language,* New York, 1993, Macmillan.
3. Bess F: *Audiology: the fundamentals,* Baltimore, 1990, Williams & Wilkins.
4. Martin F: *Introduction to audiology,* ed 4, Englewood Cliffs, NJ, 1991, Prentice-Hall.
5. National Institute of Disability and Rehabilitation Research: National Pediatric Trauma Registry: a progress report, *Rehabilitation Update* Summer/Fall, 1993.
6. Owens R: *Language development,* ed 3, Columbus, Ohio, 1992, Merrill.
7. Silva P, Williams S, McGee R: A longitudinal study of children with developmental language delay at age three: later intelligence, reading and behavior problems, *Dev Med Child Neurol* 29:630, 1987.
8. Ylvisaker M: Communication outcome following traumatic brain injury, *Seminars in Speech and Language* 13:239, 1992.

20 Screening

ONE

General Considerations

Paul H. Dworkin

By virtue of their access to young children and families, pediatric providers are well positioned to participate in the early detection of childhood problems and conditions. Within the context of child health supervision, screening refers to the process of testing whole populations of children at various set ages to detect those at high risk for significant, unexpected deviations from normal. The emphasis is on distinguishing between children at high and low risk for certain problems, rather than on diagnosing such conditions; this typically involves the application of rapidly administered tests, examinations, or other procedures.

During the past decade, several factors have contributed to an increase in the number of conditions for which screening is recommended or mandated. Research has better delineated the adverse effects of certain childhood conditions, such as the neurobehavioral and intellectual deficits associated with moderate lead poisoning and iron deficiency anemia. Technological advances, such as the development of automated equipment to measure auditory brainstem response for the diagnosis of hearing loss in young infants, have enabled affected individuals to be distinguished more effectively from those nonaffected following an abnormal screening test. Changing morbidity within pediatric practice has emphasized the importance of the early identification of behavioral, developmental, and psychosocial problems and suggests the need for revised screening policies for certain conditions such as tuberculosis. Societal changes, including demands for confidentiality of test results, concerns with the stigma associated with certain diagnoses, and legislative mandates requiring early intervention for children who have developmental problems and other chronic conditions, have influenced the scope and content of screening programs. The continuing debate over health care reform, with its emphasis both on primary prevention and cost containment, has contributed to an increased scrutiny of screening practices.

Despite the time-honored tradition of performing screening tests during child health supervision visits, the effectiveness of many such practices is uncertain. The U.S. Congress Office of Technology Assessment, in a critical review of the value of child health supervision services, concluded that the only cost-effective and cost-saving screening procedure is newborn testing for metabolic disorders.[13] Because recommendations for screening practices typically are determined by a combination of limited scientific data, empiricism, and good intentions, they often provoke considerable debate. Recent examples include the 1991 recommendation by the Centers for Disease Control and Prevention that blood lead screening be performed for all 1-year-old and probably all 2-year-old children,[2] the 1993 recommendation of the U.S. Department of Health and Human Services that all infants should be screened for sickle cell disease regardless of race or ethnic background,[11] and the 1993 National Institutes of Health Consensus Statement, which recommended screening of all infants for hearing impairment within the first 3 months of life and preferably before discharge from the hospital newborn nursery.[9]

The goal of this chapter is to review the criteria by which conditions are judged appropriate for screening and tests are selected for use in screening programs. Examples of screening recommendations that have generated debate and controversy will illustrate the extent to which conditions and tests fulfill such criteria. In addition, screening will be compared with other approaches to early detection during child health supervision services.

CRITERIA FOR CONDITIONS TO BE SCREENED

Conditions are judged appropriate for the screening process if they fulfill certain well-accepted criteria:

1. *The condition must have significant morbidity or mortality with serious consequences if not detected early on and remediated.* Recommendations for universal lead screening have been supported by evidence that some adverse effects may occur at blood lead (BPb) levels as low as 10 μg/dl in children. (However, critics of universal screening emphasize that there is no conclusive evidence that BPb levels less than 20 μg/dl at age 1 year cause a clinically important decrease in intelligence and an increase in behavioral problems by the time of school entry.) The adverse effects of early sensorineural hearing loss on language development and subsequent academic achievement and on social and emotional development are cited to support recommendations for universal screening for hearing impairment among infants.
2. *The condition must be sufficiently prevalent to justify the cost of screening programs.* Determining the true prevalence of certain conditions is difficult. For example, recommendations for universal lead screening were influenced by data indicating that 17% of all American preschool children have BPb levels greater than 15 μg/dl. However, more recent surveys from various parts of the country found that 2% to 10% of children have BPb levels greater than 10 μg/dl.[5]
3. *The screening program must include the entire population, especially those at particular risk for the condition.* Screening programs optimally are implemented within a comprehensive system of preventive child health care directed at the entire population. The lack of access of many young children and families to child health supervision services and a medical home is well recognized. Disadvantaged children at increased risk for conditions such as iron deficiency anemia, lead poisoning, and tuberculosis are less likely to receive recom-

mended screening tests because of their limited access to health care.

4. *Diagnostic tests must enable affected individuals to be distinguished from nonaffected persons or those who are "borderline."* Screening should be performed only for conditions that can be diagnosed with certainty. Concerning universal screening for hearing impairment in infants, some have criticized the test that measures evoked otoacoustic emissions (EOAEs) because the diagnostic auditory brainstem response (ABR) equipment available in hospitals often is difficult to operate and is time consuming, and test results are often difficult to interpret.[1]
5. *The condition, after detection, must be treatable or controllable.* Developmental screening is based on the premise that identification will result in intervention that will benefit the child. Although the benefits of early intervention for children who have physical handicaps (e.g., sensory impairment, Down syndrome, cerebral palsy) or marked cognitive impairment are reasonably well established, there is only limited evidence to support the benefits of early identification and intervention for young children who have learning disabilities, mild mental retardation, and delayed speech or language. Although blood lead can be reduced by house dust control, whether such intervention benefits children who have initial BPb levels less than 20 μg/dl is uncertain.
6. *Detection and treatment during the asymptomatic stage must improve prognosis, and early treatment must have significant advantage.* Newborn screening for phenylketonuria (PKU) clearly is beneficial in that early treatment prevents later brain damage and neurological impairment. Similarly, prophylactic penicillin has been shown clearly to reduce both morbidity and mortality from pneumococcal infections in infants who have sickle cell anemia. Screening for cystic fibrosis has been supported by evidence that treatment before the development of severe pulmonary disease may increase the chance of survival.
7. *Adequate resources must be available for the definitive diagnosis and treatment of disorders identified by screening.* A major criticism of the Early Periodic Screening, Diagnosis and Treatment (EPSDT) component of Medicaid has been the failure to ensure that all children whose findings on screening are suspect receive appropriate diagnostic and treatment services. The lack of adequate diagnostic and therapeutic resources for developmental, behavioral, and psychosocial problems hampers efforts at early identification. Universal screening for hearing impairment in infants is problematic because follow-up diagnostic testing and treatment of hearing loss are difficult to carry out in rural or remote areas.
8. *The cost of screening must be outweighed by the savings in suffering and alternative expenditure that would occur if the condition were not diagnosed until the symptomatic stage.* Costs of screening programs must include not only the direct cost of the procedures themselves but also the cost of diagnostic evaluation, monitoring, and intervention as a consequence of screening, as well as the costs of false positive and false negative results. For example, the cost of universal screening for hearing impairment in infants has been estimated to be \$200 million per year.[1] In contrast, the lifetime economic cost of a single case of congenital deafness is estimated to exceed \$1 million.[10] Screening for developmental delay defies simple cost-benefit analysis, and the cost of screening has yet to be justified by either the savings in alternative expenditures (such as special educational programs or services) or a quantifiable lessening of anxiety or suffering. Furthermore, such screening is not without risks, such as the dangers of labeling and creating a self-fulfilling prophecy.

CRITERIA FOR SCREENING TESTS

There also are widely accepted criteria by which specific tests are judged appropriate for use in screening programs:

1. *Tests must be simple, practical, convenient, and safe.* That newborn babies who have cystic fibrosis have abnormally high levels of immunoreactive trypsin (IRT) in serum has been the basis for a screening test for this disorder. The relative ease and simplicity of performing EOAE testing facilitates universal screening for hearing impairment in infants. However, the decrease in specificity of this test during the first 48 hours of life poses logistical problems in that hospital discharge could be delayed.
2. *Tests must be acceptable, with assurance of informed parental consent and confidentiality of findings.* Children should not be subjected to screening procedures without prior parental approval. Informed parental consent includes a discussion of potential false positive and false negative findings, the possible need for time-consuming and often expensive follow-up evaluations, and the anxiety generated by positive screening results. Confidentiality of screening results must be maintained because positive findings for disorders such as HIV infection and sickle cell disease may be socially stigmatizing and result in discrimination by insurance companies and potential employers.
3. *Tests must be accurate and reliable.* Although anodic stripping voltimetry and graphite furnace atomic absorption spectroscopy may yield BPb results having a ± 4 μg/dl accuracy, some 10% to 20% of clinical laboratories do not meet proficiency standards.[5] Furthermore, capillary screening may include skin contamination that falsely elevates BPb. Although a wide variety of developmental screening tests are used in health programs during infancy and early childhood, all suffer to varying degrees from problems of reliability and validity and from the need for well-established norms. The validity of screening tests consists of two components: sensitivity, the proportion of individuals who have a disorder whose test result is positive; and specificity, the proportion of individuals who haven't the disorder whose test is negative. Of particular clinical importance is the probability of an individual having the disorder when the test is positive—the test's positive predictive value—as well as the probability of not having the disorder when the test is negative—negative predictive value. The predictive value of a test depends greatly on

the prevalence of the disorder in the population being tested. The low prevalence of approximately 1 of every 1000 newborns being born deaf contributes to the reported low specificity and positive predictive value of ABR and EOAE testing.[1]

4. *Tests should be economical.* The costs of newborn screening for metabolic disorders such as congenital hypothyroidism, galactosemia, and maple syrup urine disease are minimal because such tests are incorporated within established screening programs for PKU. The cost of screening for such rare disorders in isolation would be prohibitive.
5. *Tests should lend themselves to easy interpretation.* Screening test results may be complex. For example, reports of screening for sickle cell disease should include the hemoglobin phenotype and the diagnostic possibilities associated with the phenotype. The screening program must ensure the availability of appropriate education and genetic counseling for parents. The test results from ABR equipment available in hospitals for screening for hearing impairment in infants may be difficult to interpret, even by trained professionals.

ALTERNATIVE APPROACHES TO EARLY DETECTION

Early detection is considered desirable for certain conditions that do not fulfill criteria for screening. For example, neither the types of developmental delays for which screening is performed nor the screening tests themselves fulfill standard criteria for acceptance.[3] Nonetheless, early identification of and intervention for developmental delays are goals of child health supervision. Alternative approaches to early detection should be considered for such conditions.

Selective Screening

Selective as opposed to universal screening may be performed for certain conditions. For example, reported differences in BPb levels between children living in urban and suburban areas have been cited to support a strategy of geographical targeting.[5] An alternative approach to selective lead screening is the use of a five-item questionnaire to identify children who are at increased risk and therefore should receive BPb testing.[2]

Screening programs may target a specific racial or ethnic group that has an increased prevalence of a particular disorder. For example, screening programs for Tay-Sachs disease target Ashkenazi Jews. However, selective screening undoubtedly will fail to identify certain affected individuals. For example, screening programs targeting a specific racial or ethnic group will not identify all infants who have sickle cell disease because it is not possible to define reliably an individual's racial or ethnic background by surname, self-report, or physical characteristics. Because prophylactic administration of penicillin has been demonstrated to reduce morbidity and mortality in children who have sickle cell anemia, universal screening of all newborns is recommended, regardless of race or ethnic background.[11]

High Risk Register

The Joint Committee on Infant Hearing has favored the use of a register to identify infants at risk for hearing impairment.[7] The Registry lists those conditions that place a newborn at increased risk for hearing loss, for example, a family history of hearing loss, anomalies of the head and neck, and a birthweight less than 1500 g. Listing these high-risk factors in the form of a questionnaire and asking parents to complete the form after delivery may be followed by ABR screening for infants considered at risk.

Questionnaires

A limited number of questionnaires have been developed to aid in the early detection of children's behavioral, emotional, and psychosocial problems. Parents may be asked to complete these brief questionnaires before meeting with the pediatric provider. Examples include the Pediatric Symptom Checklist (PSC), designed for screening the emotional well-being of school-age children in pediatric practice,[6] and a self-administered questionnaire for structured psychosocial screening.[8] Results from small-scale validation studies have been encouraging and suggest that such questionnaires deserve further study to assess their value in pediatric office practice.

Surveillance

The approach currently practiced by primary care pediatricians to the early detection of developmental problems is most consistent with the process termed "developmental surveillance." Surveillance is a flexible, continuous process whereby knowledgeable professionals observe children during the provision of child health supervision.[3] The components of developmental surveillance include eliciting and attending to parents' concerns, obtaining a relevant developmental history, observing children accurately and informatively, and sharing opinions and concerns with other relevant professionals, such as preschool teachers. Parent-completed developmental questionnaires, such as the Infant and Child Monitoring Questionnaires, also may be used to involve parents in the monitoring of their infants' and childrens' development.[12] To improve the accuracy of surveillance, pediatric providers may choose to supplement their subjective impressions occasionally by administering a test such as the Denver II, or may selectively use a test such as a "second-stage" screening instrument when suspicions arise.[4]

TWO

The Physical Examination as a Screening Test

Robert A. Hoekelman

The physical examination is a composite of individual screening tests that assess the structure and, in part, the function of the human body. It includes a series of specific measurements, as well as many objective observations, that the examiner makes by using the senses of sight, smell, hearing, touch, and, occasionally, taste. Judgments as to the normality or abnormality of these measurements and observations are then made on the basis of predetermined standards. The methodology for conducting the physical examination and some of the standards of normality are discussed in Chapter 7, The Pediatric Physical Examination.

When performed on a healthy child as part of a well visit, the physical examination is more of a screening test than it is when it is performed as one aspect of the evaluation of a specific complaint. The physical examination is an extremely sensitive and specific screening test for some conditions (e.g., strabismus, umbilical hernia, and dental caries), but not for most others. The yield from all or parts of the physical examination varies with the prevalence of abnormal conditions in the population screened. For instance, tonometric and proctoscopic examinations are not performed for infants and children except under unusual circumstances, whereas auscultation of the heart and lungs and otoscopic examination are performed routinely.

In the screening of healthy children, certain parts of the physical examination ordinarily need to be performed only once to determine the presence or absence of a specific condition (e.g., undescended testicle, choanal atresia, or color blindness). Once height, weight, head circumference, and blood pressure initially have been determined to be in the normal range for the infant's or child's age, they are highly unlikely to become abnormal without specific signs or symptoms that bring the child to the physician's attention. Nevertheless, they need to be measured periodically. Other procedures, however, do require repeated performance inasmuch as illnesses are acquired and many congenital or genetically determined conditions may not be evident on examinations performed early in life (e.g., pyloric stenosis, scoliosis, patent ductus arteriosus, and Marfan syndrome). Indeed, a normal finding may be only an assurance of normality for very brief periods (e.g., absence of an abdominal mass, presence of normal mobility of the tympanic membrane, or normal skin turgor).

There is a yield from the physical examination beyond the determination of normality or abnormality. Certain benefits accrue from "a laying on of hands" in terms of strengthening the physician-patient-parent relationship. The thoroughness, deftness, gentleness, and consideration shown to the patient by the physician in conducting the examination can be as reassuring as the results of the examination itself.

Pronouncement by the physician that the examination results show no negative findings and the child is normal may lead the parents to sense that all is well even though many aspects of health and normality have not been confirmed simply by the child's "passing" a physical examination. Periodic examinations also may lead the parents to cease using their own powers of observation and judgment regarding their children's health and often to delay seeking care for observed deviations from normal because the examination is scheduled in the near future. On the other hand, parents may misinterpret the meaning of variations in normal findings discovered in the routine physical examination (e.g., the innocent heart murmur), which can cause undue alarm and far-reaching consequences.

The actual yield of abnormal findings (not known to be present beforehand) on routine, periodic physical examinations of presumably well children is extremely small (1.5% in infants during their first year,[1] 2.5% in preschool children,[5] and 4% in primary school children[10] and high school students[9]). Because most of these findings are minor and can be detected by other means, periodic routine physical examinations of well children is considered to be an inefficient use of medical personnel and of little value from a case-finding (screening) perspective.[3,6]

Many of the elements of the physical examination—specifically, determination of height, weight, head circumference, vital signs, and hearing and visual acuity—involve measurements that physicians usually delegate to others. These are apt to yield more in terms of early detection of disease than are the remaining elements of the physical examination. However, specific conditions at certain ages might go unrecognized by parents or teachers or might remain undiscovered through routine screening measures but are detectable on the physical examination:

Cataract
Congenital heart disease
Congenital hip dysplasia
Cryptorchism
Genetic syndromes
Glaucoma
Lymphadenopathy
Scoliosis
Strabismus
Tumors (benign and malignant)

Screening generally is believed to be important in two of these conditions: congenital hip dysplasia (CHD) during infancy and scoliosis during late childhood and early adolescence. However, a study conducted in Birmingham, England, casts serious doubts on the effectiveness of screening for CHD in terms of reducing the frequency of late discovery and poor outcome of the anomaly; it suggests that the screening tests used (the Barlow and Ortolani maneuvers) and early management of "unstable" hips by holding them in an extended and flexed position may in themselves cause CHD.[7] Studies of ultrasound screening for CHD among newborns who have repeat ultrasonographic examination throughout infancy indicate that the Barlow and Ortolani maneuvers can lead to false negative results and that positive ultrasound results in the neonatal period are not highly predictive of eventual CHD requiring treatment.[2]

Although screening for scoliosis has a low yield—2 in 100 children require follow-up and 2 in 1000 require active treatment[8]—it generally is regarded as a cost-effective screening test despite the large numbers of children who are referred, on the basis of screening, for radiographic assessment and orthopedic consultation. The use of moiré topography (a photographic technique that defines the body contours) as a secondary screening procedure may reduce the number of these referrals.[4]

For the 10 diagnoses listed above and the amount of medical time spent on the physical examination, we need to ask two questions. First, in which of these 10 conditions will waiting until signs and symptoms of the disease become evident to the parents, with the ensuing delay in making the diagnosis, change the outcome? Second, can those elements of the physical examination that must be performed to detect these conditions be taught adequately to persons other than physicians, that is, in a way that ensures a sufficiently high degree of sensitivity and specificity?

The frequency with which physical examinations for purposes of screening need to be performed in infants and children should reflect the risk of abnormality that each child runs. That risk is determined by a number of variables that must be assessed by the physician. The risk is not the same for all children; therefore the scheduling of physical examinations for the purpose of screening depends on the patient.

For the well child at low risk, "screening" physical examinations probably need to be performed only at birth, 1 and 6 months, and 1, 2, 5, 10, and 14 years of age.

THREE

Recognition of Genetic-Metabolic Diseases by Clinical Diagnosis and Screening

Neil A. Holtzman and Nancy E. Braverman

Rapid progress in mapping disease-related genes to specific chromosomes and identifying the disease-causing mutations has increased the number of single-gene (mendelian) disorders for which genetic testing is available. Many of these tests will be used only when clinical suspicion is aroused. Prompt diagnosis is important for two reasons. First, early therapy will result in a better outcome for a number of conditions. Therapeutic interventions are now available for some genetic disorders. Second, diagnosis is followed by genetic counseling, which informs parents about recurrence risk and future reproductive options. In the first part of this chapter, we consider early clinical manifestations of inherited metabolic disorders and how they should be evaluated by primary care providers. In the second part, we consider population-wide screening, that is, testing without regard to occurrence in a family.

SUSPECTING METABOLIC DISEASE

Although the inborn errors of metabolism individually are rare, their collective incidence is not: about 1 in 1000 live births and about 1 in 5 sick full-term newborns who have no risk factors for infection and 1 in 100 children who have a serious medical problem will have a metabolic disease.[4,28] Thus, over the course of practice, a pediatrician can expect to see several patients who have these disorders. The primary care physician often will be the first person to evaluate these children and should be familiar with the clinical presentations and how to proceed with the initial laboratory evaluation. Formal diagnosis and treatment usually are done in consultation with a specialist.

The first disorders of metabolism to be discovered were specific enzyme defects in major catabolic or biosynthetic pathways in cells. Their symptoms result from the buildup of toxic precursors and/or the inability to produce a necessary product. Occasionally the defects were found to involve cofactors, such as certain vitamins. With recent advances in understanding cellular processes, we are recognizing defects in transport proteins,[20] membrane proteins,[16] organelle assembly,[39] intracellular processing and trafficking of molecules,[33] and many other biological processes that result in biochemical disturbances with clinical expression. A scheme for classifying these disorders is presented in Table 20-1.

Diagnostic suspicion that a patient has a metabolic disorder does not require comprehensive knowledge of the various biochemical pathways involved. Such disorders have typical clinical presentations, specific historical clues, and pertinent findings on clinical examination that should lead to their consideration. Some of the laboratory tests that are taken routinely in ill children can help to determine the presence of metabolic disease.

Characteristic Presentations

Many common pediatric illnesses present with similar symptoms. Such high-risk scenarios are considered by symptom complex and age in this section and in Table 20-2. Unfortunately, metabolic disease often is not considered until other disorders are excluded. Diagnostic delay is particularly common for metabolic disorders with a nonacute presentation, especially when slow development is the major initial finding. For optimal outcomes, metabolic disease should be included in the earliest differential diagnosis.

Acute or Recurrent Episodes of Illness. Serious acute illness in a previously well newborn or recurrent episodes of illness in a child are classic presentations of metabolic disease. The disorders characterizing this group include aminoacidopathies, organic acidemias, urea cycle defects, disorders of fatty acid oxidation, and carbohydrate metabolism.

NEONATAL PRESENTATIONS. Sudden deterioration of a full-term normal neonate within the first few days of life is a hallmark of metabolic disease. Many infants remain symptom-free for the first 24 hours of life. When feeding begins, toxic metabolites accumulate, vomiting may occur, and the infant becomes increasingly lethargic. Neurological abnormalities, respiratory distress, and shock highlight the progression of many severe illnesses in a neonate, who has a limited repertoire of responses. The differential diagnosis often includes sepsis, congenital heart disease, neurological insults, gastrointestinal obstruction, and metabolic disease. The provider should pay particular attention to the possibility of metabolic disease when risk factors for infection are absent or when the infant deteriorates in spite of antibiotic therapy. The documentation of infection, however, or cardiomyopathy or brain abnormalities does not exclude underlying metabolic disease. Serious infection occurs in metabolically debilitated patients; for example, untreated infants who have galactosemia are at higher risk for developing *Escherichia coli* sepsis.[41] Cardiomyopathies develop in several categories of metabolic disease and may present during infancy.[60] Metabolic crisis may result in diffuse cerebral swelling and stroke. Seizure activity predominates in certain disorders, and others are associated with developmental brain abnormalities.[59]

Some disorders (peroxisomal defects, disorders of pyruvate metabolism, and respiratory chain defects) present within the first 24 hours of life. They may be associated with dysmorphic features and congenital abnormalities. Hydrops is an unusual presentation of some lysosomal storage diseases.[69]

The infant who has a metabolic disorder also may present less fulminantly within the first few months of life with poor feeding, recurrent vomiting, and generalized hypotonia. In one third of patients who have inborn errors of metabolism, disease does not become apparent clinically until childhood or even later.

LATE-ONSET PRESENTATIONS. These are more variable and frequently involve precipitating factors. Associated findings of poor growth, developmental delay, or other underlying chronic abnormalities may be present, but illness due to a metabolic disorder also can occur acutely in a previously well

Table 20-1 Classification of Genetic-Metabolic Disorders

Biochemical pathways	Subgroups	Examples
Amino acid catabolism		Phenylketonuria, homocystinuria, tyrosinemia, maple syrup urine disease, nonketotic hyperglycinemia
	Amino acid transport	Lysinuric protein intolerance, cystinuria
	Urea cycle disorders	Ornithine transcarbamylase deficiency (X-linked), citrullinemia, arginosuccinic aciduria
Organic acid metabolism		Propionic acidemia, methylmalonic acidemia, isovaleric acidemia, glutaric acidemia 1, biotinidase deficiency
Fatty acid oxidation		SCAD, MCAD, LCAD
	Fatty acid transport disorders	Carnitine transport defect, carnitine palmitoyl transferase deficiencies
Carbohydrate metabolism	Carbohydrate intolerances	Galactosemia, hereditary fructose intolerance
	Disorders of glycogen breakdown (glycogen storage disorders)	*Hepatic forms:* glucose-6-phosphatase deficiency (GSD1), debrancher enzyme deficiency (GSD 3) *Muscle form:* muscle phosphorylase deficiency (GSD 5) *Lysosomal form:* Pompe disease (GSD 2)
	Disorders of glucose catabolism (glycolysis) and synthesis (gluconeogenesis)	Pyruvate dehydrogenase deficiency, pyruvate carboxylase deficiency, fructose diphosphatase deficiency
Protein glycosylation		Carbohydrate-deficient glycoprotein syndromes
Organelles	**Subgroups**	**Examples**
Peroxisomal disorders	Disorders of peroxisome assembly	Zellweger syndrome, neonatal adrenoleukodystrophy, infantile Refsum disease, rhizomelic chondrodysplasia punctata
	Single enzyme defects	X-linked adrenoleukodystrophy
Lysosomal storage disorders	Lysosomal enzyme deficiencies	*Mucopolysaccharidoses:* Hurler/Scheie (MPS 1), Hunter (MPS 2, X-linked), Sanfilippo (MPS 3) *Sphingolipidoses:* Tay-Sachs, Krabbe, metachromatic leukodystrophy, Niemann-Pick, Gaucher, Fabry (X-linked) *Glycoprotein degradation:* mannosidosis, fucosidosis
	Disorders of lysosomal enzyme transport	*Mucolipidoses:* I-cell disease (ML 2)
Mitochondrial disorders	Defects in respiratory chain complexes	Leigh syndrome (one of several causes), primary lactic acidoses, multiple acyl-CoA dehydrogenase deficiency (glutaric acidemia 2) *Mitochondrial encoded defects:* MELAS, MERRF (maternal inheritance)

All disorders are autosomal recessive unless otherwise noted.
LCAD, Long chain acyl-CoA dehydrogenase deficiency; *MCAD,* medium chain acyl-CoA dehydrogenase deficiency; *SCAD,* short chain acyl-CoA dehydrogenase deficiency; *MPS,* mucopolysaccharidosis; *GSD,* glycogen storage disease; *ML,* mucolipidosis, *MELAS,* mitochondrial encephalomyopathy, lactic acidosis, strokelike episodes; *MERRF,* myoclonic epilepsy, ragged red fibers.

individual. The clinical picture often involves an encephalopathy with progression to coma. Psychiatric symptoms, ataxia, muscle weakness, and strokelike episodes should raise suspicion for metabolic disease.[59] Recovery may be slow, with permanent or transient neurological dysfunction. Nongenetic diagnoses usually considered include Reye syndrome, toxic ingestion, and encephalitis. Presentations with common problems, such as vomiting, lethargy, and dehydration resembling viral illness, also occur. However, the course is usually more protracted than that seen in children who have no metabolic disease, and improvement often requires parenteral fluids. The recurrence of similar episodes of illness predicts metabolic disease. Abdominal pain, vomiting, and evidence of pancreatitis (e.g., elevated serum amylase) occurs in about 8% of patients who have organic acidemia and may be the presenting finding. Organic acidemias constitute a significant

Table 20-2 High-Risk Scenarios for the Consideration of Metabolic Disorders

Clinical picture	Disorders to consider
Acute illness in a previously normal newborn	Aminoacidopathies, organic acidemias, urea cycle defects, galactosemia
Neonatal seizure disorder	Pyridoxine-dependent seizures, nonketotic hyperglycinemia, sulfite oxidase deficiency
Recurrent episodic illness (lethargy, vomiting, ataxia, encephalopathy, strokelike episodes, myopathy, "near miss" SIDS)	Aminoacidopathies, organic acidemias, urea cycle defects, defects in fatty acid metabolism, disorders of carbohydrate metabolism, mitochondrial disorders
Neurological regression	Lysosomal storage disorders, X-linked adrenoleukodystrophy
Chronic, progressive symptomology (poor feeding, poor growth, slow development, neurological and other organ system dysfunction)	Aminoacidopathies, organic acidemias, disorders of carbohydrate metabolism; mitochondrial and peroxisomal diseases

proportion of otherwise unexplained pancreatitis in children.[35]

Neuropsychological Regression. Neuropsychological regression is a characteristic feature of lysosomal storage disorders such as Tay-Sachs disease. Typically a child demonstrates either normal development or slow developmental progress and then loses developmental milestones. Progressive deterioration ensues at variable ages and rates. Certain associated physical findings can narrow the differential diagnosis in this group.

Chronic, Progressive Symptoms. Metabolic disease can affect any of the major organ systems chronically and progressively. Specific organ system dysfunction or nonspecific growth and developmental delay can accompany many metabolic disorders.

Historical Clues

Dietary History. For disorders in which protein catabolism is defective (amino acid and organic acid disorders), high protein intake precipitates symptoms such as vomiting, lethargy, and coma. An infant who vomits, who improves on glucose feeding, and in whom vomiting recurs within a few days of reinstitution of milk feeding could have a metabolic disease. History may reveal the onset of illness upon weaning from breast milk, which has a lower protein content than commercial formulas, or the association of illness with high protein meals. Some older patients are found to be "protein avoiders" who limit their protein intake. Carbohydrate intolerances manifest with the introduction of fructose (fruit juices) in hereditary fructose intolerance[7] or lactose (human or cow milk) in galactosemia.

Response to Infection, Fever, and Fasting. Obtaining a history of unusual lethargy during mild illness or intolerance of fasting is a significant historical clue for metabolic disease. Infections, fever, and fasting result in an overall catabolic state.[14] Under these conditions, disorders involving impaired glucose production and fatty acid catabolism are exacerbated, and endogenous protein catabolism may precipitate expression of amino acid and organic acid disorders. Glycogen storage disease may present within the first few months of life, when time between feedings is lengthened. Medium chain acyl-CoA dehydrogenase deficiency, a disorder of fatty acid oxidation, classically presents during an episode of intercurrent illness with prolonged fasting.[67] Immunizations, which may produce mild illness in normal children, can cause metabolic decompensation in children who have inborn errors of metabolism. (If a diagnosis has been established, immunization should not be avoided; rather, children who have such metabolic disorders should be followed up carefully after immunization. Flu vaccines are recommended yearly at some genetic centers.)

Adverse Reactions to Anesthesia and Surgery. Other situations that stress metabolic systems, such as general anesthesia and surgery, can precipitate illness in patients who have metabolic disease. Patients who have homocystinuria are prone to thromboembolism during surgery.[50]

Family History. It is essential to obtain a thorough family history for all patients suspected of having metabolic disease. The majority of these disorders are inherited in an autosomal recessive fashion. Parental consanguinity, similarly affected siblings, or early death of a sibling increases the likelihood of autosomal recessive disease. However, consanguinity is uncommon in this country, and nuclear families are small. Thus a negative family history does not exclude the possibility of a metabolic disorder. The finding of similarly affected male relatives on the maternal side is consistent with X-linked disorders.

Pertinent Physical Findings

Metabolic disease affects multiple organ systems and produces a variety of physical findings. Table 20-3 lists common signs, including classic radiological findings. Some general themes can be summarized. In the disorders that present with episodic illness, significant findings may be present or exacerbated only during the acute illness. Neurological abnormalities predominate in episodic presentations, but hepatomegaly, cardiomyopathy, and muscle weakness also can be present. Tachypnea and hyperpnea often are overlooked as signs of metabolic acidosis or respiratory alkalosis. Other disorders feature a characteristic pattern of findings that develop over time. Coarse facial features, corneal clouding, hepatosplenomegaly, macrocephaly, and skeletal changes suggest mucopolysaccharidoses, disorders of glycoprotein degradation, and mucolipidoses.[31] The constellation of alopecia, chronic dermatitis, ataxia, and seizures is seen with biotinidase deficiency.[78] Lens dislocation, long extremities, and vascular occlusion secondary to thrombosis are found in homocystinuria.[56] When physical examination reveals abnormali-

Table 20-3 Pertinent Clinical Findings in Genetic-Metabolic Disorders

System	Findings
Neurological	Encephalopathy
	Strokelike episodes
	Macrocephaly
	Developmental delay
	Ataxia
	Choreoathetosis
	Dystonia
	Hypotonia or hypertonia
	Seizures
	Myoclonus
	Deafness
	Brain malformations
Ophthalmological	Cataracts
	Corneal opacities
	Macular cherry red spot
	Lens dislocation
	Retinal pigmentary changes
Respiratory	Tachypnea
	Hyperpnea
Cardiovascular	Cardiomyopathy
	Pericardial effusion
	Rhythm disturbance
	Thrombosis
Abdominal	Hepatomegaly
	Cirrhosis
	Jaundice
	Splenomegaly
	Nephrolithiasis
	Renal Fanconi syndrome
	Renal cysts
	Pancreatitis
Muscular	Hypertrophy
	Myopathy
	Myalgias
	Recurrent myoglobinuria
Skin	Eczematous rash
	Ichthyosis
	Photosensitivity
	Angiokeratomas
Hair	Sparse
	Brittle, dry
Skeletal	Scoliosis
	Kyphosis
	Joint contractures
	Dysostosis multiplex
	Epiphyseal calcifications
Other	Dysmorphic features
	Coarse facial features

ties in more than one organ system, metabolic disease should be suspected.

Initial Laboratory Evaluation

Routine laboratory investigations can provide useful diagnostic clues. The key laboratory abnormalities in many of these disorders are metabolic acidosis, hypoglycemia with or without ketosis, and hyperammonemia. The particular combination present can help predict which biochemical pathway is affected and thus which group of disorders to consider. Metabolic acidosis is assessed routinely by reviewing serum electrolytes for bicarbonate level and blood gas for pH. If the serum bicarbonate level is low, the anion gap is calculated [Na − (HCO_3 + Cl)]. An increased anion gap (>16) with a normal chloride concentration reflects the presence of unmeasured anions, such as organic acids, lactate, and ketones. These compounds accumulate in amino acid and organic acid disorders. Accumulation of lactic acid predominates in mitochondrial defects and some disorders of carbohydrate metabolism.[75] A normal anion gap with an elevated chloride concentration reflects bicarbonate wasting secondary to intestinal dysfunction or renal tubular defects and can be seen in galactosemia.[19] It is important to note that a normal blood pH does not rule out a mild metabolic acidosis because neutrality is maintained by various buffer systems. Low serum sodium concentration with normal or high serum potassium suggests the salt-losing form of congenital adrenal hyperplasia.

Hypoglycemia occurs either because of a primary defect in the generation of glucose (disorders of glycogen breakdown and gluconeogenic pathways) or because of toxic interference with these pathways (organic acidemias). Carbohydrate depletion or impaired glucose metabolism stimulates lipid catabolism, providing ketones as an alternative fuel and resulting in ketosis. Hypoglycemia without significant ketosis is the hallmark for disorders of fatty acid oxidation in which the pathway is blocked before the formation of ketones[24] or for excessive insulin secretion. Hyperglycemia occasionally is seen in organic acidemias.[59]

Ammonia is produced normally from protein catabolism and detoxified in the liver through the urea cycle. Ammonia levels are elevated in urea cycle disorders and also in some of the organic acidemias, disorders of fatty acid oxidation, and liver disease. Hyperammonemia induces central hyperventilation, resulting in respiratory alkalosis.[6]

Leukopenia and thrombocytopenia have been found in patients who have organic acidemias.[10] Patients who have methylmalonic acidemia develop evidence of renal dysfunction.[58]

A recommended primary laboratory evaluation is delineated in Table 20-4. Ancillary tests that may provide additional clues also are listed. When the results suggest a metabolic disorder, more specific testing is done. These secondary tests often are available on site or through an experienced reference laboratory; they are shown in Table 20-5. In disorders that have episodic symptoms, laboratory values may be abnormal only at the time of acute illness. Furthermore, partial treatment with intravenous fluids, transfusions, or dietary changes can mask abnormalities. Drug metabolites can result in false positives.[5] By testing for metabolic disease early in the course of illness, diagnostic results are more likely to be obtained. A practical approach consists of collecting specimens (urine, heparinized plasma, spinal fluid) early, storing them frozen, and sending them later for analysis if warranted.

Treatment

Treatment of metabolic disease can be divided into two categories: acute therapy and chronic management.

Acute Therapy. In treatment during episodes of metabolic decompensation (before or after the diagnosis has been es-

Table 20-4 Initial Blood and Urine Tests for Suspected Genetic-Metabolic Disorders

Blood tests	Abnormal finding	Disease
Blood gases, electrolytes	Metabolic acidosis, elevated anion gap	Organic acidemias, maple syrup urine disease, disorders of carbohydrate metabolism, mitochondrial defects
	Respiratory alkalosis	Urea cycle defects
Glucose	Low with ketosis	Disorders of carbohydrate metabolism, organic acidemias
	Low without ketosis	Fatty acid oxidation defects
Ammonia	High	Urea cycle defects, organic acidemias, fatty acid oxidation defects, nongenetic disorders that have significant liver dysfunction
Lactate, pyruvate	High	Disorders of carbohydrate metabolism, respiratory chain defects, severe tissue hypoxia
Uric acid	High	Glycogen storage disorders, fatty acid oxidation defects, organic acidemias
Urea nitrogen	Low	Urea cycle disorders
Liver transaminases	High	Tyrosinemia, galactosemia, hereditary fructose intolerance, fatty acid oxidation defects
Phosphate	Low	Hereditary fructose intolerance, fructose 1,6 diphosphatase deficiency
Creatine kinase	High	Primary carnitine defects, fatty acid oxidation disorders, mitochondrial myopathies, muscular dystrophies
Blood count	Neutropenia, thrombocytopenia	Organic acidemias
Urine tests	**Abnormal finding**	**Disease**
Odor (assess by opening a closed container left at room temperature for 3 hours)	Sweaty feet, musty, tomcat urine, maple syrup*	Organic acidemias, aminoacidopathies
Ketones—essential test whenever hypoglycemia is documented	Positive	Organic acidemias, maple syrup urine disease, disorders of carbohydrate metabolism
Reducing substances (requires urine glucose determination for interpretation)	Positive with glucose, galactose, fructose	Galactosemia, hereditary fructose intolerance

*See Chapter 156, Odor (Unusual Urine and Body).

Table 20-5 Specific Laboratory Tests for Genetic-Metabolic Disorders

Type	Diseases
Blood	
Quantitative plasma amino acids	Aminoacidopathies, abnormalities also found in organic acidemias and disorders of carbohydrate metabolism
Carnitine levels (total, free, and esterified), acylcarnitine profile	Disorders of fatty acid metabolism
Very long chain fatty acids, plasmalogens, phytanic acid	Peroxisomal disorders
Urine	
Quantitative amino acids	Specific amino acid transport defects, Fanconi syndrome
Organic acids	Organic acidemias
Oligosaccharide thin layer chromatography	Lysosomal disorders of glycoprotein degradation
Screens (ferric chloride, dinitrophenylhydrazine, sulfite oxidase, mucopolysaccharide spot)	Aminoacidopathies, organic acidemias, mucopolysaccharidoses (frequent false positives and negatives)
Spinal fluid	
Amino acids (glycine)	Nonketotic hyperglycinemia (requires simultaneous plasma amino acids)
Enzyme assays	
Blood, skin, or other tissue	Required for diagnosis of all lysosomal storage disorders, definitive diagnosis of most metabolic disorders

Note: In the event the child dies before a definitive diagnosis is made, a small piece of muscle and liver should be quick frozen and held at −70°. A skin biopsy for cultured fibroblasts should be obtained premortem.

tablished), the ill child is approached as usual, with attention paid to respiratory, cardiovascular, fluid, and neurological status. Intake of all potentially offending compounds (protein, lactose, fructose) is stopped, and further catabolism is inhibited by providing high caloric intake. About 60 calories/kg/day should be provided from glucose to prevent proteolysis.[26] Bicarbonate is useful in cases of severe acidosis. If a vitamin-responsive disorder is suspected, a trial of vitamin cofactors (cobalamin, biotin, thiamin, riboflavin, pyridoxine, and folate) can be instituted. Carnitine may be added in organic acidurias and disorders of fatty acid oxidation to promote excretion of toxic metabolites.[4] Hyperammonemia is treated with intravenous phenylacetate, sodium benzoate, and arginine, which help detoxify and remove ammonia.[8] These medications can be obtained through contact with a specialist in inherited metabolic diseases. Progressive hyperammonemia, or comatose states secondary to hyperammonemia or other toxic metabolites, requires prompt institution of hemodialysis.[57] Acute therapy (as well as chronic treatment) should be managed in consultation with a physician skilled in treating metabolic disease. Careful monitoring of laboratory parameters and clinical status is required, with attention being given to complications that may occur secondarily to the biochemical abnormalities and therapy.

Chronic Management. Long-term therapy is disease specific and involves several strategies. To reduce the accumulation of toxic metabolites, the intake of offending compounds is limited to the minimal amount needed for growth and development. This often requires an artificial diet that includes special formulas and caloric supplementation. Regular monitoring of amino acids and other laboratory values is required so that adjustments can be made to optimize the diet for each individual patient. For some disorders, the offending compound is nonessential and can be eliminated entirely from the diet. When the enzyme defect involves binding of a cofactor (usually a vitamin) or defective synthesis of the cofactor itself, therapy centers on dietary supplementation of the cofactor. Other strategies include the stimulation of alternative biochemical pathways to detoxify and remove the offending substance.[42] In disorders that are accompanied by fasting intolerance, treatment consists of frequent meals, which may require the use of complex carbohydrates such as cornstarch between meals to allow prolonged absorption of glucose and nocturnal nasogastric feeding. None of these interventions constitutes a cure, and most are only partially successful in alleviating clinical symptoms. With better understanding of the pathophysiology of these disorders, better therapies will become available. Liver and bone marrow transplantation has been done in several disorders, with mixed results.[36] Enzyme and gene replacement therapies are being developed for some disorders.[70]

Illustrative Case

The following case is included to illustrate some of the principles discussed in the previous sections.

J.S. was the full-term product of a normal pregnancy and delivery. His birthweight was 3.2 kg. The infant was started on a cow milk formula and discharged on day 2 of life without incident. From days 2 to 8, anorexia, lethargy, and vomiting became progressively worse. The formula was changed to a soy base, without clinical improvement. On day 8 the mother noted respiratory difficulties. There was no history of fever. Examination at this time revealed a dehydrated, hypothermic infant who had a weak suck and cry. Tachypnea and tachycardia were present. Perfusion was decreased in the distal extremities, but blood pressure was normal. Oxygen saturation was 98% by pulse oximetry. The abdomen was soft, without apparent hepatosplenomegaly or renal enlargement. The remainder of the examination was normal. Family history revealed two normal sisters and no history of early infant deaths or parental consanguinity. The initial clinical impression was that of a septic infant. Intravenous fluids and antibiotics were given, and the infant was warmed. Initial laboratory evaluation revealed the following: WBC 3500; platelets 192,000; venous blood gases—pH 7.03, Pco_2 31, Po_2 98; electrolytes—Na 146, K 4.4, Cl 103, HCO_3 5 (anion gap 38); glucose—25 mg/dl; urine—pH 5; ketones 2+ (obtained after rehydration); spinal fluid—normal chemistries and cell counts; chest radiograph—right upper lobe pneumonia.

The primary diagnosis was sepsis with aspiration pneumonia. All cultures were negative, but this was thought to be the result of antibiotic administration just before the obtaining of cultures. The hospital course was protracted, requiring several days for the acidosis to improve on IV fluids containing bicarbonate. Persistent vomiting and severe acidosis recurred upon reintroduction of formula feedings. A barium swallow test did not reveal gastrointestinal obstruction. On day 14 of life the infant became increasingly lethargic, and laboratory investigation showed the following: WBC 4300; platelets 7800; arterial blood gases—pH 7.1, Pco_2 33, Po_2 97; electrolytes—Na 141, Cl 103, HCO_3 9 (anion gap 29); glucose—50 mg/dl; ammonia—191 uM; urine—ketones 4+.

The infant was transferred to a tertiary care hospital for diagnosis and management of suspected metabolic disease. Plasma amino acids showed elevated glycine, and measurement of urine organic acids revealed elevated levels of propionic acid and methylcitrate. These findings are suggestive of propionic acidemia.[40] The defective enzyme is propionyl CoA carboxylase, a biotin-dependent enzyme. The enzyme defect was confirmed later on tissue samples. The patient responded to intravenous fluids with appropriate amounts of glucose provided through a central line. He was not responsive to a trial of megavitamin therapy with biotin. With clinical and laboratory improvement, oral feedings were instituted first with a glucose polymer solution and then advanced to a low protein diet supplemented with a special formula deficient in the precursors of propionic acid: valine, isoleucine, methionine, threonine, and odd chain fatty acids. If the patient had not improved quickly or had continued to deteriorate, hemodialysis would have been indicated for urgent removal of toxic metabolites.

Discussion. Several indicators of metabolic disease were overlooked in the initial presentation of this patient. A history of acute illness in a normal newborn represents a typical high-risk scenario for the consideration of metabolic disease. The initial laboratory findings provide further evidence consistent with metabolic disease: metabolic acidosis with an elevated anion gap, hypoglycemia, and ketosis. Ketosis, an unusual finding in a neonate, indicates metabolic disease in this age group. Recurrence of symptoms when milk feedings were resumed also is characteristic. The elevated ammonia level finally led to the suspicion of an underlying metabolic disorder. Ammonia levels should be determined in the initial evaluation of a lethargic infant. Poor response to therapy also should have prompted an investigation for metabolic disease. In retrospect, the evidence for a metabolic disorder is clear. If this possibility was considered in the primary differential diagnosis, then plasma amino acids and urine organic acids would have been requested early on, providing a diagnosis and more timely institution of therapy.

SCREENING FOR GENETIC AND SOME OTHER DISEASES

By the time symptoms of some disorders appear, it is too late to intervene with maximum effectiveness. This is the case, for instance, for phenylketonuria (PKU); although nonspecific signs occasionally appear early in infancy (such as eczema), by the time of developmental delay the infant has sustained irreversible damage. For other disorders, such as galactosemia and maple syrup urine disease, symptoms appear early, but the diagnosis often is delayed. This is also the case in some infants who have congenital hypothyroidism (CH). Newborn screening can speed up the diagnosis, provided that specimens are analyzed quickly and abnormal results are reported promptly. A sine qua non of newborn screening is that the prognosis can be improved by the *prompt* institution of therapy. As we have accumulated experience with screening, we find that the outcome is not always as good as anticipated, and for some disorders a few infants may be started on therapy unnecessarily.

A few single-gene conditions only cause trouble following exposure to environmental agents that are not harmful to most people in the doses encountered. Screening for such susceptibilities could result in treatment that ameliorates the harmful effects or warns people at risk to avoid exposure. Among people who develop cancer (retinoblastoma and breast and colon cancer have been studied the most thoroughly), a small proportion (less than 10%) has inherited alleles at single loci that greatly increase their susceptibility to malignant transformation as a result of spontaneous or environmentally induced mutations of other genes. The benefits of screening the entire population for these genetic susceptibilities remain to be established. (In conjunction with genetic counseling, tests should be made available to high-risk cancer families, usually as part of investigational protocols.) Recent claims of inherited risk factors for complex disorders such as Alzheimer disease need thorough assessment before population screening should even be considered. Genetics plays a role in adult onset coronary artery disease. Cholesterol screening is discussed in Part Four of this chapter.

Most single-gene disorders are not treatable, but those at risk for them, as well as heterozygous carriers, can be detected by genetic tests. Carrier testing before or early in pregnancy provides couples the option of avoiding the conception (by adoption, artificial insemination of donor sperm, or in the case of X-linked disorders, ovum donation or surrogacy) or birth (by prenatal diagnosis and selective abortion) of children who have severe, untreatable, inherited disorders, such as Tay-Sachs or thalassemia. Prenatal cytogenetic and biochemical testing can avoid, respectively, the birth of children who have Down syndrome or neural tube defects.

The primary health care provider will be involved increasingly with neonatal, carrier, and prenatal screening and presymptomatic testing for adult-onset disorders. In some cases she or he will inform patients about the availability of tests and will counsel them about having the test and, when they decide to be tested, about the meaning of the results.

False Positives and False Negatives

Very few people being screened, whether newborns, nonpregnant, or pregnant women, will be at risk of disease in themselves or their offspring. With the exception of DNA tests, many of the techniques used in screening yield positive results in the absence of the condition of interest. These false positives often occur more often than the condition of interest in the population being screened. The immunoreactive trypsinogen (IRT) test used in a few places to screen newborns for cystic fibrosis (CF) yields over five times as many false positive as true positive results. Because the blood phenylalanine concentration may only exceed normal levels minimally in infants who have PKU during the first few days of life, the cutpoint for phenylalanine elevations (and other metabolites) must be set lower than the minimum phenylalanine concentration needed to establish a diagnosis of PKU. Consequently, false positive results often will exceed true positive results. When the screening test entails enzyme assays, as for one type of testing for galactosemia and for biotinidase deficiency, heat denaturation (by prolonged mailing time in hot weather or letting samples dry on a radiator) greatly increases the percentage of false positives. When DNA tests are performed appropriately for single-gene disorders, false positive results seldom are encountered. For multifactorial disorders, however (such as colon cancer or Alzheimer disease), in which a single-gene mutation increases the risk of disease but is insufficient to cause it, positive DNA test results do not always mean that disease will occur. Other factors, many unknown, also are operative.

False negative results are a problem with DNA as well as with more traditional tests. In the case of DNA tests, they occur when the test does not detect all of the different mutations capable of causing disease.

The increasing tendency, driven by third party reimbursement policies, to discharge healthy newborns no later than 1 day of age also will increase the number of infants who have false negative and false positive test results. Infants who have PKU have near-normal levels of phenylalanine in cord blood, and in some the levels may not rise rapidly in the first day after birth. When a galactose test is used to screen for galactosemia, galactosemic infants screened before or shortly after they start milk feedings will be "missed." Approximately 10% of infants who have CH will have normal thyroxine levels when screened early, and most of these also have normal thyroid-stimulating hormone (TSH) levels.[9] When TSH is used as the initial screening test (common in European countries but not in the United States), as many as 25% of infants discharged early may have elevated levels.[17] In screening for congenital adrenal hyperplasia, samples collected before 36 hours of age are much more likely to yield false positive elevations of 17OH-progesterone than are samples collected after 48 hours.[2] Although the chance of misclassification is greater the earlier an infant is screened, most infants (but not all) who have the disorders for which screening usually is provided will be detected when tested after 24 hours of age. In view of difficulties of *guaranteeing* that a screening test will be performed soon after discharge, *no infant* should be discharged from the newborn nursery, even if under 24 hours old, without first being screened. Raising the cutpoint to reduce the number of false positives or lowering it to reduce the number of false negatives for infants screened before 48 hours has the problem of increasing, respectively, the number of false negatives and false positives. Using a different cutpoint for early and late screened infants requires the laboratory to treat the two groups of infants separately. *The best solution is not to discharge infants until they are at least 48 hours old.*

False positive and false negative test results are both dangerous and costly. Parents of infants who have false positive test results may become anxious until the result is proven to be false; even then anxiety may linger in a small number of parents, particularly when their infants had low Apgar scores.[66] The parent-child relationship could be influenced adversely as a result of this stress in the neonatal period.

With a high false positive rate, more infants have to be followed up, which adds to the cost of screening. The affected infants missed by screening suffer severely, usually at great cost to their families and society. Health care providers have been found financially liable for infants missed by screening. No provider should ever assume that an infant who has symptoms of a disorder for which screening was performed cannot have that disorder.

Screening tests can give erroneous results because of the presence of other substances that interfere with the analysis. Most important for genetic screening is the presence of a donor's blood products as the result of recent transfusion. Certain antibiotics can interfere with the bacterial inhibition assays used in newborn screening. Spilling of milk or other substances on the specimen also can lead to erroneous results.

In the absence of rigorous quality control programs, of which there are few in the United States, laboratory error probably is the most common cause of false positive and false negative newborn screening test results. Errors include misidentification of specimens and failure to transmit the results properly, as well as erroneous assays.

Newborn Screening

All states and Puerto Rico and the Virgin Islands routinely screen newborns for PKU (1 in 13,000 live births) and CH (1 in 4000 live births). Forty-five states screen for sickle cell anemia (1 in 500 live births of African-Americans) and other hemoglobinopathies and 43 for galactosemia (about 1 in 100,000 live births). Fewer than half of the states screen for maple syrup urine disease (less than 1 in 100,000 live births), homocystinuria (less than 1 in 100,000 live births), biotinidase deficiency (about 1 in 70,000 live births) and congenital adrenal hyperplasia (1 in 15,000 live births), and CF (1 in 2500 Caucasian live births).[52] Because states differ in the tests that are required, it is incumbent on health care providers to be familiar with the policies of their own state. In at least one state, providers were not notified when new tests were introduced. Whether this contributed to the failure of a few of them to act when notified of a positive test result is unknown, but their failure to act could have resulted in an infant's death.[43] Providers should document screening test results and any follow-up on the child's medical record.

Because screening tests can be falsely negative, practitioners should not place undue faith in a negative result. A repeat test, or a more definitive one, should be obtained in infants who have suspicious findings. Because of the problem of false positive test results, treatment should not be started merely on the basis of one positive screening test result. Consultation with someone experienced in the evaluation of metabolic disorders is highly recommended. When treatment is indicated, the response may vary; careful monitoring and expert evaluation are needed. Furthermore, consultation is reassuring to the family.

Some infants may escape screening. The largest group are infants born at home. They should be screened at their first visit for pediatric care. Sick infants transferred from one hospital to the other fall through the cracks when each hospital believes that screening was done by the other. If there is any doubt, the receiving hospital should rescreen the baby.

Screening for PKU and hypothyroidism is cost effective. The addition of other tests from which infants will benefit usually involves only marginal cost increments. The economics of sickle cell screening, as discussed below, depends on the proportion of infants at high risk in a state's population. Centralization of laboratories and more stringent regulations for quality control reduce laboratory error, increase cost effectiveness, and reduce cost to the patient.

Phenylketonuria. Infants who have PKU show few signs until they develop mental retardation, which may not be appreciated until the second year of life and is irreversible. Screening early in infancy, followed by administering a low phenylalanine diet promptly, is the only way to improve the outcome of those born with the condition. There is good evidence that intellectual performance correlates with the age at which dietary treatment is started and with the success of dietary control.[30] Studies to confirm positive test results should be performed promptly to permit the initiation of the low phenylalanine diet as soon as possible but no later than the third week of life.

The American Academy of Pediatrics recommends that every infant in the United States be screened before discharge from the nursery but that infants initially screened before 24 hours of age should be rescreened before the third week of life. Premature and sick infants should be screened by the seventh day.[12] A few states recommend that all infants have a second screen between 2 and 4 weeks of age, and a few infants who have PKU with negative first test results have been detected by the repeat screen. The second screen costs much more per infant who has PKU detected than the first screen.

In addition to the predominant phenylalanine hydroxylase deficiency, defects in the synthesis or regeneration of biopterin cofactors for the conversion of phenylalanine to tyrosine also result in positive screening test results and clinical disease. Dietary restriction of phenylalanine is insufficient to prevent mental deterioration and other signs, such as seizures, in these infants. The use of biopterin or neurotransmitter precursors offers hope of improving the outcome. Infants who have these disorders will be discovered by neonatal screening for PKU; they represent fewer than 3% of all infants in whom elevations of phenylalanine persist. Tests for these variant forms should be performed in any infant who persistently has elevated blood phenylalanine levels, even in the moderate range of 10 to 20 mg/dl while on a normal diet.

Congenital Hypothyroidism. The etiology of CH is multiple and complex, including transplacental passage of maternal antibodies that interfere with fetal thyroid development or thyroid function.[17] Maternal antibodies also can cause transient hypothyroidism. Mothers receiving antithyroid medication (propylthiouracil) also may have babies who have transient hypothyroidism. Genetic factors are suggested in families that have more than one affected infant, although such findings do not rule out environmental or maternally acquired etiologies. For unknown reasons, females are twice as likely to have CH as males, and the birth prevalence is somewhat higher in Hispanics and Native Americans than in Caucasians or Asians, in whom it is higher than in African-Americans.[45]

Infants who have the most profound deficiencies of thyroxine, usually due to thyroid agenesis, are more likely to have symptoms in the neonatal period, of which persistent jaundice, feeding difficulty, and lethargy are most frequent.[17,22] Nevertheless, even infants who have agenesis may be asymptomatic when they are examined as part of the evaluation of their abnormal screening test result. Placental transfer of thyroxine (T_4) and some fetal production of T_3 in the brain may explain this. The 10% of infants who have CH that is found on a second screen (in states that screen twice) are less often symptomatic and have lesser elevations of TSH. Negative newborn screening test results are no guarantee against hypothyroidism developing in infancy or childhood.

The incidence of CH detected by neonatal screening is higher than by clinical diagnosis in the prescreening era. This suggests either that infants who have milder disease escaped diagnosis or that some infants being diagnosed today do not really have CH. Because of this latter possibility, the need to ensure that CH persists in equivocal cases, as discussed below, is important.

In most laboratories in the United States, T_4 is measured on the screening specimen, and, if it is low, thyroid-stimulating hormone (TSH) is measured on the same specimen. If it is elevated and the findings are confirmed on another specimen, treatment with thyroxine is started. Most infants who persistently have low T_4 levels but who have normal TSH levels will prove on further study to have normal free T_4 concentrations and thyroid-binding globulin deficiency; they do not require treatment. A few infants who have low T_4 and normal TSH levels will have hypopituitary gland failure, but it is encountered much less frequently than thyroid-binding globulin deficiency. Occasionally an infant who has initial low T_4 and normal TSH levels will have a delayed rise in TSH level and symptoms of hypothyroidism. In an infant who has an initial low T_4 level and a normal TSH level, TSH should be retested if symptoms appear.

The motor and cognitive development of infants who have CH at 7½ years of age correlates with the age at which thyroxine treatment is started.[37] Although the vast majority of infants treated early have IQs in the normal range,[17] many of them are at the low end compared with matched controls.[37]

The need for long-term thyroid replacement can be assumed if scans or other studies reveal absent or ectopic thyroid or goiter caused by an enzyme defect. In the absence of these findings but when low T_4 and elevated TSH levels indicate the need for early treatment, therapy should be discontinued for 30 days, or until signs and symptoms of CH appear, when the child is between 3 and 4 years of age. At that time serum should be obtained for T_4 and TSH assays. If findings are normal, no further treatment is needed. Such transient cases usually are those in which the TSH level was elevated only moderately (20 to 100 μ/ml) in the newborn period.

Sickle Cell Anemia. Because of a randomized controlled trial demonstrating that penicillin prophylaxis reduces the incidence of pneumococcal infections in sickle cell anemia,[21] several states have added sickle cell to their newborn screening programs. Before screening was initiated, approximately 10% of infants in the United States who had sickle cell disease died by 10 years of age, most from pneumococcal sepsis. The effectiveness of screening in reducing morbidity and mortality depends on ensuring that infants detected by screening are referred to a continuing source of care from which they can receive prophylactic penicillin and their parents can learn how to manage situations that increase the chance of sickle cell crises. As yet there is no specific treatment for sickle cell anemia.

The tests used for screening—hemoglobin electrophoresis or isoelectric focusing—will discover hemoglobinopathies in addition to sickle cell anemia, not all of which will result in symptoms. The test also identifies infants who have sickle trait who will remain healthy. However, a couple who delivers an infant with "trait" may be at risk for having an infant who has sickle cell anemia if both partners are carriers of the sickle cell gene. A screening program will have 40 times more carriers to notify than parents of infants who have sickle cell anemia, raising the costs of the program. The purpose of notifying the parents of a trait is to determine, by offering to have them both tested, whether they are both carriers and, consequently, at risk of having an affected offspring. They then can be offered prenatal diagnosis in any subsequent pregnancies. The infant who has trait, who triggers this process, has nothing to gain from it. Moreover, in the vast majority of couples who have an infant with trait, only one partner will be a carrier, and the couple will not be at risk. Recently, an Institute of Medicine panel recommended that parents be informed that newborn screening might provide information about their future risks of having a child with a serious hemoglobinopathy and be given the opportunity of requesting the results.[3]

Recently the Agency for Health Care Policy and Research published guidelines calling for universal screening of newborns for hemoglobinopathies.[1] Currently about 35 states screen all newborns for hemoglobinopathies, and about 10 base screening on the race of the infant or the mother. Although this selective approach is far more cost effective than universal screening in states that have a small percentage of African-American births, an infant's race may not be determined accurately, and a cost is involved in determining if the specimen should be screened.[38] A recent analysis, on which AHCPR based its guidelines, suggests that universal sickle cell screening could be at least as cost-effective as PKU screening, provided that states that have a small percentage of African-American births, in whom screening would be much more costly, could have their tests performed in states that have a large proportion of such infants.[63]

Galactosemia. In contrast to PKU, serious manifestations of classical galactosemia occur soon after milk feedings are started. Consequently the diagnosis can be, and often is, made clinically before screening test results are reported. The prompt administration of a lactose-free diet in the newborn will save the lives of patients who have this disorder, but it may not prevent retardation or other developmental problems. The age of starting the galactose-free diet is not associated significantly with the magnitude of developmental delay, physical growth, or speech problems.[15,71]

It is not certain that all infants found by screening to have galactosemia would have developed symptoms had they not been started on a lactose-free diet. Some infants discovered by screening have variant forms of galactosemia, in which residual amounts of galactose-1-phosphate uridyl transferase, the enzyme that is absent in classical cases, are found. Although infants with some of these variants have acute neonatal symptoms, they generally are milder than in the classical cases. Other infants manifest no symptoms. Whether they are less likely to have long-term manifestations, such as developmental delay, is not clear.

We have much to learn about the pathogenesis of galactosemia and the development of effective therapy. Until we do, the value of neonatal screening for galactosemia is questionable. The principal goal is to ensure prompt intervention in those who have early onset of symptoms whose lives are threatened. These infants can be diagnosed clinically.

Maple Syrup Urine Disease (MSUD). Infants who have the classic form of MSUD usually show signs within 2 weeks of birth. The course can be fulminant and rapidly fatal, but early treatment can prevent or ameliorate the acute symptoms. If the special diet (low in branched chain amino acids) is started very early, the long-term outcome can be good. One of the problems with routine screening is the inherent delay in obtaining results. A specimen collected on day 2 may not be reported back until day 10. By that time, most infants who have the classic form will be severely ill or dead. Starting the special diet usually will save those infants still alive at this point, but the outcome often will be marred by retardation and neurological problems. Sometimes confirmation of a diagnosis of MSUD in sick infants can be accelerated by contacting the laboratory responsible for performing newborn screening; a positive result may have been obtained already. Often, the laboratory will process the specimen more quickly when it receives a special request.

The enzyme that is defective in MSUD is complex,[55] and multiple different mutations have been characterized. Except in a North American Mennonite community, where one mutation accounts for a high prevalence of the condition, several different mutations have been found.[53] Many patients are compound heterozygotes. As a result of screening and the immediate institution of the special diet, it has been difficult to establish genotype-phenotype relations. Some infants started on the diet may have forms of the disorder that would have appeared only later in infancy or childhood with episodes of ataxia, failure to thrive, and mild ketoacidosis, particularly following infection or high protein ingestion.

Congenital Adrenal Hyperplasia. In 21-hydroxylase deficiency, which accounts for more than 90% of those who have congenital adrenal hyperplasia (CAH), and in 11-hydroxylase deficiency, accounting for about 5% of cases, cortisol production is impaired. As a result of the deficiency, feedback inhibition of adrenocorticotropic hormone (ACTH) is lacking, and cortisol precursors, including those that have androgenic activity, are overproduced.

In girls, ambiguous genitalia should permit clinical diagnosis in the neonatal period. Because the diagnosis is not always made, however, screening could increase recognition of females, permitting them to be raised as girls. The diagnosis is much more difficult to establish in newborn males. About two thirds of infants who have 21-hydroxylase deficiency are salt "losers"; they may suffer severe dehydration and vascular collapse accompanied by hyponatremia during the first 2 weeks after birth. Several different mutations in the gene for 21-hydroxylase have been found. The presence of salt-losing depends on the particular mutation.[54]

By accelerating the diagnosis and instituting mineralocorticoid therapy promptly, screening can prevent life-threatening episodes in males and females. Salt-losing crises, however, often can occur before the results of screening are known. Screening also offers an advantage to affected boys who do not lose salt; steroid therapy will prevent virilization, rapid early growth, and premature closure of the epiphyses with resultant short adult stature.

The finding of more living females than males who have this autosomal recessive disorder suggests that males may die in the neonatal period before they are diagnosed.[65] By screening, an almost equal number of males and females are detected, and the birth prevalence is considerably higher than by clinical diagnosis.[54]

17-Hydroxyprogesterone is increased in the blood in both 21- and 11-hydroxylase deficiency and is measured by the screening test. Examined retrospectively, laboratory or administrative error has accounted for the handful of false negatives. When these are excluded, the test detects over 98% of infants who have CAH.[54] There are about 30 false positive results for every infant who has a true positive result. In females, the presence of ambiguous genitalia establishes a true positive, but in the absence of such findings and in most males, additional studies are needed. Measuring serum electrolytes, which are readily available, is the most important immediate follow-up to determine the presence of salt loss, in which case treatment should be started promptly. Because of the fulminant nature of salt-losing CAH, laboratories providing serum electrolyte levels should report the results promptly.

Symptom-free adults who have genetic variant forms of 21-hydroxylase deficiency have been identified. The possibility arises, therefore, that clinical problems will not develop in all symptom-free infants who have a confirmed deficiency, unambiguous genitalia, and no salt-losing.

Prenatal diagnosis in high-risk females now is possible; prenatal treatment by administering dexamethasone orally to the mother prevents or reduces intrauterine virilization in some, but not all, infants. The safety for both the mother and the fetus has not been fully established.[54]

Biotinidase Deficiency. Biotin is a cofactor of a number of carboxylases. Its availability through recycling is reduced in inherited deficiencies of biotinidase. The manifestations and age of onset of biotinidase deficiency vary, possibly because of differences in the completeness of the deficiency and the amount of biotin available to the infant. Symptoms usually appear between 2 weeks and 3 years. Ataxia, alopecia, hearing loss, decreased vision, optic atrophy, and seizures have been observed. It is not yet known whether some infants who have the disorder remain free of symptoms and, consequently, how many of the infants detected by screening would develop symptoms if left untreated. In view of the recent observation that significantly more infants found by screening have higher levels of residual biotinidase than those diagnosed clinically,[27] it seems possible that not all infants discovered by screening will ever develop symptoms. Nevertheless, the treatment—providing supplemental biotin—is simple and inexpensive. Although biotin reverses some of the symptoms after they appear, this is not always true for the hearing and visual impairments and developmental delay. Moreover, it is by no means clear that clinical diagnosis always will be made promptly. Infants treated as a result of screening have so far remained symptom-free.

Cystic Fibrosis. Immunoreactive trypsin (IRT) is elevated in the blood of most newborns who have cystic fibrosis (CF). Colorado and Wisconsin currently are performing the test. In Wisconsin, a long-term randomized controlled trial is being conducted to determine whether neonatal detection improves the health of children who have CF. Preliminary findings indicate that early identification and intervention prevents malnutrition, but whether infants discovered by screening will ultimately be better off nutritionally remains to be established. In Australia, one study showed a marked decline in hospitalizations after newborn screening, but in another the number of hospital admissions did not change.[18] In the most common CF genotype (delta f508 homozygotes), but not in a few others, pulmonary function is reduced in infants tested between 0.9 and 4.5 months of age,[49] suggesting that aggressive respiratory management could be beneficial. The few reports thus far generally are supportive of early medical intervention.[18,77] There is no treatment yet available that prevents the clinical manifestations, but earlier therapy may ameliorate the condition.

Infants who have meconium ileus and CF often have false negative IRT results, as may 3% to 10% of other infants who have the disorder. In Colorado, only 6% of the infants with positive IRT test results proved to have CF.[25] In an effort to reduce recall of infants with positive results, most newborn screening programs for CF now perform DNA tests for the most common CF mutations on specimens from infants that reveal elevated IRT. This will result in missing those infants who do not have at least one of these common mutations; they probably constitute about 10% of all infants who have CF.[18]

Homocystinuria. Although vitamin B_6–dependent forms of homocystinuria are treated easily and effectively, newborn screening will not detect all affected infants. The detection rate after the first week of life, using tests that measure blood or urine homocystine, will be higher than that of neonatal screening, which detects hypermethioninemia. In view of this, as well as the rarity of the disorder, newborn screening is hard to justify.

Screening for Genetic Susceptibilities

In a few genetic conditions, disease is likely to appear only in certain environments. Screening of infants or young children provides warning that certain exposures will be harmful and should be avoided. If harmful exposures occur, awareness of the genetic susceptibility could speed appropriate management. In the United States, no state currently screens newborns for such genetic susceptibilities. This may reflect a lack of confidence in the ability of the health care system or parents to ensure that the harmful exposures will be avoided. Screening workers or prospective employees for genetic susceptibilities (including the two conditions discussed below), in which the harmful agent may be encountered on the job, is of interest to some employers.[29]

Glucose-6-Phosphate Dehydrogenase (G6PD) Deficiency. A number of different alleles result in this X-linked genetic susceptibility. The usual manifestations are hemolytic anemia accompanied by jaundice and hemoglobinuria. Approximately 10% of African-American males inherit the mild A^- form. With the exception of some sulfur compounds (e.g., sulfamethoxazole), the drugs that trigger reactions seldom are used in Americans (e.g., primaquine), although some may develop hemolysis following heavy exposure to naphthalene (moth balls). In the more severe Mediterranean variant (but only occasionally in the A^- variant), hemolytic anemia ("favism") is encountered following ingestion of fava beans, a staple of diets in many Mediterranean countries. The initiation of a newborn screening program for G6PD deficiency in Sardinia, together with more education about the deficiency, was associated with a marked decline in the occurrence of favism and the need for blood transfusions.[48]

Alpha-1-Antitrypsin (AT) Deficiency. Individuals who have severe AT deficiency, usually the result of inheriting Z alleles from both parents, are at increased risk of chronic obstructive pulmonary disease (COPD), although in population-based surveys many people who have severe deficiency remain asymptomatic throughout life.[61] Those who have the deficiency and who smoke are likely to encounter pulmonary problems between 20 and 40 years of age, approximately 15 years earlier than nonsmokers.[79] Not all nonsmokers with AT deficiency get COPD. Severe AT deficiency accounts for about 1% of all COPD. Presymptomatic screening could alert those who have AT deficiency to the especially harmful consequences of smoking. Treatment of AT-deficient, emphysematous adults with human AT elevated their serum and lung AT levels but did not improve their pulmonary function.[32] Whether such treatment would prevent COPD remains to be established.

Because adolescents who have AT deficiency have normal pulmonary function,[74] screening of newborns or young children is of questionable value in improving outcome. A pilot program involving 200,000 newborns in Sweden was stopped when pediatricians reported adverse psychological effects on parents and on the parent-child relationship. Both short- and long-term effects were confirmed in a systematical study. In addition, although parents were told of the harm of exposing their children who had AT deficiency to cigarette smoke, there was as much parental smoking as in a control group.[47]

About 10% of infants who have AT deficiency develop cholestasis, and 2% to 3% later develop cirrhosis. There is no specific treatment or known means of preventing the liver manifestations, although human milk may be protective.[68] Consequently, newborn screening would not be expected to alter the prognosis. AT deficiency should be included in the differential diagnosis of persistent jaundice in young infants. Screening adolescents or young adults might be of benefit.

Carrier Screening

Carrier screening is undertaken for severe untreatable inherited disorders to provide those identified as carriers with options for avoiding the conception or birth of affected children. Carrier screening for Tay-Sachs has resulted in a significant decrease in the disease in many Jewish communities.[34] Carrier screening for thalassemia in Sardinia[11] and elsewhere in the Mediterranean basin has lowered its incidence. Most American couples found by carrier screening to be at risk of having a child who has sickle cell anemia decide not to terminate the pregnancy.[44] With nondirective counseling, they may not view the disorder as severe as do those at risk of having children with Tay-Sachs or thalassemia.

School-based screening programs for sickle cell and Tay-Sachs carriers probably recruit a much higher proportion of the at-risk population than do community programs or office or clinic screening programs. However, they may lead to the stigmatization of students identified as carriers unless all those being screened understand the reasons for the screening and the significance of the results. Nor is it clear that adolescents whose carrier status is identified will retain this information or act on it when they consider having children.[80] If prenatal diagnosis of a condition is available and abortion of an affected fetus acceptable, there is less reason to offer screening before mating. Couples could be screened before the woman becomes pregnant or early in pregnancy, although the latter may require more expensive testing and preclude certain options, such as artificial insemination of sperm from a donor who is not a carrier.

It now is possible to detect approximately 90% of the mutations responsible for cystic fibrosis in Caucasian populations. Questions have been raised about the merits of carrier screening because not all mutations can be discovered and the prognosis of the disorder is improving steadily.[51] A number of pilot programs have explored consumer interest in carrier screening.[64]

Screening young women to determine if they are carriers of X-linked disorders, such as fragile X, hemophilia, and Duchenne muscular dystrophy, is becoming technically feasible with DNA analysis. Because of new mutations, not all births of infants who have these disorders could potentially be avoided.

Prenatal Screening

Practitioners who provide care to the young usually do not have primary responsibility for managing pregnancies; however, they often will have prior contact with the mother and the father and can contribute to the parents' understanding of the indications for screening in pregnancy. They also may be contacted by obstetricians to assist in counseling or in anticipation of high-risk newborns. A review of *Prenatal Genetic Diagnosis for Pediatricians* has been published recently.[13] Only prenatal screening tests will be discussed here.

Neural Tube Defects. Although periconceptional dietary supplementation with folic acid will prevent some neural tube defects,[76] they are likely to remain one of the most frequent congenital malformations, at least until adequate dietary intake of folate by women contemplating pregnancy can be assured. (Supplementing bread products with folate soon may be required.) Maternal serum screening of alpha-fetoprotein (AFP) between the fifteenth and twenty-first weeks of pregnancy provides women an opportunity to avoid the birth of most infants who have anencephaly and open spina bifida by prenatal diagnosis and abortion or, if they chose to carry to term, of possibly improving the outcome. Identifying fetuses affected with open spina bifida before delivery permits prelabor cesarean section, which may improve their sensorimotor function.[46]

The maternal serum AFP test is capable of detecting 90% of fetuses that have anencephaly and about 80% of those that have open spina bifida.[72] For every true positive result, however, approximately 30 women who do not have affected fetuses will have false positive results. In women who have elevated maternal serum AFP, sonographic examination is needed to determine the accuracy of the gestational age estimate; the normal maternal serum AFP concentration is highly dependent on gestational age. If sonography confirms the gestational age, amniotic fluid is obtained by amniocentesis. If the amniotic fluid AFP is elevated, the likelihood of an open neural tube defect exceeds 90%. Further assurance that a defect is present is obtained by performing acetylcholinesterase determinations[73] and high detail (level 2) ultrasound. Although high level ultrasound *performed by expert sonographers* detects most fetuses who have open spina bifida, it should not replace AFP screening.

Down Syndrome. Until recently, prenatal diagnosis for Down syndrome (DS) was offered routinely only to pregnant women 35 years and older. The lower risk to younger women of having a fetus with DS and the risk to the fetus of chorionic villi sampling or amniocentesis, as well as the costs, could not justify testing all pregnant women. Nevertheless, most infants who have DS are born to women younger than 35 years of age. In 1984 an association between low concentrations of maternal serum AFP and DS in pregnant women regardless of their age was reported, but only about 20% of infants who had DS born to women under 35 years were detected. The detection rate has now been demonstrated to be substantially improved by measuring human chorionic gonadotropin, which is elevated in pregnancies that have DS (but not trisomy 18), and unconjugated estriol, which is reduced in pregnancies that have DS, as well as AFP. When measurements of these three substances are combined with the maternal age, women can be provided with an estimate of their risk of having DS. Currently, risks greater than 1 in 190 to 1 in 270 (depending on the center) are the basis for offering amniocentesis for karyotypic diagnosis. Using this protocol, it is possible to detect almost 60% of pregnancies that have DS. For every pregnancy in which DS is diagnosed, 37 amniocenteses in women found not to have a DS fetus must be performed. Over 80% of pregnant women under age 35 years who were at high risk accepted amniocentesis, but only 59% of women 35 and over did.[23]

AVAILABILITY OF SCREENING TESTS

Health departments usually can provide information about newborn screening and hemoglobinopathy screening. Community groups for sickle cell anemia, thalassemia, Tay-Sachs disease, and cystic fibrosis often know where carrier screening for these conditions can be obtained. The Alliance of Genetic Support Groups (Washington, D.C.) also can provide information. "Helix," operating out of the Children's Hospital in Seattle, maintains an up-to-date list of laboratories providing DNA tests as well as some biochemical tests.

ETHICAL AND LEGAL ISSUES IN SCREENING

In view of the reproductive implications of most genetic screening tests, as well as respect for the autonomy of individuals, there is widespread agreement that genetic screening, with the possible exception of newborn screening, requires informed consent.[3] The disclosure should include the nature of the disease, the probability that the condition will occur, the nature, benefits, and risks of the interventions should the result be positive (including pregnancy termination in the case of prenatal screening), the probability of test error, and other possible deleterious effects.

Some have argued that newborn screening for untreatable disorders—for instance, Duchenne muscular dystrophy (DMD), fragile X, or cystic fibrosis (CF) (for which the benefits of newborn screening have not been fully established)—is appropriate because the prompt diagnosis affords parents the opportunity of avoiding the birth of another affected child. Others have argued that the infant found to be affected by newborn screening derives no benefit from the test and may even be harmed, for instance, interference with parental bonding.[3] With current DNA test technology, some of those at high risk of having affected children can be identified by carrier screening either before or early in pregnancy. Couples at risk then have the opportunity of avoiding the conception or birth of *any* affected offspring, whereas only second or additional affected children can be avoided by newborn screening.

Third parties, such as insurers and employers, may have an interest in learning the results of genetic tests in order, for instance, to deny coverage or employment to those who have positive results. It is widely agreed that test results should not be released to such third parties without explaining to the screenee, or his or her parents in the case of newborn screening, the implications of releasing the results and obtaining consent. Except in very unusual circumstances, health care providers are not obliged to notify relatives of a patient who has a positive test result but who refuses to inform relatives that they are at risk.[3]

One reason for screening newborns in hospitals is that they are a "captive" population. Unless screening confers a benefit not otherwise attainable, such a reason is ethically suspect. For disorders for which treatment is effective only before symptoms appear, and when those symptoms appear early in childhood, newborn screening does confer a benefit not otherwise attainable. This is not true for conditions that manifest later in childhood, or not until adulthood, and for which intervention in infancy or childhood is of no proven benefit. This issue is likely to emerge if and when it becomes possible to screen for genetic predispositions to cancer and, perhaps, other mainly adult-onset disorders. Telling children or their parents that they are at risk for a late-onset condition for which intervention after childhood is adequate could alter child-rearing patterns and generate considerable anxiety. In some cases, parents and their children might differ on having the child screened. Older children should be informed of such screening and assent to it.

FUTURE OF GENETIC SCREENING

The Human Genome Project will continue to increase the identification of genes that play a role in disease. The major advances of DNA technology will make it possible to test a small specimen containing nucleated cells for genetic variants that increase the risk of many different disorders. The ethical and legal challenges to this multiplex testing may prove more difficult than the technological hurdles. The different disorders that might be included in multiplex testing will be markedly different in their age of onset, their severity, and in the interventions available to treat, ameliorate, or avoid their occurrence. How will prospective testees, or their parents, be able to decide whether they want any or all of the tests available?

The discovery of genes that play a role in complex (polygenic or multifactorial) disorders holds great appeal, but much needs to be learned of the role of alleles at these loci in the general population, as well as in high-risk families, before screening is even considered.

Many mutations of a single gene are capable of causing or predisposing to disease. One drawback of current DNA technology is not being able to detect all of these mutations or to distinguish mutations that result in disease from those that do not. Advances in DNA technology will overcome these problems. In addition, it will be possible to examine gene products in readily accessible cells by amplifying the protein synthesized by the gene of interest and examining its structure or function. Alterations in structure or function are likely to indicate the presence of more disease-causing or susceptibility-conferring mutations than could DNA analysis.

Intensive efforts are being made to isolate fetal cells from maternal circulation to be able to perform prenatal diagnosis without placing the fetus at risk.[62] If successful, it will be possible to use fluorescent DNA probes to determine the presence of extra chromosomes (as in Down syndrome) on the fetal cells as well as to perform DNA analysis for disease-causing mutations. Within a few years, this technique might make the screening of every fetus for several congenital and hereditary disorders feasible. Once again, the ethical and legal issues may be more difficult to solve than the technical.

The marked expansion of genetic testing and screening has increased commercial interest in manufacturing test reagents and providing genetic testing services. Health care providers can expect pressures from companies offering tests to provide these services. Unfortunately, tests can be made available without adequate assessment of their safety and effectiveness. Providers would do well to go beyond material in the lay press and in company-sponsored brochures before offering these tests to their patients.

FOUR

Cardiac Screening

Michael A. LaCorte
Rakesh Menon

Many forms of adult cardiovascular disease have their origin in childhood. Recent attention has been focused on diet, cholesterol, and blood pressure in the pediatric population. The purpose of this chapter is to outline screening strategies in the pediatric population that will be of value in identifying existing cardiovascular disease and identifying those individuals who have predisposition to cardiovascular disease as an adult.

For a screening program to be deemed worthwhile, the disease or potential disease must be of sufficient severity or prevalence. Screening tests should be reliable and reasonably easy to perform. The test must have acceptable sensitivity, specificity, and predictive value. A *new* screening procedure also must show benefit over current practice and be acceptable to practitioners and patients. In light of escalating health care costs, the cost effectiveness of any screening test is important.

The screening strategies outlined in this chapter are intended to supplement a good history and physical examination to optimize the identification of those children and adolescents who are at risk for cardiac disease and, thereby, to promote improved ongoing health care.

BLOOD PRESSURE SCREENING

Routine blood pressure (BP) screening in the pediatric age group *may* serve two purposes: (1) identifying children who have actual, fixed hypertension due to a variety of ongoing diseases (secondary hypertension) and (2) providing a marker for the development of essential (primary) hypertension as an adult.

An appropriate size cuff (i.e., width approximately 75% of the upper arm), proper position of the child (sitting except for infants), and a satisfactory examining area (quiet and reassuring environment) are important components in measuring an accurate blood pressure in children. In addition, the K4 (muffling) phase should be used as the diastolic blood pressure in young children because K5 (disappearance of sound) may not occur in this age group.

A particular problem in the pediatric age group is the delineation of normative BP data. To date, the definitive publication of normal pediatric BP measurements is the Report of the Second Task Force on Blood Pressure Control in Children published in *Pediatrics*.[17] The Task Force defines three levels of BP measurement. In general, systolic and diastolic BPs <90th percentile for age and sex are considered *normal*. BP measurements between the 90th and 95th percentile that are not explainable by body habitus are considered *high normal* and remain under surveillance. If an infant, child, or adolescent has three BP readings >95th percentile for age and sex, the individual is noted to have high blood pressure. Elevated BP is qualified as clinically significant (95th to 99th percentile) and severe (above 99th percentile for age and sex). Diagnostic evaluation is based on age-specific causes of secondary hypertension. In the infant and young child, renal parenchymal disease, coarctation of the aorta, and renal vascular anomalies predominate. In the older child and adolescent, renal artery stenosis and chronic renal parenchymal disease are most common. A careful physical examination, including evaluation of femoral pulses (coarctation), abdominal examination for masses and bruits (polycystic kidneys, renovascular disease), and funduscopic examination are important to the pursuit of the causes of secondary hypertension. Laboratory data in a hypertension workup include basic studies such as urinalysis and urine culture, complete blood cell count, electrolytes, and blood urea nitrogen and creatinine levels. In selected cases, specialized radiological studies (e.g., renal sonogram, intravenous pyelography, computed tomography, renal radionuclide studies), and hormonal studies (e.g., plasma catecholamine and renin) are indicated.

The role of mass blood pressure screening for the purpose of identifying children at risk of developing high blood pressure (essential hypertension) as an adult has been controversial. Because secondary hypertension in children is uncommon and because, in general, these children are identified as having BP readings well over the 95th percentile as well as other physical signs and symptoms, routine mass BP screening for the purpose of detecting secondary hypertension is difficult to advocate. The real question is whether elevated BP in childhood predicts the presence of high BP in adults. The Task Force on Blood Pressure in Children[17] advocates routine yearly BP recordings beginning at 3 years of age. However, one needs to ask whether there should there be nationwide screening in schools for hypertension. Is it cost effective? In the Bogalusa Heart Study,[19] only one third of children at the 90th percentile in BP recording remained at the 90th percentile or greater 3 years after the initial measurement; in other words, if a cutoff of the 90th percentile were used to predict hypertension in the future, 67% would be misdiagnosed. Gilman et al.[6] also report a modest correlation between elevated BP in childhood and hypertension in later life. They, too, raise the question of the cost effectiveness of mass BP screening for the purpose of identifying individuals at risk of developing essential hypertension later in life.

CARDIOVASCULAR SCREENING IN THE YOUNG ATHLETE

Sudden death in a young competitive athlete is rare but tragic and is often well publicized. It affects local school athletic programs significantly and raises questions concerning the feasibility of screening child and adolescent participants who may be at risk for sudden death.

Structural cardiovascular abnormalities account for almost all sudden deaths in young athletes, and hypertrophic cardiomyopathy is the most common cardiovascular abnormality in this group. Other entities such as Marfan syndrome and anomalies of the coronary arteries account for a significant number of the remaining causes of sudden death in young athletes. In the case of Marfan syndrome, a careful family history of early cardiovascular disease or sudden death and a thorough physical examination to reveal stigmata of the Marfan syndrome (i.e., arachnodactyly, pectus deformity, lens abnormality) can alert the physician to the possibility of the presence of this disease. Mitral valve prolapse and aortic root dilatation on echocardiography are additional evidence of the presence of Marfan syndrome and should result in restriction of competitive athletics and prophylactic treatment with beta-blockers.

Ideally, 2D echocardiography is a useful screening test to identify individuals who have Marfan syndrome who are at risk of sudden death during competitive athletics. It also is valuable in identifying individuals who have hypertrophic cardiomyopathy. The cost of 2D echocardiography makes it a prohibitively expensive screening test. However, routine ECG screening of all young competitive athletes has been suggested as a potential cost-effective means of detecting life-threatening cardiac abnormalities.[5,16] Unfortunately a resting ECG is of no value in detecting Marfan syndrome and certain anomalies of the coronary arteries in which ischemic changes are only exercise induced. However, the rest-

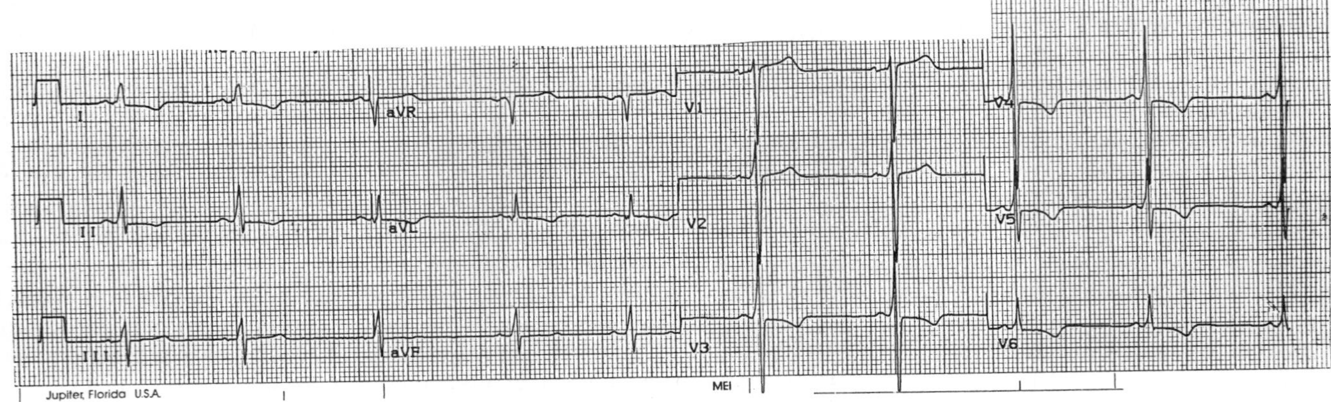

FIG. 20-1 Resting EKG of a 15-year-old male athlete who has hypertrophic cardiomyopathy. There is left ventricular hypertrophy (LVH), accompanied by some T-wave inversion ("strain"). All leads are at half standard. The patient has been restricted from competitive athletics and prescribed calcium channel blockers.

ing ECG is abnormal in over 90% of individuals who have hypertrophic cardiomyopathy who are at risk of sudden death[12] (Fig. 20-1). Because the incidence of hypertrophic cardiomyopathy in school athletes is no greater than 1 in 1000, the cost of performing ECGs is prohibitive in most school systems.

However, in some communities that have active school health programs administered collaboratively by the school district and a local hospital, a screening ECG program may be cost effective and provide valuable reassurance to families and athletic directors. Such a program has been in effect since 1986 in school districts in Nassau County, N.Y., in conjunction with the Division of Pediatric Cardiology and the Health Education Department at North Shore University Hospital.[8] To date, although almost 5000 screening ECGs have been performed without a single case of hypertrophic cardiomyopathy having been identified, approximately 5% of the young athletes screened have ECG abnormalities ranging from atrial premature contraction and right ventricular conduction delay to the more significant abnormality of preexcitation syndrome (0.5%).[8,11] Knowledge of these abnormalities is useful to the athlete, the family, and family physicians and is a major benefit of an ECG screening program. Despite the lack of detecting any cases of hypertrophic cardiomyopathy in this large series, such a screening program is reassuring to athletes and their families and to school officials. In addition, the study shows that a close working relationship between a large health care facility and well organized school districts can result in an effective ECG screening program.

CHOLESTEROL SCREENING

Coronary heart disease (CHD) is the leading cause of death in the United States. Despite much success in reducing mortality due to this disease in the past 2 decades, CHD is responsible for more than 500,000 deaths annually. Several million more Americans have symptomatic CHD, accounting for many office visits and hospitalizations per year. Estimates of the annual cost of CHD in the United States range from $41.4 to $56 billion.[13]

Many studies present substantial evidence that the process of atherosclerosis begins in childhood and progresses slowly into adulthood,[4,18] at which time CHD frequently develops. Studies also indicate that this atherosclerotic process is related to elevated levels of blood cholesterol in childhood and that these levels are predictive of elevated blood cholesterol in adulthood.[9,10,15] High blood cholesterol levels clearly play a role in the development of CHD in adults.[7,14]

The issue of cholesterol screening in childhood and adolescence abounds with controversy, with researchers and clinicians arguing for and against screening, while still others debate the appropriate time for screening and what form such screening should take. The American Academy of Pediatrics (AAP) published its recommendations regarding cholesterol and dietary fat in 1986[2] and suggested indications for cholesterol testing in children and adolescents in 1989.[1] In 1991 the *Expert Panel on Blood Cholesterol in Children and Adolescents of the National Cholesterol Education Program (NCEP)* produced a comprehensive report addressing this volatile issue and made recommendations based on an extensive review of existing knowledge and recent studies.[13] Following the NCEP report, the AAP released a statement on cholesterol based on its earlier recommendations as well as the recommendations of the NCEP report.[3]

Several authors[9,10,14,15] have dissected and analyzed these recommendations and offered their own thoughts on pediatric cholesterol screening. Despite such scrutiny, the pediatric approach to the primary prevention of CHD in adults remains controversial.

In spite of existing differences of opinion regarding cholesterol screening in the pediatric age group, it is our opinion that selective cholesterol screening (see below) indeed is a requirement that will lead to a healthier adult population.

Why Screen?

1. American children and adolescents have higher blood cholesterol levels and higher intakes of saturated fatty acids and cholesterol than their counterparts in most other countries. American adults also have higher mortality and morbidity due to CHD than these other countries.
2. Autopsies show that early coronary atherosclerosis or precursors of atherosclerosis often begin in childhood or adolescence.

3. High blood total cholesterol, low-density lipoprotein (LDL) cholesterol, very-low-density lipoprotein (VLDL) cholesterol, and low high-density lipoprotein (HDL) cholesterol levels are correlated with the extent of early atherosclerotic lesions among adolescents and young adults.
4. Children and adolescents who have elevated blood cholesterol levels, particularly LDL cholesterol levels, frequently come from families in which there is a high incidence of CHD among adult members.
5. High blood cholesterol in families results from both shared environments and genetic factors.
6. Children and adolescents who have high cholesterol levels are more likely than the general population to have high levels as adults.

Who Should Be Screened?

Universal screening is *not* recommended by both the AAP and NCEP. Selective screening seeks to identify children and adolescents who are at the greatest risk of having a high blood cholesterol level as adults and an increased risk of CHD.

Absolute Indications

1. Family history of premature cardiovascular disease
   - Parents or grandparents 55 years of age or younger found to have coronary atherosclerosis by diagnostic coronary arteriography or who have undergone balloon angioplasty or coronary artery bypass surgery
   - Parents or grandparents 55 years of age or younger who had a documented myocardial infarction, angina pectoris, peripheral vascular disease, cerebrovascular disease, or sudden cardiac death

Or

2. At least one parent with high blood cholesterol ≥240 mg/dl

Optional Indications. Especially for those children and adolescents whose parental and grandparenteral history is unavailable, the pediatrician may choose to measure cholesterol levels based on other risk factors:

1. Obesity, ≥130% ideal body weight
2. High blood pressure
3. Cigarette smoking
4. Dietary history—excessive amounts of saturated fatty acids, total fat, or cholesterol
5. A sibling who has an elevated blood cholesterol level
6. Physical inactivity
7. Exogenous causes of hypercholesterolemia, for example, drugs such as corticosteroids, oral contraceptives, anabolic steroids, and anticonvulsants
8. Diseases resulting in secondary hypercholesterolemia, for example, diabetes mellitus, hypothyroidism, nephrotic syndrome, collagen disease, glycogen storage disease, obstructive liver disease, anorexia nervosa, progeria, and Klinefelter syndrome.

Children and adolescents who have several of these risk factors should undergo cholesterol screening.

What Age To Screen?

The age at which cholesterol screening should be done also is controversial. The NCEP recommends that a blood sample be obtained any time after the age of 2 years. If cholesterol levels are acceptable then, they may be repeated after 5 years.

In general, we agree with the NCEP regarding testing after the age of 2 years; certainly testing should be done during the adolescent years (≥10 years) and again at the age of 20 to 25 years. Testing should be repeated annually or more often depending on the levels obtained.

Studies show that cholesterol levels during adolescence are predictive into adulthood. These studies indicate that it may be more appropriate to screen for hypercholesterolemia during adolescence than in early childhood. Diet tends to vary among those 2 to 5 years of age, and infrequent visits are made to the pediatrician by those 6 to 12 years of age. This reinforces the need for testing during adolescence, which also is an influential time for these emerging young adults, as they may be educated to follow a healthier life-style and to seek continued health care.

Because tracking of cholesterol through childhood and adulthood is less than perfect, it cannot be stated that every child who has an elevated blood cholesterol level will have an elevated level as an adult. Therefore multiple measurements through adolescence should be obtained before labeling a child as being hypercholesterolemic.

How To Screen?

The NCEP has outlined algorithms for screening and initiating therapy that involve the measurement of total blood cholesterol and LDL cholesterol. These have been reviewed and accepted by the American Academy of Pediatrics. In general, a persistent LDL cholesterol greater than 130 mg/dl requires evaluation for familial disorders and secondary causes of hypercholesterolemia. Those children will require appropriate intervention in the way of dietary modification and long-term follow-up of cholesterol levels. Pediatricians also will be responsible for providing advice related to identification and avoidance of other risk factors, as well as encouraging behavior changes including diet. Failure to lower blood cholesterol levels through dietary and behavior modification should prompt referral to physicians experienced in the management of lipid disorders in children.

Drug therapy to lower cholesterol levels, as recommended by NCEP, is for children over 10 years of age who, after an adequate trial of diet therapy for 6 months to a year, have either (1) LDL cholesterol levels >190 mg/dl or (2) LDL cholesterol levels ≥160 mg/dl *and* (3) a strong family history of premature CAD, or two or more adult cardiovascular disease risk factors (low HDL cholesterol level, smoking, high blood pressure, obesity, or diabetes). If drug therapy is being considered, referral to physicians experienced in the management of lipid disorders in children is advised.

FIVE

Screening for Anemia

Robert F. Reiss

Screening for anemia in infants and young children should be undertaken at 6 to 12 months and again at 2 years of age because at these ages the more common congenital anemias and iron deficiency anemia may become apparent.

Until recently, offices screened for anemia by determining the microhematocrit—using blood obtained by skin puncture, collected in a capillary tube, and then spun in a small centrifuge. The hematocrit determined by this method was compared with reference values obtained from age-matched normal children. Infants and children found to have a hematocrit less than the lower reference level (2 standard deviations below the population mean) were defined as anemic.

Recently, the older microhematocrit procedures have been replaced partially by the in-office determination of whole blood hemoglobin concentration. Although simple to perform, determinations of microhematocrits by using the previously available centrifuges were associated with the creation of blood aerosols and bloody glass fragments when the capillary tubes broke during centrifugation. These are believed to pose an infectious risk to the instrument operator. In addition, the continued accurate and precise performance of the centrifuge had to be validated periodically with time-consuming checks and calibrations. On the other hand, the whole blood hemoglobin concentration, a determination that had been performed previously as a stand-alone test or as part of an electronic complete blood count (CBC) in a hematology laboratory, now can be performed quickly, simply, and fairly accurately and precisely in the physician's office. Now available are small portable photometers that measure the hemoglobin concentration in a drop of blood obtained by skin puncture. The 1-minute procedure consists of allowing the drop to flow into a small cuvette and subsequently inserting the cuvette into the photometer and reading the digital display on the instrument. Ongoing quality control also is simple and consists of reading the display after inserting a control cuvette supplied with the photometer.

Determination of anemia through these simple screening tests must be confirmed and further information about the morphological characteristics of the patient's blood cells obtained before deciding on further diagnostic workup. These data usually are obtained by submitting a venous blood sample to the hematology laboratory for a CBC and microscopic examination of a Wright-stained peripheral blood smear.

A CBC can be performed on small samples of EDTA-anticoagulated blood (350 μL) by the modern electronic particle counters. These instruments not only measure the red cell count, mean corpuscular volume (MCV), and whole blood hemoglobin concentration directly, but also calculate the hematocrit, mean corpuscular hemoglobin (MCH), and mean corpuscular hemoglobin concentration (MCHC). In addition, these counters measure the total white blood cell and platelet counts directly. Finally, the most sophisticated cell counters perform white cell differential and reticulocyte counts.

On the basis of the reticulocyte count and the red cell indices (MCV, MCH, and MCHC), the anemia presumptively can be categorized by mechanism as either hypoproliferative (inappropriately low reticulocyte count for the degree of anemia) or hemolytic (significantly increased reticulocyte count) and by its principal morphological features as microcytic—usually hypochromic (decreased MCV and MCHC), normocytic—usually normochromic (normal MCV and MCHC), or macrocytic (increased MCV). The interpretation of the reticulocyte count and red cell indices and their use in the classification of anemias are discussed fully in the chapter on diseases of the hematopoietic system.

Examination of the peripheral smear for red cell size and the degree of cell hemoglobin content permits validation of the indices by determining whether these mean values are representative of a rather monomorphic cell population or of multiple cell populations. The finding of a wide disparity of red cell sizes on the smear is known as anisocytosis and is reflected in an increased red cell volume distribution width (RDW), an additional red cell index reported by the newer cell counters. In addition, the finding of numerous grayish-staining (polychromatophilic) macrocytes, a feature known as polychromasia, suggests increased reticulocytosis. Finally, the red cells themselves may have specific morphological abnormalities of diagnostic significance (e.g., sickled red cells and red cell fragments), or the smear may contain abnormal numbers of types of white cells or platelets, which often helps explain the etiology of the anemia.

It is important to note that with only modest formal training and subsequent ongoing experience, the practicing physician can gain considerable expertise in the interpretation of peripheral blood smears. Acquisition of this skill permits office examination of a smear of blood drop from a skin puncture. This information, together with that gained from a physical examination and history, including family history of anemia, permits an initiation of specific diagnostic testing at the time the venous CBC sample is submitted to the hematology laboratory.

Among the most common anemias detected in such screening programs are those that have microcytic indices resulting from defects in hemoglobin synthesis. The vast majority of these are due to iron deficiency and thalassemia trait. Although it has been observed that the RDW tends to be increased in the former and normal in the latter, the definitive differential diagnosis will rest on the results of iron studies, free erythrocycte porphyrin measurements, and in older children, hemoglobin A_2 levels.

Congenital hemolytic anemias are characterized by increased reticulocytosis, usually have normocytic and normochromic indices, demonstrate polychromasia, and often have diagnostically important red cell morphological abnormalities in the peripheral smear.

The finding of a microcytic anemia and the suspicion of iron deficiency requires a search for a source of blood loss, including gastrointestinal bleeding and intestinal parasites. In the absence of evidence for blood loss, iron replacement therapy can be initiated pending the results of definitive laboratory tests. Increased polychromasia in the peripheral smear after 5 to 7 days and a subsequent rise in whole blood hemoglobin concentration confirm the diagnosis of iron deficiency anemia and require the continuation of treatment to replace tissue stores.

In summary, performance of the whole blood hemoglobin concentration and examination of the peripheral smear from a drop of whole blood can be office procedures that not only detect the presence of anemia, but often permit its preliminary classification and facilitate expeditious determination of its etiopathogenesis. Finally, the availability of these office tests allows the treating physician to monitor the patient's response to therapy.

SIX

Screening for Lead Poisoning

Sergio Piomelli

The clinical symptomatology of lead (Pb) poisoning in children often is vague and ill defined. Extremely elevated blood lead levels cause frank neurological disturbances. However, neurological toxicity, even at high levels, may not be preceded by any premonitory signs, and once it occurs it may be irreversible. To prevent permanent sequelae, it is necessary to detect lead poisoning before its effects become clinically evident. In addition, subtle neurological toxicity can occur at low levels of exposure, and this may result in preventable impairment of neuropsychological function. For these reasons, asymptomatic children who potentially may be exposed to lead should be screened periodically to prevent neurological toxicity (see the box below). Because lead poisoning occurs most frequently in children between the ages of 12 months and 6 years, screening should be focused on children in these age groups who are at greatest risk.

Efforts at screening should be more intensive in areas where many homes were built before World War II, when lead-based paint was used. It is important to recognize that many children may be exposed to lead outside their primary residence in day care settings, babysitters' homes, or the homes of other family members or friends. Screening should be conducted every 6 months for those children between 12 and 36 months of age and every year thereafter. A screening test indicates the status of lead intoxication only at a given moment. Severe lead poisoning may develop over 2 to 3 months; therefore, despite a history of previously normal findings, testing should be repeated if symptoms suspicious of lead poisoning are present.

The main source of lead for children is dust in the home due to deteriorated paint. In recent years, as a consequence of the reduction in the use of lead-based gasoline, atmospheric contamination with lead has declined progressively. This decline has been paralleled by a profound decline in the average blood lead level in the entire American population, from 13 μg/dl in 1980 to <3 μg/dl in 1991. This is no minor change, considering a blood lead level of 3 μg/dl has been measured in children living in the pristine air of the highlands of the Himalayas, far from any source of atmospheric pollution.

This drastic reduction in the average blood lead level in the United States has had dramatic effects on the incidence of childhood lead poisoning; lead encephalopathy has essentially disappeared. Most children detected by the screening programs today have blood lead levels well below 40 μg/dl. Current screening programs therefore are directed toward the detection of children who have much lower blood lead levels.

FACTORS PREDISPOSING CHILDREN TO LEAD EXPOSURE

- Living in or regularly visiting a home that was built before 1960 and has deteriorated paint or is being renovated
- Living with a sibling or house-mate being followed up for lead poisoning (blood lead ≥15 μg/dl)
- Living with an adult whose job or hobby involves exposure to lead
- Living near any industry likely to release lead in the atmosphere

UNIVERSAL SCREENING: THE CONTROVERSY

Screening children for lead poisoning is the subject of great controversy. A committee of experts convened by the Centers for Disease Control and Prevention (CDC) has recommended that all American children age 6 months to 6 years be screened and that a threshold of 10 μg/dl be used as a definition of lead poisoning. The need for universal screening and the reduced threshold have been questioned. Lead essentially has been eliminated from the air and from canned food; the main source of lead for children today remains lead-based paint and contaminated dust in the home. Because homes built in the post–World War II era often are essentially lead free, it does not appear necessary (or cost effective) to screen all children who live in newer homes. Efforts to screen every child may detract from screening those children who live in high-risk areas. Many pediatricians favor screening directed to children living in those areas where lead paint is known to be present. The CDC has realized the problems associated with universal screening and is developing criteria to identify those communities where universal screening is unnecessary.

An additional point of controversy is the establishment of 10 μg/dl as the threshold of lead poisoning. Lead is an extremely toxic metal. Any atom of lead that enters the body produces some effect; the greater the number of atoms, the more severe the effect. Because lead is a nonessential metal, the natural blood lead level is 0 μg/dl.

Because the natural blood lead level is 0 μg/dl and adverse effects are measurable at infinitesimal levels of exposure, in theory we should aim at reducing children's blood lead levels to 0 μg/dl. In reality, it is necessary to set a pragmatic goal based on a reasonable estimate of the blood lead level at which adverse effects become relatively insignificant. With the refinement of techniques to detect neurophysiological damage, adverse effects have been identified at progressively lower blood lead levels. On the basis of many studies, a level of 10 μg/dl has been chosen as the threshold of lead poisoning. (In the schema of screening recommended by the CDC, however, it is recognized that no intervention is needed or possible for children whose blood lead levels are between 10 and 15 μg/dl; these children are identified to decide whether universal screening should be continued in their area and to ascertain the need for environmental intervention.)

The problems are compounded in that even in the best of laboratories measurements of blood lead in the 10 μg/dl range are accurate only within ±2 to 3 μg/dl. Thus for many of the children who are classified as having blood leads of 10, 11, or 12 μg/dl on initial screening, values above the threshold often are the result of laboratory inaccuracy. Based on 1987 data, 17% of American children had blood lead levels ≥15 μg/dl. However, the situation has improved greatly since then. The Third National Health and Nutritional Survey reported that in 1991 the prevalence of children ages 1 to 5 years having blood lead levels ≥10 μg/dl was 8.9% and that of children having blood lead levels ≥20 μg/dl was 1.1%. These figures refer to the entire population of children; great differences in the percentages between different socioeconomic groups still persisted. Thus universal screening is going to detect very few children who have blood lead levels ≥20 μg/dl, for whom intervention is useful, and thousands of children who have blood lead levels 10 to 15 μg/dl, for whom intervention is neither possible nor of proven effectiveness. This generates unnecessary anxiety among many parents, since a level above 10 μg/dl is defined as lead poisoning by the CDC. On the other hand, proponents of universal screening argue that the adverse effects of minimal lead exposure are significant and that it is necessary to prevent them. They base this judgment on the data that suggest that every increase in blood lead by 10 μg/dl corresponds to a decrease in IQ of 2 to 3 points. Moreover, they believe that it is important to detect those children who have blood lead levels ≥10 μg/dl and that universal screening and counseling will protect them from further exposure.

SCREENING: THE CDC RECOMMENDATIONS AND STATE LAWS

The CDC recommendations of 1991 were endorsed by the American Academy of Pediatrics and also have become law in several states. Thus pediatricians, whatever they may think of the controversy, are obliged by their state law to screen all children ages 6 months to 6 years, as recommended by the CDC.

Screening for lead can be done effectively by finger puncture, but only if rigorous standards are followed. With excellent technique, the percentage of false positives is quite low using this method. However, when the sampling is obtained by finger puncture, a value <15 μg/dl can be trusted, but *a value ≥15 μg/dl should be confirmed by venipuncture* before deciding on and implementing treatment.

The recommendations of the CDC are based on a definition of lead poisoning as a blood lead level ≥10 μg/dl. The lowest category includes children who have a blood lead level of 10 to 14 μg/dl. These children do not need referral for medical attention but do need periodic testing.

For children who have blood lead levels of 15 to 19 μg/dl, educational and dietary advice are recommended. Parents are to be instructed about the risk of lead poisoning and about means to reduce exposure, particularly to household dust. At higher blood lead levels the recommendations, essentially unchanged, are indicated in the box below.

Among children who have a blood lead level of 45 to 66 μg/dl a possible alternative is oral administration of DMSA (dimercaptosuccinic acid [Chemet or Succimer]). However, this oral drug regimen should be considered only if the child is in a *lead-safe environment.* This must be established either through appropriate efforts to remove the source of lead (paint or any other) or by moving the child to a safe home.

CDC guidelines are intended to set priorities for environmental and medical intervention, not to replace sound clinical judgment. For instance, a 9-month-old child with a blood lead level of 31 μg/dl is at a much greater health risk than a 6-year-old with a blood lead level of 38 μg/dl, although both would be in the same CDC category.

Because screening is directed at the detection of low blood lead levels, measurements of erythrocyte protoporphyrins can no longer be used as the primary screening tool. In fact, 50% of children have an abnormally elevated erythrocyte protoporphyrin level at a blood lead level of 32 μg/dl, but below this blood lead level the proportion of abnormally elevated erythrocyte protoporphyrins levels progressively declines. Measurements of erythrocyte protoporphyrin levels remain useful to ascertain the degree of biochemical damage by lead and to evaluate the coexistence of iron deficiency, as well as to follow the efficacy of therapy and the abatement of lead from the environment.

RECOMMENDATIONS FOR TREATMENT OF ASYMPTOMATIC CHILDREN WHO HAVE HIGH BLOOD LEAD LEVELS

Blood lead level	Treatment
20-25 μg/dl	Environmental screening for removal of the lead source
25 to 44 μg/dl	Chelation therapy, if the $CaNa_2$ EDTA provocation test is positive
45 to 69 μg/dl	Treatment with $CaNa_2$ EDTA alone
≥70 μg/dl:	Emergency hospitalization; treatment with BAL/$CaNa_2$ EDTA

$CaNa_2$ EDTA, Calcium disodium versenate, calcium disodium ethylenediaminetetraacetic acid; *BAL*, British antilewisite.

SEVEN

Screening for Drugs

Deborah E. Campbell
S. Kenneth Schonberg

Drug use and abuse occur across all cultural and socioeconomic strata; however, urban disadvantaged and underserved populations, particularly minority groups, have been affected greatly. The severity of the drug epidemic, its effect on the developing fetus, child, or adolescent, and the ramifications for society have engendered much public debate and recommendations for criminal prosecution, incarceration, and forced rehabilitation of drug abusers, in particular, pregnant substance users. Drug abuse during pregnancy is a major health problem because of frequently associated perinatal complications contributing to significant neonatal mortality and morbidity. As a result of improved methods of detecting drugs and their metabolites in body fluids, mass screening of pregnant women, newborns, and adolescents has been proposed. This has caused controversy within the pediatrics, obstetrics, and bioethics communities. Although much could be gained from early detection of substance use at either end of the pediatric patient-care spectrum, both ethical and practical considerations suggest caution about imposing drug screening on unwilling patients and parents.

METHODS

Several techniques can be used to detect the metabolites of drugs of abuse in urine, other body fluids, hair, and meconium. In general, the less expensive and less complex methods generate a greater incidence of false positive and false negative results than do more costly and sophisticated tests. Such methods range from simple litmus spot tests, which can be performed in the physician's office, to gas chromatography–mass spectrometry (GC-MS) tests, which require highly technical and expensive equipment. The most commonly employed drug screen used in clinical practice is the enzyme multiplication immunoassay technique (EMIT). This test is available at most laboratories and is reasonably accurate and affordable.[10] False positive tests do occur; thus positive results should be confirmed through more sophisticated techniques (e.g., GC-MS).

The length of time since the last drug use that test results remain positive varies with the drug, the extent of its abuse, and the sensitivity of the test employed. With the EMIT technique, most drugs can be detected for at least 2 to 3 days after their last use. The metabolites of phencyclidine (PCP), however, may be detected for up to 1 week, and cannabinoids can be found for up to 3 to 4 weeks in heavy users.[2] Among neonates the detection of drug metabolites in urine is limited because of dependence on the time of the last maternal drug intake or on when the infant's urine was collected. Maternal abstention from drug use for several days before delivery or the inability to obtain a urine sample from the infant soon after birth contributes to false negative results. In prospective studies, urine testing alone would miss nearly 50% of drug-exposed infants. The hair of neonates has been analyzed, but technical difficulties make the analysis impractical. Testing of meconium from neonates of drug-dependent women for a variety of drugs (cocaine, morphine, cannabinoids) has demonstrated high concentrations of one or more of these drugs for up to 3 days after birth.[9] Meconium testing has been used as a tool in various prevalence studies and has been suggested for use in mass screenings.

The major issues concerning drug screening do not relate to the expense of the testing, the accuracy of the results, or the number of days that testing will show a positive reaction. Rather, the controversies center on the ethical and practical implications of such screening procedures. Seeking evidence of substance abuse differs greatly from other screening procedures, in which patient and physician share a mutual concern in detecting a condition previously unknown to either.

PERINATAL ISSUES

It has been estimated that between 100,000 and 375,000 infants (3% to 11%) are born annually in the United States after prenatal exposure to illicit drugs.[5,8] In a survey conducted by the National Institute on Drug Abuse (NIDA) in 1988, 8.8% (approximately 5 million) women of child-bearing age admitted to illicit substance use in the month preceding delivery.[7] Use of other substances (alcohol, tobacco, and other drugs) are far more common but difficult to quantitate. The greatest concern regarding perinatal drug exposure involves the potential teratogenic and developmental effects of particular drugs: alcohol, opiates, and cocaine/crack. Drug-exposed infants are more likely to suffer from a range of health and developmental problems and require prolonged neonatal hospitalization due to low birth weight and prematurity, neonatal abstinence syndromes, and birth complications; they also need long-term developmental support and habilitative care for the remediation of cognitive and behavioral sequelae.

It often is difficult to ascribe causality to a particular agent because pregnant substance abusers seldom use a single agent. The high prevalence of substance use among inner-city minority populations adds confounding factors related to life-style, environment, and resources. In addition, not all infants experience detrimental effects from perinatal drug exposure. Genetic and maternal characteristics, differences in the chemical structure of drugs, and patterns of use interact to influence fetal vulnerability.

Continuing parental drug abuse after the infant's birth is a significant concern and has been associated with (1) an increased frequency of physical abuse of their infants, (2) their diversion of limited family resources and their involvement in criminal activity to enable them to buy drugs, and (3) their high risk for mental and physical illness.[3] Thus the desire to use all means to detect parental drug abuse is most understandable; however, the use of maternal or neonatal drug screening for such detection raises a series of ethical and practical concerns.[4]

Mandatory or coerced testing of pregnant women stands in contrast to traditional adherence to ethical principles of informed voluntary consent for all physician-patient interactions. Similarly, testing a neonate for the presence of drugs is, in fact, an assessment of maternal drug use. Thus many find it ethically difficult to justify testing either the baby or the mother without appropriate consent. Identical concerns have been raised regarding testing for human immunodeficiency virus, and most jurisdictions forbid such testing without informed parental consent.

A second concern is that the practice of screening mothers for drugs will cause pregnant women to delay or to avoid prenatal care. Although this avoidance of care because of fear of detection remains unproved, it is logical to expect that pregnant women who use drugs would not want this known, for social and legal reasons.

Finally, there are concerns regarding how best to use the information gathered from drug screening. There would be little concern if it were used only to provide support services to families in difficulty and to facilitate drug abuse treatment. Unfortunately, this is not the case in many areas of the country, particularly in those communities in which drug abuse is common. Often the mandatory or voluntary reporting of positive findings to child protective agencies results only in (1) punitive actions that, although motivated by the presumed best interest of the infant, separate the mother and her newborn and (2) occasionally in other interventions that do not serve the needs of the family or the child well. This is of particular concern owing to evidence of racial and cultural biases that make it more likely that, despite similar rates of substance abuse, African-American women and poor women are more likely to be reported to state authorities than are others.[6]

Infants born to mothers who have clinical indicators of drug use should be screened. Social indicators such as low income, race, and ethnic origin are *not* sufficient reasons for selective screening. When clinical indicators are present and the screening test results are positive, caretakers have the opportunity to intervene positively for the benefit of the family and the infant. These interventions include the following:

1. Exercise influence for early enrollment of the mother and father in comprehensive local drug treatment centers.
2. Observe the infant carefully for signs of drug with-

GUIDELINES FOR NEWBORN URINE DRUG SCREENING

1. The following neonates should have their urine sent for toxicology screens:
   a. Neonates of mothers who have admitted substance abuse
   b. Neonates of mothers who have a past or present history of maternal drug use
   c. Neonates whose mothers exhibit behaviors indicative of substance abuse during labor or delivery, including drug-related or bizarre behavior such as slurred speech, unsteady gait, inappropriate affect, and confusion
   d. Neonates who evidence symptoms of drug intoxication or withdrawal (e.g., sneezing, jitteriness, irritability, high pitch cry, seizure or other neurological symptoms)
2. The following neonates also may have urine sent for toxicology upon assessment and review by a physician:
   a. Neonates of mothers who have had no prenatal care
   b. Neonates not delivered in-hospital.
   c. Cases of abruptio placenta
   d. Cases of congenital syphilis or those whose mother has had a positive syphilis screening test (e.g., VDRL, RPR, FTA)

From the Division of Neonatology, Department of Pediatrics, Albert Einstein College of Medicine/Montefiore Medical Center, Bronx, NY.

drawal and initiate early treatment upon the occurrence of symptoms.

3. Discourage breast-feeding, which can cause the infant further toxicity.
4. Monitor the infant for signs of central nervous system and renal dysfunction, including the use of central nervous system and renal ultrasound testing, when indicated.
5. Involve parents in parenting and family support programs that guide, support, and coordinate services to optimize parent-child interactions and child health and developmental outcomes.

Guidelines for newborn urine drug screening currently recommended are shown in the box above.

Screening for drug abuse with informed voluntary consent or when clinically indicated in a particular newborn (with parental or court-ordered consent) is not at issue. What is debated vehemently is the routine screening of *all* newborns or their mothers without consent, and it must be viewed as ethically questionable because of its unproved benefits and its potential to affect other aspects of perinatal care adversely.

ADOLESCENT ISSUES

More than 90% of high school seniors have had some experience with alcohol; 67% report use during the previous month, and nearly 5% report drinking daily. Approximately 20% of these adolescents use marijuana at least once per month; fewer abuse opiates, cocaine/crack, and other drugs. Such substance abuse emerges as a leading cause of direct or indirect death among adolescents; it also is a cause of major morbidity and social and educational disruption.

There may be a great temptation to screen all youths for substance abuse, both to intercede on their behalf and to diminish the effects of drug abusers on society. Despite such arguments, there are ethical and practical concerns regarding routine, nonconsensual drug screening of adolescents.[1]

Although parental consent most often is sufficient for performing any procedure in the younger child who lacks the capacity to make informed judgments, parental permission alone is not sufficient for performing diagnostic or therapeutic procedures on competent adolescents. Despite the temptation to apply a different ethical standard to adolescents when investigating the potential for drug abuse, it is treacherous to adhere to principles of informed consent only when such adherence is convenient or expedient.

Beyond ethical issues are concerns regarding the effect on the physician-adolescent relationship inherent in the practice of nonconsensual (and even discreet) screening for drugs—such a practice would not remain discreet for long. The major concerns are that (1) adolescents who use drugs know they are using drugs and, wishing to keep that behavior a secret from their physician and parents, would not seek care if involuntary screening was a part of that care; (2) adolescents would abstain from drug use for the few days necessary to produce a clean and deceptively reassuring urine specimen; (3) pediatricians would not be willing to collect urine specimens under direct observation to prevent the adulteration or substitution techniques available to knowledgeable young drug abusers; and (4) the information gained from such involuntary screening would not add sufficiently to the knowledge acquired from interview to justify the risk of establishing an adversarial relationship with the teenager.

Certainly, requisites for consent and voluntary screening may be waived when there is reason to doubt competency or when information gathered by interviewing the parent or adolescent suggests that the adolescent is out of control or at high risk to self and others. However, both ethical and practical questions strongly indicate that routine involuntary screening of all adolescents is not essential. The advancing technology of drug screening should be applied selectively to monitoring the therapeutic progress of known drug abusers and to testing young persons who have been identified to be at special risk for drug abuse.

EIGHT

Use of Urinalysis and the Urine Culture in Screening

Edward J. Ruley

Examination of the urine is a simple office procedure that may provide clues to specific urinary abnormalities or more generalized diseases. For the results to be meaningful, a clean-caught, midstream specimen should be examined as soon as possible after it is obtained.

Urinalyses and urine cultures have been used to screen children and adolescents for proteinuria, hematuria, glucosuria, and bacteriuria. Investigations of large populations have defined the prevalence of urinary abnormalities in symptom-free children and determined the cost effectiveness of early detection and treatment. The prevalence of urine abnormalities in any population depends on (1) the definition of the amount and frequency of urine aberrations that are considered abnormal, (2) the presence of concomitant clinical factors that may increase the number of false positive results, and (3) the age and gender distribution of the study population. The cost effectiveness of mass urine screening depends on the total monetary and psychosocial cost of performing the screening test compared with the value of early detection in ameliorating or preventing subsequent progression of disease. Of significance is a study by Dodge and associates,[1] who determined a cumulative occurrence of bacteriuria, proteinuria, and hematuria (i.e., having one or more of these findings) to be 6475 cases per 100,000 children ages 6 to 12 years. This occurrence greatly exceeds the number of persons expected to have significant morbidity from progressive renal disease and is considerably greater than the predicted number of deaths resulting from renal disease in the United States (28 per 1 million population per year). Such a finding reflects the high degree of sensitivity and the lack of specificity of current urine tests in detecting significant renal or urinary tract disease in symptom-free children. In contrast, in a 1988 report, extensive urine screening of symptom-free schoolchildren in Japan detected a small number who were then shown to have biopsy-proved glomerular disease.[4] Although the early discovery of a symptom-free child who has renal disease may prove to be important, the cost effectiveness to society of mass screening remains unproved. In otherwise healthy children, a single complete urinalysis performed before school entry should be sufficient screening for health maintenance purposes. The American Academy of Pediatrics, however, recommends that a complete urinalysis be performed during infancy (the first year of life), during early childhood (1 through 4 years), during late childhood (5 through 12 years), and during adolescence (see Chapter 3, Child Health Supervision).

PROTEINURIA

Proteinuria is detected most easily by the dipstick method, which makes use of a paper or plastic strip to which is affixed the indicator, tetrabromophenol blue. The presence of protein causes a change in color from yellow to blue-green that is proportional to the amount of protein present. False positive findings can occur in highly alkaline urine (pH >6.5) or in urine contaminated by skin antiseptics such as chlorhexidine or benzalkonium chloride. The small quantity of protein that healthy persons excrete normally usually is not detected by this method, although the reading may show a "trace" amount if the urine is concentrated (specific gravity >1.025). In contrast, the presence of a trace amount of protein in a dilute urine may reflect significant losses and should be investigated. Detection of protein by acid precipitation with sulfosalicylic acid is more specific and can be used for urine with an alkaline pH. (The clinical approach to children who have proteinuria is discussed in Chapter 159, Proteinuria.)

The prevalence rate for proteinuria in the symptom-free pediatric population varies, depending on the degree and frequency of proteinuria that is considered abnormal. Gutgesell[2] found the prevalence of proteinuria to be 6.3% in 2309 symptomatic and asymptomatic children who made their first visit to a neighborhood clinic. Screening was performed by a dip-and-read strip and 1+ or greater on a single urine specimen was the criterion for proteinuria. When Silverberg[6,7] applied a more stringent criterion for proteinuria (2+ or greater on two urinalyses) to more than 50,000 schoolchildren, he found the prevalence to be only 0.45% for boys and 1.6% for girls. Several investigators have noted a direct relationship of proteinuria to age during childhood, the incidence peaking at adolescence and then declining rapidly only to rise progressively thereafter into adulthood. Furthermore, proteinuria is more common at each age in girls during childhood, with the occurrence rates in boys lagging 3 to 5 years behind. It has been hypothesized that these gender differences are due to the earlier onset of adolescence in girls. No differences in prevalence have been noted by ethnic group or socioeconomic level. From Silverberg's data it is not surprising that the highest prevalence was found in the adolescent population (14.8%) when less rigorous criteria for screening were used. The prevalence of proteinuria (alone or in combination with glucosuria or hematuria) determined by urinalysis on routine hospital admission has been reported to be 2.5%, which is similar to values in outpatient studies. When the criterion was made more stringent by requiring two consecutive abnormal urinalysis results, the prevalence decreased to 2%. Finally, if the number of false positive results was minimized by collecting samples only from patients who were afebrile and not menstruating, the prevalence decreased to 0.6%. The influence of such clinical factors must be considered when any data on the prevalence of proteinuria are considered.

Although screening for proteinuria as part of well-child health care has become a hallowed tradition for many practitioners, there is no evidence that this procedure benefits the population being screened. At least 75% of symptom-free patients found to have protein in a single urinalysis will have a normal urine on repeat testing. Furthermore, of those having several positive random urinalysis results, 60% will have orthostatic proteinuria. This transient form of proteinuria resolves before adulthood and does not recur. The fixed and reproducible form of orthostatic proteinuria often persists into adulthood but is not considered to be a harbinger of clinically significant renal disease. In one 10-year follow-up study of young men who had persistent orthostatic proteinuria, none developed renal insufficiency, including the 53% who had nonspecific glomerular abnormalities on renal biopsy.[8] Regular follow-up, however, remains important for these children so that any changes in the pattern of protein excretion can be detected and appropriately investigated. Follow-up care of children determined by screening tests to have proteinuria has shown an incidence of identifiable renal disease in only 1 child per 1000 children screened. Furthermore, large studies have shown that children who have been identified as having renal disease by screening usually (1) are already known to have renal disease by their parents and physicians (e.g., nephrotic syndrome), (2) have an abnormality that requires no additional management (e.g., a hypoplastic kidney), or (3) have a renal disease for which no specific treatment is available (e.g., membranoproliferative glomerulonephritis). Even in urinary tract infections, proteinuria often is not present in the symptom-free child. It is important to note that most children who have significant renal disease will have other signs and symptoms (e.g., edema, poor weight gain, or hypertension) that will cause them to seek medical care and thus to be identified even in the absence of screening programs.

Besides the lack of a positive effect on the population, screening can have a negative effect in producing undue anxiety in patients and parents and in serving as an impetus for the practitioner to perform more invasive testing, which often provides no new information. Such factors may detract from the overall well-being of the population. In our current state of knowledge there is no indication for mass screening for proteinuria in *symptom-free children,* although this may change as new tests are developed. The nonproductiveness of screening symptom-free patients, however, does not apply to children who have symptoms. Urinalysis is an important tool in evaluating the child who has renal symptoms and should also be employed in patients who have vague signs and symptoms, such as failure to thrive, or recurrent diarrhea, inasmuch as some renal diseases may present in such nonspecific ways.

HEMATURIA

Hematuria can be detected by chemical tests for blood or by microscopic examination for erythrocytes in urine specimens. The commercially available dipstick tests depend on the color change that results from the oxidation of orthotolidine and cumene hydroperoxide, which is catalyzed by the presence of hemoglobin (or myoglobin) in the urine. False positive tests for blood in the urine may result from the presence of contaminating oxidizing cleansing agents (e.g., povidone-iodine or hypochlorite) or microbial peroxidases. False negative tests result from the presence of ascorbic acid in the urine from orally ingested vitamin C preparations. A positive dipstick result for blood does not discriminate between hemoglobin and myoglobin; differentiation requires spectrophotometric analysis. Furthermore, the dipstick test does not differentiate hemoglobinuria from hematuria or give clues to whether the blood originates from the upper or lower urinary tracts. For these questions the microscopic examination of the centrifuged urine sediment is necessary (see Chapter 139, Hematuria).

The number of erythrocytes per high-power field in a centrifuged urine sediment that is abnormal is variable. This variability occurs because the concentration of erythrocytes in the centrifuged sediment depends primarily on the volume of urine centrifuged and the amount of supernatant decanted from the centrifuge tube before microscopic examination. The results are affected to a lesser degree by the centrifuge speed and duration. Another source of variation is the practice of reporting the average number of erythrocytes in each field inasmuch as few observers take the time to count each cell in several fields and then average them. Meticulous technique minimizes these methodological problems but significantly increases the labor intensiveness of the urinalysis. Dodge and associates[1] have suggested that five or more erythrocytes per high-power field in at least two or three consecutive urine specimens be considered abnormal. The prevalence of microscopic hematuria in an ambulatory setting varies from 4% when a single urinalysis is abnormal to 0.07% when two urinalyses are abnormal. As with proteinuria, the point prevalence (number of existing cases) of hematuria increases with age among children of both genders and is greater at each age for girls than for boys, although one recent study failed to find such differences. Whereas one study found no differences in prevalence among ethnic groups or socioeconomic classes, another found a higher prevalence among Caucasian and Asian children than among African-American and Mexican-American children. The prevalence of hematuria (alone or in combination with glucosuria or proteinuria) in children admitted to the hospital for medical illnesses was 5.3%. When sources of false positivity (fever or menstruation) were eliminated and the criteria were made more stringent by requiring two consecutive abnormal specimens, the prevalence decreased to 2.2%.

Few of the children detected in screening programs to have hematuria are found to have significant renal or urological disease. Thus, for much the same reasons as those advanced for proteinuria, it has been suggested that mass screening for hematuria is not justified.

GLUCOSURIA

Glucosuria can be screened for by use of the highly specific glucose oxidase–impregnated dipsticks. Normally, 99% of the glucose in the glomerular ultrafiltrate is reabsorbed by the proximal tubules. Glucosuria may occur (1) at high blood glucose levels when the glucose concentration in the ultrafiltrate exceeds the capacity of the proximal tubular reabsorptive mechanism or (2) at normal blood glucose levels when tubular reabsorption is dysfunctional. Measurement of blood glucose will differentiate these two mechanisms. Rarely, early diabetes mellitus or Fanconi syndrome will be detected in a child by means of urinalysis screening. The cost effectiveness, however, is so low that routine screening of well children for glucosuria is not recommended.

BACTERIURIA

In the past it was considered to be cost effective to screen symptom-free girls for bacteriuria, ostensibly (1) to prevent the morbidity and complications of symptomatic infection and (2) to identify individuals in whom urological investigation to prevent renal parenchymal damage was indicated. Subsequent studies showed that nontreatment did not increase the frequency of pyelonephritis, interfere with renal growth, or cause renal insufficiency.[5,9] Moreover, the incidence of significant structural abnormalities was remarkably low.[3] Furthermore, more recent studies suggest that treatment of asymptomatic bacteriuria may be associated with a greater risk for pyelonephritis because of the development of resistant organisms. Therefore, because most current research suggests that children who have asymptomatic bacteriuria do not have a high frequency of associated urinary structural abnormalities and treatment of asymptomatic bacteriuria is contraindicated, there is no reason to screen the pediatric population for its occurrence. It must be emphasized that these caveats apply only to children who are overtly healthy; they do not apply to children who are sick, even those whose symptoms are poorly defined, in whom a renal evaluation may be indicated.

NINE

Auditory Screening

David R. Cunningham

JUSTIFICATION

Routine screening for hearing loss is justified on the basis of the prevalence of this disorder in both the general pediatric population and in at-risk groups. The prevalence of profound sensorineural hearing loss in the well-baby population is 1 in 1000 births. This estimate, however, fails to account for the greater prevalence of sensorineural hearing loss among infants at risk for developmental disabilities and the greater number of well-babies who have mild, moderate, or severe sensorineural hearing loss than who are profoundly deaf. Adjusting the prevalence rate for infants at risk for developmental disabilities and for well-babies who have lesser degrees of sensorineural hearing loss yields a prevalence of approximately 6 babies who have hearing loss for every 1000 births.[11] (Compare this with 1 in 14,000 who have phenylketonuria at birth.) By 2 years of age, 1 in 25 children will have a mild to moderate (20 to 50 decibel) hearing loss resulting from ear disease. Nearly 20% of public schoolchildren in disadvantaged neighborhoods fail auditory screening tests.

The first 18 to 24 months of life are crucial for the acquisition of normal speech and language. Undetected hearing loss in this period of life leads to irreparable communicative and learning problems. Early intervention in the form of audiological management, otological treatment, amplification, parental counseling, and special education is vitally important. Regular hearing screening for toddlers and school-age children is important not only because of the seriousness of the medical sequelae of active otopathology, but also because of the negative consequences that even mild (15 to 20 decibel) hearing loss (either conductive or sensorineural) has for language growth, academic success, and behavioral development.

GOALS

The goal of auditory screening programs is to identify hearing loss cost efficiently as early as possible, regardless of its degree. The screening strategies must have high sensitivity and specificity to reduce both false positive and false negative rates. The methods of achieving this goal are adjusted for each age group. In the recent past, infant screening programs were designed to identify primarily those neonates who had profound sensorineural hearing loss. Current techniques and technologies make it feasible to detect not only severe and profound hearing loss, but also milder degrees of hearing loss. In the toddler and preschool period, the screening protocol is modified to identify otopathology (especially otitis media with effusion), milder conductive hearing loss, as well as unnoticed acquired or progressive sensorineural hearing impairment. Routine periodic auditory screening of school-age children is designed to maintain educationally optimal hearing. Although the method of screening children in the school-age group has not changed significantly in the last decade or so, there is a far greater awareness of and sensitivity to the effects of hearing loss on skills development and educational achievement. Clinicians must be especially vigilant for those children who are academic underachievers. These children may have no peripheral hearing loss but may exhibit signs of a specific auditory learning disorder. What follows here is a discussion of feasible, reliable, and cost-efficient auditory screening protocols in three age groups.

NEONATAL AND EARLY INFANT PERIOD

Much of the information presented in this section is available in greater detail in the NIH Consensus Statement on Early Identification of Hearing Impairment in Infants and Young Children published by the National Institutes of Health in 1993.[9] This panel recommends that auditory screening be implemented for *all* infants, those both of high and low risk, within the first 3 months of life, but preferably before discharge from the hospital nursery. The panel emphasizes that comprehensive intervention and management for those infants identified with hearing loss must be an integral part of a universal screening program.

The NIH panel rejects the notion of using a "high-risk register" to limit the number of infants screened. Screening only those who satisfy one or more high-risk factors identifies only 50% of infants who have significant hearing loss.[3,8,13] Failure to identify the remaining 50% of children who have hearing loss results in an unacceptably late age of diagnosis and intervention.

The NIH panel recommends that evoked otoacoustic emissions (EOAE) and auditory brainstem response audiometry (ABR) be used as the screening tools. EOAE should be used to screen *all* newborns.[12] Those who pass the EOAE screen are discharged from the process; those who fail the EOAE screen are given a second stage, or confirmatory screen, using ABR. Babies who pass the ABR screen are discharged but should be "flagged" for rescreening within 3 to 6 months. Babies who fail the ABR screen are referred for a complete diagnostic evaluation, the purpose of which is to determine the type and degree of hearing loss and to initiate a remediation program for the child and family.

The acoustic stimulus for ABR screening should include the frequency band important for speech recognition. The most important portion of the "speech frequency range" lies between approximately 500 Hertz (Hz) and 4 kHz. Acoustic "clicks," which generate their primary energy in the 2 kHz to 4 kHz region, often are used as stimuli in large-scale infant screening programs. (Although it also is possible to use tone pips or tone bursts to obtain more frequency-specific responses, these acoustic stimuli generally are used in comprehensive audiological evaluations rather than in screening programs.) The "pass" criterion for ABR infant screening is a response from both ears at intensity levels of 40 dB referenced to normal hearing level (NHL), that is, 40 dB NHL. Infants who pass the ABR screen but who are at risk for progressive hearing loss periodically should be monitored audiologically throughout the preschool years.[10]

The largest study to date to report on the feasibility of using EOAE as an infant screening method is the Rhode Island Hearing Assessment Project (RIHAP).[19] By the end of 1993, more than 23,000 infants had been screened using "transient" EOAE. EOAE screening of all infants in the regular care and special care nurseries yielded an average "pass" rate of 91.6%. The sensitivity for transient EOAE was 100%; its specificity was 82%. This is compared with sensitivity and specificity rates for ABR of approximately 94% and 89%, respectively. Thus the two screening technologies are complementary when used in a two-stage screening protocol.

Transient EOAE are low-intensity sounds produced by the cochlea in response to acoustic clicks. They are by-products of normal cochlear function. EOAE appear to be associated with the motility of the outer hair cells, which seem to be responsible for "amplifying" low-level sounds within the cochlea. This mechanical response creates motion patterns within the cochlear duct that are transmitted outward from the cochlea and through the middle ear. Motion of the tympanic membrane, which normally occurs in response to sound, now produces sound that can be detected in the ear canal by a sensitive microphone.[4] EOAE are recorded by using a computer averaging technique similar to ABR instrumentation. Because transient EOAE tend not to occur in people who have peripheral hearing loss greater than about 30 dB HL,* they appear to serve as a valuable method for identifying those who have normal or near-normal peripheral hearing sensitivity. Research is ongoing to discover the optimal EOAE stimulus/response patterns and pass/fail criteria for large-scale neonatal screening programs. Another type of EOAE, the "distortion-product" EOAE, also is under investigation as a possible screening tool.

EOAE screening will fail approximately 10% of all babies tested. It is a rapid, highly sensitive, cost-effective method of identifying those infants who have normal hearing and limiting the size of the population that is carried over to the second stage ABR screening protocol. Northern and Hayes[11] report that using a two-stage EOAE-ABR screening protocol will result in only 1.7 infants who have normal hearing being referred for a complete diagnostic evaluation for every baby who has hearing loss (based on a prevalence rate of 6 hearing-impaired infants per 1000 births). Bess and Paradise[1] question the validity and predictive value of the two-stage EOAE-ABR screening protocol recommended by NIH. Using a prevalence rate of 1 hearing-impaired infant per 1000 births, Bess and Paradise calculated that nearly 10 infants who have normal hearing would be referred for full diagnostic evaluations for every baby who has a hearing loss. They argue that the NIH protocol would result in an unacceptably high overreferral rate. Their conclusions do not appear to have wide support in the professional community, and their prevalence rate estimate (1 : 1000) generally is regarded as too low in that it applies only to those infants who are profoundly deaf and not to those who have lesser degrees of handicapping hearing loss.[11] Indeed, much evidence supports the NIH EOAE-ABR auditory screening consensus statement in literature from the United States and abroad.[2,7,15-19]

Although the NIH panel endorses the two-stage EOAE-ABR infant auditory screening protocol, they recognize that adopting its recommendations will take time. Additionally, they acknowledge that many infant screening programs already are in place that use only ABR (either automated or conventional) as a screening tool. Some of these existing screening programs use ABR technology only for NICU babies or for babies who have one or more at-risk "indicators" associated with congenital or acquired conductive or sensorineural hearing loss. The panel encourages all centers to adopt the two-stage EOAE-ABR protocol as soon as possible, but would encourage existing programs to continue using the ABR-only protocol in the interim. The Joint Committee on Infant Hearing recommends that screening programs that are based on at-risk indicators continue to provide screening services to those infants identified by use of those indicators.[6] The lists of indicators that follow are those associated with sensorineural or conductive hearing loss. These indicators might be used to reduce the size of the population screened using ABR until universal screening of infants using EOAE and ABR is achieved.

Indicators associated with sensorineural or conductive hearing loss: for use when universal screening (NIH consensus model) is not available

1. Family history of hereditary childhood sensorineural hearing loss
2. In utero infection such as cytomegalovirus, rubella, syphilis, herpes, or toxoplasmosis
3. Craniofacial anomalies, including those who have morphological abnormalities of the pinna and ear canal
4. Birth weight less than 1500 gs (3.3 lbs.)
5. Hyperbilirubinemia at a serum level requiring exchange transfusion
6. Ototoxic medications including but not limited to the aminoglycosides used in multiple courses or in combination with loop diuretics
7. Bacterial meningitis
8. Severe depression at birth with Apgar scores of 0 to 4 at 1 minute or 0 to 6 at 5 minutes
9. Prolonged mechanical ventilation lasting 5 days or longer (e.g., persistent pulmonary hypertension)
10. Stigmata or other findings associated with a syndrome known to include a sensorineural or a conductive hearing loss

Not all hearing loss in infancy or early childhood will be present at birth or acquired before the baby is discharged from the hospital. Such hearing loss may be acquired as a result of other medical conditions or from progressive hereditary etiologies. Clinicians must be vigilant for the possibility of these situations. The following indicators will help identify those infants and very young children who should be monitored carefully for hearing loss and reevaluated as necessary to rule out acquired or progressive hearing loss.

Indicators associated with sensorineural or conductive hearing loss: health conditions that may develop and require hearing evaluations every 6 months until age 3 years (infants 29 days old to 3 years old):

1. Parental concern regarding hearing, speech, language, or developmental delay
2. Bacterial meningitis and other infections associated with sensorineural hearing loss
3. Head trauma associated with loss of consciousness or skull fracture

*HL refers to hearing level referenced to American National Standards Institute (ANSI) S3.6-1989: Specifications for audiometers.

4. Stigmata or other findings associated with a syndrome known to include sensorineural or conductive hearing loss
5. Ototoxic medications including but not limited to chemotherapeutic agents, or aminoglycosides used in multiple courses or in combination with loop diuretics
6. Recurrent or persistent otitis media with effusion for at least 3 months
7. Family history of hereditary childhood hearing loss
8. History of in utero infection such as cytomegalovirus, rubella, syphilis, herpes, or toxoplasmosis
9. Neurofibromatosis type II and neurodegenerative disorders
10. Persistent pulmonary hypertension in the newborn period
11. Anatomical deformity and other disorders that affect eustachian tube function

A comprehensive universal infant auditory screening program has a number of administrative elements. Parents and caregivers should be offered educational materials pertaining to the signs and symptoms of hearing loss in infants and toddlers. This should include an overview of speech, language, and auditory developmental milestones by age in months. Parental concern about a baby's hearing or speech-language development is justification for an audiological evaluation. Data amassed in large-scale infant auditory screening programs should be forwarded to a central repository for analysis and tracking of those children who are suspected of having hearing loss. In states where auditory screening programs are mandated by law, these data are managed by agencies such as the public health department and the commission for handicapped children. Infant screening programs generally are supervised by audiologists or neonatologists associated with the hospital nurseries. The actual screening (EOAE and ABR protocols) may be carried out by well-trained nursing personnel or closely monitored paraprofessionals or volunteers. Per-patient cost always is a consideration in large-scale screening programs. Each hospital needs to determine its costs based on personnel, time, supervisory and training needs, durable equipment purchases, expendable supplies, test interpretation services, report preparation, and overhead.

PRESCHOOL PERIOD

The primary goal of screening in the 2- to 5-year-old period is the detection of medically remediable otopathology associated with a very mild (<15 dB HL) to moderate (~40 dB HL) conductive hearing loss. The screening focuses on this objective on the assumption that more severely handicapping hearing losses will have been found by 2 years of age. The principal cause of hearing loss in this age range is otitis media—a pathology capable of producing subtle, but significant, auditory learning disorders and permanent middle ear damage.[10]

Auditory screening of preschoolers often is performed at the time of well-child visits to the primary physician's office, Head Start programs, day care centers, preschool programs, or kindergartens. Although the screening procedures might differ from site to site depending on the availability of equipment and trained personnel and on the level of background noise in the screening environment, the "ideal" protocol would include four elements: (1) pure tone hearing screening, (2) acoustic immittance testing (tympanometry), (3) otoscopic "inspection" of the ear canal (as performed by the supervising professionals), and (4) an elicitation of parental/caregiver concern about the child's hearing and speech and language development.

Northern and Downs[10] described the following procedure for conducting pure tone auditory screening for children in the preschool age range:

Play-conditioning procedure for testing the 3- and 4-year-old child:

1. Have available a peg board, a ring tower, plain blocks, or other simple toys that appeal to young children.
2. With headphones on your ears, take a block (or peg) and hold it up to one ear as if listening. Make believe you hear a sound, say "I hear it," and put the block on the table.
3. Put the phones on the child's ear and hold his or her hand with the block up to the child's ear.
4. Present a 50 dB tone at 1000 Hz and guide the child's hand to build the block tower. Repeat once or twice and then see if he or she can do it alone. If he or she can, go on.
5. Decrease the hearing level to 20 dB and repeat the test. If the child responds, go on to the other frequencies (2000 and 4000 Hz) and repeat the procedure. Praise him or her for each correct response. After each presentation, place another block in the child's hand.
6. Switch to the opposite ear and repeat the test, starting at 4000 Hz, then to 2000 Hz and 1000 Hz.

A criterion for referral is failure to respond to 20 dB HL at any frequency in either ear or failure on immittance screening (tympanometry). Children who fail the screen should be retested in 2 weeks. If the rescreen also is failed, the child should be referred for a comprehensive audiological evaluation.

Screening children younger than 3 years of age presents a greater challenge to the busy clinician. Tympanometry generally is tolerated well by this group of children and should be done routinely. Auditory screening, however, is more problematic in that it requires the tester to be not only skillful in the presentation of auditory stimuli, but also familiar with the developmental hierarchy of auditory alerting and localization behaviors in young children. During the 4- to 24-month period, behavioral responses to quiet noisemakers include alerting, orienting toward the acoustic stimuli, crude head-turning for visual observation of the noisemakers, and finally brisk and precise localizing of the source of the acoustic stimuli by the time the child is 24 months of age. The 2- to 3-year-old who has normal hearing should have no difficulty localizing a sound source in any plane around the head. The absence of a localization response constitutes a failed screening test, as does a positive tympanometric test. Those who fail the screen, and those whose caregivers express concern about hearing or speech and language development should be referred for a complete audiological evaluation.

Tympanometry is (1) an essential element of a screening protocol for the preschool group and (2) an objective method of determining the status of the tympanic membrane and the middle ear mechanism. Tympanometry can reliably detect the presence of middle ear effusion and eustachian tube dysfunction that often is a precursor to otitis media with effusion

(OME). Tympanometry is especially helpful in detecting OME in children who "pass" the auditory screen because their hearing loss is so slight. The American Speech-Language-Hearing Association (ASHA) has published guidelines pertaining to tympanometric screening for hearing loss and middle ear disorders,[5] but these are more appropriate for large-scale screening programs than for "screening" at periodic intervals in the physician's office. For this reason, a discussion of the ASHA guidelines will be presented in the subsequent section on strategies for screening the school-age population. A scaled-down but rational approach to "in-office tympanometric screening" is required. The practitioner or his or her assistant can perform basic tympanometric measurements on all preschool-age children as part of routine examinations. Figure 20-2 describes the five major tympanogram types. Easy-to-use, automated tympanometers can discriminate between normal and abnormal middle ear systems reliably and inexpensively. Children whose tympanometric screening reveals one or more of the following "fail" criteria should be examined more fully in the physician's office or referred for a complete audiological evaluation:

1. Normal tympanic membrane–ossicular compliance with middle ear pressure that is more negative than −200 mm H_2O, (type C tympanogram often associated with eustachian tube dysfunction)
2. Significantly reduced or completely absent tympanic membrane–ossicular compliance with normal equivalent ear canal volume, that is, ≤ 1.0 cm^3 (type B tympanogram often associated with middle ear fluid accumulation)
3. Abnormally large equivalent ear canal volume, that is, ≥ 1.0 cm^3 and "flat" tympanogram (associated with either tympanic membrane perforation or patent tympanostomy tube)

This "in-office" screening protocol, combining an auditory test and basic tympanometry along with otoscopy and special attention to the child's speech and language development will identify those patients who require more exhaustive evaluations.

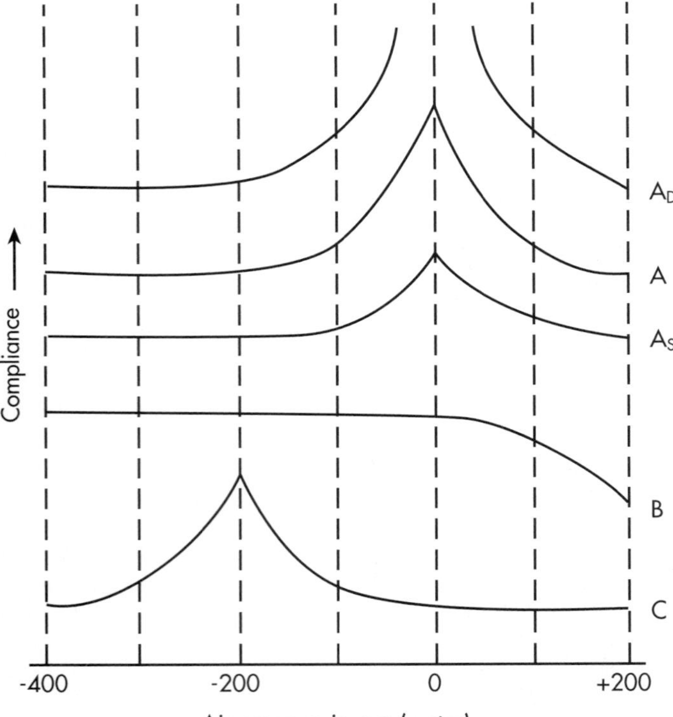

FIG. 20-2 Five typical tympanograms illustrating various conditions of the middle ear. Type A shows normal pressure-compliance functions and is typical of normal middle ears. Type A_S curves are like the A curves but are much shallower and are associated with stiffness of the stapes, the smallest of the middle ear bones. Type A_D curves are much deeper than the normal type A curves and are symptomatic of interruptions in the chain of bones or flaccidity of the eardrum membrane. Type B shows no pressure setting at which the eardrum membrane becomes most compliant and suggests fluid in the middle ear space. Type C shows the eardrum membrane to be most compliant when the pressure in the ear canal is negative, suggesting that the pressure within the middle ear is below atmospheric pressure.

(From Martin FN: *Introduction to audiology*, ed 4, Needham Heights, Md, 1991, Allyn & Bacon.)

SCHOOL-AGE PERIOD

The principal goal of screening programs for school-age populations is the maintenance of educationally optimal hearing. The secondary goal is the detection of otopathology. The physician should use the screening protocol described for 3- to 5-year-olds in the preschool section above for school-age patients who have come to the office for annual physical examinations or with otological complaints. This "in-office" procedure combines screening audiometry, tympanometry, and otoscopy and paying special attention to speech and language milestones.

What follows, however, is an explanation of a large-scale screening protocol for school-age populations, as conducted in the school (or public health facility) itself. Although the primary care physician may be called on as a consultant to these mass screening efforts, the actual management and implementation of school-based programs generally is conducted by a supervising audiologist and trained paraprofessionals or volunteers. The large-scale screening of school-age populations for hearing impairment and middle ear disorders presented here is based on the recommendations of the Working Group on Acoustic Immittance Measurements and the Committee on Audiologic Evaluation of the American Speech-Language-Hearing Association.[5] The screening protocol includes four sources of data: history, visual inspection of the ear canal, identification audiometry, and tympanometry.

History

A request for basic otological/audiological information can be obtained from the parents or caregivers (in advance) in a letter sent to them explaining the purpose of the screening program. A recent history of otalgia or otorrhea is sufficient cause for immediate medical referral.

Otoscopy

The following conditions merit medical referral without further audiological/tympanometric screening: structural defects of the ear, head, or neck; inflammation, blood, effusion, excessive cerumen, tumors, or foreign body in the ear canal; or eardrum appearance consistent with active middle ear disease, that is, abnormal color, bulging eardrum, fluid line or bubbles, perforation, or retraction. Tympanometry should not be performed when a tympanostomy tube is in place at the time of screening.

Audiometric Screening

The school-age screening protocol is given in Figure 20-3, and the referral criteria are shown in the box on p. 232.

Pure-tone stimuli presented at 20 dB HL[14] with frequencies of 1 kHz, 2 kHz, and 4 kHz should be used. Failure to respond to any frequency in either ear constitutes a screening failure. A second on-site rescreen or a rescreen at a later date is recommended. A second failure indicates the need for a more exhaustive evaluation.

Low Static Admittance

Peak admittance (Ya) is the total acoustic immittance of both the ear canal and the lateral surface of the tympanic membrane. Peak admittance is measured in millimhos—a unit that indicates the ease with which sound pressure waves flow through the outer and middle ear. A peak admittance value

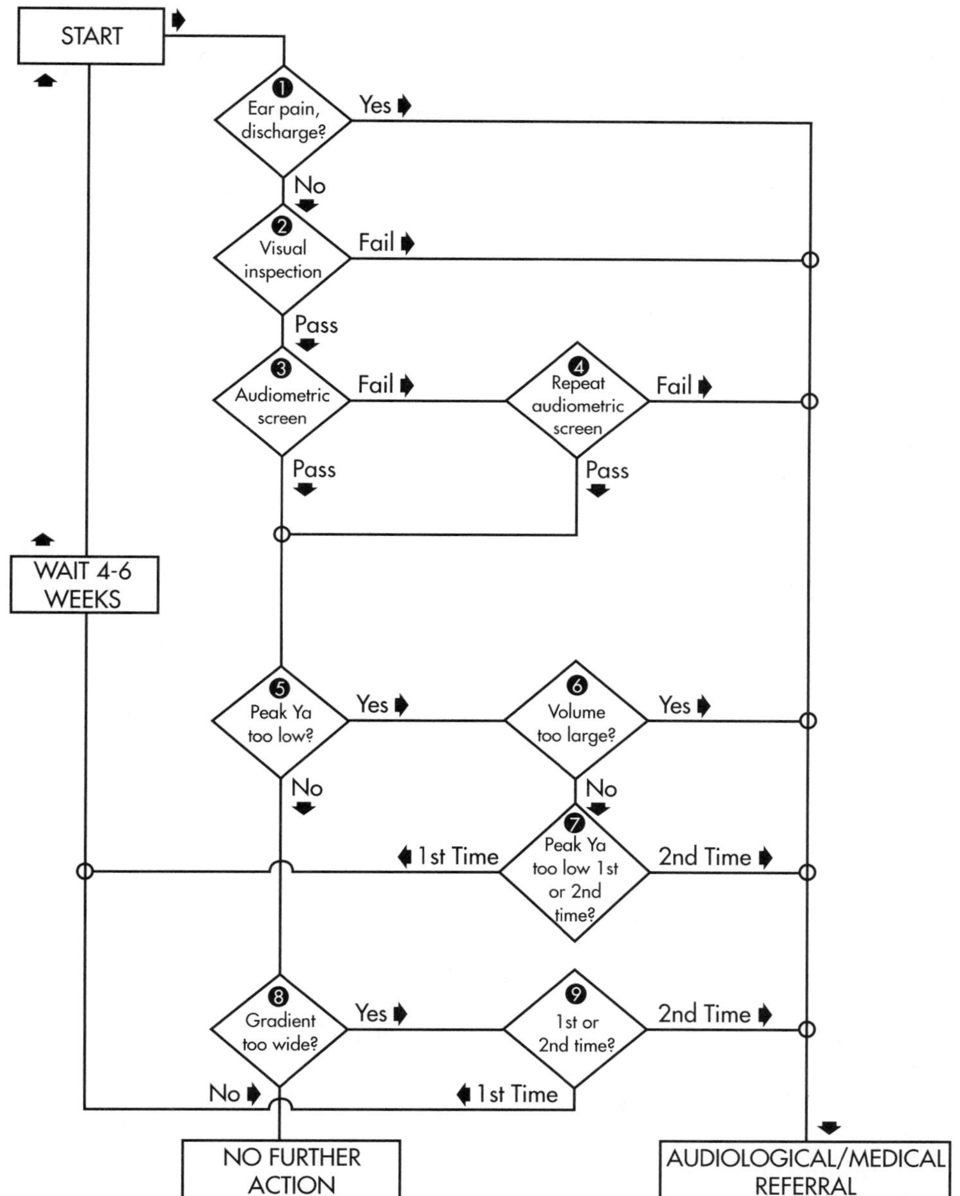

FIG. 20-3 Flow chart for determining the need for audiological/medical referral incorporating case history, visual inspection, pure-tone audiometry, and tympanometry. Each numbered box is discussed in the text. The flow chart represents the logic used to determine the need for referral. It does not indicate the order of test procedures.

(From American Speech-Language-Hearing Association: *ASHA* 32(suppl 2):17, 1990.)

REFERRAL CRITERIA

I. History

A. Otalgia
B. Otorrhea

II. Visual inspection of the ear

A. Structural defect of the ear, head, or neck
B. Ear canal abnormalities
  1. Blood or effusion
  2. Occlusion
  3. Inflammation
  4. Excessive cerumen, tumor, foreign material
C. Eardrum abnormalities
  1. Abnormal color
  2. Bulging eardrum
  3. Fluid line or bubbles
  4. Perforation
  5. Retraction

III. Identification audiometry

Fail air conduction screening at 20 dB HL at 1, 2, or 4 kHz in either ear; these criteria may require alteration for various clinical settings and populations.

IV. Tympanometry

A. Flat tympanogram and equivalent ear canal volume (Vec) outside normal range
B. Low static admittance (peak Y) on two successive occurrences in a 4- to 6-week interval
C. Abnormally wide tympanometric width (TW) on two successive occurrences in a 4- to 6-week interval

From American Speech-Language-Hearing Association: *ASHA* 32(suppl 2):17, 1990.

less than 0.2 millimhos associated with an abnormally large physical volume in front of the measuring probe is evidence of a tympanic membrane perforation and warrants immediate medical referral.

Equivalent ear canal volume is an estimated measure of the air medial to the probe tip and is measured in cubic centimeters (cm^3). An equivalent ear canal volume that exceeds 1.0 cm^3 in the presence of a "flat" tympanogram is evidence of a tympanic membrane perforation and merits a medical referral. (Note: Low static admittance, in isolation, may or may not be associated with a middle ear disorder; a "rescreening" in 4 to 6 weeks is recommended before these children are referred for medical evaluation.)

Abnormally Wide Tympanometric Width (TW)

Sometimes referred to as "tympanometric gradient," this metric is used to describe the shape of the tympanogram in the vicinity of the peak and is measured in units of air pressure called dekapascals (daPa). (Note: 1 daPa = 1.02 mm of water pressure.) A TW greater than 150 daPa is suggestive of middle ear disease in children. Those who have an abnormally wide TW and no other findings should be rescreened in 4 to 6 weeks and referred for medical evaluation only if they fail the second screen.

TEN

Vision Screening

Richard C. Wasserman

RATIONALE

Knowledge of vision screening is essential for pediatric primary care practitioners. Adequate vision is important for everyone, especially young children. The brain's developing visual cortex must receive focused images from both eyes to "learn" how to see. This process occurs over a limited time (before age 9), and conditions that interfere with the normal visual image during this time can lead to permanent vision loss (amblyopia) if not identified and corrected. Generally, the earlier these visual problems are identified, the more easily they can be remedied and amblyopia prevented.

From a public health standpoint, screening for vision problems is readily justified on the following counts:

Vision problems pose a threat to children's current and future well-being.

Vision problems are common (prevalence of 5% to 10% in preschool age and over 10% among school-age children) and can be readily defined.

Vision problems are likely to go undetected without screening.

There are acceptable, safe, and inexpensive screening procedures that identify reliably and accurately those who have (or at risk for) vision problems.

Efficacious treatments for vision problems are readily available.

Early diagnosis and treatment confer significant advantages in outcome for many vision problems (e.g., congenital cataracts, strabismus, amblyopia).

Overall, the benefits of early diagnosis and treatment of vision problems justify the costs of screening.

GOALS

The goals of vision screening are (1) to identify deficits in vision or conditions that ultimately could threaten vision before they otherwise would be discovered and (2) to ensure that appropriate diagnostic and therapeutic referrals are made so that the condition(s) threatening vision are ameliorated. To achieve the first goal, the practitioner and staff must learn the appropriate vision screening techniques and procedures and then apply them systematically in their practice. To achieve the second goal the practitioner must structure the primary care encounter so that screening results are communicated accurately to parents, appropriate referrals are made (when indicated), and proper follow-up is achieved.

Appropriate vision screening techniques and procedures vary in some degree for infants and toddlers (under age 3 years), preschool children (3 to 5 years), and school-age children and adolescents. The practitioner's physical examination provides some of the elements of vision screening (especially in infants and toddlers), but vision is tested most efficiently by ancillary personnel and apart from the physical examination. For the reasons mentioned above, vision screening is most important for children under 9 years of age. Children who have developmental problems often are at increased risk for vision problems and may require special expertise for assessment. Criteria for referral are discussed separately below.

INFANTS AND TODDLERS

Physical Examination

The eyes are first examined as part of the newborn examination and should be assessed subsequently at each health supervision visit. As part of the examination, the eyes should be inspected for any structural abnormalities. The red reflex is evaluated for abnormality or asymmetrical appearance through an ophthalmoscope. The corneal light reflex should be tested by using a penlight, and any asymmetry should be noted. Beyond the newborn period, the examiner should assess ocular motility by having the child "follow" a brightly colored object or toy. After 6 months of age, the cover/uncover test should detect any differential response to the occlusion of the eyes (which may indicate a unilateral visual defect) or ocular refixation movements (which suggest muscle imbalance).

Formal Screening

No formal screening procedures are indicated in the primary care setting for infants and toddlers.

Special Circumstances

Infants whose circumstances or family history place them at special risk for visual problems—for instance, preterm infants at risk for retinopathy of prematurity and infants who have a family history of congenital eye problems or metabolic/genetic diseases that place their eyes at risk—should be evaluated by an ophthalmologist.

Parents sometimes give a history of asymmetry of the child's eyes when none can be demonstrated at the visit. Because some problems of muscle imbalance are manifest only when the child is fatigued, it is wise to pay attention to such a history and refer to a specialist if these complaints are persistent. A family history of amblyopia, a "lazy eye," or "crossed eyes" confers a higher risk of problems and should be considered seriously for referral.

PRESCHOOL CHILDREN

Physical Examination

Inspection, red reflex, corneal light reflex, ocular motility, and cover/uncover test should be performed at each health supervision visit.

Formal Screening

Testing for visual acuity should be attempted beginning at age 3, and an interpretable result should be achieved by age 4. It is reasonable to have a child who is uncooperative or inconsistent in responses return for a repeat test. It should be remembered, however, that repeated failure to achieve an interpretable test result may itself be an indication of a visual problem. At this age, the simpler tests of acuity that do not rely on knowledge of letters are the most acceptable. Examples are Illiterate (tumbling) E and Allen Picture Cards. Detailed descriptions of these and other tests cited below have been published.[1,2] Information about test reliability and accuracy is available for most tests.[2]

Testing for binocular vision (stereoacuity) is not a substitute for assessing visual acuity, but it is a very useful adjunct and sometimes will identify a child who has vision problems that have been missed on physical examination and acuity testing. Acceptable tests for this age group include the Random Dot E test and the Stereo Fly test.

Vision testing machines (see below) may be accepted by the older children in this age group.

Special Circumstances

As mentioned above, children who have a family history of amblyopia, a "lazy eye," or "crossed eyes" are at higher risk for vision problems. Children who are developmentally delayed (e.g., trisomy 21) or who have cerebral palsy also are at higher risk for problems and may be especially challenging to test. If satisfactory results cannot be obtained on screening, a referral is indicated.

SCHOOL-AGE CHILDREN AND ADOLESCENTS

Physical Examination

Eyes should be inspected and the red reflex, corneal light reflex, ocular motility, and cover/uncover tests should be performed at each health supervision visit.

Formal Screening

Once a child knows the alphabet, the Snellen letters on a wall chart are appropriate for visual acuity screening. For school-age children and adolescents, vision testing machines that combine acuity testing with tests of binocular vision are readily accepted and require less office space.

Special Circumstances

School difficulties may be a presenting symptom of visual problems, and all children who have such troubles should have their vision evaluated if not done recently. Although the prevention of amblyopia becomes less of a concern with increasing age, the overall prevalence of vision problems increases steadily over time; therefore children should continue to be tested at health supervision visits.

PERSONNEL AND EQUIPMENT

Nonprofessional personnel who have a high school education can be trained to administer all of these formal tests. The equipment necessary for most of these tests is readily available from medical supply houses and is inexpensive. Vision testing not done with testing machines requires a well-lighted environment with at least 10 feet of available space. Vision testing machines require less space but cost over $1000.

REFERRAL

Where there is a question of strabismus or amblyopia, the child should be referred to an ophthalmologist who is skilled in working with young children. Overall criteria for referral are outlined below.

Physical Examination

A child who has a structural abnormality of the eye or its movements, any asymmetry or abnormality of the red reflex, any asymmetry of the corneal reflex, aversion to the occlusion of one eye, or any movement of the eyes on the cover/uncover test should be referred.

Visual Acuity

Preschool children failing to pass a test in either or both eyes at the 20/40 level or who display a two-line discrepancy between the eyes (e.g., 20/20 and 20/40) should be referred. In addition, any child who cannot be tested successfully by age 4 after repeated attempts should be referred. School-age children and adolescents who fail to pass at the 20/30 level in either or both eyes or who have a two-line discrepancy between the eyes should be referred. In addition, children who have developmental disabilities who cannot be tested successfully in the practice should be referred.

Binocular Vision

Children of any age who fail a test of binocular vision should be referred.

IMPROVING VISION SCREENING AND ITS OUTCOMES

In the future, new objective techniques such as photorefraction[4] may improve vision screening. Currently, however, these techniques have not been widely tested and remain prohibitively expensive for use in practice.

The practice and clinic, because they provide continuity of care, remain ideal places to carry out vision screening. Recent studies on vision screening in pediatric practice, nevertheless, have highlighted some deficiencies of the vision screening process.[3,5] Practitioners need to screen systematically (in the recommended manner at the recommended intervals) *all* of the children whom they see for health supervision visits, record and communicate the results of the screening to parents, and make sure that follow-up and referral appointments are made and kept.

ELEVEN

Sickle Cell Conditions

Charles F. Whitten

There are two distinctly different types of sickle cell conditions: (1) sickle cell disease (primarily sickle cell anemia, sickle cell–hemoglobin C disease, and sickle cell–beta-thalassemia disease) and (2) sickle cell trait, the benign "carrier" state. As with all health problems, screening for sickle cell conditions is justifiable only if those whose screening tests are positive receive some beneficial service. Beneficial services and the methodology for providing them exist for both types of sickle cell conditions.

Screening is of value with respect to the sickle cell diseases, although they are incurable, and there are no established procedures for preventing the episodic complications or the progressive damage to tissues. Because of splenic dysfunction, children who have sickle cell disease are prone to the development of bacterial infections, particularly by *Streptococcus pneumoniae,* which can proceed to septicemia and death ("sudden death") in a matter of hours. The level of red blood cell fetal hemoglobin is high enough for the first several months to prevent intravascular sickling and the resultant manifestations of sickle cell disease. After that time, although intravascular sickling is present, overwhelming bacterial infections leading to death can occur before the onset of characteristic symptoms that result in the diagnosis of sickle cell disease. A study conducted by the National Institutes of Health has demonstrated clearly the value of twice daily oral administration of penicillin in preventing pneumococcal infections and death in young children who have a sickle cell condition.[3] On the basis of results of that study, participants in an NIH consensus conference[2] recommended that all newborns be screened for hemoglobinopathies and that penicillin be given for the first 5 years of life to those who have sickle cell disease.

Subsequently the Agency For Health Care Policy and Research Sickle Cell panel recommended that infants who had documented or suspected sickle cell anemia or sickle cell–beta-thalassemia should be started on oral prophylactic penicillin as soon as possible, but no later than 2 months of age.[1] Furthermore, prophylaxis should be continued until at least 5 years of age.

APPROACH TO SCREENING

Given the scope of the problem, the consensus conference participants further recommended that state governments mandate newborn screening for hemoglobinopathies and that effective follow-up service programs be established.

For screening to be effective in reducing morbidity and mortality from infections, several services must accompany screening of the newborn:

1. A repeat test must be performed when the infant is about 3 months old because the newborn test results are only presumptive unless the hemoglobin genotypes of the biological parents are known. There is a possibility that the fetal and sickle hemoglobin (FS) pattern that is present if the newborn has sickle cell anemia also is found if the newborn has another condition, that is, sickle cell hereditary persistence of fetal hemoglobin, which is not a disease. Also, when an FS pattern is detected, it is possible that a small amount of normal adult hemoglobin (hemoglobin A) is present but not detected. The presence of small amounts of normal adult hemoglobin containing F and S hemoglobin is characteristic of sickle cell–beta-thalassemia disease at birth.
2. Parents must be taught the manifestations of sickle cell disease.
3. Parents must be told why penicillin prophylaxis is necessary and how they should respond if the early signs and symptoms of infection or acute splenic sequestration (another cause of sudden death) should occur. Symptoms include nasal congestion, cough, fever, lassitude, anorexia, pallor, and enlargement of the spleen.
4. Emergency rooms must be prepared to respond appropriately when a child who has sickle cell disease manifests the aforementioned signs and symptoms. For ex-

ample, in addition to receiving appropriate emergent medical care eventually, which consists of parenteral antibiotics (for infections) and transfusions (for acute splenic sequestration), they must be evaluated immediately. Children who have pneumococcal septicemia have died in emergency rooms while waiting to be seen by a physician.
5. The maintenance of penicillin prophylaxis must be monitored on a regular basis.
6. Efforts must be made to ensure that potential barriers to the maintenance of penicillin prophylaxis (e.g., transportation for monitoring and paying for penicillin) are removed.
7. Children must receive polyvalent pneumococcal vaccine at 2 and 5 years of age and every 5 years thereafter.

Voluntary sickle cell organizations in many communities have trained counselors and social workers who can assist in the provision of the necessary services, some of which are difficult for physicians to provide.

In those states that do not mandate hemoglobinopathy screening during the newborn period, it is incumbent upon physicians to screen all of their infants who are at risk for sickle cell disease early enough to enable affected infants to be started on penicillin prophylaxis by the second month of age.

The recommendation of penicillin prophylaxis is, of course, not restricted to children whose disease is detected through newborn screening. All children younger than the age of 5 years who are diagnosed as having sickle cell disease should be placed on penicillin prophylaxis immediately.

There are other benefits to the identification of sickle cell disease in the newborn period. A high percentage of adults who have sickle cell disease are not self-sufficient economically; that is, they depend on public assistance or their families for support despite the only limitations with respect to employment being heavy manual labor and the potential for frequent attacks of pain that result in a high level of absenteeism that is incompatible with the employer's expectations. There is considerable evidence that this discrepancy between potential for a person to be employed and that person's ability to gain and retain employment is the result of poor adjustment to the disease. Thus the early identification of sickle cell disease provides an opportunity for health care providers to begin to work with parents during their child's infancy to help them and their children make appropriate life-style adjustments to the disease. This attitude might be stated simplistically that children who have a sickle cell disease are to be treated as being ill only when they are experiencing a manifestation of the disease; at all other times they are to be treated as though they are well.

With respect to the second sickle condition, sickle cell trait, it needs to be recognized that individuals who have this condition rarely have related health problems and so usually do not discover their sickle cell trait other than through screening. These persons, however, have the potential (25% chance in each pregnancy) for having a child who has one of the sickle cell diseases if the other parent has a gene for one of the relevant hemoglobinopathies. Unless they are made aware of this potential, they may have children who have a sickle cell disease that they might have chosen not to have, or they may suffer emotional and adjustment problems through lack of preparation for handling the difficulties associated with these illnesses. Thus the purpose of screening for sickle cell trait is to provide counseling that will enable those counselled to make informed decisions that they believe are in their best interest with respect to marriage and childbearing.

Screening for sickle cell trait therefore is only of benefit for children who are approaching the childbearing age—a time at which information regarding marriage and reproduction is relevant. At that time the services consist of providing substantive information on the nature of sickle cell conditions, the risk of having a child who has sickle cell disease, and the available reproductive options.[4] Traditionally, this is termed *counseling,* but the process really is one of *education,* because persons should not be *advised* of what they should do, but simply *informed* of consequences and the options available to them.

The physician should present a balanced picture of sickle cell anemia when counseling individuals who have sickle cell trait. Presentations that underplay the potential severity can influence persons to chance having a child who has sickle cell anemia whom they would not have had if they had been informed accurately. Presentations that fail to indicate the spectrum of severity and the potential for individuals who have sickle cell anemia to live satisfying lives can influence individuals not to take the risk despite strong wishes and needs to have children.

The physician should not assume that the differences between sickle cell trait and sickle cell anemia are understood among the laity. Thus, when some individuals are told that they have sickle cell trait, they may believe that their health status is threatened, a belief that can generate severe anxiety and apprehension.

The physician should not depict sickle cell trait as a disease. Other than the rare occurrence of hematuria, it has not been documented that sickle cell trait has any influence on health status under usual physiological circumstances. Although the risk of intravascular sickling is theoretical if oxygen is deprived sufficiently during surgery, there is no reason to assume that competent surgeons and anesthesiologists would handle oxygen-deprived persons who have sickle cell trait differently from those whose hemoglobin patterns are normal.

The physician should inform the counselees that sickle cell anemia can be diagnosed prenatally by DNA analysis of cells obtained by chorionic villus sampling at about 9 weeks and by amniocentesis at about 15 weeks. This allows them to ascertain the status of their fetus and to decide whether they wish to continue or terminate the pregnancy if sickle cell anemia is present. For those parents who find termination of pregnancy an acceptable option, the availability of prenatal diagnosis enables them to have their own biological children without the possibility of having a child who has sickle cell anemia. Before prenatal diagnosis, parents had to forego having children if they wished to avoid having a child with sickle cell anemia.

As previously stated, reproductive decisions relative to the sickle cell gene should be based entirely on the potential parents' informed judgment as to what is in their best interest.

As indicated, the optimum time for sickle cell testing is at birth, a procedure that, if practiced universally, would lead to a population that would not require testing at any other time. However, because an at-risk population exists that to a large extent has not been screened for sickle cell conditions either through mandatory newborn testing programs or testing by their health care providers, it is important to decide when the unscreened should be tested/screened for sickle cell disease.

For sickle cell trait, inasmuch as the sole purpose of screening is to enable personal marriage and reproductive decisions, the procedure should be deferred until just before the childbearing age is reached. It is of no value, for example, for an 8-year-old to be tested for sickle cell trait.

For sickle cell diseases, because the purpose is to provide comprehensive care, there is no need to screen the population after the age of 5 years because by that age manifestations of the disease invariably will have led to the diagnosis.

Although from a programmatic standpoint the optimal timing for screening for sickle cell diseases and sickle cell trait is different, all of the screening methods identify both types of conditions. Thus, in screening newborns for sickle cell disease, newborns who have sickle trait are identified. This potentially is advantageous because it means that at least one and possibly both parents have sickle cell trait, which results in a highly cost beneficial detection of couples who have sickle cell trait at a time when they are having children. Among African-Americans, the incidence of sickle cell trait couples is approximately 1 in 144, whereas if a newborn has sickle cell trait the probability of both parents having sickle cell trait is 1 in 12.

In addition to implementing service programs that achieve the benefits of screening, it is equally important to institute policies, procedures, and practices that avoid potential harmful outcomes. One of these is the exposure of nonpaternity. Instances in which the putative father is not the biological father will be discovered in genetics screening in all racial groups, and this information can traumatize and even destroy previously stable families.

We can assume that when a father is told that the child he thought was his is not, it is highly likely that this will have a negative effect on his relationship with his partner and the child, particularly when the child has a chronic illness. The impaired relationship with the child might extend throughout a lifetime. This can be avoided to a large extent in newborn screening programs. Unless it is essential for the treatment of the child or for the provision of reproductive counseling, the parents need not be tested when the child has a sickle cell disease. In most instances the diagnosis is clear and the parents can be told which genes they have collectively; the service providers do not need to know which parent carries which gene. Obviously, if the parents request testing, it should be done. By the same token, if the newborn has one of the hemoglobinopathy traits, the mother should be tested for the purposes of reproductive counseling. If the mother does not have the trait in question, she can be told that the father does. There is no need for the service providers to confirm this by testing the alleged father. On the other hand, if the mother has the trait, the father then can be tested with impunity because a source of the child's gene has been identified. If the providers in a given program feel morally compelled to give all fathers their results (which means that in some cases fathers will become aware that they are not the fathers), they must implement informed consent procedures that give mothers sufficient information for them to decide whether they wish to take the risk of disclosing nonpaternity when they agree to parental testing.

Newborn screening for sickle cell conditions with the current methods also detects the presence of other hemoglobinopathies that generally do not require immediate intervention because of morbidity or mortality. Given that the racial mix and thus the incidence of the various hemoglobinopathies vary from state to state, each state must determine how this information will be handled.

Several methods currently are used to screen newborns for sickle cell disease—hemoglobin electrophoresis (cellulose acetate followed by citrate agar), ion exchange chromatography, isoelectric focusing, and high performance liquid chromatography. The methodology to be used in central laboratories for statewide programs should be selected after careful consideration of the advantages and disadvantages of each.

In the past the solubility test has been used in screening programs conducted by voluntary sickle cell organizations and by individual physicians. It is simple and inexpensive but should not be used for primary screening. Although the solubility test identifies accurately all who have inherited the sickle hemoglobin gene, it will not detect individuals who have inherited the gene for hemoglobin C. Hemoglobin C occurs in about 2% of the African-American population and gives a negative solubility test result, leading individuals screened by this procedure to assume that they cannot have a child who has a sickle cell disease. However, an African-American person who has hemoglobin C trait whose partner is an African-American has approximately an 8% chance of the partner having sickle cell trait. Should this occur, there is a 25% chance in each pregnancy for the child to have sickle cell–hemoglobin C disease, a condition that is accompanied by the same symptoms found in sickle cell anemia, although it tends to be a milder disorder. Screening programs therefore should use one of the other aforementioned tests, all of which will detect hemoglobin C trait, as well as hemoglobin C disease. Individuals who have hemoglobin C disease may have a mild hemolytic anemia.

TWELVE

Developmental Surveillance and Intervention

Rune J. Simeonsson and Nancy E. Simeonsson

While the significance of early intervention for infants and young children whose development is delayed or at risk is well established, effective identification of such children represents a challenge. At issue for pediatricians is the need for identification procedures sufficiently sensitive to detect significant variations in development and yet practical and efficient in clinical contexts. Screening tests have been recommended as the major approach to identification, but their use has been less than universally employed because of associated time demands and concerns about their limitations. A problematic result of this limited use and increased reliance on clinical judgment among pediatricians has been an underidentification of developmental, behavioral, or emotional problems in early childhood.[13] This is when pediatricians are increasingly likely to be involved with developmental problems, as documented in a study by Dobos et al.[4] comparing current practices with those 15 years ago. Pediatricians now are more likely to engage in detailed assessments, refer to other specialists, and contact schools about children. However, as Olfson[26] has noted, there is a marked discrepancy between the prevalence of children who have severe emotional disturbance seen in pediatric contexts and the estimated prevalence in the entire population. Thus there is a high likelihood that mental illness among children is underdiagnosed.

In response to these challenges, Dworkin[5] has advocated for *developmental surveillance* as an alternative approach, defined as a "flexible, continuous process that is broader in scope than screening, whereby knowledgeable professionals perform skilled observations of children throughout all encounters during child health care." This approach is comprehensive and encompasses monitoring, identifying, and assessing. As such it is consistent with the American Academy of Pediatrics[1] (AAP) recommendation for continuity of comprehensive care, as embodied in the monitoring guidelines for preventive pediatric care. Of particular relevance is the significance attached to the early years, evident in the recommendation for six visits in the first year of life and five from 1 through 4 years of age. Also relevant is the integration of effort that can be achieved by attending to the domains of the medical history, sensory screening, and developmental and behavioral guidance for both parent and child. Developmental assessment requires familiarity with developmental processes and capitalizes on opportunities for observations in all encounters with children. The results can yield information about developmental status and provide a base for parent counseling, referrals, and habilitation prescriptions.

ELEMENTS OF DEVELOPMENTAL SURVEILLANCE

Developmental surveillance should be integrated into the pediatric examination with a complete assessment of physical characteristics and laboratory studies[7]; it involves (1) a thorough history and knowledge of environmental influences, (2) familiarity with normal development, and (3) awareness of the relative significance of developmental indicators.

History

Obtaining a good history begins with a review of the family history, with particular attention to disorders of development. Details of the pregnancy, delivery, and perinatal period contribute indexes to identify children at risk. Understanding the influence of the environment on development, which includes nutrition, illness, and medication history, as well as social and psychologic variables, is important in developmental assessment. The quality of the parent-child interaction, the nature and availability of developmental stimulation, and the makeup of the social environment in terms of parents, siblings, peers, or extended caretakers may be salient.

Developmental Perspective

The importance of developmental surveillance is based on the conviction that patterns of development observed in the earliest years of life are sequential and therefore predictable. Biological maturation stimulates, as well as reflects, developmental changes in interaction with the environment. Developmental assessment of children therefore requires a perspective encompassing quantitative and qualitative aspects of development. A normative perspective views development as a sequence of milestones achieved at specific ages. In one way or another, most measures of development encompass milestones across the major streams of development of language, motor, problem-solving, and psychosocial skills.[3] Development also can be seen as a series of critical tasks to be mastered within certain stages of life, such as infancy, early childhood, middle childhood, and adolescence. Other developmental perspectives can be derived from stage-based theories, such as Erikson's theory of psychosocial stages or Piaget's stages of cognitive growth.

A basic synthesis of developmental tasks and Piaget's cognitive stages reveals infancy as a period in which the physical and social environment is understood and mastered through sensation and motor activity. This is expressed in a sequence of stages leading to independent mobility and the control involved in feeding, elimination, exploration, and initial symbol use in gestures and speech. These characteristics of infancy change in the toddler and preschool period to increasingly sophisticated language production, coordination of gross and fine motor movements for games and play, and increased awareness and conformity to peer and adult demands. The child's awareness of physical and social reality, however, is constrained by intuition and self-referenced perceptions. As the child reaches school age, a qualitative cognitive shift occurs, in which understanding no longer remains unidimensional and personally focused but can integrate several dimensions and alternative perspectives. This is reflected in the child's ability to reason logically and to classify and perform operations necessary for academic tasks.

Relative Significance of Developmental Indicators

Valid developmental assessment requires an awareness of the relative importance of developmental areas. Symbolic representation, speech, and fine motor coordination, particularly in a young child, have greater prognostic significance than more traditionally accepted indexes of development, such as acquisition of gross motor skills. The developmental points at which speech and language skills develop are perhaps the most useful clues in determining normal development. Second in importance, and closely related to speech, are appropriate social behaviors. Delayed or atypical communication and socialization behaviors are highly significant in identifying children at risk in terms of development. Of particular concern in this regard is increased alertness to emotional and behavioral difficulties. While such difficulties may reasonably be identified in school-age children, the task is made much more difficult with infants. The availability of measures to assess temperament or behavioral style in infants and toddlers, including a recent description by Medoff-Cooper et al.[20] on the assessments of infants under 4 months of age, suggests that this task can be made easier.

A final consideration is an emphasis on *rate as a principle* in developmental surveillance. Observations and assessments should be made on two or more occasions to determine developmental rate. This is particularly necessary in ruling out transient deficits resulting from normal variation or from the influence of illness or fatigue. The use of systematic procedures for assessing development can help. Although developmental status can be assessed sensitively in some domains, predicting ultimate intellectual competence is hazardous and should be avoided. Individual variations from developmental norms may be transient and, at first, simply should indicate the need for more comprehensive evaluation.

DEVELOPMENTAL DELAY OR ATYPICAL FEATURES: REPRESENTATIVE SIGNS AND SYMPTOMS BY DOMAINS

Motor domain

Hypertonicity or hypotonicity
Delayed creeping and walking
Poor coordination

Mental domain

Delayed or atypical play
Delayed or atypical use of objects
Delayed development of symbolic skills

Communication and language domain

Articulation and production errors
Immature speech
Absent or delayed speech

Social and emotional domain

Lethargy
Anxiety
Sleep difficulties
Depression
Social withdrawal
Selective attention deficits

Behavioral domain

Rhythmic habit patterns
Stereotypic behavior
Variable threshold level
Altered activity level

APPROACHES TO DEVELOPMENTAL SURVEILLANCE

For the practitioner committed to developmental surveillance, at least three complementary approaches can be used: (1) clinical observation, (2) parental involvement, and (3) screening tests.

Clinical Observation

Developmental assessment is crucial in the preschool years because growth and development in this period are particularly rapid, the pediatrician has a central role in the lives of children and their families, and qualitative developmental markers in the form of signs and symptoms can be observed clinically. These signs and symptoms can serve as indicators of at-risk status and developmental delay as well as of general school readiness. Of importance are those signs and symptoms of developmental functions associated with the identification of risk status or developmental delay.

In typical usage the terms *sign* and *symptom* are used diagnostically in regard to features or characteristics based either on objective or subjective criteria, respectively. With reference to developmental delay, consideration of signs and symptoms is complicated by several qualifications: (1) their significance is relative to development (timing); (2) their significance often is a function of temporal qualities (frequency, duration); and (3) they may be either common to developmental delay in general or associated with specific disorders. Several issues, however, are of particular importance for the pediatrician to consider. One is the diagnostic significance of rhythmic patterns such as body rocking and head rolling. Kravitz and Boehm[18] found that the onset, pattern, and decline of rhythmic habit movements can serve to document a developmental delay. Another issue is a recognition of the elements of a developmental approach to symptoms. As described by Green,[15] a developmental approach for a specific phase, such as infancy, includes a consideration of signs and symptoms, predisposing factors drawn from the history, and perinatal contingencies. A final issue pertains to signs and symptoms in emotional development, a difficult but important domain to consider. *Depression* is increasingly recognized as an entity, even in infancy and early childhood, as evident in Herzog and Rathbun's[16] description of a diagnostic system specifying criteria for symptoms by developmental stages. Another resource is Minde's[24] comprehensive view of symptoms of behavioral abnormalities in children younger than 36 months. Major developmental domains and representative signs and symptoms are summarized in the box above.

The significance in assessment lies in the discrepancies in rate of development of 25% or more likely being indicative of developmental delay. For example, a 20-month-old child whose mental, motor, or other domain of development resembles that of a 15-month-old or younger would be identified as developmentally delayed. Diagnosis of developmental delay is achieved more readily in some domains than in others. In domains for which age norms are available (e.g., motor, mental), the diagnosis can be supported objectively through motor and mental scales. In other domains (e.g., social, behavioral), clinical judgment may serve as the primary basis for diagnosis. Recognizing the central role of clinical reasoning in developmental assessment, Glascoe and Dworkin[13] have proposed that systematic attention to the process of impression formation can improve the accuracy of monitoring development.

Parental Involvement

In recent years there has been a growing recognition of the importance of parental involvement in health and education services for young children. This recognition is evident in Hutchison and Nicoll's[17] recommendation for parental partnership and interprofessional cooperation, concepts similar to the emphasis on parent involvement and the multidisciplinary approach in Public Law 99-457 (see Chapter 18, Identification of Developmental Delays and the Early Intervention System). In addition to detailing the child's history, parental contribution to developmental assessment can be enhanced productively and efficiently. An initial activity is to determine the expectations of parents about the purpose, nature, and form of developmental assessment. This can serve not only to document the extent of expectations and their realism, but also to alert providers to significant areas of concern.[27] There also is increasing evidence for the value of involving parents directly in assessing their child in terms of rating child characteristics and gathering observational data. Given the opportunity and appropriate format, parents can make reliable and valid judgments about the nature of their child's ability-disability profile.[2]

Various observation techniques (e.g., diary, interval, and time sampling) also can be used by parents to document the frequency, duration, and pattern of a particular problem (e.g., enuresis or temper tantrums), yielding a rich base of information for developmental surveillance. The efficiency and benefits of these forms of parental contributions have been documented by Glascoe and her colleagues,[10,11] who have found a high degree of correlation between parental concerns about developmental status and screening results.

Selected Screening Tests

The crux of developmental assessment is to differentiate the child who has a significant developmental problem from the one who manifests variations within a normal pattern. Appropriate measures can assist a clinician to identify developmental problems in infancy, and the preschool physical examination provides an excellent opportunity to predict school performance. Developmental status of most preschool children can be assessed validly and efficiently by use of the physical examination and selected assessment measures (Table 20-6).

The Denver Developmental Screening Test, including its most recent version (DDST-II), has enjoyed wide use.[9] The new test, the Denver II shown in Fig. 20-4, differs from the DDST with an increase of items from 105 to 125, particularly items pertaining to language (86%). The age scale of the test form conforms to the AAP's Health Supervision Visit Schedule, the norms have been updated and restandardized, and ratings of behavioral characteristics are included. The Denver II also enables identification of significant subpopulation differences attributable to race, gender, maternal education, and place of residence (rural, semirural, urban). The DDST-II is easy to administer (see sample test materials, Fig. 20-5), covers the age range of birth to 6 years, and has strong inter-rater and test-retest reliability. Only a few test items are needed, and instructions for administration of items, shown in Fig. 20-6, are printed on the back of the test form (Fig. 20-4). Of future interest is the likely availability of an abbreviated version of the DDST-II, with implications for efficient and situation-specific applications.[9] More detailed administration and scoring instructions are given in the DDST manual, which must be used to administer the test accurately. Although the old and new version of the DDST are well established as tools to monitor development in pediatric settings, concerns exist about their screening accuracy. These concerns have led Meisels[22] and Glascoe et al.[12] to caution its use and interpretation in general screening efforts. This underscores the importance of attending to the larger issue of quality control relative to the purpose and method of screening. This issue is particularly significant for children who have mild or at-risk conditions often confounded by situational factors of poverty or minority status. Because screening tests are subject to misuse in surveillance, care needs to be taken to ensure that common pitfalls are avoided and to ensure that tests are both *specific* and *sensitive*.[8] This assessment should encompass vision screening, hearing screening, and expressive and receptive language reflecting cognitive development, school readiness, self-awareness, and social awareness. Screening instruments thus should be selected in terms of their purposes and incorporated in the pediatric visit. Several screening measures are recommended as having both high specificity and sensitivity: the Early Screening Inventory (ESI), the Minnesota Preschool Screening Inventory (MPSI), and the Battelle Developmental Inventory Screening Test.[14,21] With continuing interest in the need for efficient surveillance, new screening measures are being developed. Sturner and his colleagues,[28] for example, have shown that a brief procedure (Simultaneous Techniques for Acuity and Readiness Testing, START) can be incorporated into routine pediatric procedures with strong evidence of concurrent validity.

For technical information (validity, specificity) on these and other screening instruments, see Meisels[21] and Glascoe et al.[14] (see also Appendix D).

Table 20-6 Selected Surveillance Measures

Instrument	Age (yr)
Early Infancy Temperament Questionnaire	0-4 mo
Infant Monitoring System	0-3
Denver Developmental Screening Test	0-6
Battelle Developmental Inventory Screening Test	1-8
Minnesota Child Developmental Inventory (MCDI)	6 mo-6 yr
Toddler Temperamental Scale	1-3
Peabody Picture Vocabulary Test (PPVT)[2]	2-adult
Early Screening Inventory (ESI)	3-6
Minnesota Preschool Screening Inventory (MPSI)	3½-5½
School Readiness Survey	4-6
Behavioral Style Questionnaire	4-7

DEVELOPMENTAL SURVEILLANCE AND PRIMARY PEDIATRIC CARE

Diagnosis

For those children whose developmental course is of sufficient concern to warrant one or more of the assessments described above, several outcomes are likely to involve primary pediatric care. One of these outcomes is the establishment of a diagnosis of developmental delay or disorder. Although these diagnoses have come into wide use with the early intervention mandate, the definitions may vary substantially from state to state. In general, however, developmental delay is defined as a condition in which functional aspects of the child's development are significantly delayed relative to the expected level of development. A typical criterion for developmental delay is a discrepancy of 25% or more from the expected rate in one or more domains of development. In references to standardized values, discrepancies of 1½ to 2 standard deviations also may be used. Signs and symptoms re-

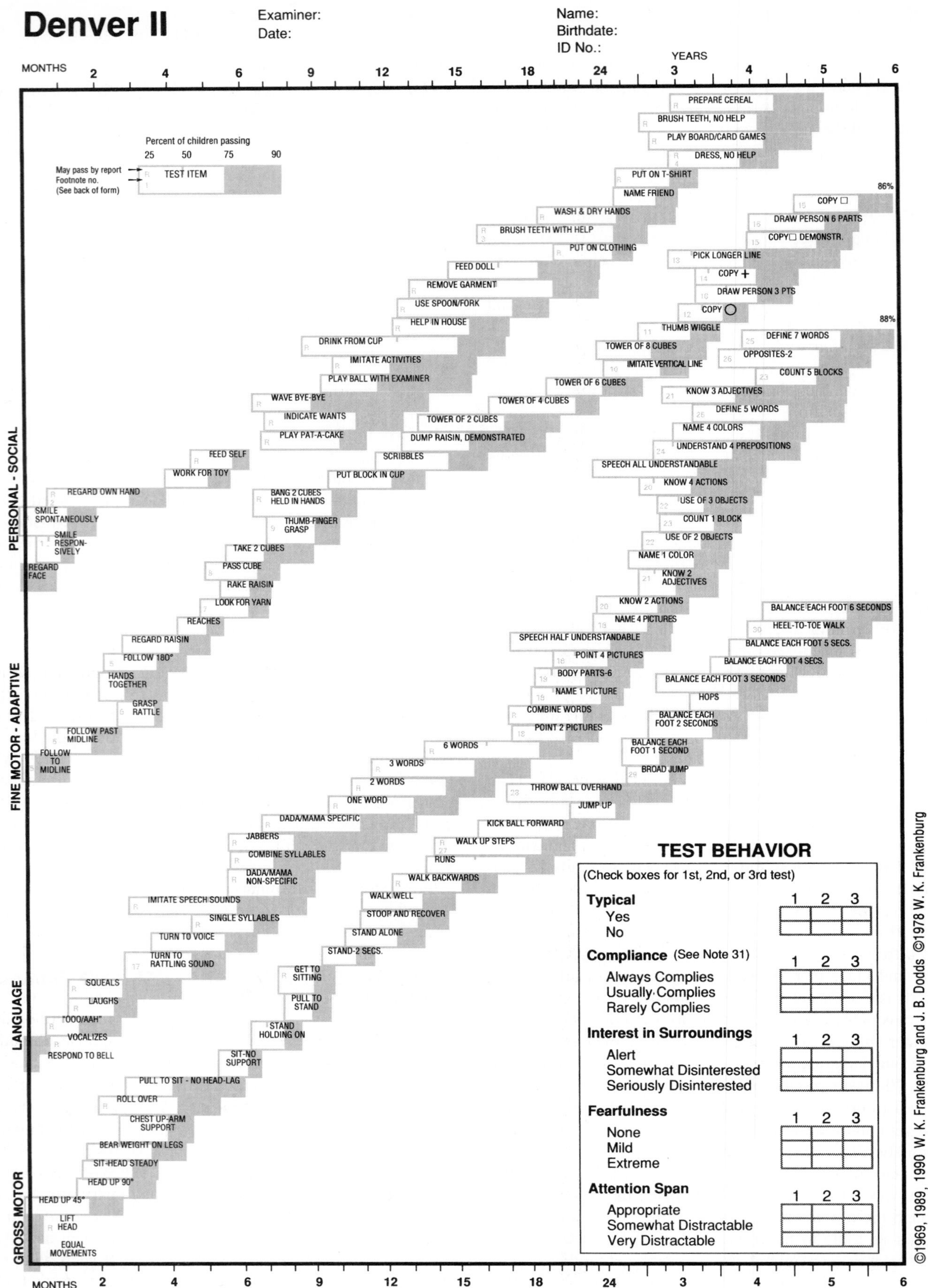

FIG. 20-4 Testing kits, test forms, and reference manuals (which must be used to ensure accuracy in administration of the test) for the DDST may be ordered from Denver Developmental Material, Inc., P.O. Box 6919, Denver, CO 80206-0919.

(Reprinted with permission from William K. Frankenburg, MD.)

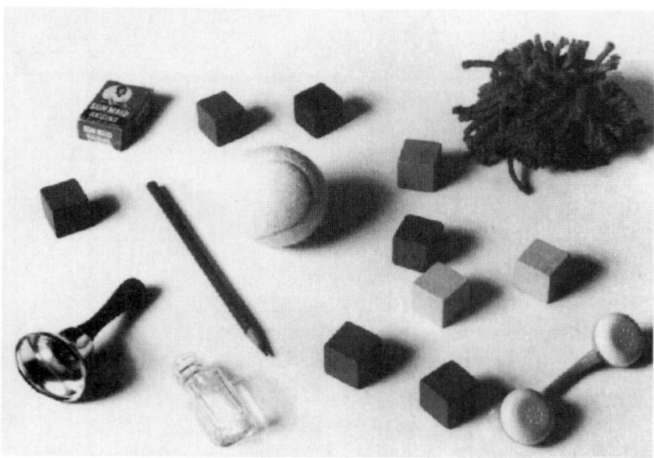

FIG. 20-5 Testing materials used in administering the Denver Developmental Screening Test.

flective of delays in functional development lead to an initial diagnosis of developmental delay. This diagnosis is either confirmed or dismissed after a consideration of the history, signs and symptoms, and associated etiological factors. In clinical contexts, "developmental delay" is a diagnostic label usually restricted to the preschool child in that neither the presenting characteristics nor assessment procedures are as specific as with older children. In the absence of findings associated with a specific developmental or behavioral disorder, the term "developmental delay" is used to define preschool children's eligibility for intervention.

Abnormal or Atypical Development

Screening for emotional and behavioral problems is difficult in that defining characteristics of atypical behavior varies in terms of sociocultural and developmental factors. Behavior considered inappropriate and deviant in a middle-class setting might not evoke concern in a lower-class environment (see Chapter 70, School Behavior Problems).

Identifying psychological problems in young children is not without difficulty. Merritt and her colleagues[23] have noted that the diagnosis of behavioral and emotional problems by pediatricians is only 25% to 33% of true prevalence rates. Caregiver-completed questionnaires and checklists, as well as interview responses, may lack accuracy, particularly when there may be reluctance to reveal a problem. The reading level of some instruments may be inappropriate for many parents, yielding questionable results. The use of psychological tests and formal observation may not be an assessment option for most practitioners, given the need for specialized training and administration time.

Presented with these difficulties, the physician who wishes to screen for psychological problems should work with mental health professionals to identify effective and efficient methods. To this end, research findings suggest that the Behavior Screening Questionnaire[6] and the Pediatric Examination of Educational Readiness[19] are useful screening instruments for the pediatrician. In a study of school-age children, Merritt et al.[23] have shown that maternal completion of behavior checklists in primary care pediatrics enhanced the accuracy of screening children who have behavioral and emotional problems. The presence of echolalia; repetitive, stereotypic mannerisms; withdrawn, uncontrollable, self-destructive, or abusive behavior; or poor or absent eye contact and social communication suggests the need for referral to a psychologist or a psychiatrist. Alone or in combination, these characteristics may reflect a variety of emotional and behavioral disturbances, ranging from acting out and testing of limits to expressions of psychopathological conditions.

Erratic or Discrepant Development

Some children demonstrate wide gaps in developmental skills. Most notably, they may experience difficulty with fine or gross motor coordination, understanding or producing language, and encoding or decoding letters and numbers. The child's developmental profile may reflect a wide range of skills that include some average abilities. A modality or functional deficit is suggested when a discrepancy of one third or more is observed in developmental skills between one area and others; such a discrepancy should be the basis for referring for further assessment and possible intervention by developmental specialists. These discrepancies may signal sensory problems, perceptual or learning disabilities, or minimal brain dysfunction. Morrison[25] and colleagues, for example, found an association between reading failure and behavior problems in children, indicating the need for focused diagnostic evaluations.

Referral

If significant speech, motor, or other developmental deficits are noted, referral to allied health specialists can provide parents and health care providers a realistic assessment of the child's needs and the development of specific plans for habilitation. Referral to the psychologist can be made when more formal evaluation of both intellectual and personal-social functioning is indicated. Such information is a valuable base for parental understanding and involvement in interventions for the child. One must not lose sight of how necessary the primary care practitioner's advocacy is when referral is made (see Chapter 93, Consultation and Referral for Behavioral and Developmental Problems). To avoid potential problems in the referral process, the information and interventions desired from the consultant should be defined clearly. Sensitivity to environmental or situational factors is particularly significant in monitoring the course of treatment for children identified as hyperactive or having attention deficits. Finally, referral for evaluation and diagnosis should be predicated on knowledge that intervention services and resources are available. Providers of special services for infants and young children who have developmental problems may take the form of private or community programs. Familiarity with available specialized resources for children who have disabilities and their families is essential if comprehensive management is to be developed and implemented.

Management

The pediatrician's role in the management of children who have developmental delays differs somewhat from that taken in the management of most illnesses. Cure with a return to normality usually is not achievable. Most of the professionals consulted about the child's assessment and treatment are nonmedical. Pediatricians who must inform parents of the

DIRECTIONS FOR ADMINISTRATION

1. Try to get child to smile by smiling, talking or waving. Do not touch him/her.
2. Child must stare at hand several seconds.
3. Parent may help guide toothbrush and put toothpaste on brush.
4. Child does not have to be able to tie shoes or button/zip in the back.
5. Move yarn slowly in an arc from one side to the other, about 8" above child's face.
6. Pass if child grasps rattle when it is touched to the backs or tips of fingers.
7. Pass if child tries to see where yarn went. Yarn should be dropped quickly from sight from tester's hand without arm movement.
8. Child must transfer cube from hand to hand without help of body, mouth, or table.
9. Pass if child picks up raisin with any part of thumb and finger.
10. Line can vary only 30 degrees or less from tester's line.
11. Make a fist with thumb pointing upward and wiggle only the thumb. Pass if child imitates and does not move any fingers other than the thumb.

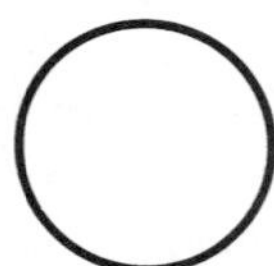

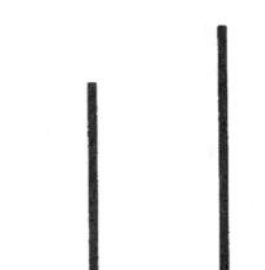

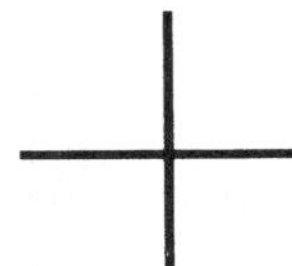

12. Pass any enclosed form. Fail continuous round motions.
13. Which line is longer? (Not bigger.) Turn paper upside down and repeat. (pass 3 of 3 or 5 of 6)
14. Pass any lines crossing near midpoint.
15. Have child copy first. If failed, demonstrate.

When giving items 12, 14, and 15, do not name the forms. Do not demonstrate 12 and 14.

16. When scoring, each pair (2 arms, 2 legs, etc.) counts as one part.
17. Place one cube in cup and shake gently near child's ear, but out of sight. Repeat for other ear.
18. Point to picture and have child name it. (No credit is given for sounds only.) If less than 4 pictures are named correctly, have child point to picture as each is named by tester.

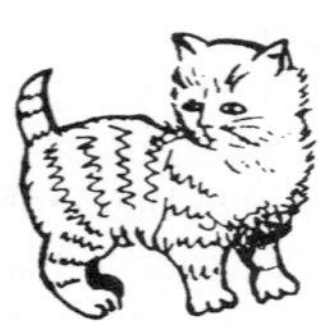

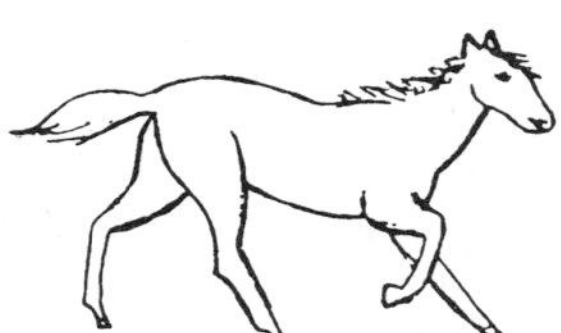

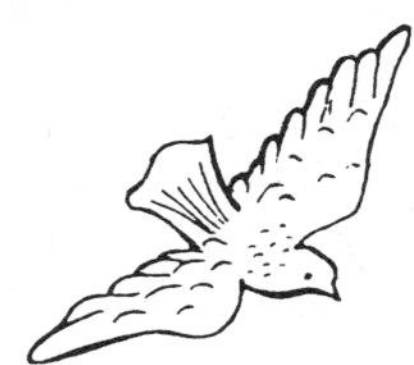

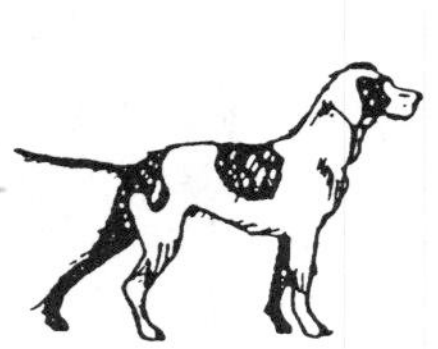

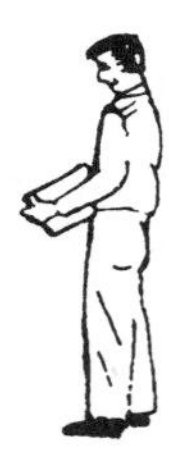

19. Using doll, tell child: Show me the nose, eyes, ears, mouth, hands, feet, tummy, hair. Pass 6 of 8.
20. Using pictures, ask child: Which one flies?... says meow?... talks?... barks?... gallops? Pass 2 of 5, 4 of 5.
21. Ask child: What do you do when you are cold?... tired?... hungry? Pass 2 of 3, 3 of 3.
22. Ask child: What do you do with a cup? What is a chair used for? What is a pencil used for? Action words must be included in answers.
23. Pass if child correctly places and says how many blocks are on paper. (1, 5).
24. Tell child: Put block **on** table; **under** table; **in front of** me, **behind** me. Pass 4 of 4. (Do not help child by pointing, moving head or eyes.)
25. Ask child: What is a ball?... lake?... desk?... house?... banana?... curtain?... fence?... ceiling? Pass if defined in terms of use, shape, what it is made of, or general category (such as banana is fruit, not just yellow). Pass 5 of 8, 7 of 8.
26. Ask child: If a horse is big, a mouse is __? If fire is hot, ice is __? If the sun shines during the day, the moon shines during the __? Pass 2 of 3.
27. Child may use wall or rail only, not person. May not crawl.
28. Child must throw ball overhand 3 feet to within arm's reach of tester.
29. Child must perform standing broad jump over width of test sheet (8 1/2 inches).
30. Tell child to walk forward, ⊂⊃⊂⊃⊂⊃⊂⊃→ heel within 1 inch of toe. Tester may demonstrate. Child must walk 4 consecutive steps.
31. In the second year, half of normal children are non-compliant.

OBSERVATIONS:

FIG. 20-6 Instructions printed on the back of the DDST form for administering some of the items contained in the Denver Developmental Screening Test.

(Reprinted with permission from William K. Frankenburg, MD.)

presence of a chronic and disabling condition should consider their initial approach carefully (see Chapter 10, Communication with Parents and Patients). This news should be shared in a quiet, private consultation with both parents present whenever possible. Sufficient time should be allocated to allow a complete and unhurried sharing of both feelings and information. It is best to clarify the parents' perceptions of the situation at the very beginning. More often than not, the pediatrician will discover that the news confirms long-standing parental suspicions. The parents are likely to be relieved that someone finally is taking them seriously. Support by the physician will do much to form a therapeutic alliance. Information given to the parents should be as complete and honest as the pediatrician is capable of providing; withholding information only builds mistrust. The pediatrician should be careful to minimize the use of technical terminology, but not to avoid developmental diagnoses if they apply. Attempting to avoid such emotionally laden terms is, in the long run, a disservice. If the parents react with anger or denial, the physician should avoid arguments or attempts to convince. The parents' perspective on their child's status can evolve in the context of an understanding relationship with a pediatrician. Management of the developmentally delayed child who hasn't a specific disorder involves monitoring progress and being supportive of the child and family. Management of children who have specific disorders (e.g., cerebral palsy, autism) involves similar activities, plus specific medical or allied treatments or interventions as indicated. Because of the complex needs of many children who have developmental problems, it is highly desirable that assessment and management be integrated into an overall plan for the child's care. Such an overall plan is implicit in the requirements of the Individualized Education Plan (IEP) for preschool and school-age children and in the Individualized Family Service Plan (IFSP) defined in Public Law 99-457. Particularly important is establishing lines of communication and accountability on behalf of the family that has a child with special needs. Given that the family may have contacts with many medical and nonmedical professionals, the pediatrician is a logical coordinator of services. Advocating for the child and family is essential to the therapeutic process and the promotion of the child's potential.

REFERENCES

General Considerations

1. Bess FM, Paradise JL: Universal screening for infant hearing impairment: not simple, not risk-free, not necessarily beneficial, and not presently justified, *Pediatrics* 93:330, 1994.
2. Centers for Disease Control: *Preventing lead poisoning in young children,* Atlanta, 1991, US Department of Health and Human Services, Public Health Service, Centers for Disease Control.
3. Dworkin PH: British and American recommendations for developmental monitoring: the role of surveillance, *Pediatrics* 84:1000, 1989.
4. Frankenburg WK et al: The Denver II: a major revision and restandardization of the Denver Developmental Screening Test, *Pediatrics* 89:91, 1992.
5. Harvey B: Should blood level screening recommendations be revised? *Pediatrics* 93:201, 1994.
6. Jellinek MS, Murphy JM: The recognition of psychosocial disorders in pediatric office practice: the current status of the pediatric symptom checklist, *J Dev Behav Pediatr* 11:273, 1990.
7. Joint Committee on Infant Hearing: 1990 position statement, *AAP News* 7:6, 1993.
8. Kemper KJ: Self-administered questionnaire for structured psychosocial screening in pediatrics, *Pediatrics* 89:433, 1992.
9. NIH Consensus Statement: Early identification of hearing impairment in infants and young children, 11:1, 1993.
10. Northern JL, Downs MP: *Hearing in children,* Baltimore, 1991, Williams & Wilkins.
11. Sickle Cell Disease Guideline Panel: *Sickle cell disease: screening, diagnosis, management, and counseling in newborns and infants,* Clinical practice guideline number 6, Rockville, Md, 1993, US Department of Health and Human Services, Public Health Service, Agency for Health Care Policy and Research.
12. Squires JK, Nickel R, Bricker D: Use of parent-completed questionnaires for child-find and screening, *Inf Young Child* 3:46, 1990.
13. United States Congress, Office of Technology Assessment: *Healthy children: investing in the future,* OTA-H-345, Washington, DC, 1988, US Government Printing Office.

The Physical Examination as a Screening Test

1. Anderson FP: Evaluation of the routine physical examination of infants in the first year of life, *Pediatrics* 45:950, 1970.
2. Castelein RM, Sauter AJM: Ultrasound screening for congenital dysplasia of the hip in newborns: its value, *J Pediatr Orthop* 8:666, 1988.
3. Del Mar CB, Miller IS: Are child surveillance clinics worthwhile? *Lancet* 2:1334, 1987.
4. Editorial: School screening for scoliosis, *Lancet* 2:378, 1988.
5. Hoekelman RA: A summer Head Start medical program, Rochester, NY, 1969: implications for change, *JAMA* 219:730, 1972.
6. Kennedy FD: Have school-entry medicals had their day? *Arch Dis Child* 63:1261, 1988.
7. Knox EG, Lancashire RJ: Effectiveness of screening for congenital dislocation of the hip, *J Epidemiol Community Health* 41:283, 1987.
8. Renshaw TS: Screening school children for scoliosis, *Clin Orthop* 229:26, 1988.
9. Rogers KD, Reese G: Health studies—presumably normal high school students. I. Physical appraisal, *Am J Dis Child* 108:572, 1964.
10. Yankauer A, Lawrence R: A study of periodic school medical examinations. II. The annual increment of new "defects," *Am J Public Health* 46:1553, 1956.

Recognition of Genetic-Metabolic Disease by Clinical Diagnosis and Screening

1. Agency for Health Care Policy and Research, Sickle Cell Disease Guideline Panel: *Sickle cell disease: Screening, diagnosis, management, and counseling in newborns and infants,* Rockville, Md, 1993, US Department of Health and Human Services.
2. Allen DB: Newborn screening for congenital adrenal hyperplasia in Wisconsin, *Wis Med J* 92:75, 1993.
3. Andrews LB et al: *Assessing genetic risks: implications for health and social policy,* Washington, DC, 1994, National Academy of Sciences Press.
4. Arn P, Valle D, Brusilow S: Inborn errors of metabolism: not rare, not hopeless, *Contemp Pediatr* 5:47, 1988.
5. Bachmann C et al: Pitfalls in amino acid and organic acid analysis: 3-hydroxyproprionic aciduria, *Eur J Pediatr* 153(suppl 1):23, 1994.
6. Batshaw ML: Inborn errors of urea synthesis, *Ann Neurol* 35:133, 1994.
7. Berghe G: Inborn errors of fructose metabolism, *Annu Rev Nutr* 14:41, 1994.
8. Brusilow SW: Treatment of urea cycle disorders. In Desnick RJ, editor: *Treatment of genetic diseases,* New York, 1991, Churchill Livingstone.
9. Buist NRM, Tuerck JM: The practitioner's role in newborn screening, *Pediatr Clin North Am* 2:199, 1992.
10. Burton B: Inborn errors of metabolism: the clinical diagnosis in early infancy, *Pediatrics* 79:359, 1987.
11. Cao A et al: Thalassemias in Sardinia: molecular pathology, phenotype-genotype correlation, and prevention, *Am J Pediatr Hemat-Oncol* 13:179, 1991.
12. Committee on Genetics: Issues in newborn screening, *Pediatrics* 89:345, 1992.
13. Committee on Genetics: Prenatal genetic diagnosis for pediatricians, *Pediatrics* 93:1010, 1994.

14. Dixon M, Leonard JV: Intercurrent illness in inborn errors of intermediary metabolism, *Arch Dis Child* 67:1387, 1992.
15. Donnell GN: Clinical aspects and historical perspectives of galactosemia. In Donnell GN et al, editors: *Galactosemia: new frontiers in research,* Washington, DC, 1993, US Department of Health and Human Services.
16. Drumm ML, Collins FS: Molecular biology of cystic fibrosis, *Mol Genet Med* 3:33, 1993.
17. Dussault JH: Neonatal screening for congenital hypothyroidism, *Clin Lab Med* 13:645, 1993.
18. Farrell PM, Mischler EH: Newborn screening for cystic fibrosis, *Adv Pediatr* 39:35, 1992.
19. Foreman JW: Acid-base physiology in health and disease. In Cohn RM, Roth KS, editors: *Metabolic disease: a guide to early recognition,* Philadelphia, 1983, WB Saunders.
20. Gahl WA: Cystinosis coming of age, *Adv Pediatr* 33:95, 1986.
21. Gaston MH et al: Prophylaxis with oral penicillin in children with sickle cell anemia: a randomized trial, *N Engl J Med* 314:1593, 1986.
22. Grant DB et al: Congenital hypothyroidism detected by neonatal screening: relationship between biochemical severity and early clinical features, *Arch Dis Child* 67:87, 1992.
23. Haddow JE et al: Prenatal screening for Down's syndrome with use of maternal serum markers, *N Engl J Med* 327:588, 1992.
24. Hale DE, Bennett MJ: Fatty acid oxidation disorders: a new class of metabolic diseases, *J Pediatr* 121:1, 1992.
25. Hammond KB et al: Efficacy of statewide neonatal screening for cystic fibrosis by assay of trypsinogen concentrations, *N Engl J Med* 325:769, 1991.
26. Hamosh A: Inherited metabolic diseases in the newborn. In Rosenstein BJ, editor: *Primary care of the newborn,* St Louis, 1992, Mosby.
27. Hart PS et al: Comparison of profound biotinidase deficiency in children ascertained clinically and by newborn screening using a simple method of accurately determining residual biotinidase activity, *Biochem Med Metabol Biol* 48:41, 1992.
28. Holtzman NA: Inherited metabolic disease. In Hoekelman RA, editor: *Principles of pediatrics: health care of the young,* New York, 1978, McGraw-Hill.
29. Holtzman NA: Proceed with caution: predicting genetic risks in the recombinant DNA era, Baltimore, Md, 1989, The Johns Hopkins University Press.
30. Holtzman NA et al: Effect of age at loss of dietary control on intellectual performance and behavior of children with phenylketonuria, *N Engl J Med* 314:593, 1986.
31. Hopwood JJ, Morris CP: The mucopolysaccharidoses: diagnosis, molecular genetics, and treatment, *Mol Biol Med* 7:381, 1990.
32. Hubbard RC et al: Biochemical efficacy and safety of monthly augmentation therapy for α1-antitrypsin deficiency, *JAMA* 260:1259, 1988.
33. Jaeken J, Hagberg B, Stromme P: Clinical presentation and natural course of the carbohydrate deficient glycoprotein syndrome, *Acta Paediatrica Scandinavica Suppl* 375:6, 1991.
34. Kaback M et al: Tay-Sachs disease: carrier screening, prenatal diagnosis, and the molecular era: an international perspective, 1970-1993, *JAMA* 270:2307, 1993.
35. Kahler S et al: Pancreatitis in patients with organic acidemias, *J Pediatr* 124:239, 1994.
36. Kelly DA: Organ transplantation for inherited metabolic disease, *Arch Dis Child* 71:181, 1994.
37. Kooistra L et al: Motor and cognitive development in children with congenital hypothyroidism: a long-term evaluation of the effects of neonatal treatment, *J Pediatr* 124:903, 1994.
38. Lane PA, Eckman JR: Cost-effectiveness of neonatal screening for sickle cell disease, *J Pediatr* 120:162, 1992.
39. Lazarow PB, Moser H: Disorders of peroxisome biogenesis. In Scriven C, editor: *Metabolic and molecular basis of inherited disease,* New York, 1995, McGraw-Hill.
40. Lehnert W et al: Propionic acidaemia: clinical, biochemical, and therapeutic aspects. *Eur J Pediatr* 153(suppl 1):S68, 1994.
41. Levy HL et al: Sepsis due to *E. coli* in neonates with galactosemia, *N Engl J Med* 297:823, 1977.
42. Levy HL: Nutritional therapy in inborn errors of metabolism. In Desnick RJ, editor: *Treatment of genetic diseases,* New York, 1991, Churchill Livingstone.
43. Listernick R, Frisone L, Silverman BL: Delayed diagnosis of infants with abnormal neonatal screens, *JAMA* 267:1095, 1992.
44. Loader S et al: Prenatal hemoglobinopathy screening. IV. Follow-up of women at risk for a child with a clinically significant hemoglobinopathy, *Am J Hum Genet* 49:1292, 1991.
45. Lorey FW, Cunningham GC: Birth prevalence of primary congenital hypothyroidism by sex and ethnicity, *Hum Biol* 64:531, 1992.
46. Luthy DA et al: Cesarean section before the onset of labor and subsequent motor function in infants with meningomyelocele diagnosed antenatally, *N Engl J Med* 324:662, 1991.
47. McNeil TF, Sveger T, Thelin T: Psychological effects of screening for somatic risk: The Swedish α1-antitrypsin experience, *Thorax* 43:505, 1988.
48. Meloni T, Forteleoni G, Meloni GF: Marked decline of favism after neonatal glucose-6-phosphate dehydrogenase screening and health education: the Northern Sardinian experience, *Acta Haematol* 87:29, 1992.
49. Mohon RT et al: Relationship of genotype to early pulmonary function in infants with cystic fibrosis identified through neonatal screening, *J Pediatr* 122:550, 1993.
50. Mudd SH et al: The natural history of homocystinuria due to cystathionine B-synthase deficiency, *Am J Hum Genet* 37:1, 1985.
51. National Institutes of Health: Statement from the workshop on population screening of the cystic fibrosis gene, *N Engl J Med* 323:70, 1990.
52. National screening status report: *Infant Screen* 17:5, 1994.
53. Nobukuni Y et al: Heterogeneity of mutations in maple syrup urine disease (MSUD): Screening and identification of affected E1α and E1β subunits of the branched-chain α-keto-acid dehydrogenase multienzyme complex, *Biochim Biophys Acta* 1225:64, 1994.
54. Pang S, Clark A: Congenital adrenal hyperplasia due to 21-hydroxylase deficiency: newborn screening and its relationship to the diagnosis and treatment of the disorder, *Screening* 2:105, 1993.
55. Peinemann F, Danner DJ: Maple syrup urine disease 1954 to 1993, *J Inherit Metab Dis* 17:3, 1994.
56. Pyeritz RE: Homocystinuria. In Beighton P, editor: *Heritable disorders of connective tissue,* St Louis, 1993, Mosby.
57. Rutledge SL et al: Neonatal hemodialysis: Effective therapy for the encephalopathy of inborn errors of metabolism, *J Pediatr* 116:125, 1990.
58. Rutledge SL et al: Tubulointerstitial nephritis in methylmalonic acidemia, *Pediatr Nephrol* 7:81, 1993.
59. Saudubray JM, Charpentier C: Clinical phenotypes: diagnosis/algorithms. In Scrivner C, editor: *Metabolic and molecular basis of inherited disease,* New York, 1995, McGraw-Hill.
60. Servidei S, Bertini E, DiMauro S: Hereditary metabolic cardiomyopathies, *Adv Pediatr* 41:1, 1994.
61. Silverman EK et al: Variability of pulmonary function in alpha-1-antitrypsin deficiency: clinical correlates, *Ann Intern Med* 111:982, 1989.
62. Simpson JL, Elias S: Isolating fetal cells from maternal blood: advances in prenatal diagnosis through molecular technology, *JAMA* 270:2357, 1993.
63. Sprinkle RH, Hynes DM, Konrad TR: Is universal neonatal hemoglobinopathy screening cost-effective? *Arch Pediatr Adolesc Med* 148:461, 1994.
64. Tambor ES et al: Offering cystic fibrosis carrier screening to an HMO population: factors associated with utilization, *Am J Hum Genet* 55:626, 1994.
65. Thompson R, Seargeant L, Winter J: Screening for congenital adrenal hyperplasia: distribution of 17 alpha-hydroxyprogesterone concentrations in neonatal blood spot specimens, *J Pediatr* 114:400, 1989.
66. Tluczek A et al: Parents' knowledge of neonatal screening and response to false-positive cystic fibrosis testing, *J Dev Behav Pediatr* 13:181, 1992.
67. Touma EH, Charpentier C: Medium chain acyl-CoA dehydrogenase deficiency, *Arch Dis Child* 67:142, 1992.
68. Udall JN et al: Liver disease in α1-antitrypsin deficiency: a retrospective analysis of the influence of early breast- vs bottle-feeding, *JAMA* 253:2679, 1985.
69. Ullrich K: Screening for lysosomal disorders, *Eur J Pediatr* 153(suppl 1):S38, 1994.

70. Valle D: Treatment and prevention of genetic disease. In Wilson JD, editor: *Harrison's principles of internal medicine,* New York, 1994, McGraw-Hill.
71. Waggoner DD, Donnell GN, Buist NRM: Long-term prognosis in galactosemia: results of a survey of 350 cases. In Donnell GN et al, editors: *Galactosemia: new frontiers in research,* Washington, DC, 1993, US Department of Health and Human Services.
72. Wald NJ, Cuckle HS: Open neural-tube defects. In Wald J, editor: *Antenatal and neonatal screening,* Oxford, 1984, Oxford University Press.
73. Wald N, Cuckle H, Nanchahal K: Amniotic fluid acetylcholinesterase measurement in the prenatal diagnosis of open neural tube defects, *Prenat Diagn* 9:813, 1989.
74. Wall M et al: Long-term follow-up of a cohort of children with alpha-1-antitrypsin deficiency, *J Pediatr* 116:248, 1990.
75. Ward JC: Inborn errors of metabolism of acute onset in infancy, *Pediatr Rev* 11:205, 1990.
76. Werler MM, Shapiro S, Mitchell AA: Periconceptional folic acid exposure and risk of occurrent neural tube defects, *JAMA* 269:1257, 1993.
77. Wilcken B: Newborn screening for cystic fibrosis: its evolution and a review of the current situation, *Screening* 2:43, 1993.
78. Wolf B, Heard GS: Biotinidase deficiency, *Adv Pediatr* 38:1, 1991.
79. Wulfsberg EA, Hoffmann DE, Cohen MM: Alpha-1-antitrypsin deficiency: impact of genetic discovery on medicine and society, *JAMA* 271:217, 1994.
80. Zeesman S et al: A private view of heterozygosity: eight-year follow-up study on carriers of the Tay-Sachs gene detected by high school screening in Montreal, *Am J Med Genet* 18:769, 1984.

Cardiac Screening

1. American Academy of Pediatrics, Committee on Nutrition: Indications for cholesterol testing in children, *Pediatrics* 83:141, 1989.
2. American Academy of Pediatrics, Committee on Nutrition: Prudent lifestyle for children: dietary fat and cholesterol, *Pediatrics* 78:512, 1986.
3. American Academy of Pediatrics, Committee on Nutrition: Statement on cholesterol, *Pediatrics* 90:469, 1991.
4. Enos WF, Holmes RH, Beyer J: Coronary disease among United States soldiers killed in action in Korea, *JAMA* 152:1090, 1953.
5. Epstein SE, Maron BJ: Sudden death and the competitive athlete: perspectives on preparticipation screening studies, *J Am Coll Cardiol* 7:220, 1986.
6. Gilman MW et al: Identifying children at high risk for the development of essential hypertension, *J Pediatr* 122:6, 1993.
7. Kannel WB et al: Serum cholesterol, lipoproteins and risk of coronary heart disease: the Framington Study, *Ann Intern Med* 74:1, 1971.
8. LaCorte MA et al: EKG screening program for school athletes, *Clin Cardiol* 12:42, 1989.
9. Lauer RM, Lee J, Clarke WR: Factor affecting the relationship between childhood and adult cholesterol levels: the muscatine study, *Pediatrics* 82:309, 1988.
10. Lauer RM, Lee J, Clarke WR: Use of cholesterol measurements in childhood for the prediction of adult hypercholesterolemia: the muscatine study, *JAMA* 264:3034, 1990.
11. Maron BJ et al: Results of screening a large group of intercollegiate competitive athletes for cardiovascular disease, *J Am Coll Cardiol* 10:1214, 1987.
12. Maron BJ et al: Sudden death in young athletes, *Circulation* 62:218, 1980.
13. National Cholesterol Education Program. Report of the expert panel on blood cholesterol levels in children and adolescents, *Pediatrics* 89(suppl):525, 1992.
14. Newman WP III et al: Relation of serum lipoprotein levels and systolic blood pressure to early atherosclerosis: the Bogalusa heart study, *N Engl J Med* 314:138, 1986.
15. Orchard TJ et al: Cholesterol screening in childhood: does it predict adult hypercholesterolemia? The Beaver County experience, *J Pediatr* 103:687, 1983.
16. Pearl W et al: Electrocardiogram value in routine adolescent physical examinations, *Intern Pediatr* 2:342, 1987.
17. Report of Second Task Force on Blood Pressure Control in Children, *Pediatrics* 79:1, 1987.
18. Strong JP: Coronary atherosclerosis in soldiers: a clue to the natural history of atherosclerosis in the young, *JAMA* 256:2863, 1986.
19. Voors AW et al: Studies of blood pressure in children, ages 5-14 years in a total biracial community—the Bogalusa heart study, *Circulation* 54:319, 1976.

Screening for Drugs

1. American Academy of Pediatrics: Screening for drugs of abuse in children and adolescents, *Pediatrics* 84:396, 1989.
2. American Medical Association, Council on Scientific Affairs: Scientific issues in drug testing, *JAMA* 257:3110, 1987.
3. Bays J: Substance abuse and child abuse, *Pediatr Clin North Am* 37:881, 1990.
4. Campbell DE, Fleischman AR: Ethical challenges in medical care for the pregnant substance abuser, *Clin Obstet Gynecol* 35:803, 1992.
5. Chasnoff IJ et al: Temporal patterns of cocaine use in pregnancy: perinatal outcome, *JAMA* 261:1741, 1989.
6. Chasnoff IJ, Landress HJ, Barrett ME: The prevalence of illicit-drug or alcohol use during pregnancies and discrepancies in reporting in Pinellas County, Florida, *N Engl J Med* 322:1202, 1990.
7. National Institute on Drug Abuse: *National household survey on drug abuse: 1988 population estimates,* Pub No 89-1636, Washington, DC, 1989, US Department of Health and Human Services.
8. Office of Substance Abuse Prevention: *Alcohol, tobacco and other drugs may harm the newborn,* Washington, DC, 1990, US Department of Health and Human Services.
9. Ostrea EM et al: Drug screening of newborns by meconium analysis: a large scale, prospective, epidemiologic study, *Pediatrics* 89:107, 1992.
10. Schwartz JG et al: Accuracy of common drug screen tests, *Am J Emerg Med* 9:166, 1991.

Use of Urinalysis and the Urine Culture in Screening

1. Dodge WF et al: Proteinuria and hematuria in schoolchildren: epidemiology and natural history, *J Pediatr* 88:329, 1976.
2. Gutgesell M: Practicality of screening urinalysis in asymptomatic children in a primary care setting, *Pediatrics* 62:103, 1978.
3. Hansson S et al: Untreated bacteriuria in asymptomatic girls with renal scarring, *Pediatrics* 84:964, 1989.
4. Kitagawa T: Screening for renal disease in schoolchildren: experience in Japan, *Indian J Pediatr* 55:481, 1988.
5. Newcastle Covert Bacteriuria Research Group: Covert bacteriuria in schoolgirls in Newcastle upon Tyne: a 5-year follow-up, *Arch Dis Child* 56:585, 1981.
6. Silverberg DS: City-wide screening for urinary abnormalities in schoolgirls, *Can Med Assoc J* 109:981, 1973.
7. Silverberg DS: City-wide screening for urinary abnormalities in schoolboys, *Can Med Assoc J* 111:410, 1974.
8. Thompson AL et al: Fixed and reproducible orthostatic proteinuria. VI. Results of a 10-year follow-up evaluation, *Ann Intern Med* 73:235, 1970.
9. Verier Jones K et al: Glomerular filtration rate in schoolgirls with covert bacteriuria, *Br Med J* 285:1307, 1982.

Auditory Screening

1. Bess FH, Paradise JL: Universal screening for infant hearing: not simple, not risk-free, not necessarily beneficial, and not presently justified, *Pediatrics* 98:330, 1994.
2. Bonfils P, Uziel A, Pujol R: Screening for auditory dysfunction in infants by evoked oto-acoustic emissions, *Arch Otolaryngol Head Neck Surg* 114:887, 1988.
3. Elssman S, Matkin N, Sabo M: Early identification of congenital sensorineural hearing impairment, *Hear J* Sept 1987, p 13.
4. Glattke TJ, Kujawa SG: Otoacoustic emissions, *Am J Audiol* 1:29, 1991.
5. Guidelines for screening for hearing impairments and middle-ear disorders, ASHA 32(suppl 2):17, 1990.
6. Joint Committee on Infant Hearing: 1993 position statement (draft copy), Rockville, Md, Sept 28, 1993, American Speech-Language-Hearing Association.
7. Kennedy C et al: Otoacoustic emissions and auditory brainstem responses in the newborn, *Arch Dis Child* 66:1124, 1991.
8. Mauk GW et al: The effectiveness of high-risk characteristics in early identification of hearing impairment, *Ear and Hear* 12:312, 1991.

9. NIH Consensus Statement: Early identification of hearing impairment in infants and young children, 11:1, March 1-3, 1993, Office of Medical Applications of Research, National Institutes of Health, Federal Bldg Room 618, Bethesda, Md 20892.
10. Northern JL, Downs MP: *Hearing in children,* ed 4, Baltimore, 1991, Williams & Wilkins.
11. Northern JL, Hayes D: Universal screening for infant hearing impairment: necessary, beneficial, and justifiable, *Audiology Today* 6:10, 1994.
12. Norton S: Infant screening/pediatric testing with otoacoustic emissions, Richmond, Va, April 27, 1994, American Academy of Audiology.
13. Pappas DG: A study of the high-risk registry for sensorineural hearing impairment, *Head Neck Surg* 91:41, 1983.
14. Specifications for audiometers: ANSI S3.6-1969, New York, 1970, American National Standards Institute.
15. Stevens J et al: Click evoked otoacoustic emissions compared with brainstem electric response, *Arch Dis Child* 64:1105, 1989.
16. Stevens J et al: Click evoked otoacoustic emissions in neonatal screening, *Ear and Hear* 11:128, 1990.
17. Uziel A, Piron J: Evoked otoacoustic emissions from normal newborns and babies admitted to an intensive care baby unit, *Acta Otolaryngol Suppl* 482:85, 1991.
18. White KR et al: Neonatal hearing screening using evoked otoacoustic emissions: the Rhode Island hearing assessment project. In Bess FH, Hall J, editors: *Screening children for auditory function,* Nashville, Tenn, 1992, Bill Wilkerson Center Press.
19. White KR, Behrens TR, editors: The Rhode Island hearing assessment project: implications for universal newborn hearing screening, *Seminars in Hearing* 14:1, New York, 1993, Thieme.

Vision Screening

1. American Academy of Pediatrics Section on Ophthalmology Executive Committee: Proposed vision screening guidelines, *AAP News* 11:25, 1995.
2. Barker J, Barmatz H: Eye function. In Frankenburg WK, Camp BW, editors: *Pediatric screening tests,* Springfield, Ill, 1975, Charles C Thomas.
3. Campbell LR, Charney E: Factors associated with delay in diagnosis of childhood amblyopia, *Pediatrics* 87:178, 1991.
4. Hoyt CS: Photorefraction: a technique for preschool visual screening, *Arch Ophthalmol* 105:1497, 1987.
5. Wasserman RC, Croft CA, Brotherton SE: Preschool vision screening in pediatric practice: a study from the pediatric research in office settings (PROS) network, *Pediatrics* 89:834, 1992.

Sickle Cell Conditions

1. Agency for Health Care Policy and Research, Sickle Cell Disease Guideline Panel: *Sickle cell disease: screening, diagnosis, management and counseling in newborns and infants,* Pub No 93-0562, Rockville, Md, 1993, US Department of Health and Human Services.
2. Consensus Conference: Newborn screening for sickle cell disease and other hemoglobinopathies, *JAMA* 258:1205, 1987.
3. Gaston MD et al: Prophylaxis with oral penicillin in children with sickle cell anemia, *N Engl J Med* 314:1593, 1986.
4. Whitten CF, Thomas J, Nishiura EN: Sickle cell trait counseling: evaluation of counselors and counselees, *Am J Hum Genet* 33:802, 1981.

Developmental Surveillance and Intervention

1. American Academy of Pediatrics: Recommendations for preventive pediatric health care, *Pediatrics* 81:466, 1988.
2. Bailey DB et al: Reliability of an index of child characteristics, *Dev Med Child Neurol* 35:806, 1993.
3. Blasco PA: Pitalls in developmental diagnosis, *Pediatr Clin North Am* 38:1425, 1991.
4. Dobos AE, Dworkin PH, Bernstein BA: Pediatricians' approaches to developmental problems: has the gap been narrowed? *J Dev Behav Pediatr* 15:34, 1994.
5. Dworkin PH: Developmental screening—expecting the impossible? *Pediatrics* 84:619, 1989.
6. Earls F et al: Concurrent validation of a behavior problems scale for use with 3-year-olds, *J Am Acad Child Adolesc Psychiatry* 21:47, 1982.
7. First LR, Palfrey JS: The infant or young child with developmental delay, *N Engl J Med* 330:478, 1994.
8. Frankenburg WK, Chen J, Thornton SM: Common pitfalls in the evaluation of developmental screening tests, *J Pediatr* 113:1110, 1988.
9. Frankenburg WK et al: The Denver II: a major revision and restandardization of the Denver Developmental Screening Test, *Pediatrics* 89:91, 1992.
10. Glascoe FP, Altemeier WA, MacLean WE: The importance of parents' concerns about their child's development, *AJDC* 143:955, 1989.
11. Glascoe FP: Can clinical judgment detect children with speech-language problems? *Pediatrics* 87:317, 1991.
12. Glascoe FP et al: Accuracy of the Denver-II in developmental screening, *Pediatrics* 89:1221, 1992.
13. Glascoe FP, Dworkin PH: Obstacles to effective developmental surveillance: errors in clinical reasoning, *J Dev Behav Pediatr* 4:344, 349, 1993.
14. Glascoe FP, Martin ED, Humphrey S: A comparative review of developmental screening tests, *Pediatrics* 86:547, 1990.
15. Green M: A developmental approach to symptoms based on age groups, *Pediatr Clin North Am* 22:571, 1975.
16. Herzog DB, Rathbun JM: Childhood depression: developmental considerations, *Am J Dis Child* 136:115, 1982.
17. Hutchison T, Nicoll A: Developmental screening and surveillance, *Br J Hosp Med* 39:22, 1988.
18. Kravitz H, Boehm JJ: Rhythmic habit patterns in infancy: their sequence, age of onset, and frequency, *Child Dev* 42:399, 1971.
19. Levine M et al: The pediatric examination of educational readiness: validation of an extended observation procedure, *Pediatrics* 66:341, 1980.
20. Medoff-Cooper B, Carey WB, McDevitt SC: The early infancy temperament questionnaire, *J Dev Behav Pediatr* 14:230, 1993.
21. Meisels SJ: Developmental screening in early childhood: the interaction of research and social policy, *Annu Rev Public Health* 9:527, 1988.
22. Meisels SJ: Can developmental screening tests identify children who are developmentally at risk? *Pediatrics* 83:578, 1989.
23. Merritt KA et al: Screening for behavioral and emotional problems in primary care pediatrics, *J Dev Behav Pediatr* 14:340, 1993.
24. Minde K: Behavioral abnormalities commonly seen in infancy, *Can J Psychiatry* 33:741, 1988.
25. Morrison D, Mantizicopoulos P, Cart E: Preacademic screening for learning and behavior problems, *J Am Acad Child Adolesc Psychiatry* 28:101, 1985.
26. Olfson M: Commentary: diagnosing mental disorders in office-based pediatric practice, *J Dev Behav Pediatr* 13:363, 1992.
27. Simeonsson RJ: Family expectations, encounters, and needs. In Brambring H, Rauh HB, Beelman A, editors: *Intervention in early childhood: theory, evaluation, and practice,* Hawthorne, NY, 1996, Walter de Gruyter.
28. Sturner RA, Funk SG, Green JA: Simultaneous technique for acuity and readiness testing (START): further concurrent validation of an aid for developmental surveillance, *Pediatrics* 93:83, 1994.

SUGGESTED READINGS

General Considerations

Dworkin PH: Detection of behavioral, developmental, and psychosocial problems in pediatric primary care practice, *Curr Opin Pediatr* 5:531, 1993.

Frankenburg WK: Periodic screening, *Adv Pediatr* 20:149, 1973.

Meisels SJ, Provence S: *Screening assessment: guidelines for identifying young disabled and developmentally vulnerable children and their families,* Washington, DC, 1989, Zero to Three/National Center for Clinical Infant Programs.

Whitby LG: Screening for disease: definition and criteria, *Lancet* 11:819, 1974.

Recognition of Genetic-Metabolic Diseases by Clinical Diagnosis and Screening

American Academy of Pediatrics Committee on Genetics: New issues in newborn screening for phenylketonuria and congenital hypothyroidism, *Pediatrics* 69:104, 1982.

American Academy of Pediatrics Committee on Genetics: Newborn screening fact sheets, *Pediatrics* 83:449, 1989.

American Academy of Pediatrics Committee on Genetics and American Thyroid Association: Newborn screening for congenital hypothyroidism: recommended guidelines, *Pediatrics* 80:745, 1987.

American Academy of Pediatrics Committee on Nutrition: Indications for cholesterol testing in children, *Pediatrics* 83:141, 1989.

Consensus conference: Newborn screening for sickle cell disease and other hemoglobinopathies, *JAMA* 258:1205, 1987.

Holtzman NA: *Proceed with caution: predicting genetic risks in the recombinant DNA era,* Baltimore, 1989, The Johns Hopkins University Press.

Holtzman NA, Leonard CO, Farfel MR: Issues in antenatal and neonatal screening and surveillance for hereditary and congenital disorders, *Annu Rev Public Health* 2:219, 1981.

March of Dimes Birth Defects Foundation: *International directory of genetic services,* White Plains, NY, 1986, The Foundation.

National Center for Education in Maternal and Child Health: *State treatment centers for metabolic disorders,* Washington, DC, 1986, The Center.

New England Regional Genetics Group Prenatal Collaborative Study of Down Syndrome Screening: Combining maternal serum alpha-fetoprotein measurements and age to screen for Down syndrome in pregnant women under age 35, *Am J Obstet Gynecol* 160:575, 1989.

Rhoads GG et al: The safety and efficacy of chorionic villus sampling for early prenatal diagnosis of cytogenetic abnormalities, *N Engl J Med* 320:609, 1989.

Scriver CR et al: *The metabolic basis of inherited disease,* ed 6, New York, 1989, McGraw-Hill.

Screening for Anemia

Bessman JD, Gilmer PR, Gardner FH: Improved classification of anemias by MCV and RDW, *Am J Clin Pathol* 30:322, 1983.

Yip R, Johnson C, Dellman PR: Age-related changes in laboratory values used in the diagnosis of anemia and iron deficiency, *Am J Clin Nutr* 39:427, 1984.

Screening for Lead Poisoning

Binder S, Matte T: Childhood lead poisoning: the impact of prevention, *JAMA* 269:1679, 1993.

Centers for Disease Control: Preventing lead poisoning in young children, Washington, DC, 1991, US Department of Health and Human Services.

Hoekelman RA: A lead balloon, *Pediatr Ann* 21:335, 1992.

Piomelli S: Childhood lead poisoning in the '90's, *Pediatrics* 93:508, 1994.

Pirkle JL et al: The decline in blood lead levels in the United States: the National Health and Nutritional Examination Surveys (NHANES), *JAMA* 272:294, 1994.

Screening for Drugs

Campbell DE, Fleischman AR: Ethical challenges in medical care for the pregnant substance abuser, *Clin Obstet Gynecol* 35:803, 1992.

Chasnoff IJ, Landress HJ, Barrett ME: The prevalence of illicit drug or alcohol use during pregnancy and discrepancies in mandatory reporting in Pinellas County, Florida, *N Engl J Med* 322:1202, 1990.

Committee on Substance Abuse, American Academy of Pediatrics: Drug-exposed infants, *Pediatrics* 86:639, 1990.

Halstead AC et al: Timing of specimens is crucial in urine screening of drug-dependent mothers and infants, *Clin Biochem* 21:59, 1988.

Mayes LC et al: Neurobehavioral profiles of neonates exposed to cocaine prenatally, *Pediatrics* 91:778, 1993.

Osterloh JD, Lee BL: Urine drug screening in mothers and infants, *Am J Dis Child* 143:791, 1989.

Ostrea EM, Romero A, Yee H: Adaptation of the meconium drug test for mass screening, *J Pediatric* 122:152, 1993.

Vega WA et al: Prevalence and magnitude of perinatal substance exposures in California, *N Engl J Med* 329:850, 1993.

Volpe JJ: Effect of cocaine use on the fetus, *N Engl J Med* 327:399, 1992.

Use of Urinalysis and the Urine Culture in Screening

Bee DE, James GP, Paul KL: Hemoglobinuria and hematuria: accuracy and precision of laboratory diagnosis, *Clin Chem* 25:1696, 1979.

Corman LI et al: Simplified urinary microscopy to detect significant bacteriuria, *Pediatrics* 70:133, 1982.

Glassock RJ: Postural proteinuria: no cause for concern, *N Engl J Med* 305:639, 1981.

Hermansen MC, Blodgett FM: Prospective evaluation of routine admission urinalyses, *Am J Dis Child* 135:126, 1981.

Jaffe RM et al: Inhibition by ascorbic acid (vitamin C) of chemical detection of blood in urine, *Am J Clin Pathol* 72:468, 1979.

Jodal U: The natural history of bacteriuria in childhood, *Infect Dis Clin North Am* 1:713, 1987.

Kiel DP, Moskowitz MA: The urinalysis: a critical approach, *Med Clin North Am* 71:607, 1987.

Norman ME: An office approach to hematuria and proteinuria, *Pediatr Clin North Am* 34:545, 1987.

Rytand DA, Spreiter S: Prognosis in postural (orthostatic) proteinuria, *N Engl J Med* 305:618, 1981.

Vehaskari VM, Rapola J: Isolated proteinuria: analysis of a school-age population, *J Pediatr* 101:661, 1982.

Vision Screening

American Academy of Ophthalmology: *Comprehensive pediatric eye evaluation: preferred practice pattern,* San Francisco, Calif, 1992, The Academy.

Trobe JD: *The physician's guide to eye care,* San Francisco, Calif, 1993, American Academy of Ophthalmology.

Developmental Surveillance and Intervention

Carey WB: Clinical use of temperament data in pediatrics, *J Dev Behav Pediatr* 6:137, 1985.

Drillien CM, Pickering RM, Drummond MB: Predictive value of screening for different areas of development, *Dev Med Child Neurol* 30:294, 1988.

Frankenburg WK, Camp BW, editors: *Pediatric screening tests,* Springfield, Ill, 1975, Charles C Thomas.

Kaplan BJ et al: Physical signs and symptoms in preschool-age hyperactive and normal children, *J Dev Behav Pediatr* 8:305, 1987.

Meisels SJ, Provence S: *Screening and assessment: guidelines for identifying young disabled and developmentally vulnerable children and their families,* Washington, DC, 1989, National Center for Clinical Infant Programs.

21 Counseling Families on a Healthy Life-style

R. Joseph Jopling

A "healthy life-style" is the product of numerous decisions a person must make about health-related fitness, diet, and psychosocial issues that allow the individual to maximize his or her genetic potential for a healthy life.[14]

Many people have misguided notions about these components. Health-related fitness, for example, is related neither to athletic ability nor to physical appearance. The decline in health-related fitness parameters among children, adolescents, and young adults in the United States is well documented,[36] and the relationship between those parameters and many preventable diseases of adulthood has been strongly suggested if not proved.* The problem is pervasive and has seemed refractory to change. This chapter suggests how primary care physicians can discuss the problem with their patients and then help them devise a healthy life-style plan for the whole family.

HEALTHY LIFE-STYLE PARAMETERS AND PREVENTABLE DISEASES

Cardiovascular diseases (myocardial infarction, hypertension, and stroke), obesity, and some types of cancer (e.g., lung and colon cancer) not only are major sources of morbidity and mortality, also are thought to be preventable, at least in part, by life-style changes.[27,31] A life-style is learned in childhood and tends to become more difficult to change as the individual grows older. Therefore the younger the patient, the more easily life-style changes can be made, and the more likely it is that those changes will help prevent, or at least reduce, the effects of the above-mentioned diseases later in life. It should be easier and more cost effective to prevent inherently active children from becoming sedentary adults than to try to change this habit once adulthood has been reached.[31]

Most experts agree that the decline in healthy life-style parameters correlates directly with an increase in the risk factors for cardiovascular disease such as obesity, hypertension, high serum cholesterol, smoking, psychosocial stress, and physical inactivity. Sometimes the tale is best told in numbers.

Obesity. Sixty percent of adults are overweight, and more than 25% are obese (more than 20 pounds overweight); 12% of prepubertal children and 16% of adolescents are considered overweight—worse yet, the number of overweight children is increasing.[10]

Hypertension. Ten percent of adults and 5% of children are considered hypertensive. This statistic, coupled with those for obesity, is particularly sobering because the risk of dying of cardiovascular disease appears to be greater in the families of children who are persistently obese, especially those with persistent high blood pressure.[4]

High serum cholesterol. Ten percent to 20% of adults have high serum cholesterol levels; however, this is not just a disease of adulthood—the problem begins in childhood. Atherosclerotic fatty streaks have been found in children as young as age 3. By age 22, anywhere from 45% to 77% of individuals may have evidence of atherosclerosis.

Smoking and psychosocial stress. Most cigarette smokers begin smoking before age 20, and psychosocial stress is more intense and more prevalent at earlier ages than ever before.

Physical inactivity. An epidemiological study reported in 1987 by the Centers for Disease Control and Prevention (CDC) has shown that physical inactivity is as strong a risk factor for coronary heart disease as are the traditional risk factors (smoking, hypertension, and high serum cholesterol).[28] Even more important, physical inactivity was shown to be three to six times more prevalent than any other risk factor. Only 20% of adults exercise adequately, and 60% do not exercise at all. Only 36% of schoolchildren have daily physical education classes. The 1984 National Children and Youth Fitness Study found that only 66% of children and adolescents 10 to 17 years of age were participating in physical activity at the recommended level.*

Not surprisingly, the U.S. Public Health Service's 1990 goal of having more than 90% of schoolchildren participating in physical activity at the recommended level was not met, and budgetary constraints in school systems across the country pose a definite risk of a decline in participation. Even when offered, physical education classes often emphasize team sports rather than individual lifelong activities (i.e., aerobic activities that can be done alone, such as walking, jogging, swimming, or cycling).

And, aggravating the inactivity problem, children in the United States average 25 hours a week watching television, often while munching some kind of less than healthy snack food.

Physical inactivity is not a recently identified issue. As early as the 1940s, Kraus and Hirschland[18] recognized a health-related physical fitness problem. When their findings for American children were compared with those for European children, American children were found to be signifi-

*References 6, 19, 21, 22, 26, 42.

*To meet the recommended level, the children had to be exercising three or more times a week for 20 minutes or longer per session, at an activity that was likely to be pursued as an adult, that used 60% or more of cardiorespiratory capacity, and that involved large muscle groups in dynamic contraction (e.g., walking, swimming, or cycling).

COMPONENTS OF A HEALTHY LIFE-STYLE

Cardiorespiratory endurance

Cardiorespiratory endurance is achieved by performing any one of a number of aerobic exercises while maintaining the heart rate at 60% to 80% of a calculated maximum for at least 30 minutes at a time, at least three times a week, for at least 6 consecutive months.

Muscle strength and endurance

Leg muscle strength enables a person to perform aerobic exercise. Abdominal muscle strength aids in proper breathing technique and helps protect the lower back. Upper body strength is important to overall muscle balance and aids in many everyday activities.

Flexibility

Flexibility helps prevent musculoskeletal injuries and makes a person feel more spry. Without warm-up and cool-down stretching periods, an exercise program can lead to loss of flexibility.

Body composition

Baseline and follow-up measurement of body composition (ratio of fat to muscle) is one of the best methods of tracking progress in health-related fitness. Using only body weight or the height to weight ratio can be misleading in assessing the fitness level.

Healthy diet

A diet high in carbohydrates, low to moderate in protein, low in fat, and moderate in total calories is essential to any fitness program.

Stress management/communication skills

In today's fast-paced world, techniques for managing stress and improved communication skills have become increasingly important components of good health.

Modified from Jopling RJ: *Pediatr Rev* 10:141, 1988.

cantly less fit than their European counterparts. In an effort to change that trend, the President's Council on Youth Fitness was formed, known today as the President's Council on Physical Fitness and Sports. In 1988 Kraus reported that fewer than half of the children who took the council's fitness test passed. Only 60% of boys 6 to 12 years of age and 30% of girls 6 to 17 years of age could do more than one chin-up; similarly, only 64% of boys and 50% of girls ages 6 to 12 could run or walk a mile in less than 10 minutes.[17]

As mentioned previously, almost all experts agree that the best way to resolve these fitness problems is to change people's life-styles. One of the best ways to accomplish this is to develop a program for the whole family. This program should focus on cardiorespiratory endurance, strength and endurance of the large muscle groups, flexibility, body composition, a healthy diet, and development of stress management techniques and improved communication skills (see the box above).

CARDIORESPIRATORY ENDURANCE

Cardiorespiratory endurance is best achieved by performing aerobic exercise for at least 30 minutes per session while maintaining the heart rate at 60% to 80% of a calculated maximum. The minimum exercise time thought to be needed for an aerobic effect initially was 15 minutes, and then 20 minutes; now it is 30 minutes. An inactive person should start at whatever level and duration of continuous activity he or she can tolerate safely and gradually work up to 30 minutes.

In the adult literature, whenever a positive relationship is found between exercise and a decline in serum cholesterol, the correlate seems to be that the more vigorous and sustained the exercise, the greater its effect.[10] This implies that "more is better" with regard to intensity, but as with duration, the recommendations for intensity level have changed. Initially, exercise physiologists proposed that a person had to reach a target heart rate to achieve an aerobic exercise threshold that led to improved aerobic fitness. Most exercise physiologists and cardiologists now believe that unless an individual already is relatively fit, it is a mistake even to discuss target heart rates. Initially, it is much more important to stress becoming physically active at any level and then begin to increase that level gradually.[1] Borg[2] has proposed a "perceived exertion" scale as an adequate measure of heart rate, a concept that has been validated more than once.[7] A common rule of thumb for finding the proper intensity is to exercise at least enough to perspire while maintaining the ability to carry on a conversation.

For those ready to use the heart rate as a guide, the recommendation is that a person who has been relatively active should aim for a target rate of about 60% when starting an aerobic exercise program. It is unwise at any time to exceed 80% of the maximum heart rate. People who are already active and who want more specific information should consult published guidelines for heart rates during exercise (Table 21-1). It cannot be over emphasized that *these numbers are based on suggestions for training athletes and should not be thought of as hard-and-fast rules.* Gradually warming up before exercising and cooling down afterward help to ensure a safe workout by allowing muscles, joints, and the cardiovascular system to adapt to the changes of exercise. The optimal times to stretch, and thereby to help maintain flexibility, are just after the warm-up and cool-down periods.

When talking about intensity, the pediatrician should discuss overuse syndromes and well-meaning adults who put undue pressure on children. Exercising to the point of pain should be discouraged because it eventually leads to injury and can exacerbate a previous chronic injury. It is important to emphasize that "slow but sure" most often achieves the goal when trying to make long-term changes. Before starting any type of exercise program, adults over age 40 or those with a family history of cardiovascular disease should see their physician.

Exercising at least three times a week helps to maintain an aerobic fitness level; exercising five times a week usually ensures a change in a person's aerobic fitness level. These training guidelines are well established for adults, and although there is less documentation for children, they have been applied to children as young as age 6. Most people need a commitment of at least 6 months to any exercise program (and some more than 12 months) to see any significant changes in the parameters of their health-related fitness. The reverse also is true in that the positive changes gained from physical activity are lost if the activity is not maintained. Some of the benefits and risks of physical activity are presented in Table 21-2.

Numerous activities can qualify as aerobic (see the box on p. 251). Brisk walking deserves special mention because it is an aerobic activity that can be done by almost everyone right from the beginning of any fitness program. Few exercises enable a family to exercise as a unit and at the same time allow all of the members to achieve an aerobic intensity level, but walking at a brisk pace usually can be done aerobically at the same time by all, or at least by most, family members. It can be done around the neighborhood for convenience or as a hike for variation. If inclement weather is a problem, one can walk inside a shopping mall or a gym.

Jump ropes, stationary bicycles, cross-country ski machines, and rowing machines are a reasonable investment to ensure a family access to aerobic exercise day or night year round. With a little insistence, one of these activities could replace snacking as the activity that accompanies TV viewing most frequently.

LARGE MUSCLE STRENGTH AND ENDURANCE

Large muscle strength and endurance are related to aerobic exercise in two ways: large muscle groups usually are the ones used in aerobic activities, and repetition of the large muscle relaxation-contraction cycle for a sufficient length of time increases the mitochondrial mass of the muscle tissue and thus increases the amount of aerobic enzymes per unit of tissue mass. Muscle contraction tends to occlude local circulation when the muscle is contracting at greater than 30% of its maximum capacity. As muscles become stronger, they can perform more work before interfering with local circulation and therefore stay aerobic longer whether performing intense exercise or everyday activities.

Abdominal muscles help in proper breathing and protect the lower back muscles. The safest way to strengthen the abdominal muscles is to increase gradually the number of modified sit-ups one can do. Modified sit-ups are done with the knees flexed and the feet on the floor or with the lower legs resting on the seat of a chair. The lumbar spine is kept in contact with the floor during the sit-up (Fig. 21-1).

Upper body strength also is important because it is helpful in everyday activities and balances the person's overall fitness. Push-ups, modified push-ups, pull-ups, or flexed arm hangs are easy ways to improve upper body strength (Fig. 21-1). If free weights or weight machines are used to strengthen muscles, relatively low weights and a high number of repetitions (20 or more) are recommended for health-

Table 21-1 Suggested Training Heart Rates*

	Heart rate (beats/min)		
Age (yr)	Maximum	80%	60%
5-9	220	176	132
10	210	168	126
11	209	167	125
12	208	166	125
13	207	165	124
14	206	165	123
15	205	164	123
16	204	163	122
17	203	162	122
18	202	162	121
19	201	161	121
20	200	160	120
22	198	158	118
24	196	157	117
26	194	155	116
28	192	154	115
30	190	152	114
32	189	151	113
34	187	150	112
36	186	149	111
38	184	147	110
40	182	146	109
45	179	143	107
50	175	140	105
55	171	137	102
60	160	128	96
65	150	120	90

From Jopling RJ: *Pediatr Rev* 10:141, 1988.

*These numbers are taken from a variety of sources and are suggested guidelines initially developed for training athletes. Individuals will vary. If the target heart rate seems too hard to maintain, a lower one should be accepted; conversely, if the target heart rate does not seem high enough to produce a sweat, the individual should work harder.

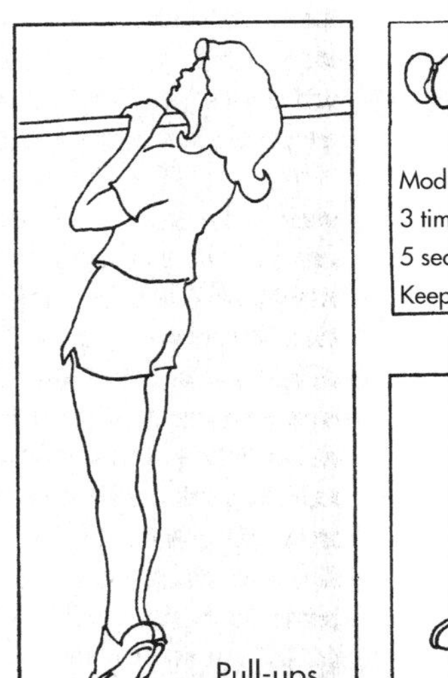

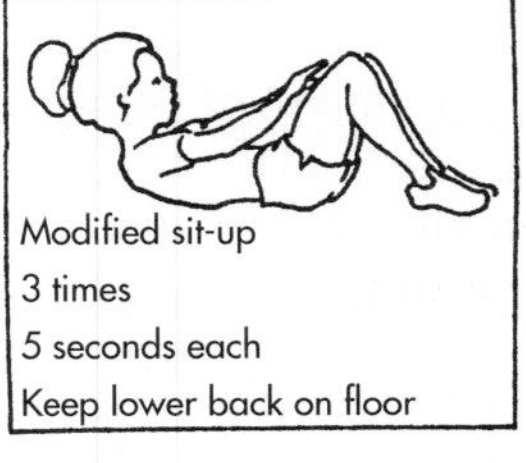

Modified sit-up
3 times
5 seconds each
Keep lower back on floor

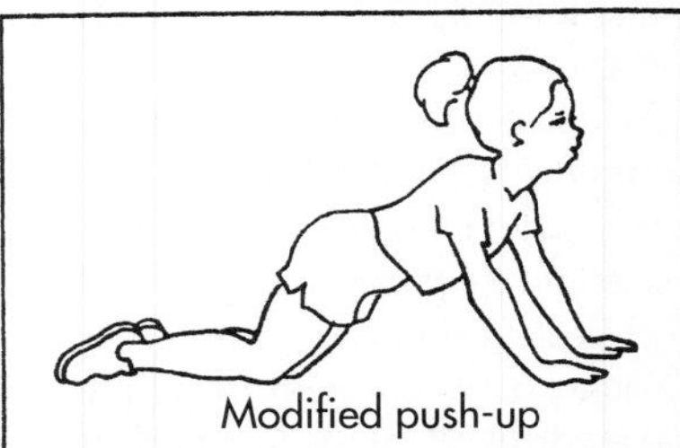

FIG. 21-1 Suggested exercises to increase muscular strength. (From "Youth Fitness," an educational handout from Ross Laboratories.)

related fitness, since this regimen will develop muscle endurance strength rather than muscle bulk.

FLEXIBILITY

Flexibility helps prevent musculoskeletal injuries and makes a person feel more spry. Stretching at the end of the warm-up period can help prevent injury during exercise; stretching at the end of the cool-down period can help prevent muscles from tightening after exercise, which reduces flexibility and increases muscle soreness.

Static stretching involves stretching a muscle group to the point where a sense of tightness first is felt, holding the stretch for 20 to 30 seconds, and then releasing the stretch. This is repeated several times for each muscle group being stretched. Ballistic stretching, which involves bouncing during the stretch, can be dangerous because it can lead to muscle or tendon damage.

The book *Stretching* by Bob Anderson (Shelter Publications, Bolinas, California) is an excellent resource for information about stretching. Its many illustrations of the techniques for everyday stretches and sports-specific stretches can be referred to for patient education. Figure 21-2 shows some examples of everyday stretches.

BODY COMPOSITION

Before any health-related fitness program is started, the percentage of body fat should be measured or the body mass index (BMI) calculated, and these values should be rechecked regularly to help assess progress. Determining body composition is a more accurate reflection of health-related fitness

Table 21-2 Benefits and Risks of Physical Activity

System and benefit	Surety rating*	Risk	Surety rating
Cardiovascular			
Blood pressure	2+	Cardiac arrest	2+
Improved serum lipid profile	1+		
Smoking cessation/prevention	0+		
Weight control	2+		
Independent effect	2+		
Psychological			
Improved affect	1+	Exercise addiction	1+
Increased self-esteem	2+		
Positive personality change	0		
Improved cognition	0		
Musculoskeletal: Prevention of postmenopausal bone loss	2+	Amenorrhea/bone loss	2+
		Trauma	2+
Central nervous system: Improved sleep	0		
Endocrine: Decreased risk of type II diabetes	0	Decreased libido	0
Gastrointestinal tract: Increased colonic motility	0	Diarrhea	1+

From Phelps JR: *West J Med* 146:200, 1987.

*The surety rating is derived from a review of the literature and is a subjective judgment of Dr. Phelps. The ratings indicate: *0*, the current literature presents mixed data claiming benefit or risk; *1+*, most but not all data in the literature support the claim; *2+*, data in the current literature establish the benefit or risk.

SUGGESTIONS FOR FITNESS ACTIVITIES*

- Brisk walking
- Cycling
- Swimming
- Aerobic exercise class
- Dancing
- Basketball
- Tumbling
- Skating
- Playground activities
- Cross-country skiing
- Racquet sports
- Jogging
- Hiking
- Soccer
- Jumping rope
- Strength training
- Volleyball
- Stretching
- Martial arts
- Tag games
- Other ______________________

____

NOTE: Stretch before and after every activity. For a more balanced fitness program, include activities for stomach muscles (modified sit-ups) and upper body muscles (push-ups/pull-ups).

From the Governor's Family FUN Award Program, Utah Governor's Council on Health and Physical Fitness, Salt Lake City, Utah.

*Minimum of 30 minutes daily.

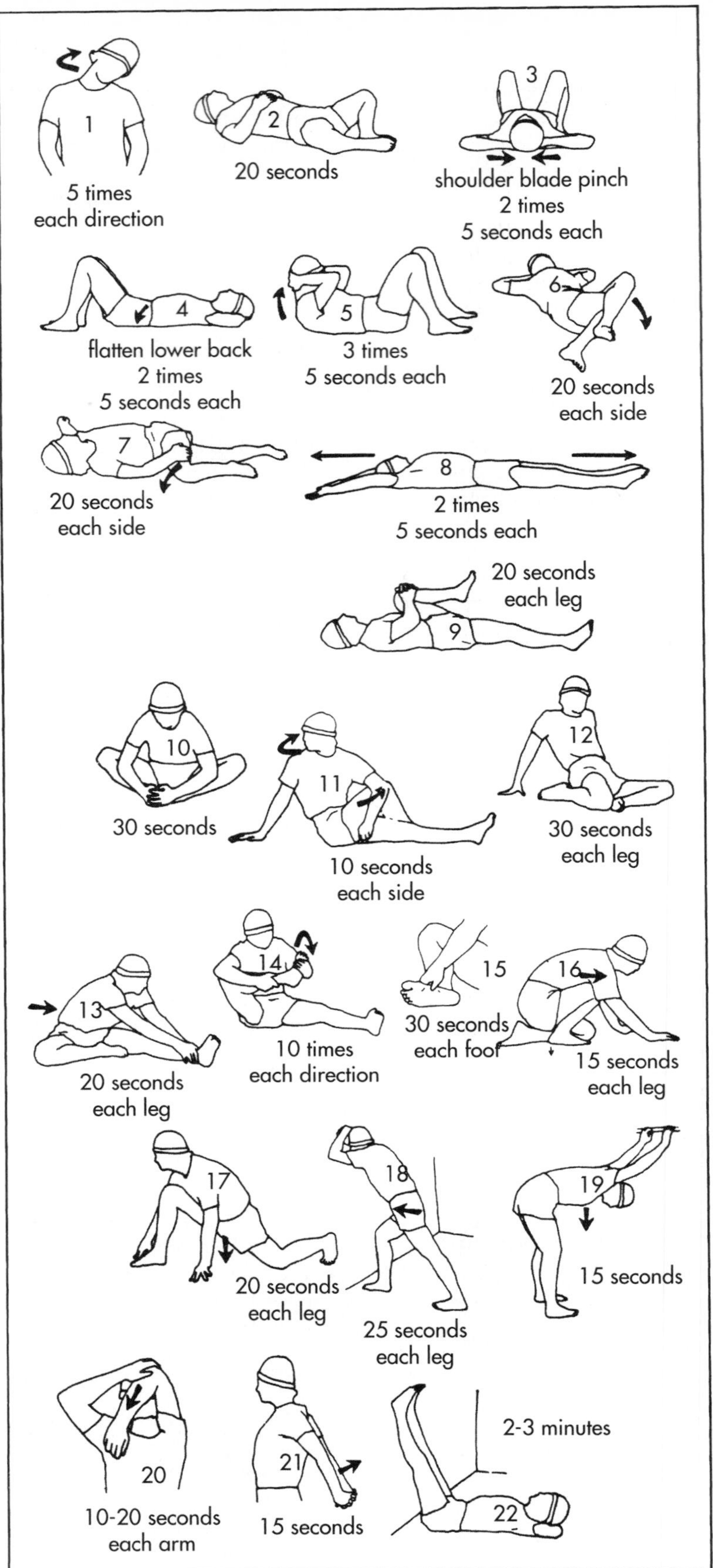

FIG. 21-2 Everyday stretches—approximately 10 to 15 minutes. These stretches should be done every day to fine-tune the muscles. This is a general routine that emphasizes stretching and relaxing the muscles more frequently used during normal day-to-day activities. In simple tasks of everyday living, the body often is used in strained or awkward ways, creating stress and tension. A kind of muscular rigor mortis sets in. Setting aside 10 to 15 minutes every day for stretching will offset this accumulated tension so that the body can be used with greater ease.

(From Anderson B: *Stretching*, Bolinas, Calif, 1980, Shelter Publications [Random House].)

than is using weight or weight to height percentile comparisons. The weight and height percentile comparisons of growth charts do not take body habitus into consideration. A muscular or large-framed person with a low percentage of body fat may have a weight percentile greater than his height percentile.

When first starting a fitness program, a person actually may gain weight, although the percentage of body fat will be the same or even lower. This phenomenon is explained by the fact that muscle is denser than fat; therefore, as a person starts to exercise, muscle may be added faster than fat is lost, which would make for an overall weight gain. This

Table 21-3 Percentile Values of Body Mass Index*

Age (yr)	Percentile 5	10	25	50	75	90	95
Males							
1	14.6	15.4	16.1	17.2	18.5	19.4	19.9
2	14.4	15.0	15.7	16.5	17.6	18.4	19.0
3	14.0	14.6	15.3	16.0	17.0	17.8	18.4
4	13.8	14.4	15.0	15.8	16.6	17.5	18.1
5	13.7	14.2	14.9	15.5	16.3	17.3	18.0
6	13.6	14.0	14.7	15.4	16.3	17.4	18.1
7	13.6	14.0	14.7	15.5	16.5	17.7	18.9
8	13.7	14.1	14.9	15.7	17.0	18.4	19.7
9	14.0	14.3	15.1	16.0	17.6	19.3	20.9
10	14.2	14.6	15.5	16.6	18.4	20.3	22.2
11	14.6	15.0	16.0	17.2	19.2	21.3	23.5
12	15.1	15.5	16.5	17.8	20.0	22.3	24.8
13	15.6	16.0	17.1	18.4	20.8	23.3	25.8
14	16.1	16.6	17.7	19.1	21.5	24.4	26.8
15	16.6	17.1	18.4	19.7	22.2	25.4	27.7
16	17.2	17.8	19.1	20.5	22.9	26.1	28.4
17	17.7	18.4	19.7	21.2	23.4	27.0	29.0
18	18.3	19.1	20.3	21.9	24.0	27.7	29.7
19	19.0	19.7	21.1	22.5	24.4	28.3	30.1
Females							
1	14.7	15.0	15.8	16.6	17.6	18.6	19.3
2	14.3	14.7	15.3	16.0	17.1	18.0	18.7
3	13.9	14.4	14.9	15.6	16.7	17.6	18.3
4	13.6	14.1	14.7	15.4	16.5	17.5	18.2
5	13.5	14.0	14.6	15.3	16.3	17.5	18.3
6	13.3	13.9	14.6	15.3	16.4	17.7	18.8
7	13.4	14.0	14.7	15.5	16.7	18.5	19.7
8	13.6	14.2	15.0	16.0	17.2	19.4	21.0
9	14.0	14.5	15.5	16.6	18.0	20.8	22.7
10	14.3	15.0	15.9	17.1	19.0	21.8	24.2
11	14.6	15.3	16.2	17.8	19.8	23.0	25.7
12	15.0	15.6	16.7	18.3	20.4	23.7	26.8
13	15.4	16.0	17.1	18.9	21.2	24.7	27.9
14	15.7	16.4	17.5	19.4	21.8	25.3	28.6
15	16.1	16.8	18.0	19.9	22.4	26.0	29.4
16	16.4	17.1	18.4	20.2	22.8	26.5	30.0
17	16.9	17.6	18.9	20.7	23.3	27.1	30.5
18	17.2	18.0	19.4	21.1	23.7	27.4	31.0
19	17.5	18.4	19.8	21.4	24.0	27.7	31.3

*National Health and Nutrition Examination Survey, 1971 to 1974 (NHANES I).

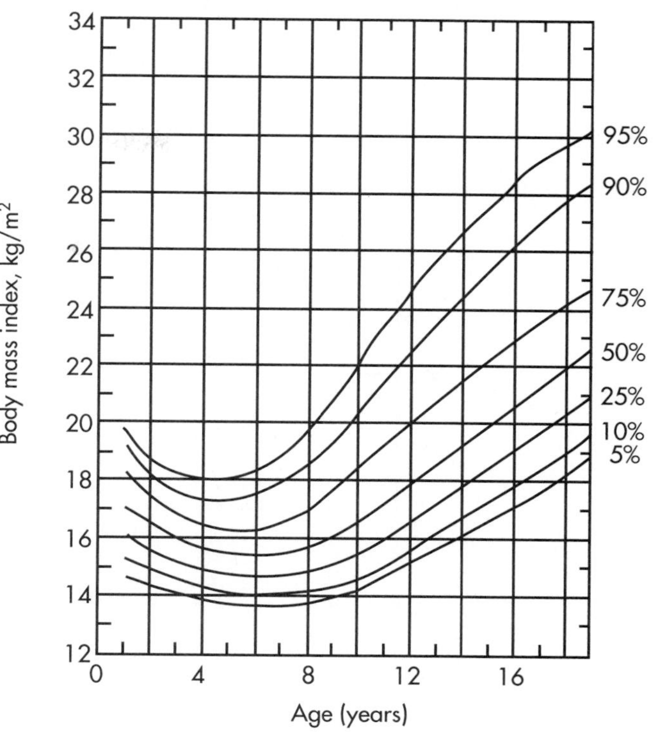

FIG. 21-3 Body mass index for white males ages 1 to 19 years. The percentiles were computed using data from the First National Health and Nutrition Examination Survey, 1971 to 1974.
(From Hammer LD et al: *Am J Dis Child* 145:260, 1991.)

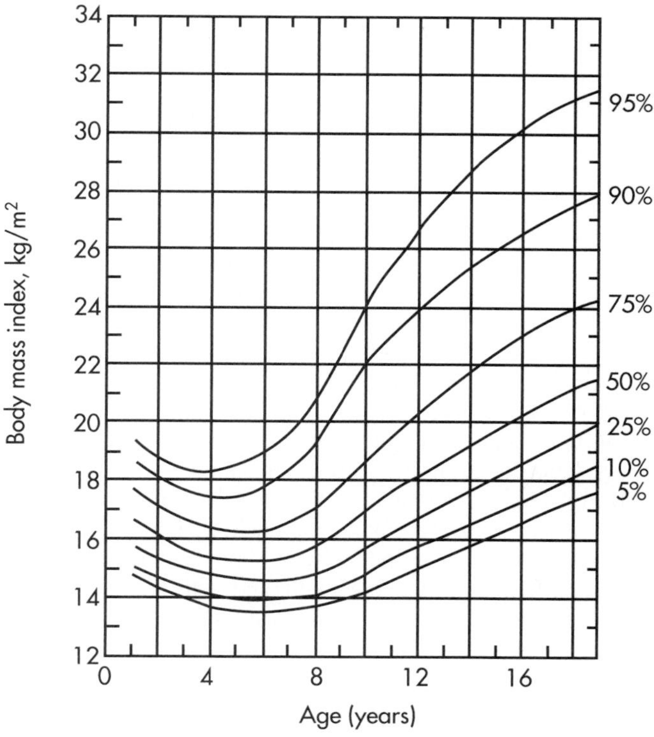

FIG. 21-4 Body mass index for white females ages 1 to 19 years. The percentiles were computed using data from the First National Health and Nutrition Examination Survey, 1971 to 1974.
(From Hammer LD et al: *Am J Dis Child* 145:260, 1991.)

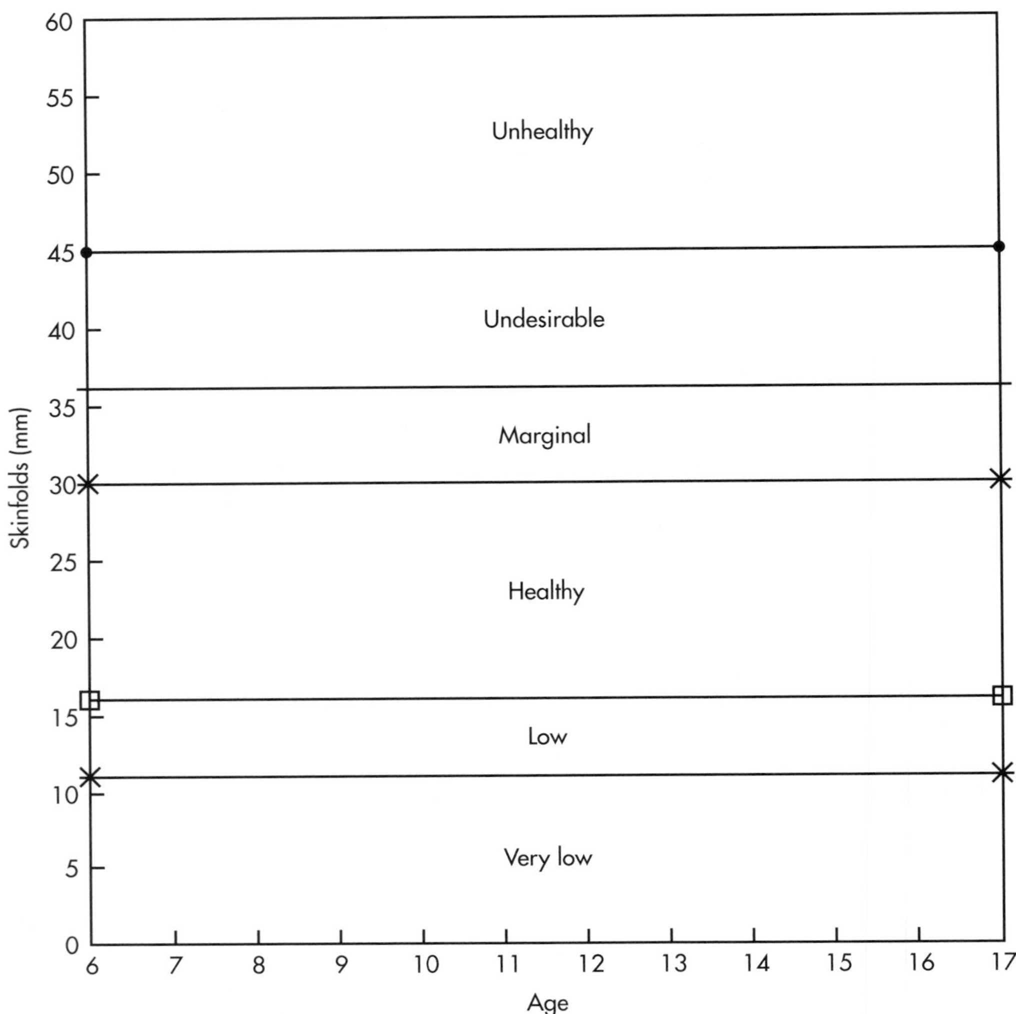

FIG. 21-5 Skinfold measurement ranges for the triceps and calf combination.

(Adapted from Lohman TG: Appraising and monitoring body composition. In Eisenman PA, Johnson SC, Benson JE, editors: ***Coaches' guide to nutrition and weight control,*** Salt Lake City, 1990, Human Kinetics Publishers.)

Continued.

seems to be especially true for individuals who were not very active before starting an exercise program.

Hydrostatic (underwater) weighing is considered the most accurate way to measure body composition; it has a 1% to 3% error factor. It also is the most inconvenient method. Skin calipers are much more convenient and with practice can approach a 3% to 5% error factor. Methods using laser techniques are becoming more reliable and in time may become the most commonly used method of measuring the percentage of body fat. Whatever method is used, the final numbers are most helpful when comparing a person's progress over time, much as growth charts or blood pressure charts are used.

The body mass index is based on the calculation of kilograms per meter squared.[11] This number is plotted on a percentile graph based on the person's age and sex and compared with figures for others of the same age and sex (Table 21-3, Figs. 21-3 and 21-4). The body mass index is recommended when hydrostatic or skin caliper methods are not available for the determination of the percentage of body fat.

When skin calipers are used, the more skin sites measured, the more accurate the final determination of percentage of body fat. The triceps and calf are the sites most often used by school systems when mass testing is done and for that reason should be used if only two sites are selected. The proper techniques for using skin calipers can be found in many references. Fig. 21-5 presents a graph of suggested ranges for the body fat percentage of the triceps and calf sites. Percentile graphs for age and sex for triceps and subscapular measurements were determined a number of years ago in England.[40]

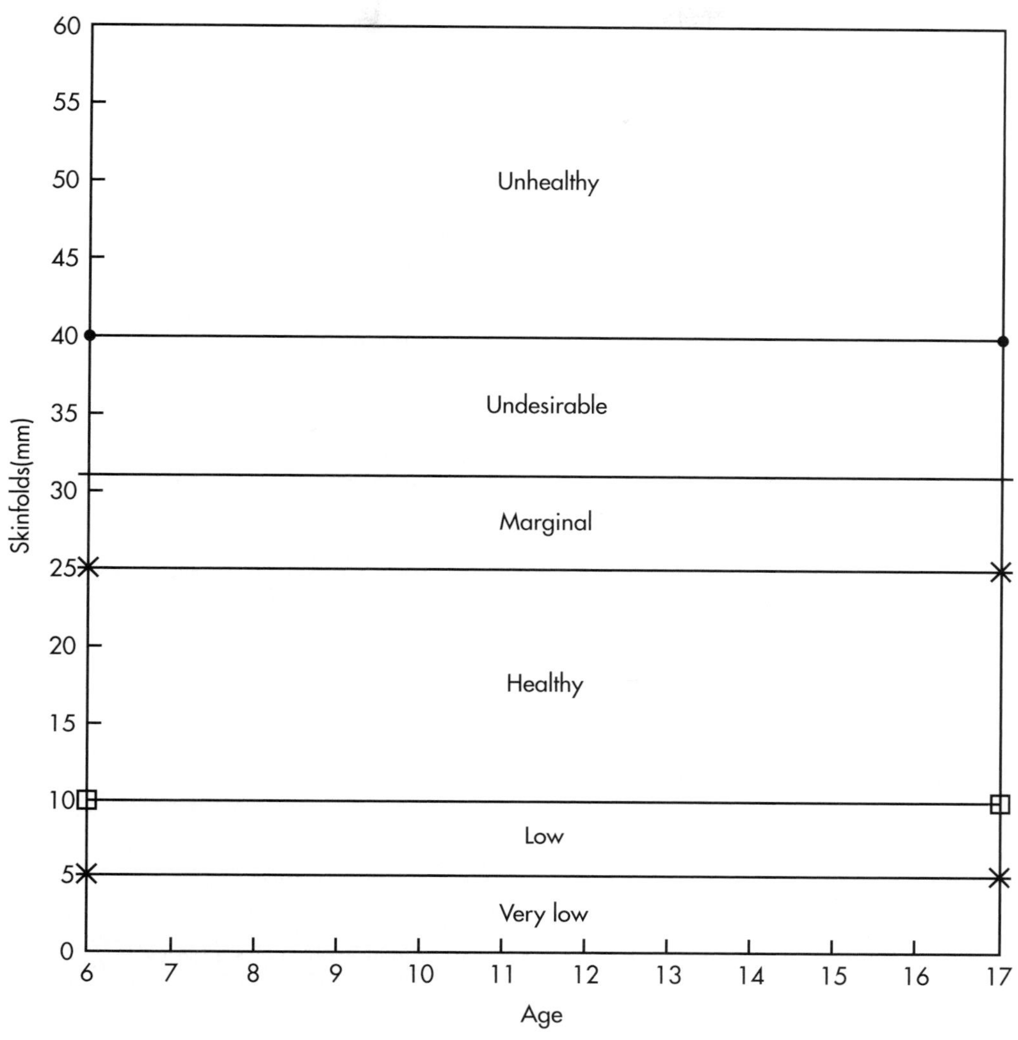

FIG. 21-5—cont'd

HEALTHY DIET

Sustaining weight loss and improving health-related fitness parameters are difficult if not impossible without making use of a proper diet as well as routine exercise.[3] It would seem logical that to lose weight, a person must make sure that the total caloric intake for 1 day is less than the total caloric output for that day. However, it must be emphasized that crash diets and ketogenic diets are essentially starvation diets and are impossible to sustain. This usually is attempted repeatedly and leads to loss of muscle tissue while sparing fat tissue.

Proper dietary recommendations are fairly simple. For growing children and adolescents, a safe and practical starting point is to worry less about total calories and more about total dietary fat. Table 21-4 shows the total number of calories recommended per day in relation to age in years. It has been shown that even when the total number of calories remains unchanged, eating the largest meal of the day at breakfast instead of at night helps people lose weight. Other dietary recommendations include increasing dietary fiber, reducing the use of salt in the diet, and increasing daily water intake. Some specific suggestions for improving dietary habits are listed in the box on p. 256 and in Figure 21-6.

Carbohydrates should be the main source of calories. Current recommendations for carbohydrates in relation to total daily calories range from 55% to 70%. Complex carbohydrates, such as those found in fruits, vegetables, legumes, and whole grain cereals, are preferable to the refined carbohydrates found in candy.

For adults and for children over age 2, it is recommended that no more than 30% of total daily calories come from fats, with vegetable fats (except palm oil and coconut oil) recommended over animal fats.[20] How much fat is appropriate for

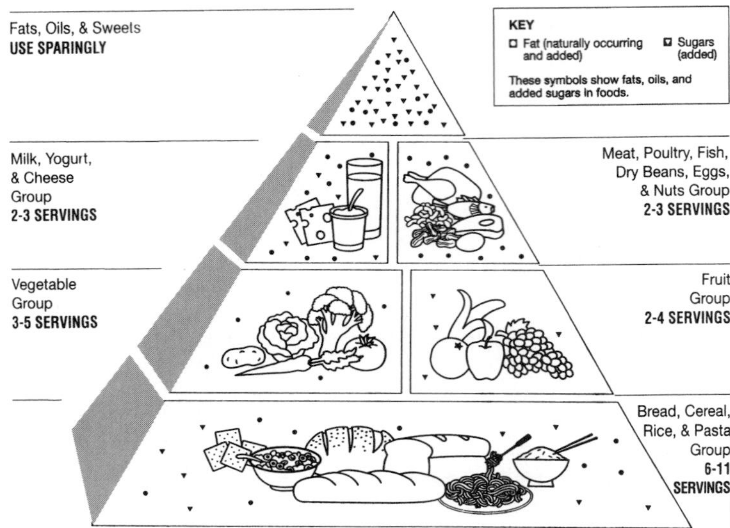

FIG. 21-6 The U.S. Department of Agriculture's Food Guide Pyramid emphasizes foods from the five food groups shown in the three lower sections of the pyramid. Each of these food groups provides some, but not all, of the nutrients a body needs. Foods in one group cannot replace those in another, and no one food group is more important than any other.

Table 21-4 Recommended Total Daily Calories* (Moderate Activity Level)

Group and age (yr)	Wt (kg [lb])	Height (cm [in])	Energy needs (kcal [range])
Children			
1-3	13 (29)	90 (35)	1300 (900-1800)
4-6	20 (44)	112 (44)	1800 (1300-2300)
7-10	28 (62)	132 (52)	2000 (1650-3300)
Males			
11-14	45 (99)	157 (62)	2500 (2000-3700)
15-18	66 (145)	176 (69)	3000 (2100-3900)
19-22	70 (154)	177 (70)	2900 (2500-3300)
23-50	70 (154)	178 (70)	2900 (2300-3100)
51-75	70 (154)	178 (70)	2300 (2000-2800)
76+	70 (154)	178 (70)	2050 (1650-2450)
Females			
11-14	46 (101)	157 (62)	2200 (1500-3000)
15-18	55 (120)	163 (64)	2200 (1200-3000)
19-22	55 (120)	163 (64)	2200 (1700-2500)
23-50	55 (120)	163 (64)	2200 (1600-2400)
51-75	55 (120)	163 (64)	1900 (1400-2200)
76+	55 (120)	163 (64)	1600 (1200-2000)

Modified from the Food and Nutrition Board: *Recommended Dietary Allowances,* ed 10, Washington, DC, 1989, National Academy of Sciences, National Research Council.

*These recommendations may vary significantly up or down for specific sports and for very active children and adolescents.

the diet of a child under 2 years of age is still controversial. The American Academy of Pediatrics currently recommends 30% to 40% to ensure adequate fat for myelination of the nervous system.[26] Although most dietary recommendations start after age 5, some experts believe that age 2 is an appropriate time to begin to expand children's taste experience to lower fat foods. When fat is removed from the diet, energy levels fall; therefore moderation in fat reduction is important for children. If any effort is made to reduce fat in the diet of a preschooler, it would be wise to limit the change to switching to 2% milk from whole milk. School-age children should drink skim milk, and both age groups would do well to be given low-fat luncheon meats.[34] (For a detailed review of the role of dietary cholesterol in cardiovascular disease, refer to Kwiterovich.[19])

SUGGESTIONS FOR PRACTICING GOOD NUTRITION

Develop a weekly meal plan
Eat balanced meals from the four food groups
Bake, boil, or broil rather than fry
Reduce sugar intake
Eat fruit for a snack
Use high-fiber cereals, grains, and breads
Use low-fat dairy products
Eat more chicken and fish
Eat low-fat meals
Cut use of butter and gravies in half
Don't add salt to food
Don't add sugar to food
Eat more raw and fresh fruits and vegetables
Drink more water
Place a copy of the Food Guide Pyramid on the refrigerator door for visual reinforcement of good nutrition

Modified from the Governor's Family FUN Award Program, Utah Governor's Council on Health and Physical Fitness, Salt Lake City, Utah.

Protein should make up the remaining 15% to 20% of the total daily caloric intake. Fish and poultry, because they have a lower percentage of fat than many cuts of beef and pork, are considered safer from a cardiovascular standpoint.

A new concept in understanding and following proper nutrition has been presented in the books *Nutripoints* (Vartabedian and Matthews) and *The New American Diet* (Conners and Conners). These are two excellent books for families seeking a more extensive reference on diet (see Suggested Readings). Recommending the counsel of a registered dietician is important in some cases such as familial hyperlipidemia.

In 1991 the Report of the Expert Panel on Blood Cholesterol Levels in Children and Adolescents[26] stated that: (1) high levels of serum total cholesterol, low-density lipoprotein (LDL) cholesterol, and very-low-density lipoprotein (VLDL) cholesterol, and low levels of high-density lipoprotein (HDL) cholesterol are linked to the extent of early atherosclerotic lesions in adolescents and young adults; (2) children and adolescents who have an elevated serum cholesterol, particularly LDL cholesterol, often come from families with a high incidence of coronary heart disease among adult members; (3) high blood cholesterol aggregates in families as a result of shared environments and genetic factors; and (4) children and adolescents who have high cholesterol levels are more likely than the general population to have high levels as adults. The panel has recommended a strategy to lower blood cholesterol levels in children over age 2 and adolescents by using a population approach coupled with an individual approach.

The population approach attempts to effect a change in the entire population of the country. It includes the general recommendation that the American diet be well balanced, chosen from a variety of foods, and adequate in total calories to support growth and development (see Fig. 21-6 for the pyramid concept of proportions of the different food groups). It also includes the specific recommendations that saturated fatty acids be less than 10% of total calories, that total fat be less than 30% of total calories, and that total cholesterol be less than 300 mg/day. The population approach is meant to be a cooperative effort among parents, health professionals, schools, government, the food industry, and the mass media.

The individualized approach is an effort to identify and treat children and adolescents who are at greatest risk of having high serum cholesterol as an adult and at subsequent risk of coronary heart disease. The panel recommends using a family history of high serum cholesterol as the basis for obtaining a serum cholesterol value for people under age 20. Specifically, the panel suggests screening of children and adolescents whose parents or grandparents, at age 55 or younger, underwent diagnostic coronary arteriography and were found to have atherosclerosis. The panel also suggests screening a child or adolescent if (1) the parents or grandparents, at age 55 or younger, suffered a documented myocardial infarction, angina pectoris, peripheral vascular disease, cerebrovascular disease, or sudden cardiac death, and (2) one parent has had a blood cholesterol level of 240 mg/dl or higher. Finally, the panel suggests screening when the family history is unknown, particularly if other risk factors are present. For individuals over age 20, obtaining a baseline serum cholesterol level is recommended, followed by repeat serum cholesterol determinations every 5 years.

Potential for error exists in this screening format,[9,29,41] which has led some to propose mass screening, beginning as early as age 2 years. However, mass screening also has several potential problems[12]:

1. The tracking of individuals from children with high cholesterol levels to adults with high cholesterol levels has enough variation to make exact prediction for any one person more difficult than expected.
2. Overzealous use of low-fat diets and cholesterol-lowering drugs can have significant side effects.
3. Serious psychological consequences may result in children labeled "at risk" for an early death.
4. "Labeling" can affect insurability and employment opportunities.

STRESS MANAGEMENT/COMMUNICATION SKILLS

The psychological components of a healthy life-style actually are fairly familiar. Pediatricians have been presenting aspects of stress management, behavior modification, and improved communication skills for years when they discuss a wide variety of anticipatory guidance topics with parents and patients.

Stress management is incorporated because many of the diseases targeted for prevention are related to psychological stress. Common examples of stress management techniques include deep breathing, ascending muscle relaxation, body awareness, positive mental imagery, meditation, priority setting, time management, and even the simple body stretches mentioned earlier. Examples of family activities that can aid in stress management are listed in the box on p. 258. The book *Handbook of Stress: Theoretical and Clinical Aspects* (see Goldberg and Breznitz under Suggested Readings) is an extensive reference on stress management.

COMPLIANCE

The most important factor in the ultimate success or failure of all life-style changes is compliance; compliance is the basis of success or failure in any effort at prevention or intervention by medical care providers. The keys to compliance are education and motivation.[23,24] The first step is to establish a rapport by listening carefully as the concerns of the patient and family are discussed. Active involvement of the patient and parents should be elicited by developing a plan based on the common understanding of the issues of the visit. The plan is implemented by offering the family opportunities to learn new behaviors, develop new experiences, and modify their environment.[14] Realistic goals should be set that are achievable by incremental change. The plan is evaluated by identifying strategies for tracking the patient's progress. Teaching the patient when possible, and the family about the problem may be motivation enough for starting a change in life-style. Long-term compliance, however, is more difficult. The physical and mental benefits of the program, when they become noticeable, may provide a self-sustaining motivation. It is during the gap between starting a program and reaching

SUGGESTED FAMILY ACTIVITIES FOR STRESS MANAGEMENT

Keep a family calendar
Keep a family job list
Hold a family meeting
Have a family game night
Attend a health fair
Read together
Keep a stress diary
Get involved in service projects
Set aside meditation and quiet time
Prepare a meal together
Keep a journal
Engage in family outdoor adventures
Have a family picnic
Get adequate sleep
Cut television time in half
Discuss family budgeting
Attend cultural events
Play new games together

Modified from the Governor's Family FUN Award Program, Utah Governor's Council on Health and Physical Fitness, Salt Lake City, Utah.

a point where the benefits are tangible (as early as the third month or as late as the twelfth month) that the drop out rate is greatest. The average dropout rate in the first 6 to 12 months of starting a fitness program frequently is 50% or higher.[35] As was stated earlier, the beneficial changes achieved through any health-related fitness program are not sustained if the program is discontinued; this is why it is important that the family comprehend the concept of a life-style change.

Many factors have been studied in efforts to solve the compliance problem. Some of the important findings in an adult survey included scheduling the time, accessibility to facilities, weather, time of year, and an interested friend or family member.[33] In a survey of diabetic children and adolescents who participated in an exercise program, the most important factors involved with compliance were enthusiastic leadership, individual attention, and parental support.[32] It also has been shown that children of physically active parents are more physically active themselves.[25] A study on the prevention of progression to severe obesity by use of family therapy showed some effectiveness when the program was started in childhood (before age 11).[8] Therefore the help of a motivated and involved adult is essential for children to acquire positive life-style habits. That role is most likely to be filled by one or both parents. The next most likely individual may be a teacher or organization leader (scouts, YMCA/YWCA, or church group).

A study of previously sedentary adults showed that subjects who exercised at home were more likely to achieve long-term compliance than those who attended exercise classes if both groups received the benefit of planning and encouragement from experts.[16] The same study showed that the home-based group tended toward moderation in intensity. Two thoughts arise from that study—that the convenience of home is certainly important and that many people may not stay with an exercise program because well-meaning trainers push them too hard.

By instructing the patient and family to keep a daily log of all areas of life-style changes and to return with the log in 1 month, the physician can provide an incentive to comply and a basis for discussion at the follow-up visit. For example, if one day the patient walked for 30 minutes, participated in a family meeting, and had broiled chicken (instead of hamburgers) for one of the day's meals, then that person could write the following on his or her individual calendar: F (for fitness): walked 30 minutes; U (for unity, or family communication): had a family meeting; N (for nutrition): ate broiled chicken. Everyone needs motivation and encouragement to stay with any life-style change, and one of the keys to achieving this is to make the process fun. This is important for adults, but it is critical for children. Spelling out FUN on the calendar helps reinforce the importance of making the program enjoyable.

Use of age- and time-appropriate rewards is essential. For example, the family could go out for frozen yogurt (instead of ice cream) if one week's goal is met; each family member could buy a desired article of clothing if one month's goal is met; and a family vacation to a favorite spot could be the reward if a 6- or 12-month goal is met. Each family member should be allowed to help decide what reward is important for him or her.

Varying the selection of exercise activities makes for a more interesting exercise program and helps prevent overuse injuries, both of which will aid in compliance. For example, one could walk twice a week, ride a stationary bike twice a week, and play games at the park as part of a family outing once a week.

For many individuals as well as families, lack of time to begin or maintain a fitness program is a major obstacle. A good starting point is to divide the day into 30-minute increments, then make the program a priority to be worked into one of those increments. Specific suggestions for getting in the desired exercise time include getting up 30 minutes earlier in the morning, taking 30 minutes of the lunch break, or allotting 30 minutes after dinner. It now is evident that even three 10-minute episodes of activity over the day may be as beneficial from a health standpoint as one 30-minute activity.

The specific topic of quitting smoking is one in which it has been difficult to obtain long-term compliance for almost everyone. Evidence shows that pediatricians are the physicians most commonly in touch with adolescents (and with young parents for that matter). It obviously would behoove the pediatrician to be familiar with antismoking techniques and strategies.[13]

EATING DISORDERS AND EXERCISE

The pediatrician should always keep in mind that some patients may have the hidden agenda of an eating disorder when they seek information on diet and exercise. A recent study suggested that more than half of all adolescent girls are extremely diet and weight conscious, if not phobic.[5] Adoles-

EXAMPLES OF HEALTH-RELATED FITNESS PROGRAMS

School programs

1. The Comprehensive School Health Programs Database

   An information source and a network, the database contains information on 150 school districts that have at least one of the elements of a comprehensive school health program and that are actively working on additional elements. The database can provide information on which districts have particular program elements, as well as statistics on the characteristics of each district and the staffing of the health program. It also provides the names of people in the programs to contact. For the database, contact: Betty Poehlman, Manager, Comprehensive School Health Programs Project, National School Boards Association, 1680 Duke St., Alexandria, VA 22314; telephone: 1-703-838-6717.
2. "Feeling Good"

   A program that appears to be the most extensive in depth (it covers all the areas mentioned in this chapter and more) and in breadth (books are available for children from kindergarten through high school, for parents, and for administrators). The emphasis in the exercise segment is on noncompetitive cardiovascular movement through "fun" games. A "homework" section helps to get families involved. Contact: Charles T. Kuntzleman, Ph.D., Fitness Finders, 133 Teft Road, Spring Arbor, MI 49283.
3. "Know Your Body"

   A plan developed as a school-based program that focuses on teaching decision making skills in the areas of nutrition, exercise, and preventing smoking. The program has been used in all socioeconomic settings. Contact: The American Health Foundation, 320 East 43rd St., New York, NY 10017.
4. "Growing Healthy"

   A comprehensive school-based program that covers many areas, including exercise and nutrition. Contact: The National Center for Health, 30 East 20th St., New York, NY 10016.

Personal and family programs

1. The Body Shop

   A program originally developed at a hospital in Minnesota and now marketed to other hospitals. It calls for intense, direct adult supervision by hospital personnel to lead children 8 to 18 years of age and their parents through 10 weeks of behavior modification and experiential skill building, which will enable them to take control of their eating and exercise behaviors and to improve their self-esteem. Contact: The Body Shop, Methodist Hospital, 6500 Excelsior Blvd., St. Louis Park, MN 55426.
2. *The Reader's Digest* Guide to Family Fitness

   A program developed for *The Reader's Digest* by several nationally recognized experts. It includes an introduction, information on testing a family's fitness level, and suggestions for starting a family exercise program. It does not include diet or stress management. Contact: Reprint Editor, The Reader's Digest, Pleasantville, NY 10570.
3. *The Well Family Book*

   Written by Charles T. Kuntzleman, Ph.D., this is a good resource for specific examples of fitness, nutrition, and stress management for families. Contact: Here's Life Publishers, P.O. Box 1576, San Bernardino, CA 92402.
4. Shapedown

   A weight-loss program of diet and exercise that uses behavior modification techniques and is available in versions for three age groups—6 to 8, 9 to 12, and 13 to 18. The program includes a 200-page section for parents, "Guide to Supporting Your Child," which is based on setting weekly goals. This program is offered at approximately 400 medical centers, health maintenance organizations, and clinics in various parts of the country. The fee is $200 for a program lasting 12 to 16 weeks. Contact: Balboa Publishing; telephone: 1-415-453-8886.
5. Publications from the American Academy of Pediatrics

   "Better Health Through Fitness," a brochure for teens ($20/100 copies) and *Sports Medicine: Health Care for Young Athletes*, a comprehensive manual on physical fitness ($35 for AAP members, $40 for nonmembers) both are available from the American Academy of Pediatrics, P.O. Box 927, Elk Grove Village, IL 60009. For information on these and other AAP publications on fitness, call 1-708-981-7389.

cents and older children who seem involved in unusual amounts of exercise or unusual diets may be at risk for or may already have started the bulimarexia process (bulimia-purging-anorexia sequence). Gymnastics, wrestling, long distance running, dancing, drill team performing, and cheerleading are activities in which weight loss not only is encouraged but actually may be demanded by adult sponsors, parents, or peers. If the patient has a psychological susceptibility to the bulimarexia process, adult prodding or peer pressure may precipitate the syndrome. If necessary, a psychological evaluation can help determine whether the patient is indeed at risk. Newman and Halverson's *Anorexia Nervosa and Bulimia: A Handbook for Counselors and Therapists* (see Suggested Readings) is an extensive reference on this topic (see also Chapter 98, Anorexia and Bulimia Nervosa).

SPECIFIC FITNESS PROGRAMS

Although health-related fitness should be based first on family life-style changes, it ideally is supplemented by comprehensive school health education programs and physical education classes. Unfortunately, school may be the only source of exercise and health information for any one child. In the past physical education classes consisted mainly of competitive sports and were the beginning of negative connotations about exercise for people who were less athletically inclined. The schools have recognized this problem and have been

SPECIFIC PROGRAMS FOR DEVELOPING A HEALTH-RELATED FITNESS PROFILE*

1. Physical Best program of the American Alliance for Health, Physical Education, Recreation and Dance (AAHPERD), 1900 Association Drive, Reston, VA 22091.
2. President's Physical Fitness Award Program of the President's Council on Physical Fitness and Sports, Washington, DC 20001.
3. The Fitness Gram of the Institute for Aerobics Research, the Aerobics Center, 12330 Preston Road, Dallas, TX 75230.

*These programs apply national standards according to age and sex.

making efforts to emphasize enjoyable "lifetime" physical activities for all children.

Totally new ideas are needed from schools and the com munity at large. Schools could sponsor physical activities and/or study halls during the after-school period before most parents get home, which may help prevent latchkey children from developing the problem behaviors that have been described in this group.[30] Sports programs for young people can accomplish the same goal and should be supported by the community.

Health-related fitness programs for schools and families already are available in a variety of forms. The box on p. 259 lists some of these programs, as well as addresses for obtaining further information. This list is not meant to be all encompassing, nor is it necessarily an endorsement of the programs mentioned.

The concept of comprehensive health education deserves special mention. Some programs in various parts of the country address all the factors mentioned earlier, as well other topics such as sex education, drug abuse education, and decision making skills, all packaged for grades K through 12. To help local school boards implement comprehensive school health programs in their districts, the National School Boards Association has established a Comprehensive School Health Programs Database. It identifies districts that have health education issues similar to those districts seeking program models. See the box on p. 259 for more information and an address for the database.

OPPORTUNITIES FOR DISCUSSING HEALTH-RELATED FITNESS

One of the best times to broach the topic of health-related fitness is a consultation for a specific problem (e.g., obesity, reactive airway disease). At these times the parent and/or patient may be especially receptive to specific therapeutic or preventive measures.[37,38] Obesity is especially difficult to treat without the team approach, which usually is offered through various hospitals and private clinics. Preventive health care visits such as well-child checkups, camp physicals, and sports preparticipation physicals are some of the other physician visits that promote discussion of this topic. The kindergarten checkup often is the last time a pediatrician can uniformly count on seeing a patient for a preventive health care visit, and it probably is the earliest age at which a program that includes exercise recommendations can be introduced. For these reasons, it should be considered as a time to routinely discuss a healthy life-style.

Height, weight, and blood pressure measurements can be obtained easily and can be plotted on an age- and sex-appropriate graph before the patient sees the pediatrician on any of the above-mentioned visits. BMI or skin caliper measurements can be determined with relative ease and proficiency by the nurse or examining physician. This information then can be compared with age- and sex-appropriate graphs to be used as a baseline for future reference and can serve as the basis for introducing this topic to the patient and parents.

The pediatrician usually cannot impart all the information needed to begin changing a family's life-style in the 20 or 30 minutes generally allotted for preventive health care visits. It is important to remember to introduce the topics of discussion personally by quickly going over the major points already listed in a brochure that the patient or parent can take home, to make specific suggestions to get the family started, and to set up a follow-up visit for 2 to 4 weeks later. At the follow-up visit, the daily log can be reviewed, measurements can be repeated, and the program can be reinforced and clarified.

Primary care physicians could try to collaborate with the local school system to create a "health-related fitness profile" for all the children in that particular school system.[39] The school can test the students in the areas of cardiovascular endurance capacity (1 mile run), muscle strength and endurance (flexed arm hang/pull-ups in 1 minute and sit-ups in 1 minute), and flexibility (sitting on the floor and reaching as far as possible past the feet). The child's pediatrician or school personnel could measure body composition (triceps and calf skin caliper measurements), height, weight, and blood pressure. When the child's test results are known, the child's physician or one appointed by the school could work with the parents and teachers to improve any one child's deficient areas (details on specific programs already available are given in the box above).

With all the problems facing medicine today, is all of this actually important enough to take up the pediatrician's time? Can we afford financially to educate our patient population, to fight for insurance reimbursement, and to encourage schools to include this topic in their curriculum? Some believe that the answers await longitudinal studies yet to be done, but most professionals in the interrelated areas of medicine, nutrition, and exercise believe that adopting a healthy life-style can enhance the quality and duration of life within the framework of any one person's genetic potential for health.

REFERENCES

1. Blair SN, Kohl HW: Physical activity or physical fitness: which is more important for health? *Med Sci Sports Exerc* 20(suppl):S8, 1988.
2. Borg GAV: A category-ratio perceived exertion scale: relationship to blood and muscle lactates and heart rate, *Med Sci Sports Exerc* 15:523, 1983.
3. Brownell KD, Nelson Steen S: Modern methods for weight control: the physiology and psychology of dieting, *Physician Sports Med* 15:122, 1987.

4. Burns TL, Moll PP, Lauer RM: Increased familial cardiovascular mortality in obese schoolchildren: the Muscatine Ponderosity Family Study, *Pediatrics* 89:262, 1992.
5. Casper RC, Offer D: Weight and dieting concerns in adolescents: fashion or symptom? *Pediatrics* 86:384, 1990.
6. Consensus Conference: Lowering blood cholesterol to prevent heart disease, *JAMA* 253:2080, 1985.
7. Dunbar CC et al: The validity of regulating exercise intensity by ratings of perceived exertion, *Med Sci Sports Exerc* 24:94, 1992.
8. Flodmark CE: Prevention of progression to severe childhood obesity in a group of obese schoolchildren treated with family therapy, *Pediatrics* 91:880, 1993.
9. Garcia RE, Moodie DS: A case for routine cholesterol surveillence in childhood, *Pediatrics* 84:751, 1989.
10. Geitmaker SL, Dietz WH: Increasing pediatric obesity in the United States, *Am J Dis Child* 141:535, 1987.
11. Hammer LD et al: Standardized percentile curves of body mass index for children and adolescents, *Am J Dis Child* 145:259, 1991.
12. Hoekelman RA: A pediatrician's view: cholesterol mania, *Pediatr Ann* 19:229, 1990 (editorial).
13. Irons TG, Kennay RD: Let's get parents to stop smoking, *Contemp Pediatr* 3:107, 1988.
14. Jopling RJ: Health-related fitness as preventive medicine, *Pediatr Rev* 10:141, 1988.
15. Jopling RJ: Let's make fitness a family affair, *Contemp Pediatr* 4:23, 1992.
16. King AC et al: Group- vs home-based exercise training in healthy older men and women: a community-based clinical trial, *JAMA* 266:1535, 1991.
17. Kraus H: Unfit kids: a call to action, *Contemp Pediatr* 5:18, 1988.
18. Kraus H, Hirschland RP: Minimum muscular fitness tests in schoolchildren, *Res Q* 25:178, 1954.
19. Kwiterovich PO Jr: Biochemical, clinical, epidemiologic, genetic, and pathologic data in the pediatric age group relevant to the cholesterol hypothesis, *Pediatrics* 78:349, 1986.
20. LaRosa J, Finberg L: Preliminary report from a conference titled "Prevention of adult atherosclerosis during childhood," *J Pediatr* 112:317, 1988.
21. Lauer RM, Clarke WR: Childhood risk factors for high adult blood pressure, *Pediatrics* 84:633, 1989.
22. Lipid Research Clinics Population Studies Data Book, vol 1, *The prevalence study,* US Department of Health and Human Services, National Institutes of Health Pub No 80-1527, Washington, DC, 1980, US Government Printing Office.
23. Martin AR, Coates TJ: A clinician's guide to helping patients change behavior, *West J Med* 146:751, 1987.
24. McCann DP, Blossom HJ: The physician as a patient educator: from theory to practice, *West J Med* 153:44, 1990.
25. Moore LL: Parents' physical activity levels and those of their young children, *J Pediatr* 118:215, 1991.
26. National Cholesterol Education Program: Report of the Expert Panel on Blood Cholesterol Levels in Children and Adolescents, NIH Pub No 91-2732, Washington, DC, 1991, US Dept of Health and Human Services.
27. Phelps JR: Physical activity and health maintenance: exactly what is known? *West J Med* 146:200, 1987.
28. Powell KE et al: Physical activity and the incidence of coronary heart disease, *Annu Rev Public Health* 8:253, 1987.
29. Resnicow K, Cross D: Are parents' self-reported total cholesterol levels useful in identifying children with hyperlipidemia?: an examination of current guidelines, *Pediatrics* 92:347, 1993.
30. Richardson JL: Relationship between after-school care of adolescents and substance use, risk taking, depressed mood, and academic achievement, *Pediatrics* 92:32, 1993.
31. Rippe JM: The health benefits of exercise, *Physician Sports Med* 15:115, 1987.
32. Rowland TW: Motivational factors in exercise training programs for children, *Physician Sports Med* 14:122, 1988.
33. Shepard RJ: Motivation: the key to fitness compliance, *Physician Sports Med* 13:88, 1985.
34. Sigman-Grant M: Dietary approaches for reducing fat intake of preschool-age children, *Pediatrics* 91:955, 1993.
35. Song TK, Shepard RJ, Cox M: Absenteeism, employee turnover and sustained exercise participation, *J Sports Med Phys Fitness* 22:392, 1983.
36. Status of the 1990 physical fitness and exercise objectives, *MMWR* 34:521, 1985.
37. Strong WB: You are a preventive cardiologist: the scope of pediatric preventive cardiology, *Am J Dis Child* 143:1145, 1989.
38. Strong WB, Dennison BA: Pediatric preventive cardiology: atherosclerosis and coronary heart disease, *Pediatr Rev* 9:303, 1988.
39. Strong WB, Wilmore JH: Unfit kids: an office-based approach to physical fitness, *Contemp Pediatr* 5:33, 1988.
40. Tanner JM, Whitehouse RH: Revised standards for triceps and subscapular skinfolds in British children, *Arch Dis Child* 50:142, 1975.
41. Wadowski SJ et al: Family history of coronary artery disease and cholesterol: screening children in a disadvantaged Inner City population, *Pediatrics* 93:109, 1994.
42. Webber LS et al: Cardiovascular risk factors from birth to 7 years of age: the Bogalusa Heart Study, *Pediatrics* 80:767, 1987.

SUGGESTED READINGS

Anderson B: *Stretching,* Bolinas, Calif, 1980, Shelter Publications (Random House).

Connor SL, Connor WE: *The new American diet,* New York, 1986, Fireside Books (Simon & Schuster).

Dietz WH, Robinson TN: Assessment and treatment of childhood obesity, *Pediatr Rev* 14:337, 1993.

Dishman RK: *Exercise adherence: its impact on public health,* Champaign, Ill, 1990, Human Kinetics Publishers.

Eisenman PA, Johnson SC, Benson JE: *Coaches' guide to nutrition and weight control,* Champaign, Ill, 1990, Human Kinetics Publishers.

Fish HT, Fish RB, Golding LA: *Starting out WELL: a parents' guide to physical activity and nutrition,* Champaign, Ill, 1989, Human Kinetics Publishers.

Goldberger L, Breznitz S: *Handbook of stress: theoretical and clinical aspects,* New York, 1982, Free Press (Macmillan).

Jopling RJ: Getting families to "eat right," *Contemp Pediatr* 9:97, 1992.

Linder CW, DuRant RH: Exercise, serum lipids, and cardiovascular disease: risk factors in children, *Pediatr Clin North Am* 29:1341, 1982.

Newman P, Halverson P: *Anorexia nervosa and bulimia: a handbook for counselors and therapists,* New York, 1983, Van Nostrand Reinhold.

Rowland TW: *Exercise and children's health,* Champaign, Ill, 1990, Human Kinetics Publishers.

Suskind RM, Varna RN: Assessment of the nutritional status of children, *Pediatr Rev* 5:195, 1984.

Vartabedian RE, Matthews K: *Nutripoints: the breakthrough point system for optimal nutrition,* New York, 1990, Harper & Row.

22 Prevention of Dental Caries

Robert J. Berkowitz and Pamela K. Den Besten

Dental caries is one of the most common bacterial infections afflicting children and adolescents. The disease may be defined as a localized, progressive destruction of the tooth structure by bacterial activity. The formation of dental caries depends on critical interrelationships between the tooth, dietary carbohydrate, saliva, and specific oral bacteria. The decay process is initiated by demineralization of the outer tooth surface as a result of organic acids formed during bacterial fermentation of dietary carbohydrates. Simultaneously, saliva functions as a remineralizing and buffering solution to counter the effect of demineralization. Should bacterial-derived demineralization exceed saliva's remineralization and buffering capacity, caries lesions form. Incipient lesions first appear as opaque white spots, and as loss of tooth mineral progresses, cavitation occurs.

Over the past 3 to 4 decades, dental research has had a significant effect on the prevention of dental caries.

ETIOLOGY

Microbial Factors

Studies in laboratory animals have demonstrated clearly that dental caries can be characterized as an infectious and transmissible disease. In such models the infection is quite specific and usually involves a group of oral streptococci collectively designated mutans streptococci. Strains of these species isolated from dental plaque and caries lesions in humans routinely exhibit a high level of pathogenicity when tested under the optimal conditions of the rodent model. The cariogenicity of these bacteria derives from their ability to synthesize insoluble dextrans from dietary sucrose. These extracellular dextrans mediate attachment of the microbes to each other and to the tooth surface. In addition, these bacteria's acidogenic and aciduric characteristics contribute significantly to their odontopathic potential. Implications for the involvement of mutans streptococci in human dental caries also come from clinical studies that demonstrate a positive correlation between caries activity and the degree of infection with these organisms. The etiological potential of mutans streptococci in human dental caries further is illustrated by their preferential association with the initial caries lesion, or "white spot." Clinical studies on the bacteriology of "radiation" caries also demonstrate that a significant increase in the level of oral mutans streptococci routinely precedes the onset of dental caries. Accordingly, several investigators have used salivary levels of mutans streptococci to predict the risk of caries. Collectively, the evidence indicates that mutans streptococci are a primary etiological agent in human dental caries. (For a review of this topic see Loesche.[3])

One important approach in preventing dental caries is to reduce intraoral levels of mutans streptococci. Epidemiological, chemotherapeutic, and immunological strategies to achieve this are under investigation.

Salivary Factors

Observations in desalivated experimental animals and xerostomic humans clearly indicate that saliva is the primary host defense against dental caries. The relationship between salivary gland hypofunction and dental caries involves several factors. First, the physical flow of saliva, augmented by the activity of the oral musculature, removes a large number of bacteria from the teeth. Second, saliva possesses numerous antibacterial systems. A group of salivary proteins (lysozyme, lactoferrin, and lactoperoxidase), working in conjunction with other salivary components, has an immediate effect on oral bacteria, interfering with their ability to replicate or killing them directly. Salivary peroxidase exerts an anticaries effect through a mechanism that reduces the acidogenic potential of cariogenic bacteria. Saliva also can interfere with bacterial attachment by means of molecular interactions. The ability to inhibit bacterial attachment is a major characteristic of the secretory IgA system. Besides antibodies, saliva contains a variety of macromolecules that interfere with bacterial attachment through several mechanisms, such as aggregation, masking of bacterial adhesins, and competition for attachment sites. Finally, saliva has properties that directly protect the tooth surface from demineralization. Salivary bicarbonate, phosphate, and histidine-rich peptides diffuse into plaque and act directly as buffers. Besides helping to counter plaque acidity, saliva helps protect the teeth from demineralization through a mechanism called *remineralization,* which is defined as the deposition of salivary minerals into enamel defects. The presence of fluoride in trace quantities is critical to the remineralization process. Fluoride enhances enamel crystal growth and hence makes remineralization more rapid and effective. Because remineralization is promoted by the frequent introduction of a low concentration of fluoride into the mouth, the small amount of fluoride in fluoridated drinking water is sufficient to promote remineralization. (For a review of this topic, see Mandel[4].)

Salivary hypofunction can be a consequence of a variety of factors, such as radiotherapy when the salivary glands are within the radiation ports; chronic administration of anticholinergic or parasympatholytic drugs; and salivary gland disease (e.g., Sjögren syndrome). Accordingly, these patients should be referred for aggressive caries preventive measures.

Dietary Factors

Most dietary sugars, carbohydrates, and starches are readily metabolized to organic acids by mutans streptococci. Thus such dietary substances are called *cariogenic substrates.* Numerous investigations in humans and laboratory animals demonstrate that frequent, prolonged oral exposure to cariogenic substrates facilitates dental caries activity.[2,10] Stated differently, it's not how much "sugar" you eat but how you eat the "sugar" that determines the "sugar's" relative cariogenic potential. For example, the cariogenic potential of apple juice in a nursing bottle that is sampled throughout the night or nap times, or both, is quite different from that of the same volume of apple juice consumed at a single meal. Similarly, the sugars in food products retained orally for a long time (e.g., caramel candies) are more cariogenic than those in food products retained for a short time (e.g., ice cream).

PREVENTION

Fluoride

Water Fluoridation. The relationships between natural water fluoride concentrations, the prevalence of caries, and enamel fluorosis were determined in classic epidemiological studies by H. Trendley Dean in the 1930s and 1940s. Through these studies, as well as through subsequent community trials with artificial water fluoridation, the level of 1 ppm of fluoride in drinking water was determined to be optimal for preventing caries with a minimal risk of fluorosis. This recommendation later was refined to a range of 0.7 to 1.2 ppm of fluoride, depending on the amount of water intake as a function of the annual average maximum daily air temperature in a community. Since these early studies, fluoridation of public water supplies has proved to be the most effective, convenient, and economical measure available for preventing dental caries.[5]

Fluoride Supplements. The dramatic reduction in caries susceptibility in populations drinking fluoridated water led to recommendations that fluoride be administered as a dietary supplement to those who did not receive it in their drinking water. Fluoride was assumed to have a systemic mode of action that resulted in the formation of a more caries-resistant enamel structure, an assumption that led to the conclusion that fluoride supplements should mimic previous estimates of dietary fluoride intake. Fluoride supplements, therefore, were proposed for the period during which teeth are developing.

More recent research has shown that the most important mechanism by which fluoride prevents caries is its topical effect. Fluoride promotes salivary remineralization of demineralized enamel. This effect is enhanced by exposing the teeth frequently to relatively low levels of fluoride, as occurs with drinking fluoridated water.[1] The realization that systemic fluoride ingestion is not fluoride's major mechanism of action, and reports of increased dental fluorosis have prompted a reassessment of fluoride supplementation recommendations.

Dental fluorosis is a hypomineralization of enamel that occurs when higher than optimal levels of fluoride are ingested during the period of enamel formation. Fluorosis can range from very mild to severe. Very mild to mild cases appear as chalky whitening of the enamel; severe fluorosis manifests as mottled enamel that is pitted and brown. Recent reports have shown a trend toward a higher prevalence of dental fluorosis, relative to historical data from earlier studies. This increase has been found to correlate with ingestion of fluoride from sources other than drinking water (e.g., fluoride supplements and fluoridated toothpaste).[6] Therefore, because fluoride's major mechanism of caries prevention is topical and because enamel fluorosis is becoming more prevalent, the Council on Dental Therapeutics of the American Dental Association has endorsed a new fluoride supplementation schedule (see Table 22-1).[7] Fluoride supplements are not recommended prenatally or during the first 6 months of life. In addition, breast-fed infants living in optimally fluoridated communities should not receive fluoride supplements.

Table 22-1 Fluoride Supplement Dosage Schedule*

	Concentration of fluoride in drinking water (ppm)		
Age	<0.3	0.3-0.6	>0.6
Birth-6 mo	0	0	0
6 mo-3 yr	0.25	0	0
3-6 yr	0.5	0.25	0
6-16 yr	1	0.5	0

*Dosage regimen accepted by the American Academy of Pediatrics, the American Academy of Pediatric Dentistry (1994), and the American Dental Association (1994).

As shown in Table 22-1, the dosage is based on the patient's age and the fluoride content of the water supply. The fluoride level of a water supply usually can be learned by calling the local water board. If the patient uses a private water supply, a fluoride analysis is indicated. The patient's parents should be instructed to use a plastic container for the water specimen (a glass container, which may have fluoride in it, could impair the accuracy of the assay). No fluoride prescription should exceed 120 mg. At this amount, even if a child ingested the entire supply, probably only mild gastric upset would ensue. However, in such an event, a poison control center should be contacted immediately.

Fluoride Dentifrice. Fluoride-containing dentifrices are highly effective in preventing dental decay. However, before age 6, children tend to swallow rather than expectorate toothpaste, and nearly all the ingested fluoride is absorbed, primarily from the small intestine. Furthermore, fluoride dentifrice constitutes approximately 95% of all dentifrice sold. The ingestion of toothpaste containing fluoride is responsible for the strong association between early use of fluoride dentifrice and an increased risk of dental fluorosis. To reduce the risk of dental fluorosis from toothpaste ingestion, a small (pea-sized) amount of toothpaste should be used for brushing a young child's teeth, and the parent should dispense the toothpaste.

Fluoride Rinses. Fluoride rinses containing 0.05% fluoride have proved highly effective in reducing dental decay. These products are available without a prescription and should be recommended for children over age 6 who are at risk for dental decay because of conditions such as compromised salivary flow rates, orthodontic therapy, and a high caries experience. These rinses are not recommended for children under age 6 because of the young child's inability to expectorate properly, which leads to excessive fluoride ingestion.

Oral Hygiene

Thoroughly brushing and flossing the teeth daily will help prevent dental caries and periodontal disease. Parents should be given professional instruction in oral hygiene techniques for their children. Clinical studies demonstrate that most children age 8 or younger do not have the hand-eye coordination required for adequate oral hygiene; therefore the parents must assume that responsibility. The degree of parental involvement should reflect the child's level of competency.

Sealants

Even excellent oral hygiene and optimal fluoride exposure have a minimal effect in preventing dental caries in the pits and fissures on the occlusal (biting) surfaces of the posterior teeth. However, sealants have proved effective in preventing pit and fissure caries.[8] Sealants are plastic coatings that are professionally applied to the occlusal surfaces of the posterior teeth. A 1989 survey conducted by the National Institute of Dental Research indicated that relatively few U.S. schoolchildren have sealants on their teeth.[9] Unfortunately, despite their proven clinical efficacy, sealants are not routinely used to prevent dental caries.

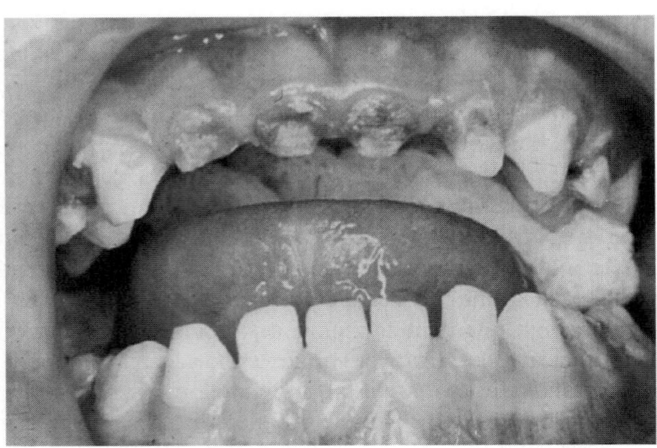

FIG. 22-1 Nursing bottle caries in a 2½-year-old child.

Diet

Cutting back on how often cariogenic substrates are ingested can prevent dental caries. Parents and children should be encouraged to avoid between-meal snacks that contain cariogenic substrates. Instead, a child with a "sweet tooth" may be offered gum, candy, and soft drinks made with sugar substitutes (mannitol, sorbitol, xylitol, and aspartame). Chewing "sugarless" gum has been clinically proven to enhance the salivary flow rate and neutralize plaque pH. Also, bottle-fed infants should be weaned by 1 year of age to eliminate the risk of nursing bottle caries (Fig. 22-1). Otherwise, bedtime and naptime nursing bottles should contain only water. Finally, chronic use of sweetened elixirs of medications can increase oral exposure to cariogenic substrates and thereby the risk of caries. Patients with this risk factor should be referred for aggressive caries prevention measures.

REFERENCES

1. Beltran ED, Burt BA: The pre- and posteruptive effects of fluoride in the caries decline, *J Public Health Dent* 48:233, 1988.
2. Bibby B: Influence of diet on the bacterial composition of plaques. In Stiles HM, Loesche WJ, O'Brien TC, editors: *Microbial aspects of dental caries,* vol 2, London, 1976, Information Retrieval.
3. Loesche WJ: Role of *Streptococcus mutans* in human dental decay, *Microbiol Rev* 50:353, 1986.
4. Mandel ID: The functions of saliva, *J Dent Res* 66(special issue):623, 1987.
5. Newbrun E: Effectiveness of water fluoridation, *J Public Health Dent* 49(special issue):279, 1989.
6. Pendrys DG: Dental fluorosis in perspective, *J Am Dent Assoc* 122:63, 1991.
7. ADA Council on Access, Prevention, and Interprofessional Relations: Caries diagnosis and risk assessment, *J Am Dent Assoc* 126(special supplement), 1995.
8. Ripa LW: The current status of pit and fissure sealants: a review, *J Can Dent Assoc* 51:367, 1985.
9. Sealant Use Low, *Am Dent Assoc News* 20:24, 1989 (editorial).
10. Van Houte J: Dental caries, *Int Dent J* 30:305, 1980.

23 Injury Prevention

Howard C. Mofenson and Joseph Greensher

CASUALTIES, CAUSES, AND CURES[45]

This chapter, formerly titled Accident Prevention, updates the challenge laid down to pediatricians by Dietrich in 1954,[17] that "accident prevention in childhood is your problem, too." In the past, accidents were regarded as product-related or behavioral problems rather than public health problems. However, as is evident from the National Safety Council (NSC) statistics cited here,[47] the casualty count both in lives lost and children maimed warrants the concerted action of primary care physicians. Considerable progress has been made in understanding the environmental situations and circumstances that contribute to the occurrence of injuries. A better knowledge of the causal factors will result in a more rational approach to solving this problem.

The first organized effort to obtain information on product-related injuries in children began with the establishment in 1952 of the AAP's Accident Prevention Committee, recently renamed the Committee on Injury and Poison Prevention. This committee has cooperated with many other organizations, manufacturers, and government to improve the safety of products, an effort that has resulted in safety education, identification of environmental hazards, voluntary compliance, and passage of legislation establishing safety standards.

Casualties

Injuries are the leading cause of death among all people from 1 to 38 years of age. In 1992, the death toll from injuries was approximately 83,000 (the lowest since 1922); disability injuries numbered approximately 17.1 million, including 350,000 that involved some degree of permanent impairment; and the cost of these injuries amounted to about $399 billion.

Among children and young people 1 to 24 years of age, injuries accounted for almost 40% of the 54,100 total deaths in 1990. This disproportion becomes even more dramatic when viewed in terms of the years of potential life lost with each death that occurs before age 65. The aggregate loss to society is staggering.

In the 1 through 14 age group, injuries account for more deaths than the next five most commonly reported causes (cancer, congenital anomalies, infectious diseases, homicide, and cardiovascular diseases). Although no accurate statistics are available, child abuse also is a significant cause of death in children.

It is estimated that each year 40,000 to 50,000 children are injured permanently and at least 1 million seek medical care because of unintentional injuries. Accurate gathering of statistics is hampered because only injuries that cause a high number of fatalities are listed. The kinds of injuries that cause fatalities are not necessarily the type that cause a large number of nonfatal injuries.

Over the past 3 decades, unintentional injuries rose to become the leading cause of death in children. Ironically, this can be attributed indirectly to the medical profession and in no small part to pediatricians, whose work in public health, medical practice, and research sharply reduced the incidence and consequences of many formerly fatal diseases; it was through this decline in other causes of death that unintentional injury achieved its dubious distinction. In 1920 only 10% of childhood deaths were caused by unintentional injury; by 1990, however, the figure was 40%. The statistical breakdown for the various types of injuries is presented in the individual discussions.

Causes[28,35,41]

The term *accident* proved a barrier to elucidating the causes of these problems, and most physicians no longer use it. The label "accident" implies a "bad break" or an "act of God" that is not understandable in terms of the usual causes of disease. Also, people often attribute avoiding an accident to "sheer luck" or "a miracle." The terms *injury* and *injury control* are preferable. Through research and experience in injury control, many of those at risk for certain kinds of injuries have been identified, as have preventive strategies that can save lives, health, and resources.

The three prime components of an injury are the host (who is affected by the injury), the agent (the direct cause of the injury), and the environment (where and when the injury occurred).

The importance of the *host* as a factor in causing injuries is evident from the difference in incidence at various ages. The preschool child is endangered by poisoning, the school-age child by drowning and firearm accidents. The immobile child under 1 year of age faces different hazards on becoming a toddler. These factors are important in planning prevention.

Some children are more susceptible, and boys, generally, are more likely to be injured than are girls (the male death rate from injury is twice that of the female). A child who has had a poisoning episode is more likely to have a second than a matched control is to have a first.

Recognizing the *agent* (e.g., flammable fabrics or refrigerators [entrapment]) allows some preventive measures to be taken, but many of these items are integral parts of modern everyday life, and it would be impossible to control injuries completely by abolishing them.

The physical and social *environments* play important roles in the occurrence of an injury; they are the settings in which the host and agent interact. The time of year, the time of day, the child's health, relocation, and frequent injuries in other family members all are factors associated with the occurrence of injuries.

A Boston study[29] showed that injuries occur when additional stress is present. The stressful situations found included:

1. Hunger or fatigue. Injuries occurred more often during the hour before a scheduled meal, in the late afternoon, or before bedtime. Maternal tension probably is an important factor at these times.
2. Hyperactivity
3. Maternal illness
4. Recent change in the caretaker of the child
5. Illness or death of a family member
6. Tense relationship between the child's parents
7. Sudden changes in environment, such as those that occur when relocating or at vacation time
8. Maternal preoccupation (rushed or too busy). The study found that most injuries occurred on Saturday, and most between 3 and 6 PM.

Another study suggested that childhood injuries are recurring symptoms of maladjustment to environment or family. Poor housing, marital disharmony, and physical or mental ill health among family members were found in significant number in the study. Using poisoning as an example of childhood injuries, it was found that repetitive poisoning was not related to environmental hazards or lack of supervision but rather to marital tension and a tense and distant parent-child relationship.[53]

It is essential that the pediatrician understand the various concepts used in the literature and research on injuries. *Injury proneness* implies personality characteristics that predispose an individual to injury; however, this implication tends to exclude further investigation of the environment. Most researchers are skeptical of the concept of injury proneness. *Injury repetitiveness* is an observed pattern of behavior that lasts for varying periods. *Injury liability* views the individual in relation to the environment. With children, this implies that not only the child but also the family and the environment are involved in the injuries. Liability arises from personality characteristics and many other factors such as sensory, motor, and neural functioning, exposure to hazards, capacity to make judgments, degree of experience and training, and exposure to social and other stresses.

Certain behavioral characteristics have been found to increase exposure to injury liability or to reduce a child's ability to cope with hazards. Most of these features are present at 1 year of age, and knowing them may help the pediatrician identify a child at risk.

A child's exposure to injury liability is likely to be increased if he or she (1) is very active, daring, curious, and happy-go-lucky, (2) mimics the behavior of older people, and (3) has exaggerated oral tendencies.

Often, a child has a reduced ability to cope with hazards if he or she (1) is high-strung, hot-headed, stubborn, and easily irritated or frustrated, (2) is careless at play, (3) lacks self-control, (4) is aggressive, and (5) has poor concentration or poor ability to pay attention.

Family life-style also has been found to be a factor in injuries. Men who have dull jobs appear to have a greater need for instant gratification. They seek recreational thrills and surround themselves with more dangerous devices, and the children in their families tend to have more injuries.

Hospitalization that requires separating infants from parents has been correlated with an increase in the incidence of childhood injuries and child abuse. Child abuse or neglect may be a significant cause of injuries; estimates vary from 10% to 50% (see Chapter 56). *When any child has two or more significant injuries in a 12-month period, an in-depth investigation of the circumstances is warranted.*

Cures

In 1970 Sobel[53] stated that if any progress was to be made in preventing injuries, practitioners must broaden their perspective and consider the parents' mental health and capacity to provide a milieu in which the child's needs are met. It is not unreasonable to believe that a profile of the family and child at risk can be developed to help identify individuals in need of behavior modification and other techniques to reduce injuries.

Parents are more likely to perform the one-time or occasional task needed to prevent injury (e.g., buying a smoke detector); these occasions, therefore, lend themselves to effective counseling. The physician can gain insight into potential problems by obtaining a history of the family that includes the parents' occupations, education, and income and their attitudes toward the children and each other, as well as use of medications, alcohol, and tobacco, television viewing patterns, previous automobile accidents, and the availability of guns in the home. Clues to the family's life-style may be found in family recreational activities and hobbies.

The pediatrician also can attempt to gauge parent-child rapport. Levy,[37] for example, found that when something complimentary was said about a baby while the mother was holding the child, the average mother would look down at her baby. Failure to do this often indicated a lack of good rapport. Observing the way the parent or parents stand beside an infant who is on the examining table also may indicate the degree of awareness of the baby's safety and comfort.

Parents, particularly mothers, should be alerted to the signals of increased risk of injury and should take extra precautions during stressful times, simplifying family life and doing only those things necessary to maintain health and comfort.

PHYSICIANS' ROLE IN PROMOTING CHILD SAFETY

What can a pediatrician do in the office to help prevent childhood injuries? Recognition that injuries are the foremost public health problem affecting children already has spurred a great deal of activity to identify injuries as amenable to study and prevention. However, too many parents still believe that drugs and kidnapping, for example, are the greatest threats to the life of their developing child. Many experts have strongly advocated that pediatricians provide preventive counseling and that they emphasize a developmental approach; until recently, however, no system was available to inform the practitioner of the necessary content and for making materials available for parent education.

Responding to the need for an office-based, pediatrician-initiated counseling program that would help reduce the risk of injuries by *influencing* behavior, the AAP in cooperation with the government and private industry, developed The Injury Prevention Program (TIPP). In its policy statement on

Table 23-1 Safety Counseling for Parents, Children, and Adolescents

Period	Topics
Perinatal	Cribs, other furniture, faucets, smoke detectors, infant car seats
1-4 mo	Furniture, falls, toy safety
4-7 mo	Ingestions, scalds, aspirations
7 mo-1 yr	Syrup of ipecac, poison control telephone number, safety packaging, poison proofing
1-3 yr	Car seats, mimicking adult behavior
3-5 yr	Supervised play; water, street, and yard safety
5-10 yr	Car seat belts, water and bicycle safety, fire and burn prevention
10-14 yr	Motor vehicle, water, fire, and firearm safety
Adolescents	Drugs, alcohol, cigarettes, sports safety, cardiopulmonary resuscitation

injury prevention, the AAP's executive board declares: "Anticipatory guidance for injury prevention should be an integral part of the medical care provided for all infants and children." Initially the program focused on children from birth to age 5, emphasizing the use of car restraints, smoke detectors, safe hot water temperatures, window and stairway guards and gates, and the availability of syrup of ipecac. TIPP has been extended to cover children to age 12, and for these older children a strong emphasis has been placed on bicycle, pedestrian, and water and sports safety. The program offers a structured approach to both advocacy and education, roles that should be uniquely suited to physicians who care for children.*

A critical review of the scientific literature on the effectiveness of primary care–based counseling to prevent childhood unintentional injury supports the AAP's recommendation to include injury prevention counseling as part of routine health supervision.[10]

THE VICTIMS

The stages of childhood development can serve as a guide for teaching parents and, eventually, children themselves about injury prevention. In a Boston study,[29] 87% of the parents whose children had injuries did not understand developmental expectations. The pediatrician should understand and be able to give an overview of the developmental stages, the hazards common to each, and precautions that can be taken to prevent the injuries typical in each age group. Table 23-1 provides a useful guide to the safety counseling necessary at the various stages of development.

The Infant from Birth to 4 Months

These infants can wiggle and squirm, but they are completely helpless. The parents should be instructed to buy and use the proper automotive restraint equipment and flame-retardant garments and to avoid the dangers of pillows, filmy plastics, and harnesses. They should be taught crib safety measures and how to prevent drowning, burns, falls, and aspiration injuries.

The Infant from 4 to 7 Months

These infants are becoming more active and are learning to reach, roll over, and sit. A crib or playpen is the safest area for this age group. The parents need advice on infant furniture and toy safety, and proper automotive restraints and flame-retardant garments are still required.

The Infant from 7 Months to 1 Year

These mobile infants are in increasing danger of falling as they begin to crawl, stand, and walk. Parents must be made aware that as children pull themselves erect, they pull everything down. There is danger in hanging tablecloths, hot pots on the stove, dangling electrical cords, electrical sockets, unguarded staircases, and reachable dangerous household products and medicines. Flame-retardant clothing and proper automotive restraints are essential.

An infant under 1 year of age needs 100% protection. The major injuries to be prevented are mechanical suffocation, ingestion or inhalation of food or foreign objects, motor vehicle injuries, fire and burn injuries, and falls. Mechanical suffocation has been listed as the leading cause of death in this age group, but this category is suspect because it also may include cases of sudden infant death syndrome (SIDS) and infection.

The Toddler 1 to 2 Years of Age

Parents should be alerted to this curious investigator, who opens doors, windows, and drawers. Toddlers' climbing ability is excellent; they like to play in water and to take everything apart. They can stoop and recover, mimic the behavior of adults and older children, and push, pull, lift, and carry—and they have no sense of danger. Parents must be aware of thermal and electrical hazards and the perils of water. They should buy safe toys and should supervise the child's play. Syrup of ipecac should be available in the home for emergency treatment of poisonous ingestions. The safest area for this age group is a playpen or blocked-off play area, with free periods of supervised house roaming.

The 2- and 3-Year-Old Child

This hurrying child is lightning fast and runs much of the time. The same precautions as for the toddler apply.

The 3- to 5-Year-Old Child

These children are teachable, and they should be taught their full names, traffic safety, obedience, and responsibility. At this age children begin to develop skills and can throw objects, ride tricycles, climb trees, and explore the neighborhood. Parents should supervise the areas where their children play and remove potential hazards. These children should not be relied upon to protect themselves; supervised play is advised until age 5. The major injuries to be prevented in this age group are motor vehicle, fire and burn injuries, drownings, and poisoning.

The 5- to 10-Year-Old Child

Daring and adventurous activity characterizes children in this age group. These children often are part of a group and will

*The complete TIPP program can be found in *A Guide to Safety Counseling in Office Practice*, available from the American Academy of Pediatrics, Department of Publications, 141 Northwest Point Blvd., P.O. Box 927, Elk Grove Village, IL 60009.

"try anything." They should be taught water safety, bicycle safety, and fire and burn prevention. Appropriate care should be taken if firearms are kept in the home. These children should be taught how to treat pets and other animals and how to avoid animal bites. By age 6, the safety of a child in this age group depends on his or her own judgment and actions 90% of the time.

The 10- to 14-Year-Old Child

Strenuous physical activity marks those in this age group. Supervised recreational facilities should be available, and a good example should be set in preparation for automobile driving. The major injuries in this age group are motor vehicle injuries, drowning, and fire, burn, and firearm injuries.

ANIMAL BITES[43]

The pet population has kept pace with our own. Since 1945 the number of animals kept as pets has more than tripled. It is estimated that there are more than 110 million cats and dogs, 20 million birds, and many more exotic pets in the United States. As the number of pets grows, so does human contact with them, which increases the potential for injuries caused by animals.

Every year approximately 1 million Americans require medical attention for animal bites. Of these, 75% are children. More than 60,000 of these bites result in loss of sight, facial disfigurement, or other serious physical or psychological problems. To reduce the number of biting incidents, all members of the community must become involved in a prevention program. The community must establish laws; the veterinarian must treat animals and advise their owners; the pediatrician must educate the parents; and the parents must educate the child.

The Community's Role

All pet dogs should be licensed and leashed or confined. Routine vaccination and immunization should be done, and reservoirs of rabies—particularly bats, skunks, and foxes—should be eliminated. Homeless or stray animals must be confined or killed. The resurgence of rabies requires increased vigilance.

The Veterinarian's Role

Pet immunizations should be kept current. New owners should be taught about bite prevention and zoonoses (diseases communicable from animals to humans). Facilities should be available for the care of "veterinarian indigent" pets.

Cooperative Efforts

By working together, veterinarians and physicians can accomplish a great deal in a prevention program. They can advise parents on pet ownership, teach owners how to prevent bites and zoonoses, encourage immunization of all animals, and instruct people in how to report bites to the proper authorities. The pediatrician must emphasize to the parents that most of the responsibility for the care of pets (walking, bathing, feeding, and nursing) is theirs.

The child's maturity level is a very important factor in the decision to get a pet. Can the child differentiate between the animal as a live being and a toy? Does the child know that the animal's tail is not a "leash" by which the animal is pulled? It must be recognized that some parents and children should never have pets.

Prospective owners should be informed that most animal bites occur when the pet is young; therefore a more mature and placid animal is better for a child. Zoonoses also are more common among young animals.

A thorough understanding of animal behavior and an honest respect for all animals will go a long way in preventing animal bites. *It is imperative that animal owners and, especially, all children be taught how to treat animals and how to react to them.* The boxes on p. 269, which provide this information in instructional form, can be photocopied and handed out to pet owners, parents, and older children.

Animal bites are addressed further in Chapter 182; rabies associated with animal bites is discussed in Chapter 17.

ASPIRATION INJURIES

Aspiration is a common cause of home-injury deaths in children under age 4. Originally, safety pins most often were involved in aspiration by infants from birth to 1 year of age, with coins and peanuts more common in the 2 to 4 age group. The NSC reported approximately 2700 deaths in 1992 as a result of suffocation caused by ingested foreign objects; 190 of these episodes occurred in children under age 5. In their review of more than 3000 incidents involving foreign bodies found in the air and food passages, Jackson and Jackson[34] noted a frequent history of eating too fast, chewing improperly, laughing, running with food in the mouth, or just holding a foreign body (e.g., pin, nail, nut, or small toy) in the mouth. Peanuts and peanut candy were very common offenders.

Conditions that reduce the gag or cough reflex are predisposing factors to aspiration. Drugs, alcohol intoxication, seizures, anesthesia, head trauma with unconsciousness, and uncommon conditions such as familial dysautonomia or certain types of cerebral palsy may facilitate aspiration.

Because foreign body aspiration is a common hazard among young children, pediatricians should emphasize this danger (see the box on p. 270).

The treatment of foreign body aspiration is determined by the location of the object. Foreign bodies in the upper airway are life threatening and require immediate treatment when the child is choking.

"Blind sweeps" of the forefinger in the posterior pharynx should be avoided in young children because this may push the foreign body posteriorly, worsening the obstruction. If a foreign body can be seen, it can be removed with a finger. If the child can speak or breathe and is coughing, the foreign object may dislodge spontaneously; therefore first aid action is unnecessary and may be dangerous. Immediate relief is required for partial obstruction with poor air exchange or with cyanosis, as well as for complete obstruction.

In children, the abdominal thrust (Heimlich maneuver) is recommended as the single procedure to be performed.[31] In infants under 1 year of age, a combination of back blows and chest thrusts is recommended because this technique increases pressure in the blocked respiratory passages, forcing expulsion of the foreign body.

The back blow–chest thrust maneuver is performed in this

HOW TO HAVE SAFE CONTACT WITH ANIMALS

1. Avoid all strange animals, especially wild, sick, or injured ones. The same techniques used to teach children not to talk to strangers should be used to teach them not to approach strange animals.
2. Notify the health department or police of any wild, sick, or injured animals.
3. Never allow a child to break up an animal fight, even when his or her own pet is involved. Use a rake, broom, or garden hose to separate the animals.
4. Become aware, and make children aware, of the danger and cruelty of mistreating or teasing pets. Never pull an animal's tail or take away food, a bone, or a toy with which an animal is playing. Pets are not toys; they are living creatures that will bite if mauled, annoyed, or frightened.
5. Alert children to dangerous and nervous animals in the neighborhood and do not permit them to enter a yard or house that harbors such animals.
6. With children who can ride bikes or tricycles, stress the importance of avoiding routes where dogs are known to chase vehicles.
7. Have children make friends, under adult supervision, with pets with which the children will be in contact in the immediate neighborhood.
8. Do not allow children to disturb an animal that is eating or sleeping. Set a good example by your own behavior.
9. Do not let pets come into indiscriminate contact with other animals.
10. Do not buy or obtain a pet for children until they demonstrate their maturity and ability to handle and care for the pet. This ability is rare in a child under age 4 and unusual in a child under age 6. Factors to consider at any age are the maturity and disposition both of the child and the animal. Some people never develop this maturity.
11. Teach children that each animal has the right to a free existence and freedom from human-inflicted pain. Set a good example by your own behavior.
12. Never put your face close to an animal, and never allow children to do so, either.
13. Do not allow a child to lead a large dog.
14. Do not run, ride a bicycle, or skate in front of a dog; it will startle the animal.
15. Do not touch a dog that is asleep or unaware of your presence. Always speak to any dog that has not seen your approach so that the animal becomes aware of your presence and will not be startled.
16. Do not overexcite an animal, even in play.
17. Do not keep an animal confined with short ropes or chains; this may make the animal aggressive and vicious, especially if teased.
18. Have children avoid a dog raised in a home without children. Such an animal may resent children.
19. Do not allow an inexperienced child or adult to feed a dog. Such a person may pull back when the animal moves to take the food, frightening the dog.

SAFETY RULES FOR MEETING A STRANGE DOG

Meeting a strange dog can be a very frightening and potentially dangerous situation. It is important to try to remain calm and, if possible, to follow these suggestions:

1. Stop, stand still, and speak softly.
2. Wait to see what the dog is going to do.
3. Look for the signs of a dangerous unsafe dog: rigid body; stiff tail at "half mast"; shrill, hysterical bark; crouching or slinking position, with head lowered and nose close to the ground; staring expressions and an attempt to circle behind you.
4. Pivot slowly if the dog tries to circle behind you. Wait until the dog stops moving, then move slowly; stop when the dog moves again.
5. Never turn your back on a dog moving toward you.
6. Never touch a strange dog.
7. Never strike, kick, or make any threatening gesture.
8. Do not hand a person a package or shake hands when the person's dog is nearby. The dog may misinterpret the move.
9. Do not make the first overture of friendship with a dog. Allow the dog to do this, which he will not do until he smells you.

way: The infant is held face down with the head lower than the trunk. Five back blows are delivered with the heel of the hand, and then five chest thrusts are delivered as for external cardiac compression. Physicians, health professionals, and the general public should familiarize themselves with recommended resuscitation techniques.

If these emergency measures fail, the victim must be transported immediately and quickly to a medical facility.

AUTOMOTIVE INJURIES[16,48]

In 1992, 20.8 million accidents occurred among the 194 million motor vehicles registered in this country; 2.2 million Americans, or more than 1 in 100, suffered a disabling injury, and 40,300 died (the lowest number in more than 30 years).

This staggering death toll actually was a significant reduction from the 1972 high of 56,278 fatalities. This is thought to be attributable in part to the energy crisis that began in the spring of 1973, which resulted in a lowering of the speed limit to 55 mph on main roads and concomitant changes in driving habits. The number of fatalities for children from birth to age 14 was 2800 in 1992; children were pedestrians in 950 of these deaths. Approximately 175,000 children are injured each year as passengers in vehicles.

Safety belts are now available for nearly all occupants of passenger cars. It is estimated that 12,000 lives could be

HOW TO PREVENT ASPIRATION

1. Young children should not be allowed to play with small objects. As a guide, the government has proposed a small-parts standard that requires toys for children under age 3 to be at least 1¼ inches in diameter and unable to fit into a truncated circular cylinder 2¼ inches long. This standard is under review; an increase in the dimensions of the small parts covered under the regulations is being considered. "Testing" tubes often are available to parents through mail-order toy catalogs.
2. Older children should be taught not to hold foreign bodies in their mouths.
3. Hard, smooth, vegetable-type foods (e.g., peanuts), or smooth, round foods (e.g., hot dogs and grapes) that require a grinding motion should be avoided as foods for children. The chewing habit is not well established until age 4. Therefore chewable tablets should not be given until that time.
4. Children should not be given coins as rewards or play items.
5. Infants and toddlers should not put large pieces of food in their mouths. Food should be cut or broken into bite-size pieces, and children should be encouraged to chew slowly and thoroughly.
6. Children should be kept quiet while eating food or candy. Excitement or activity, such as running and walking, predisposes them to inhalation of food. Speaking when eating should be forbidden.
7. Safety pins should be kept closed and pinned to the caretaker's clothing to keep this very serious aspiration or ingestion hazard out of the child's reach.
8. An uninflated balloon is an aspiration hazard because it may be sucked into the posterior pharynx or even the larynx or trachea. The federal Consumer Product Safety Commission reviewed 21 death certificates related to toy aspiration and found that 13 reported balloons as the cause of death.
9. A dry cleaner's plastic bag is not a true aspiration hazard, but it can cause suffocation if it clings to the face of a small child or infant.

Table 23-2 Child Passengers Killed in Motor Vehicle Accidents (Washington State, 1970-1980)*

	Number killed	Total number of passengers	Ratio of number killed/passengers
Unrestrained	146	33,200	1/227
Restrained	2	6300	1/3150

From Scherz RG: Auto safety: "The first ride . . . a safe ride" campaign. In Bergman AB, editor: Preventing childhood injuries. Reprinted with permission of Ross Laboratories, Columbus, OH 43216, from The Report of the Twelfth Ross Roundtable on Critical Approaches to Common Pediatric Problems, 1982, Ross Laboratories.
*Age group birth to 4 years.

saved annually if all passengers used belts at all times and that 6000 to 9000 more lives could be saved if air cushion restraint systems were installed in all passenger cars. Scherz[50] conducted a study on the effectiveness of seat belts in reducing morbidity and mortality in Washington state between 1970 and 1980 (Table 23-2). Other studies have demonstrated that restraining devices could reduce fatalities by 45% and prevent 50% of moderate to critical injuries.

Standard safety belts usually should not be worn by small children because they cause abdominal injuries in a collision. Special restraining devices are needed to protect children under 4 to 5 years of age.[52]

Infants especially are vulnerable to fatal injuries in motor vehicle accidents. In one study,[4] infants under 6 months of age had the highest occupant death rate: 9.1/100,000 compared with 4.8/100,000 for children 6 months through 12 years of age. Infants held on the laps of passengers are particularly vulnerable to serious injury. In response to these findings, the AAP initiated "The First Ride . . . A Safe Ride" campaign in October 1980 to involve pediatricians in educating the public in the use of safety seats.

Encouraged by the passage of a child passenger protection law in Tennessee in 1978 and by the positive effect of an educational and police enforcement campaign in reducing fatalities and injuries, all states had passed child restraint laws by 1985.

AUTOMOTIVE RESTRAINTS FOR INFANTS AND SMALL CHILDREN

The Federal Standard for Automotive Restraining Devices in Children went into effect in April 1971 under Motor Vehicle Safety Standard 213, Child Seating Systems. Unfortunately, the standard was based on static rather than dynamic testing.

To provide effective protection, restraining devices must distribute deceleration forces over a large area of the body and must be secured to the vehicle by a standard lap belt or by anchoring the device itself. They should be made of strong, energy-absorbing material and should not have any parts that could cause injury. It should be emphasized that the previously used child restraint seats that merely hooked over the back of the car seat or harnesses that were secured by looping a strap around the back of the car seat were *not* designed to protect in a collision.

In January 1981 a new regulation, Federal Motor Vehicle Safety Standard 213-80, replaced static testing with 20 and 30 mph dynamic testing that more closely represented car crashes. This regulation covers all types of systems used to restrain children in motor vehicles, such as infant carriers, child seats, harnesses, and car beds.

To meet the dynamic testing standard, a restraint device may not collapse, and it must retain a test dummy within its confines during the test. The standard also sets a minimum level of safety performance for restraints equipped with top tether straps or armrests, even if the top tether is not used or if the armrest is in place but the restraint system's belts are not buckled (the armrest must function as a protective barrier). The new standard also specifies padding requirements for restraints used by children who weigh less than 20 pounds and limits the force exerted on the head and chest of a test dummy during testing of restraints for children who weigh more than 20 pounds. This regulation also specifies the force needed to open buckles on the restraint belts so that young children cannot unbuckle them but adults can do so easily. Instructions for proper use must be posted on the child restraints.

Periodically, the AAP publishes a list of the crash-tested devices available (Table 23-3). The pediatrician should emphasize to parents that proper installation is vital.

Children 4 to 5 years of age or those who weigh more than 40 pounds may use a standard lap belt if necessary. The child should be placed on a firm cushion and should sit up straight against the seat back. The belt then should be adjusted to fit snugly *across the hips;* it must not be allowed to ride up across the stomach. Abdominal injuries can result from improperly adjusted belts. A lap/shoulder belt combination provides better protection than a lap belt alone. The shoulder belt should fit across the shoulder and should not cross the face and neck; if it does cross the face and neck, it should be placed behind the child's back.

Children less than 55 inches in height should *not* use a shoulder strap, and no one should use a shoulder strap without a lap belt.

In 1985 the Insurance Institute for Highway Safety[21] published its findings from a study of 8893 children under age 10 who were passengers in 5050 cars; the study found that only 7% were restrained properly against possible crash injuries. Other studies have reported higher percentages of restraint system use, but as many as 75% of those children were not protected adequately.

Parents fail to use seat belts and restraints for children for the following reasons:

1. Inconvenience or discomfort for the child
2. Prohibitive cost
3. Fear of entrapment
4. Faulty reasoning ("It just can't happen to me.")
5. Belief that it is safer to hold a child on one's lap
6. Belief that restraints are needed only on long trips or express highways
7. Forgetfulness

Physicians perhaps do not counsel parents about automotive safety devices for children because they are not well-informed about the proper restraining devices available and do not know where to buy them. There also is a lack of gratification in not actually seeing improvement in the community's health status as a result of advice given. Bass and Wilson[11] demonstrated that personal contact in a pediatric practice, followed by letters, produced a considerable increase in the use of seat belts, whereas a saturation campaign of television commercials urging use had no effect. Pediatricians and other health care workers can combine several of the following suggestions in an effort to increase the use of automotive restraining devices:

1. List restraint use as "an immunization" on the child's record.
2. Explain to the parents the danger of holding an infant if an emergency stop or collision occurs: the weight of the infant times the speed of the car is the weight that must be restrained by the person holding the child.
3. Explain to parents that studies have shown that children who travel in car seats are better behaved than those who are unrestrained; restrained children cannot stand up or climb around, and they do not cry or fuss as much as unrestrained children.
4. Arrange for physicians and hospitals to encourage the parents of newborns to take their infants home in a safe restraining device.
5. Establish a lending or swapping scheme for the devices as infants and children outgrow them.

Temporary measures for children as passengers should include the following:

1. Children are safer if restrained in adult seat belts when riding in the back seat (which is recommended for children over age 5) than if allowed to ride unrestrained. The lap belt should be worn across the hips, not the abdomen. A pillow will help to elevate the child to the proper position.
2. Children are safer in the back seat of the car standing on the floor and holding onto the back of the front seat than sitting in a front seat.

Air bag caution: The proven effectiveness of driver's side air bags has resulted in their increased installation in the front passenger side of automobiles. An unexpected consequence has been air bag–associated injuries and fatalities to infants and children riding in the front passenger seat. The highest risk is to unrestrained or improperly restrained children, who can be propelled against a deploying air bag, and infants riding in rear-facing safety seats. The National Transportation Safety Board has recommended that infants riding in rear-facing safety seats should never be placed in the front seat of vehicles with a passenger side air bag and that infants and children should always be properly restrained in a child safety seat or lap-shoulder belt in the rear seat whenever possible. Sensors are being considered that will deactivate the air bag if the seat is occupied by an infant or child; a simple air bag deactivation switch is another proposed alternative.

Children as Pedestrians

A pedestrian injury is twice as likely to be fatal as a passenger injury. These injuries essentially are an urban problem, with two thirds of the fatalities occurring between sunset and dawn. More than 950 children are killed each year as a result of nighttime pedestrian injuries. Fatalities are highest in the 5 to 9 age-group; the fatalities in the older children of this group often result from darting out into traffic. Children under age 6 have difficulty distinguishing right from left, and their peripheral vision is not as well developed as that of adults.

The National Highway Traffic Safety Association has developed pedestrian safety education programs for use in primary schools. These programs address the problems of mid-block "dart-outs" and intersection dashes. Pediatricians should encourage the schools to use these programs.

Children who are exposed to the danger of roadways at night should wear retroflective material.* It may be purchased as an integral part of garments to be worn at night, as strips of tape that can be sewn on a garment, or as an adhesive tape. The AAP's Committee on Injury and Poison Prevention supports the concept of "reflecting" pedestrians and

*Retroreflective material is produced by the 3M Company and is available from many retailers, such as the J.C. Penney Co.

Table 23-3 1994 Shopping Guide to Child Restraint Devices*

Manufacturer/Name	Harness type or belt position	Safety features	Price range
Infant seats (birth to 20 lbs unless noted)			
Century 565 series	3-pt harness	Correct recline indicator; labels in Eng/Sp/Fr; harness adjustor located on back of seat	$40-$60
Century 590 series	3-pt harness	Detachable base; can be used without base in second car; correct recline indicator; labels in Eng/Sp/Fr; harness adjustor located on back of seat	$50-$70
Cosco Dream Ride	3-pt harness	To 17-20 lbs (depending on mfg date); can be used as car bed side-facing or as car seat rear-facing; harness adjustor located on top back of seat	$59
Cosco TLC	3-pt harness	Harness adjustor located on front of seat	$25
Evenflo Dyn-O-Mite	3-pt harness	Shoulder belt wraps around front of seat; harness adjustor located on back of seat; labels in Eng/Sp	$25-$35
Evenflo Joy Ride	3-pt harness	Shoulder belt wraps around front of seat; harness adjustor located in compartment behind seat	$30-$45
Evenflo Travel Tandem	3-pt harness	Detachable base; can be used without base in second car; harness adjustor located in compartment behind seat	$45
Fisher-Price Infant Car Seat	T-Shield	Correct recline indicator; padded shield, less suitable for very small infants; harness adjustor located on back of seat	$50
Gerry Guard With Glide	3-pt harness	Can be used as glider in the house; must be converted to in-car position; harness adjustor located on back of seat	$49-$59
Gerry Secure Ride	3-pt harness	Correct recline indicator; harness adjustor located on back of seat	$39-$49
Infant Rider Car Seat (Kolcraft)	3-pt harness	To 18 lbs only; harness adjustor located on back of seat	$50-$60
Kolcraft Rock 'N Ride	3-pt harness	To 18 lbs only; no harness height adjustment; optional detachable base; can be used without base in second car; harness adjustor located on back of seat	$29-$50
Convertible seats (birth up to approximately 40 lbs)			
Babyhood Mfg Baby Sitter	5-pt harness	Harness adjustors located on sides of base	$79
Century 1000 STE	5-pt harness	One-strap harness adjustor located on front of base; labels in Eng/Sp/Fr; adjustable crotch buckle position	$50-90
Century 2000 STE	T-Shield	One-strap harness adjustor located on front of base; labels in Eng/Sp/Fr; adjustable crotch buckle position	$60-90
Century 3000 STE	Tray Shield	One-strap harness adjustor located on front of base; labels in Eng/Sp/Fr; adjustable crotch buckle position	$70-100
Century 5000 STE	Tray Shield	One-strap harness adjustor located on front of base; labels in Eng/Sp/Fr; adjustable crotch buckle position	$70-100
Century Nexus	5-pt/Tray Shield	Adjustable shield grows with child; labels in Eng/Sp/Fr	$80-110
Cosco 5-pt, Luxury 5-pt	5-pt harness	One-strap harness adjustor located on front of seat	$49-89
Cosco Comfort Ride	Tray Shield	One-strap harness adjustor located on front of seat	$69-89
Cosco Soft Shield	T-Shield	One-strap harness adjustor located on front of seat	$69
Cosco Touriva 5-pt	5-pt harness	Overhead shield/harness with 2-piece harness retainer	$49-59
Cosco Touriva LXS	T-Shield	2-piece harness retainer	$99
Cosco Touriva DXO, Luxury Touriva LXO	Tray Shield	2-piece harness retainer; adjustable shield (luxury model)	$69-119
Evenflo Champion	Tray Shield	Optional tether available; one-strap harness adjustor located on front of base	$50-70
Evenflo Scout	T-Shield/5-pt harness	Comes in either 5-pt or T-Shield; optional tether available; one-strap harness adjustor located on front of base	$40-60
Evenflo Trooper	Tray Shield	Harness adjustor located on front of base	$50-70
Evenflo Ultara I, Premier	Tray Shield	One-strap harness adjustor located on front of base; adjustable shield	$65-110
Evenflo Ultara V, Premier	5-pt harness	One-strap harness adjustor located on front of base	$60-90

Modified from the American Academy of Pediatrics: *1994 Family shopping guide to infant/child safety seats,* Elk Grove Village, Ill, 1994, The Academy.
*All products listed meet the current requirements of Federal Motor Vehicle Safety Standard 213-80 (new restraint models are in *italics*).

Table 23-3 1994 Shopping Guide to Child Restraint Devices*—cont'd

Manufacturer/Name	Harness type or belt position	Safety features	Price range
Convertible seats (birth up to approximately 40 lbs)—cont'd			
Fisher-Price Bolster	Tray Shield	Automatic harness adjustment	$97
Fisher-Price Car Seat With T-Shield	T-Shield	Automatic harness adjustment	$87
Gerry Guard Securelock	Tray Shield	Automatic harness adjustment; buckle on stalk that opens forward	$69-89
Gerry Pro-Tech	5-pt harness	Automatic harness adjustment	$59-69
Kolcraft Auto-Mate	5-pt harness	Harness adjustment knobs on both sides, requires 2-handed operation	$50-70
Kolcraft Traveler 700	Tray Shield	Harness adjustment knobs on both sides, requires 2-handed operation	$50-100
Renolux GT 2000	5-pt harness	Harness adjustors on back of seat	$60
Renolux GT 3000	5-pt harness	Harness adjustors on back of seat	$80
Renolux GT 4000	5-pt harness	Harness adjustors on back of seat	$70
Renolux GT 5000, 5500 Turn-a-Tot	5-pt harness	Harness adjustors on back of seat; seat swivels on base	$90-100
Safeline Sit 'N Stroll	5-pt harness	Harness adjustors located on back of seat; labels in Eng/Sp/Fr/Jpn; converts to stroller	$139-159
Vests and integral seats (20-25 lbs and up)			
E-Z-On Vest (25 + lbs)	4-pt harness	Tether strap must be installed in vehicle	$62
Little Cargo Travel Vest (25-40 lbs)	5-pt harness	Simplified strap-buckle system; auto lap belt attached through padded stress plate	$39-49
Chrysler Integral Child Seat (20-40 lbs; Booster 40+ lbs)	5-pt harness	Two built-in seats optional in minivans, one converts to a belt-positioning booster for larger child; one seat available in some sedans, 5-pt harness adjusts to fit child 20-65 lbs	$100-200
Ford Built-In Child Seat (1 yr-60 lbs)	5-pt harness	Two built-in seats optional in minivans	$224
GM Integrated Child Seat (20-40 lbs; booster 40-60 lbs)	5-pt harness	Manual harness adjustment; rear seat safety belt comfort guide available in some models	$125-225
Booster seats† (After convertible/toddler seat is outgrown)			
Century Breverra	Belt through base when used with shield	Removable shield for use as a belt-positioning booster seat with a lap/shoulder belt; shield for use with lap belt; high-back style; labels in Eng/Sp/Fr	$60-80
Cosco Explorer	Wrap around	Shield for use with lap belt; two seat heights	$25-35
Fisher-Price T-Shield Car Seat	Wrap around	Removable shield for use as a belt-positioning booster seat with a lap/shoulder belt, 30-60 lbs; shield with crotch post for use with a lap belt, 40-60 lbs	$44
Gerry Double Guard	Belt through base when used with shield	Removable shield for use as a belt-positioning booster seat with a lap/shoulder belt; shield for use with lap belt; internal lap strap with shield	$45-55
Kolcraft Tot Rider II	Wrap around	Removable shield for use as a belt-positioning booster seat with a lap/shoulder belt; shield with crotch post that opens forward for use with a lap belt	$25-35

†List does not include belt-positioning booster seats without shields for children over 50 pounds.

bicycle-riding children, and these measures deserve implementation.

Driveway Injuries

Pedestrian fatalities in children under age 5 are most likely to result from a parent backing over a child in the driveway. The pediatrician should emphasize to the parents the danger in allowing children to play in driveways. Following are some *family automotive safety tips:*

1. Before the car moves:
   a. All seat belts should be fastened and all restraining devices secured.
   b. All doors should be locked.
   c. All children not in approved restraining devices should be in the back seat.
   d. No heavy or sharp objects should be placed on the seat with children. Groceries should be put in the trunk.
2. Nothing should be carried on the shelf under the back window.
3. Children should never be left alone in the car and should never be allowed to play in one.
4. Rules for behavior in the car should be made to ensure that the driver is not distracted. A toy, book, or some other item should be taken along to keep children quietly occupied.
5. Children should not be allowed to put their arms, legs, or heads out the window.
6. If the driveway is the only play area for children, a car may be parked at the entrance to prevent other drivers from pulling in quickly without noticing the children (e.g., drivers turning around or a parent coming home).

Drinking and Driving

It is estimated that half of all automobile fatalities are related to ethanol consumption. Although ethanol is not a stimulant, it may appear to have such action because it relaxes the individual by depressing the central nervous system's higher centers, resulting in uninhibited behavior; however, it also depresses the reflexes vital to driving.

Although ethanol reactions vary depending on the rate of consumption, the presence of food in the stomach, and the person's mood at the time of consumption, guidelines can be used to convey to drivers the dangers of ethanol consumption and driving (Table 23-4). At a blood ethanol level of 80 mg/dl (now being considered for the legal limit in many states), the chance of a fatal crash increases dramatically; at 100 mg/dl, the probability of such a crash is 5 to 12 times that for the nondrinking driver.

Ethanol is metabolized at a rate of 12 to 20 mg/dl/hr; drinking coffee, taking a cold shower, or exercising will not increase this rate or decrease the ethanol impairment or depression resulting from consumption. Before driving it is wise to wait at least 1 hour for each drink consumed. Driver education programs in schools have not succeeded in reducing injury rates among teenage drivers. Collisions occur 2½ times more often among drivers under age 18 than among those over age 18. Drinking may play a role in this fact.

BICYCLE INJURIES[13,27,57]

The bicycle heads the list of hazardous products in the United States, according to the Consumer Product Safety Commission's National Electronic Injury Surveillance System (NEISS). NEISS' data indicate that 1 million bicycle-related injuries occur each year; the agency estimated that in 1991 more than 600,000 bicycle injuries were seen in hospital emergency departments.

In 1992, 110 million bicycles were in use in the United States. Of the 700 deaths reported in association with their use, 39% occurred in the birth to 14 age group. The proportion of deaths among children under age 14 has declined steadily from 78% in 1960 to 39% in 1992, reflecting a change in the use and ownership of bicycles. However, this fact offers little comfort, inasmuch as the total number of deaths has risen because of the greater number of bicycles in use. Approximately 90% of bicycle deaths result from collisions with motor vehicles.

Estimates of the annual number of bicycle injuries that require medical attention or that result in one or more days of restricted activity have ranged from 180,000 to as high as 1 million; the largest proportion of those injured are children. The accident rate for young riders 5 to 12 years of age averages 2% annually, and it is estimated that 20% of the accidents result in fractures and 5% in concussions.

In a study of 107 bicycle mishaps involving children[27] (20% of which resulted from collision with an automobile), head trauma was found to be the most common injury. This finding prompted the authors of the study to suggest passage of laws requiring bicycle riders to wear helmets similar to those used by motorcycle riders, and many states have passed such laws.

National advocates for children's safety have urged that bicycle helmets become standard equipment for every ride and that parents buy the helmet along with the bike. Lightweight helmets approved by the American National Standards Institute or the Snell Memorial Foundation are available for children at reasonable prices.

Table 23-4 Effects of Alcoholic Drinks

Blood ethanol level (mg/dl)	Physical effect	Number of drinks: Cocktail (1½ oz) (50% ethanol)	Beer (12 oz) (5% ethanol)	Wine (5 oz) (12% ethanol)	Hours needed to metabolize alcohol
20	Pleasant feeling	1	1	1	1-2
50	Relaxed	1½	1½	1½	2-3
100	Impaired (legal definition)	3	3	3	5-7
150	Intoxicated	4	4½	4½	7-10
300	Drunk	8	9	9	15-20
500	Dead	14	15	15	—

A community-wide bicycle helmet campaign in Seattle increased helmet use among school-age children from 5.5% in 1987 to 40.2% in 1992. In one health maintenance organization, the number of head injuries declined by 66.6% in the 5 to 9 age group and by 67.6% in the 10 to 14 age group.[49]

Factors Involved in Bicycle Injuries

Three factors account for most bicycle injuries:

1. *Horseplay.* Daredevil feats by young boys imitating Evel Knievel's exploits have led to an increase in injuries.
2. *Riding double* with a passenger on the handlebars, the crossbar of the frame, or the rear fender with no support for the feet results in a large number of "bicycle spoke" injuries, which deserve special mention. In this type of injury, the tissue is lacerated from the knifelike action of the spokes, the foot is crushed between the wheel and the frame, and a shearing injury results from a combination of these two forces. The injury may not be fully recognized on initial examination because damage to the underlying structures can take several hours to appear. This type of injury needs careful observation, as with wringer arm injuries.[33]
3. *Poor-fitting bicycles* are overrepresented in injuries involving a motor vehicle and bicycle collision. The bicycle seat should be no higher than the rider's hips so that the feet can touch the ground without causing the bicycle to lean.

Remedies to Reduce Injuries

Bicycles need design changes in the wheels (e.g., shields to prevent contact with the spokes), flat surfaces where the handlebars join the fork to prevent loosening, and professional assembly rather than do-it-yourself kits. Use of reflective paint would make the entire bicycle more visible at night.

Requiring riders to prove their proficiency through an examination and licensing before being allowed on public roads should be considered, and children under age 9 should not be allowed to use public highways. Laws or regulations requiring helmets would reduce the number and severity of head injuries.

The Consumer Product Safety Commission (CPSC) has set bicycle safety standards for brakes, seats, tires, reflectors, front fork frames, and steering systems, and the agency recommends a predelivery road test.

Safe Bicycling

Bicycle riders require education and training to avoid injuries. Loss of control by the rider has been found to be a factor in 63% of injuries. Violation of traffic rules (e.g., turning across the path of a car, disregarding signals and signs, riding against traffic, and riding into the path of a car from a driveway, alley, or intersection) plays a part in 80% of injuries.

A composite of safety suggestions from the AAP and the CPSC is shown in instructional form in the box below.

MINIBIKE, MOPED, MOTORCYCLE, AND ALL-TERRAIN VEHICLE INJURIES[6]

The CPSC estimates that 63,000 minibike-related injuries are treated in hospital emergency departments each year. Nearly half of these injuries happen to children 10 to 15 years old and 20% to those 15 to 20 years old. Males suffer 80% of the injuries. The leg is the body part most often injured (52%), followed by the arm (19%) and the head (18%).

Minibikes are particularly dangerous because of their poor handling, the product of a short wheelbase and small tires, insufficient acceleration, inadequate brakes, and small size, which reduces visibility and protects the driver in a collision inadequately. Life-threatening injuries to the larynx caused by cables and fence wire have been reported.[2] Lack of safety

SUGGESTIONS FOR SAFE BICYCLING

1. Always wear a helmet when riding a bicycle.
2. Learn and obey all traffic rules, signs, and signals.
3. Use bicycle paths when possible. Do not ride on streets that have heavy automobile traffic. When riding on the sidewalk, give pedestrians the right of way. Until age 7, ride with adult supervision and off the street.
4. If it is necessary to ride in the street, ride on the right side with the flow of traffic, not against it.
5. Walk, do not ride, the bicycle across busy intersections and around left-turn corners. Do not ride in wet weather.
6. Do not ride double. Balancing is difficult, and vision may be blocked. Spoke injuries to the foot and leg are common in passengers.
7. Do not ride barefoot; wear rubber-soled shoes and keep both feet on the pedals while riding. Avoid plastic pedals; use rubber-treated or metal pedals with serrated edges.
8. Use retroflective tape on all bikes, front and rear. For night riding, a headlight and a taillight or a red reflector on the rear are necessary, and the rider should wear light-colored clothing. Retroflective tape (white in front and red in rear) and retroflective clothing also will help the rider to be seen at night.
9. For children over 9 months of age, choose carrier seats with foot rests, foot guards, foot straps, and seat belts to prevent injuries.
10. Keep the bicycle in good condition. Be familiar with and check the brakes. Regular expert maintenance is essential for safe riding. Complicated work should be done by an experienced repairman.
11. Carefully choose a bicycle to suit the child's size and age. The seat should be no higher than the rider's hips, the feet should reach the pedals without the use of blocks, and the handlebars should be within easy reach. When sitting on the seat with hands on the handlebars, the child must be able to place the balls of both feet on the ground. Straddling the center bar, the child should be able to keep both feet flat on the ground with 1 inch of clearance between the crotch and the bar. Younger children's bicycles should have coaster brakes; hand brakes require too much strength and coordination for beginners.

devices or defective and poorly constructed components were factors in one third of 21 in-depth investigations by the CPSC.

The AAP's Joint Committee on Physical Fitness, Recreation, and Sports Medicine has urged parents to refuse to allow their children to own or operate a minibike.

Mopeds (from *mo*tor plus *ped*als) are low-speed, lightweight motorcycles that share the operating characteristics of bicycles and motorcycles. Mopeds are commonplace in Europe, and their popularity grew in the United States when fuel became scarce and expensive. Because a moped has little horsepower, its acceleration often is inadequate for city traffic, resulting in a dangerous situation. Because of its low speed, it also is inappropriate (and often illegal) for use on arterial highways and bridges and in many tunnels.

According to data from the Kentucky Department of Public Safety and the Ohio Department of Highway Safety, 83% of accidents involving mopeds cause injuries, 16% cause property damage, and 1% are fatal. Injury patterns reveal that head and lower extremity injuries are the most serious type that occur. Helmets protect the head but do not alter the incidence or severity of neck injuries. When riding on streets, moped riders can be expected to encounter the same hazards as motorcycle riders.

Most European countries now require moped riders to wear safety helmets. Both Great Britain and France, which have helmet laws, have reported a one third reduction in serious head injuries. This parallels the results of helmet use by motorcycle riders in the United States. Most states and the District of Columbia have a variety of laws governing moped use or banning them from the road. Few states, however, require the rider to wear a helmet.

Approximately 4,081,000 *motorcycles* were registered in the United States in 1992; 2700 fatalities and 135,000 injuries were estimated to be associated with their use that year. The 1992 death rate for motorcycle riders was estimated to be about 31 deaths per 100 million miles of motorcycle travel, compared with the overall motor vehicle death rate of 1.8 per 100 million miles. Accidents involving motorcycles tend to occur during the warm months, on weekends, and between noon and 4 PM and 6 and 11 PM. About 90% of the motorcyclists are male, 60% of whom are under age 25.

As a result of a federal requirement, all but three states had mandatory helmet-use laws for motorcyclists by 1975. When the federal requirement was repealed in 1976, a steady repeal of state laws began. In 1992 three states had no helmet laws and 23 had limited usage laws, which required helmets only for teenage drivers. Between 1976 and 1980, the death toll from motorcycle accidents increased 49%; more than 30% of the fatal accidents involved individuals under age 20. The protective effect of helmets has been shown at all levels of injury. Compared to riders with helmets, a rider without one is twice as likely to incur a minor head injury and five times as likely to suffer a severe or critical injury.[15]

All-terrain vehicles (ATVs) are three- or four-wheel recreational vehicles intended for off-road use on rough terrain; they originally were promoted for use by children and adolescents. More than 2.5 million of these vehicles are in use, but they are linked to more than 1000 deaths since 1982 and are associated with approximately 86,000 injuries annually. The AAP found these vehicles to be a major hazard to children and backed demands for a sales ban on and recall of the three-wheeled type. In 1983 the U.S. Justice Department and manufacturers reached an agreement that banned the sale of all three-wheeled vehicles and restricted the purchase of four-wheeled vehicles to riders over age 16.[26] However, these bans often are not enforced.

BURNS*

Burns and fires injure 1.4 million Americans each year; 40% of these are children under age 15. At least 5900 people die annually from burns, and 25% are children under age 15. House fires cause 75% of all burn-related deaths, with young children and older adults at highest risk. About 50% of all fires involve cigarettes, often with associated alcohol consumption.

Burns rank second as the cause of death (behind motor vehicle deaths) in the 1 to 4 age group and third behind motor vehicle accidents and drowning in the 5 to 14 age group. The annual death rate from fire in the United States reached a low of 1.6 per 100,000 population in 1992, but it still exceeds that of every other industrialized nation.

The vectors of burn injury have been classified as combustible materials, hot substances, electrical sources, and chemical compounds. According to Galveston Shriner's Burn Institute,[12,24] combustible substances such as flammable fabrics are the leading cause of major burn injuries. Flammable fabrics, usually cotton dresses or nightgowns, are a factor in 54% of burns and flammable liquids in 35%. A Duke University study[14] classified the causes of burns thus: 55% resulting from clothing ignition, 25% from direct contact with fires, 15% from gasoline or kerosene ignition, and 5% from scalds. Older adults and the very young are the most thin-skinned individuals, and what might produce only a second-degree burn in a hairy young man may well produce a third-degree burn in them. The young (under age 10) and older adults (over age 65) were injured in 1 out of 7 burn incidents in which they were involved, but those in the 11 to 65 age group were injured in only 1 out of 25 such incidents.

Flammable Fabrics[8]

Clothing ignition now causes only about 200 deaths a year, mostly among older adults. The importance of clothing ignition burns lies in their severity; the mortality is four times as high, the surface area burned is twice as large, the hospital stay is 50% longer, and the medical expenses are twice those of burns that do not involve clothing ignition. As a result of legislation covering flammable fabrics and a change in the style and fabrics used for sleepwear and children's clothing, the incidence of clothing ignitions that cause significant burns in children has been reduced markedly—this is one of the success stories in injury prevention. However, the pediatrician should continue to remind parents that the risk of burns is much greater with clothing that is not made out of flame-retardant material.

Most fire-related deaths occur at night and are caused by inhalation of smoke or toxic gas. Smoke detectors, which save lives, should be installed on each floor, particularly in furnace and sleeping areas. Those living in the house should

*References 7, 8, 12, 20, 24, 55.

PREVENTION OF BURN INJURIES

The pediatrician should:

1. Urge parents to "fireproof" their children. Ask the parents, "How safe are the clothes your children wear?" and encourage them to buy flame-retardant clothing. Also ask, "How safe are the fabrics on the windows, walls, furniture, and floors in your home?"
2. Emphasize that steps must be taken to protect those most likely to get burned—the very young, the handicapped, and older adults.
3. Inform the parents that cotton is the fabric most often involved in clothing ignition mishaps; they also should know the time (3 to 9 PM), season (winter), and place (kitchen) that burns are mostly likely to occur.
4. Evaluate for situations that make certain children more vulnerable (e.g., hyperactivity, separated or divorced parents, large family, working mother, crowded living conditions). Obese boys are reported to be more vulnerable to severe burns than nonobese ones.
5. Warn parents that smoking in bed and improper disposal of ashes or butts are dangerous to children sleeping in adjacent rooms because they may be trapped in a fire.

The pediatrician should instruct the parents to:

1. Install smoke detectors in every sleeping area and at the head of every stairway.
2. Make sure the house has several fire escape routes and that every family member knows what he or she should do in case of a fire. Never leave children under age 10 alone in the house; they are helpless victims.
3. Store and use flammable materials properly. Never use flammable liquids near a source of flame. In starting a charcoal fire, use only labeled charcoal starters and ensure good ventilation. Do not store gasoline in the trunk of a car. Buy minimal amounts of flammable liquids, keep them tightly capped (*never* use glass containers), and store them out of children's reach.
4. Inspect electrical equipment periodically for defective wiring.
5. Do not use defective heating equipment or improper cooking utensils.
6. Use extreme caution with steam vaporizers or pots, which can cause severe burns if overturned. Steam vaporizers heat the water to 176° F (80° C). Cool mist vaporizers (which have a central core that heats only a small amount of water) are safer but must be kept very clean to prevent the spread of water-borne bacteria.
7. Keep electrical cords out of children's reach. Pulling over automatic coffee makers, electrical skillets, and other equipment with cords is a common cause of burns in children.
8. Never leave a child alone in a bathtub; drowning or scalding could occur.
9. Do not drink hot beverages while holding or caring for a baby.
10. Make sure camping tents are made of flame-retardant material.
11. Modify igniters or combustibles as shown in the table below. Household appliances were the major source of more than 373,500 fires.

Hazard	Modification
Matches	Devise childproof containers and striking surfaces
Gasoline	Store safely and use appropriately
Space heaters	Guard, vent, maintain, and locate safely
Water heaters	Make sure no flammable liquids are stored nearby
Scalding tap water	Modify thermostats so that scalding temperatures cannot be reached; keep water heater temperature between 120° and 130° F (49° and 55° C).
Stoves	When buying a stove, look for (1) recessed burners, which keep pots more stable; (2) controls located at the back of the range rather than on the front; (3) burners located near the back of the range so that pan handles do not overhang and reaching across lighted burners is unnecessary If buying such a stove is not possible, use back burners as much as possible and keep pan handles turned away from the edge of the stove
Clothing and furnishings	Use flame-retardant fabrics for people of all ages.

know all escape routes well so that it takes no more than 4 minutes after a fire alarm sounds to get out of the house. (The box above presents, in instructional form, tips for preventing burn injuries.)

Scalds

Scalds often are the cause of children being hospitalized with burns. Most scalds are caused by spilled coffee or tea, tipped-over stove pots, splattered hot grease, and other hot foods. Prevention of these scalding burns depends predominantly on informed parents and adequate supervision of children. Turning pot handles so that they cannot be reached is part of burn prevention.

Each year an estimated 3500 people require treatment in the emergency department for tap water scalds. The most common victims are infants and toddlers, and these burns result in a high incidence of hospitalization, scarring, and death. At 150° F (65° C), deep second- or third-degree burns occur within 2 seconds. Tap water temperature is related to the burn hazard, which rises sharply with water temperatures above 130° F (55° C). The CPSC has developed a voluntary *new* tub and shower installation standard that requires antiscald devices that limit water flow at temperatures above 120° F (49° C); existing plumbing fixtures cannot be so equipped. One fourth of tap water burns, however, do not occur in the bathtub or shower.[7,55]

The CPSC has been petitioned to approve regulations limiting new home water heaters to a maximum temperature of

130° F (55° C). If a family has infants or toddlers, the pediatrician should recommend setting the water heater thermostat between 120° and 130° F (49° and 55° C).

Electrical Burns and Injuries[56]

In 1987 760 accidental deaths were attributed to contact with an electrical current. In 1972 the federal Department of Health, Education, and Welfare analyzed 212 electrical injuries and found that 103 cases (48.6%) involved burns, 19 cases (8.9%) involved electric shock, and 90 cases (42.5%) involved mechanical injuries. Of the total, 122 cases (57.5%) involved children under age 14.

In young children, electrical injuries most often are caused by mouthing of a plugged-in extension cord's recipient end; the second most common cause of injury is chewing on a poorly insulated wire. In a series of 54 cases reported by Gifford and colleagues,[23] 83% required revision of the burns through plastic surgery. High-voltage injuries most often occur among boys between the ages of 7 and 16 years and frequently involve risky activities.

The number of fatal injuries involving electricity begins to rise in the late spring and reaches its peak in the summer months, with more than 40% occurring from June to August. It is believed that perspiration, which occurs more in the warmer weather, increases the body's conduction of electrical energy. More than 25% of deaths from contact with an electrical current occur in the home.

Prevention. The following precautions can help prevent electrical burns and injuries:

1. An extension cord that is not in use should never be left plugged into a socket.
2. Plastic caps should cover all unused electrical outlets.
3. Wiring should be inspected periodically and broken plugs or poorly insulated wires replaced.
4. Older children should be taught about the hazards of an electrical current, particularly with regard to water.
5. All holiday lights should be placed out of the reach of toddlers, who tend to bite on them.

Treatment. The unique feature of electrical mouth burns is the serious bleeding that can occur from erosion of the labial artery in the first 3 weeks after the injury (seen in 25% of the cases). This condition demands very careful observation, preferably in a hospital, to prevent exsanguinating hemorrhage. Suture ligatures may be needed to control the bleeding.[23,56]

EYE INJURIES[3,32,38] (see Chapters 236 and 237)

It is estimated that 50,000 needless eye injuries occur each year; home, recreation, and automobile accidents pose the greatest danger. Sixty-six percent of ocular injuries occur in children age 16 or younger. More eyes are lost in the first decade of life than in any subsequent decade; a third of these losses arise from injuries that are largely preventable.

In 1972 the government mandated protection for the 100 million Americans who wear prescription glasses and the many millions more who wear sunglasses. The Food and Drug Administration (FDA) issued a regulation requiring all eyeglass and sunglass lenses manufactured after January 1972 to be impact resistant. A lens is considered impact resistant if it passes the "drop-ball test," which consists of dropping a ⅝-inch steel ball weighing approximately 0.5 ounce on the lens from a height of 50 inches.

Physicians can offer important guidance in this injury-conducive area. They can promote safety programs that stress the importance of proper use of safety glasses in school chemistry and industrial laboratories; encourage hobby shops not to sell hobby products that can cause eye injury unless safety glasses are sold also; and urge that sunlamps be sold only with protective glasses.

Program planning can include meetings with ophthalmologists, optometrists, school authorities, school nurses, and representatives from the National Society for the Prevention of Blindness. At these programs, speakers can distribute educational pamphlets; suggest modification of potentially dangerous products; seek the banning of specific hazards, such as fireworks; and advance good first aid treatment of eye injuries in the home, emergency department, and physician's office. (The box on p. 279 presents, in instructional form, preventive measures the pediatrician can discuss with parents and older children, as well first aid measures for physician treatment of eye injuries).

FALLS AND INFANT AND JUVENILE INJURIES CAUSED BY FURNITURE[36,51]

The NSC reported 12,400 deaths from falls in 1992. Of these, 140 involved children under age 14. Falls are the second highest cause of injury-related death in the general population and the sixth highest cause in children.

In infancy, falls most often start to occur at 7 to 7½ months of age, when infants begin to roll from a prone to a supine position, to sit up, to pull up to a standing position, and to climb.

A recent study of 536 infants showed an incidence of falls of 47.5% in the first year of life. If this incidence were found in the national population, about 1.75 million infants could be expected to sustain at least one fall during the first year of life. The most common preventable fall involved a baby climbing out of a crib.[36] Lyons and Oates[40] reviewed the hospital records of 207 children under age 6 who were documented as having fallen from a crib or bed. They found that falls from short distances are unlikely to cause serious injury, and that the reliability of the history should be assessed carefully if such a fall does produce a significant injury.

Crib Injuries and Prevention

The CPSC estimates that more than 100 infants die every year of injuries involving nursery equipment. About 40,000 infants are injured seriously enough to require treatment in a hospital emergency department. Most of these injuries occur when infants fall while climbing out of their cribs. Others occur as a result of poor crib design. (The box on p. 280 presents, in instructional form, a list of safety tips the pediatrician can urge parents to keep in mind when choosing, setting up, and equipping a crib.)

Nearly all fatalities result from strangulation, which occurs when the baby's head and neck become wedged between the crib slats.

An infant should never be left in a crib with the side rails down. The mattress should be lowered before the baby can sit unassisted and should be set at its lowest position as soon

EYE INJURIES: PREVENTION AND FIRST AID

Prevention

1. Emphasize that safety glasses should be worn for work or recreational activities that may endanger the eyes, especially in school laboratories and shops and for certain sports. Special protective glasses are particularly important for arc welding, metal hammering, tanning (using either sunlight or a sunlamp), and activities in which snow-reflected sunlight will be a factor.
2. Warn parents and children about the dangers of pointed sticks, pellet guns, bows and arrows, BB guns, air rifles, slingshots, and fireworks. Urge parents to teach their children never to point things at one another or at other people.
3. Advise parents to make sure their children's eyeglasses have safety lenses and frames; this rule applies to all types of glasses, including those worn for recreation (e.g., sunglasses).
4. Teach parents to warn their children against gazing at the sun. An eclipse is especially dangerous because the sunspot blocks out the visible rays, which usually deter people from looking at the sun; however, the infrared rays, which are just as damaging, are still present. Media attention to this hazard has reduced the number of retinal burns in children and adults, but safe viewing techniques should be publicized before and during each occurrence.
5. Warn parents against placing young babies in direct sunlight.
6. Urge parents to teach their children the proper use of potentially hazardous items, such as glass doors. When children are old enough to use hazardous equipment (e.g., lawn mowers, power tools), they must be taught the proper use of these items as well.

First aid

1. If possible, do not use a topical anesthetic, which may delay healing. If one must be used, warn the parents about loss of the protective reflex (blinking).
2. Always evaluate vision after an eye injury that requires first aid.
3. Always refer to an ophthalmologist any patient who has an abnormality of the pupil.
4. Bear in mind that corneal injuries are serious; fluorescein staining often is needed to determine the extent of injury.
5. Use fluorescein strips instead of bottles of fluorescein dye, which may act as a culture medium for bacterial growth.
6. For chemical burns of the eye, immediately irrigate the eyes with copious amounts of tap water or normal saline, and continue to irrigate for 15 minutes to 1 hour; then seek ophthalmological consultation.

as the infant can stand. No toys or other articles that can be used as steps in climbing out should be left in the crib.

No crib toys in which the child could get tangled should hang within reach, and an infant should not wear necklaces of any type. The crib should not be used as a playpen, and the child should be transferred to a juvenile bed once the height of the side rail is less than three fourths of the child's height or when the child is 35 inches tall.

Other Furniture Safety

It is important to be aware of the hazards and safety features of juvenile furnishings other than the crib.

Selection and Safe Use of Bunk Beds. Bunk beds should have rounded edges, tight-fitting mattresses, a ladder that grips the frame firmly without slipping, and a secured guardrail without open spaces. The beds should be placed in a corner of the room so that there are walls on two of the four sides, the guardrails should be in place at all times, and the ladder always should be used. Younger children should use the lower bunk, and rough play should be forbidden. A low-wattage nightlight should be kept on so that children can see the ladder if they need to get up to go to the bathroom.

Dressing Tables. Stable, concave dressing tables that have guardrails are preferred.

High Chairs. According to the CPSC, in 1974 an estimated 7000 children fell from high chairs and required treatment in a hospital emergency department; most were under age 4, and 25% were under 1 year of age.

A high chair should be stable and not easily pushed or tipped over; it also should not fold up while the child is in the chair. The child should be properly and securely strapped in the chair and should not be allowed to stand in it. Children should not be left unattended, and older brothers and sisters should not climb on the high chair. The chair should not be kept near counters and tables from which the child could push and tip over the high chair.

Infant Carriers (Plastic-type Seat). The carrier must be stable; it should have a wide base and a nonskid surface on the bottom. Also, it should be wide enough to allow separation of the infant's thighs. The carrier should never be placed on a chair, counter, or table or be used as a car seat; however, many of the car seats recommended by the AAP have a base that can be detached, allowing the seat to be safely used as an infant carrier. The belts or restraining devices provided should be used, and the infant should never be left unattended. The carrier should have a label warning against leaving the seat on an elevated surface and also specifying the maximum weight and age for its use.

Note: A young infant is safest in the parent's arms except when traveling in a vehicle. Mothers have been known to fall and completely protect the baby in their arms, whereas they have reflexively dropped the carrier, with the baby in it, to protect themselves.

Jumpers and Walkers. More than 55% of infants in the United States are placed in walkers before they begin to walk. However, walkers have not been shown to enhance walking, and the risk of serious injury associated with their use is significant. In 1980, baby walkers accounted for an estimated 23,900 injuries that required treatment; most of the victims were under age 2. Half of the infants who used walkers had at least one accident involving a tipover, a fall down stairs, or finger entrapment. In one 15-month observation period,

RECOMMENDATIONS FOR CRIB SAFETY

1. Make sure both side rails have 12 slats, which are no more than 2⅜ inches apart. The side rails should have no crossbars or toeholds, and when fully lowered, they should extend 4 inches above the mattress. The side rails also should have a safe, hand-operated locking latch that cannot be released accidentally. Corner posts (finials) should be less than ⅝-inch high, and a new crib should have a label stating that it meets federal crib standards. (Many of these recommendations became law on Feb. 1, 1974.)

   Make sure that cribs received as hand-me-downs or family heirlooms, which may not conform to the current standards, are modified to ensure the child's safety.
2. Test the crib mattress to make sure it fits snugly; if more than two fingers can be inserted between it and the sides of the crib, the mattress is too small. The side rails should be at least 22 inches high from the top of the rail to the mattress.
3. Check to be sure wood surfaces are free of splinters and cracks and that no lead paint was used anywhere on the crib. Any metal parts must be safe and have smooth, blunt edges. Make sure no plastic bells or balls are used as ornaments, and that the crib has no decorative cut-out spaces that could entrap the baby's limbs or head.
4. Use bumper pads (with at least six straps or ties) inside the crib around all four sides until the baby starts to pull up to a standing position—at which point the pads should be removed.
5. Buy the crib with the greatest distance between the top of the side rail and the mattress. Extenders, if used, should have narrowly spaced slats (i.e., 2⅜ inches apart or less), should extend no higher than the end panels, and should not have nuts and bolts that can be easily removed.
6. Do not place the crib near windows, where the child might grasp or become entangled in the pull cords for drapes or venetian blinds.

coil spring–activated devices were reported to have caused 21 amputations or near-amputations of fingers.

In view of the risks, pediatricians should strongly advise parents not to use walkers. If walkers are used, they should have covered coil springs and locking devices that prevent collapse. The wheelbase should be longer and wider than the frame, and the walker should be used only on flat surfaces away from carpets, door thresholds, and stairways.

Safety Gates. Installation of firmly attached, permanently mounted safety gates at the top and bottom of all stairways is recommended to deter toddlers from dangerous explorative forays. However, accordion-style gates or expandable enclosures with large, V-shaped openings along the top edge or diamond-shaped openings within are dangerous, posing the risk of head entrapment, and should never be used.

Falls from Windows. In 1967, falls from heights accounted for 20% of accidental deaths among children in New York City; 67% of these children were under age 5. Between 1965 and 1969, 125 children under age 15 were killed by a fall from a window. Of these, 113 were under age 5.[51] To prevent such falls all screens should be secure, but this should not be depended upon as the sole measure. Handles should be removed from windows. Windows should be opened only from the top or only 4 to 5 inches from the bottom and secured at the desired height with a window "burglar lock," which can be obtained at any hardware store. Window guards are the most effective tools. In 1970, New York City enacted an ordinance requiring installation of window guards in apartments housing children under age 10. This law produced a marked decline in deaths from falls from windows. A recent resurgence of falls, however, indicates a need for compliance surveillance.

A child's bed, crib, or other furniture should never be placed next to or under a window. Balconies and fire escapes should be secured.

FIREARM INJURIES[5]

In the United States in 1992, 1400 people were killed accidentally by firearms. Of these, 200 were children under age 15, and 500 were 15 to 24 years of age. Firearms injure 8000 children and teenagers each year, leaving 25% permanently disabled. Prevention programs for firearm accidents often emphasize the hazard to hunters, but fewer than 600 of the deaths were in this category; 700 deaths occurred at home, many while children were cleaning or playing with guns.

Educational efforts emphasizing safer use of firearms have not proved very effective. Efforts to keep guns from young children are not likely to succeed if widespread public ownership of guns continues at the current rate, with approximately 200 million guns in American homes.

The death rate from unintentional shootings is highest for teenage boys 14 to 18 years of age. For all ages combined, the male death rate is 6½ times the female rate. The death rate from unintentional shootings is four times higher in remote rural areas than in central cities, whereas the homicide rate is more than twice as high in central cities. Protection is the major reason given for gun ownership, but studies indicate that handguns in the home are more likely to be used in unintentional shootings, homicides committed by relatives and acquaintances, and suicides.

Preventive measures must address the issues of reducing the availability and accessibility of firearms, altering the characteristics of ammunition and weapons, and making guns more difficult to fire. Prevention of firearm injuries should not have to wait for shameful events such as mass shootings or the assassination of a president to highlight the carnage occurring daily; firearm injuries often involve the vital organs, leaving the victim little chance of survival.

Home Safety Precautions

All guns should be kept unloaded and under lock and key, and they should be equipped with trigger locks. They should be stored out of sight of casual visitors and away from children's play areas. All ammunition should be locked up in a location separate from the firearms. During handling, guns always should be checked carefully to make sure they are unloaded, and the muzzle always should be pointed in a safe direction. Horseplay with firearms is strictly forbidden. Gas, air, and spring-operated guns also are hazards to children.

Air Gun Injuries

When used by children, air guns are potentially lethal. Regulations are ineffective, and parents know little about these weapons. Multiple-pump air rifles have a muzzle velocity far exceeding the power of the old BB guns.

Approximately 30,000 persons each year are treated in hospital emergency departments for BB and pellet gun–related injuries. An estimated 3.2 million nonpowder guns are sold in the United States each year; 10 deaths were recorded between 1972 and 1980. Those injured usually are boys between 10 and 14 years of age.

The classic Daisy single-lever action (spring compression type) has an average muzzle velocity of 83.8 to 106.7 ft/sec, which limits serious injury to the eye. On the other hand, the multiple-pump rifles, BB guns, and pellet guns that use compressed air to propel steel BBs or lead pellets can attain a compression muzzle velocity of more than 650 ft/sec.

Most of the deaths caused by air guns result from intracranial injury caused by penetration of the orbit or the child's thin frontal bone. Penetrations of the thorax and other anatomical areas also have caused death.

The air gun must be regarded as a lethal weapon and should not be used by children without direct supervision. Stricter laws are needed to regulate the sale and use of air rifles by children.

PREVENTION OF SLEDDING INJURIES

1. Sleds should be sturdy and have no sharp, jagged edges or rivets. They should have a protective guard or bumper, a good steering mechanism, and rounded runners without sharp end hooks.
2. Communities should set aside supervised areas that are reserved for sledding. If special areas are not available, parents should select safe locations that are free of holes, large rocks, stumps, trees, fences, or posts; they should not allow their children to sled on streets, driveways, or highways.
3. A safe time should be chosen for sledding.
4. Children should be taught how to handle a sled. Both arms and legs should be on the sled. Knowing how to stop is essential; this can be accomplished by dragging the feet, dropping a hat under the runner, rolling off the sled onto the ground while cradling the face and head, steering into a snowbank, or making a sharp right turn.
5. When using sled runs, children should keep to the right, wait for a clear path before starting, and move quickly off the slope and out of the path of others.
6. Sleds should be kept in good condition by drying them before storing, rubbing the runners and metal parts with candle wax, and lubricating metal bolts with oil.
7. Sleds should never be used near or with automobiles. Hitching rides on automobiles should be illegal.
8. No sledding should be allowed on ice ponds.

FIREWORKS INJURIES

An estimated 11,390 injuries associated with fireworks occurred in 1991. More than half of these injuries were burns or lacerations, and many occurred in children under age 15. The most frequently injured part of the body was the arm, including the hand and fingers. Some injuries were quite severe, involving loss of hearing, sight, or a limb. Approximately five deaths annually result from fireworks injuries.

Since 1972, the AAP has been on record as supporting the petition by the National Association for the Prevention of Blindness to ban all fireworks except those used for public displays. This ban should include the popular sparkler, which often is erroneously considered a safe alternative to fireworks. An ignited sparkler can reach a searing temperature of 1800° F (982° C); and sparklers account for 6% of fireworks injuries.

SLED, SNOW DISK, AND SNOWMOBILE INJURIES

Each year approximately 23,000 people require treatment in hospital emergency departments for sled injuries; snow disks cause about 1200 injuries. As many as 300 children are killed each year in sledding accidents, and many more are seriously injured. These injuries are associated with mechanical and structural design problems (e.g., poor or no steering devices, flimsy materials), coupled with poor riding conditions, loss of control, and collision (without protection) with automobiles, other sleds, or stationary objects.

The first snowfall often brings with it an influx of injured people into hospital emergency departments and physicians' offices. Plans for safe sledding should be made before the snow appears (see the box above), along with plans for snow removal.

In 1985 the CPSC recorded 12,687 injuries related to use of snowmobiles; 2200 occurred in children under age 14. Collisions with fixed objects and other moving vehicles and drownings were the most common causes of fatalities; in nonfatal injuries the most common causes were collisions and "overturns." Most victims died of head injuries, with drowning a close second. Frostbite also is a major risk with this activity.

Safety features have been suggested to reduce accidents and the extent of injury, such as wearing a helmet, face shield, snowmobile suit, and ear protection against noise. The snowmobile should be prohibited on highways, and a minimum age should be set for drivers. Paradoxically, the injury rate appears to increase with the driver's experience.

TOY INJURIES[39,54]

The CPSC estimated that in 1991, 163,000 people required emergency department treatment for toy-related injuries. However, toy injuries account for only 1% of accidental deaths.

The CPSC has legislative authority to ban hazardous toys, including those having the potential for electrical, mechanical, or thermal injury. The law has been updated so that a toy or article intended for use by children can be designated

TOYS APPROPRIATE FOR VARIOUS AGE GROUPS

Infants need toys that produce *sensory stimulation*—visual, auditory, and tactile:
- Bright moving objects suspended over the baby (out of reach)
- Cradle gym
- Rattles (doughnuts, dumbbells)
- Soft balls
- Soft, washable dolls and animals
- Floating bath toys
- Music boxes or animals
- Small plastic or wooden blocks
- Pots and pans

Toddlers (1 to 2 years) use toys for *investigation*:
- Cloth, plastic books (illustrations of familiar objects, preferably one to a page)
- Nested blocks and cups of soft plastic or wood
- Kiddy car
- Push-and-pull toys
- Toy telephone
- Dolls (beware of eyes or nose that can become detached)
- Musical top
- Pots and pans

Preschoolers (2 to 5 years) should have toys that *imitate* parents' and older children's activities and that are *experimental* in nature:
- Record players, nursery rhymes
- Large wooden beads for stringing
- Housekeeping toys
- Transportation toys (tricycles, trucks, cars, wagons)
- Building blocks
- Floor trains
- Blackboards and chalk
- Easels and brushes
- Clay, crayons, fingerpaints (nontoxic)
- Outdoor toys (sandbox, swing, small slide)
- Hammers and peg benches
- Drums and bells
- Books (short stories, action stories)

Kindergarten and first-grade children (5 to 6 years) are in a phase of *creativity* and *skill:*
- Blocks
- Dolls
- Housekeeping toys
- Dress-up clothes, eating utensils
- Medical kits
- Outdoor toys
- Easels, blackboards, paints
- Doll houses
- Blunt scissors, simple sewing sets, paste, colored paper
- Simple puzzles
- Matching card games
- Hand puppets
- Small trucks
- Books, records

Older children (6 to 9 years) have greater *dexterity* with their hands:
- Paper dolls
- Table games
- Electric trains
- Crafts
- Bicycles
- Workbenches with good tools and materials
- Puppets and marionettes
- Books (for reading alone)

Middle childhood (9 to 12 years) is the period for starting *hobbies* and *scientific activities*:
- Hobby collections
- Model cars, boats, planes
- Microscopes
- Table and board games
- Sewing, knitting, needlework
- Outdoor sports
- Checkers, chess, dominoes

a hazard if it presents an unreasonable risk of personal injury or illness in normal use or when subjected to reasonably foreseeable damage or abuse. Despite the laws and volunteer consumer deputies, who canvass the marketplace regularly, especially during the Christmas season, the responsibility for choosing safe toys remains with parents. The Toy Manufacturers Association (TMA) has been working with the federal government to establish toy safety standards, but there are 1500 toy manufacturers (many of which do not belong to the TMA), 150,000 different kinds of toys, 5000 new toys produced each year, and 83,000 toys imported annually.

The pediatrician should advise parents to buy toys appropriate to their child's age, sex, development, and temperament, rather than buying impulsively what persuasive television advertisements peddle. Parents usually consider their child's chronological age, but the maturity level also must be considered[39] (see the box above). Parents should buy toys with the least potential for misuse. They should read the instructions and labels carefully and should check the packaging for the minimum age for use. Play should be supervised according to the situation, particularly among children under age 5. Children should be taught to play safely, with the parents setting a good example. They also should be taught to store toys in their proper place to avoid tripping over them.

Some toys that are appropriate for older children can be dangerous for younger brothers and sisters (e.g., the toys may have small parts that could be swallowed). The parents should ensure that any such toys are kept out of the little ones' reach, and they should teach the older children to put the toys away in these appropriate places. Toys should be inspected periodically and broken ones either repaired or discarded (see the box on p. 283).

INJURIES FROM PLAYGROUND EQUIPMENT

It is estimated that more than 250,000 people a year receive emergency treatment for injuries associated with public and

THIRTEEN TOY HAZARDS*

1. *Aspiration or ingestion.* Toys should not be too small, come apart, or be easily shattered. They should be larger than 1¼ inches in diameter and should not fit into a truncated circular cylinder 2¼ inches long.
2. *Burns.* Toys should not be made of flammable materials or have surfaces that can reach high temperatures. Hobby items, such as wood-burning kits, are *not* recommended for children under age 12.
3. *"Catch" injuries.* Toys should not have exposed gears, springs, or hinged parts that can pinch fingers or catch clothing or hair.
4. *Crumple or collapse injuries.* Children have fallen on rubber and plastic toys with metal axles that have penetrated their skulls. This type of accident would be less likely to occur if toys were made so that the chassis would not collapse or so that the axle would collapse.
5. *Electrical shock.* Battery-operated toys are preferred. Electric plug-in toys with heating elements should not be purchased for children under age 8. The minimum age recommendation should always be checked.

   Electrical toys require supervision and instruction in their proper use. Children should be taught to disconnect an electrical appliance by grasping the plug, *not* by pulling the cord. Parents should use the toy a few times together with the child to make sure the child understands how the toy is used. The wires on these toys should be checked monthly for wear.

   Electrical toys should bear the *UL label*. However, this label ensures only that the cord and the electrical device are engineered to electrical safety standards for any household equipment. It does *not* indicate that the toy is safe for use by a child or is safe in the event of misuse.
6. *Explosion injuries.* Chemistry sets and rocket-fuel kits must be selected for the appropriate age levels, usually for children over age 12. Dry ice in a stoppered bottle, match heads in a pipe or bottle, or weed killer mixed with sugar can explode. Parents should be alert for unsupervised scientific activity in the attic or basement.
7. *Lacerations.* Toys should not have sharp edges, glass, or rigid plastic that will shatter.
8. *Poisoning.* Parents should *not* buy toys composed of toxic or poisonous materials.
9. *Eye injuries.* Projectile-type toys can injure the eyes and therefore should be used under adult supervision.
10. *Strangling.* Ropes or loops can cause strangling. Strings on pull toys should be less than 10 inches long. Cradle gyms should be removed when the infant is able to sit.
11. *Abrasions.* These can be caused by rough surfaces.
12. *Punctures.* Because sharp points can cause punctures, suction tips covering such points must not be removable.
13. *Hearing damage.* Toys should not produce sound levels that can damage the hearing; the noise level should be under 100 dB. The label on caps for toy cap guns now states that they should not be used indoors or closer to the ear than 1 foot.

*Displaying this list on a bulletin board in the waiting room will remind parents of these dangers.

home playground equipment. Most of the injured children are between 5 and 10 years of age. About 25% of these injuries occur at school and another 25% on other public playgrounds; the remainder occur predominantly at home. Twenty thousand preschool children are injured annually while in day care; 72% of emergency department visits for these injuries involve falls to the ground.

NEISS did an in-depth analysis of 61 reports of injuries in children under age 15. Seven cases required hospital admission, and in two cases the victim died. Nearly 40% of the injuries occurred between 5 and 7 PM, more than 40% involved fractures, and 33% involved lacerations. The face and head were involved in 43% of the cases. Horizontal bars and jungle gyms were involved in the biggest proportion of the more serious injuries.

If parents are contemplating buying playground equipment, the pediatrician should advise them to check the stability of the equipment and to make sure that any protrusions (e.g., screws or bolts) are capped or taped over. Other features that should be avoided are open-ended S-hooks, moving parts that can pinch or crush fingers, sharp edges, and rough surfaces. If the gymnastic-type hanging rings are part of the set, they should be larger than 5 inches but less than 10 inches in diameter to prevent head entrapment.

The equipment should be installed at least 6 feet from fences, walls, and other obstructions and should not rest on a concrete or other hard surface unless a resilient covering is used. The equipment should be checked every 2 weeks for wear and necessary repairs made. Children should be taught that playing roughly (e.g., twisting swing chains and swinging empty seats) will not be allowed.

WRINGER INJURIES[22,42]

Wringer injuries occur predominantly in young children; 65% are reported in children under age 10 and 51% in children under age 5. A wringer injury is caused by a twisting force to an extremity that crushes the soft tissues. This type of injury is less common nowadays, since fewer people use the old-style washing machines with a wringer attachment; however, an identical injury can be caused by the spinning wheel of a vehicle (e.g., spoke injuries from bicycles) or by a fan belt. Severe spinning injuries also have been reported from spin clothes dryers. Estimates of the number of antiquated wringers still used (and capable of producing injury) range from 9 million to 17 million.

Clinical Signs

The severity of the injury is determined by the speed and tightness of the roller and by how long the extremity is trapped. Because the roller often gets stuck at the elbow or axilla, these areas are the most seriously injured. In the initial few hours, most victims may show only abrasions and ecchymoses and may not manifest significant external signs despite severe soft tissue injury and closed-space compression. *All wringer injuries should be considered severe until proved otherwise with the passage of time.*

An analysis by Allen and colleagues[1] showed that surgical procedures were required in 32 patients who had wringer injuries. Other series have reported lacerations in 20% of cases; fractures, usually of the phalanges, in 3%; a need for skin grafting in 10%; and some degree of motion limitation in 7%.

Treatment. Most authorities recommend hospital admission and close observation until the natural course of the injury is determined. Others recommend outpatient observation and close follow-up. Following are symptoms to look for in wringer-type injuries:

1. Edema that may become massive after the first 4 to 6 hours
2. Hemorrhage and discolored abrasions
3. Avulsion of the skin with a distally based flap
4. Pain
5. Anesthesia of the skin
6. Absent pulses in fingers or major arteries

The extent of necrosis or edema cannot be predicted from the initial appearance.

The steps to take with wringer-type injuries are:

1. At least every 30 minutes to 1 hour, observe for arterial pulses, pallor of the extremity, pain, paresthesia (numbness and cold), and paralysis; record the findings.
2. Débride all wounds and treat the skin as for a thermal burn, using topical antimicrobials such as silver sulfadiazine and povidone-iodine antiseptic.

Surgeons disagree over whether the dressing should be a standard compression dressing or a bulky, loose dressing; in either case the extremity should be elevated and the distal portion left exposed for inspection. The dressing should be changed in 24 hours. Edema ensues in 4 to 6 hours, and in rare cases a fasciotomy may be required to relieve pressure on nerves and blood vessels. The primary care physician should recognize that this type of injury is potentially serious and requires close observation and experienced care.

MISCELLANEOUS INJURIES

The following are hazards that may not be recognized as such by parents or a casual observer.

Baby Powder Aspiration

Both talc and zinc preparations have been implicated in severe and occasionally fatal inhalation episodes from containers that are deceptively similar to nursing bottles; the look-alike appearance is an invitation to trouble. Medicated powders containing calcium undecylenate also may be toxic if aspirated. Baby powders must be considered potentially harmful if aspirated. Their use should be discouraged until a drastic change is made in the appearance of the containers and a safety cap is developed that prevents accidental spills.

Digit Tourniquets

Hairs or thin fibers can become tightly wrapped around the digits or penis, resulting in gangrene and amputation. There also have been reports of leotard garments causing tourniquet-like constriction of the digits. Any infant who is crying uncontrollably should have the digits and, in boys, the penis examined for a possible tourniquet injury. Mothers or caregivers with long hair should tie it back when dressing or bathing babies.

Glass Door Injuries

It is estimated that more than 190,000 people require treatment in the emergency department each year for injuries associated with glass doors and windows. Of these, 50% are children. Thirty states have passed laws requiring installation of safety glass in all new homes. There are four types of safety glass: tempered, laminated, wired, and rigid plastic. Ideally, all regular glass doors should be replaced with safety glass. If this cannot be done, precautions such as those mentioned below should be instituted.[19]

Furniture or planters can be placed in front of doors that open to the exterior. Decals or colored tape will show the presence of glass, and a safety bar at handle level will prevent contact. The area in front of glass doors should be clear of loose rugs, toys, and other materials that could cause a person to trip or fall. Nonskid mats should be used in bathrooms, and unmounted glass should not be left unprotected.

Lawn Mower Injuries

More than 30 million lawn mowers are in use in the United States, and they cause an estimated 60,000 injuries a year. Injuries occur when children stick their fingers in the mower or fall into the path of a mower. Injuries also can be caused by objects hurled by the blades. Improvements in design must be made, and proper, careful use must be stressed.[25]

Cotton Swab Injuries

Cotton applicators should not be used in or around the auditory canal of infants or children. Older children can cause themselves severe auditory injury by using swabs.[9]

Refrigerator Entrapment

Between 1946 and 1962, 237 suffocations, with 35 fatalities were reported. Entrapment occurred primarily in children 2 to 7 years of age. More than two thirds of the 1962 fatalities involved appliances that were not in use. With the support of the AAP's Committee on Accident Prevention, Public Law 930 was enacted in 1956 and went into effect in 1958, mandating inside safety releases for refrigerator doors. Since then no fatalities have occurred involving a refrigerator with the safety release, but some of the old types still are in use and can cause suffocation. If a refrigerator or freezer is discarded, the door should be removed or padlocked.

Skateboard Injuries

In the late 1970s skateboard riding had a resurgence of popularity among children. In 1975 the CPSC reported an incidence of 27,500 injuries that required treatment in hospital emergency departments.[18] The Hawaii chapter of the AAP reported an alarming increase in severe injuries during 1975 and one death in early 1976.[30] Injuries in 1977 reached 140,000, and 25 deaths were reported in a 30-month period from February 1975 to July 1977. An analysis of accidental injuries involving skateboards revealed structural problems (e.g., improper modifications and repair and excessive wobbliness), poor skateboarding surfaces, inexperience, and skateboarding in traffic as contributors to severe injury.

Parents and retailers of skateboards must be made aware that riders under age 13 may not have adequate muscle coordination to maintain their balance or sufficient maturity to exercise judgment about types of maneuvers to attempt.

Children must be taught the proper and safe use of skateboards; they must wear protective equipment (helmet, gloves, and elbow and knee pads), and supervised areas must be made available for skateboard use to avoid the high toll of injury associated with this sport. The popularity of this activity declined in the early 1980s, dramatically reducing the use of skateboards and the associated injuries. In 1982 only 14,700 injuries were reported, and it appeared that skateboarding would be just another fad. However, the movie *Back to the Future* resurrected the glamor of daring skateboarding, and riding resurged. The CPSC reported 81,000 skateboard injuries for 1986 and 56,000 for 1991.

Toilet Seat Trauma

A small boy's penis can be injured if a toilet seat or its lid drops on it. This injury can be prevented by applying high rubber washers to the underside of the seat and the lid.[44]

SAFETY IN THE PHYSICIAN'S OFFICE, CLINIC, AND EMERGENCY DEPARTMENT

If physicians hope to instruct parents to set good examples for their children, then offices and clinics should be models of safety.

1. Is a *fire extinguisher* nearby?
2. Are *toxic agents* properly identified and kept out of the reach of small children?
3. Are *syringes and needles* disposed of safely?
4. Are "patient pleasers" safe for children, even if misused?
5. Are "harmful" *instruments* stored safely?
6. Is the *lighting* adequate?
7. Are *drug samples* disposed of safely?
8. Are the *electrical circuits* and *electrical equipment* safe?
9. Has a member of the staff been assigned the task of *checking for safety?*
10. Are *stools* available for reaching high places?
11. Are *rugs* kept in good condition? Are nonskid preparations used on highly waxed *floors?*
12. Do the nurse and aide instruct the parents to *stand close* while their children are on elevated surfaces and to *hold* onto them?
13. Are parents instructed to *supervise* their toddlers and preschool-age children during waiting time?

It really comes down to safe storage, safe disposal, periodic checks of furniture and equipment to be sure there are no sharp corners or edges, and supervision of children.

EMERGENCY MEDICAL SERVICES: TRAUMA CENTERS[46]

Trauma is a national problem of huge magnitude. It is essential to have not only programs to prevent trauma but also local systems of emergency medical service to provide optimum prehospital care and prompt, effective in-hospital care. Regional categorization of hospitals has been proposed, based on capability to receive and treat the critically injured, and regional trauma centers already have been developed.

The Emergency Medical Service Systems Act of 1973 added a section to the Public Health Services Act of 1944 "to provide assistance and encouragement for the development of comprehensive area-wide emergency medical systems." This law has effected profound changes in the handling of trauma cases.

Data are necessary to identify problems and review the performance of emergency facilities. A trauma registry was developed at the Children's Regional Trauma Unit at the Johns Hopkins University School of Medicine to gather objective data on children who have major injuries. The registry was designed to include events that occur during management from the scene of the accident, through resuscitation, and throughout in-hospital care. Problems highlighted by studies such as this have helped determine the most efficient transportation, the level of training needed by personnel, the number of centers needed in a region, and the type of back-up facilities required in a regional trauma center.

It became obvious that a traumatized child has special needs. Blunt-impact trauma accounts for 80% of multiple injuries, and head injuries are extremely common. Physicians need patience, experience, and sensitivity in dealing with pediatric trauma to lessen the impact of these experiences.

Because children are different from adults, resources and skills must be available to meet their needs. Consideration should be given to the following essential resources:

1. Rescue personnel with special training, protocols, and equipment for pediatric patients
2. Emergency rooms designed to meet the needs of pediatric injury victims
3. A community-designated pediatric trauma center or centers to provide care for severely injured children
4. An interhospital transport system with established protocols that minimize delay

Pediatricians should help organize community resources and responses to the needs of injured children.

FIRST AID MEASURES

The basic principles of treating traumatic injury can be easily remembered with the mnemonic ICE: *I*—immobilize (do not use or move the injured area), *C*—compress (apply pressure to stop bleeding and cool compresses to stop swelling), *E*—elevate (raise the injured area to stop bleeding and reduce swelling). Any rings, bracelets, or constricting garments should be removed before swelling occurs.

To facilitate first aid and to ensure proper care for their patients, pediatricians should require that a Medic-Alert bracelet* be obtained and worn by all patients who have any medical condition that cannot be seen (e.g., allergy, diabetes, epilepsy, heart condition).

Parents should be advised to prominently display the telephone numbers of the pediatrician (and other family physicians) poison control center, police, fire department, ambulance or taxi service, and hospital. These numbers should be readily available to baby-sitters, as should a first aid kit. Par-

*These can be obtained from the Medic-Alert Foundation, P.O. Box 1009, Turlock, CA 95380.

ents should be advised to use baby-sitters who are trained in first aid and who know what to do in case of an emergency. Latchkey children should be instructed in what they can and cannot do when are left alone, as well as in what to do in emergencies (see Chapter 63).

REFERENCES

1. Allen JE, Beck AR, Jewett TC Jr: Wringer injuries in children, *Arch Surg* 97:194, 1968.
2. Alonso WA: Minibike accidents lead to severe neck injury, *JAMA* 224:1344, 1973.
3. American Academy of Pediatrics, Committee on Accident Prevention: *Ocular hazards in injury control for children and youth,* Elk Grove Village, Ill, 1987, The Academy.
4. Baker SP: Motor vehicle occupant deaths in young children, *Pediatrics* 64:860, 1979.
5. Baker SP et al: *The injury fact book,* ed 2, New York, 1992, Oxford University Press.
6. Balcerak JC, Pancione KL, States JD: Moped, minibike, and motorcycle accidents: associated injury problems, *NY State J Med* 78:628, 1978.
7. Baptiste MS, Feck G: Preventing tap water burns, *Am J Public Health* 70:727, 1980.
8. Barnako D: Flammable fabrics, *JAMA* 221:189, 1972.
9. Barton RT: Q-Tip otalgia, *JAMA* 220:1619, 1972.
10. Bass JL et al: Childhood injury prevention counseling in primary care settings: a critical review of the literature, *Pediatrics* 92:544, 1993.
11. Bass LW, Wilson TR: The pediatrician's influence in private practice measured by a controlled seat belt study, *Pediatrics* 56:271, 1975.
12. Berman W Jr et al: Childhood burn injuries and deaths, *Pediatrics* 51:1069, 1973.
13. Bicycle-related injuries: data from the National Electronic Injury Surveillance System, *MMWR* 36:269, 1987.
14. Black EE: Causes of burns in children, *JAMA* 158:100, 1955.
15. Carr WP, Brandt D, Swanson K: Injury patterns and helmet effectiveness among hospitalized motorcyclists, *Minn Med* 64:521, 1981.
16. Charles S, Shelness A: Children as passengers in automobiles: the neglected minority on the nation's highways, *Pediatrics* 56:271, 1975.
17. Dietrich HF: Accident prevention in childhood is your problem, too, *Pediatr Clin North Am* Nov 1954, p 759.
18. Fact Sheet: Roller skates, ice skates, and skateboards, US Consumer Product Safety Commission Pub No 84, Washington, DC, 1976, US Government Printing Office.
19. Feinberg SN: Storm door hazards, *Pediatrics* 46:936, 1970.
20. Feldman KW: Prevention of childhood accidents: recent progress, *Pediatr Rev* 2:75, 1980.
21. Few children protected in cars, Insurance Institute for Highway Safety 10(10):1, 1985.
22. Galasko CS: Spin dryer injuries, *Br Med J* 4:646, 1972.
23. Gifford GH Jr, Marty AT, MacCollum DW: The management of electrical mouth burns in children, *Pediatrics* 47:113, 1971.
24. Goldman AS, Larson DL, Abston S: The silent epidemic, *JAMA* 221:403, 1972.
25. Graham WP III, DeMuth WE Jr, Gordon SL: A summer warning: lawnmowers can maim, *JAMA* 225:355, 1973.
26. Greensher J: Recent advances in injury prevention, *Pediatr Rev* 10:171, 1988.
27. Guichon DMP, Miles ST: Bicycle injuries: one-year sample in Calgary, *J Trauma* 15:504, 1975.
28. Haddon W Jr, Suchman EA, Klein D: *Accident research: methods and approaches,* New York, 1964, Harper & Row.
29. Haggerty RJ: Emotions and childhood accidents, *Mod Med* 31:58, 1963.
30. Hawaii Chapter, American Association of Pediatrics: The hazards of skateboard-riding, *Pediatrics* 46:793, 1976.
31. Heimlich HJ: A life-saving maneuver to prevent food choking, *JAMA* 234:398, 1975.
32. Helveston EM: Eye trauma in childhood, *Pediatr Clin North Am* 22:501, 1975.
33. Izant RJ Jr, Rothmann BF, Frankel VH: Bicycle spoke injuries of the foot and ankle in children: an underestimated "minor" injury, *J Pediatr Surg* 4:654, 1969.
34. Jackson C, Jackson CL: *Diseases of the air and food passages of foreign body origin,* Philadelphia, 1907, WB Saunders.
35. Klein D: The influence of societal values on rates of death and injury, *J Safety Res* 3:1, 1971.
36. Kravitz H et al: Accidental falls from elevated surfaces in infants from birth to one year of age, *Pediatrics* 44(suppl):869, 1969.
37. Levy D: Observations of attitudes and behavior in the child health center, *Am J Public Health* 41:182, 1951.
38. Low MB: The significance of vision problems of children and youth: eye safety in pediatric practice, *J Pediatr Ophthalmol* 6:223, 1969.
39. Lund DH: *Choosing toys for children of all ages,* New York, 1972, American Toy Institute.
40. Lyons TJ, Oates RK: Falling out of bed: a relatively benign occurrence, *Pediatrics* 92:125, 1993.
41. Matheny AP, Brown AM, Wilson RS: Assessment of children's behavioral characteristics: a tool in accident prevention, *Clin Pediatr* 11:437, 1972.
42. McCulloch JH, Boswick JA Jr, Jonas R: Household wringer injuries: a three-year review, *J Trauma* 13:1, 1973.
43. Mofenson HC, Greensher J: How to avoid animal bites, *Med Times* 100:92, 1972.
44. Mofenson HC, Greensher J: Penile trauma, *JAMA* 225:1038, 1973.
45. National Committee for Injury Prevention and Control: Injury prevention: meeting the challenge, *Am J Prev Med* 5(suppl):1, 1989.
46. National Committee for Injury Prevention and Control: Injury prevention: meeting the challenge. Trauma care systems, *Am J Prev Med* 5(suppl):271, 1989.
47. National Safety Council: Accident facts, 1993 edition, Itasca, Ill, The Council.
48. Pless IB, Roghmann K, Algranati P: The prevention of injuries to children in automobiles, *Pediatrics* 49:420, 1972.
49. Rivera FP et al: The Seattle children's bicycle helmet campaign: changes in helmet use and head injury admissions, *Pediatrics* 93:567, 1994.
50. Scherz RG: Auto safety: "The first ride . . . a safe ride" campaign. In Bergman AB, editor: Preventing childhood injuries. Report of the Twelfth Ross Roundtable on Critical Approaches to Common Pediatric Problems, Columbus, Ohio, 1982, Ross Laboratories.
51. Sieben RL, Leavitt JD, French JH: Falls as childhood accidents: an increasing urban risk, *Pediatrics* 47:886, 1971.
52. Snyder RG, O'Neill B: Are 1974-1975 automotive belt systems hazardous to children? *Am J Dis Child* 129:946, 1975.
53. Sobel R: The psychiatric implications of accidental poisoning in childhood, *Pediatr Clin North Am* 17:653, 1970.
54. Swartz EM: *Toys that don't care,* Boston, 1971, Gambit.
55. Thomson HG: Bathtub burn: pediatric disaster, *Can J Surg* 14:399, 1971.
56. Thomson HG, Juckes AW, Farmer AW: Electric burns to the mouth in children, *Plast Reconstr Surg* 35:466, 1965.
57. Weiss BD: Bicycle helmet use by children, *Pediatrics* 77:677, 1986.

SUGGESTED READINGS

Centers for Disease Control and Prevention: Air bag–associated fatal injuries to infants and children riding in front passenger seats, *MMWR* 44:845, 1995.

Centers for Disease Control and Prevention: BB and pellet gun–related injuries—United States, June 1992–May 1994, *MMWR* 44:909, 1995.

Rodriguez JG: Childhood injuries in the United States, *Am J Dis Child* 144:625, 1990.

24 The Ill Child

Marianne E. Felice and Stanford B. Friedman

Although great strides have been made in the prevention, diagnosis, and treatment of childhood illnesses in the past half century, children continue to become ill. Illnesses today, however, are different from those of former years. For example, children now have chronic illnesses that in the past were fatal, and they now have fatal diseases that in the past were not known. Sick children and their families continue to consume a major portion of the pediatrician's time, talents, and energy. It is important that the specific knowledge and skills of pediatricians reflect the changing patterns of childhood disease.

A discussion of the management of the ill child must encompass a variety of topics, including the degree and duration of illness, hospitalization and the medical delivery system, family support systems, the emotional components of physical illness, and finally, the plight of the dying child.

THE ACUTELY ILL CHILD

Treatment at Home

Whenever possible, the acutely ill child should be treated at home surrounded by a familiar environment and tended by a responsible, caring adult who knows the child well. Fortunately this is the usual case, rather than the exception, because most youngsters are only mildly to moderately ill for a brief period and have their parents, extended family members, or reliable, familiar baby-sitters to tend to them. The pediatrician, however, should not always presume that adults are in attendance. When deciding whether to treat a child at home, the physician should specifically seek answers to the following questions: Who will assume responsibility for the child during the illness? Is a telephone easily available? Are medical facilities relatively nearby? Above all, do the parents understand the nature of the child's illness and the instructions that have been given? The answer to the last question should be verified by having one or both parents repeat the instructions to the physician.

In two-parent households, fathers should be encouraged to participate actively in their children's health care. Often mothers assume full responsibility for the children's health and fathers are ignored; thus fathers cannot support either the mother or the child. This leaves the mother in the difficult position of having not only to tend to the child but also to repeat the physician's explanations and directions to her husband, a situation that can be the source of misunderstanding, misinterpretation, and resentment for both parents. When a child has a significant illness, the pediatrician should encourage *both* parents to bring the child to the physician whenever possible, and the physician should relate directions and explanations to both parents simultaneously. In this way parents can share the task of caring for their sick child and support each other.

Not all families are established two-parent households; currently, more women are employed outside the home than in previous years, including nearly 60% of mothers who have preschool children.[19] The proportion of children being reared by fathers alone now is about 20%. Consequently, physicians always should be aware of and sensitive to the household composition and problems, particularly in giving directions concerning at-home care. For example, single-parent fathers may be new to the primary caretaker role; surrounded by experienced mothers in the pediatrician's office, they may feel uncomfortable. They may be unsure of details concerning the child's birth or immunizations. This parent may need more detailed information than do other parents about the treatment of an acute illness. Working mothers may feel caught between the demands of their job and the demands of their sick child and feel guilty about asking the physician for advice. In fact, it has been shown that at least some pediatricians are biased against working mothers.[12] Physicians will serve the child's needs best by being attuned to these psychosocial and societal issues.

Treating an ill child offers an opportunity for the pediatrician to teach parents about medications. If a drug is prescribed, the physician should name the drug and explain why it is being given and what side effects should be anticipated. Antibiotic therapy frequently results in low compliance; parents begin to give antibiotics to their child and then stop when the child starts to feel better, usually after 24 to 48 hours of treatment. Parents may need to be told that many types of infections require a full course of antibiotic therapy. When a medication is discontinued by a physician before all the liquid, pills, or capsules are finished, the parents should be advised about what to do with the unused portion. For example, those medications that decompose with time, such as tetracycline, should be discarded; other medications, such as antihistamines, may be used again at a later date. Parents also should be taught which over-the-counter drugs they should have available, such as acetaminophen for children and ipecac syrup, and how to use them. Physicians also can educate parents by teaching them the proper administration of medications. The familiar "1 teaspoon 4 times a day" may result in varied quantities of medicine being administered if careful directions are not given. Some parents may need practical hints for helping a child take an unpalatable medicine—for example, crushing a tablet in applesauce.

In most families there is a tradition of myths and home remedies for common acute illnesses, and parents often turn to these ideas when their children are ill. Again, this provides the opportune time for parent education. For example, when talking to the parents of a child who has an upper respiratory tract infection, the physician can explain that the youngster did not "catch cold" because of failure to wear galoshes in the rain. In explaining the management of fever, a physician may wish to emphasize certain *do nots* in an effort to dispel misconceptions: *do not* give enemas to bring down fever; do not give cold baths to bring down fever (see Chapter 25). Some myths and home remedies are peculiar to certain communities and cultures, and each pediatrician should become familiar with the traditions of the locality (see Chapter 11).

In this age of widespread immunization programs, issues of contagion often are neglected. Parents should be informed of the infectious nature of certain childhood illnesses in order to protect other siblings, pregnant relatives, and elderly persons. The most common examples are protecting pregnant relatives from German measles or warning those taking steroids or immunosuppressive drugs to avoid contact with children who have chickenpox.

Acutely ill children at home often pose problems for the parents caring for them. Parents unaccustomed to seeing their normally active toddler listless may feel compelled to entertain the child without realizing that the child may need rest and may not be in the mood for entertainment. On the other hand, many parents may try to restrain a child and insist on bed rest when the child feels well enough to play. Parents need to be reminded that children restrict their own activity when they are ill. Parents also have a tendency to overfeed a sick child, and they must be reassured that if a child drinks appropriate fluids, this is sufficient intake during a brief illness.

It is natural for parents to become anxious when their children are ill; this anxiety may result in frequent telephone calls to the pediatrician. The pediatrician may perceive such calls as unneeded and annoying without appreciating how frightened parents may be. New parents in particular require support during their child's illnesses, and the pediatrician should teach parents patiently when it is and is not appropriate to call. The pediatrician should not frighten parents into not calling and reporting on their child's progress. When a physician decides to treat a child at home, arrangements should be made for a follow-up check, either in terms of a telephone conversation or another office visit, and the importance of such follow-up visits should be explained and emphasized to the parents.

Indications for Hospitalization

It is not always feasible or safe to treat an acutely ill child at home; hospitalization may become necessary. *Whom* to hospitalize and *when* to hospitalize are not always clear-cut issues. But, in the last decade, there has been a definite trend toward decreased hospitalizations for children.[19] Children who are critically or seriously ill are obvious candidates for inpatient care. Children who are not seriously ill also must be considered for hospitalization if the circumstances at home are such that the child will not receive adequate care. Some hospitalizations, however, can be averted by the tapping of available community resources such as public health nurses, homemaker services, and medical home care programs. Such alternate arrangements not only may be far more economical but also will allow the child and parents to remain in their home.

In teaching hospitals it is not uncommon that children who have unusual diseases be admitted for the purpose of teaching or research, in addition to receiving specific therapy. This situation can result in a child receiving more than the customary services and laboratory tests. Even though a child usually receives excellent medical care at a teaching hospital, physicians should carefully weigh the advantages of medical research and medical education against the psychological trauma a youngster may experience and any added expense to parents.

It sometimes is necessary to hospitalize children for diagnostic workups. Most diagnostic procedures can be accomplished on an outpatient basis and should be done so as often as possible. Occasionally children require numerous or complicated tests or clinical observation, and it may be more efficient to admit them for a few days for evaluation. When this is necessary, the pediatrician should schedule the admission carefully, keeping the hospital stay as short as possible; the pediatrician, for example, should postpone an admission from Friday to Monday if no tests or only a few tests can be performed over the weekend. In the age of uncertain health care reform,[16] admissions to or discharges from hospitals often are monitored or authorized by clerical staff who may not be trained in pediatric issues and who are instructed to follow guidelines designed for cost and not care. Pediatricians should always ensure that decisions concerning a child's health are based on the child's medical needs and not on financial restraints.

Some children require elective surgical procedures. The pediatric literature has reflected an emphasis on the timing of these procedures based on the observation that between the ages of 4 and 7 years children seem to be dramatically concerned about body integrity. Psychiatrists refer to this as *mutilation anxiety* or *castration anxiety.* Some authorities have recommended that elective surgery not be done during these particular years of psychosocial development. In actual clinical practice, however, it usually is not feasible to postpone surgical procedures for 3 to 4 years. An alternative approach is to delay surgery only long enough to explain to the child what is going to happen to him or her. This should be explained gradually, using age-appropriate language, and the parents should be the primary supportive resources.[7]

Unfortunately, children sometimes are admitted to the hospital primarily for the convenience of the physician. After receiving a call from the parents at night, the pediatrician may have the child admitted at a late hour and attended by a pediatric house officer on call, thus avoiding having to examine the child at that time. The pediatrician should look into the "real" reason for ordering the hospitalization and avoid doing so for personal convenience.

Care of the Child in the Hospital

When a child is admitted to the hospital, the child and the family become enmeshed in an unfamiliar and often frightening web known as the *medical delivery system.* To the lay person, hospital activities are unpredictable, and families lack control over this environment. In such a milieu both the child and the parents may express their fear in several ways. For instance, the child may cry and be uncooperative. The child is afraid of separation from the parents, of pain, of the unfamiliar environment and strange people, and of the unknown. Parents may become hostile or agitated or may constantly question the health team. They realize that their child's care is being usurped from them, and they fear that they no longer can care for or protect their child. They, too, are afraid of the strange people and the unknown environment.

There may be no facilities for parents on the pediatric floor, not even a waiting area. Nevertheless, the supportive role of the parents in helping their child get well must be emphasized, and the parents should be assured that they are needed and welcomed on the pediatric floor. It has been demonstrated that parental involvement in the lives of hospitalized children is beneficial to the child.[6] Furthermore, in the complicated network of hospital personnel who encounter the youngster, the parents should have one person consistently available to them for communication concerning their child's care. This person, usually the primary care physician, should report at least daily to the parents and more often if the child is critically ill. Whenever possible, information should be given to both parents at the same time. They then have the opportunity to ask questions, and neither parent needs to interpret the physician's remarks to the other.

It is common for a youngster to have one or even multiple consultants during hospitalization. It is vital that the child and the parents be notified that a consultation has been requested and the reasons for it explained. Communication between the pediatrician and the consultant should be made clear before the consultant sees the child so that the parents do not receive conflicting or confusing reports. The following case vignette illustrates the confusion that can occur in the process of consultation:

Gary was an obese 10-year-old admitted to the hospital for a diagnostic workup of recent "spells" consisting of dizziness and falling down. The degree of consciousness after each episode was unclear. On the day of hospital admission, Gary appeared to vacillate between a state of near coma and insensitivity to pain and aggressive fighting behavior. The physical examination disclosed no abnormal findings. All study results were negative except those of an equivocal electroencephalogram. Neurological consultation was requested without Gary's or his parents' knowledge. The neurologist told the mother that Gary probably had a form of seizure disorder and that medication would be recommended to the pediatrician. The nurses noted that Gary seemed quiet and did not play with other children, and a child psychiatric consultation was requested. Because the pediatrician feared the mother would object to psychiatry, she was simply told that "another doctor" would be talking to her son. The child psychiatrist arrived on the ward and introduced himself to the mother as a psychiatrist. The mother said that she was confused. While the psychiatrist talked to Gary, the mother was told to wait in the hall until the interview was over. A few minutes later the mother went to the nurses' station and demanded to see her son's pediatrician, who was paged but did not answer. The child psychiatrist returned to the mother and said that Gary appeared to be depressed and that he would return the next day to take the boy to the playroom to complete the evaluation. The mother began shouting at the nurses about the quality of care in the hospital.

Problems illustrated by the above vignette can be avoided easily if, before the consultant sees the patient, the primary care physician and the consultant decide together who will discuss the consultant's findings with the child and the family (Fig. 24-1). Just as it is important for the pediatrician to communicate with parents, it is necessary for the pediatrician to communicate with the child in a developmentally appropriate manner, no matter what the child's age.[23] This communication may take the form of actions rather than words. For example, it is more comforting for a toddler to be held for reassurance than to hear words of reassurance. When speaking to a child, the pediatrician should remember to sit down at the child's eye level and use age-appropriate words to ensure that the child understands what is to be done and to allow the child an opportunity to ask questions. To help the youngster trust hospital personnel, procedures should be explained honestly: If a child is to have blood drawn, for instance, and asks whether it will hurt, the pediatrician should admit that it will hurt for a few moments. All painful procedures should be performed as quickly and gently as possible. Often it is appropriate to perform any painful procedures in a special treatment room so that the ward or hospital room is not associated with unpleasant experiences.

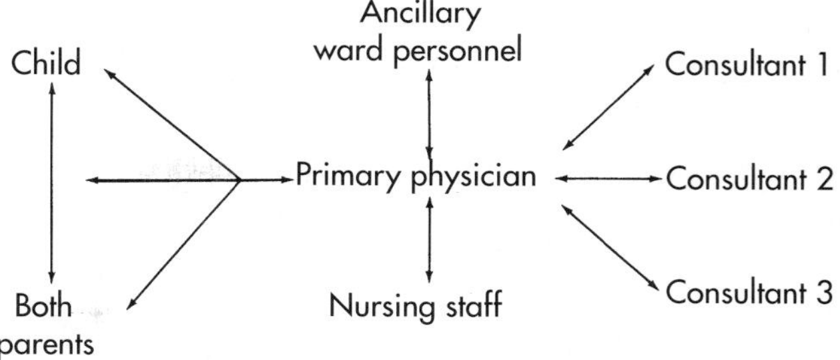

FIG. 24-1 Relationship between the primary care physician and all consultants.

Children who must undergo surgery should have the surgical procedure explained to them.[7] The physician can use a doll and a bandage to show where the patient's bandage will be. Children should be told where they will be when they awaken and who will be there. If a child is expected to be returned to an intensive care unit after major surgery, the nurses from that unit should visit the child before the surgery so that the child will feel more at ease in the new surroundings after surgery.

In preparation for anesthesia the child should be forewarned about the anesthesia mask and the odor of the gas. Many physicians find that the presence of parents during the induction and recovery phases of anesthesia helps to alleviate much of the fear and fantasy for both parents and child.

It generally is accepted that children admitted to hospitals should be placed in pediatric units especially designed for children and staffed by personnel trained to care for children. In large children's centers children may be assigned to wards by age and type of medical problem; in community hospitals children usually are assigned to wards according to age alone; and in smaller hospitals children of all ages may be assigned to one pediatric ward. Any of these arrangements is appropriate. Many hospitals have no facilities for adolescent patients, and teenagers are admitted to the adult wards. For a few older adolescents this may be acceptable, but for younger adolescents and for some older ones, such an arrangement may be detrimental to their emotional health. Whenever possible, adolescents should be placed together in a setting designed for their needs.[8]

For young children in particular, separation from their parents is painful. In these instances, rooming-in arrangements are strongly recommended until the child adjusts to the hospitalization. In fact, rooming-in may result in a shorter hospital stay for the child[26] and lower anxiety for both child and parents.[2]

The issues of visiting hours and who may visit are important in pediatrics. Policies regarding these issues should be based on what is best for the child and the family and not on what is most convenient for the hospital personnel.

The question of whether it is more beneficial for a child to have a private room than to be with other children often is raised. The answer depends on the patient's particular needs and illness. Parents often believe that their child will receive better care if placed in a private room; if this is not true, the pediatrician should communicate this to the parents. Generally, children should have as much contact with other children as is medically feasible.

When hospitalized, children often regress in development, commonly in toilet training. Parents need reassurance that this phenomenon may occur because of the strange and frightening hospital environment. Neither children nor adolescents are accustomed to using medical terminology to describe urination and defecation; thus they may hesitate to express these needs to nurses. Parents can be invaluable in clarifying these terms to their children. It is important to respect a child's or an adolescent's need for privacy in completing his or her toilette, in dressing or undressing, or in being examined. Hospital personnel should be sensitive to a child's embarrassment and pull curtains around the bed when the child is undressing or draw a sheet over the child's naked genitalia when the abdomen is being examined in full view of the hall.

Although isolation may be medically necessary, pediatric personnel must remember that it does affect the child. Children in isolation receive fewer visits from the nurses, may rarely see their physician, and spend less time with their parents. When someone does come into the room, the visitor is gowned and often masked. This can be frightening, stressful, and depressing. One such youngster portrayed her feelings in a drawing (Fig. 24-2). Isolation should be kept as brief as medically feasible, and the physician in charge should ensure that all steps are completed to avoid unnecessary days in isolation—for example, obtaining proper specimens for cultures and checking culture reports frequently. Parents of children in isolation also may need additional support during those days.

A common practice in teaching hospitals is to rotate all medical students through the pediatric service. All students, regardless of their career interests, are then taught pediatric procedures (e.g., starting IVs, drawing blood, performing spinal taps, and aspirating bone marrow) by practicing on young patients. Although students interested in pediatrics must learn these procedures, they will have ample opportunity to do so as first-year house officers. Pediatric teaching programs should be reevaluated to determine whether *all* students need to master pediatric procedures and if alternative methods are available to acquire these skills, such as the use of mannequins and animal models. Current New York State Department of Health regulations severely limit medical student involvement in performing these procedures. It is likely that other states will follow suit.

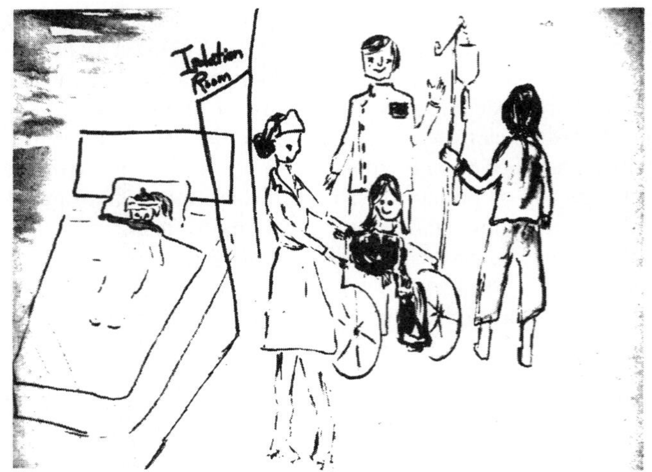

FIG. 24-2 Drawing by a 13-year-old girl in isolation.

Siblings of Hospitalized Children

When a child is hospitalized, siblings should not be neglected by the parents.[1,14] Some children resent the attention being paid to the hospitalized child and begin to misbehave at home. Other children, particularly those of school age, are confused by their brother's or sister's absence from home and may even fantasize that they caused the hospitalization in some way. Parents may need to be reminded that *all* the children should be informed of their sibling's hospitalization and told the reason for it. It sometimes helps the children at home feel included and needed if each one has a special chore to do for the hospitalized youngster—for example, feeding the patient's goldfish or painting a picture to decorate the hospital room. Whenever practical, the nonhospitalized siblings should speak to their hospitalized brother or sister by telephone and be encouraged to visit the hospital. Siblings told that the hospitalized child has a minor problem (e.g., anemia or the flu) when indeed the medical situation is serious or potentially fatal may be psychologically vulnerable in later life when they have these same minor medical problems.

Activities for the Young Patient

A major component of a child's life is school. School-age children admitted to the hospital miss their usual classroom instruction.[3,9] Obviously, children who are critically or seriously ill cannot be expected to study, but children who are convalescing should be given as much schooling as possible to prevent their falling too far behind their peers. If a child is hospitalized for a short time (i.e., 7 to 10 days), the parents can serve as liaison between the classroom and the child and can work with the child's teacher to ensure that the youngster keeps abreast of classes. Children whose anticipated hospitalization is for a longer period should receive as soon as possible instruction through the school system by a hospital or home tutor. In many school systems, hospital instruction cannot be requested until the child has been out of school for 6 weeks or more. This is too much time for a child

RIGHTS OF PATIENTS AND PARENTS

You have the right, consistent with law, to:

1. Understand and use these rights. If for any reason you do not understand or you need help, the hospital must provide assistance, including an interpreter.
2. Receive treatment without discrimination as to race, color, religion, sex, national origin, disability, sexual orientation, or source of payment.
3. Receive considerate and respectful care in a clean and safe environment free of unnecessary restraints.
4. Receive emergency care if you need it.
5. Be informed of the name and position of the doctor who will be in charge of your care in the hospital.
6. Know the names, positions, and functions of any hospital staff involved in your care and refuse their treatment, examination, or observation.
7. A no smoking room.
8. Receive complete information about your diagnosis, treatment, and prognosis.
9. Receive all the information that you need to give informed consent for any proposed procedure or treatment. This information shall include the possible risks and benefits of the procedure or treatment.
10. Receive all the information that you need to give informed consent for an order not to resuscitate. You also have the right to designate an individual to give this consent for you if you are too ill to do so. If you would like additional information, please ask for a copy of *"Do Not Resuscitate Orders—A Guide for Patients and Families."*
11. Refuse treatment and be told what effect this may have on your health.
12. Refuse to take part in research. In deciding whether or not to participate, you have the right to a full explanation.
13. Privacy while in the hospital and confidentiality of all information and records regarding your care.
14. Participate in all decisions about your treatment and discharge from the hospital. The hospital must provide you with a written discharge plan and written description of how you can appeal your discharge.
15. Review your medical record and obtain a copy of your medical record, for which the hospital can charge a reasonable fee. You cannot be denied a copy solely because you cannot afford to pay.
16. Receive an itemized bill and explanation of all charges.
17. Formulate an advance directive and appoint a health care proxy.
18. Participate in the consideration of ethical issues that arise in your care.
19. Complain without fear of reprisals about the care and services you are receiving and to have the hospital respond to you and, if you request it, issue a written response. You first should speak to the nurse or doctor caring for you and, if you remain dissatisfied, to Patient Relations. If you are not satisfied with the hospital's response, you can complain to the state health department. The hospital must provide you with the health department phone number.

If you have any questions about your rights, please speak with a staff member, especially the doctor or nurse caring for you.

Modified from University of Rochester Strong Memorial Hospital Medical Center, Statement on patients' rights, Rochester, NY, April, 1993.

to miss school work, and whenever possible the physician should protest such a policy.

Another valuable component to any child's life is play. For the hospitalized child, play also is important, and most pediatric floors are well stocked with age-appropriate toys and games. A structured activities program now is common in most pediatric wards and is known by various names in different hospitals—for example, the child-life program, play program, or children's activities program. Physicians should make use of a child-life program in caring for their patients and welcome the observations made of the child at play. Such observations often can add insight to a child's progress or lack of progress in the hospital. Children should be encouraged to act out or "draw out" their feelings about their illness or hospitalization.[22] Where there are structured activities, as many children as possible should participate. Youngsters who have intravenous lines should have the tubing anchored in such a way that walking is possible. Children in traction or restricted to bed often can have their beds moved to the playroom so that they too can take part in the activities.

While recuperating from a long illness in the hospital, children should be able to receive "leave" or passes. Pediatric health care personnel sometimes neglect the importance of children attending significant and meaningful events in their lives, such as a school occasion or a family celebration. Often a child can be allowed to leave the hospital for a few hours without detriment to his or her health, particularly for the adolescent struggling to maintain peer group acceptance during the illness.

Patients, parents, and members of a hospital staff are partners in the healing process. Each has rights and responsibilities (see the box above). The primary care physician, as the patient's advocate and a member of the hospital staff, should ensure that all concerned understand and respect these rights and responsibilities.

Indications for Discharge from the Hospital

It sometimes is as difficult to decide when to discharge children from the hospital as it is to decide when to admit them. Children should not be kept in the hospital unnecessarily, but what constitutes an unnecessary length of time is not always clear. Fortunately, most children are admitted for a given symptom, diagnosed, treated, and then sent home within a brief period. Some children require extended convalescence with minimal nursing care; for these children, alternatives to traditional hospitalization should be sought, such as convalescent homes for children, chronic illness hospitals, and visiting nurse programs. If parents are expected to perform nursing tasks for the child at home, such as injections, gavage, or dressing changes, they should be taught the procedure gradually, and the child should be discharged only when the parents and physician both feel comfortable that proper care can be given at home. Again, public health nurses can be invaluable in helping such families.

Often children are admitted to the hospital having suspected primary psychosocial problems, such as those caused by child abuse. In these cases social work consultation should be requested as early as possible so that the child will not spend extra days in the hospital while such a consultation and disposition are implemented. Pediatric health care personnel must be innovative and imaginative to minimize the length of hospitalization and to encourage comprehensive rehabilitation of the child.

THE CHRONICALLY ILL CHILD

Chronically ill children pose many issues for pediatric health care personnel.[20] Sometimes these youngsters have complex medical problems and thus require the services of several physicians or clinics. These children may have psychosocial problems concomitant with or as a result of their illness. They often require frequent checkups and characteristically have thick, illegible medical records. Their families need and deserve much support, understanding, and guidance concerning the disease and its effect on the total family.[13] Finally, children who have a chronic disease evoke a vast array of feelings in the staff members who work with them. These feelings often are ignored, suppressed, or displaced.

The number of children who have chronic illnesses is increasing rapidly, as advances in technology are enabling physicians to change the natural history of many diseases and prolong life.[19,20] This advancement, however, has resulted in some new problems. For example, before the era of antibiotics, children who had cystic fibrosis usually died before adolescence; now these patients live to young adulthood. When adolescents, they usually depend on several medications simultaneously and may resent this dependence. Boys who have cystic fibrosis nearly always are sterile; adolescent girls who have it must grapple with their fears of having children when their own life expectancy is so uncertain. Therefore physicians must focus on the psychosocial and psychosexual problems related to these issues of sterility and pregnancy.

Effects of Chronic Illness on the Child's Development

How a chronic illness influences a child's development is contingent on several questions: Was the child born with the illness? Is the illness an inherited disorder, or was it acquired? How old was the child when the illness was acquired or when it was diagnosed? The importance of these answers relates to children's beginning development of a body image even in infancy. Five-month-old infants explore their own bodies, including their fingers, toes, genitalia, and faces, and they incorporate their findings into their developing self-images. By the age of 2 or 3 years, these youngsters have some concept of their own bodies that they identify as "mine." If in their exploration they discover that an arm or a leg is absent or that they have some other abnormality, they incorporate that abnormality into their self-image. Later, at age 3, 4, or 5 years, they begin to compare their body with other children's bodies and recognize that they are different from other children. The child growing up with an abnormality appears to be better adjusted and more accepting of his or her self-image than the child who acquires a disability during later years.

After children who have a chronic illness or physical deformity have accepted their self-image, they must learn to cope with their peers' perceptions. Young children are adaptive and generally will play with other children to the best of their abilities in spite of their deformities. Although youngsters can be cruel and tease one another about their differences, usually children accept other children, particularly if the disabled children accept themselves. Parents, however, often become anxious about their disabled or chronically ill children being in the presence of "normal" children and may try to shield them from their peers. Physicians should reassure and support the parents so that the child is given the opportunity to relate to normal peers.[11,21]

Children whose disabilities are visible often receive more attention and support than do children with "hidden" ones. For example, the child who has rheumatoid arthritis and visibly swollen joints and difficulty moving often will evoke much support from family, teachers, and friends. On the other hand, the child who has juvenile diabetes, whose disability is not visible, often will not receive similar support.[10,15]

A major problem for children who have chronic illnesses is the difficulty that physicians and parents have in allowing them to develop independence. Parents tend to overprotect their chronically ill child,[11] and physicians contribute to that overprotectiveness by emphasizing restrictions. It is helpful to both parents and child if the physician lists those activities the child should and should not do.

When treating a chronically ill child over several years, the physician can attend to vocational planning for the youngster, either personally or through staff members. Each child should be encouraged to develop socially and intellectually as completely as possible, but the physician also must recognize a child's limitations and encourage realistic aspirations. One problem peculiar to pediatricians is their reluctance to terminate the physician-patient relationship when a youngster reaches adulthood, particularly if the pediatrician has cared for the child from infancy. Whenever possible, chronically ill children, on reaching adulthood, should be transferred to internists or family practitioners; such a transfer supports the patient's striving for independence. The patient should be prepared for this change over several visits.

Effects of Chronic Illness on the Family

The parents of chronically ill children often feel guilty about their child's illness.[21] If a child has an inherited disorder, both parents may scrutinize their family backgrounds to see how the disease was inherited. If the illness is acquired, the parents may feel that they did not adequately protect their child from getting the disease. If an infant is born having a congenital but not inherited disorder, the mother may become obsessed about her prenatal activities and wonder if some action of hers caused the disorder.

Guilt often leads to anger (Fig. 24-3). Guilt feelings cause discomfort, and the parents become angry at feeling uncom-

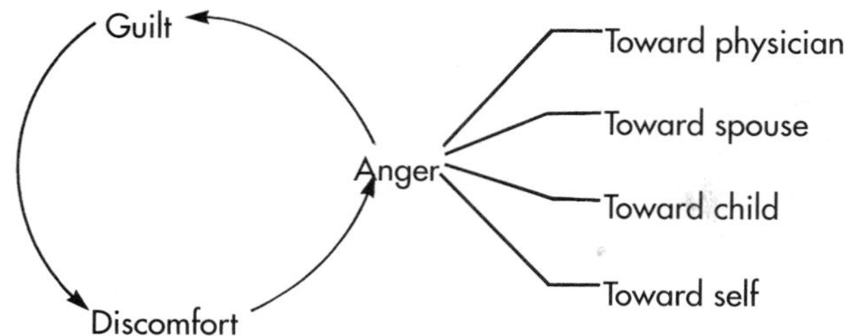

FIG. 24-3 Parental guilt over a child's illness often leads to anger.

fortable. This anger may be directed toward the physician who initially diagnosed the child's illness, toward each other, toward themselves, and even toward the afflicted child.

The marital relationship between parents of a chronically ill child may either improve remarkably or disintegrate shortly after the illness is diagnosed. Being told that one's youngster has a chronic illness is a crisis and imposes stress on most marriages. If the marriage is stable and the parents are mutually supportive, the marital bonds grow stronger. If the marriage is unstable, the child's illness serves as a final stress that may sever marital ties.

To the family, the monetary cost of having a child with a chronic illness may be astounding,[5] in which case the parents will need help finding financial aid. Most families are not able to carry the financial burden of their child's illness alone, but they may be too proud to ask for help. Physicians should be sensitive to these needs and offer their help or the services of their staff whenever possible.

To society, the cost of children who are chronically ill can be immeasurable. These children often require expensive medications and repeated hospitalizations, and some require long-term institutional care.

The siblings of children who have a chronic illness also require attention.[14] Siblings often worry about whether they will have the same disease if it is congenital or inherited. If the disorder is inherited and they have been spared, they often feel guilty. If the disease is acquired, these children may think or fantasize that their brother or sister did something to deserve the illness. Often in sibling rivalry a child may wish that the brother or sister were dead. When that brother or sister acquires an illness, the sibling may then feel tremendous guilt and responsibility for "causing" the illness. The primary physician caring for the child who has a chronic illness should always inquire as to the health, well-being, and psychological state of the youngster's siblings and may be able to provide insight to the parents concerning the siblings' behavior.

The Medical Delivery System

Children who have chronic illnesses often receive fragmented health care.[13] Frequently a primary care physician suspects an illness and requests a consultation at a children's hospital or service, where the child is taken, a workup is completed, and a diagnosis is made. The child then is assigned to a specialty clinic, returning regularly for care. Usually this clinic is attended by full-time staff specialists, but at each visit the child is seen by a different house officer who does not know or recognize either the child or the family. The contribution to the overall care by the primary care physician who referred the child originally often is ignored.

Whether a child who has a chronic illness should receive care from specialty clinics or from a primary care physician may be controversial. Often a child can be seen once or twice a year at the specialty clinic and have other checkups through the regular pediatrician. This arrangement is suitable if communication is good between the specialist and the primary care physician. During adolescence children who have chronic illnesses often continue to be treated in pediatric clinics, where they now feel uncomfortable, and their dependency is reinforced. Whenever possible, adolescents should be treated in a setting designed for teens.[8] If this is not possible, it may be appropriate to have adolescents treated by adult medical groups, if those physicians are sensitive to the issues of development.

When to hospitalize the chronically ill child is a difficult question to answer. Usually the parents are able to cope with innumerable medical problems at home simply through years of experience.[13] Hospitalization often takes on special meaning to the child who is a regular visitor to the physician or hospital; the child may view hospitalization as being followed by death if the reasons for hospitalization are not carefully explained.

Pediatricians and their staff must be aware of their own emotional responses to the chronically ill child. This child, more than any other youngster, is able to evoke mixed feelings and frustration in the staff. The staff members often are angry while caring for the child, frustrated because their patient does not get better. Often the care of a chronically ill child involves several consultants, and each consultant may give different messages to the child and the family. Complicated cases, especially those involving mental retardation, often are rejected by all members of the medical delivery system. When such children are hospitalized, they and their families frequently spend much time in the admissions office while house officers and administrative clerks decide where the children belong. The 15-year-old mentally retarded patient who has cerebral palsy may be rejected by the staff responsible for adolescent care because the patient looks like an 8-year-old child; the same patient may be rejected by the ward for school-age children because the child "is really an adolescent."

Counseling

Chronically ill children and adolescents and their parents should have opportunities to receive counseling.[11,13,31] Usually parents need this help early in the disease, shortly after it is diagnosed. Youngsters generally need this assistance as they approach adolescence. Not all chronically ill children and their parents will require counseling, but all should be given this option.

Usually the counseling can be provided by a sensitive and understanding physician willing to spend time with the family. Social workers and psychologists also are resources for handling these problems and can work closely with the physician who cares for the child. A group of adolescents who have similar problems may wish to meet regularly with an interested physician or staff member to share their common problems. In many areas parents of chronically ill children meet to support one another.

Role of the School

Children who have chronic illnesses frequently are absent from school because of their illness, clinic or physician visits, or hospitalization.[9] Absence from school should be minimized. In some communities children who have chronic illnesses attend special schools, particularly when they are severely handicapped. However, many children whose chronic illnesses are moderately severe attend regular schools. According to Public Law 94-142, children must receive (1) education in the least restricted environment compatible with their condition and (2) related services to facilitate their education. In either situation the school should be made aware of the children's medical problems.

Teachers may be helpful as objective observers of a child's condition. When medications are changed, teachers can be instructed to look for untoward side effects. With the parent's and child's permission, a physician may contact the school and notify the teacher, principal, or school nurse of changes in a youngster's illness. Often parents prefer to communicate this information themselves. Not all teachers are medically knowledgeable, and they may welcome information the medical profession can given them about a youngster in their classroom. In this way the school system and the medical system can collaborate to benefit the chronically ill youngster.

THE DYING CHILD

To care for the dying child properly, the physician must recognize that children have different concepts concerning death that depend on many factors, including chronological age, cognitive development, other experience with death, and religious and cultural beliefs.[27] All these factors should be considered when caring for the dying child.

Developmental Aspects of Death

To understand a child's concept of death, it is useful to apply Piaget's theory of sequential cognitive development[24] (Table 24-1). Infants and toddlers (2 years of age or younger) are in the *sensorimotor* stage of cognitive development. They learn through their senses (seeing, hearing, touching, and tasting) and they use their advancing motor skills to find new

Table 24-1 Development of the Concept of Death

Range (years)	Piagetian developmental stage	Concept of death	Approximate age
0-2	Sensorimotor *Preverbal* Reflex activity Purposeful activity Rudimentary thought	Expresses discomfort with separation	Infancy
2-6	Preoperational *Prelogical*	Uses word *dead* but only to distinguish "not alive"	3 yr
	Development of representational or symbolic language	Limited notion; may express no personal emotion but may associate death with sorrow of others	4 yr
	Initial reasoning	Avoids dead things; imagines death as a personified being; believes he or she will always live, only other people (especially older ones) die	5 yr
		Associates death with "old age"; may be violent and emotional about death, including representations (e.g., magazine pictures), or may display intense curiosity about dead things	6 yr
6-12	Concrete operational		
	Logical	Morbid interest in details (e.g., graveyards, coffins, possible causes); seeks answers through observation of decomposition, etc.; suspects he himself may die	7 yr
	Problem-solving restricted to physically present, real objects that can be manipulated	Less morbid, more expansive; interested in what happens after death; accepts, without emotion, that he too will die	8 yr
	Development of logical functions (e.g., classification of objects)	Understands logical and biological (e.g., absence of pulse) essentials of death; can accept full and rational explanation of death process	9-10 yr
12+	Formal operational *Abstract* Comprehension of purely abstract or symbolic content Development of advanced logical functions (e.g., complex analogy, deduction)	Meaning of death appreciated, but reality of personal death not accepted	Adolescence

From Sahler OJZ, Friedman SB: *Pediatr Rev* 3:160, Nov 1981.

objects and experiences to see, hear, touch, or taste. Although young infants are developing language, they essentially are preverbal, and the word *death* has no meaning for them. As they realize differences in individuals around them, however, infants can experience separation from loved ones (parents) and "know" the feelings of separation anxiety.

The next stage of cognitive development, described as *preoperational,* is characteristic of most children between 2 and 6 years of age. In this stage of development children have verbal skills but cannot yet think logically. Thus the preschooler has a very limited concept of death. By age 2 to 6 years youngsters generally have had some contact with death; a pet or a grandparent may have died. It is believed that these young children consider death a reversible phenomenon, as demonstrated in movies and television. For example, it is common to see a cartoon character flattened like a pancake with a steamroller and the next moment up and about and racing down the road. Such activity is completely plausible in the mind of the preschooler.

The school-age child 6 to 12 years old usually is in the *concrete operational* stage, when logical thought about the physical world is developing. Children's concepts of death undergo many changes during this time. For example, by the age of 6 to 8 years, the youngster often views death as a prolongation of sleep: Dead people's eyes are closed as though they were asleep; therefore they must be asleep, and they simply do not wake up. After accepting the concept of irreversibility, the child who views death as a prolongation of sleep generally asks questions such as: What happens when you die and you get put in the ground? Who does Jackie play with? Doesn't he need some cookies and milk? Won't he get cold? Isn't it dark down there? How can somebody be in the ground and in heaven at the same time? Later, when 8 to 10 years old, the youngster may see death personified, usually as a monster who sneaks in at night and kills the living. This fantasy often is "substantiated" by movies and television.

The final stage of cognitive development, known as the *formal operational* stage, is marked by the ability to understand and verbalize abstract concepts. Sometime during adolescence, usually by the midpoint, the teenager is able to perceive the concept of death as an irreversible phenomenon. This recognition may occur at the same time that most adolescents begin to deal with various philosophies, such as those concerning the purpose of life and the meaning of existence. Sometime in late adolescence or early adulthood, most people begin to grapple with the concept of their own death.[17]

Children, as well as adults, have fears concerning death; frequently physicians do not recognize or acknowledge these fears. Dying children, whose concept of death is poorly defined, exhibit a fear of abandonment and are concerned that while they are dying their parents will leave them alone. The child who is terminally ill and has experienced innumerable medical tests and studies usually is more afraid of bodily harm than of death. How much children know about their impending death is not completely understood.

A comparative study[25] of chronically ill school-age children who were not terminally ill and children who had leukemia who were terminally ill but in remission revealed much higher anxiety levels in the children who had leukemia. This study suggests that school-age children are more aware of the seriousness of their illnesses than physicians previously believed.

In managing the care of the dying child, medical personnel and parents must be aware that in addition to the normal developmental concepts of death, a child's perceptions can be affected by other experiences with death: the death of a sibling, a parent, or a grandparent. How the family reacted to the death of another family member may be reflected in the dying child's behavior. The child who has seen a torturous death of a very sick grandparent or sibling may be more frightened of the pain or bodily harm associated with dying than of death itself. Children from religious families also will be influenced by the family's religious attitude toward death.

The Family of the Dying Child

Parents of terminally ill children typically react to the information that their child has a fatal illness with initial disbelief and shock, which may take days or several weeks to subside. This disbelief may not necessarily be intellectual denial. The parents usually can accept the diagnosis intellectually but cannot absorb the full emotional impact. Parents may desire a second opinion, as a result of denial or in the hope that the diagnosis is incorrect. They can be warned that these feelings may occur.

After the initial disbelief and shock, the parents frequently experience anger.[17] The anger may be directed toward the physician who made the diagnosis, toward staff members caring for the child, toward each other, or toward themselves for not having protected their child from contracting the terminal illness. After anger, parents may experience the "bargaining" stage when they say to themselves, "If I give up such and such, perhaps my child will be cured." After going through the bargaining stage, parents generally feel depressed and only then perhaps begin to deal with their feelings about the illness. Some parents actually grieve over the loss while their child is still alive, particularly if they are parents of children who have leukemia at the terminal stages of the disease.

As part of their "anticipatory grieving," some parents have experienced what may be described as the *Lazarus syndrome.* A child is expected to die and is quite ill, and the parents actually grieve as though the death had already taken place, psychologically preparing themselves for it. The child then recovers unexpectedly and the parents are not always equipped psychologically to deal with the child. The physician can help the parents deal with their feelings at this time.

The marriage of parents who have a terminally ill or dying child often is stressful.[21] In traditional two-parent families it may be typical for the husband to support his wife emotionally early in the course of their child's illness and to make the important family decisions, thus allowing his wife to experience more emotion than he. In fact, the husband truly may feel the impact of the diagnosis only some days or weeks later, when his wife no longer needs such intensive support. In some instances, of course, these roles are reversed. Parents' support for each other is extremely important for the child, for the parents themselves, and for the other siblings. When children are hospitalized, mothers may be more comfortable than fathers in caring for them. Because of their inexperience in caring for a child and their work schedules, fathers may spend significantly less time with the child in the ward and have little contact with the physician. The mother then has to tell the father what the physician has said. Also, both parents may work. In estranged families, one parent may shoulder major responsibility for the child and feel little support from the other parent, or the other parent may feel "left out" of decision making and resent the former spouse or the physician, or both. To avoid such a situation, the physician should inform both parents about their child's condition, preferably at the same time.

The siblings of the dying child often are ignored by the parents and the physician. To decide what to tell siblings and how to tell them, parents must take into account their children's ages, development, and past experiences. They should be told that their brother or sister is dying, but with words that are in a manner that is comfortable for the family. They should be made to feel that they still are part of the family and can help deal with this family crisis. If the siblings are old enough, issues such as heredity or contagion should be brought up to reassure them that they themselves do not have the same illness.

The parents also may ask for help coping with extended family members and deciding what to tell grandparents, aunts, and uncles. What information parents give depends on the relationship with family members and how close they feel to them. All family members, however, should be told the same thing so that they do not hear conflicting information. Parents also should be warned that extended family members and neighbors may unintentionally add more stress to their lives. Relatives may say things such as "Johnny can't have leukemia, he looks too healthy," or they may send newspaper and magazine articles that contradict what the physician has told the family. Well-meaning grandparents or relatives may not allow the parents to lead normal lives when their child is terminally ill or shortly after their child's death. They may make statements such as "How can you have a party when one of your children is dying?," or "How can you go away on a trip when your son just died a few months ago?" If parents are forewarned of these possibilities, they may be better equipped to deal with them.

The role of religion in helping families deal with a dying child also must be considered. Ministers, priests, and rabbis can be greatly supportive to the parents and the dying child, and religious families often contact their pastor for help. In some hospitals there is a ministry devoted to dying patients and their families, and even though these clergy may not be of the same faith as the family, they can be of help to them. Most studies and written discussions to date concerning terminally ill children have been about parents of children whose deaths followed a terminal illness. Parents who lose a child suddenly or unexpectedly may not respond to the child's death in the same manner as parents who have had time to prepare themselves psychologically for the loss. They often experience disbelief that can last for several weeks. Parents may deny the death of the child for some time and often dream of the deceased youngster. Parents who endure the sudden, unexpected loss of a child experience intense, disruptive, and at times, almost intolerable grief reactions.

Death by accident deserves special attention because the parents or an older sibling may feel indirectly responsible for the death. The resulting guilt may persist, particularly if the accident might have been prevented by better judgment or supervision by the parent or sibling responsible for the child's safety. Guilt arising under such circumstances often is not resolved by the usual grief process.

The Medical Delivery System

Open communication should be maintained among the staff members caring for the dying child to determine ahead of time who will be responsible for telling the parents that the child is dying or has died. When a child has multiple consultants, the physician with the closest rapport with the family and the child should inform the parents of the death.[4] This responsibility should be shouldered by the primary care physician and not left to an unfamiliar intern.

How to tell parents that their child has died is another concern. In talking about the diagnosis of terminal illness or about death, privacy for the parents and the physician is needed. Most physicians are sensitive to parents' needs, yet often parents are told about the diagnosis or the death in the hallways and in the presence of other people. By *sitting down* with the parents, the physician assures the parents that he or she plans to spend some time with them and is not eager to leave as soon as possible. The physician should keep explanations as simple as possible. Parents often complain that they do not understand the medical situation. What they primarily want is only enough information to comprehend the situation, to understand the recommendations of the physician, and to know what is expected of them as parents.

The parents should be spoken to every day, and the same information usually should be repeated several times because they may not hear what the physician says the first time. The various details of the illness should be conveyed in a series of discussions rather than all at once. During these discussions the parents can be forewarned about the questions they may be asked by relatives and friends, and they also can be told to anticipate the desire to shift to a different hospital or a different physician. Then if and when they actually have these feelings, they will be relieved to know that this is what their physician had expected.

Staff members who care for a dying child often are depressed, and the morale of the nurses, house staff, and medical students suffers. On "losing" a child, the staff may experience feelings of failure and loss; often it is desirable for them to meet to discuss a child's death as soon as possible after the event. Blame should not be placed by one group of professionals on another; rather, a supportive attitude should be maintained by those in charge. Staff members in intensive care nurseries and other intensive care units are particularly susceptible to feelings of depression and low morale. To be constantly in the presence of severely ill children and to cope with the reactions of strained parents is stressful; therefore the programs of such units always should include outlets for emotional release and discussion of feelings concerning the death of infants and youngsters.

Whenever medically appropriate, permission for a postmortem examination should be obtained. This request should come from the physician who has the closest rapport with the family, and the responsibility should not be shifted from attending physician to house staff to student. Ideally it would be best not to ask for the autopsy at the same time that the physician is informing the parents of their child's death. Unfortunately the postmortem examination must be done within a brief time after death, and the time the parents first learn of their child's death may be the only chance that the physician has to ask the parents. Regardless of when the subject is broached, the physician should be as frank as possible, explain the reasons for the postmortem examination, and reassure the parents that mutilation and maiming will not result.

Follow-up after Death

The physician should try to contact the parents about 2 to 3 months after the child's death and offer to talk with them,[4] giving the parents an opportunity to ask the physician those questions they did not ask earlier. Parents often relive the illness and ask questions they had asked previously to assure themselves that their understanding of the child's disease was correct. As one mother said, "Talking later put a period on the whole episode." The physician also has the opportunity to see how the parents and siblings are adjusting and to inform them about the postmortem examination. Such actions assure the parents that the physician still cares about them and their adaptation to the stress of their child's death.

A family naturally grieves after a child has died, and the physician should support the grief reaction.[17] Lindemann[18] describes the process of mourning in detail, distinguishing features of acute grief such as frequent sighing respirations, waves of somatic distress, exhaustion, and digestive symptoms. The period of mourning cannot be sharply defined because there are marked differences among individuals. In general, however, feelings related to the loss are intense for 3 to 4 months after the death of a child. Birthdays, the date of the child's death, and holiday seasons all may remind parents of their loss and even years later may be associated with renewed periods of grieving. In the normal mourning process, however, parents return more or less to their previous level of psychological and social functioning approximately 4 to 6 months after their child's death.

After parents have lost a child through death, they may wonder whether they should have another child. After discussing this possibility with the parents, the physician generally can recommend that they have another child but should also forewarn them that the new baby is not to be a replacement. A phenomenon known as the *replacement child syndrome* occasionally occurs in which parents attempt to have another child as soon as possible after the death of a child and to make the new child into the one who has died.[22] In some extreme cases the same name is given to the second child. A sensitive physician who maintains contact with the parents can help them avoid this potential problem and realize that no child can truly replace another and that a subsequent child might be emotionally damaged in the attempt.

Everyone involved finds caring for dying children difficult and painful. The parents and siblings of these children need support from the physician during the terminal illness as well as after the death, and pediatric staff members, particularly nurses and house staff members, need opportunities to express their feelings of failure and loss when an infant or child dies.

REFERENCES

1. Adams DW, Deveau EJ: When a brother or sister is dying of cancer, *Death Studies* 11:279, 1987.
2. Alexander D et al: Anxiety levels of rooming-in and nonrooming-in parents of young hospitalized children, *Matern Child Nurs J* 17:79, 1988.
3. Bossert E: Stress appraisals of hospitalized school-age children, *Child Health Care* 23:33, 1994.
4. Brent DA: A death in the family: the pediatrician's role, *Pediatrics* 72:645, 1983.
5. Butler JA et al: Health care expenditures for children with chronic illnesses. In Hobbs N, Perrin JM, editors: *Issues in the care of children with chronic illness,* San Francisco, 1985, Jossey-Bass.
6. Cleary J et al: Parental involvement in the lives of children in hospital, *Arch Dis Child* 61:779, 1986.
7. Edwinson M, Arnbjornsson E, Erkman R: Psychologic preparation program for children undergoing acute appendectomy, *Pediatrics* 82:30, 1988.
8. Fisher, M: Adolescent inpatient units, *Arch Dis Child* 70:461, 1994.
9. Fowler MG, Johnson MP, Atkinson SS: School achievement and absence in children with chronic health conditions, *J Pediatr* 106:683, 1985.
10. Goldberg R: Adjustment of children with invisible and visible handicaps: congenital heart disease and facial burns, *J Counseling Psychol* 21:428, 1974.
11. Hausenstein EJ: The experience of distress in parents of chronically ill children: potential or likely outcome? *J Clin Child Psychol* 19:356, 1990.
12. Heins M et al: Attitudes of pediatricians toward maternal employment, *Pediatrics* 72:283, 1983.
13. Hobbs N, Perrin JM, Ireys HT: *Chronically ill children and their families,* San Francisco, 1985, Jossey-Bass.
14. Janus M, Goldberg S: Sibling interactions and empathy among siblings of chronically ill children: maternal versus children's reports, *J Dev Behav Pediatr* 15:296, 1994.
15. Jarman FC, Starr MC: "Unrecognized" chronically ill children in school: a group at risk for psychosocial difficulties, *Am J Dis Child* 143:416, 1989.
16. Jellinek MS: Managed care: good or bad news for children? *J Dev Behav Pediatr* 15:273, 1994.
17. Kubler-Ross E: *On death and dying,* New York, 1969, Macmillan.
18. Lindemann E: Symptomatology and management of acute grief, *Am J Psychiatry* 101:141, 1944.
19. Maternal and Child Health Bureau: *Child health USA '93,* Washington, DC, 1993, US Department of Health and Human Services.
20. Perrin EC et al: Issues involved in the definition and classification of chronic health conditions, *Pediatrics* 91:787, 1993.
21. Phillips S et al: Parent interview findings concerning the impact of cystic fibrosis on families, *J Dev Behav Pediatr* 6:122, 1985.
22. Poznanski EO: The "replacement child": a saga of unresolved parental grief, *J Pediatr* 81:1190, 1972.
23. Rasnake KL, Linscheid TR: Anxiety reduction in children receiving medical care: developmental considerations, *J Dev Behav Pediatr* 10:169, 1989.
24. Sahler OJZ: Grief and bereavement. In McAnarney ER et al, editors: *Textbook of adolescent medicine,* Philadelphia, 1992, WB Saunders.
25. Spinetta JJ, Maloney LJ: Death anxiety in the outpatient leukemic child, *Pediatrics* 56:1034, 1975.
26. Taylor MR, O'Connor P: Resident parents and shorter hospital stays, *Arch Dis Child* 64:274, 1989.
27. Wass H, Corr CA: *Children and death,* New York, 1984, Hemisphere.

25 Management of Fever

Henry M. Adam

There is a long history, at least in Western cultures, of viewing fever both as a response to illness and as a disease in itself. Hippocrates perceived fever as a defense mounted by the body against an underlying disorder; the Galenic and medieval traditions understood fever to be a means of restoring balance among the humors by burning off an excess of phlegm (water) with yellow bile (fire).[38] On the other hand, the writers of the Gospels saw fever itself as the disease that Jesus "rebuked," miraculously curing Simon's mother-in-law.[25,26]

This "double vision" of fever has persisted despite our relatively sophisticated understanding of the physiology of temperature control, still blurring how we as physicians and as parents see the febrile child. Although our science teaches us that fever, as part of the inflammatory response, is only a sign or symptom of the real pathological process, we seem to have the need to "treat" fever with a drug and a sponge, as if it were the noxious culprit itself. Fever, as opposed to hyperthermia, rarely poses a threat to a child's well-being; in fact, the argument has been made that as an energy-expensive phenomenon, it is not likely to have weathered evolution without conferring some survival benefit.[19] Considering that fever is the most common signal of illness in children, serving as the chief complaint for as many as a third of all pediatric office visits, we would do well to clarify our approach to its management distinct from the illnesses that cause it.

FEVER AND THERMOREGULATION

Fever is a regulated elevation of body temperature, mediated by the anterior hypothalamus, that occurs in response to any insult that stimulates the body's inflammatory defenses. Like a thermostat, the hypothalamic *set-point* controls the temperature the body tries to maintain. Some provocation, in children most commonly a viral infection, induces macrophages to release low-molecular-weight proteins called cytokines, among them interleukin-1 and interleukin-6 and probably tumor necrosis factor, that function as *endogenous pyrogens*. They circulate to the anterior hypothalamus, where, by increasing local levels of prostaglandin E_2, they induce a rise in the set-point.[18] With the body's thermostat now "upregulated," several mechanisms come into play to bring the *core temperature,* (defined as the temperature of blood within the pulmonary artery[23]) up to the new set-point. Because the core temperature, even as it begins to elevate, is lower than the thermostat setting, a person developing fever feels chilled. Physiologically the body's response is to generate more internal heat, setting skeletal muscles to shivering and stimulating cellular metabolism while minimizing heat loss to the environment by vasoconstricting the skin and turning off sweat glands. The one strategy is analogous to heating up the furnace, the other to closing the windows.

Hyperthermia, on the contrary, is an unregulated rise in core temperature to a level above the hypothalamic set-point, either from overproduction of heat (thyroid storm), a reduced ability to dissipate heat (a bundled-up baby) or, as with heat stroke from overexertion on a hot and humid day, a combination of the two.[45] The body's response to hyperthermia is in fact the opposite of its response when a fever is induced: instead of an initial chill, intense flushing ensues as blood vessels in the skin vasodilate and sweat glands activate in an attempt to lose as much heat as possible to the outside. The furnace is burning out of control; the only strategy is to try to open the windows wide.

Whereas hyperthermia may raise body temperature to dangerous, even deadly, levels, fever appears to be a homeostatic process, physiologically regulated within benign limits. Dubois[13] first noted how unusual it was even for patients who had an untreated serious infection to have fever exceeding 106°F (41.1° C). Two studies, one retrospective[31] and the other prospective,[35] that looked at large numbers of children who came to emergency departments were consistent in finding that in only 0.05% of visits did the child have a temperature of 106° F or higher. Although the pediatric literature is conflicting about whether a temperature over 106° F (frequently called *hyperpyrexia*) is a marker for particular risk for serious underlying infection,[1,8,31,35,49] no study suggests that the elevated temperature itself poses a threat to an otherwise healthy child except in the extraordinarily rare event fever exceeds 107° F (41.7° C). In fact, a child who has a temperature over 106° F is likely to have an element of hyperthermia, such as dehydration, in addition to fever. Evidence is accumulating that as an intrinsic feature of the febrile response, the body releases *endogenous cryogens*—peptides that counterbalance pyrogens and modulate how high the hypothalamus sets its thermostat.[18] Vasopressin and melanocyte-stimulating hormone, as well as some of the cytokines that also may act as pyrogens, appear to help limit the height fever generally can reach.[18]

As a centrally regulated response to an inflammatory insult, fever may well serve as a helpful component of the body's acute phase reaction. A growing number of studies are demonstrating that fever is an adaptive response widely present in the animal kingdom, among cold-blooded as well as warm-blooded species.[6,11,18,54] At least some species of fish and lizards, when infected, move to a warmer part of their environment, thus raising their body temperatures. This behaviorally induced fever has demonstrable survival benefit, which can be negated with antipyretic agents that lower temperature and increase mortality.[6,11,54] Fever can retard the growth and reproduction of many pathogenic microorganisms, both bacterial and viral, and it appears to lower the amount of iron available to invading bacteria, many of which have a greater iron requirement at higher temperatures.[20]

Among its other effects on human physiology, fever enhances neutrophil migration and the production of superoxides; it promotes T cell proliferation and increases the release and activity of interferon.[18,39] Interestingly, some of fever's apparently beneficial stimulation of immunological function may be reversed at very high temperatures, in the hyperpyretic range.[24]

Unfortunately, no conclusive experimental information is available to prove that fever benefits humans clinically in the course of an infection, and some data suggest that at least within the context of endotoxemia, the metabolic cost of fever contributes to mortality. But in a teleological sense, its metabolic cost argues for fever generally playing some protective role in the infected host; a process that results in a 7% to 10% increase in energy expenditure for every 1° C rise in temperature is not likely to have persisted so widely in nature, among invertebrates, fish, amphibians, and reptiles, as well as among birds and mammals, for so many millions of years without conferring some survival advantage.[18,19]

FEVER PHOBIA

If, then, fever itself only rarely poses a threat to a child and may even be of benefit, why are parents and pediatricians so generally aggressive about treating it? Schmitt[42] coined the phrase "fever phobia" when he described the prevalence of misunderstanding about fever among parents bringing their children to an inner city clinic. He found that 58% of parents defined fevers below 102° F (39° C) as "high," and 16% actually believed that if left untreated, fever could rise to 110° F (43.3° C) or higher. Almost every parent thought fever could cause harmful side effects, with 46% fearing permanent brain damage. Given these responses, it is not surprising that 63% of all the parents worried "lots" about the harm fever might cause their children and that 56% gave an antipyretic agent for a temperature within the normal range. For temperatures below 102° F (38.9° C), 85% of parents treated with a drug and 62% with sponging.

The population Schmitt described consisted mainly of medically indigent, poorly educated families. Kramer et al.[22] essentially repeated Schmitt's study in a private practice with middle-class parents. Almost half defined temperatures in the normal range as fever; 43% thought that temperatures under 104° F (40° C) could be dangerous, and 15% believed that untreated fevers could rise above 107.6° F (42° C). Death, brain damage, and stroke were among the complications of fever these educated parents feared, with 20% believing that such complications could occur at temperatures below 104° F and 95% believing that they could occur below 107.6° F. One in five of these parents would treat normal temperatures, and virtually all (97%) would treat a temperature below 104° F.

It's no wonder the use of medication to treat fever is so widespread. The English, for example, administer an estimated 68 million child-days of antipyretic drugs each year.[41] Half of the parents in Schmitt's study[42] stated that physicians or nurses were their most important source of information about fever. This claim was given credence by a survey of members of the American Academy of Pediatrics in Massachusetts,[27] in which two of three believed fever itself can pose a danger to children, and 25% of the responding physicians cited death and brain damage as potential complications of fever as low as 104° F (40° C). Almost three fourths of the pediatricians always or often recommended treatment for fever, two thirds of them for temperatures under 102° F (38.9° C). It may be the children who swallow the medicine, but the therapy seems aimed more at the anxiety of their parents and physicians than at any real danger fever holds for them.

DEFINITION AND MEASUREMENT

As would be expected with any physiological parameter, no single normal value represents the gold standard for body temperature. Rather, a range of normal values must take into account variations from person to person, fluctuations that reflect both a circadian pattern and age-related differences, and disparities arising from the method and site of temperature measurement. A reading of 98.6° F (37° C) traditionally has been considered the "norm"; however, the average mean daily oral temperature, measured every 6 hours for 41 to 108 days, of nine healthy young adult volunteers was 97.9° F (36.61° C), with a range of 97.5° to 98.4° F (36.41° to 36.9° C).[12] Young children tend to have higher normal body temperatures than older children or adults, yet infants in the first month or two of life are less likely than older children to develop fever with an infectious illness. Normally, body temperature is higher in the late afternoon and early evening than late at night or early in the morning, with a swing of as much as 3° F (1.7° C).[12,19,23,30] Probably the temperature cited most frequently as defining fever is 100.4° F (38° C), measured rectally. However, given all the variables that affect a particular person's body temperature, any specific number used to define fever is arbitrary.

In most clinical settings, where access to the pulmonary artery obviously is not a consideration, rectal temperature offers the best, although not a perfect, approximation of core temperature. To obtain this measurement, the child lies prone and a rectal thermometer lubricated at its tip is inserted to a depth of 1 inch. The thermometer is held there for 3 minutes with a mercury-in-glass thermometer or until the equilibration tone sounds with an electronic thermometer. The presence of stool in the rectum or poor perfusion of the bowel with hypovolemia can affect the accuracy of the measurement, as can improper technique.[7,23] More commonly, the problem with rectal temperature taking is the psychological discomfort, even more than physical, that it evokes.

With older children and adolescents, oral measurement is the standard method for determining body temperature. The great majority of children can learn to use an oral thermometer, with adult supervision, before they reach school age.[33] Particularly with oral measurement, electronic units have a tremendous advantage over mercury-in-glass thermometers; whereas it may take a glass thermometer at least 5 and possibly as long as 12 minutes to equilibrate in the mouth, electronic measurement usually is completed within 30 seconds. When the two methods are used simultaneously to measure temperature, the oral temperature on average will be 1° F (0.6° C) lower than the rectal temperature, but the relationship is not at all consistent. Often the oral temperature will be more than 1° F below the rectal temperature, and occasionally it may be higher. Perhaps because oral measurement is more difficult to standardize, it varies more than rectal measurement. With a glass thermometer, the time needed to reach steady state may be too long for a child to maintain proper placement of the thermometer in the posterior sublingual area; with an electronic unit, exact placement of the probe is crucial because the time to equilibration is so brief. Oral thermometers obviously are affected by either hot or cold foods eaten shortly before the measurement is taken, as well as by tachypnea, which can increase evaporative cooling in the mouth and lower the oral temperature.[50]

The appeal of axillary temperature measurement is apparent: It is less uncomfortable than rectal measurement and more convenient than oral measurement. Unfortunately, except possibly for newborn infants,[28] the correlation between axillary and rectal temperatures is too unpredictable to be clinically useful in most circumstances.[2,34] Only when no reasonable alternative is available, as in a child with an illness that contraindicates rectal manipulation and who is too young to cooperate with oral measurement, does axillary temperature measurement have a place outside the nursery. Even then, the reading should be interpreted with caution.

As a result of the development of infrared thermometry, the tympanic membrane temperature now can be measured. Theoretically, because of its proximity to the central nervous system, the tympanic membrane ought to have a temperature close to that of the hypothalamic thermostat. The procedure is fast, taking only a few seconds, and is both less invasive than rectal measurement and more convenient than oral measurement. However, to date the literature evaluating tympanic membrane temperatures has been at best equivocal.* The correlation between tympanic membrane and rectal temperatures appears to be better in the normal than in the febrile range,[15,44] thus sensitivity for detecting fever can be poor. Tympanic membrane temperatures also seem to be even less reliable at identifying febrile infants under 3 months of age than older children who have fever.[47] Until these instruments correlate more predictably with the rectal temperature or, even better, with body core temperature, tympanic membrane thermometers should not be used in routine clinical practice.

If it were reliable, skin measurement of body temperature would be the method of choice. Unfortunately, it is not reliable. Neither palpation nor temperature-sensitive crystal strips are accurate enough to replace rectal and oral measurements as the clinical standards.[4,36] The problem with palpation is the opposite of the shortcoming of skin strips. The strips are not appropriately sensitive, too often failing to detect fever,[36] but mothers tend to be too sensitive, not missing many fevers but mistakenly identifying many afebrile children as having an elevated temperature.[4] It is doubtful that pediatricians or nurses would have sufficient success with palpation to allow it to replace the thermometer. The skin itself is part of the body's temperature-regulating mechanism: With the onset of fever, it vasoconstricts to conserve heat and so may feel cool; as the body defervesces, it loses heat through vasodilation and thus may feel particularly warm.

MANAGEMENT

The management of fever rightly begins well before a child becomes febrile. As a first step, we pediatricians must recognize the part we have played in creating "fever phobia" in our patients' parents. Our almost ritualistic dependence on measuring a child's temperature, even at routine encounters where illness is not an issue, as well as our readiness to recommend antipyretic therapy for any elevation of temperature, certainly must confuse parents when we tell them not to worry about fever itself. Offering counseling about fever when a child already is ill is not as likely to be effective as introducing the subject routinely in the course of a health maintenance visit.[9,40] We need to explain that fever is one of the body's natural responses and not a threat in itself and that temperature will not spiral out of control to dangerous heights without treatment other than sensible care (e.g., maintaining hydration and not overbundling).[14] In identifying the underlying illness as the possible danger to the child, we would do well to educate parents about the symptoms and behaviors that should alert them to trouble and signal the need for medical attention.

Hyperthermia is different from fever, posing a real and immediate threat to any child suffering from heat illness. Successful treatment depends on restoring the core temperature to normal as rapidly as possible. Antipyretic agents, which work by lowering the hypothalamic set-point, are not helpful because the set-point already is below a rising body temperature that has escaped regulation; physical cooling is the mainstay of therapy.[45]

Treating fever, on the other hand, is a question of judgment. If the source of the fever poses a threat, obviously it must be addressed specifically. But intervening against fever per se should be a decision individualized to each febrile child. By far the commonest reason for treating fever is that it makes the child uncomfortable. Although on an evolutionary scale fever surely must be beneficial, its benefit during the course of an acute illness is not so well proven as to override concern for the child's comfort. The decision to treat for comfort's sake ought not be based on any particular temperature threshold, but on how the child looks and behaves; many children tolerate fevers to 104° F (40° C) without apparent ill effect, whereas others become cranky and restless with a temperature barely above 100.4° F (38° C). In some cases concern for a child's comfort may have to be balanced against the usefulness of a fever's pattern or persistence when making a diagnosis. At least one study[21] has even suggested that acetaminophen's efficacy in improving a febrile child's comfort is more presumption than fact. In a randomized, double-blind, placebo-controlled trial of 225 children 6 months to 6 years of age who had acute fever, those treated with acetaminophen were somewhat more active and alert than the control group but were no different in mood, comfort, appetite, or fluid intake. The acetaminophen group's fever and other symptoms lasted as long, and at the end of the trial parents were unable to tell with any reliability whether their child had received the drug or the placebo.

Particularly when comfort is the issue for an infant in the first few months of life, two factors weigh against routine use of medication for fever. The half-lives of all available antipyretics are significantly prolonged early in infancy, making inadvertent overdosage more of a problem. With their larger surface area relative to volume, infants also are more responsive to physical interventions that reduce body heat, such as removing clothing and blankets, keeping the room temperature moderate, and improving air circulation.

*References 15, 16, 32, 37, 44, 47, 52.

Some also believe that reducing fever with a dose of antipyretic can distinguish children who appear ill only because they are febrile from children who have a seriously threatening infection. In fact, neither the magnitude of fever reduction nor a child's clinical appearance after receiving antipyretic medication can reliably distinguish serious from trivial infectious disease.[3,53]

Although fever itself is benign in an otherwise healthy child who has a self-limited viral illness, the metabolic stress it entails may be more than an already compromised child can tolerate. Increased oxygen consumption and insensible water loss, along with tachycardia and tachypnea, can further threaten a child who is significantly anemic, septic, or in shock, as well as a child rendered vulnerable by cardiac, pulmonary, renal, or any other systemic disease that strains homeostasis. Fever also may exacerbate an acute brain injury, either infectious or traumatic, and its effect on the sensorium may be confounding in a child who has a neurological disorder.

More troublesome is defining the role of antipyretic medication in preventing febrile seizures. Children most at risk for febrile seizures (those 3 months to 3 years of age) are also the children who most frequently have self-limited viral illnesses. Urging parents to treat their young children's every fever with an antipyretic agent likely will promote fever phobia, as well as an unwarranted fear of the risk a febrile seizure poses. Undeniably a convulsive episode in a young child is terribly frightening, but only very rarely is it dangerous.[29] Aggressive attention to the possibility of a seizure with any fever will only magnify the anxiety parents already feel about both—and without any convincing evidence the strategy will work. The relationship between fever and seizures is neither clear nor predictable. Parents often are not aware that their child has a fever until after the seizure has occurred. Some children "seize" with low-grade fever and not again when their temperature is high. The lower the child's temperature with the first febrile seizure, the greater the risk of a second seizure[5]; this makes it more difficult for parents to have a sense of control because lower fevers are harder to detect. Parents overcall fever when they use palpation,[4] which may lead either to excessive dosing with an antipyretic drug or confirmatory rectal probes that become part of too many children's routine. Lastly, it has even been questioned whether around-the-clock administration of acetaminophen can prevent early recurrence of febrile seizures.[43] Although no approach seems perfect, a reasonable compromise might be using antipyretics prophylactically only for the approximately 3% of children who have had a first febrile convulsion, where the risk for recurrence is 1 in 3.[5] Even then, parents deserve reassurance that another seizure is neither their fault nor a real threat to their child's well-being. In fact, the threat may come from the treatment if prophylaxis becomes too aggressive. The use of alternating antipyretics, given every 2 hours, has worked its way into practice without real evidence to give it support, but certainly with the potential to generate more toxic reactions.

If a fever is to be treated beyond routine attention to hydration and ambient conditions, the most sensible approach follows from understanding how the brain controls the body's temperature. When the hypothalamic set-point rises, fever follows. Acetaminophen and nonsteroidal antiinflammatory drugs (NSAIDs), particularly aspirin and ibuprofen, are all effective antipyretic agents because they lower the hypothalamic set-point back toward normal by inhibiting the synthesis of prostaglandin E_2.

In most circumstances aspirin should not be the drug of choice for children because of its reported association with Reye syndrome.[10,48] Whether this association is unique to aspirin or generic to NSAIDs, which all have similar modes of action, remains unclear. When reducing fever is the principal concern, acetaminophen has the advantage of a long record of safety; it has almost no side effects, other than allergic reactions, unless ingested in toxic amounts (more than 140 mg/kg), which is at least tenfold greater than its therapeutic dose (10 to 15 mg/kg).[51] Children under age 6, the group most frequently febrile, are significantly less susceptible than older children and adults to liver destruction, the major toxicity of acetaminophen poisoning.

At its optimal dose (10 mg/kg) ibuprofen reduces fever as effectively as acetaminophen, and because its duration of action is moderately longer, it can be given every 6 hours rather than every 4 hours.[17,55] But there is a cost to ibuprofen's less frequent dosing; typically of antiinflammatory agents, it can cause gastritis and gastrointestinal bleeding, and it inhibits platelet function. The clinical situation determines whether ibuprofen's suppression of inflammation is a benefit or potentially an undesirable side effect. In a child febrile with rheumatoid disease, ibuprofen offers relief that acetaminophen cannot; a child whose fever arises from infection may well do better with the inflammatory response left intact.

As an alternative to medication, physical cooling can lower the body temperature of a febrile child, but the physiology of fever explains why the result may paradoxically make the child feel worse. With fever the hypothalamic thermostat is set above normal, dictating that the body generate heat. Whereas acetaminophen or NSAIDs push the thermostat back down, damping the impulse to produce heat, physical measures such as sponging work the opposite way; in effect, they open the windows to let heat escape without adjusting the thermostat at all. As cooling begins, the hypothalamus senses wider divergence between its own set-point and the body's actual temperature; to close the gap, it sends out the directive to generate still more heat, with muscular shivering and a rise in the general metabolic rate. Aside from how uncomfortable the child may feel, with the set-point remaining high once the sponging is finished, the temperature is likely to renew its climb.

Of course, under some circumstances physical cooling has a place. Some fevers that warrant intervention clinically may not respond to antipyretic drugs, as in a neurologically impaired child whose temperature control is aberrant. If an underlying illness gives special urgency to reducing the metabolic stress that comes with a fever, the combination of an antipyretic medication and cooling not only works more quickly than either alone[46] but also makes physiological sense; while cooling physically draws heat off, the drug lowers the set-point to avert a rebound temperature rise. The same holds for the rare fever high enough to be a concern itself, or for a fever that is complicated by some element of hyperthermia. When sponging a child, tepid water (about 90° F [32° C]) probably is best. It sets a moderate but effective gradient down from body temperature, rather than the precipitous decline colder water would induce, and it is less likely to distress the child who has a shivering response. Alcohol solutions have no place at all in the management of a febrile child because alcohol can be absorbed through the skin.

Hippocrates saw it right when, without the insights of our science, he somehow appreciated fever as part of the body's natural defense. Often, we do best to let nature have its way.

REFERENCES

1. Alpert G, Hibert E, Fleisher GR: Case control study of hyperpyrexia in children, *Pediatr Infect Dis J* 9:161, 1990.
2. Anagnostakis D et al: Rectal-axillary temperature difference in febrile and afebrile infants and children, *Clin Pediatr* 32:268, 1993.
3. Baker RC et al: Severity of disease correlated with fever reduction in febrile infants, *Pediatrics* 83:1016, 1989.
4. Banco L, Veltri D: Ability of mothers to subjectively assess the presence of fever in their children, *Am J Dis Child* 138:976, 1984.
5. Berg AT et al: A perspective study of recurrent febrile seizures, *N Engl J Med* 327:1122, 1992.
6. Bernheim HA, Kluger MJ: Effect of drug-induced antipyresis on survival, *Science* 193:237, 1976.
7. Bonadio WA: Defining fever and other aspects of body temperature in infants and children, *Pediatr Ann* 22:467, 1993.
8. Bonadio WA et al: Relationship of fever magnitude to rate of serious bacterial infections in infants aged 4-8 weeks, *Clin Pediatr* 30:478, 1991.
9. Casey R et al: Fever therapy: an educational intervention for parents, *Pediatrics* 73:600, 1984.
10. Committee on Infectious Diseases, American Academy of Pediatrics: Special report: aspirin and Reye syndrome, *Pediatrics* 69:810, 1982.
11. Covert JB, Reynolds WW: Survival value of fever in fish, *Nature* 267:43, 1977.
12. Dinarello CA, Wolff SM: Pathogenesis of fever in man, *N Engl J Med* 298:607, 1978.
13. DuBois EF: Why are fever temperatures over 106° F rare? *Am J Med Sci* 217:361, 1949.
14. Fruthaler GJ: Fever in children: phobia and facts, *Hosp Pract* (Off/Ed) 20(11A):49, 1985.
15. Hooker EA: Use of tympanic thermometers to screen for fever in patients in a pediatric emergency department, *South Med J* 86:855, 1993.
16. Johnson KJ, Bhatia P, Bell E: Infrared thermometry of newborn infants, *Pediatrics* 87:34, 1991.
17. Kauffman RE, Sawyer LA, Scheinbaum ML: Antipyretic efficacy of ibuprofen vs acetaminophen, *Am J Dis Child* 146:622, 1992.
18. Kluger MJ: Fever revisited, *Pediatrics* 90:846, 1992.
19. Kluger MJ: Fever, *Pediatrics* 66:720, 1980.
20. Kluger MJ, Rothenberg BA: Fever and reduced iron: their interaction as a host defense response to bacterial infection, *Science* 203:374, 1979.
21. Kramer MS et al: Risks and benefits of paracetamol antipyresis in young children with fever of presumed viral origin, *Lancet* 337:591, 1991.
22. Kramer MS, Naimark L, Leduc DG: Parental fever phobia and its correlates, *Pediatrics* 75:1110, 1985.
23. Lorin MI: Measurement of body temperature, *Semin Pediatr Infect Dis* 4:4, 1993.
24. Lorin MI: Rational, symptomatic therapy for fever, *Semin Pediatr Infect Dis* 4:9, 1993.
25. Luke, 4:38-39.
26. Matthew, 8:14-15.
27. May A, Bauchner H: Fever phobia: the pediatrician's contribution, *Pediatrics* 90:851, 1992.
28. Mayfield SR et al: Temperature measurement in term and preterm neonates, *J Pediatr* 104:271, 1984.
29. Maytal J, Shinnar S: Febrile status epilepticus, *Pediatrics* 86:611, 1990.
30. McCarthy PL: Fever in infants and children. In Machowiak PA, editor: *Fever: basic mechanisms and management*, New York, 1991, Raven Press.
31. McCarthy PL, Dolan TF: Hyperpyrexia in children, *Am J Dis Child* 130:849, 1976.
32. Muma BK et al: Comparison of rectal, axillary and tympanic membrane temperatures in infants and young children, *Ann Emerg Med* 20:41, 1991.
33. Norris J: Taking temperatures: the changing state of the art, *Contemp Pediatr* Nov 1985, p 22.
34. Ogren JM: The inaccuracy of axillary temperatures measured with an electronic thermometer, *Am J Dis Child* 144:109, 1990.
35. Press C, Fawcett NP: Association of temperature greater than 41.1° C (106° F) with serious illness, *Clin Pediatr* 24:21, 1985.
36. Reisinger KS, Kao J, Grant DM: Inaccuracy of the Clinitemp skin thermometer, *Pediatrics* 64:4, 1979.
37. Rhoads FA, Grandner J: Assessment of aural infrared sensor for body temperature measurement in children, *Clin Pediatr* 29:112, 1990.
38. Richards DW: Hippocrates and history: the arrogance of humanism. In Bulger RJ, editor: *Hippocrates revisited*, New York, 1973, Medcom Press.
39. Roberts NJ Jr: Impact of temperature elevation on immunologic defenses, *Rev Infect Dis* 13:462, 1991.
40. Robinson JS et al: The impact of fever health education on clinic utilization, *Am J Dis Child* 143:698, 1989.
41. Rylance GW et al: Use of drugs by children, *Br Med J* 297:445, 1988.
42. Schmitt BD: Fever phobia: misconceptions of parents about fevers, *Am J Dis Child* 134:176, 1980.
43. Schnaiderman D et al: Antipyretic effectiveness of acetaminophen in febrile seizures: ongoing prophylaxis versus sporadic usage, *Eur J Pediatr* 152:747, 1993.
44. Selfridge J, Shea SS: The accuracy of the tympanic membrane thermometer in detecting fever in infants 3 months and younger in the emergency department setting, *J Emerg Nurs* 19:127, 1993.
45. Simon HB: Hyperthermia, *N Engl J Med* 329:483, 1993.
46. Steele RW et al: Evaluation of sponging and of oral antipyretic therapy to reduce fever, *J Pediatr* 77:824, 1970.
47. Stewart JV, Webster D: Reevaluation of the tympanic thermometer in the emergency department, *Ann Emerg Med* 21:158, 1992.
48. Surgeon General's advisory on the use of salicylates and Reye syndrome, *MMWR* 31:289, 1982.
49. Surpure JS: Hyperpyrexia in children: clinical implications, *Pediatr Emerg Care* 3:10, 1987.
50. Tandberg D, Sklar D: Effect of tachypnea on the estimation of body temperature by an oral thermometer, *N Engl J Med* 308:945, 1983.
51. Temple AR: Pediatric dosing of acetaminophen, *Pediatr Pharmacol* 3:321, 1983.
52. Terndrup TE, Wong A: Influence of otitis media on the correlation between rectal and auditory canal temperatures, *Am J Dis Child* 145:75, 1991.
53. Torrey SB et al: Temperature response to antipyretic therapy in children: relationship to occult bacteremia, *Am J Emerg Med* 3:190, 1985.
54. Vaughn LK, Bernheim HA, Kluger MJ: Fever in the lizard *Dipsosaurus dorsalis*, *Nature* 252:473, 1974.
55. Walson PD et al: Comparison of multidose ibuprofen and acetaminophen therapy in febrile children, *Am J Dis Child* 146:626, 1992.

26 Management of Acute Pain in Children

Myron Yaster, Sabine Kost-Byerly, and Lynne G. Maxwell

We must all die. But that I can save (a person) from days of torture, that is what I feel as my great and ever new privilege. Pain is a more terrible lord of mankind than even death itself.

Albert Schweitzer, M.D.

I will use my power to help the sick to the best of my ability and judgement; I will abstain from harming or wronging any man by it.

Hippocrates

Even when their pain is obvious, children frequently receive no treatment or inadequate treatment for pain or painful procedures.[18,20] The common "wisdom" that children neither respond to nor remember painful experiences to the same degree that adults do simply is untrue.[2] Unfortunately, even when physicians decide to treat children in pain, they rarely prescribe potent analgesics or adequate doses because of their overriding concern that children may be harmed by the use of these drugs. This is not at all surprising because physicians are taught throughout their training that opiates cause respiratory depression, cardiovascular collapse, depressed levels of consciousness, vomiting, and with repeated use, addiction. Rarely, if ever, are the appropriate therapeutic uses of these drugs, or rational dosing regimens, discussed.

Nurses are taught to be wary of physicians' orders (and patients' requests) as well. The most common prescription order for potent analgesics, "to give as needed" *(pro re nata, "prn")*, has come to mean "to give as infrequently as possible." The prn order also means that either the patient must ask for pain medication or the nurse must identify when a patient is in pain. This is particularly difficult when dealing with children because it may be impossible for the very young to tell us when or where they hurt. Many children withdraw or deny their pain in an attempt to avoid yet another terrifying and painful experience—the intramuscular injection, or "shot." Finally, several studies have documented the inability of nurses and physicians to identify and treat pain correctly even in postoperative pediatric patients.[19]

PAIN NEUROPHYSIOLOGY

The physiology of pain is very complex and is more than simply the transmission of pain from peripheral receptors to the brain.[17] It probably is best understood in terms of Wall and Melzack's "gate theory of pain," which can be summarized as follows.[24] After an injury, peripheral pain receptors transmit sensory information to the spinal cord through relatively small diameter (A delta and C) sensory nerves whose cell bodies are located within the dorsal root ganglia. A delta fibers are associated with sharp, well-localized pain, whereas C fibers are associated with dull, burning, diffusely localized pain. The C fibers also include efferent sympathetic nerve fibers that increase the sensitivity of peripheral pain receptors. In the periphery, local release of prostaglandins, serotonin, bradykinin, norepinephrine, hydrogen ion, potassium ion, and substance P (a peripheral pain transmitter) can increase the responsiveness of the peripheral receptors to painful stimuli. Pharmacological manipulations of these local factors by prostaglandin inhibitors (e.g., aspirin, acetaminophen, or ibuprofen) thereby can blunt the transmission of pain.

The pain receptor impulse is transmitted to the dorsal horn of the spinal cord, where diverse synapses occur with essentially all incoming sensory input. In the dorsal horn of the spinal cord, interneurons are activated and release multiple neurotransmitters, including substance P, an 11-amino acid peptide pain transmitter. Alternatively, the pain impulse may be inhibited or completely blocked at the interneurons of the dorsal horn if the interneurons are overwhelmed by innocuous, nonpainful information from other peripheral nerve fibers. Stimulation of large-diameter peripheral nerve fibers can thereby blockade painful information effectively from the periphery. This is the underlying principle behind transcutaneous electrical nerve stimulation (TENS). Descending fibers also synapse at the interneurons to inhibit or modulate sensory input related to an injury via the release of neuropeptides. Of these neuropeptides, the opioid peptides (e.g., endorphins and enkephalins) are the best known and most extensively studied. Indeed, the identification of a variety of opioid receptors in the dorsal horn of the spinal cord explains the effects of intrathecal and epidural narcotic administration in the management of pain.

If unblocked, pain reception is transmitted to the brain through the classic spinothalamic and spinoreticular nerve pathways. Several areas within the brain may further modulate or abolish pain transmission, including the brainstem's medial and lateral reticular formations, the medullary raphe nuclei, the periaqueductal gray matter, the thalamus, and the cerebral cortex. Binding of either endogenous or pharmacologically administered opiates to receptors in these central locations initiates the modulation of pain transmission.[16] The gate theory therefore depends not only on peripheral stimulation and transmission of pain but also on modulation of the transmission within the spinal cord and higher central nervous system structures.

Thus pain or the transmission of pain receptor impulses requires intact neuroanatomical pathways from the peripheral origin of pain to the central nervous system. These pathways and receptors develop in early fetal life and essentially are mature and completely developed by birth.[1] The development of descending pathways for inhibiting pain receptor neurons and interneurons in the dorsal horn of the spinal cord and within the brainstem occurs during the final third of gestation and is completed during infancy and early childhood.

Pain management therefore can be best understood or designed in terms of afferent pain pathways and descending pain modulation pathways. Pain can be relieved by (1) reducing the sensory input from damaged tissue (by prostaglandin inhibitors or local anesthetics administration), (2) modulating the transmission of the pain receptor input to the central nervous system (by TENS, pharmacological opioid administration, or the administration of local anesthetics), and (3) altering the patient's emotional responses to such actual or perceived sensory input (by antidepressants, hypnotics, or amnestics). However, before one can treat pain effectively, one must be able to accurately measure and assess pain and the therapies used in treating it.

PAIN ASSESSMENT

The International Association for the Study of Pain (IASP) defines pain as "an unpleasant and emotional experience associated with actual or potential tissue damage, or described in terms of such damage."[15] Pain is a subjective experience; operationally it can be defined as "what the patient says hurts" and exists "when the patient says it does." Infants, preverbal children, and children between the ages of 2 and 7 years (Piaget's "preoperational thought stage") may be unable to describe their pain or their subjective experiences. This has led many to conclude that children don't experience pain in the same way that adults do. Clearly, children do not have to know or be able to express the meaning of an experience in order to have the experience. On the other hand, because pain is essentially a subjective experience, it is becoming increasingly clear that the child's perspective of pain is an indispensable facet of pediatric pain management and an essential element in the specialized study of childhood pain. Indeed, pain assessment and management are interdependent; one is essentially useless without the other. The goal of pain assessment is to provide accurate data about the location and intensity of pain as well as the effectiveness of measures used to alleviate or abolish it.

Validated, reliable instruments exist to measure and assess pain in children over the age of 3 years.[7] These instruments, which measure the quality and intensity of pain, are "self-report measures" and make use of pictures or word descriptors to describe pain. Pain intensity or severity can be measured in children as young as 3 years by using picture scales, for example, Wong's "smiley" face scale, which has a smiling face on one end, a distraught, crying face on the other, and several gradations in between or the "Oucher" scale, a two-part scale that has vertical numerical gradations (0 to 100) on one side and six photographs of a young child on the other (Fig. 26-1, *A* and *B*).[7,25] Pain has been assessed in infants and newborns by measuring physiological responses to painful stimuli; typically, blood pressure, heart rate, heart rate variability, vagal response, and levels of adrenal stress hormones are measured.[13] Alternatively, behavioral approaches have used facial expression, body movements, and the intensity and quality of crying as indices of response to painful stimuli. Finally, it is important to define the location of pain accurately. This is readily accomplished by using either dolls or action figures or by using drawings of body outlines, both front and back.

PAIN MANAGEMENT

Nonopioid (or "Weaker") Analgesics

The "weaker" or "milder" analgesics, of which acetaminophen (Tylenol), salicylate (aspirin), and ibuprofen (Motrin) are the classic examples, constitute a heterogenous group of nonsteroidal antiinflammatory drugs (NSAIDs) and nonopioid analgesics. They provide pain relief primarily by blocking peripheral prostaglandin production. These analgesic agents are administered enterally via the oral or, on occasion, the rectal route and are particularly useful for inflammatory, bony, or rheumatic pain. New parenterally administered NSAIDS, such as ketorolac, now are available for use in children in whom administration through oral or rectal routes is not possible. Unfortunately, regardless of dose, the nonopioid analgesics reach a "ceiling effect" above which pain cannot be relieved by these drugs alone (Table 26-1). Indeed, because of this, these weaker analgesics often are administered in combination with other more potent opioids such as codeine or oxycodone.

Aspirin, one of the oldest and most effective nonopioid analgesics, has largely been abandoned in pediatric practice because of its possible role in Reye syndrome, its effects on platelet function, and its gastric irritant properties. Despite these problems, a new salicylate product, choline-magnesium trisalicylate (Trilisate) is being used increasingly in pediatric pain management, particularly in the management of postoperative pain and in the child who has cancer. Choline-magnesium trisalicylate is a unique aspirin-like compound that does not bind to platelets and therefore has no effect on platelet function. It is a convenient drug to give to children because it is available in both liquid and tablet form and is administered only twice a day (Table 26-1). The association of salicylates with Reye syndrome will limit its use, even though the risk of developing this syndrome postoperatively or in cancer is extremely remote.

The nonopioid analgesic most commonly used in pediatric practice remains acetaminophen. Unlike aspirin and the NSAIDs, acetaminophen has minimal, if any, antiinflammatory activity. When administered in normal doses (10 to 15 mg/kg, PO or PR), acetaminophen has very few serious side effects, is an antipyretic, and like all enterally administered NSAIDs, takes about 40 to 60 minutes to provide effective analgesia. Dosage guidelines for the nonopioid analgesics most commonly used are listed in Table 26-1.

Opioids

Terminology. The terminology used to describe potent analgesic drugs is constantly changing. They commonly are referred to as "narcotics" (from the Greek *narco,* "to deaden"), "opiates" (from the Greek *opion,* "poppy juice," for drugs derived from the poppy plant), "opioids" (for all drugs that have morphinelike effects, whether synthetic or naturally occurring), or euphemistically as "strong analgesics" (when the physician is reluctant to tell the patient or the patient's family that narcotics are being used).[27,28] Furthermore, the discovery of endogenous endorphins and opioid receptors has necessitated the reclassification of these drugs into agonists, antagonists, and mixed agonist-antagonists on the basis of their receptor-binding properties.

The differentiation of agonists and antagonists is funda-

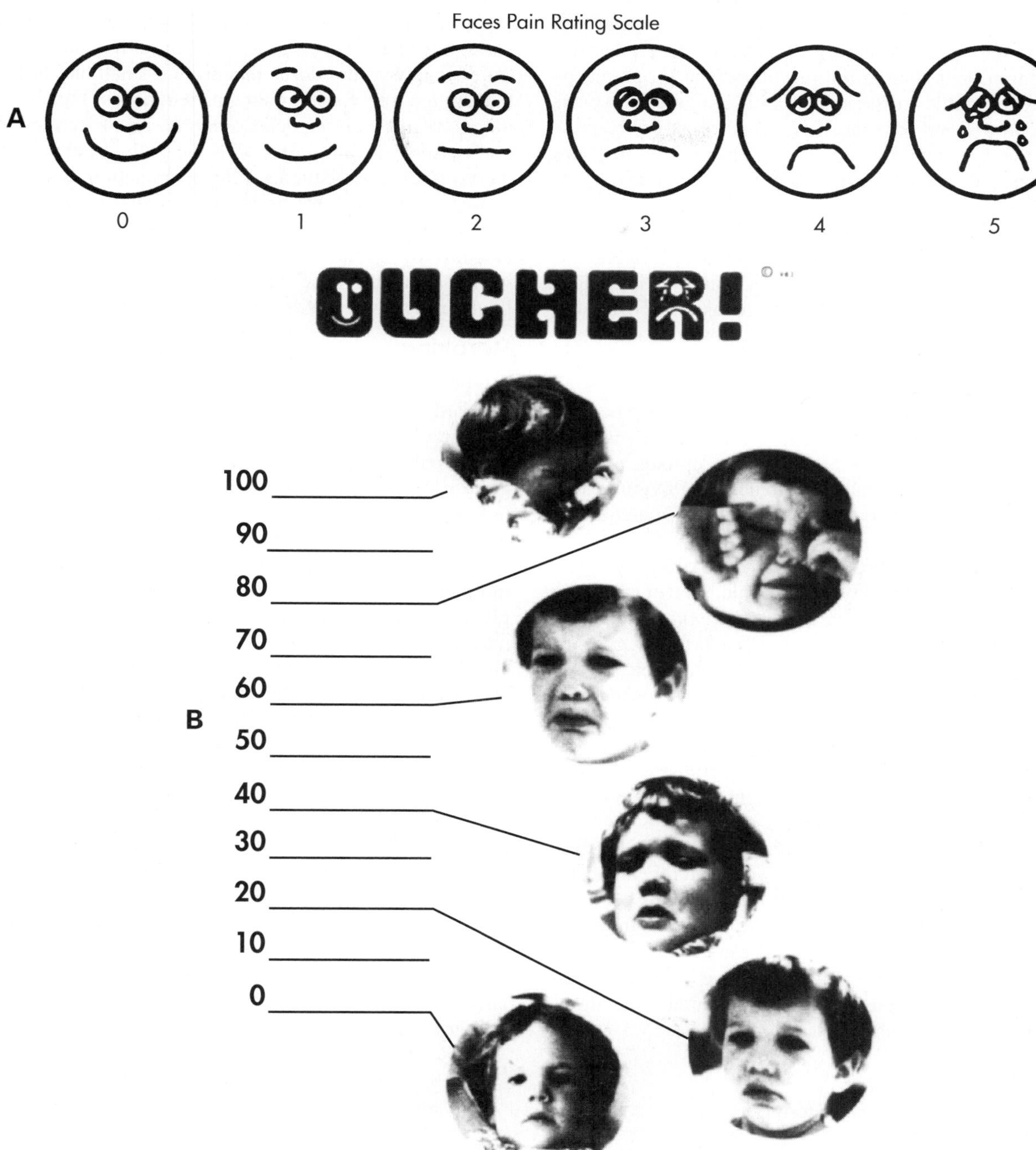

FIG. 26-1 Visual analog scales used in pain assessment in children are depicted. Note that the higher the score, the greater the child's pain. **A,** Six face interval scale. **B,** The Oucher scale.
(**A** from Wong DL, Baker CM: *Pediatr Nurs* 14:9, 1988; **B** courtesy Dr. Judith Beyer.)

mental to pharmacology. A neurotransmitter is defined as having agonist activity, whereas a drug that blocks the action of the neurotransmitter is an antagonist. By definition, receptor recognition of an agonist is "translated" into other cellular alterations, whereas an antagonist occupies the receptor without initiating the transduction step. Morphine and related opiates are agonists; drugs that block the effects of opiates, such as naloxone, are designated antagonists.

Opioids interact with specific receptors that are distributed widely throughout the central nervous system. Different effects, sensitivities, and anatomical localization have been ascribed to these various receptors. Although there are as many as eight different opioid receptors, four are of major importance in terms of pain management. These are designated as the mu, delta, kappa, and sigma receptors. The mu receptor and its subspecies and the delta receptor are related to analgesia, respiratory depression, euphoria, and physical dependence. Morphine is 50 to 100 times weaker at the delta than at the mu receptor. By contrast, the endogenous opiate-like neurotransmitter peptides known as enkephalins tend to be more potent at delta than at mu receptors. The kappa receptor, located primarily in the spinal cord, is related to spinal analgesia, miosis, and sedation. The sigma receptor is responsible for the psychotomimetic effects observed with some opiate drugs, particularly the mixed agonist-antagonist drugs. These effects include dysphoria and hallucinations.

A number of studies suggest that the respiratory depression and analgesia produced by opiates involve different receptor subtypes. These receptors change in number in an age-related fashion and can be blocked by naloxone. Zhang and Pasternak,[30] working with newborn rats, showed that 14-day-old rats are 40 times more sensitive to morphine analgesia than are 2-day-old rats.[30] Nevertheless, morphine depresses the respiratory rate in 2-day-old rats to a greater degree than in 14-day-old rats. Thus the newborn is particularly sensitive to the respiratory depressant effects of the opioids in what may be an age-related receptor phenomenon. Obviously this has important clinical implications for the use of narcotics in the newborn (see below).

Myths and Misconceptions Concerning Opioids. Despite the confusion of terminology and the plethora of available drugs, it is essential to realize that at *equipotent* analgesic doses all commonly used opioids produce similar degrees of respiratory depression, sedation, euphoria, nausea, biliary tract spasm, and constipation. Mixed agonist-antagonist drugs such as pentazocine (Talwin), nalbuphine (Nubain), and butorphanol (Stadol) produce significantly less respiratory depression and biliary spasm than do pure agonist drugs such as morphine. However, they also are significantly less potent analgesics than are the pure agonists and reach a "ceiling" above which no further analgesia can be achieved. Furthermore, they can reverse previously induced narcotic analgesia and should never be used in patients who are long-term users (or addicts) of opioids. Although an enormous number of opioids are available for clinical use, each with some purported advantage (typically "more effective," "less respiratory depression," or "less addiction" potential), the drugs listed in Table 26-2 are the most commonly used.

Opioids usually are administered at fixed intervals despite enormous variability in patient response. It is not uncommon for doctors to order doses that are too small and at intervals that are too long for individual patient needs (Fig. 26-2). Furthermore, nurses often delay administering narcotics for several reasons: unfamiliarity with the child's pain symptoms, demands of other patients, fear of addiction, and difficulty in finding the keys to the locked narcotic cabinet. Rational use of opioids requires a flexible, patient-oriented approach to allow for variability in individual pain and tolerance, as well as both the beneficial and adverse effects of the particular drug being used.

Morphine

Morphine (from Morpheus, the Greek god of sleep) is the standard for analgesia against which all other opioids are compared. When small doses, 0.1 mg/kg (IV, IM), are administered to otherwise unmedicated patients in pain, analgesia usually occurs without loss of consciousness. The relief of tension, anxiety, and pain usually results in drowsiness and sleep. Older patients suffering from discomfort and pain usually develop a sense of well-being or euphoria after morphine administration. Interestingly, when morphine is given to pain-free adults, they may show the opposite effect, namely, dysphoria and increased fear and anxiety. Mental clouding, drowsiness, lethargy, and an inability to concentrate and sleep may occur after morphine administration, even in the absence of pain. Less advantageous central nervous system effects of morphine include nausea and vomiting, miosis, and at high doses, seizures. Seizures are a particular problem in the newborn because they may occur at commonly prescribed doses (0.1 mg/kg). The nausea and vomiting that are seen with morphine administration are due to stimulation of the chemoreceptor trigger zone in the brainstem.

Morphine (and all other opioids at equipotent doses) depresses respiration, principally by reducing the sensitivity of the brainstem respiratory centers to arterial carbon dioxide content. Infants less than 1 to 2 months of age are particularly sensitive to this depression. *Indeed, this is of such great concern that the use of any narcotic in children less than 2*

Table 26-1 Dosage Guidelines for Commonly Used Nonsteroidal Antiinflammatory Drugs (NSAIDs)

Generic name	Brand name	Dose (mg/kg); frequency	Maximum adult daily dose (mg)	Comments
Salicylates	Aspirin—many brands (e.g., Bayer, Bufferin, Anacin, Alka-Seltzer)	10-15 q 4 h	4000	Inhibits platelet aggregation, GI irritability, Reye syndrome
Acetaminophen	Many brand names (e.g., Tylenol, "aspirin-free," Panadol, Tempra)	10-15 q 4 h	4000	Lacks antiinflammatory activity
Ibuprofen	Many brand names (e.g., Motrin, Advil, Medipren)	6-10 q 6-8 h	2400	Available as an oral suspension
Naproxen	Naprosyn	5-10 q 12 h	1000	Available as an oral suspension
Indomethacin	Indocin	0.3-1.0 q 6 h	150	Commonly used in NICUs to close a patent ductus arteriosis
Ketorolac	Toradol	0.2-0.5 q 6 h	150	May be given IV, IM, or PO
Choline-magnesium trisalicylate	Trilisate	8-10 q 8-12 h	3000	Does not bind to platelets; see salicylate above

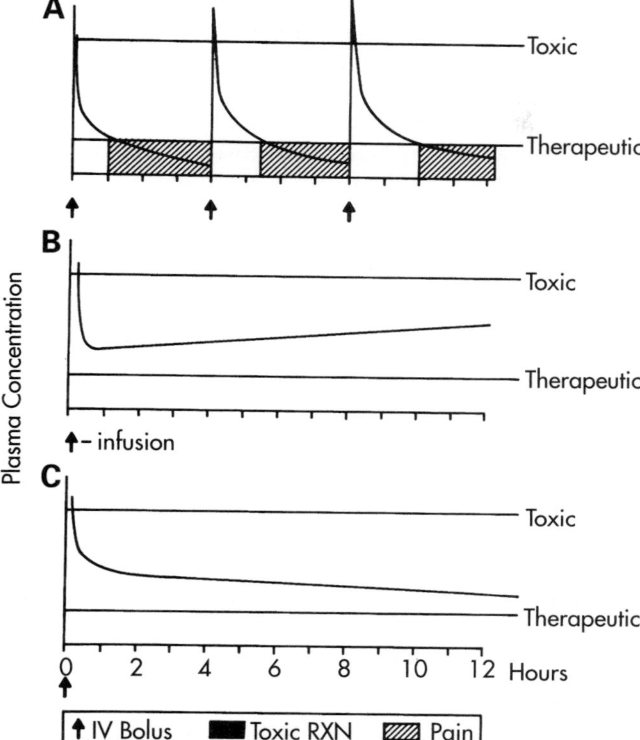

FIG. 26-2 Simulated blood concentration–dose relationships for opioids by different administration regimens. **A,** IV bolus administration of morphine sulfate (elimination half-life, 4 hours) every 4 hours. **B,** IV bolus administration of morphine sulfate followed by continuous IV infusion. **C,** IV bolus infusion of methadone (elimination half-life, 19 hours). Note the absence of pain periods in **B** and **C.** (Arrows, time of IV bolus administration, *RXN,* reaction.)

months of age must be limited to a monitored, intensive care unit. Possible explanations for this increased sensitivity include differences in opiate receptors (see above), the blood-brain barrier, and pharmacokinetics.

Way et al. suggested that an incomplete blood-brain barrier (as demonstrated in newborn rats) allows greater penetration of morphine to central nervous system receptor sites.[23] Presumably this would allow more drug to enter the central nervous system and produce a more profound effect. Several studies have demonstrated a prolonged elimination half-life (6.8 versus 2.9 hr) and decreased clearance (6.3 versus 23.8 ml/kg/min) of morphine in infants less than 1 month of age when compared with older infants and adults. Nevertheless, the half-life of elimination and clearance of morphine in children older than 1 month is similar to adult values. Thus infants less than 1 month of age will attain higher serum levels that will decline more slowly than those in older children and adults, and this may account for the increased respiratory depression seen in this age group. Conversely, on the basis of its relatively short half-life (2.9 hr), one would expect older children and adults to require morphine supplementation every 2 to 3 hours when being treated for pain, particularly if the morphine is administered intravenously. This has led to the recent use of continuous infusion regimens of morphine and patient-controlled analgesia (see below), which maximize pain-free periods (see Fig. 26-2).

Although morphine produces peripheral vasodilation and venous pooling, it has minimal hemodynamic effects in normal, euvolemic, supine patients. The vasodilation associated with morphine is due primarily to its histamine-releasing effects. Significant hypotension may occur if sedatives such as diazepam are administered concurrently with morphine. Otherwise, it produces virtually no cardiovascular effects when

Table 26-2 Commonly Used Mu Agonist Drugs

Agonist	Equipotent IV dose (mg/kg)	Duration (hr)	PO absorption (%)	Comments
Morphine	0.1	3-4	20-40	• May cause seizures in newborns; also in all patients at high doses • Causes histamine release, vasodilation, so avoid in asthmatics and in circulatory compromise • MS-contin; 8-12 h duration
Meperidine	1.0	3-4	40-60	• Catastrophic interactions with monoamine oxidase (MAO) inhibitors • Tachycardia; negative inotrope • Metabolite produces seizures • **Not recommended for routine analgesic therapy** • Low dose (0.25 mg/kg) stops shivering
Methadone	0.1	6-24	70-100	• Can be given IV even though the package insert says SQ or IM
Fentanyl	0.001	0.5-1		• Bradycardia; minimal hemodynamic alterations • Chest wall rigidity (>5 μg/kg rapid IV bolus). R_x naloxone, succinylcholine, or pancuronium • Oral transmucosal preparation 10 μg/kg
Codeine	1.2	3-4	40-70	• PO only • Prescribe with acetaminophen
Oxycodone (Tylox)	0.1	3-4	60-80	• PO only, less nauseating than codeine • Usually prescribed with acetaminophen

used alone. It will cause significant hypotension in hypovolemic patients; its use in trauma, therefore, is limited.

Morphine (and all other narcotics at equipotent doses) inhibits intestinal smooth muscle motility. This decrease in peristalsis and increase in sphincter tone explains the historical use of narcotics in the treatment of diarrhea as well as its "side effect" when treating chronic pain, namely, constipation. In fact, we routinely prescribe laxatives for patients expected to be treated with narcotics for more than 2 or 3 days. Obviously, morphine will potentiate biliary colic by causing spasm of the sphincter of Odi and should be used with caution in patients who have, or are at risk for, cholelithiasis (e.g., sickle cell disease). Finally, to minimize the complications associated with the administration of intravenous morphine (or any opioid), we always recommend titration of the dose at the bedside until the desired level of analgesia is achieved.

Morphine and most mu agonists (meperidine, methadone, and fentanyl) are biotransformed in the liver before excretion. Many of these reactions are catalyzed in the liver by microsomal mixed-function oxidases that require the cytochrome P_{450} system, NADPH, and oxygen. Morphine primarily is glucuronidated into two forms—an inactive form, morphine-3-glucuronide, and an active form, morphine-6-glucuronide. Both glucuronides are excreted by the kidney. In patients who have renal failure, the morphine 6-glucuronide can accumulate and cause toxic side effects, including respiratory depression. This is important to consider not only when prescribing morphine but also when administering other opioids that are metabolized into morphine, such as methadone and codeine.

Finally, only about 30% of an orally administered dose of morphine reaches the systemic circulation. In the past, this led many to believe that morphine was ineffective if administered orally. This is not true and was the result of failing to provide sufficient morphine. When converting a patient's intravenous morphine requirements to oral maintenance, one needs to multiply the intravenous dose by 3 to 4. Oral morphine is available as a liquid (20 mg/ml), tablet, and sustained-release preparation (MS-contin) (Table 26-2).

Fentanyl

Because of its rapid onset and brief duration of action, fentanyl has become a favored analgesic for short procedures, such as bone marrow aspirations, fracture reductions, suturing of lacerations, endoscopy, and dental procedures. Fentanyl is approximately 100 times more potent than morphine (the equianalgesic dose is 0.001 mg/kg, Table 26-2) and largely is devoid of hypnotic or sedative activity. Its ability to block painful stimuli with concomitant hemodynamic stability is excellent and makes it the drug of choice for trauma, cardiac, or intensive care unit patients. Furthermore, in addition to its ability to block the systemic and pulmonary hemodynamic responses to pain, fentanyl also prevents the biochemical and endocrine stress (catabolic) response to painful stimuli that may be so detrimental in the seriously ill patient. Fentanyl does have a serious side effect, namely, the development of chest wall rigidity after rapid infusions of 0.005 mg/kg or greater. This may make ventilation difficult or impossible. Chest wall rigidity can be treated with either muscle relaxants, such as succinylcholine or pancuronium, or with naloxone.

Fentanyl is a highly lipophilic drug and rapidly penetrates all membranes, including the oral mucosa and skin. Indeed, this has made transmucosal and transdermal preparations of this drug possible (see below). Fentanyl is eliminated rapidly from plasma as the result of its extensive uptake by body tissues. Its pharmacokinetics differ between newborn infants, children, and adults. The total body clearance of fentanyl is greater in infants 3 to 12 months of age than in children older than 1 year or adults (18.1 ± 1.4, 11.5 ± 4.2, and 10.0 ± 1.7 ml/kg/min, respectively), and the half-life of elimination is longer (233 ± 137, 244 ± 79, and 129 ± 42 min, respectively). The prolonged elimination half-life of fentanyl from plasma has important clinical implications. Repeated doses of fentanyl for maintenance of analgesic effects will lead to accumulation of fentanyl and its ventilatory depressant effects. Very large doses (0.05 to 0.10 mg/kg, as used in anesthesia) may be expected to induce long-lasting effects because plasma fentanyl levels would not fall below the threshold level at which spontaneous ventilation occurs during the distribution phases. On the other hand, the greater clearance of fentanyl in infants older than 3 months produces lower plasma concentrations of the drug and may allow these children to tolerate more drug without respiratory depression.

Meperidine

Meperidine (Demerol) is a synthetic narcotic most commonly used in children as either a premedicant for anesthesia (or sedation) or a treatment for postoperative pain. It is a potent analgesic that has pharmacokinetic properties similar to those of morphine. Meperidine is a mu agonist that binds to opioid receptors in the central nervous system and can produce analgesia, sedation, euphoria, dysphoria, miosis, and respiratory depression. At equianalgesic doses (1.0 mg/kg, Table 26-2), there is little quantitative difference between meperidine and morphine in producing these effects. It stimulates the chemoreceptor trigger zone in the brainstem to the same degree that morphine does and thereby may produce either nausea, vomiting, or both. Its effects on respiration and on gastrointestinal motility are similar to those of all the other mu-agonist opioid analgesics; thus it is a potent respiratory depressant and antitussive. Meperidine depresses intestinal smooth muscle motility and exerts a spasmogenic effect on intestinal smooth muscle. Some studies suggest that meperidine exerts less of an effect on the biliary tract, including the common bile duct, than morphine. Other studies dispute this. Indeed, in our opinion, there is *no* evidence to substantiate the belief that at *equianalgesic* doses, biliary tract pressure rises to a lesser extent after meperidine administration when compared with morphine. Thus there is no reason to prescribe meperidine preferentially for patients at risk for, or who are experiencing, biliary colic pain (e.g., sickle cell vasoocclusive crisis).

Meperidine differs from morphine in that large doses (toxic levels) may produce slow waves on the electroencephalogram. Additionally, high levels of meperidine's principal metabolite, normeperidine, may produce tremors, muscle twitches, hyperactive reflexes, and convulsions. Because of the accumulation of this metabolite, the prolonged use of meperidine should be discouraged, if not avoided completely. Indeed, we have abandoned the routine use of meperidine in our pain management practice. On the other hand, we do prescribe meperidine for *shivering*. When administered at low doses (0.25 to 0.5 mg/kg) intravenously, meperidine has the unique property of abolishing shivering. Indeed, it will stop shivering regardless of its cause (e.g., transfusion or drug [amphotericin] reactions, hypothermia, and so on).

Meperidine is effective whether administered orally or parenterally. The drug is extremely well absorbed from the gastrointestinal tract and has a bioavailability of approximately 50%, making it among the most popularly prescribed oral narcotics. It is available in both liquid (syrup) and tablet. Typically, it can exert analgesic effects within 15 to 30 minutes of oral administration and achieves peak plasma concentrations within 1 to 2 hours of ingestion. Intramuscular injection provides a more rapid onset of analgesia (approximately 10 minutes) and reaches a peak effect within 60 minutes of administration. Obviously, plasma concentrations may vary markedly after intramuscular injection, on the basis of an individual patient's state of peripheral perfusion.

Meperidine commonly is administered intramuscularly for moderate to severe pain or as part of a "lytic" (sedative) cocktail (meperidine, promethazine, and chlorpromazine) in a dose of 1 to 2 mg/kg; the frequency of administration should range between 3 and 4 hours. We *do not recommend* intramuscular administration of analgesics (or any drug) in children, nor do we advocate the use of the lytic cocktail. *In fact, we consider the lytic cocktail to be an archaic and, frankly, dangerous sedative combination.* We mention it only to condemn its continued use! For oral administration, meperidine is available in tablet and syrup; the usual dose is 1 to 2 mg/kg.

Methadone

Primarily thought of as a drug to treat (narcotic) addicted patients, methadone increasingly is being used for postoperative pain relief and for the treatment of intractable pain. It is noted for its slow elimination, very long duration of effective analgesia, and high oral bioavailability.

Methadone has the longest half-life of elimination ($t_{1/2}$ beta) of any of the commonly available opiates and provides 12 to 36 hours of analgesia following an intravenous injection. In children (ages 1-18), the $t_{1/2}$ beta of methadone averages 19.2 hours and the clearance averages 5.4 ml/min/kg. Pharmacokinetically, children, therefore, are indistinguishable from young adults. Finally, because methadone is extremely well absorbed from the gastrointestinal tract and has a bioavailability of 80% to 90%, it is extremely easy to convert intravenous to oral dosing regimens.

Because a single dose of methadone can achieve and sustain a high drug plasma level, it is a convenient way to provide prolonged analgesia without requiring an intramuscular injection (see Fig. 26-2). Indeed, when administered either orally or intravenously, it may be viewed as an alternative to the use of continuous intravenous opioid infusions. Berde et al. recommend "loading" patients with an initial dose of intravenous methadone, 0.1 to 0.2 mg/kg, and then titrating in 0.05 mg/kg increments.[6] Supplemental methadone can be administered in 0.05 to 0.1 mg/kg increments administered by slow intravenous infusion every 6 to 12 hours as needed.

Codeine and Oxycodone

Codeine and oxycodone (the opioid in Tylox and Percocet) are opiates frequently used to treat pain in children and adults. Although effective when administered either orally or parenterally, they most commonly are administered orally, usually in combination with acetaminophen or aspirin. In equipotent doses (Table 26-2), codeine's and oxycodone's efficacy as analgesics and respiratory depressants approaches that of morphine. In addition, codeine and oxycodone share with morphine and the other narcotics common effects on the central nervous system, including sedation, respiratory depression, and stimulation of the chemoreceptor trigger zone in the brainstem. Indeed, the latter particularly is true for codeine. Codeine is very nauseating, and many patients claim that they are "allergic" to it because it induces vomiting. There are much fewer problems from nausea and vomiting with oxycodone. Both drugs delay gastric emptying and can increase biliary tract pressure. Finally, codeine, like all mu-agonist opioids, has potent antitussive properties and commonly is prescribed for this effect.

Codeine and oxycodone have a bioavailability of approximately 60% after oral ingestion. The analgesic effects occur as early as 20 minutes after ingestion and reach a maximum at 60 to 120 minutes. The plasma half-life of elimination is 2.5 to 3 hours. Codeine metabolizes completely almost in the liver before its final excretion in urine. Approximately 10% of codeine is metabolized into morphine, and it is this 10% that is responsible for codeine's analgesic effect. Interestingly, approximately 10% of the population cannot metabolize codeine into morphine.

Oral codeine and oxycodone almost always are prescribed in combination with either acetaminophen or aspirin. Although conventional pediatric teaching is to prescribe single agent drugs, this is not wise with codeine and oxycodone. When prescribed as a single agent, these drugs are not readily available in liquid form at most pharmacies and are almost twice as expensive as their combined forms. Furthermore, acetaminophen (or aspirin) potentiates the analgesia produced by these drugs and allows the practitioner to use less narcotic and yet achieve satisfactory analgesia. Progressive increases in dose are associated with a similar degree of respiratory depression, delayed gastric emptying, nausea, and constipation as with other opioid drugs. Although it is an effective analgesic when administered parenterally, intramuscular codeine has no advantage over morphine or meperidine. Intravenous administration of codeine is associated with serious complications, including apnea and severe hypotension, probably secondary to histamine release. Therefore we do not recommend the intravenous administration of this drug in children.

Codeine and oxycodone are available in liquid, tablets, and capsules. Typically, codeine is prescribed in a dose of 0.5 to 1 mg/kg and oxycodone is prescribed in a dose of 0.05 to 0.1 mg/kg. Both are administered concurrently with acetaminophen (10 mg/kg).

Opioid Antagonists

A discussion of narcotic analgesics would be incomplete without mentioning the opioid antagonists. As mentioned previously, a drug that blocks the action of a neurotransmitter is an antagonist. By definition, receptor recognition of an agonist is "translated" into other cellular alterations, whereas an antagonist occupies the receptor without initiating the transduction step. Naloxone is a pure opioid antagonist that has virtually no agonist activity. It antagonizes the effects of the pure agonist drugs, such as morphine, as well as the mixed agonist-antagonist drugs, such as butorphanol. In fact, it is the most commonly used opioid antagonist in clinical practice.

Naloxone is extremely potent and nonselective in its opioid reversal effects. It reverses not only the sedation, respiratory depression, and gastrointestinal effects of the opioid agonists but also the analgesia. Indeed, the antagonism of narcotic agonist effects must be accomplished with great caution, particularly in patients who have been receiving prolonged opioid therapy, who exhibit opioid dependence, or who are in extreme pain because it may be accompanied by overt withdrawal symptoms. Occasionally a life-threatening "overshoot" phenomenon may occur in these patients, with the development of tachypnea, tachycardia, hypertension, nausea and vomiting, and sudden death. In healthy young adults this phenomenon may be accompanied by the onset of pulmonary edema. Indeed, it is our practice to employ mechanical ventilation as a safer treatment for narcotic-induced respiratory depression in dependent patients or patients in severe pain. Obviously, the magnitude of the withdrawal syndrome depends on the dose of naloxone administered as well as on the degree of the patient's physical dependence and needs. On the other hand, when naloxone is administered to patients who have not received opioids, it produces minimal to no effects (except in patients in shock; see below) and has no inherent properties that induce physical dependence or tolerance.

Naloxone metabolizes rapidly in the liver **(conjugation with glucuronic acid)** and is best given parenterally because of its rapid first-pass extraction through the liver after oral administration. After intravenous administration it reverses opioid effects virtually instantaneously. Unfortunately, it has a plasma half-life of elimination of only 60 minutes and a duration of action that is much shorter than the agonists it is used to antagonize ("reverse"). Therefore, when naloxone is used to reverse narcotic-induced respiratory depression, patients must be monitored for return of the depression on the basis of the half-life of the opiate agonist. This may require repeat intravenous doses, intramuscular (depot) injection, or a continuous intravenous infusion of naloxone.

Naloxone is supplied as a parenteral solution (1.0 mg/ml, 0.4 mg/ml, or 0.02 mg/ml). The usual initial dose in children (and adults) is 0.01 to 0.10 mg/kg given intravenously. If an intravenous route is not available, naloxone may be administered intramuscularly or subcutaneously. Doses as low as 0.001 to 0.002 mg/kg may be effective at reversing opioid-induced respiratory depression (or other unwanted side effects such as pruritus or biliary spasm) without reversing analgesia. If the initial dose of naloxone does not result in the desired degree of clinical improvement, subsequent doses of 0.02, 0.04, 0.08, and 0.1 mg/kg may be administered in a step-wise manner. The highest doses, 0.1 mg/ml, are used to treat cardiopulmonary arrest. When used to antagonize neonatal respiratory depression (from narcotics administered to the mother in labor), the usual initial dose is the same dose as used in older children (0.01 mg/kg of the 0.02 mg/ml solution).

Patient-Controlled Analgesia

Because of the enormous individual variations in pain perception and opioid metabolism, fixed doses and time intervals make little sense. On the basis of the pharmacokinetics of the opioids, it should be clear that intravenous boluses of morphine or meperidine may need to be given at intervals of 1 to 2 hours to avoid marked fluctuations in plasma drug levels (see Fig. 26-2). Continuous intravenous infusions can provide steady analgesic levels and are preferable to intramuscular injections; however, they are not a panacea because the perception and intensity of pain is not constant. Indeed, the most common method of opioid administration in adults and children is intramuscular injection. It is well known that children will suffer in silence and under-report their level of pain rather than ask for yet another painful stimulus, namely, the "shot." Thus rational pain management requires some form of titration to reach the desired effect whenever an opioid is administered. To give patients some measure of control over their pain, demand analgesia, or patient-controlled analgesia (PCA), devices have been developed. These are microprocessor-driven pumps with a button that the patient presses to self-administer a small dose of opioid.

PCA devices allow patients to administer small amounts of an analgesic whenever they feel a need for more relief. The opioid, usually morphine, is administered either intravenously or subcutaneously. The dosage of opioid, number of boluses per hour, and the time interval between boluses (the "lock-out period") are programmed into the equipment to allow maximum patient flexibility and sense of control with minimal risk of overdosage (Table 26-3). Generally, because patients know that if they have severe pain they can obtain relief immediately, many prefer dosing regimens that result in mild to moderate pain in exchange for fewer side effects such as nausea or pruritus. Typically, we initially prescribe morphine, 20 μg/kg/bolus, at a rate of 5 boluses/hour, with a 6 to 8 minute lock-out interval between each bolus (Table 26-3). Variations include larger boluses (30 to 50 μg/kg), shorter time intervals (5 min), and so forth. Hydromorphone has fewer side effects than morphine and often is used when pruritus and nausea complicate morphine PCA therapy. The

Table 26-3 Intravenous Patient-Controlled Anesthesia (PCA) Treatment Guidelines

Drug (concentration mg/ml)	Basal rate range (mg/kg/hr)	Bolus rate range (mg/kg)	Lock-out interval range (minutes)	Number of boluses/hr range
Morphine (1.0)	0.01-0.03	0.01-0.03	5-10	2-6
Fentanyl (0.01 in children <20 kg; 0.05 in children >20 kg)	0.0005 (0.5 μg)	0.0005-0.001 (0.5-1.0 μg)	5-10	1-6
Hydromorphone (0.2 in children <50 kg; 0.5-1.0 in children >50 kg)	0.003-0.005 (3.0-5.0 μg)	0.003-0.005 (3.0-5.0 μg)	5-10	2-6

PCA pump computer stores within its memory the number of boluses the patient has received and the number of attempts the patient has made at receiving boluses. This allows the physician to evaluate how well the patient understands the use of the pump and provides information to program the pump more efficiently. Many PCA units allow low "background" continuous infusions (morphine, 20 to 30 μg/kg/hour) in addition to self-administered boluses. This sometimes is called "PCA-Plus." A continuous background infusion is particularly useful at night and often provides more restful sleep by preventing the patient from awakening in pain. It also increases the potential for overdosage. Although the literature on pain does not support the use of continuous background infusions, it has been our experience that continuous infusions are essential for both the patient and the physician (fewer phone calls, problems, and the like). Indeed, in our practice, we almost always use continuous background infusions when we prescribe IV (or epidural) PCA.

PCA requires a patient who has enough intelligence and manual dexterity and strength to operate the pump. Thus it initially was limited to adolescents and teenagers, but the lower age limit at which this treatment modality can be used continues to fall. In fact, it has been our experience that any child able to play Nintendo (age 5 to 6 years) can operate a PCA pump. Furthermore, in our practice we empower nurses and parents to initiate PCA boluses and use this technology in children less than even a year of age. Difficulties with PCA include its increased costs, patient age limitations, and the bureaucratic (physician, nursing, and pharmacy) obstacles (protocols, education, storage arrangements) that must be overcome before its implementation. Contraindications include inability to push the bolus button (weakness, arm restraints), inability to understand how to use the machine, and a patient's desire not to assume responsibility for his or her own care.

Intrathecal/Epidural Opioid Analgesia

The presence of high concentrations of opioid receptors in the spinal cord makes it possible to achieve analgesia, in both acute and chronic pain, by using small doses of opioids administered in either the subarachnoid or epidural spaces. By bypassing the blood and the blood-brain barrier, small doses of agonist are effective because they can reach the receptor by the "back-door."[9] Indeed, cerebrospinal fluid (CSF) opioid levels, particularly for morphine, are several thousand times greater than those achieved by the parenteral route (see below). These high levels produce the profound and prolonged analgesia that accompanies intrathecal/epidural opioid administration.

The passage of epidurally administered agonists across the dura into the CSF depends on the lipid solubility of the drug. Additionally, once in the CSF, opioids must pass from the water phase of the CSF into the lipid phase of the underlying neuraxis to reach the receptor. This, too, depends on lipid solubility. Hydrophilic agents such as morphine will have a greater latency and duration of action than more lipid soluble agents such as fentanyl. On the other hand, the lipid-soluble agonists (e.g., fentanyl) produce more segmental analgesia with less rostral spread than do the less lipid-soluble agonists.

Even when administered caudally, epidural morphine has been shown to provide effective postoperative analgesia after abdominal, thoracic, and cardiac surgery. Krane et al. reported that 0.03 mg/kg of caudal-epidural morphine is equally effective as 0.1 mg/kg in providing postoperative analgesia, although the higher dose provides a significantly longer duration of analgesia (13.3 ± 4.7 versus 10.0 ± 3.3 hours, respectively).[11] The incidence of side effects was the same in both groups, although one patient receiving 0.1 mg/kg developed late respiratory depression. Therefore these investigators suggest starting with the lower dose when using this technique. Whether even lower doses are effective is unknown.

Spinal opiates produce analgesia without altering autonomic or neuromuscular function. Additionally, both light touch and proprioception are preserved. Thus, unlike local anesthetics, spinal opioids allow patients to ambulate without orthostatic hypotension. Common side effects of intrathecal/epidural narcotics include segmental pruritus, urinary retention, nausea and vomiting, and respiratory depression. These side effects occur with greater frequency when opioids are administered intrathecally as opposed to epidurally. Except for urinary retention, adverse side effects, with maintenance of adequate analgesia, can be reversed through the use of a low-dose (0.001 to 0.002 mg/kg) naloxone infusion. Pruritus and nausea also can be treated with intravenous or oral diphenhydramine (Benadryl), 0.5 to 1.0 mg/kg, or hydroxyzine (Vistaril, Atarax). Urinary retention has not been a reported complication in children because the majority of pediatric patients studied to date have had bladder catheters as part of their postoperative management regimen.

Although rare, respiratory depression is a major risk when intrathecal/epidural opioids are used. Attia et al.[4] demonstrated that the ventilatory response to CO_2 is depressed for as long as 22 hours after the administration of 0.05 mg/kg of morphine epidurally. Nichols et al.[14] demonstrated, in children varying between 3 months and 15 years, significant depression of the ventilatory response to carbon dioxide for up to 18 hours after intrathecal morphine administration (0.02 mg/kg). The greatest respiratory depression correlated with the highest CSF morphine levels (2863 ± 542 ng/ml), which occurred 6 hours after administration. This depression persisted despite a fall in CSF morphine levels 12 (641 ± 219 ng/ml) to 18 (223 ± 152 ng/ml) hours later. This confirms the clinical impression that respiratory depression usually occurs within the first 6 hours after the administration of epidural or intrathecal morphine but may occur as long as 18 hours afterward.

In clinical practice, respiratory depression occurs most commonly when IV or IM narcotics have been administered to supplement the intrathecal opioid. The risk of respiratory depression can be minimized if smaller doses of supplemental narcotics are used, or through the epidural use of shorter-acting, more lipid-soluble agents (fentanyl, sufentanil), which produce more segmental analgesia, with little rostral spread. On the other hand, because of its shorter duration of action, fentanyl and sufentanil increasingly are being administered by continuous epidural infusion, either alone or in combination with very dilute bupivacaine (1/16%, [0.0625 mg/ml]) or lidocaine (3 to 5 mg/ml) solutions. Typically, the epidural solution contains 1 to 5 μg/ml of fentanyl and is administered at rates ranging between 0.5 and 1.0 μg/kg/hr. This provides effective analgesia for both postoperative, acute, and chronic medical (e.g., cancer, sickle cell anemia) pain. Higher doses usually result in pruritus.

Regardless of the opioid and route of administration, a regular system of monitoring for respiratory depression is required. Clinical signs that predict impending respiratory depression include somnolence, small pupils, and small tidal volumes. We also insist on the use of oxyhemoglobin saturation monitoring ("pulse oximetry"), especially in the first 24 hours of instituting this therapy.

Transmucosal Fentanyl

Because fentanyl is extremely lipophilic, it can be absorbed readily across any biological membrane, including the skin. Thus it can be given painlessly by new, nonintravenous routes of drug administration, including the transmucosal (nose and mouth) and transdermal routes. The transdermal route frequently is used to administer many drugs chronically, including scopolamine, clonidine, and nitroglycerin. A selective semipermeable membrane patch that has a reservoir of drug allows for the slow, steady-state absorption of drug across the skin. Transdermal fentanyl is contraindicated for acute pain management in children and is applicable only for patients who are in chronic pain (e.g., cancer) or in patients who are opioid dependent. The use of this drug delivery system for acute pain has resulted in death. Additionally, the safety of this drug delivery system is compromised even further because fentanyl will continue to be absorbed from the subcutaneous fat for almost 24 hours after the patch is removed. On the other hand, the transmucosal route of fentanyl administration is extremely effective for acute pain relief and heralds a new era in the management of acute pain management in children. In this novel delivery technique, fentanyl is manufactured in a candy matrix (Fentanyl Oralet) attached to a plastic applicator (it looks like a lollipop); as the child sucks on the candy, fentanyl is absorbed across the buccal mucosa and is rapidly (10 to 20 min) absorbed into the systemic circulation. The Fentanyl Oralet has just been approved by the FDA for use in children for premedication before surgery and for procedure-related pain (e.g., lumbar puncture, bone marrow aspiration). When administered by this route, fentanyl is given in doses of 10 to 15 μg/kg, is effective within 20 minutes, and lasts approximately 2 hours. This product will be available only in hospital pharmacies and will, like all sedative/analgesics, require vigilant patient monitoring.

LOCAL ANESTHETIC AGENTS AND TECHNIQUES

Pharmacology and Pharmacokinetics of Local Anesthetics

The local anesthetics are tertiary amines and are of two types: either "esters" (e.g., tetracaine [Pontocaine], procaine [Novocain], chloroprocaine [Nesacaine], cocaine) or "amides" (lidocaine [Xylocaine], prilocaine, bupivacaine [Marcaine, Sensorcaine])[29] (Table 26-4). Both the ester and amide local anesthetics are weak bases that block nerve conduction primarily at the sodium channel when they are in their ionized (cation) form. To reach the sodium channel, the local anesthetic must cross the nerve membrane, and only the nonionized (base) form of the drug can do this. How much drug is available to cross the nerve membrane depends on the pKa of the drug and the pH of the fluid surrounding the nerve. Thus the lower the pKa of the drug, the more nonionized drug is available to cross the nerve membrane at physiological pH. For example, 28% of lidocaine exists in the base form at pH 7.4 compared with only 2.5% for chloroprocaine, because the pKa of these drugs are 7.9 and 9.0, respectively. Acidosis and hypercapnia, by significantly affecting tissue drug uptake, also increase the toxicity of local anesthetics. Indeed, studies in rats have shown that both hypercarbia and acidosis drastically lower the convulsive threshold of local anesthetics and elevate total plasma and tissue concentrations of drug.

Table 26-4 Comparative Pharmacology of Local Anesthetics

Classification	Potency*	Onset	Duration after infiltration (min)
Esters			
Procaine	1	Slow	45-60
Chloroprocaine	4	Rapid	30-45
Tetracaine	16	Slow	60-180
Amides			
Lidocaine	1	Rapid	60-120
Mepivacaine	1-2	Slow	90-180
Bupivacaine	4-8	Slow	240-480
Etidocaine	4-8	Slow	240-480
Prilocaine	1	Slow	60-120

*Related to procaine (for esters) and lidocaine (for amides).

The standard of local anesthetic potency is Cm, or the minimum concentration of local anesthetic necessary to block impulse conduction along a given nerve fiber. A variety of factors affect Cm, including fiber size and degree of myelination of the nerve to be blocked, pH, local calcium concentration, and the rate at which a nerve is stimulated. Relatively unmyelinated fibers such as the A delta and C fibers carry pain receptive information and have a lower Cm than heavily myelinated fibers that control muscle contraction. Because of the lower Cm, less local anesthetic is necessary to block the transmission of pain than is necessary to produce muscle paralysis. Thus one can block pain sensation and not motor function by using dilute concentrations of local anesthetics. In fact, concentrated local anesthetic solutions (e.g., 2% lidocaine versus 1.0%) increase the quality of sensory blockade only minimally. On the other hand, a concentrated local anesthetic will increase the incidence of motor blockade and systemic toxicity. (Concentrated solutions of local anesthetics can be diluted with *preservative-free* normal saline.) Furthermore, since the process of myelinization of the central nervous system is not completed until approximately 18 months after birth, Cm may be reduced in younger children. Thus newborns and infants may develop complete analgesia and even motor blockade when even dilute concentrations of local anesthetics are used.

Other factors also influence the quality and duration of a nerve block, such as the addition of a vasoconstrictor to the anesthetic mixture, the use of mixtures of local anesthetics, and the site of drug administration. Vasoconstrictors, particularly epinephrine, frequently are added to local anesthetic solutions. Epinephrine decreases the rate of vascular reabsorp-

Table 26-5 Suggested Maximal Doses of Local Anesthetics (mg/kg)*

Drug (concentration)†	Caudal/lumbar epidural	Peripheral‡	Subcutaneous‡
Esters			
Chloroprocaine (1.0% infiltration) (2%-3% epidural)	8-10§	8-10§	8-10§
Procaine	NR	8-10§	8-10§
Amides			
Lidocaine (0.5%-2.0%) (0.5%-1.0% infiltration) (1%-2% peripheral, epidural, subcutaneous) (5% spinal)	5-7§	5-7§	5-7§
Bupivacaine (0.0625%-0.5%) (0.125%-0.25%)	2-3§	2-3§	2-3§
Prilocaine (0.5%-1% infiltration) (1%-1.5% peripheral) (2%-3% epidural)	5-7§‖	5-7§‖	5-7§‖

*These are suggested safe upper limits; direct intraarterial or intravenous injection of even a fraction of these doses may result in systemic toxicity or death.
†Concentrations are in mg percent; e.g., a 1% solutions contains 10 mg/ml.
‡Epinephrine should never be added to local anesthetic solution administered in area of an end artery (e.g., penile nerve block).
§The higher dose is recommended only with the concomitant use of epinephrine 1:200,000.
‖Total adult dose should not exceed 600 mg. Should be used with caution in neonates.
NR, Not recommended.

tion of local anesthetic from the site of administration and thereby lengthens the duration of sensory blockade. By causing local vasoconstriction, epinephrine also reduces bleeding at sites of injury. Interestingly, epinephrine also improves the intensity of anesthesia achieved and increases the effectiveness of dilute concentration of local anesthetics. *Epinephrine should never be injected into areas supplied by end arteries, such as the penis or digits.* Injection of an epinephrine-containing solution into these areas may lead to tissue ischemia or necrosis. Finally, epinephrine most commonly is added to local anesthetic solutions in concentrations of 0.005 mg/ml (1:200,000).

The site of an injection also alters the duration of a nerve block depending on the nerve's anatomy, differences in the rate of drug absorption, and the amount of drug deposited. Bupivacaine, for example, has a 4-hour duration when injected epidurally, but a 10-hour duration when injected into the brachial plexus.

Toxicity

The systemic effects of local anesthetics are determined by the total dose of drug administered and by the rapidity of absorption into the blood. This belies the idea of accepted "maximum" doses of these drugs, because even small fractions of the accepted "maximum" dosages of local anesthetics will produce toxic systemic effects if the local anesthetic is injected intraarterially or intravenously or into any highly vascular location (Table 26-5). In general, peak absorption of local anesthetic depends on the site of the block. The order of absorption from highest to lowest is:

intercostal, intratracheal > caudal/epidural
> brachial plexus > distal peripheral > subcutaneous

Peak local anesthetic blood levels are directly related to the total dose of drug administered, regardless of the injection site or the volume of solution used. Thus the most dilute concentration of a local anesthetic should be used. At recommended clinical dosages, plasma levels usually remain well below recognized toxic concentrations. A continuum of toxic effects exists and depends on the rapidity of rise and the total plasma concentration achieved after drug administration. Mild side effects (tinnitus, light-headedness, visual and auditory disturbances, restlessness, muscular twitching) occur at low plasma concentrations; severe side effects (seizures, arrhythmias, coma, cardiovascular collapse, respiratory arrest) occur as plasma levels increase.

Cardiovascular and central nervous system toxicity rarely have been observed in children after local anesthetic administration. The hemodynamic response to regional anesthesia, even after fairly extensive epidural blockade (cutaneous analgesia below T4 to T5 dermatome, the nipple line) is minimal among children compared with adults. Convulsions are rarely noted because they may be masked or the seizure threshold may be increased by the use of sedatives, particularly the benzodiazepines. Alternatively, children may be less sensitive to the toxic effects of local anesthetics than are adults; however, this is unlikely. Several animal studies have demonstrated that there are no significant differences in the sensitivity to the toxic effects of local anesthetics between newborn and adult animals.

The treatment of toxic responses to local anesthetics is the same as for any emergency, namely, maintaining a patent *a*irway, ensuring adequate *b*reathing, and supporting *c*irculation—in other words, the ABCs. Patients who are seizing for even brief periods of time become acidotic and have ineffective ventilation. Thus emergency airway and resuscitative equipment must be available for immediate use before the administration of any local anesthetic agent (see the box on p. 314). Finally, bupivacaine as a cause of arrhythmias and cardiovascular collapse is particularly worrisome because it has been relatively refractory to treatment. The ventricular arrhythmias caused by bupivacaine that precede the cardiovascular collapse may be treated effectively with intravenous phenytoin or bretylium.[12]

Drug allergy is very uncommon with amide local anesthetics but does occur with the ester family of drugs. Usually, a previous history of allergies to local anesthetics or to suntan lotions that contain PABA can be obtained. In our experience though, local anesthetic allergy is rare and often is attributed mistakenly to adverse experiences occurring during dental anesthesia. In the dentist's office, many patients experience tachycardia and a sense of flushing and dizziness fol-

EMERGENCY DRUGS AND EQUIPMENT REQUIRED FOR SEDATION AND ADMINISTRATION OF LOCAL ANESTHETIC

I. Personnel
  A. The practitioner performing the procedure
  B. A qualified person to monitor and administer drugs
    1. Training in basic life support (CPR)
    2. Knowledge of emergency cart inventory
II. Equipment for intravenous access
  A. Catheters (various sizes)
  B. Administration sets
  C. Fluids
    1. Lactated Ringer solution
    2. D_5W + NaCl (0.2, 0.45, 0.9%)
III. Emergency cart
  A. Suction (large bore device, e.g., Yankauer suction device)
  B. Oxygen and oxygen delivery system
  C. Airway
    1. Oral airways (various sizes)
    2. Masks (various sizes)
    3. Laryngoscope and appropriate size blades
    4. Endotracheal tubes (various sizes)
    5. Stylets
  D. Drugs
    1. Epinephrine
    2. Bicarbonate
    3. Atropine
    4. Lidocaine, bretylium
    5. Calcium
    6. Glucose
    7. Naloxone, physostigmine
    8. Anticonvulsants (thiopental, diazepam or midazolam)
IV. Monitoring equipment*
  A. EKG
  B. Sphygmomanometer
  C. Pulse oximeter

Modified from American Academy of Pediatrics Committee on Drugs: *Pediatrics* 89:1110, 1992.
*Monitoring equipment should be available, particularly if the child is sedated for the procedure.

lowing nerve root infiltration with procaine and epinephrine. This usually is caused by direct intravascular injection of epinephrine and does not mean that the patient is allergic to local anesthetics.

Pharmacokinetics

The ester local anesthetics are metabolized by plasma cholinesterase. Neonates and infants up to 6 months of age have less than half of the adult levels of this plasma enzyme. Clearance thereby may be reduced and the effects of ester local anesthetics prolonged. Amides, on the other hand, are metabolized in the liver and bound by plasma proteins. Neonates and young infants (less than 3 months of age) have reduced liver blood flow and immature metabolic degradation pathways. Thus larger fractions of local anesthetics are unmetabolized and remain active in the plasma than in the adult. More local anesthetic is excreted in the urine unchanged. Furthermore, neonates and infants may be at increased risk for the toxic effects of amide local anesthetics because of lower levels of albumin and alpha-1 acid glycoproteins, which are proteins essential for drug binding. This leads to increased concentrations of free drug and potential toxicity, particularly with bupivacaine. On the other hand, the larger volume of distribution at steady state seen in the neonate for these (and other) drugs may confer some clinical protection by lowering plasma drug levels.

The metabolism of the amide local anesthetic prilocaine is unique in that it produces oxidants that can lead to the development of methemoglobinemia. This occurs in adults who take doses of prilocaine greater than 600 mg. Because premature and full-term infants have decreased levels of methemoglobin reductase, they are more susceptible to methemoglobinemia. An additional factor rendering newborns more susceptible to methemoglobinemia is the relative ease by which fetal hemoglobin is oxidized compared with adult hemoglobin. Because of this, prilocaine cannot be recommended for use in neonates and thereby may limit the use of EMLA (see below) in this patient population.

REGIONAL ANESTHETIC TECHNIQUES

Subcutaneous Injection

Subcutaneous infiltration of the skin with a local anesthetic solution is the most commonly performed regional ("local") anesthetic technique in pediatric practice. Local anesthetics, particularly lidocaine, are commonly injected subcutaneously before the performance of many painful medical and surgical procedures to minimize procedure-related pain. Examples of procedures that benefit from prior local anesthetic infiltration include repair of minor surgical wounds (traumatic lacerations or deliberate incisions, e.g., before a cutdown for venous access), insertion of an arterial or an intravenous catheter (e.g., routine percutaneous intravenous access or cardiac catheterization), bone marrow aspiration, thoracostomy tube placement, and lumbar puncture. When used in this way, the local anesthetic agent blocks nerve conduction at the most terminal branches of the sensory nerves.

Local anesthetic infiltration of traumatic lacerations requires special attention. Commonly, the wound is dirty and requires extensive scrubbing and irrigation. Should the local anesthetic be administered before the cleansing, which would make it painless, or after, to avoid introducing dirt and bacteria into the surrounding tissue? It is our practice to inject the local anesthetic through intact skin adjacent to the wound before the wound is cleaned (Fig. 26-3). Alternatively, we block the peripheral nerve supplying the injured area more proximally because smaller amounts of local anesthetic are used and it requires fewer injections.

Because local anesthetics are manufactured at a pH of 4 to 5 and are administered by injection, they are painful in and of themselves. This pain can be minimized by using buffered anesthetic solutions and small needles. Buffering a local anesthetic solution, such as lidocaine or bupivacaine, with sodium bicarbonate (9 ml of lidocaine combined with 1 ml of bicarbonate, or bupivacaine 2.9 ml with 0.1 ml bicarbonate) may make the injection painless and shorten the onset of analgesia.[5,26] Local anesthetics are not manufactured with

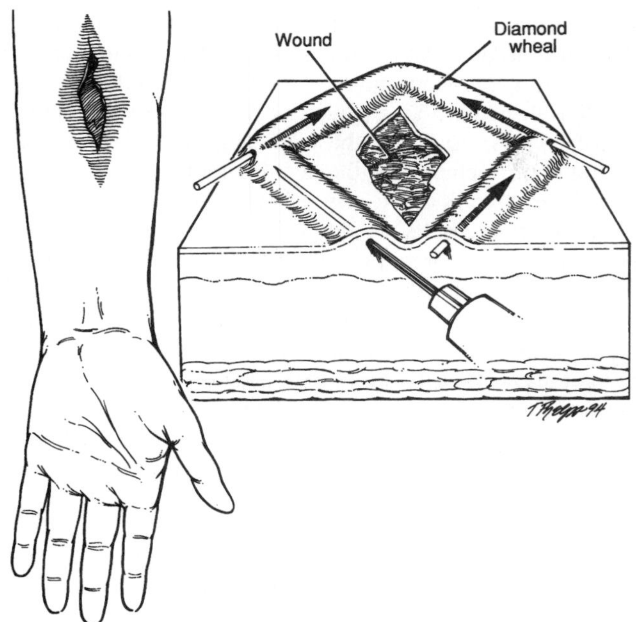

FIG. 26-3 Technique of infiltration of local anesthetic.

buffer because the buffering affects the shelf life of the drug. Obviously, using small gauge needles affects the amount of pain produced when infiltrating local anesthetics. We use either 26- or 30-gauge needles and inject the local anesthetic immediately as the needle punctures the skin. We do *not* aspirate first. Rather, we inject local anesthetics as the needle is advanced. Aspirating first is unnecessary because the amount of local anesthetic injected is so small (0.1 to 0.2 ml) that even an intravascular injection would be inconsequential.

Topical Local Anesthetic Techniques

TAC Solution. A useful and increasingly popular topical anesthetic mixture for laceration repair is known by its acronym, TAC. This solution consists of a mixture of tetracaine, epinephrine (adrenalin), and cocaine. A stock solution is prepared in the pharmacy by mixing 7 g of cocaine, 300 mg of tetracaine (15 ml of a 2% solution), 30 mg of epinephrine (30 ml of a 1:1000 solution), and saline to bring the total volume to 60 ml. The resulting mixture can be kept refrigerated and dispensed as needed. This method of topical anesthesia avoids the use of a local anesthetic injection. It is most effective when used on lacerations of the face and scalp and less effective on lacerations of an extremity. It does not penetrate unbroken skin well. Typically, a 3 ml solution of TAC provides analgesia for an approximately 3 cm long laceration. Half of the solution is instilled directly into the wound, and the other half is applied to a gauze pad held on the wound surface for 10 to 15 minutes. Blanching of the surrounding tissue indicates effective penetration. Failure to keep the TAC solution in contact with the wound surface for 10 to 15 minutes usually accounts for most cases of TAC's ineffectiveness and provides inadequate analgesia. In the 10% to 25% of patients in whom TAC is not completely effective, the subsequent injection of lidocaine required to complete the procedure is much less painful. Use of TAC also avoids the swelling and distortion of the wound edges that may be caused by injections. This painless method of application enhances patient compliance and results in briefer suturing times for minor lacerations. Gloves must be worn by all personnel coming into contact with TAC solution because it can cause vasoconstriction even in intact skin.

Because this mixture contains very high concentrations of its components, toxicity is a major concern.[10] Three ml of TAC contains the equivalent of 1.5 ml of 1:1000 epinephrine and 350 mg of cocaine, the latter being unique among local anesthetics because of its sympathomimetic actions. It impairs the reuptake of catecholamines at adrenergic nerve endings and blocks muscarinic cholinergic receptors, resulting in the promotion of hypertension and cardiac dysrhythmias, the most common causes of toxic deaths due to cocaine abuse. In the central nervous system, cocaine affects transmission by several monoamines such as norepinephrine, serotonin, dopamine, and tryptophan. Toxic reactions include dysphoria, anxiety, convulsions, and fever and do not necessarily correlate with blood levels.

Although some systemic absorption of cocaine occurs with the proper use of TAC, toxic reactions usually result from the rapid systemic absorption after unintentional contact with mucosal membranes. Case reports have documented prolonged seizures when TAC was applied to the buccal mucosa and death when excess solution dripped into the nares and mouth from a sponge that was applied to the upper lip.[10] Other fatalities and neuropsychological reactions have been reported, leading some authors to condemn the use of this solution.

In addition, because of its mechanism of monoamine oxidase action, cocaine should not be used concurrently with tricyclic antidepressants or monoamine oxidase (MAO) inhibitors (which also inhibit the reuptake of catecholamines at nerve endings) or in patients who have hypertension or cardiac conduction disturbances. Finally, because of its systemic absorption, patients should be advised that urinary drug screens for cocaine and its metabolites will be positive for 48 to 72 hours after an application of TAC.

Interactions among the components of TAC have been suspected of enhancing the potential for toxic reactions. Cocaine and epinephrine both act at adrenergic receptors; cocaine and tetracaine both compete for plasma cholinesterase for metabolism. Thus attempts to reduce the toxic potential of the mixture have focused on removing one of the components. However, use of either tetracaine alone, tetracaine with epinephrine, or cocaine alone was found to be far less effective than the complete mixture.

The most serious local adverse reaction is ischemia of end-arterial tissues due to the potent vasoconstrictive properties of TAC. Thus it should not be applied to the digits, nose, pinna of the ear, penis, or a skin flap. Despite concerns about serious toxicity, during the past decade, TAC has continued to enjoy widespread use and strong advocacy of its safety when used selectively and prudently.

EMLA Cream. EMLA (eutectic mixture of local anesthetics) cream, a topical emulsion composed of prilocaine and lidocaine, produces complete anesthesia of intact skin after application. Unfortunately, for best effect, EMLA cream must be applied and covered with an occlusive dressing (such as Saran wrap) for 60 to 90 minutes before a procedure is performed. This limits its use in the emergency room or office unless the site is prepared well in advance of anticipated use. Furthermore, if the procedure is a venipuncture, multiple sites must be prepared, in case the initial attempt is unsuccessful.

Unfortunately the effectiveness of EMLA cream (like all other methods) in reducing pain depends on who makes the assessment. Soliman et al.[21] studied the efficacy of EMLA cream compared with injected lidocaine at reducing the pain associated with venipuncture. Both an observer and a physician performing the procedure judged pain relief to be virtually complete in both groups. The children involved in the study were not so sanguine and were equally dissatisfied with both methods, particularly if the needle used for venipuncture was visible to them. Thus, despite two observers feeling that the child was pain-free, the child's cooperation with venipuncture did not improve. Therefore it is not clear whether the delay involved in the use of EMLA (60-minute wait for effect) is justified. On the other hand, EMLA may be more effective in children accustomed to frequent medical procedures (e.g., oncology patients) or for procedures in which the child cannot see the needle, such as lumbar puncture or bone marrow aspiration.

Peripheral Nerve Blocks. As mentioned previously, emergency airway and resuscitative equipment, as well as individuals trained in using it, must be available for use before the performance of a peripheral nerve block. Additionally, if a patient is to be sedated during a nerve block, one member of the health care team must be responsible for the patient's overall well-being.[3] This person is responsible for monitoring vital signs, assessing the adequacy of the airway, and alerting other members of the health care team if a problem is occurring (see the box on p. 314).

Digital Nerve Blocks. The digital nerve block provides excellent anesthesia for surgery performed on either the fingers or toes. It particularly is useful for incision and drainage of an abscess (paronychia). The alternative, local anesthetic infiltration, may fail because the acidic pH of infected tissue may not allow the active (nonionized base) form of the local anesthetic to reach the nerve membrane.

PERFORMANCE OF THE DIGITAL NERVE BLOCK. Digital nerve block is performed similarly for both the fingers and toes. Each digit is supplied by two pairs of nerves (palmar and dorsal), which travel on either side of that digit (Fig. 26-4). *Epinephrine-free* local anesthetic (0.5 to 1.0 ml) is injected between the metacarpal (or metatarsal) heads on either side of the digit. The 25-gauge needle is kept perpendicular to the plane of the hand or foot and advanced from the dorsal to

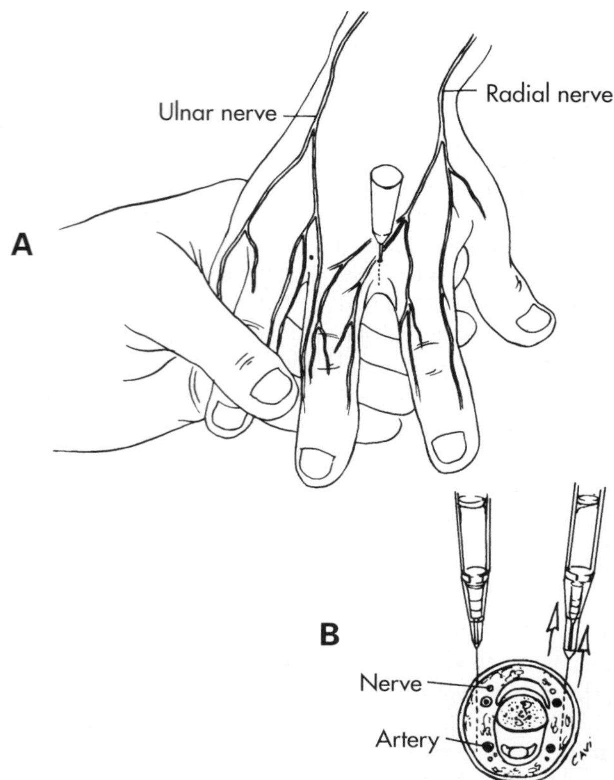

FIG. 26-4 Anatomy of the digital nerves of the hand and of the digital nerve block. **A,** A 25-gauge needle is inserted between the heads of the metacarpals (or metatarsals) on either side of the digit to be anesthetized. Both dorsal and ventral branches are blocked by continuously injecting during advancement of the needle from the dorsal surface to the palm. **B,** One can see the anatomical relationship of the digital nerves and arteries at the level of the metacarpal head in this cross section view.

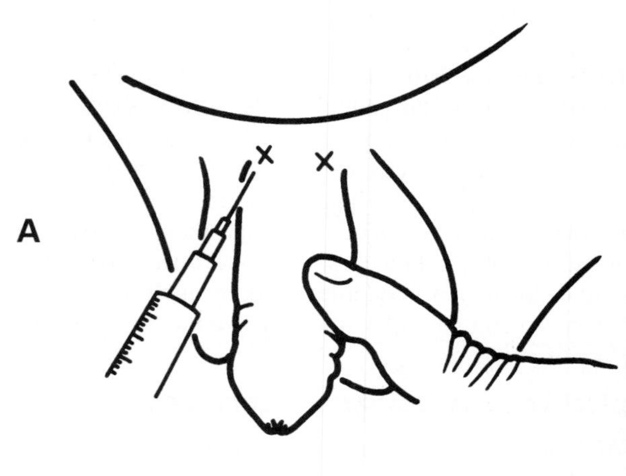

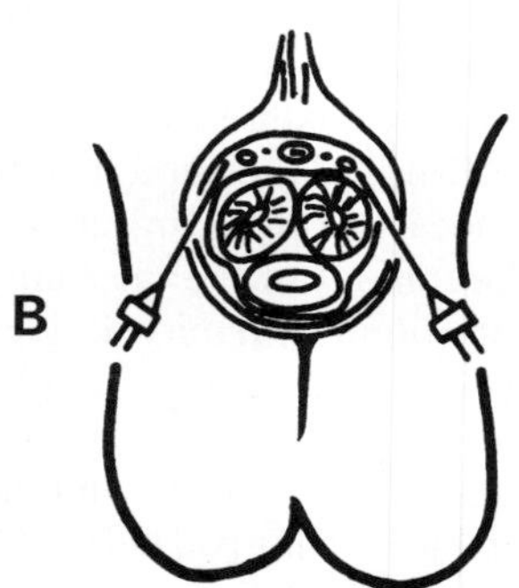

FIG. 26-5 Penile nerve block. **A,** A 25-gauge needle is inserted at the 10:30 and 1:30 positions at the penile base. The fascia is entered approximately 3 to 5 mm below the skin surface. **B,** One can see the dorsal vein of the penis, the two dorsal arteries, and the two nerves lying in Buck's fascia. Directly below this fascia, one can see the corpora of the penis.

(From Maxwell LG et al: *Obstet Gynecol* 70:415, 1987.)

the palmar surface. Local anesthetic is injected continuously. Aspiration before injection is unnecessary because the volume of local anesthetic is small.

Complications are few. Obviously, the digital nerve block should never be performed when there is any question of the digit's blood supply. Indeed, even when epinephrine is not used, the most serious complication of this block is caused by the use of too large a volume of local anesthetic. A large volume within a closed fascial space may result in vascular compression ("compartment" syndrome).

Penile Nerve Block. Although routine circumcision of newborns has been condemned by various groups, it remains a common practice. Active campaigns by pediatricians and obstetricians to discourage the procedure in the newborn period has resulted in increasingly large numbers of older children being presented for this surgery. These older children obviously require general anesthesia for their surgery. In both the newborn and older child, the penile nerve block can be used either for complete anesthesia or for postoperative pain relief. The efficacy and safety of this block for newborn circumcision has been demonstrated in several studies and requires very little time to perform (<60 sec).[13] Whether this extremely safe and effective block should be performed *routinely* before newborn circumcision is controversial. *It is our belief that it should be.* In both the older child and the newborn, profound postoperative analgesia also can be provided by the topical application of 2% lidocaine jelly.[22]

PERFORMANCE OF THE PENILE NERVE BLOCK. In the newborn we use 0.8 ml of 1% lidocaine and in older children from 1 to 3 ml of 0.25% bupivacaine.[13] Peak plasma lidocaine levels in the newborn averaged less than 0.6 μg/ml. In either case, it is vital that *epinephrine-free solution* be used because the artery supplying the penis is an end artery and vasoconstriction by epinephrine can cause catastrophic consequences. The dorsal nerves of the penis (Fig. 26-5) lie on either side of the dorsal artery and vein of the penis. They are deep to Buck's fascia but are superficial with respect to the skin at the penile base. Following aseptic preparation of the skin, two injections of local anesthetic solution are made by using either a 25- or 26-gauge needle. The anesthetic solution is injected at the 10:30 and 1:30 positions at the penile base just beneath Buck's fascia. This fascia is approximately 3 to 5 mm below the skin surface. Alternatively, a single midline injection may be used. In this technique the needle is advanced to the lower surface of the pubic symphysis in the midline. Local anesthetic (approximately 1 to 3 ml) is injected slowly as the needle is withdrawn. As the needle passes through Buck's fascia, the local anesthetic is spread to both sides, anesthetizing the nerves. Broadman et al. described a

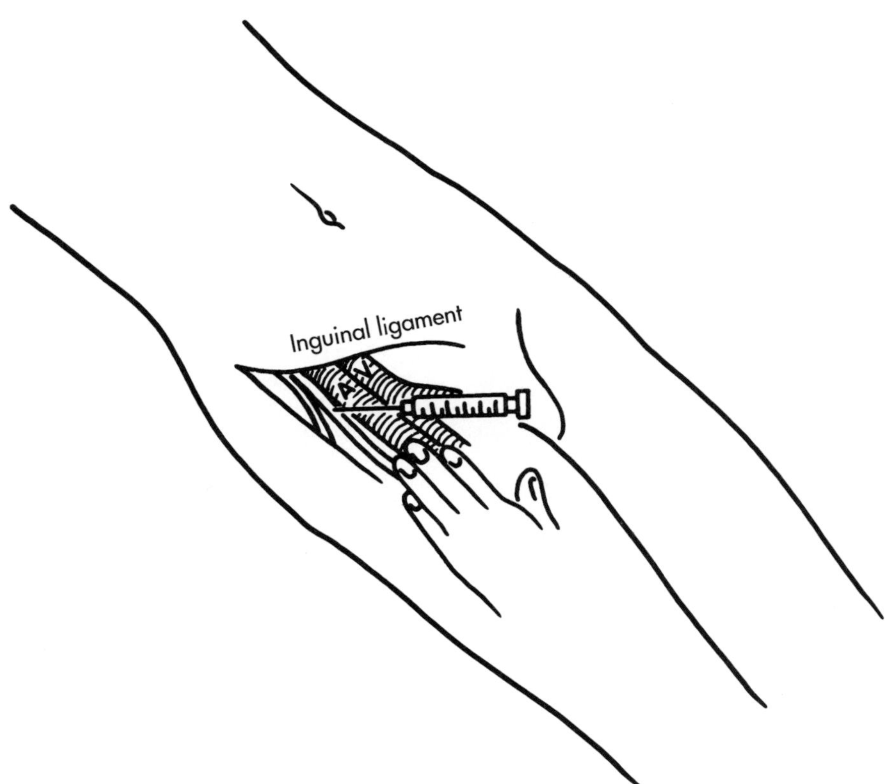

FIG. 26-6 Femoral nerve block. After placing a skin wheal, the physician's nonoperative hand compresses the femoral artery and nerve against the underlying tissue and bone immediately below the inguinal ligament. A 22- or 25-gauge needle then is inserted perpendicularly, approximately ½ to 1 cm lateral to the pulsation of the femoral artery *(A)* into the perineural fascia of the femoral nerve.

(From Maxwell LG et al: *Obstet Gynecol* 70:415, 1987.)

ring block of the penile base in which no attempt was made to inject below Buck's fascia.

Complications are rare.

Femoral Nerve Block. The femoral nerve block (L2, 3, 4) is the quickest, easiest, and most effective technique for relieving the pain of a femoral shaft fracture. The femoral nerve block provides fracture patients with adequate anesthesia for the application of traction as well as for the necessary (and usually painful) manipulations that occur during radiological examinations. The duration of analgesia for bupivacaine without epinephrine is 3 hours, and peak plasma levels of bupivacaine average less than 1 μg/ml.

PERFORMANCE OF THE BLOCK. Following aseptic preparation of the skin, a 22- or 25-gauge needle is inserted perpendicularly, approximately 3 to 5 mm lateral to the pulsation of the femoral artery at the level of the inguinal ligament (Fig. 26-6). The needle is inserted to a depth clearly deeper than the artery. The feeling of penetration of the fascia over the nerve (a distinct "pop") helps in judging the depth of penetration. Following a negative aspiration for blood, 5 to 10 ml of local anesthetic solution (0.25% bupivacaine with 1:200,000 epinephrine) is injected. Local anesthetic solution then is injected in a fanlike manner lateral and deep to the femoral artery. The dose of 0.25% bupivacaine used is 1 ml/kg, up to 10 ml.

REFERENCES

1. Anand KJ, Carr DB: The neuroanatomy, neurophysiology, and neurochemistry of pain, stress, and analgesia in newborns and children, *Pediatr Clin North Am* 36:795, 1989.
2. Anand KJ, Hickey PR: Pain and its effects in the human neonate and fetus, *N Engl J Med* 317:1321, 1987.
3. American Academy of Pediatrics Committee on Drugs: Guidelines for monitoring and management of pediatric patients during and after sedation for diagnostic and therapeutic procedures, *Pediatrics* 89:1110, 1992.
4. Attia J et al: Epidural morphine in children: pharmacokinetics and CO_2 sensitivity, *Anesthesiology* 65:590, 1986.
5. Bailey PL et al: Differences in magnitude and duration of opioid-induced respiratory depression and analgesia with fentanyl and sufentanil, *Anesth Analg* 70:8, 1990.
6. Berde CB et al: Comparison of morphine and methadone for prevention of postoperative pain in 3- to 7-year-old children, *J Pediatr* 119:136, 1991.
7. Beyer JE, Wells N: The assessment of pain in children, *Pediatr Clin North Am* 36:837, 1989.
8. Broadman LM et al: Post-circumcision analgesia: a prospective evaluation of subcutaneous ring block of the penis, *Anesthesiology* 67:399, 1987.
9. Cousins MJ, Mather LE: Intrathecal and epidural administration of opioids, *Anesthesiology* 61:276, 1984.
10. Dailey RH: Fatality secondary to misuse of TAC solution, *Ann Emerg Med* 17:159, 1988.
11. Krane EJ, Tyler DC, Jacobson LE: The dose response of caudal morphine in children, *Anesthesiology* 71:48, 1989.
12. Maxwell LG, Martin LD, Yaster M: Bupivacaine-induced cardiac toxicity in neonates: successful treatment with intravenous phenytoin, *Anesthesiology* 80:682, 1994.
13. Maxwell LG et al: Penile nerve block for newborn circumcision, *Obstet Gynecol* 70:415, 1987.
14. Nichols DG et al: Disposition and respiratory effects of intrathecal morphine in children, *Anesthesiology* 79:733, 1993.
15. Pain terms: a list with definitions and notes on usage. Recommended by the IASP Subcommittee on Taxonomy, *Pain* 6:249, 1979.
16. Pasternak GW: Multiple morphine and enkephalin receptors and the relief of pain, *JAMA* 259:1362, 1988.
17. Phillips GD, Cousins MJ: Neurological mechanisms of pain and the relationship of pain, anxiety, and sleep. In Cousins MJ, Phillips GD, editors: *Acute pain management,* New York, 1986, Churchill Livingstone.
18. Schechter NL: The undertreatment of pain in children: an overview, *Pediatr Clin North Am* 36:781, 1989.
19. Schechter NL, Allen DA, Hanson K: Status of pediatric pain control: a comparison of hospital analgesic usage in children and adults, *Pediatrics* 77:11, 1986.
20. Schechter N, Berde C, Yaster M: *Pain in infants, children, and adolescents,* Baltimore, 1993, Williams & Wilkins.
21. Soliman IE et al: Comparison of the analgesic effects of EMLA (eutectic mixture of local anesthetics) to intradermal lidocaine infiltration prior to venous cannulation in unpremedicated children, *Anesthesiology* 68:804, 1988.
22. Tree-Trakarn T, Pirayavaraporn S, Lertakyamanee J: Topical analgesia for relief of post-circumcision pain, *Anesthesiology* 67:395, 1987.
23. Way WL, Costley EC, Way EL: Respiratory sensitivity of the newborn infant to meperidine and morphine, *Clin Pharmacol Ther* 6:454, 1965.
24. Wall PD, Melzack R: *Management of pain,* New York, 1985, Churchill Livingstone.
25. Wong DL, Baker CM: Pain in children: comparison of assessment scales, *Pediatr Nurs* 14:9, 1988.
26. Yaster M et al: Hemodynamic effects of primary closure of omphalocele/gastroschisis in human newborns, *Anesthesiology* 69:84, 1988.
27. Yaster M, Deshpande JK: Management of pediatric pain with opioid analgesics, *J Pediatr* 113:421, 1988.
28. Yaster M, Maxwell LG: *Opioid agonists and antagonists.* In Schechter NL, Berde CB, Yaster M, editors: *Pain in infants, children, and adolescents,* Baltimore, 1993, Williams & Wilkins.
29. Yaster M, Tobin JR, Maxwell LG: *Local anesthetics.* In Schechter NL, Berde CB, Yaster M, editors: *Pain in infants, children, and adolescents,* Baltimore, 1993, Williams & Wilkins.
30. Zhang AZ, Pasternak GW: Ontogeny of opioid pharmacology and receptors: high and low affinity site differences, *Eur J Pharmacol* 73:29, 1981.

27 Hypnosis and Biofeedback Therapy

Laurence I. Sugarman

Since Milton Erickson[6] published his pioneering work, *Pediatric Hypnotherapy,* in 1958, more and more pediatricians have been teaching their patients relaxation, self-hypnosis, and biofeedback to manage pain, the irritating side effects of medication, behavior problems, and physiological responses (Fig. 27-1). This growth in application and research indicates that these methods of therapy have a fundamental value for patients and practitioners. The term *cyberphysiology* has been coined as a name for this emerging discipline of self-regulation strategies. Derived from the Greek *Kybernan,* the prefix *cyber-* means "to steer" or "take the helm." Cyberphysiology refers to a person's ability to steer or regulate physiological response.[3,25,27]

PERSPECTIVES

Five "urges," described by Olness and Gardner as thematic in child development, form the foundation for hypnosis with children; experience, mastery, social interaction, wellness, and imagination.[27] These urges steer the inner world of the child and are influenced profoundly by developmental stages.[5] Children use imaginative processes to consider their options for behavior, to modify threatening situations, to gratify unmet needs, and for pleasure. Many of a child's interactions with the outer world, at home, in school, and especially when confronting the harsh reality of illness, tend to depreciate the power of fantasy as a coping tool.[5,27] The purposes of a child's imaginative world seem the least appreciated in medical therapeutics.

How a child's nature is valued in health and illness is important. The attitudes and belief systems that practitioners present to youngsters can and do affect their behavior, including their response to therapeutic interventions.[34] In an effort to provide prompt, effective treatment, physicians particularly are apt to ignore urges for personal experience and autonomy; the child is told that the inhaled medication will control the asthma and that he or she should sit still and cooperate with the physical examination. Restraint and sedation are the primary treatments for controlling discomfort. Such approaches do not encourage active participation by the young patient. The child gains no personal mastery in these situations.

Training in cyberphysiological skills provides a bridge between the child's innate imagery and therapeutic change, reinforcing the power and effectiveness of the child's imaginative capabilities.[3] Children and adolescents benefit from learning to regulate their own physiological processes by assuming a more central role in resolving health their problems. The child's perception of "locus of control" affects his or her response to therapy.[3,24,34] The confidence and ability achieved through applying cyberphysiological training enhances self-esteem. Young people learn to apply this technique to engage future challenges better. The benefits extend to family members and other caregivers, who are reassured that the youngster has an inherent ability to cope.

Primary care practitioners are well suited to apply these strategies. Noting cyberphysiological aptitude in daily encounters with children reinforces the child's and family's awareness of mind-body linkages. These techniques can be introduced to diminish acute anxiety and pain during injections, minor surgery, and other procedures. Psychophysiological disorders are estimated to show up in 15% to 20% of primary care pediatric visits. Thus the primary care physician often is the first to diagnose the problems for which cyberphysiological skills will be useful as primary or adjunctive therapy. Finally, success in facilitating self-regulation training rests on understanding a patient's developmental stage, strengths, and needs, all of which are familiar to the primary care practitioner.

MISCONCEPTIONS, DEFINITIONS, AND CONCEPTS

The notion that "hypnotists" magically exert "mind control" over passive subjects is rampant in the mass media, fairy tales, and cartoons. This belief not only is incorrect but also impedes the success of these strategies. To teach cyberphysiological skills, the pediatrician first must dispel this misconception for colleagues, parents, and patients. Hypnosis is not magic. The person in hypnosis actually experiences more control than in usual states of awareness.[21] All hypnosis is self-hypnosis.

Hypnosis

Hypnosis is an alternative state of awareness, usually but not always involving relaxation, in which one has an enhanced receptivity to suggestions for controlling specific physiological or behavioral reactions.[25,27] Narrowly focused attention and primary process thinking are common features of the hypnotic state, or trance. Children enter similar mind states quite naturally when they pretend, listen to stories, or play video games. These phenomena may be indistinguishable from physical relaxation, since they manifest decreases in muscle tone, blood pressure, and heart rate and an increase in peripheral skin temperature. However, hypnotic phenomena such as analgesia and amnesia cannot be explained by relaxation alone.[27]

There is no unified theory of hypnosis. The theoretical bases divide into two main currents: (1) hypnosis is a form of dissociation, "an interference with or loss of familiar associative processes," and (2) hypnotic responding is a sociocultural construct derived not from an altered state of consciousness but from "an interrelated set of ideas that provide guidelines concerning how hypnotists and hypnotized sub-

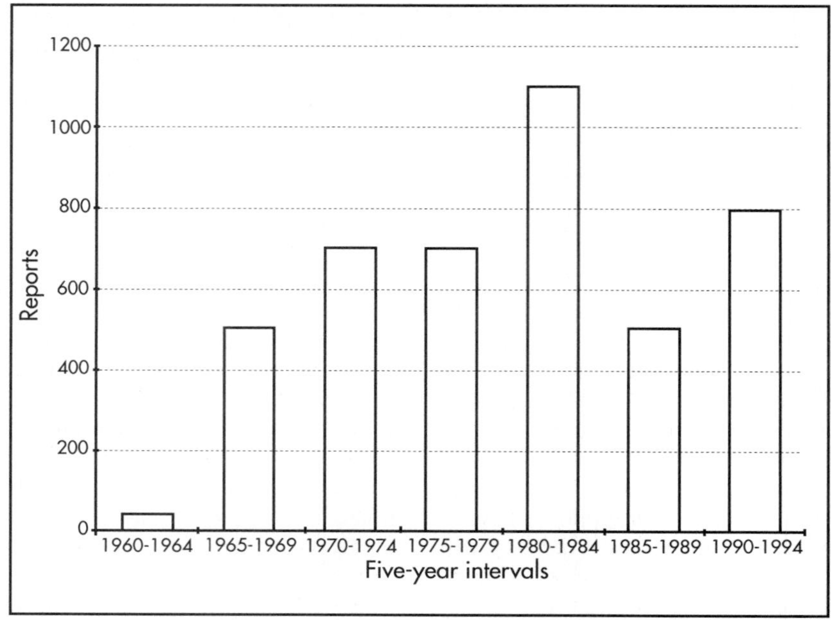

FIG. 27-1 Cumulated *Index Medicus* listings for hypnosis and biofeedback in children and adolescents for the past 35 years by 5-year intervals.

jects are supposed to act and feel while enacting their respective roles in those social situations defined as hypnotic."[21]

It is likely that *both* dissociative and sociocultural phenomena are keys to the complex set of interactions called hypnosis.

Hypnotherapy

Hypnotherapy is a method of treatment that uses hypnosis. Achieving a hypnotic state can be therapeutic in itself. As with any learning process, the youngster's personal practice with hypnosis can facilitate the development of his or her coping skills. The child or adolescent may discover his or her ability to relax and reduce tension, even tension-associated pain; this affirms the power of the individual's own self-regulation. In this regard, teaching the process of self-hypnosis is like teaching relaxation or meditation.[27]

Therapeutic learning in hypnosis may involve: (1) development of imagery as a means to help change symptoms, (2) acceptance of suggestions for changing behavior, and (3) exploration of feelings and relationships. It long has been observed that hypnosis seems to confer an enhanced aptitude for transforming the idea received into action.[1] The purpose of hypnosis in therapy is to foster the mental activity that allows change to occur.[11]

It is impossible to be certain that therapeutic outcomes attributed to hypnosis are not due to something else. However, the same can be said of psychotherapy and medical therapeutics.[32] Growing amounts of data support the validity of hypnotherapy. Until the limits of the domain called hypnosis and the mechanisms of physiological alteration attained through hypnosis are defined, doubts will remain about the validity of clinical use of hypnosis.

Biofeedback

Biofeedback provides a mechanical link to the skills of physiological self-regulation. It uses equipment to measure and feed back to the patient information about specific physiological functions. The patient then uses this information (or feedback) to manipulate the physiological variable toward a desired therapeutic outcome.[3] The responses most commonly measured are peripheral temperature changes and electromyographic (EMG) and electrodermal activity (EDA). The latter two modalities increase with heightened sympathetic tone and decrease with relaxation. Muscle tension and migraine headaches have been well documented to respond to biofeedback protocols that employ peripheral skin temperature or muscle activity.[29] Anorectal manometry and electromyograms have been shown to assist in the sensory discrimination necessary to resolve encopresis.[31] Although not commonly viewed as biofeedback, nocturnal enuresis alarms are highly effective.[2,4] Autonomic nervous system (ANS) disorders such as Raynaud disease and reflex sympathetic dystrophy can be treated effectively with biofeedback methods that cultivate enhanced sympathetic nervous system (SNS) control over the peripheral skin temperature, heart rate, and breathing patterns.[3] Electroencephalographic (EEG) biofeedback is being explored as a treatment for children who have attention deficit disorders.[20]

Integration of Strategies

The cyberphysiological strategies of self-hypnosis and biofeedback have several common characteristics, which are listed in the box on p. 321. Four "application paradigms" integrating biofeedback and self-hypnosis have been described: (1) Biofeedback can be applied for the purpose of teaching and strengthening a person's awareness of the mind-body link, introducing cyberphysiological phenomena; (2) it can be used to apply advanced biofeedback instrumentation that responds simultaneously to different physiological variables so that specific markers of a given individual's stress responses can be determined in a "physiological stress profile"; (3) for some young people, hypnotic imagery, suggestions,

CHARACTERISTICS COMMON TO SELF-HYPNOSIS AND BIOFEEDBACK TRAINING

- Cultivation of a lower state of arousal
- Enhanced and narrowed focus of attention
- Facilitation of a sense of curiosity
- Facilitation of imagery/fantasy abilities
- Development of an internal locus of control
- Fostering of themes of empowerment and self-mastery, both concretely and metaphorically
- Reinforcement of awareness of mind-body linkages
- Enhanced access to unconscious information
- Heightened suggestibility

and metaphors (likening one thing to another) can enhance biofeedback training; and (4) biofeedback can be used to facilitate a lowered state of arousal and a narrowly focused attention as well as an ego-strengthening technique that can motivate a person to explore new things and thereby better engage in hypnotherapy.[3]

No controlled studies have shown that one cyberphysiological method is superior to another for a given problem. Rather, the most appropriate strategy probably stems from the interplay between the young person's capabilities and needs and the practitioner's flexibility and skill.

TOOLS

The utilization approach described by Erickson[7] is part of any skilled clinician's work with children. The practitioner uses the youngster's natural reflexes (in the case of an infant) or fantasies and interests (in the case of an older child) to encourage responsiveness and build rapport. The method can be carried one step farther if the examiner provides stimuli that can facilitate the child's curiosity.[9] This technique is a critical part of training young people in cyberphysiological skills in that it legitimizes and values their abilities and interests. The primary tool the practitioner needs is a sound understanding of child development. Many toys, books, and biofeedback devices are available to help the practitioner teach self-regulation.

Breathing control is a fundamental method of focusing and relaxing. Blowing pinwheels, hanging mobiles, playing with balloons and using wands for blowing bubbles encourage the child to breathe with purpose and control. Pop-up books, puppets, stuffed animals, and dolls are means of distraction and imagery. They also can be the child's allies during procedures.[18]

Children can listen to favorite stories and songs on an audiotape with headphones during procedures. This often is an unexpected and enjoyable way for older children and adolescents to focus their attention quickly on what they are hearing and away from the procedure. When practical, patients may bring their own audiotapes. Hypnosis sessions in the office also can be recorded for home use.

Videotapes of other youngsters using self-hypnosis are an efficient way to demonstrate techniques. Written informed consent must be obtained before videotaping youngsters for

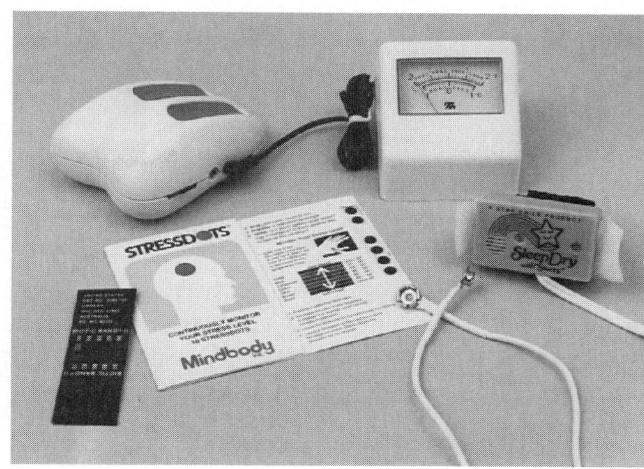

FIG. 27-2 Biofeedback devices (clockwise from top left): (1) GSR/TEMP-2 Biofeedback System, (2) peripheral temperature meter, (3) StarChild Sleep Dry enuresis alarm, (4) Stressdots, and (5) Biotic Band II.

(Photograph by William Rhinehart.)

this purpose. It is the author's experience that young people are pleased with the opportunity to "teach."

Dr. Leora Kuttner of Vancouver Children's Hospital, British Columbia, has prepared two videotapes for educating families and practitioners. "No Fears, No Tears"* introduces parents, children, and health care providers to various nonpharmacological techniques to assist young people who have cancer. "Children in Pain"* can augment a professional training program in hypnotic and behavioral pain management.

Various inexpensive biofeedback devices are available and practical for use in the pediatric office (Fig. 27-2). The Biotic Band II and Stressdots display peripheral skin temperature as color changes in a liquid crystal medium.† Analog display temperature devices are more expensive but more accurate and can be combined with EDA monitors. EDA devices such as the GSR/TEMP-2 Biofeedback System come with instructional materials for the patient and practitioner.‡ For home enuresis monitoring, the Star Child Sleep Dry alarm comes with excellent instructions for parents as well as a motivational "Star Chart" on which to track progress.§ The wireless Potty Pager has a vibrating buzzer that can be worn day or night.||

More expensive and complex office-based biofeedback devices also are available. Models such as the J&J I-330 Physiologic Monitoring System process physiological responses for child-friendly display on an IBM-compatible computer to engage the child in games such as "Traffic Light" and "River

*Available from the Association for the Care of Children's Health, 7910 Woodmont Ave., Bethesda, MD 20814; telephone: 1-301-654-6549.

†Available from Magic Lantern Film Distributors, Vancouver, BC, Canada; telephone 1-604-273-8111.

‡These devices are available from Bio-Medical Instruments, Inc., 2387 East Eight Mile Road, Warren, MI 48091; telephone 1-800-521-4640.

§StarChild/Labs, P.O. Box 404, Aptos, CA 95001-0404; telephone 1-408-662-2659.

||Ideas for Living, Inc., 1285 N. Cedarbrook, Boulder, CO 80304; telephone 1-303-440-8517.

Rafting."* This equipment requires advanced training to operate but can be worthwhile because it uses appealing displays for children, allowing them to engage in a "video game for your body."[3]

One final biofeedback device deserves mention. Dr. Karen Olness, a leader in the field of cyberphysiological training, has developed a biofeedback demonstration product designed for use in institutional and educational settings.† This "Mind Over Body" device uses an EDA sensor to demonstrate for children how their feelings and thoughts create changes in the body. A high-resolution graphic monitor with touch-screen access displays animated images that change their behavior in coordination with the child's EDA. This 8-minute experience demonstrates that how a child thinks and feels affects his or her body and others as well.

SKILLS

Just as the domain of hypnosis is poorly defined, so are the limits of its therapeutic applications. It has been said that, although "not all hypnosis is therapy . . . all therapy is hypnosis."[22] That is, all effective therapeutics have some elements of the knowledge and responsiveness that underlie hypnotherapy. Application of cyberphysiological skills training to primary care is similar to the use of any other therapeutic methodology such as diet, exercise, medication, or adaptive equipment. The practitioner must understand the methodology and limitations, gain experience in the art and science of its use, and know his or her patient.

As with other therapeutic skills, training and continual evaluation are crucial. The practitioner beginning education in cyberphysiological skills training should enroll in a basic workshop sponsored by the Society for Developmental and Behavioral Pediatrics,‡ The Society for Clinical and Experimental Hypnosis,§ the American Society of Clinical Hypnosis,‖ or classes offered by a university school of medicine or psychology department. After completing this training, practitioners should apply their new skills to limited areas of treatment and should review literature specific to these areas. Continual self-evaluation is vital. Videotaped patient encounters should be critiqued by faculty and peers. Intermediate and advanced workshops afford the practitioner the opportunity to hone his or her skills and to focus on the specific problems of children.[25,27]

The American Board of Medical Hypnosis (ABMH)¶ is the only organization sanctioned by the Society for Clinical and Experimental Hypnosis and the American Society of Clinical Hypnosis to certify competency in Medical Hypnosis. This is the highest credentialing available for physicians skilled in hypnosis. Applicants must be licensed physicians in good standing, board certified in their specialty, and have at least 2 years of experience in clinical hypnosis. The three-part examination comprises written and oral segments and a practical clinical demonstration.

It is crucial that the practitioner restrict cyberphysiological skill training to patients whose problems lie within their therapeutic expertise. The role of hypnosis or biofeedback as part of the treatment for chronic conditions (e.g., asthma and migraine syndromes) should be defined at the outset, although its potential usefulness is unlimited. A careful medical evaluation is necessary before considering cyberphysiological strategies as primary treatment of a disorder. In one study of children referred for hypnotherapy, 20% had a previously undiagnosed biological etiology for their condition.[28] Olness and Gardner have suggested indications and contraindications for cyberphysiological therapy with children[12,26] (see the box below).

Successful use of cyberphysiological strategies depends largely on the practitioner's understanding of the patient's developmental level and learning abilities, as well as the family context of the youngster's problems. A younger child responds best to concrete suggestions, becomes animated with open eyes, and may be comfortable having his or her parents present during hypnotic imagery. In contrast, an adolescent requires suggestions for relaxation and prompting to use mental imagery and often is inhibited by the parents' presence. Therapists need to shift their approach if a desired response is to be achieved.

Practitioners must be sensitive to the pace and tone of their language and actions, modifying them to reinforce the young person's innate abilities. Phrases such as "I want you to" and "you should" are too directive and do not facilitate self-control. Distraction techniques (e.g., pinching the contralateral arm while an injection is given) may diminish the sensation of the needle momentarily, but they do not teach the child about his or her own potential for self-regulation. Semantics must support a child's curiosity and mastery by suggesting that he or she is in control of the process, as in "You know, it's neat how you don't know that you already know

INDICATIONS AND CONTRAINDICATIONS FOR CYBERPHYSIOLOGICAL THERAPY WITH CHILDREN

Cyberphysiological methods are indicated if:
- A child is responsive to hypnotic suggestions
- The problem has been demonstrated to be treatable with hypnosis or biofeedback
- The therapist has a positive relationship with the child
- The child is motivated to remedy the problem
- No iatrogenic harm is foreseen from using such methods

Cyberphysiological methods are contraindicated if:
- They would lead to physical endangerment
- They might aggravate existing problems or create new ones
- They are used for "fun" or entertainment
- The problem could be addressed more effectively and appropriately through a different method (e.g., medication or family therapy)

*Performance Concepts, Inc., 7855 Division St., Mentor, OH 44060; telephone 1-216-974-9550.

†Contact Noreen M. Spota, administrative director, 19 Station Lane, Philadelphia, PA 19118-2939; telephone 1-215-248-9168.

‡Contact Marge Degnon, American Psychological Association, executive director, 6728 Old McLean Village Drive, McLean, VA 22101.

§Contact Sandy Kappel, 2200 East Devon Avenue, Suite 291, Des Plaines, IL 60018; telephone 1-847-297-3317.

‖Contact Steven F. Bierman, M.D., secretary-treasurer, 143 8th Street, Del Mar, CA 92014; telephone 1-619-481-9537.

how to help your arm feel numb so the needle poke can't bother you."[13]

These general skills—understanding the social and developmental context of a child's problem, performing thorough medical evaluations, knowing the limits of one's expertise, being responsive to the child's feedback, and using therapeutic language carefully—are well within the expertise of the primary care practitioner. Although all physicians may not be inclined to expend the time and effort needed to learn these skills, those who do so are rewarded by an enriched experience in pediatric practice. The child health practitioner trained in hypnotherapeutic methods grows increasingly sensitive to the value of language in therapy, the connections between the child's state of mind and physiological response, and the benefits of having the child join in therapy.[25]

PRACTICAL ASPECTS

The past 35 years have seen the application of cyberphysiological techniques across the spectrum of pediatric care (see the box below). Within the primary care pediatric setting, such strategies can permeate every encounter. They can be divided into (1) **contextual/informal applications,** in which self-regulation methods are used to create comfort, diminish anxiety, and strengthen a youngster's self-control as adjunctive therapy in a variety of settings (e.g., the examination room, emergency department, or hospital procedure room); and (2) **problem-based/formal strategies,** in which a child or adolescent learns cyberphysiological skills explicitly, often as primary therapy, as part of the treatment of a given problem.

PEDIATRIC PROBLEMS THAT RESPOND TO CYBERPHYSIOLOGICAL METHODS

Anxiety associated with procedures or illness
Asthma
Attention deficit disorders
Cerebral palsy
Conditioned nausea and vomiting
Diabetes mellitus
Dysfluencies
Encopresis
Enuresis
Habit coughs
Insomnia
Irritable bowel syndrome
Migraine syndromes
Nail biting
Nightmares
Pain associated with acute problems (injuries, procedures)
Pain associated with chronic disease (malignancy, hemophilia, sickle cell disease)
Performance anxiety
Pruritus
Psychogenic seizures
Reflex sympathetic dystrophy
Thumb sucking
Tongue thrusting
Tourette syndrome
Trichotillomania
Warts

Contextual/Informal Applications

Erickson established that children use imagery, dissociation, and hypnotic states quite naturally. He observed, "There is seldom, if ever, a need for a formalized or ritualistic technique" when using hypnotic methods with children.[6] Whether ill or well, children who come to see the pediatrician seem already to be in an altered state of awareness and heightened suggestibility conditioned by previous, usually uncomfortable, experiences in health care settings.[15,17,33] This trance state, often typified by regression, withdrawal, and lack of communication, arises from an increased sense of vulnerability and becomes an adaptive response.[17] Health care practitioners have an important opportunity to optimize positive therapeutic suggestions for self-control and personal mastery early in their relationships with young patients. Children are likely to act on these suggestions immediately. Inadvertent negative suggestions are equally powerful. The author often comments on the value of cyberphysiological skills in the course of health supervision visits. In this context, rapport and trust are established, and the youngster's understanding of self-regulation is explored for the future.

Hypnotherapeutic methods can facilitate physical examination of the child by replacing the traditional, painful frame of reference of the doctor's office with one of comfort, trust, and positive interest in which the child's interesting physical reflexes and power to control his or her body become the focus of the encounter.[9] Such statements as "I wonder how soft your tummy might get as my hand touches it?" or "It's amazing how much your body relaxes when you breathe out" reinforce the child's innate capability for self-regulation. Challenging the child with "You can't get up on that examination table, can you? It's way too high for you, isn't it?" playfully enhances mastery. Used throughout the encounter, these techniques provide the youngster with an enjoyable set of achievements summarized by the examiner with, "You certainly have showed me all the things you know how to do and how in charge of yourself you are!" For parents, this demonstrates the child's cooperation and competency.

With infants and toddlers, more kinesthetic, behavioral, or nonverbal auditory techniques are useful. Rocking, singing, and blowing a pinwheel or bubbles can engage the attention of infants, young children, and their parents.[18] Parental anxiety is so instantly transmitted to these youngsters that the guidance provided by the practitioner is therapeutic for both parents and child.

Anxiety and pain related to procedures, such as injections and suturing of wounds, can be diminished by teaching self-regulation skills in the context of the procedure. "Blowing away shot pain"[8] and "blowing out imaginary birthday candles" can be explained to children as a way to "keep the needle from bothering you as much." Reframing the sensation of pain acknowledges the child's experience and supports his or her innate ability to find a more comfortable frame of reference from which to respond. Instead of announcing that "this might hurt" or it is "just a little pinch," the practitioner should calmly explore the experience—"Some kids say this feels like a kitten scratching, some say it's like a little bird pecking, others say it feels sharp. I wonder how it feels to you? Please tell me."[25]

Simply accepting the child's desire not to be in the office or emergency department for a painful procedure is an effective method to establish therapeutic rapport and invite the use of imagination to diminish anxiety and pain responses.[15] As the suture set and sterile drapes are unwrapped, the practitioner can say "I am sure you want to be somewhere else right now, I wonder where?" Most youngsters will respond with an activity or a place they would prefer, such as a playground. The conversation continues: "Well, you certainly can pretend to go there now and leave this cut on your forehead here for me to take care of. You can play much better there than here. If you go on the swings, can you pump yourself very high? Really? All by yourself?! You are good at that!" This theme can be maintained throughout the procedure, ending with implications for healing and recovery, such as "Now, when you are done here, perhaps your parents can take you there, tomorrow or the next day. You can swing higher and higher there as you heal this cut and your skin grows stronger."[25]

Problem-Based/Formal Usage

Most published reports of cyberphysiological skills training describe explicit use for primary or adjunctive therapy of defined problems. A study of migraine therapy comparing propranolol, placebo, and self-hypnosis found that the latter was most effective in reducing the frequency of migraine episodes.[30] In the largest published series of pediatric hypnotherapeutic encounters to date, Kohen et al[16] reported on 505 children and adolescents with a variety of problems, including pain, habit disorders, and chronic disease. The authors found that 83% had more than 50% reduction of symptoms; 50% showed complete resolution. Most (84%) required four or fewer visits to improve clinically. The study showed an inverse correlation between clinical success and the number of visits. Most children acquired usable skills in two visits.

Many studies of cyberphysiological training have involved children who have cancer. They demonstrate that training is more effective if begun shortly after diagnosis than if started after fearful responses have become conditioned.[19] In a prospective, single-blind study of hypnosis used to prevent chemotherapy-induced nausea and vomiting, children were randomized to perform self-hypnosis as primary therapy, using antiemetic medication as a supplement, or to undergo a standardized regimen of antiemetic medication. Children in the hypnosis group used less antiemetic medication and experienced less anticipatory nausea.[14]

When cyberphysiological strategies are to be learned explicitly for adjunctive or primary therapy, a more formalized protocol is effective. During an initial visit for the problem, the following elements should be explored:

- The history, physical findings, and laboratory evaluation
- The therapy to date and its efficacy
- The limitations imposed on the youngster by his or her symptoms
- A method for understanding symptom intensity (a scale from 1 to 10, a visual analog scale)
- The significance of the symptoms for the family
- The child's likes, dislikes, and fears
- The child's and family's understanding of cyberphysiological concepts

After gathering these data, the practitioner can explain how "thinking and feeling affect our bodies" and that people regulate these subconsciously. Examples include:

- How our brain takes care of us even during sleep (an especially useful example for children who have nocturnal enuresis)
- How a youngster can "turn off his parent's voice" when focusing his attention on a television show or video game (meaningful when parents have been frustrated by their inability to change a child's habit behavior)
- How a sleeping mother can remain asleep despite the familiar sounds of cars at night but awakens to the cries of her baby (a reassuring illustration for parents)[10]

A brief example of relaxation and mental imagery or demonstration of biofeedback devices can close the session. This experience demystifies the process and stimulates curiosity. The practitioner can provide written materials on hypnotherapy and biofeedback, and the youngster can be handed a personal calendar for recording symptom frequency, intensity, and therapy before the next visit.

The timing of the next encounter depends on the characteristics of the symptom and its meaning for both the child and family. At this point, self-monitoring is reviewed while the symptom is further described and reframed. Hypnotic trance induction or biofeedback training is taught through a variety of techniques. This is followed by intensifying the trance, using appropriate imagery, and reinforcing the patient's ability with ego-strengthening suggestions. After this, the young person's understanding of the experience is assessed. The practitioner can explain to the youngster that, as in other learning experiences, practicing self-hypnosis or biofeedback will enhance symptom control. Follow-up is important, whether by telephone, letter, or more visits. No studies have been done investigating the correlation between follow-up interval, method, and outcome.

This entire program needs to be an agreement between the practitioner and the patient, with parental consent. It is recommended that the young person learn self-regulation techniques without the parents present. Parents must come to understand that they cannot learn their son's or daughter's skills for them. When parents remind their child to "practice," the efficacy of cyberphysiological skills training can be clouded by issues of dependency. With seriously ill youngsters, parents may join the child to work for their own stress reduction as well as for further attachment. Credit for success needs to go to the youngster. The outcome is due to the child's innate ability and unique imagination; the mastery is the child's alone.[10]

CLINICAL VIGNETTES

The following examples illustrate concepts of self-regulation training. Each youngster is a different age and learns with different techniques. In all cases the young patient suggests his or her own imagery, to which the practitioner responds.

The children in the following examples are patients in the author's general pediatric practice. Rapport, a history of the current problem, and some knowledge of the young person's interests are derived from that prior relationship. No visit was longer than 30 minutes; most were less.

A.R. is a 6½-year-old boy who has cerebral dysgenesis with motor, visual-perceptive, language, and cognitive delays. He was born with syndactyly of his right first-second and third-fourth fingers and mild left arm paresis. Surgical correction of his syndactyly and left thumb tendon transfers have improved his fine motor capabilities. More surgical intervention will improve his dexterity.

His parents' advocacy and early intervention programs have allowed him to flourish developmentally. He was to be "mainstreamed" in first grade with occupational therapy and language resources. His mother requested a consultation just before he started school in the fall because he habitually sucked his right thumb. This behavior had attracted some attention in kindergarten, but the mother was concerned about A.R.'s self-esteem if he were teased about the habit in first grade. Also, his younger sister, already more adept in motor and language skills, had begun to tease him.

A.R. was accompanied by his mother for the first visit. She explained that her efforts to remind him when he sucked his thumb by quietly saying "thumb," placing a bandage on his thumb, and rewarding him with attention when he stopped, had not changed his behavior over 6 months. I recommended that she stop all reminders because it "was not her thumb."

A.R. was reluctant to talk about the reason for this visit. I discussed the nature of habits, "things we do without thinking much about them," including "habits that we do really well, like walking, running, riding a two-wheeler, using the toilet, and sleeping well all night." He nodded in response to the question, "Isn't it neat how your body figured out how to do these things without your thinking much about it?" He then helped me "think up some baby habits," such as baby talk, using baby bottles, and thumb sucking. He admitted to having a problem with the latter. I presented him a "menu" of reasons why thumb sucking might be a problem. He chose four: "It's not what big brothers do," "It makes you feel sad," "You don't feel grown up," "It can make your teeth stick out."

I asked him if he would like to help his thumb learn how not to go in his mouth. He nodded in agreement. Kneeling very close to A.R., I asked him to show me how and where his mother put a bandage on his thumb. He rubbed the thumb and then put it in his mouth, smiling. With his permission I asked to see his thumb. He agreed, then focused his gaze on the thumb as I examined it, rubbed it, and repeatedly asked if the bandage "felt like this?" He smiled and nodded as he stared intently at his thumb. I stated that there were many different colors of bandages he might put on his thumb. Rubbing his thumb in rhythm with my voice, I began naming different colors and patterns. He smiled at notions of "polka dot band-aids" and "squiggly purple band-aids"; then, without prompting, he closed his eyes and sank back in his chair as if to imagine the different bandages better. I suggested that "imaginary band-aids were the best kind" because they could be anything he wanted and they could best remind his thumb not to go in his mouth. He opened his eyes and stared again at his thumb, still smiling.

He said that he liked the imaginary "band-aids better than real ones." He agreed that this was a "fun visit" and would come back to learn how to use "pretend band-aids to help his thumb not go in his mouth."

He happily walked to the consultation room without his mother for the second visit 3 weeks later. His mother had noticed no change in his thumb sucking in the interim. She had stopped reminding him, as requested. When asked who was the "boss of his thumb and its sucking," he replied, "Me! Me! Me!" He liked the idea of pretending with bandages again. He closed his eyes and laid back in the chair as I rubbed an imaginary "band-aid that could be any color he wanted" on his thumb. I then suggested that "big kids who go to school and play fair" would want to be equally fair to other fingers and so placed imaginary bandages on all his other fingers and wondered what colors he might find them to be. He smiled, sitting quietly with his eyes closed, imagining as I spoke. In this state of relaxation and focused attention, he participated in the forming of four messages: (1) He was the "boss of his mouth and thumb"; (2) he could put his own special bandage on his own thumb whenever "it wanted to go in his mouth"; (3) his mouth would tell his thumb, quietly, "stop, don't go in me" (A.R.'s words); and (4) each time he helped them stay apart it would get easier. A.R. spontaneously acted out each of these steps: first rubbing his thumb, then whispering to it as it came to his mouth, then putting it down and smiling proudly. He rehearsed this a few more times.

He picked up a large ball of rubber bands on the floor of the room and marveled at it, saying "look at all the rubber *band-aids!*" I said that this "rubber band-aid" ball started out very small but grew bigger, little by little, with the addition of each new rubber band. As it got bigger, it could bounce higher and higher. With this he threw the ball against the floor with a loud "boom" and, to his delight, it bounced nearly back to his height. I asked if he would like to start a ball of his own. He nodded "yes." Together we removed some rubber bands and rolled them into a small ball for him.

We walked back to his mother in the waiting room. She asked me what she might expect of him. He announced that she did not need to put a bandage on his thumb any more, his "band-aid" ball would serve that purpose now.

A.R. accompanied his sister to her office visit 1 week later. He proudly showed me a red rubber band loosely encircling his right wrist. His mother explained that the rubber band indicated the color of the pretend "band-aid" on his thumb. He had not sucked his thumb in school since the last office visit and had a growing rubber band ball of different rubber band-*aids* at home.

A.R.'s first visit allowed him to listen to his mother's review and then participate in reframing his habit. The formation of this new perspective included his acknowledgment that he was growing and capable of change while choosing reasons why he might want to change. He engaged in "pretending" that linked the pleasure of rubbing his thumb with imagery that internalized the locus of control of his habit: imaginary band-aids are better than real ones. The language and kinesthetic imagery were developmentally appropriate. The second visit built on this playful technique, leading to a more image-filled hypnotic experience, including concrete, direct suggestions for altering his behavior and for finding that change easier with practice. Finally, he selected a creative symbol to remind himself of his imagery and suggestions for change.

A.R. already had overcome much adversity with the support of others and his own creativity, and he will face increasing demands in school, more surgery, and social pressures. The skills he has developed with this significant step can evolve to meet these challenges.

K.H. is an 8-year-old girl who has end-stage renal disease due to obstructive uropathy. She was well until just before her seventh birthday, when, as part of an evaluation for anemia and short stature, her renal failure was discovered. She had a frightening 8-week hospital course that included bilateral pyeloplasties and hypertensive crises with management in the pediatric intensive care unit. She emerged from the process feeling frightened and vulnerable. The stress was heightened by her parents' separation and initiation of divorce proceedings. I became her primary care physician at this point, overseeing school adjustment issues, health supervision, and coordination of care. She was referred to a psychologist for family counseling.

One year later, having started peritoneal dialysis, she began receiving erythropoietin injections at my office. Her anticipatory fear and anxiety before the injections was extreme. It took 20 minutes of discussion and negotiation to give the injection, which K.H. felt was very painful. Nurse, mother, and child all were quite anxious each time. I recommended hypnosis to diminish K.H.'s procedure-associated pain and anxiety. An introductory pamphlet on the subject was given to the family.

K.H. came to the initial visit without her mother. All of our other encounters centered around her renal disease and its manifestations. This time, we talked about her likes and dislikes. She mentioned that her favorite pastime was playing with her new kittens. One of them was "a little wild" and would scratch her in play. We discussed how, while this hurt, she did not let it bother her because "he's just a silly kitty." I taught K.H. how to relax her body and focus her attention while staring at a coin she held at arm's length. She was intrigued by this hypnotic induction technique and learned it very well, relaxing her body and facial muscles and closing her eyes when the coin slipped from her fingers. She was less anxious during her injection immediately after the session. She agreed to return to learn more.

Her mother accompanied her for the next visit. We discussed the coin induction technique, and I suggested that this time, once relaxed, she might enjoy pretending to "play with her kitties." When she agreed, we would give her the injection, but she could let it "not bother her" in the same way her kitten's scratch did not bother her.

Using the coin, she relaxed, imagined, helped indicate where on her arm she wanted the injection, and received it without moving. I asked her to finish playing with her kittens when she was ready. She opened her eyes, stretched, smiled, and announced that she did not "feel the shot." I reinforced that she was in control of this process. She began to use her "relaxation" for her weekly injections, taking less than 5 minutes per visit.

In the next month she "relaxed" for venipuncture and during peritoneal dialysis. Her mother noticed that her blood pressure was lower after her self-hypnosis. K.H. returned for an additional session to develop imagery for blood pressure control. Finally, with the support of her psychologist, her relationship with her *"kitties"* in hypnosis became an exploration of her relationship with her *kidneys,* her altered body image, and acceptance of her disease.

K.H. transforms a needed method for relieving pain and procedure-related anxiety into a technique for blood pressure (physiological) control and then applies the imagery to her own identity issues.

D.A. is a 13½-year-old young man who has secondary nocturnal enuresis and attention deficit disorder (ADD). Medical evaluation of his enuresis revealed no endocrinological, infectious, or neurogenic etiology. His symptoms began 6 months before, coinciding with his grandfather's terminal illness and death, family financial stress, his father's myocardial infarction, and his own accelerating puberty. He takes methylphenidate to help control his ADD. His school progress has been excellent. He is proud of his work.

At his first visit for this problem, D.A. chose to come without his mother. He had a "dry bed" two nights a week. Restricting fluids after dinner, having his parents wake him at night, and using an alarm clock in the middle of the night had not changed the frequency of his enuresis. He was not interested in an enuresis alarm I had shown him at a previous visit. He was changing his own sheets in the morning and doing his laundry.

We discussed his interests. He enjoyed video games, stereo equipment, and building his own skateboards. He was proud that he had his own television in his room and watched it at bed time. I showed him an inexpensive EDA monitor that has a tone that declines with decreasing EDA and increasing relaxation. He thought that the device, with its black case and finger leads, was "cool." I helped him place the electrodes on his fingers. I explained that electrodermal activity (EDA) had to do with "the electricity and reflexes in his skin," which he could control "with his mind" through the "wires from his brain called nerves." As I talked, he succeeded in lowering the EDA monitor's tone without any instruction. I continued to explain that just as he could lower the EDA output without exactly knowing how, he could use other "nerve wires" to control his bladder at night even when he was asleep. He took the monitor home to practice with it at bedtime and "figure out how it works."

He returned 2 weeks later, proud of his ability to get the tone of the device "down to nothing" before going to bed every night while watching television. He had bought his own monitor. His enuresis had not changed except when he had spent four nights at his grandmother's house. He was dry there every night. This was the bed he had slept in whenever he visited his grandparents' home all his life. We talked of the memories that the house, the room, and the bed held for him.

I invited him to demonstrate his use of the EDA monitor. Within a few minutes he had lowered the tone and achieved a deep state of relaxation. He nodded his head in agreement when I asked if I might now suggest some ways to link the monitor to better control of his bladder at night. Using multisensory imagery, I suggested that he could recall all of the sensations about the bed in his grandparents' house and the good memories there. At my request he raised his finger to signal when he had recalled all of this. I asked him to remember being there as a little boy, when "you weren't as strong as you are now, with strong muscles and the ability to do so many new things." After talking about the growing strength of these muscles, I listed "the muscles in your mouth, muscles in your intestines, muscles that keep you from having a bowel movement when you don't want to have one, and the muscles that keep you from peeing when you don't want to pee . . . and for some reason that only you know, you are in charge of those muscles in that bed better than in any other bed." He nodded agreement to this last statement. I suggested that he could imagine himself in that bed, with that control, whenever and wherever he chose, because "you are you no matter where you are." Finally, I suggested that with nightly practice, this control would become automatic and "your bladder would know" how to control itself. After a few more minutes, he regained his usual alert state and said he felt good. He said that he understood the connections between his mind and bladder, the EDA response and his bladder control. I audiotaped the session so that he could listen, if he chose, to reinforce his self-hypnosis. We parted with an agreement that he would call me with his progress in 2 weeks.

He came to the office 9 days later to leave me a note that he had had "a dry bed for 9 straight days!" His success continued.

This adolescent uses biofeedback-assisted hypnosis to resolve his nocturnal enuresis. He had learned to lower his EDA with a biofeedback device, and this self-regulation was linked to imagery and suggestions to be therapeutic. Themes of mastery over his changing body, interest in things electronic, and autonomy are important in his therapy.

RESEARCH AND THE FUTURE

Training in self-regulation has been demonstrated to be effective therapy for a variety of pediatric biobehavioral disorders. Cyberphysiology is an emerging discipline with promising implications for preventive health care and research in physiology. Although the precise pathways by which cyberphysiological strategies mediate therapeutic change are unknown, so are the limits of the benefits. These methods are not a panacea for all psychophysiological disorders. One must maximize medical therapy and make appropriate psychological referrals.

Three broad directions for future research can be defined: (1) clarifying the roles of cyberphysiological strategies for-biobehavioral disorders and defining their efficacy, (2) elaborating upon the implications of self-regulation training for preventive care and health care economics, and (3) elucidating the mechanisms by which the mind effects physiological change.

Most research in pediatric cyberphysiology has focused on new applications in the form of case reports. Several hypnotic susceptibility scales have been developed for use with children, although none has proved able to predict the outcome in clinical settings because the average child scores high.[25,27] Few controlled studies show increased efficacy of medications, and none demonstrates prolonged survival as a result of biofeedback training or hypnotherapy. Larger series with standardized regimens reported in the mainstream literature will be required to elucidate the therapeutic roles of self-regulation. Practitioners need direction regarding indicators of success, choice of techniques, duration of effect, and measures of efficacy.

Opportunities for discovery lie in the preventive potential of self-hypnosis and biofeedback. Incorporating self-regulation training in well-child care and as part of anticipatory guidance can form the basis for teaching lifelong coping strategies in health and disease. Training children to achieve relaxation before tests in school or musical or athletic performances may foster the development of adults who meet challenges with more poise and competence. It is conceivable that teaching cyberphysiological skills to youngsters at risk for familial disease such as hypertension, asthma, and ADD may delay their onset or diminish morbidity. Assessing each youngster's ability to use cyberphysiological skills upon admission to the hospital would allow nursing and medical staff to facilitate training and enhance both the child's and family's comfort and response to therapy. Certainly such training could reduce the amount of medications used for treatment as well as the sociocultural dependence on stress-reducing drugs.[25]

Exciting breakthroughs are being made in our understanding of the mechanisms by which psychological processes affect the autonomic, immune, and endocrine systems.[32] In structured settings, children have been able to vary salivary IgA content and increase neutrophil adherence, compared with matched controls, without cyberphysiological training.[12,26] In another experimental design, children who had asthma were shown to have cholinergically mediated airway reactivity in response to emotional stimuli.[23]

These paths of discovery are intertwined. Methods of cyberphysiological therapy in childhood asthma, for example, have great preventive potential while shedding new light on the neurophysiological mediators of reactive airways. This comingled research forges new coalitions between the physiologist, psychologist, subspecialist, and primary care practitioner—all aligned to rediscover and facilitate the child's innate ability to engage the future with equanimity.

REFERENCES

1. Bernheim H: *Suggestive therapeutives: a treatise on the nature and uses of hypnotism,* Westport, Conn, 1886 (reprinted 1957), Associated Booksellers.
2. Butler RJ, Forsythe WI, Robertson J: The body-worn alarm in the treatment of childhood enuresis, *Br J Clin Pract* 44:237, 1990.
3. Culbert TP, Reaney JB, Kohen DP: "Cyberphysiologic" strategies for children: the clinical hypnosis/biofeedback interface, *Int J Clin Exp Hypn* 42:97, 1994.
4. Devlin JB, O'Cathain C: Predicting treatment outcome in nocturnal enuresis, *Arch Dis Child* 65:1158, 1990.
5. Dixon SD, Stein MT, editors: *Encounters with children: pediatric behavior and development,* ed 2, St Louis, 1992, Mosby.
6. Erickson MH: Pediatric hypnotherapy, *Am J Clin Hypn* 1:25, 1958.
7. Erickson MH: Further techniques of hypnosis: utilization techniques, *Am J Clin Hypn* 2:3, 1959.
8. French GM, Painter EC, Coury DL: Blowing away shot pain: a technique for pain management during immunization, *Pediatrics* 93:384, 1994.
9. Gall JC: The art of examining a child: use of naturalistic methods in the pediatric physical examination, *Ericksonian Monogr* 7:69, 1990.
10. Gardner GG: Parents: obstacles or allies in child hypnotherapy?, *Am J Clin Hypn* 17:44, 1974.
11. Haley, J: *Uncommon therapy: the psychiatric techniques of Milton H. Erickson, M.D.,* New York, 1993, WW Norton.
12. Hall HR et al: Voluntary modulation of neutrophil adhesiveness using a cyberphysiologic strategy, *Int J Neurosci* 63:287, 1992.
13. Hammond DC, editor: *Handbook of hypnotic suggestions and metaphors,* New York, 1990, WW Norton.
14. Jacknow DS et al: Hypnosis in the prevention of chemotherapy-related nausea and vomiting in children: a prospective study, *J Dev Behav Pediatr* 15:258, 1994.
15. Kohen DP: Applications of relaxation/mental imagery (self-hypnosis) in pediatric emergencies, *Int J Clin Exp Hypn* 34:283, 1986.
16. Kohen DP et al: The use of relaxation-mental imagery (self-hypnosis) in the management of 505 pediatric behavioral encounters, *J Dev Behav Pediatr* 5:21, 1984.
17. Kuttner L: Management of young children's acute pain and anxiety during invasive medical procedures, *Pediatrician* 16:39, 1989.
18. Kuttner L: Helpful strategies in working with preschool children in pediatric practice, *Pediatr Ann* 20:120, 1991.
19. LeBaron S, Hilgard JR: *Hypnotherapy of pain in children with cancer,* Los Altos, Calif, 1984, William Kaufman.
20. Lubar JF: Discourse on the development of EEG diagnostics and biofeedback for attention-deficit/hyperactivity disorders, *Biofeedback Self Regul* 16:201, 1991.
21. Lynn SJ, Rhue JW, editors: *Theories of hypnosis: current models and perspectives,* New York, 1991, Guilford Press.
22. Maddock J: Trance: a generic model for clinical interaction. Paper presented to the Minnesota Society for Clinical Hypnosis, April 14, 1994.
23. Miller BD, Wood BL: Psychophysiologic reactivity in asthmatic children: a cholinergically mediated confluence of pathways, *J Am Acad Child Adolesc Psychiatry* 33:1236, 1994.
24. Nowicki S, Strickland BR: A locus of control scale for children, *J Consult Clin Psychol* 40:148, 1973.
25. Olness K: Hypnosis and relaxation therapy. In Levine MD, Carey WB, Crocker AC, editors: *Developmental-behavioral pediatrics,* ed 2, Philadelphia, 1992, WB Saunders.
26. Olness K, Culbert TP, Uden D: Self-regulation of salivary immunoglobulin A by children, *Pediatrics* 83:66, 1989.
27. Olness K, Gardner GG: *Hypnosis and hypnotherapy with children,* ed 2, Philadelphia, 1988, Grune & Stratton.
28. Olness K, Libbey P: Unrecognized biologic bases of behavioral symptoms in patients referred for hypnotherapy, *Am J Clin Hypn* 30:1, 1987.
29. Olness K, MacDonald J: Self-hypnosis and biofeedback in the management of juvenile migraine, *J Dev Behav Pediatr* 2:168, 1981.
30. Olness K, Macdonald J, Uden D: A prospective study comparing self-hypnosis, propranolol, and placebo in management of juvenile migraine, *Pediatrics* 79:593, 1987.
31. Olness K, MacParland F, Piper J: Biofeedback: a new modality in the treatment of children with fecal soiling, *J Pediatr* 96:505, 1980.
32. Rossi EL: *Psychobiology of mind-body healing: new concepts of therapeutic hypnosis,* New York, 1986, WW Norton.
33. Spiegel H, Spiegel D: *Trance and treatment: clinical uses of hypnosis,* New York, 1978, Basic Books.

34. Taylor S et al: Self-generated feelings of control and adjustment to physical illness, *J Soc Issues* 47:91, 1991.

SUGGESTED READINGS

Haley, J: *Uncommon therapy: the psychiatric techniques of Milton H. Erickson, M.D.*, New York, 1993, WW Norton.

Hammond DC, editor: *Handbook of hypnotic suggestions and metaphors*, New York, 1990, WW Norton.

Olness K (guest editor): *Pediatr Ann* 20:113, 1991.

Olness K, Gardner GG: *Hypnosis and hypnotherapy with children*, Philadelphia, 1988, Grune & Stratton.

Rossi EL: *Psychobiology of mind-body healing: new concepts of therapeutic hypnosis*, New York, 1986, WW Norton.

28 Fluid Therapy

Alice D. Ackerman

Regulation of body water, solute concentration, and acid-base parameters is important to the preservation of health in humans. Because almost every disease process results in some alteration of input, output, or amount of water or solute needed, a thorough understanding of these aspects of physiology is mandatory to enable physicians to approach the care of their patients rationally.

This chapter reviews some basic homeostatic mechanisms that enable the human body to maintain relative stability despite large fluctuations of intake, metabolism, and excretion. Specific instances in which those mechanisms are inadequate and the physiological responses that occur to meet the challenge of alterations in body fluid chemistry also are addressed. Finally, ways to correct various derangements are examined, and specific and unusual situations concerning fluid administration are discussed.

ONE

Theory: Body Fluid, Electrolyte Concentration, and Acid-Base Composition

BODY FLUID COMPARTMENTS

The entire body mass is composed of total body water (TBW) and body solids (fat, skeletal muscle, and cellular solids). Traditionally TBW has been viewed as a composite of intracellular fluid (ICF) and extracellular fluid (ECF).[47] ECF is composed of intravascular fluid (plasma) and interstitial fluid (ISF). Although further subdivisions of extravascular fluid have been devised, it is sufficient for the purposes of most clinical situations to view the body fluid compartments as depicted in Figure 28-1.

The size of the body's fluid compartments changes significantly with age. TBW makes up nearly 75% of the newborn's weight but only 60% of an adult man's weight[47] (Fig. 28-2). By about 1 year of age the proportionate distribution of body water begins to approximate that of the adult, and only minor changes occur thereafter.[47] At puberty, characteristic sex differences become apparent. Females have less body water than males because females have a larger proportion of body fat. Plasma volume remains nearly unchanged throughout the growth process, although this is not noted specifically in Figure 28-2.

Another fluid compartment not explicitly represented in Figures 28-1 or 28-2 is transcellular fluid, which is secreted by cells surrounding certain body spaces. This includes fluids within the gastrointestinal, pleural, peritoneal, joint, ocular, cerebrospinal, and pericardial spaces. Even though transcellular fluid in the healthy body accounts for only 2% to 3% of TBW, in certain disease processes it can increase dramatically (e.g., ascites secondary to portal hypertension or pleural and pericardial effusions caused by inflammatory processes in those areas).

SOLUTE CONCENTRATIONS

Clinically the only available measurements of solute concentration involve quantitating the various electrolyte concentrations and other solute particles found in the plasma. Most solutes are electrically charged particles. In plasma, sodium is the major cationic (positively charged) particle, with smaller concentrations of calcium, magnesium, and potassium present. To maintain electroneutrality an equal number of anionic (negatively charged) particles need to be present. These primarily are chloride, bicarbonate, and protein. However, there also are the unmeasured anions that constitute the "anion gap"—phosphate, sulfate, and various organic acids. Figure 25-3 depicts a "Gamble-gram," in which solute concentrations are presented in milliequivalents per liter of water. For each body fluid compartment the cations are on the top and the anions on the bottom. As seen in Figure 28-3 the major difference between plasma and ISF is the protein component because the two compartments are separated by a capillary membrane that is permeable to all except the largest of the charged particles (i.e., proteins).

However, the composition of ICF is different from that of ISF and plasma. Potassium is the major intracellular cation, followed by magnesium and a relatively small amount of sodium. The anions are led by organic phosphates and proteins, with smaller concentrations of bicarbonate and sulfate. The exact composition of intracellular contents is difficult to determine and probably varies substantially from one tissue type to another.

As depicted in Figure 28-3 there is a large concentration gradient between ICF and ECF for sodium, potassium, and chloride. These gradients are maintained by active transport mechanisms essential for the preservation of cellular integrity.[47]

Although the solute concentrations present in plasma are measured readily, the values reported by some clinical laboratories are in milliequivalents per volume of *plasma,* not water.[46] The total volume of plasma includes any suspended solids such as lipids or proteins, which usually constitute about 7% of the total volume. If the concentrations of these substances are abnormally elevated, the resultant measured electrolyte values will fall relatively, although their actual concentration in plasma *water* essentially will remain unchanged. Because of its predominance in ECF, the plasma solute most commonly affected is sodium, and the expected reduction of its concentration can be calculated easily if the concentra-

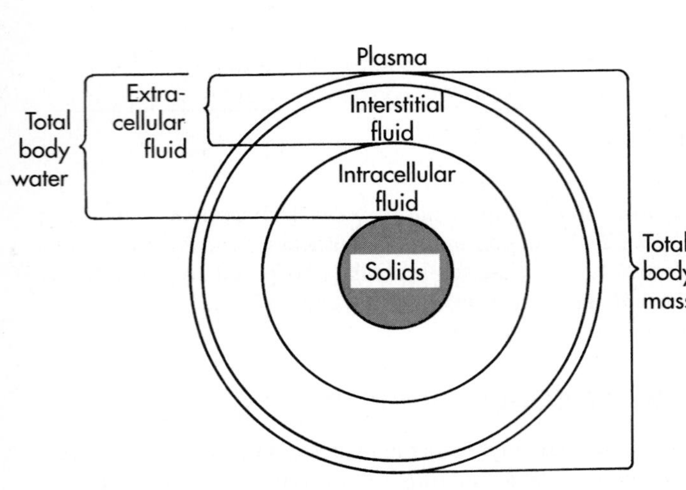

FIG. 28-1 Fluid compartments of the body.

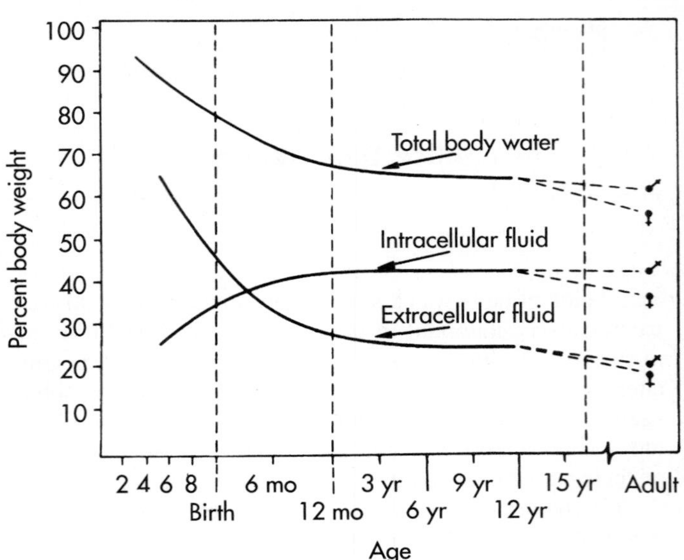

FIG. 28-2 Changes in body fluid compartments with age. Total body water remains relatively stable after 1 year of age, with the exception of changes that occur at puberty.

(From Winters RW, editor: ***The body fluids in pediatrics,*** Boston, 1973, Little, Brown.)

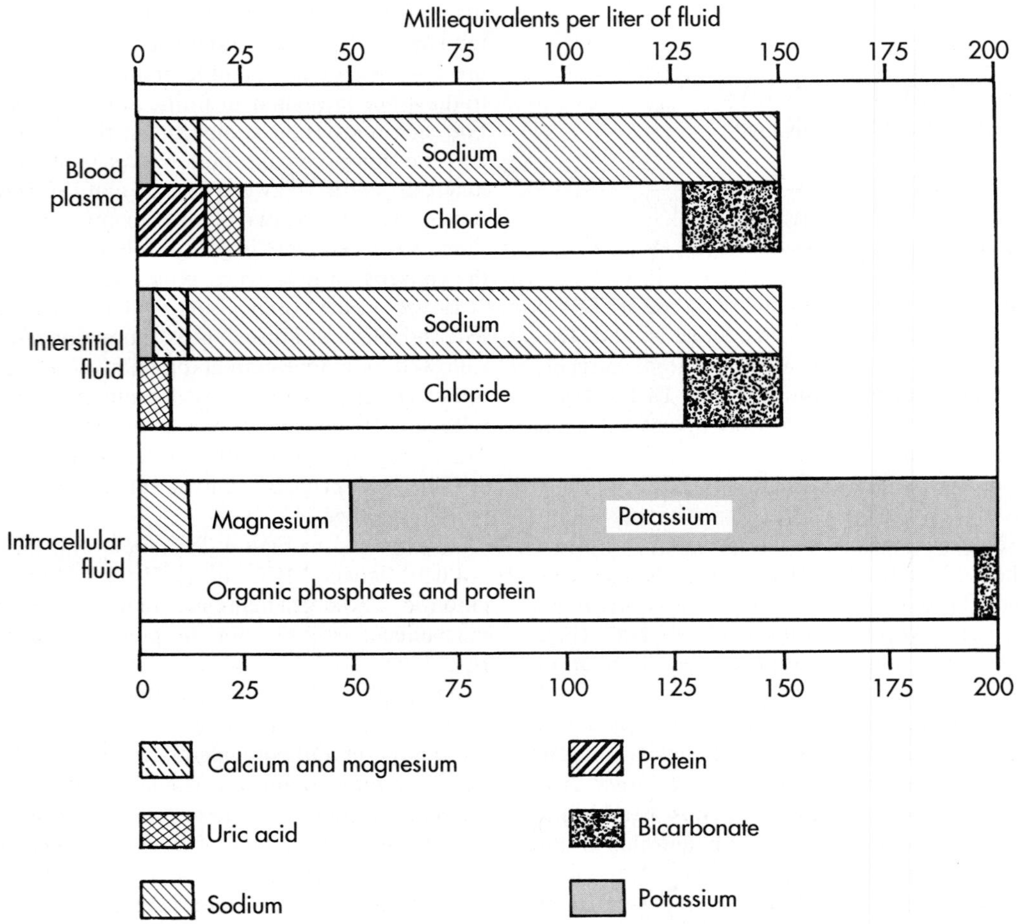

FIG. 28-3 "Gamble-gram" showing the various body fluid compartments and their electrolyte makeup.

(Modified from Winters RW, editor: ***The body fluids in pediatrics,*** Boston, 1973, Little, Brown.)

tion of the offending serum solid is known. In the presence of hyperlipidemia, multiplying the plasma lipid concentration (expressed in milligrams per deciliter) by 0.002 will yield the reduction (in milliequivalents per liter) of serum sodium as a result of displacement by this solid. The same information (milliequivalents per liter reduction in serum sodium) resulting from hyperproteinemia can be obtained by dividing the plasma protein concentration in excess of 8 mg/dl by 4. For example, if the serum total protein concentration is 12, the measured sodium concentration will be 1 mEq lower than its actual concentration in plasma water:

$$\frac{12 - 8}{4} = 1$$

These calculations are only necessary or appropriate if the clinical laboratory uses an *indirect* method to measure the serum sodium concentration (i.e., flame emission spectrophotometry or indirect-reading potentiometry). Measurement of the sodium concentration in a nondiluted serum sample by the ion-selective electrode method (termed *direct* potentiometry) will not be affected by alterations of lipid and protein concentrations, and the results will represent the "true" serum sodium concentration.[46]

OSMOLALITY AND OSMOTIC PRESSURE

The osmolality of any aqueous solution is a function of the total number of solute particles within it, regardless of their size or charge. When two solutions of different osmolality are separated by a membrane permeable only to water, water moves through that membrane to equalize the osmolality or tonicity of the two solutions. The force enabling this water movement (*osmotic* pressure) is proportional to the difference in osmolality between the two solutions. The resultant measured *hydrostatic* pressure of water in each compartment reflects the osmotic pressure of the particles that resulted in the transmembrane movement of water. The portion of osmotic pressure exerted by the plasma proteins represents the *oncotic* pressure present in the intravascular space.

Clinically it is simpler to look directly at the osmolality (number of particles per kilogram of water) or osmolarity (number of particles per liter of fluid) by actual measurement (most laboratories use freezing point depression) or by calculation rather than by measurement of hydrostatic pressure. The unit of osmolality used most commonly is the milliosmol, defined by:

$$\text{Milliosmol} = \text{Millimol} \times n$$

where n equals the number of particles produced by dissociation of a millimol of a given solute.[39] Because it does not dissociate, a millimol of glucose would represent 1 mOsm. The number of particles for sodium chloride would be 2, for calcium chloride 3, and so on.

By far the most substantial contribution to normal plasma osmolality is made by sodium and its associated anions. Under most circumstances the plasma osmolality is approximately equivalent to twice the concentration of plasma sodium. However, under unusual circumstances or for precision the osmolality can be calculated via the following formula:

$$\text{Osmolality (mOsm/kg body water)} = 2\,[\text{Na}^+]\ \text{mEq/L} + \frac{[\text{Glucose}]\ \text{mg/dl}}{18} + \frac{[\text{BUN}]\ \text{mg/dl}}{28}$$

Osmolality is normally maintained between 286 and 294 mOsm/kg of body water. The measurement of plasma osmolality is a fairly good estimate of the osmolality of other body fluids. However, plasma osmolality is slightly higher than that of ISF because plasma contains a slightly greater concentration of nondiffusible protein. This difference accounts for 1 to 1.5 mOsm/kg water, but it exerts a pressure known as *plasma protein osmotic pressure,* which is between 20 and 30 mm Hg.

To understand the control of the flow of fluid across capillary membranes, it is necessary to consider the three Starling forces that determine fluid movement. *Hydrostatic pressure*—the pressure exerted by the water of plasma—is determined both by the force with which it is being pumped (mean arterial pressure) and by the distensibility of the vessel. Therefore plasma hydrostatic pressure changes from arteriole to capillary to venule, but in general it favors the movement of plasma fluid into the interstitial space. Hydrostatic pressure is opposed by *ISF pressure* and *plasma osmotic pressure,* both of which tend to move fluid into the intravascular space. Although in health these bulk fluid movements are small and remain in equilibrium, they become more significant in several pathological conditions, most notably in peripheral edema formation and other processes described later.

CONTROL OF BODY FLUID VOLUME AND OSMOLALITY

Although the remarkable consistency of plasma osmolality has been mentioned already, it is important to reiterate that both plasma volume and osmolality remain nearly constant despite wide variations of water and solute intake. Control of osmolality and volume can be viewed as two separate but related mechanisms involved in a thirst-regulating hypothalamus-pituitary-kidney feedback system that works to adjust intake or output of water rapidly in response to changes, however minor, in plasma osmolality. The feedback mechanism hinges on the action of antidiuretic hormone (ADH) on the kidney's distal and collecting tubules to increase renal reabsorption of water.

Thirst and Antidiuretic Hormone

Thirst is regulated by plasma osmolality. Normal adults begin to experience thirst at plasma osmolality levels of 290 mOsm/kg,[48] with profoundly increasing intensity as the osmolality reaches 300 to 305 mOsm/kg. At this point the person consumes large amounts of water (assuming free access, which is not the case with infants and young children) until plasma osmolality is brought back below the threshold level. Secretion of ADH occurs at a lower threshold than that for thirst and is initiated (thus inhibiting renal water loss) at a plasma osmolality level above 280. With rising osmolality, ADH secretion increases, so changes in osmolality as small as 2.9 mOsm/kg effect a measurable increase in ADH release. Maximum antidiuresis usually occurs at around the same osmolality level responsible for initiation of the thirst mechanism just described. The ADH mechanism is far more sensitive than that of thirst, but drinking is the only physiological way to replace large losses of fluid. When osmolality levels fall below 280, ADH secretion is inhibited, enabling the kidney to secrete a high volume of dilute urine. The thirst mechanism is repressed simultaneously.

Many factors may alter the usual response of the ADH-thirst system. These include individual (genetically determined) variations, pregnancy, various drugs, and the nature of the osmolar load. However, the most important variable is the hemodynamic status of the patient. Regardless of the plasma osmolality level, any short-term reduction of blood volume or arterial pressure of at least 10% increases ADH secretion, whereas similar increases in volume or pressure have the opposite effect, thereby altering the threshold or set point but not disrupting the reactions to osmolar changes previously described.

TOTAL BODY FLUID HOMEOSTASIS

In addition to the primary factors regulating water intake and output, other organs contribute to fluid gain or loss, and they must be considered when trying to understand TBW homeostasis. In health these organs or systems work together to preserve the integrity of the child; in disease, however, any or all systems may either malfunction individually or lose the ability to compensate for the instability of another system.

The gastrointestinal (GI) tract is responsible for the digestion and absorption of nutrients—calories (in the form of fat, carbohydrate, and protein), vitamins, minerals, and water—and the excretion of food-derived waste products, including water. Numerous diseases may inhibit adequate intake or stimulate large losses.

The evaporative water loss of sweat makes the skin the major organ of temperature regulation. The lungs also excrete water and may provide some component of temperature control. In addition to responding to alterations in ADH release, the kidneys adjust their water output to meet the requirements of the solutes they secrete. Finally, the exocrine glands contribute to water needs and excretion by altering the metabolic rate or the systemic blood pressure, among other means.

CONTROL OF INDIVIDUAL SOLUTE CONCENTRATIONS

Sodium

As noted above, sodium is the major osmotically active cation in plasma. The total body content of sodium approximates 60 mEq/kg, but almost 43% of this is contained in bone, most of which plays almost no role in daily regulation of sodium concentration. The majority of the remainder is concentrated in the interstitial and plasma fractions, with only a small amount in the intracellular space.

Sodium homeostasis results from the balance of sodium intake and excretion. Intake is controlled by dietary habits and cultural customs, and although there may be some higher central regulation for sodium intake as there is for thirst (many patients who lose salt seem to develop a craving for sodium), it appears to be poorly developed and has not yet been localized. The typical American adult's diet contains 100 to 170 mEq of sodium per day; the amount of sodium in the infant's diet varies according to the formula he or she receives. Most of the dietary sodium is absorbed actively in the jejunum. Aldosterone secretion increases gastrointestinal sodium absorption.

Sodium excretion is controlled primarily by the kidneys but also by the GI tract and skin. Although a large amount of sodium is presented to the kidneys during glomerular filtration, almost 99% of it is reabsorbed in the kidney tubules. In conditions of severe sodium depletion, volume depletion, or both, this amount may increase to nearly 100%; in cases of sodium and water overload, it may decrease to approximately 90%. The renin-angiotensin-aldosterone system, when stimulated by decreased renal blood flow, facilitates a greater degree of sodium reabsorption in the distal convoluted tubules and collecting ducts through the action of aldosterone at those sites.

Hypernatremia and hyponatremia are conditions usually tied closely to changes in the extracellular volume and are discussed fully in the clinical sections on dehydration and fluid overload. However, a brief overview of associated conditions is included here.

Hypernatremia (serum sodium ≥150 mEq/L) may follow dehydration if there is a greater loss of water than sodium. These losses may occur through the lungs, skin, stool, or urine (especially in the presence of diabetes insipidus). Another important although infrequent cause of hypernatremia in young children is the overuse of commercial enema preparations containing high concentrations of phosphate and sodium. Elevated sodium content of breast milk has been implicated as a cause of hypernatremia in breast-fed infants.[28]

Signs and symptoms of hypernatremic dehydration may be difficult to interpret accurately, and the severity of dehydration may not be apparent on the basis of physical examination alone. ECF volume remains relatively well preserved; therefore shock is unlikely even with marked loss of body water, and skin turgor and perfusion may remain close to normal. Notable hypernatremia results in marked changes in CNS function, especially if the electrolyte disturbance occurred rapidly (in a few hours), which is common in small children. Affected infants exhibit marked irritability alternating with severe lethargy—the hallmark of acute hypernatremia. Seizures may occur and may be followed by coma if the condition is not diagnosed and adequate therapy is not initiated. In addition, elevation of the serum sodium concentration may lead to skeletal muscle rigidity and hyperactive deep tendon reflexes. In small children one may observe fever, emesis, and respiratory distress when the onset is acute.

Hyponatremia (serum sodium <130 mEq/L) occurs whenever body sodium stores are diluted or depleted. It more often is related to failure to excrete adequate amounts of water than to simple overhydration; however, in small infants the intake of hypotonic formulas or breast milk low in sodium may lower the plasma sodium concentration substantially. Although less common than isotonic or hypernatremic dehydration, hyponatremic dehydration occurs in approximately 10% of cases of acute diarrhea and most often is encountered because large stool losses are replaced with solutions containing little or no sodium. Any situation that increases the secretion of ADH may be associated with low serum sodium concentrations. This is seen in patients who have the syndrome of inappropriate antidiuretic hormone secretion (SIADH) resulting from CNS disease, pneumonia,[7] or meningitis.[40] Addison disease and congenital adrenal hyperplasia are associated with excessive loss of sodium in the urine and with retention of potassium. Children who have obstructive uropathy and progressive renal failure are less able to reabsorb sodium from their renal tubules, and therefore they sustain large sodium losses and may exhibit mild dehydration with a borderline or low serum sodium concentration. Children treated with vasopressin or 1-deamino-8-D-arginine vasopressin (DDAVP) may develop iatrogenic hyponatremia,[2,42] as may children receiving diuretic therapy. The administration of enemas low in saline concentration also may result in hyponatremia. An excessive loss of sodium and water occurs in individuals suffering from heat-related illnesses. Also, as previously mentioned, the serum sodium concentration reported by the laboratory may be artificially low in the presence of marked hyperlipidemia and hyperproteinemia. Highly elevated concentrations of blood glucose (as in diabetic ketoacidosis) are associated with real and apparent hyponatremia.

Signs and symptoms of hyponatremia are related as much to the duration of the lowered serum sodium concentration and to the plasma volume status as to the degree of hyponatremia present. Hyponatremia associated with diminished plasma volume results in anorexia, muscle cramps, lethargy, and shortness of breath on exertion. With further decreases in sodium concentration, nausea, emesis, and muscle weakness ensue, which may proceed to delirium and seizures.[4,45] Hyponatremia associated with acute water intoxication is more likely to result in seizures and coma than in conditions in which the plasma volume remains unchanged.

Potassium

Unlike sodium, only a small fraction of total body potassium is present in the intravascular and extracellular spaces. The total potassium content is approximately 50 mEq/kg body weight, with concentrations of intracellular and extracellular potassium of 145 mEq/L and 4 to 5 mEq/L, respectively.[47]

The majority of potassium absorption occurs in the proximal portions of the GI tract. It is excreted in the colon in exchange for sodium. Increased potassium loss results from diarrhea or overuse of laxatives. Elevated levels of plasma aldosterone also increase potassium excretion from the GI tract, the skin (losses here are relatively minimal), and the kidneys. Urinary excretion of potassium results from tubular secretion rather than glomerular filtration. Aldosterone acts at the level of the distal tubule to foster sodium reabsorption and potassium secretion. Potassium frequently shifts between the intracellular and extracellular spaces, mediated mostly by alterations in the serum acid-base status. An increase in extracellular potassium concentration occurs with systemic acidosis. Alkalosis results in movement of potassium into the cell.

Cardiac toxicity is the most significant effect of hyperkalemia. Electrocardiographic changes may be seen, such as elevation and peaking of T waves, depression of ST segments, disappearance of P waves, heart block, and ventricular tachycardia or fibrillation.[37] The most severe effects are not seen until the serum potassium concentration is greater than 8 mEq/L. Most frequently the clinical findings in hypokalemia include muscle weakness and ileus. There also may be cardiac effects exhibited on the electrocardiogram by low voltage, flattening of the T waves, depression of ST segments, prominence of U waves, arrhythmias, and asystole. However, these effects usually are not seen until the serum potassium concentration falls below 2.0 mEq/L. Hypokalemia also may inhibit renal concentrating ability and worsen any existing hypochloremic alkalosis.

Calcium

The total body calcium content ranges from 400 to 950 mEq/kg body weight, increasing with advancing age. Almost all of it (99%) is contained in bone, and nearly 50% of the remainder is protein bound. Of the entire mass of calcium, only about 9/10 of 1% exists in the noncomplexed free state. This is the physiologically significant ionized fraction of body calcium. The concentration of ionized calcium is pH dependent, increasing with acidosis and decreasing with alkalosis.

Calcium homeostasis is controlled mostly through the action of 1,25-dihydroxycholecalciferol (the metabolically active form of vitamin D), which increases the intestinal absorption of calcium (1) in the presence of an elevated serum parathyroid hormone level, (2) during pregnancy, (3) when calcium intake is low, and (4) when vitamin D is ingested. Excretion of calcium through the kidney is minimal except under certain circumstances, such as with prolonged bed rest, during protracted fasting, following the administration of diuretic drugs, and in metabolic acidosis.

The other major mechanism for control of serum calcium concentration is the balance that exists between ionized calcium and bone calcium, which is influenced by parathyroid hormone (parathyroid hormone increases the resorption of calcium from bone). This regulatory mechanism may produce wide variations in the ionized fraction of serum calcium; the total serum calcium concentration remains nearly constant.

Hypercalcemia usually results from the inability of the kidneys to increase excretion adequately when calcium delivery to ECF is increased. This may occur with hyperparathyroidism, immobilization, vitamin D intoxication, various endocrine disorders, sarcoidosis, malignancies, thiazide administration, milk alkali syndrome, and familial hypocalciuric hypercalcemia. Signs and symptoms of hypercalcemia may be negligible if the condition is mild or short-lived. However, severe short-term elevations of ionized serum calcium concentration may result in acute hypercalcemic intoxication, a rare syndrome characterized by acute renal insufficiency, lethargy with progressive coma, and occasional ventricular tachyarrhythmias. It sometimes may lead to death. Less critical but more common symptoms of hypercalcemia are renal lithiasis, nausea, anorexia, constipation, polyuria, and polydipsia. In addition, rapid infusions of intravenous calcium solutions may result in bradycardia and cardiac arrest. The classic electrocardiographic findings are shortening of the QT interval, followed by widening of the T wave as the serum calcium concentration increases. With prolonged, markedly elevated serum calcium concentrations, the urine becomes hypotonic.

Vitamin D deficiency, hypoalbuminemia, hyperphosphatemia, and hypoparathyroidism produce hypocalcemia. It also is seen in some premature infants and in neonates who have polycythemia or hypoglycemia. The ionized fraction of serum calcium may decrease with alkalosis. The major clinical manifestation of hypocalcemia is tetany. In children a grand mal seizure often is the presenting symptom. There may be muscle weakness, mental confusion, decreased myocardial contractility, and sometimes congestive heart failure; classically the QT interval is prolonged.

Magnesium

As an intracellular cation, magnesium is second in concentration only to potassium. About 50% of all magnesium is contained in bone; the majority of the remainder is found in muscle. Approximately 70% of plasma magnesium is in the free or ionized form; the rest is protein bound.

Although the details are poorly understood, magnesium homeostasis is accomplished mostly in the kidneys. Excretion is 5% to 10% of the amount filtered through the glomerulus. This amount increases with elevated plasma magnesium concentrations, volume overload, hypercalcemia, and the administration of diuretics. Tubular reabsorption is enhanced by both dietary magnesium restriction and parathyroid hormone secretion, although the effects of the latter may be overshadowed by the changes it causes in the serum calcium concentration. There is little regulation of gastrointestinal magnesium absorption. Between 25% and 60% of ingested magnesium is absorbed, primarily in the ileum.

Hypermagnesemia most often is an iatrogenic disease related to the use of antacids and enemas that contain magnesium or to the intravenous administration of magnesium sulfate. Symptoms and signs rarely are observed until the serum concentration exceeds 4 to 5 mEq/L. They include diminution of deep tendon reflexes, drowsiness, coma, hypotension, and respiratory depression. Prolongation of the PR interval, sometimes progressing to complete heart block and cardiac arrest, can be seen on the electrocardiogram.

Conversely, hypomagnesemia is common and is related to a myriad of clinical situations, although it most commonly is associated with malabsorption, hypoparathyroidism, prolonged laxative abuse, and chronic alcoholism. Symptoms may mimic those of hypocalcemia, which include tetany, muscle weakness, seizures, and changes in mental status.

Phosphorus

Phosphorus is involved in a wide variety of essential physiological functions. In adults the total body phosphorus content is 700 to 800 g, 15% of which is in the soft tissues and the remainder in the bones. Available phosphorus predominantly is intracellular. It is a major constituent of phospholipid bilayer cell membranes, intramitochondrial nucleic acids, and phosphoproteins. Although its most important function is as the source of high-energy bonds in adenosine triphosphate (ATP), it also is crucial for the control of 2,3-diphosphoroglycerate (2,3-DPG) synthesis in the red cell (which regulates oxygen delivery to tissues) and to numerous other hormonal functions.

Approximately 80% of ingested phosphate is absorbed in the jejunum. The kidneys regulate most of phosphate homeostasis by tubular resorption of 85% to 90% of the amount filtered through the glomerulus under normal circumstances. Tubular resorption is increased by thyroxine, and growth hormone and is decreased by parathyroid hormone and vitamin D_3.

The level of serum phosphate may vary significantly throughout the day, reflecting shifts from cells to plasma. The levels in children normally are considerably higher than those in adults.

Hypophosphatemia most often reflects movement from plasma into muscle, liver, or fat. These shifts may occur in diabetic ketoacidosis, in association with severe burns, and with respiratory and to a lesser extent metabolic alkalosis. The transfer of phosphate into muscle and liver cells is enhanced by glucose and insulin infusions, which decrease its uptake by erythrocytes. This causes diminished levels of 2,3-DPG and shifts the oxyhemoglobin dissociation curve to the left, potentially creating tissue anoxia because of enhanced hemoglobin affinity for oxygen. In metabolic alkalosis, intracellular hydrogen ion concentration falls; this stimulates glycolysis, which results in the rapid uptake of phosphate by cells because of their increased need to produce phosphorylated compounds. Clinical situations in which body phosphate depletes totally include mostly those leading to excessive losses of phosphate through the kidney, such as the Fanconi syndrome, Wilson disease, heavy metal poisoning, and vitamin D–resistant rickets. Although rare, nutritional deprivation (usually resulting from malabsorption or vomiting) may result in clinically notable hypophosphatemia.

Symptoms of phosphate deficiency are protean and are correlated easily with two of its most important functions: maintenance of energy stores by ATP and adequate oxygen delivery by 2,3-DPG. Muscular weakness, anorexia, general malaise, decreased myocardial contractility, and ventilatory insufficiency occur with phosphate deficiency. The patient also may experience seizures or become comatose. Deficient oxygen delivery to the tissues may result in hemolysis and myolysis. Leukocyte and platelet function also may be adversely affected.

Chloride

Chloride is the predominant extracellular anion; it accounts for approximately 60% of the negatively charged ions in plasma. Although small amounts of chloride can be found in bone, connective tissue, and red blood cells, over 50% of it is found in the ECF spaces. Total body chloride has been estimated at between 30 and 50 mEq/kg body weight, being slightly higher in infancy than in adulthood.

Homeostasis of the chloride ion is related directly to sodium metabolism, and in most situations movement of chloride ions from one body compartment to another is thought to be a passive accompaniment to that of sodium ions. However, this may be reversed in portions of the renal tubule and in some other situations. Concentrations of the chloride ion also vary with changes in acid-base status.

Dietary chloride is absorbed readily in the jejunum, but over 90% is excreted, mainly in the urine. Although the usual dietary source is table salt, it also is found in foods most commonly eaten, especially eggs, milk, and red meats.

Hypochloremic conditions generally are associated with alkalosis and may result from increased gastrointestinal losses because of excessive vomiting or excretion of intestinal fluids rich in chloride. Children who have Cushing syndrome usually manifest a hypochloremic, hypokalemic metabolic alkalosis associated with normal serum sodium levels and accelerated urinary excretion of chloride and potassium. Any situation resulting in hyperaldosteronism, such as hypovolemia, excessive licorice ingestion, or Bartter syndrome, usually is accompanied by hypochloremia and a metabolic alkalosis with potassium wasting. Chloride's major physiological role appears to be to enable the kidneys to excrete bicarbonate; therefore chloride ion must be replaced to allow renal correction of alkalosis, especially when alkalosis is associated with hypokalemia.

Hyperchloremia occurs in the presence of metabolic acidosis not associated with elevated unmeasured anions (anion gap) and may result from acute expansion of the extracellular space with infused fluids that contain chloride. The specific physiological effects of chloride excess are unknown.

Hydrogen Ion and Bicarbonate (Acid-Base Parameters)

Disturbances in plasma hydrogen ion and bicarbonate concentration lead to alterations of blood pH levels and the development of alkalosis or acidosis and are important clinically because of the extreme sensitivity of all essential physiological functions to changes in the body's acid-base balance. When the blood pH level is outside the normal range (7.35 to 7.45), detrimental effects occur in the central nervous, respiratory, gastrointestinal, musculoskeletal, renal, and cardiovascular systems. The outside limits of pH levels compatible with life are 6.8 and 8.0. The body can tolerate marked deviations approaching these limits only under optimum conditions and for short periods of time.

The concentration of free hydrogen ion in ECF is lower (average 40 mEq/L) than in water (100 mEq/L). Thus ECF is more alkaline than water and has a relative "base excess." Acidosis and alkalosis can be viewed respectively as conditions in which there is a negative or a positive base excess.

Acid-base homeostasis is accomplished through a complicated set of buffering systems and by more definitive mechanisms for removal or excretion of excess hydrogen and bicarbonate ions. A *buffer* is defined as a weak acid plus its salt, or conjugate base. The acid-base pair is in equilibrium, so when any acid or base is added to the system, the resultant change in pH level is minimized. Physiologically the most important (though not the only) buffer is that formed by the bicarbonate ion-carbonic acid pair. The Henderson-Hasselbalch equation, which defines the relation between an acid and its conjugate base, is as follows:

$$pH = pK + \text{Log}\frac{[\text{Base}]}{[\text{Acid}]} \qquad \textbf{1.}$$

where *pK* represents the dissociation constant of the acid, and the square brackets indicate concentration. This equation promotes understanding of the relation between bicarbonate (HCO_3^-) and carbonic acid (H_2CO_3) as they exist in the equilibrium expressed by the following:

$$[H^+] + [HCO_3^-] : H_2CO_3 : CO_2 + H_2O \qquad \textbf{2.}$$

This relationship can be expressed in several ways. Substituting the acid-base pair into equation 1 gives the following:

$$pH = pK + \text{Log}\frac{[HCO_3^-]}{[H_2CO_3]} \qquad \textbf{3.}$$

Because carbonic acid accumulation is short-lived, and its concentration is difficult to measure, the next equation is derived by knowing that the concentration of carbonic acid is equal to the product of the partial pressure of carbon dioxide in arterial blood (Pco_2) and its solubility coefficient (a):

$$pH = pK + \text{Log}\frac{[HCO_3^-]}{[a \times Pco_2]} \qquad \textbf{4.}$$

Under usual physiological conditions pK = 6.1, a = 0.03, $[HCO_3^-] = 24$, and $Pco_2 = 40$; therefore the following substitutions can be made:

$$pH = 6.1 + \text{Log}\frac{24}{0.03 \times 40}$$

$$pH = 6.1 + \text{Log}\frac{24}{1.2}$$

$$pH = 6.1 + \text{Log } 20$$

$$pH = 6.1 + 1.3$$

$$pH = 7.4 \qquad \textbf{5.}$$

To maintain the ratio of bicarbonate to carbonic acid at 20:1 and therefore the pH level at 7.4, with any change of either the bicarbonate or the carbonic acid concentration there must be a corresponding change in the other parameter. Understanding the equations as they relate to the bicarbonate buffering system is essential to appreciating the classification of acid-base disturbances. For any buffering system to maintain blood pH levels effectively, a mechanism must exist to enable excretion of excess acid (hydrogen ion) or base (bicarbonate ion and carbon dioxide). In the bicarbonate system, this happens through the lungs (carbon dioxide) and kidneys (bicarbonate and hydrogen ions). Regardless of any compensatory mechanisms, blood pH levels rarely return to normal until the underlying problem is resolved.

Of the nonbicarbonate-related buffers, the major system is the hemoglobin-oxyhemoglobin pair. Buffering also is accomplished by small amounts of organic and inorganic phosphates and plasma proteins. A complete discussion of these systems is beyond the scope of this chapter, which focuses on further exploration of acid-base physiology as it applies to bicarbonate and its related compounds.

Acid-base disturbances have traditionally been classified as "metabolic" or "respiratory," describing abnormalities that primarily involve the kidneys or lungs, respectively. The major mechanism used to compensate for bicarbonate alterations is renal and that for carbonic acid alterations, respiratory (through carbon dioxide exchange); the terms *metabolic* and *respiratory* can be related further to the numerator and denominator of the Henderson-Hasselbalch equation, respectively.[32]

Acidemia and *alkalemia* indicate absolute alterations of blood pH levels below or above the normal range. *Acidosis* and *alkalosis,* terms used more commonly, actually refer to the relative gain or loss of each acid-base parameter (H^+, HCO_3^-, CO_2) that results in a change of pH level or a *tendency* toward such a change.

Acidosis and alkalosis also are classified as primary, secondary (compensatory), or mixed disturbances. In general, compensation for respiratory alkalosis or acidosis occurs through renal mechanisms, whereas the lungs may compensate for metabolic aberrations. All parameters return to baseline levels only when the underlying disorder is resolved.

Before making a specific etiological diagnosis, it is important to classify acid-base disorders as just described. This is accomplished easily by measuring blood pH and P_{CO_2} levels in the clinical laboratory, where a reflection of bicarbonate is expressed as the calculated value for total carbon dioxide. Once any two of the values have been generated, the third may be estimated by using one of the readily available nomograms, thereby defining the disorder. The magnitude of expected compensatory mechanisms for any primary disorder must be known in order to determine whether a mixed disturbance is present (see Table 28-1). Examination of the patient often may provide the best clues to the nature of the problem, and one should not rely solely on laboratory data. It also is important to remember that acid-base disturbances rarely occur alone but generally are associated with changes in the concentration of potassium or other electrolyte concentrates, therefore obtaining measurements of those parameters helps to make the definitive diagnosis or to find an appropriate therapy.

Metabolic Acidosis. Primary metabolic acidosis (pH usually less than 7.35, P_{CO_2} less than 35 mm Hg) occurs with the accelerated loss of bicarbonate ion, increased production of hydrogen ion, or inadequate excretion of the normal acid by-products of metabolism. Clinical classification of such disorders usually separates those that result in an elevated concentration of unmeasured anions (negatively charged ions other than bicarbonate and chloride) from those disorders in which no such elevation occurs and thus the anion gap is normal. The anion gap is easily calculated by subtracting the sum of the serum chloride and bicarbonate concentrations from the serum sodium concentration; the serum potassium concentration usually is ignored in this calculation. The normal plasma concentration of unmeasured anions ranges between 10 and 15 mEq/L. Thus an elevated anion gap occurs when such concentrations exceed 15 mEq/L.

Elevation of the anion gap indicates an acidosis related to (1) accumulation of organic acids such as ketone bodies, which occurs in diabetic ketoacidosis or starvation; (2) increased lactic acid production because of diminished tissue perfusion and oxygenation, which occurs in shock, sepsis, congestive heart failure, or pulmonary insufficiency; (3) ingestion of various toxins, including salicylates and ethanol, whose metabolism results in elevated levels of various organic acids; and (4) retention of abnormally high levels of sulfates and phosphates, as occurs in profound renal failure.

Metabolic acidosis with a normal anion gap occurs whenever there is loss of bicarbonate ion through the GI tract (as in profound diarrhea) or the kidneys (as in proximal or distal renal tubular acidosis). Distal renal tubular acidosis is associated with failure to excrete the filtered acid load appropriately or with the use of carbonic acid inhibitors that block proximal tubular resorption of bicarbonate. Metabolic acidosis also may be seen with administration of an exogenous acid load and with amino acid infusions during total parenteral nutrition. Usually the decreased bicarbonate concentration is accompanied by elevation of serum chloride, thus maintaining the anion gap at a normal level. Therefore these situations sometimes are referred to as *hyperchloremic metabolic acidoses.* Most of these disorders also are associated with hypokalemia. A normal or an elevated serum potassium concentration signals early renal failure, exogenous acid ingestion, or hyperaldosteronism as possible causes of the metabolic acidosis.

If the plasma pH is less than 7.2 in the short term, treatment of metabolic acidosis should be considered. A level of 6.9 or lower is a medical emergency. Sodium bicarbonate should be administered, *but only if the body is able to excrete the generated carbon dioxide through the lungs.* The most common complications of this therapy are hypernatremia (hyperosmolality) with volume overload and hypokalemia. Because of improved protein binding of calcium when the acidosis is corrected, tetany may result from a sudden fall in the ionized portion of the serum calcium. Too rapid correction of the body pH level may result in an "overshoot" alkalosis or in paradoxical CNS acidosis associated with cerebral edema. Although it is necessary to be aware of these potential complications and to be appropriately cautious, they should not impede adequate therapy of life-threatening acidosis.

Respiratory Acidosis. Respiratory acidosis is always related to failure of the lungs to excrete accumulated carbon dioxide. With initial elevation in the serum P_{CO_2} level (hypercapnia), excess hydrogen ion is buffered within 10 to 15 minutes and leads to an increase in blood bicarbonate concentration. In the first few hours of continued respiratory insufficiency bicarbonate may rise as much as 1 mEq/L for each 10 mm Hg rise in P_{CO_2}. However, after several days of hypercapnia bicarbonate concentration rises even more as the kidneys respond to the lowered pH level by increasing their excretion of acid. Under these circumstances bicarbonate concentration increases as much as 4 mEq/L for each 10 mm Hg rise in P_{CO_2}. By observing the degree of bicarbonate elevation it may be possible to estimate the duration of an observed respiratory acidosis.

The severity of clinical manifestations of respiratory acidosis also may be related to their duration. Although the major manifestation of hypercapnia is lethargy with a diminished sensorium, it is more profound earlier rather than later in its course.

Dysfunction of both the pulmonary and central nervous systems must be considered in determining the cause of hypercapnia. Substantial hypercapnia is never related simply to an increased production of carbon dioxide. If the brain and lungs are functioning normally, accelerated production of carbon dioxide simply results in increased alveolar ventilation (increased rate and depth of breathing).

Probably the most common disorder leading to acute retention of carbon dioxide in children is severe status asthmaticus. Other pulmonary causes include multilobar pneumonia, abnormalities of the chest wall, and neuromuscular disorders that affect the muscles of respiration. Chronic obstructive lung disease is the most common cause of respiratory acidosis in adults but is seen infrequently in children, except in those who have advanced cystic fibrosis or bronchopulmonary dysplasia. In a previously healthy child who has an acute rise in P_{CO_2}, one should always consider the presence of a compression lung injury such as hemothorax or pneumothorax or the presence of a large pleural effusion.

Conditions of the CNS that relate to hypercapnia involve inhibition of the respiratory drive and include (1) severe diffuse CNS infections such as encephalitis or meningitis, (2) trauma to the CNS, resulting in elevated cerebral pressure or vascular compromise (hemorrhage or thrombosis), and (3) ingestion of drugs known to depress the CNS (such as barbiturates, narcotics, and sedatives).

Treatment should always address the underlying pathophysiology and should increase alveolar ventilation to allow appropriate excretion of carbon dioxide. In the event of a rapidly rising P_{CO_2}, intubation with assisted ventilation may be necessary. Conversely, well-compensated respiratory acidosis usually can be treated conservatively by correcting the fundamental abnormality, unless the patient is on the verge of respiratory failure or is exhibiting substantial neurological dysfunction.

Because the kidneys continue to excrete acid for several days after correction of lowered pH levels caused by retention of carbon dioxide, one may see a notable metabolic alkalosis for as long as 36 hours after correction. This condition is self-limited and resolves without intervention.

Chronic respiratory acidosis usually does not require short-term therapy but rather a conservative approach aimed at improving air exchange. Bronchodilators to relieve airway obstruction, judicious use of oxygen (some of these patients require some hypoxia to stimulate respiration), and measures to decrease excess lung water may be helpful. Implementation of vigorous pulmonary toileting (postural drainage and percussion) helps to relieve airway obstruction caused by inspissated secretions.

Metabolic Alkalosis. In contrast to the urgency with which one must approach metabolic and respiratory acidosis, alkalosis or alkalemia is seldom of sufficient magnitude to cause alarm. A loss of hydrochloric acid or gain of bicarbonate or other forms of alkali may result in the elevation of blood pH levels. Uncommonly seen alone, these disturbances usually are accompanied by altered plasma concentrations of potassium and chloride. Therefore the clinical diseases have been divided into two categories related to those that do and do not respond to the administration of fluids that contain chloride as the major therapeutic intervention.

Chloride-sensitive conditions generally result from ongoing losses of hydrochloric acid through the GI tract, skin, or kidneys, and although the hypochloremia is associated with hypokalemia and elevated bicarbonate concentration, neither pH level nor potassium ion abnormalities can be corrected by administration of potassium if salts that contain chloride are withheld. The kidneys secrete additional bicarbonate in an attempt to return the blood pH level to normal, and with deficits of sodium and hydrogen ions, they selectively secrete potassium to maintain electroneutrality.

The most common pediatric problem associated with hypochloremic, hypokalemic metabolic alkalosis is excessive vomiting, such as is seen with pyloric stenosis; however, it also may occur in cystic fibrosis (electrolyte and acid-base imbalance infrequently may be the initial presentation of this genetically acquired disease). Treatment with potent diuretic compounds, such as the thiazides and furosemide, causes urinary losses of potassium chloride and sodium in excess of bicarbonate losses. This also generates a hypochloremic, hypokalemic metabolic alkalosis usually associated with hyponatremia.

Of the chloride-resistant metabolic alkaloses the one encountered in children most frequently is excessive mineralocorticoid activity, as seen with the adrenogenital syndrome, Bartter syndrome, Cushing disease, and excessive licorice ingestion. Contraction of the blood volume and profound potassium depletion also may lead to metabolic alkalosis and remain resistant to all measures except correction of the underlying abnormalities.

The symptoms and signs of marked alkalosis include neuromuscular irritability with muscle cramps, weakness, paresthesias, and tetany. Seizures and hyperreflexia usually precede cardiac arrhythmias, which are more common in the presence of hypocalcemia (low Ca^{++} concentration often accompanies metabolic alkalosis). Treatment almost never requires addition of acidic compounds but usually is directed at the underlying diseases and restoration of normal electrolyte and fluid status.

Respiratory Alkalosis. Primary disorders that lead to lower arterial P_{CO_2} involve an increase in alveolar ventilation, but the stimulus for such hyperventilation may stem from the CNS, the lungs, drugs, or other factors that increase the rate and/or depth of breathing. In the pediatric age group respiratory alkalosis is observed most commonly in the *hyperventilation syndrome,* which usually is a response to anxiety and is associated with tachypnea, numbness and tingling of the extremities, and other symptoms that may mimic more serious disorders. Another central cause of respiratory alkalosis is elevation of intracranial pressure; this may be seen in space-occupying lesions, head trauma, or infection. In young children and infants, hyperthermia may be sufficient to induce hyperpnea, alkalosis, and even tetany.

Pulmonary stimuli of ventilation most frequently are associated with hypoxemia. In an attempt to compensate for hypoxemia the child increases the rate and depth of breathing, thus creating a pure respiratory alkalosis. Any type of pneumonia, pulmonary inflammation, or pulmonary edema may lead to alkalosis. Severe anemia with a resultant decrease in oxygen-carrying capacity also leads to hyperventilation and respiratory alkalosis.

Specific drugs that have been implicated in respiratory alkalosis include salicylates, paraldehyde, amphetamines, and progestational agents. Ammonia is a respiratory stimulant, and accumulation of this compound in the body tissues also leads to respiratory alkalosis (as in children who have urea cycle defects or Reye syndrome).

Signs and symptoms of respiratory alkalosis are nonspecific. Treatment is based on the underlying problem; appropriate attention must be paid to associated electrolyte disturbances.

Mixed Disturbances. In clinical practice one often is faced with a combination of acid-base disturbances, and determining the primary defect or defects may not be as straightforward as the previous descriptions have made it seem. In these situations one continually must return to the basics of good medical practice and rely heavily on obtaining an adequate history and performing a thorough physical examination. Armed with these primary tools the clinician may be able to predict acid-base abnormalities and gain valuable insight into possible causative mechanisms and then use the laboratory data to confirm or reject the proposed diagnosis. At this point in the diagnostic process, it is helpful to compare available acid-base results (pH, P_{CO_2}) with any of the nomograms mentioned previously. One may consult a chart, such as Table 28-1, to look at expected compensatory mechanisms and then

Table 28-1 Primary Acid-Base Abnormalities and Their Expected Compensatory Changes

Disorder	Primary abnormality	Associated abnormalities	Expected compensatory changes if simple disorder exists
Metabolic acidosis	Elevation in hydrogen ion concentration (↓ pH)	↓ Bicarbonate concentration and total CO_2; negative base excess	P_{CO_2} will fall by 1.5 times the fall in bicarbonate concentration (maximum change is 10 mm Hg)
Respiratory acidosis	Elevation in P_{CO_2}	↑ Hydrogen ion concentration and total CO_2; ↓ pH	Bicarbonate concentration rises by 3.5-4 mEq/L for each 10 mm Hg rise in P_{CO_2} (cannot be above 30 mEq/L if the problem is short term, 45 if long term)
Metabolic alkalosis	Decreased hydrogen ion concentration (↑ pH)	↑ Bicarbonate concentration and total CO_2; positive base excess	P_{CO_2} rises by 0.5-1 mm Hg for every 1 mEq rise in bicarbonate concentration (to a maximum of 55 mm Hg)
Respiratory alkalosis	Decreased P_{CO_2}	↓ Hydrogen ion concentration and total CO_2; ↑ pH	Bicarbonate concentration falls by 2.5-5 mEq/L for each 10 mm Hg fall in P_{CO_2} (lower limit is 18 mEq/L if short term, 12-15 mEq/L if long term)

decide whether the numbers "fit" into a simple disturbance. However, two rules can be invaluable in evaluating simple versus mixed acid-base disturbances:

1. In a simple acid-base disturbance, the bicarbonate abnormality *always* is in the same direction as the P_{CO_2}.
2. Under most circumstances the body does not *over*compensate. Common sense and a lot of thinking about physiology and expected changes in acid-base disorders enable the clinician to diagnose most of these problems accurately without relying on cumbersome formulas and nomograms, which sometimes are inaccessible.

TWO
Fluids and Electrolytes in Clinical Practice

MAINTENANCE REQUIREMENTS

As described in previous sections the body's numerous homeostatic mechanisms combine to orchestrate a complex balance between gains of water and electrolytes (ingested, administered, or internally generated) and obligatory losses (through the kidneys, lungs, skin, and GI tract). Fortunately the human organism is adaptable and in health can adjust easily to most conditions of excess and can tolerate limitations to a point. However, to support vital functions, maintain health, and encourage adequate growth, the body must be supplied with water, electrolytes, nutrients, and vitamins. This chapter deals predominantly with water and solute requirements; other nutritional necessities for health maintenance are discussed under Nutritional Requirements in Chapter 16.

Knowledge of fluid and salt needs is helpful in everyday pediatric practice but becomes most important in situations in which the physician is responsible for the child's intake. Notably these situations occur when parenteral fluids are administered to a child who is unable to drink or who has experienced major losses in addition to his or her usual excretion of water and solutes. Furthermore, familiarity with basic requirements is important when physicians attempt to determine why a child loses weight or "fails to thrive." Before one can approach the fluid therapy for any of the previously described circumstances, it is essential to understand the child's needs under usual conditions and then adjust the intervention to meet his or her altered requirements.

Water

Traditionally, calculating water requirements has been done by one of three methods: body weight, body surface area, or metabolic rate. Water need per unit of body weight changes dramatically with age and size and therefore is not very useful. Body surface area once was thought to correlate well with both metabolic expenditure and fluid needs, but this subsequently has been shown not to be the case, especially in small babies during the newborn period and in children between 6 months and 3 years of age. Additionally, surface area is determined by comparing height and weight with a nomogram, which is cumbersome and depends on accurate measurements (height is notoriously difficult to measure in young children and infants). Use of the metabolic rate to calculate fluid requirements is attractive because it is based on physiological principles and is a constant number: approximately 100 ml (1 deciliter [dl]) of water is needed for every 100 calories consumed.[41]

Bedside methods of measuring caloric expenditures in children have been developed. These methods are cumbersome and are not often used in clinical practice. Fortunately, adequate estimates exist to allow one to predict the caloric expenditure of a *hospitalized patient who is receiving only parenteral fluid therapy.* These values rest nearly midway between those of a normally active, healthy individual and those of a child who has a basal metabolic rate (Fig. 28-4). The middle curve can be divided into three sections and caloric expenditure related to weight as follows: from 2 to 10 kg, 100 Cal/kg; from 10 to 20 kg, 50 calories for each kilogram over 10; and beyond 20 kg, 20 Cal/kg. Thus a child weighing 17 kg (hospitalized and confined to bed) would require 1350 Cal/day ([10 × 100] + [7 × 50]); an adult weighing 70 kg would require 2500 Cal/day ([10 × 100] + [10 × 50] + [50 × 20]). These relationships are easy to memorize and are useful in determining caloric needs and fluid requirements in the appropriate hospitalized patients, assuming there are no unusual heat or fluid losses and no net increase or loss of water, calories, or solutes.

The next step is to consider the usual modes of fluid and solute loss and to calculate the magnitude of these losses, re-

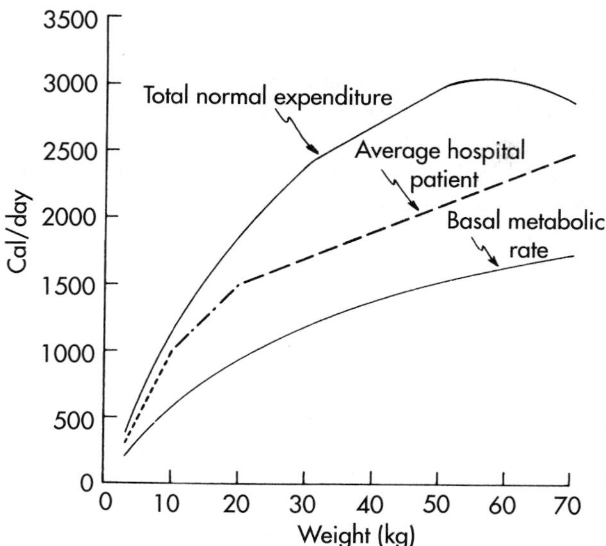

FIG. 28-4 Metabolic requirements of the average hospitalized patient. The center line represents calculated caloric requirements for average hospitalized patients. See text for explanation of the three sections of the curve.

(From Winters RW, editor: *The body fluids in pediatrics,* Boston, 1973, Little, Brown. Modified from Segar WE: *Pediatrics* 19:823, 1957.)

lating the results to units of caloric expenditure. Fluid is lost through the kidneys along with solute as urine, through the lungs and skin as "insensible" water loss, through the skin as sweat, and through the GI tract in stool (negligible in a hospitalized child who is receiving only parenteral fluids). Although the human kidney can excrete a relatively concentrated urine (1500 mOsm/kg water), the aim of maintenance fluid therapy is to provide enough water to allow excretion of the renal solute load (electrolytes and urea) without unduly taxing renal concentrating ability. Therefore the aim is to excrete a urine that has a concentration of between 200 and 400 mOsm/kg water, which is equivalent to a specific gravity of 1.010 to 1.015. To excrete the usual renal solute load of 12 to 20 mOsm/100 Cal of expended energy at a reasonable concentration, a urine volume of between 45 and 65 ml/100 Cal, or approximately 55 ml/100 Cal, is required.

Nearly 15 ml of water is lost through the lungs for every 100 calories expended. In addition insensible loss through the skin amounts to about 30 ml/100 Cal. Specific water loss caused by sweating varies with ambient temperature and in most cases equals less than 20 ml/100 Cal. Stool losses generally can be ignored because except under unusual circumstances, stool water losses rarely exceed 5 to 10 ml/100 Cal.

As the various obligatory water losses are tallied, it must be remembered that the metabolism of calories to heat and energy produces carbon dioxide and water. This "hidden" water intake is approximately 12 ml/100 Cal; therefore if we ignore stool losses and add fluid requirements for urine excretion (55 ml/100 Cal), insensible loss (45 ml/100 Cal), and sweat (10 to 20 ml/100 Cal), then subtract the unseen water intake (12 ml/100 Cal), the usual maintenance water requirement is approximately 1 dl for every 100 calories of energy expended.

Electrolytes

When determining maintenance solute requirements (sodium, chloride, and potassium primarily), the aim is to provide more than absolute minimum requirements but not to present the child with so much as to tax the body's excretory abilities. Because the diet of infants varies widely with respect to electrolyte concentration, the figures suggested for specific solutes represent average numbers based on usual intakes that allow optimum functioning of the organism. As with water requirements, these maintenance values can be expressed as milliequivalents per kilogram of body weight or of body surface area. However, caloric expenditure is used continually as the base of reference in this chapter.

The maintenance requirement of sodium for the average infant is between 2 and 3 mEq/100 Cal; potassium is closer to 2 mEq/100 Cal. Because sodium and potassium are supplied routinely in the form of chloride salt, the infant or child receives between 4 and 5 mEq/100 Cal of chloride ion, although the absolute chloride requirement probably is very small. Conversely, renal excretory ability is such that this amount does not present any particular hardship under normal conditions.

Calories

In the section of this chapter dealing with total parenteral nutrition, alternatives for providing adequate calories for patients whose oral intake is limited are considered. For short-term administration of parenteral fluids, little consideration usually is given to trying to replace caloric expenditure calorie per calorie. Rather, the reason for adding calories in the form of dextrose to parenteral fluids is to prevent ketosis and the breakdown of endogenous protein. In the average hospitalized patient this requires that approximately 25% of caloric expenditure be provided with an intravenous solution that contains glucose; therefore the aim should be 25 Cal/100 Cal expended energy. Because each gram of dextrose provides 4 calories, this equates to 5 g of dextrose per 100 calories expended. For infants and small children, the absolute glucose requirement to prevent ketosis and overt hypoglycemia is between 4 and 6 mg per kg per minute.

COMPOSITION OF MAINTENANCE FLUID FOR PARENTERAL USE

To summarize the previous sections on maintenance requirements and to determine the composition of a parenteral fluid that can be administered *under normal circumstances* to hospitalized patients for a *short period* (up to several days), it should be understood that for every 100 calories expended it is necessary to provide 1 dl water, 2 to 3 mEq sodium, 2 mEq potassium, and 5 g glucose. Because prepared intravenous fluids are formulated on a per liter basis the composition of a suitable fluid for maintenance therapy would be 20 to 30 mEq sodium, 20 mEq potassium, and 50 g glucose (values expressed per liter).

Values of sodium in parenteral fluids usually are expressed as a fraction of "normal saline solution." Normal saline (NS) is a 0.9% solution of sodium chloride that provides 154 mEq of sodium per liter of solution. The most commonly available prepared solutions contain either "half-normal" saline (77 mEq of sodium per liter) or "quarter-normal" saline (38 mEq of sodium per liter). Because of the body's ability to excrete any excess sodium, a solution containing quarter-normal (or 0.225%) saline is an acceptable preparation. This usually is formulated with 5% glucose (50 g/L), and to each liter one can add 20 mEq of potassium, yielding a solution that is slightly hypertonic (compared with plasma), with an osmolarity of 386 mOsm/L, but that is hypotonic with respect to sodium. It is possible to add sodium in any desired concentration to a liter of 5% dextrose in water if the need arises, but usually this is unnecessarily time consuming and expensive.

ADMINISTRATION

Once the appropriate concentration of each solute in the parenteral fluid has been determined, the solution is administered at a rate of 100 ml/100 Cal of expected energy expenditure through a peripheral vein (extremity or scalp). Procedures for gaining vascular access in children are described in Appendix B. Although not a new method, the technique of administering fluids and medications into the bone marrow (intraosseous infusion) recently has been demonstrated to be safe and effective in providing volume replacement and resuscitation drugs in an *emergency.* It may be used in infants and children when intravenous access cannot be obtained rapidly. Techniques for performing this procedure also are found in Appendix B.

WHEN MAINTENANCE IS NOT ADEQUATE

In the preceding sections a rational approach was developed for supplying children with maintenance fluids. Based on the physiology of the illness, the needs of any given child may differ considerably from these "maintenance" requirements. However, the calculations presented remain valid over a wide range of situations if used as a base to which unusual losses are added. Any and all of the organs normally involved in water homeostasis may be included: water lost through the GI tract in the form of diarrhea; massive renal excretion of water in diabetes mellitus or diabetes insipidus or following the administration of osmotic or other diuretics; excessive sweating caused by autonomic instability, fever, or high ambient temperature; and an increased loss of lung water with hyperpnea from any cause, including hyperpyrexia. Processes that normally do not contribute to water loss also may be involved, such as massive vomiting, losses through a nasogastric tube, and acute blood loss. In addition, increased demands for fluids exist in various conditions of elevated metabolic rate (e.g., thyrotoxicosis), in situations that create large shifts in the body's fluid compartments (usually of the vascular space), and in many perioperative conditions (third spacing) that if uncorrected may produce shock. Persistence of any of these abnormal conditions in the absence of adequate fluid intake leads to water or electrolyte deficits or both. The purpose of replacement fluid therapy is to determine a rational approach to body water and electrolyte restoration. Additionally the fluid administration scheme so devised has to take into consideration the ongoing losses that persist beyond the institution of parenteral fluid therapy and provide appropriate replacement of these lost fluids.

Fluids sometimes need to be supplied in amounts *below* those estimated for the average hospitalized patient. Any child who has a diminished urine output because of renal failure does not require as much free water as his or her normal counterpart. Children who are placed in mist tents or maintained on ventilators lose less water through their lungs and should have a lower estimate made of insensible water loss. Children whose activity levels are below those predicted for most bedridden patients (e.g., those in coma or who are paralyzed) expend fewer calories and therefore require less water (see Fig. 28-4; water requirement is closer to that for the basal metabolic rate).

ESTIMATION AND CORRECTION OF DEFICITS AND ONGOING LOSSES

The best way to estimate fluid and electrolyte deficits is to determine how much fluid has been lost from each body compartment, the electrolyte concentration of the lost fluid, and the period of time over which such losses have occurred. In most short-term situations therapy must be initiated before all of these data can be collected. In addition volumes of diarrheal or emetic losses may be extremely difficult to measure.

The first step in evaluating any child is to determine the severity and acuteness of the problem. For children who have a history of abnormal losses, the clinician's first priority must be to assess the *adequacy of the intravascular volume.* This is accomplished by evaluating the child's overall condition: Is he or she alert and awake, or has he or she suffered an alteration in CNS functioning, perhaps from diminished cerebral perfusion or electrolyte abnormalities (discussed later)? Are the pulses strong and full, or "thready," weak, and rapid? Is there normal blood flow to the skin, or is the perfusion decreased and the skin cool and clammy? What is the quality of the skin turgor—is it normally firm and moist or has it become dry and loose, with a doughy feeling to the abdomen and "tenting" of the overlying skin when pinched lightly between the fingers? If any of these indications of impending circulatory collapse exist, it is essential to begin parenteral fluid therapy *without delay.* An intravenous line should be placed and a bolus of fluid administered (20 ml/kg of expected body weight of a solution containing approximately 150 mEq/L of sodium) as rapidly as feasible while the physician completes his or her evaluation. Once the lifesaving therapy is in progress, or if the child's vital functions appear satisfactory, the child's parent or guardian should be questioned to obtain details of the history and the child examined thoroughly (including weight and length). It is helpful to inquire about the child's last known weight, for example, at the latest visit to his or her pediatrician. If recent, this information can help the physician decide on the degree of dehydration or volume depletion by using the following formula:

$$\text{Percent dehydration} = \frac{\begin{pmatrix}\text{Expected or}\\ \text{recent weight}\end{pmatrix} - \begin{pmatrix}\text{Current}\\ \text{weight}\end{pmatrix}}{\text{Expected weight}} \times 100$$

For example, a 3-year-old child who weighed 15 kg at a well-child visit to the pediatrician 2 weeks ago and who now weighs 12 kg after 3 days of vomiting and diarrhea has lost 20% of his or her body weight:

$$\frac{(15 - 12)}{15} = \frac{3}{15} = 0.2 \times 100 = 20\%$$

When an accurate recent weight is unavailable, one may substitute predicted (average) weight for age, assuming the child is of average stature and physique (Table 28-2).

Initial evaluation of the dehydrated child also should include laboratory evaluation of the serum electrolyte concentrations and measurement of the ions contained in whatever fluid is being lost. While waiting for these laboratory results, however, estimates based on the known average concentration of solutes in various body fluids can be used (Table 28-3).

The approach to definitive therapy is based on the magnitude of dehydration and the estimated solute deficit. Table 28-4 describes the expected findings at various degrees of dehydration. It is important to remember that the clinical signs relate mostly to extracellular (especially *intravascular*) volume status and may not always reflect total body fluid loss accurately.

Because in many situations loss of either water or solute may predominate, the resultant dehydration may be either hypertonic or hypotonic. In hypertonic (hypernatremic) conditions, water moves out of cells and into the extracellular spaces, thus preventing (to some extent) abnormalities of skin turgor and many of the other parameters that determine the clinical severity of dehydration. Therefore to exhibit the same signs of dehydration when plasma is hypertonic, one must have lost more total fluid than when isotonically or hypotonically dehydrated. This means that clinical assessment usually *underestimates* the magnitude of dehydration in a child who is hypernatremic. Conversely, symptoms and signs generally appear more severe in hypotonic dehydration. Therefore the table should be used to judge severity only in patients who are dehydrated isotonically, and adjustments should depend on the value of the serum sodium.

As noted previously, rehydration is accomplished in stages. Step 1 already has been mentioned: the restoration of effective circulatory volume by rapid infusion of an isotonic salt solution (normal saline or lactated Ringer solution), 20 ml/kg, if systemic blood pressure is low or if tissue perfusion is inadequate. In less severe situations one may begin with a bolus of 10 ml/kg. If this does not improve vital signs and CNS responses, it may be repeated. If it is successful, the next step is to restore ECF volume over the succeeding 24 hours. Attempts generally are made to replace 50% of the calculated deficit in the first 8 hours of this period, to restore

Table 28-2 Average Weight by Age

Age	Weight (kg)		Convenient weight to remember (kg)
	Girl	Boy	
Newborn	3.4	3.2	3
3 mo	6.0	5.9	6
6 mo	8.5	7.7	
9 mo	9.6	9.0	9
1 yr	10.8	10.0	10
2 yr	13.3	12.5	
3 yr	15.2	14.8	15
4 yr	17.3	16.9	
5 yr	19.5	19.2	20
8 yr	29.4	29.9	30
10 yr	34.9	35.5	35
15 yr	60.1	57.5	60

Table 28-3 Usual Electrolyte Composition of Abnormal Gastrointestinal Fluids

Source	Electrolytes (mEq/L)		
	Sodium	Potassium	Chloride
Stomach	20-80	5-20	100-150
Small intestine	100-140	5-15	90-130
Colon	10-90	10-80	10-110

Table 28-4 Signs and Symptoms Related to Degree of Dehydration*

Parameter	Degree of dehydration		
	Mild	Moderate	Severe
Weight loss (%)†	3-5 (2-3)	10 (7)	15 (9-12)
Skin color	Pale	Gray	Mottled
Skin turgor	May be normal	Decreased	Tenting
Mucous membranes	Slightly dry	Dry	Dry, parched, collapse of sublingual veins
Eyes	Probably normal	Decreased tears	Sunken, absence of tears, soft globes
CNS	Normal	Irritable	Lethargic
Pulse			
Quality	Strong	Somewhat decreased	Distal pulse not palpable
Rate	Probably normal	Somewhat increased (orthostatic changes)	Markedly tachycardic
Capillary refill	Normal (<2 seconds)	2-4 seconds	>4 seconds
Blood pressure	No change	Orthostatic decrease	Decreased while supine
Urine	Probably normal or slightly decreased volume	Elevated specific gravity, decreased volume	Less than 0.5 ml/kg/hr over past 12-24 hr; may be anuric

*Table is most useful for situations involving isotonic dehydration. (See text for adjustments needed for other forms of dehydration.)

†Percentage of weight loss listed applies to infants younger than 1 year of age. In older children and adults, dehydration becomes more notable with smaller losses of water (these values are listed in parentheses).

the remaining 50% over the following 16 hours, and to continue to supply fluid for maintenance and ongoing losses. A positive response is appreciated by noting return of body weight to near baseline and gradual normalization of all the other signs, symptoms, and laboratory data. Over the following days to weeks, the third step is accomplished—replacement of intracellular potassium stores and restoration of the child's nutritional status.

At this juncture it is helpful to consider a case of isotonic dehydration (the special issues of hyponatremia and hypernatremia are discussed later).

Linda is a 4-year-old girl who has no underlying health problems and who is brought to the emergency department having a 2-day history of vomiting and diarrhea. During this time she has been able to tolerate only small amounts of fluids by mouth. Her mother states that she has urinated only twice in the past 18 hours. She is irritable, but when she cries, her mother has noticed that she produces no tears. Her most recent weight, almost a year ago at her last well-child visit, was 14.5 kg. On examination she has a pulse of 140 beats/min; a systolic blood pressure of 65 mm Hg; skin that does not tent, is dry, and is pale; dry mucous membranes; and ocular globes that are not soft. Her weight is 15.8 kg. Laboratory data reveal normal sodium and potassium levels. Her blood urea nitrogen level is 36 mg/dl, and her urine specific gravity is 1.035.

This child has signs and symptoms of moderate dehydration. Although her recent weight was unknown, her weight 1 year ago was close to the average for her age; thus it may be assumed that her current weight should be close to 17 kg. This would indicate dehydration close to 7%, which correlates well with the clinical impression of moderate dehydration.

Step 1. Restoration of intravascular volume. The child is not in shock, but it still would be reasonable to administer a bolus of isotonic fluid over the first 20 to 30 minutes (10 ml/kg of ideal weight = 170 ml of normal saline solution).

Step 2. Replacement of ECF volume over the next 24 hours (to include maintenance and ongoing losses). First, the 24-hour maintenance water requirement (1 dl/100 Cal) is calculated, based on an expected caloric expenditure of:

$$(100 \text{ Cal/kg} \times 10 \text{ kg}) + (50 \text{ Cal/kg} \times 7 \text{ kg}) = 1350 \text{ Cal/day}.$$

Therefore the maintenance fluid requirement is 1350 ml/day, which is equivalent to a rate of 56 ml/hr.

Step 3. Calculation of the deficit:

$$7\% \text{ of } 17 \text{ kg} = 1.19 \text{ kg}$$

which is equivalent to 1190 ml of volume lost. However, 170 ml has already been replaced, which leaves 1020 ml of deficit to be replaced over the next 24 hours. Ideally half of the total amount should be replaced in the first 8 hours (510 ÷ 8 hr = 64 ml/hr).

Step 4. Addition of the maintenance rate (56 ml/hr) *to the deficit rate* (64 ml/hr) *and administration of the intravenous solution at this rate* (120 ml/hr) *over the next 8 hours.* Then the rate is changed so that the remainder of the solution is delivered at a rate of 88 ml/hr over the following 16 hours. Rates can be rounded to even numbers. Ongoing losses must be monitored and replaced as needed, volume for volume. The child needs glucose in her fluids because severe vomiting prohibits any oral intake initially. Therefore, although she should have a solution close in concentration to isotonic saline, a hypertonic solution is not advisable; thus her intravenous solution should be changed from normal saline to 5% dextrose in water (D_5W), containing 77 mEq/L of sodium chloride (half-normal saline solution), and it should be given at the rate determined. *Potassium should not be added until an adequate urine output is certain.* Serum electrolytes, urine output, and vital signs need to be determined at regular intervals, and the fluid therapy (content and rate of administration) should be adjusted as necessary. The volume and electrolyte content of any parenteral medications administered should be considered in these calculations (many pharmaceutical preparations, especially antibiotics, have a high concentration of either potassium or sodium).

In general two approaches to replacement therapy exist: one is to calculate the water deficit and assume isotonic losses (except in the case of extreme hypernatremia) as in the example just given; the second is to calculate specific solute needs and determine a precise formula for rehydration and repletion of electrolyte concentrations. Solute deficit is determined by calculating the total numbers of milliequivalents required and is accomplished through the use of a formula into which one must substitute values for patient weight, current electrolyte concentrations, and a plasma "distribution factor" (fraction of the body water in which the substance is distributed). However, these measurements and calculations are helpful only when dealing with predominantly extracellular electrolyte particles; they are useless in determining potassium deficiency. Table 28-5 lists normal values, distribution factors, and the desired concentration used most commonly in estimating the deficits (these usually correspond to the lower end of normal values).

The formula used to calculate solute deficit is:

$$\begin{aligned}\text{Deficit (mEq)} &= \text{Body weight (kg)} \times [\text{Desired concentration (mEq/L)} \\ &\quad - \text{Actual concentration (mEq/L)}] \times \text{Distribution factor}\end{aligned}$$

For example, the total sodium deficit in a 10 kg child who has a serum sodium concentration of 123 mEq/L is 10 kg × (12 mEq/L) × (0.6) = 72 mEq of sodium, which should be replaced similarly to water—half the deficit in the first 8 hours and the remainder in the following 16 hours.

Similar calculations can be performed for bicarbonate and chloride, and a final fluid and electrolyte prescription can be written. Only half the calculated bicarbonate deficit is replaced during the first 24 hours as a precaution against too rapid a correction, which might lead to alkalosis.

The case of dehydration presented earlier should be reconsidered and the following information added: the serum sodium concentration (125 mEq/L) and the serum bicarbonate

Table 28-5 Values Required to Calculate Solute Deficits in Children

Solute	Normal concentration range (mEq/L)	Desired corrected concentration (mEq/L)	Distribution factor
Sodium	135-145	135	0.5-0.7
Chloride	100-106	100	0.2-0.3
Bicarbonate	24-30 20-26 (neonates)	15	0.4-0.5

(12 mEq/L). With this knowledge the child's electrolyte deficits can be calculated as follows:

Sodium deficit
$$= 17 \text{ kg} \times (135 \text{ mEq/L} - 125 \text{ mEq/L}) \times 0.6 = 102 \text{ mEq}$$

However, we gave 26 mEq of sodium in our initial bolus of saline solution, leaving a residual deficit of 76 mEq.

Bicarbonate deficit
$$= 17 \text{ kg} \times (15 \text{ mEq/L} - 12 \text{ mEq/L}) \times 0.5 = 25 \text{ mEq}$$

The water deficit is unchanged from the previous calculation; therefore in the first 8 hours she needs to receive 960 ml of water—half her deficit (510 ml) plus one third daily maintenance (450 ml)—in which are dissolved 38 mEq of sodium and 12 mEq of bicarbonate (one half deficit) with additional sodium to equal one third of the maintenance requirements (approximately 3 mEq/kg/day), or 17 mEq. The formula then would call for mixing 1 L of D_5W with 43 mEq of sodium chloride and 12 mEq of sodium bicarbonate and administering this solution at the rate previously described.

Toward the end of the first 8 hours of rehydration therapy solute deficit must be recalculated based on the current values of electrolyte concentrations. It is particularly important to remember that bicarbonate deficits often are corrected much more quickly than predicted. Therefore to avoid producing an "overshoot" alkalosis when administering bicarbonate, its serum concentration must be monitored carefully.

THERAPEUTIC APPROACH TO SPECIAL SITUATIONS

Shock

Severe plasma volume deficit, with actual or impending cardiovascular collapse, is a life-threatening pediatric emergency, requiring *immediate* action; initial therapy is as above—replacing the intravascular volume depletion with *whatever appropriate solution is most available*. In most hospitals this would be either a normal saline or lactated Ringer solution; the latter formulation contains small amounts of potassium and calcium as well as base in the form of lactate. The utility of the lactate requires the liver to be able to convert it to bicarbonate. In the presence of severe lactic acidosis, which may accompany hypoxia and markedly diminished tissue perfusion, the administration of lactate may be harmful and actually worsen the metabolic acidosis. Hemorrhagic shock, which must be considered with any history of trauma or any possible internal source of bleeding (e.g., a known peptic ulcer or other gastrointestinal disease that might lead to acute blood loss), must be treated with administration of packed red blood cells. This is because administering additional electrolyte solutions to a patient who has an already diminished hematocrit further decreases oxygen-carrying capacity and may result in irreversible damage to vital organs (especially the heart and brain). Therefore most hospital blood banks keep a fairly ready supply of type O blood, which should be infused as rapidly as possible once the diagnosis of hemorrhagic shock has been considered. A sample of the patient's blood (obtained *before* transfusion) should be sent to the blood bank so that a properly matched unit of donor blood can be obtained without delay in case it is needed for further therapy. Also, if the patient's blood type is known, type-specific noncross-matched blood, which carries less risk than the use of O noncross-matched blood, may be administered. While awaiting the arrival of blood from the blood bank, normal saline or lactated Ringer solution should be given, as noted previously. The use of colloid-containing plasma expanders such as albumin or dextran remains controversial and probably provides no benefit over the use of a crystalloid solution unless the shock is on the basis of protein loss. Additionally, if the shock is cardiogenic, administration of albumin may worsen pulmonary edema. In sepsis, where volume depletion is caused by leaky capillaries and exudation of plasma into extravascular spaces, fresh-frozen plasma may be useful (because it also replaces many clotting factors) and sometimes is used in combination with other fluids.

Shock in babies and small children almost invariably is associated with depletion of glycogen stores. Thus hypoglycemia often may also be present. Administration of 2 to 4 ml/kg of a 25% dextrose solution will correct hypoglycemia and improve the results of further resuscitation efforts. For this reason rapid bedside determination of blood glucose concentration always should be part of the initial evaluation of the infant or child in shock (current or impending).

Serious Electrolyte Abnormalities

Sodium. The most commonly encountered pediatric electrolyte aberrations relate to sodium balance, and they ordinarily occur with dehydration. This section discusses the clinical conditions of hyponatremia and hypernatremia, which involve abnormalities of both the patient's volume status and plasma osmolality.

HYPONATREMIA. Hyponatremia usually is associated with hypotonicity. When it is not, the clinician must suspect either artifactual lowering of the serum sodium such as with hyperlipidemia and hyperproteinemia as described earlier or the presence of an osmotically active substance such as glucose or mannitol.[46] These compounds cause a shift of intracellular water into the extracellular space to restore osmotic neutrality, thereby lowering effective serum sodium by 1.6 mEq/L for every 100 mg/dl rise in serum glucose or mannitol concentration. Such situations almost universally are associated with preservation of intravascular volume (except in some extreme cases of diabetic ketoacidosis) and often are apparent from the history, physical examination, or a few simple laboratory tests.

The most common clinical situation leading to hyponatremia is volume loss, usually caused by diarrhea, in which the child has lost fluid with a sodium concentration higher than that of the serum. If ongoing diarrheal losses are replaced with hypotonic fluids, hyponatremia will develop, even if the volume deficit is not great. Sodium-rich fluid also is lost from the intravascular space when ascites or other abnormal accumulations of fluid occupy a body cavity. This phenomenon is known as *third spacing* and is discussed later in this chapter in the section on perioperative fluid management.

When volume status is normal one must consider situations that lead to a combination of sodium loss with water intake sufficient to maintain usual hydration. Such negative sodium balance can result from severe restriction of sodium intake or profound loss of sodium through the skin, GI tract, or kidneys (salt-losing nephropathy or diuretic use).

Mild hyponatremia (serum sodium 128 to 134 mEq/dl) with normovolemia or hypovolemia can be managed by providing isotonic sodium solutions with adequate fluid administration, thereby allowing excretion of water at an appropriate rate. It is important in these circumstances to replace ongoing losses with the correct solution (i.e., measure electrolyte concentration of the fluid lost and infuse fluid of that concentration milliliter for milliliter) so that the patient's sodium concentration returns to normal. When there are simultaneous large deficits of both water and saline solution, it is important to replace both effectively; the usual normal saline solution is sufficient at the outset.

Severe total body potassium depletion, sometimes overlooked, may lead to persistent hyponatremia. Because potassium is the major intracellular cation, sodium ions enter the cells to replace potassium ions to provide electroneutrality; therefore the concentration of sodium in the extracellular space may fall. Potassium then must be supplied to allow the restoration of normal sodium balance.

More rapid correction of the sodium deficit is necessary with serious symptoms (seizures), which may accompany a large or precipitous decline in serum sodium concentration. This can be achieved through the administration of 3% saline solution (containing 500 mEq of sodium per liter), which allows rapid replacement of sodium without infusing a large volume of water.[36]

The sodium deficit is calculated as detailed previously, but half the calculated deficit should be administered rapidly to try to resolve the seizure activity. *Once the seizures have abated, the infusion should be stopped.* If seizures continue for 10 or 15 minutes beyond the end of the initial infusion, a second serum sodium value should be obtained and the remainder of the deficit replaced (without necessarily waiting for the repeat value). It is presumed that this rapid infusion of hypertonic saline solution eases convulsions by reversing the cerebral edema that developed when, because of extracellular hyponatremia, water moved into the brain cells in an attempt to restore osmotic neutrality. Osmotic equilibrium is rapidly established once intravascular tonicity is restored, because sodium is distributed quickly throughout all body fluid compartments. Intravenous administration of hypertonic sodium chloride solutions is not without risk to the patient, however, especially one who has cardiac or renal disease. Such infusions cause a rapid shift of water into the intravascular space and may lead to acute volume overload. This therapy must therefore be reserved for potentially life-threatening situations, and the child must be monitored closely throughout the infusion. Demyelination syndromes have been noted in adults due to rapid reversal (a rise of more than 12 mEq/L in 24 hours) of long-standing or chronic hyponatremia.[4]

When hyponatremia exists with expanded vascular volume the most likely cause is excessive secretion of ADH, which may occur because of increased intracranial pressure, severe pneumonia, or the stress of certain surgical procedures. The diagnosis of SIADH is made on the basis of laboratory and physical examination data and requires the presence of hyponatremia with normal or increased intravascular volume (the diagnosis *cannot* be made if the patient has an inadequate intravascular volume) and a urine osmolality that is less than maximally dilute. Sodium excretion in the urine is variable but usually is higher than expected for the level of serum sodium concentration. Treatment of this disorder, whatever the cause, consists of *fluid restriction* and not sodium administration unless the patient is convulsing. Some authors have urged the simultaneous use of a potent diuretic such as furosemide, which is expected to induce the loss of more water than sodium.[33] In most cases, however, fluid restriction remains the safest and most efficacious mode of therapy. Once the sodium concentration returns to near normal, moderate fluid restriction (generally to two thirds of maintenance requirements) may need to be continued, usually for at least 24 hours, but sometimes for as long as the underlying disorder continues.

HYPERNATREMIA. As with decreased serum sodium concentration, hypernatremia may occur with overhydration, dehydration, or normal hydration. However, unlike hyponatremia, an elevated serum sodium level *always* is associated with hypertonicity.

Hypernatremia associated with overhydration generally is an iatrogenic problem created by (1) administering intravenous or oral solutions with high salt content and (2) not providing the requisite free water. Patients treated with large amounts of sodium bicarbonate for metabolic acidosis also are at risk of developing marked hypernatremia (there is approximately 1 mEq of sodium for every milliliter of bicarbonate solution administered). Occasionally, when infant formulas are being mixed, mistakes occur that result in markedly hypertonic solutions that may induce particularly severe hypernatremias. These patients are at risk of developing obvious signs of plasma volume overload, including hypertension, congestive heart failure, and pulmonary edema.

Under such circumstances administration of additional fluid is risky and may prove fatal. The most rational approach is to limit sodium and water input and attempt to induce sodium loss to a greater extent than water. This may be accomplished by the use of a potent loop diuretic such as furosemide, which will induce a net sodium loss if the child's renal function is adequate. One concurrently must watch closely for the development of dehydration because it is impossible to predict precisely how much water and sodium will be lost. Generally some portion of the induced urine output (50% to 75%) should be replaced with intravenous fluid that is slightly hypotonic (i.e., 66% or 75% normal saline solution) until normal hydration and tonicity have been achieved. In patients who have *severe* hypernatremia (ordinarily considered as a serum sodium value over 155 or 160 mEq/L), serious complications may occur if the sodium concentration falls too rapidly. This action produces marked shifts of extracellular water to the intracellular space and results in cellular swelling. This is most worrisome in the CNS because cerebral edema may occur, which may lead to seizures, coma, or death. Therefore when the serum sodium value is high and is accompanied by overhydration, the preferred therapeutic approach is to restrict sodium and water, thus permitting a spontaneous diuresis to occur. Serum electrolyte values must be monitored every few hours. If the patient has substantially decreased renal function, hemodialysis or peritoneal dialysis should be considered, especially in the presence of hypertension or pulmonary edema.

Hypernatremia associated with decreased plasma volume is encountered frequently in pediatric practice. It most commonly is caused by acute gastroenteritis that induces relatively larger losses of water than sodium. Although these children may have severe hypernatremia, their total body sodium content usually is depleted; they therefore present quite a therapeutic challenge.

Patients who have this condition need to be evaluated carefully. The physician must consider all the aspects of dehydration previously discussed but must remember that because ECF volume is relatively well preserved, he or she may seriously underestimate the severity of the plasma volume loss. Even with *significant* fluid losses these children rarely have signs of incipient vascular collapse. When using the signs and symptoms of dehydration shown in Table 28-4 to determine the degree of dehydration, if the serum sodium concentration is over 155 mEq/L, another 3% to 5% should be added to the predicted degree of dehydration.

Fluid therapy of hypernatremia dehydration is not nearly as straightforward as for other types of dehydration because the risk of creating major fluid shifts and cerebral edema is great. One cannot simply try to remove sodium because a decrease in the plasma tonicity without an increase in plasma water may induce circulatory collapse. Therefore a cautious rehydration scheme must be developed.

Instead of being rehydrated over a 24-hour period, as with isonatremic or hyponatremic dehydration, the child who has a serum sodium over 155 mEq/L should have his or her fluid deficit replaced over 48 to 72 hours. It is *not* possible to calculate the actual amount of sodium lost. The physician should estimate the water deficit (based on weight and clinical signs) and plan to replace that volume evenly over 48 to 72 hours. The solution used should be *slightly hyponatremic* (containing 100 to 120 mEq of sodium per liter). Glucose should be added so that the solution is not hypotonic. As soon as the urine output is judged to be adequate, potassium should be added to the intravenous solution to correct the potassium deficit and to preserve the intracellular osmolality, thus helping to prevent intracellular edema. It is particularly important to monitor serum electrolyte concentrations, serum osmolality, and urine output and osmolality as frequently as possible. Although one needs to avoid a persistent elevation of the serum sodium concentration, it also is important to ensure a slow, steady decline in the serum sodium and osmolality levels.[18] Decreases in serum tonicity should be limited to a rate of 5 mOsm/hr. Serum sodium concentration should fall at a rate no more rapid than 0.5 mEq/L/hour. In many cases it is possible to add up to 40 mEq of potassium per liter to the infused solution and thereby reduce its sodium concentration to 50 mEq/L.

Sometimes, no matter how carefully hypernatremia is handled, seizures ensue during the rehydration period. They usually can be managed successfully by infusing a solution slightly more hypertonic than the one being given (i.e., normal saline or lactated Ringer solution). If the seizures are particularly severe, or if there is evidence of brain herniation, the use of a hypertonic agent such as mannitol may be required. Unfortunately the diuresis induced by mannitol may worsen the dehydration substantially. Also, mannitol should *not* be used if urine output has not been established.

A relatively uncommon cause of hypernatremia is diabetes insipidus, which usually is evident as hypernatremia with a normal plasma volume. This presupposes an intact thirst mechanism and that the patient has access to the large volume of water required to replace renal losses. Such is not the case for small babies and certain other patients who have diabetes insipidus and hypernatremic dehydration. Large renal losses of free water may occur because of deficient ADH (central or pituitary diabetes insipidus) or impairment of the normal renal response to the hormone (nephrogenic diabetes insipidus).

In infants and children the most common cause of central diabetes insipidus is a brain tumor, such as a craniopharyngioma. The syndrome also may follow intracranial surgical procedures or trauma. Other causes include CNS diseases of vascular, infectious, or granulomatous origin or histiocytosis. The familial form of central diabetes insipidus accounts for fewer than 1% of all cases. Probably 50% of adult patients who have diabetes insipidus remain classified as *idiopathic;* that percentage is much lower in children.

Nephrogenic diabetes insipidus may be evident as a congenital disorder, but more commonly it is secondary to renal failure (particularly that caused by obstructive uropathy) or to electrolyte disorders, drug ingestions, or sickle cell disease. Laboratory findings in diabetes insipidus usually include a moderate to marked hypernatremia (depending on how adequately the lost fluid volume has been replaced) and dilute urine, usually produced in large volumes. Clinically these patients exhibit a tremendous thirst (often craving ice-cold water) and, as already mentioned, usually show signs of normal hydration. The laboratory differentiation between central and nephrogenic diabetes insipidus is unnecessary when the cause is apparent (e.g., after surgical removal of a craniopharyngioma) but in other situations is essential to help guide the therapeutic approach. This generally is determined by performing a "water deprivation test." Water is withheld from the patient until approximately 3% of the body weight has been lost, until three consecutive hourly urine samples show no further increase in osmolality, or until the serum osmolality reaches 295 mOsm. Although in the adult patient the desired effects may take 10 to 12 hours to become manifest, a child who has complete central diabetes insipidus may become notably dehydrated in just a few hours. Therefore throughout the period of water deprivation the child must be watched carefully via (1) frequent monitoring of vital signs, (2) hourly monitoring of urine volume and osmolality, and (3) measurement of serum electrolyte concentrations and osmolality every 1 to 2 hours.

When the end point is reached, a normal person exhibits maximum urinary concentration with a marked fall of urinary output but little change in the serum sodium concentration. A patient who has either total central diabetes insipidus or nephrogenic diabetes insipidus exhibits little change in urinary concentration or flow but develops an elevated serum sodium concentration and a high serum osmolality. A slight increase in urine concentrating ability that stabilizes at a fairly low level (but substantially higher than when the patient is well hydrated) indicates probable incomplete central diabetes insipidus. If further resolution of the problem is necessary, subcutaneous injection of aqueous vasopressin (5 units in adults) is performed, and the urine output and concentration are followed hourly. No further change is seen in normal individuals who previously had concentrated their urine maximally (i.e., already had high circulating levels of

ADH). Also, patients who have nephrogenic diabetes insipidus show no decrease in urine volume or elevation of urine osmolality following the vasopressin injection because the defect lies in the kidneys' inability to respond to ADH. Patients who have complete or partial central diabetes insipidus respond with a dramatic rise in their renal concentrating function. It cannot be stressed enough that *although the water deprivation test is useful, it also is dangerous and requires the utmost care, with close observation of the patient and knowledge of resuscitation maneuvers. The advice and supervision of a pediatric endocrinologist should be sought.*

Treatment of diabetes insipidus requires an accurate diagnosis and the ability to monitor the patient carefully. Postoperative central diabetes insipidus may be transient and therefore can be treated by replacing urinary losses of water and sodium. If the volume needed exceeds the physician's ability to replace it (mostly an intravenous access problem), if the condition continues for more than several days, or if the patient had signs of diabetes insipidus preoperatively, the most rational approach is hormonal replacement. In the past this was accomplished by using intramuscular vasopressin tannate in oil (a difficult product to deal with and one that has a half-life that cannot be predicted reliably) or subcutaneous aqueous vasopressin (Pitressin), but this has a short half-life and needs to be repeated every 2 to 3 hours. The most recent development in ADH replacement therapy has been the production of a synthetic analog of vasopressin, 1-desamino-8-D-argininevasopressin (DDAVP), that can be administered intranasally or intravenously. It has a long half-life and reaches peak activity within the first 30 minutes. The dose and schedule are adapted to the patient's response. The recommended starting dose is 0.3 μg/kg intravenously or 0.05 to 0.3 ml (5 to 30 μg) intranasally administered once or twice daily. The intranasal preparation can be used as easily in the hospital as in the home and is relatively free of side effects. It is effective for both partial and complete central diabetes insipidus.

Nephrogenic diabetes insipidus is more difficult to treat and generally requires chronic provision of adequate fluid volume, unless the underlying abnormality can be corrected. This usually is not a problem as long as the patient has an intact thirst mechanism and fluid is readily available. Some success has been achieved with diuretic therapy in association with low sodium intake to prevent hypernatremia. Also, prostaglandins may be useful in reducing the urine volume.

Potassium

HYPOKALEMIA. Symptoms of hypokalemia were discussed in the sections on solute homeostasis. A low serum potassium concentration seldom represents an emergency unless cardiac effects are seen, and this does not occur typically until the concentration is less than 2 mEq/L. In patients receiving digitalis preparations, however, a combined cardiac toxicity may ensue, and the typical T wave changes and arrhythmias of hypokalemia may occur at serum potassium levels closer to normal. Other patients at risk of exhibiting an exaggerated response to mild hypokalemia include those who have an acid-base disturbance or other ionic aberration that may create a cardiac conduction disturbance by substantially altering the flux of ions between the intracellular and extracellular spaces. At particular risk of developing such alterations are children receiving long-term diuretic therapy. Hypokalemia may occur following large losses of potassium from the GI tract during treatment for diabetic ketoacidosis and as a manifestation of hyperaldosteronism.

When emergency therapy for hypokalemia is necessary (in the situations just mentioned and in the preoperative patient who has a serum potassium concentration less than 3.5 mEq/L), intravenous potassium repletion should be implemented. This is accomplished either by increasing the concentration of potassium ion in the fluids given intravenously (maximum of 80 mEq/L) or by administering a bolus of potassium into a central vein. The maximum amount of potassium that may be given is 1 mEq/kg over a 1-hour period (with the physician at the bedside and continuous electrocardiographic monitoring), but it generally is safer to deliver only 20% or 25% of that amount and to repeat the dose as necessary to raise the concentration to a safe level. In nonemergent circumstances enteral potassium supplementation is safer and very effective.

HYPERKALEMIA. Substantial elevations of serum potassium concentration most frequently are encountered with renal failure or systemic acidosis, combined with an increased intake of potassium or a rapid breakdown of tissue or blood products.

When the potassium concentration reaches 8 mEq/L or more, or if characteristic electrocardiographic abnormalities are noted at any potassium concentration, the child is in grave danger of cardiac toxicity. Such a patient should have continuous electrocardiographic monitoring, and immediate steps should be taken to *protect the heart from the effects of severe hyperkalemia.* The first priority is the infusion of intravenous calcium, 0.2 ml/kg of 10% calcium chloride given over 2 to 5 minutes.[3] This should be followed by the administration of sodium bicarbonate (2 to 3 mEq/kg given within a 30-minute period) to raise the serum pH level and help move the potassium into cells, thereby decreasing (transiently) the intravascular potassium concentration. Simultaneously or immediately following the above steps, a mixture of glucose and insulin should be infused, which also induces movement of potassium ions from the extracellular to the intracellular spaces. This accelerates the usual process by which glucose moves into the cells and is converted to glycogen. A dose of 2 ml/kg of a 25% glucose solution is given along with 1 U/kg of regular insulin. This solution may be administered over 30 minutes and repeated as necessary. Serum glucose concentration must be monitored closely during and following therapy.

Salbutamol, a selective beta$_2$ agonist, has been used successfully to reduce temporarily serum potassium levels in neonates[8,15] and children.[22] It may be administered intravenously or by nebulization. The parenteral form is not yet available commercially in the United States.

Once lifesaving measures have been instituted, attention must be given to removing potassium from the body. One of the most effective means of accomplishing this is with hemodialysis or peritoneal dialysis. One or the other should be initiated without delay in patients who have hyperkalemia accompanied by congestive heart failure and volume overload. The other commonly used mechanism for removing potassium from the body is to bind potassium in the GI tract by using an exchange resin such as sodium polystyrene sulfonate (Kayexalate).[24,27] This usually is introduced through a retention enema that contains sorbitol. One can expect a decline in serum potassium of 1 mEq/L for each g/kg of resin introduced. The dose is calculated on the basis of the severity of the hyperkalemia, with a maximal adult dose of 60 g. Caution should be used in patients who have renal failure, because sodium is absorbed as potassium is excreted, and each gram of resin contains 4.1 mEq of sodium; hypernatremia and hypervolemia may result. Additionally one must monitor the patient for the development of hypocalcemia and hypomagnesemia. Metabolic alkalosis may result from repeated polystyrene sulfonate enemas. When hyperkalemia becomes a chronic but not life-threatening problem, the best approach is to restrict dietary potassium and administer potassium-losing diuretics concomitantly.

Calcium

HYPERCALCEMIA. A serum calcium concentration over 15 mg/dl constitutes a medical emergency but rarely is seen in pediatric patients. Signs and symptoms of acute hypercalcemia intoxication were reviewed earlier in this chapter. Therapy should be aimed at bringing the total calcium concentration below 12 mg/dl. If urine output is adequate, one should rapidly administer intravenous normal saline solution at a rate of 20 to 30 ml/kg over several hours. This may be combined with the use of furosemide, which increases calcium excretion through the kidneys. In addition it is essential to eliminate as much calcium from the diet as is feasible and to restrict the gastrointestinal absorption of calcium by administering a corticosteroid preparation. Patients unresponsive to these procedures may benefit from oral phosphate supplementation or rectal administration of a Fleet enema that contains phosphorus. In children who have substantially impaired renal function, hemodialysis may be necessary.

HYPOCALCEMIA. When hypocalcemia is symptomatic it requires immediate treatment with the intravenous administration of a calcium salt. The most commonly used preparations are calcium chloride and calcium gluconate. The solution chosen should be given in a dose of 0.5 to 1 mEq/kg or 10 to 20 mg of elemental calcium per kilogram. Whenever calcium is provided intravenously, the cardiac rate and rhythm must be monitored continuously because notable bradycardia may occur with an abrupt rise of the ionized fraction of calcium.

Sick neonates may benefit from the continuous administration of intravenous calcium to prevent substantial declines in the calcium concentration. This should be provided at a rate of 2 to 4 mEq/kg/day. The intravenous access site must be checked frequently because extravasated calcium causes striking necrosis of the subcutaneous tissues.

THERAPY OF CLINICAL ACID-BASE DISORDERS

Metabolic Acidosis

Previous sections have touched on the approach to the life-threatening problem of metabolic acidosis, but its importance demands reconsideration. As already described, a pH level lower than 7.2 requires immediate evaluation and probable therapy.[32] This task traditionally has been accomplished by calculating a bicarbonate deficit as:

Weight in kilograms
× (Desired concentration − Actual concentration)
× Volume of distribution

where the *desired concentration* is 15 mEq/L and the *volume of distribution* is between 0.4 and 0.6 (0.5 is used mostly for younger children, 0.4 for those over 1 year of age).[16] As noted in the section on dehydration only half the calculated deficit is administered; the acid-base status is reevaluated several hours later because in the absence of persistent acid production, the deficit usually is overestimated if this formula is used.

The most important element to remember in bicarbonate replacement is that *it is essential to follow serial electrolyte values and adjust the therapy accordingly.* The complications of bicarbonate therapy include hypokalemia (with a lessening of acid environment, potassium is shifted back into the cells), hyponatremia, volume overload, and, occasionally, tetany (caused by improved binding of calcium to protein, with a subsequent decline of the ionized fraction of calcium).[32] As mentioned previously administration of sodium bicarbonate may result in CNS acidosis and cerebral edema caused by the diffusion of CO_2 into the CSF.[49] Although it may not always be possible to prevent such iatrogenic developments, the clinician must remain aware that even well-intentioned therapy may cause undesirable results. Therefore, whenever therapy is undertaken, the patient must be adequately monitored in an area where emergency measures can be taken if indicated.

On some occasions bicarbonate administration is relatively contraindicated. Patients suffering from congestive heart failure may not be able to tolerate the rapid expansion of intravascular volume that accompanies the administration of sodium bicarbonate. Bicarbonate infusion in children who have ventilatory insufficiency will cause a decline in the level of blood pH. Neonates may be adversely affected by the elevation of plasma osmolality. Such patients may benefit from an organic amine buffer, tris(hydroxymethyl)aminomethane (THAM), also known as TRIS or tromethamine. It induces a rapid decline of Pco_2 by metabolizing carbonic acid to bicarbonate.

THAM is available as a 3.6% solution with a pH level of 10. The total dose in milliliters to be administered is the base deficit multiplied by the weight in kilograms. This dose should be spread over 1 or more hours, with 25% administered in the initial few minutes and the remainder given slowly with ongoing monitoring of serum pH levels and electrolyte concentrations. Important and possibly fatal complications associated with the use of THAM include hypoglycemia, induction of a marked diuresis, and apnea from a sudden decline of Pco_2. Therefore these parameters must be monitored frequently throughout the period of therapy. It is recommended that THAM be used only in situations where administration of sodium bicarbonate clearly is contraindicated.

Carbicarb, a preparation containing an equimolar mixture of sodium bicarbonate and sodium carbonate, which does not generate CO_2, was developed in the hopes of avoiding some of the adverse effects seen when using sodium bicarbonate alone.[11,12] It has not been proven to affect the outcome of cardiac arrest in adults, nor has it been evaluated in children.[49] Its use in critically ill children cannot be recommended at this time.

Respiratory Acidosis

When respiratory acidosis is severe (pH level less than 7 and/or Pco_2 greater than 55), the best mode of therapy is intubation and hyperventilation, unless the patient suffers from chronic respiratory failure, in which the effects of an elevated P_{CO_2} are well compensated for by an increased serum bicarbonate level, resulting in a normal or nearly normal pH. The use of bicarbonate should be avoided until adequate excretion of the generated carbon dioxide is ensured. Formulas and mechanisms to determine appropriate ventilator settings are beyond the scope of this text. When treating acidosis with assisted ventilation, it is essential to observe the patient's preintubation rate and depth of breathing. The use of standard rates and tidal volumes may be insufficient and may seriously compromise the patient. Once an artificial airway and assisted ventilation are established, arterial blood gases must be determined within 15 minutes.

Because respirator-provided air is humidified, the patient's water maintenance requirements need adjustment. As described earlier the typical hospitalized child loses up to 15 ml/100 Cal/day through the respiratory tract. Because specific amounts of water delivered by the ventilator vary in different systems and mucosal absorption varies according to the nature of the child's illness, it is impossible to predict accurately the magnitude of the reduction in water maintenance required. Therefore it is reasonable to reduce fluid administration by approximately 10%, assuming *all other variables remain the same,* but to follow the patient's weight and serum electrolyte levels closely. In rare cases, in very small babies and in persons who have severe inflammatory disease of the airways, there actually may be a *net gain* of water through respiratory tract absorption, which may lead to water intoxication and hyponatremia.

Metabolic and Respiratory Alkalosis

As already mentioned metabolic and respiratory alkaloses generally do not require specific therapy but respond to treatment of the underlying abnormalities. Most important in the clinical approach to alkalosis is the recognition of concomitant electrolyte aberrations such as hypokalemia, hypocalcemia, and hypochloremia.

CLINICAL FLUID PROBLEMS INVOLVING GLUCOSE METABOLISM

The serum glucose should be measured in all seriously ill children, especially youngsters less than 1 year of age, who are particularly prone to hypoglycemia. Because this topic is covered in detail in Chapter 285, specific issues of diagnosis and therapy are not considered here. To be successful in fluid management, baseline caloric needs (to prevent ketosis) must be provided. The requirements of a patient who needs long periods of maintenance fluid therapy are discussed later in this chapter in the section on parenteral nutrition.

Recent medical literature has raised concerns relating to provision of glucose-containing fluids in patients suffering from *or at risk for* cerebral hypoxia/ischemia.[10,13] Glucose theoretically worsens CNS injury secondary to hypoxia/ischemia caused by augmented accumulation of lactate, which may exacerbate cerebral edema and cell damage.

It has become common clinical practice to withhold glucose-containing fluids from certain groups of patients—most notably, patients undergoing open heart surgery[9] and patients who have suffered a neurological catastrophe and/or are undergoing a neurosurgical procedure. Clinical data in human infants and children to support such practices are sparse; therefore these children must be monitored carefully. The clinical goal should be to keep the serum glucose level in the normal range, regardless of the amount of glucose that must be provided in the parenteral fluids to achieve the goal.

Diabetic ketoacidosis, with notable hyperglycemia, is associated with a myriad of other fluid and solute abnormalities. The diagnosis must always be considered with a child who is in a coma of undetermined cause. The approach to this complicated problem also is presented in Chapter 275.

PERIOPERATIVE FLUID MANAGEMENT AND THE CONCEPT OF THIRD SPACING

The outcome of a surgical procedure depends on intraoperative events and the nature of the child's illness. Also of major importance is the preoperative status of the patient. Recognized only within the last half century is the concept that the presence of hypovolemia or hypervolemia in the preoperative patient may affect outcome adversely.

Most healthy children have intravascular volume and electrolyte concentrations at the proper levels. However, the preoperative assessment always should include an estimation of hydration status on physical examination and by measurement of urine specific gravity. It is imperative to obtain an accurate preoperative weight for calculating maintenance fluid requirements and drug dosages and for helping to assess postoperative changes in fluid balance. Any child who has had vomiting, diarrhea, or a substantial limitation of oral intake in the 72-hour period preceding surgery will benefit from the measurement of serum electrolyte concentrations. Young babies (especially neonates) may benefit from preoperative measurement of their glucose and calcium concentrations. If a substantially abnormal balance of water or solute is discovered, the operative procedure should be delayed until the identified problem has been corrected. Preoperative hypovolemia induced by a prolonged period of restricted fluid intake may cause a small child to exhibit notable difficulties following surgery. The neonate or young infant who must remain without oral intake for longer than 4 to 6 hours should have an intravenous line placed and maintenance fluids administered.

A more complicated situation exists when an ill child requires immediate surgery. In such cases initial steps should be taken to restore normal fluid status before inducing anesthesia. Fluid balance restoration should continue during the intraoperative and postoperative periods. Optimum care depends on frequent and detailed communication among pediatrician, surgeon, and anesthesiologist.

In some cases fluid losses are relatively easy to estimate (e.g., gastric outlet obstruction with subsequent vomiting). However, in any situation in which third spacing is likely to occur, losses from the intravascular space may be grossly underestimated. *Third spacing* is the term given to any situation in which there is movement of intravascular fluid into any of the potential or real spaces of the body. It may occur in all conditions associated with tissue injury that result in the formation of edema, a collection of extracellular, extravascular fluid having the electrolyte composition of plasma. Third space losses may be particularly marked in patients suffering from peritonitis, bowel obstruction, tissue ischemia or necrosis, perforation of an intraabdominal viscus, major crush injuries of the extremities, or ascites. Some degree of third spacing accompanies even simple uncomplicated surgical procedures. Generally, movement of fluid into tissues is preceded by movement of plasma proteins, blood, or pus. Fluid is thus retained in the extravascular space because of the elevation of tissue oncotic pressure. As healing occurs, extravascular oncotic pressure diminishes, capillary integrity is restored, and fluid returns to the intravascular space. This generally occurs between 48 and 72 hours after the injury.

The initial evaluation of a child at risk of developing notable third space losses must include consideration of the specific disease entity involved and the duration of the problem before fluid therapy is initiated. If the child is adequately hydrated when first seen, fluids can be administered at a rate of one and one-half to two times the maintenance requirement. If the underlying process has been ongoing for several hours or more, the patient almost certainly will be volume depleted and may require large amounts of a physiological electrolyte solution (normal saline or lactated Ringer solution). Occasionally such children also require administration of albumin or plasma to restore intravascular oncotic pressure.

Preoperative assessment in particularly severe cases may require the use of invasive monitoring techniques. Central venous pressures may help to determine the adequacy of preload while enabling large volumes of fluid to be administered rapidly when necessary. An indwelling arterial line permits continuous monitoring of the blood pressure while permitting easy access for frequent arterial blood gas determination. A balloon-tipped, flow-directed pulmonary artery (Swan-Ganz) catheter permits evaluation of the patient's cardiac output and calculation of oxygen consumption, which may be helpful in the child who is in significant shock. The use of any of these monitoring modalities generally requires placement of the patient in an intensive care unit.

Intraoperative control of the child's fluid volume status generally is the responsibility of the anesthesiologist, who also must ensure adequate ventilation, oxygenation, temperature control, analgesia, immobility, and muscle relaxation in the patient. Decisions regarding fluid needs made during surgery depend on many complex variables, the discussion of which is beyond the scope of this chapter. Paramount are the adjustments required to maintain vital signs and urine output within the normal range.

Postoperatively, communication between the surgeon and the pediatrician becomes essential because postoperative fluid management depends on both the events that transpired in the operating room and an estimation of expected ongoing losses. Those depend to a great degree on the nature of the surgery and the intraoperative findings. Prediction of third space losses is based primarily on experience and on knowledge of the anatomy and physiology of the tissues involved.

Where possible, external losses should be measured accurately and replaced with suitable solutions. The frequency with which such measurements are made depends on the child's size, general health, and volume of fluid lost.

In the immediate postoperative period, the goal is to stabilize the vital signs and avoid or correct any major fluid, electrolyte, or acid-base derangement. General monitoring in this situation relies on the principles previously discussed. In evaluating the child's general condition, there is no substitute for a thorough physical examination. Careful monitoring of laboratory data (serum electrolytes, blood gases, blood glucose, and hematocrit) is also essential. This needs to be coupled with close attention to the patient's vital signs, mental status, peripheral perfusion, urine output, and weight. Placement of a central venous or a Swan-Ganz catheter may be necessary for children who have substantial cardiac, renal, or respiratory dysfunction.

The child who has had a relatively straightforward surgical procedure that has not been accompanied by ongoing tissue damage caused by a persistent infection or leakage of intraabdominal contents may be expected to begin diuresis on the third postoperative day. Third spacing generally stops by that time, and the extravasated fluid returns to the intravascular space. To prevent fluid overload and its cardiorespiratory and renal effects, the pediatrician must watch for the onset of such diuresis and alter fluid therapy accordingly. If the anticipated rise of urine output does not occur at this time, one must suspect a perioperative complication. The appropriate studies to exclude infection and hyponatremia should be performed in consultation with the surgical team.

Pain, anxiety, and the stress of surgery can lead to an accelerated secretion of ADH. Before considering the diagnosis of postoperative SIADH, however, it is essential to correct any underlying hypovolemia. Some authors assert that the additional secretion of ADH is appropriate with the intravascular volume depletion associated with third spacing, as already discussed. If the syndrome does occur in the postoperative period, its duration usually is short, and fluid restriction often is not required. Its presence, however, may make using urine output to help judge volume status unreliable.

Surgery places a person in negative nitrogen balance. If the operation is simple and if oral intake can be resumed within several days, simple electrolyte solutions may be used for parenteral hydration. After several days, however, it becomes imperative to establish a positive nitrogen balance to aid wound healing and the return of normal function. Provision of adequate calories, protein, vitamins, and essential fats is more important in children than in adults because of a child's need for continued growth and development. These goals can be achieved through the use of parenteral nutrition when oral intake is not possible. A later section deals with the indications for and the composition and administration of such fluids. A significant infection in the postoperative period adds to the patient's metabolic requirements and must be considered in the physician's treatment plan if healing is to continue and metabolic acidosis is to be prevented.

CLINICAL APPROACH TO FLUID MANAGEMENT OF BURNS

Despite recent advances in legislation and education aimed at fire prevention, burn injuries to children remain a serious problem in our society. Estimates of numbers of affected children vary widely, but as many as 150,000 youngsters are moderately to severely burned each year. Of the close to 8000 deaths per year in the United States attributed to burns or smoke inhalation, nearly 30% occur in children younger than 15 years of age.

The skin, as the body's largest organ, serves a variety of physiological functions. Most important, it serves as a barrier that prevents large losses of body fluids and prohibits invasion by microorganisms. Its sweat glands are important in temperature regulation, and it is the organ of sensation and of vitamin D metabolism. The epidermis is a thin outer layer of dead cornified cells that serves as a tough and protective shell; the dermis, or corneum, is the thicker area that lies beneath the epidermis and contains all the cutaneous nerves, blood vessels, hair follicles, and sweat glands. The dermis may be only half as thick in children as in adults.

The physiological effects of a burn depend on the depth to which tissue has been destroyed (i.e., just epidermis or all or part of the dermis) and the area of the body that is burned. Although burns traditionally have been classified as first, second, and third degree, this distinction is not always apparent on initial evaluation. It is probably more reasonable from a functional standpoint to classify a burn as being of partial thickness (which, although it may be severe, heals with time) or full thickness (which usually requires grafting).

Simple first-degree burns involve only the epidermis and are characterized by pain and redness that last up to 72 hours, followed in 5 to 10 days by peeling of the involved area. Superficial second-degree burns involve all the epidermis and variable parts of the dermis. They are characterized by pain, erythema, and blisters that enlarge for several hours after exposure. These burns also, in the absence of infection, usually heal without scarring. A deep second-degree burn injury extends far into the dermis. The injured skin looks tough and usually is red but blanches with pressure. Although there is no permanent anesthesia, the sensation of pain may be lost for the first 48 hours. Healing is slow and occurs by the epithelium of the sweat glands and hair follicles regenerating. Generally the patient is left with deep scars. These burns can become full-thickness burns if infection occurs. Third-degree burns are full-thickness burns, with complete necrosis of the skin and all of its elements. The color usually is brown, tan, black, or white. Occasionally the burned skin looks red, but it does not blanch with pressure.

The size of a burn generally is described in terms of percentage of body surface area (BSA) affected. The rule of nines, sometimes employed in adults, is not helpful in small children, in which the most useful determination is made with the use of a burn chart. If such a chart is not available, one can assume that the skin overlying the patient's closed fist represents 1% of his or her BSA, as does the skin of the perineum. Table 28-6 presents the percentage of BSA of various body parts as a function of age.

Generally the first question to be considered in evaluating the burned child is whether hospitalization is required and, if so, whether admission to a specialized burn center or to a community hospital is more appropriate. Outpatient management of a child may be considered if (1) superficial, second-degree burns involving no more than 10% of the BSA or (2) third-degree burns of less than 2%, but not involving the hands or face, are present. Second-degree burns involving 10% to 20% of the BSA may be managed in a community hospital if parenteral fluid and electrolyte support can be provided. Most full-thickness burns and all partial-thickness burns greater than 30% of the BSA, as well as any substantial burns of the face, perineum, hands, or feet, are best referred to a specialized burn center. Additionally any child who has evidence of inhalation injury complicating the burn (respiratory distress, wheezing, stridor, sooty oral or nasal secretions, deteriorating blood gas values, or any abnormality seen on a chest roentgenogram) needs specialized care, as does any youngster who has a notable underlying medical problem. Significant burns in a child who is younger than 2 years of age and most electrical and chemical burns require admission to an intensive care unit. Any situation in which the physician suspects child abuse or neglect is an indication for hospitalization.

Table 28-6 Percentage of Body Surface Area (BSA) in Relation to Age

Body part	Percent BSA by age				
	Infant	1-4 Years	5-9 Years	10-14 Years	Adult
Parts that change with age					
Head	19	17	13	11	7
Each thigh	5.5	6.5	8	8.5	9.5
Each leg	5	5	5.5	6	7
Parts that do not change with age					
Neck	2				
Anterior trunk	13				
Posterior trunk	13				
Buttocks	5				
Genitalia	1				
Both arms	14				
Both hands	5				
Both feet	7				

Outpatient therapy of minor burns requires observation of the wound at least every other day to ensure that adequate healing occurs and that infection is avoided. A 1% silver sulfadiazine cream is applied to the burned area, which is wrapped with a gauze dressing (susceptible patients should be screened for glucose-6-phosphate dehydrogenase deficiency). Fresh cream should be applied every 24 to 48 hours until adequate healing has taken place.

Optimum initial fluid therapy for critical burns is essential in reducing mortality and must be begun immediately, even when there are plans to transfer the patient to a tertiary care facility. Large amounts of fluid may be required in the first several days after the thermal injury. Markedly increased capillary permeability occurs in the layers of tissue immediately beneath the burned skin, with concomitant losses of water and protein. Although normal intact skin loses up to 15 ml/hr/m^2, the patient who has a partial- or full-thickness burn may lose up to 300 ml/hr/m^2 of burned skin. These losses are accompanied by elevated oxygen and calorie consumption with profound loss of heat. There also are chemical mediators at work in the damaged areas that increase capillary permeability further—not only in the affected places but also systemically. In general, fluid losses are at their maximum immediately after the injury, and by 24 to 48 hours after the burn has occurred, capillary permeability approaches normal, and the extravasated fluid begins to resorb.

General resuscitative efforts should commence as soon as possible. As with any other acute injury, the first step is to evaluate the adequacy of the child's airway and assess the possibility of an accompanying inhalation injury. This possibility is suspected in cases of a fire within an enclosed space, of thermal injuries on the upper torso or face, and when the physical findings previously listed are present. If smoke inhalation is suspected, humidified oxygen should be administered by mask, and blood gases and a carboxyhemoglobin level should be measured (to evaluate the possibility of carbon monoxide poisoning). A child who is dyspneic or critically ill should be intubated as soon as possible; increasing airway edema makes the procedure more difficult later. As soon as the airway is ensured, the circulatory status of the patient should be assessed and the depth and severity of the burn evaluated. In a severe or large burn, at least two large-bore intravenous lines should be established and a Foley catheter inserted.

Over the years multiple regimens have been developed to guide fluid and electrolyte replacement, but the most important aspect of fluid therapy in the management of burn injuries is *monitoring* the patient's vital signs and other important physiological parameters.

As a helpful starting point, however, the most favored regimen uses the Parkland formula. This requires the administration of 4 ml of fluid per kilogram per percentage of BSA burned during the first 24 hours, giving 50% of the total in the first 8 hours. Some centers prefer to administer the initial resuscitation fluids more rapidly and therefore provide the first half of the first day's requirement in the initial 2 to 4 hours of care.[29] A balanced salt solution such as lactated Ringer solution should be used. *Glucose should not be given.* Severe burns induce a marked outpouring of catecholamines and steroids, which raises the serum glucose concentration and renders the child relatively resistant to insulin. Exogenously administered glucose concentrates in the burned area, increasing the likelihood of infection. The need for glucose is best determined by measuring the blood glucose frequently, especially in young children.

Although the initial rate of intravenous fluid administration is guided by the Parkland formula, one should ensure that sufficient fluid is given to maintain a urine output of 0.5 to 2.0 ml/kg/hr. In this situation, more is not better, because too much fluid worsens peripheral edema, delays healing, and may lead to heart failure when the extravasated liquid begins to resorb.[26] The best indicator of optimum fluid therapy is a normal cardiac output. However, a pulmonary artery catheter must be placed to measure cardiac output accurately. Blood pressure, heart rate, and weight measurement may be helpful in estimating cardiac output indirectly, but each of these can be affected by a number of other factors. Maintenance requirements should be added to the daily fluids suggested by the Parkland formula in children who have burns of less than 30% BSA and in all infants.

Colloid (such as plasma or 5% albumin) generally is withheld until 24 hours after the burn has occurred, although some authors advise the use of colloid in the initial resuscitation phases.[6,14] Because children show some evidence of earlier healing of the capillary bed, colloid may be useful at 12 to 18 hours. The usual dose is 0.5 ml/kg/% of burned BSA given over 24 hours, with D_5W added to reach a total of approximately 50% of the previous day's requirement. Measuring electrolyte concentrations carefully and frequently (especially potassium, because with burns there can be massive losses of this ion through the kidneys) determines whether and how much electrolyte solution is necessary.

Care of the burn wound may require excision, escharotomy, or eventual grafting and is best left in the hands of an experienced surgical team. Tetanus prophylaxis should be administered. Routine use of low-dose penicillin prophylaxis is no longer recommended.

After the first several days a fluid rate of an amount close to maintenance may be sufficient (at approximately 72 hours maximum resorption of edema has taken place). If the burn is of major proportions, parenteral nutrition or early enteral feeding should be initiated once the electrolyte balance is stable.[6,23] Attention also must be paid to the social and psychological needs of the child and the family. Recovery from a major burn injury is slow, is fraught with complications, and leaves substantial scars. If the child's emotional well-being is not tended to adequately, the psychological scars may outweigh any physical disability that results.

PARENTERAL NUTRITION

In previous sections of this chapter many situations have been noted in which provision of maintenance fluid and electrolyte concentrations in the standard glucose solutions is insufficient to meet caloric or nutritional requirements. Such situations occur whenever oral intake is limited or impossible for prolonged periods of time (over 1 week in older children, 2 to 3 days in the infant or neonate) or the body's metabolic demands exceed those that can be supplied orally. The box below lists some of the major indications for parenteral nutrition in the pediatric population.

Intravenous provision of nutrients and calories may be in the form of total parenteral nutrition (TPN) or partial parenteral nutrition. For the majority of children who are able to tolerate at least small amounts of oral intake, partial parenteral nutrition is preferred. The choice between TPN and partial parenteral nutrition depends on the nature of the child's illness and the length of time nutritional support is required. Parenteral nutrition fluids consist of the following components.

Calories

The basic goal of parenteral nutrition is the prevention of protein breakdown. In long-term pediatric users an additional goal is the promotion of normal growth and development. Caloric needs vary with age. The neonate requires 130 to 140 Cal/kg/day; the 1-year-old child, 100 Cal/kg/day; and the adult, 30 Cal/kg/day. Between 1 year of age and adulthood,

MAJOR PEDIATRIC INDICATIONS FOR USE OF PARENTERAL NUTRITION

- Gastrointestinal lesions preventing adequate oral intake
  - Congenital: anterior abdominal wall defects, intestinal atresia
  - Acquired: necrotizing enterocolitis, chronic fistulas, intestinal obstruction
- Gastrointestinal lesions precluding adequate absorption
  - Status after bowel resections, chronic diarrhea, inflammatory bowel disease
- Severe hypermetabolic or catabolic conditions
  - Multiple trauma, malignancies, major burns, extensive surgery
- Severely undernourished patients
  - Malnutrition, anorexia nervosa
- Acute and chronic renal failure
- Small premature infants

the drop in caloric requirements is approximately 10 Cal/kg/day for each 3-year increment. After 10 years of age, girls require fewer calories than boys. It is impossible to predict the precise caloric requirements of an individual patient. Preexisting nutritional deprivation, recent weight loss, and hypermetabolic conditions increase caloric needs. Bedside determination of the metabolic rate by indirect calorimetry may provide important information in individual patients.

Calories may be supplied as carbohydrate (usually dextrose), as protein (amino acid mixtures), or as fat (usually an isotonic soybean emulsion). Calories derived from different sources are not equivalent in their ability to generate a positive nitrogen balance. Amino acids generally are incorporated into the lean body mass unless a positive nitrogen balance already exists, in which case they yield 4 Cal/g administered. In the calorically deprived patient, carbohydrate exerts a much better protein-sparing effect than does fat on a calorie-for-calorie basis. Nitrogen balance is best preserved under these circumstances when at least 80% of the administered calories consists of carbohydrate. However, because the metabolism of glucose results in thermogenesis and increases the metabolic rate, providing such a high percentage of the calories as carbohydrate may lead to an elevation of the respiratory quotient and potentiate existing or imminent respiratory failure. High glucose loads also increase circulating levels of endogenous catecholamines, and patients may become insulin resistant.

Protein

Children beyond the neonatal period require between 1 and 3 g of protein per kilogram per day. This usually is supplied as a mixture of amino acids in which the final concentration of protein is between 1.7% and 2.75%. Whatever solution is used should provide adequate amounts of the essential amino acids — lysine, threonine, tryptophan, phenylalanine, methionine, leucine, isoleucine, and valine. Most solutions also contain the nonessential amino acids. Protein is administered primarily to provide adequate material for the repair of tissues and the synthesis of new cells, *not* to provide calories per se. In general, at least 30 nonprotein calories should be provided for every gram of protein delivered in a 24-hour period.[44]

Because the majority of nitrogen losses occur through the urinary tract, the child whose renal function is marginal or failing usually requires an adjustment in the type and amount of protein given to avoid worsening azotemia.

Carbohydrate

Carbohydrate in the form of glucose is the major source of calories in standard parenteral nutrition solutions. Although carbohydrates ordinarily provide 4 Cal/g, most parenteral nutrition solutions contain hydrated glucose, which provides only 3.4 Cal/g. Glucose concentration depends primarily on the *method* of administration. Although concentrated glucose solutions (20% or 25%) provide a large number of calories, they present a high osmotic load (1120 and 1400 mOsm/kg, respectively) and cannot be administered through a peripheral vein because of problems with phlebitis and thrombosis. To deliver such glucose solutions, a central venous catheter must be placed. The catheter should be placed so that the tip is near the junction of the superior vena cava and right atrium; intraatrial placement should be avoided because of the risk of the catheter perforating the atrial wall.

Central venous catheters are difficult to place in small children. For this reason and for long-term use, most pediatric centers are using a soft Silastic catheter placed in the operating room and tunneled several centimeters beneath the skin. The Hickman and Broviac catheters are designed specifically for this purpose. Each has a Dacron cuff that, when placed in the skin tunnel, allows growth of fibrous tissue, thus fixing them in place and obviating the need for sutures. Such lines may remain in place for a year or longer, provided they are cared for properly.

If a central line cannot be placed or is deemed unnecessary, glucose and amino acid solutions may be infused through a peripheral vein. The glucose concentration of solutions used in this situation generally is limited to 10% to 12%. The caloric content is limited by the volume of fluid the child can tolerate. In the majority of cases, adequate calories cannot be provided by such glucose–amino acid mixtures alone.

Fat

Currently the lipid solutions used are derived from an emulsion of soybean oil in water to which egg yolk–phospholipid and glycerol are added, resulting in an isotonic solution containing linoleic, oleic, palmitic, and linolenic acids. The most widely used fatty acid mixture (Intralipid) is available in 10% and 20% solutions, containing 1.1 Cal/ml and 2.2 Cal/ml, respectively. Daily administration of Intralipid provides an isotonic solution high in calories, which can be presented through a peripheral vein, thereby improving the usefulness of peripheral parenteral nutrition. The maximum tolerance for fat given in this way is 4 g/kg/day; in no case should the fat administered exceed 60% of the daily nonprotein caloric intake.[44]

Children receiving large doses of lipid may have difficulty "clearing" the emulsion from their serum. This may result in deposition of fat droplets within pulmonary capillaries, with a concomitant decrease in pulmonary diffusion capacity. Another consequence of lipid administration is the binding of free fatty acids to albumin, in competition with bilirubin; therefore this is considered hazardous in infants who have total bilirubin concentrations greater than 8 to 10 mg/dl. Long-term administration of fat emulsions also leads to deposition of an unusual pigment within the reticuloendothelial cells of bone marrow, lymph nodes, liver, and spleen. The significance of this pigment is unknown, but no disruption of normal function has been documented.

Essential fatty acid requirements can be met by providing between 2% and 4% of the child's caloric needs as lipid. However, because of the above-noted problems from too much glucose administration and because of amino acid tolerance limitations, 30% to 60% of the total calories generally are delivered in the form of fat.

Electrolyte Concentrations

The electrolyte content of each solution varies according to the source of amino acids. The sodium content, for example, ranges from less than 10 to more than 50 mEq/L, with other common minerals varying just as widely. Electrolyte concentrations may be added to each solution so that daily requirements are met.

Trace Minerals

Trace elements known to be essential for pediatric growth and development include copper, zinc, chromium, manganese, selenium, iodine, and iron. The first five are available as a premixed pediatric trace element additive. When needed, generally in patients receiving TPN for greater than 30 days, iron can be added separately at a dose of 1 to 2 mg/day.[1] Iodine is not generally administered parenterally.

Vitamins

A standard mixture of vitamin supplements is available for addition to TPN solutions in infants and children (M.V.I. Pediatric—multivitamin infusion). The product comes as a powder; after reconstitution with sterile water, each 5 ml contains the following:

Vitamin A (retinol): 0.7 mg (2300 USP units)
Vitamin C (ascorbic acid): 80 mg
Vitamin D (ergocalciferol): 10 μg (400 USP units)
Vitamin E (alpha-tocopherol acetate): 7 mg (7 USP units)
Vitamin B_1 (thiamine): 1.2 mg
Vitamin B_2 (riboflavin): 1.4 mg
Vitamin B_6 (pyridoxine): 1 mg
Vitamin B_{12} (cyanocobalamin): 1 μg
Vitamin K_1 (phytonadione): 200 μg
Biotin: 20 μg
Dexpanthenol: 5 mg
Folic acid: 140 μg
Niacinamide: 17 mg

For children under 11 years of age who weigh more than 3 kg, the entire 5 ml should be administered (dissolved in the TPN solution). Infants weighing between 1 and 3 kg receive 3.25 ml; neonates weighing less than 1 kg receive 1.5 ml of the reconstituted solution. It no longer is necessary to administer vitamins K or B_{12} as weekly intramuscular injections, as was the case until recently.

Parenteral Nutrition in Clinical Practice

It is cumbersome and expensive to personalize fully the parenteral solution administered to each patient; therefore most hospitals have devised standard solutions of protein, glucose, electrolyte concentrations, and minerals. Generally these are determined by a group of professionals (physician, nurse, pharmacist, nutrition specialist) who have a special interest and expertise in parenteral nutrition). In some hospitals the duties of such a team may be assumed by a single person (physician or pharmacist). Such specialists are available for consultation regarding the best mode of parenteral nutrition, the delivery systems, and the makeup of solutions to be used. Use of standardized TPN formulations and TPN order forms decreases both the costs of TPN preparation and the risks of errors.[25]

The use of parenteral nutrition requires careful monitoring of the patient's blood glucose levels, serum protein, albumin, and electrolyte values, hematocrit, liver enzyme levels, and renal function. Results of laboratory determinations should be maintained on a flow sheet, which also lists the daily weight, urine output, and calories and fluid administered (including the type and glucose content of each). Some major centers with large nutritional support teams are able to manage chronically ill patients on a home parenteral nutrition program.

FLUID THERAPY OF THE NEONATE

The provision of adequate fluid replacement therapy for newborn infants depends on perinatal alterations in body composition and the infant's size and gestational age. Hydration of sick premature babies who weigh less than 1500 g is beyond the scope of this chapter. Specific issues relating to the health of the neonate are presented in Part Five.

TBW content decreases progressively throughout gestation and the first year of postnatal life. This is accompanied by increases in the body's content of protein and fat. Shrinkage of the ECF compartment accounts largely for the decrease in TBW. In the first few days of extrauterine life, both term and premature babies normally lose up to 10% of their body weight. Although this is considered a physiological reduction, failure to replace such losses may lead to substantial dehydration.

All newborns show a progressive increase in their metabolic rate. The metabolic rate for full-term infants approximates 32 Cal/kg/day at birth and reaches close to 43 Cal/kg/day within 3 days. Following this there is a slow, steady increase over the first 2 weeks of life. Premature infants maintain a higher metabolic rate than full-term babies, even when they achieve a similar weight.

In addition to the baseline metabolic expenditure of calories, newborns use energy with cold, stress, and muscular activity. The growth rate is rapid during this period, and the average newborn requires 25 to 35 Cal/kg/day for growth. Therefore the total caloric need of an infant over 3 days of age is between 100 and 125 Cal/kg/day.

Water requirements are governed by losses through the skin, respiratory tract, and kidneys. Evaporative losses through the skin generally average 20 to 30 ml/kg/day, whereas respiratory losses account for approximately 15 ml/kg/day. Both parameters are affected by ambient humidity, and respiratory losses actually may be reduced by 50% with provision of high humidity to the baby's immediate environment.

The newborn's kidneys are limited in their ability to concentrate urine because of the relative shortness of the loops of Henle and the absence of a notable concentration gradient. Thus they are able at best to excrete urine with an osmolality that approaches 300 mOsm/kg. As the solute load increases the free water requirement rises, so for a formula-fed infant urinary water loss may be as high as 120 ml/kg/day. However, the average range probably is closer to 60 to 75 ml/kg/day.

Electrolyte requirements for infants have not been fully established, but they seem to tolerate a fairly wide range of electrolyte provisions. Fluids that have been used successfully yield between 1 and 3 mEq of sodium per 100 calories per day, and this has become the recommended starting range for maintenance fluid therapy.

When preparing a maintenance parenteral fluid formula for newborns it is important to ensure adequate monitoring, which will indicate whether fluid estimates have been adequate. It also is important, especially with the sick neonate, to record weights once or twice a day and to record intake, output, vital signs, urinary osmolality, electrolyte concentrations, and other indications of optimum cardiac and respiratory homeostasis frequently. Frequent changes may be needed; therefore the physician must never become "locked into" a particular formula but rather must apply the basic rules of fluid therapy to the situation logically and be ready to compensate for failing systems or increasing losses when necessary.

HYDRATION OF THE AMBULATORY PATIENT: ALTERNATIVES TO PARENTERAL FLUID THERAPY

It is fairly common practice for pediatricians in the United States to recommend oral fluids for young patients who have mild diarrhea or vomiting. Such therapy has been suggested for many years on totally empirical grounds, and most physicians have urged the use of a dilute solution that contains sodium and potassium in concentrations of 30 and 20 mEq/L, respectively, and 5% to 7% glucose. When diarrhea leads to moderate or severe dehydration, or if substantial emesis accompanies the illness, the standard teaching had dictated hospitalization of such children and "resting" the GI tract with the use of parenteral therapy, as outlined in previous sections.

Through the efforts of scientists working with the World Health Organization (WHO) in an effort to curb the large diarrhea-associated mortality seen in developing countries, data concerning gastrointestinal function in diarrhea have been accumulated.[34,35]

Sodium absorption in the small intestine depends on the presence of glucose or small neutral amino acids such as glycine or alanine. Likewise the absorption of glucose is enhanced by the presence of sodium salts. Movement of salt and glucose across the mucosal border is accompanied by an influx of water and other electrolyte concentrations. Maximum rates of absorption are achieved when (1) sodium and glucose are present in a 1:1 to 1:2 molecular ratio, (2) glucose concentration is between 110 and 140 mmol (2% to 2.5% solution), and (3) sodium concentration is not substantially less than that of normal jejunal fluid.

Based on this and other information WHO derived a formula for use with all patients suffering from diarrheal illness regardless of its cause. It contains 90 mmol of sodium, 20 mmol of potassium, 30 mmol of bicarbonate, 80 mmol of chloride, and 111 mmol of glucose per liter. This formulation provides a solution that has an osmolality of 331. When given ad lib to patients who have diarrhea, it corrects dehydration rapidly and can return electrolyte concentrations to the normal range regardless of the presence of hyponatremia or hypernatremia on initial evaluation. Large field studies have documented its successful use in patients who have ongoing emesis. There has been no evidence to suggest that the use of such fluid prolongs the duration of diarrhea; just the reverse appears to be the case. In addition children given this oral rehydration therapy (ORT) seem to tolerate resumption of a regular diet earlier than those treated solely with intravenous fluids. Use of a solution with lower osmolality (224 mOsm/L) has been shown to result in superior water absorption and patient weight gain.[31]

In 1985 the American Academy of Pediatrics (AAP) Committee on Nutrition published recommendations for the use of the WHO solution or similar solutions in developed countries.[21] The Committee concluded that the WHO oral rehydration solution (WHO-ORS) is appropriate for use in the initial phases of rehydration and should be used for the first 6 hours to replace acute volume loss. After this time the Committee recommends that the solution be replaced with one containing 40 to 60 mEq of sodium per liter, for maintenance of hydration in the child who continues to have stool losses, or as the only solution administered to a child who is not acutely dehydrated. Alternatively, as used in the developing countries in the maintenance phase, children may be given the ORS on a 1:1 basis with fluid low in sodium content, such as breast milk or water, to avoid potential hypernatremia.

There are commercially available preparations that meet WHO and AAP guidelines, as indicated above. Because such preparations are available in ready-to-use form, the bicarbonate found in the WHO powder has been replaced with citrate.[34] Studies have documented equivalent efficacy of the two bases in correcting the mild acidosis that accompanies mild-to-moderate diarrhea. Most of the large-scale evaluations that have been performed in developed countries have excluded the use of ORS in patients in shock who are treated initially with intravenous fluids.[30,43] Research is ongoing to determine the optimal composition of oral rehydration solutions. Some formulations have replaced glucose with carbohydrates derived from rice, or with synthetic glucose polymers; others have replaced glucose with glycine or alanine.[1,5,19,20,38]

In summary, oral rehydration therapy provides a cost-efficient approach to the problem of childhood diarrhea for the patient who is able to drink, is not in shock, and has a relative or other responsible person who can understand the instructions for using the ORT formula. Such a therapeutic approach avoids the hospitalization of a child and the consequent disruption in the lives of the family members. More important, this treatment approach eliminates the potential complications of intravenous therapy.

REFERENCES

1. Ament M: Trace metals in parenteral nutrition. In Chandra RK, editor: *Trace elements in nutrition of children—II,* New York, 1991, Raven.
2. Beach PS, Beach RE, Smith LR: Hyponatremic seizures in a child treated with desmopressin to control enuresis: a rational approach to fluid intake, *Clin Pediatr* 31:566, 1992.
3. Broner CW et al: A prospective, randomized, double-blind comparison of calcium chloride and calcium gluconate therapies for hypocalcemia in critically ill children, *J Pediatr* 117:986, 1990.
4. Cheng JC et al: Symptomatic hyponatremia: pathophysiology and management, *Acute Care* 14-15:270, 1988-1989.
5. Cunha Ferreira RM et al: Dominant role for osmolality in the efficacy of glucose and glycine-containing oral rehydration solutions: studies in a rat model of secretory diarrhoea, *Acta Paediatr* 81:46, 1992.
6. Derganc M: Present trends in fluid therapy, metabolic care, and prevention of infection in burned children, *Crit Care Med* 21:S397, 1993.
7. Dhawan A, Narang A, Singhi S: Hyponatraemia and the inappropriate ADH syndrome in pneumonia, *Ann Trop Pediatr* 12:455, 1992.
8. Dilmen U et al: Salbutamol in the treatment of neonatal hyperkalemia, *Biol Neonate* 62:424, 1992.
9. Ellis DJ, Steward DJ: Fentanyl dosage is associated with reduced blood glucose in pediatric patients after hypothermic cardiopulmonary bypass, *Anesthesiology* 78:812, 1990.
10. Emergency Cardiac Care Committee and Subcommittees, American Heart Association: Guidelines for cardiopulmonary resuscitation and emergency cardiac care. Part VI. Pediatric advanced life support, *JAMA* 268:2262, 1992.

11. Filley G, Kindig N: Carbicarb, an alkalinizing ion-generating agent of possible clinical usefulness, *Trans Am Clin Climatol Assoc* 96:141, 1984.
12. Gazmuri RJ et al: Cardiac effects of carbon dioxide–consuming and carbon dioxide–generating buffers during cardiopulmonary resuscitation, *J Am Coll Cardiol* 15:482, 1990.
13. Ginsberg MD, Welsh FA, Budd WW: Deleterious effect of glucose pretreatment on recovery from diffuse cerebral ischemia in the cat, *Stroke* 11:347, 1980.
14. Gomez-Cia T, Roa L: A burn patient resuscitation therapy designed by computer simulation (BET). Part 2. Initial clinical validation, *Burns* 19:332, 1993.
15. Greenough A et al: Salbutamol infusion to treat neonatal hyperkalemia, *J Perinat Med* 20:437, 1992.
16. Hazard PB, Griffin JP: Calculation of sodium bicarbonate requirements in metabolic acidosis, *Am J Med Sci* 283:18, 1982.
17. International study group on improved ORS: Impact of glycine-containing ORS solutions on stool output and duration of diarrhoea: a meta-analysis of seven clinical trials, *Bull World Health Org* 69:541, 1991.
18. Jacobson J, Bohn D: Severe hypernatremic dehydration and hypokalemia in an infant with gastroenteritis secondary to rotavirus, *Ann Emerg Med* 22:1630, 1993.
19. Khin-Maung U, Greenough WB III: Cereal-based oral rehydration therapy. I. Clinical studies, *J Pediatr* 118:S72, 1991.
20. Khin-Maung U et al: Comparison of glucose/electrolyte and maltodextrin/glycine/glycyl-glycine/electrolye oral rehydration solutions in acute diarrhea in children, *J Pediatr Gastroenterol Nutr* 13:397, 1991.
21. Mauer AM et al: American Academy of Pediatrics Committee on Nutrition: use of oral fluid therapy and posttreatment feeding following enteritis in children in a developed country, *Pediatrics* 75:358, 1985.
22. McClure RJ, Prasad VK, Brocklebank JT: Treatment of hyperkalemia using intravenous and nebulised salbutamol, *Arch Dis Child* 70:126, 1994.
23. McDonald WS, Sharp CW Jr, Deitch EA: Immediate enteral feeding in burn patients is safe and effective, *Ann Surg* 213:177, 1991.
24. Meyer I: Sodium polystyrene sulfonate: a cation exchange resin used in treating hyperkalemia, *ANNA J* 20:93, 1993.
25. Mitchell KA et al: Standardized TPN order form reduces staff time and potential for error, *Nutrition* 6:457, 1990.
26. Murison MS, Laitung JK, Pigott RW: Effectiveness of burns resuscitation using two different formulae, *Burns* 17:484, 1991.
27. Noerr B: Sodium polystyrene sulfonate (Kayexalate), *Neonatal Netw* 12:77, 1993.
28. Peters JM: Hypernatremia in breast-fed infants due to elevated breast milk sodium, *J Am Osteopath Assoc* 89:1165, 1989.
29. Puffinbarger NK, Tuggle DW, Smith EI: Rapid isotonic fluid resuscitation in pediatric thermal injury, *J Pediatr Surg* 29:339, 1994.
30. Rautanen T, el-Radhi S, Vesikari T: Clinical experience with a hypotonic oral rehydration solution in acute diarrhoea, *Acta Paediatr* 82:52, 1993.
31. Rautanen T et al: Randomised double-blind trial of hypotonic oral rehydration solutions with and without citrate, *Arch Dis Child* 70:44, 1994.
32. Riley LJ, Ilson BE, Narins RG: Acute metabolic acid-base disorders, *Crit Care Clin* 5:699, 1987.
33. Rossi NF, Cadnapaphornchai P: Disordered water metabolism: hyponatremia, *Crit Care Clin* 5:759, 1987.
34. Salazar-Lindo E et al: Bicarbonate versus citrate in oral rehydration therapy in infants with watery diarrhea: a controlled clinical trial, *J Pediatr* 108:55, 1986.
35. Santosham M et al: Oral rehydration therapy for acute diarrhea in ambulatory children in the United States: a double-blind comparison of four different solutions, *Pediatrics* 76:159, 1985.
36. Sarnaik AP et al: Management of hyponatremic seizures in children with hypertonic saline: a safe and effective strategy, *Crit Care Med* 19:758, 1991.
37. Satlin LM, Schwartz GJ: Disorders of potassium metabolism. In Ichikawa I, editor: *Pediatric textbook of fluids and electrolytes,* Baltimore, 1990, Williams & Wilkins.
38. Sazawal S et al: Alanine-based oral rehydration solution: assessment of efficacy in acute noncholera diarrhea among children, *J Pediatr Gastroenterol Nutr* 12:461, 1991.
39. Segel IH: *Biochemical calculations,* ed 2, New York, 1976, John Wiley & Sons.
40. Shann F, Germer S: Hyponatremia associated with pneumonia or bacterial meningitis, *Arch Dis Child* 60:963, 1985.
41. Simmons CF, Ichikawa I: *External balance of water and electrolytes.* In Ichikawa I, editor: *Pediatric textbook of fluids and electrolytes,* Baltimore, 1990, Williams & Wilkins.
42. Smith TJ et al: Hyponatremia and seizures in young children given DDAVP, *Am J Hematol* 31:199, 1989.
43. Tamer AM et al: Oral rehydration of infants in a large urban US medical center, *J Pediatr* 107:14, 1985.
44. Warner BW: Parenteral nutrition in the pediatric patient. In Fischer JE, editor: *Total parenteral nutrition,* ed 2, Boston, 1991, Little, Brown.
45. Wattad A, Chiang ML, Hill LL: Hyponatremia in hospitalized children, *Clin Pediatr* 31:153, 1992.
46. Weisburg LS: Pseudohyponatremia: a reappraisal, *Am J Med* 86:315, 1989.
47. Winters RW, editor: *The body fluids in pediatrics,* Boston, 1973, Little Brown.
48. Yared A, Ichikawa I: Regulation of plasma osmolality. In Ichikawa I, editor: *Pediatric textbook of fluids and electrolytes,* Baltimore, 1990, Williams & Wilkins.
49. Zaritsky A: Pediatric resuscitation pharmacology, *Ann Emerg Med* 22:445, 1993.

29 Blood Products and Their Uses

Eva G. Radel

The ability to separate blood into its components, store them appropriately, and administer them as needed has resulted in markedly improved supportive care, particularly in the areas of oncology and neonatology. However, the unfortunate occurrence of blood-transmitted acquired immune deficiency syndrome (AIDS) has made the medical profession and the public aware of the hazards of blood products and, in some cases has led to excessive fear of transfusion. As a result, the indications for transfusion have been reassessed, and more effort is being devoted to a search for alternatives to the use of blood products.

GENERAL INDICATIONS FOR BLOOD TRANSFUSION

The general indications for transfusion of blood or blood products are (1) restoration of blood volume when it has been acutely depleted, (2) restoration of oxygen-carrying capacity, (3) restoration of a particular blood component (cellular or humoral) to a level allowing adequate function, (4) replacement or supplementation of an abnormally functioning component with a normal one, and (5) replacement after removal of large amounts of plasma or blood cells (exchange transfusion or apheresis).

The level of a blood component almost never has to be restored to the normal range; instead, the goal should be a level that will correct pathological processes and allow normal physiological functioning for the patient's current condition. In deciding whether component replacement is necessary, physicians should ask themselves two questions: (1) Is it essential to correct the particular deficit immediately through replacement? and (2) Is there no other method that would effectively restore an adequate physiological state? The necessary component should be administered selectively, if possible. An increasing number of non-blood-product medications, such as erythropoietin, granulocyte colony–stimulating factor (G-CSF), and desmopressin (DDAVP), are available for some situations in which previously only blood components could be used.

BLOOD DONORS AND HANDLING OF BLOOD PRODUCTS

In recent years public demand has been high for directed donations from family members and friends; this allows an individual to avoid receiving blood from routine donors, whom many consider unsafe. However, a higher incidence of hepatitis B and C has been found among first-time directed donors than among volunteer donors.[13] With directed transfusions, the risk arises of graft-versus-host disease (GVHD) developing in immunocompetent blood recipients who have been transfused with blood products from relatives who are homozygous for one of the patient's HLA haplotypes. This problem can be prevented by irradiating the blood product. Although the risk is greatest for donors who are first-degree relatives, it recently was recommended that blood products from all blood relatives be irradiated.[9]

All possible precautions must be taken to avoid clerical errors when drawing and labeling blood specimens to be used for preparation of blood, as well as when starting transfusions. Inadvertent infusion of incompatible blood could cause a fatal hemolytic transfusion reaction. Blood products must be stored and handled properly. Once blood has been taken out of the blood bank, it should be used promptly and not refrigerated. If administration will be delayed, the blood should be returned to the blood bank. Improper refrigeration can cause blood to freeze, resulting in lysis of the red cells, hemoglobinuria, and poor response to transfusion.

RED CELL TRANSFUSIONS

In some situations (e.g., exchange transfusions, massive bleeding) use of whole blood is desirable. However, many blood banks no longer store whole blood and have only packed red cells (PRBCs) available. These can be reconstituted, if indicated, with saline, albumin (or another colloid), or fresh-frozen plasma (FFP). FFP rarely is needed in these situations, and using it exposes the recipient to the risks of receiving another unit of blood. RBC preparations are described in Table 29-1.

Acute Blood Loss

Acute loss of more than 20% of the blood volume usually requires transfusion of PRBCs. If the patient is actively bleeding, rapid administration may be necessary.

Massive bleeding involving the loss of more than one blood volume over several hours can give rise to some unique problems:

1. A bleeding tendency may develop due to dilution and inadequate replacement of platelets and coagulation factors (particularly factors V and VIII). If the platelet count is below 50,000 to 75,000/μl, platelets should be administered. If the results of coagulation studies are abnormal (i.e., prothrombin time [PT] over 15 seconds, partial thromboplastin time [PTT] over 45 seconds, and fibrinogen under 100 mg/dl), FFP should be given as well. Occasionally, administering cryoprecipitate can be helpful in replacing fibrinogen.
2. Excess citrate (from the anticoagulant in the donor blood) may produce hypocalcemia, alkalosis, and hypokalemia. Hypotension may ensue as a result of the hypocalcemia, leading to additional—and inappropriate—transfusion, which can exacerbate the problem.[5]

Table 29-1 Red Blood Cell Preparations

Product	Preparation	Hematocrit (%) or cell count	Volume/unit (ml)	Indications/comments
Whole blood	450 ml blood, plus anticoagulant	40%	500	Massive bleeding, exchange transfusion
Packed RBCs	Centrifuged or sedimented to remove about two thirds of plasma	80%	250	Most RBC transfusions
Buffy coat–depleted RBCs	Centrifuged to remove white cell layer	90% Contains 15%-30% of original WBCs	200	Chronically transfused patients; patients who have severe febrile reactions
Washed RBCs	Several manual and automated techniques available to remove plasma; must be used within 24 hours	90% Contains <1% of original plasma, <10% of WBCs	200	Repeated febrile and allergic reactions
Frozen RBCs	Frozen in glycerol, thawed, and washed; must be used within 24 hours of thawing; 10%-15% loss of original RBCs	Contains <0.025% of original plasma, 1%-5% of original WBCs and platelets	200	Rare blood types, multiple severe febrile/allergic reactions, IgA deficiency, autologous blood donations

Monitoring ionized calcium and electrolytes and preventing abnormalities can prevent this problem.

Restoration of Oxygen-Carrying Capacity

Transfusion often is recommended for a variety of indications to improve oxygen delivery in anemic patients, but frequently there is no scientific basis for such recommendations. The patient's general clinical condition is very important when determining the need to correct mild degrees of anemia. Transfusions often are given to small premature newborns or to older children who are critically ill and have cardiovascular compromise. The indications in these situations are controversial.[14]

Careful consideration must be given to the risks of transfusion versus those of a low hemoglobin concentration. In many situations treating the underlying cause of the anemia can avert the need for transfusion. The volume of PRBCs given for anemia usually is about 10 ml/kg, which can be given over 2 to 3 hours to a patient who is clinically stable. With severe chronic anemia, the risk of congestive heart failure from transfusion may be greater than the risk of treating the patient medically. In this situation the volume transfused should be no more than 4 to 5 ml/kg given over 4 hours, and a diuretic may be needed. If the anemia must be corrected rapidly (e.g., for emergency surgery), a partial exchange transfusion can be done.

Chronic Transfusion

Several precautions that are not relevant to a patient receiving short-term transfusions are advisable for a child who is likely to undergo prolonged and repeated transfusion therapy:

1. *Red cell phenotyping:* Typing for several common red cell antigens should be done to prevent transfusion of blood containing antigens against which the patient is likely to form antibodies. This has been a particular problem for patients with sickle cell disease.[10]
2. *Leukocyte depletion:* Because most "minor" transfusion reactions are caused by leukocytes or plasma proteins, patients who are transfused frequently should receive buffy coat–depleted red cells.
3. *Hemosiderosis:* Serum ferritin should be monitored, and chelation therapy may be required.
4. *Hepatitis:* Although the incidence of hepatitis transmission has been markedly reduced by routine donor screening, the hepatitis B vaccine should be given to individuals likely to receive repeated transfusions.

Surgery

Children with significant anemia develop more complications from surgery and anesthesia. In the past a hematocrit of 30% was recommended as the minimum requirement for patients undergoing anesthesia. Recent observations indicate that otherwise healthy patients may tolerate hemoglobin values as low as 7 g/dl.[15] However, the extent of surgery, the probability for massive blood loss, and coexisting factors such as impaired pulmonary function or inadequate cardiac output must be considered. The combination of anemia and hypovelemia must be avoided.[14]

With adults there has been an increasing tendency to use autologous blood donations for elective surgery. This also has been done successfully in adolescents and children as young as age 8, particularly for those having orthopedic procedures in which the expected blood loss is quite significant and for prospective bone marrow donors. Several phlebotomies can be performed over a period of a few weeks just before surgery, or the process can be carried out over a longer period and the blood can be frozen and stored. Salvaging blood during surgery, collecting it with special equipment, and reinfusing it also has been attempted to reduce the use of banked blood; to date, experience with children has been limited.[4]

Special Circumstances in Red Cell Transfusion

Newborns. Maternal blood is used, if possible, to crossmatch blood for the infant's transfusion. However, the blood used should be ABO-specific for the baby or type O with a low titer of isoagglutinins. If the infant is Rh-negative, the blood should be Rh-negative as well. An infant who has hemolytic disease of the newborn, whether for simple transfusion or exchange transfusion, should receive blood that does not contain the antigen to which the mother is sensitized. With ABO incompatibility, the blood should be type O. With a small premature infant who is transfused frequently, it no longer is considered necessary to perform a cross-match procedure for each transfusion unless plasma, platelets, or granulocytes have been administered. Many blood banks now designate certain blood units, which are drawn into four small bags, to be used for repeated transfusions for specific neonates to limit the number of donor exposures.[14]

Sickle Cell Disease. Patients who have sickle cell disease often are transfused to replace cells capable of sickling in the circulation with cells that are more deformable and will not participate in a vasoocclusive process. The blood used should be from sickle-negative donors.

Potential Bone Marrow Transplant Recipients. Children who may require bone marrow transplantion should not be given blood products from genetically related family members because it may lead to sensitization to HLA antigens and subsequent bone marrow rejection.

Immunosuppressed Patients. This category includes (1) patients being treated for a malignancy, (2) bone marrow or organ transplant recipients, (3) premature infants weighing less than 1250 g and other severely ill neonates, (4) fetuses receiving intrauterine transfusions, and (5) children who have severe congenital immune deficiency disorders. These children are susceptible to GVHD because of their failure to eliminate viable lymphocytes from the transfused blood. Leukodepletion does not prevent this complication. Irradiation of all blood products with a minimum of 15 to 20 Gy is recommended for these children.[12]

Cytomegalovirus (CMV) infection also is a risk in immunosuppressed patients. If the child (or the mother of a newborn) does not already have antibodies to CMV (indicating preexisting infection), blood products from CMV-seronegative donors should be given. If this is not possible, the product should be administered with a leukofilter that can remove 99.9% of the white cells.[8] CMV-negative blood also should be given to pregnant women who are seronegative.

PLATELET TRANSFUSION

Platelet transfusions are useful primarily in situations in which there is a lack of production of platelets by the bone marrow. If thrombocytopenia is due to peripheral destruction, transfusion is unlikely to raise the platelet count. Spontaneous hemorrhage usually does not occur with a platelet count above 10,000/μl, but it often is standard procedure to maintain the count above 20,000/μl. Patients who have chronically low platelet counts are less likely to bleed spontaneously than those whose platelets are diminishing rapidly. Traumatic or surgical bleeding may require platelet counts above 30,000 to 60,000/μl. Dysfunctional platelets (e.g., those that may result from a congenital platelet disorder, after extracorporeal perfusion, or after massive blood replacement) may result in bleeding at somewhat higher levels of platelet counts.

The half-life of transfused platelets is about 24 hours under normal circumstances, but survival may be shortened by fever or infection, platelet antibodies, splenomegaly, massive bleeding, or any condition that results in peripheral destruction or the consumption of platelets. Variations in donor platelet count and collection or storage techniques, as well as increased manipulation of platelets, also may result in decreased platelet recovery.

Platelets are not cross-matched for transfusion, but ABO-compatible platelets should be used when possible. For patients who need a single transfusion or a brief period of platelet transfusions, random donor platelets are satisfactory. For patients who have a malignancy or aplastic anemia, who likely will require repeated platelet transfusions, single donor platelets are preferable (Table 29-2). Patients who have aplastic anemia have a particularly high incidence of alloimmunization[11] and may benefit from having a limited number of designated platelet donors who are apheresed regularly. For patients who have malignancies or are immunosuppressed, the precautions recommended above for red cell transfusions should be followed. Patients who have become refractory to random donor platelets and who are not candidates for bone marrow transplantation may benefit from receiving platelets from family members who are at least partly HLA-matched. Unrelated but HLA-matched donors also may be good platelet donors for sensitized patients.

GRANULOCYTE TRANSFUSIONS

White blood cells (WBCs) are the most difficult blood cellular components to transfuse because of problems with yield,

Table 29-2 White Cell and Platelet Preparations

Product	Preparation	Cell count	Volume/unit (ml)	Indications/comments
Random donor platelets	Separated from single whole blood units	5-7 × 10^{10} platelets/unit	50	Infants, short-term need; 1 unit/10 kg increases platelet count by 50,000
Single donor platelets	Collected by apheresis	Equivalent to 6-10 random units	200-400 usually in two bags	Patients who require repeated transfusions
Buffy coat granulocytes	Separated from single whole blood units	0.35-5 × 10^9/unit	25	? usefulness; must be ABO-compatible; must be used within 24 hours of collection
Apheresed granulocyte concentrates	Various techniques to increase donor neutrophil count and yield	0.5-3 × 10^{10}/unit	500	Contains RBCs, must be ABO-compatible; must be used within 24 hours of collection

recovery, and complications. The use of granulocyte transfusions has been controversial; some centers use them regularly and others rarely. Studies have shown conflicting results and have been difficult to compare and interpret, both in neonatology and oncology.

Febrile reactions and pulmonary infiltrates often are seen with granulocyte transfusion and may be associated with alloimmunization to both HLA antigens and granulocyte-specific antigens. Simultaneous administration of granulocytes and amphotericin has been implicated in severe pulmonary decompensation with intraalveolar hemorrhage.[5] CMV transmission is a risk (see above).

EXCHANGE TRANSFUSION AND THERAPEUTIC APHERESIS

One unit of whole blood is equivalent to approximately twice the blood volume of a full-term neonate (i.e., a double volume exchange) and will replace about 85% of the infant's RBCs. PRBCs can be reconstituted with FFP. The blood used should be less than 3 to 5 days old, and the recommendations for transfusion of newborns (see above) should be followed. Although manual exchange transfusion often is done in older children for a variety of indications, this can be difficult and time-consuming. Automated cell separators simplify the process, and some can be adapted for use in young children. Whole blood is removed, and plasma, platelets, leukocytes, and red cells are separated, and the desired component is removed. Except with erythrocytapheresis, the red cells are returned to the patient. Volume can be replaced with saline, albumin, or FFP.[10]

Erythrocytapheresis (partial exchange transfusion) may be done for polycythemia in neonates or in older children who have cyanotic heart disease using volume replacement with saline or albumin. The volume of exchange can be calculated:

$$\text{Volume exchanged} = \frac{\text{Total blood volume} \times (\text{Observed Hct} - \text{Desired Hct})}{\text{Observed Hct}}$$

In sickle cell disease, red cells may be removed and replaced with normal ones; formulas are available for calculating the required volume.[3] Leukocytapheresis may be done for patients who have leukemia and very high WBC counts to reduce viscosity and leukostasis until chemotherapy takes effect. Plasma exchange can be done for thrombotic thrombocytopenic purpura or hemolytic-uremic syndrome using FFP for replacement. Many autoimmune disorders in adults also have been treated with plasmapheresis, using albumin for replacement.

PLASMA PRODUCTS

Plasma products used to treat coagulation disorders are described in Table 29-3. Commercial lyophilized coagulant concentrates have the advantage of being assayed so that the physician knows exactly how much of a desired factor is being administered. Several very effective methods for inactivating viruses have made commercial concentrates much safer in recent years, although some viral agents still cause concern, such as parvovirus and hepatitis A. The treatment of hemophilia is described in Chapter 211.

Albumin

Albumin is available as a 5% or 25% solution, the latter being advantageous for patients who have hypoproteinemia and

Table 29-3 Products for Coagulation Disorders

Product	Content	Dose or concentration	Indications/comments
Fresh-frozen plasma	200-240 ml whole plasma	5-15 ml/kg; 1 u factor/ml	Contains all plasma factors; for multiple factor deficiency, DIC, reversal of coumadin effect, HUS, or TTP, unknown coagulation defect; not virus inactivated
Cryoprecipitate	Factor VIII, VWF, factor XIII, fibrinogen, fibronectin	± 75-100 u. factor VIII or VWF/bag; volume ±20 ml	From single donor units; not virus inactivated
Prothrombin complex	Factors II, VII, IX, and X	Preassayed for factor IX; factor VII content varies among products (high and assayed in Proplex); dose for inhibitor 100-150 u/kg	Hemophilia B; mild bleeding in hemophilia A with inhibitor; congenital deficiency of factor II, VII, or X; danger of thrombosis (including MI and DIC) with liver disease, vascular disease, prolonged use; virus inactivated*
Factor VIII	Factor VIII; VWF in Humate P	Preassayed; up to 100 u/ml	Hemophilia A; Humate P for VWD†; recombinant product available; virus inactivated; DDAVP is preferred for type I VWD and mild hemophilia when possible
Factor IX	Factor IX	Preassayed	Hemophilia B; virus inactivated*
Activated prothrombin complex	Factors II, VII, IX, and X; factor VIII "bypassing" activity	50-100 u/kg up to q6-8h	Cannot evaluate response by measuring factor VIII activity; risk of thrombosis
Hyate:C	Porcine factor VIII	Preassayed	Hemophilia A with inhibitor that is not cross-reactive

*Virus attenuation processes may not inactivate parvovirus, hepatitis A, and possibly other viruses.
†Has not been approved by the FDA for use in VWD.
DDAVP, Desmopressin; *DIC*, disseminated intravascular coagulation; *MI*, myocardial infarction; *VWD*, von Willebrand disease; *VWF*, von Willebrand factor.

need large amounts of albumin and who would get a much larger sodium load with the less concentrated product. Albumin is fractionated from pooled plasma and is pasteurized to inactivate viruses.

Immune Globulin

Two types of immune globulin preparations are available, one for intramuscular (IM) administration and another for intravenous (IV) use. Special products prepared from individuals who have high titers for specific infectious agents (varicella-zoster, hepatitis, and tetanus) also are available for IM administration. Intravenous gamma globulin is used to treat hypogammaglobulinemia, idiopathic thrombocytopenic purpura (ITP), Kawasaki disease, and a variety of immune disorders.

Anticoagulants

Pediatric patients who have thrombotic disease are more likely than adults to have a congenital deficiency of one of the normal anticoagulants, antithrombin III (ATIII), protein C, or protein S. ATIII concentrate is available, and protein C is awaiting FDA approval in the United States.

COMPLICATIONS OF TRANSFUSION

Immediate Hemolytic Transfusion Reaction

Severe, immediate hemolytic transfusion reactions almost always are related to ABO-incompatibility and clerical errors, such as incorrect labeling of a tube or administration of another patient's unit of blood. An acute onset of fever and chills may be accompanied by nausea, abdominal and lower back pain, dyspnea, and hypotension. Renal failure, disseminated intravascular coagulation (DIC), and shock may rapidly ensue. If such a reaction is suspected, the transfusion must be stopped immediately. Blood from the patient should be sent to the blood bank immediately, together with the remainder of the unit of donor blood or the empty bag and any attached blood tubing. A rapid screening test can be performed by obtaining a blood specimen (with care taken to avoid artificial hemolysis) and centrifuging it; pink, red, or brown plasma indicates intravascular hemolysis. A urine sample should be checked for the presence of hemoglobin at the same time. If there is evidence of a hemolytic reaction, fluid, steroids, and mannitol should be administered to induce diuresis, and pressors should be given as needed. Treatment of DIC and renal dialysis may be needed, and red cell transfusions should be given as indicated.[6]

Delayed Hemolytic Transfusion Reaction

Delayed reactions may develop 3 to 21 days after transfusion in patients who may have had prior sensitization to red cell antigens with titers too low to be detected before the recent transfusion. An anamnestic reaction may increase antibody production so that hemolysis ensues, and the patient becomes anemic, with or without hyperbilirubinemia and hemoglobinuria. Usually no specific therapy is required, but additional transfusion may be needed.

Febrile Transfusion Reaction

Fever is the most common transfusion reaction, occurring most often in patients who are multiply transfused and those who receive platelet transfusions. The fever usually is associated with antibodies directed against leukocytes, or with cytokines in the blood product.[2] The onset usually occurs 30 minutes to 2 hours after the transfusion is begun, and the patient also may have chills. If the reaction is mild and the patient has been multiply transfused and has had previous febrile reactions, it is not necessary to stop the transfusion, but it should be slowed. In more severe reactions, temporary interruption or discontinuation of the transfusion is indicated. If chills and back or abdominal pain accompany the reaction, the transfusion *must* be stopped immediately and the precautions for a hemolytic transfusion reaction taken. Treatment with acetaminophen and, for more severe reactions, corticosteroids is helpful; for future transfusions, pretreatment may prevent such reactions. If they continue to occur, leukodepleted blood should be used.

Allergic Reactions

The etiology of urticarial reactions usually is not clear, although they may be associated with antigens in donor plasma. Allergic donors' plasma also may result in an allergic reaction if the recipient is exposed to the corresponding antigen. Individuals who have congenital IgA deficiency have a 20% to 25% incidence of antibodies directed against IgA. These patients may develop severe anaphylactic reactions to any blood product containing plasma proteins. Anti-IgA antibodies also may develop in normal individuals and result in urticarial or anaphylactic reactions.[10] People who have repeated minor allergic reactions should be pretreated with an antihistamine or corticosteroids. Frozen washed RBCs may be effective and may be available from IgA-deficient donors. Urticarial reactions cannot be prevented by leukodepletion.

Transfusion-Transmitted Infections[1]

Routine screening of donors for antibodies to the human immunodeficiency virus (HIV) has been in effect in the United States since 1985, when 27 per 100,000 donations were found to be HIV positive. Currently it has been estimated that failure to detect HIV in a donor might occur in only 1 in 100,000 to 1 in 1 million donations. The greatest danger is posed by products containing pooled plasma that have not been treated for virus inactivation.[10]

Groups at risk for CMV infection have been discussed previously. Individuals who have been infected carry the virus in their leukocytes indefinitely. In a normal recipient, infection is asymptomatic or associated with a mild, mononucleosis-like illness 3 to 4 weeks after transfusion. Epstein-Barr virus (EBV) also can be transmitted by transfusion but has much less clinical significance than CMV.

Routine screening of blood donors for hepatitis B has reduced the incidence to 1 in 10,000 units (usually due to donation during the incubation period). In the United States, donor blood has been tested for antibody to hepatitis C virus since 1990. This agent previously was the major cause (90%) of non-A, non-B transfusion-associated hepatitis.[7]

Malaria and babesiosis also can be transmitted by contaminated blood. The latter resembles malaria and is a problem only for patients who have undergone a splenectomy or who are immunocompromised. Bacterial contamination of blood is quite rare but most often is associated with transfusion of platelets.

REFERENCES

1. Barker LF, Dodd RY: Viral hepatitis, acquired immunodeficiency syndrome, and other infections transmitted by transfusion. In Petz LD, Swisher SN, editors: *Clinical practice of transfusion medicine,* ed 2, New York, 1989, Churchill Livingstone.
2. Brand A: Passenger leukocytes, cytokines, and transfusion reactions, *N Engl J Med* 331:670, 1994.
3. Breiter SN, Luban NLC: Transfusion formulas. In Kasprisin DO, Luban NLC, editors: *Pediatric transfusion medicine,* vol 2, Boca Raton, Fla, 1987, CRC Press.
4. DePalma L, Luban NLC: Autologous blood transfusion in pediatrics, *Pediatrics* 85:125, 1990.
5. Dutcher JP: Granulocyte transfusion therapy in patients with malignancy. In Dutcher JP, editor: *Modern transfusion therapy,* Boca Raton, Fla, 1990, CRC Press.
6. Holland PV: The diagnosis and management of transfusion reactions and other adverse effects of transfusion. In Petz LD, Swisher SN, editors: *Clinical practice of transfusion medicine,* ed 2, New York, 1989, Churchill Livingstone.
7. Kevy SV: Red cell transfusion. In Nathan DG, Oski FA, editors: *Hematology of infancy and childhood,* ed 4, vol 2, Philadelphia, 1993, WB Saunders.
8. Lane TA et al: Leukocyte reduction in blood component therapy, *Ann Intern Med* 117:151, 1992.
9. McMilin KD, Johnson RL: Transfusion-associated graft-versus-host disease, *Trans Med Rev* 7:37, 1993.
10. Mollison PL, Engelfriet CP, Contreras M: *Blood transfusion in clinical medicine,* ed 9, Oxford, 1993, Blackwell.
11. Nugent DJ: Platelet transfusion. In Nathan DG, Oski FA, editors: *Hematology of infancy and childhood,* ed 4, vol 2, Philadelphia, 1993, WB Saunders.
12. Pisciotto P: Irradiated blood. In Kasprisin DO, Luban NLC, editors: *Pediatric transfusion medicine,* vol 2, Boca Raton, Fla, 1987, CRC Press.
13. Starkey JM et al: Markers for transfusion-transmitted disease in different groups of blood donors, *JAMA* 262:3452, 1989.
14. Wilson SM, Levitt JS, Strauss RG, editors: *Improving transfusion practice for pediatric patients,* Arlington, Va, 1991, American Association of Blood Banks.
15. Perioperative red cell transfusion, National Institutes of Health Consensus Development Conference Statement, vol 7, June 27-29, 1988.

30 Clinical Pharmacology

Therese K. Schmalbach

Pharmacology is the field of science concerned with the physiological effects of organic substances that are foreign to the body (xenobiotics). This discipline encompasses the design, testing, clinical application, and biochemistry of drugs, as well as their metabolism, excretion, and toxicity and the methods for monitoring drug levels in patients. Pediatric pharmacology applies these scientific principles to the pediatric patient.

The recognition of pharmacological differences in the pediatric population was dramatized by several tragedies in the 1950s. Administration of accepted doses of chloramphenicol to premature infants resulted in vascular collapse — the "gray baby syndrome." Subsequent investigation revealed that because of their incompletely developed renal and hepatic systems, newborns, especially premature infants, are unable to metabolize and excrete chloramphenicol as rapidly as are adults. Thus the use of modified adult dose regimens resulted in the accumulation of lethal levels of the drug.[27] Similarly the treatment of suspected neonatal sepsis with sulfisoxazole caused death from kernicterus because this drug binds to albumin, displacing bilirubin.[22] The epidemic of phocomelia following the widespread use of thalidomide emphasized the risk maternal drug use poses to the developing fetus.

One consequence of these disasters is the extensive preclinical and clinical drug testing regulations currently enforced by the U.S. Food and Drug Administration (FDA). The FDA regulations require data demonstrating the safety and efficacy of a medication before approval of its use; however, federal regulations did not routinely require information regarding the use of a new drug in children. The complex ethical and medicolegal issues of experimentation on children have hindered pediatric experimentation and the development of new pediatric drug regimens.[26] Theoretically this results in restricting potentially efficacious therapy. It has been estimated that 75% of the drugs marketed in the United States do not carry the FDA indication for pediatric use.[5] In actuality children are receiving medication that is not labeled for pediatric use; one study revealed that 7% of the drugs prescribed for pediatric inpatients during a single 19-day period were not designated specifically for use in the pediatric population.[24]

The hazards of this situation are recognized. The American Academy of Pediatrics has published guidelines for the ethical conduct of drug studies among children and encourages such investigation.[5] More recent FDA rules clarify how data from adequate and well-controlled trials performed in adult populations may be applied to support the use of a drug in the pediatric population (defined as including children from birth to 16 years of age). Data from rigorously conducted adult trials together with other information supporting pediatric use, such as pharmacokinetic, pharmacodynamic, and safety data, may be used to support approved use of the product for children. Labeling for pediatric use also may be based on controlled trials in the pediatric population. This new rule is intended to provide more information about pediatric use, thereby providing the practitioner with more reliable information for prescribing to the pediatric population. Additionally, if a drug's label carries information for prescribing to the pediatric age group, any limitations of the trials performed (e.g., studies not carried out in patients below the age of 2 years), specific hazards for a pediatric subgroup, or lack of the establishment of substantial evidence to support a pediatric indication must be provided. Finally the agency has reserved the right to determine that pediatric studies are needed before or after approval for a new drug.[1] Thus the objective of the new ruling is to provide practitioners with more pediatric dosing information while ensuring the safe introduction of new drugs for this age group.

The additional information will result in safer and more efficacious drug therapy, both by increasing pediatricians' armamentarium of drugs and by clarifying proper doses and dosing regimens for our patients. As the chloramphenicol experience illustrated, adult drug doses cannot be extrapolated routinely to children. Average pediatric doses are calculated most accurately on the child's body surface area or weight, and drug doses frequently may need to be adjusted to the individual's unique response and medical condition. Thus individualization of drug doses often is required to achieve the desired therapeutic response. An understanding of the basic principles of pharmacology therefore is imperative for safe and effective pediatric prescribing practices.

DRUG DISPOSITION

The production of a physiological response requires that a therapeutic concentration of a drug or its active metabolite be present at its site of action. Physiochemical characteristics of the drug, such as lipid solubility, the degree of ionization at physiological pH, the molecular weight (i.e., size) of the drug, and the affinity to biological proteins, will affect the movement of the drug through body membranes. However, these are properties of the drug itself and will not vary significantly among patients.

Pharmacokinetic parameters play an integral role in the therapeutic or toxic effects of drugs; growth and maturation are associated with numerous physiological changes that influence drug handling. Thus the pediatrician is confronted with a variety of patients who have differing physiological capabilities and medicinal needs. An understanding of basic pharmacokinetics will optimize drug therapy and increase the safety with which drugs are used. Four pharmacokinetic factors — absorption, distribution, metabolism, and excretion — can be used to describe the movement of a drug through the body.

ABSORPTION

One primary consideration of drug therapy is absorption, the translocation of a drug from its site of administration into the circulation. This process depends on the physical and chemical properties of the individual drug, as previously mentioned, and on the route of administration. The term *bioavailability* refers to the rate and extent of absorption of a drug. Many drugs have incomplete bioavailability when given orally. The absolute bioavailability of a drug is determined by administering the drug to the same individual orally and intravenously, on two separate occasions. The serum or plasma concentration of the drug is measured after each administration. The ratio of the area under the serum or plasma concentration curve from time zero to infinity by both routes defines the absolute bioavailability of the oral dosage.

This can range from zero, in the case of a drug that does not reach the systemic circulation at all following oral dosing, to 1 for a drug that has complete bioavailability and completely enters the circulation. Proportionately higher doses must be given orally for drugs that have a bioavailability significantly less than 1.[10] Because it is a measure of the amount of the drug that is actually absorbed and available to interact with drug receptors, the principle of bioavailability allows the comparison of different pharmaceutical formulations and dosages of the active compound. The peak plasma concentration of a drug depends on the rate and extent of absorption. The time required to reach this peak concentration depends only on the rate of absorption.[12]

A drug's route of administration affects its bioavailability. Commonly the intravenous (IV) route is used for efficient and controlled (e.g., either rapid or slow) delivery of a medication directly into the circulation. This method eliminates the absorptive process common to other methods of drug administration and allows the provider to stop or start drug delivery immediately. However, other factors may affect the bioavailability of drugs administered intravenously. The absorption of medication onto filter surfaces of the infusion apparatus may decrease the dose that the patient receives. The IV flow rate and the volume of drug suspension affect blood levels of the drug. This can be especially problematic with pediatric patients, for whom IV fluid rates on the order of a few milliliters per hour are common. For example, injection of a drug at a site in the infusion line somewhat removed from the patient may result in approximately 5 to 10 ml of intervening fluid volume. At an infusion rate of 3 ml/hr, it takes approximately 1.7 to 3.3 hours before the drug actually begins to reach the patient. A quick bolus injection followed by a "flush" will deliver the entire dose to the patient, resulting in higher peak blood levels rapidly. Typically the larger the volume of the drug solution, the longer the administration time. In a fluid-restricted patient or in an infant receiving minimal fluids, administration of numerous medications, each of which is suspended in a certain volume of fluid, may provide for the total daily fluid requirement.[14] Thus intravenous administration of drugs circumvents the absorptive process, but the bioavailability of a drug may still be affected by the rate of infusion and the quantity of drug actually delivered to the patient.[15,19]

Pediatric patients receive many drugs orally. Although the stomach is not the major site of drug absorption, the rich blood supply, the potential for prolonged contact of a drug with the gastric epithelium, and the relatively large epithelial surface facilitate the entry of drugs into the circulation. The changing pattern of gastric acidity, the relatively slow gastric emptying time seen in neonates and premature infants, and the nearly continuous presence of milk in the stomach of formula-fed babies all affect the gastric absorption of medication.[15,18]

The major site of drug absorption is the small intestine because of its large surface area and the presence of specialized absorptive cells within this organ. The intestinal motility, enzymatic activity, permeability and maturation of the mucosal membrane, the ileal bile salt pool, bacterial flora, and the presence and type of food in the gastrointestinal (GI) tract play a role in drug absorption and may alter the dose requirement, efficacy, and toxicity of the drug. In addition, certain common childhood diseases such as diarrhea of viral, bacterial, or genetic origins (e.g., cystic fibrosis or celiac disease) affect the intestinal absorption of drugs.[7,15]

Intramuscular absorption in neonates, infants, and young children may be unpredictable because of vasomotor instability, decreased muscle tone and contraction, and diminished muscle oxygenation.[3,18] The absorption of a topically applied medication is related inversely to the thickness of the stratum corneum and related directly to hydration of the skin and therefore is increased in the newborn and young infant.[18] The ratio of surface area to body weight in the full-term neonate is much greater than that of an adult. If a newborn received the same percutaneous dose of a medication as an adult, the systemic availability per kilogram of body weight would be approximately 2.7 times greater in the neonate.[3] Tissue perfusion also is an important variable affecting the absorption of a medication applied subcutaneously, intramuscularly, or topically; absorption from these sites may be decreased because of circulatory insufficiency.

Medication administered per rectum (PR) may be absorbed very rapidly, depending on the formulation of the compound. This has been exploited clinically in several instances, such as in the use of diazepam PR to suppress seizure activity rapidly or in the administration of antiemetics to patients who have nausea and vomiting. The disadvantages of this method of administration include a lack of patient acceptability, an interruption of absorption by defecation, and the much smaller absorptive surface area of the rectum compared with that of the small intestine.[6]

Not all medications require absorption for activity. Some drugs, such as cholestyramine or bulk laxatives, are formulated specifically to remain within the GI tract with little or none of the drug entering the general circulation.

DISTRIBUTION

After absorption into the bloodstream drugs are distributed to the body tissues. The specific distribution of a drug within the body can be determined only by direct tissue analysis. However, relating the concentration of the drug in the plasma to its concentration in the remaining areas of the body (the volume of distribution [V_d]) provides some insight into drug distribution. The V_d is the hypothetical fluid space needed to contain the total body store of a drug if the concentration throughout the whole body equals that measured in the plasma. V_d is calculated by dividing the total amount of drug

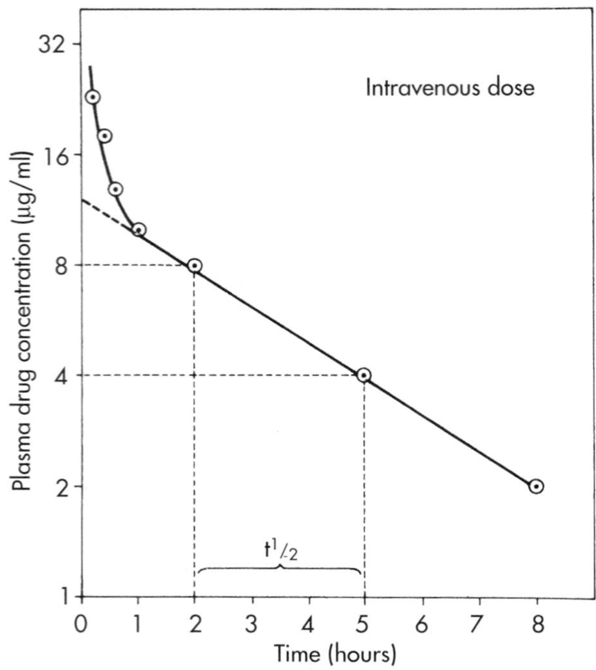

FIG. 30-1 Fundamental pharmacokinetic relationships for single doses of drugs. A drug (500 mg) is administered intravenously, and plasma samples are obtained for determination of drug concentration. The concentration falls rapidly initially, as distribution occurs. First-order elimination kinetics follows. Extrapolation of this line indicates a hypothetical plasma concentration of 12 µg/ml at zero time. The volume of distribution (V_d) is thus 500/0.012, or 41.7 L. The half-time of drug elimination (when the plasma concentration is 6 µg/ml) is estimated to be 3 hours.

(Modified from Goodman LS, Gilman A: *The pharmacological basis of therapeutics*, ed 6, New York, 1980, Macmillan.)

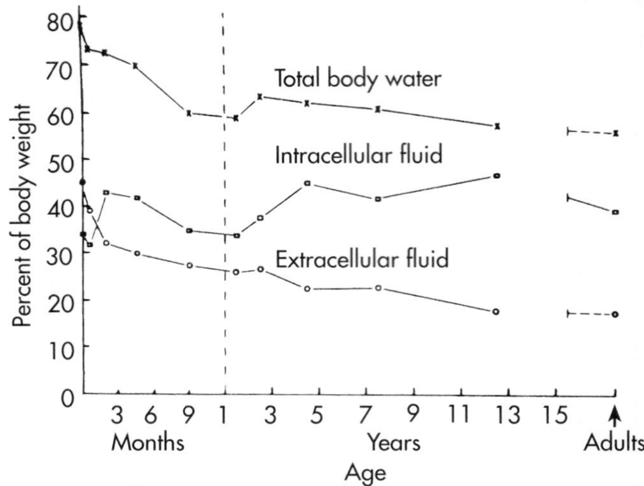

FIG. 30-2 Developmental changes in total body water, intracellular water, and extracellular water in infants and children. The changes are expressed as percentages of body weight.

(From Rane A, Wilson JT: *Clin Pharmacokinet* 1:2, 1976; data from Friis-Hansen B: *Pediatrics* 28:169, 1961.)

in the body by the plasma concentration that would exist, assuming instant equilibration, at time zero following a bolus intravenous injection (Fig. 30-1).

$$V_d \text{ (liters)} = \frac{\text{Total drug in body (mg)}}{\text{Plasma concentration (mg/L)}}$$

Because the V_d often exceeds the plasma volume it is also referred to as the *apparent volume of distribution*. The larger the V_d, the greater the tissue concentration of the drug.[3,7] The concept of the V_d is useful in calculating drug doses (see further discussion under Drug Dosing Regimens) and in comparing different age groups or disease states in which intrinsic patient variables alter the distribution of drug.

One variable that affects drug distribution is the change in the relative volumes of the water constituting the body mass (Fig. 30-2). Neonates have a much higher proportion of body mass in the form of water (85% in premature infants, 75% in full-term infants) than does the older child (59% at 1 year of age) or adult (55%). The ratio of extracellular to intracellular water also is higher in neonates, infants, and children. Total body water declines rapidly during the first year of life, and adult levels are reached by 12 years of age.[7] Higher doses of drugs, on a per kilogram of body weight basis, that distribute into the extracellular fluid must be given to infants and children to achieve plasma and tissue concentrations comparable to adult concentrations.[3]

The relative amount of adipose tissue also fluctuates during growth. At birth adipose tissue makes up 10% to 15% of the total body mass and at 1 year of age accounts for 20% to 25% of body weight. This percentage declines between 1 and 2 years of age with the onset of walking and the development of greater muscle mass and remains unchanged until puberty. In girls there is a rather sudden increase in adipose tissue at puberty; the increase is less prominent in boys, in whom growth of muscle and skeletal mass predominate.[15]

Another factor affecting the V_d of a drug is the affinity of the drug for plasma proteins. The degree of protein binding is related inversely to the V_d because the large protein-drug complexes do not leave the vascular compartment readily. Renal clearance of the drug is decreased because only free drug is filtered at the glomerulus. Protein binding also increases the half-life of the drug (i.e., the time required for the concentration of drug in the plasma to decline to half the original level). The bound complexes slowly dissociate, resulting in the prolonged release of free drug into the circulation.[15]

Albumin is the protein primarily responsible for binding acidic drugs (e.g., salicylate, phenobarbital), and basic drugs are bound by a variety of plasma proteins such as lipoproteins, alpha-1-acid glycoproteins, and beta-globulins. In addition to diminished levels, neonatal albumin also exhibits a decreased affinity for many drugs (e.g., phenytoin). The full plasma-protein levels are not reached until approximately the end of the first year of life.[7]

One additional variable affecting protein binding is competition of endogenous molecules for binding sites. Endogenous molecules may displace drugs from binding sites, creating a transient rise in free drug and intensifying the pharmacological response. This effect is transient because the free drug is excreted, restoring a steady-state level. Alternatively the drug may displace an endogenous molecule.[3] In the case of sulfisoxazole, bilirubin is displaced, increasing the risk of kernicterus.[22]

Cardiac output, blood flow to individual organs and tissues, variations in pH, and the acid-base balance all influence the distribution of drugs within the body. These factors are variable during the first days of life and also may vary depending on the medical condition of the patient.[18]

In summary, the V_d is influenced by the blood volume, the tissue volume and perfusion, the fraction of unbound drug in the blood, and the fraction of unbound drug in body tissues. For example, the aminoglycoside antibiotics are highly water soluble, exhibit poor penetration of lipid membranes, and have minimum tissue and protein-binding. The mean V_d is 0.25 to 0.45 L/kg for children and 0.50 L/kg in neonates, reflecting the extracellular fluid (ECF) volume. Disease states that increase the ECF volume (e.g., ascites) increase the distribution of these drugs. In contrast, theophylline is partially lipid and water soluble and is approximately 60% protein bound. Theophylline's V_d is greater in newborns because of decreased protein binding and increased total body water than in children or adults (0.6 to 0.9 L/kg versus 0.3 to 0.7 L/kg, respectively).[12]

DRUG METABOLISM

Metabolism and excretion are the primary mechanisms of drug elimination. The relatively high lipophilicity of most drugs inhibits their elimination in the unchanged form because intestinal and renal reabsorption are very efficient for lipid-soluble compounds. Renal excretion is facilitated by the biotransformation of drugs into more water-soluble metabolites. Lipophilic compounds generally are less toxic, although also usually less pharmacologically active, so metabolism also has been described as drug detoxification.[15] However, biotransformation reactions often can activate a xenobiotic (drug or poison), initiating or potentiating physiological responses to the compound.

The liver is quantitatively the most important organ for drug metabolism, although the kidneys, gut, and skin possess a variety of drug-metabolizing functions.[15] Uptake of the drug is the first step in hepatic biotransformation. Drugs are delivered to the liver through the portal vein following gastric or intestinal absorption. A drug that is exposed to hepatic metabolism before reaching the general circulation is subject to substantial hepatic biotransformation, and the resulting moiety that enters the systemic circulation may be predominantly in the form of inactive metabolites. Thus this initial "pass" through the liver may result in a drug that is substantially inactivated, causing a significant decrease in the pharmacologically active species. This process is known as the *first-pass effect*. Lidocaine, propranolol, meperidine, and morphine are drugs subject to substantial first-pass effects.[17]

After delivery to the liver, carrier proteins transport the drug into the hepatic cell. The neonate has a lower concentration of transport proteins than does the adult.[1,5,10] For example, the level of ligandin, a basic protein that binds organic anions and bilirubin, is low at birth but reaches adult levels by 5 to 10 days of age.[3]

Once the drug is within the cell it may be biotransformed by one or more of the phase I reactions, which may in turn be followed by a phase II reaction. Phase I reactions change a drug into a more active metabolite (e.g., chloramphenicol succinate to chloramphenicol) or into an equally active, less active, or inactive metabolite; phase II reactions generally result in inactive products. Biotransformation also may result in the transformation of a drug into a metabolite whose activity qualitatively differs from that of the parent compound.[3,15] For example in neonates theophylline is methylated to caffeine; in older children and adults this elimination pathway is insignificant.

Phase I reactions include oxidation, reduction, hydrolysis, and hydroxylation. The chemical structure, configuration, and presence of functional groups determine the type of reaction a particular drug undergoes. The hepatic mixed-function oxidases (cytochrome P-450 and NADPH cytochrome C reductase) are responsible for most of the phase I reactions catalyzed by the human liver. Low levels of these enzymes also are present in the kidneys and lungs. Most phase I enzymes at gestation are present at low levels and remain low at birth, but the oxidative enzymes exhibit rapid postnatal maturation. At birth hepatic clearance of drugs is reduced, but within the first several weeks of life hepatic clearance equals or exceeds adult rates.[3] Drugs administered to the mother, either prepartum or during labor, may induce hepatic enzyme activity in the fetus or neonate. Examples of such drugs include phenytoin, phenobarbital, diazepam, and tricyclic antidepressants.[15]

Phase II reactions involve the combination of the drug with an endogenous molecule, thereby rendering the drug more water soluble and facilitating renal excretion. A relatively small number of such synthetic reactions are known in human beings. They include *conjugation* with glucuronide, glycine, glutathione, and sulfate, as well as *methylation* and *acetylation*.[3,15] Glucuronidation is depressed at birth and reaches adult levels by 3 years of age. Thus agents that are eliminated almost entirely by this pathway are potential toxins in neonates and infants because alternate pathways of metabolism are not available. In contrast sulfate conjugation is more efficient in neonates than in adults. In children acetaminophen is excreted predominantly through sulfate conjugation; in adults the glucuronide conjugate is the major metabolite.

Variations in biotransformation should not be assumed always to result in impaired drug elimination. Oral quinidine, for example, is cleared significantly faster by pediatric patients than by adults.[7]

EXCRETION

There are a variety of routes through which xenobiotics can be eliminated. Drugs may be excreted in the bile, feces, urine, or by exhalation through the lungs.[17]

Most drugs and their metabolites are excreted from the body by the kidneys. In the newborn the ratio of kidney weight to body mass is approximately twofold higher than in the adult. However, the organ is anatomically and functionally immature, and all aspects of renal function are reduced.[18]

Renal excretion depends on glomerular filtration, tubular reabsorption, and tubular secretion. At birth the glomerular filtration rate (GFR) is directly proportional to gestational age, and adult GFRs are not reached until 2.5 to 5 months of age.[3,7] This increase is most likely the result of the combination of increased cardiac output, decreased peripheral vascular resistance, increased mean arterial pressure, increased surface area for filtration, and increased membrane pore size.[1] In the preterm infant the GFR is further reduced, and the rate of increase in renal function lags behind that observed in the full-term neonate. Low clearance rates for aminoglycoside antibiotics and indomethacin, both of which depend on glomerular filtration for excretion, are common. For example, the administration of gentamicin according to guidelines established for full-term newborns resulted in extremely high plasma concentrations in premature neonates. Digoxin is another drug primarily eliminated by glomerular filtration. Renal clearance of digoxin is low in the neonate and increases progressively until it reaches adult levels by the first year of life.[7] However, glomerular function is more advanced than tubular function. This imbalance may persist until 6 months of age and is reflected in functional differences of secretion in the proximal tubular cells. Many drugs rely on either the organic anion or cation transport systems present in the proximal tubule for renal excretion (e.g., penicillins, sulfonamides, and furosemide).[3] Elimination of these drugs exhibits an age-related alteration, and adjustments in drug doses are essential to prevent toxicity.

Some factors that contribute to alterations in pharmacokinetics in infants and children are summarized in Table 30-1.

Table 30-1 Factors That May Contribute to Variations in Pharmacokinetics in Infants and Children

Parameter	Newborns	Older children
Absorption	↓ Intestinal motility	
	↓ Gastric acidity	
	Delayed intestinal enzyme development	
Distribution	Relative fat content, blood flow	Relative fat content, blood flow
	Alteration in body water compartments	Alteration in body water compartments
	↓ Serum albumin	
	Variations in albumin drug-binding capacity	
Metabolism	Enzyme immaturity	
Excretion	↓ Glomerular filtration rate	
	↓ Tubular function	

KINETICS OF DRUG ELIMINATION

Following drug administration, plasma levels are determined by the pharmacokinetic characteristics of the drug. The drug is absorbed and distributed into various tissues, and the amount of drug remaining in the body is determined by the rate of elimination. *Clearance* refers to the overall rate of drug removal and thus is the sum of the clearance of drug by various routes, including the liver, kidneys, lungs, and skin.[17] Clearance of a drug cannot exceed the rate of blood delivered to the clearing organ; the organ blood flow therefore sets an upper limit of clearance.[10] Clearance does not decrease significantly with age.[2] The total body clearance (TBC) is the volume of body fluid from which a drug is completely removed per unit time. It also may be thought of as the rate of drug removal per unit of plasma concentration and may be calculated by:

$$\text{TBC} = \text{K}(\text{V}_d)$$

where V_d is the volume of distribution and K is the elimination rate constant for a given drug.

It is simpler to consider drug disappearance following intravenous injection because other drug delivery modes may have prolonged absorption times.[9] Initially there is a rapid decrease in the plasma concentration as the drug distributes throughout the body (Fig. 30-3). As the drug is cleared, a slower decline ensues, reflecting the elimination of drug from the body. Most drugs are eliminated from the body following first-order kinetics — that is, a constant fraction of the drug in the plasma is eliminated per unit of time. This implies that the amount of drug eliminated per unit of time is proportional to the plasma drug concentration and gradually declines as the plasma concentration decreases. This relationship is depicted graphically in Fig. 30-3, *A*. Note that the rate of elimination of the drug (represented by a tangent to the curve) varies continuously depending on its concentration at any given time. The decline in plasma concentration is exponential, and the results usually are plotted on a semilogarithmic scale (Fig. 30-3, *B*). This representation demonstrates that a constant fraction of the drug in the plasma is eliminated per unit of time.[9]

Further analysis of the semilogarithmic graph yields useful information about the biological half-life, represented by $t_{1/2}$. The half-life is the time required for the concentration of drug in the plasma to decline to half its original level. Note that a constant fraction — that is, 50% — of the drug is eliminated per unit of time regardless of the plasma concentration. Half-life can be calculated as:

$$t_{1/2} = \frac{0.693\ (\text{V}_d)}{\text{Plasma clearance}}$$

The half-life reflects the efficiency of drug removal and is determined by the clearance as well as by the volume of distribution. A change in half-life may not necessarily reflect a change in clearance. For example, the clearance of kanamycin by neonates is approximately half that observed in adults. The half-life, however, is four times longer, reflecting the approximately twofold increase in the V_d in neonates.[17] Both parameters must be considered for proper dosing.

Some drugs are eliminated following zero-order kinetics. Elimination of these drugs occurs at a constant rate regardless of the plasma concentration; a constant amount (as opposed to a fraction, as with first-order kinetics) of the drug is eliminated per unit of time (see Fig. 30-4). The half-life, then, depends on the plasma concentration of the drug.

In some instances the elimination may follow zero-order kinetics because of saturation of the elimination processes. This is significant because ingestion or absorption of a drug at a rate exceeding the elimination can raise plasma drug concentrations, increasing the risk of toxicity. Ethanol, aspirin, and phenytoin all exhibit this phenomenon. At low doses elimination proceeds according to first-order kinetics. At high

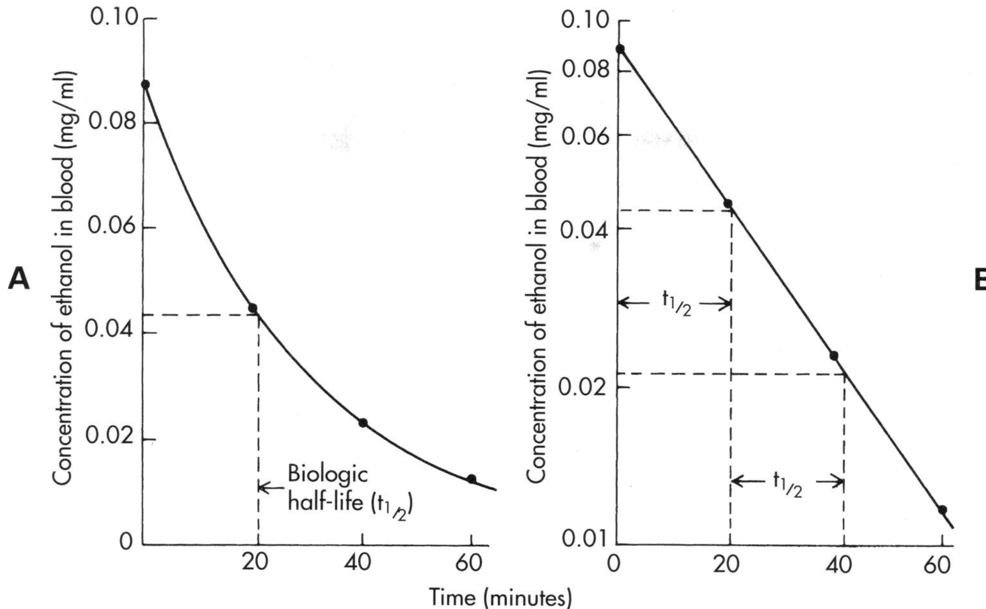

FIG. 30-3 First-order rate of elimination. Decline of ethanol content in blood after intravenous administration of a *small* dose to a dog. The ordinate reflects the concentration of ethanol in blood (mg/ml) on an arithmetic scale **(A)** and on a logarithmic scale **(B).** Biological half-time ($t_{1/2}$) is about 20 minutes on both scales.

(Modified from Marshall EK Jr, Frity WF: *J Pharmacol Exp Ther* 109:431, 1953.)

doses saturation of renal transport occurs, and elimination follows zero-order kinetics. Once saturation occurs, continued intake of the drug at a rate exceeding elimination will raise plasma concentrations to potentially toxic levels. The threshold at which first-order kinetics changes to zero-order kinetics varies in each individual. Once this threshold has been exceeded, small changes in drug dose may cause unanticipated increases in the plasma concentration.[9]

Drugs may enter organs or other body tissues in addition to distributing within the general circulation. These other areas are referred to as *compartments,* and the presence of drugs within these various compartments alters the kinetics of elimination. For example, the concentration of a drug within the plasma equilibrates with the concentration of drug in the second compartment. As elimination from the plasma occurs, the drug moves from the second compartment back into the plasma (from a higher concentration to a lower concentration). The rate of elimination is determined by the concentration of drug within the plasma, but the presence of drug within the second compartment provides a reservoir that maintains plasma levels of the drug, thereby prolonging elimination. To complicate matters further, reentry of the drug into the plasma may occur slowly, thus extending the half-life of the drug.[4] These factors affect the dose and frequency of drug administration.

PHARMACODYNAMICS

The term *pharmacodynamics* describes the action of drugs within the living system. At the cellular level xenobiotics may function outside the cell membrane, at the cell membrane, or at an intracellular organelle such as the nucleus.

Generally drugs that act outside the cell membrane react with some constituent of the extracellular fluid or within the gastrointestinal or renal tubular lumen. For example, antacids such as sodium bicarbonate act outside the cell by neutralizing gastric acidity directly. The chelators penicillamine and desferrioxamine also are effective without cellular interaction. Developmental differences are evident with the latter two drugs. Lead is deposited in the bone of children to a greater extent than in the bone of adults. Thus chelation of the lead in circulation may produce a greater efflux of lead from bone in children, aggravating the symptoms of plumbism.[15]

The volatile general anesthetics are examples of drugs that interact with cell membranes. There is evidence that these compounds act at specific areas of membranes and produce conformational changes in membrane proteins and lipids. Similarly the osmotic diuretics function by establishing an osmotic gradient between the two sides of a cell or cell membrane.[15]

The most common interaction between drugs and body tissues involves the reaction with a cellular receptor. The important features of a drug-receptor interaction include the specificity and affinity of a drug for certain receptors, the reversibility of the interaction, and the proximity of the drug to the receptor.

The affinity and concentration of receptors are not static but can be modulated by the ligand. The affinity of insulin for its receptor varies inversely with the number of receptors occupied, a process known as *negative cooperativity.* Hyperinsulinemia may decrease or "downregulate" the receptor concentration at the cell surface. Downregulation of receptors may explain tachyphylaxis, the phenomenon of a de-

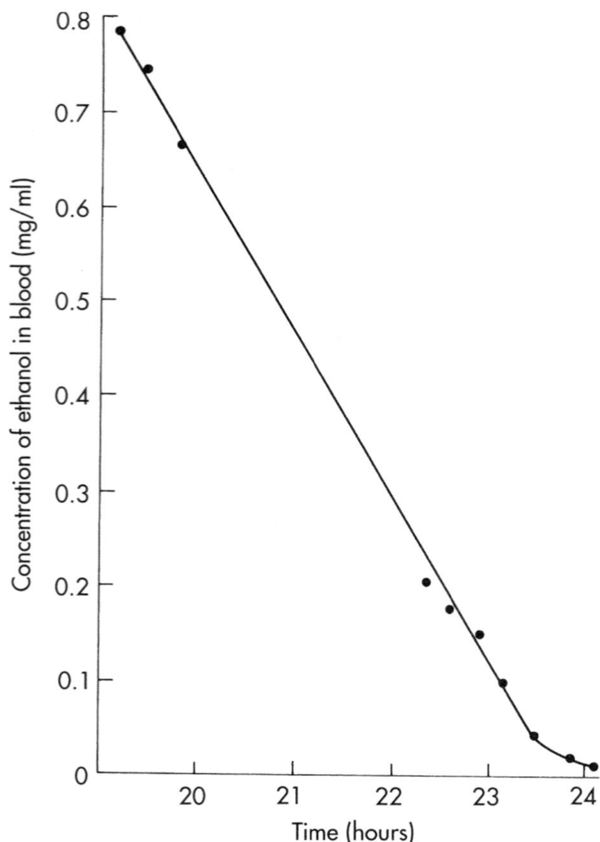

FIG. 30-4 Zero-order of elimination. Curve illustrating decline of ethanol content in blood after intravenous administration of a *large* dose to a dog. The ordinate is concentration of ethanol in the blood (mg/ml) on an *arithmetic* scale. The plotted data show the change from zero-order to first-order kinetics when low concentrations are reached between 23 and 24 hours after administration.

(From Marshall EK Jr, Frity WF: *J Pharmacol Exp Ther* 109:431, 1953.

creased physiological response to a drug over time. "Upregulation" of receptors occurs when the receptor concentration increases in the presence of low levels of ligand.[15]

Most of the developmental studies of receptor levels and function have been performed in animals, and careful interpretation of these data is necessary. However, age-related modulation of receptor sites has been reported. The binding of insulin has been observed to be greater in neonates than in adults. The larger digoxin doses required by neonates can be partially explained by receptor differences. Digoxin receptor sites are twice as numerous in the neonate per unit of tissue than in the adult, but the receptor affinity for digoxin is less in the neonate. Thus higher doses of digoxin are required to achieve physiological effects comparable to those in adults.[7,15]

Pharmacological effects of drugs can be altered by the interaction between two or more drugs. Pharmaceutical incompatibility is one of the simpler types of drug interactions. Physiochemical properties of two or more drugs (or their excipients) or of a drug and the infusion fluid may result in a diminished or absent therapeutic effect. Some incompatibilities are obvious, such as the precipitation of a compound in the infusion fluid (e.g., mixing amphotericin B with amikacin sulfate). Others may not be easily visualized, such as the decomposition of ampicillin and gentamicin sulfate when combined.[28]

Drug interactions can alter absorption by altering either the amount of drug absorbed or the relative rates of absorption. Antacids containing polyvalent cations chelate tetracyclines, forming an insoluble, inactive, and nonabsorbable complex. Alterations in the pH, typically by antacids, also can affect drug delivery. The concomitant administration of an antacid with an enteric-coated preparation can cause undesired side effects; the enteric-coated drug begins to dissolve in the elevated gastric pH produced by the antacid.[25,28] The administration of drugs that affect gastrointestinal motility also has been observed to affect the absorption of other, concomitantly administered drugs. However, many of the effects that have been described are of little clinical significance because of the large therapeutic indices and rapid absorption of most drugs. The profound effect of opioids on gastric emptying may delay absorption significantly, resulting in a clinically relevant change in therapeutic effect of concomitantly administered agents (e.g., in the postoperative patient).[11]

Administration of two or more drugs that compete for protein-binding sites may increase, decrease, or have no effect on the amount of drug at the receptor site. The concomitant administration of methotrexate with either aspirin or sulfisoxazole, which increases the displacement of methotrexate from its binding site, can significantly potentiate toxicity because of elevated levels of methotrexate.[28]

Drug interaction at receptor sites is another area of clinical significance. Administration of diuretics can cause hypokalemia, which in turn may induce digitalis toxicity. It is proposed that digitalis acts by inhibiting the enzyme regulating the sodium potassium pump. If extracellular potassium is decreased, more digitalis binds to this enzyme, lowering the amount of potassium entering the myocardial cell. Myocardial contractility therefore is increased, and arrhythmias can occur.[28]

The induction or inhibition of metabolic enzymes by one drug can significantly affect concomitantly administered drugs. A toxic reaction to phenytoin has been reported as a result of the inhibition of metabolism by isoniazid. The induction of hepatic enzymes has been exploited by clinicians, as previously mentioned, to speed excretion.[15,28]

Renal excretion of drugs depends on the net effect of glomerular filtration, tubular secretion, and tubular reabsorption. Glomerular filtration is not altered markedly by other drugs. Tubular secretion can be altered by drug interactions, a fact that has been used to therapeutic advantage. The use of probenecid to inhibit tubular secretion of penicillin is well known. Manipulating tubular reabsorption also has clinical significance. For example, alkalinizing the urine prevents the reabsorption of weak acids, such as phenobarbital and aspirin, and has been used in the treatment of overdoses with these medications.[25,28]

Drug interactions can be potentially hazardous *or* can increase the therapeutic efficacy of drugs. The number of possible drug interactions has resulted in the publication of lists of potentially hazardous drug combinations. More recently, computer programs exist that can perform similar functions. Drug interactions are less common in the pediatric population, because few patients receive several drugs, but such interactions still pose a risk that the informed physician can easily prevent.

PHARMACOGENETICS

Pharmacogenetics identifies the part that heredity plays in clinically significant variations in drug response. This science is the study of inherited traits that cause atypical responses to xenobiotics. Generally, genetic variation has been revealed after observations of significant intersubject variability in drug response during early clinical trials of new compounds. These differences can result in accumulation of the parent compound, reduced formation of an active metabolite, accumulation of an active metabolite, or accumulation of both the parent drug and an active metabolite. Many of the pharmacogenetic disorders that have been characterized are at the level of drug metabolism. Generally, adverse reactions to drugs are more frequent in patients who are poor metabolizers, but if the xenobiotic forms an active metabolite, risks are greater for patients who exhibit extensive metabolism; poor metabolizers may show decreased therapeutic efficacy.[16]

Genetic variation of N-acetylation is one of the most widely recognized pharmacogenetic differences of drug metabolism. Approximately 50% of Caucasians are slow acetylators and achieve a higher parent drug blood concentration after typical therapeutic doses of acetylated drugs such as isoniazid, sulfamethazine, or procainamide. Toxic effects of elevated levels can include sulfasalazine-induced hemolysis and hydrazine-induced peripheral neuropathy. One of the best characterized genetic polymorphisms is that associated with the debrisoquine and sparteine metabolism. This difference in a cytochrome P-450 enzyme has the potential to affect a large number of drugs, including beta-blockers, antiarrhythmics, tricyclic antidepressants, and neuroleptics, among others. There can be as much as a ten- to twentyfold difference in the disposition of some of these xenobiotics.[16] Several drugs can induce hemolysis of red blood cells in patients who have glucose-6-phosphate dehydrogenase deficiency, one of the commonest hereditary enzymatic abnormalities.[15,28]

The clinician usually handles pharmacogenetic variation in the elimination of drugs by recognizing that such variation exists and by the use of therapeutic drug monitoring. In practical terms the cause of the variation often is not important, but the appropriate individualization of the drug dose is imperative. The example of succinylcholine sensitivity, however, exemplifies one extreme genetic variability. Shortly after use of this drug became widespread, extreme sensitivity to succinylcholine was observed in some patients, and several deaths associated with its use were reported. The rapid hydrolysis of succinylcholine by pseudocholinesterase typically limits the duration of action of this drug to 2 to 3 minutes. However, genetically inherited variants of this enzyme are responsible for prolonging the half-life of succinylcholine, thereby increasing the pharmacological action of the drug.

Awareness of pharmacogenetic differences in drug disposition enables the astute clinician to maximize the therapeutic benefit of medications and minimize patient risk.

DRUG-DOSING REGIMENS

The goal of drug therapy is to produce the desired pharmacological response. This requires administration of the proper type and amount of drug at an appropriate frequency. In many cases there is a need to individualize therapy by altering the amount of drug administered, the frequency of doses, and the route of administration. For most drugs there is a plasma concentration below which subtherapeutic responses occur. Higher concentrations of the drug elicit the desired therapeutic effect, and still higher concentrations may result in adverse side effects. The goal of drug-dosing regimens is to maintain the plasma concentration of the drug within the therapeutic range.[15]

Several factors must be considered in selecting the appropriate drug dose. The condition being treated and any other potentially complicating medical conditions are of foremost importance. As previously discussed, other drugs that the patient may be taking can influence the current therapy. The child's age, size, and development, as well as the status of organs responsible for drug elimination, are important in the pharmacokinetics of the medication.

Many empirical rules and formulas have been published for pediatric drug dosing, reflecting the complexity of prescribing. The most acceptable general guide to drug dosing in children is based on the child's body surface area. Nomograms are available in several references, along with tables of recommended drug doses.[8,15,20,23]

In some situations the observed response is used readily as a therapeutic end point (e.g., as with antihypertensives and diuretics); for other drugs such an objective response is not readily available. Monitoring drug plasma levels may facilitate the modification of therapeutic regimens.[17] This therapeutic monitoring can be very useful if a strong correlation exists between the plasma concentration of a drug and its pharmacological effect. A therapeutic level can be determined within which the majority of patients will have the desired therapeutic response without sustaining undesired side effects. Above this range the risk of adverse reactions increases, and below this range optimum therapy is not achieved.[15] The method of drug analysis must be reliable and relatively rapid for effective drug monitoring. Therapeutic monitoring is typically used with drugs that exhibit a low therapeutic index — that is, the ratio of the plasma concentration providing therapeutic effects to that causing toxicity is low.

To use this method of determining an effective drug dose, peak plasma drug concentrations are obtained shortly after infusion of the medication. However, pharmacokinetic parameters of the individual drug must be considered when obtaining drug levels. If the peak plasma level is subtherapeutic, the dose is increased. Trough levels (or minimum plasma concentrations) typically occur immediately before the subsequent dose.[15] Low trough levels signal a need either to increase the dose, increase the frequency of drug administration, or both to maintain the plasma concentration within the therapeutic range.

Many clinical situations require continuous drug administration over a period of time. In this situation plasma drug levels are determined by the efficiency rather than the rate of drug elimination. Administration of a drug either by continuous infusion, which provides a smooth plasma level-time curve, or by intermittent dosing, which yields a sawtooth profile, results in drug accumulation until a steady-state level is reached (Fig. 30-5). The ultimate average steady-state concentration achieved with either dosing pattern is directly proportional to the dosage rate (D/τ, where *D* represents dose and τ represents time) and inversely related to the efficiency of the systemic clearance (i.e., the drug removal from the plasma). Thus,

$$\text{Concentration steady state} = \frac{\text{Dosage rate}}{\text{Plasma clearance}}, \textit{ or}$$
$$= \frac{D/\tau}{\text{Systemic clearance}}$$

Individual variability in systemic clearance requires modification of the dosing rate to provide the desired steady-state plasma level; therefore if systemic clearance is altered because of disease or developmental maturation, an inversely proportional change in the steady-state level results. For example, the faster elimination of theophylline observed in children necessitates more frequent dosing.[15]

Although the plasma elimination half-life is not useful in individualizing therapy, it is important in determining the length of time required to achieve steady state or to change from one steady-state level to another. Approximately four to five half-lives are required to attain a steady-state condition after beginning or altering the dose rate. The half-life also is used in determining the frequency of drug administration following an intermittent, repetitive regimen. For any given steady-state plasma level, the fluctuations between the peak and trough levels depend on the ratio of the half-life to the dosage interval. The smaller the dosage interval relative to the half-life, the smaller the fluctuations. Large doses given at greater intervals cause greater fluctuations in the plasma level and increase the risk of potentially toxic drug levels occurring soon after drug administration. Subtherapeutic levels may occur at the end of these long dosing intervals.[15]

In some situations it may be undesirable to wait for drug accumulation to reach therapeutic levels, especially if the drug's half-life is prolonged. In this case a loading dose may be administered to achieve the desired plasma level and pharmacological response immediately. The loading dose is larger than the usual maintenance dose and hence carries a risk of toxicity. The loading dose may be divided and given as multiple doses over a short period of time to avoid this risk. The size of the loading dose depends on the desired plasma level and the volume of distribution of the drug.

$$\text{Loading dose (mg/kg)} = V_d \text{ (L/kg)} \times \text{Desired drug concentration (mg/L)}$$

Maintenance doses then are instituted to keep the plasma level within the therapeutic range. The maintenance dose interval is determined primarily by the drug's half-life, as previously discussed.[15]

The plasma concentration of drugs, and therefore the therapeutic efficacy, can be affected by the drug formulation, time of sampling, absorption, metabolism, and patient compliance.

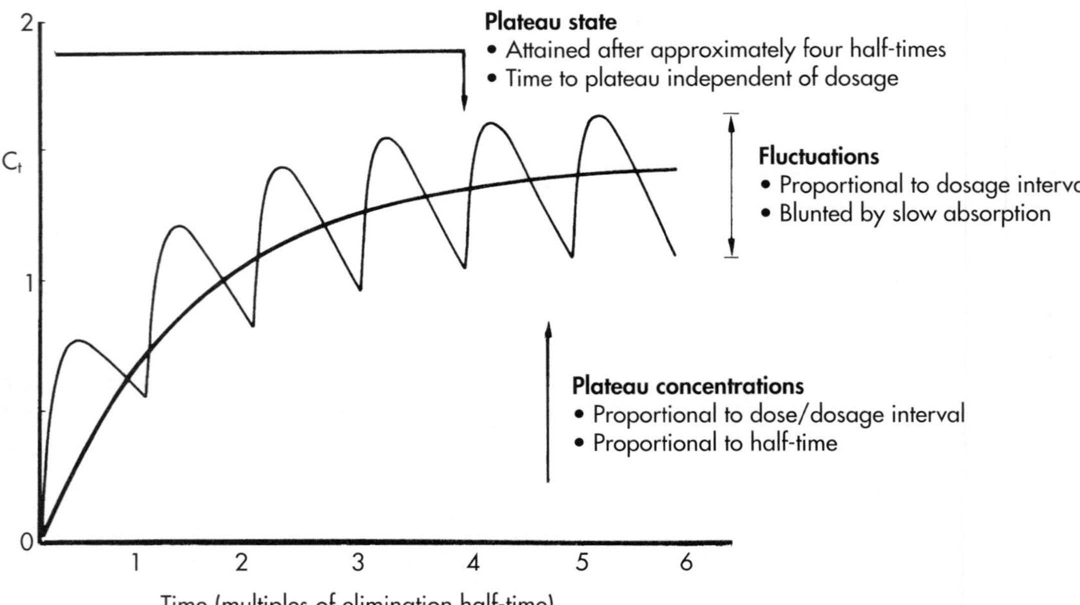

FIG. 30-5 Fundamental pharmacokinetic relationships for repeated administration of drugs. The light fluctuating line represents the pattern of drug accumulation during repeated administration of a drug as intervals equal to its elimination half-time. The heavy nonfluctuating line depicts the pattern during administration of equivalent dosage by continuous IV infusion. C_t, Concentration of a drug in plasma at time t.

(From Goodman LS, Gilman A: *The pharmacological basis of therapeutics,* ed 6, New York, 1980, Macmillan.)

Compliance can adversely affect even the most optimum drug regimen. It is estimated that the noncompliance rate in the pediatric clinic population is approximately 50%, with a range from 20% to 80%[28]; noncompliance rates in private practices are slightly lower.[21] Compliance can be improved by minimizing the number of drugs prescribed, by prescribing a palatable form of the drug that is easy to administer, and by simplifying drug regimens.

Whenever possible the frequency of drug administration should be amenable to the family's regular schedule. In addition, careful instructions to the patient and parent and a positive interaction among the health care providers and the parents and patient increase compliance.[21] Sufficient amounts of the medication should be prescribed for treatment so that no significant amount will be left after therapy is completed, and parents should be instructed to discard any surplus medication. Parent and patient perception of the therapy, method, and goals of treatment critically affect the outcome, and the time the pediatrician spends understanding these perceptions and educating the parents and patient will be amply rewarded. (See Chapter 12, Compliance with Pediatric Health Care Recommendations, for further discussions of compliance.)

Pediatric dosing can be complicated by the very individualization that promotes efficacy and that is required by the diverse age range being treated. Many pediatric dosing regimens require the preparation of small volumes of stock solutions. Thus significant calculation errors may still result in drug amounts that appear quite normal. Several cases of tenfold errors in drug dosing have been described and can be attributed to health care providers' calculation errors, communication difficulties with the parents, or illegibility, among other reasons. Dosing calculations require meticulous attention, and independent verification of patient doses is being increasingly practiced.[13]

SPECIAL CONDITIONS

Almost every drug is capable of eliciting an adverse reaction if sufficient quantities are administered. Idiosyncratic toxicity may be caused by an altered response to or metabolism of a drug or its metabolic products. A variety of drugs can induce hemolytic anemia in patients who have glucose-6-phosphate dehydrogenase deficiency. Drug metabolites can act as haptens, inducing secondary immunological responses. Often a detailed family history will reveal a pattern of toxicity to a particular class of drugs, thus guiding therapeutic choices.[15]

In a growing child, additional considerations about drug toxicity arise because some medications interfere with the normal growth process. Corticosteroid therapy, for example, can halt growth, particularly linear growth. Tetracyclines interfere with calcium metabolism; enamel hypoplasia can result in permanent dental staining in addition to a temporary inhibition of bone growth.[9]

Breast milk represents one potential source of drugs for the newborn. Drug passage into breast milk is favored if the drug has a low molecular weight, is present in an un-ionized (lipid-soluble) form, and has low affinity for plasma proteins.[15] Social drug use, including nicotine and ethanol, should be considered in addition to the mother's use of prescription medication. Although the list of drugs that are absolutely contraindicated for the breast-feeding mother is short and the relative concentration of a given drug within the breast milk may be so low that adverse effects for the infant are unlikely, it is prudent to minimize maternal drug exposure.[15,28] If maternal medication is unavoidable, drug exposure for the nursing child can be minimized by scheduling maternal drug dosing around nursing times. For most medications this can be achieved by instructing the mother to ingest the medication just after nursing or at least 4 hours before the next nursing period.[28] (See Chapter 16, Nutrition, Part Two, Feeding of Infants and Children.)

PRACTICAL APPLICATION OF PHARMACOLOGICAL PRINCIPLES

From the preceding discussion it is clear that significant differences exist between children and adults, and these differences determine optimum medical therapy. The overview of the use of theophylline in the pediatric patient[28] provided below highlights many of the pharmacological parameters previously discussed in this chapter and exemplifies a systematic approach to optimizing one drug regimen.

Absorption

Theophylline is absorbed rapidly, completely, and consistently when it is administered in liquid or uncoated tablets. Enteric-coated tablets and rectal suppositories have been associated with slow and incomplete absorption. Although sustained-release formulations may exhibit variable bioavailability, this limitation may be superseded by their therapeutic advantage in children in whom elimination is rapid and fluctuations in the plasma concentration between doses can be excessive.

Distribution

Once absorbed, theophylline is distributed throughout the body water rapidly; plasma levels equilibrate with interstitial fluids within 1 hour after IV injection. The apparent volume of distribution shows age-dependent changes. The V_d in a newborn is approximately 0.6 L/kg, reflecting the newborn's larger fraction of extracellular fluid; in children and adults the V_d is approximately 0.45 L/kg. Protein binding of the drug varies as well, with approximately 40% of the absorbed drug bound in the neonate versus approximately 60% in older children. Theophylline passes freely into breast milk, where the concentration approaches that of the plasma, and crosses the placenta. However, no serious consequences have been reported resulting from the transplacental passage of therapeutic theophylline levels or ingestion of breast milk containing theophylline.

Elimination

Renal excretion accounts for 10% of the drug clearance, and theophylline appears in unchanged form in the urine. The majority of the drug is metabolized in the liver by oxidation and demethylation reactions. Demethylation varies among individuals, and because the enzyme has a limited capacity, increasing plasma concentrations of theophylline result in a decreasing fraction of the drug being eliminated by this pathway. Thus changes in the drug dose may result in disproportionately large changes in the plasma concentration. The variability in clearance of theophylline therefore is a function of the rate of biotransformation, which is influenced by age, physiological abnormalities of the patient, and concomitant use of other medications.

Clinical Use and Dosing

The bronchodilatory effect of theophylline has been shown to be proportional to the log of the plasma concentration over the range of 5 to 20 μg of theophylline per milliliter of plasma. Similarly, symptoms associated with chronic asthma have been prevented when plasma theophylline levels are maintained within 10 to 20 μg/ml. The potential for serious toxicity also correlates well with increasing plasma concentration. These observations have prompted monitoring of theophylline plasma concentrations to provide safe and optimum drug-dosing regimens.

When theophylline is used as an acute bronchodilator, the therapeutic goal is to relieve symptoms as rapidly as possible. A therapeutic concentration can be achieved quickly by administering an initial or loading dose of the drug in a form that provides rapid and reliable absorption (e.g., intravenous or oral preparation). Because of theophylline's rapid absorption and distribution, the resulting plasma concentration is related more closely to the V_d than to the rate of elimination. The plasma concentration (C) subsequently approaches a value equal to the administered dose (D) divided by the volume of distribution, $C = D/V_d$. Assuming a V_d of approximately 0.5 L/kg, each milligram of theophylline administered in rapidly absorbable form results in a 2 μg/ml increase in the plasma concentration. For example, a 7.5 mg/kg dose would be expected to result in a peak plasma theophylline concentration of approximately 15 μg/ml, assuming the patient has had no other medication containing theophylline. If a patient has an initial theophylline level of 10 μg/ml and the desired concentration is 15 μg/ml, the loading dose can be estimated as follows:

$$D = C \times V_d \text{ therefore,}$$

$$\text{Estimated loading dose} = (15\ \mu g/ml - 10\ \mu g/ml)(500\ ml/kg)$$
$$= 2500\ \mu g/kg = 2.5\ mg/kg$$

Excessively rapid intravenous administration results in transiently higher-than-predicted plasma concentrations because a finite period of time is required for distribution of the drug. Delayed gastric emptying (e.g., as a result of food in the stomach) may result in lower peak plasma levels because of slower absorption of the medication. During this lag period elimination of the drug begins and the expected peak levels may not be achieved. Interpatient variability in the V_d also will cause variation in peak plasma concentrations; aiming for initial peak levels of approximately 15 μg/ml should result in safe, therapeutic drug levels for most patients.

The therapeutic level of theophylline achieved with the loading dose is maintained by administering a continuous IV infusion at a rate that matches the patient's rate of drug elimination. This infusion rate is based on the age and clinical condition of the patient. Monitoring plasma theophylline levels will help to determine the appropriate infusion parameters. This maintenance dose then can be used to determine the appropriate oral dose for the patient. The same total daily dose, in milligrams administered per 24-hour period, is divided by the desired dosing interval to determine the intermittent medication regimen. The dosing interval is a function of the absorption rate of the particular theophylline preparation used and the individual patient's rate of elimination.

If theophylline is started on an outpatient basis and therefore no IV infusion is planned, the dose titration can be followed by periodic measurement of the plasma theophylline concentration. Reevaluation of therapy is important because children tend to "outgrow" their doses, and frequent reassessment of therapeutic regimens is necessary during periods of rapid growth.

Trough levels may not provide essential therapeutic information. For example, if trough levels are low but the patient is symptom free, no adjustment of dose is needed. If the patient is symptomatic before the next drug dose, the peak-trough differential may be too great. This can be reduced by giving the same total daily dose at shorter intervals or by administering a preparation that is more slowly absorbed.

SUMMARY

The numerous physiological changes that occur during the development and maturation of the human body create the unique challenges faced by the pediatrician. Clinical pharmacology has a unique role in the physician's daily practice. An understanding of basic pharmacological principles ensures that these challenges are successfully met and that optimum therapy is provided to the patient.

REFERENCES

1. 21 CFR Part 210 "Specific Requirements on content and format of labeling for human prescription drugs; revision of 'pediatric use' subsection in the labeling; final rule," *Federal Register* 59:63239, 1994.
2. Benet LA: The role of pharmacokinetics in the drug development process. In Yoacobi A et al, editors: *Integration of pharmacokinetics, pharmacodynamics, and toxicokinetics in rational drug development,* New York, 1993, Plenum.
3. Besunder JB, Reed MD, Blumer JL: Principles of drug biodistribution in the neonate, *Clin Pharmacokinet* 14:189, 1988.
4. Clark B, Smith DA: *An introduction to pharmacokinetics,* Oxford, 1981, Blackwell Scientific Publications.
5. American Academy of Pediatrics Committee on Drugs: Guidelines for the ethical conduct of studies to evaluate drugs in pediatric populations, *Pediatrics* 60:91, 1977.
6. de Boer AG et al: Rectal drug administration: clinical pharmacokinetic considerations, *Clin Pharmacokinet* 7:285, 1982.
7. Evans WE, Jusko WJ, editors: *Applied pharmacokinetics: principles of therapeutic drug monitoring,* Spokane, Wash, 1986, Applied Therapeutics.
8. Gellis SS, Kagan BM, editors: *Current pediatric therapy,* vol 12, Philadelphia, 1986, WB Saunders.
9. Gilmar AG et al, editors: *The pharmacological basis of therapeutics,* ed 7, New York, 1985, Macmillan.
10. Greenblatt DJ: Presystemic extraction: mechanisms and consequences, *J Clin Pharmacol* 33:650, 1993.
11. Greiff JMC, Rowbotham D: Pharmacokinetic drug interactions with gastrointestinal motility modifying agents, *Clin Pharmacokinet* 27:447, 1994.
12. Kelly HW: Pharmacotherapy of pediatric lung disease: differences between children and adults, *Chest Med* 8:681, 1987.
13. Koren G, Haslam RH: Pediatric medication errors: predicting and preventing tenfold disasters, *J Clin Pharmacol* 34:1043, 1994.
14. Leff RD, Roberts RJ: Problems in drug therapy for pediatric patients, *Am J Hosp Pharm* 44:865, 1987.

15. MacLeod SM, Radde IC, editors: *Textbook of pediatric clinical pharmacology,* Littleton, Mass, 1985, PSG-Wright.
16. May DG: Genetic differences in drug disposition, *J Clin Pharmacol* 34:881, 1994.
17. Mirkin BL, editor: *Clinical pharmacology and therapeutics: a pediatric perspective,* Chicago, 1978, Mosby.
18. Morselli PL, Franco-Morselli R, Bossi L: Clinical pharmacokinetics in newborns and infants, *Clin Pharmacokinet* 5:485, 1980.
19. Roberts RJ: Intravenous administration of medication in pediatric patients: problems and solutions, *Pediatr Clin North Am* 28:23, 1981.
20. Rowe PC: *The Harriet Lane handbook: a manual for pediatric house officers,* Chicago, 1987, Mosby.
21. Shope JT: Medication compliance, *Pediatr Clin North Am* 28:5, 1981.
22. Silverman WA et al: A difference in mortality rate and incidence of kernicterus among premature infants allotted to two prophylactic antibacterial regimens, *Pediatrics* 18:614, 1956.
23. Tendler C, Grossman S, Tenenbaum J: Medication dosages during pediatric emergencies: a simple and comprehensive guide, *Pediatrics* 84:731, 1989.
24. Thompson DF, Heflin NR: Frequency and appropriateness of drug prescribing for unlabeled uses in pediatric patients, *Am J Hosp Pharm* 44:792, 1987.
25. Valman HB, editor: *Pediatric therapeutics,* Oxford, 1979, Blackwell Scientific Publications.
26. Ward RM, Green TP: Developmental pharmacology and toxicology: principles of study design and problems of methodology, *Pharmacol Ther* 36:309, 1988.
27. Weiss CF, Glazko AJ, Weston JK: Chloramphenicol in the newborn infant, *N Engl J Med* 262:187, 1960.
28. Yaffe SJ, editor: *Pediatric pharmacology: therapeutic principles in practice,* New York, 1980, Grune & Stratton.

31 Antimicrobial Therapy

Keith R. Powell

The use of antimicrobial agents to treat diseases caused by bacteria is part of the day-to-day practice of pediatrics. Antimicrobial therapy has advanced and continues to advance at a rate unparalleled in medicine; even experts on infectious diseases have trouble staying abreast of new agents and their pharmacology and pharmacodynamics. Developing a rationale for the use of antimicrobial agents should help prevent overuse and allow consistent evaluation of the merits and drawbacks of new antimicrobial agents. For the practitioner, it is more important to know how to use a limited number of antimicrobial agents well than to have a meager knowledge of many.

APPROACH TO ANTIMICROBIAL THERAPY

Three important questions should be answered before antimicrobial therapy is begun: (1) where is the infection (anatomical site)? (2) what pathogens usually cause infections at this site? and (3) which antimicrobial agents, given by what route of administration, will achieve effective concentrations at that site? The answers to the first two questions usually are addressed critically by the practitioner. However, selection of an antimicrobial agent is more likely to be based on a "bug-drug" relationship than on knowledge about the ability to achieve an effective concentration at the site of infection.

The anatomical site of most bacterial infections can be identified by a combination of historical information and findings on physical examination. When the site of infection is more obscure, diagnostic studies such as roentgenograms, radionucleotide scans, computed tomography (CT) scans, magnetic resonance imaging (MRI), and ultrasound evaluation often are helpful.

Based on the site of infection and the patient's age, habitat, history of exposures, and clinical signs and symptoms, the pediatrician usually can develop a list of potential bacterial pathogens. Knowing the site of infection and possible causative agents helps the clinician to decide what (if any) specimens should be cultured for bacteria, as well as whether the laboratory should be alerted to use special culture media or techniques. Selecting an antimicrobial agent based on its ability to achieve effective concentrations at the site of infection requires a working concept of what an effective concentration is. To define an "effective concentration," it first is necessary to review some of the basic pharmacodynamics of antimicrobial agents.

PHARMACODYNAMICS

The term *pharmacodynamics* describes the relationship between antimicrobial activity and the pharmacokinetics of an antimicrobial agent.

Minimal Inhibitory and Minimal Bactericidal Concentrations

An antimicrobial agent's activity against a particular bacterium in vitro is expressed as the agent's minimal inhibitory concentration (MIC) or minimal bactericidal concentration (MBC). To determine the MIC, bacteria are grown in broth to a concentration of 100,000 (10^5) microorganisms per milliliter. The broth containing bacteria, which is clear to the naked eye, is then placed in a series of test tubes, and a decreasing amount of antimicrobial agent is added to each test tube. The broth containing the bacteria and antimicrobial agent is incubated overnight and then examined for visible turbidity, since turbidity represents bacterial growth. The test tube with the smallest amount of antimicrobial agent that remains clear to the naked eye is the MIC. To determine whether the antibiotic is bactericidal, the tubes that remained clear are quantitatively subcultured onto agar plates. After overnight incubation, bacterial colonies are counted. Each colony represents one bacterium that survived, or one colony-forming unit (CFU). The smallest amount of antibiotic that results in the death of 99,900 (99.9%) of the original 100,000 microorganisms per milliliter inoculum (a 1000-fold reduction) is the MBC. MIC and MBC results are reported in micrograms of antimicrobial agent per milliliter of broth required to inhibit or kill, respectively.

Serum Inhibitory and Bactericidal Titers

Antimicrobial activity in vivo can be approximated by determining the inhibitory or bactericidal titers. Although the test usually is performed using serum, it can be done with most body fluids that are clear, except urine. The test is performed by growing organisms to 10^5 CFU per milliliter of broth, as in determining the MIC. However, instead of adding known concentrations of antimicrobial agent to each test tube, serial twofold dilutions of serum (or other body fluids) are added to sequential tubes (i.e., undiluted serum is added to the first tube, serum diluted 1:2 to the second tube, 1:4 to the third, and so on). After incubation overnight, the tubes are examined for visible turbidity; the most dilute sample that has no visible turbidity is the serum inhibitory titer. To determine if the bacteria are being killed, the broth is cultured quantitatively as for the MBC, and the most dilute specimen that results in the death of 99.9% of the original inoculum is the serum bactericidal titer.

The outcome of bacterial infections usually is associated with the peak serum bactericidal titer. In general, a peak serum bactericidal titer at a 1:8 dilution correlates with a clinical and microbiological cure. To measure peak activity, blood sampling must be timed based on when the drug is given, the route by which it is given, and the time after administration that peak serum concentrations are reached. Table 31-1

Table 31-1 Times That Peak Serum Concentrations Are Reached After Administration of Antimicrobial Agents

	Route of administration	Time of peak concentration*
Penicillins	IV	5 min
Cephalosporins	IV	5 min
Penicillin V	PO	30 min - 1 hr
Amoxicillin	PO	2 hr
Cephalexin	PO	1 hr
Aminoglycosides	IV	30 min
	IM	1 hr
Trimethoprim-sulfamethoxazole	PO	1-2 hr
Sulfisoxazole	PO	2-3 hr
Erythromycin (estolate or ethylsuccinate)	PO	2 hr
Clindamycin	PO	1-2 hr
Chloramphenicol	PO/IV	2 hr
Vancomycin	IV	2 hr
Rifampin	PO	2 hr

*For drugs given intravenously, the time of peak serum concentrations is stated in minutes or hours after *completion* of the infusion.
IV, Intravenous; *PO*, oral; IM, intramuscular.

shows the times that peak serum concentrations are reached with selected antimicrobial agents.

Tolerance

Tolerance to an antimicrobial agent describes the situation in which organisms are inhibited by the normal concentration of a bactericidal agent but require much higher concentrations of the agent to achieve a bactericidal effect. The clinical significance of tolerance is still controversial, but it appears that this phenomenon may be important with infections that require bactericidal activity to effect a cure.[5]

Bacteriostatic Versus Bactericidal

Most infections in normal children do not require a bactericidal antimicrobial agent. In general, bactericidal agents are needed for optimal treatment of bacterial endocarditis, meningitis, and osteomyelitis. The effectiveness of bacteriostatic agents depends on the host's ability to opsonize and phagocytize bacteria that have been inhibited; thus bactericidal agents usually are necessary to treat bacterial infections in a neutropenic host.

Pharmacokinetics

Because blood samples are easily obtained, the pharmacokinetics of antimicrobial agents usually are described as serum concentrations over time. Once administered, an antimicrobial agent initially is distributed throughout the intravascular volume and the extracellular fluid of tissues with high perfusion rates. The drug enters tissues that are not highly perfused at a slower rate. Some antimicrobial agents, such as the beta-lactams, are distributed only in extracellular fluid, whereas others distribute intracellularly as well (rifampin, trimethoprim-sulfamethoxazole [TMP-SMX]).

The pharmacokinetic parameter that best correlates with microbiological cure is the length of time the serum concentration of the antimicrobial agent exceeds the MIC. Therefore it is important to know not only the antimicrobial agent's specific activity against the infecting organism, but also the serum concentration above this activity that can be reached (peak serum concentration) and how long the activity will be sustained (serum half-life). The peak serum concentration that can be achieved is determined by the antimicrobial agent's rate of absorption and rate of excretion. Higher peak serum concentrations are achieved with antibiotics that are absorbed readily and excreted slowly. When a drug is given intravenously, absorption does not play a role in peak serum concentrations. Some of the relationships between pharmacokinetics and antimicrobial activity are illustrated in Fig. 31-1.

The route by which an antibiotic is administered depends on the patient's condition and the pharmacokinetics of the antibiotic. For some antimicrobial agents (e.g., chloramphenicol and TMP-SMX), the peak serum concentrations after oral (PO) and intravenous (IV) administration are equivalent. For others (e.g., ampicillin), the peak serum concentration is 100-fold higher after IV administration. Any time oral antimicrobial therapy is considered, the patient's ability to take, retain, and absorb the drug also must be considered.

Inhibitory Quotient

One way to express the relationship between antimicrobial activity and pharmacokinetics is the inhibitory quotient (IQ). The IQ is found by dividing the concentration of antibiotic that can be achieved at the site of infection by the MIC of the agent required for the causative bacteria[2]:

$$IQ = \frac{\text{Concentration of antimicrobial agent}}{\text{MIC for causative bacteria}}$$

If the concentration of the antibiotic exceeds the MIC by a factor of 10, the outcome is likely to be a clinical and microbiological cure. In treating infections in well-perfused tissues, a favorable outcome can be expected when the peak serum concentration exceeds the MIC tenfold. For infections in sites such as the central nervous system (CNS), it is necessary to know how well antimicrobial agents reach these sites.

Role of the Laboratory in Antimicrobial Therapy

For the vast majority of bacterial infections treated in the ambulatory setting, little or no laboratory testing is necessary to use antimicrobial agents rationally. For example, otitis media is the most common infection of children that is treated with antimicrobial agents in the ambulatory setting. The site of infection is determined by physical examination. The bacterial pathogens that cause otitis media have been well established, and several antimicrobial agents have been shown to produce a clinical and microbiological cure when given orally. Only if empirical therapy fails does it become necessary to perform a tympanocentesis to obtain a specimen for isolating the bacteria and performing susceptibility tests. Likewise, by knowing the usual pathogens and their susceptibility to antimicrobial agents, the practitioner can manage common infections such as impetigo, cellulitis, cervical adenitis, local abscesses, and conjunctivitis without obtaining specimens for culture.

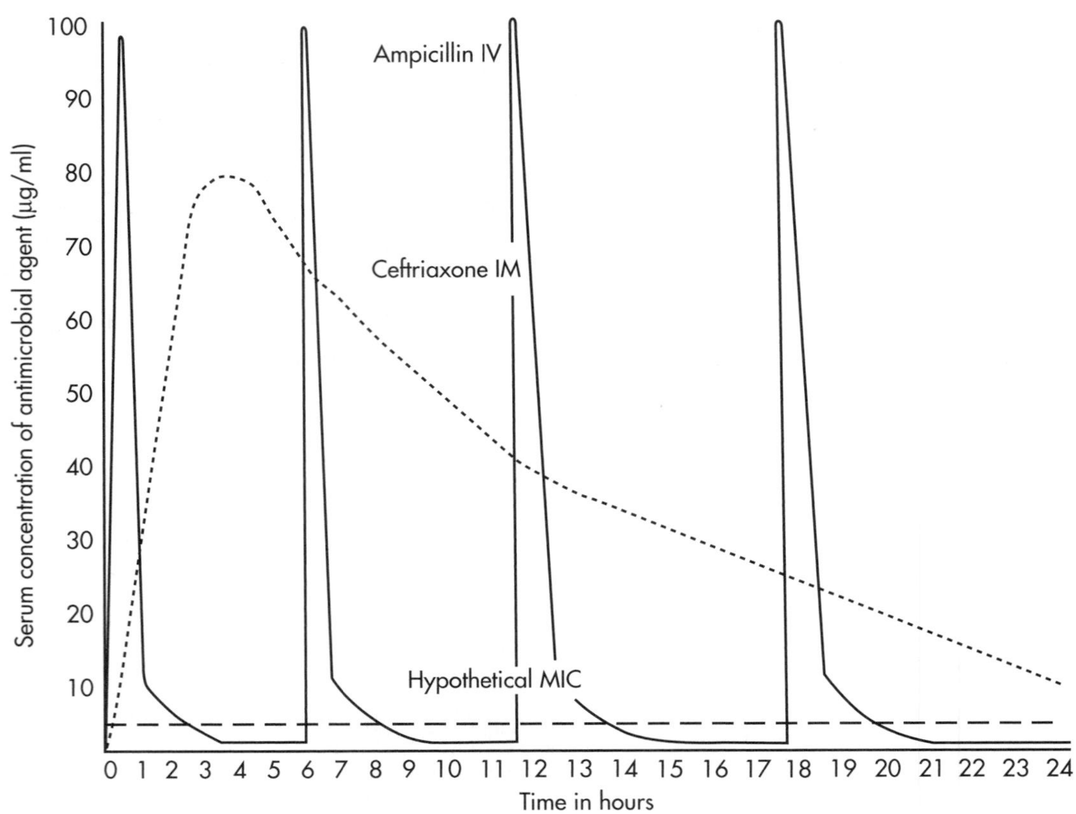

FIG. 31-1 The solid line represents serum concentrations of an antimicrobial agent with a short serum half-life (e.g., ampicillin), given by rapid intravenous infusion. The peak serum concentration is achieved during the infusion; then concentrations fall rapidly. The length of time the serum concentration remains above the minimal inhibitory concentration (MIC) depends on the actual value of the MIC. The dotted line represents serum concentrations of an antimicrobial agent with a long half-life, given by the intramuscular route (e.g., ceftriaxone). Reaching the peak serum concentration takes longer after intramuscular administration because the antimicrobial agent must be absorbed from the muscle before it can be excreted. As a result of this slow excretion, serum concentrations remain above the MIC of susceptible organisms for a longer period. When a rapidly excreted antimicrobial agent such as ampicillin is given intramuscularly, peak serum concentrations are not very high because the drug is excreted almost as quickly as it is absorbed.

Culture and Susceptibility

When the usual therapy fails, when the patient is more seriously ill or is immunocompromised, or when the clinical situation is unusual, the first step is to obtain appropriate specimens to culture for bacterial pathogens. When bacterial pathogens are isolated from a normally sterile specimen, antimicrobial susceptibility is tested. Susceptibility is tested by either determining the MIC as described previously or by using the disk diffusion method.

In the disk diffusion method, a culture plate is inoculated with the bacteria to be tested, and paper disks containing standardized concentrations of antimicrobial agents are placed on the surface of the culture medium. The culture plates are incubated, and the moisture from the medium allows the antimicrobial agents to diffuse out of the paper disks. The farther from the disk the diffusion reaches, the lower the concentration of antimicrobial agent. If the bacteria are inhibited by the antibiotic, a zone around the disk forms in which the bacteria do not grow. The zone of inhibition is measured after overnight incubation and, based on its diameter, the organism is determined to be "susceptible" or "resistant." A report of "intermediate" or "indeterminant" should be interpreted to mean that the microorganism is resistant or that the MIC should be determined. The diameter of the zone of inhibition has been correlated to MIC determinations so that "susceptible" actually means that the MIC will be equal to or less than a certain concentration of the antimicrobial agent.

When an organism is reported to be susceptible by disk, it means that 95% of the strains of this bacteria are *inhibited* by concentrations of the antimicrobial agent that can be achieved in the *serum* if the antimicrobial agent is given at the usual dose by the usual route of administration for an infection with that organism. This concentration is called the *MIC_{95}*. The MIC_{95} of selected antimicrobial agents for bacteria reported as susceptible by disk are listed in Table 31-2. Clearly, the site of infection, the proposed antibiotic's activity against the pathogen, and the concentration of the antibiotic that can be achieved at the site of infection all must be considered.

For example, "susceptible to ampicillin" has very different meanings, depending on the organism being tested. When gram negative organisms or enterococci are reported as susceptible to ampicillin (see Table 31-2), it means that 95% of these organisms are inhibited by 8 μg/ml or less of ampicillin.[9] For gram positive cocci, susceptible means that 95% are inhibited by 0.2 μg/ml or less, or 40 times less ampicillin than it takes to inhibit gram negative enterics.[9] For *Haemophilus influenzae,* susceptible means that it takes 2 μg/ml or less to inhibit 95% of all strains.[9] Unless the MIC has been determined for the individual isolate, the clinician must assume that MIC_{95} must be achieved at the site of infection to inhibit the isolate. Thus, to treat pyelonephritis caused by *Escherichia coli* with ampicillin, the practitioner ideally would achieve concentrations of ampicillin 10 times the MIC in renal parenchymal cells. Because susceptible means that 95% of *E. coli* are inhibited by 8 μg/ml or less, the concentration of ampicillin required in renal parenchymal cells should be assumed to be 80 μg/ml ($IQ = \frac{80}{8} = 10$) unless the actual MIC for the isolate is known.

SPECIFIC ANTIBACTERIAL AGENTS

Because of the large number of antimicrobial agents currently available, several usually are equally effective for a given infectious disease. The antimicrobial agents preferred by a practitioner reflect the drugs' cost and availability as well as the physician's training and local practices. In general, it is far better to know how to use a small number of antimicrobial agents well than to know all of the possible alternatives. Table 31-2 presents the antimicrobial agents physicians use most frequently and selected pharmacological and pharmacodynamic information about them. This table is intended to serve as an example of the information a practitioner should have at hand when using antimicrobial agents; the specific antimicrobial agents that should be used for selected infections are discussed later in this chapter, following some general information about classes of antimicrobial agents.

Penicillins

Mechanism of Action. Although the general mechanism of action of penicillins is to inhibit cell wall synthesis, precisely how they do this is unknown. Current evidence, however, points to inhibition of transpeptidation. Most bacteria have penicillin-binding proteins (PBP) in their cell membranes. There are a number of penicillin-binding proteins, and the number and type vary from bacteria to bacteria. The activity of penicillins generally correlates with the number of high-affinity PBP the organism has.

Resistance of Bacteria to Penicillins. Resistance to penicillins can be based on several factors. Bacteria that lack appropriate PBP will be resistant. However, for penicillins to reach the PBP, they first must pass through the protein layers on the outer surface of the organism's membrane. Some bacteria are resistant because, as a result of shape or electronic charge, the penicillin cannot reach the binding sites. The most important mechanism of resistance is bacterial production of beta-lactamases. These enzymes hydrolyze the beta-lactam structure, rendering the penicillin inactive. Some organisms bind penicillin and are inhibited but do not undergo autolysis and death; these organisms are penicillin tolerant.

Classification. Based on their specific antibacterial activity, penicillins can be loosely classified as (1) natural, (2) penicillinase resistant, (3) amino, (4) antipseudomonad, and (5) extended-spectrum penicillins. The practitioner should be well versed in the use of one penicillin from each class, as presented in the section below, Use of Selected Penicillins.

Pharmacological Properties. Penicillins vary greatly in absorption after oral administration, with penicillin V, amoxicillin, cloxacillin, and dicloxacillin having the greatest absorption. Food reduces the absorption of oxacillin and dicloxacillin but not of penicillin V or amoxicillin. Procaine penicillin G and benzathine penicillin G are absorbed slowly after intramuscular injection and are given every 12 to 24 hours and every 15 to 20 days, respectively. Penicillins are excreted by renal tubular cells and have a very short half-life, ranging from less than 30 minutes to slightly over 1 hour. Penicillins are distributed to most areas of the body if inflammation is present. However, they are poorly lipid soluble and do not enter the CNS well even if inflammation is present. Penicillins do not enter cells well. Passage of penicillins from the serum of a pregnant woman to her fetus depends on the degree of protein binding present; little of highly protein-bound penicillins reaches the fetus.

Side Effects. The most important adverse reactions to penicillins are caused by hypersensitivity; they range from skin rashes to anaphylaxis. Anaphylactic reactions to penicillin are IgE mediated and occur in about 2 in every 1000 courses of treatment; about 1 in every 100,000 courses results in a fatality. The morbilliform rashes seen during therapy with penicillins probably are IgM mediated and often disappear even when therapy is continued. Less common reactions include serum sickness, exfoliative dermatitis, and Stevens-Johnson syndrome.

Penicillin Desensitization. When it is deemed important to use penicillin in a patient who may have an anaphylactic reaction, immunotolerance to penicillin can be achieved by starting with very small doses. An effective protocol is to administer 5 U of penicillin G intracutaneously, in the forearm and then, at 60- to 90-minute intervals, increase the dose to 10, 100, 1000, 10,000, and 50,000 U. If the intradermal doses are tolerated, IV penicillin can be instituted.

Use (See Table 31-2). The natural penicillins listed in Table 31-2 are penicillin G (aqueous, procaine, and benzathine) and penicillin V. These antimicrobial agents are most active against both aerobic and anaerobic gram positive cocci, *Neisseria meningitidis, Neisseria gonorrhoeae, Fusobacterium* species, *Eikenella* species, *Listeria monocytogenes,* and *Borrelia burgdorferi.* Penicillins are still the mainstay of treatment for infections caused by group A beta-hemolytic streptococci, group B streptococci, *Streptococcus pneumoniae, N. meningitidis,* and *L. monocytogenes.* Penicillin also is the drug of choice for acute infections with *B. burgdorferi* (Lyme disease) in children and for infections caused by anaerobes normally found in the mouth.

The potassium salt of penicillin G usually is used and is almost exclusively given intravenously. When given intramuscularly, aqueous penicillin G is excreted very rapidly; when given by mouth, it is poorly absorbed. Either procaine

Table 31-2 Dosage, Peak Serum Concentrations, and MIC_{95} for Selected Antimicrobial Agents

Antimicrobial agent	Route of administration	Age: <1 wk* (<2000 g) mg/kg/dose/interval	Age: 1 wk-1 mo* (<2000 g) mg/kg/dose/interval	Age: >1 mo mg/kg/dose/interval	Age: Adult dose† g/dose/interval	Peak serum concentration (μg/ml)	Susceptibility (MIC_{95}) (μg/ml)‡
Penicillin G	IV	50,000 U q8h	50,000 U q6h	25,000-50,000 U	25,000-50,000 **U/kg**	400	≤0.1
		(50,000 U q12h)	(50,000 U q8h)	q4-6h	q4-6h		*L. monocytogenes* ≤2
Procaine penicillin	IM	50,000 U q24h	50,000 U q24h	25,000-50,000 U	25,000-50,000 **U/kg**	5-6	≤0.1
		(50,000 U q24h)	(50,000 U q24h)	q12-24h	q12-24h		
Benzathine I penicillin	IM	50,000 U; 1 dose	50,000 U; 1 dose	50,000 U; 1 dose	2.4×10^6 U; 1 dose	0.2	≤0.1
		(50,000 U; 1 dose)	(50,000 U; 1 dose)				
Penicillin V	PO	Not recommended	Not recommended	6.25-12.5 q6h	0.25-0.5 q6h	3-5	≤0.1
Ampicillin	IV	25-50 q8h	25-50 q6h	25-75 q4-6h	1-2 q4-6h	40	Gram negative ≤8
	IM	(25-50 q12h)	(25-50 q8h)			8	Streptococci ≤0.1
							H. influenzae ≤2
Amoxicillin	PO	Not recommended	Not recommended	10-15 q8h	0.25-0.5 q8h	4.7-7.5	As for ampicillin
Nafcillin	IV	20 q8h	37.5 q6h	25-50 q6h	0.5-1.5 q4-6h	11	≤1
		(25 q12h)	(25 q8h)				
Methicillin§	IV	25-50 q8h	25-50 q6h	—	—	—	—
		(25-50 q12h)	(25-50 q8h)				
Dicloxacillin	PO	Not recommended	Not recommended	3-6.25	0.25-0.5 q6h	15-18	≤1
Mezlocillin	IV	75 q12h	75 q8h	50-75 q4-6h	3-4 q4-6h	200-300	≤64
	IM	(75 q12h)	(75 q8h)			15	
Cefazolin	IV	20 q12h	20 q8h	8.3-25 q6-8h	0.5-1.5 q6-8h	188	≤8
	IM	(20 q12h)	(20 q12h)				
Cephalexin	PO	Not recommended	Not recommended	6.25-12.5 q6h	0.25-1 q6h	8-40	≤8
Cefoxitin	IV	Not recommended	Not recommended	20-26.6 q4-q6h	1-2 q4-q6h or 3 q8h	110-125	≤8
	IM						
Cefotaxime	IV	50 q12h	50 q8h	25-50 q6h	1-2 q4-q12h	1 g 40	≤8
		(50 q12h)	(50 q8h)			2 g 80-90	
Ceftriaxone	IV	50 q24h	50-80 q24h	50 q24h	0.5-2 q24h	1 g 150	≤8
	IM	(50 q24h)	(50 q24h)	CNS: 80 q24h		1 g 50	
Ceftazidime	IV	30 q8h	50 q8h	25-50 q6h	0.5-2 q8-12h	1 g 85	≤8
	IM	(50 q12h)	(50 q8h)			1 g 34	

Amikacin	IV IM	10 q12h (7.5 q12h)	10 q8h (7.5 q8h)	5 q8h or 7.5 q12h	5 **mg/kg** q8h or 7.5 **mg/kg** q12h	20-40 20	≤16
Gentamicin	IV IM	2.5 q12h (2.5 q12h)	2.5 q8h (2.5 q8h)	1-2.5 q8h	1-1.7 **mg/kg** q8h	4-10 7	≤4
Tobramycin	IV IM	2 q12h (2 q12h)	2 q8h (2 q8h)	1-2 q8h	1-1.7 **mg/kg** q8h	4-14 4	≤4
Trimethoprim-sulfamethoxazole (TMP-SMX)	PO IV	Not recommended	Not recommended	3-6 TMP/15-30 SMX q12h 5 TMP/25 SMX q6h for pneumocystosis	0.16 TMP/0.8 SMX q12h	2-4/80-100	≤2/38
Sulfisoxazole	PO	Not recommended	Not recommended	30-37.5 q6h	0.5-1 q6h	40-50	≤100 (urinary tract infection only)
Erythromycin estolate	PO	10 q12h (10 q12h)	10-12.5 q8h (10 q8h)	10 q8h or 15 q12h	0.25-0.5 q6h	4.2	≤0.5
Erythromycin ethylsuccinate	PO	10 q12h (10 q12h)	10 q8h (10 q8h)	10 q6h	0.25-0.5 q6h	1.5	≤0.5
Clindamycin	PO IV	5 q8h (5 q12h)	5 q6h (5 q8h)	2.5-7.5 q6h	0.15-.45 q6h	2.5-3.6	≤0.5
Chloramphenicol	IV PO	25 q24h (25 q24h)	25 q24h (25 q24h)	12.5-18.75 q6h 18.75-25 q6h (meningitis)	12.5-25 **mg/kg** q6h	19 25	*H. influenzae* ≤4 Others ≤12.5
Tetracycline	IV PO	Not recommended	Not recommended	Children >8 yr 6.25-12.5 q6h	0.25-0.5 q6h	8 4	≤4
Vancomycin	IV	15 q12h (10 q12h)	10 q8h (10 q8h)	10-15 q6h	15 **mg/kg** q12h or 6.5-8 **mg/kg** q6h	30-40	≤5
Metronidazole	PO IV	7.5 q12h (7.5 q12h)	15 q12h (7.5 q12h)	5-12 q8h 7.5 q6h	7.5 **mg/kg** q6h	11.5 20-25	≤4
Rifampin	PO	Not recommended	Not recommended	10-20 q24h	0.6 q24h	7	≤1

*Doses and intervals shown in parentheses are for infants with a birth weight <2000 g; doses and intervals shown without parentheses are for infants with a birth weight >2000 g.

†Maximum recommended dose (units other than grams are in **boldface**).

‡μg/ml of the antimicrobial required to inhibit isolate reported to be susceptible to disk diffusion method.

§Methicillin is preferred for newborns when kernicterus is a concern.

or benzathine preparations are used for intramuscular administration. It must be remembered, however, that very low serum concentrations are achieved with these preparations; they can be used only for exquisitely sensitive organisms and generally should not be used to treat CNS infections. Procaine penicillin can be used in a newborn to treat neurosyphilis. Penicillin V is well absorbed from the gastrointestinal tract and therefore is preferred for oral administration. Peak serum concentrations and MIC_{95} equivalents for susceptibility by disk are listed for individual penicillins in Table 31-2.

Ampicillin has the same general activity as penicillin, but it is also active against *E. coli, Proteus mirabilis, Salmonella* species, and *Shigella* species and is more active against group D streptococci and *L. monocytogenes.* Amoxicillin differs from ampicillin in molecular composition only by the presence of a hydroxyl group. Because amoxicillin is absorbed much better than ampicillin, peak serum concentrations of amoxicillin after oral administration are equal to those achieved with an equivalent dose of ampicillin given intramuscularly. The antimicrobial activity of amoxicillin is virtually identical to that of ampicillin, except that it is not useful in the treatment of shigellosis.

Clavulanic acid is a beta-lactamase inhibitor that is available in a fixed combination with amoxicillin and marketed as Augmentin. The beta-lactamase inhibitor extends the activity of amoxicillin to include organisms that produce beta-lactamases. The MIC_{95} of Augmentin for beta-lactamase-producing *Staphylococcus aureus, H. influenzae, N. gonorrhoeae,* and *Moraxella catarrhalis* is 2 μg/ml, and its MIC for *E. coli, Klebsiella sp., Proteus sp.,* and *Bacteroides fragilis* ranges from 8 to 16 μg/ml. Ampicillin in a fixed combination with sulbactam (another beta-lactamase inhibitor) is marketed as Unisyn for intravenous use. Ampicillin-sulbactam's activity is similar to that of ampicillin-clavulanate, and it is widely used for adults. Ampicillin-sulbactam has not been approved by the FDA for use in children.

Nafcillin is one of several penicillinase-resistant penicillins used primarily to treat infections caused by *S. aureus.* Most strains of *S. aureus* are inhibited by concentrations of 2 to 3 μg/ml. Because nafcillin is highly protein bound, methicillin is preferred for newborns when the possibility of kernicterus is a concern, since the amount of albumin for binding bilirubin will be diminished. Absorption of nafcillin from the GI tract is erratic; it should not be given orally. Dicloxacillin is absorbed from the GI tract more consistently and is a good oral agent for treating *S. aureus* infections. The oral suspension of dicloxacillin has a very bitter taste, which can create problems with compliance.

Several antipseudomonad and extended-activity penicillins currently are available. In general, *Pseudomonas* infections should be treated with a combination of one of these agents plus an aminoglycoside, both for synergy and to reduce the emergence of resistant bacteria. Mezlocillin has the antipseudomonad activity of carbenicillin and ticarcillin, plus it is more active against enterococci, *Klebsiella* species, *H. influenzae,* and *B. fragilis.* It is important to remember that a report of "susceptible to mezlocillin" means that concentrations as high as 64 μg/ml will be needed to inhibit 95% of the strains tested; this is compensated for by the high serum concentrations achieved when the drug is given intravenously (the peak serum concentration is 300 μg/ml after a dose of 4 g).

Cephalosporins

Mechanism of Action. Like penicillins, cephalosporins are beta-lactam antibiotics that interfere with cell wall synthesis. However, the precise mechanism is not known, and the effects of cephalosporins on bacteria range from lysing the organism to producing bacteria with unusual morphologies.

Resistance of Bacteria to Cephalosporins. Resistance to cephalosporins can arise if the cephalosporin is inactivated by beta-lactamase, if it is unable to reach antibiotic binding proteins, if the bacteria does not have appropriate binding sites, or if tolerance develops (see Penicillins above).

Classification. In the past 15 years, more new cephalosporins have been introduced for general use than any other type of antimicrobial agent.[8] The usual classification system for cephalosporins is based on antibacterial activity and is divided into a first, second, and third generation (see the box below). In general, the first generation cephalosporins have good activity against gram positive cocci except enterococci, coagulase negative staphylococcal species, and methicillin-resistant *S. aureus;* they have limited activity against gram negative organisms except *E. coli, Klebsiella pneumoniae,* and *P. mirabilis.* The second generation cephalosporins have the general activity of the first generation but are somewhat more active against gram negative organisms, including *H. influenzae.* Third generation cephalosporins are more active than second generation drugs against gram negative organisms but are less active against gram positive organisms than the first generation drugs.

Pharmacological Properties. Because of the number of cephalosporins and the wide variations in pharmacology, each drug should be considered individually.

CEPHALOSPORINS

First generation

Cefadroxil*
Cefazolin
Cephalexin*
Cephalothin
Cephapirin
Cephradine†

Second generation

Cefaclor*
Cefamandole
Cefmetazole
Cefonicid
Cefotetan
Cefotiam
Cefoxitin
Cefprozil*
Cefuroxime
Cefuroxime axetil*

Third generation

Cefepime
Cefixime*
Cefmenoxime
Cefoperazone
Cefotoxime
Cefpodoxime proxetil*
Cefpiramide
Cefsulodin
Ceftazidime
Ceftizoxime
Ceftriaxone
Moxalactam

*Oral.
†Oral and parenteral.

Side Effects. The side effects seen with cephalosporins generally are those seen with penicillins. Hypersensitivity reactions are the most common side effects. Although immunological studies have shown about 20% cross-reactivity between penicillins and cephalosporins, in practice only 5% to 10% of those who have hypersensitivity reactions to penicillins have them with cephalosporins. In general, if a patient has had only a nonurticarial rash as the manifestation of penicillin hypersensitivity, it is safe to use cephalosporins. In patients who have had urticaria or an anaphylactic reaction in response to penicillins, cephalosporins should be used with great caution or not at all. Less common side effects with cephalosporins are nephrotoxicity (cephaloridine should not be used), diarrhea, alcohol intolerance, and bleeding.

Use

FIRST GENERATION CEPHALOSPORINS. First generation cephalosporins are useful to treat infections caused by gram positive cocci when penicillin cannot be used, to treat infections caused by methicillin-sensitive *S. aureus,* and to provide coverage against *E. coli, K. pneumoniae,* and *P. mirabilis*. Cefazolin is preferable to cephalothin because it has greater activity against *E. coli* and *Klebsiella* species, achieves higher peak serum concentrations, and has a longer half-life. The peak serum concentration of cefazolin after a dose of 1 g given intravenously is 188 μg/ml; the serum half-life is 1½ to 2 hours. Susceptible by disk means that 95% of the bacteria tested are inhibited by 8 μg/ml or less. Cephalexin (Keflex) is a first generation cephalosporin that can be given orally. A peak serum concentration of 16 μg/ml can be achieved with a dose of 0.5 g. The antibacterial activity of cephalexin is similar to that of cefazolin. Cefadroxil achieves peak serum concentrations and has antimicrobial activity similar to that of cephalexin but is excreted more slowly, allowing administration at 12- to 24-hour intervals.

SECOND GENERATION CEPHALOSPORINS. Although several second generation cephalosporins enjoy widespread use, there usually is a penicillin or a first or third generation cephalosporin that will have advantages in either cost or specific activity. The most useful exceptions are the aphamycins (cefoxitin, cefotetan, and cefmetazole).[4] Cefoxitin is highly resistant to beta-lactamases and is more active against anaerobes, especially *B. fragilis,* than other cephalosporins. It is not as active as other second generation cephalosporins against *H. influenzae* and Enterobacteriaceae, nor is it as active against gram positive cocci as are first generation cephalosporins. Cefotetan is more active against aerobic gram negative bacilli than cefoxitin but is less active against aerobic gram positive cocci. Cefmetazole appears to be more active against *S. aureus* than either cefoxitin or cefotetan but is less active than cefotetan against Enterobacteriaceae and less active than cefoxitin against *B. fragilis*.[4] Because of its activity against anaerobes plus some gram positive and gram negative aerobes, cefoxitin has proved useful in the treatment of pelvic inflammatory disease and lung abscesses. The peak serum concentration after a dose of 1 g given intravenously is about 22 μg/ml, and the serum half-life is about 50 minutes. Susceptible by disk means that the MIC_{95} for the organism is 8 μg/ml or less.

Cefuroxime is the only second generation cephalosporin that achieves therapeutic concentrations in cerebrospinal fluid (CSF). For a period of time cefuroxime was advocated as single-drug therapy for bacterial meningitis in infants and children over 2 months of age. However, cefuroxime does not sterilize the CSF as rapidly as ampicillin plus chloramphenicol or selected third generation cephalosporins and should not be used to treat meningitis. Cefuroxime can be used when parenteral coverage for both *S. aureus* and *H. influenzae* is desirable in a patient who has no CNS infection.

Second generation cephalosporins available for oral administration include cefaclor (Ceclor), cefuroxime axetil (Ceftin), cefprozil (Cefzil), and loracarbef (Lorabid). Loracarbef technically is a carbecephem rather than a cephalosporin.[16] The main rationale for using oral second generation cephalosporins is to treat upper respiratory infections (e.g., otitis media or sinusitis) in patients unable to take amoxicillin/clavulanate or trimethoprim/sulfamethoxazole (TMP-SMX). The structure and spectrum of activity of loracarbef are very similar to those of cefaclor.

THIRD GENERATION CEPHALOSPORINS. Third generation cephalosporins can be thought of as those that have a role in treating *Pseudomonas* infections and those that do not. Cefotaxime, the first third generation cephalosporin to be widely used in the United States, is still useful clinically. Ceftriaxone is very similar to cefotaxime in antibacterial activity but has a much longer half-life. Both cefotaxime and ceftriaxone are active against most gram positive aerobes except enterococci and *L. monocytogenes*. Neither is active against methicillin-resistant *S. aureus* or coagulase negative staphylococci. Both are active against most gram negative aerobic bacteria, except for *Pseudomonas* species. The disacetyl breakdown product of cefotaxime also has a broad range of activity, but specific activity is less than that of cefotaxime itself. The peak serum concentration after IV administration of 1 g of cefotaxime is about 40 μg/ml, compared with 150 μg/ml for ceftriaxone. The serum half-life of cefotaxime is about 1 hour, compared with 8 hours for ceftriaxone. Because ceftriaxone is excreted slowly, a peak serum concentration of 50 μg/ml is achieved in adults after a dose of 0.5 g is given intramuscularly. Susceptible by disk means that the MIC_{95} of either drug for the bacteria tested is 8 μg/ml or less.

The two third generation cephalosporins that have good antipseudomonad activity are cefoperazone and ceftazidime. Ceftazidime is more active than cefoperazone against *Pseudomonas* in vitro but is less active than cefotaxime against gram positive organisms. Whether ceftazidime should be used as a single agent to treat *Pseudomonas* infections still is controversial. In adults, the peak serum concentration of ceftazidime after 1 g is given intravenously is 85 μg/ml; the serum half-life is about 1 hour and 48 minutes. About 90% of *Pseudomonas* isolates are inhibited by 8 μg/ml or less of ceftazidime.

Two third generation cephalosporins currently are available for oral use, cefixime (Suprax) and cefpodoxime proxetil (Vantin).[16] Cefixime is active against most of the bacteria that cause otitis media, although its activity against *S. pneumoniae* is questionable. Cefixime also is active against the gram negative bacilli most often responsible for urinary tract infections. Because *S. pneumoniae* coverage is spotty, cefixime is recommended for treatment of otitis media only if treatment with an antimicrobial that has good antipneumococcal activity fails. Not enough data are available to support the use of cefixime to treat urinary tract infections in children. The usual dose of cefixime is 8 mg/kg/day given as a single dose. Cefpodoxime proxetil has a spectrum of activity similar to that of cefixime, but it also has excellent activity against *S. pneumoniae*. Cefpodoxime achieves higher tissue concentrations in the lungs and tonsils than other cephalosporins. The usual dosage is 5 mg/kg every 12 hours, with a maximum dose of 400 mg/day for otitis media and 200 mg/day for pharyngitis or tonsillitis. Although the third generation cephalosporins are effective in treating bacterial pneumonia, otitis media, tonsillitis, and pharyngitis, equally effective and less expensive alternatives are available.

Other Beta-Lactam Antibiotics

Two other beta-lactam antibiotics, imipenem and aztreonam, have a limited role in the treatment of bacterial infections in children. Imipenem has an extremely broad spectrum of activity that covers most gram positive organisms, including enterococci, *Listeria* species, and methicillin-susceptible staphylococci, including coagulase negative staphylococci. Imipenem also inhibits most Enterobacteriaceae, *Pseudomonas aeruginosa,* and *Pseudomonas maltophilia,* as well as most anaerobic bacteria. Because imipenem is rapidly destroyed by a renal peptidase, it is supplied in a fixed combination with a dehydropeptidase inhibitor called cilastatin. In adults, 500 mg of imipenem with cilastatin given intravenously produces an average peak serum concentration of 33 μg/ml, and the serum half-life is about 1 hour. The MIC_{95} of bacteria susceptible by disk is 4 μg/ml or less. Imipenem's broad spectrum of antimicrobial activity seldom is required in clinical practice.

Aztreonam, a monobactam, has little activity against gram positive or anaerobic bacteria because these bacteria have little PBP 3, which is the primary binding site for aztreonam. On the other hand, aztreonam is very active against Enterobacteriaceae (MIC, 0.5 μg/ml or less) and moderately active against *P. aeruginosa* (MIC, 16 μg/ml or less). In adults, 1 g of aztreonam given intravenously results in a peak serum concentration of about 125 μg/ml, and the serum half-life is 1 hour and 42 minutes. Susceptible by disk means that the MIC_{95} will be 8 μg/ml or less. There is very little experience with the use of aztreonam in children.

Aminoglycosides

MECHANISMS OF ACTION. It is known that aminoglycosides inhibit bacterial protein synthesis, but a second mechanism appears to be necessary to explain bacterial killing, and this second mechanism is not yet known. Protein synthesis is inhibited through interaction with bacterial ribosomes at the interface between the smaller and larger ribosome subunits.

RESISTANCE OF BACTERIA TO AMINOGLYCOSIDES. There are three known mechanisms of resistance to aminoglycosides. The first, ribosomal resistance, is known to occur only with streptomycin, when alteration in the protein of the smaller ribosomal subunit results in inability to bind streptomycin.

The most common mechanism of resistance is the production of enzymes that inactivate the aminoglycosides. Because aminoglycosides are similar in structure, certain enzymes can inactivate more than one aminoglycoside. The capacity to produce aminoglycoside-inactivating enzymes is inherent among gram negative anaerobic bacteria and seldom occurs by induction. The number and types of enzymes vary among places and populations. As an aminoglycoside becomes more widely used, bacteria that produce inactivating enzymes become more prevalent. The ability to produce inactivating enzymes can be carried by plasmids and transferred among gram negative bacteria.

The third mechanism of resistance is bacterial impermeability to aminoglycosides. This mechanism is not very common, and it has been observed that permeability mutants generally are not very virulent. When an organism is susceptible to tobramycin or gentamicin (or both) but is resistant to amikacin, the amikacin resistance must be based on amikacin's inability to enter the organism. This must be the case because the only enzyme produced by gram negative organisms that inhibits amikacin also inhibits tobramycin and gentamicin.

PHARMACOLOGICAL PROPERTIES. Aminoglycosides are absorbed poorly or not at all after oral administration. Absorption after intramuscular administration is excellent, with the peak serum concentration occurring 30 to 90 minutes after administration. The serum concentration after intravenous administration over 20 to 30 minutes is about the same as after intramuscular administration. Aminoglycosides do not cross cell membranes well and therefore achieve poor concentrations inside most cells except renal tubular cells, which actively transport these agents. In general, only low concentrations of aminoglycosides are achieved in the CNS, eyes, biliary tract, or prostatic fluid. Aminoglycosides do enter synovial fluid well.

Because aminoglycosides are excreted by glomerular filtration, care must be taken to adjust the dosage for patients with renal failure. After filtration some of the aminoglycoside is reabsorbed by the proximal renal tubular cell, which probably plays a role in nephrotoxicity. By convention, the drug is infused over a 30-minute period, and the peak serum concentration is measured 30 minutes after the infusion is completed. With intramuscular administration, the peak serum concentration is measured 1 hour later. Because the therapeutic-to-toxic index is very low for aminoglycosides, the serum concentration should be monitored.

SIDE EFFECTS. The two most common toxicities of aminoglycosides are ototoxicity and nephrotoxicity. Ototoxicity is caused by destruction of the outer hair cells in the organ of Corti and possibly is related to the concentration of aminoglycoside in the endolymph or perilymph that bathes these cells. Transient elevations in aminoglycoside concentrations probably do not affect hearing. Nephrotoxicity results in a decrease in the glomerular filtration rate. Both ototoxicity and nephrotoxicity seem to occur less often in children than in adults. Nonetheless, it is important to measure the serum concentration to make sure it is both safe and therapeutic. Aminoglycosides also can cause neuromuscular paralysis, particularly with curare-like drugs, in the presence of botulinus toxin, and in patients who have myasthenia gravis. Neuromuscular paralysis usually does not occur if aminoglycosides are given intramuscularly or if they are infused over 30 minutes. Neuromuscular paralysis can be treated by administering calcium.

USE. Streptomycin, the first aminoglycoside used clinically, is used almost exclusively to treat tuberculosis, but it also is used to treat tularemia, plague, and brucellosis. Neomycin is used primarily to reduce the number of bacteria in the large bowel. It is given by mouth, and very little reaches the bloodstream.

Three aminoglycosides—gentamicin, tobramycin, and amikacin—currently are used systemically to treat serious infections caused by gram negative aerobic bacteria. In general, there is no evidence that one of these aminoglycosides is clinically superior to another in the treatment of susceptible bacteria. Tobramycin is more active against *P. aeruginosa* than is gentamicin or amikacin, but differences in clinical effectiveness have not been observed. Tobramycin and amikacin are somewhat less nephrotoxic than gentamicin. Amikacin is susceptible to inactivation by one aminoglycoside-inactivating enzyme, whereas tobramycin and gentamicin are inactivated by at least six enzymes. Thus organisms are less likely to be resistant to amikacin than to either tobramycin or gentamicin. Because amikacin is less toxic on a weight basis, a larger dose is given and a higher peak serum concentration is achieved. With a dose of 7.5 mg/kg of amikacin given intravenously, the peak serum concentration averages 38 μg/ml. At a dose of 2 mg/kg of tobramycin or gentamicin, the peak serum concentration ranges from 3 to 12 μg/ml. All three drugs have a serum half-life of 2 to 2½ hours. The MIC_{95} of amikacin for bacteria reported susceptible by disk is 16 μg/ml or less; the MIC_{95} of gentamicin or tobramycin is 4 μg/ml or less.

Once-daily dosing of aminoglycosides has been found to have several advantages over dosing every 8 to 12 hours, the customary practice. Once-daily dosing results in a higher peak serum concentration, an acceptably low trough concentration, and a lower incidence of nephrotoxicity and ototoxicity. Dosing once daily also facilitates administration and reduces costs. Gentamicin and tobramycin are dosed at 4 to 7 mg/kg/day, producing a peak serum concentration that ranges from 10 to 20 μg/ml and a trough concentration below 2 μg/ml. Amikacin is dosed at 15 mg/kg/day with a resulting peak serum concentration of 54 μg/ml and a trough concentration below 5 μg/ml. Despite studies showing an efficacy equivalent to divided daily doses, once-daily administration of aminoglycosides has not become widespread in pediatrics.

Sulfonamides and Trimethoprim

MECHANISMS OF ACTION. Sulfonamides inhibit bacterial growth by reducing bacterial synthesis of folic acid, resulting in a decrease in bacterial nucleotides. Trimethoprim inhibits bacterial dihydrofolate reductase, which is the step in folic acid synthesis that follows the one inhibited by sulfonamides. The combination of trimethoprim and sulfamethoxazole results in a synergistic, sequential blockage of folic acid.

RESISTANCE OF BACTERIA TO SULFONAMIDES AND TRIMETHOPRIM. Resistance to sulfonamides can be based on overproduction of substrate by the bacteria or a change in enzyme structure to one with diminished sulfonamide binding. Trimethoprim resistance also may be caused by a decline in the bacteria's capacity to bind the drug or to a change in dihydrofolate reductase. Resistance to both drugs can result if an organism shows decreased permeability to the drugs. Resistance occurs less often when the combination trimethoprim-sulfamethoxazole (TMP-SMX) is used.

PHARMACOLOGICAL PROPERTIES. The sulfonamides currently used in the United States, either alone or in combination with trimethoprim, are sulfisoxazole (Gantricin), sulfamethoxazole, and sulfadiazine. Sulfonamides usually are given orally, but intravenous preparations of sulfadiazine and sulfisoxazole are available. These sulfonamides are quickly and completely absorbed from the stomach and small intestine. Sulfonamides are distributed throughout the body, including the CSF. They readily cross the placenta and are found in fetal blood. Sulfonamides are partially metabolized in the liver, and free drug metabolites are excreted by glomerular filtration.

Trimethoprim also is usually given orally and is readily absorbed. It is well distributed throughout the body, with the CSF concentration reaching about 40% of the serum concentration. Excretion is primarily by renal tubular secretion.

SIDE EFFECTS. A wide variety of toxicities are associated with sulfonamides, ranging from GI upset, headache, and rash to serum sickness and hepatic necrosis. Severe hypersensitivity reactions can occur, such as toxic epidermal necrolysis, Stevens-Johnson syndrome, erythema nodosum, vasculitis, and anaphylaxis. Blood cell disorders, including aplastic anemia, granulocytopenia, thrombocytopenia, and leukopenia, have been attributed to sulfonamides. Patients who have glucose-6-phosphate dehydrogenase (G6PD) deficiency are at risk for aplastic anemia. Sulfonamides should not be taken during the last month of pregnancy because they cross the placenta and compete for bilirubin-binding sites, increasing the risk for kernicterus. All the side effects associated with sulfonamides can occur with trimethoprim as well, the most common being GI upset and hypersensitivity reactions. With prolonged use trimethoprim can interfere with folate metabolism, resulting in a megaloblastic anemia. This can be prevented by administering folinic acid.

USE OF TRIMETHOPRIM-SULFAMETHOXAZOLE AND SELECTED SULFONAMIDES. The combination of trimethoprim and sulfamethoxazole initially was introduced to treat urinary tract infections. However, because of its wide range of antibacterial activity, it has proved useful in a number of bacterial infections. Gram positive organisms susceptible to TMP-SMX include both coagulase positive and coagulase negative staphylococci, *S. pneumoniae,* enterococci, *Listeria* species, and *Streptococcus pyogenes.* However, TMP-SMX is not as effective as penicillin in the treatment of *S. pyogenes.* TMP-SMX also is inhibitory for a wide range of gram negative aerobic organisms, including *E. coli, Klebsiella* species, *Salmonella* species, *Shigella* species, *H. influenzae,* and *N. meningitidis.*

Trimethoprim-sulfamethoxazole is useful in the treatment of acute urinary tract infections and for long-term suppression in patients who have chronic or recurrent urinary tract infections, respiratory tract infections, otitis media, sinusitis, prostatitis, orchitis, and epididymitis. TMP-SMX is the drug of choice for treating *Pneumocystis carinii* infections and has proved effective in preventing *P. carinii* infection in children who have malignancies. Many adults infected with the human immunodeficiency virus (HIV) do not tolerate TMP-SMX well. To date, however, this has not been a major problem in HIV-infected infants. The peak serum concentrations for both drugs, reached about 2 hours after an oral dose, average 2 μg/ml for trimethoprim and 60 μg/ml for sulfamethoxazole. After repeated doses the peak serum concentration of trimethoprim approaches 9 μg/ml. The MIC_{95} for bacteria susceptible to the combination is 2 μg/ml or less for trimethoprim and 38 μg/ml or less for sulfamethoxazole. However, the combination usually is synergistic in vivo.

Sulfisoxazole primarily is used to treat acute urinary tract infections or to effect long-term suppression in patients who have chronic or recurrent urinary tract infections. Sulfadiazine is effective prophylaxis for close contacts of patients who have *N. meningitidis* infections if the strain is known to be susceptible (see Chapter 287). The peak serum concentrations after an oral dose of 2 g range from 30 to 60 μg/ml for sulfadiazine, 40 to 50 μg/ml for sulfisoxazole, and 80 to 100 μg/ml for sulfamethoxazole.

Topical sulfonamides are used primarily in two settings. Ophthalmic preparations of sulfacetamide are used to treat acute conjunctivitis and as adjunctive therapy in the treatment of trachoma. Silver sulfadiazine is used in the topical treatment of burns. In this combination the sulfadiazine serves principally as a vehicle for the release of silver ions, which have an antibacterial effect.

Macrolides and Azalides: Erythromycin, Clarithromycin, and Azithromycin

Mechanism of Action. Macrolides inhibit RNA-dependent protein synthesis at the step of chain elongation.

Resistance of Bacteria to Macrolides. Bacteria that lack the appropriate binding site are resistant to erythromycin, as are bacteria that are less permeable to the drug.

Erythromycin

PHARMACOLOGICAL PROPERTIES. A number of erythromycin preparations are available for oral administration. Erythromycin base is destroyed by gastric acid and therefore is useful only when given as an enteric-coated tablet. Pediatric preparations use the ester or ester salt derivatives of erythromycin because they are acid stable, soluble, and tasteless. Preparations vary in their rate and degree of absorption from the GI tract. The best absorbed is the estolate ester, which results in a peak serum concentration of about 4 μg/ml. The ethylsuccinate and stearate preparations produce peak serum concentrations that range from 0.4 to 1.9 μg/ml when given at a dose equivalent to the estolate. Erythromycin is distributed throughout the body and persists in tissue longer than in the blood. Therapeutic concentrations are reached in middle ear fluid, paranasal sinuses, tonsils, and pleural fluid. Therapeutic concentrations of erythromycin do not enter the CSF even when the meninges are inflamed. Limited data suggest that entry into synovial fluid is poor.

Erythromycin's route of elimination is not clear. A small percentage of a dose of erythromycin can be found in the urine, and erythromycin is known to be concentrated in and excreted with bile. However, most of an administered dose cannot be recovered.

SIDE EFFECTS. The most common side effect of erythromycin is GI upset. Allergic reactions occur but are relatively uncommon. Cholestatic hepatitis has been reported after treatment with the estolate ester; this side effect has been seen primarily in adults. The better absorption characteristics of the estolate probably outweigh the slight risk of cholestatic hepatitis in children.

USE. Erythromycin has a broad range of antibacterial activity and is the drug of choice for infections caused by *Mycoplasma pneumoniae, Legionella* species, *Corynebacterium diphtheriae, Bordetella pertussis, Chlamydia trachomatis,* and *Campylobacter jejuni.* Erythromycin is an alternative drug for the treatment of streptococcal and staphylococcal infections and as prophylaxis for syphilis, urinary tract infections, rheumatic fever, and bacterial endocarditis. The MIC_{95} of erythromycin required to inhibit bacteria reported as susceptible by disk is 0.5 μg/ml or less. Lactobionate and gluceptate preparations are available for parenteral administration but are not used often. The peak serum concentration after intravenous administration is about equal to that achieved when estolate is given by mouth.

Clarithromycin

PHARMACOLOGICAL PROPERTIES. Clarithromycin is stable in gastric acid, is well absorbed from the GI tract, and its bioavailability is not affected by food.[6,11] A peak serum concentration of 4 to 5 μg/ml is reached in 2½ to 3 hours, and concentrations in middle ear fluid and lung tissue exceed serum concentrations. The major route of excretion is in bile, but about one third of an administered dose can be recovered in the urine. A metabolite of clarithromycin, 14-hydroxyclarithromycin, achieves a serum concentration that is about 60% that of clarithromycin, and 14-hydroxyclarithromycin is about twice as active against *H. influenzae*.

SIDE EFFECTS. Clarithromycin causes much less gastric upset than erythromycin, but diarrhea (6% of cases), vomiting (6%), abdominal pain (3%), and nausea (1%) are the most common side effects.

USE. Clinical trials have demonstrated efficacy in the treatment of otitis media, pharyngitis, skin and soft tissue infections, and MAC infections. In general, clarithromycin can be used for infections traditionally treated with erythromycin. Because of the activity of the 14-hydroxy breakdown product, clarithromycin may prove useful in *H. influenzae* infections.

Azithromycin

Azithromycin differs structurally from erythromycin and clarithromycin by having a 15-member rather than a 14-member ring.[6,17] Because of its unique structure, azithromycin has a much larger volume of distribution, a longer half-life, and greater penetration at the cellular level. In vitro studies show antimicrobial activity that equals or exceeds that of erythromycin and clarithromycin.

Clindamycin

MECHANISM OF ACTION. Clindamycin shares binding sites with erythromycin and chloramphenicol on the 50S ribosomal subunit and interferes with protein synthesis by inhibiting the transpeptidation reaction.

MECHANISMS OF RESISTANCE. These are the same as for erythromycin.

PHARMACOLOGICAL PROPERTIES. Clindamycin usually is given orally, but preparations for intramuscular and intravenous administration are available. About 90% of a dose of clindamycin is absorbed after oral administration, and peak serum concentrations are reached in 1 hour and are dose dependent. Clindamycin palmitate (oral suspension) and clindamycin phosphate (preparation for intravenous administration) are inactive but are rapidly hydrolyzed in vivo to the active free base. Clindamycin is well distributed throughout the body except for the CSF. Clindamycin is one of the few antimicrobial agents that is concentrated in polymorphonuclear neutrophils. The serum half-life of clindamycin is about 2 hours and 24 minutes. Most clindamycin is metabolized in the liver to products that have variable antibacterial activity. Antibacterial activity in the bile and GI tract is very high and results in a dramatic decline in sensitive bowel flora.

SIDE EFFECTS. The most highly publicized side effect of clindamycin is the occurrence of colitis secondary to the toxin of *Clostridium difficile* (pseudomembranous colitis). This complication now has been associated with many other antimicrobial agents and seems to occur less often in children than in adults. Other side effects include allergic reactions, rashes, and minor elevations in transaminase concentrations.

USE. Clindamycin is highly active against most gram positive aerobic bacteria and most anaerobic bacteria. The major clinical use of clindamycin is the treatment of anaerobic infections. Clindamycin is used routinely when intraabdominal spillage of fecal material has occurred, and it also is used to treat anaerobic bronchopulmonary infections. Clindamycin also is used as alternative therapy for groups A and B streptococcal infections and as oral therapy to complete a course of antibiotics for *S. aureus* osteomyelitis. Clindamycin does not enter the CSF in useful concentrations. A peak serum concentration of 2.5 to 3.6 μg/ml is achieved about 1 hour after oral administration, and a concentration of 6 to 9 μg/ml can be reached after intravenous infusion. The MIC_{95} of clindamycin for bacteria reported as susceptible by disk is 0.5 μg/ml or less.

Chloramphenicol

MECHANISM OF ACTION. Like erythromycin and clindamycin, chloramphenicol binds to the 50S ribosomal subunit and inhibits protein synthesis.

RESISTANCE OF BACTERIA TO CHLORAMPHENICOL. Mechanisms of resistance include (1) bacterial production of an acetyltransferase that inactivates chloramphenicol and (2) inability of chloramphenicol to enter bacteria.

PHARMACOLOGICAL PROPERTIES. Chloramphenicol can be given orally as the free base or as chloramphenicol palmitate, which is hydrolyzed in the intestine to free base. Because chloramphenicol is extremely bitter, oral palmitate suspension is given to patients who cannot take capsules containing free base. The intravenous preparation is chloramphenicol succinate, which also is hydrolyzed to free base. Because the palmitate is hydrolyzed more completely than the succinate, the peak serum concentration generally is higher after oral administration. Chloramphenicol distributes well throughout the body, including the brain and CSF. Chloramphenicol is conjugated by the liver and excreted in an inactive form in urine.

SIDE EFFECTS. The major side effects of chloramphenicol are dose-related bone marrow suppression, which is reversible; aplastic anemia, which is idiosyncratic and usually fatal; and gray-baby syndrome. Gray-baby syndrome was first described and most commonly occurs in infants, but it has been reported in all age groups. The syndrome, which is characterized by cyanosis, circulatory collapse, and death, occurs when the chloramphenicol concentration becomes very high.

USE. Chloramphenicol's importance in the treatment of infectious diseases has waxed and waned since its introduction in the late 1940s. Because of its side effects, practitioners have tended to use alternative antimicrobial agents whenever possible. However, because of its antibacterial and pharmacological properties, it often must be included to optimize treatment. With the introduction of the third generation cephalosporins, use of chloramphenicol in the United States again is on the decline. Some experts on infectious diseases still maintain that chloramphenicol is the drug of choice to treat brain abscesses, bacterial meningitis in infants and children over 2 months of age, typhoid fever, and salmonellosis. Others prefer metronidazole for anaerobic coverage in brain abscesses, ceftriaxone for bacterial meningitis, and either TMP-SMX or ceftriaxone to treat typhoid fever and salmonellosis. Chloramphenicol, rather than tetracycline, is the drug of choice for rickettsial infections in children under age 8 because the side effects of tetracycline preclude its use in this age group.

When chloramphenicol must be used, the peak serum concentration should be measured after four or five doses to ensure that the concentration is safe and therapeutic and that the drug is not accumulating in the patient. A complete blood count and differential count should be done twice a week while the patient is receiving chloramphenicol to check for dose-related bone marrow suppression. The peak serum concentration is reached 1 to 2 hours after oral or intravenous administration and averages 25 μg/ml (PO) and 19 μg/ml IV.[9] The serum half-life of chloramphenicol is about 4 hours. The MIC_{95} of chloramphenicol for bacteria reported as susceptible by disk is 4 μg/ml or less for *H. influenzae* and 12.5 μg/ml or less for other organisms. Although chloramphenicol is bactericidal for *H. influenzae, S. pneumoniae,* and *N. meningitidis,* it is bacteriostatic for most other bacteria. When used with a beta-lactam to treat organisms inhibited only by chloramphenicol, antagonism may occur.[12]

Tetracycline

MECHANISM OF ACTION. Tetracycline binds to the 30S ribosomal subunit and blocks aminoacyl-tRNA binding to the receptor site; this inhibits protein synthesis.

RESISTANCE OF BACTERIA TO TETRACYCLINE. Tetracycline's entry into bacterial cells is energy dependent; resistance usually is based on interference with entry into the cell. In general, tetracycline is not altered by resistant bacteria.

PHARMACOLOGICAL PROPERTIES. A number of analogs of tetracycline have been produced, but the range of antibacterial activity is similar for each. The semisynthetic analogs, minocycline and deoxycycline, are the most active tetracyclines but are used less often than other tetracyclines because they are considerably more expensive.

Tetracycline has a broad spectrum of activity that includes inhibition of *Streptococcus* species, *Neisseria* species, *E. coli,* and many common anaerobic bacteria. Tetracyclines are well absorbed from the intestinal tract, and the peak serum concentration is achieved 1 to 3 hours after oral administration. Tetracycline distributes in varying concentrations throughout most of the body, with concentrations in synovial fluid, urine, and the maxillary sinuses approaching the serum concentration, whereas the CSF concentration reaches only 10% to 20% of the serum concentration.

SIDE EFFECTS. The side effects of tetracycline essentially precludes its use in children under age 8 and in pregnant women. Tetracycline causes a permanent gray-brown to yellowish discoloration of the teeth and can be associated with hypoplasia of the enamel. Skeletal growth can be depressed when the drug is given to premature infants. Although bone and tooth defects are associated with the total dose of tetracycline given and occur more often after repeated courses, it is safest to avoid using the drug during pregnancy and in young children. Other side effects of tetracycline are allergic reactions and skin toxicity.

USE. For individuals over age 8, tetracycline is considered the drug of choice for brucellosis, chlamydial infections, lymphogranuloma venereum, epididymitis, granuloma inguinale, infections with spirochetes (Lyme disease, relapsing fever, leptospirosis), pelvic inflammatory disease, plague, prostatitis, and rickettsial infections. Tetracycline also is an effective alternative for many other infectious diseases.

In adults, the peak serum concentrations after oral administration of 500 mg of tetracycline or 200 mg of doxycycline or minocycline are 4 μg/ml, 2.5 μg/ml, and 2.5 μg/ml, respectively. The peak serum concentration is reached 1 to 3 hours after administration. The serum half-life of tetracycline is 8 hours, compared with 16 hours for minocycline and 18 hours for doxycycline. Intravenous administration of tetracycline results in a peak serum concentration about twice that achieved when the same dose is given by mouth. The MIC_{95} of tetracycline for bacteria reported as susceptible by disk is 4 μg/ml or less.

Vancomycin

MECHANISM OF ACTION. Vancomycin inhibits cell wall synthesis and alters the permeability of the cytoplasmic membrane of protoplasts.

RESISTANCE OF BACTERIA TO VANCOMYCIN. To date, no cross-resistance between vancomycin and other antimicrobial agents has been observed. However, enterococci resistant to vancomycin (and all other approved antimicrobial agents) have become a clinical problem in some regions. As the use of vancomycin increases, the number of resistant bacteria probably will increase.

PHARMACOLOGICAL PROPERTIES. Vancomycin is minimally absorbed after oral administration and is given orally only to treat pseudomembranous colitis caused by the toxin of *C. difficile.* After intravenous administration, vancomycin is distributed throughout the body, except for the aqueous humor of the eye and the CSF when the meninges are not inflamed. A bactericidal concentration can be achieved in the CSF in cases of meningitis caused by susceptible organisms. Sometimes vancomycin must be administered intraventricularly to treat meningitis adequately with or without ventriculitis. Vancomycin is excreted unchanged in the urine by glomerular filtration. It therefore is important to monitor the serum concentration and adjust the dosage based on renal function.

SIDE EFFECTS. When vancomycin initially became available for clinical use, commercial preparations contained as much as 20% of another substance, and its use was limited by toxicity. Currently available preparations are more highly purified and less toxic. The most common side effects are fever, chills, and pain at the injection site or, less often, flushing and tingling of the face, neck, and thorax (red neck syndrome). These side effects can be largely avoided by infusing vancomycin slowly in a large volume of fluid. Auditory nerve damage is common when the serum concentration exceeds 80 μg/ml but is uncommon if the serum concentration is kept below 30 to 40 μg/ml. Nephrotoxicity occurs infrequently with current preparations of vancomycin, but a high incidence of nephrotoxicity has been reported when vancomycin and an aminoglycoside are used together.

USE. In recent years infections caused by methicillin-resistant *S. aureus,* coagulase negative staphylococci (e.g., *Staphylococcus epidermidis*), and ampicillin-resistant enterococci have become major clinical problems for which vancomycin is the drug of choice. Vancomycin is active against most aerobic gram positive cocci, including most *Streptococcus* species and *L. monocytogenes* and, in combination with streptomycin or gentamicin, is synergistic against enterococci. Many anaerobic streptococci also are susceptible to vancomycin, whereas most gram negative bacteria are resistant. Some methicillin-resistant staphylococci have demonstrated tolerance to vancomycin killing, and rifampin or TMP-SMX must be added to kill bacteria. Vancomycin is the drug of choice to treat serious infections with methicillin-resistant staphylococci or coagulase negative staphylococci and to treat enterococcal endocarditis in patients allergic to penicillin. The initial dose of vancomycin should be a full therapeutic dose, even in patients in renal failure. Subsequent doses and intervals should be adjusted to achieve a peak serum concentration of 30 to 40 μg/ml. The MIC_{95} of vancomycin for bacteria reported as susceptible by disk is 5 μg/ml or less.

A concentration of 20 μg/ml of vancomycin in a heparin flush or hyperalimentation solution has been shown to prevent line-related infections in children with cancer who have tunneled central venous catheters[14] and in premature infants.[15]

Metronidazole

MECHANISM OF ACTION. After being taken up by bacteria, metronidazole is reduced to intermediate products that are toxic to the bacteria; the organism then releases inactive end products.

RESISTANCE OF BACTERIA TO METRONIDAZOLE. Resistance to metronidazole develops only infrequently and has been associated with decreased entry of the drug into bacteria and a decreased rate of reduction once in the cells.

PHARMACOLOGICAL PROPERTIES. Metronidazole is active against most anaerobic bacteria, *Treponema pallidum, Campylobacter fetus,* and *Trichomonas vaginalis,* as well as certain parasites. After oral administration, metronidazole is absorbed rapidly and completely, with the peak serum concentration being proportional to the dose administered. Metronidazole is distributed well throughout the body, including the CNS and the aqueous humor of the eye. The serum half-life is about 8 hours. After being metabolized, metronidazole is excreted primarily in the urine.

SIDE EFFECTS. The most common side effect of metronidazole is GI upset. Metronidazole also has been associated with

CNS dysfunction (seizures, encephalopathy, ataxia) and peripheral neuropathy, and it can potentiate the effects of warfarin and cause a disulfiram reaction when alcohol is consumed. A major concern with the use of metronidazole has been its carcinogenic potential. Although rats and mice that have received metronidazole for a long period have shown an increase in neoplasms, mutagenicity for human cells has not been demonstrated in vitro, and follow-up studies on women who received metronidazole for trichomonal infections have shown that they did not have an increased frequency of tumors up to 10 years later.

USE. Originally introduced to treat *T. vaginalis,* metronidazole also has proved effective in the treatment of amebiasis and giardiasis. More recently it has gained widespread use in the treatment of anaerobic bacterial infections; it is not effective in treating actinomycosis or *Propionibacterium acnes* infections. Metronidazole also is not optimally effective in the treatment of anerobic lower respiratory tract infections, perhaps because of the presence of aerobic bacteria; the outcome generally is good if penicillin or ampicillin is given concomitantly.

The peak serum concentration achieved in adults after 0.5

Table 31-3 Initial Empirical Therapy for Selected Infections*

Clinical diagnosis	Most likely offending organisms	Antimicrobial agents
Meningitis	**Neonate:** group B streptococci, *E. coli, L. monocytogenes*	Ampicillin and cefotaxime (or ceftriaxone)
	Child: *S. pneumoniae, N. meningitidis, H. influenzae* type b	Ceftriaxone or cefotaxime (plus vancomycin if *S. pneumoniae* is suspected)
Brain abscess	Streptococcal species, anaerobes, *S. aureus*	Penicillin and metronidazole (plus nafcillin if *S. aureus* is suspected)
Orbital cellulitis	Streptococcal species, *S. aureus, H. influenzae* type b	Ceftriaxone or cefotaxime plus clindamycin
Epiglottitis	*H. influenzae* type b	Ceftriaxone or cefotaxime
Pneumonia (lobar or segmental)	**Neonate:** group B streptococci, *S. aureus,* gram negative organisms	Ampicillin plus an aminoglycoside
	Child: *S. pneumoniae, H. influenzae* type b, *S. aureus, S. pyogenes, M. pneumoniae*	Penicillin or nafcillin, or erythromycin
Infective endocarditis	*Streptococcus viridans, S. aureus*	Nafcillin plus an aminoglycoside
Acute diarrhea (fecal WBC present)	*Salmonella, Shigella* species	If patient is systemically ill, very young, or immunocompromised, cefotaxime or ceftriaxone
Abdominal sepsis	Anaerobes, aerobic enterics, enterococci	Clindamycin, aminoglycoside, and ampicillin
Urinary tract infection	**Acute:** *E. coli, Klebsiella* species	Gentamicin or trimethoprim/sulfamethoxazole (TMP-SMX)
	Chronic: *E. coli, Proteus* species, *Pseudomonas* species	Await culture and sensitivity results
Osteomyelitis	**Neonate:** group B streptococci, *S. aureus, S. pyogenes, S. pneumoniae*	Nafcillin plus an aminoglycoside
	Child: *S. aureus, S. pyogenes*	Nafcillin
Pyogenic arthritis	**Neonate:** group B streptococci, *S. aureus, S. pyogenes, N. gonorrhoea*	Nafcillin and an aminoglycoside
	Child: *H. influenzae* type b (<5 yr), *S. aureus, S. pyogenes, N. gonorrhoea*	Ceftriaxone or cefotaxime (test MIC for *S. aureus*) plus nafcillin
Suspected sepsis	**Neonate:** group B streptococci, *L. monocytogenes,* gram negative enteric organisms	Ampicillin plus an aminoglycoside
	Infant (1-6 wk): as for neonate plus as for child	Ampicillin plus ceftriaxone
	Child: *S. pneumoniae, H. influenzae* type b, *N. meningitidis*	Ceftriaxone
Compromised host		
Fever only	*S. aureus, E. coli, Pseudomonas* species	Cefotaxime or aminopenicillin
Pneumonia	As under pneumonia above, and *P. carinii, Candida albicans,* other fungi	As under pneumonia above plus TMP-SMX; if patient's condition deteriorates, bronchoalveolar lavage (BAL) or lung biopsy is needed to direct therapy
Shock (sepsis without source)	**Neonate:** group B streptococci, enterics	Ampicillin plus an aminoglycoside
	Child: *N. meningitidis, S. pneumoniae*	Ceftriaxone or cefotaxime

*For most clinical diagnoses, an acceptable alternative choice of antibiotics could be proposed.

Table 31-4 Antimicrobial Prophylaxis Against Specific Pathogens

Pathogen	Disease to be prevented	Antimicrobial agent	Dose	Duration of therapy
Bacteria				
Bordetella pertussis	Secondary cases of pertussis in household contacts	Erythromycin estolate	40-50 mg/kg/day in 4 doses (not to exceed 2 g/day)	14 days
*Chlamydia trachomatis**	Urogenital infections in exposed individuals	Doxycycline (>8 yr) **or** azithromycin (adolescents) **or** erythromycin	200 mg/day in 2 doses 1 g 40-50 mg/kg/day in 4 doses (not to exceed 2 g/day)	7 days 1 dose PO 7 days
*Corynebacterium diphtheriae**	Diphtheria in unimmunized contacts	Benzathine penicillin **or** erythromycin	*<30 kg:* 600,00 U *>30 kg:* 1.2 million U 40-50 mg/kg/day in 4 doses (not to exceed 2 g/day)	1 dose IM 7 days
Haemophilus influenzae	Secondary cases of systemic infection in close contacts <1 yr of age and in children 12-47 mo who are not fully immunized	Rifampin	*≤1 mo:* 10-20 mg/kg *>1 mo:* 20 mg/kg (maximum 600 mg)	Once a day for 4 days
Mycobacterium tuberculosis	Overt pulmonary or metastatic infection	Isoniazid	10-20 mg/kg (not to exceed 300 mg)	Once a day for 9 days
Neisseria meningitidis	Meningococcemia in exposed susceptible individuals	Rifampin	*≤1 mo:* 5-10 mg/kg *>1 mo:* 10 mg/kg (maximum 600 mg)	q12h for 4 doses
Neisseria gonorrhoeae	Gonococcal infection in exposed individuals; ophthalmia neonatorum	Ceftriaxone **or** cefixime **or** zofloxicin (≥18 yr)	250 mg 400 or 800 mg 400 mg	1 dose IM 1 dose PO 1 dose PO
Streptococcus pneumoniae	Fulminant pneumococcal infection in individuals with asplenia or sickle cell disease	Penicillin V	125 mg	2 times/day for life
Group A streptococcus	Recurrent rheumatic fever	Benzathine penicillin **or** penicillin V **or** sulfadiazine	1.2 million U 125-250 mg *<27 kg:* 0.5 g *>27 kg:* 1 kg	Every 4 wk 2 times/day Once a day for life Once a day for life
Group B streptococcus	Neonatal infection	Ampicillin	*Mother:* 2 g IV given intrapartum, followed by 1 g q4h until delivery *Infant:* 50 mg/kg IM q12h for 2 days	
Treponema pallidum	Syphilis in exposed individuals	Benzathine penicillin	2.4 million U	1 dose IM
*Vibrio cholerae**	Cholera in close contacts	Tetracycline or trimethoprim-sulfamethoxazole	250 mg q6h (>8 yr) 5 mg/kg as trimethoprim 2 times/day	3 days 3 days
*Yersinia pestis**	Plague in household contacts or individuals exposed to pneumonic disease	Tetracycline (>8 yr) **or** sulfonamide	15 mg/kg/day in 4 doses 40 mg/kg/day in 4 doses	7 days 7 days
Parasites				
Plasmodium species (malaria)	Overt infection in endemic areas	Chloroquine	5 mg/kg base once a week (maximum 300 mg base), beginning 2 wk before entering endemic area, while in area, and for 6 wk after leaving area	
Viruses				
Influenza A	Influenza in individuals at risk of complications	Amantadine	*1-9 yr:* 2-4.4 mg/kg q12h (maximum 150 mg/day) *>9 yr:* 100 mg q12h	Duration of influenza outbreak
Other				
Pneumocystis carinii	Pneumonia in a compromised host	Trimethoprim-sulfamethoxazole	5 mg trimethoprim/25 mg sulfamethoxazole	Once a day while patient is undergoing chemotherapy

Modified from Peter G et al, editors: Report of the Committee on Infectious Diseases: *1994 Red Book,* ed 23, Elk Grove Village, Ill, 1994, The American Academy of Pediatrics.

*Efficacy of treatment has not been established.

g of metronidazole is given orally averages 11.5 μg/ml; after an intravenous dose of 0.5 g, the serum concentration ranges from 20 to 25 μg/ml. The MIC_{95} of metronidazole for susceptible bacteria usually is 4 μg/ml or less. Most diagnostic microbiology laboratories do not routinely test anaerobic bacteria for susceptibility.

Rifampin

MECHANISM OF ACTION. Rifampin works by inhibiting DNA-dependent RNA polymerase at the B subunit, preventing chain initiation but not elongation.

RESISTANCE OF BACTERIA TO RIFAMPIN. Resistance to rifampin develops rapidly by mutation of the DNA-dependent RNA polymerase. The rates of mutation are so high they preclude use of rifampin as monotherapy except for very short courses of prophylaxis.

PHARMACOLOGICAL PROPERTIES. Rifampin usually is administered orally and is completely and rapidly absorbed, with the peak serum concentration achieved 1 to 4 hours after ingestion. An intravenous form of rifampin also is available. Rifampin is distributed throughout the body, deacetylated by the liver, and excreted in the bile. The serum half-life is 2 to 5 hours early in therapy, but it declines over time because of increased biliary excretion. Rifampin also can enter phagocytes and kill viable intracellular organisms, which may explain why rifampin is better able to enter and sterilize abscesses than other antimicrobial agents.

SIDE EFFECTS. When rifampin is given daily, the most common side effects are a mild, self-limited rash and mild GI complaints. When rifampin is used intermittently at high individual doses, a flulike syndrome with fever, aches, and chills develops in up to 20% of patients. Because rifampin crosses the placenta and teratogenic effects have been observed in rodents, it should not be used during pregnancy except in severe cases of tuberculosis. Patients or parents should be warned that urine, feces, saliva, and tears may turn a red-orange color while they are taking the drug. The patient should not wear contact lenses, which can become permanently discolored.

USE OF RIFAMPIN. Rifampin is extremely active against a wide range of organisms. Most strains of *S. aureus* and coagulase negative staphylococci are exquisitely sensitive to rifampin, which also is active against most other gram positive cocci. *H. influenzae*, *N. meningitidis*, and *N. gonorrhoeae* are exquisitely susceptible to rifampin, but other aerobic gram negative pathogens are less susceptible. Rifampin also is active against *Legionella* species and *Mycobacterium tuberculosis*.

Despite its widespread use for treating tuberculosis and as prophylaxis for *N. meningitidis* and *H. influenzae*, no pediatric preparation of rifampin is available. Instructions for preparing a suspension for pediatric use are detailed in the *Physicians' Desk Reference*.[13] Internationally, rifampin most commonly is used to treat tuberculosis and leprosy. Rifampin also is recommended for prophylaxis of close contacts of patients who have meningococcal disease and for household contacts of children who have systemic *H. influenzae* type b disease. When another antimicrobial agent is used with rifampin for the last 4 days of treatment of group A beta-hemolytic streptococcal infections, the microbiological failure rate falls to almost zero. Rifampin in combination with other antistaphylococcal agents has been used to treat severe staphylococcal infections such as *S. aureus* endocarditis, osteomyelitis, and CSF shunt infections caused by coagulase negative staphylococci.

The peak serum concentration of rifampin after oral ad-

Table 31-5 Clinical Situations in which Prophylaxis with Antimicrobial Agents Has Proved Effective

Body site	Infection to be prevented	Agents	Recommended dosage
Conjunctivae	Neonatal gonococcal ophthalmia	1% silver nitrate, 0.5% erythromycin, 1% tetracycline, penicillin	Applied topically once shortly after delivery
Abnormal heart valve	Bacterial endocarditis (e.g., after dental extraction)	Penicillin, ampicillin	*Standard-risk patients, oral procedures:* penicillin V, 2 g PO, then 1 g 6 hours later; *high-risk patients, dental, or all patients, GU or GI tract procedures:* ampicillin, 2 g IM or IV plus gentamicin, 1.5-2 mg/kg 30 min before and 8 hours after procedure
Surgical wound	Serious postoperative wound infection	Appropriate for expected contaminants	See Kaiser AB: *N Engl J Med* 315:1129, 1986.[3]
Middle ear	Recurrent otitis media	Amoxicillin, sulfisoxazole	5-10 mg/kg given q12h 40-50 mg/kg given q12h (given during winter and spring)
Urinary tract	Recurrent infection	Trimethoprim/sulfamethoxazole, nitrofurantoin	2 mg TMP and 10 mg SMX/kg once daily 1-2 mg/kg once daily Duration: months to years, depending on clinical situation
Human/animal bite wound*	Wound infection, cellulitis	Amoxicillin/clavulanate	40 mg of the amoxicillin component/kg/day given q8h for 5-7 days

Modified from Peter G et al, editors: Report of the Committee on Infectious Diseases: *1994 Red Book*, ed 23, Elk Grove Village, Ill, 1994, The American Academy of Pediatrics.

*Efficacy of treatment has not been established.

Table 31-6 Antiviral Drugs

Generic (trade name)	Indication		Normal recommended dosage
Acyclovir* (Zovirax)	Genital herpes simplex virus (HSV) infection, first episode	PO IV	1200 mg/day in 3 divided doses for 7-10 days† 15 mg/kg/day in 3 divided doses for 5-7 days
	Genital HSV infection, recurrence	PO	1200 mg/day in 3 divided doses or 1600 mg/day in 2 divided doses for 5 days†
	Recurrent genital HSV episodes in patient with frequent recurrences:		
	Chronic suppressive therapy	PO	800-1000 mg/day in 2-5 divided doses for as long as 12 continuous months†
	HSV in immunocompromised host (localized, progressive, or disseminated)‡	IV	*Children <1 yr except neonates:* 15-30 mg/kg/day in 3 divided doses for 7-14 days (some experts also recommend this dosage for children ≥1 yr)
		IV	*Children ≥1 yr:* 750 mg/m^2/day in 3 divided doses for 7-14 days (some experts recommend 1500 mg/m^2/day in 3 divided doses)
		PO	1000 mg/day in 3-5 divided doses for 7-14 days†
	Prophylaxis of HSV in immunocompromised HSV-seropositive patient‡	PO IV	600-1000 mg/day in 3-5 divided doses during risk period† 750 mg/m^2/day in 3 divided doses during risk period
	HSV encephalitis	IV	*Children <1 yr:* 30 mg/kg/day in 3 divided doses for a minimum of 14 days (some experts also recommend this dosage for children ≥1 yr)
		IV	*Children ≥1 yr:* 1500 mg/m^2/day in 3 divided doses for 14-21 days (some experts also recommend this dosage for children <1 yr)
	Neonatal HSV‡	IV	30 mg/kg/day in 3 divided doses for 14-21 days (some experts recommend 45-60 mg/kg/day in 3 divided doses for term infants; for premature infants, 20 mg/kg/day in 2 divided doses is recommended for 14-21 days)
	Varicella or zoster in immunocompromised host	IV	*Children <1 yr:* 30 mg/kg/day in 3 divided doses (some experts also recommend this dosage for children ≥1 yr)
		IV	*Children ≥1 yr:* 1500 mg/m^2/day in 3 divided doses for 7-10 days
	Zoster in immunocompetent host‡	IV PO	Same as for zoster in immunocompromised host 4000 mg/day in 5 divided doses for 5-7 days for patients ≥12 yr†
	Varicella in immunocompetent host	PO	80 mg/kg/day in 4 divided doses for 5 days; maximum dose is 3200 mg/day
	Prophylaxis of cytomegalovirus (CMV) infection in immunocompromised host (e.g., transplant recipient)‡	PO IV	800-3200 mg/day in 1-4 divided doses during risk period*† 1500 mg/m^2/day in 3 divided doses during risk period
Amantadine (Symmetrel)	Influenza A: treatment and prophylaxis	PO	*>20 kg:* 100 mg/day in 1 or 2 divided doses for duration of exposure *<20 kg:* 5 mg/kg/day in 1 or 2 divided doses for duration of exposure
Ribavirin (Virazole)	Treatment of respiratory syncytial virus (RSV) infection	Aerosol	Given by a small particle generator, in a solution of 6 g in 300 ml of sterile water (20 mg/ml), for 12-20 hours/day for 1-7 days; longer treatment may be necessary for some patients
Rimantadine (Flumadine)	Influenza A: treatment and prophylaxis	PO	*>20 kg:* 100 mg/day in 1 or 2 divided doses for duration of exposure *<20 kg:* 5 mg/kg/day in 1 or 2 divided doses for duration of exposure
Vidarabine (Vira-A)	Neonatal HSV	IV	15-30 mg/kg/day in 1 dose over 12-24 hr for 10-21 days
	Varicella or zoster in immunocompromised host‡	IV	10 mg/kg/day in 1 dose over 12-24 hr for 5-10 days

Modified from Peter G et al, editors: Report of the Committee on Infectious Diseases: *1994 Red Book,* ed 23, Elk Grove Village, Ill, 1994, The American Academy of Pediatrics.

*Dose should be reduced if the patient's renal function is impaired.

†In children, oral dose of acyclovir should not exceed 80 mg/kg/day.

‡As of June 1994 the drug had not been licensed for this use or was investigational.

Table 31-7 Recommended Doses of Parenteral and Oral Antifungal Drugs

Drug	Route	Dose (per day)	Adverse reactions*
Amphotericin B	IV	0.25 mg/kg (after test dose†) initially, increase as tolerated to 0.5-1 mg/kg; infuse as single dose over 4-6 hr	Fever, chills, phlebitis, renal dysfunction, hypokalemia, anemia, cardiac arrhythmias, anaphylactoid reaction, hematological abnormalities
	Intrathecal (IT)	0.025 mg, increase to 0.1-0.5 mg twice weekly	Radiculitis, sensory loss, foot drop
Clotrimazole (troches)	PO (topical)	10 mg tablet 5 times/day (dissolved slowly in the mouth)	Nausea, vomiting, increase in serum transaminase
Fluconazole	IV PO	*Children*‡: 3-6 mg/kg/day *Adults:* 200 mg once, followed by 100 mg/day for oropharyngeal, esophageal candidiasis; 400 mg once, followed by 200-400 mg/day for cryptococcal meningitis (200 mg/day for maintenance in patients with acquired immune deficiency syndrome [AIDS])	Rash, nausea, abdominal pain, diarrhea, headache, possibly hepatotoxicity
Flucytosine	PO	50-150 mg/kg in 4 doses at 6-hr intervals (adjust dosage with renal dysfunction)	Bone marrow suppression; renal dysfunction can lead to drug accumulation; nausea, vomiting, increases in transaminases, blood urea nitrogen (BUN), and creatinine
Griseofulvin	PO	Ultramicrosize: 7.3 mg/kg, single dose; maximum dose, 375-750 mg Microsize: 15-20 mg/kg/day divided in 2 doses; maximum dose, 500-1000 mg	Rash, leukopenia, proteinuria, paresthesia, GI symptoms, mental confusion
Itraconazole	PO	*Children:* dose has not been established; a dose of 100 mg/day has been reported for children 3-16 yr *Adults:* 200 mg once or twice daily	Nausea, epigastric pain, headache, edema, hypokalemia, increased serum aminotransferase, hypertension, adrenal insufficiency
Ketoconazole	PO	*Children:* 3.3-6.6 mg/kg, once daily§ *Adults:* 200-400 mg once daily	Rash, anaphylaxis, nausea, vomiting, abdominal pain, fever, gynecomastia, thrombocytopenia, hepatoxicity, and depression of endocrine function (dose dependent, reversible); should not be given concurrently with the antihistamine terfenadine
Miconazole	IV	20-40 mg/kg/day divided into 3 infusions 8 hr apart; maximum 15 mg/kg per infusion; infuse over 30-60 min	Phlebitis, rash, fever, nausea, anemia, hyponatremia, thrombocytopenia, hyperlipemia
	IT	20 mg per dose for 3-7 days	
Nystatin	PO	*Infants:* 200,000 U 4 times/day *Children and adults:* 400,000-600,000 U 4 times/day	Nausea, vomiting, diarrhea

*See the package insert or the listing in the current edition of the *Physicians' Desk Reference,* Montvale, NJ, Medical Economics.
†Test dose is 0.1 mg/kg, with a maximum dose of 1 mg/kg.
‡The daily dose has not been established for children ≤2 yr.
§Efficacy has not been established for children. A small number of children 3 to 13 years of age have been treated safely with this dose.

ministration of 600 mg to an adult or 10 mg/kg to a child averages 7 μg/ml. Because of rifampin's long half-life, the peak serum concentration and bioavailability are better if the drug is given once a day. The MIC_{95} of bacteria reported as susceptible by disk to rifampin is 1 μg/ml or less.

INITIAL THERAPY OF SELECTED ACUTE INFECTIONS

In most clinical situations the physician must decide which antimicrobial agent or agents to use before the offending organism has been positively identified through culture results, serological tests, or microscopical examination of material obtained from the infected site. The practitioner should consider the following points before starting treatment:

- The patient's age and immune status
- Whether concomitant disease is a factor
- The patient's history of exposure to infectious agents
- Current or recent administration of antimicrobial agents
- The findings on physical examination

Appropriate specimens for bacterial and viral cultures and specimens for serological tests and microscopical examinations should be obtained before antimicrobial therapy is started, and specific adjunctive, supportive therapy should be instituted concomitantly. Table 31-3 lists the most likely offending organisms and the antimicrobial agent or agents that could be used empirically for various diagnoses under these circumstances. Local susceptibility patterns and other special circumstances always should be considered.

PROPHYLAXIS

Antimicrobial agents can be given to prevent colonization, to eradicate carriage, to prevent bacteria that colonize one body site from causing disease at a usually sterile site, or to prevent bacteria that have been introduced into a usually sterile site from causing disease.[3] In general, an antimicrobial agent with the narrowest spectrum that is effective against the most likely pathogen or pathogens should be used at the lowest dosage and for the shortest period that will prevent infection. Prophylaxis also should be restricted to situations in which prophylaxis is known to be effective and the risk of infection exceeds the potential risks of the antimicrobial agent or the emergence of resistant bacteria. Specific bacterial pathogens for which prophylaxis has proved effective are shown in Table 31-4, and clinical situations in which prophylactic antimicrobial agents might be effective are listed in Table 31-5.[4] The reader is referred to the *1994 Red Book* (Report of the Committee on Infectious Diseases, American Academy of Pediatrics) for regularly updated recommendations for prophylaxis in specific situations, such as prevention of bacterial endocarditis.[12]

ANTIMICROBIAL THERAPY FOR VIRAL, FUNGAL, AND PARASITIC INFECTIONS

Currently there are only a limited number of agents and a limited number of indications for systemic treatment of viral, fungal, and parasitic infections in the United States, and because of this, most primary care pediatricians are unlikely to be familiar with the use of these agents. Therefore it is recommended that the pediatrician consult a specialist in pediatric infectious diseases before treating a patient with these drugs. The antiviral drugs currently available, along with their indications and dosages, are presented in Table 31-6; antifungal drugs (and their dosages and adverse reactions) are listed in Table 31-7. Treatment of parasitic infections is discussed in the appropriate chapters in this text and in the AAP's *1994 Red Book,* in the *Pocketbook of Pediatric Antimicrobial Therapy,*[10] and in *The Medical Letter Handbook of Antimicrobial Therapy.*[1] Use of topical antifungal and antiviral preparations also is discussed elsewhere in this text.

REFERENCES

1. Abramowicz M, editor: *The Medical Letter handbook of antimicrobial therapy,* New Rochelle, NY, 1990, The Medical Letter.
2. Ellner PD, New HC: The inhibitory quotient: a method of interpreting minimum inhibitory concentration data, *JAMA* 246:1575, 1981.
3. Kaiser AB: Antimicrobial prophylaxis in surgery, *N Engl J Med* 315:1129, 1986.
4. Karam GH, Sanders CV, Aldridge KE: Role of newer antimicrobial agents in the treatment of mixed aerobic and anaerobic infections, *Surg Gynecol Obstet* 172(suppl):57, 1990.
5. Kim KS: Clinical perspectives on penicillin tolerance, *J Pediatr* 112:509, 1988.
6. Klein JO: Clarithromycin: where do we go from here? *Pediatr Infect Dis J* 12:S148, 1993.
7. Moellering RC Jr, editor: Proceedings of symposium, tissue-directed antibiotic therapy, *Am J Med* 91(suppl 3A):1S, 1991.
8. Molavi A: Cephalosporins: rationale for clinical use, *Am Fam Physician* 43:937, 1991.
9. National Committee for Clinical Laboratory Standards: *Performance standards for antimicrobial disk susceptibility tests,* ed 3, 1984.
10. Nelson JD: 1991-1992 *Pocketbook of pediatric antimicrobial therapy,* ed 9, Baltimore, 1991, Williams & Wilkins.
11. Neu HC: The development of macrolides: clarithromycin in perspective, *J Antimicrob Chemother* 27(suppl A):1, 1991.
12. Peter G et al, editors: Report of the Committee on Infectious Diseases: *1994 Red Book,* ed 22, Elk Grove Village, Ill, 1994, The American Academy of Pediatrics.
13. *Physicians' Desk Reference,* ed 48, Oradell, NJ, 1994, Medical Economics.
14. Schwartz C et al: Prevention of bacteremia attributed to luminal colonization of tunneled central venous catheters with vancomycin-susceptible organisms, *J Clin Oncol* 8:1591, 1990.
15. Spafford PS et al: Prevention of central venous catheter–related coagulase negative staphylococcus sepsis in neonates, *J Pediatr* 125:259, 1994.
16. Stamos JK, Yogev R: Oral cephalosporins: the newest of the new, *Contemp Pediatr* 10:28, 1993.
17. Whitman MS, Tunkel AR: Azithromycin and clarithromycin: overview and comparison with erythromycin, *Infect Control Hosp Epidemiol* 13:357, 1992.

SUGGESTED READINGS

Donowitz GR, Mandell GL: Beta-lactim antibiotics, *N Engl J Med* 318:419, 1988.

Kucers A, Bennett N: *The use of antibiotics,* ed 4, Philadelphia, 1987, JB Lippincott.

Mandell GL, Douglas RG Jr, Bennett JE, editors: *Principles and practice of infectious diseases,* ed 3, New York, 1990, Churchill Livingstone.

Moellering RC, editor: Antibacterial agents: pharmacodynamics, pharmacology, new agents, *Infect Dis Clin North Am* 3:375, 1989.

32 Minimally Invasive Surgery

George W. Holcomb III

Minimally invasive surgery (MIS) is an attempt to achieve the same surgical results as open surgery but with added benefits such as fewer days of hospitalization, reduced discomfort, faster return to regular activities, and improved cosmesis. The two primary techniques employed in MIS are laparoscopy (MIS in the abdomen) and thoracoscopy (MIS in the chest).

The technology for widespread application of MIS in patients has only recently become refined for application to a broad spectrum of diseases. Although a surge in the use of this technology in adults has occurred over the past 4 years, its utilization in infants and children has been slower to evolve. The purpose of this chapter is to introduce the principles of MIS in pediatric patients and to describe indications for its use.

HISTORY

The first attempt at endoscopy was made in the early 19th century by Bozzinni, who devised a waxed candle with a mirror reflection to illuminate shallow orifices for examination and manipulation.[7] In 1867 Desormeau designed an open tube endoscope that was used to examine the urethra and bladder.[14] He used the light of a small flame from a mixture of alcohol and turpentine for illumination. He noted that a properly placed lens could condense the light to a narrower and brighter focal spot. Kussmaul learned of Desormeau's instrument and wanted to use it for esophagoscopy. Before that time the obstacle to esophagoscopy was overcoming the oropharyngoesophageal angle (the angle made by the horizontal axis of the mouth and the vertical axis of the pharynx and the esophagus). By chance a sword swallower was observed by one of Kussmaul's assistants and subsequently observed personally by Kussmaul. Kussmaul noted that the oropharyngoesophageal angle could be overcome by positioning the head and neck properly and he had a local instrument maker fashion a suitable tube by using Desormeau's principles. In 1868 Kussmaul began to perform esophagoscopy—a notable accomplishment of the time.[42]

Over the next 100 years small refinements were made in the lens system. Reasonable optics were developed for endoscopy in adults, but the size of the instrument remained the limiting factor for use in children. The field of view was too small and the light too dim with smaller scopes, making orientation difficult and image clarity less than satisfactory. Therefore procedures were prolonged, repeated, or abandoned, even in skillful and experienced hands.

In 1902 Kelling introduced the use of laparoscopy on dogs; in 1910 Jacobaeus first described laparoscopy in the human.[32,36] By 1950 advances had been made in endoscopy such that Kalk and Bruhl were able to conduct a series of 2000 laparoscopic procedures in adults without a fatality.[35] However, acceptance of this modality was slow, and it was used mainly by gynecologists.

The development of the rod-lens telescopic system by Hopkins allowed the construction of smaller endoscopes.[3] These telescopes used glass rod lenses with small interspaces; in traditional telescopes the lenses were placed in air channels. The new telescopes had a much larger viewing angle which provided a wider field of view and made orientation easier. In 1971 Gans and Berci first reported laparoscopy in children.[15] They verified a contralateral patent processus vaginalis using an endoscope introduced through the known inguinal hernia sac. Following this procedure there was a succession of reports involving liver and pelvic conditions.[16] However, despite many presentations and demonstrations, laparoscopy failed to be accepted widely in pediatric surgery.

Years later the rapid spread of MIS began with the description of laparoscopic cholecystectomy by Phillippe Mouret in 1987 and the report of its use in 25 adult patients by Reddick and Olsen in 1989.[9,55] The latter report initiated an explosion in the use of MIS in adults. Some interest has developed recently in the use of these newer endoscopic techniques in infants and children. However, the use of these techniques will surely extend to pediatric patients as medical personnel gain more experience with endoscopy.

PRINCIPLES OF MIS

The basic principle of MIS is the utilization of small (5 mm to 10 mm) incisions through which hollow tubes (cannulas) are inserted into a body cavity such as the abdomen or thorax (Fig. 32-1). A telescope, similar to the ones employed for esophagoscopy, bronchoscopy, and cystoscopy, is introduced through one of the cannulas for visualization (Fig. 32-2). The telescope then is connected to a camera, which also is connected to one or several video monitors (Fig. 32-3). By placing instruments through the hollow cannulas and observing on the video monitor their manipulation by the surgeon, it is possible to perform various surgical procedures.

Laparoscopy requires that the abdomen be distended in order to develop an adequate space to perform the procedure. If the abdomen is not distended, the underlying abdominal visceral and intestinal organs are at risk for injury. However, in the chest, with intubation of the contralateral mainstem bronchus and desufflation of the ipsilateral lung, adequate working space is obtained and insufflation usually is not necessary.

The number of incisions required for a laparoscopic procedure usually is proportional to the difficulty of the procedure. For example, diagnostic laparoscopy may require only a single incision. This usually is placed in the umbilicus because the incision can be hidden well and results in a satisfactory cosmetic appearance. In infants a 3-mm incision is

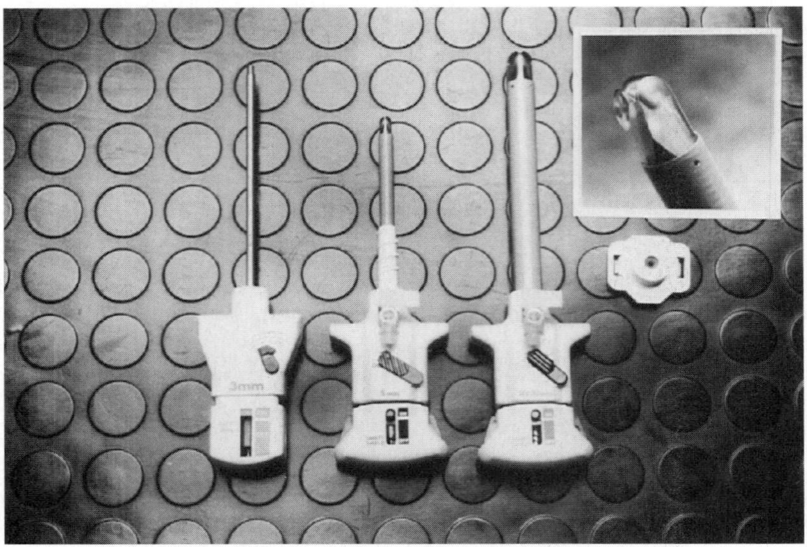

FIG. 32-1 Three disposable cannulas and trocars of different sizes are shown. A 3-mm cannula is shown on the left and 5-mm and 10/11-mm cannulas are shown on the right. Inset shows the safety shield surrounding the sharp stylet.

(From Holcomb GW III, editor: *Pediatric endoscopic surgery,* Norwalk, Conn, 1993, Appleton & Lange.)

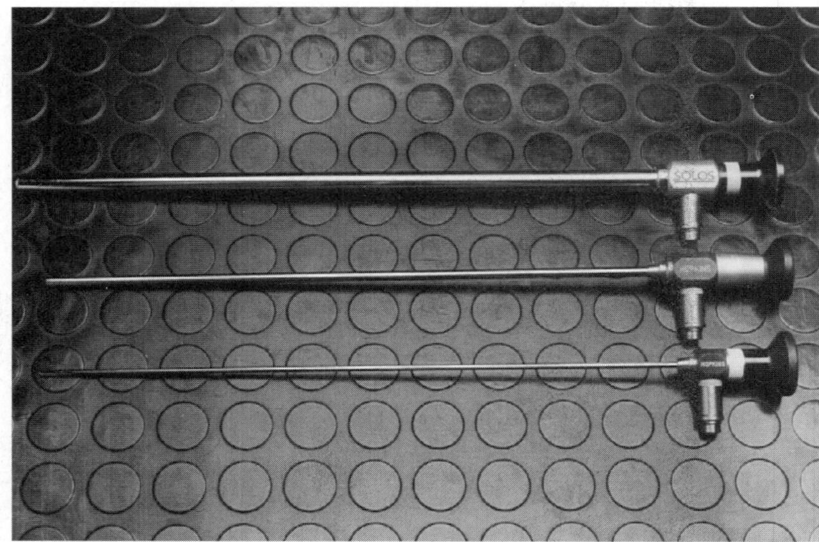

FIG. 32-2 Three telescopes are identified: a 10-mm telescope, a 5 mm telescope, and a 2.8-mm telescope. These can be introduced through a 10-, 5-, and 3-mm cannula, respectively.

(From Holcomb GW III, editor: *Pediatric endoscopic surgery,* Norwalk, Conn, 1993, Appleton & Lange.)

all that is needed for diagnostic laparoscopy because a 3-mm cannula and telescope can be inserted with adequate visualization. However, as the size of the patient increases, the size of the telescope usually increases as well—a 5-mm telescope usually is employed in young preschool children, whereas a 10-mm telescope is utilized in school age, adolescent, and adult patients.

For procedural laparoscopies such as appendectomy and cholecystectomy, two and sometimes three other incisions are required. For appendectomy a 5-mm incision customarily is placed in the left lower abdominal quadrant and a 5-mm incision in the suprapubic area. Therefore by using a total of three incisions, including one in the umbilicus, laparoscopic appendectomy usually can be performed. For cholecystectomy, an additional cannula is needed for retraction purposes.

As the complexity of the laparoscopic procedure increases, more cannulas are needed for retraction. Procedures such as fundoplication and splenectomy usually require four and sometimes five small incisions.

Thoracoscopic procedures necessitate three incisions. One incision is employed for insertion of the telescope, one for placement of an instrument for retraction, and another as the working "port" for the surgeon. Placement of the thoracoscopic incisions should be individualized according to the disease process. For instance, placement of the incisions for

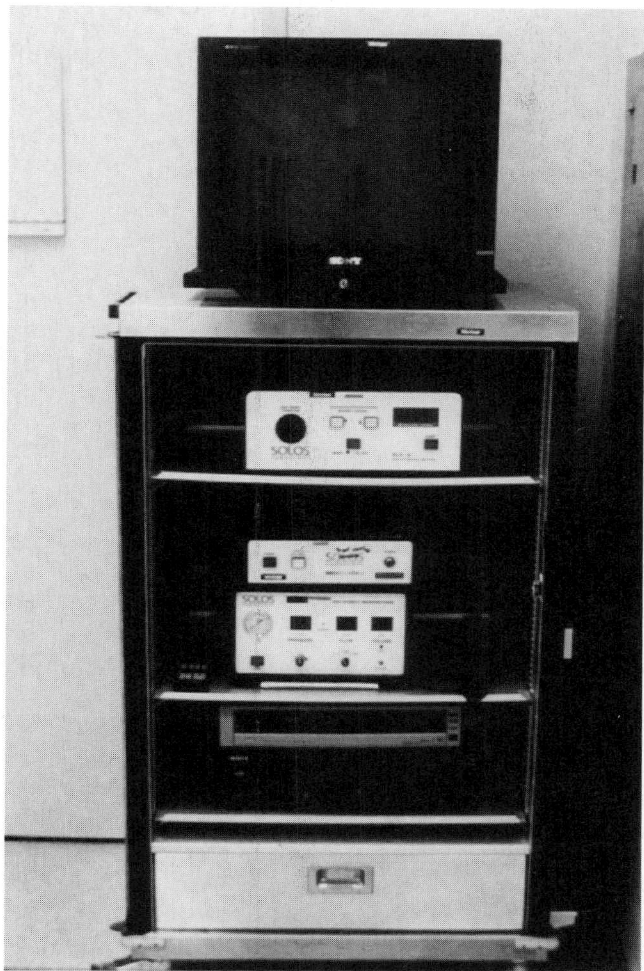

FIG. 32-3 A case cart has been designed that contains the video monitor *(top)*, telescope light source, camera light source and pressure monitor, and VCR/printer *(bottom)*.

(From Holcomb GW III, editor: *Pediatric endoscopic surgery*, Norwalk, Conn, 1993, Appleton & Lange.)

evaluation of an anterior mediastinal mass would be different from that for a posterior mediastinal mass.

Different instruments have been developed specifically for laparoscopic and thoracoscopic procedures. Vascular ligation usually is accomplished with endoscopic clip appliers using stainless steel clips or by endoscopic staplers similar to those used with open surgical procedures. Other instruments such as curved dissectors, scissors, grasping forceps, and cautery are also standard for both laparoscopic and thoracoscopic procedures (Fig. 32-4).

DIAGNOSTIC LAPAROSCOPY

Diagnostic laparoscopy is performed easily in infants and children and can be quite useful in solving certain surgical problems (see the box above). It has been used since 1991 at Children's Hospital–Vanderbilt University Medical Center (CH-VUMC) for evaluation of boys who have a nonpalpable testis.[24] The vexing question facing surgeons who treat boys who have a nonpalpable testis is the uncertainty regarding its location. It is known that some nonpalpable testes have atrophied during in utero descent into the scrotum. However, in other boys the descent of the testis has been arrested within the abdomen or in the upper inguinal canal, accounting for the testis not being palpable (Fig. 32-5). It is in this latter group that orchiopexy can be technically difficult because of the very short length of the testicular artery and vein. Thus, when shortened, these vessels can become the limiting factor in whether the testicle can be brought into the scrotum. If the length is insufficient and the testicle is placed forcefully in the scrotum with undue tension, vascular spasm will result in ischemia and testicular infarction.

INDICATIONS FOR DIAGNOSTIC LAPAROSCOPY IN CHILDREN

Nonpalpable testes
Contralateral patent processus vaginalis
Chronic abdominal pain
Diagnostic evaluation for appendicitis
Evaluation of possible traumatic injury
Evaluation of infants with ambiguous genitalia
Staging evaluations in children with cancer

To overcome the problem of short testicular vessels in a child who has an intraabdominal testis, the Fowler-Stephens orchiopexy was developed. The basic principle of this procedure is to divide the testicular artery and vein, thus allowing the testicle to be nourished through collateral vessels along the vas deferens. Because the vas deferens originates in the pelvis and has a lengthy course along the lateral pelvic wall into the inguinal canal, it usually is of sufficient length to reach into the scrotum. The success rate for a Fowler-Stephens orchiopexy when performed as a single stage varies between 50% to 70%.[4]

A more favorable experience with a two-stage approach was reported by Ransley et al. in 1984 in which the testicular vessels were divided at the first stage followed by orchiopexy several months later.[54] The rationale for this approach is that preliminary ligation of the testicular vessels allows augmentation of the collateral vessels and thereby improves the chances that the collateral vasculature will be sufficient to nourish the testis. In 1988 this initial ligation using laparoscopy was described by Bloom.[5] Following that report, several other investigators have described successful endoscopic ligation of the testicular vessels in an attempt to enhance the vasal collaterals before orchiopexy.[6,8,10,22,26]

Diagnostic laparoscopy is performed on boys who have a nonpalpable testis as an outpatient procedure by using a 3-mm or 5-mm umbilical incision to determine if an intraabdominal testis exists. When there is no evidence of an intraabdominal testis but viable testicular vessels and vas deferens are seen entering the inguinal canal, inguinal exploration is required. In this circumstance either a very small, atrophic testicular remnant is encountered in the canal and should be excised, or a small testicle is found and orchiopexy is performed. However, if there is no laparoscopic evidence of an intraabdominal testis and the testicular vessels clearly end before entering the inguinal canal, an inguinal exploration is unnecessary. At diagnostic laparoscopy, however, if an intra-

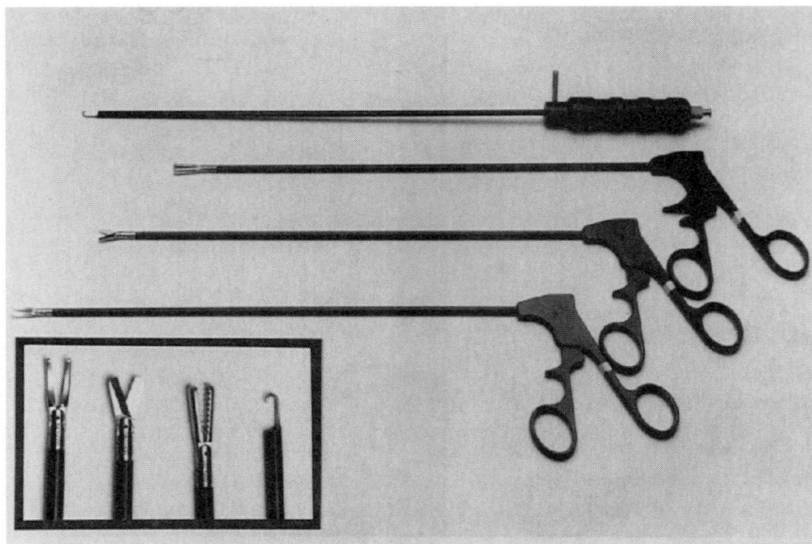

FIG. 32-4 Several different reusable instruments, including a curved dissector, scissors, atraumatic grasper, and hook cautery, are shown.

(From Holcomb GW III, editor: *Pediatric endoscopic surgery,* Norwalk, Conn, 1993, Appleton & Lange.)

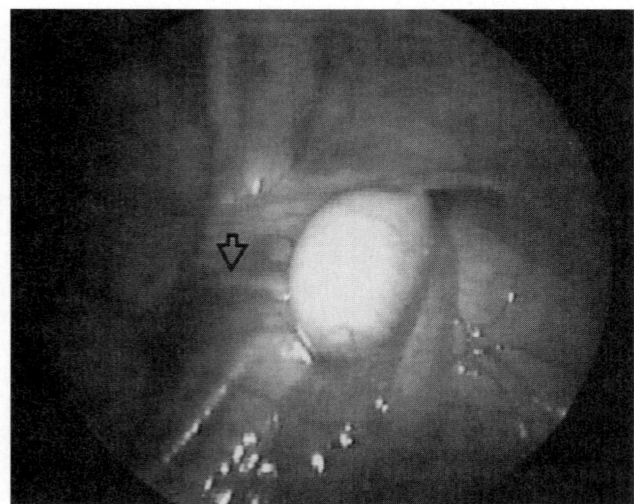

FIG. 32-5 Diagnostic laparoscopy was used in this 18-month-old infant with a nonpalpable right testis. An intraabdominal testis was identified at laparoscopy. Note the vas deferens *(open arrow)* as it is coursing toward the intraabdominal testis.

(From Holcomb GW III: *Pediatr Ann* 22:678, 1993.)

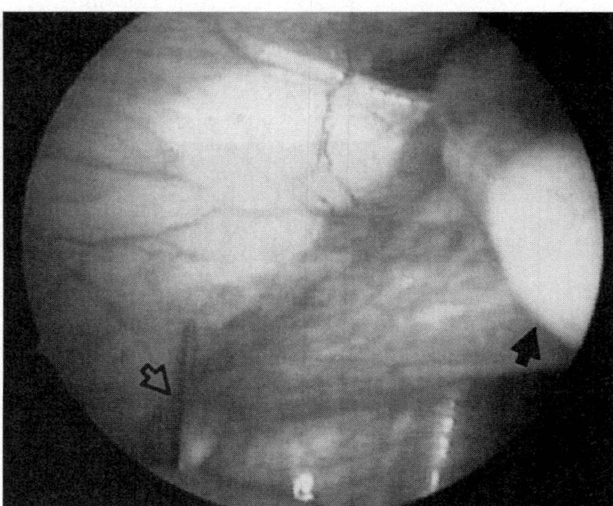

FIG. 32-6 The testicular vascular leash appeared to be short and could not reach into the scrotum in this boy with a nonpalpable right testis. Therefore a two-stage Fowler-Stephens orchiopexy was planned. At laparoscopy, the initial stage was accomplished by endoscopically placing a clip *(open arrow)* across the testicular vessels. Note the testicle *(solid arrow)* on the right side of the photograph.

(From Holcomb GW III: *Pediatr Ann* 22:678, 1993.)

abdominal testis is found and the testicular vasculature appears too short for performance of a tension-free orchiopexy, the testicular vessels are ligated by using a 10-mm suprapubic incision through which an endoscopic clip applier is inserted for ligation of the vessels (Fig. 32-6). As mentioned previously this will allow improvement in the collateral vasculature along the vas deferens and, it is hoped, will enhance the success of a second-stage orchiopexy several months later. In teenagers who have an intraabdominal testis, laparoscopic orchiectomy is preferred because there is little evidence to suggest that this gonad will have adequate testicular function. This can also be performed using a 10-mm suprapubic incision and a 5-mm lower-quadrant incision.

Diagnostic Laparoscopy for Contralateral Inguinal Hernia

Diagnostic laparoscopy in infants and children also is used to evaluate the contralateral inguinal region in children who have a known unilateral inguinal hernia. The reason for diagnostic laparoscopy in this setting is to identify patients who need contralateral exploration while undergoing anesthesia

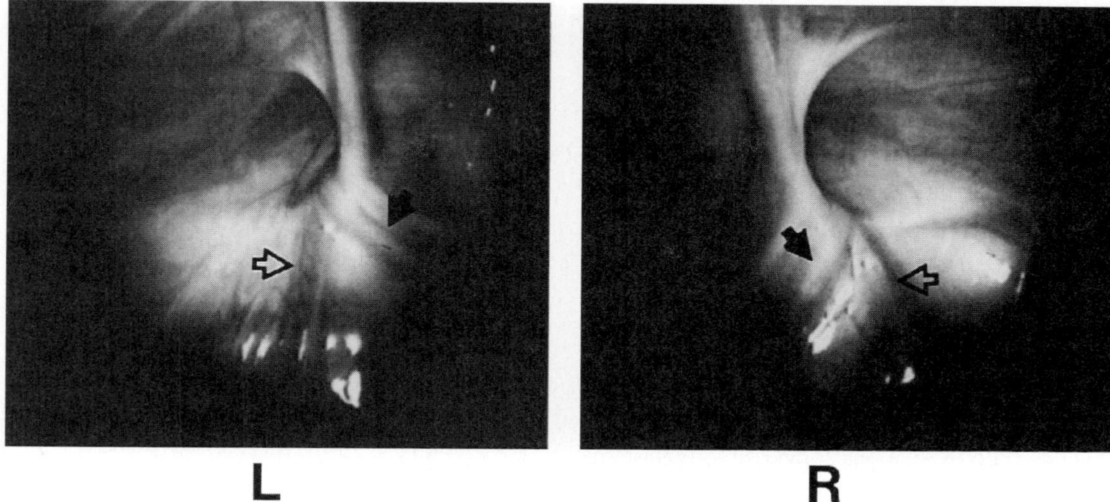

FIG. 32-7 This 3-year-old child had a known right inguinal hernia *(right)*. At laparoscopy an equally large left inguinal hernia was documented *(left)*. Note the vas deferens *(solid arrow)* and the testicular vessels *(open arrow)* coursing through the internal opening of the hernia sac.
(From Holcomb GW III: *Pediatr Ann* 22:678, 1993.)

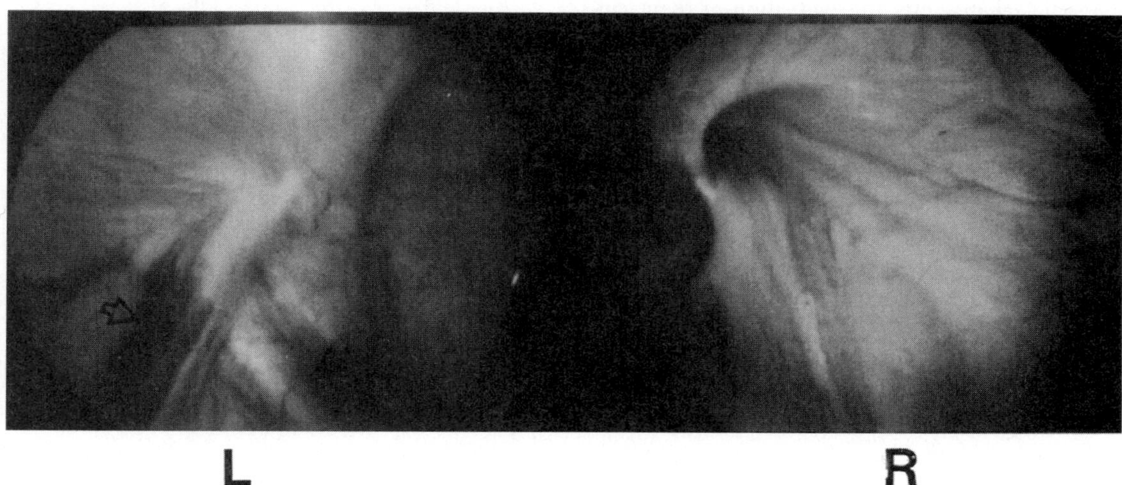

FIG. 32-8 This 6-month-old infant had a known right inguinal hernia *(right)*. However, at laparoscopy there was no evidence of a hernia on the left side *(left)* and unnecessary contralateral exploration was avoided. The vas deferens *(solid arrow)* and testicular vessels *(open arrow)* are best seen on the left side.
(From Holcomb GW III: *Pediatr Ann* 22:678, 1993.)

for a unilateral hernia repair. An alternative technique would be routine blind contralateral inguinal exploration for the same purpose. However, there is a negative exploration incidence of 40% to 60% in several series in which such contralateral inguinal exploration was used.[19,40,61,62,67] For this situation diagnostic laparoscopy can be performed using a 3-mm telescope and cannula and requires approximately only 5 to 10 minutes of additional operating time. With this information, the surgeon knows with certainty which contralateral inguinal region needs exploration (Figs. 32-7 and 32-8).

Other Indications

Another indication for diagnostic laparoscopy in the pediatric age group is evaluation for chronic abdominal pain. Previously, laparotomy often was required despite multiple radiographic and physical examinations in selected circumstances when abdominal pain recurred. The incidence of positive findings accounting for the etiology of the pain varies among pediatric surgeons. Telander reports an incidence of positive findings in 60% of 40 cases of laparoscopy for chronic abdominal pain.[70] In addition, 30% of these patients have had an abnormal appendix on pathological examination. Stafford[68] recently described his experience in Philadelphia with 20 patients. In that report 60% of the children were free of abdominal pain 3 months after laparoscopic evaluation and management, which included appendectomy and lysis of adhesions.

Other indications include diagnostic evaluation for patients who have appendicitis, evaluation of traumatic injury in children in whom radiographic evaluations are equivocal, and evaluation of infants who have ambiguous genitalia.

Laparoscopy also is being used to evaluate resectability and for staging purposes when the radiographic evaluations are not diagnostic in children who have cancer. Rather than performing an extensive initial laparotomy, this evaluation can be performed endoscopically. If resectability is possible, an open laparotomy can be performed; otherwise, treatment with adjuvant therapy is initiated and followed later by either repeat laparoscopy or laparotomy, depending on the results of the repeat radiographic studies. In a recent review of institutions participating in Children's Cancer Group (CCG) protocols, 24 children were found to have undergone laparoscopy as part of their surgical management for a variety of indications. Included are evaluations for possible metastatic tumor or recurrent disease, consideration of a new mass for suspected cancer, and evaluation of hepatoblastoma for resectability. In addition, second-look laparoscopy was performed in four patients following chemotherapy to evaluate if resection was now possible. Five patients underwent diagnostic staging laparoscopy, including four who had Hodgkin disease. No complications were noted within this group of patients undergoing laparoscopy for evaluation of their cancer.[28]

PROCEDURAL LAPAROSCOPY

Cholecystectomy

Laparoscopic cholecystectomy has become the preferred technique for removing the gallbladder in adults. Descriptions of its use in children, however, have been limited to small series because cholelithiasis and gallbladder disease are much less prevalent in children than in adults.[24,27,49,50,66] The incidence of cholelithiasis, however, has increased dramatically in the last two decades, and gallstones should now be considered in the differential diagnosis of every child or adolescent who has vague or colicky upper abdominal pain.

The percentage of children who have cholelithiasis caused by hemolytic disease is likely to be greater in institutions that have an active pediatric hematology department than in hospitals that do not have such a program. The early reports of cholelithiasis in children indicate that most patients who have gallstones have associated hemolytic disease; for a long time the diagnosis usually was not considered in children who had not had hemolysis.[20,41,64,69] However, in two earlier reports from our institution the growing incidence of nonhemolytic cholelithiasis has been emphasized and recently observed by other investigators.[1,13,23-25,56]

For laparoscopic cholecystectomy, four cannulas are required. Two 5-mm incisions and one 10-mm incision are used. In addition, the final incision either is 5 mm or 10 mm depending on the size of the patient (Figs. 32-9 and 32-10). Following isolation of the cystic duct, cholangiography will identify the cystic and common ducts correctly and help prevent inadvertent injury to these structures in small patients (Fig. 32-11). Following cholangiography the gallbladder is dissected from its liver bed and extracted through one of the 10-mm cannulas.

Thirty-one children ranging in age from 25 months to 19 years underwent laparoscopic cholecystectomy at CH-VUMC between June 1990 and December 1993.[27] Only six children had hemolytic diseases. The mean age was 12.3 years and the median age was 13 years. Five patients presented with acute cholecystitis and underwent laparoscopic cholecystectomy within 5 days of admission, with a mean postoperative hospitalization of 2.5 days. The remaining 26 children underwent elective laparoscopic cholecystectomy, with a mean postoperative stay of 1 day and no complications (Table 32-1).

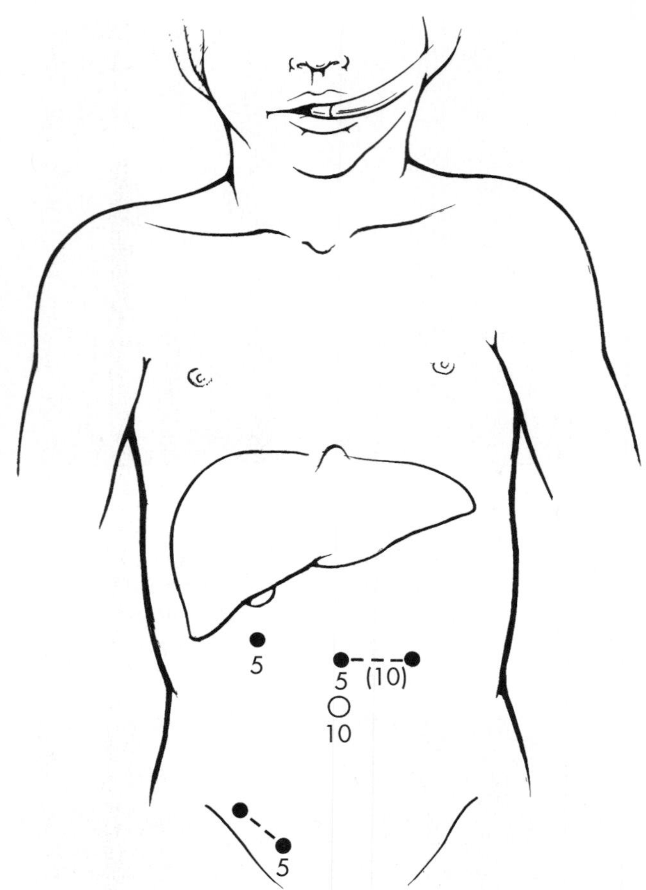

FIG. 32-9 Placement of the ports for laparoscopic cholecystectomy will depend on the size of the patient. The 5-mm epigastric port should be placed laterally in small children. In addition, the right lower port can be placed in the inguinal crease in smaller children.

(From Holcomb GW III: *Semin Pediatr Surg* 2:159, 1993.)

During the same period seven patients underwent open cholecystectomy. The mean age in this group was 11.5 years, and two patients had hemolytic disease. The average postoperative hospitalization was 3.71 days; no short- or long-term complications have been noted.

Appendectomy

Appendicitis is a common pediatric surgical problem. In 1980 Leape and Ramenofsky[45] reported the use of diagnostic laparoscopy to reduce the number of appendectomies in which a noninflamed appendix was removed; 3 years later Semm[65] described incidental laparoscopic appendectomy during gynecological procedures but did not think that laparoscopy should be employed for the acutely inflamed appendix. How-

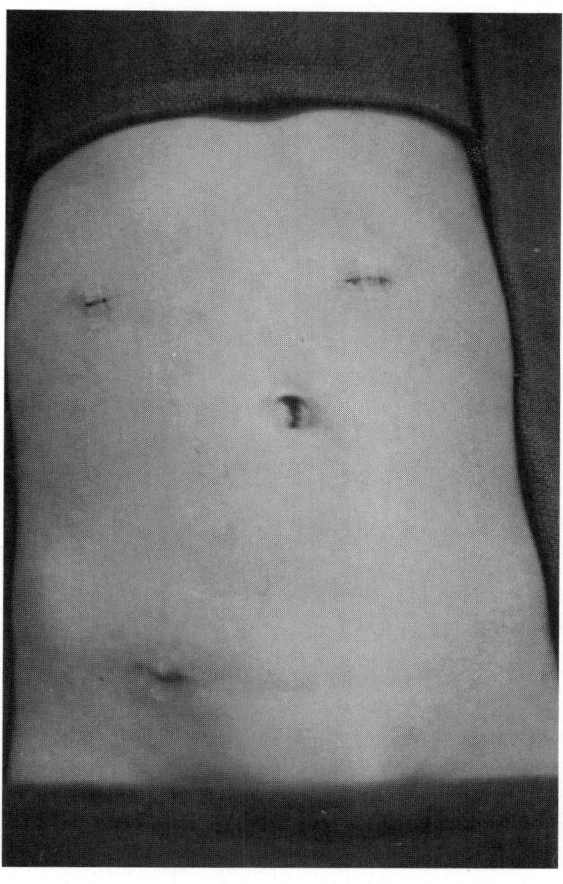

FIG. 32-10 The cosmetic result following laparoscopic cholecystectomy is seen in this 4-year-old patient. A 10-mm cannula was placed through the umbilicus. The other three incisions are 5 mm in length.

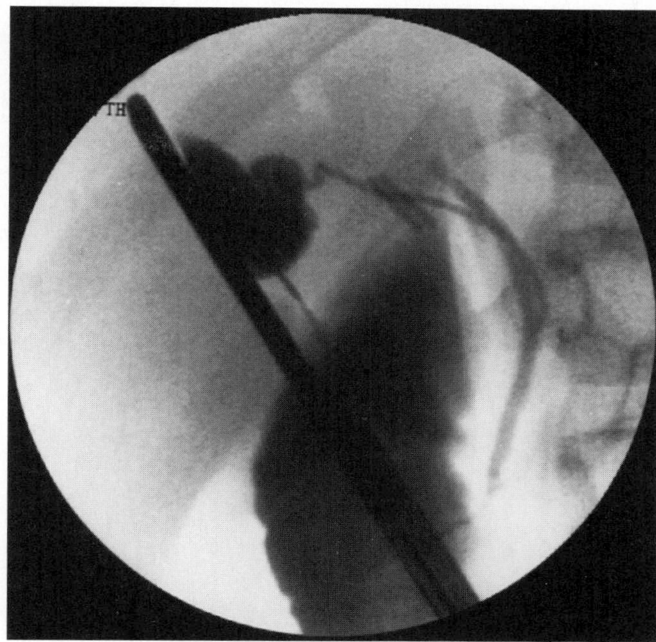

FIG. 32-11 Cholangiography is now being performed using fluoroscopy. The clamp *(solid arrow)* is placed across the gallbladder with the sclerotherapy needle *(open arrow)* inserted into the infundibulum. A small, long cystic duct is seen to enter the common duct with free flow of dye into the duodenum. There is no evidence of stones. Two clips have been previously placed on the cystic artery because it coursed on top of the cystic duct and needed to be divided before dissection of the cystic duct.
(From Holcomb GW III et al: *J Pediatr Surg* 29:900, 1994.)

Table 32-1 Comparison of Children Undergoing Laparoscopic and Open Cholecystectomy at CH-VUMC, 1990-1993

	Elective laparoscopic cholecystectomy	Elective open cholecystectomy
Number of patients	26	7
Hemolytic disease	6	2
Mean age (years)	12.3	11.5
Mean postoperative hospitalization (days)	1	3.71

ever, with the evolution in laparoscopic technology, the laparoscopic approach is increasingly being used to treat acute appendicitis in children.

A three-cannula technique is used, with a 10- or 12-mm cannula being placed in the umbilicus. A 5-mm cannula is located in the left lower abdominal quadrant and a 5-mm cannula in the suprapubic region (Fig. 32-12). A 5-mm telescope then is inserted through the left lower quadrant cannula for visualization. The working port is the umbilical port and needs to be 12 mm wide for insertion of an endoscopic stapler, which is used to ligate and divide the mesentery and the appendiceal stump (Fig. 32-13); the appendix then can be removed through the 12-mm cannula.

An alternative technique uses endoscopic clips rather than a stapling device to ligate the mesentery, and pretied suture ligatures to ligate the appendiceal stump. Either technique is equally effective and successful.

Laparoscopic appendectomy appears to be the preferential approach in certain selected circumstances (see the box on p. 400). In thin children less than 7 or 8 years of age an appendectomy generally can be performed through a 2-cm right lower abdominal incision with minimal resulting morbidity and brief hospitalization. However, in older children in whom a longer incision is required, the laparoscopic approach is preferred because of reduced postoperative discomfort. Also, in obese children who require a long incision for exposure, in athletes who desire a quick return to participation in their athletic activity, and in adolescent females in whom the differential diagnosis between gynecological or appendiceal origin is not completely clear, the laparoscopic approach has advantages over the open approach.

One area of controversy is the child who has suspected or known perforation. It has been estimated that 30% of children who have appendicitis are perforated before an appendectomy is performed. Therefore management of suspected perforative appendicitis is a frequent pediatric surgical dilemma. One advantage of the laparoscopic approach for perforated appendicitis is the opportunity for a more thorough irrigation and debridement of the abdominal cavity than can be obtained through a small right lower quadrant incision. On the other hand these patients often require 5 to 8 days of hospitalization to recover from the complications of perfora-

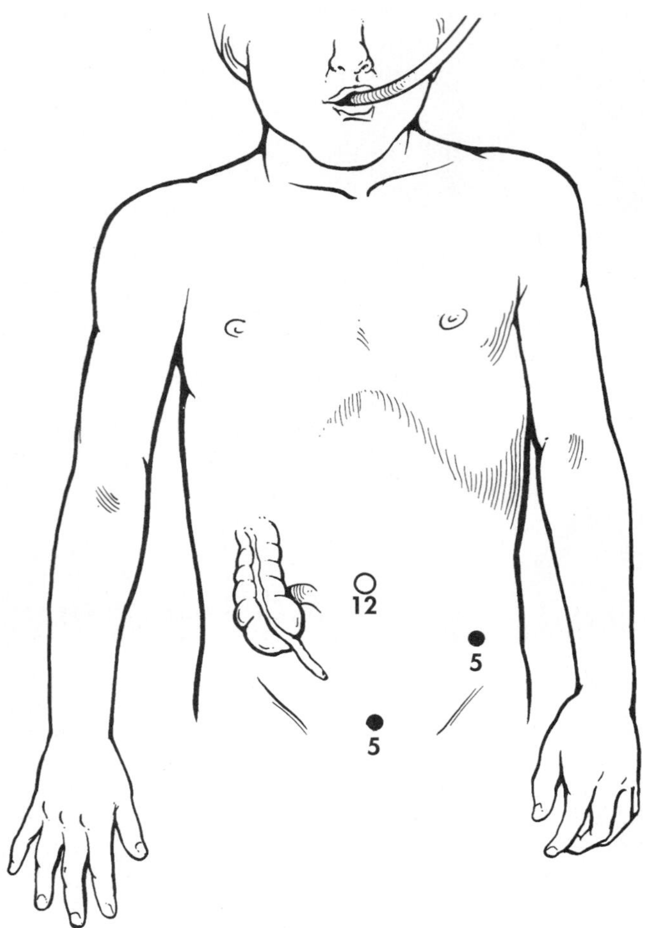

FIG. 32-12 This diagram depicts the location of the cannulas used in the three-port technique for laparoscopic appendectomy. A 10- or 12-mm cannula is inserted through the umbilicus for laparoscopic visualization and insertion of an endoscopic stapler. Two 5-mm cannulas are placed in the left lower quadrant and suprapubic area.

SELECTED INDICATIONS FOR LAPAROSCOPIC APPENDECTOMY IN CHILDREN

Patient older than 8 to 10 years
Obese patient
Athletes
Adolescent females with unclear diagnosis

tion including sepsis and ileus; therefore reduced hospitalization is not an advantage of the laparoscopic route. In addition, laparoscopic management for perforated appendicitis usually requires longer operating time than for nonperforated appendicitis; therefore the cost of the operative procedure itself is increased.

In a small series of 35 patients undergoing laparoscopic appendectomy at CH-VUMC, patient age ranged between 5 and 16 years. Four patients had developed abscesses from perforation, but the abscess cavity was opened laparoscopically and appendectomy was accomplished in three; one patient required conversion to an open appendectomy.

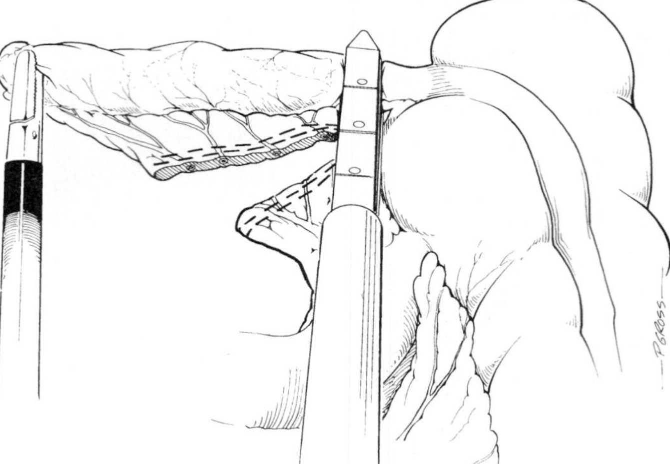

FIG. 32-13 The mesoappendix has already been divided with the stapler, and the proximal appendix is now being ligated and divided with an endoscopic stapler.

(From Holcomb GW III: *Laparosc Surg* 1:145, 1993.)

Of the remaining patients 29 had acute nonperforated appendicitis. Of two children who did not have appendicitis, one had terminal ileitis and the other had no pathology to account for the symptoms. No intraoperative complications occurred, and long-term complications have not developed.

Fundoplication and Splenectomy

The laparoscopic approach is becoming a useful alternative to the open operation for fundoplication and splenectomy in children. Advantages of the laparoscopic technique for these two procedures include reduced discomfort compared with that of an upper abdominal incision, reduced respiratory complications, and an improved return of pulmonary function. The resulting postoperative ileus also may be reduced by the laparoscopic approach. In addition, the endoscopic procedure has a cosmetic advantage.

The principles of the endoscopic procedure are very similar to those of the open operation.[46,47,72] In a splenectomy the peritoneal attachments to the spleen are divided, exposing the splenic vessels and pancreas within the hilum of the spleen. The vessels can be ligated and divided by using either intracorporeal or extracorporeal knot-tying techniques before division or by placing an endoscopic stapler across the vessels for ligation and division. Following mobilization of the spleen within the abdominal cavity, the major obstacle remains removing the spleen. The spleen is placed in a reinforced nylon bag, the neck of the bag is exteriorized through the largest incision, and the resulting splenic tissue is morcellated or diced into small pieces until the entire sac can be removed from the abdomen. Lobe et al.[48] have performed laparoscopic splenectomy on 11 children after failing to control their hematological disease with medical therapy. The operative time ranged from 2½ to 4 hours, and 8 of the 11 patients left the hospital on the second postoperative day; the other three required longer hospitalizations because of postoperative ileus.

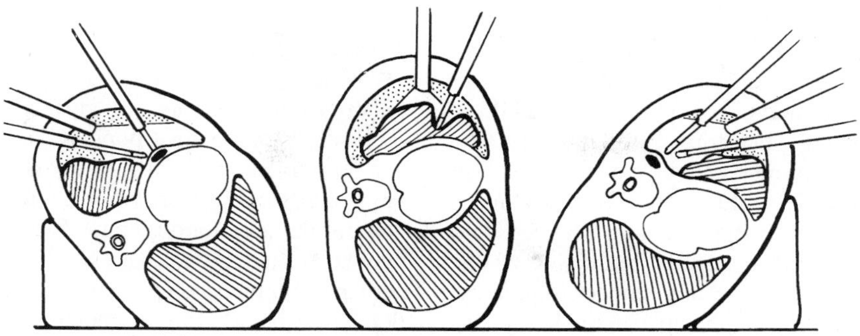

Anterior lesions: relative face up

Lung biopsy: lateral decubitus

Posterior lesions: relative face down

FIG. 32-14 Patient positioning for the thoracoscopic approach to mediastinal and pulmonary lesions in children is important. The relative positions of the three cannulas are also illustrated for these lesions.

(From Rodgers BM: Thoracoscopy. In Holcomb GW III, editor: *Pediatric endoscopic surgery,* Norwalk, Conn, 1993, Appleton & Lange.)

For laparoscopic fundoplication four cannulas are required. The diaphragmmatic crura are approximated as in to the open procedure, the gastric fundus is mobilized, and a 360 degree Nissen fundoplication usually is performed by using either silk sutures or staples. Alternative procedures such as the Thal anterior fundoplication also can be performed laparoscopically. A gastrostomy can be established if required, either endoscopically (percutaneous endoscopic gastrostomy) or laparoscopically at the time of fundoplication. Georgeson[18] recently reviewed the first 60 children to undergo laparoscopic fundoplication and/or gastrostomy at Birmingham Children's Hospital and compared these with a similar group of 60 consecutive children undergoing the open procedure. The most notable difference between the two groups was the median postoperative stay, which averaged 3 days less in the laparoscopic group as compared with those undergoing the open procedure. In addition, the patients who underwent the laparoscopic procedure were able to receive feedings sooner than the open group. However, it will be important to compare the outcomes of the laparoscopic procedure to those of the open fundoplication over a longer period of time before one approach is deemed better than the other.

Other Indications

Other indications for procedural laparoscopy in children include laparoscopic gastrostomy without fundoplication, assistance with insertion and removal of ventriculo-peritoneal shunts, gonadectomy for intersex abnormalities, ovarian cystectomy, and testicular vein ligation for management of varicoceles. In addition, laparoscopy may play an larger role in intestinal resection in the future. Laparoscopic Meckel diverticulectomy has been reported and an endoscopic Soavé, Duhamel, and Swenson procedure has been performed in children for the management of Hirschsprung disease.[31]

A final area of potential application for this evolving technology is fetoscopic surgery. The major difficulty to date with fetal surgery is that preterm labor can be induced because of the long uterine incision required for exposure. Physicians at the fetal treatment center at the University of California in San Francisco have developed fetoscopic techniques in research animals for repair of fetal cleft lip and creation of a vesicocutaneous fistula for managing obstructive uropathy. Studies in primates for the development of this technology are ongoing, with the ultimate goal of human applicability.[11,12] Quintero et al.[53] recently reported successful fetoscopic ligation of the umbilical cord to an acardiac twin—a healthy twin was born at 36 weeks' gestation.

THORACOSCOPY

The first description of thoracoscopy came in 1921 when five cases of intrathoracic malignancy were described by Jacobaeus.[33] Over the next two decades this technique was widely accepted in Europe and North America for "closed intrapleural pneumolysis," which was being performed for the treatment of pulmonary tuberculosis. However, the frequency of its use for this indication diminished with the development of effective antimicrobial therapy for tuberculosis in North America. In Europe, however, thoracoscopy continued to be used by medical pulmonologists to evaluate occult pleural effusions. In 1976 Rodgers and Talbert[59] first described the use of thoracoscopy for pulmonary and pleural biopsy in nine children who ranged in age from 17 months to 16 years. However, only a few pediatric surgeons were persuaded to use this technology. As the technique of laparoscopy has become refined, interest in the application of endoscopy to thoracic conditions has been renewed.

Principles of Technique

The patient's position on the operating table depends on the site of pathology. Unlike laparoscopy, in which the patient is placed supine, the patient is placed in the decubitus position similar to that used in open thoracotomy. For lesions located in the anterior mediastinum the patient is placed in a somewhat lateral decubitus position, allowing the lung on the side to be thoroscoped to fall posteriorly, resulting in improved visualization of the anterior mediastinum. For posterior mediastinal masses the patient is placed in an exaggerated decubitus position—the lung is allowed to fall forward, allowing improved visualization of the posterior mediastinum (Fig. 32-14).

If possible, it is helpful to collapse the ipsilateral lung to improve visualization and increase the working space within the thoracic cavity. Unlike the abdominal cavity, which is distended with carbon dioxide to achieve improved visualization and working space, the thoracic cavity is rigid and does not expand with insufflation. Therefore insufflation usually is not required but may be used selectively to compress the underlying lung when selective intubation of the contralateral lung is not possible. The ipsilateral lung may be collapsed in older children who have selected intubation of the contralateral main stem bronchus and in younger children by inserting a Fogarty catheter down the ipsilateral bronchus, which will occlude ventilation to the ipsilateral lung.

Indications

Indications for thoracoscopy in children are different from those in adults (see the box below). In adults the most compelling reason is the evaluation or treatment of pleural effusions and pleural masses. However, the most frequent indication in children is for the evaluation of mediastinal masses. Both the anterior and posterior mediastinum are readily available for endoscopic visualization, especially if the patient is positioned properly. Biopsy of anterior mediastinal masses and resection of benign posterior mediastinal masses can be performed. In addition, small neuroblastomas located in the posterior mediastinum may be amenable to resection in se lected circumstances. Diagnostic accuracy for thoracoscopy in children who have mediastinal masses has ranged from 88% to 100%.[38,60,63]

COMMON INDICATIONS FOR THORACOSCOPY IN CHILDREN

- Biopsy of mediastinal mass
- Lung biopsy for diagnosis
- Evacuation of empyema
- Pleural mass biopsy
- Resection of pulmonary bleb (recurrent pneumothorax)

The second most common indication for thoracoscopy in children is the diagnosis of diffuse or localized pneumonia. Included in this patient population are those who are immunocompromised with diffuse interstitial pneumonia and children with localized pneumonic processes not responding to appropriate antibiotic therapy. Diagnostic accuracy has been over 90% in reported series.[34,57] Most of the morbidity in pediatric thoracoscopy occurs in immunocompromised patients who have diffuse parenchymal involvement. In one report two patients required transfusion; however, a secondary open procedure was not necessary. The 30-day mortality was 11%, although the procedure itself was not thought to have directly influenced the deaths of these critically ill children.[58] No mortality has been reported in patients who have localized inflammatory processes who undergo thoracoscopic biopsies.[34,58,60]

Another reason for thoracoscopy in children is for the evaluation and treatment of pleural diseases. At CH-VUMC there has been an interest in early surgical intervention for children who have empyema.[29,30] An extension of the concept of mini-thoracotomy for evacuation and debridement of the pleural space in children who have empyema is the use of thoracoscopy for this purpose. In a report of nine patients its use was described with very good results.[37] This technique has been used at CH-VUMC, resulting in striking improvement in the child's clinical course and early hospital discharge (Figs. 32-15 and 32-16).

Thoracoscopy also is advantageous for localized or diffuse pleural-based masses in children who have suspected malignancy. Thoracoscopic biopsy can be performed, obviating the need for an open thoracotomy for diagnosis.

Thoracoscopy has been used extensively in adult patients for recurrent pneumothoraces and is being used increasingly in children. In thoracoscopy the entire visceral pleural surface is examined and the bullous disease identified. Usually there is a fibrin peel caused by an inflammatory response

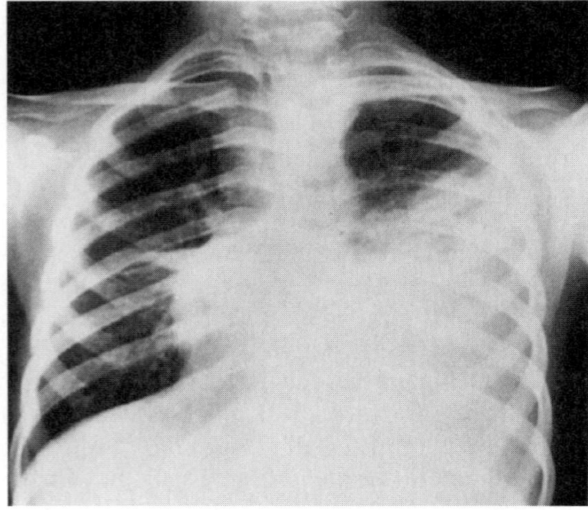

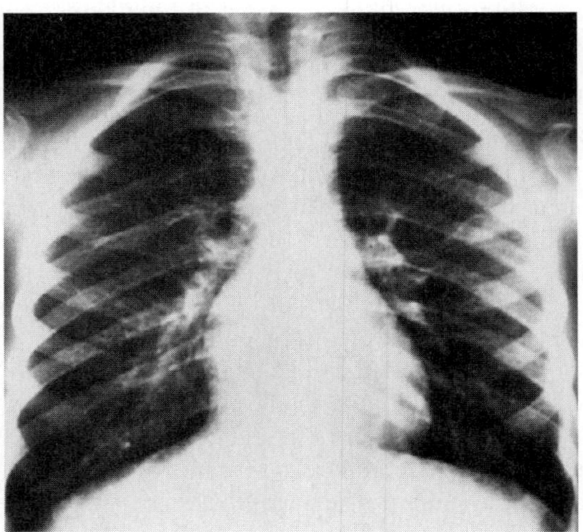

FIG. 32-15 A 6-year-old girl presented with fever, respiratory distress, and a large left thoracic empyema *(left)*. Following thoracoscopic debridement and evacuation of her left pleural space, she was discharged on the fifth postoperative day. A chest radiograph *(right)* 1 month postoperatively documents almost complete resolution.

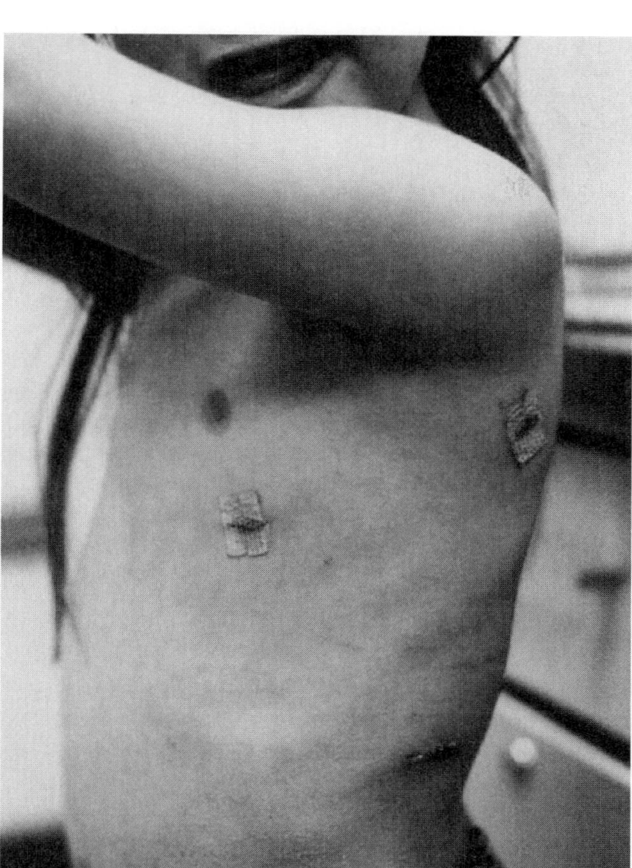

FIG. 32-16 Postoperative photograph of the 6-year-old girl described in Fig. 32-15. Note the three small incisions for her thoracoscopic procedure.

from the ruptured bulla, which can be resected by using the endoscopic stapler or pretied surgical ligature. Another technique uses the CO_2 laser for the treatment of bullous disease, but this has been described only in adults.[73]

Recurrent pneumothoraces are seen fairly frequently in children who have cystic fibrosis. Thoracoscopy is ideal for this fragile patient population. Tribble and Rodgers[71] reported on five patients with cystic fibrosis undergoing thoracoscopic management.[71] They also performed pleurodesis in these patients by dusting the pleural surface with dry talc or by mechanical abrasion. Although the use of talc has been successful in most cases, using this substance in patients with cystic fibrosis who later may be candidates for lung transplantation is controversial.

Other Indications

Thoracoscopy has been used for a wide variety of other reasons both in adults and in children. However, these indications have not been as common as those previously mentioned. Many of these indications that have been employed in adults also may apply to children, although their efficacy has not been reported. For instance, thoracoscopy has been used in adults who have chest trauma to differentiate between diaphragmmatic rupture and phrenic nerve palsy with eventration.[39] It also has been reported for resection of esophageal leiomyomata and for esophageal myotomy for achalasia in adults.[2,52] Moreover, its use for creation of a pericardial window in patients who have chronic pericardial effusions has been described.[51]

Other reported indications include thymectomy, truncal vagotomy, and sclerosis for malignant effusions. In addition, thoracoscopy for ligation of a patent ductus arteriosus in infants and children has been reported.[17,44] It also has been reported for pleurodesis in a child who had a chylothorax and for sympathectomy in patients who had palmar and axillary hyperhidrosis.[21,43]

THE FUTURE

It is unknown what the future holds for laparoscopy and thoracoscopy in children. It is likely, however, that a number of open procedures will have an endoscopic counterpart in the future. It will be necessary for both pediatricians and pediatric surgeons to review this new technology critically to ensure that the endoscopic approach is beneficial and not harmful to the patient. Only through additional experience will we gain appreciation for which diseases the laparoscopic or thoracoscopic approach is preferable and for which diseases the open approach is more desirable.

REFERENCES

1. Bailey PV et al: Changing spectrum of cholelithiasis and cholecystitis in infants and children, *Am J Surg* 158:585, 1989.
2. Bardini R et al: Videothoracoscopic enucleation of esophageal leiomyoma, *Ann Thorac Surg* 54:576, 1992.
3. Berci G, Kont LA: A new optical system in endoscopy with special reference to cystoscopy, *Br J Urol* 41:564, 1969.
4. Bloom DA: Two-step orchiopexy with pelviscopic clip ligation of the spermatic vessels, *J Urol* 145:1030, 1991.
5. Bloom DA, Ayers JWT, McGuire EJ: The role of laparoscopy in the management of nonpalpable testes, *J d'Urol* 94:465, 1988.
6. Bloom DA, Ritchey ML, Manzoni G: *Laparoscopy for the nonpalpable testis*. In Holcomb GW III, editor: *Pediatric endoscopic surgery*, Norwalk, Conn, 1993, Appleton & Lange.
7. Bozzinni PH: Lichtleiter, eine erfindung zur anschauung innerer teile und krankheiten, *J Prak Heilk* 24:107, 1806.
8. Diamond DA, Caldamone AA: The value of laparoscopy for 106 impalpable testes relative to clinical presentation, *J Urol* 148:632, 1992.
9. Dubois F, Berthelots G, Levard H: Cholecystectomy par coelioscopie, *Presse Med* 18:980, 1989.
10. Elder JS: Laparoscopy for the nonpalpable testis, *Semin Pediatr Surg* 2:168, 1993.
11. Estes JM, Adzick NS, Harrison MR: Fetoscopic surgery. In Holcomb GW III, editor: *Pediatric endoscopic surgery*, Norwalk, Conn, 1993, Appleton & Lange.
12. Estes JM et al: Fetoscopic surgery for the treatment of congenital anomalies, *J Pediatr Surg* 27:950, 1992.
13. Frexes M, Neblett WW III, Holcomb GW Jr: Spectrum of biliary disease in childhood, *South Med J* 79:1342, 1986.
14. Gans SL: Historical development of pediatric endoscopic surgery. In Holcomb GW III, editor: *Pediatric endoscopic surgery*, Norwalk, Conn, 1993, Appleton & Lange.
15. Gans SL, Berci G: Advances in endoscopy of infants and children, *J Pediatr Surg* 6:199, 1971.
16. Gans SL, Berci G: Peritoneoscopy in infants and children, *J Pediatr Surg* 8:399, 1973.
17. Geiger A et al: Thoracoscopic closure of patent ductus arteriosus in premature infants in the intensive care unit, Third International Congress

on Endoscopy and Laparoscopy in Children, Münster, Germany, Feb 1-2, 1994 (abstract).
18. Georgeson KE: Laparoscopic gastrostomy and fundoplication, *Pediatr Ann* 22:675, 1993.
19. Gilbert M, Clatworthy HW: Bilateral operations for inguinal hernia and hydrocele in infancy and childhood, *Am J Surg* 97:255, 1959.
20. Hagberg B, Svennerholm L, Thorén L: Cholelithiasis in childhood, *Acta Chir Scand* 123:307, 1962.
21. Hejgaard N, Olsen P: Massive Gorham osteolysis of the right hemipelvis complicated by chylothorax: report of a case in a 9-year-old boy successfully treated by pleurodesis, *J Pediatr Orthop* 7:96, 1987.
22. Holcomb GW III: Laparoscopic evaluation for a contralateral inguinal hernia or a nonpalpable testis, *Pediatr Ann* 22:678, 1993.
23. Holcomb GW Jr, Holcomb GW III: Cholelithiasis in infants, children, and adolescents, *Pediatr Rev* 11:268, 1990.
24. Holcomb GW III, Olsen DO, Sharp KW: Laparoscopic cholecystectomy in the pediatric patient, *J Pediatr Surg* 26:1186, 1991.
25. Holcomb GW Jr, O'Neill JA Jr, Holcomb GW III: Cholecystitis, cholelithiasis and common duct stenosis in children and adolescents, *Ann Surg* 191:626, 1980.
26. Holcomb GW III et al: Laparoscopy for the nonpalpable testis, *Am Surg* 60:143, 1994.
27. Holcomb GW III et al: Laparoscopic cholecystectomy in infants and children: modifications and cost analysis, *J Pediatr Surg* 29:900, 1994.
28. Holcomb GW III et al: Minimally invasive surgery in children with cancer, *Cancer* 76:121, 1995.
29. Hoff SJ et al: Parapneumonic empyema in children: decortication hastens recovery in patients with severe pleural infections, *Pediatr Infect Dis J* 10:194, 1990.
30. Hoff SJ et al: Postpneumonic empyema in childhood: selecting appropriate therapy, *J Pediatr Surg* 24:659, 1989.
31. Huang CS, Lin LH: Laparoscopic Meckel's diverticulectomy in infants: report of three cases, *J Pediatr Surg* 28:1486, 1993.
32. Jacobaeus HC: Kurze ubersicht uber meine erfahrungen mit der laparoskopie, *Munchen Med Wochenschr* 58:2017, 1911.
33. Jacobaeus HC, Key E: Some experiences of intrathoracic tumors, their diagnosis and their operative treatment, *Acta Chir Scand* 53:573, 1921.
34. Janik JS, Nagaraj HS, Groff DB: Thoracoscopic evaluation of intrathoracic lesions in children, *J Thorac Cardiovasc Surg* 83:408, 1982.
35. Kalk H, Bruhl W: *Leitfaden der laparoskopie und gastroskopie*, Stuttgart, 1951, Thieme.
36. Kelling G: Uber oesophagaskopie, gastroskopie und celioskopie, *Munchen Med Wochenschr* 49:21, 1902.
37. Kern JA, Rodgers BM: Thoracoscopy in the management of empyema in children, *J Pediatr Surg* 28:1128, 1993.
38. Kern JA et al: Thoracoscopic diagnosis and treatment of mediastinal masses, *Ann Thorac Surg* 56:92, 1993.
39. Kern JA et al: Thoracoscopy: a potential role in the subacute management of patients with thoraco-abdominal trauma, *Chest* 104:27, 1992.
40. Kiesewetter WB, Oh KS: Unilateral inguinal hernias in children: what about the opposite side? *Arch Surg* 115:1443, 1980.
41. Kirtley JA, Holcomb GW Jr: Surgical management of diseases of the gallbladder and common duct in children and adolescents, *Am J Surg* 111:39, 1966.
42. Kussmaul J: Über magenspiegelung. Verh naturforschenden, *Ges Freiburg* 5:112, 1870.
43. Kux M: Thoracic endoscopic sympathectomy in palmar and axillary hyperhidrosis, *Arch Surg* 113:264, 1978.
44. Laborde F et al: A new video-assisted thoracoscopic surgical technique for interruption of patent ductus arteriosus in infants and children, *J Thorac Cardiovasc Surg* 105:278, 1993.
45. Leape LL, Ramenofsky ML: Laparoscopy for questionable appendicitis. Can it reduce the negative appendectomy rate? *Ann Surg* 191:410, 1980.
46. Lobe TE, Schropp KP, Lunsford K: Laparoscopic Nissen fundoplication in childhood, *J Pediatr Surg* 28:358, 1993.
47. Lobe TE, Schropp KP, Rogers DA: Laparoscopic management for inguinal and hiatal hernia (Nissen fundoplication). In Holcomb GW III, editor: *Pediatric endoscopic surgery*, Norwalk, Conn, 1993, Appleton & Lange.
48. Lobe TE et al: Laparoscopic splenectomy, *Pediatr Ann* 22:671, 1993.
49. Moir CR, Donohue JH, VanHeerden JA: Laparoscopic cholecystectomy in children: initial experience and recommendations, *J Pediatr Surg* 27:1066, 1992.
50. Newman KD et al: Laparoscopic cholecystectomy in pediatric patients, *J Pediatr Surg* 26:1184, 1991.
51. Ozuner G et al: Creation of a pericardial window using thoracoscopic techniques, *Surg Gynecol Obstet* 175:69, 1992.
52. Pellegrini C et al: Thoracoscopic esophagomyotomy, *Ann Surg* 216:291, 1992.
53. Quintero RA et al: Brief report: umbilical-cord ligation of an acardiac twin by fetoscopy at 19 weeks of gestation, *N Engl J Med* 330:469, 1994.
54. Ransley PG et al: Preliminary ligation of the gonadal vessels prior to orchidopexy for the intra-abdominal testicle: a staged Fowler-Stephens procedure, *World J Urol* 2:266, 1984.
55. Reddick EJ, Olsen DO: Laparoscopic laser cholecystectomy, *Surg Endosc* 3:131, 1989.
56. Reif S, Sloven DG, Lebenthal E: Gallstones in children: characterization by age, etiology and outcome, *Am J Dis Child* 145:105, 1991.
57. Rodgers BM: Thoracoscopy in children, *Poumon-Coeur* 37:301, 1981.
58. Rodgers BM, Moazam F, Talbert JL: Thoracoscopy in children, *Ann Surg* 189:176, 1979.
59. Rodgers BM, Talbert JL: Thoracoscopy for diagnosis of intrathoracic lesions in children, *J Pediatr Surg* 11:703, 1976.
60. Rogers DA et al: Thoracoscopy in children: an initial experience with an evolving technique, *J Laparoendosc Surg* 2:7, 1992.
61. Rothenberg RE, Barnett T: Bilateral herniotomy in infants and children, *Surgery* 37:947, 1955.
62. Rowe MI, Copelson LW, Clatworthy HW: The patent processus vaginalis and the inguinal hernia, *J Pediatr Surg* 4:102, 1969.
63. Ryckman FC, Rodgers BM: Thoracoscopy for intrathoracic neoplasm in children, *J Pediatr Surg* 17:521, 1982.
64. Seiler I: Gallbladder disease in children, *Am J Dis Child* 99:662, 1960.
65. Semm K: Endoscopic appendectomy, *Endoscopy* 15:50, 1983.
66. Sigman HH et al: Laparoscopic cholecystectomy: a treatment option for gallbladder disease in children, *J Pediatr Surg* 26:1181, 1991.
67. Sparkman RS: Bilateral exploration in inguinal hernia in juvenile patients, *Surgery* 51:393, 1962.
68. Stafford PW: The evaluation of chronic abdominal pain in children—a role for diagnostic laparoscopy? 3rd International Congress on Endoscopy and Laparoscopy in Children. Münster, Germany, Feb 1-2, 1994 (abstract).
69. Swenson O, *Pediatric surgery*, New York, 1958, Appleton-Century-Crofts.
70. Telander R: Personal communication.
71. Tribble CG, Selden RF, Rodgers BM: Talc poudrage in the treatment of spontaneous pneumothoraces in patients with cystic fibrosis, *Ann Surg* 204:677, 1986.
72. Tulman S et al: Pediatric laparoscopic splenectomy, *J Pediatr Surg* 28:689, 1993.
73. Wakabayashi A: Expanded applications of diagnostic and therapeutic thoracoscopy, *J Thorac Cardiovasc Surg* 102:721, 1991.

33 Physical Disability and Chronic Illness

Gregory S. Liptak and Beverly A. Myers

DEFINITION AND DEMOGRAPHICS

Children who have chronic health conditions and physical disabilities (frequently termed children who have special health care needs) include those who have physical conditions that affect daily functioning for more than 3 months in a year, cause hospitalization of more than 1 month (total) in a year, or are likely to do either of these. Chronic disabling conditions include (but are not limited to) asthma, bronchopulmonary dysplasia, cerebral palsy, cystic fibrosis, congenital heart disease, diabetes mellitus, hemophilia, HIV infection, meningomyelocele, inflammatory bowel disease, renal failure, epilepsy, cancer, juvenile arthritis, and red cell disorders (such as sickle cell disease).

Although each condition taken individually is uncommon, taken together they affect approximately 5% to 10% of all children and constitute an important part of pediatric practice.[9] Over the past 20 years disease-specific survival rates have improved dramatically; however, many of these survivors have severe limitations of activity and function.[12]

COMMON CHARACTERISTICS

Although these children differ from each other in various ways, they and their families share common characteristics, which are shown in the box on p. 406.[9] A widely held generalization is that 85% of the issues with which children and families must deal are common to all chronic conditions, whereas 15% of the issues are specific to the child's particular condition.

The negative impact of a chronic condition, which can manifest as behavioral problems and psychopathology, such as depression, poor socialization, and family disruption,[4] is worsened at all periods of development by low socioeconomic status.[8]

DEVELOPMENTAL CONSIDERATIONS

In addition to understanding the medical condition and commonalities cited above, the health care provider caring for a child who has a chronic disability also must understand the interactions between the condition and the developing child and family.[16]

Infancy

Conditions that affect the physical appearance of an infant, such as cleft lip and palate or hydrocephalus, can affect the bonding and attachment between child and caretakers.[10] In addition, once a chronic condition has been diagnosed, the parents will begin to grieve for the lost "normal" child. This bereavement includes shock, denial, anger, sadness/depression, guilt, and anxiety. Parents may go through these stages of mourning at any time in the child's development, especially during transitions—for example, when the child begins kindergarten or the family moves to a new community.[20] One parent may be primarily experiencing one set of feelings such as guilt while another experiences feelings such as anger. This makes communication between them difficult and decreases their ability to support each other. This grief also may interfere with their ability to become attached to the chronically ill child. Parents may direct their feelings of anger toward the pediatrician or seek multiple opinions because of their denial.

The behavior of pediatricians during this period can have a major influence on the family's acceptance of their disabled child. The words that are used and the actions that are shown, such as holding the infant or encouraging the parent to do so, can improve acceptance. Discussion of parental feelings and counseling about financial assistance and community support can be invaluable to the family's coping.

Whenever a pediatrician informs a family of the presence of a chronic disability in their child, care must be taken to ensure that the family understands the condition and that their needs (including those of siblings) are met.[7] This requires the ability to listen nonjudgmentally, even to negative opinions and feelings, without providing false reassurances or premature suggestions (before the family feels they understand or have received empathy from the physician). Patience and repetition of information often are required, as is sensitivity to verbal and nonverbal communication.

Preschool

The normal development of preschool children includes the achievement of a sense of autonomy and initiative. One way that children show autonomy is by literally walking away. If a child is physically disabled and cannot walk or is bedridden because of illness, he or she cannot express autonomy by walking away and must express it in some other way. This may manifest as negative verbal behavior or disobedience.[6] Allowing the child to show autonomy in acceptable ways—for example, by having the child choose clothing or food items on a menu or the arm into which the intravenous line will go—can decrease the occurrence of unacceptable behaviors.

The demands of the chronic condition placed on the family, as well as feelings of sympathy for the child (e.g., "She has suffered enough") may make consistent limit-setting difficult for parents and can lead to behavior problems in the

COMMON FEATURES OF CHRONIC DISABILITY IN CHILDHOOD

Child
- Chronic, often unpredictable course
- No cure
- Pain and discomfort
- Restricted growth and development
- Frequent hospitalizations and outpatient visits
- Painful, embarrassing treatments
- Inability to participate in peer activities
- Daily burden of care

Family
- Loss of "ideal" child
- Daily burden of care
- Expense (financial, time)
- Lost opportunities
- Neglected siblings
- Confusing systems of health and other care
- Social isolation

Community
- Poor understanding of chronic illness
- Inconsistent policies and funding
- Inadequate facilities (including barriers to access)
- Poor communication and coordination within the health care system and with other agencies

child. One parent (often the mother) may become overinvolved with the child, thus blurring normal family relationships. The father may become isolated from health care decisions or the care of the child, a process that is promulgated by the typical Monday through Friday, 9:00 AM to 5:00 PM office hours of most pediatricians and paternal work schedules. Encouraging parents to achieve a balance in their roles as parents, spouses, and workers by helping them find support in the community (e.g., for spending time as a couple away from the children) can help families cope.

Referring a young child to an early intervention program may provide support for the family and educational and therapeutic treatments that will assist the child's development. It also may encourage the family to increase their contact with their child. Public Law 99-457 and subsequent legislation are increasing the availability of preschool programs for children at risk for developmental delay.[2] Unfortunately day care and nursery programs for disabled children who are not at risk for developmental delay, such as those who have asthma, are woefully insufficient to meet the demand.

Young children are especially vulnerable to the effects of separation that occur when they are hospitalized. The pediatrician should encourage rooming-in for parents during hospitalizations, as well as frequent visits from all family members. This includes helping the family obtain transportation, child care, or other nonmedical services.

The pediatrician needs to be aware of the child's temperament, as well as his or her abilities and motivations. Children who are intense, persistent, irregular in day-to-day rhythm, and negative in mood can be especially difficult for families, even without the added stress of a chronic illness.[5] Providing insight to families about the nature of their child's temperament can decrease their guilt and can provide them with more effective ways of coping with their child's behavior.

School Age

Problems with autonomy and initiative from the previous period may become manifest during school age. The dependent, disabled child may have serious difficulty separating from his or her parents in order to attend school. Separation anxiety can affect the parents, who may impose unreasonable restrictions on their child's activities or who may have unreasonable expectations of their child's abilities.

Some chronic conditions such as hydrocephalus, cerebral palsy, lead toxicity, or brain injury impair the child's cognitive or motor abilities directly. Other conditions, such as cyanotic heart disease and sickle cell anemia, which do not affect the brain directly, also have been shown to impair cognition. Children who have chronic conditions often miss more school than do other children.[19] These outcomes of chronic illness can hinder a child's ability to achieve a sense of industry at school. A wide array of educational and health-related services are mandated by Public Law 101-476, the Individuals With Disabilities Education Act (IDEA), which requires children from ages 3 years to 21 years to receive an appropriate education in an inclusive, least restrictive environment (see Chapter 39). This law authorizes the provision of "related" services such as physical therapy, occupational therapy, speech therapy, audiology, transportation, psychological services, assistive technology, social work services, and nursing services, including clean intermittent catheterization. Taking children away from their classrooms to perform these services, however, may affect their academic performance and socialization adversely. IDEA also entitles every child to a written Individualized Education Plan (IEP); parents are guaranteed the right to question decisions about placement and the right to due process in settling differences.

According to social learning theorists[1] a child's conviction that he or she can execute successfully a behavior required to produce a certain outcome (self-efficacy) determines how much effort will be expended in that activity. Because chronically disabled children may look or act different from others, they frequently are rejected by peers despite their best efforts at socialization. Their repeated lack of success in this regard will lead to decreased efforts in the development of social relations (learned helplessness) and may produce deviant social and personality development as they grow older. Children who are deficient in physical and self-help skills have been shown to have fewer coping skills and more difficulty establishing satisfactory social relations than their peers.[3]

If the child's teacher or the school nurse is not knowledgeable about the child's condition, the child's care at school may be impaired. The pediatrician should inform and regularly update school personnel about the child's condition and expectations for achievement must be available for intervention during a crisis. Providing a written assessment of the child's needs and a plan for the school to follow during an emergency and clarifying roles and responsibilities can greatly decrease the discomfort of school personnel, improve communication, and enhance care.[15] Parents also should be encouraged to collaborate with school personnel.

During this period the pediatrician also can increase the child's responsibility to manage his or her condition—for example, the child can be made responsible for ensuring that medications and treatments are received as scheduled and can keep a diary of illness-related events.

Adolescence

Chronic disabilities can affect the social and emotional development of the adolescent profoundly. Issues of major concern during this period are shown in the box on the right. The presence of a chronic condition significantly increases the risk for behavior problems and psychiatric disorders such as depression. The pediatrician should be aware of the signs and symptoms of depression, which may be subtle, including a sad or flat affect, loss of interest in usual activities, lowered self-esteem, social withdrawal, impaired school work, fatigue, and irritability. Behavioral problems and emotional distress are not directly correlated with the physiological severity of the condition, however. Children who are marginally affected — for example, those who have low-level spina bifida or minimal arthritis[17] — may have greater difficulty adjusting during adolescence than those more severely affected. Minimally affected children cannot identify with the world of "normals" because they cannot accomplish many normal activities (such as running or achieving continence), nor do they identify with the world of the severely impaired individual, such as a child in a wheelchair.

The adverse effects of chronic conditions are modified by the gender of the child as well as by socioeconomic status.[6] For example, delayed sexual maturation is more likely to lead to depression and social isolation in boys than in girls.

Adolescents develop a sense of identity by emulating role models. Disabled adolescents often have few role models. The normative values for concepts such as "beauty," which assail adolescents through the print media and television, often are widely discrepant from their own self-images. The lack of role models, isolation from peers, poor self-image, and a pervasive culture that stresses physical appearance make the development of a positive identity difficult at best.

The pediatrician should address the issues outlined in the box above and address the feelings of the adolescent related to his or her self-concept and condition. Most authorities recommend that the adolescent be evaluated by the pediatrician without the parents present in order to build a trusting relationship that inspires independence.

ISSUES OF SPECIAL RELEVANCE FOR ADOLESCENTS

- Physical appearance (actual and perceived)
- Social isolation
- Sexual development
  - Physical maturation, including onset of puberty
  - Heterosexual relationship ideations
  - Sexual behavior and contraception
- Vocational planning
- Genetic counseling

SYSTEMS OF CARE

The goal for the management of the child who has chronic disabilities should be to *achieve maximum functioning*. For example, the goal of a specific orthopedic intervention should be to help a child walk, not to straighten his or her feet. It is ironic that the specialization that has improved the health and longevity of children who have chronic conditions has resulted in fragmentation of care within the health care system. Also, communication between medical personnel and other agencies, such as the educational and legal systems, often is inadequate. Access to services still is difficult for many families, especially those who have no health insurance, and preventive services may be unavailable.[18] This has resulted in duplication of some services and gaps in others.

Case Management

Achieving optimum functioning requires an organized, coordinated approach to care, which is embodied in the concept of case management.[11] Comprehensive case management includes (1) *assessing needs*—identifying and assessing the needs of the child and family, including their financial needs[13]; (2) *planning comprehensive care*—planning and arranging for medical and nonmedical services; (3) *facilitating and coordinating services* (including training community providers); (4) *following up*—monitoring services and patient progress; and (5) *empowering*—counseling, educating, training, and supporting the child and family. Successful implementation requires knowledge of the child, the family, and the community in which they function.

Possible case managers for children who have chronic conditions have been suggested, including the primary care physician, the specialty program, the community health nurse, and governmental programs. However, any professional who cares for a child who has special health care needs must ensure that *someone* is providing this service. Without it these children will receive less than optimum care, and families will face an even greater burden.

The pediatrician who attends the child who has a chronic condition can foster the child's development and functioning in the community. Achieving this goal requires knowing the needs of the child's family and the resources in the community. This does not necessitate the provision of all services by that single provider. It does, however, require time, which frequently is not reimbursed, thoughtful coordination of effort, support of other professionals, and advocacy.

SUMMARY

The physician who cares for the child or adolescent who has a physical disability or chronic condition is in a particularly advantageous position to foster the child's psychological development. He or she can do this both at the time of the "informing" interview[14] with the parents and throughout the patient's infancy, childhood, and adolescence. Even when the physician is not in a position to carry out this process directly, his or her support of others, such as social workers, psychiatrists, and psychologists, in their interactions with the parents and the child will help the parents to recognize the importance of psychosocial issues in their child's development. In this way it may be possible to reduce the high prevalence of behavioral and emotional problems that reflect maladaptation to a physical disability or chronic illness.

REFERENCES

1. Bandura A: *The social foundations of thought and action: a social theory,* Englewood Cliffs, NJ, 1986, Prentice Hall.
2. Blackman JA, Healy A, Ruppert ES: Participation by pediatricians in early intervention: impetus from Public Law 99-457, *Pediatrics* 89:98, 1992.
3. Breitmayer BJ et al: Social competence of school-aged children with chronic illnesses, *J Pediatr Nurs* 7:181, 1992.
4. Cadman D et al: Chronic illness, disability and mental and social well-being: findings of the Ontario Child Health Study, *Pediatrics* 75:805, 1987.
5. Carey WB: Temperament issues in the school-aged child, *Pediatr Clin North Am* 39:569, 1992.
6. Eiser C et al: Adjustment to chronic disease in relation to age and gender: mothers' and fathers' reports of their childrens' behavior, *J Pediatr Psychol* 17:261, 1992.
7. Faux SA: Siblings of children with chronic physical and cognitive disabilities, *J Pediatr Nurs* 8:305, 1993.
8. Gortmaker SL et al: Chronic conditions, socioeconomic risks, and behavioral problems in children and adolescents, *Pediatrics* 85:267, 1990.
9. Hobbs N, Perrin JM, Ireys HT: *Chronically ill children and their families,* San Francisco, 1985, Jossey-Bass.
10. Klaus MG, Kennell JH: *Parent-infant bonding,* St Louis, 1982, Mosby.
11. Martinez NH, Schreiber ML, Hartman EW: Pediatric nurse practitioners: primary care providers and case managers for chronically ill children at home, *J Pediatr Health Care* 5:291, 1991.
12. McCormick MC, Gortmaker SL, Sobol AM: Very low birthweight children: behavior problems and school difficulty in a national sample, *J Pediatr* 117:687, 1990.
13. McManus MA, Newacheck P: Health insurance differentials among minority children with chronic conditions and the role of federal agencies and private foundations in improving financial access, *Pediatrics* 91:1040, 1993.
14. Myers BA: The informing interview: enabling parents to "hear" and cope with bad news, *Am J Dis Child* 137:572, 1983.
15. Palfrey JS, Haynie M, Porter SN: *Children assisted by medical technology in educational settings: guidelines for care,* Boston, 1989, Project School Care, The Children's Hospital.
16. Revell GM, Liptak GS: Understanding the child with special health care needs: a developmental perspective, *J Pediatr Nurs* 6:258, 1991.
17. Stein RE, Jessop DJ: Measuring health variables among Hispanic and non-Hispanic children with chronic conditions, *Pub Health Rep* 104:377, 1989.
18. Stein R, Jessop DJ, Riessman CK: Health care received by children with chronic illnesses, *Am J Dis Child* 137:225, 1983.
19. Weitzman M et al: High-risk youth and health: the care of excessive school absence, *Pediatrics* 78:313, 1986.
20. Worthington RC: The chronically ill child and recurring family grief, *J Fam Pract* 29:397, 1989.

34 Mental Retardation

Thomas J. Kenny and Katherine Nitz

The prevalence of mental retardation is such that all primary care physicians will confront it eventually. In 1992 the American Association on Mental Retardation (AAMR) adopted a new definition of mental retardation, as follows:

> Mental retardation refers to substantial limitations in present functioning. It is characterized by significantly subaverage intellectual functioning, existing concurrently with related limitation in two or more of the following applicable adaptive skill areas: communication, self-care, home living, social skills, community use, self-direction, health and safety, functional academics, leisure, and work. Mental retardation manifests before age 18.[16]

Considerable controversy surrounds this new definition. Critics point out that it could increase the number of persons identified as mentally retarded, in that the definition is less exact and raises the IQ cutoff to 75 from the previous 70. Others note that the 10 areas of adaptive behavior specified in the diagnosis are difficult to define and measure.[17] Jacobson believes that the new diagnosis expands the social or political aspects of the problem, which can be seen as humanistic, but it does so at the expense of science: "Foundation in science has been replaced by referendum and affirmation."[11] For the purposes of this chapter and to keep the focus on the issues that concern the primary care physician, we will simplify the definition and stress the broader elements that are shared by the old and new definitions.

It is noteworthy that in both definitions, subaverage general intellectual functioning and deficits in adaptive behavior must coexist for diagnostic criteria to be fulfilled.[8] *Subaverage intelligence* has been defined as a score that is at least 2 standard deviations below the mean on a standardized intelligence test. This statistically based definition indicates that 2.5% of a given population will be classified as mentally retarded; in the United States this definition encompasses about 5 million individuals. Actually, however, the number of individuals who are identified as mentally retarded at any given time is far lower.[19] *Adaptive behavior* means the effectiveness or degree with which individuals meet the standard of personal independence and social responsibility expected of their age or cultural group. Thus it is possible that a given individual could be considered mentally retarded in one setting (or one age group) but not at another age or in another environment — one that is perhaps less competitive or more relaxed, permissive, and accepting. Such a circumstance is much more likely to occur with "educable" or mildly retarded persons, who account for 75% of the total population of those who are or may be retarded.

In the old definition the AAMR defined four official levels of mental retardation (Table 34-1); the new definition eliminates these levels, despite a strong feeling that significant differences are associated with the levels of retardation. In the old definition mild retardation (encompassing those who are educable) is the most prevalent and is significantly more so among persons of lower socioeconomic status. In this group the incidence of overt neurological problems and multiple handicaps is not markedly elevated. In fact no specific etiology is identified for 75% to 80% of those at this level. In contrast the more pronounced types of retardation, although less common, are found equally across all socioeconomic groups. Generally these more markedly handicapped individuals are more likely to be identified early, are more likely to have an identifiable etiology and diagnosis, and are more likely have other overt neurological handicaps (e.g., seizures, cerebral palsy).[14,15,18]

The 10 areas of adaptive behavior listed in the AAMR definition are similar to those the federal government adopted in defining developmental disabilities. In PL-100-146, the Developmental Disabilities Bill of Rights and Assistance Act amendments of 1987, the law defines seven areas of life function — thinking, economic self-sufficiency, communication, locomotion, capacity for independent living, self-care, and motivation; deficiencies in three or more of these functions caused by physical or verbal impairment that occurred before 22 years of age constitute a developmental disability. Studies have demonstrated that this definition tends to include only some of those persons who would fit the AAMR categoric definition. Because such definitions often dictate eligibility criteria for services, the disparity may create problems for some children in states that have adopted the federal definition.[3]

A number of causal factors have been linked with mental retardation. In most cases, particularly in the mildly retarded range, specific etiological mechanisms are unknown. Risk of mental retardation is associated with a number of contributing social and physiological factors that have been linked to developmental outcome. In recent years children known to have one or more of these risk factors have been monitored in an effort toward early identification of delays. Various early intervention programs have been designed to stimulate these children and to offset or modify the effects of deleterious social and physiological factors. These programs have demonstrated varying degrees of success and have not always had the broad and long-lasting effects that theorists predicted. In general, however, they appear to affect developmental outcome positively.[14,18]

Generally it is not possible to confirm a diagnosis of mental retardation during the newborn period; Down syndrome (with an incidence of 1 in 800 births) and primary microcephaly are two exceptions. In most other clinical circumstances the diagnosis of retardation is first suspected because the child does not reach developmental milestones when expected rather than because of any specific positive findings. Because developmental differences in early childhood can be difficult to assess, the physician's responsibility in this regard can be burdensome.

Table 34-1 Official Levels of Mental Retardation and Some Developmental Characteristics*

Level and title	IQ range	Estimated percentage of total retarded	Adaptive and developmental characteristics		
			Preschool age 0-5 (maturation and development)	School age 6-20 (training and education)	Adult ≥ 21 (social and vocational adequacy)
1. Profound	<20	5	Gross retardation; minimum capacity for functioning in sensorimotor areas; may need nursing care	Some motor development present; may respond to minimum or limited training in self-help	Some motor and speech development; may achieve very limited self-care; may need nursing care
2. Severe	20-35		Poor motor development; minimal speech; able to profit from training in self-help; little or no expressive skills	Can talk or learn to communicate; can be trained in elemental health habits; can profit from systematic habit training	May contribute partially to self-maintenance under complete supervision; can develop self-protection skills to a minimum useful level in controlled environment
3. Moderate	36-51	20	Can talk or learn to communicate; poor social awareness; fair motor development; profits from training in self-help; can be managed with moderate supervision	Can profit from training in social and occupational skills; unlikely to progress beyond second-grade level in academic subjects; may learn to travel alone in familiar places	May achieve self-maintenance in unskilled or semiskilled work under sheltered conditions; needs supervision and guidance when under mild social or economic stress
4. Mild	52-68	75	Can develop social and communication skills; minimal retardation in sensorimotor areas; often not distinguished from normal until later age	Can learn academic skills up to approximately sixth-grade level by late teens; can be guided toward social conformity; "educable"	Can usually achieve social and vocational skills adequate to minimum self-support but may need guidance and assistance when under unusual social or economic stress

*Definition of mental retardation: "Significantly subaverage general intellectual functioning existing concurrently with deficits in adaptive behavior and manifest during the developmental period."

Individuals who are mildly mentally retarded frequently are not identified as such during the preschool years. The first real concern about their developmental status may be raised when they encounter academic problems.[12] After leaving school many of these individuals are assimilated into society. They may obtain jobs, raise families, and be self-sufficient, at least to some degree. Mildly retarded individuals may demonstrate their handicaps most prominently in the academic area and may function quite well in nonacademic activities. Some observers have even charged that mildly retarded children are "manufactured" by the school system. Speech and language problems are characteristic of persons who are mentally retarded. In general the greater the degree of retardation, the higher the incidence and the more marked the degree of speech problems. It is estimated that about 50% of mildly retarded persons and over 95% of severely retarded persons have speech problems; about 50% of profoundly retarded persons are nonverbal.

PHYSICIAN'S ROLE

The primary care physician has a four-part role in the care of the person who is mentally retarded: (1) identification and diagnosis, (2) provision of comprehensive health care, (3) counseling, and (4) continuity of care, case management, and advocacy. The most effective way to identify children at risk for mental retardation is to assess developmental status at each health care visit. This assessment should include a history of motor, language, and social development. A screening tool that measures cognitive and behavioral development also can be useful. One standard tool for such screening is the Denver Developmental Screening Test, presented in Chapter 20. Repeated studies have demonstrated that this instrument is highly effective and easily administered. Another option is to use the combined vision/developmental screening procedure developed by Sturner,[24] which is both brief and valid.

After identification, the physician's role in health care remains important. Although there is no specific medical treatment for most types of mental retardation, children who are mentally retarded are at increased risk for many medical problems. For example, the child who has Down syndrome is at risk for congenital heart disease, thyroid dysfunction, visual problems, obesity, and leukemia. As a group, mentally retarded persons have a higher incidence of delayed speech development, decreased visual acuity, and seizures. Therefore it is vital that the physician provide comprehensive health care to the affected youngster or see that it is provided.

The third role of the physician involves counseling parents of the child who is mentally retarded. First, simple, clear, effective communication with the parents about their child and issues of mental retardation is needed (see Chapter 33). A frequent issue the physician may face pertains to the developmental course of mental retardation. This is one of the most difficult and frequently asked questions by parents. In general it is difficult to predict developmental outcome for any individual child who is mentally retarded, except for those children who are functioning within the range of severe to profound retardation. Parents especially may benefit from anticipatory guidance to help them adjust to the transitions they may face in the future regarding developmental milestones and life skills. Issues that may necessitate anticipatory guidance by various professionals cover the entire lifespan. They include (1) toilet training, (2) peer relations, (3) puberty, (4) sexual relationships, and (5) job training. The physician should refer parents to health professionals who can address these issues. Another issue that surfaces eventually is that of sexual development and related behavior, often a difficult area for parents to face. Specific issues, such as the management of menstruation, or the general problems of adolescence itself can be difficult to deal with in those who are mentally retarded. Similarly, retarded persons have sex drives; their more limited social heterosexual contacts, however, provide fewer reasonable outlets for these feelings.

The parent or professional who has concerns in these areas should contact local agencies, including the local Association for Retarded Persons, that are likely to have a spectrum of help available. Possibilities include educational programs and appropriate literature. Two very useful books for parents or professionals are Kempton's *A Teacher's Guide to Sex Education for Persons with Learning Disabilities*[13] and Monat's *Sexuality and the Mentally Retarded*.[20] A new book by Monat, *Understanding and Expressing Sexuality: Responsible Choices for Individuals with Developmental Disabilities*,[21] has current information relating to the issue of AIDS as well as a helpful directory of resources.

The fourth role for the physician is that of case manager or advocate. The physician therefore should be ready to refer the child for appropriate evaluations (including psychological evaluation) to establish basic data about the child's developmental status, especially in the areas of cognition and social skills. The results of this evaluation should help the physician and parents plan for the child's needs; thus the child should be evaluated as early as possible. A reasonably accurate assessment usually can be conducted at about 2 years of age, and a comprehensive evaluation should be performed before the child starts school.

The primary care physician's role in care coordination has increased dramatically with the increasing number of mentally retarded children who do not live in institutions and remain with their families until adulthood. Health care for children who are mentally retarded often does not exceed the level of care necessary for children who do not have disabilities. Mentally retarded children require coordination of allied health, educational, and family support services, which the physician may be in a unique position to provide.[9]

Other evaluations that may be necessary include those for speech and language development; audiometric evaluation also may be called for. In addition, ophthalmological and neurological consultations frequently are indicated.

BEHAVIORAL PROBLEMS

As a group mentally retarded persons have a greater incidence of behavioral problems than do those in the general population. Foale[7] found the incidence of psychoneurosis in retarded persons to be twice that of the general population. Pervasive emotional problems such as psychosis and autism also are more frequent among retarded children.[10,18] In an excellent review of the prevalence of psychopathology in people who are mentally retarded, Borthwich-Duffy[4] cited studies estimating the range from under 10% to more than 80%. The more severely retarded person often has poor communication abilities and frequently has increased motor activity (i.e., hyperactivity). Mentally retarded persons also tend to have short attention spans and problems focusing their attention. Their behavior tends to be impulsive, repetitive, or stereotypic, and they are at increased risk of engaging in self-stimulatory or self-injurious behaviors.

Mildly retarded children have many of the characteristics of children who have an attention deficit disorder. They usually are overactive, have a poor attention span, and are impulsive; they also tend to be aggressive and to "act out" their frustrations. Management of these problems is similar to that for nonretarded children. Medications such as methylphenidate hydrochloride (Ritalin) or dextroamphetamine sulfate (Dexedrine) can be useful if used judiciously and monitored carefully and behavior management techniques have been demonstrated to be effective. A number of books can be used by parents to develop behavior management programs, including *Parents Are Teachers* by Wesley Becker,[1] and Gerald Patterson's book, *Families: Application of Social Learning to Family Life*.[22]

Cromwell[5] sees the behavior of retarded persons as a consequence of the frustration related to the many failures they experience. He proposes that this causes the retarded person to (1) perform in a new situation below the level of his or her constitutional ability, (2) be less likely to be motivated by failure, and (3) be less likely to try harder after a minor failure — that is, to give up more easily. Cromwell thus describes the retarded child as a "failure-avoider" as opposed to a "success-striver."

MANAGEMENT

Current trends in the management of mentally retarded persons will require increased services from the primary care physician. Improved medical care has extended the life span of such people, which has resulted in a greater need for ongoing health maintenance by the physician as well as for expanded efforts in case management, especially in the psychosocial area.

The current emphasis on "deinstitutionalization" and "normalization" of living experiences requires a comprehensive and sustained social support system. More attention must be devoted to vocational training and the development of occupational opportunities. The deinstitutionalization effort necessitates helping the family and the mentally retarded person prepare for alternate living arrangements. Greater numbers of mentally retarded persons are moving into group homes and apartments in the community, which requires a support system that meets their physical, social, and occupational needs.[6] Available data on the effectiveness of such programs are conflicting but suggest that much remains to be done to facilitate the optimum adjustment of mentally retarded persons and to match settings to individual needs.[2,14,23] The physician can help the family and the child prepare for entry into this system of independent living and working.

REFERENCES

1. Becker WC: *Parents are teachers: a child management program,* Champaign, Ill, 1971, Research Press.
2. Birenbaum A, Re M: Resettling mentally retarded adults in the community — almost 4 years later, *Am J Ment Defic* 31:323, 1979.
3. Boggs E, Henney RL: *A numerical and functional description of the developmental disabilities population,* Philadelphia, 1979, EMC Institute.
4. Borthwich-Duffy SA: Epidemiology and prevalence of psychopathology in people with mental retardation, *J Consult Clin Psychol* 62:17, 1994.
5. Cromwell RL: Personality evaluation. In Baumeister A, editor: *Mental retardation: appraisal, education, and rehabilitation,* Chicago, 1967, Aldine.
6. Eyman RK, Arndt S: Life-span development of institutionalized and community-based mentally retarded residents, *Am J Ment Defic* 86:342, 1982.
7. Foale M: The special difficulty of high-grade mental defective adolescents, *Am J Ment Defic* 60:867, 1956.
8. Grossman HJ: *Classification in mental retardation,* Washington, DC, 1983, The American Association on Mental Deficiency.
9. Guralnick MJ, Bennett FC: *The effectiveness of early intervention for at-risk and handicapped children,* Orlando, Fla, 1987, Academic Press.
10. Jacobson J: Problem behavior and psychiatric impairment within a developmentally disabled population. I. Behavior frequency, *Appl Res Ment Retard* 3:121, 1982.
11. Jacobson J: Mental retardation: definition, classification, and systems of support, *Am J Ment Retard* 98:539, 1994.
12. Kappelman M, Kenny T, Clemmens R: Mild mental retardation: clinical characteristics in early and late identification, *Md Med J* 23:83, 1974.
13. Kempton W: *A teacher's guide to sex education for persons with learning disabilities,* North Scituate, Mass, 1975, Duxburg Press.
14. Landesman-Dwyer S: Living in the community, *Am J Ment Defic* 86:223, 1981.
15. Lazar I, Darlington RB: Lasting effects of early education, *Monogr Soc Res Child Dev* 47:1, 1982.
16. Luckasson D et al: *Mental retardation: definition, classification, and systems of supports,* Washington, DC, 1992, American Association on Mental Retardation.
17. MacMillan DZ, Gresham FM, Lipnstein GN: Conceptual and psychometric concerns about the 1992 AAMR definition of mental retardation, *Am J Ment Retard* 98:325, 1993.
18. McKey RH et al: Impact of Head Start on children, families, and communities, Pub No (OHDS) 85-31193, Washington, DC, 1985, Department of Health and Human Services.
19. Mercer J: The myth of 3% prevalence. In Tarjan G, Eyman RK, Meyers CE, editors: *Sociobehavioral studies in mental retardation,* Monograph No 1, Washington, DC, 1973, The American Association on Mental Deficiency.
20. Monat RK: *Sexuality and the mentally retarded,* San Diego, 1982, College-Hill Press.
21. Monat-Haller RK. *Understanding and expressing sexuality: responsible choices for individuals with developmental disabilities,* Baltimore, 1992, Paul H Brookes.
22. Patterson GR: *Families: application of social learning to family life,* Champaign, Ill, 1975, Research Press.
23. Reiss S: Psychopathology and mental retardation: survey of a developmental disabilities mental health program, *Ment Retard* 20:128, 1982.
24. Sturner RA et al: Simultaneous screening for child health and development: a study of visual/developmental screening of preschool children, *Pediatrics* 65:614, 1980.

SUGGESTED READINGS

Clarke ADB, Clarke AM: Research on mental handicap, 1957-1987: a selected review, *J Ment Defic Res* 31:317, 1987.

Hill BK, Lakin KC, Bruininks RH: Trends in residential services for mentally retarded people, 1977-1982, *J Assoc Persons with Severe Handicaps* 9:243, 1984.

35 Children Assisted by Medical Technology

Marilynn Haynie and Judith S. Palfrey

SCOPE OF THE PROBLEM

Over the past two decades advances in pediatric medical and surgical techniques have allowed children who have chronic illness and disabilities to live longer, more functional lives.[12] Children who have spina bifida, congenital heart disease, and leukemia live at least twice as long as they did a few decades ago. Children who have cystic fibrosis have a sevenfold higher chance of surviving to age 21 than previously.[19] Extremely premature infants and children who have congenital anomalies also are surviving longer.[2,18]

This is due in part to an increasing reliance on the use of medical technologies, such as oxygen therapy, ventilators, tracheostomies, central venous lines, urinary bladder catheterization, renal dialysis, enterostomies, and gastrostomy tubes to replace or augment a physiological function.[6,8,9,25-27] As a result a new population of children who have special health care needs has evolved—children assisted by medical technology. This group of children is becoming increasingly visible in the community as they leave tertiary care medical centers to live at home.[13]

Children assisted by medical technology are defined as those children who have a chronic condition that requires daily assistance by a medical device to replace or augment a body function in order to sustain life.[28] Examples of such conditions include an 18-year-old boy who has a high cervical cord injury and is ventilator dependent; a 2-year-old girl who has spastic quadriplegic cerebral palsy and a gastrostomy tube, and a 1-year-old boy who has a craniofacial abnormality and a tracheostomy.

Estimates of the number of children assisted by medical technology are sparse. A study in Massachusetts reported the prevalence rate to be 1 to 2/1000 children.[20] Other resources only provide ranges of estimates of the size of the population nationwide.[28,29] Future trends in the size of this population of children will depend on the extent to which the individual technologies are used, as well as the reasons for their use. For instance, with the availability of artificial surfactant, the prevalence of severe bronchopulmonary dysplasia may be decreasing, resulting in decreased use of oxygen and ventilators among infants.[1] However, ease in placement of percutaneous gastrostomy tubes[10] and improved nutritional outcomes in children who have severe cerebral palsy and have gastrostomy tubes[24] may result in an increase in the use of this technology.

ETIOLOGY

Some technologies are used temporarily to enhance or replace a physiological function until the child is old enough to undergo corrective surgery or "outgrows" the need. Children born with severe congenital malformations of the head and neck such as those who have Pierre Robin syndrome, craniosynostosis syndromes, and lymphatic malformations frequently need their airways protected via tracheotomies for several months to years; many subsequently are able to be decannulated. Infants who have necrotizing enterocolitis may require enterostomies that are closed in a few months to a year.

Children who are unable to eat by mouth because of anatomical problems such as esophageal atresia may require gastrostomy tubes for several months until their atresia has been repaired. Children on long-term parenteral chemotherapy frequently have central venous lines that are removed once their course of chemotherapy is completed. Continuous ambulatory peritoneal dialysis may be used by a small child who is awaiting a renal transplant.

Other technologies are necessary for long-term use by children who will never gain the function that the technology performs. A gastrostomy tube may be required as a result of dysphagia secondary to severe neuromuscular involvement in cerebral palsy. Children who have neurogenic bladders from myelodysplasia or cervical cord injuries require bladder catheterization several times daily. Children who have AIDS increasingly are being treated with feeding tubes and central lines for hyperalimentation.[4] Children who have high cervical spinal cord injuries or muscular dystrophy may require permanent ventilatory assistance.

PSYCHOSOCIAL ISSUES

The psychosocial issues facing children assisted by medical technology and their families are the same as those encountered by children who have other forms of chronic illness.[18] Children who are dependent on medical technology may or may not be obviously "different" from their peers as a result of their underlying condition. Some technology is relatively easy to conceal, such as enterostomies, g-tubes, and central venous lines; ventilators are not. Being different from one's peers is quite stressful for adolescents. Issues concerning body image, independence, and self-identity may be exacerbated for adolescents assisted by medical technology.

For little children assistance by medical technology does not seem to be as stigmatizing. However, the underlying condition or the technology may make participation in regular childhood activities difficult. For instance the child who has a tracheostomy may not be able to play in a sandbox or use glitter unless the tracheostomy is covered by an appropriate device. For some children, dependence on caregivers may hamper development of independence and interpersonal skills.

Having children assisted by medical technology who live at home contributes to increased levels of stress among the families of those children.[13,22] Parental burnout occurs as a result of physical and emotional exhaustion, lack of recreational opportunities with and without the children, and increased financial burdens; for those who have ventilator-assisted children, burnout appears to increase with the duration of ventilator use.[23]

As children are living at home with their technology and going to school, adults and children in the community are more and more confronted with the child who is "different" by virtue of being assisted by medical technology. Teachers may be frightened by medical conditions with which they are not familiar. Procedures once only done in hospitals are now being done in schools, which seems to highlight the child's problems. The term *medically fragile* serves to increase anxiety about the stability and oddness of children whose medical needs are complex. Playmates and peers may not understand the equipment used or the child's need for privacy in order to perform a procedure such as catheterization.

MANAGEMENT

Caring for a child assisted by medical technology can be both challenging and rewarding for the primary care pediatrician. In addition to providing routine pediatric well-child care, the pediatrician must work with the child's parents to provide family-centered care.[14] This means not just referring the child to specialists in the tertiary care center, but managing the care in the community with input from the specialist. This involves coordinating community services such as home care agencies, equipment vendors, and early intervention services to ensure that all the child's needs are met as well as working with the local school to ensure a safe educational environment through the use of special health care and emergency treatment plans.[21]

Specific medical management revolves around the child's underlying condition and issues specific to the technology used. For instance, a child who has a tracheotomy because of subglottic stenosis may be more prone to respiratory infections secondary to organisms bypassing the defense mechanisms of the upper airway, as well as to the slightly increased risk of aspiration of secretions around the tracheostomy tube. He or she may be at risk for the tracheostomy becoming plugged if secretions are not humidified adequately. Reactive airways disease may result from frequent aspiration or contact with airborne particles that are normally filtered from the upper airway. Children who have uncuffed tracheostomy tubes are at risk for aspirating secretions and food. Accidental decannulation could be life threatening, depending on the degree of stenosis.[7]

For a child who has a gastrostomy tube (g-tube), gastroesophageal reflux often is a confounding issue. This especially is true for children who have neuromuscular impairment, such as cerebral palsy. Although gastrostomy feedings result in improved weight gain and possibly a better developmental outcome, in the child who has severe spastic quadriplegic cerebral palsy, aspiration pneumonia and/or severe esophagitis often occurs secondary to reflux of the gastrostomy feedings.[17] Children who have g-tubes but do not have fundoplications frequently require prokinetic agents and H_2 blockers to manage the reflux. If a gastrostomy tube falls out or is pulled out, it must be replaced within a few hours because of the risk of the stoma and tract closing.

Central venous catheters provide excellent access for frequent blood drawing and administration of parenteral nutrition or chemotherapy. However, they are sites for infection and thrombosis, both of which can be life threatening. Fevers require investigation. Lines can break or become plugged with blood clots, requiring surgical replacement or chemical thrombolysis.[3]

Children assisted by mechanical ventilators frequently are recipients of multiple technological devices, including tracheostomies, gastrostomies, and catheters. Although ventilator settings may be adjusted by the pulmonary specialist, frequent monitoring of the child's respiratory status is required, with treatment of intercurrent infections. A high level of home nursing care may be necessary to maintain good pulmonary "toilet."[11,16]

PROGNOSIS

The prognosis for children dependent on medical technology depends largely on the underlying medical condition. Children who have Pierre Robin syndrome and have a tracheostomy and a g-tube placed at birth likely will not need either by 1 to 2 years of age and will go on to enjoy "normal" good health.[5] The use of technology gives their mandibles time to grow while preserving normal cognitive functioning.

Children who have spina bifida require clean intermittent catheterization four or five times daily and are likely to need this for the rest of their lives. However, the risk of developing end stage renal disease from recurrent infections is significantly lower than when this is not done.[15] A ventilator-dependent adolescent who has high cervical cord trauma requires permanent ventilator support but may be able to hold a job. Adolescents and young adults who have muscular dystrophy and anterior horn cell disease may live for several years with ventilator assistance.

CONCLUSION

Children assisted by medical technology are a relatively new subgroup of the chronically ill and disabled. It is not clear whether the prevalence of this group of children is increasing. As advances in surgical techniques and technology applications continue, technologies such as gastrostomy tubes, tracheotomies, central venous catheters, and ventilators will continue to be used for a small group of children, both temporarily and chronically. The goal of these technologies should be to enhance the quality of life for the children and their families. This group of children presents primary care pediatricians with the opportunity to coordinate and manage the care of those who require frequent contact with specialists and tertiary care medical centers but who thrive at home and in the community.

REFERENCES

1. Abman SH, Groothius JR: Pathophysiology and treatment of bronchopulmonary dysplasia: current issues, *Pediatr Clin North Am* 41:277, 1994.
2. Alward GP et al: Outcome studies of low birth weight infants published in the last decade: a meta-analysis, *J Pediatr* 115:515, 1989.
3. Bagnall HA, Gomperts E, Atkinson JB: Continuous infusion of low-dose urokinase in the treatment of central venous catheter thrombosis in infants and children, *Pediatrics* 83:963, 1989.

4. Beaver BL et al: Surgical intervention in children with human immunodeficiency virus infection, *J Pediatr Surg* 25:79, 1990.
5. Bull MJ et al: Improved outcome in Pierre Robin sequence: effect of multidisciplinary evaluation and management, *Pediatrics* 86:294, 1990.
6. Cairo MS et al: Long-term use of indwelling multipurpose Silastic catheters in pediatric cancer patients treated with aggressive chemotherapy, *J Clin Oncol* 4:784, 1986.
7. Duncan BW et al: Tracheostomy in children with emphasis on home care, *J Pediatr Surg* 27:432, 1992.
8. Fine RN, Salusky IB, Ettinger RB: The therapeutic approach to the infant, child, and adolescent with end-stage renal disease, *Pediatr Clin North Am* 343:789, 1987.
9. Gauderer MWL: Gastrostomy techniques and devices, *Surg Clin North Am* 72:1285, 1992.
10. Gauderer ML: Percutaneous endoscopic gastrostomy: a ten-year experience with 220 children, *J Pediatr Surg* 26:288, 1991.
11. Goldberg AI, Monahan CA: Home health care for children assisted by mechanical ventilation: the physician's perspective, *J Pediatr* 114:378, 1989.
12. Hendren WH, Lillehei CW: Pediatric surgery, *N Engl J Med* 319:86, 1988.
13. Hobbs N, Perrin JM, Ireys HT, editors: *Chronically ill children and their families,* San Francisco, 1985, Jossey-Bass.
14. Hostler SL: Family-centered care, *Pediatr Clin North Am* 36:1545, 1991.
15. Klose AG, Sackett CK, Mesrobian HG: Management of children with myelodysplasia: urological alternatives, *J Urol* 144:1446, 1990.
16. Mallory GB, Stillwell PC: The ventilator-dependent child: issues in diagnosis and management, *Arch Phys Med Rehab* 72:43, 1991.
17. Mollitt DL, Golladay ES, Seibert JJ: Symptomatic gastroesophageal reflux following gastrostomy in neurologically impaired patients, *Pediatrics* 75:1124, 1985.
18. Morbidity and Mortality Weekly Reports Centers for Disease Control Surveillance Summaries, 39:19, 1990.
19. Newacheck PW, Taylor WR: Chronic childhood illness: prevalence, severity, and impact, *Am J Public Health* 82:364, 1992.
20. Palfrey JS, Haynie M, Porter S: Prevalence of medical technology assistance among children in Massachusetts in 1987 and 1990, *Public Health Rep* 109:226, 1994.
21. Palfrey JS et al: Project School Care: integrating children assisted by medical technology into educational settings, *J School Health* 62:50, 1992.
22. Patterson JM, Leonard BJ, Titus JC: Home care for medically fragile children: impact on family health and well-being, *J Dev Behav Pediatr* 13:248, 1992.
23. Quint RD et al: Home care for ventilator-dependent children: psychosocial impact on the family, *Am J Dis Child* 114:1238, 1990.
24. Rempel GR, Colwell SO, Nelson RP: Growth in children with cerebral palsy fed via gastrostomy, *Pediatrics* 82:857, 1988.
25. Schreiner MS, Donar ME, Kettrick RG: Pediatric home mechanical ventilation, *Pediatr Clin North Am* 34:47, 1987.
26. Selzman AA, Elder JS, Mapstone TB: Urologic consequences of myelodysplasia and other congenital abnormalities of the spinal cord, *Urol Clin North Am* 20:485, 1993.
27. Swift AC, Rogers JH: The changing indications for tracheostomy in children, *J Laryngol Otol* 101:1258, 1987.
28. Task Force on Technology-Dependent Children: Fostering home and community-based care for technology-dependent children, Washington, DC, 1988, Maternal and Child Health Task Force.
29. *Technology-dependent children: hospital v home care.* A technical memorandum, Washington, DC, 1987, Office of Technology Assessment, US Congress.

SUGGESTED READINGS

Cardoso P: A parent's perspective: family-centered care, *Child Health Care* 20:258, 1991.

Farrell PM, Fost NC: Long-term mechanical ventilation in pediatric respiratory failure: medical and ethical considerations, *Am Rev Resp Dis* 140:536, 1989.

Healy A, Lewis-Beck JA: *Improving health care for children with chronic conditions: guidelines for physicians,* Iowa City, 1987, University of Iowa.

Lantos JD, Kohrman AF: Ethical aspects of pediatric home care, *Pediatrics,* 89:920, 1992.

Wesenberg F et al: Central venous catheter with subcutaneous injection port (Port-A-Cath): clinical experience with children, *Pediatr Hematol Oncol* 4:137, 1987.

36 Cystic Fibrosis

Jeffrey M. Ewig

Cystic fibrosis (CF), the most common lethal inherited disease of the Caucasian population, follows an autosomal recessive mode of inheritance. Carriers are asymptomatic. The majority of CF patients are Caucasian (95%), with an estimated incidence of 1 in 3100.[12] This disease does occur among all races, with an estimated incidence of 1 in 14,000 live African-American births and 1 in 11,500 live Hispanic births.[12] The main characteristics are recurrent pulmonary infection, pancreatic insufficiency, increased salt loss in sweat, and male infertility.

Cystic fibrosis was first described as a clinicopathological entity in 1938.[2] Since that time the survival rate has improved steadily as a result of better nutritional support and antibiotic therapy. The major cause of death is from respiratory insufficiency secondary to chronic recurrent pulmonary infection. The median age of survival is approximately 29 years, with males having a slight survival advantage. It is hoped that the recent discovery of the CF gene and its protein product will lead to an improved understanding of the pathophysiology of this debilitating disease and be translated into physiological and/or genetic "cures" for the pulmonary sequelae, thus reducing morbidity and improving survival. Because pulmonary disease is the major cause of death (>95%), this chapter focuses on this aspect of CF.

RESPIRATORY PATHOPHYSIOLOGY AND MANIFESTATIONS

The CF gene was identified in 1989.[16,26,28] It consists of 250 kilobases located on the long arm of chromosome 7. It codes for a 1480 amino acid protein product known as the cystic fibrosis transmembrane conductance regulator (CFTR). The most common mutation in North America and Europe is a deletion of three base pairs, resulting in the deletion of phenylalanine (F) at position 508 (ΔF_{508}). This deletion is present in approximately 70% of Caucasians who have CF; however, over 400 mutations have been identified. Certain populations (e.g., Ashkenazi Jews) have a relatively low frequency of ΔF_{508} and a high frequency of other mutations. This factor must be considered when screening individual patients and when devising larger scale screening programs.

Current understanding about the pathophysiology of CF focuses on the role of CFTR as a cAMP-regulated chloride channel in the apical cell membrane; however, other functions, such as the acidification of intracellular organelles, may be important in the pathogenesis.[3] The consequence of the genetic defect is abnormal electrolyte transport (Fig. 36-1). Chloride secretion from the apical respiratory epithelial cell to the airway lumen is impaired, and sodium reabsorption from the airway lumen is increased two to three times the normal amount. Water passively follows sodium away from the airway lumen leading to dehydration of airway secretions, making them more viscous and more difficult to clear, thus predisposing the patient to infection. This explanation probably oversimplifies the pathophysiology of CF. Recent work suggests that the abnormalities in surface electrolyte composition described above may increase the viscosity of mucus by altering mucin side chain interactions without significant dehydration of airway surface fluid.[31]

Chronic bronchopulmonary infection leads to progressive damage, lung dysfunction, and death. The most common initial bacterial isolates in the first years of life are *Staphylococcus aureus* (SA) and *Haemophilus influenzae*.[1] By contributing to airway inflammation, epithelial injury, and altered production of mucus, SA colonization may create an environment favorable to *Pseudomonas aeruginosa* (PA) adherence and colonization. Over time PA becomes the prominent bacterial pathogen in CF, with a prevalence of 70% to 80%.[15] The mucoid variant rarely is found in non-CF patients, and its presence strongly suggests the diagnosis of CF. Some patients are colonized with other *Pseudomonas* species, such as *Pseudomonas cepacia*.

The question haunting patients and caregivers has been, "Why PA?" because the host systemic immune response to PA is intact, if not excessive. Certain features of the host-microbe relationship contribute to the ability of PA to evade host defense in CF.[23] PA exoproducts promote colonization and impair local host defense. The expression of these exoproducts may be increased in hyperosmolar conditions that exist in the lungs of CF patients.[6] It is not PA, but the immune-mediated inflammatory response that is responsible for the progressive lung damage of CF. PA exoproducts stimulate the recruitment of neutrophils. Neutrophil and PA elastase overwhelm the host antiprotease defense and injure the respiratory epithelium directly. In addition, elastase excess interferes with host defense by cleaving IgG, thus rendering phagocytosis ineffective.[10] Another important consequence of the influx of neutrophils is the release of large amounts of DNA from damaged and disintegrating cells, which greatly increases the viscosity of airway secretions.

Recurrent and persistent lower respiratory tract colonization and infection lead to the symptoms of chronic cough, bronchiectasis, hemoptysis, and pneumothorax. Classically cough is productive of purulent sputum that is worse on arising in the morning or following activity: however, some patients may have intermittent symptoms and a nonproductive cough. Physical findings may include an increased anteroposterior diameter of the thorax, persistent crackles or wheezing, and digital clubbing.

The upper respiratory tract commonly is involved as well. Between 10% to 20% of patients have nasal polyps, often multiple and recurrent, that require surgical removal if associated with refractory sinusitis or severe obstruction. Chronic pansinusitis is present radiographically in 90% to 100% of

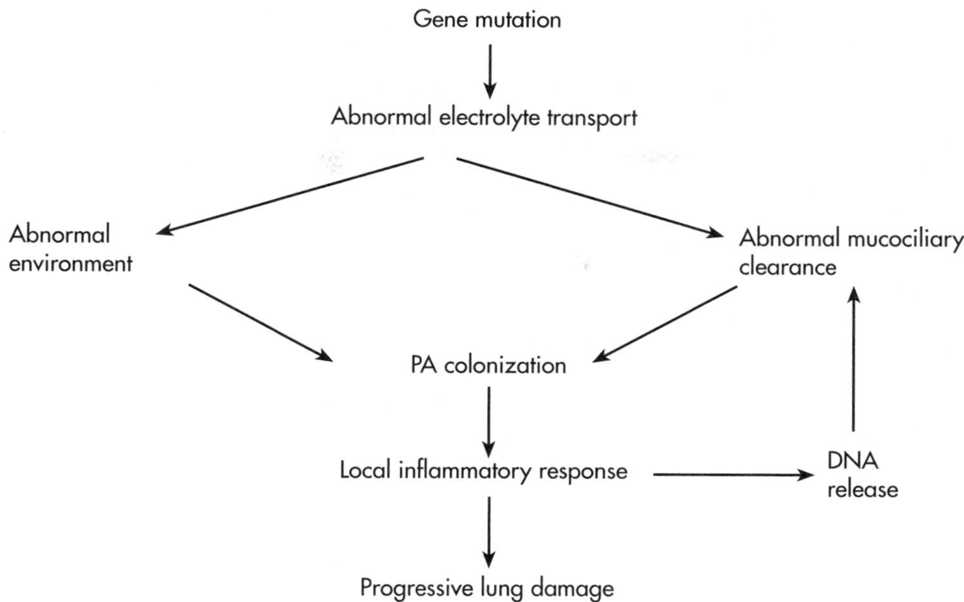

FIG. 36-1 The pathogenesis of cystic fibrosis. *PA, Pseudomonas aeruginosa.*

patients; the degree of symptomatology from sinus disease varies among patients.

GASTROINTESTINAL MANIFESTATIONS

Pancreatic exocrine deficiency is present in 85% to 90% of patients. Similar to the pathology in the lungs, dehydrated secretions lead to pancreatic duct obstruction and poor secretion of digestive enzymes and bicarbonate, leading to malabsorption of protein, fat, and fat-soluble vitamins (A, D, E, and K). Presenting symptoms and signs include frequent bulky, greasy stools, failure to thrive, rectal prolapse, hypoproteinemia, edema, and delayed puberty. Droplets of fat may be seen in the stool. Because of the increased fat content, stools often are malodorous. Presentation caused by vitamin deficiency alone is rare but does exist, and includes bleeding diathesis from vitamin K deficiency. Pancreatic sufficiency is associated with certain genotypes (R117H)[14] and an improved prognosis. Supplementation with pancreatic enzymes, fat-soluble vitamins, and increased caloric intake are the mainstays of therapy for pancreatic insufficiency.

Pancreatic fibrosis leads to the destruction of the endocrine pancreas (decreased density of islet cells), resulting in glucose intolerance (40% to 60%) and insulin dependent diabetes (15%).[27] Ketoacidosis and ketonuria rarely are seen because patients may have enough residual endogenous insulin to turn off ketone production. Alternatively, reduced glucagon levels may fail to stimulate ketone production.

Meconium ileus syndrome is associated almost exclusively with CF and is the presenting symptom in 10% to 15% of cases in newborns. Extremely viscid meconium causes intestinal obstruction and occasionally is complicated by volvulus, atresia, and/or meconium peritonitis. The presence of meconium ileus seems to be related to intestinal gland involvement rather than to pancreatic insufficiency. Infants who have meconium ileus who survive beyond 6 months have the same prognosis as other CF patients. Meconium plug syndrome is more common in CF, but it is less specific for CF than is meconium ileus.

Some patients suffer from recurrent episodes of crampy abdominal pain with partial or complete bowel obstruction known as *distal intestinal obstruction syndrome* (DIOS). The etiology of DIOS includes some combination of pancreatic insufficiency, inspissated intestinal secretions, undigested food residues, fecal stasis, and dehydration. This syndrome must be distinguished from other causes of acute abdomen, including cholecystitis, pancreatitis, and appendicitis.

Recently, some patients have developed colonic strictures (fibrosing colonopathy) that seem to be associated with large quantities of pancreatic enzyme supplements. This diagnosis should be considered in patients who present with evidence of obstruction, bloody diarrhea, or chylous ascites.[5]

Intussusception occurs in 10% of patients. The diagnosis of CF should be considered in patients who have intussusception after infancy. Rectal prolapse is present in approximately 20% of patients and usually occurs before CF is diagnosed (before pancreatic enzyme replacement therapy).

HEPATOBILIARY MANIFESTATIONS

Focal biliary fibrosis is seen in 20% of patients; the more severe multilobulated biliary cirrhosis occurs in fewer than 5%. A small percentage of patients (2%) may progress to clinically apparent liver disease. Symptoms include hypersplenism, ascites, icterus, and hematemesis from esophageal varices. The gallbladder is abnormal in up to a third of patients; the most common finding is a microgallbladder.

OTHER MANIFESTATIONS

The elevated electrolyte concentration of sweat is present in 99% of patients and formed the basis for the diagnostic sweat test. The abnormally functioning chloride channel reduces the amount of chloride and sodium normally reabsorbed from the

Table 36-1 Indications for Sweat Testing

Respiratory	Gastrointestinal	Other
Lower respiratory	**Neonatal**	Aspermia
Chronic cough	Meconium ileus	Absent vas deferens
Recurrent/chronic pneumonia	Meconium plug	Metabolic alkalosis
Recurrent wheezing	Intestinal atresia	Salty taste
Atelectasis	Prolonged jaundice	Salt crystals
Bronchiectasis	Malabsorption	Positive family history
Clubbing	Steatorrhea	Hypoprothrombinemia
Colonization with mucoid PA	Edema and hypoproteinemia	
Hemoptysis	Failure to thrive	
Pneumothorax	Rectal prolapse	
Upper respiratory	Recurrent intussusception	
Nasal polyps	Recurrent pancreatitis	
Pansinusitis	Recurrent ABD obstruction	
	Cirrhosis	
	Cholecystitis	

resorptive duct and leads to elevated levels of these ions in sweat compared with normal patients. Excessive chloride loss has led to development of hypochloremic metabolic alkalosis, especially in infants and young children who cannot regulate their salt intake independently.

The majority of male patients (98%) have obstruction of the vas deferens with resultant azoospermia and sterility. Although fertility in females is decreased because of thickened cervical mucus, many women who have CF have had children. Pregnancy is well tolerated in women who have good pulmonary function but may accelerate pulmonary decline in those who have moderate to severe disease.

DIAGNOSIS

It is important to realize that there is no such thing as a child who "looks too healthy" to have CF. Other misconceptions are that CF is a such rare disease that it is not a consideration or that the patient *must* have pancreatic insufficiency. Pediatricians often hesitate to refer a child for a sweat test for fear of alarming the parents about the possibility that their child might have a fatal disease. On the contrary once parents become educated about CF, they often become quite angry about delays in the diagnosis and lose faith in the pediatrician as a primary caretaker for that child and/or other non-CF siblings. One should strongly consider referring children for a sweat test if they have any of the following symptoms: chronic/recurrent pulmonary infection, wheezing or productive cough, clubbing, positive sputum cultures for SA or PA (especially mucoid PA), failure to thrive, malnutrition, or malabsorption. For a more complete list of indications for a sweat test see Table 36-1.

Early recognition of CF avoids costly diagnostic workups. The diagnosis of CF is confirmed or ruled out in 98% of patients by a sweat test (quantitative pilocarpine iontophoresis). The sweat test should be done at a CF center to avoid erroneous results from inexperienced laboratories. Sweat chloride levels >60 meq/L in the presence of signs or symptoms suggestive of the disease confirm the diagnosis. Adequate sweat collection is a minimum of 50 mg, preferably 100 mg. Testing in the first few weeks of life may be unreliable because of low sweat rates. Positive tests at this time should be confirmed, and negative tests should be repeated without hesitation if suspicion about the diagnosis persists. Some patients who have typical clinical symptoms of CF and repeatedly borderline sweat chloride levels (40 to 60 meq/L) have been reported. In these cases genetic analysis is indicated.

PSYCHOSOCIAL

Patients who have CF should be followed up by their general pediatrician and at a CF center that offers a multidisciplinary approach to this complex disease. The team includes the CF specialist, a nurse, a social worker, a nutritionist, a physical therapist, and a geneticist. The CF specialist, usually a pulmonologist, is able to optimize current medical treatment, enter patients into ongoing clinical trials, and alert patients appropriately to the most recent and relevant developments in the field. Although all team members provide emotional support, the nurse and social worker have major input in this regard. Social workers help the patients and families through the various stages of the disease from diagnosis to adulthood—hospital admissions, pulmonary deterioration, genetic counseling, and death. Social workers are invaluable in helping families cope with the emotional and financial burden of CF. The nutritionist may be able to give valuable insights to maximize caloric intake.

Patients often are referred to a CF center after having a positive result on a sweat test at an institution that is not a CF center. After learning of a positive sweat test result, the pediatrician should contact a CF specialist who will make every effort to see the patient and family within 24 hours of the diagnosis to evaluate the child and confirm the diagnosis. Despite increasing publicity, many parents of newly diagnosed patients have not heard of the disease. The initial approach to the family at the CF center is crucial. Cystic fibrosis is presented as a chronic disease primary involving the lungs and digestive tract. The genetic basis of CF is explained and the parents are told clearly that no one is to blame, nor is there any way to have prevented its occurrence. Life expectancy issues are discussed, and survival into adulthood with current treatment and the hope of further improvements

Table 36-2 Approach to the Treatment of Cystic Fibrosis

Lesion	Standard therapy	Future therapy
Abnormal CF gene		Gene therapy
Abnormal CFTR protein		Protein replacement
Epithelial defect		Amiloride
		Chloride secretagogues
Infection	Antibiotics—IV, PO, aerosol	Anti-PA vaccine
Airway inflammation	Corticosteroids	Antiproteases
Viscous secretions	CPT, DNase inhalation	DNase, amiloride
Airflow obstruction	Bronchodilators	DNase
Bronchiectasis	Chest physiotherapy	
Respiratory failure	Oxygen	Lung transplantation

Adapted from Collins FS: *Science* 256:774, 1992; and Fiel SB: *Lancet* 341:1070, 1993.

given the rapid progress in CF research is emphasized. The goal is to paint a picture of cautious optimism. Genetic counseling and prenatal diagnosis should be offered to the parents and other close family members. All siblings should have sweat testing to rule out CF. If the result is negative, they have a two thirds risk of being a carrier; absolute carrier status can be determined by genetic analysis.

Parents will forget most of this initial discussion; various aspects should be reintroduced at regularly scheduled clinic visits. In the past all newly diagnosed patients were hospitalized for medical treatment and to help the family adjust to the diagnosis; currently this decision is individualized. If the decision is made to forego admission, frequent follow-up and phone contacts are made to ensure appropriate understanding of the disease. Appropriate reading materials are provided to the family, and they are encouraged to meet, for emotional and practical support, other families of patients who have CF who are coping well. Often, after diagnosis and treatment with dietary supplementation, pancreatic enzymes, and/or antibiotics, patients do well and have a "honeymoon" phase. Many parents may deny the presence of CF or think that the major sequelae will somehow skip over them. "My child is no different from other children; he just needs to take some pills before he eats," is a common theme of denial. The first hospitalization for a pulmonary exacerbation therefore may have the same devastating impact on the family as the initial diagnosis.

During late childhood and adolescence the responsibility for care should be transferred gradually to the patient. Genetic and vocational counseling are mandatory. Most men (98%) who have CF are sterile; however, this topic is not discussed often by the family. The difference between sterility and penile virility (not impaired in CF) needs to be addressed. Adult males contemplating fatherhood should have semen analysis. Female fertility is only mildly impaired, and most women are capable of bearing children. They need to be counseled concerning the risk of having a child who has CF, the role of genetic screening of their spouse for the most common mutations, the availability of prenatal screening, and the potential negative effects of a pregnancy on their health.

GENETICS

Accurate prenatal diagnosis and carrier status have been a goal of caretakers and affected families for many years. In the early 1980s prenatal diagnosis was limited to analysis of microvillar intestinal enzymes (reduced activity caused by transient meconium ileus in utero). A high rate of false positive and false negative results limited use to families at high risk.[4] The discovery of DNA markers tightly linked to the CF gene further improved prenatal diagnosis through linkage analysis.[32] In most families linkage of these markers can be followed and restriction fragment length polymorphisms (RFLPs) of affected and unaffected chromosomes can be analyzed. With this technique virtually all families can receive accurate information. The major limitation of linkage analysis is that a sample of DNA from the deceased patient who has CF must be available. Cloning of the CF gene has improved genetic screening, even in families where no DNA is available from the index case. Current prenatal testing involves the use of one or more molecular genetic techniques, including direct detection of the most common known mutations. Carrier screening of the general population is limited by the large number of CF mutations.

MANAGEMENT

The management of the patient who has CF can be categorized as standard therapy, treatment of respiratory complications, and novel approaches targeted toward various stages of the pathophysiological process (Table 36-2).

Standard Therapy

Once acquired, PA infection rarely is eradicated. Patients have periods of relative stability, with intermittent "exacerbations" of disease. Pulmonary exacerbations often have a subacute presentation. Triggers are multifactorial and include viral or bacterial infection and exposure to allergens, airway irritants, and pollutants. Classic signs of lung infection such as fever, leukocytosis, and chest radiograph changes usually are absent; the diagnosis often is made on the basis of subjective findings (see the box on p. 420). Management includes some combination of antibiotics, chest physiotherapy, bronchodilators, and nutritional support. Pulmonary exacerbations are treated with a combination of intravenous antibiotics (an aminoglycoside and penicillin derivative) effective against PA for approximately 2 weeks. Recommended doses are higher for CF patients because of their higher clearance rates for many antibiotics and the difficulty in achieving adequate drug levels in their pulmonary secretions. Aerosolized

PULMONARY EXACERBATION: SIGNS AND SYMPTOMS*

Change in sputum volume, color, and appearance
Deterioration in pulmonary function test results
Increased cough, dyspnea, and tachypnea
New chest examination findings
New chest radiographic findings
Fever
Fatigue
Decreased exercise tolerance
Decreased appetite
Weight loss

*Often insidious onset.

antibiotics are used for patients with chronic PA colonization who continue to decline significantly or relapse despite aggressive IV treatment.

Another controversy concerns the use of daily, prophylactic anti-SA therapy. Some CF specialists advocate its use with the rationale that the presence of SA in the respiratory tract "paves the way" for the acquisition of PA; others feel that eliminating SA may encourage colonization with PA. A recently completed yet to be published placebo-controlled, double-blind trial of cephalexin as anti-SA prophylaxis in healthy children who have newly diagnosed CF did not demonstrate any advantage in the active treatment group. Although patients in the treatment group had reduced SA colonization, an increase in PA colonization was seen. It is unclear if sicker patients would benefit from anti-SA prophylaxis.

Prevention of disease in CF patients is essential in routine health care maintenance. Parents should be warned about the dangers of secondhand smoke. In addition to routine immunizations, all CF patients should be vaccinated yearly for influenza virus.

Chest physiotherapy (CPT) continues to be a component of therapy for lung disease. The rationale is that the airway secretions of CF are difficult to expectorate and that these techniques facilitate clearance of mucus. Unfortunately CPT is one of the most time-consuming aspects of therapy and constitutes a frequent area of noncompliance. Alternative methods, such as the forced expiration technique, use of a positive expiratory pressure mask, self-positional drainage, use of mechanical percussors, and the Flutter device have been developed to meet the need for patient independence. Currently CPT is individualized to meet the patient's needs.

Wheezing and airflow obstruction are major features of CF. The rationale for the use of bronchodilators (BD) seems clear; however, many patients have an inconsistent response to BD.[22] Some patients may have a paradoxical response to BD because of the collapse of bronchiectatic central airways and reduced cough efficacy. Cystic fibrosis patients who have classic symptoms of asthma benefit from the use of bronchodilators. For the remainder of patients careful and frequent evaluation is necessary to ensure optimum bronchodilator use. Corticosteroids may be used for patients who have symptoms of asthma.

Therapy for Pulmonary Complications

Pneumothorax (PTX) most often is caused by rupture of subpleural blebs through the visceral pleura; 5% to 8% of patients eventually will experience a PTX. The incidence increases with disease severity and age. Pneumothorax should be suspected in patients who present with sudden onset of chest pain and respiratory distress. Every CF patient who has a PTX, even if asymptomatic, should be hospitalized for a minimum of 24 hours. A chest tube should be inserted if the PTX is greater than 20% of the hemithorax volume or if the patient is symptomatic. A large PTX initially is managed best by letting the lung slowly expand without applying suction in order to reduce the incidence of reexpansion pulmonary edema. Removal of the chest tube is recommended for PTX that resolves with simple chest tube drainage. Excision of blebs and a limited surgical pleurodesis (production of adhesions) are recommended for most patients with persisting air leak. Chemical pleurodesis with quinacrine or tetracycline should be reserved for poor surgical candidates. Pleurodesis is not an absolute contraindication for lung transplantation; however, for those patients experiencing a PTX while on a transplant list, the transplant team should be contacted before pleurodesis in initiated.[29]

Blood streaking of sputum is common (50% to 60%) and requires no specific treatment. Major hemoptysis (240 ml/24 hr or 100 ml/day × 3 to 7 days) may be life threatening because of asphyxiation or, more rarely, exsanguination. The bleeding usually is from dilated and tortuous bronchial (systemic) arteries and often is associated with pulmonary infection. Hemoptysis should be differentiated from bleeding originating from other sites (gastrointestinal, upper airway). Drugs that interfere with coagulation should be discontinued and any coagulation defects should be corrected. An episode of major hemoptysis does not change the long-term prognosis. The major risk is during the acute bleeding. Although the bleeding may respond to bedrest and antibiotics, bronchial artery embolization is indicated for major hemoptysis. This procedure should be performed by an interventional radiologist who has experience with this procedure, and the patient should be transferred to a facility that has experienced personnel, if necessary.

Newer Therapies

Lung transplantation is a final option for patients who have end-stage pulmonary disease. Suitable candidates for referral are patients who have a FEV_1 <30% of predicted.[17] The procedure is heart-lung or double lung transplantation. The 3-year survival rate of 60% is similar to that among non-CF patients. Shortage of supply, sepsis, and rejection are the main obstacles.

Large amounts of DNA released from neutrophils add greatly to the viscosity of mucus. Recombinant human DNase (Pulmozyme) by inhalation (2.5 mg daily) has been shown to reduce rates of respiratory tract infection and improve pulmonary function and patient perception of well-being.[13,24] No allergic or anaphylactic responses were seen; voice alteration is a potential, self-limited side effect. The currently recommended dosage is 2.5 mg/day using one of the nebulizer systems studied during clinical trials (Hudson T/Updraft II Nebulizer/Pulmo-aide DeVilbiss Compressor, Marquest Acorn II Nebulizer/Pulmo-aide DeVilbiss Compressor, Pari LC

Nebulizer/Pari Proncb Compressor). Pulmozyme should not be mixed with other drugs in the nebulizer.[25]

In an attempt to reduce the inflammatory response that is responsible for progressive lung damage, various antiinflammatory agents are being assessed, including corticosteroids, ibuprofen, and antiproteases.[21] High-dose alternate-day prednisone (2 mg/kg qod) was associated with unacceptable side effects in a multicenter trial. The group of patients that received a lower dose (1 mg/kg qod) showed a mild improvement in pulmonary status; however, adverse effects developed after 24 months.[9] High dose ibuprofen when taken consistently over 4 years slowed significantly the progression of lung disease without serious adverse effects.[20] Adequate dosing and close monitoring for adverse effects are essential.

Attempts to alter ion transport with amiloride, a sodium channel blocker that blocks the reuptake of sodium from the airway surface, have shown a slowed rate in decline of vital capacity, reduced sputum viscosity, and increased mucociliary clearance.[18] Chloride secretagogues, such as ATP and UTP, may be useful in correcting the ionic environment toward normal after pretreatment with amiloride.[19] In patients who are homozygous for ΔF_{508}, CFTR is "trapped" intracellularly. In certain experimental conditions mutant CFTR functions appropriately as a chloride channel once at the cell surface. Therefore experimental work on cell protein transport of functional but trapped protein is being undertaken. The possibility of protein replacement through aerosol is being investigated.

A variety of approaches to gene replacement are being investigated.[7] Some vectors for gene transfer (adenovirus, liposomes) do not integrate into the host genome and are likely to have a transient effect, requiring multiple reapplications. The use of retrovirus as a vector offers the potential for longer-lasting treatment because the gene product is incorporated into the host. Many questions of safety, efficacy, and cell type requiring treatment need to be addressed. Early phase I trials are under way.

The discovery of the gene also has led to the development of animal models[8,30] that should help in evaluating the multiple therapeutic approaches mentioned above.

SUMMARY

Most of the current therapy of CF has involved the treatment of preexisting disease. Although the life expectancy of CF patients has improved steadily, it is clear that new approaches to therapy are necessary to achieve further significant improvement in patient survival. The discovery of the CF gene has led to an evolving concept and understanding of the pathophysiology of the disease and an explosion in research and promising therapeutic modalities. The accessibility of the target tissue by the aerosol route makes the possibility of genetic transfer feasible. The approach to CF will represent a model approach for other genetic diseases in the future.

REFERENCES

1. Abman SH et al: Early bacteriologic, immunologic, and clinical courses of young infants with cystic fibrosis identified by neonatal screening, *J Pediatr* 119:211, 1991.
2. Anderson DH: Cystic fibrosis of the pancreas and its relation to celiac disease: a clinical and pathological study, *Am J Dis Child* 56:344, 1938.
3. Barasch J et al: Defective acidification of intracellular organelles in cystic fibrosis, *Nature* 352:70, 1991.
4. Beaudet AL, Buffone GJ: Prenatal diagnosis of cystic fibrosis, *J Pediatr* 111:630, 1987.
5. Borowitz DS et al: Use of pancreatic enzyme supplements for patients with cystic fibrosis in the context of fibrosing colonopathy, *J Pediatr* 127:681, 1995.
6. Cacalano G et al: Production of *Pseudomonas aeruginosa* neuraminidase is increased under hyperosmolar conditions and is regulated in genes involved in alginate expression, *J Clin Invest* 89:1866, 1992.
7. Collins FS: Cystic fibrosis: molecular biology and therapeutic implications, *Science* 256:774, 1992.
8. Dorin JR et al: Cystic fibrosis in the mouse by targeted insertional mutagenesis, *Nature* 359:211, 1992.
9. Eigen H et al: A multicenter study of alternate-day prednisone therapy in patients with cystic fibrosis, *J Pediatr* 126:515, 1995.
10. Fick Jr RB: Pathogenesis of the *Pseudomonas* lung lesion in cystic fibrosis, *Chest* 96:158, 1989.
11. Fiel SB: Clinical management of pulmonary disease in cystic fibrosis, *Lancet* 341:1070, 1993.
12. FitzSimmons SC: The changing epidemiology of cystic fibrosis, *J Pediatr* 122:1, 1993.
13. Fuchs HJ et al: Effect of aerosolized recombinant human DNase on exacerbations of respiratory symptoms and on pulmonary function in patients with cystic fibrosis, *N Engl J Med* 331:637, 1994.
14. Hamosh A, Corey M: Correlation between genotype and phenotype in patients with cystic fibrosis, *N Engl J Med* 329:1308, 1993.
15. Isles A et al: *Pseudomonas cepacia* infection in cystic fibrosis: an emerging problem, *J Pediatr* 104:206, 1984.
16. Kerem B et al: Identification of the cystic fibrosis gene: genetic analysis, *Science* 245:1073, 1989.
17. Kerem E et al: Prediction of mortality in patients with cystic fibrosis, *N Engl J Med* 326:1187, 1992.
18. Knowles MR et al: A pilot study of aerosolized amiloride for the treatment of lung disease in cystic fibrosis, *N Engl J Med* 322:1189, 1990.
19. Knowles MR et al: Activation by extracellular nucleotides of chloride secretion in the airway epithelia of patients with cystic fibrosis, *N Engl J Med* 325:533, 1991.
20. Konstan MW et al: Effect of high dose ibuprofen in patients with cystic fibrosis, *N Engl J Med* 332:848, 1995.
21. McElvaney NG et al: Modulation of airway inflammation in cystic fibrosis. In vivo suppression of interleukin-8 levels on the respiratory epithelial surface by aerosolization of recombinant secretory leukoprotease inhibitor, *J Clin Invest* 90:1296, 1992.
22. Pattishall EN: Longitudinal response of pulmonary function to bronchodilators in cystic fibrosis, *Pediatr Pulmonol* 9:80, 1990.
23. Pier GB: Pulmonary disease associated with *Pseudomonas aeruginosa* in cystic fibrosis: current status of the host-bacterium interaction, *J Infect Dis* 151:575, 1985.
24. Ramsey BW et al: Efficacy and safety of short-term administration of aerosolized recombinant human deoxyribonuclease in patients with cystic fibrosis, *Am Rev Respir Dis* 148:145, 1993.
25. Ramsey BW et al: Consensus conference: practical applications of Pulmozyme, *Pediatr Pulmonol* 17:404, 1994.
26. Riordan JR et al: Identification of the cystic fibrosis gene: cloning and characterization of complementary DNA, *Science* 245:1066, 1989.
27. Rodman HM, Doershuk CF, Roland DM: The interaction of two diseases: diabetes mellitus and cystic fibrosis, *Medicine* 654:389, 1986.
28. Rommens JM et al: Identification of the cystic fibrosis gene: chromosome walking and jumping, *Science* 245:1059, 1989.
29. Schidlow DV, Taussig LM, Knowles MR: Cystic Fibrosis Foundation Consensus Conference Report on pulmonary complications of cystic fibrosis, *Pediatr Pulmonol* 15:187, 1992.
30. Snouwaert JN et al: An animal model for cystic fibrosis made by gene targeting, *Science* 257:1083, 1992.
31. Tomkiewicz RP et al: Amiloride inhalation therapy in cystic fibrosis: influence on content, hydration and rheology of sputum, *Am Rev Respir Dis* 148:1002, 1993.

32. Tsui L-C et al: Cystic fibrosis locus defined by a genetically linked polymorphic DNA marker, *Science* 230:1054, 1985.

SUGGESTED READINGS

Berger HA, Welsh MJ: Electrolyte transport in the lungs, *Hosp Pract* March 1991, p 53.

Koch C, Hoiby N: Pathogenesis of cystic fibrosis, *Lancet* 341:1065, 1993.

Park RW, Grand RJ: Gastrointestinal manifestations of cystic fibrosis: a review, *Gastroenterology* 81:1143, 1981.

Tizzano EF, Buchwald M: Cystic fibrosis: beyond the gene to therapy, *J Pediatr* 120:337, 1992.

37 Muscular Dystrophy

Richard T. Moxley III

The muscular dystrophies represent a group of slowly progressive inherited diseases that usually have a very specific pattern of muscle wasting and weakness (Tables 37-1 and 37-2). These disorders occur infrequently in childhood; a busy pediatrician may follow only a few patients during his or her career. However, breakthroughs in molecular biology have provided direct genetic tests for these diseases and have created opportunities for the pediatrician to recommend and coordinate family counseling and prenatal testing. Primary care physicians play important roles by coordinating care with specialists in neuromuscular disease, by helping with genetic testing, and by monitoring patients for the various complications of these muscular dystrophies.

Duchenne dystrophy is the most common muscular dystrophy in childhood, and major advances have been made in its diagnosis and treatment. For these reasons, this chapter focuses on Duchenne dystrophy. However, Tables 37-1 and 37-2 provide useful information about other muscular dystrophies that occur in childhood, and the last section of the chapter includes a short commentary on these other muscular diseases, as well as suggestions for further reading on these disorders.

DUCHENNE DYSTROPHY

Duchenne dystrophy is a slowly progressive muscle-wasting disease marked by symptoms that develop before age 5. Early in its course, Duchenne dystrophy affects the proximal hip and shoulder girdle muscles as well as the anterior neck and abdominal muscles.[6,7,11,15,24] The symptoms arise from an absence or extreme deficiency of a large cytoskeletal protein, dystrophin, that attaches to the inner surface of the muscle fiber membrane as a part of a complex of glycoproteins.[1,15,23] Dystrophin also is part of the inner membrane structure of smooth and cardiac muscle and of certain cells in the central nervous system and in specialized connective tissues, such as the myotendinous junctions.[1] This distribution of dystrophin corresponds closely to those tissues that have major clinical manifestations in Duchenne dystrophy.

The mechanism by which dystrophin deficiency causes dysfunction in some muscle groups while sparing others is a puzzle. Some have speculated that dystrophin protects and strengthens the muscle membrane to withstand the stresses of repeated muscle contractions and that it helps prevent excessive influx of calcium and to speed effective repair of tears in the muscle membrane that occur with vigorous exercise.[1,7,23] But this puzzle still remains: Why do heavily used muscles, such as the extraocular and laryngeal muscles or the gastrocnemius muscles, maintain their strength despite the lack of dystrophin? Some researchers have wondered if another large cytoskeletal protein, such as utrophin, can take the place of dystrophin and help maintain muscle function.[23] Further research is in progress to clarify the role that such alternative proteins may play in rescuing muscle fibers from destruction in diseases involving dystrophin deficiency. The findings will help in developing new strategies for treatment.

Genetics

The gene for dystrophin in the Xp21 region is among the largest known, occupying 1% of the entire X chromosome.[1,7,11] It contains 79 exons, and five different promoters control production of isoforms that are cell type specific (e.g., muscle, cerebral cortex, Purkinje, glial, and Schwann cells).[1,7] Large deletions occur in 60% to 65% of cases of Duchenne dystrophy and in an even higher percentage of cases of Becker dystrophy (a later onset X-linked dystrophy also caused by a deficiency of dystrophin).[1,7] In addition to large deletions, smaller point mutations occur in approximately 30% of patients who have Duchenne dystrophy and 15% of those who have Becker dystrophy.[7] No consistent relationship has been established between clinical severity (Duchenne dystrophy versus the milder Becker dystrophy) and the size of the gene mutation. However, deletion of the first muscle exon and the adjoining muscle promoter region appears to produce two somewhat consistent phenotypes, cases that have either mild muscle involvement or cases that have mild muscle involvement but severe cardiomyopathy.[7]

Clinical Presentation and Course

As outlined in Table 37-1, Duchenne dystrophy typically manifests between 2 and 4 years of age. Parents notice weakness of forward head flexion that persists beyond infancy, accompanied by slowed motor development. Patients never run normally and usually put their hands on their knees to arise from the floor (Fig. 37-1) and to assist in climbing steps. These patients have difficulty keeping up with their peers, which becomes more apparent as they enter nursery school and kindergarten. Often the teacher observes a problem and helps the parents decide to bring the child to the pediatrician. It becomes clear that their son has a real problem and is not just normally clumsy, that poor motivation is not the cause for his tendency to fall easily and for his complaints of tiredness and calf cramps. A busy pediatrician has to be sensitive to the protean nature of these early complaints in Duchenne dystrophy.

Because Duchenne dystrophy has an increased frequency of mild cognitive deficits,[7,11] the patient may appear to be mentally retarded, and the pediatrician may not consider Duchenne dystrophy. Because of the gradual development of hip and knee extensor weakness in mid-childhood, patients often toe-walk to use the power of the gastrocnemius to help stabilize knee extension. Reliance on the calf muscles during ambulation contributes to the hypertrophy of the calf muscles that is so typical for most patients who have Duchenne dys-

Text continued on p. 428.

Table 37-1 Muscular Dystrophies in Childhood: Symptoms, Genetics, and Diagnostic Testing

	Duchenne dystrophy	Becker dystrophy	Myotonic dystrophy	Facioscapulohumeral dystrophy	Severe childhood autosomal recessive muscular dystrophy	Fukuyama-type congenital muscular dystrophy	Emery-Dreifuss muscular dystrophy
Onset	Before age 5, typically between 2 and 4 yr	After age 5; can begin in adult life	Infancy, childhood, or adult life	Rare cases in infancy, occasionally in childhood, usually in adult life	Between 5 and 10 yr	Infancy	Middle to late childhood
Initial symptoms	Cannot run or keep up with peers; can take only one step at a time	Fatigue or marked high weakness; trouble climbing steps; occasional calf or thigh cramps; patients can ambulate beyond age 15	*Congenital form:* floppy infant, poor suck; weak respiratory effort; talipes *Childhood form:* bifacial weakness, slurred speech, impaired hearing, mental retardation	*Congenital form (rare):* bifacial weakness, sometimes ophthalmoparesis, occasionally floppy, deafness *Childhood form (more common):* mild facial weakness and weakness of scapular fixator muscles	Thigh muscle weakness; trouble climbing stairs or arising from a squat	Floppy infant, slow improvement up to 6-8 yr, then a decline	Mild elbow contractures and mild weakness of triceps, biceps, and scapular fixator muscles
Incidence	1:3500 male births	1:35,000 male births	1:8000	1:20,000	Unknown	1:18,000	1:100,000
Genetics	X-linked recessive/XP21 region of gene for dystrophin	X-linked recessive/XP 21 region of gene for dystrophin	Autosomal dominant chromosome 19	Autosomal dominant, most cases localize to chromosome 4	Autosomal recessive, forms on chromosomes 13 and 17	Autosomal recessive, chromosome 9, q31-33 region	X-linked recessive, q 28 region
Gene lesion	Absence of dystrophin	Marked deficiency of dystrophin	Abnormal expansion of CTG trinucleotide repeat in 3 prime nontranslated region of a gene coding for a serine/threonine kinase	Unknown	Deficiency of a 50 kd glycoprotein associated with a complex of proteins that bind dystrophin to the inner surface of muscle membrane	Probable deficiency of dystroglycan, a glycoprotein combination regulated by a single gene (dystroglycan is part of the large complex that binds dystrophin to the muscle membrane)	Deficiency of emerin, a novel protein that resembles membrane proteins involved in vesicular transport

Serum creatine kinase	10× above normal		Normal or mildly elevated	Mildly elevated		>10× above normal	2-5× above normal
Electrodiagnostic testing	Normal nerve conduction; myopathic EMG	Normal nerve conduction; mildly myopathic EMG	Normal nerve conduction; myotonic discharges present in children and adults, but often absent in infants (EMG should be performed on the mother)	Normal nerve conduction; EMG occasionally myopathic, often within normal limits	Normal nerve conduction; myopathic EMG	Normal nerve conduction; myopathic EMG	Normal nerve conduction, EMG often normal in early stages
Muscle biopsy	Active myopathy, absence of dystrophin, severe reduction in dystrophin-associated proteins	Moderately active myopathy, absence or deficiency of dystrophin, reduction in dystrophin-associated proteins	Increased central nuclei, atrophy of type 1 fibers, ringbinden and subsarcolemmal masses	Variable changes, often shows moderately active myopathy	Active myopathy, dystrophin normal, deficiency of dystrophin-associated glycoprotein	Active myopathy, dystrophin normal, reduced dystoglycan, glycoprotein complex	Increased variation in fiber size; type A fiber atrophy; increased connective tissue
Leukocyte DNA testing	If biopsy shows deficiency of dystrophin, patient's DNA is screened for deletions (60%-70% have them); if deletion is found, deletion tests are performed in at-risk family members; if no deletion is found, linkage analysis can be used to screen the family	Same as Duchenne dystrophy	If this diagnosis is suspected, a Southern blot analysis is done to identify an abnormally large expansion of CTG repeats in the DM gene; if the Southern blot test is normal, a polymerase chain reaction test is done to search for smaller expansions of the repeat; most childhood cases show very abnormal CTG repeat enlargements (e.g. 500-4000 repeats), whereas normal alleles have 5-30 repeats	Linkage analysis is possible in some families; discovery of the gene is likely in the near future	Not yet available	Not yet available	Not yet available

Table 37-2 Muscular Dystrophies in Childhood: Complications and Treatment

	Duchenne dystrophy	Becker dystrophy	Myotonic dystrophy	Facioscapulohumeral dystrophy	Severe childhood autosomal recessive muscular dystrophy	Fukuyama-type congenital muscular dystrophy	Emery-Dreifuss muscular dystrophy
Muscle weakness	Treatment with prednisone slows or stabilizes muscle strength; Lightweight long leg bracing maintains ambulation in later stages	No controlled studies of prednisone treatment; bracing is helpful in late stages	No specific therapy; braces for foot drop; children usually can participate in gym in school	No specific treatment; patients should avoid lifting with arms fully extended and abducted; braces are sometimes needed	No specific treatment; lightweight bracing may help in some cases; patients often are wheelchair bound early in childhood	No specific treatment; bracing and physical therapy are useful in some patients	No specific treatment; skeletal muscle weakness often is relatively mild compared with cardiac problems and does not limit function
Respiratory problems	Forced vital capacity is monitored (in later stages, atelectatic pneumonitis is common); colds are treated aggressively; if signs of respiratory failure develop, nasal ventilation should be considered	Uncommon until late stages; management then is as with Duchenne dystrophy	For congenital cases, ventilatory care often is needed; the prognosis for survival is very poor if the patient is ventilator dependent >4 wk; other management is as for Duchenne dystrophy	Uncommon	Similar to that described for Duchenne dystrophy	As with Duchenne dystrophy; patients often succumb to respiratory failure late in childhood or in early teens	Mild other than symptoms related to cardiac dysfunction
Cardiac problems	Occasionally cardiomyopathy leads to congestive heart failure—afterload-reducing therapy often helps; the role of digoxin is uncertain; patient should be monitored for intracardiac clots	Occasionally severe cardiomyopathy develops; treatment is the same as for Duchenne dystrophy	Occasionally tachyarrhythmias or heart block develop in childhood forms, and pacemaker treatment is indicated	Uncommon	Cardiomegaly and arrhythmias in later stages	Uncommon	Frequent cardiac conduction defects; atrial paralysis, cardiac arrest, and sudden death are common; pacemaker treatment and preventive therapy for cardiac emboli often are necessary-

Orthopedic problems	Achilles tendon contractures respond to stretching in early stages, later tendon release surgery often is necessary; contractures at the hips, knees, elbows, and wrists usually develop after the patient becomes wheelchair bound; scoliosis often develops when patients stop ambulating, and spinal stabilization surgery helps maintain use of the arms and preserves pulmonary reserve	Uncommon; contractures are much less common than in Duchenne dystrophy	Talipes deformity requires treatment with stretching; occasionally surgery is necessary	Occasionally knee effusion and low back pain develop secondary to weakness; conservative care measures are effective; in late stages some surgeons have reported good results with procedures to stabilize the scapula; surgery is uncommon	As the patient becomes wheelchair bound, contractures occur at the ankles, hips, knees, and elbows; scoliosis also develops; treatment is as for Duchenne dystrophy	Contractures develop in late stages at the ankles, knees, hips, and elbows	Contractures, especially in the elbows, occur early and respond somewhat to physical therapy; some patients develop a rigid spine syndrome, for which there is no effective therapy
Nervous system symptoms	Increased incidence of cognitive and behavioral problems; some patients improve with small doses of methylphenidate	Uncommon	Mental retardation is common, especially in congenital cases, and special classroom care is needed; hearing deficits are common and may require hearing aids; facial weakness, dysarthria, and hearing problems exaggerate the impression of mental retardation	Uncommon; in rare cases, the infant-onset form of the disease occurs in association with hearing loss and/or retinal disease	Uncommon	Generalized or focal seizures occur in most patients; anticonvulsant therapy is necessary; mental retardation is common; most patients have microcephaly, as well as polymicrogyria, pachygyria, and heterotopias, in the brain on postmortem examination	Due only to stroke from heart block or cardiac emboli
Gastrointestinal dysfunction	Constipation is common, especially late in the disease; careful dietary monitoring, stool softeners, and good water intake (urine specific gravities 1.007-1.010) usually are effective; occasionally acute gastric dilation occurs; it resolves over 2-3 days with NG tube decompression of the stomach and intravenous hydration	Uncommon	Spastic colon–type complaints with abdominal pain are common; occasionally these symptoms improve with antimyotonia therapy with phenytoin; eating small portions at each meal diminishes tendency to aspirate	Uncommon	Uncommon	Uncommon	Uncommon

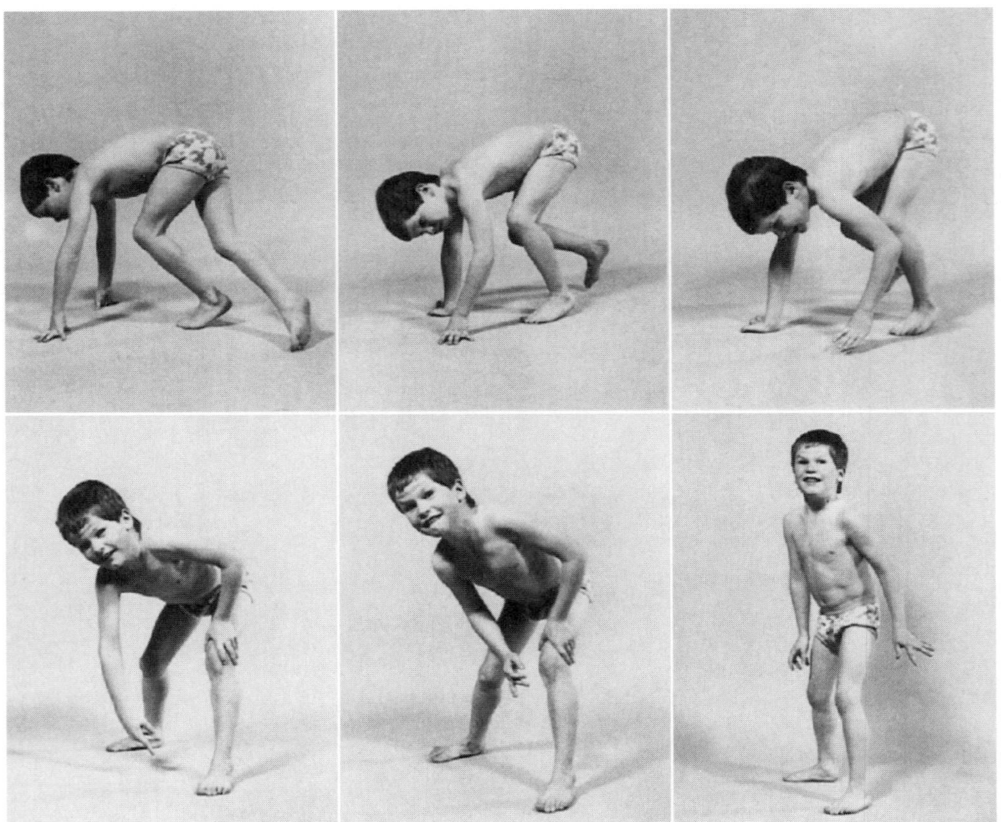

FIG. 37-1 A boy who has Duchenne muscular dystrophy demonstrates the sequence of maneuvers that constitutes Gowers sign. The child pushes off the floor with all four extremities, then prepares to push up by moving his hands along the floor closer to the feet, and finally placing the hands on the thighs and pushing up to the erect position. The maneuver is necessary primarily because of marked weakness of the hip extensors.

(From Swaiman KF: *Pediatric neurology principles and practice,* ed 2, St Louis, 1994, Mosby.)

trophy. However, the pattern of walking in these patients and the presence of a dull intellect sometimes can lead to the incorrect diagnosis of cerebral palsy, delaying an effective treatment plan.

A careful history almost always distinguishes patients who have Duchenne dystrophy from those who have other conditions that cause proximal weakness without sensory findings in childhood. Hypothyroidism usually has more generalized symptoms, as does carnitine deficiency. Blood tests can exclude these two conditions from the differential. Neither causes the marked elevation of creatine kinase that occurs in Duchenne dystrophy. Variants of spinal muscular atrophy and early onset cases of facioscapulohumeral dystrophy (FSH) may resemble Duchenne dystrophy. Hypertrophy of the calf muscles may be a feature of either condition. Spinal muscular atrophy produces no elevation or only a mild rise in creatine kinase; FSH causes only a mild to moderate elevation. As outlined in Table 37-1, electrodiagnostic testing and subsequent muscle biopsy are the appropriate diagnostic tests to establish the diagnosis of Duchenne dystrophy.

Other, more acute conditions, such as childhood myasthenia gravis and inflammatory myopathy, usually are not confused with Duchenne dystrophy. The more rapid evolution of weakness, along with the presence of ptosis, ophthalmoparesis, and facial weakness, distinguish myasthenia gravis from Duchenne dystrophy. The more generalized weakness that occurs in inflammatory myopathy, along with a skin rash, helps to separate these patients from those who have Duchenne dystrophy. In rare cases chronic demyelinating polyneuropathy may be confused with Duchenne dystrophy, but the absence of ankle reflexes, more generalized weakness, a more rapid course, and abnormally slowed nerve conduction identify these patients.

The combination of a careful history and judicious use of the tests outlined in Table 37-1 will establish the diagnosis of Duchenne dystrophy in virtually all cases. In rare cases a "floppy" infant will have a markedly elevated serum creatine kinase, and physicians will wonder if the baby has a variant of Duchenne dystrophy. Newborns or infants who have Duchenne dystrophy *do* have a marked elevation of creatine kinase, but they are not floppy infants. Some other problem must be present as well if a Duchenne dystrophy patient is floppy. Floppy infants who have a markedly elevated creatine kinase usually do not have Duchenne dystrophy. If such a patient does not have an infectious, toxic, or metabolic disorder that causes muscle destruction to account for the marked elevation of creatine kinase, usually he has one of the two relatively rare childhood muscular dystrophies noted in Tables 37-1 and 37-2. These diseases are the severe childhood autosomal recessive form of muscular dystrophy and the Fukuyama type of congenital muscular dystrophy. The workup and treatment of these disorders are summarized in Tables 37-1 and 37-2, and the reader may wish to consult other reviews for more detailed discussion of these two conditions.[3,17,23,32] Other recent reviews provide a thorough commentary on muscle diseases that fit into the broad category of congenital myopathies.[4,8] Certain congenital myopathies may be marked by floppiness, but these infants do not have a significant elevation of creatine kinase.[4,8]

Evaluation and Workup

Once the physician suspects the possibility of Duchenne (or Becker) dystrophy, it is helpful to measure the serum creatine kinase. A marked elevation (tenfold or more above normal) excludes most other disorders and strongly suggests the diagnosis of Duchenne dystrophy. At this point it is appropriate to raise with the parents the possibility that the child has a muscular dystrophy. However, it is important to refer the patient for further evaluation by a neurologist skilled in the care of patients who have neuromuscular disease. It also is useful to mention that the neuromuscular specialist may want to perform other diagnostic tests, such as electromyography, a nerve conduction evaluation, and a muscle biopsy. A detailed discussion of the natural history of Duchenne dystrophy or of the procedures for screening the mother and other at-risk family members for carrier status can be postponed; this discussion is best initiated after the neurological consultation and after specific information from the muscle biopsy is available (see Table 37-1). The neuromuscular specialist should assume responsibility for the initial description of the course of Duchenne dystrophy and should discuss the treatment options.

The absence of dystrophin on the muscle biopsy specimen establishes the diagnosis of Duchenne dystrophy; leukocyte DNA testing of the patient's blood is the next step in the detection of deletions. If deletions are noted, they can be used to identify any women in the family who are carriers. If deletions are not detected and dystrophin is absent on the muscle biopsy specimen, linkage analysis can be used to identify carriers. This analysis involves more extensive DNA testing of family members and is more expensive.

If the biopsy tissue shows an absence of dystrophin, the results should be discussed with the patient and parents, and the family physician should arrange a referral for genetic counseling. This aids development of a coordinated care plan for the patient and family. The geneticists can discuss different options for preventive therapy with female carriers, and the pediatrician and neuromuscular specialist can focus on supportive care for the patient.

MANAGEMENT

Supportive Care

The overall goals in managing patients who have Duchenne dystrophy are to maintain ambulation for as long as possible, to optimize the development of the patient's cognitive abilities, and to anticipate the occurrence of complications, such as excessive weight gain, joint contractures (especially of the Achilles tendons), respiratory insufficiency, scoliosis, and gastrointestinal hypomotility. Table 37-2 summarizes the principal problems and treatment options.

The patient and his family need to work closely with the physicians, schoolteachers, physical educators, and physical and occupational therapists to develop an individualized care plan for the patient for each stage of his disease. Early in the illness the patient usually can play with his peers in most activities, but by the first or second grade some adaptation of physical education requirements becomes necessary. The natural history of Duchenne dystrophy predicts that the patient will become wheelchair bound between 10 and 12 years of age.[6] Often, lightweight long-leg bracing is helpful at this stage to prolong weight bearing and ambulation, both of which delay the development of joint contractures and scoliosis. Contractures and scoliosis both develop when the patient becomes wheelchair bound. They do not appear at a specific age but depend on the patient's functional status. Once contractures begin to develop, usually at the ankles and elbows (flexion), it is important to obtain physical therapy (PT) and occupational therapy (OT) consultations. Follow-up care can be coordinated with PT and OT, and patients usually can receive this care in their schools. Once significant heel cord contractures develop, it also is useful to obtain an orthopedic consultation. The orthopedist can help guide the timing of the use of long-leg bracing and can discuss the possible need for surgery to lengthen the Achilles tendons. The orthopedic care, PT, OT, and neurological care often are coordinated by the neuromuscular specialist and typically are provided in a clinic financed partly by the Muscular Dystrophy Association (MDA).

Although MDA clinics provide an excellent opportunity to offer multiple services to patients, the role of the primary care physician remains critical. The pediatrician usually provides routine care of upper respiratory infections, as well as treatment for other common medical problems. In the middle and late stages of Duchenne dystrophy, minor medical problems can provoke major complications. A mild cold may lead to atelectatic pneumonitis and acute respiratory insufficiency. Such a problem, if treated aggressively, is fully reversible. Even chronic constipation can produce respiratory compromise in the later stages of Duchenne dystrophy, due to abdominal distention and upward pressure on the diaphragm. An effective regimen to maintain regular bowel movements becomes very important in routine care. Respiratory insufficiency often develops in the late stages of Duchenne dystrophy. Forced vital capacity declines, usually into the range of 600 to 1000 ml. One recent review describes the management options, which include nasal ventilation rather than positive pressure ventilation via tracheostomy.[28] Ventilatory care usually is coordinated among the pediatrician, neuromuscular specialist, pediatric pulmonologist, and the patient and his family. All have to participate if the treatment plan is to be effective. Considerable discussion is necessary to educate the patient and his family at this stage and to help to decide which options are most appropriate for them. Often physicians and nurses who have special training in neuromuscular diseases are the individuals who educate the family, and the roles of the pediatric pulmonologist and pediatrician have to be tailored to each medical care setting.

Occasionally, in the late stages of Duchenne dystrophy, patients develop cardiomyopathy.[7,11] A chest roentgenogram reveals a dilated heart, and the cardiac ejection fraction falls to 10% to 20% of normal. Heart failure often is exacerbated by coexisting respiratory insufficiency. In all these cases simultaneous ventilatory support must be considered if the patient and his family have decided to pursue a vigorous course of treatment. The heart failure is difficult to manage, and afterload reduction therapy often is more effective than digoxin. Occasionally ventricular and/or atrial clots are present, and long-term anticoagulant therapy is necessary.

Acute gastric dilation is another infrequent complication in the late stages of Duchenne dystrophy. This typically occurs in association with an idiopathic metabolic acidosis and responds rapidly to nasogastric tube decompression of the stomach and intravenous hydration. Caution must be used with intravenous repletion of potassium because in the late stages of the disease the patient's muscle mass is considerably diminished and is not available to buffer an acute rise in extracellular potassium.

The cause of the gastric dilation is unknown, but this problem, as well as the chronic intestinal hypomotility (constipation), probably result from the deficiency of dystrophin in the smooth muscle of the gastrointestinal (GI) tract. Good hydration, a balanced dietary intake, and regular bowel habits are the mainstays of treatment for these problems.

PREDNISONE TREATMENT

The only effective therapy for Duchenne dystrophy is prednisone. Double-blind, randomized, controlled studies have shown that prednisone in a daily dose of 0.75 mg/kg maintains muscle strength and function for at least 18 to 36 months[9,10,15,24]; these studies also have demonstrated that daily treatment is more effective than alternate-day therapy.[10,24] Some benefit occurs at doses as low as 0.3 mg/kg/day,[14] and prolonged improvement of strength has occurred at doses ranging from 0.5 to 0.6 mg/kg/day.[9] The mechanism responsible for the beneficial effect of prednisone is unknown. However, there are several clues about the process involved. The increase in strength begins to develop after only 10 days of treatment[14] and reaches a maximum response after 3 months of therapy.[14,15,24] Muscle mass increases 10% after 3 months of prednisone treatment,[15,24,30] and the rate of muscle breakdown declines in association with maintenance of a normal rate of muscle protein synthesis.[30] One investigation compared the efficacy of 12 months of azathioprine immunosuppressive therapy with that of prednisone; no beneficial effect occurred with azathioprine.[15] This result argues against the possibility that an immunosuppressive effect accounts for the improvement in muscle strength with the use of prednisone.

Patients have been treated with prednisone at only a small number of specialized neuromuscular centers.[15,24] Prednisone treatment preferably is monitored by or coordinated with one of these centers. The protocol for monitoring side effects and for assessing muscle strength and function have been published previously.[9,14,15,24] The most common side effects are excessive weight gain, mood disturbances (more aggressive, more tearful), and cushingoid facial appearance.[9,10,15,24] More serious side effects (compression fractures of the spine, high blood pressure, GI bleeding, severe infections, or diabetes) have not occurred. Some patients have developed small, dot-shaped cataracts; others, as expected, have had decreased linear growth, which probably has helped maintain ambulation.

To allow monitoring for the development of side effects, patients are seen every 3 months for weight, blood pressure, pulse, and forced vital capacity checks, urinalysis, and assessment of neuromuscular functioning. At each visit the patient undergoes timed function tests (time needed to travel 30 feet, to arise from supine to standing position, and to climb four standard steps) and a muscle strength evaluation (shoulder abductors, elbow flexors and extensors, knee extensors, hip flexors and extensors). These measures help guide the physicians in adjusting the dosage of prednisone. The blood count and serum electrolyte levels are measured at 6-month intervals.

With close follow-up, patients have been kept stable or showed only very mild progression of muscle weakness for periods exceeding 5 years. Even in the late stages, prednisone appears to maintain respiratory muscle power and has reduced the number of patients who develop respiratory failure.

The recent discovery of the gene in Duchenne dystrophy and the ability to manufacture small segments of DNA containing the normal gene for dystrophin has raised hopes that direct gene therapy, either by local injection or by viral vector, will prove feasible. Currently gene therapy is the subject of intensive investigation, but as of now there is no immediate plan for its use. Recent reviews provide a good update on this promising area of research.[7,20]

OTHER MUSCULAR DYSTROPHIES IN CHILDHOOD

Myotonic dystrophy, or dystrophica myotonia (DM), is due to an abnormal enlargement of a trinucleotide repeat in the 3 prime nontranslated regions of the DM gene on chromosome 19.[5,12,13,22,25] Discovery of the gene has led to the development of gene probes to identify both symptomatic and asymptomatic carriers.[27,31] Genetic counseling and prenatal testing now can be done with a high degree of accuracy, an important advance in preventive therapy.[29,31] One recent article provides a detailed review of management of the problems that occur in the neonatal and childhood forms of DM.[25] It includes comments about the complications that occur when patients receive anesthetics and describes the problems involved in pregnancy and delivery.[25]

Facioscapulohumeral dystrophy is not common in childhood and usually does not pose significant management problems. Many are optimistic that the gene for this disease soon will be isolated from its localization on chromosome 4, which would provide a more accurate means of establishing the diagnosis in suspected cases and would lead to improvements in genetic counseling.[26]

The infant-onset muscular dystrophies, severe childhood autosomal recessive muscular dystrophy, and Fukuyama-type congenital muscular dystrophy are rare disorders and already have been mentioned in the discussion of the differential diagnosis of Duchenne dystrophy. For more detailed discussion of these diseases, the reader should refer to the recent literature on genetic and neuromuscular diseases.[3,17,23,32]

Emery-Dreifuss muscular dystrophy is a rare X-linked disorder distinct from but occasionally confused with Becker dystrophy. It can have severe cardiac complications that require urgent treatment. For that reason, it has been included in Tables 37-1 and 37-2. For more detailed discussion of this disease, the reader should consult two recent reviews one by Grimm and Janka[16] and the other by Hopkins and Warren.[18]

In closing, it should be mentioned that the category of limb girdle muscular dystrophy largely has restructured. New molecular genetic research indicates that there is a rare autosomal recessively transmitted limb girdle dystrophy that localizes to chromosome 15, but there is still considerable uncertainty about the general use of the term "limb girdle muscular dystrophy." This diagnosis currently represents a cluster of different syndromes, many of which have different chromosomal locations and differences in their natural history. In fact, many patients who have dystrophin deficiencies have manifested symptoms late in childhood or in adulthood and previously have carried the diagnosis of limb girdle dystrophy. Males diagnosed with limb girdle dystrophy now are having their muscle biopsies tested for dystrophin, and many physicians have been surprised to discover that dystrophin is absent.[7] For a discussion of the limb girdle syndrome, the reader should consult the recent review by Shields.[21]

REFERENCES

1. Ahn AH, Kunkel LM: The structural and functional diversity of dystrophin, *Nat Genet* 3:283, 1993.
2. Ashizawa T, Anvret M, Baiget M: Characteristics of intergenerational contractions of the CTG repeat in myotonic dystrophy, *Am J Hum Genet* 54:414, 1994.
3. Banker BQ: The congenital muscular dystrophies. In Engeland AG, Franzini-Armstrong C, editors: *Myology: basic and clinical,* ed 2, vol 2, New York, 1994, McGraw-Hill.
4. Bodensteiner JB: Congenital myopathies, *Muscle Nerve* 17:131, 1994.
5. Brook JD et al: Molecular basis of myotonic dystrophy: expansion of a trinucleotide (CTG) repeat at the 3′ end of a transcript encoding a protein kinase family member, *Cell* 68:799, 1992.
6. Brooke MH et al: Clinical investigation in Duchenne dystrophy. II. Determination of the "power" of therapeutic trials based on the natural history, *Muscle Nerve* 6:91, 1983.
7. Engel A et al: *Dystrophinopathies, DMD myology,* ed 2, vol 2, New York, 1994, McGraw-Hill.
8. Fardeau M, Tome FM: Congenital myopathies. In Engeland AG, Franzini-Armstrong C, editors: *Myology: basic and clinical,* ed 2, vol 2, New York, 1994, McGraw-Hill.
9. Fenichel GM et al: Long-term benefit from prednisone therapy in Duchenne muscular dystrophy, *Neurology* 41:1874, 1991.
10. Fenichel GM et al: A comparison of daily and alternate-day prednisone therapy in the treatment of Duchenne muscular dystrophy, *Arch Neurol* 48:575, 1991.
11. Fischbeck KH, Griggs RC: X-linked muscular dystrophies. In Vinken PJ et al, editors: *Handbook of clinical neurology,* New York, 1992, Elsevier Science.
12. Fu YH et al: Varying expression of myotonin-protein kinase mRNA and protein levels in the adult form of myotonic dystrophy, *Science* 72:971, 1993.
13. Fu YH et al: An unstable triplet repeat in a gene related to myotonic muscular dystrophy, *Science* 255:1256, 1992.
14. Griggs RC, Moxley III RT, Mendell JR: Prednisone in Duchenne dystrophy: a randomized, controlled trial defining the time course and dose response, *Arch Neurol* 48:383, 1991.
15. Griggs RC et al: Duchenne dystrophy: randomized, controlled trial of prednisone (18 months) and azathioprine (12 months), *Neurology* 43:520, 1993.
16. Grimm T, Janka M: Emery-Dreifuss muscular dystrophy. In Engeland AG, Franzini-Armstrong C, editors: *Myology: basic and clinical,* ed 2, vol 2, New York, 1994, McGraw-Hill.
17. Hamida MB, Fardeau M, Attia N: Severe childhood muscular dystrophy affecting both sexes and frequent in Tunisia, *Muscle Nerve* 6:469, 1993.
18. Hopkins LC, Warren ST: Emery-Dreifuss muscular dystrophy. In Vinken PJ et al, editors: *Handbook of clinical neurology,* New York, 1992, Elsevier Science.
19. Jansen G et al: Gonosomal mosaicism in myotonic dystrophy patients: involvement of mitotic events in (CTG)n repeat variation and selection against extreme expansion in sperm, *Am J Hum Genet* 54:575, 1994.
20. Karpati G, Acsadi G: The potential for gene therapy in Duchenne muscular dystrophy and other genetic muscle diseases, *Muscle Nerve* 16:1141, 1993.
21. Limb girdle syndrome. In Engeland AG, Franzini-Armstrong C, editors: *Myology: basic and clinical,* ed 2, vol 2, New York, 1994, McGraw-Hill.
22. Mahadevan M et al: Myotonic dystrophy mutation: an unstable CTG repeat in the 3′ untranslated region of the gene, *Science* 255:1253, 1992.
23. Matsumura K, Campbell KP: Dystrophin-glycoprotein complex: its role in the molecular pathogenesis of muscular dystrophies, *Muscle Nerve* 17:2, 1994.
24. Mendell JR et al: Clinical investigation of Duchenne muscular dystrophy: a methodology for therapeutic trials based on natural history controls, *Arch Neurol* 44:808, 1987.
25. Moxley III RT: Myotonic dystrophy. In Vinken PJ et al, editors: *Handbook of clinical neurology,* New York, 1992, Elsevier Science.
26. Munsat TL, Serratrice G: Facioscapulohumeral and scapuloperoneal syndromes. In Vinken PJ et al, editors: *Handbook of clinical neurology,* New York, 1992, Elsevier Science.
27. Neville CE et al: High-resolution genetic analysis suggests one ancestral predisposing haplotype for the origin of the myotonic dystrophy mutation, *Hum Mol Genet* 3:45, 1994.
28. Normand M et al: Management of respiratory problems in neuromuscular disease. In Lane RJM, editor: *Handbook of muscle disease,* New York, 1996, Marcel Dekker (in press).
29. Redman JB et al: Relationship between parental trinucleotide CTG repeat length and severity of myotonic dystrophy in offspring, *JAMA* 269:1960, 1993.
30. Rifai Z, Welle S, Moxley III RT: Effect of prednisone on protein metabolism in Duchenne dystrophy, *Am J Physiol* 268:67, 1995.
31. Shelbourne P et al: Direct diagnosis of myotonic dystrophy with a disease-specific DNA marker, *N Engl J Med* 328:471, 1993.
32. Toda T et al: Localization of a gene for Fukuyama-type congenital muscular dystrophy to chromosome 9q31-33, *Nat Genet* 5:283, 1993.

38 Cerebral Palsy

Gregory S. Liptak, Geoffrey Miller, and Steven Couch

The cerebral palsies are a clinically heterogeneous group of conditions classified according to the type and distribution of motor abnormality. They are defined as a group of *disorders of movement and posture caused by a nonprogressive lesion of the developing brain.*[2] Although the cerebral palsies are neither distinct neuropathological, nor etiological conditions, their specific diagnosis is important because it determines the clinical course, treatment, and prognosis.[18]

EPIDEMIOLOGY

The incidence of cerebral palsy is about 2 to 2.5 cases per 1000 live births in developed countries. The prevalence has increased 15% to 20% over the past 20 years, coinciding with the increased survival rate of infants of very low birth weight.[15] In a recent survey of infants, 28% of cases of cerebral palsy occurred in children born weighing <1500 g; 20% occurred in children born weighing between 1500 and 2500 g. Children born weighing less than 1000 g constituted 0.2% of the survivors but accounted for 8% of the children who had cerebral palsy.[8]

Obviously, cerebral palsy has a significant impact on the lives of children. For example, in a national survey, 59% of children who had cerebral palsy attended a special school, compared with 0.5% of those who did not have cerebral palsy. Use of health care services is much higher, too; in the 12 months before the survey, children who had cerebral palsy (compared with those who did not) had 16 visits to a physician (versus 3), 29 hospital episodes per 100 children (versus 4), and 108 hospital days per 100 children (versus 20).[3]

ETIOLOGY AND PREDICTION

Since Little's description[20] in 1862 of the influence of prematurity and abnormal birth on the development of spasticity and developmental delay, health care providers have attributed the cause of cerebral palsy to these perinatal events. However, in 1897 Freud[13] argued that it was impossible to identify the timing or nature of the events that caused cerebral palsy and that many factors operating in the prenatal, perinatal, and postnatal periods could damage the infant's brain.

A definite cause cannot be identified for most cases of cerebral palsy, and when a cause can be identified, it usually is of prenatal origin.[23] Intrapartum events play a limited role[12] and often are influenced by a preexisting abnormality.[3,4,21] Neither sophisticated fetal monitoring nor a higher rate of cesarean sections has reduced the occurrence of cerebral palsy.[27] Isolated risk factors such as fetal bradycardia, neonatal acidosis, intraventricular hemorrhage in the absence of periventricular leukomalacia, and low Apgar scores are poor predictors of cerebral palsy, especially in full-term infants. However, a low birth weight (2000 g or less), periventricular leukomalacia (necrosis of white matter near the lateral ventricles), hydrocephalus, congenital malformations, and newborn encephalopathy (recurrent seizures, hypotonia, coma) all are associated with cerebral palsy.[17]

In about 10% of children who have cerebral palsy, the etiology of the condition is thought to be postneonatal (after 28 days).[28] The most common of these causes are infections (e.g., meningitis and encephalitis), asphyxia, and accidental injury. In some cases cerebral palsy may be prevented by devising strategies to reduce the occurrence of injuries during childhood and by measures to minimize periventricular leukomalacia in premature infants, such as improving circulation and countering the effects of excitatory neurotransmitters.

CLASSIFICATION AND DIAGNOSIS

Cerebral palsies may be classified according to the type and distribution of motor abnormality (see the box on p. 433). This classification system can be simplified into three categories: spastic (involving the pyramidal tracts), athetoid (involving the extrapyramidal tracts), and mixed (involving both). Spasticity is defined as velocity-dependent passive resistance of muscle to stretch. It is associated with neurological signs of upper motor neuron damage such as hyperreflexia, clonus, and extensor plantar response. These abnormalities impair normal movements, such as gait and the manipulation of objects, in complex ways. Diplegia is defined as greater involvement of the legs than the arms, quadriplegia as an equal involvement of all four limbs, hemiplegia as involvement of one side of the body, and double hemiplegia as greater involvement of the arms than the legs. Dyskinesia is characterized by the involuntary movements of athetosis, chorea, and dystonia, which are most pronounced when the child initiates a movement. Dysarthria commonly occurs with dyskinesia. Ataxia involves incoordination of movement and impaired balance and may be associated with an intention tremor. Children who have mild ataxia appear to have normal coordination but are apraxic; that is, they are unable to initiate acts such as hopping, skipping, or buttoning. Because the fibers in the corticospinal tract that control the legs are closest to the ventricles, mild periventricular leukomalacia is most likely to lead to spastic diplegia. Children who have spastic quadriplegia generally have more extensive lesions, and they are more likely to be mentally retarded (64% have an IQ below 50) and have seizures (56%) than are children who have other kinds of cerebral palsy.[10] Children with spastic quadriplegia also are more likely to have feeding difficulties, severe joint contractures, and scoliosis.

Each form of cerebral palsy can be caused by a multitude of conditions, and a single etiological factor (e.g., meningi-

CLASSIFICATION OF CEREBRAL PALSY

Spastic
- Diplegic
- Quadriplegic
- Hemiplegic
- Double hemiplegic

Athetoid
- Dyskinetic
  - Hyperkinetic
  - Dystonic
- Ataxic

Mixed

tis) can lead to different forms of cerebral palsy. Therefore a direct link between the type of cerebral palsy and its etiology cannot be established without using diagnostic evaluations such as ultrasonography or magnetic resonance imaging (MRI).

Early and Differential Diagnosis

Although the brain lesion in cerebral palsy is not progressive, the clinical signs change, especially in the first several years of life. Abnormal patterns emerge as the damaged nervous system matures. For example, the child who is destined to have spastic quadriplegia often will be hypotonic in early infancy. At 6 months of age, as his tone increases, he may develop adduction of the thumb (palmar thumb) followed in a month or two by scissoring of the legs when he is held upright. By 9 months of age, he may have diffuse spasticity and hyperactive deep tendon reflexes. Dyskinetic patterns generally are not obvious until about 18 months of age. Ataxia, as opposed to the incoordination and motor delay of mental retardation, may not be apparent until even later. In a large sample of children, the mean age at which cerebral palsy was diagnosed was 10 months.[24] Early diagnosis of cerebral palsy is aided by a history of an abnormal pregnancy, labor, delivery, or neonatal period or by the occurrence of a serious acute illness and trauma.

The diagnosis is further aided by evaluation of the child's primitive reflexes (e.g., the asymmetrical tonic neck response), postural responses (righting the head when tilted to the side), muscle tone, motor milestones, and neurobehavioral responsiveness.[7] Early signs that suggest cerebral palsy include difficulty feeding because of abnormal oral-motor patterns (tongue thrusting, tonic bite, oral hypersensitivity), irritability, and delayed milestones such as head control. Exaggerated or persistent infantile reflexes such as the asymmetrical tonic neck response, hyperreflexia, and asymmetry may be seen. Delayed milestones, primitive or exaggerated reflexes, abnormal muscle tone, abnormal posture, and an abnormal neurological examination suggest the diagnosis of cerebral palsy.

A diagnosis of cerebral palsy implies that no active disease is present and that the disorder is in the brain. The differential diagnosis includes neurodegenerative disorders, inborn errors of metabolism, developmental or traumatic lesions of the spinal cord, severe neuromuscular disease, movement disorders, spinocerebellar degeneration, neoplasms, hydrocephalus, and subdural hematoma. Repeated examination is necessary to rule out a degenerative condition. Recurring subclinical seizures or adverse reactions to anticonvulsants may worsen the clinical condition of children who have cerebral palsy. Hypotonia in association with weak muscles and depressed tendon reflexes suggests a neuromuscular disease. Extrapyramidal signs in early infancy or marked worsening during periods of illness also make the diagnosis of cerebral palsy suspect. If a child diagnosed as having dyskinetic cerebral palsy has symptoms that worsen significantly as the day progresses, Dopa-responsive dystonia should be considered.[16] This rare but treatable form of dystonia may begin with toe-walking and difficulties with gait, and it responds dramatically to administration of levodopa. There usually is no history of a preexisting condition that would be consistent with cerebral palsy. Other unusual inborn errors of metabolism such as arginase deficiency and glutaric aciduria may mimic cerebral palsy. However, these conditions cause progressive deterioration, whereas cerebral palsy does not.

ASSOCIATED DISORDERS

Table 38-1 lists disabilities and impairments associated with cerebral palsy. All types of language abnormality may be encountered, from aphasia to poor articulation. Abnormal speech may be related to hearing, intelligence, experience, language development, the integration of motor mechanisms of the oropharynx, and coordination of breathing patterns. Nearly 75% of individuals who have cerebral palsy are cognitively impaired. About 60% are mentally retarded (mildly so in about one third of cases and moderately or worse in another third). In the remainder, who function in the normal range, specific learning disabilities such as visual-spatial impairment are common. Impaired mobility also is common and may result from spasticity with or without joint contractures and scoliosis. Self-care and hygiene may be impaired by gross motor and fine motor abnormalities and problems such as drooling. Defects in gastrointestinal functioning and growth are common. In general, physical growth is inhibited. Many of these patients fail to thrive, especially those who have dyskinesia or spastic quadriplegia. Feeding difficulties caused by oropharyngeal incoordination and recurrent vomiting occur and may be associated with aspiration and gastroesophageal reflux. Dental disease (malocclusion and caries) is common. Seizures are common, as are impaired vision and hearing. Roughly 40% of these children develop seizures, which most often have their onset in the first 2 years of life. Oculomotor anomalies include strabismus, refractive error, and nystagmus.

Sociocultural risk factors have a profound effect on development and interact with biological risk factors. Perinatal and other biological risk factors that can lead to intellectual impairment do not have the same detrimental consequences for middle- or upper-class children as they do for poor children.

Children who have cerebral palsy have much in common with children who have other chronic conditions. Cerebral palsy is a lifelong disorder with no cure. The treatments used, such as bracing, often are difficult and sometimes embarrassing. Children who have cerebral palsy often appear different

Table 38-1 Disabilities and Impairments Associated with Cerebral Palsy in Children and Possible Interventions

Disability/impairment	Possible intervention	Possible consultation
Impaired communication	Augmentative communication aids	Speech therapist, audiologist
Impaired cognition	Early intervention, special education program	Education specialist, psychologist, school advocate
Impaired mobility	Orthoses (braces), walker, wheeled mobility	Orthopedist, orthotist, physical therapist, specialty program, gait laboratory
Spasticity	Medications, selective dorsal rhizotomy, intrathecal baclofen, botulinum toxin injection	Orthopedist, neurodevelopmental specialist, physiatrist, neurologist
Joint contractures	Range of motion, orthoses, surgery	Physical therapist, orthopedist, orthotist
Scoliosis	Orthoses, surgery	Orthopedist, orthotist
Impaired self-care and hygiene	Assistive technological devices, home modifications, training	Occupational therapist, rehabilitation engineer
Drooling	Scopolamine patch, surgery	Otolaryngologist
Sexual functioning	Education, adaptive devices	Gynecologist, urologist, psychologist
Impaired nutrition/ feeding	Education, monitoring, medical evaluation, medication, surgery	Nutritionist/dietician, gastroenterologist, speech therapist, occupational therapist
Dental caries, malocclusion	Repair of caries, orthidonture	Dentist, pedodontist, orthodontist
Seizures	Medication, surgery	Neurologist
Impaired vision or hearing	Assistive device, surgery	Ophthalmologist, otolaryngologist
Impaired access to care	Financial counseling, care coordination, transportation	Financial counselor, care coordinator, specialty program
Adverse effects on family	Parent support group, counseling, support	Social worker, psychologist, specialty program, care coordinator
Impaired transition to adulthood	Counselling, adult-oriented health care, care coordination, transportation, recreation, vocational services	Internist, family physician, care coordinator, vocational specialist, independent living specialist, attorney, psychologist

from their peers and have restricted physical development, which makes them unable to engage in peer-related activities. Many children who have cerebral palsy experience pain and physical discomfort as well as psychological distress. Access to care may be a problem. These children visit numerous health care professionals and require services from others such as those in the educational and social services fields. Characteristically, communication is poor within the health field and among professionals and agencies in different arenas. Policies affecting chronically ill children often are erratic. For example, the rules in one county for obtaining money from the state's program for physically disabled children may be very different from those in another county.

For the family, cerebral palsy means the loss of the ideal child—the loss of a dream. This may lead to mourning characterized by denial, anger, guilt, sadness, and depression. In addition, care of a child who has cerebral palsy may be extraordinarily expensive. The burden of daily care falls on the family, and families may feel isolated because of the lack of understanding of cerebral palsy in the community. Siblings may be neglected and have behavioral and other problems. Facilities such as play areas and public facilities (transportation, libraries) often are inaccessible to wheelchair users. Schools may be inaccessible to children who have special mobility needs or may be unable to provide the "adapted" facilities that they require. Because cerebral palsy is considered a *pediatric problem,* transition to adulthood is difficult because physicians who care for adults, social service agencies, and other care providers are unfamiliar with the care of adults who have cerebral palsy.

INVESTIGATION

Neuroimaging techniques such as ultrasonography, computed tomography (CT), and magnetic resonance imaging (MRI) have increased our understanding of the structural abnormalities associated with cerebral palsy and may help clarify the timing of a lesion.[31] Neuroimaging may demonstrate periventricular leukomalacia, postischemic necrosis, cerebral dysgenesis, hydrocephalus, porencephaly, tumor, prenatal ischemic injury, or leukodystrophy. The information gained with brain imaging, although usually not helpful in directing therapy, can be useful to the physician in explaining (or demonstrating) the specific cause of a child's cerebral palsy to the parents. The electroencephalogram (EEG) is an important part of the diagnosis and management of associated seizures; continuous EEG monitoring with videography may help differentiate seizures from other movement disorders. The presence of dysmorphic features may trigger a search for a chromosomal abnormality. However, an increase in minor congenital anomalies is common in cerebral palsy in the absence of any genetic cause for them. Evaluation of complications such as altered gait and feeding disorders may require special diagnostic studies, such as gait analysis and videofluoroscopic swallowing studies.

INTERVENTION

Pathophysiological abnormalities of the brain such as leukomalacia lead to impairments such as spasticity. Spasticity then leads to alterations in functioning, such as shortened stride length, which leads to disabilities, such as slow gait.

The disabilities may lead to adverse social consequences, or handicaps, such as inability to use public transportation. Adults who have cerebral palsy have identified communication skills, self-care activities, and mobility as the three most important functional outcomes of care.[14] The goals of intervention are to prevent adverse functional outcomes, disabilities, and handicaps. Thus, although spasticity occurs, muscle relaxation or surgery around a joint will not be worthwhile if it does not improve the child's ability to function.

Table 38-1 lists some possible interventions and referrals to address the complications of cerebral palsy. No single professional can fulfill the multiple medical, social, psychological, educational, and therapeutic needs of a child who has cerebral palsy.[30] Comprehensive management requires a multidisciplinary team, such as those found in a specialty program, whose members instruct and support parents to enable them to achieve maximal potential for self-help and care for their child and to understand their child's ability and potential for development. Public Law 99-457 mandates access to early intervention services for infants at risk for handicapping conditions. These services include special education, physical, occupational, and speech therapies, adaptive equipment, training for mobility and living skills, and communication. Physical therapy does not change the basic disorder significantly.[25] However, physical therapists may help the families by teaching them how to position and handle their child, by providing more opportunity for play and learning, and by facilitating feeding and the parent/child relationship. Whether or not formal early intervention services are provided, the family should have early social support to help them cope with the crisis of diagnosis.[29]

The care provided should be integrated. For example, children whose legs are spastic often have dorsiflexion at the ankle, flexion at the knee, and flexion and adduction of the hip. Repair of only one or two of these problems may leave the child unimproved or worse off—all three problems must be addressed. Gait analysis using videography, EMG, and sensors has improved the orthopedic care given to these children. After orthopedic surgery, therapy should be started to maximize range of motion and skills.

Medications are used to reduce spasticity (e.g., diazepam, oral baclofen, and dantrolene), but all have potential adverse effects and produce no documented improvement in functioning. Various casting and splinting techniques that may maintain muscle length and inhibit increased tone may be helpful. In many cases orthopedic procedures such as tenotomies and tendon transfers are necessary. Selective dorsal rhizotomy and intrathecal baclofen can reduce spasticity and increase range of motion, and some patients' sitting and gait may improve functionally.[1,26]

Intramuscular botulinum toxin has been used experimentally in children who have mild cerebral palsy to reduce spasticity in individual limbs; this demonstrates promise for future therapy.[6] Drooling has been managed with the transdermal scopolamine patch[19] and with surgery of the salivary glands.[5] Because children who have cerebral palsy are at increased risk for nutrition and feeding problems, careful monitoring of their physical growth is critical. Reliable measures of height or length in children who have cerebral palsy often are impossible to obtain because of the scoliosis, fixed joint contractures, involuntary muscle spasms, and poor cooperation stemming from cognitive deficits. Tibial length has been used as a proxy for height. Evaluation of the child whose growth is impaired includes evaluation of dietary intake for calories and content, evaluation for gastroesophageal reflux (using barium swallow, pH probe, radionuclide gastric emptying study, or endoscopy with biopsy). A clinical feeding evaluation includes assessment of the child's seating and posture during "feeds" as well as assessment of the swallowing mechanism, which can be aided by a videofluoroscopic swallow study using foods of different consistencies. The assistance of feeding specialists is invaluable in this evaluation. Treatment options may include providing special seating devices to maintain the child in an upright, neutral position, or insertion of a gastrostomy tube with or without fundoplication. This usually improves weight gain and general health but may not improve longitudinal growth. The primary care physician should act as an advocate to ensure that a child with cerebral palsy has access to first-rate care. In addition to the individual child and family, advocacy includes ensuring that the community provides access to services so that disabilities do not become handicaps.

PROGNOSIS

More than 90% of infants who have cerebral palsy survive into adulthood. Those who are so severely affected that they cannot move their extremities or bodies voluntarily are at increased risk for early death.[11] Prognostication before the child's second birthday may be difficult, except at the extremes of involvement. In general, the prognosis is related to the clinical type of cerebral palsy, pace of motor development, evolution of infantile reflexes, intellectual abilities, sensory impairment, and emotional-social adjustment.[22] Patients who sit unsupported by 24 months of age and crawl by 30 months of age are more likely eventually to walk independently.[9] Most of those who sit between 3 and 4 years of age walk only with aids or braces or have restricted functional ambulation. Retention of obligatory primitive reflexes at 18 months of age makes independent ambulation unlikely. Virtually all children who have hemiplegia learn to walk, as do many with athetosis or ataxia. Those who walk before age 2 are more likely to have a normal or borderline IQ. Individual achievement is related to many factors, such as intelligence, physical functioning, ability to communicate, and personality attributes. The availability of training, jobs, sheltered employment, and counseling is a major factor in the adjustment of affected adults. A supportive family and the availability of specialist medical care are other important factors.

Long-term planning and preparation are required to help these patients make the transition from adolescence to adulthood, particularly when a patient has multiple needs. A variety of mechanical devices, such as switches that improve the individual's ability to control the environment, computers, and small electric motors, which may replace some motor activities, are available. Using speech synthesizers, symbol charts, or spelling boards can enhance an individual's ability to communicate effectively. Simple environmental enhancements, such as ramps or accessible showers, and assistive devices, such as a pencil holder or mouth-activated switch, can improve dramatically the quality of life of individuals who have cerebral palsy. Gaining access to these services requires coordination of care, knowledge of the resources available in the community, referral to experts, and financial assets. The physician who cares for patients with cerebral palsy has the ability and the obligation to ensure that these services are available both to the patient and the family.

REFERENCES

1. Albright AL, Cervi A, Singletary J: Intrathecal baclofen for spasticity in cerebral palsy, *JAMA* 265:1418, 1991.
2. Bax M: Terminology and classification of cerebral palsy, *Dev Med Child Neurol* 6:295, 1964.
3. Boyle CA, Decoufle P, Yeargin-Allsopp M: Prevalence and health impact of developmental disabilities in U.S. children, *Pediatrics* 93:399, 1994.
4. Brann AW: Factors during neonatal life that influence brain disorder. In Freeman JM, editor: Prenatal and perinatal factors associated with brain disorders, NIH Pub No 85-1149, Washington, DC, 1985, US Government Printing Office.
5. Burton MJ: The surgical management of drooling, *Dev Med Child Neurol* 33:1110, 1991.
6. Calderon-Gonzalez R et al: Botulinum toxin A in management of cerebral palsy, *Pediatr Neurol* 10:284, 1994.
7. Capute AJ et al: Primitive reflex profile: a quantitation of primitive reflexes in infancy, *Dev Med Child Neurol* 26:375, 1984.
8. Cummins SK et al: Cerebral palsy in four northern California counties, births 1983 through 1985, *J Pediatr* 123:230, 1993.
9. dePaz AC Jr, Burnett S, Bragga LW: Walking prognosis in cerebral palsy: a 22-year retrospective analysis, *Dev Med Child Neurol* 36:130, 1994.
10. Edebol-Tysk K: Epidemiology of spastic tetraplegic cerebral palsy in Sweden. I. Impairment and disabilities, *Neuropediatrics* 20:41, 1989.
11. Eyman RK et al: Survival of profoundly disabled people with severe mental retardation, *Am J Dis Child* 147:329, 1993.
12. Freeman JM, Nelson KB: Intrapartum asphyxia and cerebral palsy, *Pediatrics* 82:240, 1988.
13. Freud S: *Infantile cerebral paralysis* (1897) (Translated by Russin LA), Coral Gables, Fla, 1968, University of Miami Press.
14. Goldberg MJ: Measuring outcomes in cerebral palsy, *J Pediatr Orthop* 11:682, 1991.
15. Hagbery B et al: The changing panorama of cerebral palsy in Sweden, *Acta Paediatr Scand* 78:283, 1989.
16. Iivanainen M, Kaakkola S: Dopa-responsive dystonia of childhood, *Dev Med Child Neurol* 35:362, 1993.
17. Kuban KC, Leviton MD: Cerebral palsy, *N Engl J Med* 330:188, 1994.
18. Levine MS: Cerebral palsy in children over 1 year: standard criteria, *Arch Phys Med Rehabil* 61:385, 1980.
19. Lewis DW et al: Transdermal scopolamine for reduction of drooling in developmentally delayed children, *Dev Med Child Neurol* 36:484, 1994.
20. Little WJ: On the influence of abnormal parturition, difficult labour, premature birth, and asphyxia neonatorum on the mental and physical conditions of the child, especially in relation to deformities, *Transactions of the Obstetrical Society of London* 3:293, 1862.
21. Miller G: Minor congenital anomalies and ataxic cerebral palsy, *Arch Dis Child* 64:557, 1989.
22. Molnar GE, Gordon SU: Cerebral palsy: predictive value of selective clinical signs for early prognostication of motor function, *Arch Phys Med Rehabil* 57:153, 1976.
23. Nelson KB, Ellenberg JH: Antecedents of cerebral palsy: multivariate analysis of risk, *N Engl J Med* 315:81, 1986.
24. Palfrey JS, Singer JD, Walker DK: Early identification of children's special needs: a study in five metropolitan communities, *J Pediatr* 111:651, 1987.
25. Palmer FB et al: The effects of physical therapy on cerebral palsy: a controlled trial in infants with spastic diplegia, *N Engl J Med* 318:803, 1988.
26. Peacock WJ, Staudt LA: Spasticity in cerebral palsy and selective posterior rhizotomy procedure, *J Child Neurol* 5:179, 1990.
27. Stanley FJ: The changing face of cerebral palsy, *Dev Med Child Neurol* 29:263, 1987.
28. Stanley FJ, Blair E: Postnatal risk factors in the cerebral palsies. In Stanley FJ, Alberman E, editors: *The epidemiology of the cerebral palsies,* Philadelphia, 1984, JB Lippincott.
29. Taylor DC: Counselling the parents of handicapped children, *Br Med J* 284:1027, 1982.
30. Vining PG et al: Cerebral palsy: a pediatric developmentalist's overview, *Am J Dis Child* 130:643, 1976.
31. Volpe JJ: Value of MR in definition of the neuropathology of cerebral palsy in vivo, *AJNR* 13:79, 1992.

39 The Chronically Ill and Disabled Child in School

Linda J. Juszczak and Marcie B. Schneider

It is estimated that 10% to 40% of children have a chronic health problem; the wide range in estimates is due to differing definitions of chronic illness.[10] The American Academy of Pediatrics estimates that in a school with 1000 students, 20 to 40 will have a severe chronic illness.[2] School-age children and adolescents who have physical handicaps, chronic illnesses, or long-term transient health problems have the same basic educational and developmental needs as their healthy peers. Well-organized and collaborative efforts among school personnel, health professionals, and families will enhance the education and development of chronically ill and disabled children and should be the basis for addressing their needs in the school.

School systems vary greatly in how they put special education laws into practice. The need for chronically ill and disabled children to participate in educational programs appropriate for their abilities in the "least restrictive" physical setting possible is recognized by the Education For All Children Act of 1975 (Public Law [P.L.] 94-142). This law, which went into effect in 1977, defines as handicapped children who are mentally retarded, hearing impaired, deaf, speech impaired, visually handicapped, seriously emotionally disturbed, orthopedically impaired, or multihandicapped and those who have specific learning disabilities. As a result of this law, an individualized education program (IEP) must be prepared for each child identified as handicapped, outlining the special education and related services the child needs and will receive. Chronically ill and disabled children whose educational performance is impaired by their illness clearly are eligible for special education and related services under Public Law 94-142. It is less evident to what extent services should be provided for children whose health problems may require support services but who are able to function in a regular classroom. In 1986 the Education of the Handicapped Act Ammendents (P.L. 99-457) were passed. The Act again was amended in 1990 (P.L. 101-476) and became known as the Individuals with Disabilities Education Act (IDEA). In addition to recognizing the importance of early intervention, these laws identify the need to address in school the various transitions that face children who have disabilities. The ambiguities regarding the provision of related health services persist in this legislation. Purvis[11] presents an excellent overview of the public laws concerning the education of those who have disabilities.

PROBLEMS OF CHRONICALLY ILL AND DISABLED CHILDREN IN SCHOOL

School is important not only as a place where a child develops academic skills, but also as a major socialization experience. Furthermore, the school-related problems and concerns that all children have can be exacerbated for a child who has a chronic illness or disability. For example, the child's medical condition may require frequent and occasionally long absences, illness and medications may affect cognitive functioning, and physical limitations may restrict participation in school activities. These obstacles, combined with unreasonable expectations of teachers and parents and social isolation from peers, can cause these children to miss opportunities for academic achievement, psychosocial development, and vocational placement.

Medical Issues

The medical problems of children who have chronic illness and disabilities are diverse. Questions school personnel often ask about the effects of a child's health problem include restrictions on physical activity; delineation of medications and their side effects; need for a special diet, preferential seating, counseling, special equipment, or toileting assistance; need for physical, occupational, or speech therapy; guidelines for emergencies; prognosis; and the child's understanding of his or her disability.[14]

Examples of common health problems that require guidelines for participation in activities include asthma, seizure disorders, and heart conditions. Children who have asthma may require medication in order to exercise. Provided that wheezing is controlled, they should be allowed to participate in all sports. Children who have petit mal, psychomotor, or frequent seizures should refrain from contact sports. Children who have well-controlled, generalized seizures may participate in contact sports, although they should be encouraged to focus on noncontact sports. Children who have heart murmurs should have medical clearance to participate in sports. In most cases an innocent murmur can be diagnosed by a primary care provider; those who have innocent murmurs can participate fully in sports. The cardiac diagnoses that may preclude participation in collision or contact sports include mitral stenosis, aortic stenosis, aortic insufficiency, coarctation of the aorta, cyanotic heart disease, and recent carditis.[4]

For those who have infectious diagnoses, such as tuberculosis or hepatitis, there are clear precautions and rules for school attendance. Acquired immune deficiency syndrome (AIDS) is an infectious disease that is spread only through *intimate* contact. Although children who have AIDS cannot spread the disease through casual contact in school, the subject of children who have AIDS and are attending school can be emotional and controversial. The American Academy of Pediatrics Task Force on Pediatric AIDS states that these children should be "admitted freely to all [school] activities, to the extent that their own health permits."[13]

A recent survey of the nation's largest school districts on the subject of schoolchildren infected with HIV found that schools were responding to the need to accommodate these children and adolescents.[9] The authors concluded that despite the small number of children infected with HIV, these circumstances call for a major effort on the part of all the disciplines involved.[9] The *Journal of School Health* has published "Best Practice Guidelines" for children infected with HIV, which address preparation of the school, the enrollment process, assurance of appropriate services, and other elements.[3] Clearly, most health problems do not require severe restriction of activity. Participation in physical education programs should not be denied because of overprotectiveness or assumed limitations; rather, it should be encouraged. Schools are protected by insurance against injuries that occur during sports participation and thus are covered if a chronically ill child who is "medically cleared" to participate in a sport sustains a sports-related injury.

The focus in the classroom and in recreation programs should be on what these children can do as opposed to what they cannot do. This emphasis helps the child develop a positive self-image and gain the respect of his or her peers, and fosters a sense of independence.

School Achievement

Although many children who have chronic illnesses and disabilities are of normal intelligence, they may not achieve as well as their healthy peers in school.[5,12] Several factors, including the child's economic, physical, emotional, and intellectual status, contribute to this diminished achievement. Children who have chronic illnesses and disabilities may have limited physical endurance. If they must take a 2-hour test but tire within 1 hour, they will not score up to their potential. If endurance is taken into consideration and the test is given in two 1-hour blocks, such children would have a better opportunity to score at their best level.

These children often miss extended periods of school. The absence rate reportedly is highest among teenagers.[7] Reasons for absence may include physical fatigue or acute physical illness that requires visits to the physician and/or hospitalization. In most states, special education departments require that children be hospitalized for longer than 2 weeks to be eligible for tutoring. Obviously, if they are hospitalized several times for intervals of less than 2 weeks, they will miss a great deal of schooling. Furthermore, those hospitalized for a 3-week period usually receive only 1 week of tutoring.

A child's anxiety about a disability also may contribute to diminished academic performance. A large but not easily measured factor is the expectations of parents and teachers. Anxiety about a child's potentially unstable medical condition may lead to lower expectations for academic performance, unnecessary restrictions, and tolerance of inappropriate social behavior. The child, in turn, increasingly may use the illness for secondary gain, which compounds the problem. This cycle may begin at an early age and may contribute to lowered self-esteem and the child's low expectations of his or her own performance.[8,14,15]

Health professionals can contribute significantly to improving attitudes toward the child's abilities. It is hoped that attitudes can be changed by educating parents and school staff members about the child's assets and strengths, as well as about his or her limitations. Testing situations can be changed to ensure optimal test-taking conditions in keeping with the disabled child's individual limitations. Last, school absence may decline with better anticipatory guidance, medical care, and compliance with medical regimens.

Job Achievement

Each year 650,000 chronically ill and handicapped individuals are graduated from or terminate eligibility for special education programs. Only 31% of students in high school special education classes have prevocational or vocational objectives in their individual programs. Of the 650,000, 21% will have full-time jobs, 40% will be underemployed and exist at the poverty level, 8% will stay in their homes "idle," 26% will be unemployed and receive public assistance, and 3% will be institutionalized.[6]

Employment or further educational opportunities available to chronically disabled young adults are varied. The largest number of chronically disabled young adults (100,000) enter workshops. Vocational rehabilitation, a federally funded, state-operated program, helps approximately 60,000. Other programs include vocational education, higher education, public employment, and training programs.[6] Although legislation is in place and training programs are available, disabled young adults need to avail themselves of the opportunities, and more employers need to be open to hiring them. Both tasks are formidable. It is essential that schools encourage the achievement of goals from the earliest stages, including thought to future employment. Parental support also is essential. Health care workers who are in contact with these youths from birth can encourage them, their families, and schools to attend to future planning from the earliest years.

COLLABORATION OF SCHOOL STAFF AND HEALTH PROFESSIONALS

Collaboration among school staff, community-based medical providers, and school health personnel is essential in the management of the chronically ill child in school. It is only through well-coordinated efforts that educators are aware of the child's medical needs and that health providers are aware of the child's learning needs. States and school districts vary widely in the way health services are delivered in the school and the extent to which the primary care providers' active participation is sought in evaluating and modifying services for the disabled child.

Teacher's Role

Teachers are in a unique position to address the issues that confront chronically ill and disabled children in school, inasmuch as they can implement the recommendations of special education evaluators and health professionals. They also can be objective about the child's school performance, including academic and social achievements and difficulties. Meeting the needs of these children poses many obstacles. Teachers may be unaware of the implication of the child's medical condition for school performance. Lack of adequate information can result in misunderstanding of the child's condition, which can lead to denial of services, misinterpretation of behaviors, or undue restrictions on the child. On the other hand, with adequate information, teachers can foster not only academic achievement but also social confidence. As the best judge of the appropriateness of the child's educational placement, the teacher can facilitate the child's full academic and vocational potential. Health professionals in the school and in the community should seek teachers' input in the ongoing evaluation and implementation of medical care for these children.

Primary Care Provider's Role

Primary care providers potentially can play a vital role as advocates for their chronically disabled patients. The Committee on Children with Disabilities of the American Academy of Pediatrics recognizes the inequalities in the interpretation and provision of related health services and has made recommendations to increase physician involvement in this area.[1] The provider's role also encompasses direct medical care to patients and guidance about medical issues. With chronically disabled patients whose illnesses may cause school absence, the provider should strive to arrange nonacute medical care after school hours. The primary care provider also can guide the patient to anticipate acute crises and thus prevent school absences to the greatest extent possible. As the professional who knows the patient medically and psychosocially, the primary care provider can encourage the child's academic achievement and socialization. An important function of this role is to provide medical information, including a clear explanation of the child's disability, to the school staff so that they can concentrate on teaching the child rather than worrying about his or her medical state.

Primary care providers are not subspecialists and thus do not have the final word on what patients who have particular diagnoses can or cannot do; however, they often are the ones who fill out school physical examination forms. They should not assume that the list of restricted activities will enable the child to participate in more appropriate sports; allowable activities should be listed specifically.

The American Academy of Pediatrics' sports medicine handbook contains a chapter that addresses recommendations for participation in competitive sports for children with health problems[4]; also, individual subspecialists can help set guidelines for children with particular limitations.

School Nurse's Role

The school nurse usually coordinates health services in the school. As previously mentioned, how and what health services are provided varies widely. In most school districts the nurse is responsible for contacting physicians and parents about a child's medical needs. In the case of chronically ill and disabled children, the nurse's role as liaison among community health providers, educators, and parents often forms the core of collaborative efforts to meet these children's medical needs. The school nurse, who usually is responsible for implementing the recommended medical regimens during the school day, is in an excellent position to assess a child's medical status and the need to modify treatment. The role of the school nurse and models of school health service are discussed in greater detail in Chapter 68.

School-based Clinics

The number of school-based clinics is growing rapidly, an effort to address children's comprehensive health needs in the school. These clinics often are located in medically underserved areas to increase access to health services for high-risk populations. Although there are many different models for these health centers, most often they have a multidisciplinary staff (e.g., a physician, nurse practitioner, social worker, and health educator) that provides a myriad of ambulatory health services. The controversy that surrounds school-based clinics, especially those in senior high schools, relates to matters of teaching and dealing with the outcome of sexuality and often eclipses the value of the primary care, acute care, health education, counseling, and referral services that they provide. The potential of these clinics to contribute to the care of chronically ill and disabled children can be overlooked as a result of the assumption by physicians and educators that these children's health needs are being met.

Staff members of a school-based clinic are in an excellent position to communicate with school personnel and to function as the patient's advocate. They may serve as the primary care provider for children who do not have access to health services, or they may supplement the role of the community-based provider by making health services for acute problems available in the school. Thus acute medical care (e.g., treatment of acute exacerbations of asthma), ongoing care (e.g., chest physical therapy for patients who have cystic fibrosis), and routine care (yearly physical examinations) can be provided with minimal school absence and maximal communication with the school staff. Adolescents, in particular, appreciate school-based services, inasmuch as they are designed to be responsive to their needs and respectful of their confidentiality.

REFERENCES

1. Committee on Children with Disabilities, American Academy of Pediatrics: Provision of related services for children with chronic disabilities, *Pediatrics* 92:879, 1993.
2. Committee on School Health, American Academy of Pediatrics: Children with chronic illness. In Nader PR, editor: *School health: policy and practice,* ed 5, Elk Grove Village, Ill, 1983, The Academy.
3. Crocker AC et al: Supports for children with HIV infection in school: best practice guidelines, *J Sch Health* 64:32, 1994.
4. Committee on Sports Medicine, American Academy of Pediatrics: *Health care for young athletes,* Evanston, Ill, 1983, The Academy.
5. Fowler MG, Johnson MP, Atkinson SS: School achievement and absence in children with chronic health conditions, *J Pediatr* 106:683, 1985.
6. Hippolitus P: Employment opportunities and services for youth with chronic illness. In Hobbs N, Perrin JM, editors: *Issues in the care of children with chronic illnesses,* San Francisco, 1985, Jossey-Bass.
7. Klerman LV: School absence: a health perspective, *Pediatr Clin North Am* 35:1253, 1988.
8. Mearig JS: Cognitive development of chronically ill children. In Hobbs N, Perrin JM, editors: *Issues in the care of children with chronic illness,* San Francisco, 1985, Jossey-Bass.
9. Palfrey JS et al: Schoolchildren with HIV infection: a survey of the nation's largest school districts, *J Sch Health* 64:22, 1994.
10. Perrin JM, MacLean WE Jr: Children with chronic illness: the prevention of dysfunction, *Pediatr Clin North Am* 35:1325, 1988.
11. Purvis P: The public laws for education of the disabled: the pediatrician's role, *J Dev Behav Pediatr* 12:327, 1991.
12. Rutter M, Tizard J, Whitmore K, editors: *Education, health and behavior,* London, 1970, Longman Group.
13. Task Force on Pediatric AIDS, American Academy of Pediatrics: Pediatric guidelines for infection control of human immunodeficiency virus (acquired immunodeficiency virus) in hospitals, medical offices, schools, and other settings, *Pediatrics* 82:801, 1988.
14. Walker DK: Care of chronically ill children in schools, *Pediatr Clin North Am* 31:221, 1984.
15. Weitzman M: School and peer relations, *Pediatr Clin North Am* 31:59, 1984.

PART FOUR

The Reproductive Process

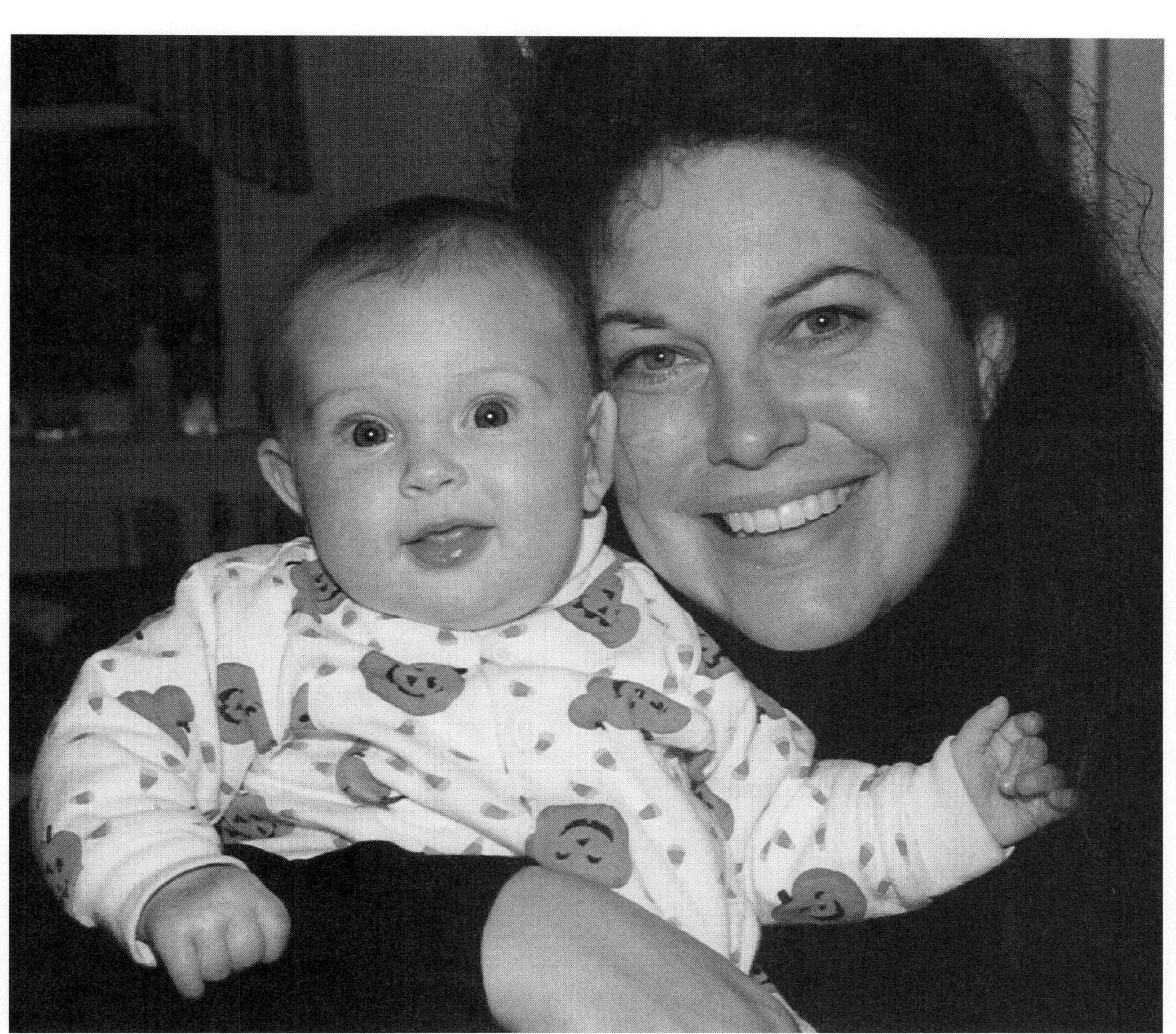

40 Approaches to Genetic Diseases

Marvin E. Miller

Physicians who care for children need to be aware of how genetic diseases and congenital malformations can be diagnosed, which individuals are at increased risk for these disorders, and the various laboratory tests available to help determine the diagnosis. For almost 30 years chromosome analysis has made accurate diagnosis of most chromosomal disorders possible. More recently, application of molecular genetics has resulted in remarkable advances in the diagnosis of common genetic diseases. The alpha- and beta-hemoglobin genes, the cystic fibrosis gene, and the dystrophin gene have been cloned and sequenced, which permits molecular diagnosis of the various hemoglobinopathies, cystic fibrosis, and Duchenne muscular dystrophy. Significant advances also have been made in prenatal diagnosis of congenital malformations and genetic disease through amniocentesis, chorionic villus sampling, maternal serum alpha-fetoprotein screening, and ultrasound. However, in spite of all these scientific and technological advances, the family history and an understanding of the types of genetic disease and their inheritance patterns still form the foundation for the diagnosis of genetic disease.

TYPES OF GENETIC DISEASE

The human genome consists of 23 pairs of nuclear chromosomes and a much smaller mitochondrial genome. The nuclear chromosomes consist of 22 pairs of autosomes that are the same for males and females and a sex chromosome pair that is different in the two sexes. Females have two X chromosomes (XX); males have one X chromosome and one Y chromosome (XY). There are about 50,000 genetic loci in the human genome. The X chromosome contains several thousand loci and thus is similar to the autosomal chromosomes. The Y chromosome, however, contains only one or perhaps only a few genetic loci that determine male gonadal differentiation.

The 24 different nuclear chromosomes (22 autosomes, X, and Y) can be readily distinguished from each other by their size, centromere location, and banding pattern. Each of the 22 autosomes is designated by a number. Chromosomal disorders can be diagnosed by a karyotype, which is a photographic enlargement of the chromosomes arranged by their numbered pairs.

One chromosome of each chromosomal pair is inherited from the father; the other chromosome of that pair is inherited from the mother. Thus at each genetic locus an individual has two genes, which are more properly called *alleles.*

Genetic disorders can be divided into four categories:

1. *Chromosomal disorders,* which involve an excess or a deficiency of chromosomal material
2. *Mendelian disorders,* which involve an abnormality (mutation) at a single genetic locus in one or both of the alleles at that locus
3. *Polygenic disorders,* which involve mutations at two or more genetic loci
4. *Multifactorial disorders,* which involve mutations at one or more genetic loci that interact with an environmental factor, such as exposure to a drug, an infectious agent, or a xenobiotic (a foreign substance).

The mitochondrial genome recently has been sequenced and encodes a number of genes that have been associated with specific disorders.

Chromosomal Disorders

Chromosomal abnormalities occur in 0.5% of newborns; almost all arise from meiotic nondisjunction (i.e., abnormal splitting of homologous chromosomes so that one daughter cell receives both and the other receives none) in one of the parental gametes (sperm and egg). This produces a fertilized egg with a chromosomal number that is different from the normal diploid number of 46 chromosomes, a condition called aneuploidy (i.e., any numerical deviation from the normal 46-chromosome human karyotype). Most aneuploidy abnormalities have 47 chromosomes, such as trisomy 13, 18, and 21. Although the etiology of nondisjunctions is unclear, there is an association with advanced maternal age in some chromosomal disorders, such as in the autosomal trisomies. This association is the reason that prenatal diagnosis with amniocentesis is offered to pregnant women 35 years of age and older. The recurrence risk for aneuploidy abnormalities is small—1% or less.

The karyotypes of parents who have had a child with an aneuploidy abnormality are normal and thus need not be obtained. However, parents who have had a child with an unbalanced karyotype, in which 46 chromosomes are present but additional material is attached to another chromosome (duplication) or is deleted from one chromosome (deletion), should have their karyotypes determined. In these situations one of the parents could be a "balanced" carrier and at increased risk for having another child with a chromosomal abnormality.

Mendelian Disorders

There are four mendelian, or single-gene, inheritance patterns: autosomal dominant, autosomal recessive, X-linked recessive, and X-linked dominant (Table 40-1). Determination of the pattern involved is based on whether the genetic locus is on an autosome or on the X chromosome and whether a single dose of the mutant allele causes the disease (dominant) or a double dose of the mutant allele causes the

Table 40-1 Characteristics of Mendelian Inheritance Patterns

	Autosomal dominant	Autosomal recessive	X-linked recessive	X-linked dominant
Sex	M = F	M = F	Only M	F > M (2:1)
Genotype of affected individual	AN	AA	X^A Y	X^A Y; X^A X^N
Generations affected	Successive	Single	Successive; through carrier females	Successive
Recurrence risk for parents with affected child	50% if parent affected; negligible if parents unaffected	25%	25% if mother is carrier; negligible if new mutation	If M affected, all daughters affected; no sons affected. If F affected, 50% offspring affected
Male-to-male transmission	Yes	NA	No	No
Other features	Advanced paternal age with new mutations in some disorders; variable expressivity	Consanguinity sometimes found	—	Rare inheritance pattern

A, Abnormal allele on autosomal chromosome; *F*, female; *M*, male; *N*, normal allele on autosomal chromosome A; *NA*, not applicable; *X*, abnormal allele on X chromosome.

disease (recessive). There are no known Y-linked human diseases.

Autosomal Dominant Inheritance. Individuals who have an autosomal dominant disorder have one normal (N) and one abnormal (A) or mutant allele at the genetic locus in question. Thus an affected individual has the genotype of NA and has a 50% chance of passing the N allele and a 50% chance of passing the A allele to each child. Because an affected person's mate almost always has two normal alleles (NN) at the same locus, there is a 50% chance that their children will inherit the A allele and thus have the disorder.

Pedigrees of autosomal dominant disorders often show successive generations of affected individuals in which affected children have an affected parent. An individual who has an autosomal dominant condition, however, sometimes can have normal parents who do not have the condition, which illustrates the concept of a *new mutation*. In this situation the risk of the normal parents having another affected child is negligible, whereas there is a 50% risk that the person with the new mutation will have an affected child.

Achondroplasia is a well-documented autosomal dominant condition that most likely represents new mutations; 90% of affected individuals are born to parents of normal stature. Advanced paternal age has been associated with new mutations in a number of autosomal dominant conditions, including achondroplasia, Apert syndrome, and myositis ossificans.

On average, equal numbers of males and females are affected; male-to-male transmission also occurs. These two characteristics help distinguish autosomal dominant inheritance from X-linked recessive inheritance. In X-linked inheritance, females almost never are affected and male-to-male transmission cannot occur (see X-Linked Recessive Inheritance below).

Variable expressivity is another feature of some autosomal dominant disorders in which a spectrum of clinical manifestations can appear in affected individuals. This principle is illustrated in the autosomal dominant condition of Marfan syndrome, in which any combination of the following can occur: musculoskeletal abnormalities, including long, thin fingers, high arched palate, pectus excavatum, and scoliosis; the eye abnormality of dislocated lenses; and cardiac abnormalities, including mitral valve prolapse and a dilated aortic root.

Autosomal Recessive Inheritance. Individuals who have an autosomal recessive disorder have two mutant alleles at the genetic locus in question; thus they have the genotype AA and are homozygous for the mutant allele. Most individuals, however, are homozygous for the normal allele (NN) at this locus, although the occurrence of the heterozygote or carrier (NA) can be as high as 5% for some common autosomal recessive disorders such as cystic fibrosis. Persons who have the NA genotype are entirely normal and show no evidence of the disease in question.

Couples who have had a child with an autosomal recessive condition are both carriers (NA) of one abnormal allele; the other allele is normal. Each parent has a 50% chance of passing the A allele to subsequent children. Thus the probability that both will pass on the A allele to produce an affected child is 50% × 50%, which is 25%. On average, equal numbers of males and females are affected. Pedigrees almost always show the disease confined to one sibship without transmission of the disease from generation to generation. The probability that an affected individual will have an affected child is negligible because the mate of this individual also would have to be a carrier of the same abnormal allele, which is relatively unlikely. Consanguinity sometimes is found in pedigrees of autosomal recessive diseases, especially in very rare conditions, because inbreeding increases the likelihood of two individuals having the same mutant allele at a genetic locus that they can pass on to their children.

X-Linked Recessive Inheritance. X-linked recessive disorders are caused by a mutation at a genetic locus on the X chromosome. Because females have two X chromosomes, it is highly unlikely that they will have mutant alleles at a given locus on both X chromosomes. Males, however, have only one X chromosome; if they inherit an X chromosome from their mother with a mutation at a disease-associated locus, then they will have the disease. Thus females rarely are af-

Table 40-2 Polygenic/Multifactorial Diseases

Disorder	General population frequency (%)	Recurrence risk after one affected child (%)
Neural tube defects	0.1	4
Congenital heart disease	0.6	3
Cleft lip ± palate	0.1	4
Juvenile diabetes	0.1	4

fected with X-linked recessive disorders; for all practical purposes, only males are affected. Males can inherit an X-linked disorder from a carrier female, or the X chromosome that the mother passes on can mutate and give rise to the disorder.

Male-to-male transmission in X-linked recessive inheritance never occurs because the genetic locus is on the X chromosome, and a man has to pass the Y chromosome, not the X chromosome, to his male child. The sons of carrier females have a 50% chance of being affected with an X-linked recessive disorder; the daughters of carrier females have a 50% chance of being carriers. In those X-linked conditions in which males can reproduce, such as hemophilia, none of the male children of affected fathers will be affected, but all female children will be carriers.

X-Linked Dominant Inheritance. X-linked dominant inheritance is a rare type of inheritance pattern. Twice as many females are affected as males, there is no male-to-male transmission, and all female children of affected males are affected.

Polygenic and Multifactorial Inheritance

Because it is difficult to distinguish between polygenic and multifactorial inheritance in human genetic diseases, they will be discussed together. These disorders are characterized by a recurrence risk that is greater for the development of the disorder than the general population's risk but that clearly is lower than that of the 25% autosomal recessive or 50% autosomal dominant mendelian disorders.

Table 40-2 lists some of these disorders, with general population frequency and recurrence risk if a couple already has had an affected child. These disorders are important in pediatrics because they are common and because many are associated with significant morbidity and mortality. It has been difficult to define the specific genetic loci and environmental factors that cause these disorders. Etiological heterogeneity is one explanation for the observation of an intermediate risk after a couple has an affected child. This means that there could be distinctly different causes of the same clinical phenotype. For example, some cases of congenital heart disease may result from an environmental cause such as a congenital infection, whereas others may result from a single gene disorder such as Holt-Oram syndrome. Thus the recurrence risk for each is different. In the former case, the risk would be negligible, in the latter, which is an autosomal dominant disorder, it would be 50% if a parent is affected.

Mitochondrial Disorders

Mitochondrial DNA is maternally inherited. The hallmark of mitochondrial inheritance is that disease transmission is never through the father and is always through the mother or occurs as a fresh mutation. Examples of mitochondrial disorders include the MELAS (*m*itochondrial *e*ncephalomyopathy with *l*actic *a*cidosis and *s*trokelike episodes) syndrome, the MERRF (*m*yoclonic *e*pilepsy and *r*agged-*r*ed *f*ibers) syndrome, and Leber's hereditary optic neuropathy.

Table 40-3 Populations at Increased Risk for Specific Genetic Diseases

Population	Disease	Disease frequency/10,000 births
African American	Sickle cell	20
Ashkenazi Jew	Tay-Sachs	3
Mediterranean	Beta-thalassemia	20
Southeast Asian	Alpha-thalassemia	20
Caucasian	Cystic fibrosis	5
Innuit	Congenital adrenal hyperplasia	20

FAMILY HISTORY

A family history should be part of the medical record of every pediatric patient. It should consist of a three-generation pedigree that shows the age and state of health of all living individuals and the age and cause of death of all deceased individuals (see Fig. 6-1 with accompanying text). Spontaneous and induced abortions should be listed, as well as stillbirths. The ethnic backgrounds of both sides of the family should be noted, as should consanguinity, if present.

As shown in Table 40-3, certain ethnic groups have an increased incidence of disease-associated alleles and thus are at increased risk for some genetic diseases. Consanguinity increases the risk that an child will be homozygous for a disease-associated allele and thus for autosomal recessive diseases. For example, first-cousin matings have a twofold greater risk (4% to 6%) for a congenital disorder, compared with the background risk of unrelated matings (2% to 3%).

PRENATAL SCREENING

Amniocentesis

Amniocentesis is the process of removing amniotic fluid from the amniotic cavity by a needle puncture through the abdominal wall and anterior portion of the uterus. It is a safe procedure that typically is performed at about 16 weeks of gestation, although it can be done as early as 12 to 13 weeks. The amniotic fluid contains fetal cells that can be karyotyped or used for biochemical and DNA analysis.

The most common indication for amniocentesis is advanced maternal age because older mothers are at increased risk for chromosomal disorders. Pregnant women 35 years of age and older are offered amniocentesis and fetal chromosome analysis as part of their prenatal care. Couples with a child who has a chromosomal abnormality or who are balanced translocation carriers also should be offered amniocentesis and fetal karyotyping.

Couples who have had a child who has a genetic disease may choose to have amniocentesis if the condition can be diagnosed by enzyme analysis of fetal cells or by biochemical analysis of amniotic fluid. For example, Hurler syndrome, an autosomal recessive disorder that has a 25% recurrence risk, causes severe mental retardation; most affected children die by adolescence. The disease is caused by a lack of production of the enzyme iduronidase. The disorder can be diagnosed by determining the iduronidase activity in fetal cells obtained by amniocentesis.

Molecular genetics has paved the way for prenatal diagnosis of some of the more common and severe genetic disorders. DNA analysis of fetal cells obtained from amniocentesis can be used to diagnose cystic fibrosis, Duchenne muscular dystrophy, sickle cell anemia, beta-thalassemia, and alpha-thalassemia. Couples who have a child with one of these disorders have a 25% risk of having another affected child. Because DNA diagnosis is highly accurate, many couples who have an affected child choose to have amniocentesis and DNA analysis in subsequent pregnancies.

Amniotic fluid also can be analyzed for alpha-fetoprotein, which is significantly elevated in neural tube defects. The alpha-fetoprotein concentration usually is determined when an amniocentesis is performed for advanced maternal age. Couples who are at increased risk for having a baby with a neural tube defect may choose to have amniocentesis, including the determination of alpha-fetoprotein, as well as fetal ultrasound. Couples who have had a baby with a neural tube defect are at increased risk for having another child with this defect; other risk factors are maternal diabetes and maternal use of valproic acid during pregnancy.

Chorionic Villus Sampling

Chorionic villus sampling (CVS) is another technique for procuring fetal tissue that can be used for chromosomal, biochemical, or DNA analysis. Fetal tissue is obtained transcervically by means of a catheter that can retrieve small pieces of chorionic villus. The procedure is relatively safe, although there is not as much experience with CVS as with amniocentesis. Because CVS can be performed earlier in a pregnancy, couples who are extremely anxious about having a child with a particular condition may choose to undergo CVS rather than amniocentesis.

Ultrasound

Significant advances in fetal ultrasound have resulted in the diagnosis of many congenital abnormalities during pregnancy. These conditions include major central nervous system abnormalities (hydrocephalus, anencephaly, myelomeningocele, and holoprosencephaly), gastrointestinal abnormalities (duodenal atresia and diaphragmatic hernia), many types of congenital heart disease, genitourinary abnormalities (polycystic kidney disease and hydronephrosis), and many types of skeletal disorders. Ultrasound has been helpful to couples who have had children who have congenital abnormalities and who want reassurance that subsequent children will be unaffected.

Maternal Serum Alpha-Fetoprotein Screening

Because elevated levels of alpha-fetoprotein in maternal serum are associated with an increased risk for neural tube defects, pregnant women now are offered maternal serum alpha-fetoprotein screening (MSAFP). Although the test is not as accurate as amniotic alpha-fetoprotein determination, it requires only a maternal blood specimen. If the levels are high, then ultrasound or amniocentesis and amniotic alpha-fetoprotein analysis can be considered. Recently, low levels of MSAFP have been associated with Down syndrome; however, this association is weak and the test was not designed to detect Down syndrome. Couples whose MSAFP reveals low levels of alpha-fetoprotein may consider having amniocentesis and fetal karyotyping to detect Down syndrome.

It should be noted that prenatal screening for genetic diseases is designed to provide accurate information about the likelihood of an child being affected by one of these diseases. Parents are advised of the consequences of such an outcome so that they may make an informed decision as to whether they wish to continue the pregnancy.

NEWBORN SCREENING

All states have mandatory newborn screening programs. Although the tests vary from state to state, all states test for phenylketonuria and congenital hypothyroidism because they are relatively common, easily treated, and clearly cost effective. Some states mandate testing for maple syrup urine disease, homocystinuria, cystic fibrosis, hemoglobinopathies, biotinidase deficiency, congenital adrenal hyperplasia, and galactosemia. The results of newborn screening tests usually are available 1 to 2 weeks after an infant is discharged from the hospital; the pediatrician always should ascertain that the newborn screening test has been performed and is normal. Obviously, any abnormal values should be investigated further.

DNA-BASED DIAGNOSIS OF GENETIC DISEASES

Molecular genetic advances now allow for DNA-based diagnosis of several common pediatric genetic disorders and have changed the diagnostic evaluations of these conditions.

Fragile X Syndrome

Laboratory diagnosis of fragile X syndrome used to be done by cytogenetic-based evaluation of cells for the fragile X chromosome. The gene for fragile X syndrome was characterized in 1992 and has been called FMR-1 (fragile X mental retardation syndrome; the 1 designates the first X-linked mental retardation gene to be characterized). A novel form of mutation has been found in affected individuals who have fragile X syndrome in which the trinucleotide repeat CGG (cytosine-guanine-guanine) is amplified in the FMR-1 gene. Males and females who have fragile X syndrome have more than 230 copies of the CGG repeat; normal individuals have fewer than 50 copies. Carrier females have between 50 and 230 copies.

Laboratory evaluation of an individual suspected of having fragile X syndrome because of autism, mental retardation, or the physical features of fragile X syndrome (large testes, large ears, or a prominent jaw) should be done with the DNA-based test and not the more expensive and less reliable cytogenetic-based test.

Duchenne Muscular Dystrophy

The diagnosis of Duchenne muscular dystrophy (DMD) has been made by muscle biopsy. In 1987 the gene that causes

Table 40-4 Common Genetic Disorders

Disorder	Manifestation	Frequency/10,000 births
Chromosomal		
Trisomy 21	Congenital heart disease, Brushfield spots, short hands, clinodactyly, simian crease, hypotonia, dysmorphic facies	16
Trisomy 18	Congenital heart disease, small for gestational age (SGA), clenched fist, rocker-bottom foot, dysmorphic facies	3
Trisomy 13	Congenital heart disease, SGA, polydactyly, holoprosencephaly, dysmorphic facies	2
XO	Congenital peripheral edema, webbed neck, short stature, primary amenorrhea	3
XXY	Behavior problems, small testes, infertility, clinodactyly	5
Autosomal recessive		
Sickle cell disease	Anemia, infection	20 (African American)
Beta-Thalassemia	Anemia	20 (Mediterranean)
Cystic fibrosis	Failure to thrive, malabsorption, cough, recurrent pneumonia	5 (Caucasian)
Autosomal dominant		
Familial hypercholesterolemia	Family history of early coronary artery disease	20
Neurofibromatosis	Café-au-lait spots	3
X-linked recessive		
Fragile X	Mental retardation, large testes, dysmorphic facies	5
Duchenne muscular dystrophy	Muscle weakness, pseudohypertrophy of calf	1

DMD was characterized and named dystrophin. About two thirds of cases of DMD are from large intragenic deletions in the dystrophin gene that can be detected by the molecular methods of either Southern blotting or polymerase chain reaction. In most cases the diagnosis of DMD can be made using DNA-based methods and thus avoiding a muscle biopsy. In cases in which there is no deletion, a muscle biopsy is required.

Spinal Muscular Atrophy

The gene for spinal muscular atrophy (SMA) was characterized in 1995. Microdeletions of this gene are a common cause of SMA, and DNA-based diagnosis is now possible.

Cystic Fibrosis

In 1989 the gene for cystic fibrosis was characterized and found to encode for a transmembrane protein of epithelial cells that controls chloride transport; this gene was named CFTR (cystic fibrosis transmembrane regulator). One common mutation has been found at the CFTR locus, which accounts for about 70% of the CF alleles in the Caucasian population; it has been named ΔF 508 (deletion of a phenylalanine residue at the 508 position of CFTR). It now is possible to perform mutational analysis on individuals to determine their genotype at the CFTR locus. This approach commonly is used in families that have had cystic fibrosis, particularly to determine the carrier status of at-risk individuals. Typically, a panel of CF alleles is evaluated, which will detect 85% to 90% of CF alleles. The initial diagnostic test for cystic fibrosis in an individual suspected of having the disease still is the sweat chloride test. In situations in which it is difficult to obtain sweat, such as in very young infants, or in equivocal sweat tests, mutational analysis of CFTR may be especially helpful.

Fragile X syndrome, DMD, and cystic fibrosis all can be diagnosed prenatally with great accuracy using molecular genetic techniques on a chorionic villus sample or on amniocytes obtained by amniocentesis.

SCOPE OF PEDIATRIC GENETIC DISORDERS

It is beyond the intent of this chapter to describe in any detail the numerous genetic diseases. Table 40-4 lists some of the more common genetic disorders that manifest in children. Two excellent references that may help pediatricians to establish a genetic diagnosis or a dysmorphology syndrome are Jones' *Smith's Recognizable Patterns of Human Malformation*[1] and McKusick's *Mendelian Inheritance in Man*.[2]

REFERENCES

1. Jones KL: *Smith's recognizable patterns of human malformation,* ed 4, Philadelphia, 1988, WB Saunders.
2. McKusick VA: *Mendelian inheritance in man,* ed 10, Baltimore, 1992, Johns Hopkins University Press.

SUGGESTED READINGS

Johns DR: Mitochondrial DNA and disease, *N Engl J Med* 333:638, 1995.

Thompson MW: *Genetics in medicine,* ed 4, Philadelphia, 1986, WB Saunders.

41 Contraception and Abortion

Eric A. Schaff

Major advances have been made recently in contraception and early induced abortion. Subdermal 5-year implants became available in 1991 and the 3-month injection depomedroxyprovera in 1992. Postcoital contraception (the "morning-after" pills), if more widely available, potentially can reduce unintended pregnancies significantly. Medical abortifacients, RU 486 and methotrexate, are under study in the United States. These alternatives to surgical abortion will increase access to safe, early abortions, thereby reducing maternal morbidity and mortality worldwide.

CONTRACEPTION

Use of contraceptive practices can help reduce the medical and social morbidity associated with unplanned, premature pregnancy in adolescents. National studies have shown that almost 50% of 15- to 19-year-old teenage females are sexually active, ranging from 20% of 15-year-olds to more than 70% of 19-year-olds.[9] The rates among teenage males are higher. Whereas 25% of teenage women seek family planning services before or at the time of becoming sexually active, 75% have been active an average of almost 2 years before making a family planning health visit.[11] Approximately 1 million teenagers become pregnant each year, and most of these pregnancies are unintended. Two thirds of these young women have a child, and one third have abortions. The United States has the highest teen pregnancy rate in the Western world, and infection with the human immunodeficiency virus (HIV) has added a deadly new dimension to teen sexuality.

Health care providers are in a unique position to offer anticipatory guidance to parents, preteens, and teenagers about puberty, abstinence, female contraception, and use of condoms to reduce the risks of pregnancy and sexually transmitted diseases (STDs). Practitioners should provide family planning services and screening for and treatment of STDs.

The theoretical and typical effectiveness (or failure rates) of different contraceptive methods should not be confused. For example, if oral contraceptives are used correctly and consistently, their *theoretical failure rate* of 0.1% (that is, 1 of 1000 couples who use the method perfectly for 1 year will experience an accidental pregnancy) is dramatically better than the theoretical failure rates of both condoms and diaphragms (3%). Unfortunately, the typical failure rates for oral contraceptives in a teenage population (teens often stop using them because of minor problems) can be as high as the typical failure rates of condoms and diaphragms, 10% to 20%. The message is clear: *It does not matter what method you use as long as you use it correctly and consistently.* Using two methods simultaneously and having a backup method available significantly reduce the chance of an unintended pregnancy.

Teenagers have had legal access to family planning services since the Supreme Court decision in *Belotti v. Baird* in 1976. Confidential care also can be inferred from Public Health Law 7896 regarding treatment of STDs and "related services."

Condoms

Condoms must be recommended strongly to sexually active teenagers because of their effectiveness in preventing pregnancy (if used consistently and correctly) and in reducing the spread of all STDs, including HIV. Even if teenagers prefer another method for preventing pregnancy, they also should be encouraged strongly to *use condoms to prevent disease.* Condoms are (1) inexpensive, (2) available over the counter, (3) a means to involve the male in sharing responsibility for contraception, (4) lubricated (and therefore reduce dyspareunia), (5) associated with no side effects, (6) simple to use, and (7) a remediable method—if they break, postcoital contraception (discussed later in the chapter) can be used.

The disadvantages are the diminished genital sensation for both partners and the lack of 100% protection against STDs (lesions on the external genitalia and genital secretions on the pubic area, hands, and mouth can lead to infection).

For optimum compliance, the following information should be offered to teenagers verbally and, ideally, in writing:

1. Condoms are highly effective at preventing pregnancy when used consistently and correctly.
2. Condoms are highly effective at preventing sexually transmitted diseases and the virus that causes acquired immune deficiency syndrome (AIDS).
3. Lubricated latex condoms with or without the spermicidal nonoxynol-9 offer the best protection. "Natural" condoms (made from lamb intestine) provide significantly less protection because of their greater permeability to viruses and therefore are not recommended.
4. Condoms should be placed on the erect penis just before insertion into the vagina.
5. To prevent condom breakage, (a) do not store condoms in warm places (e.g., a wallet) for long periods, (b) do not use petroleum-based lubricants such as Vaseline, (c) use lubricated condoms, (d) allow room at the condom's end for the ejaculate, and (e) do not reuse condoms.
6. To avoid accidental spillage, remove the penis shortly after ejaculation while holding the rim of the condom on the penis.
7. If spillage occurs or a condom breaks, insert spermicidal vaginal foam, which may help, or consult your health care provider about postcoital contraception ("morning-after" pill).

Oral Contraceptives

As new, lower dose oral contraceptives become available, studies indicate fewer serious health problems[8] and more beneficial side effects from their use. Oral contraceptives consist of estrogen and progestin. All low-dose pills contain ethinyl estradiol as the estrogen and one of many progestational agents. Oral contraceptives (1) suppress luteinizing- and follicle-stimulating hormones, thereby inhibiting ovulation, (2) thicken cervical mucus, making it less penetrable by sperm, and (3) alter the endometrium, making it less receptive for implantation of a fertilized ovum.

The new progestins are *desogestrel* and *norgestimate*. Because they are potent progestins but weak androgens, they have fewer androgenic side effects, increase high-density lipoprotein (HDL),[4] which protects against atherosclerosis, and have a longer half-life, so spotting and pregnancy are less likely if a pill is missed.

Advantages. The advantages of oral contraceptives are (1) low failure rate if taken correctly, (2) safety, (3) ease of reversal if pregnancy is desired, (4) low cost of generic formulations, (5) regular menses, (6) protection against pelvic inflammatory disease because of the thickened cervical mucus, (7) less anemia, (8) improvement of acne, (9) decrease in benign breast disease, and (10) protection against ovarian[10] and endometrial[8,10] cancer.

Disadvantages. The disadvantages of oral contraceptives are (1) the need for daily compliance, (2) the cost, (3) the "minor" side effects of nausea, headaches, breakthrough vaginal bleeding, mood changes, and weight gain, (4) the increased risk of chlamydia infection after exposure, possibly due to endocervical columnar cell eversion, (5) the decreased effectiveness with rifampin and antiseizure medications, (6) oral contraceptives' possible role as a promoter in breast cancer in women under age 35,[8] and (7) the increased risk of thromboembolic disease.

Oral contraceptives are contraindicated in women who have a history of thromboembolic diseases and must be prescribed cautiously for women who have risk factors such as smoking, high blood pressure, diabetes, and sickle cell disease. Oral contraceptives also are contraindicated with active liver disease, uterine bleeding of unknown cause, estrogen-dependent tumors, and suspected pregnancy.

Prescribing Oral Contraceptives. Healthy teenage girls who have or who anticipate having sexual intercourse are excellent candidates for use of oral contraceptives. Before prescribing them, the health care provider should obtain a medical history and perform a complete physical and gynecological examination. A Pap smear should be obtained, and vaginal secretions should be examined and cervical secretions tested for STDs. Determining the hematocrit level is recommended because of the high prevalence of iron deficiency in this age group. Those who have not had documented rubella and/or a second rubeola immunization should receive a measles-mumps-rubella (MMR) injection and be advised to avoid pregnancy for 3 months. A yearly serological test for syphilis is indicated if the prevalence in the community is high. A lipid profile may be done when a teenager has a family history of early coronary artery disease.

With a very young sexually active teenager, the health care provider must weigh the theoretical risks of hormonal contraception on future growth and fertility against the real medical and social risks of a premature pregnancy. *There is no current clinical evidence that early use of oral contraceptives either limits growth or affects future fertility.*

To reduce side effects and complications, all women should be started on low-dose 30 to 35 μg estrogen pills. The low-dose estrogen preparations have been as effective as the higher dose 50 μg pills in preventing pregnancy. Most often, oral contraceptives are prescribed on a 28-day cycle: 21 days of taking active ingredients and 7 days of taking either inert pills or no pills at all. The estrogen and progestin compounds in the pill can be fixed, or the concentrations of either hormone may vary during the 21-day period (multiphasic pills). The advantage of the multiphasic pills over most fixed combination pills is the lowering of the total amount of hormone administered during each cycle. The stronger progestin pills that have this component are reduced proportionately; therefore there are few clinically noticeable differences among pills.

Three alternative prescribing strategies include choosing (1) an inexpensive generic brand, (2) a low hormonal preparation (e.g., ethinyl estradiol, 35 μg, and norethindrone, 0.4 mg [Ovcon-35]), or (3) a progestin preparation.

Return appointments can be scheduled in 1 to 3 months to reinforce compliance and to measure blood pressure. Future appointments can be scheduled every 12 months or, if clinically indicated, more often.

Health care providers rarely will need to prescribe progestin-only pills; they usually are recommended for women in whom estrogen is contraindicated.

Compliance. To increase compliance with oral contraceptive pills, the health care provider should provide the following anticipatory guidance verbally and, ideally, in writing:

1. Oral contraceptive pills should be started on the first Sunday after the onset of menses to ensure that pregnancy has not occurred.
2. If started correctly and taken daily, oral contraceptives should inhibit ovulation effectively in the first month, but using a backup contraceptive method during the first week provides additional security.
3. Pills should be taken at the same time each day for 21 days, followed by the seven placebo pills. Withdrawal bleeding usually occurs on day 2 or 3 after the last hormonal pill has been taken.
4. Ovulation (and therefore pregnancy) is possible if a pill is missed, particularly during the first 7 days. Take the missed pill as soon as possible to "catch up." If two pills are missed, take two tablets as soon as you remember and two the following day, and use a backup contraceptive method during this month. If three pills are missed, toss out the pack and restart a new pack the first Sunday after the next menses. A backup contraceptive method is necessary for that cycle when any pills are missed. If pills are missed frequently, consider using the 3-month contraceptive injection Depo-Provera.[11]
5. Mild side effects such as vaginal bleeding (spotting), nausea, bloating, and irritability are likely to resolve after several cycles. If not, the prescription can be changed.
6. Menses usually become lighter and occasionally are absent while taking oral contraceptive pills. If there are

no menses, the pills should be continued, but a pregnancy test should be obtained for reassurance and to detect the rare possibility of pregnancy.

7. The major side effect of oral contraceptives is blood clots (thrombosis.) These are significantly more likely to occur in women over age 40, women over age 35 who smoke, and women who have additional risk factors for thrombosis (e.g., hypertension, diabetes, hypercholesterolemia, and obesity). A warning sign that requires immediate medical care is severe head, chest, or leg pain. The risks to a healthy teenager are extremely low.
8. The major disadvantage of oral contraceptives is the lack of protection against STDs, including the AIDS virus. Condoms are strongly encouraged to prevent STDs.
9. Oral contraceptives are less effective when taken with certain medications such as antibiotics (e.g., amoxicillin and doxycycline) and certain anticonvulsants (e.g., phenobarbital and phenytoin). Simultaneous use of condoms or other barrier methods provides additional protection.

Subdermal Implants and Injectable Contraceptives

More than 1.8 million women have used the 5-year *subdermal implants* (Norplant) worldwide. Norplant consists of six Silastic capsules containing levonorgestrel. They are about the size of match sticks and are placed under the skin inside the upper arm, with one skin puncture made using local anesthesia. Levonorgestrel is released slowly over the 5-year period, providing continuous protection from pregnancy.

Depo-medroxyprovera (Depo-Provera) has been used by more than 15 million women worldwide. It comes in a single 150 mg dose vial, which is shaken vigorously before the drug is given as a deep intramuscular injection in the deltoid or gluteal muscle. The injection area should not be massaged. Depo-Provera provides 3 months of continuous protection and an additional 1 week "grace" period (13 weeks).

Both of these methods work primarily by (1) inhibiting ovulation, (2) thickening cervical mucus, and (3) producing an atrophic endometrium. Both have failure rates of less than 1% (fewer than 1 woman in 100 who use this method for 1 year will become pregnant), and success is not user dependent. Both methods should be started within 5 days of the onset of normal menses.

The advantages of these progesterone-only medicines include (1) no estrogen and therefore no risk for thromboembolic diseases, (2) decreased anemia, (3) decreased risk for ovarian and endometrial cancer and pelvic inflammatory disease, (4) reversibility, (5) no interference with breast-feeding, (6) possible reduction in the incidence of seizures and sickling episodes (with Depo-Provera), and (7) amenorrhea occurring in 30% to 50% of women in the first year of Depo-Provera, which occurs in a higher percentage of women thereafter.

The disadvantages of these medicines include (1) menstrual cycle disturbances, (2) weight gain, (3) side effects such as hair loss, nausea, mood changes, and aching and tenderness at the site of the subdermal implant, (4) decreased effectiveness with most antiseizure medications and rifampin with implants but not with Depo-Provera, (5) low estrogen state, with Depo-Provera causing a decrease in bone density that has not been significant clinically, (6) a possible role as a promoter of breast cancer in women under age 35, and (7) delay in clearance of Depo-Provera for as long as 12 months. There have been a few reports of pseudotumor cerebri (headaches, blurred vision, and papilledema) with the implants—this necessitates removal.

The initial cost of the implants is high—$370 plus the insertion fee. The lack of any additional costs before removal makes them cost effective. Depo-Provera costs about $30 per injection, plus the office visit fee.

Managing side effects is important in supporting continued use of these methods. Prolonged uterine bleeding can be managed by adding one to two cycles of oral contraceptives or a month's supply of exogenous estrogens (Premarin 0.625 mg tablets, twice a day for 20 days). With support, continuation rates in the first year are over 70%.[2,6]

Postcoital "Morning After" Contraception

Postcoital contraception is underused and could reduce unintended pregnancies significantly. It can help when other methods fail, when no other contraception was used, or when rape has occurred. These methods are most helpful during the mid-menstrual cycle, when ovulation occurs, but can be used at any time if pregnancy is possible. Postcoital contraception must be used as soon after intercourse as possible, but no later than 72 hours afterward. The most common treatment consists of two tablets of ethinyl estradiol (50 μg) and norgestrel (0.5 mg) (Ovral), followed by two more tablets 12 hours later.[14] Alternatively, to achieve the same doses, four tablets of low-dose pills containing norgestrel or levonorgestrel (Lo/ovral, Nordette, Levlen, Triphasyl, or Tri-Levlen) can be given, with four more tablets taken 12 hours later. Medication may be necessary for nausea. Menses should begin 2 to 3 weeks later. If this does not happen, the patient should be instructed to return for a pregnancy test. The mechanism of action for the postcoital contraceptives is thought to be related to luteal phase dysfunction, endometrial changes that make implantation less likely, and alterations in fallopian tube mobility that adversely affect the movement of the fertilized ovum to the uterus.

Although postcoital contraception has not been approved by the U.S. Food and Drug Administration (FDA), it has been used extensively in Europe and for rape victims in the United States. Mifepristone (RU 486)[7] is an alternative effective treatment that has minimal side effects, but it has not been approved by the FDA.

Diaphragm, Female Condom, and Cervical Cap

The diaphragm is a thin rubber dome that is inserted into the vagina, where it blocks sperm from entering the cervix. It must be used with a spermicidal contraceptive jelly whose active ingredient is nonoxynol-9. The diaphragm's typical failure rate varies from 6% to 16%. It also offers some protection from STDs and has minimal side effects. Occasionally it is chosen by an older, more motivated teenager. The disadvantages of the diaphragm include (1) the technical skill needed for correct placement, (2) the need to leave it in place 6 hours after intercourse, (3) the need for a second application of spermicidal jelly if intercourse is repeated, and (4) the association with vaginitis, urinary tract infections and, in rare cases, toxic shock syndrome. Disadvantages for the health care provider include keeping a set of diaphragm rings for sizing and learning and maintaining the skill to fit one when the requests are likely to be few.

The female condom is available but not widely used. It is made from polyurethane, with two flexible polyurethane rings. One ring is placed inside the vagina to cover the cervix; the open ring remains on the outside to protect the perineum from STDs. The female condom, which costs about $2.50, should not be used with latex condoms, nor should it be reused.

The cervical cap is a thimble-shaped rubber device that fits over the cervix and can be left in place for continuous protection up to 48 hours. Its advantages and rates of effectiveness are similar to those of the diaphragm. Disadvantages include (1) the skill needed for insertion and removal (significantly more than that for the diaphragm), (2) the association of cervical dysplasia in the early months of use, and (3) the inability to fit the cervix of some women.

Spermicidals: Vaginal Sponge, Vaginal Foam, and Vaginal Suppository

The vaginal sponge, vaginal foam, and vaginal suppository use nonoxynol-9, which has in vitro and in vivo properties against some STDs. All these methods are relatively simple, effective, and inexpensive and can be obtained without a prescription. They have the same pregnancy failure rates as the diaphragm and tend to have similar actions, advantages, and disadvantages. The spermicidals are important complementary methods (1) when used with condoms, (2) when intercourse is infrequent, and (3) when used as a backup for other birth control methods.

The vaginal sponge, which first is moistened with water, can be inserted several hours before intercourse and remains effective for 24 hours. Vaginal suppositories must be left in place 10 to 30 minutes before intercourse to allow them to dissolve.

Natural Family Planning

Natural family planning methods include (1) charting of menstrual cycles on the calendar, (2) recording basal body temperatures, and (3) monitoring cervical mucus to detect when ovulation occurs. Advantages include the lack of side effects, acceptance by religious groups opposed to medicinal and barrier methods, and the knowledge gained about reproductive physiology. Disadvantages for young teenagers include their irregular menstrual cycles, which make predicting ovulation difficult, and the high degree of motivation required for effective use.

Intrauterine Device

Exactly how the intrauterine device (IUD) works is not known. It probably irritates the endometrium, making it unsuitable for implantation of a fertilized egg. However, the IUD is contraindicated in adolescents because of the increased risk of pelvic inflammatory disease and its associated risk of infertility. A marked decline in IUD availability is due to its increased initial cost as a result of the expenses incurred by pharmaceutical companies in defending the large number of lawsuits related to IUD use. The major advantage of an IUD is that once in place, it requires no effort for continued effectiveness and no ongoing cost.

Abstinence

Abstinence is the safest contraceptive method for teenagers. Half of all teenagers choose abstinence, and they should be offered support and encouragement, as well as contraceptive information if and when they choose to have intercourse.

ABORTION

An induced abortion is a purposeful termination of a pregnancy before extrauterine viability. At least 1.5 million legal abortions are reported each year in the United States, and 90% are surgical terminations done in the first trimester of pregnancy. Approximately 26% of abortions are performed on women age 19 or younger; 67% of the women are Caucasian, 80% are unmarried, and more than 50% have not been pregnant previously.[1] Only when contraceptive services become universally available will the need for abortion be reduced significantly.

Abortion became legal in the United States in 1973 when the Supreme Court set the following guidelines in *Roe v. Wade:*

1. In the first trimester (up to 13 weeks from the onset of the last menstrual period), a woman, in consultation with her physician, is free to choose an abortion.
2. In the second trimester (from 13 to 24 weeks of gestation), the state can regulate the abortion procedure to promote the pregnant woman's health.
3. After viability, the state has interests in promoting fetal life and can regulate or ban the abortion procedure except to preserve the pregnant woman's life or health.

A brief review of legal decisions regarding teenagers and abortion is included here to help health care providers understand issues of parental consent and laws of notification. In 1976, in *Planned Parenthood of Central Missouri v. Danforth,* the Supreme Court decided that a teenager has a legal right to abortion in consultation with her physician and without parental consent. In 1979, in *Belloti v. Baird,* the Supreme Court reaffirmed a minor's right to an abortion and found that a Massachusetts parental consent law was unconstitutional. The Court, however, left open the possibility that parental consent law might be permissible if a judicial or an administrative bypass was included in order for the minor to demonstrate her maturity or to serve her best interests and not involve her parents. In 1990, in *Hodgson v. Minnesota,* the Supreme Court affirmed that two-parent notification and a 48-hour waiting period following parental notification before the abortion can be performed were acceptable if a judicial bypass was provided. In 1992, in *Planned Parenthood of Southeastern Pennsylvania v. Casey,* the Supreme Court affirmed that a 24-hour waiting period, state-mandated information about abortion, and a minor's abortion conditioned upon one-parent or guardian consent in person at the clinic or a judicial waiver were acceptable.

Medical evaluation of a pregnant teenager should include a urine pregnancy test and a gynecological examination to estimate uterine size and to obtain cultures for gonorrhea and chlamydia. Dating the pregnancy and detecting and treating diseases are important, regardless of the outcome of the pregnancy. When dating is not clear, an ultrasound scan can determine gestational age accurately.

When considering her pregnancy alternatives, each teenager considers many aspects of her life, such as her age, marital status, health, education, financial situation, religious upbringing, family support, and future plans. Pregnant teenagers should receive counseling about their options, including keeping the infant, adoption, and abortion. The health care provider should provide nonjudgmental support and explore whether the teen can involve family members or other potential sources of advice, such as relatives, siblings, clergy, teachers, counselors, and boyfriend. Some teenagers are unable to involve their parents in a discussion of their pregnancy. Health care providers should be aware of state laws concerning public funding for abortion through Medicaid and parental notification or consent requirements. Health care providers who are morally unable to support a decision for abortion should refer their patient to a colleague who can.

First Trimester and Early Second Trimester Abortions

Suction curettage initially was used only in first trimester pregnancies. With additional experience, gynecologists have used this procedure up to 20 weeks of gestation—that is, in almost 98% of all abortions. This procedure often involves the insertion of laminaria to dilate the cervix 6 to 24 hours before the procedure, local cervical anesthesia, dilation of the cervix using dilators, and introduction of an appropriately sized cannula to suction fetal and placental parts. Products of conception should be identified and examined microscopically by a pathologist.

All women whose blood type is Rh negative should receive anti-$Rh_O(D)$ immunoglobulin (RhoGAM). Contraceptive methods should be discussed and prescribed if appropriate. Oral contraceptive pills and the new progesterone-only implants and injections can be started in the first week after abortion. The teenager should be reexamined within 2 to 3 weeks to ensure that she is doing well and that the abortion is complete.

The average incidence of complications from suction abortion is 1% and failure is 0.5%. Complications include uterine perforation, hemorrhage, cervical lacerations, and anesthetic mishaps. The maternal mortality rate for early abortions is 0.5 to 0.7/100,000 procedures,[1] mainly from infection (23%), thromboembolic phenomena (23%), hemorrhage (20%), and anesthetic complications (16%). Complications increase when skilled surgeons are unavailable (as often happens in developing countries).

RU 486

Surgical abortions are not available in 80% of the counties in the United States[5]; therefore women in these areas must travel long distances to obtain an abortion. The availability of a safe medical abortifacient would reduce significantly the number of women who would have to travel for a surgical abortion.

RU 486, mifepristone, is an antiprogestin agent that initially was studied in France and is 95% effective as an early abortifacient.[13] It is taken orally up to 7 weeks (in France) and up to 9 weeks (in Great Britain and Sweden) after the last menses in conjunction with misoprostol, a prostaglandin. Because this is not an invasive procedure, there is no risk of infection or perforation. Side effects may include mild gastrointestinal problems and excessive uterine bleeding. Five percent of women require suction abortion for completion. RU 486 also has potential benefit in the treatment of Cushing syndrome, breast cancer, endometriosis, and glaucoma. The drug is under study in the United States as an alternative to surgical abortion.

Methotrexate

Methotrexate with misoprostol also represents a potential major development for first trimester abortions.[3,12] Methotrexate currently is used in the treatment of cancers, as an immunosuppressive agent, and for both gestational trophoblastic neoplasia and ectopic pregnancy. Methotrexate has been studied extensively in humans, and its safe dosing schedules are well documented. Advantages of methotrexate for early abortions include its safety/risk ratio, low cost, and availability. Methotrexate currently is under study for early induced abortion in the United States.

Late Second Trimester Abortions

Later abortions involve injection of a hypertonic saline solution or prostaglandin, often in combination with laminaria to dilate the cervix and oxytocin to augment contractions. *Later abortions are more dangerous,* with a mortality rate of about 3/100,000 procedures. Fewer than 2% of abortions are performed by these methods. Complications include those seen with earlier abortions, in addition to embolism, hypernatremia, disseminated intravascular coagulation, and cervical laceration.

Most studies on abortion conclude that there is no evidence that infertility, spontaneous miscarriages, or a propensity to deliver babies prematurely are late sequelae. Neither is there evidence that psychiatric problems after abortion are more common than those after childbirth.

SUMMARY

There have been recent major advances in the areas of contraception and abortion that will affect the health of adolescent and adult women positively worldwide. Primary health care providers should become familiar with these new methods.

REFERENCES

1. Abortion surveillance, United States, 1984-85, *MMWR* 39(SS-2):11, 1989.
2. Alvarez-Sanchez F, Brache V, Faundes A: The clinical performance of Norplant implants over time: a comparison of two cohorts, *Stud Fam Plann* 19:118, 1988.
3. Creinin MD, Darney PD: Methotrexate and misoprostol for early abortion, *Contraception* 48:339, 1993.
4. Crook D et al: A comparative metabolic study of two low-estrogen-dose oral contraceptives containing desogestrel or gestodene progestins, *Am J Obstet Gynecol* 169:1183, 1993.
5. Darney PD: Maternal deaths in the less developed world: preventable tragedies, *Int J Gynaecol Obstet* 26:177, 1988.

6. Glantz S et al: Contraceptive implant use among inner city teens, *J Adolesc Health Care* 16:389, 1995.
7. Glasier A et al: Mifepristone (RU 486) compared with high-dose estrogen and progesterone for emergency postcoital contraception, *N Engl J Med* 327:1041, 1992.
8. Grimes DA: The safety of oral contraceptives: epidemiologic insights from the first 30 years, *Am J Obstet Gynecol* 166:1950, 1992.
9. Hofferth SL, Kahn JR, Baldwin W: Premarital sexual activity among U.S. teenage women over the past three decades, *Fam Plann Perspect* 19:46, 1987.
10. Jick SS, Walker AM, Jick H: Oral contraceptives and endometrial cancer, *Obstet Gynecol* 82:931, 1993.
11. Mosher WD, Horn MC: First family planning visits by young women, *Fam Plann Perspect* 20:33, 1988.
12. Schaff EA et al: Combination methotrexate and misoprostol for early induced abortion, *Arch Fam Med* 4:774, 1995.
13. Silvestre L et al: Voluntary interruption of pregnancy with mifepristone and a prostaglandin analogue: a large-scale French experience, *N Engl J Med* 322:645, 1990.
14. Yuzpe AA, Smith RP, Rademaker AW: A multicenter clinical investigation employing ethinyl estradiol combined with dl-norgestrel as a postcoital contraceptive agent, *Fertil Steril* 37:508, 1982.

SUGGESTED READING

Hatcher RA et al: *Contraceptive technology,* ed 16, New York, 1994, Irvington.

42 The Fetus at Risk

George A. Little

In the past pediatricians first saw their newly born patients most often in the nursery, where a philosophy to intervene with sick patients as little as possible often dominated. Today pediatricians often are involved in preconception and interconception counseling, fetal risk identification, and peripartum decisions and are present at high-risk deliveries to assume primary responsibility for resuscitation and stabilization of the newly born infant.

Knowledge of fetal health includes appreciation of the interaction of the fetus with the mother, family, health professional, and society. The pediatrician uses knowledge of fetal medicine frequently, including genetic counseling and perinatal care. Although major scientific strides have made a broader understanding of fetal well-being possible, the fund of knowledge remains inadequate.

Prospective parents and professionals have good reason to be concerned about the immediate and long-term effect of agents or processes on the fetus. There are too many well-documented examples of negative impact and increasing evidence of ability to prevent or treat to deny the value of fetal medicine as part of preconception and prenatal care. Infections such as rubella can result in fetal loss or multisystem disease. The magnitude and seriousness of manifestations of maternal alcohol consumption or abuse of cocaine and its derivatives during pregnancy may be evident in the infant's physical appearance or behavior at the time of birth. The effects of diethylstilbestrol (DES) given to mothers for threatened abortion may not manifest until the appearance of clear cell carcinoma of the vagina in female offspring 10 to 20 years later; there is legitimate concern that grandchildren may be at risk, leading some to advise third-generation screening and follow-up.[11] Growth and development are as much a key to fetal medicine as they are to pediatrics. One must regard human growth and development as a continuum that begins with conception. This section depicts some of the normal physical and interactive aspects of fetal existence, followed by a discussion of selected pathophysiological states that may affect that existence adversely.

FETAL LIFE SPAN

The human product of conception *technically becomes a fetus at the end of the eighth week* after fertilization and remains so until birth. The normal human pregnancy lasts 36 to 40 weeks from fertilization or 38 to 42 weeks from the last menstrual period (by menstrual dating). Fetal development begins at fertilization, when a sperm combines with an oocyte (immature ovum) to form a zygote. The fetal life span is defined here in the broad sense to include the entire gestational interval (Fig. 42-1).

The process from conception to birth has three stages: (1) the zygote and preembryo, (2) the embryo, and (3) the fetus. The conceptus, or product of conception, is made up of all structures that develop from the zygote, both embryonic and extraembryonic (i.e., the embryo or fetus and the membranes, including the placenta).

The *stage of the zygote and preembryo,* illustrated in Figure 42-1, begins with fertilization wherein a single haploid sperm (23 chromosomes) penetrates the oocyte (immature haploid female ovum). This usually takes place within the ampulla of the fallopian tube. The complicated fertilization process takes up to 24 hours after initial penetration by the sperm, before the genetic material from the two haploid cells in the stage of syngamy fuses to form a diploid cell, the *zygote,* with a full complement of genetic material.

The *preembryo* consists of the developing cells produced by division of the zygote and lasts until the formation of the "primitive streak," approximately 14 days after the beginning of fertilization. The preembryonic stage has been of special interest clinically and ethically because of the ability to sustain human preembryos in vitro for up to 6 to 9 days after fertilization.

Preembryo development, during the interval before implantation in the uterine lining, includes a series of morphological changes. Progression proceeds from blastomeres or individual cells to a tightly compacted group of cells called the *morula.* The blastocyst, a mass of cells having a fluid-filled inner cavity, appears at about 4 days after syngamy. Early mitotic divisions lead to totipotential cells that are able to produce all the products of conception. It is during this time that "twinning" becomes possible; by approximately day 7, differentiation leads to cells becoming individualized. The multicellular blastocyst with a tropoectoderm and an inner cell mass initially attaches to the maternal endometrial lining at day 8 or 9 and over the next several days becomes embedded, thereby completing the process of implantation.

By the time of the first missed menstrual period (Fig. 42-2), the primitive streak has been formed in the embryonic disc, embryogenesis is beginning, and a critical time has passed during which up to 50% or more of fertilizations do not complete preembryonic development and implementation successfully. This obviously is a period when the product of conception is at very high risk.

The embryonic period encompasses approximately weeks 3 to 8 and is characterized by the differentiation of all major organs that will be present in the fetus, the newborn, and the adult. Near the beginning of this interval the mother usually becomes aware of cessation of menstruation. Laboratory tests are available that can confirm pregnancy by this time.

During the preembryonic period adverse conditions may cause the death of the products of conception. This often occurs around the time when a menstrual period would have been expected, and fertilization may not be recognized. *Adverse influences during the embryonic period can cause ma-*

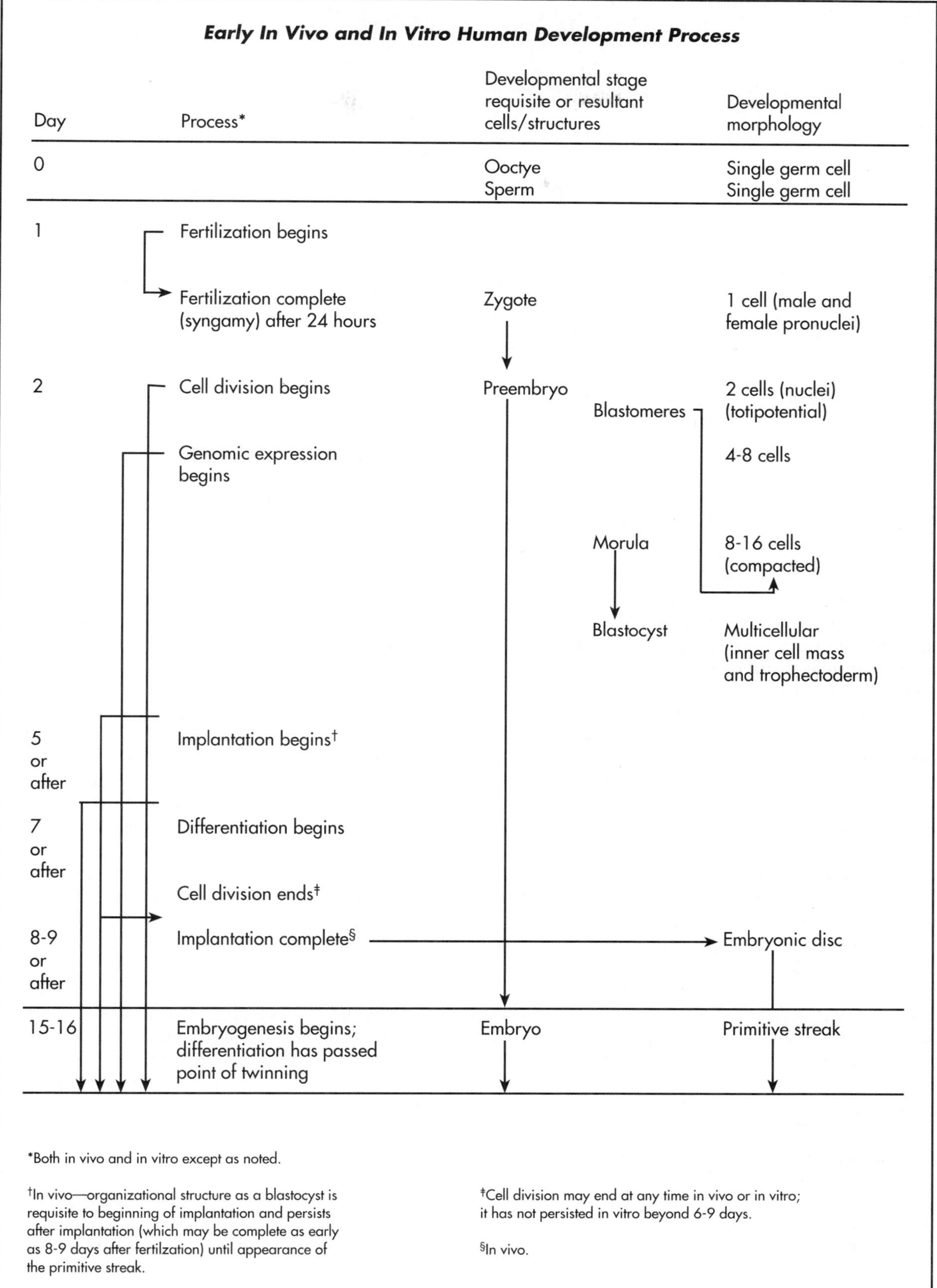

FIG. 42-1 Early in vivo and in vitro human development process.

(From American College of Obstetricians and Gynecologists Preembryo Research: ***History, scientific background, and ethical considerations,*** ACOG Committee Opinion No. 136, Washington, DC, 1994, ACOG.)

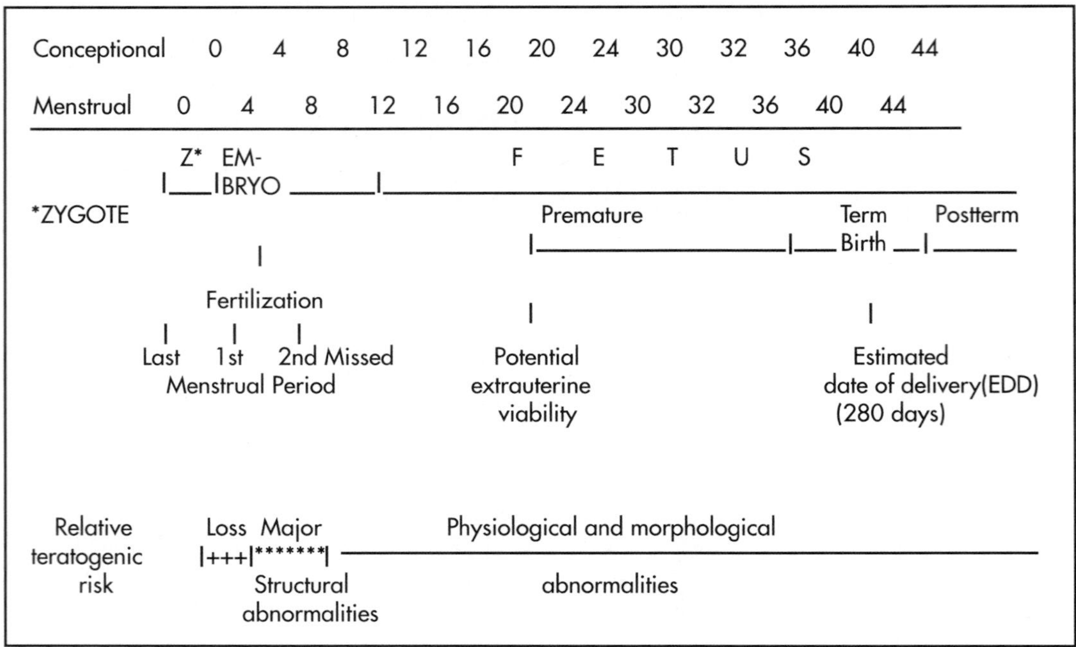

FIG. 42-2 Pregnancy dating and relative teratogenic risk by weeks.

jor and severe interruptions in the pattern of system development, resulting in major congenital anomalies in a surviving fetus. The embryo is recognizable as humanoid toward the end of this period; malformations, such as those of the limbs, resulting, for example, from maternal ingestion of thalidomide, are readily identifiable.

The *fetal period,* the longest of the three periods of the fetal life span, ends with delivery. Growth in size is the most apparent change during this interval, but maturation of organ systems and bodily processes is equally important. The high incidence and problems of premature birth make the degree of organ and enzyme systems maturation of compelling interest to the pediatrician. *The development of pulmonary surfactant probably is the single most important maturational process directly affecting survival in premature infants.*

The late fetal period is the focus of increasingly sophisticated diagnostic techniques. Ultrasonography not only provides images of the fetus but also facilitates invasive procedures, such as amniocentesis, with the result that specimens of amniotic fluid or fetal cells can be obtained with little risk. The pediatrician needs to keep pace with developments in this area, such as intrauterine treatment and, eventually, the addition or modification of genetic material.

INTRAUTERINE GROWTH AND NUTRITION

The physician dealing with the newborn must have a firm conceptual framework of intrauterine growth to evaluate and treat the normal and abnormal newborn effectively. In particular the common clinical problem of prematurity can be managed more appropriately if one appreciates growth patterns as they relate to gestational age.

The growth rate of the fetus is especially rapid during the period from 12 to 16 weeks and again during the final months. Both rapid-growth phases are associated with events of immediate concern for the practitioner. By the end of the sixteenth week after fertilization the size and activity of the fetus have reached a point that both multiparous and primiparous women are able to feel fetal motion. This event, known as *quickening,* is a valuable tool in assessing fetal age and well-being. The late-growth phase can be monitored by several means, including physical examination or the measurement of the height of the fundus above the symphysis.

The period from 8 to 12 weeks after fertilization begins with a fetus whose head makes up almost half of the total length. By 12 weeks the total length has doubled, but the head represents a smaller proportion. The 12- to 16-week interval is characterized by extremely rapid growth in length. In the 17- to 20-week interval growth slows somewhat, but extremities assume their relative proportions. The 21- to 25-week interval after fertilization is characterized by significant gains in both length and weight.

Twenty-one weeks after fertilization, or 23 weeks from the last menstrual period, represents an extremely important milestone. *The potential for extrauterine viability now is recognized to occur at approximately 23 weeks* (by menstrual gestational dating), with neonatal intensive care necessary to sustain the potential.[7,14]

Many studies have attempted to quantify fetal growth through the use of postnatal data. Such growth curves, derived from measuring live-born infants, can give an approximation of intrauterine growth, but they have shortcomings. The fact is that the baseline population is by definition abnormal because the babies were born before term. In addition, the population of premature live births is very difficult to standardize for factors such as race, parity, socioeconomic level, maternal smoking, and maternal disease states.

In spite of all this, intrauterine growth curves derived from

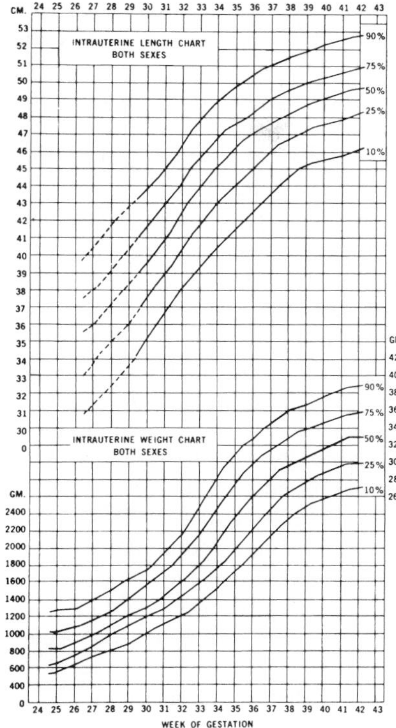

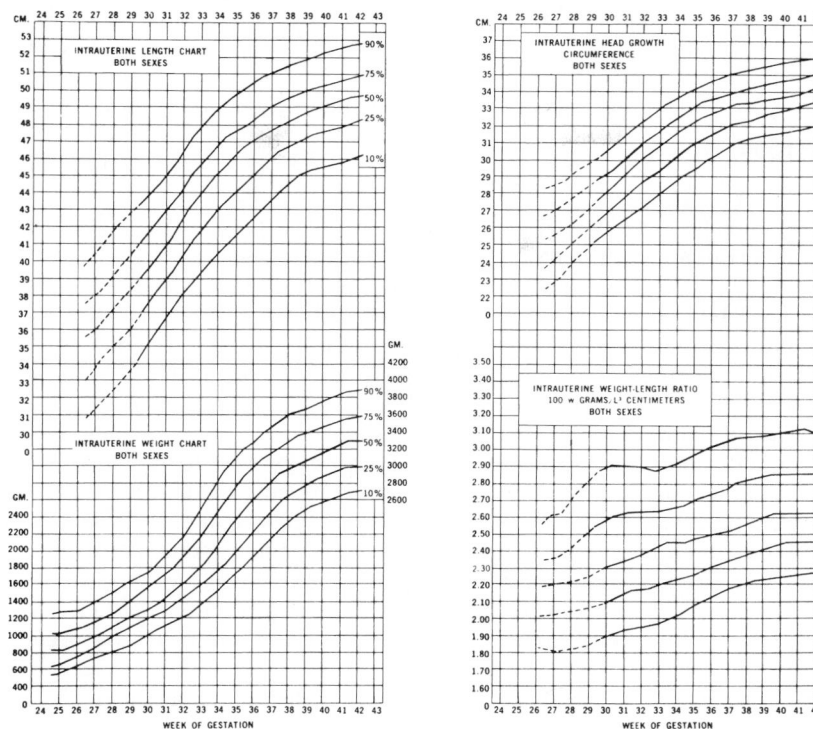

FIG. 42-3 Colorado intrauterine growth charts.
(From Lubchenco LO et al: *Pediatrics* 37:403, 1966.)

postnatal data can be of great clinical assistance. The *Colorado Intrauterine Growth Charts* depicted in Figure 42-3 are among the better known. Percentiles of intrauterine growth for weight, length, and head circumference are given. In addition, a weight-to-length ratio is shown. From weight and length data a *ponderal index* can be derived to depict proportionality. The growth curves in Figure 42-3 were derived from a population of inborn and outborn infants who had mixed racial backgrounds and were living at an altitude of 5000 feet. Intrauterine growth curves derived from live births from other populations show significantly different values, particularly at some of the higher percentiles. However, the basic sigmoid shape of the curve persists.

Intrauterine growth curves for the last trimester of pregnancy can be very helpful in both fetal and neonatal medicine. One cannot assume without reservation that intrauterine growth is a steady process; it is conceivable that growth occurs in bursts of undetermined length. However, monitoring individual fetuses for growth against the baseline of an intrauterine growth scale can be helpful. These graphs also are used widely for risk identification in the immediate neonatal period.

Fetal nutrition can be conceptualized in basic parameters that are quite familiar to the pediatrician. As with the child, two basic processes are under way: accretion of substance for growth or new tissues and oxidation or energy production for metabolism. Growth and development occur as a continuum from fetal to extrauterine existence, but the physiology of nutrition for that continuum changes abruptly at birth when the principal fetal organ for respiration and nutrition (the placenta) gives way to other organs and systems.

Glucose is a primary nutrient for the fetus, with transplacental passage leading to material for energy and for contributions to the fetal carbon pool. Initially, tissue growth is the main location for carbon and other constituents, with the 20-week fetus having little or no fat and about 90% water in its body composition. By term, fetal body water has decreased to about 76%, a figure high by adult standards; fat, a material of high carbon content, approximates 16%. These observations, coupled with the instability of neonatal glucose metabolism when the baby is stressed by infection or other problems, should reinforce the importance of glucose metabolism in the perinatal period and particular respect for the relatively depleted stores of energy in the small premature infant.

Amino acids, both essential and nonessential, are important as building blocks for fetal protein synthesis. The uptake of essential amino acids through the placenta seemingly serves as a basic requirement for growth, yet the fetal ability to synthesize nonessential amino acids leaves the point unclear. Maternal nutritional state and placental function are crucial to fetal well-being and growth; in the neonate amino acids and nitrogen originate with digestion of milk and uptake through the portal venous route.[1]

The clinician dealing with the newborn has to consider the prior fetal nutritional state. Fortunately, if the digestive system of the neonate is unable to function at a level to provide energy and growth, today's physicians have the knowledge and technology available to approximate the fetal state. Total parenteral nutrition effectively returns the baby to the fetal state, where all necessary nutrients, including essential and trace substances, enter directly into the circulation. Although this can be maintained for reasonable intervals, such therapy does have complications, including infection and liver disease, making very long-term parenteral nutrition of the child much more problematic than it is for the fetus.

FETAL SYSTEM FORMATION AND MALFORMATION

Teratology is the study of the etiology, development, structure, and classification of fetal abnormalities. Modern prenatal diagnosis provides information about the presence of structural abnormalities in a large portion of cases well before birth. The pediatrician and other health care providers must be prepared to discuss the teratological process with parents; that discussion increasingly includes management during pregnancy and the peripartum period.

During the first trimester, or in the interval up to 12 weeks after conception or 14 weeks from the last menstrual period, basic organogenesis and system development takes place. Major structural abnormalities can result from adverse influences during this early interval, as seen in congenital heart disease. During later pregnancy more subtle physiological and morphological abnormalities, such as fetal cardiac arrhythmias, may appear.

The causal factors for the vast majority of major malformations and disruptions of system function can be categorized as genetic, intrauterine, maternal conditions, and drugs or other agents. *Genetic factors* have their origin in parental cell lines or in aberrations of initial cellular division after fertilization and are discussed in Chapter 40. Evaluation of risk for genetic disease has advanced rapidly as the techniques for prenatal diagnosis (including fetal cell or tissue sampling) have become increasingly sophisticated. *Intrauterine* factors include problems such as uterine abnormalities, amniotic bands, and umbilical cord or placental problems; resulting structural conditions are said by some to be deformations. *Maternal conditions,* such as diabetes, can be teratogenic (see p. 468); problems with maternal nutrition are of major concern, with the relationship between folic acid deficiency and neural tube defects now well recognized.[4] *Drugs and other agents* are a major concern because of the recognition that practically any drug potentially is teratogenic and the observation that chemical, radiation, or infectious agents may vary in degree of expression, depending on genetic predisposition or gestational age at time of insult. (See discussion in Maternal and Familial Environment and Life-style.)

The major systems are discussed in the following sections, with attention drawn to the gestational time of origin and major types of abnormalities.

Central Nervous System

The central nervous system starts from an ectodermal origin at about day 18 of gestation, and development continues through delivery and long after birth. It is susceptible to teratogenic agents throughout the embryonic and fetal periods and is most susceptible during the first half to two thirds of the embryonic period.

The original neural plate develops into a neural tube that has cranial and caudal ends. The neural tube walls develop to become the brain and spinal cord; the inner part evolves into the ventricles of the brain and the central canal of the spinal cord. Brain development is very complex and passes through stages of a forebrain, midbrain, and hindbrain, with subsequent development of the cerebrum, midbrain structures, pons, and cerebellum. Cells that originally separated from the neural plate and became the neural crest develop into cranial, spinal, and autonomic ganglia, as well as the autonomic nervous system and chromaffin tissue, especially the adrenal medulla.

Malformations of the central nervous system confront the clinician frequently. Some of these defects are among the most grotesque, such as the *anencephalic* baby or infants who have very large *encephaloceles.* Application of technology in the form of assisted ventilation and nutrition to babies who have such problems has been subject to public debate, as has the issue of organ donation.[17] Other anomalies, such as *microcephaly* or cystic lesions in the brain, may be compatible with life for variable lengths of time, but carry extremely bleak prognoses. Congenital malformations of the spinal column, especially those that have defects in overlying tissue, also pose major moral and ethical dilemmas to parents and health professionals, when potentially treatable complications are superimposed on a poor prognosis. Some central nervous system lesions are of known origin, but others, such as *meningomyelocele,* may be the result of interactions between genetic predisposition and extrinsic factors.

Of major concern is the evidence that intrauterine exposure of the developing nervous system to substances such as "crack" cocaine or alcohol results in permanent functional morbidity as well as structural changes. Although morphological and behavioral changes often appear together, thus inviting the postulation of cause and effect, there is no reason to think that the two always are related. Theoretically there may be long-term effects on higher cerebral function and behavior that have no morphological effects, and vice versa.

Cardiovascular System

The cardiovascular system is the first to function, with a rudimentary blood circulation beginning in the third week. Initially two tubes fuse to form a single tube that evolves into the four-chambered heart and great vessels. By the end of the fourth or fifth week partitioning of the chambers is completed, with two atria and two ventricles. Equally complex is the initial formation of a truncus arteriosus, aortic sac, and aortic arches, which evolve by the eighth week into a fetal circulatory pattern. This system undergoes changes in flow patterns during adjustment to extrauterine existence.

Schematic representations of the process whereby the initial pair of tubes forms a single tube with subsequent twisting and formation of chambers and very complex vascular structures—some of which become atretic whereas others become dominant—can help in understanding spatial relationships and the reasons why specific lesions develop. The lymphatic system, which develops in a similar time frame, initially is seen somewhat later than the cardiovascular system. The lymphatics have connections with the venous side of the developing cardiovascular system. *Malformations of the cardiovascular system occur in approximately 7.5 of 1000 live births.* The critical period for teratogenic effects is over relatively early in the intrauterine period, but the process of formation is so complex that a multitude of possibilities for maldevelopment exists. The degree of severity varies considerably.

Some structural malformations, such as the patent foramen ovale type of *atrial septal defect,* may be functional only when another pathological condition exists. The *patent ductus arteriosus (PDA)* as a pathological entity occurs when closure fails after birth; in the fetal state PDA is normal. Early malrotation of the fused cardiac tubes can result in *dextrocardia.* This can occur with an otherwise normal heart and great vessel structures and may not be a clinical problem if complete situs inversus of the viscera also is present. Dextrocardia without situs inversus often is a major problem because of a tendency for associated complex intrinsic abnormalities.

Intracardiac malformations, such as *septal defects,* are very common, especially in the ventricle. Complex problems, with formation of the great vessels evolving from an inappropriate partitioning of the *truncus arteriosus,* also are fairly common. *Coarctation of the aortic arch* is an example of a malformation that may be some distance from the heart itself. Manifestations of malformations can occur in utero and are believed in some instances to result in large-for-gestational-age infants (Fig. 42-4). In severe and relatively rare instances they can produce a form of nonimmune hydrops fetalis.

The pediatrician, pediatric cardiologist, and neonatologist increasingly are becoming involved with cardiac dysfunction before birth. The evaluation of fetal well-being includes that of cardiac status, with the result that problems such as cardiac arrhythmia or cardiac failure can be detected in utero. Fetal echocardiography now can detect specific structural defects. Pregnant women who are themselves healthy are admitted to hospitals for treatment of fetal cardiovascular disease; maternal digitalization of fetal cardiac arrhythmias is an example of fetal treatment through maternal and placental circulation.

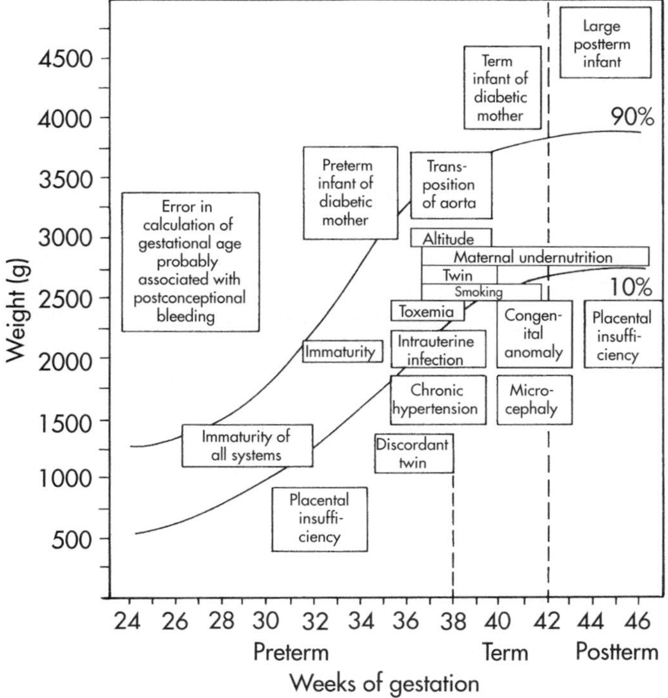

FIG. 42-4 Birth weight and gestational age groupings of selected neonates affected by intrauterine pathophysiological processes.

(From Lubchenco LO: *Major problems in clinical pediatrics,* vol 11, *The high-risk infant,* Philadelphia, 1976, WB Saunders.)

Musculoskeletal System

Formation of the musculoskeletal structures becomes grossly apparent in the embryo by at least the fourth week, when limb buds—first the upper and subsequently the lower—become obvious. Muscle structures originate from mesoderm, much of which arises directly from the somites. Bone evolves from mesoderm that undergoes a process of chondrification. Cardiac muscle and other smooth muscles have a different origin in the splanchnic mesoderm of the primitive gastrointestinal tract. The origin of some muscles, such as those of the iris and extrinsic eye, is unclear. The limb buds elongate while forming bone and large-muscle masses. A process of rotation and growth, in which upper and lower extremities rotate in different directions, results in the muscle groupings and dermatome patterns of the child and adult.

Malformations of the limbs are relatively common; otherwise skeletal and muscular abnormalities are rare. The health professional providing newborn care often is struck by the significant attention paid by parents to the extremities, particularly the hands of newborns. For this reason relatively minor defects can have major emotional significance. *Polydactyly* or *syndactyly* are among the more common human malformations.

Many limb abnormalities are genetic in origin, but some malformations result from genetic predisposition interacting with environmental factors. The thalidomide deformities are a specific and perhaps relatively isolated example of limb teratogenesis.

Gastrointestinal System

The alimentary tract, developing from a primitive anlage seen initially at the fourth week, has three main divisions: foregut, midgut, and hindgut. Each of these has its own specific blood supply in the celiac, superior mesenteric, and inferior mesenteric arteries. Because development of each tract can be traced, abnormalities of the individual divisions are seen. The *foregut,* from the pharynx to the insertion of the common bile duct, develops into various structures, including the intestine and the liver and pancreas. *Midgut* structures include all the small intestines (with the exception of the duodenum before the insertion of the common bile duct) plus the cecum, appendix, ascending colon, and about two thirds of the proximal transverse colon. The midgut structures go through a complex rotation during development, whereby an initial loop develops outside the fetal abdomen and rotates approximately 90 degrees at that time. At approximately the tenth week these midgut intestinal structures return to the abdomen and go through a further complex rotation of 180 degrees, leading to the final anatomical relationships of the intestine. *Hindgut* structures include the transverse, descending, and sigmoid colon and rectum through the final portion of the anal canal, which develops from an anal pit. The cloaca, or early expanded end of the hindgut, and tissues of other origin lead to the perineal structures.

Alimentary tract malformations are fairly common and often are associated with other anomalies. The foregut has an initial tracheoesophageal common origin, with subsequent separation. *Tracheoesophageal fistulas* resulting from errors in formation of the tracheoesophageal septum occur in four basic patterns (see Chapter 48, Critical Neonatal Illnesses); early detection is important to prevent extensive aspiration pneumonitis. Errors of midgut development and malrotation lead to many problems, the most spectacular of which is the lack of return of the bowel to the abdominal cavity, with a resultant *omphalocele*. Other malrotation presentations include acute intestinal obstruction and ischemia in utero or at varying lengths of time after birth, often after initial feedings. Malformations of the intestinal tube in the form of *stenosis, duplication,* or *atresia* are of unclear origin but may result from problems with recanalization or from a compromised vascular supply. Hindgut malformations occur most commonly at the most distal portion, resulting in lack of continuity or *imperforate anus,* stenosis, or membranous conditions. Many other intestinal malformations can be seen. Of special interest is *Meckel diverticulum* (an outpouching in the ileum), representing the remnant of the yolk stalk.

Respiratory System

Respiratory system formation is noteworthy for development that begins at approximately 26 days and goes on long after birth. Initial cell lines arise on the floor of the primitive pharynx and produce a laryngotracheal tube. Endoderm of this tube becomes the lining and glands of the lower respiratory system; connective tissue and cartilage of the respiratory system arise from splanchnic mesoderm.

Further growth of the endotracheal tube results in two lung buds that divide further into two sections on the left and three on the right; these correspond to the adult lobes. Branching continues after this point from the pulmonary segment system. At approximately 5 to 7 weeks after fertilization, a pseudoglandular period exists during which there is major growth of the bronchi and terminal bronchioles.

During an overlapping canalicular period beginning at 13 weeks and continuing to approximately 25 weeks, bronchioles and alveolar ducts develop, and significant vascularization occurs. From 24 weeks until birth, terminal sacs arise and become alveoli. These initially are lined by a cuboidal epithelium, which changes to a squamous form at about 26 weeks of gestation. Alveolar development continues through early childhood.

The enzymatic maturation of systems leading to the production of surfactant does not take place until alveoli are formed. Complex cell types lining the alveoli have been described. A vacuolated cell, the type II pneumocyte, appears to have a secretory function and to be involved in alveolar stabilization through surfactant elaboration.

Anatomical malformations of the respiratory system are unusual but include many dysplastic and cystic abnormalities. The clinician often is confronted with functional problems related closely to the formative status of the lung. For example, an immature lung that is not well into the stage of alveolar formation may be able to support life for only several hours until the immature infant dies from pulmonary insufficiency refractory to present-day treatment. Whether respiratory distress syndrome is present after the birth of a premature baby depends largely on the stage of fetal maturity, with treatment including administration of exogenesis surfactant until endogenous production occurs (see Chapter 48).

Abnormalities in development of the diaphragm, the most common of which is *diaphragmatic hernia,* are most common on the left and often are associated with severe restriction of lung development on one or both sides. Some babies who have diaphragmatic hernia develop pulmonary hypertension, a complication that includes elevated vascular resistance similar to that seen in the fetal state.

Hematopoietic System

Initial red cell formation is seen as early as day 14 after conception, when cells containing embryonic hemoglobin arise from the endothelium of primitive vessels of the yolk sac. Hematopoiesis within the embryo begins in the liver at approximately the sixth week. The liver is the most active site of hematopoiesis for the early part of the fetal life span. The bone marrow assumes the primary role at about the sixth month, and other sites, especially the spleen and lymph nodes, play a contributory role.

Fetal hemoglobin (Hb F) predominates for much of intrauterine existence and under normal circumstances is seen to a small degree in early infancy. Beginning at about the third month some hemoglobin A (Hb A) (5% to 10%) is present, and the proportion of Hb A to Hb F increases rapidly from about 35 weeks to term, when blood is approximately 50% to 65% Hb F. Hb F has an increased oxygen affinity compared with Hb A; this probably is the result of a differing action of 2,3-diphosphoglycerate (2,3-DPG), which facilitates oxygen saturation in the intrauterine environment. Blood group antigens are familial in their determination and can be identified as early as the second month of fetal life. Platelets also are seen at approximately the second month. The presence of hematopoietic abnormalities is important for the clinician to recognize. In the first place, certain *hemoglobinopathies* may result in intrauterine disease. Alpha-thalassemia results in hemoglobin Bart (tetrameric gamma chains), which has a very high oxygen affinity, resulting in intrauterine distress and nonimmune hydrops fetalis. Other hemoglobinopathies, such as homozygous thalassemia and sickle cell disease, can be diagnosed antenatally through analysis of fetal blood. Hemolytic anemia secondary to *maternal-fetal blood group incompatibilities* and transplacental passage of antibody is an immune disease; however, it has a marked effect on hematopoiesis, resulting in erythroblastosis fetalis, an extensive proliferation of hematopoietic tissue. Fetal *thrombocytopenia* may be primarily of fetal origin, or it may be associated with some form of extrinsic agent or process, such as immune antibody of maternal origin or intrauterine infection. Many fetal intrauterine hematological manifestations are part of disease processes involving other systems.

Percutaneous umbilical blood sampling (PUBS) (see p. 465) is clinically useful in many fetal hematological disorders.

Immune System

Immune system components function very early in fetal life, with some parts present as early as the eighth week and with a total rudimentary system capability by the twelfth week. Activation usually does not occur before birth. The cellular immune system originates in liver or spleen stem cells that migrate to the thymus at about the eighth week. These T cells enter the bloodstream and are distributed to the body, mainly to lymph nodes and spleen. The antibody immune system generates IgM in lymphoid tissues as early as the eleventh week and IgG at about the twelfth week. IgA, IgD, and IgE are seen in the fetus in small amounts toward the end of pregnancy. Current thinking suggests that specific immunoglobulin synthesis occurs in a stem or B cell. Passive transfer of maternal antibody has been demonstrated very early in fetal life. Maternal IgG is detectable as early as the fortieth day, and practically all cord IgG is maternal in origin, arising from both passive and active enzymatic transplacental passage. IgM is not transferred passively. The complement system has some fractions present during the embryonic period at the eighth week, and by 12 to 14 weeks of gestation a considerable complement fraction is present. Malformations of the fetal immune system, either of familial or developmental origin, have been described and have contributed to an understanding of the adult system. Abnormalities are believed to exist in all parts of the immune system, and it is important that the clinician understand the basic possibilities because of fetal and neonatal diseases that result. *Fetal graft-versus-host reactions* have been documented after intrauterine transfusions. Congenital infections activate the immune system, with an elevated cord IgM level possibly being evidence of such infections. Transplacental antibody passage with effects on the fetus, as seen in isoimmunization (erythroblastosis fetalis), is the classic clinical example of fetal disease resulting from activation of a maternal immune system response.

Urogenital System

A close interrelationship exists between the development of two basic systems: the urinary (or excretory) system and the genital (or reproductive) system. There are three separate excretory organs in the human embryo: the pronephros, the mesonephros, and the metanephros. The metanephros appears at approximately the fifth week after fertilization, functions 2 to 3 weeks later, and remains as the permanent kidneys. The other two systems involute, with the mesonephros remaining as a few ducts in the male genital tract and as a vestigial remnant in the female. There are two main divisions in the final excretory system. The entire collecting system from the kidney to the bladder originates from the ureteric bud; nephrons arise from the mesodermic-metanephric mass. The kidney tissue appears originally in the early pelvic region and ascends into the abdomen. The bladder develops from the urogenital sinus and splanchnic mesenchyme. Excretory system function is present by approximately the ninth week; theoretically, contributions to amniotic fluid become possible at this time and are definitely a major component later in gestation.

The prospective phenotype of the genital system is determined at fertilization. However, there is an indifferent stage of genital development ending at approximately the seventh week, with the gonads showing specific sexual characteristics. By the twelfth week after fertilization the genitals are distinctly male or female. The Y chromosome appears to be responsible for the differentiation of testes. Masculinizing hormones from the testes stimulate development of mesonephric ducts into genital components and result in the external genitals forming a penis and scrotum. Feminization of the external genitals seemingly occurs in the absence of androgens. Gonadal tissue has its origin in the lateral abdominal wall, with the testes descending into the scrotum late in fetal life.

Malformations of the urogenital system are relatively common and result in a myriad of morphological and microscopical manifestations. Some entities, such as *renal agenesis,* result in intrauterine manifestations, including oligohydramnios, and in morphological changes in the fetus. Other problems may present in the immediate neonatal period. For example, renal abnormalities that result in cystic lesions of the kidneys initially may be detected in the newborn period as abdominal masses found on physical examination or as abnormalities in renal function. Malformations in the vascular supply to the kidneys or the collecting system result in congenital problems such as obstructive uropathy that predispose the person to renal disease that manifests in infancy and childhood. Malformations arising from problems of formation of the urogenital sinus and urachus may be severe, as in *exstrophy of the bladder* or, less obviously, as in fistulas between perineal structures.

Malformations of the genitals also can be complex in origin. Those resulting from errors in the sex-determining mechanism can result in *hermaphrodites,* but such errors are rare. Errors in sexual differentiation, producing *pseudohermaphrodites,* are somewhat more common. The presence of neonatal ambiguous genitalia is a true medical emergency; the *adrenogenital syndrome,* with fetal adrenal androgen excess resulting in masculinization of a female genotype, is one cause of ambiguous genitalia.

Special Considerations

Certain situations of fetal formation and malformation deserve special mention. The special senses, specifically those of *the eyes and ears, are very sensitive to teratogenic activity* and result in profound effects on the developing infant and child. Eye formation begins at the fourth week and proceeds very rapidly, especially through the sixth week. Malformations of the eye and ear may be associated with errors in genetic material; some syndromic conditions have readily identifiable eye and ear malformation patterns. Intrauterine infections, particularly rubella, can affect the eye and inner ear. The external ear migrates up to its final location on the head; errors in position or morphology often are associated with other malformations.

Malformations of the face and palate are of major concern. These have their origin in the embryonic branchial apparatus from which the face, pharynx, and attendant structures develop. Cleft lip often is associated with cleft palate but arises from distinctly different origins. Difficulties in these areas are probably of mixed genetic and environmental causation. The branchial arch merging in the formation of palate structures is most susceptible to teratogenic factors between 6 and 10 weeks of gestation.

FETUS, MOTHER, AND FAMILY

The fetus influences both the mother and the family. Expectations regarding conception and childbearing vary, but the overall viewpoint should be positive. Psychological factors involved in the decision to become pregnant are extremely complex and heavily influenced by the reproductive instinct. More than 50% of all pregnancies in the United States, and a much higher portion of teenage and unmarried pregnancies, are unintended at conception. Psychosocial situations that detract from optimum health before conception should be interpreted as *the beginning of potential fetal risk.*

Many maternal and familial situations of unfortunate familiarity to the physician provide such a negative start for the fetus. A common example is pregnancy in the younger adolescent, who is both physically and emotionally immature and who may not have a stable interpersonal relationship with her male partner. Preconceptual factors interact once fertilization occurs, with a progression of biochemical, physical, and emotional changes that influence mother, father, and family.

These changes, some subtle and some not, alter the previous life. New situations demand behavioral adaptations and a process of coping. If this coping process is successful, major developmental progress has been made, especially by the mother; this usually is true to a lesser extent in the father and to varying degrees in people further removed. But if attitudes and the coping process are unsatisfactory, then in certain situations abortion might be considered.

The first missed menstrual period, an overt sign of change to many women, does not occur until after the period of the dividing zygote essentially is complete. By the time of the second missed menstrual period, the embryonic period is half over. Apparently the *zygotic period is relatively unaffected by teratogens, but the embryonic period is one of very high risk.* Maternal and familial habits potentially injurious to the fetus are difficult to alter under any circumstances and are even more so when the mother does not yet know that she is pregnant. Pregnancy often is not confirmed in the present medical system until after the second missed menstrual period.

The *first trimester* may be the most important phase of adjustment to the fetal presence. Many physical symptoms such as fatigue, nausea, headache, and changes in emotional status may reflect emotional tension. However, there also are complex interactions of psychological stress and physiological change that can involve the autonomic nervous system and produce discomfort. These can alter prior life-style and, if very disruptive, might produce untoward effects because the fetus at this early time has the potential of establishing a very negative set within its future family.

Biochemical relationships between the fetus, its placenta, and the mother are of major interest to the clinician. They form the basis for many tests confirming pregnancy and assessing fetal well-being. The placenta, a fetal organ, plays a very active metabolic role. Theoretically, placental hormones can supply much of the endocrine support that ordinarily originates in the woman's pituitary glands, adrenal cortex, and ovaries. The rare appearance of panhypopituitarism in the postpartum period supports this phenomenon.

Many of these endocrinological processes are of major practical interest to the clinician. *Human chorionic gonadotropin* is produced by trophoblastic cells within a few days of implantation. Concentrations of this substance in maternal blood and urine are highest during the first trimester and decrease through the remainder of pregnancy. Most current early pregnancy tests take advantage of this phenomenon. *Human placental lactogen,* a polypeptide also produced by trophoblastic cells, appears in the serum of pregnant women at about the sixth week of gestation and is present throughout pregnancy. The placenta plays a very active role in the synthesis and metabolism of progesterone and estrogen. End products of estrogen metabolism in the form of maternal *estriol* are the basis for an important test of fetal well-being.

The *second trimester* usually is marked by less overt signs of physical and emotional adjustment. System development in the fetus basically is complete, and major growth is occurring. This leads to the phenomenon of "quickening," when a woman feels fetal movements for the first time. This usually occurs at about week 18 in the primigravida; in the multigravida such movement may be felt 1 to 2 weeks earlier. Quickening undoubtedly represents a major milestone in the relationship between a mother and her fetus. This is the first overt or direct sign of independent fetal activity. Quickening can provide important information about fetal or gestational age. For some women it also serves as a milestone after which abortion is less acceptable.

The *third trimester* is marked by an acceleration of the fetal alteration of life-style. Maternal physical activity, previously undertaken easily, may become increasingly difficult. Sexual activity between parents may be subject to changes or even cessation. Preparation for delivery becomes more of a part of everyday life; childbirth education, financial planning, and other aspects of preparation and emotional adjustment should be in progress. Initially in the third trimester the maternal emotional state largely is oriented toward the fetus; however, as labor and delivery approach, a mother's concern, and very often the father's, tends to become more centered on maternal well-being.

FETUS, HEALTH PROFESSIONAL, AND SOCIETY

There is great concern about the influence of factors such as smoking, alcohol consumption, radiation, and pesticides on the fetus, and researchers continue to develop an objective data base. Societies that advocate preconception care and the introduction of employment, nutritional, and life-style changes for women as soon as they miss a period (or even before conception), may be the most enlightened in terms of fetal advocacy.

Amniocentesis, chorionic villus, and percutaneous umbilical cord sampling (see p. 465) represent procedures of major interest to individuals and society because they enable physicians to detect conditions incompatible with what is considered normal human existence. Moral and ethical concerns over these procedures are related to those associated with an abortion. The debate over abortion and its legalization has brought to the fore concerns about the legal and interpersonal status of the fetus. Health professionals are embroiled in this debate, especially over whether a practitioner of perinatal medicine can oppose abortion personally by not mentioning all alternatives to patients.

Viability, or the capability of a fetus to assume an independent extrauterine existence, is a concept that demands attention and thought. We do know that 22 completed weeks from the last menstrual period is the time at which a few fetuses, if born into an environment where neonatal intensive care is available, can survive.[7,14]

The clinician must be aware of the close approximation of potential viability, gestation limits on legal abortion, and the worrisome, significant variations in clinical estimates of fetal age; under *Roe v. Wade* abortion can be performed legally until 24 weeks, the beginning of viability, but it is not unusual for joint appraisals by mother and physician of gestational age to be erroneous by 2 and perhaps 4 weeks. This is more likely to occur in patients who receive little prenatal care or who have menstrual irregularities.

THE IDENTIFICATION AND MANAGEMENT OF FETAL AND MATERNAL RISK

Any factor that increases the possibility of an adverse outcome for a pregnancy contributes to risk. Medical risk includes physiological, nutritional, obstetrical, and genetic factors. Psychosocial risk includes psychological, social, environmental, and behavioral factors and personal habits. These two broad categories of risk often act concurrently, and individual risks may overlap, accompany, or follow each other.[2] The relationship between risk factors and adverse outcome may be obvious, as with a specific toxic agent such as mercury; more often, however, risk is subtle and cumulative.

Preconception Care

Health before pregnancy has become increasingly recognized as an important determinant of pregnancy outcome. Preparation for pregnancy should begin before conception, including assessment of risk and preventive or therapeutic intervention. The box on the right illustrates the general categories and some specific problems that should be addressed in preconceptional care.

The concept of care before conception is related to, but not exactly the same as, family planning; more is involved than the spacing of pregnancies. Wider acceptance of this concept within society may have a major affect on the outcome of pregnancy in such specific populations as adolescents. The role of the pediatrician in preconception and interconception care recently has been emphasized.[9]

PRECONCEPTION CARE INVENTORY

Family history

Diabetes
Hypertension
Epilepsy
Multiple pregnancies

Genetic history

Disease related to ethnic background (e.g., Tay-Sachs)
Muscular dystrophy
Hemophilia
Cystic fibrosis
Birth defects
Mental retardation

Parental medical history

Diabetes, hypertension, epilepsy
Anemia
Rubella
Specific medical and surgical problems
Possible exposure to sexually transmitted diseases, including AIDS
Immunizations
Allergies
Medications, including over-the-counter
Substance use and abuse
- Alcohol
- Caffeine
- Smoking
- Drugs

Nutrition

Environmental

Occupational exposures
Pets

Modified from American Academy of Pediatrics, American College of Obstetricians: *Guidelines for perinatal care* (Appendix B), ed 2, Elk Grove Village, Ill, 1988, The Academy.

Prenatal Care

A report entitled *Caring for Our Future: The Content of Prenatal Care* published by the U.S. Department of Health and Human Services (HHS) in 1989 defines the three basic components of prenatal care as (1) early and continuing risk assessment, (2) health promotion, and (3) medical and psychosocial interventions and follow-up.[2]

Previous discussion has emphasized that during the prenatal period the fetus is undergoing rapid and continuous growth and development. Anything that jeopardizes that process must be recognized as a fetal risk factor and subjected to assessment. Major contributors to fetal risk are listed in the box on p. 464.

There is little doubt that prenatal care results in healthier babies and mothers. Much of the original interest in and emphasis on prenatal care involved pregnancy-induced hypertension (PIH) and the use of periodic blood pressure determinations. Standardized schedules (with details such as number and timing of visits, procedures, and studies) are available. In addition, the aforementioned HHS report offers suggestions, including the addition of preconception care to traditional prenatal care.

Assessing Fetal Status Before Labor

The clinician is obligated to make every effort to identify risk and practice *expectant fetal medicine.* Pediatricians must be familiar with the basic principles of techniques used to gather information concerning high-risk pregnancies and deliveries in which they are involved as members of the perinatal care team. Fetal history, structure and growth, heart rate, and amniotic fluid and fetal blood analyses provide the basis for the majority of these methods. Some are noninvasive; they have been included in obstetrical practice for years and provide statistically valid information—for example, history taking and measurement of uterine size. They are used as screening procedures that may indicate a need for other investigative techniques, such as those discussed next.

Fetal Activity. Quickening can be valuable in confirming length of pregnancy. *The duration, amplitude, and frequency*

MAJOR CONTRIBUTORS TO FETAL RISK

Genetic

Chromosome abnormalities
Inherited traits

Maternal-familial environment and life-style

Socioeconomic status
Social environment
Physical environment
  Radiation
  Teratogens
Nutrition
Smoking or secondary exposure to smoke
Drugs or alcohol abuse
Lack of prenatal care

Maternal reproductive capability and health

Age, weight, height
Reproductive tract abnormalities
Maternal medical disorders
  Cardiac
  Respiratory
  Renal
  Hematological (e.g., sickle cell disease)
  Metabolic (e.g., diabetes, thyroid disorders, phenylketonuria)
  Epilepsy
Emotional status

Placenta and membrane disorders

Implantation (abdominal, tubal, previa)
Vessel and cord complications
Abruption
Premature rupture of membranes (PROM) and infection

Maternal-fetal unit

Multiple gestation
Obstetrical complications
  Malposition and malpresentation
  Cephalopelvic disproportion
Abnormal fetal growth and gestation
Isoimmunization (erythroblastosis fetalis)
Intrauterine infections
Pregnancy-induced hypertension

of fetal movement after quickening and in the third trimester can provide important information about fetal well-being. An inactive fetus may be chronically compromised. Rapid onset of inactivity in a previously active fetus can be ominous. Assessment of fetal activity lacks standardization and specificity for cause but is of clinical value.

Fetal Heart Rate. The normal fetal heart rate (FHR) settles in the 120 to 160 beats/min range by the last trimester and is monitored easily by use of a stethoscope (fetoscope) or an electronically amplified device. Electronic fetal monitoring is used widely but has not been shown conclusively to be more efficacious than listening, despite many studies. FHR monitoring most commonly is used for evaluation of fetal status during labor but can help in prenatal assessment.

Bradycardia, especially less than 100 beats/min, is of concern because of an association with acute or chronic distress. Explanation for its presence must be sought. The list of possible causes is long and includes many that have a poor outcome, such as placental insufficiency. An intrinsic fetal cause, heart block, is not as ominous. *Tachycardia* usually occurs as an autonomic response to stimulation and can indicate fetal normality. It may be associated with a maternal condition, such as pyrexia. Intrinsic fetal arrhythmias, such as supraventricular tachycardia, can result in secondary manifestations, including hydrops fetalis.

Uterine Size. The uterus and the products of conception are monitored closely during prenatal care. Measurements of fundal height above the symphysis are obtained and plotted. The umbilicus is reached by 20 to 22 weeks. Deviations from the expected curve may indicate a number of abnormal and high-risk states.

Fundal height at a level greater than expected may be the result of a miscalculation of dates, with the pregnancy being further along than anticipated. Another relatively straightforward cause of unexpectedly large uterine size is multiple pregnancy. Conversely, fetal causes of smaller than expected uterine size include pregnancy less advanced than anticipated and many problems that lead to *intrauterine growth retardation* (IUGR).

Amniotic fluid volume deviations, in the form of oligohydramnios or polyhydramnios, may be detected initially by abnormal uterine size or fundal height. Confirmation and further study by ultrasonography should follow, because imaging by ultrasound can estimate the volume of fluid present and assess fetal structures.

Under normal circumstances amniotic fluid volume increases until 40 weeks and then decreases. *Oligohydramnios* thus can be associated with postterm and postmature pregnancies. The pediatrician also needs to be alert to situations in preterm pregnancies in which oligohydramnios occurs, inasmuch as this may be associated with a number of disease processes, including IUGR and renal abnormalities in which renal excretion is severely compromised. Renal agenesis (Potter syndrome) or dysplasia and structural and functional renal problems may not become evident until after birth.

Polyhydramnios may result from maternal problems, such as eclampsia or diabetes, or from fetal causes. The pediatrician immediately should suspect fetal and neonatal abnormalities of the gastrointestinal tract, such as esophageal or intestinal obstruction. Normal circulation of amniotic fluid is interrupted on the absorptive side of the loop in these conditions, and the baby will require special attention at birth and probably surgical intervention.

Ultrasonography. Clinical ultrasound has had a profound effect on all aspects of perinatal medicine. A transducer, acoustically linked to the skin surface by a gel, transmits ultrasonic vibrations, and the returning sound echoes are processed electronically to produce a two-dimensional pictorial "slice" of the organs being imaged.

Types of ultrasound used in obstetrics are listed in Table 42-1. B-scan systems with their pulsed cross-sectional images of tissue are assuming remarkable clarity. When images

Table 42-1 Types of Obstetrical Ultrasound

Type	Wave	Use
A-scan	Unidirectional	Historical interest; displays distance (e.g., fetal biparietal diameter)
B-scan	Cross sectional, pulsed	Displays composite image (e.g., fetal skull or placenta)
Real-time imaging	As in B-scan	Displays continuous changes in spatial configuration (i.e., fetal motion)
Doppler	Usually continuous	Detects and measures blood flow or heart rate; energy input may be high with prolonged use

are presented sequentially faster than the flicker rate of the eye, real-time "movie" imaging occurs, documenting motion. Doppler ultrasound usually is used clinically to monitor fetal heart rate.

All areas of reproductive medicine have been influenced directly by ultrasound technology. *Fetal growth and development* can be monitored for *structural abnormalities* and growth rate. Structural normality of maternal reproductive organs can be documented, as can placental site. The potential medical and economic benefits of ultrasound in pregnancy are so extensive that many individual authorities and some European health care systems advocate routine screening in all pregnancies.

Although no clinically significant untoward effects have been documented in humans, biological effects might be structural (morphological) or functional, and at the energy levels used in most clinical imaging, the possibility of risk cannot be eliminated. Doppler ultrasound theoretically has greater potential for harm because of the continuous, rather than pulsed, wave and the amount of time such devices may be used.

Indications for use of diagnostic ultrasound imaging in pregnancy were addressed by a National Institute of Health Consensus Development Conference in 1984.[5] The panel concluded that when there is an accepted medical indication, ultrasound improves pregnancy management and outcome. A large number of specific clinical situations were mentioned. Routine screening, identification of fetal sex, educational purposes, and parental desire to see their fetus were not considered appropriate reasons for imaging because of possible risk and ethical concerns.

Amniocentesis. Amniotic fluid bathes the fetus, is swallowed by the fetus, and contains fetal cells, urine, and other substances. The technique for obtaining a specimen of this fluid by percutaneous aspiration has been made safer and more successful by the use of real-time ultrasonography.

Diagnostic amniocentesis at 14 to 15 weeks of gestation in conjunction with ultrasonography confirms placental localization, fetal size, and gestational age, in addition to providing information obtained from fluid analysis. Evaluation of fetal cells through *karyotyping* can detect chromosomal abnormalities before potential extrauterine viability, and abortion can be considered. Molecular genetic studies on DNA extracted from fetal cells are expanding so rapidly that the pediatrician is advised to contact a genetic center to determine if prenatal testing has become available for a specific disorder.[13] Neural tube defects can be diagnosed by evaluation of maternal serum and amniotic fluid *alpha-fetoprotein*.

Chorionic Villus Sampling (CVS). This technique involves ultrasound-directed aspiration of trophoblastic tissue surrounding the gestational sac during the first trimester. The approach can be transcervical, vaginal, or abdominal. Transcervical sampling commonly is done at 10 to 12 completed gestational weeks, thereby providing information earlier than does amniocentesis.

A study of the safety and efficacy of transcervical CVS for early prenatal diagnosis of cytogenetic abnormalities concluded that it may have a somewhat higher risk of procedure failure, maternal complication, and fetal loss than does amniocentesis.[15] There are, however, major advantages (e.g., *rapid karyotyping*) to first- versus second-trimester diagnosis if intervention is contemplated. Furthermore, the additional risk associated with CVS seemingly is small and may decrease as experience with the technique expands. There is some concern that CVS conducted before 9 weeks may be of higher risk.

Percutaneous Umbilical Blood Sampling (PUBS or Cordocentesis). Direct aspiration of fetal blood by means of a needle placed transabdominally through maternal skin and into a fetal blood vessel is another technique facilitated by ultrasound that has improved fetal diagnosis and therapy significantly. Sampling is possible from about 17 weeks to term with greater apparent safety than with other techniques. *Fetoscopy* has a complication rate of 4% to 5%, *fetal scalp sampling* requires labor and cervical dilation, and placental aspiration results in contamination with maternal blood in more than 50% of attempts.

Common diagnostic indications for PUBS are the need for *rapid fetal karyotype* and evaluation of fetal isoimmune hemolytic disease. The main treatment is *transfusion for fetal anemia*. The PUBS technique is useful because it provides immediate fetal blood specimens for study of hemoglobin, platelets, blood gases, and other parameters in the same fashion as studies in the neonate. Risk is a concern, with fetal loss a possibility. Currently, this is a technique that requires sophisticated technology and expertise.[8]

Nonstress and Contraction Stress Tests. The pediatrician or other provider of newborn care frequently is confronted with information obtained during evaluation of fetal well-being. Tests that record FHR and the presence, absence, or temporal sequence of uterine contractions are used extensively. The FHR is driven by neurogenic reflex mechanisms similar to those seen in newborns.

The nonstress test (NST) is used when a pregnant patient is not in labor. The interrelationship between FHR and movement or spontaneous uterine contractions is observed. Such testing can begin at 26 to 28 weeks but usually is performed closer to term and if a risk factor has been identified. This simple, easily repeated test can provide valuable information. A normal or reactive NST has two or more accelerations of the FHR in 10 to 20 minutes along with normal baseline rate and variability (120 to 160 beats/min, 5 to 15 beats/min). A nonreactive or abnormal NST is defined as one that does not meet standardized criteria and that may show decelerations.

The *contraction stress test (CST)*, or *oxytocin challenge test (OCT)*, uses oxytocin-stimulated uterine contractions and FHR response. The NST is used more commonly; the CST is employed by some physicians only after a nonreactive (abnormal) NST result. The presence of repeated late decelerations is considered problematic. Interpretations can be difficult, and there are relative and absolute contraindications for performing CST, along with an appreciable high false positive rate. Interpretation requires experience. Nipple stimulation rather than oxytocin challenge is used by some practitioners to induce uterine contractions.

Fetal Biophysical Profile. Fetal well-being can be assessed through the use of multiple parameters collated in a standardized fashion. Items such as muscle tone, body movement, breathing movement, amniotic fluid volume, and results of the NST can be identified, and a score can be derived in a fashion similar to that for determining an Apgar score. The use of multiple noninvasive procedures to assess fetal status is being refined constantly.

Fetoscopy. This technique involves introduction of a small optical viewing instrument into the amniotic cavity, using real-time ultrasound to assist the physician in the procedure. Fetoscopy is difficult, and its place in clinical medicine currently is diminishing as other techniques prove efficacious.

MATERNAL NUTRITION, FAMILIAL ENVIRONMENT, AND LIFE-STYLE

Many authorities have pointed to socioeconomic status and social environment as causes of fetal risk. Delineation of specific influences is difficult, but *poverty* undoubtedly is important, as are *nutrition* and *hygiene*. Intrauterine infection is more frequent in mothers of lower socioeconomic status. Emotional influences on fetal wastage have been discussed, and the possibility that medical or socioeconomic deprivation contributes cannot be discounted.

Maternal Nutrition

Maternal nutritional disorders represent a definite risk to the fetus, including situations in which gross deprivation is not apparent. The supply of substrate to the fetus for growth originates with the maternal circulation and passes through an interface with fetal tissue at the placenta. Placental insufficiency can result in intrauterine growth retardation (IUGR) that is not of maternal origin. The relation between maternal and fetal nutrition is complex. Maternal dietary changes usually do not directly or rapidly influence fetal well-being; thus the positive or negative effects of changes in maternal nutrition are not recognized easily. Maternal weight is an important but not overriding concern.[16]

Traditionally two types of nutritional deficiency have been conceptualized: *general caloric or energy-related deficiency states* and *specific deficiencies*. Deprivation of maternal caloric intake to the point where fetal growth is markedly impaired also may be associated with specific deficiencies. If maternal caloric deprivation is severe, fertility is decreased.

Women whose prepregnancy weight is below standard for height tend to have babies whose weight is less than expected. Women who are obese tend to have babies of higher weight. Problems such as hyperemesis gravidarum can be sufficient to result in fetal caloric deprivation. The expression during reproductive years of eating disorders that often start during late childhood and adolescence, such as anorexia, is a possible fetal risk.

Specific deficiencies are well-recognized, and their risk to the fetus can be reduced through public health and individual clinical interventions. Vitamin deficiency has been of interest, and problems such as congenital beriberi (lack of thiamin) and infant calcium disorders (maternal vitamin D lack) are of historic and decreasing incidence. Recent studies have confirmed that neural tube defects can be reduced by consuming folic acid, with the best protection being achieved when 0.4 mg is ingested from at least 1 month before conception through the first month of pregnancy.

Minerals are a major concern in pregnancy. Iodine deficiency is said to be the most common cause of preventable mental deficiency in the world; treatment during pregnancy protects the fetal brain, with later treatment being much less beneficial to neurological status.[18] Zinc deficiency also may be associated with anomalies. Maternal anemia caused by reduced availability of iron is well known; the fetus and infant as a result can have low iron stores, making the infant susceptible to iron deficiency if intake after birth is inadequate.

Environmental factors, such as radiation, chemicals, and drugs, affect all socioeconomic classes. *Radiation* exposure in mammals causes fetal death, growth retardation, and congenital malformation, with the central nervous system commonly affected. The relationship between embryonic or fetal irradiation and carcinogenesis is unclear. Effects are both dose and rate related. Death during the preimplantation period, malformation during early organogenesis, and cell deletion and hypoplasia during fetal life form a general pattern in animal studies. There are guidelines for limiting radiation to the embryo and fetus during occupational exposure or elective diagnostic techniques; however, dilemmas often arise as a result of lack of foreknowledge about pregnancy, nonelective medical evaluations, and emotional factors. When necessary, a radiation therapist should be consulted.

Chemicals in the environment are of natural and synthetic origin, with the latter being of greater concern. Certain substances, such as pesticides and mercury, have received publicity, but a hidden teratogenic potential exists that needs further elucidation. Many agents are potentially more toxic to the embryo, fetus, and neonate than to older children and adults.

Drugs and Other Substances

Drug use during pregnancy is extensive and may be on the rise. The physician must be concerned about all types: legitimate (nonprescription and prescription), social, illegal, and abusive. All health care providers and especially the primary care physician should recognize that the concept of the placenta as an effective barrier between maternal and fetal circulation has been discarded.

Maternal-fetal pharmacology is complex (Fig. 42-5), with the placenta serving as an organ of exchange. Placental diffusing capability or permeability of the simple variety is operative for many substances with facilitated diffusion (car-

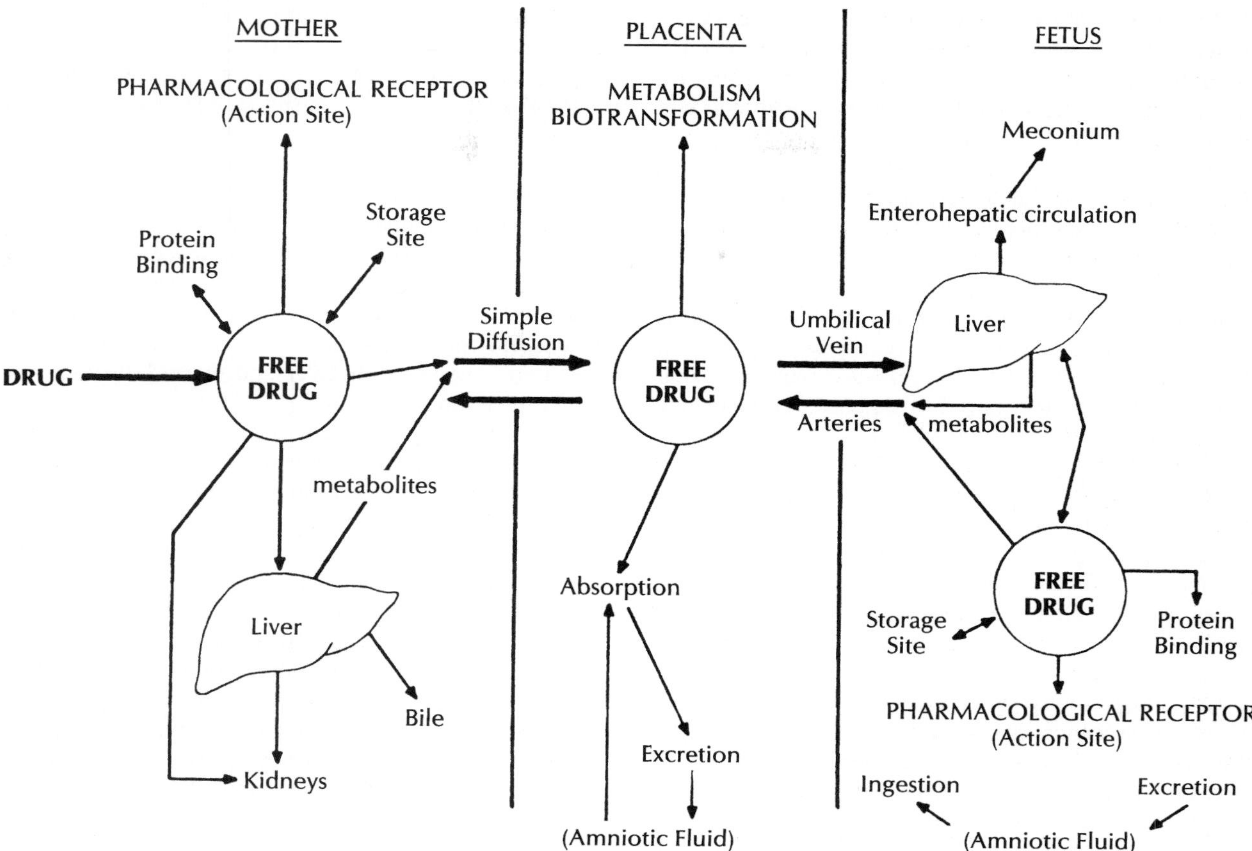

FIG. 42-5 Schematic diagram of movement of drugs between maternal and fetal circulations.
(From Rayburn WF, Anderson BD: *Principles of perinatal pharmacology.* In Rayburn WF, Zuspan FP, editors: *Drug therapy in obstetrics and gynecology,* Norwalk, Conn, 1982, Appleton-Century-Crofts.)

rier dependent); energy-utilizing transport is also important. Virtually all drugs in the maternal circulation should be assumed to cross the placenta and all should be considered potentially teratogenic. The risk to the fetus depends on a number of factors, including concentration, length of exposure, and time of exposure during gestation.

Therapeutic agents, both prescribed and nonprescribed, may be taken before pregnancy is recognized, thereby placing the products of conception at risk during the period of organogenesis in early gestation. An important benefit of preconception or interconception care is the opportunity to identify medication uses that are necessary, such as anticonvulsants, or desirable, such as nonnarcotic analgesics, and monitor or modify exposure. Examples of problems include fetal hydantoin syndrome and the potential effects on the mother and fetus of aspirin, including clotting abnormalities and disruption of prostaglandin synthesis.

Many of the therapeutic agents indicated during the course of pregnancy and delivery require judicious use because of known and potential risks. Antimicrobials are necessary when treating maternal conditions, such as urinary tract or gynecological conditions, but must be used with the knowledge that well-recognized fetal problems can result, such as bone and dental problems associated with fetal tetracycline exposure and the potential hearing problems of fetal aminoglycoside toxicity. Cardiovascular medications that cross the placenta readily, such as digitalis, can be used to treat the fetus and can cause fetal problems. Pediatricians must know the effects of obstetrical drugs including narcotics, oxytocin, and magnesium sulfate, which can cause depression of respiration, hyperbilirubinemia, and hypotonia, respectively.

Socially used and abused drugs are very well known to pediatricians for their deleterious effect on the fetus, newborn, child, and adult. Mothers who smoke have babies that are smaller than those of nonsmokers by an average of 200 g. Varied active agents in smoke, such as carbon monoxide and nicotine, have physiological effects; although studies to document long-term negative neurodevelopmental outcomes have given mixed results, the clear medical consensus is that smoking must be considered a health hazard for the fetus and newborn. Alcohol has been mentioned elsewhere for its association with fetal alcohol syndrome (FAS). Alcohol consumption during pregnancy should be discouraged, especially during the first trimester, although it is difficult to demonstrate deleterious effects of small amounts.

Addictive drug use during pregnancy creates major medical and societal problems of seemingly increasing and endlessly complex proportions. Many if not most users have risk factors, such as poor nutrition or lack of prenatal care, that present risk irrespective of the agent. Heroin is known to reach the fetus soon after maternal use, with intrauterine dependency and withdrawal recognized. Cocaine is considered to be responsible directly or indirectly for many admissions to NICUs. It can result in maternal and placental problems such as abruption that compromise the fetus as well as directly affect fetal and neonatal systems, including the cardiovascular and neurological. Investigative efforts to characterize and quantify long-term neurodevelopmental effects are ongoing (see Chapter 49, Neonatal Drug Abstinence Syndrome).

Identification of environmental and life-style risk relies largely on the maternal medical history. When specific factors such as radiation or chemical exposure are detected, assessment of fetal well-being, especially growth and morphology, might be helpful. In many situations, however, decisions to continue, interrupt, or enhance pregnancies are made on the basis of nebulous possible fetal effects, involve parental emotions, and require "art" more than science in the practice of fetal medicine.

Maternal Reproductive Capability and Health

Certain maternal factors result in risk to the fetus, regardless of the nature of the products of conception. Pregnancy can produce physiological changes in the mother that may affect preexisting maternal conditions adversely, thereby jeopardizing the fetus.

Maternal biological factors such as age, weight, height, race, parity, and previous obstetrical history affect fetal risk directly. Age in particular has been demonstrated to relate to perinatal mortality, with minimal risk occurring between 20 and 30 years of age. Weight and height are related to maternal nutrition, socioeconomic status, and other variables; they may jeopardize the fetus by increasing the incidence of prematurity or intrapartum complications. Race is a complex factor having socioeconomic determinants; some congenital anomalies and medical conditions may be racially predisposed. Maternal reproductive tract abnormalities, such as congenital malformations, frequently are associated with fetal wastage by spontaneous abortion or prematurity. *Cervical incompetence* occurs in 1 of 500 to 600 pregnancies and can result in premature delivery. The interval between pregnancies is an important contributor to the risk of low birth weights.

Maternal medical disorders carry a significant risk to fetus and mother. Cyanotic congenital heart disease in a mother has a clear relationship to fetal problems, with intrauterine growth retardation and premature delivery resulting frequently. Elective abortion is a consideration, if maternal cardiac decompensation later in pregnancy is anticipated. Asthma in pregnancy can threaten mother and fetus. Tuberculosis demands aggressive management of maternal disease and of potential fetal exposure to drugs. Pregnancy is being seen more frequently in women who have cystic fibrosis, with the fetus being exposed to medications, maternal pulmonary insufficiency, and atypical labor and delivery.

Renal disease is a frequent occurrence in pregnancy. Fetal risk increases markedly in the presence of infection or hypertension. Hypertension can result in placental changes and in intrauterine growth retardation. Fetal mortality and morbidity, resulting from second-trimester abortion and prematurity, are associated with urinary tract infections. The risk to the fetus in the event of renal transplantation is not clear; many do very well, even if the mother is being treated with corticosteroids.

Hematological maternal problems are very common. In developing countries *anemia* has been demonstrated to correlate with low birth weight; the effect of moderate maternal iron and folic acid deficiency on the fetus is unclear. Some hemoglobinopathies can increase fetal mortality and morbidity profoundly, either as a result of maternal health status or of fetal disease. Pregnant patients who have sickle cell disease have a fetal wastage rate of one in three. Sensitization problems (Rh, ABO) are discussed in Chapter 40.

Maternal metabolic disorders can be significant for the fetus. The interaction of mother and fetus seems limitless; compounds are metabolized actively on both sides of the placenta. In addition, fetal organogenesis and development may be affected, and end organs may respond to maternal abnormalities. Two conditions, diabetes and thyroid disorder, deserve special mention.

Diabetes in pregnancy causes a myriad of fetal complications, including death (stillbirth), increased frequency of congenital anomalies, macrosomia (a large-for-gestational-age [LGA]) state characterized by an increase in fat but not in total body water), and conversely, growth retardation in a small number of infants. Evidence suggests that fetal pulmonary and neurological maturity may be delayed in these pregnancies. In addition, obstetrical problems, including preeclampsia, hydramnios, and intrapartum complications resulting from excessive size, increase risk further. As discussed previously glucose is a primary metabolite of the fetus. Pregnancies complicated by diabetes probably cause fluctuations in maternal-fetal glucose and potential fetal hyperinsulinism and hypoglycemia. These fetuses have an increase in pancreatic islet tissue. Fetal hyperinsulinism may have a growth hormone effect that results in macrosomia. More severe degrees of maternal diabetes may result in smaller fetuses because of placental insufficiency and fetal nutritional deficit rather than macrosomia. Close control of maternal diabetes results in a better overall perinatal outcome.

Maternal thyroid disease is much less common than diabetes but also has profound fetal effects. Fetal thyroid function appears by 12 weeks of gestation; thyroxine and triiodothyronine probably can cross the placenta in small amounts in either direction. The effect of maternal hypothyroidism on the fetus is unclear, but evidence suggests that fetal nervous system development may be affected negatively; IQs in offspring also are lower. Abortions, stillbirths, anomalies, and prematurity are associated with hypothyroidism. Hyperthyroidism, when untreated, increases fetal wastage. In addition, treatment carries a definite fetal risk because antithyroid drugs may affect the fetal thyroid, and surgical intervention carries an operative risk to fetus and mother. Postoperative treatment with thyroid-replacement therapy may minimize fetal complications.

Although *seizure disorders* are common, their course during pregnancy is difficult to predict with certainty. The status of approximately half of those affected is unchanged, and of the remaining number, half improve and half become worse. Destabilizing seizure manifestations, as in status epilepticus, are an emergency for the mother and fetus. Unfortunately there appears to be an increased incidence of congenital anomalies among infants of mothers who have seizure disorders, even with cessation of an anticonvulsant medication. Some anticonvulsants, such as trimethadione and valproic acid, clearly seem teratogenic. Phenytoin has been linked with a fetal hydantoin syndrome, although the actual incidence is much debated. Phenobarbital, carbamazepine, and other medications may increase risk because of their possible broad-based impact on fetal enzymatic systems.

Seizures that appear de novo in pregnancy must be evaluated thoroughly. *Eclampsia* usually manifests with other signs and symptoms but is associated with a high incidence of fetal and neonatal complications (see Pregnancy-induced Hypertension).

Maternal emotional status has too complex a relationship with physical and familial status to be used as a specific fetal risk factor in most situations. Whether maternal emotional illness, not related to pregnancy, can affect the fetus directly is unclear. Pregnancy-caused or pregnancy-aggravated crises leading to abortion, drug abuse, or poor maternal nutrition can generate obvious fetal consequences. *Hyperemesis gravidarum,* an entity of unclear but perhaps emotional origin, can result in profound maternal malnutrition and fetal growth retardation.

Placenta and Membrane Disorders

The placenta and associated membranes are fetal tissue on which the fetus depends for respiration, nutrition, protection, and other functions. Manifestations of placental disease are diverse and severe and include fetal death, distress, hypoxia, shock, anemia, polycythemia, infection, congenital anomalies, and neoplasia.

The *implantation site* normally is in the upper uterus but may be in the lower segment, in the tubes, or rarely in the abdominal cavity. Maternal anatomical factors may contribute to abnormal implantations. Abdominal and tubal (ectopic) pregnancies are potential disasters for both mother and fetus; with the exception of a rare surviving abdominal fetus, fetal wastage nearly is uniform, and maternal mortality and morbidity are common.

Placenta previa is associated with multiparity and places the fetus at risk in the event of hemorrhage; premature delivery, often by cesarean section, is necessary. *Abruption of the placenta* often is associated with maternal problems, including toxemia, hypertension, renal disease, and multiparity. Sudden fetal demise may occur in extensive separation, with lesser degrees resulting in hypoxia and acute fetal stress. Bleeding from placenta previa and abruption usually is maternal, but in a minority can be fetal and sufficient to cause fetal hypovolemia and anemia.

Cord abnormalities are unusual but may have severe consequences. A short umbilical cord may be complicated by abruption. True knots are present in 2% of deliveries and increase perinatal losses twofold. *Vasa previa, velamentous insertion,* or *circumvallate placenta* are difficult to identify before labor and can result in fetal exsanguination. Vascular abnormalities within the main placental structure occur rarely; fetal risk in monozygous multiple pregnancy includes the possibility of *twin-to-twin transfusion syndrome,* in which arteriovenous vascular anastomoses result in blood flow between fetuses and in severe circulatory problems for one or both, recipient and donor.

Vascular abnormality of the cord itself frequently is observed (1% of pregnancies) as a two-vessel cord with a single umbilical artery. Contrary to prior opinion no particular fetal abnormalities currently are thought to be associated with a two-vessel cord.

Premature, or prolonged, rupture of membranes (PROM) is a major contributor to perinatal mortality and morbidity. It often is defined as rupture that occurs an hour or more before onset of labor; it usually is spontaneous but may be accidental during an examination or artificial for induction of labor. Regardless of classification, the perinatal care team must be aware that an inevitable process of increased fetal risk begins soon after rupture and that prospective treatment protocols are desirable. Most protocols stipulate evaluation and treatment in relation to intervals since rupture. Many authorities consider 24 hours after rupture of membranes to be the beginning of accelerated risk.

The primary cause of fetal and maternal morbidity and mortality in PROM is sepsis. At term, labor occurs within 24 hours of rupture in 80% of pregnancies; in preterm pregnancies, labor begins within 24 hours in less than 50%. Prolonged rupture of membranes with 24 hours or more elapsed before delivery is much more common in preterm pregnancies. The cause of spontaneous rupture often is not clear, and with the exception of entities such as incompetent cervix, statistical correlation and prior risk identification are unsuccessful.

The frequency and degree of inflammation of membranes, cord, or fetus vary directly with time and onset of labor. Infection apparently ascends to the fetus through the cervix, with labor accelerating the process. Antibiotics are of uncertain effectiveness before delivery.

A dilemma in fetal risk assessment occurs in the PROM pregnancy that is significantly preterm. The fetus in this situation is at risk not only from infection but also from premature birth and its complications, especially respiratory distress syndrome (RDS). On the other hand there is an unresolved debate about whether PROM results in acceleration of fetal lung maturity and therefore decreased RDS. The clinician has available prepartum agents (corticosteroids) that seem to accelerate pulmonary maturity in certain situations and improve postpartum status overall in certain populations. A 1994 NIH Consensus Development Conference recommended antenatal treatment with corticosteroids for all fetuses between 24 and 34 weeks at risk for preterm delivery.[6]

Maternal-Fetal Unit

Fetal risk and poor perinatal outcome frequently are associated with pathophysiological processes in which both mother and fetus play an integral role. Causality in some situations is well understood, as in, for example, isoimmunization. There also are situations such as toxemia in which causality is not yet clear.

Premature Birth. Prematurity and its complications are the prime contributors to perinatal mortality and morbidity. Only birth asphyxia challenges this entity as a common cause for prompt skilled intervention by providers of newborn care. These providers must understand the relationship between prematurity (gestational age) and low birth weight. The problems of prematurity and low birth weight are similar but not identical (see Chapter 44, Three, Recovery Period).

Prevention and management of premature birth has been and remains a primary objective of perinatal care providers. Prematurity probably is multifactorial in origin, and causality will remain unclear for the foreseeable future, inasmuch as the precise mechanisms that cause labor have yet to be elucidated. Many of the factors listed in the box on p. 464 as contributors to fetal risk precipitate adverse outcomes directly or indirectly through premature birth.[3,12]

Pharmacological Intervention. Tocolysis, or inhibition of uterine activity, is therapy directed at preventing premature birth once labor has begun. Pharmacological agents have been used with this intent for some time but with limited or minimal success. Progesterone and ethanol once were used extensively but have been replaced by more promising agents.

The theoretical basis for the use of *beta-mimetic drugs* as tocolytics is their inhibitory effect on uterine contractions through activation of beta-adrenergic receptors. Alpha-receptor stimulation causes uterine contractions. Beta-receptors are subdivided into beta-1 and beta-2 groups, with the latter dominant in blood vessels and uterus.

Isoxsuprine hydrochloride, a derivative of catecholamine, *ritodrine* hydrochloride, and *terbutaline* sulfate have been used and are believed to be effective in depressing uterine contractions. A beta-mimetic that has a narrow impact on only the uterus has yet to emerge. Thus maternal and fetal or neonatal side effects do occur, with cardiovascular, pulmonary, and metabolic complications documented. For example, neonatal hypoglycemia is a recognized complication of isoxsuprine therapy.

Calcium antagonists may be useful in the future but as yet are unproved. Magnesium sulfate is no more effective than other agents. Prostaglandin synthetase inhibitors may have a future role, but their use at present cannot be recommended because of their potential vasoactive effect on the fetus, especially on the ductus arteriosus.

Tocolytic therapy continues to be controversial; however, such intervention appears beneficial in some preterm labors. Analysis of neonatal and maternal care suggests that in certain situations, especially between 26 and 33 weeks of gestation, such therapy is cost effective.[10]

Prevention of Prematurity. Certain authorities, especially Papiernik et al.[12] in France, and Creasy[3] in the United States, along with Canadian leaders in maternal-fetal medicine,[7] have documented and promoted comprehensive programs to *prevent prematurity through alteration of patient and professional behavior.* Key to such efforts is identification of risk factors associated with prematurity. Subsequent intervention to alter risk might be medical, but social and behavioral interventions may be equally important. Unfortunately studies of such intervention have had, at best, mixed results.

Health professionals such as nurse coordinators can play a major role in programs because they ensure that the need for intervention is documented and that intervention occurs. In addition to management of problems such as elevated blood pressure, alterations in life-style, work environment, and behavior patterns may be necessary. Good prenatal care and early work leave may be very important. Countries where such policies exist, such as Sweden, have low prematurity rates.

Multiple Gestation. Multiple gestation is relatively common (twins occur in about 1 in 80 births) and increases risk. This results from a host of complications ranging from those that are placental in origin, such as twin-to-twin transfusion, to fetal malformations that can be obscure and spectacular, as in compound twins, to much more frequent problems, such as prematurity and obstetrical complications. Multiple gestation is one of the three most common causes of prematurity. Complications of labor and delivery increase the risk of hypoxia or trauma markedly, with the second-born twin being more susceptible than the first. The incidence of multiple gestation may be increasing because of the application of reproductive technology to treat infertility.

Obstetrical Complications. Obstetrical complications jeopardize the fetus, with the most overt manifestation being intrapartum fetal demise. Even the most ideally healthy fetus is at increased risk during labor and delivery. Stress to the fetus may be documented retrospectively by low Apgar scores, poor recovery after birth, and subsequent complications. A fetus chronically compromised by adverse factors, such as diabetes in pregnancy, is at even greater risk when obstetrical problems arise.

Abnormal presentations, such as breech and transverse lie, greatly increase fetal risk, as does cephalopelvic disproportion (a mismatch between the maternal pelvis and the fetal head). Malproportion can be predominantly fetal, as in congenital hydrocephalus, or maternal when congenital pelvic bone abnormalities exist.

Abnormal Growth and Gestation. Discrepancies between fetal growth and gestation often are manifestations of an underlying disease process but may occur without apparent cause. A general discussion of intrauterine growth and nutrition, including growth curves, was introduced earlier (see Fig. 42-3). Regardless of cause, discrepancies in growth and gestation often can result in such severe risk to the fetus as to be more worrisome than the underlying problem. Prematurity is considered to be the leading cause of perinatal mortality and morbidity. Postmaturity occurs much less frequently but presents a greatly increased risk because little or no growth occurs in the human fetus after term, and many postterm fetuses and infants are dysmature and tolerate the stress of labor and delivery poorly. They have a significantly increased chance of neonatal problems such as hypoglycemia and aspiration pneumonia.

Deviations of growth and gestation can be cumulative for fetal risk. The premature infant who is affected by intrauterine growth retardation tolerates intrauterine stress poorly, may manifest RDS or gestationally related apnea after birth, and is at risk for the development of hypoglycemia. The clinician should appreciate that evaluation of the fetus or newborn by birth weight and gestational age can provide specific information that facilitates diagnosis and treatment (see Fig. 42-4).

Isoimmunization. Isoimmunization is a disease of the maternal-fetal unit that is decreasing in incidence because of efforts to prevent Rh disease with Rh_o globulin (RhoGAM). Passage into the maternal circulation of fetal red cells, which possess antigens not present in the mother, stimulates production of antibodies. Maternal antibodies of the IgG class cross the placenta, resulting in a hemolytic process in the fetus that can be severe. Variations on this basic theme occur. The initial isoimmunization can occur with blood transfusions, with an abortion, or with the first or subsequent pregnancy. Small amounts of antigen on amounts of blood of 1 ml or less, especially if repeated, can cause antibody response even in normal pregnancies. Sensitization incidence is increased by complications such as toxemia or cesarean section.

Rh incompatibility is associated with a variable but often severe sensitization that can cause stillbirth, massive fetal erythropoiesis or erythroblastosis, anemia, hydrops fetalis (a syndrome with edema and anasarca), and other systemic manifestations. Hyperbilirubinemia occurs in the newborn and to a lesser degree in utero, where the placenta clears bilirubin.

The incidence of Rh disease varies with the prevalence of Rh negativity. Rh negativity rarely occurs in Orientals and Native Americans; however, it occurs in 15% of American whites, resulting in the possibility of approximately 9% of their pregnancies involving an Rh-negative woman carrying an Rh-positive fetus.

Since the delineation of the cause of Rh-sensitization, a wide range of diagnostic and therapeutic methods has become available, to make Rh treatment a paradigm for intensive perinatal care. Routine procedures for the disease today include initial screening for possible "setups"; maternal serum and amniotic fluid analyses for severity of sensitization; intrauterine fetal transfusions when indicated; planned delivery, taking into consideration fetal well-being and maturity; and aggressive neonatal intensive care, including exchange transfusions and cardiopulmonary support. Complicating the Rh story is the major Rh antigen group (D antigen), being but one of several causes for isoimmunization; C and E antigens also exist, but at much lower frequencies. Most clinical tests and screening efforts involve the D antigen.

Incompatibilities of the ABO system result from the presence of maternal anti-A or anti-B antibodies when the fetus' blood type is group A or B and the mother's group O. Severe hemolysis is less common, even though ABO incompatibility potentially is present in about 20% of pregnancies. Fetal erythrocytes appear to have fewer antigenic loci, and maternal antibody appears as IgA, IgM, and IgG, with only the latter crossing the placenta. These facts may explain why ABO isoimmunization usually is of greater concern in the newborn than in the fetus. Stillbirths and hydrops fetalis are rare, but prolonged neonatal hyperbilirubinemia occurs frequently. Other incompatibilities, such as *anti-Kell sensitization,* are of low frequency (less than 1% of newborn hemolytic disease) but do on rare occasions present significant fetal and newborn risks.

Intrauterine Infections

Understanding of the scope of the problem of intrauterine infections and their fetal effects has broadened considerably but probably is far from complete. Expression ranges from fetal loss with spontaneous abortion and stillbirth, through very severe teratogenic structural change, to subtle systemic manifestations—including those of the central nervous system not detected until later in childhood as problems with higher cerebral function and behavior.

Agents include viruses, bacteria, spirochetes, and protozoa. The route of infection varies with the agent and can be transplacental, ascending through the cervix with or without the rupture of membranes, which provide a protective cover, and direct contact with the fetus during passage through the birth canal.

The student and practitioner of pediatrics needs to have a basic appreciation for the variety of agents and pathophysiological processes as well as knowledge of specific problems, especially those of high prevalence and morbidity. Table 42-3 is a modification of an acronym that has served well for several decades, as a reminder, even though new knowledge and agents, such as the intrauterine manifestations of *Parvovirus* (fetal hydrops and death) and human immunodeficiency virus (HIV), have emerged. A detailed discussion of a few specific infections follows, to outline the magnitude of the problem.

Human Immunodeficiency Virus (HIV). Fetal, intrauterine, and peripartum considerations are but a small part of the story of this agent; a complete discussion appears in Chapter 180. Given the magnitude of the HIV/AIDS problem and the fact that of the three predominant modes of transmission in the United States (sexual contact, percutaneous contact with contaminated sharps, and fetal or infant contact with an infected mother before or after birth) two involve reproduction, recognition of some specifics is important.

The fetus apparently can be infected in utero, although the exact timing is uncertain; possibilities include transplacental or peripartum, as well as immediately postpartum (through breast-feeding). Fetal manifestation of the infection is unusual and correlates with expression of disease in the child

Table 42-3 Maternal-Fetal Infections: the TORCH Acronym

Infection	Agent	Comment
T—Toxoplasmosis	Protozoa	Transplacental passage; mild maternal illness, variable fetal or neonatal manifestations; maternal antibody test available
O—Other	Virus, bacteria, parasite	HIV, *Listeria,* syphilis, gonococcus, group B streptococcus, varicella-zoster, malaria
R—Rubella	Virus	Prototype for transplacental viral infections; severe and chronic fetal or neonatal disease; antibody test and immunization available
C—Cytomegalovirus	Virus	Transplacental passage, ubiquitous agent; broad spectrum of fetal or infant manifestations
H—Herpes simplex	Virus	Rare transplacental passage, usual intrapartum transmission from maternal genitalia; severe neonatal disease; antiviral treatment available

Modified from Nahmias AJ: *Hosp Pract* 9:5, 1974.

and adult being variable and occurring months and years after birth. While less than 50% of babies born to HIV-seropositive mothers appear to develop infection, the percentage is large, and evidence suggests that risk and clinical course of the infection can be altered by treatment, making knowledge of maternal seropositivity important. Most babies born to HIV-positive mothers are positive because of placental passage of maternal antibody.

Rubella. Rubella virus is recognized as a potent teratogen. Infections during the first trimester result in approximately 20% of fetuses being severely damaged or malformed, with second-trimester involvement damaging 10%. Third-trimester infection has presented few clinical problems. Manifestations of first-trimester fetal disease can be severe (e.g., abortion, stillbirth, and the findings of severe rubella syndrome). Severe rubella syndrome includes growth retardation; eye defects, including cataracts and microphthalmia; congenital cardiac defects; deafness; thrombocytopenic purpura; hepatosplenomegaly; bone lesions; pneumonitis; and cerebral defects, including microcephaly, encephalitis, mental retardation, and spastic quadriparesis. Infections in the second trimester are more variable and tend to be less severe. It now is apparent that the classic fetal presentation, with the severe manifestations listed above, is at one end of a spectrum that extends to documented infection with little or no apparent disease; the expression of rubella syndrome is variable and unpredictable. The 1964 rubella epidemic affected thousands of infants.

The high fetal risk and potentially devastating consequences of intrauterine rubella have stimulated aggressive efforts toward preventing maternal rubella and, when this fails, termination of pregnancies. Congenital rubella is a reportable disease. Vaccination of children between the ages of 1 and 12 years is routine, but administration of vaccine to women of childbearing age has been controversial because of potential teratogenic effects of the vaccine virus on the fetus. *Antibody screening can establish whether an individual woman is among the 85% who are immune.* Obstetricians should monitor their patients for risk of rubella infection. When probable rubella infection occurs in early pregnancy, abortion is an alternative.

Cytomegalovirus (CMV) Infections. The cytomegaloviruses may be the most common cause of congenital infections, occurring in somewhat fewer than 1% of births. This group of viruses is widespread and produces various apparent and inapparent infections in the general population. Among pregnant women, 3% to 5% have this virus in their cervix or urine. Fetal infection usually occurs transplacentally, although intrauterine transfusion has been documented as a cause.

The fetal disease has been called *cytomegalic inclusion disease (CID)* because of the large inclusion-bearing cells found in urine and many organs. Severe CID includes hepatosplenomegaly, microcephaly, cerebral calcifications, mental and motor manifestations, and chorioretinitis. Reviews suggest that expression of intrauterine infections is quite variable and that full recognition of incidence is yet to come. Serological tests for CMV are available and can provide presumptive evidence for infection; however, reliability is not as good as with rubella titers, and a vaccine is not available.

Herpes Simplex Virus Infections. Herpes simplex virus (HSV) infections in humans are from two strains, types 1 and 2, with distinct serotypes but some cross-reactivity. *Perinatal disease usually is associated with type 2,* although type 1 is more common in the general population. Type 2 produces genital lesions and is transmitted venereally in most instances. Herpetic disease in the fetus or newborn is relatively rare but potentially devastating. Transmission occurs by direct contact at birth or by ascending transcervical infection after rupture of membranes. Transplacental infection early in pregnancy with fetal manifestations similar to those of CMV infection has been documented in at least one case. Whether transplacental transmission is a frequent problem is unclear, as is the severity of manifestations.

Newborn manifestations of intrapartum contact are well known. They range from vesicular lesions of the skin to encephalitis and severe systemic disease, with a mortality of more than 90% without treatment and severe central nervous system morbidity in those who survive. Expression probably is linked to primary versus recurrent maternal disease, being more intense in the latter.

A major recent development is the *success of antiviral agents* in the treatment of systemic herpes infection—in particular, encephalitis. Early diagnosis and treatment are essential. Prevention is desirable and possible. (See discussion of venereal diseases in Chapter 258 and of herpes infections in Chapter 214.) Current recommended management for a pregnant mother who has genital lesions is a *cesarean section* to prevent fetal inoculation by contact. This should be done within 4 hours of rupture of the membranes.

Toxoplasmosis. Toxoplasmosis is caused by an intracellular protozoan parasite, *Toxoplasma gondii.* Infection is widespread, is congenital or acquired, and varies in expression from almost asymptomatic to generalized and fatal. The fetus is at risk for death when the infection occurs early in pregnancy or may be born with fully developed disease indicative of a long intrauterine course. *Chorioretinitis, cerebral calcification, hydrocephalus or microcephaly, hepatosplenomegaly, and a host of systemic manifestations* are observed. Long-term sequelae, especially involving the central nervous system, are present in the majority of infants who have severe infection and who survive.

It is believed that pregnant women become infected through exposure to cat feces or incompletely cooked meat. Incidence of the perinatal disease is higher in certain locales. Antibody detection by means of the Sabin-Feldman dye test and a complement-fixing test can document the onset of infection, but antibodies remain high for several years. Thus high initial titers without subsequent change do not necessarily indicate current fetal infection. Children born to mothers who have a prior congenitally affected child are rarely, if ever, infected. Prospective antibody studies on children, for disappearance of transplacentally acquired dye antibody at 4 months of age, can help to rule out congenital infection. Congenital infection may be inapparent at birth and produce central nervous system signs late in infancy.

Other Intrauterine Infections. Fetal *syphilis* is caused by transplacental passage of *Treponema pallidum.* Fetal infection has been thought not to occur before the eighteenth week of gestation, but this may be subject to dispute. Pregnancy in a woman who has primary- or secondary-stage disease may terminate in stillbirth. Other manifestations vary from presentation in the newborn to those appearing in the first 2 years of life or later. In general the earlier the infection, the more severe the lesions. Severe fetal infection manifests in early infancy by osteochondritis and periostitis, rhinitis (snuffles), rash, and mucosal fissures or patches. Premarital and prenatal screening for syphilis, in conjunction with antibiotic treatment, has decreased the incidence of intrauterine disease effectively, especially that with the more severe or classic manifestations. Unfortunately, somewhat of a resurgence may be occurring. Recently trained clinicians have not had the experience in recognizing congenital syphilis that many of their older compatriots have had, sometimes resulting in a delayed diagnosis.

Listeria monocytogenes is a gram positive bacillus that probably plays an important role in overall fetal wastage. Incidence varies widely. Fetal death may occur after a relatively mild systemic maternal disease. Neonatal manifestations include systemic disease at birth or a delayed appearance as meningitis in the second to fifth week of life, with a characteristic monocellular cerebrospinal fluid manifestation.

Group B streptococcal disease has many similarities in presentation to that of the *Listeria* organisms and is a more common problem (see Chapter 48, Critical Neonatal Illnesses). A fulminant hemorrhagic pneumonitis in the first hours of life and a delayed meningitis cause very high mortality. Fetal infection probably occurs in the intrapartum period from organisms in the birth canal. Maternal immune status may play a role. An effective protocol involving prenatal detection and treatment is needed.

Other known intrauterine infections include agents of all classes, and undoubtedly many others will be discovered. Many viruses can cause fetal infection or manifestations, including varicella, coxsackievirus, mumps, rubeola, echovirus, hepatitis, and others. *Mycoplasma* may be an important perinatal agent, and malaria is a significant fetal threat in many areas of the world.

Assessment of fetal well-being in suspected intrauterine infection follows the precepts set out above. Serological tests have been alluded to in the discussion of individual entities and may be helpful, as in rubella. Unfortunately, although diagnostic certainty often is quite satisfactory for the newborn, it is less reliable for the fetus.

Pregnancy-induced Hypertension. Hypertension of pregnancy is a major contributor to fetal risk. A group of diseases seen only in pregnancy and presenting with acute and chronic manifestations of hypertension, edema, and proteinuria may be lumped together in this category. *Preeclampsia* is another term for the basic process, which can be severe; when convulsions or coma occurs, *eclampsia* is present. Chronic hypertensive vascular disease with pregnancy is believed by many to be a separate disease state that can have superimposed toxemic manifestations.

Spontaneous labor occurs frequently in all hypertensive gestations (for unclear reasons), leading to a risk of premature birth, which is increased further in incidence because early delivery frequently is employed. As the severity of the disease increases and particularly when eclampsia intervenes, stillbirth and maternal death become much more frequent. Intrauterine growth retardation is seen in a third of perinatal deaths associated with toxemia. From the fetal viewpoint, this disease process presents a bleak perspective; prenatal stress is significant, labor and delivery often are premature and timed for maternal rather than fetal well-being, and neonatal complications are many and severe.

Risk identification and evaluation in hypertension rely heavily on prenatal detection. When the process is discovered, intensive perinatal care may be necessary, with sedatives and anticonvulsants, especially magnesium sulfate, a mainstay of therapy. Fetal well-being and maturity can be assessed by regular observation of fetal heart rate, uterine growth, estriols, and ultrasound and by amniotic fluid parameters. Oxytocin for stress testing or induction may cause fluid retention. The physician responsible for the infant may be confronted by unfavorable test results of fetal well-being and maturity plus the need for imminent delivery. In addition, medication such as magnesium sulfate used before delivery may complicate neonatal management, adding to risk.

REFERENCES

1. Battaglia F, Meschia G: *An introduction to fetal physiology,* Orlando, Fla, 1986, Academic Press.
2. Caring for our future: the content of prenatal care, Report of the Public Health Service Expert Panel on the Content of Prenatal Care, US Public Health Service, Washington, DC, 1989, Department of Health and Human Services.
3. Creasy RK: Preterm birth prevention: where are we? *Am J Obstet Gynecol* 168:4, 1223, 1993.
4. Czeizel AE, Dudas I: Prevention of the first occurrence of neural-tube defects by periconceptional vitamin supplementation, *N Engl J Med* 327:1832, 1992.
5. Diagnostic ultrasound imaging in pregnancy, Report of a Consensus Development Conference, Feb 6-8, 1984, NIH Pub No 84-667, Washington, DC, 1984, Department of Health and Human Services.
6. Effect of corticosteroids for fetal lung maturity on perinatal outcomes, Consensus Development Conference Statement, March 1994, National Institutes of Health.
7. Fetus and Newborn Committee, Canadian Paediatric Society; Maternal-Fetal Medicine Committee, Society of Obstetrics and Gynaecologists of Canada: Management of the woman with threatened birth of an infant of extremely low gestational age, *Can Med Assoc J* 151:547, 1994.
8. Hobbins JC et al: Percutaneous umbilical blood sampling, *Am J Obstet Gynecol* 152:1, 1985.
9. Klerman L et al: Interconception care: a new role for the pediatrician, *Pediatrics* 93:327, 1994.
10. Korenbrot CC, Alto LH, Laros RK Jr: The cost effectiveness of stopping labor with beta-adrenergic treatment, *N Engl J Med* 310:691, 1984.
11. Mittendorf R, Herbst AL: DES exposure: an update, *Contemp Pediatr* 11:59, 1994.
12. Papiernik E et al: Prevention of preterm babies: a perinatal study in Haguenau, France, *Pediatrics* 76:154, 1985.
13. Prenatal genetic diagnosis for pediatricians, American Academy of Pediatrics, Committee on Genetics, *Pediatrics* 93:1010, 1994.
14. Report from the Committee on Fetal Extrauterine Survivability to the New York State Task Force on Life and the Law, Fetal Extrauterine Survivability, January 1988.
15. Rhoads GC et al: The safety and efficacy of chorionic villus sampling for early prenatal diagnosis of cytogenetic abnormalities, *N Engl J Med* 320:10, 1989.
16. Rosso P: A new chart to monitor weight gain during pregnancy, *Am J Clin Nutr* 41:644, 1985.
17. Stumpf DA et al: The infant with anencephaly: the Medical Task Force on Anencephaly, *N Engl J Med* 322:669, 1990.

18. Xue-Yi C et al: Timing of vulnerability of the brain to iodine deficiency in endemic cretinism, *N Engl J Med* 331:1739, 1994.

SUGGESTED READINGS

American College of Obstetricians and Gynecologists Preembryo Research: History, scientific background, and ethical considerations, ACOG Committee Opinion No. 136, Washington, DC, 1994, ACOG.

Beckman DA, Brent RL: Mechanisms of known environmental teratogens: drugs and chemicals, *Clin Perinatol* 13:649, 1986.

Chalmers I, Enkin M, Keirse M, editors: *Effective care in pregnancy and childbirth,* Oxford, 1989, Oxford University Press.

Dorris M: *The broken cord,* New York, 1989, Harper & Row.

Fetal Research and Applications—A Conference Summary, Institute of Medicine, National Academy Press, Washington, DC, 1994.

Freeman RK, Poland RL: *Guidelines for perinatal care,* ed 3, American Academy of Pediatrics, American College of Obstetricians and Gynecologists, Washington, DC, 1992, ACOC.

Hetzel BS: Iodine deficiency and fetal brain damage, *N Engl J Med* 331:1770, 1994.

Moore KL, Persaud TVN: *The developing human: clinically oriented embryology,* ed 5, Philadelphia, 1993, WB Saunders.

Report of the Human Embryo Research Panel, National Institutes of Health, Bethesda, Md, 1994, NIH.

43 Perinatal Medicine

ONE

Overview

Nicholas M. Nelson

PERINATAL MEDICINE

The sharper inflection of the general and continuing downward trend in neonatal mortality in the United States beginning around 1970 (Fig. 43-1) has engendered much discussion because it is chronologically coincident with the rise of modern perinatal-neonatal medicine. This field has been characterized by a level of intense obstetrical and pediatric collaboration on the needs of the fetus and newborn that was unknown a generation ago.

Figure 43-2 shows that much of this progress has been achieved through better management of the obstetrical aspects of the perinatal period, particularly near or at term gestation. This has been associated with a reciprocal rise to prominence of premature labor (which precipitates immature but genetically sound fetuses) as the major unyielding problem of modern obstetrics. If that issue were resolved, most neonatologists could retire from active duty and instead observe and support the progress of geneticists, teratologists, and others in addressing the bedrock problems of congenital malformations and heritable diseases.

Scientific and technological advances (Table 43-1) have formed a necessary, but not sufficient, foundation for this achievement. Just as the entrepreneur must have channels for the distribution of his or her product from factory through dealership to consumer, neonatal and perinatal care providers must establish ways of identifying the high-risk target population likely to need such care and then bringing that population to the site for its provision, inasmuch as multidisciplinary human services are not as easily distributed as are products.

Meeting this requirement has necessitated assessing the risk of perinatal morbidity or mortality as far in advance of the anticipated risk event as possible (Table 43-2). Pregnant women identified as being at risk of having a complicated pregnancy, labor, or delivery (about 15% of the total) are managed best under the supervision of an obstetrician at a level II or level III facility. In some locales about 50% of these high-risk mothers are delivered safely in their own community (level I) hospital following consultation with a perinatologist. Nearly 1 in 15 of these patients probably will have an unanticipated stillbirth; of the 80% of pregnant women initially identified as being at low risk, however, about 1 in 30 will develop an unanticipated problem during pregnancy (e.g., toxemia, vaginal bleeding, or premature labor) and require referral. The delivered infant also may develop unanticipated problems requiring referral, but most neonatal morbidity and mortality risk factors (e.g., maternal age, diabetes, abortion, gestational age, or birth weight) can be anticipated well before delivery.

Although the obstetrician or perinatologist (the only physicians who always attend two patients) is first concerned with the mother, the near-total conquest of maternal mortality in developed countries has allowed him or her to focus at least equal attention on fetal health—both prepartum and intrapartum (Tables 43-3 and 43-4).

Fetal growth, and therefore accurate gestational age, is monitored by abdominal ultrasound techniques with considerable accuracy (even to the point of identifying "catch-up" growth in some growth-retarded fetuses) by measuring the fetal crown-rump length (at 6 to 12 weeks) and later the biparietal diameter (at 14 to 26 weeks). The frequency and intensity of fetal breathing movements also are used as indices of fetal well-being. The perinatologist uses a Doppler-shift measuring device to assess fetal heart rate patterns when seeking evidence of healthy variability in the basal fetal heart rate in association with normal fetal movements (nonstress test). If such variability is lacking (nonreactive nonstress test), or if there is evidence of fetal growth failure the perinatologist may want to stress the fetoplacental unit by mimicking labor, using sufficient oxytocin to produce at least three uterine contractions within 10 minutes. A positive test result, indicating uteroplacental insufficiency, is one in which two thirds of the induced contractions are followed by a late (10-second delay) deceleration of the fetal heart rate (Table 43-5). This evidence then is weighed against that of fetal pulmonary maturity and the availability of neonatal special care, among other factors, in deciding whether to continue or terminate the pregnancy. When assessing fetal health many practitioners likewise consult the mother regarding fetal activity. Indeed, some have incorporated her observations into a simple and effective plan for surveillance, despite an acknowledged lack of reproducibility of such observations.

NEONATAL MEDICINE

The major problems faced in neonatal special care units are indicated in the typical experiences shown in Figure 43-2. Problems of the perinatal process include birth trauma, asphyxia, and aspiration. Developmental diseases include prematurity, immaturity, and hyaline membrane disease. Overall survival is exquisitely sensitive to gestational age (Fig. 43-3), and hyaline membrane disease of the newborn often imposes an added burden that can be fatal.

The major intellectual advance in neonatal medicine over the last three decades probably has been the description of the appropriately grown (or inappropriately grown) infant

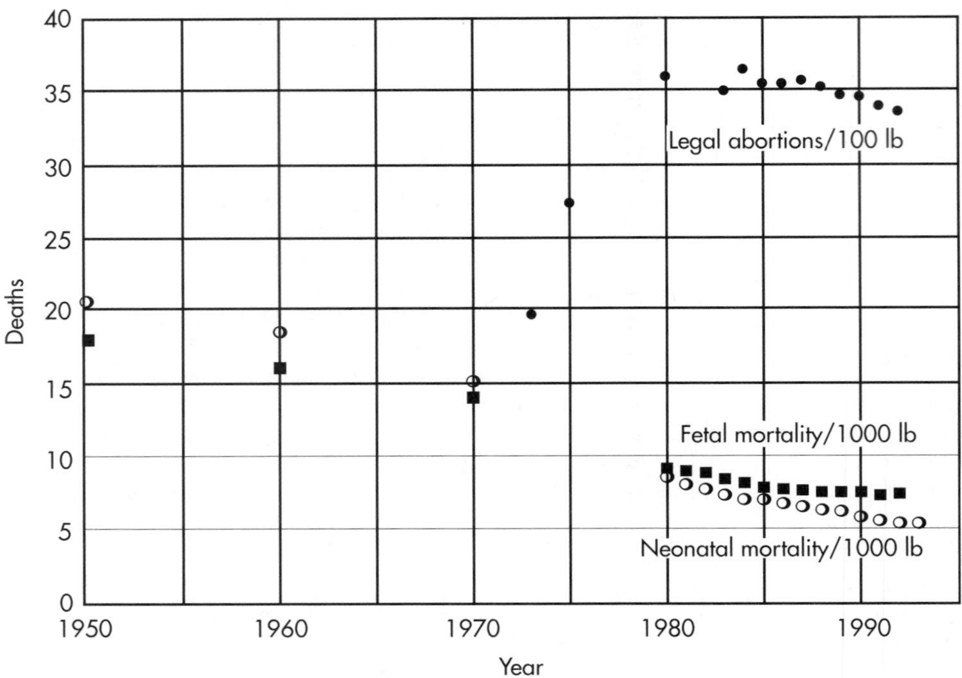

FIG. 43-1 Fetal and neonatal mortality in the United States. *lb,* Live births.

(Data from Health, United States, 1994. US Department of Health and Human Services—Public Health Service, Centers for Disease Control, National Center for Health Statistics, Hyattsville, Md, 1995, DHHS Publication No. (PHS) 95-1232.)

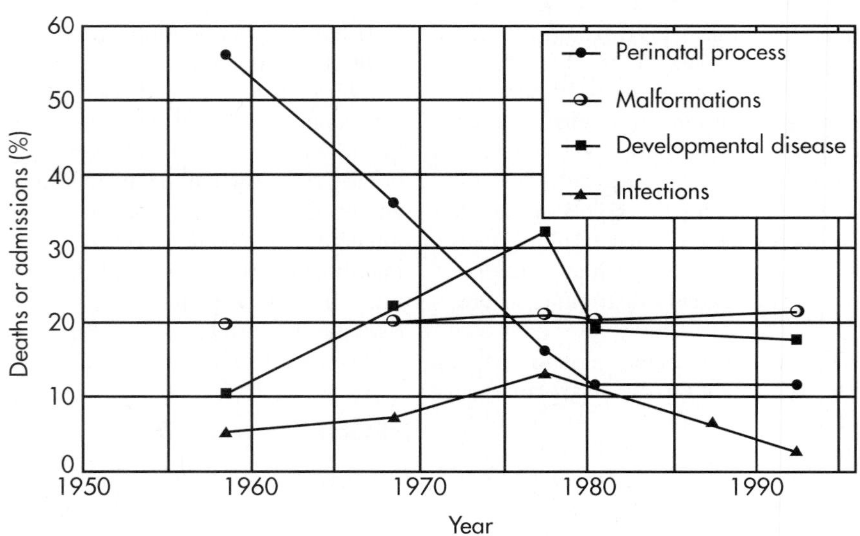

FIG. 43-2 Incidence and fatality rates of certain perinatal conditions. Experience at Milton S. Hershey Medical Center, Hershey, Pennsylvania (1973-1987), the United Kingdom (1950-1970), and the United States (1980-1992). *HMD,* Hyaline membrane disease.

(Modified from Vuilliamy DG: *The newborn child,* ed 2, Boston, 1967, Little, Brown.)

Table 43-1 Advances in Perinatal-Neonatal Medicine

Years	Mortality/1000 live births		Basic science	Obstetrics	Anesthesia	Pediatrics
	Fetal	Neonatal				
1940-1950	18	21	Blood grouping, antibiotics	Elimination of maternal mortality		Umbilical venous catheterization, exchange transfusion
1950-1960	16	18	Human karyotyping, surfactant, blood gas measurements, pulmonary function tests	Elimination of mid forceps and high forceps	Apgar score, local anesthesia	Phototherapy
1960-1970	15	15	Lecithin/sphingomyelin ratio, shake test, ultrasound	Liberalized abortion practices, RhoGAM, fetal heart rate monitoring		Umbilical artery catheterization, regionalization of care
1970-1980	10	10	Rubella vaccine, steroid induction of surfactant	Liberal use of cesarean section, deferred labor, regionalization of care, stress testing	Constant positive airway pressure, positive end-expiratory pressure	Total parenteral nutrition
1980-1990	6	6	Prostaglandins cause of onset of labor (?)	Real-time fetal ultrasound	High-frequency ventilation	Neonatal ultrasound, surfactant replacement
1990-2000	(?)	(?)		Arrest premature labor (?)	(?)	(?)

Table 43-2 Prenatal Risk Factors

	Major	Moderate	Minor
Fetal	Premature (Hx*)		
	Postmature (Hx)	Infant >10 lb (Hx)	Congenital malformation (Hx)
	Stillbirth (Hx)	Intrauterine growth retardation (Hx)	
	Neonatal death (Hx)		
	Exchange transfusion (Hx)	Rh sensitization	
Obstetrical	Uterine malformation	Small pelvis	
		Infertility	
	Abnormal cytological findings	Vaginal spotting	
	Incompetent cervix	Habitual aborter (Hx)	
	Multiple pregnancy	Grand multiparity (>5)	
	Abnormal presentation	Cesarean birth (Hx)	
	Polyhydramnios	Uterine dystocia	
	Toxemia, moderate to severe	Toxemia, mild	Toxemia (Hx)
		Eclampsia (Hx)	
Medical	Endocrine ablation (Hx)	Thyroid disease	Small stature (<60 in)
	Sickle cell disease	Hemoglobin <9 g/dl	Hemoglobin 9-10.9 g/dl
	Heart disease, severe (II-IV)	Heart disease, moderate (I)	
	Renal disease, moderate to severe	Pyelitis (present or Hx)	Cystitis (present or Hx)
	Hypertension, chronic diabetes (≥class A-II)	Prediabetes (Class A-I)	Diabetes (family Hx)
		Viral disease	
		"Flu" syndrome, severe	
		Pulmonary disease	
		Positive tuberculosis skin test (Hx)	
		Epilepsy (Hx)	
Psychosocial		≤15 yr, ≥35 yr age	
		<100 lb, >200 lb	Emotional problems
		Uneducated	
		Unmarried	
		Unregistered (prenatal care)	
		Medically indigent	
		Drug abuse (including alcohol)	Moderate alcohol use
			Smoker

From Hobel CJ et al: Prenatal and intrapartum high-risk screening, *Am J Obstet Gynecol* 117:1, 1973.
*Hx, History of.

Table 43-3 Assessment of Fetal Health—Prepartum

	Biochemical	Biophysical
Genome	Karyotype by chorionic villus sampling*	
Well-being	Alpha-fetoprotein	Electronic monitoring of fetal heart rate
	Human chorionic gonadotropin	Nonstress test
	Fetal blood sampling from cord vessels*	Oxytocin challenge test
		Ultrasound monitoring of fetal breathing
Maturity	Renal and muscular by amniotic creatinine*	Ultrasound monitoring of crown-rump length (early) and fetal biparietal diameter (late)
	Pulmonary by amniotic lecithin/sphingomyelin ratio,* shake test*	
Semiqualitative		Maternal notation of fetal activity

*Invasive procedure.

(Fig. 43-4). Once grasped, this concept enhances the practitioner's approach to the newborn patient by focusing attention on those problems most likely to be encountered in the patient experiencing normal growth, undergrowth, or (more rarely) overgrowth. This approach depends critically on assessing gestational age accurately; in this assessment the fetal sonographic data, physical examination, and the mother's opinion all should be accorded approximately equal importance. Note also, in Figure 35-3, that overall *mortality decreases by approximately 50% with each biweekly advance in gestation* beyond the onset of viability (currently around 25 weeks of gestation).

Some have questioned the wisdom and even the morality of investing precious societal resources in the effort to achieve survival in infants weighing less than 1500 or 1000 g at birth, in whom the incidence of chronic and crippling diseases (e.g., necrotizing enterocolitis and bronchopulmonary dysplasia) and crushing disappointments (e.g., intraven-

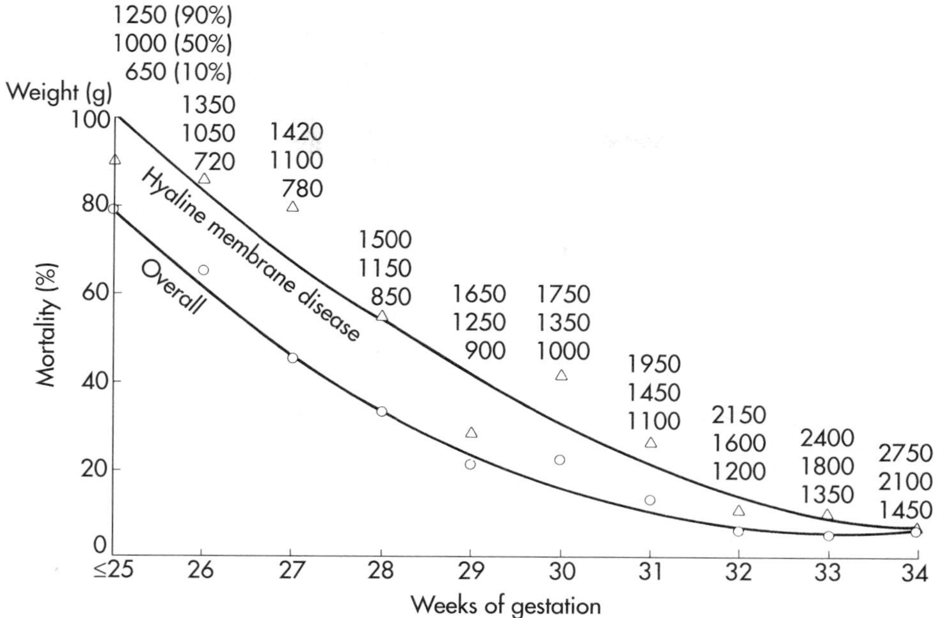

FIG. 43-3 Neonatal mortality in 1114 admissions at Milton S. Hershey Medical Center (1976-1980), caused by hyaline membrane disease and overall factors. The 90th, 50th, and 10th percentiles for grams birth weight at each week of gestation are taken from the Denver data.
(From Battaglia FC, Lubchenco LO: *J Pediatr* 71:159, 1967.)

Table 43-4 Assessment of Fetal Health—Intrapartum

Observation	Significance
Monitoring of fetal heart rate during and after uterine contractions (stages I, II)	
Early deceleration	Compression of fetal head
Variable deceleration	Compression of umbilical cord
Late deceleration	Uteroplacental insufficiency
Sampling of fetal scalp pH (stage II)	Anticipate postpartum difficulties if pH <7.20

Table 43-5 Neurological Outcome among Very Low–Birth-Weight Infants: Results from a 2-Year Follow-up Study

Outcome	90 Infants, 501-1000 g (%)	201 Infants, 1001-1500 g (%)
Normal	27.8	53.7
Impaired	7.8	10.0
Died	60.0	23.9
Lost to follow-up care	4.4	12.4

From Hack M, Fanaroff AA, Merrkatz IR: *N Engl J Med* 301:1162, 1979.

tricular hemorrhage and the attendant neurological catastrophe) begins to rise dramatically. These critics should study the data in Table 43-5 and be challenged to present 28% to 54% *normal* survivors of comparably devastating illnesses occurring at any other stage in life. Similarly criticized in 1913 regarding his efforts on behalf of marasmic infants in New York City's foundling hospitals, Dr. L. Emmett Holt, Sr., insisted, "These infants are *not* unfit, they are merely unfortunate!" Nonetheless, it would appear that 24 to 25 weeks of gestation is the current floor for fetal viability, regardless of birth weight.

REGIONALIZATION OF CARE

The advent of neonatal intensive care around 1960 presaged and somewhat catalyzed similar developments in obstetrics in such a manner that around 1975, neonatally oriented pediatricians and fetally oriented obstetricians began engaging in close daily therapeutic collaboration over the needs of their patients. This and other forces led to the development of subspecialty boards of examiners in each discipline and culminated in the joint production in 1983 (by the American Academy of Pediatrics [AAP] and the American College of Obstetricians and Gynecologists [ACOG]) of *Guidelines for Perinatal Care,*[1] supplanting the AAP's preceding 5-yearly revisions of *Standards and Recommendations for Hospital Care of Newborn Infants.* This publication properly celebrates recent achievements in lowering perinatal mortality (see Figs. 43-1 to 43-4), particularly in the under–1500 g birth weight group, and codifies many of the means that have brought it about, especially the process of regionalization in perinatal health care. This process is defined as a systems approach in which program components in a geographical area are defined and coordinated.

The phrase *defined and coordinated* implies more centralized planning than historically was the case. Rather, pioneering efforts in improving neonatal mortality were undertaken spontaneously and separately in Montreal, Toronto, New York, Denver, San Francisco, Boston, and many other sites beginning around 1960. These efforts attracted the attention of obstetricians, pediatricians, primary care physicians, parents, medical equipment developers, and later, hospital

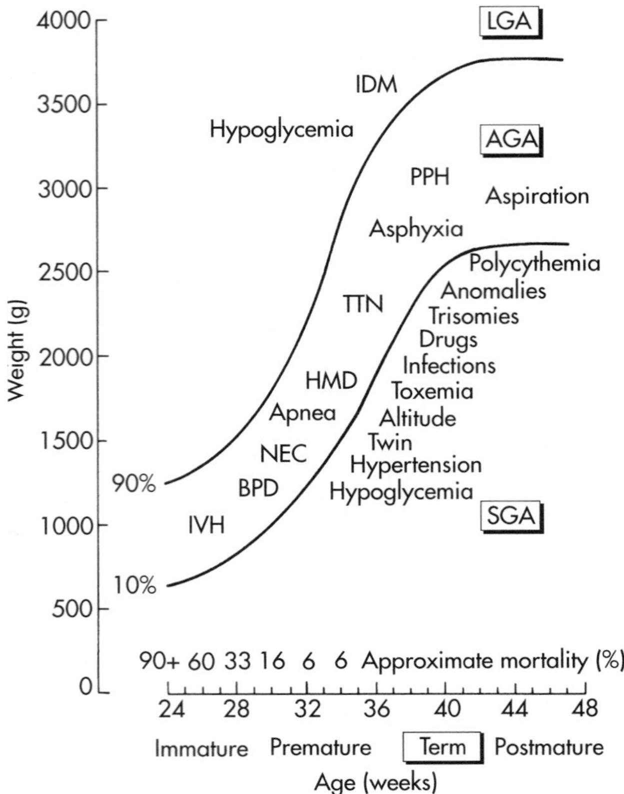

FIG. 43-4 Specific perinatal clinical entities encountered frequently in the three major developmental channels: (1) large for gestational age *(LGA)*, (2) appropriate for gestational age *(AGA)*, and (3) small for gestational age *(SGA)*. Expected approximate overall mortality is superimposed on the abscissa. *IDM*, Infant of a diabetic mother; *IVH*, intraventricular hemorrhage; *BPD*, bronchopulmonary dysplasia; *NEC*, necrotizing enterocolitis; *HMD*, hyaline membrane disease; *TTN*, transient tachypnea of the newborn; *PPH*, persistent pulmonary hypertension or persistent fetal circulation.

(From Battaglia FC, Lubchenco LO: *J Pediatr* 71:159, 1967.)

boards of trustees, partly because they were glamorous, but mostly because they were successful. In a process of healthy and natural self-selection, hospitals began to identify themselves as providing what has come to be known as (level I, II, or III) perinatal-neonatal care. Given the size, demographics, and medical history of North America, a certain amount of natural geographical coalescence was inevitable. Also given the tendency for medical personnel to congregate in attractive urban and suburban environments, compounded by a certain amount of entrepreneurial spirit, some conflict over turf and duplication of services was equally inevitable—especially under a system of unlimited reimbursement in the United States that automatically paid back to hospitals nearly every dollar expended (cost reimbursement). The prospective hospital payment system (diagnosis-related group [DRG]) inaugurated in the United States in July 1984 has not yet reversed unnecessary proliferation of perinatal services, despite their being expensive and many of the most needy consumers lacking medical insurance. The perinatal effects of "managed care" currently are quite uncertain.

Nevertheless, regionalization of perinatal services has been remarkably effective in reducing perinatal mortality and has now been embraced officially as policy by the two most pertinent professional groups—the AAP and ACOG. How the concept develops in a given geographical area begins with the definition of the pregnant patient's status and needs by her primary care provider as she enters the health care system. That definition, once displayed against local availability of the requisite services, helps her physician determine the level of the institution that can best serve her needs.

To the physician in a given local community who would contend that the infant in respiratory distress or the laboring woman having ineffectual contractions is "within my level of competence," the proper response is "Agreed, but is the problem within your level of availability?" *A patient's medical outcome is not affected by the expertise of the physician who is not present.* The particular medical and surgical skills employed most frequently by the perinatologist and neonatologist were learned by nearly every general obstetrician and pediatrician during his or her residency. However, the neonatologist and perinatologist are hospital-based and have no medical commitment other than the high-risk pregnant mother or sick newborn; it is these attentions of time (as well as expertise) that have been the most important factors in reducing perinatal mortality.

Thus, based on the presumption that appropriate expertise is constantly available at each institutional level, the AAP-ACOG *Guidelines*[1] for institutional responsibility are shown in Tables 43-6 to 43-8. These guidelines imply and demand a high level of bidirectional and tridirectional communication, education, and, where necessary, transportation (including return transportation of the infant to his or her hospital of birth once the need for intensive care has subsided). *Education and communication frequently diminish the need for transportation of the infant.* Some primary care practitioners may feel that taking responsibility for a level I unit provides insufficient professional gratification or challenge. They should inspect the experience, set out in Table 43-9, from a large and unselected maternal population and note how many of the problems listed they are likely to encounter in their own primary care practice. They also should note how many of these conditions they alone have the first opportunity to prevent or correct. Indeed, many feel that the major portion of the recent reduction in perinatal mortality is attributable solely to improved monitoring of the fetus, better timing of the termination of the threatened pregnancy, and careful attention to the oxygen, thermal, and nutritional needs of the "large" 1500 to 2500 g infant.

TWO

Perinatal Transport

George A. Little

Transportation of the perinatal patient is an essential service in the systematic application of perinatal care. Perinatal regionalization and system development involves applying resources in an organized fashion following need identification and risk assessment. Because not all services can be provided

Table 43-6 Perinatal Care Programs—Ancillary Services*

Services	Level I	Level II	Level III
Laboratory			
(microtechnique for neonates)			
Within 15 min	Hematocrit		
Within 1 hr	Glucose, BUN, creatinine, blood gases, routine urinalysis	Blood type, and Rh, electrolytes, coagulation studies, blood available from type and screen program	Special blood and amniotic fluid tests (creatinine, lecithin/sphingomyelin ratio, shake, karyotype)
Within 1-6 hr	CBC, platelet appearance on smear, blood chemistries, blood type and cross-match, Coombs' test, bacterial smear	Coagulation studies, magnesium, urine, electrolytes, and chemistries	
Within 24-28 hr	Bacterial cultures and antibiotic sensitivity	Liver function tests, metabolic screening	
Within hospital or facilities available	Viral cultures		All laboratory facilities available
Radiography and ultrasound	Technicians on call 24 hr/day available in 30 min Technicians experienced in performing abdominal, pelvic, and obstetrical ultrasound examinations Professional interpretation available on 24-hr basis Portable x-ray and ultrasound equipment available to labor and delivery rooms and nurseries	Experienced radiology technicians immediately available in hospital (ultrasound on call) Professional interpretation immediately available Portable x-ray equipment Ultrasound equipment may be in labor and delivery or nursery areas Sophisticated equipment for emergency GI, GU, or CNS studies available 24 hr/day	Computed tomography Magnetic resonance imaging
Blood bank	Technicians on call 24 hr/day, available in 30 min, for routine blood banking procedures	Experienced technicians immediately available in hospital for blood banking procedures and identification of irregular antibodies Blood component therapy readily available	Resource center for network Direct line communication to labor and delivery area and nurseries

*All ancillary services listed for level I nurseries should be available at level II and III nurseries, and those listed for level II nurseries should be available at level III nurseries.

in every location where births occur and babies receive care, movement of some patients is necessary. Pregnant women and babies who have clinical problems often require special attention in preparation for and during transport.[3]

HISTORICAL PERSPECTIVE

The early literature regarding perinatal transport describes the transfer of stable, pregnant women to hospitals, but little mention is made of critically ill newborns. With the development of regional centers for the care of premature infants and the improvement in mortality and morbidity at these centers, transfer of neonatal patients became increasingly important. Early transport services were primitive by today's standards, involving the use of equipment such as wood or tin boxes heated with hot water bottles. In 1948 the New York City Department of Health and Hospitals instituted a service staffed by five nurses to transport infants to centers caring for premature infants; Denver instituted a similar program at about the same time.

With the emergence of improved critical care capability and perinatal regionalization, transport services became increasingly sophisticated. The Canadian Pediatric Society published the first manual devoted to neonatal transport in the early 1970s[4] at a time when North American pediatricians were debating aspects of neonatal transport.[2] Later in the decade the benefits of maternal and neonatal transport were documented, while concerns and risks were evaluated.[1,5] The American College of Obstetricians and Gynecologists' and the American Academy of Pediatrics' technical advisory committees have assumed an active role in supporting and standardizing transport.[6,8]

Table 43-7 Levels of Program Development (I, II, III)

Levels of basic perinatal network	Functional activities	Usual locations	Usual physician leadership (practice and style)
I	Usual focus of patient entry into system Assess risk Carry out uncomplicated perinatal care Stabilize unexpected problems Initiate maternal, neonatal transport Accept return neonatal transport Collect data Sponsor local education	Community hospital or co-located at level II, III facilities	Primary care physician or specialist (solo practitioner)
II	Initiate and receive maternal, neonatal transport Initiate return neonatal transport Diagnose and treat selected high-risk pregnancies and neonatal problems Educate part of network	Large community hospital with many support services or colocated at level III facility	Specialist or subspecialist (monodisciplinary group practice)
III	Receive maternal, neonatal transport Initiate return neonatal transport Diagnose and treat most perinatal problems Research and outcome surveillance Educate regionally Administer regionally	Large academic medical centers with comprehensive residency programs	Subspecialist (multidisciplinary team practice)

Table 43-8 Perinatal Care Programs—Medical Personnel

Personnel	Level I	Level II	Level III
Chief of service	One general physician responsible for perinatal care (or codirectors from obstetrics and pediatrics)	Ob: Board-certified obstetrician with subcertification, special interest, experience, or training in maternal-fetal medicine Ped: Board-certified pediatrician with subcertification, special interest, experience, or training in neonatology	Ob: Full-time obstetrician board-certified in maternal-fetal medicine Ped: Full-time pediatrician board-certified in neonatal-perinatal medicine
Other physicians	Physician (or certified nurse-midwife) at all deliveries Anesthesia services Physician care for neonates	Board-certified director of anesthesia services Medical, surgical, radiological, pathological consultation	Anesthesiologists with special training or experience in perinatal and pediatric anesthesia Obstetrical, pediatric, surgical subspecialists
Supervisory nurse	RN in charge of perinatal facilities	Ob: Supervisory RN with education and experience in normal and high-risk pregnancy Ped: Supervisory RN with neonatal specialist certification or equivalent experience	Supervisor of perinatal services with advanced skills Separate head nurses for maternal-fetal and neonatal services, master's degree level certification
Staff nurse/patient ratio	Normal labor—1:2 Delivery in second stage—1:1 Oxytocin induction—1:2 Cesarean delivery—2:1 Normal nursery—1:6-8	Complicated labor, delivery—1:1 Intermediate nursery—1:3-4	Intensive neonatal care—1:1-2 Critical care of unstable neonate—2:1
Other personnel	LPN, assistants under direction of head nurse	Social service, respiratory therapy, biomedical laboratory as needed	Designated full-time social service, respiratory therapy, biomedical engineering, laboratory technician Nurse-clinician and specialists Nurse program and education coordinators

Ob, Obstetrician; *Ped*, pediatrician.

Table 43-9 Morbidity among Premature Infants*

Causes	Percent affected
Metabolic	
Acidosis	43
Glucose (outside 40-150 mg/dl range)	26
Calcium (<7 mg/dl)	24
Body temperature on admission (<96° F [<36° C])	24
Sodium (outside 130-150 mEq/L range)	15
TOTAL	132†
Cardiorespiratory	
Asphyxia at birth (Apgar 0-6)	54
Apnea	29
Respiratory distress syndrome	20
Patent ductus arteriosus	19
Bronchopulmonary dysplasia, air leak	10
TOTAL	132
Hematological	
Hemoglobin (outside 10-21 g/dl range)	64
Platelets (<100,000/mm^3)	11
TOTAL	75
Infection	
Premature rupture of membranes	25
Localized systemic	16
Sepsis	5
TOTAL	46
Gastrointestinal	
Hyperbilirubinemia (>12 mg/dl)	12
Necrotizing enterocolitis	11
Cholestatic jaundice	10
TOTAL	33
Neurological—Convulsions	5

Data from Usher RH: The special problems of the premature infant. In Avery GB, editor: *Neonatology,* ed 3, Philadelphia, 1987, JB Lippincott.
*Data from 110 preterm infants (<34 weeks of gestation) from an unselected maternal population.
†Cumulative frequencies may exceed 100% because of multiple occurrences.

CURRENT STATUS

There are three types of perinatal transport: maternal-fetal transport, neonatal transport, and return transport of the neonate. Maternal-fetal transport is initiated for an identified high-risk condition in the mother (e.g., poorly controlled diabetes, preeclampsia) or for fetal risk (e.g., premature rupture of membranes at less than 34 weeks of gestation). The concept of maternal-fetal transport evolved more slowly than that of neonatal transport. Issues in the establishment of maternal-fetal transport have included uncertainty about the level of risk, cost containment, and the reluctance of local physicians to refer patients. With increasing documentation favoring maternal-fetal transport, many hospitals that have neonatal intensive care units (NICUs) now receive the majority of their neonates in utero.

Maternal-fetal transports often use local ambulances. Most clinical situations necessitate attendance in transport by a professional—the referring physician, nurse-midwife, or obstetrical nurse. A complicated delivery or the birth of a high-risk infant en route is thus anticipated and the risks minimized. Maternal-fetal and neonatal transports that originate at a community hospital and do not involve the center transport team are known as *one-way transports.* These transports can shorten the time it takes for the patient to arrive at the regional center. In less acute situations, when little or no risk of delivery en route is involved, the pregnant patient may be referred and responsible for her own travel. In all situations direct communication between the referring physician and the physician who will be attending the patient at the center is mandatory before departure.

Neonatal transports are initiated by the referring physician. Most often the physician calls the regional center to ask for transport when a problem is identified after birth; however, the request may be made before the birth. For example, if a woman who is at 28 weeks of gestation arrives at the hospital in active labor and delivery is imminent, nurses and physicians should consider requesting the regional center's transport team to be present for the delivery or to arrive soon thereafter. The *two-way transport,* in which an ambulance and team from the regional center travel to the community hospital to pick up the neonate, is the most common type of neonatal transport. Some community hospitals have the equipment and trained personnel necessary for one-way transports to their regional center.

The request for a neonatal transfer to the regional center should prompt the initiation of an established protocol that immediately alerts the provider of the transport vehicle, the transport personnel, and the responsible neonatologist. Telephone communication with the referring physician enables the regional center's neonatologist to define a plan for stabilization of the infant and meeting his or her immediate needs. Depending on the capabilities of the local hospital, this plan may include studies and interventions such as placing an arterial or a venous catheter, expanding fluid volume, determining serum electrolytes and blood gases, obtaining appropriate roentgenograms, and initiating antibiotic or oxygen therapy. Communication should be continuous to allow for management changes according to a neonate's needs. The regional center's transport team usually assumes responsibility for care of the infant on their arrival at the community hospital but works closely with the referring physician, who should be present when the team arrives. Samples of maternal and umbilical cord blood, roentgenograms, and copies of records should accompany the newborn to the regional center. The transport team should obtain the placenta for examination.

Optimal transport of a newborn is best achieved when stabilization of the newborn is as complete as possible before departure to the referral NICU. *The neonate's stable condition is more important than a quick return to the regional center.*

Parents should have the opportunity to see, to touch, and, if possible, to hold their newborn before transport and to receive information from the transport team members about how to communicate with regional center personnel. A brochure listing names of center personnel and telephone numbers can be helpful. A photograph of the baby taken before transport can be a comfort for the parents during the stressful period of separation from their infant. A telephone call soon after arrival at the neonatal unit from the transport team to the parents and the referring physician is important to bring them up-to-date on the neonate's status. NICU personnel should make subsequent contact with the parents or the referring physician at least daily and more frequently if the neonate's condition is critical.

It often is possible to transfer the mother to the postpartum floor of the tertiary center so that she can be close to her newborn. Parents should be encouraged to visit the NICU at any hour to see, touch, and hold their baby and to participate in his or her care as soon as possible. Perinatal care providers are aware that parental grief and stress reactions develop when a pregnancy is abnormal and that parents may express their grief verbally or behaviorally. Transport and distance add to stress.

Return transport is indicated as soon as the infant can be treated appropriately at the community hospital and the services of a regional center are no longer needed. The timing of the return depends on the facilities and the capabilities of the staff of the local hospital. The infant may be growing well but may still require special care such as gavage feedings, monitoring for occasional apneic episodes, or completion of antibiotic therapy. Communication between the staffs of the community hospital and the regional center and with the parents regarding plans for return transport must be established well before the return is scheduled. A NICU nurse who can discuss the neonate's problems and needs with the nursing staff of the community hospital should accompany the neonate on the return transport to ensure the greatest continuity of care. A return transport places the infant in his or her own community near the parents and frees space and resources at the regional center for treatment of other critically ill newborns. A specific benefit is the return of direct responsibility for the infant's care to the primary care physician.

TRANSPORT VEHICLES

Improved technology of two types, the vehicle itself and the mobile equipment used to stabilize and treat in transit, has expanded transport capability and alternatives. Discussions of transport include comparisons of the advantages and disadvantages of alternatives.[8] Specially equipped ground ambulances ensure optimum care during transport and are adequate for distances of up to 200 to 300 miles. When distances are greater or when physical barriers or time are problematic, air transport has advantages. Fixed-wing aircraft have the speed and space for distances from several hundred to over a thou-

Table 43-10 Physician Responsibility in Perinatal Transport

Physician base	Maternal-fetal transport (MFT)	Neonatal transport	Return neonatal transport
Referring	Understand benefits of MFT Identify high-risk situations at earliest moment Communicate with regional center Assume proper transport including appropriate professional accompaniment Assume care of the patient on return to the community	Understand benefits of neonatal transport Identify problems and initiate communication with regional center Initiate stabilization of the infant and provide appropriate therapy until transport team arrives, then assist the transport until departure Provide appropriate documentation, including hospital record, maternal and cord blood, and roentgenograms Participate in case discussion at follow-up conferences	Assess local resources and provide optimal neonatal care at community hospital Accept the infant in transfer as soon as medically indicated Understand importance and support of continuity of care, including parental participation
Receiving	Educate regional physicians about benefits of MFT Establish and maintain a 24-hour telephone consultation and referral system Establish and maintain data collection for evaluation and educational purposes Provide tertiary care for the mother and the fetus Maintain communication with community health care providers Discuss the case with local physicians at all stages, including a follow-up conference and case-based transport conferences	Educate regional physicians on benefits of neonatal transport Establish and maintain a 24-hour telephone consultation referral system Ensure immediate availability of an experienced transport team Assess responsibility for the infant at community hospital and direct the continuing stabilization process before transport Communicate with the family and their physicians at all stages of care Discuss case with local physicians in a follow-up conference and case-based transport conferences	Maintain knowledge of local hospital capabilities Communicate with local physicians, nurses, and parents in anticipation of transfer Provide documentation, including a written discharge summary, to accompany the patient

sand miles and can be pressurized. Rotary-wing aircraft (helicopters) are being utilized increasingly with their obvious advantages of speed and ability to land near the sites of care, but have internal environmental concerns such as space, noise, and vibration. Prior planning and an appropriate decision-making process at the time of transport, which takes into consideration the needs of the patient and the safety of the crew, are indicators of a well-managed transport service.

PERSONNEL

The transport team must have the capability to stabilize the infant at the referring hospital and provide care during each phase of the journey. Traditionally the team consists of an experienced physician and a neonatal nurse.

More recently, programs have used a specially trained neonatal nurse practitioner as the primary transport specialist. An emergency care nurse, a respiratory therapist, or an emergency medical technician also may complement the team.

A NICU nurse, preferably the newborn's primary care nurse, usually accompanies the newborn on the return transport to communicate the neonate's current status, including the feeding routine, the presence of apneic episodes, and any special family problems, to the receiving nurse at the community hospital.

The importance of primary care physicians in the care of the neonate cannot be overemphasized. The identification of the newborn at risk, the initial resuscitation and stabilization of the newborn, the communication with the regional center before transport and thereafter, and the management of the neonate on return from the regional center are their special responsibilities (Table 43-10).

EQUIPMENT

Neonatal transport equipment should be adequate to provide full intensive care and should include a transport incubator, a portable ventilator, an oxygen mixing and measuring system, a cardiorespiratory monitor, blood pressure monitors, infusion pumps, and essential drugs and supplies such as chest tubes. All electrically powered equipment should have "stand-alone" capability with batteries as an alternative power source. Batteries must have sufficient longevity for the duration of the transport, should electricity not be available. Critical care equipment should be adaptable to 12- and 24-volt DC and 110-volt AC power for use in a hospital or an ambulance to avoid excessive use of batteries.

EDUCATION

The responsibility of the regional perinatal center does not end with the successful transport and treatment of the patient. Most referral centers assume direct responsibility for the continuing education of perinatal care professionals in their region. These activities should include didactic presentations and the distribution of related printed materials.

Case-based transport conferences at the community hospital can be educationally effective.[7] These conferences also should involve physicians and nurses from the regional center to promote interaction with referring community hospital staff members. Open discussion of all aspects of care, including management at the community and center levels, is important. Such discussion facilitates development of improved clinical skills, decision making, and continuity of care.

REFERENCES

Overview

1. American Academy of Pediatrics and the American College of Obstetricians and Gynecologists: *Guidelines for perinatal care,* ed 3, Elk Grove Village, Ill, 1992, The Academy.

Perinatal Transport

1. Boehm FH, Haire MF: One-way transport: an evolving concept in patient services, *Am J Obstet Gynecol* 134:484, 1979.
2. Chance GW, O'Brien MJ, Swyer PR: Transportation of sick neonates, 1972: an unsatisfactory aspect of medical care, *Can Med Assoc J* 109:847, 1973.
3. Committee of Perinatal Health: *Toward improving the outcome of pregnancy: the 90s and beyond,* White Plains, NY, 1993, March of Dimes Birth Defects Foundation.
4. Segal S, editor: *Manual for the transport of high-risk infants: principles, policies, equipment, techniques,* Vancouver, 1972, Canadian Pediatric Society.
5. Harris TB, Isamen J, Giles HR: Improved neonatal survival through maternal transport, *Obstet Gynecol* 52:294, 1978.
6. *Interhospital care of the perinatal patient.* In Freeman RK, Poland RL, editors: *Guidelines for perinatal care,* ed 3, Elk Grove Village, Ill, and Washington, DC, 1992, American Academy of Pediatrics and American College of Obstetricians and Gynecologists.
7. Philip AGS, Little GA, Lucey JF: The transport conference as a teaching strategy: evaluation in the Vermont/New Hampshire regional perinatal program, *Perinatatology/Neonatology* 8:63, 1984.
8. Task Force on Interhospital Transport, American Academy of Pediatrics: *Guidelines for air and ground transport of neonatal and pediatric patients,* Elk Grove Village, Ill, 1993, American Academy of Pediatrics.

SUGGESTED READINGS

Overview

Avery GB, Fletcher MA, MacDonald MG, editors: *Neonatology—pathophysiology and management of the newborn,* ed 4, Philadelphia, 1994, JB Lippincott.

Budin P: *The nursling—the feeding and hygiene of premature and full-term infants,* London, 1907, CEEPI, Ltd (translated by WJ Maloney).

Clifford SH: Postmaturity with placental dysfunction; clinical syndrome and pathological findings, *J Pediatr* 44:1, 1954.

Curran JS: Birth-associated injury, *Clin Perinatol* 8:111, 1981.

Davis JA, Dobbing J, editors: *Scientific foundations of pediatrics,* ed 2, Baltimore, 1982, University Park Press.

Fanaroff AA, Martin RJ, editors: *Neonatal-perinatal medicine: diseases of the fetus and infant,* ed 5, St Louis, 1992, Mosby.

Klaus MH, Fanaroff AA, editors: *Care of the high-risk neonate,* ed 4, Philadelphia, 1993, WB Saunders.

Ledger WJ: Bacterial infections complicating pregnancy, *Clin Obstet Gynecol* 21:455, 1978.

Lubchenco LO: *The high risk infant,* Philadelphia, 1976, WB Saunders.

Lubchenco LO et al: Intrauterine growth as estimated from liveborn birthweight data at 24 to 42 weeks gestation, *Pediatrics* 32:793, 1963.

Monheit AG, Resnik R: Cesarean section: current trends and perspectives, *Clin Perinatol* 8:101, 1982.

Painter MJ, Bergman I: Obstetrical trauma to the neonatal central and peripheral nervous system, *Semin Perinatol* 6:89, 1982.

Parmalee AH: *Management of the newborn,* ed 2, Chicago, 1959, Mosby.

Toeusch HW, Ballard RA, Avery ME: *Schaffer and Avery's diseases of the newborn,* ed 6, Philadelphia, 1991, WB Saunders.

von Reuss AR: *The diseases of the newborn,* New York, 1922, William Wood.

Vulliamy DG: *The newborn child,* ed 5, New York, 1982, Churchill Livingstone.

PART FIVE
The Newborn

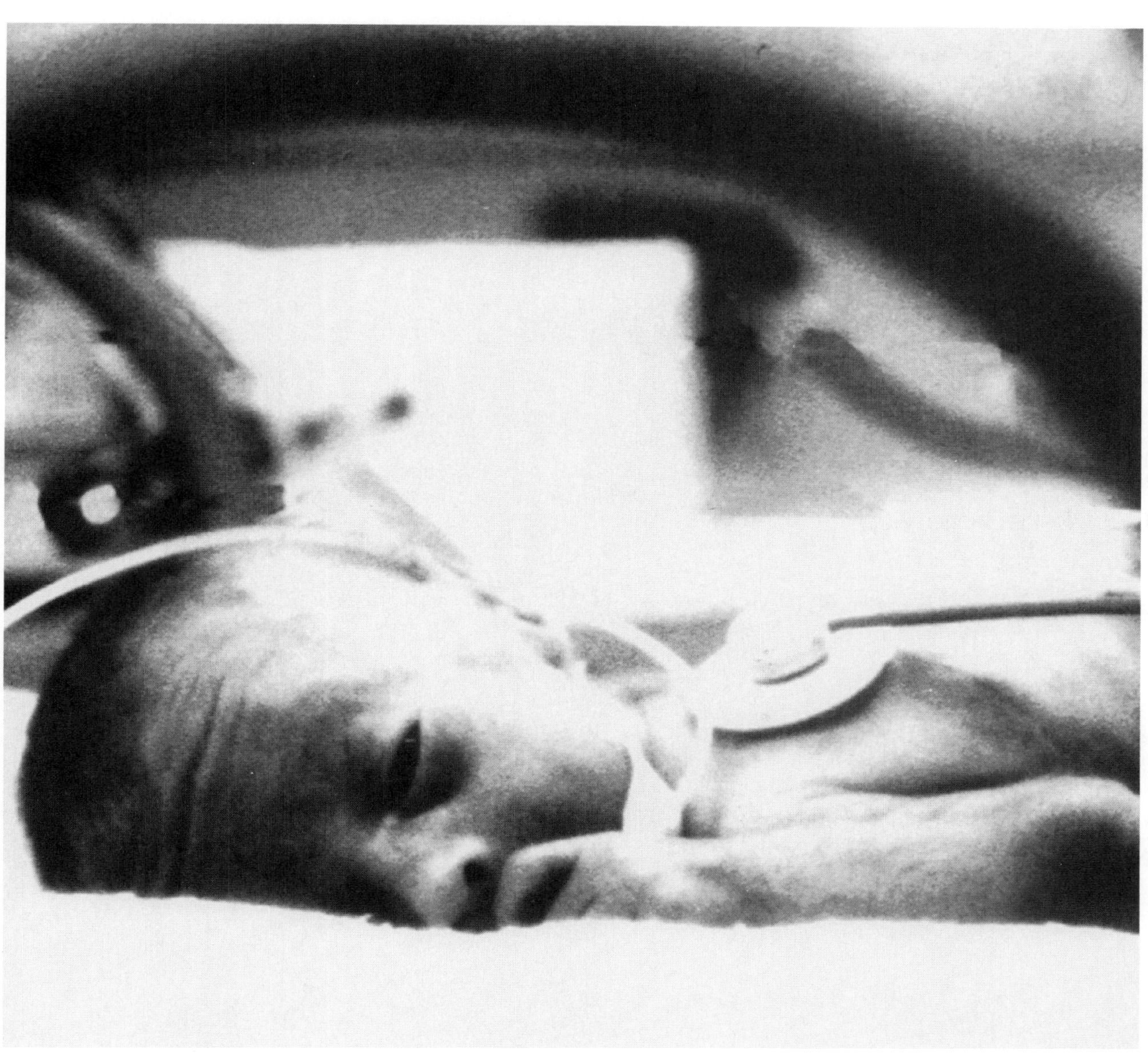

44 Neonatal Adaptations

The fundamental objective of the component of pediatric practice involving neonatal adaptations is the healthy transition of the fetus from intrauterine to extrauterine life. The most effective strategy for achieving this objective calls for the physician to enlist the parents (and their extended family) in a continuous collaboration designed to stimulate, form, and enhance their developing parenting skills.

It often has been noted—accurately—that no human activity of comparable responsibility is more often undertaken with so little preparation or training than parenthood. Somewhere in the past millennia, humans, as a species, appear to have lost many of those instinctual elements of parenting behavior so clearly designed to foster thriving survival of the young—elements that we observe daily, for example, in the parenting behavior of house pets. The possible role of the health professions in contributing to this loss of skills is a matter outside the scope of this chapter, but evidence is found throughout this book (e.g., failure to thrive and the abused child) to support the contention that many pediatric problems stem from the misfortune of a child's being unwelcome on arrival. Conversely, there are few better guarantees for a child's health or even for optimal adjustment to ill health than that his or her birth be happily and lovingly anticipated by both parents—a blessing that far outweighs any material support, public or private. Equally blessed are the obstetrician and pediatrician who have the good fortune to work with parents motivated by such love to seek and sustain their child's health.

The best tactic for optimizing parenting skills is a staged approach to anticipatory guidance and problem management, marked by continuing obstetrical-pediatric collaboration extending throughout gestation and the puerperium (Table 44-1). Each stage is typically pursued in a different site, addresses different processes, pursues different objectives, requires different observations, and may require different interventions.

ONE

Peripartum Considerations

Nicholas M. Nelson and M. Jeffrey Maisels

The performance sites for the peripartum stage of management of the newborn (from 0 to 40 weeks of gestation) are principally the obstetrician's office but also the community hospital's prenatal, labor, and birth classes and its high-risk pregnancy clinics. The main biological processes supervised are organogenesis in the first trimester and maternal and fetal nutrition in the second and third trimesters (focusing on more strictly obstetrical concerns in the third trimester). The embryo is largely unavailable for scrutiny in the first trimester but, chiefly through amniocentesis and ultrasonography, it becomes accessible during the second trimester, when its activity, breathing, growth, and general well-being can be observed. Medicine has developed a considerable capability to diagnose structural defects, particularly during the last trimester—a capability nearly as sophisticated as that for diagnosing genetic defects in the second trimester. However, our ability to repair specific genotypical or phenotypical defects in utero still is rudimentary, and the fundamental decision to be made concerning a pregnancy so threatened is whether it should be terminated well before the threshold of viability (currently around 25 weeks' gestation) or as far beyond that threshold as is consonant with reasonable fetal health.

More and more often specialists are deciding that a fetus threatened by any of several conditions (e.g., intrauterine growth retardation, uteroplacental insufficiency, hemolytic disease, maternal diabetes, hydronephrosis, hydrocephalus, and ileal atresia) stands a better chance for effective intervention by early delivery and management in a neonatal intensive care unit than by continuing in utero much beyond the stage of fetal pulmonary maturation (about 32 weeks).

In developed nations for the past 50 years, birth has taken place nearly exclusively in the hospital, to which most attribute the near-total conquest of maternal death. However, the benefits for the term infant, the mother-infant pair, and the nuclear family increasingly have been called into question. Overly rigid hospital "routines," established under the rubric of safeguarding the mother and infant (and often serving only to maximize hospital efficiency and staff convenience), reduced the "lying-in" period from 2 weeks to 2 days, placed fishbowl glass between infant and parents (with occasional excursions to the breast of that relatively rare mother who bravely defied hospital pressure to the contrary), and generally depersonalized the central human event that is birth.

The inevitable counterrevolution of the last generation has seen the medical profession yield significantly on its more pompous stances regarding the management of the birth process—to the extent that fathers in labor classes and labor and delivery rooms, infant and mother rooming-in (both enjoying visits from brothers and sisters), breast-feeding (replete with hospital support), and "birthing rooms" (née delivery rooms) have become happy commonplaces. These advances still are almost exclusively in the hospital (although it is more homelike), and maternal mortality remains near zero, with perinatal (fetal plus neonatal) mortality approaching the zero level, provided that gestation has proceeded beyond about 36 weeks. The major dinosaurs left in this evolution are the unsolved problems of premature labor and whether the rapidly increasing recourse to electronic fetal monitoring and cesarean birth (which now accounts for more than 20% of all deliveries in some hospitals) should be regarded as merely the current medical means of dehumanizing the birth process or as instruments of fetal salvation.

Table 44-1 Management of the Newborn*

Stage	Age	Obstetrics	Pediatrics
Prenatal	0-40 wk	*****	*
Birth	0-1 hr	****	**
Recovery	1-8 hr		***
Adjustment	8-48 hr		****
Establishment	48 hr-6 wk		*****

*Asterisks indicate the degree of involvement of obstetricians and pediatricians in management decisions.

CONVERSION FROM PLACENTAL TO PULMONARY RESPIRATION

The biological processes involved at this stage are the nonnegotiable demands placed on the fetus for rapid and successful conversion from placental to pulmonary respiration and the ability to support its metabolic needs (to defend body temperature and create new tissue) through its own, rather than the mother's, organs of digestion and excretion.

The first breaths (the fetus actually has been "panting" in utero for some weeks) are taken in response to many stimuli—sound (beyond the maternal souffle), light, chilling (from 98.6° to 71.6° F [37° to 22° C]), pressure, and probably pain. This "sensory overload" has been compared to that of weightless astronauts returning from orbit and modulates the fundamental respiratory regulation by the chemoreceptors of the carotid and aortic bodies and by the medullary centers.

Every normal labor is, to a degree, an asphyxiating event, because each uterine contraction interrupts umbilical venous flow. This brief and intermittent asphyxia often is reflected in simultaneous and brief slowing of the fetal heart rate. Indeed, many infants at cesarean delivery not preceded by labor are notably slow to take their first breath until submitted to that ultimate asphyxiating event, the clamping (or natural constriction) of the umbilical cord vessels. If excessive prenatal asphyxia (as from placental infarction) or intranatal asphyxia (as from a "nuchal," or knotted, umbilical cord) occurs, agonal or preagonal responses may well lead to passage of meconium, aspiration, and inspissation in utero.

As the fetal thorax is compressed by passage through the birth canal and the head emerges on the perineum, a certain amount of fetal lung liquid may be expressed through the airways to the exterior. As the chest wall recoils to its natural proportions after emergence of the thorax, some small amount of air may then be drawn into the airways, thus establishing an air-liquid interface. Next, the first breaths and cries are taken, and the airless (but liquid-filled) alveoli begin to establish air-liquid interfaces under the counterforces of increased surface tension tending toward atelectatic collapse. It is the special function of the alveolar phospholipoprotein complex (pulmonary surfactant, produced by alveolar pneumocytes) to reduce surface tension at the air-liquid interface, thus promoting alveolar stability. Once the lung is expanded, usually within one or two breaths, its vascular resistance (as high as the systemic resistance in utero) begins to decline rapidly, as pericapillary alveolar pressure diminishes and arteriolar resistance relaxes, under the influence of the rapid rise in PaO_2 from the normal fetal level of about 25 torr to that of the newborn (about 80 torr). This done, pulmonary blood flow (only about 5% of total cardiac output in utero) increases vastly, such that the left atrium, receiving increased pulmonary venous return, begins to distend its walls to their compliant limits and left atrial pressure rises to exceed that of the right (which is decreasing with diminishing umbilical venous return); thus the foramen ovale (basically a one-way flutter valve barring egress from the left atrium) closes. Meanwhile, the placental circulation (formerly a low-resistance shunt during fetal life) shuts down, as its vessels are either constricted naturally or clamped artificially.

Thus birth converts the systemic circulation to one of higher total vascular resistance than that of the pulmonary circulation; blood returning to the right side of the heart from the superior and inferior venae cavae now preferentially flows through the pulmonary circulation, whereas in fetal life the right ventricular output had largely bypassed the high-resistance pulmonary artery by flowing through the ductus arteriosus directly into the aorta, which bathes the coronary and carotid vessels with the best-oxygenated blood available to the fetus—that from the umbilical vein, which crosses the liver through the ductus venosus, coursing to the inferior cava and the right atrium. Two thirds of this fetal blood crosses the foramen ovale directly into the left atrium; the remainder passes through the right ventricle and ductus arteriosus (from the right to the left circulations) to the aortic isthmus. However, as these respective circulations' vascular resistances reverse after birth, blood returning from the lungs to the left atrium is pumped by the left ventricle to the aortic root, where again it confronts an open ductus arteriosus and a now higher systemic than pulmonary resistance; thus it preferentially passes through the ductus (from left to right) to *recirculate* through the lungs. At this stage of life (within the first 1 or 2 hours after birth), the circulation is "transitional" in that the foramen ovale is functionally closed, while the ductus arteriosus is still open and is recirculating blood from the left to the right circulatory systems through the lungs. Moreover, during this period the volume and pressure load on the left ventricle nearly triples compared with fetal life, during which the right ventricle was dominant in both load and size and both ventricles worked "in parallel," connected by the foramen ovale and the ductus arteriosus.

The terminal phase in conversion of the fetal circulatory pattern to the neonatal pattern is marked by closure of the ductus arteriosus in a process of interaction between the increasing oxygen content of the blood coursing through it and decreasing levels of circulating or local tissue prostaglandins. This usually occurs somewhere in the second 12 hours of the first day of life, when early systolic murmurs at the base of the heart often are heard, presumably related to the process.

OBSERVATIONS DURING AND IMMEDIATELY AFTER LABOR AND DELIVERY

Observations during the perinatal period should be directed toward ensuring that the fetus remains well oxygenated, the chief evidence for which is sought during labor through monitoring of the fetal heart rate by either acoustic or electronic means. Meconium staining of the amniotic fluid (in vertex deliveries) is taken as evidence of significant fetal hypoxia, acute or chronic, and should alert the attending physician to the potential need for aspiration of meconium from the nasopharynx and trachea before the infant has the opportunity to aspirate and inspissate that viscous material into the airways with the first few breaths.

After full cervical dilation, the fetal scalp becomes available for microsampling of fetal blood gases; the pH is a more reliable indicator of hypoxia than is oxygen tension under these circumstances. At delivery the cord blood becomes available for the same purpose.

However, immediately after delivery, the entire infant should be assessed to establish the success of oxygenation throughout labor by means of the Apgar score (see Chapter 7, Table 7-1), which includes a grading of neuromuscular reactivity (muscle tone and reflex irritability), as well as of heart rate, respiration, and color. The 1-minute assessment has not nearly the overall prognostic power of the 5-minute score, but most serious decisions for resuscitative intervention are or should be made for the child whose respiratory effort is absent or failing at 1 minute after birth and certainly if the heart rate is decreasing.

PHYSICAL EXAMINATION

With an uncomplicated delivery of a low-risk fetus, the responsibility for the delivery room examination of the newborn most often falls to the person performing the delivery. With a high-risk delivery, resuscitation, if required, and the initial delivery room assessment normally are in the hands of the pediatrician in attendance. Whether an elective cesarean birth at term constitutes a high-risk delivery requiring the attendance of a pediatrician is more a matter of individual circumstance and local custom than actual likelihood of resuscitative intervention.

Once the decision can be made that active resuscitation from birth asphyxia is unnecessary, or after its successful completion, the infant should receive a brief and "directed" physical examination in the delivery room (if possible, before formal introduction to the parents) under circumstances promoting maximum visibility while preventing chilling (an overhead radiant warmer or floodlight illumination is simple and effective). The principal objectives of this examination are to seek evidence of obstetrical trauma, particularly in the

DELIVERY ROOM (OR SUBSEQUENT) ASSESSMENT

A. General
  1. Whole
     a. Proportions
     b. Symmetry
     c. Facies
     d. Gestational age (approximate)
  2. Skin (color, subcutaneous tissue, and imperfections), bands, and birthmarks
  3. Neuromuscular
     a. Movements
     b. Responses
     c. Tone (flexor)

B. Head and neck
  1. Head
     a. Shape
     b. Circumference
     c. Molding
     d. Swellings
     e. Depressions
     f. Occipital overhang
  2. Fontanelles, sutures
     a. Size
     b. Tension
  3. Eyes
     a. Size
     b. Separation
     c. (Cataracts)
     d. (Colobomas)
  4. Ears
     a. Placement
     b. Complexity
     c. (Preauricular tags or sinuses)
  5. Mouth
     a. Symmetry
     b. Size
     c. Clefts
  6. Neck
     a. Swellings
     b. Fistulas

C. Lungs and respiration
  1. Retraction
  2. Grunt
  3. Air entry (breath sounds)

D. Heart and circulation
  1. Rate
  2. Rhythm
  3. Murmurs
  4. Sounds

E. Abdomen
  1. Musculature
  2. Bowel sounds
  3. Cord vessels
  4. Distention
  5. Scaphoid shape
  6. Masses

F. Genitalia and anus
  1. Placement
  2. Testes
  3. Labia
  4. Phallus

G. Extremities
  1. Bands
  2. Digits (number and overlapping)

H. Spine
  1. Symmetry
  2. (Scoliosis)
  3. (Sinuses)

Table 44-2 Obstetrical Situations in Which Delivery Trauma May Occur

Type of injury	Normal vertex	Cesarean	Premature	Precipitate	Difficult: Breech extraction	Difficult: Large infant	Difficult: High midforceps
Hemorrhage							
Cerebral							
Subdural							X
Subarachnoid				X	X	X	X
Intraventricular			X				
Abdominal							
Liver					X	X	
Spleen					X	X	
Adrenal gland					X	X	
Cutaneous, presenting part	X				X		
Conjunctival	X						
Fracture or dislocation							
Clavicle						X	
Humerus					X		
Femur					X		
Skull							X
Nerve injury							
Brachial plexus						X	
Spinal cord					X		
Facial	X						
Laceration		X					

instance of a "difficult delivery" (e.g., shoulder dystocia, aftercoming head of the breech delivery, and any operative delivery more challenging than simple "outlet forceps") and unanticipated gross congenital anomalies (many of these are now detected by ultrasound in utero) and to assess gestational age. Most of the important information at this stage is gathered by careful observation, along with brief palpation and auscultation, with an emphasis on the points listed in the box on p. 491. Obstetrical situations in which the physician should be especially wary of possible delivery trauma are listed in Table 44-2.

The infant who displays good flexor muscle tone, who is properly reactive to tactile stimuli, who is unarguably "pink" in midface and trunk (as opposed to the often still blue extremities) by about 5 minutes of age, who has a perforate anus, whose genitalia are unambiguous, and whose neural tube and palate are closed can be presented to his or her parents as "normal," after auscultation of the chest and palpation of the abdomen (see description of the physical examination in Part Two, Physiological Status of the Healthy Infant).

Infants who are tachycardic or who have grunting expirations and flaring alae nasi at about 10 minutes of age may be regarded with some suspicion but not yet alarm because much fetal lung fluid (about 20 ml/kg) must be absorbed into the circulation. If air entry into the lungs is satisfactory, the outlook may well be sanguine. The heart examination may reveal an early systolic murmur that merits continuing observation. The second sound usually is single until increasing pulmonary blood flow leads to its normal splitting some hours later.

The more detailed physical examination can safely wait until after the infant is admitted to the "recovery room" (nursery), where prophylactic eye ointment and vitamin K may also be given. Apart from sharing in the parents' joy and relief, the primary physician's remaining time in the delivery room might more profitably be devoted to study of the placenta, which usually is available for inspection about the time the initial examination of the infant is completed. The placenta should be searched for gross areas of infarction, marginal separation, velamentous insertion of vessels, meconium staining, and purulence, as clues to the infant who may be pallid (from occult blood loss) or subsequently septic. The cord vessels (two arteries and one vein) also should be confirmed as normal because there appears to be an association (of arguable validity) between the presence of a single umbilical artery and other anomalies, most of which are obvious (e.g., trisomies).

INTERVENTIONS AT BIRTH

Placental Transfusion

Even before the infant's attendant has had an opportunity to wipe away the greasy vernix, the initial intervention (or decision not to intervene) has been taken by the obstetrician regarding management of the cord. Some clamp the umbilical cord immediately, some wait until the pulsations have ceased, and others prefer to wait until the infant has breathed

PERINATAL CONDITIONS THAT INCREASE THE RISK OF NEONATAL ASPHYXIA

Antepartum conditions

1. Diabetes
2. Toxemia
3. Hypertension
4. Rh sensitization
5. Previous stillbirth or neonatal death
6. Third trimester bleeding
7. Maternal infection
8. Polyhydramnios
9. Oligohydramnios
10. Postterm gestation
11. Multiple gestation
12. Intrauterine growth retardation

Intrapartum conditions

1. Operative delivery
   a. Cesarean section
   b. Midforceps delivery
2. Breech or other abnormal presentation
3. Premature labor
4. Ruptured membranes (>24 hr)
5. Chorioamnionitis
   a. Maternal fever, tachycardia, or both
   b. Ruptured membranes (>24 hr)
   c. Tender uterus
   d. Foul-smelling amniotic fluid
6. Prolonged labor (>24 hr)
7. Fetal distress
   a. Fetal tachycardia (>160 beats/min)
   b. Fetal bradycardia (<120 beats/min)
   c. Persistent late decelerations
   d. Severe variable decelerations without baseline variability
   e. Scalp pH ≤7.25
   f. Meconium-stained amniotic fluid
   g. Cord prolapse
8. General anesthesia
9. Narcotics administered during labor
10. Abruptio placentae
11. Placenta previa

and cried *or* placental artery pulsations have ceased (whichever is later), with the infant kept below the introitus and thus ensured of the maximal "placental transfusion" of blood (nearly 150 ml in term deliveries) within about 2 minutes.

Perinatal scientists have yet to achieve consensus on the proper management of the placental transfusion, since it is not yet clear whether the "extra" blood presents an intended advantage or whether the documented increase in blood pressure and cardiac load presented by such transfusion presents a significant cardiopulmonary disadvantage. Recollecting that the primeval delivery posture probably placed the mother on her knees or in a squatting position, so as better to attend the infant and afterbirth *before* the cord was cut, may suggest nature's (as opposed to medicine's) intent in the matter.

EQUIPMENT REQUIRED FOR RESUSCITATION

Ventilation

1. Oxygen source—oxygen, warmed and humidified
2. Suction—De Lee suction trap, wall suction with adjustable pressure gauge; suction catheters; sizes 6, 8, 10, 12 Fr
3. Ventilation bag—500 ml self-inflating type with reservoir (capable of delivering 100% O_2) or 500 cc anesthesia type
4. Face masks—infant sizes, premature and term
5. Laryngoscope—blade sizes 0 and 1, spare batteries, and bulbs
6. Endotracheal tubes—sizes 2.5, 3, and 3.5 mm with plastic adapters attached
7. Soft metal stylets for endotracheal tubes
8. Stethoscope
9. Feeding tube—8 Fr tubes to evacuate stomach contents

Temperature control

1. Evaporation—warm towels
2. Conduction—mattress covered with prewarmed towels
3. Convection—air conditioning turned down; delivery room temperature 75° F (23.9° C) minimum
4. Radiation—radiant warmer

Circulation and biochemical resuscitation

1. Umbilical catheterization tray
2. Drugs and volume expanders

Other

50 ml syringe with three-way stopcock and 21-gauge butterfly needle for evacuation of pneumothorax

Resuscitation from Asphyxia

Perinatal asphyxia is the most common example of acute respiratory failure in the neonatal period. It occurs in the delivery room when the infant fails to initiate adequate respiration or when respirations simply are insufficient to provide adequate gas exchange. It arises nearly always as the result of intrauterine asphyxia, during which the fetus becomes hypoxic and hypercarbic and may develop metabolic acidosis. The sine qua non of its management is to provide immediate ventilatory assistance.

Planning for Resuscitation. Obstetrical events usually herald the arrival of an asphyxiated infant in sufficient time to allow for preparation. However, organization and preplanning are essential to ensure appropriate action for an unanticipated problem. The "disaster plan" for delivery room resuscitation should be the primary responsibility of a physician and should be reviewed periodically. The delivery room staff should have on permanent and prominent display a list of maternal and fetal complications that require the presence in the delivery room of a professional qualified specifically in newborn resuscitation (see the box above, left).

Equipment Required. All equipment should be checked regularly (as well as before any delivery) for readiness and appropriate function. Is the laryngoscope light bright? Does the bag and mask ventilation system provide adequate flow? Is it free of leaks? A list of suggested equipment is provided in the box on p. 493.

Personnel. Proper resuscitation cannot be performed alone. Two people (e.g., physician and nurse) must be solely responsible for the infant's care directly after birth, undistracted by the needs of the mother.

Apgar Score. The Apgar score should be determined 1 and 5 minutes after birth (see Table 7-1). If the 5-minute score is less than 7, additional scores should be obtained every 5 minutes up to 20 minutes, unless and until two successive scores are 8 or higher. Ideally the Apgar score should be compiled by a person not directly involved in the resuscitation (e.g., a nurse).

Resuscitation Procedure. Figure 44-1 outlines the initial steps.

1. *Temperature control.* Immediately after delivery, the infant should be placed under a previously heated radiant warmer and completely dried with prewarmed towels to prevent excessive evaporative heat loss.
2. *Suctioning.* Suctioning is not essential for all infants; however, if necessary, it should be gentle. In particular, vigorous suctioning of the posterior pharynx must be avoided because this frequently produces significant bradycardia. If the amniotic fluid is meconium stained, the mouth and pharynx should be suctioned thoroughly using a De Lee trap to prevent meconium aspiration before delivery of the shoulders. With thick or particulate meconium, the larynx should be visualized and direct suction applied by means of an endotracheal tube. This procedure is repeated as often as necessary to remove as much material as possible. Guidelines for endotracheal tube sizes and suction catheters are provided in Table 44-3.
3. *Establishing respiration.* A normal infant should breathe within a few seconds of delivery and establish regular, effective respirations by 1 minute of life. An infant who at any age is not breathing spontaneously and whose heart rate is less than 100 beats/min requires immediate ventilation without recourse to a precise Apgar score. Figure 44-2 provides a flowchart for positive pressure ventilation.

With few exceptions, bag and mask ventilation, correctly performed, will provide adequate ventilation for most infants. The few infants in whom it should not be used include those who have meconium-stained amniotic fluid and those who have a diaphragmatic hernia. In addition, it may be very difficult to achieve adequate lung expansion by means of bag and mask ventilation in small premature infants whose lungs are noncompliant. *These exceptional cases require endotracheal intubation.*

Table 44-3 Guidelines for Endotracheal Tubes and Suction Catheters

Infant's weight (kg)	Endotracheal tube internal diameter (mm)	Depth of insertion from upper lip (cm)	Suction catheter size (Fr)
1	2.5	7	5
2	3	8	6
3	3.5	9	8

Critical to the success of bag and mask ventilation are a good facial seal and a nonobstructed airway, obtained by positioning the infant with his or her neck slightly extended and by lifting the infant's face to the mask by using the fingers of the left hand (Fig. 44-3). The little finger actually should elevate the angle of the jaw, thus bringing the tongue forward and opening the airway. Pushing the mask into the baby's face pushes the tongue back to obstruct the airway. The neck must *not* be hyperextended—this narrows the airway.

There are two kinds of bags: the open-ended *anesthesia bag,* which requires continual gas flow for inflation, and the *self-expanding (Ambu) bag,* which remains inflated with or

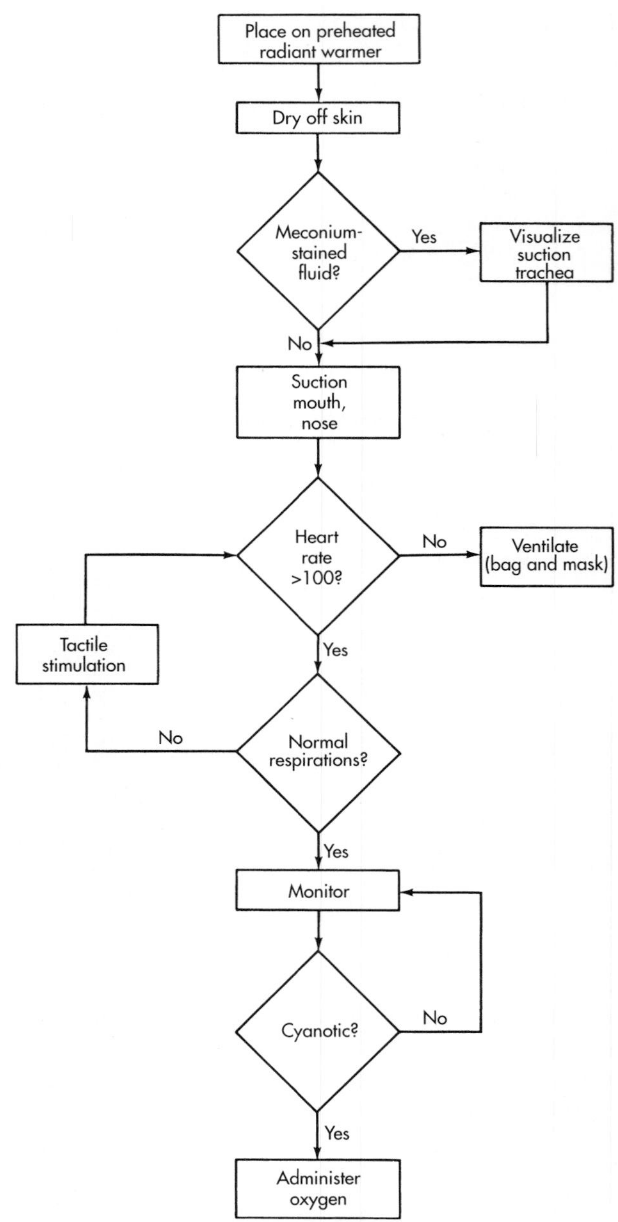

FIG. 44-1 Protocol for initial steps in resuscitation of an infant in the delivery room.

(Modified from Klaus MH, Fanaroff AA: *Care of the high-risk neonate,* ed 4, Philadelphia, 1993, WB Saunders.)

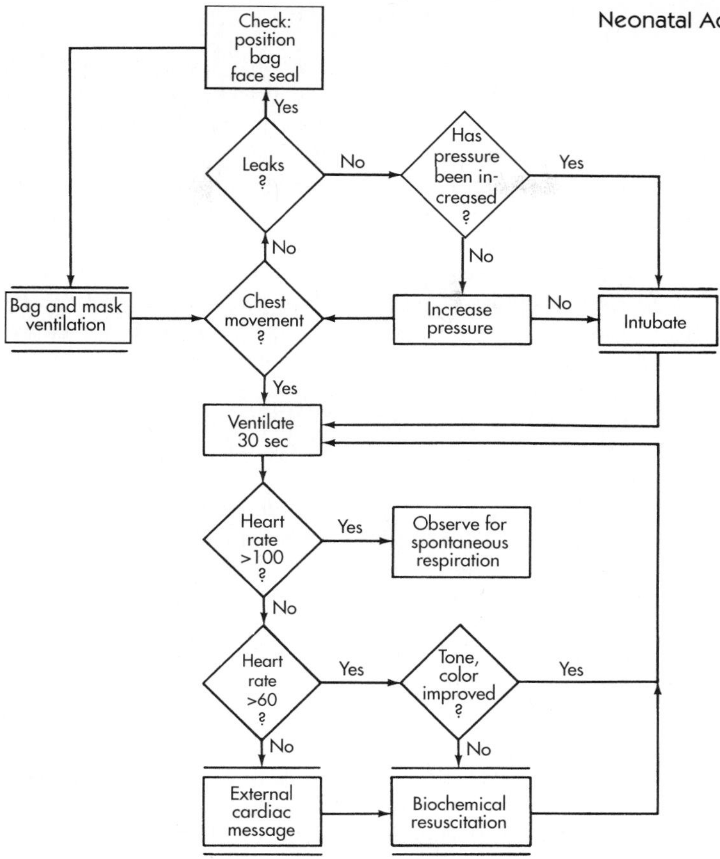

FIG. 44-2 Protocol for positive pressure ventilation in resuscitation of an infant in the delivery room.

(Modified from Klaus MH, Fanaroff AA: *Care of the high-risk neonate,* ed 4, Philadelphia, 1993, WB Saunders.)

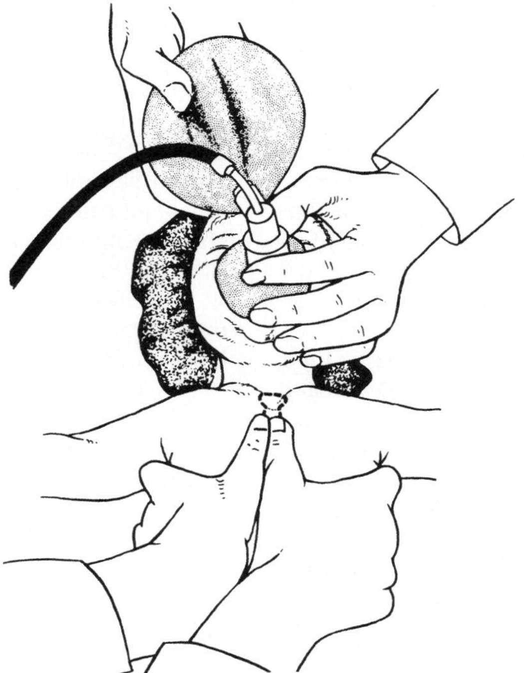

FIG. 44-3 Technique for bag and mask ventilation and external cardiac massage.

(From the American Academy of Pediatrics and the American Heart Association: *Textbook of neonatal resuscitation,* Dallas, 1994, American Heart Association.)

without gas flow. The latter is the more convenient to use, particularly for less experienced resuscitators, and several models are available. However, these bags must be fitted with an oxygen reservoir to deliver high concentrations of oxygen. The absence of a reservoir limits oxygen delivery to only 40% to 50%, a level grossly inadequate for delivery room resuscitation. Also, the valve assembly in most self-inflating bags permits oxygen flow *only when the bag is being compressed;* thus these bags cannot be used to provide free-flowing oxygen to the baby's face.

With successful ventilation, the chest should rise and fall while the infant's heart rate and color rapidly improve. If this does not occur, the seal between mask and face must be checked; continued inability to obtain adequate chest movement by bag and mask ventilation mandates endotracheal intubation.

Whether ventilation is provided via mask or endotracheal tube, *the appropriate inflating pressure is that which is required to expand the chest and improve gas exchange.* It is not to be determined solely by reference to a manometer. If the manometer indicates that high pressures are necessary to expand the chest, then the possibilities of airway obstruction, severe hyaline membrane disease, and hypoplastic lungs should be considered. Although overinflation entails a risk of producing a pneumothorax, this is relatively rare. Underventilation, on the other hand, is far more common and usually results from the unwise choice of a predetermined pressure limit, as shown by a manometer rather than by observation of the chest wall.

Effective assisted ventilation is the *only* intervention required in the overwhelming majority of severely asphyxiated neonates. With few exceptions, asphyxiated infants respond promptly to adequate ventilation.

The infant's heart rate should be monitored continuously by an assistant during the resuscitation procedure because this is the most useful and readily measurable criterion of the effectiveness of resuscitation. After intubation, the chest should be observed to ensure that it expands well and symmetrically and that equal breath sounds are heard in both axillae (not over the apices). Improvement in heart rate, color, and muscle tone confirms that ventilation is adequate. If any doubt exists about the position of the endotracheal tube, it should be checked by visualizing the larynx directly with a laryngoscope.

Meconium Aspiration

If thick particulate meconium is present in the amniotic fluid, the nose and pharynx should be suctioned by the obstetrician using a De Lee catheter as soon as the head is delivered. If possible, the physician who resuscitates should suction the baby's larynx before spontaneous breathing occurs. Whether or not the baby has breathed, the larynx should be visualized, and meconium should be removed directly by suction through an endotracheal tube. The process is repeated until the larynx is clear. If bradycardia has occurred, it may be necessary to ventilate the infant between suctioning.

External Cardiac Massage

If the heart rate does not increase above 80 beats/min after effective ventilation with oxygen, external cardiac heart massage should be instituted immediately while ventilation is continued; the technique is shown in Figure 44-3. The thumbs should be positioned over the midportion of the sternum, the chest encircled with both hands, and the sternum compressed ½ to ¾ inch (1.5 to 2 cm) 120 times per minute. Ventilation should continue while cardiac massage is administered. The actual timing of ventilation during cardiac massage probably is not critical, although some authorities recommend that a breath be provided after every third compression. If cardiac massage does not produce rapid improvement in the heart rate, appropriate drug therapy and volume expansion (if indicated) should be initiated.

Drugs

Drugs are rarely needed for resuscitation in the delivery room. They certainly should never be administered until after adequate ventilation has been established. If possible, drugs should be administered via the umbilical vein; however, if this route is unavailable, epinephrine and naloxone, as well as other necessary drugs, can be administered via the endotracheal tube. A list of drugs and appropriate doses is provided in Tables 44-4 and 48-2.

Asphyxiated infants usually have a combined metabolic and respiratory acidosis, which is properly treated by correcting the cause. Respiratory acidosis, the result of hypoventilation, is treated by intermittent positive pressure ventilation. Some experimental evidence indicates that metabolic acidosis has a specific detrimental effect on myocardial function in the hypoxic heart, but it also has been shown that the performance of the ischemic heart is related more closely to tissue P_{CO_2} than to the pH and that nonischemic cardiac muscle performance also is depressed by increases in P_{CO_2}. These observations further emphasize the primary role of ventilation in acid-base adjustments during resuscitation—adequate ventilation is the sine qua non, but if bradycardia or poor perfusion persists despite adequate ventilation, 1 to 2 mEq/kg of sodium bicarbonate may be given as a last resort. It should be diluted 1:1 with sterile water to a concentration of 0.5 mEq/ml and infused at a rate no faster than 1 to 2 mEq/min.

Hypovolemia

Most asphyxiated neonates are not hypovolemic. Moreover, it is important to recognize the potential hazards (e.g., intracranial hemorrhage) involved in overzealous volume expansion. On the other hand, certain conditions (e.g., vasa previa or fetal-maternal bleeding) may produce significant hemorrhage from the fetoplacental unit. Compression of the umbilical cord during labor, compounded by failure of the obstetrician to allow for the normal placental transfusion, may also be associated with hypovolemia. If significant hypovolemia is suspected (clinical signs of shock are usually not apparent until 20% to 25% of the blood volume has been lost), small infusions of volume expanders (10 to 20 ml/kg) may be given (see Table 44-4). The infant's response should be assessed after each infusion, and volume expansion should be discontinued as soon as tissue perfusion is adequate.

Respiratory Depression Caused by Narcotics

Respiratory depression caused by narcotics can be managed by assisted ventilation alone; however, if respiratory depression persists despite adequate assisted ventilation, naloxone (0.1 mg/kg) may be given.

Table 44-4 Indications for Drugs in Resuscitation of the Newborn

Indication	Drug	Dose
Metabolic acidosis	Sodium bicarbonate	1-2 mEq/kg initially and cautiously
Bradycardia	Epinephrine hydrochloride	0.1 ml/kg of 1:10,000 solution
Low blood volume	Albumin, human (Albumisol)	10 ml/kg of 5% solution
	Lactated Ringer	10 ml/kg
Respiratory depression secondary to narcotics	Naloxone	0.25 mg/kg

TWO

Physiological Status of the Healthy Infant

Nicholas M. Nelson

Throughout fetal life the placenta is at once the necessary and sufficient organ for respiration, nutrition, metabolism, excretion, and immune defense, whereas certain endocrine functions (likely including growth itself), as well as the events of parturition, require more active fetal effort. The fetal lung, gut, liver, kidney, thymus, and even the brain have no functional assignment, other than to grow, differentiate, and be ready to assume function at birth. Thus it is perfectly possible for nature to carry many of her human "experiments" to term with no kidneys, gut, liver, lungs, or brain. However, a fetal circulatory system, comprising pump and "exchange" vessels (capillaries), is necessary very early in gestation for all placental mammals, although a single ventricle will do.

CIRCULATORY SYSTEM

The major cardiorespiratory events that attend birth (discussed previously) sever the parallel connections of the greater (systemic) and lesser (pulmonary) circulations through the foramen ovale and ductus arteriosus, resulting in a serial circulatory pathway from right ventricle to pulmonary circulation to left ventricle to systemic circulation and guaranteeing that 100% of cardiac output (rather than about 5%, as in the fetus) passes through the lungs. This, perhaps paradoxically, results in a decrease in load on the right ventricle because pulmonary vascular resistance diminishes concomitant with an increase in left ventricular load, which occurs when the low-resistance placental shunt is removed by birth. This simultaneously converts a low-flow, high-resistance circuit (the pulmonary) to its inverse and a higher flow, lesser resistance circuit (the systemic) to its inverse. The result is that the right ventricular preponderance characteristic of fetal and early neonatal life begins to give way to the left ventricular dominance of later life; these events are most obvious in the changing QRS and T vectors on an electrocardiogram of the developing infant's heart. All these alterations in hemodynamics set the conditions that place the two ventricles (especially the left) high on their respective function curves—that is, producing relatively high cardiac outputs but with little further reserve for emergencies.

The infant myocardium appears to be less able than that of an adult to sustain tension against the loads imposed by high-volume (preload) or high-pressure (afterload) work loads. This possibly results from a level of sympathetic innervation that is as yet incomplete, even by term gestation, so myocardial beta-receptors are insufficiently stimulated. In any case, and especially in a premature newborn, there appears to be a parasympathetic/sympathetic innervational imbalance with parasympathetic dominance and frequent bradycardia, which often responds to atropine. Moreover, for a time the pulmonary arterioles retain their thick fetal musculature, which renders them supersensitive to any vasoconstrictive stimuli, such as hypoxia. The condition known as persistent pulmonary hypertension of the newborn (or as persistent fetal circulation) is characterized by such vasoconstriction, which forces blood right to left across the anatomically still-open shunts of the foramen ovale and ductus arteriosus to produce cyanosis and a general clinical picture quite difficult to distinguish clinically from true cyanotic congenital heart disease.

HEMATOPOIETIC SYSTEM

Certainly the earliest fetal organ function to become established, hematopoiesis (and later hemostasis), is sited first in the yolk sac (0 to 2 months), then the liver (2 to 6 months), and finally, the bone marrow (6 to 9 months).

The ontogeny of the hemoglobin chains is such that at birth fetal hemoglobin (hemoglobin F) is dominant. During the chronic hypoxic insult that is fetal life (with an average oxygen tension of perhaps 35 mm Hg), renal production of erythropoietin is stimulated; this in turn stimulates production of red cells to maximize oxygen-carrying capacity—at birth the red cell mass is at a maximum (hematocrit level of 55% to 65%), beyond which increasing blood viscosity would so impede blood flow as to actually diminish oxygen transfer. With birth these largely young red cells (abetted by an extra supply provided by a "placental transfusion" of up to 150 ml of whole blood, which occurs when the infant is kept below the vaginal introitus and the cord is left unclamped until after the first breath) rapidly begin to be torn down to add to the infant's bilirubin load. Oxygen transfer from placenta to red cell in the relatively hypoxic fetus is aided by hemoglobin F, which displays greater affinity for oxygen than does adult hemoglobin and a reduced affinity for its reciprocally binding coenzyme, 2,3-diphosphoglycerate (DPG). Immediately after birth the concentration of DPG rises sharply, and the oxygen affinity of the infant's blood conveniently falls, because now, after birth, the infant is operating at an oxygen pressure of about 100 mm Hg (rather than at 30 mm Hg) and needs not so much to be able to snatch precious oxygen molecules from a "hypoxic" placenta into the death grip of fetal hemoglobin as to be able graciously to give up the oxygen so carried to the harder-working peripheral tissues of his or her newly born and better-oxygenated body.

The several components of reliable hemostasis (blood vessels that can constrict, aggregatable platelets, and a functioning coagulation cascade of clotting proteins) appear largely intact in the term newborn, with the likely exception of the vitamin K–dependent factors (II, VII, IX, and X). These factors are present but at levels 50% or less of those of adults; they may decline even further, to as low as 5% to 20% of adult levels, and pose the risk of hemorrhagic disease unless vitamin K is given.

RESPIRATORY SYSTEM

During fetal life the infant's respiratory system, made up of gas-exchanging alveoli and air-conducting pathways, prepares developmentally to take on (very quickly after ligation of the cord) the awesome responsibility for gaseous metabolism previously assumed by the placenta.

From about 25 to 35 weeks of gestation, the alveoli, complete with their integrated perfusing blood supply, develop from "glandular" to more acinar structures. Concomitantly, the alveolar pneumocytes (type II cells) elaborate a complex of phospholipids and protein (pulmonary surfactant) and store it against the moment of the first breaths of life, when surfactant is spread in a thin layer over the alveolar epithelium, there to stabilize the alveoli by diminishing the surface tension established at the air-liquid interface. A somewhat leisurely process of absorption of fetal lung liquid occurs during the first hour of life (principally through the lymphatics), after the lungs have fully expanded and after the vast initial decline in pulmonary vascular resistance and reciprocal increase in pulmonary blood flow (described in the previous section) has occurred. Disruptions in this process of liquid resorption are thought to play a role in the condition called transient tachypnea of the newborn.

By the time of birth at term, the neuromuscular and skeletal apparatus that constitutes the thoracic bellows (ribs, intercostal muscles, and diaphragm) has had considerable intrauterine practice at breathing through a paroxysmal form of rapid panting (oscillatory movement of only very small amounts of amniotic fluid in the airways). These paroxysms (at least in fetal sheep) temporally coincide with episodes of "active sleep" (see Part Three of this chapter, Recovery Period). The only significant inefficiency of the thoracic bellows occurs during active sleep, when there is widespread inhibition of motor neurons, particularly those responsible for ongoing intercostal muscle tone. As a consequence, the chest wall becomes rather less fixed and stiff (i.e., more "compliant," like a loose-fitting glove); thus the tendency of the underlying stretched lung to collapse is less opposed by a firm chest wall than is the case in quiet sleep; the descending diaphragm is able to pull the lower rib cage counterproductively inward during inspiration ("paradoxical" respiration). Therefore the mechanical situation for an infant's lung is a bit more tenuous than is the case for an adult—specifically, the infant's lung tends to operate at a level rather close to its "collapse volume"; this tendency must be counteracted by increasing inspiratory muscle tone and laryngeal tone during expiration.

Nonetheless, the newborn's ability to ventilate and perfuse his or her alveoli and thereby permit exchange of carbon dioxide for oxygen within them is (relative to his or her metabolic needs) quite on a par with that of an Olympic runner. Indeed, the reason for the characteristic mild hypoxemia of the newborn (arterial PO_2 of 70 to 85 torr) is not that arterialization of venous blood within the lung is imperfect, but rather that a certain amount of right-to-left "fetal" shunting of desaturated venous blood continues to occur across the foramen ovale and ductus arteriosus until vascular resistance and pressure within the pulmonary circulation decline to more nearly adult levels. It remains uncertain whether the mild hypocapnia typical of neonatal life (arterial Pco_2 of 35 torr) results from a progesterone-mediated lowering of the respiratory center's threshold for carbon dioxide or whether it simply reflects the result, in the form of a lowered serum and cerebrospinal bicarbonate level, of the prolonged fluid volume expansion of fetal life.

RENAL FUNCTION

It has been suggested of the perinatal kidney that it emerges at birth from a primeval, water-rich swamp into an extrauterine desert, because the fetus and newly born infant behave in many ways as does a chronically volume-expanded subject with decreased tubular resorption of water and sodium (leading to "wasting" into the fetal urine), bicarbonate, glucose, and phosphate. The teleological and metaphysical question arises whether the fetus sustains such polyuria to maintain amniotic fluid volume. This question has not been answered yet, but certainly the fetus that has renal agenesis (Potter syndrome) exists in a dry intrauterine desert (called *amnion nodosum* to describe profound oligohydramnios).

Renal vascular resistance, like that of the lung, is great in the fetus and diminishes after birth, although not so rapidly and possibly under the influence of the prostaglandins. Partly because of this, glomerular filtration and renal plasma flow are reduced relative to what they shortly become. The interim effect is an infant who easily can be overloaded with water despite his or her difficulty conserving it. Strikingly, these problems seem to occur at the hands of physicians, not mothers.

DIGESTIVE SYSTEM

The newborn at term is neuromuscularly equipped to create the successively caudad sequence of intraluminal pressure gradients that constitute a sufficient peristalsis for movement of an ingested bolus from mouth to anus. These pressure gradients begin at the mouth in the form of the primeval act of deglutition, which requires cooperative intermingling of motor and sensory effectiveness throughout the hindbrain (cranial nerves IX, X, and XII) working in concert with the midbrain (cranial nerves V and VII). Although gastrointestinal motility immediately postpartum may appear uncoordinated by adult standards, it nevertheless is extremely effective in moving swallowed air from mouth to rectum by 2 to 4 hours of age. By histological criteria, all the requisite structures (e.g., microvilli) for efficient absorption from the small bowel would appear to be in place by the time of term birth. The biochemical necessities for absorption also would appear to be satisfied for digestion of carbohydrates (amylase, lactase, and other disaccharidases) and proteins (gastric acid and pepsin, trypsin, and other pancreatic peptidases).

Fat absorption, on the other hand, is more tenuous. Lipase and bile salts are present by term; their rate of functional appearance is a linear function of gestational age. However, some significant doubt has long surrounded the question of which form of exogenous nutritional fat is the best to offer a newborn. Currently the best answer to this appears to be that the optimum ratio of unsaturated to saturated fatty acids and the optimum distribution of carbon chain lengths of saturated fatty acids are provided each species by its own mother's milk.

The microbiological sterility of the newborn gut at birth (gnotobiosis) begins to change immediately after birth through invasion of the mouth and anus by ambient microorganisms. This is a necessary act of matriculation as a human (or other terrestrial) being, which is best handled by the newborn's unhurried introduction only to those benign microbial species that will dominate the intestinal tract and eventually aid in the production of vitamin K to reduce the likelihood of the infant's contracting hemorrhagic disease of the newborn.

HEPATIC FUNCTION

During fetal life most hepatic duties are assumed by the maternal liver via the placenta. Indeed, most fetal blood flow returning from the placenta actually is shunted through the liver via the ductus venosus, which collapses after birth (as umbilical and placental venous return collapses), thus forcing perfusion of the liver by the portal circulation.

The liver's stores of glycogen are depleted rapidly after birth to supply energy until effective oral feeding is established. Stored fat is used next, after the supply of liver glycogen becomes depleted. Liver and cardiac glycogen and the energy these stores contain are the likely basis for the newborn's greater resistance to hypoxia.

However, the major lifetime job of the liver is to produce proteins—the plasma proteins (albumin and globulins), enzymes, and clotting factors—and it is in this area that the neonatal liver appears most immature, for reasons not yet clear. Many drug or other detoxifying reactions under enzymatic control are slow in infants, leading to prolonged half-lives for many drugs compared with adults.

The best known example of this enzymatic torpor in the newborn is the conjugation of free bilirubin (lipid soluble) with glucuronic acid to form excretable (water-soluble) bilirubin diglucuronide. The reaction is controlled by glucuronyl transferase, an enzyme whose activity is diminished at birth (which helps account for the common occurrence of jaundice in newborns) but which rises rapidly to adult levels thereafter.

IMMUNE SYSTEM

B cell functions (the production of antibody) develop relatively late in fetal life. Moreover, the bacteriologically sterile fetus normally receives no stimulus from foreign antigen to produce antibodies. Why maternal cells leaking into this system are not soon rejected as immunological invaders is one of the great mysteries of reproductive biology. In any case, the only significant antibody level normally mounted at birth is IgG, passively obtained transplacentally from the mother; however, the infant shortly will (or should) receive a good deal of IgA and macrophages from the mother's colostrum and breast milk. These facts can be diagnostically useful, in that elevations of cord blood IgM may be taken as evidence for preexisting (long enough to mount an antibody response) intrauterine infection.

Cellular immunity (T cell function) is largely intact in a newborn and, along with the borrowed maternal IgG, is the bedrock of the infant's immune competence. Phagocytosis is depressed, however, and, in the face of large bacterial inocula, sometimes critically so. The problem is that although the newborn's macrophages and neutrophils are quite capable of ingestion and digestion, the particles and bacteria to be attacked are insufficiently opsonized by the low serum complement levels. Thus, although the infant inevitably must learn to deal with microorganisms through exposure, it would be most prudent to arrange that all such exposures occur in moderation.

ENDOCRINE SYSTEM

The *thyroid* gland is operative early in fetal life and by term has stored sufficient triiodothyronine (T_3) and thyroxine (T_4) to sustain the infant's metabolism against thermal and nutritional stress, by virtue of the miniature thyroid storm precipitated by his or her eviction from the womb.

The *parathyroid* gland is similarly functional, but perhaps not robustly so. The relatively high serum calcium level of fetal life drops rapidly at birth from about 11 to 8.5 mg/dl, as phosphorus rises, and yet apparently does not elicit a reactive resorption of bone to defend serum calcium or enhanced excretion of phosphorus. Precise explanations are not at hand but may deal in part with a high ingested phosphorus load, especially in the infant who is fed cow milk–based formula.

The *adrenal cortex* of the normal infant is quite capable of mounting a suitable glucocorticoid and mineralocorticoid response to stress. On the other hand, the *adrenal medulla* (and the paraspinal chromaffin organ of Zuckerkandl) is almost totally devoted to the production of norepinephrine (an alpha-agonist) rather than to epinephrine (an alpha- and beta-agonist). Perhaps these organs sense that the heart is at the peak of its function curve and may not be able to respond to further beta-stimulation without decompensation. In addition, norepinephrine is the facilitator of thermogenesis within dark adipose tissue ("brown fat"), an important factor in helping infants maintain their body temperature after birth. The hormones of the pancreatic islet cells, *insulin* and *glucagon* (and, just as important, their receptors in the body's tissues) are functional at birth, although, in the case of insulin, somewhat sluggishly released.

NEUROLOGICAL SYSTEM

Through most of the last half of fetal life, glial and neuronal cells differentiate in the paraventricular germinal matrix, with the neuronal axons developing dendrites that, through a prolonged process of arborization, develop many thousands of synapses. The process of neuronal migration distributes these neurons throughout the neuraxis (cord, hindbrain, midbrain, forebrain) in the form of compact nuclei or looser reticular formations or the laminated sheets (six in all) of the cerebral gray matter.

The axonal pathways are formed when neurons and glial cells are combined and become myelinated, but differentially (caudad to cephalad), so at birth the forebrain and midbrain are still largely unmyelinated. Although unmyelinated pathways have slower conduction times, the shorter interneuronal and neuromuscular distances to be traveled in the newborn result in reflex arcs not much different in duration of action from those of adults.

The behavior of reflexes is much influenced by the (behavioral) state of consciousness. Proprioceptive reflexes, which generate postural body tonus, are abolished during active (rapid eye movement) sleep, which strongly inhibits motor neurons. Similarly, quiet sleep diminishes the exteroceptive reflexes whose efferent arcs come from skin, retinal, and aural receptors, rather than from the muscle stretch receptors of proprioception.

The higher cortical functions just now are being investigated through both biophysical and psychological techniques. It already appears that newborn humans are a great deal more involved with and occasionally manipulative of their environment and caregivers than previously supposed.

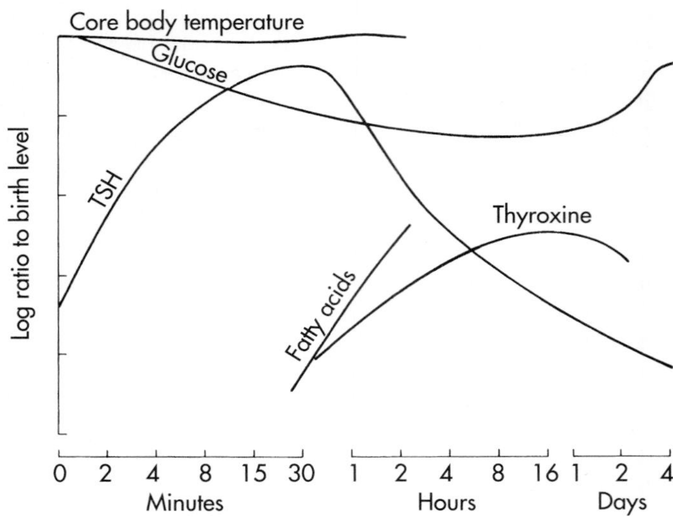

FIG. 44-4 Metabolic changes at birth. Data are shown as the approximate log (value at time/value at birth), which ranges from 0 *(bottom tic)* to 1 *(top tic)*. *TSH*, Thyroid stimulating hormone.

(Data from Smith CA, Nelson NM: *The physiology of the newborn infant*, ed 4, Springfield, Ill, 1976, Charles C Thomas.)

THREE
Recovery Period

Nicholas M. Nelson

The most complex modern surgical procedure is unlikely to equal the physiological strain on an infant of a normal birth—massive head trauma, asphyxiation, massive blood transfusion with cardiopulmonary bypass and, often resuscitation, all followed by major hypothermic insult—no wonder the infant cries! Clement Smith[1] has called this "the valley of the shadow of birth," but it is a normal event experienced by every human being (just as is death) and may be regarded as the disease from which *nearly* everyone recovers. However, where should the "recovery room" be?

Important observations need to be made in these first few hours, and it is not easy in either home or hospital (however homelike) to make them without untoward medical intrusion on what many would wish were more of a private family affair. The solution is to begin early in pregnancy to build toward expanding the parents' "family" to include the hospital's perinatal personnel to the point that it becomes almost immaterial whether these observations are made in the mother's room or in a contiguous recovery room (observation nursery).

CONVERSION FROM PLACENTAL TO ORAL ENERGY ASSIMILATION

The eviction from the womb that is birth may be compared, metabolically speaking, with forceful ejection from one's warm and friendly neighborhood "pub" into the cold, midwinter streets—naked and without a free lunch. The sober adult in such circumstances immediately would seek clothing—not out of civilized modesty, but from primal necessity to prevent excessive loss of body heat through convection by surrounding the skin with layers of insulating dead air. He simultaneously would vasoconstrict his skin ("blue with cold"—acrocyanosis), shiver to produce muscular heat, and begin to generate an increased amount of chemical heat by releasing thyroxin (to energize all cells) and catecholamines (to release the energy stored in fat by its lipolysis into glycerol and free fatty acids). The newborn child does precisely the same (but does not shiver) and with at least as great efficiency (Fig. 44-4).

Thoughtful medical attendants to the newborn will supply warm clothing or warmth by radiant warmer, incubator, or other thermal device and arrange the ambient temperature so that minimal thermal energy demands (the "neutral temperature," Fig. 44-5) are made of the infant, who must concentrate most of his or her stored energy investment on the principal continuing task of growth and development, at least until ingestion, digestion, and excretion are well established.

TRANSITION AND ESTABLISHMENT OF VITAL FUNCTION

The initial hours of recovery have been characterized clinically as *alert* (0 to 30 minutes), then *unresponsive* (30 minutes to 2 hours) and, finally, *reactive* (2 to 8 hours), as shown in Fig. 44-6, during which time the infant displays signs of general sympathetic discharge (tachycardia, tachypnea, and vasomotion) and then parasympathetic discharge (peristalsis), probably in response to the sensory overload that attends birth, particularly chilling. The onset of peristalsis heralds the first defecation and micturition, the timing of which should be carefully noted, since untoward delay in either (Fig. 44-7) may signal significant gastrointestinal or genitourinary abnormalities.

With a normal birth, the pediatrician is likely to make first physical acquaintance with the newborn in the nursery rather than in the delivery room. Therefore, after a period of observation by the nursery ("recovery room") staff, those elements calling for special surveillance (Table 44-5) need to be gleaned from the obstetrical history and brought to the pediatrician's attention as a confirmation of previous alerts from the obstetrical staff.

TECHNIQUES FOR ASSESSMENT OF NEUROMUSCULAR MATURITY

Posture

With the infant supine and quiet, score as follows:
- Arms and legs extended = 0
- Slight or moderate flexion of hips and knees = 1
- Moderate to strong flexion of hips and knees = 2
- Legs flexed and abducted, arms slightly flexed = 3
- Full flexion of arms and legs = 4

Square window

Flex the hand at the wrist (exert pressure sufficient to get as much flexion as possible); do not rotate the wrist. Measure and score the angle between the hypothenar eminence and the anterior aspect of the forearm according to Fig. 44-8.

Arm recoil

With the infant supine, fully flex the forearm for 5 seconds, then fully extend by pulling the hands and releasing. Score the reaction according to the following:
- Remains extended or random movements = 0
- Incomplete or partial flexion = 1
- Brisk return to full flexion = 2

Popliteal angle

With the infant supine and the pelvis flat on the examining surface, use one hand to flex the leg on the thigh and then fully flex the thigh; use the other hand to extend the leg. Score the angle attained as in Fig. 44-8.

Scarf sign

With the infant supine, take the infant's hand and draw it across the neck and as far across the opposite shoulder as possible (assistance to the elbow is permissible by lifting it across the body). Score according to the location of the elbow:
- Elbow reaches beyond the opposite anterior axillary line = 0
- Elbow reaches to the opposite anterior axillary line = 1
- Elbow is between opposite anterior axillary line and midline of thorax = 2
- Elbow is at midline of thorax = 3
- Elbow does not reach midline of thorax = 4

Heel-to-ear maneuver

With the infant supine, hold the infant's foot with one hand and move it as near to the head as possible without forcing it. Keep the pelvis flat on the examining surface. Score as in Fig. 44-8.

From Amiel-Tison C: *Arch Dis Child* 43:89, 1968; Dubowitz LMS, Dubowitz V, Goldberg C: *J Pediatr* 77:1, 1970.

tainty (date of birth). Practicing these principles is more difficult in the perinatal period because time is measured in weeks and the date of conception cannot be fixed with any real certainty. Nonetheless, fetal and neonatal examinations of many infants from many different populations by many observers have produced a number of acceptable norms and have standardized the assessment of gestational age.

Assessment of Gestational Age

The combined assessment of neuromuscular maturity (presented in instructional form in the box above) and certain physical features of genitalia, ears, skin, breast, plantar creases, and hair has proved to be a reliable means for estimating gestational age (Fig. 44-8). Further corroboration may be sought by examining the vascularity in the anterior capsule of the lens (Fig. 44-9). Thus armed with a working knowledge of gestational age in comparison with birth weight against established norms (e.g., the Colorado intrauterine growth charts), the examiner next should judge whether the infant is large, appropriate, or small for his or her gestational age (LGA, AGA, and SGA, respectively) and thus become appropriately alerted to diagnostic possibilities (see Fig. 43-4).

Behavioral Assessment

Although not often part of the routine surveillance of the normal newborn infant, a Brazelton score awarded by a skilled observer of newborn behavior has proved to be a reproducible and valid means of evaluating infant behavior (see the box on the right) and of detecting behavioral changes imposed by birth injury or maternal analgesics.

Through this and other means, it recently has become apparent that term newborns regularly indulge in considerably more environmental interaction (and even manipulation) than heretofore suspected; they prefer human faces to other faces, listen to high-pitched voices, and respond to speech cadences; they are soothed by resumption of the intrauterine "position of comfort," and they can smell their mother's milk.

BRAZELTON BEHAVIORAL SCALE

Environmental interactions

Alertness
Consolability
Cuddliness
Orientation

Stress responses

Skin color lability
Startle reaction
Tremulousness

Motor processes

Activity
Defensive reactions
Hand-to-mouth movement
Maturity
Reflex
Tone

Physiological state

Habituation to stimuli
Self-quieting

Neuromuscular Maturity

	-1	0	1	2	3	4	5
Posture							
Square Window (wrist)	>90°	90°	60°	45°	30°	0°	
Arm Recoil		180°	140°-180°	110° 140°	90° -110°	<90°	
Popliteal Angle	180°	160°	140"	120°	100°	90°	<90°
Scarf Sign							
Heel to ear							

Physical Maturity

	-1	0	1	2	3	4	5
Skin	sticky friable transparent	gelatinous red, translucent	smooth pink, visible veins	superficial peeling &/or rash, few veins	cracking pale areas rare veins	parchment deep cracking no vessels	leathery cracked wrinkled
Lanugo	none	sparse	abundant	thinning	bald areas	mostly bald	
Plantar Surface	heel-toe 40-50 mm:- 1 <40 mm: -2	>50 mm no crease	faint red marks	anterior transverse crease only	creases ant. 2/3	creases over entire sole	
Breast	imperceptible	barely perceptible	flat areola no bud	stippled areola 1-2 mm bud	raised areola 3-4 mm bud	full areola 5-10 mm bud	
Eye/Ear	lids fused loosely: -1 tightly: -2	lids open pinna flat stays folded	sl. curved pinna: soft: slow recoil	well-curved pinna: soft but ready recoil	formed & firm instant recoil	thick cartilage ear stiff	
Genitals male	scrotum flat, smooth	scrotum empty faint rugae	testes in upper canal rare rugae	testes descending few rugae	testes down good rugae	testes pendulous deep rugae	
Genitals female	clitoris prominent labia flat	prominent clitoris small labia minora	prominent clitoris enlarging minora	majora & minora equally prominent	majora large and minora small	majora cover clitoris & minora	

Maturity Rating

score	weeks
-10	20
-5	22
0	24
5	26
10	28
15	30
20	32
25	34
30	36
35	38
40	40
45	42
50	44

FIG. 44-8 Assessment of gestational age in weeks, using a combination of neuromuscular and physical maturity criteria. The box on the bottom describes methods used to assess neuromuscular maturity. The assessment is quickly and easily performed because the box includes measures of physical maturity and of passive but not active tone. Physical maturity is most accurately assessed in the minutes or hour or so after birth. The score for each item is indicated at the top of the vertical column. However, neuromuscular maturity may be spuriously retarded in an asphyxiated neonate or in a neonate obtunded by anesthetic agents or drugs. Thus the neuromuscular maturity rating should be repeated after a day or two. The sum of the scores on all the items of physical and neuromuscular maturity provides an estimate of maturity in weeks *(see lower right).* (From Ballard JL: *J Pediatr* 119:417, 1991.)

How much of this behavioral display may be available for viewing depends on the infant's behavioral "state," which includes several states of sleep, variously graded on a scale of 4 points (awake, active sleep, indeterminate sleep, and quiet sleep) or 6 points (awake-crying, awake-active, quiet-alert, drowsy, rapid eye movement [REM] sleep, and deep sleep). They are at their most behaviorally competent in the quiet-alert state and at their most physiologically interesting in REM sleep (Fig. 44-10). During REM sleep, for instance, breathing becomes irregular and "paradoxical," as intercos-

RAPID ASSESSMENT OF GESTATIONAL AGE[1]

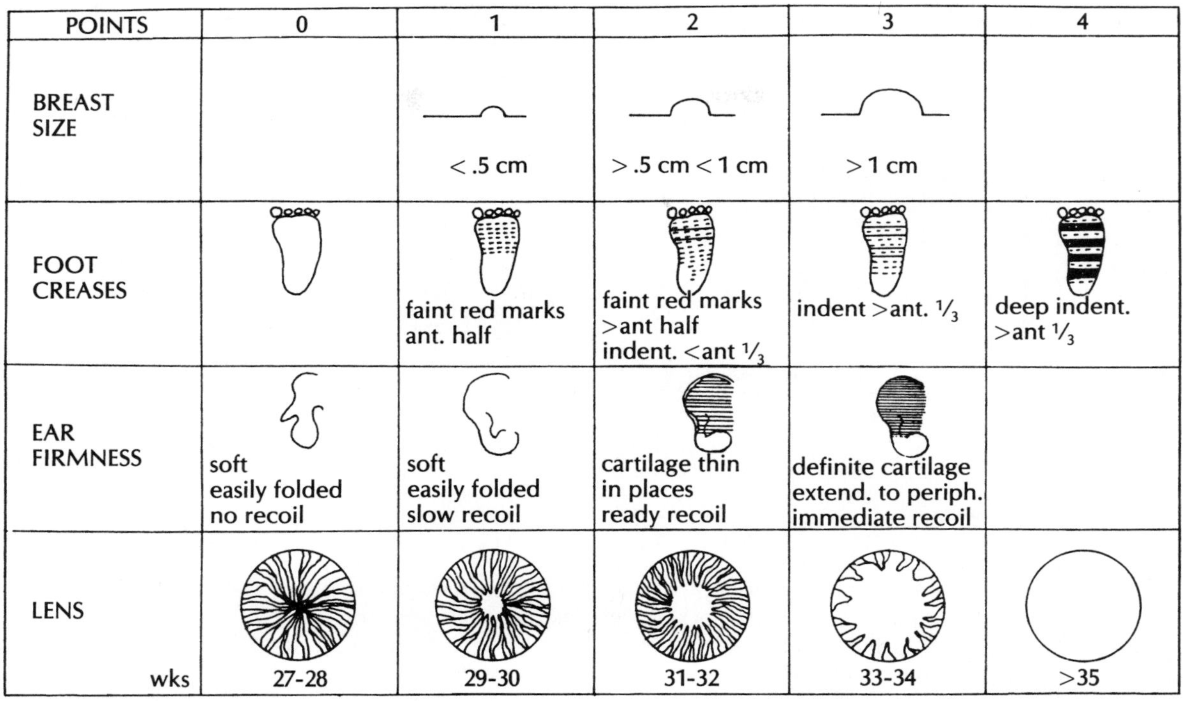

POINTS	0	1	2	3	4
BREAST SIZE		< .5 cm	> .5 cm < 1 cm	> 1 cm	
FOOT CREASES		faint red marks ant. half	faint red marks >ant half indent. <ant 1/3	indent >ant. 1/3	deep indent. >ant 1/3
EAR FIRMNESS	soft easily folded no recoil	soft easily folded slow recoil	cartilage thin in places ready recoil	definite cartilage extend. to periph. immediate recoil	
LENS					
wks	27-28	29-30	31-32	33-34	>35

Total Score	Gestational Age Weeks
1	28
2	29
3	29½
4	30½
5	31

GESTATIONAL AGE

For scores >5: Score + 26 = weeks gestational age (example: score = 6 (+ 26) = 32 weeks gestational age).

FIG. 44-9 Rapid assessment of gestational age.

tal muscle tone collapses (thus weakening the chest wall) to allow the diaphragm to pull the thorax inward during its inspiratory descent.

General Physical Examination

As is implicit from the preceding discussion, the newborn's first formal and complete physical examination (Fig. 44-11) occurs during the period of transition in a setting of continuous and intense scrutiny by both the delivery room and nursery staffs, not to mention the parents. Moreover, observations and interventions overlap considerably during the nursery stay.

The nursing staff observes the vital signs (Fig. 44-12). These traditionally have not included blood pressure because of the difficulty in auscultating Korotkoff sounds, but the increasing availability of oscillometers and Doppler devices should make this important measurement routine. The most cooperative infant is one who is 1 to 2 hours postprandial, in the quiet-alert *behavioral state,* and examined under thermal conditions not too far from his or her neutral thermal environment (see Fig. 44-5). The infant's *general appearance* will have been noted during the assessment of gestational age, but particular attention now should be directed to his or her apparent *nutritional state* (especially subcutaneous tissue and muscle mass) and *postural tone.* The more mature the infant, the greater the flexor tone displayed as part of the resting posture.

The most productive physical (and neurological) examination is one conducted on an infant who is 1 to 2 hours postprandial, at a reasonably normal ambient temperature, and in a quiet-alert state of consciousness.

Much of the normal (or normal variant) findings of the newborn's physical examination are presented in Chapter 7; here we focus on those aspects that should raise the suspicion of abnormality. Nevertheless, those portions of Chapter 7 dealing with the physical examination of each of the organ systems under the heading "Newborn" also should be consulted.

The Skin and Its Appendages (Table 44-7). The naked infant should be observed most carefully for skin color; *pallor, jaundice,* and *cyanosis* each may become an indication for alarm, depending on the time of onset, duration, and intensity. *Excoriations* of the epidermis can be a normal result of long fingernails, but when observed in a yawning or "jittery" baby, they also may indicate neonatal abstinence syndrome (withdrawal from maternal narcotics; see Chapter 49). A *lum-*

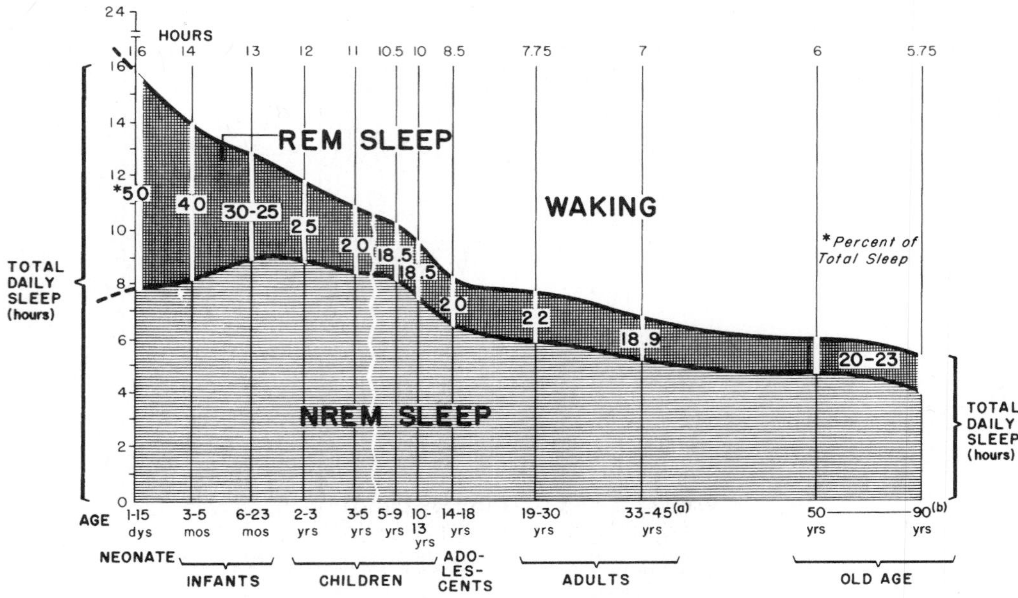

FIG. 44-10 Graph showing changes (with age) in total amounts of daily sleep, daily rapid eye movement *(REM)* sleep, and percentage of REM sleep. Note sharp diminution of REM sleep in the early years. REM sleep falls from 8 hours at birth to less than 1 hour in old age. The amount of nonrapid eye movement *(NREM)* sleep throughout life remains more constant, falling from 8 hours to 5 hours. In contrast to the steep decline of REM sleep, the quantity of NREM sleep is undiminished for many years. Although total daily REM sleep falls steadily during life, the percentage rises slightly in adolescence and early adulthood. This rise does not reflect an increase in amount; it is caused by the fact that REM sleep does not diminish as quickly as total sleep.

(From Roffwarg HP, Muzio JN, Dement WC: *Science* 152:604, 1966.)

NEONATAL RECORD (2)—NURSERY

BIRTH

BORN AT		HOSPITAL	CITY	STATE
TIME	DATE	REFERRING PHYSICIAN		M.D.
LMP	EDC	GESTATIONAL AGE WKS	VIT K₁ GIVEN AT	HRS OF AGE

INTERVAL HISTORY

NURSERY EXAMINATION

DATE	TIME	AGE HRS	WGT GMS	SEX	RACE
LENGTH CMS	BIP CMS	SKULL CMS	CHEST CMS	ABDOMEN CMS	
[KEY ✓= NORMAL, 0 = ABSENT, X = ABNORMAL]		EFFECTS OF FETAL POSTURE		GENERAL APPEARANCE	
SKIN	SC TISSUE	FACIES	MASSES	SPLEEN	HIPS
VERNIX	EDEMA	EYES	THORAX	KIDNEYS	CNS-REFLEXES
PALLOR	NODES	EARS	BREATHING	CORD	CRY
ICTERUS	HEAD	NARES	LUNGS	ANUS	TONE
CYANOSIS	FONTANELLES	MOUTH	HEART	GENITALIA	PARALYSIS
BIRTHMARKS	SUTURES	NECK	ABDOMEN	SKELETON	MORO
BRUISING	CPHLHMTOMA	THYROID	LIVER	CLAVICLES	GRASP

GESTATIONAL AGE ASSESSMENT = WEEKS

ABNORMAL FINDINGS

IMPRESSION

SIGNED M.D.

FIG. 44-11 Data relevant to the neonatal physical examination.

NEWBORN NURSING ASSESSMENT

Admission: Date ____ Time ____ Birth: Date ____ Time ____ Weight ____ Length ____ Head ____
Gestation: By Dates ____ By Dubowitz ____ AGA/LGA/SGA ____
Relevant OB History

Ears & Eyes — $AgNO_3$ 1% Crede ☐ 2 gtts each eye
Nose — Nares Patent: By occlusion ☐ catheter ☐
Mouth
Skin
Head
Chest
Abdomen, Umbilical Vessels
Genitals — Anus Patent: By appearance ☐ catheter ☐
Extremities, Skeleton
Nervous System
Activity

Transitional TPR			General Comments
Time	Comments	Initials	
			Signature:

Six Hour Assessment

Skin ____
Chest ____
Abdomen ____
Nervous System ____
Activity ____

Comments:

Signature: ____

FIG. 44-12 Nursing surveillance of a normal newborn infant.

Table 44-7 Levels of Surveillance of the Newborn Based on the Examination of the Skin and Its Appendages

Characteristic	Level of surveillance: Normal	Alert	Alarm
Color (age of occurrence)			
Cyanosis	Acrocyanosis (<12 hr)	Central (<1 hr)	Central (>1 hr)
Jaundice	>24 hr	18-24 hr	<18 hr
Pallor			>30 min
Epidermis	Dermatoglyphics	Excoriations	Sloughing
Hair	Lanugo	Lumbosacral tuft and scalp defect	
Texture	Soft and moist	Dry and scaling	Thickened and crusting
Vascular pattern	Harlequin, mottling (cold)	Persistent mottling	
Cysts	Milia and Epstein pearls		
Papules	Acne and miliaria		
Desquamation	Delicate scaling (>2 days)	Peeling (<2 days)	Denuded sheets (anytime)
Hemangiomas	Telangiectatic (forehead, lids, lips, and nape)	Telangiectatic (trigeminal) and angiomatous (few)	Angiomatous (multiple)
Hemorrhage	Petechiae (head or upper body)	Petechiae (elsewhere)	Ecchymoses and purpura
Macules	Mongolian spots	Café-au-lait spots (fewer than 6)	Café-au-lait spots (6 or more) and "mountain ash" leaf
Pustules	Erythema toxicum		Large and dermal
Vesicles			Any
Nodules		Subcutaneous fat necrosis	Sclerema

bosacral tuft of hair may point to pilonidal sinus, diastematomyelia, or teratoma, and it should be established that a *scalp defect* is not accompanied by other signs of trisomy 18. The skin's texture normally is soft and moist ("as a baby's bottom") at term, but it lacks fullness of subcutaneous tissue in a preterm infant and is dry, cracked, or peeling in a vernix-deprived postmature or undergrown infant. The skin is grotesquely thickened and crusted ("collodion baby") in various rare types of *ichthyosis.* An apparently normal phenomenon of vascular reactivity is the mottled ("marbled") vascular pattern of dilated venules in the (usually chilled) newborn. When persistent, this mottled *cutis marmorata* may be associated with trisomy 18 (see Chapter 40) or trisomy 21 (see Chapter 201). A phenomenon of the late neonatal period (1 month) is *acne* (true comedo), seen mostly over the cheeks and chin as tiny, coalescing, erythematous papules that usually disappear over a few weeks.

The clay-colored greasy *vernix caseosa* that covers a healthy term newborn at birth evaporates almost magically within hours after birth and is sparse to absent in a postmature infant, whose superficial epidermal layers soon are cracked and peeling. However, this is quite different from the full-thickness denudation that marks the *scalded skin syndrome* (toxic epidermal necrolysis) of staphylococcal sepsis.

Probably the most common tumors in humans (or, certainly, in infants), hemangiomas range from the telangiectatic ("capillary") nevi, or "salmon patch," so common on the lids, forehead, and nape ("stork bite") of the newborn, to the multiple or massive and often grotesque angiomatous ("cavernous") lesions (see Chapter 45). Diffuse neonatal *hemangiomatosis* is the rare but fatal maximum expression of this spectrum, often marked by cardiac failure to manage the vast volume overload presented by multiple arteriovenous fistulas, often in major organs such as the liver and brain. Between these extremes is *Sturge-Weber syndrome* (venous angiomatosis of leptomeninges, atrophic cerebral cortex, buphthalmos, seizures, hemiparesis, and mental retardation), suggested by an ipsilateral facial port-wine stain in the trigeminal distribution. However, the linkage of cerebral and cutaneous venous angiomatosis is not firm, because many children who have a *port-wine stain* have perfectly normal cerebral function.

A cutaneous *hemorrhage* in any form is justifiable cause for concern that some form of bleeding diathesis may be at hand. Yet some *petechiae* (and *subconjunctival hemorrhage*) may well be observed within the superior vena caval drainage system after a normal vertex delivery, as an expression of the significant pressure differentials to which the fetus is subject upon rupture of the forewaters.

The very common, completely mysterious, and completely benign perifollicular eruption known as *erythema toxicum* ("flea-bite dermatitis") appears on the second or third day of life as 1 to 3 mm white or pale yellow papules or pustules on a small erythematous but uninflamed base. They can become much larger and even confluent, risking confusion with bacterial pyoderma; however, smears of the sterile contents of these lesions reveal eosinophils rather than neutrophils. The infants are well, and the pustules resolve simultaneously within hours to days.

Vesicles may be associated with benign conditions (e.g., transient neonatal pustular melanosis) but must always raise concern that a serious disease is involved, whether infectious (e.g., herpes, syphilis, toxic epidermal necrolysis) or inherited (e.g., epidermolysis bullosa or incontinentia pigmenti). These lesions demand expert consultation.

Nodules are perhaps the least common primary cutaneous lesion seen in newborns. *Subcutaneous fat necrosis* (pseudosclerema) appears in the first few days as localized areas of induration over the buttocks, cheeks, or back, with blotchy, reddened overlying skin. Its definitive cause is unknown, but it is attributed to poor perfusion caused by cold stress or asphyxia, and it resolves spontaneously over weeks to months.

Sclerema neonatorum is a presumably related process of induration in adipose tissue, formerly seen in hypothermic and usually moribund premature infants.

The Head and Neck (Table 44-8). *Caput succedaneum* is subcutaneous edema over the presenting part of the head; it is far more common than cephalohematoma, usually is situated over the occiput, and crosses suture lines. Caput tends to feel soft and lacks a well-defined outline, but it is not fluctuant (as is a cephalohematoma). The edema is most pronounced at birth and subsides within 2 or 3 days. It is particularly common after delivery by vacuum extraction.

Cephalohematoma, on the other hand, is a subperiosteal collection of blood and as such is bounded by suture lines. It occurs in full-term healthy babies, most often in the parietal region. Cephalohematoma may not be obvious at birth but may increase in size over the first few hours or days of life, giving rise to a firm mass with a well-defined edge. The center of the swelling may liquify, giving a feel of fluctuance or an erroneous impression of a depressed skull fracture. The mass occasionally calcifies and persists for weeks to months. Complications include hyperbilirubinemia and underlying skull fracture, the latter being associated with about 20% of cephalohematomas.

A *subgaleal hemorrhage* is sometimes mistaken for cephalohematoma. However, the subgaleal space is not limited by suture lines, and the blood tends to collect in dependent positions. Moreover, the space is large; thus a newborn may lose a large amount of blood, leading to hyperbilirubinemia and anemia or even shock.

Molding refers to the overriding of sagittal, coronal, or lambdoid sutures in a normal newborn delivered vaginally from the vertex position. Molding serves as benign testimony to the forces of labor, not shared by the infant delivered by cesarean section or from the breech position; the latter often is characterized by a pronounced occipital "overhang" in the skull contour. The molded head often is irregular in shape, with the parietooccipital region prominent; the forehead tends to slope backward. Molding is especially likely to be seen in first babies, in a large infant after prolonged labor, or with an element of cephalopelvic disproportion. The abnormal skull features usually return to normal by 5 or 6 days after birth.

A *large anterior fontanelle* should alert the examiner to the possibility of a defect in membranous bone formation (e.g., achondroplasia, hypophosphatasia, or cretinism) or increased intracranial pressure. *Small or absent fontanelles,* if associated with a pronouncedly misshapen skull or facies, may indicate a number of cosmetically threatening but treatable bony abnormalities, such as Crouzon disease or craniosynostosis, although the latter usually is not evident in the immediate neonatal period. The uninformed observer often is too willing to attribute a unilateral *facial palsy* to "misapplied" forceps, which often leaves a blade mark temporarily over the eye or cheek. Most such infants have a shoulder that neatly tucks under the ear (and into the stylomastoid foramen) of the palsied side. In any case, these palsies tend to resolve quickly after birth.

Two of the most threatening observations to be made of the skull are also two of the most subtle: (1) the examiner must specifically listen for a *bruit,* which may indicate a cerebral arteriovenous fistula, and (2) positive *transillumination* ("candling") of the head (using a flashlight in a darkened room or a high-intensity "Chun gun" beam in a lighted room) may be the only clinical indication of hydranencephaly—massive liquefaction of cerebral tissue.

After noting the presence of a retinal *red reflex* and palpebral fissures of normal size, the examiner also should ensure that the eyes do not have a *mongoloid slant* (as in Down syndrome) and that the iris is present, because of the high correlation between Wilms tumor and aniridia. An *enlarged or cloudy cornea* may be the only visual indication of *congenital glaucoma.*

A *high-arched palate,* described as a frequent accompaniment of many complex malformation syndromes, usually is simply short and hypoplastic. An observation of *macroglossia* should stimulate the search for other signs of cretinism or Beckwith-Wiedemann syndrome, whereas *micrognathia* suggests, among other things, Treacher Collins and Pierre Robin syndromes. Although *cleft lip or palate* may occur singly, the examiner should determine whether other signs of trisomy 13 are present (i.e., low-set or malformed ears, webbed neck, scalp defects, microphthalmia, and micrognathia). Similarly, any ear that is apparently low set (i.e., whose upper attachment to the scalp is below an imaginary line connecting the inner and outer canthi and extended to the occiput), particularly if the foldings of pinna and tragus appear "simplified," should prompt a search for bilateral renal agenesis (Potter syndrome) and other markers of genetic disease (e.g., webbed neck, "rocker-bottom" feet, and hypoplastic and incurved fifth digit).

Table 44-8 Levels of Surveillance of the Newborn Based on the Head and Neck Examination

	Level of surveillance		
Location	Normal	Alert	Alarm
Skull	Caput succedaneum, molding, or occipital overhang	Cephalohematoma, craniotabes, large fontanelle, or forceps mark	Craniosynostosis, transillumination, or bruit
Facies		Hypoplasia or palsy	
Eyes		Mongoloid slant	Aniridia and enlarged cornea
Nose		Nasal obstruction	
Mouth		High-arched palate or macroglossia	Cleft palate and/or lip or micrognathia
Ears		"Simple" structure or low set	
Neck	Rotation ±90 degrees	Dimple or webbing	

The neck should be freely rotatable and free of dimples or masses, which could suggest a *thyroglossal duct cyst* (midline) or *branchial cleft cyst* (anterolateral).

The Chest (Table 44-9). Apart from inspecting the newborn's breasts for engorgement or discharge, the thoracic wall is observed most closely in the attempt to characterize respiration. *Paradoxical respirations* are those in which inspiratory efforts are accompanied by protuberance of the abdomen and a sinking in of the lower ribs as the diaphragm descends, unopposed by adequate intercostal muscle tone. Although this phenomenon is characteristic of normal active (REM) sleep in the newborn, it also can signify abnormal respiration. Inspiratory *retractions* of the lower sternum and intercostal spaces, particularly if accompanied by use of accessory respiratory muscles (alae nasi and sternocleidomastoids), imply a decrease in lung compliance (stiffening), often caused by atelectasis or accumulation of fluid within the lung. Expiratory *grunting* (actually, an explosive Valsalva maneuver) is the hallmark of loss of alveolar volume and most frequently is displayed in pediatric experience by the small premature infant whose lungs are atelectatic shortly after birth because of insufficient amounts of stabilizing pulmonary surfactant (i.e., hyaline membrane disease). However, other causes of respiratory distress (e.g., transient tachypnea, meconium aspiration, and congenital pneumonia) may be impossible to distinguish clinically on the basis of the physical characteristics alone.

Diminished auscultatable *air entry* on inspiration is difficult to evaluate during quiet breathing. However, when observed in situations in which greater respiratory effort is seen yet not heard, this means that the tidal volume of airflow is reduced, potentially because of atelectasis or airway obstruction. When *bowel sounds* are clearly audible within the chest, especially the left hemithorax and particularly when accompanied by a displacement of heart sounds to the right, a diaphragmatic hernia must be ruled out instantly by chest roentgenogram, regardless of whether respiratory distress is obvious.

Indeed, although its use cannot be advocated routinely for newborns who do not have symptoms, *the chest roentgenogram should be the diagnostic supplement of first resort* in the physical examination (especially of the chest and abdomen) of an ill infant. If it is used, maximum advantage should be extracted from it, particularly by inspecting last those areas of prime interest; this policy prevents many embarrassing omissions of such "incidental" findings as a fractured clavicle or rib, a hemivertebra or spina bifida, or a paralyzed diaphragm. The character of the lung parenchyma should be noted, as well as the presence or absence of fluid or effusion, an "air bronchogram," or a distinct cardiac border (an indistinct border signifies lack of alveolar air). In an infant who has any cardiovascular symptoms, the examiner should be especially careful to estimate the cardiac size and determine if the vascularity of the lung fields is oligemic, normal, or plethoric.

The physician should be concerned by a *cardiac impulse* that lifts rather than taps at the examining palm or fingertips, since this implies a more generously developed left ventricle than should be the case at the immediate conclusion of fetal life, during which the right ventricle is dominant in both pressure and volume work. Any diminishment of *peripheral pulses* (especially femoral) is evidence of impeded left ventricular outflow (e.g., coarctation of the aorta) and demands measurement of blood pressure in all four extremities. Sinus *bradycardia* may be precipitated, presumably by vagal reflex, during suctioning or other stimulations of the nasopharynx. Some immature infants may sustain alarming but transient episodes of bradycardia with no apparent stimulus (or symptoms, including apnea), but bradycardia is seen most often during the episodes of prolonged apnea so common in a premature newborn. Indeed, many authorities believe that cardiac (rather than cardiorespiratory) monitoring is a perfectly

Table 44-9 Levels of Surveillance of the Newborn Based on the Chest Examination

	Level of surveillance		
Characteristic	**Normal**	**Alert**	**Alarm**
Respiration		Paradoxical, periodic, or retractions	Apnea, expiratory grunt, flaring alae nasi, stridor
Auscultation		Diminished air entry	Bowel sounds
Chest roentgenogram		Enlarged heart	Oligemia or plethora
Cardiac			
Impulse	Tapping	Heaving, lifting	
Pulses	Full	Decreased	Absent (femoral) and lag (cardiac-radial)
Rate and rhythm	110-165, sinus arrhythmia	Sinus bradycardia	Persistent sinus tachycardia
Sounds	"Tic-toc"	S_2 widely split	S_2 fixed split
Murmurs	Systolic (<24 hr)	Systolic (>24 hr)	Diastolic
Electrocardiograph (QRS)			
Vector	+35 to +180 degrees		0 to −90 degrees; −90 to −180 degrees
Amplitude			
V_1	Rs	Rs	rS
V_6	qrS	qRs	qRs

Table 44-10 Levels of Surveillance of the Newborn Based on Examination of the Abdomen

	Level of surveillance		
Characteristic	**Normal**	**Alert**	**Alarm**
Shape	Cylindrical	Scaphoid	Distended
Muscular wall	Diastasis recti		Absent
Umbilicus	Amniotic navel or cutaneous navel	Exudation or leakage, granuloma, hernia, inflammation, or less than 3 cord vessels	Gastroschisis, omphalitis, or omphalocele
Liver	Smooth edge, 2-3 cm below ribs	>3 cm below ribs	Enlarged
Spleen	Nonpalpable	<1 cm below ribs	Enlarged
Kidneys	Lobulated or palpable (lower poles)	Horseshoe	Enlarged

adequate means of monitoring vital signs in the newborn special care unit. Unameliorated paroxysmal auricular *tachycardia* can lead to cardiac exhaustion and failure.

The normal tic-toc quality of the *heart sounds* results from the near-equal duration of systole and diastole. The high (but subsiding) pulmonary vascular resistance of the first hours and days of life normally accentuates the intensity of the pulmonary component of S_2, at first difficult to distinguish from the preceding aortic component. However, as pulmonary vascular resistance decreases (and, hence, pulmonary flow increases), the "splitting" of S_2 widens because closure of the pulmonary valve is delayed by the longer time required to eject the increased right-sided stroke volume. Similarly, the widened and "fixed split" in the S_2 of critical pulmonary stenosis denotes the increased time required to force blood past the obstructed outflow tract of the right ventricle.

An acute and undistracted ear may often (about 20% to 30% of the time) hear transient *systolic ejection murmurs* at the base of the heart during the first day, presumably associated with flow through the closing ductus arteriosus. Later-developing murmurs have more significance because the increasing resistance (and pressure) differential between the pulmonary and systemic circulations allows the expression of murmurs caused by increasing flow across abnormal connections (e.g., septal defects) between the two circulations. Systolic ejection murmurs heard early (even in fetal life) and that persist throughout the neonatal period may well result from flow across a stenotic valve (i.e., pulmonary or aortic stenosis). *Diastolic murmurs* should alarm the examiner whenever heard, but they rarely are solitary.

Apart from specific diagnostic aid regarding the type and probable origin of an arrhythmia, the electrocardiogram, like the chest roentgenogram, is a helpful supplement to the physical examination in assessing the volume *(preload)* and pressure *(afterload)* presented to the ventricles. Indeed, knowledge of three major data points alone—whether the right or left ventricle is electrically dominant, whether plethora or oligemia of the pulmonary vasculature is seen on a chest roentgenogram, and whether cyanosis is present or absent clinically, with application of a suitable diagnostic algorithm ("recipe" for systematic assessment of clinical data)—can narrow the likely cardiac diagnosis to two or three entities before echocardiographic or catheter confirmation and without reference to murmurs. For instance, the "adult progression" of precordial QRS complexes (rS in V_1, qRs in V_6) suggests an abnormally dominant left ventricle (or abnormally diminished right ventricle). Combined with cyanosis and oligemic lung fields, these data might well suggest pulmonary atresia.

The Abdomen (Table 44-10). A significantly *distended* abdomen is usually distinctly tense and accompanied by signs of obstruction (vomiting, no stool). The traditional *scaphoid* (empty) abdomen of a diaphragmatic hernia perhaps is more the exception than the rule, depending on the amount of intestinal gas. Generally, the normal infant abdomen is pleasingly round, soft, and full in the flanks. It often appears to lack a muscular wall, until it becomes rigid during the expiratory phase of crying (or, less fortunately, it displays the "prune belly" appearance of truly absent abdominal musculature).

Although drainage of clear liquid from the navel can accompany a simple (and cauterizable) *umbilical granuloma,* the examiner must be careful not to miss a *urachal fistula.* The grosser umbilical malformations *(omphalocele* and *gastroschisis)* are impossible to miss and demand immediate intervention. Any sign of inflammation must be watched closely; however, use of "triple dye" for cord care may so discolor the skin (while exerting bacteriostatic action) that inspection becomes quite difficult. Finding less than the normal complement of one large-diameter, thin-walled central vein and two smaller-diameter, thicker-walled arteries at about the 4-o'clock and 8-o'clock positions (facing the infant) in the freshly cut surface of the umbilical cord (best done in the delivery room) should alert the examiner to the likelihood of other developmental anomalies, especially genitourinary ones.

Detection of true enlargement of either the *liver* or the *spleen* must be regarded with suspicion. However, the upper borders of both organs should be located by percussion before conclusions are drawn about enlargement because they are easily displaced downward by the diaphragm under a lung often distended during the early hours after birth by the "wet lung" conditions (e.g., transient tachypnea).

The *kidneys* are easier to evaluate at this time than perhaps at any subsequent period in life because the infant abdomen offers little resistance to a gentle yet deep bimanual paraspinal exploration, which easily should yield the impression of at least the (often lobulated) lower poles of the kidneys. Any apparent malformation or enlargement should be confirmed immediately by ultrasonographic examination, as should any frank intraabdominal mass.

The Perineum (Table 44-11). Examination of the perineum is straightforward and mainly involves ensuring that the *anus* is patent and puckers, that the male *phallus* is well formed

Table 44-11 Levels of Surveillance of the Newborn Based on Examination of the Perineum

Location	Level of surveillance		
	Normal	Alert	Alarm
Anus	Coccygeal dimple		Imperforate, fistula, patulous
Female			
Clitoris		Enlarged, hooded	
Vulva	Bloody secretion, edema, gaping labia, or hymenal tags		Hydrometrocolpos
Male			
Gonad	Edema, hydrocele	Bifid scrotum	Cryptorchidism, inguinal hernia
Phallus	Phimosis	Chordee, hypospadias	Microphallus

Table 44-12 Levels of Surveillance of the Newborn Based on Examination of the Musculoskeletal System

Characteristic	Level of surveillance		
	Normal	Alert	Alarm
Fetal posture	Flexor, position of comfort	Frank breech	Extensor
Hand	Webbing	Cortical thumb, overlapping fingers, short, incurved little finger	Polydactyly, syndactyly
Foot	Dorsiflexion 90 degrees, plantar flexion 90 degrees, abduction or adduction of forefoot 45 degrees, inversion or eversion of ankle 45 degrees	Decreased range of motion	Fixed
Extremities	Tibial bowing		Constriction bands, amputations
Neck	Rotation ±90 degrees		
Joints		Reluctance to use	Subluxation (hips), contracture

and accompanied by palpable gonads, and that the female *vaginal vault* is patent and contains no extraneous tissues. An incorrect assignment of sex is extremely difficult to retract; therefore any initial ambiguities must be faced with the parents carefully and courageously while the ambiguities are explored.

The Musculoskeletal System (Table 44-12). All late fetuses spend considerable periods of time (when not kicking their mothers) in one rather cramped *position of "comfort,"* which can be restored easily and visibly during the nursery examination by enfolding the infant's feet, tibias, and femurs with gentle pressure placed on the soles of the feet. Everything then seems to fall magically into place as it was in utero, and the infant becomes soothed (and the origin of the *tibial torsion* of infancy becomes obvious). Given current obstetrical trends away from vaginal delivery of the breech presentation, the splayed and extended legs (and hematomas and edema of the buttocks and perineal parts) of the frank breech delivery are increasingly rare. Although a dominantly extensor posture of the extremities is characteristic of the premature infant (and a fundamental part of gestational age assessment by physical examination), its appearance in a newborn at term should suggest significant neuromuscular abnormality.

A certain amount of digital webbing can be familial and normal, but true *syndactyly* and *polydactyly* are common in many complex congenital syndromes of malformation; they also occur singly. Similarly, although normal infants frequently (but transiently) manipulate their digits into strange positions, a persistent and almost obligatory grasping of the thumb within the "fisted" fingers suggests the *cortical thumb* of corticospinal tract malformation. A shortened, curved little finger *(clinodactyly),* just as a "simple" ear, can be a general marker of genetic disease. The foot that can display the normal range of motion outlined in Table 44-12 cannot be a *clubfoot,* whereas one more restrained may be. General joint contractures *(arthrogryposis)* suggest neuromuscular disease, but an infant's reluctance to use a normal-appearing joint should suggest trauma. However, subluxated hips are congenital and should be treated forthwith.

The Nervous System. Recent discoveries regarding the behavior of newborns, particularly their responses to visual and auditory stimuli, have made it clear that it is no longer appropriate to consider them, at least in their quiet-alert state, as "thalamic" animals. The *exteroceptive reflexes* (rooting, grasping, plantar, and superficial abdominal), involving touch receptors, are emphasized in the quiet-alert state, whereas the *proprioceptive reflexes* (deep tendon, Moro, and ankle clonus) are accentuated during quiet sleep.

Depressive changes in mental status, if occurring early (less than 1 to 2 days of life), most often are related to the birth process (oxygenation, trauma, or drugs); if they occur later, metabolic processes probably are involved. For instance, an infant who is normal at birth but days later (after digestion of milk and assimilation of its protein and carbohydrate) develops lethargy, stupor, coma, or convulsions (and may have a peculiar odor of, say, maple syrup) might very well have an *inborn error of metabolism.*

The less flexor and symmetrical the posture, the less wise it is to accept a term infant as neurologically normal. It can be difficult to distinguish between *neuro*muscular tone and neuro*muscular* strength as being responsible for the *floppy*

Table 44-13 Levels of Surveillance of the Newborn Based on Examination of the Nervous System

Characteristic	Level of surveillance: Normal	Alert	Alarm
State	Awake: crying, active, quiet-alert Asleep: active, indeterminate, quiet	Hyperalert, lethargic	Stupor, coma
Motor			
Posture	Flexor, symmetrical	Extensor, asymmetrical	Obligatory, decerebrate
Tone	Obtuse popliteal angle	Limp in upright suspension	Limp in ventral suspension
Movement	All extremities, nonrepetitive, random, symmetrical	Jitteriness, tremor	Seizures
Reflexes	Deep tendon, grasp, Moro, placing and stepping, sucking, tonic neck	Asymmetrical, does not habituate	Absent
Sensory	Pinprick response slow (2-3 sec)	Pinprick response equivocal	No response

Table 44-14 Levels of Surveillance of the Newborn Based on Examination of the Cranial Nerves

Cranial nerves	Level of surveillance: Normal	Alert	Alarm
Forebrain: II	Fix and follow (visual evoked potential)	Equivocal (arc <60 degrees)	No response
Midbrain: III, IV, VI, and VIII	Pupillary response, "doll's eye" response	Unequal, disconjugate, nystagmus	Absent, fixed position
Hindbrain			
VIII	Auditory evoked potentials, evoked otoacoustic emissions	Diminished	No response
V, VII, and XII	Sucking	Weak	Unequal
IX and X	Swallowing	Uncoordinated	
XI	Sternocleidomastoid muscles	Weak	

baby who slides between the examiner's opposing palms in upright suspension or who droops over the examiner's uplifting palm in ventral suspension. Beyond the purely neuromuscular causes of hypotonia (hypoxic, metabolic, or genetic encephalopathies; traumatic, toxic, and infectious myelopathies and neuropathies; and congenital, structural, and metabolic myopathies) can lurk a bewildering and poorly understood array of connective tissue, endocrine, and totally idiopathic causes of floppiness.

The jittery, tremulous baby is a common sight in nurseries, and such movements occasionally raise concern that the infant may be sustaining a convulsion. However, unlike "jitters," a true *seizure* tends to be asymmetrical and stimulus insensitive. The tremors of *jitteriness* most often are precipitated by noise or motion and usually can be obliterated, unlike the seizure, by manual restraint of the involved limb.

The most useful and diagnostically informative *reflexes* to be elicited from the newborn are listed in Table 44-13. As in most other aspects of the neurological examination, the reflex responses normally are symmetrical and tend to diminish in intensity (habituate) on repetition. Because of the newborn's slow nerve conduction relative to an adult, sensory responses can be quite slow. Yet a definite response to a pinprick, and certainly to more noxious stimuli, must be elicitable from all areas of the body.

Table 44-14 should make clear that all the cranial nerves, possibly excluding the olfactory, are easily tested in a newborn. The visual and auditory responses require the most patience and equipment (including, if necessary, formal evaluation of evoked electroencephalographic potentials); yet one dealing with a seeing and hearing infant can gain considerable confidence in the baby's possession of those abilities by presenting a red ball or human face to determine his or her ability to fix and follow and a human voice or loud noise to assess aural attention.

Interventions: Measures to Ensure the Integrity of the Newborn

Measures to ensure the integrity of a newborn infant are enumerated in the box on p. 513 and are quite straightforward. Although effective for the prophylaxis of gonorrheal ophthalmitis, 1% silver nitrate uniformly produces a brief *chemical conjunctivitis* (which may distress uninformed parents), and any drops spilled on the skin will discolor it temporarily. For these reasons, the antibiotic ointments have gained favor as prophylactic agents.

Apart from strictly cosmetic issues, skin and cord care is addressed to controlling the rate at which and the microorganisms with which the gnotobiotic infant's skin is to become colonized, as it inevitably must. Previous efforts to prevent establishment of a staphylococcal flora through use of hexachlorophene baths and the like were doomed to failure. The current emphasis is on permitting controlled colonization with what one hopes are benign bacterial strains. This is complemented by rigidly excluding any staphylococcal "carriers" from contact with the newborn and by minimal handling of the infant by all involved in his or her care. However, because it affords a direct route to the bloodstream, ex-

INITIAL CARE OF THE NEWBORN DESIGNED TO DETECT OR AVERT DIFFICULTIES DURING THE NEONATAL PERIOD

At delivery

Cord blood—*saved* for possible ABO typing, Rh typing, or Coombs test
Identification of infant as belonging to mother

At nursery admission

If not previously done in the delivery room:
- Eye care—1% silver nitrate drops or 1% tetracycline or 0.5% erythromycin ointments
- Hemorrhagic prophylaxis—0.5 to 1 mg vitamin K_1 oxide (phytonadione [Pholloquinone]), administered parenterally

Subsequent care

Skin care—"dry" (after initial cleansing with sterile water and cotton sponges)
Cord care—triple dye or bacitracin ointment

Diagnostic care

If indicated by:
- Premature rupture of membranes
- Temperature instability
- Small or large for gestational age
- Pallor

Then:
- Search for leukocytes and bacteria in gastric aspirate
- Perform blood glucose screen
- Obtain hemogram (hemoglobin, hematocrit, red blood cell count, white blood cell count, differential)

cessive infestation of the cord stump is discouraged with application of a bacteriostatic agent.

Premature rupture of the membranes places the fetus at risk for ascending *amnionitis* and the physician in a quandary as to just how aggressively to approach prevention or treatment of what often may turn out not to be a problem. Many find it helpful to be guided by the presence of leukocytes or bacteria (usually dead or otherwise nonculturable) in the gastric aspirate or ear canal.

Hypoglycemia is sufficiently common and threatening that it must be aggressively sought out and treated. *Occult hemorrhage* is less common, but failure to detect and treat it can be instantly tragic.

FOUR

Adjustment Period

Kathleen L. Gifford, M. Jeffrey Maisels, and Nicholas M. Nelson

The next sequential but overlapping stage in management of the newborn is replacing the maternal-fetal unit with the mother-infant pair; this pairing encompasses tactile and emotional factors as well as biological and nutritional concerns. Beyond this, and as important as the obvious processes of feeding, stooling, burping, and weighing, are the mystical, magical, and arguable processes of "bonding" and extending the family to include father, brothers and sisters, and grandparents, as well as medical personnel. Much of this already will have been achieved during a properly managed pregnancy, but reinforcement always is in order.

ONSET OF ORAL NUTRITIONAL INTAKE AND PARENTING

The first few days (or hours, in hospitals practicing early discharge) are devoted largely to mutual patterning by mother and child, as their schedules for sleeping, eating, relaxing, and playing begin to mesh. This prolonged and productive process seems easier and certainly more natural if managed in a rooming-in setting, whether at home or in the hospital.

As the new or experienced mother establishes or refines her skills at mothering during this period, she should expect and receive from hospital personnel nothing but the warmest, most enthusiastic support, regardless of how many tiresome and routine deliveries were managed that day without morbidity or death. In teaching hospitals these personnel often include young pediatric house officers who typically are terrified by (and therefore avoid) the daily duty of confidently answering the normal questions of normal mothers about their normal infants. The place to learn this aspect of the art of medicine is not in a book, but in the mother's room.

OBSERVATIONS AND EXAMINATION

Although in the absence of specific symptoms no particular examination of the infant is called for, the processes of feeding, growing, and excreting are monitored with particular care—the amount (of formula) ingested, the amount regurgitated, the quality and strength of sucking, the frequency and type of stooling and voiding, and the daily weight gain or loss.

A loss of 6% to 8% of birth weight is expected over the first 3 or 4 days, largely because of normal fluid shifts but also because of the decreased oral (as opposed to placental) fluid and nutritional intake in the first days of life. This weight loss tends to be somewhat more pronounced and prolonged in a nursing infant. Weight usually begins to increase after the fourth day, and the birth weight should be regained by 1 to 2 weeks of age; however, the outline offered here is purposefully vague because there is much normal variation.

FEEDING

The decision for breast-feeding or bottle-feeding will have best been made by the unpressured mother well before her delivery (see Chapter 16). Her decision should be supported without undue proselytizing in either direction. On the other hand, the mother who is undecided can be apprised without prejudice or commitment of the advantages of nursing (simplicity, certainty, safety, nutritional equality, and immunological and economic superiority).

A strictly biochemical comparison of breast and formula feeding is presented in Table 16-5, wherein it is noted that breast milk is lower in protein and higher in fat, lower in calcium and much lower in phosphorus. The various commercial formulas have been fortified with vitamins (particularly vitamin D), and a nursing infant probably should receive vitamin supplementation. Although a well-mothered, well-fed normal infant in North America certainly can expect to receive adequate nutritional iron by the appropriate age (4 to 6 months) as his or her diet expands to include fortified cereals, meats, and egg yolks, it still is unfortunate that not all infants are so lucky. In addition, many if not most of these latter babies probably are not breast-fed. In any case, the recommendation has been made and implemented that all infant formulas be supplemented with iron to improve infant health (similar to the fluoridation of water). There seems to be little question that both forms of supplementation have been effective passive health supports. Iron supplementation for the nursing infant is optional but probably wise.

ESTABLISHMENT OF LACTATION

Human milk is the ideal food for human infants, and breast-feeding is the most natural and practical way to feed a baby. It is emotionally satisfying, provides the closest possible contact between mother and infant, and should produce a unique sense of fulfillment. Unfortunately, breast-feeding in the Western world is no longer instinctive, and mothers who want to nurse their infants require guidance and emotional support. At no time is this more important or the mother more receptive than in the immediate postpartum period. However, the psychological and physical preparation for nursing should begin well before delivery, with information about nursing and a detailed discussion of its benefits.

Given an uncomplicated delivery and a vigorous infant, the baby should be nursed within the first hour of life during the first stage of transition, when he or she is alert and shows an interest in sucking. "Test feeds" of water are unnecessary because patency of the esophagus can be confirmed on examination in the nursery. Babies should be nursed on demand and no less than eight times a day to ensure establishment of adequate lactation; some infants require nursing as often as every 2 hours. This is normal and thus to be encouraged. Frequent nursing (more than eight times a day) has been shown to reduce serum bilirubin levels in the newborn, produce good letdown, and help prevent breast engorgement.

A schedule of 5 minutes on each breast for each feeding the first day, 5 to 10 minutes on each breast for each feeding the second day, and 10 to 15 minutes on each breast for each feeding thereafter is said to prevent nipple soreness, although satisfactory data to support this contention are lacking. However, it has been shown that most infants can empty a breast in about 7 minutes, so additional sucking, however pleasant for either or both parties, is nonnutritive and may lead to sore nipples. These time limits are not sacrosanct, and mothers should be encouraged not to nurse "by the clock." To ensure adequate emptying and stimulation of both breasts, the mother should be instructed to alternate the breast with which she begins each feeding.

Good technique involves washing the hands, finding a comfortable position and support, using the rooting reflex (placing the infant's cheek against the warm, naked breast, which stimulates him or her to turn the face into the breast) to encourage the baby's grasp of the entire nipple and areola, and breaking suction by putting a finger in the corner of the baby's mouth (see Fig. 16-8).

An explanation of the anatomy and physiology of lactation and suckling helps the mother respond naturally to the process and avoid complications. Hormonal changes immediately after delivery enhance the process that provides colostrum. The production of milk occurs secondary to the release of prolactin and oxytocin in response to a number of stimuli, including the tactile stimulus of the suckling infant. In fact, the milk ejection (letdown) reflex and the release of oxytocin occur in most women before actual suckling begins, and further release of oxytocin follows in response to the suckling. Oxytocin causes the smooth muscle cells around the alveolar cells (milk glands) to contract, leading to a release of milk, which flows via the ducts into the lactiferous sinuses (milk pools) situated behind the areola. The release of oxytocin is readily affected by the mother's emotional state and her ability to relax before and during nursing.

The letdown reflex is of utmost importance because its failure can lead to congestion, engorgement, a diminished milk supply, and a hungry baby. Mothers recognize the letdown when they feel a tingling sensation in the breasts or start to leak milk from the unused breast. To encourage letdown, mothers should practice relaxing in a quiet room and should feed their infant on demand. Warm showers, warm compresses, and warm beverages also may be helpful.

Technique

When the infant grasps the nipple, he or she uses the tongue to pull it into the mouth and press it against the palate. This brings the lactiferous sinuses into a position where they are accessible to pressure from the gums and facial muscles. It is the baby's pressure on these sinuses and *not* the sucking that squeezes milk from the breast and is necessary for adequate emptying (see Fig. 16-5).

Establishing a good nursing pattern should be the major goal during the first few weeks; supplementation with formula or water, which disrupts this pattern, should be avoided. Offering a bottle confuses the infant, diminishes his or her desire to suckle, and may cause the mother concern about her ability to provide adequate nutrition. Contrary to popular belief, water supplementation does not lower serum bilirubin levels in a breast-fed baby.

Common Complications

Sometime during the first 24 hours the mother is likely to complain of a "lazy" baby who refuses to suckle. She can be reassured that the baby does not require large amounts during the first day. Despite lack of vigorous suckling, each session at the breast provides experience in position and technique for both mother and child. By the second day the baby's appetite and technique should begin to improve.

Mothers often develop sore nipples when the baby begins to suckle with vigor, but this can be prevented or minimized by feeding the baby on demand and by good technique (see the box below).

Sometime between 48 and 96 hours postpartum, when true (i.e., noncolostrum) milk production starts, most mothers experience some degree of engorgement caused by venous and lymphatic stasis in the breast tissue and the presence of milk in the alveolar cells (and therefore merit congratulatory reassurance that milk production has begun). This lasts for several days and diminishes as the breast adjusts to the nursing pattern. Frequent suckling is the most effective means of preventing and treating engorgement and helps ameliorate discomfort by relieving pressure from the presence of milk. A badly engorged breast prevents the baby from drawing the nipple well into the mouth and makes it difficult for him or her to nurse. Manual or mechanical expression of a little milk before nursing, sufficient to soften the breast and extend the nipple, allows the infant to grasp it easily.

Special Situations

Inverted Nipples. Nongraspable or nonprotractile nipples may be manipulated in the prenatal or postpartum periods to loosen adhesions and improve protractility. A breast pump, stretching techniques, milk cups, and nipple shields will draw the nipples out so that the infant can grasp them.

Cesarean Section. The processes of postoperative recovery require only slight variations in the initial breast-feeding routine. Comfort techniques, analgesics, and appropriate positioning help improve the nursing experience.

Twins. Mothers can produce sufficient milk for twins and sometimes for triplets. The babies may be fed either simultaneously or separately. Various positions are possible.

Jaundice. Breast-feeding has been associated with an increased incidence of jaundice in the first week of life. The increase in the bilirubin level generally is small and of no clinical importance. Frequent nursing (at least eight times a day) may ameliorate this problem. If the bilirubin level approaches 20 mg/dl ("true" breast milk jaundice syndrome), nursing should be interrupted for 24 to 48 hours, the mother pumping her breasts in the interim. Invariably the serum bilirubin level declines, and breast-feeding can be resumed. The mother needs positive support and reinforcement to reassure her that it is desirable and safe for her to continue nursing. After breast-feeding is resumed, the bilirubin level may rise slightly, but it rarely returns to the previous concentration.

Prematurity. Recent experience shows that premature infants thrive on breast milk and can suckle adequately at the breast by about 34 weeks of gestation. Expressed breast milk can be given to the more premature infant. To succeed, the mother needs instruction in breast pumping and milk collection, accompanied by continued support and, obviously, a strong personal motivation. The milk from the mother of a premature infant has a higher protein content than that from the mother of a full-term infant. Thus the infant's own mother's milk is more desirable than either pooled or "banked" breast milk.

Cleft Lip and Palate. Nursing may be difficult when a cleft in the lip or palate prevents the infant from maintaining sufficient suction to seal the nipple in the mouth. If the infant has a cleft lip but intact palate, the mother's soft breast tissue should help occlude the cleft and improve the seal. However, a palatal cleft complicates the infant's attempt to press the nipple against the palate and "milk" it. In the case of a unilateral cleft, placing the nipple may avoid this problem. Highly motivated mothers have maintained breast-feeding by holding the nipple in place, by manually expressing directly into the infant's mouth, or by pumping the breasts and then bottle-feeding the expressed milk.

AID FOR SORE NIPPLES

1. Air-dry nipples after each feeding.
2. Change bra and breast pads when they become moist.
3. Clean nipples with water only. Excessive soap dries the nipples.
4. Nurse every 2 hours, but for only 5 to 7 minutes on each breast, and offer the least sore nipple first.
5. Apply a small amount of breast cream, anhydrous lanolin, or hydrophilic ointment to the nipples after each feeding. (The efficacy of this therapy is questionable.)
6. Change the baby's nursing position to alter the mouth-to-nipple pressure points.
7. As a last resort, use a nipple shield for 24 to 48 hours to allow for healing before commencing the toughening process again.

Additional Concerns

Additional concerns about breast-feeding include the following:

1. Milk may leak for several months; this can be controlled by applying pressure to the nipple and using an absorbent, not plastic, breast pad.
2. During the first weeks, engorgement diminishes as the baby's demands increase. Thus the mother may be concerned about a lack of milk. Reassurance, a discussion of supply and demand, and an explanation of physiology will help.
3. The baby is "getting enough" when six or seven moderately wet diapers must be changed each day.
4. A periodic replacement bottle may be offered after the first 2 to 3 weeks, but only after consistent feeding patterns and a steady milk supply have been established.
5. A plugged milk duct is seen as a small, tender lump in the breast that persists after a feeding. Massage, frequent feedings, and cleansing of caked milk from the nipple usually resolve this problem.
6. Mastitis produces flulike symptoms and a reddened, tender area on one or both breasts. It should be treated with rest, warm compresses to the affected breast, frequent nursing to prevent stasis, and antibiotics (if symptoms persist). Left untreated, mastitis can progress to a breast abscess, requiring surgical drainage and discontinuation of feeding at the affected breast until it heals.

Vitamins, Iron, and Fluoride

Whether the diet of breast-fed infants needs to be supplemented with vitamins, iron, and fluoride is a matter of controversy. However, based on the estimated needs of growing infants, many feel it wise to provide additional vitamin D and iron. Because the fluoride content of breast milk is low, fully breast-fed infants also require supplemental fluoride.

Maternal Medication and Diet

Almost all drugs ingested by the mother are excreted in breast milk, but very few in amounts large enough to be hazardous to the infant (Table 16-7). To minimize risk, however, maternal drugs should be avoided whenever possible. If maternal medication is absolutely necessary, the *infant should be nursed before each dose*. The mother requires a well-balanced diet during pregnancy, plus approximately 200 calories in high-protein food while breast-feeding. The nursing period is no time for "crash" or fad dieting.

FIVE
Establishment of Equilibrium

Nicholas M. Nelson and Dennis M. Super

In this final phase of management of the newborn, the practitioner pursues the twin objectives of completing the infant's perinatal adjustments and integrating the mother-infant pair into an ongoing program for their health supervision. Precisely where this begins or is implemented (hospital, home, private office, or clinic) varies with local facilities, resources, and expectations, but the principal expectation to be instilled before discharge is that continuing health supervision is the best guarantee for maintaining the healthy process already begun.

In these later days of the infant's hospital course, *jaundice* especially is sought out and, if excessive (more than 10 to 12 mg/dl total bilirubin), investigated. In addition, the various requirements for statewide screening programs (e.g., phenylketonuria and hypothyroidism) need to be fulfilled and a decision reached (not imposed) concerning the *circumcision* of a baby boy.

The benefits of neonatal circumcision remain controversial in North America. In the United States, more than 70% of male infants are circumcised, whereas in Europe, neonatal circumcision is rare.[13] Proponents state that neonatal circumcision reduces the risk of penile carcinoma, prevents balanoposthitis, phimosis, and paraphimosis, has a lower anesthetic risk than does circumcision performed later in life, and eliminates the need for penile hygiene. Opponents state that it subjects the neonate to additional stress and that the procedure has a definite complication rate. They also argue that proper penile hygiene will prevent phimosis, paraphimosis, balanoposthitis, and penile cancer and that the foreskin protects the delicate urethral meatus from the irritation of soiled diapers. In 1989 the American Academy of Pediatrics Task Force on Circumcision stated that neonatal circumcision has potential medical benefits as well as disadvantages and risks.[9]

An association between urinary tract infections and the uncircumcised neonate has been noted in numerous retrospective studies.[13] A possible explanation for this association may be that the urethra of an uncircumcised neonate is readily colonized with uropathogenic organisms, in contrast to the urethra of a circumcised infant.[14] An alternative to circumcision in preventing infantile urinary tract infections may be to foster more natural colonization of the infant's urethra by promoting strict rooming-in of the mother and baby or by active colonization of the baby with the mother's nonpathogenic, anaerobic gut flora.[12] Future studies are needed to determine which of these interventions may best prevent urinary tract infections.

In 1976 Gee and Ansell[5] reviewed the risks of a neonatal circumcision. In their study of 5882 male births at the University of Washington from 1963 to 1972, 5521 (94%) infants were circumcised. Almost 2% developed a complication from the procedure, including hemorrhage (1%), postcircumcision infection (0.4%), wound dehiscence (0.16%), strangulation of the glans from a tight plastic bell (0.13%), and circumcision of children who had hypospadias (0.15%, or 36% of all children with hypospadias). The percentage of severe complications was 0.2%; these included life-threatening hemorrhage (one case), systemic infection (four cases), circumcision of a child who had hypospadias (eight cases), and denudation of the shaft of the penis (one case). The only significant difference between the complication rates of the Gomco and the Plastibell techniques was a lower incidence of wound infection with the Gomco technique. Other complications include urethral cutaneous fistula, penile amputation, recurrent pneumothorax, transient hypoxia, penile lacerations, postcircumcision phimosis, and death.[6] The contraindications for neonatal circumcision are (1) any type of congenital anomaly (especially hypospadias), (2) bleeding diathesis, (3) prematurity, and (4) any neonatal illness.

The physician should perform a circumcision only after a complete physical examination has been performed and after the child has urinated. Circumcision should be delayed until after the first day of life because the infant may not have recovered fully from the stress of delivery. Also, some illnesses may take some time to become clinically evident during the neonatal period.

Infants undergoing elective circumcision without analgesia feel pain, as evidenced by increases in heart rate, respiratory rate, blood pressure, and plasma cortisol levels.[1] After the procedure, these infants are also more irritable and display altered behavior that may last for up to a day.[7] Hence, the clinician should consider analgesia for the neonate in the same way as one would for an older patient.[1] Some methods of relieving pain include a dorsal penile nerve block, infiltration of the foreskin with 1% lidocaine, topical anesthesia (30% lidocaine in an acid mantle base or an eutectic mixture of 2.5% lidocaine and 2.5% prilocaine), and a pacifier saturated with 24% sucrose solution.[2,4,7,11] Local infiltration with lidocaine produces better analgesia than a dorsal penile nerve block.[7] Special care is needed in administering analgesia to neonates because of the prolonged pharmacological half-lives in infants, increased skin permeability, and susceptibility to apnea (opiates). Some of the potential rare side effects of these medications include allergic reactions, intravascular injection of local anesthetics (irritability, lethargy, convulsions, bradycardia, hypotension, and cardiac arrest), and methemoglobinemia (prilocaine).[3] In addition, a hematoma from a dorsal penile nerve block could compromise the blood supply to the penis, resulting in gangrene of the glans. Until clinical trials can determine which of the above methods produce the best analgesia, the clinician should discuss these various options with the parents who have elected to have their son circumcised.

The parents' desire for their son to be circumcised should be discussed during a prenatal visit during which they can reflect calmly and rationally on the risks and benefits of the procedure.[9] If they decide against circumcision, the physician should include proper foreskin hygiene in their anticipatory guidance during subsequent health maintenance visits. Once the foreskin is easily retracted, the parents should be instructed to gently retract it each day, to wash the glans and foreskin with soapy water, and to dry the area thoroughly.[8]

Perhaps no wiser words have ever been spoken on the subject of infant circumcision than the following[10]:

> My dear C.,
>
> Your patient, C.D., at age 7 months, has the prepuce with which he was born. You ask me, with a note of persuasion in your question, if it should be excised. Am I to make this decision on scientific grounds, or am I to acquiesce in a ritual that took its origin at the behest of that arch-sanitarian Moses?
>
> If you can show good reason why a ritual designed to ease the penalties of concupiscence amidst the sand and flies of the Syrian deserts should be continued in this England of clean bed linen and lesser opportunity, I shall listen to your argument, but if you base your argument on anatomical faults, then I must refute it.
>
> The anatomists have never studied the form and evolution of the preputial orifice. They do not understand that Nature does not intend it to be stretched and retracted in the Temples of the Welfare Centres or ritually removed in the precincts of the operating theatres. Retract the prepuce and you see a pin-point opening, but draw it forward and you see a channel wide enough for all the purposes for which the infant needs the organ at that early age. What looks like a pin-point opening at 7 months will become a wide channel of communication at 17. Nature is a possessive mistress, and whatever mistakes she makes about the structure of the less essential organs such as the brain and stomach, in which she is not much interested, you can be sure that she knows best about the genital organs.

Despite such wisdom and its frequent reiteration, many parents expect, some insist on, and not a few physicians and hospitals seem too anxious to support the continuing North American medical ritual of circumcision.

On the day of discharge a careful physical examination needs to be repeated, particularly emphasizing the baby's behavioral state, the appearance (or disappearance) of any cardiac murmurs, and a close inspection of the cord. These findings and a recapitulation of the infant's progress since birth need to be recorded in a form (Fig. 44-13) easily transmissible to the physician or facility assuming responsibility for the infant's continuing care.

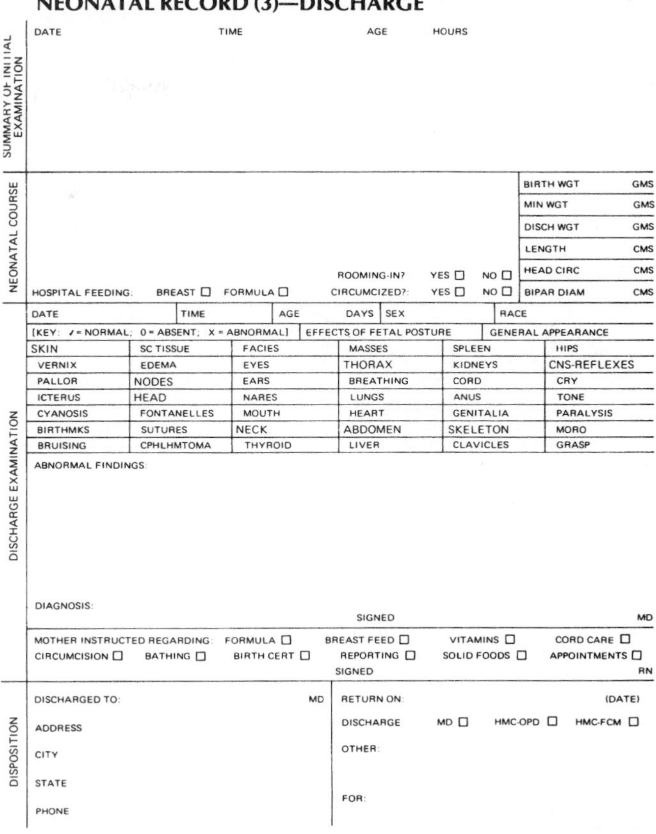

NEONATAL RECORD (3)—DISCHARGE

SUMMARY OF INITIAL EXAMINATION

DATE TIME AGE HOURS

NEONATAL COURSE

BIRTH WGT GMS
MIN WGT GMS
DISCH WGT GMS
LENGTH CMS
HEAD CIRC CMS
BIPAR DIAM CMS

ROOMING-IN? YES ☐ NO ☐
HOSPITAL FEEDING: BREAST ☐ FORMULA ☐ CIRCUMCIZED?: YES ☐ NO ☐

DISCHARGE EXAMINATION

DATE | TIME | AGE DAYS | SEX | RACE

[KEY: ✓ = NORMAL; 0 = ABSENT; X = ABNORMAL] | EFFECTS OF FETAL POSTURE | GENERAL APPEARANCE

SKIN	SC TISSUE	FACIES	MASSES	SPLEEN	HIPS
VERNIX	EDEMA	EYES	THORAX	KIDNEYS	CNS-REFLEXES
PALLOR	NODES	EARS	BREATHING	CORD	CRY
ICTERUS	HEAD	NARES	LUNGS	ANUS	TONE
CYANOSIS	FONTANELLES	MOUTH	HEART	GENITALIA	PARALYSIS
BIRTHMKS	SUTURES	NECK	ABDOMEN	SKELETON	MORO
BRUISING	CPHLHMTOMA	THYROID	LIVER	CLAVICLES	GRASP

ABNORMAL FINDINGS:

DIAGNOSIS:

SIGNED MD

MOTHER INSTRUCTED REGARDING: FORMULA ☐ BREAST FEED ☐ VITAMINS ☐ CORD CARE ☐
CIRCUMCISION ☐ BATHING ☐ BIRTH CERT ☐ REPORTING ☐ SOLID FOODS ☐ APPOINTMENTS ☐
SIGNED RN

DISPOSITION

DISCHARGED TO: MD
ADDRESS
CITY
STATE
PHONE

RETURN ON: (DATE)
DISCHARGE MD ☐ HMC-OPD ☐ HMC-FCM ☐
OTHER:
FOR:

FIG. 44-13 Data relevant to the entire neonatal course that should be conveyed from the hospital of birth to the physician assuming responsibility for continuing health supervision.

By 2 to 3 weeks of age, weight gain should be well established, the mother's breast milk abundantly flowing, the father back to work, and the infant's real impact on the household readily apparent.

SIX

Pediatric Support for Parents

John H. Kennell and Marshall H. Klaus

Experiences during pregnancy, labor, and delivery and events shortly after birth may greatly affect an infant's later development. We explore here what is known about this period in the life of the infant, the parents, and the family and emphasize what interventions may aid the maturation of the family.

It has been difficult to assess which factors determine the parenting behavior of human beings and how pediatric support can alter the process. Parents' actions and responses toward their infant derive from a complex combination of their own genetic endowment, the way the baby responds to them, the long history of interpersonal relations within their own families and with each other, their experiences in this or previous pregnancies, the practices and values of their respective cultures, and—probably most important—how each was raised by his or her own mother and father. The mothering or fathering behavior of each woman and man, their ability to tolerate stress, and their need for support may differ greatly and will depend on a mixture of all these factors. Strong evidence for the importance of the effect of the mother's own mothering on her caretaking comes from an elegant 35-year study by Engel et al.[8] that documented the close correspondence between how Monica (an infant who had a tracheoesophageal fistula) was fed during the first 2 years of life, how she then cared for her dolls, and how as an adult she fed her own four children.

Figure 44-14 presents our current conception of the major influences on parenting behavior and the resulting disturbances that we postulate as arising from them. Included under parental background are the following:

1. Parent's care by his or her own mother
2. Parents' endowment or genetics

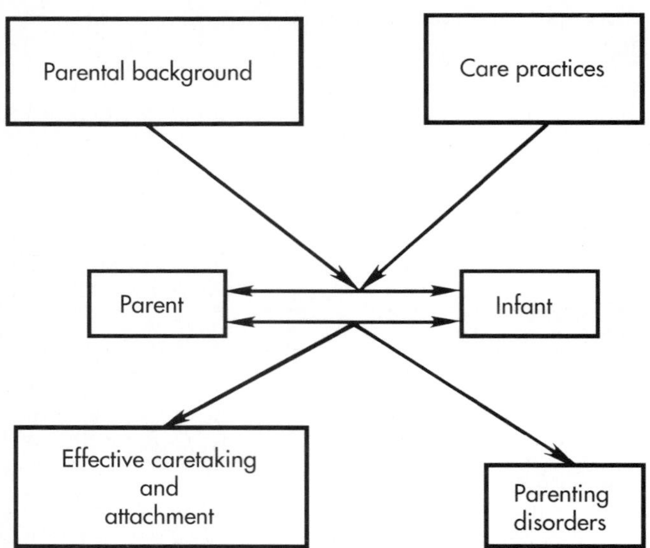

FIG. 44-14 Major influences on parent-infant attachment and the resulting outcomes.

(From Klaus MH, Kennell JH: *Parent-infant bonding,* ed 2, St Louis, 1982, Mosby.)

3. Practices of the culture
4. Experiences with previous pregnancies
5. Planning, course, and events during pregnancy

Although the effects of these particular determinants once were thought to be fixed and unchangeable, it has been observed that their impact may be altered, both favorably and unfavorably, during the experience of birth. Parenting behavior and the parent-child relationship also may be influenced significantly by factors such as the parents' observation of attitudes, statements, and practices of the nurses and physicians in the hospital, whether the mother is alone for short periods during her labor, whether the mother and father are separated from their infant in the first few days of life, the infant's nature and temperament, and whether the infant is healthy, sick, or malformed. Included under parenting disorders are the following:

1. Child abuse and neglect
2. Nonorganic failure to thrive
3. Vulnerable child syndrome
4. Disturbed parent-child relationship
5. Some developmental and emotional problems among high-risk infants

The following questions are helpful in focusing on the special needs of each member:

1. How long have you lived in this area, and where do most of your own family live?
2. How often do you see your mother and other close relatives?
3. Has anything happened to you in the past (or do you have any condition) that causes you to worry about the pregnancy or the baby?
4. What was your husband's reaction to your becoming pregnant?
5. What other responsibilities do you have outside the family?

Table 44-15 Levels of Functioning for Infants

Prechtl and Beintema[24]	Wolff[34]
1. Deep sleep: eyes closed, regular respiration, no movements	1. Same
2. Active sleep (REM): eyes closed, irregular respiration, small movements	2. Same
3. Quiet-alert: eyes open, no movements, no crying	3. Drowsy
4. Active-alert: eyes open, gross movements, no crying	4. Quiet-alert: no movements, eyes open
5. Crying (vocalization), eyes open	5. Active-alert: gross movements, no crying
	6. Crying (vocalization)

It is important to inquire about how the pregnant woman herself was mothered: did she have a neglected, deprived infancy and childhood, or did she grow up in a warm, intact family?

In addition to those who received inadequate or disturbed mothering in their own early life, other mothers who have special needs are single, young, or adoptive parents. We will consider the needs of all these women who have healthy full-term newborns, together with those of healthy parents from "normal" backgrounds.

INFANT STATE

For parents to begin to understand and meet their infant's needs, it is important that they understand the infant's differing states of consciousness. The "state" or "pattern" of behavior refers to the infant's overall level of functioning at any given time, ranging from deep sleep to wakefulness, activity, or crying. Wolff[34] originally designed the descriptive scale for rating the state of the full-term infant. He defined six states, but Prechtl and Beintema[24] omitted the "drowsy" state, regarding it as a transition between states, thus defining five states (Table 44-15). These states can be differentiated by physiological measurements, including respiration, heart rate, eye movements, and electromyography, or by behavioral observation.

These states appear to form a continuum that differs qualitatively and with distinct types of organization. They are relatively stable and recur in regular cycles during day and night. Practically every behavior and body function of the newborn depends on his or her state and on the stability and control of this state. Cognitive functions in the newborn period, for instance, can best be assessed in the quiet-alert state. Each of these six states is accompanied by quite specific and individual behaviors. For the human infant there are six ways of being or acting in the world. One can liken these states of consciousness to the changing of sets for acts in a play. Each act has its own setting, time, and mood, and the action makes sense only with the appropriate scenery. Likewise for the newborn, each state of consciousness has a specific set of behaviors. In the *quiet-alert state* (state 4), which is very similar to conscious attention in adults when they are listening closely to us, babies rarely move. Their eyes are wide open, bright, and shiny. In this state they can follow a red ball, select pictures they prefer, and even imitate their mother's facial expression. Right after birth, within the first hour of life, normal infants have a prolonged period of quiet-alertness, averaging 40 minutes, during which they can look directly at their mother's and father's face and respond to voices. It appears to be a perfect time to meet their parents. In this state, motor activity is suppressed and all the baby's energy seems to be channeled into seeing and hearing.

LABOR AND DELIVERY FOR PARENTS OF NORMAL FULL-TERM INFANTS

In 1959 Bibring[3] wrote, "What was once a crisis with carefully worked-out traditional customs of giving support to the woman passing through this crisis period has become at this time a crisis with no mechanisms within the society for helping the woman involved in this profound change of conflict-solutions and adjustive tasks." This deficiency may account for the recent development of the many support systems in our society, such as the wide assortment of childbirth classes.

A recent review of ethnographical material has shown that in 127 of 128 representative, nonindustrialized societies, another woman was present with the mother during labor—in only one society did the mother labor alone. The significance of this almost universal custom of support has been revealed in seven randomized, controlled studies, which have shown that the presence of a supportive woman companion (a "doula") during labor and delivery reduced the cesarean delivery rate 50%, reduced the length of labor 25% (and oxytocin use by 40%), and reduced pain medication by 30%, the need for forceps by 40%, and requests for epidurals by 60%.[19] In one study, mothers who had received doula support shortly after birth were awake most of the time, and when they were with their newborns after delivery, they showed more affectionate interaction with their babies than did mothers without a doula. Interestingly, fewer infants born after a doula-supported labor in the United States had a prolonged hospital course.

We believe that supportive management of labor and delivery should adhere to the following principles:

1. The less anxiety the mother experiences during delivery, the better will be her immediate relation with her baby. Thus she and her husband (or other support person) should visit the maternity unit to see where labor and delivery will take place and to learn about delivery routines. What will happen should be presented in detail, realistically but tactfully, if not previously covered in the childbirth class.
2. It is essential that parents be involved in the many decisions associated with labor and birth. A birth "plan" should be developed in the third trimester.
3. The mother and father ought to have one experienced woman for guidance and reassurance (midwife, nurse, or doula) who is continuously present at the mother's side throughout labor and birth to help the couple.[19] *No woman should ever labor alone.*
4. Once delivery has been completed, it is important for the mother to have a few seconds to regain her composure before she proceeds to the next task. It is best not to present her with her baby before drying and examining the infant briefly to confirm that he or she is completely normal and before the mother indicates that she is ready to take her baby; it should be her decision.
5. It is valuable for the mother, father, and infant to be together for at least 1 hour. The mother and father usually never forget these significant and stimulating shared experiences. It helps some parents to begin the process of attaching themselves to the real infant. We wish to emphasize that this should be a private, "executive" session and that many normal parents take many days to fall in love with their infants.
6. The mother and father should stay together continuously or have long periods together in the days after the birth. The postpartum period should be a time when the mother interacts with her infant, becoming acquainted and gaining confidence in her own abilities. It is suggested that the infant stay in a small bassinet at the mother's side for a minimum of 5 hours aday (Fig. 44-15). After a cesarean delivery it will be painful for the mother to pick up, feed, and manage her infant without assistance. The father or another family member should be encouraged to stay with the new mother throughout the day to provide this assistance. Help at home with household tasks is especially valuable.
7. Whenever possible, infants who require additional heat in an incubator should be allowed to remain with the mother, and phototherapy for hyperbilirubinemia should take place in the mother's room. A mother may become extremely anxious about the health of her baby when they are apart and is reassured by the baby's presence. This is a common example of Winnicott's proposal of primary maternal preoccupation.[33]
8. Breast-feeding mothers should be encouraged to feed their babies during the first hour and then on demand. This can mean between 8 and 18 feedings in a 24-hour period. Studies by deCarvalho[5,6] reveal that women who feed this often in the first 14 days are more successful at breast-feeding, have a larger milk output at 2 weeks, have minimum nipple soreness, and have infants with significantly lower bilirubin levels than do women who nurse fewer than eight times a day in the first 2 weeks.
9. After giving birth the mother needs the emotional support of close contact with her husband or chosen companion, as well as with her children, especially those under 3 years of age. Even under a policy of early discharge 24 to 48 hours after delivery, sadness on separation from husband and children may compel a woman to leave the hospital before she is ready physically. The first few days at home usually go more smoothly for the siblings and mother if they have had daily visits during the hospitalization.
10. We strongly recommend that nurses, physicians, and other maternity staff consistently be optimistic and avoid criticism in their interaction with new mothers. In the postpartum period even a perfectly normal woman may be extremely sensitive to physicians' and nurses' opinions and statements about her baby or herself.

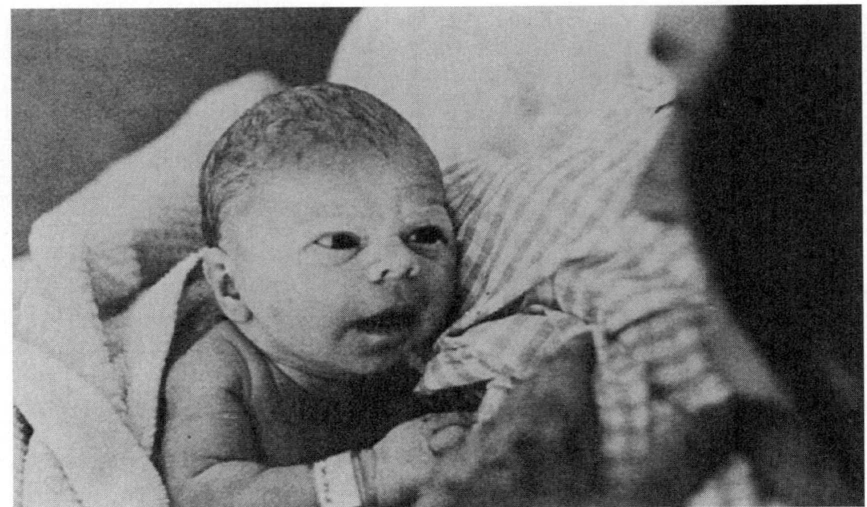

FIG. 44-15 What the mother sometimes sees.
(From Klaus MH, Kennell JH: *Parent-infant bonding,* ed 2, St Louis, 1982, Mosby.)

STUDIES OF A SENSITIVE PERIOD

The question of whether additional time for close contact between the mother and her full-term infant in the first minutes and hours of life can alter the quality of the mother-infant bonding over time has been the subject of numerous studies and extensive debate. Because hospital practices recently have been altered on the basis of these studies, it is essential to explore their design, ecology, and outcome measures. Thirteen separate studies have looked at the effect of additional mother-infant contact in the first hour of life, with contact after this period being similar in both the experimental and the control groups.[20] In 9 of the 13 studies, differences in the behavior of both mother and infant were noted in the experimental group.

In six of those nine studies, breast-feeding was more successful and continued for a significantly longer period for mothers who had contact that involved suckling their babies in the first hour after birth than for those whose suckling occurred later. It is difficult to know whether it was the early contact per se or, more specifically, the early suckling that altered the length of time that these mothers continued to breast-feed. It may be argued that the length of breast-feeding is not a valid assessment of the strength of the mother-infant bond because breast-feeding is determined to a great extent by culture.

When additional time is given for close mother-infant contact after the first 8 hours after delivery, differences in later mothering behavior also occur. In a study of 301 mothers, O'Connor and others[23] noted that increasing the time by 12 hours (6 hours on days 1 and 2) significantly reduced the number of mothering disorders that lead to child abuse or neglect; there were 10 such occurrences in the control group, but only 2 in the group of mothers that received extra time with their infants (Table 44-16). Using a similar design, Siegel et al.[26] studied a group of new and multiparous mothers and found differences in parenting at 4 and 12 months but no difference in mothering disorders. A woman was defined as having a mothering disorder if her infant was battered, had nonorganic failure to thrive, was abandoned, or was given up for an unplanned adoption.

Table 44-16 Relationship Between Extended Early Mother-Infant Contact and Child Abuse and Neglect

Study	Number of subjects	Number of cases
O'Connor et al.[23] (1980)		
Extended contact	134	2
Control	143	10*
Siegel et al.[26] (1980)		
Extended contact	97	7
Control	105	10

Modified from Klaus MH, Kennell JH: *Parent-infant bonding,* St Louis, 1982, Mosby.
*$p < 0.05$.

Because of the relatively small number of patients studied, the negative finding by Siegel and coworkers does not answer the important question of whether extended contact for all mothers in the United States would prevent child abuse in some of the 100,000 infants abused each year. It can be calculated that a study of about 1600 patients would be needed to detect a reduction in child abuse from 3% to 1.5% 80% of the time, performance criteria that have not yet been met. Thus, although most studies of additional early or extended contact do show changes in maternal and paternal behavior in the first days and weeks of life, the question concerning the clinical significance of the long-term effects remains.*

Feelings of love for the infant are not necessarily instantaneous with initial contact. Many mothers have shared with us their distress and disappointment that they did not experience the feelings of love for their baby in the first minutes or hours after birth. It should be reassuring for them to learn

*References 10-12, 14, 15, 18, 28, 29, 32.

of the following study of normal, healthy mothers in England. MacFarlane and associates[21] asked 97 Oxford mothers, "When did you first feel love for your baby?" The replies were as follows: during pregnancy, 41%; at birth, 24%; first week, 27%; and after the first week, 8%.

A review of a representative ethnographical sample shows that 183 of 186 nonindustrial societies expect mothers and babies to "nest" together for days or weeks after delivery (a rooming-in equivalent); virtually none permits the degree of separation that has been routine in maternity hospitals in many "developed" nations. This early rooming-in usually is followed by extensive mother-infant contact and prolonged, frequent breast-feeding during the early months. This almost universal practice of protecting and supporting the mother-infant pair together in the first weeks has evolved over thousands of years. Does it have significance for the industrialized societies of today, particularly in view of the widespread shift to early hospital discharge and the absence of a public health nursing system of support for mothers and infants and of legislated maternity or paternity leave with pay in the United States?

In 1957 Winnicott[33] made remarkably perceptive observations that appear to describe what we call the sensitive period. He proposed that a healthy mother goes through a period of "primary maternal preoccupation" that "gradually develops and becomes a state of heightened sensitivity during, and especially toward the end of, the pregnancy. It lasts for a few weeks after the birth of the child." According to Winnicott, "The mother who develops this state . . . provides a setting for the infant's constitution to begin to make itself evident . . . and for the infant to . . . become the owner of the sensations that are appropriate to this early phase of life." He notes further that this is true only if a mother is sensitized in the way described and can identify with her baby's needs and thus be better able to meet them. As a result of recent changes in American society and modified expectations of young parents, some might consider the roles of the father and the mother as increasingly indistinguishable in relation to their newborn. We, however, tend to agree with Winnicott that each parent has a separate and unique role. He noted that fathers "can provide a space in which the woman has elbow room." When so protected, the mother does not have to deal with her surroundings just at the time that she wants to be "concerned with the inside of the circle she can make with her arms, in the center of which is the baby." This period does not last long, but "the mother's bond with the baby is very powerful at the beginning, and we must do all we can to enable her to be preoccupied with her baby at this time—the natural time."

Several studies[25,31] have shown that when the father is more supportive of the mother, she evaluates her maternal skills more positively and is more effective in feeding her baby. But it also might be the case that competent mothers generally elicit more positive evaluation and support from their husbands; therefore it is important to avoid fitting the data to expectations. However, the facts seem to indicate that increased paternal contact and involvement at the time of early infancy can provide important benefits to the newborn, to the mother, and to the father himself.[13,25,35] For this reason it seems particularly important to support and encourage both parents during labor, delivery, and the postpartum period. It also is beneficial to provide for early and extended mother-infant contact, especially for single and teenage parents.

Anisfeld and Lipper[2] have reported that mothers who have poor social supports (i.e., two or more of the following: unmarried, on public assistance, not a high school graduate, no father or other support person in the delivery room) showed greatly reduced affectionate interaction with their infants when they received routine care that separated mother and infant after delivery. On the other hand, mothers from the same background who were given their infants for the first hour showed a high level of affectionate interaction, even higher than mothers who had better social supports. At the 3-month checkup, 69% of the low-social-support mothers who had early contact returned with their infants for the scheduled appointment, in contrast to 26% in the group of women who had received only routine care.

No studies specifically have considered the effects of early or delayed contact between infants and adoptive parents. Most adoptive parents, of course, achieve a satisfactory attachment to their infant, but this may take extra time, effort, patience, and motivation. On the basis of the evidence now available, we believe that parents and adoptive infants should be brought together as soon as possible after birth and that the parents should be encouraged to take over full responsibility for care and planning for the infant, just as other parents do.

In summary, although evidence is increasing that a sensitive period exists that is helpful in parenting, this does not imply that every mother and father develop a close tie to their infant within a few minutes of the first contact.[20] Parents do not react in a standard or predictable way to the complex environmental influences that occur in this brief period. However, rather than considering this as evidence against the concept of a sensitive period, we think that it represents only the multiple individual differences among mothers and fathers.

THE PARENTS OF A SICK, PREMATURE, OR HIGH-RISK INFANT

When talking to the parents of an infant in the neonatal intensive care unit (NICU) or to the mother before her first NICU visit, it is best to describe what the infant looks like and how the infant will appear physically to the mother. Rather than talking about chances of survival, rates, or percentages, we stress that most babies survive despite early and often worrisome problems. There is no need to emphasize problems that may occur in the future; however, we do try to anticipate common developments (e.g., the need for bilirubin reduction lights for jaundice in small premature infants). The following guidelines may be helpful:

1. A mother's room arrangements should be adjusted to her needs—does she or does she not wish to be with other mothers who have healthy, full-term infants?
2. If at all possible, mother and infant should be kept near each other, and the mother should be able to visit whenever she wishes.
3. It is best to talk with the mother and father together, whenever possible. At least once a day discuss with the parents how the infant is doing; talk with them at least

twice a day if the baby is critically ill. It is necessary to find out what the mother believes is going to happen and what she has read about the problem. Any discussion should move at her pace.
4. The physician should not relieve his or her own anxiety by unburdening to the parents; once mentioned, for instance, the thought of death or brain damage can never be erased completely.
5. During the mother's first NICU visit, a chair always should be nearby so that she can sit down. A nurse can stay at her side during most of the visits, describing in detail the procedures being carried out.
6. It is important to remember that feelings of love for the baby often are elicited through eye-to-eye contact. Therefore, if an infant is under bilirubin lights, the lights should be turned off and the eye patches removed so that mother and infant can see each other.
7. It may be possible to enhance normal attachment behavior as late as several days or weeks after birth by permitting a special "nesting" period of 2 or more days and nights of close physical contact, with privacy and virtual isolation during which the mother provides complete care for her small infant, with help and nursing support readily available.[17] Because providing care enhances maternal attachment, it is best to involve the mother in tasks appropriate for the infant's condition as early as possible (e.g., stroking the baby's extremities to reduce apnea and enhance weight gain, changing the diaper, or assisting with nasogastric feedings).

Allowing a mother to hold the infant skin to skin for prolonged periods in the hospital appears to have beneficial effects. It has been shown in several trials that if the usual precautions are taken, such as hand washing, there is no increase in the infection rate or problems in oxygenation, apnea, or temperature control. Although the most significant medical benefit appeared to be increased success of maternal lactation, several studies showed that the mother's own confidence in her caretaking improved along with an eagerness for discharge, and many women reported feeling an increased closeness to the infant compared with a control group of mothers.

Another approach for the mother who is severely distressed emotionally after the birth of a small premature infant is to alter the responses of the developing infant, an area of intense study by Als and associates.[1] In a series of creative studies, they demonstrated that their individualized nursing care plans for high-risk, low-birth-weight infants, which took into account the babies' behavioral and environmental needs, altered the infants' outcome remarkably. The babies' requirements for light, sound, positioning, and nursing care were developed only after a detailed behavioral assessment.

In two randomized trials using the preceding procedure, infants receiving individualized behavioral management required fewer days on a respirator and fewer days on supplemental oxygen; their average daily waking time increased; they were discharged many days earlier; and they also had a lower incidence of intraventricular hemorrhage. In addition, their behavioral development after discharge progressed more normally and their parents more easily developed ways of sensing their needs and responding and interacting with them pleasurably. Parents have an easier time adapting to premature infants who are more responsive.

Minde and colleagues[22] have reported a randomized trial in which parents of premature infants who participated in self-help groups rated themselves as being more competent in infant care measures, as visiting their infants more often, and as more often touching, talking to, and looking at their infants en face. This interest in the infant persisted at home until at least 3 months after discharge.

At the Ramon Sarda Mother and Infant Hospital in Buenos Aires, Argentina,[16] an exemplary program has been developed based on extensive research of premature infants and their parents. The program applies those features that have been shown to enhance the attachment of mothers to sick and premature infants and reduces or removes factors, such as mother-infant separation, that interfere with it. Mothers are invited to stay at the Residence for Mothers when discharged from the obstetrical unit. The poorer mother usually stays until her baby is discharged. Beds and meals are provided. The mothers rest and are well fed, and collectively they make up a community with common concerns—their children's premature birth or illness. There are formal and informal group meetings to develop maternal abilities and to teach mothers how to care for special infants. At the human milk bank, a mother extracts colostrum and breast milk to be given to her infant. The mother has access to the NICU, with no time restrictions. She is involved in the care of her infant, usually from the time of admission. She learns from experience by sharing ideas and by "imitating" within the group of resident mothers.

In contrast to most neonatal intensive care centers, the poor mothers living in the residence usually develop a solid relationship with their infants and the hospital (Fig. 44-16). This is shown by the excellent rate of breast-feeding, continuous attendance at follow-up evaluations, and the disappearance of preventable diseases or problems such as malnutrition and diarrhea, child abuse, neglect, or desertion of children.

Further emphasizing the importance of the home and family in the final result is a very large, randomized, well-carried out trial (985 premature infants) in eight centers in the United States.[9] The study demonstrated that a comprehensive program with weekly home visits in the first year of life, group meetings for mothers during all 3 years, and daily attendance by the child at a developmental center from 1 to 3 years of age resulted in a significant improvement in intelligence quotient (IQ) scores as well as reports by mothers of fewer developmental problems.

It is important to remember that over half the variance in IQ can be accounted for by social conditions such as parental occupation, education, minority status, anxiety, and mental illness. As we improve the social conditions for the entire population, we will significantly improve the outcome for the low-birth-weight infant.

THE PARENTS OF AN INFANT WHO HAS A CONGENITAL ANOMALY

Although previous investigators[4,7,30] agree that the birth of an infant who has a congenital malformation often precipitates major family stress, Solnit and Stark's conceptualiza-

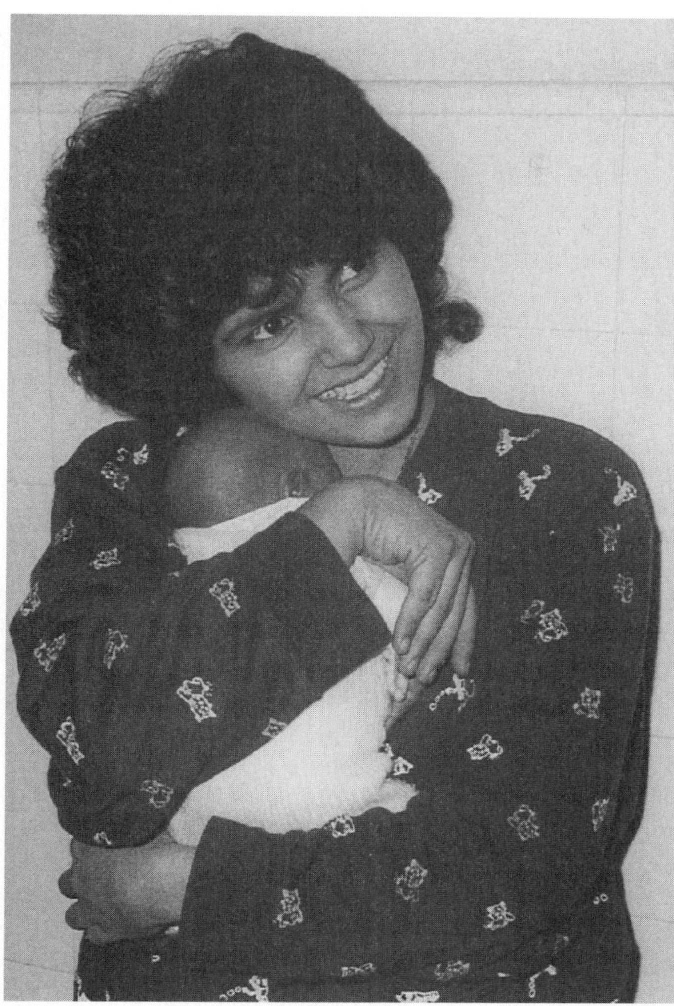

FIG. 44-16 A mother who has lived in the Residence for Mothers and cared for her premature infant from birth.

(From Klaus MH, Kennell JH: *Parent-infant bonding,* ed 2, St Louis, 1982, Mosby.)

tion[27] of parental reactions is most valuable. They note that the malformed infant is a distortion of the ideal infant that was dreamed of and planned for. The parents first must mourn the loss of the normal child they had expected before they can become fully attached to their living, defective infant. This significant aspect of adaptation may take many months. Parental reactions to the birth of a child who has a congenital malformation appear to follow a predictable course (Fig. 44-17). Most parents experience initial shock, disbelief, and a period of intense emotional upset (including sadness, anger, guilt, and anxiety), followed by a period of gradual adaptation that is marked by a lessening of intense anxiety and emotional reaction. This adaptation is characterized by an increased satisfaction with and ability to care for the baby.

These stages in parental reactions are similar to those reported in other crises, such as having a terminally ill child. The intense emotional turmoil described by parents who have produced a child who has a congenital malformation is a period of crisis (defined as "an upset in a state of equilibrium caused by a hazardous event that creates a threat, a loss, or a challenge for the individual"[7]). During such crises, a person is unable, at least temporarily, to respond with his or her usual problem-solving activities.

The sequence of parental reactions to the birth of a baby who has a malformation differs from that following the death of a child in one important respect: the mother must become attached to her living but damaged child. The task of becoming attached to the malformed infant and providing for his or her physical care can be overwhelming to parents at just the time around birth when they are physiologically and psychologically depleted. The mother's initiation of the relationship with her child is a major step in reducing the anxiety and emotional upset associated with the trauma of birth.

1. The parents' mental picture of the anomaly often may be far more severe and distorted than the actual defect. Any delay in seeing and touching the baby greatly heightens this anxiety. Therefore we suggest bringing the baby to both parents when they are together as soon after delivery as possible.
2. Parents should not be given tranquilizers, which tend to blunt responses and slow adaptation to the problem.
3. Parents who become very involved by trying to find out what the best corrective procedures are and who ask many questions about the care of their baby and his or her abnormality often adapt best. It is important to be more concerned about parents who ask few questions and who appear stunned or overwhelmed by the problem.
4. It is best to move at the parents' pace. If the physician moves too quickly, he or she runs the risk of losing the parents along the way. It is beneficial to ask the parents how they view their infant. We try to show parents one problem at a time or to wait until several can be put together logically.
5. Each parent moves through the process of shock, denial, anger, guilt, and adaptation at his or her own pace. If they are unable to talk with one another about the baby, their own relationship may be disrupted. During our discussions with parents we ask the mother how she is doing, how she feels her husband is doing, and how he feels about the infant. We then reverse the questions and ask the father how he is doing and how he thinks his wife is progressing. Thus they start to think not only about each other but also about their own adaptation. Often communication between the parents improves after one or two of these sessions. Some couples who did not seem to be close previously may move closer together over the next weeks and months. As with any painful experience, the parents may emerge much stronger after they have gone through the ordeal together.

STILLBIRTH OR NEONATAL DEATH

When the diagnosis of stillbirth is established in utero, both parents should be fully informed and the events surrounding labor and delivery explained thoroughly. As much as possible, an atmosphere of understanding and mutual support should be established between the bereaved parents and the medical staff.

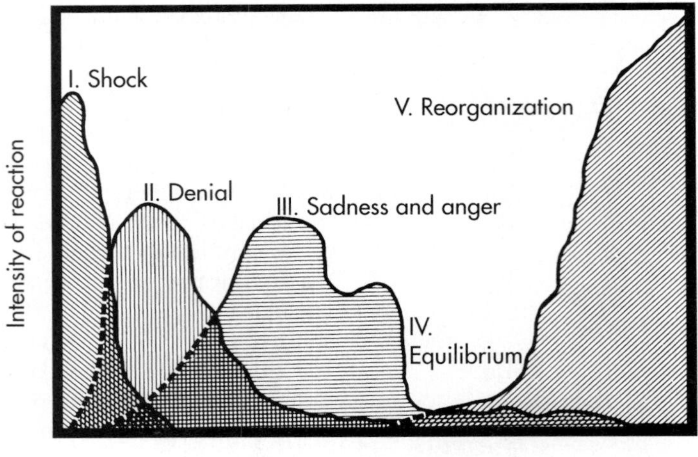

FIG. 44-17 Hypothetical model of the sequence of normal parental reactions to the birth of a child with congenital malformations.
(From Drotar D et al: *Pediatrics* 56:710, 1975.)

Many have emphasized the importance of establishing the stillborn infant's identity. A death without a body that has been seen by a family member seems unreal. Grief after stillbirth is susceptible to distortion because there are no postpartum experiences with the baby to remember, and the infant often is perceived as someone who did not exist, a person without a name. This sense of nonexistence is exaggerated in women who are heavily sedated or anesthetized during delivery and thereby deprived of the memories necessary for normal grief. The infant's identity can best be established if the bereaved parents are encouraged to look at, touch, and hold their child.

The parents sometimes may find the idea of holding a dead baby abhorrent at first, but once the baby is dead, there is no need to rush. We have found that parents frequently change their minds; to facilitate this, we may keep the baby on the delivery floor for a few hours. Parents who have held their stillborn infant or dead neonate report that this was a meaningful experience that they "never would have wanted to miss."

We gradually have come to appreciate that almost no baby is so deformed that the parents will not benefit from viewing the infant—if they so wish. It often is possible to present such babies (e.g., a baby who has anencephaly) to parents, using receiving blankets in such a way as to minimize any shock that might arise on seeing the malformation.

If a mother loses an infant anytime after she has felt movement, she usually goes through a long period of intense mourning. To help with the mourning process after a neonatal death or stillbirth, mothers should be encouraged to see and handle the infant after death, in privacy, if they desire. Some parents choose to hold the dying baby when intensive resuscitation efforts are no longer appropriate. Some mothers have cleaned, diapered, and dressed their dead baby. At first one might think that it only is good to remember the baby as a normal, active infant, but it is important for parents to see the dead infant so that they have clear, visual proof that the baby really died. Also, if the baby had been rushed away right after birth, it is particularly valuable for the mother and father to see that they really did produce a baby that was normal in most respects. Many mothers report having lost a baby in the past and wishing for years that they could have seen, touched, handled, or even just seen a picture of the baby before he or she was taken away. Most have had none of these opportunities. If the mother is still confined in another hospital, there should be no reason that the infant's body cannot be held until the mother is discharged and ready to see the baby and participate in the funeral. The experience of seeing and holding a stillborn infant may temporarily deepen the sadness of both parents, but it provides concrete memories that will facilitate normal mourning. It is highly desirable to obtain a photograph of every stillborn infant or live-born infant who dies, even if the parents do not wish to see it at the time.

Our general plan is to meet with the parents at least three times after a neonatal death or stillbirth. The first time is right after the death. At this moment they are so overwhelmed that they are unable to hear or retain anything other than the event of death. However, we describe the details of the mourning process in simple terms. For example, we explain to the parents that they may have physical symptoms, such as chest pains. Waves of intense sadness may come over them for the first few weeks, but these gradually diminish up to 6 months and stop after 1 year. At times the parents may find themselves angry with each other and their friends and may feel guilty about the death of their infant, believing that actions they could have taken would have saved the infant or prevented the illness in the first place. At times they may imagine that they see their baby alive and hence believe they are going crazy.

We meet with the parents together for a second time (sometimes with their own parents), usually within the first 3 days but at least within the first week. At this meeting it is much easier to review the grieving process. It is helpful for the parents to understand what the usual reactions are so that they will not worry that they are ill. The most important action is to listen and listen again. We stress that the parents meet with us together to maintain rapport and communication. The third meeting with the parents occurs 3 to 6 months after the death. We meet with them to ensure that their grieving is progressing normally and that there is no persistently high level of mourning or other sign of pathological grief. If such symptoms are noted during the interview, the parents should be referred to a psychiatrist.

Our attendance over 2 decades at monthly meetings of parents who have experienced a perinatal loss has shown the great value of parents supporting, understanding, and listening to other parents who have experienced a similar loss. This monthly little window into the lives of bereaved parents has progressively broadened our own view of the "normal" range and duration of mourning reactions. Helping parents through these experiences is, to be sure, taxing and difficult; it is important, however, and this essence of "physicianship" can be quite rewarding.

REFERENCES

Recovery Period

1. Smith CA: The valley of the shadow of birth, *Am J Dis Child* 82:171, 1951.

Establishment of Equilibrium

1. American Academy of Pediatrics, Committee on Fetus and Newborn, Committee on Drugs: Neonatal anesthesia, *Pediatrics* 80:446, 1987.
2. Benini F et al: Topical anesthesia during circumcision in newborn infants, *JAMA* 270:850, 1993.
3. Berde CB: Toxicity of local anesthetics in infants and children, *J Pediatr* 122:S14, 1993.
4. Blass EM, Hoffmeyer LB: Sucrose as an analgesic for newborn infants, *Pediatrics* 87:215, 1991.
5. Gee WF, Ansell JS: Neonatal circumcision: a 10-year overview with comparison of the Gomco clamp and the Plastibell device, *Pediatrics* 58:824, 1976.
6. Kaplan GW: Complications of circumcision, *Urol Clin North Am* 10:543, 1983.
7. Masciello AL: Anesthesia for neonatal circumcision: local anesthesia is better than dorsal penile nerve block, *Obstet Gynecol* 75:834, 1990.
8. Osborn LM, Metcalf TL, Mariani EM: Hygienic care in uncircumcised infants, *Pediatrics* 67:365, 1981.
9. Schoen EJ et al: Report of the Task Force on Circumcision, *Pediatrics* 84:388, 1989.
10. Spence J: Letter of 1950 to a general practitioner, *Lancet* 2:902, 1964.
11. Weatherstone KB et al: Safety and efficacy of a topical anesthetic for neonatal circumcision, *Pediatrics* 92:710, 1993.
12. Winberg J et al: The prepuce: a mistake of Nature? *Lancet* 1:598, 1989.
13. Wiswell TE et al: Declining frequency of circumcision: implications for changes in the absolute incidence and male-to-female sex ratio of urinary tract infections in early infancy, *Pediatrics* 79:338, 1987.
14. Wiswell TE et al: Effect of circumcision status on periurethral bacterial flora during the first year of life, *J Pediatr* 113:442, 1988.

Pediatric Support for Parents

1. Als H et al: Individual behavioral and environmental care of very low-birth-weight infants at risk for bronchopulmonary dysplasia: neonatal intensive care unit and developmental outcome, *Pediatrics* 78:1123, 1986.
2. Anisfeld E, Lipper E: Early contact, social support, and mother-infant bonding, *Pediatrics* 72:79, 1983.
3. Bibring GL: Some considerations of the psychological processes in pregnancy, *Psychoanal Study Child* 14:113, 1959.
4. Daniels LL, Berg GM: The crisis of birth and adaptive patterns of amputee children, *Clin Proc Child Hosp DC* 24:108, 1968.
5. DeCarvalho M, Klaus MH, Merkatz RB: Frequency of breast-feeding and serum bilirubin concentration, *Am J Dis Child* 136:737, 1982.
6. DeCarvalho M et al: Effect of frequent breast-feeding on early milk production and infant weight gain, *Pediatrics* 72:307, 1983.
7. Drotar D et al: The adaptation of parents to the birth of an infant with a congenital malformation: a hypothetical model, *Pediatrics* 56:710, 1975.
8. Engel GH, Reichsman F, Harvey VT: Infant feeding behavior of a mother gastric fistula fed as an infant: a 30-year longitudinal study of enduring effects. In Anthony EJ, Pollock GH, editors: *Parental influences in health and disease,* Boston, 1985, Little, Brown.
9. Gross R et al: Enhancing the outcomes of low-birth-weight premature infants, *JAMA* 263:3035, 1991.
10. Hemminki E et al: A trial on continuous human support during labor: feasibility, interventions, and mothers' satisfaction, *J Psychosom Obstet Gynecol* 11:239, 1990.
11. Hodnett ED, Osborn R: Effect of continuous intrapartum professional support on childbirth outcomes, *Res Nurs Health* 12:289, 1989.
12. Hofmeyer GJ, Nikodem VC, Wolman WL: Companionship to modify the clinical birth environment: effects on progress and perceptions of labour and breast-feeding, *Br J Obstet Gynaecol* 98:756, 1991.
13. Keller WD, Hildebrandt KA, Richards M: Effects of extended father-infant contact during the newborn period, *Infant Behav Dev* 8:337, 1985.
14. Kennell JH, Klaus MH, McGrath S: Continuous emotional support during labor in a U.S. hospital, *JAMA* 265:2197, 1991.
15. Kennell JH et al: Labor support: what's good for mother is good for baby, *Pediatr Res* 25:15, 1989.
16. Kennell JH, Klaus MH: The perinatal paradigm: is it time for a change? *Clin Perinatol* 15:801, 1988.
17. Klaus MH, Kennell JH: Interventions in the premature nursery: impact on development, *Pediatr Clin North Am* 29:1263, 1982.
18. Klaus MH et al: Effects of social support during parturition on maternal and infant morbidity, *Br Med J* 293:585, 1986.
19. Klaus MH, Kennell JH, Klaus PH: *Mothering the mother: how a doula can help you have a shorter, easier, and healthier birth,* Reading, Mass, 1993, Addison-Wesley.
20. Klaus MH, Kennell JH: *Parent-infant bonding,* St Louis, 1982, Mosby.
21. MacFarlane JA, Smith DM, Garrow DH: The relationship between mother and neonate. In Kitzinger S, Davis JA, editors: *The place of birth,* New York, 1978, Oxford University Press.
22. Minde K et al: Self-help groups in a premature nursery: a controlled evaluation, *J Pediatr* 96:933, 1980.
23. O'Connor S et al: Reduced incidence of parenting inadequacy following rooming-in, *Pediatrics* 66:176, 1980.
24. Prechtl H, Beintema D: The neurological examination of the full-term newborn infant. In Lavenham L, editor: *Little club clinics in developmental medicine,* no 12, London, 1964, Heinemann.
25. Rödholm M: Effects of father-infant postpartum contact on their interaction 3 months after birth, *Early Hum Dev* 5:79, 1981.
26. Siegel E et al: Hospital and home support during infancy: impact on maternal attachment, child abuse and neglect, and health care utilization, *Pediatrics* 66:183, 1980.
27. Solnit AJ, Stark MH: Mourning and the birth of a defective child, *Psychoanal Study Child* 16:523, 1961.
28. Sosa R et al: The effect of a supportive companion on perinatal problems, length of labor, and mother-infant interaction, *N Engl J Med* 303:597, 1980.
29. Sosa R et al: The effect of early mother-infant contact on breast-feeding, infection, and growth. In *Breast-feeding and the mother,* Ciba Foundation Symposium 45 (new series), Amsterdam, 1976, Elsevier.
30. Voysey M: Impression management by parents with disabled children, *J Health Soc Behav* 13:80, 1972.
31. Westbrook MT: The reactions to childbearing and early maternal experience of women with differing marital relationships, *Br J Med Psychol* 51:191, 1978.
32. Whitelaw A et al: Skin-to-skin contact for very low-birth-weight infants and their mothers: a randomized trial of "kangaroo care," *Arch Dis Child* 63:1377, 1988.
33. Winnicott DW: *The child, the family, and the outside world,* New York, 1964, Penguin Books.
34. Wolff PH: Observations on newborn infants, *Psychosom Med* 21:110, 1959.
35. Yogman MW: Development of the father-infant relationship. In Fitzger-

ald HE, Lester BM, Yogman MW, editors: *Theory and research in behavioral pediatrics,* vol 1, New York, 1980, Plenum Press.

SUGGESTED READINGS

American Academy of Pediatrics and the American College of Obstetricians and Gynecologists: *Guidelines for perinatal care,* ed 3, Washington, DC, 1992, The Academy.

American Academy of Pediatrics and American Heart Association: *Textbook of neonatal resuscitation,* ed 2, Dallas, 1994 American Heart Association.

Avery GB, editor: *Neonatology: pathophysiology and management of the newborn,* ed 4, Philadelphia, 1994, JB Lippincott.

Fanaroff AA, Martin RJ, editors: *Neonatal-perinatal medicine,* ed 5, St Louis, 1992, Mosby.

Jones KL: *Smith's recognizable patterns of human malformation,* ed 4, Philadelphia, 1988, WB Saunders.

Klaus MH, Fanaroff AA, editors: *Care of the high-risk neonate,* ed 4, Philadelphia, 1993, WB Saunders.

Polin RA, Fox WW, editors: *Fetal and neonatal physiology,* Philadelphia, 1992, WB Saunders.

Seidel HM, Rosenstein BJ, Pathak A: *Primary care of the newborn,* St Louis, 1993, Mosby.

Volpe JJ: *Neurology of the newborn,* ed 3, Philadelphia, 1995, WB Saunders.

45 Skin Lesions of the Neonate

Marvin E. Miller

Birthmarks are common, and many newborn babies exhibit some type of skin lesion that may arouse parental concern. Fortunately, the overwhelming majority of these skin lesions are benign. It is important for the practicing physician who evaluates newborns to be familiar with these benign birthmarks and also to recognize the much less common birthmarks that may indicate a significant underlying condition. Listed in Table 45-1 are the birthmarks discussed in this chapter and their approximate frequency in newborns.

SKIN LESIONS

Transient Lesions

Several common, transient skin abnormalities occur in the newborn.[3,6,8] Because they are self-limited, no medical treatment is indicated.

Milia. Milia are multiple, small (1 to 2 mm) pearly white papules found on the forehead, cheeks, and nose. When found on the oral mucosa, they are called Epstein pearls. Milia are found in about 50% of newborns and represent cystic inclusions of keratin and sebaceous material in the pilosebaceous apparatus. They disappear spontaneously during the first month of life and require no treatment.

Miliaria. Miliaria, or neonatal "prickly heat," are clear, thin-walled vesicles, 1 to 2 mm in diameter, that are filled with fluid. They are very fragile and rupture when light pressure is applied. Miliaria result from eccrine duct occlusion and sweat retention. These lesions occur when an infant is placed in a warm and humid environment, and they disappear when a dry and cooler environment is provided or when the infant is dressed in lighter clothing. Topical medications should not be used because they often exacerbate these lesions.

Erythema Toxicum. Erythema toxicum consists of yellow-white papulopustules surrounded by erythema. Erythema toxicum is seen in 50% of full-term newborns but only rarely in premature babies. The lesions can be seen on any part of the body except the palms and soles. They usually appear at 1 to 2 days of age and rarely are present at birth or after 5 days. The lesions persist for several hours to as long as a few days. Smears of the papular contents show numerous eosinophils but no organisms. The cause of erythema toxicum is unknown. These babies are well while they have the lesions, and no treatment is necessary.

Transient Neonatal Pustular Melanosis. The lesions of transient neonatal pustular melanosis are present at birth and consist of superficial vesiculopustules that are easily ruptured to leave a collarette of white scales around a central pinhead-sized macule of hyperpigmentation. This hyperpigmentation remains for several weeks to several months. The clusters of lesions most often are seen on the forehead, under the chin, on the back of the neck, on the lower back, and on the shins.

The pustules last from 1 to 2 days, but cultures of the lesions are sterile, and smears of the pustules show cellular debris with variable numbers of neutrophils. Small numbers of eosinophils sometimes are present but never in such abundance as in erythema toxicum. Babies who have transient neonatal pustular melanosis are healthy, and no treatment is needed. This condition is less common than the other transient lesions and is found in 4% of African-American newborns and 0.3% of Caucasian newborns.

Nevi

Nevi constitute a group of common birthmarks that result from the local proliferation of any of the following three major cell types that make up the skin[1,3-5,8]:

1. *Cells that line the vascular channels* of either capillaries (hemangiomas) or lymph vessels (lymphangiomas)
2. *Cells that produce pigment* (pigmented nevi)
3. *Cells from the epidermis* (epidermal nevi), including those that make keratin or those that compose the epidermal appendages

Vascular Nevi

Salmon Patch (Nevus Simplex, Telangiectatic Nevus). The salmon patch is the most common vascular lesion of infancy and is found in about 40% of all newborns. This lesion is flat and light pink, with poorly defined borders; it commonly is seen on the nape of the neck, glabella, forehead, upper eyelids, or the nasolabial region. The salmon patch is not a true nevus because there is not an actual proliferation of vascular elements, which is seen in the flat hemangiomas. Histopathological examination of the salmon patch reveals *distended dermal capillaries,* representing a persistent, localized fetal capillary bed that usually matures into the normal vasculature.

Within the first year of life, 95% of salmon patches fade, although portions can persist, particularly those found on the nape of the neck. Salmon patches are not associated with any malformation syndromes. No treatment is necessary, and parents can be reassured that the salmon patch is a benign lesion that almost always will fade and disappear.

Flat Hemangiomas (Nevus Flammeus). The flat hemangioma, or *port wine stain,* is similar in appearance to the salmon patch but is darker and has a deep red or purplish red hue. Port wine stains usually involve the face or the extremities and usually, but not always, are unilateral. These stains commonly are present at birth and grow in proportion to the child's growth. Microscopic examination shows proliferation of dilated dermal capillaries. Flat hemangiomas usually do not fade completely or involute. Various treatments such as cryosurgery and Ganz rays have not been very successful. In cosmetically sensitive areas a tinted, opaque, waterproof cream (such as Covermark) helps mask the hemangiomas.

Table 45-1 Birthmarks and Their Frequency[1,6,8]

Birthmark	Frequency
Transient lesions	
Milia	50%
Miliaria	Common
Erythema toxicum	50%
Transient neonatal pustular melanosis	Uncommon
Nevi	
Vascular nevi	
Salmon patch	40%
Flat hemangiomas	0.3%
Raised hemangiomas	3%
Hemangiomas associated with malformation syndromes	Rare
Lymphangiomas	Uncommon
Hyperpigmented lesions	
Café-au-lait spots	Common*
Pigmented nevi	Common*
Mongolian spots	Common*
Hypopigmented lesions	Uncommon
Epidermal nevi	Uncommon
Miscellaneous	
Cutis marmorata	Common
Birthmarks from delivery trauma	Common
Cutis aplasia	Rare
Purpura	Rare

*There is a significant difference in the frequency of hyperpigmented lesions between African-American and Caucasian newborns: the frequency of café-au-lait spots, 12% versus 0.3%; pigmented nevi, 20% versus 2%; and Mongolian spots, 90% versus 10%, respectively.

Raised Hemangiomas. The raised hemangiomas, also called *strawberry hemangiomas,* can be divided histologically into capillary hemangiomas and cavernous hemangiomas, although the distinction has no important clinical relevance. The cavernous hemangioma consists of larger capillaries that empty into sinusoidal blood spaces; the capillary hemangiomas merely show capillary proliferation. Strawberry hemangiomas may be present at birth but more commonly become apparent within the first weeks of life; 90% are noted by 1 month of age. They usually begin as a circumscribed area of grayish white discoloration, then grow rapidly and develop into red, raised, well-defined lesions that are lobulated and compressible, although they usually do not blanch. Strawberry hemangiomas can occur on any part of the body; about 38% occur on the head and neck and 29% on the trunk (80% of affected individuals have an isolated lesion; 20% have more than one).

Strawberry hemangiomas grow rapidly during the first 6 months of life and then begin to involute by 15 months of age. Most strawberry hemangiomas grow to 3 to 4 cm in diameter, with some as small as a few millimeters and others as large as 20 cm. At least 90% of strawberry hemangiomas resolve by 9 years of age without treatment. Although various modes of treatment have been used to remove strawberry hemangiomas, the rational approach is to let these lesions regress on their own because the cosmetic appearance is much better than those treated by surgery or radiotherapy. Parents should be reassured that time is the best treatment for the majority of these lesions.

Life-threatening hemangiomas that impinge on vital structures such as the esophagus or trachea are rare but require aggressive therapy to reduce the size of the tumor and to relieve the compromise of the vital structure. Until recently, corticosteroid therapy was the only medical approach to reduce the size of large hemangiomas.[7,8] Laser therapy and interferon alfa-2a are two promising new therapeutic modalities in the treatment of life-threatening hemangiomas. Laser therapy also is being used to treat flat and raised hemangiomas of the skin for cosmetic reasons.[2]

There are several malformation syndromes in which flat or raised hemangiomas are seen; the features of these syndromes are listed in Table 45-2. The vast majority of hemangiomas are not associated with any other malformations.

Lymphangiomas. Lymphangiomas are much less common than hemangiomas; sometimes elements of both are found in one lesion. Lymphangiomas usually manifest as (1) a cluster of circumscribed gelatinous papules 2 to 4 mm in diameter, containing clear lymph fluid (lymphangioma circumscription), (2) a larger cavernous nodule (cavernous lymphangioma), or (3) a large mass (cystic hygroma). There is no satisfactory treatment. Surgical removal can be attempted, but recurrences are common.

Hyperpigmented Nevi. Several common hyperpigmented lesions manifest at or shortly after birth. As shown in Table 45-1 and demonstrated in the discussions that follow, African-American newborns have a greater frequency of each of the three common hyperpigmented lesions than do Caucasian newborns.

Café-au-Lait Spots. Café-au-lait spots are flat, sharply bordered, uniformly light brown pigmented lesions of varying shape and usually are less than several centimeters in their greatest dimension at birth. An isolated café-au-lait spot has no medical implications. However, the presence of multiple café-au-lait spots that have smooth (rather than ragged) borders is diagnostic of *neurofibromatosis,* and such individuals are susceptible to the complications of this genetic condition. A striking difference has been noted in the frequency of café-au-lait spots in Caucasian versus African-American newborns. Only 0.3% of the former will have one café-au-lait spot, as opposed to 12% of the latter; 1.8% of African-American newborns will have three or more café-au-lait spots without evidence of neurofibromatosis during follow-up care or by family history. Thus the finding of several café-au-lait spots in an African-American newborn is not, in itself, indicative of neurofibromatosis.

Café-au-lait spots are not always present at birth and may appear during infancy. Histologically, café-au-lait spots result from increased melanogenesis in a group of melanocytes and thus are not true nevi. In adults, more than six café-au-lait spots greater than 1.5 cm in diameter are diagnostic of neurofibromatosis. In children who have neurofibromatosis, however, the café-au-lait spots may be fewer in number and smaller in size because the spots increase in number and size over time. Thus among children under 5 years of age, the finding of five café-au-lait spots greater than 0.5 cm in diameter is strongly suggestive of neurofibromatosis. Café-au-lait spots also can be seen in *McCune-Albright syndrome* (polyostotic fibrous dysplasia and pubertal precocity), but the

Table 45-2 Malformation Syndromes Associated with Congenital Hemangiomas[3,4]

Condition	Nature of hemangioma	Other features
Sturge-Weber syndrome	Large, flat hemangioma over face; usually involves ophthalmic branch of trigeminal nerve; usually unilateral	Seizures Glaucoma Mental deficiency
Kasabach-Merritt syndrome	Usually large cavernous hemangiomas, although small ones have been reported	Thrombocytopenia from platelet sequestration
Klippel-Trenaunay-Weber syndrome	Large, flat hemangioma on an extremity	Hemangioma overlies area of soft tissue and bone overgrowth Macrocephaly
Diffuse neonatal hemangiomatosis	Multiple hemangiomas that can involve skin and internal organs	High-output cardiac failure; poor prognosis

café-au-lait spots in this condition are larger and have irregular borders.

Pigmented Nevi (Pigmented Moles, Melanocytic Nevi, Neurocellular Nevi). Pigmented nevi are very common in adults (most adults have an average of 30 lesions), and many people call them birthmarks because they believe they were born with them. However, this usually is not the case because almost all pigmented nevi are acquired and do not appear until later in infancy; some do not appear until adolescence. Only 2% of Caucasian newborns and 20% of African-American newborns are born with pigmented nevi. These congenital, pigmented moles are flat, dark brown or black, irregularly pigmented, and sharply demarcated. They tend to be larger than the acquired moles, and the major concern about congenital pigmented moles is their potential for malignant transformation, which is significantly greater than that of acquired moles. There are no firm guidelines as to when a congenital pigmented mole should be removed, although the large congenital pigmented moles ("bathing trunk nevus" or "garment nevus") usually are removed surgically.

Mongolian Spots. Mongolian spots are large, flat, diffuse, and poorly circumscribed areas of hyperpigmentation that are blue, black, or slate-colored and are located over the buttocks or lumbosacrum. Once again, there is a striking ethnic difference in the frequency of this hyperpigmented lesion. Although it is noted in over 80% of Oriental, Native American, and African-American newborns, it is seen in fewer than 10% of Caucasian newborns. The natural history of Mongolian spots is benign, with most disappearing by late childhood. They result from pigment-producing cells in the dermis. When a similar-appearing lesion is seen in the periorbital region, it is called an *Ota nevus;* when seen on one side of the neck and shoulder, it is referred to as an *Ito nevus.*

Hypopigmented Lesions. Hypopigmented lesions are uncommon in newborns; their presence may be the first sign of a more serious condition. There are two important neurocutaneous conditions (phacomatoses) in which hypopigmented areas that appear at birth or in early infancy usually are found—tuberous sclerosis and hypomelanosis of Ito. It is important for the physician to recognize these conditions because of the likelihood of some neurological dysfunction.

Almost 90% of individuals who have *tuberous sclerosis* will have multiple white macules present at birth or in early infancy. These white macules usually are 1 to 3 cm in diameter and have irregular leaf-shaped margins. They almost always are the first manifestation of tuberous sclerosis, other features of which include developmental delay, seizures, cutaneous angiofibromas, and intracranial calcifications.

Hypomelanosis of Ito (incontinentia pigmenti achromiens) is a recently described and poorly understood condition in which irregular swirls and whorls of hypopigmentation appear at birth or in infancy. Like tuberous sclerosis, the association with neurological abnormalities such as developmental delay and seizures is high. In addition, ocular and musculoskeletal abnormalities can be seen.

Epidermal Nevi. Epidermal nevi are skin lesions appearing at birth or in the first few weeks of life. They are composed of aggregates of epithelial cells (keratinocytes) or cells of any of the epidermal appendages (apocrine, eccrine, sebaceous gland, or hair follicle). Although lesions of mixed histology are common, there usually is one predominant cellular element.

The verrucose nevus represents a proliferation of the epidermal cells and their product, keratin. These lesions are raised, yellow-brown, velvety or rough and warty, and often pigmented. They usually are found as a cluster of lesions and frequently are arranged linearly when on the limbs. Surgical excision is indicated for cosmetic reasons, and the tendency for malignant degeneration is small.

Sebaceous nevi are elevated, granular, waxy, orange plaques found on the face and scalp. Surgical excision is the treatment of choice because these nevi can develop into basal cell carcinomas during adulthood.

Miscellaneous Lesions

The physician should be familiar with several other congenital skin abnormalities.[3,8]

Cutis Marmorata. Cutis marmorata is a reticulated bluish mottling of the skin, which is the normal newborn response to chilling. When the infant is warmed, the cutis marmorata disappears. The tendency may persist for several months, and usually there is no medical significance. However, cutis marmorata may be a persistent feature in the dysmorphic conditions of de Lange syndrome, congenital hypothyroidism, or in Klippel-Trenaunay-Weber syndrome.

Birthmarks from Delivery Trauma. Birthmarks from the mechanical trauma of forceps or suction are common. Ecchymoses of the face where forceps have been placed often are distressing to parents. The marks themselves will disappear, but when they are present, the physician should be certain that no neurological deficit in ocular or facial muscle function is present. Suction marks on the vertex of the scalp almost always are seen when suction is used to augment delivery. These are benign and indicate no underlying brain lesions. The parents should be reassured that they will disappear.

Cutis Aplasia. Cutis aplasia is a congenital absence of skin that occurs most commonly on the vertex of the scalp. The lesion appears as a punched-out ulcer that may be "weeping" or covered by a thin membrane. Management is directed at prevention of infection until healing is complete. Cutis aplasia can be seen in any one of several settings. First, it can be transmitted as an autosomal dominant condition with variable expression; thus a family history is important. Second, it can be an isolated lesion that has an unremarkable family history. Third, it can be seen in association with other birth defects such as brain malformation, limb anomalies, and gastrointestinal defects; in this group, a vascular origin is likely. Scalp defects also can be seen in infants who have trisomy 13.

Purpura. Purpura are flat bluish purple lesions of variable size that represent subcutaneous bleeding and can be present at birth. If they are very small, they are called petechiae; if large areas are involved, they are called ecchymoses. The differential diagnosis of neonatal purpura includes congenital infection, coagulation defects, autoimmune disorders, and hemangioma with platelet trapping.

REFERENCES

1. Alper J, Holmes LB, Mihm MC Jr: Birthmarks with serious medical significance: nevocellular nevi, sebaceous nevi, and multiple café-au-lait spots, *J Pediatr* 95:696, 1979.
2. Ezekowitz RA, Mulliken JB, Folkman J: Interferon alfa-2a therapy for life-threatening hemangiomas of infancy, *N Engl J Med* 326:1456, 1992.
3. Hurwitz S: *Clinical pediatric dermatology,* Philadelphia, 1981, WB Saunders.
4. Jacobs AH: Birthmarks. I. Vascular nevi, *Pediatr Rev* 1:21, 1979.
5. Jacobs AH: Birthmarks. II. Melanocytic and epidermal nevi, *Pediatr Rev* 1:47, 1979.
6. Jacobs AH, Walton RG: The incidence of birthmarks in the neonate, *Pediatrics* 58:218, 1976.
7. Tan OT, Gilchrest BA: Laser therapy for selected cutaneous vascular lesions in the pediatric population: a review, *Pediatrics* 82:652, 1988.
8. Weinberg S, Hoekelman RA: *Pediatric dermatology for the primary care practitioner,* New York, 1978, McGraw-Hill.

46 Signs and Symptoms of Neonatal Illness

Kristi Watterberg and Keith J. Gallaher

The term *clinical signs* refers to objective evidence of disease, whereas the term *symptoms* refers primarily to subjective descriptions. The newborn and infant, although unable to verbalize complaints, are able to relay information in ways that are equally informative to the astute clinician. The recognition of neonatal illness therefore relies primarily on the correct interpretation of objective findings. The clinical assessment of newborn infants emphasizes the basic skills of assessment. Much of the information relevant to evaluating the health of a newborn or infant can be obtained simply by looking, without palpation or auscultation. The determination of vital signs and growth measurements provides further clues to health status. Although it is not possible to get a history directly from the newborn infant, one must not underestimate the diagnostic value (and courtesy) of speaking with the parents and reviewing the maternal chart.

In this chapter, signs commonly noted in full-term newborns are described and correlated with more specific clinical diagnoses. In most cases, more information related to specific diagnoses can be found in subsequent chapters. The material is organized in the fashion by which most newborns and infants actually are monitored in the normal newborn nursery.

VITAL SIGNS

Heart Rate

Abnormalities of the heart rate (HR) or rhythm are quite common in the newborn period and, if isolated, usually are benign. In some instances these abnormalities first may be noted prenatally or during labor and delivery. During the first few days of life, the normal heart rate is from 120 to 160 beats per minute. Abnormalities of heart rate fall into two main groups: tachycardia (HR over 180 beats per minute) or bradycardia (HR under 80 beats per minute). The initial evaluation of heart rate or rhythm abnormalities includes a 12-lead electrocardiogram and "rhythm strip."

Tachycardia

Sinus Tachycardia. The differential diagnosis of a narrow QRS complex tachycardia is between sinus tachycardia and paroxysmal supraventricular tachycardia (SVT). Sinus tachycardia usually can be differentiated from SVT on the following basis: (1) the heart rate usually is less than 200 beats per minute; (2) the beat-to-beat interval varies; and (3) vagal stimulation slows the heart rate gradually. Sinus tachycardia is a common manifestation of a wide variety of both physiological and pathological factors. It may be caused by an elevated temperature, an early warning of infection, or inappropriate environmental heat regulation. It also may be a sign of the newborn's attempt to increase cardiac output in response to situations such as severe anemia, congestive heart failure, or shock.

Supraventricular Tachycardia (SVT). SVT usually is associated with a more rapid heart rate (220 to 320 beats per minute) than is seen with sinus tachycardia. P waves may or may not be visible, preceding the narrow QRS complexes. Newborns can tolerate this rate for variable periods of time but often have associated irritability, poor feeding, tachypnea, and poor perfusion. Although SVT is associated with structural anomalies less than 20% of the time, newborns who have SVT need an echocardiographic assessment of this possibility. Other causes include underlying abnormalities of the conducting system, such as Wolff-Parkinson-White syndrome (WPW), and conditions that increase myocardial irritability, such as infectious or metabolic cardiomyopathies.

Ventricular Tachycardia. Ventricular tachycardia is an unusual problem in the newborn period. When seen, it usually is associated with severe underlying electrolyte disturbances or structural heart disease. The ECG usually shows wide QRS complexes. By definition, it is abnormal and potentially life threatening.

Bradycardia

Sinus Bradycardia. Sinus bradycardia is the most common form of slow heart rate seen in the neonatal period. The heart rate usually is less than 80 beats per minute, with a well-formed P wave preceding each QRS complex. The episodes usually are transient and associated with feeding or sleeping. The heart rate speeds up readily with stimulation. Persistent bradycardia not responding to stimulation should be evaluated further. Abnormalities occasionally associated with persistent sinus bradycardia include increased intracranial pressure, hypoxemia, and hypothyroidism.

Congenital Heart Block. Congenital heart block, on the other hand, is diagnosed on ECG by varying degrees of incoordination between atrial and ventricular depolarizations. The most serious form of congenital heart block is third-degree block (complete atrioventricular [A-V] dissociation). Approximately 30% of infants who have a complete A-V dissociation will have underlying structural heart disease (e.g., atrial septal defect, corrected transposition). It frequently is caused by connective tissue disorders in the mother and may be the first manifestation of the maternal disease. The heart rate usually is in the range of 50 to 80 beats per minute, and the newborn frequently is asymptomatic, whereas symptomatic newborns usually have rates of <50 beats per minute.

Irregular Heart Rate

The most common cause of irregular heart rate in the newborn is an extrasystolic arrhythmia, such as premature atrial or ventricular contractions. Both should be considered benign in the absence of underlying heart disease and if they disappear with increasing sinus heart rate (i.e., upon stimulation of the newborn). They usually disappear within a few days or weeks. Newborns who have very frequent extra beats or extra beats associated with cardiopulmonary symptoms deserve further evaluation to rule out electrolyte abnormalities or cardiomyopathies.

Blood Pressure

It is unusual to have blood pressure (BP) abnormalities as isolated findings in neonatal illness. Low blood pressure (systolic pressure less than 60 mm Hg for a full-term infant) most often is associated with tachycardia and signs of poor cardiac output. Hypertension (systolic BP greater than 90 mm Hg; diastolic BP greater than 60 mm Hg) also is unusual in the otherwise healthy newborn infant. Coarctation of the aorta often is diagnosed by the combination of increased blood pressure in the upper extremities with low blood pressure and/or poor pulses in the lower extremities. Renovascular occlusion also may manifest initially as persistently elevated blood pressure—this especially should be considered if the newborn or older infant has had umbilical artery catheterization. Determination of serum electrolytes, as well as evaluation of renal structure and perfusion, often is helpful in evaluating the infant whose blood pressure is persistently elevated.

Temperature

Meticulous attention to the thermal status of the newborn is a hallmark of good newborn care. The increased relative surface area characteristic of newborns makes them extremely sensitive to environmental conditions, especially immediately after delivery when they are wet. The infant should be dried carefully and placed in a heat-gaining environment until stabilized and should not be bathed until thermal stability is assured. Term infants should be dressed and blanketed and the room temperature maintained at 24° C to 26.5° C in the normal newborn nursery.

In the sick infant, fluctuations in body temperature (T) are more common than is stable pyrexia; therefore, persistent hyperthermia >37.5° C axillary usually is a manifestation of poor environmental heat control. One clue to whether a fever is disease-related is the core temperature (rectal)-to-leg temperature (midthigh) gradient. A rectal temperature more than 1° to 2° C greater than midthigh temperature suggests a disease-related fever.

Hypothermia is a prominent finding in neonatal illness, especially sepsis. Hypothermia caused by the environment increases the metabolic demands on the newborn and can have disastrous consequences, including metabolic acidosis, pulmonary hypertension, and hypoxemia.

Respiration

Given the dramatic physiological changes associated with transition from the aqueous fetal environs to the air-breathing newborn state, it is not surprising that respiratory compromise is common in the newborn period. Both abnormalities in respiratory rate and the quality of respiratory effort often are associated with neonatal illness. The normal respiratory rate of the term newborn is 30 to 60 breaths per minute.

Tachypnea

Infants commonly attempt to increase their minute ventilation through increases in respiratory rate. Tachypnea is defined as a respiratory rate of more than 60 breaths per minute. A primary pulmonary cause of tachypnea is suggested by the presence of other signs of respiratory distress, including expiratory grunting, nasal flaring, inspiratory crackles, or rales. Evaluation of neonatal respiratory distress includes chest roentgenography, which should be considered part of the physical examination of the sick newborn. This study can eliminate from consideration congenital malformation, such as diaphragmatic hernia or cystic adenomatoid malformation, as being the underlying cause. The diagnosis of tracheoesophageal fistula (with a proximal esophageal pouch and a distal fistula) should be suspected when copious oral secretions and tachypnea are associated with the presence of a nasogastric tube coiled in the proximal esophagus.

Transient Tachypnea. Transient tachypnea of the newborn (TTN) is the most common cause of neonatal tachypnea in the term infant and probably represents delayed clearing of the normal fetal lung fluid. TTN is especially common following cesarean section delivery without labor. The onset is at birth; typically gradual improvement is noted with resolution generally occurring by 3 to 5 days of age. Because TTN can be difficult to distinguish from other entities, such as pneumonia or aspiration, the clinician must maintain a high index of suspicion for these possibilities.

Pneumonia. The most worrisome cause of tachypnea is infection, and concerns over this possibility largely have dictated our approach to all newborns who evidence respiratory compromise. Congenital pneumonia is an ominous cause of respiratory distress in the infant, and group B beta-hemolytic streptococcus probably is the best-known pathogen. Often the clues to the diagnosis are subtle, and death can result even if the pathogen is treated promptly.

Aspiration Syndrome. Aspiration syndromes also are relatively common. This category includes both blood and amniotic fluid aspirations. Newborns who have aspiration pneumonitis typically have a barrel-shaped, hyperexpanded chest and rapid, shallow respirations. If the aspirated amniotic fluid is meconium stained, clinical management may become especially difficult. In addition, pulmonary "air leaks," such as pneumothorax or pneumomediastinun, often accompany aspiration pneumonitis. In the case of suspected meconium aspiration, attention also should focus on determining why the infant passed meconium in the first place (e.g., resulting from asphyxia or sepsis). Often the answer to this question has a greater bearing on the baby's long-term outcome than does the aspiration itself.

Spontaneous Pneumothorax. Spontaneous pneumothoraces are relatively common occurrences in otherwise healthy infants and also may manifest initially as tachypnea. Usually, auscultation of the lungs helps in the clinical diagnosis because decreased breath sounds over the involved lung may be noted. In addition, the chest often is hyperresonant to percussion on the side of the air leak. The diagnosis is confirmed by transillumination and chest roentgenogram. Treatment is dictated by the degree of cardiopulmonary compromise.

Metabolic Acidosis. Metabolic acidosis may elicit an increase in respiratory rate as the baby attempts to provide respiratory compensation. An arterial blood gas analysis will assist in the recognition of this possibility. The differential diagnosis of metabolic acidosis is extensive and can be divided broadly into two groups: bicarbonate wasting (most commonly in the urine) or acid gain. Lactic acidosis signifies either tissue hypoxia (most commonly) or an inborn error of metabolism. Other circulating acids (e.g., pyruvic or methylmalonic acid) may cause a metabolic acidosis as a sign of an inborn error of metabolism.

Irregular Respiration

Apnea. In contrast to breathing too rapidly, some ill infants may breath too slowly or not at all. Apnea is defined as the cessation of air flow and may result from decreased respiratory drive, airway obstruction, or a combination of the two (mixed apnea). Symptomatic (prolonged) apnea is defined as apnea lasting for 20 seconds or longer or as shorter periods of apnea associated with cyanosis, marked pallor, hypotonia, or bradycardia. A wide variety of disorders display the common sign of apnea, so this sign deserves a meticulous search for cause. Symptomatic apnea never is a normal finding in the term or near-term (over 35 weeks' gestation) infant. Perhaps the most ominous cause is *infection;* however, any metabolic disturbance or airway anomaly may result in apnea. Certain drugs administered to the mother, especially narcotics and magnesium sulfate, also may depress the newborn's respiratory drive. Although specific antidotes may be available in certain instances (e.g., naloxone for narcotic depression), the first treatment is to ensure adequate ventilation.

Periodic Breathing. Periodic breathing is a breathing pattern in which three or more respiratory pauses lasting longer than 3 seconds are separated by less than 20 seconds of respiration. Most commonly, periodic breathing is a normal event, especially in infants born prematurely. However, it also may be a manifestation of instability of the brainstem respiratory control center, a condition induced by disease.

GROWTH

Body Weight

One of the first questions asked by new parents is, "How much does my baby weigh?" The answer to this question may give the clinician valuable clues to the health of the infant. Abnormalities in growth may reflect effects of fetal nutrition, environmental toxins, systemic infections, chromosomal or syndromic influences, or family heritage. The adequacy of growth usually is assessed by comparing a newborn's measurements with normal values obtained from published standards. This involves accurate determination of gestational age so that the appropriate standards can be used. *The gold standard for determination of gestational age is good obstetrical dating;* physical examination of the newborn may confirm the age.

Macrosomia. The term *macrosomia* refers to newborns whose weight places them above the 90th percentile, compared with other newborns of similar gestational age (large for gestational age, or LGA). Newborns born to mothers who have either preexisting or gestational diabetes often are macrosomic. This is believed to represent the effects of increased fetal insulin levels, which result from exposure to a chronically elevated blood glucose level. Acute complications may include hypoglycemia, hyperbilirubinemia, hypocalcemia, and polycythemia. Preexisting maternal diabetes, but not gestational diabetes, also is associated with an increased incidence of congenital anomalies. Macrosomia may result from intrinsic hyperinsulinemia, resulting from unusual disorders characterized by early onset of hypoglycemia and elevated glucose requirements. The best-known of these uncommon problems is Beckwith-Wiedemann syndrome. Infants who have this syndrome also have macroglossia and may have omphalocele. Macrosomic newborns may be difficult to deliver and thus predisposed to birth trauma.

Microsomia. Microsomia (small for gestational age, or SGA), on the other hand, most often is defined as a birth weight below the 10th percentile compared with other newborns of the same gestation. Other growth measurements, such as length or head circumference, may or may not be similarly affected. Asymmetrical growth retardation (underweight for length and head circumference) often suggests a problem extrinsic to the baby, such as decreased uteroplacental blood flow, whereas symmetrical growth retardation suggests either a long-standing cause or a problem intrinsic to the infant, such as a congenital viral infection or a chromosomal abnormality. Of note is that certain ethnic groups (e.g., East Asian) have newborns who "plot" as being small compared with normal American standards but are appropriate relative to other infants of their heritage. Microsomic infants may have hypoglycemia because glycogen and fat stores often are very minimal. Therefore close attention must be directed to maintaining adequate blood glucose levels.

Head Growth

Macrocephaly. Newborns whose head circumference exceeds 2 standard deviations above the mean, or the 97th percentile, are said to be macrocephalic. It is critical to search for evidence of neurological impairment. Macrocephaly may be caused by volume increases in any of the normal components of the cranial vault—namely brain, blood, or cerebrospinal fluid. Increases in the cerebrospinal fluid compartment, either intraventricular or external to the ventricles around the surfaces of the brain, are referred to as hydrocephalus. This finding often is associated with a rapid rate of increase in the head circumference. The shape of the cranium may give clues as to whether fluid collections are intraventricular (frontal bossing) or external to the brain (biparietal enlargement). Hydrocephalus may or may not be a progressive finding and is relatively easily diagnosed by cranial ultrasonography or computed tomography.

Increases in brain volume also may be noted. This may represent either a normal brain (as in benign familial megalencephaly), accumulation of abnormal metabolic products (e.g., lipidoses, mucopolysaccharidoses), a generalized growth disorder (e.g., achondroplasia), or, in rare cases, tumors.

Blood collections either in or around the brain may result in macrocephaly. Auscultation of the head may reveal a bruit, which is a sign of an arteriovenous malformation. Intracranial hemorrhage is an unusual primary cause of increased head size, but frequently leads to hydrocephalus.

Microcephaly. Microcephaly refers to a head circumference less than the 3rd percentile. It is an ominous finding and often indicates a severe underlying abnormality of brain growth or development or both, caused either by primary brain dysgenesis or by secondary insults such as teratogens, an infection, or hypoxic-ischemic encephalopathy.

Body Length

Abnormally short or long newborns usually fit into the classification of the connective tissue or skeletal disorders. Unfortunately, body length is one of the most notoriously inaccurate measurements made in the nursery. If a newborn's length seems inappropriate, further measurements, such as long bone or upper-to-lower segment ratios, may be beneficial, along with a skeletal survey.

TONE, POSTURE, AND ACTIVITY

The normal term infant assumes a flexed posture of all limbs and, when awake, is active on gentle stimulation. Limbs often move in an alternating fashion. When pulled to sit, the head should be righted, then held in the same plane as the rest of the body for several seconds. Muscle tone is evaluated best by passive limb manipulation.

Hypertonia

Hypertonia can be a prominent manifestation of hypoxic-ischemic brain injury, meningitis, or intracranial hemorrhage. Arching of the back (opisthotonos) is a manifestation of extensor hypertonia.

Hypotonia

Hypotonia perhaps is the most common motor abnormality noted in the neonatal period. Any acutely ill infant may demonstrate some degree of mild hypotonia. Most often hypotonia is associated with at least some degree of weakness, although significant disproportion may be noted. The hypotonic newborn often assumes a "spread-eagle" posture, with little to no resting limb flexion. Certain patterns of tone and weakness are associated with specific disorders.

Increased Activity

Increased activity clearly is a subjective finding, based to a great extent on the past clinical experiences of the observer. Unfortunately, an important diagnostic consideration in our society is neonatal abstinence syndrome (drug withdrawal). The importance of recognizing this syndrome cannot be overemphasized. If drug withdrawal is suspected, the newborn's behavior can be monitored with a neonatal abstinence scoring system (see Coen and Koffler, Suggested Readings). The syndrome usually is diagnosed by the demonstration of illicit drugs in the newborn's urine or stool.

Decreased Activity

Decreased activity may represent the effects of pharmacological agents administered in the peripartum period, such as narcotics or magnesium sulfate. Both of these agents also may result in transient but significant respiratory depression. Once again, sepsis remains a possibility in any newborn who persistently has decreased activity. An underlying neurological abnormality also needs to be considered.

Jitteriness

Jitteriness is defined as rhythmical tremors of equal amplitude and probably is the most common involuntary movement of the healthy infant. The movements of jitteriness (or tremors) are provoked easily in susceptible neonates by external stimuli, such as handling or loud noise, and can be stopped simply by holding the affected extremity gently. Although these tremors usually occur in healthy infants, jitteriness may be caused by hypoglycemia, hypocalcemia, or perinatal asphyxia, and these diagnoses should be investigated. In addition, neonatal jitteriness may be seen in association with maternal use of marijuana, cocaine, and narcotics.

Seizures

Seizures in the newborn rarely occur as dramatic, well-organized, symmetrical, generalized tonic-clonic episodes. More frequently, seizure episodes appear as focal abnormalities or as subtle findings such as repetitive staring, blinking, or sucking movements. Because seizures in the newborn usually are a sign of an underlying abnormality, including primary central nervous system disease, systemic illness, or metabolic abnormality, they must be diagnosed and treated as relative medical emergencies.

COLOR

Cyanosis

Peripheral cyanosis involving the hands and feet (acrocyanosis) is a common normal finding in the first 1 to 2 days of life. In contrast, persistent central cyanosis always is abnormal. The ability to detect it, however, depends on the skill of the observer. Its presence suggests an abnormality in blood oxygen content resulting in 3 to 5 g of unoxygenated hemoglobin. Cyanosis resulting from a respiratory origin usually occurs with associated signs of respiratory distress. *Cyanosis without respiratory distress suggests an anatomical right-to-left shunt caused by a congenital cardiac anomaly.* This right-to-left shunt can be confirmed by a minimum increase in pO_2 (pO_2 less than 100) with administration of 100% oxygen. In rare instances cyanosis may be caused by an abnormal hemoglobin, such as methemoglobin.

Jaundice

Visible jaundice in the first 24 hours of life is abnormal and usually suggests an increase in red blood cell turnover and production of bilirubin. Hemolysis on an immune or an infectious basis is the most frequent cause. Inherited red cell membrane and enzymatic defects are less common problems that often are difficult to diagnose in the first few days of life. Aggressive treatment aimed at keeping levels of indirect bilirubin from climbing too rapidly is important in preventing the central nervous system complications of hyperbilirubinemia. Although some degree of jaundice is normal in healthy newborns, direct or conjugated hyperbilirubinemia is not. Levels of direct bilirubin persistently above 1.5 mg/dl require further evaluation, including but not limited to assessments of liver function.

Petechiae/Purpura

Petechiae are pinpoint hemorrhages into the skin that do not blanch with pressure, whereas purpura denotes larger, nonblanching areas of bleeding into the skin. Petechiae may appear on the presenting part for a vaginal delivery without signifying an underlying pathological condition. Extensive, generalized petechiae, on the other hand, may be the initial manifestation of an underlying platelet abnormality. The differential diagnosis includes infectious, immunological, hematological, or a myriad of miscellaneous causes.

Pallor

The term *pallor,* or *paleness,* describes a decrease in the normal rosy skin color of the Caucasian newborn. It may result from anemia or a generalized vasoconstriction.

Anemia. Anemia that appears in the newborn (hematocrit under 45) may have multiple causes, which can be subdivided into two main categories—excessive losses of red blood cells (e.g., acute or chronic hemorrhage, hemolysis) or inadequate red cell production (red cell hypoplasia). The first group is much more common. Diagnostic evaluation includes assessment of cardiovascular stability because hypotension, tachycardia, and delayed capillary refill may be seen in cases of acute blood loss. Determination of central hematocrit, red blood cell indices, indices of red blood cell production, and adequacy of other blood cell lines (white blood cells, platelets) may give other clues. The detection of acid-stable fetal hemoglobin in maternal blood (Betke-Kleihauer test) is diagnostic of fetal bleeding into the maternal circulation (fetomaternal hemorrhage). Anemia in the newborn is discussed more thoroughly in Chapter 113.

Vasoconstriction. Pallor caused by vasoconstriction may represent a normal response to cold stress, which requires attention to thermoregulatory management. On the other hand, this finding may be a clue to underlying hemodynamic compromise most commonly related to hypovolemia or cardiac dysfunction. In this case, pallor often accompanies tachycardia, weak pulse, and low blood pressure. A history of blood loss (or tight nuchal cord resulting in occult blood loss) during delivery may provide an additional clue to the diagnosis of hypovolemia; a therapeutic response to volume expansion confirms this diagnosis. If cardiac dysfunction is the underlying cause, then other physical findings may be present, including a "gallop" heart rhythm, pulmonary rales, and hepatomegaly. In this situation, volume expansion actually may exacerbate the problem. A chest roentgenogram may help differentiate between these two possibilities.

Plethora

Plethora usually is caused by polycythemia, and a venous hematocrit reading of greater than 65% confirms the diagnosis. Polycythemia occurs more frequently among infants who are postmature, who demonstrate intrauterine growth retardation, or who are born to mothers who smoke or have diabetes or preeclampsia. Twin-to-twin transfusion and chromosomal anomalies (e.g., trisomies 13, 18, and 21) are other causes. The main clinical concern related to polycythemia is that a high hematocrit often is associated with an elevated blood viscosity, which may impede tissue blood flow. Therefore a wide variety of clinical signs also may be associated with plethora, including respiratory distress and cyanosis, central nervous system (CNS) signs, poor feeding, hypoglycemia, and many others. The treatment for symptomatic polycythemia is a partial exchange transfusion aimed at decreasing the hematocrit to approximately 50 and thus eliminating hyperviscosity.

SOUNDS

Crying

Abnormalities of an infant's cry have long been recognized as markers for a variety of neonatal disorders. More recently, advances in electronics have enabled investigators to characterize individual cry patterns. High-pitched cries may herald CNS abnormalities, whereas hoarse or low-pitched cries can be associated with upper airway abnormalities.

Breathing

Noisy breathing often is a clue to underlying airway problems and is associated with clinical evidence of increased work of breathing. Inspiratory stridor implicates extrathoracic airway obstruction due to entities such as laryngomalacia, laryngeal web, and vocal cord trauma or paralysis. Accurate diagnosis requires direct visualization of the larynx and upper airway by someone trained in airway management of the newborn. Less invasive methods of evaluation include fluoroscopy or measurement of air flow–volume loops. Expiratory grunting often is noted in infants who have poorly compliant lungs and represents a compensatory maneuver that increases end-expiratory lung volume. Expiratory stridor and wheezing implicate intrathoracic obstruction involving the small and midsize airways.

ODORS

The astute clinician uses all senses in the evaluation of newborns, including the sense of smell. Inborn errors of metabolism often are associated with unusual odors of the urine or of the infant. Although individual inborn errors of metabolism are rare, as a group they are not uncommon. Unusual odors have been described, for example, as mustiness (phenylketonuria), sweaty feet (isovaleric acidemia), and maple syrup (maple syrup urine disease). Screening of urine and plasma for specific metabolic compounds provides an initial step toward diagnosis.

ABDOMINAL DISTENTION

Although mild gastric distention can be a normal finding, moderate distention that persists or is associated with other systemic signs of illness should be evaluated. Abdominal distention can result from gas, fluid, or an abdominal mass.

Gaseous Distention

Gaseous distention can be diagnosed by hyperresonance to percussion. Functional decreases in bowel motility (ileus) can accompany a wide variety of systemic illnesses in the neonate. Usually there is no associated tenderness. Mechanical bowel obstruction often is associated with bilious emesis and delayed passage of stools. Free intraabdominal air resulting from a perforated viscus usually is accompanied by signs of peritonitis, which may include erythema of the abdominal wall, marked tenderness to palpation, and absence of bowel sounds.

Fluid Distention

Intraabdominal fluid is diagnosed by a fluid wave on palpation or by shifting dullness to percussion. Hemoperitoneum occasionally is noted after a difficult delivery or in association with disorders characterized by massive splenomegaly (e.g., erythroblastosis). Urinary ascites occasionally is noted in association with obstructive uropathy. The most common cause of fluid distention (ascites) is transudation, resulting from conditions such as hemolytic disease, congestive heart failure, or nonimmune hydrops.

Distention Caused by Abdominal Mass

Urogenital. Most abdominal masses in the newborn are urogenital in origin. Palpation of the abdomen may give clues as to location and consistency; however, the preferred method for diagnosis is an abdominal ultrasound examination. Flank masses (either unilateral or bilateral) usually are caused by cystic dysplasia of the kidneys or by hydronephrosis. Cystic ovary may appear as a lower abdominal mass in female infants.

Hepatomegaly. Hepatomegaly also may appear as an enlargement of the abdomen. The liver may normally be palpable 2 cm below the right costal margin with the upper border typically percussed at the fifth intercostal space. Liver enlargement can be seen with a wide variety of systemic illnesses, including infections, primary hepatic disease, congestive heart failure, hematological disorders, storage disorders, trauma, and, in rare cases, tumors.

Splenomegaly. The tip of the spleen occasionally may be palpable in normal infants during the first days of life. A prominent spleen may be associated with congenital viral infection, inborn errors of metabolism, or, more commonly, in association with the increased extramedullary hematopoiesis noted with hemolytic disease.

Adrenal Hemorrhage. Massive adrenal hemorrhage may manifest as a flank mass in a stressed infant after a difficult delivery. Risk factors include macrosomia, breech presentation, and perinatal asphyxia.

Gastrointestinal Enteric Duplication Cysts. Gastrointestinal enteric duplication cysts may be palpable and can lead to bowel obstruction. Intrauterine meconium peritonitis may result in formation of a palpable pseudocyst. An olive-size mass in the epigastrium can be caused by the hypertrophied pylorus of pyloric stenosis.

Tumor. Wilms tumor, neuroblastoma, and congenital mesoblastic nephromas are uncommon; however, their usual presenting sign is abdominal swelling or a palpable abdominal mass.

INTAKE AND OUTPUT

Feeding Problems

Oral feeding, although often taken for granted, represents a very complicated neuromotor process involving coordination of sucking, swallowing, and breathing. Indifference to feeding may be noted in conjunction with other systemic illnesses. As a result, difficulties in feeding are seen in association with a wide variety of disorders. Although this group of disorders is nonspecific, it commonly is seen in newborns born prematurely or in those who have CNS and neuromuscular disorders. Less commonly, the cause may be an anatomical abnormality, such as tracheoesophageal fistula.

Oliguria

Most infants (more than 90%) void by 24 hours of age and 99% do so by 48 hours; they maintain adequate output thereafter (more than 1 ml/kg/hr). Failure to pass urine by 48 hours suggests either primary renal dysfunction or obstructive uropathy.

Polyuria

Polyuria is uncommon in the newborn. It is considered pathological when the infant is unable to achieve normal total body water and electrolytes because of persistent passage of unconcentrated urine. Most commonly this represents renal tubular dysfunction, as can be seen after acute tubular necrosis or in association with a partial obstruction of the renal collecting system. Less common causes include other renal parenchymal disease and inadequate antidiuretic hormone response.

Hematuria/Hemoglobinuria

Red urine usually indicates hematuria; however, other possible causes include the presence of hemoglobin, uric acid, or porphyrins. Examination of a freshly voided urine sample will aid in the diagnosis. If intact red blood cells are detected, extraurinary sources (e.g., rectal or vaginal bleeding) must be excluded. If red cell or other types of renal cast are present, then parenchymal kidney disease is the likely cause. The differential diagnosis of hematuria in the newborn includes asphyxial kidney injury (e.g., acute tubular necrosis, cortical necrosis), renovascular accident (e.g., renal vein thrombosis), obstructive uropathy, cystitis, nephritis, or underlying coagulopathy.

Hemoglobinuria is seen most commonly in association with intravascular hemolysis. Urate crystals may give a reddish orange cast to the urine in infants who otherwise are healthy.

Proteinuria

A small amount of protein normally may be detected in the urine of healthy newborns; however, most term newborns excrete less than 25 mg in 24 hours. If excessive proteinuria is suspected, then a timed urine collection should be obtained. Proteinuria may be seen in association with nearly any form of renal disease.

Delayed Passage of Meconium

Most term infants (94%) pass their first meconium stool by 24 hours of age; 99% pass meconium by 48 hours. Delays in passage may represent significant underlying bowel pathology, including Hirschsprung's disease, atresias, meconium ileus, or meconium plug syndrome.

Melena/Hematochezia

The most common source of blood in the newborn infant's stool is maternal blood swallowed at delivery. These infants typically are not ill. This cause can be diagnosed quickly at the bedside by the Apt-Downey test for the presence of adult hemoglobin. Neonatal gastrointestinal (GI) hemorrhage may be acute and life threatening or may be detected only in trace amounts by stool heme testing. GI hemorrhage may be the presenting sign of a generalized bleeding disorder, such as vitamin K deficiency, disseminated intravascular coagulation, thrombocytopenia, or hereditary coagulopathy. Upper GI trauma, such as from vigorous suctioning or placement of a nasogastric tube, usually results only in occult blood in the stool; lower GI pathology typically results in more obvious hematochezia. The differential diagnosis includes, but is not limited to, peptic ulcers, necrotizing enterocolitis, malrotation and volvulus, Meckel diverticulum, and intussusception. Hematochezia with mucus may result from infectious enteritis, which can be diagnosed by appropriate cultures.

Vomiting

Although the spitting up ("posseting" in British infants) of small amounts of formula occurs frequently in otherwise healthy newborns, large or persistent emesis may herald underlying pathological conditions. Vomiting of non-bile-stained fluid usually represents anatomical or functional obstruction at or above the first portion of the duodenum. Causes include esophageal atresia, gastric web, pyloric stenosis, or severe gastroesophageal reflux (GER). Anatomical obstruction should be ruled out before linking the diagnosis of vomiting to GER alone. Obstruction below the opening of the bile duct may produce bilious vomiting. This may result from a functional ileus caused by systemic disease (such as hypokalemia, adrenal hyperplasia, or elevated intracranial pressure) or may represent a structural abnormality (e.g., atresia or malrotation with volvulus). Diagnostic tests start with anteroposterior and horizontal beam abdominal roentgenograms.

Diarrhea

Diarrhea is the passage of frequent stools. Newborn infants may have up to five or six stools per day, especially if breastfed. Persistent passage of watery stools, however, is abnormal and may be a sign of enteric or systemic disease.

Gastroenteritis. Bacterial gastroenteritis is unusual in the newborn period; however, nursery epidemics, as well as isolated cases, do occur. The diagnosis is suggested by the presence of blood and mucus in the stools and is confirmed by appropriate cultures. Viral gastroenteritis, especially that caused by rotavirus, has been described in newborns.

Lactose Intolerance. Lactose intolerance is a very common cause of diarrhea in the newborn. Stools are watery and test positive for reducing sugars. The diagnosis is suggested further when these findings resolve after a lactose-free formula is begun. Most commonly, this represents a transient lactase deficiency. Therefore lactase-containing formula can be reinstituted after several weeks.

Other Causes. Other, less common causes include phototherapy, neonatal abstinence syndrome, thyrotoxicosis, and other specific malabsorption syndromes, such as cystic fibrosis.

OTHER FINDINGS ON EXAMINATION

Leukokoria

Leukokoria literally means white pupil and is not a normal finding in the newborn. The observation of a white pupil requires immediate, further revaluation by an ophthalmologist experienced in examining newborns. The most common cause is a cataract, of which nearly 50% have diagnosable and potentially treatable causes. Other causes include persistent hyperplastic primary vitreous, cicatricial retinopathy of prematurity, retinal dysplasia, tumor (retinoblastoma), glaucoma, and numerous other conditions.

Red Eye

Ophthalmia neonatorum, or neonatal conjunctivitis, often manifests as a red eye with exudate (see Chapter 164). The cause is chemical (silver nitrate), bacterial, viral, or chlamydial in nature. All cases should be examined thoroughly with appropriate culture work performed and appropriate therapy instituted promptly, especially when the eyelids are markedly swollen and a purulent discharge is present, most likely representing infection with *Neisseria gonorrhoeae.*

Heart Murmur

A large number of normal, healthy newborns have a soft, short systolic murmur heard in the first few days of life, relating to ductal closure. The absence of a murmur, on the other hand, does not eliminate the diagnosis of serious cardiac anomaly. Falling pulmonary vascular resistance over the first few days of life also affects the presence and the quality of the murmur. A significant murmur heard on the first day of life is more likely to be caused by an obstructive lesion, such as aortic stenosis, pulmonic stenosis, or coarctation. A significant murmur first heard after the day of birth suggests a shunt lesion, such as a patent ductus arteriosus or ventricular septal defect. Loud, persistent systolic murmurs, especially if accompanied by other cardiopulmonary findings, require further evaluation.

SUGGESTED READINGS

Catalano DJ: Leukokoria: the differential diagnosis of a white pupil, *Pediatr Ann* 12:498, 1983.

Coen RW, Koffler H: *Primary care of the newborn.* Boston, 1987, Little Brown.

Fanaroff AA, Martin RJ: *Neonatal-perinatal medicine diseases of the fetus and infant,* St Louis, 1991, Mosby.

Jones KL: *Smith's recognizable patterns of human malformation,* ed 4, Philadelphia, 1988, WB Saunders.

Klaus MH, Fanaroff AA: *Care of the high-risk neonate,* ed 4, Philadelphia, 1993, WB Saunders.

Long WA: *Fetal and neonatal cardiology,* Philadelphia, 1990, WB Saunders.

Parker S et al: Jitteriness in full-term neonates: prevalence and correlates, *Pediatrics* 85:17, 1990.

Volpe JJ: *Neurology of the newborn,* Philadelphia, ed 2, 1987, WB Saunders.

47 Common Neonatal Illnesses

Charles Palmer

APNEA

Irregularity in the pattern of breathing is common among newborn infants. The preterm infant responds to a decline in inspired oxygen concentration with a transient increase in ventilation, preceding a sustained depression of ventilation. In addition, infants at fewer than 33 weeks of gestation exhibit reduced ventilatory responses to inspired carbon dioxide. A similar response has been observed in the term infant during the first week of life, when a progressive decrease in inspired oxygen concentration results in reduced carbon dioxide responsiveness.

Apnea is defined as a cessation of respiratory air flow. The respiratory pause may be central (i.e., no respiratory effort), obstructive, or mixed. Short (<15 seconds) central apnea can be normal at all ages. *Periodic breathing* is seen commonly among premature infants and is defined as a breathing pattern in which three or more respiratory pauses of more than 3 seconds' duration are separated by less than 20 seconds of respiration. *Pathological apnea* is defined as a prolonged (>20 seconds) respiratory pause or a shorter period associated with cyanosis, marked pallor, hypotonia, or bradycardia.[6] *Apnea of prematurity* is defined as pathological apnea in a premature infant.

Apnea of prematurity is more frequent during rapid eye movement sleep than during quiet sleep. It usually starts after the first day of life and resolves by 37 weeks of gestation but occasionally persists to several weeks postterm. It is a common finding in preterm infants and, if the apneic periods are prolonged, can lead to hypoxemia and bradycardia.

Although uncomplicated apnea of prematurity is common, apnea may be symptomatic of an underlying disorder, even in the preterm infant. Specific causes for apnea include the following:

1. Septicemia (e.g., meningitis or necrotizing enterocolitis)
2. Impaired oxygenation, hypoxemia, severe anemia, and shock or marked systemic to pulmonary circulatory shunt (e.g., patent ductus arteriosus)
3. Metabolic disorders (e.g., hypoglycemia, hypercalcemia, hyponatremia, hypernatremia, and hyperammonemia)
4. Drugs (e.g., narcotics or central nervous system depressants taken by the mother)
5. Central nervous system disorders (e.g., intracranial hemorrhage, seizures, or malformations of the brain)
6. Thermal instability (i.e., a rapid increase or decrease of temperature)

Investigation for an underlying cause should be pursued vigorously in any one of these cases: (1) apnea occurs within 24 hours of delivery; (2) apnea occurs in infants born after 36 weeks of gestation; (3) apnea requires vigorous resuscitation; (4) apnea is preceded by or is associated with marked cyanosis; and (5) existing apneic episodes increase in severity.

The preterm infant should be monitored for apnea, and, because bradycardia usually follows within 30 seconds of obstructive apnea, heart rate monitoring also should be included. This is important because obstructive apnea (in which breathing effort continues but air flow ceases because of obstruction in the upper airways) will not trigger the usual form of respiratory monitor, which relies on changes in the chest wall electrical impedance. Convenient monitors of both respiration and heart rate are available.

Treatment of neonatal apnea should address its underlying cause. Several treatments are available for apnea of prematurity, including the following:

1. Tactile stimulation. Gentle tapping on the infant's heel usually suffices. A pulsating waterbed sometimes is used for recurrent episodes.
2. Pharmacological intervention with methylxanthines (theophylline or caffeine). A loading dose of theophylline (5 mg/kg) is followed by maintenance at 1 to 2 mg/kg/dose (twice a day). Caffeine usually is given as 20 mg/kg loading dose orally, followed by 5 mg/kg/day.
3. Continuous positive airway pressure by nasal prongs.
4. Small increases in inspired oxygen from 21% to 25%, with monitoring of the response to maintain the arterial oxygen pressure (PaO_2) between 50 and 90 mm Hg.
5. Endotracheal intubation with positive end-expiratory pressure may be required for a short period in some cases.

When pharmacological therapy is used, age-related variations in theophylline metabolism necessitate the monitoring of the plasma theophylline concentration. The concentration required for apnea is less than that required for bronchodilation; thus levels should be maintained between 6 and 13 μg/ml. Because caffeine, in contrast, has a broad therapeutic index, its concentration usually does not need to be monitored if it is given in the prescribed dose. Physicians who administer methylxanthines should be aware that the hepatic metabolism of these drugs is slowed by macrolide antibiotics, such as erythromycin, and by intercurrent viral illnesses. The toxicity of theophylline is related to its serum level; clinical manifestations usually begin with tachycardia, succeeded by jitteriness, irritability, and signs of gastrointestinal dysfunction. Occasionally, if apnea of prematurity does not cease by 37 weeks, the infant may be discharged home with an apnea monitor. In these cases the parents are expected to be skilled in cardiopulmonary resuscitation and the use of the monitor.

The term *apnea of infancy* applies to the occasional infant who has an unexplained respiratory pause for at least 20 seconds or a shorter respiratory pause associated with bradycardia, cyanosis, pallor, and/or marked hypotonia. The term generally refers to infants who are greater than 37 weeks postconception at the onset of pathological apnea. An *apparent life-threatening event* is an episode that is frightening to the observer and characterized by some combination of apnea (central or obstructive), color change (cyanosis or pallor), marked change in muscle tone (usually marked limpness), choking, or gagging. In some cases the observer fears that the infant has died. These incidents should be investigated for an underlying cause, especially gastroesophageal reflux, a tracheoesophageal fistula, and possible seizures. When the diagnosis of such apnea is in question, the simultaneous recording of respiratory electrical impedance, nasal air flow, esophageal pH, and the electrocardiogram for prolonged periods ("pneumograms") can document the occurrence of apnea and bradycardia. After diagnostic evaluation of an apparent life-threatening event, the patient should be discharged home with a cardiorespiratory monitor.

The outcome of apnea of prematurity usually is good, provided appropriate monitoring and treatment are ensured to prevent long periods of hypoxia. Among apneic newborns and infants, pneumograms cannot predict which infants will require resuscitation to terminate a subsequent apneic spell. When compared with a control group, however, infants who have apnea of infancy have significantly higher respiratory and heart rates.

HYPERBILIRUBINEMIA

Hyperbilirubinemia occurs commonly during the first week of life. It usually is physiological, and appropriate management includes reassurance, with avoidance of unnecessary investigations and maternal-infant separation. Occasionally, hyperbilirubinemia is symptomatic of an underlying pathological condition. These cases need identification and an etiological workup. Select cases may require specific management to prevent the harmful effects of excessive unconjugated bilirubin on the central nervous system.

Physiological Jaundice

Clinical jaundice is visible at serum bilirubin levels of approximately 5 to 7 mg/dl (85 to 120 μmol/l). Approximately 50% of all normal newborns and a higher percentage of premature infants appear jaundiced during the first week of life. Nearly all newborns have some degree of mild hyperbilirubinemia that disappears after a few days; this transient hyperbilirubinemia has been called *physiological jaundice*. Mechanisms involved in producing physiological jaundice include an interaction between an increased load of bilirubin (from the high fetal hematocrit) and a decreased ability of the newborn liver to clear bilirubin. The clinician can recognize the presence of physiological jaundice by certain criteria. It is evident clinically *after* the first 24 hours of life. It peaks between days 3 and 5, and in normal full-term infants it does not rise higher than 12.7 to 12.9 mg/dl.[4] The bilirubin is almost all unconjugated. Jaundice usually is not detectable after 10 days. Deviation from this physiological pattern generally signifies a pathological process and requires special investigations to define a cause.

Breast-Feeding and Jaundice

Breast-feeding has been associated with increased levels of bilirubin and prolongation of hyperbilirubinemia. The association between breast-feeding and jaundice in the healthy, full-term newborn can be considered in terms of two categories: (1) the jaundice that is *associated* with breast-feeding and (2) true breast-milk jaundice.

Jaundice Associated with Breast-Feeding. Prolonged hyperbilirubinemia in association with breast-feeding occurs in about 30% of breast-fed babies. There is some indication that frequent feeding may reduce the incidence of hyperbilirubinemia and that breast-feeding should not be withheld. An association between decreased frequency of nursing and higher bilirubin levels has been found. Hence, breast-feeding mothers should be encouraged to nurse their infants as frequently as possible. If it appears that the bilirubin concentration will rise above 20 mg/dl, feeding should be stopped temporarily for 48 hours and then resumed.

True Breast-Milk Jaundice. The syndrome of true breast-milk jaundice in which the bilirubin concentration rises progressively from the fourth day of life, reaching a maximum of 10 to 30 mg/dl (171 to 153 μmol/l) by 10 to 15 days, develops in approximately 1% to 2% of breast-fed neonates. If breast-feeding continues, the bilirubin may continue to rise before declining after about 4 to 10 days to reach normal levels by 3 to 12 weeks of age. Finally, if breast-feeding is interrupted at any stage, the bilirubin concentration declines markedly within 48 hours. With resumption of nursing, bilirubin concentrations may rise moderately by 1 to 3 mg/dl but usually do not reach the previous level.

If breast-feeding needs to be withheld temporarily, mothers should be given enthusiastic support and encouraged to resume breast-feeding after a 48-hour interruption. They also should be encouraged to maintain lactation by breast pump or manual expression.

Pathological Jaundice

Pathological jaundice refers to a pattern of hyperbilirubinemia that falls outside the limits defined for physiological jaundice. It may occur earlier, last longer, or reach higher levels. In these cases, jaundice should be regarded as symptomatic of an underlying pathological condition. The following criteria, modified from Maisels,[4] help identify pathological hyperbilirubinemia:

1. Clinical jaundice in the first 24 hours of life
2. Total serum bilirubin concentrations increasing by more than 5 mg/dl (85 μmol/l/day)
3. Total serum bilirubin concentrations exceeding 12.9 mg/dl (221 μmol/l) in full-term infants or 15 mg/dl (257 μmol/l) in premature infants
4. Direct (conjugated) serum bilirubin concentration exceeding 1.5 to 2 mg/dl (25 to 34 μmol/l)
5. Clinical jaundice persisting for more than 1 week in full-term infants or 2 weeks in premature infants

Deviations from these guidelines should be investigated.

In such patients, physiological jaundice will reach levels above 12.9 mg/dl, and a higher level may be tolerated before special investigations are initiated. In a recent study,[6] only 6% of infants admitted to a well-baby nursery had serum bilirubin levels that exceeded 12.9 mg/dl. Serum bilirubin levels above 12.9 mg/dl were significantly associated with breast-feeding, maternal diabetes, oxytocin-induced labor, prematurity, Oriental race, and male gender. Appreciation of these factors permits a more rational approach to the level of bilirubin at which to initiate special studies. In these patients a peak bilirubin level of 15 mg/dl can be tolerated as the upper range of normal before investigation is warranted. In the absence of these factors, values higher than 12 mg/dl should be used as the level at which jaundice should be investigated.[6]

Causes of Pathological Jaundice in the Neonate. The newborn who has jaundice should have total and direct (conjugated) bilirubin estimated as soon as jaundice is diagnosed. Jaundice first is evident clinically after 48 hours. That occurring during the first 24 hours usually is caused by an excessive load of bilirubin, resulting from hemolysis caused by maternal antibodies against fetal red cell ABO or Rh antigens. Nonimmune causes of hemolysis also should be considered, including hereditary spherocytosis and deficiency of glucose-6-phosphate dehydrogenase.

Infants of mothers who have diabetes are prone to increased bilirubin production, as are patients who have increased intrahepatic circulation of bilirubin secondary to small or large bowel obstruction. Clearance of bilirubin also can be hindered in premature infants by breast-feeding and by certain inborn errors of metabolism such as hypothyroidism. Essential investigations for nonphysiological jaundice include (1) serum bilirubin concentration including a determination of the direct bilirubin if jaundice is prolonged, (2) blood typing of both mother and infant, and (3) direct Coombs test on the infant. A peripheral blood smear for red cell morphology, reticulocyte count, and hematocrit are optional. An increased direct bilirubin level exceeding 1.5 to 2 mg/dl (or one third of the total serum bilirubin) requires diagnostic evaluation. This should proceed rapidly because patients who have biliary atresia (a possible cause of elevated direct bilirubin) require early surgical intervention for optimal outcome.

The presence of pathological jaundice should provoke a review of the maternal and infant history and a thorough examination of the infant. A family history of jaundice or liver disease and a maternal history of illness, diabetes, or drug ingestion during pregnancy should be excluded. The labor and delivery history should be reviewed for documentation of oxytocin administration, delayed cord clamping, and vacuum extraction, because all of these may lead to increased red cell mass and thus an elevated serum bilirubin level from hemolysis. The maternal history should be evaluated further for evidence of bacterial or viral infection (fever, premature rupture of membranes), and the mother's blood needs to be analyzed for ABO and Rh blood groups and the presence of isoantibodies. Any maternal history of hepatitis or family history of anemia or glucose-6-phosphate dehydrogenase deficiency should be noted.

The infant who has nonphysiological (pathological) jaundice (especially if jaundice is prolonged or associated with an elevated direct fraction) should be examined carefully for signs of sepsis such as lethargy, temperature instability, a change in feeding pattern, cutaneous petechiae, and poor capillary perfusion. Signs of extramedullary hematopoiesis, including hepatosplenomegaly may reflect a congenital infection. The presence of a hematoma, extensive bruising, plethora, polycythemia, or ingested maternal blood may provide an additional hemoglobin source and lead to an elevated serum bilirubin level.

Conjugated Hyperbilirubinemia. An increase in direct (conjugated) bilirubin greater than 1.5 to 2 mg/dl (or more than 33% of the total serum bilirubin concentration) almost always is pathological. Causes include liver inflammation and obstruction to bile flow. Hepatitis can be caused by sepsis, intrauterine infection, inborn errors of metabolism (alpha-1-antitrypsin deficiency, galactosemia) or pyloric stenosis and upper gastrointestinal obstruction (e.g., annular pancreas). Inflammation of the liver and cholestasis also can be produced by prolonged parenteral nutrition.

Cholestasis in the infant also can result from biliary atresia, either intrahepatic or extrahepatic, a choledochal cyst, or inspissated bile. The presence of bile pigment in the stool or duodenal aspirate excludes complete biliary atresia. Such patients should be examined carefully for signs of hepatosplenomegaly (which would support a congenital infection), and the urine should be cultured so that a urinary tract infection can be excluded; blood cultures should be drawn so that septicemia can be excluded. An ultrasound examination of the liver can demonstrate the presence of a choledochal cyst and dilated biliary structures. Bile flow also can be evaluated by radioisotopes excreted through the hepatobiliary system. Finally, a liver biopsy and cholangiogram may be necessary to determine the specific pathology.

Patients who have conjugated hyperbilirubinemia should be investigated at a referral center where facilities permit full investigation of this disorder. The Kasai procedure of hepatic enterostomy (portoenterostomy) can improve bile drainage for patients who have extrahepatic biliary atresia; the earlier the procedure is performed, the better the results. Thus every effort should be made to arrive at a diagnosis and to begin appropriate intervention early.

Treatment of Neonatal Hyperbilirubinemia

Observations made some 30 years ago established a strong association between severe (hemolytic) hyperbilirubinemia and the clinical syndrome of kernicterus among patients who have erythroblastosis fetalis. Kernicterus refers to the finding at autopsy of yellow discoloration and neuronal degeneration of the brain, particularly the basal ganglia, hippocampus, and cerebellum. Survivors often manifest severe neuropathological sequelae, including athetoid cerebral palsy, deafness, and failure of upward gaze. Kernicterus was not seen in full-term infants if the serum bilirubin concentration was maintained below 20 mg/dl (342 μmol/l). Despite the regrettable absence of randomized clinical trials, a serum unconjugated bilirubin level of 20 mg/dl has been adopted widely as the maximum acceptable for full-term infants who have *hemolytic jaundice*. Levels above this are lowered by performance of an exchange transfusion; this practice diminished the incidence of kernicterus dramatically.

The precise mechanism of bilirubin neurotoxicity is not known, although animal and human experiments demonstrate that hyperbilirubinemia can disrupt neurotransmission, producing lethargy, disturbances in the cry, and impairment of the brainstem auditory-evoked response, even at levels of serum bilirubin below 20 mg/dl. These changes, however, are reversible and may not reflect permanent neuronal injury. Theoretically, bilirubin must be "free" (from binding with albumin) to cross the blood-brain barrier. Animal studies have shown that when the normal blood-brain barrier is disrupted by exposure to hyperbilirubinemia, both bound and unbound bilirubin can cross it. Recent studies have shown that in addition to imparting a yellow color to the brain tissue, disruption of the blood-brain barrier in the presence of hyperbilirubinemia also can impair cellular energy metabolism. Other experiments indicate that acidosis exacerbates bilirubin neurotoxicity further.

Although both exchange transfusion and phototherapy can lower serum bilirubin effectively, the indications for their use remain hotly debated. With the exception of the infant who has hemolytic jaundice, most current recommendations for use of these therapies developed out of consensus and have not yet been validated by properly designed studies.

Phototherapy. Phototherapy is effective in lowering serum bilirubin levels and may reduce the need for exchange transfusion. There are no data, however, to indicate that phototherapy used to lower serum bilirubin will enhance developmental outcome. As a general guideline, phototherapy is started at a bilirubin level of about 5 mg/dl lower than the threshold level for exchange transfusion. For ABO incompatibility, phototherapy can be started when there is evidence of a rapidly rising bilirubin level, as defined by an increase of .5 mg/dl/hour or more. The *routine use of phototherapy for ABO incompatibility is not necessary* because hyperbilirubinemia develops in only a minority of these infants, even when the Coombs test shows a positive reaction.

For healthy full-term newborns who have no hemolysis, phototherapy should start at a total serum bilirubin level between 17 to 22 mg/dl (290 to 325 μmol/l), and an exchange transfusion should be performed if the bilirubin level reaches 25 mg/dl (430 μmol/l) despite intensive phototherapy.[3,5] For infants of low birth weight, phototherapy often is started at 5 mg/dl below the exchange threshold. Some authorities use phototherapy prophylactically for newborns weighing less than 1500 g because the exchange threshold recommended is lowered in proportion to birth weight. An exchange should be performed at a total serum bilirubin level of 13 to 16 mg/dl (220 to 275 μmol/l) for infants less than 1500 g, 16 to 18 mg/dl (275 to 300 μmol/l) for infants between 1500 and 1999 g, and 18 to 20 mg/dl (300 to 340 μmol/l) when the birth weight is between 2000 and 2499 g. These recommendations[5] represent ranges currently used in neonatal intensive care units and do not take into account all possible situations.

Bilirubin absorbs light maximally in the wavelengths near 460 nm, which can be found in the blue-green part of the visible spectrum. During phototherapy the bilirubin molecule undergoes isomerization. The photo-isomers are hydrophilic and are excreted directly in bile and urine. Although blue light delivers the optimal wave length for phototherapy, it also obscures the infant's skin color and can induce headaches and nausea among nursing staff. This problem can be alleviated by combining three or four "special blue" narrow spectrum lamps (Westinghouse 20W F20T12BB) with daylight lamps placed on the outside of the phototherapy unit.

To achieve the maximum therapeutic effect from phototherapy, it is necessary to provide the highest intensity irradiance over the largest surface area of the baby. The response to phototherapy increases with irradiance until a saturation point is reached at an irradiation of approximately 25 to 30 $\mu W/cm^2/nm$ in the blue spectrum. Because irradiance is inversely proportional to the square of the distance from the light source, free-standing phototherapy units should be as close to the baby as possible without incurring the risk of burn. This may be as close as 15 to 20 cm from the infant.

Another way to improve phototherapy is to increase the surface area exposed. This can be achieved by removing the diaper, surrounding the infant by more than one bank of lights, placing reflective material strategically, and also by placing the infant on a fiberoptic phototherapy blanket. The infant should be kept well hydrated, preferably with milk because it inhibits the enterohepatic circulation and therefore will facilitate excretion of bilirubin.

Phototherapy can be discontinued when the bilirubin level falls below 14 to 15 mg/dl in full-term infants. A rebound of less than 1 mg/dl (17 μmol/l) can be expected, provided that the infant does not have hemolytic disease. Additional follow-up of serum bilirubin is necessary if phototherapy is discontinued before its normal peak at 3 to 5 days of age in full-term newborns or if the infant has (or is suspected of having) hemolytic disease.

Whenever phototherapy is used, serum bilirubin measurements must be followed because the skin is bleached by phototherapy, making it an unreliable indicator of the degree of jaundice. Side effects of phototherapy include increased insensible water loss, frequent loose stools, occasional abdominal distention, lethargy, and skin erythema. Skin erythema can be reduced by placing an acrylic plastic shield between the patient and the light source. This is used to filter out damaging ultraviolet and infrared rays. Patients who have an elevated conjugated bilirubin level and who receive phototherapy develop a dark green-brown discoloration ("bronze baby"). Because retinal damage has occurred in animals during phototherapy, the *infant's eyes must be shielded* with opaque patches. These patches need constant attention to ensure that they do not obstruct the nostrils. No long-term harmful complications of phototherapy have been identified.

Home Phototherapy. Equipment designed for delivering phototherapy in the home has become available in the past few years. This service was developed to reduce costs of hospitalization and to prevent separation of the mother and infant. The service is appreciated especially by lactating mothers because it facilitates continuation of breast-feeding. The physician should limit the use of home phototherapy to infants who have the following characteristics (as amended from the recommendations outlined by the Committee on Fetus and Newborn of the American Academy of Pediatrics[2]:

1. Full-term, older than 48 hours, and otherwise healthy
2. Serum bilirubin concentrations greater than 14 mg/dl but less than 18 mg/dl
3. No elevation in direct-reacting (conjugated) bilirubin
4. No pathological causes of hyperbilirubinemia

A candidate for home phototherapy should have caretakers who can follow instructions regarding use of the equipment, correct application of eye patches, and provision of adequate hydration. Therapy should be under the supervision of a physician who should contact the caretakers daily and ensure that arrangements are made for serum bilirubin to be measured at least every 12 to 24 hours. The committee suggests that the newborn be removed from phototherapy during feedings and diaper changes and when the parents are asleep. Phototherapy should be discontinued once the serum bilirubin concentration falls below 14 mg/dl. If phototherapy is discontinued before 5 days of age, the serum bilirubin concentration should be remeasured 12 to 24 hours after cessation of phototherapy because a rebound in bilirubin concentration may occur.

Exchange Transfusion. Bilirubin can be toxic to the central nervous system under certain circumstances. Thus far, the association between increasing levels of serum bilirubin concentration below 20 mg/dl and developmental outcome in both full-term and preterm infants remains unresolved. A recent review in which the published literature regarding hyperbilirubinemia and its neurological effects was reviewed concluded that *at levels below 25 mg/dl in full-term infants who have no hemolysis, there is good evidence that hyperbilirubinemia does not cause significant cognitive, neurological, or hearing impairment.* Accordingly, for well, healthy full-term newborns who have no hemolysis, exchange transfusion should be performed if, despite intensive phototherapy, the bilirubin level remains between 25 and 29 mg/dl (425 to 500 μmol/l). For sick full-term infants or those in whom hemolysis is likely, an exchange transfusion should be performed at a lower total serum bilirubin level of 17 to 22 mg/dl (290 to 375 μmol/l).[3,5]

Diagnosis of hemolysis often is difficult without the advantage of special investigations. An infant who has hyperbilirubinemia within 24 hours should be considered to be hemolysing or ill and is not to be regarded in the same category as a well infant. A negative Coombs test does not rule out nonimmune causes of hemolysis. For instance, diagnosis of glucose-6 phosphate dehydrogenase deficiency requires an awareness of genetic background and should be considered in geographical regions in which the disease is prevalent and in certain ethnic groups including Sephardic Jews, or families of Middle Eastern, Nigerian, Chinese, or Mediterranean origin. In cases of G6PD deficiency, clinical jaundice often manifests initially after the first 24 hours of life, which is relatively late for the immune causes of hemolysis.

Much concern has been expressed regarding the risk of kernicterus in sick, low-birth-weight infants. Yellow-stained brain tissue has been reported at autopsy among premature neonates in whom the serum bilirubin concentrations were below 10 mg/dl. *In premature infants, serum bilirubin levels alone do not predict kernicterus accurately.* Thus decisions regarding the initiation of phototherapy and exchange transfusion should include consideration of possible risk factors contributing to bilirubin neurotoxicity, such as acidosis, hypoglycemia, and birth asphyxia, as well as those factors that promote delivery of bilirubin to the brain, such as displacement of bilirubin from albumin-binding (unbound bilirubin) or impairment of the blood-brain barrier.

Bilirubin normally binds with the serum protein albumin tightly in a one-to-one molar ratio because there is one primary binding site per molecule of albumin. If the molar concentration of bilirubin exceeds the molar concentration of albumin, then bilirubin can distribute beyond the intravascular albumin space, cross the blood-brain barrier, and produce neurotoxicity. Accordingly, unbound bilirubin possibly is a better predictor of long-term neurological outcome among jaundiced infants than is the serum-indirect bilirubin concentration.

The binding sites for bilirubin on albumin are saturated theoretically when a molar ratio of 1.0 is reached. This occurs when the *bilirubin/albumin ratio* is 9.0 (bilirubin expressed mg/dl divided by albumin in g/dl). Thus the lower the serum albumin level, the lower the bilirubin level required to reach saturation. Albumin levels are lower among sick and among premature infants. In addition to the absolute level of bilirubin, consideration must be given to the compounds that can compete against bilirubin for the albumin-binding sites. Sepsis and hemolysis reduce binding affinity and free fatty acids, and some drugs, including sulfonamides and diuretics, compete for bilirubin binding.

Some authorities have recommended using the bilirubin/albumin ratio as an indirect surrogate for the unbound bilirubin concentration. In 1994 Ahlfors[1] showed that if the bilirubin/albumin ratio was greater than 6.7, there was a greater than 65% chance of having a serum-unbound bilirubin level of greater than 20 nmol/l. When the bilirubin/albumin ratio reaches 8.0, approximately 95% will have more than 20 nmol/l unbound bilirubin in the serum. At that level of unbound bilirubin, nearly 90% of neonates will have an abnormal auditory brainstem response. Recommended exchange criteria extend over a broad range of total serum bilirubin levels at all gestational ages. Some authorities recently have recommended considering the bilirubin/albumin ratio to assist the decision whether to do or delay an exchange transfusion. Accordingly, when the bilirubin/albumin ratio is added to help fine tune established exchange criteria, a decision to perform an exchange transfusion is recommended if the bilirubin/albumin ratio exceeds 7 and is not declining upon intensive phototherapy. (The technique for performing an exchange transfusion is presented in Appendix B.)

THE INFANT OF THE MOTHER WHO HAS DIABETES

Maternal diabetes during pregnancy encompasses a range of metabolic disturbances involving carbohydrate intolerance with an elevation of serum glucose levels. Included with the mother who has long-standing insulin-dependent diabetes is the one who manifests glucose intolerance only during pregnancy (gestational diabetes).

Maternal hyperglycemia imposes a continuous glucose load on the fetus, since glucose readily crosses the placenta. In the face of continuing hyperglycemia, the fetal pancreatic islet cells undergo hypertrophy and hyperplasia, and the fetus produces large amounts of insulin from about 12 to 14 weeks of gestation. This hyperinsulinemia stimulates the intracellular transport of glucose and is the main mechanism of the diabetic fetopathy that produces infants who have enlarged and immature organs. The reported incidence of gestational diabetes varies from 0.15% to 12.3%. The highest prevalence rates are found among young African-American women. It now is recognized that *all pregnant women should be screened for gestational diabetes at least once during the course of their pregnancy.* The screening procedure consists of a 50 g glucose load that is administered orally and venous plasma glucose assessment 1 hour later. A serum glucose level ≥140 mg/dl (7.8 mmol/l) is considered a positive finding. This screening procedure has a sensitivity of 79% and a specificity of 11% for all pregnant women. A positive screening test result is followed by the oral glucose tolerance test.

Control of maternal diabetes is important to the outcome

of the fetus. Mothers who have diabetes who have good metabolic control before conception have a spontaneous abortion rate approximating that of the general population, whereas women who have poorly controlled diabetes have a significantly higher rate of pregnancy loss at all stages of gestation. Pregnancy loss correlates with the degree of hyperglycemia and with glycosylated hemoglobin levels in the first trimester. When adequate control of diabetes is not achieved, the pediatrician often must deal with complications among infants of affected mothers. These complications include congenital malformations, birth injury, neonatal asphyxia, hypoglycemia, respiratory distress, polycythemia, hyperbilirubinemia, hypocalcemia, and renal vein thrombosis.

Structural Abnormalities

At birth the infant of a diabetic mother (IDM) may have the classic appearance of being large for gestational age and lethargic. The head appears small because adipose tissue is concentrated around the trunk. Occasionally the infant is appropriately grown or even small for gestational age and is at great risk for teratogenesis with major organ system malformation. The major defects occur within four systems: *central nervous, cardiovascular, urinary tract, and gastrointestinal.*

The *caudal regression syndrome* comprises the classic central nervous system abnormality. This syndrome consists of absence or maldevelopment of the sacrum and coccyx, with hypoplastic femurs, dislocated hips, and defects in the tibias or fibulas. It occurs in 0.5% of diabetic pregnancies. *Neural tube defects* also are reported more frequently in diabetic pregnancies, as are hydrocephaly and microcephaly.

The incidence of *congenital heart disease* in IDMs is five times that of the general population. The most common malformations are septal defects, transposition of the great vessels, coarctation of the aorta, and situs inversus. The IDM also is susceptible to a cardiomyopathy secondary to asymmetrical septal hypertrophy from glycogen deposition in the myocardium. Hypertrophic changes may occur in the ventricular septum or in the subaortic valve area to produce a self-limiting idiopathic hypertrophic subaortic stenosis. Treatment with digoxin or other inotropic agents worsens the obstruction, but myocardial wall tension can be decreased with propranolol. Cardiomegaly with or without congestive heart failure can be seen on chest roentgenogram and may reflect prior hypoxia, hyperglycemia, hypocalcemia, or current hypertrophic cardiac disease.

Management

The pediatrician should be prepared to resuscitate the IDM, especially because delivery may be complicated by vigorous attempts to deliver a large infant vaginally. Thus birth injury commonly is encountered in the macrosomic infant; this takes the form of shoulder dystocia and associated fracture of the clavicle or humerus, or brachial plexus injury. Because polycythemia and hyperviscosity are common complications in the IDM, the umbilical cord should be clamped early to prevent an excessive placental transfusion.

Hypoglycemia. The hypoglycemia that occurs in the IDM largely is related to fetal hyperinsulinemia and can be aggravated by maternal hyperglycemia immediately before delivery. Hypoglycemia in the infant usually occurs within the first 1 to 3 hours of age, and the diagnosis is based on a blood glucose determination below 30 mg/dl (1.7 mmol/l) in term infants or below 20 mg/dl (1.1 mmol/l) in preterm infants. *Hypoglycemia often manifests no symptoms* because newborns have the capability to utilize alternative substrates, such as ketone bodies. Blood glucose screening should begin within the first hour of delivery and continue at least hourly for 6 hours; if the baby is stable, the screening is continued less frequently for the first 3 days. Glucose levels can be monitored in drops of whole blood obtained from heel pricks and a glucose oxidase enzyme method (Chemstrip or Dextrostix). If the infant shows symptoms or if the glucose screen shows a level of less than 45 mg/dl, the blood glucose should be measured directly.

Expectant management of the IDM should include an intravenous glucose infusion begun as early as possible, despite lack of symptoms. These newborns, apart from having hyperinsulinemia, are unable to produce glucose because they lack the normal neonatal surge in circulating free fatty acids, and they also have depressed glucagon levels. They should receive an infusion of glucose via peripheral vein at a dose of 4 to 6 mg/kg/min to bring and maintain the blood glucose levels to normal. Because it can be difficult to cannulate peripheral veins, the umbilical vein may provide convenient access, provided that the catheter is placed within the ductus venosus or in the inferior vena cava (with radiological confirmation). Symptomatic hypoglycemia can be prevented by this management, and early feeding should be initiated within the first 2 to 6 hours of life if the cardiorespiratory status allows it. Small feedings, starting with 5% glucose in water followed (importantly) by advancement to milk formula or breast milk, can be provided every 2 hours, and the intravenous infusion of glucose can be tapered once feeding is established and the patient's condition is stable.

Symptomatic hypoglycemia can have a wide range of clinical manifestations that include jitteriness, tremors, seizures, apathy, apnea, difficulty in feeding, and an abnormal cry. Because these symptoms may be caused by other life-threatening conditions, such as sepsis and asphyxia, it is imperative that the diagnosis of symptomatic hypoglycemia be confirmed by a blood glucose estimation and that the symptoms promptly disappear after parenteral glucose administration. Symptomatic hypoglycemia warrants immediate treatment with an intravenous infusion of 10% to 12.5% glucose that delivers 6 mg/kg/min. The response to treatment should be monitored every 15 minutes until the blood glucose level has normalized. Treatment should *not* be instituted with a rapid infusion of 25% to 50% glucose because of its high osmolality and because it also stimulates insulin secretion, resulting in "rebound" hypoglycemia. If hypoglycemia persists despite glucose infusion of 12 mg/kg/min, then glucagon administered intramuscularly (0.3 mg/kg) generally will maintain the blood glucose at normal levels for 2 to 3 hours.

Refractory hypoglycemia can be treated with hydrocortisone (5 mg/kg/day divided into three doses), which usually will stabilize the glucose level. The physician should ensure that hypoglycemia has not been induced by inappropriate treatment with hypertonic glucose infusion and that an umbilical arterial catheter does not deliver glucose above the level of the diaphragm because this circumstance may stimulate pancreatic insulin secretion. In rare cases, refractory hypoglycemia is caused by hyperinsulinism accompanying disorders of the pancreas.

The IDM is at increased risk for several other neonatal problems. Among these is respiratory distress syndrome, which may be caused by an inhibition of surfactant production secondary to fetal hyperinsulinemia. The synthesis of phosphatidylcholine and phosphatidylglycerol (PG) is inhibited in the IDM. Monitoring of fetal lung maturity during the diabetic pregnancy calls for the assessment of both the amniotic fluid lecithin/sphingomyelin (L/S) ratio and the amniotic PG. An L/S ratio of less than 2:1 indicates a high potential risk for respiratory distress syndrome. Because of the delay in the appearance of PG among IDMs, the usually adequate L/S ratio of 2:1 does not completely ensure a low risk for respiratory distress syndrome, because low PG itself also is associated with respiratory distress syndrome, despite a normal L/S ratio. Therefore an amniotic PG measurement also should be obtained, in addition to the L/S ratio; in the absence of a biochemical assay for PG, an L/S ratio greater than 3:1 generally correlates with an adequate PG level.

The IDM also is prone to respiratory distress from causes other than surfactant deficiency (hyaline membrane disease). The infant is at increased risk for transient tachypnea of the newborn, which can be related to such conditions as asphyxia, hyperglycemia, retained lung fluid, congestive heart failure, and polycythemia. The incidence of physiological hyperbilirubinemia is increased in the IDM (see previous section). Management should include the usual modalities of phototherapy and exchange transfusion.

Chronic intrauterine hypoxia often occurs in the IDM. This stimulates erythropoietin production, resulting in an increased incidence of polycythemia (central hematocrit >65) and hyperviscosity. In addition, the IDM is susceptible to an excessive placental transfusion at delivery. Because this adds to the polycythemia, the cord should be clamped immediately after delivery of the body to minimize further postnatal placental transfusion.

The appropriate treatment for polycythemia and hyperviscosity is a partial exchange transfusion. This consists of the removal of the patient's blood and its isovolemic replacement with a volume expander, usually 5% albumin or saline. Most authors agree that such treatment of polycythemia should be begun only when signs become detectable. These include arterial and venous thromboses, pulmonary hemorrhage, apnea, lethargy, transient tachypnea (with evidence of interlobar fluid on chest roentgenogram), jitteriness, and hypoglycemia. There also may be signs of impending congestive heart failure and necrotizing enterocolitis. Patients who have central hematocrit values in excess of 65% who display the foregoing symptoms should receive a partial exchange transfusion. The indications for treatment in symptom-free patients who have hematocrit values *below* 65% to 70% are not pressing. When the hematocrit level is above 70% to 75% at less than 12 hours after birth, it also is best to treat with a partial exchange transfusion, even in the absence of symptoms.

TRANSIENT TACHYPNEA OF THE NEWBORN

Transient tachypnea of the newborn (TTN) refers to one of the commonest causes of respiratory distress in the neonatal period. It is believed to be caused by a delay in the absorption of the normal fetal lung fluid. Between 2 and 6 hours after birth, tachypnea, grunting, chest wall retractions, and (often) cyanosis in room air develop. Typically the symptoms are mild and resolve within 72 hours after birth. The terms *wet lung* and *transient tachypnea* refer to the same condition.

The fetal lung secretes fluid that fills the airways. During vaginal delivery some of this fluid is squeezed out of the major airways, but the remainder takes between 2 and 6 hours to be reabsorbed from the alveoli. This fluid passes into the interstitial space and then into the perivascular lymphatics and venules. According to hypothesis (the Starling equilibrium), this resorption can be impeded by (1) decreased capillary or lymphatic oncotic pressure (e.g., low serum protein, often found in premature infants), (2) increased capillary or lymphatic hydrostatic pressure (e.g., hypervolemia and polycythemia, which may occur with delayed cord clamping), (3) increased alveolar or interstitial fluid osmotic pressure, or (4) decreased alveolar or interstitial fluid hydrostatic pressure.

Thus, as normal lung fluid is being absorbed during the first 4 hours of life, mild respiratory symptoms may be accepted as a variant of normal; the diagnosis of TTN should not be made unless symptoms persist or progress beyond 4 hours. Infants born by cesarean section are not subjected to a thoracic squeeze and the resultant expulsion of lung fluid that occurs during passage through the birth canal. Consequently, with increased lung fluid present, they commonly manifest mild transient tachypnea. Birth asphyxia and premature labor also predispose to TTN.

Transient tachypnea (wet lung syndrome) usually occurs in the more mature preterm infant (34 to 37 weeks) and in term infants born by cesarean section. Tachypnea usually persists beyond the first few hours, peaks by 6 to 36 hours, and resolves in 5 or 6 days. The clinical picture is characterized by signs of air-trapping with widening of the anteroposterior diameter of the chest. The liver often is palpable well below the right costal margin because it is pushed down by pulmonary hyperaeration. Tachypnea shortly after birth in the full-term or more mature preterm infant must be differentiated from pneumonitis (e.g., meconium aspiration and bacterial infection), air leak (e.g., pneumothorax and pneumomediastinum), pulmonary vascular congestion resulting from congestive heart failure or polycythemia, and the respiratory restriction imposed by congenital diaphragmatic hernia or cystic adenomatoid malformation of the lung. Last, tachypnea in the face of a normal-appearing chest roentgenogram may be symptomatic of a central nervous system disorder (such as drug withdrawal) or a metabolic derangement (such as acidosis, hyperthermia, or hypoglycemia).

Newborns who have mild TTN usually do not need more than 40% oxygen to maintain adequate oxygenation (PaO_2 of 50 to 70 mm Hg), but the severity may vary and rarely may require intermittent positive pressure ventilation for respiratory failure. TTN is nonprogressive, and supplemental oxygen usually is not necessary for longer than 1 to 3 days. Treatment of the excess lung water is not required. Because bacterial pneumonia cannot practically be excluded from the initial diagnostic presentation as a primary cause or secondary complication, antibiotics should be given after blood cultures have been obtained. Oral feedings should be suspended because the ability to suck and swallow may be impaired by the respiratory difficulty. Intravenous fluids should be minimized to equal only insensible fluid losses and to maintain serum glucose concentration.

The radiological changes of transient tachypnea are characteristic and help to differentiate it from hyaline membrane disease. According to Wesenberg[8]:

> The earliest radiographs usually are taken at age 2 to 6 hours, when the tachypnea becomes evident clinically. In infants having the most lung fluid, the initial radiographs show a pattern of diffuse bilateral alveolar edema with concomitant hyperaeration of the lungs, sternal retraction, and an air bronchogram effect. In the next 8 to 10 hours, there is progressive clearing of the alveoli, with some patients developing a bilateral granular or miliary pattern suggestive of hyaline membrane disease. This is a transitory stage, usually lasting only several hours. The lung fields remain hyperaerated. The pulmonary vascularity becomes prominent during this stage. This then progresses to complete clearing of the alveoli, with congestive pulmonary vascularity secondary to interstitial edema, engorged perivascular lymphatics, and the standard pulmonary capillaries. Occasionally, a small amount of pleural fluid is present. The lower lobes are last to clear. The clearing pattern of the lung fluid is thus from peripheral to central and upper to lower lung fields. By 48 to 72 hours, the chest radiographs are within normal limits.

Occasionally the fetus will inhale a small amount of amniotic fluid into the already fluid-filled upper airway. Amniotic fluid has more protein than does fetal lung fluid, and the increased protein concentration lowers the oncotic gradient between the alveoli and the pulmonary lymphatics. Amniotic fluid also contains desquamated cellular debris and lanugo. After delivery, this debris is transported into the alveoli and may produce a syndrome indistinguishable from TTN. Such aspiration of amniotic fluid occurs more frequently in breech deliveries because the thoracic squeeze occurs while the head is still within the uterine cavity and the cord is compressed between the infant and the pelvic brim. These asphyxiated infants are more likely to gasp in utero and inhale their amniotic fluid. If the fetus has passed meconium, it also will be inhaled into the upper airway. Such *aspiration of meconium must be prevented* because it can cause a life-threatening pneumonitis, usually accompanied by severe pulmonary air trapping, respiratory failure, and pulmonary hypertension. Therefore, when delivery is imminent and thick (particulate) meconium is present in the amniotic fluid, attendants should prepare to suction the oropharynx of the infant as soon as the head delivers and before the first breath; immediately after delivery of the infant the trachea should be suctioned with an endotracheal tube to clear the meconium.

Intrauterine passage of meconium increases with advancing gestation to a frequency as high as 30% by 42 weeks. In addition to meconium aspiration, postmature infants (older than 42 weeks of gestation) are at risk for hypoglycemia and intrauterine asphyxia as a result of uteroplacental insufficiency. These three potential problems should be anticipated in postmature infants. Hyperaeration may persist for 4 to 5 days in infants who aspirate clear amniotic fluid.

LOW BIRTH WEIGHT

The commonest causes of low birth weight are prematurity and intrauterine growth retardation.

Prematurity

Accurate assessment of gestational age is critical to the appropriate care of the mildly to moderately premature infant, because knowledge of gestational age guides management, helps one to anticipate potential problems, and provides a standard by which to assess developmental changes related to postconceptional age (gestational age at birth plus postnatal age). Traditionally, many problems of the premature infant have been related to the more easily and accurately measured birth weight rather than to gestational age because, for a large population of appropriately grown infants, the two are closely related. In the individual patient, however, the use of birth weight alone may lead to overestimating or underestimating potential problems often related to immaturity. Considering only newborns who are appropriately grown for gestational age (AGA), a birth weight of 1700 g may be associated with a gestational age of 30 to 35 weeks; yet a baby who weighs 2500 g at birth may have a gestational age of 33.5 to 39 weeks. Thus the infant born weighing more than 1700 or even more than 2500 g still may be at significant risk for perinatal problems that relate to prematurity, not size.

Standard criteria have been developed to assess gestational age in the first 3 days after birth. Physicians who care for newborns must become skilled in the use of these methods because maternal dates may not be accurate and birth weight per se may not accurately reflect the perinatal problems likely in the individual patient; *the frequency of most neonatal problems decreases as gestational age increases.*

Premature Infant: Birth Weight 1700 g or More. Despite the major physiological differences between infants of equal birth weight but of different gestational age, most countries maintain neonatal mortality statistics according to birth weight. Thus, in what follows, we consider the gestational age of the infant who weighs 1700 g or more. For the fetus whose gestation has progressed 32 to 38 weeks, a small risk remains for development of severe neonatal problems related to prematurity (e.g., hyaline membrane disease, persistent patent ductus arteriosus, necrotizing enterocolitis, sepsis and pneumonia, symptomatic apnea, and intracranial hemorrhage). Fortunately, however, the problems of the premature infant beyond 32 to 33 weeks of gestation and weighing more than 1700 g most often are not severe or life threatening and are limited mainly to simple apnea, hyperbilirubinemia, and an inability to feed orally or to maintain body temperature outside an incubator. Management of these infants ordinarily is well within the competence of most primary care facilities (i.e., level I or level II nurseries). Nonetheless, physicians who accept responsibility for the care of these infants must be aware of the signs of more serious disorders that should be recognized promptly if they are to be managed optimally.

The cause of premature onset of labor should be determined, inasmuch as a small portion of cases may occur because of placental abruption, a multiple gestation, or a uterine abnormality. Spontaneous and *premature rupture of membranes* has been associated with an increased incidence of neonatal infection. The risk of neonatal septicemia increases when membranes have been ruptured for longer than 24 hours.

Obstetrical management of the preterm fetus that has had its membranes ruptured prematurely can be assisted by daily fetal biophysical profile assessment. The first manifestations of impending fetal infection usually are a nonreactive nonstress test result and the absence of fetal breathing movements. Loss of fetal movements and fetal tone are later and more ominous signs of fetal infection. A poor fetal biophysical profile in patients whose membranes have ruptured prematurely may be an early predictor of fetal infection and can help determine obstetrical management.

Management of infants born after prolonged rupture of membranes should include careful observation for such subtle signs of infection as lethargy, poor feeding, hyperthermia, hypothermia, early hyperbilirubinemia, jitteriness, poor skin perfusion, diarrhea, or abdominal distention as a result of ileus. Prematurity may mask some signs of the nonspecific origin of sepsis.

Examination of placentas from a large group of premature infants frequently reveals evidence of chorioamnionitis. Therefore clinical signs of amnionitis, such as uterine tenderness or maternal fever, indicate the need to obtain a culture specimen from the neonate and to initiate antibiotic treatment. Prophylactic antibiotics administered to the mother before delivery will not treat fetal infection effectively and actually may impair accurate cultures of the newborn (false negative culture results). Any clinical sign of infection in a premature newborn warrants cultures of blood and cerebrospinal fluid, followed by treatment with appropriate antibiotics. It is the usual practice to culture blood, cerebrospinal fluid, and urine specimens and treat with ampicillin and gentamicin for 3 to 4 days while definitive culture results are pending. Significant systemic signs of infection, such as pneumonia, seizures, apnea, or shock, may mandate active treatment of sepsis for 7 to 10 days, even in the absence of positive culture results.

Certain laboratory tests are helpful in the diagnosis of chorioamnionitis. A gram stain of a gastric aspirate taken before the first feed, showing more than five cells per high-powered field and the presence of organisms, indicates chorioamnionitis, but not necessarily fetal infection. Histopathological examination of the placenta is the definitive method of diagnosis.

Management. For infants whose birth weight is between 1700 and 1900 g (less than 36 weeks), respiration and heart rate should be monitored during the first 10 days at least because there is some risk of apnea. Until consistent weight gain is established, these infants should remain in incubators kept at the "neutral temperature" to maintain body heat and to prevent excessive caloric expenditure. Some newborns of very low birth weight in this weight range may grow rapidly in a bassinet, but they are exceptions to the rule.

Management of feedings and fluids is the most important aspect of care for the healthy, mildly to moderately premature infant. Feedings can be initiated within the first 24 hours after birth in the infant who is stable and has experienced no preceding perinatal distress or birth asphyxia (which may have compromised intestinal perfusion). During the first 8 hours of life, little is to be gained by initiating feeds with sterile water. Breast milk or dilute proprietary formula may be given orally or by a gastric tube in an initial volume of 2 to 4 ml/kg every 3 hours. Newborns whose gestational age is less than 34 weeks are fed initially by nasogastric tube. Proprietary formulas that have a 60:40 whey:casein ratio more closely resemble human milk and are better suited for the preterm infant. Unmodified cow milk is not suitable for the preterm newborn because its predominant casein content is not well tolerated.

Breast milk may be fed to any preterm newborn whose mother wishes to do so and who can supply it. The milk is collected individually into a sterile container after careful washing of the breast and nipple. When possible, the milk is given immediately to the infant. Otherwise it is refrigerated for up to 24 hours and either used or immediately frozen. Once full-volume feedings are well tolerated, breast milk needs to be fortified with carbohydrate, protein, and essential minerals to provide optimal nutrition for the growing premature newborn. Special powdered preparations for breast milk fortification are available that, when added to breast milk, bring up the caloric density to that of standard premature formulas (80 Cal/dl).

If feeding must be delayed or is not well tolerated, 10% dextrose in 25% normal saline should be infused intravenously. Fluid and caloric intake should be calculated daily, and growth measurements of length, weight, and head circumference should be plotted weekly so that caloric intake can be assessed adequately. Feeding volumes should be increased slowly from 60 to 80 ml/kg/day but only if tolerated without emesis or increasing gastric residual volumes of formula before feedings. A total fluid volume of 150 to 180 ml/kg/day or 100 to 120 kcal/kg/day should be reached by 7 days of age. Fluid requirements depend largely on environmental conditions. The newborn receiving phototherapy, for instance, may well require increased fluid.

When the newborn is ready to progress from tube to oral feeding, the tube may be used for an extra 12 to 24 hours to measure gastric residual. A residual of more than 3 to 4 ml immediately before the next feeding suggests intolerance; this situation may require a reduction in the feeding volume but only after systemic illness is carefully considered and excluded. Abdominal distention or bile-stained gastric drainage from a properly positioned gastric tube (not in the duodenum) warrants immediate cessation of feedings and evaluation of the intestinal tract. Examination of the stool for macroscopic and microscopic blood should be performed. Microscopic blood (positive occult blood test result) may not in itself suggest a pathological condition unless it becomes more severe or represents a recent change.

Although coordination of sucking and swallowing develops around 33 to 34 weeks of gestation, the care of each infant should be managed individually and cooperatively between physician and nurse. The nurse experienced at feeding premature infants can provide helpful guidance concerning the infant's tolerance of the workload imposed by oral feeding. No more than 30 minutes ordinarily should be spent coaxing an infant to take a feeding if he or she lacks sufficient endurance to persist in sucking. Infants should be cuddled comfortably and securely in the feeder's lap: great benefit can be derived from cuddling and close body contact during feeding. The bottle should be held so that air rises in the upturned bottle and the infant sucks in milk and not air through the nipple. The bottle should never be propped unattended for a young infant.

Patients are discharged from the hospital when they can maintain body temperature in a bassinet, feed sufficiently on demand, and show evidence of normal growth.

The overall prognosis for the premature infant between 33 and 38 weeks of gestation is good because of an inherently lower incidence and a better tolerance of severe neonatal problems. For the healthy premature newborn weighing more than 1700 g, survival and outcome approach those of full-term infants. Intellectual function generally is normal.

The Infant Who Is Small for Gestational Age

The infant whose birth weight is at or below the tenth percentile for gestational age is considered small for gestational age (SGA). Poor fetal weight gain results from aberrant maternal, placental, or fetal circumstances that restrain growth. Other categories in which these infants may be placed include *light-for-date, intrauterine growth retardation,* and *dysmaturity.* These infants show an increase in perinatal mortality (both fetal and neonatal) that is four to eight times that of the appropriately grown infant of equal gestational age.

Early diagnosis is difficult, and most patients are diagnosed after birth. A high index of suspicion, accompanied by serial physical examinations, during which progressive growth of the uterine fundus is palpated through the abdominal wall, aids early diagnosis. A fundal height less than 4 cm or less than that for the estimated gestational age suggests poor intrauterine growth. This clinical impression can be confirmed by careful fetal ultrasound examination. Ideally, serial ultrasound measurements of fetal growth parameters should be obtained. The head/abdominal ratio (as defined by the head circumference divided by the abdominal circumference) is used to detect asymmetrical (abdomen undergrown relative to head) forms of intrauterine growth retardation. The normal ratio is approximately 1 from 32 to 36 weeks and less than 1 from 36 weeks to term.

Etiological Factors. Growth of the fetus is determined by genetic, nutritional, and environmental factors. Fetal factors that can compromise growth potential include (1) congenital abnormalities, (2) congenital infections—for example, toxoplasmosis, rubella, cytomegalovirus, herpes, and syphilis (TORCH infections), (3) chromosomal defects, and (4) inborn errors of metabolism. Inherent fetal conditions usually result in early growth retardation and an actual reduction in the number of fetal cells. These patients appear symmetrically growth retarded (head and abdomen equally undergrown). Maternal factors include low maternal weight (less than 50 kg), poor weight gain during pregnancy, and chronic maternal disease, especially conditions that produce hypoxemia or reduce placental blood flow (e.g., chronic hypertension, preeclampsia, toxemia, cyanotic congenital heart disease, and sickle cell disease). Drug ingestion, including alcohol, cigarette smoke, and heroin, can affect the quality of fetal growth adversely. Phenylketonuria often results in decreased fetal growth and microcephaly; thus the maternal diet must be controlled strictly during pregnancy.

During the third trimester, less than adequate maternal-placental transport becomes the major growth-limiting factor, despite normal fetal growth potential. Optimal fetal growth depends on the placenta for nutrient and gaseous exchange. The placenta promotes fetal growth by actively transporting amino acids and synthesizing chorionic somatomammotropin, which is responsible for mobilizing maternal substrate for the fetus. Diminished placental function thus will affect total nutrient and gaseous transfer adversely, resulting in fetal growth retardation. Placental insufficiency is associated classically with postmaturity; it therefore is understandable that placental abnormalities, such as chronic abruption, infarction, single umbilical artery, and multiple fetuses, affect the transfer of fetal nutrients directly during the third trimester. The box below lists factors associated with poor intrauterine growth.

Clinical Presentation. The SGA infant may be "symmetrically" growth retarded in some cases; in others, birth weight may be reduced relatively more than length and head circumference. Fetuses subjected to third trimester "starvation" may be of normal length but appear wasted at birth. The skin is parchmentlike, and the head appears too large for the body. These infants often are termed *asymmetrically growth retarded.* These various presentations offer some insight into etiological factors because symmetrical growth retardation

FACTORS ASSOCIATED WITH POOR INTRAUTERINE GROWTH

Maternal

1. Prepregnancy weight <50 kg
2. Poor nutrition; poor weight gain during pregnancy; socioeconomic factors
3. Maternal illness:
   a. Associated with uterine ischemia: hypertensive vascular disease, preeclampsia, diabetes mellitus, sickle cell anemia, autoimmune vasculitis
   b. Associated with chronic hypoxia: cyanotic congenital heart disease, high altitude
4. Drug ingestion:
   a. Drugs that affect fetal growth directly, e.g., ethanol, methadone, heroin
   b. Drugs that inhibit placental blood flow (nicotine)
5. Multiple gestation, primiparity, grand multiparity

Placental

1. Villitis associated with congenital infections (TORCH infections)
2. Ischemic villous necrosis or infarction
3. Chronic separation (abruptio placentae)
4. Diffuse fibrinosis
5. Abnormal insertion
6. Umbilical vascular thrombosis

Fetal

1. Syndromes associated with diminished birth weight; e.g., Cornelia de Lange syndrome, Potter disease, anencephaly, and dwarfism
2. Metabolic disorders (inborn errors of metabolism)
3. Chromosomal disorders: trisomies 13, 18, 21; XO
4. Congenital infections: TORCH infections, malaria, varicella

usually implies a more chronic problem—for example, chromosomal or congenital infection.

If based on physical criteria alone, gestational age assessment of the SGA infant may be misleading. Because less vernix is produced in these infants, the skin is exposed continuously to amniotic fluid and will begin to desquamate after birth. Sole creases are more mature and breast tissue markedly reduced as a result of the diminished estriol levels. Ear cartilage also may be diminished. In contrast, neurological criteria are affected less by intrauterine growth retardation than are physical criteria, inasmuch as organ maturation continues despite diminished somatic growth. Moreover, stress in utero may even promote the maturation of some organ systems, such as the lung. This may explain why respiratory distress syndrome is less frequent among SGA infants.

Because the SGA infant is prone to perinatal asphyxia and its sequelae, optimal management should begin with antenatal assessment. Expert resuscitation must be provided for these infants in the delivery room, with strict attention paid to the prevention of possible meconium aspiration, because decreased placental reserve and decreased cardiac glycogen stores put the fetus at risk for perinatal asphyxia. The fetus should be delivered if at or near term, but even earlier if tests of placental function, such as stress and nonstress monitoring, indicate fetal compromise. When gestational age is not known, the risks of preterm birth can be defined better by assessing pulmonary maturity by use of amniocentesis (lecithin/sphingomyelin ratio). Occasionally, maternal disease will necessitate delivery of a preterm, growth-retarded infant who will be prone to all the complications of both immaturity and growth retardation (see the box below).

The SGA newborn, especially when showing evidence of third trimester wasting with low ponderal index, is more prone to fasting hypoglycemia because of decreased glycogen stores and impaired gluconeogenesis. Thus blood glucose values must be determined frequently in the first few days after birth. Hourly recordings are recommended in the first 4 hours of life. Thereafter, if the newborn is stable, measurements of blood glucose levels can be spaced more widely. If asymptomatic hypoglycemia occurs (whole blood glucose concentrations less than 30 mg/dl during the first 3 days in term or 20 mg/dl in preterm newborns), a glucose infusion of 4 to 8 mg/kg/min should be started. If symptomatic hypoglycemia—especially concomitant with seizure activity—has occurred, an intravenous bolus of 10% dextrose in water at 200 mg/kg (2 ml/kg) should be given, followed by constant infusion of glucose. As a consequence of their increased metabolic rate, these infants often need a higher caloric intake.

Attention to thermoregulation is required because decreased subcutaneous fat stores impair conservation of body heat. This is important in delivery room management where these patients frequently are compromised by perinatal asphyxia. Radiant heat and warm, dry towels will help to maintain the newborn's body temperature during neonatal resuscitation.

A thorough examination for clinical stigmata of congenital infection is indicated in all SGA babies, as is appropriate screening for intrauterine infection. This should include estimation of total IgM and a urine culture for cytomegalovirus. A urine (and especially stool) "screen" for illicit drugs may provide evidence of maternal drug exposure otherwise denied. Because chronic fetal hypoxia stimulates erythropoietin production, polycythemia and hyperviscosity also should be excluded.

Prognosis. The growth and developmental outcome for the SGA infant depend on the cause of the growth failure. The prognosis is poorest for infants who have congenital infections, chromosomal disorders, and severe congenital abnormalities. Intellectual development in the remaining infants depends on the presence or absence of adverse perinatal events, in addition to the specific etiological factors of the growth retardation. Even when perinatal problems are minimal, the SGA infant may have developmental handicaps. Developmental problems should be looked for beyond infancy and may not become manifest until 2 to 5 years of age or even later. Term SGA infants may exhibit little difference in developmental quotient during infancy, but their school performance is poor, in part because of behavioral and learning disabilities. SGA infants who demonstrated decreased fetal head growth earlier than 26 weeks of gestation have diminished developmental quotients in infancy. SGA infants, however, are a heterogeneous group; in some follow-up studies of both term and preterm SGA infants, they have compared well developmentally with appropriate-for-gestational-age (AGA) infants. Perhaps this discrepancy in developmental outcome is related to obstetrical and early neonatal management and to the quality of home care and parental involvement.

With regard to postnatal growth, the cause of the intrauterine growth retardation and the time of its onset during gestation will dictate the infant's growth potential. Newborns who have early-onset intrauterine growth retardation (because of an intrauterine infection, teratogen, or chromosomal abnormality) will remain small throughout life. Those who have late-onset third trimester intrauterine growth retardation, however, may show evidence of catch-up growth in the first 6 months of life and usually catch up to their AGA counterparts.

NEONATAL PROBLEMS IN INFANTS OF LOW BIRTH WEIGHT

Preterm

Respiratory distress syndrome
Patent ductus arteriosus
Retinopathy of prematurity
Hyperbilirubinemia
Necrotizing enterocolitis
Intraventricular hemorrhage

Small for gestational age

Perinatal asphyxia
Meconium aspiration
Polycythemia

Common to both groups

Fasting hypoglycemia
Temperature instability
Hypocalcemia

REFERENCES

1. Ahlfors CE: Criteria for exchange transfusion in jaundiced newborns, *Pediatrics* 93:488, 1994.
2. American Academy of Pediatrics, Committee on Fetus and Newborn: Home phototherapy, *Pediatrics* 76:136, 1985.
3. American Academy of Pediatrics, Subcommittee on Hyperbilirubinemia: *Management of hyperbilirubinemia in the healthy term newborn,* 1994 (in press).
4. Maisels MJ: Jaundice in the newborn, *Pediatr Rev* 3:305, 1982.
5. Maisels MJ: Jaundice. in Avery GB, Fletcher MA, MacDonald MG, editors: *Neonatology: pathophysiology and management of the newborn,* ed 4, Philadelphia, 1994, JB Lippincott.
6. National Institutes of Health Consensus Development Conference Statement in Infantile Apnea and Home Monitoring, NIH Pub No 87-2905 6:3, 1986.
7. Newman TB, Maisels MJ: Evaluation and treatment of jaundice in the term newborn: a kinder, gentler approach, *Pediatrics* 89:809, 1992.
8. Wesenberg RL: Wet lung disease and aspiration of clear amniotic fluid. In Wesenberg RL, editor: *The newborn chest,* Hagerstown, Md, 1973, Harper & Row.

SUGGESTED READINGS

Cornblath M: Hypoglycemia. In Nelson NM, editor: *Current therapy in neonatal-perinatal medicine,* vol 2, Philadelphia, 1990, BC Decker.

Dickinson JE, Palmer SM: Gestational diabetes: pathophysiology and diagnosis, *Semin Perinatol* 14:2, 1990.

Kliegman RM, Hulman SE: Intrauterine growth retardation: determinants of aberrant fetal growth. In Fanaroff AA, Martin RJ, editors: *Neonatal-perinatal medicine: disease of the fetus and infant,* ed 4, St Louis, 1987, Mosby.

Lawrence S, Yeomans ER, Rosenfeld CR: Intrauterine growth retardation: pediatric aspects. In Nelson NM, editor: *Current therapy in neonatal-perinatal medicine,* vol 2, Philadelphia, 1990, BC Decker.

Maisels MJ: Hyperbilirubinemia. In Nelson NM, editor: *Current therapy in neonatal-perinatal medicine,* vol 2, Philadelphia, 1990, BC Decker.

Meyer BA, Palmer SM: Pregestational diabetes, *Semin Perinatol* 14:12, 1990.

Vintzileos AM, Campbell WA, Nochimson DJ: Premature rupture of the membranes. In Nelson NM, editor: *Current therapy in neonatal-perinatal medicine,* vol 2, Philadelphia, 1990, BC Decker.

48 Critical Neonatal Illnesses

Keith H. Marks and M. Jeffrey Maisels

It is important for the physician who is called on to treat the newborn in a critical situation to be able to make a diagnosis, institute immediate management, and plan for appropriate continuing consultation in caring for the patient. Errors or omissions may result in permanent damage or death, so recognition and immediate resuscitation of a baby in distress require an organized plan for the actions of immediately available and qualified personnel, supported by the proper equipment.

The emergence throughout the Western world of regionalized systems for neonatal care has played a crucial role in the general improvement in neonatal outcome and has made it possible and desirable for almost all critically ill infants to be cared for in a tertiary care neonatal center. Assuming that most primary care physicians embrace this approach, the following discussion deals mainly with those conditions that require recognition, initial management, and stabilization preceding the transport of infants to such centers.

Safe and efficient transport of an infant requires an organized approach.* Here we deal specifically with the preparation and stabilization of the infant before transport. In doing so we will cover those critical situations with which the primary care physician must deal immediately.

The resources available at the hospital of birth will determine the need for transport. In general, therefore, transport should be considered when those resources immediately available (equipment, support services, expertise, and available *time* of the attending physician) are inadequate to deal with the infant's current or anticipated medical and surgical problems. Note, however, that the decision to transfer a newborn should be made only *after* consultation with the neonatologist at the receiving hospital so that bed availability can be confirmed and preparations undertaken.

STABILIZATION

Certain basic laboratory investigations should be performed on every critically ill infant (see the box on p. 551); every hospital should be capable of performing these tests rapidly. The information so gained frequently provides an accurate diagnosis (e.g., the chest roentgenogram reveals evidence of hyaline membrane disease or of cardiomegaly; the hematocrit reading indicates polycythemia as the cause of respiratory distress) and leads to appropriate intervention.

By far the most frequent reason for referral of an infant to a neonatal intensive care facility (ICU) is the onset of respiratory distress soon after birth. Such infants most often demonstrate tachypnea, retractions, expiratory grunting, nasal flaring, and, frequently, cyanosis. However, they may show only apnea or shock. An approach to the differential diagnosis of respiratory distress is shown in the box on p. 551.

In some cases the suddenness and severity of the distress make it apparent that immediate referral to an ICU is necessary. In others, the major challenge to the primary care physician is to separate those infants whose respiratory distress or cyanosis may only be transient and are likely to improve, from those whose condition almost certainly will deteriorate and necessitate further investigation and intervention.

Changes in clinical status can occur with frightening rapidity; thus constant vigilance is necessary to anticipate and prevent potentially disastrous deterioration. Infants who have respiratory failure require immediate referral to a neonatal center. *Respiratory failure can be anticipated as imminent or actual when any of the following signs is present:*

- Increasing tachypnea, retractions, and grunting
- Persistent tachycardia with minimal variability in heart rate
- Poor peripheral perfusion (shock)
- Congestive heart failure
- Cyanosis unresponsive to the administration of oxygen at 40% or greater concentrations
- Apnea
- Rising $Paco_2$, falling pH, and falling Pao_2

Any infant who is cyanotic and does not respond to the administration of oxygen requires immediate attention. Central cyanosis (as opposed to peripheral acrocyanosis) should never be disregarded in the hope that it will disappear. Such infants inevitably get worse, and their cyanosis requires urgent investigation and treatment. Many cyanotic infants also have significant respiratory distress, so their referral tends to be effectively mandated; others, however, may appear merely "dusky" and not suffer from respiratory distress, thus inviting an unwise expectant temporization before eventual emergent transfer. By definition, cyanosis reflects the presence in the circulation of at least 3 g of reduced (desaturated) hemoglobin. *Central* cyanosis (as opposed to *peripheral* acrocyanosis) implies cyanosis of the lips, tongue, and oral mucous membranes. Because cyanosis is produced by a definitive amount (not relative concentration) of desaturated hemoglobin, it may be detected even at high arterial oxygen saturations, should the total hemoglobin concentration be sufficiently elevated (polycythemia). In other words, polycythemic infants actually may have normal Pao_2 levels yet be clinically cyanotic. Conversely, when the hemoglobin concentration is low, as in severe anemia, significant central cyanosis may not be visually apparent, despite substantial arterial desaturation. The *immediate investigations required in all cyanotic infants* are as follows:

- Chest roentgenogram
- Measurement of O_2 saturation by pulse oximetry

*Discussed in detail in American Academy of Pediatrics and the American College of Obstetricians and Gynecologists: *Guidelines for perinatal care*, Elk Grove Village, Ill, 1992, The Academy.

- Measurement of arterial Po_2, Pco_2, and pH
- Response of the Pao_2 or O_2 saturation to breathing 100% oxygen
- Hematocrit, blood glucose determinations
- Electrocardiogram

Any infant who is cyanotic and whose Pao_2 does not respond promptly to the administration of 100% oxygen should be referred immediately to an appropriate center for treatment. Such infants are likely to have *cyanotic congenital heart disease, persistent pulmonary hypertension* (persistent fetal circulation), or *severe respiratory disease*.

The approach to all critical situations is similar—namely, to establish and maintain vital functions. Thus the *maintenance of oxygenation, perfusion, blood glucose, and body temperature is the cornerstone of successful initial management*.

LABORATORY INVESTIGATIONS TO BE PERFORMED ON ALL ACUTELY ILL NEWBORN INFANTS

- Venous or arterial hematocrit
- Rapid reagent strip glucose screening (Dextrostix or Chemstrip) and quantitative laboratory blood glucose determination
- Portable chest roentgenogram
- Measurement of O_2 saturation by pulse oximetry
- Arterial (or arterialized capillary*) Po_2, Pco_2, and pH
- White cell count and differential
- Blood culture
- Response of infant's Pao_2, and Sao_2 to breathing oxygen

*These measurements are unreliable in the presence of shock or when the Pao_2 exceeds 50 to 60 mm Hg.

Ventilation

The first thing to consider is that *oxygen should be provided in whatever concentration (including 100%) is necessary to keep the baby pink.* This point cannot be overemphasized! The legacy of the alleged association between hyperoxia and retinopathy of prematurity (ROP) continues to haunt us, with the fear of litigation subverting reasoned judgment. However, no clear relation between *brief* periods (several hours) of hyperoxia (Pao_2 levels >150 mm Hg) and ROP has ever been documented. Moreover, recent data suggest that there may be an association of ROP with episodes of *hypoxemia* (Pao_2 <40 mm Hg). Thus, although emphasis historically has been placed on the necessity for avoiding hyperoxia, it may be equally if not more important to avoid periods of hypoxia, as well as of compromised perfusion.

Degrees of "pinkness" cannot be used to estimate Pao_2 levels reliably; therefore actual measurements of arterial blood gases or oxygen saturation by pulse oximetry are necessary for optimal management. The wide availability of pulse oximetry has removed much of the guesswork from the assessment of oxygenation. Pulse oximetry is simpler and more reliable than capillary blood gas measurement. Supplemental oxygen should be given sufficient to maintain the baby's Pao_2 within the range of the normal newborn (50 to 100 mm Hg) or the oxygen saturation (Sao_2) to >90%. Oxygen should be warmed, humidified, and delivered using an oxygen hood. If, despite breathing 100% oxygen, the baby remains cyanotic, or if the Pao_2 is less than 50 mm Hg, or the Sao_2 is less than 90%, then the infant should receive artificial ventilation. The use of early nasal constant positive airway pressure (CPAP) at 5 cm H_2O pressure may obviate the subsequent need for mechanical ventilation.

Assisted ventilation also is indicated if respiratory failure is evidenced by recurrent apnea, a $Paco_2$ greater than 50 to

CAUSES OF RESPIRATORY DISTRESS IN THE NEWBORN

Pulmonary causes

Common

- Hyaline membrane disease
- Transient tachypnea of the newborn (TTN)
- Meconium aspiration
- Primary pulmonary hypertension

Occasional

- Pulmonary hemorrhage
- Pneumonia
- Pneumothorax
- Pulmonary dysmaturity

Rare

- Airway obstruction
  - Choanal atresia
- Space-occupying lesion
  - Diaphragmatic hernia
  - Cysts
  - Tumors

Nonpulmonary causes

Cerebral

- Hemorrhage
- Edema

Metabolic

- Acidosis
- Hypoglycemia
- Hypothermia

Hematological

- Hypovolemia
  - Acute blood loss
  - Twin-to-twin transfusion
- Hyperviscosity

60 mm Hg (and rising), and a pH of less than 7.25, with a rising $Paco_2$ or Pao_2 of less than 50 mm Hg in 70% to 100% oxygen. Infants meeting these criteria should receive ventilation, preferably through an endotracheal tube. Should someone skilled in infant intubation not be immediately available, then bag and mask ventilation must be used.* The bag used must be capable of delivering 100% oxygen (see section on delivery room management in Chapter 44, and Fig. 44-3 for the technique of bag and mask ventilation). An orogastric tube should be in place to prevent gastric distention.

The correct management of respiratory acidosis is ventilation, not "buffering" with intravenous (IV) sodium bicarbonate. Among infants who have severe hyaline membrane disease, it invariably is necessary to perform endotracheal intubation (see Appendix B for technique to be used) to ensure adequate ventilation. Intubation also allows the application of positive end-expiratory pressure (PEEP), which is critical to maintaining adequate oxygenation by overcoming atelectasis. The instillation of exogenous pulmonary surfactant can lower the risk of complications of mechanical ventilation.

Perfusion

Infants who are in shock have a low effective circulating blood volume and show all the signs of poor perfusion: paleness, mottled skin, and poor capillary filling. Adequate capillary filling is present when normal pink color returns to the toes within 3 seconds after squeezing. In practice, capillary filling time has only limited accuracy in newborns, and the information must be interpreted with caution. Recent studies suggest that in older infants and children capillary refill is a highly unreliable measurement and almost totally dependent on ambient room temperature. In the premature infant who is several hours to days old, and in a controlled thermal environment, delay in capillary filling may be useful in the assessment of peripheral perfusion. When applied to full-term infants who normally are much more acrocyanotic in the first several hours, a prolonged capillary refill time may be present in those who are perfectly normal.

The infant in shock also frequently has cyanosis, tachycardia, and acidosis but may or may not have low blood pressure. The blood pressure should be determined by the oscillometric technique (e.g., DynaMap). Table 48-1 shows normal systolic and diastolic levels for newborns at various birth weights. The oscillometric method, used carefully, is quite accurate for the noninvasive determination of arterial blood pressure, but two important conditions must be met: (1) the width of the cuff must be at least 50% to 60% of the limb circumference and (2) the infant must be quite still during the measurement to prevent motion artifact in the readings. The physician should note, however, that *many infants, despite severe underperfusion, may maintain normal blood pressure by means of vasoconstriction. Thus a normal blood pressure by no means rules out the diagnosis of shock* (hypoperfusion of the peripheral tissues).

Hypovolemia is the single most important cause of shock and always should be considered when metabolic acidosis exists. Shock is treated by expanding the circulating blood volume by use of 10 to 20 ml/kg of normal saline, lactated Ringer, or a 5% albumin solution and, if necessary, packed red blood cells given over 5 to 10 minutes.

*Diaphragmatic hernia is one situation in which bag and mask ventilation should not be used (see p. 553).

Table 48-1 Blood Pressure in Newborns

Birth weight (g)	Systolic (mm Hg)		Diastolic (mm Hg)	
	5%	95%	5%	95%
1000	35	58	16	36
1500	40	62	19	39
2000	43	67	22	41
2500	48	70	25	43
3000	50	73	28	48
3500	54	78	30	49
4000	58	81	31	51

Data from Versmold HT et al: *Pediatrics* 67:607, 1981.

Metabolism

Blood glucose concentration should be determined on all sick infants by a semiquantitative screening technique (Dextrostix or Chemstrip). If the screening test indicates a blood glucose level of less than 45 mg/dl, then quantitative laboratory analysis of blood glucose should be performed. If hypoglycemia is thus documented as present (quantitative blood glucose level of <40 mg/dl), it is treated by administration of a continuous IV infusion of 10% dextrose in water solution. An initial bolus of 3 to 4 ml/kg should be given slowly over about 5 minutes and the infusion then continued at a rate of 5 ml/kg/hr—this provides 8 mg/kg/min of glucose. Another Dextrostix test should be performed within 15 minutes. If the blood glucose level remains persistently low, 15% glucose in water solution should be infused. If there still is no response, hydrocortisone (5 mg/kg) should be given every 12 hours (see Persistent Neonatal Hypoglycemia, p. 553).

All sick infants, and particularly those of very low birth weight, require meticulous attention to thermoregulation. The body temperature should be maintained in the neutral thermal environment (see Fig. 44-5) so these newborns should be swaddled in plastic wrap or similar insulating material.

Most sick infants have some degree of ileus and should not be fed by mouth. All require IV fluids. An appropriate IV solution is 0.2% saline in 10% dextrose in water administered initially at a rate of 50 to 60 ml/kg/day. Adjustments to this rate of fluid administration may be required if the infant has hypoglycemia or evidence of gastrointestinal obstruction, when large amounts of fluid may be lost into the bowel lumen.

Metabolic acidosis occurs when organic acids accumulate in tissues that are hypoxemic or underperfused. Other causes are loss of bicarbonate (which does not occur in the first hours or days of life) and some rare inborn errors of metabolism. The proper treatment of metabolic acidosis is directed to its cause rather than to its effect (i.e., adequate oxygenation and perfusion should be provided rather than bicarbonate given). The administration of sodium bicarbonate should be limited to those very few infants in whom metabolic acidosis is not self-corrected by the time the Po_2 is normal and adequate perfusion has been ensured. Respiratory acidosis is, by definition, an elevation of the $Paco_2$ and therefore can be treated only by the use of assisted ventilation; bicarbonate administration is not indicated in this situation.

SPECIFIC CONDITIONS

Abstinence Syndrome

Infants born to mothers who are users of narcotics have withdrawal symptoms in the first days of life. When the symptoms include severe irritability and tremors (which prevent normal feeding), vomiting and diarrhea, seizures, hypothermia or hyperthermia, or severe tachypnea, then treatment is indicated. Phenobarbital, paregoric, diazepam, and methadone all have been used to treat neonatal narcotic withdrawal. Paregoric is a useful and easy drug to use and is administered orally in a dose of 0.05 to 0.1 ml/kg body weight every 6 hours. If there is no improvement, the dose is increased by two drops per dose until clinical improvement is apparent (see Chapter 49, Neonatal Drug Abstinence Syndrome).

Ambiguous Genitalia

The finding of ambiguous genitalia must raise the suspicion of congenital adrenal hyperplasia, which can produce convincing masculinization of the female external genitalia, leading to unfortunate (and difficult to retract) misassignment of sex in the delivery room. Some of these infants have a salt-losing syndrome and develop profound hyponatremia with vascular collapse. Congenital adrenal hyperplasia therefore should be suspected in all infants whose genitalia are ambiguous, as well as in all those who are vomiting or have dehydration or failure to thrive in the first weeks of life. Treatment involves expansion of the circulating volume with isotonic saline and subsequent administration of glucocorticoids. Diagnosis is confirmed by serum and urinary electrolyte patterns, hormonal measurements, and occasionally, karyotyping.

Diaphragmatic Hernia

Diaphragmatic hernia occurs in 1 in 2200 live births and almost always (90%) is found on the left side. The infant may show very little respiratory distress or may be profoundly distressed with severe cyanosis that is unresponsive to ventilation. The diagnosis should be considered if the infant has a flat or scaphoid abdomen or if bowel sounds are heard in the chest. Because the hernia usually is on the left, heart sounds may be displaced to the right. The diagnosis is confirmed by a chest roentgenogram. All these infants should be given 100% oxygen and have a large-bore (10 or 12 Fr) orogastric tube inserted into the stomach, to which intermittent suction at low pressure is applied. If respiratory distress is significant, endotracheal intubation and intermittent positive pressure ventilation must be performed. This is one of the few situations in which bag and mask ventilation is contraindicated because this forces gas into the intestinal tract, thus increasing distention of the intestine that lies within the thorax and compromising pulmonary function further.

Gastroschisis or Omphalocele

Infants who have gastroschisis or omphalocele may suffer from severe evaporative fluid loss and hypothermia. They are managed best by placing the entire body below the shoulders in a bowel bag (a clear sterile plastic bag). A drawstring permits the bag to be tightened at the level of the axillae, preventing both heat and fluid loss. A large-bore (10 to 12 Fr) orogastric tube should be inserted and intermittent suction applied to decrease intestinal distention. Intravenous fluids should be administered at a rate of 8 to 10 ml/kg/hr while the baby is transported to a tertiary care pediatric facility where definitive corrective surgery can be performed.

Hydrops Fetalis

The care of women likely to deliver infants who have severe erythroblastosis should be managed exclusively in perinatal centers capable of the full range of obstetrical and neonatal intensive care. The successful management of these previously doomed infants demands a comprehensive team approach that includes intensive monitoring and vigorous treatment of asphyxia, acidosis, hypoglycemia, and hypothermia. Assisted ventilation frequently is required.

Hypoglycemia

The maintenance of a normal blood glucose concentration in the newborn is important because glucose is the primary energy substrate for the brain. Thus hypoglycemia may result in central nervous system (CNS) damage. Newborns have brain weights that are greater in relation to body weight than is the case in adults and thus are at greater risk from the effects of hypoglycemia. Long-term follow-up studies regarding the neurological impairment of infants who have had symptomatic hypoglycemia in the newborn period indicate that *hypoglycemia represents a critical situation for the newborn.* This requires that all nurseries have a plan to screen newborns for hypoglycemia and to institute immediate therapy when it is diagnosed.

Glucose should be monitored on all premature infants and newborns who are either large for gestational age (LGA) or small for gestational age (SGA) until the plasma glucose is stable within the normal range.

We recommend that any infant, term or preterm, who has a Dextrostix determination of blood glucose of 45 mg/dl or less have an immediate quantitative blood glucose level (glucose oxidase method) determined in the laboratory. Infants with (1) a whole blood glucose level of less than 35 mg/dl in the first 24 hours or 40 mg/dl thereafter or (2) a plasma glucose level of less than 40 mg/dl in the first 24 hours or 45 mg/dl thereafter require immediate intervention and subsequent glucose monitoring.

Transient Neonatal Hypoglycemia. CNS abnormalities—for example, septooptic dysplasia associated with agenesis of the septum pellucidum, malformation of the optic chiasma, agenesis of the corpus callosum, and growth hormone deficiency—all can cause transient neonatal hypoglycemia. Other causes include SGA and LGA infants, asphyxia, anoxia, respiratory distress syndrome, sepsis, cold injury, prolonged starvation, and abrupt cessation of IV hypotonic glucose solution. Infants of diabetic mothers (IDMs), as well as those whose mothers have been given certain drugs (e.g., propranolol) and those who have erythroblastosis fetalis also are prone to develop symptomatic transient hypoglycemia of the newborn. Finally, this difficulty may develop in some infants without apparent predisposing causes.

Persistent Neonatal Hypoglycemia. Any of the following conditions can give rise to persistent hypoglycemia in the newborn:

1. Pancreatic defects
    a. Hyperinsulinism
    b. Nesidioblastosis
    c. Islet cell adenoma
    d. Focal adenomatosis

e. Microadenomatosis
f. Beta-cell hyperplasia
g. Beckwith-Wiedemann syndrome
h. Idiopathic leucine sensitivity
2. Hereditary defects of carbohydrate metabolism
a. Glycogen storage diseases
b. Deficiencies of enzymes important to gluconeogenesis
c. Other enzyme defects such as galactosemia and hereditary fructose intolerance
3. Hereditary defects in amino acid and organic acid metabolism
a. Maple syrup urine disease
b. Propionic acidemia
c. Methylmalonic aciduria
d. Tyrosinosis
e. 3-hydroxy-3-methylglutaric aciduria
f. Glutaric aciduria type II
4. Hereditary defects of fat metabolism
a. Systemic carnitine deficiency
b. Carnitine palmitoyl transferase deficiency
5. Hormone deficiencies
a. Congenital hypopituitarism
b. Hypothalamic abnormalities that lead to diminished production of growth hormone, cortisol, adrenocorticotropic hormone (ACTH), glucagon, thyroid hormone, and catecholamines.

Although the clinical manifestations of neonatal hypoglycemia are varied, they may include episodes of tremor (jitteriness), apnea, cyanosis, irregular respirations, limpness, twitching, sweating, hypothermia, weak cry, refusal to feed, eye rolling, and convulsions. Among infants at risk for hypoglycemia it is common practice to estimate the plasma glucose concentration by Dextrostix as soon as possible after birth, at 2 hours, and again at 4 to 6 hours of age. In all infants at increased risk for hypoglycemia, including those small for gestational age and of diabetic mothers, it is advisable to monitor blood glucose levels more frequently until the plasma glucose is stable within the normal range and oral milk feedings have been well established. In the event of a confirmed blood glucose reading of less than 45 mg/dl, the infant should be started immediately on a feeding of 5% glucose, followed by standard formula feedings at intervals of 2 to 3 hours. The blood glucose level should be monitored before each feeding. Adequate glucose concentrations usually can be maintained by this regimen; however, if plasma glucose values remain below 40 mg/dl, an IV infusion of 10% glucose should be started to provide 5 to 8 mg/kg/min of glucose. On rare occasions when hypoglycemia persists despite such an infusion of glucose, hydrocortisone may need to be administered intravenously or intramuscularly at intervals of 12 hours (5 mg/kg body weight/dose). On this regimen the blood glucose level in most infants should stabilize rapidly. The IV infusion of glucose can be tapered after 48 hours and the cortisone therapy gradually eliminated during the subsequent 4 to 5 days. Should the hypoglycemia persist for more than 72 hours on this regimen, other causes must be sought (see Chapter 285, Hypoglycemia).

Meningitis

For a discussion of meningitis, see Chapter 230.

Pneumothorax

Spontaneous pneumothorax occurs in 0.5% to 2% of all newborns but with much greater frequency among infants who have severe hyaline membrane disease or aspiration pneumonia. The clinical diagnosis may be entertained when an infant shows signs of respiratory distress with breath sounds that are decreased on one side. This physical sign, however, may be very difficult to elicit, particularly in the small premature infant; a more reliable technique therefore is to transilluminate the chest with a high-intensity fiberoptic light. Increased lucency on one side of the chest suggests the presence of a pneumothorax. Ultimately, however, the gold standard for diagnosis is the chest roentgenogram, which reveals lucency in one hemithorax, partial collapse of the lung, and displacement of the mediastinum to the opposite side of the chest. Indeed, a roentgenogram of the chest should be part of the routine assessment of all ill newborns.

A small pneumothorax in a full-term infant, which produces only mild distress, may well require no therapy other than observation. On the other hand, in an infant who is severely distressed and has cyanosis or bradycardia (as signs of cardiovascular compromise by a tension pneumothorax), immediate evacuation of the accumulated intrathoracic air is essential. This is performed by inserting a no. 21 scalp vein needle through the chest wall, usually at the superior edge of the third or fourth rib, in the anterior axillary line. The needle is connected to an airtight stopcock and a 50-ml syringe. As the needle is advanced into the chest, negative pressure is applied to the syringe until air enters it. This procedure, which may at first appear intimidating, actually is remarkably simple and relatively safe; because the intercostal blood vessels course along the inferior border of the rib, there is no danger of producing a hemorrhage by inserting the needle over its superior rim. Furthermore the presence of the pneumothorax tends to prevent inadvertent puncture of the lung. Even if a lung puncture or a hemorrhage does occur, rarely is either severe.

Persistence of a significant pneumothorax requires insertion of a chest tube, although an Intracath may be used as a temporary device for transporting the baby to a neonatal ICU. If an Intracath or a chest tube is left in place, it should be connected to underwater drainage. If no underwater seal is available, a one-way Heimlich flutter valve may be used (Bard-Parker No. 3460).

Respiratory Distress

For a discussion of respiratory distress, see Chapters 46, Signs and Symptoms of Neonatal Illness, and 47, Common Neonatal Illnesses.

Seizures

For a complete discussion of neonatal seizures, see Chapter 256, Seizure Disorders.

Shock, Including Sepsis

Shock may be defined as an acute hemodynamic disturbance that causes significant and generalized reduction of capillary blood flow throughout the body, with consequent decreased tissue perfusion and anoxia, which, if prolonged, leads to a generalized impairment of cellular function. The major causes of shock in the newborn are hypovolemia, sepsis, severe congestive heart failure with low cardiac output (e.g., the hypoplastic left heart syndrome), and rarely endocrine failure (hypoadrenocorticism) (see also Chapter 292, Shock).

Hypovolemic Shock. Shock caused by hypovolemia most often is attributable to (1) hemorrhage associated with obstetrical accidents or malformations of the placenta and cord, (2) occult hemorrhage from the fetus into the maternal circulation or into a twin fetus, and (3) internal hemorrhages (e.g., ruptured liver or spleen, intracranial hemorrhage, or adrenal hemorrhage—see the box below).

Loss of plasma (rather than whole blood) from the circulatory system sometimes can be severe enough to cause hypovolemic shock (e.g., the exudation of severe extensive peritonitis, necrotizing enterocolitis, or gastroschisis).

Loss of fluid and electrolytes also may cause dehydration sufficient to reduce the circulating blood volume and result in hypovolemic shock similar to that caused by actual hemorrhage. Causes in the newborn include fluid losses in severe diarrhea or vomiting, inadequate intake of fluid and electrolytes (particularly with the use of potent diuretics), or inadequate replacement of large insensible water losses from the very premature infant.

The relation between cardiac output and hypovolemia depends not only on the amount of blood or fluid lost but also on the rate of that loss; during slow bleeding compensatory mechanisms come into play for which there is insufficient time if the bleeding is acute. Clinical signs of shock may not become apparent until 10% to 25% of the blood volume has been lost, if that loss is sufficiently slow. The immediate reaction of the body to oligemia from acute, unreplaced blood loss is to maintain circulation to vital areas (brain, heart, adrenals, and lungs) by sacrifice of perfusion (vasoconstriction) of less vital vessels in the skin, muscles, and splanchnic bed. Initiated by powerful sympathetic reflexes that stimulate the release of circulating epinephrine, this compensatory mechanism increases the peripheral resistance and raises the blood pressure but decreases the tissue perfusion. This emergency increase in peripheral sympathetic activity is manifested clinically by tachycardia and rapid, shallow, and irregular respirations, as well as by pale and cold skin that frequently appears mottled because capillary filling is slow. The low peripheral venous pressure also manifests clinically by empty peripheral veins; thus it may be difficult to introduce a transfusion needle.

Reflexes from pressure receptors initially maintain total body perfusion to some extent in the early shock state by increasing cardiac output. When blood loss exceeds this compensation, however, shock ensues. With the decrease in venous return to the heart and consequent poor cardiac filling, poor cardiac output results eventually in a further drop in blood pressure. Ischemic damage to the myocardium then may produce myocardial failure, which further reduces cardiac output and aggravates the fall of arterial blood pressure. At this state the infant usually will display gasping respirations and an altered state of consciousness. The peripheral pulses are weak, and the blood pressure is low or unobtainable.

When the blood volume lost is more than that which can be compensated, blood pressure falls to produce what is known as *uncompensated oligemic shock*. If the oligemia is not severe, circulating blood volume may be restored partially by absorption of fluid from interstitial tissues and gradual replacement of red cells so that blood pressure is reasonably well maintained; this is known as *compensated oligemic shock*.

TYPES OF HEMORRHAGE IN THE NEWBORN

Obstetrical accidents and malformation of the placenta and cord

- Rupture of a normal umbilical cord
  - Precipitous delivery
  - Entanglement
- Hematoma of the cord or placenta
- Rupture of an abnormal umbilical cord
  - Varices
  - Aneurysm
- Rupture of anomalous vessels
  - Aberrant vessel
  - Velamentous insertion
  - Communicating vessels in multilobed placenta
- Incision of placenta during cesarean section
- Placenta previa
- Abruptio placentae

Occult hemorrhage before birth

- Fetoplacental
  - Tight nuchal cord
  - Cesarean section
  - Placental hematoma
- Fetomaternal
  - Traumatic amniocentesis
  - Following external cephalic version, manual removal of placenta, or use of oxytocin
  - Spontaneous
  - Chorioangioma of the placenta
  - Choriocarcinoma of the placenta
- Twin-to-twin transfusion
  - Chronic
  - Acute

Internal hemorrhage

- Intracranial
- Giant cephalohematoma, subgaleal, or caput succedaneum
- Adrenal
- Retroperitoneal
- Ruptured liver, ruptured spleen
- Pulmonary

Iatrogenic blood loss

- Blood sampling

Modified from Oski FA, Naiman JL: *Hematological problems in the newborn,* ed 3, Philadelphia, 1982, WB Saunders.

Diagnosis. In the evaluation of acute blood loss from the fetus at the time of delivery, the bleeding site, appearance of the blood, signs of blood loss, and evidence for disordered hemostasis all should be considered. The sites and common causes of bleeding are listed in the box on p. 555.

A mandatory part of the diagnosis is to examine the placenta and cord carefully in an attempt to ascertain the site of blood loss. Factors in the obstetrical history that should arouse suspicion of hemorrhage include placenta previa, abruptio placentae, and antepartum hemorrhage occurring in the third trimester. A traumatic delivery should arouse suspicion of possible internal bleeding (e.g., intracranial hemorrhage, ruptured liver or spleen, and hemorrhage into the retroperitoneal space). Hemorrhage into the adrenal glands may manifest as enlarging abdominal masses. This also may occur with subcapsular hematoma of the liver or spleen.

The appearance and intensity of signs and symptoms depend on the amount and rate of bleeding. The blood pressure may be normal, whether indirectly measured by the oscillometric technique or by a pressure transducer connected directly to an umbilical artery catheter. The hemoglobin concentration and hematocrit reading often are normal initially but may be low if measured immediately after hemorrhage. It must be emphasized that if the infant is in shock, capillary hemoglobin and hematocrit levels may be misleadingly high because of peripheral sludging and stasis, so hemoglobin and hematocrit levels should be determined only on central venous blood samples obtained as blood is drawn for crossmatching. If the hemoglobin level initially is high, then the determination should be repeated and the level followed closely during the next 12 to 24 hours of life to observe the fall expected as hemodilution occurs.

Fetomaternal hemorrhage is diagnosed by demonstrating the presence of fetal red cells in the maternal circulation (Kleihauer-Betke test). A twin-to-twin transfusion should be suspected when a hemoglobin difference greater than 5 g/dl exists between identical twins. Hemoglobin and hematocrit levels should be determined on venous blood to prevent sampling errors that might lead to misinterpretation of results.

The metabolic response to acute blood loss also depends on the degree of the hemorrhage. If recruitment of extracellular fluid and contraction of the great veins are sufficient to compensate for the loss of circulating blood volume, then the metabolic response will be slight and signs and symptoms transient. With further blood loss the increased glycolysis and lipolysis are manifested by increased blood glucose, fatty acid, and lactate levels in the blood. A respiratory alkalosis can be detected in the arterial blood gas levels, and decreased urinary sodium and volume are noted. With more severe blood loss a severe lactic acidosis occurs, and severe oliguria is noted.

Optimal treatment has but four goals:

1. *Ensure adequate ventilation and oxygenation.* Poor tissue perfusion results in anoxia and anaerobic metabolism with metabolic acidosis, which may be aggravated in the presence of hypoxia. Therefore oxygen should be administered and an adequate airway ensured. An endotracheal tube may be necessary for intermittent positive pressure ventilation.
2. *Stop the hemorrhage.* An infant who has a ruptured liver generally appears to be well for 24 to 48 hours and then suddenly goes into shock, coinciding with that time when the gradually increasing hematoma finally ruptures the hepatic capsule and hemoperitoneum occurs. The spleen also may rupture after a difficult delivery, particularly if it already is enlarged as a result of severe erythroblastosis. Both these situations may require an operation after adequate resuscitation by blood transfusion.
3. *Restore the circulating blood volume by transfusion.* Treatment should be directed toward restoration of cardiac output and tissue perfusion to prevent the ongoing effects of continuing anoxia. If significant hypovolemia is suspected, it should be treated with repeated small infusions of volume expanders given over 5 to 10 minutes (5 to 10 ml/kg). The neonate's response should be assessed after each infusion. Therapy is stopped only when tissue perfusion is judged adequate (improved mental state, urinary output, skin color, and temperature). Group O, Rh-negative packed red cells crossmatched against the mother's blood are best to use but may not be available. For unanticipated shock the infant's own heparinized placental blood may be used in an emergency. This is obtained from the umbilical cord after sterilization with a solution of 1% iodine and 70% alcohol. Blood is withdrawn into a 20-ml syringe containing 1 ml of 50 U/ml heparin and administered by use of the filter from an IV blood administration set. Alternatively 5% albumin, lactated Ringer, or normal saline may be used.

   The amount of blood, plasma, or lactated Ringer solution that should be infused must be determined by the response of the infant to a satisfactory circulatory blood volume: the pulse rate should come down; the skin should become pink, warm, and dry; the urinary volume should increase; the central venous pressure should rise to normal; and the blood pressure should rise. Note that the hemoglobin level should be estimated only with caution in assessing the amount of blood to be transfused, particularly if whole blood is administered, inasmuch as normal transfused blood has a low hematocrit; any attempt to restore a neonate's hemoglobin level to normal by using transfused blood may result in overtransfusion; total blood volume (not red cell mass) is critical in these situations.
4. *Improve cardiac function with external cardiac massage and appropriate drugs when indicated.** If the heart rate is less than 100 beats/min and does not increase to normal with ventilation, then closed-chest cardiac massage should be instituted at a rate of 120 chest compressions per minute (see Appendix A). Drug therapy rarely is necessary for resuscitation of infants in the delivery room. When cardiotonic agents are needed, they should not be administered until adequate ventilation has been established; the preferred route for administration is the umbilical vein. Epinephrine and naloxone also can be administered through an endotracheal tube (Table 48-2).

*This is discussed in detail in American Academy of Pediatrics: *Textbook of neonatal resuscitation*, Dallas, 1990, American Heart Association.

Table 48-2 Medications for Neonatal Resuscitation

Medication	Concentration to administer	Preparation (ml)	Dosage/route*	Total dose/infant			Rate/precautions
				Weight (kg)	**Total ml**		
Epinephrine	1:10,000	1	0.1-0.3 ml/kg	1	0.1-0.3		Give rapidly
				2	0.2-0.6		
			IV or IT	3	0.3-0.9		
				4	0.4-1.2		
Volume expanders	Whole blood	40	10 ml/kg	1	10		Give over 5-10 min
	5% Albumin		IV	2	20		
	Normal saline			3	30		
	Lactated Ringer			4	40		
Sodium bicarbonate	0.5 mEq/mL	20	2 mEq/kg		**Total dose (mEq)**	**Total ml**	Give *slowly,* over at least 2 min
		or		1	2	4	
	(4.2% solution)	two 10 prefilled syringes	IV	2	4	8	Give only if infant being effectively ventilated
				3	6	12	
				4	8	16	
Naloxone	0.4 mg/ml	1	0.25 ml/kg		**Total ml**		
				1	0.25		
			IV, IM, SQ, IT	2	0.50		
				3	0.75		
				4	1.00		Give rapidly
	1.0 mg/ml	1	0.1 ml/kg	1	0.1		
				2	0.2		
			IV, IM, SQ, IT	3	0.3		
				4	0.4		
Dopamine	$\frac{6 \times \text{weight (kg)} \times \text{desired dose (µg/kg/min)}}{\text{desired fluid (ml/hr)}}$ = mg of dopamine per 100 ml of solution		Begin at 5 µg/kg/min (may increase to 20 µg/kg/min if necessary) IV		**Total µg/min**		Give as a continuous infusion using an infusion pump
				1	5-20		
				2	10-40		Monitor HR and BP closely
				3	15-60		Seek consultation
				4	20-80		

From American Academy of Pediatrics: *Textbook of neonatal resuscitation,* Dallas, 1990, American Heart Association.
**IM,* Intramuscular; *IT,* intratracheal; *IV,* intravenous; *SQ,* subcutaneous.

The immediate and obvious effects of hemorrhage are on the general circulation, but virtually all vital organs (lungs, kidneys, liver, gut, muscle) are likely to display evidence of impaired perfusion. Less frequently considered, but often altered, are body chemical composition, the hormonal settings that control fluid, fuel, and electrolyte balance, neurological function, circulating inflammatory mediators, and the antibacterial defense systems.

After resuscitation the infant may become irritable and have involuntary muscular movements, often resulting from electrolyte abnormalities. Many of these infants have hypoglycemia, hypokalemia, and hypocalcemia in the first days after birth. They often require 10% glucose administered intravenously to keep blood glucose levels above 45 mg/dl, as well as additional calcium gluconate (200 to 400 mg/kg/24 hr).

Increased pulmonary capillary permeability often persists, even after perfusion pressure is restored to normal, so transient pulmonary edema with worsening respiratory distress should be anticipated by frequent monitoring of arterial blood gases. The patient may suffer from increased susceptibility to pulmonary infection after a major hemorrhage, which increases pulmonary insufficiency. The effect of severe hemorrhage on the gastrointestinal tract also is significant: small ulcerations may occur in the stomach and progress to necrotic ulcers; alterations in the distribution of blood flow combined with the general decrease in blood flow, producing ischemic injury to the mucosa, can result in enterocolitis. The liver often is damaged by severe hemorrhage; jaundice with an elevation of liver enzymes is a frequent finding, and centrilobular necrosis with fatty infiltration of the liver is found at autopsy. Disorders of hemostasis with bleeding are common after hemorrhagic shock and generally are associated with a deficiency of coagulation products caused by disseminated intravascular coagulation.

Septic Shock. A complex form of shock can result from bacterial infection. The most common bacteria that cause septic shock in neonates include *group B streptococci* and gram negative *Escherichia coli* (which may produce endotoxic shock). The physician should suspect overwhelming herpesvirus infection in infants in whom an acute shocklike state develops within 7 to 10 days after delivery, particularly when there is a history of exposure to maternal genital herpesvirus infection.

Septic ("hot") shock is characterized by vasodilation of peripheral vessels with the loss of peripheral resistance, a drop in the blood pressure, poor tissue perfusion, diminished venous return, and reduced cardiac output. Damage to the capillary endothelium results in an increase in capillary permeability, edema, and loss of fluid from the intravascular space into the extravascular tissues, resulting in hypovolemia and a shocklike state. A direct toxic effect on the heart with cardiac failure may occur, as well as toxic effects in other vital organs noted above.

The onset of respiratory distress or apnea together with shock in full-term or preterm infants ominously heralds group B streptococcal disease. Signs include low blood pressure, congested mottled skin, and the effects of the toxin on other vital organs. The underlying illness, such as peritonitis or necrotizing enterocolitis, may modify the vascular response because of superimposed hypovolemia.

The diagnosis of neonatal septicemia ultimately depends on a positive blood culture, but cerebrospinal fluid and urine cultures also should be obtained. Indirect evidence of the presumptive diagnosis of overwhelming sepsis includes abnormally elevated or depressed neutrophil band counts with thrombocytopenia. Disseminated intravascular coagulation with generalized bleeding may complicate the shock.

Treatment for presumed neonatal septicemia must be instituted immediately after appropriate diagnostic studies have been performed, including a blood culture, spinal tap, and urine culture. Antibiotics must be administered before final or even initial identification of the responsible microorganism. The choice of antibiotic depends on the location of the infection, as well as on the timing of the onset of septic shock. When the presumed septicemia occurs within the first 48 to 72 hours of life (perinatal infection), antibiotic coverage with ampicillin and gentamicin (or cefotaxime) most often is used. In late septicemia, secondary to hospital-acquired infection, a penicillinase-resistant penicillin or vancomycin should be given in combination with an aminoglycoside such as amikacin or gentamicin. Once the specific pathogen has been identified, the best combination of drugs is selected on the basis of susceptibility of the organism in vitro.

Although correct antibiotic therapy is the key to successful management of neonatal septic shock, competent supportive measures also are essential. These include increasing the circulating blood volume by transfusion of packed red cells, 5% albumin, or lactated Ringer, as necessary. An attempt to improve cardiac function and vasomotor tone with use of cardiotonic drugs should be considered. Careful monitoring of fluid balance is necessary, with intake and output measurements taken while monitoring fluid and electrolyte status. Gastric dilation, increased gastric secretion, and ileus are common; the stomach and bowel should be decompressed to prevent aspiration. In severe, overwhelming sepsis the use of an exchange transfusion and infusion of granulocytes may be effective, although more knowledge needs to be gained in this area.

Cardiogenic Shock. Cardiogenic shock usually is associated with underlying severe congestive heart failure, with low cardiac output states secondary to an obstructive lesion of the left ventricular outflow tract, such as severe coarctation of the aorta or hypoplastic left heart syndrome. Because there is no output from the left ventricle, the venous blood returning to the left atrium must pass through the atrial septum to the right atrium. The smaller the atrial opening, the greater the pulmonary venous hypertension and congestion—hence the earlier the appearance of symptoms. These infants generally have poor pulses (although they may be normal early in life), mild to moderate cyanosis, characteristic mottling of the skin, and hepatomegaly. Diagnosis is made by clinical, radiographical, electrocardiographic, and especially echocardiographic procedures, followed rapidly by cardiac catheterization and surgery in selected infants. Prostaglandin E_1 (0.05 μg/kg/min IV) should be infused to maintain the patency of the ductus arteriosus (to bypass the obstructed left ventricular outflow) before surgical correction of the lesion.

Shock Resulting from Hypoadrenocorticism. In the neonatal period bilateral adrenal hemorrhage after a traumatic delivery can lead to shock from blood loss and adrenal insufficiency. A mass may be palpable in each flank and visible on abdominal ultrasound examination. The disorder occurs most often in large infants who have had a traumatic delivery, and it must be differentiated from renal vein thrombosis. The latter is associated with gross hematuria, whereas in an adrenal hemorrhage the hematuria usually is microscopic. Infants who have unilateral adrenal hemorrhage do not have symptoms of adrenal insufficiency, but they may experience shock from blood loss.

Congenital adrenal hyperplasia is a group of inherited autosomal recessive disorders caused by the absence of essential enzymes in the pathways for synthesis of cortisol and aldosterone. The interruption of the normal negative-feedback systems stimulates excessive release of ACTH and overactivity in the biosynthetic steps preceding the block, with a resultant accumulation of androgenic steroids. The most common variety is 21-hydroxylase deficiency, which may be seen in affected females as virilization at birth, including clitoral hypertrophy and variable fusion of the labia minora. *These masculinized girls may tragically be misdiagnosed as males with hypospadias and cryptorchism.* Prompt recognition of this problem is less easy in males, who may not be diagnosed easily before an adrenal crisis, which usually occurs in the second week of life. The crisis often is preceded by vomiting and poor weight gain and is characterized biochemically by low serum sodium and high serum potassium levels.

A salt-losing crisis demands urgent therapy with IV saline, glucose, and hydrocortisone, whereas the aim of long-term management must be to suppress the hyperplastic adrenal glands and provide replacement hydrocortisone and a salt-retaining steroid such as fluorocortisone. Elevation of the plasma 17-hydroxyprogesterone level confirms the diagnosis of 21-hydroxylase deficiency, and cortisol is the drug of choice for replacement of glucocorticoid action in adrenal insufficiency. Acutely the use of desoxycorticosterone (DOCA), 1 mg intramuscularly, is indicated and will not interfere with the measurement of the 17-hydroxyprogesterone. Hydrocortisone (Solu-Cortef) is given intravenously as a 50-mg bolus, with an additional 25 mg placed in the IV maintenance solution. Should the patient decompensate further, 5% albumin (10 ml/kg), instead of isotonic saline, should be given. The use of morphine, barbiturates, or other sedatives is contraindicated. Potassium should not be added to any of the IV fluids. A prompt and complete endocrinological evaluation and maintenance therapy are required for these infants.

Esophageal Atresia and Tracheoesophageal Fistula

The diagnosis of esophageal atresia with or without a tracheoesophageal fistula should be suspected whenever there is a history of *polyhydramnios* during the pregnancy (because amniotic fluid cannot be swallowed by the fetus). Eight types of these anomalies have been described and are illustrated in Figure 48-1. More than 85% of these infants have a blind

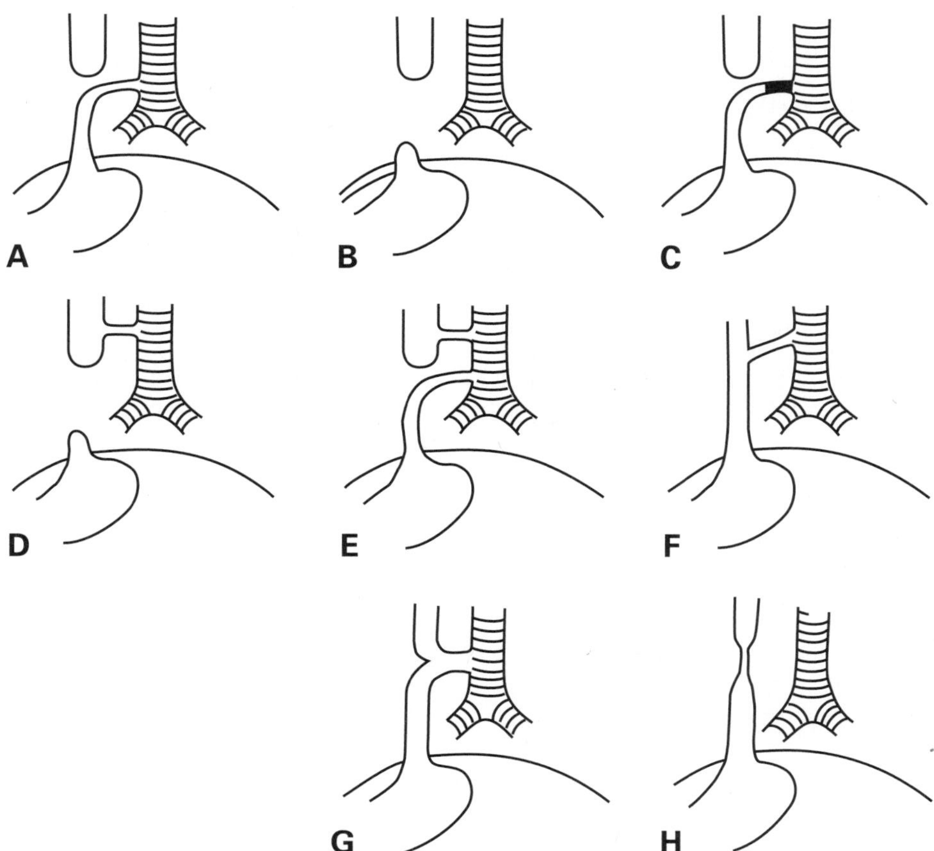

FIG. 48-1 Types of esophageal atresia and stenosis with and without tracheoesophageal fistula.

(From Avery ME et al: *The lung and its disorders in the newborn infant,* ed 4, Philadelphia, 1981, WB Saunders.)

proximal esophageal pouch and a fistulous connection from the distal esophagus to the trachea (type A). Type B is the next most common and is distinguished from type A by absence of air in the intestinal tract on roentgenogram. In types A, B, and C the infant is unable to swallow secretions, giving rise to the clinical presentation of excessive oral secretions, with or without aspiration pneumonia soon after birth. The diagnosis is suspected when a nasogastric tube cannot be passed into the stomach and the contents aspirated. It is confirmed by a roentgenogram of a radiopaque tube curled up in the short, blind esophageal pouch. These infants should be kept with head up (45-degree angle) and a Replogle tube inserted into the upper esophageal pouch; suction should be maintained constantly. If a Replogle tube is not available, a large-bore (10 to 12 Fr) catheter will suffice. Immediate transfer to a regional NICU is mandatory for definitive diagnostic testing and surgical correction of the defect.

A flat or gasless abdomen suggests an esophageal atresia without tracheoesophageal fistula. Rarely, when a tracheoesophageal fistula is proximal to the esophageal atresia (types D and E), severe aspiration is likely to occur soon after birth. Those infants who have the H-type fistula (type F) may have minimal symptomatology initially but subsequently develop respiratory distress with feedings or manifest recurrent pneumonias.

SUGGESTED READINGS

American Academy of Pediatrics: *Textbook of neonatal resuscitation,* Dallas, 1990, American Heart Association.

American Academy of Pediatrics and American College of Obstetricians and Gynecologists: *Guidelines for perinatal care,* ed 3, Evanston, Ill, 1992, the Academy.

Avery GB, Fletcher MA, MacDonald MG, editors: *Neonatology: pathophysiology and management of the newborn,* ed 4, Philadelphia, 1994, JB Lippincott.

Fanaroff AA, Martin RJ, editors: *Neonatal-perinatal medicine,* ed 5, St Louis, 1992, Mosby.

Nelson NM, editor: *Current therapy in neonatal-perinatal medicine,* ed 2, Philadelphia, 1990, BC Decker.

Taeusch HW, Ballard RA, Avery ME, editors: *Diseases of the newborn,* ed 6, Philadelphia, 1991, WB Saunders.

49 Neonatal Drug Abstinence Syndrome

Enrique M. Ostrea, Jr., and Daisy Capistrano Garcia

The problem of drug abuse has reached epidemic proportions during the past 2 decades, increasing both the number of drug users and the types of drugs abused. The increase in the proportion of drugs users who are pregnant is equally alarming because the effects of drugs on the pregnancy and fetus can be significant. In the household surveys conducted by the National Institute on Drug Abuse, drug abuse among women of childbearing age (15 to 44 years of age) was estimated to be 25.4% in 1985, 18.1% in 1988, and 17.3% in 1990.[44] In one study that surveyed predominantly urban hospitals, drug use among pregnant women was estimated to be 0.4% to 27%.[12] More important, meconium drug analysis showed a 44% prevalence of illicit drug use in pregnant women, in contrast to the 11% derived from maternal self-report.[57]

Most drugs a pregnant woman ingests cross the placenta and enter the fetal circulation; there is very little barrier to transport or to biotransformation in the placenta.[62] Thus the fetus chronically is exposed to the drugs that the pregnant woman uses throughout gestation, which can lead to a number of complications in the pregnancy or the infant, such as stillbirth, meconium-stained amniotic fluid, premature rupture of the membranes, abruptio placentae or placenta previa, and fetal distress.[8,48,55,58] In a newborn infant, mortality as well as morbidity are high.* Long-term sequelae also have been reported.† This chapter is confined solely to neonatal drug withdrawal, or the so-called neonatal abstinence syndrome, as a complication of gestational drug exposure.

As a pregnant woman develops a tolerance for or addiction to a drug, her fetus develops a passive dependence on the drug. The mechanism by which withdrawal occurs is not well understood, but it has been shown that stimulation of noradrenergic cells in the brainstem elicits signs similar to those of opiate withdrawal. Furthermore, in experimental animals morphine has been shown to inhibit activation of these cells; thus chronic exposure to morphine results in an increase in the number of brainstem adrenergic binding sites.[2,84] It has been postulated that withdrawal is a consequence of the development of adrenergic supersensitivity, which occurs secondary to prolonged inhibition of the adrenergic cells.

For the infant, withdrawal from drugs may occur in utero or soon after birth. The former circumstance manifests as an increase in fetal movement or activity, an increase in catecholamine in the amniotic fluid,[86] or signs of fetal distress (e.g., meconium staining of the amniotic fluid). Therefore it is unwise for a pregnant addict to undergo withdrawal, such as can occur in abrupt detoxification, because this invariably leads to drug withdrawal in her fetus.

*References 9, 11, 32, 53, 59, 86.

†References 10, 15, 16, 70, 81, 82.

DRUGS ASSOCIATED WITH NEONATAL DRUG ABSTINENCE SYNDROME

For both mother and infant, withdrawal from drugs can occur from gestational exposure to narcotics or to nonnarcotic hypnosedatives (see the box on p. 562). Although addiction to drugs in both groups can occur, there are some important differences[60]:

- With nonnarcotic hypnosedatives—unlike with narcotics—the rate at which an adult develops physical dependence does not increase with the dosage. With adults, large, partly incapacitating doses must be administered continuously for several months to years to induce addiction to nonnarcotics, especially if the drugs are taken orally. The neonate, on the other hand, can become passively addicted to nonnarcotics, even to therapeutic doses the mother may take during pregnancy. For example, treating the mother for epilepsy with phenobarbital can induce passive addiction in her fetus—without evident addiction in the mother.
- The manifestations of withdrawal from nonnarcotics frequently are more intense than those seen with narcotics, and convulsions occur more often with nonnarcotics.
- With narcotics, withdrawal signs commonly are seen within the first 3 days of life because of the short half-life of these drugs. Withdrawal from the nonnarcotics (e.g., phenobarbital) may not become evident until 7 to 10 days after birth.
- Addiction to nonnarcotic hypnosedatives may well be induced by physicians who mistakenly believe that these drugs are not addictive.

Narcotics

The term *narcotics* (opiates) refers to a family of natural or synthetic drugs that have a morphinelike pharmacological action. These drugs include the natural opiates (morphine and codeine) and the many synthetic opiates. Regular use of narcotics, even in therapeutic dosages, can result in addiction characterized by psychological and physical dependence on the drug.

Barbiturates

Although barbiturates have been used in clinical medicine for more than 50 years, their addiction potential has been recognized only recently. It may be that adults' frequent use of barbiturates with alcohol prevented earlier recognition of these drugs' potential for addition.[29,40] Nonnarcotic abstinence in newborns most often involves the barbiturate phenobarbital.

A fetus can passively acquire physical dependence on a barbiturate through prolonged intrauterine exposure to the drug.[6,21] Barbiturates readily cross the placenta and establish high levels in cord blood. Relatively high levels of barbitu-

DRUGS THAT CAN CAUSE WITHDRAWAL IN THE NEONATE

Narcotics or opiates

Codeine
Fentanyl (Innovar, Sublimaze)
Heroin
Hydromorphone (Dilaudid)
Meperidine (Demerol)
Methadone
Morphine
Oxycodone (Percodan, Tylox, Percocet)
Pentazocine (Talwin)
Propoxyphene (Darvon)

Nonnarcotic hypnosedatives

Barbiturates
Nonbarbiturate sedatives and tranquilizers
- Bromide
- Chloral hydrate
- Chlordiazepoxide (Librium)
- Diazepam (Valium)
- Ethchlorvynol (Placidyl)
- Glutethimide (Doriden)

Alcohol (ethanol)

Cocaine

rates have been found in the fetal brain, liver, and adrenals.[65] The manifestations of barbiturate withdrawal in the neonate are similar, regardless of which barbiturate was used, but the onset of withdrawal may differ; it occurs within a day after birth with intermediate-acting barbiturates[56] and about 3 to 7 days after birth with long-acting barbiturates.[6,21]

Barbiturates are metabolized principally by the liver, although a significant portion may be excreted unchanged by the kidneys. In adults, for instance, up to 30% of the total dose of phenobarbital is excreted unchanged in the urine.[75] When phenobarbital is administered prenatally to infants, its half-life is almost twice that in an adult and varies inversely with the degree of prenatal exposure to the drug.[41] Phenobarbital's prolonged half-life in neonates is due to infants' lower glomerular filtration rate and to the reduced capacity of the neonatal liver to metabolize the drug.

Infants experience withdrawal from barbiturates even at therapeutic, nonaddicting maternal doses. Phenobarbital withdrawal has been reported in infants born to epileptic mothers who took the drug in doses of 60 mg/day.[21]

Bromide and Chloral Hydrate

Bromides and chloral hydrate were popular hypnosedatives for many years until they gradually were replaced by the barbiturates and other hypnosedative agents. Addiction to chloral hydrate has been described in adults, and many cases of bromide intoxication could have been due partly to chloral hydrate because it was not unusual to combine the two drugs.[50] A withdrawal syndrome and growth retardation have been reported in newborn infants whose mothers took bromides during pregnancy.[54,71]

Benzodiazepines

Chlordiazepoxide (Librium) and diazepam (Valium) are used widely for their hypnosedative effects. During pregnancy, benzodiazepines cross the placenta with relative ease, resulting in significant levels of the drug in the fetal serum and tissue.[28] An acute withdrawal syndrome has been observed in these newborns.[3,67]

Ethchlorvynol

Ethchlorvynol (Placidyl) was introduced in 1955 as a nonbarbiturate hypnotic for the treatment of insomnia. Like other nonbarbiturate sedatives, claims were made about its nonaddictive property.[20,77,83] Most individuals found it useful for relieving anxiety and inducing sleep.[33] As with the barbiturate and nonbarbiturate sedatives, tolerance to ethchlorvynol develops with continued use; thus the person tends to increase the dose to obtain the desired effect. Cases of addiction to ethchlorvynol have been reported.[4,31,36,38,49] The drug crosses the placenta readily, and studies in animals indicate that it achieves rapid equilibration between the maternal and fetal blood. It also can be detected in the chorionic and amniotic fluids,[39] and the inevitable occurrence of an abstinence syndrome in newborns has been duly reported.[72]

Glutethimide

Glutethimide (Doriden) was introduced in 1954 as a nonbarbiturate hypnosedative allegedly free of addicting properties. As with other nonbarbiturate hypnosedatives, this led to widespread use, particularly as a substitute in the treatment of alcohol addiction.[74] Unfortunately, in adults numerous reports have emerged of acute and sometimes fatal intoxication with the drug, and as well as physical dependence.[27,43,51] A possible case of neonatal withdrawal has been observed.[68]

Alcohol

Ethanol is an anxiolytic analgesic that depresses the central nervous system.[63] It is absorbed rapidly by diffusion in the mucosa of the stomach (20%) and intestines (80%). The absorption rate is not affected by pregnancy, but blood alcohol levels may be higher in pregnancy.[1] Alcohol usually is cleared from the bloodstream within 1 hour in adults and 2 hours in newborns. Approximately 95% is metabolized by the liver, and 5% is eliminated by the kidneys and lungs. Ethanol is metabolized to acetaldehyde, then to acetate. Acetaldehyde is more toxic than ethanol itself.

Infants undergo withdrawal from alcohol, but it rarely is recognized as such because the symptoms may be confused with withdrawal from a narcotic or other drug. Withdrawal from ethanol, which may be noted in the period from birth to 12 hours of life, may cause abdominal distention, opisthotonus, convulsions, tremors, hypertonia, apnea, and cyanosis. These infants are irritable, sleep restlessly, and display exaggerated mouthing behavior.[19,69]

Cocaine

Neurobehavioral abnormalities have been observed in newborns exposed to cocaine before birth. These infants are marked by tremulousness, irritability, hypertonicity, high-

MANIFESTATIONS OF NEONATAL DRUG WITHDRAWAL

Central nervous system signs

Exaggerated reflexes
Hyperactivity
Hyperirritability (excess crying, high-pitched cry)
Increased muscle tone
Short, nonquiet sleep
Sneezing, hiccups, yawning
Tremors

Respiratory signs

Excess secretions
Tachypnea

Gastrointestinal signs

Abdominal cramps (?)
Diarrhea
Disorganized, poor sucking
Drooling
Hyperphagia
Sensitive gag reflex
Vomiting

Vasomotor signs

Flushing
Stuffy nose
Sudden, circumoral pallor
Sweating

Cutaneous signs

Excoriated buttocks
Facial scratches
Pressure point abrasions

Fever

pitched crying, abnormal sleep patterns, and seizures,* manifestations similar to those of opiate withdrawal. It is difficult to distinguish the overlapping effects of cocaine and opiate withdrawal because women who abuse drugs commonly use several types. However, the central nervous system manifestations in infants exposed to cocaine generally are significantly milder than those seen with narcotic withdrawal.[32,73] Neonates exposed to cocaine have shown abnormal cardiorespiratory patterns (more episodes of apnea and periodic breathing),[11] electroencephalographic (EEG) abnormalities (bursts of sharp waves and spikes),[25] and abnormal neonatal behavior as assessed by the Brazelton test (impaired orientation, motor, and state regulation).[8,11] These same abnormalities are seen in infants exposed to opiates alone.

ONSET AND DURATION OF NEONATAL DRUG WITHDRAWAL

Withdrawal often begins within the first 72 hours after birth, commonly within the first 24 to 48 hours. In a few instances it may begin soon after birth, if the mother already has begun to experience withdrawal before delivery. There have been reports of withdrawal occurring after the first or second week of life with drugs that have a longer half-life, such as phenobarbital.[21] Delayed manifestations of withdrawal (as late as 1 week after birth) also have been reported for the narcotic methadone.[42]

The onset and severity of withdrawal are affected by a number of factors such the amount of a drug the mother has taken (as is seen with methadone[23,59]), the timing of the last dose before delivery, the character of the labor, the type and amount of anesthesia or analgesia given to the mother, and the maturity and nutrition of the infant.*

*References 5, 8, 17, 18, 25, 35, 52.

*References 24, 34, 45, 61, 64, 66.

Withdrawal signs in an infant usually peak by about the third day of postnatal life and subside by the fifth to seventh day. The duration of withdrawal is related to its severity.[59] If drugs are used to treat the withdrawal, they should not be discontinued abruptly because relapse may occur. It should be noted that although withdrawal manifestations subside within 1 to 2 weeks, they do not disappear completely. Tremors and irritability may persist until 8 to 16 weeks of age.[14]

SIGNS OF NEONATAL DRUG WITHDRAWAL

Neonatal drug withdrawal may involve the central nervous, respiratory, gastrointestinal, vasomotor, and cutaneous systems (see the box above).

Central Nervous System

Neurological signs predominate and appear early. The findings are those of CNS excitability (hyperactivity, irritability, tremors, and hypertonicity). Occasionally fever may accompany this increase in neuromuscular activities.

Hyperactivity manifests as almost incessant movement of the extremities. When the infant is supine and unrestrained, these movements assume a jerky, purposeless, "en masse" nature, apparently perpetuated by unchecked proprioceptive stimuli. When the infant is placed in the prone position, the motor behavior becomes more organized, appearing as crawling movements and other motions such as chin lifting, head movement from side to side, chest elevation, and hand-to-mouth placement. The last-mentioned movement usually quiets the infant, indicating the usefulness of pacifiers.

Hyperirritability manifests as almost incessant crying with shrill, high-pitched outcries. The infant's muscle tone is exaggerated, sometimes leading to opisthotonic positioning. This makes the infant hard to hold because he or she cannot mold to the body of the holder. Tremors and myoclonic jerks are common and sometimes sustained. In contrast to true seizures, tremors can be abolished by restraining the tremulous extremity. Infantile automatisms (Moro, traction response, weight bearing, placing, stepping, crawling, and Landau re flex) all are exaggerated. The infant's response to sound and light also is increased disproportionately. The EEG tracings of an addicted neonate may be abnormal and show high-frequency dysynchronous activity suggestive of CNS irritability.

In premature infants the neural hyperexcitability is more episodical. The infant appears restless and overactive for short periods and then lapses into periods of lethargy and inactivity. Sustained tremors usually are not seen until the infant reaches the gestational age when tonicity increases in the upper and lower extremities.

The normal patterns of active and quiet sleep periods also are disturbed. Chronic maternal abuse of opiates has been shown to significantly reduce an infant's sleep periods, from a normal 3 to 4 hours to less than 1 hour. Heroin- and methadone-addicted babies also have fewer periods of quiet sleep.[66] Initially these observations were thought to be related to withdrawal. However, because the abnormal sleep patterns persist beyond the period of withdrawal, some believe that they result from the addiction process itself rather than from the general distress caused by withdrawal and that they may arise from the direct effects that chronic exposure to opiates has on the opiate receptors in the brain involved in regulating sleep.[64]

Cardiorespiratory Signs

Ventilation abnormalities, including longer and more frequent episodes of apnea and periodic breathing, have been described in infants whose mothers abused narcotics. During withdrawal these infants also may exhibit tachypnea, with concomitant respiratory alkalosis.[34] In animals, morphine has been shown to have a dual effect on fetal breathing—apnea initially followed by respiratory stimulation. It has been postulated that this dual action is the result of the effects of the drug and its concentration on two different sites involved in controlling respiration. Morphine inhibits the respiratory neurons in the medulla and the neurons located more rostrally, which act to inhibit respiration.

Abnormal heart rate tracings associated with an elevated serum creatine phosphokinase (CPK) were found among infants of drug-dependent mothers.[61] These changes were more intense in infants undergoing moderate to severe withdrawal. The elevated serum CPK is thought to occur secondary to the excess muscular activity of an infant undergoing withdrawal.

Gastrointestinal Signs

Swallowing is poorly coordinated.[45] Both sucking rate and nutrient consumption are low. Often milk drools around the corners of the infant's mouth. The infant appears incessantly hungry and, when unfulfilled, displays mounting agitation, persistent crying, hyperactivity, and exhaustion. Vomiting and diarrhea also are observed often.

Vasomotor Signs

Significant vasomotor instability manifests as a stuffy nose, flushing, mottling, sweating, and episodes of sudden circumoral pallor.

Cutaneous Signs

Because of the infant's hyperactivity, facial scratches and abrasions on pressure points may be observed on the skin. Diarrhea may cause excoriation of the buttocks.

PERSISTENCE OF DRUG WITHDRAWAL

With narcotic withdrawal, symptoms may persist up to 8 to 16 weeks of age.[14] The later manifestations, which usually are milder than those of the initial withdrawal period, consist of irritability, tremors, hypertonicity, sneezing, hiccups, and regurgitation. The persistence of withdrawal is related directly to its initial severity; it is more prolonged with severe withdrawal. Infants treated for withdrawal with medications also have a prolonged withdrawal period; thus drug treatment may ameliorate the manifestations of withdrawal, but it does not shorten the duration. The mother must be made aware that her infant's withdrawal will persist even after discharge from the nursery; otherwise she may become alarmed when the infant continues to manifest some withdrawal signs at home. The unwarned mother also may misinterpret the infant's irritability as hunger and overfeed the child, leading to diarrhea and vomiting. The mother also should be instructed in how to reduce the infant's discomfort by swaddling and cuddling. In addition, she should be reassured that the infant's withdrawal eventually will subside without the use of medications. In most instances a well-informed mother can cope with the situation successfully.

DIAGNOSIS

The diagnosis of drug withdrawal in an infant is based on the clinical manifestations and the verification of gestational exposure to drugs. However, identifying drug exposure in an infant is not easy; pregnant women significantly underreport drug use out of fear of the consequences of such an admission. Even with maternal cooperation, information about the type and extent of drug use often is inaccurate.[57] Similarly, many of the drugs to which the fetus is exposed in utero do not produce immediate or recognizable effects in neonates.[42] Currently a number of laboratory tests are used to detect gestational drug exposure, including toxicological analysis of the infant's urine, hair, and meconium.

DIFFERENTIAL DIAGNOSIS

Withdrawal from narcotic and nonnarcotic drugs should be distinguished from other conditions that cause similar symptoms, such as hypoglycemia, hypocalcemia, hypomagnesemia, sepsis, meningitis, intracranial hemorrhage, infectious diarrhea, and intestinal obstruction.

Infants whose mothers took *tricyclic antidepressants* and *lithium* during pregnancy may manifest signs and symptoms of toxicity similar to those of withdrawal (e.g., irritability, tachycardia, respiratory distress, sweating, and convulsions).[26,76,78-80] Likewise, maternal ingestion of *phenothiazines* (e.g., chlorpromazine) may induce extrapyramidal dysfunctions in a newborn (e.g., tremors, facial grimacing, increased muscle tone, cog-wheel rigidity, increased reflexes, and torticollis), all of which can resemble drug abstinence syndrome.[32,37,46] The elements needed to establish the diag-

Table 49-1 Assessment of the Clinical Severity of Neonatal Narcotic Withdrawal

	Mild	Moderate	Severe
Vomiting	Spitting up	Extensive vomiting for 3 successive feedings	Vomiting associated with imbalance of serum electrolytes
Diarrhea	Watery stools <4 times/day	Watery stools 5-6 times/day for 3 days; no electrolyte imbalance	Diarrhea associated with imbalance of serum electrolytes
Weight loss	<10% of birth weight	10%-15% of birth weight	>15% of birth weight
Irritability	Minimal	Marked but relieved by cuddling or feeding	Unrelieved by cuddling or feeding
Tremors or twitching	Mild tremors when stimulated	Marked tremors or twitching when stimulated	Convulsions
Tachypnea	60-80 breaths/min	80-100 breaths/min	>100 breaths/min associated with respiratory alkalosis

From Ostrea EM, Chavez CJ, Stryker JS: *The care of the drug-dependent woman and her infant,* Lansing, Mich, 1978, Michigan Department of Public Health.

nosis are the history and identification of the offending drug's metabolites in the infant's serum or urine.

ASSESSMENT OF THE SEVERITY OF NEONATAL DRUG WITHDRAWAL

Neonatal drug withdrawal can vary from none to severe. With heroin it has been shown that the severity of the newborn's withdrawal is not related to the infant's gender, race, or Apgar score nor to the mother's age, parity, or duration of drug abuse.[59] Similarly, manipulating the environment (e.g., reducing the amount of light or noise in the nursery) does not ameliorate the severity of withdrawal. Adults experience abdominal cramps, palpitation, nausea, and other discomforts while undergoing withdrawal; the infant probably endures similar discomforts, which may nullify any potential benefit from dimming lights or reducing noise.

On the other hand, the severity of the infant's withdrawal appears to correlate significantly with the mother's methadone dose.[23,59] The infant's withdrawal tends to be more intense if the mother has been taking more than 20 mg/day before delivery.

After birth, the infant of a drug-dependent mother should be observed closely for withdrawal and for a possible need for treatment with drugs. However, only about 25% of infants who undergo withdrawal need drug treatment[59]; the remainder can be successfully managed conservatively (i.e., swaddling, placing the infant in a prone position, and frequent cuddling). Swaddling, particularly with the newborn's extremities flexed and the hands placed in front of the mouth, enhances the infant's hand-to-mouth facility for soothing. A similar soothing action can be achieved with a pacifier.

The frequency of diarrhea and vomiting should be noted and the infant's weight checked at least every 8 hours. Temperature, heart rate, and respiratory rates should be measured every 4 hours. Laboratory examinations to detect serum electrolyte or pH imbalance should be done as needed.

The severity of the withdrawal can be assessed by several clinical scoring systems,[7,30,47] some of which are significantly detailed.[30] The system we use is simple and evaluates the infant principally for the need for treating withdrawal signs with drugs. Thus the system focuses essentially on withdrawal manifestations that can be life threatening if left unresolved, such as irritability, tremors, weight loss, vomiting, diarrhea, and tachypnea (Table 49-1). Drugs are used to treat (1) any severe condition or (2) significant vomiting, diarrhea, or weight loss.

Table 49-2 Drugs Commonly Used To Treat Neonatal Drug Abstinence Syndrome

Drugs	Dosage
Paregoric	3-6 drops q4-6h PO
Laudanum (0.4%)	3-6 drops q4-6h PO
Chlorpromazine	2-3 mg/kg/day q6h PO
Phenobarbital	3-6 mg/kg/day q6h PO

PHARMACOLOGICAL TREATMENT OF WITHDRAWAL

Narcotic or nonnarcotic drugs are used to treat drug withdrawal in the infant (Table 49-2). However, narcotics are preferred if withdrawal is from narcotics because the action is more physiological for such an abstinent state. The neurological manifestations of withdrawal from narcotics can be controlled successfully by a nonnarcotic drug; however, narcotics are more effective in relieving the non-CNS manifestations of withdrawal (e.g., diarrhea).

The narcotics paregoric, tincture of opium, and methadone have been used for this treatment. We prefer tincture of opium (laudanum, USP) over paregoric because the latter contains camphor, which also is a CNS stimulant. (*Caution:* Laudanum, USP, is available in a standard 10% solution containing 1% morphine. *Laudanum must be diluted 25-fold to a concentration of 0.4%* to reduce its morphine content to the equivalent of that of paregoric. At this dilution, 0.4% laudanum can be given at the same dose as paregoric.)

A cross-reaction exists between the different nonnarcotic hypnosedatives (see Table 49-2)—each drug is effective in treating withdrawal from any drug belonging to the same group. That is, barbiturates can be used to treat withdrawal from nonbarbiturates (including alcohol), or vice versa. Drugs that have been used for this purpose in the neonatal period are *phenobarbital,* 3 to 5 mg/kg/24 hr in divided doses every 6 hours; *chlorpromazine,* 2 to 3 mg/kg/day every 6 hours; and *diazepam* (not commonly used because of reported side effects such as bradycardia and respiratory depression).

Although chlorpromazine does not belong to the group of nonnarcotic drugs that can cause withdrawal manifestations, its amelioration of the signs of withdrawal may occur secondary to its ability to suppress the exaggerated REM sleep of withdrawal.[22]

During treatment of withdrawal, attention also should be focused on the infant's nutrition and fluid and electrolyte balance, particularly if vomiting, diarrhea, hyperpyrexia, and hyperhidrosis occur. Appropriate intravenous fluids may be required to correct deficits or prevent imbalances.

The aim of treatment with drugs is to keep the infant comfortable but not obtunded. Therefore the drug should be titrated, starting with the smallest recommended dose and increasing accordingly until the desired effect is achieved. Once the infant has been asymptomatic for 3 to 5 days, the drug can be tapered slowly, first in dose and then in frequency, until it is discontinued. The total detoxification period from the point of initial treatment can take 2 to 3 weeks. After the drug is discontinued, the infant should be observed for 1 to 2 days for possible recurrence of withdrawal (rebound phenomenon). Once the infant is discharged from the nursery, the mother should be instructed to anticipate some mild jitteriness and irritability, which may persist for 8 to 16 weeks, depending on the initial severity of the withdrawal.

COMPLICATIONS

The complications of neonatal drug withdrawal are related to the severity of the symptoms. Aberrations in serum electrolytes, pH, and dehydration may occur secondary to vomiting and diarrhea. Weight loss may be profound not only because of excess fluid losses, but also because of poor and ineffective oral intake. Aspiration pneumonia may occur secondary to vomiting and incoordinated sucking and swallowing. Respiratory alkalosis can occur as a result of tachypnea. Convulsions are a rare manifestation of narcotic withdrawal but are common in withdrawal from nonnarcotic drugs.

OTHER SUPPORTIVE MEASURES

An addicted woman faces serious impediments to successful mothering. She probably has meager past mothering experience to rely on and there is often little or no support from a father or husband. The neurobehavioral abnormalities and withdrawal signs in her infant may hamper gratifying feedback. The mother and infant should have early and repeated contact. A staff member also should have repeated and relatively brief contacts with the mother to describe her infant's status and to reassure her that, with the disappearance of withdrawal, her baby will feed more vigorously and respond better to her ministrations.

Breast-Feeding

Most drugs taken by the mother cross into her breast milk (see Chapter 16, Two, The Feeding of Infants and Children). The concentration of illicit drug in the breast milk depends on the amount of the drug the mother takes and when she takes it. In general, breast-feeding is not recommended if the mother has been shown to abuse drugs continuously during her pregnancy or is HIV-antibody positive.

Decisions About the Caregiver

A drug-addicted woman's ability to perform her maternal functions and provide adequate care for her infant has been questioned seriously on many occasions. These women often have been denied their maternal rights and responsibilities soon after the infant's birth on the basis of their unstable homes, life-styles, and emotional and psychological weaknesses. Current evidence suggests that such a practice may be unnecessary and counterproductive. A study that determined the outcome of infants on the basis of the type of caregiver[13] showed that the outcome (growth, development, and frequency of medical illnesses and child abuse) for an infant under its mother's care, with the help of a husband or relative, was better than that seen in foster care. Thus with proper guidance and supervision the addicted mother is capable of caring for her infant adequately. Similarly, although a high incidence of problems suggestive of child abuse (cigarette burns or hematoma) was noted among infants cared for exclusively by the mother, very few of these complications were noted in infants whose mothers had help available. Besides allowing the mother to care for her infant, it is important that someone help her at home.

Social Service Referral

All infants of drug-dependent mothers must have a social service referral to assess the adequacy of parenting. Discharge of the infant to the mother's care is the primary objective unless serious conditions dictate otherwise. In our experience, the best outcome for the infant is achieved when he or she is cared for by the mother, with help from a support person such as the grandmother or a relative. The infant should be discharged to a person other than the mother only when it is apparent that the infant will be neglected, poorly cared for, or abused. Most mothers hesitate to admit to using drugs during pregnancy because they fear their infants will be taken away from them. They should be assured otherwise; in fact, they should be encouraged to be responsible for the primary care of their infants. The social worker and physician also should advise the mother on medical and social services available in the community that she can consult in caring for her infant and herself.

REFERENCES

1. Abel EL: *Fetal alcohol syndrome,* Montvale, NJ, 1990, Medical Economics.
2. Aghajanian GK: Tolerance to locus coeruleus neurons to morphine and suppression of withdrawal response by clonidine, *Nature* 276:186, 1978.
3. Athinarayanan P et al: Chlordiazepoxide withdrawal in the neonate, *Am J Obstet Gynecol* 124:212, 1976.
4. Aycrigg JB: Two cases of withdrawal from ethchlorvynol, *Am J Psychiatry* 120:1201, 1964.
5. Bingol N et al: Teratogenicity of cocaine in humans, *Pediatrics* 110:93, 1987.
6. Bleyer W, Marshall RE: Barbiturate withdrawal syndrome in a passively addicted infant, *JAMA* 221:185, 1972.
7. Chasnoff IJ, Burns WJ: The Moro reaction: a scoring system for neonatal narcotic withdrawal, *Dev Med Child Neurol* 26:484, 1984.
8. Chasnoff IJ et al: Cocaine use in pregnancy, *N Engl J Med* 313:666, 1985.
9. Chasnoff IJ et al: Perinatal cerebral infarction and maternal cocaine use, *J Pediatr* 108:456, 1986.

10. Chasnoff IJ, Hatcher R, Burns WJ: Polydrug and methadone addicted newborns: a continuum of impairment, *Pediatrics* 70:210, 1982.
11. Chasnoff IJ et al: Prenatal cocaine exposure is associated with respiratory pattern abnormalities, *Am J Dis Child* 143:583, 1989.
12. Chasnoff IJ, Landress HJ, Barrett ME: The prevalence of illicit drug or alcohol use during pregnancy and discrepancies in mandatory reporting in Pinellas County, Florida, *N Engl J Med* 322:1202, 1990.
13. Chavez CJ, Ostrea EM: Outcome of infants of drug-dependent mothers based on the type of caregiver, *Pediatr Res* 11:375A, 1977.
14. Chavez CJ et al: Prognosis of infants born to drug-dependent mothers: its relation to the severity of the withdrawal during the neonatal period, *Pediatr Res* 10:328A, 1976.
15. Chavez CJ et al: Sudden infant death syndrome among infants of drug-dependent mothers, *J Pediatr* 95:407, 1979.
16. Chavez CJ et al: Ocular abnormalities in infants as sequelae of prenatal drug addiction, *Pediatr Res* 12:367A, 1979.
17. Cherukuri R et al: A cohort study of alkaloidal cocaine ("crack") in pregnancy, *Obstet Gynecol* 72:147, 1988.
18. Chouteau M, Namerow PB, Leppert P: The effect of cocaine abuse on birth weight and gestational age, *Obstet Gynecol* 72:351, 1988.
19. Coles CD et al: Neonatal ethanol withdrawal: characteristics in clinically normal, nondysmorphic neonates, *J Pediatr* 105:445, 1984.
20. Cuthburt KJR: Two hypnotics, *Practitioner* 190:509, 1963.
21. Desmond MM et al: Maternal barbiturate utilization and neonatal withdrawal symptomatology, *J Pediatr* 80:190, 1972.
22. Dinges DF, Davis MM, Glass P: Fetal exposure to narcotics: neonatal sleep as a measure of nervous system disturbance, *Science* 209:619, 1980.
23. Doberczak TM, Kandall SR, Friedmann: Relationship between maternal methadone dosage, maternal-neonatal methadone levels, and neonatal withdrawal, *Obstet Gynecol* 81:936, 1993.
24. Doberczak TM et al: Neonatal neurologic and electroencephalographic effects of intrauterine cocaine exposure, *J Pediatr* 113:354, 1988.
25. Doberczak TM, Kandall SR, Wilets I: Neonatal opiate abstinence syndrome in term and preterm infants, *J Pediatr* 118:933, 1991.
26. Eggermont E: The adverse influence of imipramine on the adaptation of the newborn infant to extrauerine life, *Acta Pediatr Belg* 26:197, 1972.
27. Eidelman JR: Doriden intoxication, *Mo Med* 53:194, 1956.
28. Erkkola R, Kangas L, Pekkarinen A: The transfer of diazepam across the placenta during labour, *Acta Obstet Gynecol Scand* 52:167, 1973.
29. Essig CF: Addiction to barbiturate and nonbarbiturate sedative drugs, *Res Publ Assoc Res Nerv Ment Dis* 68:188, 1968.
30. Finnegan LP: Neonatal abstinence. In Nelson NM, editor: *Current therapy in neonatal-perinatal medicine,* Philadelphia, 1990, BC Decker.
31. Flemenbaum A, Gunby B: Ethchlorvynol (Placidyl) abuse and withdrawal, *Dis Nerv Syst* 32:188, 1971.
32. Fulroth R, Phillips B, Durand D: Perinatal outcome of infants exposed to cocaine and/or heroin in utero, *Am J Dis Child* 143:905, 1989.
33. Garetz FD: Ethchlorvynol: addiction hazard, *Minn Med* 52:1131, 1969.
34. Glass L et al: Effect of heroin withdrawal on respiratory rate and acid-base status of the newborn, *N Engl J Med* 286:746, 1972.
35. Hadeed AJ, Siegel SR: Maternal cocaine use during pregnancy: effect on the newborn infant, *Pediatrics* 84:205, 1989.
36. Harenko A: On special traits of acute ethchlorvynol poisoning, *Acta Neurol Scand* 43:141, 1967.
37. Hill RM, Desmond MM, Kay JL: Extrapyramidal dysfunction in an infant of a schizophrenic mother, *J Pediatr* 69:589, 1966.
38. Hudson HS, Walker HI: Withdrawal symptoms following ethchlorvynol dependence, *Am J Psychiatry* 118:361, 1961.
39. Hume AS, Williams JM, Douglas BG: Disposition of ethchlorvynol in maternal blood, amniotic fluid, and chorionic fluid, *J Reprod Med* 6:229, 1977.
40. Isbell H: Addiction to barbiturates and the barbiturate abstinence syndrome, *Ann Intern Med* 33:108, 1950.
41. Jalling B et al: Disappearance from the newborn of circulating prenatally administered phenobarbital, *Eur J Clin Pharmacol* 6:234, 1973.
42. Kandall SR, Gartner LM: Late presentation of drug withdrawal symptoms in newborns, *Am J Dis Child* 127:58, 1974.
43. Kanter DM: The acute toxicity of Doriden overdosage, *Conn Med J* 21:314, 1957.
44. Khalsa JH, Gfroerer J: Epidemiology and health consequence of drug abuse among pregnant women, *Semin Perinatol* 15:265, 1991.
45. Kron R et al: Neonatal narcotic abstinence: effects of pharmacotherapeutic agents and maternal drug usage on nutritive sucking behavior, *J Pediatr* 88:637, 1976.
46. Levy W, Wisniewski K: Chlorpromazine causing extrapyramidal dysfunction in newborn infant of psychotic mother, *NY State J Med* 74:684, 1974.
47. Lipsitz PJ: A proposed narcotic withdrawal score for use with newborn infants, *Clin Pediatr* 14:592, 1975.
48. MacGregor SN et al: Cocaine use during pregnancy: adverse perinatal outcome, *Am J Obstet Gynecol* 157:686, 1987.
49. Magness JL: Ethchlorvynol intoxication and severe abstinence reaction, *Lancet* 1:80, 1965.
50. Margetts EL: Chloral delirium, *Psychiatry* 24:278, 1950.
51. McBay AJ, Katsas GG: Glutethimide poisoning: a report of four fatal cases, *N Engl J Med* 257:97, 1957.
52. Neerhof M et al: Cocaine abuse during pregnancy: peripartum prevalence and perinatal outcome, *Am J Obstet Gynecol* 161:633, 1989.
53. Oleske J et al: Immune deficiency syndrome in children, *JAMA* 249:2345, 1983.
54. Opitz JM, Grosse FR, Heneberg B: Congenital effects of bromism, *Lancet* 1:91, 1972.
55. Oro AS, Dixon SD: Perinatal cocaine and methamphetamine exposure: maternal and neonatal correlates, *J Pediatr* 111:571, 1987.
56. Ostrea EM Jr: Neonatal withdrawal from intrauterine exposure to butalbital, *Am J Obstet Gynecol* 143:597, 1982.
57. Ostrea EM et al: Drug screening of newborn infants by meconium analysis: a large-scale prospective epidemiologic study, *Pediatrics* 89:107, 1992.
58. Ostrea EM, Chavez CJ: Perinatal problems (excluding neonatal withdrawal) in maternal drug addiction: a study of 830 cases, *J Pediatr* 94:292, 1979.
59. Ostrea EM Jr, Chavez CJ, Strauss ME: A study of factors that influence the severity of neonatal narcotic withdrawal, *J Pediatr* 88:642, 1976.
60. Ostrea EM: Neonatal addiction to narcotic drugs. In Ostrea EM, Chavez CJ, Stryker JS, eds: In *The care of the drug-dependent woman and her infant,* Lansing, Mich, 1978, Michigan Department of Public Health.
61. Ostrea EM Jr et al: Abnormal heart rate tracings and serum creatine phosphokinase in addicted neonates, *Neurotoxicol Teratol* 9:305, 1987.
62. Ostrea EM et al: The effect of chronic maternal drug addiction on placental drug (xenobiotic) metabolism, *Dev Pharmacol Ther* 12:42, 1989.
63. Pietrantoni M, Knuppel RA: Alcohol in pregnancy, *Clin Perinatol* 18:93, 1991.
64. Pinto F et al: Sleep in babies born to chronically heroin-addicted mothers: a follow-up study, *Drug Alcohol Depend* 21:43, 1988.
65. Ploman L, Persson BH: On the transfer of barbiturates to the human fetus and their accumulation in some of its vital organs, *J Obstet Gynecol Br Empire* 64:706, 1957.
66. Reddy A, Harper R, Stern G: Observations on heroin and methadone withdrawal in the newborn, *Pediatrics* 48:353, 1971.
67. Rementeria JL, Bhatt K: Withdrawal symptoms in neonates from intrauterine exposure to diazepam, *J Pediatr* 90:123, 1977.
68. Reveri M, Pyati S, Pildes RS: Neonatal withdrawal symptoms associated with glutethimide (Doriden) addiction in the mother during pregnancy, *Clin Pediatr* 16:424, 1977.
69. Robe LB, Gromisch DS, Iosub S: Symptoms of neonatal ethanol withdrawal, *Curr Alcohol* 8:485, 1981.
70. Rosen TS, Johnson HL: Children of methadone-maintained mothers: follow-up to 18 months of age, *J Pediatr* 101:192, 1982.
71. Rossiter EJR, Rendle-Short TJ: Congenital effects of bromism, *Lancet* 2:705, 1972.
72. Rumack BH, Walravens PA: Neonatal withdrawal following maternal ingestion of ethchlorvynol (Placidyl), *Pediatrics* 52:714, 1973.
73. Ryan L, Ehrlich S, Finnegan L: Cocaine abuse in pregnancy: effects on the fetus and newborn, *Neurotoxicol Teratol* 9:295, 1987.

74. Sadwin A, Glen RS: Addiction to glutethimide (Doriden), *Am J Psychiatry* 115:469, 1968.
75. Sharpless SK: The barbiturates. In Goodman LS, Gilman A, editors: *The pharmacological basis of therapeutics,* London, 1970, MacMillan.
76. Stothers J: Lithium toxicity in the newborn, *Br Med J* 3:233, 1973.
77. Tsapogas MJC, Modle J, Wheeler T: A comparison between two hypnotics: ethchlorvynol and dichloralphenazone, *Br J Clin Pract* 17:407, 1963.
78. Tunnessen W: Toxic effects of lithium in newborn infants, *J Pediatr* 81:804, 1972.
79. Webster PAC: Withdrawal symptoms in neonates associated with maternal antidepressant therapy, *Lancet* 2:318, 1973.
80. Wilbanks B: Toxic effects of lithium carbonate in a mother and newborn infant, *JAMA* 213:865, 1970.
81. Wilson GS: Clinical studies of infants and children exposed prenatally to heroin, *Ann NY Acad Sci* 562:183, 1989.
82. Wilson GS et al: The development of preschool children of heroin-addicted mothers: a controlled study, *Pediatrics* 63:135, 1979.
83. Wood-Walker RB: A clinical evaluation of a nonbarbiturate hypnotic: ethchlorvynol, *Br J Clin Pract* 17:201, 1963.
84. Wuster M, Schultz R, Herz A: Opioid tolerance and dependence: re-evaluating the unitary hypothesis, *Trends Pharmacol Sci* 6:64, 1985.
85. Zuckerman B et al: Effects of maternal marijuana and cocaine use on fetal growth, *N Engl J Med* 320:762, 1989.
86. Zuspan FB et al: Fetal stress from methadone withdrawal, *Am J Obstet Gynecol* 122:43, 1975.

50 High-Risk Follow-up

Dennis J. Mujsce and Nicholas M. Nelson

Discharge from the neonatal intensive care unit (NICU) does not terminate the problems faced by high-risk infants, their families, medical care providers, and our society. Although the special needs of seriously ill neonates usually abate during the course of hospitalization, their follow-up home care often remains formidable. These survivors have markedly higher rates of serious illness, rehospitalization, and death in the first years of life than do infants who did not need intensive care. Their high-risk status is reflected in persistently high mortality after discharge, which is five to nine times greater than postneonatal mortality of other infants.[1,18] Care of a high-risk infant at home may create large demands on time, energy, and money. Unfortunately, many of these infants are discharged to severely disadvantaged homes, which are poorly equipped to manage a normal infant, much less one who has such extensive needs.

CHARACTERISTICS OF HIGH-RISK INFANTS

The term *high risk* can be applied appropriately to any infant who has an unusual perinatal course or a greater than normal likelihood of morbidity or mortality, or who requires other than standard newborn care. Recognizing the infant's high-risk status is the important first step toward anticipating defined problems and giving optimal care.

Population

Premature Neonates. The cornucopia for high-risk infants is the premature population. Over the past 3 decades, mortality related to birth weight has been reduced remarkably in this group.[15] In 1960, for newborns weighing less than 1500 g, the mortality rate was 70%; for those weighing less than 500 g, it was 90%. By 1985 those figures had been cut to 30% and 50%, respectively.[25] Unfortunately, the advances in neonatal care that improved these survival rates did not eradicate many of the serious sequelae that handicap NICU survivors. Furthermore, the number of infants born weighing less than 1500 g (40,000 to 50,000 annually in the United States) has not declined significantly during the past decade. As a result, larger numbers of both well and handicapped infants from this high-risk population are being seen in follow-up clinics today.

Other Neonates. Although prematurity and its attendant complications contribute most heavily to the high-risk pool, numerous other causes of neonatal morbidity and mortality (see the box on p. 569) are now being treated in the NICU. Indeed, expanded diagnostic and therapeutic capabilities (see the box on p. 569) allow aggressive management of a growing number of disorders, some of which were once considered fatal. Survivors of these newborn conditions may well have follow-up needs that equal or exceed those of the tiniest premature infants.

Special Needs

Each high-risk infant is an individual who brings a unique mix of problems and needs to the health care system. All these patients require standard well-baby care, but few will move smoothly and quickly through a pediatric office or clinic because they represent extraordinary medical illnesses, treatments, and altered family dynamics that demand considerable time and attention. Physicians who care for high-risk infants therefore must be prepared to allocate a disproportionate amount of effort to this minority of patients.

Comprehensive care of these infants often is best accomplished as a team effort involving the follow-up group of the tertiary care center and the infant's own primary care physician. To be effective members of the high-risk follow-up team, however, all health care providers need to become familiar with many treatments that originally were confined to the hospital, such as administration of supplemental oxygen, ventilator support, tracheostomy care, gastrostomy and nasogastric tube feedings, intravenous hyperalimentation, peritoneal dialysis, and home apnea monitoring. In addition to such technical forms of therapy, physicians also are called upon to stay abreast of the wide range of medications and services now incorporated into outpatient care of high-risk infants. Finally, the physician must understand the disease processes themselves so that serious changes or deteriorations in an infant's condition can be detected and addressed promptly. Perhaps most important, the primary health care provider must recognize subtle impairments of motor development, cognition, and behavior that can appear beyond the neonatal period and adversely affect the infant's quality of life.[22]

DISCHARGE PLANNING

Follow-up care begins with discharge planning, one of the least dramatic aspects of neonatal intensive care, but a truly important one. Continued success of even the most spectacular NICU story requires a comprehensive plan at the time of discharge that has been developed continuously throughout the infant's hospital stay.

The first step is to identify infants who will benefit from high-risk follow-up. Opinions vary, but the box on p. 569 lists some conditions that most agree warrant special attention after discharge. Besides these infants, who can best be followed up by primary care practitioners working with high-risk clinics, many neonates who have specific problems (e.g., imperforate anus, congenital heart defects, ventriculoperitoneal shunts) require services now available only in certain subspecialty clinics. Follow-up care for these babies is best achieved through collaboration of the primary care physician and the appropriate subspecialists.

Development of a discharge plan early in the infant's hospitalization helps to ensure that discharge occurs at the ap-

MAJOR NEONATAL ILLNESSES TREATED IN THE NICU

- Sepsis
- Altered growth and gestation
  - Infants of extremely low birth weight (<750 g)
  - Severe intrauterine growth retardation
- Pulmonary disorders
  - Hyaline membrane disease (respiratory distress syndrome)
  - Meconium aspiration syndrome
  - Pneumonia
  - Pulmonary hemorrhage
- Cardiovascular disorders
  - Acyanotic heart diseases (e.g., hypoplastic left-heart syndrome)
  - Arrhythmias and heart blocks
  - Cyanotic heart disease (e.g., transposition, pulmonary atresia)
  - Persistent pulmonary hypertension
- Renal/genitourinary disorders
  - Obstructive uropathy
  - Renal dysplasias
- Gastrointestinal disorders
  - Necrotizing enterocolitis
  - Biliary atresia
  - Diaphragmatic hernia
  - Malformations (e.g., gastroschisis, omphalocele, bowel atresias)
- Central nervous system (CNS) disorders
  - Developmental anomalies (e.g., hydrocephalus, Arnold-Chiari malformation, neural tube defect)
  - Hypoxic-ischemic encephalopathy
  - Intracranial hemorrhage
- Inborn errors of metabolism
- Genetic and chromosomal disorders

CURRENT NICU TREATMENT OPTIONS

Diagnostic modalities

- Cardiac catheterization and angiography (heart, blood vessels)
- Computed tomography (brain, abdomen, body)
- Magnetic resonance imaging (brain)
- Nuclear medicine scans (renal, hepatobiliary)
- Positron emission tomography (brain)
- Real-time and Doppler ultrasonography (brain, heart, abdomen)

Therapeutic interventions

Medical management

- Continuous prostaglandin E_1 infusion (to maintain ductus arteriosus patency)
- Conventional and high-frequency ventilation (respiratory failure)
- Exogenous surfactant administration (hyaline membrane disease)
- Immunoglobulin and antibiotic therapy (infection)
- Nitric oxide therapy (pulmonary hypertension)
- Steroid therapy (bronchopulmonary dysplasia)

Surgical management

- Cardiopulmonary bypass, hypothermic circulatory arrest (cardiac repair)
- Dialysis and hemofiltration (renal failure)
- Extracorporeal membrane oxygenation (diaphragmatic hernia, pulmonary hypertension)
- Neurosurgical procedures (to correct CNS anomalies)
- Organ transplantation (biliary atresia)

CRITERIA FOR NEONATAL HIGH-RISK FOLLOW-UP PROGRAMS

- Birth weight ≤1500 g
- Bronchopulmonary dysplasia
- Extracorporeal membrane oxygenation
- Hydrocephalus/microcephaly
- Hyperbilirubinemia requiring exchange transfusion
- Intracranial hemorrhage/periventricular leukomalacia
- Meningitis and sepsis
- Persistent pulmonary hypertension
- Severe intrauterine growth retardation (birth weight <25% for gestation)
- Severe meconium aspiration syndrome
- Symptomatic hypoglycemia
- Symptomatic perinatal asphyxia

propriate time, that all the infant's needs will be met, and that parental anxiety is kept to a minimum. Parents require a great deal of time and repetition of explanations and instructions to assimilate all the necessary information. Logistical barriers to the exchange of information (e.g., early discharge of the mother and large distances separating the family from the infant in the tertiary care center) make early communication imperative. A truly multidisciplinary plan must be formulated, one based on the opinions of parents, nurses, social workers, neonatologists, subspecialists, and the infant's primary care physician.

A primary goal of discharge planning is to ensure a smooth transition of the infant's care from the well-staffed, specialized NICU to the home, where adequate support mechanisms have been put in place. A successful discharge plan must outline the support network clearly, must match the infant's needs with appropriate resources, and must define the responsibilities of all follow-up participants precisely. An effective plan is kept as simple as possible to prevent delay, duplication, absences, or fragmentation of necessary services. Sound discharge planning also must provide for continual reevaluation of the plan itself and for alternative measures in the event of unforeseen emergencies. The timing of the actual discharge will depend on the readiness of the infant, the family, the home, and the follow-up team. Therefore each must be assessed thoroughly before discharge.

Most contemporary neonatal staffs no longer insist on achievement of a minimum body weight for discharge, provided the infant's medical problems have been stabilized and several criteria are met. The infant should competently maintain body temperature while in a bassinet, feed regularly by mouth (or gastrostomy tube in selected cases), maintain consistent growth, and breathe regularly without frequent or severe apnea.[6] Recent pressures to reduce health care costs and provide more services in an ambulatory setting have challenged these "traditional" criteria for discharge of high-risk preterm infants. For example, insurers are investigating the feasibility of managing convalescing premature infants at home, rather than in the NICU or step-down nursery. Care at home might include an incubator to maintain a thermoneutral environment, nasogastric tube feedings, and electronic surveillance of the heart and respiratory rates. Insurance providers are contracting with home nursing agencies to administer this care, along with the infant's parents, to assess the infant's condition, and to provide feedback to the responsible physician. Increasingly, primary care physicians, the "gatekeepers" of tomorrow's health care system, will be expected to manage these high-risk infants as they are discharged ever-earlier from the NICU.

Nevertheless, before any high-risk infant is discharged, it is essential to document the infant's physiological stability, the caretaker's competence, and the adequacy of the home environment. Although most NICU patients are discharged directly into the care of their parents, stable high-risk infants increasingly are being transferred from a distant tertiary care center to a local "level II" NICU or lower level nursery near their home for further treatment before being sent home. Proximity to home allows the parents and extended family to bond with the infant, to perform routine caretaking procedures, and to participate in medical management. These internursery transfers reduce health care costs and open NICU beds for new acutely ill patients. Thus the receiving health care providers must share responsibility for discharge planning with the referring NICU staff.

GOALS OF HIGH-RISK FOLLOW-UP

The benefits of a comprehensive follow-up program are important to the health care system and to the patients and families it serves. Longitudinal studies of high-risk patients are the gold standard source for information to guide and gauge the effectiveness of NICU care. Educators, politicians, and policymakers at all levels require such follow-up data to allocate funds and resources on the basis of the special medical and educational needs of NICU graduates. Parents, of course, need the best information available to understand what may lie in store for their child and family and to plan their lives accordingly. Although short-term neonatal mortality and morbidity can be estimated from acute NICU statistics, many effects of neonatal intensive care are appreciated only through the data gathered in long-term follow-up studies; such effects include later mortality and health problems, incidence of rehospitalization, neurodevelopmental outcome, academic achievement, quality of life, effects on the family and society, costs, and use of resources. For example, we now know that the incidence of neurological abnormalities in very low-birth-weight (VLBW) infants jumps from 10% to 30% to 30% to 60% if learning disabilities are added to the list of sequelae (such as cerebral palsy, developmental delay, and seizures) that classically are identified at an earlier age.[20] In addition, high-risk follow-up studies recently demonstrated that the incidence of cerebral palsy in VLBW survivors (<1500 g) in Australia,[28] Great Britain,[26] and Sweden[16] has increased from 1967 to 1985. Such findings have obvious implications for those treating pregnant women and neonatal patients, as well as the caretakers and educators of these surviving children.

Parents often are reluctant to return with their infants to high-risk follow-up programs for a variety of real or perceived reasons, such as extra cost, inconvenience, time away from the job, distance between the home and clinic, a previous unpleasant NICU experience, fear of uncovering new abnormalities, and the conviction that the clinic staff benefits more from the visit than does the infant or family. Primary care physicians, concentrating on immediate infant care needs, may unintentionally reinforce the belief that little is to be gained from return visits to the follow-up clinic. Such "dropouts" can skew outcome figures seriously. One report[29] found that only 4.4% of "easy to review" patients were severely disabled, whereas in the "hard to review" group, the figure was 35%!

Most medical students and pediatric residents learn about management of acute neonatal problems in the NICU setting, but few receive sufficient exposure to a structured high-risk follow-up clinic to realize that each critically ill infant is a person who is part of a family and that most of these infants ultimately will thrive. Most recently graduated pediatricians regard their residency training as their primary source of information about the care of high-risk infants. Therefore a residency curriculum that encourages and guides house staff in attending a high-risk clinic should produce better-prepared pediatricians.

Thriving high-risk infants who are brought to the follow-up clinic for return visits can rejuvenate the morale of NICU personnel, who spend long, stressful hours attending sick infants whose outcome is uncertain. Additionally, this forum is a good opportunity to review instructions, dispel misconceptions, and address the new questions that invariably crop up once the parents have brought their infant home.

ORGANIZATION OF HIGH-RISK FOLLOW-UP

In some clinics the neonatologists who cared for the infants in the NICU maintain a strong presence in the follow-up program, whereas in other facilities outpatients are transferred to teams that specialize in high-risk follow-up. When an organized neonatal follow-up program is not available, the infant is discharged from the NICU directly to his or her primary care physician without scheduled high-risk follow-up. Thus primary care physicians should be aware of several public health, community, and ancillary health services available (see the box on p. 572) and should use them to the benefit of their high-risk patients.

Successful strategies for high-risk follow-up all have several elements in common. First, each infant has an individual discharge plan that is specifically tailored to provide routine pediatric care while attending to the child's particular needs. Second, continuity of care is maintained when the infant is discharged home and when different people assume new roles in that care. Third, all those participating in the follow-up plan make sure that the other team members are kept up to

RESOURCES AVAILABLE TO FAMILIES OF HIGH-RISK INFANTS

Ancillary health care services

Dietitians and nutrition specialists
Home health equipment and services vendors
Home nursing services
Physical, occupational, and hearing and speech therapy
Social services

Community resources

Churches and religious organizations
Community health nurses
Departments of public health
County and state financial support programs
Early intervention programs
Hospice and respite services
Parental support groups
Schools and special educational programs
Specialized foster care parents

Family support network

Extended family
Significant friends

date, and all clearly understand who holds coordinating responsibility for the infant's care.

The Neonatal Intensive Care Unit

Because the NICU staff has weeks or months to become familiar with the infants it manages, it generally is in the best position to identify the patient's needs, initiate discharge planning, and ensure that the required components of the follow-up team are in place. Responsibility for identifying an infant as high risk is assumed by the infant's primary nurse, the neonatologist, or a neonatal follow-up coordinator, who might be either a nurse or a physician. High-risk infants are identified as quickly as possible, their parents are notified, and an immediate attempt is made to enroll the patient into the comprehensive follow-up program. Early discussion with the parents is essential, inasmuch as it allows them to contribute to and understand the objectives of the follow-up plan.

As the day of discharge from the NICU approaches, neonatal staff members must be satisfied that the infant's condition is stable and that the family is capable of assuming his or her care. Any major medical problems should have been either resolved or stabilized. Medication regimens should be rechecked to determine that each has been simplified to the extent possible, that all dosages are correct, that appropriate blood levels have been obtained, and that adverse reactions or side effects have been explained to the parents. The final days of hospitalization also provide time to ensure that all necessary testing has been completed (e.g., hematocrit levels, hearing screening, ophthalmological examination for retinopathy of prematurity, head ultrasonography, or echocardiography). The infant's medical history is reviewed with family members, their questions are answered, and their residual concerns are addressed and, if possible, assuaged.

Unfortunately, evidence persists that when many infants leave the NICU, their parents do not have a good understanding of what has transpired or of what they can expect, and the primary care physician has not even been notified of the discharge through a formal narrative summary of the infant's hospital course, much less included in the discharge planning by a telephone call from the neonatologist. Even with the practitioner's busy schedule, the telephone (and electronic mail) can be invaluable tools for exchanging information. Such a call allows each party to participate in discharge planning and to discuss issues of concern; it also provides an opportunity to update the primary care physician on new treatment modalities, fosters a feeling of collaboration, and encourages future discussion. Despite the availability of such avenues of communication, in one survey 55% of pediatricians believed that they had been inadequately informed about the NICU discharge status of their high-risk patients before the first office visit.[17]

High-Risk Follow-up Programs

High-risk neonatal follow-up clinics are not meant to provide primary care or in any way to replace the community physician. Indeed, most high-risk clinics prefer to work in conjunction with the infant's primary care physician, assisting wherever possible and offering supplemental services. A typical neonatal high-risk follow-up schedule might include an initial visit 2 to 6 weeks after the infant's discharge, followed by visits at 6 months, 1 year, and 2 years of age. The strengths of a neonatal high-risk clinic include its multidisciplinary composition and its links to other health care resources. During a clinic visit an infant may be evaluated by any combination of the following: neonatologists, nurses, physical therapists, social workers, developmental specialists, and child psychologists. Using this team of experts allows a look beyond the child's more immediate medical problems to such long-range issues as infant development and behavior, family stresses, and financial problems.

Subspecialty Clinics

Among the services neonatal patients and their illnesses attract into the NICU are cardiology, neurology, endocrinology, genetics, hematology, surgery, orthopedics, urology, cardiothoracic surgery, neurosurgery, and ophthalmology. Dietitians, physical therapists, audiologists, nurses specializing in wound care, and many others also participate in the care of NICU patients. The neonatal high-risk follow-up clinic is the natural coordinating center in which the efforts of these individuals and their communication with the primary care physician and parents can occur in single rather than multiple visits.

Ancillary Health Services

A number of nonphysician personnel can enhance considerably the care given high-risk infants in the NICU and in their homes.

Neonatal nurses, who bond with the infants they care for day after day, develop relationships with the families that persist beyond the day of discharge. Social workers are consulted frequently in the NICU, since families of high-risk infants often are at high risk—single-parent households, young and uneducated parents, inadequate home environment, unemployment and financial stress, child abuse and neglect, drug abuse, and other difficulties that have major implications for the well-being of discharged infants. These problems often are magnified during the hospital course in the NICU.

Physical and occupational therapists and feeding specialists strengthen follow-up and enhance the quality of life for high-risk infants. Physicians, also, rely on therapists to perform serial assessments of gross and fine motor development, reflexes, muscle tone, strength, range of motion, posture, ambulation, sensory perception, feeding abilities, phonation, and adaptational skills. After a thorough evaluation, these therapists are able to counsel parents and physicians, suggest management strategies, and instruct parents in how to perform specific therapies. As treatment proceeds, the therapists should participate in the reevaluation of both the patient and the treatment plan.

Commercial home health care companies are burgeoning, and all physicians need to be familiar with and use them. They supply a wide range of services and home health care equipment that are especially appropriate for high-risk infants, such as home oxygen supplies, ventilators, pulse oximeters, apnea monitors, and suction machines. The equipment is backed by 24-hour maintenance and service, as well as professionals with experience in pediatrics who can go into the home and teach the parents or perform physical assessments at the physician's direction. These companies rely on physician referrals, and usually they are conscientious about reporting problems within the home or changes in the infant's condition. Thus they can serve as an essential local link of expertise between the high-risk follow-up staff and the primary care physician.

Community Resources and Public Health Services

A comprehensive review of all community resources and public health services is beyond the scope of this chapter, but knowledge of regionally available programs will assist the physician greatly in the management of high-risk infants. Such programs include visits from community health nurses or special services for children, special educational programs, early intervention programs with evaluation and rehabilitation, specialized foster care, parental support groups, respite or hospice care, and financial assistance for food, supplies, and medical needs. In considering community resources, the physician should not neglect friends, relatives, and individuals with religious or social significance to the family. Physicians should learn to take advantage of these types of resources because they can affect the immediate health and long-term development of their patients significantly.

Parents of High-Risk Infants

By necessity, the parents of a high-risk infant become immediate members of the follow-up team. These are the people with the heaviest emotional investment in their baby; ultimately, they will assume the greatest share of the caretaking responsibilities. A major prerequisite for adequate parenting (sadly, not always satisfied) is that the parents have a genuine interest in the infant and his or her well-being. Once it is established that this basic requirement has been fulfilled, the neonatal staff must begin the rigorous preparation that these parents need most.

During the hospitalization the parents should have developed a reasonable idea of their infant's illnesses, symptoms, treatments, and prognoses. This information provides the groundwork for the observational skills the parents will use in the home to monitor their infant's medical condition. Because they will have the most extensive contact with the baby, the parents must be capable of detecting deterioration or significant alteration in their infant's health and bringing these findings to medical attention. Parents who will be expected to administer medications must demonstrate understanding and competence regarding dosages, timing, routes of administration, adverse effects, and precautions. Parents of infants who are discharged with special equipment (e.g., nasal cannula oxygen, nasogastric tube feeding, intravenous hyperalimentation, home apnea monitors) must be completely and explicitly schooled in their use. They also must understand what to do and whom to notify when malfunctions occur.

Parents often are required to learn certain basic or even "high-tech" nursing functions, as well as cardiopulmonary resuscitation. Nonetheless, time spent demonstrating how to feed, bathe, dress, and simply enjoy their baby will enhance the quality of care rendered and boost the parents' self-esteem. The neonatal team also should ascertain whether the parents can procure food, clothing, a car seat, and a crib for their infant and if they have access to a telephone and transportation.

Although these requirements must be fulfilled before an infant is discharged from the NICU, it is equally important to ensure that circumstances do not deteriorate over time after discharge. The primary care physician must assume principal responsibility for continued monitoring of these aspects of the infant's family and home.

The Primary Care Physician

The distribution of high-risk infant survivors is such that any primary care practitioner today can expect to be called upon to manage these infants. Whether that involvement occurs during or subsequent to the NICU stay is very much a function of local custom, as well as the practitioner's interest, training, available time, and geography relative to the NICU.

The practitioner's fundamental role, however, is to serve as the family's principal assimilator and translator of the onslaught of often-confusing information presented by an army of nurses, neonatologists, pediatric subspecialists, dietitians, technologists, and students, all encountered during the NICU stay or subsequent visits to the high-risk follow-up clinic. As the only person in this vast array who may have known the family before and after the added stress of its high-risk infant, the primary care physician is the natural "case manager" for this child. In this setting the practitioner must serve as the link between the family and the NICU and its follow-up staff.

MEDICAL MANAGEMENT OF HIGH-RISK INFANTS

A comprehensive catalog of common and critical neonatal illnesses and treatments is provided in Chapters 47 and 48; the review presented here concentrates on VLBW infants (those whose birth weight is less than 1500 g) and their diverse problem lists.

Primary Health Care Considerations

In addition to monitoring the identified medical problems of high-risk infants, primary care physicians also must promote normal growth and development, anticipate normal age-appropriate problems, and educate parents about routine pediatric issues, just as they do with their low-risk patients. For example, the parents should receive anticipatory counseling about preventing injuries, even though they may not realize initially that their NICU graduate eventually will encounter the same hazards as other children. Likewise, pediatricians need to emphasize that infants must be secured adequately whenever traveling by automobile. All states now enforce seat belt laws, which were meant to prevent the 500 deaths and 53,000 injuries that occur each year in the United States among children under age 4 as the result of automobile accidents. Parents taking VLBW infants home need to know that most infant restraint systems are marketed for babies weighing more than 7 pounds. Some of these devices may be inappropriate for tiny infants because they do not provide enough support to prevent airway compromise with decreases in arterial oxygen saturation when the infant is seated upright. Any medical equipment also must be secured and, if an apnea monitor has been recommended for the infant, it should function properly during any automobile travel. Helpful guidelines are available from the American Academy of Pediatrics' Committee on Accident and Poison Prevention.

Growth

Growth, an exquisitely sensitive marker of health, must be monitored and documented frequently. Weight, length, and head circumference must be measured and plotted against "corrected age" (postnatal age in weeks less the number of weeks by which the infant was prematurely born) on appropriate growth curves. Although there are specific growth charts for sick, tiny premature infants while they are in the NICU, these generally are not required after an infant is discharged; standard growth charts are suitable. *Weight should be plotted against the infant's corrected age until 24 months of age,* after which time premature infants generally follow the same weight curves as children who were born at term. Significant deviations from expected weight gain may indicate excess fluid retention or inadequate caloric intake relative to metabolic demands. Length should be similarly corrected for prematurity until the infant is 3½ years of age, whereas head circumference (as an indicator of brain growth) should be plotted against corrected age until 18 months of age. Although not entirely predictive, correlations do exist between growth failure and neurodevelopmental delays.[27] Conversely, achievement of a normal head circumference by 8 months of age is a predictor of normal psychosocial development at age 3.[14]

Many premature infants at discharge are smaller than the third growth percentiles for corrected age, either because of intrauterine growth retardation or because of serious neonatal illness. "Catch-up growth" should be expected and promoted in most of these infants in the first year of life. Generally, *head circumference reaches a normal percentile first, followed by length, and finally by weight.* Catch-up growth is maximal between 36 to 44 postconceptual weeks; most infants begin to grow along their new growth curve by 6 to 12 months. If a premature infant of birth weight appropriate for gestational age does not achieve at least the third percentile by age 3, future catch-up growth should not be anticipated. Premature infants who show severe intrauterine growth retardation usually do not achieve normal values postnatally.

Nutrition

The American Academy of Pediatrics recommends breast milk as the feeding of choice for infants, including premature ones. To achieve 1800 to 2000 g of body weight, premature infants require either calorically dense "premature formula" or mother's breast milk fortified by calories, minerals, and vitamins. The AAP's Committee on Infant Nutrition suggests that after the infant has attained a weight of 2000 g breast milk alone is a practical, nutritionally adequate source of nutrition with immunological properties that may reduce the incidence of respiratory and gastrointestinal infections. Mothers who opt not to breast-feed may use standard infant formula after the baby's weight reaches 2000 g. Certain infants, such as those who have severe osteopenia or those whose fluids must be restricted, may benefit from the increased calcium/phosphorus content and caloric density (24 Cal/ounce) of premature formula until they reach 44 to 48 weeks of postconceptual age. Breast-fed infants who are well enough to be discharged from the NICU should receive standard amounts of vitamins A, D, and C, with fluoride added, if the family's water supply is fluoride deficient. The need for vitamin E supplementation usually diminishes after 6 to 8 weeks of postnatal age, by which time the risk of hemolytic anemia has passed. Despite the osteopenia common to acutely ill premature infants, most ultimately can manage normal bone development on the usual amounts of calcium and phosphorus found in standard lactose-based infant formulas. Finally, formula-fed premature infants should receive 2 to 3 mg/kg/day of supplemental elemental iron from 6 to 8 weeks of postnatal age until approximately 6 months of age. Some believe that infants whose birth weight was less than 1000 g may benefit from supplementary doses of iron approaching 4 mg/kg/day until they are 1 year old. Finally, dietary advances in premature infants should be based on their actual, rather than "corrected," postnatal age.

The feeding of high-risk infants should be normalized to the extent possible, but there are many qualifying conditions that deserve consideration. Some infants, such as those with intrauterine growth retardation or bronchopulmonary dysplasia, have such a high metabolic rate that their bodies demand 120 to 150 Cal/kg/day for sustained growth. Ironically, many infants who have the highest caloric requirements have the misfortune also to require fluid restriction. In others, a structural or functional short bowel syndrome (secondary to conditions such as necrotizing enterocolitis, gastroschisis, bowel atresia, malrotation, meconium ileus, or Hirschsprung disease) can seriously limit enteral nutrition. Loss of gastrointestinal surface area because of such diseases or their surgical treatment also can limit absorption of other important nutrients, such as vitamins and minerals. In many cases, the amount and composition of the infant's feedings will require continual alteration and reevaluation. Protein, fat, and carbohydrate can be added to breast milk or formula to provide a more calorically dense feeding. Caloric densities as high as 30 Cal/ounce can be achieved, but care must be taken to prevent unwanted gastrointestinal or renal effects as a result of inordinate amounts of any one source of calories. If the infant's enteral caloric intake will not be sufficient for acceptable growth, intravenous total parenteral nutrition should be instituted. This route for nutrition is quite demanding and requires profound parental commitment, a central venous catheter, many monitoring laboratory determinations, and a qualified team responsible for designing and monitoring the nutritional strategy and working with the primary care physician.

Aside from monitoring growth variables, the primary care physician also should review details of the infant's feeding habits, such as schedules, amount and type of feeding, signs of gastroesophageal reflux, or other feeding difficulties. Graduates of the unnatural NICU environment who have experienced insufficient amounts of nonnutritive sucking and prolonged periods of nasogastric or endotracheal intubation can be notoriously difficult feeders. Parents often need much reassurance, coaching, and support in this regard; referral to a qualified feeding specialist occasionally is indicated. The physician also should inquire about stooling and voiding patterns, since these may be clues to underlying conditions, such as malabsorption or colonic stricture (secondary to previous episodes of necrotizing enterocolitis).

Immunizations

In general, immunization schedules for high-risk premature infants do not differ from those recommended for term infants by the American Academy of Pediatrics' Committee on Infectious Disease. Dosages should not be reduced, divided, or delayed to correct for prematurity. Moreover, these recommendations are updated continuously; thus primary care practitioners must stay abreast of revisions as they occur.

Hepatitis B is common in high-risk pregnancies, and any infant born to a mother who is seropositive for hepatitis B surface antigen (or whose hepatitis B status is unknown) is a candidate for prophylactic therapy. Such infants should receive 0.5 ml of hepatitis B immunoglobulin intramuscularly within the first 12 hours of life, followed by 0.5 ml of hepatitis B vaccine (10 μg) intramuscularly within the first day, at 1 month, and again at 6 months. The American Academy of Pediatrics currently recommends that all infants receive hepatitis B vaccine on the first day of life, at 1 to 2 months of age, and again at 4 to 6 months of age. Certain chronically ill high-risk infants, such as patients who have bronchopulmonary dysplasia or congestive heart failure, should be vaccinated annually against influenza. In the fall, before the influenza season begins, infants generally are given two doses (0.25 ml) of split virus vaccine intramuscularly at least 4 weeks apart. Recommendations for vaccination against respiratory syncytial virus (RSV) are being developed currently for premature infants and those who have chronic lung disease.

Other Primary Care Issues

As with any other children, pediatricians should screen NICU graduates for such common problems as anemia, lead intoxication, and tuberculosis. Sadly, they also must maintain awareness of the risks of HIV infection, especially among those who have disordered life-styles. Infant behavior, development, and sleep patterns, as well as parental bonding, frequently are areas of intense concern and stress for parents of high-risk infants who had a lengthy stay in a NICU. Finally, all health care providers must guard against the chronic environmental insults of malnutrition, poor hygiene, abuse, and neglect. High-risk infants appear to be more likely than others to suffer these insults.

Rehospitalization

The path back to the hospital may be well-worn during the first year or two after discharge of the VLBW child. One fourth to one third of these infants require rehospitalization, principally for exacerbations of developmental problems that derive from their prematurity—necrotizing enterocolitis, ligation of a patent ductus arteriosus, herniorrhaphies, and revisions of ventriculoperitoneal (or other) shunts for hemorrhagic hydrocephalus.[21,23] Especially wearing are the rehospitalizations for respiratory infectious disease (particularly respiratory syncytial virus) that often are necessary with children receiving home oxygen therapy for residual bronchopulmonary dysplasia during the winter season.

All these assaults easily can weaken the resolve and decimate the morale of even the most robust family network; they are infinitely more oppressive for the often-dysfunctional nonfamilies in which many high-risk infants live. An uneducated, drug-abusing, single, teenage child-mother (with or without the support of her unemployed boyfriend), recently ejected from the house of her alcoholic parents is among the more severe management challenges modern society can throw at the medical establishment, with demands for instant resolution. It is gratifyingly remarkable what often can be accomplished in such a situation by a primary physician/social worker team knowledgeable about the mother and her community and in close touch with the pertinent NICU's high-risk follow-up staff.

Specific Neonatal Problems

Hearing. The high-risk infant's situation is fraught with opportunities to sustain significant sensorineural hearing loss: asphyxia, hyperbilirubinemia, nosocomial infection (meningitis), and congenital infection (cytomegalovirus, rubella, herpes, toxoplasmosis, syphilis), as well as frequent exposure to aminoglycoside antibiotics. Moderate to profound hearing loss is two to five times more likely to develop in high-risk infants than in the general population of children, and the VLBW child is at even greater risk for severe hearing loss. The usual behavioral-observational pace of ascertaining whether a child hears is simply too slow to be of much help in this assessment. Accordingly, the recent development of the brainstem auditory evoked response (BAER), an electroencephalographic technique, has been most welcome, especially in meeting the challenge of the infant under 6 months of age.[4,24] These examinations usually are performed before the infant is discharged from the NICU, but regular reassessment often is necessary.

Retinopathy of Prematurity. The renaming of retrolental fibroplasia (RLF) to retinopathy of prematurity (ROP) has served to emphasize that this is much more a developmental than an iatrogenic phenomenon. Indeed, as VLBW infants increasingly survive, their risk for the development of ROP is nearly 50% (if the birth weight is under 1000 g), regardless of the oxygen environment sustained. This risk falls to less than 3% as the birth weight advances to over 1500 g, so the so-called second epidemic (of RLF since the original episode of the 1950s) is attributable to the increasing survival of the "tiny premature" at maximum developmental risk for ROP.[12] The principal risk factors remain immaturity of retinal vascularization and fluctuating levels of arterial oxygen saturation.

The current approach to minimizing that risk is one principally of increased ophthalmological surveillance (indirect ophthalmoscopic examination under pupillary dilation by the pediatric ophthalmologist) and early intervention (by cryotherapy or laser surgery) if the disease threatens to advance beyond the reversible early stages to irreversible, cicatricial disease. Fortunately, even some cicatricial disease eventually may resolve. Most VLBW infants will need continuing ophthalmological evaluation to monitor resolution of ROP and ascertain retinal maturity, as well as to assess refractive errors and the problems in ocular alignment so commonly found in the VLBW population.

Bronchopulmonary Dysplasia (BPD). This condition is the frustrating outcome for 20% to 30% of the VLBW survivors of hyaline membrane disease; its incidence is inversely related to gestational age and birth weight. The necessary ingredients are pulmonary immaturity (including surfactant deficiency and immature immunological/antioxidant systems), increased alveolar oxygen concentration, and the "barotrauma" imposed by prolonged periods of artificial ventilation at high airway pressures. BPD also can develop in extremely immature infants who have not had preceding hyaline membrane disease. The pathophysiological behavior of BPD is similar to that of chronic obstructive lung disease (COLD) seen in later life. These behavioral features include (1) "reactive" small airway disease, characterized by increased resistance to gaseous flow through the airways, (2) consequent "air-trapping" and mismatching of deoxygenated pulmonary blood flow with deoxygenated, rather than fresh oxygenated alveolar gas, and (3) increased vascular resistance and right-sided heart strain. Just as in adult emphysema, the gas-exchanging hallmark is one of hypercapnia and hypoxemia. The former usually is compensated by bicarbonate retention via the kidneys, and the latter can be palliated with an enriched oxygen environment. Treatment is similar to that for other reactive airway diseases (e.g., asthma) and currently involves bronchodilators, diuretics, physiotherapy and, increasingly, steroids. The primary care practitioner who assists in the home care of these infants needs to help the family deal with home oxygen therapy (chiefly by nasal cannula), apnea monitoring (impedance monitor), and pulse oximetry during the 4 to 6 months usually required for improvement (probably through remodeling of the growing and differentiating lung). Serial chest roentgenograms, ECGs, and echocardiography can be helpful in detecting early cor pulmonale during this period. It is essential that patients who have BPD receive enough calories daily (often in the face of fluid restriction) to support adequate growth and activity. During this trying time, the infant can be expected to be particularly susceptible to respiratory infections, especially respiratory syncytial virus. Exposure to such infections should be minimized wherever possible, and rehospitalization should be quickly considered for possible respiratory support, should such prevention not succeed. Such attentions eventually are rewarded by normalization of the chest roentgenogram at about 2 years of age; yet abnormal small airways are detectable by certain pulmonary function tests well into adolescence, evidently more related to the degree of prematurity than to the duration of artificial ventilation therapy.[8,11,13]

Developmental Delays. Despite the numerous insults that plague premature infants during their stay in the NICU, a happy developmental outcome for most (at least those VLBW infants over 1000 g at birth) has been the gratifying norm. However, certain complications, such as intraventricular hemorrhage, periventricular leukomalacia, and advanced cicatricial ROP, contribute to poor, even devastating, neurodevelopmental outcome. The development of significant BPD may itself be a marker of poor neurodevelopmental outcome, even where no specific injury to the brain can be documented. The current biological threshold for reasonable expectation of a healthy viability appears to be about 25 weeks of gestation and a birth weight of 750 g, if the infant is appropriately grown for gestational age.[2,15] Major handicaps (mental retardation, cerebral palsy, hydrocephalus, seizure disorders, sensorineural impairments) can be expected in about 30% of surviving infants below this threshold.[9,20]

The most recent study exploring the limits of viability reports *intact* survival rates of 2%, 21%, and 69% for infants born at 23, 24, and 25 weeks' gestation, respectively.[2] The screening and more definitive tools available for assessing the extent and impact of such disabilities in these infants are the same as those developed for the general evaluation of gross and fine motor function, language skills, and social adaptation (see Chapter 20).

Even the more horrendous developmental disabilities, once sustained, tend to be stable, rather than progressive. However, infants with hydrocephalus who have shunts in place are susceptible to shunt malfunction and infection. These events may dictate that the neurosurgeon share with the primary care physician the role of maintaining the shunt. Indeed, the ongoing management of shunts in these children is a paradigm for the multidisciplinary approach required to best serve all multiply handicapped children. The government also plays a role in the multidisciplinary approach. Public Law 94-142 (Education for All Handicapped Children, 1975) stipulated the provision of special education within the school system for handicapped children; this law was extended by Public Law 99-457 (1986) to include infants and preschool children. It thus supports the extension of appropriate early intervention services directly to NICU graduates as they are enrolled in high-risk follow-up clinics.

Apnea/Bradycardia. Prolonged apnea has been defined operationally as a cessation of breathing for at least 20 seconds, or as a briefer episode of apnea that is associated with bradycardia, cyanosis, or pallor. Briefer episodes, as well as frank periodic breathing are normal respiratory patterns of preterm infants; the severity and frequency of these immature respiratory patterns are inversely related to gestational age. Many otherwise thriving premature infants now are discharged from the NICU to their homes to continue the same sort of cardiorespiratory monitoring that characterized their NICU stay (heart rate, impedance pneumography, and pulse oximetry) until their respiratory function matures, as documented by 8 alarmless weeks of monitoring. A recent Consensus Statement by the National Institutes of Health does not endorse the use of "pneumograms" to decide when home apnea monitoring can be discontinued safely. Impedance pneumography is the most commonly used (but not always the most reliable) of these several monitoring modes, with frequent false alarms being related simply to poor electrode-skin contact.

For some years, much emotion but little information has swirled around the presumption that infantile apnea (long or short) is related to sudden infant death syndrome (SIDS). Parents (but not their physicians) may be excused for confusing a very large population of normal premature infants with immature respiratory systems from the (probably) very different and immensely smaller population of infants at true risk for SIDS. These latter infants include (1) the siblings of infants who died of SIDS, (2) babies who have suffered an acute life-threatening event (ALTE) of sudden apnea, pallor or cyanosis, limpness, and unconsciousness, and (3) babies who suffer from severe bronchopulmonary dysplasia.

The infant who has an ALTE merits particular investigation to rule out gastroesophageal reflux, upper airway obstruction, seizure disorder, anemia, or other remedial disorders before he or she is automatically placed on a regimen of home apnea monitoring. More than a decade of such monitoring efforts have not appeared to have prevented many SIDS deaths; however, many episodes of less severe apnea may have been prevented.[3,19]

SUMMARY

As difficult as the VLBW infant may have been to care for within the protective shell of the NICU, the challenge presented to the family does not slacken quickly after discharge. These children are more expensive, more temperamentally "difficult,"[23] and often perceived as more vulnerable than a child of term birth. The emotional and fiscal burdens they present often are unloaded on a shaky family structure. Simple tools for examining this structure—the Pediatric Review and Observation of Children's Environmental Support and Stimulation (PROCESS) inventory and the Home Observation for Measurement of the Environment (HOME) inventory[7] or its office equivalent, Home Screening Questionnaire (HSQ)[10]—recently have become available to assess and follow the success of the interventional strategies used to maximize the full development of each infant's potential.[5]

The happy photographic "rogues' gallery" of NICU graduates that adorns the entrance to most such units bears smiling testimony to the level of success that can be anticipated to reward this effort.

REFERENCES

1. Allen DM et al: Mortality in infants discharged from neonatal intensive care units in Georgia, *JAMA* 261:1763, 1989.
2. Allen MC, Donohue PK, Dusman AE: The limit of viability: neonatal outcome of infants born at 22 to 25 weeks' gestation, *N Engl J Med* 329:1597, 1993.
3. American Academy of Pediatrics' Committee Statement, Task Force on Prolonged Infantile Apnea: Prolonged infantile apnea 1985, *Pediatrics* 76:129, 1985.
4. American Academy of Pediatrics' Joint Committee on Infant Hearing: Position statement 1982, *Pediatrics* 70:496, 1982.
5. Barrera ME, Cunningham CE, Rosenbaum PL: Low birth weight and home intervention strategies: preterm infants, *J Dev Behav Pediatr* 7:361, 1986.
6. Brooten D et al: A randomized clinical trial of early hospital discharge and home follow-up of very-low-birth-weight infants, *N Engl J Med* 315:934, 1986.
7. Casey PH et al: The clinical assessment of a child's social and physical environment during health visits, *J Dev Behav Pediatr* 9:333, 1988.
8. Fiascone JM et al: Bronchopulmonary dysplasia: review for the pediatrician, *Curr Probl Pediatr* 19:169, 1989.
9. Field TM et al: Teenage, lower class black mothers and their preterm infants: an intervention and developmental follow-up, *Child Dev* 51:426, 1980.
10. Frankenburg WK, Coons CE: Home Screening Questionnaire: its validity in assessing home environment, *J Pediatr* 108:624, 1986.
11. Galdès-Sebaldt M et al: Prematurity is associated with abnormal airway function in childhood, *Pediatr Pulmonol* 7:259, 1989.
12. Gibson DL et al: Retinopathy of prematurity-induced blindness: birth weight–specific survival and the new epidemic, *Pediatrics* 86:405, 1990.
13. Goldson E: Severe bronchopulmonary dysplasia in the very-low-birth-weight infant: its relationship to developmental outcome, *J Dev Behav Pediatr* 5:165, 1984.
14. Hack M, Breslau N: Very-low-birth-weight infants: effects of brain growth during infancy on intelligence quotient at 3 years of age, *Pediatrics* 77:196, 1986.
15. Hack M, Fanaroff AA: Outcomes of extremely-low-birth-weight infants between 1982 and 1988, *N Engl J Med* 321:1642, 1989.
16. Hagberg B et al: The changing panorama of cerebral palsy in Sweden, *Acta Paediatr Scand* 78:283, 1989.
17. Hurt H: Continuing care of the high-risk infant, *Clin Perinatol* 11:3, 1984.
18. Kulkarni P et al: Postneonatal infant mortality in infants admitted to a neonatal intensive care unit, *Pediatrics* 62:178, 1978.
19. Light MJ, Sheridan MS: Home monitoring in Hawaii: the first 1000 patients, *Hawaii Med J* 48:304, 1989.
20. McCormick MC: Long-term follow-up of infants discharged from neonatal intensive care units, *JAMA* 261:1767, 1989.
21. McCormick MC, Shapiro S, Starfield BH: Rehospitalization in the first year of life for high-risk survivors, *Pediatrics* 66:991, 1980.
22. Medoff-Cooper B: Temperament in very-low-birth-weight infants, *Nurs Res* 35:139, 1986.
23. Mutch L et al: Secular rehospitalization of very-low-birth-weight infants, *Pediatrics* 78:164, 1986.
24. Nield TA et al: Unexpected hearing loss in high-risk infants, *Pediatrics* 78:417, 1986.
25. Office of Technology Assessment: Neonatal care for low-birth-weight infants: costs and effectiveness, Health Technology Case Study 38, Pub No OTA-HCS-38, Washington, DC, 1987, US Government Printing Office.
26. Phavoah P et al: Birth-weight–specific trends in cerebral palsy, *Arch Dis Child* 65:602, 1990.
27. Saigal S et al: Follow-up of infants 501 to 1500 gm birth weight delivered to residents of a geographically defined region with perinatal intensive care facilities, *J Pediatr* 100:606, 1982.
28. Stanley F, Watson L: Trends in perinatal mortality and cerebral palsy in Western Australia, 1967 to 1985, *Br Med J* 304:1658, 1992.
29. Wariyar UK, Sam R: Morbidity and preterm delivery: importance of 100% follow-up, *Lancet* 1:387, 1989.

SUGGESTED READINGS

Hurt H: Continuing care of the high-risk infant, *Clin Perinatol* 11:1, 1984.

Taeusch HW, Yogman MW: *Follow-up management of the high-risk infant,* Boston, 1987, Little, Brown.

PART SIX
Psychosocial Issues in Child Health Care

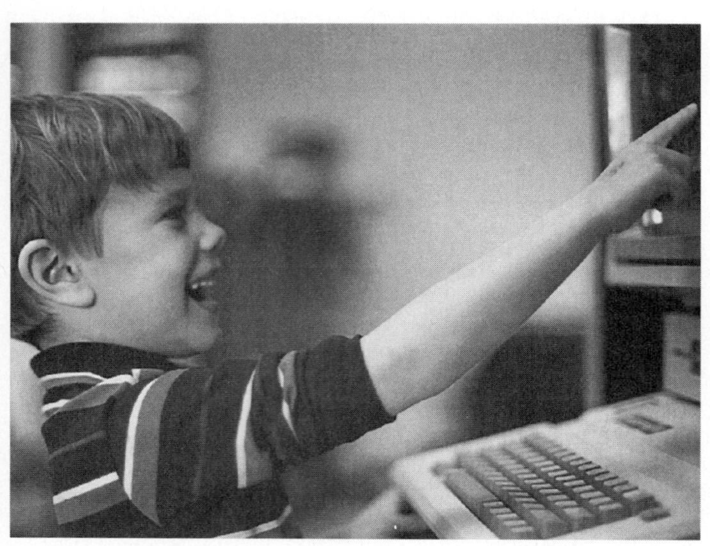

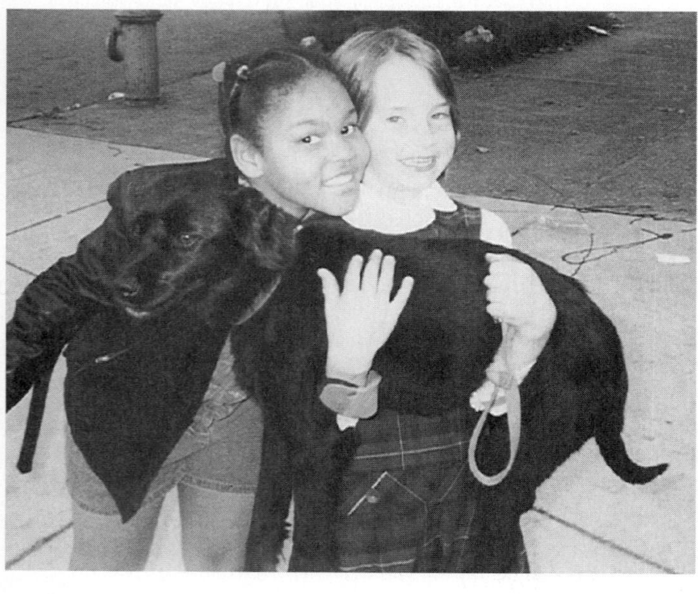

SECTION ONE

PSYCHOLOGICAL DEVELOPMENT

SECTION TWO

THE FAMILY

51 Theories and Concepts of Development As They Relate to Pediatric Practice

Olle Jane Z. Sahler and Beatrice L. Wood

This chapter focuses on the psychological development of the child from fetal life through adolescence. For the purposes of this discussion, *psychology* is defined as that branch of science devoted to the study of emotion, cognition, and social conduct. Because the individual is part of a larger psycho-social-biological system, the chapter incorporates discussions of the effects of heredity, environmental influences, and biological maturation on development. Finally, three specific issues are examined: the development of moral judgment, the development of gender identity, and the psychobiology of stress.

No unified developmental theory, by itself, explains or defines all the behaviors that can be observed in any particular child. Thus several theories are presented that, taken collectively, enable us to understand and interpret behaviors common to a particular developmental age. With this framework it becomes possible to interpret a child's behavior to parents in a developmental context and to devise strategies that can help children and their families cope effectively with common stressful situations.

The ever-developing personality style and cognitive functioning of the pediatric patient add the requirement of constant reevaluation and renegotiation to any treatment regimen, regardless of whether a child's problem is physical or the result of a combination of physical and emotional elements. However, this very fluidity and malleability often make substantive intervention possible with a pediatric patient when it would be impossible with an adult patient. The practitioner's ability to help rechannel and refocus the child's emotional energy along more constructive paths before undesirable habits or other maladaptive behaviors become fixed is one of the rewards of working with children. Primary prevention is a realistic goal. Conversely, the child's relatively unformed and fragile sense of self is particularly vulnerable to outside influences that might have little or no effect on the adult. Thus the practitioner has an obligation to evaluate the social network surrounding the child to identify and help eliminate impediments to the child's realization of his or her fullest potential. In this context, the practitioner, as developmentalist, can become a knowledgeable and effective advocate for someone who is too young, too inexperienced, and too politically naive to speak as an independent individual.

FACTORS THAT INFLUENCE PSYCHOLOGICAL DEVELOPMENT

Although it still is unclear how innate capacities and inclinations (heredity) and learning and experience (environment) influence who and what a child becomes as an adult, we do know that both act as observable and measurable factors.

Heredity

Temperament and Personality. Several years ago, investigators such as Thomas and Chess[46,47] identified a complex system of idiosyncratic differences in the responsiveness of infants and young children to their environment. These individual tendencies have been shown to be stable from infancy through early adulthood; thus they appear to be innate behavioral tendencies that shape later personality. This collection of personal attributes has been labeled *temperament,* and nine elements have been found to be useful descriptors of how a child behaves: (1) activity level, (2) rhythmicity, (3) approach and/or withdrawal from a new stimulus, (4) adaptability, (5) intensity of reaction, (6) threshold of responsiveness, (7) mood, (8) distractibility, and (9) attention span and persistence. These temperamental traits lead to parental perceptions that a particular child is "easygoing" or "difficult." Such judgments are based on the parents' observations of how the child responds to various environmental stimuli and on the degree to which the child is self-sufficient in meeting his or her own needs for contentment. These early studies spawned a robust and far-ranging area of investigation in developmental psychology, and the concept has been refined through empirical validation studies. Currently, constructs of temperament emphasize psychophysiological reactivity[24] and self-regulation, particularly of arousal level and emotion.[36,37] There is strong support for the heritability of temperament and even personality,[16,31] although only about half of the influence seems to be of genetic origin. Thus even the so-called innate or constitutional characteristics of temperament are influenced by environmental factors.

Intelligence. Data suggest that the capacity to perceive and understand facts and to reason about them is, in large measure, genetically determined. *Intelligence,* as defined in our culture, is a composite of specific abilities, including verbal ability (use of language), quantitative ability (use of numbers), spatial ability (discrimination of objects in space), disembedding (separation of an element from its background), analytical ability (problem solving), reasoning (formulation and testing of hypotheses), and mastery of concepts. Individuals are not born with all these skills, nor are they all learned during infancy. Rather, skills are acquired gradually over a period that extends into adolescence and even adulthood. Thus the concept of the intelligence quotient (IQ), or ratio of the cognitive maturational age (MA) to the chronological age (CA)

$$IQ = \frac{MA}{CA} \times 100$$

has become a popular device for comparing the abilities of a particular child with those of other children at a similar age. Although test interpretations and score distributions vary somewhat, IQs in the range of 90 to 110 usually are considered average. The most widely used tests are composed of subscales that measure both verbal and performance intelligence (see Appendix D).

Studies of the contribution of inherited or genetic factors to intelligence have focused primarily on gender and racial differences uncovered by analyzing scores attained on standardized tests across various population groups.[33] Although there are no consistent gender differences in total IQ scores on tests that present a balanced contribution from all the skill groups, beginning in adolescence gender differences appear in certain specific areas of ability. Females, in general, have greater verbal ability than males; conversely, males have greater visual-spatial and quantitative abilities than females. Whether these differences are the result of learning (i.e., greater emphasis on developing verbal skills in girls and manual skills in boys) or genetic predisposition remains controversial. However, it has been hypothesized that the rate of brain maturation is linked to verbal and visual-spatial ability; thus the verbal superiority of females may be due to their relatively fast rate of development, whereas the spatial advantage seen in males may be due to their slower rate of maturation. This gender difference is thought by some to be due to the effect of the Y chromosome in prolonging the process of maturation. Support for the hypothesis that specific skills are related to the length of the maturation process is provided by studies showing that early maturers, irrespective of gender, have greater verbal than spatial ability, whereas later maturers have greater spatial than verbal ability.

Studies of children and adolescents reared in single-parent homes have shown that boys raised in father-absent homes may have more "female" cognitive traits, whereas girls raised in mother-absent homes may have more "male" cognitive traits compared with gender-matched controls raised in traditional two-parent families.[6,21,25] This finding is somewhat inconsistent and appears to depend on the child's age at the time of separation and the degree to which the same-gender parent or a replacement figure interacts with the child. However, the finding that these differences occur even to a limited extent is important, because it points to the role of the environment in modifying what once were thought to be inherited gender-specific traits and further highlights the interaction between nature and nurture in psychological development.

Racial differences in intelligence testing also have been found. International studies have shown that members of Oriental populations originating in Japan and China and Caucasian populations originating in Northern Europe tend to score highest on IQ tests. These findings should be interpreted with caution. Although "global" intelligence tests have been designed to equalize the relative contributions of each of the specific skill areas in which scores vary by gender, psychologists have been less successful in devising "culture-fair" tests that can measure mental ability separately from learned cognitive skills and independently of social or economic effects. Thus it still is arguable whether differences in test scores among various population groups obtained to date reflect true superior racial ability or merely greater cultural emphasis on training in the particular skills measured.

Environment

The contribution of genetic makeup to temperament, personality, and cognitive function as a factor influencing development undoubtedly is important. However, in recent years developmentalists have become more sophisticated in the way they view the nature-versus-nurture conflict. Indeed, the most important implication of their recognizing that heritability explains only a portion of behavioral outcome is that the other portion must be accounted for by other factors, most notably the environment. For children and adolescents the most likely environmental influences come from the family, school, and peer systems.

Family. The family is the first social unit to which the child belongs. Cultural changes that have increased the diversity of caregiving systems necessitate redefinition of the term "family." In this context, perhaps the most useful definition of "family" is "that group of people, living together or in close contact, who take care of one another and provide guidance for their dependent members." Membership in a family helps to ensure that the child is physically and emotionally nurtured. In addition, the family's cultural beliefs are transmitted to the child. The ultimate goal of the family is to produce an autonomous adult who can individuate from the family of origin and live a meaningful and generative life.

Traditional approaches to studying the relationship between a child's environment and his or her development assume that children in the same family experience or "share" similar environmental influences, such as socioeconomic opportunities and child rearing attitudes. However, current research in behavioral genetics has shown that siblings are surprisingly different from one another despite their upbringing in the "same" family environment. In a study of personality, Scarr and Grajek[41] assert, "Lest the reader slip over these results, let us make explicit the implications of these findings: upper middle-class brothers who attend the same school and whose parents take them to the same plays, sporting events, music lessons, and therapists, and use similar child rearing practices on them are little more similar in personality measures than they are to working class or farm boys, whose lives are totally different." Other studies support the observation that siblings are strikingly different from one another in personality, cognitive function, and psychopathology—far more different than expected, given their genetic relatedness.[22] One factor that may contribute to these sibling differences is the differential ("nonshared") experiences siblings undergo, both within and outside the family. For example, within families, siblings differ in how they receive and perceive parental affection, parenting practices, and sibling relationships; outside the family, siblings experience different relationships with teachers and peers. These differential experiences appear to outweigh the similarities in family environment in determining developmental outcomes.

School. The two basic functions of the school are education and socialization. For some children, the first regular and routine experiences outside the home are provided by attending school.

In its role as an agent of socialization, school provides a graded transition from the circumscribed environment of the home to the world at large. This role is less well defined but is as important as cognitive instruction. The most crucial social goals of early schooling are individuation from the family, subordination of gross motor activity to achieve decorum in the classroom, mastery of the fine motor skills that are prerequisites to learning to read and write, and initiation of certain habits that are important to the educational process, such as cooperation, successful completion of tasks, and respect for others.

By late elementary grades, competition and achievement become prominent aspects of school life. Innate ability and degree of motivation (derived both from self and the environment), as well as environmental resources, determine a student's achievement level.

Peer Group. Although the family and school undoubtedly are important sources of environmental influence on development, the peer group also exerts a strong influence. Peers model behavior, help determine value systems, and provide the security of group identity, not only for children and adolescents but also for adults.

The earliest peer interactions occur at about 6 months of age, when infants placed together look at and approach and explore one another for a few seconds.[20] These interactions increase in duration and complexity as the child matures. Complementary and reciprocal social play emerge at about 1 year of age; social pretend play appears at about age 2. Most children have developed a characteristic way of relating to their peers, independently seeking friendships and engaging in social activities, by about age 3. Early friendships are based on proximity (the child next door). Later, the classroom is the source of friends. Finally, friendships become defined by mutual interests.

As might be expected, friendship becomes more enduring as children grow older. For example, it is common for friendships of older school-age children to remain stable over the course of one or more school years.[5] Friendships perceived as intimate are most likely to endure, and good friends tend to be of similar age, gender, and peer status. The key determinants of friendship formation include common interests and the clarity of the intent of both verbal and nonverbal communication. Self-disclosure of feelings and private thoughts, especially among girls, contributes to the bond between friends. Children also come to value mutual respect and loyalty. Whereas younger friends, especially boys, tend to be competitive with one another, older friends seek equality through sharing.

During adolescence the peer group becomes more influential than the family with regard to social activity and the development of value systems. In some instances adolescents deliberately choose a peer group with social values that are antithetical to those of their parents so that through the process of strong group identification they can individuate from the family—a major goal of late adolescence. This period is conflict ridden; some habits adopted by youth can be antisocial and self-destructive (see Chapter 79, Conduct Disorders).

Research and clinical observation clearly indicate that questioning whether a behavioral trait is due to genetic factors versus environmental factors is an unprofitable task. Instead, data strongly support the necessity of an interactional perspective that appreciates the interplay between heritable predispositions and specific environmental conditions (family, peers, and social group) in shaping the individual throughout development. Most developmentalists have adopted an interactional perspective.[39,40] In so doing, the important question now becomes *how* do heritable predispositions interact with environmental factors to influence the developmental trajectory.

Examples of Heredity-Environment Interaction

Gender. Gender has been associated with certain behavior patterns in infants. For example, in general, infant boys are more irritable and become calm less easily than do infant girls. The nature-nurture interactional model of development provides an interesting explanation for these findings: The greater neurological maturity of the girl at birth (nature) may result in less spontaneous random activity, distractibility, and intensity of reaction and greater attentiveness, persistence, and rhythmicity in baseline behavior; parental response (nurture) may then reinforce some of these behaviors in accord with culturally defined gender-specific expectations (see the section on gender identity in Chapter 80). In other words, quiet, demure, compliant girls and alert, aggressive, intense boys may be rewarded with parental attention. Indeed, parents have been observed to treat their male and female offspring differently from birth, usually being more physically active with boys.[28,34] Thus over time gender differences evident at birth are reinforced differentially by the environment (parent) and eventually become a significant part of the gender role behaviors adopted by the child.

Temperament and Attachment. Chess and Thomas[9] suggested that the "match" or mismatch of a child's temperamental style with the demands and expectations of the environment may influence the functional outcome of that child, with mismatches being associated with increased risk of behavioral and emotional disorders. Mismatches can occur when the expectations placed on the child chronically exceed his or her current developmental capacities. Mismatches between expectations and capacities also may occur when a parent's temperament differs dramatically from that of the child. For example, easygoing, quiet parents may have an energetic and highly excitable child whom they try to teach to be like them because that is what they expect a child to be like. This situation is even more likely to arise if the child has a quiet sibling whose disposition is similar to that of the parents. On the other hand, if the expectations and demands of the environment do not exceed or even meet the child's level of development, the child may not be challenged to change and develop new levels of mastery, reorganization, and growth.

It has been suggested that temperament influences the quality of attachment between a parent and child.[12] That is, some parents, depending on their temperament, are unable to respond sensitively to a highly irritable or "difficult" baby, resulting in an insecure attachment relationship. For example, an anxious parent may respond inappropriately to an infant who is highly emotionally reactive or prone to distress, leading to insecure attachment on the part of the infant. Such findings lend support to Chess and Thomas' "goodness of fit" model.

Pediatricians need to be aware of temperament as a factor influencing behavior so that the patient's behaviors can be evaluated in the context of the family and the parents counseled accordingly. Furthermore, it is highly likely that temperamental "goodness of fit" also will affect the nature of the relationships the pediatrician establishes with patients and their families. On occasion, allowances and adjustments must be made, if possible, when temperamental differences affect these personal and professional relationships negatively.

In summary, the factors that influence psychological development are understood best in the fullest interactive sense of the biopsychosocial model. That is, it is unlikely that some elements of development are driven purely by genetics and others determined solely by environment. Furthermore, it is not sufficient to ask what portion of certain elements of development are influenced by genetics versus environment. Rather, psychological development should be viewed as a series of processes by which genetically based individual tendencies interact with particular environmental factors to shape the path of a given child's developmental trajectory.

THEORIES OF DEVELOPMENT

Even seemingly bizarre behavior can become understandable when we know why a child acts as he or she does. Because no single theory explains all aspects of psychological development (emotional, cognitive, and social), it has become customary to examine behavior from the perspective of several viewpoints. Although cumbersome at times, this approach is analogous to that of physiological systems, in which an observable process may occur as a result of a combination of biochemical and anatomical events; each can be explained but only in terms defined by its own particular basic science.

In psychology there are many schools of thought or basic scientific approaches to development. We will focus on three major theoretical frameworks: psychodynamic theory (Freud and psychosexual development, Erikson and psychosocial development), cognitive-intellectual theory (Piaget), and learning theory (Skinner and conditioning, Sears and social learning). Each model approaches human development from different perspectives (psychodynamic: relationship and motivation; cognitive-intellectual: thought process and content; learning theory: observable behavior). Each approach has its own vocabulary and set of assumptions and hypotheses. It is noteworthy, however, that each of these theories relies on the presence of certain primitive instinctual behaviors that are operative at birth and later modified by the environment. Given our original definition of psychology as the study of emotion, cognition, and social conduct, we immediately see that each theory is incomplete; taken collectively, however, they complement each other. Table 51-1 provides a summary of psychological development from these perspectives from childhood through young adulthood.

Psychodynamic Theory

Freud and Psychosexual Development. The theory of psychosexual development is derived from Freud's in-depth examination and retrospective analysis of childhood behaviors he thought might have contributed to the neuroses for which his patients, as adults, were seeking treatment. Based on the content of memories supplied by his patients, Freud theorized that personality formation results from those intrapsychic struggles between polar forces experienced by an individual as he or she matures. This particular approach and the theoretical framework derived from it are limited in that (1) objective observations of current behavior are lacking and (2) heavy focus is placed on explanations for the development of undesirable adult behaviors rather than on behavior in general. Despite these shortcomings, Freud and his work have had a formidable influence on generations of developmental psychologists.

The family triad of mother-father-child and, in particular, the early mother-child dyad were central to Freud's investigation, interpretation, and explanation of later adult behaviors. Although pediatric psychology currently focuses largely on the individual in relation to a broader social unit than the family and on coping mechanisms (positive management strategies in stressful situations) rather than on defense mechanisms (often interpreted as negative management strategies), elements of freudian theory are represented in or are the foundation of a variety of other major developmental theories. Similarly, Freud's discussions of both conscious and unconscious factors that motivate observable behavior provide a unique framework for understanding otherwise apparently inexplicable conduct.

The total personality as conceived by Freud consists of three parts or motivating forces—the id, the ego, and the superego. The *id* is the foundation of the personality; its aim is to avoid pain, find satisfaction or pleasure, and maintain constancy in the midst of internal or external disturbance.

The *ego,* that part of the personality most visible to the external world, is the intermediary system between the id and reality; it provides the individual with an accurate perception of what exists in the environment. On some occasions, fulfillment of pleasure as desired by the id may be suspended temporarily by the ego in acknowledgment of reality.

The *superego* is the moral function of the personality; it is concerned with strivings for perfection rather than for pleasure or for responses to reality. Freud further divided the superego into the *ego ideal,* the conception of what is morally good, and *conscience,* the conception of what is morally bad. To the superego, thought is synonymous with action; therefore feelings of guilt or satisfaction may be experienced merely by thinking something "bad" or "good." Clinically, this has relevance to psychosomatic illness, which is considered in this theoretical framework to be an example of pain or dysfunction resulting from the superego's displeasure with the individual.

Although behavior can be motivated by the drive to fulfill a variety of needs (e.g., food, sleep), the major motivational system according to the psychosexual theory of development is libido, which is based in the instinctual (sexual) drive to preserve the species. Satisfaction of the sexual instinct is derived from stimulation or manipulation of both genital and nongenital body regions that have been called *erogenous zones.* Three primary erogenous zones, each with its associated vital need and presented in the chronological order in which each gains prominence, are (1) the mouth and eating,

Table 51-1 Psychological Development from Infancy to Young Adulthood

	Psychosexual				
Period	**Stage**	**Erogenous zone**	**Source of libidinal pleasure**	**Conflict**	**Resolution**
Infancy	Oral	Mouth	Tough; incorporation; biting	Weaning	Independence; emergence of the ego
	Anal	Anus	Expulsion; retention	Toilet training	Self-control
Toddlerhood, preschool age	Phallic	Genitalia	Masturbation	Oedipal complex	Identification with same-sex parent; emergence of the superego
School age	Latency	—	—	—	—
Adolescence/ adulthood	Genital	Genitalia	Sexual stimulation	Incest taboo; frustration of genital impulses	Selection of a hetero-sexual partner

*Modified from Erikson EH: *Childhood and society,* ed 2, New York, 1963, WW Norton.

Continued.

Table 51-1 Psychological Development from Infancy to Young Adulthood—cont'd

Psychosocial		Cognitive		Social learning	
Stage	**Description***	**Stage**	**Distinguishing characteristics of cognitive functioning**	**Phase**	**Description**
Basic trust versus basic mistrust	"Trust . . . implies not only that one has learned to rely on the sameness and continuity of the outer providers, but also that one may trust oneself. . . ."	Sensorimotor	Preverbal Reflexive activity to purposeful activity Development of object permanence and rudimentary thought	I Rudimentary behavior: initial behavioral learning	Basic need requirements met by parents Positive reinforcement is primary socializing agent
Autonomy versus shame and doubt	"From a sense of self-control without loss of self-esteem comes a lasting sense of good will and pride. . . ."				
Initiative versus guilt	". . . the child is . . . ready . . . to become bigger in the sense of sharing obligation and performance . . . (he moves) toward the possible and the tangible, which permits the dreams of early childhood to be attached to the goals of an active adult life."	Preoperational	Prelogical Inability to deal with several aspects of a problem simultaneously Development of representational language and use of symbols	II Secondary motivational systems: family-centered learning	Socialization within larger family environment Negative reinforcement introduced as socializing agent
Industry versus inferiority	". . . he now learns to win recognition by producing things."	Concrete operational	Logical Problem solving restricted to physically present or real objects and imagery Development of logical operations (e.g., classification, conservation)	III Secondary motivational systems: extrafamilial learning	Social penetration into neighborhood and beyond Controls universally defined and internally enforced
Identity versus role confusion	"The sense of ego identity, then, is the accrued confidence that the inner sameness and continuity prepared in the past are matched by the sameness and continuity of one's meaning for others, as evidenced in the tangible promise of a career."	Formal operational	Abstract Comprehension of purely abstract or symbolic content Development of advanced logical operations (e.g., complex analogy, induction, deduction, higher mathematics)		
Intimacy versus isolation	". . . the young adult, emerging from the search for and the insistence on identity, is eager and willing to fuse his identity with that of others. He is ready for intimacy. . . ."				

(2) the anus and elimination, and (3) the genitalia and reproduction. According to Freud, the action an individual takes to reduce tension (derive pleasure) in an erogenous zone may or may not actually fulfill the vital need associated with that area (e.g., both eating and nonnutritive thumb-sucking may produce pleasure in the oral area).

Activities involving the erogenous zones may bring the child into conflict with the parents. The resulting frustrations and anxieties associated with these conflicts lead to the development of a number of adaptive maneuvers or defense mechanisms, such as repression, regression, denial, projection, intellectualization, and sublimation. Resolution of the conflict associated with a given stage allows the individual to progress to the next developmental stage. Freud conceptualized five psychosexual stages: oral, anal, phallic, latency, and genital. Full maturation of psychosexual development is thought to occur in late adolescence or early adulthood with the establishment of a stable heterosexual relationship.

Erikson and Psychosocial Development. Whereas Freud focused on the intrinsic development of the individual, especially as it is shaped by the triadic relationship of the child with his or her parents, Erikson focused on the development of the individual within the wider context of his or her historical-cultural-social milieu. For Erikson, unconscious motivation (id) exists, but it is the process of socialization that facilitates development and determines an individual's outcome. Unlike Freud, Erikson studied individuals and their families within the spheres of their everyday lives and at a particular moment in their cultural history. Also, unlike freudian theory, Erikson's theory focuses with optimism on an individual's potential for mastery by successfully resolving developmental crises, rather than with pessimism on the potential for dysfunction from persistent psychological conflict.

Two assumptions underlie Erikson's construction of the theory of psychosocial development[13]: (1) that the human personality develops according to steps predetermined in the growing person's readiness to be driven toward, to be aware of, and to interact with a widening social radius, and (2) that society tends to be so constituted as to meet and invite this succession of potentialities for interaction and attempts to safeguard and encourage the proper rate and the proper sequence of their unfolding.

Thus Erikson proposes that a close, sequentially patterned mutual relationship exists between individual capabilities and environmental demands. An individual cannot develop outside of or beyond the readiness of his or her social context, nor can society progress independent of the individual.

Erikson conceptualized eight ages in human life that represent a reformulation and extension of Freud's five psychosexual stages of development. However, whereas psychosexual theory postulates that the individual attains full developmental maturity at entry into the genital stage, which begins during adolescence or young adulthood, psychosocial theory postulates the continuation of substantial developmental change throughout the life cycle. The first six Eriksonian ages are easily associated with their corresponding freudian stages: basic trust versus basic mistrust (oral), autonomy versus shame and doubt (anal), initiative versus guilt (phallic), industry versus inferiority (latency), and the combination of identity versus role confusion and intimacy versus isolation (genital). The last two Eriksonian ages, generativity versus stagnation and ego integrity versus despair, have no one-to-one correspondence in freudian theory, but instead deal with the specific developmental transitions of middle and old age.

Cognitive-Intellectual Theory

Piaget and Cognitive Development. Cognition, as studied most notably by Piaget, is defined as the means by which an individual accumulates organized knowledge about the world and uses that knowledge to solve problems and modify behavior. Whereas the psychodynamic schools of developmental theory are concerned primarily with issues of motivation as a force for change, the cognitive-intellectual theory is centered almost exclusively on the process of acquiring and using knowledge. Piaget, although influenced by Freud and tacitly subscribing to the notion that *why* a child learns is a valid question, did not himself investigate this issue critically. Rather, his research largely ignores emotion and motivation and concentrates on the organizational structure of cognitive functioning and how it influences understanding and, therefore, behavior.

According to piagetian theory, cognitive development is the result of neurophysiological maturation, environmental stimulation, experience, and continual internal cognitive reorganization. Two major principles form the framework for Piaget's theory: (1) all species tend to *organize* or order their activities hierarchically, and (2) all species tend to *adapt* through *assimilation* (incorporating new information or unfamiliar objects into an already existing idea about the world) and *accommodation* (changing ideas about the world and behavior in response to new knowledge or situations). For example, when infants are handed a set of small blocks for the first time, they are likely to bite or shake them. That is, they use age-specific behaviors to learn about new objects that they assume are similar to other more familiar objects, such as nipples and rattles, that they have experienced before (assimilation). Once being shown or discovering that blocks can be used to build a tower, the child changes his or her behavior and tries to stack the blocks each time they are presented (accommodation).

As is true of all developmentally based psychological theories, Piaget's theory is premised on a stepwise, ordered sequence of learning in response to experience. He defined four discrete stages of cognitive development from birth to adulthood: sensorimotor, preoperational, concrete operational, and formal operational. The exact chronological age at which certain abilities are attained depends on factors such as individual differences in physiological functioning, experience, and environment. Transitional periods, during which children exhibit some but not all characteristics of the next stage of thinking, exist between developmental phases. Targeted teaching during these times may result in rapid acquisition of new cognitive skills characteristic of the next stage of thinking. Although the concept of transitional periods is not unique to piagetian theory, Piaget's framework lends itself to investigational techniques that are more clearly defined than those that can be employed to test psychoanalytical theory. Thus Piagetian theory allows more precise empirical analysis and identification of developmental processes and stages.

Learning Theory

Learning theory is an outgrowth of behaviorism, or stimulus-response psychology. Following are some basic principles of learning theory:

1. Behavior is learned; however, genetic factors and innate, involuntary reflexive behaviors influence this learning.
2. All types, patterns, and combinations of behavior can be learned as long as they are not incompatible physically.
3. Behavior can be conditioned.
4. Behavior can be shaped.
5. Behavior is learned through reinforcement, which may be internal or external and positive or negative.
6. Learning results from many independent processes, including observation and imitation.

Behavior can be conditioned in two ways. In the process of classical conditioning, discovered by the Russian physiologist Pavlov, a reflex response associated in nature with one stimulus can be modified in such a way that it can be evoked by another stimulus. In Pavlov's original experiment, reflexive salivation in a dog at the sight of food could be induced eventually merely by the sound of a ringing bell, which over a period of time had been "paired" with eating. (Interestingly, the saliva evoked by the ringing bell differed slightly in chemical content from naturally occurring saliva.)

In the process of instrumental conditioning, a nonreflexive behavior is learned because it is reinforced positively. For example, in an experiment, a rat in a cage might, by chance, depress a lever. If a pellet of food is released each time this occurs, the rat will "learn" to depress the lever and will do so with increasing frequency, especially when hungry.

Several features of conditioned behavior are important clinically. Conditioned behavior can be *extinguished,* or unlearned, if it is not reinforced; it can be *inhibited,* or counteracted, if it is followed by negative reinforcement or punishment; it can be *partially reinforced* by inconsistent or random reinforcement; it can be *generalized* so that similar stimuli will elicit the same response; and it can be made *discriminatory* so that by selective reinforcement only one (or a few) specific stimuli elicits the response.

Reinforcement is the key element in learning theory. According to this theoretical framework, an individual can be motivated to perform a certain behavior because of the positive effect (reward) derived from it. Furthermore, an individual can be motivated to *not* perform a certain behavior because of the negative effect (punishment) derived from it or because some other behavior gives more benefit. Thus giving a neutral response (not reinforcing, ignoring) or reinforcing a behavior negatively leads to the behavior's being extinguished. A consistent response, whether it is positively or negatively reinforcing, leads to the most rapid learning.

Shaping is the process of molding a given behavior to be more like a desired behavior. This is accomplished by positively reinforcing successive approximations of the desired behavior. A classic example of this has been described by Baldwin in his recounting of the work of B.F. Skinner[3]:

> When Skinner wants to teach a pigeon to hit a ping pong ball through a pair of goal posts by pecking at it, he can't wait until the pigeon just happens to do so. He begins by reinforcing the pigeon whenever it is within a certain distance of the ball. The pigeon gradually learns to stay close to the ball. The experimenter now reinforces the pigeon only when he is close to the ball and looking in its direction, thus teaching the pigeon to keep his eye on the ball. In the next stage, the experimenter requires the pigeon to peck at the ball to receive a reinforcement. Finally, the pigeon must peck the ball in the right direction.

In the strictest sense, learning theory, in and of itself, is not a developmental theory because there is no intrinsic sequential order or hierarchical staging to learning behavior, as long as the individual has the neurophysiological maturation to be physically able to perform the desired task. However, a group of early workers in the field sought to incorporate psychoanalytical hypotheses (both psychosexual and psychosocial) into explanations for certain observable behaviors. This group became known as the *school of social learning theory.*

An important aspect of social learning theory is its attention to the dyadic nature of human behavior. Thus the child is in constant interaction with his or her environment and other individuals in that environment. The child's response to an environmental stimulus acts as a stimulus itself, thus evoking a response from the environment, and so on. In turn, the child's development of new levels of functioning depends on the ability of the environment to shape the child's behavior so that it conforms with increasing regularity to what will be expected eventually from him or her as an adult.[42]

This transactional scheme is in keeping with current general psychological theories that highlight the interactional quality of developmental processes, and the individual-society dyad is highly reminiscent of Erikson's psychosocial theory.

In the foregoing discussion of learning theory, desired behaviors were viewed as being obtained through some direct effect on the performer. Learning also occurs indirectly through observation and imitation. In *observational learning* the individual watches others and modifies his or her behavior in accord with the rewards and punishments others receive. *Imitative learning* is rooted in the process of identification (Freud). The child acts like (i.e., copies) a desired model (e.g., mother or father) and is positively reinforced with rewards that either are internal (being proud of oneself) or external (being praised by others). Both observational and imitative learning are particularly common in social groups.

If the individual learns by observational imitation, then modeling (demonstrating) is a particularly important element in the production of behavior. Models can be used to demonstrate everything from simple one-step behaviors to entire life-styles (role models). Children and youth observe the behaviors of others and, based on how much they wish to identify with these others, will imitate their actions. Indeed, the adage "actions speak louder than words" may have preceded the formulation of learning theory by centuries but still is the most profound basis for those behaviors that are perpetuated within families from generation to generation, despite parental admonitions to the contrary. For example, modeling helps explain successive generations of child or spouse abuse. If the only template for interactions is within the family and provided by the parents, the children will come to believe that whatever behaviors they observed in their parents, their earliest teachers, are normative and acceptable. Thus intervention aimed at altering child rearing practices, for example, can be difficult, if not impossible, because change requires not only learning new behaviors but also abrogating the teaching of those to whom conscious or unconscious allegiance can be exceedingly strong.

RELATIONSHIP BETWEEN PHYSIOLOGICAL AND PSYCHOLOGICAL DEVELOPMENT

In this section we examine the child at different chronological ages, beginning with the parents' response to the pregnancy and its potential effects on the child's later psychological development.

Because a basic premise of the developmental theories presented is that innate, involuntary reflexive, and instinctual behavior is the foundation on which all future behaviors are built, psychological development depends heavily on physiological maturation. Thus an individual's physical capacities at any point in time help to determine the extent of his or her interaction with the environment.

Several important principles of physical development that bear directly on psychological development can be summarized as follows:

1. Development is a continuous process that begins at conception. Birth is merely an event in the natural course of development, although it signals the beginning of the individual's ability to cope independently with the environment.
2. The sequence of development of the individual as a whole and of each of the organ systems is relatively fixed. However, the rate at which development occurs varies considerably, and different systems may mature at different times.
3. Development of both involuntary (autonomic) and voluntary activity is related intimately to the maturation of the nervous systems.
4. Certain primitive reflexes (e.g., stepping, grasping) must be "lost" before the corresponding voluntary (learned) movement is acquired.
5. Development occurs cephalocaudally.

Pregnancy

The bonds of attachment that eventually will be formed between the infant and his or her parents are initiated during pregnancy. According to Mary Ainsworth,[2] attachment is a long-lasting emotional tie that one person has with another that persists even when they are apart. Attachment also implies emotion. Although the emotions of attachment are complex and vary from time to time, in general, positive feelings toward the other person predominate, and attachment is thought of as implying affection or love.

"Precursors of attachment" are physical and psychosocial changes that occur in couples anticipating and preparing for the birth of their child. These changes have been researched best in pregnant women, but studies of men suggest that expectant fathers also experience emotional change and psychological readjustment and share many of the same feelings as expectant mothers.[48]

Both conscious and unconscious expectations may begin well in advance of conception and may be heightened by family and social factors. More commonly, however, anticipatory or expectant behavior begins, at least consciously, at the time the pregnancy first becomes known. Examples of such behavior include changes in social patterns associated with the physical demands of pregnancy, alterations in the family's economic planning, and preparation for the child by the accumulation of various material goods. On another level, many expectant parents report a heightened sense of responsibility to keep the mother (and therefore the fetus) well and fit (e.g., as abstaining from tobacco, drugs, or alcohol) and to protect the father (e.g., reducing or eliminating risky behavior). Planning for the future of someone who will depend totally on them becomes a major preoccupation of the pregnant couple.

During pregnancy a woman concurrently experiences two types of developmental change: physical and emotional changes within herself and the growth of the fetus. The woman faces two adaptive tasks: acceptance of the pregnancy and perception of the fetus as an individual.

Most women report strong emotional swings that vary from positive to negative anticipation; frequently they feel ambivalent about the pregnancy. Perceiving the fetus as an individual usually commences with the first sensation of fetal movement, or "quickening." If the original reaction to the pregnancy was predominantly negative (unplanned, unwanted), many women report heightened acceptance and noticeable changes in attitude when fetal movement is first felt. After quickening, women usually begin to have fantasies about the infant, including those of physical and personality characteristics they hope or are afraid the child will have.[26]

Most likely every couple has some fantasies, regardless of how vehemently they deny them or how carefully they attempt to avoid them. Gender preference probably is the most common, but inherent in all individuals is the wish to have progeny who will be a credit to them, carry on tradition, excel in some activity, and be attractive, good, and healthy. As the time of delivery approaches, this last concern, to have a healthy baby, increases in importance. Thus, should a child be born with a congenital defect, life threatening or not, the parents actually suffer the loss of their "expected" child, and some time may pass before they can reorganize their expectations and fully accept their child.

Birthing Process

Data relating to the birthing process suggest that mothers who are relaxed during labor and who have a supportive person (family member, friend, or lay volunteer helper) assisting them are more likely to have a shorter labor and to be more alert and interactive with their infant on first sight.[43] Being unconscious during birth does not appear to cause rejection of the infant, although systematic studies in this important area are lacking. What is known, however, is that the more difficult the labor, the less likely the mother is to breast-feed.

Certain delivery procedures and administration of anesthetics can affect both the mother and child at birth. For example, an infant who is in a physiologically depressed state because the mother was given a narcotic during delivery is more likely to respond poorly on initial contact or during feedings and thus is less stimulating to the mother.

Research on the behavior of fathers toward the newborn has shown that engrossment, absorption, and preoccupation with the infant occur in men as well as in women. A sense of increased self-esteem also has been reported among new fathers.[17]

Immediate Postpartum Period

The interval immediately after birth has been called the *maternal sensitive period*.[26] Mother-infant interaction is truly reciprocal. The mother supplies touch, eye-to-eye (en face) contact, high-pitched voice, heat, and odor; the infant supplies eye-to-eye contact, odor, entertainment, and if nursing at the breast, stimulation of maternal production of prolactin and oxytocin.

The mother's behaviors match certain infant needs. For example, the female voice is naturally high pitched, and the mother consciously makes it more so. This fits the infant's sensitive auditory perception and attraction to speech in the high-frequency range. The mother's odor also appears to affect the infant. It has been found that infants can discriminate their own mother's axillary odor[8] and the smell of their own mother's breast milk from those of other women.

The infant's reflexive behaviors (suckling, clinging) are care-eliciting; that is, they serve the function of ensuring the survival of the individual by bringing the caregiver closer to the child and helping to maintain physical and emotional contact between them by mutual reinforcement. Thus parental reinforcement behaviors (feeding, fondling) in response to the child's care-eliciting behaviors lead to further suckling and clinging. In this way the infant's innate behaviors and the responses they generate in the caregiver form the basis of that special relationship that eventually becomes true attachment.

Certain factors impede the development of attachment. For example, the provocative stimulus of the young infant's intense gaze is missing if the child is blind. Variations of normal behavior, such as an infant who does not cling but rather stiffens on being held, may be a response to anxiety in the caregiver or a demonstration of a particular type of temperament. A psychological impediment to attachment is the tendency of some parents to identify their own or another's undesirable traits in the infant, thus hindering formation of bonds.

Infancy

The period of infancy, which extends from birth to 24 months of age, is divided most logically at 12 months. The first year is marked by tremendous physical growth and the development of rudimentary skills, culminating in the ability to walk several steps unassisted and to speak about three to six intelligible words.

The second year is characterized by skill refinement to the point where some children can pedal a tricycle and speak in relatively complete, although syntactically poor, sentences. Infants also learn that other individuals inhabit their world and that these individuals, most notably family members, come and go and return again. Lastly, they learn that they have a will and can manipulate their environment purposefully rather than merely be its captive.

Intricately interwoven with somatic growth is the differentiation and beginning emotional maturation of the individual. Of the many changes taking place, two principal emotionally relevant psychological tasks are mastered within the period of infancy: attachment (first year) and separation (second year).

Attachment does not depend on the infant's perceiving the attachment figure as separate from self and actually is facilitated by the newborn's earliest perception of the caregiver as an extension of self.[2] Indeed, *bonding,* an early manifestation of attachment, usually is discussed with reference to mother-child interactions in the newborn period.[26] Thus recognition of potential impediments to bonding (use of anesthesia or narcotics, separation of mother and infant) have led to major changes in obstetrical and newborn care. However, true attachment is such an important element for successful growth and development that it is "overdetermined"—that is, many opportunities, over time, are available to facilitate and cement the formation of attachment, not only with the mother but with the father and other significant caregivers as well.[29]

Interestingly, it has been found that as the infant becomes able to discriminate between caregivers, his or her expectations for the father's behavior are different from those for the mother; and fathers do, in fact, act differently, providing less predictable and rhythmic and more exciting physical and auditory stimulation than do mothers.[29,30] Despite such differences in interaction, however, attachment between the infant and any consistent caregiver is strengthened by continued mutual reinforcement.

If we assume that object permanence (out of sight but not out of mind) is a prerequisite for the formation of true attachment, attachment between the infant and caregiver probably does not occur before 6 to 8 months of age. At this age, however, the infant and caregiver can derive enough positive reinforcement from each other that periods of being apart do not interrupt the essential tie—that is, true attachment is considered to have taken place when the bond remains strong despite periods of absence.

Separation is a direct extension of attachment because without attachment, there is no separation; rather, there merely is movement from one more or less contiguous relationship to another. Just as positive affect usually is associated with attachment, negative affect usually is associated with separation.

Separation anxiety occurs after the child becomes able to recognize and discriminate among individuals. It is manifested by various degrees of crying and withdrawal when the attachment figure is not present. Closely allied with separation anxiety is *stranger anxiety*—fear of someone unfamiliar to or not closely associated with the infant. A stranger, however, is reasonably well tolerated when a familiar, safe caregiver also is present.

Psychosexual Development: Oral and Anal Stages. In freudian or psychosexual terms, the child less than 12 months of age is considered to be in the *oral phase* of development, so called because the mouth is the primary source of tension and pleasure. Satisfaction of hunger, as well as many of the comforting maneuvers provided by both the child and the caregiver (e.g., finger-sucking and object-sucking), center on stimulation of the mouth.

The mouth has at least five primary modes of functioning that, in analytical theory, are prototypes for certain later personality types: (1) taking in (acquisitiveness), (2) holding on (tenacity), (3) biting (destructiveness), (4) spitting out (rejection), and (5) closing (negativism). The theory proposes that the extent to which any of these traits becomes part of the mature personality depends on the amount of anxiety or frustration the individual experiences in his or her original encounter with a particular function. For example, abrupt weaning may lead to a strong tendency to hold onto things; or a child who is oral-aggressive because of inconsistent nursing and bites with his or her teeth may become an adult who is oral-aggressive and "bites" with sarcasm.

Typically, food becomes equated with love and the mother's approval. That is, the infant depends on someone else, usually the mother, to relieve oral distress and fulfill oral pleasure. The mother can control the infant's conduct by giving or withholding food. Weaning from the breast or bottle, a natural developmental stage, is a point of conflict because the infant can experience it as rejection or disapproval by the mother. In psychoanalytical theory, this conflict is resolved successfully when the infant, developing a sense of separate individuality, learns to satisfy needs through his or her own personal effort. This is in contrast to the so-called oral-dependent character style, which theoretically arises when this conflict is not resolved adequately; it is typified by the person who expects others to provide things when he or she is good and withhold or take away things when he or she is bad.

During the second year of life the infant moves into the *anal stage* of psychosexual development. Tensions arise in the anal region as the result of accumulation of fecal material; expulsion brings relief. It is hypothesized that as a consequence of experiencing a pleasant reduction in tension from elimination, the infant may use this action to reduce tension arising in other parts of the body. Expulsive elimination thus is considered the prototype for emotional outbursts, temper tantrums, rages, and other primitive discharge reactions.

Usually, during the second to fourth year of life, involuntary expulsive reflexes are brought under voluntary control through a set of experiences known as toilet training. This usually is the first crucial experience the child has with discipline and external authority. It represents a conflict between instinct and an external barrier.

The methods caregivers use in training the child and their attitudes about defecation, cleanliness, control, and responsibility are thought to leave indelible imprints on the child's development. For example, if the training method is strict and punitive, the child may react by soiling intentionally. When older, the child may react to authority figures by being messy, disorderly, or irresponsible.

Psychosocial Development: Basic Trust Versus Basic Mistrust and Autonomy Versus Shame and Guilt. In psychosocial or eriksonian terms, the infant faces the tasks of the first two of the eight stages of human development. The first task, occurring during the first year, is *developing a sense of basic trust and overcoming a sense of mistrust.* According to Erikson, to do this the young infant needs to experience a mutually satisfying relationship based on familiarity, regularity, and predictability. The development of trust initially requires a feeling of physical comfort, which then promotes emotional comfort. If this feeling of comfort is achieved, the infant becomes trusting even in new situations because of his or her confidence that the environment will be supportive and helpful in meeting new challenges. If, however, the infant experiences physical discomfort or is uncertain about whether needs will be met (because responses elicited from the environment are unpredictable), he or she will face new experiences with apprehension or mistrust. Thus developing a sense of confidence in the well-intentioned motives of others (motives that he or she eventually learns to emulate) is the foundation for success in future relationships and endeavors.

Basic trust is mutual and, according to Erikson,[13] "implies not only that one has learned to rely on the sameness and continuity of the outer providers, but also that one may trust oneself and the capacity of one's own organs to cope with urges; and that one is able to consider oneself trustworthy enough so that the providers will not need to be on guard lest they be nipped."

Thus, unlike Freud, who emphasizes food and physical nurturance, Erickson emphasizes the sense of trust the child develops. Such a sense of trust depends on the overall physical and emotional quality of the maternal or, more broadly, caregiving relationship that the infant has with the total environment.

Basic trust is the foundation of true attachment, and basic trust cannot be complete until there has been significant and sufficient testing. Erikson describes this vividly: "The constant tasting and testing of the relationship . . . meets its crucial test during the rages of the biting stage, when the teeth cause pain from within and when outer friends either prove of no avail or withdraw from the only action which promises relief: biting."[13]

The second eriksonian stage of psychosocial development, *autonomy versus shame and doubt,* is analogous to the anal stage of freudian psychology. It begins in infancy but is not realized fully until toddlerhood. Erikson notes that muscular maturation during this time is an important element for experimentation with two simultaneous sets of social modalities, holding on and letting go.

With increasing control over both self and the environment, the child begins to experiment with manipulation and control. At times he or she is successful and at other times not. The manner in which successes and failures are met by caregivers becomes decisive in the early formation of freedom of self-expression and its suppression. "From a sense of self-control without loss of self-esteem comes a lasting sense of good will and pride; from a sense of loss of self-control and of foreign overcontrol comes a lasting propensity for doubt and shame."[13]

Cognitive Development: Sensorimotor Period. According to piagetian theory, the child from birth to approximately age 2 is in the *sensorimotor stage,* manifested by sensory exploration, the attainment of purposeful movement, repetition of activities, manipulation of the environment, and imitation. Although the infant largely is preverbal throughout this period, instrumental language (use of words to indicate wants or needs or to identify objects) develops toward the end of this phase.

The sensorimotor period can be divided into six stages: stage 1: the infant initially depends heavily on reflex activity, which is modified by experience (e.g., rooting evolves into active searching for the nipple); stage 2: the infant can anticipate (e.g., making sucking movements at the sight of the bottle); stage 3: the infant attempts to imitate familiar behavior (e.g., clapping hands in imitation of the someone); stage 4: the infant can act purposefully (e.g., remove an obstacle to a goal); stage 5: the infant is interested in producing novel behaviors (e.g., trying new methods to remove an obstacle to a goal); and stage 6 (transition phase): the infant or child begins to think about problems, to imitate an absent model from memory, and to use words to designate ongoing events, immediate desires, or objects that are present. In addition, the child has a fully developed sense of object permanence; that is, he or she will look for a vanished object even if it has been displaced. Thus the child appears to understand that things exist independently of the self.

Social Learning Development: Rudimentary Behavior Phase. The social learning theorists describe infancy as the period during which basic needs are met and initial learning takes place within the intimate environment of the home. Positive reinforcement in the form of attention (feeding, comforting) is the predominant mode used by the family to shape the infant's behavior. Reflexive activities (grasping in response to a parental finger in the infant's palm) are rewarded (parent plays with the infant's hand, talks, and coos—i.e., gives attention). In time, true grasp is learned and is followed by lifting the arms as a signal to be played with or to be held. In this way a naturally occurring primitive reflex evolves into a purposeful activity. A further step takes place during later infancy, when the child begins to be able to modify behavior in response to signals that are not directly or immediately physically rewarding (e.g., a smile rather than actually being held). Sensitivity to nonphysical as well as physical cues is the foundation for the social component of human learning. In freudian and eriksonian terms, such responsiveness to the environment and acknowledgment that we are only part of it mark the *development of the ego.*

Toddlerhood and Preschool Age (2 to 5 Years)

During the toddler stage, the growth rate slows, personality develops further, and important strides are made in cognitive ability. Bowel and bladder control usually evolve during the third year, although the range extends from 15 months to 4 years and sometimes beyond.

The various aspects of development interact clearly during this period. For example, what the child can do physically influences his or her perception of self, which in turn influences social development and independence. The positive feedback loop of testing leading to success, leading to confidence, leading to further testing is of particular significance during this stage of rapid achievement of milestones.

Psychosexual Development: Phallic Stage. According to Freud, during the late preschool period, the child is preoccupied with his or her genitalia as a body area from which pleasure is derived through self-stimulation. This masturbatory drive is different from the sexual drive of the later genital stage characteristic of adolescence and adulthood, even though the same erogenous zone is involved. The basic innocence of this behavior in both boys and girls deserves repeated emphasis, especially to parents who may be unduly concerned or disturbed by it.

According to Freud, during the *phallic stage* both boys and girls experience a period of intense attachment to the parent of the opposite sex and hostility toward the same-sex parent. This situation has been called the *Oedipal complex* after the mythological Greek character who killed his father and married his mother. The sex-specific rivalries are the Oedipal conflict (males) and the Electra conflict (females).

Before the phallic stage the mother is the primary love object for both boys and girls. During the phallic stage the boy develops a more intense relationship with his mother and becomes jealous of and rivalrous with his father for his mother's attention. Conversely, the girl begins to pursue her father, relying on him to be her ally against the mother. Such behavior can produce consternation within the family unit if the parents do not appreciate the reason for—indeed, the universality of—such alliances. Conflict resolution begins when the child recognizes the futility of his or her desires and, instead of wishing to take the place of the same-sex parent, moves in the direction of trying to become more like him or her. This process, by which boys desire to become more like men in their self-concept and girls desire to become more like women, has been called *identification.* It includes the incorporation of many of the same-sex parent's qualities into the child's own personality.

Freud assumed that all people are constitutionally bisexual and that the tendencies of both sexes are inherited by each child. Furthermore, he also hypothesized that a child experiences some degree of identification with each parent. Ultimately, the degree of masculinity or femininity that the child displays in later life depends on the relative strengths of his or her innate masculine or feminine tendencies, the degree to which these tendencies are rewarded or inhibited, and the strength of identification he or she has with each parent.

This stage has resolved completely when incorporation of parental qualities (internalization of parental controls) is sufficient for what Freud has called *superego formation,* or the development of conscience; that is, the child develops a rudimentary sense of right and wrong based on instruction by and modeling by the parents.

Psychosocial Development: Initiative Versus Guilt. Erikson perceived children in the *initiative versus guilt stage* to be moving into a larger social environment in which they are able to initiate new activities. Occasionally, the sense of personal autonomy they had developed previously is challenged or frustrated by the autonomous activity of others. The ensuing conflict may lead to a sense of guilt for having gone too far in striving for initiative. This sense of guilt is overcome by learning self-modulation through the development of a conscience that reflects parental and societal values. Thus, without denigrating themselves, children begin to learn to put personal and social needs into perspective and to modify the one to be in concert with the other.

Cognitive Development: Preoperational Period. Extending from 2 to 7 years of age, the *preoperational period,* as defined by Piaget, is distinguished by the appearance of representational language and rudimentary reasoning. Problem solving during this period is intuitive rather than logical, and the child cannot explain his or her reasoning strategies.

The thought processes of the preoperational child are limited by centration (inability to consider several aspects or dimensions of a situation simultaneously), syncretism (the tendency to group several apparently unrelated things or events into a confused whole), juxtaposition (failure to perceive the real connection among several things or events), irreversibility (inability to understand successive changes or transformations), egocentrism (perception of the world only from his or her own point of view or the belief that he or she is the origin of all actions in the world), and magical thinking (equation of thought and fantasy with action—i.e., feeling that a wish can cause some external event).

The thought content of the preoperational child is influenced by animism (the belief that inanimate objects are alive as people are alive), artificialism (the belief that all things are made for a purpose), and participation (the belief that there is some continuing connection or interaction between human actions and natural processes).

Social Learning Development: Secondary Motivational Systems; Family-Centered Learning. As the child becomes able to move within a larger environment, a greater number of individuals are available to serve as models and reinforcers of behavior. In addition, negative reinforcement (punishment) is introduced as an agent for modifying the child's behavior. Discipline that is either too prescriptive or too indulgent can produce a child who has no internal sense of responsibility for personal actions. In the first instance, the child relies on the environment to provide all cues as to what is or is not acceptable. In the latter instance, excessive indulgence provides such insufficient cueing that the child does not learn to distinguish right from wrong.

It is at this age that negative attention-seeking behaviors become common. These are seen most often in situations in which the child, who has become accustomed to reinforcement as a method of guiding behavior, becomes frustrated by persistent nonreinforcement (such as might occur if a new infant is born into the family, diverting much of the parents' time and attention away from the preschooler). Frustration at a lack of positive reinforcement for good behavior may lead to bad behavior that demands attention, negative though it is. The child may learn, in time, to use even violent behavior to meet needs for attention, even though the attention elicited is disapproving, deprecating, or punitive. Although some children may fear the punishment they receive for their behavior, such punishment may seem preferable to feeling neglected, unimportant, or even nonexistent in their parents' lives.

School Age (6 to 12 Years)

Freud called the developmental stage between the end of toddlerhood and the onset of adolescence *latency* to describe the relatively quiescent period of sexual activity between the resolution of the Oedipal conflict and the emergence of the sexual drives of adolescence. Actually, the child's sexual drive is not really latent (present but not visible or active—i.e., dormant) at all. Nor, as we shall see, is sexual drive absent; it is, however, channeled differently.

During latency there is no qualitative change in the external genitalia, which retain their infantile appearance. In general, the hypothalamus and pituitary gland are highly sensitive participants in a negative feedback system that results in suppression of any gonadal activity. At the point of late latency and early adolescence, however, the sensitivity of the hypothalamus and pituitary gland declines, permitting increased synthesis of luteinizing hormone and follicle-stimulating hormone. With higher circulating levels of these hormones, the physical changes of sexual development begin. Enlargement of the breasts and rounding of the contours of the hips are the first discernible changes in girls. Increasing size of the testes and penis and the appearance of pubic hair at the base of the penis are the first changes noted in boys. Although these changes can occur as early as age 8 in girls and age 10 in boys, the average age of onset of adolescence usually is 10 and 12 years, respectively.

Lack of outward physical change and diminution of sexually oriented drives do not mean that children are uninterested in sex, especially sex differences. Curiosity is common among 5- to 7-year-old boys and girls. Because children have been taught (sometimes through shaming) to keep themselves clothed in the presence of others, especially members of the other gender, "playing doctor" becomes a relatively socially acceptable way of satisfying natural curiosity. Girls and boys of middle latency often "kiss and run"; snapping the bra strap of a more developed girl in the group is common in late latency. "Crushes," often intense and frequently focused on some unattainable hero or idol, occur with regularity. Parents sometimes need reassurance that these practices are widespread and represent normal behavior.

The first major task of the latency-age child is to enter into school and achieve independence from the strict confines of home. Teachers, who at first are parent surrogates and then independent role models and authority figures, become important resources for the developing child. Teachers join with parents in setting expectations and goals for behavior and achievement.

The child of 6 years of age has the ability to perform most rudimentary gross and fine motor tasks. Therefore latency is the time when skills are refined. Progress, then, is tested not so much by the acquisition of new skills as by the rapidity and accuracy with which old skills are performed.

Indeed, skill plays a critical part in the development of the emerging personality. For the child for whom physical activity is easy and therefore filled with positive reinforcement, playing games and being a member of the team bring pleasure and friendship. For the child for whom physical activity does not come easily, there is less, if any, positive reinforcement from these activities, and the individual looks for other areas in which strengths may lie. Some children who are not good with their hands can turn to books and receive the praise of their parents and teachers. However, it should be noted that peer group emphasis, especially in boys, is on athletic prowess, and academic distinction is less prized, especially in early latency. There is tremendous pressure on the 8-year-old boy to play sports well; if he is clumsy, he can be at a decided disadvantage in making and retaining friends.

The child who cannot do anything well, sports or schoolwork, presents a special problem and becomes a prime candidate for acting-out behavior. For this child, like the toddler who is displaced by a new baby in the family, attention (usually reprimand) comes primarily from negative attention-seeking devices, and approbation comes from a peer group that either baits him or joins him in these activities, marveling at his prowess at getting into trouble and his apparent lack of concern about inviting punishment.

In previous generations, girls often were categorized as belonging to one of two groups during latency. The first group comprised girls who demonstrated characteristics known as *tomboyism*. These girls tended to be athletically aggressive and, because of their greater physical maturity as contrasted with boys of the same age, they could be as or more skilled than their male counterparts in physical activities. The second group was made up of girls who displayed little proclivity toward athletics. During latency these girls tended to enjoy activities and games that were much more gender specific in the traditional sense and revolved around playing house and other more strictly "feminine" activities (see Chapter 80).

In more recent time, as social roles have become less categorized and restrictive for both boys and girls, there has been a move toward less competition and more cooperation, resulting in greater acceptance of all individuals into any given activity. In addition, a new value system for social roles has emerged that encourages both athleticism in girls and relational interests in boys.

Psychosexual Development: Latency. Freud has described the *latency stage* as that period of development when the previously active libidinal and aggressive drives of the Oedipal stage become latent, and a truce ensues between the id and the ego until the true sexual drive emerges in the genital stage. At the beginning of latency, the superego (conscience) becomes more firmly internalized. The child derives comfort from the representations of parental values and outlooks contained within his or her own being, as embodied in the superego. These internalized parental values not only have resolved the otherwise intolerable Oedipal conflict from within but also continue to offer definite answers to troublesome moral and ethical problems from without. The outlook of the latency-age child is fairly black and white; notions about good and bad are clear and absolute and follow the guidelines set by the family.

Psychosocial Development: Industry Versus Inferiority. Erikson[13] has called the latency period the *age of industry versus inferiority,* stating that the child:

> has mastered the ambulatory field and the organ modes. He has experienced a sense of finality regarding the fact that there is no workable future within the womb of his family and thus becomes ready to apply himself to given skills and tasks, which go far beyond the mere playful expression of his organ modes or the pleasure in the function of his limbs. He develops a sense of industry; that is, he adjusts himself to the inorganic laws of the tool world. He can become an eager and absorbed unit of a productive situation. To bring a productive situation to completion is an aim which gradually supercedes the whims and wishes of play.

The issue of the status of one's self and one's possessions has its beginning in latency and intensifies during the period of strong peer group identity of adolescence. According to Erikson, the potential danger to the child at this stage lies in acquiring a sense of inadequacy or inferiority. If the child does not feel that he or she has adequate tools or skills, it may not be possible to become a successful member of the group. Failure to become a member of the group may result in withdrawal into the family and social isolation.

Systematic instruction occurs in all cultures during this time, although not all learning takes place within the confines of school. Much is learned about the world through experience and manipulation rather than by explanation; perhaps the greatest amount is learned from older children, who are perceived as "touchable" heroes. Society's contribution to the successful navigation of this stage is support for questing, gentle guidance, and perhaps most important, praise for achievements, even if small.

Cognitive Development: Concrete Operational Stage. Piaget has characterized the cognitive processes in the latency-age child as *concrete operational.* The child is able to view the world from an external point of view; logic and objectivity are increased over previous stages. Thinking becomes dynamic, decentralized, and reversible. It becomes possible to understand the intermediate steps between two states. It also becomes possible to "conserve." In Piaget's classic experiment about conservation, a clay ball is rolled into (i.e., becomes) a clay sausage. If the child can think about the transformation in such a way that he or she appreciates that shape does not alter quantity, the child is described as able to conserve, or to recognize that certain changes (e.g., physical rearrangement) do not necessarily alter other properties (e.g., quantity) of a substance. Conservation is the result of the child's ability to focus on several aspects of a problem or situation at one time and relate them. Thus, as exemplified in the ball-sausage experiment, the child who can *conserve* mass can understand the reciprocity of length and width in the problem presented.

A child in the early concrete operational period can solve a problem only if the elements of the problem are physically present, and often they must be actually manipulated for full understanding. By the late concrete operational period, the child can solve problems of space and time; can conserve substance, quantity, weight, and volume; and can classify objects into hierarchical systems. Physical manipulation remains helpful but is not essential to problem solving.

Social Learning Development: Secondary Motivational Systems; Extrafamily Learning. Beginning with entrance into school and extending throughout the remainder of life, individuals are influenced increasingly by the social values and customs of those outside their family. The dependency on family that the child has developed must be unlearned; instead, he or she must learn to act independently and in compliance with expectations made by nonfamily members of the larger social group. The child's identification with models among adults or peers in school or in the community provides initial instruction through imitation or observation. Reinforcement, such as admiration or approval, serves to perpetuate socially acceptable behaviors. If desirable behaviors are not reinforced consistently or if the only attention the child receives is through participation in socially unacceptable behaviors, undesirable behaviors will be learned at this stage just as they were at earlier ages within the confines of the home. Thus the basic principles of learning are invariant and independent of the individual's age and setting.

Adolescence and Young Adulthood

The term *adolescence* is derived from the Latin, *adolescere* (to grow up), and refers to the psychological, biological, and sociological aspects of development that occur during the second decade of life. *Puberty* refers to the condition of becoming sexually mature and being capable of sexual reproduction.

The age of onset of puberty has varied considerably over the centuries, a phenomenon known as the *secular trend.*[45] For example, earlier maturation was noted over a period of

150 years during the nineteenth and early twentieth centuries but reached a plateau in American teenagers beginning in the 1960s. Reasons for such changes have been related to a variety of environmental factors such as nutrition and global temperature cycles.

Adolescence usually is divided into three stages: early, middle, and late. During early adolescence most of the individual's physical and emotional energy is centered on physical change and its consequences, during middle adolescence on separation from parents, and during late adolescence on preparation for an adult identity.

Important gender-specific differences exist in both the timing of growth and final adult size. The female growth spurt occurs about 2 years earlier than the male growth spurt, but the final adult height of women is less than that of men because of the shorter growth period. Muscle growth appears to be influenced primarily by androgenic stimulation. Thus there is greater muscle mass and strength in the mature man than in the mature woman.

Increase in body size and maturation of neuronal pathways contribute to the child's and adolescent's increasing ability to perform complex motor tasks. Large muscles develop before small muscles. Therefore younger children are more skillful in activities involving gross motor movements than they are in activities requiring fine motor coordination. In early adolescence differential bone and muscle growth can result in transient increases in awkwardness, particularly in gross motor functioning. During middle and late adolescence, the diminution in growth rate over time leads to greater stability in body proportions; motor awkwardness gradually decreases.

Throughout infancy and childhood, circulating levels of pituitary follicle-stimulating hormone and luteinizing hormone are low. Although growth of both the internal and external genitalia parallels increases in body size, the genitalia retain their infantile appearance and function until the onset of pubertal change.

Pubertal change can be divided into three stages. During the first, prepubescence (prepuberty), the gonadotropin and sex steroid levels remain low; however, secondary sexual characteristics begin to appear. In girls, the earliest sign of the initiation of sexual maturation often is widening of the pelvic girdle. This is followed by breast and pubic hair development and the onset of the height spurt. In boys, testicular growth precedes penile growth, development of pubic hair, and the onset of the height spurt.

For reasons that are not completely clear but that may be related to critical body weight, the hypothalamus begins to become less sensitive to negative feedback from circulating gonadotropin. Luteinizing hormone–releasing factor is produced and gonadotropin secretion is enhanced, rising progressively toward adult levels.

During the second stage, pubescence (puberty), the reproductive organs (primary sexual characteristics) become functional, and the secondary sexual characteristics become more evident. The last stage, postpubescence (postpuberty), includes a 1- to 2-year period of relative reproductive infertility. Skeletal growth is completed during this time.

Psychosexual Development: The Genital Stage. According to freudian theory, sexual impulses reemerge during adolescence, marking the onset of the *genital stage*. Whereas pleasure-seeking through oral, anal, and genital stimulation was the aim of the infantile form of sexuality, during puberty another sexual aim arises: reproduction, through a mature heterosexual relationship with a love object.

During early adolescence there is thought to be a partial recrudescence of the Oedipal conflict or a regression to the psychosexual stage characteristic of the preschool child. This may occur because the adolescent feels safer expressing some of his or her new and confusing sexual feelings within the familiar environment of the family. However, the adolescent recognizes that emotional closeness to the parent of the other gender is both unrealistic and unacceptable. The adolescent also has learned from experiences during the phallic stage that real competition with the parent of the same gender is hopeless.

In addition to whatever sexual overtones may be associated with movement into the genital stage, the process of renewed competition with the parent of the same gender also stirs in the adolescent a questioning of the behavior, values, and judgments of the parent. To explain this phenomenon, it is important to recall that resolution of the Oedipal phase in early childhood brought with it acceptance of the parental value system and a desire to be like the parent. The value system that was accepted, however, was primitive and rudimentary because the child was not cognitively capable of full understanding; for example, the preoperational child cannot comprehend that although behavior sometimes is modified depending on the situation, such modifications do not necessarily impair the basic underlying value system. That is, for the young child, judgments are black and white; very little, if any, gray area exists. But, as we shall see as we discuss cognitive growth during adolescence, the ability to understand hypothetical situations and to argue both for and against certain points of view renders the teenager's previous value system inadequate to deal with larger moral and philosophical issues. However, rather than turn to the parent for explanation and clarification, the adolescent assumes that the parents' value system is exactly as he or she conceived of it as a young child (e.g., parents of adolescents often comment, "My teenager thinks I don't know anything."); thus the adolescent turns to peers or adults outside the family, looking for a new, expanded set of values. In the process the adolescent is likely to reject the parents' values to some extent. Eventually the adolescent seeks independence from both parents, not just the parent of the same gender. In some cases a period of significant alienation from the family may be necessary to attain sufficient distance for independence to be truly attained. During the resolution of the parent-child conflict of the genital stage, the boy completes his (adult) identification with his father by choosing a female partner. Similarly, the girl completes her (adult) identification with her mother by seeking a male partner. Thus full sexual maturity, in freudian terms, is attained when feelings directed toward the parent of the other gender are transferred successfully to a love object that is not taboo.

The genital stage is the longest phase in the psychosexual developmental framework, lasting from adolescence to senility, when regression to the pregenital stage is thought to be common. However, attainment of the genital stage does not necessarily preclude continuing to derive pleasure from satisfaction of pregenital as well as genital drives. In addition, the personality constructs and defense mechanisms developed during the pregenital stages continue as part of the individual's permanent character structure and are manifested throughout life.

Psychosocial Development: Identity Versus Role Confusion and Intimacy Versus Isolation. Identity formation is thought by many to involve answering three questions: who am I as a physical being? Who am I as a sexual being? Who am I as a vocational being? Of these, the major focus of this phase of development in Eriksonian terms is the task of choosing an occupational identity (i.e., selecting a role to play within the adult community, including investment in the choice of work and the work itself and involvement in the community for the community's sake).

The process of general identity formation begins in early adolescence. The individual becomes determined to be the same as other members of his or her peer group, which usually is composed of members of the same gender and often is an extension or continuation of a latency-age "chum" group. Often cruel in its exclusion of others, the "in" group attempts to establish its identity as a separate social unit in and of itself. The security of the small group permits individual members to clarify their particular roles within the group and thus eventually to move toward a sense of personal identity as members of society as a whole.

Through the rigidity of their structure and customs, cliques serve the sometimes useful purpose of guarding the individual from a sense of confusion about role. Thus, as the adolescent moves out of the known environment of family into the world, he or she passes through a transitional phase as a member of a closely knit peer group. In much the same way as parents did, this group helps to define acceptable and unacceptable behavior. However, to facilitate separation from family, the rules and values of the group the adolescent chooses often are different from, if not antithetical to, those of the family. In this way teenagers try to demonstrate that they are their own persons, doing their "own thing" (see Chapter 86).

Part of developing identity is (1) recognizing specific personal strengths and weaknesses, (2) aspiring to goals that are realistic and attainable, and (3) working toward those goals. The potential danger is never achieving clarity of role; closely allied is having too many nebulous or halfhearted roles (identity diffusion) or choosing a role without sufficiently exploring options (identity foreclosure).

Some adolescents may choose a negative identity (i.e., an identity counter to that suggested by society) because they see conformity as the route to being a nonentity. The positive role of the individual who has a negative identity can be social change. In such situations, even though overcoming the inertia of the status quo may require great energy and commitment, the result of such deviance can have such a major effect on social mores that the individual perceives the effort as worthwhile. For example, many of the characteristics of the hippie of the late 1960s could be found in conventional youth by the mid-1970s; similarly, the antiwar sentiments of young people who were ostracized in the 1970s became common in the 1980s. For those who advocated such changes, assuming an identity outside the mainstream may have appeared to be the only option for changing the system. The danger of assuming a counterculture identity, however, is permanent ostracism—never achieving sufficient reintegration to effect desired change or to derive a satisfying sense of self from society.

During late adolescence and young adulthood, the individual moves into the stage of *intimacy versus isolation.* Once personal identity becomes established, the young adult is eager to fuse his or her identity with that of another—to develop intimacy or the capacity to commit oneself to a partnership despite personal sacrifice and compromise. Although often thought of in sexual terms, intimacy includes close friendships, inspiring teacher-student relationships, and other affiliations in which personal vulnerability and true glimpses of the self are permitted. The antithesis of intimacy, in eriksonian terms, is the state of *distantiation*—isolation from or the destruction of those who appear to be a danger to oneself or to one's intimate relations (i.e., prejudices against those who are unfamiliar or foreign and thus threatening).

True genitality, a term borrowed from Freud, develops during this phase. Erikson states that to be of lasting social significance, true genitality should include a heterosexual love relationship that ultimately produces children.

The danger of this adolescent/young adult phase is selection of an inappropriate "permanent" partner for reasons of expediency rather than for complementary elaboration or fulfillment of mutual purposes.

Cognitive Development: Formal Operational Period. Beginning in early adolescence and extending throughout adulthood, the period of *formal operations* is distinguished by the ability to use abstract thought. Characteristics of formal operational thought include flexibility, complex reasoning, and hypothesis formation.

Not all adolescents or all adults apply formal operational thinking to all aspects of reality, nor are they "formal operational" under all conditions and circumstances. Rather, use of formal operations often is restricted to cognitive functioning in areas of particular personal interest or professional concern and is applied most productively at times of low stress and anxiety. In addition, there are gender-specific differences; thus females are more likely than males to apply formal operations to interpersonal matters; males are more likely to apply formal operations to scientific matters.

The development of formal operational or abstract thought allows the adolescent to understand certain moral, political, and philosophical ideas and values for the first time. With the emergence of the ability to deal with concepts such as liberty and justice, adolescents become preoccupied with social, religious, and political issues. Because they can conceive of the ideal, be it society, religion, or family, they become aware of the contradictions, falsehoods, and shortcomings embedded in their previously accepted beliefs.

Adolescents can think about thinking; they understand the thought processes of others and wonder how individuals see them and what these individuals really think about them. A belief that others may dwell on or constantly evaluate their appearance and behaviors results in the egocentrism or self-centeredness particularly characteristic of the early and middle adolescent. Self-consciousness is a direct reflection of this self-centeredness. As formal operational thinking becomes better established (in middle to late adolescence), the individual begins to distinguish between personal preoccupation and the thoughts of others. Once this distinction can be made, the adolescent can enter into an intimate emotional relationship with others.

Stress, such as illness, can have a profound influence on the individual's ability to use higher order cognitive skills in solving a problem. The general physical and emotional regression seen in a hospitalized child, regardless of his or her usual functional ability, often also is accompanied by a cognitive regression. Such phenomena as magical thinking (my wish equals action) or egocentrism (my action caused some external unrelated event) are common. The ability to think futuristically when considering the potential consequences of current actions can be impaired. Conversely, long-term illness in some individuals results in increased learning and adultlike understanding of related issues. Because this can occur in children of all ages, it is not unusual for children who have long-term, fatal malignancies, for example, to have an understanding of body function or a conception of death that is surprisingly mature. This finding is in keeping with Piaget's premise that cognitive functioning is highly dependent on and molded by experience.

Social Learning Development: Secondary Motivational Systems; Extrafamilial Learning. As the individual matures, the nature and scope of interactions with others broaden. Reinforcement of particular behaviors becomes less critical because participation in the large class of socially acceptable behaviors has become habitual. Rewards and punishments are based largely on internal rather than external controls. Thus the adolescent is able to enter into relationships based on the mutuality of needs of two or more independent people.

SPECIFIC DEVELOPMENTAL ISSUES

Research that has focused on the development of the child's understanding of certain concepts has provided the opportunity for practical application of certain developmental theories. Three examples of such applications are (1) development of moral judgment, (2) gender identity, gender role behavior, and sexual behavior, and (3) response to stress.

Development of Moral Judgment

Parents often ask pediatricians to explain why a child appears to have little concept of right and wrong or why conflicts arise (between a parent and child or between two children) that cannot be reconciled, even though the solution appears straightforward to the parent. Many parents find it burdensome and feel guilty when they resort to time-out or the threat of no bedtime story to induce their children to do what is "right" rather than use the logic of some higher moral authority to persuade the child.

Although frustrating at times, it is clear that children's moral judgments are qualitatively different from those of adults. Furthermore, the ability to make moral judgments based on an internal rather than external value system evolves during childhood and adolescence through a series of stages. Kohlberg[27] has done pioneering work in this field, basing his model on the cognitive-intellectual principles Piaget described. According to Kohlberg's theory, thinking about moral issues depends on and represents the individual's general cognitive stage at any point in development. He also suggests that there is a "cultural universality" to the sequencing of moral development, although the chronological ages at which certain stages appear may be different in various cultures—and within a culture, they may depend on particular social experiences. Kohlberg's scheme describes three overall levels of moral judgment: *preconventional* (premoral), *conventional,* and *postconventional* (principled). Each level is subdivided into two stages; that is, level I, stages 1 and 2; level II, stages 3 and 4; and level III, stages 5 and 6.

In the discussion that follows, these stages are presented and then related to the freudian, eriksonian, and social learning theory stages that occur simultaneously. These associations among theories illustrate the wide variety of simultaneously occurring events and challenges the child experiences that shape how he or she will respond to situations that require judgment about appropriate behavior.

Level I. The *preconventional level* is characteristic of children in the sensorimotor and preoperational periods of cognitive development. Judgments about right and wrong are determined by the external physical consequences of the actions; that is, by whether the actions elicit punishment or rewards.

In stage 1, moral judgment clearly is based on the principle of punishment and obedience. Stage 2 behavior is instrumental and relativistic; this stage is exemplified by the child who acts to satisfy his or her own needs, although occasionally the needs of others may be satisfied incidentally. Fairness, reciprocity, and sharing are based on pragmatism ("I help you; you help me") rather than on an understanding of loyalty or gratitude.

These stages are analogous to the oral and anal stages of freudian theory and the trust versus mistrust and autonomy versus shame and doubt stages elaborated by Erikson. In stage 1, the child depends entirely on the external cues of the caregiver for decisions about right and wrong behavior, and compliance is motivated by a desire to obtain love and nurturance. In stage 2, the child is able to take some responsibility for satisfying personal needs but behaves out of a sense of pleasing himself or herself primarily and others secondarily.

In early level I, behavior first is conditioned and then shaped (in learning theory terms) by rewarding desirable behaviors through positive reinforcement and punishing undesirable behaviors through nonreinforcement (withholding attention). Restraint and redirection are other successful strategies in modifying behavior. Late in this stage, punishment is introduced as a form of negative reinforcement, because the child lacks experience to *understand* that some poor judgments (e.g., sucking on an electrical cord) could have lasting negative consequences. Punishment (such as yelling and spanking) often is used to denote the more serious outcomes that could occur if the child persisted in the behavior. Thus the child learns to not suck on electrical cords, not because he or she understands the consequences of being electrocuted, but because of the consequence of being verbally or physically reprimanded.

Level II. At the conventional level, moral judgments are based on two objectives: (1) wanting to perform a desired role (and thus fulfilling the expectations of others who will give praise), and (2) wanting to maintain order (and thus following the rules). Unlike judgments characteristic of level I, those characteristic of level II are based on a consideration of the desires of others and can function independently of any actual physical consequences of the action.

Stage 3 behavior is that which pleases or helps others, who then show their approval by designating the child a "good boy" or a "nice girl." Stage 4 behavior, based on the principles of "law and order," is determined by respect for authority and the rules of the social group, which are seen as unchangeable. That is, rules are fixed and independent of circumstance or situation.

In Freudian and Eriksonian terms, this is the stage that develops in concert with resolution of the Oedipal conflict and occurs during the stages of initiative versus guilt and industry versus inferiority.[19] Thus the child is learning to sublimate his or her own immediate aims and desires and to incorporate the values of others into a personal value system (through the process of identification as defined by Freud). Desire to be like the parent helps the child to internalize parental qualities that please others. With this process comes the emergence of the superego, or conscience. Similarly, in Eriksonian terms, the child learns to modulate both wishes and behavior to please others. Part of pleasing others is to play by the rules: construct products, attend to learning, and refine skills; in other words, to become a person who is perceived by society as being industrious.

According to social learning theory, the child who is moving into the community learns through observation and imitation of an increasingly large pool of individuals who act as models. Conformity to rules and respect for authority are particularly important attributes for successful participation in large group activities and therefore are strongly reinforced as socially acceptable behaviors.

Level III. At this level, moral judgments are based on personal conformity to principles that are valid apart from social authority and convention. This level of reasoning requires full formal operational thinking.

In stage 5, sometimes known as the social contract or legalistic stage, the individual recognizes that personal rights and standards exist, but that such personal values and opinions are relative. Procedural rules for reaching consensus are exercised; laws are recognized as changeable to meet the needs of the common good rather than as rigid and inflexible. Stage 6 judgments are based on broad abstract moral principles (e.g., the Golden Rule) rather than on concrete moral imperatives (e.g., the Ten Commandments). Universal principles of justice, reciprocity, equality of human rights, and respect for human dignity are applied to moral decision making.

Again, there are striking similarities in the way Kohlberg conceptualizes this stage and the major characteristics identified in the genital stage of freudian theory and the identity versus role confusion stage of eriksonian theory. Thus knowledge of and respect for oneself as an individual allow the adolescent or young adult to engage in mutual and reciprocal relationships with other people (the basis of "true genitality" as well as of "identity" and "intimacy"). This process also forms the basis for postconventional moral reasoning.

Finally, in terms of social learning theory, participation in broad extrafamilial learning systems in which the motivations for behavior are secondary and derived from nonimmediate reinforcement permits the individual to obtain satisfaction from behavior that is conducive to some higher social goal, even though it may be unsatisfying personally in the short term. Certainly there can be little argument that the ability to delay gratification, or even suffer personally, is a key element if adherence to such stage 6 principles as justice and equality is to be successful.

In keeping with other general developmental theorists, Kohlberg states that individuals who have attained certain levels of moral judgment still have available to them, and occasionally use, lower levels of judgment.[27] He has called this regression a *judgment of ease* as opposed to a *judgment of preference* because he assumes that an individual would, under all circumstances, prefer to use the highest level of moral reasoning available to him or her. Kohlberg also suggests that the motivation for a given behavior may not always be clear from the behavior itself. For example, if the driver of a car decelerates to the speed limit when a police car appears ahead on the road, such behavior may represent a judgment of ease based on stage 1 (obedience and punishment) reasoning or higher order stage 4 (law and order) reasoning. (Interestingly, it is possible that someone operating at stages 5 or 6 might not slow down at all if traffic were light and the driving conditions excellent, arguing that speed limits are arbitrary and the spirit of the law [safe driving] and not the letter of the law [55 mph speed limit] is the more valid ethic on which to base behavior.)

Although the Kohlberg model provides a reasonable framework for understanding moral development in general, its applicability is limited by its reliance on boys and men as the major subject pool from which his observations were drawn. Gilligan[15] and others who have studied girls and women have questioned whether the intense focus on competitiveness and following rules is as valid in the development of moral reasoning and judgment in females as it may be in males. Indeed, it has been suggested that compared with boys, girls are more pragmatic about rules, more contextual in their application (e.g., factoring relational variables into the reasoning process to promote harmony within the group), and more adaptable to innovation. These characteristics of female decision making are thought to reflect society's traditional tendency to socialize girls so that they will view "playing the game" as subordinate to keeping friends—a tradition that, in the past, has placed them at substantial disadvantage when seeking the time-honored version of corporate success. However, the trend in current American society is toward less gender role stereotyping, and although the influence on both male and female moral judgments remains to be seen, the effects of some recent changes in corporate structure, especially in the direction of such management strategies as shared decision making, are already evident.

Development of Gender Identity, Gender Role Behavior, and Sexual Behavior

The relationship between physiological and psychological growth and development is particularly well illustrated by the development of gender identity, or the individual's own self-concept of male or female. The final expression of adult gender identity is preceded by a series of events, some biological and others social or psychological in nature.

Initial biological differentiation is determined on the basis of chromosomal composition, which directs primordial gonadal development.

Although most families are unaware of the gender of the fetus, the parents' conscious or unconscious expectations, wishes, and anxieties, as noted earlier in this chapter, play a role in their developing attachment to the unborn child.

The morphology of the newborn's external genitalia has an immediate psychological effect on the family that persists for the remainder of the individual's life. On first contact with the infant after birth and determination of the child's gender, a set of cultural expectations influences all communication to and about the child, including choice of the child's name and of external reinforcers (blue versus pink clothes, types of toys). There are subtle differences in parental voice inflection and handling of the infant, depending on the gender of the child and of the particular parent. Different temperamental characteristics in the infant are reinforced, depending on gender. Thus clinging by baby girls and active play by baby boys may be reinforced selectively from birth. This is consistent with the biases of most cultures, which designate aggressive, assertive behavior as masculine and dependent and socially compliant behavior as feminine.[38]

As the child matures, both the behavior of others and the child's image of his or her physical self in comparison with others serve as cues about how to internalize a concept of self through adoption of certain gender role behaviors. For example, children between 2 and 4 years of age can identify themselves as boys or girls (although they may not yet be able to identify the gender of other people correctly). Although certain personality characteristics already may have developed in a given child because of selected gender-determined environmental reinforcements, actual behavior is less stereotyped than it is likely to become later. Thus much of the earliest imitative behavior in children of both genders revolves around housework, which usually (but not always) is modeled by the mother, the first "identificatory" object, as defined by Freud. As children experience and resolve the Oedipal conflict and identify more strongly with the parent of the same gender, they adopt an increasing number of behaviors they perceive to be appropriate to their biological gender (e.g., "When I grow up, I want to do 'man things,' like Daddy."). Thus, for example, for boys, behaviors that are culturally masculine and those that are culturally feminine are available to him through observation and imitation. As he moves out of toddlerhood, he generally does not adopt behaviors that are perceived as specific for the female gender role. Instead, he incorporates behaviors that are masculine into his behavioral repertoire. In learning theory terms, it can be hypothesized that "appropriate" role behaviors are being reinforced and "inappropriate" role behaviors are being inhibited. Such reinforcements may be extremely subtle. In a study of children attending a day care center that specifically deemphasized gender role stereotyping in play, it was found that even when given free selection, boys still were likely to choose traditionally masculine toys (cars, trucks) and girls still were likely to choose traditionally feminine toys (baby dolls, cooking utensils).[11] Interestingly, the stereotypically determined selection rate for girls tends to be less pronounced than that for boys. This finding supports the notion that cues about gender role behaviors are highly ingrained and pervasive in our society and that, to date, Western culture has been more successful in providing latitude in the definition of acceptable behavior for girls than it has for boys.

As children mature, they undergo somatic and pubertal changes that affect their psychological development directly. However, cultural tradition prescribes how they will express their sexuality, and this behavior is highly age dependent. *Sexual behavior* is a broad term and ranges from the sex-related activities of the infant and young child to the truly genital behaviors of the adolescent and adult. Much of the child's early sexual behavior occurs because it satisfies curiosity and is pleasurable although not necessarily erotic. However, it is behavior that to some degree is an expression of masculinity or femininity. Sexual behavior is an integral part of the developmental process, and certain types of behaviors are particularly common at certain ages.

Penile erections have been noted on ultrasonography of the developing male fetus. Vaginal lubrication occurs at least from birth. During the first year of life, boys become aware of their penis and girls become aware of their clitoris as sources of pleasurable and painful sensations. Masturbation is common among children between 2 and 5 years of age.

Young children's natural inquisitiveness about their bodies leads them to touch not only themselves but their parents and siblings as well. Older children "play doctor" or "family" with their peers, games that often entail some undressing and mutual touching.

By early school age, humor or conversation involving "dirty" words and giggled references to body functions is used as a way of responding to parental admonitions about modesty and what constitutes socially acceptable conversation about sexuality. In some children, modesty is taken so literally that it can lead to such a strong generalized sense of privacy that even a physical examination by a physician is vigorously opposed. This extreme desire for personal physical privacy can extend into adolescence unless parental guidance is available to help the child learn to judge those circumstances under which the definition of modesty is appropriately subject to modification.

Many children express their sexuality through increased masturbatory behavior in early adolescence. Many also engage in homosexual behaviors. Actually, homosexual experimentation, especially in the early genital stage, is common enough to be considered a normal developmental phase that may or may not give rise to an eventual homosexual orientation.

Sexual activity typically occurs initially within the context of group dating, with little or no actual pairing. A transitional stage of double dating may occur before the adolescent enters into a phase of individual dating, in time with an exclusive partner. The most common initial sexual activity during adolescence is holding hands. This is followed, usually in order, by kissing, petting, and finally, intercourse.

In summary, boys and girls appear to be reared differently from the moment their particular morphological gender is known, or even before, through conscious or unconscious expectations. Children develop a sense of their own gender identity through selective environmental inhibition or reinforcement of certain kinds of behaviors that have been deemed by their culture to be consistent with the expression of male or female roles. Gender identity, the objective perception of oneself as male or female, is the sum total of one's feelings and behaviors. It is displayed in a variety of ways in daily living, beginning in earliest childhood. The most intimate expression of gender identity is mature sexual activity within the confines of a stable mutual relationship.

Developmental Aspects of the Psychobiology of Stress

Current times are highly stressful for children and adolescents. Socioeconomic disadvantage, divorce, and child abuse and neglect are at an all-time high. Furthermore, racism and class distinction continue to be strong negative influences on a growing number of children. Although stress has been recognized for some time as a risk factor for mental and physical illness in adults, only recently has it become recognized as a risk factor for childhood morbidity as well.

Temperament appears to be an important factor in determining the degree of individual vulnerability to stress, which carries with it increased risk for various childhood diseases.[7] Studies have documented a pattern of physiological hyperreactivity, consisting of elevated heart rate, sympathetic adrenomedullary activation, and a rise in plasma cortisol or corticotropin levels, among both behaviorally inhibited infant monkeys[44] and human children.[24] These characteristics of psychobiological reactivity persist into later periods of development and are related to social withdrawal in group settings. Developmental studies focused on cardiovascular responsivity suggest that exaggerated reactivity is at least partly genetically determined and persists into adult life,[14] possibly contributing to increased risk of cardiovascular disease and other chronic health problems.[7]

Psychobiological hyperreactivity also has been implicated in the development of subsequent anxiety disorders.[23] In addition, Miller and Wood[32] found that emotional and physiological reactivity was related to the degree of airway compromise induced in certain asthmatic children who were exposed to emotional challenge under laboratory conditions. These findings suggest that certain temperamental patterns may place some children at risk for later health problems, if they grow up in stressful environments or if they have a particular physiological vulnerability, such as asthma.

In a similar vein, Porges[35] identified and documented the importance of parasympathetic (vagal) activation in mediating the impact of stress on the individual. He demonstrated that high-risk preterm neonates have lower vagal tone than do full-term neonates, and that these differences are related to later dimensions of clinical risk, such as low weight gain and inability to habituate to stimuli and to sustain attention. This work suggests that children who were high-risk preterm neonates may be more vulnerable to stress-related physical or emotional illnesses later in development.

The influence of stress on the organism's ability to mount an effective immune response is well documented.[1,10] Current research with infant primates indicates that the nutritional and psychological effects of separation from the mother may have long-lasting effects on some immune responses in the developing infant. These findings suggest that the quality of parent-child attachment may have far reaching implications for the physical well-being of the child.

In addition to impeding adaptation, psychobiological reactivity and other aspects of temperament also can enhance adaptation. For example, Gunner[18] cites research indicating that children who have greater elevations of cortisol in response to stressors such as academic examinations, hospitalization, and surgery tend to be children who are more competent with peers, more involved in their school work, more positive and cooperative in the clinic, and more realistic in their appraisals of the importance of the stressor. Interestingly, studies attempting to correlate level of anxiety and degree of distressed behavior among both infants and older children have been inconclusive.

It is important to recognize that there are both risks and benefits associated with particular temperamentally based individual differences in psychobiological reactivity. Pediatricians will find themselves caring for children who are unusually shy and withdrawn or emotionally reactive, and parents or teachers may ask whether such behaviors are normal. It is critical to remember that high psychobiological reactivity is not abnormal, nor necessarily prodromal for any abnormal physical or emotional condition (see Barr[4] for a discussion of "normal"). Rather, children who have such a temperament might best be considered as highly sensitive individuals who will thrive in facilitating environments but will be more vulnerable when stressed. It most likely is the interaction of temperament and environment that will determine the child's developmental outcome, not one factor or the other alone.

SOME FINAL THOUGHTS ON "IT'S JUST A STAGE"

Although, theoretically, children and adolescents achieve biopsychosocial maturity in a predictable, specific fashion, in reality, human variability and dissonance between growth and development make predictions about a given individual difficult, frustrating, and challenging. When the pediatrician can offer reassurance about the temporary nature of a particular undesirable or anxiety-provoking stage of development, children and their families often are better able to cope, knowing that minor changes in parenting expectations or interpersonal relationships will result in a better adjustment to the current stage and a smoother transition to the next stage.

Although the spectrum of variability is broad, not all deviations from average expected development are normal. The greatest challenge to the practitioner is to distinguish between adequate, although not necessarily perfect, development and true dysfunction. Passing a situation off as merely "a stage" is justified only when the true limits of acceptable behavior for that stage are clearly understood, the reasons for the behavior can be explained in such a way that the parents and/or child can understand what they are experiencing and why, and appropriate guidance to help them master the stage is provided.

REFERENCES

1. Ader R, Felton DL, Cohen N: *Psychoneuroimmunology*, ed 2, San Diego, 1991, Academic Press.
2. Ainsworth MDS: Object relations, dependency, and attachment: a theoretical review of the infant-mother relationship, *Child Dev* 40:969, 1969.
3. Baldwin AL: *Theories of child development*, New York, 1967, John Wiley & Sons.

4. Barr RG: Normality: a clinically useless concept—the case of infant crying and colic, *J Dev Behav Pediatr* 14:264-270, 1993.
5. Berndt TJ, Hawkins JA, Hoyle SG: Changes in friendship during a school year, *Child Dev* 57:1284, 1986.
6. Biller HB: Father absence and the personality development of the child, *Dev Psychol* 2:181, 1970.
7. Boyce WT, Barr RG, Zeltzer LK: Temperament and the psychobiology of childhood stress, *Pediatrics* 90:483, 1992.
8. Cernoch JM, Porter RH: Recognition of maternal axillary odor by infants, *Child Dev* 56:1593, 1985.
9. Chess S, Thomas A: *Origins and evolution of behavior disorders: from infancy to early adult life,* New York, 1984, Brunner/Mazel.
10. Coe CL et al: Early rearing conditions alter immune responses in the developing infant primate, *Pediatrics* 90:505, 1992.
11. Cole HJ, Zucker KJ, Bradley SJ: Patterns of gender-role behavior in children attending traditional and nontraditional day care centers, *Can J Psychiatry* 27:410, 1982.
12. Eder R, Mangelsdorf SC: The emotional basis of early personality development: implications for the emergent self-concept. In Hogan R, Johnson J, Briggs S, editors: *Handbook of personality psychology,* Orlando, Fla, 1994, Academic Press.
13. Erikson EH: *Childhood and society,* ed 2, New York, 1963, WW Norton.
14. Falkner B, Ragonesi S: Psychosocial stress and reactivity as risk factors of cardiovascular disease, *J Am Acad Child Adolesc Psychiatry* 25:779, 1986.
15. Gilligan C: *In a different voice: psychological theory and women's development,* Cambridge, Mass, 1982, Harvard University Press.
16. Gottesman II: Heritability of personality: a demonstration, *Psychological Monographs* 77 (No 9, Whole No 572), 1963.
17. Greenberg M, Morris N: Engrossment: the newborn's impact upon the father, *Am J Orthopsychiatry* 44:520, 1974.
18. Gunner MR: Reactivity of the hypothalamic-pituitary-adrenocortical system to stressors in normal infants and children, *Pediatrics* 90:491, 1992.
19. Hall CS: *A primer of freudian psychology,* New York, 1954, World.
20. Hay D, Nash A, Pedersen J: Interactions between 6-month-old peers, *Child Dev* 54:557, 1983.
21. Hetherington EM: Effects of natural absence in sex-typed behaviors in Negro and white preadolescent males, *J Pers Soc Psychol* 14:87, 1966.
22. Hetherington EM, Reiss D, Plomin R: *Separate social worlds of siblings: the impact of nonshared environment on development,* Hillsdale, NJ, 1994, Lawrence Erlbaum.
23. Hirshfeld DR et al: Stable behavioral inhibition and its association with anxiety disorder, *J Am Acad Child Adolesc Psychiatry* 31:103, 1992.
24. Kagan J, Reznick JS, Snidman N: The physiology and psychology of behavioral inhibition in young children, *Child Dev* 58:1459, 1988.
25. Kestenbaum CJ, Stone MH: The effects of fatherless homes upon daughters: clinical impressions regarding paternal deprivation, *J Am Acad Psychoanal* 4:171, 1976.
26. Klaus MH, Kennell JH: *Parent-infant bonding,* ed 2, St Louis, 1982, Mosby.
27. Kohlberg L: Moral development. In Sills DL, editor: *International encyclopedia of the social sciences,* New York, 1968, Macmillan.
28. Korner AF: The effect of the infant's level of arousal, sex, and ontogenetic stage on the caregivers. In Lewis M, Rosenblum LA, editors: *The effect of the infant on its caregiver,* New York, 1974, John Wiley & Sons.
29. Lamb ME: Father-infant and mother-infant interaction in the first year of life, *Child Dev* 48:167, 1977.
30. Lamb ME: The role of the father: an overview. In Lamb ME, editor: *The role of the father in child development,* New York, 1981, John Wiley & Sons.
31. Loehlin JC, Rowe DC: Genes, environment, and personality. In Caprara G, Van Heck GL, editors: *Modern personality psychology: critical reviews and new directions,* New York, 1992, Harvester Wheatsheaf.
32. Miller BD, Wood BL: Psychophysiologic reactivity in asthmatic children: a cholinergically mediated confluence of pathways, *J Am Acad Child Adolesc Psychiatry* 33:1236, 1994.
33. Osborne RT, Noble CE, Weyl N: *Human variation: the biopsychology of age, race and sex,* Orlando, Fla, 1978, Academic Press.
34. Parke RD: Perspectives on father-infant interaction. In Osofsky JD, editor: *Handbook of infant development,* New York, 1979, John Wiley & Sons.
35. Porges SW: Vagal tone: a physiologic marker of stress vulnerability, *Pediatrics* 90:498, 1992.
36. Rothbart MK, Derryberry D: Development of individual differences of temperament. In Lamb ME, Brown AL, editors: *Advances in developmental psychology,* vol 1, Hillsdale, NJ, 1981, Lawrence Erlbaum.
37. Rothbart MK, Posner MJ: Temperament and the development of self-regulation. In Hartlage H, Telzrow CG, editors: *The neuropsychology of individual differences: a developmental perspective,* New York, 1985, Plenum Press.
38. Rubin JZ, Provenzano FJ, Luria Z: The eye of the beholder: parents' views on sex of newborns, *Am J Orthopsychiatry* 44:512, 1974.
39. Sameroff AJ: Early influences in development: fact or fantasy? *Merrill-Palmer Q* 21:267, 1975.
40. Sameroff AJ: Models of developmental regulation: the environtype. In Cicchetti D, editor: *The emergence of a discipline: Rochester Symposium on Developmental Psychopathology,* vol 1, Hillsdale, NJ, 1989, Lawrence Erlbaum.
41. Scarr S, Grajek S: Similarities and differences among siblings. In Lamb ME, Sutton-Smith B, editors: *Sibling relationships: their nature and significance across the life span,* Hillsdale, NJ, 1982, Lawrence Erlbaum.
42. Sears RR: A theoretical framework for personality and social behavior, *Am Psychol* 6:476, 1951.
43. Sosa R et al: The effect of a supportive companion on perinatal problems, length of labor, and mother-infant interaction, *N Engl J Med* 303:597, 1980.
44. Suomi SJ: Genetic and maternal contributions to individual differences in rhesus monkey biobehavioral development. In Krasnagor N, editor: *Psychobiological aspects of behavioral development,* New York, 1988, Academic Press.
45. Tanner JM: *Fetus into man: physical growth from conception to maturity,* Cambridge, Mass, 1978, Harvard University Press.
46. Thomas A, Chess S: An approach to the study of sources of individual differences in child behavior, *J Clin Exp Psychopathol Q Rev Psychiatry Neurol* 18:347, 1957.
47. Thomas A, Chess S: *Temperament and development,* New York, 1977, Brunner/Mazel.
48. Yogman MW: Development of the father-infant relationship. In Fitzgerald H et al, editors: *Theory and research in behavioral pediatrics,* New York, 1980, Plenum.

52 Mental Health of the Young: An Overview

William R. Beardslee and Julius B. Richmond

Advances in knowledge of child development, gained through the in-depth study of healthy infants and children as well as through observations of deviations or delays in development, have provided the pediatrician with the conceptual framework needed to deal effectively with the mental health needs of children. Recent advances within child psychiatry also have contributed substantially, including, for example, the development of reliable, standardized interview instruments, a criterion-based diagnostic system (Diagnostic and Statistical Manual-IV of the American Psychiatric Association), more effective pharmacological treatments for affective and attention-deficit disorders, and the description of the epidemiology of a number of childhood mental disorders. A more sophisticated understanding of the prevalence and nature of neurodevelopmental and neuropsychiatric difficulties also has substantially expanded the information available to the pediatrician. An expanding knowledge base in the neurosciences, including molecular biology and molecular genetics, already has strengthened our understanding of the etiology and treatment of childhood psychiatric disorders and undoubtedly will continue to expand in the years to come. For example, in both Tourrette syndrome and childhood depression, evidence of interference with neurotransmitter function leading to the behavioral manifestations of the disorder is increasing.

Advances in the development of preventive and therapeutic agents over the past 40 years have brought about major reductions in infant mortality and childhood morbidity and mortality. No longer is the practicing pediatrician's time consumed by rickets, scurvy, or the acute infectious diseases such as measles, pertussis, diphtheria, and poliomyelitis. Rather, more time and energy are available to focus on the prevention of disease and the early detection and care of children who have chronic disorders, including developmental disabilities.

In addition, the past decade has been characterized by an increasing awareness by organized consumers of the desirability of high-quality child health and child care services. Pressure from communities for improved child health services has increased, a concern reflected in the development of such programs as Head Start; maternal and infant care (M&I); children and youth (C&Y) early periodic screening, diagnosis, and treatment (EPSDT) for Medicaid-eligible children; and community mental health centers. The new approaches to more comprehensive services for the handicapped also reflect intensified community sophistication, such as the Education for All Handicapped Children Act (Public Law 94-142), which emphasizes the need to "mainstream" such children. Public Law 99-457 has mandated adequate services for younger handicapped children.

Recently attention to cost effectiveness and the need for broadening the base of medical and psychiatric coverage to include all Americans also has led to a reexamination of the service delivery system. A recent report from the Carnegie Foundation[2] has emphasized the need for a wide array of services for children, as has current interest in the expansion downward of the Head Start Program to include youngsters 0 to 3 years of age. These and other policy changes can have wide-ranging and positive changes on children's health.

The increasing interest in child health undoubtedly will result in an effort to reorganize services and generate local initiatives to reflect local needs and priorities. The emphasis increasingly will be on the enhancement of health and the prevention of disease. Thus competence in the assessment and guidance of growth and development needs to be among the pediatrician's clinical skills.

The pediatrician must have a firm grasp of the child development field. Piaget's work[6] provides the most useful framework within the cognitive sphere because of its emphasis on the child's actions as necessary for the acquisition of knowledge and on the predictable sequence of stages through which a child passes in developing intelligence. Skinner's work[10] in the area of behavior modification and its applications have proved valuable both in helping children to learn and in suggesting ways to manage difficult or troublesome symptoms. Several workers in the area of early infant and child behavior, including Thomas, Chess, and Birch,[11] have helped to focus attention on the importance of temperament as an early influence. Expansion of developmental frameworks to include moral development[4] and interpersonal development[9] have further contributed to the understanding of normal development. In addition, large scale epidemiological studies have provided valuable data about prevalence and incidence of both physical and mental disorders.[4]

Psychoanalytic theory and formulations have contributed to our understanding of all aspects of the development of the child.[10,11]

The work of Erikson[3] probably provides the best integrative framework through which pediatricians can understand the different factors shaping the mental health of the child and then best meet the needs of their patients. Erikson stresses the importance of all three major factors—biological, intrapsychic, and cultural—in the child's mental health. He sees the child as going through a series of stages in development and formulates the essential task or critical area to be mastered for each stage. Thus, as one example, the dilemma for the very young infant is basic trust versus mistrust; firm patterns for the solution of this dilemma must be successfully established for the infant to develop in a healthy way. As another example, the dilemma for the adolescent is identity versus role diffusion. Youths in this stage must come to understand their own physical endowments, experiences, and opportunities in a way that allows them to function in the world and have a sense of certainty about themselves. Specifically, youths must come to grips with three areas: (1) relationships with others, both sexual and nonsexual, (2) independence from family, and (3) choice of work or career. Familiarity with each stage, both with its task and the signs of its successful resolution, provides the pediatrician with knowledge of the principles of child mental health.

Common to a series of recent investigations of youngsters at risk because of poverty or parental mental illness or other stressors is the finding that no matter how great the risk, a significant number of children turn out to do well and, indeed, function very effectively. Rutter[8] has indicated a variety of conceptual areas to be reviewed in studying the sources of resiliency and looking for explanations. These include genetic effects, individual differences, particularly the role of temperament, inner psychological processes, and the role of influences outside of the home, especially the schools. The presence of close confiding relationships that provide support and direction has been found crucial in all of the studies of resilient individuals. Of particular relevance to pediatric practice are a number of studies of resilient individuals that have emphasized the importance of the way these individuals understand themselves and what they have accomplished—their self-understanding.[1] This self-understanding involves adequate appraisal of the stresses to be dealt with, realistic assessment of the capacity to act, and actions congruent with the assessment and has characterized people in such diverse circumstances as survivors of cancer, civil rights workers, and children of parents who have an affective disorder. The recognition and characterization of resilient behavior in pediatric practice in high-risk families is important and emphasizes the need to assess a child or family's strengths and capacities to adapt and to identify a pathological condition.[7]

Increasing attention has been paid to the prevention of mental disorder and psychological difficulty in addition to the treatment of disorder once it occurs. This requires an understanding of the developmental pathways of both psychopathology and healthy development and the positioning of interventions at the times of greatest likelihood of success—for example, enhancing the bond between caregiver and child early in life or assisting in developmental transition in adolescence. A number of well-validated intervention strategies exist that can contribute strongly to the mental health of children across the life span.[5]

Knowing the cultural and psychological background of a child's family is important for understanding the mental health needs of that child. The emotional climate in which a child is reared reflects the personality development of the parents or parent substitutes. Therefore the pediatrician must know about the developmental background of each parent and the immediate environmental factors that are significant in the child's life. Because different families impose different roles on children, it is important for the pediatrician to know how the child fits into the family constellation. Just as the physiological structure and function of an infant have determinants that antedate birth, the practices and attitudes that determine how the child will be cared for have comparable antecedents. The pediatrician may develop an understanding of these factors as they become apparent during the prenatal period or after birth, as he or she comes to know the family as a unit.

The pediatrician can regard the family as carrying the "chromosomes" that perpetuate the culture and also that form the cornerstone of emotional development. Cultural influences are like a mainstream with many tributaries: each varies from time to time in depth, rate of flow, and course; the mainstream is modified by its tributaries, but also influences them.

In the United States many variations exist in cultural patterns relating to childbearing attitudes and practices. These are determined in part by geographic, religious, educational, social, and economic backgrounds. For example, in some communities a great premium is placed on the first child being male. Religious backgrounds definitely tend to influence the size of families. Higher educational backgrounds of parents have been correlated with a later childbearing age and with limitation in family size.

The relative rapidity of social movement tends to confuse young parents in terms of their basic group identification. Also, increasing educational opportunities usually generate upward social mobility for many young parents. The pediatrician should know how much parents identify with their old and how much with their new social grouping and its culture. Either of these identifications (usually some of both) involves some reintegration on the part of the parents, who may require professional assistance. Moreover, changes in the structure of the American family have led to a large increase in the number of single-parent families and to a marked decrease in the availability of the extended family for assistance in child care. Therefore parents are relying more and more on pediatricians and other practitioners for guidance.

The pediatrician should learn to adjust his or her cultural background and attitudes toward childbearing and child rearing with the cultural backgrounds and attitudes of parents who seek advice. It then becomes easier to understand that there is no "right" attitude or practice. A certain practice may be effective for one family and yet its objectives fail with another. Thus the pediatrician can help by being objective rather than judgmental in viewing the family. This requires the capacity to observe, listen, and, as a consequence, understand.

The pediatrician can develop an objective attitude by remembering that it is the culture and not the physician that, within certain limits, defines mental health. For example, Erikson[3] and others have pointed out that children brought up in one Native American culture might not be considered capable of performing the developmental tasks required of children in another tribe living in a different climate with significantly different cultural demands. Many similar cross-cultural comparisons can be made. Although the pediatrician generally deals with more subtle contrasts, they nevertheless are real and significant for each family. In a country of people who have such varied origins and so much educational, social, economic, and geographic movement, it is unlikely that any one stable tradition of child-rearing practices will emerge in the next several decades. Therefore the objective in each instance is to help each family attain its goal in child rearing in its unique and most effective manner.

Schools, families, child care centers, and hospitals are all concerned with the mental health of children. The pediatrician can combine medical findings with observations of children within their families and perceptions of larger cultural influences to evaluate and meet the mental health needs of children. The evaluation of psychological health is a vital part of the comprehensive pediatric assessment of children. Such evaluations provide the basis for helping parents become more effective in rearing their children through helping them to articulate and realize their own goals for them. Because of the increasing numbers of health professionals and disciplines that work with children, the pediatrician's role has become even more integrative. He or she is the one who brings together the different disciplines and different kinds of knowledge—biological, psychological, and social—in a comprehensive understanding of the treatment program for the child.

When the pediatrician approaches the management of illness as one aspect of the total care of the child and is interested in the interpersonal relations between the pediatrician and family, each child can provide an intriguing study. The pediatrician also has the opportunity to help foster the psychological development of the child. In this regard, and in dealing with the child and parents, the pediatrician's attitudes, interest, and curiosity about human behavior and relations are important, probably more so than formal knowledge in this area. The pediatrician's receptivity and alertness in recognizing psychologically charged situations will extend, condition, or limit his or her effectiveness in the care of many children.

Assuming the primary responsibility for all physical and medical care of the child also provides pediatricians with responsibility and opportunity to learn about and care for the psychological and mental health needs of children. Pediatricians who wish to provide total care should be interested in children not only in intellectual terms but also in emotional terms. Those pediatricians are in a favorable and unique position from which to encourage wholesome attitudes of child rearing during each contact with the family. Concomitantly they can detect unwholesome attitudes and disturbances early in a child's life and endeavor to provide a more favorable setting for the child through interviews and counseling with the parents. In situations of severe distress, the pediatrician may decide that more extensive psychological treatment through psychotherapy or other means is needed and make a referral for psychiatric consultation. But fundamentally, he or she remains the key professional who evaluates comprehensively the overall health of the child, including the child's mental health, while serving as the central person in the parents' eyes for counseling and guidance.

REFERENCES

1. Beardslee WR: The role of self-understanding in resilient individuals: the development of a perspective, *Am J Orthopsychiatry* 59:266, 1989.
2. Carnegie Task Force: *Starting points: meeting the needs of our youngest children: the report of the Carnegie Task Force on meeting the needs of our youngest children,* New York, 1994, Carnegie Corporation of New York.
3. Erikson EH: *Childhood and society,* ed 2, New York, 1963, WW Norton.
4. Kohlberg L: *Stage and sequence: the cognitive-developmental approach to socialization.* In Goslin D, editor: *Handbook of socialization theory and research,* Chicago, 1969, Rand McNally.
5. Mrazek PJ, Haggerty RJ, eds: *Reducing risks for mental disorders: frontiers for preventive intervention research,* Report of the Committee on Prevention of Mental Disorders, Division of Biobehavioral Sciences and Mental Disorders, Institute of Medicine, Washington, DC, 1994, National Academy Press.
6. Piaget J: *The origins of intelligence in children,* New York, 1963, WW Norton.
7. Richmond JB, Beardslee WR: Resiliency: research and practical implications for pediatricians, *J Dev Behav Pediatr* 9:157, 1988.
8. Rutter M: Meyerian psychobiology, personality development, and the role of life experiences, *Am J Psychiatry* 143:1077, 1986.
9. Selman RL, Schultz LH: *Making a friend in youth: developmental theory and pair therapy,* Chicago, 1990, The University of Chicago Press.
10. Skinner BF: *Science and human behavior,* New York, 1953, Macmillan.
11. Thomas A, Chess S, Birch H: *Temperament and behavior disorders in children,* New York, 1968, New York University Press.

SUGGESTED READINGS

Richmond JB: Child development: a basic science for pediatrics, *Pediatrics* 39:649, 1967.

Richmond JB: An idea whose time has arrived, *Pediatr Clin North Am* 22:517, 1975.

53 Foster Care and Adoption

Mark D. Simms

Foster home care and adoption are two means of providing care for children who, for many different reasons, cannot remain in their parents' custody. Foster care is intended to be temporary, until the child can return to the family of origin; adoption is the permanent joining of a child with a new family unit. Both foster care and adoption reflect society's social, political, and moral values, and both fields are undergoing great change.

During the past 2 decades new types of fostering and adoptive arrangements for children have emerged, and every pediatrician probably will care for children who are in foster care or who have been adopted. This chapter will familiarize readers with the structure and organization of these systems, common problems encountered, and current issues and trends in these related fields. In-depth discussion of many controversial or complex aspects of these topics can be found in the excellent reviews and references supplied at the end of this chapter.

FOSTER CARE

From the Middle Ages through the American colonial period, poor and dependent children often were indentured or placed in public institutions. By the mid-nineteenth century the unique needs of children began to be recognized, and, as the twentieth century began, social policies were created to protect children from abuse and exploitation and to provide state-supported foster family care for those who could not live with their parents. During the period of economic growth following the Second World War, the number of children placed in foster care declined. However, in the 1960s increased recognition of child abuse led to dramatic growth in the number of children placed in foster care. Because the child welfare system was not prepared to meet the needs of growing numbers of children and their parents, many children remained in "temporary" placements for much of their childhood. Reform focused on finding permanent families for children.

In 1980 Congress passed the Adoption Assistance and Child Welfare Reform Act (PL 96-272), which mandates agencies to prevent unnecessary placement whenever possible, to track children while they are in state custody, and to move them expeditiously through the foster care system toward a permanent setting. However, record numbers of children entered the foster care system during the mid-1980s, a development attributable in part to inadequate federal funding for social programs and preventive family services and the combined social epidemics of crack cocaine abuse, HIV infection, and homelessness. In just 5 years, from 1986 to 1991, the number of children in placement increased by 53% to 429,000. At the end of fiscal year 1993, the most recent date for which reported data exist at this writing, 445,000 children were residing in foster homes in the United States.[9] Based on current trends it is estimated that this number will surpass 600,000 children at some point during 1995.[8] Yet, over the past decade, as the number of two-parent working families increased, the numbers of families willing to serve as foster parents has declined steadily. For practical and philosophical reasons, therefore, child welfare policy is shifting toward increased efforts to prevent unnecessary placement and to recruit extended family members to care for children in what are called "kinship care homes."

How Children Enter Foster Care

All states have statutes protecting children under 18 years old from physical, sexual, and mental injury and from abandonment and neglect by parents or caretakers. State child protection service agencies are authorized to remove children from their parents' care and to place them in state custody if they are thought to be at great risk of harm. In all cases placement must be sanctioned by court order within a 10-day period. By law a child cannot be committed to state custody for more than 18 months without further court review. Frequently, state agencies seek to avoid the traumas arising from involuntary placement by attempting to persuade parents to place their children in foster care voluntarily. Under this arrangement parents may revoke the placement at anytime; however, if the parents fail to cooperate with the plan for reunification, the agency may pursue court-ordered commitment.

Foster Parents

Foster parents are the cornerstones in the foster care system because they provide all the immediate care and largely determine childrens' experience in placement. A diverse group, foster parents often are middle-aged individuals who have stable marriages and older children. They are fairly representative of the general population in many respects, although their incomes are skewed toward the lower range. The majority own their own homes and move less often than the average American family. Many foster parents were raised in large families. Individuals who engage in "fostering" frequently have had contact with other foster or adoptive parents. Foster parents are paid a monthly board rate to care for and support children in their homes. However, in many areas these payments do not cover the costs of raising a child, as estimated by U.S. Department of Agriculture; additional expenses for transportation, recreation, respite, and clothing often are not covered.

Biological Parents

Parents of children who enter placement often live in poor, inner-city neighborhoods. A majority are single parents whose incomes are below the poverty line; a disproportionate number are minority group members. Many grew up in impoverished and chaotic families, and as many as one third lived in foster homes at some time during childhood. They suffer from high rates of emotional and physical illnesses, which often contribute to their inability to care for their children. Many such families are known to protective service agencies, the police, or the courts for extended periods before their children are placed.

Children in Foster Care

The vast majority of children in foster care have experienced some degree of neglect or abuse before placement. Approximately 10% are placed because a serious behavioral problem or disability has overwhelmed their parents' ability to care for them. Since the mid-1980s, especially in large urban areas, increasing numbers of infants and young children have been placed because of parental drug addiction and homelessness. At the time of placement more than 50% of the children are developmentally delayed in one or more domains of functioning, most of the older children are achieving one or more grades below age level, and nearly one in three suffers from a chronic medical condition. Nearly all children manifest some behavioral and emotional stress reaction as a result of their removal from their families. In addition, more than 50% suffer from significant underlying emotional disturbances, most often related to experiences and events that occurred before placement. Frequently these involve depression, an attachment disorder, an eating disturbance, and antisocial or aggressive behavior. Unfortunately, very few children receive comprehensive psychosocial, medical, mental health, or educational evaluations during placement, and, because there is little coordination between health, mental health, and social service systems, many children in need of special services fail to receive appropriate help. Furthermore there usually are no formal programs to screen and evaluate children for these problems and to formulate a management plan as they enter care or after they have been placed.

Visits with Parents

Because foster care is intended as a temporary measure for children and families in crisis, maintaining the parent-child relationship through regular visits is extremely important. Indeed, visiting patterns are the strongest predictor of whether a child eventually will return home. Paradoxically, however, visiting with parents often is very stressful for children in foster care; when children react strongly to visits with their parents, it often is not immediately clear whether their best interests are served by continuing or suspending these contacts.

Role of the Pediatrician

In recent years the Child Welfare League of America[6] and the American Academy of Pediatrics[1] have emphasized the importance of integrating health and social service systems for children. Child welfare agencies also are turning to pediatricians increasingly to help in program and policy development.

Pediatricians can play a crucial role in helping child welfare agencies, foster parents, and biological families while children are in out-of-home placement. Caring for these children takes considerably more time than usual, and physicians must be prepared to be primary care providers even when little or no information is available during the initial health visit. Whenever possible, biological parents should participate in the care of their children's health during placement. Current efforts are under way to develop health information systems in the form of paper-based or electronic medical "passports" to ensure continuity of health care, even when children change foster homes or physicians.

All children should receive an initial physical examination before or soon after placement so that acute medical conditions can be identified and foster parents given information to enable them to care properly for the children placed in their home. Within 1 month of a child's placement, and at regular intervals while in foster care, he or she should receive comprehensive multidisciplinary medical, developmental, mental health, and educational evaluations so that therapeutic needs and specific interventions can be recommended and progress monitored. The results of these evaluations should be incorporated into the child's social service case records and become an integral part of the case plan.

Impact of Placement on Children

For a significant minority of these children, a projected brief, temporary placement may extend over many months or years as the agency or courts struggle to support the biological family in the hope that the children may be returned to them. During this time the children may change foster homes several times and experience the stress of prolonged separation and the lack of a predictable future. Inadequate attention to their physical, emotional, and educational needs may compound preexisting disturbances. Yet, for children who have suffered significant abuse or neglect or whose families cannot care for them adequately, foster care potentially provides an opportunity for appropriate intervention and rehabilitation. Despite the psychosocial stresses inherent in separating children from their families, evidence is convincing that when services are made available, many children show improvement in physical development, health status, intellectual ability, and school performance and experience decreased emotional and behavioral problems during placement. Pediatricians, through their own efforts and advocacy, can help these children significantly by ensuring that their needs are identified and appropriately addressed by all involved in their care.

ADOPTION

In ancient times legal adoption frequently was a means for adults to consolidate wealth and power or provide continuity for a family line. On the other hand, informal arrangements to raise orphaned or dependent children always have been very common. In the United States, along with other reforms in child welfare in the latter half of the nineteenth century, individual states passed laws to regulate adoptions. It was not until the beginning of this century, when advances in nutrition and health care improved survival rates of infants separated from their mothers, that the adoption of young children became feasible.

Currently an estimated 1 million children in the United States live with adoptive parents, and between 2% and 4% of American families have adopted children. Although data on adoption are not now collected systematically by the government, several private sources provide estimates from which trends are followed. Based on data gathered from state social service agencies, bureaus of vital records, and state court administrative offices, the Adoption Information Improvement Project estimates that 118,559 children were adopted in the United States in 1990. Approximately 50% of these adoptions were by related individuals, most often stepfathers. Of those adopted by unrelated adults, 16% were children brought to the United States from other countries and 26% were categorized as having "special needs" because of a developmental disability, serious health impairment, emotional disturbance, being of a minority or mixed race, being older (greater than 6 years of age), or because of their sibling group status in which two, three, or more children from the same family require placement. Furthermore the Voluntary Cooperative Information System estimated that nearly 19,000 children moved from foster homes into adoptive homes in 1988. Approximately 40% of these were adopted by people unrelated to them, an additional 37% were adopted by unrelated former foster parents, and 13% were adopted by relatives.

Adoption practice is changing significantly. Efforts have been increased to recruit families for children waiting for adoption. A wider range of postadoption services are becoming available to support adoptive families and to help adopted adults deal with their adoption experience, including in some instances assistance in searching for their birth family. Thus adoption, which was once regarded as a simple solution to an immediate problem at the time of the infant's birth, now is recognized as a lifelong process for all members of the adoption triad: adoptee, adoptive parents, and birth parents.

Adoptive Parents

In 1988 the National Survey of Family Growth[3] found that of the more than 2 million women 15 through 44 years of age who had ever contacted an agency or lawyer about adoption, only 620,000 (31%) successfully had adopted and 204,000 (10%) currently were seeking children. Although many are infertile married couples in their twenties and thirties, the number of older and single adoptive parents has increased in recent years. Approximately 40% of adoptive placements of unrelated children are made through public agencies, 30% by private agencies, and 30% by independent arrangements.

Infant Adoption

Approximately 50% of the children adopted by unrelated adults are less than 2 years old at the time of placement. Most have little or no memory of their lives or relationships before adoption. It is important for adoptive parents to recognize and acknowledge the uniqueness of their family's origin throughout the child's developing years. Introduction of the terms "adoption" and "adopted" should occur early and in a matter-of-fact manner because discovery or disclosure of adoption information when the child is older may lead to mistrust and anger. As the children enter latency and become more aware of the meaning of adoption, they may feel grief over the loss of their birth parents. They are likely to be curious about the conditions under which the adoption took place, and some adopted adolescents or young adopted adults may want to search for their birth parents. This usually suggests healthy emotional development and should not be viewed as a sign of rejecting the adoptive parents or their values.[2] If such curiosity is not expressed by the adopted child, parents need to take the initiative in offering information about the child's adoption and assuring the child that it is normal to be curious. Laws regarding confidentiality of adoption records have been modified during the past 2 decades, and many states have established mutual consent registries to help adoptees and birth parents who wish to establish contact after the child has reached the age of majority. Anecdotal evidence suggests that over the long run the adoptees' adjustment may be improved because of these efforts, whatever their outcome. However, the child, the birth parents, and the adoptive parents may need support and assistance during this process.

Independent Adoption

As the availability of healthy infants has decreased in recent years, many couples have turned to private attorneys in attempts to avoid long waiting periods and seemingly arbitrary standards associated with agency adoptions. Such proceedings are made possible when a birth mother chooses to have her child's adoption arranged by an independent attorney rather than an agency. In this process her role in the choice of adoptive parents and the terms and conditions of the adoption is increased.

Open Adoption

An increasingly common term and arrangement is "open adoption," which involves a variable but mutually agreed upon degree of contact between adoptive parents, birth parents, and child before and, in most cases, after placement. Research on the impact of such arrangements is limited to descriptions of the experiences of adoptive and birth parents. Very little actually is known about open adoption's long-term consequences on family relationships or the psychological adjustment of the children adopted.

International Adoption

Adoption of children from abroad has been the subject of much controversy. In many ways a more complicated and expensive route to adoption, international adoption provides an alternative for families to fulfill their desire to raise children. For many years a small number of countries have supplied the vast majority of the children brought to the United States. However, in many countries the internal political climate may fluctuate over time, and previously "open" countries may "close" to foreign adoption without warning. Countries also "close" because of periodic scandals or perceived abuses of international adoption.

It is helpful for the physicians who care for children adopted from abroad to appreciate the long and complex path their parents have taken and to be sensitive to their feelings and anxieties. This should be combined with a thorough understanding of any medical problems the children may have when they arrive. Excellent guidelines exist to assist physicians in caring for newly arrived adopted children.[2,7] Although the prevalence of particular infections varies according to the country of origin, a baseline set of screening tests is recommended, including the following: a hepatitis B profile, a Mantoux test with *Candida* control for tuberculosis, tests for fecal ova and parasites, a complete blood count with red cell indices for hemoglobinopathy, a urine culture for cytomegalovirus, a syphilis serology, and HIV testing, as well as physical, developmental, and sensory examinations. In addition, immunization status should be reviewed and updated.

Transracial Adoption

Transracial adoption, primarily of African-American, Hispanic, and Native American children by Caucasian families, was common from the 1960s until the mid-1970s, when a group raised strong opposition to stop this practice. The National Association of Black Social Workers (NABSW) voiced concern that children raised in a cross-racial setting would fail to learn social skills necessary to survive in a "racist" society and would be cut off from their cultural heritage.[5] Under the pressure of disproportionate numbers of African-American and mixed-race children in the foster care system awaiting adoptive placements, public and private agencies have increased their efforts to identify and support same-race adoptive homes in preference to transracial placement. While the NABSW continues to support this position, there is little empirical evidence to support their concerns or conclusions, and children whose adoptive parents are of another race generally do as well as other adopted children. Moreover, U.S. civil rights law prohibits policies that tie adoption to same-race placements; nevertheless there are relatively few transracial placements of American-born children today. With the passage of the Indian Child Welfare Act in 1978, responsibility for Native American child custody matters was put under the jurisdiction of the child's tribe, significantly reducing mixed-race placements for this population.

Adoption of Children with Special Needs

Because of increasing numbers of children entering the foster care system and the strong emphasis on family preservation and reunification of children with their families of origin, children eligible for adoption tend to be older and in out-of-home placement for considerable periods. As previously noted, many of these children are significantly disabled medically and psychologically, and a disproportionate number belong to minority or sibling groups. Experience has shown that adoptive placement is possible for virtually any child and that no child should be considered "unadoptable." Although disruption rates (i.e., termination of placement before finalization) for children having special needs generally are higher than those of healthy infants, the vast majority do well. Furthermore even one or more disrupted placements do not appear to preclude the chances of a successful adoption. The strongest factor associated with increased risk for disruption is an emotional or behavioral problem, especially in boys placed at an older age. Other factors include lack of extended family supports for the adopting family, noninvolvement by the adoptive father, and single-parent adoption. Not surprisingly children adopted during adolescence are at especially high risk for disruption (10% to 24%). On the other hand, children who have serious medical and developmental problems and transracially adopted children are not at increased risk for disruption. It is ironic that those adults whom agencies generally consider "least desirable" for adopting infants because of low income and education or minority or single-parent status frequently are the most successful in adopting children who have "special needs."

Pediatric Roles in the Adoption Process

Pediatricians can play valuable roles at each stage of the adoption process. By reviewing existing medical and genetic information accompanying the child and performing a comprehensive physical and developmental examination, physicians can help adoptive parents understand the potential significance of any factors that may place the child at risk for immediate or future problems. During the initial adjustment period after placement of a child with his or her adoptive family, the pediatrician can provide the family with information about the child's medical needs, help the parents understand behavioral problems, and suggest ways to help the child settle into the adoptive family. After the adoption has been finalized, the pediatrician should remain a close support to the family by providing expert advice and guidance and, when necessary, referring appropriate community resources for assistance.

Outcomes for Adopted Children

For the overwhelming majority of children and families involved, adoption is beneficial. It is remarkable that despite many children's unfavorable early experiences, the love, nurture, and support they receive from their adoptive families have a strong, ameliorative effect.[4] Although adopted children are more likely to suffer from certain types of emotional distress and often are overrepresented in mental health settings, as adults they are as well adjusted as nonadopted individuals. Thus the simple fact of being adopted rarely is, by itself, the principal cause of dysfunction. Similarly there is little research to support concerns that transracially or internationally adopted children may have identity crises as a result of growing up in mixed ethnic and cultural family settings. On the contrary, considerable anecdotal experience continues to support these placements. It is important for pediatricians to understand the problems and appreciate the benefits of adoption and to be supportive to children and families at each stage in the adoption process.

REFERENCES

1. American Academy of Pediatrics, Committee on Early Childhood, Adoption and Dependent Care: Health care of children in foster care, *Pediatrics* 93:335, 1994.
2. American Academy of Pediatrics, Committee on Early Childhood, Adoption and Dependent Care: Families and adoption: the pediatrician's role in supporting communication, *Am Acad Pediatr News* Feb 21, 1992.
3. Bachrach CA, London KA, Maza PL: On the path to adoption: adoption seeking in the United States, 1988, *J Marriage Fam* 53:705, 1991.
4. Bohman M, Sigvardsson S: Outcome in adoption: lessons from longitudinal studies. In Brodzinsky DM, Schechter MD, editors: *The psychology of adoption,* New York, 1990, Oxford University Press.
5. Chestang L: The dilemma of biracial adoption, *Soc Work* 17:100, 1972.
6. Child Welfare League of America: *Standards for health care services for children in out-of-home care,* Washington, DC, 1988, Child Welfare League of America.
7. Hostetter MK et al: Medical evaluation of internationally adopted children, *N Engl J Med* 325:479, 1991.
8. Select Committee on Children, Youth and Families: *No place to call home: discarded children in America,* Washington, DC, 1989, US Government Printing Office.

9. Tatara T: US child substitute care flow data for FY 1993 and trends in the state child substitute care populations. Voluntary Cooperative Information Service (VCIS) Research Notes 11 (August) 1995, Washington, DC, American Public Welfare Association.

SUGGESTED READINGS

Behrman RE, editor: *Adoption: the future of children,* ed 1, vol 3, Center for the Future of Children, Los Altos, Calif, 1993, David and Lucille Packard Foundations.

Brodzinsky DM, Schechter MD, editors: *The psychology of adoption,* New York, 1990, Oxford University Press.

Simms MD: Foster children and the foster care system. I. History and legal structure, *Curr Probl Pediatr* 21:297, 1991.

Simms MD: Foster children and the foster care system. II. Impact on the child, *Curr Probl Ped* 21:345, 1991.

54 Changing American Families

Shirley A. Smoyak

Pediatrics is best practiced with a solid groundwork in the family, which includes its biological, cultural, socioeconomic, and demographic dimensions. The family contexts in which infants, children, and adolescents are raised set the patterns for response to illness and the expectations of caregivers. Families' beliefs about health and illness—what is preventable, what is treatable, what is natural, what is good, and what is to be avoided—are communicated to upcoming generations both subtly and directly.

Scientists who attempt to study the family are faced with a peculiar dilemma. Something familiar to all of us growing up in a family somehow eludes the grasp of the scientific method. Because most of us have experienced childhood and adolescence in a family setting, and because most of us as adults create families of our own, the temptation is great to view our experiences as normal and to use them as a standard for understanding others. This ethnocentric tendency leads to assumptions that the familiar must be the correct or better way and that other styles or patterns at best are strange and at worst are wrong or deviant. The "family" is an elusive concept; its shape, character, and functions have been interpreted differently by historians, sociologists, psychologists, and anthropologists.

Privacy about matters of family life has produced what sociologists call *pluralistic ignorance*. Each of us knows what goes on in our own bedrooms and bathrooms and how we handle a sassy 2-year-old at bedtime or an adolescent who comes home drunk or smelling of pot, but we really do not know how the neighbors do it. Systematic, rigorous research on the intimacies of family life is in its infancy, although the study of marriage and the family can be traced back several centuries.

Despite the less-than-adequate funding for research on the family, the literature has grown voluminously. Today there are nearly two dozen professional journals that deal with the family, some specializing in theory and research, some on family issues and policy matters, and many on clinical and therapeutic concerns. Family agendas are addressed at conferences convened by prominent professional associations in the major social science disciplines, and the field is not lacking in newsletters, monographs, audiotapes and videotapes, and books.

Research on the family conducted at the Rand Corporation, spanning more than a decade, now is available in a readable report, entitled *New Families, No Families? The Transformation of the American Home*.[4] This report has provided one of the most complete analyses of how families have responded to social change by creating new rules and structures for family and nonfamily living.

This chapter provides an overview of changing patterns of family structure and the associated changes in functions. It attempts to explode some cherished myths about "the American family" and to provide clinicians who treat sick, injured, or well children a more realistic understanding about families. In this chapter a family will be viewed as a married couple or other group of adult kinsfolk who cooperate economically and psychosocially in bringing up children and who share a common dwelling.

FAMILY ORIGINS

According to Gough,[6] "The trouble with the origin of the family is that no one knows." She provides evidence that it is not known *when* the human family originated (probably between 2 million and 10,000 years ago) or whether some kind of embryonic family came before, with, or after the origin of language. Although varying significantly in structure and function, some kind of family exists in all known human societies. "Family" implies several universals: (1) that sexual relations between close relatives are forbidden, (2) that men and women cooperate through a division of labor based on gender, and (3) that marriage is a durable although not necessarily lifelong arrangement. Another universal, that men in general have higher status and authority than the women in their families, has generated much controversy between feminist scholars and other historians. Although feminist writers persuasively have demonstrated the long-standing, erroneous bias of earlier male "scholars," they disagree among themselves about the exact nature of past relationships among men and women in families.

The exact nature of family structure and gender relationships is shrouded in many layers of conjecture and scientific guesswork. Since the beginning of recorded history, no fixed pattern across cultures has been found.[7] Culture, not biology, determines the rules of organization within families. In most primitive, nomadic, communal societies, family descent was traced through the mothers, possibly because maternity could be verified, whereas paternity often was a mystery. Roughly 5000 years ago, when the development of agriculture so drastically changed how people lived and organized themselves, patrilineal groups emerged. As the concept of private property developed, the transfer of such property from father to son influenced not only economic but also social patterns.

Historians of the family, notably Aries,[2] have taught us that much of what we take as familiar and commonplace is a relatively recent invention. Childhood as a concept to us is real; Aries maintains that it did not exist as an idea before the Middle Ages. In medieval days, as soon as a child could live without the constant attention of its mother, he or she was accorded adult status. According to Sagan, no institution has been changed so remarkably by modernization as has the family. Until the late eighteenth century, families were primarily economic units.[12] Marriages were arranged for the purpose of preserving property, and children were a cheap source of labor or a hedge against poverty in old age.

Historically all the work necessary for safety and survival was done within family units. Within the boundaries of the family, functions performed were educating the young, ensuring safety from invaders, praying to God or a superior being, providing nurturance, clothing, and shelter, and caring for the sick, infirm, young, or disabled. Every family textbook includes a discussion of the "erosion of family functions," and it has been popular from time to time to predict the eventual demise of the family as we know it because all the reasons for its existence have been reassigned to institutions outside the family, such as schools, hospitals, welfare boards, and churches.

There actually have been several experiments in alternative forms of living in human groups, but none has survived. Although there is no general societal law that people must live in families, most do. Historical perspectives help in understanding social contexts and institutions. Present patterns, when the observer can see their roots, make more sense. More important, such understanding eliminates or dampens the tendency toward emotionality over issues of intimacy, closeness, and human relationships. Perceptions of American family life are full of myths, such as the belief that a three-generational household is and was the norm. Such beliefs generate a false nostalgia—a longing for what never was. In popularizing a picture of the American family as three generations in one household, Norman Rockwell actually did a disservice to the American public—there had never been a time when three generations living in one household was typical. Given the short life span (an expected 49 years at the turn of the century), most parents could not have expected to live with their grandchildren. Although the three-generation family of the past largely was mythical, today more grandparents are alive than ever before.

For the first time in history families may have four or five generations alive. Children today may have not only living grandparents, but also great-grandparents and perhaps great-great grandparents. This increased longevity poses problems for families that they have never faced before.[12] On a simple level there is the question of what the "layers" of grandparents should be called by their grandchildren. On a more complex level, great economic and psychosocial concern faces middle-aged persons who see their retirement years not as golden but as burdened by financial and social support of several elder generations.

There are two major reasons for the difficulty in tracing accurate patterns and structures for families. First, upper-class or high-status families were grossly overrepresented in the literature. Second, until about the last 60 years writers tended to describe families as they *should* be, rather than as they really were. This led to what Goode has so aptly labeled "the classical extended family of Western nostalgia."[5] For instance, some accounts of colonial families in America are so steeped in nostalgia that the reader concludes that those times were not so rough at all and that if they were, the close, warm family ties healed all wounds.

Families have turned over many of their previous functions, already noted, to institutions, organizations, and professionals outside the family, but they have maintained the functions of childbearing, primary socialization of children, and psychosocial validation or "refueling" for all their members. This last function, the provision of psychosocial verification, worth, and meaning, probably is the most important. Standards for its performance have increased tremendously in recent years, with the popular press reporting all types of help available to meet increased expectations, from individual psychotherapy and counseling to retreats and renewals, self-help books and groups, and high-priced encounters with marriage and family specialists. At the turn of this century the only interpersonal, behavioral requirement between husbands and wives was that they be civil to one another. The new requirement is that they love one another and continue to express this love unfailingly, even into their elder years. An associated new requirement is for increased intimacy through sexuality. Since those who marry for economic purposes have few reasons to terminate marriage, the current high rate of divorce is an indication that marriage as an economic arrangement is definitely a thing of the past.

The high divorce rates in the United State have been viewed by some as symptomatic of an erosion of the American family and its associated value systems. An alternative view, however, is to interpret these statistics as indicating that Americans today place a higher value on forming *successful* marriages than did earlier generations. The new requirement that marital partners "love each other" carries with it the expectation that irreconcilable differences can be settled by divorce. The consequences of divorce for children is a separate issue and will be discussed later.

"THE AMERICAN FAMILY"

Everyone (even non-Americans) knows what the stereotypical American family is. It is thought to be a white, middle-class mother and father living together in a suburban home with their boy child and girl child (and an optional third child of either sex). The father leaves for work daily and is successful in his career; the mother transforms the house into a home and is not expected to work full time until the last child is in school.

Although this stereotype is changing rapidly, to a great extent it is still thought to be true, even among minorities or those who live in dual-career families or single-parent families. The stereotype excludes more than half the population in the United States today. It is a tribute to American advertising to realize how pervasive this "ideal type" of picture is despite the fact that census data provide contradictory evidence.

The old notions of family life span are dysfunctional, considering so many families today change their structures repeatedly by marriage, divorce, and remarriage, interspersed with varying lengths of time alone or as single parents. For instance, in the first half of this century the sequence described was courtship, marriage, childbearing and rearing, "empty nest," retirement, and death of one or both spouses. Today there are many departures from this sequence. Among alternative family forms are unmarried couples living together (with or without children); homosexual couples (with or without children); deliberately childless couples, married or not; single-parent families with either a father or a mother as the parent; middle-aged couples whose divorced adult children return home with their young children; middle-aged couples living in very crowded situations because of the former pattern, and in addition, with their elderly parent or parents living with them; various types of blended families created by divorced or widowed parents remarrying; and group families, in which several unrelated families share a large space. Within each of these varied structures the rules of organization for carrying out the chores of daily living differ widely.

Marriage, divorce, widowhood, remarriage, and childbearing patterns have changed dramatically since the 1950s and have altered the size and composition of the American family radically. According to Ahlburg and DeVita,[1] "Family patterns are so fluid that the U.S. Census Bureau has difficulty measuring family trends. Most large-scale, nationally representative surveys cannot tell us readily what proportion of husband-wife families are stepfamilies or how adopted or foster-care children are faring; distinguish roommates from couples who are living together as unmarried partners; or measure the extent of family support networks for elderly persons who live alone." Families today often have two or fewer children. Mothers are likely to be employed outside the home, even when children are under 6 years of age. Young people are marrying at older ages. Men and women alike continue to delay marriage, with the median age at first marriage rising in 1993 to 26.5 years for men and 24.5 years for women.[11] Many people even are exercising the option of never marrying. Although marriage is less permanent today (the number of people divorced rose to 16.7 million in 1993 from 4.3 million in 1970), it still is highly likely that marriage will be part of the future for better than 90% of Americans. A very drastic recent trend is that more births are occurring outside of marriage and that more children are being raised in single-parent homes.

For pediatricians the relevance of these different arrangements is that children being raised within them experience very different levels of support and nurturance and are socialized to value, challenge, or to reject them.

One trend in American families of which most physicians certainly are aware is that families are smaller than they were just a decade ago. They may not be aware, however, that the number of children in families is related to the family's general physical and mental health. The obvious inverse correlation of the more children, the fewer the resources for each reveals some surprises when social class is added. Infant and childhood mortality rates fell for both upper and lower classes when fewer children were born into the families. Young children of large families continue to have more infections, more accidents, and higher overall mortality than do the children of small families, regardless of social class.[12] An only child in a poor family has about the same chance of surviving the first year of life as a child who is born into a professional family but who has four or more siblings. Small families, however, are more prone to violence. One possibility for the increased likelihood of violence in small families is that fewer resources are available when a crisis occurs. For instance, if a single mother of two children younger than 5 years old becomes ill, she is likely to be less tolerant of noise or even simple demands of the children. If they do not sleep, or even if they remain relatively quiet when she is trying to rest, they are more likely to be hit or punished. Divorced fathers, trying to make every moment of their visits count, often lose their tempers and end up verbally or physically abusing their children. Spouse abuse also is more common in smaller than in larger families.

CHANGING FAMILY STRUCTURES AND FUNCTIONS

Although the myth of the American family as a married couple with two or more children, the father as breadwinner, and the mother as homemaker, remains an ideal type in popular media, the demographic reality is that in 1991 just over one third of all families (37%) consisted of a married couple with children, regardless of the number of children or the employment status of the wife; only 20% of married couples fits the popular stereotype.[1]

The Census Bureau distinguishes between a "household" and a "family." Households consist of units occupied by persons. A household may consist of one person living alone or several people sharing the dwelling. A family is two or more persons related by birth, marriage, or adoption who reside together. Relatives who may be involved with the family very integrally, but who do not share the dwelling, are not counted. Although 70% of U.S. households contain a family unit, family composition is quite diverse. Families include married couples with and without children, single-parent families headed by a woman or a man, siblings living together, and many other arrangements. Just under half of all families have children, but their structures, the number of generations, and the number of people in each generation varies considerably.

Married couples that have children (including the whole array of arrangements, such as biological and adopted children and stepfamilies) continue to be a prominent family pattern. Most married-couple families that have children are intact biological families (77% in 1985, the last available estimate), but 19% had one or more stepchildren and 2% had one or more adopted children.[1] Although over 80% of stepfamilies are Caucasian, the odds of being in a stepfamily are double for African-Americans. Demographer Paul Glick estimates that a third of all Americans are stepparents, stepchildren, stepsiblings, or some other member of a stepfamily. If current trends continue, the share will rise to nearly half by the year 2000.[9]

Single-parent families have doubled since 1970; in 1991 nearly one in eight families was headed by a single parent. Women are five times more likely to be the single parent than men, and African-Americans are almost three times more likely than Caucasians to be single parents. Single parents rearing children head one in five Caucasian families, one in three Hispanic families, and six in ten African-American families. The rise in births to unmarried women has contributed to the growth of single-parent families. The Census Bureau[11] reported in July 1994 that births to unwed women soared by more than 70% from 1983 to 1993. According to the Bureau, in 1993 6.3 million children, or 27% of all children under the age of 18, lived with a single parent who had never married—up from 3.7 million in 1983. In 1960 only 243,000 children lived with one parent who had never married. Minority children are more likely to live in those families; 57% of African-American children are living with one parent who never married, compared with 21% of Caucasian children and 32% of Hispanic children. About half of America's children will spend some time in a one-parent family, mostly as a consequence of divorce.

One quarter of homeless individuals are in family units. Of these, 60% are children, 32% are their parents (overwhelmingly single mothers), and 8% are couples that have no children.

Another new pattern is the increasing involvement of grandparents in childrearing. Adult children, both divorced and married, when faced with tough economic times are doubling up households by returning to their parents' homes. This trend is more likely in minority families. In 28% of households grandparents become the sole caretakers of the children, with neither parent present.[13]

In past generations pediatricians were surprised if anyone other than the child's mother brought the child for visits to the office or was the caretaker during minor and major crises. Today pediatricians encounter grandmothers, grandfathers, fathers, and even babysitters in increasing numbers. Pediatricians used to dealing with mothers face the challenge of adjusting their psychosocial style as they encounter men as caretakers.

Although contraception has been available to teens, the increase in birth rates among women under 20 is rising steadily. In 1970 there were 21 births per 1000 unmarried teenagers; by 1993 this rate had doubled. However, teenagers account for less than a third of all unmarried mothers, African-American teenagers for less than 12%. Out-of-wedlock childbearing has risen fastest among women 20 and older. Furthermore, married women are having fewer children, thus inflating the share of out-of-wedlock births.

Working mothers are creating pressures for social change both inside and outside the family. The willingness of men to adjust their priorities and to shift energies from work to family is critical for producing the expected "home as haven." Their unwillingness to change in the direction of more family involvement often produces stress, even chaos, for their wives and children. Goldscheider and Waite[3] have analyzed the effects of fathers' changing roles and functions as breadwinners and homemakers. In 1991 58% of mothers who had children under 6 years were employed full time. In 1960 the figure was 20%. By 1995 a projected two thirds of preschool children and three fourths of school-aged children will have mothers working outside the home.[7]

DISTINGUISHING NORMAL FROM ABNORMAL FAMILIES

Clinical theory about dysfunctional families has not kept pace with the dramatic changes that have occurred in family structures and associated functions and ways of living. As Walsh[15] points out, "Most clinical theory explicitly or implicitly upholds the ideal model of the family as intact, with father as primary wage-earner and instrumental leader and mother as primary parent, homemaker, and socioemotional caretaker." However, fewer than 20% of American families fit this pattern. Still, deviation from this standard is regarded in much of the literature as unquestionably pathogenic. Current textbooks used in clinical training virtually ignore alternative arrangements as possibly being more normative. Even when divorce or separation are acknowledged as occurring in half the marriages, the normal sequence of dissolution of ties, emotional upset, management of stress, and adaptations to community demands are not given appropriate consideration.

According to Walsh clinicians thus lack knowledge about what is and is not normal in family life.[15] She describes two types of errors frequently made: the first is to identify mistakenly as pathological a family pattern that is normal; the second is to assume normality because of failure to recognize a dysfunctional pattern. An example of the first error is the reaction of a clinician, reared in a family in which adults did not demonstrate affection openly and children were supposed to follow the directions of adults, who encounters a family that is noisy, affectionate, and open in expressions of joy and anguish. This clinician, seeing the solicitous concern of a mother for her child—to the point of her bringing homemade lasagna to her hospitalized child—might view this behavior as enmeshment or symbiosis instead of normal caring. Of course, clinicians do not always assume that what they experienced at home was normal. Some, instead, see their own upbringing as departing from normal and then apply this view to the families they see; when they encounter one like their own, they view it suspiciously and diagnose the behavior as pathological.

An example of this second error according to Walsh is acceptance of the myth that healthy families are free of conflict. Such a view would preclude the clinician from exploring further an assertion by a couple that they have not disagreed in 20 years of marriage. What is common also may be accepted as normal. For instance, noncustodial fathers are so frequently cut off from their children after a divorce that clinicians may fall into the trap of seeing this as normal and thus fail to explore ways that the father and his children might be together.

Pediatricians who feel uncomfortable about exploring the psychosocial aspects of their patients' families miss opportunities to suggest repairs and to help families rethink destructive relationships. Recent research demonstrates a positive association between continued supportive contact with the noncustodial parent and long-term adjustment of children. Such contact also affects the custodial mothers positively. Even when previous contact had negative consequences, continuing paternal detachment produces poorer functioning and more symptomatic behavior, especially in boys. Fathers who had negative relationships with their children before divorce have been able in many cases to develop improved relationships after divorce. Citing several long-term studies, Walsh[15] concludes that a clinical imperative in cases of nonparticipating parents is to assess and build the coparenting alliance in postdivorce families. The degree to which pediatricians feel comfortable in adding psychosocial exploration to their "history taking" or ongoing assessments of treatment depends on the messages they received from their mentors or subsequent attempts to change practice habits, which might come from colleagues or the families themselves. Some are reluctant to suggest that psychiatric consultation be sought, even when there is clear evidence of the need either in the child or in the parent. Some are reluctant to discuss behavior that is willful or that reflects a life-style rather than an illness. Drug and alcohol abuse are examples of problems that, even when noticed, are not mentioned by many clinicians.

Early research in family behavior tended to overrepresent Caucasian, Anglo-Saxon, Protestant, middle-class families.

Comparative studies have included the differences in structures and styles of relating among varied ethnic groups.[10] Other recent studies focus on alternative family forms, such as single-parent and blended family systems. Wallerstein[14] has contributed an insightful and clinically relevant study of the children of divorce, tracing the lives of families 5 to 10 years after breakup. An emergent theme is that no single pattern distinguishes well-functioning from pathological families. Something that looks like intrusiveness to a less-than-careful observer may simply be caring, expressed in a particular ethnic style. Also no single family structure is "healthier" than other arrangements. If the stresses and the available resources are more or less equivalent, children in single-parent families or children raised by a homosexual couple can do just as well as those in families having two biological parents.

Walsh[15] cautions that "too often, families with the same presenting problem are presumed to have a similar dysfunctional style, when research, albeit limited to date, reveals a good deal of diversity among families with similarly diagnosed members." Clinicians need to remind themselves that there is no one-to-one correspondence between symptom and system. In the past, rigid application of theories, unsubstantiated by adequate research, created additional strains for families who already were burdened by caring for a sick child. For instance, about 40 years ago, it was fairly popular to remove children who had asthma from their families as a therapeutic strategy; this was called a "parentectomy," the reasoning being that overinvolved, enmeshed, emotionality between parent (mostly mothers) and child precipitated asthma attacks. Just as there is no single pattern that demarcates a normal family clearly, families cannot be typed by the diagnosis of a family member, whether that is asthma or alcoholism or cancer. Keeping in mind that families are tremendously complex and that a wide array of variables is operative at any moment prevents jumping to faulty conclusions. A better stance is to form a tentative hypothesis and then engage the family in its mutual exploration.

CHANGING SOCIALIZATION NORMS

Generations ago parents simply bore and raised children, with almost no input from strangers and generally little, depending on ethnicity, from extended family members. Today there are specialists for every dimension of these functions, from how to be healthy in pregnancy to how to respond to an adolescent's bad manners. Americans generally are the greatest consumers of advice on children and health in the world. Depending on their social class and culture, parents choose different authorities to consult. The appropriate resource for parents' questions is determined very much by their social group, their level of education, and their general sense of assuredness about parenting. All of us, parents or not, tend to hear and believe what we *want* to hear and believe. Most parents measure the advice not against a standard of good research but rather against a more pragmatic one of whether the advice giver is trustworthy or has a track record of sensible prior advice.

Fifty years ago no profession identified as one of its functions how to teach parents to be parents. Parents were supposed to know how to be good parents either intuitively or because they learned it from growing up in large extended families. Today, advice, counseling, and teaching about parenting are considered part of the work of pediatricians, pediatric nurse practitioners, child study specialists, health educators, child psychologists, and behavior modifiers. Courses on effective parenting can be found in high school, college, and graduate school curricula, as well as on public television. Failure at socialization might be treated by an educational course or by a stay at a psychiatric hospital; some parents still see the military as a solution for offspring who fail to adopt parental values and norms. When a younger child behaves badly in the classroom or resists going to school entirely, the tendency now is to treat this as a "system" difficulty and to use a range of strategies to involve the parents in some type of parenting program. There even are programs for parents whose teenagers abuse drugs or alcohol and for other comparable sibling support groups.

Goldscheider and Waite[4] state that two revolutions currently face families. One revolution is under way inside families, where changes in sex roles, resulting in increased participation in the work force, are challenging traditional marital rules. Wives who work two jobs every day, one outside the home and one inside the home, resent the noninvolvement of their husbands in the tasks necessary to make a house a home. The second revolution is going on outside the family, where unmarried people now can experience the privacy, dignity, and authority (and some times the loneliness) of living in their own home. There now is a choice available, and some adults are choosing not to live within a family.

The first revolution is creating significant pressure to change the normative order between husbands and wives, with fathers being much more involved in homemaking and childrearing and mothers being more involved with careers and contributing economically to families. Changes in how family roles and rules are carried out, departing drastically from the traditional norms, produce "new families." The second revolution, where adults choose not to marry and instead to live independently away from families produces the alternative, or "no families." Although the outcomes are quite different, both revolutions have the same origin—our social priorities valuing the work place over the home. Men, while acknowledging the importance of families and the necessity to do family tasks to provide a comfortable environment, do not see themselves as the primary workers in this arena. Women increasingly spend more of their time and energy on issues in the work place rather than on family matters. These new directions are leading to a new generation of children who know less and less about what it takes to run a family, whether that includes inside tasks such as cleaning and meal preparations, or outside chores such as lawn-cutting or snow removal. The allocation of their energies mirrors that of their parents: they spend more time on school work, after-school activities, friends, and recreation than on domestic responsibilities.[3]

FAMILY TIES

Sagan[12] has suggested that the real reason we live longer is related directly to changes in how children are treated within families rather than to advances in medicine and science. It is well known that life expectancy has risen dramatically in most societies over the past few centuries. As noted earlier, as recently as 1900 the typical American lived only 49 years, and one child in five died in infancy. Today, the life expectancy for Americans is 75 years, and infant mortality has declined to less than 1 in every 100 births. Both physicians and the public credit modern medicine for these bold achievements, assuming almost reflexively that people who lack expert medical care die earlier and that providing more care is the key to longer life. Sagan's plea is that we look more carefully at these assumptions, which largely are unfounded. He provides compelling data for our rethinking of the assumptions we tend to make about the relationship between our efforts at health care on the one hand and our actual health on the other. He shows that although America spends more on health care than does any other nation in the world, in many respects Americans are not actually healthier. He does not deny that modern medicine has accomplished much that is of great value, such as alleviating suffering and developing useful surgical treatments for illnesses or trauma, but he shows clearly that neither saving individual lives nor alleviating suffering has contributed to overall life expectancy. Most therapy is not aimed directly at prolonging life, nor do the vast majority of missed physician's appointments endanger life. He reminds the reader that too often what physicians do is not necessary or is based on poor research or no research at all and that they prescribe too many medicines often without justification for their use.

Having described many compelling instances of how medicine has saved or improved individual lives, Sagan concludes that it has had little effect on the overall health of large populations.[12] What remains is a need for an explanation of why life expectancy has increased spectacularly during the nineteenth and twentieth centuries. There is no question that sanitation and nutrition, the other factors most often cited, have been beneficial. Neither of these, however, accounts fully for the leaps in longevity. Sagan attributes family ties as the key variable in longevity: "It is, in a word, impossible to trace the hardiness of modern people directly to improvements in medicine, sanitation, or diet. There is an alternative explanation for our increased life expectancy, however—one that has less to do with these developments than with changes in our psychological environment."[12] According to Sagan, growing up and living surrounded by scarcity and ignorance and constant loss is to endure a special misery—that which is a consequence of forces beyond one's control. By extension, a kind of personal powerlessness prevails, in which one's best efforts are not enough to ward off disaster. There is ample evidence that such a sense of helplessness often is associated with apathy, depression, and death—whether in laboratory animals or in prisoners of war. The reader is reminded of Martin Seligman's classic experiments with dogs, which resulted in the concept of learned helplessness as an explanation for why animals and human beings give up, endure pain, and die rather than act to prevent pain and death. People in poverty now share a feature of most premodern societies.

Modernization, with its associated community supports such as fire departments, building codes, social insurance, and emergency medical care, cushions most of us from physical, psychic, and economic disaster. These supports have created circumstances in which few of us feel utterly powerless or unable to take control over our lives. We generally feel like the masters of our own destinies, "and that, in itself, leaves us better equipped to fight off disease."[12]

Sagan directly connects the sources of such a sense of personal efficacy and self-esteem to the changed family. Until the late eighteenth century families primarily were economic units. Marriages were arranged for the purpose of preserving property, and children were cheap labor. Beating and whipping were commonplace, even among royalty, as approved tools to teach or extract conformity and obedience. Then during the Enlightenment the standards and goals of child rearing began to change. Philosophers argued, eloquently and at length, that if children were to survive in a disorderly and unpredictable world, they could not rely passively on traditional authority. They needed reasoned judgment. To develop such judgment children needed affection and guidance rather than harsh unreasoned discipline and brute force. Gradually, as these ideas took hold, childhood came to be recognized as a special stage of life.[2] Affection and nurturing replaced obligation and duty as the cohesive elements among family members.

Childhood mortality fell as a direct consequence of families having fewer children. Starting with the upper classes, families came to see that children had needs of their own and did not exist to serve the family. This revolutionary idea resulted in curtailing the numbers of births. Children were seen as individuals in their own right, to be paid attention to and nurtured rather than always to do for others. As lower classes also had fewer children, mortality fell among them as well. Family size is an excellent predictor of childhood survival, even today. Children in small families are strengthened by the extra nurturance and resources available to them; several studies of infants in institutions during World War II and after demonstrated that infants who receive only physical care do not survive.

The new field of psychoneuroimmunology is pursuing the connections between emotional and physical health. Whatever the mechanism that produces greater physical health during periods of emotional well-being needs to be understood. Affection and security may be thought of as natural vaccines. Children who receive consistent love and attention—who grow up in situations in which self-reliance and optimism are nurtured and expected—are better equipped to survive.

THE FUTURE

The future of the family cannot be predicted without placing it squarely in its social context. The trends toward equality of the sexes within families and the larger society certainly have increased self-esteem for women but may cause new stress for men and for women. Careful watching of morbidity and mortality trends will provide a clue to the effect of this important social movement. Divorce rates have leveled, and marriage again is gaining in popularity. The number of dual-career or dual-job marriages and unions is growing each year. Although such arrangements improve the family's economic assets, child care becomes complex and costly, especially in the preschool years. Considering recent trend analyses and surveys, it seems likely that the following future directions for American families might be possible:

1. Increasing value will continue to be placed on human potential, tenderness and warmth, and psychosocial

needs being met, rather than on material pursuits as a primary goal for families.
2. The trend toward decreasing numbers of children per family will continue and will result in greater attention being paid to parent-child relationships and an increased use of professionals as parenting advisers.
3. Neighborhoods will reemerge along with increased numbers of community support systems.
4. Extended families will gain the attention of researchers, as will grandparent-grandchild relationships.
5. The new American ideal—strength without domination—will gain impetus and influence in socialization patterns of families.

The challenge for pediatricians will be to keep abreast of changes in family patterns and dynamics and to use this knowledge in providing humanistically oriented and enlightened patient care and advice regarding parenting.

REFERENCES

1. Ahlburg DA, DeVita CJ: New realities of the American family, *Pop Bull* 47:2, 1992.
2. Aries P: *Centuries of childhood,* New York, 1962, Random House.
3. Chapman V: Working hard or hardly working? An examination of children's household contributions in the 1990s, doctoral dissertation, Princeton, NJ, Nov 1994, Princeton University.
4. Goldscheider FK, Waite LJ: *New families, no families? The transformation of the American home,* Berkeley, Calif, 1991, University of California Press.
5. Goode WJ: *World revolution and family patterns,* New York, 1963, The Free Press.
6. Gough K: *The origin of the family.* In Skolnick A, Skolnick J, editors: *Family in transition: rethinking marriage, sexuality, child rearing and family organization,* Boston, 1986, Little, Brown.
7. Hareven T: *American families in transition: historical perspectives on change.* In Walsh F, editor: *Normal family processes,* New York, 1982, Guilford.
8. Hofferth SL, Phillips DA: Child care in the United States, 1970 to 1985, *J Marr Fam* 49:559, 1987.
9. Jarson J: Understanding stepfamilies, *American Demographics,* July 1992, p 36.
10. McGoldrick M, Pearce J, Giordano J, editors: *Ethnicity and family therapy,* New York, 1982, Guilford.
11. *New York Times:* Birthrate for unwed women up 70% since '83, study says, p 1 and A8, July 20 1994.
12. Sagan L: *Family ties: the real reason that people are living longer.* In *Annual editions: Health, 1989-1990,* Guilford, Conn, 1989, Dushkin Press.
13. Smoyak S: Assessing aging caretakers and their families. In Wright L, Leahey M, editors: *Families and chronic illness,* Springhouse, Penn, 1987, Springhouse Corp.
14. Wallerstein J: *Second chances: men, women, and children a decade after divorce,* New York, 1989, Ticknor & Fields.
15. Walsh F: The clinical utility of normal family research, *Psychotherapy* 24:496, 1987.

55 Gay- and Lesbian-Parented Families

Melanie A. Gold and Ellen C. Perrin

American family structures are undergoing change. The traditional structure of a married couple with a working father, homemaker mother, and one or more children no longer describes the majority of American families. According to the 1990 U.S. Census 37% of United States families consist of a married, two-parent couple who have children; only 7% of those families report a pattern in which the father works and the mother stays home full time.[5] Alternative forms of family are quite diverse. For example, unmarried couples live together (either with or without children), and some couples choose to remain childless. Single mothers and fathers, stepparents, and "blended" families can be created by divorce, death, and remarriage. Gay men and lesbians can form stable families with or without children. Children can flourish in various family environments as long as these include adequate nurturance and guidance for optimal development.

Current estimates suggest that there are about 5 million lesbian mothers, 3 million gay fathers, and 6 to 14 million children of gay or lesbian parents in the United States. These figures probably underestimate the true total because many gay and lesbian parents are reluctant to reveal their sexual orientation. Gay- and lesbian-parented families themselves exist in a wide range of constellations. Until recently the majority of gay men or lesbian women became parents in the context of a heterosexual relationship before they recognized or acknowledged their homosexuality. Such parents may continue to live with their heterosexual spouse and children, or they may divorce and live as single parents or form stable relationships with a gay partner. These parents may have full or joint custody or regular visitation with their children.

As gay men and lesbian women choose increasingly to "come out" in their youth, growing numbers are becoming parents in the context of an ongoing homosexual relationship. Gay men may father children through arrangements with friends or surrogates, and lesbians may become parents by using insemination techniques with a known or unknown donor. When the donor is known, he may or may not choose to have an acknowledged, active role as the child's parent. Gay men and lesbians also can become parents by adoption or foster parenting. In most states only one member of the same-sex couple may be designated the child's legal parent, by birth or adoption. This convention results in formidable obstacles to both parents' having legal status consistent with their joint parental responsibilities.

RESEARCH ON CHILDREN WHO HAVE HOMOSEXUAL PARENTS

Research on children reared by homosexual parents has been limited by small sample sizes, nonrandom subject selection, a narrow range of demographic variables, and lack of long-term follow-up. The majority of studies were not double-blinded and have been done by gay researchers, who may be perceived as biased. Most research has focused on demonstrating the absence of a pathological situation rather than on elucidating patterns of strength and resilience.

Much of the research has been on children whose gay or lesbian parents divorced after a heterosexual marriage. For the children who have lived through parental discord, separation, and divorce, these experiences may be of more concern to them and have greater effect on their emotional and social development than the sexual orientation of their parents. Consciously planned families are different from those that occur from the loss of a parent or through divorce. The circumstances for children whose same-sex parents were not previously in a heterosexual marriage require far more research.

In a recent review Patterson[4] found that children who have gay or lesbian parents did not differ from children who have heterosexual parents in terms of psychological health and social relationships. Patterson reviewed 12 studies whose sample sizes ranged from 12 to 56 children whose parents are gay or lesbian and equal numbers of children who have heterosexual parents. No differences were found in the development of sexual or gender identity or gender role behavior between children who have homosexual parents and those who have heterosexual parents. Adolescent sexual orientation was similar, with about 5% to 8% of teenagers in both groups reporting homosexual attraction or behavior. No differences were found in personality characteristics, locus of control, moral maturity, intelligence, or the incidence of psychiatric disturbance or behavioral problems.

These studies also report that children whose mothers are part of a lesbian couple spend more time with their mothers' male friends and relatives and have more contact with their biological fathers than do children whose mothers are heterosexual and single. Children do not become confused or have difficulty relating to two same-sex parents but will easily create names to address their same-sex parents (e.g., Daddy and Papa, or Mommy Sue and Mommy Jane), just as they do routinely to identify grandparents and other relatives. Children growing up having homosexual parents have been shown to be more tolerant of diversity in general and more open to discussions on topics such as sexuality and interpersonal relationships than children having heterosexual parents. Children in a gay- or lesbian-parented family are less likely to be victims of parental sexual or physical abuse than are children in a heterosexual-parented family.

Children growing up having gay fathers have been studied less extensively than those having lesbian mothers. In a review of the literature that included over 20 studies, Bozett[1] compared characteristics of parenting among gay and heterosexual fathers and found no differences between the two groups in problem solving, providing recreation for children, or in encouraging autonomy. Gay fathers were found to be less traditional, to demonstrate greater nurturance, and to have more investment in their paternal role and to view it more positively than did heterosexual fathers. Gay fathers who have disclosed their homosexuality to their children tended to be less authoritarian and to use less corporal punishment with their children than did gay fathers living with wives. Gay fathers who did not have physical custody of their children maintained contact with them more consistently than did divorced or separated heterosexual fathers.

SOCIAL RELATIONSHIPS AND DISCLOSURE

It is important for all children, especially as they reach school age, to develop a wide range of relationships outside their nuclear family. Children who have gay or lesbian parents may be assumed to be homosexual and experience stigmatization by peers when their parents' sexual orientation becomes known. Casper et al.[2] described the conflict raised for children who have gay or lesbian parents when the dominant cultural values reflected in the school define "family" in ways that are different from what the children experience in their own homes. This discrepancy may be distressing to children and add to their social isolation and uncomfortable relationships with peers. Gay and lesbian parents frequently fear that school staff will treat their children differently if they disclose their sexual orientation and family constellation. As a result many parents help children to learn "differential disclosure"—to be open about their parents' homosexuality to some people but not to others—so that harassment and social isolation can be minimized. Parents should understand that both secrecy and disclosure represent potential burdens for their children.

Pediatricians and other health professionals may act as intermediaries between the family and the school to help make the educational environment more supportive. They can talk to child care providers and teachers and can encourage schools to include information about diverse family structures in their libraries and curricula. Pediatricians also can encourage families to develop a social support network in the interest of their children. In many larger cities there is an active network of gay and lesbian parents who work to create an environment of peer support in which their children feel accepted and less "different" than they may in their other social contexts. Parent-child discussion or play groups, "story hours," and periodic communal meals have helped some parents and children seeking mutual support.

LEGAL ISSUES

There is a growing trend toward legal security of parental rights for gay and lesbian parents. Still, in most states only one parent in a same-sex couple can be a child's legal parent, and ambiguity in laws governing custody, compounded by vast differences in state laws, have left decisions in the hands of individual judges. Despite court precedents declaring that parents cannot be deprived of child custody based *solely* on parental sexual orientation, a heterosexual parent still is more likely than a homosexual parent to be granted custody and visitation rights unless the heterosexual parent is unavailable or obviously unfit.

Because courts have continuing legal authority to "protect" children until they reach majority (18 years of age), custody questions can be reopened in any state in which the child resides, leaving the family vulnerable if they move to another state. If a court finds it to be in the child's "best interest," it can remove the child from the home if parental custody is challenged (e.g., by former spouse or grandparents), particularly when a parent's homosexuality was unknown in a previous custody decision.

In the frequent circumstance that only one of the same-sex couple is legally recognized as a child's parent, the pediatrician should clarify how responsibility for medical decisions and consent for treatment for the child will be shared. In the event of serious illness, injury, death, or voluntary separation of the legal parent, a prior written agreement giving the other parent power of attorney in making medical decisions for the child is necessary.

In general, when gay and lesbian couples first contemplate raising a child together, they should agree in writing on issues concerning child custody, support, and consent for treatment. Curry et al.[3] give guidelines for writing agreements that specify parental rights and responsibilities. Without a written agreement, a nonbiological/nonadoptive parent may have difficulty proving his or her status as the child's parent.

ISSUES IN PROVIDING PEDIATRIC CARE

Pediatricians should convey their support of all forms of caring families and not assume that all parents are heterosexual. Pediatricians who care for children who have gay or lesbian parents should communicate trust and respect, be sensitive and aware of the special needs, expectations, and concerns of these parents, and focus on the family's strengths and resources as they pertain to the child's care and development. Pediatricians should be wary of giving unintentional signals of negative feelings toward homosexuality, which can interfere with the supportive and helpful role expected by parents. Those physicians who cannot reconcile their personal beliefs with their professional obligation to provide supportive, understanding, and respectful care to gay- and lesbian-headed families should recognize this limitation and refer these families to a physician who can meet their needs.

Gay or lesbian parents may choose not to identify their sexual orientation to their pediatrician. They may worry that latent homophobia or bias in professional and nonprofessional staff will jeopardize the care their children receive or that the pediatrician will not honor their confidentiality, particularly if the parents are concerned about legal challenges to their custody rights. Pediatricians should discuss consent for medical care and clarify in writing any power of attorney granting the nonbiological/nonadoptive parent the right to make medical decisions. They should discuss issues of confidentiality with parents—with whom parents will confide and from whom will they withhold disclosure of their family structure (e.g., school officials, hospital and office personnel).

Pediatricians should create a safe and inclusive environment for same-sex parents and their children. Part of creating that environment entails an awareness among professional and nonprofessional staff about issues of concern to lesbian and gay parents and the problems presented by homophobia, heterosexism, and bias. Discussion of nontraditional family structures can be facilitated by evidence of the pediatrician's acceptance of diverse families (see the box

QUESTIONS TO CLARIFY THE FAMILY CONSTELLATION

Is there anything about your family that would be helpful for me to know?
Who are the adults who make up your family?
Who are the important people in your child's life?
Who lives at home? What is your relationship with each child caretaker?
By what name does your child call each family member?
Who are the other important members of your family or support system who help care for your child?
Do you share parenting responsibilities with anyone else?
Who helps you with parenting?
Is there anyone else who participates in parenting?
Do(es) the biological parent(s), if not part of the current constellation, have any involvement in child care?
Which of your child's caretakers can give legal consent for medical care?
Do any of your child's biological relatives have any medical conditions?

above). Questions on standardized office intake forms using gender-neutral terms such as "parent" or "family member" (instead of mother/father), pictures of diverse families in the waiting room, and brochures, books, and magazines that acknowledge same-sex parents, communicate the pediatrician's availability to assist *all* families in their parenting challenges. Pediatricians can create and implement a policy against lesbian and gay slurs, jokes, and put-downs in the office, which might be hurtful or offensive to patients, parents, and staff. Such office modifications also will help adolescents questioning their sexual orientation to discuss their concerns with the pediatrician.

As with any family, the pediatrician should discuss the parents' histories, as individuals and as a couple, and their plans for partnership in the care of their children. Knowledge about the family provides the pediatrician with valuable information in helping parents to care for their children. Asking questions sensitively about each parent's family background, perhaps including the creation of a genogram (see Chapter 54), helps to establish a fuller understanding of the family's sometimes complex relationships.

Pediatricians in communities in which there are many gay- or lesbian-headed families may want to know more about the specific concerns and issues surrounding these families. This perspective can be achieved by talking to friends, the spouse or partner, or members of the gay or lesbian communities; attending relevant continuing medical education courses; reading professional literature on the effect of family structure and sexual orientation on child development; attending gay or lesbian support groups; and reading both fiction and nonfiction that address issues about homosexuality and gay and lesbian parenting.

Medical Access and Experiences of Gay and Lesbian Parents

One of the authors (ECP) investigated the experiences of gay and lesbian parents in obtaining pediatric care for their children. In a questionnaire survey sent to lesbian and gay parents in the Boston area, 75% reported that their pediatrician knew of their sexual orientation and family constellation, nearly all having made it a point to inform the pediatrician at the initial visit. Nevertheless, many parents reported fears related to their pediatric care, including that their child's health care might suffer, that there might be potential negative implications for custody and adoptive decisions, that negative attitudes might be transmitted to their children, and that any difficulties their children might have would be attributed to the parents being gay. Indeed several parents described experiences in which their family constellation had been presumed to be the etiology of their child's growth failure or behavioral and school difficulties. Of the parents whose children had been hospitalized, 21% reported difficulties with hospital policies that did not recognize the nonbiological parent as a legitimate parent.

This preliminary study included primarily Caucasian, middle-class, suburban parents. Pediatricians should keep in mind that lesbian and gay parents who are poor, live in rural areas, or are members of a racial or ethnic minority are likely to have less choice in the selection of a pediatrician and thus may be faced with the dilemma of working with a health care provider who may be insensitive or unsympathetic to their family constellations. Pediatricians should recognize that gay and lesbian parents, even those who are open about their orientation, may have a number of fears that should be addressed. Pediatricians also should work within hospitals to change policies that exclude nonbiological/nonadoptive parents from participating in their child's medical care.

Physician Advocacy

There is no evidence to suggest an obstacle to the healthy development of a child who has gay or lesbian parents. Nevertheless, because of the extent of homophobia and bias, these children may be faced with criticism and isolation, which may affect their self-esteem. Pediatricians have an opportunity, and perhaps an associated responsibility, to help change social attitudes and restrictive legal codes that are damaging to gay and lesbian parents and their children. Pediatricians should be informed community resources and may choose to be available as consultants to gay or lesbian support groups. They may be able to foster community understanding by participating in parent-teacher association meetings and various community programs. They can learn which programs are receptive and supportive of alternative family life-styles and can provide guidance to gay and lesbian parents regarding child care and school selection. Pediatricians also can provide a bibliography of books for children and parents and a list of local and national resource groups. Above all, pediatricians have the opportunity and the responsibility to support and advise all families in achieving their maximal nurturing potential.

REFERENCES

1. Bozett FW: Gay fathers: a Review of the literature, *J Homosex* 18:137, 1989.
2. Casper V, Schultz S, Wickens E: Breaking the silences: lesbian and gay parents and the schools, *Teachers College Record,* 94:109, 1992.
3. Curry H, Clifford D, Leonard R: *A legal guide for lesbian and gay couples,* ed 7, Berkeley, Calif, 1993, Nolo Press.
4. Patterson CJ: Children of lesbian and gay parents, *Child Dev* 63:1025, 1992.
5. US Bureau of the Census Current Population Report: Series P20, No

486, 467, *Statistical Abstract of the U.S.:1992,* ed 112, 1992, Washington, DC, the Bureau.

SUGGESTED READINGS

Gold MA et al: Children of gay or lesbian parents, *Pediatr Rev* 15:354, 1994.

Martin A: *The lesbian and gay parenting handbook: creating and raising our families,* New York, 1993, Harper Collins.

NATIONAL ORGANIZATION

Gay and Lesbian Parents Coalition International (GLPCI) PO Box 50360, Washington, DC 20004 Telephone: (202) 583-8029. *This national organization can assist physicians and families in locating local support and information in their own or neighboring communities. It also provides an extensive reference list of books, articles, and videotapes for a nominal fee.*

56 Child Abuse and Neglect

Howard Dubowitz and Martin Finkel

Almost 3 million reports for child maltreatment were made in 1993, over half of them for child neglect. The Second National Incidence Study of Child Abuse and Neglect in 1986 found that professionals identified 9.4/1000 children as abused and 14.6/1000 as neglected. In another study approximately 3% of parents reported using very severe violence (e.g., hitting with fist, burning, using gun or knife) against their child in the prior year.[16] Studies suggest that approximately one in three girls and one in six boys have been sexually abused.[3] It is probable that all these estimates are low; clearly child abuse and neglect are not rare.

There can be serious sequelae for maltreated children, ranging from subtle neurological signs to death; in 1991 1383 children are estimated to have died as a result of maltreatment.[12] Approximately half the fatalities result from neglect, usually involving children left unsupervised and dying in fires or drowning. Other effects of maltreatment include cognitive and language delays, poor social skills, diminished self-esteem, aggressive behavior, and serious emotional problems. There are many potential negative effects of child maltreatment, and these may be long term.

Every state has a law mandating pediatricians to report suspected maltreatment to a designated public agency. Failure to do so may lead to legal action or professional censure.

Pediatricians typically enjoy trusting relationships with their patients' families and do not have the stigma often associated with the child welfare and mental health systems. Thus we are in a position to be knowledgeable about a child's and family's situation and their strengths and difficulties and to intervene appropriately. We may be the only professionals in contact with preschoolers.

DEFINITIONS

A consensus in defining abuse and neglect has been elusive. However, that *abuse* refers to acts of commission, and *neglect* to acts of omission generally is agreed upon. Debate surrounds whether potential harm (or endangerment) should be included in the definition, as well as actual harm. The federal model definition (a guideline for states) does include endangerment. Including potential harm allows consideration of consequences that may be uncertain or long term.

Physical abuse includes severe beatings, scalding, and an uncommon form of abuse termed *Munchausen by proxy,* wherein a parent induces or feigns illness in a child to attract medical care. Given that corporal punishment is widely accepted in the United States, what is the threshold for defining abuse? One approach is to discourage all hitting (and provide preferable alternatives) and to consider any injury beyond immediate redness of the skin as abuse. In addition, acts of severe violence (e.g., throwing a rock at a child) are abusive even if no injury ensues; there is significant risk of harm.

Child neglect refers to omissions in caregiver obligations to provide adequate child care in the areas of health, education, supervision, physical needs (e.g., clothing, food), and emotional support, with abandonment being the most severe form of neglect. Most state laws exclude cases where these needs are unmet because of poverty. In many areas the threshold for Child Protective Services (CPS) accepting a report of neglect is very high.

An alternative view to focusing on caregiver behavior is instead to consider the basic needs of children (i.e., adequate food, clothing, shelter, health care, education, and nurturance); neglect occurs when one of these needs is not met, whatever the reasons. This broader perspective encompasses the role of caregivers as well as other factors (e.g., lead in the environment, lack of access to health care, costs of medications) that may contribute to the neglect of children, and it demonstrates the need for broad strategies to target these factors.

Emotional abuse has been difficult to define and so it is even more difficult to identify it and intervene. This partly is inherent in the nature of emotional abuse that its manifestations (e.g., low self-esteem) frequently are not overt or specific to abuse. Emotional abuse includes verbal abuse and belittlement and acts that terrorize a child. Although this form of abuse may be extremely harmful to children, CPS seldom becomes involved in these cases. Indeed the emotional aspect of all forms of maltreatment may be the most damaging aspect, particularly in the long term.

ETIOLOGY

There is no single cause of child maltreatment; rather, there are multiple and interacting contributory factors.[13] At the *individual* level a child's difficult temperament or a parent's poor impulse control may increase the risk of maltreatment. At the *familial* level, spousal abuse or desertion by a father poses risks for children. Influential *community* factors include stressors such as dangerous neighborhoods or a lack of recreational facilities. There also are broad societal factors that may contribute to maltreatment; examples include the wide acceptance of corporal punishment and violence explicitly portrayed in the media.

Resources and strengths can help buffer the effects of these problems. Examples of protective factors include a parent's recognition of a problem and interest in help, a supportive grandparent, good, affordable child care, and a federal program to make fathers pay child support. Child abuse and neglect results from the complex interplay among many of these positive and negative factors. For example, a single mother who has a colicky baby and who recently lost her job is at high risk, but a loving grandmother may be a protective influence.

SCREENING

The *review of systems* is a standard part of child health supervision. The psychosocial situation of the child and family is part of this screening interview and should include a few questions pertaining to such areas as the parent's feelings about the child, any problems with the child and how the parents cope with them, the relationship with the spouse, supports and stresses, and recent changes in the family's circumstances. If a response to any of these questions emerges as a "red flag," further clarification is needed. *Direct observation* of parent(s), children, and their interaction can reveal useful information about their affect, functioning, and relationship. For example, does a parent appear involved in the child's issues? Does the child seem afraid of the parent and reluctant to talk forthrightly? Does the parent hit the child? Does the relationship between them appear warm and comfortable or is tension or anger evident? These observations may serve as cues for further investigation.

Further screening is needed when physical or behavioral signs or symptoms suggest maltreatment. A thorough history, including gathering comprehensive psychosocial information and performing an examination, are needed. Past medical history may reveal several noninflicted injuries suggestive of poor supervision, injuries that raise suspicions of abuse, or questionable compliance with medical recommendations. If one is not the child's primary care provider, it would help to get that person's impressions of the family.

PREVENTION

Pediatricians can help prevent child maltreatment in a number of ways.[2] *Anticipatory guidance* during child health supervision visits may be valuable in assisting parents to cope with the challenges of raising children. This support can enhance their competence and confidence, thereby diminishing the likelihood of child abuse and neglect.

Careful *screening* through an expanded review of systems and direct observation should alert the sensitive clinician to family difficulties that might lead to maltreatment. Unfortunately efforts to predict child abuse have not been successful for clinical purposes. Nevertheless, if screening for risk factors associated with child abuse leads to beneficial interventions, then it is valuable.

Pediatricians may implement a variety of interventions. *More frequent office visits* could be scheduled to offer support and counseling. *Other key family members* could be invited in and informal supports encouraged. Practices could arrange *parent groups* where problems and solutions are shared. Pediatricians need to recognize their limitations and when *other professional intervention* is indicated. Knowledge of community resources is essential, and pediatricians can facilitate referrals. Their knowledge of the family and their position of trust may help encourage parents and children to accept recommended services (see Chapter 93).

DIAGNOSIS

Pediatricians frequently must decide whether a child's injury is inflicted. To differentiate with some degree of certainty, an understanding of the manifestations of trauma and the context in which maltreatment occurs is essential. Before reaching a conclusion, it is necessary to consider alternative explanations for the problem.

Just as pediatricians are accustomed to viewing subspecialists as consultants, so should they consider physician experts in child maltreatment, social workers, police officers, and mental health colleagues as consultants. Multidisciplinary intervention is helpful to determine whether maltreatment has occurred and the therapeutic needs of the child and family. For example, law enforcement officers or CPS workers who have visited the home may provide valuable information concerning the circumstances surrounding the injury and insight into the functioning of a family. Such information can help determine the likelihood of maltreatment and the risk of further abuse or neglect.

When attempting to find out what has happened to a child, it is important to do so in a nonjudgmental and empathic manner. It may be necessary to control one's outrage at a child's maltreatment. Pediatricians should be nonaccusatory and nonconfrontational. It is the pediatrician's responsibility to consider all available information objectively to explain an injury. Maintaining a position as a concerned, helping professional who has a mandate to protect children ultimately will serve the child's and family's best interests. Most maltreated children are not removed from their caretakers, and if they are, the placement usually is temporary. Thus it is important to maintain a positive relationship with the caretaker as well as to follow the statutory requirements to report suspected maltreatment.

When obtaining a history it is advisable to interview the child alone. In an emotionally supportive and safe environment, children frequently are able to explain their injuries. The physical finding may be nonspecific, and the history is extremely important. A history that does not explain an injury reasonably is key to determining abuse. Caretakers may attempt to avoid providing any history, stating that they did not witness the injury and do not know how an injury occurred; this may be the truth. In spite of great skill on the part of all involved professionals, how an injury occurred may never be known.

Just as great care must be used when obtaining a history, the physical examination must be comprehensive and meticulous, with detailed and legible documentation. Whenever possible, documentation should be supplemented by photography so as to create a permanent record of an injury. This serves as objective evidence of an injury and enables a second opinion, if necessary.

Cutaneous Manifestations of Maltreatment

The integument is the first line of protection that absorbs the impact of trauma. The location, age, shape, and pattern of an injury assists in determining its cause. There should be an attempt to date the injury and corroborate this information with the history. As blood breaks down, contusions change color, providing a rough guide to the age of the injury.[17] During the first 1 to 2 days, bruises usually are red-blue or purple-violet, tender, and swollen. They then turn greenish, and by 7 to 10 days they are yellowish. Finally they turn brown and fade.

Some injuries have distinct configurations that suggest a hand or implements such as belt buckles, electric cords, hangers, switches, paddles, or hot metal objects. Injuries that have clearly delineated borders suggest abuse.[8] Bruises over hard bony surfaces such as the shin generally are noninflicted; those in the axilla and the folds of the neck and groin are more likely to be inflicted. Circumferential marks around wrists, ankles, and the neck may result from squeezing, grabbing, or use of a ligature. These injuries seldom are unintentional.

Contusions and erythema can be seen following the cultural practices of "coining" and "cupping" in the treatment of illness.[6] These injuries frequently are seen along the rib margins and spine. These cultural practices, deemed appropriate in their native environment, may be construed as maltreatment in the United States. Mongolian spots can be confused with bruises. If an underlying bleeding disorder is suspected as the cause of easy bruisibility, a platelet count, prothrombin time, partial thromboplastin time, bleeding time, and assay of specific clotting factors should be considered. Henoch-Schönlein purpura (HSP) is the most common vasculitis seen in young children and may be confused with inflicted trauma. Lacerations seldom result from abuse.

Bite Marks

The oval impression of a pair of crescentic bruises following a bite varies depending on the location, degree of force, and movement of the jaw and victim.[5] A bite by a child under approximately 8 years of age who does not have permanent teeth has a distance of less than 1 inch between the canines. Thus it generally can be determined if a bite was inflicted by a young child or an adult. A forensic odontologist may be consulted to assist in documenting and preserving bite mark evidence. Police photographers are capable of photographing these injuries precisely for their size for later study to determine the identity of the person who bit the child.

Burns

Hot liquids are the most common cause of burns. Scalding burns generally are of two types: immersion and splash. An immersion burn pattern that has a stocking and glove distribution, and burns of the buttocks and perineum with or without the "donut" pattern (circle of burned skin from hot water with the central area spared where child was pressed down against the cooler tub) strongly suggest abuse. Splash patterns are seen most commonly in noninflicted injuries. Liquids naturally flow downward and as they flow they cool; thus the more proximal area tends to be more severe and broader than the most distal narrower injury, conferring an "arrowhead" pattern. The depth of a burn is a function of the temperature, exposure time, and thickness of the exposed skin.[15] Water at a temperature of 150° F may cause a second degree burn in 1.5 seconds, whereas water at 120° F may take 300 seconds.[7] Burns from hot objects such as curling irons, hot plates, radiators, steam irons, metal grids, hot knives, and cigarettes generally are distinct and mirror the implement that was used. When children accidentally brush against such objects, the burns generally are superficial and not extensive. Second-degree burns must be differentiated from blistering skin disorders that can mimic burns. For example, impetigo may be confused with a cigarette burn. The diameter of a cigarette is 7 to 8 mm; impetiginous lesions tend to vary in size and may exceed the diameter of a cigarette burn.

Skeletal Trauma

Fractures strongly suggestive of inflicted injury in children under 2 years old are those involving the metaphyseal-epiphyseal plate, thoracic cage, scapula, and vertebra. These fractures all require substantial force (twisting, rotational, and shearing), which would not be anticipated from minor falls or routine handling of a child. Metaphyseal-epiphyseal fractures, rib fractures, and fractures of the sternum rarely are seen following unintentional injuries or cardiopulmonary resuscitation.[4] These fractures usually are caused by the violent compression and shaking of a young child's thorax.

Clavicular, femoral, supracondylar humeral, and distal extremity fractures in children older than 2 years of age are most likely noninflicted unless multiple or accompanied by other stigmata of inflicted injury. Multiple fractures in various stages of healing are considered to be child abuse unless proven otherwise, although underlying bone disease must be considered.[9] This differential diagnosis includes osteogenesis imperfecta, metabolic and nutritional disorders such as scurvy and rickets, renal osteodystrophy, osteomyelitis, congenital syphilis, and neoplasia.

A skeletal survey should be obtained following any fracture in a child less than 2 years of age. If the survey is negative yet suspicion remains of an occult injury, then a radionucleotide scan can be helpful.[14] A scan generally will be positive within 24 to 48 hours after an injury and remain positive throughout the stage of callous formation.

The age of a fracture should correlate with the history, even though fractures cannot be "aged" with great precision. Soft tissue swelling generally subsides in 2 to 5 days. Periosteal new bone can be seen as early as 4 days after injury. Callus on a long bone can first be observed 8 to 10 days after an injury. The soft callus stage lasts approximately 3 to 4 weeks. Hard callus and remodeling of bone occur over a few months. These time frames are shorter in infancy and longer when the child's nutritional status is poor or there is a chronic underlying disease. Fractures of flat bones such as the skull cannot be aged.

Central Nervous System (CNS) Injury

Of all inflicted injuries, those to the CNS result in the most significant morbidity and mortality. Injury results from either direct impact, asphyxia, or shaking. Direct trauma may be the result of punching, slapping, or an object being thrown at a child's head. Choking and suffocation result in asphyxial injury, often with minimal external signs. Shaking can result in a constellation of injuries that are intracerebral and intraocular (particularly retinal hemorrhages) and involve the cervical spine. A fall from a height of 4 feet or less by children under 2 years of age rarely results in simple or complex skull fractures. Any skull fracture that has a history of a minor fall or any child who has retinal hemorrhages may be suspected to have suffered an inflicted injury. "Raccoon eyes" may be observed in association with subgaleal hematomas following traction on the hair and scalp. Bruises from attempted strangulation may be visible on the neck. The differential diagnosis of an infant presenting with a CNS injury includes noninflicted trauma, spontaneous bleeds of vascular anomalies, or signs of a ventricular injury. Radiographs are best to identify skull fractures. CT scans are best suited for screening CNS injury and are useful to detect subarachnoid hemorrhages; MRI is of greatest value for identifying and dating parenchymal injury and subdural hematomas.

The history provided by caretakers frequently is incomplete. Symptoms may be insidious in onset, and as in all forms of maltreatment, the seeking of medical attention often is delayed. Severe CNS injury in the absence of clear accidental injury must be considered inflicted until proven otherwise. Thus in CNS-inflicted injury it is the objective CNS findings that may be pivotal in determining whether the injury was inflicted.

Visceral Injuries

Although only 5% of physically abused children have intra-abdominal injuries, 90% of blunt trauma in children is inflicted. Abdominal trauma is the second most common cause of death in abused children. Children most vulnerable to blunt trauma are those under 3 years of age because of the limited protection afforded by their small rib cages and their small abdomens, which are unable to dissipate the massive energy of blunt trauma. Infants who were crying before the blunt trauma may have swallowed large volumes of air, increasing the potential for perforation at the time of impact. Most children who have intraabdominal trauma do not have external injuries. Children who have a ruptured viscus and bleeding may present insidiously, with nonspecific complaints, or with signs and symptoms of an acute abdomen.

When solid viscera are injured, bleeding may result from trauma to the organ or from shearing of the vascular supply. Duodenal hematomas virtually are diagnostic of inflicted blunt trauma in young children, unless they follow bicycle or motor vehicle accidents. Unexplained bilious vomiting in the absence of fever or peritoneal irritation suggests a duodenal hematoma.

Laboratory and radiological evaluation can help to define the nature and extent of injury. Liver enzymes and serum amylase help to identify hepatic and pancreatic trauma. An elevated CPK and myoglobin reflect muscular trauma. Acute renal failure may be secondary to myoglobin in the absence of direct renal trauma. Serial hematocrits help determine the degree of blood loss; a urinalysis helps to evaluate renal trauma. Plain films of the abdomen or with water-soluble radiopaque dye are valuable in identifying hollow viscus injury. A CT scan with both oral and IV contrast is of value in assessing solid visceral injuries. Renal and pancreatic trauma can be assessed readily with ultrasound.

Oral Facial Injuries

Injuries to the head, neck, and oral cavity are commonly seen in physically abused children. Fractures of the facial bones and subluxation of the mandible are far less common. In cases of significant trauma a dentist should be consulted to assist in managing the obvious injuries and detecting the sometimes subtle injuries such as fractured teeth. Soft tissue injuries to the maxillary lip or the frenulum are seen in force feeding but also can occur when a toddler trips with a hard object in his or her mouth. The forceful introduction of objects into a child's mouth or scalding and caustic substances may result in intraoral lacerations or mucosal injury.[1]

The "tin ear syndrome" results from blunt trauma to the ear. It manifests with subperichrondral hematoma and associated intracerebral injury as a result of the rotational acceleration of the head. Noninflicted trauma to the forehead, lower lip, chin, and nose are common in toddlers and should be differentiated from inflicted injuries. More insidious is chronic dental neglect, which may result in eating difficulties, chronic pain, and infection.

Ocular Trauma

Direct trauma may result in abrasions, subconjunctival hemorrhages, globe fractures, and orbital edema. Orbital edema and globe fractures may lead to extraocular entrapment and an altering of the visual axis and amblyopia. Anterior chamber injuries such as a hyphema reflect severe direct trauma.[10]

Indirect trauma may lead to retinal or vitreous hemorrhages, most commonly the result of "shaken baby syndrome." Retinal hemorrhages may resolve within days, whereas vitreous hemorrhages may persist and can help to date the injury.[11] The postmortem examination may demonstrate patterns of posterior orbital hemorrhage and intraorbital optic nerve injury, which helps to differentiate noninflicted head injury from shaken baby syndrome. In shaken baby syndrome the presence of ocular injury (e.g., optic nerve injury, retinal hemorrhage), CNS injury, and skeletal trauma strongly suggests an inflicted etiology.

Behavioral Manifestations of Child Maltreatment

Many emotional and behavioral effects have been associated with child maltreatment, such as depression, anger, poor self-esteem, developmental delays, poor cognitive abilities and poor school performance, and aggressive and delinquent behavior. None of these problems is specific to child abuse or neglect. Consequently pediatricians encountering children who have such problems should consider the *possibility* of maltreatment, but be cautious not to jump to conclusions.

Manifestations of Child Neglect

The manifestations of child neglect are varied. For example, infants of depressed mothers who are emotionally unresponsive to their needs might not feel securely attached and may be very anxious in unfamiliar situations. Older children who are neglected emotionally might be sad, withdrawn, and depressed.

Neglect of physical needs may be quite apparent. Inadequate food might manifest as hunger and poor growth. Inadequate clothing may be obvious when, for example, children lack appropriate clothing for cold weather. Poor hygiene similarly may be overt. Recurrent noninflicted injuries or ingestions suggest that poor supervision may be a factor. Inadequate or delayed health care may lead to children presenting at a relatively late stage having a disease or problem. Obvious dental problems might reflect neglect.

The assessment of child neglect hinges on the identification of a child's basic need not being met, resulting in actual or potential harm. As suggested earlier, while CPS is concerned with omissions in parental care, children will be served best when all the factors that compromise their health and well-being are considered. In this way pediatricians can recommend services from an array of options.

REPORTING

State laws mandate pediatricians to report *suspected* child abuse or neglect to the designated public agency. It remains a "judgment call" whether the level of suspicion transcends the threshold for reporting. Consultation from an interdisciplinary team expert in child maltreatment or from CPS may be very helpful.

Reporting child maltreatment is never easy (Table 56-1). Parental inadequacy or culpability is at least implicit, and considerable anger may result. Pediatricians should inform families directly of the report, supportively and sympathetically. It can be explained as an effort to clarify the situation and provide help, or as a professional (and legal) responsibility. It is useful to explain what the ensuing process is likely to entail (e.g., a visit from a CPS worker and a police officer) and what will *not* happen (e.g., that their child will definitely be removed from their care).

LEGAL ISSUES

Whenever a physician is involved in a case of possible abuse or neglect, there is always the potential for legal involvement, although only a small percentage of cases are tried in court. It is important to be aware of the nuances of differentiating inflicted from noninflicted injury, to describe the findings, and to interpret them for the court. The astute diagnostician who explains the basis for the diagnosis clearly should not feel intimidated by the adversarial court system.

Most physicians provide their opinion in their capacity as the diagnosing and treating physician. This is important because much of what the child tells the physician may be admissible in criminal court proceedings as one of the few exceptions to hearsay rules of evidence. Hearsay rules, which apply primarily to the clinician, are fresh complaint disclosures, excited utterances, and statements made relative to diagnosis and treatment.

Table 56-1 Common Issues for Pediatricians When Faced with a Potential Case of Child Abuse or Neglect

Issue	Considerations
Unsure of the diagnosis	Law requires reporting *suspected* maltreatment All the data should be weighed and the likelihood of maltreatment assessed; consultation should be obtained Terms such as "probable" or "possible" may be used
Discomfort confronting parents	Convey concerns forthrightly and compassionately; avoid being confrontational Goal is to protect child and help family
Public agencies are ineffective	Recognize agencies' resources (e.g., to visit home) and work with them
Prefers to handle the matter alone	This assumes an immense responsibility; better to report to and work with agencies
Neglect less serious than abuse	Morbidity and mortality caused by neglect are substantial
Cases are so time consuming	Time demands often are unavoidable Needs to adjust practice, as for other complex cases
Reluctant to testify	Understandable; see references on documentation and legal system Consult with expert colleague in this field Legal system *can* protect children Most cases do *not* require medical testimony

Documentation is crucial to the admissibility of all evidence. Verbal evidence in cases of child abuse may be as important as physical evidence. Both the questions asked and the responses must be recorded verbatim. This allows objective interpretation of the degree of suggestibility and the content of the verbal evidence. Questions preferably should be open-ended and not leading. A comprehensive and legible record may diminish the need to testify.

Pediatricians may be called to testify before a grand jury, which in many states is a preliminary step to indictment. It is an opportunity for the prosecution alone to present their case. A grand jury indictment implies that evidence is sufficient to justify a trial, and it determines what charges will be filed.

A subpoena often is the physician's first indication of the need for involvement in the legal system. Different subpoenas are generated on behalf of the state, the child, or the defendant. When a subpoena is received, one should consult with the person who issued the subpoena for help in preparing for trial. Prosecutors and the court generally respect and accommodate the time constraints of physicians.

Any information a physician has should be considered privileged and confidential. Confidential information should be disclosed only when the client or legal guardian consents or a subpoena requires such disclosure. Each state varies as to specific laws concerning confidentiality and reporting responsibility in suspected child abuse and neglect. Physicians need to know their state's statutes regarding confidentiality and reporting. In the pretrial process of "discovery," both the prosecutor and defense attorney have an opportunity to learn what evidence the other possesses. The defense attorney may contact the examining physician directly to discuss the case as part of discovery. The physician is not legally obligated to comply unless the request is accompanied by a subpoena. During cross examination, failure to have met with the defense attorney if previously requested may be used to demonstrate a lack of objectivity. It is well to note that the defense is responsible for representing the accused; the interests of the child are secondary. This is the essence of the adversarial process.

Lastly, all reporting statutes supersede any ethical duty to protect confidentiality. As long as the physician's statutory obligation to report suspected abuse and neglect is made in good faith, he or she is immune from both civil and criminal liability. Although this does not mean that physicians cannot be used to establish the case against the accused perpetrator, every state has a law protecting physicians from liability.

TREATMENT

Pediatricians are responsible for treating any *medical* problem. They should be a liaison between the family and the public agencies, and they should make every effort to remain involved after reporting. Families typically are under great duress following a report, and the involvement of the different professionals and agencies can be very confusing. With more frequent office visits, practitioners can offer *support and guidance*.

In families in which maltreatment occurs, the parents may need to be nurtured before they are able to nurture their children. Therefore it is important that a treatment strategy consider the *needs of the family.* The use of *informal supports* such as family members, neighbors, and friends (e.g., inviting the father or a grandparent to an office visit) should be encouraged. Families also may benefit from other professional interventions (e.g., family therapy), and practitioners can help with *referrals.*

ADVOCACY

Advocacy should target the factors contributing to child maltreatment. At the *individual* level, explaining to a parent that a "hyper" toddler is behaving normally albeit being a challenge, and the child is "not out to get you" is advocating on behalf of that child. Encouraging a mother to seek help dealing with a violent spouse, saying "you and your life are very important" is advocacy on behalf of someone feeling powerless.

Pediatricians advocate on behalf of *families* when they try to enhance the functioning of families. Encouraging the involvement of fathers in child care, strengthening ties with extended family, and referring for family therapy all are forms of advocacy. Remaining involved after reporting to protective services and helping to ensure the implementation of appropriate interventions is another.

In the *community,* practitioners can be influential advocates for resources for children and families. These may include parenting programs, services for battered women and their children, and recreational facilities. Other efforts might attempt to combat violence in a neighborhood or the sale and use of drugs.

Finally, pediatricians can advocate at the *state* and *national* levels for policies and programs that benefit children and families. Such efforts include writing to one's congressman or supporting effective advocacy groups. Child maltreatment is a complex problem with no easy solutions, but enough is known that interested professionals can make a difference.

REFERENCES

1. Ambrose JB: Orofacial signs of child abuse and neglect: a dental perspective, *Pediatrician* 16:188, 1989.
2. Dubowitz H: Pediatrician's role in preventing child maltreatment, *Pediatr Clin North Am* 37:989, 1990.
3. Faller KC: *Understanding child sexual maltreatment,* Newbury Park, Calif, 1990, Sage Publications.
4. Feldman KW, Brewer DK: Child abuse, cardiopulmonary resuscitation and rib fracture, *Pediatrics* 73:339, 1984.
5. Furners J: A general review of bite mark evidence, *Am J Forensic Med Pathol* 2:49, 1981.
6. Gellis S, Feingold M: Cao Gio, pseudo-battering in Vietnamese children, *Am J Dis Child* 130:857, 1976.
7. Hobbs CJ: When burns are not accidental, *Arch Dis Child* 61:357, 1986.
8. Johnson CF, Sahuers J: Injury variables in child abuse, *Child Abuse Negl* 9:207, 1985.
9. Kleinman PK: *Skeletal trauma: general considerations in diagnostic imaging in child abuse,* Baltimore, 1987, Williams & Wilkins.
10. Levin AV: Ocular manifestations of child abuse, *Ophthal Clin North Am* 3:249, 1990.
11. Massicotte SJ et al: Vitreoretinal traction and perimacular retinal folds in eyes of deliberately traumatized children, *Ophthalmology* 98:1124, 1991.
12. McCurdy K, Daro D: Current trends in child abuse reporting and fatalities: results of the 1991 state survey. Paper presented at the Ninth International Congress on Child Abuse and Neglect, Chicago, August 31, 1992.
13. Newberger CM, Newberger EH: The etiology of child abuse. In Ellerstein NS, editor: *Child abuse and neglect: a medical reference,* New York, 1981, John Wiley & Sons.
14. Pickett WJ et al: Comparison of radiologic and radionucleotide skeletal surveys in battered children, *South Med J* 76:207, 1983.
15. Raine PA, Azmy A: A review of thermal injuries in young children, *J Pediatr Surg* 18:21, 1983.
16. Wauchope BA, Straus MA: Physical punishment and physical abuse of American children. In Straus MA, Gelles RJ, editors: *Physical violence in American families: risk factors and adaptions to violence in 8145 families,* New Brunswick, NJ, 1990, Transaction Publishers.
17. Wilson EF: Estimation of the age of cutaneous contusions in child abuse, *Pediatrics* 60:750, 1977.

SUGGESTED READINGS

American Medical Association: *Diagnostic and treatment guidelines on child physical abuse and neglect,* Chicago, 1992, AMA.

Cicchetti D, Carlson V, editors: *Child maltreatment,* New York, 1989, Cambridge University Press.

Kleinman PK: *Diagnostic imaging of child abuse,* Baltimore, 1987, Williams & Wilkins.

Ludwig S, Kornberg AE, editors: *Child abuse—a medical reference,* New York, 1992, Churchill Livingstone.

Myers JEB: *Legal issues in child abuse and neglect,* Newbury Park, Calif, 1992, Sage Publications.

Reece RM, editor: *Child abuse—medical diagnosis and treatment,* Philadelphia, 1994, Lea & Febiger.

57 Child Custody

Elizabeth Meller Alderman

Child custody arrangements at the time of a divorce have evolved over a long period, being a judicial issue only since the early nineteenth century. Changes in child custody laws reflect the social mores of the times. This chapter reviews the history of child custody statutes, different custody arrangements, and the role of mediation. The pediatrician often is called to court to assess the family and child's situation in determining custody arrangements and thus should be familiar with these aspects of family law.

HISTORY

Roman law dictated that the wife and children were under the absolute control of the father. This also was the case in feudal England, British common law, and courts in the United States until the nineteenth century. With the advent of developmental and psychological studies of infants and children that highlighted the importance of the mother-child bond, the concept of *parens patriae,* or judicial consideration of the best interest of the child, became the law. Both parents received equal consideration in cases of child custody.

The "tender years doctrine" subsequently evolved and was first introduced in the United States in the 1900s. This interpretation of the law gave custodial preference to the mother because of the perceived notion that mothers were the best caretakers for young children. The growing women's rights movement also advocated for maternal custody. However, this concept has fallen out of favor in the last 20 years, with laws forbidding discrimination on the basis of gender and because it violates the father's rights. Thus, according to judicial standards, the pendulum has swung back. *The best interests of the child* now are given the greatest consideration. Current laws and court decisions try to preserve the parenting rights of both parents and provide for their ongoing commitment.

Over the last 3 decades the total number of children under the age of 18 involved in a divorce has tripled, and it is projected that in the 1990s only 59% of American children will be living with both natural parents.[1,2] This increased divorce rate has forced the courts, as well as pediatricians and mental health professionals, to evaluate the impact of different custody arrangements on children and adolescents. Additionally, new considerations in awarding child custody have surfaced as life-styles and the definition of family have changed. In 40% of all cases mothers receive custody.[3] However, fathers are now more likely to demand a greater role in the child's life. Issues that may have impeded a parent receiving custody in the past, such as sexual orientation, parental health, psychiatric history, life-style, religion, and cohabitation out of wedlock, now are being scrutinized. Grandparents and nonbiological parents also may wish to obtain some degree of custody or visitation privileges.

CUSTODY ARRANGEMENTS

Many different custody or parenting arrangements exist. *Sole custody* had been the traditional settlement in the past and still exists if one parent deserts a family or is judged to be unfit or if the parents cannot agree on what is best for the child. The custodial parent is legally responsible for all major decisions regarding the child.

Split custody—in which each parent assumes custody of one or more of their children—rarely is awarded. This arrangement usually is not considered because it is important to keep children together to provide consistency and mutual support.

Joint custody—which encompasses either joint legal or joint physical custody—is becoming a more common arrangement. Joint legal custody is the most popular and allows both parents equal responsibility in important decisions regarding the child's life. One parent is awarded physical custody of the child, with the other receiving liberal visiting privileges. Joint physical custody provides for the child to live with both parents for significant amounts of time, but not simultaneously.

Thirty-three states in the United States have enacted joint custody laws.[4] Some states have ordered joint custody as the preferred arrangement; others have the legal assumption of joint custody if agreed upon by both parents. Advocates of joint custody, such as fathers' rights activists and family mediators, believe that children living solely with mothers have less paternal contact and that mothers are overburdened physically and financially if they are the sole caretakers.

Research examining whether joint custody is preferable to sole custody has shown mixed results. Joint custody provides the best continuity for the child with both the parents. Parents in joint custody arrangements have better cooperation with former spouses and greater financial resources than those who obtain sole custody. However, increased access and visitation may be related to greater emotional and behavioral problems in the child and greater parental dispute. Joint custody is a more expensive option, as each parent must provide full physical facilities for the child. However, most parents demonstrate high satisfaction with joint custody. Success of such an arrangement depends on geographical proximity, valuing the other parent as the child's parent, lack of guilt, and low levels of anger.

Contrary to popular belief, only a small percentage of child custody decisions are made occur in the courtroom; most cases are settled by attorneys and clients or go to mediation. Those cases that do go to court result from different motivations. A parent may wish to establish the incompetency of the other in a public forum such as the courtroom. Custody of the child may be a way to seek revenge on a former spouse or fulfil a parent's emotional needs after the divorce. From a financial standpoint, the parent providing child support may wish to have full custody to have greater control over the child's life as well as decreased support payments. In addition, a continued court battle may allow former spouses to maintain a relationship although their marriage has been dissolved. Child custody may become a bargaining chip in a divorce settlement. Unfortunately some parents use desperate measures, such as allegations of child abuse, to obtain custody of a child. If abuse does exist, then it is important for the courts to know of it. However, if it is an unfounded allegation, it will lengthen the proceedings and may cause undue emotional harm to an already fragile family constellation.

In the past decade there has been a movement in the legal system away from litigation as a method of resolving child custody disputes and toward mediation. In fact many states have statutes that mandate mediation as the first step in determining child custody to facilitate communication and conflict resolution and encourage exploration of all alternatives to reach a compromise that is acceptable to both parties. The benefits of mediation are: both parties get their needs heard, the spouse feels more competent because a third party (lawyer or judge) is not relied on to arrive at a decision, it is less expensive, and the process is shorter. Mediated settlements usually are stable because they have been obtained by consensus rather than mandate from the courts. The majority of couples who use mediation are able to reach a mutually acceptable agreement, which usually is joint custody. The key variables that predict successful conflict resolution are commitment, communication, and the experience of the mediator. A situation of great conflict, such as, allegation of child abuse or domestic violence, is less likely to be resolved by mediation. Mediation also is not appropriate if a spouse has a serious psychiatric illness or mental retardation.

THE ROLE OF THE PEDIATRICIAN

The pediatrician may be asked by the attorney to evaluate the family and by the court to help determine the best custody arrangement. In fact evaluation by a health or mental health professional is one of the most influential factors considered by judges in disputed child custody cases. There are several considerations in determining the best custody arrangement: health, safety, and welfare of the child, maintenance of a consistent living arrangement, quality of the parent-child relationship, degree to which a parent has been a caretaker, the child's preference, the parent's physical and mental health, and the parent's ability to provide emotional support for the child. It is important for the health professional to consider all aspects of a child's life. This should be done by interviewing the child and the parents and observing their interactions. The physician also may need to gather information from the child's school, friends of the family, relatives, and other community organizations with which the family may be involved. Medical records also may be very important.

The pediatrician should reassess custody situations periodically; the child's needs may change as he or she changes physically and developmentally. The physician may need to refer some children and families for psychological support. The pediatrician also is in the unique position to offer developmentally appropriate advice to parents who are helping their child cope with divorce and a new living situation.

REFERENCES

1. Veltcamp LJ, Miller TW: Family mediation: clinical strategies in mediating child custody, *Fam Med* 18:301, 1986.
2. Wallerstein JS, Johnston JR: Children of divorce: recent findings regarding long-term effects and recent studies of joint and sole custody, *Pediatr Rev* 11:197, 1990.
3. Kunin CC, Ebbesen EB, Konecni VJ: An archival study of decision-making in child custody disputes, *J Clin Psychol* 48:564, 1992.
4. Coller DR: Joint custody: research, theory, and policy, *Fam Process* 27:459, 1988.

SUGGESTED READINGS

American Psychiatric Association Task Force on Clinical Assessment in Child Custody: *Child custody consultation,* American Psychiatric Association, 1400 K Street NW, Washington, DC, 20005, 1988.

Emery RE: *Marriage, divorce and children's adjustment,* London, 1988, Sage.

Fidler AJ et al: Joint custody: historical, legal, and clinical perspectives with emphasis on situation in Canada, *Can J Psychiatry* 34:561, 1989.

Griffith DB: The best interest standard: a comparison of the state's *parens patriae* authority and judicial oversight in best interests determinations for children and incompetent patients, *Issues in Law and Medicine* 7:283, 1991.

Hlady LJ, Gunther EJ: Alleged child abuse in custody access disputes, *Child Abuse Negl* 14:591, 1990.

Johnson JR, Kline M, Tschann JM: Ongoing postdivorce conflict: effects on children of joint custody and frequent access, *Am J Orthopsychiatr* 59:576, 1989.

Kappelman MM, Black J: Children of divorce: the pediatrician's responsibility, *Pediatr Ann* 9:50, 1980.

Wallerstein JS, Kelly JB: *Surviving the breakup—how children and parents cope with divorce,* New York, 1980, Basic Books.

58 Children of Divorce

Robert E. Emery

The concept of *resilience* best captures the experience of children of divorce.[5] This conclusion is based on three observations that are well grounded in research. First, both children and parents experience considerable emotional distress, relationship conflict, and changes in their everyday life as a result of divorce. Second, children from divorced families are on average only slightly more troubled on various measures of their mental health as compared with children from married families. Third, many children and adults nevertheless harbor feelings of longing, sadness, or anger about divorce and its effects on their past and present. These observations are consistent with Garmezy's definition of resilience as "the maintenance of competent functioning despite an interfering emotionality."[6]

In addition to summarizing and integrating the research literature accurately, the resilience perspective offers a helpful clinical framework. Parents and children from divorced families appreciate the clinician's awareness of their past turmoil and lingering uncertainties—especially when this understanding is combined with the recognition of their competence in overcoming adversity. Stereotypical images of overwhelmed mothers, deadbeat dads, and troubled children dominate popular discussions of divorce. Parents and children from divorced families do not want to be treated as stereotypes, and sensitive clinicians note both their struggles and their strengths.

PREVALENCE: NATIONAL TRENDS

Statistics on divorce rates are cited widely in the popular media, but a few broad demographic trends are worth highlighting. First, divorce rates have leveled off since about 1980, but they have stabilized at a high level. Nearly one of every two children born to married parents will experience a divorce before the age of 18.[2] Second, childbirth outside of marriage is another major contributor to single-parent families. (At any one point in time about 40% of American families are headed by a single parent.) Approximately 16% of Caucasian children, 32% of Hispanic children, and 61% of African-American children are born to unmarried mothers.[9] Third, about 50% of divorced people remarry within 5 years, and informal live-in partnerships also are frequent before, or as an alternative to, remarriage. (Formal remarriage is more common among Caucasians than African-Americans.) It is important to note that, with the exception of improved finances, remarriage is *not* a return to the two-parent family. Instead, remarriage is another major transition, especially for children who initially may view stepparents as outsiders or intruders.

CHILDREN'S PSYCHOLOGICAL HEALTH

The findings of research on the psychological consequences of divorce for children have been debated considerably. Much of this debate has taken place in the popular media, and many parents and professionals have the misperception that scientific research documents profoundly negative outcomes for children. This simply is not the case. A metaanalysis (combining the results of 92 separate studies) found an average difference of only a 0.14 standard deviation (SD) between all measures of the psychological functioning of children from married and divorced families. This roughly is equivalent to the difference between an IQ of 100 and an IQ of 102, a notable but modest difference. The largest effect (0.23 SD) was found for children's conduct problems, but this difference still is comparatively equal to only about 3 IQ points.[1]

Even these relatively small differences in the average psychological functioning of children from married and divorced families must be interpreted with caution. Recent studies have found that many of the psychological problems found among children after divorce actually begin *before* divorce.[4] This longitudinal research demonstrates that many of children's emotional difficulties are not consequences of divorce. Rather the troubles more likely result from conflict or poor parenting predating divorce or of nonrandom selection of individuals who divorce. (For example, some people who have antisocial tendencies may be more likely both to divorce and to have children who have conduct problems.)

CAUTIONS AND CONCERNS ABOUT EXISTING RESEARCH

These conclusions about the functioning of the average child from a divorced family are scientifically accurate and should be reassuring to worried or misinformed parents (and children). However, the rather optimistic conclusions must be tempered with several cautions. First, divorce has devastating *economic* consequences for children and their single mothers. We should be concerned by family living standards falling by an average of 15% to 20% as a result of divorce, and many children live in poverty as a result of more substantial declines in living standards. Second, psychological measurement is far from perfect. Existing evidence is based on parent and teacher checklist scores, grades, achievement tests, and observational assessments, but these measures often fail to capture children's subtle and important feelings of turmoil, pain, longing, and unhappiness. In fact the relative insensitivity of objective psychological measurement to more elusive emotions may be a cause of the vehement debates about the consequences of divorce for children. Sensitive clinicians note children's distressing emotions. This discrepancy between research and practice is another appealing aspect of the concept of resilience. This perspective highlights children's strengths as measured by their objective functioning, but when viewed appropriately it also acknowledges the emotional struggles that children go through in "overcoming the odds."

A third caution about existing research is that it focuses on the average functioning of children of divorce. Many individual children suffer substantially as a result of divorce and as a consequence of the continued tensions that surround a difficult divorce. The perceived increased risk for significant psychological distress among a subset of children is demonstrated by children from divorced families being two to three times more likely to be referred to a mental health professional than are children from married families.[11]

INADEQUATE PARENTING AND PARENTAL CONFLICT

When the clinician conveys information about the effects of divorce on children, it is essential to recall the norm and to present accurate and reassuring information to parents about the modest effects, on average, on children's psychological well-being. Clinicians typically are asked questions about children who are facing problems. Thus we must be prepared to focus on children who are having troubles coping with their changed family circumstances.

Most children who are notably distressed by their parents' divorce are *not* suffering because of their own internal confusion. Rather, the much more common problem among troubled children from divorced families is being caught in their parents' own ongoing struggles. Inadequate parenting and continued conflict between parents are the two most consistent risk factors for children's psychological problems after divorce.[3,4]

Psychologists have demonstrated that the most effective style of child rearing is *authoritative parenting,* an approach that combines rich and responsive love with firm, *consistent,* and democratic discipline. Unfortunately, both parental love and parental discipline can be undermined by divorce. Custodial (residential) parents who assume primary responsibility for rearing their children may not be emotionally available to the children because of their own inner struggles and the demands of parenting alone. For similar reasons, residential parents may become less firm or consistent in disciplining children; alternatively they may become more harsh and dictatorial. Fortunately these problems typically diminish within a year or two as residential parents resume earlier patterns of authoritative parenting.[7]

A different set of problems occurs in noncustodial (nonresidential) parent-child relationships. Contact between children and nonresidential parents often is erratic and unpredictable shortly after a separation. Moreover the frequency of contact diminishes as time passes. Thus nonresidential parent-child relationships deteriorate as residential parent-child relationships improve over time. Ninety percent of nonresidential parents are fathers, and only about 25% of nonresidential, divorced fathers see their children once a week or more. Approximately one third of nonresidential, divorced fathers see their children once a year or not at all.[10] This startling lack of involvement usually is a major change in the love in father-child relationships. Other evidence indicates that nonresidential parents also tend to discipline ineffectively.

Children often appear to be quite distressed by their distant relationships with their nonresidential parents particularly at two points in time: when the separation first occurs and contact is unpredictable, and again in late adolescence as young people struggle with forming their own identity. Nevertheless researchers have demonstrated only weak links between contact with nonresidential parents and children's mental health. (The same cautions noted earlier hold in interpreting this research.) In contrast, continued inadequate parenting by the residential parent—lack of love or lack of discipline—is a consistent and significant risk factor for children's mental health problems.

JOINT CUSTODY AND PARENTAL CONFLICT

Joint custody is one much-discussed solution to increasing contact between children and their nonresidential parents, as well as easing the burdens of parenting alone. Like many issues related to divorce, joint physical custody is controversial. (Joint *legal* custody involves continued sharing of legal parental rights and responsibilities, and it is considerably less controversial; joint *physical* custody occurs when children spend approximately equal time with each parent.) Recent research indicates the reason for the debate about joint physical custody: it is at once the best and the worst arrangement for children. When parents cooperate after divorce, children fare better in joint physical custody than in sole custody. When parental conflict continues, children fare worse in joint physical custody than in sole custody.[8]

This brings us back to the important point that continued parental conflict is a significant risk factor for children from divorced families (joint physical custody exposes children to more of these distressing disputes). A particular problem occurs when children are caught in the middle of their parents' conflict. There is little that children can do to ameliorate or resolve their parents' problems, but children often are thrust into the role of mediator, ally, or caretaker. Children may take on these responsibilities themselves because of their concern for their parents' well-being, or children may have these developmentally inappropriate roles foisted on them by parents who are blinded by their fury. Many clinicians who work with children from divorced families encourage them to take on less responsibility for their parents' conflict (or for one of their parent's individual emotional struggles). The message that a child's job is to "be a kid" also can be brought out in support groups for children of divorce, which may be run in schools, courts, or mental health centers.

New interventions are available to help divorced parents deal directly with their disputes and get their children out of the middle. The most notable of these is *divorce mediation,* an approach where the parents meet with a neutral third party who helps them resolve their financial and child rearing conflicts.[4] Many parents see a mediator or a family therapist after a divorce. However, both legal and mental health professionals have recognized increasingly that the traditional legal methods of obtaining a divorce or deciding custody exacerbate rather than ameliorate children's emotional problems. Thus divorce mediation is used increasingly as an alternative to adversarial legal negotiations at the time of divorce (see Chapter 57, Child Custody).

OTHER RISK AND PROTECTIVE FACTORS

Other factors also are related to lesser or greater risk for psychological problems among children of divorce. There is no "right" or "wrong" age for children to experience a divorce;

evidence is inconsistent in documenting relations between children's age at divorce and their long-term psychological adjustment. Nevertheless children's age at the time of divorce clearly influences their immediate reactions. Separation distress and related issues of attachment dominate the reactions of infants and toddlers, who benefit from shorter, more frequent contact with nonresidential parents and stable, responsive relationships with residential parents. A lack of cognitive understanding, including self-blame, is common among preschoolers, who benefit from frequent reassurance, consistent relationships with both parents, and simple, practical explanations about divorce and their new family circumstance. Early school-aged children may be torn by strong loyalties to both parents; older school-aged children can be more angry and embarrassed by divorce. Parents can help by offering school-aged children age-appropriate explanations, listening to children's feelings, and accepting their relationship with the "other parent." Not surprisingly teenagers have varied reactions to their parents' divorce, including anger, sadness, embarrassment, disgust, and indifference. Parents are wrong to assume that an adolescent's coolness indicates an absence of inner turmoil. Nor is it developmentally appropriate for teenagers to become their parents' confidant.

Some research has indicated more problems among boys than girls from divorced families, but contradictory evidence also exists. It probably is true that sons and daughters are equally likely to experience psychological distress as a result of divorce, but boys are likely to show obvious external (behavior) problems, whereas girls harbor subtle internal concerns. Initial findings have demonstrated more positive outcomes among African-American than Caucasian children, perhaps as a result of the increased acceptance of and social support for single-parent families in African-American communities. In general, social support from other children and adults (including caring physicians) benefits children from divorced families. Ironically one positive effect of the increased divorce rate is that children have more social support from many of their friends who are in or who have gone through similar circumstances.

INTERVENTIONS

Numerous interventions have been developed for children and families during the process of divorce; surprisingly, however, there is little research on the effectiveness of treatment. Evidence does indicate that divorce mediation can keep parents out of court and increase their satisfaction with the results.[4] In addition, self-help and other group approaches for children and parents have been found to facilitate psychological adjustment. With respect to psychotherapy, most experts recommend some form of family therapy (or mediation) for former parents or for residential parents and their children, as opposed to individual psychotherapy. This is a very reasonable recommendation; however, there is no research on the relative effectiveness of these treatments.

Education and referral probably are the primary and most useful interventions that can be offered by the pediatrician. Many concerned parents will find solace in the pediatrician's confident reassurance or in a brief discussion of the research (especially given the many and often frightening reports in the media). The availability of educational pamphlets and self-help books also can be an important resource in the pediatrician's office. For other parents the pediatrician's education may be more direct: the pediatrician may suggest that the parent improve his or her relationship with the children's father or mother or raise specific concerns about a given parent's relationship with a child.

Pediatricians also can use and post a referral list of agencies and professionals who specialize in divorce and of community resources for divorce, single-parenting, and remarriage. In compiling the list, courts, schools, self-help organizations, and women's centers should be contacted in addition to mental health centers and professionals who specialize in divorce (including lawyers and mediators as well as psychologists). Many mental health professionals specialize in dealing with divorce; they are a preferred source of referral when children or parents are having problems.

Finally, pediatricians can help children and parents from divorced families by being careful about language and attitudes. Terms such as "broken home," "intact family," "custody," "visitation," and "child of divorce" are offensive and hurtful to many parents and children. "Divorce," "married family," "residence," and "contact" are preferred. Stereotypes can be avoided. Many divorced fathers are very involved in their children's lives; many divorced mothers continue to be effective "super moms"; and many children from divorced families remain much more concerned with "being a kid" than about their parents' divorce. Finally, we all need to consider our personal beliefs about marriage, child rearing, and divorce to ensure that these values help rather than hinder our patients and their families.

REFERENCES

1. Amato PR, Keith B: Parental divorce and the well-being of children: a meta-analysis, *Psychol Bull* 110:26, 1991.
2. Cherlin AJ: *Marriage, divorce, remarriage,* ed 2, Cambridge, Mass, 1992, Harvard University Press.
3. Emery RE: *Marriage, divorce, and children's adjustment,* Beverly Hills, Calif, 1988, Sage Publications.
4. Emery RE: *Renegotiating family relationships: divorce, child custody, and mediation,* New York, 1994, Guilford.
5. Emery RE, Forehand R: *Parental divorce and children's well-being: a focus on resilience.* In Haggerty RJ et al, editors: *Risk and resilience in children,* London, 1994, Cambridge University Press.
6. Garmezy N: Resilience in children's adaptation to negative life events and stressed environments, *Pediatr Ann* 20:459, 1991.
7. Hetherington EM: Coping with family transitions: winners, losers, and survivors, *Child Dev* 60:1, 1989.
8. Maccoby EE, Mnookin RH: *Dividing the child: social and legal dilemmas of custody,* Cambridge, Mass, 1992, Harvard University Press.
9. Select Committee on Children Youth and Families (SCCYF): *U.S. children and their families: current conditions and recent trends, 1989,* Washington, DC, 1989, US Government Printing Office.
10. Seltzer JA: Relationships between fathers and children who live apart: the father's role after separation, *J Marriage Fam* 53:79, 1991.
11. Zill N, Morrison DR, Coiro MJ: Long-term effects of parental divorce on parent-child relationships, adjustment, and achievement in young adulthood, *J Fam Psychol* 7:91, 1993.

59 Child Care and Early Education Programs

Susan S. Aronson

In the United States most families supplement maternal care with other types of child care. By the time 4- to 5-year-old children are ready to enter school, 80% have received care regularly in a nonmaternal arrangement. Many families use more than one type of care for the same child or for siblings during the same day, for different days, and for parts of the year. When mothers work outside the home, relatives provide 41% of the child care; child care centers and nurseries provide 30%, and nonrelatives provide 17% of care in their homes. In-home caregivers and mothers who take their children to work care for the rest. Many school-aged children are in after-school arrangements or in self-care.[4,5]

Increasing use of out-of-home, nonparental early care parallels the rise in labor force participation by mothers of young children. More mothers are working outside the home for the same reasons men work outside the home: economic gain, personal satisfaction, and societal recognition. Parents also use child care at other times when their children cannot be with them. As a result children spend many hours with caregivers other than their parents.

Increasingly, child care workers have formal training in early childhood education. Although the amount of preparation varies widely, the average education for the child care work force is 2 years of college. Early childhood education training focuses on child development and curriculum design, but also includes preventive health care and safety. Collaboration between competent early childhood professionals and child health providers can foster developmentally appropriate, comprehensive, coordinated, continuous, holistic care.

Options for out-of-home child care facilities include small family child care homes (6 or fewer children in the caregiver's home), large family child care homes (7 to 12 children in a caregiver's home that has more than one caregiver), and center-based care. Any of these arrangements may be used for part-day, part-week, or seasonal care. The names given to out-of-home child care programs do not define the type of service provided or the professional competence of the staff who work there. Babysitting, nursery schools, preschools, Head Start programs, play groups, and child development or early learning centers may take place in safe or hazardous environments. The staff may be loving or neglectful, culturally competent or culturally incompatible, unskilled or developmentally sophisticated.

PSYCHOSOCIAL OUTCOMES

For the Child

Science does not support the prevailing fantasy that exclusive early maternal experiences are necessary for optimum later performance of children. This fantasy feeds maternal guilt and public ambivalence about child care as a necessary family support service. Although the sum of early experiences does affect later development, the majority of children are remarkably resilient. They thrive in a wide variety of reasonably nurturing child care arrangements.

Reasonably nurturing child care supports parent-child relationships and fosters the physical, social, and intellectual development of children. In all settings and circumstances, children are learning. Children's emotional security, social skills, cognitive development, and physical health and safety must be addressed whenever and wherever they are in care.

Good child care and early education programs benefit children whether their parents work or seek child care for other reasons. Participation in group care usually is the child's first socialization experience outside home. Good programs provide many opportunities for enriching children's growth and development. Programs of poor quality can expose children to significant risks and diminish their enthusiasm for learning.

Researchers have looked at several psychosocial outcomes for children in a wide variety of types of group care.[10] One of the most crucial influences on psychosocial outcomes is maternal comfort with child care arrangements. Studies of children at risk for developmental disability found that those in child care and education centers of good quality scored higher on tests of cognitive competence than did those cared for only at home. Studies of healthy children in a wide variety of child care arrangements found no influence of the type of child care on intelligence scores. Some research on socio-emotional development found that children who were in early group care were less polite, less compliant, and more aggressive than other children. However, they also were more self-confident, assertive, self-sufficient, cooperative, and verbally expressive. In later childhood, differences between children who have been in early group care and other children disappear.

For the Family

Good child care and early education programs support families. Early childhood professionals serve as extended families for young parents. In a child care program information about community resources often is shared among parents and staff. Early education professionals and peer groups help parents find services and share their burdens. Good early childhood programs also help identify and care for children who have special needs and provide daily parent education by modeling and sharing strategies for healthy development of children.

HEALTH AND SAFETY

Infection

Close contact in child care facilitates the spread of many respiratory, gastrointestinal, systemic, and skin infections.[8] The incidence of common respiratory disease is nearly doubled for infants but decreases as children grow older or spend more time in group care. By the time children are 3 years of age, researchers find little difference in the incidence of infectious disease for children in group care compared with those cared for only at home. Three-year-old children who enter care as infants and stay in the same group as they grow older have fewer common respiratory infections than their peers who were never in group care.

One consequence of increased frequency of respiratory infections at younger ages is more episodes of otitis media and lower respiratory tract illnesses among children in group care. Although group care makes work force participation by both parents possible, frequent illness of children in child care is a burden for children, parents, employers, and the community. Many diseases that are transmitted in group care also can infect others in the community, including caregivers, parents, and family members. The most important infections transmitted to adult contacts of children in group care are hepatitis A, cytomegalovirus, and parvovirus B19.[9]

The risk of infectious disease in group care can be reduced by caring for children in age cohorts and by practicing good hygiene. Caregivers must pay particular attention to hand washing, diaper changing, and sanitizing of contact surfaces. As in health facilities, these practices must be taught and monitored continuously or they are ignored.

Child care workers need advice about treatment and exclusion of ill adults and infants who have infectious diseases in group care. An infected child does not need to be excluded unless the child cannot participate in activities, requires care that exceeds caregiver resources, or puts the other children at increased risk with continued exposure. For example, children who have diarrhea must be excluded from ordinary child care until their stools are contained by their diapers or by their ability to use the toilet. Guidelines for handling specific types of infections in group care are available from the American Academy of Pediatrics and the American Public Health Association.[1,2]

Injury

Children in child care centers have fewer injuries during the hours they are at the center than do children who receive care only at home. However, children who use child care centers suffer more injuries during the hours they are at home than do children who are cared for only at home. In family child care homes children have a higher incidence of injury while in child care than either children in child care centers or those cared for only in their own homes. Table 59-1 summarizes the incidence of injury by type of child care arrangement reported from a national study conducted by the Centers for Disease Control and Prevention.[6]

Table 59-1 Injury Rates/100,000 Hours by Type of Child Care

Type of Child Care Setting	Number of injuries per 100,000 hours in care
Child care center	2.18
Care only in child's own home	2.31
Care in own home (for child who also receives care in child care center)	3.40
Care in family child care home	3.95

From Gunn W et al: *Am J Dis Child* 145:779, 1991.

Falls from climbing equipment mounted over surfaces that do not absorb impact cause the most common and most severe injuries. Grass, carpeting, packed earth or sand, cement, or asphalt are hazardous. Both indoor and outdoor climbing equipment should be installed over cushioning materials such as 9 to 12 inches of bark mulch or a manufactured pad rated for the maximum fall height. Child health professionals can encourage parents and licensing inspectors to identify and help child care providers correct hazards wherever children play. Special vigilance to prevent injuries is needed in family child care homes and in children's own homes during the sometimes hectic hours when children come home from child care.

Health Promotion

Child care professionals have many opportunities to promote healthy medical, dental, and mental health behavior, as well as sound nutrition. All states have regulatory requirements for immunization of children in some group settings. Some states still do not require Hib vaccine; many states require immunization checks only in licensed child care centers, but not in nursery schools or family child care homes. Some states require child care providers to keep records that show enrolled children are up to date with all routinely recommended preventive health services. These requirements make child care providers natural allies of child health professionals. When children are found lacking preventive health services, child care providers can refer them to a source of primary health care to obtain needed services. Child health professionals can work with early childhood educators to link families to primary health care providers.

Early childhood educators need specific instructions from pediatric practitioners to provide appropriate care for children who have special health care needs. Teachers also have valuable daily observations to contribute to the health provider's understanding of the child's and family's functioning. Health professionals and early childhood educators have a mutual responsibility to share information with each other to enrich their ability to support the family. Because many educators believe that the child's health professional is inaccessible to them, the health professional may have to initiate contact with the child care provider for children with special needs.

Community Surveillance and Training of Early Childhood Educators

Performance requirements for facilities that serve young children are regulated by states through facility licensing and teacher certification. Regulatory control varies widely from state to state. The requirements may be stringent but often are lax. Surveillance through inspections may be done as often as quarterly but often are superficial or delayed because of inadequate staffing. Some regulators are skillful professionals; others are civil servants who have no appropriate training for the job. In the last few years national professional child care organizations for centers and family child care homes have developed systems of accreditation by self-study and peer validation. The number of accredited programs is small but growing steadily.

Some states have a designated agency to provide advice and training on health and safety for early childhood professionals; many do not. Because few child care programs have a nurse on staff, most seek health and safety advice from the health providers of children enrolled in the program, from overburdened health departments, or from no one at all. As a group, caregivers usually will remove hazards and follow safe practices called to their attention, if they have the means.

State regulations generally address three types of training requirements for caregivers: preservice training before employment for a given role, orientation for the tasks of a new position, and ongoing training while employed. The most common type of requirement is for ongoing training in child development and curriculum planning for caregivers. Although many directors of center-based early care and education programs have a master's degree or higher, in some states, caregivers are not required to have any early childhood training before they start taking care of children. The vast majority of training is entry level and repetitive. Caregivers need specialized training to work competently in programs for infants and toddlers, after-school care, mixed-age groups, and children who have special needs.[7]

First aid training is the most common requirement specified by licensing agencies. Usually it is provided by nurses, emergency medical technicians, or paraprofessionals. Some teach approaches that are not appropriate for children. The American Red Cross offers a good basic child care course developed in cooperation with the American Academy of Pediatrics.

ROLES FOR CHILD HEALTH PROFESSIONALS

Child health professionals can support quality education and care for children by:

- Seeking good care and education for their own children
- Asking and advising families about child care arrangements
- Providing consultation to child care and early education programs in their communities
- Advocating for social policy to improve the quality of child care and early education programs

Provider-Family Interactions

Families face difficult choices. Some parents can work less and thereby accept reduced means and limited career opportunities to spend more time with their children. Some couples will work split shifts so that they can share child care between them. Some have relatives who provide good care; some have relatives who constantly disagree with the parents about how to care for their children. Some parents buy low-quality, minimally regulated, unregulated, or illegal care. Some leave their children unattended. Some find good-quality affordable child care but worry about losing it. Many parents take their ill children to child care because they feel unable to take time off from work to stay with them at home. Some take their ill children to work with them or leave them home under "telephone" supervision.

Whatever their choices, balancing the care of their offspring and the demands of their job, while also meeting their own needs as individuals, is a tough challenge. Often young parents are too stressed to raise and weigh the issues of quality against affordability of child care. Convenience and cost are priorities; decisions about how much to spend often are weighed against the mother's income rather than against the wages of both parents. The portion of family income spent on child care can be substantial and still be grossly insufficient to purchase good care.

In 1990 the economics department of the University of Colorado at Denver estimated the full production cost for infant care (if caregivers were paid comparable wages) at $1,148 per month, the market cost (fees) at $613, and the net cost to parents after income tax credits at $573. [3] Tax credits favor families that have higher incomes. Even though low caregiver wages subsidize child care fees, many low- to middle-income families spend nearly 25% of their income on child care. The supply of quality child care is greatest in affluent areas where parents can afford to pay and in urban areas where government subsidies increase supply for those living in poverty. However, subsidized care is available only to a small percentage of those who are eligible for it.

Child health providers can focus parents' attention on issues related to quality care and help parents make good choices. From the first contact with the family, the child's health history should include information about who will be involved in the child's care when the child is well and ill. By asking parents about the experience and training of the caregivers, the child-to-staff ratio, the group size, and the facility where care is provided, the child health professional helps parents to evaluate these arrangements. Beginning with the prenatal visit, questions about child care arrangements should be part of the history-taking routine. When asked to complete a health form for enrollment in a child care program, the child health professional can revisit these issues in greater detail. Before commenting on the child care arrangement the child health provider should find out what options the parent has explored, what the parents have observed about how the child care program actually operates, and how the child is responding to that care.

Many communities have child care resource and referral agencies (R&Rs) where parents can find out about child care. These agencies help to inform parents on what to look for in a child care facility. R&Rs keep track of vacancies, size of waiting lists, complaints about service, local sources of subsidy, requirements for providers to operate legally, and many other policy issues related to child care. Some also provide training for child care providers. A call to the local licensing agency will locate local R&R agencies and yield information on how much public supervision of child care exists in the community.

Group size and staff-to-child ratio are related to the quality of care; Table 59-2 shows the recommended limits. Each group should have at least two caregivers. Because two caregivers are not available in a small family child care home, reliable and familiar backup arrangements should exist for emergencies and times when the caregiver cannot work.

Young children need consistency of caregivers during the day and from day to day to foster the intimate, trusting relationships essential for healthy development. These relationships can form only in small groups where few caregivers share child care responsibility. Within the group, quality of

Table 59-2 Staff/Child Ratio and Group Size

Age group	Staff/child ratio*	Maximum group size
Birth to 24 months	1:3	6
25 to 30 months	1:4	8
31 to 35 months	1:5	10
3 years	1:7	14
4 to 5 years	1:8	16
6 to 8 years	1:10	20
9 to 12 years	1:12	24

From American Public Health Association and the American Academy of Pediatrics: *Caring for our children, national health and safety performance standards: guidelines for out-of-home child care programs,* Washington, DC, & Elk Grove Village, Ill, 1992.

*For mixed age groups, the recommended ratio is the one consistent with the requirement of the majority of the children in the group except when infants and toddlers are in the group, when the recommended ratio is 1:3.

care improves when each child is assigned to a specific caregiver who provides most of that child's routine daily care and comforts the child during times of stress. Primary caregiver assignments also help foster supportive relationships between the child's caregiver and parents.

The curriculum of an early childhood education and care program should encourage children to be involved in learning. Children need a variety of experiences, including independent and group play, gross and fine motor activities, reading and language development, music, and art. The daily schedule of activities should include going outdoors once or twice a day, alternating quiet and active play, having more child-initiated than adult-initiated activities, and having planned transitions between activities. Television watching should be limited. Except for older school-aged children who are able to move around the community on their own, children should always be under direct adult supervision.

The Child Health Professional as a Parent

No matter how well-educated they are, few parents objectively evaluate their child care arrangements. They tend to deny the presence of clearly evident health and safety hazards, even though they will agree that such hazards are intolerable. With high expectations for job performance, many parents who are professionals suppress doubts about the quality of the care they arrange for their children. Some health professionals prefer in-home care for their own children because these arrangements provide coverage for irregular and long hours. However, competent caregivers who are carefully selected, trained, and supervised in the home are rare. Many caregivers who provide in-home care lack training and experience for this role. In addition, they may be culturally incompatible with the family or may not communicate well in the family's language. All need close supervision, which is hard to arrange in the isolated setting of a private home.

Parents who are health professionals have a special responsibility as community role models. They should seek good care and help to improve the care they find. When they find sanitation problems and safety hazards, they should call attention to these problems. In addition to focused problem solving, child care programs need help from health professionals to plan health and safety training for staff and to review their program's policies and procedures.

The Child Health Professional as a Program Consultant

Child health professionals can become involved as paid or volunteer program consultants. One of their most common roles is as advisors on health problems that have implications for the group. Many standard medical liability insurance policies provide coverage only when a physician-patient relationship exists. However, some carriers will issue a letter that amends the standard language to indicate that the policy will cover advising a child care program as part of the insured physician's consultative role. Before becoming a regular advisor, visit a child care program during the most active time of day (usually early morning until midafternoon) to develop a context for the advice you will give. Watch how well caregivers manage the needs of the equivalent of triplets, quadruplets, and more, while nurturing each child. A visit helps the child health professional to put health and safety issues into perspective and to give advice that fits program constraints.

As a consultant a child health professional also can help plan and provide training for child care providers. Good training materials are available from the American Red Cross, the American Academy of Pediatrics, and Head Start. Child care providers welcome open-ended question-and-answer sessions that require little preparation and build the relationship of the consultant with the staff for later communication and referrals. The children's nap time often may be the only time when caregivers can participate in training activities.

The Child Health Professional as an Advocate for Quality of Care

Research shows that the key determinants of the quality of care are trained teachers, group size, and adult-child ratios that are based on the age and needs of the children served. In 1992 the American Academy of Pediatrics and the American Public Health Association published health and safety performance standards for child care.[1] To improve the quality of care these standards must be disseminated and implemented widely.

Without affordable and accessible early education and child care programs of good quality, children will not come to school eager to learn. The quality of early childhood programs can be improved by systematic planning to set appropriate requirements, good surveillance systems to measure performance, use of surveillance data to design interventions (technical assistance, training, linkages, resource development), ongoing surveillance to determine whether the interventions improve performance, and allocation of societal resources to these activities. Child health professionals can help improve the quality of care in their communities by becoming involved as practitioners, parents, consultants, and advocates.

REFERENCES

1. American Public Health Association and the American Academy of Pediatrics: *Caring for our children, national health and safety performance*

standards: guidelines for out-of-home child care programs, Washington DC and Elk Grove Village, Ill, 1992, American Public Health Association and the American Academy of Pediatrics.
2. Committee on Infectious Diseases of the American Academy of Pediatrics: *Report of the Committee on Infectious Diseases,* ed 23, Elk Grove Village, Ill, 1994, American Academy of Pediatrics.
3. Culkin ML, Helburn S, Morris J: Current price versus full cost: an economic perspective. In Willer B, editor: *Reaching the full cost of quality,* Washington, DC, 1990, National Association for the Education of Young Children.
4. Dawson DA, Cain VS: Child care arrangements: health of our nation's children. In *Advance data from vital and health statistics No 187,* 1990, National Center for Health Statistics.
5. Casper LM: What does it cost to mind our preschoolers? Current Population Reports No P70-52, 1995, Census Bureau.
6. Gunn W et al: Injuries and poisonings in out-of-home child care and home care, *Am J Dis Child* 145:779, 1991.
7. Morgan G et al: *Making a career of it: the state of the states report on career development in early care and education,* Boston, 1993, The Center for Career Development in Early Care and Education at Wheelock College.
8. Osterholm M et al: *Pediatr Infect Dis J* 11:S31, 1992.
9. Reves R, Pickering L: Impact of child day care on infectious diseases in adults, *Infect Dis Clin North Am* 6:239, 1992.
10. Scarr S, Phillips D, McCartney K: Facts, fantasies and the future of child care in the United States, *Psychol Sci* 1:26, 1990.

SUGGESTED READINGS

American Academy of Pediatrics, Committee on Early Childhood, Adoption and Dependent Care: The pediatrician's role in promoting the health of patients in early childhood education and/or child care programs, *Pediatrics* 92:489, 1993.

American Academy of Pediatrics: Part-time care for your child. In *Caring for your baby and young child: birth to age 5,* New York, 1993, Bantam Books.

American Public Health Association and the American Academy of Pediatrics: *Caring for our children, national health and safety performance standards: guidelines for out-of-home child care programs,* Washington DC, and Elk Grove Village, Ill, 1992, American Public Health Association and the American Academy of Pediatrics.

Chehrazi S, editor: *Psychosocial issues in day care,* Washington, DC, 1990, American Psychiatric Press.

Thacker S et al: Infectious diseases and injuries in child day care, *JAMA* 268:1720, 1992.

60 Family Interactions: Children Who Have Unexplained Physical Symptoms

John Sargent

Illness and physical symptoms are physical, psychological, and social events. The family, as the child's primary social context, is affected significantly by a child's physical condition; in turn, the family affects both the child's physical status and psychological well-being.[8] The family, in collaboration with health care providers, is responsible for managing appropriate treatment and promoting the child's psychosocial adaptation. Because of the importance of the family, the investigation and treatment of unexplained physical symptoms should include examination of the interaction between the family and the child.

CHARACTERISTICS OF FAMILIES THAT HAVE CHILDREN WITH PSYCHOSOMATIC DISORDERS

Liebman et al.[4] and Minuchin and colleagues[5,6] investigated the influence of a child's family in maintaining the symptoms of chronic illness and functional physical symptoms. Their work involved children who had recurrent diabetic ketoacidosis and intractable asthma and adolescents who had anorexia nervosa. They studied the patterns of interaction of these families and identified five specific characteristics of family interaction that typified their daily responses and manner of reacting to the child's physical symptoms: (1) enmeshment, (2) overprotection, (3) rigidity, (4) lack of resolving family conflict, and (5) involvement of the symptomatic child in unresolved parental conflict.

Enmeshment refers to an extremely high degree of involvement and responsiveness among family members. Members are exquisitely sensitive to one another, and minor upsets of one individual may lead to rapid attempts of another to restore calm. Relationships can be overly close to the point that individuation and autonomy are sacrificed. Family members report that they feel for one another and that they know what other family members are thinking. Where parents and infants are concerned, enmeshment is an appropriate and necessary quality. However, as a child grows and develops, more distance in family relationships and independence for the child are required. Pathological enmeshment always entails excessive parental involvement for the child's developmental stage. Enmeshment between parents and child also interferes with the child's development of problem-solving skills, since the parents act rapidly to relieve the child's distress rather than require the child to respond to stressful situations. Family members also excessively accommodate viewpoints of others, even when they disagree. Therefore family cohesion is based on submerged and denied family conflict rather than on negotiation, compromise, and agreement.

A child who has a chronic illness, such as diabetes, may become angry about the need for medical treatment and dietary discretion. Parents in "adaptive" families learn to allow the child to become upset while continuing to require necessary adherence to the treatment regimen. In the pathologically enmeshed family, the parents become upset when the child attempts to deny his or her disease and need to comply with its treatment regimens, and the parents attempt to rationalize their nonadherence to the restrictions of the illness and its treatment.[1] The parents also may carry out illness management tasks that the child can perform. Finally, one or both parents may become so involved with the ill child that they recognize the symptoms before the child does. In sum, these family responses seriously inhibit the child's acceptance of the illness and autonomy in learning to manage and control his or her body.

The *overprotectiveness* seen in these families refers to an overly high degree of concern of all family members for one another. Although the ill child is the most obviously vulnerable member of the family, all members are perceived as vulnerable and in need of protection. Evidence of distress in any one family member induces protective responses from the rest of the family. The father may be perceived as explosive and in need of calming, the mother as depressed and in need of paternalistic treatment, and the ill child as sick and weak and in need of care and attention. Immature behavior on the child's part is allowed, and any difficulties that the child might experience at school or with peers lead to pity and excuses from the parents. The parents may try to shield the child from unpleasant events, such as medical procedures, even to the child's physical detriment.

The *rigidity* of these families is demonstrated not only in their attempts to deny family problems and to repeat the same ineffective solutions over and over but also in their desire to maintain fixed relationships among one another, even when development or stress requires change. Each family member states steadfastly that he or she cannot alter how he or she or others behave, regardless of the need for change. A mother will report that she cannot bring her husband to the doctor's office or hospital no matter how ill the child is. A father will insist that he cannot assist his wife in following through with illness treatment for their child (e.g., giving insulin injections by himself). The child will state that he cannot help his parents understand his feelings about his chronic illness. These protestations of incompetence persist, thereby increasing the overall family stress and leading to a deterioration in the child's condition and further ineffective family responses, resulting in a circular pattern. These families appear to be in a tenuous balance, with any change seen as highly threatening.

Disagreement and conflict exist in all families. However, in those families in which a member has a psychosomatic disorder, to maintain these rigid patterns of extreme closeness and protectiveness, *conflict is denied* and therefore unresolved. Family members contradict themselves to maintain a facade of agreement, and an immediate consensus develops concerning even small issues of disagreement. If a consensus cannot be achieved immediately, distractions occur that dissipate the conflict, or the disagreeing family members avoid one another until the situation calms. There is an air of chronic tension in the family, which is reinforced by avoidance, denial, or outright capitulation by one member. These unresolved disagreements may involve any aspect of family life; however, the physician should note in particular that the parents do not resolve differences of opinion about the ill child and management of his or her disease.[1]

Finally, when conflict occurs between the parents, the ill child becomes involved in the disagreement, distracting attention to himself or herself and thus reducing the disagreement significantly. The balance of harmony and consensus is then restored. The child often is asked to mediate between the parents; at times he or she sides with one parent against the other; at other times the parents unite (leaving their disagreement) either to protect and nurture the sick child or to attack the child and blame him or her for all family troubles. Chronic marital strife is reinforced as more and more disagreements remain unresolved. Yet, often because of the child's illness or symptoms, neither parent leaves the family. The ill child remains highly vigilant to future family disagreements and experiences, increasing stress as family tension persists. It is precisely at the point of parental disagreement and personal stress that the child becomes symptomatic, requiring medical care and hospitalization. The cycle then begins again.

Thus the child's participation in parental conflict reduces physical and psychological distress in the parents but induces symptoms in the labile child. The family's patterns of interaction induce symptoms in the child, while the child's symptoms assist the family in maintaining stability. Minuchin and colleagues[5,6] found that these family characteristics occurred in families who had children with unexplained (functional) physical symptoms, regardless of the child's primary diagnosis. Although all families engage in enmeshed, protective, and conflict-avoiding interactions, some families engage in these patterns inordinately, even when such patterns are unproductive. This does not mean that the family causes the insulin deficiency of diabetes or the reactive airway diathesis of asthma. The physiological differences in these children are specific vulnerabilities that are affected by the family and other factors to become repeatedly symptomatic. Thus functional or unexplained symptoms become a circular process, reinforcing and reinforced by the child's vulnerability and the family's characteristic patterns of interaction.

Criticisms of this model have pointed out the lack of consistent data supporting the existence of all of these features in families of children who have unexplained physical symptoms.[2,3] Minuchin's description of the family also has been interpreted as blaming parents for the child's physical difficulties and psychosocial problems. These authors have emphasized that the family does not cause the child's symptoms and that unexplained symptoms in a child often cause significant stress for a family and worsen any interactional difficulties a family might have.

Wood[11] has suggested that families who have children who have unexplained physical symptoms have two factors that highlight their situation: (1) biobehavioral reactivity among members, which renders them exquisitely sensitive, physically and emotionally, to one another and (2) poor collaboration among parental figures, leading to marked difficulty dealing with the uncertainty, stress, and confusion associated with persistent unexplained physical symptoms.

IMPLICATIONS FOR THE PEDIATRICIAN

Diagnosis

Assessment of the family, including both parents, is essential in evaluating situations in which a child's illness becomes repeatedly symptomatic at home and yet is controlled easily in the hospital.[7,10] The pediatrician should note how family members behave with one another and should question each member directly about his or her impressions of the causes of the child's frequent symptoms. The pediatrician can suggest to family members that they discuss the problem together and can observe their nonverbal responses when other members are talking. The pediatrician will need to attend to the process of family interaction, as well as to the content of their statements.

These families typically are well informed about their child's medical condition, and they understand and carry out treatment. However, they often appear helpless and defeated, relating to the physician in a dependent and demanding fashion. Parental overprotectiveness is common, and the enmeshment within the family is demonstrated as parent and child constantly maintain eye contact, speak for one another, and sit very close together. Therefore the physician often will find it difficult to develop an interdependent relationship with the child. The father also may be devalued and thus may appear disinterested and unsympathetic. The parents may present differing views of the situation, and when asked to reconcile these different perceptions, they are unable to do so. The child often is immature or pseudomature and frequently clings to one parent. He or she usually has limited peer relationships and is the primary focus of parental attention because of the symptoms. The child's lack of insight and general sense of helplessness often are striking. Finally, both family and symptomatic child readily deny psychological difficulties, and all maintain a strongly somatic orientation.

Pediatric Interventions

The pediatrician's primary goal in these situations is to gain the family's trust and collaboration in the evaluation and with treatment. The physician should not challenge the reality of the child's physical symptoms and should ensure that the appropriate medical evaluation is completed. Results of medical evaluations should be presented clearly and directly and with compassion and support. Through honesty and empathy the pediatrician can enlist the family's trust, accept family difficulties, and create, with family and child involvement, a treatment plan for further assessment that will foster the child's development.

When caring for a physically symptomatic child, the pediatrician, noting significant parental involvement and protectiveness, can help the parents require more independence from their child. If the physician determines that the parents disagree about how to accomplish this and thus are rendered ineffective, he or she can stress the need for them to act cooperatively. The pediatrician also can ensure that the child is participating in school and in activities with peers. Regular follow-up will be necessary to determine if the parents can cooperate and encourage more maturity from their child and also if that maturity leads to improvements in the child's physical condition.[9] If the child improves, the pediatrician will need to watch for signs of marital distress in the parents. He or she then can discuss with the parents the need to resolve their differences either independently or through psychotherapy. Three principles should guide the pediatrician's efforts: (1) attend first to the physical and psychological difficulties of the ill child before attempting to address stress in the marriage directly; (2) in working with the family, develop and maintain an attitude that places responsibility on them to ensure their child's physical and psychosocial adjustment; and (3) pursue regular follow-up care with the family to ensure that progress is maintained.

Referral for family psychotherapy is indicated in situations in which the ill child demonstrates serious emotional and behavioral immaturity or in which his or her illness is so labile that he or she is hospitalized repeatedly, which leads to school absence, further social isolation, and worsening parental concern.[7,9] Referral also is indicated when the parents are unable to decrease overinvolvement and overprotectiveness with the physician's assistance or to develop and carry out cooperative methods of dealing with the ill child. Before referral, the pediatrician must identify the child's physical condition accurately and outline appropriate medical treatment. All physicians involved in the child's care must agree on the diagnosis, treatment, and recommendation for family therapy. The therapist should be familiar and comfortable with family-oriented treatment of serious physical and emotional disorders in children.[10] In the treatment of these disorders, the physician and family therapist collaborate. The therapist can best be introduced to the family as a professional who will help them manage their child's illness or symptoms more effectively and assist them in reducing the stressful effects of the child's symptoms on both child and family. The physician further can state that therapy is a highly important part of treatment and that without therapy the physician will continue to be ineffective in reducing the symptoms. The family should not perceive the referral for therapy as implying blame for their problems. Rather, it can be described as an opportunity for the family and physician to improve the child's condition.

Pediatrician-Therapist Collaboration

The pediatrician actively assists the course of therapy by answering the medical questions of the family directly and by informing the family of the improvements that should be achieved through their work with the therapist. Both professionals will need to support each other's efforts and encourage the family to resolve differences straightforwardly with each of them. The physician should avoid answering psychological questions that the family raises and should inform the family that these issues will need to be addressed with the therapist. This support enables the family to work directly with the therapist and resolve any disagreements they may have with him or her straightforwardly. It also prevents the family from pitting the therapist against the physician during treatment. The therapist, in turn, refers any medical questions the family raises to the physician. During the initial phases of family treatment, the child's medical condition may worsen, and short-term emergencies may develop at stressful points during the therapy. Both the therapist and the physician need to be available to the family at these times. By maintaining a mutually supportive relationship and open communication, the pediatrician and the family therapist can assist one another through difficult phases of treatment. Working together, pediatrician, therapist, and family can improve the child's physical and psychological condition dramatically.

REFERENCES

1. Baker L et al: Psychosomatic aspects of juvenile diabetes mellitus: a progress report, *Mod Probl Paediatr* 12:332, 1975.
2. Coyne JC, Anderson BJ: The "psychosomatic family" reconsidered. I. Diabetes in context, *Marital Fam Ther* 14:113, 1988.
3. Coyne JC, Anderson BJ: The "psychosomatic family" reconsidered. II. Recalling a defective model and looking ahead, *J Marital Fam Ther* 15:139, 1989.
4. Liebman R, Minuchin S, Baker L: The use of structural family therapy in the treatment of intractable asthma, *Am J Psychiatry* 131:535, 1974.
5. Minuchin S et al: A conceptual model of psychosomatic illness in childhood, *Arch Gen Psychiatry* 32:1031, 1975.
6. Minuchin S, Rosman BL, Baker L: *Psychosomatic families: anorexia nervosa in context*, Cambridge, Mass, 1978, Harvard University Press.
7. Sargent J: The family and childhood psychosomatic disorders, *Gen Hosp Psychiatry* 5:41, 1983.
8. Sargent J: The sick child: family complications, *J Behav Develop Pediatr* 4:50, 1983.
9. Sargent J: Physician-family therapist collaboration: children with medical problems, *Family Systems Medicine* 3:454, 1985.
10. Sargent J, Liebman R: Childhood chronic illness: issues for psychotherapists, *Community Ment Health J* 21:294, 1985.
11. Wood B: Proximity and hierarchy: orthogonal dimensions of family interconnectedness, *Fam Process* 24:487, 1985.

61 Family-Centered Care in Pediatric Practice

W. Carl Cooley

CHANGING VIEW OF FAMILIES

Pediatricians, like most physicians, have been taught to watch for deviations from normal and to recognize the occurrence of pathology. Pediatric training concentrates on the abnormal functioning of biological or behavioral systems, etiological identification, and the interventions necessary to correct or ameliorate altered function. This is, to some degree, appropriate, for there is much to know, and competence is the first expectation that parents have of their child's pediatrician. But even with its emphasis on the prevention of disease, pediatric practice should extend beyond pathology to embrace the strengths that individual children and families possess and to promote their health. Advocating for healthy life-styles, supporting behaviors that protect children from exploitation or abuse, teaching self-care for children who have chronic conditions, and facilitating the development of self-confidence and self-esteem are important pediatric endeavors that now are finding a place in curricula and textbooks.

Pediatricians long have recognized that most children live in the context of families. Family ecology has been portrayed as a homeostatic system in which the interrelationships among the elements (parents, siblings, extended family) exert complex, but to some degree predictable, tensions on each other. The theory of family systems viewed families like biological systems, seeking balance and equilibrium but disturbed by the stresses introduced when one family member is ill, disabled, or behaviorally disruptive. Though helpful in emphasizing the need to attend to the status of all family members, family systems theory and related therapeutic interventions extend to the family the same focus on pathology that has been overemphasized in our approach to individual patients.

Just as pediatricians should identify and nourish sources of strength and resilience in the individual children for whom they care, they also must understand families in the same light. Newer research about families that are stressed by poverty, isolation, or raising a child who has a chronic illness has abandoned hypotheses that assume pathological outcomes. Using open-ended, qualitative methodologies, studies have found that most families use healthy strategies to cope with stress, that the characteristics of resilient families can be identified (see the box on p. 641) and even taught to other families, and that families often identify different stressors than those predicted by clinicians or researchers.[5,7] Pediatricians can help families by inquiring about major stressors from the family's perspective, coping strategies the family has used in the past, obstacles to coping or stress reduction, and sources of social support (extended family, friends, church) upon which the family relies. Evidence of poor coping with past crises or the absence of social supports is predictive of low resilience and potential breakdown when multiple stressors accumulate.

DEFINITION OF FAMILY

The family is defined in many ways and clearly has taken many forms in contemporary life. The definition of family that we choose not only determines what we mean by family-centered care, but also incorporates the values by which we provide pediatric care. The New Mexico Coalition for Children, Youth, and Families developed the following definition of family*:

> We all come from families. Families are big, small, extended, nuclear, multi-generational, with one parent, two parents, and grandparents. We live under one roof or many. A family can be as temporary as a few weeks, or as permanent as forever. We become part of a family by birth, adoption, marriage, or from a desire for mutual support. As family members, we nurture, protect, and influence each other. Families are dynamic and are cultures unto themselves, with different values and unique ways of realizing dreams. Together, our families become the source of our rich cultural heritage and spiritual diversity. Each family has strengths that flow from the individual members and from the family as a unit. Our families create neighborhoods, communities, states, and nations.

Families who seek pediatric care usually do so in the pursuit of better health for their children. This may mean for the treatment of a worrisome condition (fever, headache, diarrhea), for a better understanding of confusing symptoms, for advice about behavioral or educational problems, or for the prevention of illness. In most instances, families seek reduction of stress and worry about their child and reassurance that they are doing the best they can under the circumstances. However, each family enters the relationship with a pediatrician with its own personal and cultural history, its own set of perceptions about health and health care, and its own expectations about outcomes. It is unlikely that these characteristics will always be the same as those of the physician or in every way consistent with the physician's perceptions and values. Pediatricians must be able to define families in a way that acknowledges and respects their diversity without subordinating responsibility for the well-being of each child.

FAMILY-CENTERED CARE

In the late 1970s and early 1980s, the child life movement began fostering new ways of caring for children in hospitals. These new methods involved making the hospital experience less threatening by incorporating age-appropriate activities into the hospital environment, providing for the rooming-in of parents and involving them in a child's hospital care, and acknowledging and responding to the fears and confusion experienced by hospitalized children. The evolution of these methods eventually led to the formulation of the Elements

*From New Mexico Coalition for Children, Youth, and Families and New Mexico Young Children's Continuum, 1990.

THE NINE ASPECTS OF RESILIENT FAMILY PROCESS

1. Balancing illness or other stressors with other family needs
2. Maintaining clear family boundaries
3. Developing communication competence
4. Attributing positive meanings to difficult situations
5. Maintaining family flexibility
6. Maintaining a commitment to the family as a unit
7. Engaging in active coping efforts
8. Maintaining social integration
9. Developing collaborative relationships with professionals

Adapted from Patterson JM: *Pediatr Ann* 20:492, 1991.

of Family Centered Care by the Association for the Care of Children's Health in 1987.[4] In the same year, the Surgeon General of the United States published his report on children who have special health care needs, which mandated a commitment to family-centered care.[8] Since then, family-centered practice has become the standard of care among many health, mental health, early intervention, and education professionals. The elements outlined in the box on the right provide benchmarks against which pediatricians should measure their own behaviors, the organization of their offices, and the operation of the hospitals in which they practice.

During the 1980s a convergence of consumerism, policy developments, and research led to the formulation of a new relationship between child care professionals and families. The essence of this new relationship is *partnership*. When families feel like active participants in their children's care, their sense of competence in providing care increases. Characterized by some as empowerment, the process of building a caring partnership between families and professionals is seen by some as being as important as the outcomes of care.[3] Pediatricians are ideally placed to empower families by involving them as partners rather than as passive recipients of care.[2]

PRIMARY CARE SETTINGS

Translating the Elements of Family Centered Care into day-to-day practice in a primary care setting involves thoughtful planning and self-conscious effort. Every pediatric practice should design and implement a method of quality assurance and consumer feedback. This may take the form of consumer satisfaction surveys on a periodic basis or comment forms enclosed with bills or other mailings to patients. Some practices may choose to organize a family council that meets periodically to formulate suggestions for physicians and office staff. Since 10% to 15% of the children in any pediatric practice are affected by chronic conditions, efforts should be made to hear the concerns of specific families who experience the added health care needs of such children.

Families who are new to a primary care practice should be offered an initial visit in which family information is gathered and roles and expectations are made explicit. In this process, parents can define their needs for pediatric care, and the physician can explain his or her interpretation of the primary care physician's role. This meeting offers an opportunity to reconcile differences between a family's expectations and a physician's capacities and practice style. When a child is found to have a chronic illness or disability, an explicit redefinition of roles may be necessary to avoid confusion, for example, about the division of responsibility between specialists and primary care providers, about procedures for communication with schools and other agencies, and about the provision of care coordination or case management services.

THE KEY ELEMENTS OF FAMILY-CENTERED CARE

- Recognizing that the family is the constant in a child's life, while the service systems and personnel within those systems fluctuate
- Facilitating family/professional collaboration at all levels of health care
- Honoring the racial, ethnic, cultural, and socioeconomic diversity of families
- Recognizing family strengths and individuality and respecting different methods of coping with stressors
- Sharing with parents complete and unbiased information on a continuing basis and in a supportive manner
- Encouraging and facilitating family-to-family support and networking
- Understanding and incorporating the developmental needs of infants, children, and adolescents and their families into health care systems
- Implementing comprehensive policies and programs that provide emotional and financial support to meet the needs of families
- Designing accessible health care systems that are flexible, culturally competent, and responsive to family-identified needs

From Johnson BH, Jeppson ES, Redburn L: *Caring for children and families: guidelines for hospitals,* Bethesda, Md, 1992, Association for the Care of Children's Health.

Physicians in primary care need to be knowledgeable about resources for families in their communities and states. State agencies responsible for special services such as clinics for children who have special health care needs, early intervention services, special education, family support services for children who have disabilities, Medicaid programs and other entitlements should be contacted for current information about eligibility and intake procedures. Physicians should be aware of parent support organizations in their state or region and of the availability of parent-to-parent services that link parents of children with special needs to one another. Most states are now required to have an accessible resource guide for family services under each state's plan for early intervention services.

THE PEDIATRICIAN AS RELIABLE ALLY FOR FAMILIES

Families who cope successfully with challenges, such as the prolonged hospitalization of a prematurely born infant or the occurrence of a disability in a child, usually have a number of strengths in common. Most important among those strengths is access to social support.[6] Families without social supports become not only socially and emotionally isolated, but also fail to access tangible aid such as financial assistance and respite care and informational supports that enhance their self-confidence and mastery over their circumstances. The social supports that families require begin with the informal, natural supports of extended family, friends, and community, extending when necessary to include the formal supports of professionals and social service agencies.[1]

Families who have strong social support systems usually identify individuals among both their formal and informal networks upon whom they depend as resources. The relationships with these dependable resources may be described as reliable alliances. Reliable alliances are characterized by mutual respect, mutual trust, common goals and visions, sharing of information, and a shared stake in the outcomes. Though families will naturally identify those who are reliable allies within their support systems, pediatricians who aspire to this sort of relationship with families not only will provide more effective care, but also will nourish themselves in the process.

REFERENCES

1. Cooley WC: The ecology of support for caregiving families, *Journal of Behavioral and Developmental Pediatrics* 15:15, 1994.
2. Cooley WC: Pediatric training and family-centered care. In Darling R, Peter M, editors: *Families, physicians, and children with special health care needs: collaborative medical education models,* Boston, 1994, Greenwood Press.
3. Dunst C, Trivette C, Deal A: *Enabling and empowering families: principles and guidelines for practice,* Cambridge, Mass, 1988, Brookline Books.
4. Johnson BH, Jeppson ES, Redburn L: *Caring for children and families: guidelines for hospitals,* Washington, DC, 1992, Association for the Care of Children's Health.
5. Patterson JM: Family resilience to the challenge of a child's disability, *Pediatr Ann* 20:491, 1991.
6. Singer GHS, Irvin LK: Family caregiving, stress, and support. In Singer GHS, Irvin LK, editors: *Support for caregiving families,* Baltimore, 1989, Paul Brookes.
7. Summers JA, Behr SK, Turnbull AP: Positive adaptation and coping strengths of families who have children with disabilities. In Singer GHS, Irvin LK, editors: *Support for caregiving families,* Baltimore, 1989, Paul Brookes.
8. *Surgeon General's report on children with special health care needs,* DHHS Pub No HRS/D/MC87-2, Rockville, Md, 1987, United States Department of Health and Human Services.

SUGGESTED READINGS

Brewer EJ et al: Family-centered, community-based, coordinated care for children with special health care needs, *Pediatrics* 83:1055, 1989.

Liptak GS, Revell GM: Community physician's role in the case management of children with chronic illness, *Pediatrics* 84:465, 1989.

Sia CCJ: Medical home and child advocacy in the 1990s, *Pediatrics* 90:419, 1992.

62 Health Needs of Parents

Henry M. Seidel

The health needs of parents, like those of children, are determined by physical, social, and emotional factors. Because pediatric practitioners basically are advocates of the child, they do not, as a rule, view the parent in isolation—that is, as an individual who has needs that may not always include the child as a prime factor. It is essential to the care of the child, however, to understand the differing characteristics of the various groupings possible within a family. For example, given a family of three—mother, father, and child—the various "units" include each of them as individuals, the group of three, and the three dyads—mother-father, mother-child, father-child—a total of seven combinations. Thus a family of four would have 13 such units. The characteristic of a given unit varies with infinite subtlety, depending on the particular combination and the basis of the interaction in which it may be involved at any given time. Thus appropriate care of the child requires an understanding of the parent and that parent's own health needs.

Among the physical, social, and emotional needs of the parent, primary care practitioners are most likely to become involved with the emotional. Within their individual practices and in the broader public arena, pediatricians often have acted as "experts," suggesting "principles" to parents regarding their relationship with their children and their life-styles. One effect of this advice in recent decades has been a diminution in the self-confidence of parents, a loss of their ability to resort to common sense, and a consequent breach in their composure and naturalness. In the latter part of the twentieth century, their sense of direction often has been confused by the dizzying impact of the audiovisual media and increasing evidence of disruptions in the family.

The care of children might be improved if we, as a society, took greater advantage of the resources inherent in the intelligence, humor, and judgment of parents. To work with and presume to advise parents, pediatricians must seek to exploit these resources, putting aside value judgments and the occasional impulse to preach. Perhaps their major contribution to the health needs of parents can be to make available an objective listening ear and provide the opportunity to achieve a balanced viewpoint together.

Determining the extent to which pediatricians should become involved with the health needs of parents is a problem. For example, should pediatric practitioners take care of the sore throat of a child but not of that child's parent? Is it appropriate, when both are in the office, to send the older person off to another setting at the cost of convenience, dollars, and delay? Much of the response will depend on factors such as the following:

An objective assessment of one's experience and competency. Much in the primary care of the adult requires a technical sophistication that a pediatrician may not be able to invoke with appropriate confidence.

The circumstance of the particular family and the individual parent's access to care. The burdens of additional cost or an unreasonable wait for care elsewhere should be alleviated if possible. Often, transportation is a problem.

The equipment and the physical setting available. One is not likely to diagnose and treat a vaginal discharge in a parent if the appropriate examining table is not at hand.

The practitioner's concern over the possibility of a malpractice action. The risk is greater if the boundaries of one's specialty are extended.

It is practical to limit involvement to those aspects of parental health that are immediately relevant to the child. There is a gray area, an unspoken constraint on going beyond the limits of one's certified area of competence, the constraint imposed by the generally accepted apportionment of medical responsibilities *and* economic rewards to the various health care specialties. The practitioner then is left to judge the parent's need and decide accordingly. That judgment is easier in the following instances.

THE ADOLESCENT PARENT

The adolescent parent has needs that require total care from a professional who has a sound perspective on the young. A poignant example is that of the teenage, unmarried mother who elects to raise her child and who sees and treats that child as a "baby doll." The professional can provide a sensitive understanding of the interdependencies of that dyad and a ready availability both to the mother when she needs reassurance about her own self-worth when her baby does not behave perfectly and also to the baby when the mother "acts out" in frustration.

THE ABUSED PARENT OF THE BATTERED CHILD

The origins of child abuse are set most often in the socially disorganized childhood experience of the parent. To end the abuse and preserve the family, the parent must be included within the caring and the curing efforts of the professionals involved. The parent should be "gathered in" rather than "referred out" as much as possible. Fragmentation of service to the individuals concerned, with the consequent requirement of a difficult to achieve, sensitive communication among too many persons, lessens the likelihood of successful treatment.

THE PARENTS OF FIRSTBORNS

Anticipatory guidance is a major responsibility of primary care practitioners and reflects a common need in parents, especially those who are parents for the first time. For example, the emotionally nourishing interdependence of the man-woman dyad before the birth of a child easily may be threatened by the mother's diminishing ability to attend to the care and feeding of the father. Resentment and a strain on the bond between the parents may develop.

THE SICK OR POTENTIALLY SICK PARENT

Many instances arise in which pediatricians can extend care to parents as a result of their involvement with the child. Depression in the parent is a good example. If depression can be described as a feeling of helplessness resulting from a wide gap between one's perception of who one is and who one should be, then it is easy to understand the stress imposed by child rearing and the role of the pediatrician in reacting sensitively to parental symptoms.

While depression is discussed more completely elsewhere (see Chapter 103), it is important to note here that the impact of maternal mood on infants and children has been well documented. An infant given to extended periods of distressed crying may provide a clue to stress in a mother who needs attention and counseling. Indeed, a wide range of child behaviors—for example, breath-holding, failure to thrive, many visits to the doctor for hard to define illness, temper tantrums, disturbed sleep—should prompt an inquiry that includes both parents. If they, individually or together, seem to derive no fun from life or pleasure in the child, express unreasonable guilt, find it difficult to make decisions, are withdrawn and without spontaneity—among many other possible clues—the possibility—indeed the *probability*—of depression should be considered.

Although the day of the house call largely is past, it still is possible in the office or clinic (without observing the home) to sense the presence of alcoholism or inappropriate dependency on drugs as a problem within some families. In addition, illness detected in the child should alert one to the possibility of a related condition in the parent. Obviously, for genetically determined diseases, access to genetic counseling and discussions aimed at resolving parental guilt must be sought. In fact, a sensitivity to the potential of parental guilt must be a common denominator in the development of a management plan for all childhood illness. Clinical evidence of physical abnormality in a child should initiate appropriate screening for similar findings in the parent. Obvious environmental and genetic examples are tuberculosis, venereal disease, streptococcal disease, lead poisoning, hearing loss, and glucose-6-phosphate dehydrogenase deficiency. The less obvious circumstance includes increased susceptibility to major psychic disturbance in the relatives of children who have phenylketonuria.

PARENTS INVOLVED IN MARITAL CONFLICT OR DIVORCE

Marital conflict is a major source of "morbidity" among children today. Statistically, nearly one divorce occurs for every two marriages each year. There is, on average, one child per divorce; therefore, divorce is a factor in many children's lives. Moreover, because the median duration of marriage is slightly more than 7 years, most divorces affect young children. The father becomes the noncustodial parent 90% of the time; however, the tendency in this direction is shifting somewhat, and there currently are arrangements in which parents attempt to share the care of the child equally. We must remember that divorce is a process and not a discrete pathological entity to which psychological disturbances in children can be neatly ascribed. It is in the precursors of divorce that one finds the psychopathological root in the child and the parents. There are competing priorities for the attention of health professionals, who must walk a fine line, recognizing the priority of the child and the imperative that, in serving that priority, they do not "take sides" with one or the other parent. Although they cannot ignore parental need, they must cooperate in the search for an outcome that provides the optimum nurturance for the child with appropriate support for each parent.

Thus the responsibility that the pediatric practitioner may have to the health needs of parents often is significant and recurrent. The degree of need and the practitioner's consequent involvement may depend on a judgment based on some of the variables already mentioned and on an assessment of the psychosocial competence of the parents involved. There may at times be a competition for loyalties. It is likely that most practitioners will choose in favor of the child. In this regard, the practitioner would do well to ponder, for example, the development of a therapeutic plan for the child born having a meningomyelocele, or the content of subpoenaed testimony in a divorce action when each adult has legal representation but the child has none, or that due process is not extended fully to children in our society. There is a point, then, when the pediatric practitioner must refer the parent elsewhere for medical assistance and emotional support if for no other reasons than the requirement of technical skills or the priority of child advocacy.

SUGGESTED READINGS

Beardslee WR, McMillan HL: Psychosocial preventive intervention for families with parental mood disorders: strategies for the clinician, *J Dev Behav Pediatr* 14:271, 1993.

Green M: Maternal depression: bad for children's health, *Contemporary Pediatrics* 10:28, 1993.

Guyer B et al: Annual summary of vital statistics: 1994, *Pediatrics* 96:1029, 1995.

Miller AR, Barr RG, Eaton WO: Crying and motor behavior of 6-week-old infants and postpartum maternal mood, *Pediatrics* 92:551, 1993.

Zuckerman BS, Beardslee WR: Maternal depression: a concern for pediatricians, *Pediatrics* 79:110, 1987.

63 Latchkey Children: Children in Self-Care

Rickey L. Williams

An estimated 8 to 10 million American children younger than 18 years of age are in self-care (i.e., the child is by himself or herself) before or after school; 2 to 5 million of these "latchkey" children are grade schoolers 6 to 13 years of age.[4] Even greater numbers of children are cared for by older siblings. In this era of single-parent families and families that have two employed parents, many children must return to an empty home after school. In many communities affordable, conveniently located care programs are unavailable or have long waiting lists; parents in such communities might leave a child in self-care because they have no alternative. Some parents simply may be unwilling to pay for child care or feel that self-care (i.e., the child is by herself or himself) is acceptable. In addition, many parents fear that baby-sitters or program personnel may abuse their children; they may feel more comfortable leaving their child home alone than at a center or with a baby-sitter. And, of course, there will never be enough centers and personnel to permit every child to be supervised adequately in a program.

Even if adequate child care is arranged, children might at times take care of themselves, especially during minor illnesses. Working parents may find it difficult to leave their jobs for each mild communicable illness that their children acquire; day care centers frequently exclude children who have a fever, are vomiting, have diarrhea, or have other communicable diseases.[9]

Pediatricians may not be familiar with self-care. In a publication for pediatricians entitled "Child Care and the Pediatrician," almost no mention was made of self-care.[1] In contrast to the amount of attention and research focused on day care centers, virtually no research has been carried out on the various informal care arrangements for school-age children, even though there are far more children in such arrangements than in formal day care centers.[8] Research on children in self-care is difficult because the self-care status of a particular child may not remain stable over time because of several factors, including parental employment, economic necessity, and the availability of other types of care. Parents responding to surveys regarding children in self-care may not be willing to admit that their children are or were left alone.[4]

EFFECTS OF SELF-CARE

The effects of self-care on children are unknown and depend on many factors, including the child's age and maturity level, the circumstances surrounding the reason for the child being in self-care, and the community in which the child lives. Hypothesized benefits of self-care include increased maturity, self-reliance, decision making, freedom, and responsibility.[6] Negative aspects of self-care include feeling or actually being neglected, in danger, isolated, or at medical risk.[4] One report suggests that many children in self-care fear attack from intruders and from other children, particularly siblings.[7] Children in sibling care may be at greater risk for negative effects on self-esteem and social development. Children in self-care also may experience more social isolation after school than children in other forms of after-school care.[2] Some children in self-care will thrive, some will just manage to cope with the situation, and others actually will be harmed in some way.[3]

Studies of academic achievement and school adjustment among children in self-care have yielded mixed results. Some studies reported social problems and lower academic achievement among children in self-care compared with other children of working mothers who had adult supervision[13]; other studies found no differences in academic achievement, self-competence, or school adjustment between those children in self-care and those in adult care.[5,8,11] One study found that the less directly supervised children were, the more susceptible they were to peer pressure.[10]

Are children in self-care less physically fit or less healthy than those in adult care? One can postulate that children in self-care are at especially high risk for obesity, since they are less likely to be permitted to play outside after school than are children in adult care or sibling care.[7] However, one study found no differences in weight or body mass index between children in self-care and those in adult care.[12] In addition, there were no differences between the two groups of children in the number of school days missed or in the number of visits to the school health office.

Parents of children in self-care might feel guilty that they are leaving their children alone, and articles in the lay press suggest that being in self-care has negative consequences. For example, a majority of parents and teachers in one poll believed that students would perform better in the classroom if adults did not leave the youngsters by themselves routinely after school.

THE PEDIATRICIAN'S ROLE

Pediatric health professionals cannot reverse maternal employment and child care trends. They can, however, advocate for children by counseling individual parents about self-care of their children and by supporting the establishment of affordable, after-school, high-quality care programs in their communities.

In addition, anticipatory guidance during health supervision visits for those children identified as being in self-care could include age-appropriate advice on safety issues such as personal protection, guns, fires, cooking, and basic first aid. The pediatrician also should recommend that the child have appropriate telephone numbers (including the physician's office number) available in case of emergency.

REFERENCES

1. Aronson S: Child care and the pediatrician, *Pediatr Rev* 10:277, 1989.
2. Berman BD et al: After-school child care and self-esteem in school-age children, *Pediatrics* 89:654, 1992.
3. Coolsen P, Seligson M, Garbarino J: *When school's out and nobody's home,* Chicago, 1985, National Committee for Prevention of Child Abuse.
4. Fosarelli PD: Latchkey children, *J Dev Behav Pediatr* 5:173, 1984.
5. Galambos NL, Garbarino J: Identifying the missing links in the study of latchkey children, *Child Today* 12:2, 1983.
6. Garbarino J: Latchkey children: getting the short end of the stick, *Vital Issues* 30:1, 1980.
7. Long T, Long L: Latchkey children: the child's view of self care, *ERIC Doc ED* 211229, 1981.
8. Rodman H, Pratto DJ, Nelson RS: Child care arrangements and children's functioning: a comparison of self-care and adult-care children, *Dev Psychol* 21:413, 1985.
9. Shapiro ED: Exclusion of ill children from day-care centers: policy and practice in New Haven, Connecticut, *Clin Pediatr* 23:689, 1984.
10. Steinberg L: Latchkey children and susceptibility to peer pressure: an ecological analysis, *Dev Psychol* 22:433, 1986.
11. Vandell DL, Corasaniti MA: The relation between third graders' after-school care and social, academic, and emotional functioning, *Child Dev* 59:868, 1988.
12. Williams RL, Boyce WT: Health status of children in self-care, *Am J Dis Child* 143:112, 1989.
13. Woods M: The unsupervised child of the working mother, *Dev Psychol* 6:14, 1972.

SUGGESTED READING

Padilla M, Landreth G: Latchkey children: a review of the literature, *Child Welfare* 68:445, 1989.

64 Teaching Parents about Effective Discipline

Ellen C. Perrin

WHAT IS DISCIPLINE?

The word discipline has its root in the Latin word *disciplinare,* which means to teach. Discipline refers to the structure created by parents to teach their children how they are expected to behave. The term discipline often is used in a much more limited fashion to refer only to punishment. Punishment, however, is only a very small part of the total parenting environment that helps children feel safe, capable, and lovable and helps parents feel effective.

Pediatricians are in an important position to help parents create a constructive pattern of discipline, fostering optimal interaction and teaching. The pediatrician may be the only, or at least the most accessible, professional who knows children and their families during the preschool period. Even later in children's development pediatricians remain important anchors for parents as they negotiate the ever-changing challenges of parenting. Thus pediatricians have the opportunity (and thereby the responsibility) to help parents in their efforts to provide the best possible context for growth.

The longitudinal role of primary care pediatricians dictates their continuing involvement from initial guidance about effective parenting through help with the management of any serious dysfunction. Pediatricians can empower parents and provide anticipatory guidance and advice about methods to structure the family environment to avoid difficulties.[1,2,6,7]

Pediatricians also have the opportunity to monitor children's behavior and development and to recognize and advise parents about observed or described problems with children's behavior early in their course, thus preventing more serious behavioral or emotional dysfunction. In addition, they are critical participants in the management of more serious behavioral or emotional dysfunction; some pediatricians may be able to provide some counseling themselves, and all pediatricians can help families by referring them to respected colleagues in the mental health professions (see Chapter 93).

WHEN SHOULD DISCIPLINE BE DISCUSSED?

Because effective discipline is so central to parenting, its discussion should be a part of every health supervision visit. The earliest discussions about discipline can occur within the first few months of life. Parents' attempts to organize the family's schedule around the infant's eating and sleeping routines are among their earliest efforts at defining and agreeing on a set of rules or limits. Another opportunity to help parents discuss and agree on appropriate rules occurs as children become mobile and parents begin to create and maintain safety guidelines. The requirement to keep their child safe is accepted by parents quite universally, encouraging a discussion of optimal limits that must be set and a structure by which they can be taught and enforced. The pediatrician can point out to parents that in determining methods of keeping their child from falling down the stairs, poking objects into electrical outlets, or pouring hot liquids on himself or herself, they have defined their expectations and some of their earliest rules. When parents recognize that they must discuss and agree on rules to create a safe structure, they begin to recognize their own power in communicating their expectations for their child's behavior. This empowerment is one step along the arduous trail by which parents create a safe, nurturing environment and help their children to learn the appropriate standards of adult behavior. Table 64-1 provides some guidelines of other developmental periods when discussion about discipline can be woven usefully into the context of health supervision visits.

BASIC PRINCIPLES AND TECHNIQUES

Parents generally want to do what's best for their children. They may be limited by inadequate knowledge of appropriate strategies and techniques, by depression or anxiety, by overwhelming challenges of their own life situations, anger, or psychopathology. The box on p. 648 outlines several basic principles underlying effective discipline. It is important to remember that each child exists in the context of a complex family that is an interactive system. The behavior of any member of the family affects in complicated ways the behavior of all members of the family. A family can be imagined to be carrying out its life on a waterbed: each time one member moves, complicated ripples and counter-ripples affect the movements of everyone else. It also is important to remember that parents work primarily on intuition and on the basis of their experiences as children. While parenting is among the most difficult and the most important jobs we have as adults, it is the one for which we have the least training and support. Pediatricians can be very important in providing support for parents, some direction to parents' observations, and guidance if they need help.

Parents can use several specific strategies to help their children feel loved and capable. The first is "alone time" with the child (see the box on p. 648). This refers to a short but structured period of time, 15 to 30 minutes, that each parent has with each child on a predictable schedule. During this time, the parent and child interact one-on-one, and no interruptions are tolerated. The parent and child engage in an activity that is pleasurable for both of them, and the time allotted to this activity is monitored by an alarm clock or a kitchen timer. This predictable, promised time is not contingent on the child's behavior or on the parent's mood; it occurs at its scheduled time under all circumstances.

Parents also do well to learn the skill of "catching them being good." Parents should attend to and praise their children liberally when they are playing appropriately, relating well with another adult or child, trying to be helpful, or at-

Table 64-1 Recommended Contexts for Discussions About Discipline at Various Ages

Age	Contexts to frame discussions about discipline
1-4 months	Sleeping and eating schedules/routines
6-9 months	Rules to ensure safety of the environment
12-18 months	Emerging autonomy and independence
2 years	Toileting; perhaps new sibling
3 years	Entering preschool
4 years	Doing household chores
5 years	Entering a more formal school setting
6-12 years	Increasing peer activities and orientation
Adolescence	Observing curfews, guidelines for alcohol use, driving, and sexual behavior

UNDERLYING PRINCIPLES OF DISCIPLINE

1. Parents want to do the best they can for their children.
2. Parents learn to parent from their experience as children.
3. Families are complex systems in continuous transaction.
4. Behavior is learned primarily from its consequences.
5. *Something* is keeping the problematic behavior in place.
6. Punishment only teaches children what's *not* OK.

RULES FOR "ALONE TIME"

1. Predictable
2. One-on-one, with *no* interruptions
3. Time marked with a clock or timer
4. Interactive activity the child enjoys
5. Noncontingent on child's behavior or parent's mood.

tempting to do what the parent asks. The most effective praise takes the form of short, direct verbal messages, preferably referring directly to the parent's feelings rather than the child's behavior. An evaluative statement such as, "You did a good job," admits the possibility that the child will do a *bad* job the next time. In contrast, statements like "I really like how you cleaned up that pile of blocks," or "It makes me feel very proud when I see how well you play with Johnny," refer only to the speaker's *response* to the behavior and don't predict potential criticism. Nonverbal messages are powerful as well, such as a hug, a smile, or a pat on the back.

A third strategy involves giving children appropriate choices. In encouraging children to make and take part in appropriate decisions, parents teach them that they are responsible for their own behavior. The opportunity to make effective choices empowers children and enhances their growth. Choices must be appropriate to the child's developmental abilities, and parents must be careful to offer choices only when there actually is time to choose among options that are *all* acceptable to the parents.

Table 64-2 Basic Rules for Effective Discipline

Reward behavior you like	Rewards can be tangible or symbolic Rewards should be immediate Hugs and praise are powerful rewards
Use natural and logical consequences as your ally	*Natural* consequences are what would happen if you did nothing *Logical* consequences are those you impose as a reasonable outcome of the specific behavior
Punish behavior you don't like	Take away something the child values or impose something the child dislikes Punishment should be immediate Frequent small punishments are more effective than occasional big ones Spanking is effective only for the moment and has undesirable side effects

SHAPING CHILDREN'S BEHAVIOR

All behavior is learned, shaped primarily by its consequences. Behavior that is reinforced is likely to be repeated, whereas behavior that results in an unpleasant consequence is much less likely to be repeated. Removing reinforcement (i.e., ignoring) of a particular behavior also decreases its frequency. However, even *occasional* reinforcement prevents the extinction of an undesirable behavior. It also is important to note that what a parent intends as punishment may have some reinforcing characteristics to the child. A common example of this paradox is yelling at or even spanking a child; although these are not *pleasant* consequences, they do reflect intense emotional involvement on the part of the parent toward the child, which may be very valuable. Table 64-2 outlines a summary of the use of behavioral consequences to shape children's behavior.

Increasing Desirable Behavior

Parents are the most important people in children's lives, and pleasing their parents is an important goal. Furthermore, children, like the rest of us, appreciate being attended to and considered valuable company. Thus parents' attention, recognition, and praise are important reinforcers of their children's behavior. Behaviors that are rewarded or reinforced are likely to continue and even to increase in frequency. Reinforcement provided by parents may be intentional or inadvertent, and the behavior reinforced may be desirable or undesirable. Examples of intentional reinforcement of behavior are a parent's praise for appropriate play or accomplishment of a task, a planned gift, or a joint activity contingent on the child's completion of a particular assignment. Inadvertent rewards for good behavior may include a smile on the mother's face as she watches her child create a high tower and take pleasure in knocking it down, or a child overhearing her speaking on the telephone with pride about her daughter's accomplishments in school. Unfortunately, however, inadvertent reinforcement also occurs in relation to *undesirable* behavior. A child who receives a cookie to head off a temper tantrum, or one whose parents feed her each time she awakens during the night, is receiving unintentional rewards for behavior the parents would rather see disappear. Similarly, some attempts by parents to punish their children's unacceptable behavior may in some way reinforce it. Even negative attention from parents is better than none at all—"yelling" at least is intense interaction.

Decreasing Undesirable Behavior

All humans learn faster and more effectively when they are rewarded for good behavior than when they are punished for bad. Nevertheless, because all children at some time behave inappropriately, their parents must find a way to indicate that this behavior is not acceptable and to decrease its frequency.

Several mechanisms can be used to decrease the likelihood of undesirable behavior. Reinforcement for the behavior can be withdrawn (i.e., ignoring), or it can have an unpleasant consequence, either naturally occurring or imposed by adults in the environment (i.e., punishment). Given enough time, behaviors that are not reinforced either intrinsically or by others will fade. However, behaviors that are intrinsically rewarding, such as taking cookies from the cookie jar or splashing in the toilet bowl, will not diminish simply as a result of the parents ignoring them.

Punishment. Active punishment can take two forms: (1) privileges or pleasurable activities can be denied the child, or (2) painful, uncomfortable, or undesirable circumstances or activities can be imposed on the child. Examples of the restriction of privileges include decreasing the amount of time the child may watch television, decreasing the number of books a parent will read at bedtime, or forbidding the child to eat dessert with the family. Examples of the imposition of undesirable circumstances include spanking, requiring certain chores to be done, or imposing separation from the activities of the family, such as "time out."

The most powerful punishers are consequences that occur naturally as a result of the child's behavior, for example, dawdling in the morning results in being late for school; if a child does not eat at mealtime, he or she may be hungry at bedtime; if the goldfish aren't fed, they will die. Parents need only refrain from interfering with the natural consequences that follow upon the child's behavior. If no negative consequences would follow *naturally,* parents can create some that follow *logically:* scribbling on the wall might result in no crayons for a week or in the assignment of washing the walls; if toys are not put away by a prescribed time, they are removed for several days.

Some forbidden behaviors require parents to create a more contrived intervention. For example, hitting or biting do not result in any acceptable, immediately occurring, logical, or natural negative consequence; thus a punishment such as "time out" needs to be imposed. For maximal effectiveness, time out should be instituted in a planned and carefully specified manner after it is described to the child (see the box above).

RULES FOR "TIME OUT"

1. Offending behavior(s) described in *concrete* statement(s)
2. Maximum of *three* offending behaviors
3. Occurs *immediately* after the behavior occurs
4. Occurs *each time* the behavior occurs
5. Plans and place arranged in *absence* of problematic behavior
6. One minute per year of age, marked with a *timer*
7. Welcome child back to *"time in"* without lecturing

Corporal Punishment. In spite of the prevalent experience and beliefs of many parents and pediatricians,[3-5] *spanking and other forms of physical punishment have no place in the discipline of children.* Although spanking may at first appear effective as a result of children's surprise, pain, and fear, it seldom is effective in the long run and is used at tremendous cost.

Children learn more effectively by watching their parents' behavior than by listening passively to their words. Parents who spank model a type of behavior that they generally do not allow for the child; how can young children understand that their parents may hit them while they themselves are punished for hitting other children? Furthermore, spanking reduces the opportunities available for using more effective disciplinary strategies.

Physical punishment undermines parents' attempts to maintain effective, cooperative, and nurturing relationships with their children. Children who are spanked learn aggressive and violent forms of conflict resolution based on power and strength. When adults are hit, they feel violated, shamed, hurt, and angry; children, too, will experience these feelings when being hit. That this action and these feelings come from the adults they trust and love most makes them even more destructive. There is evidence that adolescents and adults who were physically punished as children are more likely to engage in violent behavior as adults.[8]

Another reason spanking generally is not effective is that most parents are reluctant to spank their children. This reluctance is a result of two factors: (1) parents don't like to hurt their children, and (2) most parents come to recognize that spanking is, at best, inconsistently effective in changing children's behavior. In addition, physical punishment is difficult to modulate. It generally is carried out when the parent is angry and carries with it the risk of excessive anger and unintentional abuse.

Basic Principles for Using Rewards and Punishments

Certain principles should be followed in deciding on strategies for rewarding or punishing children's behavior.

1. The target behaviors to be rewarded or punished should be specified clearly in short, concrete sentences.
2. A maximum of three behaviors should be systematically targeted for rewards and three for punishment.
3. The reward or punishment must follow immediately upon the recognition of the behavior.
4. The particular reinforcement or punishment to be applied must be individualized in order to determine (a) that it is acceptable to all members of the family and (b) that it is, in fact, punishing or reinforcing for the child.

Common pitfalls summarized in the box on p. 650 include inadvertently rewarding undesirable behavior, failing to notice and reward desirable behavior, a family environment that is so busy or stressed that the child does not experience suf-

COMMON PITFALLS LEADING TO INEFFECTIVE DISCIPLINE

Inadvertent rewarding of undesirable behavior
Failure to notice and reward desirable behavior
Insufficient "time in"
Inconsistent rules from day to day, situation to situation
Too many punishable behaviors

PREVENTIVE STRATEGIES

1. Empowerment of parents
2. Discipline = *rules* and *consequences*
3. Praise and attention
4. Alone time
5. Effective choices

ficient positive interaction with the parents ("time in"), and inconsistency in the consequences that follow behaviors.

It is very important to remember that *punishment is never enough.* At best, punishment only teaches children what behavior is *not* acceptable, but cannot teach what behavior is desirable. Thus punishment should constitute only a small part of an overall disciplinary strategy. Effective discipline results from parents' creation of an environment in which children feel *safe* by virtue of predictable rules and consequences, *lovable* as a result of adequate attention and praise, and *capable* of making decisions and taking responsibility for their own behavior. These basic preventive strategies are outlined in the box above.

Pediatricians can model for parents, teaching them the importance of empowerment in the context of a respectful and emotionally safe and nurturing environment, and teach them some of the skills that will help their children know that they are lovable, capable, and responsible. There are many helpful books available to help parents learn effective strategies for discipline and for parenting in general.

REFERENCES

1. Christophersen ER: Discipline, *Pediatr Clin North Am* 39:395, 1992.
2. Howard BJ: Discipline in early childhood, *Pediatr Clin North Am* 38:1351, 1991.
3. Larzelere RE: Moderate spanking: model or deterrent of children's aggression in the family? *Journal of Family Violence* 1:27, 1986.
4. Larzelere RE et al: Relationship of spanking and other parenting characteristics to self-esteem and perceived fairness of parental discipline, *Psychol Rep* 64:1140, 1989.
5. McCormick KF: Attitudes of primary care physicians toward corporal punishment, *JAMA* 267:3161, 1992.
6. Schmitt BD: Discipline: rules and consequences, *Contemp Pediatr* June 1991, p 65.
7. Smith EE, Van Tassel E: Problems of discipline in early childhood, *Pediatr Clin North Am* 29:167, 1982.
8. Straus MA: Discipline and deviance: physical punishment of children and violence and other crime in adulthood, *Social Problems* 38:133, 1991.

Helpful Books for Parents

Brazelton T: *Touchpoints,* Reading, Mass, 1992, Addison-Wesley.
Clark L: *The time-out solution,* Chicago, 1989, Contemporary Books.
Dreikurs R: *Children: the challenge,* New York, 1964, Penguin Books.
Dreikurs R, Grey LA: *Parent's guide to child discipline,* New York, 1970, Hawthorn Books.
Faber A, Mazlish E: *How to talk so kids will listen and listen so kids will talk,* New York, 1980, Avon Books.

65 Sexual Abuse of Children

John M. Leventhal

Although sexual abuse of children has existed for centuries, only in the last 20 years have clinicians begun to recognize the scope of the problem, including its epidemiology, clinical characteristics, approaches to management, and consequences to children and families.

DEFINITION AND EPIDEMIOLOGY

Sexual abuse of children is defined as the involvement of children or adolescents in sexual activities that they do not understand fully, to which they cannot give informed consent, and that violate the social taboos of families or society.[15] It includes activities such as the sexual touching of a child's genitals by an adult or adolescent, sexual intercourse between an adult and child, exposure of children to pornography, or involvement of children in prostitution. Sexual abuse should be distinguished from sexual play or exploration by preschool or young school-age children and from sexual activities between consenting adolescents.

Child protection laws passed in the 1960s in each state initially required the reporting of cases of suspected abuse or neglect; shortly after, they were broadened to include children suspected of being sexually abused. Since 1976, when national statistics of cases reported to each state's child protection agency were compiled, cases of maltreatment have increased yearly. The most dramatic increase in reports of sexual abuse occurred in the 1980s owing to increased publicity and increased recognition by parents and clinicians. In 1994 approximately 11% of 3 million reports of maltreatment to child protective service agencies were due to sexual abuse. About 45% of cases reported to protective services are considered substantiated, meaning that protective services had enough evidence to believe that sexual abuse occurred. This rate of substantiation for sexual abuse is somewhat higher than for other forms of maltreatment. The failure to substantiate an allegation does not necessarily mean that the abuse did not occur but rather that protective services did not have enough evidence. About 75% of children evaluated for suspected sexual abuse are female; the age range is from 6 months to 18 years with a median age of about 6 years.

While such cases represent those reported to child protective services, sexual abuse of children continues to be underrecognized and underreported. An alternative approach to estimating the frequency of the problem has been to interview adults about their childhood experiences of sexual abuse. These studies provide information about a lifetime prevalence; the rates of adults indicating that they had been sexually abused during childhood vary from 7% to 62% for females and 3% to 19% for males.[17] These rates vary in part because of the population studied, the number and types of questions asked, and the definition of sexual abuse used. Reasonable estimates in this country are that 20% to 25% of adult women and 10% to 15% of adult men report having been sexually abused before age 18 years.

Unlike cases of physical abuse or neglect, which are much more commonly reported in families who are poor and have limited education, cases of sexual abuse occur in families from all social classes and educational backgrounds. Perpetrators of sexual abuse are almost all males, and 25% of them are juveniles. Most children who have been sexually abused know the perpetrator, who may be the father, stepfather, another male relative, family friend, or an adult in the child's community. Approximately 15% of sexually abused children do not know the perpetrator; these victims usually are older children or adolescents who are victims of forceful sexual assault or "rape."

ETIOLOGY

Clinicians are able to understand how a parent might lose control and physically abuse a child, but it is much more difficult to understand how an adult can move from close bodily contact and even sensual feelings toward actually sexually abusing a child. Two prerequisites for sexual abuse to occur include the offender's sexual arousal to children and the willingness to act upon this arousal.[13] Recent studies have attempted to examine adults' sexual attraction to children. For example, 21% of male college students in an anonymous questionnaire indicated that they felt sexual attraction toward children.[10] Some offenders may focus their attention on children of a certain age or gender; others may find themselves aroused only by children in certain circumstances. Factors that influence the offender's willingness to act on the aroused feelings toward the child include a lack of conscience about such behaviors, a lack of empathy for the child, a belief that such sexual behaviors are acceptable and not harmful to the child, poor impulse control, and the use of drugs or alcohol that might further decrease the ability to control one's behavior.[13] Additional contributors to the likelihood that sexual abuse may occur include the history of the perpetrator (e.g., having been sexually abused during childhood), circumstances that allow the perpetrator to have increased contact with the child (e.g., a mother hospitalized for a lengthy period), and the particular vulnerabilities of the child (e.g., mental retardation).

Children who are sexually abused often are selected because they seem particularly vulnerable or needy. Such children initially may enjoy and appreciate the attention that they receive from the offender, who may begin by giving the child gifts, attention, and special hugs and touches. These behaviors may progress to special secrets and eventually from nonsexual to sexual activities, eventually leading to sexual intercourse. This process has been labeled the "child sexual abuse accommodation syndrome,"[24] which describes five stages that occur in the sexual abuse of children: (1) secrecy, (2) helplessness, (3) entrapment and accommodation, (4) delayed, unconvincing disclosures, and (5) later retraction of the alleged abuse.

CLINICAL MANIFESTATIONS

Like other forms of family violence, sexual abuse of children often occurs in the privacy of a home or in a setting that involves only the abused and abuser and thus seldom is witnessed by another person. A child who has been sexually abused may have been maltreated in other ways, including physical abuse or neglect, and certainly has been emotionally abused as well.

A clinician's concerns about the possibility of sexual abuse surface because of reports of specific statements made by the child, usually to a parent or other adult, about uncomfortable experiences such as being touched on the genitalia; reports of specific behaviors of the child, such as sexualized behaviors with a sibling; symptoms, such as encopresis or vaginal discharge or bleeding; or a genital or anal abnormality noted on physical examination.

Clear statements by the child (or, occasionally, accidental direct observations of the sexual abuse) are the best indicators that sexual abuse has occurred. These usually are told to a parent or trusted adult, such as a school teacher. Young children, however, may not have the necessary vocabulary to describe what has happened to them. They may use words that the perpetrator used to encourage their participation (e.g., "we played the hugging game") or words that describe their experience of what happened or what it felt like, but are confusing to the adults (e.g., "he stuck a knife in my pee-pee"). Older children may begin by offering a guarded, vague disclosure (e.g., "My uncle kisses too hard"). If the adult reacts in a concerned manner with appropriate exploratory questions, more details may follow. The older child may be embarrassed about what happened, feel partially responsible, have experienced pleasurable feelings, or be concerned about the threats that the perpetrator made (e.g., "If you tell your mother, I will punch you"). Even after a clear disclosure, once the child realizes how upsetting the information is to the family, he or she may retract the statement. Older children also may feel responsible for holding the family together: if the child tells, the father will go to jail, the house will be sold, and everyone will be angry at the child; on the other hand, if nothing is said, the sexual abuse will continue, but at least the family will be saved. Some children consciously or unconsciously sacrifice themselves for their family.

Children who have been sexually abused may demonstrate a variety of symptoms and behaviors. Some may be relatively asymptomatic and be able to function reasonably well in social settings and in school. Many children exhibit nonspecific symptoms, such as sleep problems, generalized anxiety, suicidal gestures, or poor school performance, which are seen in response to other childhood stresses as well. Sexualized behaviors, such as excessive masturbation, using adult words associated with sexuality, or simulating sexual intercourse with another child, animal, or doll are more suggestive of sexual abuse. Other concerning symptoms include vaginal pain, bleeding, or discharge or rectal bleeding. Even a symptom such as a vaginal discharge, however, has a low likelihood of being caused by sexual abuse. Several studies of premenarcheal girls with vaginal discharge have shown that sexual abuse occurs infrequently (less than 5% to 10%) and that the most common cause is poor hygiene.[23]

Approximately 15% to 20% of sexually abused children will have an abnormal genital or anal finding suggestive of sexual abuse. The absence of physical findings, however, does not rule out sexual abuse because there may have been no injury to the genital area or, if an injury did occur, it may have healed without leaving any physical signs.

Over the last few years, there has been increasing research to define normal and abnormal genital and anal anatomy in prepubertal children and adolescents. Several studies have described the variations in the anatomy of the hymen in female newborns and have concluded that the hymen is present in all normally developed newborns.[7] The appearance of the hymen often is thickened early in life because of the effects of maternal estrogen in utero; in preschool and school-age girls, the hymenal tissue becomes thinner until the effects of estrogen during puberty result in a thickening of the tissue and the development of redundant folds. Studies of normal prepubertal girls have described the shapes of the hymen as crescentric (or posterior rim), concentric (or annular), and fimbriated (or redundant) and have noted the frequency of normal variations, including hymenal bumps, vaginal ridges, and adhesions of the labia minora.[6,20] Important findings have been derived from these studies. For example, data are available on the means and ranges of the vertical and horizontal diameters of the hymenal orifice in different age groups and on the variations in diameter depending on how the genitalia are examined (e.g. separation vs. traction of the labia majora).[19]

Children who have been sexually abused may have acute injuries of the genitalia, including acute lacerations, abrasions, or hematomas.[3] Most children who have been sexually abused, however, do not disclose the abuse until weeks or months after its occurrence. Among such children, findings suggestive of past abuse include U- or V-shaped notches of the posterior rim of the hymen (which occur in the healing process after an acute laceration), decreased hymenal tissue posteriorly (that also is noted when the child is examined in the prone, knee-chest position), and scarring, such as of the posterior fourchette.[1,3] Although investigators have considered an enlarged horizontal diameter of the hymen of greater than 4 mm to be suggestive of previous sexual abuse in prepubertal children, studies of normal children have indicated that this demarcation is incorrect and that the size of the opening varies with the child's age and different examination techniques,[19] as well as with the child's state of relaxation. A horizontal diameter of greater than 10 mm may concern a clinician about the possibility of sexual abuse but should not by itself be used to make a diagnosis.

Data about the size of the hymenal orifice in adolescence have been collected in a recent study comparing three groups of adolescent females: (1) those who denied sexual intercourse and used only pads for menses, (2) those who denied sexual intercourse and used tampons, and (3) those who had experienced sexual intercourse.[11] Although there were significant differences in the median horizontal diameters of the hymenal orifice in the three groups (1.2, 1.5, and 2.5 cm, respectively), there certainly was overlap among the groups.

In addition, a striking difference among the groups was that of the sexually active teenagers; 81% had a complete cleft (or V-shaped notch) between the 2 o'clock and 10 o'clock positions on the hymenal border compared with 11% in tampon users and 5% in pad users.

Abnormalities of the male genitalia caused by sexual abuse are unusual. Acute abrasions, lacerations, or bruises caused by physical abuse, however, can be seen.

Acute anal findings, such as lacerations caused by anal penetration or injury, have been noted in sexually abused children, but there have been few systematic studies of perianal findings in chronically abused children. Worrisome findings include thickening of the rugae, distorted anatomy secondary to scarring, and dilation greater than 2.0 cm (when the child is in the prone, knee-chest position and no stool is visible in the rectal ampulla). A study of normal prepubertal children highlighted common normal findings that were noted when the child was examined in the prone, knee-chest position; these included skin tags in the midline, fan-shaped areas in the midline superiorly, perianal erythema, venous congestion, and anal dilation up to 2.0 cm.[21]

Children who have been sexually abused may acquire a sexually transmitted disease (STD). How children acquire such diseases is controversial in part because of the social and legal implications and because of the difficulty in believing that a young child's disease is from sexual contact. The most commonly occurring STDs in sexually abused children are due to *Neisseria gonorrhoeae, Chlamydia trachomatis,* and human papilloma virus (HPV). Each of these organisms can be transmitted perinatally. In a study of young children who acquired *Chlamydia* perinatally and were followed from birth, the organism was recovered from the throat or nasopharynx up to 28 months of age and from the vagina or rectum up to the first birthday.[5] Although systematic data have not been collected regarding the isolation of HPV from a child after transmission of the organism at birth, the range of the incubation period in adults is 3 weeks to about 8 months.[14] Condylomata that are noted in 12- to 24-month-olds are believed to be caused by perinatal transmission, but because of the child's age it is difficult to be certain about the cause. There is some suggestion that HPV also can be transmitted nonsexually. Other diseases such as syphilis or HIV infection also have been reported in victims of sexual abuse.

It should be noted that female adolescent victims are at risk of pregnancy from sexual abuse.

ASSESSMENT AND DIAGNOSIS

The evaluation of children for suspected sexual abuse should include a history from the parent(s) and child, a physical examination, appropriate laboratory tests, and careful documentation of the findings. In addition, data may be collected from other professionals who know the child and family. This evaluation often is conducted by a multidisciplinary team; a social worker or psychologist interviews the parents and child, and a physician, nurse practitioner, or physician's associate conducts a medical examination. As part of the evaluation, the clinicians should consider alternative explanations, including an unintentional injury (or "accident"), a medical problem, or a false allegation.[8] Because evaluations for suspected sexual abuse usually include the child protection and legal systems, care should be taken to provide an unbiased assessment and one that provides documentation that can be reviewed by professionals outside the medical system.

History

The purpose of the history is to understand what may have happened to the child. This history should include the events that led to the evaluation, the child's health status and development, and the family's strengths and weaknesses. The parents (or guardian) should be asked what the child has said, how the child reacted when telling about the abuse, and whom the child told. Information should be obtained about (1) the child's behaviors, such as changes in behaviors or attitudes toward a specific person or situation, recurrent fears or nightmares, or sexualized behaviors; (2) specific symptoms, such as vaginal bleeding or discharge, rectal bleeding, constipation, and encopresis; and (3) where the child spends his or her time and who takes care of the child. Also, it should be determined who the alleged perpetrator is, the relationship with the child, and the amount of time spent with the child. In preparation for interviewing the child, it is important to know about the child's developmental history—for example, whether there is a language delay or impaired cognition.

The family history should include information about the parents' physical and mental health (including a history of any sexual abuse during childhood), the health and developmental status of the siblings, the presence of family violence, substance abuse, or recent stresses, and the resources and supports available to the family. It is important to understand how family members view the allegations and how they have reacted. Because allegations that arise during a custody fight between parents often are difficult to sort out, the clinician should determine whether the parents are separated or divorced, what the custody arrangements are, what kind of visitation schedule exists, and whether there is a dispute about custody or visitation. It is helpful to distinguish whether the allegations of abuse occurred before the separation or divorce, during the process of separation and divorce, or after the divorce had been finalized.

A child who is old enough to be interviewed directly should be asked about what may have happened.[18] This interview or series of interviews should be conducted with the child alone, if possible. The interviewer should be comfortable and skilled at interviewing young children about the possibility of sexual abuse, use simple questions, and be aware of the child's nonverbal responses, as well as direct statements. Leading questions such as "Didn't he touch your peepee?" should be avoided, when possible. Nonleading questions are preferable, such as "Can you tell me what happened?" or "Where did he touch you?" Often, however, children are reluctant to talk because of a variety of reasons, including fear and embarrassment; in such cases, questions that have forced choice responses, "Was it your mother or father or teacher who did that?" or "Was his pee green or pink or white?" can be helpful.

To help young children, anatomical drawings or anatomically detailed dolls can be used. Considerable controversy exists about the sexual nature of the dolls and whether their use suggests to children that they can talk about sex, thus leading to false allegations. Research, however, indicates that few nonsexually abused children respond in sexual ways with the dolls and that the dolls can be helpful to children in describing what happened.[12] Because of the controversy around the dolls, many interviewers prefer to use them to help the child identify body parts and explain the details of what happened only after the child has indicated verbally that sexual abuse has occurred.

Physical Examination

The purposes of the physical examination are to determine whether there are (1) signs of physical abuse or neglect, (2) anogenital injuries consistent with or suggestive of sexual abuse, and (3) conditions that need medical treatment. In addition, the examination provides an opportunity for the clinician to reassure the child and family about the child's physical condition. In premenarcheal girls, the genital examination is performed best in both the supine and prone and knee-chest positions; a speculum seldom is used. In many centers, a colposcope is used during the anogenital examination to provide 5× to 30× magnification and allow documentation of injuries through photographs or video recordings. A study comparing examinations with and without the use of the colposcope indicated that over 95% of physical findings can be detected without its use.[22] A hand-held magnifying lens that provides 2.5× to 3× magnification or an otoscope head can provide adequate magnification.

Laboratory Tests

When the child is at risk of acquiring an STD from suspected sexual contact, appropriate tests should be obtained for gonorrhea, chlamydia, syphilis, HIV infection, and hepatitis B. Tests for gonorrhea and chlamydia should be cultures for the organisms. In many medical settings, however, obtaining swabs for cultures no longer is routine practice because of the availability of other tests, such as for the organism's DNA (e.g., Gen Probe). In such settings, positive results should be confirmed via cultures. In a child who has a vaginal discharge, additional studies may be done to test for trichomonas or *Gardnerella vaginalis.* In children who have genital or perianal condyloma, it may help to obtain information about HPV typing, which is based on characteristics of the viral DNA. Certain types, such as 6 or 11, are associated with genital diseases in adults; occasionally type 2, which causes common warts, can produce condyloma in the anogenital region.

When a child is evaluated within 72 hours of an episode of suspected sexual abuse, appropriate forensic samples, such as swabs to detect semen, should be collected[2] (see Chapter 290). In an adolescent, a pregnancy test may be necessary.

Documentation

Documentation of the evaluation should include direct quotations, when appropriate, from the parents and the child and a clear description of the findings from the physical examination, with diagrams if necessary. In many states the information is recorded on a specific form for suspected sexual assault. A videotape of the child's interview and photographs of the examination provide additional detailed information; these should be labeled with the date, child's name, and record number.

DIFFERENTIAL DIAGNOSIS

Conditions that need to be considered depend on the child's symptoms and physical findings.[4] Some of the physical findings that can be seen in sexually abused children also are nonspecific, such as erythema of the vulva or introitus. Bruises to the genital or anal area should raise concern about physical abuse, but if bruising is more widespread, medical conditions, such as bleeding disorders, need to be considered. Straddle injuries, which can affect the genitalia, usually are witnessed, so the history is clear. These types of injuries usually are unilateral or anterior and produce obvious bruising and swelling of the external genitalia; it is unusual for such injuries to affect the hymen because of the protection provided by the labia and bones of the pelvis.

An important dermatological condition that may occur with genital soreness and subependymal hemorrhages is lichen sclerosis.[4] This condition usually affects the vulva and perianal region and produces an hourglass appearance with areas of subependymal hemorrhage, decreased pigmentation, and tissue friability. Another condition that may be mistaken for sexual abuse is a streptococcal infection that can cause marked redness of the perianal region and a vaginal discharge. In children who have a foul smelling vaginal discharge, a foreign body should be considered in the differential diagnosis.

The possibility of a false allegation also should be considered in the differential diagnosis.[8] Although false allegations seem to occur infrequently, there is increasing controversy about the accuracy of young children's memory, under what research circumstances they can be asked leading questions that result in false reports of what happened, and how relevant these studies are to children's reports of sexual abuse. False allegations should be considered carefully if the child (1) has a serious mental health problem, (2) is part of a bitter dispute between the parents (e.g., a custody fight), or (3) provides statements that lack detail about the event, have important inconsistencies, or appear rote in nature, and the child seems minimally affected by telling what happened.

MANAGEMENT AND TREATMENT

Management of children who are suspected of having been sexually abused includes action in three domains: (1) providing appropriate medical care, (2) reporting the case to protective services, (3) and ensuring mental health services for the child and family.

Guidelines for the treatment of STDs are highlighted in Chapter 290; in addition, counseling may be necessary about the implications of certain infections, such as human papilloma virus or HIV. Occasionally, surgical repairs of genital or anal injuries are necessary, and adolescents may need counseling about terminating a pregnancy that was due to sexual abuse. A major purpose of the physical examination is to reassure the child and family that his or her body is intact physically. When abnormalities are noted on the physical examination, reassurance often can be provided by indicating that these will likely heal and be of little functional importance to the child.

Clinicians who suspect sexual abuse are mandated to report their findings to the state child protection agency. Because sexual assault is a criminal offense, the local police also participate in the investigation. Issues that need to be considered include to what extent the child should be interviewed further, by whom, and in what setting; where the child should go to ensure his or her safety; and whether other children in the home need to be evaluated.

The period after the child's disclosure can be upsetting for all involved and especially confusing to the child. Repeated interviews of the child (by well-meaning professionals, such as police or a protective service worker) may upset the child, who may be confused about why so many people are asking questions, embarrassed about talking about private parts, and worried about the family's reactions. Family members may blame themselves for allowing the abuse to happen and be furious at the suspected perpetrator. If the abuser is a relative, the family may be divided, with the child's side believing the child and the abuser's side believing that the abuse could not happen and that the child is lying. If the abuser is in the immediate family, the psychological issues are even more complicated. A mother will have to decide between siding with and supporting her daughter or believing that her daughter lied and supporting her husband. If her husband did sexually abuse their child, the mother may question her own sexuality and her ability to protect her child and choose a partner; at the same time, she may be concerned about how the family will be supported with the father in jail.

The clinician can be helpful by maintaining contact with the family, advocating for a reasonable approach by protective services (e.g., having the alleged abuser leave the home rather than place the child in foster care), and helping the family recognize and discuss the various emotional issues that surface. In many communities, multidisciplinary teams have been developed to coordinate the evaluation of children suspected of having been sexually abused in order to minimize the interviewing of the child and to help the family through the initial crisis period.

Many sexually abused children and their parents need short- or long-term counseling to come to terms with what happened to the child. Important issues for the child's treatment include self-blame for allowing the abuse to happen, the child's sexuality and sexual awareness, poor self-esteem and feelings of powerlessness, and mistrust of adults. For example, school-age and adolescent boys may be very concerned about their own masculinity and whether, because they were abused by an older male, they are gay. At the same time, because of changes in the family (e.g., the child no longer visits the grandfather), the child has to come to terms with the losses created by the disclosure and the upset and anger in the family.

Because sexual abuse of a child is a criminal offense, the child and family often are involved in the criminal justice system. Despite this involvement, however, most cases do not result in a trial in criminal court because of a variety of reasons, including lack of clear evidence that abuse has occurred, the young age of the victim, a confession of the perpetrator, or the willingness of the perpetrator to plea bargain for a lighter sentence. In only approximately 3% to 5% of cases is a criminal trial held in which the child actually testifies. Additionally, sexual abuse cases often are tried in family court when allegations of sexual abuse occur as a part of a divorce or custody proceeding or in juvenile court when protective services is concerned about the child's safety in the home.

PSYCHOSOCIAL CONSEQUENCES

Sexual abuse can have a long-lasting and devastating impact on the development of children, adolescents, and adults.[9,16] Domains of functioning that can be affected include the survivor's emotional state (e.g., depression, anxiety, suicide), sense of self (e.g., feeling worthless or powerless and viewing oneself as a victim), and relationships with others (e.g., poor boundaries, increased promiscuity, use of sexual behaviors inappropriately, and lack of trust). Teenage girls and women appear to be at an increased risk of other mental health problems, such as eating disorders, multiple personality disorders, and posttraumatic stress disorder. They also are more likely to be revictimized. Less research has been conducted on the consequences for males who were sexually abused as children, but they do appear to be at an increased risk of becoming perpetrators.

PREVENTION

Attempts to prevent sexual abuse have been directed toward developing programs to teach children, usually at school, about "good" and "bad" touches and what to do if bad touches occur. Children as young as 4 to 6 years old are able to learn these concepts and retain them, at least over a short period. In general, evaluations have focused on the children's increased knowledge resulting from participation in a teaching program; it is important to note that these evaluations have not been able to provide systematic data about whether such programs actually have resulted in the prevention or earlier recognition of sexual abuse.

REFERENCES

1. Adams JA, Harper K, Knudson S: A proposed system for the classification of anogenital findings in children with suspected sexual abuse, *Adolesc Pediatr Gynecol* 5:73, 1992.
2. American Academy of Pediatrics, Committee on Adolescence: Sexual assault and the adolescent, *Pediatrics* 94:761, 1994.
3. American Academy of Pediatrics, Committee on Child Abuse and Neglect: Guidelines for the evaluation of sexual abuse of children, *Pediatrics* 87:254, 1991.
4. Bays J: Conditions mistaken for child sexual abuse. In Reece RM, editor: *Child abuse: medical diagnosis and assessment,* Philadelphia, 1994, Lea & Febiger.
5. Bell TA et al: Chronic *Chlamydia trachomatis* infections in infants, *JAMA* 267:400, 1992.
6. Berenson A, Heger A, Andrews S: Appearance of the hymen in newborns, *Pediatrics* 87:458, 1991.
7. Berenson AB et al: Appearance of the hymen in prepubertal girls, *Pediatrics* 89:387, 1992.
8. Bernet W: False statements and the differential diagnosis of abuse allegations, *J Am Acad Child Adolesc Psychiatry* 32:903, 1993.
9. Briere J: *Child abuse trauma: theory and treatment of the lasting effects,* Newbury Park, Calif, 1992, Sage.
10. Briere J, Runtz M: University males' sexual interest in children: predicting potential indices of pedophilia in a nonforensic sample, *Child Abuse Negl* 13:65, 1989.
11. Emans SJ et al: Hymenal findings in adolescent women: impact of tampon use and consensual sexual activity, *J Pediatr* 125:153, 1994.
12. Everson MD, Boat BW: Putting the anatomical doll controversy in per-

spective: an examination of the major uses and criticisms of the dolls in child sexual abuse evaluations, *Child Abuse Negl* 18:113, 1994.

13. Faller KC: *Understanding child sexual maltreatment,* Newbury Park, Calif, 1993, Sage.
14. Gutman LT, Herman-Giddens ME, Phelps WC: Transmission of human papilloma virus disease: comparison of data from adults and children, *Pediatrics* 91:31, 1993.
15. Kempe CH: Sexual abuse, another hidden pediatric problem: the 1977 C Anderson Aldrich lecture, *Pediatrics* 62:382, 1978.
16. Kendall-Tacket TA, Williams LM, Finkelhor D: Impact of sexual abuse on children: a review and synthesis of recent empirical studies, *Psychol Bull* 113:164, 1993.
17. Leventhal JM: Epidemiology of child sexual abuse. In Oates RK, editor: *Understanding and managing child sexual abuse,* Syndney, Australia, 1990, Harcourt Brace Javonovich.
18. Leventhal JM et al: What to ask when sexual abuse is suspected, *Arch Dis Child* 62:1188, 1987.
19. McCann J et al: Comparison of genital examination techniques in prepubertal girls, *Pediatrics* 85:182, 1990.
20. McCann J et al: Genital findings in prepubertal girls selected for nonabuse: a descriptive study, *Pediatrics* 86:428, 1990.
21. McCann J et al: Perianal findings in prepubertal children selected for nonabuse: a descriptive study, *Child Abuse Negl* 13:179, 1989.
22. Muram D: Child sexual abuse: genital findings in prepubertal girls: comparison of colposcopic and unaided examination, *Am J Obstet Gynecol* 160:333, 1989.
23. Paradise JE et al: Vulvovaginitis in premenarcheal girls: clinical features and diagnostic evaluation, *Pediatrics* 70:193, 1982.
24. Summit RC: The child sexual abuse accommodation syndrome, *Child Abuse Negl* 7:177, 1993.

SUGGESTED READINGS

Behrman RE, editor: Sexual abuse of children. In *The future of children,* vol 4, no 2, Palo Alto, Calif, 1994, The Packard Foundation.

Ceci SJ, Bruck M: *Jeopardy in the courtroom: a scientific analysis of children's statements,* Washington, DC, 1995, American Psychological Association.

Chadwick DL et al: *Color atlas of child sexual abuse,* Chicago, 1989, Mosby.

Finkel MA, DeJong AR: Medical findings in child sexual abuse. In Reece RM, editor: *Child abuse: medical diagnosis and management,* Philadelphia, 1994, Lea & Febiger.

Heger A, Emans SJ, editors: *Evaluation of the sexually abused child: a medical textbook and photographic atlas,* New York, 1992, Oxford University Press.

Krugman RD, Leventhal JM, editors: *Child sexual abuse: report of the twenty-second Ross roundtable on critical approaches to common pediatric problems,* Columbus, Ohio, 1991, Ross Laboratories.

66 Violence in Television and Video Games: Influence on Children and Adolescents

Leonard D. Eron

Over the last 40 years, research results have accumulated that leave little doubt that the continued viewing of violence on the television screen by young children influences their behavior and has a long-lasting effect. The likelihood of their acting violently is increased not only at that time but also in the future. A new dimension has been added to the problem by the advent of video games, which were introduced into the arcades in the 1970s but did not invade the home market with hand-held displays and controls until the second half of the 1980s. Thus the video game phenomenon is new, and a body of evidence has not yet developed from both laboratory and longitudinal studies to assess its full effect on the behavior of children and adolescents. However, by extrapolation from results with standard television, it seems that the influence of the video games would be even greater.

Television programs have great influence on children because of their constant repetition and because the youngster is bombarded by two senses at the same time—visual and auditory. With video games, the same or even more constant repetition plus the involvement of a third sense—the kinesthetic—applies. The player not only sees and hears what is going on, but also engages in muscular activity by moving a lever or pressing a button, which brings on the mayhem by one's own activity and skill.

This review examines the evidence implicating violence on television programs in the aggressive behavior of the young observer, discusses the psychological processes that are implicated in this relation, reviews research on the impact of video games that has appeared thus far, and discusses what parents can do to counteract these effects.

First, it is essential that the terms *media violence* and *aggressive behavior* be defined clearly. For the purpose of this review, *media violence* refers to graphic visual portrayals of acts of physical aggression by one or more persons against others. This definition does not include acts of violence that may have been carried out off screen and merely are implied. Aggressive behavior, either by a child or an adult, refers to an act intended to injure or irritate another person.[9]

TELEVISION VIOLENCE

In the United States today it is almost impossible to escape the influence of television. An estimated 98% of American households have television, and many of these homes have multiple sets.[16] Within these homes the television is on about 28 hours a week for children ages 2 to 11 years and 23 hours for teenagers. Television occupies more time than any other nonschool activity. Also, there is more viewing among African-American and Hispanic children, regardless of socioeconomic status,[23] and the poorest and most vulnerable groups in society are the heaviest viewers of television for want of alternative activities.[17,23]

Within these total hours of exposure to television, how much time is taken up by displays of violence? According to research done at the University of Pennsylvania, 5 to 6 violent acts are shown per hour on prime time, and 20 to 25 are shown on Saturday morning children's programs.[11] This accounts for almost 188 hours of violent programs per week, or 15% of program time.[12] These figures refer only to network television. The introduction of cable TV has added to the level of violence by introducing new, more violent programs and recycling older violent programs. In 1 day in Washington, D.C., observers identified 1846 violent scenes on TV and cable TV between 6 AM and midnight. The most violent periods were between 6 and 9 AM and 2 and 5 PM, when children are most likely to be watching television.[18]

What has been the effect of this immersion in televised violence on the children who have been observing it? After 40 years of research, there is little doubt that televised violence is a cause of aggression. The evidence comes from both laboratory and other studies. Television violence affects youngsters of all ages, of both genders, at all socioeconomic levels, and of all levels of intelligence. The effect is not limited to children who are already disposed to being aggressive and is not restricted to the United States. That this same finding of a relation between television violence and aggression in children was found in study after study, in one country after another, cannot be ignored.

The causal effect of television violence on aggression, even though it is not very large, exists and has been demonstrated among many different children. The results indicate that a vicious cycle exists in which television violence makes children more aggressive, and these more aggressive children turn to watching more violence to justify their own behaviors.

One long-range study carried on over 22 years exemplifies both the contemporaneous and long-range effects of exposure to violence at a young age.[8,14] In 1960 a survey was conducted of all third-grade school children in a semirural county in New York State. A total of 875 boys and girls were interviewed in school, and separate interviews were completed with 80% of their parents. The question to be answered was how aggressive behavior, as it is manifested in school, is related to the kinds of child rearing practices parents use. An unexpected finding was that for boys there seemed to be a direct positive relation between the violence of the television programs they preferred and how aggressive they were in school. Because this was no more than a contemporaneous relation, it was impossible to tell by these data alone whether aggressive boys liked violent television programs, whether the violent programs made boys aggressive, or whether aggression *and* watching violent television were both due to some other third variable. However, because these findings fit in well with certain theories about learning by imitation and the results of laboratory studies,[2] a cause-and-effect relation was certainly plausible.

Ten years later in 1970, however, over 50% of the original sample was reinterviewed. The most striking finding then was the positive relation between the viewing of violent television at age 8 years and aggression at age 19 among the male subjects. Actually the relation was even stronger than it was when both variables were measured when the children were age 8 years.

By use of a variety of statistical techniques, it was demonstrated that the most plausible interpretation of these data was that early viewing of violent television caused later aggression. For example, if boys' aggressiveness is controlled at age 8, the relation does not diminish. In fact, those boys who at age 8 scored "low aggressive" but watched violent television were significantly more aggressive 10 years later than boys who originally scored "high aggressive" but did not watch violent programs. Similarly, every other third variable that might account for this relation was controlled—IQ, social status, parental aggression, social and geographical mobility, and church or synagogue attendance. None of these variables affected the relation between violence of programs preferred by boys at age 8 and how aggressive they were 10 years later.

When the subjects were 30 years old, they were interviewed again and archival data such as criminal justice records were consulted. It was found that the more frequently the subjects watched television at age 8, the more serious were the crimes for which they were convicted by age 30, the more aggressive was their behavior while under the influence of alcohol, and the harsher was the punishment they administered to their own children. A variety of television viewing behaviors at age 8 and a composite of aggressive behaviors at age 30 were strongly correlated. These relations held up even when the subjects' initial aggressiveness, social class, and IQ were controlled. Further, measurements of the subjects' own children, who were now the same age as the subjects were when we first saw them, showed that the subjects' aggressiveness and viewing of violence at age 8 related to their children's aggressiveness and their children's preferences for viewing violence 22 years later, when the subjects themselves were 30 years old. What one learns about life from the television screen seems to be transmitted even to the next generation.

Now, it is not claimed that the specific programs these adults watched when they were 8 years old still directly affected their behavior; the continued viewing of these programs probably contributed to the development of certain attitudes and norms of behavior and taught these subjects, when they were youngsters, ways of solving interpersonal problems—ways that remained with them over the years.

This causal link between the watching of violent television and subsequent aggressive behavior is not an isolated finding among a unique or nonrepresentative population in one area of the United States at a particular time. Seventeen years after the original data collection, another large group of youngsters was studied in a different geographical section of the U.S.—a heterogeneous suburb of Chicago. They were studied for 3 years, and essentially the same results were obtained.[15] Further, this 3-year follow-up was replicated in four other countries—Australia, Finland, Israel, and Poland.[13] The data from all five countries investigated in the study clearly indicate that more aggressive children watch more television, prefer more violent programs, identify more with TV characters, and perceive violence as more like real life than do less aggressive children. Further, it became clear that the relation between TV habits and aggression was not limited to boys, as had been found in the original study. Girls, too, are affected. Generally the causal relation was bidirectional, with aggressive children watching more violent television and the violent television making them more aggressive.

These findings of a causal relation between the watching of television violence and later aggressive and violent behavior are not unique. Since 1970 there have been at least three major national commissions composed of recognized scholars that have issued reports implicating television violence as a cause of aggression and violence in society. These reports are (1) the 1972 *Surgeon General's Report on Television and Social Behavior,*[22] (2) the 1982 *National Institute of Mental Health Report on Television and Behavior,*[20] and (3) the 1992 report of the *American Psychological Association Task Force on Television and Society.*[16] Further, in a 1991 report by the Centers for Disease Control and Prevention,[5] concerns about exposure to violence in the media as a factor in the development of aggression in children were reinforced once again. Among its recommendations for reducing violence, the CDC called on parents to avoid exposing their children to mass media depictions that "aggrandize" violence and to look for programs that educate children and families in the use of nonviolent alternatives for solving interpersonal problems. To date, at least four professional organizations have issued position papers endorsing the reduction of violence in the mass media—American Medical Association, American Academy of Pediatrics, American Academy of Child Psychiatry, and the American Psychological Association.

PSYCHOLOGICAL PROCESSES

Why do televised and film violence have such deleterious effects? Researchers have identified a number of psychological processes involved in producing the effect. First, young children imitate what they see others do, particularly if the "other" is a desirable hero with whom the youngster can identify. It is well established that observational learning is one of the most powerful mechanisms through which children acquire social skills and learn how to behave in society. If a boy is surrounded by aggressive family members and peers who solve problems violently, then that boy is likely to learn violent ways to solve problems—what have been termed *violent scripts* for social behavior. Similarly, if a boy is exposed constantly to television and film heroes solving problems aggressively, the boy will mimic those behaviors. Second, repeated exposure to media violence changes attitudes about the acceptability of violence. Viewers become more tolerant of violence in themselves because they come to believe that the world is a more violent place. The youngsters who are experiencing the frustrations and rage that today's urban life may engender are less likely to inhibit aggressive and violent actions because the mass media have taught them that aggression and violence are typical ways of behaving and are acceptable. Moreover, research has shown that attitudes and beliefs that specifically endorse aggression as a response to being disrespected or that make aggression against females seem acceptable can be taught by media portrayals. Third, continuous habitual exposure to media violence desensitizes children and adults to the negative emotional reactions that aggression and violence normally produce. After enough exposures, the physiological signs of unpleasant emotions disappear and the viewer becomes relatively unaroused by violence. This, of course, makes the viewer less affected by the viewer's own violent acts. Finally, the very frequency of aggressive cues in the media stimulates viewers to think of aggressive ways of responding that they otherwise might ignore. For example, numerous studies have shown that simply the sight of a gun stimulates children to think about aggressive actions.[3]

VIDEO GAMES

Interactive video games are one of the most popular forms of entertainment, particularly among adolescents. In the United States, video game revenues total $5.3 billion, about $400 million more than is spent at the movies.[7] Video games are now played in 42% of American homes.[19]

Surveys have indicated that most young adolescents play video games either at home or in arcades or both, with boys being more frequent players than girls in both settings.[10] Of the 21 most popular games in urban video arcades, 15 featured violent content or property destruction of objects or individuals. Either war, sports, or criminal activity (e.g., an escape from jail) were the most common themes for violent video games.[4]

As indicated at the beginning of this review, very little research has been done on the impact of video games on the aggressive behavior of the players. What studies there have been primarily are laboratory type experiments in which children and adolescents have been observed before and after playing a violent video game under controlled laboratory conditions. For example, in one study, 28 children ages 4 to 6 years were observed playing before and after watching a violent cartoon and before and after playing a violent video game, "Space Invader." Results indicated significant differences in aggressive behavior relative to preexposure behavior after watching the cartoon and after playing the video game. There was no difference between the television and video game conditions. It would appear that violent video games have much the same effect as violent television cartoons.[21] It is interesting that in a questionnaire study completed by 250 tenth and eleventh graders, it was reported that those respondents who watch more violent television also spend more time playing violent video games at arcades.[6]

OTHER BEHAVIOR

Although this report has focused on the effects of television and video games on the aggression of young viewers, the effects of television on other domains of behavior should not be overlooked. Television can encourage positive behaviors in children; indeed, this has been demonstrated. For example, watching programs such as "Sesame Street" and, in the past, "The Electric Company" has been shown to improve the cognitive skills of youngsters watching them. Prosocial behavior and values (e.g., nurturance, empathy, and task persistence) can be learned from such programs as "Mr. Rogers' Neighborhood."[16] Unfortunately, in the past, the violent content has overshadowed these positive achievements.

WHAT PARENTS CAN DO

After 30 years of facing such findings, the television industry still balks at taking steps to curb the level of violence being broadcast. Unfortunately, this leaves parents and other caretakers to protect children against this potent teacher; indeed, parents can do some things to counteract the influence of violent video, interactive or otherwise.

As recommended by the American Psychological Association Commission on Violence and Youth in its 1993 summary report:[1]

> Children can learn to distinguish between fictional portrayals and factual presentations. In addition, children can be taught to recognize ways in which violence is portrayed unrealistically (e.g., when it is portrayed without any negative consequences). Children can also learn to think about alternatives to the violence portrayed, a strategy that is particularly effective when an adult viewing the violence with the child expresses disapproval of violence as a means of solving problems and then offers alternatives. The availability of such protective measures for some parents, however, does not absolve the film and television industries from their responsibility for reducing the level of violence portrayed on the screen.

Television, of course, is not all bad. It can be an effective and persuasive teacher of prosocial attitudes and behavior and make an important contribution toward reducing violence in society. To achieve this goal, the APA Commission on Violence and Youth recommends including more prosocial messages and nonverbal problem-solving examples in television productions. Broadcasters also are urged to comply with laws requiring them to serve the educational needs of children by providing programs that educate children to prevent violence. The introduction of child viewing hours (e.g., 6 AM to 9 PM) during which excess violence in programs is banned would be helpful, as would meaningful rating systems based on a program's potential for damage to a child rather than on what is offensive to the parents.

REFERENCES

1. American Psychological Association Commission on Violence and Youth: *Violence and youth: psychology's responses,* Washington, DC, 1993, American Psychological Association,
2. Bandura A, Ross D, Ross SA: Imitation of film mediated aggressive models, *Journal of Abnormal and Social Psychology* 66:3, 1963.
3. Berkowitz L: Words and symbols as stimuli to aggressive responses. In Knutson J editor: *Control of aggression: implications from basic research,* Chicago, 1973, Aldine-Atherton.
4. Braun CM, Giroux P: Arcade video games: proxemic, cognitive and content analyses, *Journal of Leisure Research* 21:92, 1989.
5. Centers for Disease Control: Position papers from the Third National Injury Conference: setting the national agenda for injury control in the 1990s, Washington, DC, 1991, US Government Printing Office.
6. Dominick JR: Videogames, television violence and aggression, *Journal of Communication* 34:136, 1984.

7. Elmer-Dewitt P: The amazing video game boom, *Time* Sept 27, 1993, p 688.
8. Eron LD et al: Aggression and its correlates over 22 years. In Crowell D, Evans I, O'Donnell C, editors: *Childhood aggression and violence: sources of influence, prevention, and control,* New York, 1987, Plenum Press.
9. Eron LD, Walder LO, Lefowitz MM: *Learning of aggression in children,* Boston, 1971, Little, Brown.
10. Funk JA: Reevaluating the impact of video games, *Clin Pediatr* 32:86, 1993.
11. Gerbner G, Signorelli N: Violence profile, 1967 through 1988-1989: enduring patterns, Unpublished manuscript, University of Pennsylvania, Annenberg School of Communication, 1990.
12. Huesmann LR: Violence in the mass media. Paper presented at the Third International Conferences on Film Regulation, London, 1992.
13. Huesmann LR, Eron LD, editors: *Television and the aggressive child,* New York, 1986, Erlbaum.
14. Huesmann LR et al: The stability of aggressive behavior over time and generations, *Developmental Psychology* 20:1120, 1986.
15. Huesmann LR et al: Intervening variables in the television—aggression relation: evidence from two countries, *Developmental Psychology* 20:746, 1984.
16. Huston AC et al: *Big world, small screen: the role of television in American society,* Lincoln, Neb, 1992, University of Nebraska Press.
17. Kuby RW, Csikszentmihalyi M: *Television and the quality of life: how viewing shapes everyday experience,* Hillsdale, NJ, 1990, Erlbaum.
18. Lichter RS, Amundson D: A day of television violence, Washington, DC, 1992, Center for Media and Public Affairs.
19. Menn D: Rating violence ratings, *Multimedia World* Jan 1994, p 8.
20. National Institute of Mental Health: *Television and behavior: ten years of scientific progress and implications for the eighties* (vol. 1) *summary report,* Washington, DC, 1982, US Government Printing Office.
21. Silvern SB, Williamson PA: The effects of video game play on young children's aggression, fantasy and prosocial behavior, *Journal of Applied Developmental Psychology* 8:453, 1987.
22. Surgeon General's Scientific Advisory Committee on Television and Social Behavior: *Television and growing up: the impact of televised violence,* Washington, DC, 1972, US Government Printing Office.
23. Tangney JR, Feshbach S: Children's television viewing frequency: individual differences and demographic correlates, *Personality and Social Psychology Bulletin* 14:145, 1988.

67 Overview of School Health and School Health Program Goals

Philip R. Nader

School health programs and school-linked and school-based primary health care clinics are receiving increasing attention as logical ways to assist families in accessing health care, providing coordinated social and health services, and promoting health through preventive programs. Over 500 school-linked or school-based clinics exist (usually at the high school level) because of the problem of adolescents' access to health care services. However, a number of programs also are developing at the elementary level.

This proliferation of school-linked services is a direct outgrowth of the educational, health, and welfare reform movements. They develop most frequently in urban settings and target disadvantaged populations. However, one rural state, Vermont, is developing private-public partnerships to coordinate a wide range of human services for children and their families. Historically, school health is intended to link school-based services to an ongoing medical care home for the child.

SCHOOL HEALTH PROGRAM GOALS

The American Academy of Pediatrics' School Health Committee has suggested seven major school health program goals:

- Goal 1: Ensure access to primary health care
- Goal 2: Provide a system for dealing with critical medical situations
- Goal 3: Provide mandated screening and immunization monitoring
- Goal 4: Provide systems for identifying and solving students' health and educational problems
- Goal 5: Provide comprehensive and appropriate health education
- Goal 6: Provide a healthful and safe school environment that promotes learning
- Goal 7: Provide a system for evaluating the effectiveness of the school health program

Goal 1: Ensure Access to Primary Health Care

For school health programs to be effective, linkages must be formed between the school and the source of primary care for the child. Major difficulties arise when there is no regular source of care. The school health service plays an important role in the well-being of children by linking children and families to community primary care resources.

Providers of primary care would be wise to examine ways to utilize midlevel practitioners and other school-based personnel to provide cost-effective services at school sites when it is deemed desirable for a given community. Although a school-based clinic could become a medical home for a family—given no other resources in a community—it would be preferable to develop additional resources so that each family could have an ongoing medical home that would be available over the long term. All school-based services should include provision for 24-hour, 7-day-a-week back-up extending beyond the school day and the school year. Newer systems of managed care need to examine the potential benefits of linking services to families through the schools.

Goal 2: Provide a System for Dealing with Critical Medical Situations

In addition to expected instances of trauma requiring immediate medical attention (e.g., crisis episodes of asthma or seizures), the school health service must be prepared to deal with life-and-death situations of medically fragile children who may be located on school campuses, as well as the unfortunate eruption of violence, shootings and suicide, and community disasters. Trained personnel, standing policies and procedures, and key decision makers need to be identified. Most urban schools are readily accessible to emergency 911 systems. The American Academy of Pediatrics (AAP) has published suggested guidelines and procedures for school health programs.[3]

Goal 3: Provide Mandated Screening and Immunization Monitoring

Pediatric care providers need to know the required immunizations and screening procedures and also when these are supposed to be carried out in the schools. Guidelines and recommendations vary among the states, and adherence to these regulations varies depending on local resources. Guidelines for establishing screening mandates often are created by the state legislature. Primary care providers can lobby for more reliance on scientific evidence and whether a proposed screening procedure meets scientific criteria for establishing screening programs. These criteria include having a reliable and valid method of screening, as well as having accepted, effective treatment or remediation available to students in need of services.

Immunizations are required for school attendance in all 50 states. With recent initiatives for improving immunization rates among both school-age and preschool-age children, some schools are providing immunizations directly to school-age children and their preschool siblings.

Goal 4: Provide Systems for Identifying and Solving Students' Health and Educational Problems

The completeness and effectiveness of problem identification and solution depends to a large degree on the numbers and quality of school health personnel. The more trained and sophisticated the personnel, the more they can be expected to achieve. Differentiated staffing with appropriate utilization of aides, nurses, nurse practitioners, and physician consultant back-up is likely to be the most cost-effective way of responding to the identified needs of a population. Problems may be self-identified by parents and children themselves, or difficulties may be detected through observation in classrooms or consultation with teachers. Analysis of frequent visits to the school health room also indicates students who may need attention. Close links to community sources of care for physical and mental health resources are required to develop treatment plans effectively.

Goal 5: Provide Comprehensive and Appropriate Health Education

It is somewhat ironic that the same educational movement that is leading schools to become involved in human services delivery systems is, at the same time, decreasing the already underemphasized role of health education. Health is only referred to obliquely in recent formulations of national educational standards and goals.

Health providers can support schools to enhance health education programs and services. Collaboration and integration with community-wide health promotion efforts are helpful. This espouses the concept that schools cannot do the job alone. Within the school, attempts should be made to relate all aspects of school life with the health program. For example, classroom health curricula need to be integrated with healthful choices in the school nutrition program and activity promotion in the school's physical education program. Schools should be smoke-free environments. Teachers need work-site programs to encourage them to be healthful role models for children and youth. Teachers also need information and skills to communicate and answer children's questions effectively. If they do not know the answers, teachers need to know where questions about health can be answered.

Human sexuality education programs are needed on a much wider basis than currently are provided to children and youth in this country. Health care providers can help communities see the value of comprehensive health education programs, including education about sexuality. One way to introduce such programs gradually is to develop them jointly with the school. The program can be located in school, but the instruction can be provided by health personnel and teachers. Courses for parents and children will increase acceptability.

Goal 6: Provide a Healthful and Safe School Environment that Promotes Learning

In addition to the environmental aspects of comprehensive school health education mentioned above, other environmental conditions need to be guaranteed. Teachers should be as knowledgeable as possible about principles of child development. Teaching strategies need to be matched to the developmental and cognitive capabilities of children. Research has shown that systems that espouse noncoercive discipline and high academic expectations have the best educational outcomes.

Attention must be given to the physical safety of the school environment. This includes the presence of possible toxic agents, as well as the potential spill-over of neighborhood violence onto school campuses.

Goal 7: Provide a System for Evaluating the Effectiveness of the School Health Program

Because school health programs in the future will be linked more closely to existing and new systems of health care delivery in a community, evaluation will become an integral part of program planning and assessment. A community-needs assessment can determine the needs and resources present in a particular community. The needs assessment should involve all key child health, education, and social services leaders in the community and be broadly based across both private and public sectors. The needs assessment will guide the development of the extent of school-linked or school-based health services to be used.

As mentioned previously, selection of outcome indicators to be measured at periodic intervals will demonstrate to program planners and funders the usefulness of the programs established. It will be important to include outcome indicators for all seven goals for school health programs. Potential outcomes for each goal are listed in Table 67-1. For example, monitoring problem identification and outcomes can be useful by providing rationale and justification for services, as well as assessing needs for additional services.

INTEGRATED SERVICE SYSTEMS

Pediatric primary and secondary care providers need to take an active role in the development and implementation of so-called integrated service systems. These "one-stop" programs propose to streamline and make social, health, and family support services more cost effective and user friendly. Often, these services are placed in (or near) a school and include multiple human services in one easily accessible place. Health services often rank high among perceived needs in these systems. Exactly how to link the various services, and the much greater need for mental health services with such programs, often presents significant barriers.

A recent consensus conference of over 90 national child-related health, educational, and social professional associations came together and created basic principles that were designed to guide policymakers in setting administrative and professional practice objectives.[1]

These principles include (1) the structure and function of the basic elements of preventive and effective strategies, (2) "financing" guidelines for integrated services, (3) the role of needs assessment and evaluation, and (4) the importance of stronger coordinating structures for integrated service systems.

Role of the Pediatrician in School-Linked Services

Pediatric primary care providers may serve as consultants to or be directors of comprehensive school-based or school-linked health programs. In these roles, the provider will (1) have had experience in planning, managing, and evaluating systems of care, (2) be knowledgeable about funding and pro-

Table 67-1 Potential Outcome Measures for School Health Program Goals

Goal	Outcome measure(s)
One: Access to primary care	Number (%) of students who have an identifiable medical care home (ongoing source of primary health care) Decrease in use of emergency departments for nonemergent care
Two: Critical medical situations	Number (%) of staff who have active CPR certification Presence of standing emergency medical orders No preventable deaths Reduction in school accidents
Three: Mandated screening and immunization	Number (%) of vision referrals made, confirmed to need correction, and fitted (using corrective lenses) Number (%) of false positive screening results (referred but found to not have needed referral) Number (%) referred and not reaching a source of care Number (%) of students up-to-date on required immunizations
Four: Identification/solution of problems	Number (%) of problems identified that are corrected or being dealt with Absenteeism rates; dropout rates Number (%) at risk of academic failure (retention)
Five: Health education	More healthful school lunches (decreased fat and salt) More aerobic/active PE classes Existence of parental programs in health Existence of comprehensive sexual education course(s)
Six: School environment	Smoke-free school No incidents of violence in school Soap, water, and toilet paper available
Seven: Evaluation	Existence of a plan for evaluation and publication of an annual report

Table 67-2 The Physician's Role in Schools

Clinical issue/problem	Examples of physician's activities as child's primary care provider	Examples of physician's activities as consultant to school or school system
Learning disability	1. Requests teacher's perception of child's learning and behavior; results of individualized testing 2. Shares results of medical evaluation of child with the school 3. Works cooperatively with school personnel and parent(s) to develop educational and behavioral management plan for child (may include school visit) 4. Sets up mechanism for follow-up on behavioral and educational progress of child	1. Serves on district committee to accomplish biannual review of handicapped children's progress 2. Assists in setting up mechanism for providing follow-up behavioral and academic information to physicians who have placed students on psychoactive medication 3. Provides in-service session for classroom teachers on new concepts in attention deficit disorder 4. Advises school board on need for movement training for children who have learning disabilities
Asthma (school-age)	1. Requests school information on absenteeism, visits school nurse, obtains evidence of nonparticipation in physical education activities 2. Sets up mechanism for regular administration of bronchodilator at school 3. Sets up follow-up mechanism for continued monitoring of school attendance, medication-taking compliance, and participation in appropriate physical activities	1. Reviews absenteeism data to identify groups of students who have excessive absences that might be amenable to some intervention 2. Assists curriculum director and nurse in developing educational program for children who have asthma and their parents 3. Helps publicize program and communicates directly with students; solicits primary care physician's input and support for the educational program by reinforcing concepts in their patient visits

From Nader P: *Pediatr Rev* 4:82, 1982.

grammatic requirements in both health and education, and (3) be able to establish quality assurance programs. These skills will build on a solid clinical expertise in child and youth health issues, as well as first-hand knowledge and expertise with schools and educational systems.

The role of the primary or special care provider requires less expertise in program development and evaluation, but does require knowledge of the educational system and how to access the system for the benefit of the patient. These roles may be related to the school by nurse practitioners or other physician-extender personnel who are stationed in or visit the school regularly.

Guidelines for physicians as school consultants have been suggested.[3] Table 67-2 and the three boxes that follow illus-

GUIDELINES FOR PHYSICIAN AS CHILD'S CARE PROVIDER

1. Always inform parents and obtain permission to communicate with the school. Keep them informed of progress.
2. Approach all school personnel as coprofessionals who have skills and interests that complement your expertise and that can provide you with information you do not have. Recognize their interest in helping the children in their charge.
3. When contacting a school for the first time, contact the principal initially.
4. When calling a teacher, find out the best time for him or her to talk.
5. Encourage direct school-parent and parent-school communication.
6. Be willing to attend a school meeting, if necessary, to share information and develop treatment plans.
7. Listen carefully to ascertain the school personnel's main concerns and questions and attempt to respond to them.

GUIDELINES FOR PHYSICIAN AS SCHOOL HEALTH CONSULTANT

1. Distinguish between roles of a primary health care provider and those of a school consultant.
2. Become aware of laws and regulations affecting schools, including those related to school finance, education for handicapped children, bilingual education, and other education mandates.
3. Become knowledgeable about the formal and informal decision-making processes in schools regarding "regular" and "special" education of children (including health education).
4. Be a liaison to the rest of the medical community.
5. Establish a contract with the school that defines mutually agreed upon expectations and objectives.
6. Provide a regular report on your consultation to the school district.
7. Attempt to establish relationships with all levels and departments of the school system to permit access from the board and superintendent level to that of the classroom teacher.
8. Become aware of group process dynamics and decision making in groups.

trate examples of activities and suggested guidelines and approaches to be used by primary or secondary care providers interested in working with schools in their locale.

School Health Content for Pediatric Primary Care Providers

First, pediatric care providers must be current with new approaches and use school-linked human services programs to reach families in need. They should understand the basic principles of community organization and the need for increased

A CHECKLIST

State policies and programs

Have you apprised yourself of state policies and programs related to comprehensive school health programs?
Have you checked to see whether health outcome objectives exist, and if so, how they are assessed?

Local policies and programs

Have you apprised yourself of district policies and programs related to comprehensive school health programs?
Have you determined what health curriculum, textbooks, and materials actually are being used in the schools?
Have you ascertained

- policies and programs that need strengthening?
- serious gaps or deficits?
- opportunities for health professionals to contribute meaningfully?

Influencing local policies and programs

Do you know how the local education system works? Who makes decisions? Who has authority? Who actually does the work?
Do you know who supports (and who is concerned with) various aspects of comprehensive school health programs and their reasons for doing so?
Have you contacted appropriate officials about your ideas and obtained their support for working with schools?
Have you refined your ideas in consultation with key parties—teachers, administrators, school health professionals, public health professionals, school board members, and parents?
Have you provided for periodic progress reports and changed direction or emphasis based on their results?

From National Association of State Boards of Education: *How schools work and how to work with schools,* Alexandria, Va, 1989.

public policy support for school-linked preventive care. Second, pediatric providers need to be aware of the seven major goals of a comprehensive school health program. Third, pediatric providers need to be aware of the multitude of health and nonhealth personnel that play key roles. Unless pediatric providers are aware of the child development principles from preschool through adolescence, they cannot help implement comprehensive school health programs effectively.

A wide variety of clinical problems that are encountered commonly in school health practice, including the following:

1. School attendance and school avoidance problems
2. Psychosomatic complaints
3. Learning problems
4. Attention-related disorders
5. Behavioral and disciplinary problems
6. Medically fragile, technologically dependent students
7. Various communicable diseases, in adolescents and teachers
8. Sexually transmitted diseases, including HIV
9. Substance use and abuse

Because medications, including psychoactive drugs, sometimes are needed to keep children in school and "on task," the provider should master ways to ensure medication compliance. Standardized procedures for medication administration in schools are available.[2]

Objectives for Educating Physicians in School Health

Many methods of teaching about school health are available. One of the best ways is to expose trainees to experiences in community-based programs. Those responsible for developing educational experiences need to use faculty and staff who have had experience in school health services and schools. Objectives have been developed for medical students, residents, and fellowship trainees in community and school health. They have been published in the American Academy of Pediatrics' manual entitled *School Health: Policy and Practice,* ed 5, 1993.[3]

CONCLUSION

School health programs are rapidly developing to a point where they may more likely reach their potential in ensuring access to care, as well as provide a good system of preventive health care. Pediatric care providers need to become integral parts of these systems; only in this way will they continue to play a major role in improved health and health educational outcomes for children.

REFERENCES

1. American Academy of Pediatrics: Principles to link by: integrated service systems that are community-based and school linked. Presented at the National Consensus Building Conference on School-Linked Integrated Service Systems, Washington, DC, January 23-24, 1994.
2. American Academy of Pediatrics, Committee on School Health: Guidelines for the administration of medication in school, *Pediatrics* 92:499, 1993.
3. American Academy of Pediatrics, Committee on School Health: *School health: policy and practice,* ed 5, Elk Grove Village, Ill, 1993, American Academy of Pediatrics.
4. Nader PR: A pediatrician's primer for school health activities, *Pediatr Rev* 4:82, 1982.
5. National Association of State Boards of Education: *How schools work and how to work with schools,* Alexandria, Va, 1989.

68 School Health Education

Guy S. Parcel and Laura K. McCormick

Our increased awareness of the limitations inherent in the curative aspects of health care has made for greater emphasis on the importance of health maintenance and preventive medicine. Through the years health education has been used to help individuals prevent illness and maintain the best state of health possible for them. The underlying assumption has been that an informed public is better prepared to make decisions that will promote health.

Within this framework, health education in the schools has become particularly attractive. Almost all children go to school and while in school constitute a "captive audience." Thus schools have been suggested as the logical place for children to learn about health and to develop the abilities needed to make effective decisions about health-related behavior. However, it has yet to be demonstrated that schools can meet this objective. As the search continues for ways to improve the effectiveness of school health education, it is becoming increasingly clear that success must involve a cooperative effort between educational and health care personnel. For example, the pediatrician's knowledge of child health and development is much greater than that of most educational personnel in the schools. Therefore the child health care professional has an essential role in school health education programs. On the other hand, most educational personnel have more refined and effective skills in teaching and a greater opportunity to reach more children than do pediatricians.

Including health education as part of the instructional program in schools is by no means a new concept. Through the involvement of a school nurse or school physician, health education activities have become part of school health services. For example, while screening for vision and hearing, the school nurse can discuss with the children, either individually or in groups, the purpose of the screening and the importance of health care in terms of sight and hearing. The school nurse also could go into the classroom and instruct the students in particular health habits, such as dental health (brushing teeth) or nutrition (good eating habits). When health instruction is incorporated into the curriculum of the regular classroom teacher or the special health education teacher, it is referred to as *curricular health education.* Health education is either integrated into the classroom curriculum or established as a separate curriculum within the school's total instructional program.

TRENDS IN SCHOOL HEALTH EDUCATION

Early approaches to curriculum development in health education focused primarily on specific types of health problems, particularly those associated with risky or illicit behavior. In the 1950s it was recognized that drinking had become a serious health and social problem. In an attempt to solve this problem, school personnel were called on to provide instruction, pointing out the dangers and health hazards associated with alcohol consumption. It was assumed that if students knew about these dangers and were told about the health hazards, they would avoid alcohol abuse. Some states went so far as to enact laws requiring public schools to instruct students in the prevention of alcohol abuse.

It has been demonstrated, however, that even when information is presented effectively, it does not necessarily lead to a change in behavior. Many drug education programs were developed that effectively taught the pharmacological aspects, legal penalties, and physical risks of drug abuse; however, evaluations of these programs revealed that they had a limited effect on alcohol abuse and other drug use.[2] Similar results from nutrition and tobacco education programs in the late 1960s, 1970s, and early 1980s further demonstrated the weaknesses of health education programs based primarily on a cognitive approach.[6,16]

This failure reinforced what many educators had been suggesting for years—that health behavior is related not only to knowledge but also to factors such as expectations and values associated with health behavior. It also became apparent that health-related problems could not be resolved effectively on a "crisis" basis; if health problems were to be prevented through education, a means of addressing these problems had to be developed long before they reached a state of crisis. Teaching methods that focus on the learners' attitudes and feelings fall into the realm of *affective education.* Teaching in this area is related more to personal development than to learning facts and concepts. Affective education programs hypothesize that children who feel good about themselves, who can develop effective relationships with others, and who clearly understand what is important to them are less likely to have problems with drug abuse. For the teacher, this approach involves helping students to build self-esteem, to learn interpersonal skills, and to develop effective decision-making and problem-solving techniques.

As an outgrowth of the increased interest in affective education, in the 1970s many school health education programs were expanded or redirected to focus more on attitudes, feelings, and values. Some suggested programs tended to deemphasize the importance of information, whereas others emphasized an integration of cognitive and affective learning. However, a review of affective approaches to preventing substance abuse concluded that, in general, they made no significant impact on substance use.[7]

In the 1980s school-based interventions were grounded in social learning, which typically involved training students to resist social pressure to engage in unhealthy behavior (e.g., smoking), as well as creating a social environment that encouraged the development of healthy behavior.[12,18]

Social learning methods were expanded to health education curriculum, which led to development of the *social in-*

fluences approach. This approach recognized the importance of preparing students to resist the pressures of an environment that encouraged risk-taking behavior. Teaching strategies in this approach include augmenting students' knowledge about the short-term consequences of risky behavior, training in resisting peer pressure, "inoculation" against mass media messages, establishing normative expectations for healthful behavior, using peer leaders as role models, and having students make a personal commitment to avoid risk-taking behavior or to engage in healthy behavior. These methods have been applied successfully to smoking prevention[17] and drug abuse prevention,[15] and evaluations have indicated a significant effect in reducing risk-taking behavior.

Another approach that emerged recently in school health education is the use of skill development methods to prevent risky behavior. The *skills approach* assumes that a set of social and behavioral skills is essential for making effective decisions about health behavior. Furthermore, if students are able to develop these skills, if they know the consequences of risky behavior, and if they have opportunities to practice these skills, they will be more likely to avoid risk-taking behavior and develop healthier patterns. The skills usually addressed in these types of programs involve decision making, problem solving, communication, and stress management or relaxation. The skills approach has been shown to be especially effective when applied to smoking; it also has proved effective in other areas of health behavior.[3]

Besides the health education curriculum, the concept of school-based health promotion and disease prevention has been expanded to include other components of the school that influence or facilitate healthy behavior.[9] Such programs have been developed to coordinate classroom health instruction with changes in school food services and physical education, thus improving the diet and amount of physical activity of elementary schoolchildren.[13] Efforts also have been made to involve parents and to focus on the family as a critical component in influencing changes in health behavior through school-based programs.[10,17] Linking school-based programs with community programs and agencies also has shown potential for improving the effectiveness of existing programs concerned with promoting healthy behavior and preventing health problems.[14,15,19]

Most state guidelines for health education in the schools are organized around content areas, such as nutrition, safety, substance abuse, chronic disease, infectious diseases, mental health, growth and development, and family living. The term *comprehensive school health education* has been used to describe a curriculum that provides a sequence of activities at each grade level to address each designated content area. Thus the predominant approach to health education in the schools today is to present health-related information within each content area, with increasing complexity at each grade level.

THE PHYSICIAN'S ROLE IN SCHOOL HEALTH EDUCATION

The goal of health education is to help people develop skills and confidence that will enable them to make good choices about their health behavior and about appropriate use of health care resources. If this goal is to be achieved through a school health program, it will require a cooperative effort by health care and educational personnel. In structured classroom activities and in noncurricular health education activities, the physician can contribute to school health education in five distinct ways: (1) by reviewing the content and process of health education for accuracy and age appropriateness, (2) by conducting health education activities for children and parents through the school program, (3) by assisting with the training of personnel involved in health education, (4) by helping to collect data to evaluate the outcomes of health education activities, and (5) by encouraging community support for school health education activities.

The physician can play an important role in the development of a health education curriculum by identifying the health concerns related to specific age groups. Physicians are aware of the health concerns of and needs expressed by their patients. These concerns and needs can be identified and interpreted for educational personnel in planning health education activities. With the physician's help, critical skills can be identified for the various age groups, and once these skills have been identified, activities can be developed to help children develop them.

Physicians also can help teachers understand the normal processes of child development and help them identify children's developmental needs. Teachers are required to master a broad spectrum of information related to health behavior, and it is difficult for them to stay abreast of current knowledge in all these areas. The physician can be especially helpful by alerting teachers to recent information about specific areas of health and by suggesting resources for additional information. There almost always is a gap between data generated by the health sciences and the information available for use in instructional programs. The physician can help narrow this gap.

Physicians may be called on to serve as guest lecturers in classrooms. When a teacher is faced with complicated or sensitive material, such as information on HIV or AIDS, contraception and family planning, or specific diseases, the physician may be asked to talk to students. The easiest way for physicians to handle such a request is to visit the classroom. However, there are some obvious drawbacks to this approach. The physician may not be prepared to present the material at a level appropriate for the students, and the physician's time will be limited. A better approach is for the physician to work with the teacher to identify the information students need. Together the physician and teacher can plan an ongoing program that the teacher can then present. In this way a larger number of students can benefit from the physician's contribution over a longer period.

The time, effort, and resources devoted to the school health education curriculum depend on the priority a school district places on health education. When it comes to health, physicians obviously enjoy considerable influence and prestige in a community. Spending time with school board members and administrators can encourage a high priority for the school health education curriculum. The following section outlines a strategy for physicians and other community members to follow in developing a comprehensive school health education program in their communities.

AN APPROACH TO DEVELOPING HEALTH EDUCATION PROGRAMS

Planning Committees

An initial group consisting of the top school administrators and school staff likely to have responsibility for the health program should be formed to establish the guidelines and process for program planning. Regardless of the level of community enthusiasm and support for health education, school administrators and staff always should be included at the highest levels of the decision-making process to approve and support program development officially. A second group then is organized to develop the program. This program planning group should be made up of administrators, teachers, students, parents, and resource people or consultants from the community and should establish strong communication links with the decision-making group.

Assessment of Needs and Resources

The planning group will need information to determine the scope and direction of the proposed program. Useful information can be obtained from a review of the literature and of programs from other school districts. However, information about the local situation is essential to direct the program toward local needs. Standardized survey questionnaires can be used to measure students' current health knowledge, attitudes, and behaviors. This information can be useful in setting priorities for the program.

Information also should be obtained about the resources available for a health education program. Individuals who have training and experience in health education, in effective educational techniques, in the development of interpersonal skills, and in methodologies of social learning are invaluable resources. It also is important to identify potential sources of funding (local, state, and federal) and available instructional materials and consultants.

Development of Program Goals and Objectives

Goals, the outcomes expected to result from the program, should be realistic and achievable. The goals preferably should be stated in such a way that the extent of their achievement can be measured. For example: (1) at the end of 5 years, the number of youths under age 19 arrested for driving under the influence of alcohol or drugs will be reduced by 30%; or (2) at the end of 3 years, the number of youths who begin smoking in the eighth grade will be reduced by 50%. Goals that include statements about "when," "how much," "of what," and "by whom" add specificity that provides more direction and focus for the education program.

The next step is to state specific objectives for each goal by student grade level. Objectives are accomplished by *students* and therefore usually are stated in behavioral terms and address what the student is expected to be able to do as a result of this instruction. For example, the student will be able to (1) demonstrate how to use techniques to resist peer pressure, (2) apply steps in decision making to resolve a conflict about food selection in a social situation, and (3) use relaxation techniques to cope with feelings of stress.

Program Activities

Activities are the experiences that will provide the knowledge, skills, practice, reinforcement, and confidence for performing the behaviors stated in the objectives. Activities are linked to objectives and should not be developed until after the specific goals and objectives for the health education program have been identified. Attention also should be given to activities outside the classroom that will support and reinforce classroom learning. Activities for parents, teachers, and other school staff are valuable in providing the social support and environment for reinforcing the learning of new behaviors.

It is helpful to conduct a pilot program in one school or a few schools to test ideas and techniques and to make changes before a district-wide program is implemented. Once a pilot program has worked effectively and has been shown to be acceptable, it usually is easier to implement in other schools in the district. It is essential that the pilot program be evaluated in such a way that components that may require modification can be identified.

Teacher Preparation

In-service training for teachers is essential for implementing a new curriculum. Such training should include attitudinal support for the curriculum and specific teaching skills. Attention also should be given to involving other school personnel who might not teach the curriculum but whose support for it is important. For example, the school principal, nurse, counselor, or social worker should be involved in planning the implementation of the program.

IMPLEMENTATION OF CHANGE

Change in school systems tends to occur slowly, often because of the lack of a systematic approach to effect change. This phenomenon is especially relevant to the introduction of innovative programs to promote school health, an area in which change often needs to occur within several components of the total school program. The model for implementing change in schools has four phases: (1) organizational commitment, (2) change in policies and practices, (3) alteration of roles and actions of staff, and (4) implementation of learning.[11] This model is intended to provide a systematic approach to change that includes school components that support and facilitate behaviors addressed by health education programs in the classroom.

In the first phase, commitment is obtained from key decision makers in the school system to proceed with the planning of a new or modified health promotion program. A top-down approach would involve school board members, superintendents, and program directors arriving at a decision to commit to the proposed program. The proposal for the new program can come from an agency outside the district, such as a health department or voluntary health agency, or from inside groups, such as curriculum planning committees or task force groups appointed to address specified problems. Commitment usually is obtained through a series of meetings with key decision makers. These meetings typically involve a written or verbal presentation on the importance of and need for the proposed program. Physicians can provide information to help establish a high priority for proposed health promotion programs.

Commitment also needs to be obtained from a bottom-up, or grassroots, approach, in which the individuals who implement the program (teachers and staff members) are involved in making decisions about planning new or modified programs. One method for obtaining this type of commitment, the "seaside" model (named for a seaside retreat in Oregon), has been implemented in several states. The seaside model involves teams from school districts coming together in a conference to explore their own personal health promotion needs, as well as those of their students. The process involves planning a health promotion program or activity for their district. Recently the seaside model has been expanded to include community representatives. This experience often results in a strong personal and professional commitment for health promotion programs.

Once commitment is demonstrated, a policy planning group composed of the program directors and key administrators should be established to develop and define policies. The policies then are given to a second planning group to address changes that will be needed in current practices to follow through on the intent of the policies necessary to the new program. This second planning group usually consists of program directors and representatives of teachers and staff members who will be implementing the program.

The third phase focuses on preparing the teachers and staff members to implement the program. In-service training, technical assistance, and monitoring and feedback can be used to alter roles and actions of personnel to implement new programs. Finally, with these changes in place, the school program is ready to provide activities that will help the students develop healthy behavior. Student activities should include classroom instruction, practice in school, practice at home, and reinforcement and social support from the school for practicing the healthy behaviors.

REASONABLE EXPECTATIONS FOR SCHOOL HEALTH EDUCATION

The health professional may expect that, to be effective, health education must influence behavior to reduce the risk of disease or to improve health status. The educator, however, might argue that the role of the school is to increase knowledge and develop critical thinking and not necessarily to change student behavior, which may be greatly influenced by factors outside the classroom. Both perspectives could be considered correct, and each will influence how programs are designed and evaluated.

School health education programs can help students learn about their health. Evaluations of school health education programs have demonstrated their effectiveness in influencing a variety of outcomes, including knowledge, attitudes, health practices, behavior, and physiological factors.* The program's effect on learning, and eventually on behavior, depends on the quality of the planning and the input of sufficient resources, including teacher training and adequate classroom instructional time.[5] Behavioral change, however, is complex, and simplistic approaches that do not effectively use what has been learned both in research and in the field are unlikely to succeed.

It is unreasonable to expect school-based educational programs alone to influence behaviors that are not supported by the child's larger social environment. For example, how can a child change to a low-fat diet when the other family members continue their same eating patterns? How can an adolescent be expected to avoid the social use of drugs or alcohol when the larger social environment not only supports but also encourages the use of alcohol and drugs? How can an adolescent be expected to prevent an unwanted pregnancy when the appropriate counseling and health services are difficult to find and use? School health education programs should be planned with a consideration of reasonable outcomes and the type of program necessary to accomplish those outcomes.

One of the major obstacles to health promotion and disease prevention for children and adolescents is the fragmentation of health education and preventive services. The Centers for Disease Control and Prevention (CDC) recommends a model for school health that integrates several components of the school and community to address risky behaviors. These components include school health services, school health education, school health environment, integrated school and community health promotion efforts, school physical education, school food services, school counseling, and school site health promotion programs for faculty and staff.[9]

The CDC's Division of Adolescent and School Health has further identified six health risk areas to be targeted by school and community programs: HIV and sexually transmitted diseases, injuries, nutrition, physical activity, alcohol and illicit drug use, and tobacco use. They are supporting this effort by developing a series of guidelines for schools to assist in the planning, implementation, and evaluation of school health programs. The CDC also has supported the American Medical Association in the development of the AMA's Guidelines for Adolescent Preventive Services (GAPS),[1] which are designed to set priorities and establish standards for the provision of preventive services by primary care physicians. Although these efforts target different segments of the community (schools and primary care physicians), they have the same long-range goal: improving the health of adolescents. Ultimately, this goal will be realized only when various segments of the community exist within a larger framework of coordinated services.

It is unreasonable to expect that a single unit on health education placed within the total curriculum will accomplish the development of skills needed to adopt healthy behaviors. A comprehensive approach that provides knowledge, the development of skills, and practice in a developmental sequence through each of the grade levels is necessary. It also is important to relate the health education program to other parts of the school curriculum and programs. Students need numerous opportunities to experience personal development, and the social environment of the school should be structured to support students in their practice of decision making and related skills.

*References 4, 5, 8, 13, 15, 17, 19, 20.

REFERENCES

1. American Medical Association, Department of Adolescent Health: *Guidelines for adolescent preventive services,* Chicago, Ill, 1992, The Association.
2. Bangert-Drowns RL: The effects of school-based substance abuse education: a meta-analysis, *J Drug Educ* 18:243, 1988.
3. Botvin GJ: Prevention of adolescent substance abuse through the development of personal and social competence. In Glynn T, editor: *Preventing adolescent drug abuse: intervention strategies,* NIDA Research

Monograph Series, No 47, Washington, DC, 1983, US Government Printing Office.

4. Bush PJ et al: Cardiovascular risk prevention in black school children: the "Know Your Body" evaluation project, *Health Educ Q* 16:215, 1989.
5. Connell DB, Turner RR, Mason EF: Summary of findings of the school health education evaluation: health promotion effectiveness, implementation, and costs, *J Sch Health* 55:316, 1985.
6. Contento IR, Manning AD, Shannon B: Research perspectives on school-based nutrition education, *J Nutrition Educ* 24:247, 1992.
7. Hansen WB: School-based substance abuse prevention: a review of the state of the art in curriculum, 1980-1990, *Health Educ Res* 7:40, 1992.
8. Killen JD et al: The Stanford Adolescent Heart Health Program, *Health Educ Q* 16:263, 1989.
9. Kolbe LJ: Increasing the impact of school health promotion programs: emerging research perspectives, *Health Educ Q* 17:47, 1986.
10. Nader PR et al: A family approach to cardiovascular risk reduction: results from the San Diego Family Health Project, *Health Educ Q* 16:229, 1989.
11. Parcel GS, Simons-Morton BG, Kolbe LJ: Health promotion: integrating organization change and student learning strategies, *Health Educ Q* 15:435, 1988.
12. Parcel GS et al: School promotion of healthful diet and physical activity: impact on learning outcomes and self-reported behavior, *Health Educ Q* 16:181, 1989.
13. Parcel GS et al: Translating theory into practice: intervention strategies for the diffusion of a health promotion innovation, *Fam Community Health* 12:1, 1989.
14. Pentz MA: Community organization and school liaisons: how to get programs started, *J Sch Health* 56:382, 1986.
15. Pentz MA et al: A multicommunity trial for primary prevention of adolescent drug abuse, *JAMA* 261:3259, 1989.
16. Perry CL, Kelder SH: Models for effective prevention, *J Adolesc Health* 13:355, 1992.
17. Perry CL et al: Parent involvement with children's health promotion: a one-year follow-up of the Minnesota home team, *Health Educ Q* 16:171, 1989.
18. Perry CL et al: The Child and Adolescent Trial for Cardiovascular Health (CATCH): overview of the intervention program and evaluation methods, *Cardiovascular Risk Factors* 2:36, 1992.
19. US Department of Health and Human Services: Preventing tobacco use among young people: a report of the surgeon general, Atlanta, 1994, Centers for Disease Control and Prevention.
20. Walter HJ: Primary prevention of chronic disease among children: the school-based "Know Your Body" intervention trials, *Health Educ Q* 16:201, 1989.

69 Attention Deficit/Hyperactivity Disorder

Esther H. Wender and Mary V. Solanto

The behavioral syndrome known as attention deficit/hyperactivity disorder (AD/HD) is actually a cluster of behaviors (i.e., an excessively high level of motor activity, plus problems with concentration, attention, and impulsivity) that emerges early in a child's life and persists over time.[6] Although broadly defined and associated with several etiological agents, AD/HD is thought to arise from a combination of biological factors and environmental influences, which produce the typical clinical features.

AD/HD has been known by a variety of names, each reflecting a different focus on symptoms or etiology. Among these names were "hyperactivity," "hyperkinetic syndrome," and "minimal brain dysfunction." With the publication of the third edition of the *Diagnostic and Statistical Manual of Mental Disorders* (DSM III)[7] in 1980, the focus shifted to attention deficits as the feature that unified all aspects of the syndrome, and it was named attention deficit disorder (ADD). At that time the syndrome was said to occur either with hyperactivity (ADD-H) or without (ADD–non-H). When the nomenclature was revised in 1987, it was felt that the evidence was insufficient to support the existence of two different syndromes; the name was changed to attention deficit hyperactivity disorder, and the symptoms of attention deficits, hyperactivity, and impulsivity were lumped together. The criterion for diagnosis was exhibiting 8 of 14 total behaviors.

The current criteria, established in 1994 with the publication of the fourth edition of the *Diagnostic and Statistical Manual of Mental Disorders* (DSM-IV),[6] again separate the symptoms of inattention and those of hyperactivity/impulsivity. This nomenclature recognizes three separate syndromes: attention deficit/hyperactivity disorder, predominantly inattentive type; attention deficit/hyperactivity disorder, predominantly hyperactive/impulsive type; and attention deficit/hyperactivity disorder, combined type. Yet another category, attention deficit/hyperactivity disorder, not otherwise specified, is used when the patient does not quite meet diagnostic criteria but nonetheless experiences significant difficulty. The current criteria are listed in the box on p. 672.

RELATED PROBLEMS

It long has been recognized that other common behavioral and emotional problems are seen with the symptoms of AD/HD. Some of the most common are learning disabilities, oppositional defiant and conduct disorders, and mood and anxiety disorders.

With regard to learning disabilities (LD), many children identified as having these problems seem to display the behaviors of AD/HD and qualify for that diagnosis. In one study, 25% of a group of children initially identified as learning disabled also qualified for the diagnosis of AD/HD.[14] In another study, 45% of a group of children identified as having AD/HD also qualified for a diagnosis of specific learning disability.[15] Most children who have learning disabilities also demonstrate impaired attention. However, the diagnosis of AD/HD is used only when the inattention is sufficiently significant to warrant a diagnosis of AD/HD, combined type, or AD/HD, predominantly inattentive type (see the box on p. 672). A significant problem in identifying the overlap between specific learning disabilities and AD/HD is distinguishing between the underachievement that results from the perceptual problems of LD and the poor school performance that stems from the behavioral issues of AD/HD (i.e., failure to follow through, difficulty persisting in a task, and disorganization).

Oppositional defiant disorder (ODD) and conduct disorder (CD) are two disruptive behavior disorders commonly seen in conjunction with AD/HD. ODD is characterized by negativistic, hostile, and defiant behaviors, which are specifically described in the box on p. 673. CD is a more serious disorder in which the basic rights of others are violated. Specific diagnostic criteria for CD are discussed in Chapter 79, Conduct Disorders.

The relationships among ODD, CD, and AD/HD remain controversial.[17,18] It is clear that many children who have AD/HD also have disruptive behavior problems and qualify for ODD when they are younger. A smaller but unknown percentage qualify for CD when they are older. Some investigators have proposed that certain behaviors (e.g., emotional lability and impaired response to conditioning) are part of the core symptomatology in a subgroup of AD/HD children and lead to disruptive behaviors. Others argue that AD/HD leads to poor self-esteem and, in some families, to inadequate parenting, which in turn results in conduct problems.

Another issue is the overlap of AD/HD symptoms with those of anxiety and mood disorders.[3,4] Studies that describe this overlap have focused either on the early histories of children who have mood or anxiety disorders or on extensive family histories that reveal AD/HD and mood and anxiety problems in the same or closely related individuals.

PRESENTING PROBLEMS

The key to diagnosis is an accurate, comprehensive history. However, because the practitioner usually is overwhelmed by a barrage of complaints about many behaviors and has difficulty sorting out those that contribute to the diagnosis, it is important to group specific behaviors into broader categories that may then suggest the presence of AD/HD. The three broad categories of behavior that characterize AD/HD are (1) hyperactivity, (2) impulsivity, and (3) inattentiveness. The behaviors that suggest oppositional and conduct disorders are (1) emotional lability and (2) resistance to conditioning. Finally, poor peer relationships and poor school performance are common consequences of all these traits.

ATTENTION DEFICIT/HYPERACTIVITY DISORDER: DIAGNOSTIC CRITERIA*

I. Either (A) or (B)
—Lasting 6 months or more longer
—Severe enough to be maladaptive and inconsistent with normal development

(A) Inattention (at least six of the following nine symptoms):

1. Often fails to give close attention to details or makes careless mistakes in schoolwork, work, or other activities
2. Often has difficulty sustaining attention in tasks or play activities
3. Often does not seem to listen when spoken to directly
4. Often does not follow through on instructions and fails to finish schoolwork, chores, or duties in the work place (not due to oppositional behavior or failure to understand instructions)
5. Often has difficulty organizing tasks and activities
6. Often avoids, dislikes, or is reluctant to engage in tasks that require sustained mental effort such as schoolwork or homework
7. Often loses things necessary for tasks or activities (e.g., toys, school assignments, pencils, books, or tools).
8. Often is easily distracted by extraneous stimuli
9. Often is forgetful in daily activities

(B) Hyperactivity/Impulsivity (at least six of the following nine symptoms):

Hyperactivity

1. Often fidgets with hands or feet or squirms in seat
2. Often leaves seat in classroom or in other situations in which remaining seated is expected
3. Often runs about or climbs excessively when it is inappropriate (may be limited to subjective feelings of restlessness in older individuals)
4. Often has difficulty playing or engaging in leisure activities quietly
5. Often is "on the go" or acts as if "driven by a motor"
6. Often talks excessively

Impulsivity

7. Often blurts out answers before questions have been completed
8. Often has difficulty waiting for his or her turn
9. Often interrupts or intrudes on others (e.g., butts into conversations or games)

II. Symptoms (at least some of those noted above) present before 7 years of age

III. Some impaired function in two or more settings (e.g., school, work, and home)

IV. Clear evidence of impairment in social, academic, or occupational functioning

V. Symptoms are not exclusively associated with
Pervasive developmental disorder
Schizophrenia or other psychoses and are not better accounted for by
Mood disorder
Anxiety disorder
Dissociative disorder
Personality disorder

*From the *Diagnostic and statistical manual of mental disorders,* ed 4, Washington, DC, 1994, American Psychiatric Association.

Hyperactivity

Hyperactive children are excessively active even in inherently active situations (i.e., during active play), especially when they are younger (3 to 10 years of age). For instance, instead of running, they run headlong. Instead of dropping objects, they throw them. They tend to talk excessively. When engaged in activities that require sitting still, such as doing schoolwork or watching television, they stand out as exceptionally restless and fidgety. There also is a difference in the quality of motor behavior. From early in life, children who have this condition shift more than usual from one activity to another; this apparently is secondary to their difficulty or unwillingness to sustain attention. Parents often say that their child is bored easily, and they may attribute this boredom inaccurately to high intelligence. Studies of highly intelligent children reveal that they usually are exceptionally attentive and persistent.

Impulsivity

The younger child who has AD/HD frequently is described as one who touches everything or rushes to explore things without concern for likely danger or displeasure from others. In the laboratory these children have difficulty delaying their response to a task and thus make errors based on a failure to reflect. In the classroom, they often do written work quickly and erroneously or messily, just to be finished. As they get older, these children frequently get into trouble because they act quickly without thinking of the consequences. Some studies have shown that these children have more accidents than do their non-AD/HD peers.

Inattentiveness

Parents and teachers describe children with AD/HD as having a short attention span and being easily distracted. However, adults also may observe that the child can concentrate and "attend" in some situations, typically when the activity is one that he or she especially likes. Also, concentration often improves strikingly when the teacher or parent gives the child individual attention. Variability in attention, depending on the surroundings and the nature of the task, also has been found in laboratory investigations of this trait. This leads to speculation that attention problems are closely tied to motivation; in other words, children who have AD/HD are less likely to be motivated by tasks that engage the attention of most children their age. Activities that particularly provoke inattention are household chores and classroom work. Because these tasks are not inherently interesting to most children, an important element of motivation in the average child

CRITERIA FOR OPPOSITIONAL DEFIANT DISORDER*

A. A pattern of negativistic, hostile, and defiant behavior lasting at least 6 months, during which four (or more) of the following are present:
   1. Often loses temper
   2. Often argues with adults
   3. Often defies or refuses to comply with adults' requests or rules
   4. Often annoys people deliberately
   5. Often blames others for his or her own mistakes or misbehavior
   6. Often is touchy or easily annoyed by others
   7. Often is angry and resentful
   8. Often is spiteful or vindictive

   Note: A criterion is considered met only if the behavior occurs more often than is typically observed in individuals of comparable age and developmental level.

B. The disturbance in behavior causes clinically significant impairment in social, academic, or occupational functioning.

C. The behaviors do not occur exclusively during the course of a psychotic or mood disorder.

D. Criteria are not met for conduct disorder and, if the individual is 18 years of age or older, criteria are not met for antisocial personality disorder.

*From the *Diagnostic and statistical manual of mental disorders*, ed 4, Washington, DC, 1994, American Psychiatric Association.

seems to be fear of punishment or a desire to please; these feelings appear to be deficient in children who have AD/HD.

Emotional Lability

Many children who have AD/HD tend to experience both positive and negative emotions more intensely and with less provocation than do other children of the same age. Parents and teachers report frequent and poorly controlled temper outbursts and overexcitement in response to new or pleasurable activities. The child's easily provoked and intense anger, combined with a relative lack of fear, leads to excessive fighting, aggressiveness, and impulsive responses to stimulating situations. This troublesome trait may be the earliest precursor of antisocial behavior seen later in many adolescents who have AD/HD. Excessive excitability often is perceived as positive by these children. Stimulant medication frequently subdues this excitability, a result older children and adolescents often dislike. This reaction may explain why many older patients resist taking medications.

Resistance to Conditioning

Conditioning refers to the general process of reinforcing desirable behaviors and extinguishing undesirable ones. Parents and teachers more commonly refer to this process as discipline. Many children who have AD/HD are more difficult to discipline, relative to their age. One component of this resistance seems to be the relative lack of fear and the lack of desire to please others described earlier. Misbehavior is repeated often, despite punishment. The child avoids household chores, and discipline often is not helpful. Teachers report that the children fail to complete classroom work despite loss of privileges and other punishment. These children require special behavior modification techniques, consisting of close monitoring and immediate and consistent responses; the average child, in contrast, responds to less intensive measures.

Poor Peer Relationships

All of the characteristics already described lead to poor peer relationships. Typically children with AD/HD are outgoing and eager to make friends. However, because of their impulsive behavior, they often knock others down or push them aside. Because of their emotional lability, they overreact to normal teasing and taunting, and others then pick on them because they are easily riled. At play, children who have AD/HD often are described as "wanting to be boss." At the other extreme, in large groups they often allow themselves to be led. Often these children display social interests that are normal for younger children, a characteristic that also impairs social relationships.

Poor School Performance

All the above behavioral characteristics interact to cause poor school performance. The most important factor appears to be the lack of motivation to persist in the tiresome and repetitive tasks required of children when they are learning new skills. Despite the lack of attention and failure to complete work, these children often do learn, as indicated by their performance on individually administered achievement tests. However, as they become older, lack of persistence also begins to affect achievement adversely. Children who have AD/HD also characteristically approach academic tasks impulsively. Rather than analyze a problem, they respond to the component that first attracts their attention or put down any answer just to finish tasks they find tiresome.

Children who have these behavioral characteristics also may have learning disabilities. If so, academic achievement, by definition, will be poor. Some children who have AD/HD have specific problems with handwriting, including poor spacing between words, irregular size and placement of letters, and slow, awkward letter formation. This writing difficulty appears to result from coordination deficits that affect the ability to reproduce language-related written material, in contrast to the ability to draw pictures or copy geometrical shapes, which may be normal. Eye-hand coordination also may be normal.

DIAGNOSIS

History

The most important aspect of diagnosis is obtaining a careful history from the parents and from teachers who know the child well. If either of these two perspectives is missing, the history should be viewed cautiously, and supplemental information should be obtained (e.g., from relatives or babysitters).

It should be emphasized that the behavioral characteristics of AD/HD are situationally dependent, meaning that there is an important interaction between the biologically determined disorder and the child's immediate environment. The physician's task, therefore, is vastly complicated because the sought-after, nonbiased observer is nonexistent. Teachers and parents frequently vary in their descriptions of and information about the same child. Knowing how to synthesize these accounts is part of the art of behavioral evaluation. The clinician should ask about each of the behavioral characteristics of AD/HD and adapt the questions to the behavioral repertoire typical of the child's age. For example, inattentiveness in a child of nursery school age typically might be seen in play or when the child is being read to; in 9-year-olds, such symptoms are likely to be noted when the child is doing class work or homework. Since the publication of *DSM-III* and *DSM-IV,* specific behaviors have been listed as criteria for the disorder. These behaviors can be transformed into specific questions that can be asked of the parent or older child. This technique has been used in developing structured, diagnostic interviews such as the Diagnostic Interview for Children and Adults (now revised DICA-R),[13] and the Diagnostic Interview Schedule for Children-Revised (DISC-R),[19] developed at the National Institutes of Mental Health. The clinician can use the same approach, taking care to confirm that the child shows more of any specific behavior than do other children of the same age. To establish the chronicity of the condition, it should be determined when each behavior first appeared. This information tells the clinician whether the behaviors are more likely an acute response to stress (e.g., the birth of a sibling or a divorce) or a temperamental profile present since early childhood.

It would not be necessary to depend on the parents' or teachers' perceptions if these behaviors could be measured objectively. Equipment designed to test attention and impulsivity recently has become available to the practitioner, but because inattentiveness and impulsivity vary depending on the nature of the task and the testing situation, such office-based measurements should be viewed cautiously. Even in the research laboratory, no single objective measure reliably indicates the diagnosis in an individual child, although differences between AD/HD children as a group and normals often are seen.[2] Behaviors such as emotional lability and resistance to conditioning are difficult to quantify because the manifestations of these behaviors depend on the complexity of interaction between the child and others. The best information comes from behavior observed over long periods and under many circumstances. Teacher observations are particularly helpful because the teacher can compare this child with a classroom of other children of the same age. However, if either the parents or teacher appears to have a negative or positive bias toward the child, the information obtained from that source should be viewed cautiously.

Questionnaires

Questionnaires that have been standardized (i.e., have been administered and scored on large populations of normal and deviant children) provide useful supplements to the history. A number of such questionnaires have appeared in recent years. The best standardized questionnaire is Achenbach's Child Behavior Checklist (CBCL),[1] but this questionnaire focuses on a broad range of behaviors, and a profile typical of AD/HD has not been validated, although a recent study begins to accomplish this.[20] One of the most useful questionnaires in the diagnosis and management of AD/HD was developed by Conners and revised and standardized in 1978 by Goyette and colleagues.[11] The revised questionnaire comes in a 48-question version for parents and a 28-question version for teachers. Ten questions common to both versions are referred to as the Conners Abbreviated Parent-Teacher Questionnaire and can be scored to produce what is known as the Hyperkinesis Index. These questions, the scoring instructions, and the cut-off scores are shown in Table 69-1.

It should be noted that these 10 questions include items identifying disruptive behaviors and emotional lability. The clinician who uses questionnaires should remember that results can be affected by observer bias and distorted by responders who know little about normal children. Also, they do not provide important information about how long the symptoms have been present.

Neurodevelopmental and Other Testing

The usual neurological examination is not helpful in diagnosing AD/HD. However, a neurological examination that focuses on skills acquired with development frequently reveals developmental delays that have implications for the diagnosis and management of AD/HD. For example, physical coor-

Table 69-1 Conners Abbreviated Parent-Teacher Questionnaire*

Behavior	Rating			
	0 Not at all	1 Just a little	2 Pretty much	3 Very much
1. Restless in the "squirmy" sense	_______	_______	_______	_______
2. Demands must be met immediately	_______	_______	_______	_______
3. Temper outbursts and unpredictable behavior	_______	_______	_______	_______
4. Distractibility or attention span a problem	_______	_______	_______	_______
5. Disturbs other children	_______	_______	_______	_______
6. Pouts and sulks	_______	_______	_______	_______
7. Mood changes quickly and drastically	_______	_______	_______	_______
8. Restless, always up and on the go	_______	_______	_______	_______
9. Excitable, impulsive	_______	_______	_______	_______
10. Fails to finish things that he or she starts	_______	_______	_______	_______

From Goyette CH, Conners CK, Ulrich RF: *J Abnorm Child Psychol* 6:221, 1978.
*Score by adding the ratings points. Maximum score = 30; usual cut-off score for diagnosis = 15.

dination often is poor for the child's age. A finding of poor coordination should lead to altered expectations for the child's performance in competitive sports and games, and such altered expectations may help prevent the loss of self-esteem that often results when children are pushed into competition in these areas during elementary school. Another characteristic finding is motor overflow, meaning that the child is less able to inhibit motor activity unrelated to the specific motor skill being examined. For example, hopping on one foot may be accompanied by an excessive amount of associated movements for that age. This finding suggests neurological immaturity, which many, but not all, children who have AD/HD display. The child who has AD/HD also is frequently inattentive during this type of neurological examination, providing the physician the opportunity to observe the dysfunction characteristic of this syndrome directly. However, the developmentally oriented neurological examination requires skill to administer and experience to interpret.

All children suspected of having AD/HD should have their vision and hearing tested because deficits in these primary senses can affect behavior and academic performance markedly. An individually administered IQ test is necessary to establish realistic expectations for learning performance. For children between 3 and 5 years of age, the Stanford-Binet-Revised test or the Wechsler Primary Preschool Scale of Intelligence–Third Edition (WPPSI-III) are the most appropriate tests; after age 6, the Wechsler Intelligence Scale for Children-Revised (WISC-R) test should be used (see Appendix D, Common Psychological and Educational Tests). A physical examination is necessary to rule out other illnesses or disorders that may affect behavior or learning.

PREVALENCE

Results of prevalence studies of AD/HD vary widely, depending on the particular method of assessment, the informant (the parent, teacher, child, physician, or some combination of these), and the distribution of ages in the sample. All studies are in agreement in indicating greater prevalence of AD/HD in boys than girls. Studies that rely solely on a score above the traditional cut-off of 15 on the Conners Teacher Questionnaire yield the highest prevalence rates. For example, an overall rate of 15% was reported in a study in the United States,[16] and percentages of 20.6% and 7.5% for boys and girls, respectively, were seen in a study in Canada.[22] By contrast, Szatmari, Offord, and Boyle (1989)[21] reported an overall prevalence of 9% of boys and 3.3% of girls ages 4 to 16, based on a questionnaire tailored to DSM III-R symptom criteria. A diagnosis was assigned if parent or teacher (for the age group 4 through 11) or parent or youth (for ages 12 through 16) achieved sufficient criteria on the questionnaire. If *both* types of informants for each age group were required to confirm the diagnosis, the prevalence was much lower. This discrepancy between observers has been noted frequently and is a source of controversy in establishing a diagnosis (see Diagnosis section earlier in this chapter). Costello[5] used yet a third approach; on the basis of a structured diagnostic interview (the DISC) conducted with 300 children ages 7 through 11 and their parents, she reported a prevalence of 3.4% of boys and 1.1% of girls. Diagnostic criteria in this study could be achieved on *either* the parents' or the child's report. The DSM-IV states, conservatively, that "as many as 3% of children" may meet the diagnostic criteria for AD/HD.

ETIOLOGY

Many retrospective studies have demonstrated an increase in behavior disorders, including hyperactivity, following a disease or insult that affects the functioning of the central nervous system (CNS).[26] However, prospective studies that specifically assess AD/HD syndromes are lacking.[30] Although there appears to be an association between CNS insult and a hyperactive behavior disorder, such a relationship probably accounts for only a small proportion (fewer than 10%) of children identified as having this problem.

Much evidence suggests that genetic factors play an important role in the etiology of these problems.[9] Speculation on the biological mechanism underlying genetic causation centers on dysfunctions in monoamine neurotransmitters that are active in the limbic brain and the reticular activating system. Positron emission tomography (PET) scans have been used recently to examine differences between AD/HD and normal brains in glucose utilization during performance of tasks requiring attention. Although one widely publicized study[29] reported reduced levels of glucose metabolism in the premotor cortex and superior prefrontal cortex in adults who have hyperactivity of childhood onset, these findings were not replicated in a subsequent study of teenagers who have AD/HD.[8] The earlier results may represent chance findings stemming from a high number of test comparisons between groups.

Another recent, widely publicized study ascertained that generalized resistance to thyroid hormone, a rare genetically determined thyroid condition, was associated with AD/HD.[12] It is important to bear in mind, however, that this rare condition may account for only an extremely small number (fewer than 0.1%) of AD/HD cases.

NATURAL HISTORY AND PROGNOSIS

AD/HD usually is detected during the elementary school years. Hyperactivity, as described in this chapter, persists but changes in quality as the child enters adolescence. For example, the activity level diminishes and the ability to concentrate improves. However, when compared with matched control subjects, the hyperactive traits are still present, although less prominent and disruptive.[25] Antisocial and acting-out behaviors become more salient during adolescence. Emotional immaturity becomes more of a concern to adults, probably because it is a more distressing symptom during adolescence. School performance often is worse because close supervision of academic work diminishes, which increases the adolescent's failure to complete work, resulting in an adverse affect on achievement. There also is a cumulative effect on academic performance, resulting from a prolonged period of failure to complete work and practice skills. Adolescents are particularly vulnerable to low self-esteem and problems in peer relations; these are exacerbated in individuals whose AD/HD symptoms were not recognized and treated earlier in development. These problems may be manifested in adolescence as poor social skills, lack of friends, a feeling of not being liked, low self-confidence, frequent fighting, and, in some cases, delinquent behavior.

Prospective longitudinal studies of individuals diagnosed in childhood as having AD/HD reveal that approximately 50% continue to have disabling symptoms of the disorder as young adults and continue to merit the diagnosis.[10,24] Approximately 25%, including some individuals in the persistent AD/HD group, exhibit antisocial behavior such as lying, stealing, and aggressive outbursts of the type characteristic of adults who have antisocial personality disorder. More than 50% of the individuals in this second group also are substance abusers.[10] Individuals who do not qualify for diagnosis may have continued concentration difficulties, distractibility, or restlessness; however, in this group these problems do not interfere significantly with daily functioning.

A recently published follow-up of one cohort, now in their mid-20s, found that the rate of AD/HD diagnoses had dropped to 11%. Antisocial personality and drug abuse disorders occurred in 18% and 16% of all cases at follow-up, respectively, which significantly exceeded rates in the comparison group. It is particularly interesting that adults who had continuing AD/HD symptoms were seven times more likely to have an antisocial personality or substance use disorder at follow-up than were those whose AD/HD symptoms had remitted.[10]

Follow-up research[23] has revealed that the long-term prognosis in AD/HD is better for children who have higher IQs and for those from families of higher socioeconomic status. On the other hand, the triad of aggressiveness, emotional instability, and low tolerance of frustration in the child and the presence of a psychopathological condition in the parent (especially parental antisocial behavior) have been found to be associated with a poor long-term outcome. The impact of pharmacological and psychosocial treatment on the long-term outcome of AD/HD is a subject of continuing investigation.

TREATMENT

AD/HD is a complex behavioral syndrome that stems from biological differences but is influenced by environmental factors and the child's underlying temperament. In recognition of the importance of biological and environmental factors, treatment should be multifaceted. The physician should be competent in the management of medication, especially since only the physician is legally empowered and medically trained to prescribe drugs. However, it is a mistake for the physician to rely exclusively on medication to treat this disorder. Some physicians will want to pursue aspects of psychological management; others will not. At the very least, the physician should coordinate care with special educators and mental health professionals.

Medication

CNS-stimulant medication has a striking, beneficial effect on behavior in 60% to 80% of children who have AD/HD. In children who have AD/HD and ODD or CD, stimulant medication often improves all aspects of the disorder. Activity become less frenetic and more goal directed, and children begin to concentrate more and complete their work. Their emotions also are less labile, resistance to discipline is reduced, and the parents may report, for instance, that a scolding that previously would have been ignored now produces tears.

The effects of stimulant medication on academic performance are less clear. The visual and auditory perceptual problems characteristic of LD appear to be unaffected. However, handwriting often improves. A short-term improvement in mathematics performance often is seen, presumably because learning mathematics depends particularly on the ability to concentrate. Follow-up studies to date have not demonstrated beneficial effects of stimulant medication on long-term academic or occupational outcome. It may be that medication must be combined with other treatments, such as remedial tutoring and training in social skills, to reverse both the primary and secondary deficits associated with AD/HD.

Medication Management

It has proved impossible to predict which patients will respond favorably to stimulant medication, although many attempts have been made to do so. Therefore, once AD/HD has been diagnosed and contraindications to medication have been ruled out, a trial of stimulant medication should be arranged. Parents, who often are fearful of psychopharmacological medications, may be reassured by a trial of medication preceding any decision to pursue long-term treatment. The medications used most frequently, suggested starting doses, and the frequency of administration are listed in Table 69-2.

Short-acting stimulants usually have an immediate effect,

Table 69-2 Guidelines for Use of Stimulant Medication in Children Who Have AD/HD

Medication	Starting amount per dose	Suggested increments	Doses/day	Time of administration
Methylphenidate (Ritalin)	0.3 mg/kg*	0.15 mg/kg	2-3	8 AM, noon, 4 PM
Methylphenidate, sustained release (Ritalin-SR)†	20 mg	20 mg	1	8 AM
Dextroamphetamine (Dexedrine)				
Tablets	0.15 mg/kg*	0.08 mg/kg	2-3	8 AM, noon, 4 PM
Spansules	≤7 yr: 5 mg	5 mg	1	8 AM
	≥8 yr: 10 mg	5 mg	1	8 AM
Pemoline	≤7 yr: 37.5 mg	18.75 mg	1‡	8 AM
(Cylert)	≥8 yr: 75 mg	37.5 mg	1	8 AM

*Suggested starting dose of methylphenidate and dextroamphetamine (mg/kg) refers to the *amount per dose;* the amount per day is greater, depending on the frequency of administration.

†The sustained-release form of methylphenidate is available only in a 20 mg size. If the child's total daily dose is close to 20 mg, this form may be used.

‡Some physicians give an additional dose at 4 PM: 18.75 mg for younger children and 37.5 mg for older children.

but at least 4 days should pass before the dose is adjusted. If no response is seen at the end of 4 days, the dose should be increased gradually, and each new dosage should be maintained for 4 to 7 days until a favorable response is seen or significant side effects develop. The box below lists side effects that can be expected and managed, as well as those indicating that the dose is too high and should be reduced. Once an appropriate dose is established, treatment should continue for at least 1 month to determine the effects on behavior both at school and at home. If significant side effects are seen before benefits are noted, the medication trial should be terminated. However, some side effects may subside with time. These often can be managed by adjusting the timing of medication or changing the time of meals to reduce interference with sleep or eating.

There are few contraindications to a trial of medication in the treatment of AD/HD. First, medication should not be prescribed if there are strong indications that the patient or members of the family will abuse these drugs. In fact, abuse of the child's medication by family members might warrant removing the child from the home. If the physician is uncertain whether such abuse is taking place, he or she should keep a record of the number of pills prescribed and their rate of use to detect any overuse. Explanations that pills have been "lost" should be viewed skeptically. Second, the physician should be reluctant to prescribe medication for children under age 5. Beneficial effects have been noted in children at this age, but side effects often are more severe. Also, the diagnosis is more difficult to establish at this age because hyperactive-like behaviors are typical of the 2- to 5-year-old child and because behavior changes rapidly during this period of development. It is reasonable to delay pharmacological treatment at this age because the child interacts primarily with the parents, who, with appropriate help, can learn to manage difficult behavior. However, in extreme cases medication should be considered. Most pediatricians should refer these children for more specialized evaluation. Third, drug treatment should be delayed in adolescent patients who deny the need for medication and indicate their intention not to comply. Such patients need time and a treatment approach that will persuade them of the potential benefits of medication. Finally, if the child has any symptoms of Tourette syndrome, stimulants should not be used until a consultation is obtained, usually with a neurologist or psychiatrist. Children who come from a family with a strong history of Tourette syndrome but have no evidence of the disorder can be treated with caution.

If the child's behavior improves substantially with medication, treatment should continue until trial periods off the drug indicate that it may no longer be needed. Children will benefit most if medication is administered regularly, including on weekends and holidays, because the behaviors favorably affected by stimulants usually pose problems for the child at home and at play, as well as at school. Skipping just one or two doses usually results in an obvious return of problem behaviors, such as emotional lability, restless inattention, and resistance to discipline. However, if missed doses fail to result in deterioration, the medication could be discontinued on weekends or holidays; if no significant deterioration is noted with this type of intermittent administration, a trial period without medication is warranted. Such a trial should last at least 2 weeks because some children deteriorate at first but then improve over time, and others show no change at first but then gradually lose the ability to control their behavior. The medication can be discontinued when a trial of 2 to 3 months off the drug results in no substantial behavioral deterioration.

Once medication is begun, if beneficial effects are followed by a gradual worsening of behavior (usually over the first few weeks of treatment), the dose should be increased gradually because frequently an initial drug tolerance is noted.

When stimulant medication proves helpful, the treatment often is continued for several years. Such children should be seen by the health care provider periodically, at least every 3 to 4 months. The purpose of these visits is to (1) monitor the continued need for medication, (2) assess and manage side effects, and (3) review the child's and family's understanding and management of drug-related psychological factors (see below). The child's response to stimulants does not change suddenly when he or she reaches adolescence. If the adolescent continues to have problems, medication usually will still be helpful. However, particular attention needs to be paid to the adolescent's perception of the need for medication. If he or she understands that medication is for his or her benefit and not for the benefit of others, compliance will be assured.

SIDE EFFECTS OF STIMULANT MEDICATION

1. Often noted with appropriate doses
   a. Reduced appetite
   b. Difficulty falling asleep
   c. Pallor
2. Indicates overdose or adverse response
   a. Social withdrawal
   b. Dazed appearance
   c. Tics or stereotypical movements (if new or if increasing in severity)
   d. Increased irritability and depression
3. Often seen as dose of medication is wearing off
   a. Weepiness
   b. Rebound hyperactivity
   c. Emotionally explosive behavior

Psychological Factors

Attention also should be given to the psychological aspects of pharmacological treatment. Physicians usually discuss the proposed treatment with the parents but often fail to include the child in age-appropriate discussions. It is most helpful to explain to children that medication will be given to determine whether it helps them control some of their own behavior. Without such an explanation, children often think that the medication is being given for the benefit of their parents and teachers because it "makes me be good." This perception is reinforced when adults (or siblings) ask about or administer medication immediately after an episode of misbehavior. Parents should be advised to avoid this response and also to coach brothers and sisters, as well as teachers, to respond appropriately. If misbehavior reminds the adult that a dose has been missed, the medication should not be administered until the episode of misbehavior has passed.

Growth

The effects of stimulant medication on growth have been raised as a potential contraindication to continued therapy. It clearly has been established that some children show weight loss or a diminished rate of weight gain that may be followed, after a period of several months, by a decrement in the rate of increase in height. This effect on growth varies a great deal from child to child but appears to be most pronounced in children who are large to begin with. It also is clear that discontinuing medication results in catch-up growth, especially in weight, but also in height. It is not likely, however, that these short-term changes result in any change in long-term growth potential. For example, studies of stature in adults who were treated with stimulant medications for long periods in childhood do not show differences from population norms. Also, one study suggested that a return to a normal growth rate occurs after prolonged treatment with stimulants (2 years or more). It has been assumed that this effect on growth is due to decreased appetite and resulting weight loss. However, this causal mechanism has not been established, and some evidence suggests that these medications have a direct effect on hormones such as somatomedin and prolactin.

In the absence of evidence for any impact on ultimate stature, and because such an impact, if there is one, is likely to be very small, it seems prudent to monitor growth carefully, adjust the timing of medication and meals to minimize weight loss, and, if severe short-term effects on growth are seen, discontinue the medication during less stressful periods, such as the summertime. It also may be prudent to use a medication other than stimulants (e.g., neuroleptics) when AD/HD is seen in a child who has significant, preexisting growth problems.

Diet

The notion that sugar and artificial food additives can precipitate or exacerbate hyperactivity in children has been popularized by the media and tenaciously supported by parents who report having observed food-related behavior changes in their children. In his book, *Why Your Child is Hyperactive,* published in 1975, Benjamin Feingold originated the idea that artificial coloring, artificial flavoring, antioxidant preservatives, and all salicylates produce hyperactivity and learning disabilities in children. He claimed that eliminating these substances from the diet would improve dramatically the behavior of 60% of affected children. Controlled research has failed to substantiate these claims.[27]

The hypothesis that sugar intake contributes to hyperactive behavior also has received little support in research, even when the high sugar intake was maintained as long as 3 weeks, as in a recent study.[28]

In the absence of research validation of the purported negative effects on behavior of additives and sugar, it is well to consider other explanations of the popularity of the dietary approach and parental claims of its effectiveness. First, the diet offers a relatively simple explanation of the etiology of the child's problems and an easy treatment to effect. Second, it offers an explanation external to the child and therefore releases the child from blame for his or her misbehavior and the parents from frustration and guilt over their possible contribution to the problem. The result may be a significant reduction in the tension between parent and child and a significant increase in positive attention toward the child, both of which may bring about marked improvement in the child's behavior, at least in the short term; the parents may misperceive this as a direct response to the dietary change.

In response to parents' inquiries about dietary treatment, the physician should be truthful about the status of the scientific evidence. Some families will pursue this form of treatment anyway; if so, they may be reassured that the Feingold Diet is safe and that reducing sugar intake may be beneficial from the perspective of reducing risk for dental caries and obesity. Any improvement, even if based on psychological rather than physiological factors, is desirable as long as the family continues to pursue other recommended treatment and the child does not rebel against the dietary restrictions.

Behavioral Management

Children who have AD/HD are difficult to manage. Resistance to discipline, combined with emotional lability, leads to emotionally charged acts of disobedience. The inattention (or lack of motivation) and emotional immaturity result in failure to complete tasks. When the child is pushed to perform, emotional outbursts are common. Inattention and impulsive responses to stimulating activities often result in unintentional destructive behaviors. Unless adults are able to manage these problems effectively, their frustration will lead to negative feelings toward the child, which ultimately contributes to the child's low self-esteem. Therefore all parents of children who have AD/HD should learn both to recognize the source of the child's misbehavior and how to manage it effectively. Behavior modification should be used regularly, and the parents should learn to focus on preventing misbehavior. Finally, clear, empathic communication between parent and child is especially important.

Parents should be referred to a program that will train them in behavioral management and communication. Unfortunately, this type of training is not well reimbursed by health insurance plans. Another problem is that mental health professionals, who often are involved in such programs, might not understand the interaction between biological and psychological factors—an understanding necessary for effective management of AD/HD. For example, it is helpful for parents to understand not only the psychodynamic determinants of the child's behavior ("He got angry when teased by his sister") but also the biological or temperamental determinants ("He gets angry more easily than other boys his age, and it takes longer for him to control that anger"). Without this perspective, parents come to feel that they are responsible for all their child's misbehavior, and they may drop out of behavior management training. Therefore practitioners should identify professionals in the community who are skilled in providing behavior management counseling and who understand the biological contribution to these syndromes. They also should become skilled in persuading parents of the need for this kind of therapy. Parents may resist referral that focuses on them when they perceive that the problem is with the child. They should be advised that special skills, beyond those possessed by most parents, are needed to manage these children effectively.

Behavior management training is best begun just after the

medication trial has been started because the therapist, parents, and child then know the effect that stimulants will have on specific behaviors, a factor that helps clarify the relationship between psychological and biological determinants. This also allows the therapist to concentrate on behaviors unaffected by medication. It also is helpful for the child to become aware of the effects of medication. For example, when a child becomes aware of having greater control over emotional responses as an effect of medication, he or she also may become aware of his or her low frustration tolerance in the absence of medication and the need to learn to cope with it.

Cognitive behavior therapy is a variant of behavior therapy in which the focus is on the patient's habitual thoughts, or "self-talk," as they relate to clinical problems. This approach has been attempted to teach children to self-monitor, self-pace, and self-instruct so as to achieve greater self-control academically and socially. Disappointingly, recent research in this area concludes that this type of intervention is not effective in children who have AD/HD (see Chapter 93, Consultation and Referral for Behavioral and Developmental Problems).

Special Education

As mentioned earlier, many children who have AD/HD also show signs of learning disability. The association between AD/HD and LD is sufficiently common that both disorders should be assessed routinely. If LD is present, special education, in the form of resource room or special class placement, should be considered. The child who has AD/HD and LD may be much more amenable to special education approaches if medication is prescribed and it helps control inattentiveness and impulsivity.

The child who has AD/HD only also needs special help in school. In 1992 the federal government recognized AD/HD alone as a handicapping condition within the category of "Other Health Impaired." This change in regulation also began a study in several regional educational research centers as to how best to provide remedial education to these children. As an interim measure, special education programs are invoking Section 504 of the Rehabilitation Act of 1973 to provide individual support in the form of a paraprofessional who will provide one-to-one reinforcement to promote the completion of classroom work.

Psychotherapy

The symptoms characteristic of AD/HD frequently are viewed as arising from emotional conflict secondary to experiences that are stressful to the child. This analysis of causality leads to recommendations for individual psychotherapy. However, genetic data and the effects of stimulant medication suggest that biological factors play a key role. Therefore a different approach to psychotherapy has developed out of the recognition that in AD/HD, biology and experience interact to produce the characteristic emotional symptoms. Children who have AD/HD typically come to feel inadequate, partly because they cannot do things (e.g., schoolwork, athletics) as well as others their age. In part, they come to view the anger and frustration displayed by parents, teachers, and peers as personally threatening. The preoccupation with themes of violence in the drawings of children who have AD/HD and their choice of television shows and stories seem to be a way of compensating for a sense of vulnerability. These psychological issues, which develop as reactions to their perception of the environment, may best be dealt with in psychotherapy. Children who have AD/HD need to acquire insight not only into their own conflicts and sources of stress but also into their temperament. Learning to recognize how medication changes inner experience and outward behavior is part of this process.

Other adjunctive therapies also may help the child. Social skills training, which typically is conducted in a group, may help the child by modeling and reinforcing appropriate interpersonal behaviors. Family therapy can help address the many strains on family functioning imposed by the child who has AD/HD. For example, brothers and sisters, who may feel that their needs are being overlooked because of the attention given to the "problem" child, often welcome the opportunity to express these feelings in a supportive context. Marital therapy is indicated when the child's behavior has caused deterioration of the marital relationship. Finally, individual psychotherapy may help parents who have low self-esteem, who often view their child's misbehavior as personally directed toward them. This usually is indicated by a persistently negative reaction toward the child, despite appropriate explanation of the origins of the child's behavior.

REFERENCES

1. Achenbach TM, Edelbrock CS: *Manual for the child behavior checklist and revised child behavior profile,* Burlington, Vt, 1992, University Associates in Psychiatry.
2. Barkley RA: The ecological validity of laboratory and analogue assessment methods of ADHD symptoms, *J Abnorm Child Psychol* 19:149, 1991.
3. Biederman J et al: Evidence of familial association between attention deficit disorder and anxiety disorder and major affective disorders, *Arch Gen Psychiatry* 48:633, 1991.
4. Biederman J et al: Familial association between attention deficit disorder (ADD) and anxiety disorder, *Am J Psychiatry* 148:251, 1991.
5. Costello EJ: Child psychiatric disorders and their correlates: a primary care pediatric sample, *J Am Acad Child Adolesc Psychiatry* 28:851, 1989.
6. *Diagnostic and statistical manual of mental disorders,* ed 4, Washington, DC, 1994, American Psychiatric Association.
7. *Diagnostic and statistical manual of mental disorders,* ed 3, Washington, DC, 1980, American Psychiatric Association.
8. Ernst M et al: Reduced brain metabolism in hyperactive girls, *J Am Acad Child Adolesc Psychiatry* 33:858, 1994.
9. Faraone SV, Biederman J: Genetics of attention deficit hyperactivity disorder, *Child Adolesc Psychiatr Clin North Am* 3:285, 1994.
10. Gittleman R et al: Hyperactive boys almost grown up. I. Psychiatric status, *Arch Gen Psychiatry* 42:937, 1985.
11. Goyette CH, Conners CK, Ulrich RF: Normative data on revised Conners parent and teacher rating scales, *J Abnorm Child Psychol* 6:221, 1978.
12. Hauser P et al: Attention deficit hyperactivity in people with generalized resistance to thyroid hormone, *N Engl J Med* 328:997, 1993.
13. Herjanic B, Reich W: Development of a structured psychiatric interview for children: agreement between child and parent on individual symptoms, *J Abnorm Child Psychol* 10:307, 1982.
14. Holobrow PL, Berry PS: Hyperactivity and learning difficulties, *Journal of Learning Disabilities* 19:426, 1986.
15. Lambert NM, Sandoval J: The prevalence of learning disabilities in a sample of children considered hyperactive, *J Abnorm Child Psychol* 8:33, 1980.
16. Langsdorff R et al: Ethnicity, social class, and perception of hyperactivity, *Psychology in the Schools* 16:293, 1979.
17. Manuzza S et al: Adult outcome of hyperactive boys: educational

achievement, occupational rank and psychiatric status, *Arch Gen Psychiatry* 50:565, 1993.
18. Newcorn JH, Halperin JM: Comorbidity among disruptive behavior disorders, *Child Adolesc Psychiatr Clin North Am* 3:227, 1994.
19. Piacentini J et al: The diagnostic interview schedule for children: revised version (DISC-R). III. Concurrent criterion validity, *J Am Acad Child Adolesc Psychiatry* 32:658, 1993.
20. Steingard R et al: Psychiatric comorbidity in attention deficit disorder: impact on the interpretation of Child Behavior Checklist results, *J Am Acad Child Adolesc Psychiatry* 31:449, 1992.
21. Szatmari P, Offord DR, Boyle MH: Ontario Child Health Study: prevalence of attention deficit disorder with hyperactivity, *J Child Psychol Psychiatry* 30:219, 1989.
22. Trites RL et al: Prevalence of hyperactivity, *J Pediatr Psychol* 4:179, 1979.
23. Weiss G, Hechtman L: *Hyperactive children grown up,* New York, 1986, Guilford Press.
24. Weiss G et al: Psychiatric status of hyperactives as adults: a controlled, prospective 15-year follow-up of 63 hyperactive children, *J Am Acad Child Adolesc Psychiatry* 23:211, 1985.
25. Weiss G et al: A 5-year follow-up study of 91 hyperactive schoolchildren, *Arch Gen Psychiatry* 24:409, 1971.
26. Wender PH: *Minimal brain dysfunction in children,* New York, 1971, Wiley Interscience.
27. Wender EH: The food additive–free diet in the treatment of behavior disorders: a review, *J Dev Behav Pediatr* 7:35, 1986.
28. Wolraich ML et al: Effects of diets high in sucrose or aspartame on the behavior and cognitive performance of children, *N Engl J Med* 330:301, 1994.
29. Zametkin AJ et al: Cerebral glucose metabolism in adults with hyperactivity of childhood onset, *N Engl J Med* 323:1361, 1990.
30. Zametkin AJ, Rapaport JL: Neurobiology of attention deficit disorder with hyperactivity: where have we come in 50 years? *J Am Acad Child Adolesc Psychiatry* 26:676, 1987.

70 School Behavior Problems

William A. Shine

The primary care physician can play a major role in helping to ameliorate the effects of classroom behavior problems by (1) identifying potential difficulties as early as possible, (2) offering guidance to the parents, (3) monitoring the relationship between the school and the parents, (4) assisting school authorities in developing approaches to behavior problems, (5) assessing and treating behavior disorders, and (6) making appropriate referrals.

A child's classroom behavior is defined as a problem either by a teacher or a parent. The teacher's definition is based on internalized standards for this age group developed through his or her own experiences and conventional norms[4]; the parent's definition is concerned more with the effect of the child's current school life on his or her long-term happiness. As defined by teachers, most classroom problems involve adjustment and relate either to disruptive or withdrawn behavior. This definition is situational; teachers', schools', and parents' interpretations of behavior and its consequences differ. Most classroom behavior problems are brought to the physician's attention by parents.

School stress often provokes behavior that otherwise would go unattended. Usually, the school is the first setting outside the family in which children are evaluated. An undesirable concomitant consequence of schooling is the invidious comparison that may occur among the children, their parents, and the teachers. A primary care physician who is knowledgeable about school organization and has a reliable medical history of the child can help the school and the parents protect the child from such comparison by focusing on the child's individual needs. Early intervention offers the greatest chance for success in modifying behavior that may become socially or academically dysfunctional, or both.

EARLY CHILDHOOD

In good school practice, the nursery school or kindergarten teacher will inform the parents of problem behavior. A physician who has established a rapport with the family is better able to assess strategies for intervention. He or she may counsel a moderate "wait and see" approach or suggest a parent-teacher conference. At this point, the physician can assist the parents by delineating the problem and suggesting an approach to the teacher that will focus on resolving the problem rather than establishing causation or fixing blame. The most important point to emphasize is that the parents and the teacher should respect each other. The physician who assumes professional competence on the teacher's part will convey that assumption in his or her attitude toward the conference.

If the parent-teacher conference fails to resolve the problem, then the physician may choose to intervene directly. Otherwise, valuable time may be wasted in a clash of opinion between the school and the parents regarding the cause of the problem and, consequently, in reaching agreement on the best course of action to address it. It is here, as well as at any other point along the continuum of schooling, that the physician can provide trusted advice and counsel to break the logjam of inaction and prevent the development of an adversarial relationship between the home and the school.

It also is good school practice for the principal to view the physician as an ally in addressing the child's school-related problems. Good rapport between the school principal and the physician is vital to successful intervention. If the physician is not familiar with the school, he or she should arrange for a meeting to assess the school climate. A visit to the child's classroom often provides valuable insight into the child and the environment.

Prekindergarten and kindergarten programs are characterized by their flexibility. When behavior problems occur, they usually can be addressed by a change in the child's routine or in the quality of the teacher's interaction with the child. An accepting environment that reflects an understanding of the child's temperament and that reinforces good behavior positively often is enough to resolve the immediate problem.[15] Unless the child presents serious behavior problems such as bizarre, extremely withdrawn, or dangerous behavior, the natural maturation process should be allowed to occur. This process can be aided by good modeling by the parents and teacher and by using behavior modification techniques such as instant recognition of good behavior and time-out periods immediately after poor behavior. Because a temperamentally difficult child is vulnerable to developing a behavior disorder later in life, the length and severity of any school-related problem should be recorded by the parents and physician for future reference.[6]

ELEMENTARY SCHOOL

Elementary school places an increasingly heavier emphasis on academic skills. Throughout these grades, classroom behavior problems are closely related to a lack of academic success, for a child's self-esteem is closely tied to his or her competence at the tasks imposed. Most students encounter few academic barriers during this period, but even these can result in school adjustment problems. Very active children may find the relative physical inactivity of the classroom oppressive, and their reaction to this inactivity often disrupts the class. If the child's behavior is not affecting his or her schoolwork but is disruptive to others, then strategies to focus this excess energy should be developed collaboratively.

Some children do not complete the demanding developmental tasks of early childhood. At critical points in their school career, they may refuse to go to school. Parents should try to identify any specific events, persons, or situations that may be the cause of the problem. If no school situation is identified as a cause, the child should be assessed or referred immediately (see Chapter 71, School Absenteeism and School Refusal).

In most situations a parent-teacher conference can resolve the problem, whether it is related to academic frustration, physical inactivity, or undefined school refusal. These conferences should be planned carefully, with sufficient time and privacy provided. Because emotions tend to run high in these situations, hasty, episodical, or fragmentary encounters usually are counterproductive.[16]

Organic Bases for Behavior Problems

In exceptional cases the classroom behavior problem cannot be resolved solely through home and school collaboration. In such cases the child may have an organic problem that is unrecognized by either the parents or the teacher. Attention deficit/hyperactivity disorder (AD/HD) is receiving increasing attention as an organic disability that relates to school problems (see Chapter 69). An estimated 5% of school-age children are affected by this condition, which is considered a behavior disorder.[10] This condition should be diagnosed medically only after intensive cognitive and behavioral investigation has ruled out primary environmental causes. Behavior rating scales for children who have AD/HD can provide information important to proper diagnosis. Neuropsychological testing and psychiatric evaluation also may be required.[1]

AD/HD does not define the child; rather, it identifies a condition that probably will require some environmental modification to address associated problem behavior rationally. Many children who have AD/HD have coexisting learning problems and anxiety disorders, oppositional defiant disorder, or conduct disorder. School officials should be alert to the existence of these multiple handicapping conditions.

Symptoms of a behavior disorder commonly first appear before age 7.[10] First noticed at home, these can become disruptive behaviors in school, generally manifested by physically aggressive behavior that discounts the rights of others. Identification of a child's disability is useful only to explain his or her behavioral reaction to situations at school; judgments about the inevitability of failure or "delinquency" should be avoided. These children deserve the presumption of success.

Pharmacological therapy is considered the most effective management for AD/HD.[10] This therapy requires medical decisions and supervision. Close monitoring of the child's progress is essential to help the physician determine the success of treatment. This therapy is not a cure, but, coupled with behavior modification techniques, it is thought to offer the best hope for behavioral adjustment to academic and social norms.[1]

The most common cause of learning problems, some of which result in classroom behavior problems, is a group of specific developmental disorders known as learning disabilities (LD) (see Chapter 72, School Learning Problems and Developmental Differences). Frustration in coping with one or many of a plethora of cognitive, social, and motor skill deficiencies can cause the child to develop inappropriate strategies designed to obscure the problem and to protect himself or herself from failure. A teacher or school may focus on the inappropriate behavior and fail to address the causal academic frustration. A team of learning specialists, including a psychologist, should identify the specific learning disability and develop a plan to address it.

Unfortunately, more research is directed to the diagnosis of academic problems than to remediation. A search of the literature indicates that few "proven" methods have been verified scientifically. Behavior modification and direct, intensive early intervention, peer tutoring, and use of computers are considered to have the best nonpharmacological efficacy. To succeed, these approaches require extensive record keeping, perseverance, emotional control on the part of the parents and teacher, and a heavy time commitment.[2] However, such strategies are inconsistent with the training and belief system of most teachers, who favor higher-order thinking skills, inference, and the discovery method.[10]

For schools, categories of disabilities listed in Public Law 94-142 (The Education of All Handicapped Children Act) are as significant as those in the American Psychiatric Association's *Diagnostic and Statistical Manual of Mental Disorders.* Although the PL 94-142 categories are intended for funding rather than diagnosis, they direct resources to the school districts and as such are highly influential. Fifty percent of federal money spent under this law is for children classified as having LD. AD/HD is not listed, but because it is a medical diagnosis, some states administer the federal law to permit funding for AD/HD under the category "other health impaired."

PL 94-142 addresses many of the problems antecedent to classroom behavior problems. Its sufficiency, however, depends on its implementation by the state and by the local school district. The law is administered in the local school district by a committee on special education. Each school district has such a committee, called by different names in various states, that is responsible for evaluating children whom a teacher, parent, or physician has identified as potentially disabled. A primary care physician may request a classification with or without the parents' agreement. School districts vary in their application of this law; their attitude toward children and behavior greatly determines eligibility for treatment of behavior disorders.

Environmental Basis for Behavior Problems

When classroom behavior is closely tied to an organic problem, it is more likely to be addressed because of the legal requirements of PL 94-142. However, some cases of poor classroom behavior are primarily the result of environmental factors. At times a classroom behavior problem stems from family stress. In these cases the physician plays a unique role by virtue of his or her intimate knowledge of the family dynamics. He or she may either counsel the family or refer it to an appropriate resource. One often overlooked resource is pastoral counseling. In many cases a rabbi, minister, or priest has access to a family's emotional core that is not available to others. Although it is not appropriate for the counselor to share the details of family strife with school personnel, it is helpful for a child's school to know that there are family problems that might explain the child's behavior.

Many behavior problems are cultural in origin. When the values of the parents and community are at odds with those of the school, the clash of values often manifests itself in the child's inability to control his or her anger through appropriate behavior. Some children and young people who are culturally alienated also have problems associated with AD/HD, LD, conduct disorder, and psychiatric illness. These conditions often are undiagnosed, and the child's behavior is interpreted as being merely a reaction to social circumstances.[11] School authorities tend to generalize behavior and adopt disciplinary practices that serve only to alienate these children further. There is evidence that bureaucratic use of suspension, while expedient, results in more disruptive behavior and a higher dropout rate.[3] Many of these children and young people do not have access to a primary care physician. Their plight could be addressed through establishment of a school-based primary health care program in each school that has students whose health needs are unmet.

More boys than girls are identified as having behavior disorders; however, this does not necessarily mean that more boys than girls have such disorders. Some theorists hold that boys manifest their disorders by more disruptive behavior, whereas girls, more externally suppressed by powerful social controls, mask their disorders by withdrawn behavior. Gender bias in research and practice can blind schools and institutions to the social constraints that prevent girls from expressing their frustration as overtly as boys.[7] Teachers and physicians should be alert to these less overt classroom behavior problems.

ADOLESCENCE

In early adolescence the entire school milieu becomes the arena in which problems occur. Middle schools have been created in response to the need for a school environment that provides the necessary freedom and control to meet the early adolescent's developmental needs.[9] Children who adapted well to elementary school usually find this new environment stimulating and productive. One current theory of adolescent behavior holds that adolescent turmoil is not as pervasive as previously thought.[12,13] Although most adolescents have mood swings, only a small number experience serious emotional distress. The myth of adolescent turmoil could lead to a dangerous failure to identify serious behavior disorders.[9]

Symptoms of behavior disorders commonly appear between 6 and 8 years of age.[1] These symptoms may be suppressed by authoritarian punishment, only to appear overtly in adolescence when the child gains the physical strength and social mobility to resist authority. Low self-esteem, poor peer relationships, and increasingly poor school performance can deteriorate into physical aggression by later adolescence. A school with many "at-risk" children and limited resources lacks the capacity to identify or address behavior disorders and tends to rely on punishment as a deterrent. Only a school that has sufficient resources and child-centered values can identify behavior disorders and implement individualized approaches to help children develop appropriate social skills. However, schools in poor areas typically do not have such resources, nor can families in such deprived neighborhoods find affordable mental health care.

Violence

Although the fear of violence often is exaggerated, violence actually is a problem for many adolescents. Bullying long has been a fact of life for countless children who have suffered its physical and emotional effects. The introduction of weapons into the schools has further increased the anxiety level of children, who see themselves as potential victims. Some classroom behavior problems are the direct result of victims' efforts to mollify their tormentors by rejecting authority and adopting the oppositional style of their abusive peers. When a school climate is oppressive, this strategy often is all that remains for children who lack effective adult guidance and support.

The chronic bully requires early therapeutic intervention. Parents and teachers should not rationalize violent behavior.[8] Although anger can be useful, uncontrolled aggression cannot be tolerated. Controlling aggression can be one of an adolescent boy's most difficult developmental tasks.[12] Most learn to master their emotions through sublimation (e.g., athletics) and productive social activities. Schools must differentiate between violent behavior and other discipline problems. Recent federal legislation requires expulsion for any student determined to have brought a firearm to school (Title VIII, Gun-Free Schools Act of 1994). Treatment of the violent offender is a responsibility of the larger society (see Chapter 108).

Academic Failure

Most school behavior problems are associated with academic failure. This is even truer for adolescents than for elementary schoolchildren because this developmental period is characterized by heightened self-awareness and the need for peer group validation. For students with poor impulse control, organizational deficiencies, or weak skills, productive classroom and school participation seems impossible. There is strong evidence that most children's perception of their own ability is set by the seventh grade.[14] Sometimes the disappointment felt by some academically successful parents clouds their vision of the strengths of their mildly handicapped child. These children often struggle to achieve a good self-image bereft of authentic parental approval.[5]

A plan to address learning problems should be the focus of any attempt to deal with classroom behavior problems for two reasons: (1) it addresses the probable cause and (2) it communicates to the adolescent a sense of his or her worth. Such a plan should demystify the learning problem and thus alleviate guilt. Educational methodology should include behavior modification, as well as strategies to bypass areas of vulnerability—for example, having a student whose handwriting is poor use a computer for word processing, or using audio books to supplement and at times even supplant the reading entry into history and literature. These strategies encourage participation in peer-related learning that might otherwise be foreclosed. A deficiency in mathematics, reading, or writing skill can be addressed better within the context of the adolescent's emerging social needs than in remedial isolation.

Opportunities should be provided for the student to develop and display nonacademic skills and abilities in or out of school. The school day could be modified to encourage community service or work. In some communities, for example, membership in the fire department provides a disciplined, prestigious outlet for adolescents who crave action and recognition. School activities also can provide important cocurricular experience. Therefore it is of questionable value to deny students the opportunity to participate in athletics or other cocurricular activities as a punishment for improper behavior or academic failure. Although this practice is widely employed and often appears to be the only solution to an intractable problem, it takes away what often is the only opportunity for that student to experience the success necessary to maintain his or her self-esteem. A decision to remove a student from a valued activity should be subject to intensive review that might well include the opinion of the child's physician.

For most young people in late adolescence, college life offers a healthy moratorium from the responsibility of choosing a lifetime companion and a vocation. Ironically and unfairly, lifetime choices are thrust upon those who drop out of high school or whose lives are filled with unresolved turbulence. For centuries, military service, the farm, or the factory provided a viable occupational goal for many adolescents. The current complexity of military and civilian vocational requirements foreclose these options for a large percentage of those who have not achieved a modicum of school success. This group often lacks the social skills necessary for these positions. Society cannot afford to discount this group. Alternative training opportunities and dignified entry-level employment, coordinated with adult counseling programs directed at life skills, should be available in each community.

SUMMARY

Occasional classroom misbehavior is common for many children and young people. For most middle class children, their interaction with their environment is an exciting opportunity for growth. For the child who has a difficult temperament, a behavior or learning problem, or who is culturally deprived, the school often is a less comfortable place. For this child to achieve a healthy future, the parents and school must, as early as possible, assess his or her ability and temperament accurately to develop a program that fits. However, this early identification sometimes is impeded because (1) some parents and teachers are reluctant to identify problems in order to avoid confrontation; (2) some parents resist special education classification for fear of stigmatizing their child; and (3) some school districts constrain special education expenditures.

Tragically, for the economically and culturally deprived child, it is doubtful that sufficient resources will be made available to accomplish this goal. Physicians who lend their considerable prestige and expertise to creating an environment where the problems inherent in behavior disorders are identified early and receive long-term attention can have a positive effect on the lives of the children they serve.

REFERENCES

1. Barkley RA: *Attention deficit hyperactivity disorder: a handbook for diagnosis and treatment,* New York, 1990, Guilford Press.
2. Blechman EA: *Solving child behavior problems at home and at school,* Champaign, Ill, 1985, Research Press.
3. Bowditch C: Getting rid of troublemakers: high school disciplinary procedures and the production of dropouts, *Social Problems* 40:493, 1993.
4. Brophy J, McCaslin M: Teachers' reports of how they perceive and cope with problem students, *Elem School J* 93:3, 1992.
5. Casey R et al: Impaired emotional health in children with mild reading disability, *J Dev Behav Pediatr* 13:256, 1992.
6. Chess S, Alexander T: *Origins and evolution of behavior disorders from infancy to early adult life,* New York, 1984, Brunner/Mazel.
7. Gilligan C: *In a different voice: psychological theory and women's development,* Cambridge, Mass, 1982, Harvard University Press.
8. Greenbaum S, Turner B, Stephens RD: *Set straight on bullies,* Malibu, Calif, 1989, Pepperdine University Press.
9. Hamburg BA: Psychosocial development. In Friedman SB, Fisher M, Schonberg SK, editors: *Comprehensive adolescent health care,* St Louis, 1992, Quality Medical Publishing.
10. Ingersoll BD, Goldstein S: *Attention deficit disorder and learning disabilities: realities, myths, and controversial treatments,* New York, 1993, Doubleday.
11. McIntyre T: Reflections on the new definition for emotional or behavioral disorders: who still falls through the cracks and why, *Behav Disorders* 18:148, 1993.
12. Offer D: *The psychological world of the teen-ager,* New York, 1969, Basic Books.
13. Offer D, Ostrov E, Howard KI: *The adolescent: a psychological self-portrait,* New York, 1981, Basic Books.
14. Sandler AD, Levine MD: Learning and attention deficit disorders. In Friedman SB, Fisher M, Schonberg SK, editors: *Comprehensive adolescent health care,* St Louis, 1992, Quality Medical Publishing.
15. Turecki S, Tonner L: *The difficult child,* New York, 1989, Bantam Books.
16. Turecki S, Wernick S: *The emotional problems of normal children: how parents can understand and help,* New York, 1994, Bantam Books.

71 School Absenteeism and School Refusal

Ronald V. Marino

A major developmental task of childhood is separating from one's family and accepting the functional demands of society. One of the most obvious indicators that this process may not be occurring normally is lack of attendance at school. It is the responsibility of child health professionals to assess the child's school attendance and functioning in the context of biopsychosocial health supervision.

Nonattendance may be due to a variety of underlying reasons. *Absenteeism* generally is considered to be parentally sanctioned nonattendance, most commonly attributed to medical illness. *Truancy* is nonattendance without parental consent, in which the time allegedly spent at school often is spent engaging in antisocial behaviors or rebelling against authority. *School refusal* is characterized by inappropriate fear about leaving home, inappropriate fear of school, or both.

Excessive absenteeism is important to health professionals because it is an excellent marker for both physical and mental health problems (see the box on p. 686). It also is negatively correlated with social adjustment and academic performance. In fact, excessive absenteeism and failure to read at grade level in third grade are the two strongest predictors of subsequent dropping out of school. National surveys indicate that healthy children average four or five absences a school year, whereas children who have a chronic disease typically are absent at least twice as often. Educators believe that missing more than 10 days in a 90-day semester results in difficulty staying at grade level.

Acute physical health problems are given as the reason for nonattendance 75% of the time. However, the variability in absenteeism among children who have the same medical condition suggests that, in determining attendance, individual and family responses to the physical condition are more important than the actual condition. The decision not to attend school reflects subtle and complex relationships between the physical, social, and psychological states of the student, family, and community. Individual rates of absenteeism tend to be stable for a given child and also for a given school district.

The minor health complaints most commonly cited are upper respiratory tract infections, headaches, abdominal distress, and menstrual cramps. Parental characteristics associated with excessive absenteeism include lower socioeconomic class, cigarette smoking, chronic parental illness (including mental illness), lower educational expectations, and "vulnerable child syndrome." A plethora of nonmedical conditions, including transportation difficulties, illness of other family members, religious holidays, family vacations, inclement weather, and professional appointments, also are reasons children miss school.

Chronically ill children typically miss more school than their healthy peers. This may be because of a wide variety of causes, including acute exacerbation of the underlying condition, health care visits, side effects of medications, and parental misconceptions about the child's ability to attend school. Healthy adjustment by the child and family to the chronic condition minimizes the potential impact of the increase in school days missed. A significant increase in absenteeism over baseline is always a "red flag." It is the clinician's responsibility to explore the reasons a particular child seeks to avoid school. Sudden changes in school attendance may be the first concrete symptom of family dysfunction, mental illness, physical deterioration of the student or a family member, alcohol or drug abuse, or school refusal.

SCHOOL REFUSAL

School refusal is characterized as the child's desire to stay home from school despite the parents' support for attendance. Since it was first described in the psychiatric literature in 1941 as "school phobia," this condition has presented itself as a great imitator and challenge to parents, physicians, school personnel, and children. The term "school refusal" is used here, although other terms such as "school phobia," "school avoidance," or "separation anxiety disorder" sometimes are used.

Criteria for making this diagnosis include (1) severe difficulty in attending school or refusal to attend school, (2) severe emotional upset on attempting to go to school, (3) absence of significant antisocial disorders, and (4) staying at home with the parent's knowledge. A variety of vague physical symptoms commonly accompany the child's request not to attend school. Symptoms can be quite impressive to parents and emulate organic medical problems.

Prevalence

The prevalence of school refusal has been estimated to be 0.4% to 18%. Difficulties at the beginning of school attendance (4 to 6 years of age) are more likely to be brought to the attention of a primary care pediatrician, whereas adolescents who refuse to go to school are more commonly treated by mental health professionals. Thus readers must be mindful of the population studied when reviewing the literature. The American Academy of Pediatrics estimates that 5% of elementary school children and 2% of junior high school children have this disorder.

School refusal represents a symptom with a variety of underlying dynamics. Attempts to classify it into acute versus chronic (or anxiety type) versus characterological or secondary gain type have little to offer in the development of therapeutic strategies. Clinicians should employ a sensitive, holistic approach to data gathering because the history represents the initial therapeutic ground breaking. Factors related to the child, parents, family, and school environment must be investigated when exploring school maladaptation.

CHRONIC SCHOOL ABSENCE: DIFFERENTIAL DIAGNOSIS

School refusal
Overresponse to minor illnesses
Chronic physical disease with poor adaptation
Learning disability with poor adaptation
Truancy
Substance abuse
Psychosis
Teenage pregnancy
Family dysfunction

Modified from Nader P, editor: *School health: policy and practice,* Elk Grove Village, Ill, 1993, The American Academy of Pediatrics.

Child-related Factors

Boys and girls are affected equally and usually are reported to have at least average intelligence and academic achievement. Vague somatic symptomatology, which typically is offered as a rationale for nonattendance, belies the underlying anxiety frequently present. Symptoms may amplify in response to parental pressure to attend school. Overdependency on a parent, usually the mother, also is common. Classical descriptions refer to passive, dependent, inhibited, timid, and willful children. Numerous authors have noted depression, panic disorder, and agoraphobia. Some children have unrealistically high expectations of themselves, which is a contributing factor.

Parent-related Factors

More attention has been paid to mothers of school refusers than fathers. There appears to be a higher incidence of neurosis associated with anxiety and depression in these women, and they have been noted to have unresolved conflicts with their own mothers. Overindulgence and overprotection may reflect underlying maternal ambivalence or hostility toward the parental role. Other maternal characteristics include perfectionism, fear of illness, and an inability to set limits effectively.

Fathers commonly are professionals or skilled workers and good "material" providers. They frequently have been described as passive and ineffectual. They may be indifferent to or withdrawn from parental decision making. Conversely, some authors have described the father as firm, active, and overenmeshed. Both fathers and mothers have been noted to be older than average.

Family Factors

The family context always is a major factor in understanding the symptoms. Marital conflict or constricted communication patterns frequently are found in families who have school refusers. The child's presence at home due to physical illness may provide a cohesive force to an otherwise unstable marital relationship.

Nader has described three common patterns of communication in families in which school refusal occurs: (1) both parents are overly concerned and solicitous of the child's medical problem; (2) one parent, usually the mother, is overprotective and concerned, whereas the other overtly disagrees; and (3) one parent, typically the mother, is overinvolved in caring for the child's every need, whereas the other parent is absent emotionally.[2] Understanding and clarifying the family dynamics are important in developing an effective treatment plan.

School Environment Factors

The role of the school environment in school refusal has received little attention. Institutional factors such as changing classrooms or lack of privacy in the school bathroom have been associated with fear of school. Humiliation caused by an insensitive teacher also may be a precipitating stressor in the onset of clinical symptomatology.

Recent developments in secondary school violence have provided children a seemingly appropriate reason for refusing to attend school. A survey of 12,000 students and school personnel conducted by the New York State Education Department during the 1992-1993 academic year revealed that 26% of junior and senior high school students had been assaulted on school grounds, 20% of students admitted bringing a knife or gun to school, and 10% admitted not going to school due for fear of violence.[3] Clearly, school-associated stressors are emerging as a concern in understanding and treating school refusal.

Associated Stressors

While exploring child, parent, family, and school environment factors, the clinician also must search for a precipitating event or stress that may have tipped the balance in causing a child to refuse to attend school. Illness or injury of a family member or of the child may be the initial reason for nonattendance. Likewise, the death of a relative or close friend may precipitate the refusal. Moving to a new home, community, or school also may contribute to refusal. The longer a child has been out of school, the more potentially stressful and difficult returning becomes.

Clinical Management

The foundations of any clinical treatment plan are rapport, trust, and respect. The initial interview should serve not only as a means of gathering data but also as the start of a therapeutic alliance. The child must understand that the very fact that a physician is involved in treatment begins a change in the existing behavior.

Organic disease should be ruled out through a careful history and physical examination, coupled with *judicious* laboratory evaluation. Time spent in conducting a thorough medical examination communicates the physician's sincere acceptance of the child's presenting symptom as being real. Parents are better able to confront the lack of organic disease when it is explained to them by a clinician who is completely familiar with the child's history and physical examination. The laboratory should be used in a symptom-specific, noninvasive, cost-effective manner consistent with ruling out possible organic disease.

The parents, physician, and school personnel all must agree that returning to school as quickly as possible is the immediate goal of treatment. Allowing the child to stay home while awaiting laboratory data or using home tutors only makes the return to school more difficult. A specific plan must be de-

CRITERIA FOR MENTAL HEALTH REFERRAL

Unresponsive to pediatric management
Out of school for 2 months
Onset in adolescence
Psychosis
Depression
Panic reactions
Parental inability to cooperate with treatment plan

veloped to respond to clinical symptoms. Objective criteria such as an elevated temperature should be used consistently both at home and in school. When the parents are in doubt, they should seek the guidance of the child's physician regarding the significance of acute symptoms before keeping the child home. Also, the patient must understand that the significant attachment figures in his or her life will adhere to the therapeutic program consistently and persistently.

In most cases of school refusal, especially in the elementary years, the above program, carried out by the primary caregiver, is curative. Other treatment modalities, typically by a mental health professional, include desensitization, psychotherapy, hypnotherapy, and psychopharmacology. Suggested criteria for mental health referral are listed in the box above.

Prognosis

Pediatric experience suggests that the vast majority of children who refuse to attend school overcome the difficulty rapidly with appropriate clinical management. Intermittent relapses associated with stress or new separation experiences, such as camp or sleep-overs, occur in approximately 5% of children. Children who require psychiatric management do not fare as well. Most published series in the psychiatric literature reveal significant cohorts of patients requiring ongoing therapy and having persistent difficulties in emancipating themselves from their family.

Prevention

Anticipatory guidance is an excellent means of primary prevention, which allows the pediatrician to advise parents on developmentally appropriate "separation" guidelines. For example, by the time an infant is 6 months old, the parents should be able to spend some evenings out alone. By 1 year of age, peer contact should be encouraged. Toddlers should experience baby-sitters while awake. By age 3 the child should experience being away from home without a parent, such as in a play group or neighbor's home. Age 4 is a good time to consider preschool for the child. Such guidance can be shared in the context of routine health supervision. Parents also should be discouraged from keeping children home because of minor illness, and physicians must avoid unnecessary medical restrictions.

Preventing "vulnerable child syndrome" also is important when caring for ill children. This disorder arises when parents feel that their child's life has been threatened significantly, and it results in separation difficulties, overprotection, bodily concerns, and underachievement in school.[1] Parents need to be informed about the true significance and prognosis of any medical difficulty the child has experienced. Practitioners have a responsibility to avoid creating iatrogenic misconceptions about a child's health; they can do this by using everyday language as much as possible, rather than medical jargon, and by demystifying anxiety associated with insignificant findings such as a functional murmur. Parents need to be reassured that children who have recovered fully from an acute illness are at no increased risk for future illness. By inquiring about children's school attendance and promoting healthy parenting styles, pediatricians can help prevent school refusal.

TRUANCY AND DROPPING OUT

Truancy is a good predictor of dropping out later on. Many schools in inner cities report daily absence rates above 20%; an equal or greater percentage of these children never finish high school. Truancy is a serious social problem that has potentially lifelong consequences. Unemployment or underemployment, criminal behavior, marital problems, and chronic social maladjustment often are seen in both truants and dropouts. These same long-term outcomes have been identified in groups of children with learning disabilities. Clearly, an unrecognized learning disability is a risk factor for school failure, with subsequent disengagement and truancy. Truancy also has been noted among children who have a history of having been sexually abused. Other risk factors are low socioeconomic status, conduct disorder, gang membership, substance abuse, cigarette smoking, and family discord. Early recognition of children at risk should prompt immediate intervention to promote optimal adjustment. Mobilization of resources in the school, community, and family is critical to help prevent progression from truancy to dropping out. Creative programs to foster school attendance and success have been conducted with variable results. Practitioners must assume a leadership role in guiding and supporting therapeutic interventions in the educational and social welfare arenas.

CONCLUSION

Absenteeism is a simple symptom with multiple causes. Because success in school often is the foundation for continuing success in life, health care professionals must devote thoughtful attention to understanding and treating absentees. Using a biopsychosocial model and mobilizing multidisciplinary resources are the keys to clinical success.

REFERENCES

1. Green M, Solnit AJ: Reactions to the threatened loss of a child: a vulnerable child syndrome, *Pediatrics* 34:58, 1964.
2. Nader PR, Bullock D, Caldwell B: School phobia, *Pediatr Clin North Am* 22:605, 1975.
3. New York State Education Department, Division of Criminal Justice Services, unpublished survey data, February 1994.

SUGGESTED READINGS

Berg I: Absence from school and mental health, *Br J Psychiatry* 161:154, 1992.

Dworkin PH: *Learning and behavior problems of school children,* Philadelphia, 1985, WB Saunders.

Eisenberg L: The pediatric management of school phobia, *J Pediatr* 35:758, 1959.

Heath CP: School phobia: etiology, evaluation, and treatment, ERIC Document No 261321, Springfield, Va, 1985, CBIS Federal.

Klerman LU: School absence: a health perspective, *Pediatr Clin North Am* 35:1253, 1988.

Nader PR, editor: *School health: policy and practice,* Elk Grove Village, Ill, 1993, The American Academy of Pediatrics.

Schmitt BD: School refusal, *Pediatr Rev* 8:99, 1986.

Weitzman M et al: School absence: a problem for the pediatrician, *Pediatrics* 69:739, 1982.

72 School Learning Problems and Developmental Differences

Paul H. Dworkin

School learning problems are complex issues that defy traditional methods of pediatric assessment and management. Learning problems are not the exclusive responsibility of the pediatrician, but rather are of multidisciplinary concern. Furthermore, pediatricians neither definitively diagnose nor independently treat learning disabilities. Nonetheless, pediatricians should assume critical roles when their patients manifest learning problems. Such roles include clarifying the reasons for poor school performance and facilitating appropriate intervention. The importance of such pediatric involvement increasingly has been recognized; parents and educators regard such problems as learning disabilities to be within the pediatrician's area of responsibility and demand pediatric attention to the needs of children who perform poorly in school. Unfortunately, many pediatricians view themselves as inadequately prepared to deal with school learning problems.

REASONS FOR LEARNING PROBLEMS

The British pediatrician Martin Bax noted that a student's learning problems may result from a variety of causes, "from his school burning down to the lack of the appropriate textbook."[2] Causes of school failure may be classified somewhat simplistically into "intrinsic" and "extrinsic." Intrinsic causes comprise the inherent characteristics of the failing child, such as specific learning disabilities, mental retardation, and sensory impairment. Extrinsic causes are adverse external influences, such as family dysfunction and social stressors within the home or ineffective schooling. Actually, however, learning problems typically are the consequence of a complex interaction of variables related to the child, the family, and the school (Fig. 72-1). For example, a subtle learning disability can be particularly devastating for a child reared in poverty and attending a school of inferior quality. Furthermore, learning problems often coexist with "clusters" of adverse influences. For example, a learning-disabled child may be at a particular disadvantage if he or she has a slow to warm up style of temperament that precludes active classroom participation or if the child is confronted with the trauma of parental divorce. Thus the pediatrician's assessment of school learning problems must include the child's capabilities and weaknesses within the context of social and environmental circumstances.

Specific Learning Disabilities

Of the many causes of school learning problems, specific learning disabilities are the most prevalent and perplexing. Learning disabilities are regarded as a heterogeneous group of disorders manifested by significant difficulties in the acquisition and use of listening, speaking, reading, writing, reasoning, or mathematical abilities. These disorders are presumed to be due to central nervous system (CNS) dysfunction and not the direct result of environmental influences or other handicapping conditions.[5] The hallmark of learning disabilities is a discrepancy between a student's potential for academic achievement, as suggested by cognitive abilities, and actual performance, as documented by achievement tests. The prevalence of learning disabilities is estimated to be 3% to 5% of students.

Although no single cause of learning disabilities has been identified, research has emphasized the critical importance of language development in learning. Many learning-disabled children have experienced delayed or disordered language acquisition, supporting the belief that learning disabilities may be the expression of a more general linguistic disability. More recently, the importance of weaknesses in higher-order cognitive functions (i.e., thinking and reasoning processes and memory) has been emphasized. Deficits in so-called metacognitive skills, such as being able to access acquired knowledge when needed and knowing how to apply learned skills, may be the reason learning-disabled children are unable to focus attention on the salient features of tasks or effectively devise problem-solving strategies. Such children have been described as passive learners because of their difficulty with strategy selection and problem solving.[10]

Learning-disabled children typically display deficits in various areas of developmental functioning. When developmentally assessed, these children are more likely than their learning-normal peers to be confused by sequences and time relationships (temporal-sequential deficits), to have "right-left confusion" (directional disorientation), to fail to appreciate spatial relationships and visual detail (visuoperceptual difficulties), and to have difficulty integrating auditory and visual stimuli, such as the sounds of words and the visual configurations of letters (deficits in intersensory integration). These children also are more likely to be clumsy and awkward (motor abnormalities) and neurologically immature (i.e., to exhibit neuromaturational delay or so-called soft neurological signs). In addition, behavioral or emotional problems, such as diminished self-esteem, are more common among such students.

Except for language and cognitive deficits, the extent to which these clinical correlates contribute to, result from, or merely coexist with learning disabilities is uncertain. For example, extensive research fails to substantiate a significant causal relationship between faulty visuoperceptual skills and academic deficits. The presence of such correlates should not form the basis of a diagnosis of learning disability. Rather, findings such as temporal-sequential deficits and directional disorientation should serve as "red flags" that increase the

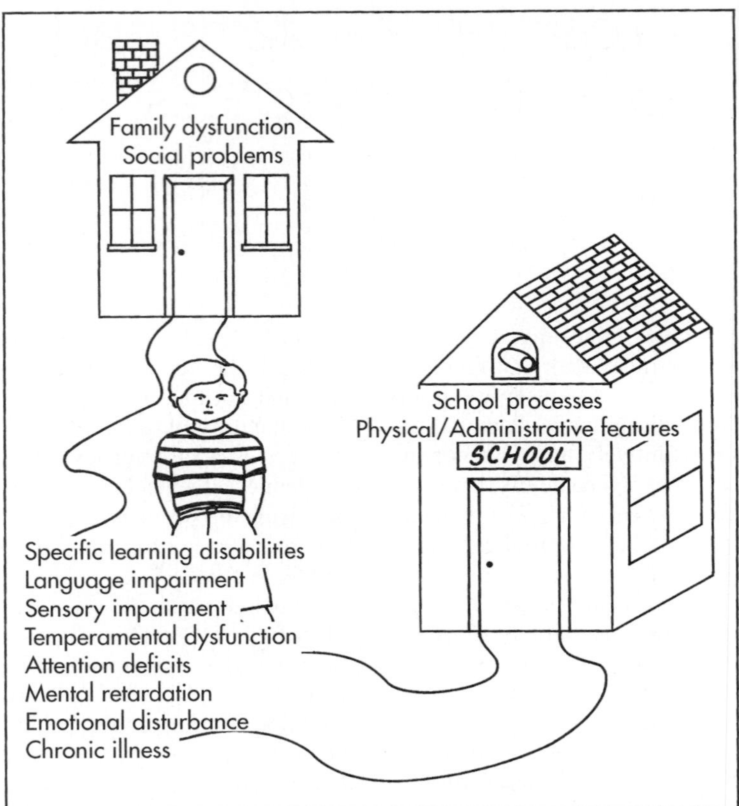

FIG. 72-1 Learning problems typically stem from a complex interaction of variables related to the child, family, and school.

(From Dworkin PH: *Pediatr Rev* 10:301, 1989.)

clinician's suspicion about the possibility of learning disabilities and prompt a referral for psychoeducational evaluation to document the potential-performance disparity required for diagnosis.

Learning-disabled children most commonly have problems with the language arts (reading, spelling, and written expression) and they also may have difficulties with arithmetic and handwriting skills, although isolated problems with arithmetic are less common. A child's pattern of academic performance may change over time. For example, some learning-disabled children may cope satisfactorily during the first 3 years of school, only to experience increasing problems with academic achievement and organization of assignments by third or fourth grade, as classroom expectations increase and demands for the rapid retrieval of information and work productivity escalate.[7]

Other Reasons for Learning Problems

Whether *attention deficit disorders* represent a specific syndrome (attention deficit/hyperactivity disorder) or result from complex interactions between child-related and environmental factors is highly controversial. Regardless, there clearly is a group of children for whom difficulties such as inattention, distractibility, lack of persistence, and impulsivity impair school functioning. These attention deficits often are associated with other causes of learning problems, such as specific learning disabilities.

Mild *mental retardation* usually is not identified until the child is confronted with the cognitive demands of school. The academic performance of such children is characterized by slow learning and acquisition of skills to at most the fifth or sixth grade level. Mental retardation and learning disabilities may coexist, and both contribute to a child's learning problems.

Sensory impairment may contribute to school learning problems. Of the five senses, hearing and vision are the most crucial for academic learning. Of these two, *hearing loss* results in the more profound educational handicap, primarily because of impaired language acquisition and communication skills. The learning problems of hearing-impaired children are characterized by difficulties in reading, as well as in mathematical reasoning and problem solving. Deaf students also may struggle with classroom maladjustment, behavioral problems, and social immaturity. Children who have *visual disturbances* usually fare better than their hearing-impaired peers in the classroom. In general, such children tend to perform rather well; thus their academic achievement has received only limited scrutiny.

Although 30% to 80% of emotionally disturbed students have problems with academic achievement and classroom behavior, *emotional illness* (e.g., depression or conduct disorders) is the primary cause of learning problems for only a small percentage of children facing school failure. Rather, emotional factors may be far more important in the exacerbation of academic difficulties caused by other problems. For example, the inevitable feelings of diminished self-esteem

Table 72-1 Role of the History in the Evaluation of School Learning Problems

Aspect	Findings suggesting specific learning disabilities
School functioning	
Academic achievement	Discrete delays in select subjects (e.g., language); adequate early performance with difficulties emerging later (e.g., mathematics, writing)
Classroom behavior	Long-standing, pervasive problems with inattention, impulsivity, overactivity; disorganization and poor strategy formation; depression, moodiness
Attendance	Excessive absenteeism; school avoidance
Past psychoeducational testing	Discrepancy between cognitive abilities and academic achievement
Special required school services	Response to "diagnostic teaching"
Perinatal history	"Clusters" of adverse events; maternal alcohol or drug intake
Medical history	Recurrent and/or persistent otitis media; iron deficiency anemia; lead poisoning; seizures; frequent accidents; chronic use of medication
Development	Delayed or disordered language acquisition and communication skills; subtle delays in select milestones; "uneven" pattern of skills and interests
Behavioral history	Long-standing, pervasive problems with attention span, impulsivity, overactivity; sadness; acting out; poor self-esteem
Family history	Learning problems, school failure among first-degree relatives
Social history	Child abuse or neglect; other stressors

and frustration that accompany school failure because of learning disabilities may serve to impair classroom functioning even further.

One fourth to one third of children who have a *chronic illness* have problems achieving academically. Chronic illness may contribute to school learning problems as a consequence of limited alertness or stamina, chronic pain, side effects of medication, absenteeism, altered or inappropriate expectations of teachers or parents, maladjustment, or inappropriate placement in special classes. Low intelligence and learning disabilities may be problems for children who have certain neurological disorders.

A child's behavioral style, or *temperament,* may contribute to school learning problems. The temperamentally "difficult" child quickly may become frustrated and angry when confronted with material not easily mastered. Or the initial reluctance of the "slow to warm up" child to participate and his or her tendency to withdraw may be misinterpreted as anxiety or a limited capability for learning. Although the "easy" child usually fares well in the classroom, problems may arise when expectations for behavior differ markedly between home and school.

Social and environmental factors also can contribute to school learning problems. These include parental divorce or separation, child abuse or neglect, illness or death of immediate family members, parental emotional illness, early parenthood, substance abuse, and poverty. Ineffective schooling itself may contribute to learning problems. Some studies have revealed that school processes (e.g., academic emphasis, use of rewards and praise, teachers' actions during lessons) are more important than physical or administrative features.[9] Factors such as school climate and social environment may be particularly important for children from disadvantaged homes who attend schools with limited resources.

For children of ethnocultural minorities, additional factors may influence school performance. *Cultural factors* include differences in concepts necessary to learn such subjects as math and science, teaching and learning styles, assumptions about interpersonal relations, and language. The influence of bilingual education is controversial. Select studies report that acquisition of English as a second language may interfere with school achievement, but other studies indicate that acquisition of a second language facilitates school achievement and cognitive development in the bilingual child.[1]

PEDIATRIC EVALUATION OF LEARNING PROBLEMS

The goal of pediatric evaluation of school learning problems depends on the specific circumstances of a child's referral. When school-based assessment has already raised the possibility of a child being learning disabled, pediatric evaluation assumes a relatively limited role in excluding medical problems that may contribute to poor school functioning. Alternatively, pediatric evaluation is far more challenging when a child is experiencing unsuspected or unexplained learning problems. The goals of such evaluation are diagnosing "medical" conditions that may contribute to school problems (e.g., sensory impairment or a seizure disorder) and identifying clinical correlates (medical, neurophysiological, and psychological) of other causes of learning problems, such as specific learning disabilities.

The pediatrician should follow certain guidelines when evaluating school learning problems. For example, the numerous factors that can contribute to school failure must be considered. Communication with school personnel is invaluable in obtaining information about classroom functioning, past assessments, and school resources. The child must be evaluated within the context of the learning environment; for example, the expectations of a 5-year-old entering an academically oriented kindergarten class are quite different from those of a child entering a more developmentally and socially oriented program.

History

Important historical information should be sought from parents, teachers, and the child (Table 72-1); questionnaires may facilitate the gathering of necessary information.[6] Certain aspects of *school functioning* should be examined in detail, including the child's academic achievement, classroom behavior, school attendance, past psychoeducational testing, and special school services provided. Findings that suggest the possibility of specific learning disabilities may include (1) discrete delays in select subjects, such as the language arts, or an adequate early performance with later emergence of difficulties, (2) behavioral problems such as long-standing, pervasive problems with inattention, impulsivity, overactivity, acting out, disorganization, and poor strategy formation, or depression, sadness, and moodiness resulting from frustration and diminished self-esteem, (3) school avoidance because of frustration, (4) a discrepancy between cognitive abilities and academic achievement on past psychoeducational testing, and (5) poor response to special teaching techniques, which suggests special learning requirements.

Other aspects of the traditional medical history also should be examined in detail. The perinatal history of learning-disabled children is characterized by a somewhat increased incidence of "clusters" of adverse events, such as anoxic encephalopathy, prematurity, and bronchopulmonary dysplasia, as well as maternal alcohol and drug intake (e.g., substance abuse and anticonvulsants). The past medical history may be significant for recurrent or persistent otitis media, iron deficiency anemia, lead poisoning, seizures, frequent accidents as a result of overactivity, or chronic use of medication (e.g., phenobarbital, theophylline, or antihistamines). The developmental history of learning-disabled children may suggest delayed or disordered language acquisition and communication skills; subtle delays in select milestones, such as speaking, sitting, or walking; or an "uneven" pattern of skills and interests, with discrete areas of strength and weakness. The behavioral history may reveal long-standing, pervasive problems with attention span, impulsivity, and overactivity; sadness; acting out; or poor self-esteem. The family history may corroborate the increased incidence of learning problems and school failure among first-degree relatives of learning-disabled children. The social history may reveal such stressors as child abuse or neglect, known to be associated with specific learning disabilities.

Physical Examination

The physical examination has a limited but important role in the evaluation of children who have learning problems (Table 72-2). The physician's general observation of the youngster may note sadness, anxiety, a short attention span, impulsivity, or overactivity. Tics may indicate Tourette syndrome, which is known to be associated in some cases with learning disabilities. Physical features may be observed that suggest syndromes associated with learning disabilities, such as fragile X syndrome, fetal alcohol effects, or Turner syndrome. Alternatively, an increased incidence of so-called minor congenital anomalies (epicanthic folds, hypertelorism, low-set ears, high-arched palate, clinodactyly, and syndactyly of the toes) has been observed among some children who have specific learning disabilities and attention deficits.

Certain specific aspects of the physical examination deserve special emphasis. Examination of the skin should include a search for multiple café-au-lait spots (neurofibromatosis), as well as "ash leaf" spots and adenoma sebaceum (tuberous sclerosis), inasmuch as both conditions are associated with learning problems. Examination of the tympanic membranes may reveal signs suggesting recurrent or chronic otitis media. Among older boys, examination of the genitalia may reveal delayed sexual maturation, which has been correlated with learning problems. Growth measurements may indicate problems such as short stature, microcephaly, and macrocephaly, which also have been associated with learning disabilities. Sensory screening should exclude hearing impairment or vision defects.

Table 72-2 Role of the Physical Examination in Evaluation of School Learning Problems

Aspect	Findings suggesting specific learning disabilities
General observations	Sadness, anxiety, short attention span, impulsivity, overactivity; tics
Phenotypical features	Stigmata of genetic syndromes (e.g., sex chromosome abnormalities, fetal alcohol syndrome); minor congenital anomalies
Skin	Multiple café-au-lait spots; "ash leaf" spots, adenoma sebaceum
Tympanic membranes	Signs of recurrent or chronic otitis media
Genitalia	Delayed sexual maturation in boys
Growth measurements	Short stature; microcephaly and macrocephaly
Sensory screening	Poor hearing or vision

Examination of Mental Status

Simple projective testing may identify emotional issues as either the cause or, more likely, the consequence of school learning problems. Techniques such as asking the child for three wishes, asking the child to draw a picture of his or her family, or playing the Winnicott Squiggle Game[3] may reveal the child's sadness, diminished self-esteem, or concerns regarding family functioning.

Neurodevelopmental Screening

Surveying the child's functioning in different areas of development may help identify factors that contribute to learning problems. As previously noted, children who have specific learning disabilities are more likely to have deficits in language functioning and cognitive abilities. Furthermore, the developmental profile of learning-disabled children is characterized by an uneven pattern, with discrete areas of relative strength and weakness.

A few tools have been developed for assessing school-age children. One is the Pediatric Early Elementary Examination (PEEX),[8] which requires about 45 minutes to administer and surveys the following areas of development: temporal-sequential organization, visuospatial orientation, auditory-language function, memory, fine motor function, and gross motor function. The PEEX also includes a search for minor neurological indicators of dysfunction ("soft" neurological signs) such as dysdiadochokinesia (difficulty with rapid alternating movements), synkinesis (mirror movements), and dystonic posturing of the upper extremities, associated with heel walking. An increased incidence of such signs has been observed among boys who have attention deficits and, to a lesser extent, specific learning disabilities.

Laboratory Studies

Laboratory tests are of limited value in assessing school learning problems and should be used only in studies of children at specific risk for conditions known to be associated with learning disabilities. Examples include *anemia screening* for children at risk because of nutritional or socioeconomic factors; *lead screening* for those at risk because of their home environment or a history of pica; *thyroid function studies* if signs or symptoms of thyroid disease are noted or if the possibility is suggested by family history; and *chromosome analysis* (including a search for the fragile X site in retarded boys and in retarded girls who have a positive family history) if the child has phenotypical features or multiple congenital anomalies that are associated with mental retardation. *Drug screening* is recommended for older children and adolescents who have shown a precipitous decline in school performance or erratic, unpredictable behavior.

Neuroanatomical and neurophysiological studies should be performed only for specific indications. For example, an *electroencephalogram* (EEG) should be reserved for children suspected of having a seizure disorder, whereas *computed tomography (CT)* or *magnetic resonance imaging (MRI)* is indicated for suspected CNS malformations, microcephaly, or macrocephaly.

Further Investigations and Referrals

Referral for *psychoeducational evaluation* is indicated when the pediatric assessment suggests the possibility of learning disabilities as a cause of learning problems. For example, learning disabilities may be suspected if (1) the pediatric history reveals difficulties with discrete subjects such as reading and spelling, (2) developmental testing indicates an "uneven" profile, with areas of strength and weakness, and (3) a child demonstrates poor self-esteem and poor self-image. The goals of psychoeducational evaluation are to examine the child's academic strengths and weaknesses, to determine cognitive ability, to assess perceptual strengths and weaknesses, to examine communicative ability, and to assess social and emotional adaptation. Ideally, such evaluations are performed by the child's school system, although specific circumstances may dictate a private referral. School personnel participating in such evaluations may include psychologists, special educators and learning disability specialists, speech-language pathologists, and social workers. Tests typically administered include those for intelligence, general learning abilities, academic achievement in reading, mathematics, and writing, perceptual and motor function, and speech and language skills. Diagnostic teaching also may be an effective test.

Pediatric assessment may indicate the need for referral to a variety of other professionals. For example, concern about language functioning may result in direct referral to a speech-language pathologist, and emotional disturbance or family dysfunction may suggest the need for referral to a mental health professional (e.g., psychologist, social worker, or psychiatrist). Concern about sensory impairment may suggest referral to an ophthalmologist, otolaryngologist, or audiologist.

PEDIATRIC INTERVENTION

A variety of actions may follow assessment of the child who has school learning problems. Although educational programming is the mainstay of treatment for specific learning disabilities, pediatric participation may involve a variety of traditional and nontraditional roles.

Examples of traditional roles include specific medical intervention for underlying conditions, such as treatment of a seizure disorder that may contribute to learning problems, as well as pharmacological management of attention deficits. Counseling is another traditional role, which may include clarifying a child's strengths and weaknesses, alleviating undue concern, guilt, and anxiety, explaining the legal rights of children and families under state and federal regulations (e.g., the Individuals with Disabilities Education Act), offering guidance on such alternative treatment strategies as diet, megavitamins, and optometric training, and, depending on the pediatrician's expertise, giving advice about such specific behavioral management strategies as positive reinforcement and "time-out." Arranging for further investigations and referrals is yet another traditional role, and it may involve coordinating indicated laboratory studies and referring the child for psychoeducational testing and other evaluations.

With their access to young children and families and their responsibility for monitoring children's growth and development during the preschool years, pediatricians are well positioned to contribute to early detection of potential school dysfunction.[4] Developmental surveillance may be the most effective process for enabling the pediatrician to predict school readiness. Surveillance has four components: (1) eliciting and attending to parents' concerns and impressions, thereby acknowledging the importance of their opinions and descriptions of their child's development, (2) observing the child's development, which may be done longitudinally by using an informal collection of age-appropriate tasks or a developmental screening test, (3) obtaining the opinion of preschool teachers, which is important because such opinions are the single best predictor of kindergarten success, and (4) interpreting findings, including social and environmental circumstances, within the context of the child's overall well-being.

A less traditional but nonetheless important pediatric role is serving as ombudsman to help students and families use community services and resources effectively. Specific measures may include facilitating communication with school systems, introducing families to helpful parent and peer support groups, and initiating referrals to mental health and social service agencies. Although pediatricians are unlikely to have the expertise to suggest educational strategies for learning disabilities, participation as a member of a multidisciplinary planning team is both helpful and feasible. Such participation often is reassuring to the parents and children, who regard the pediatrician as an effective child advocate.

REFERENCES

1. Baca L, Amato C: Bilingual special education: training issues, *Except Child* 56:168, 1989.
2. Bax M: Looking at learning disorders, *Dev Med Child Neurol* 24:731, 1982 (editorial).

3. Berger LR: The Winnicott Squiggle Game: a vehicle for communication with the school-aged child, *Pediatrics* 66:921, 1980.
4. Dworkin PH: School readiness, *Curr Opin Pediatr* 3:786, 1991.
5. Interagency Committee on Learning Disabilities: Learning disabilities: a report to the US Congress, Washington, DC, 1987, US Department of Education.
6. Levine MD: *The ANSER system,* Cambridge, Mass, 1981, Educators Publishing Service.
7. Levine MD, Oberklaid F, Meltzer L: Developmental output failure: a study of low productivity in school-aged children, *Pediatrics* 67:18, 1981.
8. Levine MD et al: The Pediatric Early Elementary Examination: studies of a neurodevelopmental examination for 7- to 9-year-old children, *Pediatrics* 71:894, 1983.
9. Rutter M et al: *Fifteen thousand hours: secondary schools and their effects on children,* Cambridge, Mass, 1979, Harvard University Press.
10. Torgesen JK: The learning-disabled child as an inactive learner, *Top Learn and Learn Disabil* 2:45, 1982.

SUGGESTED READINGS

Dworkin PH: *Learning and behavior problems of schoolchildren,* Philadelphia, 1985, WB Saunders.

Dworkin PH: School failure, *Pediatr Rev* 10:301, 1989.

Levine MD: Neurodevelopmental variation and dysfunction among school-aged children. In Levine MD, Carey WB, Crocker AC, editors: *Developmental-behavioral pediatrics,* ed 2, Philadelphia, 1992, WB Saunders.

Wender ED, editor: School dysfunction in children and youth: the role of the primary care provider for children who struggle in school, Report of the Twenty-Fourth Ross Roundtable on Critical Approaches to Common Pediatric Problems, Columbus, Ohio, September, 1993, Ross Products Division, Abbott Laboratories.

73 Nursing Roles in School Health

Mary Farren and Donna M. Hill

The school nurse is one of the key elements for implementing a viable, effective school health service. The responsibilities are diverse, and the school nurse must be able to work with a variety of people, including children and their families, school administrators, teachers, and other school personnel, school physicians, other physicians, and community agencies.

The role of the school nurse is multifaceted and complex. Although it originated in community health nursing, the work varies greatly from one school to another depending on the nurse's educational preparation and the priorities of the school board. In a few schools, licensed vocational (practical) nurses, who have up to 1 year of nursing preparation, provide limited health services; registered nurses may have 2 to 4 years of nursing preparation. School nurse practitioners, whose expanded role in school health is described later in this chapter, often are prepared in postbaccalaureate or master's degree programs that include specific preparation in school health.

The scope of the school nurse's role is related not only to the nurse's educational preparation but also to the organizational structure under which the health services are provided. Although some school health services are provided by local health departments or, in a few innovative programs, by a nonprofit corporation,[1] most school nurses are employed by boards of education. The scope of the nurse's role often indicates the school's priority in meeting the health needs of its students, as well as the resources the school can commit to that endeavor or can secure from other public and private sources. An awareness of some of the variations in the school nurse's role can help the physician establish a collaborative relationship with the nurse and become familiar with the school health program.

FUNCTIONS OF THE SCHOOL NURSE

In most schools that have a well-established traditional school health program, high priority is assigned to the three levels of prevention: health promotion and disease prevention, identification and remediation of health problems, and restoration of children who have chronic diseases to their optimal level of health. School nurses are responsible for assessing, managing, and controlling any health problems they discover in students or in the environment. According to the American School Health Association (ASHA), school nurses help children learn to use their intellectual potential to make worthwhile decisions that affect their present and future health.[11] Priority is assigned to modifying or removing health-related barriers that interfere with student learning. The school nurse ordinarily gathers a health history from parents when the child enters school and verifies the child's immunization status. The school nurse also is responsible for planning a systematical health appraisal of all schoolchildren, although some of the specific activities may be carried out by volunteers or paraprofessional personnel. Screening programs for vision and hearing problems, along with other selected assessment procedures, are conducted routinely at specified grade levels. When health problems are identified, a referral process is initiated that involves counseling the student and family about the nature of the problem, the necessity of further treatment, and the health resources available in the community. After obtaining the family's consent, the school nurse may speak directly with the family's physician about the problem and, after medical evaluation, discuss any educational implications and follow-up care indicated. The nurse can provide the physician with useful information about a child's response to the treatment and facilitate any temporary or long-term modification of the child's school milieu to meet health needs.

The school nurse works closely with parents and teachers of children who have chronic health problems. Because increasing numbers of children with major health problems are included in regular classrooms, teachers need more information, advice, and, sometimes, support to promote maximum development and academic achievement for these children. The Individuals with Disabilities Act (IDEA), Section 504 of the Rehabilitation Act, the Americans with Disabilities Act (ADA), and state laws and regulations address education of the disabled and widely broaden the scope of Public Law 94-142, which allowed many children to be enrolled in school for the first time. School nurses have provided physical and rehabilitative nursing care, as well as individual health teaching and counseling, to these students and their families to help them cope with chronic health problems.[8]

Obviously, the school considers emergency care for ill or injured pupils or staff members important. First aid policies and procedures ordinarily are developed by the school nursing staff, administration, and medical consultants. Although many school nurses are involved directly in providing some emergency care, teaching basic first aid procedures to all school personnel usually is a high priority. Often the nurse conducts in-service educational training for all staff members on emergency care; sometimes only a paraprofessional or a small group of staff members receives specific first aid training from the nurse. Many emergencies can be prevented by analyzing previous accident data, checking for health and safety hazards in the school, and ensuring that appropriate protective equipment is available for students involved in laboratories, workshops, and athletic activities. Such primary, secondary, and tertiary preventive measures usually constitute the common core of the school nurse's traditional role; most nurses view individual and group health education as important responsibilities and, time and energy permitting, become involved in a variety of such educational activities.

Virtually every contact with a student is an opportunity for incidental teaching or health counseling. The nurse also may develop special programs in the school for students who have similar health needs (e.g., teenagers who need to lose weight). Some nurses are involved in the health education curriculum, directly either as primary instructors or as collaborators with a classroom teacher or health educator in specific units of instruction.

EXPANDED ROLE OF THE SCHOOL NURSE

In recent years considerable interest has arisen in the expanded role of the nurse in various primary care settings. Designated by titles such as *nurse practitioner* or *nurse associate,* the expanded role generally involves acquiring skills that enable the nurse to provide more comprehensive health care. The notion of the nurse practitioner in the school is a natural extension of the role of the pediatric nurse practitioner in other ambulatory child health care settings.[4] Working with a pediatrician colleague, the nurse practitioner may assume a primary care role, which involves providing comprehensive well-child care, managing minor illnesses, and performing initial assessments of more serious acute and chronic conditions.

Nurse practitioner preparation is obtained within a graduate nursing education program or, alternatively, through a certificate program consisting of a minimum of 4 months of intensive study, including both theory and practice, followed by a preceptorship of 6 to 8 months with experienced nurse practitioners and physicians. In addition to acquiring new assessment techniques, nurses enrolled in practitioner programs expand their understanding of child development and behavioral problems, learn more about the common illnesses of children and adolescents, and sharpen their interviewing and counseling skills.[3] Specific attention is directed to integrating new and expanded knowledge and skills into the role of the school nurse and into the entire child health care delivery system. Contemporary school nursing demands that the practice focus on principles of epidemiology, case management for aggregates of students, and program management and evaluation.[5] Role reorientation is an important component, with emphasis placed on an interdependent, collaborative relationship with physicians and a generally more assertive approach in assuming responsibility for children's health care.

The nurse practitioner in an expanded school nurse role has a larger repertoire of assessment skills to use in evaluating a child's health status. Beginning with a health history obtained in interviews with the child and the family, the school nurse practitioner develops a complete data base by using sources of information in the school, such as teachers, and by performing a complete physical examination, including the neurological component. Diagnostic laboratory tests, as well as developmental and psychological screening procedures to identify behavioral and learning problems, are conducted as indicated. On the basis of the findings, appropriate health teaching and counseling are initiated with the student and family. If referral outside the school is indicated, a report of the nurse practitioner's findings assists in further management of the problem.

The health team concept is particularly important in the implementation of the nurse practitioner role in the school. Unless paraprofessionals are available to assume some of the more routine activities, such as minor first aid, clerical tasks, and some screening procedures, nurses may not have enough time to fulfill an expanded role. In the past this applied to school nurses in general; screening and health appraisal procedures often were dictated by tradition, if not mandated by state regulations, and nurses tended to believe that their time was consumed by activities that did not require professional nursing skill.

The school nurse practitioner also collaborates closely with the physician consultant. In fact, the physician-nurse team may provide comprehensive primary health care to a segment of the school population that has no other source of primary care.[11] In demonstration projects in several states, the school has become the base for primary health care for children in the community.[6] More commonly, in communities that have a well-established primary child health care system outside the school, the school nurse-physician team serves as the liaison between the school and the primary care physician.[7]

MODELS OF SCHOOL NURSE SERVICES

Numerous studies[2] have documented the effectiveness of nurse practitioners in improving and maintaining the health of schoolchildren. The school nurse practitioner role has received support from major professional organizations concerned with nursing and school health,[3] and many school districts have demonstrated an interest in an expanded role for the nurse, even though these services may be more costly. However, reimbursement of some costs to the school district through federal, state, and other third-party payment sources, also is more likely when school nurse practitioners provide some primary health care in the school in addition to some of the more traditional school nursing services.

Although the approximate number of nurses who work in schools has remained relatively constant in recent years, the number of students served by one nurse generally has increased, often surpassing the recommended ratio of 1 nurse to 750 students.[13] A few schools have attempted to meet basic school health needs by employing paraprofessional aides in lieu of nurses or nurse practitioners. Although less costly to the school, these personnel require careful training and supervision by a registered professional nurse to provide safe and effective care.[9] Other schools have used the nursing services provided by local public health departments. In this model of service the nurse's school-related activities may constitute only a part of his or her total community nursing role because the nurse provides care to all age groups within a geographical district and also may be responsible for health department clinics and other activities. Assigning a high priority to school health activities within the context of community health needs has been a problem because children ordinarily are the healthiest segment of the community's population. Some schools are trying to achieve an optimal mix of the services provided by the health aide, physician consultant, school nurse, and nurse practitioner to meet the health needs of a diverse school population.[12] This plan allows the services of the nurse practitioner to be concentrated in areas underserved by community primary care resources. It also frees both nurses and nurse practitioners from activities that can be delegated to health aides, yet provides backup and consultation for personnel at all levels. In times of rising educational costs and limited resources, however, many schools choose less expensive and thus less comprehensive health services. Studies of cost effectiveness and national trends in the financing of health care may well determine the composition of school nursing services in the future.[10]

PHYSICIAN AND SCHOOL NURSE COOPERATION

Although communication between the physician and the school may occur in many other contexts, more often it is the school nurse who interacts with the family physician. School and health care agencies have different "languages," priorities, and backgrounds. The school nurse can help the physician bridge the gap; at the same time the nurse may gain valuable consultation and support for health-related activities in the school. The rewards of collaboration in pursuit of common goals outweigh the occasional temporary barriers of frustration and misunderstanding. Mutual respect, open communication, and some understanding of each other's view of the world can enhance cooperation between the physician and the school nurse in improving the health of school-age children.

REFERENCES

1. Cronin G, Young WM: Poson/Robbins: a model school health care project, *Nurse Pract* 2:22, 1977.
2. Goodwin LD: The effectiveness of school nurse practitioners: a review of the literature, *J Sch Health* 51:623, 1981.
3. Guidelines on educational preparation and competencies of the school nurse practitioner: a joint statement of the American Nurses' Association, the American School Health Association, and the Department of School Nurses National Education Association, *J Sch Health* 48:265, 1978.
4. Igoe JB: Changing patterns in school health and school nursing, *Nurs Outlook* 28:486, 1980.
5. Igoe JB: What is school nursing? A plea for standardized roles, *Matern Child Nurs J* 55:142, 1980.
6. Kort M: The delivery of primary health care in American public schools, 1890-1980, *J Sch Health* 54:453, 1984.
7. Nader PR, editor: *Options for school health,* Rockville, Md, 1978, Aspen Systems.
8. National Association of State School Nurse Consultants define role of school nurse in "PL 94-142: Education for all Handicapped Children Act of 1975," *J Sch Health* 52:475, 1982.
9. National Association of State School Nurse Consultants: Delegation of school health services to unlicensed personnel, *J Sch Nurs* 11:13, 1995.
10. Passarelli C: School nursing: trends for the future, *J Sch Health* 64:141, 1994.
11. Snyder A, editor: Implementation guide for the standards of school nursing practice, Kent, Ohio, 1991, American School Health Association.
12. Sobolewski SD: Cost-effective school nurse practitioner services, *J Sch Health* 51:585, 1981.
13. *Standards of school nursing practice,* Kansas City, Mo, 1983, American Nurses Association.

SUGGESTED READINGS

Nader PR, editor: *School health: policy and practice,* Elk Grove Village, Ill, 1993, American Academy of Pediatrics.

National Nursing Coalition for School Health: School health nursing services: exploring national issues and priorities, *J Sch Health* 65:371, 1995.

Wold SJ: *School nursing: a framework for practice,* St Louis, 1981, Mosby.

74 Developmental Approach to Behavioral Problems

T. Berry Brazelton, David M. Snyder, and Michael W. Yogman

Every encounter between pediatrician and child is an opportunity for developmental assessment. The continuous, long-term relationship the pediatrician maintains with the child and family offers data about physiological and behavioral functioning under a variety of circumstances. When questions arise about the normality of a child's behavior, this data base gives the pediatrician a diagnostic and therapeutic edge, which a consultant can duplicate only with much time and effort.

The spectrum of behaviors about which parents become concerned is broad. Its range encompasses:

1. Nonproblems—concerns based on simple misinformation, which require support and corrective information only
2. "Problem behaviors," which are normal behaviors that often are difficult for the parents to deal with, such as negativism in the second year of life
3. Long-standing, relatively fixed "behavioral problems," such as continued, too-frequent night waking in 2-year-olds
4. Clearly pathological behavior based on psychopathology or organicity, such as that seen in an autistic child or a child who has lead encephalopathy or major psychiatric deviance that essentially is irreversible

This chapter takes a conceptual approach to the assessment of reversible behavioral problems as opposed to irreversible ones. The emphasis is on the center of the spectrum: problem behaviors and behavioral problems. These represent both the majority of parental concerns brought to pediatricians' attention and some of the most taxing diagnostic entities in behavioral pediatrics. This chapter shows how a conceptual approach based on normal development can be applied to these everyday problems in an office practice.

In pediatric practice it may not be possible to diagnose a behavioral problem in a single encounter; the rush to "make a diagnosis" on the first visit may well be inappropriate. It takes time to assess the dimensions of parental concern and the meaning of the behavior to the child. An early diagnosis may miss the appropriate dimensions of each of these factors. It can lead to extensive diagnostic studies or to referrals that not only may be unnecessary and costly but actually may make diagnosis and treatment more elusive by reinforcing parental concerns. This pursuit of a physical diagnosis often diverts the parents from approaching the child's problem. Frequently, the true nature and severity of the behavioral problem emerge only as we observe the parents' responsiveness to counseling or the child's reaction to altered parental approaches. This does not imply an interminable diagnostic phase. Rather, it reflects that, in managing behavioral problems, diagnosis and treatment often proceed in parallel, the diagnostic hypotheses suggesting counseling approaches, the family's response to these generating more precise diagnostic formulations, and so forth.

ETIOLOGY

Behavioral problems arise in the course of growing up as a consequence of the normal stresses of coping with new adjustments.[10] These problems must be viewed as part of the "coping process," the steps through which the child comes to terms with a challenge and successfully masters the difficulties inherent in learning about oneself and about the environment. The coping process may be modified by genetic, biological, and environmental factors, but it is always present and needs to be assessed even in those infrequent instances when a severe, underlying pathological condition is present (e.g., brain damage, autism, or parental psychosis). The progression from a limited problem behavior to a more global behavioral problem and occasionally even to a severe psychopathological condition depends heavily on how effectively the parent-child unit supports this coping process.

In those few instances when problems are becoming more severe, the parents often show excessive concern about the child's symptom rather than the underlying reason. The symptom may in fact be adaptive and represent a coping response to the stress of growing up or to illness or somatic defect. Most often the presenting symptom has had its beginning long before, and the parents' concerns have reinforced a chain of *behavior→concern→problem behavior→increasing concern→increasing behavioral problem.* To understand the cause and to achieve any change in this ever-lengthening chain, a pediatrician must understand each link in its development.[9]

EVALUATION

The most valuable clinical technique the pediatrician can use to assess developmental behavior in children is to observe the behavior of all participants as they interact. Clinical judgments about parents and children at every encounter are based on the physician's observational skills. Although formal tests of the child's intellectual and emotional functioning can structure these observations and articulate clinical judgments more clearly, tests can never entirely replace careful observation.

When parents make us, as pediatric observers, feel angry or depressed as they describe a problem, this becomes an important measure of the parent's own depth of reactions to the child and the behavioral problem. Do these feelings represent their feelings about their conflicts with the child? Why are they generating parallel feelings in us as we observe them? Moments of intense emotion may provide the best clue to the depth of underlying issues. For example, when a mother brightens and becomes animated as she talks about her child's negativism, the pediatrician can be certain that she enjoys it and can identify with it and that it will not create a serious problem for either mother or child. Similarly, when a young father begins to hold on grimly to his contention that his 5-year-old son's enuresis is punishable, the depth of tension and frustration created in us becomes our best measure of his inability to react appropriately to this symptom in the boy and indicates that a "fixed" problem area exists between them.

Mostly, pediatricians must begin by "listening with a third ear" or observing the behavior and documenting their own reactions to understand clearly what parents mean as they present their children's problem behaviors.[1] As the pediatrician attempts to gather the necessary information about a disturbing behavior (e.g., when it was first noted, the circumstances in which it occurs, how the parents react to it, and how the child responds to their reactions), he or she should be most alert to behavioral signs of deeper concerns. These deeper, often unconsciously controlled concerns usually are the real reasons the parents seek help. Parents often are reluctant to begin discussing their fears about brain damage, mental retardation, or psychological disorder in the child, and expressed concerns may, in fact, cover up their worries about these issues. These underlying concerns may not be expressed on the first visit. To the degree that they are, they signify that the parents feel the pediatrician is taking them seriously and can be trusted to accept their feelings without censure. Establishing this alliance with the pediatrician is the parents' first step toward solving the problem they are having with their child.

Evaluation of the Parents

In general, a child's behavior becomes problematical because it does not conform to the parents' expectations. Evaluation of the parents should start with the assumption that they are concerned about this dichotomy and should proceed with specification of the worrisome behavior and how it deviates from their expectations. Insofar as the parents are the focus of attention, we are interested in:

1. How realistic their expectations are
2. How rigid they are in their expectations
3. Whether the child violates these expectations in a narrow or broad area of functioning
4. Whether the violation means abnormality or "badness" in the child or their own failure in parenting

It also is important to determine the origin of their expectations; for example, their own experiences in growing up, their experiences with their older children, the grandparents' comments, or their cultural expectations.[8] Parents come to the pediatrician feeling guilty, inadequate, often isolated from their children, and defensive about the difficulties they are having. These feelings, which invariably impede problem solving, may well be the tragic result of our cultural biases that blame parents for everything "wrong" with their children. These feelings commonly raise questions about the impact of medications taken during pregnancy, genetic factors, and their own child rearing style as it affects the child's behavior. In some cases these concerns are realistic; in others, the overconcern can be a symptom and measure of the severity of the problem. However, in all cases this concern and guilt interfere with the parents' relationship with their child and therefore need to be brought out and examined in a positive and supportive manner. This entails accepting the parents' concern, validating their right to get help and, above all, feeding back to them a perception of their own basic competence and of their child's strengths, along with an assessment of the child's problem.

Occasionally, signs of markedly unrealistic expectations, such as attributing adult goals to an infant or small child, may come to the surface. Significant parental thought disorders may become apparent. A parent's own needs and concerns about his or her marriage or about another child may turn out to be the underlying motive for the visit. In any case, the degree to which the parents are conscious of their feelings about their child and his or her problematical behavior, and the ease with which they can express them, can tell us much about the kind of treatment most likely to work.

If the pediatrician's assessment of the child reveals that he or she is markedly different from the parents' description, or if their level of concern seems out of proportion to the problem they report, the physician should suspect an undiscovered parental concern. However, two alternative hypotheses also should be considered: (1) that the behavior observed is not typical of the child and (2) that the discrepancy represents an actual distortion of the child's behavior by the parents.

In the case of significant parental psychological disorder, pediatricians may first sense that their observations do not parallel the expressed complaints. Then they may realize that they cannot reach the parents to help them with their reaction to the child. This, then, may suggest that the primary problem is outside the realm of pediatrics altogether. Even in such situations, the manner in which the pediatrician talks with the parents about their feelings can influence significantly their acceptance of referral for psychiatric help. If they have learned that candidly expressing their concerns and feelings is met with acceptance and understanding rather than with censure or disinterest, it will be easier for them to make use of such psychiatric consultation.

Evaluation of the Child

In evaluating a child's behavior at any one time, pediatricians must keep in mind the following questions:

1. How is inborn individual temperament influencing the child's behavior (either overreactivity or underreactivity)?[5,11]
2. Is the symptom appropriate to the child's age?[6,9]
3. How do the child's reactions to all stress reflect either adaptive strengths or inadequate coping mechanisms?[4,10]
4. To what degree has the symptom influenced broad areas of a child's functioning (e.g., with the family or peers, or in school)?

5. What is the duration of the symptom as a sign of "fixation"?

If the child has not changed over time, one should worry; if the symptom has increased in severity, the situation becomes even more ominous.[11]

In practice the pediatrician evaluates a problem on all five levels simultaneously, but separate discussion may clarify the importance of each level.

Temperament as a Background for a Symptom. An understanding of infant temperament is helpful in assessing the child's contribution to common problems such as crying, feeding, sleeping disorders, temper tantrums, and poor weight gain.[2] Children vary in the rhythmicity of repetitive biological functions. These include sleep-wake cycles, appetite, and elimination. Interviews with the parents enable a pediatrician to assess a child's temperament in vital areas of function (activity, intensity, mood, adaptability, rhythmicity, threshold, distractibility, persistence, and approach-withdrawal), as suggested by the longitudinal studies of Thomas, Chess, and Birch.[11] Knowing patterns of individual differences such as that of the "temperamentally difficult" child (high intensity, low adaptability, low threshold) helps a pediatrician understand the child's intrinsic contributions to a sleep problem, and this understanding in turn can help the parents manage this "difficult" yet still normal child.

Age Appropriateness of Behavior. A given behavior has different meanings in children of each age. Although this is obvious in the case of motor milestones, it is equally true for behavioral problems. Temper tantrums, nightmares, phobias, stuttering, and other types of behavior are seen regularly at certain ages and usually pass without consequence. For example, temper tantrums in an 18-month-old are an appropriate indicator of the child's growing sense of independence.[3] A tantrum of similar intensity at age 4 deserves exploration for an answer to why the child's striving for autonomy does not take a more mature form. By being aware of the individual temperamental and maturational differences, a pediatrician not only can better evaluate problems when they arise, but also can use this information preventively to understand the child as an individual and, by sharing this information with the parents, establish an alliance to optimize the child's development.[6]

Child's Pattern for Coping with Stress. Because the pressures of growing up are a part of everyday life, children's behavioral problems must always be evaluated in the context of how they handle these stresses, as well as others that confront them. A pediatrician can note whether the behavioral symptoms in question provide a way for the child to cope better with the pressures of his or her environment. For example, thumb-sucking and holding onto a bottle, blanket, or beloved toy through the stressful second and third years of life seem to be healthy solutions to stress. Unless the parents' concern about such a "lovey" makes it nonadaptive, one should see such behavior as a source of strength for the child and help the parents to see it as such. Assessing a child by means of a "stress model" allows the practitioner to generalize and view the child's underlying resources for coping with any challenging situation.

A psychological testing instrument, such as the Denver Developmental Screening Test,[7] can be administered easily in the pediatrician's office, and it may be viewed as just such a stress. Such an assessment can become a way to evaluate the child's "level" of development, as well as his or her reaction to the stress of being tested. This, then, becomes a way to attend to the child's responses to the stress of testing and how the child is likely to cope with other stresses of life. In other words, we are given an opportunity to see how a child approaches any given problem or item rather than merely whether the test is passed or failed. When a 14-month-old boy turns to his mother to seek help when he is asked to stack blocks, this not only tells us about the child's response to the stress of the test, but also tells us something about the strength of his attachment to his mother and something about his level of autonomy.[10]

The idea of identifying a child's mechanisms for coping is part of the broader principle of being able to list the child's individual strengths, as well as problems, in a "problem list." When asked to stack blocks, a 2-year-old may take great delight in knocking them over rather than stacking them. Negativism is a healthy sign of the toddler's growing independence and should not be overlooked.[3]

Influence of the Symptom on Other Areas of Function. In determining the significance of any problem to a child, it is crucial to determine how isolated and discrete the problem is. A 4-year-old's bed-wetting at night may represent a discrete delay in maturation, whereas the same symptom in a 6-year-old may interfere with peer relations (e.g., the child is unable to spend the night at a friend's house). As children grow and attempt to identify with their peers, such a symptom becomes a real source of anxiety about their own adequacy. This anxiety can begin to interfere with all areas of function. They may begin to show signs of deficit in school performance and in their self-esteem in general. In a small child and in the area of feeding, the problem may range from a discrete attempt to control choices, such as refusing vegetables (a transient, self-limited problem) to a more global feeding disturbance, such as a refusal to eat any solid food. When the problem no longer is confined to feeding and involves other areas of adjustment, such as sleep and toilet problems, this suggests an even more global impairment in the parent-child relationship. The degree to which a problem is clinically significant commonly is related to the number of functional areas affected in the child's life.

Determining the degree to which any symptom affects the child's overall level of function not only has diagnostic implications, but also helps in the management of the problem. A therapeutic plan should account for and support the child's achievement and areas of success while attempting to improve any weaknesses.[8]

Chronicity of a Symptom. Since development implies change over time, any symptom that becomes chronic is worrisome. Crying, for instance, reaches a developmental peak between 3 and 6 weeks of age and tapers off by 3 months of age.[3] A 6-month-old who shows a persistent problem of "colicky" crying requires evaluation and intervention. Thus the degree of fixation in a behavior becomes a measure of the extent of the problem.

Finally, behavioral symptoms that become inflexible should arouse even more concern. If appropriate 2-year-old negativism is replaced by intense temper tantrums accompanied by persistent head-banging whenever the child does not get his or her way, this constrained, inflexible behavior pattern indicates a need for therapeutic attention to the child's relationship with the parents.

Delaying a diagnostic decision while collecting observations at several visits allows a pediatrician to assess the flexibility of any symptom by observing the parents' and child's responses to various therapeutic suggestions. Although an assessment of the parents' concerns, as well as the five areas of child behavior described, aids the pediatrician, no evaluation is complete without similarly observing the parent-child interaction.

Evaluation of Parent-Child Interaction

The pediatrician should evaluate not only the parents and the child separately, but also the interaction of parent and child over time. The essence of the parent-child interaction may be seen in the mutual request for attention and responses by parents with their children. Pediatricians should record observations of these interactions. They can distinguish the mother who sensitively shapes and shows her child how to achieve a task from one who either angrily shoves the child to a task or is completely unavailable to the child. Similarly, pediatricians can distinguish between the child who explores the surrounding environment, using a parent as a secure base, and the child whose interactions with a parent are either minimal or provocative. Value judgments should never substitute for repeated careful observations that attempt to understand the interaction of parent and child on its own terms and in its own culture.

MANAGEMENT

The therapeutic first step may be for the physician to try a simple suggestion. If the parent cannot establish a working relationship with the pediatrician and misuses the suggestion so that the behavioral problem becomes worse or reinforced, this becomes a measure of the depth of the parent's inability to accept help and of the need for more intensive therapy if the problem is to be solved. Pediatricians tend to blame themselves when a helping relationship cannot be established, instead of recognizing the diagnostic implications of the parents' inability to let down their defenses and to join in a therapeutic effort to help the child.

Pediatric management of childhood behavioral problems usually requires seeing parent and child together. By using the child's behavior as a way of communicating with parents and pointing out the child's behavior and their response to it, the pediatrician can help parents see their child as an individual who has strengths as well as weaknesses. For instance, when parents understand and accept their toddler's negativism as a striving for independence, they can pursue the goal of allowing the child the opportunity to "work out" negative struggles and to define his or her own capacities and limits. In this way the pediatrician forms an alliance with the parents that supports them in their concern, but gives them a goal that enables them to work together at finding adaptive parental responses to help the child.

A pediatrician who no longer feels able to understand or help a family should consider referral to a psychiatrist or social worker who is trained to work with more difficult parents. Because of the nature of the problem and the nature of their relationships with families, pediatricians should approach such referrals even more sympathetically than they might a referral to another physician. The parents' need for defenses against acknowledging that they have a family problem must be respected. The pediatrician may have to see a family several times to gain a clear idea of what kind of referral they will accept and to outline the questions that should be answered. The pediatrician must remain the primary health care provider for the family and must continue to support them after therapy is instituted by the consultant. The pediatrician not only should remain involved in the assessment, but also must understand clearly the consultant's assessment of the problem, because the pediatrician most often will be left to carry out the consultant's treatment and management recommendations after the diagnostic or therapeutic interval has terminated.

Pediatric management of behavioral problems and the fostering of normal development can be among the most challenging and rewarding aspects of practice. They need not be especially time consuming, but they do require a knowledge of normal development as a dynamic process, as well as concerned attention in understanding the parents' reports and in observing both the child's and the parents' behavior.

REFERENCES

1. Balint M: *The doctor, his patient and the illness,* New York, 1972, International Universities Press.
2. Brazelton TB: Crying in infancy, *Pediatrics* 29:579, 1962.
3. Brazelton TB: *Toddlers and parents,* New York, 1974, Delacorte Press.
4. Brazelton TB: *Touchpoints,* Reading, Mass, 1992, Addison-Wesley.
5. Carey WB: A simplified method for measuring infant temperament, *J Pediatr* 77:188, 1970.
6. Erikson E: *Childhood and society,* New York, 1950, WW Norton.
7. Frankenburg WK et al: Revised Denver Developmental Screening Test, *J Pediatr* 79:988, 1971.
8. Lewis M: *Clinical aspects of child development,* Philadelphia, 1971, Lea & Febiger.
9. Murphy L: *The widening world of childhood,* New York, 1962, Basic Books.
10. Murphy L, Moriarty A: *Vulnerability, coping, and growth,* New Haven, Conn, 1976, Yale University Press.
11. Thomas A, Chess S, Birch H: *Temperament and behavior disorders in children,* New York, 1968, New York University Press.

75 Interviewing Children

David I. Bromberg

In assessing pediatric problems in which psychosocial and emotional factors are particularly important, it is essential that the pediatrician have a clear understanding of these children and their relationship to their world. For each child, this relationship has three interrelated parts: the relationship with the family, the relationship with the community (mainly school), and the relationship with peers. Diagnostic interviewing is the primary method of attaining this understanding. A great deal of information is available from the parents (see Chapter 6, The Pediatric History) and the school (see Chapter 67, Overview of School Health and School Health Program Goals). However, a wealth of qualitatively unique information and insight can be obtained through a careful interview with the child.

STRUCTURE OF THE INTERVIEW

The interview can be divided into three parts: (1) establishing rapport, (2) the body of the interview (data collection), and (3) summation of the session (closure). Certainly the major goal is to collect data about the child, but other important functions also are served. For example, over the course of the interview, the pediatrician can establish himself or herself as a "helping" person by showing an understanding of the child's feelings and problems and a willingness to offer help rather than judgmental advice.

Establishing Rapport

Attempting to teach a person how to establish rapport is somewhat akin to teaching someone how to ride a bike; you have to do it to learn it. Nevertheless, several concepts are useful. Rapport is built continually throughout the interview and the ongoing relationship and is not limited to introductory remarks. Showing a sincere interest in and empathy for what the youngster has to say is essential. Verbalizing the feelings represented by a child's story can be very helpful in this regard.

Patient: (An 8-year-old boy being evaluated for school underachievement) I got sent to the principal's office yesterday.
Physician: Oh, really? What did you do?
Patient: We had a substitute, and everyone was throwing this eraser around the room.
Physician: Then what happened?
Patient: I guess I threw it last, and she yelled at me and sent me to the office.
Physician: Sometimes it doesn't seem fair to get into trouble for something the whole class is doing.
Patient: (brightening) Yeah, but I guess I shouldn't have thrown it.

Interpreting nonverbal behavior also can help by demonstrating that the pediatrician is "in tune" with the youngster. For example, 11- and 12-year-olds are seen routinely for physical examinations upon entering middle or junior high school. Sitting undressed and draped on an examining table, many of these youngsters appear angry or overly shy. They often avoid eye contact, scowl, and give brief answers. By saying, "I guess it's pretty embarrassing to have to undress and have a physical examination," the physician acknowledges the youngster's feelings, which can aid substantially in establishing rapport. Once rapport has been established, the examiner can watch the hostility wash away and the subsequent interview progress much more profitably.

"Reflecting" feelings generally is a useful way for the health care provider to display caring and a desire to communicate. This can involve responding to an "unspoken" message, for example, by commenting, "It sounds like you're pretty angry about that" or by summarizing the point of a story.

Patient: (A 10-year-old boy being seen for behavioral problems after his parents' separation) It's just not the same since my dad left.
Physician: Really? What differences have you noticed?
Patient: Well, yesterday I had soccer practice, and my dad usually takes me, but he wasn't around to do it.
Physician: Didn't your mom take you?
Patient: Oh, yeah. She's really trying hard to do all the things. But dad and I always talk about the practice, and mom just doesn't know much about soccer.
Physician: So you've really missed your dad since he moved away but don't want to say so to your mom.

The same message can be communicated by "checking back" with the child, prefaced by saying something like, "Just to be sure we're understanding each other . . ."

When doing a behavioral assessment, it is important to remember that the consultation rarely is initiated by 8- or 10-year-olds. Such children often are brought to the office with little or no explanation. Exploring their fears and expectations, as well as the activities they may be missing by being there, can help "break the ice." For younger children this may involve clarifying that they will not be undergoing any blood tests or receiving immunizations. The physician should discuss the format of the evaluation and the demands that will be placed on the youngster. Explicitly stating, "Mary, first I will be talking with you and your family about your school difficulty, and afterwards I will be meeting just with you so that we can get to know one another better; then next week I will give you a physical examination," clearly establishes the format of the sessions. For older children, recognizing how difficult it is to talk about oneself (or to be talked about) is worthwhile.

Physician: What concerns has the school expressed about John's behavior in the third grade?
Mother: The teacher is worried that he can't "stay on task" and is always out of his seat. He can be very disruptive in class.
Physician: How about at home?

Mother: Well, he leaves things all over the house, and he often annoys his younger sister and brother. He tends . . .
Patient: I do not. They always pick on me.
Physician: John, it can be pretty hard to have people talk about you, especially about things that are difficult for you. Remember, it's not that everyone is just angry at you, but rather we're trying to understand a problem in order to make it better.

Third-person techniques can facilitate conversation with a child. Rather than attributing feelings or characteristics to the patient, the interviewer can talk about these feelings in other youngsters. The statement, "Many 9-year-olds who wet the bed are embarrassed and afraid of sleeping over at a friend's house" allows a youngster to claim these same feelings but does not confront him or her directly. It also shows that the physician will not be shocked or dismayed by this information.

As with all pediatrics, the interviewer must maintain a developmental perspective in relating to the patient. Complimenting a 3-year-old on climbing the steps to the examining table would be quite appropriate, whereas the same comment to an 8-year-old would be condescending. In his book, *Childhood and Society,*[2] Erikson describes the "eight ages of man," or critical periods of development. Each "age" is presented as a task in development of the ego. The eight ages are summarized as the accomplishment of the following characteristics: (1) basic trust versus basic mistrust, (2) autonomy versus shame and doubt, (3) initiative versus guilt, (4) industry versus inferiority, (5) identity versus role confusion, (6) intimacy versus isolation, (7) generativity versus stagnation, and (8) ego integrity versus despair. Erikson's tasks of development provide a useful framework for both evaluating and relating to children. Commenting on issues of autonomy in the 3- to 4-year-old, issues of initiative in the 5- to 6-year-old, and issues of industry in the 7- to 9-year-old often successfully engages the child.

Physician: (To an 8-year-old who is being counseled for encopresis) To review, we've discussed why you soil your pants. We've also come up with a plan for helping you stop. Do you think you would be interested in this program?
Patient: Sure, it sounds easy.
Physician: Actually, it involves a lot of hard work. In talking with you today, I think that you are a pretty hard worker and I believe that you could do a very good job with this program. So, if you're willing, we could start this week.
Patient: Yeah, I think I'd like to do it.

It also is important to proceed from very concrete "here and now" discussions with the preschooler and early school-age child to more abstract explanations as the child gets older.

Data Collection

By the conclusion of the interview, the examiner ideally should have accumulated data covering three main areas: (1) the child's perceptions about the presenting problem, (2) information about the child's relationships with family, school, and peers, and (3) an assessment of the youngster's psychological and cognitive functioning.

Understanding the child's perception of the presenting problem probably is the most difficult assessment to make. Denial of emotional issues is common in school-age children. The 5- to 12-year-old frequently claims to be neither worried nor upset about the problem being evaluated. The physician must listen with his or her "third ear" and be sensitive to nonverbal cues to understand the youngster's relationship to the presenting complaint. Using third-person techniques may be helpful.

Physician: How has school been going?
Patient: Oh, I do OK. My grades are pretty good.
Physician: Your mother had mentioned that reading and phonics were sometimes difficult for you.
Patient: Well, maybe a little bit.
Physician: Many children have told me that they feel dumb when they have trouble with reading.
Patient: Yeah, I know I do. Sometimes I just get so mad.

When a child is reluctant to discuss problems, another useful approach is to ask him or her for "both sides of the coin"; for example, to state what he or she likes and dislikes about school. The same technique can be used to assess the child's feelings toward individuals or toward himself or herself—for example, "Can you brag about yourself and then run yourself down?" Social skills also can be evaluated in this manner: "What do your friends like about you? What things do you do that makes them mad at you?"

Information about the child's relationships with family, school, and peers is best obtained by using open-ended questions, which leave the respondent a great deal of latitude in interpretation. This often is information that the pediatrician will obtain during routine health supervision visits. A multidisciplinary group under the auspices of the National Center for Education in Maternal and Child Health published *Bright Futures National Guidelines for Health Supervision of Infants, Children, and Adolescents,*[5] in which they outlined the preventive and health promotion needs of youngsters. For each health supervision visit, they suggested "trigger questions" the pediatrician should ask the parents and the child. These questions form a valuable foundation for a semistructured interview with children. Below is a sample interview using these "trigger questions" *(in italics)* during a checkup for a 10-year-old girl.

Physician: *How is school going?*
Patient: Fine.
Physician: *And how are your grades?*
Patient: They're OK, straight As.
Physician: That's terrific. You should be quite proud. *What do you do to have fun and whom do you like to do it with?*
Patient: I'm interested in acting and am rehearsing for a play. Some of my friends are in acting with me.
Physician: *Are you involved in any other after-school activities?*
Patient: I wanted to play indoor soccer, but my mother doesn't want me to do it.
Physician: Why is that?
Patient: She thinks that I'm involved in too many activities.

This interview could serve as the basis for discussion of a healthy life-style, overcommittment, and balancing of physical and sedentary activities. Other "trigger questions" explore safety, health risk behaviors, including drugs, alcohol, and cigarettes, sexual activity, and pressures, and body image.

The physician should attempt to be nonjudgmental and allow the youngster maximum leeway in presenting his or her thoughts or feelings. Asking, for example, "You have lots of friends, don't you?" displays the examiner's preference for friendships and closes the subject to the child. A more effective question might be, "Do you have many friends or do you prefer doing things by yourself?" This allows the child to choose either option, without the physician prejudicing the choices.

Psychological functioning can be assessed by paying careful attention to both the content and the process of the interview. The assessment should include an estimate of intellectual functioning, an evaluation of the child's approach to problem solving (e.g., impulsivity, frustration), and the child's fears and fantasies, self-concept, and superego functioning (conscience). A useful framework for this analysis is the mental status examination. Because a complete discussion of this examination is beyond the scope of this textbook, the interested reader is referred to Simmons' *Psychiatric Examination of Children.*[6]

Numerous assessment techniques are available for gathering important data, ranging from the very unstructured "play" evaluation to the very structured questionnaire. The choice of particular tools depends on the patient's age and verbal abilities and the examiner's expertise and style. For school-age children, a semistructured interview probably is the most appropriate. This combines specific questions about the specific problem, peer relations, and related issues with the use of projective techniques. A discussion of several diagnostic techniques the pediatrician can use is included later in this chapter.

Closure

At the end of the interview, it is important to summarize for the child. A review of the session, highlighting the important points, is useful. An attempt should be made to offer the youngster honest, positive reinforcement and an optimistic outlook wherever possible. Plans for future meetings also should be discussed. A typical ending statement might be, "Bobby, I know you really worked very hard today, having to tell me all those things about yourself. It was especially hard to tell me how sad you were when your grandma died. But now I think we'll be able to make it easier for you to get back to school. I look forward to seeing you and your family next week."

The end of a session typically is the time that unanswered questions may be raised. The following excerpt is from an AD/HD summation conference with a patient and the parents:

Physician: I am glad we had the opportunity to review attention deficit/hyperactivity disorder today and to discuss James' medical treatment. I would like to see you again in 3 months.
Patient: (hesitatingly) Doctor, during the visit you told my mother that I was taking stimulants. Does that mean that I take drugs?
Physician: That must have been confusing. Let's review the differences between medications and drugs.

THE PARENTS' ROLE

The relationship binding physician, patient, and parents is a complex one. Children are brought to the physician to have a problem "fixed." As we have noted previously, the consultation rarely is initiated by the youngster. The pediatrician must define his or her relationship to the child and parents, paying careful attention to the issue of confidentiality and to the patient's therapeutic needs. What format the interview should take and in what order the practitioner will see the child and parents is the initial decision. Then the physician must decide how to share information among the parties.

Mature preadolescents and teenagers often are seen alone and first in the diagnostic process. The physician thereby demonstrates the primacy of the doctor-teenager relationship. Although establishing a similar relationship with a latency-age or preschool-age patient may be equally important, these youngsters may be frightened by an initial separation from their parents. I frequently see the child and parents together for the first diagnostic interview. This allows the youngster a chance to become more comfortable with the examiner in a less threatening setting. Parents occasionally are uncomfortable about discussing behavioral or emotional concerns with their children present. Children, however, usually are well aware of these concerns and find an honest discussion much less frightening than their fantasies about the process should they not be included. After an initial joint interview, both parents and child should be seen separately.

The issue of confidentiality is a difficult one to balance. On the one hand, the youngster has the right to tell the examiner specific things that should be held in confidence. On the other hand, the parents need information to play an effective role in the therapeutic process. It may be helpful to discuss treatment recommendations with the youngster before the final sum-up session with the family. The parents play a crucial role, both in the diagnostic process and in executing the therapeutic program. The physician should plan the consultation process carefully so as to maximize an effective relationship with both patient and parents.

PEDIATRIC PSYCHODIAGNOSTICS

Many techniques and types of questions are available to help engage youngsters in an interview as well as to uncover "defended" emotional material. Projective techniques allow the youngster to respond to loosely structured stimuli, giving answers that reflect his or her personality. Examples include, "If a genie were to come and give you three wishes, what would you wish for?" or "If you were stranded on a desert island and could have only one person with you, who would it be?" Another area involves the child's happiest, saddest, and maddest times.

Physician: What is the happiest time that you remember?
Patient: Probably when the whole family took the vacation at the beach last summer.
Physician: How about the saddest time?
Patient: I really can't think of one.
Physician: Really, no sad times?
Patient: Well, I guess when my grandma had to go to the hospital last year.
Physician: That certainly can be frightening. Have you ever been so sad that you've thought of hurting or killing yourself?
Patient: Oh, no, I've never considered that.
Physician: How about the maddest you've been? Does your temper ever get the better of you?

The responses to these questions must be evaluated in the context of what is known about the child. Other semistructured projective techniques are described below.

Sentence Completion

The physician should tell the child that they are going to play a sentence game. The physician gives the first part of a sentence, and the child has to finish it with the first thought that comes to mind. Short sentence fragments are used, such as "Boys are . . .," "Girls are . . .," "Mothers should . . .," "I feel bad when I . . ." The answers may indicate areas of conflict or may introduce other topics of interest to the child.

Drawings

Many children find it easier to express themselves through drawings than through verbal communication. Several formats can be used. The pediatrician might ask a youngster to make the best drawing of a person that he or she can. Standards are available in using the "Draw-a-Person" test to assess an IQ.[4] Kinetic family drawings are obtained by asking the child to draw a picture of his or her family doing something.[1] Family relationships and activity can be discussed using this stimulus. Figure placement, size relationships, and use of symbols all may be useful in interpreting the drawing. Allowing a child simply to draw a picture and tell you a story about it also can be very helpful.

Storytelling

Stories can be useful for talking about emotions or conflicts. A storytelling format that uses fables was developed by Despert and expanded by Fine.[3] With this technique, the physician tells the child that they are going to play a storytelling game in which the child must finish stories that the doctor begins. The child then is given a series of up to 20 fables that touch on many characteristic areas of conflict.

Physician: A boy and his mother go for a nice walk in the park all by themselves. They have a lot of fun together. When he comes home, the boy finds that his daddy is angry. Why is he angry?
Patient: Because the dinner wasn't ready.
Physician: What do you think the boy's father did when he got angry?
Patient: He yelled a lot at the mommy.
Physician: What does your father do when he gets angry?

The storytelling has offered several insights about this family that might have been difficult to obtain in other ways.

SUMMARY

Engaging children in a helping relationship is the core of pediatric practice. The formation of a close, empathic relationship with a patient begins with the diagnostic interview. It is important, therefore, to be alert to both the process and content of this interview and to select diagnostic tools that will foster development of the desired relationship between physician and child.

REFERENCES

1. Burns RC, Kaufman SH: *Actions, styles, and symbols in kinetic family drawings,* New York, 1972, Brunner/Mazel.
2. Erikson EH: *Childhood and society,* ed 2, New York, 1963, WW Norton.
3. Fine R: Use of Despert fables (revised form) in diagnostic work with children, *J Projective Techniques* 12:106, 1948.
4. Goodenough FL: *Measurement of intelligence by drawings,* New York, 1926, World.
5. Green M, editor: *Bright futures national guidelines for health supervision of infants, children, and adolescents,* Arlington, Va, 1994, National Center for Education in Maternal and Child Health.
6. Simmons JE: *Psychiatric examination of children,* ed 4, Philadelphia, 1987, Lea & Febiger.

76 Concepts of Psychosomatic Illness

Stanford B. Friedman

The notion that psychological and emotional factors influence a variety of disease states can be traced to antiquity. Only recently, however, has there been systematic observation and scientific study of such relationships. From his clinical observations of patients in the 1940s, Alexander[1] proposed that specific psychological conflicts could be identified in individuals suffering from seven disease entities: peptic ulcer, ulcerative colitis, regional enteritis, hyperthyroidism, rheumatoid arthritis, essential hypertension, and bronchial asthma. At about the same time, Dunbar[2] proposed specific personality types, rather than the nature of the existing conflicts, as being of etiological importance. Common to both theoretical formulations was a belief that *specific* psychological phenomena caused or predisposed to *specific* diseases, and thus evolved the "theory of specificity." This approach to the conceptualization of "psychosomatic medicine" has led to the common belief that some diseases are influenced significantly by psychological factors and others are "purely" physical. This "either-or" concept represents a simplistic attempt to relate disease, as it exists in a particular individual, to a single cause.

In contrast, Engel emphasized a "multifactorial" concept of etiology and, more recently, developed the "biopsychosocial model" of disease.[3,4] This model acknowledges that most diseases are the result of the complex interaction of multiple factors—biological, psychosocial, and cultural—converging at a particular point in the life of an individual.

INFLUENCE OF PSYCHOSOCIAL FACTORS

The degree to which any one etiological factor contributes to the development of disease depends on a number of considerations. First, some diseases appear to be influenced more than others by psychosocial factors. The clinical source of ulcerative colitis, for example, may be related directly to the psychological status of the patient. On the other hand, little or no evidence exists that brain tumors in children are affected by such factors. However, the lack of such a relationship *may* be a result of insufficient study of this possibility. Second, just as the virulence and dose of a microorganism affect the development and severity of an infectious disease, so may the nature and intensity of a psychosocial stimulus influence its impact on a disease. Third, individual differences attributable to genetic factors or previous experiences modify the effect of etiological factors on the health status of the individual. Fourth, some temporal and developmental factors may alter the role of psychosocial stimuli in disease. Thus an individual's vulnerability to a particular disease may change with progression from infancy to late adulthood, with biological and psychological factors interacting to account for such change.

That psychosocial factors may exert influence on certain disease processes has been observed clinically and, as reviewed by Plaut and Friedman,[5] has been supported by experimental findings in infectious diseases that traditionally are not considered "psychosomatic" in nature. Therefore no *specific* number of diseases can be identified as psychosomatic, but rather a spectrum of illnesses exists with varying degrees of susceptibility to psychosocial stimuli. Diseases such as asthma and peptic ulcer, for example, traditionally have been viewed as influenced by psychological factors, but in managing these diseases the clinician should not necessarily assign etiological importance to psychological factors in every patient who has these illnesses. Extreme biological vulnerability in a given patient may result in disease without psychological distress or conflict beyond that normally experienced in everyday life. On the other hand, the presence or absence of psychosocial factors may, in a given individual, determine whether predisposition toward a disease will later become a clinical problem. Further, psychosocial factors may influence the course of the disease, as well as the response to drugs or other forms of therapy.

ROLE OF THE PEDIATRICIAN

In the evaluation of symptoms and disease, the pediatrician always should consider psychosocial factors of *possible* etiological importance.[6] In many instances, however, the benign and infrequent nature of the illness, such as occasional upper respiratory infection, does not warrant an extensive psychosocial assessment of the patient and family. In other instances, the pediatrician would be amiss not to evaluate thoroughly the psychological status of the patient; examples include severe headaches, frequent infections, hypertension, chronic gastrointestinal symptoms, and the onset of many serious childhood diseases.

In the medical evaluation, the physician should be aware of those diseases that frequently appear to be influenced by psychosocial factors (e.g., asthma, ulcerative colitis). In addition, he or she should explore interactions between disease and environmental factors that are characteristic of some diseases, such as exacerbation of asthmatic symptoms secondary to persistent family dysfunction and conflict.

The psychological environment of the child or adolescent also should be addressed. This evaluation may be divided into the three major spheres of a child's life—namely, relationship to *peers,* functioning with the *family,* and successes and failures at *school,* work, or both. Basically, the psychological world of the child should be defined, including parental expectations and environmental pressures, as well as sources of psychological and social support. For example, within the context of the child's social and community environments, is the child feeling excessive pressure to conform? Are expectations unreasonable? Are these expectations related more to parental needs than to those of the child? The answers to these questions should be accompanied by evaluation of the child's past and current coping abilities, psychological strengths, and the existence or lack of social support systems.

The child's psychosocial and cognitive development should be assessed, with a focus on identifying biological or experiential factors that might predispose him or her to certain diseases or might make psychological adaptations more difficult. In terms of temperament, was this child's early behavior that of the "difficult child?" Is there a history of hyperactivity or learning problems in the family? Has the patient been abused or rejected by his or her parents? These merely are examples of biological and psychological factors that may interact with current experiences to predispose to disease states.

In the overall psychosocial evaluation of a child or adolescent, the developmental status is critical in interpreting the child's "psychological world" (see Chapter 51, Theories and Concepts of Development As They Relate to Pediatric Practice). Are the child's behaviors age appropriate? Of at least equal importance, are the expectations of parents (and grandparents) age appropriate for the child? The pediatrician should have an ongoing clinical impression of the "match" between the patient's chronological age and developmental status.

In conclusion, the concept of a defined number of "psychosomatic diseases" is overly limited. Rather, a spectrum of susceptibility to psychosocial factors exists that is related to the disease entity, the biological and psychological makeup of the patient, the psychological and social environment, and the developmental status of the child or adolescent. The *clinical importance* of these considerations must be individualized by the provider of primary health care, and the clinical management, including the advisability of mental health consultation, must be planned accordingly.

REFERENCES

1. Alexander F: *Psychosomatic medicine,* New York, 1950, WW Norton.
2. Dunbar HF: *Psychosomatic diagnosis,* New York, 1943, Hoeber (Harper & Row).
3. Engel GL: Selection of clinical material in psychosomatic medicine, *Psychosom Med* 16:368, 1954.
4. Engel GL: The need for a new medical model: a challenge for biomedicine, *Science* 196:129, 1977.
5. Plaut SM, Friedman SB: Psychological factors in infectious disease. In Ader R, editor: *Psychoneuroimmunology,* New York, 1981, Academic Press.
6. Prazar G: Psychosomatic disorders and conversion reactions. In Friedman SB, Fisher M, Schonberg SK, editors: *Comprehensive adolescent health care, ed 3,* St Louis, 1997, Mosby.

77 Prediction of Adult Behavior from Childhood

David S. Pellegrini

That adult psychopathology has its roots in childhood adjustment difficulties is widely assumed. By extension, earlier intervention in such difficulties generally is assumed to be better, since psychopathology is likely to crystallize over time, making subsequent remediation more difficult. Epidemiological studies suggest that a large proportion of children show some behavioral or emotional deviance at some stage of their development. However, according to Rutter and colleagues,[10] such problems prove to be transitory in the majority of cases. Moreover, a number of well-intentioned early intervention programs have yielded adverse or mixed results.

Clearly, therapeutic efforts are not without risk. Unnecessary treatment might best be avoided if children otherwise would grow out of their difficulties through the natural process of development. Therefore identifying those children prone to suffer serious lifetime maladjustment would be enormously advantageous.

Unfortunately, although childhood behavior and early life circumstances show some tendency to predict adult behavior, the correlations generally are too modest to allow useful prediction with regard to individuals.[8] For example, in a large-scale study published in 1973, West and Farrington[11] obtained a false positive identification rate greater than 50% when predicting deliquency on the basis of early family and child characteristics. Nevertheless, available findings offer some important and useful clues to guide the primary care physician in referring appropriate children for treatment.

Temperamental differences among infants and very young children frequently are noted by parents and hence are likely to be of interest to their pediatricians. Such temperamental qualities as irritability, low regularity, and low malleability are widely assumed to identify children who are likely to remain "difficult" over their life spans. However, most dimensions of temperament have proven to be elusive, and the characteristics ascribed to temperament generally appear to be unstable over time. Recently, however, Kagan and Snidman[4] have established "inhibition" as a relatively stable, potentially important temperamental contributor to social behavior. Inhibited children tend to be markedly quiet, fearful, and restrained in their approach to unfamiliar and risk-taking situations. (The physiological profile of such children is characterized by a low heart rate and a relatively low level of circulating cortisol.) Recent research suggests that temperamental inhibition may be an early marker of emotional dysregulation, of which anxiety disorder is one eventual consequence later in life.[6] Temperamental disinhibition, on the other hand, appears to be a possible risk factor in the subsequent development of conduct disorder and various forms of antisocial behavior, especially in children living under adverse social circumstances.[3]

Various symptoms of neurotic or emotional disorder also are readily observed and very common in childhood. These include nail-biting, thumb-sucking, bed-wetting, eating and sleeping difficulties, and fears of animals, situations, and places. Such symptoms appear to be of little long-term significance when they are mildly intense and when they occur in isolation, rather than as part of a general pattern of multiple symptomatology. Isolated symptoms of this kind might best be thought of as exaggerations of normal developmental trends rather than as signs of childhood disorder or as precursors of adult disorder. On the other hand, the timing of such symptoms is interesting. Manifestations of emotional distress appear to be less benign when they are age inappropriate than when they occur at ages when the conditions are more common. For example, school refusal or phobia in an 11-year-old typically has a poorer long-term prognosis than the same clinical condition in a child just starting school.

General emotional disorder, in contrast to isolated symptomatology, does appear to have some long-term risk. Rutter and his colleagues[10] observed that children who manifested emotional disorder at age 10 years were twice as likely as the general population to show such disorder at age 14. However, even those children who show severe and persistent disorders of this kind appear to have a relatively good adult prognosis, with or without treatment. Moreover, when emotional disorders do persist into adulthood, they tend to remain true to type, rather than evolving into more troubling conditions such as adult sociopathy or psychosis. Finally, emotionally troubled children seem to respond better to treatment than any other maladjusted group. Evidence suggests that appropriate and timely intervention can shorten the course of emotional disorders.

Childhood depression is one such condition for which the empirical picture is considerably less clear. Unlike most other symptoms of emotional maladjustment, depressive indicators such as sad mood, apathy, and self-deprecation become increasingly prevalent with age, especially among girls. Recent research suggests that isolated symptoms of depression are much more common among prepubertal children than was once thought.[9] Such symptoms have been recognized increasingly as common corollaries or consequences of physical illness and injury in childhood.

Less consensus is evident regarding the prevalence of depression as a syndrome in childhood, although it probably is much less common before than after puberty. Most mood disturbances appear to be so short-lived before puberty that some have argued against clinical intervention in all but the most severe cases. However, adequate long-term data particularly are sparse in this area. Although depressive illness arising in adolescence has been shown to have a relatively poor long-term prognosis, possible links between untreated depressive symptomatology in childhood and chronic mood problems or other difficulties in adulthood have not been explored adequately.

In contrast to most indicators of neurosis or emotional disorder, certain indicators of social and behavioral maladjustment in childhood have demonstrated considerable predictive power with regard to adult psychopathology. However, few such predictors exhibit clear continuity with or a direct developmental path to specific and unique outcomes. Rather, they tend to predict a range of adverse outcomes. Moreover, predictive stability of this kind does not emerge until the early school years.

One such indicator pertains to the quality of peer relations. Recent research suggests that peers play a number of important roles in child development. For example, as agents of socialization, peers help to shape sexual and aggressive behavior. They also are a major source of emotional support, while providing instruction in a variety of social, cognitive, and motor skills. It should not be surprising, then, that poor peer relations in early childhood have been linked with later emotional difficulties, deliquency, substance abuse, suicide, and psychosis. In one classic study, Cowen and co-workers[2] attempted to uncover the early signs of persistent psychiatric disturbance. Of 537 schoolchildren, 33% (180) were identified as being at risk on the basis of ineffective school performance and behavior. By the time of follow-up 11 years later, 19% of this group, compared with only 5% of nondesignated children, had received some form of psychiatric care, as indexed by appearance on a cumulative county register. Negative peer evaluations in third grade exceeded a variety of other adjustment indicators (including teacher and school nurse judgments) in predicting later mental health difficulties.

Active rejection by peers seems to be more critical in the prediction and the development of later psychopathology than is social isolation resulting from shyness and social withdrawal. Indeed, shyness alone appears not to be as closely linked to adult disorders, such as schizophrenia, as was once thought. In a long-term epidemiological study undertaken in the Woodlawn area of Chicago, Kellam and associates[5] found that shyness in first grade actually was correlated with reduced rates of delinquency and substance abuse in adolescent boys and with reduced intake of hard liquor in adolescent girls. However, shyness was related to higher levels of anxiety in adolescent boys (see Chapter 86, Peer Relationship Problems).

Early antisocial behavior and aggressiveness appear to be the sturdiest predictors of adult maladjustment. For example, in an exceptionally thorough and well-planned study, Robins[7] followed up some 500 individuals who had attended child psychiatry clinics 30 years earlier. Whereas most neurotic children went on to lead psychiatrically normal lives, children who engaged in early and repeated delinquent or aggressive acts grew up to be, with disturbing regularity, adult sociopaths. Looking backward, Robins noted that 95% of the adult sociopaths had been referred initially for antisocial and aggressive behavior.

In the Woodlawn study,[5] aggressiveness in first-grade boys clearly was linked to heavy drug, alcohol, and cigarette use in adolescence, as well as to delinquency. Although such associations were not apparent for girls, aggressiveness in conjuction with social isolation was associated with the poorest outcome for both sexes. Aggressive behavior also has emerged as a primary prognostic component of hyperactivity.

Troublesome behavior patterns appear most likely to persist into adulthood when other social, psychological, and cognitive handicaps also are present. According to Rutter and associates,[10] parental antisocial behavior or alcoholism, chronic marital discord, and poor academic achievement tend to potentiate emerging behavioral difficulties. Pervasive behavioral problems also tend to persist more than situation-specific problems. For example, those few youngsters who demonstrate hyperactivity, poor impulse control, and attentional problems in multiple settings (e.g., school, home, and the community at large) are more likely to show a variety of difficulties later in life (e.g., antisocial behavior, poor academic achievement, and depression) than are youngsters who are hyperactive in only one such setting (the majority of such cases). Similarly, children who engage in a variety of delinquent acts in multiple settings are at greater risk for adult criminality than are those who engage in isolated delinquent acts (see Chapter 102, Juvenile Delinquency).

Clearly, much more work needs to be done to determine the early precursors of, turning points in, and contextual (family, peer, and community) influences on psychopathology. In the interim we are left only with general guidelines regarding the appropriate timing of clinical intervention.[1] Available findings to date highlight the particular importance of early treatment for pervasive conduct and relational problems, especially because intervention efforts with antisocial adolescents and adults so far have proved to be singularly unsuccessful.

Early intervention also seems warranted whenever symptoms appear likely to interfere with the acquisition of social and academic skills, which could, in turn, lead to social rejection and school or work failure. Beyond that, intervention may be justified on the grounds of relieving or shortening the immediate distress caused by the symptoms themselves, even when they may bear little or no functional relationship to later difficulties.

REFERENCES

1. Coie JD et al: The science of prevention: a conceptual framework and some directions for a national research program, *Am Psychol* 48:1013, 1993.
2. Cowen EL et al: Long-term follow-up of early detected vulnerable children, *J Consult Clin Psychol* 41:438, 1973.
3. Earls F: Oppositional-defiant and conduct disorders. In Rutter M, Taylor E, Hersov L, editors: *Child and adolescent psychiatry: modern approaches,* ed 3, London, 1994, Blackwell.
4. Kagan J, Snidman N: Temperamental factors in human development, *Am Psychol* 46:856, 1991.
5. Kellam SG et al: Paths leading to teenage psychiatric symptoms and substance use: developmental epidemiological studies in Woodlawn. In Guze SB, Earls FJ, Barrett JE, editors: *Childhood psychopathology and development,* New York, 1983, Raven Press.
6. Klein RG: Anxiety disorders. In Rutter M, Taylor E, Hersov L, editors: *Child and adolescent psychiatry: modern approaches,* ed 3, London, 1994, Blackwell.

7. Robins L: Sturdy childhood predictors of adult antisocial behavior: replications from longitudinal studies, *Psychol Med* 8:611, 1978.
8. Rutter M: Pathways from childhood to adult life, *J Child Psychol Psychiatry* 30:23, 1989.
9. Rutter M, Izard CE, Read PB, editors: *Depression in young people: developmental and clinical perspectives,* New York, 1986, Guilford Press.
10. Rutter M et al: Isle of Wight studies, 1964-1974, *Psychol Med* 6:313, 1976.
11. West DJ, Farrington DG: *Who becomes delinquent?* London, 1973, Heinemann.

78 Colic

David I. Bromberg

Certain problems in pediatrics demand a multifactorial approach to etiology to be well understood. The clinician must consider biological, developmental, psychosocial, and environmental causes to appreciate fully their contributions to the clinical problem. Only in understanding the interaction of these factors can the physician evaluate the problem accurately and offer a meaningful interpretation and effective treatment plan to the patient and family. Infantile colic is such a problem.

Colic is a poorly defined syndrome of paroxysmal infant crying. The clinical picture as described by Illingworth[3] had the infant "beginning with flushing of the face, a frown, drawing up of the legs, followed in a few seconds by high pitched screaming, suddenly ending in a few minutes, and followed in a few minutes by another paroxysm. The attacks recur for up to 2 or 3 hours. . ."

These symptoms, in affected babies, begin at several days to weeks of life, increase through the fourth to sixth weeks, and often are gone by 3 to 4 months of age. The research definition used by Wessel et al. in 1954[5] defines colic as occurring in an infant who in the first 3 months cries for greater than 3 hours in a day, 3 or more days a week. Other terms for this entity include "3-month colic," "evening colic," and "paroxysmal fussing." Studies suggest that colic occurs in an estimated 10% to 30% of infants and equally in males and females.

Two major issues emerge in understanding the definition and evaluation of colic. First, crying is a behavior in infants that spans a spectrum from normalcy to pathology both quantitatively and qualitatively. When Brazelton[1] had mothers keep a detailed diary of infant behaviors, he found that crying increased over the first 6 weeks of life, peaking at a median of 2¾ hours per day. Crying then gradually decreased over the remainder of the study through 3 months of age. The descriptions of crying infants also varied from those of a hungry baby, through the crying of a bored, fussy baby, to the above description of the colicky baby. The demarcation between normal and abnormal amounts of crying and normal cries and those of pain is not clear.

Second, Carey[2] raises the issue of primary versus secondary excessive crying. Crying is a behavioral final pathway for a multitude of reasons. The infant who has a urinary tract infection who cries because of bladder spasm, or the child who is fussy because of a subdural bleed, would have crying secondary to these conditions. The otherwise healthy infant who exhibits paroxysmal crying over a protracted period of time would be the colicky infant whose excessive crying is primary. Again the demarcation between these groups is not totally clear. To many researchers and clinicians, the healthy colicky infant appears to be in pain that often is thought to be gastrointestinal, albeit of undetermined origin.

Regardless of the cause, the effect on families of having a paroxysmally crying infant is dramatic. Parents often describe feelings of guilt and inadequacy over their inability to soothe their babies. Families excited over the prospect of having a newborn at home begin to respond very dysfunctionally. One mother notes,

> When I was pregnant, I had these romantic visions. . . . The reality was quite different. I spent day after day walking this screaming baby from room to room, crying right along with her. I snapped at my husband so much that I'm amazed we're still together.

Another mother remembers,

> I used to walk up and down the hall with this screaming baby. I'd say 'Stop it Emma,' and squeeze her leg real hard. Later I'd look at her, so innocent, and I'd cry that I could have done that. How could I want to hurt her when I love her so much?[4]

ETIOLOGY

Infant Factors

Any condition causing pain in the infant may result in excessive crying. Consideration should be given to the possibility of incarcerated inguinal hernia, chronic subdural bleeds, corneal abrasion, renal disease or infection, or acute otitis media. Factors related to increased infant irritability, such as prenatal drug exposure, also must be considered.

Infant temperament has been shown to have a relationship to the development of symptoms of colic. Infants who have the temperamental cluster characterized as difficult and infants who have a low sensory threshold both are at greater risk for being colicky. These are infants who respond to environmental stimuli of a low level. At times, when they already may be "bored" or fussy, for example, during the evening, minor additional stimuli may "set them off."

The question remains open whether there is any gastrointestinal predisposition to the development of colic. Several Swedish studies have demonstrated statistical differences in the hormone levels in a colic-diagnosed group compared with a control group. These differences are demonstrable on cord blood. Similarly, differences in the absorption of lactalbumin can be shown between colic and noncolic groups. The significance of these findings is unknown. Infants who have colic appear to many observers to be experiencing abdominal pain.

The final category of infant factors relates to feeding techniques and diet. No clear pattern of feeding technique, or alteration in technique, has been clearly demonstrated to relate to colic. There is an extensive literature relating cow milk protein, both in formula and in the maternal diet for breastfeeding infants, to the course of colic. Much of this literature, however, is conflicting and does not measure the persistence of improvement when a formula change has been instituted.

Parents

Parental ability to cope with an inconsolable infant, as well as their ability to read and respond to infant cues, alters the course of colic. Parents develop "tunnel vision" in regard to their infant's crying. They feel unable to offer any comfort to their child and talk of the frustration of being out of control. This is not to say that parental anxiety or conflict is the cause of the problem; these feelings usually develop secondarily to the infant's crying pattern. They do, however, interfere with the parents interacting effectively with the child. Additional family stressors also may exacerbate the situation. These might include such issues as poor maternal support, marital difficulties, criticism from the extended family, and maternal depression.

EVALUATION

A complete pediatric history and physical examination must precede any interventions for colic. The history should be obtained empathically and optimistically. Included should be a history of any physical complaints, an evaluation of the impact of the colic on the family, a detailed psychosocial history, and a complete feeding and sleeping history. As part of the assessment the physician should evaluate the observed interaction between the mother and infant. Through the course of the evaluation the physician should attempt to identify temperamental factors that may have put this infant at greater risk for colic. This information is helpful in educating the parents about the dynamics of the problem. In most cases of colic the physical examination will be normal; however, it is essential that this be done thoroughly and carefully. Parents enter this session angry and frightened. They are sure that there is something seriously wrong with their child. Only with the reassurance of a careful normal examination can they be satisfied that the infant is healthy. Laboratory studies generally are not indicated.

MANAGEMENT

Management should be aimed at parental education, family support, and counseling about interventions for handling a crying infant. Parents come in mystified by their baby's crying. Explaining the multifactorial nature of colic, with specific reference to those features most applicable to this family, can be very helpful. Allowing parents to see the infant's contribution to the symptoms, which may include an explanation of normal crying patterns in infants or the temperamental characteristics of their child, can help alleviate their guilt. Knowing that the pediatric office will follow and share this problem with them also is very relieving. Frequent phone and office follow-up are critical. A tone of reassurance and optimism, based on the good prognosis, should be maintained.

As noted previously, parents of colicky babies often see few options in trying to calm their crying infants. Counseling should be directed at problem solving with the parents and alternatives for handling a crying infant. Many of the studies of colic suggest that doing something unique with an infant will at least temporarily calm them. Strategies might include swaddling and holding in different positions, keeping the baby in a front carrier, or using an infant swing. Reviewing with the family the reasons that infants cry may give them a logical approach to handle the crying. A sequence of feeding, changing, holding, and resting can be agreed upon. Empowering parents with these strategies is a first step. Parents also must be reminded, however, that in spite of these efforts the baby may continue crying. Under these circumstances parents must recognize that putting a crying infant down also is permissible and that no physical or psychological harm will result from the crying.

The clinician must always keep in mind the dictum of *doing no harm*. The parents' complaints must be taken seriously. Callous reassurance such as reminding the parents that "all babies cry," or advising them to just sit it out, can be destructive. Pharmacological interventions can be dangerous and should be considered only in very limited circumstances. Similarly, dangerous therapies, including enemas, should be avoided. There is no clear evidence that formula changes are an effective intervention for colic. Multiple formula changes can be discouraging to the family and suggest medical problems that do not exist. Lastly, most infants who have colic are free of symptoms by 3 to 4 months of age.

REFERENCES

1. Brazelton TB: Crying in infancy, *Pediatrics* 29:579, 1962.
2. Carey WB: "Colic": primary excessive crying as an infant-environment interaction, *Pediatr Clin North Am* 31:993, 1984.
3. Illingworth RS: Infantile colic revisited, *Arch Dis Child* 60:981, 1985.
4. Waldman W: *Coping with infant colic: a guide for parents*, Columbus, Ohio, 1982, Ross Laboratories.
5. Wessel MA et al: Paroxysmal fussing in infancy, sometimes called "colic," *Pediatrics* 14:421, 1954.

SUGGESTED READINGS

Barr RG: Normality: a clinically useless concept: the case of infant crying and colic, *J Dev Behav Pediatr* 14:264, 1993.

Pinyerd BJ: Strategies for consoling the infant with colic: fact or fiction? *J Pediatr Nurs* 7:403, 1992.

Taubman B: Clinical trial of the treatment of colic by modification of parent-infant interaction, *Pediatrics* 74:998, 1984.

79 Conduct Disorders

Linda M. Forsythe and Michael Jellinek

All children and adolescents misbehave at one time or another. Epidemiological studies indicate that disruptive, oppositional, and problematical behaviors tend to cluster at certain developmental stages. Many such behavioral problems resolve in the process of development and do not predict future patterns; some of them reemerge in a more mature form at a later stage, and a few more indicate lifelong patterns. For example, infantile temper tantrums, a manifestation of aggression, remain common during the preschool years but decrease to less than 10% of 5-year-olds and to nearly 2% of 15-year-olds.[6] Through the school-age years, most children disobey their parents at one time or another, but few break the major rules of society. Although local police become familiar with nearly one third of adolescents, only a small percentage of these youths will continue to break the law beyond adolescence.[7]

A conduct disorder—defined as a persistent pattern of behavior in which a child or adolescent violates the basic rights of others or age-appropriate rules of society—does not emerge suddenly; it evolves slowly within a context. Children and adolescents do not come into the office with organized complaints that lead easily to the diagnosis of a conduct disorder. They, or their parents, present story fragments of unexplained impairments in social and academic functioning, of altered attachments with vague explanations, and of violent or violating misconduct.

Pediatricians evaluate children daily who have a wide range of behaviors. Their clinical assessment includes attempts to recognize patterns and elicit relevant information. Throughout this process they consider whether instances of misconduct are due primarily to expectable temperamental or developmental variations or whether they are early manifestations of psychopathology. They routinely assess the severity of the behavioral pattern, attempt to predict its trajectory, and offer parents their best prognostic opinions. They search for the meaning and the quality of particular behaviors in an effort to answer such parental questions as "Why is this happening?" and "What have we done wrong?" The process of generating a differential diagnosis and of considering various management options flows naturally from a thorough clinical assessment.

CLINICAL ASSESSMENT

Statistically valid, reliable diagnostic measures of behavioral characteristics are being developed for research purposes but are impractical for the primary care setting. Instead, clinicians rely on clinical judgment and experience when addressing parental concerns about disruptive behavior, asking themselves whether the child is behaving normally for his developmental stage, what the severity of the disruptive behavior is, and why it is happening now.

Is the Child Behaving Normally for His Developmental Stage?

Some behaviors are normal for very young children but are less appropriate at later stages. Preschoolers do not understand distinctions between wanting, grabbing, and "stealing" because of their egocentric view of the world; they own everything they see or desire. The concept of "lying" is equally problematic in the young child, for he or she naturally mixes fantasy and reality in stories.

School-age children may tell lies to avoid doing something or to gain immediate favor. Older children, fearing harsh consequences, momentarily may prefer the risk of a lie to the certainty of punishment. Until a child's cognitive development reaches the abstract stage (usually not until the teen years), their moral reasoning remains organized around avoiding punishment and seeking rewards. Parents who witness their school-age children cheating on board games may worry that their child is obsessed with winning. Sometimes this cheating is an early sign of a child's neediness and insecurity and warrants concern. More often, however, it is an aspect of made-up rules and is a normal variant of play.

Adolescents may feel justified when a lie is used to avoid hurting the feelings of a friend or to maintain their privacy. These differences are key to the clinical assessment and crucial to diagnostic and management considerations. Lying that seems to occur when a child is unable to deal with overwhelming demands may be an early sign of more severe difficulties. Whereas the threats of some adolescents to run away are early signs of a lifelong pattern of truancy, drug use, or prostitution, other threats are merely temporary, clumsy attempts to counteract strongly felt attachments.

Some parents, at the time of a first, even minor, legal infraction, may become paralyzed in their fear that their child will become a menace. Parents may be tempted to compensate for their child's lack of internal controls by imposing severe external controls on all independent and self-assertive behavior. Alternatively, they may threaten to sever all emotional or supportive ties. Efforts to counter the adolescent's developmental path to autonomy are unlikely to succeed. More often, they have the unintended consequence of inhibiting further development of the youngster's appropriate internal controls or of forcing the teenager prematurely to be independent. Minor violations are most likely to become important learning experiences when parents are able to initiate age-appropriate discussions, negotiations, and consequences thoughtfully (see Chapter 97, Counseling Parents of Adolescents).

As with all pediatric care, the clinician must listen carefully to the degree of parental anxiety about such issues as dependency and control. Are both parents in agreement, or is the youngster caught in parental discord? Are other adults in the child's life (e.g., teachers and coaches) equally concerned about the path the youngster is following? Are the parents seen as overly rigid and critical? Is the child having difficulties in other areas of functioning such as with peers, at school, or in after-school activities?

What is the Severity of the Disruptive Behavior?

Severity is a complex judgment that includes separate considerations of (1) the symptomatic behavior, including developmental considerations, intensity, frequency, duration, and context; (2) the impact of the behavior on family functioning, school performance, and peer relations; (3) the cumulative effect of psychosocial risk factors in the child's life, including neglect, abuse, poverty, violence, parental illness and strife, access to guns, and the influence of cultural norms; and (4) an appreciation of the child's or family's preoccupation with the behavior and an assessment of additional psychiatric or neurological illnesses (see the box below).

The assessment of severity is made even more complicated by severity factors themselves often being interrelated. For instance, an 18-month-old child's difficult temperament, although often perceived as a sign of disobedience, is more likely to be partially biologically determined, partially a sign of emerging autonomy, partially affected by the degree of his or her mother's tolerance, goodness of fit, and empathy, and partially determined by such associated deleterious factors as poverty and frequent moving. Each of these factors affects the child-parent relationship directly and at the same time affects each of the other factors. Parental sociopathy and alcoholism may mask serious underlying parental psychopathology such as major depression, posttraumatic stress disorder, or psychosis. Similarly, parental pathology may contribute to parental denial, symptom dismissal, and the rejection of assistance.

As parental stresses increase and supportive resources decrease, children tend to adapt more slowly, function more poorly, and become more aggressive. Parental abuse toward each other and toward their children is known to promote, or may even cause, a child's or adolescent's violent behavior. Abuse incites intense levels of rage in the child, provides violent role models, and may directly cause neurological damage to impulse control. The histories of the most behaviorally disturbed children and violent adolescents typically reveal physical or sexual abuse—often by adults, including parents.

A direct interview with the child should be used to ascertain the degree of the youth's burden of suffering,[3] his or her mood state, especially depression, and any related, comorbid (coexisting) psychiatric, neurological, or cognitive vulnerabilities. For example, when facing a substance-abusing adolescent, pediatricians should consider whether a given street drug is being used as a self-medication for a psychosis, depression, an attentional deficit, or an anxiety disorder. Depressed children may exhibit sad facies or a bored and irritable demeanor. Beneath the "coolest" or most obnoxious facades may lie severely psychotic, depressed, or aggressive states.

Subtle signs of central nervous system dysfunction may give etiological clues to behavioral dyscontrol and limited affect tolerance. Perinatal difficulties, headaches, loss of consciousness, dizziness, accidents, seizures, and injuries may be revealed in the process of a careful neurological history. Neurological examinations typically show nonspecific abnormalities. EEGs may reveal equivocal electrical findings in limbic areas.

Truancy and poor school performance may indicate such cognitive difficulties as lower than normal intelligence, poor

FACTORS THAT INFLUENCE SEVERITY OF MISCONDUCT

Symptoms

- Age
- Temperament
- Developmental stage
  - Cognitive
  - Affective
  - Moral
  - Language
  - Social
- Behavior
  - Frequency
  - Intensity
  - Duration
  - Context

Impact on functioning

- Family
- School
- Peer relations
- Activities
  - Sports
  - Hobbies
  - Clubs

Psychosocial risk factors (partial list)

- Poverty
- Parental mental illness
  - Substance abuse
  - Psychosis
- Family violence
- Access to weapons
- Frequent moving
- Physical or sexual abuse
- Neglect

Burden of suffering

- Preoccupation with the behavior
- Mood disorder (especially depression)
- Other psychiatric disorders
  - Attention deficit/hyperactivity disorder
  - Substance abuse
  - Posttraumatic stress
- Neurological disorder
  - Learning disability
  - Seizures
  - Head trauma

judgment, or undeveloped abstract reasoning. Specific language disabilities may involve particular difficulties with verbal expression that lead to increased physical expression of mood states.

Why is the Disruptive Behavior Happening Now?

Specific information about the context in which the behavior surfaces may provide insights into its cause and development. Traditionally, socioeconomic pressures and peer influences were emphasized as causal factors of delinquency. More recent evidence suggests that individual characteristics, such as violent behavior before the joining of a gang, may be the most powerful predictor.[2]

An exploration of the child's character structure and internal motivations is critical, as is an understanding of the nature and context of the rules the child tends to break. For instance, are the broken rules those of his or her parents, of teachers, or of society as a whole? How violent is the behavior? Does it surface more when the child is alone or in a group? Does the child in question take on a leadership role or become a passive follower?

Inevitably, both the parents and pediatrician will wonder if the given severity and quality of the behavior are manifestations of a deeper flaw in the child's personality or character. The expression of anger and feelings of helplessness are major problems for youths who are verbally and physically aggressive with other children and with adults. Some of the most violent and aggressive youths have histories of severe neglect or serious emotional, physical, or sexual abuse. "Identification with the aggressor" may provide a temporary feeling of control and superiority in an otherwise distraught, empty, or wounded teenager.

The terms "character" and "personality" attempt to define who a person is and to predict an individual's reaction to given circumstances. The concept encompasses much of what makes our lives meaningful. It integrates genetics, temperament, child rearing, and critical life events with cognitive, affective, moral, language, and social development. As with all other behavior, most isolated or intermittent instances of misconduct (e.g., cheating, stealing, lying, or threats to run away from parents) have their roots in the child's or adolescent's developing personality style. When this style is rigid and dysfunctional, a disorder of character or personality should be considered. A character disorder is a serious, often lifelong, distortion of an individual's approach to inner feelings and the feelings of others. Because characterological defenses usually are unyielding and reality tends to have little impact, dealings are likely to be taxing and irritating. Either as a result of character pathology of their own or in response to their child, parents may be anxious, demanding, and hostile.

Characterological behavioral disorders involve rigid and relentless patterns of cheating, stealing, lying, bullying, and running away. A character-disordered adolescent may engage in repetitive stealing and bullying as an unconscious solution to feeling unworthy (of friends, favors, kindness, or gifts), as well as to satisfying the need for immediate relief. Because the gain is superficial, the relief temporary, and the satisfaction limited, the behavioral pattern continues. As long as the reasons for the disturbance of behavior remain unconscious, these behavioral solutions for dealing with extremely painful feelings are likely to continue. Once the child or adolescent is able to face the anxiety, anger, and sadness connected to relationships or expectations, the reliance on behavioral solutions may diminish and he or she may be more free psychologically to love and to work.

While most children outgrow developmental immaturities naturally, and others do so with the aid of psychotherapeutic interventions, a small percentage persist with immature patterns as a defining aspect of their adult interactions and are diagnosed with adult personality disorders. At the extreme, pediatricians may be asked to assess adolescents who have long-standing criminal records who have committed such serious acts of violence as assault, arson, and rape. These severely disturbed youngsters should raise concerns about character structure, severe psychopathology, neurological injury, and histories of extreme deprivation or abuse.

DIAGNOSIS

The American Psychiatric Association's *Diagnostic and Statistic Manual of Mental Disorders* (DSM-IV) lists specific criteria for each diagnostic category. Rather than being fully based on new research findings, however, the DSM-IV has resolved some diagnostic debates by committee consensus. For example, the manual refers to age 18 as the age at which adolescents complete child development. By convention, then, such adult character-disordered terms as "antisocial personality" or "sociopathic character disorder" do not apply to

Table 79-1 Comparative Factors in Key Disruptive Behavioral Disorders

Age	Oppositional defiant disorder under 18 years	Conduct disorder under 18 years	Antisocial disorder 18 years and over
Whose rules broken?	Parents' and teachers' rules only	Society rules/laws violating the basic rights of others and/or age-appropriate norms	Society rules/laws violating the basic rights of others
Key diagnostic features	Angry, resentful, spiteful, and/or vindictive	Bullies, threatens, harms, and/or intimidates with or without breaking any one of a number of such age-appropriate societal rules as stealing, breaking and entering, arson, and assault	Law-breaking

Note: "Juvenile delinquency" is not a medical term; it is a legal term that requires adjudication in court.

persons under age 18. Minors who have behavioral disorders are diagnosed as having attention deficit/hyperactivity disorder, oppositional defiant disorder, or conduct disorder. The terms "delinquent," "status offender," and "criminal" are legal terms (Table 79-1).

According to the DSM-IV (see the box below), conduct disorder is a disturbance of behavior lasting at least 6 months during which the basic rights of others or the major age-appropriate norms and rules of society are violated. To meet diagnostic criteria, a child or adolescent needs to demonstrate 3 of the 14 behaviors. The behavioral symptoms or individual acts of misconduct that make up the diagnosis have relatively low base rates and relatively high predictive value.[1] The American Academy of Pediatrics is modifying the DSM-IV psychiatric criteria to make them more applicable to primary care office settings.

DSM-IV DIAGNOSTIC CRITERIA FOR CONDUCT DISORDER

A. A repetitive and persistent pattern of behavior in which the basic rights of others or major age-appropriate societal norms or rules are violated, as manifested by the presence of three (or more) of the following criteria in the past 12 months, with at least one criterion present in the past 6 months:

Aggression to people and animals

1. Often bullies, threatens, or intimidates others
2. Often initiates physical fights with others
3. Has used a weapon that can cause serious physical harm to others (e.g., bat, brick, broken bottle, knife, gun)
4. Has been physically cruel to people
5. Has been physically cruel to animals
6. Has stolen while confronting a victim (e.g., mugging, purse snatching, extorting, armed robbery)
7. Has forced someone into sexual activity

Destruction of property

8. Has deliberately engaged in fire-setting with the intention of causing serious damage
9. Has deliberately destroyed others' property (other than by fire-setting)

Deceitfulness or theft

10. Has broken into someone else's house, building, or car
11. Often lies to obtain goods or favors or to avoid obligations (i.e., "cons" others)
12. Has stolen items of nontrivial value without confronting a victim (i.e., shoplifting, but without breaking and entering, or forgery)

Serious violations of rules

13. Often stays out at night despite parental prohibitions, beginning before age 13 years
14. Has run away from home overnight at least twice while living in parental or parental-surrogate home (or once without returning for a lengthy period)
15. Often is truant from school, beginning before age 13 years

B. The disturbance in behavior causes clinically significant impairment in social, academic, or occupational functioning.

C. If the individual is age 18 years or older, criteria are not met for antisocial personality disorder.

MANAGEMENT

Management of children and adolescents who have conduct disorders is difficult and time consuming; the causes of the illness are complex, and each youngster's situation requires individualized treatment. Treatment often requires the development of new attitudes and behavioral patterns. It is made more complicated by the child's or adolescent's resistant attitude and distrust of adults.

Research shows that the future of conduct-disordered youngsters is likely to be grim if they and their families do not receive early, ongoing, and comprehensive treatment. All management considerations need to include simultaneous efforts to treat existing disruptive behavioral problems and comorbid disorders while attempting to prevent antisocial behavior that has not yet developed. Because of differences in developmental stages, attempts to prevent or treat disruptive behavior in the early years should focus on altering individual and family functioning, whereas prevention and treatment of later adolescent disruptive states require more attention to alterations in the peer culture, the school system, and larger social contexts.

Mild disturbances of behavior are not likely to cause serious developmental difficulties or dysfunction. As the behavioral disorder increases in severity, more intensive evaluation, treatment planning, and possibly referral is indicated. In the most severe cases, where behavioral disturbances are causing serious developmental difficulties and dysfunction in one or more key areas of the child's life, mental health referral and comprehensive treatment planning are indicated, possibly on an urgent basis (see Chapter 93, Consultation and Referral for Behavioral and Developmental Problems).

Research findings suggest that those adolescents who terminate treatment prematurely show greater impairment at home, at school, and in the community compared with children who complete treatment. Selection factors and severity of impairment before the initiation of psychotherapy are important predictors of both attrition rates and limited response rates among patients who continue in therapy.[4]

Clinical follow-up studies of formerly incarcerated male delinquents have found little psychiatric treatment for identified vulnerabilities, inadequate supports, and the perpetuation of risk factors for violence.[5] Without earlier interventions and longer-term tracking studies, the hope to target treatment and improve the prognoses of subsequent generations is poor.

Ever-increasing numbers of young people engage in delinquency and criminal acts. Together they pose an enormous challenge to the family system, the school system, the justice system, the health care system, and to society as a whole. Currently we can categorize their behavior and suggest the multiple biological, psychological, familial, and social forces that contribute to the rising trend. For an individual child, pediatricians should work with a number of colleagues to design the best available treatment. On a broader level, pediatricians can advocate to implement programs that are known to help prevent adolescent violence and collaborate in this area of high priority for further research.

REFERENCES

1. Frick P et al: DSM-IV field trials for the disruptive behavior disorders: symptom utility estimates, *J Am Acad Child Adolesc Psychiatry* 33:529, 1994.
2. Friedman C, Mann F, Friedman A: A profile of juvenile street gang members, *Adolescence* 40:563, 1975.
3. Green M: *Personal communication,* 1994.
4. Kazdin A, Mazurick J, Siegel T: Treatment outcome among children with externalizing disorder who terminate prematurely versus those who complete psychotherapy, *J Am Acad Child Adolesc Psychiatry* 33:549, 1994.
5. Lewis DO et al: A clinical follow-up of delinquent males: ignored vulnerabilities, unmet needs, and the perpetuation of violence, *J Am Acad Child Adolesc Psychiatry* 33:518, 1994.
6. Shepherd M, Oppenheim B, Mitchell S, editors: *Childhood behaviour and mental health,* London, 1971, University of London Press.
7. Wolfgang ME, Figlio RM, Sellin T: *Delinquency in a birth cohort,* Chicago, 1972, University of Chicago Press.

SUGGESTED READINGS

Lewis DO: Conduct disorder. In Lewis M, editor: *Child and adolescent psychiatry: a comprehensive textbook,* Baltimore, 1991, Williams & Wilkins.

Robins L: *Deviant children grown up: a sociological and psychiatric study of sociopathic personality,* Baltimore, 1966, Williams & Wilkins.

Sanson A et al: Precursors of hyperactivity and aggression, *J Am Acad Child Adolesc Psychiatry* 32:1207, 1992.

80 Cross-Sex Behavior

George A. Rekers and Mark D. Kilgus

Cross-sex behavior may represent either a normal episodical exploration of sex role behaviors ("tomboyishness" in girls or "sissyishness" in boys) or a persistent and compulsively stereotyped pattern indicative of a "gender identity disorder of childhood."[1,3] Although many arbitrary sex role stereotypes for males and females increasingly are being challenged in our culture, and although values regarding fathers sharing child rearing and household duties are changing, a cultural consensus remains concerning certain sex role distinctions that children normally master in early development (e.g., females but not males normally are permitted to appear in public wearing lipstick or wearing a dress).

In 1980, "gender identity disorder of childhood" first became an official diagnosis in the third edition of *Diagnostic and Statistical Manual of Mental Disorders* (DSM-III) for prepubertal children who are persistently and intensely distressed about their gender role or anatomical sex. As of 1994, official criteria[1] for "gender identity disorder" included the following:

Strong and persistent cross-gender identification (not merely a desire for any perceived cultural advantages of being the other sex) manifested by at least four of the following:

1. Repeatedly stated desire to be, or insistence that he or she is, a member of the opposite sex
2. In boys, preference for cross-dressing or simulating female attire; in girls, insistence of wearing only stereotypical masculine clothing
3. Strong and persistent preferences for cross-sex roles in make-believe play or persistent fantasies of being a member of the opposite sex
4. Intense desire to participate in the stereotypical games and activities of the opposite sex
5. Strong preference for playmates of the opposite sex

Among adolescents and adults, the disorder is manifested by symptoms such as "a stated desire to be the opposite sex, frequent 'passing' as the other sex, desire to live or be treated as the other sex, or the conviction that one has the typical feelings and reactions of the other sex."

Another essential criterion is a persistent discomfort with one's sex or a sense of inappropriateness in assuming the gender role of that sex. This is manifested in children by any of the following:

In boys, (1) assertion that his penis or testes are disgusting or will disappear or that it would be better not to have a penis, or (2) aversion toward rough-and-tumble play and rejection of male stereotypical toys, games, and activities; in girls, (1) rejection of urinating in a sitting position, (2) assertion that she does not want to grow breasts or menstruate, or (3) marked aversion toward normative feminine clothing.

Among adolescents and adults, manifested symptoms include the following:

Preoccupation with getting rid of one's primary and secondary sex characteristics (e.g., request for hormones, surgery, or other procedures to physically alter sexual characteristics to simulate the other sex) or belief that one was born as a member of the wrong sex.

"Gender identity disorder" may not be "concurrent with a physical intersex condition." In addition, the disturbance causes clinically significant distress or impairment in social, occupational, or other important areas of functioning.

Cross-sex behavior in boys[9,17] includes dressing in feminine clothing, using cosmetics, avoiding male playmates and rough-and-tumble play, being rather rigidly and exclusively preoccupied with girls' activities,[3,9,13] taking a predominantly female role in play, talking predominantly about female topics, projecting the voice into a high femalelike voice inflection, and displaying effeminate gait and body movements ("swishing hips") or feminine-appearing gestures such as "limp wrist" (flexing the wrist toward the palmar surface of the forearm), "arm flutters" (rapid up and down movements of the forearm or upper arm or both, while the wrist remains relaxed), or "palming" (touching the palm or palms to the back, front, or sides of the head above the ear level).[12] Boys outnumber girls more than five to one in numbers of diagnosed cases of gender identity disorder.

For girls, cross-sex behavior[3,9] may include chronic rejection of feminine clothing, cosmetics, and jewelry, regular avoidance of female playmates, a stated desire to be "one of the boys," frequent projection of the voice into a low male-like voice inflection, predominant talk about male activities, and habitual attempts to stand, sit, or walk in a hypermasculine manner (e.g., sitting with legs crossed with the ankle of one leg resting on the other knee).

The gender identity disorder is a rare condition; its onset occurs before puberty, and cross-sex behavior patterns often begin before 4 years of age. In later grade school years, overt cross-sex behavior may lessen in public, even though a gender identity disorder is present. Both retrospective and prospective data[5,9,18] indicate an unusually high incidence of depression and suicide attempts in the adult years for boys who are untreated and that 46% to 64% of boys whose gender identity disorders are untreated develop homosexual or bisexual orientation during their adolescence. A small minority of girls who have a gender identity disorder retain a masculine identification, with some also developing a homosexual orientation. These reports further indicate that 5% to 12% of untreated males develop adulthood *transsexualism* accompanied by severe depression and suicide attempts, whereas approximately 1% to 5% develop heterosexual *transvestism.* The remaining 6% to 23% have a heterosexual orientation in adulthood.

The formation of gender identity is related to the child's appropriate identification with his or her sexual anatomy and its reproductive function.[7,9,17] Normal child-rearing experiences contribute to identification with the parent figure and peers of the same sex and to development of complementary role behaviors toward members of the opposite sex. Some reports suggest that excessive and extremely prolonged physical and emotional closeness between mother and infant, coupled with physical or psychological absence of the father during early childhood years, contribute to gender identity disorders in boys.[8,9] Similarly, some young girls whose mothers are "unavailable" may be at risk for a compensatory identification with the father, contributing to a male gender identity. However, children reared in a single-parent home are not necessarily at risk for a gender identity disorder, especially when the child is afforded the opportunity to develop positive and enduring attachments with adults of both sexes to compensate for the missing parent.

In only extremely rare cases are gender identity disorders associated with any detectable abnormalities in genetic constitution, gonads, external sex organ anatomy, internal accessory genital structures, sex endocrinology, or maternal health during pregnancy.[4,9,10] Except for those individuals who have anomalies of sexual differentiation, such as ambiguous genitalia resulting from congenital adrenal hyperplasia or 5-alpha reductase deficiency,[16] little support exists for brain androgenization ("testosterone imprinting") or other biological phenomena as major factors in establishing gender identity or sexual orientation.[4] Researchers have *not* discovered differences in sex steroids or gonadotropin secretion between transsexual and heterosexual females[14] or males.[6] A few reports exist of transsexuals who have an abnormal karyotype, for example, a fertile male having 47 XYY chromosomes.[15] Nonetheless, the vast majority of those who have gender identity disorder have normal chromosome numbers, external genitals, and hormone levels.

DIAGNOSTIC CONSIDERATIONS AND ISSUES

Clinicians have found it useful to assess a child who exhibits cross-sex behavior across the seven major psychosexual dimensions as outlined in Table 80-1, because a complete diagnosis must consider all these levels of assessment.[9] The evaluation of cross-sex behavior should involve notation of frequency and setting, as well as the social labeling attached to the behavior pattern.[8] The developmental context of the behavior and the child's overall emotional and psychosocial functioning also should be considered. An inquiry should be made regarding the cultural context of the sterotypic behavior, the presence or absence of a compulsive cross-sex behavior pattern, and the significance of the behavior to the child or adolescent. The cluster of behaviors should be considered because it is the ratio of masculine to feminine behavior rather than the exact number of cross-sex behaviors that is diagnostically significant.[8,13] Parents can be asked specific questions:

1. How do you categorize masculine and feminine behaviors?
2. Does your child identify with and model after the parent and peers of the same sex?
3. In what ways does your child relate to boys and girls differently?
4. To what degree does your child identify with his or her sexual anatomy and understand its future reproductive function?
5. What is the history and frequency of the following behaviors in your child: cross-dressing, masculine and feminine gestures, play with cosmetics, avoidance of play with peers of the same sex, play with girls' toys and activities, play with boys' toys and activities, feminine and masculine voice inflection, desire to be called by a name of the opposite sex, "deviant" sexual behaviors, and masturbation in association with cross-dressing articles?
6. Does your child insist on being or pretend to be a member of the other sex?
7. Has your child ever asked for a *sex change,* and if so, how often?

The parents can be asked to record the frequency of several key masculine and feminine behaviors daily for 1 or 2 weeks.[3,8,13] Parental inquiries with the school teacher on how the child relates to boy and girl classmates may be recommended.

In interviewing the child, the pediatrician simply can ask the boy or girl to draw a person or a picture of himself or herself and talk about the drawing. In some cases, this is a quick diagnostic screening test that may provide clues to the

Table 80-1 Dimensions for Psychosexual Assessment

Level of assessment	Dimension	Major categories
Sexual status	Physical sex	Male, female, or intersexed; Tanner's stages for prepubertal, pubertal, or postpubertal development
	Social assignment	Male, female, or intersexed; child, adolescent, or adult (boy, girl, man)
Intrapersonal behavior	Gender identity	Normal, undifferentiated, cross-gender, or conflicted
	Sexual role identity	Heterosexual, bisexual, homosexual, transsexual, transvestite, "queen," "fag," "drag queen," "gay," etc.
	Sexual arousal orientation	Human object choice (male, female, both); animal object choice; magnitude and frequency; fantasies
Interpersonal behavior	Gender role behavior	Masculine, feminine, undifferentiated, androgynous
	Sexual behavior	Human partner (male, female, both); animal partner; inanimate object; intrusive versus receptive roles; group versus individual partner, etc.

From Rekers GA: Psychosexual assessment of gender identity disorders. In Prinz RJ, editor: *Advances in behavioral assessment of children and families,* vol 4, Greenwich Conn, 1988, JAI Press.

child's gender identity. After establishing rapport with the child, interview questions similar to the ones that follow can help clarify progress in gender identity development.

1. What are the first names of your friends and playmates at home and school? (Note and compare the number of female and male friends.)
2. Are you more like your mom or your dad? How?
3. If you could have three wishes, what would you wish for?
4. What are your favorite subjects and activities at school?
5. How often do you feel like a boy? How often do you feel like a girl?
6. When you have free time, what are your favorite things to do?
7. Most kids are called names at some time or other; what names do the other kids call you?

Although children under 8 years of age often are open to disclosing truthful answers to such interview questions, older children and adolescents are more aware of the social significance of their gender role behavior and may have gone "underground" with their true interests at home, and they may conceal their cross-gender preferences from the physician as well.

Pediatricians also should inquire about the possible occurrence of bondage or attempted autoerotic asphyxia, which sometimes, although rarely, is associated with transvestic behavior among adolescents.[2] "Bondage" refers to tying together one's hands or feet with a rope or similar object, or having another individual tie one's hands or feet together, for the purpose of inducing a deviant sexual arousal pattern. "Autoerotic asphyxia" refers to unconsciousness resulting from oxygen deprivation and the systemic accumulation of carbon dioxide, which occurs accidentally as a result of the deviant (and potentially life-threatening) sexual practice in which an adolescent intends to induce temporary anoxia (oxygen deprivation) while masturbating, such as by tightening a plastic bag over one's own head or tightening a rope around one's own neck, in order to heighten sexual sensations during the sexual self-stimulation; adolescents often do not realize that the deviant sexual practice of autoerotic asphyxia can lead to death.

In such cases a more comprehensive evaluation with use of psychological testing by a clinical psychologist is recommended.[3,8]

If appropriate, parallel questions from the parent interview described previously should be asked. Even when the criteria for a gender identity disorder are not all present, a persisting "gender role behavior disturbance" (which can be diagnosed as an example of "gender identity disorder not otherwise specified," as defined earlier) can be detected in a child as young as 4 years of age.[8,9] In cases of chronic cross-sex behavior, evaluation should include medical and pregnancy history, physical examination (including external genitalia), chromosome analysis, and sex chromatin studies, even though these diagnostic procedures result in negative findings in the vast majority of cases.[10]

For adolescents, the pediatrician will find it necessary to assess sexual arousal patterns and frequency of specific sexual behaviors by interviewing the adolescent or by asking the patient to record the occurrence of sexual urges and sexual behaviors over a 2- to 4-week period.[8]

SUGGESTIONS FOR MANAGEMENT

If psychodiagnostic questions are raised regarding a potential gender identity disorder, refer the child *immediately* for psychological evaluation.[3,8] Early detection accompanied by early intervention is the preferred clinical strategy for optimum gender identity adjustment. In cases of cross-sex behavior lacking conclusive evidence of gender identity disorder, the following management strategies should be recommended, when appropriate:

1. Encourage the same-sex parent to invest time in positive play and interaction with the child, avoiding criticism of the child
2. Where a same-sex parent is unavailable, recommend finding a substitute same-sex adult who can be a positive role model
3. Recommend ignoring cross-sex behavior where possible
4. Advise parents to reward or praise appropriate "sex-typed" play and mannerisms
5. Provide appropriate sex education where needed
6. Inquire at regular office visits about the child's sex-typed behavior; if only limited improvement is apparent after several months, refer the child to a clinical child psychologist or child psychiatrist for behavioral therapy.

Specific child behavioral therapy techniques have been demonstrated to be effective in the successful treatment of gender identity disorders and other cross-sex behavior problems in childhood.[8,11] Positive reinforcement for normal sex-typed play, normal speech pattern, and sex-appropriate behavioral mannerisms as noted previously has been found to be effective in the clinic, home, and school in the successful treatment of deviant cross-sex behaviors in boys and girls, particularly when the parents are trained and supervised closely by a child psychologist or psychiatrist to carry out behavior-shaping programs in the child's environment.[8,11]

REFERENCES

1. American Psychiatric Association: *Diagnostic and statistical manual of mental disorders* (DSM-IV), Washington, DC, 1994, American Psychiatric Press.
2. Blanchard R, Hunker SJ: Age, transvestism, bondage, and concurrent paraphilic activities in 117 fatal cases of autoerotic asphyxia, *Br J Psychiatry* 159:371, 1991.
3. Blanchard R, Steiner BW, editors: *Clinical management of gender identity disorders in childhood and adults,* Washington, DC, 1990, American Psychiatric Press.
4. Byne W, Parsons B: Human sexual orientation: the biologic theories reappraised, *Arch Gen Psychiatry* 50:228, 1993.
5. Davenport CW: A follow-up study of 10 feminine boys, *Arch Sex Behav* 15:511, 1986.
6. Hendricks SE, Graber B, Rodriguez-Sierra JF: Neuroendocrine responses to exogenous estrogen: no differences between heterosexual and homosexual men, *Psychoneuroendocrinology* 14:177, 1989.
7. Rekers GA: Development of problems in puberty and sex roles in adolescence. In Walker CE, Roberts MC, editors: *Handbook of clinical child psychology,* ed 2, New York, 1992, John Wiley & Sons.
8. Rekers GA: Assessment and treatment methods for gender identity disorders and transvestism. In Rekers GA, editor: *Handbook of child and adolescent sexual problems,* Boston, 1995, Lexington Books/Macmillan.
9. Rekers GA, Kilgus MD: Differential diagnosis and rationale for treat ment of gender identity disorders and transvestism. In Rekers GA, edi-

tor: *Handbook of child and adolescent sexual problems,* Boston, 1995, Lexington Books/Macmillan.

10. Rekers GA et al: Genetic and physical studies of male children with psychological gender disturbances, *Psychol Med* 9:373, 1979.
11. Rekers GA, Kilgus M, Rosen AC: Long-term effects of treatment for childhood gender disturbance, *J Psychol Hum Sexuality* 3:121, 1990.
12. Rekers GA, Morey SM: Sex-typed body movements as a function of severity of gender disturbance in boys, *J Psychol Hum Sexuality* 2:2, 1989.
13. Rekers GA, Morey SM: The relationship of sex-typed play with clinician ratings on degree of gender disturbance, *J Clin Psychol* 46:28, 1990.
14. Spinder T et al: Pulsatile luteinizing hormone release and ovarian steroid levels in female-to-male transsexuals compared to heterosexual women, *Psychoneuroendocrinology* 14:97, 1989.
15. Taneja N et al: A transsexual male with 47 XYY karyotype, *All India Inst Med Sci* 161:698, 1992.
16. Zucker KJ, Bradley SJ, Hughes HE: Gender dysphoria in a child with true hermaphroditism, *Can J Psychiatry* 32:602, 1987.
17. Zucker KJ, Green R: Psychological and familial aspects of gender identity disorder, *Child Adolesc Psychiatr Clin North Am* 2:513, 1993.
18. Zuger B: Is early effeminate behavior in boys early homosexuality? *Compr Psychiatry* 29:509, 1988.

81 Encopresis

Barton D. Schmitt

Encopresis (soiling) is the voluntary or involuntary passage of feces into the clothing. Some children who have encopresis involuntarily leak fecal material from an impaction (retentive encopresis). Others simply pass normal movements into their underwear rather than use the toilet (nonretentive encopresis). Retentive and nonretentive encopresis should be separated because the treatment for each type is radically different. The minor fecal staining that occurs when children do not wipe themselves adequately after using the toilet should not be mistaken for encopresis.

Encopresis affects approximately 2% of kindergarten and first-grade students. The DSM-IV inclusion criteria for encopresis require the child to be 4 years of age or older, although any child over age 3 years who is not toilet-trained may be considered encopretic. Without professional advice for this age range, many parents mistreat encopresis with coercion or punishment, and the condition worsens.[8] Most children who have encopresis are brought in for examination by age 5, when their symptom interferes with school entry.[7] Affected boys outnumber affected girls by a ratio of 3 : 1.

ETIOLOGY

To understand retentive encopresis, one first must understand the pathophysiology of an impaction. An impaction occurs when constipation has gone unrelieved for about a week. By then, the rectum is so distended with stool that the sacrospinal defecation reflex is no longer energized and the mass is so wide that voluntary effort alone cannot force it through the anal canal. Hence, an impaction is fairly irreversible by natural events. The pressure of the impaction dilates the internal anal sphincter and makes it incompetent. Small amounts of the impaction are extruded intermittently through the external sphincter as a result of gravity, exercise, and relaxation. A few children become impacted because of organic factors. Most children hold back stool in an attempt to avoid the pain associated with passage or because they are enmeshed in a control issue with a parent.

Approximately 10% to 20% of children who are encopretic are not constipated. Frequently, preschoolers who are of this type are resisting bowel training deliberately. Most school-age children who have this type are postponing bowel movements ("waiting too long") because they don't want to leave some enjoyable activity (e.g., video games) or they don't want to use public toilets (e.g., school bathrooms).

All encopretic children (of either type) eventually develop secondary emotional problems; this embarrassing symptom takes a great toll in shame. The unpredictable nature of the symptom in retentive children causes constant fear of exposure. Many of these children are "scapegoated" at home, teased by peers (e.g., called "stinky"), and ostracized at school.

EVALUATION

History

A careful history usually distinguishes between retentive and nonretentive encopresis (Table 81-1). The clinician asks about size and consistency of stools and soiling intervals. In the retentive form, leakage occurs many times a day or even continuously. Commonly one elicits a history of periodic pain or crying with bowel movements, blood on the toilet tissue, passage of a huge bowel movement that clogs the toilet, or posturing that suggests deliberate holding back. By contrast, the child who has nonretentive soiling passes a bowel movement of normal size and consistency into the underwear once or twice a day; all symptoms of constipation are denied.

Other helpful parts of the history are diet and use of the toilet. The intake of milk products, fruit juice, and fiber should be recorded, as should information about sitting on the toilet—how many times per day and if sitting is spontaneous or prompted by parents or teachers. If the stool pattern is unknown, sending the parent home with an encopresis diary to complete can be most illuminating.

Physical Examination

The physical examination provides definitive information. In retentive soiling, an abdominal mass usually is palpable. Sometimes, the mass extends throughout the entire colon, but more commonly it involves only the rectosigmoid area. The mass is midline, suprapubic, irregular, and moveable. The mass can be missed if the rectus abdominis muscles are not relaxed. The backup of gas and stool can cause a protuberant abdomen.

A rectal examination must be performed on every patient; it can be done without any pain or distress in most children. Overlooking this procedure can lead to an erroneous diagnosis. Inspection of the anal opening often will show protruding fecal material in those children who are deliberate stool holders. The rectum in all impacted children is dilated and packed with wall-to-wall stool (often 6 to 10 cm across). The consistency of the impaction more commonly is like wet clay, rather than hard. By contrast, the child who has nonretentive soiling has a normal abdominal examination, and the rectal vault contains either a stool of normal caliber or nothing if the child recently has evacuated.

Retentive encopresis has an organic basis in less than 5% of children. Organic causes of constipation and retentive soiling often are noted on physical examination (Table 81-2).

Laboratory Studies

Children who are encopretic generally need no routine laboratory confirmation of this diagnosis. Because an impaction can cause partial bladder emptying and urine retention, a urinalysis for nitrite and pyuria may be a helpful screen for urinary tract infection, especially for any associated enuresis.

Table 81-1 Differentiation of Retentive Soiling from Nonretentive Soiling

	Retentive soiling	Nonretentive soiling
History		
Symptoms of constipation	Yes	No
Interval	Many times per day	Once per day
Size	Small	Normal
Consistency	Loose	Normal
Previous need for laxatives, suppositories, or enemas	Yes	No
Examination		
Abdominal mass	Yes	No
Abdominal distention	Often	No
Anal canal	Sometimes full	Empty
Rectum	Packed	Normal

Table 81-2 Organic Causes of Constipation and Retentive Soiling

Entity	Diagnostic criteria
Constipating medication	History positive
Constipating diet	History positive
Chronic anal fissure	Examination positive
Perianal cellulitis	Examination positive
Hypothyroidism	Linear growth delayed
Anal or rectal stenosis	Finger cannot enter rectum
Pelvic mass	Mass found on rectal examination (usually posteriorly)
Hirschsprung disease	Rectal ampulla repeatedly empty; rectum is tight

Suspicious perianal erythema should be cultured for group A *Streptococcus*. Occasionally, thyroid function tests are warranted.

Radiographic Findings

If the examiner cannot determine whether the patient is impacted, a plain postvoiding, supine abdominal radiograph can be helpful. Other indications include sexually abused children who might be emotionally traumatized by a rectal examination and those who refuse a rectal examination. A child who is impacted will demonstrate on roentgenogram a rectum grossly dilated with granular stool and increased stool in the transverse and descending colon, which is normally empty.[1] A normal child has granular stool in the ascending colon and formed stool of normal diameter in the rectosigmoid area. A barium enema or rectosigmoid manometric study is indicated only if Hirschsprung disease is strongly suspected. Children who have retentive soiling and experience repeated treatment failures occasionally may warrant a barium enema to reassure the family (and physician) that some rare diagnosis has not been overlooked.

MANAGEMENT OF RETENTIVE ENCOPRESIS (see the box above)

Most children over age 5 years want to stay clean; they don't want the embarrassment of "messing" their underwear. However, they may not understand how to become free of this disgraceful symptom. Tell them they "need to have a BM every day." They need to keep their rectum empty. Help them understand that holding back BMs is the main cause of "leaking" or "messing" their pants.

TREATMENT OF RETENTIVE ENCOPRESIS

Hyperphosphate enemas (two or three) to remove impaction
Mineral oil or lactulose for 3 months to keep the stools soft
Laxatives if stool softeners are ineffective
Sitting on the toilet for 10 minutes three times per day
Nonconstipating, high-fiber diet

Initial Disimpaction

Unless the impaction is removed, the child will be unable to maintain any bowel control. The traditional way to remove an impaction is to give two or three sodium phosphate enemas over 2 days. Warn the parents that phosphate enemas given in excessive dosage can cause tetany or dehydration. Gleghorn and colleagues[2] showed that administering 8 oz of mineral oil per day orally also can dislodge the impaction if the treatment is continued for approximately 4 days. A combination of these two approaches, starting with mineral oil orally and followed by enemas on day 3, may be useful. Inpatient enemas and therapy rarely are necessary.

Stool Softeners

As soon as the impaction is eliminated, the long-term treatment of constipation should be administered orally. Mineral oil or lactulose is prescribed (see Table 81-3 for dosages). The end point is the passage of one or two normal-size bowel movements per day. Stool softeners must be continued for 3 months because bowel diameter and tone require this long to return to normal. If the child refuses to take straight mineral oil, consider a better-tasting (though more expensive) emulsified derivative of mineral oil.

Laxatives

Stool softeners are the first line of therapy for constipation. If stool softeners such as mineral oil or lactulose are not effective, recommend laxatives (bowel stimulants) to help the child keep the rectum empty. Laxatives usually are needed for children who deliberately hold back bowel movements or for those who have acquired megarectum and megacolon[6] (for dosages, see Table 81-3).[9]

If the child is not having a daily bowel movement, the dosage should be increased. Some children temporarily require dosages that exceed the "standard" dosage recommended by textbooks and the package insert. Many parents worry unnecessarily about laxative dependency. Reassure them that children can be tapered off laxatives successfully, even after 6 months of taking them.[5]

All affected children will need stool softeners or laxatives for at least 3 months, and many for 6 months or longer. Many parents are in a hurry to stop the medications. Explain to them on the first visit that to achieve a cure, medications need to be continued until the child has gone at least 1 month without any soiling. The medications then can be tapered gradually over 1 to 2 months.

Toilet Habits

The child must sit on the toilet for at least 10 minutes three times a day. The gastrocolic reflex, which goes into effect 20 to 30 minutes after a meal (especially breakfast), should be used to advantage. Any treatment program that neglects this aspect will fail.

The child who has been impacted for many months has no urge to defecate. The defecation urge may not return until the rectum is kept empty for 2 to 4 weeks. Other important tips to impart to the child are to flex the hips to open the rectum and to use a foot stool for leverage and apply some pressure to the abdomen while pushing. If he has no bowel movement for 24 hours, he needs to sit on the toilet more often and longer each time. Soiling (leakage) also requires sitting on the toilet, as well as a cleanup.

Some preschoolers and toddlers adamantly refuse to sit on the toilet, holding back their stools when they are forced to do so. The overriding goal is to produce a daily bowel movement. Passing it into the diaper is better than holding it in. This is a case where pediatricians and parents need to lower their expectations. The child can be told that the "poop wants to come out every day and it needs your help." Going in the diaper is *fine*.

Table 81-3 Medications for Constipation and Impaction

Medication	Dosage	Comments
Stool softeners		
Mineral oil	1-2 ml/kg/dose bid Adolescents: 60 ml/dose (max 8 oz/day)	Do not use in children who have GE reflux or vomiting or who are not yet walking Emulsified types (Petrogalar, plain Agoral, Kondremul) taste better
Lactulose	0.5-1.0 ml/kg/dose bid Adolescents: 15 ml bid (max 3 oz/day)	This is a prescription item
Laxatives		
(Listed in order of increasing potency)		
Phillips' Milk of Magnesia or Haley's M-O (75% MOM, 25% mineral oil)	1 ml/kg/dose bid Adolescents: 60 ml bid	1 tablet MOM = 2.5 ml liquid
Senokot	<5 yr: 1-2 tsp syrup >5 yr: 2-3 tsp syrup Adolescents: 1 tbsp (max 2.5 tbsp or 8 tablets)	1 tablet = 3 ml granules = 5 ml syrup
Fletcher's Castoria	<5 yr: 1-2 tsp >5 yr: 2-3 tsp Adolescents: 2 tbsp max	
Dulcolax, 5-mg tablet	>5 yr: 5 mg >12 yr: 10 mg (2 tablets) Adolescents: 4 tablets max	No liquid form
Phenolphthalein	>5 years: ½ tablet Adolescents: 1 tablet	Chewable tablets (Ex-Lax) 90 mg
Rectal suppositories		
Glycerin suppository	1 or 2	
Dulcolax, 10 mg	>2 yr: 1 suppository	
Enemas		
Mineral oil enema	1-2 oz/20 lb of weight Adolescents: 4 oz	Squeeze-bottle size: 4.5 oz
Sodium phosphate enema (Fleet)	1 oz/20 lb of weight Adolescents: 4 oz (max 8 oz)	Squeeze-bottle size: 2.25 oz children, 4.5 oz adult

Modified from Schmitt BD, Mauro RD: *Contemp Pediatr* 9:47, 1992.

Nonconstipating, High-Fiber Diet

All constipated children need more fiber in their diet, as is found in such foods as popcorn, grains, fruits, and vegetables. However, diet therapy alone will cure children who have mild constipation only. The only foods that have been shown to be constipating are milk products. It is critical to identify the 10% or so of children who have impactions and who are drinking great amounts of milk (more than 32 oz per day). Milk intake can be limited to 16 oz per day in children over 1 year of age. Fluid requirements for these children can be met with fruit juices, especially those that have a high sorbitol content such as pear or peach juice. This can increase the frequency of stools.

Follow-up Visits

All children who have impactions need follow-up about 1 week into treatment; over 30% still will be impacted.[9] Repeat the abdominal examination even if the patient tells you that he is having normal bowel movements and no soiling. A child who has an impaction actually can keep himself clean temporarily by making a superhuman effort at control and sitting on the toilet several times a day. If the history and abdominal examination leave you uncertain, repeat the rectal examination.

If a child still is impacted at the follow-up examination, a more detailed explanation of the disimpaction process is called for. Some children need enemas in the office at this point.

Back-up Plan for Recurrence of Constipation or Encopresis

Back-up plans are critical for preventing all-too-frequent relapses. If the child goes more than 48 hours without a bowel movement, instruct the parents to increase the dosage of stool softener or laxative.[9] This is critical to prevent impactions from recurring.

If soiling occurs more than twice over a few days, it means that the child is becoming reimpacted. At this point, the parents should intervene vigorously by giving a double dose of laxative, a suppository, or an enema. Sometimes merely mentioning an enema results in the child sitting on the toilet and producing a bowel movement. For older children who are cooperative about sitting on the toilet, sitting there for 10 or 15 minutes out of every hour usually will relieve an early impaction. Again, make sure the family realizes that soiling always means the rectum is full and the impaction is returning.

Biofeedback Treatment

Treatment failure has been attributed to rectal hyposensitivity and inability to relax the external anal sphincter.[4] Both of these pathophysiological conditions probably are acquired, the former caused by prolonged stretching of the rectum and the latter resulting from voluntary attempts to prevent stool leakage or pain. Both of these conditions usually revert to normal after a cure. No outcome study yet has shown the advantage of biofeedback training over using stool softeners, changing toileting habits, and instituting behavior modification.

MANAGEMENT OF NONRETENTIVE ENCOPRESIS (see the box below)

For those children who simply postpone BMs, a simple admonition "to find a toilet whenever you feel rectal pressure" and "don't make your body wait" usually removes the symptom. Most of these children, however, are resistant to toilet training, and they need more intensive intervention.

Medications

Stool softeners, laxatives, and enemas clearly are not needed in any of these cases.

Reminders and Lectures

Reassure the parents that there is nothing more for them to teach. Ask the parents to stop all reminders about using the toilet. Let the child decide when he or she needs to go to the bathroom. Such children should neither be reminded to go to the bathroom nor asked if they need to go. Reminders, inquiries, and lectures are a form of pressure, and pressure doesn't work. Remove any threats of punishment. Many young children try to hold back all bowel movements to avoid punishment, such as being spanked or grounded for soiling. They are under the mistaken impression that not passing any bowel movements is the best way to avoid punishment. Talk to the parents about the importance of not punishing their child for soiling. Then reassure the child that he or she will no longer be punished for soiling.

Incentives

Give incentives for BMs into the toilet. Reassure the parents that this is how they can turn the tide. If the child has a BM into the toilet, the parents should give immediate positive feedback such as praise, a hug, and a sticker. To achieve a breakthrough with some children who have never had a bowel movement into a potty chair or toilet, the parent should offer major incentives such as going out to their favorite fast-food restaurant, watching their favorite video, or giving them treats.[8] A star chart also helps many children stay focused on the goal of using the potty chair or toilet. Incentives also are helpful in younger children who deliberately hold back BMs and refuse to sit on the potty chair.

Changing Soiled Underwear

Don't ignore soiling. The parents' only remaining assignment is to help the child change clothes when he or she is soiled. As soon as the parent notices that the child has messy pants, clean him or her up immediately. Make changing a neutral, quick interaction.

TREATMENT OF NONRETENTIVE ENCOPRESIS

Don't give medications
Stop all reminders, lectures, or punishments
Give incentives for BMs into the toilet
For soiling, insist on immediate cleanup
Refer treatment failures

PROGNOSIS

Pediatric management can cure 99% of children who have pain-related impaction. The physician will be successful with approximately 70% of children who have psychogenic impaction and will need to work in conjunction with a mental health professional for the others. Many children who require psychological intervention can be recognized initially because they are depressed, overtly angry, or over 8 years of age. Levine studied 127 encopretic children for over 1 year.[3] At that time, 51% were cured and 27% had marked improvement.

Nonretentive encopresis is much easier to treat. These children have good results if the problem is recent and poor results if the problem is long-standing (over 5 years). In mildly resistive children, primary care management can achieve a 90% to 95% cure rate. Those who have severe resistance, deliberate encopresis at school, or severely disturbed parent-child relationships need early referral.

SUMMARY

The primary care pediatrician plays a critical role in the evaluation of children with encopresis. Most nonphysicians cannot distinguish between the retentive and nonretentive types. The physician also can treat many of these children successfully by using combined therapy (stool softeners, laxatives, diet, altered toilet habits, and positive reinforcement incentives). If a child who has retentive soiling is referred to a mental health professional, the pediatrician should remain involved in titrating medications against symptoms.

REFERENCES

1. Barr RG et al: Chronic and occult stool retention: a clinical tool for its evaluation in school-aged children, *Clin Pediatr* 18:674, 1979.
2. Gleghorn EE, Heyman MB, Rudolph CD: No-enema therapy for idiopathic constipation and encopresis, *Clin Pediatr* 130:669, 1991.
3. Levine MD, Bakow H: Children with encopresis: a study of treatment outcome, *Pediatrics* 58:845, 1976.
4. Loening-Baucke V: Modulation of abnormal defecation dynamics by biofeedback treatment in chronically constipated children with encopresis, *J Pediatr* 116:214, 1990.
5. McClung HJ et al: Is combination therapy for encopresis nutritionally safe? *Pediatrics* 91:591, 1993.
6. Nolan T et al: Randomised trial of laxatives in treatment of childhood encopresis, *Lancet* 338:523, 1991.
7. Nolan T, Oberklaid F: New concepts in the management of encopresis, *Pediatr Rev* 14:447, 1993.
8. Schmitt BD: Toilet training refusal: avoid the battle and win the war, *Contemp Pediatr* 4:32, 1987.
9. Schmitt BD, Mauro RD: 20 common errors in treating encopresis, *Contemp Pediatr* 9:47, 1992.

82 Enuresis

Michael W. Cohen

The evaluation and management of an enuretic child is a frequent, challenging, and potentially rewarding task for the primary care provider. One must consider the various causes of enuresis in developing a reasonable, efficient, and successful approach to a "wetting" child and his or her family.

Enuresis is defined as the involuntary discharge of urine, although it often is used to mean wetting during nighttime sleep *(nocturnal enuresis)*. Daytime wetting is termed *diurnal enuresis*. The diagnosis of enuresis should be reserved for girls wetting beyond the age of 5 years and for boys, 6 years; the sex-related age differences reflect developmental variations.

Nocturnal enuresis affects 5 to 7 million children in the United States and occurs in approximately 15% of all 5-year-olds, 7% of 8-year-olds, and 3% of 12-year-olds. Lower socioeconomic groups, families of lower educational levels, and institutionalized populations have a higher reported prevalence of enuresis. Males predominate at all ages within all enuretic populations, with the differential being greater in older children. Somewhat fewer than 10% of all children with enuresis also wet in the daytime. Diurnal enuresis infrequently occurs without nocturnal enuresis.[1]

Primary enuresis exists when a child has never achieved consistent dryness. A child who has ssu econdary enuresis generally is considered to have had a period of dryness of at least 3 to 5 months and commonly is referred to as a "relapser" or an "onset enuretic." Among enuretic children, secondary enuresis generally increases with age, with over 50% of all enuretics being of this type by 12 years of age. Approximately 25% of children will have some relapse in bedwetting after a period of initial dryness. This form of secondary enuresis usually is self-limiting and may occur only at times of illness or emotional stress.

The strong familial aspect of enuresis is well established. If both parents have a history of enuresis, there is approximately a 75% chance that one or more of their children will be enuretic. If one parent had enuresis, the chance is 40% to 45% that a child in that family will be enuretic. If neither parent was enuretic, the risk decreases to 15%.[2,6]

ETIOLOGY

Enuresis must be considered multifactorial in etiology. Developmental "delays," organic disorders, and psychological factors all have been emphasized as causes of enuresis. Although definitive proof is lacking, many believe that a delay in the enuretic child's adequate neuromuscular bladder control is the major cause. This view is supported by (1) the primary nature of most enureses, (2) the common familial pattern, (3) the common history of frequent voiding and urgency to void as a manifestation of a small functional bladder capacity, and (4) the high incidence of spontaneous remission (or developmental maturation). Proponents of this theory argue that the persistence of enuresis after neuromuscular maturation is based on the psychological effects of the child's interaction with significant individuals in his or her environment. One investigator, using suprapubically indwelling catheters, refutes these assumptions, finding rather that enuretic children have age-appropriate bladder stability with normal bladder capacities and normal coordinated awake and sleep micturition.[5]

Sleep investigations in enuretic children have evolved with the technological advances that allow study of sleep patterns. Initial studies concluded that enuresis occurred in lighter stages of sleep. Subsequent studies described nocturnal enuresis as a "disorder of arousal," with the voiding episodes beginning in the deepest stages of sleep, from which the patients lightened their sleep but were unable to wake completely. More recent studies conclude that nocturnal enuresis is independent of sleep stage and not specifically related to the depth of sleep. Enuretic episodes occur randomly throughout the night; wetting occurs in each stage of sleep in proportion to the amount of time spent in that stage.[3,4]

Organic explanations have focused primarily on the genitourinary and nervous systems. Obstructive lesions of the distal outflow tract, such as posterior urethral valves, have received particular attention both as a cause of urinary tract infections and as an independent cause of enuresis. A current urinary tract infection or the history of previous infections may be causal factors in enuresis. However, in a primary setting, only about 3% to 4% of enuretic youngsters demonstrate significant urological pathology.[2]

Nervous system dysfunction may be associated with enuresis, either through lumbosacral disorders that affect bladder innervation or as a reflection of global mental retardation. Although true myelodysplastic disorders may affect bladder function, the radiological finding of spina bifida occulta has not been shown to be related causally to enuresis.

Recent studies of preadolescents and teenagers have focused on the contribution of polyuria and diuresis in their nocturnal enuresis. These patients were urodynamically normal. They had a sleep diuresis that exceeded their daytime bladder capacity by up to several hundred percent. In contrast to the normal nighttime increase in antidiuretic hormone (arginine vasopressin), these patients maintained constant serum levels at night. Enuresis for this group of patients appears to be related to polyuria secondary to a lack of circadian rhythm in antidiuretic hormone secretion. This information is consistent with parental reports of multiple nighttime wetting episodes and an apparent excessive urinary output in their children.[5] Diabetes mellitus, sickle cell anemia and sickle cell trait, food allergies, and ingestion of foods or medications that have diuretic actions all have been implicated as infrequent causes of enuresis.

Psychological functioning may relate to enuresis at two levels. The enuresis may be only one aspect of a child's general difficulty in behavioral adaptation, or it may be an isolated symptom in a child whose behavioral functioning otherwise is normal.

The incidence of behavioral problems in enuretic children has been estimated by behavioral inventories, interviews, and observation of children who have been evaluated for their enuresis. These surveys indicate a slight increase in behavioral problems among this population. However, it also has been shown that families who bring their enuretic child for an evaluation perceive more behavioral problems in their child than those who do not. Therefore the true incidence of behavioral problems in enuretic children is difficult to determine. It is reasonable to conclude that most enuretic children are not maladjusted or psychopathological.[2]

Enuresis has been viewed by some as the result of poor or deficient learning of a habit pattern during toilet training. The impact of these influences is unknown, although resistance to initial training efforts despite the nature of the techniques used may be relevant.

The evaluation should be considered the initial phase of therapy. The positive therapeutic value of a complete evaluation that satisfies the concerns and expectations of the enuretic child and his or her family is well documented. Potential parental guilt associated with toilet-training approaches and management failures can be alleviated by a brief explanation of the multifactorial origin of the condition and the common difficulties in management.

HISTORY

The type of enuresis (primary versus secondary, nocturnal versus diurnal) should be established. The severity of the enuresis should be estimated and expressed as the number of wet nights per week or month (e.g., 4/7, 16/30). Quantification of the enuresis allows for a relatively accurate demonstration of a trend and the effect of intervention. The effect of environmental factors on the severity of the symptoms also should be explored. Parental management techniques should be discussed, beginning with a history of initial toilet-training efforts. The age and response of the child, the attitudes and approach of the parents, and the results of such efforts are important. The child's perception of family and peer responses to the difficulty should be elicited. The presence of a significant negative emotional response by the child and whether the enuresis is limiting age-appropriate activities may influence decisions about intervention.

The medical history will reveal any perinatal difficulties that may have led to neurological trauma; the weight and gestation of the patient can alter developmental expectations. The review of systems should focus on the genitourinary and nervous systems. Delays in perceptual-motor or communication skills might coexist with a delay in bladder control. In addition to frequency and urgency of urination and symptoms of urinary tract infection, dysuria and dribbling after and between micturition have been found to be more common in enuretic children than in nonenuretic children. Approximately 1 in 10 enuretics also will be encopretic. This association is firmly established and may reflect an underlying deficiency in toilet training or organic pathology.

PHYSICAL EXAMINATION

A full examination is essential. Renal disease may be reflected in poor growth or elevated blood pressure. Examination of the genitalia should be complete and sensitive to the feelings of a developing youngster or teenager. A search for major and minor anomalies should be followed by an observation of micturition. Anomalies, including undescended testes, underdeveloped scrotum, epispadias, phimosis, and abnormalities in the urethral meatus in males, and location and characteristics of the urethral meatus in females should be observed because they may be associated with internal anomalies. Abnormalities or difficulties in voiding, such as changes in the quality (e.g., size and velocity) of the urinary stream, an inability to initiate or stop micturition voluntarily, and the presence of dysuria or dribbling, should be noted.

A neurological examination may reveal lower spinovertebral dysfunction that reflects abnormalities of bladder innervation. Gait, muscular strength and tone, deep tendon reflexes, sensory responses, and rectal sphincter tone therefore should be examined.

LABORATORY TESTS

A urinalysis provides valuable information about a wide range of organic disorders that may be associated with enuresis, including diabetes insipidus, psychogenic water drinking, diabetes mellitus, urinary tract infection, and various forms of renal pathology. Beyond the urinalysis and urine culture, the indication for further evaluation remains quite controversial.

Rushton[8] has divided nocturnal enuresis into uncomplicated and complicated, with the second category requiring additional diagnostic studies. Factors that dictate these studies include persistent secondary onset of bed-wetting, severe voiding dysfunction, associated encopresis, urinary tract infection, and abnormal findings on neurological examination. Further studies may include a renal or bladder sonogram, intravenous pyelogram (IVP), a voiding cystourethrogram (VCUG), or urodynamic measurements. If these procedures are indicated, the child must be adequately prepared in a manner that will minimize the psychological trauma, with the nature of this preparation depending on the age, sex, and developmental maturity of the child. Functional bladder capacity should be measured if bladder training is the proposed form of treatment. Unless an undiagnosed seizure disorder is strongly suspected, the presence of enuresis does not warrant an electroencephalogram.

By the end of this type of evaluation, the majority of enuretic children who have significant organic dysfunction or psychopathological dysfunction will have been discovered. When their needs exceed the expertise of the primary care physician, these patients should be referred to the appropriate specialist (urologist, neurologist, endocrinologist, nephrologist, or mental health or behavioral specialist). The remaining group, which constitutes the vast majority of children who have enuresis, will present a picture consistent with a basic developmental delay in bladder control with associated psychological factors. This population is managed best by the clinician who is most familiar with the child and the child's family and environment.

MANAGEMENT

An air of optimism is realistic and may be immeasurably therapeutic. Although a positive clinical response to the process of evaluation and intervention often has been labeled a placebo effect, the benefit of a carefully planned approach has been documented and should be considered a therapeutic response. An annual spontaneous remission rate of approximately 15% between ages 5 and 19 applies primarily to boys[9]; remission rates for girls are highest early in this age range. Optimism also may be bolstered by uncovering a history of parental enuresis.

The participation of the child enhances the efficacy of any specific mode of therapy and should be solicited. The child's involvement should begin with a demystification and an explanation of the probable cause of his or her enuresis at the child's level of understanding. A clarification of the involuntary nature of the symptoms usually removes any sense of guilt and allows the child to develop an optimistic perspective. Such involvement also decreases the chances of struggle between child and parents and promotes the child's responsibility for alleviating the symptoms.[6]

Reassurance may be the therapy of choice for younger children or for children developing transient secondary enuresis in response to an environmental stress. For parents who feel compelled to do something while awaiting a remission, various simple measures have been recommended, such as limiting the child's fluid intake, having the child empty his or her bladder at bedtime, or taking the child to the bathroom during the night. If these are suggested, it should be explained that, although they may decrease the symptoms somewhat, they have not been shown to hasten a remission. These tactics also may initiate or aggravate a struggle between parent and child.

Supportive counseling may be required as the sole mode of therapy or as an adjunct to other specific regimens. The goals of counseling could include (1) parental understanding of the multifactorial nature of enuresis, (2) parental acceptance of the child and the symptoms in a manner that allows them to provide maximum emotional support, (3) acceptance by the child of the symptom and an appreciation of "individual differences" that many children demonstrate in other areas of functioning, and (4) appreciation by the patient that he or she can have some control over the enuresis. The requirement for counseling depends on the age of the child, the child's general developmental and behavioral pattern, the family's experience with enuresis, the coexistence of emotional problems, intrafamily communication patterns, and the response to the initial management.

If the enuresis is deterring the child's social, emotional, or cognitive development, therapy beyond reassurance and supportive counseling is indicated. Because no one therapy has been consistently superior, the clinician's experience, enthusiasm, and comfort should dictate the choice. Conditioning devices, bladder training, and self-hypnosis and drug therapy all have been shown to be effective. However, both parents and child should be alerted to the potential for relapse and thus the need for a "second dose" of treatment.[1]

Enuresis-conditioning instruments involve a moisture-activated sensor, which is connected to an alarm that provides auditory or vibratory stimulation to wake the child or parent at initiation of wetting.[6] Older devices involve a mattress pad; the new ones have portable mechanisms that attach to the child's underpants. The auditory sources are contained in a wristwatch or small pin-on battery-powered alarm. Because the temporal relationship between the wetting episode and the alarm is critical for effective conditioning, a refined instrument of adequate sensitivity is required.

Cure rates have varied among studies, but several controlled studies have yielded rates between 60% and 85%. Personal resistance by the child may lead to as high as a 10% to 20% noncompliance rate. Permanent responders require an average of 60 days of therapy. A 20% to 40% relapse rate is reported in all studies, but dryness often is obtained more quickly and permanently with a second course of treatment. Foxman et al.[1] believe that the technique of "overlearning" by increasing fluid intake before bedtime to stress the bladder and increase the waking episode decreases the relapse rate. An intermittent reinforcement program, with the alarm sounding during 70% of the wetting episodes, also may lead to a lower relapse rate. They concluded that the safety and portable nature of the new devices and the reported successful results of such conditioning therapy make this an attractive therapeutic technique.

Self-hypnosis or self-conditioning has been effective in primary nocturnal enuresis.[7] The enuretic episode is viewed as a habit disorder that allows the wetting episode without the child awakening. The child is taught the technique of self-induced relaxation, to be practiced before sleep. During this "trance," the child tells himself that he *will* wake up when he experiences the need to void, thus allowing a dry bed and very happy feelings on waking in the morning. This happiness can be associated with a visual image of some warm, tranquil, and enjoyable experience in the youngster's memory to enhance the desirability of the feeling of waking in a dry bed. Significant improvement and cure rates (80%) have been reported after only a few training visits. This technique requires special therapy skills, but appears to be a potent and safe alternative treatment with much promise.

Bladder-training therapy is based on the observation that functional bladder capacity in many children who have enuresis is decreased. The goal of this training is to transform a functionally infantile bladder into one of adult volume and coordination. The procedure involves the participation of the child in holding the urine as long as possible once a day for several months. Increasing urine volumes and number of dry nights are recorded on a calendar, which serves as a reinforcement for the child. The clinician must be cautious that the discomfort caused by urine retention does not discourage the participation of the youngster and create a struggle with the parents. In addition, measured increases in bladder volume do not necessarily generalize to nighttime dryness.

Several pharmacological agents have been used to treat enuresis. Sedatives, stimulants, and sympathomimetic agents are not beneficial. Oxybutynin, an anticholinergic agent, is not significantly better than a placebo in reducing the frequency of bed-wetting but may help some children who have diurnal enuresis. Tricyclic antidepressants, particularly imipramine, have been used extensively to treat enuresis, with total dryness being achieved in 10% to 20%, a "50% improvement" in 67% of children, and the remainder receiving less or no benefit. A very high relapse rate is noted when the medication is discontinued. Three proposed mechanisms of action are (1) a direct relaxation effect on the bladder detrusor muscle, (2) an alteration in the arousal state of the nervous system during sleep, or (3) an antidepressant effect. Because there is no evidence that enuretic children are depressed and because enuretic improvement can be immediate, whereas antidepressant benefits take more than 7 to 10 days, antidepression is unlikely to be the mechanism. The arousal proposal also is questionable because the relationship between depth of sleep and enuresis has been questioned.[8] A proposed mechanism that suggests an imbalance among catecholamines that facilitate continence centrally has some pharmacological support but remains unproven. Imipramine generally is given 30 minutes to 1 hour before bedtime, with no proven advantage to multiple daily doses. The initial dose of imipramine is 25 mg for children under 12 and 50 mg for older children. Although the maximum recommended dose has been 75 mg, studies measuring plasma levels at 12 hours after the bedtime dose suggest dramatic variations in levels and in the need for and safety of higher doses in some children. Measuring plasma levels routinely is not indicated but may be useful before concluding that imipramine is unhelpful.

The child should be asked to maintain a diary of success. At the first follow-up visit, the imipramine dosage can be altered and the youngster supplied positive feedback. Once the therapeutic response is successful, the child should be maintained on the medication for approximately 3 months. At the end of this period, a gradual discontinuation of the drug may decrease the likelihood of a relapse. The drug should be tapered to once every other night and then every third night over 4 to 6 weeks. The maximum psychological benefit of dryness on "nondrug" nights can be supplied by emphasizing and praising the child's newly developed bladder control, which, it is hoped, can be sustained without medication. The most common adverse effects are nervousness, insomnia, headaches, and anticholinergic symptoms.

Imipramine is well known for its toxicity and thin margin of safety. The triad of coma, convulsions, and cardiac disturbances can occur at relatively low-dosage accidental ingestions in young children and may be fatal. School-age youngsters are vulnerable to overdosage because of magical thinking that leads them to believe that more medication might be more beneficial. A number of deaths have been reported under these circumstances. Great caution must be used in prescribing this agent, and the parents and child must be well aware of the potential dangers involved in, and their control over, its administration.[5] Drug therapy with this agent should be reserved for the older child who has not responded successfully to other modalities of therapy.

The diuresis theory of causality has led to clinical trials with desmopressin (antidiuretic hormone). This agent serves as a substitute for endogenous nocturnal vasopressin, leading to a reduction in overnight urine volume. There is a correlation between increased dose and clinical benefit. An initial dose of 20 μg can be increased gradually to 40 μg until dryness is achieved. Most studies have used intranasal administration, although the oral route appears to be just as effective and causes fewer electrolyte changes. Desmopressin has been used for 20 years in the treatment of central diabetes insipidus with few adverse effects. Water intoxication and hyponatremia are a theoretical concern but have not occurred in otherwise healthy children given only a bedtime dose. Headaches, nausea, mild abdominal cramps, and vulvar pain have been reported but disappear when the dose is reduced. The drug neither suppresses endogenous production of vasopressin nor induces destructive antibodies.

A recent literature review indicated that desmopressin reduces the number of wet nights but that only about 25% of the subjects studied achieved complete dryness.[4] The best responses were in those who had a family history of enuresis and those who could achieve a urine osmolality greater than 1000 mmol/kg before or after the administration of desmopressin. A small proportion of responders remained dry after the medication was withdrawn, independent of how long they were treated. At this point desmopressin should be viewed as a symptomatic treatment. When compared with conditioning devices, desmopressin had a more immediate benefit, but conditioning provided significantly more long-term results and less chance of relapse.[5] Long-term treatment is viewed as being well tolerated and safe, and appropriate for adults.

The specific indications for the use of desmopressin have not been defined. It may be most useful in older patients (over 10 to 11 years of age) who have not benefited from prior therapies. It also may help in conjunction with conditioning devices to achieve a rapid improvement while the conditioned response is developing, allowing eventual withdrawal of the medication. Intermittent use may be helpful in special situations in which enuretic children need to be dry to avoid embarrassment while awaiting results of other therapy or spontaneous resolution.

TREATMENT FAILURES AND RELAPSES

Relapses and treatment failures are relatively frequent for all methods of therapy. A particular therapy should not be considered a failure until it has been tried for at least 4 to 6 weeks. A failure of one type of therapy might dictate the addition of another. If combination therapy fails, the practitioner may have to tell the child and the family that the neuromuscular bladder control mechanisms still are too immature and that the symptoms must be tolerated for several more months, when the treatment can be reinstituted. Reassurance of physical and mental normality *must* accompany this message. However, if any new information concerning organic dysfunction or a psychopathological problem becomes apparent, further evaluation might be indicated. For example, a treatment failure could result from noncompliance, which reflects either (1) an underlying family interactional pattern that precludes the necessary empathy and understanding or (2) emotional needs of family members that require persistence of the symptom. This aspect should be investigated appropriately by the primary care clinician or a mental health associate. Relapses may be handled by explaining to patients that the nervous system–bladder control mechanism is developing but is not yet fully mature and that a few more months of specific therapy will be required. The previously temporary successful mode of therapy then is reinstituted. This approach allows for maintenance of an optimistic posture and, if necessary, the use of several courses of therapy.

REFERENCES

1. Foxman B, Valdez RB, Brook RH: Childhood enuresis: prevalence, perceived impact and prescribed treatment, *Pediatrics* 77:482, 1986.

2. McLorie GA, Husmann DA: Incontinence and enuresis, *Pediatr Clin North Am* 34:1159, 1987.
3. Mikkelson EJ, Rapoport JL: Enuresis: psychopathology, sleep stage and drug response, *Urol Clin North Am* 7:361, 1980.
4. Moffatt MEK, Harlos S, Kirshen AJ: Desmopressin acetate and nocturnal enuresis: how much do we know? *Pediatrics* 94:420, 1993.
5. Norgaard JP: Pathopsychology of nocturnal enuresis, *Scand J Urol Nephrol Suppl* 140:1, 1991.
6. Novello AC, Novello JR: Enuresis, *Pediatr Clin North Am* 34:719, 1987.
7. Olness K, Gardner GG: *Hypnosis and hypnotherapy with children,* Philadelphia, 1988, Grune & Stratton.
8. Rushton HG: Nocturnal enuresis: epidemiology, evaluation and currently available treatment options, *J Pediatr Suppl* 114:691, 1989.
9. Schmitt BD: Nocturnal enuresis: an update on treatment, *Pediatr Clin North Am* 29:21, 1982.

83 Fire-setting

Amy L. Suss

Childhood fire-setting is common and results in significant property damage, injury, loss of life, and other serious consequences for families and communities. In 1989, arson was suspected in 97,000 fires involving structures, causing over $1.5 billion in property loss. Arson was the third leading cause of residential fires and the second leading cause of residential fire-related injuries and deaths; it also was the leading cause of nonresidential fires.[1]

Although little definitive information is available regarding the overall extent of fire-setting among children and adolescents, reported prevalence rates among both outpatient and inpatient psychiatric populations of children and adolescents range between 19% and 35%, respectively.[4] Fire-setting is more frequent by children less than 8 years of age and during adolescence.[6] During the 1970s, approximately 55% of all arsonists arrested in the United States were less than 18 years of age, and 11% were below age 10.[6] Younger children are more likely to set fires at home, whereas older children are more likely to set fires outside the home and to cause more overall damage.

ETIOLOGY

Psychoanalytical theory has assigned unconscious meaning to fire as a symbol of sexuality. Fire-setting by children and adolescents is viewed as a substitute for masturbatory behavior in response to parental prohibitions. While some instances of fire-setting may be a manifestation of sexual problems, subsequent study has revealed more complex and diverse etiological factors. Researchers have examined the family background, the social and psychiatric history, and the stated reasons for engaging in fire-setting behavior. A high incidence of family dysfunction, including parental alcoholism, psychosis, and criminality has been noted.[1] Similarly, child and adolescent emotional disturbances, including hyperactivity, psychosis, rage reactions, and enuresis also have been described.[1] Fire-setters exhibit higher levels of aggressive and antisocial behavior than their non-fire-setting peers. Characteristics consistently attributed to child fire-setters include male predominance (females constitute less than 10% of fire-setters), absence of a parent, a history of abuse or neglect, scholastic problems, and lower than average intelligence.[6]

Although no typical profile of childhood fire-setters has been established, high risk for future fire-setting can be identified by several characteristics. Children at high risk generally are motivated out of anger or revenge and often have a history of repetitive fire-setting. High-risk children tend to have individual or family-related psychopathology, including psychosis, alcoholism, abuse, and neglect. One- and five-year prospective studies of childhood fire-setting describe recidivists as coming from less stable homes and tending to be more antisocial than children who no longer set fires.[5,7] Of particular note is the symptom triad of fire-setting, enuresis, and cruelty to animals. This syndrome has been suggested as a possible predictor of adult violent behavior.[2] Children at lower risk generally are motivated to set fires out of curiosity or experimentation (e.g., playing with matches); in these children the fire-setting frequently is an isolated event. Low-risk children tend to have intact families and no history of abuse or neglect.

MANAGEMENT

Approaches to the management of fire-setting depend on recognition and assessment of the seriousness of the problem. Physicians are in a position to facilitate early recognition by screening routinely for fire-setting behaviors. At least in theory, early detection of childhood fire-setting is critical to improving prognosis and reducing the potential for damage, injury, and death. The physician may assess the seriousness of the problem by differentiating low-risk from high-risk fire-setters on the basis of the previously described characteristics.

Low-risk fire-setters are, in general, described as being "curious" and experimenting or playing with fire in an isolated incident. They tend to be younger, show remorse or guilt after the incident, express no other deviant behaviors, and reside in intact families.[1,3] These children are suitable for brief interventions that consist of education from parents or physicians about the dangers of fire and may benefit from training in fire safety. The physician, in discussing fire-setting behavior, should attempt to prevent inappropriate parental responses such as either burning a child to teach him or her a lesson or trying to help the child get over his or her interest in fire by allowing him or her to light matches or candles. Children have difficulty discriminating between permissive and nonpermissive opportunities to light fires. Parents should be provided with guidance regarding techniques to modify the behavior by communicating clearly the inappropriateness of the behavior, supervising the child (e.g., limiting access to matches), and reinforcing appropriate behavior positively (e.g., returning found matches without lighting them).

In contrast, high-risk fire-setters tend to be older, to use fire more deliberately as an expression of anger or revenge, to be emotionally disturbed, and to reside in dysfunctional families.[1,3] In this context the physician should address the behavior as being representative of a broader pattern of disturbance that is in need of immediate attention. The possibility that the fire-setting is a response to environmental factors, including family dysfunction, needs to be explored. This exploration should be nonaccusatory, emphasizing action to help the child or adolescent. At this point, referral to a mental health professional for treatment may be appropriate. Owing to the potential dangers of continued fire-setting, the physician should make a routine call to the family to ensure compliance with any referral. Hospitalization may be necessary in cases of severe underlying psychiatric disturbances. A purpose of such hospitalization is to reestablish control if the child represents an imminent danger and the parents are unable to ensure safety or supervision.

Treatment of fire-setting by children is directed toward exploring the child's motivation, targeting therapeutic interventions toward individual/familial dysfunction, and teaching acceptable alternatives to fire-setting. Treatment should include close follow-up of the child to prevent repeated episodes. The prognosis is guarded in children and adolescents who have high-risk behaviors such as repetitive fire-setting motivated by anger or revenge. In general the prognosis is good for treated children who have low-risk fire-setting behaviors such as playing with matches out of curiosity or experimentation; complete remission in these children is a realistic goal.

REFERENCES

1. Geller JL: Arson in review: from profit to pathology, *Psychiatr Clin North Am* 15:623, 1992.
2. Hellman DS, Blackman N: Enuresis, firesetting, and cruelty to animals: a triad predictive of adult crime, *Am J Psychiatry* 12:1431, 1966.
3. Kolko DJ, Kazdin AE: Motives of childhood firesetters: firesetting characteristics and psychological correlates, *J Child Psychol Psychiatry* 32:535, 1991.
4. Kolko DJ, Kazdin AE: Prevalence of firesetting and related behaviors among child psychiatric patients, *J Consult Clin Psychol* 56:628, 1988.
5. Kolko DJ, Kazdin AE: The emergence and recurrence of child firesetting: a one-year prospective study, *J Abnorm Child Psychol* 20:17, 1992.
6. Showers J, Pickrell E: Child firesetters: a study of three populations, *Hosp Community Psychiatry* 38:495, 1987.
7. Stewart MA, Culver KW: Children who set fires: the clinical picture and a follow-up, *Br J Psychiatry* 140:357, 1982.

SUGGESTED READINGS

Fineman K: Firesetting in childhood and adolescence, *Psychiatr Clin North Am* 3:483, 1980.

Kaufman I, Henis LW: A reevaluation of the psychodynamics of firesetting, *Am J Orthopsychiatry* 31:123, 1961.

Yarnell H: Firesetting in children, *Am J Orthopsychiatry* 10:272, 1940.

84 Lying and Stealing

Gregory E. Prazar

Acts of lying and stealing by children often evoke strong emotional reactions from parents. Truthfulness and respect for property are two highly valued mores espoused by our society, even though adults frequently violate their own moral codes. Lying and stealing can represent a psychopathologic spectrum from a common transient developmental phenomenon to an ominous indication of severe psychiatric disturbance. Frequently both parents and professionals overreact to symptoms of lying and stealing before analyzing all the relevant information.

Prevalence figures for lying and stealing indicate that these behaviors occur more frequently in boys than in girls and achieve highest rates between 5 and 8 years of age. In one study by MacFarlane and colleagues[3] 49% of mothers of 5-year-old boys and 42% of mothers of 5-year-old girls reported that their children had lied; stealing among 5-year-old boys was reported for 10% and for 4% of 5-year-old girls. By age 8, 41% of the boys and 19% of the girls exhibited some lying, whereas only 9% of the boys and 5% of the girls exhibited stealing behavior.

Given the prevalence of these behaviors, the responsibility of the primary care physician is to inquire about symptoms of lying and stealing during routine visits and to help families understand and respond to these if they do occur. To identify and manage these problems adequately, a history as complete as possible should be obtained from parents and child, encompassing aspects of the home environment (patterns of child rearing, child's interaction with siblings and parents), peer relationships, and school performance.

LYING

When lying is presented as a problem to the pediatrician, either directly by the parents or indirectly from questions asked by the physician during a regular visit, several important aspects of the child's functioning should be considered before definitive action is taken: his or her maturational level; the influence of family, peers, and school, and, above all, the situation in which lying occurs.

The child's chronological age and developmental level greatly influence the extent to which lying should be evaluated. Children under 3 years are beginning to establish independence from their parents; for these children the differentiation between what Stone and Church[5] refer to as "private self and public self" is tenuous. Children at this age have no concept of deception and therefore do not lie intentionally. Their experimentation with concepts of language often is interpreted by adults as lying. The toddler, attempting to understand presence and absence of individuals, may tell the father that "Mommy is not here," when she may indeed be in the next room.[4] Emotionally painful situations are avoided by all children, especially by toddlers under 3 years. The child, whose moral code is immature, thinks nothing of denying a misdeed, because admission might bring painful consequences.

The mental life of the preschool child (3 to 7 years) is one filled with fantasy. According to Stone and Church,[5] 20% to 50% of this age group create imaginary companions, pets, or situations. The imaginary companion usually is a helpful, empathic playmate, although he or she may function as a disciplinarian for the child. By serving as a surrogate friend, the imaginary companion helps the child adapt to new social situations. By serving as a disciplinarian, the imaginary companion helps the child to develop a sense of right and wrong. The imaginary companion usually has a very short life span, generally dying of "old age" by the time the child is 5 to 7 years old. For the preschooler, fantasy and reality frequently are not well delineated, as evidenced by the existence of imaginary companions and also by the child's love for fairy tales. A 4- to 5-year-old unabashedly tells tall tales, although he or she will, when encouraged, admit to creating a make-believe situation. By the age of 6 or 7 years, children are aware of the morality of lying. Although they are quick to accuse peers of cheating and lying, they often continue to cheat, seemingly guiltlessly, while playing.

Between the ages of 6 and 12 years, the child understands the concept of lying and its moral implications. However, lying may continue in an attempt to test adult-imposed moral codes. Children may admit to lying but have many rationalizations for their behavior. Rules are more important at this age than is winning, so cheating is less important and therefore less frequent. "Half-beliefs" become a part of the child's life; children become believers of superstitions, from the dangers of walking under a ladder to stepping on sidewalk cracks. Half-beliefs may extend into adulthood, and they are invested heavily with emotion. Their level of acceptance by the individual is inversely proportional to the individual's level of intellectual development.

Aside from developmental issues, external influences (family, school, and peers) affect the incidence of lying in children. Parents unconsciously may encourage their children to lie if expectations for the children exceed their ability to fulfill them and if truthfulness is not valued by the parents (i.e., if parents frequently lie). Parents who overestimate their child's academic capabilities frequently find that their child lies about grades received. Parents who tell "white lies" to protect the feelings of others, or for personal gain, fail to realize that young children cannot discern the moral issues involved in lying. Parents demanding to know why their son hit his younger sister or why the child broke the cookie jar are unaware that the child often cannot explain these behaviors to himself, much less to them. When interrogated, the confused child, in desperation, lies. According to Ginott,[2] "awkward lies" are told to avoid "embarrassing confessions"—confessions that the child knows from experience parents do not want to hear. For example, after hitting his younger sister, the son knows that his parents do not want to hear that he hit her because he does not like her. The parents want to believe that their children love each other, and they find it difficult to accept verbalizations to the contrary.

The child who is disciplined inconsistently, receives little positive reinforcement from parents, and lives in an inflexible, demanding environment often is the child who lies. Physicians can help parents deal with childhood lying in several ways. First, by apprising parents of what behavior is normal during maturational stages, the physician helps the parents understand more easily why their 5-year-old makes up stories or why their 7-year-old cheats at games. Second, by helping parents become aware of their importance as role models for their child, the physician effectively guides the parents in explaining to their child the importance of truthfulness. Third, when specific problems arise, the physician, by counseling gently and nonpunitively, encourages parents to be as tactful and nonthreatening with the child as possible. For example, Spock[4] believes that the child who spends much time with imaginary companions may need more age-appropriate friends or may be asking indirectly for more parental involvement in play activities.

Children who cheat at games past age 7 (when rules become more important and therefore cheating becomes a form of breaking the rules) need guidance from parents. If the parent is playing with a child who is cheating, the behavior should be identified calmly. The parent should tell the child that everyone likes to win and that losing is difficult to accept. Cheating among children, when identified, should best be settled among the players, without parental "judicial" intervention. Academic cheating is a more serious problem, frequently signaling that unrealistic expectations for performance have been placed on the child. Parents should be counseled to explore with school personnel possible academic problems.

Parents should be made cognizant of their importance as role models for their child and of the child's need for reasonable and clear expectations. Similarly, physicians must understand that they are role models for the parents whom they counsel. The physician who assumes a flexible, constructive, nonthreatening approach to problems raised by parents and who has been honest with the family in the past is more likely to be successful in counseling.

Lying becomes a symptom of more severe psychopathology under several circumstances. If other behaviors exist concomitantly (such as fire-setting, cruelty to animals, sleep disturbances, hyperactivity, phobias), there is a much greater likelihood of significant emotional disturbance. Similarly, if lying or fantasizing becomes a predominant behavior for children, more serious behavior disturbances must be suspected, such as chronically poor self-esteem, endogenous depression, and sociopathic behavior. Children who have few friends and limited interest in group activities often suffer from low self-esteem and depression. Children who lie for material gain and, apparently, guiltlessly may be displaying early signs of sociopathic behavior. If these symptoms are present and if attempts at counseling fail to dissipate lying, referral to a psychiatric professional should be considered.

STEALING

Stealing often represents a much more worrisome symptom to parents than does lying because the former more often involves situations outside the home, represents a much more severe societal taboo, and affects other people more directly. Indeed, especially during school years, stealing can be an ominous sign of psychiatric disturbance. However, it may represent conformity to peer pressure and consequently a transient phenomenon. Children under 3 years of age take things because they want them and have an immature sense of "mine" and "not mine," a concept related to their beginning struggle for independence from parents. Slowly they develop a conception of their own bodies (or property) and those of their parents. By age 3, children have a firmer sense of what belongs to *them*. They become possessive of their things and jealous of those of others, although they have only a tenuous grasp of others' property rights.

Between 3 and 7 years of age, as they begin to develop peer relationships, children become more respectful of property rights. However, they frequently give away their possessions and have not developed a concept of one thing being more valuable than many things (e.g., 25 hoarded pennies may be treasured much more than one piece of paper currency). The school-age child, though not yet completely mature, has a much more sophisticated sense of property rights. Consequently an 8-year-old may pick up loose change from the table while unsupervised. However, after about age 9, respect for property should be well integrated into the child. Children who steal at this age or beyond are motivated by one or more factors. They may steal in a group, especially during adolescence, to conform to peer pressure. They may suffer from poor self-esteem because they feel unloved by parents or because they have difficulty making friends. They may steal to buy friendship, to achieve peer acceptance, or to display to themselves and their parents that they are worthwhile because they can succeed in at least one activity. Stealing as a mechanism to improve self-esteem especially is common with adolescents, who are concomitantly attempting to separate from parents and to establish satisfactory same-sex and heterosexual relationships. If adolescents feel they have failed in both tasks, they frequently steal.

Families exert an important influence with respect to childhood stealing. If parents stole as children, they are more likely to assume a permissive role to intrafamilial stealing. Their reactions to extrafamilial stealing, however, may be extremely punitive, since their child's stealing will reflect unfavorably on them as parents. This value discrepancy between intrafamilial and extrafamilial acts is recognized easily by the child, whose resentment frequently precipitates intensified stealing. Parents giving little attention, affection, or approval to their child will potentiate poor self-esteem, which may result in stealing as the child attempts to attract attention and approval. Punishment may be ineffective, since the child may rationalize that, as Fraiberg[1] states, "Any ensuing punishment will cancel the crime."

Management of stealing, as in management of lying, requires an empathic but firm approach by both physician and parents. Parents should be advised to deal with the specific incident forthrightly. The child over 3 years of age should be confronted with the evidence but should not suffer interrogative techniques (e.g., the parent should say, "I believe you took $5 from my wallet," rather than, "Why did you take $5 from my wallet?"). Immediate restitution of the stolen item is extremely important. If the article has been taken from a friend, the child should return it. If the article has been stolen from a store, the parent should accompany the child to the store and explain to the manager tactfully that the child took an item without paying for it and now wants to return it. The parents should voice their disapproval of stealing to the child but should also reinforce their belief in the child's basic integrity. A child who has stolen usually has poor self-esteem; punitive measures serve to damage self-concept further and imbue in the child the parent's mistrust.

Several specific questions should come to mind when the child steals because the answers may aid in management. Is the child receiving a reasonable allowance? If not, the child may feel the need to resort to stealing to obtain spending money. Are there unrealistic academic pressures on the child? Children who feel they cannot fulfill academic expectations of parents frequently steal to display at least transiently their success in one activity. Is the child having difficulty making friends? Stealing often occurs in situations in which the child feels that peer group acceptance can be achieved by offering peers stolen material goods. In cases of group stealing, are alternative community facilities available to occupy extracurricular hours? Although structured community activities may not obliterate all acts of group stealing, they may help to discourage such acts by offering alternative activities to occupy adolescents' time.

Stealing assumes more ominous connotations in several situations. As in lying, if other behavioral disturbances coexist, a more psychiatrically sophisticated approach may be necessary. A child who steals without guilt, who compulsively steals (kleptomania), or who seemingly steals in a setting in which apprehension is inevitable may have serious emotional problems. Frequently these are children who received little or inconsistent love and security as infants. Without psychiatric intervention, they will progress to delinquent and ultimately criminal life-styles (see Chapter 102, Juvenile Delinquency). Unfortunately, psychic damage to these children often is severe by the time psychiatric referral finally is made.

REFERRAL CRITERIA

Effective referral to mental health specialists for problems of lying and stealing requires several things of referring physicians. The family should be informed of the possible need for referral when the physician first suspects a potential for significant psychopathology. As in managing less severe cases, the referring physician should be empathic and non-punitive in the explanation given to parents. The physician should make sure that the parents do not think that their child is "crazy" because he or she is being referred. The parents also should know that the referral does not sever the physician's relationship with the family. Continued communication by the referring physician, both with the family and with the specialist, often solidifies recommendations made to parents by the therapist and encourages compliance with recommendations. The physician personally should introduce the family to the therapist. In general a team approach between the referring doctor and specialist increases the treatment plan's efficacy.

SUMMARY

Lying and stealing in childhood usually cause both parents and physicians concern and also create much worry for the involved child. The seriousness of these behaviors depends on many factors: the age of the child, the circumstances that precipitate the behavior, the psychosocial adjustment of the child (in school, with peers, and at home), and the reaction of parents. The physician's approach to the problem influences whether the behavior disappears or intensifies. In dealing with problems of lying and stealing, the physician should obtain a complete history, explain carefully to the parents and the patient the significance of the behavior, and ensure regular follow-up for the problem. If referral to psychologically trained professionals becomes necessary, the physician is obligated to prepare the family for the referral, to maintain communication with the consultant, and to offer the family emotional support before and after the consultation. In most cases lying and stealing represent transient developmental behavioral problems that resolve if an empathic approach is used by parents and physician. However, the symptoms are not to be ignored in hopes that the child will "grow out of it" or because "all children lie and steal."

REFERENCES

1. Fraiberg S: *The magic years,* New York, 1968, Charles Scribner's Sons.
2. Ginott HG: *Between parent and child,* New York, 1965, Macmillan.
3. MacFarlane JW, Allen L, Honzik MP: *A developmental study of the behavior problems of normal children between twenty-one months and fourteen years,* Berkeley and Los Angeles, 1954, University of California Press.
4. Spock B: *Baby and child care,* New York, 1985, Pocket Books.
5. Stone LJ, Church JC: *Childhood and adolescence: a psychology of the growing person,* ed 5, New York, 1984, Random House.

85 Nightmares and Other Sleep Disturbances

Thomas F. Anders

During the first 2 years of life sleep problems are the most frequent complaint of parents at the time of pediatric visits; 30% to 50% of infants manifest disrupted sleep serious enough to cause parents to seek professional assistance.[4,9,13,18] Richman[19] has defined problem sleep in 1-year-old infants as either sleep onset periods associated with fussing that regularly last longer than 30 minutes or night waking episodes that occur at least four nights a week and require parental intervention. During the toddler period the rates of disturbance increase. Sleep problems often are associated with daytime behavior disorders.[10,20,21,23]

Sleep problems continue during the preschool years. Zuckerman et al.[24] followed prospectively 8-month-old infants who had sleep problems and found that 41% still had problems when they were 3 years old. Retrospectively, only 26% of the children who had sleep problems at age 3 years did not manifest them when they were 8 months old. In another 3-year follow-up study of 2-year-olds, Kataria et al.[12] found that 84% of the children still suffered from their sleep problems. Similarly Richman et al.[21] found that almost 50% of the 3-year-old night wakers had had their problem from birth and that 40% of the children who had sleep problems at 8 years of age had had problems at least from the time they were 3 years old. These reports emphasize that sleep problems in infancy often are persistent and may lead to chronic sleep problems. They confirm some retrospective studies of adults who have sleep problems who recall disrupted sleep during childhood.[8,17,22]

With the introduction of polygraphic recording techniques in the 1950s, we have been able to investigate physiological and behavioral activities during sleep. It now is well established that sleep is not a unitary state of physiological restitution but rather two cycling states of differing physiological function and activity. A description of the adult sleep cycle provides an introduction to an understanding of developing sleep patterns in the infant and young child.

Four states of electroencephalographic (EEG) activity during adult sleep have been described by Dement and Kleitman[6]: stage I is typified by low-voltage, fast activity; stage II by the presence of sleep spindles and K complexes against a low-voltage background; and stages III and IV by varying degrees of slow, high-voltage, delta-wave activity.

Sleep spindles are defined as EEG activity of 12 to 14 Hz, at least 0.5 second in duration, occurring in runs of greater than 6. K complexes are defined as EEG wave forms having a well-delineated negative sharp wave, which is followed immediately by a positive component. The total duration of the complex should exceed 0.5 second. The K complex generally is maximal over vertex regions. Delta-wave activity is defined as waves of two cycles per second or slower, which have amplitudes greater than 75 μV from peak to peak.

Rapid eye movement (REM) sleep is defined by the occurrence of a stage I EEG pattern in association with binocularly synchronous rapid eye movements, the suppression of muscle tone as recorded from the chin electromyogram (EMG), and accelerated, irregular respiratory and heart rates. Nonrapid eye movement (NREM) sleep lacks REMs and is accompanied by the presence of tonic muscle activity recorded from the chin EMG, a stage II, III, or IV EEG pattern, and slowed, regular cardiac and respiratory rates. Alternating REM and NREM sleep states represent two distinct patterns of neurophysiological organization: the REM state is highly activated; the NREM state is basal and highly regulated. They follow each other in a periodic fashion, and together they make up the sleep cycle.

Although active REM sleep periods of infants are qualitatively similar to REM periods of adults, three important quantitative differences have been described: whereas adults spend 20% of a night's sleep in active REM sleep, sleeping full-term neonates, recorded for a 4-hour interfeeding sleep period or for an entire 24-hour period, spend 50% of their total sleep in this state. The proportionate amount of time spent in active REM sleep diminishes as the infant becomes older and as the central nervous system (CNS) matures. Second, infants frequently enter sleep through an initial active REM period, in contrast to adults, who enter their first REM period 90 minutes after the onset of sleep. Third, active REM periods emerge more frequently in infants than do REM periods in adults; thus the infant's sleep cycle is shorter than the adult's. Active REM periods recur every 50 to 60 minutes during infancy in contrast to every 90 to 100 minutes as reported in adults. The staging of quiet NREM sleep by EEG criteria into four distinct NREM sleep stages becomes possible only after the second 6 months of life.[2] The differences between sleep patterns in infants and adults are outlined in Table 85-1.

PATHOLOGICAL SLEEP PATTERNS

Certified pediatric sleep disorders centers, using modern techniques of polysomnography to record multiple physiological parameters during a night of sleep, are rapidly becoming important in the diagnostic assessment of sleep disturbances. *The International Classification of Sleep Disorders Diagnostic and Coding Manual*[1] broadly classifies three categories of disordered sleep: dysomnias, parasomnias, and sleep disorders associated with medical/psychiatric conditions.

The *dysomnias* are defined as disorders of insufficient, excessive, or inefficient sleep, characterized by either difficulty in initiating and/or maintaining sleep, or in contrast, by excessive sleepiness. The disorders of initiating and maintaining sleep (DIMS), generically referred to as the *insomnias,* comprise disorders associated with complaints of insufficient

Table 85-1 Comparison Between Infant and Adult Sleep Patterns

Parameter	Infant	Adult
Ratio of REM to NREM	50:50	20:80
Periodicity of sleep states	50- to 60-min REM-NREM cycle	90- to 100-min REM-NREM cycle
Sleep onset state	REM sleep onset	NREM sleep onset
Temporal organization of sleep states	REM-NREM cycles equally throughout sleep period	NREM stages III and IV predominant in first third of night; REM state predominant in last third of night
Maturation of EEG patterns	Low-voltage, fast EEG pattern High-voltage, slow EEG pattern 1 NREM EEG stage	K complexes Delta-waves 4 NREM EEG stages
Concordance of sleep measures (organization of sleep states)	Poor	Good

sleep to support good daytime functioning. The disorders of excessive somnolence (DOES), also known as the *hypersomnias,* are disorders in which a persistent need for sleep is excessive and leads to impaired daytime functioning.

The *parasomnias* are defined by behaviors that intrude upon the sleep process as a result of central or autonomic nervous system activation. Parasomnias are not primary disorders of sleep-wake organization; rather, they represent disruptions of sleep continuity. This presentation focuses on parasomnias—the sleep disorders characterized by episodic events that interrupt sleep. The insomnias and the hypersomnias, including narcolepsy and the sleep apnea syndrome, are reviewed extensively elsewhere.[3] An idealized version of a night's sleep is portrayed in Figure 85-1, which serves as a useful guide for locating the parasomnias and sleep disturbances described below.

Parasomnias

The NREM parasomnias include pavor nocturnus (night terrors), somnambulism (sleepwalking), somniloquy (sleeptalking), and possibly, stage IV sleep-related enuresis. The REM parasomnias include nightmares and REM behavior disorder. NREM parasomnias also have been called *disorders of arousal.* They have certain features in common: mental confusion and disorientation, automatic behaviors, relative nonreactivity to external stimuli, difficulty in being fully awakened, and fragmentary or absent dream recall. The next morning the episode is not remembered. Most characteristic of the disorders of arousal is their occurrence at a typical point in the sleep cycle, usually in the first third of the sleep period, at the point of transition from stage IV NREM sleep to REM sleep, as indicated in Fig. 85-1. Instead of the usual smooth transition to the lighter state of REM sleep, the individual who has a NREM parasomnia arouses suddenly and manifests symptoms of autonomic discharge.

Most younger children outgrow the symptoms of NREM parasomnias as they mature neurophysiologically. When these disturbances persist in adolescents and adults, however, secondary psychological conflicts frequently complicate the clinical picture. Although specific medications are available for disabling symptomatology, reassuring support to the family and child, blended with an optimistic and patient attitude, generally suffices. Medications should be prescribed only when the symptoms are so severe that they affect waking behavior, particularly school performance, peer interaction, and family relationships. Parasomnias can be diagnosed most often from a careful history. In rare cases temporal lobe seizures may mimic these disorders, but adequate study in a sleep laboratory readily differentiates epileptic disorders from a sleep disorder. Children whose presentations of symptomatology are unusual (daytime attacks or attacks between 1 AM and 6 AM when stage IV NREM sleep is absent) should be referred to a sleep disorders center.

Pavor Nocturnus. Pavor nocturnus, or night terrors, is found with greatest frequency among children 3 to 8 years of age. In some, however, symptoms may begin during the second half of the first year of life; a small number of children will continue to have severe night terror attacks into adulthood.

Night terrors must be differentiated from the more common nightmare or anxiety dream. Nightmares are associated with vivid visual imagery. They occur during REM sleep, and the child is aroused fully after the episode. Recall of the nightmare's content is excellent. In pavor nocturnus, approximately 90 to 100 minutes after going to sleep the child suddenly sits upright in bed and screams. Tachypnea, tachycardia, and other signs of autonomic activation are apparent. The child usually is inconsolable for 5 to 30 minutes, then finally relaxes and returns to sleep. If the child arouses, dream recall is fragmentary. The following morning the child has no memory of the attack. Attacks frequently occur after stressful or especially fatiguing daytime activities. The diagnosis can be made most often from the history alone. An attack occurring during the latter third of the night with vivid recall is unlikely to be pavor nocturnus (see Fig. 85-1) but rather a nightmare or a spontaneous awakening. Most night terror episodes in young children occur so infrequently that medication is not indicated. For severe cases, however, the drug of choice is diazepam (Valium).

Somnambulism and Somniloquy. Somnambulism and somniloquy present more commonly during the school-age years. According to Kales et al.[11] 15% of all children between the ages of 5 and 12 years have walked in their sleep at least once. Persistent sleepwalking occurs in 1% to 6% of the population, afflicting more males than females, and often is associated with nocturnal enuresis. A typical somnambulistic episode consists of the following behavioral sequence: a body movement during stage IV NREM sleep is followed by the subject abruptly sitting upright in bed. Although the eyes are open, they appear glassy and "unseeing." Movements are

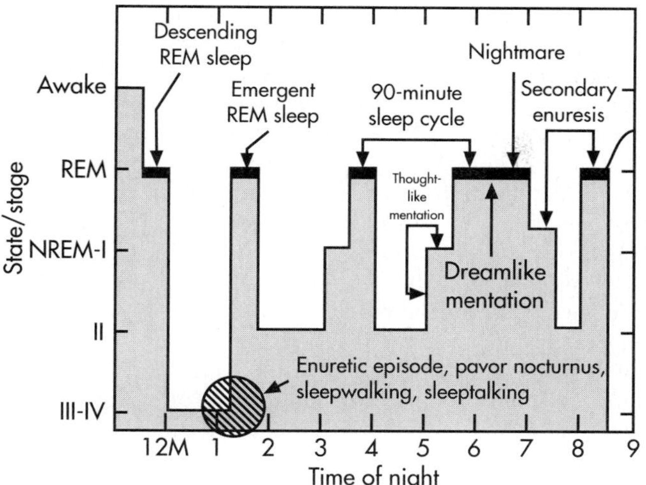

FIG. 85-1 An idealized all-night sleep state histogram. The various disorders and disturbances of sleep are depicted at their usual point of occurrence.

clumsy, and efforts to communicate with the sleepwalker usually elicit mumbled and slurred speech with monosyllabic answers. The total duration of the episode may range from 10 to 30 seconds when sitting in bed to 5 to 30 minutes or more when actually walking. The event is not remembered on awakening in the morning. Severe sleepwalkers may have one to four episodes weekly. The episode occurs most often at the transition point from stage IV NREM sleep to the first REM period. If individuals who have a predilection for somnambulism or somniloquy are aroused during stage IV NREM sleep, a walking or talking episode may be precipitated. In contrast, no such response is obtained from unaffected controls.

Several misconceptions about sleepwalking and sleeptalking need to be addressed. Sleepwalkers are not acting out dreams and are not in control of purposeful actions. Rather, sleepwalkers are in danger. They frequently hurt themselves and must be protected from self-injury by a secure environment. Similarly, somniloquists do not reveal their deepest secrets while sleeptalking. Their utterances most often are incomprehensible or monosyllabic. Meaningful speech and purposeful walking during sleep suggest psychological dissociative disorders rather than physiological NREM parasomnia symptomatology. Again, as in night terrors, temporal lobe epilepsy must be ruled out, particularly in adults. As the CNS matures somnambulistic episodes usually diminish and disappear spontaneously. For severe, intractable cases, diazepam has been used successfully.

Mixed Parasomnias

Sleep-related Enuresis. Enuresis should not be considered a syndrome, but rather a symptom of a disorder. By careful history one should determine whether the enuretic symptom has been present from birth (primary) or has occurred after a period of successful training (secondary), whether it is confined to the night or occurs during the day as well, and whether organic factors are present. In addition, an attempt should be made to localize the episode to a time of night and point in the sleep cycle. Sleep-related enuresis usually is primary and occurs only at night, often during the first third of the sleep period at the transition point from stage IV NREM sleep to REM sleep. Enuretic episodes however, may occur at any point during the night.

Sleep-related enuresis probably is the most common parasomnia of childhood. Broughton[5] has defined an enuretic episode as one that occurs generally 1 to 3 hours after sleep onset as the child shifts from stage IV NREM sleep to the first REM period. The sleep state change often is associated with a body movement and increased muscle tone, followed by tachycardia, tachypnea, erection (in males), and decreased skin resistance. Micturition occurs 30 seconds to 4 minutes after the start of the episode in a moment of relative quiet. Immediately after micturition, children are difficult to awaken and, when aroused, indicate that they have not dreamed. They also do not remember the event. Broughton[5] has demonstrated that enuretic children have higher resting intravesical pressures, especially during stage IV NREM sleep, have more frequent and spontaneous bladder contractions during stage IV NREM sleep, and have secondary contractions in response to naturally and artificially occurring increases in pressure in contrast to nonenuretic controls, whose bladder functions and capacities are normal. On the other hand Mikkelsen and Rapoport[15] report that enuresis is not limited to stage IV NREM sleep.

For children who have severe sleep-related enuresis, imipramine (Tofranil) has proved to be effective. It is unclear whether it is efficacious primarily because of its anticholinergic properties affecting bladder tone or because of its stimulant effect on the sleep-stage pattern. A flexible dosage and slow withdrawal schedule are recommended. Conditioning methods also are effective and recommended as a first choice (see Chapter 82, Enuresis, for a more complete discussion of this subject).

REM Parasomnias

The most common REM parasomnia is the nightmare. Nightmares are awakenings from REM sleep associated with dream reports that are typically anxiety-laden and frightening. Stress of various kinds, and especially traumatic experiences, increase the frequency and severity of nightmares. Certain medications, including beta-adrenergic blockers and the withdrawal of REM suppressants, can induce or increase the incidence of nightmares.

Nightmares usually start between the ages of 3 and 6 years and affect 10% to 50% of children in that age group severely enough to disturb their parents. Nightmares are easily differentiated from sleep terrors. Nightmares occur later in the night, usually in the last third of the sleep period, when REM sleep predominates. Nightmares characteristically are more organized, in terms of frightening dream reports, than sleep terrors. The child recounting a nightmare is fully awake and oriented. There usually is good recall of the nightmare in the morning. Nightmares also need to be differentiated from REM sleep behavior disorders described below. Treatment of nightmares consists of comforting at the time of occurrence and reducing precipitating daytime stresses when possible. For children who have serious behavioral disruption associated with regularly recurring nightmares, individual or family psychotherapy may be indicated.

REM Sleep Behavior Disorder. REM sleep behavior disorder (RSBD) is a rare parasomnia characterized by vigorous and sometimes violent self-directed or other-directed motor attacks that interrupt REM sleep. Typically, peripheral muscle tone is inhibited during REM sleep, causing sleep "paralysis." In RSBD, however, the tonic inhibition is interrupted episodically, which leads to motor outbursts. CNS anomalies or lesions are associated with this disorder in both children and adults.[14]

Dysomnias and Developmental Disturbances of Sleep

The disorders described in this section are characterized by normal polysomnography. Nevertheless, they may be a source of psychological suffering for the child and conflict within the family. Virtually all parents anticipate sleep disturbances in their children. These sleep disturbances are much more common than those described previously. They often reflect normal phases of development and have been loosely labeled as *insomnias* and *nightmares*. The majority are transient, and although they are a source of irritation and concern, they are inconsequential. Sometimes, when overwhelming or persistent, they may indicate a more serious psychopathological condition. Medication usually is not indicated, although the short-term use of chloral hydrate has been advocated to promote peace and quiet in the family and prevent the sleep disturbance from becoming ingrained by "positive" reinforcement. Understanding the source of a child's anxiety, the parental concerns, and the family situation most often is sufficient to enable the pediatrician to provide supportive guidance until the disturbance subsides.

These sleep disturbances may occur anytime from the imminent approach of bedtime to awakening. Ferber[7] has reviewed these disturbances extensively; they can be classified according to their most common age of appearance. This system of classification affords optimum understanding of the disturbance within the context of the child's developmental stage.

First Year of Life. During the first year of life, sleeping through the night ("settling") and night awakenings are the primary concerns of the family. In England a comprehensive investigation of sleep patterns among infants during the first year of life reported that 70% of babies slept through the night, or settled, by 3 months of age. Another 13% had settled by 6 months of age, and 10% never slept through the night without interruption. Once settling occurred, night waking recurred in 50% of the infants during the second half of the first year of life.[16] Environmental factors, such as changed sleeping arrangements, separations, minor trauma, and new family members, were associated with night waking after settling had occurred, although these factors did not seem to affect the age of initial settling.

Second Year of Life. The problems of separation and object permanence confront the immature ego of the 2-year-old child. Lacking the capacity to differentiate between absence and total disappearance of an object, the child attempts to hold on to important ties to avoid the fear of loss. A prevalent disturbance of this age therefore is reluctance to go to sleep. Substitute (transitional) objects, such as teddy bears or blankets, often tide the child over difficult separations. By the end of the second year, with the acquisition of language and the development of a sense of object permanence, these difficulties often disappear. Because children of this age also are overexcited and frightened easily by daytime experiences, nightmares also make their appearance in this age group.

Third to Fifth Years of Life. It is rare to find a child in the age group of 3 to 5 years who is not experiencing some difficulty over sleep, whether it be tardiness in falling asleep, nightmares, projective fears of ghosts and wild animals, fear of the dark, inability to sleep alone, or ritualistic presleep behaviors. These disturbances usually are associated with frightening or otherwise conflictual daytime experiences. They most often are transient and responsive to minimal environmental manipulation. If refractive, sleep disturbances may represent one symptom of a more profound psychological conflict. In such cases they usually reflect the child's inability to enter into the widening world of social relationships. Family counseling or individual psychotherapy may be indicated.

USE OF THE SLEEP LABORATORY IN THE DIFFERENTIAL DIAGNOSIS

Polysomnography in pediatric sleep disorder centers has been increasingly useful in diagnosing sleep-related pathological conditions. The following case report is exemplary:

Richard, a 7-year-old boy, was referred because of night wakening occurring several times a night, four to five times a week. These attacks started approximately 1 hour after falling asleep and were associated with disorientation, confusion, and screaming. The boy did not remember the event in the morning. Frequently, second and third attacks occurred later in the night. Sometimes these attacks were associated with sleepwalking. Complete physical and neurological examinations, including two waking EEGs, were unremarkable. A variety of medications, including phenytoin (Dilantin), diazepam, flurazepam (Dalmane), imipramine, and barbiturates, were successful for short periods of time, but then symptomatology worsened.

The sleep disorders clinic workup revealed a complex disturbance. Continuous all-night polysomnography and time-lapse video monitoring were carried out. Approximately 65 minutes after the onset of sleep, during the midst of stage IV NREM sleep, Richard sat up glassy-eyed and began screaming. He appeared in obvious distress and was inconsolable. After about 5 minutes, he lay back in his bed and returned to sleep. At 3:30 AM, some 6½ hours after he fell asleep, Richard again aroused and began to cry out. This arousal was from stage I NREM sleep. The arousal was followed by movement and was characterized by a waking EEG pattern. For the next 10 minutes Richard remained awake with his eyes closed, sobbing and crying out. Finally he returned to sleep, covered by a sheet and curled up in a fetal position. Approximately 1 hour later, another attack resembling the latter occurred. The character of the first attack was markedly different from the two later attacks. In the first attack Richard seemed disoriented and confused, whereas in the later ones he awakened and appeared depressed and anxious. Thus it was apparent from our video monitoring and our polysomnographic recording that we were dealing with two distinct types of sleep disturbances—night terror attacks and night waking episodes. Although the various medications had suppressed the night terror attacks, secondary sleep disturbances broke through repeatedly.

We recommended that, since Richard's anxiety was excessive and inhibiting, family counseling and psychotherapy be instituted. We felt that the secondary sleep disturbance was more important than the night terror attacks and therefore suggested that medications be withheld. Six months after evaluation, the family situation had improved, and the nighttime disturbances had diminished significantly without medication.

REFERENCES

1. American Sleep Disorders Association: *The international classification of sleep disorders: diagnostic and coding manual,* Lawrence, Kansas, 1990, Allen Press.
2. Anders T, Carskadon M, Dement W: Sleep and sleepiness in children and adolescents, *Pediatr Clin North Am* 27:29, 1980.
3. Anders T: *Treatment of sleep disorders.* In Gabbard G, editor: *Treatment of psychiatric disorders: the DSM-IV edition,* Washington, DC, 1994, American Psychiatric Press.
4. Beltramini A, Hertzig M: Sleep and bedtime behavior in preschool-aged children, *Pediatrics* 71:153, 1983.
5. Broughton R: Sleep disorders: disorders of arousal? *Science* 159:1070, 1968.
6. Dement W, Kleitman N: Cyclic variations in EEG during sleep and their relation to eye movements, body motility and dreaming, *Electroencephalogr Clin Neurophysiol* 9:673, 1957.
7. Ferber R: *Solve your child's sleep problems,* New York, 1985, Simon & Schuster.
8. Hauri P, Olmstead E: Childhood-onset insomnia. *Sleep* 3:59, 1980.
9. Jacklin C et al: Sleep pattern development from 6 through 33 months, *J Pediatr Psychol* 5:295, 1980.
10. Jenkins S, Bax M, Hart H: Behavior problems in preschool children, *J Child Psychol Psychiatry* 21:5, 1980.
11. Kales J, Soldatos C, Kales A: *Childhood sleep disorders.* In Gellis S, Kagan B, editors: *Current pediatric therapy,* ed 9, Philadelphia, 1980, WB Saunders.
12. Kataria S, Swanson M, Trevarthin G: Persistence of sleep disturbances in preschool children, *J Pediatr* 110:642, 1987.
13. Klackenberg G: Sleep behavior studied longitudinally: data from 4-16 years in duration, night awakening and bedtime, *Acta Paediatr Scand* 71:501, 1982.
14. Mahowald MW, Rosen GM: Parasomnias in children, *Pediatrician* 17:21, 1990.
15. Mikkelsen E, Rapoport J: Enuresis: psychopathology, sleep stage and drug response, *Urol Clin North Am* 7:361, 1980.
16. Moore T, Ucko LE: Night waking in early infancy. I., *Arch Dis Child* 32:333, 1957.
17. Monroe L: Psychological and physiological differences between good and poor sleepers, *J Abnorm Psychol* 72:255, 1967.
18. Ragins N, Schachter S: A study of sleep behavior in two-year old children, *J Am Acad Child Psychiatry* 10:464, 1971.
19. Richman N: A community survey of characteristics of one- to two-year-olds with sleep disruptions, *J Am Acad Child Psychiatry* 20:281, 1981.
20. Richman N: Sleep problems in young children, *Arch J Dis Child* 56:491, 1984.
21. Richman N, Stevenson J, Graham P: *Preschool to school: a behavioral study,* London, 1982, Academic Press.
22. Salzarulo P, Chevalier A: Sleep problems in children and their relationships with early disturbances of the waking-sleeping rhythms, *Sleep* 6:47, 1983.
23. Simonds J, Parraga H: Sleep behaviors and disorders in children and adolescents evaluated at psychiatric clinics, *Dev Behav Pediatr* 5:6, 1984.
24. Zuckerman B, Stevenson J, Baily V: Sleep problems in early childhood: predictive factors and behavioral correlates, *Pediatrics* 80:664, 1987.

86 Peer Relationship Problems

Sharon L. Foster and Heidi M. Inderbitzen

Peer relations and positive social interaction are crucial to the normal development of children. A child's relations with peers serve important functions in his or her life, including promoting the development of social skills through interaction and feedback, providing emotional support and security, enhancing feelings of self-worth; providing guidance, assistance, and companionship, and offering validation through sharing information about common situations and events during childhood and adolescence. The importance of peer relations is highlighted by the finding that by the sixth grade, children spend twice as much time with their peers as with their parents.

EPIDEMIOLOGY

Being poorly accepted by one's peer group and lacking friends are the major identifying characteristics of children who have peer relationship problems. These can be manifested in three ways: social withdrawal, social neglect, and peer rejection. Socially withdrawn children interact infrequently. Socially neglected children are those who are ignored by peers and are neither liked nor disliked. Socially rejected children are openly and actively rejected by peers.

Studies investigating peer relationship problems have indicated incidence rates between 3% and 22%. As many as 33% of all children in regular classrooms have low levels of social interaction; 3% are classified as socially withdrawn.[7] Other investigations[11,13,25] have suggested that between 6% and 22% of children in third through sixth grade have no friends in their classrooms, and an additional 12% to 22% have only one classroom friend.[11,13] Furthermore, reports indicate that 10% of elementary school children are especially lonely.[7]

There is some evidence that rejection is relatively stable, with one investigation finding that about 67% of rejected children assessed in elementary school still had peer problems 5 years later.[3] Neglected children's status was less stable, with only 25% still manifesting peer relationship difficulties over the same interval. Reports indicate that between 40% and 60% of children who have few or no friends are socially withdrawn or neglected, whereas the remainder are rejected by peers.[13] Girls are slightly more likely than boys to have classroom friends.[18]

Some evidence indicates that children who have poor peer relations (particularly peer rejection) experience short- and long-term social and emotional adjustment problems. Relative to their peers, poorly accepted children feel lonelier and less satisfied both with their peer relationships in general and with specific friendships[19] and are overrepresented in mental health referrals for concurrent problems such as attention deficit/hyperactivity disorder, conduct disorder, and anxiety and depressive disorders.[7] Problematic peer relations in childhood and adolescence have been linked to problems later in life, including juvenile delinquency, dropping out of school, adult criminality, bad conduct discharges from military services, and other mental health problems in adulthood. On the other hand, positive peer relations have been associated with academic achievement and better interpersonal adjustment in later life.[17,25] Unfortunately, causal relationships between early peer problems and later difficulties have not been established. Whether withdrawn and neglected children experience serious concurrent or future difficulties is not well documented and continues to provoke controversy. Nonetheless, the substantial number of associations noted above strongly suggests that intervening early with children who have poor peer relationships may alleviate current dysfunction and prevent dysfunction later in life.

ETIOLOGICAL FACTORS

Understanding the etiology of peer relationship problems is complicated by findings that children may lack friends for a variety of reasons. Characteristics of the child, including physical attractiveness, race, sex, and academic competence, may affect his or her social status with peers. The major hypothesis with respect to why children have difficulties in peer relationships, however, is that children who have problems possess inadequate repertoires of social skills, which result in ineffective social interaction, causing them to be ignored or actively rejected by their peers.[17] This negative experience may encourage further maladaptive responses such as increased social withdrawal or retaliatory verbal or physical aggression. These behaviors could in turn create a vicious circle by making children even less accepted by their peers.

Various theories of the development of socially skillful behavior have some empirical support, but none has unequivocal acceptance. Behavioral theories of etiology propose that early socialization by parents influences the acquisition of social repertoires through modeling, direct teaching, classical conditioning, and providing rewards as positive feedback for appropriate social behavior.[23] Others hypothesize that poor social skills result from inadequate development of information-processing skills believed to be prerequisites for effective social intervention.[8] These include (1) perceiving and interpreting social situations correctly, (2) generating and evaluating possible ways of responding, (3) selecting and performing an appropriate response, (4) and monitoring the impact of that response. Related hypotheses emphasize the role of social role-taking (the ability to view situations from others' perspectives) and empathy (actually experiencing another's feelings) in adaptive peer relationships.

Research with preschool and first-grade children highlights the relationship between family experience and children's social competence.[15,22] Children who are poorly accepted, when compared with peers who are better accepted, interact with their mothers in more negative and demanding ways. Their mothers are less positive and more negative, focus less on feelings, and participate less in play during these interactions. Fathers of unpopular children issue more commands and engage less in their child's play.[15] Parent-reported spousal and parent-child aggressive conflict also relate negatively to peer acceptance.[28] Additionally, mothers of poorly accepted children supervise their children more intrusively than mothers of better accepted children.[14] Finally, deviant maternal values and expectations (e.g., positive endorsement of aggression as a solution to interpersonal problems and mothers' reports of more coercive discipline) are associated both with how children think about social problems and with peers' and teachers' views of children's social competence in the classroom.[12,20] Together, these findings suggest that early social experiences play an important role in children's development of socially competent behavior and social cognition, which then act as proximal causes for peer acceptance and rejection.[2]

CHARACTERISTICS AND DIAGNOSIS

Observations of socially withdrawn and neglected children reveal similar behavioral characteristics. Rejected children display a different constellation of behavior, particularly during preschool and early elementary school years (see the article by Newcomb et al.[16] for a review). Children who spend little time interacting with peers at school also do not initiate interactions with peers and fail to respond to others' initiations. They tend to be less verbal than their classmates. Furthermore they spend more time in solitary activities and play submissive or deferent roles when they do interact with more sociable partners.[26] Some of these children may experience more anxiety, low self-esteem, and depression than their peers, although for what percentage of children these reactions are outside the normal range is not yet clear.[27]

In contrast, peer rejection in preschool and the primary grades has been associated with more actively negative behavior—higher rates of "off-task" behavior as well as solitary activity, greater dependence on adults, negative statements, interference with ongoing activities, aggression, and failure to conform to classroom rules. Poorly accepted children have difficulty joining ongoing play activities and are more likely than their peers to disengage from the group, to make weak demands, to engage in incoherent behavior (i.e., inaudible, ambiguous, or nonsensical), or to hover near the peer group. They interrupt the flow of social exchange by being disagreeable and demanding.[24] Once engaged in group play, rejected boys engage in more physical and verbal aggression than do their better-accepted peers.[4,6]

Rejection also has been linked to *relational aggression* (behavior such as social ostracism intended to harm another's social relationships) in both boys and girls. In general, relational aggression is more characteristic of elementary school girls than boys, whereas physical aggression is more common among boys.[5]

Children also treat rejected classmates differently than they treat their better-accepted peers. Peers initiate relatively few interactions with rejected children and may view their positive behavior less favorably than they do similar behavior by better-accepted peers. Researchers document that behavioral differences between rejected and better-accepted peers are more readily apparent during preschool and early elementary school than during later primary school years, perhaps because important social behavior is less readily observed as children grow older.

In addition, poorly accepted children differ from their better-accepted peers in how they think about and try to solve social dilemmas. When questioned about handling interpersonal problems, rejected children's responses indicate that their knowledge of appropriate behavior may be deficient. Rejected children may be able to verbalize only one or two appropriate strategies to cope with a problem, and they voice unusual or inappropriate responses when pressed for other options. Furthermore, as compared with average boys, aggressive boys are less accurate at detecting prosocial intentions but more accurate at detecting hostile intentions, generate a higher proportion of aggressive responses to hypothetical situations, and are less likely to choose appropriate responses when evaluating the possible ways of reacting to problems. Although most studies treat rejected children as a homogenous group, findings suggest that there are at least two distinct subtypes of rejected boys: aggressive-rejected and nonaggressive-rejected, with different behavioral profiles.[9,21] Peers view aggressive-rejected boys as more aggressive and disruptive than accepted boys; teachers report that these children lack self-control and academic motivation and appear anxious. Peers view nonaggressive-rejected boys as more withdrawn, inattentive, and immature than others.

Subgroups seen by peers as aggressive and nonaggressive also emerge among girls.[10] Peers see both groups as withdrawn. Teachers view the nonaggressive subgroup of girls as more deviant than nonaggressive boys and as having particular difficulties with anxiety and academic performance.

Detection of peer relationship problems by the physician is complicated by several factors. Most children's problems are first noted by teachers and peers and occur in the school. Parents may be unaware that the child has difficulties because they are uninformed, they ignore the teacher's feedback, or the child behaves differently at home. Although some rejected children recognize their difficulties and will admit to loneliness and low self-esteem, others view themselves no differently than their well-accepted peers and may deny that they have difficulties.[1] Indications that peer relationship problems may be present include reports from the child's teacher, complaints by the child that he or she has few or no friends, evidence that the child frequently is used as a scapegoat by others, or reports of excessive shyness around other children, particularly at school. In addition, interpersonal difficulties have been associated with physical disabilities, learning disabilities, obesity, conduct disorders, hyperactivity, and delinquency; thus assessment of the child's functioning with peers would seem warranted when any of these correlated problems is present.

MANAGEMENT AND INTERVENTION

The physician's direct intervention with a child having peer relationship problems is of questionable use unless the physician plans to meet with the child, teachers, or parents every week. However, the physician who sees the child only occasionally can still play an important role in educating both parents and teachers about the importance of developing good peer relationship skills. Furthermore, he or she may be able to advise them of initial strategies to ameliorate the problem. In addition, the physician may be able to identify the cases in which the child's rejection may be a result of poor physical appearance and instruct the parents and child in more appropriate dress or personal hygiene.

For the young child who has more minor or circumscribed peer relationship difficulties, advising the parents or teacher to provide the child with toys that require cooperation and sharing (e.g., seesaw, board games, flash cards) can lead to increased positive social interaction. Cooperative parents and teachers also can be advised to engineer opportunities for the child to interact positively with peers and then attend to and positively reinforce desirable social behaviors, such as cooperative play, while ignoring negative or nonsocial behaviors.

Children rejected because of off-task and disruptive behavior that results from academic problems may improve behaviorally when provided with effective tutoring so that they can keep up academically with their peers.

With children whose difficulties are pervasive or whose parents and teachers are uncooperative, more extensive intervention is advisable. Intervention methods that have documented effectiveness vary with the age of the child. With preschoolers and young primary grade-age withdrawn children, modeling can be effective in increasing positive peer interactions. Modeling procedures typically include observation of other children (usually filmed) engaged in positive interaction, followed by opportunities for the child to engage in similar activities with peers. Modeling has been shown to be effective generally, although less so for children from families of lower socioeconomic status. Alternatively, reinforcement programs can be instituted in which the teacher or parent rewards positive social participation with praise, attention, or tokens that can be exchanged later for privileges or other rewards. A variant of this procedure appropriate for withdrawn children involves verbally praising peers for interacting with the withdrawn child, which presumably leads others to get to know the withdrawn child better and to begin to include him or her in their activities. This approach, however, is contraindicated for the child whose responses to peers often are negative, as the child's annoying behavior is likely to lead to increased exclusion in other situations.

With older children intervention frequently consists of one-to-one or group training in specific social skills. Training may focus on teaching specific social interaction skills, such as helping others, conversing, and taking turns. "Coaching" procedures frequently are used to teach the child in the skill to be mastered. Coaching includes providing a rationale for the target skill, having the child rehearse the skill in a "mock" situation with an adult or child partner, providing feedback on the child's performance, and sometimes reenacting the scene. In general, social skills training programs are most effective for children who lack positive behaviors and are less effective for children who drive others away with frequent negative behavior.

Coaching usually results in the child learning the trained skills, but generalizing the new skills to ongoing social interactions is a problem for some children and requires additional intervention. Peer-mediated interventions sometimes are used in an attempt to generalize trained skills. Typically, same-sex accepted peers are recruited as "co-therapists" and trained to initiate interactions, to respond to refusals, to maintain interactions, and to respond to the target child's negative behavior in order to engage the target child in the activities of the larger peer group. This procedure needs to be conducted and monitored carefully, however, to avoid even more stigmatization of the rejected child in the peer group.

Changing the child's school is another intervention sometimes considered by parents or teachers. However, research shows that rejected boys quickly reestablish their rejected status when placed in a group of children all unknown to one another.[4] These findings suggest that simply changing a child's school, without a concomitant change in a child's social behavior, will merely perpetuate a child's negative peer relations. Changing the child's school may be indicated, however, if his or her previous negative reputation is making it difficult for the child to be accepted by peers even though the child is performing new socially appropriate behaviors.

Similar to social skills training are interventions that address more general interpersonal problem-solving skills. In this approach the child is taught (usually by means of coaching) to handle interpersonal dilemmas by defining the problem, generating several alternatives that might resolve the situation, and selecting the solution most likely to produce desirable results. Although these programs are successful at improving children's social knowledge, their effects on actual social behavior (particularly negative behavior) is less clear.

The health care worker who elects to work directly with the child is best advised to assess the effects of the intervention after approximately six sessions. If progress is not apparent, referral to a child psychiatrist, psychologist, social worker, or school counselor experienced with peer relationship problems is warranted. In addition, preschools and elementary schools (particularly in urban and academic communities) occasionally include curricula related to social development, and such classrooms are referral possibilities if available in the local area.

REFERENCES

1. Boivin M, Begin G: Peer status and self-perception among early elementary school children: the case of the rejected children, *Child Dev* 60:591, 1989.
2. Coie JD: Toward a theory of peer rejection. In Asher SR, Coie JD, editors: *Peer rejection in childhood,* New York, 1990, Cambridge University Press.
3. Coie JD, Dodge KA: Continuities and changes in children's social status: a five-year longitudinal study, *Merrill-Palmer Q* 29:261, 1983.
4. Coie JD, Kupersmidt JB: A behavioral analysis of emerging social status in boys' groups, *Child Dev* 54:1400, 1983.
5. Crick NR, Grotpeter JK: Relational aggression, gender, and social-psychological adjustment, *Child Dev* 66:710, 1995.
6. Dodge KA: Behavioral antecedents of peer social status, *Child Dev* 54:1386, 1983.
7. Dodge KA: Problems in social relationships. In Mash EJ, Barkley RA, editors: *Treatment of childhood disorders,* New York, 1989, Guilford Press.
8. Dodge KA et al: Social competence in children, *Monogr Soc Res Child Dev* 51:1, 1986.

9. French DC: Heterogeneity of peer-rejected boys: aggressive and nonaggressive subtypes, *Child Dev* 59:976, 1988.
10. French DC: Heterogeneity of peer-rejected girls, *Child Dev* 61:2028, 1990.
11. Gronlund NE: *Sociometry in the classroom,* New York, 1959, Harper & Row.
12. Hart CH, Ladd GW, Burleson BR: Children's expectations of the outcomes of social strategies: relations with sociometric status and maternal disciplinary styles, *Child Dev* 61:127, 1990.
13. Hymel S, Asher SR: Assessment and training of isolated children's social skills, ERIC Document No ED 136:930, 1977.
14. Ladd GW, Golter BS: Parents' management of preschooler's peer relations: is it related to children's social competence? *Dev Psychol* 24:109, 1988.
15. MacDonald K, Parke RD: Bridging the gap: parent-child play interaction and peer interactive competence, *Child Dev* 55:1265, 1984.
16. Newcomb AF, Bukowski WM, Pattee L: Children's peer relations: a meta-analytic review of popular, rejected, controversial, and average sociometric status, *Psychol Bull* 113:91, 1993.
17. Parker JG, Asher SR: Peer relations and later personal adjustment: are low-accepted children at risk? *Psychol Bull* 102:357, 1987.
18. Parker JG, Asher SR: Significance of peer relationship problems in childhood. In Schneider BH et al, editors: *Social competence in developmental perspective,* Boston, 1989, Kluwer Academic Publishers.
19. Parker JG, Asher SR: Friendship and friendship quality in middle childhood: links with peer group acceptance and feelings of loneliness and social dissatisfaction, *Dev Psychol* 29:611, 1994.
20. Pettit GS, Dodge KA, Brown MM: Early family experience, social problem solving patterns, and children's social competence, *Child Dev* 59:107, 1988.
21. Pope AW, Bierman KL, Mumma GH: Aggression, hyperactivity, and inattention-immaturity: behavior dimensions associated with peer rejection in elementary school boys, *Dev Psychol* 27:663, 1991.
22. Putallaz M: Maternal behavior and children's sociometric status, *Child Dev* 58:324, 1988.
23. Putallaz M, Heflin AH: Parent-child interaction. In Asher SR, Coie JD, editors: *Peer rejection in childhood,* New York, 1990, Cambridge University Press.
24. Putallaz M, Wasserman A: Children's naturalistic entry behavior and sociometric status: a developmental perspective, *Dev Psychol* 25:297, 1989.
25. Roff M, Sells SB, Golden MM: *Social adjustment and personality development in children,* Minneapolis, 1972, University of Minnesota Press.
26. Rubin KH: Social and social-cognitive developmental characteristics of young isolate, normal, and sociable children. In Rubin KH, Ross HS, editors: *Peer relationships and social skills in childhood,* New York, 1982, Springer-Verlag.
27. Rubin KH, Mills RSL: The many faces of social isolation in childhood, *J Consult Clin Psychol* 56:916, 1988.
28. Strassbourg Z et al: The longitudinal relation between parental conflict strategies and children's sociometric standing in kindergarten, *Merrill-Palmer Q* 38:477, 1992.

87 Phobias

Norbert B. Enzer and Jed G. Magen

A phobia is an extreme and persistent fear of an object, event, or situation that in reality is not dangerous to the individual and would not be of concern to most people. There are three categories of phobias—simple phobia, social phobia, and agoraphobia (often associated with panic disorder)—all of which may occur in children and adolescents.

EPIDEMIOLOGY

In large-scale population studies of adults, phobias and other anxiety disorders are the most frequent psychiatric disorders occurring in the general population.[11] Although there are no comparable studies of the frequency of psychiatric disorders in childhood or adolescence, clearly phobias are common in these age groups.[2,6] In Rutter's Isle of Wight Study, about 2.5% of children had disabling specific fears or phobias.[13] A more recent community study found simple phobias in 2.6% of children.[6]

In a study of children and adolescents who have anxiety disorders, with the exception of separation anxiety disorders, simple phobias and social phobias were the most frequent, accounting for an incidence at 20% and 15%, respectively, at the time of the study and a 32% and 42% lifetime prevalence.[7]

The most common simple phobias occurring in children and adolescents involve animals and insects and are likely to begin before the age of 7 years. Other common phobias of closed spaces *(claustrophobia)* and heights *(acrophobia)* are much less frequent and tend to have their origins in adulthood.

Certain phobias associated with injury, blood, and health care also are common and should not be dismissed as trivial. These disorders may occur in as many as 4% of children and more frequently in girls.[8] Extreme responses such as panic, bradycardia, fainting, or vomiting as a reaction to injury, venipuncture, or injection (even when such events involve another person) may interfere with a phobic person seeking any health care.

DEVELOPMENTAL ISSUES

Some fears are common and expected at various developmental levels. For example, stranger anxiety is seen at roughly 8 months and usually decreases around the middle of the second year. It also is common for toddlers to be fearful of being left alone or with babysitters and for preschool children to be afraid of the dark. Because such fears are so common and so readily recognized as part of childhood, parents often do not consult physicians about them.

Many children have experiences that technically might meet the criteria for a diagnosis of simple phobia but that disappear over time without specific intervention. However, the avoidance behavior associated with a phobia may interfere with usual activities and productive social relationships. Animal phobias may prevent a child from playing with neighbors or attending after-school activities because of a need to avoid the feared object. Even when the specific simple phobia disappears spontaneously, the consequences of the missed opportunities, embarrassment, or interference with social development may linger.

ETIOLOGY

The literature offers little in regard to the etiology of phobias. Earlier theories postulated unconscious conflicts as the source. Others suggested that phobias are learned responses in the context of a child's experience; still others relate children's fears to those of their parents.

Empirical research indicates that early correlates of anxiety disorders may be present. In very young children behavioral inhibition, the tendency to exhibit withdrawal, and autonomic arousal to challenge or novelty is correlated with the later risk for anxiety disorders. As compared with a normal group, these children are at increased risk for multiple anxiety, overanxious, and phobic disorders.[12]

SYMPTOMS

The key symptoms of phobias are a fear often associated with sweating, tachycardia, difficulty in breathing, and lightheadedness or dizziness and avoidance of the fear-provoking object or situation. In extreme cases panic may occur. The degree to which avoidance or anticipatory anxiety occurs often is the critical factor in parents' seeking help.

Although simple phobias are defined as being related to single feared objects, they may occur in multiples or at times in sequence—one phobia develops as another disappears. Such patterns, along with the lengthy persistence of a single phobia, suggest a more severe problem and the need for further evaluation.

Social phobia is more complex, potentially more disabling, and has a less optimistic prognosis. This disorder, which often begins in late childhood or early adolescence, is characterized by a fear that the patient may do or say something that will be socially inappropriate and thus humiliating. Because of the fear of social situations, children limit contacts and become at risk for social immaturity and stigmatization by other children.

A 14-year-old girl, the daughter of a minister, developed a fear that she might vomit if she ate at church suppers. This progressed to the point where she could not attend such social functions or eat in public—at school, restaurants, or at friends' homes.

A 12-year-old boy had such a fear of "making a fool" of himself that he was unable to respond verbally in school or present oral reports.

In both these cases even the thought of these activities produced severe anxiety and led to avoidance behavior sufficient for the patient to appear "ill" enough to remain at home rather than face the social situations that were so feared.

True agoraphobia, the fear of being in places from which escape may not be possible or those where help might not be available, often begins in late adolescence. It may be associated with panic disorder or fears of panic or embarrassing happenings such as the loss of bowel or bladder control. Because of these fears, individuals often will progressively limit outside activities. This disorder usually is persistent and disabling.

At age 13, one girl began to be unable to go anywhere except school without her mother. Shortly, she was unable to go to school or anywhere else where there would be numbers of people (e.g., the grocery store or a shopping mall), even with her mother. She could take rides in the car with her mother. By about 17, she was unable to leave her home unless heavily sedated.

DIAGNOSIS

A careful history usually will define the diagnosis. The report of fearful behavior, the symptoms of anxiety, or the development of avoidance behavior or compulsions (repetitive, purposeful, intentional behaviors in response to fears or obsessions) should prompt an evaluation. A detailed history of the symptoms and behaviors, the circumstances in which they occur, the responses of parents, teachers, peers, and others, and the general pattern of psychosocial development should be explored. Because children, and more commonly adolescents, may recognize that their fear is irrational, they invent another reason for their avoidance behavior. The possibility of traumatic experience with the phobic object (such as having been frightened by even a playful dog, being lost, threatened, or abused) should be explored.

Although the history may seem to define the problem clearly, particularly if the patient can describe the object of the fear, a careful physical examination should be accomplished if physical problems are likely. Hypoglycemia, hyperthyroidism, and pheochromocytoma all can present with symptoms similar to anxiety. Withdrawal from some abused substances may be associated with episodes of severe anxiety, and some substances, particularly psychostimulants, may produce some similar symptoms.

Structured interviews and questionnaires, personality inventories, and behavioral checklists address some symptoms of anxiety and phobias, but they are not any more sensitive or specific than a careful history and a clinical interview with the patient and the parents and contacts with the school. Psychological testing, although useful in estimating cognitive abilities and personality characteristics, is of little use in the diagnosis of phobic disorders.

The differential diagnosis of simple phobia in young children should include separation anxiety disorder, overanxious disorder, and avoidant disorder of childhood. Social phobia and agoraphobia must be distinguished from avoidant disorder, depression, overanxious disorder, substance abuse, and schizophrenia, as well as from certain personality disorders.

In separation anxiety children are afraid of leaving parents or others to whom they are attached and often fear that something may happen to parents when they are not present. Fear of the dark, animals, or objects may be present, but unlike a simple phobia there is the added fear of separation from loved ones. So called "school phobia" or "school refusal" is a specific manifestation of this disorder (see Chapter 71, School Refusal and School Absenteeism).

The essential feature of overanxious disorder is excessive or unrealistic anxiety or worry for a period of 6 months or longer. Although phobias often are present, this disorder is more global and has less focused fears. Children may worry about the future, about past behavior, or about many other things.

In avoidant disorder of childhood or adolescence, there is a fear of contact with unfamiliar people that is sufficiently severe to interfere with social functioning and peer relationships for at least 6 months. At the same time these children wish to have social relationships with familiar individuals. One recent study questions the distinction between social phobia and avoidant disorder in children and adolescents.[3,7]

In older children and adolescents the differential diagnosis involves the above disorders and obsessive compulsive disorder and schizophrenia. In obsessive compulsive disorder individuals may avoid objects or show intense anxiety and concern around specific stimuli. However, instead of only developing anxiety and avoidant behavior, they also will engage in some repetitive, purposeful, and intentional behavior to neutralize or prevent the occurrence of anxiety or worry.

Individuals who are developing schizophrenia may exhibit phobic avoidance behaviors. However, the behavior may be bizarre and the ideation behind the avoidance unusual, such as avoiding the kitchen because monsters live in the oven. Other symptoms common to schizophrenia will develop or will be present.

Finally, some individuals who have major depressions and those abusing substances may develop phobias and other anxiety disorders as part of their symptomatology.

TREATMENT

Decisions regarding the treatment of a child or adolescent who has a phobia depend on several issues. As noted previously, children may exhibit "phobic" behaviors that are developmentally based, common, and likely to be self-limited. The common fear of the dark may be "treated" with a night light and some comfort and reassurance from parents. There is little point in attempting to insist that the child remain in the dark when such simple intervention is effective. More likely the "phobia" will abate spontaneously over time.

Along with the intensity of symptoms and their duration, the degree to which a simple phobia interferes with daily living, relationships, and school or the presence of stigmatization are critical in treatment decisions. When specific treatment seems indicated, certain aspects apply virtually to all situations. The patient needs to be as completely informed regarding the diagnosis and treatment as age and cognitive development permit. The parents need to be partners in the treatment; their responses may be crucial to the outcome. Without intending to do so, parents can reinforce and perpetuate symptoms.

Traditional insight-oriented psychotherapy often has been used in the treatment of patients who have simple phobias. However, behavioral approaches appear to be the most effective and efficient.[8,9] Systematic desensitization is the more frequently used behavioral treatment. Patients who have simple phobias can be treated with gradual exposure to the phobic stimulus and relaxation techniques. As anxiety occurs, the relaxation techniques are invoked and the stimuli removed. The number of treatment sessions and the overall duration of therapy vary widely.[10] It should be noted that in blood injury phobias where there is any suggestion of vasovagal bradycardia and syncope, exposure to the phobic object (e.g., a needle or a scalpel) should be accomplished with the patient in a prone position.

Medications may be useful in the desensitization process if relaxation techniques are difficult for the patient or if anxiety is particularly intense. Short-acting anxiolytic agents are most helpful. Beyond this use, medications have little utility in the treatment of simple phobias because the symptoms occur only in relation to the phobic object and because of the sedating side effects.

Social phobias are more difficult to treat and often require psychological treatment and pharmacotherapy. Systematic desensitization often is difficult to establish because of the complexity of the anxiety-provoking stimuli and because there often is an associated social immaturity. Individual psychotherapy, particularly the use of cognitive-behavioral approaches, may be useful. Group therapy with age-appropriate peers can be helpful in promoting socialization and the development of social skills. Placement in structured social settings where expectations are clear and success can be expected also is useful.

Other behavioral techniques also can be useful in phobic disorders of various types. Structured systems in which rewards are given for desired behaviors are especially useful for younger children. It is very useful to involve the patient in the development of this kind of system so that he or she is invested in making it work and interested in the rewards. Physicians or nonphysician mental health professionals often will need to coach parents in negotiating these points with their children.

The treatment of agoraphobia with or without panic usually involves both cognitive-behavioral techniques and pharmacotherapy, as well as other supportive measures. Progress may be slow. Often there is a comorbid depressive disorder that benefits from antidepressants. Support from family members and friends can be crucial in helping the patient through anxiety-provoking situations. If available, participation in a support group of patients who have similar problems may be useful.

MEDICATIONS

Medications can be useful in reducing anxiety in patients who have great difficulty with or find it impossible to tolerate anxiety and to participate in other aspects of treatment. If medications are contemplated, in the vast majority of children anxiolytics or antidepressants are the medications of choice.

Benzodiazepines are the anxiolytics used most commonly. These agents treat both acute anxiety and anticipatory anxiety. Common side effects include lethargy and sleepiness, which can interfere with academic performance. The most worrisome problem is dependency, which can develop with use for more than 3 to 6 weeks. A withdrawal syndrome including rebound anxiety, tremulousness, abdominal pain, and seizures has been described. Sudden discontinuation of medication is therefore not recommended. These agents are most useful for treating acute anxiety while other treatments are being put into place and in situations in which patients are not responsive to nonsomatic treatments. Newer anxiolytic agents have not yet been shown to have greater efficacy.[4]

Antidepressants are a better choice for long-term anxiolytic therapy because they do not carry the risk of dependency and because they are quite effective. Individuals who have comorbid depressive disorders are good candidates for antidepressants. Antidepressants will decrease or block panic attacks and other severe episodes of anxiety. Traditional tricyclics can be used, although they have the usual anticholinergic and cardiac side effects. Selective serotonin reuptake inhibitors are as equally efficacious as tricyclic antidepressants in adults and have far fewer side effects. From this standpoint they are probably a better choice for children and adolescents, as well as adults. The most common side effects are sedation or sleeplessness, nausea, or diarrhea. Specific dosages still are to be established fully.

PROGNOSIS

In children and adolescents most phobias do seem to respond to treatment, at least in terms of relief of major symptoms, although the lack of controlled studies makes it difficult to attribute remission clearly to treatment. Follow-up studies are limited, but those that exist suggest a positive long-term outcome.[1,5] However, adults seeking treatment for phobias and other anxiety disorders often report a childhood onset or similar symptoms during childhood or adolescence that diminished or disappeared for some time.

The prognosis for patients who have social phobia in childhood or adolescence is less clear, but experience suggests that this disorder is less likely to remit spontaneously or as a consequence of treatment. Agoraphobia also has a more guarded prognosis, although here outcome studies and long-term follow-up information are lacking.

Clearly, more research is needed, and newer medications and other treatment approaches may prove more effective than those of the past.

REFERENCES

1. Agres WS, Chapin HN, Oliveau DC: The natural history of phobia, *Arch Gen Psychiatry* 26:315, 1972.
2. Anderson JC et al: DSM-III disorders in preadolescent children, *Arch Gen Psychiatry* 44:69, 1987.
3. Francis G, Last CG, Strauss CC: Avoidant disorder and social phobia, *J Am Acad Child Adolesc Psychiatry* 31:1086, 1992.
4. Graae F et al: Clonazepam in childhood anxiety disorder, *J Am Acad Child Adolesc Psychiatry* 33:373, 1994.
5. Haurpe E et al: Phobic children one and two years posttreatment, *J Abnorm Psychol* 82:447, 1973.
6. Kashani JH, Orvaschel H: A community study of anxiety in children and adolescents, *Am J Psychiatry* 147:313, 1990.
7. Last CG et al: DSM-III-R anxiety disorders in children: sociodemographic and clinical characteristics, *J Am Acad Child Adolesc Psychiatry* 31:1071, 1992.
8. Marks I: Blood injury phobia: a review, *Am J Psychiatry* 145:1207, 1988.

9. McDermott JF Jr et al: Anxiety disorders of childhood or adolescence. In American Psychiatric Association: *Treatments of psychiatric disorders: a task force report of the American Psychiatric Association,* vol 1, Washington, DC, 1989, The Association.
10. Ollendirk TH, Francis G: Behavioral assessment and treatment of childhood phobias, *Behav Modif* 12:165, 1988.
11. Robius LN et al: Lifetime prevalence of specific psychiatric disorders in three sites, *Arch Gen Psychiatry* 41:949, 1984.
12. Rosenbaum JF et al: Further evidence of an association between behavioral inhibition and anxiety disorders: result from a family study of children from a non-clinical sample, *J Psychiatr Res* 25:49, 1991.
13. Rutter M et al: Research report: Isle of Wight studies, 1964-1974, *Psychol Med* 6:313, 1976.

SUGGESTED READINGS

American Psychiatric Association: *Diagnostic and statistical manual of mental disorders,* ed 4, Washington, DC, 1994, American Psychiatric Association.

Baer L: *Getting control: overcoming your obsessions and compulsions,* Boston, 1991, Little, Brown.

Gitteman R, Koplewicz HS: Pharmacotherapy of childhood anxiety disorders. In Gittelman R, editor: *Anxiety disorders of childhood,* New York, 1986, Guilford Press.

Husain SA, Kushani JW: *Anxiety disorders in children and adolescents,* Washington, DC, 1992, American Psychiatric Press.

Klesges RC, Malott JM, Ugland M: The effects of graded exposure and parental modeling on the dental phobias of a four-year-old girl and her mother, *J Behav Ther Exp Psychiatry* 15:161, 1984.

Kohen DP et al: The use of relaxation mental imagery (self-hypnosis) on the management of 505 pediatric behavioral encounters, *J Dev Behav Pediatr* 5:21, 1984.

Leonard LL, Rapoport JL: Simple phobia, social phobia and panic disorders. In Wiener JL, editor: *Textbook of child and adolescent psychiatry,* Washington, DC, 1991, American Psychiatric Press.

Marks IM: *Fears, phobias, and rituals,* New York, 1987, Oxford University Press.

Morris RJ, Kratochwill TR: Behavioral treatment of children's fears and phobias, *School Psychol Rev* 14:84, 1985.

Sreenivasan, PM, Mamocha SN, Jain VK: Treatment of severe dog phobia in childhood by flooding, *J Child Psychol Psychiatry* 2:255, 1979.

88 Psychosis

Irving B. Weiner

Psychosis refers to a serious degree of psychological disturbance in which a person's grasp of reality is so impaired as to prevent him or her from meeting the demands of everyday living. A psychotic disorder causes people to perceive themselves and their experiences inaccurately. As a result of being out of touch with reality, psychotic individuals often misjudge the consequences of their actions and behave strangely, unpredictably, and sometimes destructively. Other people frequently cannot comprehend why psychotics act as they do and consider their behavior "crazy."

In young people disorders of psychotic proportion appear mainly in three patterns, distinguishable by their typical age of onset: early-onset childhood psychosis, known as *infantile autism,* which begins almost always before 3 years of age and interferes with psychological development from infancy on; late-onset childhood psychosis, now commonly called *schizophrenia in childhood,* which begins usually between 7 and 12 years of age and is continuous with adolescent and adult forms of schizophrenic disorders; and *schizophrenia in adolescence,* which begins after puberty and, like schizophrenia in childhood, constitutes a breakdown or regression in psychological functioning following some years of more or less normal development.[7,11]

INFANTILE AUTISM

The primary characteristic of infantile autism is a lack of relatedness to people. Autistic children are indifferent and unresponsive to social overtures. As infants they do not clamor for attention, they do not enjoy being picked up, and they do not cuddle or cling when someone holds them. They rarely look or smile directly at other people, and they seem happiest when left alone. For these reasons, parents of autistic children usually find little pleasure in nurturing them: "It was like taking care of an object; he never seemed to know or care whether I was around, and I never got any feeling of warmth from him." Nevertheless, because autistic infants tend to be healthy physically and to develop normally physically, their serious deficits in social attachment often go unnoticed initially or are attributed to their being placid or reserved.

During the preschool years, however, the detachment and unresponsiveness of these children become noticeably persistent, and also they begin to display a number of other unmistakable abnormalities. Most prominent in this regard are (1) a need to preserve sameness, which makes them intolerant of any change in their environment, such as moving their playpen or taking a piece of furniture out of their bedroom; (2) marked language abnormalities consisting either of failure to develop any communicative speech or of developing speech that is difficult to understand because of peculiar word usage, unusual grammatical constructions, and lack of relatedness to ongoing conversations; (3) repetitive, ritualistic behaviors, such as sitting for hours staring off into space or passing a toy back and forth from one hand to the other; and (4) indices of a developmental disorder such as strange body movements or posturing, neuropsychological abnormalities, and "soft" signs of neurological impairment.

Infantile autism is a rare condition that is found in 4 to 5 live births per 10,000 and occurs three to four times more frequently in boys than in girls. Despite its rarity, autism is noteworthy for its devastating interference with psychological development virtually from birth and for its serious long-term consequences. Some autistic children improve spontaneously, especially if they are among the few who develop near-average intellectual and communication skills. Others respond favorably to specialized treatment programs that combine behavioral, educational, and pharmacological approaches. The general prognosis for the condition is poor, however. No more than 25% of autistic children make any substantial social or educational progress, and of these, most achieve only fair academic and interpersonal functioning. As adults, only 10% of these children are likely to do well in work or family situations, and 60% will remain totally dependent on other adults for the rest of their lives[1,4-6] (see Chapter 168, Strange Behavior).

SCHIZOPHRENIA IN CHILDHOOD

Although schizophrenia can begin as early as the preschool years, many children who are first identified as psychotic between ages 3 and 7 most likely are autistic youngsters whose developmental problems dating from infancy previously were overlooked. Children who become schizophrenic develop the same features of impaired personality functioning that characterize adult schizophrenia: disorganized and illogical thinking, distorted perception of reality, inappropriate ways of relating to people, and poor control over feelings and impulses. As a result these late-onset psychotic children manifest many of the symptoms seen in infantile autism, including compulsive routines and self-preoccupied behavior, incoherent or incomprehensible speech patterns, excessive, diminished, or unpredictable responses to sensory stimulation, body rigidity and strange posturing, poor social skills, and periods of unaccountably severe anxiety or violent temper tantrums. Schizophrenic children also are likely to develop delusions or hallucinations that detach them even further from reality and from an appropriate relationship to people. Common in this regard are unrealistic fears about other children being "out to get me," bizarre fantasies about possessing special powers, and the conviction of being a machine or some kind of animal rather than a person. Schizophrenic youngsters are more likely than autistic children to have a history of poor physical health and development, but they are less likely to be intellectually or linguistically handicapped.

The distinction between schizophrenia in childhood and infantile autism is based not only on symptom patterns and age of onset but also on differences in etiology and course. Autism appears to be a biogenetic disorder resulting from prenatal, perinatal, or early postnatal damage to areas of the brain crucial to the development of language comprehension and social relationships. Psychosocial factors play no demonstrable role in whether or when autism appears, and the parents of autistic children do not differ in any psychologically significant way from parents of other handicapped children.

Schizophrenia currently is understood best as a disorder of interactive origin in which biogenetic dispositions and psychosocial stressors combine to precipitate personality breakdown. Patterns of family interaction, especially the quality of parent-child communications, bear considerably on the severity and duration of these schizophrenic breakdowns.

Once begun, the symptoms of autism run a continuous, unrelenting course, whereas schizophrenia is an episodic disorder in which periods of severe symptomatology alternate with periods of reasonably adequate functioning. Autistic children who do not improve tend eventually to develop primary features of mental retardation, epilepsy, or aphasia; by contrast approximately 90% of schizophrenic children subsequently present evidence of adult schizophrenia.[2,3,8]

SCHIZOPHRENIA IN ADOLESCENCE

Late-onset childhood psychosis occurs somewhat more frequently than infantile autism, but schizophrenia remains a rare condition until adolescence. Following puberty the incidence of the disorder increases sharply. The population prevalence of schizophrenia is approximately 1%, and most schizophrenic persons experience their first psychotic breakdown in late adolescence or early adulthood (15 to 25 years of age). Schizophrenia is diagnosed in 25% to 30% of 12- to 18-year-olds admitted to public mental hospitals and in about 15% of those admitted to psychiatric units of general hospitals. Approximately 15% of schizophrenic patients being treated in private psychiatric hospitals are under the age of 18.

In addition to these instances of overt schizophrenia, many adolescents who are destined to become schizophrenically disturbed as adults show prodromal signs of the disorder during their teenage years. This means that pediatricians who care for adolescents will see an appreciable number of young people in whom various kinds of apparently minor behavioral problems in fact constitute the early stages of a schizophrenic disorder.

The adolescent personality patterns from which schizophrenia emerges usually involve either *schizoid* or *stormy* behavior. Schizoid adolescents tend to withdraw into themselves, avoiding activities that would bring them into contact with people and sharing few interests in common with others. They express little or no emotion, and they may appear apathetic and unenthused about life, as if depressed. "Stormy" adolescents, in contrast, exercise little control over their emotions or actions. They consequently tend to be in constant conflict with their parents, peers, and teachers over such behavior as fighting, stealing, running away, being disobedient, being truant, and failing in school. Neither schizoid nor stormy personality patterns are by themselves diagnostic of schizophrenia, and both can occur in the context of numerous other behavior disorders. However, either pattern appearing in adolescence, especially if it represents a marked change from a youngster's childhood behavior, should alert the clinician to the possibility of incipient schizophrenia.[9,10,12]

Generally the older people are when they develop a psychotic disorder, the better their prospects for improvement and recovery. Hence late-onset psychosis, although often a persistent and disabling disorder, offers better prospects for improvement and marginal social adaptation than does infantile autism. Likewise, in schizophrenic disorder the earlier in life a breakdown in response to stress occurs, the greater is the constitutional disposition or vulnerability to psychosis. Thus the prognosis in schizophrenia among adolescents usually is less guarded than in cases of schizophrenia in childhood. Of adolescents hospitalized for schizophrenia, about 25% recover, 25% improve substantially but suffer lingering symptoms or occasional relapses, and the remaining 50% make little or no progress and are likely to require continuing residential care.

REFERENCES

1. Borden MC, Ollendick TH: The development and differentiation of social subtypes in autism. In Lahey BB, Kazdin AE, editors: *Advances in clinical child psychology,* vol 14, New York, 1992, Plenum.
2. Cantor S: *Childhood schizophrenia,* New York, 1988, Guilford Press.
3. Chambers WJ: Late-onset psychoses of childhood and adolescence. In Kestenbaum CJ, Williams DT, editors: *Handbook of clinical assessment of children and adolescents,* New York, 1988, New York University Press.
4. Cohen DJ, Donellan AM, editors: *Handbook of autism and pervasive developmental disorders,* New York, 1987, John Wiley & Sons.
5. Dawson G, Castelloe P: Autism. In Walker CE, Roberts MC, editors: *Handbook of clinical child psychology,* ed 2, New York, 1992, John Wiley & Sons.
6. Gillberg C: Outcome in autism and autistic-like conditions, *J Am Acad Child Adolesc Psychiatry* 30:375, 1991.
7. Rutter M, Schopler E: Classification of pervasive developmental disorders: some concepts and practical considerations, *J Autism Dev Disorders* 22:459, 1992.
8. Volkmar FR: Childhood schizophrenia. In Lewis M, editor: *Child and adolescent psychiatry,* Baltimore, 1991, Williams & Wilkins.
9. Weiner IB: Identifying schizophrenia in adolescents, *J Adolesc Health Care* 8:336, 1987.
10. Weiner IB: *Psychological disturbance in adolescence,* ed 2, New York, 1992, John Wiley & Sons.
11. Werry JS: Child and adolescent (early-onset) schizophrenia: a review in light of DSM-III-R, *J Autism Dev Disord* 22:601, 1992.
12. Westermeyer JF: Schizophrenia. In Tolan PH, Cohler BJ, editors: *Handbook of clinical research and practice with adolescents,* New York, 1993, John Wiley & Sons.

89 Self-Stimulating Behaviors

Richard M. Sarles and Alice B. Heisler

Self-stimulating behaviors, such as head-banging, head-rolling, rocking, thumb-sucking, and masturbation and habits such as hair-pulling and nail-biting are of concern to both parents and primary care practitioners. It has been suggested that there are commonalities among such behaviors, sometimes classified as *stereotypies,* and that they represent an interaction of the stage of neuromotor development with environmental influences (e.g., restrictive car seats and cribs) and are a homeostatic mechanism that serves to regulate stimulation from the environment. Several of these behaviors, such as head-banging, head-rolling, and rocking, typically appear before 12 months of age, peak soon thereafter, and subsequently decline rapidly. In general, most of these behaviors are self-limited to the preschool period and usually are viewed as normal, common, expected behaviors. As such these habits generally do not signify psychological maladjustment; thus they often require little intervention other than reassuring the parents and recommending adequate stimulation of their child.[5]

HEAD-BANGING AND ROCKING BEHAVIOR

Head-banging consists of rhythmic movements of the head against a solid object, such as the crib mattress or the headboard itself, and often is associated with rocking the head and the entire body. It most commonly is observed at bedtime or at times of fatigue or stress and may vary in duration from several minutes to hours. It has been noted that head-banging often continues even when the child is asleep. The age of onset shows wide variability, but the behavior most commonly is witnessed during the preschool years. The reported incidence of head-banging or rocking behavior varies between 3% and 20%, with a male-to-female ratio of approximately 3:1. There occasionally is a positive family history of such behavior, but only 20% of siblings of "rockers" exhibit similar or other rhythmic pattern disturbances.[4]

Various theories have been developed to understand these self-limited but often disturbing behaviors.[8] Rocking is thought to be a soothing, pleasurable experience every infant encounters in utero and most infants encounter from the neonatal period onward. The pleasure from movement is repeated throughout life, from early childhood rocking in mother's arms, for example, to childhood jump rope games, the playground swing, and dancing in adulthood. Individual constitutional patterns in childhood account for a wide variability in the amount of stimulation any particular child may require. However, in certain children, such as those who are deaf, blind, emotionally disturbed, or severely mentally retarded, marked rhythmic movements are found commonly. In these cases the movements may represent a compensatory reaction for the lack of, or the inability to integrate, stimuli. In addition, the normal child who is inactive because of physical illness generally shows a need for motor release often manifested in bed rocking or other rhythmic body movements, which generally disappear once normal mobility is restored to the child.

Physical and neurological examinations show these children to be predominantly within normal limits, and EEG studies are not indicated because they generally have been nonrevealing. It appears that these behaviors are linked to maturational patterns and correlate closely with teething and other transitions of growth and development, perhaps as a mechanism of increasing or reducing arousal and maintaining homeostasis. Even though psychosocial growth and development apparently are not disturbed in these children, and studies indicate no connection between rocking behavior and parental divorce or separation, the question of inadequate stimulation for the child should be raised, or the presence of family turmoil and stress should be investigated.

Treatment generally is directed toward assuring the parents that head-banging cannot cause brain injury and that the child will show no adverse neurological residual in later life; in fact "head-bangers" usually grow up to be coordinated and completely normal children. Padding the crib and securing the bed to prevent rolling may help during the limited rocking behavior. Sedation in the form of diphenhydramine may prove effective, but psychotropic medication generally is unnecessary and thus discouraged. Rarely, if ever, do fractures of the skull or cerebral hemorrhages result from head-banging, but soft tissue swelling and scalp contusions have been reported. A protective helmet may be advised in severe cases. Consultation with a child psychiatrist or psychologist is indicated if the head-banging or rocking behavior persists beyond 3 years of age. In the child who shows a lack of social interaction or a preoccupation with himself or herself or with self-stimulatory behavior, such as overt, compulsive masturbation, consultation also is indicated.[3]

THUMB-SUCKING AND NAIL-BITING

Thumb-sucking occurs almost universally in infancy. Infants may place virtually every object in the mouth until parents restrict certain objects for reasons of safety.

The pleasurable sensations associated with the double tactile experience of sucking and being sucked and the feelings of security and comfort that this evokes tend to reinforce this type of behavior. Many families substitute artificial pacifiers as a more socially acceptable means of oral pleasure, and children themselves often suck a security blanket, a doll, or a stuffed animal spontaneously. Thumb-sucking usually occurs during times of stress or boredom and at bedtime. Social and family pressures generally limit thumb-sucking to the preschool years. However, the habit may persist into adolescence. An incidence as high as 59% has been reported, and it is estimated that approximately 30% to 40% of American children engage in finger-sucking during the preschool years, and 10% to 20% continue past 6 years of age.

Nail-biting is an extension or permutation of the habit of thumb-sucking. Some consider this behavior a form of more overt aggression directed toward one's self, whereas others would define nail-biting simply as a variation of thumb-sucking because this behavior also is seen typically during times of stress. It is estimated that 40% of all children over 6 years of age bite their nails at some time or other, and 20% of college students continue to bite their nails. Thus nail-biting, in contrast to thumb-sucking, often continues throughout childhood and into adulthood. There appears to be a family history in most cases, but this habit is so common that such an apparent association may be of no significance. There does not appear to be any correlation with the number of children in the family, the birth order, the type of feeding or type of feeding schedule, or the age or race of the parents. However, there is a significant association with the time of weaning, in that the later the weaning takes place, the less likely the chance of thumb-sucking.[1]

Thumb-sucking, nail-biting, and cuticle-biting or picking generate an increase in the probability of dental malocclusion and an increase in the incidence of digital cutaneous infections. The probability of malocclusion in the thumb-sucker appears directly related to the age at which the habit is discontinued. Thus those children who cease the habit only after 6 years of age generally manifest malocclusion to some degree when seen at 12 years of age. In addition, thumb-sucking that persists into school age can bring on teasing from peers and criticism from teachers and family, leaving the child with decreased self-esteem and increased psychological distress.

Clarifying with parents the nature of these habits is important, as is encouraging them to avoid punishing or shaming the child for them. An underlying cause of tension always should be investigated, but often, simple behavioral therapy (based on positive reinforcement) is sufficient to alleviate this habit. The parents should be advised to avoid punishment, threats, or anger. Encouragement in the place of restrictions is helpful in engaging the child in his or her own program to decrease or eliminate this behavior.

Bitter-tasting commercial preparations applied to the fingers may be used as a reminder for the child but generally are inadequate unless supplemented by consistent positive reinforcement. This choice of reinforcement reward should be the child's and might represent a "Chinese menu" of extra television privileges, dessert, or other special treats. Friman and Leibowitz[2] found a combination of aversive taste treatment and a reward system to be effective in treating chronic thumb-sucking. Weekly visits to the physician for the first month of treatment are important to reinforce the change in behavior. Hypnosis is another treatment that often is quite successful and poses no dangers; psychotropic medications, on the other hand, are of little value. If these habits are linked to other signs of emotional distress, referral to a specialist in behavioral disorders is warranted.

MASTURBATION

Masturbatory activity in children is almost universal and often leads to great parental concern. Such activity may vary from direct manual genital stimulation to movements of the thighs against each other. Rhythmic swaying or thrusting motions of the child while straddling a hobby horse, pillow, stuffed animal, or other objects also are common methods of masturbation. Infants and children are capable of a physiological orgasmic response similar to that experienced by the adult, except for the absence of ejaculation in the male child. This was demonstrated by the common practice in Europe at about the turn of the century of masturbating an irritable child to induce relaxation and sleep. Occasionally this orgasmic response has been thought incorrectly to represent a convulsive disorder in the preschool child. Masturbatory activity generally is initiated as a response to the learned pleasure associated with touching of the genitalia first experienced in infancy during normal body exploration. Masturbation will continue as a lifelong pleasurable experience unless suppressed by parents or other adults.

It is important for the practitioner to counsel parents about masturbatory practices and emphasize that masturbation is a normal, harmless, and healthy practice that helps the child to derive pleasure from his or her own body. Myths must be dispelled concerning the belief that masturbation may cause mental retardation, physical deformity, blindness, poor physical and mental health, facial pimples, hair on the palms of the hand, homosexuality, and sexual perversions. Parents should be aware that masturbation is normal and almost universally occurs in children and should be encouraged not to punish or shame their child. If parents observe masturbatory activity in their child, they may want to suggest to the child the inappropriateness of manipulating their genitalia in public places or in front of others and inform the child that certain practices such as "toileting" and masturbation are best carried out in private.

Because local genital irritation, candidal infection, or pinworms in rare cases may cause one to masturbate, a physical examination helps to exclude such possibilities. Compulsive, overt masturbation among children and adolescents may lead to social ridicule and condemnation or may signify a deeper emotional problem. Consultation with a specialist in behavioral disorders of children and adolescents is indicated if the practitioner suspects that the masturbatory activity is excessive, compulsive, or overt or may indicate the presence of a more complicated, troublesome emotional problem.

The practitioner should be aware that even with the current trend within our society of sexual openness and enlightenment, myths and feelings concerning masturbation often are deep-seated and persistent. Thus counseling and advice given by the practitioner may be met with covert or overt resistance by parents or school authorities. The practitioner should be well prepared to educate those responsible for the growth and development of children.

HAIR-PULLING AND TWISTING

Hair-pulling and twisting *(trichotillomania)* is an uncommon form of self-stimulating behavior and often is indicative of psychological stress on the child. The scalp is the most common area affected; eyebrows and eyelashes are the next most likely sites. The obvious cosmetic damage often results in ridicule by peers and shame for the child. The possibility of a hair ball, or trichobezoar, forming in the stomach if the child ingests the hair is a serious problem that often results in hospitalization for surgical removal of the accumulated matted hair. This behavior, more frequent in females than males, has been reported in preschoolers, school-age children, adolescents, and adults. Classified as a disorder of impulse control (DSM-IV), there are suggestions that this disorder might best be grouped with the obsessive-compulsive disorder spectrum because of the common pathological compulsion of excessive grooming.[7] In general, the patient is totally unaware of the behavior during the hair pulling or twisting itself, and the patient often recognizes the action as senseless and undesirable.

Treatment usually is indicated and varies from initial behavior modification techniques, such as a positive reinforcement-reward system, to wearing a cap. Local irritation from a primary dermatological condition rarely is the cause of this disorder, but the possibility should be investigated. Referral to a mental health professional often is warranted to investigate possible underlying causes of tension, anxiety, depression, or obsessive compulsive disorder. Hypnosis or psychotherapy may be required in many of these cases. Clomipramine, fluoxetine, and selective serotonin reuptake inhibitors, but not desipramine, have proven useful in cases that are unresponsive to nonmedication treatment.

SPECIAL PROBLEMS IN DISTURBED CHILDREN

A broad spectrum of self-stimulating behaviors may be seen in the severely retarded or emotionally disturbed child. The behaviors, including body-twirling or spinning and hand- or arm-flapping, often are seen in cases of infantile autism or childhood schizophrenia.

Excessive rocking behavior is common in the severely retarded and emotionally disturbed child. In addition, severe self-mutilating behaviors such as compulsive self-biting, severe head-banging, and skin-gouging occasionally may be seen in these disorders[2] but are more characteristic of certain metabolic-genetic disorders such as Lesch-Nyhan syndrome and de Lange syndrome.

It is believed that these behaviors are part of a symptom complex in a severe disorder, quite in contrast to the generally isolated behavior discussed previously in normal children. The etiology generally is linked to the basic disorder and also may reflect the lack of, or disordered integration of, sensory stimuli.

All these cases require treatment for the basic disorder and generally demand special treatment beyond the scope and expertise of the primary care physician. Institutionalization often is required, and methods of treatment include the application of aversive behavior modification techniques, the use of arm and neck restraints, head helmets, and major tranquilizers, and the institution of psychotherapeutic programs.[6]

REFERENCES

1. Fletcher B: Etiology of fingersucking: review of literature, *J Dent Children* 42:293, 1975.
2. Friman PC, Leibowitz JM: An effective and acceptable treatment alternative for chronic thumb- and finger-sucking, *J Pediatr Psychol* 15:1, 1990.
3. Green A: Self-mutilation in schizophrenic children, *Arch Gen Psychiatry* 17:234, 1967.
4. Kravitz H et al: A study of head-banging in infants and children, *Dis Nerv Sys* 21:203, 1960.
5. Lourie R: The role of rhythmic patterns in childhood, *Am J Psychiatry* 105:653, 1949.
6. Singh NN: Current trends in the treatment of self-injurious behavior, *Adv Pediatr* 28:377, 1981.
7. Swedo SE, Leonard HL: Trichotillomania: an obsessive-compulsive spectrum disorder? *Psychiatr Clin North Am* 15:4, 1992.
8. Werry JS, Carlielle J, Fitzpatrick J: Rhythmic motor activities (stereotypies) in children under five: etiology and prevalence, *J Am Acad Child Adolesc Psychiatry* 22:329, 1983.

90 Stuttering

Harold L. Luper

Stuttering is a disorder in the continuity of speech characterized by repetitions and prolongations of speech sounds. Typically, stuttering first is observed during the preschool years as children are progressing through various stages of language development. Although all children are disfluent, only 4% to 5% demonstrate true stuttering at some point in their lives. Most children will be disfluent only for a few months and show no reaction to these temporary disfluencies. Unfortunately about 20% to 30% of those who begin to stutter will have a lifelong problem.[1] In general, the longer stuttering continues, the more likely the problem will be exacerbated and the greater the likelihood that the child will develop lowered self-esteem and fear of speaking. The pattern of stuttering described above sometimes is called *developmental stuttering* to distinguish it from the much rarer type, *acquired stuttering*. The latter usually appears suddenly, long after speech and language skills have been developed.

When developmental stuttering is treated appropriately, especially in its beginning stages, the prognosis for recovery generally is quite good. The types of behaviors typically seen in advanced stuttering (severe struggling and fear of talking) usually can be prevented. Even adults who have stuttered for years often can learn to decrease the severity of their stuttering and improve their attitudes about speaking.

The prognosis for acquired stuttering is much less certain. The small number of cases and the wide differences in type of cortical damage or psychogenic trauma make prediction of recovery much more tenuous.[6]

ETIOLOGY

Despite much research the specific causes of developmental stuttering are unknown. Findings from several studies suggest a weak genetic pattern. In many instances, however, there is no familial history of stuttering. As a consequence both physiological and environmental factors appear to play a role in the origin and progression of stuttering.[4]

There is considerable evidence that developmental stuttering is related to children's efforts to learn to talk. Children in general are disfluent between the ages of 2 and 5, when they are mastering speech and language skills rapidly. Disfluencies in all children are more likely to occur when the child is using more complicated vocabulary or syntactical structures.[3] It long has been observed that many children who stutter have a history of slow speech and language development.[2]

A current explanation of childhood stuttering, useful for counseling parents, explains etiology by a "demands and capacities" model.[7] This model states that disfluencies occur when demands (e.g., parental or internal pressures for speech performance) exceed the child's capacities for fluent speech (e.g., levels of motor speech ability or cognitive-linguistic development).

In contrast to the lack of definitive known causes for developmental stuttering, acquired stuttering usually has a neurogenic or, more rarely, a psychogenic origin. Neurogenic stuttering usually is a sequela of brain damage. No consistent pattern in type of damage (e.g., stroke, tumor, disease) or site of lesion (hemisphere or lobe) has been found.[6]

Differential Diagnosis

At its onset stuttering is difficult to differentiate from normally disfluent speech. All speakers are disfluent, and children are even more likely to have interruptions in their speech. To differentiate stuttering from normally disfluent speech it is necessary to estimate the frequency, duration, and type of disfluencies in the child's speech, observe the child's reactions to his or her stuttering, and determine the presence of struggling as the child tries to speak. Because stuttering frequently varies among those afflicted, it may be necessary to obtain much of this information by questioning the parents or parent-surrogates. The *Physician's Checklist for Referral* presented in Table 90-1 summarizes key criteria for determining if a child normally is disfluent or stutters mildly or severely. These criteria are expanded on below.

Normally Disfluent Speech. The repetitions usually are brief (typically ½ second or less) and occur infrequently (only once in 10 sentences), and there are no signs of struggle in speaking. Repetitions of a word or phrase (rather than of a sound or syllable) are considered normal and often are associated with the search for a word (e.g., "Mommy, where is my, where is my—you know, my uh, twicycle?"). Disfluencies often increase when a child is excited or tired.

Young children who stutter mildly will be disfluent more frequently than those whose speech normally is disfluent (on 3% to 5% of words spoken) and will have longer trains of repetitions ("ba-ba-ba-ball") and perhaps some prolongations of sounds. The disfluencies will tend to occur more often on the initial sound or syllable of a word; excess tension may be visible around the lips or eyes. There usually is little concern on the part of the child other than occasional embarrassment or frustration.

Stuttering is considered *severe* when the following conditions are found: stuttering is very frequent (on 10% or more of the words spoken); the repetitions are very rapid and uneven; sound prolongations or blockings typically last 1 second or longer; the child appears to struggle in his or her attempts to say a word; and fear or avoidance of speaking is evident.

Effects of Stuttering

A child's initial reactions to stuttering usually are surprise and frustration. If the stuttering continues, the frustration can change to a fear of "being stuck." Because severe stuttering occurs in only about 1% of the population, many young chil-

Table 90-1 Physician's Checklist for Referral

	Normal disfluencies Age of onset: 1½ to 7 years of age	Mild stuttering Age of onset: 1½ to 7 years of age	Severe stuttering Age of onset: 1½ to 7 years of age
Speech behaviors you may see or hear	Occasional (not more than once in every 10 sentences), brief (typical ½ second or shorter) repetitions of sounds, syllables, or short words (e.g., "li-li-like this")	Frequent (3% or more of speech), long (½ to 1 second) repetitions of sounds, syllables, or short words, (e.g., "li-li-li-like this"); occasional prolongations of sounds	Very frequent (10% or more of speech) and often very long (1 second or longer) repetitions of sounds, syllables, or short words; frequent sound prolongations and blockages
Other behaviors you may see or hear	Occasional pauses, hesitations in speech, or fillers such as "uh," "er," or "um"; changing of words or thoughts	Repetitions and prolongations begin to be associated with eyelid closing and blinking, looking to the side, and some physical tension in and around the lips	Similar to mild stutterers only more frequent and noticeable; some rise in pitch of voice during stuttering; extra sounds or words used as "starters"
When problem is most noticeable	Come and go when child is tired, excited, talking about complex/new topics, asking or answering questions, or talking to unresponsive listeners	Come and go in similar situations but more often present than absent	Tends to be present in most speaking; far more consistent and nonfluctuating
Child reaction	None apparent	Some show little concern, some will be frustrated and embarrassed	Most are embarrassed and some also fear speaking
Parent reaction	None to a great deal	Most concerned, but concern may be minimal	All have some degree of concern
Referral decision	Refer only if parents moderately to overly concerned	Refer if continues for 6 to 8 weeks or if parental concern justifies it	Refer as soon as possible

Adapted for use by permission of the Stuttering Foundation of America, Memphis, Tenn.

dren have difficulty understanding why they are different from others. In the primary grades a stuttering problem can make reading aloud difficult and interfere with the acquisition of reading skills. Stuttering may interfere with a child's learning in other ways. Many stuttering children will not ask questions of a teacher even when they want information. The psychosocial aspects of stuttering are particularly insiduous. School-age stutterers are frequent targets of teasing.[5] The embarrassment about stuttering usually increases in adolescence, and teens may begin to avoid social situations. Even adults who formerly stuttered often report feeling embarrassed and guilty about their use of tactics to avoid or conceal a problem, such as pretending to not have heard a question or substituting a word for one on which stuttering is anticipated.

Referral

Unless the parents express undue or continual concern, it usually is not necessary to refer a child whose speech is considered *normally disfluent*. Parents can be advised to avoid bringing any attention to the disfluencies, to give the child their full attention when is or she is talking, and to allow the child plenty of time to say what he or she wants to say.

Children who stutter mildly should be referred to a speech-language pathologist (SLP)* if they have stuttered for 3 months or more or if the stuttering continues for a few weeks after the parents have been trying to follow the suggestions mentioned above.

If a child's speech meets the criteria for *severe stuttering,* he or she should be referred to a qualified SLP as soon as possible. The course of treatment may well last a year or more. The pediatrician can assist teenagers who stutter by showing an understanding for the difficulty they encounter but urging them not to let the stuttering prevent them from engaging in activities they otherwise would attempt. Again, qualified speech-language pathologists can be of great value by aiding such individuals to identify their feared speech situations and supporting them as they work to develop a more positive attitude.

In the past parents concerned about their child's stuttering frequently were advised to ignore the problem and told that the child would outgrow it eventually. Although it is true that many young children who have incipient stuttering become fluent without treatment, children whose speech is diagnosed appropriately as stuttering usually require professional attention from an SLP to avoid the long-term embarrassment and frustration of a stuttering problem that gets worse rather than better as the child gets older. The type of fluency-enhancing suggestions and activities given to a child or parent would be helpful for any child, so even if there is a question as to whether the child has a fully developed stuttering problem, there appears little justification in withholding a referral.

The pediatrician often is the first professional person to recognize stuttering in a child. If a child (or his or her parents) can be seen for therapy when the problem consists primarily of easy, effortless repetitions, the chances for success are much higher than when the stuttering has become complicated by habitual struggle, fear of speaking, and avoidance behaviors. But even if the problem has already become severe, much can be done to improve the child's overall abil-

*The SLP should hold a Certificate of Clinical Competence from the American Speech-Language-Hearing Association and be experienced in working with childhood stuttering.

ity to communicate effectively and to decrease the severity of the stuttering.

REFERENCES

1. Andrews G: Epidemiology of stuttering. In Curlee RF, Perkins WH, editors: *Nature and treatment of stuttering: new directions,* San Diego, 1984, College-Hill.
2. Bloodstein O: *A handbook on stuttering,* Chicago, 1987, National Easter Seal Society.
3. Gordon PA, Luper HL: Speech disfluencies in nonstutterers: syntactic complexity and production task effects, *J Fluency Disorders* 14:429, 1989.
4. Kidd KK: Stuttering as a genetic disorder. In Curlee RF, Perkins WH, editors: *Nature and treatment of stuttering: new directions,* San Diego, 1984, College-Hill.
5. Peters TJ, Guitar B: *Stuttering: an integrated approach to its nature and treatment,* Baltimore, 1991, Williams & Wilkins.
6. Rosenbek JC: Stuttering secondary to nervous system damage. In Curlee RF, Perkins WH, editors: *Nature and treatment of stuttering: new directions,* San Diego, 1984, College-Hill.
7. Starkweather CW, Gottwald SR, Halfond MM: *Stuttering prevention: a clinical method,* Englewood Cliffs, NJ, 1990, Prentice-Hall.

SUGGESTED READINGS

Fraser J, Perkins WH, editors: *Do you stutter? A guide for teens,* 1987.

Guitar B: Is it stuttering or just normal language development? *Contemp Pediatr,* Feb 1988, p 109.

Guitar B, Conture EG: *The child who stutters: to the pediatrician,* 1991.

Materials and services available from the Stuttering Foundation of America, PO Box 11749, Memphis, TN 38111-0749. Phone 800-992-9392.

91 Temper Tantrums and Breath-Holding Spells

Gregory E. Prazar

TEMPER TANTRUMS

Temper tantrums represent a behavior that children exhibit almost inevitably during the second through fourth years of life. Therefore this is generally a "problem behavior" rather than a "behavioral problem." Displays of temper can run the gamut from a verbalized "no" to dramatic breath-holding spells, during which the child may lose consciousness. Helping parents cope with temper tantrums involves providing anticipatory guidance, sharing information on developmental psychology, and offering strategies to deal with tantrums.

Temper tantrums usually become part of the child's emotional repertoire during the second and third years of life. Early signs of the negativism that is part of tantrums can be appreciated as early as 12 months of age. Some children continue to display occasional tantrums until the age of 5 or 6 years. Tantrums typically then reappear in a slightly less intense form during adolescence, when independence once more becomes an issue for the developing child.

Several aspects of the toddler's development appear to make tantrums almost inevitable. First, because the 1-year-old can walk and climb, the child begins to achieve physical mastery over the environment. This increased physical independence and an insatiable curiosity frequently place the child in dangerous situations that require parental intervention. Imposition of adult safety limits thwarts and frustrates the child, often precipitating tantrums. Second, the child's increased exploration of the environment immediately creates a conflict because he or she must adapt to rules of an adult world. The child enters a hostile environment of adult social values, where people are expected to use the bathroom appropriately, verbalize their dissatisfactions rather than "act" them out physically, sit quietly while eating, and sometimes subjugate their own wants to those of others. This is too much for the egocentric toddler to bear, and frustration is inevitable.

Third, between the ages of 1 and 4 years the toddler begins to develop an increased awareness of how he or she is separate and different from his or her mother. The child experiences a conflict between desires for autonomy and desires to remain close to the mother. Frustration in dealing with these intense feelings frequently results in tantrums.

Tensions therefore are created in "establishing ego boundaries as separate from those of parents," as Brazelton[1] states, and in coping with physical limitations placed on exploring an adult world. Adults frequently deal with their own tensions and frustrations by verbalizing their feelings; the toddler, however, lacks a sophisticated ability to verbalize. A toddler's frustration with the adult world may be displayed in doing the exact opposite of what the adult requests, by saying "no, no" yet following through with the adult request (what Fraiberg[2] refers to as the "cheerful no"), by dawdling, or by displaying physical behavior outright (e.g., kicking, screaming, lying on the floor, hitting, throwing, biting).

Most parents probably would agree that intellectual appreciation of the cause of tantrums does not necessarily aid in coping with a screaming and inconsolable child. Reasons for parental frustration are understandable. Well-meaning relatives and friends (who likely have forgotten their experience as young parents) may propagate myths about tantrums, which intensify parental anxiety and confusion. Myths of causation suggest that children who display tantrums are overindulged, underdisciplined, or parented by inadequate adults. Myths of management suggest that tantrums should be quelled by spanking, dousing with cold water, or threats.

Anticipatory Guidance for Tantrums

It is the responsibility of the primary care physician to provide anticipatory guidance about temper tantrums. Such guidance may forestall events that precipitate tantrums and prevent future parental confusion in dealing with negative behaviors. The physician has many opportunities during the child's first 2 years to provide behavioral counseling.

At the 6-month infant visit the importance of time away from the infant should be emphasized. Parents who occasionally leave their infants and toddlers with responsible babysitters provide their children with the security that adults can leave and *will* come back, and provide themselves with important mental health holidays from the rigors of parenting.

At the 9- or 12-month infant visit, environmental engineering should be discussed. The importance of home safety (e.g., safety plugs in outlets, safety latches on drawers), the removal of valuables or breakables from the child's reach, and the availability of a safe place for the child to play (playpen or enclosed area) are examples of such engineering. Therefore this visit not only may reduce chances for childhood accidents, but also may forestall potential adult-toddler power struggles over environmental dangers.

The 15- or 18-month visit provides the physician another opportunity to offer the parent alternatives to negative interactions with the toddler. Afternoon naps (to allow for renewal of toddler and maternal energy), the importance of praising cooperative toddler efforts, and the concept of limited decision making for the toddler ("Do you want to wear the green or blue shirt today?" versus "Which shirt do you want to wear today?") represent issues that may help parents to minimize hostile encounters with their toddler.

The approach here should be one that encourages parents to describe how they believe tantrums should be handled rather than one that displays the physician's personal biases about child rearing. Several excellent books describing turbulent toddlerhood can be suggested to parents, including Brazelton's *Toddlers and Parents,*[1] Ilg and Ames's *Child Behavior,*[3] and Schmitt's *Your Child's Health.*[5] Furthermore, *general* guidelines concerning tantrums can be given. Tantrums are best ignored unless, as Fraiberg[2] states, "they encroach on rights of others or potentially endanger." If safety is the issue, either environmental engineering should take place or the child should be restricted to his or her room for 2 to 3 minutes (a kitchen timer is helpful to remind both parent and toddler of the time). If the child hits, bites, or throws in anger, room restriction for 2 to 3 minutes once again should be suggested.

Some parents are reluctant to use bedroom restriction because they worry either that the child will associate the bedroom with unpleasant experiences or that the child will not feel adequately remorseful if placed in a room full of toys. Parents should be reassured that room restriction does not cause bedroom fears. Similarly, goals of discipline are to teach rules and to help the child understand which behaviors are acceptable. Discipline does not need to be severe to be effective.

Temper tantrums occur much more frequently in the presence of parents; they are much less common in the presence of alternative care providers. Most experienced child care providers feel comfortable dealing with temper tantrums. If the child care provider expresses concern to a parent about a child's temper tantrums, several questions should be considered. Does the day care provider have adequate training to deal with such a common behavior? Is this child care setting the most appropriate for the child (in terms of adult-child ratio, philosophy of discipline used by the day care provider, and realistic developmental expectations for the child's behavior in the day care setting)? Are the child's temper tantrums much more severe or frequent than those of his or her peers? These questions should be addressed with the day care provider. Subsequently, parents and the day care provider should formulate a plan for dealing with the tantrums that is followed consistently both at home and at the day care location. If the parent and the day care provider cannot agree on such a plan, the child's primary practitioner should be consulted.

More specific guidelines for managing tantrums may be necessary in other individual situations. Parents should be encouraged by the physician to ventilate their feelings (to the physician) about tantrums and reassured that they are doing the best job they can for their toddler.

Management of Problem Tantrums

Although tantrums represent a stage of the normal developing toddler personality, several factors suggest that further professional intervention is advisable. Toddlers who display persistent negativism or tantrums may suffer from too restrictive parenting, may receive too little positive reinforcement and affection, or may have parents who place unreasonable behavioral expectations on them.

Children who display tantrums regularly past 5 or 6 years of age may be displaying signs of depression or poor self-esteem, or they may be children who live in a family in which emotional problems exist. When temper tantrums regularly occur at school, academic problems should be suspected, as peer pressure usually inhibits displays of tantrums.

Children exhibiting persistent tantrums along with other associated behaviors (e.g., inability to concentrate, stereotypic behaviors, unrealistic fears, inability to display affection) may have underlying emotional problems. Similarly, parents who verbalize persistent frustration with tantrums or an inability to cope with age-appropriate tantrums may need more comprehensive counseling than the primary practitioner can provide.

Many parenting groups are available to help parents cope with negative behaviors. Programs such as Systematic Training for Effective Parenting (STEP) and Parent Effectiveness Training (PET) provide valuable community referral sources for families. If such services are not available, or if it is obvious that more sophisticated professional counseling is warranted, the family should be referred to a psychiatrically trained counselor.

Referral should be discussed as soon as the physician anticipates its necessity and should stress the involvement of *both* parents. The physician should maintain contact with the family concerning their problem after the referral has been made. Such ongoing contact may solidify the family's commitment to obtain and comply with the counseling (see Chapter 93, Consultation and Referral for Behavioral and Developmental Problems).

BREATH-HOLDING SPELLS

Breath-holding spells represent a childhood behavior that causes particular anxiety for parents. Spells occur between ages 6 months and 5 years, with most occurring between 12 and 18 months of age. According to Menkes,[4] approximately 5% of all children display breath-holding spells. The pathophysiology of such spells, however, is unclear.

Spells are precipitated by anger, frustration, fear, or minor injury (often a very minor head injury) and are categorized as *cyanotic spells* or *pallid spells.* Both types of spells are unlikely to occur more often than once a day and apparently are not associated with an increased predisposition to epilepsy (although brief seizurelike activity can occur as a terminating event in either form of spell).

Cyanotic breath-holding spells more often are precipitated by anger or frustration than by fear or injury. The toddler emits a short, loud cry, takes a deep breath, and holds it. Cyanosis occurs after approximately 30 seconds. Either the attack terminates at this point or the toddler becomes rigid or limp and loses consciousness (loss of consciousness occurs in approximately 50% of all children who have breath-holding spells). In rare situations mild clonic movements of the extremities follow.

Pallid breath-holding spells are similar to cyanotic spells in most respects, but more often are precipitated by fear or minor injury. The initial cry is brief or silent. The spell then proceeds as with a cyanotic spell. Toddlers who suffer from pallid spells often are from families that have a history of syncope and, in fact, themselves have an increased chance of syncopal attacks as adults.

Because both forms of breath-holding spells potentially can terminate with seizurelike movements, differentiation between spells and epilepsy is important. Patients who have epilepsy, when they have seizures, display cyanosis *during* or *after* the seizures, not before seizure onset. Furthermore, electroencephalograms performed on patients who suffer from breath-holding spells are normal during non-breath-holding periods; patients who have epilepsy often have abnormal electroencephalograms during seizure-free periods.

Management of Breath-Holding

There is no effective medical therapy for breath-holding spells, although some toddlers who experience seizurelike activity along with spells are prescribed anticonvulsant therapy. However, the decision to use medication remains controversial among pediatric neurologists.

Coping with breath-holding spells can be extremely difficult for parents. Spells that terminate with loss of consciousness or with seizurelike movements obviously are frightening. Convincing parents that no harm will come to their child is important. Nevertheless, parents of a breath-holder frequently will not enforce limits for fear of precipitating the child's anger and a consequent attack. Such parents need repeated reassurance and encouragement to continue age-appropriate limits on their child's behavior. To do otherwise will create an overindulged child who subsequently may fear loss of parental love *because* limits have been rescinded.

When to refer a breath-holding patient to a neurologist or a psychiatrically trained professional may not be an easy decision for the physician. If parents request further consultation, their wish certainly should be respected, even if the physician is confident that further evaluation is unnecessary. If parents indicate agreement with the physician that spells are of no consequence yet continue to withhold appropriate limit-setting, referral to a mental health professional should take place. The physician who is unsure of the diagnosis of breath-holding (especially in situations where loss of consciousness or seizurelike activity occurs) always should refer the family to a pediatric neurologist. Referral must not end the physician-parent communication concerning the spells, however, because an ongoing dialogue may ensure compliance with the referral source.

SUMMARY

Temper tantrums and breath-holding spells usually represent benign forms of childhood behavior, evolving from the child's preverbal attempts to express feelings of frustration and anger. Unfortunately, parents frequently find it difficult to appreciate the benign course of such behaviors when they daily must face a screaming, inconsolable toddler who may even lose consciousness and then display seizurelike movements. Parents can best deal with negative behaviors when they are adequately prepared by the physician *before* such behaviors occur and when they are offered empathic guidance and positive reinforcement during regular office visits.

REFERENCES

1. Brazelton TB: *Toddlers and parents,* New York, 1979, Dell.
2. Fraiberg S: *The magic years,* New York, 1959, Charles Scribner's Sons.
3. Ilg FL, Ames LB: *Child behavior,* New York, 1955, Harper & Row.
4. Menkes JH: *Textbook of child neurology,* ed 2, Philadelphia, 1980, Lea & Febiger.
5. Schmitt B: *Your child's health,* New York, 1987, Bantam Books.

92 Options for Psychosocial Intervention with Children and Adolescents

Sheridan Phillips and Mark D. Weist

The pediatrician often is unsure about what therapeutic options exist for children and adolescents who have psychosocial problems, as well as about what actually will transpire in the course of treatment. This hampers the effort to refer the patient appropriately and to prepare the child and parents for what to expect. This chapter acquaints the pediatrician with the most common forms of therapeutic interventions available and provides a brief review of their efficacy. Discussion is focused on treatment rather than on assessment. Also, only "psychological" treatment is described (i.e., pharmacotherapy is not discussed), although it must be noted that a combination of psychotherapy and pharmacotherapy is indicated in some instances of severe psychosocial disorders.[17] We have attempted to highlight the key aspects of major *approaches* to child therapy. There are a plethora of *techniques:* Kazdin,[10] in his review of the child psychotherapy literature, identified over 230 therapy techniques from "activity-interview" therapy to "Z-process therapy."

Much of the confusion regarding psychotherapy is caused by two confounding variables: the therapist's theoretical orientation and the modality in which it is used. For example, one can take a behavioral approach with a child or with a family. Alternatively, family therapy can be conducted from a "systems" point of view. This chapter examines the five major schools of thought, or theoretical orientations, as well as the modalities in which they most commonly are applied (sometimes in adapted form), as shown in Table 92-1. Each school of thought listed at the left in the table is presented as a separate and distinct orientation. It is important, however, to emphasize that these are artificial divisions. There is much more melding and blending in the actual practice of child therapy, and combinations of approaches are both sensible and common. The modalities in which these theoretical orientations are typically applied are indicated under the appropriate column in the table.

Discussion of each therapeutic orientation includes the basic premises and goals of treatment, its typical course (e.g., length), examples of techniques or procedures used, most appropriate recipients, and a brief review of the efficacy of that approach. Evaluating the efficacy of treatment, however, is so important yet complex that a general discussion of psychotherapy research precedes the presentation of specific therapeutic orientations.

In an attempt to provide an overview, this review undoubtedly oversimplifies both theories and issues and omits much of the detail and nuance each orientation deserves. Specific discussion of when and how to refer children is not included because this is provided throughout this section of the textbook for each specific clinical problem, particularly in chapter 93, Consultation and Referral for Behavioral and Developmental Problems.

THERAPEUTIC EFFICACY: GENERAL CONSIDERATIONS

Physicians, consumers, and society at large have an abiding concern to document the usefulness of therapy. The "bottom line" questions are, "Does it work?" and "Is it cost effective?" These questions are easy to ask but extraordinarily difficult to answer. Conceptual, methodological, pragmatic, and ethical considerations appear to conspire against a clear-cut assessment of therapeutic efforts. Before discussing the apparent efficacy of specific orientations and modalities, this section reviews the general types of research strategies used to evaluate therapies and the complexity of and problems inherent in such research.

One form of psychotherapy research is focused on the *process* of treatment and examines aspects of therapy as it is unfolding (i.e., what transpires within a session). This large body of literature has yielded very useful information about treatment[3] (e.g., see Client-centered Therapy, discussed below). However, for the sake of brevity this section reviews the other major type of research, *outcome* research, which investigates change that occurs from the beginning to the end of therapy and following the conclusion of treatment. Ideally such investigations document the nature and extent of change and demonstrate that such outcomes result directly from specific aspects of the intervention.

One approach is a *within-subject* design, whereby the experimental control is internal (i.e., no control groups are used). In this approach each subject or patient serves as his or her own control. Such an evaluation typically begins with a "baseline" period, during which the patient's behavior is recorded before any attempt at intervention. Recording continues during an intervention phase, when specific therapeutic procedures are in effect. One then may cease intervention and return to the baseline condition and subsequently reinstitute treatment. Repeated alternation accompanied by substantial changes in the observed behavior is an indication that the treatment is responsible for the behavior change. A variant of this design is to introduce one component of the treatment at a time (e.g., each might be targeted at a different type of behavior) to determine whether a behavior changes when—and only when—the relevant intervention is introduced. The durability of change is assessed at various follow-up points.

The advantages of this design are the degree of experimental control and specificity it offers and its applicability with only a small number of patients or even with a single case (a

Table 92-1 Overview of Therapeutic Orientations and Therapeutic Modalities

	Therapeutic modality					
Therapeutic orientation	**Individual (child alone)**	**Parents alone**	**Parents and child**	**Family**	**Group (children and/or parents)**	**Residential**
Psychodynamic	X	Adapted		Adapted	Adapted	Adapted
Behavioral	X	X	X	X	X	X
Phenomenological						
Client-centered	X				X	
Gestalt	X				X	
Systems		X		X		
Eclectic	X	X	X	X	X	X

"single-subject" design). Although internally valid, however, it is difficult to generalize from only one case; replications and extensions thus are required to increase confidence in the efficacy of treatment. Another difficulty is the "irreversibility" of some interventions, either for pragmatic or ethical reasons. It also has been argued that a therapeutic effect should be permanent and not so easily reversible.

In *between-subject* research, the nature of change is compared for a therapy group (or groups) versus a control group (or groups), typically before and after treatment and at various follow-up points (e.g., 6 months and 1 year after treatment). If done well, such research is costly and complex. For example, studies generally include several treatment groups. One group might receive a complete treatment "package" consisting of two components; a second group might receive one component only and a third group the second component only, with appropriate "fillers" to equate time spent in treatment. (Note how a three-component package would generate seven treatment groups.) Alternatively, or in addition, another group might receive a different type of treatment (e.g., behavior therapy versus client-centered therapy). With this approach the difficulty is in controlling for therapist characteristics: using a "switch-hitter" most likely would result in differential levels of skill confounded with therapeutic orientation, whereas using different individuals would confound personal characteristics and therapeutic orientation.

Devising appropriate control groups is no easier. One option is to use a "no treatment," or "waiting list," control group. This is accomplished by collecting a large group of comparable patients who have requested treatment and then randomly assigning them to therapy conditions: (1) immediate treatment or (2) treatment following a waiting period, with a delay at least as long as therapy for the treatment group (and longer if maintenance is to be assessed). It is common for at least some patients in the waiting-list group to improve over time. This is thought to occur because the individuals who have requested treatment have come to recognize that they have a problem and have made a commitment to change; deprived of access to professional therapists, they often turn to therapists in their environment (e.g., friends, pastor, self-help groups) or simply apply for treatment elsewhere. With children, one also must consider the effect of maturation during the waiting period.

Another important control is the "placebo," or "attention-control," group, where the therapist is given the challenging task of conducting sessions with patients but not actually doing anything specific. This controls for the patient's expectation that he or she is being helped and for "nonspecific" effects of therapy. The "nonspecificity" hypothesis asserts that significant change in therapy can be attributed to four primary factors: (1) providing a trusting and caring relationship, (2) working within a "safe" atmosphere, (3) explaining confusing feelings and behaviors, and (4) implementing a set of procedures based on some conceptual scheme.[12] Such nonspecific factors are used to explain why placebo control groups typically display some improvement and why different forms of therapy can achieve equivalent results. To demonstrate its efficacy, then, a therapeutic intervention must demonstrate that it produced significantly greater change than could be accounted for by the nonspecific aspects of treatment.

A host of other difficulties beset research endeavors, such as the selection of appropriate dependent measures (behavior to be recorded) and the reliability and validity of the methods by which behaviors are assessed. Assuming that these challenges can be met and that a large enough pool of comparable patients and comparable therapists is available, the researcher still is confronted by major ethical concerns. Withholding treatment for an extended time and offering placebo intervention or a treatment hypothesized to be less than optimal all pose clear ethical obstacles. It is understandable therefore to find that some investigators have chosen to conduct *analog* research, which attempts to simulate clinical conditions in the laboratory. Participants typically are undergraduates who volunteer for course credit or monetary incentives or who have minor problems (e.g., mild fear of snakes or dogs or mild test-taking or speech-giving anxiety). The difficulty with this approach is the trade-off between internal and external validity: although greater experimental control is gained, the ability to generalize to real clinical situations is lessened.

Given the numerous and varied obstacles to be confronted, it is admirable to find investigators who remain undaunted and struggle valiantly to conduct the best possible evaluations of their therapeutic efforts. Accepting this challenge has continued to improve the level of sophistication evidenced in psychotherapy research.[5] Even the questions asked have become more sophisticated and have moved well beyond the question of "Does it work?" Gordon Paul has summarized the ultimate outcome question as, "What treatment, by whom, is most effective for this individual, with this problem, under this set of circumstances, and how does it come about?"[3]

Clearly this question cannot be answered by a single study but will represent the cumulative knowledge of multiple efforts to address the efficacy of therapy.

PSYCHODYNAMIC THERAPY

Basic Assumptions

Psychodynamic therapy covers a wide variety of approaches, from traditional analysis to neofreudian variants such as sociocultural, object relations, and ego psychology. The fundamental assumptions, however, were derived from Freud by his daughter, Anna Freud, by Melanie Klein, and by subsequent analytical theorists who specialized in work with children.[7] The concept of *unconscious conflict* is central: the child's disturbed or abnormal behavior is hypothesized to result from intrapsychic conflict in the same manner that an infection causes the overt manifestation of a fever. Therefore treatment is focused on identifying and resolving the underlying conflict among instinctual urges (id), conscious thoughtful regulation or reality orientation (ego), and self-evaluative thoughts, or "conscience" (superego). In contrast with other therapy approaches, psychodynamic therapists do not base decisions related to termination of therapy on whether presenting symptoms have improved. Instead, therapy continues until internal conflicts are brought to the surface and worked through. The belief is that, without resolution of underlying problems, other symptoms will develop to replace the original symptoms—what some dynamic therapists refer to as "old wine in new bottles."

Therapeutic Activities

The therapist first attempts to establish a relationship with the child that will enable the child to feel free to express any thoughts and feelings, such as anger and sadness. In fact this freedom of expression is seen by many theorists to be therapeutic in itself. With this relationship in place the therapist comments on the child's expressed feelings, generally interpreting the meaning of symbols revealed in the child's fantasies, dreams, or, most often, free play. Most of the therapeutic work is conducted in a playroom, using materials such as clay and sand, fingerpaints, games, and human figures and a doll house. The "depth" of interpretation provided varies among different theorists. For example, a doll thrown across the room might be seen by Anna Freud as anger toward the situation, whereas others might interpret it as hatred for the mother. Although interpretation is an important therapeutic device, it is used parsimoniously, especially at the outset of treatment. Most therapists draw on additional devices, such as developing the transference reaction (or reaction to the therapist), "working through" past interpersonal conflicts, and gratifying dependency needs. There are so many different adaptations of psychodynamic treatment and so much variation among therapists that it is difficult to provide a unitary picture of therapeutic activities. Many therapists vary the intensity of treatment and their approach, depending on the developmental stage of the child, the nature of the psychopathology, and the family situation.

Certain obvious adjustments have been made to apply psychodynamic treatment to children. Because children find it more difficult than adults to express their inner lives verbally, play is used more often than techniques based on free association (method of encouraging the patient to reveal anything that comes to mind, without censorship or guiding efforts by the therapist, in an effort to bring forth unconscious processes). Also, children generally do not seek therapy themselves; thus it is the therapist's responsibility to develop the child's insight so that he or she understands that a problem exists. Even with these modifications, however, analytical intervention generally is not attempted with children younger than 4 years of age. For the most part adolescents have not been considered to be appropriate candidates for such treatment because they are too old for play therapy and too young for the traditional analytical couch.

It should be noted that less traditional forms of psychodynamic therapy increasingly have been used with children and adolescents. Particularly when children and adolescents have experienced severe trauma such as sexual abuse, psychodynamic therapy techniques play a central role in treatment. In addition to education regarding common misperceptions of sexually abused children (e.g., feelings of self-blame, guilt, inferiority), these children are assisted in reporting on what happened to them and in expressing emotions associated with the abuse. Such processing and working through of abuse-related perceptions and emotions is viewed as central in removing threatening and disabling aspects of the abusive experience. The ultimate aim is for the child to achieve some perspective and self-acceptance such as, "Yes, that happened to me, and I can talk about it. But I know that I did nothing wrong and many other children have experienced what I have. I also know that I can cope with what happened and move on with my life."[9] Many therapists believe that for the abused child or adolescent to reach this perspective it is necessary to revisit and work through painful historical events and conflicts, the *sine qua non* of psychodynamic therapy.

As shown in Table 92-1 the traditional form of psychodynamic treatment has been conducted alone with the child. Whereas Anna Freud believed that it was the therapist's responsibility to educate parents about their child's problems, many psychodynamic therapists deliberately have little contact with the parents and other family members. Such therapists generally consider it inappropriate to work with both the child and any other family member; thus it is quite possible to find a family that uses three or more therapists: one for the child, another for a second child, and a third for the parents' marital problems. A major concern of psychodynamic therapists is that, when working with parents and the child together, the child will perceive an alliance between the adults and thus feel that his or her relationship with the therapist has been compromised. Additional rationales for this approach are the avoidance of "competition" for the therapist and "transference" problems that may arise when parents and children are seen together.

The disadvantage of separate therapists is the frequent lack of coordination among their efforts, so at times they may be working at cross purposes. The absence of contact between the therapist and the child's parents also often results in the parents' ignorance of the child's problems, of the goals and progress of therapy, and of what parents might do to assist the child's progress. Meeting only with the child may leave parents with the impression that they are expending significant money and effort, often over a period of several years, to enable the child to play with toys such as those he or she has at home. This obviously does a disservice to the therapist's efforts. Such problems have prompted adaptations of psychodynamic treatment, with some therapists seeing the entire family together or meeting with the parents separately.

The psychodynamic approach also has been adapted for use with groups of children and adolescents (usually from five to eight children). Group therapy has two major assets: it makes more efficient use of professional time and provides therapy in a different setting, where children interact with and learn from each other as well as from the therapist. Groups of younger children typically play games or engage in activities such as arts and crafts, with the therapist guiding the group indirectly (i.e., by example). Psychodrama and more "talking" techniques generally are employed with older children and adolescents. The main goals of treatment continue to be achieving insight into and resolving unconscious conflict. Such groups may be homogeneous (e.g., victims of sexual abuse) or more heterogeneous (e.g., including both aggressive and withdrawn children). It also is possible to structure residential treatment with many psychodynamic features—combining individual and group treatment in an accepting, tolerant atmosphere that highlights the use of expressive materials such as paints and clay.

The course of traditional child psychoanalysis is lengthy, typically requiring two to four sessions per week for anywhere from 2 to 5 years. The obvious expense of such treatment and the limited number of children who can receive it have led to the development of less extensive psychotherapy that incorporates many aspects of analysis. Such intervention might involve one or two sessions a week for 1 to 3 years. The more limited goals of this shorter-term treatment have been described as (1) increasing capacity for reality testing, (2) strengthening object relations, and (3) loosening fixations. The appropriate adult candidate for psychodynamic treatment has been semijokingly referred to as a "YAVIS"—young, attractive, verbal, intelligent, and salaried. The same general point can be applied to children because the typical patient is only mildly to moderately disturbed and has many assets. Aspects of the analytical approach, however, have been included in other interventions with more universal applicability (see Eclectic Therapy).

Efficacy

Although a considerable amount of study has been devoted to child psychoanalysis and new adaptations of psychodynamic therapy, the majority of these investigations represent either uncontrolled case studies or investigations of the therapeutic process. Thus there are some data available (1) regarding *process* questions such as who is an appropriate candidate for psychodynamic therapy and (2) on the effect of therapists' interpretations. However, even these studies have yielded equivocal findings.[1,6,8] As with all forms of therapy, less research has been conducted with children than with adults. For both children and adults, psychodynamic therapists have paid the least amount of attention to *outcome* research, or controlled investigation of actual change or improvement produced by treatment.

Following Eysenck's devastating 1952 critique of the outcome of psychodynamic psychotherapy with adults,[3] Levitt conducted similar analyses of traditional psychotherapy with children (one paper reviewed 17 studies; a second described another 22 studies).[13] This work, published in 1957 and 1963, failed to find any sound support for the contention that traditional psychotherapy facilitates children's recovery from mental illness. These startling reports prompted attempts to broaden approaches to the treatment of children and to develop other alternatives, notably that of behavior therapy.

In recent years investigators have used "meta-analysis" in an attempt to evaluate the effectiveness of various therapies. Meta-analysis enables quantification of the results of studies so that they are comparable with other investigations. The most common meta-analytic technique is to compute "effect size," defined as the difference between means of treatment and control groups divided by the standard deviation of the control group. A number of meta-analyses have been conducted on the adult psychotherapy literature, with findings generally indicating that treatment is better than no treatment and that alternative models of therapy have equivalent impacts, for the most part; for specific problems such as fears, behavior therapy has been shown to be superior. Very few meta-analyses have been conducted on child therapies. Casey and Berman[4] (1985) reviewed 75 psychotherapy interventions among children published between 1952 and 1983 and found that only 5 of the 75 (9%) studies used a psychodynamic approach. Effect size for these psychodynamic interventions was .21, the lowest effect size of any therapy (compared with effect sizes of .49 for client-centered therapy and .91 for behavior therapy). However, interpretation of this finding is constrained by the small number of psychodynamic studies reviewed. An additional consideration is that outcomes in psychodynamic interventions tend to be defined broadly (and subjectively), which decreases the likelihood of documenting significant change, particularly when compared with behavioral studies, which generally use specific and discrete outcome criteria (e.g., the number of fears reported on a self-report measure). Other child therapy meta-analyses have since replicated Casey and Berman's findings indicating the relative inferiority of psychodynamic techniques when compared with behavioral techniques.[16] Studies of group psychotherapies similarly have shown relatively limited impacts of psychodynamic approaches, particularly when compared with behavioral methods.[10]

This is not to say that psychoanalysis does no good; the available research merely indicates that clear evidence of efficacy is still lacking. It may be that psychoanalysis has limited applicability to children because of their level of cognitive development. It has been well established that young children have difficulty understanding adult interpretations of social interactions and in taking the other person's point of view and that often they do not understand how others perceive them. Before about 8 years of age most children have only a primitive understanding of intentions, motives, and feelings. Given these well-documented cognitive limitations, children may have difficulty understanding complex psychodynamic explanations of their thoughts and feelings. Alternatively, psychoanalysis may be useful with children but merely not as cost effective as other forms of treatment.

Part of the difficulty in conducting scientific research of psychoanalysis lies in the very nature of the concepts used. For example, how can one gain access to an unconscious that by definition is inaccessible? However, the crux of the problem is determining acceptable criteria for measuring outcome: symptom relief is viewed as being too superficial an index of the change brought about in the child. Furthermore, many analysts maintain that each situation or case is unique and therefore that no situation can be replicated and no two patients adequately matched. They also argue that it is impossible to differentiate changes caused by maturation from those resulting from therapy. Finally, most analytically oriented therapists agree with Freud in insisting that psychoanalysis can be judged only by experienced analysts. It should be noted, however, that Freud himself was not optimistic about a scientific study of psychoanalysis. One must observe that these obstacles have not hindered therapists of other orientations from at least attempting to evaluate the effectiveness of their interventions in a controlled manner. Ultimately, then, the lack of scientific study of psychoanalysis probably reflects the values of its practitioners, who typically are uninterested in research. Investigators have distinguished between statistically significant and clinically significant therapy outcomes; the latter assesses the extent to which intervention returns the patient to a normative range of functioning, with the presenting problems resolved and change perceptible by significant others in the patient's life. Perhaps use of this less rigorous standard is more appropriate for evaluating the impact of psychodynamic therapies on children.

BEHAVIOR THERAPY

The behavior approach to treatment has grown with amazing rapidity in the past 25 years. For example, the first report of a token-economy intervention was published in 1968; its use was widespread by the mid-1970s. Behavior therapists who were trained 10 years ago are surprised to find themselves no longer a rebellious, vocal minority but a part of the establishment. Surveys indicate that approximately 50% of all clinical psychologists in the United States and over 60% of clinical child psychologists identify their orientation as behavioral or cognitive-behavioral, and behavior therapy associations now exist in more than 30 countries.

Basic Assumptions

Behavior therapy is not, as often is thought, a collection of techniques. Rather, it is an *approach* to conceptualizing and changing human behavior, an approach characterized by empirical methodology.[5,8] The key assumption of behavior therapists is that they must "anchor" their understanding by reference to observable behavior. An abstract concept, such as anxiety, thus is understood by asking questions such as how the patient experiences anxiety, when it is worse and when it is better, what the "trigger" events are, how the patient responds to these anxious situations, and what the consequences are for him or her and for others. Each patient represents a "miniexperiment" in which the therapist examines the presenting problem and its development in the context of the patient's history. The therapist then searches for those variables that control the problem behavior. The resulting *functional analysis* represents a hypothesis that guides the therapist. This hypothesis is tested by the therapist and the patient as intervention proceeds. The therapist also typically relies heavily on data collection to assess the progress of treatment and the adequacy of his or her working hypothesis; thus the therapist often asks the patient to monitor and record specific behavior and will track its frequency over time.

A very early focus for behavioral analysis was a search for the stimuli that prompted the behavior and for the patient's response (hence S-R, or stimulus-response). This fairly rapidly evolved to SORC (stimulus-organism-response-consequence), which incorporates "organismic" factors such as the patient's perception of the stimulus and the consequences that the response engendered (e.g., the reaction of others). In the past 20 years growing numbers of behavior therapists have emphasized the importance of patients' thought processes or cognitions, as well as their overt behavior. This approach, referred to as *cognitive-behavior therapy,* has become the second most common therapy orientation after the "eclectic" orientation.[10] The cognitive-behavior therapist attends to factors such as the patient's expectations for himself and others, how the patient labels an event, and what kinds of statements the patient makes to himself. For example in their work with impulsive children Kendall and Braswell[11] have developed and evaluated interventions that focus on the use of behavioral principles to alter cognition (internal behavior) rather than overt behavior. These children are trained to use a series of self-statements (e.g., "What is my problem?" "What is a good plan?" "How is my plan working?" "How did I do?") in approaching, negotiating, and evaluating their performance in problematic situations. Increased understanding of such attitudinal and perceptual processes and deliberate attempts to modify them have brought behavior therapy much closer to other therapeutic approaches, such as ego psychology. In fact, the past few years have seen several laudable attempts to bring about a rapprochement between behavioral and psychodynamic formulations.[6] Even though cognitive-behavioral approaches are gaining increasing prominence, more traditional approaches (manipulating antecedents and reward and punishment contingencies for target behaviors) continue to play a central role in child behavioral interventions, particularly those used with developmentally disabled children.

In designing therapeutic interventions, the behavior therapist draws on the principles and models of experimental psychology. Many of these come from learning theory: classical and operant conditioning, observational-social learning (i.e., modeling), and the development of self-control. Other paradigms also are useful, such as research in social psychology regarding the process of attitude change and "commitment" to a specific course of action. Probably the broadest theory employed is social learning theory, which presumes a continuity between normal and abnormal behavior, implying that maladaptive behaviors are acquired through the same processes as normal behaviors. Accordingly, specific efforts to learn and use more adaptive behavior are expected to bring about changes in the way patients view themselves and in how others see and react to them. Thus intervention is a cyclical process involving change in behavior, attitudes, and cognitions. Bandura's more recent "self-efficacy" theory[2] attempts to synthesize a variety of therapeutic interventions as procedures that gradually convince the individual of his or her ability to cope with difficult and frightening situations.

Therapeutic Activities

It is difficult to state succinctly what a behavior therapist does with a patient because the hallmark of the behavioral approach is to tailor intervention to the particular needs of a given patient. Therapy therefore is very different for different problems. Although various treatment "packages" have been developed for specific problems, these are standardized largely for research and demonstration and subsequently are adapted for the individual patient. The key, as noted before, is the functional analysis or behavioral formulation of the problem. Treatment then is derived logically from assessment. For example, one important distinction is that of a behavioral *deficit* versus an *inhibition.* In the case of a deficit of the appropriate skills, the therapist would focus on acquiring skills (e.g., for social skills training: see Chapter 86, Peer Relationship Problems). Alternatively a patient might possess the appropriate skills but be inhibited in using them in certain situations because of excessive anxiety or fear of the consequences; therapy then would focus on reducing these inhibitions.

Regardless of the specific problem, there are some commonalities in behavioral and cognitive-behavioral approaches. The focus largely (although not exclusively) is on the present. There is a commitment to experimental evaluation; the behavior therapist is likely to set concrete goals to be achieved within a relatively short time, with progress then being evaluated by both the therapist and the patient. Whenever possible, targets for intervention are selected based on empirical evidence that changes in such targets will result in enhanced clinical outcomes for the patient, rather than targets being selected by subjective judgment or clinical intuition.[15] Therapy is active and involves joint planning and homework assignments for the patient (and sometimes for the therapist). It is assumed that insight almost always is insufficient for satisfactory behavioral change and that it needs to be accompanied by gradual learning and implementation of new behavior in a concrete manner. Finally, therapy obviously takes place in an interpersonal context, and practitioner characteristics are an important aspect of therapeutic change. Goldfried and Davison[8] have pointed out that a tough-minded approach to conceptualizing human problems in no way precludes a warm, genuine, and empathic interaction with patients. In fact, patients of behavior therapists who were asked to describe their therapist identified the same personal qualities that have been found to be therapeutic in other orientations, such as client-centered therapy (discussed below).

Behavior therapy initially was applied with psychotic, retarded, and autistic populations and with patients who had severe phobias—that is, people who had intractable problems that no one else wanted to treat. This approach to therapy subsequently has been applied to an enormous array of problems and situations and is not restricted by the age of the patient or the type of problem. In some cases it may be applied in conjunction with pharmacotherapy (e.g., for treatment of hyperactivity), although the goal typically is to withdraw medication whenever feasible. The same basic principles can be applied with a child who has a conduct disorder and with a group of hospitalized patients who are not functioning optimally. In fact a behavioral approach has been applied to many nontherapeutic situations (e.g., examining the voting behavior of Congress and energy conservation behaviors of the public) and thus is used in businesses and other consultative settings. For example, one could analyze a pediatric clinic to determine whether the existing contingencies promote desired behavior of its users, such as keeping appointments. Other general education efforts include self-help books (e.g., on toilet training). This broader application of behavior principles generally is referred to as *behavior modification,* with behavior *therapy* referring specifically to clinical problems.

It is important to note that behavior therapy appears deceptively simple to the neophyte therapist. In fact, the therapist is merely guided by general principles and must rely on considerable improvisation and inventiveness in the clinical situation. Many inexperienced practitioners (and teachers) have failed because of insufficient expertise both with clinical practice and with the theoretical principles on which therapy is based. Thus it is not uncommon to be told before instituting a successful behavioral program, "Oh, we tried behavior modification and that didn't work."

When using behavior therapy with individual children, therapists typically employ a combination of sessions with the child and parents and, if indicated, the school or other extrafamilial agency. With infants and toddlers the therapist typically works almost exclusively through the parents, although the child may be present for sessions when the therapist "models" a type of interaction with the child or provides feedback to parents as they attempt to interact with the child in a different manner. With older children and adolescents, the extent to which the parents and other family members are involved depends on the analysis of the problem and the focus of treatment. Seeing all family members together for all sessions is indicated in some situations, whereas in others the therapist may choose to focus on the teenager and his or her parents. In cases of multiple problems the therapist may alternate family sessions (e.g., to work on communication and problem solving) with individual sessions (e.g., to address problems with peers). Sessions typically occur once or twice a week, and the length of treatment can be as short as four sessions or can continue for over a year.

Behavior therapy also can be employed with groups of children or adolescents or with groups of children and their parents. This form of treatment, when appropriate, makes efficient use of professional time and also provides an opportunity to interact therapeutically with peers (e.g., engage in role-playing). Group therapy typically, although not necessarily, is employed with a relatively homogeneous group, such as shy and withdrawn boys, to enable treatment to focus on specific problems. A group approach also has been employed with parents; some parent-training groups are specifically therapeutic, and others are more educational and designed for a "normal" population. In any form groups generally are limited in time and rarely continue for longer than 6 months. It is not uncommon for two therapists to lead the group because they offer two models of behavior and also can model interaction with each other (e.g., a male and female therapist with a parent group). In addition, group interactions are so complex that having two therapists helps in tracking events in the group and ensuring that all patients receive therapeutic attention. Behavioral group therapies often focus on training of skills in a sequential and cumulative fashion (i.e., skills taught earlier are reviewed as new skills are taught). As each skill is taught, group leaders use a format of instruction (on the skill and when and how to use it), demonstration (leaders model the skill), rehearsal (participants take turns practicing the behavior), feedback (leaders and participants provide feedback to each other), continued rehearsal (incorporating feedback), and reinforcement (praise and encouragement from the leaders and participants). Also, considerable efforts are undertaken to ensure that the trained skills generalize to relevant settings in the child's natural environment (e.g., by incorporating realistic stimuli into training sessions, conducting training in natural environments) and maintain over time (e.g., by thinning reinforcement schedules from frequent to random).

Behavioral interventions also have had widespread use in the classroom. These range from management tips developed for use in the normal classroom to special classroom programs for children who have attention deficit/hyperactivity disorder (AD/HD) or conduct disorder.[7,13] Residential programs also have been developed for a variety of populations. Two examples are Project Re-ED and Achievement Place, the first for emotionally disturbed children and the second for delinquent children and adolescents.[7] Children are placed in an intensive treatment environment that includes sessions with parents and then are returned gradually to the home. (Achievement Place, a community-based program, even enables children to continue attending their own school during treatment.) In these residential settings, there usually is some form of token economy or behavior management system as a framework delineating behavioral expectations for residents and rewards and privileges that correspond to how well they meet these expectations. It is now difficult to find residential programs for emotionally disturbed and retarded children that do not make at least some use of behavioral principles. In fact, behavior therapy's greatest contribution may be the introduction of successful toilet training and management of retarded children, which has released an enormous amount of staff time and reoriented such programs from being almost completely custodial to emphasizing self-care and education.

Efficacy

With the possible exception of client-centered therapy for adults, no other therapeutic approach has been subjected to as much systematic evaluation as has behavior therapy. Investigations of behavior therapy thus dominate most scientific journals that report on professional treatment outcomes, and over 70% of investigations of treatment efficacy funded by the National Institutes of Mental Health are conducted by behavioral therapists. Although less research has been conducted on children than on adults, literally hundreds of outcome studies have been published in the past 20 years.

Notwithstanding the limitations of child therapy meta-analyses, evidence is strong for both the efficacy and the superiority of behavior therapy (1) for children who are retarded, autistic, aggressive, enuretic (especially those who have primary enuresis), introverted and withdrawn, hyperactive, academic underachievers, anxious about tests, or engaging in self-injurious behavior, and (2) for classroom management.[7,13] Additional evidence indicates that behavior therapy is as effective or more so than other orientations for the treatment of specific fears and phobias of children, depression, delinquency, and family problems.[7,13] It should be noted that this is based on reviews of treatment that sometimes combine behavior therapy with other forms of intervention (e.g., pharmacotherapy). Early concern regarding "system substitution" has proved to be unfounded; given appropriate problem analysis and intervention the substitution of a new symptom for the one that was treated has not been evident. Behavior therapy has had a more modest degree of success to date with problems such as obesity, addiction, and lack of assertion.[1,5-7,13] In addition, support is developing for the utility of behavioral treatment of headaches and other somatic disorders such as asthma, seizures, and persistent vomiting, as well as for helping children to cope with chronic illness and with medical and dental procedures and for promoting compliance with medical regimens.[7,13]

Although its accomplishments to date have been gratifying, much remains to be learned about behavior therapy. One prominent criticism is that behavior therapists do not understand completely why successful procedures are successful. For example, relaxation training and desensitization, although clearly efficacious, have been variously explained as counterconditioning (using a classic conditioning model), as operant conditioning, and as a process of cognitive change. Meta-analyses of child therapy efforts have shown larger-sized effects for behavioral as compared with nonbehavioral (e.g., client-centered, psychodynamic) methods. However, considering the different types of outcome measures and clinical problems and considering the relatively smaller number of nonbehavioral interventions, definitive conclusions cannot be drawn regarding the relative efficacy of the different therapeutic approaches. "Dismantling treatment designs," wherein components of treatments are reduced systematically in an attempt to identify the core therapeutic factors, could be used to address this question, but such studies are sorely lacking. An additional problem is that, whereas behavior therapists tend to be more concerned with the generalization and maintenance of treatment impacts than do nonbehavioral therapists, treatment effects that generalize across settings and maintain over time still are relatively rare.[10] This has led to attempts to identify and focus on classes of behavior that promote generalization and maintenance of more specific behaviors. For example, encouraging children to be energetic and attentive in social interaction often leads to concomitant improvement in behaviors such as smiling and initiating conversation. Other approaches to bolster and lengthen the impact of behavioral treatments include training patients to handle expected relapses (e.g., for problems such as enuresis, drug addiction), and using combined treatment approaches to address complex problems (e.g., desensitization for specific fears and relaxation training/cognitive restructuring to address generalized anxiety).

PHENOMENOLOGICAL THERAPIES

Phenomenological (or humanistic) therapy is insight oriented, as is psychodynamic therapy, and assumes that disordered behavior can best be altered by increased awareness of one's own motivations and needs. The distinction of humanistic therapy, however, is its emphasis on free will, attributing considerable freedom of choice to the patient. Phenomenological therapies focus on promoting the patient's "growth as a person," the primary vehicle for doing so being the patient-therapist relationship.

Client-centered Therapy

Basic Assumptions. The major phenomenological model is Carl Rogers' *client-centered therapy.* (Rogerians refer to "clients" rather than "patients" because they maintain that these individuals are healthy and responsible, not "sick.") This approach assumes that patients can best be understood by the way in which they construe events subjectively (a phenomenological perspective) rather than by an objective view of the events themselves.[3] The focus of therapy therefore is to attend to the client's perceptions and feelings and to let the client take the lead in the therapeutic process. Rogers postulates an innate tendency to actualize, or to realize one's potential, which is as much a human drive as the reduction of biological tensions (e.g., hunger).

Because people are assumed to be innately striving for good, total and nonjudgmental acceptance by the therapist is the key to providing an atmosphere in which the client's natural growth may proceed unhindered. Rogers assumes that maximal development will take place when the client does not need to struggle for and be concerned about approval by others. This approach is thus believed to be the appropriate remedy when people have been thwarted in their growth by the evaluations and judgments imposed on them by others, creating "conditions of worth" that force individuals to distort or become unaware of their own real feelings.

Therapeutic Activities. The key therapeutic relationship is based on three vital attitudes of the therapist: (1) *unconditional positive regard* (sometimes also referred to as "warmth"), (2) *empathy,* and (3) *congruence* (sometimes referred to as "genuineness"). To display *unconditional positive regard,* the therapist must convey the message that he or she cares about the client as a person, accepts the client, and trusts the client's ability to change. The therapist is willing to listen and avoid interpretation and value judgments. To display *empathy,* the therapist actively attempts to perceive the client's feelings and to communicate this understanding by "reflecting," or paraphrasing, what he or she believes to be the client's views. It should be emphasized that this is more than merely repeating what the client has said; it represents the distillation and "playback" of the client's feelings. Finally, in displaying *congruence,* the therapist establishes a real, human relationship by abandoning any facade and expressing himself or herself genuinely. In so doing, the therapist leaves the responsibility for the client's life with the client and indicates confidence in the client's ability to handle the therapist's feelings.

This individual, verbal form of client-centered therapy, although developed for adults, also is appropriate for many adolescents. Its course typically consists of one or two sessions weekly, for a period ranging from a few months to several years. Client-centered therapy generally is used for individuals who have a mild or moderate disturbance; Rogers himself has warned that it probably is not appropriate for those who have severe pathological conditions. The Rogerian approach also has been applied with groups, most notably with encounter groups. The goals of individual and group treatment are similar: increasing awareness, self-acceptance, interpersonal comfort, and self-reliance.

Client-centered therapy has been adapted by Virginia Axline and others for young children through the use of play therapy, using much the same setting and material as do psychodynamic therapists.[3,7] The key difference is that the Rogerian therapist does not use play to make symbolic interpretations. Analogous to treatment with adults, the therapist encourages the child to lead the session and displays unconditional positive regard by his or her words and actions.

Many aspects of client-centered therapy are used by therapists who represent other approaches. For example, behavior therapists often spend considerable time in developing a relationship with children and adolescents before specific interventions are implemented, and this relationship focus is no less important when clients are learning to modify maladaptive behaviors and cognitions and to develop skills. As such, Rogerian elements of interpersonal warmth, empathy, and genuineness toward the client commonly will be evidenced throughout therapy by the behavioral clinician. Although the therapist may express concern or unhappiness over a child's *behavior,* such a reaction would occur in the context of unconditional positive regard for the *child.* There is more variability in the presentation of these qualities by psychodynamic therapists, as some adopt a passive posture with minimal talking to avoid disruption of the child's expressed feelings, memories, and symbolic play.

Gestalt Therapy

Basic Assumptions. As with client-centered therapy, Fritz Perls' *gestalt therapy* promotes growth by increasing self-awareness and encouraging patients to assume responsibility for their actions and feelings.[3] Identifying theoretical differences between the two models is difficult, because the language used to describe gestalt therapy often is esoteric and unclear and because it seems only to be loosely related, at best, to principles of gestalt psychology (a laboratory-based study of human perception). Gestalt therapy is discriminated from client-centered therapy most easily by the methods used in treatment, which involve an active, directive therapist and often dramatic techniques.

Therapeutic Activities. A major focus of gestalt therapists is to emphasize the present; this therapy takes place in the "here and now." The therapist thus insists that the patient talk in the present tense and discuss current feelings. Use of language also is important in assisting the patient to assume direct responsibility for his or her feelings. For example, a patient who says, "It's really aggravating to hear that," might be asked to restate this as, "I am angry with you for saying that to me." Another technique is to ask the patient to project himself or herself into another person or object. For example, if a patient says that it feels like there is a wall between her and her parents, she may be asked to "become" that wall and talk about how it feels.

Possibly the most useful technique used by gestalt therapists is to externalize conflicts and feelings. For example, a patient may confront an empty chair, imagine that his father is there, and tell his father the things he has wanted to say but has been unable to say to him. Or, if the patient is stuck in her decision making (e.g., whether to go to a local college and live at home or to go away to college), she may be asked to alternate sitting in two chairs. When she is in one, she takes the side of staying at home and tells why she wants to stay at home and how she feels about it; sitting in the other chair she fully experiences and relates to the therapist the part of herself that wants to go away to college. This enables the patient to sort out the emotional aspects of the conflict, and it is fascinating to observe how the balance gradually shifts as one side predominates and the decision begins to be made.

Gestalt therapy has not been adapted systematically for children and thus is used typically only with adolescents. As with client-centered treatment, it generally is appropriate only for mildly or moderately disturbed patients. Gestalt therapy is used both with individuals and with groups. Individual therapy generally consists of one or two sessions weekly for anywhere from a few months to several years. Groups often are begun with an intensive weekend experience and then typically meet for one evening a week for 6 months to a year, although some groups continue almost indefinitely.

Efficacy. Largely at Rogers' own insistence there have been numerous attempts to study and evaluate client-centered therapy.[3,6] In fact it has been suggested that Rogers can be credited with stimulating the whole field of psychotherapy research. Much of this has been a study of the *process* of therapy, and Rogerians have been responsive to the findings. For example, Rogers no longer calls his therapy "nondirective" (the original label); a careful analysis of his own therapy transcripts has shown that the therapist does "shape" or subtly guide the client's verbal statements. Outcome studies of adults also have shown changes in clients' self-perceptions following treatment, in contrast to a normal control group (not in therapy) and a waiting-list control group. This research has been criticized, however, because it is based on clients' self-reports, with no external judgment of how clients actually behave after treatment. Also, it is not clear how much change is attributable to this form of therapy per se and how much to the nonspecific aspects of this and other forms of treatment.

As with all therapeutic modalities, less study of client-centered therapy has been directed to the treatment of children. Investigators have reported positive changes following child therapy, but some of these evaluations suffer from flaws, such as the selective assignment of children to treated and nontreated groups and the use of ratings by observers who were not "blind" to the therapeutic status of the children. The results of these evaluations currently are therefore suggestive rather than conclusive.

Gestalt therapy has been evaluated much less. Like psychodynamic therapists, many gestalt therapists are uninterested in or relatively inimical toward the collection of data. Those who have attempted to study therapeutic outcome have been hampered by the gap between Perls' concepts and his techniques. Gestalt therapy (and to some extent client-centered therapy) has been criticized for being incomplete: by deemphasizing clinical assessment and the patient's history, the therapist may miss diagnostic signs or background information that could be important in planning treatment. The danger of inadequate screening of group members, for example, can be seen in an estimated 8% "casualty" rate from phenomenological group experiences (e.g., sensitivity training, encounter groups).[3,4] Although these casualties are not all as dramatic as a psychotic episode, evidence suggests that these participants have been harmed in some way by the experience. This intervention thus may be beneficial for many but not all participants.

SYSTEMS THERAPY

Basic Assumptions

Systems therapy represents an approach to family therapy that views the family as a unit—a dynamic system—rather than a collection of individuals. The relationships among the family members are hypothesized to have developed in the specific manner in which they did so that the family could achieve *homeostasis*. This relatively stable state is disrupted periodically by external events (e.g., geographical relocation) or change within the family (e.g., birth of a child). This triggers changes in the family members' relationships and the subsequent reemergence of a homeostatic state, which may be different from the previous one, in much the same way that a mobile is affected by a gust of wind. Homeostasis sometimes may be achieved in ways that are not beneficial for all members, such as a "problem child" distracting attention from an unhappy marriage.[18]

Systems therapists therefore view the child who has behavior problems as merely the "identified patient" and believe that treatment is focused most appropriately on the entire family. This form of intervention, conjoint family therapy, treats the family as a group and includes all members who live together except for infants and toddlers. Treatment may focus initially on the "problem child," but the therapist often attempts to move fairly quickly to "reframe," or redefine, the problem as a disturbance in family process, faulty communication, or both. The therapist thus encourages all family members to see their own contribution to the problem and the positive changes that each can make.

The systems approach examines the roles played by family members and the function of the child's problem in maintaining the homeostasis of the family.[18] One goal of treatment is to identify covert family rules that produce the same maladaptive interactions consistently. For example, a stepfather believes that his marriage could be threatened by his stepdaughter, who dislikes him; he thus is overly critical of her and promotes conflict between her and her mother to diminish her influence on her mother. Another goal of treatment is to promote appropriate communication, such as providing direct messages, using noncoercive communication, and minimizing "scapegoating" of the identified patient. Note the similarity of the above to the functional analysis and skill training conducted by behavior therapists.

Therapeutic Activities

Therapeutic goals are achieved by analyzing and commenting on the verbal and nonverbal messages exchanged by family members. As the family becomes more aware of these maladaptive "rules" and messages, it is assumed that they are better able to change them. The therapist also may ask family members to relabel a behavior more positively (e.g., use the term "independent" rather than "selfish"). Another tactic might be to direct family members to exaggerate their customary style (be the ultimately critical father or ultimately martyred mother) to foster awareness and change.

Minuchin's structural family therapy is an adaptation that emphasizes family "sets" as the target for change.[3,18] These sets refer to the hierarchy, or structure, of family relations and the alliances between members. For example, an *enmeshed* family is one in which the members are overinvolved with one another. Here the therapist would attempt to strengthen the alliance between the parents and clearly designate their status as parents (e.g., he or she might even say, "You are a child—be quiet; this is a matter for your parents to settle."). The therapist would then encourage members to interact more with others of their own age and would promote more activities outside the family. With a *disengaged* family there might be an uninvolved father, kept distant by a strong "coalition" between mother and son. The therapist again would attempt to reorder these alliances and reestablish the father in the family structure.

Systems therapy has been used for a variety of problems, both with children and adolescents (although typically not with very young children). Some therapists insist that all family members always attend; others may work with the parents alone for a part of the treatment (e.g., for marital problems). The course of therapy typically consists of one session a week (although this may be longer than the usual 50-minute session), with the active participation of the family between sessions by the use of assigned homework. (Again, note the similarity to behavior therapy.) Treatment may continue for several months or several years.

Efficacy

Evaluation of "pure" systems therapy to date is inconclusive because of the lack of appropriately controlled outcome studies. A combined behavioral-systems approach has demonstrated beneficial effects for both the identified patient and other family members (e.g., siblings).[7,14] A combined approach also has been shown to be as effective or more so than individual therapy and client-centered family therapy.[1,7,13]

In general, available data indicate that *conjoint* family therapy with all members present, regardless of theoretical orientation, appears superior to other methods, such as providing individual treatment for each family member. This particularly is true when the presenting problems relate to family crises and conflicts about values, life-styles, or goals. Treatment outcomes have been found to be superior when fathers agree to participate in treatment. Interestingly, this has been shown to be the case when parents are separated as well as when they are together.[7]

ECLECTIC THERAPY

Basic Assumptions

Eclectic therapy is not so much a school of thought as the *absence* of an identified school. It has been included in this chapter because surveys of psychologists have indicated that eclecticism frequently is identified as a therapeutic orientation (eclectic, behavioral, and psychodynamic being the most common). As discussed previously, experienced therapists often employ procedures and techniques from a variety of therapies. Furthermore, they also may incorporate *concepts* from orientations other than that of their original training. With increasing borrowing and blending, a therapist may come to believe that his or her orientation no longer can be classified accurately as that of an identified school or theory; such therapists will label themselves "eclectic."

It is important to distinguish between *technical eclecticism* and *theoretical eclecticism.* The former refers to a therapist (1) who consistently is guided by a theoretical framework as he or she conceptualizes and understands a patient, the patient's problems, and his or her attempts to change, but (2) who employs techniques borrowed from other modalities when appropriate for a particular patient. For example, it is not uncommon for a behavior therapist to be guided by the principles of social learning theory and yet employ gestalt exercises to help an overly intellectual patient identify the emotional factors involved in his or her problem solving or decision making. Similarly a behavior therapist may use play materials when working with children. These techniques, however, are selected carefully to fulfill a specific purpose, which is part of an overall therapeutic strategy; in other words, the therapist uses them as a *behavior* therapist. In addition, as mentioned earlier, behavior and other therapists often use Rogerian methods to develop and maintain rapport throughout therapy. In contrast, *theoretical* eclecticism eschews the guidance of any theoretical system. It is our bias that any theory is better than no theory because successful therapy requires some purposive stance on the part of the therapist. Victor Meyer has semijokingly said that a theoretical framework is therapeutic for the therapist, because the therapist at least thinks he understands what is going on.[8]

Eclecticism also may be an appropriate label for interventions that have been developed for very specific situations or populations, even though they may be associated loosely with some theoretical system. Probably one of the clearest example of this is Synanon, an intensive, residential program developed to treat drug addiction. Although much of this program is translated readily into social learning (or behavioral) terms, it also makes extensive use of client-centered techniques and encounter group sessions. Other examples abound in community psychology, such as crisis intervention, suicide hotlines, and prevention efforts. Although some programs are explicitly behavioral, many community programs are atheoretical.

Efficacy

Given the plethora of programs and treatments that are essentially eclectic and the general absence of sound evaluative study, no pretense will be made here of discussing the efficacy of eclectic modalities.

SUMMARY

The goal of this chapter has been to increase the pediatrician's understanding of variants of psychotherapy that are available for use with children and to increase the practitioner's ability to effect an appropriate referral and prepare the patient and family for treatment. In becoming more familiar with the different therapeutic orientations described, it is hoped that the reader will appreciate the extent to which these are not completely separate and distinct. With increasing clinical experience therapists become more similar to one another, and many combine elements from different schools of thought. Therapeutic orientation is only one of several factors important in the selection of a therapist; quality of training, personal characteristics, general reputation, responsiveness, and ability to work with the pediatrician clearly are vital considerations (see Chapter 93, Consultation and Referral for Behavioral and Developmental Problems).

Finally, it is hoped that the reader will appreciate the difficulty and complexity of psychotherapy research and thus be tolerant of the therapist's inability to make categorical and unqualified claims regarding the efficacy of his or her intervention. In fact, some degree of humility should be evidenced by individual therapists and proponents of particular therapeutic approaches. Even those instances of "demonstrated efficacy" reviewed earlier represent a tentative conclusion based on a number of studies, each of which is imperfect and rarely, if ever, reports unqualified, long-term success with all patients.

REFERENCES

1. Achenbach TM: *Developmental psychopathology,* ed 2, New York, 1982, John Wiley & Sons.
2. Bandura A: *Social foundations of thought and action,* Englewood Cliffs, NJ, 1986, Prentice-Hall.
3. Bernstein DA, Nietzel MT: *Introduction to clinical psychology,* New York, 1980, McGraw-Hill.
4. Casey RJ, Berman JS: The outcome of psychotherapy with children, *Psychol Bull* 98:388, 1985.
5. Davison GC, Neal JM: *Abnormal psychology: an experimental clinical approach,* ed 4, New York, 1986, John Wiley & Sons.
6. Garfield S, Bergin AE, editors: *Handbook of psychotherapy and behavioral change,* ed 3, New York, 1986, John Wiley & Sons.
7. Gelfand DM, Jenson WR, Drew CJ: *Understanding child behavior disorders,* ed 2, New York, 1988, Holt, Rinehart & Winston.
8. Goldfried MR, Davison GC: *Clinical behavior therapy,* New York, 1976, Holt, Rinehart & Winston.
9. James B: *Treating traumatized children: new insights and creative interventions,* Lexington, Mass, 1989, Lexington Books.
10. Kazdin AE: *Child psychotherapy: developing and identifying effective treatments,* New York, 1988, Pergamon Press.
11. Kendall PC, Braswell L: *Cognitive-behavioral therapy for impulsive children,* New York, 1985, Guilford Press.
12. Parloff MB: Psychotherapy research and its incredible credibility crisis, *Clin Psychol Rev* 4:95, 1984.
13. Quay HC, Werry JS, editors: *Psychopathological disorders of childhood,* ed 3, New York, 1986, John Wiley & Sons.
14. Robin A, Foster SL: *Negotiating parent-adolescent conflict: a behavioral-family systems approach,* New York, 1989, Guilford Press.
15. Weist MD, Ollendick TH, Finney JW: Toward the empirical validation of treatment targets in children, *Clin Psychol Rev* 11:515, 1991.
16. Weisz JR et al: Effectiveness of psychotherapy with children and adolescents: a meta-analysis for clinicians, *J Consult Clin Psychol* 55:542, 1987.
17. Wiener J, editor: *Psychopharmacology in childhood and adolescence,* New York, 1977, Basic Books.
18. Zuk G: *Family therapy: a triadic-based approach,* New York, 1981, Behavioral Books.

93 Consultation and Referral for Behavioral and Developmental Problems

Sheridan Phillips, Richard M. Sarles, Stanford B. Friedman, and Joseph E. Boggs

INDICATORS FOR CONSULTATION OR REFERRAL

Certain types of behavior are such clear indicators of psychosocial problems that a single occurrence should signal the pediatrician to consider referral. For example, infantile autism usually is apparent before 30 months of age. These children generally show a lack of responsiveness to others, self-isolation, grossly deficient language development, and peculiar attachments to animate or inanimate objects. Autistic children do vary in symptomatology, and few are totally unresponsive to environmental stimuli, including people; however, their responses are characteristically unusual, variable, or inappropriate. Similarly, schizophrenic children typically display such bizarre behavior or preoccupations and such grossly impaired emotional relationships that they are readily identifiable. In fact, a major shortcoming of even relatively successful therapy is the inability to make the psychotic child socially inconspicuous.

Generally, it also is easy to identify certain acting out behaviors as clear signals for referral. These include behaviors that are dangerous to the child or others, vandalism, fire-setting, and cruelty to animals. Family intervention often is indicated, especially for problems such as child abuse and secondary enuresis. Also, a skilled therapist can help both patient and family deal with the aftermath of rape.

Unfortunately, most problems cannot be readily identified by the occurrence of a single behavior. Probably the most difficult determination to make is whether certain behaviors, such as mood swings in adolescence, represent merely the normal developmental process or are manifestations of a more serious problem. One indication, however, is any *sudden change in behavior,* such as a significant drop in grades or withdrawal from peers or family (or both); such change may be related to a change in environment (e.g., moving to a new school or neighborhood). In these cases it is important to reassess the child's status about 2 months after the change is observed. If the situation has not improved substantially at that time, the child probably needs special assistance adapting to the new environment.

In general, the difference between "normal" and "problematical" behavior is not the actual behavior (or behaviors) but rather the *quantity* (frequency of occurrences), *distribution* (different manifestations), and *duration* (generally, at least 4 weeks).[1] Two additional factors also determine when behavior warrants attention: if it is *maladaptive,* impairing social or cognitive functioning (or both) or when the concomitant *level of distress* is inappropriate (either elevated distress, or a total lack of distress when some would be anticipated).[5] For example, many young boys occasionally dress as girls or prefer girls as playmates, or say, for example, "I wish boys could have babies." These behaviors should be distinguished from genuine cross-sex behavior, which is characterized by a variety of manifestations, by the frequency and duration of each behavior, by the degree to which these behaviors interfere with other socialization, and by the level of tension the behavior causes in the patient or family.

Similarly, all five factors (quantity, distribution, duration, maladaptiveness, and level of distress) are relevant in discriminating between the normally energetic child and one who is hyperactive. In other instances, the problem behavior may be more circumscribed but still of concern because of its frequency, duration, or maladaptiveness (e.g., drug abuse, sexual promiscuity, stealing, and poor academic performance). Children often have conduct problems at home but not at school or at school but not at home.[1] The maladaptiveness of the behavior, however, may signal a need for intervention even though the behavior occurs in only one setting.

The problems most likely to be missed are the "quiet" ones that do not make life difficult for parents or teachers, such as poor peer relationships, emotional and social withdrawal, apathy, dysphoria, and poor self-esteem. Pediatricians also may not recognize "quiet" parenting problems. Some parents consistently express concern about their children's behavior or how they manage them. The specific behavior in question may be different at each visit, but the pediatrician continually may be providing brief reassurance, which often is ineffective. At such times the pediatrician should consider why these parents do not realize that their children's behavior is well within the norm. Are they isolated from other parents who have children the same age? Do they need education and anticipatory guidance? The parents' questions may indicate that they are excessively protective or concerned or that they have unrealistic expectations of their child. If so, this will continue to be a problem for the child and warrants intervention.

Admittedly, it sometimes is difficult to discriminate between problems that do and do not warrant referral. A framework for making this distinction flows naturally from a biopsychosocial treatment model. For example, in the case of a closed head injury, the pediatrician would assess for three things: (1) biological risk factors that might predispose the patient to a coexisting psychological (comorbid) disorder (e.g., Is there a significant family history of or genetic predisposition for depression?), (2) psychological risk factors that may affect the treatment course and outcome (e.g., Does this patient have previously documented cognitive deficits or behavior problems?), and (3) social stressors that may prevent the patient from achieving an optimal recovery (e.g., Will lack of financial resources or family support systems play a role?). Using this framework with every patient will not generate a referral to the behavioral specialist each time; however, it will ensure that factors that could inhibit treatment will not be missed and it will help prevent initial "treatment failure" by determining the role of these factors earlier.

When deciding whether to refer patients, the pediatrician must consider not only the current maladaptiveness of the problem but also the potential benefit of early intervention, which may prevent severe problems or significantly improve the quality of life for a child or family. Some reasons for pediatricians' hesitancy to refer children who have behavioral problems and some considerations related to determining whether to refer are discussed in the following section.

SOURCES OF RELUCTANCE TO EMPLOY BEHAVIORAL SPECIALISTS

For a variety of reasons, physicians often are reluctant to use behavioral consultation or referral. The primary care provider may feel pressured to comply with the current medical trend to treat the "total" patient. However, any individual physician may not have the time, expertise, or interest to do so. In such cases only the insecure professional fears consultation with a colleague. Generally, parents acknowledge a physician's honesty in delineating his or her own area of expertise and concomitant limitations and appreciate the concern and interest evidenced by the physician's suggesting appropriate consultation or referral.

Conversion reactions illustrate the advisability of simultaneously exploring organic and psychosocial factors (see Chapter 96, Conversion Reactions in Adolescents). First, when a patient is admitted to the hospital for diagnostic evaluation, behavioral consultation should be requested at the outset of the hospitalization. Many behavioral specialists have been frustrated by the request to evaluate such a patient on the last day of the hospital stay after no significant physical findings were obtained. Involvement of a specialist at the outset permits a more reasonable and thorough assessment. For example, it provides the opportunity to observe the child's behavior during the hospital stay, thus generating information difficult to obtain in any other way. Second, if the behavioral assessment is requested early, parents do not view it as a "last resort." Third, the specialist can consult with hospital staff when gathering data about the patient's condition. This initial contact with hospital staff is crucial in establishing a relationship that allows the specialist to offer specific recommendations about the patient's condition. Last, should the patient begin exhibiting troublesome behavior while still hospitalized, the consultant may offer valuable recommendations to the hospital staff about treating these behaviors.

The tendency to request a behavioral consultation *only after* a variety of other subspecialty consultations have been conducted poses problems not only for the child and family but also for the consultation service per se. Many insurance and medical assistance plans limit the number of reimbursable consultations per hospital stay. Delaying the request for behavioral evaluation therefore is one of the reasons consultation/liaison services typically have trouble remaining solvent and viable.

Pediatricians also may avoid referring a child who has a behavioral problem because they are reluctant to label a child or adolescent as having such a problem and fear that both parents and child will see the referral as an indication that the patient is "crazy" or seriously disturbed. Thus many physicians tend to be excessively conservative and recommend referral only for a blatant and obviously severe problem or when all else has failed. This implicit acceptance of the social stereotype of therapy is unfortunate because early intervention can be extremely advantageous. For example, it is much easier for a child to catch up, whether with academic or social skills, when the performance gap is small. Similarly, intervening with a 16-year-old who truly is out of control is a different matter from treating that same youngster at age 12. At other times, it is not clear that the problem will become progressively more serious. Many parents and adolescents survive several stormy years of teenage rebellion and ineffective parental efforts to exert control. However, family disruption and stress can be reduced by a brief series of sessions with a specialist who is skilled in teaching communication and problem-solving skills.[4] It is likely that many parents and teenagers would consider this a worthwhile investment of time and money. The same argument can be made for many other difficulties that are "problem behaviors" rather than "behavior problems" (see Chapter 74, Developmental Approach to Behavioral Problems).

Many behavioral problems reflect a child's lack of skills rather than deep-seated pathological conditions. However, it probably is the latter, historical view of behavioral problems that underlies current negative social prejudice toward psychosocial treatment. Thus many individuals avoid using behavioral services, yet they readily turn to experts in virtually every other area of life—accountants, physicians, teachers, plumbers—as a natural and clever use of specialists. A pediatrician familiar with the nature and purpose of different treatments can encourage families to use behavioral resources effectively.

Pediatricians also may hesitate to refer patients if they are concerned about the efficacy of behavioral intervention—that is, how much good it will do. A related concern, which also is appropriate, is the effort involved for physicians, parents, and children in going to a different place and person for consultation, then possibly having to adapt to yet another professional. Financial considerations may present another difficulty. In general, the question is whether a referral involves much more effort and expense than it is worth.

Although no therapeutic approach or professional can be totally effective, a skilled therapist generally is at least helpful, often very successful, and unlikely to be harmful. Many behavioral specialists now routinely generate a "treatment contract" with their patients, by which both parties agree to an initial series of sessions (usually between four and six), after which they jointly assess whether progress has been made. If the parents or patient believe that the initial experience has been productive, they may continue with the intervention plan; if not, there should be a change in either the plan or the therapist. This practice ensures that patients will not continue in a long and expensive course of treatment that is deemed unnecessary or unproductive by the therapist or the family. However, the length and intensity of appropriate intervention vary tremendously with the particular patient and problem. Even a highly effective and responsible therapist will have a range of cases, some requiring four sessions or less and others 100 sessions or more. The key is to select and use a behavioral specialist to provide optimum care while maintaining contact with the primary care physician.

GENERAL CONSIDERATIONS

The physician sometimes can select a consultant to reduce the chances of a "patient shunt," in which the child first must relate to a consultant and then adjust to another professional for intervention. When the primary care provider suspects that treatment is indicated, he or she should recommend a consultant who can both assess and intervene. In some cases this will not be possible, nor would it always represent optimum use of specialized skills. Knowledge of available behavioral resources, however, enables the physician to recommend appropriately.

Another consideration is how best to structure interaction with behavioral specialists. One possibility is to include behavioral specialists within general pediatric practices. Increasingly, pediatricians have invited mental health professionals to base their practices in adjacent offices. Even better, such professionals have become members of group practices. This approach has obvious advantages for providing many behavioral services to patients naturally and efficiently. In addition, this approach allows the behavioral specialist the opportunity to provide a variety of other services. The specialist may offer suggestions to office staff concerning aspects of patient treatment (e.g., behavioral techniques or interventions for reducing anxiety during painful procedures). One or two brief sessions with this specialist before an inpatient hospitalization for treatments or procedures, such as chemotherapy, magnetic resonance imaging (MRI), and computed tomography (CT) scans, to familiarize the patient and family with these events also would be an excellent use of the specialist's consultation skills. Another example would be short-term groups for common problems of young mothers or diabetic teenagers. Although any particular professional cannot possess the entire range of skills required, he or she can enhance the effective use of other resources in the community.

Preparing the Parents

Preparation of the parents for behavioral consultation begins during the first discussion of the differential diagnosis, when both physical and emotional factors are included as potential causes of the symptoms.[6] Even when the primary care physician has correctly introduced the possibility of emotional issues early in the diagnostic workup, parents may resist exploring emotional factors. Such resistance is most likely when the symptoms appear to have an organic origin or when no overt behavioral disruption is involved.

In some instances parents may not be aware that they foster their child's aberrant behavior; instead, they often blame the school or their child's peers. In other instances, parents may deny any problems with their child, partly to avoid revealing their own interpersonal or marital difficulties or a problem such as alcoholism. Nevertheless, the physician should present an honest appraisal of the situation (with appropriate recommendations for behavioral consultation) without trying to please or appease the parents by avoiding a discussion of his or her true assessment of the clinical situation.

If parents are reluctant to consider a behavioral consultation, it may help to address their concern for their child's health and welfare. In explaining the need for such consultation, the pediatrician should suggest that this is an important service for complete, comprehensive care of their child. It should be emphasized that behavioral consultation does not imply that the child is crazy; rather, it suggests that emotional factors may totally or partly account for their child's difficulty.

When the complaint is somatic, a useful example most parents can understand is the feeling of "butterflies in the stomach" or sweating before an examination, when speaking in public, during a marriage ceremony, or at other times of stress. A tension headache is another common symptom that can be used to demonstrate that a person can experience physical distress or pain without actual structural or physical disease being present.

If the parents agree to the consultation, the pediatrician should give them the consultant's name and detail the reasons for this selection, the consultant's credentials, and how closely the consultant works with the primary care physician. It is the pediatrician's responsibility to contact the consultant initially and to discuss the reasons for consultation.

The parents also should be informed that the consultant probably will want to see both parents together to collect important data about the child's development and a detailed family history. The number of visits generally required for a consultation and its approximate cost also should be discussed with the parents. After the consultation, the primary care physician should meet with the parents to discuss the consultant's findings and recommendations. It often is useful to include the consultant and the child in this meeting as well.

If the parents are reluctant to follow a recommendation for intervention, the primary care physician should be careful not to support the parents' hesitation. Such a stance engenders lack of faith in the consultant the physician has recommended. It also suggests expertise by the primary care physician in a field in which he or she has just recommended consultation. If, however, both parents and pediatrician drastically disagree with the findings and recommendations of the consultant, a second opinion is indicated.

Preparing the Child

The young child should be told that his or her parents and the physician are concerned about aspects of the child's behavior, such as an inability to get along with friends, anger, nightmares, or difficulty coping with a physical illness. In the case of a psychosomatic symptom, the child needs to be told that pain or illness often is caused by emotional feelings or worries. The child should be informed that he or she will be seeing a professional known to the pediatrician who is an expert in helping with these kinds of problems; it should be emphasized that the consultant may help by playing with children and by talking with them about their thoughts and feelings.

With an older child or adolescent, the pediatrician begins to prepare the patient for consultation even while obtaining a physical and psychosocial history. As the physician concentrates on social and emotional aspects, the teenager may become indignant and confront the physician about the personal nature of the questions. The physician should not retreat or become defensive, but should emphasize the need for such probing personal questions to understand the symptoms or illness troubling the patient. As with parents, relating everyday examples can help the older child or adolescent understand the connection between emotions and physical well-being. Teenagers, because they are struggling with the developmental tasks of adolescence, may be concerned about confidentiality. Also, given the normal mood swings during this period, it is common for teenagers to wonder about their own mental health. Suggesting behavioral consultation can trigger a protest that may reflect their own worst fear—that they really are different or "crazy." In most cases the pediatrician can reassure teenage patients that they indeed are not; however, the physician must convey concern if a significant psychopathological condition is suspected. Not to do so is frightening to the patient or parent, who may recognize that reassurance is premature and inappropriate. If severe problems are present, the pediatrician should explain that the teenager's behavior does signal a departure from normal and indicates some excessive stress, which may be interfering with optimum well-being. Also, it is extremely useful to identify some specific potential benefit of intervention that is likely to be meaningful to the patient (e.g., better relationships with peers) as well as the alleviation of a problem (e.g., reducing conflict with parents or feelings of anxiety).

It is essential that the physician be firm but not argumentative about the need for referral. While acknowledging the adolescent's anger or dismay, the physician needs to assert professional responsibility to render the best medical opinion, even if it is not to the patient's liking. It seems paradoxical that a sturdy posture in this regard often is reassuring, but it does convey the idea that someone is listening and hearing the patient's troubles and is concerned about his or her behavior.

In most instances the child or adolescent should be informed of the approximate number of visits usually required and the type of interaction to expect. If the patient inquires about the cost of the consultation and evidences concern, the physician can assure the patient that only the parents can make this decision. In most situations the physician can emphasize that the patient's parents are concerned enough and care enough to be willing to spend whatever it may take to obtain proper help.

In cases of overt psychosis wherein "reality testing" is seriously impaired, psychological preparation of the patient may be ineffective. However, the physician cannot assume that the patient is totally oblivious to the surroundings. In fact, the pediatrician can provide a stabilizing, reliable, and predictable influence for the patient. The physician can introduce the consultant as an expert in helping patients whose thoughts are confused or jumbled. It may even be helpful for the primary care physician to offer to be present during the first consultative session as a source of security for the patient.

Selecting a Consultant

Choosing the appropriate professional or agency probably is the most important service provided by the primary care physician to a patient who has psychosocial or learning problems. Although the common practice of suggesting a list of specialists protects the physician from any accusation of favoritism, it actually is not helpful to parents. A specific referral is preferable because it relieves the family of wondering if they made the best choice.

A common question is whether it is best to use a pediatrician interested and expert in behavioral disorders, a child psychiatrist, a clinical psychologist, a psychiatric nurse, or a social worker. Although a thorough discussion of this issue is beyond the scope of this chapter, a brief review of relevant training and credentials may be helpful.

Pediatricians well versed in managing behavioral disorders generally have had training in behavioral or developmental pediatrics (or both) after their pediatric residency. Their specialized training typically consists of a 1- to 3-year fellowship in behavioral pediatrics and/or child development, including academic and clinical experience. Such fellowships vary greatly in their emphasis, some focusing almost exclusively on infants and young children, others covering a broad range of ages and problems. The behavioral pediatrician's area of expertise, theoretical orientation, and interests obviously will reflect the specific training received.

Most physicians formally engaged in psychotherapy have been trained in psychiatry. The internship year can be the first year of a 4-year residency in psychiatry, or it can consist of a year in internal medicine, pediatrics, or neurology. Three additional years of psychiatric residency are required for board eligibility in psychiatry. Two years of child and adolescent psychiatric training (1 year of which can constitute the fourth year of psychiatric residency) are needed for board eligibility in child and adolescent psychiatry. Certification in child and adolescent psychiatry is allowed only after an individual has been certified in general psychiatry.

Psychologists vary greatly in their educational background and may have a master's or doctoral degree. Those qualified to provide clinical service, both diagnostic assessment and therapy, have received a degree in clinical psychology (as opposed to developmental, experimental, physiological, or social psychology) or have completed a formal, accredited respecialization program in clinical psychology. Such training includes, in addition to a dissertation, 3 or 4 years of graduate course work, with accompanying practicum experience, and a year of clinical internship. Graduate programs in clinical psychology and clinical internships are reviewed and accredited by the American Psychological Association (APA).[2] Also, the referring physician may wish to determine whether the consultant is listed in the National Register of Health Service Providers.[3] Finally, most states have licensing procedures for psychologists, and the physician should not use an individual who is unlicensed in those states. It should be noted, however, that such licensure typically is generic—that is, it does not distinguish areas of training in psychology (e.g., clinical, developmental, experimental, industrial).

A clinical specialist in child and adolescent psychiatry and mental health nursing (psychiatric nurses) is required to have earned a 4-year bachelor's degree in nursing, to have obtained registered nursing licensure, and to have been involved in direct clinical nursing practice. Completion of an 18- to 24-month master's degree in psychiatric nursing is then necessary; this program consists of academic and clinical work focused on children, adolescents, and families. Upon providing evidence of post-master's degree clinical experience and access to supervision, these clinicians must pass a national examination, which results in certification by the American Nurses Association. These clinicians must be recertified every 5 years.

Social workers may have a bachelor's degree (BSW), a master's degree (MSW), or a doctoral degree (DSW or PhD). Social workers are accredited nationally by the Academy of Certified Social Workers (ACSW), a component of the National Association of Social Workers (NASW), the primary professional association. The ACSW accreditation requirements include (1) a master's degree from a school of social work accredited by the Council of Social Work Education, (2) 2 years of supervised, post-master's degree social work practice, and (3) successful completion of a written examination. Many states now have licensing procedures for social workers, with requirements similar to those of the ACSW. The ACSW and most state licenses are generic, however, and do not distinguish among practitioners in clinical social work, administration, and community organization. The NASW maintains a national register of clinical social workers who have demonstrated *clinical* training and experience. As with all the disciplines discussed above, even clinical social workers vary substantially with regard to orientation and areas of expertise.

Accreditation and organizational affiliations indicate only minimum standards of professional competence. No single mental health profession has sole claim to competence; all fields have individuals who are inadequate and those who are superb. This unevenness of skill simply highlights the importance of the referring physician's systematical evaluation of consultative resources.

Knowing what behavioral resources are available in a particular community and arranging ongoing contact with appropriate individuals requires deliberate effort. Pediatricians should meet with an experienced and respected mental health professional to discuss appropriate referral resources within the community. Acquiring appropriate sophistication about available referral sources undoubtedly is time consuming, but it will ensure more meaningful referrals and, ultimately, save time.

The role of the primary care physician does not end once the referral has been made. The physician should contact the family to see that an appointment actually has been made. With the appropriate permission, he or she should provide a summary of the pertinent information to the professional or agency and, in turn, *expect periodic reports.* It is helpful if the primary care physician clearly states at the time of referral his or her expectations for feedback—how much detail is to be included and how often this feedback is to occur. Ongoing communication allows the pediatrician to maintain an integral role in providing total care to patients. Over time, it also allows evaluation of the quality of service available from a particular professional or agency.

REFERENCES

1. Evans IM, Nelson RO: Assessment of child behavior problems. In Ciminero AR, Calhoun KS, Adams HE, editors: *Handbook of behavioral assessment,* ed 2, New York, 1986, John Wiley & Sons.
2. General guidelines for providers of psychological services, Washington, DC, 1987, The American Psychological Association.
3. National Register of Health Service Providers in Psychology, published biannually by the Council for the National Register of Health Service Providers in Psychology, Washington, DC.
4. Robin A, Foster SL: *Negotiating parent-adolescent conflict: a behavioral–family systems approach,* New York, 1989, Guilford Press.
5. Sarason IG, Sarason BR: *Abnormal psychology: the problem of maladaptive behavior,* Englewood Cliffs, NJ, 1987, Prentice-Hall.
6. Sarles RM, Friedman SB: The process of consultation and referral. In Gellert E, editor: *Psychosocial aspects of pediatric care,* New York, 1978, Grune & Stratton.

94 Adolescence

W. Sam Yancy

Adolescence generally is defined as the period of psychological growth and development during the transition from childhood to adulthood. Physical growth and development, or pubescence, also occur during this period. Many of these changes can be confusing for both teenagers and the adults who care for them. "Rebellious" and "tumultuous" are terms often associated with this age group; "joyous" and "carefree" are more positive adjectives also used to describe adolescents. With such diverse feelings about teenagers, it is no wonder the health care of adolescents in the United States has been neglected for so long.

Efforts on behalf of adolescents have come about not entirely because of increasing problems in this age group and certainly not because of increasing demands by teenagers themselves, but because adolescents' unmet needs have been recognized. It was believed formerly that this was a carefree, healthy age, one that required no special interest from health care professionals. This is no longer true. Citing vital statistics data, Blum[1] reported in 1987 that violence has replaced communicable diseases as the chief cause of mortality in teenagers and that more than 75% of adolescent deaths are caused by accidents, suicide, and homicide. The latest statistics from the Centers for Disease Control and Prevention show no improvement.[2] The prevalence of sexually transmitted disease, pregnancy, substance abuse, suicide, delinquency, chronic illness, mental illness, and school problems cannot be ignored.[3,5] Equally important, if not more so, is the need for practitioners knowledgeable about normal adolescent development and about adolescent behaviors that concern these patients and their parents. Diagnosis and treatment of the physical and psychosocial problems of adolescents, as well as early recognition of risk factors and appropriate anticipatory guidance, should be incorporated into the practice of all primary care physicians.

Although attention was focused on the health care needs of adolescents in England as early as the late 1800s, it was not until the 1930s that significant reports about this age group began to appear in the U.S. medical literature. It was not until 1951 that the first separate hospital inpatient adolescent unit was established at Boston Children's Hospital. Progress in the area of adolescent medicine is outlined in the box on the right.

Pediatricians have led the way in providing health care for adolescents. In 1980, the report of the Task Force on Pediatric Education[4] called for more training in adolescent medicine. The Pediatric Residency Review Committee of the Accreditation Council for Graduate Medical Education requires all pediatric residency programs to include training in adolescent medicine. Also, 95% of all adolescent medicine fellowship training programs and divisions of adolescent medicine are based in pediatrics departments.

Teenagers, however, are cared for by professionals in many disciplines (e.g., internists, obstetrician-gynecologists, psychiatrists, psychologists, family physicians, social workers, nurses, and educators). The most effective health care programs for young people depend on collaboration among all interested disciplines to provide comprehensive care for these

PROGRESS IN ADOLESCENT MEDICINE

1938 Publication of Greulich WW et al: A handbook of methods for the study of adolescent children, *Monogr Soc Res Child Dev,* vol 3, no 2, serial no 13, Washington, DC.
1941 Publication of American Academy of Pediatrics: Symposium on adolescence, *J Pediatr* 19:289, 1941.
1951 Boston Children's Hospital establishes the first hospital adolescent unit.
1965 The *Journal of Pediatrics* lists four fellowship programs for adolescent medicine.
1968 The Society for Adolescent Medicine is founded. Also, federal funding of training programs in adolescent medicine is established, through the Division of Maternal and Child Health of the Department of Health, Education, and Welfare.
1975 The First International Symposium on Adolescent Medicine is held in Helsinki.
1977 The American Medical Association (AMA) recognizes adolescent medicine as a specialty.
1978 The National Conference on Adolescent Behavior and Health is established as part of the National Academy of Sciences' Institute of Medicine.
1979 The American Academy of Pediatrics (AAP) creates its Section on Adolescent Health.
1980 The first volume of the *Journal of Adolescent Health Care* is published (the name is changed to the *Journal of Adolescent Health* in 1992).
1987 The International Association for Adolescent Health is founded.
1988 The AMA's First Annual National Congress on Adolescent Health is held in Chicago.
1994 The first certifying examination in adolescent medicine is administered by the American Board of Pediatrics and the American Board of Internal Medicine. Also, the *Journal of Adolescent Health* lists 42 fellowship training programs in adolescent medicine.

patients (see Chapter 95, Challenges of Health Care Delivery to Adolescents).

REFERENCES

1. Blum R: Contemporary threats to adolescent health in the United States, *JAMA* 257:3390, 1987.
2. Centers for Disease Control and Prevention: Mortality trends, causes of death, and related risk behaviors among US adolescents, CDC Publication No 099-4112, Atlanta, 1993, CDC.
3. Cohen MI: Adolescent health: concerns for the eighties, *Pediatr Rev* 4:4, 1982.
4. Cohen MI: Importance, implementation, and impact of the adolescent medicine components of the report of the Task Force on Pediatric Education, *J Adolesc Health Care* 1:1, 1980.
5. Hein K: *Issues in adolescent health: an overview,* Washington, DC, 1988, Carnegie Council on Adolescent Development.

SUGGESTED READINGS

American Medical Association: *Guidelines for adolescent preventive services,* Chicago, 1992, The Association.

Cromer BA, McLean CS, Heald FP: A critical review of comprehensive health screening in adolescents, J Adolesc Health (suppl)13;3S, 1992.

Hamburg, BA: Psychosocial development. In Friedman SB, Fisher M, Schonberg SK, editors: *Comprehensive adolescent health care,* St Louis, Mo, 1992, Quality Medical Publishing.

Marks A, Fisher M: Health assessment and screening during adolescence, Pediatrics (suppl)80:135, 1987.

Neinstein LS: *Adolescent health care: a practical guide,* ed 2, Baltimore, 1991, Urban & Schwarzenberg.

Thornburg HD: *Development in adolescence,* ed 2, Monterey, Calif, 1982, Brooks/Cole.

95 Challenges of Delivering Health Care to Adolescents

Donna E. Wiener and Michael I. Cohen

Among health providers, "adolescence" is a word that often conjures up an unpleasant state of mind and even more unpleasant facial grimacing. Whether this is because it draws forth our own awkward memories of this period of the life cycle or because it paints a picture of a defiant group whose mission is to make others miserable is of little consequence. Unfortunately, as a patient, the adolescent's health needs often are not understood well; this, coupled with a fundamental professional discomfort with this population, results in significant neglect and ever-increasing morbidity. In the not too distant past, this "difficult" age group was relatively free of physiological disease compared with infants, children, and adults. Our health care system, primarily geared to quick remediation and shying away from health education and prevention, focused much of its attention and resources on dealing with other age groups in which physiological disease was more bountiful, simple to quantitate, and much easier to fix. Minimal attention was paid to adolescent health care, the training of adolescent health professionals, and the research questions that needed to be addressed to bring relief to this unique population. In addition, the adolescent patient did not fit easily into a child or an adult model, upon which our present health care system is designed. As a result, the health care of adolescents has been allowed to deteriorate to a crisis level; this is most apparent in subpopulations of teens who are disadvantaged economically and socially.

Over the past 50 years, the approach to adolescent health care has changed very little. Before the 1960s three generic modes of care were available to adolescent patients: (1) the traditional personal physician and the public clinic, which were available to all age groups but were not particularly welcoming to teens, (2) military health care programs, which were available to older teens in the service and which offered excellent care, but to an obviously very restricted group of patients, and (3) private secondary school health services, which were high quality but limited to a small population of very affluent teens.

From the 1960s to the early 1980s, the adolescent health care delivery system changed significantly. Five other venues of care specifically for adolescents emerged and expanded to virtually all geographical regions of the United States. These were (1) hospital-based clinics affiliated with large teaching institutions, organized through divisions or sections of adolescent medicine, where the adolescent could receive personal and developmentally appropriate services, (2) freestanding, community-based clinics in large urban centers, which tended to serve counterculture adolescents at no cost and which commonly were staffed by volunteer professionals, (3) prison and detention center health services, which served youngsters the courts determined to be persons in need of supervision (PINS) or juvenile delinquents, (4) categorical disease-related centers, which targeted specific adolescent health care problems (e.g., drug treatment facilities, clinics for the diagnosis and treatment of sexually transmitted diseases, family planning clinics that offered abortion and pregnancy services, and mental health centers), and (5) college health services, which expanded dramatically in the 1960s and most often were modeled after the private secondary school programs of the immediate postwar era following World War II.

In the 1980s the latest innovative method of delivering adolescent health care services emerged—the school-based or school-linked clinic, most of which were established in urban centers to serve disadvantaged and minority youngsters.

These somewhat innovative approaches, as well as the traditional model, all attempted to deliver comprehensive health services that were age-, sex-, and developmentally appropriate for adolescents. However, adolescent morbidity and mortality have continued to rise—alarmingly so in recent times. Regional and national data bases show that the health of American youngsters continues to deteriorate dramatically. Certainly, biological indicators of disease have not improved, as evidenced by the high rates of severe asthma, anemia, and numerous chronic diseases, but the overwhelming increase in morbidity and mortality has occurred in the psychosocial and behavioral domains.

Despite the numerous innovative adolescent-specific delivery systems that have emerged since the 1960s, none has been able to provide a sufficient number of services to American youngsters; thus most adolescents are forced to remain in a traditional health care system that clearly is not "user friendly" to these young patients.

To suggest a remedy to this problem, we must review the failings of the traditional system of care, which has 10 essential shortcomings.

1. The traditional health care system is designed to provide a "quick fix"—the practitioner spends a brief amount of time with each patient and attempts treatment that will produce results rapidly. Such a design leaves little room for the time-consuming preventive care adolescents require.

For example, with adolescent patients, a visit for physiological dysfunction often is coupled with exploration of psychosocial risk-taking behaviors. Some of these critical issues are (1) experimenting with illicit drugs, which leads to substance abuse and ultimately addiction; (2) sexual exploration, which can lead to unprotected intercourse, multiple partners, and adolescent pregnancy or sexually transmitted disease, possibly a lethal one; (3) drinking, which leads to compromised driving skills and automotive accidents; and (4) inability to control anger and frustration internally, which often emerges as a suicide attempt or peer-directed violence and use of guns.

2. The central theme of the current system is "first help those who help themselves." The adolescent must seek out health care to obtain treatment—a large burden for a not yet mature, not yet adult patient. Also, the traditional health care system is not very tolerant of many of the adolescent's concerns. For example, these youngsters typically have a heightened concern about body image, which may prevent them from seeking help in a setting in which they must expose their bodies. They also have feelings of immortality, which often cause them to delay seeking help for serious conditions. Adolescents have trouble trusting adults or authority figures; it may take several visits for a health care provider to earn the trust of these young patients, and only then might they come forth with their real health concerns.

3. Our current system rarely offers adolescents a personal health care provider whom they can visit regularly. Yearly health maintenance care is not encouraged and rarely is reimbursed by the current generic health care model. Also, most adolescents do not seek routine preventive care, but rather seek help only during an acute episode of distress. For disadvantaged teens, this typically means visiting an emergency department or a hospital-based clinic, both of which often are overcrowded and have little time to address anything more than the chief complaint.

4. Adolescent health problems often stem from what many consider taboo subjects. Health care providers feel uncomfortable dealing with issues such as sexuality, teen pregnancy, substance abuse, acquired immune deficiency syndrome (AIDS), and suicide.[1] Many clinicians avoid such discussions; a few occasionally feel compelled to impose their strong opinions on the adolescent patient. Neither approach is appropriate. The pediatrician must have a welcoming, nonjudgmental attitude that encourages adolescents to discuss fears, myths, and concerns openly. He or she must pay close attention to any pressing concern, and both provide and discuss with these young patients information that is current, clear, and concise.

5. The physical facility and its location may be a major obstacle to care. For example, do teenagers need to sit in a pediatrician's waiting room, one filled with screaming infants? Do they need to wait in an internist's or family physician's office, seated next to the frail and elderly? Do they have to travel out of their local community to receive health care? Do they need to go to an unwelcoming hospital clinic, and do they need to miss school to attend that clinic? All these situations are more the norm than the exception, and all tend to limit young people's access to health services.

6. Serious financial obstacles exist as well.[2] Adolescents rarely have a job, much less medical coverage or the ability to pay for medical services independently. One of seven adolescents lacks health insurance; one of three poor adolescents lacks Medicaid coverage. Even when health insurance or fiscal resources are available, they usually are attached to a family policy and thus compromise access to care because of issues of confidentiality. Adolescents may not want their families to know about certain health visits and therefore may avoid an important professional contact or may not provide appropriate and accurate information.

7. Adolescents have special psychosocial needs. Their chronological age may not be synchronous with their psychological or developmental age. Although most want to be treated as adults, the development of some may require that they receive the medically directed style necessary for a younger person. The practitioner must be prepared professionally to meet not only the physical but also the emotional needs of adolescent development so as to build trust and improve compliance with treatment. Although adolescent morbidity and mortality have increased markedly, the training of adolescent specialists has lagged behind the need.[3]

8. The issues of confidentiality and consent are murky and offer little guidance and few rules for the practitioner to follow. Obviously, any life-threatening situation should be reported to a parent or guardian, and the physician would always hope to convince adolescents to inform their parents or guardian of health problems. However, there are numerous situations in which adolescents will seek care only if they are promised confidentiality. A health care provider may rightfully refuse to promise such to teenagers but then risk adolescents' refusal to obtain needed care and guidance.

9. Our current system of care typically is organized around categorical diseases and is not structured around an array of comprehensive services. However, the major issues of adolescent health care require a multidisciplinary approach to both prevention and treatment and are undermined by this categorical approach to services. With a system heavily focused on biological diseases, research is geared toward technological improvement. Yet adolescents suffering from dysfunctional states stemming from rapidly changing biological processes coupled with peer pressure, family conflicts, educational stresses, and societal demands for greater responsibility, self-sufficiency and, ultimately, successful employment actually are disasters in the making. The result often is a lack of internal controls, overwhelming feelings of helplessness and hopelessness, and eventually the emergence of self-destructive behaviors that contribute to the following statistics for the early 1990s:

Every 47 seconds an American child is abused or neglected; about 50% are teens.
Every 22 seconds an American teenager becomes pregnant.
Every 67 seconds an American teenager has a baby.
Every day 40,000 American teenagers are in jails, lockups, or prisons.
Every day 6 American teenagers commit suicide.
Every day 626 American teenagers get syphilis or gonorrhea.

Will a newer generation MRI or PET scanner help these youngsters?

10. Accurate morbidity and mortality data are unavailable for specific groups of adolescents. The present coding system groups younger adolescents in the age category 10 to 15 years and older adolescents in the category 15 to 24 years. There also is a marginal separation of adolescents by socioeconomic, racial, and ethnic status. Without accurate data of this type, it is nearly impossible for the health care system to respond to unmet needs appropriately.

Although innovative and interesting models of adolescent care have emerged in the past 3 decades, they all are far from perfect and collectively are limited in the number of adolescents they serve. The overwhelming shortcomings of our traditional health care delivery system have become acutely apparent with the continued rise in morbidity and mortality. Clearly, a reordering of the adolescent health care delivery system is urgent. However, all recent indicators suggest that the United States is moving toward a managed care model, with cost effectiveness as a central goal—a system that does not accommodate the special needs of adolescents. All recent health care reform proposals have put forth a model that does not serve this target population because it remedies only one of the 10 previously identified shortcomings (lack of a personal health care provider). Presumably, this much-touted managed care model would allow for a readily available generalist provider. It does not ensure confidential care, a youth-oriented and user friendly environment, regularly scheduled and recurrent visits, adequate time for health promotion and health education, universal guarantees for provider reimbursement not linked to family contracts, support of significant psychosocial interventions, or extensive multidisciplinary care.

The real challenge of delivering health care to adolescents goes far beyond the current national debate over managed care, primary providers, cost containment, portability of insurance, reduction in hospital stays, extended care, and nursing home care. These may be critical issues for infants, children, adults, and the elderly, but they don't begin to meet the needs of teens, whose requirements include multidisciplinary and comprehensive services, ethnoculturally sensitive care, confidential care, encounters unconstrained by narrow time frames, and professionals properly prepared in the various disciplines of adolescent health.

We must ensure that in the ensuing debate over restructuring the national health care system along the lines of managed competition, the needed changes in adolescent health care are not sacrificed. Although it theoretically may be possible to incorporate most, if not all, of the key elements of an optimal adolescent health care system into the overriding national model, many knowledgeable observers of the adolescent health scene doubt it. An alternative approach would be to extract several critical elements from each of the successful adolescent delivery venues described earlier and marshall these resources into a multiservice center model of care. This is a structural unit that is adolescent specific, user friendly, community based, and comprehensive; its replicability nationally would be sensitive to different geographical, ethnic, racial, and socioeconomic teen populations. Such centers would have a health promotion and education focus as well as the more traditional curative and disease treatment approaches to health care. In addition, such centers would offer social, vocational, remedial, educational, and if locally appropriate, legal and recreational opportunities—a true multiservice center for young people aimed at improving total health, where hope for a better future can be restored. Access would be assured by a universal insurance coverage policy that enfranchises all teens as individuals rather than through family contracts.

The American adolescent population is diverse and has wide-ranging health needs. However, the real challenge of delivering health care to this unique segment of our citizenry is not in replicating their heterogeneity by creating multiple but different delivery systems, as has been our style for the past half century. Rather, success lies in establishing the concept of a multiservice center system with the underlying principles noted above that are unique to adolescents yet recognize regional, ethnic, and social differences. The consequences of failing to alter the current adolescent health care delivery system are awesome, yet the magnitude of the changes necessary to achieve a reversal of the extant morbidity and mortality data are equally daunting. Neither of these scenarios should paralyze us. Instead, we should take our lead from F. Scott Fitzgerald's remark, "The test of a first-rate intelligence is the ability to hold two opposed ideas in one's mind at the same time and still retain the ability to function. One should, for example, be able to see that things are hopeless and yet be determined to make them otherwise."

REFERENCES

1. Blum RW, Bearinger LH: Knowledge and attitudes of health professionals toward adolescent health care, *J Adolesc Health Care* 11:289, 1990.
2. Newacheck PW: Improving access to health services for adolescents from economically disadvantaged families, *Pediatrics* 84:6, 1989.
3. US Congress, Office of Technology Assessment: Adolescent health. Vol I. Summary and policy options, Pub No OTA-H-468, Washington, DC, 1991, US Government Printing Office.

SUGGESTED READINGS

US Congress, Office of Technology Assessment: Adolescent health. Vol II. Background and effectiveness of selected prevention and treatment services, Pub No OTA-H-466, Washington, DC, 1991, US Government Printing Office.

US Congress, Office of Technology Assessment: Adolescent health. Vol III. Cross-cutting issues in the delivery of health and related services, Pub No OTA-H-467, Washington, DC, 1991, US Government Printing Office.

96 Conversion Reactions in Adolescents

Gregory E. Prazar and Stanford B. Friedman

DEFINITION, INCIDENCE, AND ETIOLOGICAL FACTORS

The amalgamation of emotions and physical symptoms in patients challenges the primary care physician to formulate priorities in history-taking, diagnosis, and management. Some somatic complaints, such as headaches, nausea, and vomiting, can result directly from emotional upsets. Indeed, anxiety often is associated with palpitations, sweating, and tremulousness; depression often is manifested by symptoms such as fatigue and weakness. Other somatic complaints reflect organic disorders, such as a peptic ulcer, which may be associated with emotional turmoil. Still other physical problems are attributed to conversion symptoms.

Conversion reactions are a way of communicating the uncomfortable, or as Engel writes, "a psychic mechanism whereby an idea, fantasy, or wish is expressed in bodily rather than in verbal terms and is experienced by the patient as a physical symptom rather than as a mental symptom."[2] The idea or wish is psychologically threatening to the individual or is unacceptable for him or her to express directly. A conversion symptom serves as a form of decompression, whereby unpleasant affects associated with acknowledgment of the wish are dissipated through use of a somatic symptom. Because the wish is completely unconscious, the patient in no way relates any psychological stigmata to the somatic complaint. As Hollender succinctly states, "The conversion symptom is a code that conceals the message from the sender as well as from the receiver."[5]

To understand why a wish or thought is represented by a bodily symptom, it is necessary to explore patterns of everyday behavior and infant development. Body activity (i.e., gestures) is used to express ideas during verbal interaction. Common conversational phrases frequently allude, metaphorically, to the intermixing of emotion and body functioning. "I'm fed up" and "He gives me a pain in the neck" are two such examples. Developmentally, infants express feelings and communicate through visible behavior long before spoken language becomes their dominant mode of communication. Furthermore, infants explore and learn about their environment, including the people in it, by using their bodies as investigative tools (e.g., placing new objects in the mouth) and as a means of making contact. Any bodily process that can be perceived by the individual can serve as the focus for conversion symptoms. Similarly, somatic symptoms of relatives or close friends also can serve as the source of a patient's complaint. It is the patient's *interpretation* of the other person's symptom that provides a model for the somatic complaint. When the symptom is adapted from one observed in the other person, that person frequently evokes strong feelings in the patient. Because the patient feels guilty about his or her feelings or impulses toward that person, he or she may take the other person's symptoms as a form of self-punishment, while at the same time psychologically expressing his or her own forbidden idea or wish.

All body systems may be invoked in a conversion reaction. The sensory system frequently is involved (e.g., paresthesia, anesthesia, or diffuse pain), although typically these symptoms are not distributed in the correct pattern of innervation of the implicated cutaneous nerves. Motor system involvement can be represented by paralysis, tremors, or weakness of an extremity. Hyperventilation and dizziness are other common conversion symptoms, as are nausea and vomiting and visual problems.

A common conversion symptom seen in children and young adolescents is abdominal pain. After an extensive investigation of 100 children who had abdominal pain, Apley[1] found an organic cause in only eight cases. Another study, by Oster,[10] revealed abdominal pain in 14% of the children studied. The incidence was highest in those 9 years of age and lowest in those 16 to 17 years of age. Recurrent abdominal pain and its etiology remain controversial. However, it is important to remember that many patients who have recurrent abdominal pain may have emotional concerns of which they are unaware. Many of these patients may be suffering from conversion symptoms.

Although the incidence of certain individual somatic complaints has been studied, the specific overall incidence of conversion symptoms in children and adolescents is not known. Available data suggest an incidence of 5% to 13%.[4] Lack of more definitive data reflects the difficulty in ascertaining whether a somatic complaint indeed represents a conversion symptom. Conversion symptoms may appear to be more common among adolescents than among children because the former more often have alarming somatic complaints, such as chest pains and fainting spells, whereas children frequently suffer from more indolent complaints, such as sporadic abdominal pains. Conversion symptoms are two to three times more common in girls than in boys and may appear as early as 7 or 8 years of age.[2] There appears to be no correlation between the occurrence of conversion symptoms and socioeconomic status; less sophisticated patients, however, tend to have bizarre and physiologically unexplained symptoms.

Conversion symptoms can appear as a group phenomenon. Such a situation often is referred to as *epidemic hysteria*. Adolescent girls swooning and fainting at rock concerts is an easily appreciated example. In this situation the unacceptable wish relates to sexualized thoughts involving rock stars. Other examples of epidemic hysteria are explained less easily. Episodes of epidemic hysteria appear to have several characteristics in common: (1) audiovisual cues (e.g., seeing ambulances arrive to care for accident victims) seem to be important as precipitators; (2) adolescent girls are involved more often than adolescent boys; (3) the reaction is more likely if it is initiated by a group member identified either as a leader (of a large subgroup) or as an outsider; and (4) episodes are likely to involve larger numbers of adolescents if the youngsters are allowed to confer among themselves without adults present. Entire school populations may be involved in mass conversion reactions.[6,9]

Although conversion symptoms have no organic basis by themselves, their perpetuation may result in biochemical or physiological body changes, known as *conversion complications*. They can include changes such as muscle atrophy secondary to long-standing paralysis and respiratory alkalosis secondary to acute hyperventilation. It is important to differentiate conversion complications from psychophysiologically mediated lesions, such as peptic ulcers, in which physiological processes concomitant with emotions contribute to altered activity of an involuntary body function.

INTERVIEW TECHNIQUES

Because symptoms caused by conversion and somatic processes can be confused easily, the practitioner evaluating any patient with a somatic complaint always should consider the possibility of a conversion symptom. Attention to the personal history (family functioning, school performance, and peer relationships), as well as to physical functioning, demonstrates to the patient and family that the physician appreciates without prejudice the importance of all elements that may be contributing to ill health. Showing respect for the importance of emotional-physical interaction is thereby suggested so that this concept will not be foreign if it later is presented to the family in a diagnostic framework. Such an approach also contributes to the physician's understanding, as Engel[2] states, "of those personal, family, and social circumstances that are most relevant to the understanding of the illness and the care of the patient, whether or not the ultimate diagnosis is conversion."

Nondirective interviewing proves more rewarding than direct questioning. For example, asking the patient to describe the pain ("Tell me how it feels") almost always provides insight into the emotions the patient associates with the symptom. Suggesting how the symptom feels to the patient ("Is it dull or sharp pain?") limits his or her possible responses. If the patient spontaneously offers information about recent events, the interviewer should obtain further data related to such changes in the patient's life. However, care should be taken to avoid suggesting a cause-and-effect relationship between the patient's feelings and the symptoms. Because the patient who has conversion symptoms has no conscious knowledge of such an association, the suggestion of such a relationship may alienate him or her and prevent establishment of a trusting relationship.

DIAGNOSTIC CRITERIA FOR CONVERSION SYMPTOMS

The conversion symptom has a specific, but unconscious, symbolic meaning to the patient. In other words, the conversion symptom often is related to an unconscious wish, and the physical impairment serves to prevent acting out the wish. For example, the adolescent boy who has hand paralysis may have anxieties about masturbating. The physician treating children and adolescents may not always be aware of the symbolic meaning of the symptom. Indeed, the concept that conversion symptoms have a symbolic meaning to the patient was formulated only after a series of these patients had undergone extensive psychotherapy. Although it may be intellectually rewarding for the physician to be cognizant of the presence of the symbolic meaning, ignorance of the specific symbolism does not prevent adequate treatment of the patient. For example:

Jane, a 12-year-old, suddenly developed an inability to walk. Physical examination, including a neurological evaluation, revealed no abnormalities. Interviews by a psychiatrist and a pediatrician working as a team revealed no apparent symbolic etiological factor. The pediatrician formulated a system to reward Jane's progress in walking and implemented this approach; the psychiatrist was similarly supportive with the patient. Over a period of 3 weeks, the patient regained her ability to walk.

Adolescents who have conversion symptoms frequently display characteristic patterns of behavior, sometimes designated as traits of the "hysterical personality." Such characteristics include egocentricity, labile emotional states (quick shifts from sadness to elation and from anger to passivity), dramatic, attention-seeking behavior, and sexual provocativeness (displayed in gestures and in dress). Patients who have such characteristics also usually are demanding, display an air of pseudomaturity, and are dependent in personal interactions. Their personal relationships, however, rarely are intimate or satisfying. Although many aspects of the hysterical personality are seen in adolescent patients who have conversion symptoms, such characteristics also are demonstrable in adolescents who do not have such symptoms. Therefore hysterical behavior traits in adolescents are not synonymous with conversion symptoms and, in isolation, are not indicative of a psychopathological condition.

The manner in which patients who have a conversion symptom describe their problem often is distinctive. The account frequently is dramatic. A pain may be described as "thousands of burning needles thrust into my leg" or as "a giant spike being driven into my chest." Because these patients are suggestible, any symptom description alluded to by the physician may be readily adopted and thereafter reported, which again emphasizes the importance of a nondirective approach in the interview.

As previously described, conversion symptoms are adopted unconsciously in an attempt to reduce unpleasant affects, especially anxiety, depression, and guilt. Therefore, although the patient may describe incapacitating pain, he or she often affects an air of unconcern. Psychiatrists refer to this as *la belle indifference*. The extent to which the conversion symptom diminishes the unpleasant affect and symbolically communicates the forbidden wish for the patient is referred to as the *primary gain*. Patients who have conversion reactions often are stubborn in their belief that the symptom is caused by organic problems. This reflects denial of the underlying emotional problem. Conversely, insistence (especially by an adolescent) that a symptom is psychological in origin may indicate denial of a physical problem. Therefore differentiating between conversion symptoms and physical disease in adolescent patients cannot depend solely on the patient's emotional response.

Conversion symptoms not only effect a primary gain for

the patient but also help him or her cope with the environment. In this respect the conversion symptom achieves a *secondary gain* for the patient. For example, the patient who has a conversion symptom defending against homosexual thoughts may be excused from attending school, where anxiety may have been intensified (e.g., in the locker room). Limitations imposed by the symptom may contradict the patient's verbalized wish to participate in activities but, nevertheless, remove him or her from potentially threatening social interactions. Interference with daily activities also provides a secondary gain for the patient in that attention and more frequent expressions of love are elicited from concerned parents and friends. This situation may be quite resistant to change, not only because the symptom is reinforced continually, but also because the symptom meets the parents' psychological needs. In effect, the symptom may provide the parents with a reason for nurturing or infantilizing their child. Consequently the patient and his or her entire family may fall into a vicious circle of dependence on the symptom.

Demonstration of a secondary gain does not ensure a diagnosis of conversion. To an extent, all illness is involved with some secondary gain. Bedridden patients must accept increased attention to cope with their physical confinement. Therefore a degree of secondary gain is necessary for adequate adaptation to a physical disability. However, in the case of a conversion symptom, secondary gain not only intensifies symptoms but also may be associated with further occurrence of somatic complaints. Because perpetuation of secondary gain depends on concern from others, a conversion symptom is exhibited more readily in the presence of individuals meaningful to the patient.

Children and adolescents who develop conversion symptoms often are overprotected and become extremely dependent on their parents. Daily familial communication may have been invested heavily in somatic complaints, the child recognizing how often activities may have been cancelled because of father's headaches or mother's cramps. Therefore the patient's symptom may conform to the unspoken interactional rules of the family. The patient's problem is thereby reinforced indirectly by family members, who may even assume an air of indifference with respect to his or her symptoms. For example:

James was a 13-year-old who had severe abdominal pain and was referred to a pediatrician by his family practitioner. Physical examination revealed little objective evidence of abdominal pain in the physician's office. However, his return home quickly resulted in intensified pain. Abdominal pain appeared to be well controlled during a subsequent 4-day hospitalization (all organic tests were unremarkable). His return home again produced an immediate exacerbation of the abdominal discomfort. Furthermore, John, James's identical twin, began exhibiting signs of abdominal pain. The boys' mother admitted feeling trapped by the demands of her children and volunteered that in the past she had been treated for chronic abdominal pain. The appearance of abdominal pain in both twins reassured her that the pain was "probably a virus." She chose not to pursue further counseling for the boys.

Precipitation of a conversion symptom may be related to specific stressful events. A change of school, final examinations, new social experiences, and parental conflict are examples of events that may induce a conversion symptom. A study by Maloney[8] suggests that unresolved grief reactions may represent a source of stress that can precipitate a conversion symptom. Examples of grief reactions listed in the study include loss of a parent through death, divorce, or moving. Because the patient's association between conflict and the conversion reaction is unconscious, a history is helpful only if the interviewer elicits details about daily activities. Often the stressful event precipitating a conversion symptom becomes apparent only after many visits. For example:

Chip, a 13-year-old, was brought by his mother to his pediatrician because of chronic abdominal pain, which appeared to be precipitated by his competing in horse riding events. His history revealed the death of a grandparent 4 months previously, but his mother alleged that her son's pain preceded the onset of the fatal illness. Other family stresses were denied. The teenager did not appear for follow-up care but returned 6 months later, primarily because his mother wanted to discuss her son's reaction to her upcoming divorce. At this visit, the mother volunteered that marital stress had been ongoing for several years.

Symptom selection is based on the patient's unconscious remembrance of his or her own body function or on his or her understanding of symptoms in others. The patient's conversion symptom may appear quite dissimilar to that displayed by the other (often a parent or a close relative) because it is the patient's *perception* of disease that governs the display of symptoms. Parents and relatives often misinform children and adolescents about diseases, fearing that the truth would be too frightening. However, such misinformation actually may potentiate the adolescent's fantasies and result in the development of a symptom quite different from the one actually experienced by the individual serving as the model. For example:

During a routine physical examination, Jeff, a 14-year-old, mentioned that he experienced "migraine headaches," which appeared to be focused "behind my left eye" and occurred approximately once a month. Jeff's mother attached more importance to the symptoms than did Jeff. Initially, exploration of the family history proved unremarkable. Persistent questioning about stress led the mother to mention almost parenthetically that she had recently been diagnosed as having multiple sclerosis. She felt that the case was mild and therefore had not told Jeff and her other children directly about the diagnosis, although she sensed that the children knew. Her initial symptom that precipitated the diagnosis of multiple sclerosis was temporary loss of vision in her left eye.

The choice of a symptom also may be based on a physical illness the patient had suffered previously. Thus patients who have a history of seizures may, after many years of adequate anticonvulsant control, have atypical and physiologically unexplainable seizures. Unfortunately, these patients often re ceive only a physiological workup for seizures. Despite the atypical history, the physician assumes that the diagnosis rests "where the money is, or was" in the past. For example:

Terry a 15-year-old girl, recently had been treated for otitis media, which was marked by pain and some dizziness. After the ear appeared adequately healed, her dizziness persisted. By encouraging Terry to discuss her daily schedule, it became apparent that she was under significant academic pressure, having recently transferred to an extremely competitive private school. In addition, extracurricular pressures were heavy, including her fervent commitment to gymnastics and her hope to achieve professional status. On further ques-

CRITERIA FOR DIAGNOSIS OF CONVERSION SYMPTOMS

The symptom has symbolic meaning to the patient.
The patient frequently exhibits characteristic interpersonal behaviors.
Conversion symptoms are more common in girls than boys.
There is a characteristic style of reporting symptoms.
The symptom helps the patient cope with his or her environment ("secondary gain").
There often is frequent use of health issues and symptoms in family communication.
Symptoms occur at times of stress.
The symptom has a model.
History and physical findings often are inconsistent with anatomical and physiological concepts.

From Prazar G: *Pediatr Rev* 8:279, 1987.

tioning, Terry related that she had had dizzy spells in past years just before competitions.

Because the somatic complaint expressed by the patient is based on a model symptom, a physical disease often is mimicked. Close scrutiny of the symptom's history and description often reveals anatomical and physiological discrepancies. The child or adolescent who has a *stocking anesthesia,* an anesthesia confined to a specific area of an extremity without any relationship to cutaneous nerve innervation, demonstrates an example of such symptom inaccuracy. It is based on the patient's concept of his or her body rather than on anatomical principles.

A thorough history may not only elicit symptom inconsistencies in the present illness, but also may reveal a record of inexplicable or recurrent bouts of illness associated with life events. A history of chronic abdominal pain that occurs only on school days, a history of somatic complaints associated with stressful social events, or documentation of abdominal surgery with equivocal findings should raise suspicion that the patient's current problem represents conversion. A list of the diagnostic criteria for conversion symptoms appears in the box above. No one criterion can be confirmatory, and each patient who has a conversion symptom may not display every criterion listed. However, the diagnosis of a conversion symptom cannot be made solely on the basis of negative physical and laboratory findings; it is not a diagnosis of exclusion.

DIFFERENTIAL DIAGNOSIS OF OTHER PSYCHOSOMATIC DISORDERS

Other psychosomatic disorders at times may be confused with conversion symptoms. Patients exhibiting *hypochondriasis,* a common entity, especially in adolescents, view their symptoms with extreme concern. There is none of the apparent indifference seen in patients who have conversion symptoms. Patients who have conversion symptoms frequently seem relieved when an organic cause is considered; patients who have hypochondriasis become more concerned if an organic diagnosis is suggested because they suspect and fear a serious or fatal disease. However, neither type of patient is reassured more than transiently by being informed that he or she has no disease.

Malingering is an uncommon problem in adolescents, except in institutionalized adolescents or those who are in restrictive situations (e.g., military service). Malingering may even be regarded as an appropriate means of avoiding threatening or unpleasant circumstances. Attempts to feign illness often are naive, especially in younger patients. As Engel states, malingerers exhibit "an intense need to be nurtured or suffer." Many appear to be accident prone, and many submit to painful procedures readily and without objection. Malingering adolescents are aloof and hostile to the physician; thus discovery of their deception often is delayed. In contrast, patients who have conversion symptoms often are appropriately fearful of procedures and may appear charming and garrulous with the physician. Patients who have conversion symptoms and malingerers are similar in that their parents may have an unconscious psychological need to have their children be ill and therefore may reinforce their children's symptoms.

Somatic delusions are symptoms of psychosis and usually are not confused with conversion symptoms. Other signs of severe mental illness usually are present, such as an inability to relate to peers, visual or auditory hallucinations, and stereotypical behaviors. Furthermore, the symptoms described sometimes are intermittent and often are extremely bizarre. For example, a patient who has somatic delusions may express the conviction that his or her heart is shriveling or that something is wrong with the blood that is running from the head to the leg.

Psychophysiological symptoms may occur when conversion symptoms have failed to dissipate anxiety. Thus continuing anxiety activates biological systems (especially the autonomic nervous system), resulting in physiological changes such as tachycardia, hyperperistalsis, and vasoconstriction. A patient's cognizance of these changes is manifested by palpitations, diarrhea, and sweating. In this situation the symptom itself has no organic symbolic meaning and results from a reaction to actual body changes. Therefore psychophysiological symptoms can occur when conversion symptoms have failed. Similarly, conversion symptoms can replace psychophysiological symptoms.

CARE OF THE PATIENT WHO HAS CONVERSION SYMPTOMS

Adolescents who have conversion symptoms most often are seen initially and eventually managed by pediatricians or other primary care physicians. Families see this as appropriate because the obvious aspect of the problem is physical. They typically will accept a diagnosis of conversion only from a medical professional they consider an expert in physical disease. Nevertheless, when the physician undertakes a case of suspected conversion, his or her interviewing acumen and sensitivity to the patient's feelings are paramount. The initial interaction between the physician and the patient is crucial to the degree of success achieved in dealing with a conversion symptom. In essence, treatment of the patient begins before a definitive diagnosis is made. Some considerations involved in the initial evaluation of patients suspected of having conversion symptoms appear in the box on the right.

The physician should advise the patient and family that the cause of any disorder involves both physical and emotional factors. As Schmitt[12] states, the family should be told that "everyone's body has a certain physical way of responding to emotional stress." Similarly, every individual has an emotional response to physical stress. Simple examples should be given (e.g., most people have learned that headaches often are intensified when they are upset). If the physician communicates an appreciation of the role of emotions in physical disease, the family may volunteer information more readily about psychosocial functioning. Furthermore, an eventual diagnosis involving emotional aspects may be more acceptable because the family has been prepared for the possibility. Focusing only on an organic diagnosis intimates to the parents that psychological involvement is unlikely, unimportant, and improbable. Turning to psychological issues after all physical tests prove unremarkable implies to parents that this tack was chosen as a last resort because the physician was unable to ascertain an organic cause. A concurrent physical-psychological diagnostic approach not only prepares the physician to consider the problem with some psychotherapeutic intent, but also may save the family time and money because multiple laboratory tests often can be avoided.

After the evaluation has been completed, the physician must develop a treatment plan. Before embarking on this venture, the physician must be satisfied with the completeness of the medical evaluation. Common sense should dictate when he or she feels that further organic tests will be futile. The patient and family often can sense a physician's uncertainty, especially if the family is averse to accepting a psychological diagnosis. Therefore it is prudent to ask the family what additional tests they might expect to have performed and what other diagnoses they may have considered. Involvement of the patient and family in this diagnostic process frequently dissipates anxiety and allows eventual psychological counseling.

Although patients who have conversion symptoms are suggestible, reassurance that the symptom will go away rarely is effective and also does not contribute to a psychological investigation of the symptom. On the contrary, suggesting that the symptom will persist allows time to work out a therapeutic relationship with the patient and sometimes has a paradoxical effect. Because the symptom is unlikely to disappear after two or three visits, the patient retrospectively will view the physician's suggestion as sound. Trust in the physician will be reinforced, and the patient may be more comfortable communicating information about his or her feelings. Placebo medication usually is ineffective and raises questions of medical ethics. Tranquilizers may reduce attendant anxiety transiently in some cases of conversion symptoms; however, using medication as the sole therapy rarely results in lasting improvement. Because medication does not relieve the underlying conflict responsible for the symptom, another symptom eventually may appear. Furthermore, there is risk that the medication's side effects may become the model for new conversion symptoms or that new symptoms may be confused with side effects.

At the conclusion of the evaluation, the number and type of counseling sessions the physician anticipates should be discussed. The number of sessions should be flexible so that it can be renegotiated if needed. Follow-up sessions with the teenager usually can be limited to 20 to 30 minutes every 2 to 4 weeks. More frequent visits may be necessary if the symptom interferes with school attendance, peer relationships, or family functioning. During follow-up sessions, the teenager should be encouraged to talk about his or her daily life (e.g., school, friends, family, dating). If the teenager volunteers information about recurrence of the somatic complaint, the physician should inquire about events that were transpiring concurrently when the symptom occurred and how the teenager *felt* about these events. In this way the physician can help the adolescent become reacquainted with how daily events and feelings are related.

Because the physician will serve both as therapist for the teenager and provider of acute medical care, there may be occasions when the teenager has a new physical symptom or complaint. If the physician suspects a physical illness unrelated to the conversion symptom, he or she must perform whatever evaluation is indicated, including a full or partial physical examination. However, an overzealous search for disease should be avoided. Treatment goals need to be realistic. Conversion symptoms seldom disappear completely. However, adolescents often acquire increased coping skills so that their daily functioning is unimpaired and dependence on secondary gain is minimized.

Follow-up visits with parents should take place every 4 to 6 weeks. Such meetings should serve to elicit persistent or new concerns that parents may have about their teenager's progress and should attempt to assess the parents' reaction to their teenager's continuing complaints. The practitioner should emphasize the validity of the teenager's concerns so that misconceptions about the symptom being "faked" are dispelled. Furthermore, positive reinforcement needs to be offered so that parents believe they are doing what is best for their child. Selected follow-up sessions with the parents should include the teenager. Not only do such family meet-

IMPORTANT CONSIDERATIONS IN THE INITIAL EVALUATION OF PATIENTS SUSPECTED OF HAVING CONVERSION SYMPTOMS

From the outset, parents and patient should be told that every person has an emotional response to physical stress.

Parents and patient should be encouraged to suggest diagnostic tests that they may want performed and to suggest possible diagnoses for consideration by the physician.

Parents and patient should understand that the symptom may persist but that the goal is to help maintain normal daily functioning in school and with peers.

Parents and patient should understand that referral to a psychiatrically trained professional may be necessary if progress is not made in coping with the symptom.

From Prazar G: *Pediatr Rev* 8:279, 1987.

ings demonstrate to the patient that confidentiality of individual sessions is not being violated, they also offer the physician an opportunity to observe parent-adolescent interaction. These observations may provide an important index to the effectiveness of ongoing therapy.

REFERRAL

Referral to mental health professionals is indicated if symptoms continue to interfere with the patient's daily activities or functioning or when the physician or school personnel feel that the teenager's symptoms have not diminished. School officials can provide valuable information about the effect of the conversion symptom on school functioning and peer interaction. Referral is dictated if the family feels that inadequate progress has been made after an agreed-upon duration of therapy.

Referral is indicated if the patient's symptom creates uncomfortable feelings in the pediatrician. Situations involving seductive adolescent behavior in association with a conversion symptom may create feelings in the pediatrician that can prevent effective intervention. It is as unrealistic to assume that a pediatrician can treat all psychological problems adequately as it is to assume that he or she can treat all medical ones. Cognizance of one's own limitations is an important professional attribute. Another situation requiring referral involves the patient or family member who is a social acquaintance or a relative of the pediatrician. Dealing with the emotional problems of friends' or relatives' children is inappropriate. Obtaining personal details of family or sexual functioning often is indicated in the evaluation and may jeopardize the social relationship. Conversely, failure or hesitancy to obtain appropriate data may jeopardize subsequent resolution of the problem.

In all cases, when referral is suggested, parental and patient compliance with the referral is improved if the possibility has been mentioned as a contingency *early* in the evaluation. The pediatrician should always help families understand that seeing a psychiatrically trained professional does *not* connote "craziness." Rather, the pediatrician may suggest that a psychiatrist could help because a doctor trained in psychiatry can help teenagers understand feelings about unusual symptoms better than can most pediatricians. After the referral is made, continued pediatrician contact with the family concerning the conversion symptom promotes compliance with the therapy. Indications for referring patients who have conversion symptoms are listed in the box above.[11]

The prognosis for patients who have conversion reactions is unknown. In a report of 74 children who had psychogenic pain, Friedman[3] found a large number of patients who were judged to be improved after several years, regardless of whether professional intervention took place. In a 7-year follow-up of patients hospitalized with conversion, 23 of 41 patients no longer suffered from their presenting physical symptom, were free of underlying stress, and had experienced no symptom substitution or new associated complaint.[7] Patients who have conversion symptoms indeed may have an encouraging future. On the other hand, in some patients adolescent conversion symptoms mark the beginning of a lifelong career of conversion illness.

INDICATIONS FOR REFERRAL OF PATIENTS WHO HAVE CONVERSION SYMPTOMS

The symptom continues to interfere with daily functioning (school attendance, participation in extracurricular activities, involvement with peers).

Parents and patient believe that no progress is being made in dealing with the symptom.

The physician feels uncomfortable with the patient's symptom or behavior (e.g., patients exhibiting seductive behavior).

The patient's family includes a social friend or relative of the physician.

From Prazar G: *Pediatr Rev* 8:279, 1987.

SUMMARY

Conversion reactions represent an emotionally charged issue, not only literally for the adolescent but also figuratively for the physician, because patients displaying such symptoms often elicit a wide range of emotions from their physician. The physician's emotional response results from his or her frustration in dealing with such difficult patients. Every patient who has a somatic complaint has feelings about his or her symptoms. An evaluation of any somatic complaint should involve inquiry into aspects of the patient's family, school performance, and peer relationships. A better understanding of the patient's baseline emotional functioning can be achieved in this way. The physician must advise both parents and patient that it is acceptable to have feelings about somatic complaints. Both family and patient may be much more accepting of primary emotional involvement if permission for expressing feelings is given early in the physician-patient relationship. The diagnosis of a conversion reaction should never be one of exclusion and should follow specific diagnostic criteria.

Care of the adolescent patient who has a conversion reaction involves establishing a renegotiable number of regular visits, encouraging the patient to discuss daily activities and interrelated feelings, meeting with parents regularly to provide them with emotional support and counseling, and knowing that palliation rather than a cure may be the optimal goal. When the physician feels uncomfortable treating a patient who has a conversion reaction or when ongoing follow-up care appears to have made no progress in reducing the symptom, the patient should be referred to a mental health professional. However, referral should not end the pediatrician's contact with the patient because ongoing physician interest may improve patient compliance with the referral source and may increase the physician's ability to resume responsibility later for the patient's care. The patient who has a conversion symptom usually will not outgrow it and will not respond permanently to placebo medication. Such patients severely tax the primary care physician's diagnostic and therapeutic acumen. However, the physician who respects the involvement of emotions with somatic complaints can play a vital role in helping patients who have conversion symptoms cope with their disorders.

REFERENCES

1. Apley J: *The child with abdominal pains,* ed 2, Oxford, England, 1975, Blackwell Scientific.
2. Engel GL: Conversion symptoms. In MacBryde CM, Blacklow RS, editors: *Signs and symptoms: applied pathologic physiology and clinical interpretation,* ed 6, Philadelphia, 1983, JB Lippincott.
3. Friedman R: Some characteristics of children with "psychogenic" pain: observations on prognosis and management, *Clin Pediatr* 11:331, 1972.
4. Friedman SB: Conversion symptoms in adolescents, *Pediatr Clin North Am* 20:873, 1973.
5. Hollender MH: Conversion hysteria: a post-Freudian reinterpretation of nineteenth century psychosocial data, *Arch Gen Psychiatry* 26:31, 1972.
6. Levine RJ: Epidemic faintness and syncope in a school marching band, *JAMA* 238:2373, 1977.
7. Maisami M, Freeman JM: Conversion reactions in children as body language: a combined child psychiatry/neurology team approach to the management of functional neurologic disorders in children, *Pediatrics* 80:46, 1987.
8. Maloney MJ: Diagnosing hysterical conversion reactions in children, *J Pediatr* 97:1016, 1980.
9. Moffett MEK: Epidemic hysteria in a Montreal train station, *Pediatrics* 70:308, 1982.
10. Oster J: Recurrent abdominal pain, headache, and limb pains in children and adolescents, *Pediatrics* 50:429, 1972.
11. Prazar G: Conversion reactions in adolescents, *Pediatr Rev* 8:279, 1987.
12. Schmitt BD: School phobia—the great imitator: a pediatrician's viewpoint, *Pediatrics* 48:433, 1971.

SUGGESTED READING

Prazar GE: Psychosomatic disorders and conversion reactions. In Friedman SB, Fisher M, Schonberg SK, editors: *Comprehensive adolescent health care,* St Louis, 1992, Quality Medical Publishing.

97 Counseling Parents of Adolescents

Frances C. Paolini-Masucci

As a child grows, so should the pediatrician-parent partnership. Particularly with regard to psychological and behavioral issues, parents tend to see the trusted pediatrician as less threatening than a mental health provider as a person from whom to seek advice. The pediatrician's ongoing relationship with the family presents him or her with a unique opportunity to educate and support the parents as their children enter and move through adolescence.

Adolescence is notable for the dramatic, uneven integration of development characterized by a changing body image, mood swings, burgeoning sexuality, intense need for peer acceptance, increasing independence from the family, expectations to achieve and "act one's age," and fragile egos. At the conclusion of this developmental phase the emergent young adult is expected to comprehend the nuances of complex issues and arrive at decisions, develop an ethical and moral value system, prepare for a chosen field of work, and be capable of intimacy. These daunting tasks are realized largely within a family unit (see Chapter 51, Theories and Concepts of Development as They Relate to Pediatric Practice).

It is crucial to note that adolescent autonomy or independence evolves from a *fluctuating process* that progresses within an environment of continuous connectedness to parents and family. Most adolescents do not achieve independence through a sudden break with their parents; instead the process is one of gradual redefinition of their relationship. The adolescent years represent but one phase of a developmental continuum as the young person continues the process begun in childhood of increasing autonomy while continuing to use the family as a mainstay. It is well recognized that adolescents do not accept the presumed wisdom of their elders. They need to experience the tension created by going forth and experimenting with ideas and life-styles that often are in marked contrast to those of the family. It is a time of "trying on" diverse personalities, like an actor in the center of an imaginary stage. At the same time, the adolescent needs to know that return to the refuge of the family is assured.

A parent's greatest challenge is to maintain that delicate balance between enabling the adolescent's independent behavior while supporting his or her sense of trust and security in the family. Herein lies the principal source of conflicting emotional distress experienced simultaneously by parents and adolescents. The parents' pain is the result of feelings of loss of control provoked by the young person's independent behavior; the adolescent's discomfort is activated by feelings of loss of childhood security as he or she struggles to cope with greater freedom and responsibility. Unfortunately, all too often such emotional conflict and pain remain unrecognized and unarticulated and yet underlie many confrontations between parents and adolescents. Helping parents to understand the developmental basis for this inherent parent-adolescent conflict serves to reduce their frustration.

With the ever-widening array of diverse family systems and complex choices facing adolescents, what counsel can the pediatrician give parents to help them navigate the turbulent adolescent waters? Practitioners can begin by providing parents with information about the physical, cognitive, and psychosocial developmental tasks of adolescence and by helping parents realize that adolescent development is a fluctuating process that occurs within the family system. Parents should be encouraged to assume the role of facilitator and teacher for their adolescent, with two critical major goals. The first goal is to promote expression and resolution of conflict between themselves and their teenager through *mutual respect*. Parents should maintain the adolescent's trust in the family by seeing to it that their child speaks respectfully to them and that they, in turn, speak respectfully to their child. The second goal is to learn to tolerate the adolescent's differing views, thereby nurturing their teenager's self-esteem and independent growth. The parents should view themselves as leaders in a process in which collaboration and mutuality are affirmed; the ultimate goal is a partnership.

Open communication probably is the most important skill for parents to develop and maintain with their maturing child. Adolescents need a trusted sounding board before venturing forth. As facilitators, parents need to *listen* more than speak. When parents start to lecture, the adolescent's attention automatically shuts down. The axiom "Actions speak louder than words" makes a useful parental motto, far better than "Do as I say, not as I do." This latter philosophy raises the question of hypocrisy, often diminishing the adolescent's respect for the parent. Such a situation can result in more angry confrontations and a weakening of the parent-teen collaborative relationship.

Adolescents' continuing need for parental affection and acceptance, plus a not yet fully developed sense of self, leaves them highly vulnerable to self-perceived injustices, putdowns, and negative innuendos. Parents gain immeasurably when they respond to their adolescents' feelings with an emotional rather than an intellectual response. For example, during the teen years, peer relationships are experienced with intense emotions characteristic of adolescent egocentricity. Should a break occur in a heretofore close friendship, it is a wise parent who demonstrates support by empathizing with their child's hurt feelings. Statements such as "I'm so sorry that you are in such pain," "I can imagine how bad you are feeling," or "It seems that your friend has really hurt you; do you want to talk about it?" are appropriate and allow room for continued discussion. Sometimes, in an attempt to "make it better," parents tend to minimize the adolescent's pain, perceiving it as "only" a short-lived adolescent drama. They respond with statements such as "You'll find other friends," or

"Don't worry, you're young and have your whole life ahead of you." Rather than finding this helpful, the adolescent feels misunderstood and may cut off further communication by saying "You just don't understand!"

If the parent did not approve of the friend, the end of the relationship may be a source of relief for the parent. Telling a teenager to "forget about it" may be more representative of the parent's wish than of the teen's. The ultimate negative scenario is a parent who adds, "I told you so!" Few, if any, adults respond kindly to such admonishment. The thoughtful parent refrains from statements that only serve to belittle the adolescent. In fact, adolescents feel devastated when berated by a parent, despite their attempts to defend against the hurt by false bravado or an "I don't care!" response. When parents appropriately empathize with their teenagers' emotional intensity and allow their youngsters to express their emotions without restraint or embarrassment, adolescents are comforted and feel supported. This reinforces open communication with parents and minimizes the need for adolescents to act out angry or hurt feelings maladaptively.

Parents also have an obligation to clarify expectations, responsibilities, and privileges; these decisions are not made in a vacuum. Just as a parent of a 2-year-old might give the toddler a choice between a red or a blue outfit, it is imperative for the parent of an adolescent to allow him or her to participate as a member of the contractual, decision-making team. It is well known that the success of any contract between two or more parties requires that each person be allowed to express, *without dissent,* what he or she wants. It also is important that both sides negotiating the contract *gain something* from the outcome. An "all-or-nothing" result breeds discontent and nonadherence by the person who perceives no gain. *Nothing less is required between parents and adolescents.* How to "make a deal" or negotiate an agreement is a skill best learned within a family where mutual respect and trial and error are supported.

One way pediatricians can assess how families are coping with adolescent development is to ask the parents how parent-teen decision making is progressing. Curfew, the generations-old source of conflict, especially when associated with social events, is a good issue to discuss with parents. The physician should explore whether the parents are able to have an open discussion with their adolescent about his or her plans. Do the parents routinely inquire about the location of the social function and the travel plans? Are they able to easily work out an agreed-upon curfew with which everyone is reasonably satisfied? In the event of a disagreement, how are compromises negotiated? Counsel parents to avoid making arbitrarily rigid time limits. An example of the type of statement best avoided is "Your Dad and I have decided that you are to be home no later than midnight." Such unilateral decisions usually end in angry, unresolvable confrontations. Sometimes the rigidity of the curfew time is confounded by the parents' disapproval of the adolescent's choice of friends or life-style.

Not infrequently, parental disapproval of the adolescent's friends may be the *expressed* reason for parental inflexibility about the young person's curfew. However, the *real* cause for concern may have more to do with the parents' fear of adolescent sexual activity. The pediatrician might ask the parents whether they and their adolescent have been able to share their views about adolescent sexual activity and sexual relationships. If so, did such a discussion result in a consensual understanding? If not, the pediatrician can suggest that such a meeting take place "to clear the air." Although the issue of sexuality may be unexpressed, it is never far from thought.

Parents also may feel anxious because they fear adverse outcomes when they perceive their adolescent's behavior as "deviant." In particular, parents may be afraid that such behavior will be permanent and will destroy the teen's opportunity to mature into a responsible, productive adult. It may reassure the parents to know that extremes of adolescent behavior generally are transient and that most adolescents mature into adults who have life-styles, values, and mores fairly similar to those of their families. Here, it might be pointed out that the more rigid the parents' control, the greater the adolescent's rebellion. Nevertheless, parents should be supported in their efforts to protect the adolescent from accidents and other dangerous behavior that might occur during these experimental ventures. Thus flexibility and reasonableness are traits to strive for as parents negotiate behavioral limits with their teenagers.

Another important aspect of the decision-making process concerns the consequences of breaking a contract. Here, too, the process of open discussion *by all family members* should apply—that is, the reason for the infraction should be discussed and renegotiated. Many parents have little difficulty grounding their adolescent for nonadherence to an agreement, but they have more difficulty acknowledging that they, themselves, have failed to abide by an agreement. One situation involved a family in which the parents conceded that they nagged their daughter about not spending enough time on schoolwork, fearing her academic failure. The parents agreed with the physician's counsel that they respect the adolescent's privacy and give her the responsibility for her schoolwork. A "contract" was signed by the pediatrician, as mediator, the parents, and the adolescent. The terms included the adolescent's decision about the time to set aside for study, and the parents agreed to permit her to experience her decision and not to nag. If the adolescent's grades declined, she would be grounded; if the parents continued the harangue, *they* would be grounded for that weekend!

Parents also are well advised not to abdicate their authority abruptly. Rather, they need to be encouraged to maintain confidence in their authority to negotiate limits, particularly where true issues of safety are involved. A striking example was presented by a mother and her soon-to-be 14-year-old son during a pediatric visit. In response to a question about how things were going, the mother angrily reported that her son thought he no longer needed a parent. The boy silently reacted by rolling his eyes upward. Each was given an opportunity to explain. The mother focused on her son's defiant behavior after the parents had denied his request for an extended curfew to join in a friend's birthday celebration at a downtown urban center. The pediatrician encouraged the mother to give her main objection. She cited their fear for their son's safety, given the lateness of return. At this the boy blurted, "Why didn't you just say 'No' and mean it!" The parents' perceived loss of control undermined their authority, and as a result, their son's "immaturity" became the focus of their confrontation. Here, the pediatrician facilitated a reframing of the problem to highlight the safety issues, on which both the parents and the son agreed.

Some families are unable to make use of a pediatrician's counsel and require the intervention of a mental health provider. For example, some parents resist acknowledging the relevance of understanding adolescent development and the *mutuality* of the parent-adolescent interaction. Instead, they chronically respond to the adolescent's point of view with "Yes . . . but" followed by a litany of the adolescent's misdeeds. Other parents have inappropriate expectations and inappropriately rely on their adolescent for nurturance and support. The unmet needs of such adolescents generally are manifested in a chronic pattern of acting-out behaviors, such as poor school performance, loss of friends, somatic complaints and, in extreme situations, depression or suicide attempts. For the less serious behaviors, pediatricians might consider meeting with the parents to assess their willingness and capacity to understand the developmental and family communication issues. If parents are refractory to counseling after one or two meetings, the pediatrician will be in a better position to make an appropriate mental health referral than he or she would have been at the initial visit (see Chapter 93, Consultation and Referral for Behavioral and Developmental Problems).

Pediatricians who counsel parents in a mutually satisfying, working relationship can make a significant difference. By enhancing the parents' knowledge, reducing their stress, and increasing their coping abilities, pediatricians can help provide a safe familial harbor for their adolescent patients.

SUGGESTED READINGS

Cooper CR, Grotevant HD, Condon S: Individuality and connectedness in the family as a context for adolescent identity formation and role taking skill. In Grotevant HD, Cooper CR, editors: *Adolescent development in the family: new directions in child development,* San Francisco, 1983, Jossey-Bass.

Montemayor R: Parents and adolescents in conflict: all families some of the time and some families most of the time, *Journal of Early Adolescence* 3:83, 1983.

Sabetelli RM, Mazor A: Differentiation, individuation, and identity formation: the integration of family system and individual developmental perspectives, *Adolescence* 20:6, 1985.

98 Anorexia and Bulimia Nervosa

Martin Fisher

The eating disorders, a group of conditions that primarily affect adolescents and young adults, have increased dramatically in prevalence during the past 3 decades. Marked by a combination of medical and psychological factors in their etiology and outcome, they predominantly include the well-known entities of anorexia and bulimia nervosa. Anorexia nervosa, viewed most simply as the *purposeful loss of weight beyond that which is healthy,* now is said to affect 1 out of every 200 adolescent girls in the United States and Great Britain. Bulimia, which is marked by *recurrent episodes of binge eating and/or vomiting,* has been estimated to affect 2% to 20% of young women of high school and college age in these same countries, depending on the criteria used. The diagnosis and prevalence of these disorders are much debated, and many questions remain about their etiology and outcome. Nevertheless, the growing prevalence of eating disorders has made it increasingly important for the primary care physician to have some knowledge of the principles involved in evaluation and treatment of both anorexia and bulimia nervosa.

DIAGNOSIS AND PREVALENCE

Although individual cases suggestive of anorexia nervosa and cultural behaviors suggestive of bulimia have been described from antiquity, neither disorder was defined specifically as a medical condition until the 1880s. At that time, Charles Laseque in France described a condition he called "anorexia hysterica"; William Gull in England referred to the same condition as "anorexia nervosa." Although the latter term is a misnomer, since patients who have eating disorders do not simply have a loss of appetite as the name implies, this name has prevailed since that time.

Individual cases of "anorexia nervosa" appear in the medical literature from the 1880s through the 1950s. Beginning in the 1960s, possibly because of the increased emphasis on thin physiques that swept through the developed world, more cases of anorexia nervosa began to be seen. At first considered only a component of anorexia nervosa, bulimia (now more formally called "bulimia nervosa") was recognized as a separate entity in the 1970s. It now is well known that anorexia nervosa and bulimia may appear as separate syndromes, that they may occur concomitantly or sequentially in the same individual, and that both may be associated with several other entities, including laxative abuse or alternating with obesity. The growing diversity of the eating disorders has accompanied ever-improving refinements in the diagnostic criteria for these conditions.

The first officially published criteria for the diagnosis of anorexia nervosa were developed by Feighner and colleagues in 1972.[9] The original Feighner criteria stipulated that an individual considered as having anorexia nervosa must (1) be under 25 years of age, (2) have lost at least 25% of his or her initial body weight, (3) not have an alternative medical diagnosis to account for the weight loss, (4) not have an alternative psychiatric diagnosis to account for the weight loss, (5) display evidence of a distorted body image, desire for extreme thinness, and a preoccupation with food and weight, and (6) have at least two of the following signs or symptoms associated with anorexia nervosa: amenorrhea, lanugo, bradycardia, periods of hyperactivity, episodes of binge eating, and vomiting.

Changes in both the nature of anorexia nervosa and our understanding of it have occurred in the ensuing years. It now is acknowledged that in rare instances patients may develop the illness after age 25. A 25% weight loss simply may be the result of an appropriate diet for those who start out overweight, whereas a 15% to 20% weight loss may be extremely unhealthy for those already underweight. Patients who have anorexia nervosa may have other psychiatric diagnoses (e.g., depression),[13] and a few patients may manipulate the treatment of other medical conditions (e.g., diabetes mellitus or cystic fibrosis) to lose weight (i.e., a concomitant diagnosis of anorexia nervosa). Furthermore, the emergence of bulimia as a distinct entity required specific criteria for this disorder as well. The best current criteria for both disorders are those listed by the American Psychiatric Association in the fourth edition of the *Diagnostic and Statistical Manual of Mental Disorders* (DSM-IV).[2] The criteria are shown in the box on p. 793. As noted, anorexia and bulimia nervosa have separate criteria and requirements specific to each. The DSM-IV acknowledges that some patients who have eating disorders do not meet the strict criteria for either anorexia or bulimia nervosa; therefore an additional category, "eating disorders not otherwise specified," also has been established.

It has become apparent in recent years that increasingly larger numbers of adolescents, and even children, are displaying abnormal attitudes toward weight and food, and many of these adolescents are showing evidence of subclinical eating disorders.[11] Included in this category are adolescents who lose enough weight to cause irregular periods but not enough to meet DSM-IV criteria for anorexia nervosa and those who use vomiting to control their weight but do not binge and therefore do not meet specific criteria for bulimia nervosa. These adolescents often have medical and psychological difficulties similar to those described in patients whose eating disorders are more overt and generally require similar treatment.[5] Many experts who treat eating disorders in adolescents and children have called for inclusion of such patients in the DSM criteria for eating disorders.

Changes in diagnostic criteria are partly responsible for the debates about incidence that have taken place over the past several years. Most researchers in the field believe that eating disorders have increased in both incidence and prevalence

CRITERIA FOR THE DIAGNOSIS OF EATING DISORDERS

Anorexia nervosa	Bulimia nervosa
Refusal to maintain body weight at or above a minimally normal weight for age and height (e.g., weight loss leading to maintenance of body weight less than 85% of that expected; or failure to make expected weight gain during period of growth, leading to body weight less than 85% of that expected). Intense fear of gaining weight or becoming fat, even though underweight. Disturbance in the way in which one's body weight or shape is experienced, undue influence of body weight or shape on self-evaluation, or denial of seriousness of the current low body weight. In postmenarcheal females, amenorrhea, i.e., the absence of at least three consecutive menstrual cycles. (A woman is considered to have amenorrhea if her periods occur only following hormone, e.g., estrogen, administration.) *Restricting type:* during the current episode of anorexia nervosa, the person has not regularly engaged in binge-eating or purging behavior (i.e., self-induced vomiting or the misuse of laxatives, diuretics, or enemas). *Binge-eating/purging type:* during the current episode of anorexia nervosa, the person has regularly engaged in binge-eating or purging behavior (i.e., self-induced vomiting or the misuse of laxatives, diuretics, or enemas).	Recurrent episodes of binge eating. An episode of binge eating is characterized by both of the following: Eating, in a discrete period of time (e.g., within any 2-hour period), an amount of food that is definitely larger than most people would eat during a similar period of time and under similar circumstances A sense of lack of control over eating during the episode (e.g., a feeling that one cannot stop eating or control what or how much one is eating) Recurrent inappropriate compensatory behavior in order to prevent weight gain, such as self-induced vomiting; misuse of laxatives, diuretics, enemas, or other medications; fasting; or excessive exercise. The binge eating and inappropriate compensatory behaviors both occur, on average, at least twice a week for 3 months. Self-evaluation is unduly influenced by body shape and weight. The disturbance does not occur exclusively during episodes of anorexia nervosa. *Purging type:* during the current episode of bulimia nervosa, the person has regularly engaged in self-induced vomiting or the misuse of laxatives, diuretics, or enemas. *Nonpurging type:* during the current episode of bulimia nervosa, the person has used other inappropriate compensatory behaviors, such as fasting or excessive exercise, but has not regularly engaged in self-induced vomiting or the misuse of laxatives, diuretics, or enemas.

From The American Psychiatric Association: *Diagnostic and statistical manual of mental disorders,* ed 4, Washington, DC, 1994, The Association.

during the past 30 years, although others believe that mostly greater awareness and improved diagnosis account for an apparent rise. One long-term study has demonstrated a steady rise in incidence and prevalence among adolescents but smaller increases in adults.[18] More than 90% of patients who have anorexia and bulimia nervosa are girls or young women; although most cases of anorexia nervosa begin in the teenage years, bulimia is more apt to begin in the late teens and early twenties. It generally is accepted that 0.5% of all adolescent girls meet strict criteria for anorexia nervosa, although not all of these are diagnosed medically. With the criteria for bulimia nervosa being somewhat more vague, some researchers have found prevalences of binge eating and vomiting in 20% to 30% of college-age women; others, using a strict criterion, limit the diagnosis to only 2% to 3% of the same populations.[22] Both diagnoses are far less common in developing nations and among minorities and those of lower socioeconomic status in industrialized societies, although recent increases in these populations have been noted as well.

PRESENTATION AND ETIOLOGY

The patient who has an eating disorder may seek medical care in a variety of ways. Some visit their pediatrician or family physician because of concern about weight loss, vomiting, or abnormal eating attitudes noticed by family, friends, or school authorities. Others visit a gynecologist because of the menstrual irregularities that characteristically accompany the disorder. Many are seen first by a psychiatrist, psychologist, or social worker; others may be seen for the first time in an emergency department because of dehydration or other medical complications. Some patients may be seen within weeks of the disorder's onset, whereas others avoid medical care for months or even years. It is common for patients to be brought for their initial evaluation against their will, claiming, "There's nothing wrong with me," although older patients may seek help willingly, saying, "I'm sick of having this problem." Large-scale questionnaire surveys have shown that many patients who have mild to moderate eating disorders, both anorexia nervosa and bulimia, avoid medical care altogether by hiding or denying their illness.

A considerable body of literature has explored the possible etiological factors in these disorders.[12] Several key questions are addressed: Why has there been an apparent increase in these disorders during the past 3 decades? Why are women affected predominantly? What factors cause any particular individual to develop the disorder? Cultural, psychological, and biochemical factors all have been invoked in responding to these questions about etiology.

Several cultural changes that have taken place during the

past 30 years may bear directly on the increased incidence of eating disorders. Foremost among these is the strong emphasis our society places on the desirability of a thin appearance, especially for women. This factor, along with changes in clothing styles that emphasize the female figure, could explain why certain vulnerable individuals may feel it necessary to choose an unhealthy means, whether it be excessive dieting, vomiting, laxative abuse, or a combination thereof in striving for a dangerously thin weight goal. Societal changes in sexual mores, which have lowered the mean age of initiating sexual intercourse from the late teens to the mid-teens, thereby putting increased pressure on adolescent and young adult women, also are hypothesized to play a role in furthering the psychological vulnerability of some individuals. The issue of career versus family, which places added decision making pressure on young women, may create another level of vulnerability for some individuals at risk for the development of psychological difficulties. These pressures, which were not as problematical for women in previous generations and which do not affect men in the same ways, may point to why the eating disorders are increasing in frequency so dramatically and why they mostly affect girls and young women. Of further interest is the fact that issues of sexual identity have been noted in some young men who develop these disorders.

The psychological factors responsible for the development of an eating disorder in any given individual are numerous and complex.[15] When anorexia nervosa first came to prominence in the 1960s, it was found that most of the girls who had this disorder exhibited a set of similar characteristics, some of which were manifested openly, whereas others emerged with intensive therapy. Specifically, these girls were described as having been excellent students, compulsive workers, and compliant daughters before the onset of their illness. These same girls then became hostile, withdrawn, and depressed after the illness began. In therapy they revealed exceedingly low self-esteem despite their apparent outward success. Their families, outwardly healthy and often so-called pillars of society, were found to have significant hidden psychopathological disorders.

Based on these early findings, three major lines of reasoning, often overlapping, were proposed to explain the psychological basis of the eating disorders. The first concentrated on the psychopathological condition of the individual. This theory postulates that poor self-esteem in the face of outward success poses a major difficulty, which the vulnerable adolescent tries to alleviate by striving for one achievable goal—the thinnest possible body. The second theory focuses on the family. It postulates that patients who have anorexia nervosa come from families in which the natural childhood processes of separation and individuation are not allowed to proceed normally. The refusal to eat represents the ultimate rebelliousness in a teenager who previously has done "everything you've asked of me." A third, older theory was developed around a series of sexual themes. This theory hypothesized that the weight loss in anorexia nervosa serves to diminish the female figure on a young lady who is afraid of becoming a sexual adult. The basis of this fear may be sexual taboos in the family, in some cases, or sexual overstimulation in the family in other cases. In the extreme psychoanalytical interpretation of this theory, patients who have anorexia nervosa may even be refusing food intake for fear of "oral impregnation."

The concepts inherent in each of these theories have been expressed in therapy by many patients who have eating disorders. However, with more recent recognition of many cases of anorexia nervosa in which the patient does not fit the traditional "good girl" mold, and as in many cases of bulimia, a number of psychological themes may be found. For instance, although many girls who develop anorexia nervosa are very compulsive, shy, and not involved sexually, those who have bulimia may be impulsive, outgoing, and even promiscuous. Furthermore, the previous finding that most girls who have anorexia nervosa are excellent students from apparently healthy and intact families is no longer as true as in the past. In fact, increasing numbers of girls who have anorexia nervosa are noted to have learning disabilities or mental retardation or to be from broken homes and other difficult family situations. More recently, the role of sexual abuse as an etiological factor in the development of eating disorders, especially intractable bulimia, has been the focus of increased attention and debate.[6]

The possibility that a biological vulnerability may be present in the initiation and continuance of the eating disorders also has received much attention of late. Because cases of anorexia and bulimia have been associated with depression or addiction, or both, in family studies, it is surmised that a biochemical predeterminant may be present in both disorders. Changes in either dopamine or serotonin metabolism help bring on these disorders, and the cholecystokinin and endorphin systems have been implicated in maintaining them. It is very possible that the biochemical factors that may predispose an individual to begin losing weight or vomiting may be different from those that prevent reversal of these behaviors.

Most likely several factors converge in the development of an eating disorder. The adolescent girl who is culturally primed, biologically at risk, and psychologically vulnerable may begin dieting or vomiting in response to a particular precipitant (often an insult by family or friends, exposure to another individual who has an eating disorder, or a stressful situation). The positive psychological feedback that initially accompanies an "improved" appearance and the biochemical changes that occur in response to decreased nutrition may serve to perpetuate the behavior. It is at this stage that family and friends become concerned and the individual patient seeks medical care.

EVALUATION

Initial evaluation of the patient who has an eating disorder includes a determination of the diagnosis and its severity, an evaluation of other possible causes of weight loss and effects of malnutrition, an analysis of the psychological context of the illness, and a decision about treatment planning.

As presented in the box on p. 793, specific diagnostic criteria currently exist for the eating disorders. Evaluation of these criteria serves both to elucidate the diagnosis and determine the severity of the illness. Distortion of body image, a hallmark in the diagnosis of anorexia nervosa, may be evaluated by exploring the patient's views of her initial weight, current weight, and desired weight. A history of vomiting or binge eating (or both) is elicited in the patient who has bulimia. This information is used to gain insight into the severity of the eating disorder, but the physician must realize that many patients who have eating disorders will not be completely truthful. Establishing the patient's nutritional and exercise patterns and her use of vomiting or medications designed to promote weight loss (including diet pills, laxatives, diuretics, or ipecac) provides hints both to the diagnosis and the possibility of medical complications. Care must be taken to avoid being misled by the patient who is not completely forthright; often the physical examination and laboratory tests suggest the true extent of the patient's disorder.

The first steps in the physical examination of the patient who has an eating disorder are calculation of the percentage below ideal body weight (IBW) and determination of vital signs. The percentage below IBW, which may be calculated by comparing the patient's current weight with the average weight expected for height, age, and sex (as determined by standard growth charts), serves both as one of the diagnostic criteria and as a gross estimate of the degree of malnutrition. In general, body weight more than 30% below IBW represents severe malnutrition, that 20% to 30% below IBW represents moderate malnutrition, and that not yet 20% below IBW represents mild malnutrition. For example, a 16-year-old girl who is 5 feet, 4 inches tall would be expected to have a body weight of 120 pounds, plus or minus 10%; she would be 20% below IBW at 96 pounds and 30% below IBW at 84 pounds.

Vital signs provide further evidence of the degree of malnutrition because chronic malnutrition is accompanied by declines in blood pressure, pulse, and electrocardiographic (ECG) voltage.[10] Other physical changes associated with malnutrition or its concomitant hormonal changes include the findings of scaphoid abdomen, muscle weakness, lanugo similar to that seen in newborns, diminished reflexes, and dry skin. Few physical findings are associated with the vomiting of bulimia, although telltale bite marks on the knuckles (used to induce gagging) may be evident in some patients.

Laboratory tests further elucidate the severity of the illness. Most patients who have anorexia and bulimia nervosa initially have normal laboratory results, although all organ systems probably are affected by the malnutrition. The laboratory abnormalities found on routine testing generally are related to the individual's particular nutritional pattern. Thus the patient who is chronically malnourished usually has leukopenia, occasionally thrombocytopenia and, in rare cases, severe anemia (she is protected for some time from iron deficiency anemia by the concomitant amenorrhea). The patient who restricts her fluid intake may show evidence of dehydration on blood chemistry determinations (including an elevated sodium or blood urea nitrogen), whereas the patient who drinks excessive fluids to satisfy her hunger or the doctor's scale may show signs of hyponatremia and a dilute urine. Conversely, the patient who vomits or uses laxatives may show evidence of hypokalemia, which often is very severe in those who use both methods of weight control. Nutrient values, including levels of zinc, calcium, magnesium, copper, vitamin B_{12}, and folate, all may be altered in the malnourished patient; amylase levels and urinary pH may be elevated in some patients who have bulimia.[3]

Hormonal testing may produce evidence of dysfunction in endocrine systems.[19] The development of hypothyroidism, believed to be an adaptive response to inadequate nutrition, generally is evident in low-normal levels of triiodothyronine (T_3), thyronine (T_4), and thyroid-stimulating hormone (TSH). Amenorrhea, a hallmark of the disorder, generally develops when the patient's weight reaches approximately 15% below IBW but may be seen earlier; it is accompanied by low levels of luteinizing hormone (LH) and follicle-stimulating hormone (FSH). Loss of the diurnal variation in cortisol production and abnormalities in antidiuretic hormone may be noted as well, although these tests need not be performed in most patients. Evidence of abnormalities may be found on computed tomography (CT) scans of the brain or echocardiograms, but these tests generally are reserved for evaluating other possible causes when the diagnosis is in question. In general, the initial laboratory workup of eating disorders consists of a complete blood count, urinalysis, and ECG, as well as evaluation of serum electrolytes, liver function, thyroid function, and levels of LH and FSH in patients who have amenorrhea. This battery of tests generally is sufficient to provide a barometer of current status, a baseline to follow further changes, and screening for other possible causes of weight loss.

Recent data have demonstrated that patients who have eating disorders, especially those whose amenorrhea is prolonged secondary to malnutrition, show evidence of osteopenia on bone density studies.[16] Initial studies have shown that this effect may not be preventable, even with calcium supplementation or hormonal replacement, or completely reversible, even after the patient regains her normal weight.[4] Concern is growing, therefore, that patients who have eating disorders may be at significant risk for developing osteoporosis and fractures later in life. Studies are under way to determine whether the osteopenia is due solely to low levels of estrogen or also to the effects of increased cortisol production and whether hormonal replacement in fact might be able to lessen the development of this complication.[1] It now is recommended that patients whose amenorrhea is prolonged be studied for osteopenia when specialized radiological equipment is available and that hormonal replacement be used when osteopenia is expected or found.[7]

DIFFERENTIAL DIAGNOSIS

The differential diagnosis of the eating disorders includes possible medical causes of weight loss or vomiting and other psychiatric causes of poor appetite. The history, physical examination, and baseline laboratory tests should help rule out infectious, inflammatory, neoplastic, or endocrine disease; further testing may be necessary if the weight loss or vomiting cannot be explained adequately by the medical history from the patient and family. A CT scan, gastrointestinal (GI) series, or other tests may be considered in rare cases for patients who claim to be eating well or not vomiting on purpose. Case reports abound with instances of hypothalamic tumors, inflammatory bowel disease, mesenteric artery syndrome, or GI tract tumors being mistakenly diagnosed as eating disorders in patients whose weight loss or vomiting was not understood adequately. Occasionally a patient may show obvious pleasure in the weight loss or vomiting brought on by another disorder, but this must not be confused with a positive diagnosis of anorexia or bulimia nervosa.

Psychiatric causes of weight loss can include depression and psychosis (especially schizophrenia). The patient who refuses to eat because of a desire to lose weight must be differentiated from the patient who cannot eat because of depression or the patient who will not eat because of delusional fears (e.g., that the food is poisoned). Although patients may have concomitant depression or psychosis with anorexia or bulimia nervosa, separate criteria must be used to establish each entity. A full psychosocial history must be obtained as part of the initial evaluation to establish both the diagnosis and the psychosocial severity of the disorder. The patient's functioning in the family, in school, and among peers must be determined, and possible psychiatric symptoms such as sleep disorders, hallucinations, delusions, or obsessions should be elicited. It is the rare patient who has an eating disorder who does not exhibit psychosocial changes with the onset of the illness. These generally include fighting with the family, withdrawing from friends, and performing less optimally in school. If additional psychiatric symptoms are found, the possibility of an additional diagnosis should be pursued.

The results of the initial medical and psychiatric evaluation play a major role in establishing a treatment protocol for the patient.[17] Although most patients who have an eating disorder may be treated as outpatients, those whose medical findings are significant (including severe malnutrition, electrolyte disturbance, or vital sign abnormalities) require hospitalization. Patients who fail to gain weight with outpatient treatment, whose vomiting is extreme, or whose psychiatric condition is out of control also may require hospitalization. These hospitalizations may be a short term stay in an adolescent medicine unit or a long term stay in a psychiatric unit.[20] Treatment approaches, both inpatient and outpatient, are aimed at restoring more normal physical and psychological functioning.

TREATMENT

Most clinicians consider patients who have an eating disorder as some of the most difficult and frustrating patients to treat. Undoubtedly, several factors are responsible for this perception. The combination of medical and psychological care required makes it difficult for any single professional to be proficient in all aspects of a patient's care. If the patient is hostile to the physician (e.g., often chooses to ignore suggestions and tests how much she can "get away with"), the physician may find himself or herself in an uncomfortable and adversarial relationship with the patient. The difficult families within which many of these patients live often make it a challenge to establish the most rational treatment plans. For these reasons it is advisable that no single individual be responsible totally for any patient's care beyond the initial evaluation or for the most straightforward of cases.[24] Rather, a team approach should be used. The team may consist of a primary care physician, a psychiatrist, a psychologist, a social worker, and a nutritionist, with the exact combination determined by local availability and preference. Generally, each team member manages specific aspects of care, and team meetings and discussions are held frequently to avoid miscommunication that can sabotage the treatment plan. One team member serves as spokesperson to the patient and, especially, the family.

The treatment team may use several modalities, including nutritional rehabilitation, behavior therapy, individual psychotherapy, family and group therapy, and psychopharmacology. It generally is acknowledged that a "multimodality therapy" that includes aspects of each of these approaches holds the best promise for successful treatment.[25] The degree to which each of these approaches is incorporated into the treatment plan varies, both with the preferences of the treatment team and the requirements of the individual patient. Each of these approaches may be used for inpatients *and* outpatients.

NUTRITIONAL REHABILITATION

The malnutrition that accompanies anorexia nervosa is directly responsible for most if not all of the physical abnormalities noted in the disorder and also for some of the mental deterioration. Accordingly, nutritional rehabilitation is crucial in the treatment of the patient who has anorexia nervosa. Restoration of body weight, generally to an end point of within 10% of IBW, should be one of the main goals of treatment. For many patients whose malnutrition is mild to moderate, (15% to 25% below IBW), this may be accomplished on an outpatient basis; patients who have moderate to severe malnutrition (more than 25% below IBW) rarely can accomplish the required weight gain without hospitalization.

Nutritional rehabilitation generally can be achieved through oral feedings; a daily intake of three substantial meals and three to four snacks usually is sufficient to bring about the required weight gain. On inpatient units, meals generally are provided as part of a strict regimen, and snacks generally consist of high-calorie supplements, available as liquids or puddings in various brands and flavors. Care is taken not to overfeed patients whose malnutrition is severe because a too rapid weight gain has been associated with severe metabolic abnormalities in some patients. In the outpatient setting, an appropriate meal pattern may be developed based on the patient's and family's prior eating habits or on a specific dietary plan offered by the physician or a nutritionist. The dietary plan should be specific so that ambiguities that can lead to family fighting are avoided; it should provide approximately 2000 to 3000 calories a day, with up to 1000 calories supplied in the form of high-calorie supplements. The plan should be well balanced and include foods from each of the major food groups. Compliance with the dietary regimen may be evaluated by having the patient keep a diet diary; however, many patients do not always keep these accurately and honestly. Except for the high-calorie supplements, a similar dietary plan may be offered to the normal-weight patient who has bulimia because these patients generally require "nutritional adjustment" rather than nutritional rehabilitation.

BEHAVIOR THERAPY

Merely offering a nutritious diet to a patient who has either anorexia or bulimia nervosa is unlikely to result in a drastic change in the patient's status. For this reason behavioral therapy normally is a necessary component of the treatment plan. The goal of behavioral therapy in the treatment of eating disorders is to offer a set of external positive and negative reinforcements to replace those internal sensors that usually control appetite and weight gain but that currently are missing. Behavioral therapy is not intended to be definitive, but rather to accomplish specific goals in the areas of weight and diet stabilization, thus allowing the psychological modalities of treatment to proceed in a more "medically healthy" patient.

Various behavioral approaches may be used. The strict behavioral plans used on some psychiatric units involve removal of all "privileges," including use of the telephone, television, and regular clothing, if a particular weight goal is not achieved each day. A somewhat less strict plan we use on our adolescent unit involves four phases of treatment, with patients moving from one phase to another based on achievement of progressively higher weight goals. Each phase incorporates additional privileges into the patient's daily activities (e.g., mobility on the unit, exercise, meals, snacks, and passes) in such a way that improved weight and eating patterns lead to additional privileges and responsibilities. For patients unable to respond to the positive reinforcements provided by such a phased system, an all-liquid diet, provided by mouth or, more rarely, nasogastric tube, may be substituted. Use of such methods ultimately achieves the necessary weight goals in almost all patients. However, behavioral therapy alone cannot be considered an adequate treatment approach; controlled studies have been unable to distinguish between the effects of the various behavioral approaches.

Applying behavioral principles may be somewhat more difficult when treating patients with anorexia nervosa in the outpatient setting, or patients who have bulimia. For many patients with anorexia nervosa, the usual approaches to behavioral therapy in outpatient settings (e.g., use of monetary or similar rewards) may not be strong enough to overcome the fear of eating. Fear of hospitalization itself may be the sole motivation. Similarly, classic approaches may not be effective for the patient who has bulimia because the symptom of vomiting cannot be readily measured. More sophisticated cognitive-behavioral approaches have been developed, therefore, so that the patient who has bulimia may understand and participate actively in her own behavioral therapy.[8] These approaches make use of diaries and changes in daily patterns to effect change in the bulimic patient.

INDIVIDUAL, FAMILY, AND GROUP THERAPY

Individual psychotherapy remains an essential part of the treatment for most patients who have an eating disorder. Although therapeutic styles differ based on the treatment team and the individual therapist, exploration of underlying psychological features and possible mechanisms for change is appropriate for most patients who have either anorexia or bulimia nervosa. Although several common themes have been noted in many of these patients, including poor self-esteem, family conflicts, difficulties with friends, and fear of sexuality, there obviously is great individual variety in the way these themes are expressed and manifested. For many patients, it is apparent that the eating disorder serves as a defense against other difficult aspects of life; an important secondary gain also may be involved. It generally is acknowledged that psychological change is a necessary precursor to significant improvement in the disordered thinking and behavior exhibited by most patients who have an eating disorder.

Family therapy has become increasingly popular as a treatment method, especially for younger patients, as the major role that family conflicts and problems play in symptom continuation has become more apparent. Family sessions, arranged in varying combinations to include parents and siblings, generally focus on the disordered communication patterns that preceded and presumably contributed to the eating disorder. Resolving specific conflicts arising from the presence of the eating disorder itself also becomes an important area for discussion. It has been found that the course of the eating disorder is much more difficult for adolescent patients whose families are unable or unwilling to make necessary changes in their customary patterns of communication and parenting. It also has been demonstrated that family therapy is particularly important for adolescents who have eating disorders and less so for adults.[21]

Many patients who have eating disorders participate in group therapy during the course of their treatment. For some patients whose anorexia nervosa is mild and for college-age patients who have bulimia, this may be the only approach to therapy used. Groups may be organized in many different ways—some focusing on a psychotherapeutic approach, others concentrating more specifically on behavioral changes. Initial fears that patients who have eating disorders will "learn bad habits" from each other in the group have been outweighed by the apparent benefit most patients derive from group therapy. This is especially true for patients who have had social difficulties during their adolescence.

PSYCHOPHARMACOLOGY

The use of medication to treat eating disorders has a long history of decidedly mixed results. Numerous medications have been tried, from thyroid hormone and insulin in the 1940s and 1950s to phenytoin (Dilantin) and hydroxyzine (Atarax) in the 1960s and 1970s, as attempts were made to improve appetite, increase weight gain, and reverse physiological abnormalities. More recently, pharmacological treatment of the eating disorders has concentrated on psychoactive medications, including antidepressants, lithium, and antipsychotics. Two specific lines of reasoning have guided the use of these medications. In patients who are diagnosed as having an eating disorder along with or as part of another psychiatric diagnosis, medication for the associated diagnosis is offered with the expectation that the eating disorder will improve as other depressive or psychotic symptomatology is relieved. Alternately, more recent evidence has demonstrated that use of psychoactive drugs, especially the antidepressants (including tricyclics antidepressants, monoamine oxidase inhibitors [MAOIs], and the newer serotonergic medications), diminish the urge to binge and vomit in patients who have bulimia.[23] Although earlier studies failed to show definitive benefits from the use of medication in the eating disorders, recent studies have delineated subgroups of patients most likely to improve with their use.[23] Antidepressants are being used increasingly in the management of the eating disorders; however, only those very familiar with their use should consider including these medications as part of the treatment.

OUTCOME AND PROGNOSIS

Eating disorders must be looked on as a chronic illness, similar to other medical or psychiatric chronic illnesses. A wide range of outcomes can be expected.[14] Some patients improve rapidly with treatment, return to functioning normally, and show no evidence of eating disorder behavior on long-term follow-up. Other patients improve more slowly, showing partial or complete resolution of symptoms but having relapses during periods of stress. Yet others do poorly for a long time, retaining the symptoms of their anorexia nervosa or bulimia for many years and sometimes alternating between the two. Although many different approaches are used to evaluate outcome, it is estimated that approximately 25% of patients do well in the long term, 50% show varying degrees of improvement, and 25% do poorly despite adequate treatment. Patients who are younger, as well as those whose forms of the disease are milder, appear to have a better prognosis than these general numbers indicate.

Numerous personal, family, and treatment factors have been considered for their significance in predicting the course of an eating disorder. Several factors have been found to be associated with the prognosis, yet none of these may be predictive for an individual patient. For instance, a poorer outcome in anorexia nervosa has been associated with factors such as older age, vomiting, and premorbid personality problems, yet any particular patient who has this constellation of findings still may do well with treatment. Furthermore, no specific treatment has been shown by controlled studies to be more effective than others, in general or for any particular type of patient. Thus the eating disorders remain a complicated, challenging set of disorders for the patient, the family, and the treatment team.

REFERENCES

1. Abrams SA et al: Mineral balance and bone turnover in adolescents with anorexia nervosa, *J Pediatr* 123:326, 1993.
2. American Psychiatric Association: *Diagnostic and statistical manual of mental disorders* (DSM-IV), Washington, DC, 1994, APA Press.
3. Arden MR, Bidow L, Bunnell DW: Alkaline urine is associated with eating disorders, *Am J Dis Child* 145:28, 1991 (letter).
4. Bachrach LK et al: Recovery from osteopenia in adolescent girls with anorexia nervosa, *J Clin Endocrinol Metab* 72:602, 1991.
5. Bunnell DW et al: Subclinical versus formal eating disorders: Differentiating psychological features, *Int J Eat Disord* 9:357, 1990.
6. Connors ME, Morse W: Sexual abuse and eating disorders: a review, *Int J Eat Disord* 13:1, 1993.
7. Emans SJ et al: Estrogen deficiency in adolescents and young adults: impact on bone mineral content and effects of estrogen replacement therapy, *Obstet Gynecol* 76:585, 1990.
8. Fairburn CG et al: Psychotherapy and bulimia nervosa: longer-term effects of interpersonal psychotherapy, behavior therapy, and cognitive behavior therapy, *Arch Gen Psychiatry* 50:419, 1993.
9. Feighner JP et al: Diagnostic criteria for use in psychiatric research, *Arch Gen Psychiatry* 26:57, 1972.
10. Fisher M: Medical complications of anorexia and bulimia nervosa, *Adolescent Medicine: State of the Art Reviews*, 3:487, 1992.
11. Fisher M et al: Eating attitudes, health-risk behaviors, self-esteem and anxiety among adolescent females in a suburban high school, *J Adolesc Health* 12:377, 1991.
12. Garner DM: Pathogenesis of anorexia nervosa, *Lancet* 341:1631, 1993.
13. Halmi KA et al: Comorbidity of psychiatric diagnoses in anorexia nervosa, *Arch Gen Psychiatry* 48:712, 1991.
14. Herzog DB, Keller MB, Lavori PN: Outcome in anorexia nervosa and bulimia nervosa, *J Nerv Ment Dis* 176:131, 1988.
15. Johnson CL, Sansone RA, Chewning M: Good reasons why young women would develop anorexia nervosa: the adoptive context, *Pediatr Ann* 21:731, 1992.
16. Kreipe R, Forbes GB: Osteoporosis: a "new morbidity" for dieting female adolescents? *Pediatrics* 86:478, 1990.
17. Kreipe RE, Uphoff M: Treatment and outcome of adolescents with anorexia nervosa, *Adolescent Medicine: State of the Art Reviews* 3:519, 1992.
18. Lucas AR et al: Fifty-year trends in the incidence of anorexia nervosa in Rochester, Minnesota: a population-based study, *Am J Psychiatry* 148:917, 1991.
19. Newman MW, Halmi KA: The endocrinology of anorexia nervosa and bulimia nervosa, *Neurol Clin* 6:195, 1988.
20. Nussbaum M et al: Follow-up investigation in patients with anorexia nervosa, *J Pediatr* 106:835, 1985.
21. Russell GFM et al: An evaluation of family therapy in anorexia nervosa and bulimia nervosa, *Arch Gen Psychiatry* 44:1047, 1987.
22. Stein DM: The prevalence of bulimia: a review of the empirical research, *J Nutrition Educ* 23:205, 1991.
23. Walsh BT, Devlin MJ: The pharmacologic treatment of eating disorders, *Psychiatr Clin North Am* 15:149, 1992.
24. Yager J et al: American Psychiatric Association practice guidelines for eating disorders, *Am J Psychiatry* 150:207, 1993.
25. Yates A: Current perspectives on the eating disorders. II. Treatment, outcome, and research directions, *J Am Acad Child Adolesc Psychiatry* 29:1, 1990.

99 Drug, Alcohol, and Tobacco Abuse

Susan M. Coupey and S. Kenneth Schonberg

The use of drugs, or more precisely, the use of substances that alter the state of consciousness, has become nearly a universal rite of passage for American adolescents. Whereas the use of alcohol always has been widespread among youth, the past 3 decades have witnessed a dramatic rise in the amount and types of other substances abused by teenagers and young adults. Opiates, barbiturates, cocaine, hallucinogens, amphetamines, inhalants, anabolic steroids, and marijuana all have become familiar terms to those who provide care for youth. In the early 1990s data from high school students indicated a slight decrease in drug use; however, use by preadolescents has been increasing over the past several years.

The pattern of substance use by adolescents is continually evolving. New drugs, new fads, and new epidemics have been an invariable feature of substance abuse. The late 1960s and early 1970s were marked by a major concern with the abuse of opiates and barbiturates. Addiction, overdose, and medical sequelae from these drugs led to frequent hospitalizations, serious illnesses, and significant mortality. By the mid-1970s the use of these "hard" drugs had declined markedly. A variety of hallucinogens appeared, gained widespread popularity, and subsequently faded from the spotlight as their use lessened; however, hallucinogens remained readily available. Among these agents have been peyote (which contains mescaline), lysergic acid diethylamide (LSD), and phencyclidine (PCP, angel dust).

Over the decade of the 1980s, major attention focused on the use of milder intoxicants—alcohol and marijuana. Although these drugs are less likely to cause serious somatic illness during the teenage years, their widespread use and frequent association with both accidents and behavioral disruption cause the health practitioner concern. In addition, in the latter part of the 1980s, cocaine use and abuse became quite common among both adolescents and adults. The emergence of "crack" (a smokable form of free-base cocaine) as a major public health problem, especially in inner cities, was accompanied by greater public awareness of the addictive and destructive properties of the drug. As the decade of the 1990s began, cocaine use by adolescents declined, but an increase in hallucinogen and anabolic steroid use became apparent.

Traditionally, discussion of drug-related illnesses with teenagers has been approached either by outlining the physiological consequences associated with the abuse of a particular substance or by reviewing the effects of abuse on different organ systems. Such approaches, however, are at variance with the usual way most teenage drug abusers are seen for medical care. The substances now abused most commonly are not associated with frequent illness; therefore teenagers using these agents most often are encountered when they seek routine health maintenance or care for an illness unrelated to drugs. Only through routine questioning is such drug use discovered.

Even the adolescent suffering from a drug-related illness seldom seeks care because of a particular drug habit or the impairment of a specific body organ, but rather because a symptom complex mandates medical attention. In this respect, teenage drug abusers are like other patients: determining the etiological factors and the pathological conditions of their illnesses requires a comprehensive analysis of all possibilities. If drug abuse, of either one or several agents, is not considered along with other possible etiological factors to explain the symptoms, the physician may miss an opportunity for meaningful therapeutic intervention. Therefore, in keeping with the more usual method by which such adolescent patients come to medical attention, drug abuse–related illnesses are discussed as they initially appear to the primary care health professional.

THE MEDICAL HISTORY

Inquiries about the extent of drug involvement should be made to every teenager during a periodic health examination. Such inquiries should be a natural adjunct to the assessment of other psychosocial indicators, including academic progress, sexual behavior, family and peer relationships, and recreational interests. An accurate drug history can be obtained only in an atmosphere of confidentiality and privacy, with parents excluded from the interview. In the proper setting, positive responses should be expected from the majority of teenagers when queried about current or past use of alcohol and cigarettes. Information should be obtained about not only the specific type of drug used, but also the frequency of use, the setting in which use occurs, and the degree of social, educational, and vocational disruption attributable to the drug use behavior. This information is necessary for a proper appraisal of the need for further intervention. Obtaining such information depends largely on the physician's ability to listen to the adolescent without alarm or dismay, to establish an atmosphere of trust, and to direct the interview to obtain the specific information required.

Alcohol and marijuana are the substances used most commonly on a recreational basis by adolescents, and frequently they lead to problems in this age group. Although nearly 90% of adolescents will have tried alcohol and over 33% will have tried marijuana before graduating from high school, a significant percentage of whom report weekly use, teenagers seldom volunteer information on the extent of their substance use unless questioned specifically. The medical complications of chronic alcoholism or marijuana abuse, although severe, usually do not appear until after adolescence. The physician's task is to identify those teenagers who are experiencing psychosocial disruption or who are at greatest risk of becoming alcoholic or substance-abusing adults. The youngster who is doing poorly in school, is having difficulty with peer relationships, or is engaging in delinquent behavior, and who is drinking or smoking marijuana daily or weekly is not difficult to identify as one in need of special attention. In addition, a history of marijuana smoking, alcohol consumption, or the abuse of any drug by an adolescent indicates the need for further exploration into the possibility of underlying psychopathological conditions. Frequently the psychosocial problems that initiate drug-taking are more important than the specific medical complications of abuse.

The teenager who has not experienced academic or social failure but whose substance use goes beyond experimentation or occasional use represents a more difficult problem. Although no specific criteria determine who is at greatest risk of future difficulty, a history of parental alcoholism or other serious family dysfunction or widespread alcohol or marijuana abuse within the teenager's peer group are factors associated with a poor prognosis. Even for youngsters in this high-risk but still high-functioning category, no specific therapy may be indicated beyond the need for periodic reevaluation of the situation. The history of substance use by most teenagers in this category should be noted, quantitated, and used as a reference point by which to evaluate information obtained during subsequent visits.

All teenagers, including the minority who do not drink or use drugs at all, need to be counseled regarding the relationship between intoxicants and accidents. Accidents are by far the leading cause of death among adolescents. The majority of these fatal accidents are automotive, and intoxicants are involved in many if not most. A teenager who will not at some time drive while intoxicated or be a passenger in the automobile of an intoxicated driver is rare. Preventive health care for adolescents and their families must include a discussion of alternatives to such risk-taking behavior.

While the intoxicating effects of alcohol and the importance of its role in causing motor vehicle accidents are well known, the effects of marijuana are understood less widely. Because teenagers and their parents frequently raise questions about the toxicity of marijuana smoking, the physician, for appropriate counseling, should have an understanding of its physiological and behavioral effects. Although sore throats and bronchitis are frequent sequelae to marijuana smoking, the teenager seldom seeks treatment for those complications. Other respiratory effects with more prolonged exposure include bronchodilation with acute inhalation and bronchoconstriction. Thus adolescents who have asthma may experience either relief or exacerbation of symptoms. Allergic reactions to marijuana do occur and may cause asthmatic attacks. A potential long-term pulmonary consequence in the chronic marijuana abuser is carcinoma of the lungs. Bronchial biopsies of marijuana smokers who have clinical diagnoses of chronic bronchitis have revealed lesions characteristic of the early stages of cancer. Cardiovascular effects include both tachycardia and a transient low-grade elevation of systolic and diastolic blood pressure. Neither of these cardiac consequences is of clinical significance. Marijuana has been reported to have a number of effects on the endocrine system in males who have histories of prolonged and frequent use. They include depression of testosterone levels in the blood, diminished sperm counts, impaired sexual function, and gynecomastia. The associated clinical problems of impotence and infertility should respond to abstinence from marijuana. The long-term effects of these endocrine imbalances on the developing adolescent, however, as yet are unclear.

Although marijuana causes electroencephalographic changes and alterations in neurotransmitters, neither structural damage to the brain nor an increase in seizure potential has been demonstrated. In contrast, a number of acute behavioral changes are of clinical significance because of their potential to cause accidents. In addition to euphoria, the marijuana "high" causes a loss of critical judgment, distortions in time perception, impairment of tracking (the ability to follow a moving object accurately), and poor performance on "divided attention" tasks, such as driving. The infrequent correlation between marijuana intoxication and accidents probably is because the users show no specific signs of drug abuse and the authorities lack a quick, convenient method to detect marijuana. Other behavioral effects include impaired short-term memory, interference with learning, and difficulty with oral communication, all of which can affect school performance adversely. Occasionally a physician will encounter a patient who has an acute adverse reaction to marijuana manifested as a toxic psychosis with depression or panic. Both the symptoms and the treatment of these reactions are similar to those noted for hallucinogen abuse. Prolonged (and possibly permanent) personality changes have been reported in long-term marijuana users. This *amotivational syndrome* is marked by lethargy and a lack of goal-directed activity.

Although fewer teenagers use tobacco than alcohol, nearly 30% of high school seniors smoke at least monthly. The long-range cardiac, pulmonary, and carcinogenic consequences of cigarette smoking have been well publicized, and this information has not escaped the teenage population. Although the physician may have little to add in the way of warning to what has already been proffered by the schools and the press, it is negligent not to inquire about the adolescent's smoking habits and offer counsel on those health issues regarding tobacco, which have immediate relevance to the life of the teenager. The adverse effect of smoking on pulmonary function may make an impact on the adolescent who has athletic aspirations. The pregnant teenager concerned with the welfare of her unborn baby may alter her smoking habits when informed of the possible association between tobacco and low birth weight and neonatal mortality. The adolescent girl who is starting to use oral contraceptives may be counseled that although "the pill" does not cause cancer, smoking certainly does, and she may be motivated to give up cigarettes. Adolescents who have a respiratory illness, particularly asthma, must be apprised of the immediate effects of smoking on their day-to-day health. All these issues lend themselves to discussion in the give-and-take atmosphere of the personal history interview.

PHYSICAL EXAMINATION

The teenager who is heavily involved in the abuse of hard drugs is more likely to come to medical attention with a specific illness associated with drug abuse than through a routine physical examination. However, even those adolescents who use less dangerous drugs often have some concern about the potential somatic consequences of their behavior, and they may seek the reassurance of a checkup to prove to themselves that all is well. In such circumstances the teenager may deny a history of drug abuse even when questioned directly so as not to prejudice the results of the examination. The physician must be alert to those physical findings that either are pathognomonic of or associated with illicit substance abuse.

The abuser of either marijuana or the stimulants, cocaine and amphetamines, may have an accelerated pulse rate. Stimulant abuse also is associated with weight loss and may mimic the symptoms of hyperthyroidism. In contrast, anabolic steroid use is associated with a marked weight gain, particularly in muscle mass. Pinpoint pupils unresponsive to light are characteristic of opiate abuse. Barbiturates usually produce sluggish pupillary responses. Conjunctivitis and irritation or ulceration of the nasal mucosa may be found in the teenager abusing drugs by inhalation. Glue "sniffers," marijuana smokers, and "snorters" of heroin or cocaine are likely to manifest these conditions.

Dermatological Manifestations

The majority of the specific physical signs of drug abuse are found on the skin and are associated with the subcutaneous or intravenous abuse of opiates, cocaine, anabolic steroids, and less commonly, barbiturates. Subcutaneous fat necrosis, similar to that experienced by persons who have diabetes and receive insulin injections, is common in teenagers who inject heroin under their skin ("skin popping"). Cutaneous scars ("tracks") following the course of superficial veins are found in teenagers who have a prolonged history of injecting drugs intravenously ("mainlining"). They are caused by chronic inflammation associated with repeated injections or by the deposition of carbonaceous material from needles that were "flamed" briefly in an attempt at sterilization. The teenager frequently disguises these tracks by covering them with a self-administered tattoo applied with a needle and india ink. Any tattoo placed by an amateur or professional and found in the antecubital fossa should be examined closely for tracks or needle marks. Plastic surgery for the removal of tracks and tattoos should be suggested to the patient because these stigmata often interfere with later employability and thereby compromise rehabilitative efforts.

Both the intravenous and subcutaneous routes of drug administration are characterized by a lack of sterile technique. Skin abscesses and cellulitis are common among teenage addicts. When these conditions come to medical attention, drug abuse should be considered a possible cause. The presence of needle marks confirms drug abuse as an etiological factor. Localized pain is the most frequent symptom of skin abscesses, with *Staphylococcus aureus* being the most common causative organism. Fever and leukocytosis are relatively uncommon, and regional adenopathy may or may not be present. Treatment involves incision and drainage and the administration of an appropriate antibiotic as determined by isolation of the causative organism by culture. Skin abscesses and superficial skin ulcers are potential sites for the growth of *Clostridium* organisms, and tetanus has been reported in adult heroin addicts. A similar incidence of tetanus in teenagers has not been encountered, probably because of residual protection from childhood immunizations; nevertheless, the administration of a tetanus toxoid booster should be considered. Superficial thrombophlebitis, particularly of the upper extremities, is common among intravenous opiate-abusing teenagers and is a cause of both localized symptoms and systemic infection. Treatment includes local soaks and systemic antibiotic therapy. Anticoagulation is not a necessary part of the treatment for superficial thrombophlebitis.

Serious Systemic Infections and Opportunistic Infections

In the course of evaluating the teenager who has a systemic infection or a fever of unknown origin, the physician should remember that intravenous drug abuse may be an etiological factor in the development of the infectious process. The direct injection of bacteria or viruses into the bloodstream during intravenous drug administration or septic embolization from a site of superficial thrombophlebitis will give rise to the hematogenous dissemination of infectious agents to the heart, brain, osseous structures, and, less commonly, other organs.

Human immunodeficiency virus (HIV) is the most serious of such infections transmitted by contaminated injection apparatus. Because of the prolonged asymptomatic period associated with this virus, clinical illness is not expressed often during the teenage years. However, an adolescent who has a history of injecting any illicit drug, including opiates, cocaine, amphetamines, or anabolic steroids, should be offered counseling and testing for HIV. Adolescents who have an unexplained weight loss, night sweats, generalized lymphadenopathy, oral thrush, recurrent bacterial infections, severe prolonged diarrhea, tuberculosis, or *Pneumocystis carinii* pneumonia should have HIV-related illness considered in the differential diagnosis. Teenagers who are HIV-positive and asymptomatic should have their immune function assessed initially and at least twice per year thereafter. Antiretroviral treatment and prophylaxis for opportunistic infections then can be instituted according to current guidelines on the basis of significantly decreased immunocompetence. Because HIV is transmitted sexually as well as by contaminated needles, adolescent girls who are not themselves drug users but whose sexual partners use drugs intravenously require counseling and testing for HIV infection.

Endocarditis in the intravenous drug abuser may affect either the right or left side of the heart. Beyond fever and occasional pulmonary symptoms, right-sided endocarditis is associated with few if any systemic signs and almost always affects a previously undamaged tricuspid valve. *S. aureus* frequently is the causative organism. Left-sided endocarditis may involve either normal or abnormal mitral or aortic valves and usually is associated with systemic evidence of infection. *S. aureus* and streptococcal species are the organisms encountered most frequently, and fungal infections with *Candida* organisms also have been reported. The teenager who has endocarditis must be hospitalized and treated with intravenous antibiotics as determined by the isolation of the causative organism.

Central nervous system (CNS) infection may be associated with endocarditis or may be a primary manifestation of drug abuse-related septicemia. Brain abscess is rare during adolescence, so, when present, intravenous drug abuse should be suspected. Multiple microabscesses are found more frequently than a single large abscess; thus focal neurological signs may be absent. Because the only manifestation of multiple microabscesses of the brain may be fever or a personality change, lumbar puncture, electroencephalography, transaxial computed tomography, and magnetic resonance imaging may be required to reach the correct diagnosis. *S. aureus* is found most often to be the causative organism. The same organism has been associated with the increased frequency of osteomyelitis among intravenous drug abusers. The treatment and prognosis for CNS infection and osteomyelitis are the same for the user and the nonuser of drugs.

The intravenous injection of starch and talc, used as fillers for medicinal preparations designed solely for oral use, may lead to pulmonary angiothrombosis and granulomatosis. Although pulmonary hypertension and cor pulmonale eventually can result from this process, for these problems to become clinically apparent during adolescence is unusual. Nevertheless, the evaluation of teenagers manifesting unexplained compromise to respiratory function should include the consideration of intravenous drug abuse; thus chest roentgenograms, blood cultures, and tuberculin skin testing should be performed.

Sexually Transmitted Diseases (STDs) and Other Urological and Gynecological Manifestations

Because of the life-style often adopted by adolescents who use drugs frequently, STDs are common in this population and may be the reason they seek medical care. Syphilis can be acquired both sexually and through contaminated needles; therefore a serological test for syphilis always should be obtained, keeping in mind that false positive results are common in heroin users. Gonococcal and nongonococcal urethritis, cervicitis, salpingitis, proctitis, and pharyngitis often are diagnosed in adolescents who abuse a variety of illicit substances. The signs, symptoms, and treatment of these conditions are the same as for patients who do not abuse drugs.

HIV infection transmitted sexually has been noted in adolescents who abuse drugs other than by the intravenous route. Both male and female adolescent "crack" abusers are at particular risk for sexually acquired HIV infection because of the practice of trading sex for drugs. The highly addictive nature and short duration of the crack "high" encourage drug binges that often include frequent acts of sexual intercourse with multiple partners. This has resulted in an increased prevalence among crack abusers of many sexually transmitted diseases, including syphilis and HIV-related illness.

Amenorrhea occurs frequently in teenage girls who are opiate addicts. Because amenorrhea is associated with anovulation, these girls experience no increase in pregnancies despite their often increased sexual activity. Ovulation, menses, and fertility usually return to normal within a few months of cessation of opiate use; thus contraceptive counseling and prescription must be part of rehabilitation.

Unfortunately, no such protection from pregnancy occurs in girls who abuse cocaine and crack. Cocaine use during pregnancy is associated with an increased incidence of spontaneous abortion, abruptio placentae, intrauterine growth retardation, premature delivery, and irritability in newborns. Contraceptive management is particularly important for these girls during the period of assessment and treatment for their drug abuse.

Anabolic steroid use is associated with testicular atrophy, lowered sperm count, gynecomastia, and accelerated male pattern baldness in males and with menstrual irregularities, lowered voice pitch, clitoral hypertrophy, and hirsuitism in females. Both sexes experience increased libido as a result of steroid abuse.

Abdominal Pain

Many physiological and psychosomatic illnesses produce abdominal pain in teenagers. Among them are a variety of illicit drug-related conditions. Severe abdominal pain, anorexia, vomiting, and gastrointestinal hemorrhage may accompany a large and acute ingestion of alcohol. Although the chronic medical complications of alcoholism, such as cirrhosis, are not found in teenagers, acute gastritis and acute pancreatitis may accompany the consumption of a large quantity of alcohol. The pain of acute gastritis usually will subside with the administration of antacids alone. However, persistent pain or bleeding requires therapy with medications that suppress acid secretion, such as ranitidine or omeprazole. Specific diagnostic studies to determine the origin of the hemorrhage may be indicated. In addition to severe abdominal pain and profuse vomiting, acute pancreatitis usually is accompanied by elevation of serum amylase and lipase levels. An increased incidence of peptic ulcer disease has been reported in adult opiate addicts, although no such increase has been noted in adolescents.

If ulcer disease or any other cause of acute abdominal pain does occur, the addict may attribute the discomfort falsely to withdrawal symptoms and quickly administer opiates as a form of self-treatment. Having thus masked the symptoms of possible intraabdominal pathological findings, the opiate-addicted teenager may not seek medical attention until gastric perforation has occurred. Similarly, the physician faced with a patient experiencing opiate withdrawal must be cautious not to overlook other serious illness by attributing all of the patient's symptoms to the abstinence syndrome.

Constipation almost is universal among opiate abusers and, at the extreme, causes symptoms of intestinal obstruction. Hemorrhoids, otherwise uncommon during adolescence, may result and cause rectal bleeding. Constipation responds rapidly to interruption of opiate abuse. Although constipation is one of the more benign complaints, it represents the most common complaint of the young methadone-maintained patient. In most instances the drug-abusing teenager who has abdominal pain should be hospitalized for evaluation because close observation and testing are required to reach a definitive diagnosis.

Jaundice

In evaluating the teenager who has jaundice, the physician must consider the possibility of drug abuse as an etiological factor. Acute viral hepatitis is common among intravenous opiate abusers. Although primarily associated with the mainlining of heroin, hepatitis also has been reported in intravenous abusers of other substances, including cocaine, amphetamines, and anabolic steroids. In addition, the hepatitis virus can be transmitted by saliva and semen, and cases have been attributed to the sharing of marijuana joints. The inhalation of cleaning fluid fumes, an abuse practiced most often by younger adolescents and preadolescents, can cause acute toxic hepatitis. Anabolic steroid users can develop cholestatic hepatitis along with jaundice, hepatic cysts, and benign and malignant hepatic tumors.

The symptoms, signs, and serological abnormalities found

in patients who use drugs do not differ from those of non-drug users who have acute hepatitis. These include right upper quadrant tenderness, anorexia, nausea, jaundice, and hepatomegaly. Elevations of the serum transaminases and hyperbilirubinemia are expected, whereas hepatitis B surface antigen is present in over 25% of patients. The assessment of a jaundiced teenager who has acute hepatitis should include measurement of the prothrombin time because prolongation may indicate impending hepatic encephalopathy. Transaminase elevations are of little value in predicting this untoward development. Other indications of early hepatic encephalopathy are changes in sensorium and behavior. In the drug-using teenager, belligerence and lack of cooperation often are attributed incorrectly to drug withdrawal or an underlying personality disturbance rather than to hepatic encephalopathy. This error in judgment may lead to inappropriate treatment with sedatives; the administration of sedatives to patients in acute hepatic failure can precipitate coma.

Dehydration or evidence of impending hepatic encephalopathy is an indication for hospitalization in any patient, but particularly for the drug-abusing teenager who has hepatitis, because noncompliance and lack of supportive care at home are more likely. Hepatitis B immunization should be offered to adolescent drug abusers who are antibody negative and who are at high risk for infection by either the intravenous or sexual route.

LABORATORY TESTING

The teenager who is well clinically occasionally will have abnormal findings on laboratory tests that raise suspicion of covert drug use. Although neither anemia nor total peripheral white blood cell count abnormalities are associated with substance abuse, peripheral eosinophilia may be found in up to one third of heroin users. The cause of eosinophilia in heroin users is unknown. Users of anabolic steroids often will show elevated serum concentrations of low-density lipoprotein cholesterol and reduced levels of high-density lipoprotein cholesterol. These adolescents are at increased risk for accelerated atherosclerosis. The routine urinalysis yields no findings specific to drug abuse, with the rare exception of mild proteinuria associated with serum glutamic-pyruvic transaminase elevations, which may be present in heroin-abusing adolescents. These patients show evidence of focal glomerulonephritis when evaluated using renal biopsy. A false positive serological test for syphilis may be found in approximately 10% of heroin abusers. Although these false positive test results may occur for any teenager who has active liver disease, they have been observed for heroin abusers who have no evidence of hepatic dysfunction.

Liver function is not usually assessed as a part of the usual laboratory evaluation in teenagers; however, it represents the most fruitful method of screening for unsuspected opiate abuse because the liver is the best source for abnormal chemical findings in the known heroin abuser. Nearly 40% of clinically well adolescents who have a history of heroin abuse have serum elevations of glutamic-pyruvic transaminase and glutamic-oxaloacetic transaminase. Other indicators of hepatic function, including serum bilirubin and alkaline phosphatase levels, usually are normal. The transaminase abnormalities may persist for months or years after heroin abuse has been interrupted and are not associated with signs or symptoms of hepatic dysfunction. Liver biopsies performed on adolescents who have enzyme abnormalities documented over 4 months or longer have revealed histological evidence of chronic persistent hepatitis.

Technological advances have made it possible to detect specific drugs of abuse in body fluids. However, the appropriate use of this testing ability has become an issue of some controversy, especially with regard to teenagers (see Chapter 20, Part Seven, Screening for Drugs). Routine urine screening for drugs of abuse such as marijuana or cocaine of all adolescent patients without their knowledge and without clinical indicators of substance abuse is not advocated by most thoughtful authorities. Under such conditions, with an expected low prevalence of actual use, many false positive tests would result, leading to potentially harmful confrontations with adolescents who are not abusing drugs. In addition, only recent drug use would be detected, and no information about patterns and frequency of use or degrees of impairment would be obtained. However, urine drug testing may be a helpful adjunct to the treatment and rehabilitation of adolescents who are known to be drug abusers. Indeed, many drug treatment programs use random urine toxicological testing, with the knowledge and consent of the patient, as an early warning system for relapse and as an additional way of helping the adolescent to abstain from drugs. Blood and urine toxicological testing for illicit substances also can help in the assessment of an acutely ill adolescent whose mental status is altered and who is unable to give a history because of coma or psychotic behavior.

CHANGES IN SENSORIUM: INTOXICATION, ACUTE PSYCHOSIS, LETHARGY, AND COMA

The teenager who apparently is intoxicated or is disoriented, lethargic, or comatose represents a complex diagnostic and therapeutic problem. Even when head trauma, diabetic acidosis, hypoglycemia, encephalitis, and other causes of coma and confusion can be excluded and the diagnosis of intoxication is clear, the specific causative drug must be determined. Information from the patient, the family, or friends may provide a ready answer, but such information may be unavailable or unreliable. Serum and urine toxicological screening can be extremely helpful in such a situation. An attempt must always be made to determine the reason for the intoxication. Was it accidental or deliberate? If the patient is suicidal, the physician must offer appropriate protection, assessment, and treatment.

Although the overwhelming majority of mild intoxications never come to medical attention, sometimes a youngster will be brought for care for being "high." A wide variety of substances are capable of producing a high, including inhaled fumes from airplane glue or cleaning fluid, marijuana, alcohol, and cocaine. Teenagers who exhibit euphoria or minimal disorientation require only protection against self-injury. At an appropriate time after the sensorium has cleared, inquiries should be made as to the nature, frequency, and pattern of episodes of intoxication to determine the need, if any, for further psychosocial intervention.

Teenagers who have severe alcohol intoxication usually can be distinguished by their ethanolic breath and, except in instances of extremely large or mixed ingestions, are not at serious physiological risk. Treatment need only be supportive, with protection provided against the aspiration of vomitus and observation for the development of respiratory depression, hypoglycemia, or the gastrointestinal complications of a large alcohol ingestion. Even when the teenager is not at risk, a brief hospitalization while sobriety is regained may be preferable to immediate discharge to the care of distraught parents.

The adolescent who comes for medical attention as a result of an acute psychosis may be suffering from a hallucinogen ingestion or "bad trip." A wide variety of compounds are capable of producing hallucinations, including LSD, peyote, PCP, and occasionally marijuana or hashish. Hallucinations may recur weeks or months after the ingestion of a hallucinogen as part of a "flashback" phenomenon. In addition, large doses of amphetamines or cocaine may precipitate a psychotic state marked by paranoia and aggression. A similar psychotic episode may follow abrupt cessation of amphetamine abuse. Along with the hallucinations that, in contrast to the auditory hallucinations of schizophrenia, almost always are visual, the teenager who has ingested one of the previously mentioned drugs often has dilated pupils, hyperreflexia, hyperthermia, and tachycardia. Identification of the specific abused hallucinogen is difficult. Even when the substance is known, the adolescent seldom has accurate knowledge of its exact composition because the compounds frequently are adulterated and misrepresented by the seller. Detection of the presence of PCP, tetrahydrocannabinol, or cocaine in the patient's blood or urine can help in the prognosis of acute psychosis.

Regardless of the hallucinogen abused, treatment is nonspecific and directed at allaying anxiety and protecting the patient from injury to self or others. The teenager should be placed in a quiet, nonthreatening environment. Verbal contact should be established and maintained, with frequent reassurance that the hallucinogenic experience is temporary and drug related. If at all possible, physical restraints should be avoided because they are certain to increase anxiety and panic in the already frightened adolescent.

Sedatives should be administered only if verbal contact does not control behavior successfully or cannot be maintained because of limitations of time and staff. Any sedation administered will compromise sensorium further and may thereby increase the severity of hallucinations. All the most commonly used sedative medications carry additional risks. The administration of phenothiazines is potentially dangerous because hallucinogens often are adulterated with anticholinergics, and this combination of drugs may precipitate circulatory collapse. However, small doses of benzodiazepine may help to allay anxiety. Haloperidol in a dose of 2 to 5 mg may be administered intramuscularly to control the agitation of an acute drug-related psychosis. This dose may be repeated as soon as 1 hour later if severe symptoms persist or recur.

PCP is among the most toxic of the hallucinogenic agents. Toxic reactions, which may be indistinguishable from schizophrenia and include elements of paranoia, agitation, or catatonia, may last for days and, in rare cases, weeks. With high-dose ingestions, convulsions, opisthotonos, coma, and, very rarely, apnea may ensue. Treatment of overdose reactions includes (1) anticonvulsants for seizures, (2) support of respiration, and (3) enhancement of drug excretion by gastric lavage with half normal saline, the administration of furosemide, and the acidification of the urine by administering ammonium chloride or ascorbic acid.

In most instances teenagers who have an acute drug-related psychosis should be hospitalized. These adolescents may have brief periods of lucidity and then relapse into hallucinations. It is difficult to determine with certainty if the teenager has recovered fully without having an opportunity to observe behavior over at least a few hours. In addition, there always is a question of whether the drug ingestion unmasked a preexistent psychosis or simply precipitated psychotic behavior in an otherwise healthy individual. The answer to that question is gained best through an opportunity to observe and evaluate the adolescent during hospitalization.

The adolescent who has had an opiate or barbiturate overdose will have respiratory depression and constricted or sluggish pupils and be lethargic or comatose. In patients who have respiratory depression precipitated by an unknown agent, the use of naloxone has both diagnostic and therapeutic potential. Although it is of no therapeutic benefit in the teenager who has had a sedative overdose, it is free of the effects of respiratory depression common to other narcotic antagonists and therefore can be used without fear of accentuating respiratory compromise in the nonopiate intoxication. Naloxone also is useful in treating propoxyphene ingestions. Failure of the teenager to respond to naloxone given intravenously indicates that the symptoms are not due to an opiate. Pupillary dilation, an improved level of consciousness, and an increase in the respiratory rate in response to the administration of naloxone strongly suggest that an opiate produced the syndrome. The presence of clinical signs of intravenous drug use supports the diagnosis of opiate overdose. Pulmonary edema and hypoxemia may occur in the teenager who has had an opiate overdose who then requires intubation, assisted ventilation, and administration of oxygen under positive pressure. Even the adolescent who responds dramatically to naloxone alone will require hospitalization for continued observation and continuous naloxone infusion. A relapse with respiratory depression may occur if the infusion is discontinued too early. This is a particular hazard in the patient who has had a methadone overdose because its duration of action is between 24 and 48 hours.

As noted previously, the teenager who has become intoxicated on a sedative displays clinical characteristics similar to those of one who has overdosed on an opiate. The patient who has overdosed on a barbiturate has pinpoint or slowly reactive pupils unresponsive to naloxone, whereas the adolescent who has a glutethimide overdose exhibits widely dilated pupils. In either case, treatment is supportive. The respiratory rate and arterial blood gases must be monitored and mechanical ventilation instituted at the first sign of ventilatory failure. Intravenous fluids should be administered to ensure a high urine output. Analeptics have no role in the treatment of sedative overdose, and although hemodialysis may be effective, it seldom is necessary because the supportive measures described usually are adequate.

Hospitalization for observation almost always is indicated for the teenager who has a drug intoxication, although emergency room treatment may negate all immediate medical risks. Even in those instances in which self-destruction was not a motivation, an overdose may signal the loss of the adolescent's ability to control his or her drug-abuse behavior. The teenager should not be released from care until a concerted effort has been made to minimize future risk.

ABSTINENCE SYNDROMES

The opiate- or barbiturate-addicted teenager who is hospitalized involuntarily requires treatment to prevent the discomfort and danger inherent in a withdrawal syndrome. At times drug withdrawal is not imposed on the adolescent; rather, some life crises provides the motivation for voluntary detoxification. In either case, adolescents often are ambivalent regarding their abstinence and require careful, meticulous attention to their symptoms lest they become disruptive in the hospital or interrupt the attempts to free them from addiction.

A teenager must abuse opiates daily for weeks to months before the risk of suffering an opiate withdrawal syndrome develops. Within 12 hours after the last dose of heroin and 36 hours after the last dose of methadone, the addicted adolescent begins experiencing a progression of symptoms, including yawning, "gooseflesh," lacrimation, restlessness, dilated pupils, muscle cramps, diarrhea, and tachycardia. Insomnia may be severe during the first week of withdrawal and may persist to some degree for up to a month after abstinence from drugs.

Most teenagers who report less than daily heroin use are not physiologically addicted but rather are psychologically habituated. Nevertheless, they are quite fearful of becoming ill if their opiate supply is interrupted. Most often, these teenagers require no specific therapy beyond reassurance that relief for discomfort will be offered if symptoms appear. The adolescent who manifests symptoms and signs of opiate abstinence can be treated in a variety of ways. Methadone may be offered in a dosage of approximately 40 mg/day orally and then withdrawn slowly at a rate of 5 mg every 1 or 2 days over the course of 1 to 2 weeks. An alternative therapy is to administer 10 mg of diazepam every 4 to 6 hours. This medication may be given intramuscularly or by mouth. Better results can be anticipated if the intramuscular route is used at least initially because the adolescent addict has greater faith in the efficacy of needle-administered drugs.

Diazepam relieves most symptoms, except diarrhea and insomnia. Persistent or severe diarrhea can be treated with diphenoxylate hydrochloride. No satisfactory treatment for the insomnia associated with opiate withdrawal is available, and addiction-prone adolescents must be cautioned against self-medication with barbiturates in their search for sleep. Diazepam needs to be continued for 4 to 7 days after the last dose of opiate, the longer treatment being reserved for methadone addiction and the shorter course for heroin addiction.

Methadone maintenance treatment programs may be appropriate for the older, opiate-addicted teenager. This treatment modality substitutes a synthetic opiate, methadone, for the abused opiate. A single daily oral dose of methadone can both prevent opiate craving and block the euphoric effect of subsequently administered heroin. With interruption of the need to obtain illegal opiates, the adolescent now is free to take advantage of support services and make an effort toward restructuring his or her life. Therapy is aimed toward eventually withdrawing methadone treatment and preparing the patient for a drug-free existence. Unfortunately, although many adolescents do well while remaining in treatment, evidence to date indicates a high incidence of subsequent drug abuse and significant morbidity and mortality after discharge from these programs.

Unlike opiate-addicted adolescents, barbiturate addicts are at grave risk of a life-threatening withdrawal syndrome if their sedative dosage is discontinued abruptly. They become restless, develop postural hypotension, and have seizures in rapid succession, usually within 36 hours of their last dose. Occasionally a teenager may not come for medical attention until after a seizure has occurred and then may require large doses of anticonvulsants. The teenager who seeks medical attention for voluntary detoxification before seizures have occurred should be offered phenobarbital as a substitute for the abused sedative; an initial dose comparable to the barbiturate dose to which the patient is addicted should be used. This should be divided into four equal parts, with each given every 6 hours. The daily dosage then should be reduced slowly at a rate of 120 mg/day to zero. Because this method of detoxification relies on the accuracy of the original estimate by the addict of daily abuse, it is extremely difficult to judge accurately the appropriate initial dose of phenobarbital to be given. If too much medication is offered, the teenager is at risk of iatrogenically induced barbiturate overdose and coma. If too little phenobarbital is given, convulsions may ensue. To be confident that an adequate dose has been administered, it often is necessary to induce mild barbiturate toxicity, which is accompanied by nystagmus, ataxia, and dysarthria, but which stops short of respiratory depression and coma. Treatment within this narrow therapeutic range requires careful observation of the adolescent, particularly during the first few days. Because an excessive initial dose of phenobarbital may cause the teenager to become somnolent during the initial stages of treatment, a concomitant interruption of oral intake may develop. Therefore intravenous fluids should be administered routinely and the patient's fluid intake and output monitored carefully.

The high incidence of convulsions during barbiturate withdrawal and the need for frequent reevaluation and adjustment of therapy mandate in-hospital treatment of this abstinence syndrome. In many instances the guidance of a neurologist or a physician who has expertise in addictive illnesses may be necessary. The opiate abstinence syndrome can be managed on either an ambulatory or an inpatient basis. In general, greater success can be anticipated with hospitalization because this physically separates the addicted teenager from a supply of illicit opiates and provides him or her continual support and reassurance.

Stimulants such as cocaine and amphetamines are not associated with a dramatic or life-threatening withdrawal syndrome. Nevertheless, they are considered physically addictive because of the biochemical changes in the brain, induced by these drugs, that lead to the intense cravings and compulsive drug abuse behavior noted in both animal and human studies. A stimulant-abstinence syndrome has been described that follows a three-phase pattern. An initial crash after a drug-taking binge is characterized by a craving for sleep, often leading to the use of opiates, alcohol, or benzodiazepines.

After 1 to 3 days of hypersomnolence, the stimulant abuser begins to experience an increasing intensity of withdrawal symptoms, including anergia, anhedonia, limited interest in the environment, and marked drug cravings. If abstinence is sustained for 6 to 18 weeks, the anhedonia, fatigue, and dysphoric mood usually improve. In the final extinction phase of abstinence, brief episodes of drug cravings recur with gradually diminishing frequency, often provoked by circumstances or objects that cue conditioned memories of drug euphoria. Treatment for adolescent stimulant abusers is best conducted within a highly structured chemical dependency program and often does not require hospitalization because the withdrawal syndrome does not necessitate intensive medical management. Inpatient treatment may be necessary, however, if outpatient treatment fails, if the adolescent exhibits suicidal or psychotic behavior, or if he or she is addicted to alcohol, sedatives, or opiates in addition to stimulants.

Delirium tremens, the major alcohol withdrawal syndrome, is rarely if ever seen in adolescents. In contrast, a more benign withdrawal syndrome consisting of tremors, diaphoresis, agitation, disorientation, and (in rare cases) brief seizures may occur in adolescents who have drunk heavily over weeks or months. Teenagers whose drinking history suggests the possibility of a minor withdrawal syndrome should be hospitalized for observation if they become abstinent.

SUMMARY

Whether the adolescent voluntarily comes for treatment for a drug abuse problem, is compelled to seek medical attention because of a drug- or alcohol-related illness, or is discovered to be using drugs or alcohol during a routine evaluation, the physician is in an advantageous position to intercede beyond the confines of treating somatic illness. The illegality and stigma attached to drug abuse often prevent the teenager from seeking help from clergy, educators, and particularly family members. Protected by federal guidelines that ensure the confidentiality of the physician-patient relationship in drug abuse treatment, the physician who uses a nonjudgmental, sympathetic approach to these teenagers may be able to establish trust and thereby gather sufficient information to make a knowledgeable judgment as to the need for further intervention. Such information must include not only the history of past and present drug or alcohol abuse, but also the nature of peer and family relationships, the extent of involvement with law enforcement authorities, the degree of educational or vocational disruption, and the adolescent's own interpretation of the need for subsequent therapy.

Often, the extent of substance abuse and related disruption is so minimal that no further action beyond the counsel of the physician is required. Such counsel should address the potential somatic effects of the teenager's current drug practices, the potential for escalation of drug-taking behavior, and the risks of accidents and death from even occasional intoxication. Alternatives to driving while intoxicated should be discussed with the adolescent and his or her family.

At the other extreme are teenagers who have severe psychopathological conditions and who are in obvious need of psychiatric care. A variety of other therapeutic modalities, not all of which may be present in a given community, are available for treatment of substance-abusing teenagers. Group or individual counseling may be indicated for the teenager who has less than severe drug involvement but has some evidence of psychosocial disruption. Group residences are available for adolescents from unsupportive homes. They usually offer counseling and a place to stay while teenagers continue their education or employment. Therapeutic communities are appropriate for those teenagers who are involved more deeply in drugs. These programs often are operated communally and staffed by former addicts, with or without professional support. The retention rate for teenagers within these programs is poor and may reflect the adolescents' inability to tolerate the rigors of relative incarceration and abrasive therapy.

Often, limitations of time for adequate psychosocial evaluation or lack of familiarity with available therapeutic resources prevents practitioners from reaching a meaningful long-term disposition for their patients. In these instances, referrals need to be made to other professionals or agencies that have expertise and interest in the field of teenage drug and alcohol abuse. In this regard, substance abuse does not differ from certain other behavioral problems for which specific therapeutic interventions are beyond the physician's professional scope.

SUGGESTED READINGS

Anonymous: Crack, *Med Lett Drugs Ther* 28:69, 1986.

Committee on Adolescence, American Academy of Pediatrics: Alcohol use and abuse: a pediatric concern, *Pediatrics* 79:450, 1987.

Committee on Substance Abuse, American Academy of Pediatrics: Role of the pediatrician in prevention and management of substance abuse, *Pediatrics* 91:1010, 1993.

Council on Scientific Affairs: Medical and nonmedical uses of anabolic-androgenic steroids, *JAMA* 264:2923, 1990.

Gawin FH, Ellinwood EH Jr: Cocaine and other stimulants, *N Engl J Med* 318:1173, 1988.

Institute of Medicine, Division of Health Sciences Policy: *Marijuana and health,* Washington, DC, 1982, National Academy Press.

King NMP, Cross AW: Moral and legal issues in screening for drug use in adolescents, *J Pediatr* 111:249, 1987.

Kipke MD, Futterman D, Hein K: HIV infection and AIDS during adolescence, *Med Clin North Am* 74:1149, 1990.

Perry CL, Silvis GL: Smoking prevention: behavioral prescriptions for the pediatrician, *Pediatrics* 79:790, 1987.

Schonberg SK, editor: *Substance abuse: a guide for health professionals,* 1988, American Academy of Pediatrics/Pacific Institute for Research and Evaluation.

Schydlower M, Rogers PD, editors: Adolescent medicine: adolescent substance abuse and addiction. In *State of the art reviews,* Philadelphia, 1993, Hanley & Belfus.

Shedler J, Block J: Adolescent drug use and psychological health, *Am Psychol* 45:612, 1990.

100 Homosexuality: Challenges of Treating Lesbian and Gay Adolescents

Robert J. Bidwell

Lesbian and gay youths, though often unrecognized regarding their sexual orientation, make up a part of the practice of all physicians working with adolescents. In 1993 the American Academy of Pediatrics Committee on Adolescence[1] published its statement on "Homosexuality and Adolescence," which affirms the existence of lesbian and gay youth, acknowledges their special experience and needs, and provides physicians' guidelines for helping these adolescents reach a healthy, productive adulthood. Despite the greater recognition and acceptance of lesbian and gay youth, however, society still disagrees over homosexuality, especially as it relates to this age group. This controversy has presented obstacles to the development of strategies to meet the significant physical and mental health risks faced by these adolescents. This failure to address their experience and needs has led to many damaged and lost young lives over the past decades.

BACKGROUND

Human sexuality, its origins and manifestations, is an extremely complex phenomenon. Chromosomal sex, anatomical sex, gender identity, gender role behavior, sexual behavior, and sexual orientation all are interrelated aspects of an individual's sexuality. Sexual orientation generally refers to one's prevailing pattern(s) of erotic and affectional attraction to members of the same or opposite gender. Homosexuality refers to same-gender attraction, heterosexuality to opposite-gender attraction, and bisexuality to attraction to members of both genders. However, Kinsey's research in the 1930s and 1940s showed that these categories are not discrete; rather, human beings fall along a continuum of sexual orientation from same-sex to opposite-sex attraction. To add to the complexity, an individual's sexual orientation also is reflected in his or her fantasies, life-style, self-identification as gay or lesbian, and choice of friends for emotional and social, as well as erotic, fulfillment.

The origins of sexual orientation have been debated widely, often with limited scientific support for proposed theories. Some have suggested that sexual orientation is determined primarily by nature, that is, through genetic programming, brain anatomy, or prenatal hormonal influences on a developing central nervous system. Others have presented sociological or psychoanalytical theories suggesting that environment or "upbringing" are of primary importance. The preponderance of recent research, consisting primarily of anatomical studies and studies of twins, appears to support a biological explanation for sexual orientation. Whether the major determinants reflect "nature," "nurture," or a combination of the two, sexual orientation generally is believed to be not chosen and is established well before puberty; moreover, a gay or lesbian person's homosexuality is no less deeply rooted, and therefore no more amenable to change, than another person's heterosexuality. Furthermore, no scientific evidence exists that homosexuality is a matter of "something gone wrong." The lack of such evidence led the American Psychiatric Association in 1973 to accept homosexuality as simply a part of the spectrum of human sexuality.

The process of acquiring a gay or lesbian identity is long and often painful. Troiden[7] has proposed a model describing a process that begins in childhood, continues through the confusion and first explorations of adolescence, and culminates in a healthy and open self-acceptance sometime during adulthood. Remafedi's study[5] of gay male youth has reconfirmed the adolescent years as particularly tumultuous and also has demonstrated that far from being "just a phase," homosexuality is a firmly established identity for a certain proportion of adolescents. They also found that for these adolescents, homosexuality was not simply sexual behaviors but involved a broader "attraction and affinity" to other men. A small subset of lesbian and gay individuals includes those who are "nontraditional" in their gender role behaviors as children. This is made up of very effeminate boys or very masculine girls. Green's[2] longitudinal study of boys with cross-gender behavior found that two thirds of prepubertal boys labeled as "sissies" because of their interest in stereotypic girls' games and activities or their displaying feminine mannerisms were bisexually or homosexually oriented as adults.

The estimated percentage of Americans who are lesbian or gay is imprecise at best. Research techniques have been refined and sexual mores redefined since Kinsey's studies 50 years ago. Many studies have surveyed only sexual behaviors. These may be an imprecise measurement of sexual orientation, especially during adolescence. Some lesbian and gay teens have been active only heterosexually, and many have not yet become sexually active at all. Remafedi et al.[4] found that among Minnesota adolescents, the prevalence of predominantly homosexual attractions increased generally with age (6.4% by age 18). Although only a small proportion (0.8%) of 18-year-old boys labeled themselves as homosexual, 8.9% report being "uncertain" about their sexual orientation. About 3% of 18-year-old boys acknowledged homosexual activity. Most studies conclude that somewhere between 3% and 10% of the population is lesbian or gay, and perhaps a larger percentage is bisexual in orientation.

GROWING UP LESBIAN OR GAY

Gay and lesbian adolescents are ordinary teenagers in every regard except that they grow up in an environment that often is unaccepting of a deepest part of who they are—their sexual orientation. In spite of this, most of these youths grow up to be happy, healthy, and productive adults. Nevertheless, recent research has shown that for some adolescents, the experience of growing up lesbian or gay can be difficult and even dangerous.[3,6]

Many gay and lesbian youths face an adolescence of profound isolation, believing that they are the only ones in their families or among their friends with feelings of same-sex attraction. They have little access to objective information on sexual orientation, though their daily lives may be filled with antigay messages in school hallways and at home. They often have no access to informed and supportive counseling in schools or youth agencies. Accompanying this isolation is a fear of discovery; because most of these youths are "invisible," not fitting the gay or lesbian stereotypes, much of their energy is spent in "living a lie" that creates a wall between them and those they respect and love. It also prevents many of them from achieving the developmental tasks of adolescence related to self-esteem, identity, and intimacy. Harassment and violence are additional burdens faced by those gay and lesbian teenagers who identify themselves or are identified by others as homosexual. The results of isolation, fear, and violence are predictable, as they are for any group of alienated youths. Gay youth are at higher risk of dropping out of school, being kicked out of their homes, and turning to life on the streets for survival. There they often encounter violence and sexual exploitation with the attendant risks of pregnancy and sexually transmitted diseases, including HIV. Some gay and lesbian youth engage in substance use, and a significant number attempt suicide.

Many gay and lesbian youths have never had sex with another person. Some have been active heterosexually. Because of the social barriers to the exploration of their sexuality, those teenagers who are active homosexually often become so through anonymous sexual encounters in circumstances that engender feelings of guilt, self-loathing, and fear.

To date, more is known about the experience of urban white gay male youth than other groups of gay or of lesbian adolescents. Lesbian teens, gay and lesbian youth of color, and rural youths may be even more isolated and, therefore, at risk.

Unfortunately, society's response to the experience and needs of gay and lesbian youth has been one primarily of silence. Health practitioners, counselors, teachers, clergy, and other youth-serving professionals have failed to address these issues because of their own discomfort, disapproval, or fear. This failure has increased the alienation of gay and lesbian adolescents and has contributed, in part, to the significant morbidity and mortality among them.

WORKING WITH LESBIAN AND GAY YOUTH

Lesbian and gay youth come to the attention of health practitioners in a variety of ways. A small percentage will self-refer or self-identify themselves to receive appropriate medical services or counseling. More often they are brought in by concerned parents or referred by youth agencies. The stated concerns may not relate specifically to sexual orientation but rather represent "red flags," including substance use or depression. Most gay and lesbian teenagers, however, are "invisible" and will pass through clinics and counselors' offices without raising the issue of sexual orientation on their own, even if it has caused them distress and led to high-risk behaviors. Therefore health providers must be able to address issues of sexual orientation with all adolescent patients. Only if these issues are addressed can specifically targeted medical screening, medical treatment, and anticipatory guidance be provided.

Health providers are not responsible for labeling, or even identifying, each and every lesbian and gay teen. Instead, the provider should create a clinical environment where clear messages are given that sensitive personal issues, including sexual orientation, can be discussed whenever the adolescent feels ready to do so. The provider should be ready to raise and discuss issues of sexual orientation with all teenagers, particularly any adolescent in distress or engaged in high-risk behaviors. If a youth acknowledges homosexual behavior or concerns about possibly being lesbian or gay, the practitioner should be able to explore the teenager's understanding and concerns about homosexuality, dispel any misconceptions, provide appropriate medical care and anticipatory guidance, and connect the teen to appropriate supportive community resources. One of the most important responsibilities of the practitioner is to facilitate every adolescent's growth toward a healthy homosexual, bisexual, or heterosexual adulthood.

HISTORY

Clinical settings and procedures must give clear, explicit messages that sexual orientation is among the personal issues that can be discussed with the practitioner. Otherwise, most gay and lesbian youth will believe that discussion of their possible homosexual orientation or behaviors is far beyond the limits of what health practitioners might be able to address supportively and knowledgeably. This message can be given through posters and brochures in the waiting area, a teen questionnaire that asks about sexual orientation concerns among other health issues, a clearly defined confidentiality policy, and by routinely seeing adolescent patients without their parents being present. The practitioner also must be careful not to presume heterosexual or homosexual orientation based on stereotypes. *Any* teenager should be considered as possibly dealing with issues of sexual orientation. Sexual orientation should be addressed in all "well-teen" visit interviews. To explore this area is especially important when "red flags" appear, including school problems, teen-parent conflicts, substance use, runaway behavior, depression, and self-destructive behaviors of any kind including increased heterosexual or homosexual activity. How the issue is raised and explored depends on the individual teen and on the practitioner's interviewing style. Most gay and lesbian teenagers do not raise concerns about sexual orientation on their own. The practitioner therefore must open the door to discussion. If the adolescent has been referred by parents or the school, the best policy usually is to let teenagers know what you have been told, as a starting point for discussion. More commonly, the practitioner is alerted by "red flags" to the possibility of concerns regarding sexual orientation.

A practitioner can approach and explore sexual orientation in a number of ways. The practitioner might first ask if the adolescent has ever dated. Whether teenagers have dated or not, they also should be asked whether they have ever "had sex" with another person and whether their sexual partners have been males, females, or both males and females. Homosexually active youths, as well as heterosexual youths who engage only in oral or anal sex, may answer "no" to the question, "Have you ever had sexual intercourse?" Whether adolescents have been sexually active or not (and many gay and lesbian adolescents have not been so), all teenagers should be asked whether they have ever been concerned about feelings of sexual attraction to people of the same sex. Many teens with same-sex attractions or activity have not labeled themselves as gay or lesbian, and so asking "Are you gay?" may be inappropriate. If a teenager acknowledges or hints at same-sex attractions, however, asking "Have you ever been concerned you might be gay?" may be appropriate.

If an adolescent denies homosexual feelings or behavior (sometimes with an expression of disgust), the practitioner can conclude by saying, "This may or may not ever be a part of your life. But if it ever is, I want you to know that I'm someone you can come to talk with about it."

It is necessary to ask any adolescent acknowledging same-sex activity about kinds of sexual behaviors, frequency, number of partners, consensual and nonconsensual sex, sex exchanged for money or drugs, the nature of partners (anonymous versus boyfriend or girlfriend), "safer sex" practices, and symptoms of sexually transmitted diseases. All teens acknowledging homosexual attractions or activity should be asked about substance use, depression, and other risky behaviors common to alienated youths.

If teenagers believe that they might be lesbian or gay, the origins of these concerns should be explored. Homosexual feelings and experiences do not necessarily mean that one is gay. Similarily, heterosexual feelings and experience do not necessarily represent a heterosexual orientation. Certainly, to tell a teenager that homosexual feelings are "just a phase" would be a mistake. For a significant percentage of adolescents, they do, in fact, represent an emerging lesbian or gay identity.

PHYSICAL EXAMINATION

Lesbian and gay adolescents face the same health risks as their heterosexual peers. Therefore they should receive the same "well-teen" screening and acute-care examinations as any teenager. Because teenagers may fear disclosing homosexual, bisexual, or heterosexual activity, the physical examination should not be guided solely by the history given in the interview.

The incidence of sexually transmitted diseases (STDs) among lesbian adolescents who are exclusively homosexually active is low. These consist primarily of *Gardnerella vaginalis, Candida* organisms, and *Trichomonas* organisms. However, many lesbian teenagers occasionally may be active heterosexually, have female partners who are heterosexually active, or be the victims of heterosexual rape. Therefore all lesbian adolescents should be considered at risk for STDs, including gonorrhea (pharyngeal, cervical, rectal), chlamydia (cervical, rectal), genital herpes, genital warts, and HIV infection. Pregnancy, too, may be a possibility. Lesbian adolescents also should have regular Papanicolaou and breast examinations. All gay male youth, whether acknowledging sexual activity or not, should have a general screening examination with careful attention to the skin, lymph nodes, oropharynx, abdomen, genitals, and anorectal region. They should be considered for STD evaluation, including gonorrhea (oral, urethral, rectal), chlamydia (urethral, rectal), genital herpes, genital warts, and HIV infection. As with other adolescents, the content and frequency of screening examinations depends on the frequency and nature of the teenager's sexual activity. The evaluation and treatment of sexually transmitted diseases are discussed in Chapter 258, Sexually Transmitted Diseases.

LABORATORY EVALUATION

All sexually active gay male youths and heterosexually active lesbian adolescents should have serological studies performed to detect syphilis and be considered for HIV testing. All adolescents, regardless of sexual orientation, should receive hepatitis B immunization.

ANTICIPATORY GUIDANCE

Because so little information is available to lesbian and gay youth about their sexual orientation, the health practitioner should address these seven areas to ensure their safe passage into adulthood:

1. *Information about sexual orientation.* While different segments of society and various religions may view homosexuality either positively or negatively, the field of pediatrics generally accepts that homosexuality is not a choice, that its origins appear to be established early in childhood, and that it appears to be a healthy or natural outcome for perhaps 3% to 10% of the population.
2. *Feelings about sexual orientation.* A teenager's feelings about the possibility of being lesbian or gay likely will come from a mixture of societal, religious, ethnic, and familial influences. The practitioner should not attempt to argue against any of these but rather allow teenagers the time to explore the influence of these in their lives and correct any misconceptions or matters of fact related to homosexuality or what it means to be lesbian or gay.
3. *Experience of lesbian and gay adolescents and adults.* Although lesbian and gay people historically have been subjected to ridicule, harassment, and discrimination, increased understanding and acceptance has been a definite trend in large segments of society, including some religious denominations. Teenagers should understand that they can aspire to rewarding careers, long-term, loving relationships, and parenthood in their adult lives.
4. *Risk behaviors and safer-sex practices.* The practitioner should evaluate every adolescent's decision-making abilities related to risky behaviors and attempt to enhance negotiation skills related to sex and drugs. Helping the teen to postpone serious sexual involvement until older should be a goal in working with younger adolescents. All teenagers, sexually active or not, should understand in detail the rationale and techniques of safer sex, particularly the use of condoms.

5. *"Coming out" to parents and friends.* "Coming out" (revealing one's sexual orientation to others) is a strong urge some adolescents feel as they become more comfortable with their gay or lesbian identity. Many suggest waiting until one is legally and financially independent before coming out to parents. Before coming out a review of the range of possible responses from parents or friends and how the teenager will handle these is helpful.
6. *Resources for lesbian and gay teenagers.* Many larger towns have agencies that sponsor lesbian and gay teen support groups. Local gay and lesbian community organizations will know whether such groups exist in a particular area. Several excellent books have been written for lesbian and gay teenagers and their friends or parents. Teenagers in significant distress should be referred to experienced supportive counselors (social workers, psychologists, or psychiatrists). Care should be taken in making such referrals, because counselors who claim to be able to alter an adolescent's sexual orientation are engaging in an unethical and dangerous practice.
7. *Special experience of rural youth and youth of color.* Health practitioners should be sensitive to the possibility that these groups of youths may be especially isolated and, therefore, have their own unique experience and needs.

PARENTS

Most lesbian and gay teenagers will decide to postpone telling their parents of their sexual orientation. This decision should be respected by the health practitioner. At times the practitioner, at the teen's request, might facilitate the coming out process by meeting with both adolescent and parents to discuss these issues. Parents who become aware that their teenager is gay or lesbian often go through a very difficult period. Like their teen son or daughter, they may experience fear, anger, guilt, confusion, and a sense of isolation. Some may reject their child or seek out therapies to change their child's sexual orientation. The practitioner can ease parental distress by providing information and connecting them to community resources such as experienced counselors and local chapters of Parents/Friends of Lesbians and Gays. The practitioner also can acknowledge the pain and anger that parents may feel but at the same time stress that what their sons or daughters need most is renewed assurance of their continuing love.

ADVOCACY

Although much is known about sexual orientation and the experience of lesbian and gay youth, a great deal of societal ignorance and fear still is related to working openly with them. Health practitioners are well situated to dispel the myths, initiate community dialogues, and create a *network* of supportive community service for these young people. These networks must include schools, churches, youth agencies, health centers, correctional facilities, and all other youth-serving institutions. These efforts are beginning in many communities throughout the country and enable these young people to become the happy, healthy, and productive gay and lesbian adults they are meant to be.

REFERENCES

1. Committee on Adolescence, American Academy of Pediatrics: Homosexuality and adolescence, *Pediatrics* 92:631, 1993.
2. Green R: *The "sissy boy syndrome" and the development of homosexuality,* New Haven, Conn, 1987, Yale University Press.
3. Remafedi G: Adolescent homosexuality: psychosocial and medical implications, *Pediatrics* 79:331, 1987.
4. Remafedi G et al: Demography of sexual orientation in adolescents, *Pediatrics* 89:714, 1992.
5. Remafedi G: Male homosexuality: the adolescents' perspective, *Pediatrics* 79:326, 1987.
6. Seattle Commission on Children and Youth: *Report on gay and lesbian youth in Seattle,* Seattle, Nov 1992, City of Seattle Commission on Children and Youth.
7. Troiden RR: Homosexual identity development, *J Adolesc Health Care* 9:105, 1988.

SUGGESTED READINGS

Fairchild B, Hayward N: *Now that you know: what every parent should know about homosexuality,* San Diego, 1981, Harcourt Brace Jovanovich.
Gold MA et al: Children of gay or lesbian parents, *Pediatr Rev* 15:354, 1994.
Remafedi G, editor: Special section on adolescent homosexuality, *J Adolesc Health Care* 9:93, 1988.
Rench JE: *Understanding sexual identity: a book for gay teens and their friends,* Minneapolis, 1990, Lerner.
Whitlock K: *Bridges of respect: creating support for lesbian and gay youth,* Philadelphia, 1989, American Friends Service Committee.

RESOURCES

1. Parents/Friends of Lesbians and Gays, 1012 14th Street NW, Washington, D.C. 20005. Provides information on local chapters, written materials for parents, and advocacy on lesbian and gay issues.
2. Hetrick Martin Institute for the Protection of Lesbian and Gay Youth, 401 West Street, New York, NY 10014. Provides educational and social services for lesbian and gay youth. Also publishes written material for youth, including posters and brochures.
3. Lambert House: A Gay/Lesbian/Bisexual Youth Center. 1818 Fifteenth Avenue, Seattle, WA 98122. Provides a drop-in center, support groups, recreation, education, and health services.

101 Interviewing Adolescents

Esther H. Wender

The skill of interviewing is put to a strong test in the practice of adolescent medicine because the relationship between the adolescent patient and adults in positions of authority is changing rapidly and often is fragile. Yet good interviewing requires establishing a relationship that enhances communication between the interacting parties. The information most relevant and useful to both people emerges if the relationship promotes communication. Conversely, the most skillfully formulated questions do not yield useful information if the interaction between the conversing parties is tense or hostile.

WHOM TO INTERVIEW

During adolescence, a transition from dependence to independence should be made by the teenager and should be facilitated by the parents. In early adolescence the parents still are largely responsible for their teen's health care, although by late adolescence these patients often are managing their own medical needs completely. These changes occur over a relatively brief period; therefore the physician is faced with assessing the stage of transition toward independence each time the adolescent patient is seen. Whom to interview should be decided in the context of this transition, and several potential problems need to be considered.

The Adolescent's Developmental Level

Nothing is more upsetting to adolescents than feeling that they are being treated like younger children. This particularly is a problem in early adolescence when lack of sexual maturation on the part of teens causes insensitive adults to underestimate the patients' psychological age. Adolescent patients, when they feel free to comment, resent an office or hospital setting designed only for younger children. Even more upsetting, however, is the adult who talks to adolescents as though they are younger children. Therefore, to gain the respect of adolescent patients, the physician should take a genuine interest in them at the beginning of the interview.

It usually is best to greet the adolescent patient before greeting the parent. It also is helpful to chat with the patient briefly before the interview begins, being careful to gear the conversation to the appropriate level for that patient. To accomplish this, the physician should know enough about normal adolescent development to judge the appropriateness of this preinterview conversation (see Chapter 51, Theories and Concepts of Development as They Relate to Pediatric Practice).

The Parents' Role

While it is essential to make the adolescent feel comfortable, the physician should not ignore the importance of the parents' role. In early and middle adolescence, the parents' input is critical for a thorough evaluation because adolescents still have only limited insight about themselves and have inadequate perspective on the timing and importance of symptoms. During late adolescence seeing the adolescent without the parents' involvement may be appropriate, if that is the teenager's wish. When the parents are involved, the physician should allow them time to discuss their concerns without their child being present. Parents may be reluctant to discuss their concerns openly, particularly in the presence of their adolescent.

A younger (12- to 16-year-old) adolescent may request to be seen alone, particularly regarding sexual issues. The physician should be aware of the particular state's laws regarding the adolescent's rights to confidential evaluation, and these rights must be respected. However, because of adolescents' limited perspective and their need for emotional and financial support, the physician would be wise in most cases to encourage younger adolescents to involve their parents. Although the adolescent's independence should be encouraged and he or she should always have some time to see the physician alone, the appropriate role of the parents should not be ignored. In our culture parents still are responsible for their children through adolescence.

Adolescent Sensitivity to Parents-Only Interviews

Adolescent patients often are both upset and resentful when the parents and physician talk about them in their absence. This particularly is true if the adolescent disagrees with the parents' assessment of the problem or objects to consulting a physician. Therefore the need to obtain information from the parents may be in direct conflict with consideration for the adolescent's feelings. One way to solve this problem is to see the patient and parents together for the initial portion of the interview. During this session the physician should tell both the adolescent and parents that each will be able to talk to the physician alone and that these conversations will be confidential. This approach, which allows disagreements between parents and patient to be aired openly, usually reduces the natural "paranoia" that the adolescent feels when in conflict with his or her parents' assessment of the problem.

Physician Neutrality

If a significant disagreement exists between the adolescent and parents, the physician must avoid seeming to take sides on these issues. Again, this can be accomplished best by interviewing the adolescent and parents together, concentrating on understanding and clarifying their disagreements, and thus conveying an appropriately neutral attitude about the conflict. The following vignette illustrates this technique. The evaluation has been initiated by parents, concerned that their 15-year-old son has behavioral problems.

Mr. Jones: We think his choice of friends leaves a lot to be desired.
Jim: What's the matter with my friends?
Mr. Jones: Most of them have no ambition. They don't care about school and spend their time just hanging around.
Jim: It's just that we're not like you. You don't care about anything except work. At least my friends know how to have fun.
Physician: Jim, you think your father devotes too much attention to work?
Jim: Yeah.
Physician: And, Mr. Jones, you wish Jim were more ambitious and also picked friends who were?
Mr. Jones: Yes. I worry that Jim isn't going to succeed.
Jim: (to his father) I'll succeed in my own way.
Physician: What are your ideas about success, Jim?

In this interaction, the physician has facilitated communication between the father and son without stating an opinion that would appear to commit him to either's point of view.

A review of these issues before the interview helps the physician to make a reasonable decision about whom to interview first; no rigid rules apply. The choice depends on the age of the patient, the person who initiates the contact, and whether conflict exists between the adolescent and parents regarding the problem.

PHYSICAL SETTING

Adolescent patients often are quite sensitive to the atmosphere of the physician's office or hospital ward that emphasizes the interests of the young child. Therefore the pediatrician should arrange the office waiting room with a section that contains reading material and decor appropriate for adolescent patients. At least one examining room should be equipped and decorated with the adolescent patient in mind. The hospital ward also should have a section furnished and decorated specifically for adolescent patients, and an interviewing room to be used exclusively for teens should be available. The need for privacy during the interview is never more important than in the practice of adolescent medicine. If the adolescent believes that the conversation will be interrupted or overheard, important information may not be revealed. Privacy may be particularly difficult to find on the hospital ward or in the emergency room, but every effort should be made to do so.

The interview room should be arranged with physician, patient, and parents seated at the same level, at a comfortable conversational distance, and without desks between the physician and the other person or persons to whom the physician is speaking. The few moments it takes to rearrange furniture to meet these requirements are well spent.

INTERVIEWING TECHNIQUE

The key to good interviewing is building a trusting relationship between the physician, patient, and parents. This goal can be accomplished if the physician makes an effort to understand how the adolescent patient perceives the problem and relationships with important people in his or her life. Most physicians would say that they do attempt to understand their patients. However, physicians often become involved in their own agenda of obtaining answers to specific medical questions and miss important clues about their patients' feelings.

The following vignette illustrates the insensitivity that results when medical issues are pursued vigorously and the physician becomes more interested in the answers than in the relationship. The patient is a 16-year-old girl who has diabetes.

Physician: How much insulin do you take?
Susan: Sixteen units of NPH and four units of regular each morning.
Physician: Do you test your urine?
Susan: Yeah.
Physician: How often?
Susan: Every morning and in the late afternoon, when my mother doesn't bug me.
Physician: Do you ever spill sugar?
Susan: Sometimes; not too often.
Physician: How much? One plus, two plus?
Susan: Just one plus a couple of times a week. Mom's always asking me that, but I tell her to leave me alone.
Physician: Do you ever have insulin reactions?
Susan: Not for a long time.
Physician: How's school?

One can sense the physician's need to fill in the blanks of the medical history. In the process, this physician has failed to pick up the clues of the daughter-mother conflict. The physician completed the agenda and then turned to a question about the adolescent's life that probably will be perceived by the patient as a "mechanical" question, since the physician did not "hear" previous comments.

Techniques that promote the acquisition of useful information fall into two main categories: listening skills and facilitative responses (see Interviewing Techniques in Chapter 6, The Pediatric History). Component aspects of these two skills, discussed briefly in the next two sections are outlined as follows:

1. Listening skills
   a. Clarification of meaning
   b. Verbal asides
   c. Nonverbal communication
2. Facilitative responses
   a. Repetition and review
   b. Acknowledgment of feelings
   c. Periods of silence

Listening Skills

Unless physicians pay attention to the meaning of words, they often will think they understand when they really do not. Every time patients use words or phrases that are abstract or unclear, physicians should ask for *clarification.* Skilled interviewers continually ask themselves if they understand what has just been said. In the following vignette, the importance of this technique is illustrated. The patient is a 15-year-old boy who has school problems.

Physician: Your parents seem concerned about how you are doing in school. What do you think?
Gary: Sometimes I think I'm a wreck.
Physician: A wreck?
Gary: Yeah, you know, all washed up.
Physician: I don't know, Gary; what does that feel like?
Gary: Like I get these funny feelings, and I think I'm falling apart.

Physician: Tell me about one of these funny feelings.
Gary: Well . . . sometimes it's like my fingers are growing really big, or small. It's weird.
Physician: You mean like parts of your body are changing size?
Gary: Yeah.
Physician: Anything else?
Gary: Sometimes I feel like I'm walking just a little off the ground, like I was floating.

If the physician did not pursue the meaning of Gary's words, he or she might have been left with the vague statement that Gary feels he is a "wreck," which many people would assume means he thinks he is a failure. Instead, the physician now has evidence that Gary is experiencing somatic symptoms of anxiety or psychotic thinking, and he or she can pursue the source of these feelings.

Verbal asides are parenthetical statements that often reveal the patient's true feelings but that are stated as though they are unimportant. They usually reflect the adolescent's ambivalence about exposing his or her real feelings. The diabetic patient, described earlier, who said that she tested her urine twice a day "when my mother doesn't bug me" is giving a verbal aside. Statements about her mother constitute unsolicited information. Physicians often focus only on the solicited information and therefore fail to hear such asides. All that usually is required to facilitate further communication is to echo the phrase back to the patient in the form of a question.

Nonverbal communication consists of body movements and facial expressions that reveal a person's feelings. A physician who is preoccupied with asking the right questions and accumulating the answers will miss these important clues. The skilled interviewer learns to divide attention between the words that are being said and the body language of the person being interviewed. Because body language usually is outside the patient's awareness, it may be premature to immediately comment on such observations. Part of the art of interviewing is to sense when such comments may be useful.

A good rule to remember is that when body language reveals something the person seems to be trying to hide, it should be left alone. For example, a person's clenched fists may indicate tension, when his or her words suggest calm. However, when a facial expression suggests an inner thought or feeling, it often is useful to comment. The patient may say something funny, for example, and then appear sad. In this instance, it usually is helpful to say something like, "It looks as if that thought suddenly made you feel sad."

Facilitative Responses

The person who is talking usually feels good when the listener can synthesize what the speaker has just said into a summary that reflects the thoughts accurately. If, for example, the patient has had difficulty finding the right words to describe his or her symptoms and the physician then restates those symptoms briefly and accurately, the patient realizes he or she has been heard. People like to be understood, and this type of *repetition and review* greatly facilitates further communication.

An important component of repetition and review is the *acknowledgment of feelings,* as well as the recognition of facts. Often, patients make a series of statements that really are meant to build a case for the underlying feelings they are experiencing. If the physician can hear and then acknowledge these feelings, the relationship may be significantly enhanced. The following segment of an interview illustrates this interaction. The patient is a 13-year-old girl brought in by parents because of acting-out behavior.

Physician: Your parents are upset over some of the things you have done. What do you think?
Judy: They really bug me. Last week, Mom wouldn't let me go to the roller rink with my friends. She said that we were too young to go by ourselves, but all my friends' parents let them go. Then, a couple of nights ago, I wanted to stay at Sally's house for dinner and Dad made me come home. He said that it's getting too dark at night. Geez, you'd think I was a baby.
Physician: It sounds like you don't feel your parents trust you.
Judy: I *know* they don't trust me. It makes me feel like doing whatever I want, since they don't trust me anyway.

Another important facilitative response is the carefully timed use of *silences.* This is particularly important when the patient has difficulty expressing himself or herself. Physicians usually are highly verbal people and respond to such patients by asking more and more questions. When a question has been asked and the response is not immediate, the interviewer should look closely for cues that the patient is processing the question. If the patient appears to be thinking about the answer, the physician should learn to pause to allow a response. Further statements might include facilitative responses such as, "What thoughts are you having?" or "It's hard, sometimes, to find the right words." Such replies tend to encourage the response.

The periods of silence should not be so long that the patient is made to feel uncomfortable. Sometimes in psychiatric interviews, long silences are used purposefully, but this approach would be too threatening for most medical interviews. Instead, the recommended approach is to allow time for the person whose verbal responses are slow.

APPROACHING THE SENSITIVE ISSUES OF DRUGS AND SEX

Vital issues in adolescent medicine include a healthy response to emerging sexuality and the avoidance of addiction to drugs or alcohol. Health care professionals should address these issues from the perspective of prevention. This approach requires inquiring about these topics throughout the period of adolescent development. However, both adolescents and physicians often feel uncomfortable with these issues. Questions about sexual activity and the use of drugs and alcohol often seem intrusive and embarrassing. Once the adolescent is assured of confidentiality and privacy, the physician should approach the topic of sexuality beginning with appropriate medical inquiry, moving from there into issues of sexual behavior. For females, questions about menstruation can precede inquiries about avoiding pregnancy and sexually transmitted disease. For males, questions about ejaculation and penile discharge can precede questions about sexual intercourse. Current abstention from sexual activity can be supported while assuring the teen that the physician is willing and able to provide medical guidance if that should change. The physician must not assume heterosexual interest and sexual activity because homosexual preferences usually emerge first during adolescence, and these youth need an understanding approach to the prevention of disease. A good exploratory question might be, "Have you ever been worried about feelings of sexual attraction to people of the same sex?"

Inquiries about tobacco, alcohol, and drug use usually should be approached in that order, from the experimentation that is most likely to the least likely (and most dangerous) use of hard drugs. Inquiring indirectly about the substance by using activities of friends often leads more easily into the behaviors of the teen patients themselves. If any substance use is identified, it is helpful to inquire about those factors that suggest problems. A recommended format is the so-called CAGE questions:

1. Have you ever tried to *cut* down on drug or alcohol use?
2. Have you ever been *annoyed* by someone's criticism of your drug or alcohol use?
3. Have you ever felt *guilty* about your drug or alcohol use?
4. Have you ever used drugs or alcohol as an *eye-opener?*

SUMMARY

The techniques just described are only suggestions. Effective interviewing requires practice. However, the skill is well worth learning because it leads to completing better medical histories and improved patient compliance. The result is improved health care for adolescents and their families.

SUGGESTED READINGS

Felice ME, Friedman SB: Behavioral considerations in the health care of adolescents, *Pediatr Clin North Am* 29:399, 1982.

Ginott HG: *Between parent and teenager,* New York, 1969, Macmillan.

Weiner IB: *Psychological disturbance in adolescence,* ed 2, New York, 1992, John Wiley & Sons.

102 Juvenile Delinquency

Irving B. Weiner

"Juvenile delinquency" is the legal term for youthful behavior that violates the law. This broad legal definition embraces two specific questions pediatricians must address when dealing with delinquent behavior: Does the kind and extent of a patient's illegal activity call for clinical intervention? If so, what is the cause of the delinquent behavior in which he or she has been involved?

The first of these questions is important because delinquent acts, regardless of whether they have been detected by the police, can range widely in severity and frequency. Young people may have committed major felonies such as assault or armed robbery, or they may be guilty only of misdemeanors, such as running away or disturbing the peace, that have few implications for criminal tendencies. Likewise, a particular kind of delinquent act may have occurred only once or may have become a repetitive pattern of illegal behavior.

The point at which delinquent acts come to professional attention often is influenced by the tolerance level for such behavior in a particular child's family, neighborhood, or community. Generally, however, the more serious the delinquent acts and the more frequently they have been occurring, the more likely they are to require clinical evaluation and treatment.

Regarding the causes of delinquent behavior, one should not think of juvenile delinquency in a global sense, as if there were universally applicable explanations of its causes and uniformly appropriate ways of dealing with this behavior. To the contrary, delinquent youngsters are a psychologically heterogeneous group. Some are socialized delinquents who are well-integrated members of a delinquent subculture and display few if any psychological problems; others are delinquent as a result of various psychological maladjustments, some of which are characterological in nature and some of which express neurotic tendencies.

Characterological maladjustments usually begin forming early in life and crystallize into various forms of personality disorder during adolescence. Individuals who have personality disorders are satisfied with their basic nature and have no wish to be different; they feel comfortable with themselves and attribute any difficulties they encounter to external events over which they have no control and for which they bear no responsibility.

Neurotic maladjustments, on the other hand, usually do not appear until the elementary school years and may emerge at any subsequent time of life with little previous warning. They constitute immature or unrealistic ways of attempting to solve problems or to reduce anxiety and are uncharacteristic of how the affected person usually behaves. Neurotic individuals usually are concerned about how they are feeling (e.g., phobic or depressed) or acting (e.g., being compulsive or having temper tantrums) and wish they could change themselves back to what they were like before these symptoms began.[13]

DIFFERENTIAL DIAGNOSIS OF DELINQUENT BEHAVIOR

The appropriate response to delinquent behavior in a patient follows from the differential diagnosis of the origin of his or her delinquency as stemming from socialized, characterological, or neurotic patterns of behavior.

Socialized Delinquency

In socialized delinquency, illegal activity emerges among members of a subculture who share antisocial standards of conduct. In contrast to psychological forms of delinquency, which are maladaptive for the individual, socialized delinquency is adaptive behavior in that it earns delinquents praise and acceptance from their immediate social group and thereby provides them a sense of satisfaction and belonging. Socialized delinquency usually is a group or gang activity, and it seldom accounts for delinquent acts that are committed alone or without the approval of neighborhood or peer groups.[4]

Accordingly, the differential diagnosis of socialized delinquency is suggested by four findings in the clinical history: (1) the delinquent acts have been performed with valued companions rather than alone or with strangers; (2) these delinquents see themselves as accepted and integral members of their peer group and rarely exhibit feelings of personal alienation or social inadequacy; (3) unlike people suffering psychological disorders, socialized delinquents evidence little neurotic symptom formation or basic character flaws; and (4) these delinquents typically will have enjoyed close and supportive family relationships during their early years—again, in contrast to the kinds of family tensions and disruption that contribute to psychological problems—although their delinquency as adolescents may result in part from inadequate parental supervision.

Characterological Delinquency

The illegal behavior of characterological delinquents reflects a basically asocial personality orientation. These young people manifest many features of what is commonly termed *psychopathy.* Because of prominent guiltlessness (defective conscience) and lovelessness (incapacity for loyalty to others), they are highly prone to committing illegal acts against persons and property.

Characterological delinquents tend to be loners who neither trust nor expect to be trusted by others. They break the law primarily as a result of disregard for the feelings and rights of others and an inability or unwillingness to control their own behavior. Such personality impairments derive from parental rejection early in life, which deprives children of an opportunity to learn to share mutual bonds of affection and attachment with other people, and parental neglect in middle childhood, which deprives young people of the discipline and guidance necessary to inculcate self-control and internal standards of moral conduct. Lacking such parenting, future psychopaths grow from childhood into adolescence loving no one and guided by an external morality in which acceptable behavior is whatever they can get away with.[3,10]

The differential diagnosis of characterological delinquency is based on the adolescents' personality style, their behavioral history, and the nature of their past and current family relationships. The more patients appear basically to be aggressive, impulsive, and amoral, with little sympathy for others and little capacity to tolerate frustration of their own wishes, the more likely their delinquency will reflect a psychopathic personality disorder. Because the roots of psychopathy extend far back into childhood, characterological delinquents usually will have a long history of problem behaviors such as fighting, lying, stealing, being unruly in school, and being cruel to people and animals.

The diagnosis of characterological delinquency rarely is justified in the absence of this kind of history, and it also should be avoided for children who appear to have enjoyed close and supportive care from reasonably well-adjusted parents. Evidence of early affective deprivation, on the other hand, especially when combined with a family history of irresponsible behavior, considerably increases the probability that delinquent activity is characterological in origin.

Occasionally the long-term consequences of having had a childhood learning disability produce patterns of misconduct during adolescence that bear a superficial resemblance to characterological delinquency. The blows to self-esteem typically suffered by learning-disabled children at home, in the classroom, and on the playground can result in their becoming insecure, short-tempered teenagers who need to bolster their self-image and beat down unwanted criticism. Hence, like characterological delinquents, they tend at times to show the kinds of aggressive, self-centered behavior seen in psychopathic individuals. The basic nature of their difficulties, however, can be differentiated readily from psychopathy by a good clinical history. Instead of early affective deprivation or other family problems, these adolescents have demonstrated evidence of an attention deficit/hyperactivity disorder in early childhood (including hyperactivity, delayed motor and language development, and impaired perceptual-motor coordination); in elementary school they have been slow to learn (especially reading) despite having adequate intelligence and have had strained relationships with their teachers and classmates.

Neurotic Delinquency

Neurotic delinquents commit illegal acts neither as commonplace pursuits shared with their peer group nor as a reflection of a long-standing characterological disorder. Rather, their delinquency emerges without previous warning as a way of expressing needs for recognition or help. In the first case, young people who feel ignored or unappreciated by others may carry out daring or dramatic acts of delinquency to bask, even if only briefly, in the notoriety they achieve. In the second case, children and adolescents who cannot find direct ways of communicating a need for help in dealing with some problem may act delinquently as an indirect means of getting this message across. The kind of distress most frequently associated with such delinquency is underlying depression, and the onset of uncharacteristic misconduct commonly can be traced to feelings of loneliness or discouragement that a young person cannot express or get others to hear through more direct channels of communication.[1,2]

A key to identifying this pattern of delinquency is the regularity with which neurotic delinquents manage to be caught in the act or give themselves away. Because the symptomatic use of delinquency to express underlying concerns serves its purpose only if the misdeeds come to light, successful concealment of law-breaking usually contraindicates neurotic delinquency. The differential diagnosis of neurotic delinquency also is facilitated by certain elements of the history and family circumstances. Unlike psychopathic individuals, neurotic delinquents have little or no history of earlier behavioral problems. Their current misconduct deviates sharply from how they have acted before and how others have come to expect them to act.

Moreover, in their relationships with their parents, neurotic delinquents ordinarily have enjoyed both the close supervision denied socialized delinquents and the warmth and affection denied characterological delinquents. Nevertheless, specific problems in family communication often are the final factor in prompting otherwise law-abiding youngsters to resort to delinquent behavior as a means of getting their parents to recognize and respond to their needs. The more clearly these or other kinds of specific precipitating events (such as a painful rebuff from peers or loss of a parent through death or divorce) can be identified as occurring just before the onset of delinquent behavior, the more likely is the illegal activity to constitute neurotic symptom formation.

DIFFERENTIAL TREATMENT PLANNING IN DELINQUENCY

Differential treatment planning for delinquent youth depends on the type of delinquent behavior manifest. In socialized delinquency, antisocial actions are adaptive group behaviors that neither reflect nor lead to diagnosable psychological disturbance; hence little is gained from efforts at psychological intervention in the practitioner's office. Socialized delinquents need (1) supervision and control, (2) guidance and models that can encourage them to exchange their antisocial values for more conventional standards of conduct, and (3) help in preparing themselves for an adult life in which they can find ways of enjoying and supporting themselves within the law rather than by breaking it. Accordingly, the indicated treatment for adolescents displaying subcultural delinquency usually is referral to community-based activities or agencies that provide group-oriented programs for developing the talents and redirecting the energies of delinquent youth.[6,7,12]

Characterological delinquency, because of its integral relationship to psychopathic personality formation beginning early in life, constitutes a serious and usually chronic form of psychopathology. Successful intervention in characterological delinquency accordingly requires intensive, long-term psychotherapy, which even under the best circumstances offers much less hope for a favorable outcome than can be expected for most other child and adolescent behavioral problems. Pediatricians are unlikely to undertake the long and arduous treatment of characterological delinquents themselves, unless they have had extensive training in child and adolescent psychiatry or behavioral pediatrics and can commit large amounts of time to such work. Instead, their usual choice will be to refer these patients to mental health practitioners or agencies, many of whom, in turn, feel that only an extended period of residential treatment can affect these young people sufficiently to alter their chronic personality disorder.[5,9]

Recent advances in theory and practice have begun to improve this gloomy prognosis for psychopathy. The likelihood of psychopathic adolescents becoming seriously and persistently delinquent appears related to their lacking social skills that could help them find noncriminal ways of satisfying their needs. Attention, accordingly, is being directed to modifying the behavior of these delinquents not by attempting to change their character style, but by enhancing their coping capacities through a variety of training exercises designed to increase their repertoire of interpersonal skills and their capacity for judgment and self-control. Adolescents' parents frequently are brought into this type of treatment program, not for traditional family therapy but to receive training themselves in interacting with their child in ways that encourage and reward prosocial behavior.[8,11]

Neurotic delinquency, because of its specific symptomatic meaning and relatively recent onset, frequently responds promptly to brief psychotherapy. Psychotherapy in correctly diagnosed instances of neurotic delinquency offers much greater promise of altering antisocial conduct than any of the known ways of intervening in socialized or characterological delinquency, and pediatricians who conduct psychotherapy can provide the necessary treatment in the office readily. Because the deviant behavior of neurotic delinquents is motivated by needs for attention and help, the very act of hearing them out and offering to work with them can, in short order, result in their stopping delinquent activity.[14]

Beyond this immediate salutary impact, effective psychotherapy with neurotic delinquents consists mainly of (1) gaining the patient's trust and confidence and (2) adopting the stance of an interested and concerned listener who makes observations from time to time on the apparent significance of what is being said, rather than of someone who judges and advises. If these patients also can be helped to recognize connections between the onset of their delinquency and the onset of certain psychological problems they could not express in other ways, the likelihood of their resorting to such indirect channels of expression in the future will be diminished substantially.

REFERENCES

1. Bynner JM, O'Malley PM, Bachman JG: Self-esteem and delinquency revisited, *J Youth Adolesc* 10:407, 1981.
2. Chiles JA, Miller ML, Cox GB: Depression in an adolescent delinquent population, *Arch Gen Psychiatry* 37:1179, 1980.
3. Deutsch LJ, Erickson MT: Early life events as discriminators of socialized and undersocialized delinquents, *J Abnorm Child Psychol* 17:541, 1989.
4. Dishion TJ et al: Family, school, and behavioral antecedents to early adolescent involvement with antisocial peers, *Dev Psychol* 27:172, 1991.
5. Doren DM: *Assessing and treating the psychopath,* New York, 1987, John Wiley & Sons.
6. Gottschalk R et al: Community-based interventions. In Quay HC, editor: *Handbook of juvenile delinquency,* New York, 1987, John Wiley & Sons.
7. Jensen JM, Howard MO: Skill deficits, skills training, and delinquency, *Children Youth Services Rev* 12:213, 1990.
8. Kazdin AE, Siegel TC, Bass D: Cognitive problem-solving skills training and parent management training in the treatment of antisocial behavior in children, *J Consult Clin Psychol* 60:733, 1992.
9. Marohn RC: Residential services. In Tolan PH, Cohler BJ, editors: *Handbook of clinical research and practice with adolescents,* New York, 1993, John Wiley & Sons.
10. Meloy JR: *The psychopathic mind,* Northvale, NJ, 1988, Aronson.
11. Miller GE, Prinz RJ: Enhancement of social learning family interventions for childhood conduct disorders, *Psychol Bull* 108:192, 1990.
12. Nelson KE: Family-based services for juvenile offenders, *Children Youth Services Rev* 12:193, 1990.
13. Weiner IB: *Child and adolescent psychopathology,* ed 2, New York, 1992, John Wiley & Sons.
14. Weiner IB: Psychological interventions for disturbed adolescents. In McNamara JR, Appel MA, editors: *Critical issues, developments, and trends in professional psychology,* New York, 1987, Praeger.

103 Mood Disorders in Children and Adolescents

Åke Mattsson and John M. Diamond

Disorders of mood, such as depression and mania, were seldom recognized among children and adolescents in North America before 1970. Children were viewed as too "immature" to experience and communicate a depressed mood or feelings of guilt and low self-esteem.[16] Adolescents were expected to go through a period of "storm and stress" (Sturm and Drang) as a normal developmental phase characterized by frequent mood swings such as states of elation, boundless energy, and compassion, alternating with hours or days of sullenness, self-doubt, and irritability—that is, signs of a dysphoric mood.

The distinction between short-lived mood disturbances among healthy children and adolescents and persistent disturbances of mood as signs of a "true" mood disorder, either of a depressive type (unipolar disorder) or a manic-depressive type (bipolar disorder), became recognized in the early 1970s.

Major mood disorders of children and adolescents are characterized by symptoms, signs, treatment approaches, and a guarded prognosis similar to those of adults who have unipolar and bipolar mood disorders.[1,10] Recent longitudinal studies indicate a continuity between juvenile and adult forms of major mood disorders that calls for a heightened medical and public attention to the early signs of mood disturbances and disorders among children and adolescents so that adult morbidity from depression and suicidality can be ameliorated or prevented[5,10,11] (see Chapter 104, Suicidal Behavior in Childhood and Adolescence).

The primary care physician often is called on to evaluate a mood disturbance in a pediatric patient. For instance, is a sad, despairing mood in a grade schooler or in an adolescent an appropriate, adaptive response to a serious loss? Or does the dysphoric mood imply a depressive mood disorder accompanied by suicidal ideation? The evaluation of mood disturbances requires knowledge of normal cognitive and psychosocial development of children and adolescents (see Chapter 51, Theories and Concepts of Development As They Relate to Pediatric Practice) and of the clinical features of juvenile mood disorders.

DEVELOPMENTAL ASPECTS AND CLINICAL MANIFESTATIONS OF MOOD DISTURBANCES AND MOOD DISORDERS

What follows first is a note on depressive states among infants and preschoolers and then a presentation of adjustment disorders with depressed mood, depressive (unipolar) mood disorders, and manic-depressive (bipolar) disorders seen among school-age children and adolescents. Disorders related to organic causes are not included. The diagnostic criteria are those described in the latest edition (1994) of the *Diagnostic and Statistical Manual of Mental Disorders*.[1]

Infants and Preschoolers

Infants and young children have long been known to show sadness, protestation, despair, and physical deterioration as a reaction to separation from their main caregivers.[3] The similar syndromes of "anaclitic depression," "nonorganic failure to thrive," "psychosocial dwarfism," and "reactive attachment disorder of infancy and early childhood" all testify to the devastating effects on physical and psychomotor growth and development that may ensue from young children's separations from their primary caregivers[16] (see Chapter 130, Failure To Thrive). Obviously, these infants and preschoolers cannot verbalize feelings associated with a depressed mood; their countenance, postures, withdrawal, and sparse psychosocial interaction convey the depressive-like sad or empty emotional states. Consistent environmental nurturance and stimuli, encompassing the child's total senses, often result in dramatic improvement in growth and development.

School-Age Children and Adolescents

School-age children usually can recognize and verbalize major states of feelings in themselves, from sad and "blue" to happy and "great." Strides in cause-effect reasoning help them link external events, good or not-so-good ones, with changes in their mood. Observing others—peers as well as adults—allows them to compare with themselves in regard to "showing feelings" and even sharing feelings—the groundwork for the capacity of empathy and caring for others. Finally, their progress at school, in games with peers, and in "arguments" with parents, shape their sense of emerging "self," of self-reliance, and of individuality. Thus the grade-school child is vulnerable emotionally and cognitively to both dysphoric and elated mood states, which at times assume clinical criteria of true mood disorders.

Puberty and adolescence entail developmental strides in biological, psychosocial, and cognitive areas—strides that for centuries have been associated with turbulence and with common onset of major psychiatric disorders. The physiological changes, inducing rapid growth spurt and maturation of sexual organs and functions, pose a new body image to the adolescent and may cause anxiety. Psychosocially, teenagers are struggling to attain independence from their families and to establish a sense of identity in a society that tries to prolong their dependence on family and educational systems. The "breaking away" from the key persons of childhood often is associated with feelings of loneliness and sadness, like being a stranger among one's family.

In terms of cognitive development, the adolescent's

achievement of formal, abstract operational thinking implies an ability for introspection, to reflect on one's own thoughts and mental constructs. Most teenagers tend to overestimate their emotional and intellectual experiences and believe that no one else can understand the uniqueness of *their* "inner life." Their eagerness to construct ideals and ideal persons usually proves disappointing because of the unrealistic qualities assigned to the ideals. Finally, the adolescents' egocentric preoccupation with their many physical and mental changes often is accompanied by their belief and fear that others are as concerned about their new appearance and behavior as they are. These cognitive strides help to explain (1) the vulnerability of teenagers to open or implied remarks about them and (2) their proneness to react with self-derogatory, depressed moods, which often are combined with defensive, irritable attitudes toward family and peers.

MOOD DISORDERS

Adjustment Disorders with Depressed Mood

The most likely mood disorders primary care physicians encounter among pediatric patients are adjustment disorders accompanied by depressed mood. Although their prevalence rate in a general pediatric population is not documented, the rate can be estimated as high because these adjustment disorders are precipitated by common psychosocial stress factors such as loss of a family member or close friend, serious family strife or illness, change of home or school, or a natural disaster. By definition, these disorders do not show a biological, familial origin. However, some children and adolescents may be predisposed constitutionally to respond severely to environmental stressors. Common signs and symptoms of these maladaptive, depressive states are a depressed mood accompanied by feelings of sadness and hopelessness, tearfulness, a drop in academic or vocational performance, loss of interest in usual activities, indecisiveness and poor concentration, withdrawal from family and peers, appetite and sleep disturbances, and brooding over issues of life and death that may include suicidal ideation. These states usually last from 1 to a few months. Some mood disorders in this group do not subside within 6 months. They may then warrant the diagnosis of a more serious disorder, usually a unipolar depressive disorder.

Depressive Disorders

Depressive disorders also are referred to as unipolar disorders because there is no history of manic or hypomanic episodes. Currently, two depressive disorders have well-established diagnostic criteria: dysthymic disorder and major depressive disorder.

Dysthymic Disorder. Dysthymic disorder (or dysthymia) is diagnosed commonly among children and adolescents referred for psychiatric evaluation (a lifetime prevalence of at least 6%). The established criteria for juvenile forms of dysthymia[1] are a depressed mood or irritability (dysphoria; being "cranky") of at least a year's duration, never remitting for more than 2 months at a time, with at least two of the following symptoms present: poor appetite or overeating, sleep disturbance, low energy or fatigue, low self-esteem, poor concentration, and feelings of hopelessness. Dysthymia may be secondary to preexisting psychiatric conditions such as anxiety, attention deficit, substance abuse, or conduct disorders. Serious physical illness also may be associated with secondary dysthymia. The often protracted course of dysthymia carries a risk for superimposed episodes of major depression, self-destructive acts, and alcohol and drug abuse.

Major Depressive Disorder. Often referred to as major depression, major depressive disorder shares all of the diagnostic criteria for dysthymia. However, its signs and symptoms are more acute, dramatic, and functionally impairing. A few criteria have been added for the diagnosis of major depression: diminished interest or pleasure in age-appropriate activities (anhedonia), psychomotor agitation or retardation, feelings of worthlessness or excessive or inappropriate guilt, and recurrent suicidal ideation.[1] Finally, a certain number (five) of the criteria should have been present over at least a 2-week period for a conclusive diagnosis of an "episode" of major depression; an episode often lasts for several months among both pediatric and adult patients.[1]

The severely depressed child or adolescent usually shows a mixture of marked dysphoria, anhedonia, psychomotor and speech retardation, fatigue, indecisiveness, inability to study, sleep and eating disturbances, bouts of feeling worthless and hopeless, suicidal thoughts, and at times delusional, psychotic ideation of nihilism, guilt, disease, and personal "nullness," stupidity, and numbness. *And* the patient is at high risk to want "to end it all" by suicide.

A smaller but "noisy" group of depressed adolescents, temperamentally extroverted, engage in delinquent behaviors, such as truancy, substance abuse and trade, stealing, and sexual promiscuity—behaviors warranting an additional, coexisting diagnosis of conduct disorder, with antisocial traits. The self-destructive implications of such behaviors often are obvious to the teenagers themselves.

Recent surveys suggest a prevalence of major depression among preadolescents of at least 2% and among adolescents of 5%.[7,16] These are conservative rates, as they were based on DSM-IV criteria[1] and formulated on an adult clinical population. However, the symptom profiles of juvenile and adult depressive disorders remain highly similar, with but few exceptions; for example, preadolescents exhibit more somatic complaints and irritability ("crankiness") than do older cohorts.

Reliable studies of prevalence of depressive symptoms among healthy adolescents—those using validated self-rating scales—found rates as high as 30% to 35% for male and about 50% for female teenagers.[11,13] These rates *do not* translate into diagnosable mood disorders. They do confirm, however, that a high minority of North American adolescents admit to depressive features, including suicidal ideation.

There are few well-designed, longitudinal *outcome studies* of treated childhood and adolescent depressive disorders (clinic populations) and of adolescents' self-rated depressive symptoms (general populations). Yet, both types of studies convey a grim outlook: depressive states among children and adolescents become permanent or recurrent conditions for at least 20% to 30% of the subjects, through their adolescence and into adulthood. They also carry a high suicidal risk, compared with nondepressed adolescents, especially when the depressive disorder coexists (is comorbid) with conduct and substance abuse disorders[5,8,12,14] (see Chapter 104, Suicidal Behavior in Children and Adolescents).

MAJOR ETIOLOGICAL FACTORS. The factors known to contribute to major depression in childhood and adolescence can be presented as interacting within a biopsychosocial systems model. This means that youngsters who are at risk biologically for a depressive disorder are the ones most prone to show a depressive response in coping with psychosocial stressors. The biological risks reflect the evidence of genetic loadings for depression on the basis of family and twin studies, as well as on age and gender factors. Major depression rates rise steadily from prepuberty through adolescence and at a faster rate in girls than in boys. A marked psychological arousal within a youngster, caused by psychosocial stress, may influence the activity of CNS-neurotransmitter systems (e.g., adrenergic, serotonergic, dopaminergic) and trigger a behavioral response in the form of a depressive disorder, with somatic manifestations such as appetite and sleep disturbances.[9] The youngster's depression is bound to affect family functioning. Changes in the family's behavior toward its "sick" member often modify the patient's condition by reinforcing or ameliorating it. The outcome might be an alienated, suicidal teenager or a "listened to" teenager open to professional help.

Biochemical evidence of disturbed neurotransmitter systems function in major depression (involving primarily CNS-amines) has been documented in adult patients. Similar investigations of juvenile cohorts are in progress.

ADDITIONAL RISK FACTORS. Since World War II a secular increase has occurred in both juvenile and adult onset of major depression, associated with an earlier age of incidence.[15] This observation, termed a *birth cohort effect,* cannot be explained solely on genetic grounds. Moreover, being a single, adolescent mother who has an infant greatly increases the risk for a maternal depression, which also may cause developmental delay of the infant or toddler.[6] An adolescent mother often feels insecure, lonely, and helpless in her new role, even when she has elected to keep the baby. The child's symptoms and signs may include excessive crying and irritability, feeding and sleeping problems, failure to thrive, and listlessness. In these situations the primary care provider should explain the depressive disorder to the mother, arrange for any necessary psychiatric consultation, and initiate a supportive, educational program for the mother and her child aimed at improving parenting skills and maternal confidence.[2]

Bipolar Mood Disorders

Formerly named "manic-depressive disorders," bipolar mood disorders rarely are diagnosed before puberty. In adolescence the prevalence rate rises to about 1%; adults show the same rate. Gender makes no difference. The common mode of onset in adolescence is a *manic episode* of weeks' to months' duration characterized by a state of euphoric, expansive, irritable mood, associated with many or all of the following features: inflated self-esteem, at times with grandiose delusions, decreased need for sleep, pressured speech, racing thoughts, and high distractibility.[1,7] The patient usually shows poor judgment and engages in idiosyncratic activities such as buying sprees, sexual indiscretions, stealing, elopement, and heavy alcohol and substance use. The latter may serve a self-medicating, calming purpose, at times acknowledged by the patient. Many patients who have a bipolar disorder show "muted" periods of mania, named *hypomanic episodes,* because the symptoms are less severe and neither associated with marked functional impairment nor with delusions, as seen in full-blown manic episodes.

Most manic episodes require hospital admission to protect the youngster from flamboyant, careless, irresponsible behaviors including spending sprees, impulsive journeys, hypersexuality, excessive substance use, and bizarre acts in general. The admission also provides for the initiation of proper psychotropic and psychotherapeutic treatment. Even carefully monitored outpatient treatment cannot prevent recurrences of manic or hypomanic "breakthroughs." Eventually the bipolar nature of the disorder becomes clear, that is, the patient develops a major depressive episode. From then on, yearly cycles of mania and depression may recur, well into adulthood, and require long-term psychiatric management.

Because of many shared symptoms among manic episodes, attention deficit disorders, and conduct disorders, the diagnosis of a bipolar (manic phase) disorder tends to be overlooked. At times a manic episode gets superimposed upon an existing attention deficit disorder and conduct disorder.[4]

Cyclothymia

Cyclothymia is a chronic, cyclic mood disorder of at least 1 year duration for children and adolescents; it is characterized by repeated, alternating periods of hypomania and depressed, dysphoric mood. These episodes are not severe enough to meet the criteria of a bipolar disorder or a major depressive disorder because they interfere only mildly with social and school functioning. Yet clinical evidence shows that juvenile cyclothymia is underdiagnosed and often a forerunner of bipolar disorders developing in adolescence or young adulthood.

EVALUATION AND MANAGEMENT

The primary care physician evaluating a child or adolescent who has depressive or manic features must assess the depth of the mood disturbance and any presence of suicidal intentions. This requires interviewing the patient and the essential family members. The physician should inquire about the youngster's medical and psychosocial history, including child neglect and abuse, individual and family functioning, school performance, and peer relationships. In addition, the following areas should be explored: (1) any recent stressful events that might have precipitated the mood disorder, (2) signs of an organic brain syndrome resulting from central nervous system disease such as HIV infection or substance abuse, (3) the common features of major depression and mania, (4) evidence of past and present suicidal ideation and acts, (5) the possibility of a psychotic state with cognitive impairment, preoccupation with feelings of guilt and worthlessness, and delusions or hallucinations, and (6) signs of hyperactivity, manic excitement, elopement, reckless driving, delinquent acts, and substance abuse.

The physician should discuss the possibility of a mood disorder openly with the patient and inquire about any thoughts of self-destruction. Most dysphoric youngsters are relieved to find that their physician understands their painful state.

A medical evaluation is an integral part of the initial psychiatric evaluation. Somatic problems that may present symptoms similar to those of depression and bipolar illness include medication reactions, endocrine disorders, tumors, and neurological disorders.[16]

At the conclusion of the evaluation, the physician may wish to undertake the psychological counseling of the patient and the parents, provided the following conditions are met: (1) the mood disturbance is an exaggerated, normal type of juvenile mood swings or an acute depressive reaction caused by clearly recognized psychosocial stress factors; (2) the patient, the parents, and the physician all understand the major reasons for the mood disturbance and feel reasonably certain that the youngster is not contemplating suicide or engaged in high-risk behaviors such as running away or substance abuse; (3) evidence is lacking of a major depressive episode, a manic episode, psychotic features, or a conduct disorder; and (4) those in the home and school are able to provide psychosocial support. The first aim of these sessions, usually held weekly, should be to encourage trust in the physician, who then may help the patient examine the reasons for his or her mood disturbance. Whenever feasible, the emphasis should be on its "normality" and adaptive nature and on the patient's available strengths.

A psychiatric referral should be made when the primary care physician finds evidence of a serious major depression or manic disorder that is associated with suicidal behavior or hazardous manic acts or impairs social functioning, school performance, and vegetative functions. The task of the psychiatrist is then to assess the nature and seriousness of the disorder and the suicide risk and decide whether hospitalization is necessary for safety and evaluation. Any need for emergency medical care of a suicidal child or adolescent requires admission followed by psychiatric consultation (see Chapter 104, Suicidal Behavior in Children and Adolescents).

The psychiatrist usually recommends various treatment interventions (at times initiated during an admission). Frequently suggested psychosocial therapies include individual psychodynamic psychotherapy, interpersonal psychotherapy (for depressed adolescents),[11,13] cognitive-behavioral psychotherapy, and family and group therapy (for more information, see Chapter 92, Options for Psychosocial Intervention with Children and Adolescents, and Chapter 93, Consultation and Referral for Behavioral and Developmental Problems).

The indications for pharmacotherapy as an adjuvant to psychosocial therapies are clear in regard to juvenile manic episodes as part of a bipolar disorder. Mania usually responds well to mood-stabilizing drugs such as lithium carbonate. In regard to juvenile depressive disorders, the indications are less clear because still no documented evidence supports that the various antidepressant drugs are efficacious in children and adolescents.[7,11] Yet, most psychiatrists consider a trial with a tricyclic antidepressant or one of the newer serotonergic drugs, preferably after having monitored the youngster's response to one of the psychosocial therapies for several weeks. If the patient remains significantly depressed, based on clinical examination and use of valid rating scales, medication should be initiated. The optimal *and* safe usage of antidepressants and mood-stabilizing drugs requires a psychiatrist to conduct baseline medical workups and close monitoring of therapeutic effects, including a multitude of side effects—some serious, such as cardiotoxicity and seizures. Overdoses with antidepressant drugs by depressed adolescents are fairly common and should be treated as serious medical emergencies.

When a psychiatric referral is made, the primary care physician often can assist in the evaluation because of his or her knowledge of the patient's psychosocial and medical history. The physician may provide follow-up care after the psychiatrist has completed the evaluation and made psychotherapeutic and medication recommendations.

SUMMARY

Major advances have occurred in the recognition of child and adolescent mood disorders. The primary care physician can help identify depressive and manic states and prevent suicidal acts by prompt recognition of juvenile mood disorders and suicidal tendencies. Most adolescent mood disturbances are transient, adaptive, and prepare teenagers for successful mastery of the inevitable losses and disappointments of adult life. The physician-counselor may assume the role of an empathetic listener and supporter who takes an active role in explaining the reasons for the depressive condition and charting new courses for the patient and family. Together, the physician and family often find that most mood disturbances are normative, self-limited crises having a potential to promote the child's psychological and social growth, attainment of self-reliance, and beginnings of adult independence.

REFERENCES

1. American Psychiatric Association: *Diagnostic and statistical manual of mental disorders,* ed 4, Washington, DC, 1994, The Association.
2. Beardslee WR, MacMillan HL: Psychosocial preventive intervention for families with parental mood disorder: strategies for the clinician, *J Dev Behav Pediatr* 14:271, 1993.
3. Bowlby J: *Maternal care and mental health,* ed 2, Geneva, 1951, World Health Organization.
4. Bowring MA, Kovacs M: Difficulties in diagnosing manic disorders among children and adolescents, *J Am Acad Child Adolesc Psychiatry* 31:611, 1992.
5. Fleming JE, Boyle MH, Offord DR: The outcome of adolescent depression in the Ontario child health study follow-up, *J Am Acad Child Adolesc Psychiatry* 32:28, 1993.
6. Green M: Maternal depression: bad for children's health, *Contemp Pediatr* 10:28, 1993.
7. Kashani TH, Eppright TD: Mood disorders in adolescents. In Wiener JR, editor: *Textbook of child and adolescent psychiatry,* Washington, DC, 1991, American Psychiatric Press.
8. Kovacs M, Goldston D, Gatsonis C: Suicidal behaviors and childhood-onset depressive disorders: a longitudinal investigation, *J Am Acad Child Adolesc Psychiatry* 32:8, 1993.
9. Marttunen MJ, Aro HM, Lonnqvist JK: Adolescent suicide: endpoint of long-term difficulties, *J Am Acad Child Adolesc Psychiatry* 31:649, 1992.
10. McCauley E et al: Depression in young people: initial presentation and clinical course, *J Am Acad Child Adolesc Psychiatry* 32:714, 1993.
11. Mufson L et al: *Interpersonal psychotherapy for depressed adolescents,* New York, 1993, Guilford Press.
12. Pfeffer CR et al: Suicidal children grow up: suicidal episodes and effects of treatment during follow-up, *J Am Acad Child Adolesc Psychiatry* 33:225, 1994.
13. Powell JW, Denton R, Mattsson Å: Adolescent depression: effects of

mutuality in the mother/adolescent dyad and locus of control, *Am J Orthopsychiatry* 65:263,1994.

14. Rao U et al: Childhood depression and risk for suicide: a preliminary report of a longitudinal study, *J Am Acad Child Adolesc Psychiatry* 32:21, 1993.
15. Ryan ND et al: A secular increase in child and adolescent onset affective disorder, *J Am Acad Child Adolesc Psychiatry* 31:600, 1992.
16. Weller E, Weller RA: Mood disorders in children. In Wiener JR, editor: *Textbook of child and adolescent psychiatry,* Washington, DC, 1991, American Psychiatric Press.

SUGGESTED READINGS

Brent D: Major depressive disorder. In Peschel E, Peschel R, Howe JW, editors: *Neurobiological disorders in children and adolescents,* San Francisco, 1992, Jossey-Bass.

Lewis M, Cantwell DP, editors: *Child and adolescent psychiatric clinics of North America: mood disorders,* vol 1, no 1, Philadelphia, 1992, WB Saunders.

Weller EB, Weller RA: Mood disorders. In Lewis M, editor: *Child and adolescent psychiatry,* Baltimore, 1991, Williams & Wilkins.

104 Suicidal Behavior in Children and Adolescents

Åke Mattsson

Suicidal behavior includes suicidal acts, suicidal ideation, that is, a preoccupation with self-destructive thoughts, and in some instances self-injurious behavior. Suicide remains the third leading cause of death among the nation's 15- to 24-year-olds, after accidents and homicide. Self-destructive acts also are becoming more common in the 10- to 14-year age group.

EPIDEMIOLOGY

Recent surveys of mortality in the United States show that the country's annual suicide rate from 1980 to 1993 remained at about 12 persons per 100,000 population, with a ratio of four males to one female.[16] In 1992 the total number of deaths caused by suicide was 30,484. Geographically the lowest suicide rates were reported in Washington, DC, New Jersey, and New York and the highest in Nevada, Montana, and Indiana.

Among the pediatric age groups, the 10- to 14-year-olds had a suicide rate of 1.7 per 100,000 in 1992 compared with 0.8 in 1980. Ages 15 to 19 showed a similar increase: from 8.5 in 1980 to 10.8 in 1992 per 100,000 population. Finally, in 1992 the group of 20- to 24-year-olds had a suicide rate of 14.9 per 100,000 compared with 16.1 in 1980.[16]

The distribution of juvenile suicide rates according to gender and ethnicity is markedly higher for boys than for girls at all ages and among all ethnic groups. White adolescents have higher rates than African-American adolescents and adolescents of all other ethnic minorities. Unfortunately the lumping together of our nation's many minorities in mortality statistics fails to document the high suicide rates among Native American youth.

The suicide mortality rates for United States' *total* population has not changed significantly over the past 20 years. It is among the 10- to 24-year-olds that the rates rose sharply. This increase is concentrated in white and black male youth; white and black females show little change in suicide rates.[16]

When compared with suicide rates, the age-adjusted death rates caused by "homicide and legal intervention" show similar figures for most age groups over the past 20 years and actually quite close to the overall suicide rates per 100,000 population.[16] However, 15- to 24-year-old African-American males and females have considerably higher homicide than suicide rates.[16]

The increased availability of firearms during the 1990s has been cited as one major reason for the stark rise in "firearm mortality" among juveniles.[6,9] Federal data from 1992 showed a firearm suicide rate among white and black males, ages 10 to 14, of about 1 per 100,000 population.[16] Among the 15- to 19-year-old white males the rate of firearm suicide was 13.6 per 100,000 population; among black males it was 9.0. White females, ages 15 to 19, showed a firearm suicide rate of 2.1 and black females, a rate of 0.8 per 100,000 population. These figures confirm the clinical evidence of firearms becoming the leading method of successful self-destruction in the United States which in 1992 was chosen by 65% of male and 39% of female suicide victims (all ages).[16] The combination of easy access to firearms and alcohol intoxication looms significantly in the rise of suicide acts among adolescents in the 1990s.[3,9]

No reliable data reveal the number of nonfatal suicide attempts among children and adolescents. Various studies, using different sampling methods, have estimated that about 10% of high school students report at least one suicide attempt; among grade-schoolers, 1% report the same.[9] Among adolescent suicide attempters, girls outnumber boys five to one.

This chapter discourages the use of "suicidal gesture" to denote supposedly "manipulative, not seriously meant" suicidal acts. The primary care physician or mental health worker should examine each instance of child and adolescent self-destructive behavior as a potentially lethal act. Its seriousness of intent often can be known only after a thorough psychiatric evaluation.

CLINICAL AND DEVELOPMENTAL ASPECTS

Suicidal behavior among children and adolescents is a clinical syndrome, reflecting a number of underlying psychiatric disturbances of various seriousness. Even if the rates of suicide and suicidal attempts are low among preadolescent children and even if many of them lack a concept of the finality of death, their suicidal acts and ideation must be taken seriously by their families and health care providers. Preschool children at times mimic their parents' suicidal ideation and behavior as a consequence of their identifying with the parents' anguish and depressed mood. Grade school age children may experience a deep sense of helplessness and hopelessness caused by stressful life situations or psychotic thought derailment, comparable to experiences of adolescents and adults.

Suicidal behavior among adolescents is receiving considerable research attention because of its increasing prevalence, need of prompt medical-psychiatric services, and portent for adult mental health. Several studies of completed adolescent suicides, using "psychological autopsies" based primarily on interviews with persons close to the dead adolescent, have yielded valuable clinical data about adolescent suicides.[5-7,14] In these studies the male-female ratio was about 4 to 1, and the most common means of suicide were the use of firearms, hanging, drug ingestion, and jumping from heights. The prevalent lethal drug was an antidepressant prescribed to a family member. The common site was the juvenile's own home, with about 50% of the victims leaving a suicide note before the act. Major precipitating events were relational conflicts and losses, arguments and fights with relatives and peers, and acute school problems. More long-standing psychiatric risk factors were serious mood disorders, substance abuse, and conduct disorders. A high minority of suicide victims had used alcohol or illicit drugs just before their self-destructive act.

Turning from psychological autopsy studies to general studies of juvenile self-destructive acts, recent reports on suicide methods and their lethality indicate that the use of firearms has taken the lead for both sexes, while hanging is a common means for boys and jumping from heights for girls.[6,9,14] Self-poisoning, especially by drug ingestion, remains a favored suicide method among girls, which may allow for more successful rescue efforts than do violent means of self-destruction. Overdosing with psychotropic medications, such as antidepressants, is a common suicidal method. Action should be taken to monitor closely the availability of potent prescribed drugs in the homes of depressed teenagers.

Most juvenile suicide attempts are impulsive, unplanned acts precipitated by stressful events common to all children and adolescents. These events cause acute anguish accompanied by a wish "to be dead" in those youngsters whose preexisting psychiatric conditions have made them uniquely vulnerable.[6,14] An increasingly common contributory factor is the state of intoxication: the bereft, lonely, or ravingly furious, "not-listened-to" adolescent drinks or drugs himself into a state of cognitive impairment and disinhibition that precludes any rational means at seeking relief.[3,6] Only self-destruction carries a hope for relief.

PREDISPOSING RISK FACTORS

The syndrome of child and adolescent suicidal behavior usually is related to a preexisting psychiatric disorder of the patient. In addition, a family history of mood disorders, suicidal behavior, physical violence, and substance abuse often is present in suicidal youth.[9]

The common preexisting psychiatric disorders[1] are (1) major depression with a pervasive sense of worthlessness and hopelessness accompanied by suicidal ideation, at times associated with delusions of guilt, self-accusation, and deserving punishment; (2) schizophrenic disorders with psychotic features such as paranoid delusions and command hallucinations directing the youngster toward self-destruction; (3) conduct disorders with antisocial acting out often characterized by angry, assaultive, and attention-seeking behaviors where the suicide attempt represents a manipulative, often repeated act[2,14]; (4) substance abuse or dependence[3,6]; (5) borderline personality disorders, especially among female adolescents, who at times show a history of early sexual and physical abuse.[4,9] Conduct disorders alone or coexisting with depressive or substance use disorders have become leading presuicidal disturbances along with primary depressive disorders.[5,14] At times, determining whether a mood disorder preceded the onset of a conduct disorder may be impossible in youngsters who have coexisting (comorbid) psychopathology.

No measurable biological markers have been found to correlate with child and adolescent self-destructive behaviors. Yet, evidence has shown that violent suicidal acts of adult patients are associated with chronically low levels of serotonin metabolites in the spinal fluid.[2,14]

Environmental risk factors for juvenile suicidal acts include the increased availability of firearms in the United States; the "contagion effect" for youth suicidal behavior, usually seen among high school students, where one youngster's suicide attempt seems to trigger other student attempts, at times as part of a self-destructive "pact"[14]; the common media attention to adolescent suicides[9,14]; and the evidence of a post–World War II secular increase in juvenile and adult onset of affective disorders—a birth cohort effect—that seems bound to contribute to rising suicide rates among young age groups[13] (see Chapter 103, Mood Disorders in Children and Adolescents).

EVALUATION AND MANAGEMENT

When alerted to an acutely suicidal pediatric patient reported to have inflicted self-injury, the primary care physician first attends to the patient's physical condition via an immediate office or emergency room assessment (1) of signs of drug poisoning, alcohol intoxication, or other injuries, where the vital signs may require monitoring; (2) evaluation of the patient's sensorium, respiratory and cardiovascular functioning, and fluid and electrolyte balance; (3) request for drug screening and radiographs, as indicated; and (4) initiation of appropriate treatment such as gastric lavage, intravenous fluids, and antidote therapy. The physician should maintain the patient on "suicide watch" and begin to obtain a history of the circumstances preceding the suicide attempt and of the act itself.

As soon as the patient is stable medically, he or she should be interviewed alone or with a family member present by the attending physician. Pediatric patients often are open historians about the reasons for a suicidal act following their "rescue"—even when the "act" was deliberately not serious (e.g., only a few aspirin tablets or verbal threats). Most suicidal acts of children and adolescents, despite their seemingly impulsive nature, represent a "cry for help." The acts have an irrational logic and often result from escalating family dysfunction and inner emotional turmoil, at times of psychotic proportions. During the hours following their "rescue," the patients usually are fairly open about the immediate reasons for their self-destructive attempt and the antecedent psychosocial problems. Thus the attending physician should inquire early about recent and past events and ask about possible motives—what did the patient "have in mind," want to achieve, want to change? In so doing, the physician should listen calmly, be appropriately empathetic, and be nonjudgmental, reassuring the patient about the common occurrence of suicidal ideation and acts among people. Thus, the physician "normalizes" the youngster's suicidal ideation, which often reflects long-standing emotional problems. The physician has initiated a therapeutic course, gained important information to pass on to a psychiatric consultant, and relieved some of the patient's self-blame, embarrassment, and dysphoria.

When the primary care physician has concluded the initial interview and confirmed that the patient remains medically stable, he or she should already have planned the next step in the management of the suicidal patient—the request for a psychiatric consultation. It makes little difference whether the youngster "only" had threatened suicide or actually inflicted self-injury. The physician-in-charge should request expert assistance in determining the seriousness of the patient's self-destructive intent and whether the patient still poses a suicide risk, making hospital admission necessary. In addition, the physician usually requests an evaluation of the patient's possible psychopathology related to a depressive or a conduct disorder, substance abuse, or a highly dysfunctional home environment. Finally, the psychiatric consultant would be expected to recommend further evaluation and psychiatric treatment that might include psychological assessment, individual and family therapy,[8] psychotropic medication, and involvement of school and social agencies. The consultant's recommendations should include arrangement for prompt follow-up appointment for the (nonhospitalized) patient and instruction about telephone access to a psychiatrist in case of renewed acute need. (Chapter 104, Mood Disorders in Children and Adolescents, has suggestions for psychiatric management.)

Outcome and Prevention

Well-conducted follow-up studies of suicidal children and adolescents are scarce and difficult to generalize, because of different sampling methods and lack of standardized assessments. Based on her outcome studies of juvenile suicidality and a review of those of others, Pfeffer[9-11] has suggested that, from a 6- to 8-year follow-up study, prepubertal and adolescent suicidal patients are at high risk for a repeated suicide attempt (up to 10%). However, few completed suicide acts. Marked risk factors for repeated suicide attempts were the presence of a major depressive disorder, substance abuse, and poor social adjustment.[11] The reports by Pfeffer[9,10] and others[12,14] indicate that a severe depressive illness might be a stronger predictor for repeat suicide attempts among young patients than a history of previous attempts.

The major role of the primary care physician in the prevention of suicidal acts among children and adolescents is to recognize and attend to signs of psychiatric disorders—mood disorders, psychotic illness, substance abuse, and conduct disorders in particular.[15] In addition, any evidence of a youngster's poor social adjustment and problems with parents and other key family members should be explored and viewed as potential risk factors for depressive disorders and suicidal ideation and behavior.

REFERENCES

1. American Psychiatric Association: *Diagnostic and statistical manual of mental disorders,* ed 4, Washington, DC, 1994, American Psychiatric Association.
2. Apter A et al: Suicidal behavior, depression, and conduct disorder in hospitalized adolescents, *J Am Acad Child Adolesc Psychiatry* 27:696, 1988.
3. Berman AL, Schwartz RH: Suicide attempts among adolescent drug users, *Am J Dis Child* 144:310, 1990.
4. Brent DA et al: Personality disorder, tendency to impulsive violence, and suicidal behavior in adolescents, *J Am Acad Child Adolesc Psychiatry* 32:69, 1993.
5. Brent DA et al: Psychiatric risk factors for adolescent suicide: a case-control study, *J Am Acad Child Adolesc Psychiatry* 32:521, 1993.
6. Hoberman HM, Garfinkel BD: Completed suicide in children and adolescents, *J Am Acad Child Adolesc Psychiatry* 27:689, 1988.
7. Marttunen MJ, Aro HM, Lonnqvist JK: Adolescent suicide: endpoint of long-term difficulties, *J Am Acad Child Adolesc Psychiatry* 31:649, 1992.
8. Moreau D et al: Interpersonal psychotherapy for adolescent depression: description of modification and preliminary application, *J Am Acad Child Adolesc Psychiatry* 30:642, 1991.
9. Pfeffer CR: Suicide and suicidality. In Wiener JR, editor: *Textbook of child and adolescent psychiatry,* Washington, DC, 1991, American Psychiatric Press.
10. Pfeffer CR et al: Suicidal children grow up: rates and psychosocial risk factors for suicide attempts during follow-up, *J Am Acad Child Adolesc Psychiatry* 32:106, 1993.
11. Pfeffer CR et al: Suicidal children grow up: suicidal episodes and effects of treatment during follow-up, *J Am Acad Child Adolesc Psychiatry* 33:225, 1994.
12. Rao U et al: Childhood depression and risk for suicide: preliminary report of a longitudinal study, *J Am Acad Child Adolesc Psychiatry* 32:21, 1993.
13. Ryan ND et al: A secular increase in child and adolescent onset affective disorder, *J Am Acad Child Adolesc Psychiatry* 31:600, 1992.
14. Shaffer D et al: Preventing teenage suicide: a critical review. *J Am Acad Child Adolesc Psychiatry* 27:675, 1988.
15. Shaffer D et al: The impact of curriculum-based suicide prevention programs for teenagers, *J Am Acad Child Adolesc Psychiatry* 30:588, 1991.
16. U.S. Bureau of the Census: *Statistical abstract of the United States: 1993,* ed 113, Washington, DC, 1993, US Government Printing Office.

105 Runaway Youth

Gerald R. Adams

DEMOGRAPHIC ESTIMATES

In 1976 the National Opinion Research Corp. conducted the largest, most comprehensive study of the problem of runaway adolescents in the United States. This study, the National Statistical Survey on Runaway Youth,[11] was a nationwide probability study of nearly 14,000 households with teenagers. It found that 5.7% of the households surveyed had had at least one runaway incident in 1976. When extrapolated to the general population, this statistic reflects an annual incidence of 985,000 to 1,134,200 episodes.

During the 1980s, Cairns[9] tracked 695 children for 8 years. She reported that 22% of the children in her sample had run away from home; furthermore, 29% of the girls and 41% of the boys had considered running away.

The federal General Accounting Office (GAO) analyzed data on runaways for the years 1985 to 1988 (the data were obtained from the Department of Health and Human Services). The GAO study found that only 35% of boys, but 65% of girls, who run away use federally funded shelters for youths.

From all these studies and statistics we can conclude that 1 in 3 children considers running away, 1 in 5 actually does so, and girls are more likely than boys to use shelter services.

According to the National Statistical Survey on Runaway Youth, those most likely to run away are teenagers 15 through 17 years old (the median age was 16). Additional data from the GAO reveal that 71% of runaways fall in the 10 to 17 age group.[16] Slightly more than half of all runaways were boys. Racial and socioeconomic differences were not apparent, but regional differences were observed. The incidence of runaway behavior tended to be higher in the western and north central states than in northeastern or southern states.

DISTINGUISHING RUNAWAYS FROM THROWAWAYS

In the early 1970s, runaways were considered a homogeneous group.[1] However, several subsequent investigations have established that runaway adolescents are divided into several subtypes. In a study of Colorado youngsters, Brennan, Huizinga, and Elliott[8] identified two broad categories of runaways. One group (class 1) consisted of young people who were not delinquent or particularly alienated. In general, they appeared to be psychologically healthy and had nondelinquent or nondeviant friends. The second group (class 2), in contrast, were delinquent and manifested considerable alienation in their attitudes and behavior. These youngsters experienced considerable conflict with and rejection from their parents, had delinquent peers, manifested school alienation, reported low self-esteem, and behaved deviantly. The class 1 youngsters mostly were temporarily escaping from a conflict-laden home, had unrestrained peer activities without supervision, and tended to be lonely or isolated from their peers. The class 2 youngsters were rejected, rebellious, and unrestrained youths who were labeled negatively and were pushed away from their families.

In 1985 Adams, Gullotta, and Clancy[3] substantiated the theory of multiple types of runaways in a study of runaway youngsters who currently were "on the streets." Runaways were interviewed while still away from home at a YMCA facility that had a shelter program. Three classes of runaways were identified. The first group consisted of runaways who were similar to Brennan's class 1 youths. These youths left home because of family conflict (hostile, confrontative, and unpleasant but endurable), alienation from family, schools, and sometimes peers, and poor social relationships with others. A second group consisted of "throwaways," children who had been encouraged or forced to leave home and were told not to return. A third group were called societal rejects. These youngsters were rejected by their families, their neighborhood and school peers, their teachers, and even the justice and public social services. They lived independently, usually through criminal behavior, and were an integral part of street culture. The "throwaways" and societal rejects were similar to Brennan's class 2 runaways. Very little is documented empirically on class 2 throwaways and societal rejects. Because of the difficulty involved in identifying class 2 youths and obtaining their cooperation, our knowledge base about runaways is limited primarily to information obtained from class 1 youngsters. Allison[6] has provided additional information on classification and an easy to read, comprehensive review of much of the pertinent research on runaway adolescents.

UNDERSTANDING RUNAWAY BEHAVIOR

To speak authoritatively to parents and with adolescents about runaway behavior, medical professionals should be knowledgeable about the typical behaviors, psychological characteristics, social and familial circumstances, and documented negative consequences of running away.

Typical Behavioral Patterns

Reviews by Nye,[12,13] Nye and Edelbrock,[14] Allison,[6] Adams and Munro,[4] and Adams and Gullotta[2] describe the behavioral patterns of runaways similarly. About half of the adolescents who run away do not run far and stay near home. Many stay with friends, relatives, or neighborhood families (sometimes with their parents' knowledge). Most stay away just briefly (overnight absences are most common). Adams and Gullotta[2] estimate that approximately 40% of runaways return home in 1 day and 60% after 3 days. More than 80% return in 1 month or sooner. These researchers also reported that 52% of runaways stay within a 10-mile radius of home; only 18% travel more than 50 miles from home. Fewer than

5% of runaways run away more than three times, and most run away without companions. However, girls are slightly more likely than boys to run away with a partner. There is some evidence that older runaways are likely to travel greater distances and stay away longer. Cairns[9] reports that boys are more likely to run away only overnight or up to 1 week, whereas girls are more likely to run away for extended periods or permanently. Furthermore, although some runaways deliberate over their decision, most do not plan the episode substantially; usually the quick decision to leave is a result of emotional reactions.

Nye and Edelbrock[14] found that more than half of runaways reported their experience neutrally and as relatively noneventful. About 25% reported a positive adventure resulting in a sense of independence and confidence in their ability to survive on their own. Approximately 20% reported negative consequences, with 3% reporting at least one violent experience. According to Nye,[12,13] approximately 40% of runaways returned willingly and on their own initiative. Approximately 20% were found by parents and brought home, and another 20% were returned by the police. The remaining 20% were returned by relatives and friends or by other individuals the family did not know personally.

Psychological Characteristics

The American Psychiatric Association at one time classified the "runaway reaction" as a specific mental disorder. To assess the appropriateness of this decision, Adams and Munro[4] reviewed the numerous investigations comparing youngsters who ran away and those who did not. They concluded that runaways are more likely to have low self-esteem, to show more signs of depression, to feel they had less control over their environment, and to use poor judgment. They also concluded that runaways are more impulsive, easily frustrated, and less tolerant or sustaining of close interpersonal relationships. Allison[6] came to similar conclusions. However, as Walker[17] correctly cautions, we are uncertain whether these psychological characteristics are antecedents or consequences of runaway behavior.

Social and Familial Circumstances

Problems in social and family relationships are important factors in running away. Many forms of evidence indicate problems not only between parents and runaway but also between the parents themselves.[4] Family life generally is tense and conflict laden. Evidence summarized in the National Statistical Survey on Runaway Youth[11] clearly indicated that parents of runaways make few positive comments about their children, have more drinking problems, and physically abuse their children more than do parents of children who do not run away. These same parents are uninvolved in their child's community and school activities, and they show marked problems in communicating with their child. Roberts[15] reports that the severity of family conflict often is associated with an increased probability of physical or sexual abuse.

According to Wolk and Brandon,[18] parents of runaways commonly are unable to supervise effectively. Parents of runaway adolescent boys seem unable to control them, whereas parents of runaway adolescent girls tend to overcontrol and punish their daughters. According to Gottlieb and Chafetz,[10] this inability to supervise effectively tends to result in a long series of confrontations between parents and adolescent. These researchers also found that upon returning home, runaways were likely to face even worse communication problems, which are reflected in increased conflict and withdrawal.[10] According to GAO[16] data, approximately one third of runaways return home from shelters. Another third move into foster care, and the remaining third live in crisis houses, with friends, or in other unstable situations.

NEGATIVE CONSEQUENCES

Runaways leave home for several reasons; contributing factors include psychological characteristics, home environment, school and peer influence, abuse and neglect (particularly for throwaways), and delinquency. Throwaways are considerably more likely to leave for extended periods or even permanently, thus placing themselves at considerable risk, but most runaways return home within 1 to 2 weeks and consider their experience as relatively benign. However, the greater the distance from home and the longer the youngster is on the streets, the greater the risk of negative consequences. Longitudinal research shows that repeat runaways often have violent confrontations with family members and show extremely high levels of alcohol and drug abuse.[6] Young and colleagues[19] have studied the evidence concerning the potential negative consequences for runaway youngsters. Clearly, the risk factors are substantial; they include confrontation with the legal system, substance abuse, coercive sexual behavior, contraction of sexually transmitted diseases (including acquired immune deficiency syndrome [AIDS]), nutritional and general health problems, loss of educational training opportunities, pregnancy, and early parenting. Furthermore, the negative conditions that may have motivated the adolescent to run away are only likely to be exacerbated because tension in the home is likely to increase when the adolescent returns.

Of particular concern to health care providers is the greater likelihood that the runaway will be abusing drugs or will have contracted a sexually transmitted disease. Runaways are more likely to sell drugs to support their own habits, and their potential for addiction is extremely high. Furthermore, the risk of prostitution also is evident. Boyer and James[7] estimate that there are 600,000 prostitutes between the ages of 6 and 16. Most emerge from runaway and abandonment backgrounds. Unplanned pregnancies commonly result from selling sex. Not only does an early pregnancy have negative health consequences for the teenage girl, it also places the newborn at risk for numerous medical problems. Indeed, Young and associates[19] have summarized evidence indicating that children born to young adolescents are at risk of becoming socially maladjusted, commonly manifesting poor peer relationships and a propensity for temper tantrums and impulsivity during their childhood.

A final cautionary note about negative consequences. According to Allison,[6] 61% of youths in shelters are depressed; 24% of shelter users indicate they have made one or more serious suicide attempts; 82% manifest serious psychiatric impairment in their responses on the Achenbach Child Behavior Checklist. Therefore treating runaways must be seen as a potentially volatile and unpredictable situation requiring close observation and supervision during the initial period of crisis.

INTERVENTION SERVICES AND RECOMMENDATIONS

Services for runaway and throwaway youngsters are enmeshed in federal and state statutory definitions of emancipation (see Chapter 4, Legal and Ethical Issues of Pediatric Medicine). Running away is referred to as "functional emancipation" when the departure is undertaken without the benefit of legal maneuvering. In most states, statutory emancipation can occur if the minor is under a judicial order, by marrying, or upon joining the military. When treating a known runaway, most states require either parental permission or contact with a parent after a designated period. Because the laws vary considerably, interested professionals must refer to their state's laws and requirements.

Adams and Adams[5] have suggested a three-phase method for intervening with and treating runaways. The first phase consists of *crisis intervention* and *stabilized placement,* the second involves *supportive counseling* and *assessment,* and the third includes *long-term therapy, education and training, and support services.* The agency (or physician, where appropriate) that first interacts with the youngster should assume responsibility for crisis intervention and initiation of a stabilized placement. Assessment and supportive counseling should be undertaken by local mental health providers. Long-term therapy, education and training, and supportive services should be provided through family and social welfare assistance.

The purpose of crisis intervention is to defuse existing and looming physical, social, and mental crises. The agency that initially accepts responsibility for the care of the youngster should conduct the crisis intervention required. The desired outcome is to resolve immediate crises sufficiently to make stable placement possible. The purpose of stabilization is to provide security, calm the runaway, and ensure assessment of the situation. The assessment should elicit the information necessary to enhance supportive counseling and to determine appropriate long-term treatment and placement. Long-term treatment, education and training, and supportive services should be undertaken to deal with the medical, social, and mental health issues of the youngster. The desired outcome is diminution of runaway reactions, increased skill and coping abilities, and reunion of the adolescent with the family and/or the establishment of alternative care. The National Statistical Survey on Runaway Youth[11] found that few runaways use hotlines to contact their parents; nevertheless, care providers can encourage the youngster to make contact. The current national hotline number is 1-800-231-6946.

REFERENCES

1. Adams GR: Runaway youth projects: comments on care programs for runaways and throwaways, *J Adolesc* 3:321, 1980.
2. Adams GR, Gullotta T: *Adolescent life experiences,* Monterey, Calif, 1983, Brooks/Cole.
3. Adams GR, Gullotta T, Clancy M: Homeless adolescents: a descriptive study of similarities and differences between runaways and throwaways, *Adolescence* 20:715, 1985.
4. Adams GR, Munro G: Portrait of the North American runaway: a critical review, *J Youth Adolesc* 8:359, 1979.
5. Adams PR, Adams GR: Intervention with runaway youth and their families: theory and practice. In Coleman JC, editor: *Working with troubled adolescents,* London, 1987, Academic Press.
6. Allison KW: Adolescents living in "nonfamily" and alternative settings. In Lerner RM, editor: *Early adolescence: perspectives on research, policy, and intervention,* Hillsdale, NJ, 1993, Lawrence Erlbaum.
7. Boyer D, James J: Easy money: adolescent involvement in prostitution. In Weisberg K, editor: *Women and the law,* Cambridge, Mass, 1981, Schuckman.
8. Brennan T, Huizinga D, Elliott DS: *The social psychology of runaways,* Lexington, Mass, 1978, DC Heath.
9. Cairns BD: Emancipation, abdication, and running away: a longitudinal perspective. Paper presented at the biennial meeting of the Society for Research in Child Development, Kansas City, Mo, April 1989.
10. Gottlieb D, Chafetz JS: Dynamics of familial generational conflict and reconciliation, *Youth & Society* 9:213, 1977.
11. National Opinion Research Corporation: National statistical survey on runaway youth, Princeton, NJ, 1976, NORC.
12. Nye IF: Runaways: a report for parents. Extension Bulletin No 0743, Pullman, Wash, 1980, Washington State University.
13. Nye IF: Runaways: some critical issues for professionals and society. Extension Bulletin No 0744, Pullman, Wash, 1980, Washington State University.
14. Nye IF, Edelbrock C: Some social characteristics of runaways, *J Fam Issues* 1:147, 1980.
15. Roberts A: Adolescent runaways in suburbia: a new typology, *Adolescence* 17:387, 1982.
16. US General Accounting Office: Homeless: homeless and runaway youth receiving services at federally funded shelters, Washington, DC, US General Accounting Office.
17. Walker D: Suburban runaway youth in the 1970s. Paper presented at the biennial meeting of the American Psychological Association, Washington, DC, September 1976.
18. Wolk S, Brandon J: Runaway adolescents' perception of parents and self, *Adolescence* 12:175, 1977.
19. Young RL et al: Runaways: a review of negative consequences, *Fam Relations* 32:275, 1983.

106 Adolescent Sexuality

Susan M. Coupey

All of us are born with the capacity for sexual response, but it is only during adolescence that we become conscious of certain thoughts and feelings as being sexual. It is then that we begin to integrate our sexuality as part of our self-concept. Of course, we have developed gender identity as boys or girls much earlier in childhood; however, the sexual specifics of that gender identity, including sexual orientation and behaviors, become clear only during adolescence or young adulthood. Overt expression of sexuality depends on the biopsychosocial environment in which the individual exists. The biological changes of puberty prime the adolescent brain and body for reproduction, while individual and family psychodynamics influence sexual behavior choices. The larger sociocultural environment sets the norms for sexual behaviors and controls them through its institutions (e.g., churches, schools, government, and the media). As adolescents experiment with sexual expression, they inevitably make errors of judgment. Most such errors are minor, but many have significant health consequences.

Sexually transmitted diseases (STDs) are common among sexually active adolescents. Young people who begin to have sexual intercourse in early or middle adolescence are much more likely to develop an STD than are those who postpone intercourse until later adolescence or adulthood (see Chapter 51, Theories and Concepts of Development As They Relate to Pediatric Practice). Some STDs are associated with a high rate of permanent damage to the reproductive tract, especially for young girls. For example, salpingitis caused by *Chlamydia trachomatis* is the leading cause of acquired infertility in women, and genital infection caused by the human papilloma virus can cause cancer of the cervix, vulva, anus, and penis. Infection with the human immunodeficiency virus (HIV) is becoming more prevalent in certain groups of adolescents. Seroprevalence in a national sample of disadvantaged adolescents enrolled in the Job Corps was found to be 3.2/1000 in young women and 3.7/1000 in young men.[12] Unintended pregnancy, with all of the accompanying physical and psychosocial costs of either early parenthood or therapeutic abortion, is endemic in the United States. Among 15- to 17-year-old girls who are sexually experienced, nearly 1 in 5 becomes pregnant each year. For some young people the onset of adolescence stirs up feelings of uncertainty about sexual orientation or reminders of childhood sexual abuse. These psychosocial issues may be associated with significant depression and suicide attempts.

Pediatricians and other primary care providers have an essential role to play in helping adolescent patients maintain their biopsychosocial sexual health (see the box on p. 830). Monitoring pubertal changes and providing anticipatory guidance to adolescents and their parents regarding timing of the growth spurt or onset of menstruation traditionally have been viewed as appropriate tasks for pediatricians. However, with the trend toward sexual intercourse at a younger age, primary care providers now are being called on to provide preventive care related to sexual behavior, such as advising the adolescent about and prescribing contraceptives, screening for STDs, and counseling on issues of sexual orientation and abuse. In addition, because of the high prevalence of health problems stemming from sexual behavior in the adolescent age group, providers must be able to diagnose and manage such conditions as pregnancy, STDs, sexual dysfunction, and sexual victimization. Schools and other community organizations often can benefit from the expertise of health care providers in helping to design sexuality education classes, pregnancy prevention programs, or HIV/AIDS management. This expanded societal role gives clinicians a broader influence on the environment than is possible within the patient-provider-family relationship.

PUBERTAL DEVELOPMENT AND SEXUALITY

In the United States today, girls enter puberty on average at 9 or 10 years of age, reach menarche at age 12½, and achieve full fertility at age 15. Boys enter puberty somewhat later, at 11 or 12 years of age, begin to produce sperm (spermarche) and have their first ejaculation at age 13 or 14, and achieve full fertility at about age 15. Thus by middle adolescence, most boys and girls have completed the biological developmental requirements for reproduction. How do these pubertal changes affect sexuality? Udry and colleagues[14,15] have done a number of studies to elucidate the biosocial factors that contribute to sexual behavior in adolescence. Pubertal development can contribute in at least two ways: first, through hormonal effects on the brain that stimulate the adolescent's sexual interest and behaviors, and second, by changing the adolescent's outward appearance, thus signaling to others the individual's readiness for sexual intercourse (Fig. 106-1). Androgenic hormones primarily are responsible for sexual motivation (libido) in both boys and girls and for the visible pubertal increase in muscle mass in boys. Estrogenic hormones are important for skeletal growth in both sexes and for pubertal breast development and body fat redistribution in girls. Levels of these hormones increase dramatically during puberty. Udry's studies indicate that in developing adolescents, the subjective sexual state and noncoital sexual behavior (e.g., sexual fantasies and masturbation) depend on androgen levels in both boys and girls. Coital behaviors are more complex, however, and are subject to sociocultural influence. A study of the determinants of initiation of coitus among junior high school students (ages 11 to 15) conducted in the 1980s found that the coital behavior of early adolescent boys was highly hormone dependent and not much differentiated by social influences. In multiple regression analysis, once the free testosterone index was entered into the

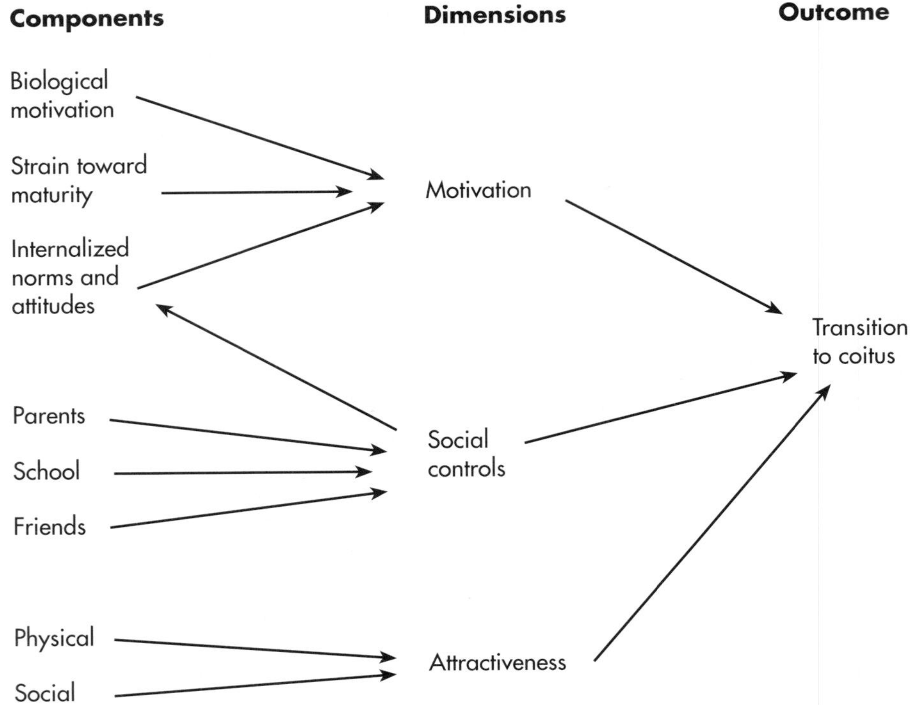

FIG. 106-1 Conceptual model of transition to coitus in adolescence.

(Adapted from Udry JR: Hormonal and social determinants of adolescent sexual initiation. In Bancroft J, Reinisch JM, editors: ***Adolescence and puberty***, The Kinsey Institute Series, vol 3, 1990, Oxford University Press.)

ADOLESCENT SEXUALITY: ROLE OF THE PRIMARY CARE PROVIDER

Anticipatory guidance

Pubertal development
Postponing coitus
Family planning
Safer sex practices
Sexual victimization
Genetic counseling

Preventive care

Screening for sexually transmitted diseases (STDs)
Prescribing contraceptives
Psychological support (sexual orientation and abuse)

Diagnosis, treatment, and referral

STDs
Pregnancy
Sexual dysfunction
Sexual victimization

model for boys, neither age, pubertal development, nor any other hormone added significantly to predicting any sexual variable, including coitus. The coital behavior of the girls, however, was not hormone dependent but was highly differentiated by social influence from diverse independent sources, including pubertal development, friends' behavior, family characteristics, and educational competence.

Adolescents who undergo late pubertal development and those who have lower secretion levels of androgens when fully developed (and thus lower libido) would be expected to respond more readily to social controls aimed at their sexual behavior. Conversely, those who have developed earlier physically and/or have higher postpubertal androgen levels would require different or more intense social controls to influence coital behavior appreciably. Factors shown to be significantly associated with postponing initiation of coitus to later adolescence or adulthood in girls include later pubertal development (menarche after age 13), careful parental supervision, good communication with parents, and high educational aspirations. No such factors have been elucidated for boys. A program devised by Howard and McCabe,[4] "Postponing Sexual Involvement: Educational Series for Young Teens," was used with all eighth grade students in 24 Atlanta city schools and was evaluated in the mid-1980s. The evaluation found that the program was helpful to both boys and girls. By the end of the ninth grade, boys who had not had sexual intercourse before they participated in the program were significantly more likely to postpone sexual involvement than were similar boys who had not participated. This result indicates that boys do respond to educational intervention aimed at helping them control their sexual behavior. Unfortunately, 44% of the eighth grade boys (ages 13 and 14) had already initiated sexual intercourse before the program was given, and they did not benefit from it.

ADOLESCENT SEXUAL BEHAVIOR

Historical Trends

Dramatic changes in the economic and sociocultural environment have taken place in most industrialized countries since the end of the World War II. This period has seen the rise of the middle class, support of the poor through the welfare state, the decline of both the extended family and the nuclear family, a reduction in the influence of religion, a vast increase in the influence of the media, and a huge "baby boom" generation whose members began to reach adolescence in the early 1960s. All these changes have had a profound influence on sexual mores in general and on adolescent sexual behavior in particular. The rising economic status of industrialized countries and improvements in medical science have allowed for better nutrition in pregnant women and children and fewer childhood infectious diseases. These, in turn, are the major causes of the downward trend in the age at which fertility is achieved in both boys and girls. At the turn of the century, the mean age at menarche in the United States was nearly 15 years, with significant socioeconomic differences in timing (wealthy adolescents matured earlier); by 1960 it had declined to about 13 years and now seems to have leveled off at 12½ years, with no significant socioeconomic differences. At the same time that puberty has been occurring at earlier ages, marriage and economic independence have been occurring at older ages. This is partly related to the need for young people to acquire more education in order to function adequately in an increasingly complex society. For young women, the interval between puberty and marriage rose from 7 years in 1890 to nearly 12 years in 1988. A similar phenomenon has occurred for young men. Earlier maturation of adolescents, in addition to looser legal and religious controls over marriage (as seen in the dramatically rising divorce rate), less supervision in the home (single parent families, more women in the work force), and a barrage of sexual imagery in the media, have contributed to a declining mean age at first sexual intercourse and an increasing interval between first intercourse and marriage.

Prevalence of Sexual Intercourse

More than half of adolescents between 15 and 19 years of age have had sexual intercourse. Nearly 20% of young people wait until after their teenage years before beginning to have sex. More boys than girls report being sexually experienced at every age. Over the past 2 decades, the transition to coitus has become more common in the middle adolescent years. According to data collected by the Centers for Disease Control and Prevention (CDC), in 1970 only 4.6% of 15-year-old girls in the United States reported premarital sexual intercourse; by 1988, 25.6% had had premarital sexual intercourse.[6] In that same year, 1988, 33% of 15-year-old boys had experienced sexual intercourse.[11] By age 19, more than 75% of young women and 85% of young men have had intercourse. Recently the CDC began collecting data on high school students through the National Youth Risk Behavior Survey. These data confirm the results of previous studies and indicate that nationally, 40% of high school freshmen (ages 14 to 15 years) are sexually experienced (32% of girls and 49% of boys) (Table 106-1).[10]

Details about the patterns of sexual behaviors among adolescents who have made the transition to sexual intercourse are only beginning to be studied, spurred on by the urgency to design effective AIDS prevention programs. Of adolescents who are sexually active, the overwhelming majority practice serial monogamy; that is, they have only one sexual partner at a time. Nevertheless, those boys and girls who begin having intercourse in early or middle adolescence often will accumulate three to five different sexual partners before they leave their teens. We do not know what percentage of young people have intercourse once or twice and then stop the behavior for months or years. Newer studies indicate that younger adolescents who are unlikely to be living with a sexual partner have intercourse relatively infrequently. For example, sexually active 15-year-old boys report spending an average of nearly 8 months of the year without a sexual partner.[11] Intercourse behaviors other than penile-vaginal intercourse, such as anal or oral intercourse, are less well studied in the adolescent age group, but indications from studies of small nonrepresentative samples are that these behaviors are practiced with some frequency.

Table 106-1 Sexual Behavior among High School Students—United States, 1990*

	All (%)	Boys (%)	Girls (%)
Students who have ever had sexual intercourse			
White	52	56	47
Black	72	89	60
Hispanic	53	63	45
Ninth grade	40	49	32
Twelfth grade	72	76	67
Students who have had sexual intercourse within the past 3 months	39	43	36

*Adapted from *MMWR* 40:885, 1992.

Masturbation

Many adolescents learn about their sexuality and their bodily responses through masturbation. Masturbation is an activity associated primarily with male adolescent sexuality; there is a paucity of information concerning this behavior in girls.

The Sarrels[8] have been gathering data from Yale undergraduates for many years. They noted that in the early 1970s, 33% of young women acknowledged masturbating. In the late 1980s, more than 80% reported this activity, a prevalence of masturbation very similar to that reported by young men at the same college. Admittedly this is a special subset of the young adult female population; nevertheless the trend likely is true for other populations of late adolescents as well. Despite the high prevalence of this sexual behavior, it still is not viewed as a normal, harmless part of sexuality by many adults. This was made dramatically clear by the firing of the U.S. Surgeon General in 1994 for appearing to sanction masturbation. Our culture seems to have an official "erotophobia," while at the same time our daily lives are permeated with erotica in the form of advertisements (e.g., Calvin Klein underwear, Guess jeans), television, popular music, and movies. Many experts in adolescent sexuality education think that to help youngsters control their sexual behavior and avoid premature intercourse, sexual pleasure must be acknowledged.[1] Ways of safely achieving sexual pleasure and satisfying sexual impulses, including masturbation, ought to be addressed by physicians and others who counsel adolescents about sexuality.

Homosexual Behavior

Only in the past few years have any systematical studies tackled the issue of sexual orientation in adolescence, although it always has been known that a portion of the population, variously estimated at between 2% and 10%, grow up to be homosexual adults (see Chapter 100, Homosexuality: Challenges of Treating Lesbian and Gay Adolescents). In 1986 and 1987 a representative sample of junior and senior high school students in Minnesota responded to survey questions pertaining to sexual attraction, fantasy, behavior, and affiliation.[7] Overall, 1.1% of students described themselves as bisexual or homosexual, and 10.7% were unsure of their sexual orientation. Boys were significantly more likely than girls to label themselves as "mostly" or "100%" homosexual. As would be expected, uncertainty about sexual orientation gradually diminished with increasing age, from 26% of 12-year-olds to 5% of 18-year-olds, with corresponding increases in heterosexual and homosexual affiliation. Nearly 5% of students reported homosexual attractions, but only 1% reported such behavior. Boys were more likely than girls to report homosexual behavior (1.6% versus 0.9%), and the prevalence of homosexual behavior increased with increasing age in boys, from 0.4% at age 12 to 2.8% at age 18. These data do not support the widely held concept that homosexual behavior is common among early adolescent boys and gradually diminishes with age. Rather, the opposite may be true—that there is a gradual unfolding of sexual orientation during adolescence and that the behavior follows the awareness of homosexual attraction.

Much less is known about the adolescence of lesbian women. The pathways by which girls develop a same-sex sexual orientation are more diverse than those of boys. Girls tend to develop a homosexual identity at an older age than boys, often not until young adulthood or even later. Because of the severe social stigma associated with homosexuality, homosexual adolescents frequently are under considerable psychological stress, and as many as 30% of gay adolescent boys attempt suicide. Initial parental reaction to disclosure of a teenager's homosexuality usually is negative. Families often need help in adjusting to the news and grieving for their lost "ideal" heterosexual child.

Sexual Victimization

Both adolescent boys and girls who have been victims of forced sex, either as young children by an adult perpetrator or as adolescents on a date or by a stranger, have higher rates of health risk behaviors as well as mental health problems. Large surveys of high school students regularly show 5% to 10% of students reporting sexual abuse. A prior history of sexual abuse in these nonclinical samples correlates significantly with young age at onset of voluntary sexual intercourse, unintended pregnancy, suicide attempts, drug and alcohol abuse, eating disorders, and violence.[5] The younger a sexually experienced girl, the more likely she is to have had forced sex. Seventy-four percent of girls who had intercourse before age 14 and 60% of those who had sex before age 15 report having had forced sex.[9] Sexual abuse always should be considered a diagnostic possibility when an adolescent has very early onset of sexual intercourse and/or has multiple behavioral problems.

Sexual Dysfunction

Sexual dysfunction is an area not well studied in adolescence, although the prevalence in both boys and girls probably is quite high. Clinical reports indicate that many sexually active adolescent girls do not enjoy sexual intercourse and have never had an orgasm. Reasons for engaging in the behavior have more to do with intimacy and closeness to the partner than with personal sexual gratification.[2] Some girls who are anxious and unsure about sexual activity or who have previously been abused develop vaginismus. Large numbers of adolescent boys are thought to have premature ejaculation, but they rarely complain of the problem. Impotence does occur in adolescence, most often due to "performance anxiety" and other psychogenic causes.[3] Heavy alcohol or marijuana use can be responsible for erectile dysfunction and should be explored in the medical history. Prescription medications often are implicated in erectile dysfunction in men and anorgasmia in women. Frequent offenders in this regard are antihypertensives, antipsychotics, and antidepressants.[13] Other drugs that cause sexual dysfunction and that may be taken by adolescents are cimetidine, ranitidine, sulfasalazine, and some anticonvulsants.

ADOLESCENT SEXUALITY AND THE PATIENT-PROVIDER-PARENT RELATIONSHIP

Even though sexual feelings and behaviors are of great concern to adolescents and their families and adverse effects of sexual behavior are common in this age group, most patients and parents will not introduce the subject at the health care visit. Primary care providers must set the stage for frank, honest discussions of feelings and behaviors that often are embarrassing, shameful, and psychologically painful. Setting the stage requires that the provider pay particular attention to privacy for both adolescent patients and parents. A seemingly innocuous question directed to the teenager when her mother is still in the room about whether she has had sex can significantly erode the patient's confidence that the provider understands the private nature of this subject. It would be equally inappropriate to ask the mother about her own sexual behavior in front of her daughter. Asking questions that do not make assumptions or presuppose certain behaviors is difficult but well worth the trouble because adolescents are more likely to disclose closely guarded information when interviewed in this way. For example, if the physician assumes that everyone is heterosexual and asks girls if they have a boyfriend and boys if they have a girlfriend, adolescents who are questioning their sexual orientation or who know they are homosexual will be unlikely to offer this information. If, on the other hand, the question asks about sexual attraction to women, men, or both men and women or includes a gender-neutral term, such as "sexual partner," the patient is more likely to understand that the provider is ready to hear nontraditional information.

In interviewing adolescents about sexual issues, it is a mistake to assume that just because a question has been asked and answered, the full story has been told. Eliciting a history of sexual abuse is a case in point. As part of their screening sexual history many physicians and nurses ask a question such as "Have you ever been sexually abused?" or "Has anyone ever done anything to you sexually that you didn't want them to do?" There is nothing wrong with these questions, but some adolescents who have been abused will answer them in the negative. They are afraid to disclose painful secrets because they have not yet developed a secure, trusting relationship with the health care provider. It is important to understand this, not to push too hard too soon for disclosure, and to explore the topic in more depth at a later visit when the relationship has had a chance to develop.

Negotiating confidentiality between adolescents and parents around sexual issues is another thorny area for the patient-provider-parent relationship. In general, the medical interview with the adolescent should take place in private. When a problem is diagnosed, the specifics of what will be disclosed to parents need to be negotiated with the patient. Providers should refuse to lie to parents; this sets a bad example and is unprofessional. However, it usually is not necessary to disclose all the details of the situation. For example, a 16-year-old girl is being seen for her annual checkup and the screening sexual history reveals that since the previous year's examination, she has become sexually active. She reports that she has had two partners in the past 8 months. She complains of a slight vaginal discharge. The clinician does a pelvic examination as part of the physical examination and discovers a mucopurulent cervicitis, most likely due to a sexually transmitted infection. Appropriate antibiotics are prescribed. What should the mother be told? Most adolescents would agree to allow the physician to tell the mother that a pelvic examination was done because of a vaginal discharge and that he or she thinks that it is a minor infection that will clear up with antibiotics. The clinician can tell the adolescent beforehand that if the mother asks directly whether the infection is sexually transmitted, she will be told that information about her daughter's sexuality is kept in confidence. However, the adolescent patient should know that the physician will encourage her mother to speak to her about her sexual behavior. The clinician must resist acting as a go-between in the mother-daughter relationship, and he or she must emphasize the necessity of direct communication between parent and child.

SUMMARY

Providing health care related to adolescent sexuality is one of the more difficult tasks of the primary care clinician. It demands in-depth knowledge of pubertal and psychosexual development, familiarity with the norms of adolescent sexual behavior, knowledge of pertinent gynecological and urological medicine, and superior communication skills. Adolescents are in great need of this type of care and are very appreciative when it is done well; the large majority of them want to be sexually healthy and eventually to have children and raise healthy families themselves.

REFERENCES

1. Brick P: Toward a positive approach to adolescent sexuality, *SIECUS Report* 17:1, 1989.
2. Cohen MW: Adolescent sexual activity as expression of nonsexual needs, *Pediatr Ann* 24:324, 1995.
3. Farrow JA: An approach to the management of sexual dysfunction in the adolescent male, *Sexually Active Teenagers* 2:39, 1988.
4. Howard M, McCabe JB: Helping teenagers postpone sexual involvement, *Fam Plann Perspect* 22:21, 1990.
5. Nagy S, Adock AG, Nagy, CN: A comparison of risky health behaviors of sexually active, sexually abused, and abstaining adolescents, *Pediatrics* 93:570, 1994.
6. Premarital sexual experience among adolescent women: United States, 1970-1988, *MMWR* 39:929, 1991.
7. Remafedi G et al: Demography of sexual orientation in adolescents, *Pediatrics* 89:714, 1992.
8. Sarrel LJ, Sarrel PM: Sexual unfolding, *J Adolesc Health Care* 2:93, 1981.
9. Sex and America's teenagers, The Alan Guttmacher Institute, New York, 1994, p 28.
10. Sexual behavior among high school students: United States, 1990, *MMWR* 40:885, 1992.
11. Sonenstein FL, Pleck JH, Ku LC: Levels of sexual activity among adolescent males in the United States, *Fam Plann Perspect* 23:162, 1991.
12. St Louis ME et al: Human immunodeficiency virus infection in disadvantaged adolescents: findings from the US Job Corps, *JAMA* 266:2387, 1991.
13. Drugs that cause sexual dysfunction: an update, *Med Lett Drugs Ther* 34:73, 1992.
14. Udry JR: Hormonal and social determinants of adolescent sexual initiation. In Bancroft J, Reinisch JM, editors: *Adolescence and puberty,* The Kinsey Institute Series, vol 3, New York, 1990, Oxford University Press.
15. Udry JR, Billy JO: Initiation of coitus in early adolescence, *Am Soc Rev* 52:841, 1987.

SUGGESTED READINGS

Bancroft J, Reinisch JM, editors: *Adolescence and puberty,* The Kinsey Institute Series, vol 3, New York, 1990, Oxford University Press.

Brooks-Gunn J, Furstenberg FF Jr: Adolescent sexual behavior, *Am Psychol* 44:249, 1989.

Coupey SM, Klerman LV, editors: Adolescent sexuality: preventing unhealthy consequences, *Adolescent medicine: state of the art reviews,* vol 3, Philadelphia, 1992, Hanley & Belfus.

107 Adolescent Pregnancy and Parenthood

Catherine Stevens-Simon and Elizabeth R. McAnarney

The true incidence of adolescent pregnancy in the United States is unknown, but it is estimated that each year more than 1 million adolescents, or approximately 1 of every 10 American teenage girls, are diagnosed as being pregnant. Studies suggest that approximately half of these young women give birth, 40% obtain abortions, and the remainder miscarry.[12] There is no way to determine how many teenage pregnancies terminate in spontaneous abortion without the teenager's knowledge. Thus many more than a million teenage pregnancies occur each year. In 1992 girls under age 20 gave birth to 517,635 infants; 12,220 of these infants were born to mothers under 15 years of age.[12]

From the mid-1970s to the mid-1980s, births to young women under age 20 declined in number and rate, but thereafter began to rise again. For 15-, 16-, and 17-year-olds, the birth rate reached an all-time high in 1991 of 30.7 per 1000, then fell slightly to 30.1 in 1992, the last year for which these data were available.

Table 107-1 shows these changes for 15- to 17-year-old young women by race and marital status. Of note is the fact that the percentage of Caucasian adolescents who have birth out of wedlock rose from 47.1% in 1980 to 71.8% in 1992, whereas the percentage among African-Americans remained constant over this period at 95.9%.

During the past 3 decades we have substantially increased our understanding of the risks associated with adolescent childbearing. Although vital statistical data still indicate that infants born to very young adolescent mothers (those under age 16 at conception) are significantly more likely to be of low birth weight and to die during the first year of life than are infants born to older mothers, evidence is minimal that this is causally related to the physiological immaturity of the young adolescent mother.[15] Rather, most investigators now believe that most of the medical risks associated with adolescent childbearing reflect the fact that young adolescent mothers are significantly more likely to encounter adverse social environments than are older mothers. Indeed, studies that control for potentially confounding psychosocial factors such as poor health habits (e.g., late prenatal care and substance abuse), poverty, and psychosocial stress find no association between young maternal age and most of the obstetrical complications traditionally associated with adolescent childbearing.[10,15]

Nevertheless, adolescent pregnancy has become a source of increasing social, economic, and political concern in this country because of substantial evidence that early childbearing seriously jeopardizes the life chances of most young parents and their children.[2,3,11] The results of studies conducted over the past 30 years suggest that by limiting the educational achievements and vocational opportunities of successive generations, adolescent childbearing both contributes to the impoverishment of one of the most socioeconomically disadvantaged segments of American society and promotes intergenerational transmission of this socioeconomic disadvantage.[2,3,11]

It is not possible to prove that adolescent childbearing and poverty are causally related because studies of the sequelae of adolescent childbearing invariably are confounded by personal characteristics and environmental conditions known to predispose nulliparous adolescents to school failure and welfare dependency. However, current data suggest that few adolescent parents are prepared adequately to assume the economic, social, and psychological responsibility of child care and child rearing.[2,3,11] Many recent reports indicate that over the past 2 decades the increased availability of alternative schools that have day care and flexible hours has enabled an increasingly large number of adolescent parents to obtain a high school education, to overcome economic and social barriers, and to become productive members of their communities. The numerous psychosocial problems still associated with youthful childbearing, however, challenge the concept that adolescent childbearing is a culturally adaptive response to socioeconomic and political disadvantage.[2-4,11]

Teenagers' ability to care for their offspring effectively has become the subject of investigation during recent years. Even though some professionals think that adolescents are more likely than adults to abuse their children, the data supporting this contention are far from conclusive. Some professionals are more concerned about adolescents' passive neglect of their children, a more benign neglect caused by their lack of child rearing experience and ability to think causally, rather than by active, aggressive abuse.

Current investigations of adolescents as parents are focusing on (1) adolescent mother–infant interaction during the neonatal period and subsequently during the first year of the child's life; (2) adolescent fathers—their strengths, needs, and behavior toward their children; (3) the intellectual, social, and emotional development of the children of adolescents; and (4) intervention programs for adolescent mothers and the effects of these programs on their offspring. These investigations will take time to complete because a methodology must be developed to study the many variables other than age that affect parenting, such as the adolescent's socioeconomic status, marital status, parity, educational level, and child rearing experience.

PSYCHOSOCIAL REASONS ADOLESCENTS BECOME PREGNANT

Teenagers become pregnant for many reasons, some conscious and some subconscious. The circumstances are unique for each individual. Although only a minority of young Americans actually state that they wish to become pregnant, many more clearly are ambivalent about postponing child-

Table 107-1 Recent Birth Rates* for 15-, 16-, and 17-Year-Olds by Race and Marital Status

	All births			Births to unmarried mothers					
Year	All	Caucasian	African-American	All	% of all births	Caucasian	% of all Caucasian births	African-American	% of all African-American births
1980	32.5	25.5	72.5	20.6	63.4	12.0	47.1	68.8	94.9
1985	31.0	24.4	69.3	22.4	71.0	14.5	59.4	66.8	96.4
1990	37.5	29.5	82.3	29.6	78.9	20.4	69.2	78.8	95.7
1991	38.7	30.7	84.1	30.9	81.7	21.8	71.0	80.4	95.6
1992	37.8	30.1	81.3	30.4	80.4	21.6	71.8	78.0	95.9

Adapted from National Center for Health Statistics: Advanced report of final natality statistics, 1992. Monthly vital statistics report, suppl 43, no 5, Hyattsville, Md, Public Health Service, 1993.
*Birth rate = number of births per 1000 women in each category (age group, Caucasians, African-Americans, unmarried status).

bearing. The results of a study of 200 teenagers who had never been pregnant, recently conducted in Denver, revealed that even though only 10% of the young women seeking routine health care in the city's teen clinics openly admitted that they wanted to become pregnant, 40% said they "wouldn't mind being pregnant."[13] Other investigators have substantiated these findings among many American teenagers.[9,17] The results of these studies are a matter of concern because they have been consistent in showing that young women who have ambivalent feelings about postponing childbearing are significantly less likely than their peers to use contraceptives and therefore are at greater risk for conception. Indeed, one study reported recently that when adolescents in the third trimester of pregnancy were asked "Why weren't you using birth control before you got pregnant?" the most frequent reply was "I didn't mind getting pregnant."[6] Thus it is imperative that we gain a better understanding of the reasons why so many American teenagers "don't mind" or want to get pregnant.

An extensive body of literature exists concerning the antecedents of adolescent pregnancy. Some young people seek pregnancy to escape from intolerable home or living situations; others seek it as part of a complex pattern of "problem behaviors" to defy parental authority. Still others may wish to become pregnant because their early sexual experiences have raised concern about their ability to conceive, and some adolescents may seek pregnancy as a rite of passage, particularly if they are doing poorly in school or living in impoverished social environments in which adolescent pregnancy is rampant and adult roles, other than parenthood, are perceived to be inaccessible.[5,7,8]

Pregnancy may be the teenager's way of trying to resolve acute or chronic depression. Acute, reactive depression may result from the loss of a loved one (parent, grandparent, or caring relative) through death, separation, divorce, or a move. The teenager may conceive in an attempt to replace the individual who has been removed from her life.

Chronic, unresolved depression may precede the pregnancy by some years. A series of problems starting in childhood (e.g., poor school attendance, running away, suicidal behaviors, or drug overdoses) may precede pregnancy. New data indicate that young women who report problem behaviors are more likely to have a child before age 19 than women who report no problem behaviors. Pregnancy, like the other behaviors, reflects the girl's chronic inability to resolve her depression. For example:

Jeannie, a 13-year-old, was 6 months pregnant when she initially was seen in the clinic. Her widowed mother worked outside the home to keep Jeannie and her two older siblings together at home. Jeannie had a history of absenteeism and withdrawn behavior at school. When she was 12 years old, she had run away and was returned to her mother by the authorities. In the year before conception, she had gone to the emergency department of the local hospital twice, the first time with acute alcoholism, the second time after a suicide gesture. Evaluation of Jeannie during the last emergency department visit revealed a depressed teenager who stated that she had been sad for as long as she could remember.

Jeannie's history indicates that she had been chronically depressed for several years and that her numerous attempts to gain attention had failed. Her history of school absenteeism, running away, alcohol ingestion, suicide gestures and, finally, pregnancy suggested a long history of unresolved depression.

Peer pressure may be another important reason some teenagers become pregnant. Peer pressure for boys may come from friends of the same sex and for girls from friends of the opposite sex. For example:

Carrie, a 15-year-old, became pregnant during the same time period as three of her classmates. She was unable to say why she had become pregnant. The four girls often had talked about having babies. Carrie's boyfriend had not wanted her to use birth control pills, and he was pleased when she told him of the pregnancy.

Pregnancy and parenthood may represent positive accomplishments for teenagers who have experienced few. For example:

Beth, an 18-year-old school dropout, had a history of school problems and also had few friends. When she was told that she was pregnant, she was very happy. During the last trimester of pregnancy, she began to talk about her baby and all she expected it would be able to do. After the baby was born, she brought her proudly to the clinic to show her to the other pregnant girls. One year later, she still talked with great pride about the baby and was trying to become pregnant again. Beth saw her child as her first real achievement and was seeking greater achievement through a second pregnancy.

In some families an adolescent is encouraged to become pregnant either through overt approval of the young woman's sexual activity or through indirect encouragement. Still other teenagers become pregnant as a direct confrontation of parental authority or as a way of showing their growing independence. The need to show independence may be most particularly intense for middle adolescents (15 to 17 years old) because they normally are in the midst of struggling for their independence and thus may be most threatened if it is challenged. Adolescents' ignorance about their sexuality and their potential for becoming pregnant also are contributing factors in teenage conception. Although some adolescents are misinformed about the details of sexuality, contraception, and pregnancy, ignorance about coitus possibly resulting in pregnancy contributes to only a limited number of teenage pregnancies.

DIAGNOSIS OF PREGNANCY

The diagnosis of teenage pregnancy poses problems for both the adolescent and the practitioner that usually do not occur with adults. Teenagers concerned about being pregnant initially may hesitate to seek help from their primary care physician. The physician may find it difficult to talk with pregnant teenagers about confidentiality, sexuality, and pregnancy if he or she and the adolescent have not discussed these topics before the pregnancy. In pediatric settings where these issues have been raised before the teenager seeks care for pregnancy, few problems arise between physician and adolescent.

Pregnant girls raise their concerns to the physician in several ways. Some (often older adolescents) who have achieved formal operational thinking state they think they may be pregnant. Others, particularly younger teenagers, may complain of vague, somatic symptoms, such as headaches, abdominal pain, or joint pains, when their real concern is pregnancy. Still others expect the physician to guess that they are pregnant and do not indicate that pregnancy even is a possibility. This belief in the physician guessing that they are pregnant may represent the magical thinking of some adolescents. If a reproductive history is included in the general history-taking procedure for all teenage women, the physician will be able to move easily into the question of pregnancy in a situation such as the one just described. Questions about the menstrual cycle, including last menstrual period (LMP) and menstrual irregularities, should be incorporated into the reproductive history. Questions about previous pregnancies, contraceptive use, sexually transmitted diseases, particularly acquired immune deficiency syndrome (AIDS), and tampon use also should be included. If pregnancy is possible, the teenager should be asked whether she may be pregnant. Most teenagers are relieved to have the question of pregnancy raised. The physician should then decide how much of the pregnancy evaluation he or she will do and when the teenager will be referred for obstetrical care.

Confirmation of pregnancy clearly is within the role of the primary care physician. In addition to the medical and reproductive history, symptoms of pregnancy should be explored; a physical examination that includes a pelvic evaluation should be performed. Unless the pregnancy is well advanced, a pregnancy test is needed to confirm the diagnosis. Serum pregnancy testing may be necessary if there still is question after the urine screen. Urine tests for pregnancy are sensitive enough to give accurate results 6 to 8 days after conception. Laboratory screening is endorsed because many teenagers inaccurately report their LMP.

When pregnancy has been diagnosed, the teenager should be referred to a special program for pregnant adolescents, if one is available. If not, the teenager can be referred to a private obstetrical office or clinic. The primary care physician then may choose to continue seeing the teenager for counseling and education throughout her pregnancy. Practitioners who have good counseling skills and knowledge of pregnancy options also can be involved in abortion or adoption counseling. Referral to agencies providing these services also is appropriate.

COUNSELING PREGNANT TEENAGERS

Counseling in the practitioner's office might concentrate on the discussion of immediate considerations, such as the course of the pregnancy, labor, and childbirth, as well as on future considerations—the effects of the pregnancy on education, vocation, and finances. Every effort should be made to work with the adolescent father-to-be if he and his partner still are in contact.

Some discussion should be directed toward the circumstances under which the teenager became pregnant and how she and her partner feel about the pregnancy. Problems may include the academic future for both, as well as the possibility of finding day care and money for day care for their child. Finances are a major concern for most teenagers, and referral to the appropriate social service agency often is helpful.

Group counseling provides an effective method of communication with and education for teenagers. If there are two or more pregnant adolescents in one practice and the health professional is knowledgeable about group processes, group counseling can be provided.

An unstructured format for groups is optimal because it allows adolescents to choose the subjects to be discussed and to exert some control in that setting. Both tasks are consistent with the developmental tasks of adolescence. Significant others, such as parents, husbands, boyfriends, or labor coaches, also can attend, allowing the group leader to help these people reorder their relationships, a task similar to altering relationships when a new baby is added to the family.

Because some teenagers are not developmentally at the level of formal operational thinking, techniques traditionally used in adult groups need modification. For example, rather than presenting didactic information on a particular subject, role playing provides an experience that teenagers enjoy. Although adolescents need to consider concrete, nonthreatening information at first, they soon become aware of their personal feelings about the meaning of pregnancy and are able to express these as the group process progresses. Although they may be unable to label their emotions abstractly, they can discuss their feelings by describing the thinking or behaviors of others. Written materials, videotapes, and movies at developmentally appropriate stages can be most helpful. Within groups, teenagers can learn to solve problems, resolve conflicts with their parents, clarify their independent, individual identities, and plan for their future.

POSTPARTUM CARE

Adolescents who become pregnant are at high risk for a repeat pregnancy during adolescence. Preventing repeat adolescent pregnancies is critical because current data indicate that the risk of adverse neonatal and maternal outcomes increases with subsequent pregnancies in this age group.[14] A major goal in providing care to teenagers during pregnancy is preparing both partners for responsible planning of their reproductive future. Ideally, responsibility for contraception after the first pregnancy is shared by both partners.

Adolescent contraception imposes many problems that do not diminish once the baby is born. Circumstances that were present before and that contributed to the initial conception may still exist, even though some teenagers are motivated to prevent a second pregnancy. Contraceptive failure caused by noncompliance in taking pills or sporadic or improper use of condoms or foam, as well as barriers to the use of these inherent in the health care system, may continue to be particular problems for teenagers seeking effective contraception.

Norplant (a subdermal implant of levonorgestrel) and Depo-provera (an injectable hormonal contraceptive agent) are particularly attractive to health care workers who provide contraceptive care to adolescents because they require less active patient participation to remain effective and thus help to bridge the gaps in contraceptive vigilance that can be created by a painful break-up with an old boyfriend or the acquisition of a new boyfriend who wants a child.[16]

For young people at risk for AIDS, special emphasis should be placed on counseling and education about condom use. The primary care practitioner may decide to assume the responsibility for contraceptive education and for prescribing birth control for adolescent parents.

TEENAGERS AS PARENTS

Teenage parents face numerous problems. Although often experienced in baby-sitting, teenagers are not prepared for the reality of round-the-clock child care. Adolescents may expect to have complacent babies who eat and sleep with regularity; they may become disillusioned easily when the child demands far more time and effort than they are prepared to give.

The attitudes of adolescent mothers suggest that they use physical punishment for discipline and have a minimal understanding of the need for stimulation. Although these attitudes may reflect sociocultural influences rather than the mother's age, professionals should be aware of this issue. Most teenagers are fond of children, want to be good parents, and are eager to learn about child rearing.

Adolescent parents frequently live with their own parents or other family members. Observing the efficiency with which their relatives care for the child may add to their own lack of confidence. The adolescents' reaction may be to give up parenting and relinquish this task to other caretakers in the home. The child, in turn, may become confused and have difficulty forming a bond with his or her own parents and may not even identify them as the actual parents. Simply teaching about child care and role modeling can help the adolescent parent. Home visits are an effective way to observe the teenage parents with the baby and help them in the care of the infant.

Many teenagers expect their baby to fulfill their own needs for love immediately and are disappointed when the infant does not respond as they had expected. Data indicate that younger adolescent mothers are less accepting of, cooperative with, and accessible and sensitive to their children during the first postnatal year than are older adolescent mothers. For example, a teenager may think her crying baby will be immediately comforted when picked up. If the infant does not respond as anticipated, the young mother may feel rejected and unloved by her child. However, with time and patience, teenagers can be taught about the needs of infants and the variety of responses that meet those needs.

Adolescent fathers who want to be actively involved with the rearing of their children should receive the same support as adolescent mothers. However, new data indicate that most adolescent boys are ill-prepared for fatherhood. In one recent study,[1] academic, drug, and conduct problems were significantly more common among adolescent fathers than among boys in general. Teenage fathers may choose to relieve the mother of total responsibility for their child by being available to provide care when the mother needs time for her education, job, or other activities. Even if the adolescent father is not available personally, he may want to ask members of his extended family to provide direct help and support for the mother.

Mixed feelings about parenthood are appropriate for teenagers. They want to be good parents and to love their children, but they also want to engage in normal teenage activities. It is important for the practitioner to remember that teenagers need to gain knowledge and expertise to fulfill their role as parents and also need to move through the adolescent period in concert with their peers. Often families will need help in effecting an appropriate balance for the adolescent mother and father between their duties as parents and their peer, school, and social activities.

LONG-TERM FOLLOW-UP

Data from a long-term follow-up study in Baltimore indicate that women who became mothers as adolescents may actually finish their education and become independent of welfare assistance. In a 17-year follow-up of a group of poor, inner city adolescents, 67% of the group had obtained their high school diplomas and 35% had graduated from college or had taken some postsecondary courses. Only 12% of those who went on welfare assistance during the first 5 years of the study continued to be on assistance nearly 2 decades later.[2]

SUMMARY

Even though fewer adolescents than in the past are choosing to become pregnant or to continue their pregnancies (primarily because of the availability of contraception and abortion), the ability of teenagers to care for their children effectively still is an area in which intensive investigation is needed. However, some professionals who have worked with adolescent parents are impressed by their strengths and their ability to learn how to be effective parents when they receive adequate instruction.

REFERENCES

1. Elster AB, Lamb ME, Tavare J: Association between behavioral and school problems and fatherhood in a national sample of adolescent youths, *J Pediatr* 111:932, 1987.

2. Furstenberg FF, Brooks-Gunn J, Morgan SP: Adolescent mothers and their children in later life, *Fam Plann Perspect* 19:142, 1987.
3. Furstenberg FF: Teenage childbearing and cultural rationality: a thesis in search of evidence, *Fam Relations* 41:239, 1992.
4. Geronimus AT: Teenage childbearing and social disadvantage: unprotected discourse, *Fam Relations* 41:244, 1992.
5. Jessor R: Risk behavior in adolescence: a psychosocial framework for understanding and action, *J Adolesc Health* 12:597, 1991.
6. Kelly L et al: Why pregnant adolescents say they didn't use contraceptives prior to conception, *J Adolesc Health* 1994.
7. Klerman LV: Adolescent pregnancy and parenting: controversies of the past and lessons for the future, *J Adolesc Health* 14:553, 1993.
8. Levinson R: Contraceptive self-efficacy: a perspective on teenage girls' contraceptive behavior, *J Sex Research* 22:347, 1986.
9. Matsuhashi Y et al: Is repeat pregnancy in adolescents a "planned" affair? *J Adolesc Health Care* 10:409, 1989.
10. McAnarney ER: Young maternal age and adverse neonatal outcome, *Am J Dis Child* 141:1053, 1987.
11. Miller BC: Adolescent parenthood, economic issues, and social policies, *J Fam Econ Issues* 13:467, 1992.
12. National Center for Health Statistics. Advanced report of final natality statistics, 1992, Monthly vital statistics report, suppl 43, no 5, Hyattsville, Md, 1993, Public Health Service.
13. Rainey DY, Stevens-Simon C, Kaplan DW: Self-perception of infertility among female adolescents, *Am J Dis Child* 147:1053, 1993.
14. Stevens-Simon C, Roghmann KJ, McAnarney ER: Repeat adolescent pregnancy and low birth weight: methods issues, *J Adolesc Health Care* 11:114, 1990.
15. Stevens-Simon C, White M: Adolescent pregnancy, *Pediatr Ann* 20:322, 1991.
16. Stevens-Simon C, Wallis J, Allan-Davis J: Which teen mothers choose Norplant? *Pediatr Res* 33:9(abstract).
17. Zabin LS, Astone NM, Emerson MR: Do adolescents want babies? The relationship between attitudes and behavior, *J Research Adolesc* 3:67, 1993.

SUGGESTED READINGS

McAnarney ER, Hendee WR: Adolescent pregnancy and its consequences, *JAMA* 262:74, 1989.

McAnarney ER, Hendee WR: The prevention of adolescent pregnancy, *JAMA* 262:78, 1989.

Unger DG, Wandersman LP: The relation of family and partner support to the adjustment of adolescent mothers, *Child Dev* 59:1056, 1988.

108 Violent and Aggressive Behavior

Trina Menden Anglin

Society's alarm over adolescent violence has escalated in recent years. The definition of interpersonal violence is based on the concept of aggression and entails a behavior that intentionally threatens, attempts, or actually inflicts physical harm on another.[9] This chapter provides clinical guidance for identifying adolescents involved in interpersonal violence, either as perpetrators or as victims, and explores health counseling and intervention strategies for them.

INCIDENCE OF VIOLENT BEHAVIOR

Nationally, 39% of adolescents report having been in a physical fight within the preceding year, and 6% report having been in more than five fights. By carrying weapons, adolescents increase the risk of causing serious physical injury or death if they become involved in a fight; in a 1-year period, 24% carried a weapon to school.[1]

Delinquency rates are a second indicator of violent behavior. The 1990 juvenile court delinquency case rate was 50 per 1000 population. Violent offenses currently account for 7.5% of all juvenile court delinquency cases and have increased by 67% since 1982.

A third major indicator of violence is the homicide rate. In 1990 homicide was the second leading cause of death among 15- to 24-year-olds in the United States (19.9 per 100,000 population).[7] The homicide rate is particularly high for African-American, Hispanic, and Native American males in this age group. Averaged over the years 1988 through 1990, the rates (per 100,000 population) for these young men were: African-Americans, 117.9; Hispanics, 45.7; and Native Americans, 27.7. Homicide accounts for more than 80% of the deaths caused by firearms among African-American adolescents and for approximately 40% of such deaths among Caucasian adolescents.[7]

THEORIES OF AGGRESSIVE BEHAVIOR

Contemporary explanations for aggressive and violent behavior are based on interactions among individuals' psychosocial development and cognitive processes, hormonal and neurological functioning, and surrounding social influences. Although information is available about the effects of each of these categories, we know little about how they interact.[9]

Psychosocial Development and Cognitive Processes

Aggressive adolescents and adults who commit acts of violence characteristically first demonstrate aggressive behaviors during early childhood. This behavioral pattern stabilizes before adolescence[2,4,8,9] (see Chapter 77, Prediction of Adult Behavior from Childhood). Aggressive and violent behaviors appear to represent children's learned responses to solving problems of frustration; their learning is facilitated by observing successful outcomes to their own and others' aggressive behaviors. One example is the child who learns that a parent can be "coerced" into giving in to a demand if the child behaves aggressively. Children subjected to harsh discipline or abuse by parents particularly may be at heightened risk for long-term aggressive behavior. Children store such successful behavioral strategies or "scripts" in their memory and retrieve them for use in future similar situations. Once behavioral "scripts" are well encoded, they may be retrieved and acted on so quickly that the behavior appears impulsive rather than reflective. In addition, based on numerous studies, there now is general agreement that intense, prolonged childhood exposure to violence portrayed on television also boosts the risk for long-term aggressive behavior[2,4,8,9] (see Chapter 66, Violence in Television and Video Games: Influence on Children and Adolescents). Children and young adolescents who display aggressive behavior usually have poor social problem-solving skills and are rejected by their conventional, nonaggressive peers.

Another psychological theory to explain aggression is adapted from Kohlberg's theory of moral development.[4,6] Aggressive adolescents who victimize others do not perceive predatory or aggressive behavior in moral terms but as a matter of personal choice.[4] They believe that the "right" behavior is the one that serves their own interests.[6] Their beliefs may bias them to disparage victims or to believe that they deserve to be attacked.

Biological Explanations

Several lines of research have explored the relationship between biological differences and aggressive behavior. However, biological causality has not been determined.[9]

Genetic Explanations. It currently is thought that genetic processes do influence the biological potential for aggressive behavior, but the level of explanatory power is controversial. However, in humans there is no clear evidence that any simple chromosomal syndrome transmits the potential for violent behavior.[9]

Hormonal Explanations. Testosterone has been linked to adolescent aggressive behavior. Male adolescents who have relatively high testosterone levels may react physically when threatened or provoked. In addition, higher testosterone levels appear to lower tolerance for frustration among younger male adolescents, which in turn is associated with the likelihood of engaging in unprovoked aggressive behavior. Other hormonal associations in aggressive, delinquent adolescent boys include relatively low testosterone/estradiol ratios, lower levels of testosterone-estradiol binding globulin, and relatively low levels of the adrenal hormone dehydroepiandrosterone sulfate (DHEAS).[9]

Neurotransmitters. Four neurotransmitters—dopamine, norepinephrine, serotonin, and gamma-aminobutyric acid (GABA)—have been studied to explore their relationships to aggressive and violent behavior. None can serve as a specific biological marker for aggression potential. However, serotonin may be more directly involved in certain human aggressive behaviors. An inverse correlation exists between the cerebrospinal fluid (CSF) serotonin concentration and its metabolites (e.g., 5-HIAA) and various measures of aggressive, impulsive, and suicidal behaviors.[9] Despite our inability to define specific roles for neurotransmitters in causing aggressive behavior, major classes of psychotropic drugs that are used to manage violent behavior and agitation (e.g., neuroleptics and anxiolytic agents) include inhibition of specific neurotransmitters as part of their spectrum of pharmacological action.

Neuroanatomical and Neurophysiological Abnormalities. Abnormalities of certain brain sites, such as structures in the limbic system, may be associated with violent behavior. For example, children who exhibit violent or aggressive behavior often have such neuropsychological problems as deficits in memory, attention, and language/verbal skills. These problems frequently follow damage to the limbic system from a head injury.[9]

Social Influences

Several community characteristics are associated with high epidemiological levels of interpersonal violence and crime. The most important are extreme poverty and its covariates, including the density of multiunit housing, residential mobility, disrupted family structures, low levels of participation in community social life and organization, and lack of legitimate employment opportunities. Community minority race and ethnicity status are not strongly associated with violence and crime rates once poverty and the other listed factors are controlled.[9]

CLINICAL APPLICATIONS

There is a broad range of involvement in interpersonal violence among adolescents. Most commonly, teenagers occasionally become involved in physical fights but otherwise appear to demonstrate adequate psychosocial adjustment. A smaller proportion of youngsters demonstrate recurrent antisocial physical aggression. For these adolescents, physically aggressive behavior usually is part of a package of deviant problem behaviors. Common associated problems include conduct disorder (see Chapter 79, Conduct Disorders) adjudication for juvenile delinquency (see Chapter 102, Juvenile Delinquency), substance abuse, bipolar disorder, poor academic performance, and rejection by conventional peers.[4,6,8] The question of gang membership also must be raised. Although overlap clearly exists among adjudicated delinquents, adolescents who have conduct disorder, and adolescents who engage in physical aggression, the three groups are not synonymous.

Primary care clinicians are the professional group most likely to encounter adolescents individually from an evaluation perspective. Given the high rate of interpersonal violence and the substantial risk it carries for death and morbidity, all adolescents deserve to be screened clinically for involvement. Adolescents should be assessed routinely as part of the following types of health care encounters and observations: visits for health maintenance and for care of acute injuries, findings of recent physical trauma and scars, and symptoms of anxiety or depression. The box on p. 841 outlines a clinically useful sequence of questions to help identify adolescents who are engaged in interpersonal violence. The screening and assessment interview should be interactive, use open-ended questions, and be low-keyed and conversational. The questions are phrased so that no assignment of blame is implied. It also is useful to ask the adolescent's parents about trouble with fighting and problems with the law or police.

In addition to determining factual information, the primary care clinician should attempt to identify issues that may help motivate an adolescent to try to change his or her violent behavior (see the box on p. 841).

Counseling Strategies for Adolescents Who Fight

Useful counseling strategies are outlined in the box on p. 842. Although adolescents who exhibit multiple, long-standing problem behaviors probably are not amenable to change through office-based counseling and may require referral for meaningful intervention, many other adolescents may benefit from interactive counseling discussions. First the primary care clinician and adolescent must together define fighting or carrying weapons as a problem behavior. The clinician may need to indicate that such behavior is dangerous and express concern for the adolescent's well-being. However, the focus should be on helping the adolescent to explore nonviolent alternatives to fighting.

Aggressive adolescents frequently have different cognitions than nonaggressive adolescents. For example, they are more likely to perceive that other people have a hostile intent toward them. It is logical, then, for them to adopt a physically aggressive solution to a problem. In addition, aggressive adolescents have a limited repertoire of ways to solve social problems without resorting to physical violence.[4,6,8] The primary care clinician can help the adolescent correct these cognitive distortions and appreciate the potential effectiveness of prosocial, nonviolent solutions to interpersonal problems.

Referral for More Intensive Intervention

Office-based counseling by the primary care clinician usually is adequate for adolescents who demonstrate normal psychosocial functioning. The clinician probably will need to refer adolescents who exhibit recurrent significant antisocial behavior (see Chapter 93, Consultation and Referral for Developmental and Behavioral Problems). The following categories of programs may be effective:

1. Parent management training, which is based on behavioral modification techniques of social learning theory. This may be helpful for families with young adolescents, and it is most effective for families that have few dysfunctional factors and are not socioeconomically disadvantaged.
2. Cognitive problem-solving skills training, a formal extension of the office-based strategy outlined in this chapter. It seeks to change how adolescents approach conflicts by teaching them a step-by-step approach to solving interpersonal problems. It also may include a sociomoral reasoning component.
3. Community-based interventions, including use of available community resources on a large scale and integra-

CLINICAL QUESTIONS TO HELP IDENTIFY ADOLESCENTS ENGAGED IN INTERPERSONAL VIOLENCE

1. How much of a problem is fighting for you?
2. About how often do you get involved in fights?
3. What happened the last time you were part of a fight?
   - How did the fight get started?
   - Was the fight more name calling, pushing/shoving/wrestling, or hitting/punching/kicking?
   - Was the fight one-on-one, or were more people involved?
   - Had anybody used alcohol or drugs before the fight broke out?
   - Did anybody use weapons such as a bat, stick, knife, or gun?
   - Did anybody get hurt or injured because of the fight? What happened? Did anybody need to get medical care?
   - Did the police get involved? What happened?
4. Have you ever gotten hurt or injured from being part of a fight? What happened? Did you need to get medical care?
5. Have you ever hurt anyone else during a fight? What happened? Did that person need to get medical care?
6. Have you ever gotten into trouble for fighting?
   - Any problems at school? Have you ever been suspended for being part of a fight?
   - Any problems with the police or law? Did you need to go to court? Were you locked up (placed in detention)? What did the court say you needed to do? (Ask about probation, house arrest, community service time, and incarceration.)
   - When you were younger, did you ever get into trouble for fighting? What happened? About how old were you the first time you got into a fight?
7. Have you ever needed to threaten someone or do something physical to get what you wanted or needed? What happened?
8. If you wanted a gun, how easy would it be for you to get it? How long would it take?
9. Have you ever carried a gun or knife? Where did you carry it? Was there any special reason for you to carry it? About how often do you carry it?
10. Have you ever shot at anyone? Have you ever shot at and hit a person? What happened?
11. Do you own a gun? What kind is it? About how often do you use it?
12. Here are some reasons why people get into fights. What do you think about them?
    - Someone calls you a name, insults you, or says something untrue about you.
    - Someone insults a member of your family.
    - Someone wants to fight you or dares you to fight.
    - Someone hits you first.
    - Someone physically hurts or kills a friend or a member of your family.
    - You want to show how tough you are, to keep up your reputation.
13. What do you think about people who get picked on by other people or who get beaten up in a fight? Do you think it's their own fault? Does it matter if they get hurt?

tion of adolescents who have antisocial behaviors into groups of adolescents who have conventional prosocial behaviors. These programs attempt to foster positive peer influences and to prevent peer modeling of deviant behaviors. It is possible that such programs best serve adolescents who appear at risk for antisocial, aggressive behaviors but who do not exhibit severe problems.[5]

Primary care clinicians can successfully refer adolescents and their families for more intensive help when either the adolescent or parents are motivated. It is important, however, for the clinician to participate actively in the referral process. The clinician should explore the following types of community resources: school-based programs (programs for disruptive students and conflict mediation curricula that the guidance department or school social worker may offer), mental health agencies (group programs for troubled youngsters), a local university's department of psychology (experimental program if a faculty member has an interest in this area), juvenile court (court diversion programs), police department's juvenile or gang unit (officers may be charismatic and often have a broad knowledge of community resources for adolescents).

JUVENILE GANGS

Although juvenile gangs are a long-standing phenomenon in the United States, they currently are receiving heightened

MOTIVATING INFLUENCES FOR AVERTING VIOLENT BEHAVIOR

1. Determine the adolescent's sense of future. Teenagers who expect to die violently at a young age may not be open to problem-solving strategies until this perception is addressed.
2. Determine the adolescent's connections to family members. Many teenagers have younger siblings or their own children whom they wish to protect from their negative life experiences. They may be persuaded that their own lives are important to members of their families and that their own behavior is a powerful model for the younger "generation."
3. Determine the adolescent's beliefs about familial attitudes toward fighting and use of weapons. Many adolescents perceive that their parents would support their fighting and using a weapon in self-defense.
4. Determine the meanings that peer status and respect have for the adolescent. How important is "toughness"?
5. Determine the adolescent's concerns about ability to control anger and impulses. Many adolescents are worried about their emotional reactivity.
6. Determine the adolescent's emotional responses to fighting. Look for thrill seeking, need to retaliate, fear, and remorse.

COUNSELING APPROACHES FOR ANGRY, IMPULSIVE ADOLESCENTS

1. Help the adolescent develop strategies to defuse anger. A combination of relaxation techniques and cognitive exercises appears to work most effectively. Teenagers can be taught that anger represents a highly charged physical state during which their body is prepared to act strongly in response to their feeling very upset; together, these sensations lead to impulsive behavior (fast physical action without thinking). They can learn to control their bodies by using relaxation techniques. Cognitive exercises consist of rehearsing four steps that correspond to the stages of a provocation sequence. Teenagers can practice scenarios with the clinician and at home.
   - Prepare for a provocation. Rehearse self-efficacy statements, such as "I can manage this situation. I know how to control my anger. I know what to do if I get upset."
   - Confront the provocation. Rehearse self-instruction, such as "Stay calm. Keep cool. Relax." Recognize that "You don't need to prove yourself."
   - Cope with the psychological arousal and agitation. "My muscles are feeling tight. It's time to relax and slow things down."
   - Reflect on the provocation. These self-statements are meant to provide perspective if the situation was not resolved and to enhance self-efficacy for anger control if the adolescent was successful.[2]

   Other strategies include purposeful diversion—allowing the course of time to exert a cooling effect and confiding angry feelings to a trusted, wise friend or adult. Teenagers who enjoy creating art may want to draw or paint their feelings. It is important not to brood about what occurred. In addition, it is not beneficial to recommend that angry feelings be released through imaginary acts of aggression, which don't purge aggressive wishes and may inflame aggressive fantasies.[2]
2. Work on effective problem-solving skills. The primary care clinician can model effective prosocial problem solving by working through specific situations with the adolescent and using the following steps: seeking alternative possible solutions, evaluating each possibility, and examining the likely consequences of each alternative before deciding on a course of prosocial action. Role playing helps to engage the adolescent and promotes exploration of perspective taking (see no. 3).
3. Help the adolescent develop sociomoral reasoning. The goal is to promote an aggressive adolescent's belief that it is morally wrong to cause harm to others and that this belief is important to hold. The adolescent learns to respect others' humanity and rights and to become sensitive to and care about others' emotions (emotional empathy) rather than to focus on one's own immediate self-interest. The clinician can use the following probes when modeling problem-solving skills: ask the adolescent to summarize the problem from the perspectives of both players, including the one who may have been victimized; clarify the meaning of moral terms (e.g., what do you mean by fair, when you say "it isn't fair"?); explain why a certain alternative was decided upon; consider an issue from a universal perspective (e.g., what would happen if everyone stole from stores?); and consider the issue's context (e.g., under what conditions would it be justifiable to break a promise?).[8]

publicity and are perceived as major threats to the community's well-being. A gang is a group of individuals that has an identifiable leadership and organizational structure and that has developed symbols of representation and engages in antisocial and criminal behaviors. Many gangs also have territorial identification. Beyond this definition, gangs are heterogeneous in their membership and level of organization, degree of involvement in aggressive violence, and use and sale of drugs. Major gangs have extensive rules and codes of conduct, as well as specialized symbols and alphabets. Although there are no accurate data on gang membership, and gang activity has been documented in rural and suburban areas in every geographical region of the United States, gangs appear to be concentrated in impoverished urban neighborhoods.

Children and adolescents join gangs for a variety of reasons. Many drift into membership because gang activities dominate the social and economic structures of their neighborhoods and provide opportunities for recognition and status, money, physical protection and safety, and a social life. Gang membership, similar to membership in conventional prosocial youth organizations, is congruent with the developmental tasks of adolescence. It offers the peer associations that allow emancipation from the family unit, and it promotes a sense of belonging through group identity. Positive gang values include respect and the forging of intimate bonds between members. However, gang membership, especially as adolescents become more deeply involved, also promotes a corruptive power from the ability to intimidate others through physical aggression. Many gang members relish the excitement brought by participation in antisocial activities and violence, as well as the quick affluence brought by selling drugs. Some gangs' formal rules and expectations have such strong and pervasive influences that they discourage independent thinking by individual members and make it virtually impossible to resign membership peacefully.

Violent behaviors by gang members occur in a variety of contexts. First, new gang members' initiations always involve ritual violence and humiliation because they need to demonstrate courage, a willingness to fight, and an ability to carry out orders. (Examples include being "beaten in," participating in a drive-by shooting, assaulting an innocent victim, and for girls, being gang raped.) Second, internal violence occurs when members who disobey rules or leaders' orders are physically disciplined. Violence between members of rival gangs is founded on the needs for territorial control and, very importantly, for maintaining or enhancing respect or honor.

Compared with other adolescents living in similar environments, youngsters who are gang members have significantly greater use of illicit drugs and engagement in a variety of violent and illegal activities. They also report higher rates of being victimized by others' physical aggression. Although male gang members are less likely to be fully integrated with their families, they are as likely as nongang youngsters to participate in conventional family, school, and neighborhood activities. It is probable that many gang members have some conventional values, but that their behavior largely is shaped by gang membership.[3]

Clinical Issues

Primary care clinicians may be able to identify individuals who belong to gangs by noting unusual tattoos, special clothing (with care taken not to confuse clothing identifiers with contemporary adolescent fashion), nicknames that have violent or seemingly bizarre connotations, stylized verbal and body language, and the appearance and demeanor of accompanying friends. Although members of major gang nations (Bloods, Crips, Folks, People) are required to disclose their affiliation when questioned, many adolescents belong to local gangs and are secretive about their involvement.

It is not necessary to confirm gang membership to determine whether an adolescent is asking for help in solving a problem or to discuss issues of personal safety, substance abuse, and expectations for the future. Although physically aggressive adolescents are likely to report anger as an emotional issue, they are less likely to report depression and anxiety.[10] However, some gang members are dismayed about the violence to which they are exposed and demonstrate mental health symptoms or request help in leaving a gang. The clinician should recognize the social complexity of these adolescents' lives and the ambivalence and disloyalty that they may experience in questioning their gang involvement. In addition, they may jeopardize their personal safety if they attempt to distance themselves from gang activities. A primary care clinician who has gained the adolescent's trust and respect eventually may be able to secure appropriate mental health counseling or be able to refer the teenager to the community's juvenile or gang control unit for assistance in leaving the gang.

ADOLESCENTS VICTIMIZED BY AGGRESSION AND VIOLENCE

A significant proportion of adolescents report being victimized. At least 14% have been robbed, 13% attacked, and 5% have been raped or the victims of attempted rape at school (see Chapter 290, Rape). An additional 34% have been threatened but not physically hurt.[1] Recurrent bullying of vulnerable children and young adolescents by aggressive agemates or older youngsters is a common phenomenon at school. Teachers and classmates perceive bullied children as shy, passive or submissive, and insecure; they do not provoke their own attacks. They report anxiety. Bullied children also may be rejected socially. As young adults they appear to function well and are not likely to be bullied at work, but are likely to be depressed and have low self-esteem.[4,8] The primary care clinician can identify bullied adolescents by assessing the quality of their peer relationships. They may benefit from programs that teach assertive social skills.

Adolescents who have been exposed to serious acts of violence report a variety of mental health symptoms, including depression, anger, anxiety, and dissociation.[10] However, many teenagers who have witnessed violence or have been victimized may not volunteer such information spontaneously. It is important clinically, therefore, to ask adolescents who have mental health symptoms about acute or recurrent exposure to violence or whether such events have happened to friends or members of their families. In particular, adolescents may show depression or recurrent somatic symptoms linked to anxiety (see Chapters 96, Conversion Reactions in Adolescents, and 154, Nervousness). They may report fear of dying and may have difficulty sleeping and concentrating, with a concomitant deterioration in school performance, or may avoid situations that arouse recollection of the trauma. They may display features of posttraumatic stress disorder. Many adolescents welcome interpretive insight into the etiology of their somatic symptoms and mental health problems. Adolescents who have significant psychological symptoms should be referred for mental health evaluation and treatment.

REFERENCES

1. American School Health Association, Association for the Advancement of Health Education, and Society for Public Health Education: *The national adolescent student health survey,* Oakland, Calif, 1989, Third Party Publishing.
2. Berkowitz L: *Aggression: its causes, consequences, and control,* New York, 1993, McGraw-Hill.
3. Fagan J: Social processes of delinquency and drug use among urban gangs. In Huff CR, editor: *Gangs in America,* Newbury Park, Calif, 1990, Sage.
4. Huesmann LR, editor: *Aggressive behavior: current perspectives,* New York, 1994, Plenum Press.
5. Kazdin AE: Treatment of antisocial behavior in children: current status and future directions, *Psychol Bull* 102:187, 1987.
6. McCord J, Tremblay RE, editors: *Preventing antisocial behavior: interventions from birth through adolescence,* New York, 1992, Guilford Press.
7. National Center for Health Statistics: Health United States 1992 and healthy people 2000 review, DHHS Pub No (PHS) 93-1232, Hyattsville, Md, 1993, Public Health Service, US Department of Health and Human Services.
8. Pepler DJ, Rubin KH, editors: *The development and treatment of childhood aggression,* Hillsdale, NJ, 1991, Lawrence Erlbaum.
9. Reiss AJ, Roth JA, editors: *Understanding and preventing violence: panel on the understanding and control of violent behavior,* Washington, DC, 1993, National Academy Press.
10. Singer MI et al: Adolescents' exposure to violence and associated symptoms of psychological trauma, *JAMA* 273:477, 1995.

SUGGESTED READING

Eron LD, Gentry JH, Schlegel P, editors: *Reason to hope: a psychosocial perspective on violence and youth,* Washington, DC, 1994, American Psychological Association.

PART SEVEN

Presenting Signs and Symptoms

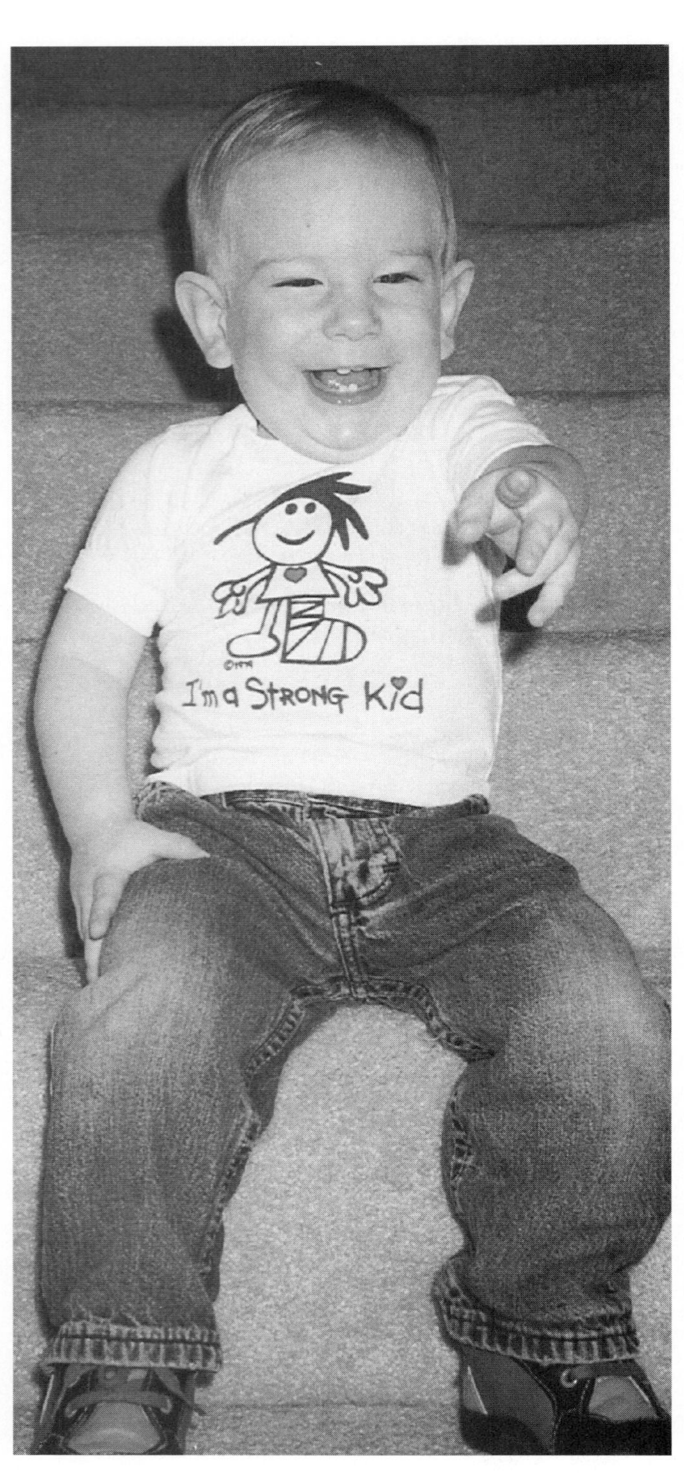

143 Hirsutism, Hypertrichosis, and Precocious Sexual Hair Development
144 Hoarseness
145 Hyperhidrosis
146 Hypotonia
147 Irritability
148 Jaundice
149 Joint Pain
150 Limp
151 Loss of Appetite
152 Lymphadenopathy
153 Malocclusion
154 Nervousness
155 Nonconvulsive Periodic Disorders
156 Odor (Unusual Urine and Body)
157 Petechiae and Purpura
158 Polyuria
159 Proteinuria
160 Pruritus
161 Rash
162 Recurrent Infections
163 The Red Eye
164 Scrotal Swelling
165 Sexual Developmental Alterations
166 Splenomegaly
167 Strabismus
168 Strange Behavior
169 Stridor
170 Syncope
171 Tics
172 Torticollis
173 Vaginal Bleeding
174 Vaginal Discharge
175 Visual Disturbance
176 Vomiting
177 Weight Loss
178 Wheezing

109 Abdominal Distention

Kenneth Kenigsberg

Cases of pediatric abdominal distention fall naturally into two groups: newborns up to 1 month of age and older infants and children. With the advent and wider use of ultrasonography, perhaps a third group should be added—fetuses with abdominal distention in utero.

NEWBORNS

Abdominal distention in newborns usually occurs as a result of an abnormality of the urinary, gastrointestinal (GI), or female genital tracts. Of these, the urinary tract is the organ system most often involved. An obstruction at the ureteropelvic or ureterovesical junction produces a unilateral, firm, nontender mass. A less common cause of distention is a multicystic kidney, which has a physical presentation almost identical to that of a hydronephrotic kidney (discussed later in this section).

In rare cases abdominal distention may be caused by bleeding from the kidney, liver, spleen, or adrenal glands as the result of trauma before or during birth. In these cases the signs of blood loss (the infant rapidly becomes tachycardic and pale) are much more obvious than the abdominal distention, and immediate treatment is necessary, involving transfusion and usually exploratory surgery.

The least common cause of abdominal distention in newborns is polycystic kidneys, which manifest as firm, noncompressible, bilateral cystic masses.

In infant boys, urinary obstruction most commonly is the result of the presence of urethral valves. If the obstruction is severe, the renal pelvis on one side may become so dilated from vesicoureteral obstruction or reflux and accompanying back pressure that it ruptures, resulting in urinary ascites and an island of intestine floating on a sea of urine. An abdominal fluid wave is easily elicited in these infants. In a way, the rupture of the pelvis is fortunate for the infant because it releases the pathological pressure on the kidney and prevents extensive damage. If the pelvis does not rupture, the infant may have bilateral flank masses very much like those in an infant with polycystic kidneys.

In the fetus, if urinary outflow is completely obstructed and the kidneys are nonfunctional, no urine is voided into the amniotic fluid and the mother will develop oligohydramnios. This can be diagnosed through ultrasonography, as can the specific site of obstruction. It originally was thought that prenatal diagnosis would salvage the function of the kidneys and reduce morbidity, and numerous attempts were made to shunt the bladder obstructed because of urethral valves, However, success has been limited. Occasionally, ultrasonographic pictures of intraabdominal fluid have led to an incorrect diagnosis.[1]

Abdominal distention resulting from renal anomalies in newborns usually can be diagnosed through physical examination and roentgenograms.

The flank mass of a multicystic kidney or of a hydronephrotic kidney that develops secondary to ureteral obstruction is apparent and can be palpated, as can the bilateral masses of polycystic kidneys or bilateral hydronephrosis that occurs secondary to the presence of urethral valves. If the kidney has ruptured, causing ascites, the bilateral bulging into the flanks and the fluid wave usually are diagnostic. In newborns contrast intravenous pyelograms usually are not very helpful diagnostically, but radionuclide and ultrasonographic scans are. When the presence of urethral valves is suspected, a voiding cystourethrogram can be confirmatory.

Abdominal distention in a newborn that arises from GI problems occurs because of obstruction or necrotizing enterocolitis. The most common obstruction in newborns is pyloric stenosis. However, this rarely manifests as abdominal distention because the infant empties the stomach by vomiting and rarely has noticeable abdominal bulging. Obstruction of the duodenum occasionally manifests with upper abdominal distention (Fig. 109-1). In these cases, also, the usual presenting sign is vomiting. The vomitus is bilious when the obstruction is distal to the ampulla of Vater, which occurs in most cases, and clear in the occasional case when the obstruction is proximal to the ampulla of Vater. The more distal the obstruction, the greater the abdominal distention.

In some cases more than one obstruction may be involved. An incarcerated inguinal hernia (Fig. 109-2) is quite common in premature infants and difficult to overlook.

The most dangerous type of intestinal obstruction that causes abdominal distention is malrotation. If the diagnosis is not made promptly and surgical treatment instituted quickly, necrosis of the entire midgut may ensue, involving all of the bowel distal to the duodenum and proximal to the transverse colon (Fig. 109-3).

Meconium ileus is the intestinal component of cystic fibrosis and usually manifests as abdominal distention with bilious vomiting. The underlying cause of the obstruction is the inspissated, agglutinated mass of nontransportable meconium in the distal ileum (Fig. 109-4). If the bowel proximal to the obstruction caused by the meconium ruptures, a condition known as giant meconium cyst peritonitis may result. This is a nonbacterial chemical peritonitis that results when the irritating meconium spews out into the free abdominal cavity, causing intense inflammation and secretion of vast amounts of fluid within the abdomen. Occasionally, in fetuses, this distention is so extreme that it calls for paracentesis before the infant can be delivered.

An insidious condition of infancy that produces abdominal distention is Hirschsprung disease. The underlying pathology of this disease is absence of ganglion cells from the distal colon and occasionally small bowel. The distention develops gradually over the first several days, when the condition is characterized by bilious vomiting and delayed passage

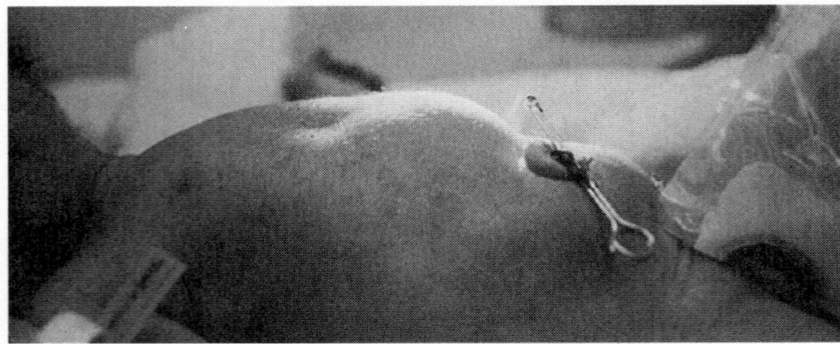

FIG. 109-1 Newborn infant with duodenal atresia and upper abdominal distention.

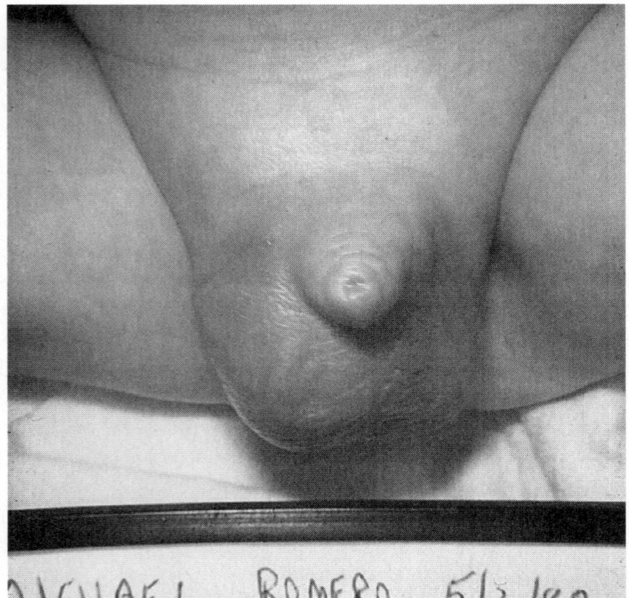

FIG. 109-2 Incarcerated right inguinal hernia in a newborn.

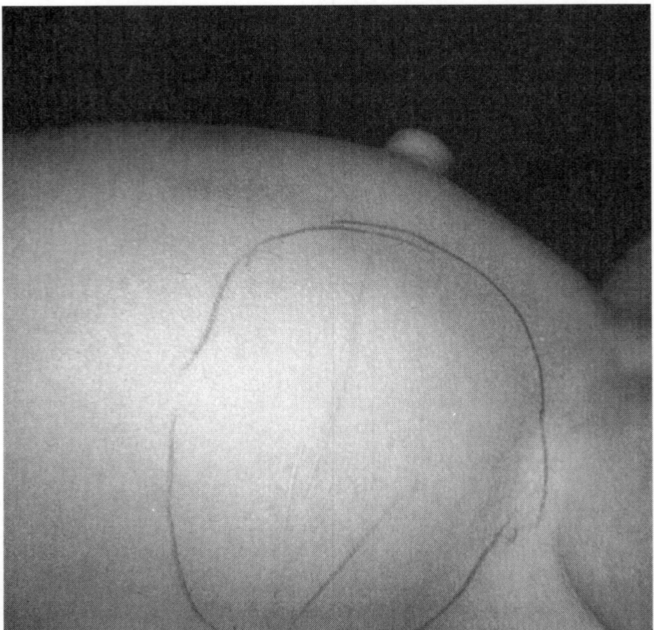

FIG. 109-3 Newborn with distention secondary to torsion.

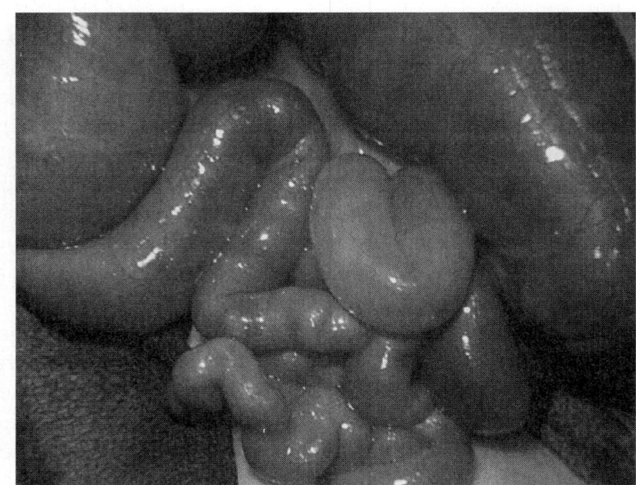

FIG. 109-4 Distal ileum with inspissated meconium secondary to meconium ileus.

of stool. Any infant who has not had a stool by 24 hours of age is likely to have Hirschsprung disease.

Necrotizing enterocolitis (NEC) currently is the most common indication for abdominal exploration in the neonatal intensive care unit. It occurs almost exclusively in stressed, premature newborns. The infant usually is on the respirator. NEC is accompanied by marked physiological deterioration and has a high mortality.

Diagnosis in the Newborn

A history, physical examination, and plain radiographs usually are all that is needed for diagnosis.[2] With bilious vomiting in a distended infant, obstruction must be considered the cause until it is proved otherwise. A history of cystic fibrosis in the family is a strong indication that meconium ileus could be the underlying cause of abdominal distention.[3] A premature infant on the respirator is at constant risk of developing necrotizing enterocolitis. An infant diagnosed as having a reducible hernia may have an incarcerated one.

Upper abdominal distention upon physical examination is characteristic of small bowel obstruction proximal to the terminal ileum. Distention that develops over several days, along with delayed passage of meconium, is strongly indicative of Hirschsprung disease; a very tight distal rectum is characteristic of this disorder. Enormous distention of the abdomen (causing it to look like a volleyball) almost always is caused by meconium cyst peritonitis. The red, tender belly in a deteriorating premature infant is the harbinger of necrotizing enterocolitis. A tender groin lump in a distended infant is pathognomonic of an incarcerated hernia.

The plain film of the abdomen usually reveals the so-called double bubble characteristic of duodenal atresia. Atresia of the bowel distal to the duodenum shows several levels of air-fluid interface. The characteristic appearance of meconium ileus is that of small bowel obstruction with several levels and a "soap bubble" appearance in the right lower quadrant. This appearance is related to a mixture of air and inspissated meconium.

Unfortunately, malrotation, the condition calling for the greatest degree of attention and prompt correction, does not

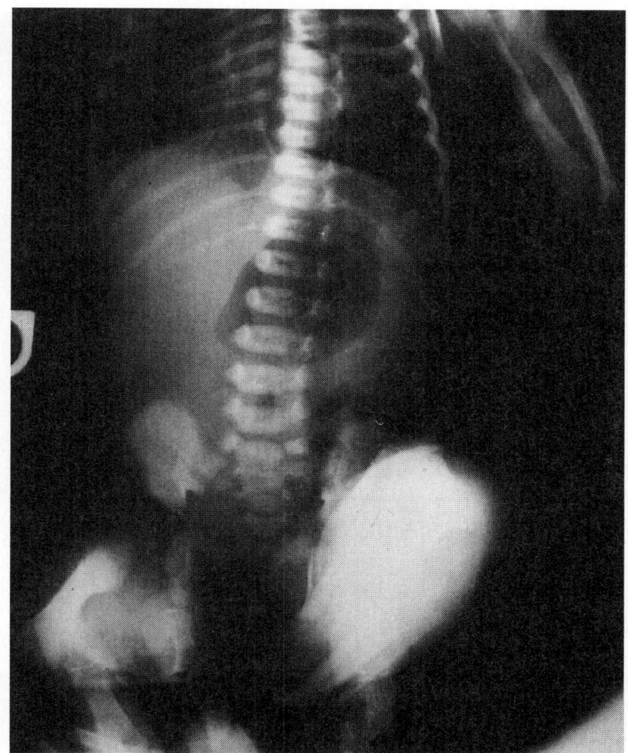

FIG. 109-5 Malrotation with distended stomach and paucity of distal gas.

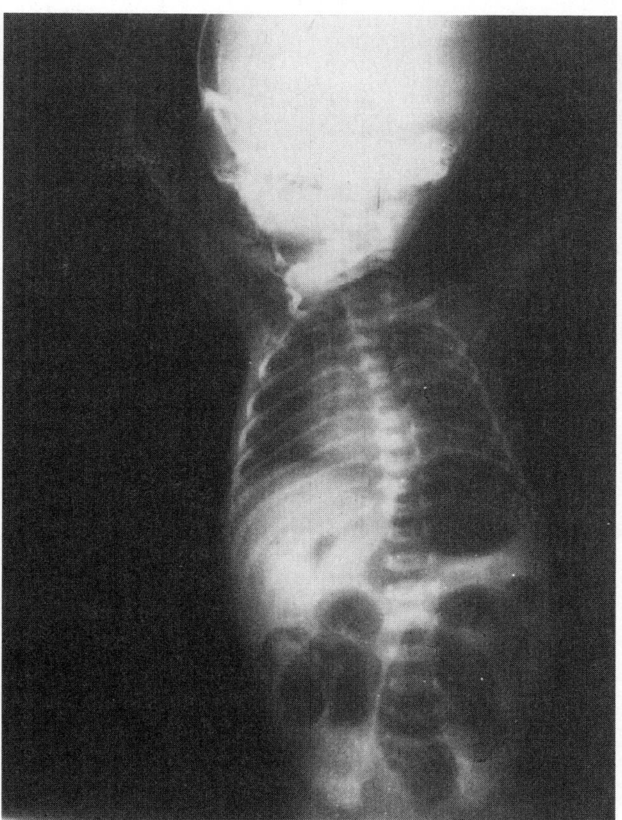

FIG. 109-6 Premature infant with necrotizing enterocolitis showing gas in the wall of the intestine and in the liver.

have a typical roentgenographic appearance. Malrotation may look like atresia, but usually some gas is present distal to the area of obstruction (Fig. 109-5). It previously was thought that a barium enema was a definitive way to diagnose malrotation, but this is not the current thinking. Some infants who have malrotation have a normally positioned cecum and appear to have normal results with a barium enema. Malrotation is diagnosed definitively by means of an upper GI series.

The plain radiograph also may not diagnose Hirschsprung disease. This condition requires a barium enema and subsequent aspiration biopsies of the distal rectum.[4] Necrotizing enterocolitis reveals gas in the wall of the intestine and later may reveals gas in the biliary tract or free air in the abdomen (Fig. 109-6).

As with prenatal obstruction of the urinary tract, obstruction of the GI tract also can be revealed by ultrasonographic scans prenatally. In utero diagnosis makes it possible to have a putative diagnosis at the time of delivery and perhaps to carry out corrective surgery a few hours earlier than would be possible without a prenatal diagnosis. However, as also is the case with prenatal renal diagnosis, early diagnosis of intestinal conditions has not resulted in any significant decline in mortality or morbidity.

The organ system least likely to cause abdominal distention in newborns is the female genital tract. If the infant has an imperforate hymen or atresia of the distal vagina, the fetal uterus, under the influence of maternal hormones, secretes enough fluid proximal to the obstruction to distend the upper vagina and the uterus. Occasionally this distention can become quite enormous. The diagnosis usually is readily made by visual inspection of the vulva and a rectal examination, which will demonstrate the mass of dilated vagina and uterus immediately above the rectal ampulla.

OLDER INFANT AND CHILD

Abdominal distention in an older infant or a child occasionally can be a continuation of a newborn condition. For instance, when missed in infancy, Hirschsprung disease can manifest at any time throughout life as abdominal distention and recalcitrant constipation. Similarly, malrotation with abdominal distention can manifest in children at any age. The child who has an imperforate hymen or vaginal atresia may not manifest hydrometrocolpos in infancy, but instead may develop signs during pubescence, after uterine bleeding without external menstruation has developed. Besides the abdominal distention, the child may appear to be pregnant and may complain of intermittent abdominal pain. Lastly, a child who has been operated on for some neonatal condition may later in childhood develop intestinal obstruction secondary to adhesions.

Abdominal distention that develops secondary to intestinal obstruction also may occur without previous surgery. The most common cause of such distention is obstruction secondary to a so-called missed appendix. In this case inflammation of the appendix causes it to rupture, and ultimately an abscess develops. The infective reaction and edema around the abscess cause obstruction of the distal small bowel, resulting in abdominal distention and vomiting.

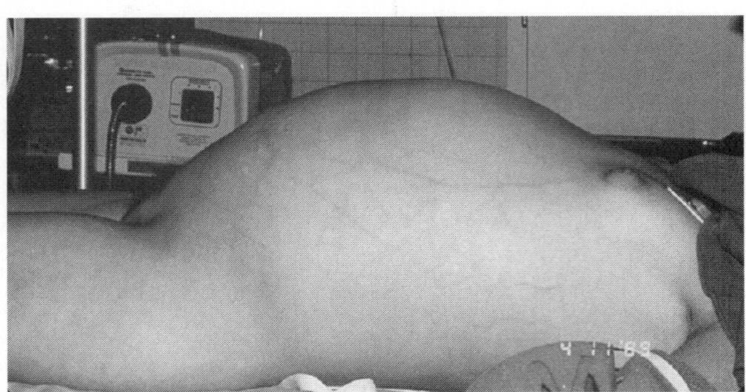

FIG. 109-7 Thirteen-year-old girl with stool withholding.

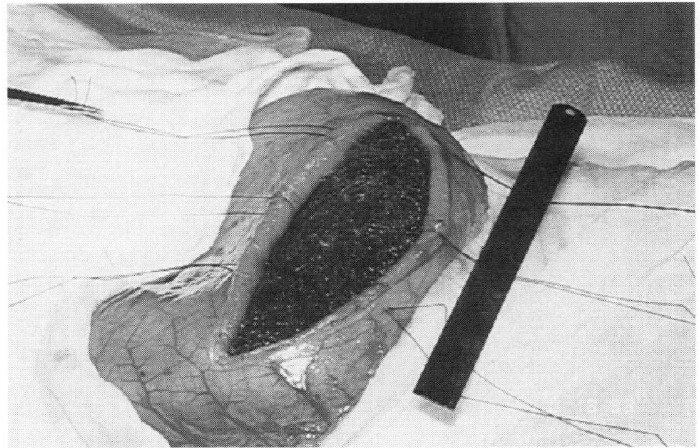

FIG. 109-8 Trichobezoar in the stomach.

Obstruction of the bowel, with subsequent distension, also may result from intussusception, but the first symptoms usually are colicky pain and rectal bleeding that usually looks like currant jelly. In most cases the intussusception occurs before age 2 and is of the so-called idiopathic variety, with hypertrophied lymphoid tissue as the lead point. Occasionally, particularly in infants over age 2, the lead point is a tumor such as a lymphoma, an inverted Meckel diverticulum, or a small bowel polyp.

The most common form of abdominal distention caused by an intestinal problem is not an anatomical problem at all. Whether it has to do with modern diets or modern stress, constipation or stool withholding is the most common form of abdominal distention. Sometimes the degree of abdominal enlargement can be quite astounding (Fig. 109-7). Another form of nonanatomical intestinal obstruction that causes distention is trichobezoar (Fig. 109-8). Children who have hairballs in the stomach and jejunum in addition to distention and vomiting usually have significant emotional problems.

The last group of distention-causing conditions are those associated with the solid organs of the stomach. In pubescent girls, any abdominal mass must be presumed to be a pregnant uterus. Tumors of the ovaries can simulate a pregnant uterus and often are confused with it because these tumors tend to lie very much in the position of a pregnant uterus (Fig. 109-9). Tumors of the liver can manifest as very large masses and often are malignant. Wilms tumors, which usually are asymptomatic, can reach considerable size before they are diagnosed (Fig. 109-10).

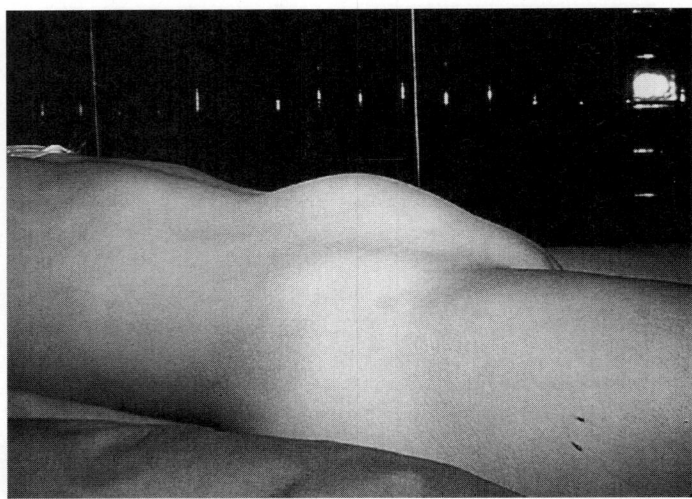

FIG. 109-9 Lower abdominal distention caused by ovarian teratoma.

Diagnosis in Older Infants and Children

As with neonatal distention, the history, physical examination, and plain radiographs usually provide the appropriate diagnosis. A history of previous surgery should alert the clinician to the possibility of intestinal obstruction. A history of frequent pain on defecation and infrequent stools should suggest constipation or stool withholding. This type of distention rarely occurs before age 2 or 3. Hirschsprung disease, however, manifests with a long history of constipation. The difference between stool withholding and Hirschsprung disease is that the former frequently involves pain upon defecation and fecal soiling, whereas the latter rarely does. The absence of menstruation in a pubescent girl who has breast and pubic hair development immediately should suggest the possibility of vaginal obstruction. An asymptomatic mass detected serendipitously should alert the examiner to the possibility of Wilms tumor, whereas a tumor in a child who has appeared ill is more likely to be associated with neuroblastoma. A child who has a habit of eating his or her own hair or the fur from a toy very well may be a child whose distention is caused by a trichobezoar.

On physical examination, an enlarged liver or spleen should be palpated readily. Similarly, the mass of a trichobezoar usually can be felt in the region between the xiphoid and the umbilicus. Abdominal enlargement caused by Wilms tumor usually is confined to one side of the abdomen, although the mass may be considerable in size and usually has a smooth edge. A neuroblastoma usually has an irregular edge and more often extends across the midline than does Wilms tumor. In the lower abdomen, the mass of an enlarged ovarian cyst or a pregnant uterus can be indistinguishable from one another upon palpation of the abdomen. However, the differential diagnosis frequently can be made upon rectal examination, in that the uterus lies in the midline and the ovarian cyst is found to be larger on one side of the pelvis than the other. An enlarged, fluid-filled abdomen that occurs secondary to liver disease often can be diagnosed because of jaundice and enlarged abdominal renal veins.

Plain radiographs usually are sufficient to confirm abdominal distention secondary to intestinal obstruction, whether it

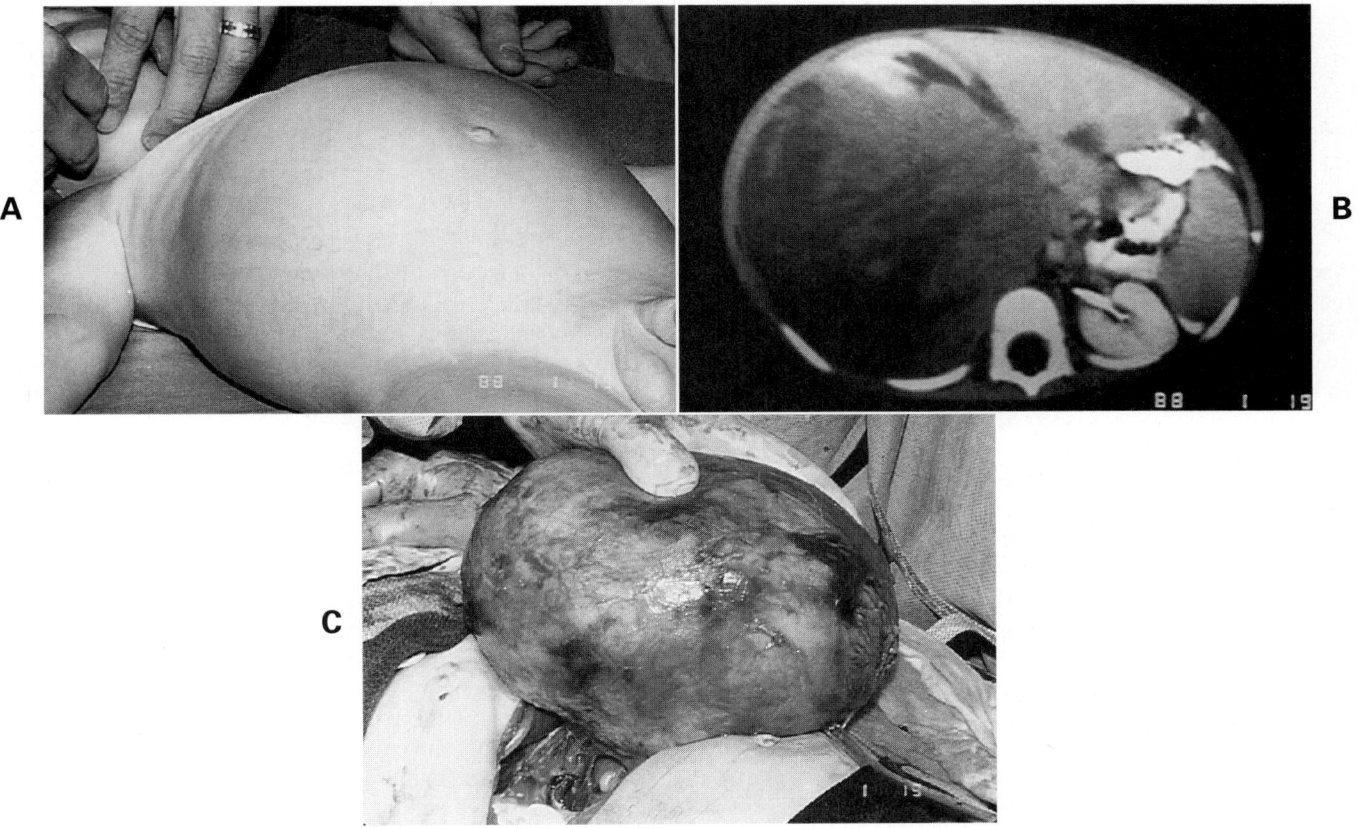

FIG. 109-10 **A,** Abdominal distention secondary to right Wilms tumor. **B,** CT scan of tumor. **C,** Tumor exposed during surgery.

be from previous surgery or from a perforated appendix. Plain films also help significantly in the diagnosis of liver tumors, an enlarged spleen, and pelvic tumors in a girl. However, further tests are necessary to establish some diagnoses firmly; that is, a computed tomography (CT) with contrast for Wilms tumors and neuroblastoma (the latter usually contain calcification), ultrasonography for ovarian cysts, liver function tests for suspected hepatic disease, human chorionic gonadotropin tests for tumors suspected of being gravid uteri, and a barium enema for Hirschspring disease.

REFERENCES

1. Petrikovsky B, Kenigsberg K, Pletcher B: Meconium peritonitis mimicking urinary ascites, *Fetus* 3:2770, 1993.
2. Rothrock SG et al: Plain abdominal radiography in the detection of acute medical and surgical disease in children: a retrospective analysis, *Pediatr Emerg Care* 7:281, 1991.
3. Schaffer AJ, Avery M: *Diseases of the newborn,* ed 3, Philadelphia, 1971, WB Saunders.
4. Welch KJ et al: *Pediatric surgery,* ed 4, vols 1 and 2, 1986, Mosby.

110 Abdominal Pain

Jean C. Smith

Abdominal pain is one of the most common presenting symptoms of children and adolescents. Acute abdominal pain may require medical or surgical intervention to prevent disability or even death. The number of children who have had acute abdominal pain is unknown, but each year 4 in 1000 children have surgery for suspected appendicitis.[6] More often, abdominal pain is recurring and is not associated with physical disability or mortality. Yet recurring abdominal pain often results in serious dysfunction for both the child and the family. Apley[2] has estimated that 10% of school-age children are affected with recurring abdominal pain at some point in their development; in pediatric office practice, 5% of the visits are for recurrent abdominal pain.

CLINICAL CLASSIFICATION

Classification of abdominal pain as simply organic or nonorganic has ceased to be helpful. A more meaningful approach is to distinguish acute conditions that may require urgent or immediate intervention from the less life-threatening but nonetheless potentially disabling chronic or recurrent abdominal pains. The boxes on p. 853 list some of the major diagnostic considerations for acute abdominal pain by pediatric age groups.[1,6] Although the diagnostic considerations clearly overlap for each age group, the child's age and physiological development can help the clinician focus the differential diagnosis. For example, Hirschsprung disease should be considered more likely in a young infant in the first weeks of life, whereas pelvic inflammatory disease clearly is in the differential diagnosis for the adolescent.

Acute Abdominal Pain

In the diagnosis of patients who have acute abdominal pain, it always is important to remember that many of the conditions that cause acute abdominal pain require immediate surgical or medical treatment. These conditions range from the infant who has intestinal malrotation or intussusception, who may develop bowel obstruction with bowel ischemia if appropriate surgical intervention is not performed, to the child or adolescent who has a urinary tract infection that requires the appropriate antibiotic treatment to prevent progression of the infection. The possibility of drug reaction or overdose, or toxins, also should be considered as a cause of acute abdominal pain that requires immediate medical intervention. Eliminating further exposure to the offending agent is crucial, and specific detoxification or supportive care should be initiated promptly.

The concept of referred pain deserves special consideration when discussing acute abdominal pain in children. In these patients, a complete history may provide crucial information that suggests that the abdominal pain may originate outside the abdomen. Thus a 3-year-old who has pneumonia may have inflammatory irritation of the diaphragm, resulting in acute abdominal pain as the presenting complaint. Also, testicular torsion can manifest as acute abdominal pain, and the physician should be sensitive to a teenager's possible reluctance to disclose a history of genital trauma or pain spontaneously.

Recurrent Abdominal Pain

Clinical studies have defined recurrent abdominal pain (RAP) as (1) occurring in children over 3 years of age, (2) involving at least three episodes of pain over a period of more than 3 months, and (2) producing pain severe enough to limit the child's usual activities. Although this definition is useful for studying outcomes and the effect of treatment on the clinical course, it is less helpful for investigating the natural pattern of RAP in a particular patient. Researchers point out that in most studies, only the children are included who themselves or whose families express a concern about the pain. Other children may have similar painful experiences but because it either does not affect their usual activities or because they do not complain, they are not included in such studies.[13] The influence of age and developmental maturation, individual differences (e.g., temperament, coping patterns), family interactions, and the community and cultural contexts are hypothesized to influence the expression of RAP. (See the box on p. 854 for a list of causes of recurrent RAP.)

For RAP, the clinical categories "organic," "psychogenic," and "dysfunctional" can be helpful with the assessment and, more particularly, with the development of a treatment plan. The traditional model of RAP was modified by Barr[3] to include the larger category of "dysfunctional," in which no specific organic or psychological *disease* is identified. However, the category of dysfunctional pain includes conditions with identifiable primary physiological disorders of the abdomen such as chronic stool retention, lactose intolerance, or dysmenorrhea. The degree to which these disorders lead to the expression of pain as a concern or interfere with the child's routine functioning varies among children.[4,9] Even within each child expression of pain may vary. For example, the child who has chronic stool retention, who generally has few or no complaints, can have significant (and possibly even acute) pain when superimposed physiological (e.g., infectious gastroenteritis) or psychological problems (e.g., parental separation) are present. Psychogenic causes of abdominal pain generally are considered to have no primary physiological initiator of the painful expression. This includes entities such as school phobia, acute reactive anxiety, or conversion reaction. All of the RAP syndromes can lead to significant dysfunction and disability, with school absences, repeated visits to several health care providers, and secondary psychological problems if assessment and initiation of treatment are either ignored or delayed inappropriately.[12]

CAUSES OF ACUTE ABDOMINAL PAIN IN INFANCY AND EARLY CHILDHOOD

Gastrointestinal causes

Meconium ileus
Hirschsprung disease
Intestinal stenosis/atresia
Infectious enteritis/gastritis
Pyloric stenosis
Malrotaion
Intestinal duplication
Inguinal hernia
Intussusception
Adhesions
Appendicitis

Genitourinary causes

Testicular torsion
Urinary tract infection
Urinary obstruction (posterior urethral valves, tumors)

Trauma

Intraluminal hematoma
Pancreatic pseudocyst

Drugs/toxins

Lead
Lactose intolerance
Salicylates
Erythromycin
Ibuprofen

Other

Sickle cell disease
Henoch-Schönlein purpura
Primary peritonitis
Pneumonia

CAUSES OF ACUTE ABDOMINAL PAIN IN LATE CHILDHOOD AND ADOLESCENCE

Gastrointestinal causes

Appendicitis
Adhesions
Infectious enteritis/gastritis
Intussusception
Obstruction
Gastroesophageal reflux
Ulcer
Inguinal hernia

Genitourinary causes

Pregnancy (tubular, incomplete/threatened abortion)
Pelvic inflammatory disease
Genital tract obstruction (imperforate hymen with menarche, bifid uterus)
Dysmenorrhea
Ovulation/ovarian cysts
Torsion of ovaries or testes
Undescended testicle
Urinary tract infection
Urinary calculi

Trauma

Intraluminal hematoma
Pancreatic pseudocyst

Drugs/toxins

Lead and other heavy metals
Lactose intolerance
Alcohol
Salicylates
Erythromycin
Tetracycline
Ibuprofen

Other

Sickle cell disease
Henoch-Schönlein purpura
Primary peritonitis
Pneumonia
Muscle strain/sprain
Cholecystitis
Pancreatitis
Familial Mediterranean fever
Porphyrias

ASSESSMENT

To identify the major diagnostic category to which further assessment and treatment recommendations can be directed, it is important to develop a systematical approach (Fig. 110-1) to the evaluation of the child or adolescent who has abdominal pain.[10,11] Because abdominal pain can be such a complex problem, systematical application of the cornerstones of medical care—history, physical examination, selected laboratory studies, and clear therapeutic recommendations based on the differential diagnosis—is essential. The history alone can account for about 80% to 90% of the data the physician uses in making a differential diagnosis. A systematical history should elicit information about the location, onset, severity, alleviating and precipitating factors, and associated symptoms. Timing of the onset of pain and the change in intensity, location, and quality of pain over time are essential factors in defining the etiology of the symptom. For children or adolescents who have recurring abdominal pain, information about the timing of the onset of the pain in relation to other events (e.g., mealtime or school days), as

CAUSES OF RECURRENT ABDOMINAL PAIN

Organic (see acute causes in the boxes on p. 853)

Infectious gastroenteritis (*Giardia lamblia, Salmonella, Shigella, Yersinia enterocolitica,* viral)
Peptic ulcer disease
Gastritis
Esophagitis
Hiatal hernia
Inflammatory bowel disease (Crohn disease, regional enteritis)

Dysfunctional

Constipation/chronic stool retention
Lactose intolerance
Intestinal gas with heightened awareness of intestinal motility
Dysmenorrhea
Mittelschmerz
Overeating
Irritable colon

Psychogenic

Acute reactive anxiety
School phobia
Conversion reaction
Depression
Complaint modeling
Hypochondriasis
Factitious

well as the duration of each episode and the frequency of recurrence, is helpful. Additional information about family (inherited disorders, concurrent illnesses, chronic pain disorders), medical history (prior surgery, chronic medication), and environmental/behavioral factors (recent changes in family or school, travel, unusual food intake) also should be obtained. In addition to the presence of specific symptoms and positive history, negative aspects of the history can provide important information to narrow the differential diagnosis. For example, the absence of dysuria in an older child or adolescent would make the diagnosis of urinary tract infection unlikely.

Laboratory and diagnostic studies that are done without any medical indications generally are unhelpful and actually may hinder the pediatrician's therapeutic recommendations. This common pitfall occurs when the pediatrician responds to the parents' initial requests to "rule everything out" by laboratory or radiographic studies.[7] The pediatrician needs to help the family how essential their history is in the assessment. The history from the child or adolescent himself or herself also is crucial and calls on the special skills of the pediatrician (see Chapter 75, Interviewing Children). The child or adolescent must feel comfortable in discussing his or her symptoms and concerns, even if these are different from those expressed by the parents. It is useful to obtain a history from the child or adolescent alone. Parents, too, may need to relate some of their concerns without the child present. In both instances important diagnostic information can be missed if the pediatrician does not give the child and parents this opportunity to give separate histories.

The historical information should serve to focus the physical examination and specific diagnostic studies. Although a complete physical examination, including an external examination of the urethra, vagina, and anus, always should be part of an initial assessment of abdominal pain, the history of the presenting symptoms will alert the pediatrician to specific aspects of the examination.

Laboratory and other diagnostic studies such as urine, stool, or genital tract cultures, serum chemistries, radiographic studies (e.g., barium swallow, upper or lower GI series, gallbladder series), and abdominal or pelvic ultrasound or computed tomography (CT) scans should be directed to clarification of a specific organic concern identified in the history and physical examination. When indicated, abdominal and pelvic ultrasound provide a safe, noninvasive way to assess bowel and pelvic organ structures and help clarify the need for urgent surgical intervention (e.g., intussusception, ovarian torsion, kidney abscess).[5] In general, the physician should consider the least invasive procedures first, while keeping in mind the cost of special studies in terms of pain, discomfort, and time.

In approaching recurrent abdominal pain, it is important to remember that dysfunctional and psychogenic causes account for most diagnoses, with organic causes identified in only about 5% to 8% of cases. When the history and physical examination indicate a dysfunctional or psychogenic cause, urinalysis should suffice as the initial laboratory study. The pediatrician should be cautious in ordering laboratory studies to reassure the family and rule out disorders because this often can lead only to considering other tests and give the impression that the diagnosis of an organic etiology is still in question.

Focusing on one particular diagnosis at the initial visit may be difficult if not impossible. At the same time, the parents want both to know what exactly is causing the pain and to obtain immediate relief for their child. The pressures to use the "shotgun" approach are great, but the pediatrician is wise to consider the long-term therapeutic effects of such an approach. The costs of not using a systematical approach to RAP are great and include expensive, unnecessary laboratory studies, multiple acute emergency visits, and delay in beginning effective treatment.

MANAGEMENT

Treatment of abdominal pain that has a specific etiology obviously is directed to the indicated therapeutic interventions. For recurrent pain, continual review of the history is important to identify a change in symptoms, which could indicate that an acute process also is occurring, superimposed on the more chronic condition. For example, an adolescent girl who has recurring abdominal pain as a result of occult sexual abuse may present acutely with the pain now caused by a tubal pregnancy.

Even though a specific cause may not be identified initially in the child who has RAP, this should not be viewed as a hindrance to developing a management plan. In the practice of medicine there are many instances of effective thera-

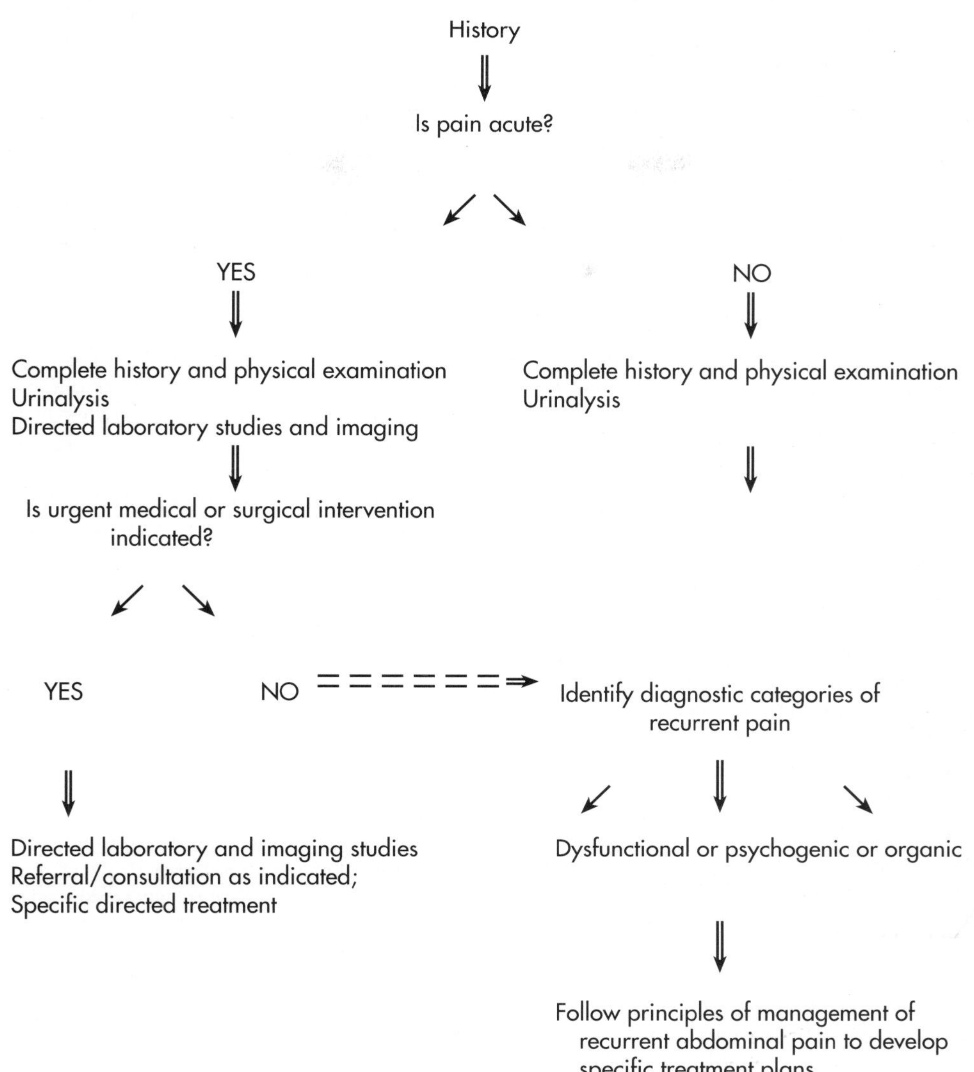

FIG. 110-1 Systematical approach to the evaluation of abdominal pain.

pies available without complete understanding of the exact diagnosis or pathophysiology of the symptom. The pediatrician should be no less willing to offer such care to the child or adolescent who has recurrent abdominal pain.

The treatment of RAP begins at the first visit to the pediatrician for assessment. This initial interaction serves as the basis for establishing clear communication with the family. Effective communication is needed to facilitate the family's cooperation with and confidence in the treatment and management recommendations.

The next step is to provide the child and family with "informed reassurance." The therapeutic relationship is fostered when the physician explains the specific factors in the presenting history and physical examination that are not consistent with urgent intervention. Until the parents have been reassured that acute or serious problems (e.g., appendicitis or tumors) have been considered seriously, they will not be able to "hear," much less understand, the treatment and assessment plans. The pediatrician should then explain the diagnostic considerations. Initially this explanation should be brief but should include the reason why the physician may be asking the family to make specific observations before the next visit.

The most important aspect of the management of recurrent abdominal pain is assuring the child and family of the commitment to continuity of care.[8] This approach helps the family feel that they have an alliance with the pediatrician to continue to assess any changes in the symptoms, as well as to monitor the effectiveness of the treatment recommendations. The pediatrician should avoid giving the message that he or she does not want to hear new or returning concerns. The family should be given a clear set of expectations and guidelines to minimize the possibility of "doctor shopping," as well as to avoid missing important symptoms not apparent initially. Such specific guidelines should address all of the following.

1. *The expected course of the painful episodes with treatment.* The child or adolescent and the parents need to hear that the pain is to be expected to improve gradually over the next 4 to 8 weeks. They also should be forewarned that any additional stresses (physiological, e.g., viral illness, or psychological, e.g., hospitalization

of a close family member) could lead to temporary exacerbation of the pain. It is important to reassure the parents that this is a transient problem rather than a worsening or more serious problem than originally explained to them. This helps avoid a renewed search for a different diagnosis and redirects attention to the treatment plan.

2. *The frequency of follow-up visits to monitor progress and adjust treatment recommendations.* The first follow-up visit should take place within 1 to 2 weeks, depending on the degree of dysfunction caused by the pain. Thus a child who has not been in school for the past 2 weeks would need an early follow-up visit to reinforce a return to school. A common mistake is asking the family to call for an appointment only if there is no improvement. Generally the pediatrician does this to minimize any more school absences for visits to the doctor and may have the mistaken assumption that he or she won't really "do" anything at a visit so close to the initial one. Because symptoms often improve immediately after the first office visit, the pediatrician is wise to take the opportunity to reinforce this positive change and avoid the hazard of the child needing more painful episodes in order to be seen. The number of subsequent visits should be tailored to the individual case, but two to four follow-up visits spaced every 2 to 3 weeks apart generally is sufficient for treating recurrent abdominal pain.
3. *The modification of pain reinforcers.* Once recurrent abdominal pain has been diagnosed, neither the parents at home nor the pediatrician in follow-up should initiate discussion about the pain with the child. When children or adolescents feel the pain, they should be encouraged to identify any precipitating stresses, should be reassured that they can deal with the pain themselves, and, if needed, should rest for a short period before resuming activities. Likewise, when children report no painful episodes, they should be praised for how well they are doing. The obvious treatment goal is to alleviate pain. A less apparent, twofold goal is to reduce the number of reports of pain and to encourage children, when they do report it, to be able to describe how they coped with it and then returned to normal activities. Parents should plan rewards for improved school attendance and resumption of usual activities. The pediatrician can explain that he or she will be checking "how well" the child is doing in follow-up and focus attention on the child's positive coping strategies.
4. *The conditions and symptoms that need to be brought to the physician's attention and the degree of urgency for reporting them.* As was mentioned before, in children and adolescents acute abdominal pain can develop superimposed on recurrent abdominal pain; thus the pediatrician should review with the family symptoms for which they should call immediately (e.g., localized pain, persistent vomiting, hematochezia) or urgently (e.g., fever, dysuria, decreased appetite). Parents should be instructed to note recurrent episodes and how their child dealt with the pain. This information is best reviewed without the child present to avoid reinforcing the reporting of pain. Parents should be encouraged to call and discuss any symptoms about which they are unsure. In this way the pediatrician can help alleviate the parents' guilt about minimizing their child's pain.
5. *The pediatrician's willingness to discuss and assist in making appropriate referrals for second opinions and treatment recommendations.* The family will be more confident in the diagnosis if they know the pediatrician can initiate consultations readily should the need arise.

Longitudinal studies have shown that 30% to 60% of children continue to have pain for years because it can take some time to "grow out of it." The goal for pediatricians should be to help the child or adolescent and the family prevent abdominal pain from interfering with their functioning and well-being by developing good communication and a systematical approach to assessment while providing clear management recommendations.

REFERENCES

1. Ammerman S, Shafer MA, Snyder D: Ectopic pregnancy in adolescents: a clinical review for pediatricians, *J Pediatr* 117:677, 1990.
2. Apley J: Pathogenesis of recurrent abdominal pain. In Apley J: *The child with abdominal pains,* ed 2, London, 1975, Blackwell Scientific.
3. Barr RG: Abdominal pain in the female adolescent, *Pediatr Rev* 4:281, 1983.
4. Barr RG, Feuerstein M: Recurrent abdominal pain in children: how appropriate are our usual clinical assumptions? In Firestone P, McGrath P, editors: *Pediatric and adolescent behavioural medicine,* New York, 1983, Springer-Verlag.
5. Bhisitkul DM et al: Clinical application of ultrasonography in the diagnosis of intussusception, *J Pediatr* 121:11182, 1992.
6. Caty MG, Azizkhan RG: Acute surgical conditions of the abdomen, *Pediatr Ann* 23:192, 1994.
7. Coleman WL, Levine MD: Recurrent abdominal pain: the cost of the aches and the aches of the cost, *Pediatr Rev* 8:143, 1986.
8. Edwards MC et al: Survey of pediatricians' management practices for recurrent abdominal pain, *J Pediatr Psychol* 19:241, 1994.
9. Feuerstein M et al: Potential biobehavioural mechanisms of recurrent abdominal pain in children, *Pain* 13:287, 1982.
10. Green M: Diagnosis and treatment: psychogenic, recurrent, abdominal pain, *Pediatrics* 40:84, 1967.
11. Poole SR, Schmitt BD, Mauro RD: Recurrent pain syndromes in children: a streamlined approach, *Contemp Pediatr* 12:47, 1995.
12. Stone RT, Barbero GJ: Recurrent abdominal pain in childhood, *Pediatrics* 45:732, 1970.
13. Zeltzer LK et al: Pediatric pain: interacting behavioral and physical factors, *Pediatrics* 90:816, 1992.

111 Alopecia and Hair Shaft Anomalies

Henry M. Seidel and Nancy K. Barnett

Perhaps one of the major lessons of the 1960s was that hair matters. It certainly does not serve an essential function, inasmuch as one can live without it. Nevertheless, the symbolism over the ages, from Samson to John Lennon, and the emotional investment everyone has in his or her hair make any of its abnormalities a matter of concern. This is particularly so with alopecia; the loss of hair is a disturbing event.

A sequence of events makes up the life of a single hair, from active growth, a busy period known as the *anagen phase,* to passivity, a resting period known as the *telogen phase.* As many as 15% of scalp hairs may be in the telogen phase at any one time. These hairs soon are lost in the constant turnover, the continuous shedding that is hardly apparent to a casual observer. Surprisingly, about 50% of the hair must be shed for loss to be noticeable.

Hair loss may increase to as much as 60% during a period known as a *telogen effluvium.* During such a period the situation is much like that of animals, which shed seasonally. In humans this change in the normal anagen/telogen ratio may occur after a high, relatively prolonged fever, a period of time after pregnancy, or after a severe illness. It may appear in either sex. The diagnosis of telogen effluvium can be confirmed simply by plucking a group of hairs and examining them microscopically. The number of resting hairs should be increased well beyond the usual 10% to 15%. This is a diffuse, nonpatterned, and nonscarring hair loss.

The constant ebb and flow of growth and shedding and the extreme activity of the hair follicle—mitotic and metabolic—put the follicle at great risk when exposed to antimetabolites and mitotic inhibitors. In addition, the constant shedding, even at the rate of 10% to 15%, sets the stage for many of the emotional problems associated with hair that the pediatrician may encounter. The ready availability and pluckability of hair, facilitated by the telogen phase, serve to some extent the need of children who are emotionally distressed.

Obviously, then, hair loss is a matter deserving careful attention. A precise, pointed history and physical examination are necessary. The pediatrician may need to consult with a dermatologist. The pediatrician must not limit the examination simply to the site of loss. The *whole* body and all hair-bearing parts of the body must be observed, and the hairs themselves must be examined microscopically. There are unusual congenital alopecias, and under the light microscope the normality of the individual hair and the ratio of anagen to telogen hairs can be judged. That ratio can be disturbed, and there may be five to six times as many telogen hairs as anagen hairs.

If a child should lose scalp hair rather suddenly, the physician should be concerned with the possibility of a toxic event. This is most common in children who have a malignancy who have been treated with antimetabolites and therefore suffer loss because of the damage done by those drugs during the anagen phase, resulting in an anagen effluvium. Occasionally, sudden hair loss is caused by accidental poisoning, as with rat poison that contains thallium or coumarin. Children must be protected from toxins, and parents must be educated in this regard. In most instances, over a period of several months, new hairs will replace those lost, unless the exposure to the toxic element is repeated or chronic.

The prognosis for the return of hair depends in large part on elimination of the toxic stimulus (when the practitioner is aware of what it might be) or on the hair loss not being accompanied by scarring. Loss with scarring (e.g., from iatrogenic scalp injury during delivery or from a burn) is permanent. In children, the various alopecias of both known and unknown causes usually occur without scarring. This is true of alopecia areata, alopecia totalis, and alopecia universalis; drug-induced, postfebrile, and postpartum alopecias; and alopecias associated with the endocrinopathies (hypothyroidism, hyperthyroidism, and hypoparathyroidism) or nutritional deficiency, particularly deficiencies of vitamins A, B, and C and the protein deficiency that causes kwashiorkor. Occasionally there can be some loss of frontal hair in sickle cell anemia or some patchy, "moth-eaten" loss in secondary syphilis. In parathyroid insufficiency the long-term calcium deficiency is associated with ectodermal abnormalities—not only alopecia and dental abnormalities but also cataracts and pitting and ridging of the fingernails. Also, hair will not grow at the site of most nevi and hemangiomas.

When there is scarring, as with the kerion associated with severe tinea capitis, keloid formation, or discoid lupus erythematosus, there is little hope for recovery. (Systemic lupus erythematosus may result in some hair loss, particularly frontally, but scarring does not necessarily occur.)

MICROSCOPIC EXAMINATION

Appropriate diagnosis requires microscopic differentiation of hair and its root in both the anagen and telogen stages. Deformities of the hair shaft are seen, particularly with aminoacidopathy and in a variety of rare syndromes, including Menkes kinky hair syndrome. One can differentiate monilethrix (usually an inherited, autosomal dominant disorder in which the diameter of the hair shaft varies) from pili torti (a disorder in which the hair is twisted on its long axis). However, the common causes of hair loss usually are innocuous, and the most common ones are distinctly age related.

PHYSIOLOGICAL LOSS OF HAIR

The first hair made by hair follicles in utero feels "silky," covers the entire body of the fetus, and is known as lanugo. It most often is shed in utero, to be replaced by hair that begins to grow on the scalp in the third trimester and continues to grow after birth. This is lost a few months after birth in a normal process that results in a temporary near-baldness. Often parents are concerned with the thinning or with a more markedly localized area of loss, usually over the occiput, the result of the movement of the head from side to side as the baby lies in the crib. Finally, however, this hair is gradually replaced by the new, which has more of a "feel" to it. It is thicker, usually darker, and more stable, growing longer before loss and shedding not quite so readily.

CAUSES OF ABNORMAL HAIR LOSS

A variety of congenital and hereditary disorders can be heralded by hair loss, either a total loss or perhaps a less obvious thinning. A true congenital alopecia may be inherited as an autosomal recessive trait. If the loss is not due to this genetic circumstance, it most often is accompanied by an equally disturbing possibility of another significant hereditary disorder. The hair may not only be thin or possibly lost but also abnormal in a variety of ways. The pediatrician must look for other signs of ectodermal dysplasia and consider radiographic exploration for skeletal defects (e.g., as with cartilage-hair hypoplasia, congenital ectodermal dysplasia, orofaciodigital syndrome), inherited metabolic disorders such as phenylketonuria or homocystinuria, or congenital problems such as hypothyroidism. These and other clinical pictures that result from serious chromosome defects (e.g., de Lange syndrome, Down syndrome) obviously provide a surfeit of signs and symptoms beyond the simple loss of hair. In addition, significant loss from telogen effluvium, occasionally even baldness, may follow intense and persistent fever, severe surgical insult, or precipitous weight loss, for any reason, with concomitant malnourishment and hypovitaminosis.

Hair Shaft Anomalies

Anomalies of the hair may result in a stubbly growth—a short, bumpy terrain most often of the scalp alone, the effect of broken hair and usually not true alopecia. There may be accompanying ectodermal defects, brittle fingernails, or perhaps cataracts and tooth anomalies. Actually, the fragility of hair and the resultant breakage (trichorrhexis) and stubble can be seen in a variety of conditions, all of which are rather rare. These may be familial or congenital, as in trichorrhexis nodosa, a familial circumstance in which the hair is fragile but in which there are no associated findings, or as with the stubbly hair associated with argininosuccinic aciduria, the stubbly hair being the least of the problems in a disease that, fortunately, is uncommon. Children who have argininosuccinic aciduria show evidence of severe mental retardation in the first year of life.

The feel of the hair may be helpful in finding the source of difficulty. In an infant who has hypothyroidism, the hair may be coarse, brittle, and without luster; in progeria and cartilage-hair hypoplasia syndrome, it may be fine and even silky. In all these circumstances the hair may break off and baldness may increase. Whenever the hair is abnormal, it becomes weakened, fragile, and fractured, and it may be lost or unevenly shortened, resulting often in a stubbly, ragged alopecia. The various abnormalities—congenital, traumatic, or endocrine—all can lead to such fragility and loss. Referral to a dermatologist is appropriate so that at the very least a specific diagnosis can be made.

Loose Anagen Syndrome. Loose anagen syndrome is characterized by anagen hairs that are quite easily and painlessly pulled from the scalp.[1] Affected children are generally, but not always, blond and female preschoolers between the ages of 2 and 5. Their hair appears sparse. The individual hairs are not fragile and on examination have misshapen bulbs with absent external root sheaths. Typically the child's hair is said to be slow growing, seldom requiring cutting. The hair over the occiput often is matted and sticky. Fortunately, the condition seems to wane as time passes. The hair grows thicker and longer, and its pigmentation increases. Still, even in adulthood it may pull out easily and painlessly. Although a hereditary factor may be involved, it is not conclusive. The diagnosis can be made on the basis of the history and examination, the painless "pull test" (when the hair is normal, it may hurt to pull), and light microscopy to view the recovered hairs. Management is limited to reassurance and allowance for the passage of time.

Trichorrhexis Nodosa. Trichorrhexis nodosa is a common abnormality of the hair shaft that becomes obvious under the light microscope. The "nodes" seen resemble the effect one observes when the ends of two brushes are pushed together. This most often is congenital and results in breakage of hair and a short stubble over the scalp. It also is probably a genetic predisposition in African-American patients who experience hair breakage over large areas of the scalp and whose hair will not grow beyond a relatively short length. There usually is an accompanying history of hair straightening or repeated vigorous brushing and combing. Avoiding this kind of steady abuse and a more gentle cosmetic approach can result in some gradual improvement. Caucasian and Oriental individuals can experience the same difficulty, probably without congenital or familial relationship, and the breakage most often occurs at the distal end of the hair. White specks may appear after some physical or chemical injury. Here again, the gentle approach and elimination of any noxious element are appropriate.

Monilethrix. Monilethrix (beaded hair syndrome) is a condition in which scalp hairs have regularly spaced differences in their circumference, suggesting a chain of beads. The cause is unknown, and there is no known treatment; however, the outlook occasionally is promising in that a degree of recovery may occur spontaneously, particularly after puberty or during pregnancy. This is a long time to wait, inasmuch as hair breakage becomes obvious during infancy. Occasionally, there are associated problems—cataracts, brittle nails, faulty teeth—suggestive of a more widespread ectodermal defect.

Pili Torti. Pili torti simply means "twisted hair," and indeed, that is the way this type of hair looks under the microscope. The color is "off," and the hair is coarse and lusterless. It is as though straight and curly hair were competing for a place in the same strand. If one looks at a straight hair in cross section, it is round—a curly hair is oval. In pili torti, both configurations may be seen in a single strand. This abnormality can be an important clue to Menkes kinky hair syndrome, an X-linked disease characterized also by progressive cerebral degeneration, arterial degeneration, and the suggestion of scurvy in the bones. There is a low serum copper level because of poor intestinal absorption of copper. This fatal disease to date has not yielded to administration of parenteral copper.

Alopecia Areata

Alopecia areata, most often seen as an acute problem, results in a rather sudden and total loss of hair in sharply circumscribed, round areas, often several centimeters in diameter, usually on the scalp but possibly anywhere on the body where there is hair. There is no evidence of inflammation. Hairs at the periphery of an area are plucked easily and may be particularly colorless and thin. "Exclamation point" hairs may appear throughout the patch. Sometimes the fingernails may look pitted and ridged, as though nature were trying to tell us that the as yet undiscovered cause goes beyond the hair to another ectodermal expression. There may be just a few patches of loss or a total absence of body hair (alopecia universalis), including eyebrows and eyelashes. The more extensive the loss and the younger the child, the less likely a full recovery. The prognosis is best when the loss is less widespread, and only one or two patches are present. Currently the pediatrician has little to offer because the cause is unknown. There has been some suggestion of an autoimmune process. Occasionally, autoimmune antibodies may be identified in patients who have alopecia areata when there is no other clinical evidence of autoimmune disease; an increased incidence of alopecia areata also occurs in persons who have acute autoimmune thyroid disease and vitiligo.

About one third of patients who have alopecia areata will regrow hair spontaneously in 6 months and about one third in 5 years, but for the remaining third, treatments such as those discussed below must be tried to stimulate hair growth.

As often is the case in a poorly understood process, cortisone applied topically has been used with some apparent success. It is possible in the older, more cooperative child to inject the hair follicles with corticosteroids. These are relatively insoluble, and the process is painful. It should be performed with a very small-gauge needle and topical anesthesia—for example, an ethyl chloride spray or EMLA cream. In any event, the primary care pediatrician should seriously question the need for this procedure, carefully assessing the impact of the disease and of the treatment on the patient and should refer the patient to a dermatologist for further consideration of this procedure. The large areas that require infiltration present obvious difficulty, and the addition of oral steroid therapy can only further complicate the treatment.

There also has been some use of irritants (dinitrochlorobenzene) and psoralen with ultraviolet light (PUVA therapy). These agents should be used only in children over age 12 and only by a knowledgeable dermatologist in controlled circumstances. PUVA treatment possibly is justified in alopecia universalis, when all hair is lost. The poor prognosis, however, suggests that although a trial is appropriate, it should not be pushed to unreasonable lengths. It is odd that when hair does regrow after alopecia areata, it may be white. This, however, is temporary, and in the long run it will be impossible for casual observers to identify the formerly affected area.

Common Baldness

There is a genetically determined loss of hair that begins most often with a receding hairline and some thinning over the occiput. This occurs most often in men, but it can happen in women. Fortunately, its fullest expression is most common in the mature adult; the pediatrician rarely is confronted with the problem except in some older adolescents. Unfortunately, there is no effective therapy.

Trichotillomania

Some children have a considerable compulsive need to pull out their hair, even their eyebrows or eyelashes. Although this may not always have important emotional significance, it may provide a major clue to an underlying psychosocial problem when there are patchy, ill-defined bizarre patterns of hair loss. The pediatrician should begin with that assumption and follow this lead gently. The family structure and the interaction with siblings and parents and with friends at home and at school should be explored. Consulting a psychiatrist also should be considered. One can paint the attacked areas with petroleum jelly in an attempt to frustrate the habit; however, without attention to the possibility of a basic emotional problem, this approach quite obviously is inappropriate.

The hair that is lost is that which is most accessible to the probing hand. Sometimes enough is pulled to simulate alopecia areata, and the patient who eats hair may accumulate it in the stomach and create a trichobezoar (hairball), which ultimately may lead to acute intestinal obstruction or, most often, to the complaint of abdominal pain. It may be possible to palpate a mass and to demonstrate it on a roentgenogram; at this point referral to a surgeon is mandatory. Both imipramine and fluoxetine have been used successfully to control trichotillomania in certain children.[2]

Traumatic Alopecia

Hair is a relatively fragile adornment. It does not respond positively to assault, and it should be handled gently and without physical or chemical importuning. It probably is best left alone, except for simple washing and, to suit the fashion, simple cutting.

For some, vanity can lead to alopecia. Constant teasing or straightening with heat or chemicals may seriously damage hair. Some hairstyles, particularly when one uses barrettes or has ponytails, braids, or corn-rows, cause traction that is constant and often tense and prolonged. The hair may then fall out, and there may be an accompanying redness and inflammation with some pustular involvement of the follicles. Generally, simply discontinuing the stress will help; the hair almost always will return. It should be remembered, however, that regrowth can be slow. The loss of any hair in this way, because of trichotillomania or a simple, excessively playful tug, will be slow to repair. Injured hair follicles do not heal quickly and often take 3 months or longer to return to an anagen phase.

Hypoparathyroidism

Sometimes hypoparathyroidism is preceded by an acute bacterial infection and sometimes by candidiasis. The nature of the association between hypoparathyroidism and candidiasis is poorly understood. Nevertheless, chronic hypocalcemia and dental abnormalities can abound in this condition, along with other ectodermal defects such as pitted and ridged fingernails, cataracts, and a stringy, patchy loss of hair.

Most likely the candidiasis does not cause the hypoparathyroidism but, rather, follows the hormonal dysfunction; an immune mechanism possibly is common to both. The pediatrician should consult with an endocrinologist to develop a firm diagnostic and management plan.

Tinea Capitis

Whenever a child has patches of alopecia or stubbly hair growth, even in the absence of crusting, scaling, redness, or other inflammatory signs, the practitioner should consider the possibility of tinea capitis, seborrheic dermatitis, or psoriasis. Obviously, if there is crusting, scaling, or redness, the likelihood of alopecia areata is diminished because inflammation is not a symptom of that condition. In any event, the practitioner should perform a mycological examination, looking particularly for the usual *Trichophyton tonsurans,* in which case the lesions tend to be more elevated than in other forms of tinea and may be characterized by black dots. In rare cases the fungi *Microsporum canis* and *M. audouinii* can invade the hair shaft and thereby cause breakage and stubbiness. *M. canis* tends to cause much more inflammation than does *M. audouinii.* The clinician can look for evidence of these fungal infections by shining the Wood lamp on the affected area in a darkened room. There may well be a greenish fluorescence, although some chemical treatments in the hair also may simulate this fluorescence, making this test less worthwhile than years ago. In any event, the absence of this finding, while not precluding the diagnosis, may suggest a source other than *M. audouinii* or *M. canis.*

On occasion, particularly with *M. canis* or after treatment with an irritant, the area may become secondarily infected and seriously inflamed, requiring treatment with an antibiotic. Kerion, a delayed hypersensitivity reaction, may develop, and the resultant scarring interferes with the regrowth of hair. Early diagnosis and treatment therefore are helpful, although the long 8- to 12-week course of oral griseofulvin may still present difficulties with compliance in a young child. The topical antifungal agents, however, do not effect a cure. Oral prednisone tapered over 10 days may help to decrease rapidly the tenderness and inflammation of a kerion and help prevent a widespread "id" reaction.

Acrodermatitis Enteropathica

Acrodermatitis enteropathica, an autosomal recessive disorder characterized by abnormal zinc absorption, has several important cutaneous manifestations, simulating, at times, psoriasis, epidermolysis bullosa, pyoderma, or candidiasis. With zinc deficiency there is abdominal pain and diarrhea; there also can be an associated "wispy alopecia" and dystrophic development of the fingernails, suggesting widespread ectodermal involvement. Zinc sulfate given orally is the treatment of choice.

Discoid and Systemic Lupus Erythematosus

Discoid lupus erythematosus can be disfiguring to the scalp, and with scarring it can cause a permanent loss of hair. Therefore early treatment is necessary. Scarring can be avoided with topical or intralesional steroids in most cases. Systemic lupus erythematosus also can cause alopecia, and the scalp itself can be erythematous; however, the loss of hair generally is temporary and does not involve the scarring characteristic of discoid lupus erythematosus.

GENERAL MANAGEMENT

Treatment for alopecia depends, of course, on the cause. Practitioners have become all too accustomed to seeing hospitalized children who have a malignancy being treated with antimetabolites and wearing baseball caps to hide their full or partial baldness. However, a noticeable loss of hair at any point may be disturbing to both patient and parent; therefore the suggestion that the child wear a baseball cap or some other unobtrusive, concealing adornment may be appropriate. Even a hairpiece can be designed for a child. These steps serve only for the interim while practitioners attend to the discovery of a potentially helpful treatment or while they wait expectantly in those circumstances in which they do not have a specific treatment and in which their role is diagnostic and supportive. The possibility that hair will not regrow cannot be discarded when loss (1) follows high fever or chronic toxicity, (2) is accompanied by scarring, or (3) occurs in the areas of nevi, aplasia cutis, or persistent hemangiomas. Therefore the supportive aspect should not be minimized because hair loss does matter. It is necessary to talk this through with the child who is old enough and also with the parents, exploring the source of emotional reaction and discomfort and, if recovery of hair is questionable, working with the patient to achieve an emotional balance consistent with reality and to adopt suitable coping mechanisms. Most often this is achievable, and the pediatrician should not back away from trying. The practitioner, sometimes frustrated by the lack of a practical, successful management regimen, should not forget the value of a willing, listening ear—in this as in all things.

REFERENCES

1. Price VH, Gummer CL: Loose anagen syndrome, *J Am Acad Dermatol* 20:249, 1989.
2. Sheika SH, Wagner KD, Wagner RF: Fluoxetine treatment of trichotillomania and depression in a prepubertal child, *Cutis* 51:50, 1993.

SUGGESTED READINGS

Atton A, Tunnessen W: Alopecia in children: the most common causes, *Pediatr Rev* 12:25, 1990.

Datloff J, Esterly NB: A system for sorting out pediatric alopecia, *Contemp Pediatr* 3:53, 1986.

Price VH: Office diagnosis of structural hair anomalies, *Cutis* 15:231, 1975.

Rasmussen JE, editor: Symposium on pediatric dermatology, *Pediatr Clin North Am* 30:417, 1983.

Solomon LM, Easterly NB, Loeffel ED: *Adolescent dermatology,* New York, 1975, McGraw-Hill.

112 Amenorrhea

Alain Joffe

Amenorrhea is a symptom, not a disease, and has a variety of causes. In terms of establishing the etiology of this symptom, it is useful to classify amenorrhea as being either primary or secondary. *Primary amenorrhea* is defined as the failure to initiate menstruation; *secondary amenorrhea* refers to cessation of menses in a girl or woman whose menstrual function previously was normal.

PRIMARY AMENORRHEA

The mean age of menarche in the United States today is 12½ to 13 years; 95% of girls will have menstruated by age 16.[3,10] Menstruation usually begins approximately 2 years after breast budding, the earliest sign of puberty in 85% of girls. However, the interval between the two can be as short as 6 months or as long as 5¾ years.

Given this broad range of individual variation in the onset of puberty, the physician first must note whether breast budding or pubic hair is present. If one or the other is absent by age 14, the patient should be evaluated for delayed puberty (see Chapter 165, Sexual Development Alterations).

If signs of puberty are present, the age at which they appeared must be determined. If fewer than 4 years have elapsed at the time the patient seeks advice and the findings of a general history and physical examination are normal, the patient should be counseled about the variability of development and reassured that hers is normal, particularly if her mother indicates that she first menstruated at a relatively late age.[5] A urine pregnancy test should first be done if there is any possibility that the patient is sexually active. Otherwise, documentation of growth and sexual development should be comforting to the patient until menarche ensues.

If more than 4 years have elapsed since the onset of puberty, the patient has true primary amenorrhea, and a thorough evaluation is warranted.[2] The major causes of primary amenorrhea are listed in the box on p. 862. In most instances a careful history and physical examination will guide the clinician in the workup.

History

The history should address the presence of significant stress in the patient's life, as well as recent weight gain or loss (anorexia nervosa). Queries about exercise or athletic participation, drug use (e.g., phenothiazines), and sexual activity also should be pursued carefully. Clues to any of the endocrine abnormalities, as well as a history of past central nervous system insults (e.g., meningitis) or symptoms of an intracranial tumor, need to be sought. The age at which the patient's mother first menstruated also is helpful information because such a pattern may be familial.[5]

Physical Examination

A complete physical examination, including a pelvic examination, should be performed. Previous growth data (both height and weight) should be plotted. Obesity or excessive thinness can result in amenorrhea.[9] Abnormalities of the visual field, smell, or cranial nerve function, papilledema, or disturbances of reflexes suggest a brain tumor. Hirsutism, a receding hairline, excessive acne, moon facies, striae, an enlarged thyroid, or buffalo hump suggests an endocrine disorder. A webbed neck, short stature,[5] or widely spaced nipples suggest gonadal dysgenesis (e.g., Turner syndrome). Physical signs and symptoms indicative of anorexia nervosa also should be sought (see Chapter 98, Anorexia Nervosa and Bulimia).

A pelvic examination is essential to ensure the presence of normal internal and external female genitalia.[8] An imperforate hymen prevents menstrual blood from escaping.[1] If the hymenal opening is patent, the examination should proceed to determine the presence of a normal vagina, cervix, and uterus. If the hymenal opening is very small, the cervix and uterus can be palpated by means of a bimanual rectoabdominal examination. The size of the clitoris should be noted because clitoromegaly indicates the presence of excess androgens (e.g., congenital adrenal hyperplasia).

Laboratory Tests

A few simple laboratory tests are helpful if the history and physical examination results are normal. A normal urinalysis would rule out diabetes mellitus and chronic renal disease. The presence of epithelial cells in a cytological smear obtained from the wall of the vagina and subsequently fixed and examined as with a Papanicolaou smear correlates with the presence of circulating estrogens. Greater than 10% superficial cells demonstrates a definite estrogen effect. Similar information can be obtained by examining the cervical mucus. The cervix is swabbed with a cotton-tipped applicator, and a small sample of cervical mucus is obtained and spread thinly onto a glass slide and air dried. The slide is examined for ferning, the presence of which indicates a definite estrogen effect. Its absence, however, does not rule out the presence of estrogen, inasmuch as circulating progesterone will prevent ferning. A pregnancy test should be performed if there is any possibility of pregnancy.

If the vaginal or cervical mucus smear shows the presence of estrogen, little else needs to be done. Thyroxine (T_4) and thyroid-stimulating hormone (TSH) levels probably should be obtained because the presence of hypothyroidism can be subtle. If these results are normal, the patient can be reassured that menstruation will begin. At this point the physician should make certain that significant stress or psychosocial problems are not a cause of the amenorrhea. If the vaginal or cervical mucus smear is equivocal, or if superficial

CAUSES OF PRIMARY AMENORRHEA*

1. Familial
2. Psychosocial stress
3. Obesity or severe weight loss (similarly, thin body habitus associated with strenuous exercise programs, as seen in ballet dancers and in patients with anorexia nervosa)
4. Endocrine
   a. Hypopituitarism
   b. Congenital adrenal hyperplasia; adrenal disease
   c. Gonadal dysgenesis (Turner syndrome or Turner mosaic)
   d. Premature ovarian failure
   e. Testicular feminization syndrome
   f. Hypothyroidism
   g. Polycystic ovary disease (rare)
5. Chronic disease
6. Pregnancy
7. Anatomical anomalies
   a. Vaginal agenesis
   b. Uterine agenesis
   c. Imperforate hymen
8. Brain tumor (e.g., prolactinoma)

*For a more detailed list, see reference 12.

cells and ferning are present, several options are open to the clinician, who at this point may wish to refer the patient to a physician skilled in adolescent medicine or to a gynecologist or an endocrinologist. Alternatively a trial of progesterone may be given (either 100 mg of progesterone in oil, given intramuscularly, or medroxyprogesterone [Provera], 10 mg twice daily given orally for 5 days). Withdrawal bleeding after this therapy indicates that the uterine lining has been stimulated by estrogens. Although no further workup, aside perhaps from obtaining T_4 and TSH levels, is necessary, these young women may need further evaluation and "cycling" with progesterone or oral contraceptives if menses are not established soon. If there is no withdrawal bleeding, referral already as noted is appropriate. Several of the diagnostic tests now indicated should be performed in laboratories that produce reliable results. Treatment with hormonal therapy consisting of estrogen and progesterone will be necessary.

An algorithm for evaluation of primary amenorrhea is shown in Fig. 112-1.

SECONDARY AMENORRHEA

By definition, secondary amenorrhea implies some previous level of normal menstrual function. Thus certain causes of primary amenorrhea, mainly abnormalities of the genitalia, are not in the differential diagnosis. However, most of the other causes of primary amenorrhea also can lead to secondary amenorrhea.

When evaluating an adolescent who appears to have secondary amenorrhea, it is important to consider her pubertal status. After the onset of menarche, many teenagers will menstruate sporadically; regular monthly cycles often are not established until 2 to 3 years after menarche.[6] Clearly, the abrupt cessation of menstruation in a teenager who has had regular cycles is of greater concern than is the absence of menses for 3 to 4 months in a teenager who has a history of oligomenorrhea (infrequent periods). The point at which the clinician elects to pursue an evaluation depends on the anxiety of the patient and her family, the possibility of pregnancy, and the physician's assessment of the likelihood that a potentially serious disease is responsible for the amenorrhea. A teenager whose menses previously were regular should be evaluated endocrinologically if amenorrhea has persisted for 3 to 6 months.

History

The history and physical examination again serve as the starting point. The hypothalamic-pituitary-ovarian axis of the teenager is more sensitive to either physical or psychological stress than is that of the adult woman. Stress, emotional upset, fever accompanying viral illness, and changes in weight or environment (e.g., going away to college) all can induce amenorrhea. More severe stresses, such as anorexia nervosa, can produce prolonged amenorrhea. The history also should include questions about drug use, particularly the use of oral contraceptives, or use of depot medroxyprogesterone acetate (Depo-Provera) or levonorgestrel implants (Norplant), all of which can cause amenorrhea. Most women who become amenorrheic while taking oral contraceptives resume menstruation within 6 months of stopping them. Whether the patient is sexually active also needs to be ascertained. If she is, pregnancy should be the primary consideration. Unfortunately, denial of sexual activity does not exclude pregnancy, inasmuch as many teenagers are reluctant to admit to something they feel will be met with condemnation from adults. Sudden cessation of menstruation is more likely to indicate pregnancy or stress as a cause, whereas a gradual cessation suggests polycystic ovarian disease or premature ovarian failure. A history of uterine surgery or abortion raises the possibility of uterine synechiae. With more and more women involved in sports, questions about exercise patterns or participation in athletics (frequency, duration, intensity) have become essential.[7]

Physical Examination

The physical examination may provide clues to the diagnosis. Hirsutism suggests polycystic ovarian disease or late-onset congenital adrenal hyperplasia[2]; receding hairline, deepening of the voice, or clitoromegaly suggests an androgen-secreting tumor. The breasts should be examined carefully; the ability to express any fluid (galactorrhea) manually strongly suggests a neuroendocrine disorder (e.g., prolactin-secreting tumor). The skin should be examined for the presence of striae, and the size of the uterus should be noted because enlargement can be an early sign of pregnancy. Enlarged ovaries suggest polycystic ovarian disease. Physical symptoms suggestive of anorexia nervosa should be sought, especially if there is a history of weight loss (see Chapter 98, Anorexia and Bulimia Nervosa).

Laboratory Tests

Again, a normal urinalysis will help to rule out diabetes or chronic renal disease. A negative urine pregnancy test result (using today's generation of sensitive tests) performed on a first-morning urine specimen makes detection of pregnancy

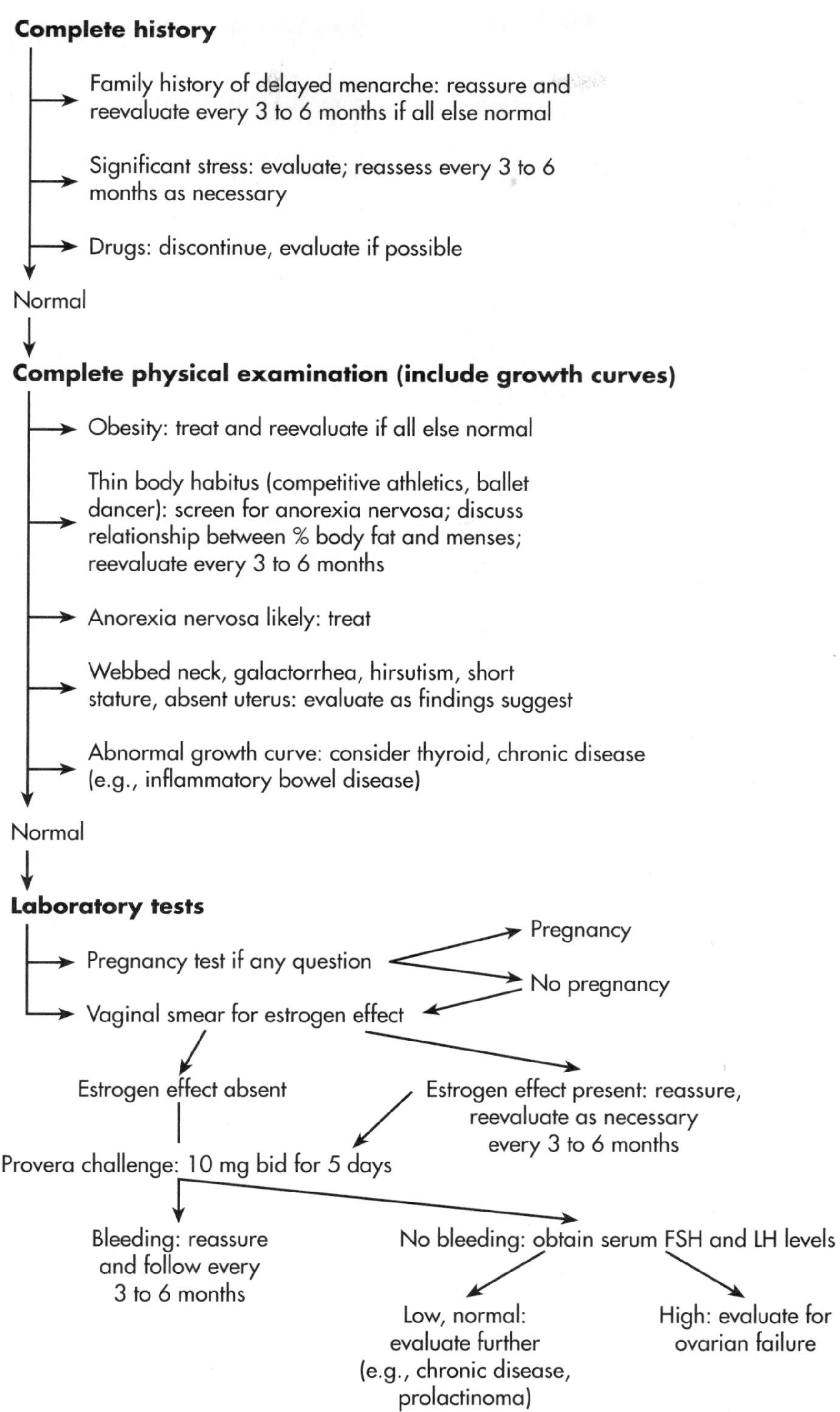

Complete history
Family history of delayed menarche: reassure and reevaluate every 3 to 6 months if all else normal
Significant stress: evaluate; reassess every 3 to 6 months as necessary
Drugs: discontinue, evaluate if possible
Normal
Complete physical examination (include growth curves)
Obesity: treat and reevaluate if all else normal
Thin body habitus (competitive athletics, ballet dancer): screen for anorexia nervosa; discuss relationship between % body fat and menses; reevaluate every 3 to 6 months
Anorexia nervosa likely: treat
Webbed neck, galactorrhea, hirsutism, short stature, absent uterus: evaluate as findings suggest
Abnormal growth curve: consider thyroid, chronic disease (e.g., inflammatory bowel disease)
Normal
Laboratory tests
Pregnancy test if any question
Pregnancy
No pregnancy
Vaginal smear for estrogen effect
Estrogen effect absent
Estrogen effect present: reassure, reevaluate as necessary every 3 to 6 months
Provera challenge: 10 mg bid for 5 days
Bleeding: reassure and follow every 3 to 6 months
No bleeding: obtain serum FSH and LH levels
Low, normal: evaluate further (e.g., chronic disease, prolactinoma)
High: evaluate for ovarian failure

FIG. 112-1 Evaluation of patients with primary amenorrhea who have secondary sex characteristics.

possible within 2 weeks of conception. Examination of the cervical mucus for ferning can indicate the presence of a normal estrogen effect. If the results of all these tests are nondiagnostic, the most likely cause of the amenorrhea lies in the hypothalamus, and the condition probably is a result of stress. However, serum T_4, TSH, and prolactin levels should be obtained to rule out hypothyroidism and a prolactinoma.

If these test results are normal and the patient is not pregnant, a progesterone "challenge" should be undertaken. Withdrawal bleeding indicates an intact hypothalamic-pituitary-ovarian axis, and no further workup is needed. The patient's condition should be monitored. If the amenorrhea continues, withdrawal bleeding should be induced to prevent endometrial hyperplasia.[7] This can be accomplished through use of progesterone alone or with oral contraceptive pills. The latter particularly is useful if the patient is sexually active.

Absence of withdrawal bleeding requires further evaluation. High FSH and LH levels indicate ovarian failure. An LH/FSH ratio greater than 3 : 1 strongly suggests polycystic ovary syndrome. Evaluation of patients who appear to have androgen excess is more complex. Useful laboratory tests include obtaining levels of serum testosterone (total and free) and dehydroepiandrosterone and its sulfate, as well as measuring 24-hour urinary excretion of 17-hydroxycorticosteroids and 17-ketosteroids. Individuals differ as to which of these tests or others are needed.

Evaluation of secondary amenorrhea can proceed along lines similar to those shown in Fig. 112-1. Particular attention should be paid to pregnancy, hypothalamic causes (weight changes, athletics,[4,11] anorexia nervosa), prior contraceptive use, a prolactinoma (especially if galactorrhea is present), endocrine causes (hypothyroidism, polycystic ovary syndrome, or late-onset congenital adrenal hyperplasia), and chronic disease (inflammatory bowel disease). Because low levels of estrogen are associated with osteopenia, it is important to treat hypoestrogenic amenorrhea.

REFERENCES

1. DeKoos EB: Primary amenorrhea, *Pediatr Ann* 5:12, 1975.
2. Emans SJH, Grace E, Goldstein DP: Oligomenorrhea in adolescent girls, *J Pediatr* 97:815, 1980.
3. Emans SJH, Goldstein DP: *Pediatric and adolescent gynecology,* ed 3, Boston, 1990, Little, Brown.
4. Frisch RE et al: Delayed menarche and amenorrhea of college athletes in relation to age of onset and training, *JAMA* 246:1559, 1981.
5. Hollingsworth DR, Kessler Kreutner AK: Gynecologic problems of adolescent girls, *Curr Probl Pediatr* 8:9, 1978.
6. Huffman JW: Diagnosis of secondary amenorrhea, *Pediatr Ann* 5:27, 1975.
7. Mansfield MJ, Emans SJ: Anorexia nervosa, athletics, and amenorrhea, *Pediatr Clin North Am* 36:533, 1989.
8. Mashchak CA et al: Clinical and laboratory evaluation of patients with primary amenorrhea, *Obstet Gynecol* 57:715, 1981.
9. McFarland KF: Amenorrhea, *Am Fam Physician* 22:95, 1980.
10. Neinstein LS: *Adolescent health care: a practical guide,* ed 2, Baltimore, 1991, Urban & Schwarzenberg.
11. Schwartz B et al: Exercise-associated amenorrhea: a distinct entity? *Am J Obstet Gynecol* 131:662, 1981.
12. Soules MR: Adolescent amenorrhea, *Pediatr Clin North Am* 34:1083, 1987.

SUGGESTED READING

Mansfield MJ: Normal female reproductive development and amenorrhea. In McAnarney ER et al, editors: *Textbook of adolescent medicine,* Philadelphia, 1992, WB Saunders.

113 Anemia and Pallor

David N. Korones and Harvey J. Cohen

Pallor and anemia are among the clinical problems encountered most frequently in pediatric practice. Pallor is a physical sign; anemia is a laboratory value. Neither is a diagnosis, and while both may be variations of normal, the pediatrician must investigate these findings thoroughly and determine their cause.

PALLOR

Pallor is pale complexion of the skin. Although it often may be a familial trait or a consequence of limited exposure to the sun, pallor also is observed in a variety of pathological conditions. Vasoconstriction of subcutaneous blood vessels causes the pallor associated with shock, exposure to cold, or syncope. Accumulation of fluid in the interstitium sometimes causes the pallor seen in edematous states such as myxedema, hypoproteinemia, and congestive heart failure. When the hemoglobin concentration is low, pallor may be due to anemia.

Assessment of skin color for pallor often is confounded by clinical and environmental factors. Fluorescent lighting, a common fixture in physicians' offices, distorts the true hue of the skin. It is particularly difficult to recognize pallor in dark-skinned patients. Assessment of pallor also may be complicated by coexistent disorders that cause changes in skin color; for example, jaundice and cyanosis may mask pallor entirely.

ANEMIA

Because most pediatricians screen children for anemia routinely in the first or second year of life and in adolescence, they frequently encounter children who have this problem. Like pallor, anemia is not a diagnosis; it is a laboratory value that alerts the health provider to a reduction in red blood cell mass. The physician or nurse practitioner therefore must be familiar with anemia and prepared to evaluate it for a broad range of etiological possibilities. Armed with a thorough history and physical examination, as well as routine laboratory data that can be obtained in the office, the pediatric health care provider in most instances can determine the cause of anemia.

Definition

Anemia is a decrease in red blood cell mass as determined by a low hemoglobin or hematocrit value. Determining whether a child is anemic sometimes is problematical. Efforts to define a normal hemoglobin level have been hampered by sampling of small or nonrepresentative groups of infants and children, by differences in the normal range of hemoglobin in various ethnic groups, and by failure to exclude patients who have mild anemia from the sample populations. In one of the most thorough studies of normal hematological values of childhood,[4] large numbers of children from different ethnic groups, socioeconomic strata, and ages were sampled. Children who had findings suggestive of iron deficiency, thalassemia, or hemoglobinopathies were excluded. It was found that normal ranges varied depending on age, gender, and race (Table 113-1). Normal hemoglobin levels in African-Americans are approximately 0.5 g/dl lower than those in Caucasians and Orientals.

Normal ranges for hematocrit and hemoglobin values usually are defined as the mean of these values ± 2 standard deviations. This definition results in the arbitrary classification of 2.5% of children as anemic. Some of these children may not be anemic, whereas others whose values fall within the normal range actually may be anemic relative to their usual value. For example, a 3-year-old whose hematocrit value has dropped from 40 to 34 still has a value that falls within the normal range, but this decrease merits further evaluation. A table of normal values serves only as a guideline for the pediatric health care provider. The hematological values of an individual child should be compared with any previous values obtained on that child and must be evaluated in the full context of the child's age, race, history and physical examination, and general state of health.

History

Because most children who have anemia are asymptomatic, a careful history may reveal clues to the existence of an anemia that otherwise would remain undetected. Demographic factors such as age, gender, and ethnic background define important risk groups for different types of anemias. Toddlers and adolescent girls are at highest risk for iron deficiency anemia. Sickle cell disease is observed almost exclusively in African-Americans. Thalassemia occurs with increased frequency in African-Americans and people of Mediterranean and Southeast Asian descent. A dietary history should be elicited. A poor or unbalanced diet may result in a nutritional deficiency, and young children who demonstrate pica are at risk of lead toxicity. Certain drugs can cause anemia; sulfa drugs can precipitate hemolysis in children deficient in the red blood cell enzyme glucose-6-phosphate dehydrogenase (G6PD). Acute infections may suppress production or accelerate destruction of red blood cells. The patient should be screened for signs of acute or chronic bleeding in the most common sites for blood loss—the gastrointestinal tract and the female genitourinary tract. Anemia also may be part of an underlying systemic disorder such as juvenile rheumatoid arthritis or Crohn disease. A family history should be taken; family members who have jaundice or who had a cholecystectomy or splenectomy at a young age may have a hereditary hemolytic anemia, such as hereditary spherocytosis, or a hemoglobinopathy.

Table 113-1 Values (Mean and Lower Limit of Normal) for Hemoglobin, Hematocrit, and Mean Corpuscular Volume Determinations

	Hemoglobin (g/dl)		Hematocrit (%)		Mean corpuscular volume (μ^3)	
Age (yr)	Mean	Lower limit	Mean	Lower limit	Mean	Lower limit
0.5-1.9	12.5	11.0	37	33	77	70
2-4	12.5	11.0	38	34	79	73
5-7	13.0	11.5	39	35	81	75
8-11	13.5	12.0	40	36	83	76
12-14:						
Female	13.5	12.0	41	36	85	78
Male	14.0	12.5	43	37	84	77
15-17:						
Female	14.0	12.0	41	36	87	79
Male	15.0	13.0	46	38	86	78
18-49:						
Female	14.0	12.0	42	37	90	80
Male	16.0	14.0	47	40	90	80

From Nathan DG, Oski F: *Hematology of infancy and childhood,* ed 3, Philadelphia, 1987, WB Saunders.

Signs and Symptoms

Children who have mild or moderate anemia show few signs or symptoms. Infants and toddlers may manifest irritability, longer periods of sleep, changes in behavior, or pallor. Older children may have similar signs or, like adults, may complain of a decrease in exercise tolerance, weakness or dizziness, fatigue, shortness of breath, or palpitations.

Signs of anemia often are subtle. It is not uncommon for a child to receive a clean bill of health at a routine health care visit, only to be called back for reevaluation because of a low hematocrit value on routine screening. Pallor may indicate anemia, but it is not appreciable in mild anemia and may not be detectable until the hemoglobin level is as low as 8 g/dl.[9] Careful examination of the conjunctivae, mucous membranes, palmar creases, and nail beds may reveal pallor when the skin does not. The presence of scleral icterus or jaundice suggests a hemolytic anemia. Frontal bossing and prominent maxillae may represent expansion of bone marrow red blood cell production caused by a chronic hemolytic anemia such as thalassemia major. Diffuse lymphadenopathy and organomegaly may indicate leukemia or lymphoma. Auscultation of the heart often reveals a pulmonary flow murmur with mild to moderate anemia, and a gallop rhythm may be heard when a profound anemia results in congestive heart failure. Splenomegaly is apparent in patients who have certain hemolytic anemias or infiltrative diseases.

Laboratory Data

In addition to the hemoglobin or hematocrit determinations, three other laboratory tests can be performed in most offices—the reticulocyte count, the peripheral blood film, and the mean corpuscular volume. These tests can provide the clinician with enough information to determine the cause of most anemias. The reticulocyte count is a measure of red blood cell production and thus provides valuable information about the bone marrow's ability to respond to an anemia. Reviewing the peripheral blood film allows the practitioner to assess the morphology and color of the erythrocytes. The mean corpuscular volume is an index of red cell size and serves as a starting point for morphological classification of anemia. Observation of the plasma in a centrifuged sample of blood is a simple test that may provide additional clues: (1) clear plasma suggests iron deficiency, (2) icteric plasma may occur secondary to extravascular hemolysis, and (3) pink plasma may develop secondary to intravascular hemolysis. Other laboratory tests may be indicated when particular causes of anemia are suspected; these are summarized in Tables 113-2 to 113-4.

CLASSIFICATION OF ANEMIA

Anemias often are classified based on decreased production or increased destruction of red blood cells. Another basis for classification is red cell morphology; the information gained from the peripheral blood film and the mean corpuscular volume enable the clinician to classify an anemia as microcytic, normocytic, or macrocytic. One then can systematically follow an algorithm to evaluate the subtype of anemia (Fig. 113-1) and minimize the number of laboratory tests done to arrive at a diagnosis.

Microcytic Anemias

In children, microcytic anemia has five causes: iron deficiency, thalassemia, lead poisoning, chronic inflammation, and sideroblastic anemia.

Iron Deficiency. Iron deficiency is by far the most common cause of anemia in children.[5] The clinician must determine whether the deficiency is due to poor dietary intake of iron, blood loss, or other less common causes. Children between the ages of 12 and 24 months are at the highest risk of iron deficiency anemia. Most of these children are no longer taking iron-containing formula but are drinking cow milk instead, and their intake of solid foods is erratic. Adolescents also may develop an anemia as a result of poor dietary intake of iron; adolescent girls may have further loss of iron from blood loss with frequent or heavy menses. Iron deficiency anemia is unusual in full-term infants in the first 6 months of life. These infants are born with sufficient

Table 113-2 Laboratory Evaluation of Hypochromic and Microcytic Anemias

Diagnosis	Laboratory test	Expected result
Iron deficiency	Serum ferritin	Low <25 μg/L
	Serum iron and total iron-binding capacity	Low/high
	% iron saturation	Low <15%
	Bone marrow iron stores	Absent
	Stool for occult blood	Positive (if gastrointestinal bleeding)
	Urine for blood, hemoglobin, or hemosiderin	Present (if renal loss)
	MCV/RBC ratio	>13
Beta-thalassemia trait	Blood film	Basophilic stippling
	Hemoglobin electrophoresis	Increased A_2 or F hemoglobin
	Biosynthetic beta/alpha-globin chain ratio	<1
	MCV/RBC ratio	<13
	Family studies	Hgb/Hct decreased Blood film Anisocysotis Poikilocytosis Basophilic stippling MCV <70 fL/cell
Alpha-thalassemia trait	No routine specific test	Normal A_2 hemoglobin
	Family studies	Hgb/Hct normal or slightly decreased Blood film Anisocytosis Poikilocytosis MCV <70 fL/cell
	Biosynthetic beta/alpha-globin chain ratio	>1
	Specific genetic probe analysis	Absent genes
Chronic inflammation	Nonspecific tests	
	Erythrocyte sedimentation rate	Increased
	Acute phase reactants	Increased
	C-reactive protein	
	Fibrinogen	
	Haptoglobin	
	Serum ferritin	Increased
	Serum iron + total iron-binding capacity	Low/low
	% iron saturation	Low
	Bone marrow iron stores	Increased
	Bone marrow sideroblasts	Decreased
Sideroblastic anemia	Serum ferritin	Increased
	Serum iron + total iron-binding capacity	Normal to increased/normal
	% iron saturation	High
	Bone marrow iron stores	Increased
	Bone marrow sideroblasts	Increased sideroblasts plus "ringed" sideroblasts
Lead poisoning	Blood film	Basophilic stippling
	Erythrocyte protoporphyrin	Increased
	Blood lead	Increased

From Segel GB: *Pediatr Rev* 10:77, 1988.
MCV, Mean corpuscular volume; *RBC,* red blood cell, *Hgb,* hemoglobin; *Hct,* hematocrit.

iron stores to maintain a normal hematocrit level for 6 months.

When children of any age have an iron deficiency anemia, it is essential to evaluate them for blood loss. Because the gastrointestinal (GI) tract is a common site of occult or chronic blood loss, patients and families should be queried about black or tarry stools, hematochezia, and bloody or coffee-ground emesis. Stool guaiac tests should be done at several different times because blood loss through the GI tract may be intermittent. Gastric or duodenal ulcers, Meckel diverticula, polyps, hemorrhoids, and aspirin-induced bleeding should be considered. Other possibilities include epistaxis and inflammatory bowel disease. Cow milk may induce GI bleeding.[17] Iron deficiency itself, through damage to iron-dependent enzymes in the intestinal mucosa, may cause occult blood loss.[10] The signs and symptoms of iron deficiency anemia do not differ significantly from those of any other slowly developing anemia. Irritability, pica, and craving for ice and unusual foods occasionally have been observed with anemia specifically caused by iron deficiency.[15]

If the deficiency of iron is enough to cause anemia, changes in other laboratory parameters will be present. The mean corpuscular volume and the absolute reticulocyte count will be low, and the peripheral blood film will show a pre-

Table 113-3 Laboratory Evaluation of Normocytic Anemias

Diagnosis	Laboratory test	Expected result
Anemias with low reticulocyte percentage		
Diamond-Blackfan anemia	Bone marrow examination	Decreased erythroid precursors
	Fetal hemoglobin and i antigen	±Increased
	Mean corpuscular volume	±Macrocytosis
Transient erythroblastopenia of childhood	Bone marrow examination	Decreased erythroid precursors
Aplastic crises	History	Underlying hemolytic disease
	Bone marrow examination	Decreased erythroid precursors
	Serology and/or viral culture	Parvovirus
Anemias with high reticulocyte percentage		
Extrinsic		
Autoimmune hemolysis	Blood film	Spherocytes
	Antiglobulin (Coombs) test	Positive
	Complement consumption assay	Positive (used if Coombs test is negative)
	Tests for underlying disease	
Fragmentation hemolytic anemia	Blood film	Fragmented RBC
	Tests for underlying disease	
Intrinsic		
Membrane disorders	Blood film	Characteristic RBC: spherocytes, stomatocytes, elliptocytes
	Incubated osmotic fragility	Increased fragility if spherocytes present
	Autohemolysis	Increased and corrected by glucose
	Membrane protein-structural analysis (investigational)	Abnormal (e.g., decreased spectrin in spherocytosis)
Hemoglobin disorders	Blood film	Irreversibly sickled cells in severe sickle syndromes: SS-, SC-, or S-thalassemia
		Targeting in CC, also in SS-, SC-, and S-thalassemia
	Hemoglobin electrophoresis	Abnormal hemoglobins
Enzyme disorders	Screening tests	Positive
G6PD	Enzyme assay	Low activity
Pyruvate kinase and other glycolytic defects	Enzyme assay	Low activity

From Segel GB: *Pediatr Rev* 10:77, 1988.

Table 113-4 Laboratory Evaluation of Macrocytic Anemias

Diagnosis	Laboratory test	Expected result
Vitamin B_{12} deficiency	Blood film	Macroovalocytes, Howell-Jolly bodies; nucleated RBC and hypersegmented granulocytes
	Serum vitamin B_{12}	Low <100 pg/mL
	Bone marrow examination	Megaloblastic erythroid and granulocyte precursors
Folic acid deficiency	Blood film	Same as above
	Serum folate	Low <3 ng/mL
	RBC folate	Low <160 ng/mL
	Bone marrow examination	Same as above

From Segel GB: *Pediatr Rev* 10:77, 1988.

dominance of hypochromic and microcytic cells. Target cells and elliptocytes also may be observed. These data usually are sufficient to diagnose iron deficiency. When the diagnosis is not certain, confirmatory laboratory tests may include determining the serum ferritin and serum iron levels (both of which will be low) and the total iron-binding capacity (elevated). The plasma of patients who have iron deficiency anemia is clear rather than the normal, straw colored, and the anemia frequently is associated with thrombocytosis.

It is reasonable to give a patient a therapeutic trial of supplemental iron (6 mg/kg of iron per day) if the patient has laboratory evidence of iron deficiency anemia and his or

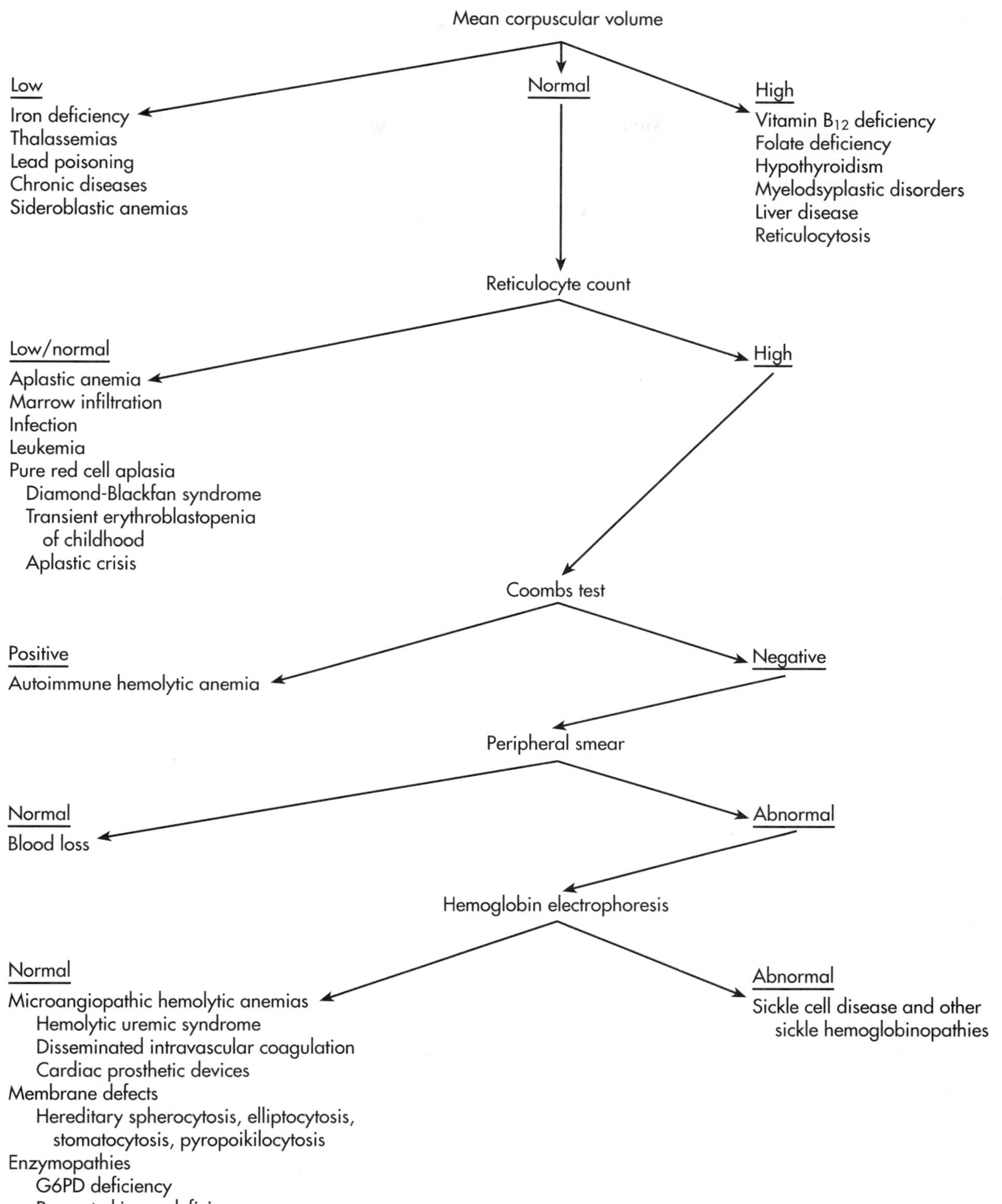

FIG. 113-1 Diagnostic approach to anemia in a child, based on the mean corpuscular volume.

her age and history suggest poor dietary iron intake. For patients who do not fall into this category or who are compliant and yet do not respond (or respond only transiently) to supplemental iron, additional evaluations for blood loss are imperative. It must be remembered that iron deficiency anemia is a pathophysiological state for which an etiology needs to be found. For individuals who have moderate to severe iron deficiency anemia, the reticulocyte count should increase within 5 to 7 days after therapy is started. The therapy for iron deficiency requires continuous iron supplementation for approximately 2 to 3 months after the anemia is corrected. For a more complete discussion of iron deficiency anemia, see Chapter 20, Part Five, Screening for Anemia.

Thalassemias. The thalassemias are a heterogeneous group of disorders of hemoglobin production. In alpha-thalassemia the synthesis of the alpha-chain is reduced; in beta-thalassemia, similar deficits occur in beta-chain production. A decrease in production of one leads to a surplus of the other. This imbalance results in precipitation of the surplus chains and destruction of the red blood cells. In general, the greater the imbalance in production of the two chains, the more severe the clinical syndrome.

BETA-THALASSEMIA. Two genes (one on each chromosome 11) direct the synthesis of the beta-chain of hemoglobin. An abnormality in one of these genes causes a mild decrease in beta-chain production. The associated clinical syndrome is called beta-thalassemia trait (or thalassemia minor) and commonly is observed in patients of Mediterranean descent. These patients are completely asymptomatic and usually are diagnosed incidentally or when undergoing routine screening for anemia. The children are mildly anemic; they have a low mean corpuscular volume (usually 60 to 70 fl), a mild increase in the number of red cells, and a peripheral blood film showing microcytosis, hypochromia, and target cells. Iron deficiency may be confused with this entity because of the similarity of laboratory findings in these two disorders. A useful guideline for distinguishing between them is the Mentzer index,[14] which is based on the premise that there are greater numbers of red blood cells in beta-thalassemia trait than in iron deficiency. Hemoglobin electrophoresis usually shows mild elevation of hemoglobin F or hemoglobin A_2. Genetic counseling is recommended for families of patients who have beta-thalassemia trait; individuals who inherit this defect from one parent and a similar or second defect from the other parent (e.g., sickle cell trait) may be afflicted with more severe hemoglobinopathies.

Severe beta-thalassemia (Cooley anemia, thalassemia major) is the result of defects in both the genes directing synthesis of the beta-chain. The marked deficiency in beta-chain production that results is reflected in the more severe clinical syndromes. Patients are severely anemic; there is brisk hemolysis, and the compensatory erythropoiesis is responsible for the characteristic prominence of the cheeks and for the frontal bossing seen in these patients.

Extramedullary hematopoiesis and red blood cell destruction cause marked hepatosplenomegaly. Effective genetic counseling has led to a dramatic decrease in the incidence of this disorder in the United States. Treatment consists of repeated blood transfusions and administration of deferoxamine to minimize iron overload from the transfusions.

ALPHA-THALASSEMIA. Four identical genes (two on each chromosome 16) code for the synthesis of the alpha-chains. Abnormalities in these genes are encountered most often in African-Americans and Asians. The silent carrier has a mutation in one of the four genes and is asymptomatic and clinically undetectable. Abnormalities in two genes causes alpha-thalassemia trait. Patients who have this mutation also are asymptomatic; their laboratory findings are similar to those of patients who have beta-thalassemia trait. However, they are even less anemic (if at all), and their hemoglobin electrophoresis result is normal. The diagnosis of alpha-thalassemia trait therefore must be based on a constellation of clinical findings: a patient who has the appropriate ethnic background and a parent having similar laboratory findings (very mild anemia, microcytosis, a normal hemoglobin electrophoresis result, and normal iron status). Hemoglobin H disease is the result of abnormalities in three of the four alpha-chain genes. Patients usually are asymptomatic but have moderate anemia (hemoglobin 7 to 10 g/dl), microcytosis, hypochromia, and red cell fragments. The hemoglobin electrophoresis shows 5% to 30% hemoglobin H (four beta-chains). Abnormalities in all four genes result in no production of alpha-chains and are not compatible with life except with extraordinary measures, such as intrauterine transfusions.

Other hemoglobinopathies associated with microcytosis and anemia include hemoglobin E syndromes (common in southeast Asians) and sickle thalassemia (a combination of beta-thalassemia trait and sickle trait).

Lead Poisoning. Although lead has no known physiological role in humans, virtually everyone has measurable levels because of the widespread use of lead in industrial societies. Lead exerts its hematological effect at low plasma levels, inactivating heme synthesis by inhibiting the insertion of iron into the protoporphyrin ring. Thus, with lead poisoning, the hematological picture is similar to that of iron deficiency anemia: microcytosis, hypochromia, and a low mean corpuscular volume. In addition, target cells and intense basophilic stippling of red blood cells may be observed. Because iron cannot be inserted into the protoporphyrin ring, the latter compound builds up in the red cell, and levels of free erythrocyte protoporphyrin (FEP) rise.

Children are exposed to lead in the air (from combustion of lead-containing gasoline), in dust, and in lead-based paint found in old houses. Approximately 4% of children ages 6 months to 5 years have lead levels over 30 mg/ml,[1] a level that can affect heme synthesis and may even result in lead encephalopathy. Even greater numbers of inner city children may be affected. Symptoms of the anemia are nonspecific, but children who have associated lead encephalopathy may show malaise or behavioral changes. Many physicians use the FEP level to screen for lead poisoning because it is a very sensitive indicator of the pathophysiological effect of the heavy metal. Children who have an elevated FEP then have the blood lead level checked. The most important aspect of treatment is removal of any known sources of lead from the child's environment. Medical treatment consists of chelation therapy with dimercaprol or calcium EDTA, both of which chelate lead and subsequently are excreted with the lead into the urine.

Chronic Inflammation. Patients who have a wide variety of chronic illnesses may have a mild microcytic anemia. This anemia can be seen in children who have cancer, collagen-vascular disease, chronic renal failure, and infection. Although the red cells of these patients more often are normocytic and normochromic, they sometimes are microcytic and hypochromic. The anemia is moderate (hemoglobin 7 to 10 gm/dl) and the reticulocyte count is normal or low. Plasma iron and total iron-binding capacity are low, and ferritin is high. This anemia is believed to be caused by a combination of decreased red blood cell survival, poor marrow response to anemia, and diminished flow of iron from the reticuloendothelial cells to the erythroblasts. The hypochromic microcytic anemia develops when the flow of iron is affected.

Sideroblastic Anemias. These rare forms of anemia are a heterogenous group of disorders caused by retention of iron in the mitochondria of developing erythrocytes. Inherited forms are extremely rare but may be seen in children. Some may respond to pyridoxine. Acquired forms of the disease are encountered more often but almost exclusively in adults.

Normocytic Anemias

Normocytic anemias can be caused by increased destruction or decreased production of red blood cells. The reticulocyte count is a valuable test for distinguishing between these two processes. It generally is high in disorders of increased destruction and low in diseases of impaired red cell production.

Normocytic Anemia with Reticulocytopenia. A normocytic anemia with a low reticulocyte count is uncommon; it may be due to either an isolated problem in the erythroid line or to a disorder that affects all hematopoietic cell lines.

PURE RED CELL APLASIA. Diamond-Blackfan anemia and transient erythroblastopenia of childhood are the most common pure red cell aplasias in children. Diamond-Blackfan anemia is a rare congenital disorder. Children usually manifest the disease in the first year of life with profound anemia and reticulocytopenia. As many as 25% of affected children have physical abnormalities such as short stature or malformed thumbs.[6] Additional laboratory features may include slight macrocytosis, persistent fetal hemoglobin, and persistence of the fetal "little i" red blood cell surface antigen. The etiology is unknown. Patients usually respond to treatment with prednisone.

Transient erythroblastopenia of childhood is a recently recognized,[13] benign, transient hypoplastic anemia that occurs most often in children between the ages of 1 and 4 years. These otherwise healthy children have marked pallor and are severely anemic, with reticulocyte counts of less than 1%. They have normal-appearing erythrocytes that show none of the fetal characteristics of the red cells of Diamond-Blackfan anemia. Although the cause is unknown, several studies suggest that there is humoral suppression of erythropoiesis.[11] Recovery is spontaneous; treatment consists only of red cell transfusions when the anemia is profound. Patients sometimes present in the recovery phase with anemia and reticulocytosis. In these instances the diagnosis may be confused with a hemolytic anemia.

PANCYTOPENIAS. Because anemia may be but one manifestation of a more global disorder of the bone marrow, a white blood cell count and differential and platelet count always should be performed when the hematocrit is low. When these other cell lines are abnormal, serious disorders must be considered in the differential diagnosis. Such disorders include leukemia, primary bone marrow failure syndromes (e.g., aplastic anemia or myelodysplasia), and infiltration of the marrow, as is seen with bone marrow metastases or granulomatous diseases. Occasionally a viral illness will cause a transient suppression of all cell lines.

APLASTIC CRISES. Children who have chronic hemolytic anemia (e.g., sickle cell anemia or hereditary spherocytosis) compensate for increased hemolysis with an increase in the rate of red cell production. Occasionally these children have transient suppression of red cell production, while the hemolysis continues at the same rate. The result is a precipitous drop in the hematocrit value, and patients may have a sudden onset of weakness, fatigue, pallor, and even shock. Laboratory values include a low hematocrit and reticulocytopenia. A patient with a known hemolytic anemia who manifests these findings must be treated immediately. The principal treatment is infusion of red blood cells. The aplasia is transient and in many instances has been associated with acute parvovirus infection.[12]

OTHER. A normocytic, normochromic anemia often is seen with chronic illness, as noted previously. Acute blood loss may be mistaken for a hypoproductive anemia when the patient is seen shortly after the blood loss but before generating a reticulocyte response.

Normocytic Anemia with Elevated Reticulocyte Count. Normocytic anemias with reticulocytosis are characterized by accelerated destruction of red blood cells and a compensatory increase in erythropoiesis. These hemolytic anemias can be classified further by the nature of the red blood cell destruction: those secondary to destruction of normal red cells by extrinsic forces and those in which intrinsic abnormalities of the erythrocytes result in their premature destruction.

HEMOLYSIS DUE TO EXTRINSIC FACTORS. Disseminated intravascular coagulation (DIC), hemolytic uremic syndrome (HUS), certain types of cardiac prosthetic devices, and immune-mediated hemolysis all cause destruction of otherwise normal red blood cells. In DIC and HUS, fibrin is deposited in the small vessels, and erythrocytes are torn apart as they attempt to flow through the maze of fibrin strands. The peripheral blood film shows red cell fragments (schistocytes). A similar morphological picture is seen when erythrocytes are destroyed by prosthetic devices such as artificial heart valves or foreign bodies such as arterial or central venous catheters.

Immune-mediated hemolysis is uncommon beyond the neonatal period; when it occurs, it usually is an autoimmune phenomenon. Autoimmune hemolytic anemia may be idiopathic or a feature of an underlying systemic disorder. Idiopathic autoimmune hemolytic anemia often is associated with an antecedent viral infection and occurs in children of all ages. In most instances the red cell destruction resolves over several months, although children under age 4 or over age 10 are more likely to develop a chronic hemolytic anemia.[2]

Symptoms of autoimmune hemolytic anemia depend on the rapidity and degree of the drop in the hematocrit level. Patients usually are jaundiced secondary to the hemolysis and often have splenomegaly. Patients who have intravascular hemolysis may have pink or red urine as a result of excretion of free hemoglobin. The hematocrit may range from normal to profoundly low, reflecting the intensity of the hemolysis. The reticulocyte count usually is elevated but is normal or low in as many as one third to one half of children,[7] presumably because autoantibodies are directed to reticulocytes as well as to the mature red blood cells. The peripheral blood film shows a preponderance of spherocytes. A positive Coombs test is diagnostic. It is imperative to evaluate the patient who has an autoimmune hemolytic anemia for an underlying systemic disorder. Autoimmune hemolysis is seen in association with malignancies, immune deficiencies, collagen vascular disease, certain drugs, and infections such as *Mycoplasma pneumoniae,* Epstein-Barr virus, and the human immunodeficiency virus (HIV). Treatment of autoimmune hemolytic anemia is directed at correcting the underlying disorder. In cases of idiopathic disease, treatment with prednisone is recommended. Patients should be maintained on a dose of 2 mg/kg/day until the hematocrit value is in the normal range and there is little or no evidence of red cell destruction. Patients who do not respond to steroids may respond to other immunosuppressives or to high doses of intravenous gamma globulin.[3]

Wilson disease must always be considered in any patient who has a nonimmune hemolytic anemia. Hemolysis in Wilson disease is due to elevated levels of serum copper. Early diagnosis leads to early treatment and prevention of severe liver disease and mental retardation associated with more advanced Wilson disease. Vitamin E deficiency also causes hemolysis. It occurs in premature infants and patients who have fat malabsorption (e.g., children who have cystic fibrosis).

HEMOLYSIS DUE TO INTRINSIC ABNORMALITIES OF RED BLOOD CELLS. Three types of intrinsic abnormalities of red cells predispose them to premature destruction: a defective red cell membrane, deficiencies in red cell enzymes, and production of abnormal forms of hemoglobin.

Membrane Defects. Hereditary spherocytosis is the most common of the membrane disorders. The membrane defect usually is due to a deficiency in spectrin, the main structural protein of the red cell membrane. This deficiency renders the red blood cell more fragile and, as a result, more susceptible to hemolysis.

Hereditary spherocytosis is transmitted as an autosomal dominant trait in 75% of cases and occurs in at least 1 in 5000 people of Northern European descent. The spectrum of disease is highly variable; classically, patients who have hereditary spherocytosis have anemia, jaundice, and splenomegaly; in fact, many are identified incidentally on routine screening. Affected patients often report family members who have a history of anemia, jaundice, and splenectomy or cholecystectomy at an early age. Laboratory studies reveal anemia, reticulocytosis, and increased numbers of spherocytes on the peripheral blood film. The osmotic fragility of the red blood cells is increased. This test is not diagnostic, however, because spherocytes or red cells in any disorder characterized by unstable membranes show increased osmotic fragility. The hemolytic anemia resolves with splenectomy, since the spleen is the sole site of red cell destruction in this disease. Most patients eventually require a splenectomy to avoid such complications of hereditary spherocytosis as aplastic crises, gallstones, or splenic trauma.

Hereditary elliptocytosis and hereditary stomatocytosis and pyropoikilocytosis are less common congenital defects of red cell membranes and are encountered infrequently in children.

Enzyme Deficiencies. Glucose-6-phosphate dehydrogenase (G6PD) deficiency is the most common enzymopathy affecting red blood cells. G6PD generates nicotinamide adenine dinucleotide phosphate (NADPH) by catalyzing the conversion of glucose-6-phosphate to 6-phosphogluconate. The NADPH is used by the red blood cell to reduce potentially toxic oxidizing agents that accumulate with exposure to certain drugs, chemicals, and infections.

Two of the most common types of G6PD deficiencies are a mild variant (Gd^{A-}) that occurs in approximately 10% of African-American males and a more severe variant ($G^{Mediterranean}$) observed in people of Mediterranean descent. The disorder is transmitted as an X-linked trait; thus males are affected more often than females. Most patients in the United States (those who have the Gd^{A-} variant) are asymptomatic, and their deficiency is not apparent unless they are exposed to an oxidant stress such as an infection. Agents that most often precipitate hemolysis include sulfa drugs and chloramphenicol, antimalarial drugs, aspirin, ascorbic acid, chemicals such as benzene or naphthalene, infection (hepatitis), and diabetic ketoacidosis.

Patients manifest jaundice and symptoms of a rapidly falling hematocrit. Because the hemolysis is intravascular, they may have hemoglobinuria. Laboratory findings include anemia and reticulocytosis. There may be pitted red blood cells on the blood film, but findings often are nonspecific. Special stains reveal the presence of precipitated hemoglobin aggregates, called Heinz bodies. A test for red cell G6PD often is normal or elevated at the time of a hemolytic episode because only the younger, more enzyme-replete cells remain. If G6PD deficiency is strongly suspected, the test should be repeated 1 to 2 months after the acute crisis or performed in the mother. Treatment is supportive and consists of eliminating exposure to the offending agent and, if necessary, giving the patient a transfusion.

Many other enzyme deficiencies predispose the red cell to hemolysis. Perhaps the most frequently occurring (excluding G6PD) is pyruvate kinase deficiency. Patients who have this rare enzymopathy suffer from a chronic hemolytic anemia. Routine laboratory studies are nondiagnostic; specific assays for pyruvate kinase must be ordered if the diagnosis is suspected.

Hemoglobinopathies. The hemoglobinopathies are a group of hemolytic disorders in which there are abnormalities in the amino acid composition of the alpha- or beta-chain of the hemoglobin molecule. Sickle cell anemia is the most prevalent disease in this group. The defect in sickle cell anemia is a single amino acid substitution of valine for glutamic acid in position 6 of the beta-chain of hemoglobin. This substitution renders hemoglobin susceptible to polymerization when it is exposed to low tensions of oxygen; as a result, the red cell "sickles" irreversibly.

Sickle cell anemia is transmitted as an autosomal recessive trait. Approximately 8% of African-Americans carry this trait. Although 30% to 45% of their hemoglobin is the sickle variant, this is not sufficient to cause their red cells to sickle under normal circumstances. These patients grow and develop normally and have normal hematocrit levels and reticulocyte counts. They occasionally may develop renal papillary necrosis, and when at high altitudes (over 10,000 feet) they are at risk of splenic infarction or other manifestations of vasoocclusive disease. For purposes of genetic counseling, it is important to identify patients who have the sickle hemoglobin trait.

Homozygous sickle cell anemia occurs in approximately 1 in 650 African-Americans. Although the vast majority of people afflicted with the disease in the United States are African-American, it occasionally has been reported in Greeks, Arabs, and natives of India.

Children who have sickle cell anemia usually do not have symptoms of the disease until they are approximately 6 months of age. From age 6 months to 3 years, however, most affected children have experienced the pain of vasoocclusive crises; by age 4 many already show delayed growth and development. Typically these children have hematocrit values ranging from the low to middle 20s, with reticulocyte counts of 5% to 15%. The mean corpuscular volume is normal. The peripheral blood film reveals some irreversibly sickled cells, but target cells, polychromasia, and Howell-Jolly bodies also are present. Hemoglobin electrophoresis is diagnostic; there usually is greater than 90% hemoglobin S and less than 10% hemoglobin F and/or hemoglobin A_2.

Most of the signs and symptoms of sickle cell anemia are a consequence of intravascular sickling and occlusion of blood vessels by the sickled cells. This vasoocclusion (often referred to as a vasoocclusive crisis) occurs episodically, usually in association with infection, dehydration, acidosis, or exposure to cold. The most common type of vasoocclusive crisis is the "painful" crisis that results from widespread ischemia and infarction of bone marrow, bone cortex, or other organs. Infants may have dactylitis; older patients complain of excruciating extremity, back, or chest pain and usually have a paucity of physical findings. Treatment consists of hydration, pain control, and careful monitoring for other complications of vasoocclusion. Patients may have focal rather than diffuse bone pain. When this occurs in association with a high fever, it often is difficult to distinguish whether the patient is experiencing a bone infarction or an osteomyelitis.

Patients also may have chest pain, respiratory distress, a high fever, and an infiltrate on the roentgenogram of the chest. This constellation of signs and symptoms is called the "acute chest syndrome" and may be caused by pneumonia, pulmonary infarction, or both. Patients who have acute chest syndrome are particularly vulnerable to severe, widespread vasoocclusive crises because the pulmonary involvement can cause hypoxia and exacerbate the sickling. Treatment should include vigorous hydration, supplemental oxygen, antibiotics to treat the presumed pneumonia and, if the patient is hypoxic, exchange transfusion to lower the amount of hemoglobin S and increase the oxygen-carrying capacity of red blood cells. Other complications of vasoocclusion include stroke, priapism, and splenic infarction.

Younger patients (ages 6 months to 3 years) are susceptible to splenic sequestration, a sudden accumulation of blood in the spleen. The result is rapid enlargement of the spleen and a precipitous drop in the hematocrit level. Treatment consists of blood transfusions and volume expanders. Patients who experience splenic sequestration are at increased risk of subsequent episodes. Some physicians advocate splenectomy for patients who have two or more episodes.

As noted previously, patients who have sickle cell anemia also are at risk of aplastic crises. The etiology, presentation, laboratory values, and treatment are similar to aplastic crises with other chronic hemolytic anemias.

Perhaps the gravest threat to patients who have sickle cell anemia is their susceptibility to serious bacterial infection. This increased risk of infection is due largely to a hypofunctional spleen; defects in opsonization of bacteria also may play a role.[8] These children are at great risk of overwhelming sepsis, meningitis, and pneumonia secondary to infection with *Streptococcus pneumoniae* or *Haemophilus influenzae* type b. They also may experience severe *Mycoplasma* pneumonia and are unusually susceptible to osteomyelitis secondary to *Salmonella* organisms.

So great is the risk of serious bacterial infection in children who have sickle cell anemia that in most centers they are started on penicillin prophylaxis at age 3 months. It also is recommended that they receive the pneumococcal, *H. influenzae* type b, and influenza virus vaccines. Patients who have sickle cell anemia who develop a fever should be carefully evaluated; if no simple cause is found, they should be admitted to the hospital and treated empirically with intravenous antibiotics. Some investigators advocate initial treatment of well-appearing febrile children with ceftriaxone and subsequent management as outpatients.[16]

Several other hemoglobin defects can occur in combination with the sickle hemoglobin trait and cause a syndrome similar to sickle cell anemia. Patients heterozygous for both hemoglobin S and hemoglobin C may have signs and symptoms of sickle cell anemia, although generally they are less affected than children who have homozygous sickle cell disease. Patients who inherit both the sickle and beta-thalassemia traits may have signs and symptoms of mild or severe sickle cell disease. Patients who have any of these sickle syndromes (as well as those who have the more rare types such as hemoglobin SD or SO^{Arab}) should be managed similarly to patients who have homozygous sickle cell disease; they should receive penicillin prophylaxis and the appropriate vaccines and should be treated similarly for any clinical manifestations of sickling.

Macrocytic Anemias

Macrocytosis is very unusual in children. It can be seen with deficiencies in folic acid or vitamin B_{12}. Folate deficiency may occur secondary to inborn errors of metabolism, poor dietary intake, malabsorption, increased requirements for folate (as in chronic hemolytic anemias), and drugs that inhibit the metabolism of folate (e.g., methotrexate). Vitamin B_{12} deficiency also may be due to inborn errors of metabolism, poor dietary intake, or malabsorption.

The anemia associated with either of these vitamin deficiencies can be severe, and the MCV often is 100 to 140 fl. The peripheral blood film shows numerous normochromic macrocytes and hypersegmented neutrophils. The diagnosis can be confirmed with a serum folate or vitamin B_{12} level; as with iron deficiency, once the deficit is documented, the cause must be determined.

Macrocytosis also is observed in hypothyroidism, myelodysplastic disorders, dyserythropoietic disorders, and liver disease and in patients who have a significant reticulocytosis. It frequently is seen in patients taking valproic acid, and it is a normal finding in the red blood cells of newborns.

ANEMIA IN THE NEWBORN

The approach to anemia in the newborn must be considered apart from that of anemia in an older infant or child. Many of the etiologies of anemia in the newborn (e.g., isoimmune disease) are unique to this age group. Conversely, some common causes of anemia in older children, such as iron deficiency anemia, are rare in infants. Furthermore, some of the etiologies of anemia common to both newborns and older children may manifest themselves quite differently in the newborn period than at an older age. A useful algorithm for evaluation of anemia in the newborn is illustrated in Fig. 113-2.

The normal hematological parameters of a newborn are markedly different from those of older children (Table 113-5). The mean hemoglobin of term infants at birth is approxi-

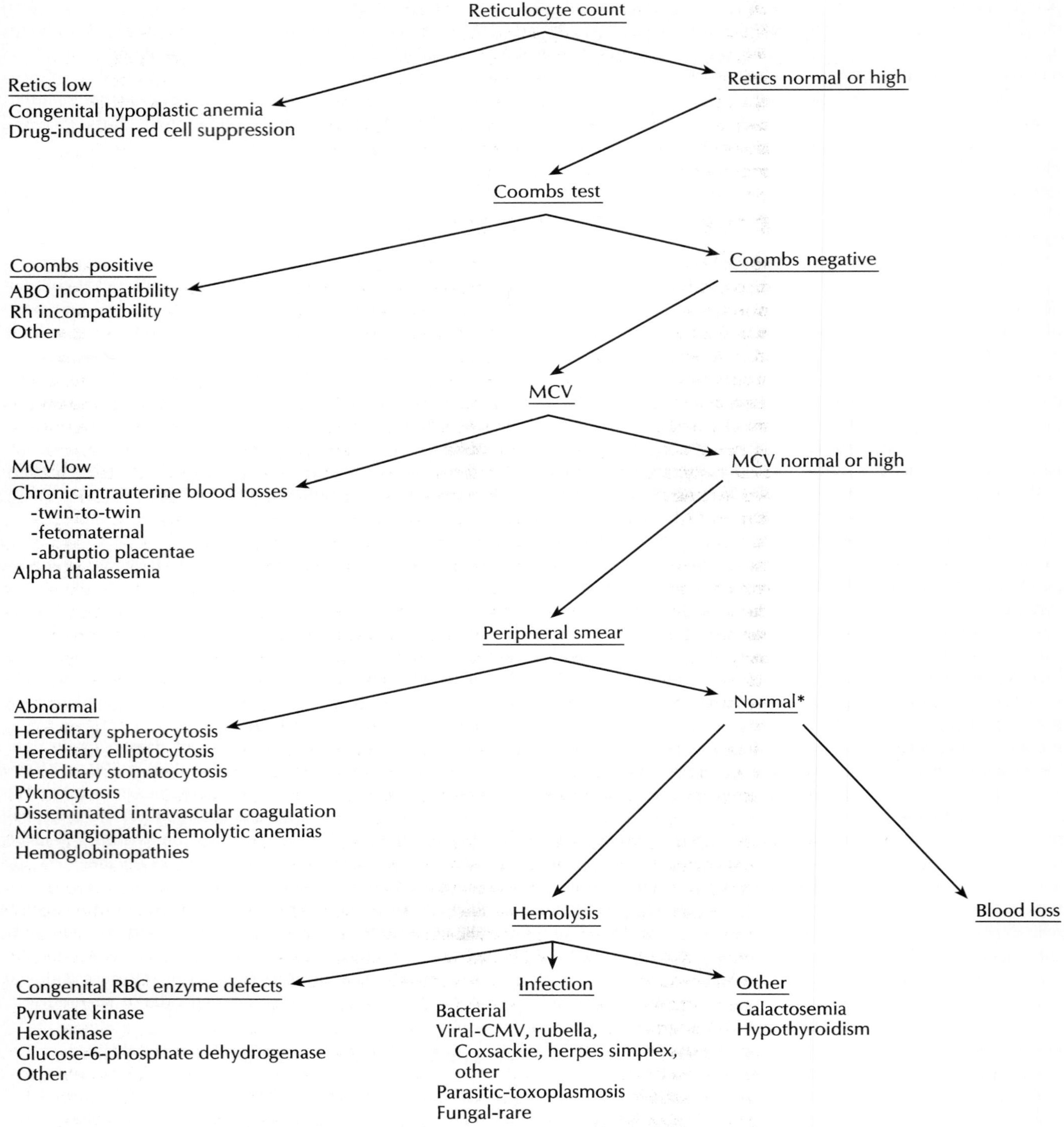

FIG. 113-2 Diagnostic approach to anemia in a newborn, based on the reticulocyte count. The asterisk indicates a peripheral blood smear that shows no specifically diagnostic abnormalities. (From Nathan DC, Oski F: *Hematology of infancy and childhood*, ed 3, Philadelphia, 1987, WB Saunders.)

mately 19 g/dl, but the level falls gradually over 8 to 12 weeks to a nadir of 10 to 11 g/dl. This phenomenon is known as the "physiological anemia of infancy." The drop is even more pronounced in premature infants, in whom hemoglobin levels may fall to 7 to 8 g/dl. This "physiological anemia" is normal in premature and term infants, and despite the low hemoglobin levels, blood transfusion is not necessary in an asymptomatic, otherwise healthy infant.

There are three broad classifications for the etiology of anemia in the newborn: blood loss, hemolysis, and decreased red blood cell production. Blood loss may occur prenatally or perinatally. Common causes include fetomaternal or twin-

Table 113-5 Normal Hematological Values During First 2 Weeks of Life in Term Infant

	Cord blood	Day 1	Day 3	Day 7	Day 14
Hemoglobin (g/dl)	16.8	18.4	17.8	17.0	16.8
Hematocrit (%)	53.0	58.0	55.0	54.0	52.0
Red cells (mm^3 × 10^6)	5.25	5.8	5.6	5.2	5.1
MCV (fL)	107.0	108.0	99.0	98.0	96.0
MCH (pg/cell)	34.0	35.0	33.0	32.5	31.5
MCHC (g/dl RBCs)	31.7	32.5	33.0	33.0	33.0
Reticulocytes (%)	3-7	3-7	1-3	0-1	0-1
Nucleated RBC/(mm^3)	500	200	0-5	0	0
Platelets (1000/mm^3)	290	192	213	248	252

From Nathan DG, Oski F: *Hematology of infancy and childhood,* ed 3, Philadelphia, 1987, WB Saunders.
MCV, mean corpuscular volume; *MCH,* mean corpuscular hemoglobin; *MCHC,* mean corpuscular hemoglobin concentration; *RBC,* red blood cells.

to-twin transfusion, placenta previa, placental abruption, and internal hemorrhage due to cephalohematoma, caput succedaneum, or intracranial hemorrhage. Fetomaternal hemorrhage can be confirmed by the Kleihauer-Betke test, which detects the presence of fetal red cells in maternal blood. (The test may result in a false negative if the mother has type O blood and the child does not.) The clinical presentation depends on the rapidity and degree of blood loss. Infants who have experienced chronic blood loss are hemodynamically stable but pale and have a microcytic, hypochromic anemia. Infants who have acute blood loss often are pale and floppy and have tachypnea, tachycardia, and hypotension. The initial hematocrit may be normal, but the infant soon develops a normocytic normochromic anemia with a reticulocytosis.

Isoimmune disease (erythroblastosis fetalis) is the most common cause of hemolytic anemia in newborns. It is caused by an incompatibility between fetal and maternal Rh, ABO, or minor blood group antigens. In Rh incompatibility, the mother's red blood cells are Rh negative, and those of the infant are Rh positive. If the Rh-negative mother previously was sensitized to Rh-positive blood (from a previous pregnancy), she may have developed antibodies to the Rh antigen; these antibodies cross the placenta and destroy the Rh-positive red cells of the infant. The result is a brisk hemolytic anemia, which occurs in utero and continues after the birth of the child. The hematocrit may fall quickly, and the associated hyperbilirubinemia can cause kernicterus. Rh disease can be prevented by prenatal administration of Rh immune globulin to Rh-negative mothers. Life-threatening Rh incompatibility is rare today, largely because of the routine use of Rh immune globulin. ABO incompatibility (a mother who has type O blood and her infant who has type A, B, or AB) is common, but the hemolysis is mild and infrequently causes hyperbilirubinemia or anemia. Hemolysis occasionally occurs when the mother has been sensitized to one of the minor blood groups, such as the Kell or Duffy antigen. An alloimmune hemolytic anemia or drug-induced hemolysis also may occur in the newborn secondary to passive transfer of maternal autoantibody or maternal drug.

Hemolytic anemia in the newborn is associated with many types of infection. Bacterial sepsis and cytomegalovirus, toxoplasmosis, herpes, and rubella infections all can cause hemolysis. A microangiopathic hemolytic anemia can occur secondary to DIC, cavernous hemangiomas (as in Kasabach-Merritt syndrome), and localized thrombi.

Hemoglobinopathies rarely cause symptoms in the neonatal period. Beta-chain defects, such as sickle cell syndromes, are not apparent until later in infancy, when appreciable concentrations of the beta-chain of hemoglobin have been produced. Similarly, beta-thalassemias are not detectable clinically at birth. Newborns who have alpha-thalassemia major present with erythroblastosis fetalis. Infants with red blood cell membrane defects or enzymopathies occasionally are diagnosed in the newborn period but more often manifest symptoms at a later age.

Disorders of red cell production are rare in the newborn. Hypoproduction of red cells most often occurs secondary to drugs or infection. Diamond-Blackfan syndrome is a rare congenital pure red blood cell aplasia, but infants who have this disease are not anemic at birth. They usually are not diagnosed until the anemia is apparent clinically, sometime between the ages of 3 and 12 months; they may be diagnosed earlier if they have one of the characteristic physical anomalies. Congenital leukemia and osteopetrosis are other very rare causes of red cell aplasia and are associated with abnormalities in other cell lines.

REFERENCES

1. Annest JS et al: Blood lead levels for persons 6 months–74 years of age: United States, 1976-80, PHS 82-1250, Hyattsville, Md, 1982, US Department of Health and Human Services.
2. Buchanan GR et al: The acute and transient nature of idiopathic immune hemolytic anemia in childhood, *J Pediatr* 88:780, 1976.
3. Bussel JB, Cunningham-Rundles C, Abraham C: Intravenous treatment of autoimmune hemolytic anemia with very-high-dose gammaglobulin, *Vox Sang* 51:264, 1986.
4. Dallman PR, Siimes MA: Percentile curves for hemoglobin and red cell volume in infancy and childhood, *J Pediatr* 94:26, 1979.
5. Dallman PR, Yip R, Johnson C: Prevalence and causes of anemia in the United States, *Am J Clin Nutr* 39:437, 1984.
6. Glader BE: Diagnosis and management of red cell aplasia in children, *Hematol Oncol Clin North Am* 1:431, 1987.
7. Habibi B et al: Autoimmune hemolytic anemia in children: a review of 80 cases, *Am J Med* 56:61, 1974.
8. Johnston RB, Newman SL, Struth AG: Increased susceptibility to infection in sickle cell disease: defects of opsonization and of splenic function, *Birth Defects* 11:322, 1975.

9. Kay R, Oski FA, Barness LA: *Core textbook of pediatrics,* ed 3, Philadelphia, 1988, JB Lippincott.
10. Kimber C, Weintraub LR: Malabsorption of iron secondary to iron deficiency, *N Engl J Med* 279:453, 1968.
11. Koening HM et al: Immune suppression of erythropoiesis in TEC, *Blood* 54:742, 1979.
12. Lefrere JJ et al: Six cases of hereditary spherocytosis revealed by human parvovirus infection, *Br J Haematol* 62:653, 1986.
13. Lovric VA: Anemia and temporary erythroblastopenia in children, *Aust Ann Med* 1:34, 1970.
14. Mentzer WC: Differentiation of iron deficiency from thalassemia trait, *Lancet* 1:449, 1973.
15. Schorin MA: Pallor and anemia. In Ziai M, editor: *Bedside pediatrics,* Boston, 1983, Little, Brown.
16. Williams JA et al: A randomized study of outpatient treatment with ceftriaxone for selected febrile children with sickle cell disease, *N Engl J Med* 329:472, 1993.
17. Wilson JF et al: Studies on iron metabolism. V. Further observations on cow's milk–induced gastrointestinal bleeding in infants with iron deficiency anemia, *J Pediatr* 84:335, 1974.

SUGGESTED READINGS

Pearson HA: Sickle cell diseases: diagnosis and management in infancy and childhood, *Pediatr Rev* 9:121, 1987.

Segel GB: Anemia, *Pediatr Rev* 10:77, 1988.

114 Back Pain

Robert A. Pendergrast, Jr.

Back pain is an uncommon presenting symptom in pediatric practice. Among adults 45 years or less, back pain or spine problems are the most common chronic conditions that limit activities.[7] Population-based data on back pain in children are extremely limited, although some estimate that as many as 26% of adolescents (down to age 10) have experienced low back pain.[8] Clearly, most of those experiencing such pain do not seek medical care, and in preadolescent children back pain is not only unusual, but also very likely to indicate serious underlying illness. One 6-year study in a tertiary orthopedic setting found that back pain constituted less than 2% of referrals in children age 15 or less, but that roughly 50% of these children had serious underlying disease.[11] From early adolescence onward back pain not only becomes more common as a presenting complaint, but also is more likely to be a benign condition related to acute injury or repetitive stress. The clinician presented with a child or adolescent complaining of back pain may use a careful history and physical examination to guide any further laboratory or radiological evaluation, but should be aware of the relatively higher risk of serious underlying disease in younger children, even without specific physical findings.

DEFINITION AND CHARACTERISTICS

For purposes of this discussion the back encompasses the region from the upper thoracic vertebra (T1) and shoulder girdle to the sacrum and surrounding musculature. The patient who complains of pain in this region may have a specific sense of localization to a muscle group or vertebral body, for example, or the pain may be more diffuse or sensed by the patient as "deep" and difficult to localize. Allowing the patient to define in his or her own words the nature, location, and duration of the pain is an important first step in arriving at a clinical assessment. Pain that is acute, lasting less than 3 weeks, especially with a history of musculoskeletal injury, may be managed expectantly in many cases, whereas more chronic pain in a child or adolescent demands more immediate attention.[3] The degree of disability that accompanies pain is an important defining characteristic as well, and the corroboration of other observers, such as parents, coaches, and school personnel, can lend urgency to the diagnostic evaluation.

ASSOCIATED SIGNS AND SYMPTOMS

A variety of additional signs and symptoms may provide diagnostic clues to the etiology of back pain. Young children or adolescents who have fever and back pain must be considered to have an infectious, inflammatory, or neoplastic process until proven otherwise; examples include discitis, vertebral osteomyelitis, ankylosing spondylitis, pyelonephritis, pelvic inflammatory disease in a sexually active female, vasoocclusive crisis in a patient who has sickle cell anemia, acute lymphoblastic leukemia, Ewing sarcoma, or Hodgkin lymphoma.[1,3] Dysuria, urgency, or urinary frequency, especially if accompanied by fever, warrants consideration of pyelonephritis; vaginal discharge in a sexually active female should prompt collection of cervical gram stain and cultures for *Neisseria gonorrhea* and *Chlamydia trachomatis* in evaluating for pelvic inflammatory disease. Weight loss, bone pain in other locations, and adenopathy should prompt aggressive diagnostic evaluation for malignancies such as leukemia, lymphoma, or sarcomas. Accompanying neurological symptoms, including radicular pain down the leg, bowel or bladder problems, sexual dysfunction, or loss of sphincter tone on neurological examination,[3] may indicate disc herniation in adolescent athletes. Low back pain associated with excessive lordotic curvature, especially in an athlete subjected to repetitive extension loading (e.g., gymnasts or football linemen) may indicate spondylolysis or spondylolisthesis. Low back pain associated with scoliosis should not be assumed to be caused by the scoliosis; rather the scoliosis and the pain may be secondary to a neoplasm in the region of the spine, such as a benign osteoid osteoma.[1] Stigmata of Marfan syndrome found during the physical examination, such as joint hyperextensibility, pectus deformities, pes planus or pronated feet, hernias, arachnodactyly or scoliosis, may indicate a dural ectasia or widening of the subarachnoid space in the lumbar area, which has been associated with low back pain in adolescents and young adults.[9] Thoracic kyphosis developing in an adolescent who has back pain may indicate Scheuermann disease.

CIRCUMSTANCES SURROUNDING PRESENTATION

The type of diagnostic evaluation and the therapeutic modalities chosen depend on several key factors at presentation. The age of the patient perhaps is the most critical of these, with the extent and urgency of evaluation usually being greater for preadolescent patients.[3] Another factor is the duration of symptoms; chronic pain, even in adolescent patients, is uncommon and may indicate structural or serious underlying disease. Chronic back pain in an adolescent should prompt a diagnostic evaluation to include rectal examination for sphincter tone loss, roentgenograms (anteroposterior, lateral, and oblique views), blood count and sedimentation rate, and urinalysis and culture. In the adolescent patient who can date the onset of pain to a specific event or injury, whose pain lasts less than 3 weeks, and whose pain clearly is exacerbated by mechanical factors such as lifting, stooping, or exercise, a diagnosis of mechanical low back pain is most likely, and these symptoms in most cases will resolve in 2 to 3 weeks regardless of therapeutic approach.[3] Other presentations in adolescents often are sport specific: gymnasts whose lumbar spines are subject to hyperextension and repetitive microtrauma should be highly suspect for spondylolysis or spondylolisthesis; ballet dancers as a group have great flexibility but may be predisposed to lumbar lordosis by postural demands and relatively weak abdominal musculature; they also are prone to spondylolysis as well as to disc disease.[2] Competitive swimmers can present with Scheuermann disease, or "butterflyer's back." The classic presentation of Scheuermann disease is thoracic kyphosis and wedging of three or more contiguous vertebrae shown on plain spine films.

DIFFERENTIAL DIAGNOSIS

Infants

From infancy through the second year of life the patient will not be capable of localizing or complaining of pain in the back. Disease in that area may present as refusal to walk, fever, or other systemic signs of illness.[10] Leukemias, lymphomas, vasoocclusive crisis or vertebral osteomyelitis in a child who has sickle cell disease, or trauma (especially intentional injury) may present as disease localized to the back in this age group.

Children

As children mature and become more capable of localizing symptoms, a specific history of the duration, quality, associated symptoms, and radiation of back pain becomes possible. The differential diagnosis in this age group includes discitis, an inflammatory process presumed to be a bacterial infection in the intervertebral disc space, which typically is associated with an elevated erythrocyte sedimentation rate and a high white blood cell count. It is most common in children less than 10 years of age (mean age, about 6 years). Magnetic resonance imaging (MRI) generally is thought to be a sensitive test in evaluating for discitis.[1,10] A family history of rheumatoid disease should prompt consideration of ankylosing spondylitis, which presents in the majority of cases with back pain.[3] In the presence of sickle hemoglobinopathy a vasoocclusive crisis is a strong consideration. Especially in the presence of fever or other systemic signs and symptoms such as adenopathy, bruising, or organomegaly, acute leukemia must be ruled out by complete blood count and evaluation of the peripheral smear, and the possibility of lymphoma must be evaluated further by lymph node biopsy if available or by MRI of the chest, abdomen, and spine. Primary vertebral tumors almost always will be visible on routine radiographs; these tumors include Ewing sarcoma, aneurysmal bone cyst, benign osteoblastoma, and osteiod osteoma.[1] It is only after a thorough diagnostic evaluation such as described above that one should consider a diagnosis of idiopathic or mechanical back pain in younger children.

Adolescents

In adolescent patients a diagnostic consideration of mechanical back pain without underlying cause becomes reasonable. The typical presentation for this diagnosis is an adolescent who has low back pain of 3 weeks' duration or less, with or without recollection of an acute injury, and whose pain is exacerbated by postural changes or specific movements; associated signs and symptoms such as neurological defects of the lower extremities, limited straight leg raising, sciatic pain, bowel, bladder or sexual dysfunction, fever, weight loss, adenopathy, urinary urgency or frequency, scoliosis, or Marfanoid habitus should be absent.[11]

The adolescent who has chronic (greater than 3 weeks) pain still may have idiopathic or mechanical low back pain, but stronger consideration should be given at this point to plain films of the spine to rule out spondylolysis or spondylolisthesis. Spondylolysis is a defect of the pars interarticularis of the spine, thought to be acquired through repetitive extension loading such as when a gymnast lands from a vault. It is visible as a break in the "neck of the Scotty dog" on oblique lumbar spine films. It may be unilateral or bilateral. Spondylolisthesis is a forward slippage of one vertebral body on top of the other, resulting from bilateral spondylolysis. It may be accompanied on physical examination not only by excess lumbar lordosis but also by the sensation of a shelf at the base of the lordotic curvature, where the lower of the two affected vertebra has held its position while the upper vertebral body slipped forward. In rare cases radiographs will reveal congenital absence of a lumbosacral articular process.[6]

Chronic low back pain, especially in adolescent athletes, may indicate lumbar disc disease. A positive straight leg raising test is highly suggestive of a herniated disc. In adolescents disc herniation is thought to be an acute traumatic event rather than a signal of degenerative disc disease. [1] Using cervical flexion to accentuate the patient's symptoms during straight leg raising may add to the test's sensitivity, and any reproduction of the patient's usual symptoms during testing, or marked asymmetry in symptoms, should be considered a positive test.[4]

Chronic low back pain without any of these signs may be a disorder of the soft tissues of the low back, perhaps secondary to repetitive strain coupled with genetic predisposition and environmental factors such as prolonged seated posture or forward bending of the spine, such as in studying or reading for long periods.

PSYCHOSOCIAL CONSIDERATIONS

Although malingering or the use of pain symptoms for secondary gain may be relatively common in adults, it should not be a strong consideration in the diagnosis of back pain in children or adolescents. However, whereas back pain is not as common a somatoform symptom in clinical practice of adolescent medicine as is headache, abdominal pain, or chest pain, if a thorough diagnostic evaluation of chronic back pain in an adolescent is unrevealing and the usual management involving exercise and stretching is not beneficial, a psychological evaluation should be considered. In these cases the pain should not be assumed to be feigned or "in the patient's head," but rather a very real physical symptom rooted in psychological or emotional distress. At the very least, chronic pain and its accompanying disability can of itself lead to psychological distress, and this should be addressed openly by the clinician.

MANAGEMENT

In cases in which back pain is secondary to an underlying disorder, treatment of the pain itself, though important, is secondary to treatment of its etiological condition. This discussion focuses on treatment of pain and its associated weakness or disability in the adolescent patient who has acute mechanical back pain or whose chronic pain is idiopathic and thought to be a disorder of the soft tissues of the low back.

When the adolescent presents with back pain acutely after an injury and there is no indication of fracture or intraabdominal trauma, the RICE mnemonic (rest, ice, compression, elevation) is useful, as in other acute injuries, for the first 48 to 72 hours. Pain-free activity may be resumed gradually after that point, and low back and hamstring flexibility, as well as the strengthening of abdominal muscles and back extensors, should be emphasized.

The scientific evidence supporting these measures as effective rehabilitation is marginal, but evidence strongly associates inflexibility of hamstrings and low back, as well as weakness of abdominal and back extensor muscles, with low back pain, so the rationale for supporting such exercises seems sound.[5] Full sit-ups with the feet fixed and the knees bent should be discouraged, as this utilizes hip flexors rather than the abdominal muscles to complete the sit-up; evidence indicates that this type of sit-up is associated with higher intervertebral disc pressure. A partial curl or "crunch" is the preferred method of abdominal muscle strengthening, the goal of which is to reduce pelvic tilt and its accompanying tendency toward lordosis and low back strain. Research also has shown that decreased strength and endurance of spinal extensor muscles is associated with low back pain; thus extensor exercises such as raising the torso and head off the floor while lying prone are recommended.[8] These same exercises, and stretching after warming the muscles by gentle exercise or heat, are recommended for chronic low back pain thought to be musculoskeletal in origin.

REFERENCES

1. Afshani E, Kuhn JP: Common causes of low back pain in children, *Radiographics* 11:269, 1991.
2. Bryan N, Smith BM: Back school programs: the ballet dancer, *Occup Med* 7:67, 1992.
3. Dyment PG: Low back pain in adolescents, *Pediatr Ann* 20:170, 1991.
4. Farrell JP, Drye CD: Back school programs: the young patient, *Occup Med* 7:55, 1992.
5. Harvey J, Tanner S: Low back pain in young athletes, *Sports Med* 12:394, 1991.
6. Ikeda K, Nakayama Y, Ishii S: Congenital absence of lumbosacral articular process: report of three cases, *J Spinal Disord* 5:232, 1992.
7. Kelsey JL et al: The impact of musculoskeletal disorders on the population of the United States, *J Bone Joint Surg Am* 61:959, 1979.
8. Plowman SA: Physical activity, physical fitness, and low back pain, *Exerc Sport Sci Rev* 20:221, 1992.
9. Schlesinger EB: The significance of genetic contributions and markers in disorders of spinal structure, *Neurosurgery* 26:944, 1990.
10. Staheli LT: Pain of musculoskeletal origin in children, *Curr Opin Rheumatol* 4:748, 1992.
11. Turner PG, Green JH, Galasko CSB: Back pain in childhood, *Spine* 14:812, 1989.

115 Cardiac Arrhythmias

Edward B. Clark

Abnormalities of cardiac rhythm or conduction are a common pediatric cardiac problem. Arrhythmias in children are caused by disturbances in impulse formation or conduction, or both.

DEFINITIONS

Tachycardia is a persistent increase in heart rate greater than required to meet the activity state of the child. Tachycardias occur more frequently in newborns because of the immaturity of the cardiac conduction and autonomic nervous systems. Bradycardia is an abnormally slow heart rate most often caused by congenital heart block. Acquired heart block is exceedingly rare in childhood, usually occurring as a complication of viral myocarditis or of heart surgery.

DIAGNOSTIC METHODS

Children often are unaware of their abnormal cardiac rhythm. However, the physician can recognize this condition by using the following methods:

1. Examination. Arrhythmias are detected at the time of a physical examination by a heart beat that is irregular, too slow, or too fast.
2. Electrocardiogram. Electrocardiograms (ECGs) taken when the child is at rest and after exercise often document an arrhythmia. However, an individual who has intermittent episodes may have a normal ECG between attacks.
3. Monitoring. A 24-hour ECG tape recording (Holter monitor apparatus) can document infrequent arrhythmias. An event monitor can transmit intermittent episodes by telephone to an ECG recorder.

ASSOCIATED SIGNS AND SYMPTOMS

Many children who have cardiac arrhythmias are asymptomatic, or the physician notes only occasional skipped beats. In other children syncope, dizziness, or lightheadedness can occur with the sudden decrease in cerebral blood flow that accompanies the onset of either paroxysmal tachycardia or sudden bradycardia. Congestive heart failure may be precipitated in infants who have sustained tachycardia of 250 to 300 beats per minute. Older children may complain of chest discomfort or of the heart racing when they have paroxysms of tachycardia; however, they rarely develop congestive heart failure.

CIRCUMSTANCES SURROUNDING PRESENTATION

Most episodes of paroxysmal tachycardia occur in the absence of heart disease or detectable electrolyte imbalance. They are found more commonly in males than in females, especially during the first few months of life, and are being detected increasingly in utero by fetal ultrasonic monitoring. Children who have heart disease are more prone to arrhythmias than are their normal counterparts. Arrhythmias also may be a late postoperative complication following heart surgery.

ANATOMY AND FUNCTION OF THE CARDIAC CONDUCTION SYSTEM

The cardiac impulse is generated by the sinus node and conveyed by sequential components of the conduction system to depolarize the myocardium. The cardiac conduction system includes the sinus node innervated by the parasympathetic and sympathetic nerve fibers located at the junction of the superior vena cava and the right atrium. Fibers from the three atrial internodal pathways converge at the atrioventricular (AV) node, which is located at the mouth of the coronary sinus just above the insertion of the tricuspid valve. From the AV node, fibers form the His bundle, which branches into left- and right-ventricular bundles. The two fascicles of the left bundle, the broad posterior fascicle and the slender anterior fascicle, fan out over the endocardial surface of the left ventricle. The right bundle branch extends directly from the His bundle to the right side of the ventricular septum. The Purkinje network of the left and right ventricles is innervated by the left and right bundle branches and is the terminal portion of the conduction system that connects with the myocardial fibers.

TYPES OF DISORDERS

Supraventricular Arrhythmias

Supraventricular rhythm with normal conduction is characterized on the ECG by a narrow QRS complex. The origin of the impulse is indicated by the P wave and by the PR interval. The supraventricular pacemaker normally is the sinus node. An ectopic atrial focus generates an abnormal P-wave axis. With some supraventricular arrhythmias the QRS complex is abnormal because of aberrant conduction below the His bundle.

Sinus Node. *Normal sinus arrhythmia* is the most common cause of an irregular heartbeat in a child (Fig. 115-1). The rate periodically slows and accelerates as respiration modulates vagal tone. Sometimes a sinus arrhythmia is so exaggerated that an ECG is needed to clarify the normal P-QRS relationship as the rate changes. *Sinus tachycardia* (Fig. 115-2) during exercise is normal, but during rest and in the absence of fever or cardiac failure it suggests the possibility of hyperthyroidism, ingestion of an atropine-like agent, or myocarditis. The smaller the baby, the higher the normal heart rate at rest. The usual range for a newborn is 110 to 150 beats per minute; for a toddler, 85 to 125; for a preschool

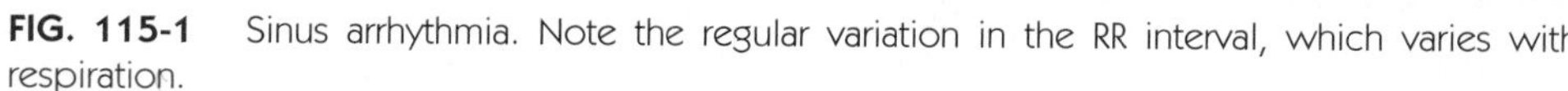

FIG. 115-1 Sinus arrhythmia. Note the regular variation in the RR interval, which varies with respiration.

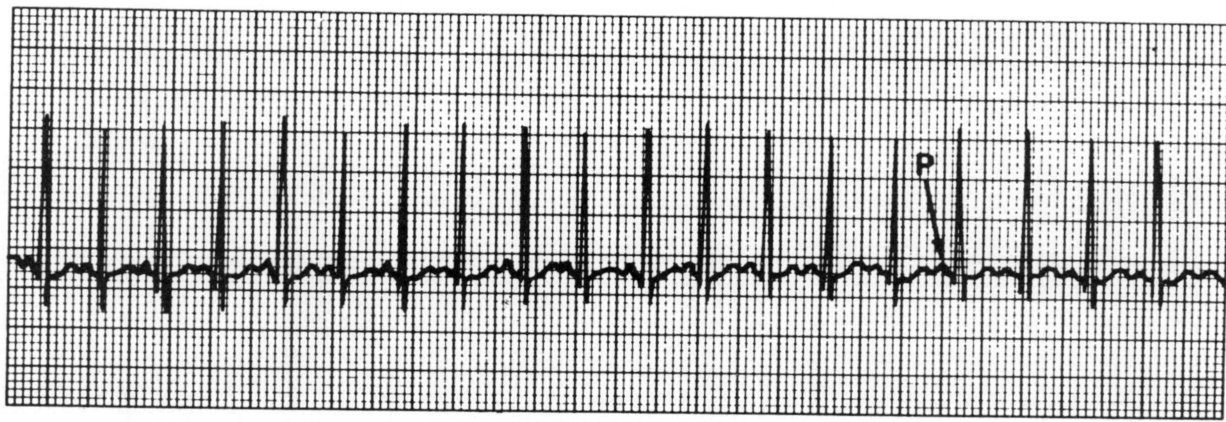

FIG. 115-2 Sinus tachycardia. Each QRS is preceded by a P wave and has a normal PR interval. (From Clark EB: In Cohen SA, editor: ***Pediatric emergency management,*** Englewood Cliffs, NJ, 1982, Prentice Hall.)

child, 75 to 115; and for a child over 6 years of age, 60 to 100.

Sinus bradycardia is normal for a trained athlete but sufficiently unusual in children that possibilities such as hypothyroidism or increased intracranial pressure should be considered. Drugs such as propranolol produce sinus bradycardia by depressing the sinus pacemaker.

A *sinus pause* is an abrupt cessation of sinus node activity characterized on the ECG by the absence of the P wave and QRS complex. *Sinus node dysfunction* (Fig. 115-3) is a disorder in which the sinus node is an unstable pacemaker. During long sinus pauses, a lower atrial focus escapes at a slower rate or with bursts of tachycardia. The patient may have symptoms either with the period of asystole or tachycardia. Treatment may include an artificial pacemaker to prevent extreme bradycardia and antiarrhythmic therapy to control the tachycardia.

Atrium and Junctional Region (AV Node, His Bundle). The atrium and junctional region possess latent pacemaker properties. They can be a focus of isolated beats or ectopic rhythm.

Ectopic Contractions. *Ectopic contractions* arise in atrial muscle (Fig. 115-4, *A*) or junctional tissue (Fig. 115-4, *B*). With atrial ectopic beats the P-wave axis is abnormal. Junctional ectopic beats show no P wave or a P wave with a short PR interval. The ectopic beats occur as escape beats when the sinus node slows, or they may occur prematurely. Although a premature atrial beat may trigger a reentry tachycardia, treatment usually is not necessary.

Supraventricular Tachyarrhythmias. *Supraventricular tachycardia* (SVT) is the most common tachyrhythmia in children (Fig. 115-5). The heart rate usually is regular and too fast to count (220 to 280 beats per minute), and all leads of the ECG show a narrow QRS and regular RR interval. Treatment depends on the duration of the tachycardia and the child's symptoms. SVT often can be terminated by an increase in vagal tone from a Valsalva maneuver or by the application of an ice-cold washcloth to the face. For tachycardias unresponsive to vagal maneuvers, the child can be treated with adenosine to interrupt transiently the conduction through the AV node. Infants in shock or congestive heart failure should have immediate direct current (DC) cardioversion.

Some infants and children who have supraventricular tachycardia have *Wolff-Parkinson-White (WPW) syndrome* (Fig. 115-6). After conversion to sinus rhythm their ECG shows a short PR interval and a prolonged QRS complex, with a delta wave initiating the QRS. An anomalous connection between the atrium and ventricle serves as a bypass tract for the reentry tachycardia. Children may be treated with digoxin or propranolol to reduce their episodes. Patients whose recurrent attacks are unresponsive to medical manage-

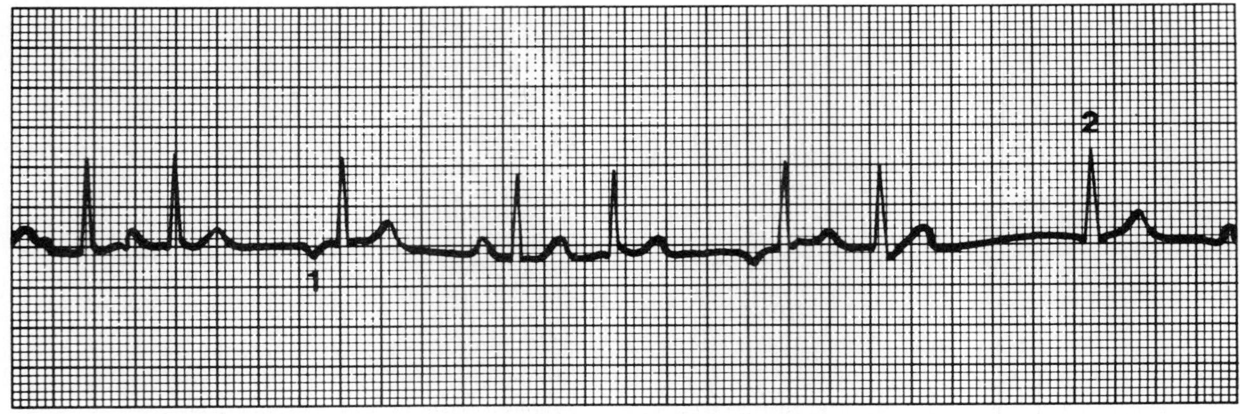

FIG. 115-3 Sinus node dysfunction is characterized by *(1)* ectopic atrial beats and *(2)* junctional escape beats.

(From Clark EB: In Cohen SA, editor: *Pediatric emergency management,* Englewood Cliffs, NJ, 1982, Prentice Hall.)

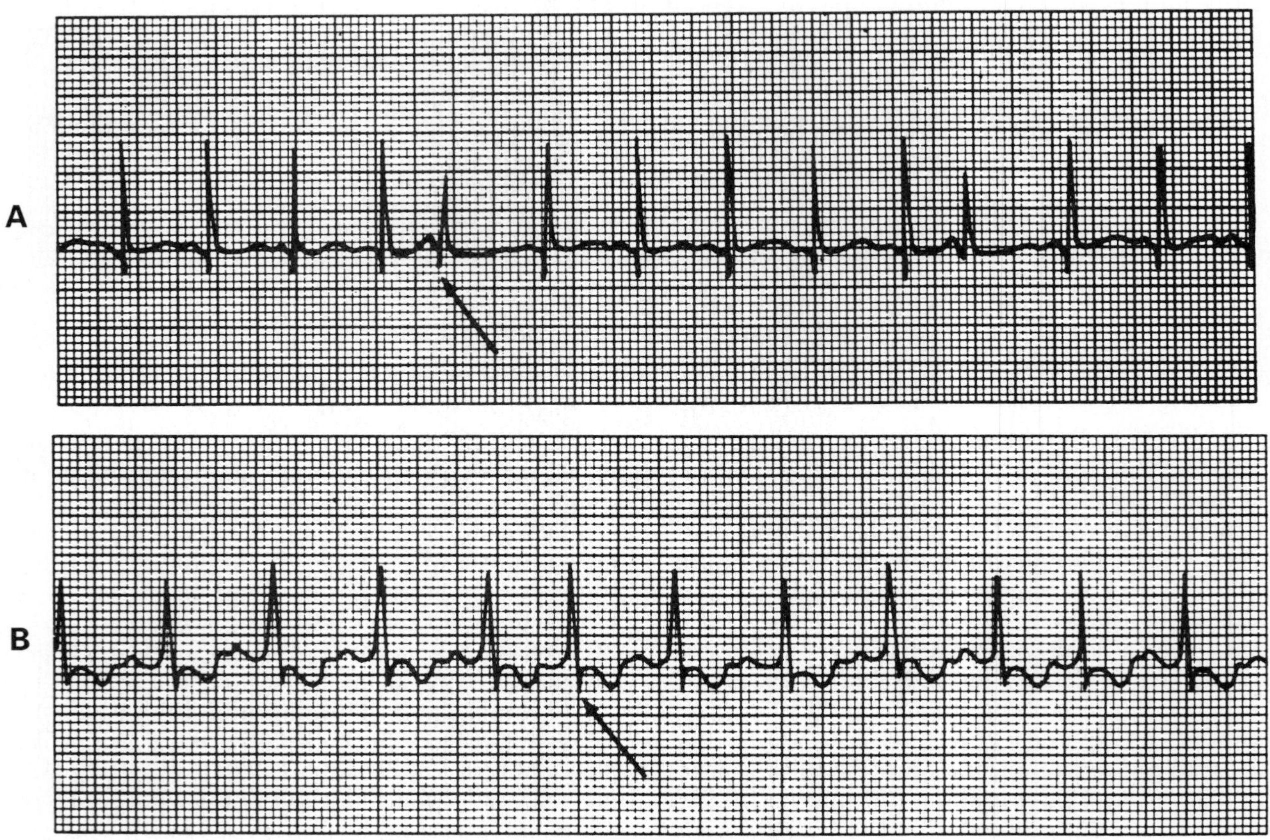

FIG. 115-4 **A,** Premature atrial contraction has an abnormal P wave *(arrow)* preceding the QRS. **B,** Premature junctional contraction *(arrow)* has no preceding P wave.

(From Clark EB: In Cohen SA, editor: *Pediatric emergency management,* Englewood Cliffs, NJ, 1982, Prentice Hall.)

ment may require interruption of the bypass tract. *Atrial flutter* (Fig. 115-7) is a combination of very rapid atrial activity (280 to 300 beats per minute) and variable AV block. The degree of block may vary but often ranges from 2:1 to 4:1 in the ratio of atrial to ventricular impulses. The ECG shows large sawtoothed flutter waves that undulate along the baseline. *Atrial fibrillation* (Fig. 115-8) is disordered, rapid atrial activity with a slower ventricular rate because of varying AV block. It is the least common of the supraventricular tachyarrhythmias in pediatric practice. No P wave is visible in an ECG, but the baseline may show small, irregular, rapid fibrillary waves and an irregular RR interval. These rhythms can

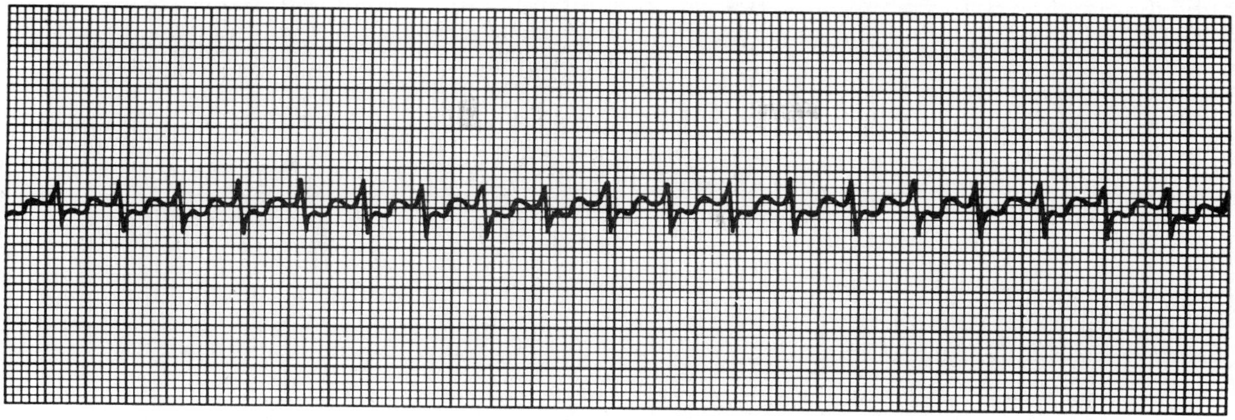

FIG. 115-5 Supraventricular tachycardia is characterized by a narrow QRS complex and no identifiable P wave.

(From Clark EB: In Cohen SA, editor: ***Pediatric emergency management,*** Englewood Cliffs, NJ, 1982, Prentice Hall.)

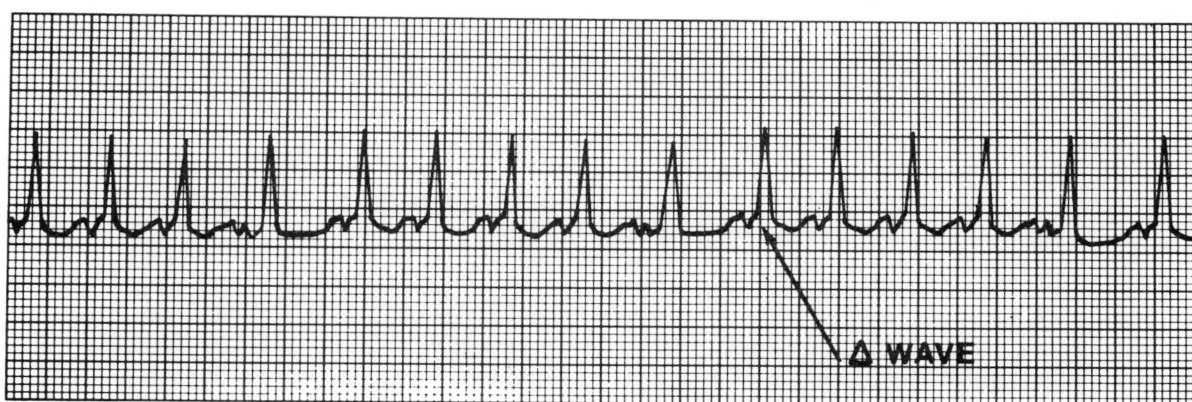

FIG. 115-6 Preexcitation syndrome has a short PR interval and a delta wave *(arrow)*, reflecting early activation of the ventricular myocardium.

(From Clark EB: In Cohen SA, editor: ***Pediatric emergency management,*** Englewood Cliffs, NJ, 1982, Prentice Hall.)

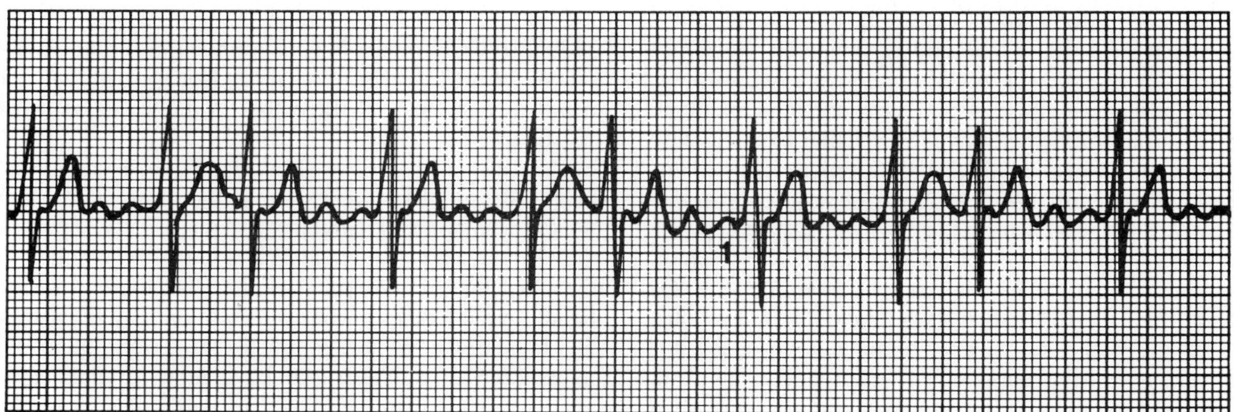

FIG. 115-7 Atrial flutter has coarse, sawtoothed flutter waves (1).

(From Clark EB: In Cohen SA, editor: ***Pediatric emergency management,*** Englewood Cliffs, NJ, 1982, Prentice Hall.)

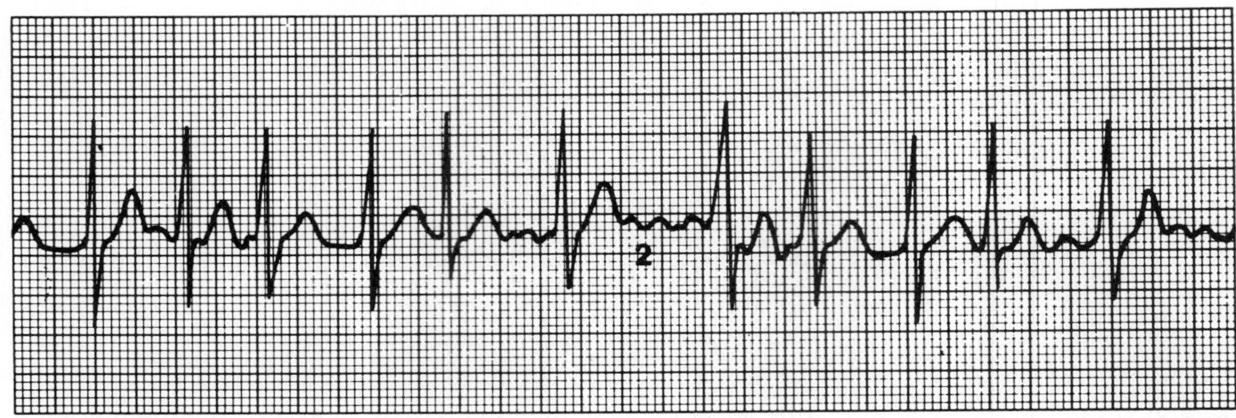

FIG. 115-8 Atrial fibrillation has fine fibrillation waves (2).

(From Clark EB: In Cohen SA, editor: *Pediatric emergency management*, Englewood Cliffs, NJ, 1982, Prentice Hall.)

be treated by slowing conduction at the AV node with digoxin and quinidine or by cardioversion.

Ventricular Arrhythmias. Ventricular arrhythmias are almost as common as arrhythmias of supraventricular origin. Most ventricular premature beats are benign when cardiac function is normal.

Ventricular Ectopic Beats. Premature ventricular contractions (PVCs) are usually unifocal (Fig. 115-9); if multifocal, the prognosis is less favorable. Typically the QRS complex is wide and the ST segments and T waves of the repolarization phase are abnormal. Premature ventricular contractions usually are benign if they (1) are unifocal, arising from the high right ventricle, (2) are suppressed with exercise, and (3) have a fixed coupled RR interval. Premature ventricular contractions may be serious if they (1) are multifocal in origin, (2) increase with exercise, (3) occur in patients with a history of heart surgery, (4) have a variable PR coupling, (5) have an R wave that falls on the T wave, and (6) occur in pairs or triplets. Benign PVCs require no treatment. Multifocal PVCs require investigation and treatment with phenytoin or propranolol.

Ventricular Tachycardia. Ventricular tachycardia is defined as four or more ectopic beats occurring in sequence. Ventricular tachycardia may come and go in bursts (repetitive tachycardia) or may be sustained, usually at a rate of about 150 to 180 beats per minute. A child may notice palpitations, may faint, or become hypotensive. Ventricular tachycardia is life threatening because of the possible progression to ventricular flutter or fibrillation. Diagnosis of ventricular tachycardia by ECG is based on wide, bizarre QRS complexes and the absence of P waves preceding each QRS complex. Ventricular tachycardia is one complication of long QT syndrome (Fig. 115-10). Patients who have delayed repolarization of the ventricle have a prolonged corrected QT interval and may have episodes of ventricular tachycardia that manifest as syncope and atypical seizures. Long QT syndrome may be isolated or familial and sometimes may be associated with sensorineural hearing loss. A child who has unexplained syncope or an atypical seizure should have an ECG analyzed for abnormalities of the QT interval. Treatment includes using a beta-blocking agent and sometimes a pacemaker.

Ventricular Fibrillation. Ventricular fibrillation is a chaotic, disorganized, ineffective ventricular rhythm. A patient who has ventricular fibrillation must be defibrillated immediately with a direct current precordial shock because this rhythm is rapidly fatal without therapy.

DISTURBANCES OF CONDUCTION

AV Block

First-degree AV block (Fig. 115-11, *A*) occurs when the impulse is abnormally delayed in junctional tissue so that the PR interval is prolonged, but each impulse is conducted to the ventricles. AV conduction is prolonged if the PR interval exceeds 0.116 second in an infant, 0.18 second in a child, and 0.20 second in an adolescent or adult.

Second-degree AV block (Fig. 115-11, *B*) occurs when some of the impulses fail to conduct to the ventricles. This rhythm can occur with rheumatic carditis, digoxin toxicity, electrolyte disturbance, and in complex heart defects. Mobitz type I block exhibits Wenckebach periodicity—that is, the PR interval gradually lengthens until a beat drops out. Mobitz type II block is an abrupt block, usually of every second beat (2:1 block), resulting from a disturbance in the conduction system distal to the AV node (in or below the His bundle).

Third-degree AV block (Fig. 115-11, *C*) is complete heart block. The atrial rate is faster than the ventricular rate. When the QRS complex is narrow, the block usually is proximal to the AV node and His bundle. When the QRS complex is wide, the block may be proximal to the His bundle (in a case of bundle-branch block) or the interruption may be distal to the His bundle. Congenital complete heart block often is noted in children of mothers who have lupus erythematosus. In some cases the maternal diagnosis is not made until decades after an affected child's birth. Complete heart block can be a complication of the intracardiac repair of congenital heart defects. Symptomatic patients are treated with a permanent transvenous pacemaker.

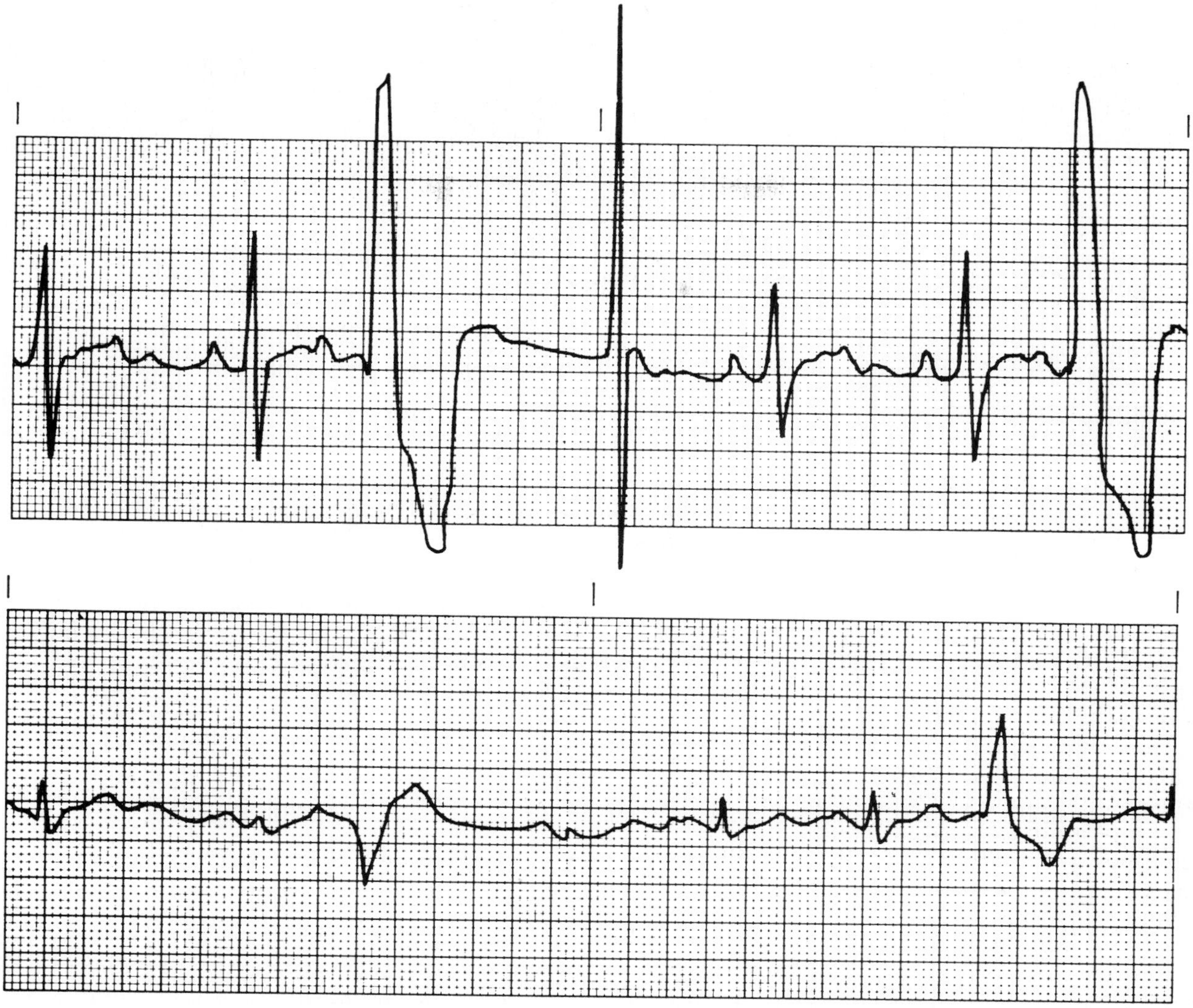

FIG. 115-9 Premature ventricular contractions. Benign unifocal PVC *(top)* and multifocal PVC *(bottom).*

(From Clark EB: In Cohen SA, editor: ***Pediatric emergency management,*** Englewood Cliffs, NJ, 1982, Prentice Hall.)

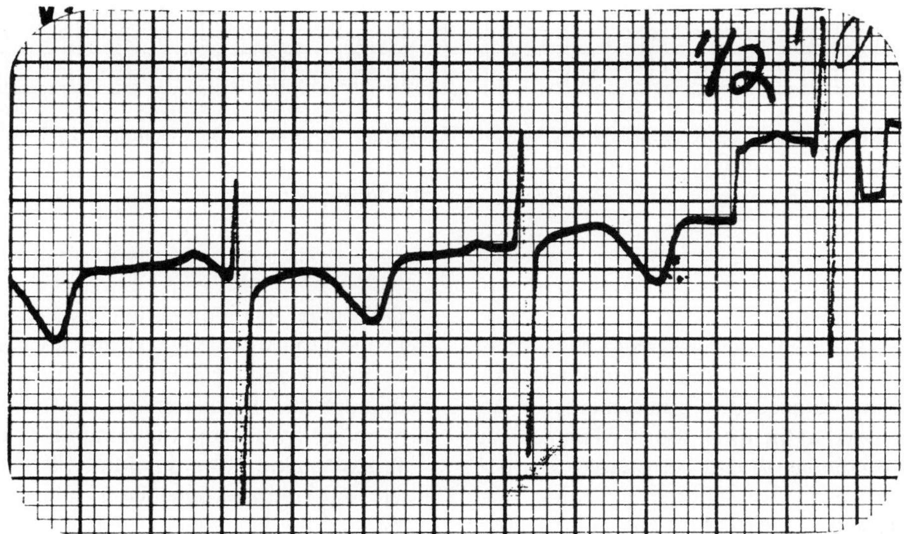

FIG. 115-10 Long QT syndrome has a prolonged recovery of ventricular myocardium.

(From Clark EB: In Cohen SA, editor: ***Pediatric emergency management,*** Englewood Cliffs, NJ, 1982, Prentice Hall.)

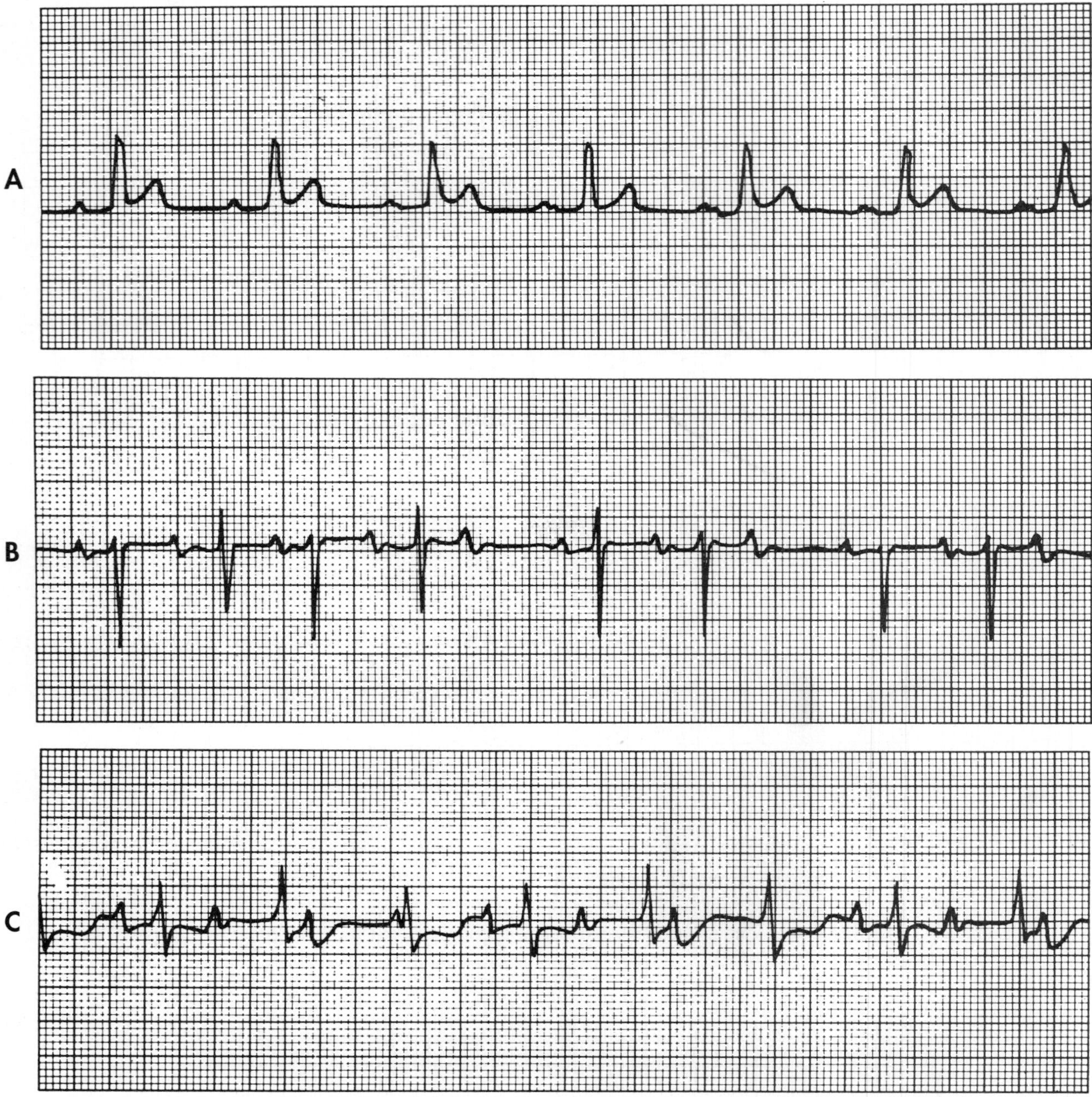

FIG. 115-11 AV heart block. **A,** First degree. **B,** Second degree. **C,** Third degree. See text for details.

(From Clark EB: In Cohen SA, editor: *Pediatric emergency management*, Englewood Cliffs, NJ, 1982, Prentice Hall.)

Management

Table 115-1 summarizes the drugs, dosages, and toxic effects of the most commonly used antiarrhythmic drugs. Electrophysiological studies may be needed to guide therapy if an arrhythmia does not respond to the usual drugs. Management of complex cardiac arrhythmias should be referred to a pediatric cardiologist.

Digoxin. Digoxin is used to treat supraventricular tachycardia, atrial flutter, or atrial fibrillation. Owing to its narrow margin of safety, extreme care must be taken in calculating drug doses and administration frequency.

Quinidine. Quinidine reduces conduction by inhibiting diastolic repolarization; it decreases conduction velocity by lowering the resting membrane potential and decreasing the maximum rate of depolarization. It also prolongs the refractory period by altering the duration of the action potential.

Procainamide. This quinidine-like agent increases the refractory period and conduction time in the atrium, the ventricle, and the junctional region.

Lidocaine. Intravenous lidocaine can be used in the initial treatment of ventricular tachycardia. It converts the rhythm to normal and maintains it that way until the cause can be

Table 115-1 Common Antiarrhythmic Agents

Drugs	Initial therapy	Maintenance therapy	Toxic effects
Digoxin	Digitalization 20-40 μg/kg divided in four equal doses	PO, 1/4 digitalizing dose/day	Heart block, ectopy
Quinidine	PO, 2 mg/kg every test dose	PO, 4-10 mg/kg every 6 hr	Rash, fever, gastrointestinal (GI) symptoms, purpura, hemolytic anemia, hypotension
Procainamide	IV, 2 mg/kg of 1:10 dilution over 5 minutes	PO, 5-15 mg/kg every 6 hr	Lupuslike syndrome, hypotension, urticaria, GI symptoms
Lidocaine	IV, 1 mg/kg of 1:1000 dilution over 3-5 minutes; up to 5 mg/kg	IV, 0.03 mg/kg/minute of dilute solution of 5 mg/ml; decrease rate as arrhythmia continues to be controlled	Convulsions, drowsiness, euphoria, muscle twitching
Phenytoin	IV, 10-15 mg/kg over 5 minutes	PO, 2 mg/kg tid	Hypotension, ataxia
Propranolol	IV, 0.01-0.15 mg/kg over 3-5 minutes	PO, 0.05-1 mg/kg/day divided, every 6 hr	Bradycardia, hypotension, cardiac failure, asthma
Isoproterenol	IV, 0.1-1.0 μg/kg/minute	Infusion adjusted to maintain stable rhythm and rate	Ventricular ectopic beats, tachycardia
Atropine	IV, 0.01-0.03 mg/kg (0.15 mg minimum; 0.5 mg maximum flushing)		Mydriasis, dry mouth
Adenosine	IV, 0.05-0.25 mg/kg/dose IV push	None	Blocks AV node conduction to convert SVT

corrected or until maintenance therapy with another drug in the group of myocardial depressants is instituted.

Propranolol. Propranolol, a beta-adrenergic blocking agent, reduces the heart rate and the contractile force of the heart; thus it is contraindicated in patients who have cardiac failure. Propranolol is effective against ventricular and supraventricular tachyarrhythmias, but its special usefulness is in situations in which there is (1) a central nervous system component to the arrhythmia, (2) a digitalis-toxicity rhythm, or (3) recurrent tachycardia associated with Wolff-Parkinson-White syndrome.

Phenytoin. Phenytoin (Dilantin) is used to treat ventricular arrhythmias and may counteract the depressant effect of procainamide. It depresses ventricular automaticity and enhances AV conduction.

Adenosine. Adenosine produces a transient complete block at the AV node, interrupting reentry tachycardia. Adenosine is the drug of choice for the conversion of supraventricular tachycardia in children.

Increased Vagal Tone

For children whose supraventricular tachycardia is repetitive or sustained, increasing vagal tone may terminate the attack. Vagal tone can be increased by Valsalva maneuver or ice water dive reflex. Older children and adolescents who have attacks infrequently can be taught to manage their attacks themselves. Pressing on the eyeball as a means to increase vagal tone should never be done because it can produce retinal detachment.

Direct Current (DC) Cardioversion

A direct current precordial shock terminates chaotic atrial and ventricular arrhythmias. Elective cardioversion should be accomplished by a team familiar with the cardioverter and with equipment that is checked regularly for proper performance. Patients should be anesthetized while the shock is delivered. Once the tachyrhythmia has been converted, antiarrhythmic medication often is needed to prevent recurrence.

Catheter Pacing

A cardiac pacemaker can be used to control cardiac arrhythmias. A transvenous pacing catheter is positioned in the atrial or ventricular chamber, or both, to stimulate the heart sequentially. Indications for permanent cardiac pacing include complete heart block, ventricular tachycardia, and sinus node dysfunction.

Radiofrequency Ablation

Radiofrequency ablation of accessory bypass tracts or ectopic foci is effective for managing patients unresponsive to the usual methods of control described above.

SUMMARY

The practitioner plays an important role in identifying children who have arrhythmias and directing them to the pediatric cardiologist for evaluation and treatment. The pediatrician also supports the family and reassures those whose arrhythmias are benign.

SUGGESTED READINGS

Adams FH, Emmanouilides GC, Riemenschneider TA: *Heart disease in infants, children, and adolescents,* ed 4, Baltimore, 1989, Williams & Wilkins.

Emmanouilides GC et al: *Heart disease in infants, children and adolescents,* ed 5, Baltimore, 1994, Williams & Wilkins.

Neill CA, Clark EB, Clark CI: *The heart of a child,* Baltimore, 1992, Johns Hopkins University Press.

116 Chest Pain

Beryl J. Rosenstein

Although not as common or bothersome as abdominal pain or headache, chest pain frequently is encountered in pediatric patients, particularly among preadolescents and adolescents.[1,7,10,14,15] It accounts for 1% of pediatric emergency department visits and approximately 5% of adolescent outpatient visits. The major causes are benign; chest pain in children rarely is associated with serious organic disease. However, parents and often the patient are concerned that chest pain indicates heart trouble; if only for this reason, a careful evaluation is indicated. It is important to strike a balance between a cursory evaluation that is less than reassuring to the family and an overly elaborate work-up that tends to reinforce the idea of underlying organic disease. In the evaluation of the patient who has chest pain, a careful history and physical examination provide the most information. Laboratory procedures usually are not indicated and rarely are helpful.[11,14,15]

HISTORY AND EXAMINATION

The history should include an accurate description of the pain, including the duration, character, intensity, location, radiation, relation to meals, and precipitating and modifying factors. Pain of pleural origin usually is sharp, stabbing, and superficial. It is accentuated by deep breaths, cough, or movement of the upper portion of the body and tends to disappear when the breath is held in expiration. Parietal pleural pain usually is localized over the involved area, whereas diaphragmatic pleural pain may be referred to the base of the neck or to the abdomen. Pain of pericardial origin may be of three distinct types: pleuritic pain, which is aggravated by a deep breath or cough; steady crushing substernal pain similar to that of a myocardial infarction; or pain along the left heart border and left shoulder that is synchronous with the heart beat. Information should be elicited regarding other somatic complaints, drug use (including cocaine and oral contraceptives), sleep disturbances, school problems, syncope, shortness of breath, history of choking, vomiting, dysphagia, Kawasaki disease, decreased exercise tolerance, and interferences with usual activities. A history of recent trauma or a temporal relationship to sports activities or exercise often is helpful. A description of psychosocial and environmental factors and family illnesses also is pertinent. The physical examination should focus on the heart, lungs, and musculoskeletal structures of the chest wall. Findings that help to determine the cause of chest pain include abnormal breath sounds, heart murmurs, tender breast masses, chest splinting, bruising, pericardial and pleural friction rubs, subcutaneous crepitus, swelling of chest wall articulations, the rash of herpes zoster, and the ability to reproduce the pain by palpation over the chest wall.

ETIOLOGY

Although it is unusual for serious disease to manifest as chest pain in children and teenagers, chest pain may be associated with pneumothorax, pneumomediastinum, gastritis, esophagitis, peptic ulcer disease, thoracic outlet syndrome, esophageal foreign bodies, Fitz-Hugh-Curtis syndrome, asthma, pneumonia, pulmonary embolus, tumors, hemoglobinopathies, and cardiac abnormalities. In these cases the underlying disease often is diagnosed readily. In about 50% of the patients who seek medical care for chest pain, an underlying cause will be found (see the box on p. 889).

CHEST WALL ABNORMALITIES

The most common identifiable causes of chest pain are related to chest wall abnormalities, including traumatic injuries, a breast mass, muscle strain, a hypersensitive xiphoid bone, and costochondritis.[4,6,11] *Costochondritis* is most common in female adolescents.[4] There is sharp pain that originates in the anterior chest, may radiate, and may persist for several months; no relationship to position, respiration, or activity exists. Most important, the pain can be reproduced by firm palpation over the involved rib cartilage. Treatment includes reassurance, avoidance of strenuous activity, analgesics, and local heat. In patients whose pain is severe, local injection of lidocaine or administration of corticosteroids, or both, may help. *Slipping rib syndrome* is an unusual cause of chest pain, probably related to trauma to the costal cartilages of the eighth, ninth, and tenth ribs.[12] The patient feels a slipping movement of the ribs, sometimes accompanied by a clicking or popping sound. The pain can be reproduced by grasping the affected rib margin and pulling it anteriorly. *Tietze syndrome,* a form of costochondritis, usually occurs in teenagers; it is characterized by chest pain, which often is intense, and a firm, tender, fusiform swelling of one or more of the upper costal cartilages or sternoclavicular joints for which no specific cause can be found.[5] A biopsy of the involved area reveals normal cartilage. The course is prolonged, and recurrences are common. It is important to reassure the patient as to the benign, self-limited nature of the disorder.

PULMONARY DISORDERS

Pulmonary causes of chest pain include pneumonia, pneumothorax, pneumomediastinum, asthma, and pulmonary embolus. A chest roentgenogram is the most helpful diagnostic procedure. *Pleurodynia,* caused chiefly by group B coxsackie virus, usually occurs with sudden onset of severe stabbing paroxysmal pleuritic pain over the lower rib cage and substernal areas. The pain is aggravated by deep breathing, moving, and coughing. It usually is preceded or accompanied by fever,

CAUSES OF CHEST PAIN IN CHILDREN AND ADOLESCENTS

Cardiac disease

Anomalous coronary artery, coronary arteritis
Cardiomyopathy, myocarditis, pericarditis
Left ventricular outflow obstruction
Mitral valve prolapse
Tachyarrhythmias

Chest wall syndrome

Costochondritis, Tietze syndrome
Hypersensitive xiphoid
Muscle strain, trauma
Slipping rib syndrome
Tender breast masses

Gastrointestinal conditions

Esophageal burns, foreign bodies
Esophageal dysmotility
Esophagitis, gastritis, peptic ulcer disease

Miscellaneous

Cigarette smoking, cocaine
Fitz-Hugh-Curtis syndrome
Hemoglobinopathy with vasoocclusive crisis
Tumors

Precordial catch syndrome
Psychogenic factors
Pulmonary conditions

Asthma, cough
Pleuritis, pleurodynia, pneumonia
Pneumomediastinum
Pneumothorax
Pulmonary embolism

headaches, malaise, anorexia, myalgias, and an unproductive cough. With the exception of a pleural friction rub, which is present in 25% of patients, examination of the chest reveals no significant findings. The clinical course of the disease takes from 1 to 14 days, and treatment is directed at the symptoms. Chest pain that occurs in association with exertional dyspnea or chest tightness suggests exercise-induced asthma.[17] A positive history for indicators of airway reactivity, that is, night cough, cough with exercise, recurrent pneumonia, and recurrent croup, may be helpful. These symptoms may occur in the absence of wheezing. Exercise testing and response to nebulization of a beta$_2$-agonist are helpful clues to the diagnosis.

A pulmonary embolus should be suspected in the patient who has an acute onset of dyspnea, pleuritic chest pain, and tachypnea. Hemoptysis may be present. Predisposing factors include use of oral contraceptives, pregnancy, recent trauma to a lower extremity, presence of a central venous catheter, intravenous drug abuse, prolonged immobilization, and collagen vascular disease. A ventilation-perfusion scan that shows normal ventilation but decreased perfusion is the most useful diagnostic procedure. In equivocal cases, pulmonary angiography should be carried out.

GASTROINTESTINAL DISORDERS

In patients whose chest pain is unexplained it is important to consider a gastrointestinal cause, including esophagitis, antral gastritis, peptic ulcer disease, hiatal hernia, cholecystitis, and abnormalities of esophageal motility.[8] The pain often is described as an uncomfortable burning sensation below the sternum and in the left precordial area. There may be associated vomiting or dysphagia. The symptoms of gastrointestinal-related chest pain often are nonspecific, however, and the underlying cause may be uncovered only by esophageal manometry, esophageal pH probe monitoring, and fiberoptic endoscopy.[8] Even in patients who have asthma or mitral valve prolapse, esophageal disorders often are the cause of chest pain.[2,19] Before an extensive gastrointestinal evaluation is embarked upon, a therapeutic trial of an antacid or a histamine-2 (H_2) blocker usually is indicated.

CARDIAC DISORDERS

Chest pain in pediatric patients infrequently is caused by clinically significant *cardiac disease,* but this has become a major reason for pediatric cardiology referrals.[3] Adolescents often equate chest pain with a heart attack or heart disease and may restrict their physical activity voluntarily.[10] Organic cardiac disease that produces chest pain can be categorized into three major groups: (1) structural abnormalities such as left-ventricular outflow obstruction, aortic stenosis, anomalous coronary artery, coronary arteritis (Kawasaki disease), and mitral valve prolapse; (2) acquired myopericardial inflammatory disease; and (3) rhythm disturbances such as supraventricular tachycardia. Pain that occurs fairly consistently with exercise but not at other times suggests heart disease, but it also may be a manifestation of *exercise-induced asthma.*[17] Although chest pain may occur in patients who have *mitral valve prolapse* (Barlow syndrome), this does not always indicate a causal relationship. In these patients a psychogenic, behavioral, or esophageal origin for the pain often can be established. Except in the case of paroxysmal arrhythmias, the history and physical examination usually will exclude most cardiac causes of chest pain. Indications for additional investigation and referral to a cardiologist include syncope, cardiomegaly, ECG abnormalities, a heart murmur, gallop rhythm or friction rub, suspicion of an arrythmia, and pain that radiates to the left shoulder. Echocardiographic examination, Holter monitoring, and exercise stress testing may be necessary in the evaluation of a patient in whom cardiac lesions are suspected, but in general these procedures supply little additional diagnostic information. It is important to note that even in patients who have a cardiac disease, associated chest pain may not be attributable to it.

MISCELLANEOUS DISORDERS

Adolescents may experience recurrent brief episodes of sudden, sharp, but not distressing pain localized near the cardiac apex. The pain usually occurs along the left sternal border or beneath the left breast, does not radiate, may have a pleuritic component, and typically occurs at rest or during mild exercise. It may be relieved by shallow breathing, a single deep inspiration, or a change in posture. This symptom complex has been referred to as the *precordial catch syndrome*, or *Texidor twinge*.[16] Treatment consists of reassurance as to the benign nature of the episodes. In adolescents, chest pain may be related to *cigarette smoking*. Severe chest pain of sudden onset may occur in association with the use of *cocaine*.[18] A urine toxicology screen will help clarify the diagnosis. Patients who have *sickle cell disease* often have episodes of chest pain secondary to pneumonia, pulmonary embolus, pulmonary infarction, and rib infarcts. There rarely have been reported cases of *chest epilepsy* presenting as daily episodes of severe nonradiating chest pain associated with sweating.[9] The diagnosis is based on an abnormal electroencephalogram and response to anticonvulsant therapy.

PSYCHOGENIC DISORDERS

In some cases where chest pain is of undetermined origin, there is undoubtedly a psychogenic basis for the complaint.[1] In these patients a specific stressful situation causally related to the onset of the complaint usually is identified. There often is a history of other recurrent somatic complaints, school problems, or significant sleep disturbances, along with a history of chest pain or serious illness in other family members. The pain may be associated with hyperventilation that, by itself, may lead to chest pain. The diagnosis of psychogenic chest pain should not be arrived at on the basis of exclusion, but rather on a history of a precipitating event along with evidence of significant underlying psychopathological factors. Therapy consists of appropriate counseling for the patient and other involved family members.

IDIOPATHIC DISORDERS

Even after a complete history, physical examination, and pertinent laboratory procedures, a specific cause will not be found in 30% to 50% of cases of chest pain in children.[1,7,11,14] A cardiorespiratory cause for chest pain is more common in younger children, whereas a psychogenic origin, including hyperventilation, is more likely in adolescents, especially girls.[14,15] The presence of pain that awakens a child, pain of acute onset, fever, and abnormal findings on physical examination suggests underlying organic disease. Constant pain usually is more significant than brief intermittent episodes of pain. The presence of chronic pain of more than 6 months' duration and a family history of chest pain or heart disease suggests nonorganic disease.[14] In general, the longer the complaint of chest pain has been present, the less likely one is to find a specific underlying disorder. Idiopathic chest pain tends to be very specific and usually is localized to the precordium. Laboratory tests generally are not helpful in establishing a specific diagnosis.[14] They usually reveal previously known or clinically suspected problems or confirm abnormalities uncovered by the history and physical examination. A chest roentgenogram and an electrocardiogram should not be obtained unless indicated by the history and physical examination. In cases in which a specific cause is not identified, management consists of reassurance and observation. The prognosis for these patients is excellent.[13] Most will become symptom-free. It is unusual for organic disease to appear after an initial assessment reveals negative findings, and the appearance of new functional symptoms is uncommon.

REFERENCES

1. Asnes RS, Santulli R, Bemporad JR: Psychogenic chest pain in children, *Clin Pediatr* 20:788, 1981.
2. Berezin S et al: Esophageal chest pain in children with asthma, *J Pediatr Gastroenterol Nutr* 12:52, 1991.
3. Brenner JI, Berman MA: Chest pain in childhood and adolescence, *J Adolesc Health Care* 3:271, 1983.
4. Brown RT: The adolescent with costochondritis, *Compr Ther* 14:27, 1988.
5. Calabro JJ, Marchesano JM: Tietze's syndrome: report of a case with juvenile onset, *J Pediatr* 68:985, 1966.
6. Calabro JJ et al: Classification of anterior chest wall syndromes, *JAMA* 243:1420, 1980.
7. Driscoll DJ, Glicklich LB, Gallen WJ: Chest pain in children: a prospective study, *Pediatrics* 57:648, 1976.
8. Glassman MS et al: Spectrum of esophageal disorders in children with chest pain, *Digest Dis Sci* 37:663, 1992.
9. Gulati S, Kumar L: 'Chest epilepsy' in a child, *Postgrad Med J* 68:369, 1992.
10. Kaden GG, Shenker IR, Gootman N: Chest pain in adolescents, *J Adolesc Health* 12:251, 1991.
11. Milov DE, Kantor RJ: Chest pain in teenagers: when is it significant? *Postgrad Med* 88:145, 1990.
12. Porter GE: Slipping rib syndrome: an infrequently recognized entity in children—a report of three cases and review of the literature, *Pediatrics* 76:810, 1985.
13. Rowland TW, Richards MM: The natural history of idiopathic chest pain in children, *Clin Pediatr* 25:612, 1986.
14. Selbst SM: Evaluation of chest pain in children, *Pediatr Rev* 8:56, 1986.
15. Selbst SM et al: Pediatric chest pain: a prospective study, *Pediatrics* 82:319, 1988.
16. Sparrow MJ, Bird EL: "Precordial catch": a benign syndrome of chest pain in young persons, *NZ Med J* 88:325, 1978.
17. Wiens L et al: Chest pain in otherwise healthy children and adolescents is frequently caused by exercise-induced asthma, *Pediatrics* 90:350, 1992.
18. Woodward GA, Selbst SM: Chest pain secondary to cocaine use, *Pediatr Emerg Care* 3:153, 1987.
19. Woolf PK et al: Noncardiac chest pain in adolescents and children with mitral valve prolapse, *J Adolesc Health* 12:247, 1991.

117 Constipation

T. Emmett Francoeur

The term *constipation* refers primarily to a diminished frequency of defecation. In this chapter *stool retention* is used as a synonym inasmuch as it implies both low frequency of bowel movements and incomplete evacuation. The tendency to retain feces may develop very early in life, may lead to persistent distress through childhood and into adult life, and may predispose the person to a variety of psychological and medical sequelae. The phrase *dysfunctional stool retention* is used to refer to the "problem" of constipation, which includes both the symptom itself and the negative secondary psychosocial consequences. Early identification and successful treatment of this problem may reduce morbidity during later years.

PREDISPOSING FACTORS

A small proportion of children who have chronic stool retention have an underlying anomaly or disease. In encountering this symptom pediatricians most often and primarily are concerned with ruling out aganglionic megacolon (Hirschsprung disease). With increasing age, the likelihood that stool retention is the result of aganglionic megacolon becomes increasingly small. Table 117-1 summarizes the clinical differences between aganglionic megacolon and chronic dysfunctional stool retention.

Other congenital abnormalities, however, can predispose a patient to stool retention. Anal strictures and stenoses (very uncommon) may appear early in life and lead to considerable pain and retention of feces. Stool retention, fecal incontinence, or both, may develop in patients who have undergone surgery for imperforate anus. This complication may result from congenital anatomical abnormalities or may be introduced by surgery.

Anal fissures (very common) or hemorrhoids cause pain during defecation and lead a child to retain stool, which in turn makes defecation painful and encourages stool retention. Pain during defecation also can be caused by diaper rashes, dermatitis, and other irritations around the anogenital area. Some young children who have diarrhea have strong negative feelings associated with defecation, which may then proceed toward chronic fecal retention, with dehydration often a contributing factor.

In some cases systemic disorders may predispose a child to stool retention. These include celiac disease, hypothyroidism, hypocalcemia, multiple endocrine neoplasia, and lead intoxication. In addition, motility can be reduced by certain medications (especially those containing codeine or phenothiazines). Children who have neuromuscular disease (e.g., cerebral palsy, spinal dysraphism, muscular dystrophy) commonly have refractory chronic stool retention, mostly because of immobility and poor control of the abdominal musculature or the anal sphincter. More recently, primary rectal myopathy[10] and neuropathy (neuronal intestinal dysplasia)[8] have been proposed as rare causes of chronic severe constipation.

Emotional problems may potentiate stool retention. A child who is chronically anxious, depressed, or agitated may exhibit psychogenic constipation. Such a youngster may be unable to persevere at or attend to the need for defecation. In some cases more deeply set negative feelings may be associated with the need to retain stool. Failure to defecate may constitute a quiet protest or expression of anger or maladaptive behavior in a toddler of parents who are ambivalent about codes of discipline. Genetic and constitutional factors, as well as developmental processes, underlie most cases of stool retention. In some families there is a tendency toward ineffective defecation; concordance for stool retention is four times more frequent in monozygotic twins than in dizygotic twins.[1] The British have used the term *primary colonic inertia* to describe young infants who, from the earliest days in life, have difficulty with complete evacuation of the rectum.

Specific events or situations that occur during development may interfere with normal defecation. Chronic retention may result from overzealous efforts to facilitate an infant's defecation. A newborn who has hard stools may be "assaulted" with gloved fingers and suppositories, thus establishing early conflicts over issues of withholding and elimination. Training for stool incontinence may trigger withholding. Parents who train children too early or use methods that are overly coercive may promote reluctance to defecate, although this has not yet been confirmed in large-scale epidemiological studies. If family stresses such as the birth of a new baby or the loss of a family member occur during training, retentive behavior may be engendered.

For reasons that often are unclear, some youngsters develop a phobia about toilets. Some may fantasize about being flushed down the drain. Others may overreact to the odor and be unable to face the reality that they have produced such unattractive waste. School bathrooms may predispose older children to stool retention. Becoming trained to defecate on a toilet is a major developmental achievement; learning to use a second toilet may represent an even greater challenge. More commonly, absence of doors, toilet paper, and sanitary conditions or the presence of potential pranks and fights results in children postponing defecation until they are safely at home.

Among children who have developmental handicaps of low severity, such as hyperactivity and learning disabilities, there appears to be a high occurrence of dysfunctional bowel disorders.

Usually more than one factor leads to stool retention. Often it is the final result of an interplay of genetic, psychological, cognitive, and physiological factors. The box on p. 892 summarizes some of the recognized predispositions to chronic stool retention.

Table 117-1 Comparison of Aganglionic Megacolon and Chronic Dysfunctional Stool Retention

Characteristic	Aganglionic megacolon	Stool retention
Prevalence	1 in 25,000 births	1.5% of 7-yr-old boys
Sex ratio	90% males	86% males
Retention as newborn	Almost always	Rare
Problems with bowel training	Rare	Common
Late onset of symptoms (after 2 yr)	Rare	Common
Toilet avoidance	Rare	Common
Incontinence	Rare	Common
Stool size	Often thin "ribbons"	Often large caliber
Frequency of defecation	Greatly diminished	Variable
Abdominal pain	Rare, except in obstruction	Common, especially in cases of recent onset
General appearance	Often chronically ill	Usually healthy
Failure to thrive	Common	Rare
Obstruction	Common	Rare
Abdominal distention	Common	Variable
Stool in ampulla	Often diminished	Often increased
Plain roentgenograms	Narrow rectum	Often dilated, distended rectum
Rectal manometry (internal sphincter)	Contraction or no response	Relaxation
Barium enema	Localized constriction with proximal dilation may be seen	Often diffuse megacolon

CLASSIFICATION OF PREDISPOSITIONS TO CHRONIC STOOL RETENTION

Altered anatomy or physiology

- Congenital
  - Aganglionic megacolon
  - Anal stenosis or atresia
- Acquired
  - Postoperative lesion
  - Fissure
  - Celiac disease
- Metabolic
  - Hypothyroidism
  - Hypocalcemia
  - Multiple endocrine neoplasia
  - Drug effects (especially codeinelike medications and phenothiazines)
- Neurogenic (myelodysplasia)

Dysfunctions

- Developmental
  - Associated with cognitive handicap
  - Attentional disorders or hyperactivity
- Situational
  - Associated with difficult training
  - School bathroom induced
  - Negative defecation-related experience (e.g., gastroenteritis)
- Psychogenic—associated with significant psychopathology
- Constitutional
  - Primary colonic inertia
  - Genetic predisposition

DIAGNOSIS

Chronic retention of stool can be an elusive diagnosis. Both parent and child may be unaware of the existence of constipation and may report a daily bowel movement. In many cases of stool incontinence the parents are unaware of the existence of long-standing stool retention or incomplete defecation, especially in school-age children. As a result parents may incorrectly interpret soiling episodes as being related to concurrent stressful events, making diagnosis more difficult. Clues helpful in detecting associated occult stool retention are listed in the box on p. 893. Stool retention can be suspected in infants and toddlers when a parent complains that the child has infrequent defecation or appears in distress while having a bowel movement. With legs hyperextended, fists clenched, and a reddish, nearly plethoric facial expression, the infant may be struggling to inhibit a bowel movement rather than to have one.

The problem of physical diagnosis is complicated further when a child who has marked retention has normal findings on physical examination. Palpation of the abdomen and a rectal examination often reveal no abnormal findings because children may retain enormous amounts of pasty soft stool that fail to present rocklike formations to the palpating hand or the inserted finger. Similarly an easily palpable sigmoid colon or cecum does not necessarily signify stool retention inasmuch as it is normal for stool transit to be slower through the distal colon and for stool to be stored in the cecum. In questionable cases demonstration of delayed whole gut[7] and segmental[4] transit times delineates underlying stool retention further. A roentgenogram of the abdomen with the patient lying supine may reveal retained stool that is granular or rocklike in appearance. There may be a distended rectal ampulla or diffuse megacolon, especially when associated symptoms are present[2] (see following section). For the small percentage of children who have clinical features more typical of

POSSIBLE CLUES TO STOOL RETENTION

1. A period longer than 3 or 4 days without a bowel movement
2. A history of blood-streaked stool (fissure)
3. Straining with small, hard stools (pellets)
4. Occasional presence of very large stools (filling the toilet or requiring mechanical breakup)
5. A child's feet suspended in air when having a movement
6. A child who stays on the toilet for less than 1 minute at a time
7. Enuresis (especially daytime and late onset)
8. History of soiling underwear
9. History of use of laxatives and enemas
10. Onset of recurrent abdominal pain

aganglionic megacolon (see Table 117-1), the initial diagnostic procedure is rectal manometry.[11] Based on the results of the sphincter's response a small number of these children require a rectal biopsy (to prove the diagnosis) and a barium enema (to measure the length of colonic involvement) before surgical intervention. Rectal and colonic manometry tests also are indicated in patients who have myelodysplasia, patients who have had rectal surgery, and children who have severe retention and are unresponsive to an adequate medical therapeutic trial.[6]

ASSOCIATED SYMPTOMS

A wide range of associated symptoms in the school-aged child may accompany chronic stool retention. The presence of such symptoms should elicit a high index of suspicion for dysfunctional problems with defecation. Many children who have recurrent abdominal pain have associated chronic stool retention. Often this bowel problem is the source of pain. The stool retention in these children may be occult in that their tendency to be retentive is not easily elicited during a routine history and physical examination. Some children who have enuresis also are found to have significant stool retention, which may cause or aggravate a child's urinary incontinence; the enuresis subsides when a normal stool pattern is restored. This is more likely to be the case in children who have secondary enuresis and daytime wetting. In addition, persistence of recurrent urinary tract infections has been related to underlying stool retention. Perhaps the most common and troublesome symptom associated with chronic stool retention is fecal incontinence, also known as *encopresis* (see Chapter 81, Encopresis).

TREATMENT

The problem of constipation provides an excellent example of the potential role for prevention within pediatric practice, because often it can be prevented by anticipatory guidance from the physician in working out with the parents an appropriate schedule for bowel "training." It is not uncommon for boys to remain untrained until after 3 years of age.

If uncomplicated dysfunctional stool retention develops, its management depends largely on its severity, the child's age, and the degree of parental anxiety. The clinician needs to achieve a happy medium between overindulgence in reassurance and an excessively aggressive approach; either extreme may aggravate the disorder.

Stool retention early in infancy should be treated gently. When underlying organic conditions have been ruled out, the physician should proceed to relatively straightforward dietary manipulations. Increasing the osmotic load in the baby's formula with the addition of liquid sugar preparations can be effective. A titrated quantity of prune juice (determined by observation of stool consistency) each day is practical and effective for infants and toddlers. Along with ad libitum water and fruit juices, toddlers can be offered raisins, raw vegetables, and oatmeal cookies at snacktime. The toddler, school-aged child, and adolescent should eat only whole-wheat bread, adequate daily portions of high-fiber vegetables (broccoli, Brussels sprouts, cabbage, corn, and so on), and fruit snacks and should avoid cakes, candies, chips, and soft drinks. Regular exercise is recommended.

In infancy, dioctyl sodium sulfosuccinate may be used in special cases. It is best to avoid the rectal administration of medications. Dilation with a finger, the use of suppositories, and the administration of enemas should be reserved for only the most resistant cases, because these interventions may generate negative feelings about defecation and promote further stool retention. In infants older than 3 months a small amount of a laxative may be administered orally (such as ¼ teaspoon of senna syrup [Senokot] daily, increased to ½ teaspoon per day in toddlers) until soft, easily passed stools occur daily.

Any perianal dermatological problems or fissures need treatment. In some cases warm baths twice daily with the addition of an emollient solution (e.g., Alpha Keri Lotion or Vaseline Intensive Care Lotion) may alleviate perianal soreness. Steroid creams in infancy tend to make the mucosa even more friable and should be avoided. Simple anal fissures in infants often are alleviated by the anal dilation that occurs when a rectal examination is performed. In rare cases chronic fissures need to be excised. Parents may need a great deal of support, and clinicians may need to exercise restraint in the management of this problem.

In older children who have chronic stool retention, treatment may be implemented in several stages.[5] The degree of retention should be estimated first. If a considerable amount of feces is retained, an initial cleanout is desirable. This is accomplished by (1) administering an adult Fleet hypophosphate enema on the morning and evening of the first day of treatment, (2) administering a bisacodyl (Dulcolax) suppository on the morning and evening of the second day of treatment, and (3) administering a bisacodyl tablet orally on the third day of treatment. This entire process may need to be repeated two to four times. In milder cases a child might benefit from 1 to 2 weeks of oral laxative therapy (using danthron, senna, or bisacodyl tablets once or twice daily). If an older child does not respond to these standard medical interventions, and if either external anal contraction or decreased rectal sensation is demonstrated on anorectal manometry, biofeedback training should be considered.[3] After the child has been relieved of retained feces, light mineral oil may be administered daily in appropriate dosage (1 to 6 tablespoons per day), with increments in dosage depending on the "daily soft stool." School-aged children, whose pants can become stained by mineral oil, may prefer senna syrup. Such treatment should continue for at least 3 months. In many cases stool softeners will be required for a year or longer. Prolonged combined laxative therapy in otherwise normal children is nutritionally safe.[9]

While the child is receiving treatment, appropriate patterns of toilet use should be encouraged. The child should be encouraged to sit on the toilet twice a day, at the same times each day, for at least 5 minutes each time. A kitchen timer in the bathroom may be helpful, and books or magazines can be offered. The child is welcome to use the bathroom at other times of the day, but such supplementary excursions do not replace the two regular sittings. It is crucial to emphasize to the child and parents that these activities do not represent punishment or criticism. If the child reverts and becomes retentive while taking mineral oil, a short course of laxatives by mouth may be reinstituted. As a general therapeutic and preventive measure, a high-roughage diet is recommended for the entire family.

PROGNOSIS

Although many youngsters who have dysfunctional bowel disorders tend to improve with time, evidence is increasing that these dysfunctions may lead to lifelong disabilities. What begins as simple "colonic inertia" in infancy may progress to chronic stool retention and to fecal incontinence in the school years. These symptoms may resolve and reappear later as the irritable or spastic colon, which is a major cause of morbidity in adults. The early recognition and comprehensive continuing management of childhood disorders of defecation must be a seriously regarded component of preventive pediatric care.

REFERENCES

1. Bakwin H, Davidson M: Constipation in twins, *Am J Dis Child* 121:179, 1971.
2. Barr RG et al: Chronic and occult stool retention: a clinic tool for its evaluation in school-aged children, *Gastroenterology* 18:674, 1979.
3. Benninga MA et al: Biofeedback training in chronic constipation, *Arch Dis Child* 68:126, 1993.
4. Casasnovas AB et al: Measurement of colonic transit time in children, *J Pediatr Gastroenterol Nutr* 13:42, 1991.
5. Davidson M, Kugler MM, Bauer CH: Diagnosis and management in children with severe and protracted constipation and obstipation, *J Pediatr* 62:261, 1963.
6. Di Lorenzo C et al: Use of colonic manometry to differentiate causes of intractable constipation in children, *J Pediatr* 120:690, 1992.
7. Dimson SB: Carmine as an index of transit time in children with simple constipation, *Arch Dis Child* 45:232, 1970.
8. Koletzko S et al: Is histological diagnosis of neuronal intestinal dysplasia related to clinical and manometric findings in constipated children? Results of a pilot study, *J Pediatr Gastroenterol Nutr* 17:59, 1993.
9. McClung HJ et al: Is combination therapy for encopresis nutritionally safe? *Pediatrics* 91:591, 1993.
10. Murray RD et al: Rectal myopathy in chronically constipated children, *Pediatr Pathol* 12:787, 1992.
11. Rosenberg AJ, Vela AR: A new simplified technique for pediatric anorectal manometry, *Pediatrics* 71:240, 1983.

118 Cough

William A. Durbin, Jr.

Cough is one of the most common symptoms that pediatric practitioners are asked to evaluate and manage. Fortunately, as a symptom cough generally is innocuous; furthermore the underlying disease process that produces cough rarely is serious and usually is self-limited. Despite its generally benign nature, however, a cough may be disruptive to the child and annoying and anxiety-provoking for parents.

PATHOPHYSIOLOGY

From a pathophysiological point of view, cough is a forceful expiration. This "convulsion of the lungs," as Samuel Johnson put it, along with airway cilia and macrophages, serves to remove secretions and foreign material from the respiratory tract. The cough reflex can be triggered either voluntarily or by stimulation of cough receptors located throughout the respiratory tract—in the nose, the sinuses, the pharynx, the larynx, the trachea, the large bronchi, and the terminal bronchioles. Afferent impulses from these airway cough receptors travel through cranial nerve pathways to the brainstem "cough center"; from there, efferent stimuli activate *coordinated* closure of the glottis and contraction of diaphragmatic, chest wall, abdominal wall, and pelvic floor musculature.

The cough sequence is composed of three phases. In the *inspiratory* phase there is an initial deep inspiration, followed by closure of the glottis. During the second, brief *compressive* phase intrathoracic pressure increases following contraction of all the expiratory muscles. At the end of this phase the glottis opens suddenly, leading to the cough caused by a sudden, explosive release of intrathoracic air. It is during this *expiratory* phase that material from the respiratory tract is eliminated. Children often do not expectorate such secretions; they swallow them instead.

CLASSIFICATION

A number of classification schemes of cough have been developed. These focus on aspects such as the duration and descriptive qualities of the cough, the age of the child, and the various types of anatomical lesions and stimuli that can induce cough. The most basic classification is by duration, with cough being characterized as *acute* or *chronic* (3 weeks or longer). In evaluating acute coughs the physician considers infection and foreign body inhalation; in chronic cough structural, allergic, irritative, and psychiatric causes become more important, as do chronic infections such as tuberculosis.

A second classification scheme is based on the characteristics of the cough. Thus a staccato coughing paroxysm in an infant suggests pertussis or chlamydial infection; a barking or brassy cough and voice changes are associated with laryngotracheal disease; a "hawking" or throat-clearing sound suggests postnasal drip; a ringing or grunting cough may be heard with asthma; and a "honking" or "foghorn" cough may suggest a psychogenic origin. Children who expectorate purulent sputum may have bacterial pneumonia, a lung abscess, bronchiectasis, or cystic fibrosis. Nighttime coughs suggest the possibility of postnasal drip related to sinus infection or allergy, whereas coughs that cease at night may be psychogenic in origin; productive morning coughs suggest bronchiectasis; coughs associated with feeding suggest aspiration; coughs induced by cold air or exercise may indicate reactive airway disease; and seasonal coughs suggest reactive airway disease or allergic rhinitis with postnasal drip. Hemoptysis raises concern about diseases such as tuberculosis, cystic fibrosis, bronchiectasis, and pulmonary hemosiderosis; it also occurs occasionally with foreign body aspiration or severe nasopharyngitis. Not infrequently, blood arising from the gastrointestinal tract is thought mistakenly to be pulmonary in origin.

A third approach to classifying cough is based on age. Infections are a prime concern in all age groups. In small infants physiological or structural alterations should also be considered—for example, gastroesophageal reflux, tracheobronchomalacia, tracheoesophageal fistula, vascular ring, and other airway anomalies. In toddlers foreign body aspiration, irritation of airways (e.g., passive smoking[2]), and reactive airway disease are important causes of cough. For school-age children asthma, sinusitis, and allergic rhinitis with postnasal drip assume greater importance, whereas in adolescents smoking and psychogenic cough should be considered.

A fourth classification is strictly anatomical, in which the practitioner considers lesions at all levels of the respiratory tract that can stimulate cough. This includes diseases of the larynx, pharynx, nose, and sinuses (infections, irritations, allergies, foreign bodies, structural anomalies); the trachea and bronchi (infections, irritations, foreign bodies, structural anomalies, asthma, cystic fibrosis); the lung parenchyma (pneumonia, lung abscess, congenital malformations, pulmonary edema); the pleura (effusion, empyema); and the mediastinum (great vessel malformations, adenopathy, tumors). In addition, nonrespiratory tract causes (external auditory canal irritation, diaphragmatic and subdiaphragmatic lesions, and cough tic) should be considered. Perhaps the most satisfactory classification is one in which the types of stimuli that can produce cough are considered. *Mechanical* stimuli include intraluminal secretions and foreign bodies (including gastric contents, i.e., gastroesophageal reflux or other causes of aspiration). In addition, extraluminal lesions that compress the airway must be considered—both extramural (e.g., vascular rings and other anomalies) and intramural (e.g., the contraction of bronchial smooth muscle, manifested by asthma). *Inflammatory* stimuli include all the infectious conditions of the respiratory tract in which edema or exudate involves either the airway or the alveoli. *Chemical* stimuli include irritative gases, such as cigarette or wood stove smoke or allergens, which cause cough on inhalation. *Thermal* stimuli—that is, hot or cold air—also can produce cough, as can *psychogenic* stimuli.[4] Lastly, toxic reactions (e.g., to latex[12] or drugs[3]) should be considered.

These classification schemes provide the physician with a general framework with which to guide the evaluation of a coughing child. Implicit in the evaluation is the knowledge that most coughs of short duration are related to acute respiratory tract infections, whereas the most common causes of chronic cough are reactive airway disease (classical or cough variant asthma[9,11]), postnasal drip (resulting from recurrent upper respiratory tract infections, sinusitis, allergic and vasomotor rhinitis), and airway irritants (e.g., smoke, dust, chemicals, and aspirated food or gastric contents).

HISTORY

The history should include a description of the cough, including its duration, frequency, quality, timing, and sputum productivity. A history of episodes of cough, respiratory infections, and allergies should be sought. The family history may be helpful in identifying children who have diseases such as asthma, cystic fibrosis, and tuberculosis. The environmental history will help identify those children whose symptoms are related to passive smoking or other chemical inhalation, to a respiratory virus that has affected a household, or to an exotic pathogen acquired while traveling. An awareness of family setting and home dynamics may aid in recognizing children at risk for foreign body aspiration or development of a cough tic. It also is important to elicit a history of associated clinical findings. Fever usually suggests an acute infectious process; rhinorrhea may indicate an upper respiratory tract infection, sinusitis, or allergy. Wheezing suggests that asthma or a foreign body is the cause of cough; a history of atopic dermatitis or allergic rhinitis provides evidence for the former. Shortness of breath is associated with asthma, upper airway obstruction, pleural effusions, pneumothorax, pneumonias, and congestive heart failure.

PHYSICAL EXAMINATION

In performing the physical examination the physician is looking for signs of an acute process (fever, tender adenopathy, pharyngitis, or a rash), as well as for signs of a chronic or recurrent process (growth failure or clubbing seen in children who have severe asthma, cystic fibrosis, immunodeficiency, or congenital heart disease). The physician also is interested in defining the level of involvement of the respiratory tract; crackles, wheezes, rhonchi, altered breath sounds, and changes in resonance signify lower respiratory tract involvement; stridor and dysphagia indicate laryngeal involvement; and changes in the mouth, nose, ears, and sinuses signify upper airway disease. Observation of color, state of hydration, respiratory rate, chest movement, retractions, flaring of the chest, and handling of oral secretions indicates the severity of the process. It also is useful to have the child demonstrate the cough! Last, inspection for stigmata of allergic disease (e.g., eczema, pale boggy nasal mucosa, clear rhinorrhea, shiners, allergic nasal crease) and for posterior pharyngeal wall cobblestoning (hypertrophic lymphoid follicles seen in chronic postnasal drainage) is important.

LABORATORY TESTS

Most children who have coughs do not require any laboratory testing. For those children in whom the cough is chronic or associated with respiratory distress, some investigations may be undertaken. A complete blood count may provide evidence of acute infection, atopy (eosinophilia), or polycythemia. Examination of the sputum, including its macroscopic appearance, cellular composition (polymorphonuclear leukocytes, eosinophils), and bacterial content (gram stain, culture), may be useful in children who are capable of expectoration. A similar examination of the nasal discharge also may help to distinguish allergic rhinitis from purulent rhinitis or sinusitis. Roentgenograms of the chest (including fluoroscopy in children who may have inhaled a foreign body), neck, or sinuses may yield useful information, as might a barium swallow test in an infant thought to be aspirating or having an obstruction. Pulmonary function testing may be carried out in children who have suspected restrictive or obstructive airway disease; reversible reactive airway disease (asthma) is indicated either by improvement in an obstructive pattern after bronchodilator administration or by the development of an obstructive airway pattern after exercise or inhalation of such agents as cold air, methacholine, histamine, or specific allergens. Such testing may identify children who have cough-variant asthma, whose reactive airway disease is manifested clinically by coughing rather than by wheezing. The performance of pH probe monitoring, sweat testing, tuberculin skin testing, and immunoglobin and alpha-1-antitrypsin measurements may be indicated in children who have chronic or recurrent cough and demonstrable pulmonary disease. Bronchoscopy is useful in searching for a foreign body, investigating persistent collapse, confirming anatomical malformations, or obtaining tissue from children who have undiagnosed infiltrates or suspected ciliary dyskinesia syndrome.

MANAGEMENT

Having completed the assessment of the coughing child, the physician is faced with the problem of management. Several caveats are in order. First, the physician often needs to defuse parental anxiety about a cough, particularly when it is part of an acute respiratory infection. An explanation of the normalcy of a cough as part of the disease process, of the protective role that it may play, and of the usually self-limited nature of coughs may be necessary. The physician must acknowledge that the cough may be annoying and disruptive but also should reassure the child and parent that coughs in children in and of themselves rarely are harmful.

Second, treating the underlying disorder, thereby reducing the stimulation to cough, is more important than providing nonspecific cough medication. Thus the child who has the productive cough of postnasal drip may benefit from antihistamines or decongestants; the child who has the barking cough of croup should receive humidification; and the child who has allergen- or irritant-induced cough may need environmental alteration, bronchodilators, or corticosteroids.

Third, the physician who prescribes cough medicines should explain their therapeutic purpose carefully—for example, expectorants to loosen (not diminish) the cough or antitussives to partially suppress (not eliminate) the cough. Such discussion helps avoid unrealistic expectations. Cough medicines generally are contraindicated in the first few months of life because of their potential toxicity. Antitussives generally are avoided in patients who have productive coughs.

There are three categories of cough medicines: expectorants, mucolytics, and antitussives.[1,6] *Expectorants* are drugs that increase sputum volume and thus promote removal of secretions from the airways. Water is the expectorant used most commonly, given both systemically and by inhalation, methods that probably work because of their demulcent effect in the upper airway; whether administration of water actually affects lower airway secretions is unclear. Another expectorant, guaifenesin (glyceryl guaiacolate), is used commonly in cough preparations; however, although it may reduce sputum thickness, it has not been shown to reduce coughing in children. Ammonium chloride and potassium iodide rarely are prescribed for children, in part because of untoward side effects associated with effective dosages.

Mucolytic agents are drugs, such as acetylcysteine, that liquify tenacious secretions. They usually are administered by inhalation for children who have bronchiectasis (e.g., cystic fibrosis). Poor taste, the potential for inducing airway reactivity, and uncertain clinical benefit limit their use.

Antitussives are drugs that suppress coughing; they are the most effective cough modifiers. Peripherally acting antitussives work by coating or by anesthetizing irritated oropharyngeal receptors. This group includes the demulcents (e.g., throat lozenges, cough drops, lollipops, honey), as well as topical anesthetics administered by swallowing or spraying. These local measures generally are safe and well tolerated and may be useful in a cough related to upper respiratory tract infections or other pharyngeal irritation; their duration of efficacy is limited, however, because they are washed away quickly. Centrally acting antitussives include both narcotic and nonnarcotic agents that suppress the cough reflex at the brainstem level. Narcotic agents are of proved efficacy in suppressing cough; codeine and hydrocodeine are the most widely used and in children have minimum potential for abuse and associated adverse effects. Among the nonnarcotic drugs, dextromethorphan is the most commonly prescribed; unfortunately, objective clinical trials have not demonstrated a clinical benefit.[10,13] Antihistamines such as diphenhydramine sometimes are classified as centrally acting antitussives, perhaps on the basis of their sedative effect; however, much of their effect stems from their drying up tracheobronchial secretions. Questions have been raised about the efficacy[8] and safety[5,7] of antihistamines and decongestants.

Most available cough preparations contain several agents, including antitussives, expectorants, sympathomimetic decongestants, and antihistamines. Such combinations generally are untested and often are irrational. Clinicians who choose to use these drugs may prefer to seek specific pharmacological effects by using preparations that contain agents from just one of these groups.

REFERENCES

1. *AMA drug evaluations,* ed 5, Philadelphia, 1993 WB Saunders.
2. Bartecchi CE, MacKenzie TD, Schrier RW: The human cost of tobacco use, *N Engl J Med* 330:907, 1994.
3. Bianchetti MG, Caflisch M, Oetliker OH: Cough and converting enzyme inhibitors, *Eur J Pediatr* 151:225, 1992.
4. Cohlan SQ, Stone SM, Zimmerman SS: Coughing and bed-sheet wrapping, *Pediatrics* 88:1077, 1991.
5. Gadomski A, Horton L: The need for rational therapeutics in the use of cough and cold medicine in infants, *Pediatrics* 89:774, 1992.
6. Hatch RT, Carpenter GB, Smith LJ: Treatment options in the child with a chronic cough, *Drugs* 45:367, 1993.
7. Hendeles L: Efficacy and safety of antihistamines and expectorants in nonprescription cough and cold preparations, *Pharmacotherapy* 13:154, 1993.
8. Hutton N et al: Effectiveness of an antihistamine-decongestant combination for young children with the common cold: a randomized controlled clinical trial, *J Pediatr* 118:125, 1991.
9. Johnson D, Osborn LM: Cough variant asthma: a review of the clinical literature, *J Asthma* 28:85, 1991.
10. Korppi M et al: Antitussives in the treatment of acute transient cough in children, *Acta Paediatr Scand* 80:969, 1991.
11. McKenzie S: Cough—but is it asthma? *Arch Dis Child* 70:1, 1994.
12. Schneck FX, Bellinger MF: The "innocent" cough or sneeze: a harbinger of serious latex allergy in children during bladder stimulation and urodynamic testing, *J Urol* 50:687, 1993.
13. Taylor JA et al: Efficacy of cough suppressants in children, *J Pediatr* 122:799, 1993.

SUGGESTED READINGS

Beardsmore CJ, Simpson H: Cough in children, *J Asthma* 28:309, 1991.

Holinger LD, Sanders AD: Chronic cough in infants and children: an update, *Laryngoscope* 101:596, 1991.

Kamei RK: Chronic cough in children, *Pediatr Clin North Am* 38:593, 1991.

Parks DP et al: Chronic cough in childhood: approach to diagnosis and treatment, *J Pediatr* 115:856, 1989.

Pratter MR et al: An algorithmic approach to chronic cough, *Ann Int Med* 119:877, 1993.

Rogers AR, O'Connell EJ, Sachs HR: Chronic cough in children: what to do, and why, *Am J Respir Dis* 12:891, 1991.

Urbach AH et al: What's behind that chronic cough? *Contemp Pediatr* 10:106, 1993.

119 Dental Stains

Lindsey K. Grossman

Parental concerns about changes in tooth color, often the cause of much anxiety, frequently are first brought to the pediatrician. It is important to remember that normal tooth color varies greatly from one tooth to another, from one individual to another, and between the usual blue-white of the primary dentition and the yellowish ivory of the permanent teeth.

EXTRINSIC STAIN

Teeth often are discolored as a result of staining from external deposits on their surface layer. These extrinsic stains usually are removable by careful daily brushing and professional oral prophylaxis (scaling). Chromogenic bacteria in plaque can result in green, orange, or black stains along the gingival margin of the teeth. Although in most cases this is associated with poor oral hygiene, black stains may be associated with good hygiene and a low incidence of caries. Excessive use of certain foods or beverages and smoking can stain the teeth, but the discoloration usually will disappear with oral prophylaxis and avoidance of the staining substance. Children who are receiving certain liquid medications, especially iron preparations, may have teeth with a dark stain. This also resolves with professional scaling after the medication is discontinued but may be completely prevented if the medication is administered through a straw from the onset.

INTRINSIC STAIN

When a staining substance is incorporated into the deep structures of the tooth (i.e., the enamel or dentin, or both), it cannot be removed by scaling and is referred to as an *intrinsic stain.* Certain problems of the neonatal period, such as erythroblastosis fetalis, biliary atresia, neonatal hepatitis, or other conditions resulting in high serum concentrations of bilirubin pigments, can cause yellow-green or blue-green staining of primary teeth, resulting from pigment deposition in the structures of these teeth. As many as 50% of children who have cyanotic congenital heart disease may have dull, pale, bluish-white teeth whose color resembles skim milk. This is believed to be caused, at least in part, by the hypoxemia associated with these conditions.

Intrinsic stains may be associated with certain rare childhood conditions. The erythrodontia of porphyria caused by deposition of red-brown porphyrin pigments into the tooth structure is readily apparent in ultraviolet light if not in daylight. The inherited disorders amyelogenesis imperfecta and dentinogenesis imperfecta are associated with hypoplastic enamel and a yellow, opalescent blue-gray or brown-violet tooth color. Major dental work is required to restore normal appearance in those who have any of these disorders.

Common pedodontic problems often result in a change in tooth color. Tooth trauma and associated bleeding into dentin can cause a pink color that fades, first to gray as pulp degenerates, and eventually to yellow. In certain cases the dentin resorption will result in a permanent pink hue. Active caries in teeth may appear chalky white or yellow but gradually converts to shiny black as the caries converts to the arrested state. An unusual secondary complication of certain childhood infections is Turner tooth. This is a brown or yellow-brown discoloration of a single tooth and is associated with hypoplasia of the enamel in a tooth undergoing odontogenesis at the time of the illness.

Persons who reside in areas in which the water contains fluoride have been noted to have increased resistance to caries. However, as the fluoride content rises over 1.5 ppm (parts per million), many individuals in the area will begin to demonstrate hypoplastic enamel, with the characteristic dull, opaque white mottled patches in the permanent teeth. If the amount of fluoride consumed is extremely high (>5 ppm), the teeth will show a blotchy brown or black-brown color that is highly disfiguring and requires extensive restoration of the dental surfaces.

A similarly involved course of treatment often is required for the severe intrinsic staining problems caused by tetracycline. This is a dose-dependent and duration-linked problem caused by the incorporation of tetracycline itself into the mineral complex at the dentinoenamel junction during odontogenesis. If the tetracycline was ingested by the mother before birth or by the child in the first months after birth, the primary teeth will be affected. Permanent teeth will be stained if drug ingestion occurs between 3 months and 7 to 8 years of age. The result may be yellow, gray, or brown tooth discoloration in a linear pattern that, without restoration, may be quite disfiguring. For this reason tetracycline should be avoided in pregnant or lactating women and in young children.

MANAGEMENT

After allaying parental anxieties, the pediatrician should consider referring any child who has extrinsic or intrinsic stains. Simple office dental procedures and preventive education can resolve all extrinsic staining problems, and esthetic improvement is possible with the vast majority of intrinsic discoloration problems. Table 119-1 should be helpful in identifying the cause of any staining problem.

SUGGESTED READINGS

Abrams RG, Josell SD: Common oral and dental emergencies and problems, *Pediatr Clin North Am* 29:681, 1982.

Acosta F, Carrel R, Binns WH: Dental stains and their relationship to periodontal diseases in children, *Acta Odontol Pediatr* 3:13, 1983.

Table 119-1 Common Colorations of Primary and Permanent Teeth

Color	Distribution and pattern	Causes	Treatment
Green	Several teeth; gingival third of crowns; extrinsic stain	Chromogenic bacteria in plaque, associated with poor oral hygiene	Oral prophylaxis; preventive education
Orange	Several teeth; gingival third of crowns; less common than green stain; extrinsic stain	Chromogenic bacteria in plaque, associated with poor oral hygiene	Oral prophylaxis; preventive education
Black	Several teeth; gingival third of crowns; less common than green and orange stains; extrinsic stain	Chromogenic bacteria in plaque, associated with poor oral hygiene	Oral prophylaxis; preventive education
	Several teeth; extrinsic stain	Oral medications, especially iron	Oral prophylaxis after discontinuing medication
	One or several teeth; occlusal or interproximal surfaces; hard, shiny	Arrested caries	Dental evaluation, observation, or restoration
Brown-black	Several teeth; occlusal pits and fissures or smooth surfaces	Accumulation of tin or staining of demineralized enamel after strontium fluoride (SrF_2) topical treatment	None or esthetic restoration
Pink	Single tooth; entire crown	Posttraumatic change	
		Within 1-2 days—bleeding into dentin; changes to gray in 1-3 wk	None or observation
		After several months—internal resorption of dentin	Minor resorption—endodontics; severe resorption—extraction
Gray	Several teeth; linear pattern or entire crown, depending on stage of tooth development	Tetracycline incorporation in tooth and subsequent oxidation by sunlight; exhibits other colors	Esthetic improvement—endodontic therapy and bleaching and/or esthetic restoration
	All primary and permanent teeth; entire crown	Dentinogenesis imperfecta (autosomal dominant)	Esthetic improvement and protection from wear—prosthetic coverage
	Single tooth; entire crown	Posttraumatic change	
		Within 1-3 wk—hemosiderin pigment in dentin	Observation
		After several months—pulpal necrosis	Endodontic treatment or extraction
Yellow	Several teeth; entire crown	Natural color of permanent compared with primary teeth	None necessary
	Several teeth; linear pattern or entire crown	Tetracyclines; systemic infections	Esthetic restoration
	All primary and permanent teeth; entire crown	Amelogenesis imperfecta (various inheritance patterns)	Esthetic restoration and protection from occlusal wear
	Single tooth; entire crown	Posttraumatic change—pulpal obliteration by dentin	Observation or esthetic restoration
	Several teeth; gingival third of crown; extrinsic stain	Food debris and chromogenic bacteria in plaque, associated with poor oral hygiene	Oral prophylaxis; preventive education
	Several teeth; extrinsic stain; part of or entire crown	Tea, coffee, cola, tobacco	Oral prophylaxis; avoid excessive use of substance

Modified from Abrams RG, Josell SD: *Pediatr Clin North Am* 29:705, 1982.

Continued.

Dayan D et al: Tooth discoloration—extrinsic and intrinsic factors, *Quintessence Int* 14:195, 1983.

Faunce F: Management of discolored teeth, *Dent Clin North Am* 27:657, 1983.

Pindborg JJ: *Pathology of dental hard tissues*, Philadelphia, 1973, WB Saunders.

Sweeney EA: Pediatric dentistry, *Curr Probl Pediatr* 11:1, 1980.

Vogel RI: Intrinsic and extrinsic discoloration of the dentition, *J Oral Med* 30:99, 1975.

Table 119-1 Common Colorations of Primary and Permanent Teeth—cont'd

Color	Distribution and pattern	Causes	Treatment
Yellow-brown	Several teeth	Premature birth; enamel disturbance—hypoplasia and hypocalcification	None
	One or several teeth; one or more surfaces with cavitations	Advanced active caries	Restoration
Brown	Several teeth; entire crown	Amelogenesis imperfecta; dentinogenesis imperfecta; premature birth; jaundice	As suggested above under gray and yellow colorations
	Individual teeth; localized area	Turner hypoplasia secondary to infection	None or esthetic restoration
		Hypocalcified or hypoplastic area—traumatized primary tooth affecting permanent crown	None or esthetic restoration
	Several teeth; linear or generalized distribution; associated hypoplasia	Fluorosis; systemic infections, especially with high fever; nutritional deficiencies	None or esthetic restoration
	Several teeth; generalized or linear	Tetracycline	Esthetic restoration
	Several teeth; one or more surfaces; loss of tooth structure	Advanced active caries	Restoration
Red-brown	Several teeth; primary and permanent; generalized	Porphyria	None or esthetic restoration
Blue	Several teeth; extrinsic stain; part of or entire crown	Berries	Oral prophylaxis; avoid excessive use of substance
Blue-green or yellow-green	All primary teeth; entire crown	Bilirubin pigments incorporated into dentin—erythroblastosis fetalis, biliary atresia, neonatal hepatitis	None; generally fades; permanent teeth not affected if condition does not continue
White or cream	Several teeth; linear or entire crown	Fluorosis; systemic infections	None; generally fades; permanent teeth not affected if condition does not continue
	All primary and permanent teeth; entire crown	Amelogenesis imperfecta	None; generally fades; permanent teeth not affected if condition does not continue
	Individual teeth; localized area	Turner hypoplasia	None; generally fades; permanent teeth not affected if condition does not continue
	One or several teeth; occlusal or gingival third of smooth surface	Early active caries—demineralization of enamel	Preventive therapy
	Several teeth; any surface; extrinsic stain	Plaque and food debris (materia alba)—removed easily with gauze	Oral hygiene instruction

120 Diarrhea and Steatorrhea

Martin H. Ulshen

Diarrhea, much like vomiting, is a common symptom in the young child, especially during infancy. Therefore it is surprising that it has been difficult to establish rigid criteria regarding what truly constitutes diarrhea. Loosely defined, diarrhea is characterized by an increase in the frequency and water content of stools. The normal daily stool volume varies with the size of the child. Adults and older children have a normal daily stool weight in the range of 100 to 200 g (consisting of 60% to 85% water); infants weighing less than 10 kg can have approximately 5 g/kg/day of stool. An intermediate range of 50 to 75 g/day is an appropriate approximation for the preschool child. In infancy the frequency and quality of "normal" stools depend very much on diet. During the first weeks of life, the breast-fed infant commonly has up to eight loose stools per day, which at times may contain mucus. These stools frequently follow feedings (as a result of the "gastrocolic reflex") and do not constitute diarrhea. Infants receiving cow milk formula usually have firmer and somewhat less frequent stools. After the first few weeks of life the normal breast-fed infant tends to have less frequent stools, which even may be infrequent (i.e., less than once a week), although they remain soft. Commonly the stool of the nursing infant becomes firm when solids or cow milk is introduced into the diet.

Steatorrhea signifies an excess of fat in the stool and is a symptom of malabsorption. However, disorders associated with malabsorption (e.g., gluten-sensitive enteropathy) do not always produce steatorrhea. Stools that contain an increased quantity of fat can be greasy, bulky, and foul smelling; however, with mild steatorrhea the stool may appear normal. The stool can be evaluated quickly for fat content using Sudan staining. Fat excretion can be measured more precisely with a 72-hour collection of stool. A record of the diet is kept during this period, and fat intake is calculated. The percentage of the ingested fat that is absorbed equals (Fat intake − Fat output)/Fat intake × 100; this is called the *coefficient of absorption*. Absorption of fat by young infants varies with the type of fat that is fed and with the maturity of the infant. A normal premature infant may absorb as little as 65% to 75% of dietary fat, but this improves to 90% in the full-term infant. Furthermore the neonate absorbs vegetable fat much more efficiently than butterfat. Children and adults typically absorb at least 95% of the fat in a normal diet.

PATHOPHYSIOLOGY

Advances in the understanding of the pathophysiology of diarrhea allow a more rational approach to diagnosis and treatment. Normally, large volumes of fluid are processed by the gastrointestinal tract, as illustrated for adults in Figure 120-1. It is not difficult to see how an infant can rapidly become fluid depleted from diarrhea when such large gastrointestinal fluid shifts take place each day. Under normal circumstances about 90% of fluid absorption takes place in the small bowel. However, the colon has a reserve capacity for fluid absorption that must be overcome before diarrhea will result. In adults as much as 2 liters of ileal fluid can be reabsorbed by the colon daily without diarrhea occurring.

Movement of water across the gastrointestinal tract mucosa is passive, following osmotic gradients created by electrolytes and other osmotically active solutes (such as glucose and amino acids). Nutrients are absorbed by active transport or passive diffusion; some first require digestion to simpler compounds. There is a bidirectional flux of electrolytes across the mucosa. The net result of absorption and secretion of these osmotically active solutes is net water retention or loss in the stool. In this sense diarrhea can be thought of as the result of either malabsorption or net secretion of osmotically active substances.

Many nutrients (including glucose and most amino acids) are absorbed by active, carrier-mediated transport, which is coupled with sodium transport. The osmotic gradient created promotes the absorption of water. Movement of water, in turn, also carries small solutes, such as sodium and chloride. This process is known as *solvent drag* and appears to be an important route for sodium absorption during normal digestion. As noted below these mechanisms of sodium movement associated with carrier-mediated nonelectrolyte transport are important to preserve normal fluid and electrolyte balance during some episodes of diarrhea. Active absorption of chloride in exchange for bicarbonate (HCO_3^-) takes place in the ileum. Potassium moves passively along electrochemical gradients in the small intestine, but there is both active absorption and secretion of potassium in the colon and probably the small bowel as well. The permeability of the intestinal mucosa to passive fluid and electrolyte movement is high in the duodenum and proximal jejunum and decreases distally to the ileum and colon, which are poorly permeable. This feature allows the proximal intestinal contents to equilibrate rapidly with the isotonic extracellular fluid and facilitates the rapid absorption of water and small solutes by diffusion. Conversely the ileum and colon are poorly permeable and are able to absorb water and sodium against high electrochemical gradients.

The pathophysiological mechanisms for diarrhea fall into three basic categories, popularized by Phillips[41]: (1) osmotic diarrhea, (2) diarrhea resulting from secretion or altered absorption of electrolytes, and (3) diarrhea resulting from abnormal intestinal motility. Each mechanism has unique clinical characteristics and requires a different therapeutic approach. Therefore, for the physician considering an individual patient who has diarrhea, this framework provides a rational approach for both diagnosis and treatment. Frequently more

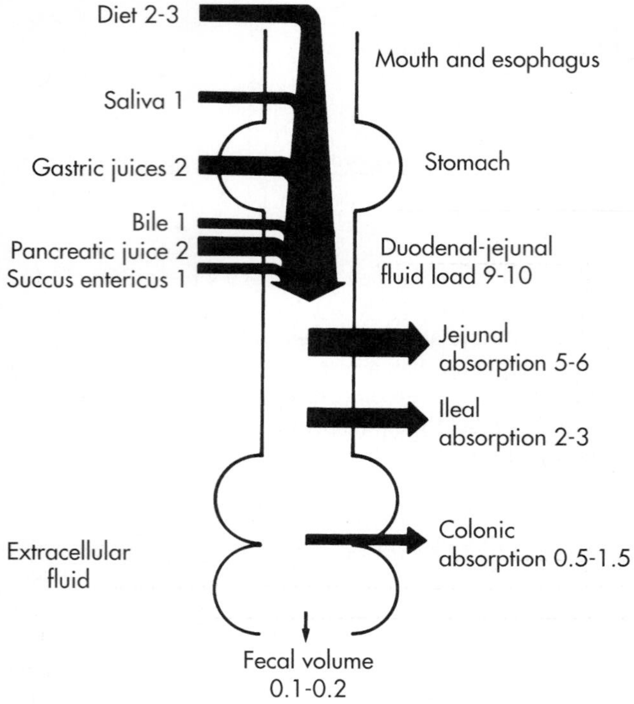

FIG. 120-1 Ingestion, secretion, and absorption of water in the gastrointestinal tract of an adult. Numbers refer to liters of water.

than one mechanism of diarrhea will be involved in an episode of diarrhea, but this will be apparent.

Osmotic Diarrhea

The ingestion of a poorly absorbable, osmotically active substance and its presence in the bowel lumen create an osmotic gradient that encourages movement of water into the lumen and subsequently into the stool. Electrolyte losses increase because electrolytes will follow water into the lumen through solvent drag and will tend not to be reabsorbed because of unfavorable electrochemical gradients.

There are two main groups of poorly absorbed solutes, the ingestion of which results in osmotic diarrhea. The first group includes normal dietary components that may be malabsorbed either transiently or permanently. For example, disaccharides usually are hydrolyzed to monosaccharides before they are absorbed. If a mucosal disaccharidase (such as lactase) is deficient, the disaccharide (in this case lactose) will be malabsorbed and will represent an osmotic load that will produce diarrhea. Similarly monosaccharides at times may be poorly absorbed. Medium-chain triglycerides (MCTs) also are osmotically active and may lead occasionally to diarrhea when ingested in high concentration, such as when infants who have compromised mucosal function are given an elemental formula containing MCTs. Malabsorption of long-chain triglycerides (LCTs) does not lead to osmotic diarrhea because LCTs are large hydrophobic molecules and therefore have little osmotic activity. Malabsorption of LCTs, however, may lead to diarrhea by mechanisms described below. In addition, any osmotically active solute may produce diarrhea in normal persons if given in quantities great enough to surpass the intestinal capacity for absorption. Thus some infants whose bowel function is normal will not tolerate the high osmolality of an elemental formula, especially if it is undiluted. Similarly, older children may develop functional gastrointestinal symptoms, including diarrhea, from ingestion of large amounts of fructose in fruits and juices. Patients who have decreased mucosal surface area may have decreased functional capacity and resultant osmotic diarrhea. This problem is seen in infants after small bowel resection. Protein malabsorption does not appear to be associated with diarrhea except in the rare instance of congenital trypsinogen or enterokinase deficiency. For example, Hartnup syndrome is a syndrome with malabsorption of primary amino acids that nevertheless is *not* associated with diarrhea.

The second group of poorly absorbed solutes includes substances that are transported in limited amounts, even by normal individuals. This group includes magnesium, phosphates, and sulfates. Because these ions invariably lead to diarrhea when given in large enough quantities, they are used as cathartics. The introduction of lactulose in the treatment of hepatic encephalopathy takes advantage of its being a nondigestible disaccharide that leads to acidification of colonic contents by bacterial fermentation of nonabsorbed sugar. Its side effect is diarrhea. In fact in recent years lactulose has become a popular alternative for the treatment of constipation because it tastes better than most other stool softeners.

The key characteristic of an osmotic diarrhea is its association with the oral ingestion of the offending solute. When a patient who has an osmotic diarrhea is given nothing by mouth, the diarrhea will stop dramatically within 24 hours or less. If the agent is reintroduced (as in a lactose tolerance test), the diarrhea will reappear. The diarrhea is of a moderate volume compared with that in secretory diarrhea. The sodium and potassium ion concentrations and osmolality in the stool fluid are very useful in establishing a diagnosis. As ileal and colonic sodium absorption continues to function against a concentration gradient, stool sodium concentration will be lower than in the plasma. The electrolyte concentration in the stool is roughly twice the combined sodium and potassium concentration. When this value is much less than the osmolality of the stool (which can be assumed to be about 280 milliosmoles), there must be osmotically active nonelectrolytes in the stool, and an osmotic diarrhea is present.[13] In some instances one may be able to find the osmotic component in the stool (such as a reducing substance in lactose malabsorption).

Diarrhea Secondary to Secretion or Altered Electrolyte Absorption

Net movement of an electrolyte across the intestinal mucosa (i.e., into or out of the bowel lumen) is the sum of the simultaneous bidirectional electrolyte flux across the mucosal surface epithelium. Thus under normal circumstances opposing secretory and absorptive processes (both active and passive) take place, and the resulting balance is reflected in normal luminal electrolyte and water content. Secretory diarrhea occurs when there is pathological stimulation of a physiological electrolyte secretory process. Under such circumstances there is a net increase in luminal electrolytes and therefore a secondary increase in water. In addition, an associated decrease in absorptive processes may occur. The electrolytes that have been implicated are sodium, chloride, and perhaps bicarbonate. Diarrhea also may result from a decrease in active electrolyte absorption in the absence of any change in secretory function. It should be mentioned at the outset that it is very difficult clinically to distinguish increased electrolyte secretion from decreased absorption; the results are similar. The prototype for a secretory diarrhea has been cholera. Cholera enterotoxin has been shown to lead to increased intestinal secretion of chloride and, possibly, bicarbonate, as well as to inhibition of the absorption of sodium. Cholera enterotoxin appears to stimulate surface epithelial adenylate cyclase, leading to an increase in cellular levels of cyclic 3′5′-adenosine monophosphate (AMP). An important observation has been the normal histological appearance of the intestinal mucosa during cholera infection or in vitro exposure to cholera enterotoxin. Specifically there is no evidence of cell necrosis, inflammation, or local bacterial invasion; other cell absorptive functions remain normal. The normal absorption of glucose provides a route for secondary sodium absorption; oral glucose- and electrolyte-containing solutions have gained wide use in the management of cholera.

It now is known that a growing number of infectious agents may be associated with secretory diarrhea. Toxigenic *Escherichia coli* produces an enterotoxin antigenically distinct from cholera enterotoxin, which also activates adenylate cyclase. Infantile diarrhea resulting from this toxin is well known. Other bacteria that have been associated with stimulation of intestinal secretion are strains of *Shigella dysenteriae, Salmonella typhimurium, Klebsiella pneumoniae, Clostridium perfringens, Staphylococcus aureus,* and *Pseudomonas aeruginosa*. Experimental work with viral enteritis suggests that there is a significant secretory component to this diarrhea.[21] Secretion is the result of viral damage to villous epithelial cells in the small intestine and repopulation of the villi with immature crypt cells, rather than toxin production.

Secretory diarrhea has several noninfectious causes. Malabsorbed bile acids and long-chain fats both have been shown to stimulate a colonic secretory diarrhea. Certain prostaglandins have been shown to activate adenylate cyclase and produce intestinal secretion in experimental models. Because prostaglandins are released during inflammation, it has been hypothesized that diarrhea associated with certain inflammatory states may be caused by these hormones. This is a particularly appealing hypothesis to explain the small bowel secretion that may take place with chronic inflammatory bowel disease. Prostaglandins also have been suggested as possible mediators for the activation of adenylate cyclase by *Salmonella* organisms in the absence of an enterotoxin. Secretory diarrheas may occur in association with increased levels of certain gastrointestinal hormones, most notably vasoactive intestinal polypeptide (VIP).

An isolated decrease of electrolyte absorption is seen much less frequently. The best known example, although extremely rare, is congenital chloride-losing diarrhea.[20] This abnormality results from the apparent lack of normal, active chloride absorption by the distal small intestine. Great quantities of chloride are lost in the stool and lead to diarrhea from birth onward.

The stool in secretory diarrheas tends to be watery and large in volume. As opposed to osmotic diarrhea, secretory diarrhea persists despite discontinuing oral intake. The stool water osmolality is approximately equal to the electrolyte concentration (i.e., twice the sum of the sodium and potassium concentrations) because there is no significant osmotic nonelectrolyte component.[13]

Motility Diarrhea

The intestine has a cyclic, orderly pattern of motility. Increased, decreased, or disordered movement can lead to diarrhea. Rapid intestinal transit often occurs in association with osmotic and secretory diarrheas. Increased intraluminal volume has been implicated in stimulating increased peristaltic action. Increased motility may cause diarrhea by allowing less time for the contact of intraluminal contents with absorptive surfaces. When bowel function is compromised (as with the short bowel syndrome), the time of contact with the limited functioning surface may be a crucial factor. In irritable bowel syndrome disordered motility also may play a role.[11]

Slowed transit and severely disordered motility lead to intraluminal stasis. In normal bowel, steady, progressive movement of chyme is one of the protective mechanisms that prevents the development of bacterial overgrowth, whereas stasis encourages overgrowth. Certain bacteria deconjugate bile acids when present in the upper small bowel and produce fat malabsorption secondarily. In addition, bacterial proteases may damage the small bowel surface. Stasis may result from an anatomical obstruction (e.g., blind loop or stricture), as well as from functional motor disorders. Motility disorder frequently is an associated factor in chronic inflammatory bowel disease. Stools associated with motility disorder, except those secondary to fatty acid malabsorption, tend to be small in volume. The response to feeding is variable, and the gastrocolic reflex may be heightened. Patients with chronic inflammatory bowel disease may find that meals stimulate intestinal activity, resulting in postprandial abdominal cramps and bowel movements.

ACUTE DIARRHEA

Acute diarrhea is common in children, is transient and usually self-limited, and most often is caused by infection. In the United States children average about one or two episodes per year.[15] The role of the physician is to rule out causes that require specific treatment, to advise the parents in supportive management, and to provide follow-up for possible complications. The box on p. 904 lists some of the more frequent causes of acute diarrhea. Day care centers are likely sites for the spread of enteric pathogens. Pathogens that have been associated with epidemics include *Giardia lamblia* and rotavirus, *Shigella, Campylobacter,* and *Cryptosporidium* organisms; and *Clostridium difficile*.[1,4,5] Asymptomatic fecal shedding of *Giardia* organisms is common in this setting.

The neonate who has acute diarrhea must be considered different from the older infant and child, both because of lower tolerance to the associated fluid shifts and because of the greater likelihood of severe infection or congenital anomaly. In addition, signs that suggest necrotizing enterocolitis must be sought, including gastric retention (frequently bilious), distention, and occult or bright red blood in the stool. Although this disease usually occurs in premature infants, it also has been reported in ill full-term infants. The presence of pneumatosis intestinalis, gas in the portal vein, or free in-

CAUSES OF ACUTE DIARRHEA

Usually without blood in stool

Viral enteritis—reovirus (rotavirus[4,48] and orbivirus), Norwalk agent, enteric adenovirus,[58] calicivirus, and astrovirus[36]

Enterotoxin—*Escherichia coli,*[24] *Klebsiella* organisms, cholera, *Clostridium perfringens, Staphylococcus* organisms, and *Vibrio* species

Parasitic—*Giardia*[5] and *Cryptosporidium*[1,57] organisms

Extraintestinal infection—otitis media and urinary tract infection

Antibiotic-induced and *Clostridium difficile* toxin (without pseudomembranous colitis)

Commonly associated with blood in stool

Bacterial—*Shigella, Salmonella,* and *Campylobacter* organisms, *Yersinia enterocolitica,* invasive *E. coli,*[24] gonococcus(venereal spread), enteroadherent *E. coli,*[54] *Aeromonas hydrophilia,* and *Plesiomonas shigelloides*[54]

Amebic dysentery

Hemolytic-uremic syndrome

Henoch-Schönlein purpura

Pseudomembranous enterocolitis (*C. difficile* toxin)[8,47]

Ulcerative or granulomatous colitis (acute presentation)

Necrotizing enterocolitis (neonates)

traperitoneal gas seen on abdominal roentgenograms supports this diagnosis. Epidemics of diarrhea associated with rotavirus, enteropathogenic *E. coli,* salmonellae, and other organisms, including klebsiellae, have been reported in nurseries. If the onset of diarrhea is associated with early feedings, one must consider congenital digestive defects, especially sugar intolerance. Hirschsprung disease may manifest with acute diarrhea and enterocolitis in the neonatal period and should especially be suspected in the infant who has not passed meconium in the first 24 hours. Bloody diarrhea that results from cow milk or soy protein intolerance may develop in infants still in the nursery. Resolution and exacerbation on removal and reintroduction of formula, as well as an atopic family history, are clues to this diagnosis.

In the older infant and child the usual episode of acute diarrhea is transient and benign. On the initial visit the physician must evaluate the course in terms of both possible causes and the status of hydration. The diarrhea usually is the result of viral enteritis, typically occurring with low-grade fever, vomiting, and frequent watery stools. Generally the stools are without blood or white blood cells. Enterotoxin-producing organisms (such as toxigenic *E. coli*) are associated with watery stools and are without evidence of mucosal invasion (no high fever or blood in the stool). *Giardia lamblia* produces watery diarrhea associated with intestinal gas and crampy abdominal pain. Diarrhea may be present in association with extraintestinal infections, most notably otitis media and pyelonephritis. This has been called *parenteral diarrhea,* and its mechanism is obscure. There may be an associated viral enteritis in some cases of otitis media. Certain antibiotics, especially ampicillin, have been associated with transient diarrhea. Less common but of greater danger is the association of pseudomembranous colitis with most antibiotics, most commonly clindamycin.[8] In childhood, pseudomembranous colitis may occur acutely or as a more chronic illness of 1 or 2 months' duration.[47] *C. difficile* toxin, which is considered the cause of most cases of pseudomembranous colitis, also may be associated with chronic childhood diarrhea in the absence of colitis.[49]

The presence of blood in the stool, especially with symptoms of colonic involvement (tenesmus, urgency, and crampy lower abdominal pain), should make one think of infection with *Shigella* and *Salmonella* organisms. These symptoms of dysentery typically are more striking with *Shigella* species; however, both may be associated with a significant secretory component. When the *Shigella* is an enterotoxin-producing organism, watery diarrhea actually may precede the onset of dysentery. Patients who have *Shigella* organisms tend to appear severely ill and may have meningismus or seizures. The stools tend to be foul smelling. *Yersinia* and *Campylobacter* enterocolitis also may be associated with blood in the stool, but *Yersinia* appears to be incriminated less commonly as an etiological agent in the United States. *E. coli* can produce diarrhea by a number of pathogenic mechanisms; the enteroadherent, enteroinvasive, and enterohemorrhagic forms all can be associated with blood in the stool.[24] Enterohemorrhagic *E. coli* is a common cause of hemolytic-uremic syndrome. Amebiasis is unusual in the United States, but *Entamoeba histolytica* can produce a picture of acute colitis. Causes of bloody diarrhea that are not obviously infectious include intussusception, immune deficiencies, and chronic inflammatory bowel disease. The last may present with an initial episode of acute dysentery, although the history may reveal previous episodes, and arthralgia or growth failure may have preceded the diarrhea. The history of recent similar diarrheal illness in family members or friends suggests an infectious diarrhea.

At the initial evaluation (see box on p. 905), the physician should establish the quantity of the diarrhea, the child's ability to maintain oral intake, and the presence of associated vomiting. On physical examination the state of hydration should be estimated. The presence of tears and saliva usually is evidence of adequate hydration. A simple guideline to hydration is that the absence of tears and the presence of a dry mouth suggest 5% dehydration, whereas the addition of sunken eyes, sunken fontanelle, and poor skin turgor suggests 10% dehydration. In the presence of hypernatremia the state of dehydration typically is more severe than suggested on physical examination inasmuch as extracellular fluid volume tends to be preserved at the expense of intracellular volume. A recorded weight is essential; it can be compared with previous weights and also will be available to reevaluate hydration during the illness. Information about the frequency and quantity of urine is useful, especially if there is a history of good urine output. Parents may underestimate urinary frequency, however, especially when urine becomes mixed with liquid stool.

A stool culture should be obtained if blood or leukocytes are noted in the stool and the child is severely ill. Examination of the stool for leukocytes is helpful in establishing the presence of colitis. A small sample of stool is placed on a microscope slide and mixed with a drop of methylene blue. Multiple fields then are scanned. In the presence of both in-

EVALUATION OF ACUTE DIARRHEA

History

1. Length of illness
2. Stools—frequency, looseness (watery versus mushy), and presence of gross blood
3. Oral intake—diet, quantity of fluids and solids taken, and presence of vomiting
4. Associated symptoms—fever, rash, and arthralgia
5. Urine output
6. Contacts with diarrhea or other infectious illness (including day care exposure)

Physical examination

1. Hydration status—moist mucosa, presence of saliva and tears, skin turgor, weight, and vital signs
2. Alertness
3. Infant—vigor of suck

Laboratory

1. Stool culture (as indicated), smear for white blood cells, and evaluation for occult blood
2. Stool ova and parasites and reducing substances (as indicated)
3. Complete blood count (as indicated)
4. If hydration status is in question—blood urea nitrogen (BUN) and serum electrolyte levels
5. Urinalysis
6. If child is lethargic or has had a seizure, culture for sepsis: measure the BUN and serum electrolyte levels and examine and culture the cerebrospinal fluid (as indicated)

fectious and noninfectious colitis, white blood cells (WBCs) usually are found in high numbers—frequently in sheets. Polymorphonuclear leukocytes may account for 60% to 80% of the cells; the presence of only occasional cells is considered a negative finding. The absence of WBCs in grossly bloody diarrheal stool occurs with enterohemorrhagic *E. coli* infection but also should direct attention to entities such as intussusception and Meckel diverticulum when these diagnoses seem clinically appropriate. Amebic colitis also may not be associated with WBCs in the stool, although the trophozoites and numerous RBCs may be visible on a saline wet mount preparation of the stool. Invasive bacterial diarrhea frequently is associated with a peripheral blood leukocytosis.

The cornerstone of treatment in acute gastroenteritis is good fluid and electrolyte management (see box on p. 906). When the patient is less than 5% dehydrated and is able to retain fluids adequately by mouth, outpatient treatment without specialized rehydration solutions is indicated. Gastroenteritis is less common in the breast-fed infant; however, it usually is possible to continue nursing even if diarrhea occurs. Human milk contains low amounts of sodium (6 to 7 mEq/L); therefore when diarrhea is persistent or severe, a regimen of a clear liquid that has a higher sodium concentration than milk should be instituted for rehydration to avoid hyponatremia (e.g., an oral maintenance or rehydration solution). A transient secondary lactose intolerance also may have developed, an indication to discontinue breast milk temporarily.

The goal of treatment for an infant receiving cow milk formula has been to provide a lactose-free oral fluid with low renal solute load (i.e., high free water) and adequate but not excessive electrolyte content. This requires the temporary discontinuation of milk and solids and the initiation of oral clear liquids. Grandmothers, as well as clinicians, traditionally have recommended a diverse group of fluids that have wide-ranging electrolyte and carbohydrate concentrations. It is clear that the electrolyte content in diarrheal stool varies widely, with the highest concentrations occurring in secretory diarrheas (e.g., cholera). Fecal sodium levels may range from 40 to 100 mEq/L and occasionally may be as high as 150 mEq/L. Commercial oral hydration solutions provide more sodium than traditional clear liquids.

At least 40% to 50% of epidemic diarrhea may be of viral origin (in winter this proportion probably is higher). Viral enteritis has been shown to result in a transient, patchy, mucosal lesion of the small intestine, which may be associated with temporary lactose and fat malabsorption. Decreased mucosal lactase levels may be seen. In experimental viral diarrhea in piglets (transmissible gastroenteritis), intestinal glucose-stimulated absorption of sodium (and therefore water) is impaired because of villus damage.[29] Abnormal glucose absorption also has been observed in infants who have rotavirus enteritis. Nevertheless, secretion can be converted to net absorption in most children by providing oral glucose electrolyte solution, because of the patchy nature of the lesion in viral gastroenteritis.

Oral rehydration solutions have been used safely and successfully to treat acute diarrhea with dehydration.[42,46,50] Infants who have diarrhea usually will drink large volumes of liquids ad libitum, appropriate for the stool output. Most episodes of diarrhea in previously healthy, well-nourished children are mild, and the use of clear liquids is not of crucial importance. Liquids can be offered ad libitum, although frequent, smaller amounts may be tolerated better when diarrhea is associated with vomiting. If the episode is more severe, an oral rehydration solution as described in the box on p. 906 should be used. Commercial rehydration solutions are available (e.g., Rehydralyte). The contents of these solutions have evolved in conjunction with advances in the understanding of optimal absorption during oral rehydration, so the clinician should consult current manufacturer specifications before choosing a product. The timing of advancement from oral fluids to formula is controversial, although recent studies suggest that rapid progression, supplemented with oral rehydration solution, is well tolerated and usually leads to quicker recovery. Vomiting usually is not a contraindication for oral rehydration. This treatment appears to be associated with shorter hospitalization and lower medical costs. Infants who have hypernatremic dehydration seem to have fewer problems with seizures during oral, as compared with intravenous, rehydration.[42,46] Oral rehydration therapy, however, requires the nearly constant presence of a caretaker, although this individual does not need to have previous medical experience. Currently the use of starches in oral maintenance or rehydration solution is being evaluated in an effort to improve sodium and water absorption (an example is Ricelyte).

MANAGEMENT OF ACUTE DIARRHEA

I. Less than 5% dehydration without significant vomiting
  A. Nursing infant may continue breastfeeding—supplement with clear fluids as necessary; discontinue solids.
  B. Formula-fed infant
    1. Discontinue formula and solids.
    2. Begin clear liquids (e.g., carbonated beverages, Kool-Aid, Jell-O water, Gatorade, Pedialyte, Ricelyte, Resol). If intake is good without vomiting, offer fluids every 3 to 4 hours; otherwise, offer small quantities more frequently.
    3. As diarrhea resolves, reinstitute formula half strength at first.
    4. If child tolerates half-strength formula for 12 to 24 hours, then go to full strength.
    5. Solids may be introduced as diarrhea resolves (rice, cereal, bananas, crackers, and mashed potatoes without butter).
    6. If reinstitution of formula is not tolerated, continue clear liquids and then try half-strength lactose-free formula (soy formula).
    7. After improvement in diarrhea, increase solids as tolerated.
    8. Reintroduce lactose in patients on lactose-free diet several days to weeks after resolution, depending on severity of original diarrhea; if not tolerated, continue lactose-free diet for several months.
  C. Avoid diphenoxylate (Lomotil), loperamide (Imodium), paregoric, and anticholinergics.

II. Greater than 5% dehydration: either oral or intravenous rehydration
  A. Oral rehydration therapy
    1. Offer rehydration solution *hourly ad libitum:* 50 to 75 mEq/L sodium, 20 to 25 mEq/L potassium, 30 mEq/L bicarbonate or citrate, remainder of anion as chloride, and 20 g/L glucose.
    2. As the diarrhea slows (usually within 24 to 48 hours), begin one-half strength formula (can be lactose free) and advance to regular diet within 24 hours. For ongoing diarrheal losses, supplement with oral hydration solution.
    3. Infants with signs of shock should be given intravenous Ringer lactate (20 ml/kg body weight per hour) until the blood pressure is normal, followed by oral rehydration solution.
    4. Initial vomiting is not a contraindication to the use of oral rehydration; however, persistent vomiting to the extent of interference with rehydration should lead to the use of intravenous fluids.
  B. Intravenous fluids
    1. Replacement of deficit is based on estimated percentage of dehydration or known weight loss and serum sodium.
    2. There may be ongoing loss through stool and vomitus.
    3. Maintenance should be appropriate for size.
  C. Give half of fluids in first 8 hours, then remainder over next 16 hours (except with hypernatremia, when fluids should be given uniformly with gradual correction over 48 hours; hypotonic fluid should not be used for hypernatremia).
  D. If severe dehydration or shock is present, give isotonic fluid or a colloid (10 to 20 ml/kg body weight, over 1 to 2 hours).
  E. Delay giving intravenous potassium until urine output is established.
  F. As diarrhea resolves, begin treatment as in those patients with less than 5% dehydration, except avoid lactose.

Indications for medications in the treatment of acute gastroenteritis in infants and children are limited. As already noted, the key mechanisms involved are intestinal secretion and transient malabsorption. Therefore, although medications frequently are used, there is no apparent rationale regarding the pathophysiology of the disorder for medications that slow gut motility—diphenoxylate, loperamide, paregoric, and anticholinergics. In fact, pooling of fluid in the intestinal lumen after treatment may give a false impression that the diarrhea has improved. Diphenoxylate also has been implicated in accidental overdosage and respiratory arrest. This drug is not approved in the United States for children younger than 2 years of age. In the study by Portnoy et al.[43] children who had acute gastroenteritis (3 to 11 years of age) were given diphenoxylate; no difference in the amount of change in stool weight or water content could be found during the 2 days after onset of treatment when these children were compared with others who had received a placebo.[43] Although Kaopectate does not carry the hazards of these drugs, it has not been shown to be efficacious in slowing fluid output and also may lead to a false impression that the diarrhea has resolved. Slowing intestinal transit with drugs may allow greater mucosal contact with pathogens and thereby allow for local mucosal invasion. Bismuth subsalicylate, which decreases the duration of diarrhea, has been shown to be a safe adjunct to oral rehydration.[14] Antibiotics are useful in specific situations: *Shigella* dysentery, *Yersinia* or *Campylobacter* gastroenteritis, pseudomembranous colitis, *Salmonella* infections in infants younger than 6 months old, and *Salmonella* infections in older patients with enteric fever, typhoid fever, or complications of bacteremia. [56] For the individual patient the presence of an *E. coli* serotype previously labeled enteropathogenic correlates poorly with the presence of diarrhea and alone is not an indication for antibiotic treatment.[24]

Most episodes of gastroenteritis are self-limited and of short duration. Symptoms of rotavirus enteritis typically last 4 to 10 days. The current approach to treatment is to restart the previous formula and solids (especially rice, cereal, bananas, apples, and dry toast) early after the onset of diarrhea. It often is best to begin with half-strength formula. If this is tolerated for 1 to 2 days, the use of full-strength formula may be resumed. If diarrhea recurs on the introduction of lactose-containing formula, the child may have acquired a transient lactose intolerance. In this situation half-strength soy formula may be offered (the sugar in this formula can be either sucrose or a glucose polymer). As noted in the section on disaccharide intolerance, sugar malabsorption can be identified by the determination of reducing substance in the stool (sucrose must be hydrolyzed first with hydrochloric acid). A secondary lactose intolerance usually lasts only a week or less but at times can persist for months.

If the degree of dehydration is greater than 5%, either oral or intravenous rehydration solution should be instituted in the manner presented in the box on p. 906. For severe dehydration or shock, rapid intravenous administration of 10 to 20 ml/kg of isotonic fluid or colloid is required initially. Hyponatremia and hypernatremia must be corrected slowly to prevent complications of the central nervous system (CNS). Oral solutions are better tolerated and result in fewer CNS complications than intravenous solutions in infants who have hypernatremia.[42,46] Potassium should not be added to intravenous fluids until adequate urine output is established. Urine specific gravity may be misleading inasmuch as kidney concentration may be poor with reduced renal urea or whole body potassium. Inability to acidify the urine during acute diarrhea occurs commonly in infants despite the presence of metabolic acidosis.[25] This finding is thought to be secondary to sodium deficiency and the resulting inadequate delivery of sodium to the distal nephron. Complete discussion of intravenous treatment is presented in Chapter 28, Fluid Therapy.

CHRONIC DIARRHEA

Chronic diarrhea occurs in children of all ages; however, it is most frequent and often most challenging to diagnose in infants. Both healthy and ill infants seem to develop diarrhea in response to a variety of stresses. The younger the infant, the more likely he or she is to enter the cycle of diarrhea and secondary malnutrition that leads to further diarrhea, malnutrition, and susceptibility to infection. Many of the causes of chronic diarrhea may appear at any time during childhood. Certain diseases, however, occur much more commonly in infancy; others are more likely to begin in later childhood. This section addresses the illnesses of infancy and older childhood separately. This division is somewhat artificial, but it is a helpful guide in evaluating the child who has chronic diarrhea. All the causes discussed are listed in the box above.

CAUSES OF CHRONIC DIARRHEA

More common causes

Chronic nonspecific diarrhea (toddler's diarrhea, irritable colon of childhood)[35]
Disaccharide intolerance[53]
Chronic constipation with overflow diarrhea
Cystic fibrosis
Gluten-sensitive enteropathy (celiac disease)[34]
Inflammatory bowel disease—Crohn disease and ulcerative colitis
Hirschsprung disease
Immunodeficiency states
Chronic enteric infection—*Salmonella* organisms, *Yersinia enterocolitica, Campylobacter* and *Giardia* organisms, *C. difficile* toxin,[47,49] enteroadherent *E. coli*,[54] rotavirus (in immunodeficient patients), cytomegalovirus, and HIV
Monosaccharide intolerance
Eosinophilic (allergic) gastroenteritis
Cow milk protein intolerance[6]
Short bowel syndrome
Urinary tract infection
Factitious causes

Less common causes

Hormonal—adrenal insufficiency and hyperthyroidism
Vasoactive intestinal polypeptide–secreting tumor
Neural crest tumor and carcinoid
Intestinal lymphangiectasia[55]
Acrodermatitis enteropathica[37]
Intestinal stricture or blind loop
Pancreatic insufficiency with neurotropenia[19]
Trypsinogen or enterokinase deficiency
Congenital chloride-losing diarrhea[20]
Abetalipoproteinemia
Microvillus inclusion disease[10]
Intestinal pseudoobstruction

Infants

The physician confronted with an infant who has a history of chronic diarrhea must decide first whether the stool pattern is abnormal. A nursing mother who has not been forewarned may become concerned about the appearance and frequency of her child's transitional stools. The infant's weight gain and healthy appearance, combined with an explanation about stools of breast-fed infants, should dispel these concerns. In the latter half of the first year and in the second year, the most common cause for persistent diarrhea is chronic nonspecific diarrhea (also called *toddler's diarrhea*).[35] Affected infants have intermittent loose stools for no apparent rhyme or reason. Often the stools occur early in the day and typically not overnight. These infants appear healthy and are thriving according to weight and length growth curves. This condition represents a stool pattern rather than a pathological state and requires minimal or no laboratory evaluation. Symptoms may begin initially after an apparent acute enteritis (postenteritis irritable bowel). Treatment may include (1) restricting the frequency of feedings, whether liquids or solids, in an effort to decrease stimulation of the gastrocolic reflex (in the older infant, three meals and a bedtime snack with nothing by mouth in between), (2) restricting the volumes of fluids ingested, which often are excessive, (3) avoiding excessive intake of juices,[22,35] and (4) reassuring the parents of the benign nature of this entity. A high-fat diet may be helpful in some children, although probably is of less importance.[9] Cholestyramine (2 g by mouth one to three times daily) also is effective at times; however, the duration of use should be restricted because of the potential for interference with fat-soluble vitamin absorption. In any event this is a self-limited condition that typically resolves by 3½ years of age. The only danger is that well-intentioned parents may restrict oral intake to clear liquids repeatedly in an effort to treat the child, and this may result in poor weight gain. Bile acid malabsorption has been described as an occasional sequela of gastroenteritis that can produce persistent diarrhea. This condition also will respond to cholestyramine therapy.

Protracted Diarrhea of Infancy. This syndrome of chronic diarrhea occurring during infancy is understood poorly[33]; it is defined somewhat arbitrarily as occurring in infants younger than 3 months of age and persisting for more than 2 weeks. Historically this syndrome, previously called *intractable diarrhea of infancy,* has been associated with a high mortality secondary to irreversible diarrhea and related malnutrition. However, the outcome has been improved markedly with the advent of total parenteral nutrition and oral elemental diets. Protracted diarrhea of infancy probably is the final pathway for multiple causes, including gastrointestinal infection and, perhaps, food intolerances. Generally, malnutrition develops and in concert with the persistent diarrhea leads to alteration of gastrointestinal flora sometimes associated with bacterial overgrowth of the small intestine. Altered mucosal function of the small intestine and pancreatic function may occur with malnutrition and intractable diarrhea. Bile salts may be deconjugated as a result of bacterial overgrowth. Commonly the initiating cause of protracted diarrhea is not found, and it is likely that it may no longer be present when the diarrhea has become chronic. The small bowel biopsy specimen may show patchy villous shortening with a decreased villus/crypt ratio and marked inflammation, as well as a damaged surface epithelium. However, the results of the small bowel biopsy also may be normal. Likewise a rectal biopsy specimen may show evidence of inflammation, including crypt abscesses, or may be normal. The presence or absence of these biopsy findings may not correlate with the severity of the clinical syndrome.[16] Affected infants are severely malnourished and have low serum protein, albumin, and hemoglobin levels. Frequently they have had repeated treatment with oral clear liquids and peripheral intravenous fluids, all of which provide inadequate caloric intake.

In evaluating a young infant who has protracted diarrhea the physician must rule out those causes that require urgent treatment while correcting hydration and nutrition. Acute rehydration is similar to the intravenous treatment of acute diarrhea, although it is more difficult to estimate the level of dehydration accurately in the presence of malnutrition. Stool output should be measured. If the urine is collected in a urine bag, diapers can be weighed before and after stools to give an accurate measure. Urine specific gravity and volume may be deceptive because of poor concentration by the kidneys in the presence of malnutrition and total body hypokalemia. The infant should be weighed at least daily. It is important to rule out infection as a cause early in the evaluation. Several stool cultures, as well as blood and urine cultures, should be taken initially. The diagnosis of Hirschsprung disease with enterocolitis should be considered early because infants who have this disorder are prone to perforation of the colon unless a decompression colostomy is performed. In such babies it usually is possible to elicit a history of the absence of stools in the first 24 hours of life and of early obstipation.

In Hirschsprung disease a flat plate roentgenogram of the abdomen may show a dilated colon, although toxic megacolon also may be seen in infectious colitis or in chronic inflammatory bowel disease in infancy. Air-fluid levels throughout the bowel are common in infants who have gastroenteritis, and this sign is not helpful in defining a cause. A barium enema under low pressure in the unprepared patient may show the narrow distal segment of rectum; however, this finding may not be present in neonates. Hirschsprung disease often is more obvious on a delayed roentgenogram (24 to 48 hours after the barium enema).

In a child who has chronic diarrhea and has been fed recently, the levels of stool pH and reducing substance should be determined to evaluate sugar malabsorption. The stool pH is not a good measure of the effect of diarrhea on total body acid-base balance. If stool concentration of sodium and potassium minus chloride is greater than the plasma bicarbonate, the infant is losing bicarbonate. An acid stool pH suggests carbohydrate malabsorption.[13] White blood cells in the stool suggest colonic inflammation, whereas occult blood in the stool suggests loss of blood across the mucosa in the small or large intestine.

It is important to begin nutritional rehabilitation at once. Currently the best choices in treatment are either enteral alimentation with an elemental or modular formula[31] or total parenteral nutrition (TPN; peripheral or central—see Chapter 28, Fluid Therapy). Often enteral nutrition is best tolerated by the continuous drip method. Recent studies suggest that recovery may be more rapid when enteral alimentation is used.[39] Nevertheless, unsuccessful attempts at enteral feeding necessitate initiation of TPN therapy in some infants. Initial treatment with TPN and a gradually increasing, continuous enteral drip is a good approach to patients who do not tolerate elemental diet alone. Elemental formulas are composed of predigested components in fixed proportions, whereas modular formulas allow one to vary the components. A small bowel biopsy for diagnosis may help in planning therapy. Severe mucosal damage would make one less inclined to persist with unsuccessful enteral alimentation. Stool output and weight gain may be measured to assess the infant's response. If disaccharidase levels are abnormal, the specific disaccharides should be avoided. During the treatment a further workup, including an upper gastrointestinal series with small bowel roentgenogram, barium edema, proctoscopy, the measurement of sweat electrolytes, and other specific tests to rule out the entities noted below, should be carried out as indicated.

Malabsorption Syndromes. Infants and children who have malabsorption syndromes typically have diarrhea, steatorrhea, growth failure, or a combination of these. Cystic fibrosis is the most common chronic disease that causes malabsorption in children in the United States. Steatorrhea results from pancreatic insufficiency and secondary maldigestion. Infants who have cystic fibrosis who nurse or are fed soy formula (but not cow milk formula) may present in the first months of life with protein malabsorption. Although cystic fibrosis is thought of primarily as a respiratory disease, some infants and children will have malabsorption and little history of respiratory symptoms; these patients typically have voracious appetites. The diagnosis must be confirmed by sweat electrolyte studies. Other diseases much less common than cystic fibrosis may be associated with prominent steatorrhea in early infancy, including congenital pancreatic insufficiency with cyclic neutropenia *(Shwachman-Diamond syndrome),*[19] *intestinal lymphangiectasia,*[55] and *abetalipo-*

proteinemia. Transient steatorrhea may follow an acute enteritis.[26] Measurement of serum trypsinogen appears to be a useful screening test for pancreatic insufficiency.[12] Values are low in Shwachman-Diamond syndrome but may be high, normal, or low in cystic fibrosis, depending on the stage of the pancreatic disease.

In infancy the age at which celiac disease becomes apparent (gluten-sensitive enteropathy) varies with the age of dietary introduction of gluten-containing products (wheat, rye, oats, and barley).[34] Usually the onset is 1 to several months later. Infants who have celiac disease typically are irritable and have loose stools, a poor appetite, and poor weight gain. They also may have recurrent vomiting. The presentation, however, is quite variable. Steatorrhea often is not present, and results of absorptive studies such as the D-xylose tolerance test may be normal. Gluten-free dietary trials and antigliadin antibody studies may be misleading.[52] The presence of antiendomysial antibody in the serum appears to be a much more reliable predictor of celiac disease and may be useful in evaluating compliance with diet.[28,45] A diagnosis of celiac disease should be confirmed by small bowel biopsy. A later challenge with gluten and a repeat biopsy may be necessary to confirm the diagnosis. *Giardia* infection can produce small bowel malabsorption that mimics celiac disease.[7]

Carbohydrate (monosaccharide or disaccharide) intolerance may be primary or more commonly secondary to other gastrointestinal disorders.[53] The congenital form of lactase deficiency is much less common than is congenital sucrase-isomaltase deficiency. The latter disorder typically appears after introduction of sucrose into the diet in solids. In carbohydrate intolerance the extent of symptoms varies directly with the quantity of the offending sugar in the diet. Similarly, the age at presentation varies with the age at which the sugar is introduced into the diet. The diagnosis may be established by conducting standard sugar tolerance tests, measuring hydrogen excretion in the breath, and assaying the enzymes present in tissue obtained by a small bowel biopsy. Examination of the stool for reducing sugars is an imprecise screening test for stool carbohydrate content.[2] Sorbitol,[21] an artificial sweetener, as well as fructose,[44] may produce diarrhea when ingested in large amounts.

The congenital deficiency of trypsinogen, the zymogen precursor of the pancreatic protease trypsin, has been reported to be a very rare cause of congenital diarrhea. The absence of trypsin in the stool suggests the diagnosis (in the absence of cystic fibrosis and congenital pancreatic insufficiency), but evaluation of the pancreatic proteases in the duodenal aspirate is necessary to confirm this impression. Congenital deficiency of enterokinase, the intestinal enzyme that activates trypsinogen to trypsin, appears in a similar fashion to that of congenital trypsinogen deficiency and is diagnosed by testing the duodenal aspirate for enterokinase activity.

Infection. It has been mentioned that acute bacterial or viral enteritis may be an important initiator of protracted diarrhea in infancy. If the initial infection is no longer present at the time of evaluation for chronic diarrhea, this association will be difficult to prove. Infections at distant sites, especially urinary tract infections, also have been incriminated as a cause of chronic diarrhea in infancy. A urinalysis and urine culture should be obtained routinely in the evaluation of children who have chronic diarrhea. *Salmonella* enteritis commonly is associated with a chronic asymptomatic carrier state, especially in infancy. *Salmonella* infection, however, also may be associated with persistent diarrhea in infants. *Y. enterocolitica* enteritis has been associated with a chronic relapsing diarrhea. *Yersinia* organisms do not appear to be common pathogens in the United States; however, one must be sure that the microbiology laboratory specifically looks for this organism or it will be missed. *Campylobacter* enteritis also can have a protracted course.

Parasites. The principal parasite associated with diarrhea in the United States is *G. lamblia.*[7] It may be associated with watery diarrhea and crampy abdominal pain and may manifest in epidemic form. This protozoon may be difficult to detect in stools, and the best yield of organisms comes from a duodenal fluid aspirate or a small bowel biopsy. Recent serological tests and stool antigen studies for *Giardia* appear to be very promising. Amebic dysentery may be indistinguishable from the colitis of inflammatory bowel disease and must be ruled out along with bacterial colitis before a diagnosis of inflammatory bowel disease can be made. Diarrhea secondary to *Cryptosporidium* occurs in immunocompetent individuals but should be considered along with giardiasis in immunosuppressed patients.[40] *Blastocystis hominis* and *Dientamoeba fragilis* have both been considered potential causes of persistent diarrhea. *Candida* has been described as a rare cause of persistent diarrhea in immunocompetent individuals.[27] However, the incidental finding of *Candida* is so common that one must be cautious before identifying it as the cause of diarrhea. A dramatic response to treatment with oral nystatin would support this diagnosis.

Hirschsprung Disease. This congenital abnormality involving the submucosal and myenteric plexuses of the colon (rarely small intestine as well) accounts for about 25% of intestinal obstructions in newborns. Such neonates almost invariably fail to pass meconium and have persistent obstipation and recurrent abdominal distention. These features may be overlooked, however, and the infants subsequently may have chronic diarrhea. The diarrhea is secondary to enterocolitis, which can be a surgical emergency that demands rapid diagnosis and treatment. A barium enema in the neonate may reveal false negative findings; anorectal manometric examination may be helpful, but an adequate rectal biopsy specimen showing absence of ganglion cells will confirm the diagnosis. Properly performed, suction biopsy of the rectum is highly reliable.[3]

Food Intolerance. Dietary protein intolerance, especially cow milk intolerance, is a well-known entity in pediatric practice.[6] The frequently inappropriate use of this diagnosis to justify formula changes has made its actual incidence difficult to determine. More objective criteria for the diagnosis are being sought. The syndrome must be considered when an infant who has chronic diarrhea has any of the following manifestations: occult or gross blood in the stool (colitis), protein-losing enteropathy, peripheral eosinophilia, or other extraintestinal manifestations of allergy such as eczema, hives, or asthma. Continued manifestations when the infant is fed a soy formula diet (free of cow milk) do not rule out the diagnosis, inasmuch as 20% of patients intolerant to cow milk protein also will be intolerant to soy protein. Bloody diarrhea develops in some infants while nursing, which then resolves when they are given a protein hydrolysate formula.[32]

Some but not all of these infants respond to the reinstitution of nursing with the removal of dairy products from the mother's diet.

Short Bowel Syndrome. This syndrome of chronic malabsorption and diarrhea follows extensive resection of the small intestine.[17] Short bowel syndrome begins most commonly in the newborn period in association with necrotizing enterocolitis or a congenital anomaly of the small intestine (e.g., intestinal atresia, gastroschisis, or malrotation with secondary midgut volvulus). Recovery may be prolonged, requiring the use of TPN for the first several years of life. The factors that appear to contribute to this entity include a decrease in intestinal absorptive surface, altered intestinal motility, intraluminal bacterial overgrowth (with secondary deconjugation of bile salts and hydroxylation of fatty acids), malabsorption of bile salts secondary to terminal ileal resection, disaccharidase deficiency, and an increase in gastric acid secretion. Symptoms of colitis often are noted during the initiation of enteral feedings.[51]

Intestinal Lymphangiectasia. This syndrome of dilated intestinal lymphatic vessels is associated with protein-losing enteropathy, steatorrhea, lymphocytopenia, and chronic diarrhea.[55] As a result of the bowel protein loss, affected children may have hypogammaglobulinemia and hypoalbuminemia, usually with peripheral edema. Primary intestinal lymphangiectasia appears to be a developmental anomaly of unknown origin and frequently is associated with lymphatic abnormalities of the extremities. Secondary lymphangiectasia may result from chronic volvulus secondary to malrotation with malfixation of the bowel, constrictive pericarditis, tumor, malformation, or any other factor that leads to obstruction of intestinal lymphatic flow. The diagnosis is suggested by a history of chronic diarrhea and poor growth and the presence of peripheral edema, hypoalbuminemia, hypogammaglobulinemia, and lymphocytopenia. The latter two abnormalities may lead to a decreased immune defense and an increased risk for infections. A radiological small bowel follow-through study may show generalized thickening of the intestinal folds. The diagnosis is confirmed by the presence of characteristically dilated lymphatics on a small bowel biopsy specimen. The treatment includes the dietary use of medium-chain triglycerides and avoidance of long-chain fat. Protection from and early treatment of infection also are important.

Acrodermatitis Enteropathica. This rare familial disease of poorly understood etiology frequently appears when breast-fed infants are weaned.[37] Typically the infant has chronic diarrhea, intermittent vomiting, and an intractable erythematous, raw, crusty rash, which is most prominent in the perianal and perioral regions. The rash also may be seen on the extremities and responds poorly to local therapy. Alopecia characteristically is present, and conjunctivitis and dystrophic changes of the nails may occur. Infants who have acrodermatitis enteropathica usually are irritable and unhappy. Results of the small bowel biopsy have been described as normal, although this has been questioned. The response to therapy is dramatic, with a relapse occurring when treatment is discontinued. The earliest treatment was a breast-milk diet; subsequently, iodoquinol was used. Intravenous infusion of polyunsaturated fats has been associated with temporary improvement. However, the disorder is associated with a zinc deficiency (perhaps secondary to malabsorption) and responds dramatically to zinc salts given orally; this appears to be the treatment of choice.[38]

Factitious Diarrhea

Factitious diarrhea is more common than pediatricians prefer to recognize. It is reasonable to screen a stool specimen for laxative abuse in the case of an infant who has persistent diarrhea that does not seem to fit any known pattern. Inappropriate administration of laxative to an infant most likely is a symptom of the caretaker's psychosocial dysfunction; problems in other areas often become apparent during the social history. Parents who administer laxatives surreptitiously frequently are medically knowledgeable persons (e.g., nurse or laboratory technician background) and often seem to prefer staying in the hospital with their child rather than being at home. They tend to be very helpful to the nursing staff, often to the degree of excessive involvement in the nursing care, and commonly are described by the nurses as caring and concerned parents. The pediatrician may note that the parent seems to encourage invasive diagnostic studies and treatment even beyond the medical plan and does not show an appropriate degree of hesitancy.

Hormone-related Diarrhea. Several entities may be included in this group. Adrenal insufficiency secondary to either adrenogenital syndrome or adrenal hemorrhage may be associated with significant diarrhea, as may congenital thyrotoxicosis. Vasoactive intestinal polypeptide (VIP)-secreting tumors of the pancreas have been reported as a rare cause of diarrhea in adults and an even less common cause in children.

Ganglioneuroma, as well as the more malignant ganglioneuroblastoma, has been associated with chronic secretory diarrhea. The tumors usually are abdominal but also have been reported in the mediastinum. Although these are catecholamine-secreting tumors, prostaglandins or VIP may be the mediator of the diarrhea. A workup of the infant who has persistent diarrhea of unknown cause that clearly is secretory in nature should include urinary catecholamine studies, abdominal and chest roentgenograms, and an intravenous pyelogram. Even when the findings of these studies are negative, one must strongly consider a CT scan or arteriographic examination and surgical exploration if a severe secretory diarrhea persists. Knowing plasma prostaglandin and VIP levels may be useful. When a tumor is found and is completely excised, the diarrhea usually resolves abruptly.

Immune Disorders. Immunodeficiency should be considered in any child who has chronic diarrhea. AIDS has become a major cause of immunodeficiency in childhood and its first manifestation may be diarrhea. The two inborn disorders associated with diarrhea in early infancy are severe combined immunodeficiency (SCID) and Wiskott-Aldrich syndrome. The most common primary disorder seen in later childhood is late-onset, variable hypogammaglobulinemia. Pure T cell abnormalities (DiGeorge syndrome and other T cell deficiencies) also are associated with diarrhea. The incidence of celiac disease is increased among persons who have selected IgA deficiency; therefore measurement of immunoglobulin levels should be a routine part of the workup of any patient who has chronic diarrhea. If the diagnosis remains unclear, a T cell evaluation should be carried out. Chronic *Giar-*

dia or rotavirus infection can be seen with immunodeficiencies. Diarrhea in association with granulomas of the intestinal tract has been noted in chronic granulomatous disease of childhood. These children may have perianal fistulas; the disorder may be mistaken initially for Crohn disease.

A number of mechanisms of diarrhea have been described in infants and children who have AIDS. In addition to the organisms one usually considers in individuals who have persistent diarrhea (especially *Giardia*), one also must consider cytomegalovirus, *Mycobacterium avium-intracellulare, Cryptosporidium parvum, Isospora belli,* and *Enterocytozoon bieneusi. E. bieneusi* also has been associated with cholangitis in patients who have AIDS. Astrovirus, calicivirus, and adenovirus recently have been associated with diarrhea in HIV-infected individuals and may be more important than rotavirus as agents of AIDS diarrhea.[18] HIV may be a primary pathogen in the bowel of these patients as well. Lactose intolerance occurs commonly in individuals who have AIDS, presumably occurring secondary to injury to small bowel mucosa. Pancreatic insufficiency with steatorrhea also has been noted in these patients.

One must consider the range of enteric infections that occurs in immunosuppressed patients in children who have received organ transplants. Diarrhea may also be the presentation of FK-506 toxicity or of lymphoproliferative disease.

Idiopathic Intestinal Pseudoobstruction

Idiopathic intestinal pseudoobstruction constitutes a group of rare disorders characterized by widespread gastrointestinal dysmotility.[23] When this syndrome occurs in early infancy, vomiting and diarrhea often are major components. Diarrhea may alternate with constipation. In older children the presentation frequently is more insidious—a long history of constipation may precede the onset of diarrhea. Persons who have this syndrome usually have intermittent or constant abdominal distention. The syndrome is characterized by the roentgenographic findings of bowel dilation with disordered motility; urinary bladder dysfunction often is also present. These disorders can be sporadic or transmitted in an autosomal dominant fashion. They can result from a visceral myopathy or neuropathy or from a combination of both. Bacterial overgrowth is an important cause of diarrhea in this disorder.

Microvillus Inclusion Disease

Microvillus inclusion disease (familial enteropathy) is a disorder that occurs at birth and causes severe intractable secretory diarrhea with malabsorption.[10] These infants have small bowel villous atrophy and crypt hypoplasia. The villous surface epithelial cells lack a normal brush border, and on electron microscopic examination the microvilli are absent or severely abnormal. These defective cells contain intracytoplasmic inclusions, which in turn contain the components of the brush border, suggesting that the cells are either unable to assemble normal brush borders or that they rapidly dismantle them. There are reports of a number of families who have more than one child having this disorder. Microvillus inclusion disease, although rare, perhaps is the most common cause of intractable diarrhea in the newborn.

Congenital Chloride-Losing Diarrhea. This very rare, familial, persistent diarrhea results from congenital absence of the normal ileal mechanism for active absorption of chloride in exchange for bicarbonate. These infants have a chronic metabolic alkalosis instead of the metabolic acidosis usually seen in chronic diarrhea. Stool chloride concentration is high, usually exceeding the sum of concentrations of Na^+ and K^+. The stool chloride of children who have this disorder may be in the range of 100 to 150 mEq/L, although in infants it may be 30 to 100 mEq/L (normally adult stool chloride is less than 20 mEq/L). There is no satisfactory treatment. Support with oral fluids and potassium chloride is recommended.

Infant of a Drug-Addicted Mother. The syndrome of neonatal drug abstinence syndrome has become a more common problem, especially in urban areas. Diarrhea may be a prominent manifestation, and this diagnosis should be entertained in newborns who have persistent diarrhea, especially when other symptoms of neonatal drug withdrawal are present (see Chapter 49, Neonatal Drug Abstinence Syndrome).

Older Children

A pediatrician will see fewer older children who have chronic diarrhea than infants, but older children are more likely to have chronic diarrhea associated with significant underlying disease (as compared with toddler's diarrhea in young children). As in infancy, the association of poor growth, weight loss, or other systemic manifestations suggests a serious organic cause. There is a common tendency in older children to deny symptoms, and the true impact of the disorder may not be apparent except in retrospect after initiation of appropriate treatment. Subtle changes in personality, sense of well-being, and appetite, as well as other systemic clues, should be sought. Children may hesitate to talk about their stooling pattern, and the degree of deviation from the norm may become apparent only after improvement occurs.

The etiological focus differs somewhat after infancy. Many of the causes seen in infancy, even congenital anomalies, may manifest first in childhood and therefore must still be considered. Factors that determine the age at diagnosis include (1) the objective variation in presentation of signs and symptoms, (2) the parental expectations of normality, and (3) the index of suspicion of the physician consulted. However, certain diseases, including inflammatory bowel disease and chronic constipation with encopresis, are much more likely to be seen in childhood than in infancy. Celiac disease clearly may occur throughout life. Cystic fibrosis may be associated with only mild manifestations in infancy and may be overlooked until frequent, bulky, foul-smelling stools become intolerable at home. AIDS is seen in older children as well as in infants.

Irritable Bowel. Irritable bowel similar to that occurring in adults may be seen in older children and adolescents.[11] Stools may alternate from diarrhea to constipation. In addition, the patient may have recurrent, crampy, abdominal pain. It is important to rule out late-onset lactose intolerance and fructose or sorbitol ingestion as causes of symptoms that may mimic irritable bowel.

Inflammatory Bowel Disease (IBD). The manifestations and presentation of both Crohn disease and ulcerative colitis are so variable that this group of diseases must be thought of and ruled out whenever one sees an older child who has chronic diarrhea.[30] Systemic evidence of inflammation (fever, weight loss, and leukocytosis), abdominal pain, blood in the stool (gross or occult), perianal disease, anemia, or extraintestinal manifestations (arthralgia, arthritis, and erythema nodosum) are helpful in making a diagnosis. Growth failure can occur with or precede other symptoms. An elevated sedimentation rate also is a clue; however, normal sedimentation rates may occur in as many as 50% of patients who have IBD. Thrombocytosis has been associated with IBD and may be present in the absence of an elevated sedimentation rate. Suggestive signs and symptoms require evaluation, including a complete blood count, platelet count, erythrocyte sedimentation rate, serum protein levels, roentgenographic contrast studies of the upper or lower bowel (including good views of the terminal ileum), and sigmoidoscopic or colonoscopic examination with rectal biopsy. The absorptive function of the gastrointestinal tract should be quantitated if indicated.

Chronic Constipation. Occasionally, chronic constipation with overflow incontinence is mistaken for diarrhea. A thorough history and physical examination, including a rectal examination, should make the diagnosis apparent. If one goes back in the history, it is often found that the problem began with constipation. A large amount of stool may be palpable in the abdomen, but a hard mass of stool usually is found in the rectal ampulla. This presentation is treated in the usual fashion of chronic constipation (as noted in Chapter 117, Constipation).

REFERENCES

1. Alpert G et al: Outbreak of cryptosporidiosis in a day-care center, *Pediatrics* 77:152, 1986.
2. Ameen VZ, Powell GK, Jones LA: Quantitation of fecal carbohydrate excretion in patients with short bowel syndrome, *Gastroenterology* 92:493, 1987.
3. Andrassy RJ, Isaacs H, Weitzman JJ: Rectal suction biopsy for the diagnosis of Hirschsprung disease, *Ann Surg* 193:419, 1981.
4. Bartlett AV, Reves RR, Pickering LK: Rotavirus in infant-toddler day care centers: epidemiology relevant to disease control strategies, *J Pediatr* 113:435, 1988.
5. Bartlett AV et al: Diarrheal illness among infants and toddlers in day care centers. I. Epidemiology and pathogens, *J Pediatr* 107:495, 1985.
6. Bock SA: Prospective appraisal of complaints of adverse reactions to foods in children during the first 3 years of life, *Pediatrics* 79:683, 1987.
7. Burke JA: Giardiasis in childhood, *Am J Dis Child* 129:1304, 1975.
8. Buts JP et al: Pseudomembranous enterocolitis in childhood, *Gastroenterology* 73:823, 1977.
9. Cohen SA et al: Chronic nonspecific diarrhea: dietary relationships, *Pediatrics* 64:402, 1979.
10. Cutz E et al: Microvillus inclusion disease: an inherited defect of brush-border assembly and differentiation, *N Engl J Med* 320:646, 1989.
11. Drossman DA, Powell DW, Sessions JT: The irritable bowel syndrome, *Gastroenterology* 73:811, 1977.
12. Durie PR et al: Plasma immunoreactive pancreatic cationic trypsinogen in cystic fibrosis: a sensitive indicator of exocrine pancreatic dysfunction, *Pediatr Res* 15:1351, 1981.
13. Eherer AJ, Fordtran JS: Fecal osmotic gap and pH in experimental diarrhea of various causes, *Gastroenterology* 103:545, 1992.
14. Figueroa-Quintanilla D et al: A controlled trial of bismuth subsalicylate in infants with acute watery diarrheal disease, *N Engl J Med* 328:1653, 1993.
15. Glass RI et al: Estimates of morbidity and mortality rates for diarrheal diseases in American children, *J Pediatr* 118:S27, 1991.
16. Goldgar CM, Vanderhoof JA: Lack of correlation of small bowel biopsy and clinical course of patients with intractable diarrhea of infancy, *Gastroenterology* 90:527, 1986.
17. Goulet OJ et al: Neonatal short bowel syndrome, *J Pediatr* 119:18, 1991.
18. Grohmann GS et al: Enteric viruses and diarrhea in HIV-infected patients, *N Engl J Med* 329:14, 1993.
19. Hill RE et al: Steatorrhea and pancreatic insufficiency in Shwachman syndrome, *Gastroenterology* 83:22, 1982.
20. Holmberg C et al: Congenital chloride diarrhea, *Arch Dis Child* 52:255, 1977.
21. Hyams JS: Sorbitol malabsorption: an unappreciated cause of functional gastrointestinal complaints, *Gastroenterology* 84:30, 1983.
22. Hyams JS et al: Carbohydrate malabsorption following fruit juice ingestion in young children, *Pediatrics* 82:64, 1988.
23. Hyman PE et al: Antroduodenal motility in children with chronic intestinal pseudo-obstruction, *J Pediatr* 112:899, 1988.
24. Infectious Diseases Committee, Canadian Paediatric Society: *Escherichia coli* gastroenteritis: making sense of the new acronyms, *Can Med Assoc J* 136:241, 1987.
25. Izraeli S et al: Transient renal acidification defect during acute infantile diarrhea: the role of urinary sodium, *J Pediatr* 117:711, 1990.
26. Jonas A et al: Disturbed fat absorption following infectious gastroenteritis in children, *J Pediatr* 95:366, 1979.
27. Kaupuscinska A et al: Disease specificity and dynamics of changes in IgA class antiendomysial antibodies in celiac disease, *J Pediatr Gastroenterol Nutr* 6:529, 1987.
28. Kerzner B et al: Transmissible gastroenteritis: sodium transport and the intestinal epithelium during the course of viral enteritis, *Gastroenterology* 72:457, 1977.
29. Kirschner BS: Inflammatory bowel disease in children, *Pediatr Clin North Am* 35:189, 1988.
30. Klish WJ et al: Modular formula: an approach to management of infants with specific or complex food intolerances, *J Pediatr* 88:948, 1976.
31. Kane JG, Chretien JH, Garagusi VF: Diarrhea caused by *Candida*, *Lancet* 1:335, 1976.
32. Lake AM, Whitington PF, Hamilton SR: Dietary protein-induced colitis in breast-fed infants, *J Pediatr* 101:906, 1982.
33. Larcher VF et al: Protracted diarrhea in infancy, *Arch Dis Child* 52:597, 1977.
34. Lebenthal E, Branski D: Childhood celiac disease—a reappraisal, *J Pediatr* 98:681, 1981.
35. Lifshitz F et al: Role of juice carbohydrate malabsorption in chronic nonspecific diarrhea in children, *J Pediatr* 120:825, 1992.
36. Mitchel DK et al: Outbreaks of astrovirus gastroenteritis in day care center, *J Pediatr* 123:725, 1993.
37. Moynahan EJ: Acrodermatitis enteropathica: a lethal inherited human zinc-deficiency disorder, *Lancet* 2:399, 1974.
38. Neldner KH, Hambridge KM: Zinc therapy of acrodermatitis enteropathica, *N Engl J Med* 292:879, 1975.
39. Orenstein SR: Enteral versus parenteral therapy for intractable diarrhea of infancy: prospective, randomized trial, *J Pediatr* 109:277, 1986.
40. Phillips AD, Thomas AG, Walker-Smith JA: Cryptosporidium, chronic diarrhoea and the proximal small intestinal mucosa, *Gut* 33:1057, 1992.
41. Phillips SF: Diarrhea: a current view of the pathophysiology, *Gastroenterology* 63:495, 1972.
42. Pizarro D et al: Oral rehydration in hypernatremic and hyponatremic diarrheal dehydration, *Am J Dis Child* 137:730, 1983.
43. Portnoy BL et al: Antidiarrheal agents in the treatment of acute diarrhea in children, *JAMA* 236:844, 1976.
44. Ravich WJ, Bayless TM, Thomas M: Fructose: incomplete intestinal absorption in humans, *Gastroenterology* 84:26, 1983.
45. Rossi TM, Albini CH, Kumar V: Incidence of celiac disease identified by the presence of serum endomysial antibodies in children with chronic diarrhea, short stature, or insulin-dependent diabetes mellitus, *J Pediatr* 123:262, 1993.
46. Santosham M et al: Oral rehydration therapy of infantile diarrhea: a controlled study of well-nourished children hospitalized in the United States and Panama, *N Engl J Med* 306:1070, 1982.
47. Schwarz RP, Ulshen MH: Pseudomembranous colitis presenting as mild, chronic diarrhea in childhood, *J Pediatr Gastroenterol Nutr* 2:570, 1983.
48. Steinhoff MC: Rotavirus: the first five years, *J Pediatr* 96:611, 1980.
49. Sutphen JL et al: Chronic diarrhea associated with *Clostridium difficile* in children, *Am J Dis Child* 137:275, 1983.

50. Tamer AM et al: Oral rehydration of infants in a large urban U.S. medical center, *J Pediatr* 107:14, 1985.
51. Taylor SF et al: Noninfectious colitis associated with short gut syndrome in infants, *J Pediatr* 119:24, 1991.
52. Tucker NT et al: Antigliadin antibodies detected by enzyme-linked immunosorbent assay as a marker of childhood celiac disease, *J Pediatr* 113:286, 1988.
53. Ulshen MH: Carbohydrate absorption and malabsorption. In Walker WA, Watkins JB, editors: *Nutrition in pediatrics—basic sciences and clinical applications,* Boston, 1985, Little, Brown.
54. Ulshen MH, Rollo RL: Pathogenesis of *Escherichia coli* gastroenteritis in man—another mechanism, *N Engl J Med* 302:99, 1980.
55. Vardy PA, Lebenthal E, Shwachman H: Intestinal lymphangiectasia: a reappraisal, *Pediatrics* 55:842, 1975.
56. Wolfe DC, Giannella RA: Antibiotic therapy for bacterial enterocolitis: a comprehensive review, *Am J Gastroenterol* 88:1667, 1993.
57. Wolfen JS et al: Cryptosporidiosis in immuno-competent patients, *N Engl J Med* 312:1278, 1985.
58. Yolken RH et al: Gastroenteritis associated with enteric type adenovirus in hospitalized infants, *J Pediatr* 101:21, 1982.

SUGGESTED READINGS

Bishop WP, Ulshen MH: Bacterial gastroenteritis, *Pediatr Clin North Am* 35:69, 1988.

Esteban MM: Adverse reactions to foods in infancy and childhood, *J Pediatr* 121:S1, 1992.

Ghishan FK: The transport of electrolytes in the gut and the use of oral rehydration solutions, *Pediatr Clin North Am* 35:35, 1988.

Lifshitz F: Management of acute diarrheal disease, *J Pediatr* 118:S25, 1991.

Seidman E et al: Nutritional issues in pediatric inflammatory bowel disease, *J Pediatric Gastroenterol Nutr* 12:424, 1991.

Targan SR, Shanahan F, editors: *Inflammatory bowel disease: from bench to bedside,* Baltimore, 1994, Williams & Wilkins.

121 Dizziness and Vertigo

Diane L. McDonald

Dizziness as described by adults is a disturbance in one's sense of relationship to the surrounding environment, characterized by feelings of unsteadiness, of random movement within the head, of total loss of concentration and awareness of ongoing activity, and of lightheadedness or confusion.

Dizziness can be difficult for children to describe; it is a vague term that can represent a variety of symptoms. Lightheadedness often is associated with high fever or the ingestion of medications (e.g., antihistamines or decongestants), or it may occur as a presyncopal event. Visual distortion, disequilibrium, and vertigo also can accompany dizziness. Differentiating among the various symptoms will help establish the diagnosis.

The ability to maintain balance depends on the interconnections of the visual, sensory, proprioceptive, and vestibular systems. Dysfunction in any of these can produce a sense of imbalance, or "dizziness." For example, a visual disturbance such as diplopia may not be recognized as such by a child. Instead, the child may appear to have difficulty walking or may seem confused. Cerebellar dysfunction, associated with ataxia, also can be perceived as dizziness by both the child and the parents. Dizziness experienced as vertigo makes one feel as if one is in motion when stationary. In the nonverbal child this may appear to be clumsiness and, in some cases, may result in expressions of fear or in vomiting. A thorough history should be obtained of the present illness, of past and family illnesses, and of possible drug use. A complete physical examination with special attention to the neurological, cardiac, and otological systems assists in establishing the diagnosis.

DIFFERENTIAL DIAGNOSIS

Children who complain of *lightheadedness* may be experiencing decreased cerebral perfusion, hypoxia, or hypoglycemia. This may be a presyncopal event. Also, upper respiratory tract infections (or "the flu") may make the child feel somewhat lightheaded.

Impaired vision or *diplopia* may be interpreted as dizziness. Refractive errors or tumors involving the optic chiasm (e.g., optic gliomas or craniopharyngiomas) alter vision. Double vision can occur as a result of trauma or a sixth nerve palsy. When problems of this magnitude are suspected, referral to an ophthalmologist or neurologist most often is necessary.

The symptom and sign of *unsteadiness* or *disequilibrium* can indicate the initial presentation of a pathological condition of the cerebellum—for example, a posterior fossa tumor, such as an astrocytoma or a medulloblastoma. Acute cerebellar ataxia can follow a viral illness—for example, varicella or mycoplasma infection. Ataxia also may be caused by drug intoxication, trauma, or an inherited disease, such as Friedreich ataxia.

Vertigo is the sensation of spinning or whirling within one's environment or of the environment doing the spinning or whirling. It may be caused by dysfunction in the vestibular system or of the eighth cranial nerve. The evaluation of vertigo therefore should include a thorough examination of the central nervous system and of the ear. Consultation with a neurological or otological specialist usually is required. Vertigo may be acute, recurrent, or persistent.

Acute vertigo can be caused by middle or inner ear infections. A middle ear effusion may transmit pressure to the inner ear, leading to a sense of imbalance or vertigo. Chronic otitis media can result in labyrinthitis or mastoiditis and, with severe protracted infections, is associated with cholesteatoma formation. In this event the labyrinth may be seriously damaged, even destroyed. A viral labyrinthitis, vestibular neuronitis, frequently is associated with an upper respiratory tract infection or otitis media. The symptoms of vertigo in this situation last 2 to 3 weeks and usually resolve spontaneously.

Trauma and toxic ingestions also must be included in the differential diagnosis of acute vertigo. Salicylate or alcohol ingestion can cause the sudden onset of vertigo. Ototoxic drugs (e.g., streptomycin and gentamicin) slowly damage the inner ear, and vertigo (and deafness) may result.

Recurrent vertigo is characterized by episodes that usually last less than 30 minutes and can be associated with *basilar artery migraine* or *temporal lobe epilepsy*. A *brainstem glioma* or an *acoustic neuroma* can affect the eighth cranial nerve, causing recurrent vertigo. Trauma that results in a fracture through the temporal bone, hemorrhage into the middle ear, or a perilymph fistula often leads to recurrent vertigo. Although *benign paroxysmal vertigo* is an entity of unknown cause, it may be associated with migraines. It affects children between the ages of 1 and 3 years. Attacks occur in clusters, with symptoms of crying and vomiting and signs of pallor and nystagmus. Although these attacks may occur over a period of months or even years, this disease is self-limited (see Chapter 155, Nonconvulsive Periodic Disorders, for further discussion of benign paroxysmal vertigo). *Meniere disease* is caused by increased endolymphatic pressure in the inner ear and may result in recurrent vertigo. Dizziness may be the presenting symptom of the demyelinating disease, multiple sclerosis. Congenital syphilis can cause a labyrinthitis.

Chronic persistent vertigo is characterized by episodes of vertigo, each lasting as long as 1 week. Structural lesions—for example, brainstem glioma or acoustic neuroma or a variety of demyelinating diseases—must be considered. A computed tomography (CT) scan, magnetic resonance imaging (MRI), or an electronystagmogram may help establish the diagnosis. Psychogenic causes such as hysteria or malingering should be considered if the findings are inconsistent with an organic cause.

MANAGEMENT

The approach to the patient who is experiencing dizziness depends on the diagnosis. Dizziness that occurs as a presyncopal event is discussed in the section on syncope. To determine if refractive error or a visual disturbance is the cause, a vision test and funduscopic examination are needed. Differentiating between cerebellar and vestibular pathology can be difficult. Ataxia and a positive Romberg test reaction commonly are seen with both. However, difficulty in performing rapid alternating movements and an intention tremor suggest a cerebellar abnormality and should prompt a CT scan or an MRI study. Consultation with a neurologist is indicated.

Dizziness associated with the sensation of motion—vertigo—frequently has a benign origin. Special attention should be given to the otological and neurological examination. The otological evaluation should include tympanometry or pneumatic bulb otoscopy examination and also a hearing test. If a middle ear effusion is noted, antibiotic therapy may be indicated. If the symptoms persist, referral to an otolaryngologist for a possible myringotomy and tube placement is advised. Other pathological conditions of the middle ear, such as a cholesteatoma, warrant similar referral for possible surgical exploration and excision.

The neurological examination should assist in differentiating vestibular disease from other central nervous system causes. If there is evidence of neurological dysfunction, a CT scan and neurology consultation are advised. Recurrent or persistent episodes of vertigo or vertigo *preceding* trauma also require a referral. An electroencephalogram should be obtained if vertigo is associated with a loss of consciousness or with seizure activity.

The Nylen-Bárány test is used to provoke nystagmus. It may help to distinguish a peripheral from a central vestibular lesion. This test is performed with the child seated on an examination table. From the sitting position the child's head and trunk are lowered backward quickly so that the head is dropped 45 degrees below the edge of the table. Then it is turned 45 degrees to one side. The entire test is repeated, turning the child's head 45 degrees in the other direction. Inner ear lesions will result in nystagmus appearing after a short (20 second) delay, with the rapid phase in the same direction regardless of the direction of gaze. With central lesions the onset of nystagmus is immediate and the direction of the nystagmus changes with gaze. Electronystagmographic examination is a more specific but less frequently used procedure to locate the vestibular lesion. Finally, if the otological and neurological examinations are unrevealing and the episode is of acute onset, the most common cause is vestibular neuronitis. These children may be treated symptomatically and if necessary reevaluated frequently. Meclizine (Antivert), 25 mg every 4 to 6 hours for children older than 12 years of age, may provide symptomatic relief.

SUGGESTED READINGS

Busis SN: Dizziness in children, *Pediatr Ann* 17:648, 1988.

Dunn DW: Dizziness: when is it vertigo? *Contemp Pediatr* 4:67, 1987.

Eviatar L: Dizziness in children, *Otolaryngol Clin North Am* 27:557, 1994.

Farmer TW: *Pediatric neurology,* Philadelphia, 1983, Harper & Row.

Neuro
Ophth
ENT

122 Dysmenorrhea

Alain Joffe

Dysmenorrhea, generally meaning painful menstruation, is a syndrome associated with varying degrees of crampy lower abdominal pain and other symptoms such as nausea, vomiting, urinary frequency, low back pain, diarrhea, fatigue, and headache. The pain may radiate to the anterior thighs. These symptoms may last from 1 to 3 days.[8] The prevalence of this syndrome is not established, but the majority of surveys indicate that at least 40% to 60% of adolescent girls suffer some degree of discomfort during menstruation, and many miss school as a result. Most affected teenage girls have primary dysmenorrhea, that is, a syndrome not associated with pelvic pathological conditions; however, before this diagnosis can be made, causes of secondary dysmenorrhea should be excluded. The physician also should ensure that the pain described is not indicative of premenstrual tension syndrome, characterized by irritability, fluid retention, edema, and a sensation of bloating, which occurs in the week before menstruation.

SECONDARY DYSMENORRHEA

The causes of secondary dysmenorrhea—such as pelvic inflammatory disease (PID) or endometriosis—usually can be excluded by a history and physical examination. Organic pathological conditions should be suspected in a woman whose pain begins after 20 years of age, who has a history of surgery related to the genitourinary or gastrointestinal tract, or whose pain is dull and constant rather than crampy.[6] Endometriosis and PID generally are characterized by pain that begins 2 or 3 days before menstruation and often is relieved by the onset of menses. Endometriosis may be associated with dyspareunia, tenesmus, and rectal pain.

Endometrial polyps or fibroids are rare in women younger than 20 years of age but should be suspected if the menstrual bleeding is heavy or prolonged or associated with the passage of clots. Whether these entities alone cause dysmenorrhea is unclear. Teenagers who have a history of genital tract surgery (including abortions) may have outflow tract obstruction.

A pelvic examination that reveals cervical motion tenderness, adnexal masses, or fixation of the ovaries strongly suggests PID. If the cervical os is stenotic or the cervix or uterus feels atretic or abnormally shaped, outflow obstruction is possible (e.g., uterus with a "blind" horn). Small fixed nodules in the rectovaginal septum or cul de sac, fixation or enlargement of the ovaries, or fixation of the uterus indicated by the sensation of pain on stretching of the uterosacral ligaments suggests endometriosis.[11] However, endometriosis can be extremely difficult to detect on clinical grounds alone.

If a secondary cause of dysmenorrhea is suspected, consultation with an adolescent medicine specialist or a gynecologist is warranted. Pelvic inflammatory disease should be treated according to standard antibiotic regimens (see Chapter 258, Sexually Transmitted Diseases). Follow-up is critical because these young women are at risk for further episodes of PID as well as for chronic pelvic pain, ectopic pregnancy, and infertility.

Confirmation of endometriosis or other causes of secondary dysmenorrhea may require laparoscopy. Endometriosis may be difficult to manage, and women with this condition are at increased risk for infertility.

PRIMARY DYSMENORRHEA[5,14]

Although psychosocial and cultural factors may play some role in the pathogenesis of primary dysmenorrhea,[4,10,11] the preponderance of current research indicates that this symptom complex is caused largely by increased amounts of prostaglandins E_2 and $F_{2\alpha}$ in the endometrium of women who have dysmenorrhea as compared with women who do not have painful menses.[1,13] Such a biological explanation correlates with clinical observation: women who have anovulatory cycles usually do not have dysmenorrhea. The incidence of dysmenorrhea increases with chronological and gynecological age (as does the percentage of ovulatory cycles), and the increase in prostaglandin synthesis may be related to changes in serum progesterone levels not seen in anovulatory women. Additional confirmation comes from the dramatic response women experience with the use of either prostaglandin synthetase inhibitors or oral contraceptives (which inhibit ovulation). The increased levels of prostaglandin activity produce myometrial contractions and ischemia, both of which result in pain.

A careful history usually excludes most pathological causes of dysmenorrhea. Physicians differ in their opinions regarding what examination is necessary to evaluate the patient who has true dysmenorrhea. Some contend that for a teenager who has mild to moderate menstrual cramps relieved by nonsteroidal antiinflammatory drugs (NSAIDs), only an external genital examination to rule out hymenal abnormalities is indicated. For any sexually active teenager or for one who is having significant pain unresponsive to NSAIDs, a thorough pelvic examination is necessary. When a vaginal examination is not possible (which should be rare if the patient is prepared properly), a rectoabdominal examination usually can exclude pelvic disease.

Although treatment of primary dysmenorrhea is likely to include drug therapy, other considerations are pertinent. To what extent is the pain interfering with the patient's activity? Is she missing school, and if so, how often? Does she miss valued activities because the pain and nausea prevent her from participating? The physician also should determine what the mother and daughter's understanding of menstruation is; many teenagers do not understand the physiology of

etry is required to establish the diagnosis of scleroderma. It is important to note that gastroesophageal reflux cannot be diagnosed by manometry or by measuring LES pressure.

Esophagoscopy

Flexible fiberoptic esophagoscopy can be performed on children on an ambulatory basis. Inspection, biopsy, and photography of suspected lesions can be performed rapidly and safely.

CAUSES AND MANAGEMENT OF DYSPHAGIA

The many causes of dysphagia are listed in the box below.

Oral-Pharyngeal Dysphagia

Dysphagia in children most commonly occurs secondary to central nervous system (CNS) injury or disease. The primary disorder usually is brain injury, cerebral palsy, or a neurodegenerative disorder. Treatment, particularly when dysphagia is associated with aspiration, involves inserting a gastrostomy tube and avoiding oral feeding.

CAUSES OF DYSPHAGIA

Structural-mechanical disorders

- Esophageal atresia
- Esophageal web
- Foreign bodies
- Hiatal hernia
- Paraesophageal hernia
- Stricture
  - Caustic
  - Congenital
  - Inflammatory
- Tumor
- Vascular ring

Motor disorders

- Achalasia
- Diffuse spasm
- Gastrointestinal reflux
- Scleroderma

Neuromuscular disorders

- Acquired central nervous system disease
  - Tumor
  - Infection
  - Trauma
- Cerebral palsy
- Dysautonomia
- Muscular dystrophy
- Myasthenia gravis

Inflammatory disorders

- *Candida albicans* infection
- Cytomegalovirus infection
- Epidermolysis bullosa
- Esophagitis
- Herpes simplex infection
- Ingestion of a caustic substance

Structural-Mechanical Disorders of the Esophagus

Congenital strictures and esophageal webs, usually in the proximal esophagus, are uncommon and may be difficult to detect on a roentgenogram. Typically the patient can point to the level of the obstruction. Esophageal foreign bodies are common in children and easily removed.[2] A hiatal hernia (Fig. 123-1) may be associated with gastroesophageal reflux and esophagitis, which are the true causes of the dysphagia and odynophagia. Hiatal hernias usually are asymptomatic. Peptic strictures resulting from symptomatic or asymptomatic gastroesophageal reflux cause dysphagia by obstructing the esophageal lumen (Fig. 123-2). Dysphagia typically is greater for solids than liquids. The diagnosis of peptic stricture is readily made roentgenographically. The stricture is treated with dilation, but the underlying reflux also must be treated. Even after esophageal atresia is repaired, swallowing problems usually persist.[16] Peristalsis nearly always is abnormal, and symptomatic gastroesophageal reflux with or without esophagitis is found nearly universally. Anastomotic strictures may occur. Esophageal tumors are rare in children. In rare cases mediastinal tumors may cause esophageal obstruction. Although vascular rings are not rare, mechanical obstruction of the esophagus by an aberrant vessel is extremely rare.[8]

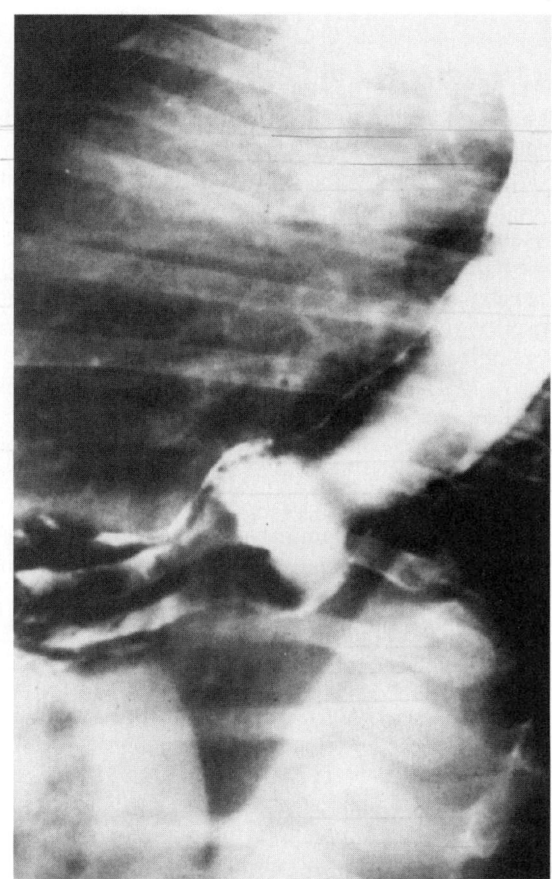

FIG. 123-1 A clearly defined small hiatal hernia.

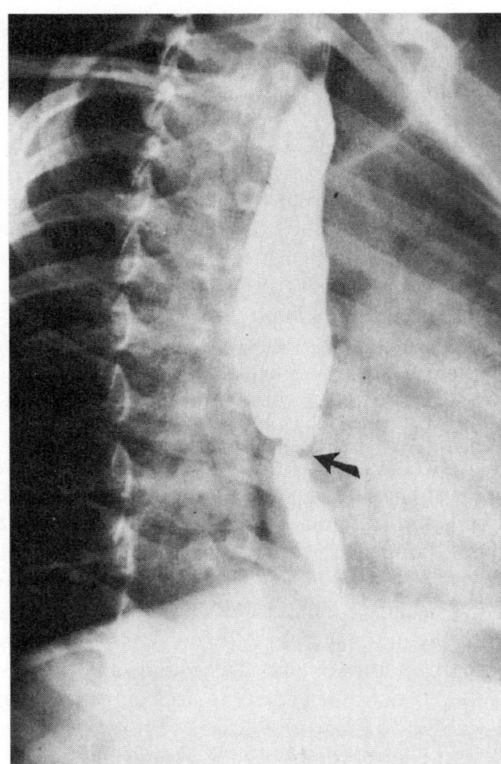

FIG. 123-2 Peptic esophagitis with stricture. Dilation is seen proximal to the tight stricture *(arrow).* Note the irregularity of the distal esophageal mucosa.

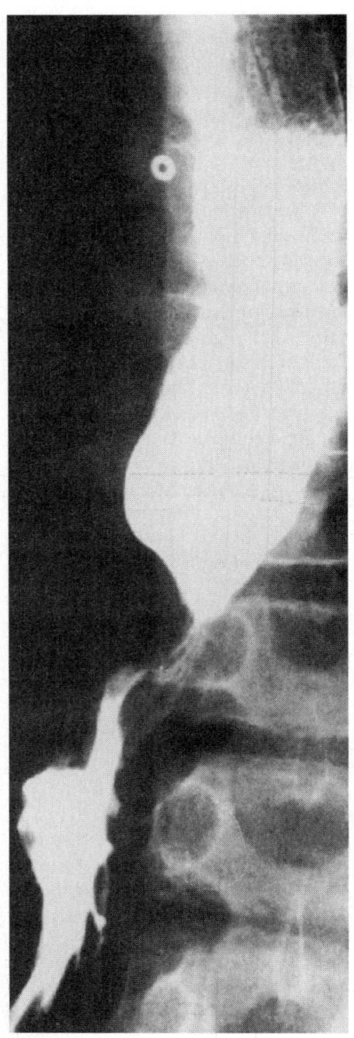

FIG. 123-3 Classic appearance of achalasia of the esophagus. The dilated esophagus ends in a narrow segment.

Motor Disorders of the Esophagus

Achalasia, a rare cause of functional obstruction of the distal esophagus, occurs when the LES fails to relax and the peristaltic wave does not propagate.[3,9] Its prevalence is about 1:100,000; 10% of cases arise during childhood. It is functionally and pathologically similar to Hirschsprung disease; in both conditions the distal myenteric ganglion cells are absent, causing functional obstruction and proximal dilation. The onset of dysphagia usually is gradual but progressive, until weight loss and aspiration occur in neglected cases. The symptoms often are surprisingly mild. Intermittent substernal pain also may be present.

A characteristic J-shaped megaesophagus, with a tapered distal beak, is seen on a barium swallow examination (Fig. 123-3). Peristalsis is absent, but sporadic aperistaltic contractions may be seen. Intraluminal manometry documents the absence of peristalsis, as well as high resting pressure in the LES and failure of the sphincter to relax after a swallow. The esophagus responds to an intramuscular injection of methacholine with spastic, high-pressure contractions conforming to Cannon's law of denervation hypersensitivity. This test can be quite painful and is not recommended for routine use. In achalasia, cholecystokinin paradoxically increases LES pressure.

Although medical therapy with the calcium channel blocker nifedipine may relieve symptoms in some patients, the current treatments of choice are pneumatic dilation and surgical myotomy, which successfully relieve the symptoms in nearly all patients.[3,9] Pneumatic dilation may need to be repeated. The long-term outlook is good, although there may be an increased risk of carcinoma of the esophagus in late adulthood.

Diffuse esophageal spasm is even less common than achalasia. Both dysphagia and pain are present.[15] Symptoms typically wax and wane, often with long symptom-free intervals. Cold beverages frequently exacerbate symptoms (this is seen readily on manometry.) The spastic contractions may be seen with a barium swallow. Medical therapy with nitroglycerin occasionally is successful. Otherwise, either pneumatic dilation or surgical myotomy is necessary; neither approach is totally satisfactory.

Dysphagia may be the presenting symptom in a small but significant number of patients who have scleroderma. Roentgenographic or manometric examination may show aperistalsis in the distal esophagus. A manometric study can be used to confirm a suspected diagnosis of scleroderma.

Gastroesophageal reflux may be associated with esophagitis, disordered peristalsis, and dysphagia. Dysphagia resolves when the esophagitis is treated.

Inflammatory Disorders

It now is recognized that normal function of the LES is the crucial factor in preventing reflux of gastric contents.[7] If the LES responds normally to swallowing and is otherwise intact, reflux esophagitis does not occur.

The presence of a hiatal hernia, demonstrated by roentgenographic studies, is not an indication for surgical repair. Rather, appropriate diagnostic studies as described above should be instituted. There has been a great deal of confusion about which patients who have reflux should have surgery. On the basis of current knowledge, it can be stated without hesitation that more than 85% of neurologically intact children referred for evaluation of reflux will respond to medical therapy. In the past children who had neurological disorders have required surgical therapy more often than neurologically intact children. This may change with the availability of the proton pump inhibitor omeprazole and the prokinetic agent cisapride.

Gastroesophageal reflux can be demonstrated in many normal infants. Normally, reflux and benign regurgitation disappear by the age of 9 to 18 months. Infants who regurgitate chronically should be observed closely and, if symptomatic, evaluated for esophagitis. Esophageal inflammation and even stricture may occur in the absence of symptoms.

Although the diagnosis of gastroesophageal reflux may be confirmed by a barium swallow study, radiographic studies may not document reflux in as many as 40% of children (even in patients who have known esophagitis) because of the intermittent nature of symptoms and the brief period of fluoroscopic observation. Esophagitis usually is not seen roentgenographically. Although intraluminal esophageal pH recording and scintigraphic techniques can assist the physician in making the diagnosis of reflux, only esophagoscopy and biopsy can document the presence of esophagitis definitively.[15] A complete blood count and serum ferritin and stool guaiac determinations are useful in documenting bleeding from an inflamed esophagus. A chest roentgenogram may be obtained because chronic reflux has been implicated as a cause of recurrent aspiration pneumonia and chronic obstructive pulmonary disease.

Although esophagitis is considered uncommon in children, pediatricians are recognizing an increasing number of patients who have the classic symptoms of heartburn, foul taste in the mouth, bad breath, and vomiting.[14,15] Symptoms increase when the patient reclines. Infants may only regurgitate, although this finding, accompanied by failure to thrive and irritability, often is an indication of esophagitis.[4]

An important factor in the development of esophagitis is the rate at which refluxed material is cleared from the esophagus. In patients who have esophagitis, the normal stripping action of the lower esophagus is impaired, and the distal esophagus remains acidic longer after reflux than in normal patients.

Although a recent study suggests that the prone position may be more effective in infants, traditional medical therapy consists of using the upright position and feedings thickened with cereal.[12] Bethanechol and metoclopramide have been beneficial in the treatment of infants; cisapride (0.2 to 0.4 mg/kg four times a day) is superior to both.[5] H_2-blockers must be administered when esophagitis is documented. In neurologically normal children surgery rarely is needed for medical failure or stricture formation.

Inflammatory lesions of the esophagus are particularly common in association with infection by *Candida albicans*, cytomegalovirus, and herpes simplex virus. Although these agents may appear spontaneously, most pediatric patients are immunosuppressed. The roentgenographic appearance of *C. albicans* and herpes may be suggestive in the appropriate clinical setting, but the roentgenographic appearance may not be typical, and endoscopy and biopsy usually are required. The possibility of an infectious agent is not always considered in the uncompromised host.

Although not truly esophagitis, the esophageal lesions that occur in cases of epidermolysis bullosa may be recognized roentgenographically.

The most effective medical treatment for esophagitis involves avoiding foods that reduce LES pressure (e.g., coffee, alcohol, and fatty foods) and elevating the head of the bed at least 8 inches.[15] Anticholinergic drugs, which reduce LES pressure, should be avoided. Cisapride diminishes both reflux and symptoms. H_2-blockers may need to be given at higher doses than required for ulcer healing. Omeprazole is even more effective in healing esophagitis than are H_2-blockers and may be successful if the latter fail.[10] Surgery is indicated only for intractable symptoms and stricture development.

When infection by *C. albicans* is documented, the therapy just described should be supplemented by the appropriate dosage of nystatin or ketoconazole. Amphotericin B frequently is required. Herpes esophagitis is treated with acyclovir. Cytomegalovirus esophagitis may be treated with ganciclovir.

Ingestion of caustic agents, especially liquid alkali, causes intense pain and dysphagia.[13] Symptoms commonly resolve after 3 or 4 days, but stricture formation associated with return of dysphagia may follow after 3 to 8 weeks. Early esophagoscopy, preferably 12 to 24 hours after the caustic ingestion, is essential to establish the extent and degree of the burn. If the burn is limited to the mouth, no therapy is necessary. The most recent literature suggests that steroids do not reduce stricture formation.[1] Strictures are treated by bougienage. Esophagectomy and colon interposition rarely are necessary.

REFERENCES

1. Anderson KD, Rouse TM, Randolph JG: A controlled trial of corticosteroids in children with corrosive injury of the esophagus, *N Engl J Med* 323:637, 1990.
2. Berggreen PJ et al: Techniques and complications of esophageal foreign body extraction in children and adults, *Gastrointest Endosc* 39:626, 1993.
3. Berquist WE et al: Achalasia: diagnosis, management, and clinical course in 16 children, *Pediatrics* 71:798, 1983.
4. Catto-Smith AG et al: The role of gastroesophageal reflux in pediatric dysphagia, *J Pediatr Gastroenterol Nutr* 12:159, 1991.
5. Cucchiara A et al: Cisapride for gastrooesophageal reflux and peptic oesophagitis, *Arch Dis Child* 62:454, 1987.
6. Dodds WJ: Instrumentation and methods for intraluminal esophageal manometry, *Arch Intern Med* 136:515, 1976.
7. Dodds WJ et al: Pathogenesis of reflux esophagitis, *Gastroenterology* 81:376, 1981.

8. Eklof O et al: Arterial anomalies causing compression of the trachea and/or oesophagus, *Acta Paediatr Scand* 60:81, 1971.
9. Emblem R et al: Current results of surgery for achalasia of the cardia, *Arch Dis Child* 68:749, 1993.
10. Gunasekaran T, Hassall EG: Efficacy and safety of omeprazole for severe gastroesophageal reflux in children, *J Pediatr* 123:148, 1993.
11. Leonidas JC: Gastroesophageal reflux in infants: role of the upper gastrointestinal series, *Am J Roentgenol* 143:1350, 1984.
12. Orenstein SR, Whittington PF, Orenstein DM: The infant seat as treatment for gastroesophageal reflux, *N Engl J Med* 29:760, 1983.
13. Previtera C, Giusti F, Guglielmi M: Predictive value of visible lesions (cheeks, lips, oropharynx) in suspected caustic ingestion: may endoscopy reasonably be omitted in completely negative pediatric patients? *Pediatr Emerg Care* 6:176, 1990.
14. Richter JE: Heartburn, dysphagia and other esophageal symptoms. In Sleisenger MH, Fordtran JS, editors: *Gastrointestinal disease,* ed 5, Philadelphia, 1993, WB Saunders.
15. Vandenplas Y et al: A proposition for the diagnosis and treatment of gastrooesophageal reflux disease in children: a report from a working group on gastrooesophageal reflux disease, *Eur J Pediatr* 152:704, 1993.
16. Werlin SL et al: Mechanisms of gastroesophageal reflux in children, *J Pediatr* 97:244, 1980.
17. Werlin SL et al: Esophageal function in esophageal atresia, *Dig Dis Sci* 26:796, 1981.

124 Dyspnea

Jay H. Mayefsky

Dyspnea is the uncomfortable feeling of not being able to satisfy "air hunger"; patients may complain of not being able to catch their breath or of a suffocating feeling. Dyspnea is a symptom, a subjective complaint by the patient, that describes the sensation caused by an underlying disorder. As with any subjective complaint, the diagnosis of dyspnea and its cause in an infant or young child can be problematical. Therefore, to evaluate fully a child in respiratory distress, the pediatric health care provider must be familiar with the pathophysiology, signs, and common causes of dyspnea. With the aid of the medical history, physical examination, and appropriate laboratory tests, the proper diagnosis can be made and therapy initiated.

PATHOPHYSIOLOGY

Dyspnea is most commonly seen with exercise. In this instance the increased work of breathing necessary to keep up with the body's increased metabolic demands causes the dyspnea.[10] The sensation probably is transmitted from stretch receptors in the chest wall muscles to the central nervous system (CNS). Chemoreceptors, sensing changes in arterial pH, oxygen, and carbon dioxide concentrations, as well as chest wall proprioceptors, lung stretch receptors, and mechanoreceptors in the heart and skeletal muscles, also may play a role.[2,12,28] The transmission is processed in the CNS, and the individual experiences the sensation of dyspnea. In the example of exercise, the person who has dyspnea is aware of an increased ventilatory effort. A person who has obstructive or restrictive lung disease also experiences difficulty breathing. A person who has neuromuscular disease feels that he or she is not getting enough air.

To satisfy their oxygen needs, children who have dyspnea must either increase their minute ventilation ($\dot{V}_E$) or must work harder than normal to maintain their usual $\dot{V}_E$. Minute ventilation, the product of tidal volume and frequency of respirations per minute ($\dot{V}_E = V_T \times f$), is helpful in diagnosing dyspnea and its causes. In normal breathing, respiratory muscles work only during inspiration, and the diaphragm does most of the work. The work of inspiration is the sum of the work necessary to overcome the elastic forces of the lung, the tissue viscosity of the lung and chest wall, and airway resistance.[9] When any of these is increased (e.g., elastic force and tissue viscosity in restrictive pulmonary disease or resistance in obstructive airway disease), the work of inspiration must increase to maintain an adequate $\dot{V}_E$. The accessory muscles of inspiration (the sternocleidomastoid, anterior serratus, and external intercostal muscles) are recruited to accomplish this. Contraction of these muscles causes forceful expansion of the thorax, resulting in an unusually large negative intrathoracic pressure. This negative pressure draws in the soft tissues of the chest wall and creates one of the classic signs of dyspnea—retractions. Retractions may be seen in the suprasternal, infrasternal, intercostal, subcostal, and supraclavicular areas. An alternative way to maintain an adequate $\dot{V}_E$ is to increase the rate of breathing; hence the second classic sign of dyspnea—tachypnea. Nasal flaring and grunting are other signs seen and heard during inspiration.

Little energy is expended during normal expiration. Relaxation of the diaphragm, elastic recoil of the lungs and chest wall, and compression of the lungs by the intraabdominal organs force air from the lungs. In obstructive airway disease the force generated by these processes may not be great enough to effect adequate expiration. In a child who has tachypnea the elastic recoil may not be fast enough to allow adequate exhalation between breaths. In either instance the accessory muscles of expiration are used. The abdominal recti muscles contract and force the abdominal contents against the diaphragm to compress the lungs, and the internal intercostal muscles contract to pull the ribs downward and to create a positive intrathoracic pressure to force the air from the lungs. The contractions of these muscles provide the most important expiratory sign of dyspnea.

Although dyspnea is a respiratory symptom, it may be caused by primary disorders in other body systems. Cardiac, hematological, metabolic, circulatory, and psychogenic causes must be considered in the differential diagnosis of dyspnea. The child's age also is important, because various disorders occur with different frequency at different ages. The history is essential, including information about associated signs and symptoms, other known illnesses, medication or toxin exposure, and the duration of the current illness. A thorough physical examination always is indicated, with special attention paid to the aforementioned systems. The most useful laboratory tests are the complete blood count (CBC) and peripheral blood smear, arterial blood gas measurement, and roentgenographic studies of the airways and lungs. Measurement of arterial oxygen saturation by pulse oximetry is invaluable for its ability to assess oxygenation status quickly and noninvasively. Pulmonary function tests are very helpful as well, but usually they are not available for evaluation of an acutely ill patient.

ETIOLOGY AND CLINICAL PRESENTATION

Pulmonary Disease

Pulmonary disease that causes dyspnea can be classified as obstructive, restrictive, or vascular.

Obstructive Pulmonary Disease. Obstructive disease is characterized by airway narrowing that can be caused by intraluminal objects (mucus, foreign bodies, or tumor), intramural factors (smooth muscle contraction, edema, or bronchomalacia), or extramural compression (tumor or lymph nodes). The narrowing increases both airway resistance and

CAUSES OF OBSTRUCTIVE PULMONARY DISEASE

Newborns

Choanal atresia or stenosis
Dermoid cyst
Encephalocele
Hemangioma
Vocal cord paralysis
Pierre Robin syndrome
Ankyloglossia (Tongue tie)[16]
Pertussis

Infants

Foreign body
Vascular ring
Tracheal web
Bronchiolitis
Asthma
Cystic fibrosis
Bronchomalacia
Pyogenic thyroid[13]
Accessory thyroid[13]

Children and adolescents

Foreign body
Asthma
Adenopathy
  Lymphoma
  Systemic lupus erythematosus
  Tuberculosis
  Sarcoidosis
Croup
Epiglottitis
Retropharyngeal abscess
Enlarged tonsils or adenoids
Cystic fibrosis
Anaphylaxis
Laryngeal tumor
Vocal cord tumor
Tracheal tumors
Vocal cord polyp
Laryngeal trauma
Supraglottitis
Diphtheria
Bacterial tracheitis
Ingestion of caustic substance
Crack cocaine[19]

turbulent flow in the airways. If a fixed obstruction is present, affected areas of the lungs will become atelectatic. With a ball valve type of obstruction (i.e., air can get into the lungs but not out), air is trapped and affected areas become hyperinflated. In either case an imbalance occurs between pulmonary ventilation and perfusion, and oxygen exchange is adversely affected.[26] All these processes force the patient to work harder to maintain adequate ventilation; hence dyspnea ensues.

During normal respiration, inspiration and expiration are of equal length. With a fixed degree of obstruction, both are equally prolonged. If the obstruction varies and is extrathoracic (i.e., above the vocal cords), inspiration is affected more because the negative intraairway pressure during inspiration tends to collapse the extrathoracic airway. The characteristic sign of such an obstruction is inspiratory stridor.

If the obstruction varies and affects the intrathoracic airways, expiration is prolonged because the positive intrathoracic pressure tends to collapse these airways during expiration. If larger airways are involved, rhonchi are present. Airflow across an obstruction in smaller airways generates wheezing.

A paradoxical pulse and cyanosis are sensitive but nonspecific signs of severe obstruction. Patients who have chronic obstructive disease may be barrel chested and have signs of chronic hypoxia, such as clubbing. Children who have a systemic disease, such as cystic fibrosis, also will show the extrapulmonary manifestations of that disease. The common causes of obstructive airway disease in childhood are shown in the box above. Obstruction in the nose or nasopharynx, especially in infants, should not be overlooked.

Blood gas values may be normal with mild obstructive disease. As the disease progresses, hypoxemia is the first abnormality seen. Hypocapnia, initially seen as a reflection of increased $\dot{V}_E$, is replaced by hypercapnia as the maldistribution of ventilation and perfusion increases (increasing dead space), the patient tires, and respiratory failure occurs.

The chest roentgenogram may reveal whether the cause of the obstruction is inside or outside the airway. Often hyperinflation with an increased anteroposterior chest diameter and flattened diaphragm are seen. Atelectasis may appear with a fixed obstruction. Fluoroscopic examination or inspiratory and expiratory roentgenograms may be useful in localizing a ball valve type obstruction.

Restrictive Pulmonary Disease. The cardinal features of restrictive pulmonary disease are a reduction in lung volume and pulmonary compliance secondary to pathological changes in the lung parenchyma or the pleura, deformities of the chest wall, or neuromuscular disease. Decreased volume necessitates an increase in respiratory rate to maintain a normal $\dot{V}_E$. The work of breathing must be increased to overcome the reduced compliance. Because it is more energy efficient to breathe rapidly with small tidal volumes than to breathe slowly and attempt to expand the chest against great restrictive forces, children who have restrictive diseases characteristically have rapid, shallow respirations.[26] The common pediatric causes of restrictive pulmonary disease are listed in the box on p. 925.

Observation of the child often reveals skeletal and neuromuscular causes. Pleural and parenchymal diseases are detected best by palpation, percussion, and auscultation of the chest. Tactile fremitus can demonstrate pulmonary consolidation or pleural effusion. Careful percussion reveals effusions, consolidation, and abnormal diaphragmatic excursion.

CAUSES OF RESTRICTIVE PULMONARY DISEASE

Newborns

Hyaline membrane disease
Hypoplastic lungs
Eventration of the diaphragm
Meconium aspiration
Pneumonia (group B streptococci or gram negative organisms)
Diaphragmatic paralysis
Osteogenesis imperfecta
CNS depression
  Hypoxia
  Congenital
  Maternal drugs
Congenital myasthenia gravis
Aspiration
Pulmonary edema
  Septicemia
  Congenital heart disease

Infants

Pneumonia
  Bacterial
  Viral
  Aspiration
Bronchopulmonary dysplasia
Wilson-Mikity syndrome
Hamman-Rich syndrome
Pulmonary edema
Infantile botulism
Congenital lobar emphysema

Children and adolescents

Skeletal
  Kyphoscoliosis
  Ankylosing spondylitis
  Pectus excavatum
  Crush chest injury
Parenchymal
  Pneumonia
  Hypersensitivity pneumonitis
  Systemic lupus erythematosus
  Scleroderma
  Fibrosis
  Toxin inhalation
  Granulomatous disease
  Drugs (e.g., antineoplastic agents and narcotics)[21]
  Carcinoma
  Fat embolus
  Pneumothorax
Smoke inhalation
Pulmonary infarction
Pulmonary edema
  Congestive heart failure
  Sepsis
  Intracranial disease[6]
  Croup[11]
  Epiglottitis[11]
Neuromuscular
  Cord transection
  Myasthenia gravis
  Muscular dystrophy
  Multiple sclerosis
  Guillain-Barré syndrome
  Pickwickian syndrome
  Toxins
Pleural effusion
  Pneumonia
  Hypoproteinemia
  Renal failure
  Tumor
  Pulmonary infarction

On auscultation, rales characteristic of alveolar disease may be heard, and changes in whispered pectoriloquy and egophony can be detected.

The CBC may be helpful in diagnosing an infectious cause. Arterial blood gases have a characteristic pattern of hypoxemia and hypocapnia. The chest roentgenogram is useful in that it can demonstrate decreased lung volume, pleural thickening and effusions, increased interstitial markings, parenchymal consolidation, skeletal deformities, and abnormal movement of the diaphragm.

Vascular Pulmonary Disease. Vascular lung disease is characterized by a decrease in the size of the pulmonary vascular bed. In the newborn this most often is due to "persistent pulmonary hypertension of the newborn."[7] Microemboli also have been reported in the lungs of infants who are in severe respiratory distress.[14] In older children the most common cause of vascular pulmonary disease is intimal hyperplasia after persistent left-to-right shunting and resultant pulmonary hypertension. The size of the pulmonary vascular bed also can be reduced by obstruction caused by thromboembolic disease, obliteration (e.g., vasculitis),[8] or destruction, as in emphysema. The reduced blood flow through the lungs results in arterial hypoxemia and hypercapnia, which in turn lead to the symptoms and signs of dyspnea. In addition to the common signs of dyspnea, the child who has vascular lung disease may have signs of pulmonary edema and pleural effusion. Systemic signs of right-sided heart failure secondary to pulmonary hypertension or left-sided failure that was the cause of the pulmonary hypertension may be present. The cardiac findings observed with pulmonary hypertension are an accentuated P_2, paradoxical splitting of S_2, an S_3, a pulmonary ejection click, and a right ventricular heave. An electrocardiogram is helpful in the diagnosis of right ventricular hypertrophy. A chest roentgenogram may reveal increased right ventricular size, enlargement of the pulmonary artery silhouette, decreased pulmonary blood flow in advanced disease, or increased flow early in the course of disease, with a left-to-right shunt.

Cardiac Disease

Dyspnea occurs with cardiac disease when insufficient blood is being pumped to the lungs as a result of congenital structural anomalies in the heart, pump failure (myocarditis or cardiomyopathy), or as already described, secondary pulmonary hypertension. Heart disease must be considered in all dyspneic newborns and older children who have a history of congenital heart disease. In the neonate, pulmonary disease often can be differentiated from cyanotic heart disease through a hyperoxia test. The nature of the cardiac defect can be delineated with the help of a thorough cardiac examination, an electrocardiogram, a chest roentgenogram, and an echocardiogram.

It must be remembered that what would be a trivial respiratory infection in a normal child may cause severe respiratory insufficiency in a child who has cardiopulmonary disease. Indeed, the mortality of infants who have respiratory syncytial viral pneumonia and congenital heart disease has been shown to exceed significantly the mortality of children who have normal hearts.[15]

Hematological Disease

If the oxygen-carrying capacity of the blood is sufficiently reduced, tissue hypoxia ensues. The resultant drop in arterial pH signals the CNS and stimulates the onset of dyspnea. Severe anemia, whether chronic or acute, congenital or acquired, is an example of this. The oxygen-carrying capacity also can be lowered when the hemoglobin's ability to bind oxygen is reduced. This is seen most commonly with carbon monoxide poisoning, but it also occurs with cyanide poisoning and methemoglobinemia. In any of these cases the child will not be cyanotic. The blue color of cyanosis is caused by a level of at least 5 g/dl of reduced hemoglobin in the blood.[26] Such a concentration of reduced hemoglobin is not found in anemia uncomplicated by other diseases or in the other conditions cited. Conversely, a polycythemic infant whose blood is hyperviscous may have dyspnea because of poor perfusion. Because such an infant has an increased hemoglobin concentration and removes more oxygen from the hemoglobin because his or her flow is decreased, this child may be cyanotic (having over 5 g/dl unsaturated hemoglobin) and not hypoxic. An extreme elevation of leukocyte or platelet counts also can cause blood hyperviscosity and dyspnea.

It should be noted that even though an anemic child may be hypoxic and dyspneic, he or she probably will not be hypoxemic—that is, the arterial oxygen tension (Pao_2) measured by blood gas analysis will be in the normal range.

Metabolic Disease

Disorders that increase the body's rate of metabolism and therefore oxygen consumption can cause dyspnea. Examples are hyperthyroidism and fever. Metabolic disorders associated with an increased production of hydrogen ion and carbon dioxide cause a dyspnea-like breathing pattern to help rid the body of the carbon dioxide. The classic example is Kussmaul breathing of those who have diabetic ketoacidosis. Aspirin poisoning can manifest similarly. In addition, children who have various muscle enzyme deficiencies, especially those affecting the mitochondria, may have dyspnea as part of their clinical presentation as a result of their increased acid production and decreased work tolerance.[20,22] In chronic renal failure the kidney's inability to remove acid from the blood adequately is the underlying cause of dyspnea. The history, physical examination, and appropriate laboratory tests should facilitate the proper diagnosis of these diseases.

If oxygen cannot reach the tissues, the body responds with dyspnea, cardiovascular collapse, and shock. This is a medical emergency and should not present a diagnostic problem.

Obesity

Dyspnea, especially with exertion, is a common complaint of obese children. An obese child is prone to dyspnea because his or her metabolic requirement for a given amount of work is increased.[29] In addition, the diaphragm of an obese child must move against increased abdominal pressure, and the chest wall is heavier; thus more energy must be expended to maintain $\dot{V}_E$. Treatment should include dietary regulation and an exercise program graded to keep pace with the child's level of exercise tolerance.

Pregnancy

Dyspnea is normal during pregnancy.[31] The onset occurs during the first or second trimester, and 76% of women complain of dyspnea by the thirty-first week of gestation. The sensation is due to a subjective awareness of the hyperventilation normally present during pregnancy.

The normal dyspnea of pregnancy can be easily differentiated from dyspnea arising from heart or lung disease. First, the woman who has dyspnea of pregnancy has no other symptoms of cardiac or pulmonary disease. Second, dyspnea of pregnancy begins early and plateaus or improves as term approaches. Dyspnea due to heart disease begins during the second half of pregnancy and is worst during the seventh month. Finally, dyspnea of pregnancy rarely is severe, rarely occurs at rest, and does not interfere with the activities of daily life.

Psychogenic Cause

Stress or hysteria may cause dyspnea.[27] A thorough history, when available, and a physical examination make the diagnosis easy. These patients are tachypneic and complain of air hunger. When dyspnea is caused by pulmonary or cardiac conditions, the shortness of breath worsens with increasing activity and improves with rest. However, when dyspnea is due to hysteria, it does not improve with rest and may worsen. The patients also often complain of chest pain and sigh more often. Contrary to previous belief, tetany is an uncommon accompaniment of hysterical dyspnea.

The physical examination usually is normal. However, stress-induced paradoxical adduction of the vocal cords during inspiration has been reported.[17] Patients who have this disorder may have either stridor or wheezing. In this instance the diagnosis of hysterical dyspnea is one of exclusion—it can be made only after pathological lesions in the airways and lungs have been ruled out.

Normally the only laboratory abnormality found with hysteria-induced dyspnea is a diminished arterial carbon dioxide tension.

Treatment consists of calm reassurance and, occasionally, mild sedation. If the condition is chronic, psychotherapy may be required. When paradoxical vocal cord motion is the cause, the patient also should be taught laryngeal relaxation techniques.

MANAGEMENT

Severe dyspnea is a medical emergency. If not treated promptly, a child who has dyspnea may progress rapidly to respiratory failure and death. First, the adequacy of the airway must be assessed. Foreign bodies must be removed and anatomical obstructions bypassed with endotracheal intubation or, in rare cases, tracheotomy. Bronchospasm, when present, should be treated with beta-agonistic drugs.

Subsequently, the efficacy of the child's ventilation must be evaluated. Normally, breathing uses 2% to 3% of the total body energy expenditure. When the work of breathing is increased during dyspnea, this amount may rise to 30% or more.[8] Such a degree of energy expenditure cannot be continued indefinitely, and the child tires. Even after an obstruction is removed, the child still will be unable to effect adequate ventilation. In this instance, or in the case of neuromuscular disease, the child requires mechanical ventilation. Once ventilation is established, the cardiovascular system's ability to deliver oxygen to the tissues must be appraised. This involves evaluating the heart, peripheral circulation, intravascular volume status, and the blood's oxygen-carrying capacity. Therapy with vasopressors, fluids, blood transfusions, or diuretics should be initiated when indicated. Although not all children who have dyspnea require supplemental oxygen, every child should have oxygen administered until the cause of the dyspnea is known. Once the patient's condition has stabilized, the search for the underlying cause of the dyspnea should progress urgently but calmly. At this point a detailed history can be elicited, a full physical examination can be performed, and a chest roentgenogram and appropriate blood tests can be obtained. When the diagnosis is made, specific therapy can be initiated.

When dyspnea is caused by a chronic illness, no satisfactory therapy may be available to treat the underlying disease. However, simply relieving the dyspnea can improve the child's functional ability and quality of life significantly.[1] Several modalities can be used to treat the symptom of dyspnea in a chronically ill child.[3,25] Sedatives and narcotics reduce $\dot{V}_E$ and thereby diminish the intensity of the breathless feeling. Prostaglandin inhibitors and beta-agonists may blunt the perception of dyspnea without affecting ventilation.[24] Theophylline may improve diaphragmatic contractility. Continuous supplemental oxygen with or without continuous positive airway pressure reduces ventilatory drive.[30] Children who have chronic obstructive pulmonary disease may be taught to breathe through pursed lips. This reduces the respiratory rate, increases the tidal volume, and diminishes the sensation of dyspnea. Hypnosis has proved useful in treating the symptoms of dyspnea. Patients also have reported a decrease in dyspnea when seated next to an open window or a blowing fan.[23]

Exercise and proper nutrition are helpful in maintaining or increasing inspiratory muscle mass and thereby in reducing the perceived magnitude of dyspnea.[1,4,18] Finally, because dyspnea is a subjective complaint, there is a significant psychological contribution to its perceived severity.[5] Therefore the child's emotional state, behavior, and personality must be monitored because psychosocial intervention may be indicated.

REFERENCES

1. Altose MD: Assessment and management of breathlessness, *Chest* 88(suppl 2):77, 1985.
2. Angelillo VA: Evaluation of dyspnea, *Postgrad Med* 73:336, 1983.
3. Belman MJ: Factors limiting exercise performance in lung disease: ventilatory insufficiency, *Chest* 101:253S, 1992.
4. Carter R, Coast JR, Idell S: Exercise training in patients with chronic obstructive pulmonary disease, *Med Sci Sports Exerc* 24:281, 1992.
5. Cherniak NS, Altose MD: Mechanisms of dyspnea, *Clin Chest Med* 8:207, 1978.
6. Drucker TB, Simmons RL, Martin AM: Pulmonary edema as a complication of intracranial disease, *Am J Dis Child* 118:638, 1969.
7. Fox WW, Duara S: Persistent pulmonary hypertension in the neonate: diagnosis and management, *J Pediatr* 103:505, 1983.
8. Goffman TE, Bloom RL, Dvorak VC: Acute dyspnea in a young woman taking birth control pills, *JAMA* 251:1465, 1984.
9. Guyton AC: *Textbook of medical physiology,* Philadelphia, 1981, WB Saunders.
10. Howell JB, Campbell EJM, editors: *Breathlessness,* Oxford, 1966, Blackwell Scientific.
11. Kanter RK, Watchko JF: Pulmonary edema associated with upper airway obstruction, *Am J Dis Child* 138:356, 1984.
12. Killian KJ, Campbell EJM: Dyspnea and exercise, *Annu Rev Physiol* 45:465, 1983.
13. Leigh M, Holman G, Rohn R: Dyspnea as the presenting symptom of thyroid disease, *Clin Pediatr* 19:773, 1980.
14. Levin DL, Weinberg AG, Perkin RM: Pulmonary microthrombi in newborn infants with unresponsive persistent pulmonary hypertension, *J Pediatr* 102:299, 1983.
15. Macdonald NE et al: Respiratory syncytial virus infection in infants with congenital heart disease, *N Engl J Med* 307:397, 1982.
16. Mukai S, Mukai C, Asaoka K: Ankyloglossia with deviation of the epiglottis and larynx, *Ann Otol Rhinol Laryngol* 153:3, 1991.
17. O'Hollaren MT: Masqueraders in clinical allergy: laryngeal dysfunction causing dyspnea, *Ann Allergy* 65:351, 1990.
18. Olopade CO et al: Exercise limitation and pulmonary rehabilitation in chronic obstructive pulmonary disease, *Mayo Clin Proc* 67:144, 1992.
19. Reino AJ, Lawson W: Upper airway distress in crack cocaine users, *Otolaryngol Head Neck Surg* 109:937, 1993.
20. Robinson BH et al: Clinical presentation of mitochondrial respiratory chain defects in ADH–coenzyme Q reductase and cytochrome oxidase: clues to pathogenesis of Leigh disease, *J Pediatr* 110:216, 1987.
21. Rosenow EC: The spectrum of drug-induced pulmonary disease, *Ann Intern Med* 77:977, 1972.
22. Scholte HR et al: Defects in oxidative phosphorylation: biochemical investigations in skeletal muscle and expression of the lesion in other cells, *J Inherit Metab Dis* 10(suppl 1):81, 1987.
23. Schwartzstein RM et al: Cold facial stimulation reduces breathlessness induced in normal individuals, *Am Rev Respir Dis* 136:58, 1987.
24. Stark RD: Dyspnoea: assessment and pharmacological manipulation, *Eur J Respir Dis* 1:280, 1988.
25. Sweer L, Zwillich CW: Dyspnea in the patient with chronic obstructive pulmonary disease: etiology and management, *Clin Chest Med* 11:417, 1990.
26. Tisi GM: *Pulmonary physiology in clinical medicine,* Baltimore, 1980, Williams & Wilkins.
27. Tobin MJ: Dyspnea: pathophysiologic basis, clinical presentation, and management, *Arch Intern Med* 150:1604, 1990.
28. Wasserman K, Casaburi R: Dyspnea: physiological and pathophysiological mechanisms, *Annu Rev Med* 39:503, 1988.
29. Wasserman K et al: *Principles of exercise testing and interpretation,* Philadelphia, 1987, Lea & Febiger.
30. Younes M: Load responses, dyspnea, and respiratory failure, *Chest* 97:59S, 1990.

31. Zeldis SM: Dyspnea during pregnancy: distinguishing cardiac from pulmonary causes, *Clin Chest Med* 13:567, 1992.

SUGGESTED READINGS

Burki NK: Dyspnea, *Lung* 165:269, 1987.

Cohen MH et al: Treatment of intractable dyspnea: clinical and ethical issues, *Cancer Invest* 10:317, 1992.

Downes JJ, Fulgencio T, Raphaely RC: Acute respiratory failure in infants and children, *Pediatr Clin North Am* 19:423, 1972.

Gandevia SC: Neural mechanisms underlying the sensation of breathlessness: kinesthetic parallels between respiratory and limb muscles, *Aust NZ J Med* 18:83, 1988.

Harun MH, Yaacob I, Mohd Kassim Z: Spontaneous pneumothorax: a review of 29 admissions into Hospital Universiti Sains Malaysia 1984-90, *Singapore Med J* 34:150, 1993.

Heyse-Moore LH: Symptom control in palliative medicine: an update, *Br J Clin Pract* 43:273, 1989.

Litam PP, Loughran TP Jr: Exertional dyspnea and headache in a 16-year-old girl, *Hosp Pract* 29:112, 1994.

Mahler DA: Dyspnea: diagnosis and management, *Clin Chest Med* 8:215, 1987.

Poole-Wilson PA, Buller NP, Lindsay DC: Blood flow and skeletal muscle in patients with heart failure, *Chest* 101:330S, 1992.

Rebuck AS, Slutsky AS: Control of breathing in diseases of the respiratory tract and lungs. In Geiger SR, editor: *Handbook of physiology,* Bethesda, Md, 1986, American Physiological Society.

Schwartzstein RM et al: Dyspnea: a sensory experience, *Lung* 168:185, 1990.

Shayevitz MB, Shayevitz BR: Athletic training in chronic obstructive pulmonary disease, *Clin Sports Med* 5:471, 1986.

125 Dysuria

Fred J. Heldrich

Dysuria is painful or difficult urination. Although this symptom occurs with some frequency in pediatric patients, it is interesting that the term rarely can be found in the index of standard pediatric texts and cannot be found in the *Cumulative Index Medicus*. The reason is that dysuria rarely occurs as an isolated symptom; far more often it occurs with other signs or symptoms of a pathological urinary tract condition and is discussed in concert with them. Although occasionally dysuria is the only complaint, it often is easier to identify the cause of the dysuria by considering the associated symptoms.

Identifying the cause of dysuria requires a thorough history, a careful physical examination, and a planned laboratory evaluation.[1] Failure to follow this routine usually leads to unnecessary expense, incorrect diagnosis, and improper management.

CLINICAL MANIFESTATIONS

Although older patients usually can tell the physician that urination is painful or difficult, infants and young children give other evidence of dysuria. Infants indicate pain on urination in a variety of ways (see the box on p. 930). Crying, the most typical sign, is associated with micturition. Just as voiding provokes crying, cessation of voiding provides relief, and the crying may stop. Characteristically, infants who cry because of discomfort associated with voiding flex their thighs. This combination of crying and drawing up of the legs frequently is described as colic. At times the association between crying and voiding is not appreciated, and the infant is thought merely to be hyperirritable. As a result of the frequent urination that usually accompanies painful urination in infants, these babies' diapers are seldom dry.

Young children unable to state accurately that urination is painful or difficult indicate dysuria by other signs (see the box on p. 930). At this age the crying that occurs because of the pain experienced with urination is identified more readily. Because of the discomfort occasioned by voiding, the child may delay urination as long as possible. This can lead to bladder distention, suprapubic discomfort, and irritability or further crying. Difficulty in either initiating or continuing urination may produce a hesitant or an episodic urine stream, which may be seen or heard when the child is seated on a potty chair or commode. In an attempt to overcome resistance to urine flow, the child may assume a squatting position or sit with each voiding. Older children use terms such as "burn," "tingle," or "hurt" to express pain, and "strain," "bear down," or "It's hard to start" to indicate discomfort and difficulty in voiding.

Although dysuria may be the only symptom, other signs and symptoms that often occur concomitantly are extremely important and helpful in establishing the cause of dysuria. Regardless of the patient's age, there is considerable similarity in the associated signs and symptoms, and they can be placed in one of two major categories: (1) other specific urinary symptoms (e.g., hematuria, malodorous urine, or frequency) or (2) nonspecific symptoms (e.g., fever, abdominal pain, diarrhea, or vomiting). Thus dysuria may be either the primary complaint or simply an associated symptom that often occurs with other symptoms of greater significance.[3]

PHYSICAL FINDINGS

The physical examination often yields no positive findings. However, anomalies of the external genitalia may be seen. An obstructive uropathy may be discernible as an abdominal mass (enlarged bladder, ureters, or kidneys). Palpation may elicit pain at the costovertebral angles, above the symphysis pubis, or over the abdomen in general. In baby boys a small meatal opening, frequently ulcerated, may be seen. A rectal examination may identify a fecal mass or, in boys, a tender, swollen prostate. In girls, inspection of the perineum may reveal excoriation of the skin, labia, or meatal opening. Urethral prolapse is identified by a doughnut-shaped, red, swollen mucosa protruding from the urethral orifice. In addition to erythema, vesicles and a serous, serosanguineous, or purulent discharge may be found in the vagina.

DIFFERENTIAL DIAGNOSIS

Any condition that leads to inflammation or irritation of the urinary tract or obstructs the flow of urine may cause dysuria.[4] Dysuria as the dominant symptom suggests the diagnostic possibilities shown in the box on p. 930.

Urinary Tract Infection

Urinary tract infection is the most common cause of dysuria. Pain on urination also may lead to urgency, frequency, hesitancy, and enuresis. The urine may be clear, cloudy, bloody, or foul smelling. Dysuria typically is associated with infection of the lower urinary tract, but it also may occur with upper tract disease. Although it is not always possible clinically to differentiate an upper urinary tract infection from a lower urinary tract infection, symptoms can be helpful. Systemic symptoms such as chills, fever, or abdominal or costovertebral angle pain usually indicate pyelonephritis. Suprapubic discomfort is more consistent with cystitis.

Upper urinary tract infection could be identified by ureteral catheterization, collection of urine by use of the bladder washout technique, or renal biopsy, but these are invasive techniques that require anesthesia. Nuclear imaging with technetium-labeled dimercaptosuccinic acid (DMSA) is a superior, noninvasive way of identifying upper tract infection.[2] Bacteria are the most common cause of both upper and lower

INDICATORS OF DYSURIA

Infants

Crying
Colic
Irritability
Flexing of legs
Diaper that is wet more often than usual

Young children

Crying when voiding
Hesitant stream
Straining
Squatting or sitting to void
Refusing to urinate

CAUSES OF DYSURIA

Urinary tract infection
Urethritis
Prostatis
Balanoposthitis
Meatal lesions
Vulvovaginitis
Kidney or bladder stones
Obstruction
Foreign bodies
Tumors
Drugs
Trauma
Sexual abuse
Hematological disorders
Perineal dermatitis (primary)
Masturbation
Psychogenic factors

urinary tract infections. Gram negative organisms predominate, and *Escherichia coli* is found most frequently. A mixed bacterial flora, although unusual, is most apt to exist if infection occurs in a urinary tract that has structural abnormalities or if the patient has had persistent reinfections.

In adolescent girls who have both frequency and dysuria, persistent recovery of a single organism at colony counts below 10^5/ml of a clean-caught, midstream specimen is consistent with the diagnosis of infection.[5]

Viruses, particularly coxsackieviruses A11 and A12, have been identified as a cause of hemorrhagic cystitis. Dysuria usually is pronounced, and blood clots pass frequently. *Ureaplasma urealyticum, Mycoplasma hominis,* and anaerobes are other potential pathogens.[5]

Tuberculosis is an uncommon cause of urinary tract infection today, but when it is the cause, it often is accompanied by dysuria and hematuria. Both the upper and lower urinary tracts may be affected. Fungi, especially *Candida albicans,* are an unusual cause of urinary tract infection, but they may occur, usually as a superimposed infection in a patient undergoing antibiotic therapy.

Pinworms *(Enterobius vermicularis)* may lead to perineal irritation and discomfort on urination.

Urethritis

Neisseria gonorrhoeae is a major cause of urethritis in sexually active adolescent boys. A profuse, creamy urethral discharge accompanies the dysuria. In prepubertal boys, urethritis often is nonspecific—that is, no etiological agent is recovered. *Chlamydia trachomatis,* yet another organism that has been identified as a cause of urethritis, frequently appears as a recurrent infection after the patient has been treated for gonorrhea. Burning on urination is a common symptom in nongonococcal forms of urethritis.

Prostatitis

Prostatitis is confined almost exclusively to sexually active patients. In addition to dysuria, the patient often has a sensation of deep, suprapubic discomfort, and he may urinate more frequently than usual. A rectal examination will reveal a tender prostate, which after massage yields a urethral discharge. The bacteria involved vary and are determined by culturing the discharge.

Balanoposthitis

Balanoposthitis, infection of the glans penis and prepuce, is an unusual infection that may occur in uncircumcised boys. The diagnosis is readily made by inspection, and the bacterium responsible is isolated by culturing the prepucal discharge.

Meatal Lesions

In a baby boy who is still in diapers (and most often circumcised), a meatal ulcer may develop as a result of irritation by the wet diaper. An ammoniacal diaper rash also is present in most instances. Bleeding at the site of the meatal ulceration may produce a spot of blood on the diaper covering the area.

Diaper rash also may be associated with dysuria in baby girls. A unique lesion of the female urethra is prolapse, which appears as a circumferential ring of red or bluish mucosa protruding from the urethral orifice.

Vulvovaginitis

Various organisms can cause vulvovaginitis; those most often encountered are *N. gonorrhoeae, Haemophilus vaginalis, C. trachomatis, Trichomonas vaginalis,* and herpes progenitalis. A discharge of varying degree is present in all instances. Herpes, an infection that is associated with severe dysuria, is characterized further by the presence of vesicles, or ulcerations after rupture of the vesicles, on the vulva and vagina. All these infections are sexually transmitted. In prepubertal girls, although any of the aforementioned agents may be identified, the infection usually is nonspecific. Gonococcal infection in a prepubertal girl should be considered as evidence of child abuse until proved otherwise.

Kidney Stones/Hypercalciuria

The pain caused by kidney stones usually is "colicky," with associated hematuria. The passage of the stone down the ureter or through the urethra is most apt to produce pain that frequently radiates to the urethral meatus. Bladder stones typically produce pain at the end of micturition. Approximately 80% of kidney and bladder stones are radiopaque and contain calcium. The family history may be positive for nephrolithiasis. Hypercalciuria without stone formation may produce dysuria and hematuria.[6] Diseases associated with renal stones include hyperparathyroidism, gout, renal tubular acidosis, idiopathic hypercalciuria, cystinuria, inflammatory bowel disease, and immobilization hypercalcemia.

Obstruction

Lesions below the bladder (posterior urethral valves, urethral strictures, urethral diverticula, or meatal stenosis) almost always are found in boys and may cause difficulty with initiating urination. Obstruction in this area may produce bladder and bilateral ureteral dilation, which can lead to overflow incontinence and suprapubic discomfort. In mild forms of urethral obstruction, dysuria may be the most important symptom. Obstructive lesions of a ureter (ureteral stricture, ureteroceles, ectopic ureters, ureteropelvic obstruction) lead to unilateral hydronephrosis, which may remain silent or cause dysuria.

Either bilateral or unilateral hydronephrotic changes increase the probability of urinary tract infection, which can then produce dysuria. Hydronephrotic urinary tracts may also be traumatized, resulting in subsequent hematuria and dysuria.

Either infection or hematuria may lead to stone formation. Finally, hydronephrotic changes may produce ptosis of urinary tract structures and can be associated with pain that radiates toward the urethra and leads to an urge to urinate. In this instance the pain may be related to changes in body position.

Other Causes of Dysuria

Children may insert foreign bodies into their own urethras or those of their playmates. Evidence of trauma at the urethral orifice and discovery of a foreign body by roentgenography confirm the diagnosis. Bladder tumors are rare in children and usually are associated with bleeding. Wilms tumor, the most common renal tumor in children, may cause dysuria with hematuria, but this presentation would be most unusual.

Use of the following drugs has been associated with dysuria: amitriptyline, chlordiazepoxide, imipramine, isoniazid, sulfonamides, cyclophosphamide, heparin, dicumarol, and antihistamines.

Trauma that produces hematuria may result in dysuria. Direct trauma to the perineum or external genitalia may be an obvious cause of dysuria. Irritation of the urethra by a catheter or a cystoscope is a self-limited cause.

A special form of trauma, sexual abuse, deserves consideration in all instances in which the history and physical findings are not compatible with the symptoms or when the accusation is made by the child or a person who brings the child for treatment.

Dysuria may occur as a result of pain caused by the flow of urine over an irritated perineum. Local lesions may be caused by soap or bubble bath, by local infections (e.g., varicella or candidiasis), or by masturbation. Wet diapers can cause perineal irritation if they are not changed frequently.

Cystoscopic examination should be avoided in the management of most urinary tract infections. It may be useful, however, in identifying bladder lesions, which often cause hematuria and dysuria. Other tests may be indicated to determine renal function and to rule out hematological disorders and rare forms of renal disease.

MANAGEMENT

The major cause of dysuria is a urinary tract infection, which the pediatrician usually can manage effectively. The principles of management are precise diagnosis, adequate evaluation of the genitourinary tract, appropriate antibiotic therapy, and long-term follow-up. Details are discussed in Chapter 269. Sexually transmitted diseases should be treated as discussed in Chapter 258. Drugs that cause dysuria should be discontinued. Patients who have idiopathic hypercalciuria may be managed with chlorothiazide. Offending irritants such as soaps, powders, or bubble bath should be removed. Tight-fitting diapers that restrict the entrance of air should be avoided. Local medications may be indicated for a candidal infection. If oxyuriasis (pinworm infestation) is present, mebendazole should be effective. (Other family members also must be treated.) After catheterization or cystoscopic examination, sitz baths in warm water may temporarily relieve acute symptoms of dysuria.

When evidence supports the diagnosis of functional dysuria, a positive approach to management begins with minimizing the laboratory workup. For example, imaging studies may not be required initially. Counseling to ensure understanding of the dynamics involved and methods to eliminate factors contributing to the symptom are of greatest importance. The patient, when old enough, should be reassured that organic disease does not exist but that the symptom of dysuria is real and steps will be taken to alleviate it. Pediatricians can manage functional dysuria effectively when they are willing and able to spend the time necessary and show appropriate concern for the problem. Suspicion of sexual abuse requires prompt protection of the child and warrants hospitalization pending adequate evaluation. Appropriate agencies should be notified.

Urological consultation occasionally is required, notably when the diagnosis of obstructive uropathy, renal calculi, foreign bodies, tumors, or urethral prolapse is suspected or confirmed.

REFERENCES

1. Carlton CE Jr: Initial evaluation: including history, physical examination, and urinalysis. In Harrison JL et al, editors: *Campbell's urology,* ed 5, Philadelphia, 1986, WB Saunders.
2. Heldrich FJ: 99^{m} Technetium dimercaptosuccinic acid scan in evaluating patients with urinary tract infection, *Maryland Medical Journal* 41:215, 1992.
3. Kaplan GW, Brock WA: Voiding dysfunction in children, *Curr Probl Pediatr* 10:41, 1980.
4. Rubin MI, Barratt TM, editors: *Pediatric nephrology,* Baltimore, 1975, Williams & Wilkins.
5. Sobel J, Kaye D: Urinary tract infections. In Gillenwater JY et al, editors: *Adult and pediatric urology,* Chicago, 1987, Mosby.
6. Stapleton FB et al: Hypercalciuria in children with urolithiasis, *Am J Dis Child* 136:675, 1982.

126 Edema

Robert H. McLean

RECOGNITION AND SIGNIFICANCE OF EDEMA

Recognizing edema can be a clinical challenge. Edema, the swelling of tissues caused by excessive fluid accumulation, often is labeled many other things before it is recognized as just what it is. Parents often notice weight gain, chubbiness, outgrown shoes, or irritability in their child, whereas the physician may diagnose allergic problems before the fundamental cause of swelling is determined.

Recognizing edema is important because any disturbance of salt and water homeostasis in the body is significant. Water makes up 65% of the adult's body weight and 75% of the newborn's. When edema is detected early, the clinical circumstances usually are dramatic enough to determine its cause. However, when it is clinically more subtle, the diagnosis can be delayed, often with serious consequences.

Edema reflects a profound abnormality in body fluid homeostasis because so much metabolic energy is spent regulating the body's water and sodium content. The patient's age and sex, as well as the organs involved and the duration of the edema, influence its ultimate importance. Edema usually is not idiopathic in children.

PATHOPHYSIOLOGY

Under normal circumstances the movement of water between the extracellular and the intracellular body compartments is regulated carefully, with the largest quantity of water located within the intracellular spaces. The appearance of edema results from disturbances in the distribution of fluid between the two extracellular space subcompartments—the intravascular and the interstitial spaces.

At the end of the nineteenth century, Starling[3] proposed the following hypothesis to explain the movement of water between the intravascular and the interstitial spaces: at the capillary and precapillary level, two types of forces cause water to leave the intravascular space (plasma)—hydrostatic pressure (blood pressure) and oncotic pressure within the interstitium. (The forces that cause oncotic pressure are discussed below.) Opposing this movement of water out of plasma are two forces: the plasma oncotic pressure and tissue turgor. The forces that create egress of water from plasma slightly outweigh the opposing ingress forces at the arterial end of the capillary bed, but the reverse is true at the venule end of the capillary bed. The result is movement of water, nutrients, and electrolytes through the interstitium at both ends of the network, but no net change occurs in intravascular and interstitial fluid exchanges. Any slight accumulation of water in the interstitial spaces is carried away in the lymphatic system.

In quantitative terms, the most important force opposing movement of water into the interstitium is the oncotic pressure.[4] Plasma contains charged electrolytes (crystalloids such as sodium and chloride) and electrically charged proteins (colloids, such as albumin). The osmotic pressure is the function of the total number of such charged particles in any given fluid. A sodium molecule is osmotically as effective as an albumin molecule, even though the latter is much larger. The sum of the positive and negative particles in each compartment containing body fluid must balance, but the exact composition of these charges varies considerably. For example, because the capillary membrane is semipermeable rather than fully permeable, the protein content of plasma normally is much greater than that of the fluid in the interstitial spaces. Because of the high plasma protein concentration and the characteristics of the capillary membranes, the total number of osmotically active particles in plasma normally is higher than the number in the interstitium. This slight difference between the osmolarity of the plasma and the osmolarity of the interstitium creates the oncotic pressure. Because this difference is caused primarily (but not exclusively) by the protein content of plasma, determining the status of protein metabolism is important in evaluating edema. For example, mechanisms that reduce oncotic pressure, such as excessive loss of protein in the urine or gastrointestinal tract, may lead to edema.

Despite this, the role of body sodium in edema is paramount in most clinical situations. Several forces control sodium balance, including the rates of glomerular filtration and aldosterone production. Simply put, continued intake of the usual amount of sodium will lead to sodium retention if the sodium-controlling factors do not respond appropriately to maintain a proper balance between the intake and output of sodium.

Sodium moves freely throughout the plasma and extracellular water spaces. It constitutes the largest cationic (positively charged) crystalloid and thus exerts the greatest osmotic force for movement of water between these spaces. Therefore it is not surprising that excessive accumulation of sodium in the body leads to accumulation of excessive body water.

The amount of sodium in the body is regulated primarily through the process of glomerular filtration, the renin-angiotensin-aldosterone hormonal axis, and atrial natriuretic factor (ANF).[2] Normally, most sodium filtered through the glomerulus is reabsorbed through the renal tubules before it reaches the pyelocaliceal system by a precisely controlled mechanism that responds to the amount of sodium consumed each day.

Total body sodium levels become abnormal when the glomerular filtration of sodium is so reduced that sodium balance no longer can be controlled through renal tubular resorption or nonresorption. Such is the case in renal failure, in which glomerular filtration is too low to excrete sodium to any significant degree. Aldosterone excess, which may occur in intravascular volume–depleted states (e.g., nephrotic syndrome), may be a primary cause of edema.

Edema confined to a single extremity or a well-circumscribed area of the body is a special situation. This can arise from obstruction of the vascular or lymphatic system of a limb through trauma, tumor, embolization, or thrombus formation. Local release of vasoactive substances that cause locally increased vascular permeability may occur in allergic individuals and in patients who lack a particular complement system inhibitor.

The pathophysiology of edema formation in congestive heart failure develops secondary to stimulation of the kidneys to retain sodium. Many investigators previously attributed the cause of edema in cirrhosis and idiopathic nephrotic syndrome (INS) to hypoproteinemia, with the hypoproteinemia being a consequence of the formation of ascites in cirrhosis and of urinary loss in INS. In the presence of hypoproteinemia, the patient who has INS is predicted to have reduced renal cortical perfusion, which results in increased renin/aldosterone and catecholamine production. The result of increased aldosterone production is sodium resorption, which leads to edema formation (see underfill theory in Fig. 126-1).

However, considerable evidence now suggests that, as with congestive heart failure, edema formation in cirrhosis and INS is due primarily to augmented retention of sodium by the kidneys (see overfill theory in Fig. 126-1). When children who have INS have their blood volume measured, only about half have decreased values; the rest are normal or increased. In addition, plasma renin levels have been noted to increase rather than decrease with remission of nephrotic syndrome. The presence of pure hypoalbuminemia, such as with congenital analbuminemia, is not associated with edema. Experimental studies document a "blunted" response by the nephrotic kidney to ANF.[2] Because of such observations, many investigators have concluded that the pathophysiology of edema in nephrotic syndrome may be due to a primary defect that results in increased sodium retention by the kidneys.

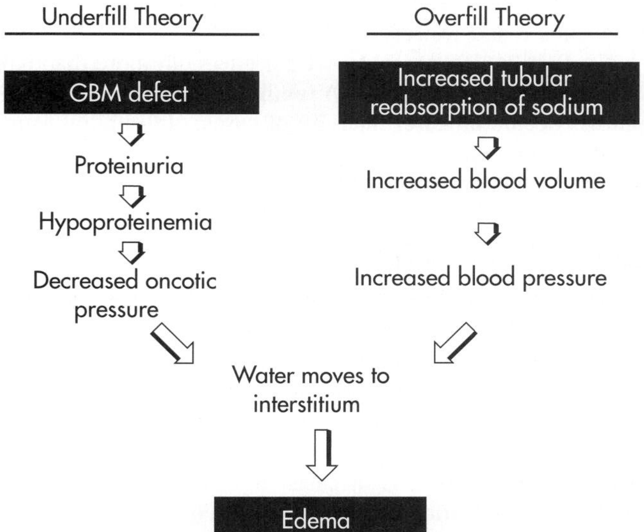

FIG. 126-1 Formation of edema in idiopathic nephrotic syndrome (INS) of childhood. Shown are the two current hypotheses for the formation of edema in INS. According to the ***underfill theory (left),*** fluid retention occurs secondary to the primary glomerular basement membrane (GBM) defect that produces proteinuria. According to the ***overfill theory (right),*** increased tubular resorption of sodium is the primary defect. Sodium retention leads to renal water resorption and the formation of edema.

CAUSES OF EDEMA

Various disorders can lead to edema[1] (see the box below). The history, physical examination, and some simple laboratory tests can point to the most likely cause, although more sophisticated procedures may be indicated.

It particularly is helpful to classify the cause of edema according to the usual age of onset (Table 126-1). In this regard the pediatrician has an advantage over the internist because this information often is less useful for diagnosis in adults.

The most common cause of chronic renal failure in children is either a congenital renal abnormality or glomerulonephritis. Signs of renal failure, such as edema, usually have their onset during infancy and childhood (unlike congenital heart disease, which so often causes edema and other symptoms at or soon after birth).

CAUSES OF EDEMA IN CHILDREN

Cardiovascular

Congestive heart failure
Acute thrombi or emboli
Vasculitis of many types

Renal

Nephrotic syndrome
Glomerulonephritis of many types
End-stage renal failure

Endocrine or metabolic

Thyroid disease
Starvation
Hereditary angioedema

Iatrogenic

Drugs (diuretics and steroids)
Water or salt overload

Hematological

Hemolytic disease of the newborn

Gastrointestinal

Hepatic cirrhosis
Protein-losing enteritis
Lymphangiectasis
Cystic fibrosis
Celiac disease
Enteritis of many types

Lymphatic abnormalities

Congenital (gonadal dysgenesis)
Acquired

Table 126-1 Causes of Edema and Age of Onset

Etiological factor	Fetal or neonatal	Infancy	Childhood	Adolescence
Hemolytic anemias	X			
Congenital heart disease	X	X	X	
Congenital kidney disease	X	X	X	X
Gastrointestinal disease	X	X	X	X
Vasculitis			X	X
Drug reactions				X
Infections	X	X		
Acute or chronic glomerulonephritis			X	X
Excessive salt and water administration	X	X	X	X
Hereditary angioedema			X	X

Certain forms of gastrointestinal disease cause edema early in life because of protein losses, but some congenital diseases (e.g., hepatic fibrosis associated with autosomal recessive diffuse cystic disease of the kidneys) cause signs of fluid retention only as the child grows older. Hepatic cirrhosis is an uncommon but important consideration in the evaluation of an edematous infant or child.

Vasculitis is a general term that includes anaphylactoid purpura, systemic lupus erythematosus, and a spectrum of inflammatory vascular diseases and syndromes. These diseases are rare in newborns or infants. Similarly, drug abuse and overuse of prescribed drugs, such as diuretics (a rare cause of edema), are confined largely to adolescents. Abuse of narcotics or other drugs can produce nephrotic syndrome and glomerulonephritis. Idiopathic glomerulonephritis and acute poststreptococcal glomerulonephritis are far more common among children and adolescents than among infants. At all ages the most common cause of edema in hospitalized patients is excessive parenteral administration of sodium and water. In the confusion of caring for a sick, postoperative, or traumatized child, inappropriate fluid management continues to be an important cause of edema in hospitalized children.

HISTORY AND PHYSICAL EXAMINATION

In trying to establish the cause of edema, some important aspects of the medical history to consider are the rate of fluid accumulation, the patient's age and sex, the location of the swelling, and the association of other medical conditions, including acute intercurrent illness.

The rate of accumulation of edema caused by significant organ damage may be so low as to go unnoticed by the parents or the child. The associated weight gain often is attributed to other causes. A change in shoe size or clothing size may be dismissed as compatible with changes that occur in a growing child.

Knowing the child's age when the edema first began is extremely helpful. The cause of edema in a newborn often can be clarified by weighing the placenta. With infants who have congenital nephrotic syndrome, the placenta is large and boggy and may weigh twice as much as normal. The appearance of edema in a newborn or infant is reason for concern because significant organ damage may be involved. Hematological and infectious disease in utero must be considered when evaluating an edematous newborn, whereas diseases of the heart, liver, and gastrointestinal tract are more common causes of edema in older infants or child.

Edema caused by nephrotic syndrome usually becomes noticeable early in the course of the disease (after a few weeks). Careful questioning can establish that subtle signs of fluid accumulation had been present for some time. Periorbital edema often is the first sign parents notice. This is more noticeable in the morning because of nighttime dependency during sleep. Similarly, prolonged bed rest or sitting is the primary cause of presacral edema in a nonambulatory child. The potbelly so characteristic of nephrotic syndrome is a late sign of fluid accumulation within the peritoneum (ascites).

Although edema caused by heart disease and chronic renal failure occurs about as frequently in boys as in girls, INS is twice as common in boys. The peak age of onset is between 3 and 4 years. Attacks of hereditary angioedema appear in adolescents and adults, but abdominal pain and swelling also may occur in a preadolescent child who has this disease. An acute intercurrent illness often precedes attacks of angioedema and exacerbations of INS.

The family history is positive for edema in more than half of the cases of angioedema. A family history positive for nephrosis occurs in fewer than 4% of cases, but familial forms of glomerulonephritis that lead to kidney failure constitute an identifiable cause of edema.

LABORATORY TESTS

The initial steps in the evaluation of edema must include a urinalysis. The presence of protein or abnormal cellular elements immediately focuses attention on a renal cause for the edema. The presence of large amounts of protein in a random urine specimen showing little or no blood strongly supports the diagnosis of nephrotic syndrome. The presence of red or white blood cells or casts suggests glomerulonephritis. Further evaluation of renal disease requires tests of renal function, including determining the serum urea nitrogen, creatinine, and total protein and albumin serum concentrations. If the results are abnormal, the (corrected) creatinine clearance and quantitative urine protein should be measured. Consultation with a pediatric nephrologist would be appropriate at this point. Normal urinalysis and renal function tests associated with a low serum protein concentration should lead the physician to consider contrast studies of the gastrointestinal tract. Protein-losing enteropathies may be expected to be accompanied by significant symptoms of gastrointestinal aberrations (diarrhea and weight loss).

A complete blood count (CBC) and serological studies for red cell antibodies are emergency procedures in the evaluation of an edematous newborn. With chronic renal disease, anemia and an elevated sedimentation rate are expected findings; in acute infectious processes, the white blood cell (WBC) count should be elevated or the differential count should be shifted to the left.

Heart failure can be confirmed quickly as the cause of edema with chest roentgenograms or through electrocardiography or echocardiography. Unlike nephrotic syndrome or protein-losing enteropathy, congestive heart failure demands rapid corrective measures. The particular combination of abdominal cramps and localized edema (e.g., edema of the hands, feet, or larynx) should prompt the physician to consider measuring the concentration and function of the serum C1 esterase inhibitor (C1 INH). In 80% of individuals with hereditary angioedema, the levels of C1 INH are reduced; however, in the remaining 20% of cases, the levels are normal or elevated, but the *functioning* of the C1 INH is reduced. Because of this, a special effort must be made to measure C1 INH function (some commercial laboratories offer this test.)

MANAGEMENT

After the cause of the edema has been determined, treatment begins with management of the causative disorder. For example, if surgical correction of a cardiac lesion is possible, the appropriate corrective procedure becomes the primary therapeutic maneuver. Supportive care before specific therapy for a cardiac, renal, or other cause of edema is begun depends on the consequences of the edema collection. Generalized edema with dependency accumulation of fluid in the legs or abdominal or genital areas is not by itself reason for treatment. Slow accumulation of edema in nephrosis or cirrhosis generally is well tolerated. Treatment with diuretics or aldosterone inhibitors has only transient benefit in many of these chronic diseases, although such drugs may be tried if the situation demands such action. For example, if edema involves the lungs, as in heart failure, or if it may lead to a skin breakdown, as may occur in the scrotum in nephrotic syndrome, then even the temporary relief provided by diuretics is indicated. In situations in which the "effective" vascular volume may be reduced, diminishing that volume further may produce acute renal failure. Use of plasma volume expanders with colloid, followed by diuretics, often is appropriate when the plasma volume is low, but this obviously should be avoided in cases involving heart failure.

Sodium requirements should be assessed carefully. Sodium and fluid restriction may be all that is required to correct the edema and is essential in iatrogenic cases. For chronic edema, patients and parents should be taught about the sodium content of foods so that the minimum sodium necessary for palatability of food is ingested. It is good practice to maintain this diet between episodes of edema, inasmuch as patients can adjust well to a low-sodium diet, but switching back and forth is difficult. Acute episodes of edema associated with nephrotic syndrome occasionally are accompanied by irritability and changes in behavior. The self-image of the child who has chronic edema can be affected seriously, either because the edema may be interpreted as obesity in an adolescent or because the underlying disease may require changes in the patient's activities and life-style. The physician and parents should be alert for such secondary effects of edema so that they can minimize the consequences for the child.

Several of the diseases that may cause significant edema require the assistance of a specialist. However, because these patients eventually return home, the primary care physician must be available for proper continuous care. The specialist should ensure that the patient and family are familiar with the early signs of recurrence or worsening of the process. The importance of keeping accurate records of weight, urine protein excretion, and blood pressure must be explained. Most parents and patients become more comfortable with a chronic disease when they acquire a working knowledge of the disorder and can participate in the required care. With such education, the primary physician can rely more fully on the parents' observations, which are of immeasurable help in home management of edema.

REFERENCES

1. Fisher DA: Obscure and unusual edema, *Pediatrics* 37:506, 1966.
2. Perico N, Remuzzi G: Edema of the nephrotic syndrome: the role of the atrial peptide system, *Am J Kidney Dis* 22:355, 1993.
3. Starling EH: On the absorption of fluids from the connective tissue spaces, *J Physiol* 19:312, 1985.
4. Valtin H: *Renal function: mechanisms preserving fluid and solute balance in health,* ed 2, Boston, 1983, Little, Brown.

127 Epistaxis

David R. Edelstein

Epistaxis, which occurs frequently in childhood, can be a frightening experience for a parent or child. Fortunately, most nasal bleeding in childhood is minor. Severe, prolonged, or recurrent bleeding, however, can indicate a more critical problem such as a bleeding disorder or nasal tumor. Epistaxis is rare in neonates and infants, increases in incidence in childhood, and again becomes less common during adolescence.[2] It is more common in boys than in girls.[11]

The nose is a highly vascular organ with a large surface area and therefore is predisposed to bleeding. Its functions are to move air, to filter pollutants, to humidify, warm, and serve as a buffer for central structures during trauma, and to act as a resonance box in speech. Its relatively high vascularity serves to increase local blood volume, which helps to warm the temperature of inspired air, to move critical cells (e.g., like leukocytes or immunoglobulins), and to provide an expansile surface area that aids in filtration and cleaning. The most vascular areas are near the front of the nose, in the Little area, which is the site of a plexus of vessels with branches from the internal and external carotid arteries (Table 127-1). Two other critical areas of the nose are the posterolateral portion, which contains large branches of the internal maxillary artery, and a portion high in the lateral nasal vault that contains other branches of the internal carotid artery.

There are many possible causes for nasal bleeding. Fortunately, most are benign. These include mucosal irritation from weather changes and allergies, simple trauma from nose picking,[4] chronic rhinitis with nose blowing, chronic usage of nasal sprays or drying agents such as decongestants, and viral or bacterial infections. More serious epistaxis may occur as a result of blunt trauma from accidents or nasal surgery. In some cases severe or recurrent bleeds may represent a bleeding diathesis such as von Willebrand disease or a neoplasm such as nasopharyngeal angiofibroma. Distinguishing local from systemic causes is very important in order to institute early treatment and to avoid the need for a blood transfusion. The correct diagnosis may have implications for the patient's family or community because some causes of epistaxis may be genetic or result from environmental problems.

CHARACTERISTICS

The type, location, and frequency of nasal bleeding may help the physician understand its cause and danger. In 1988 Katsanis and colleagues[12] devised an epistaxis scoring system to help identify children who may need elaborate workups. This system is based on the frequency, duration, amount, and site of bleeding. Children who had high scores had a much greater chance of having a clotting abnormality.[12] Standard criteria are important in deciding whether to proceed with an elaborate evaluation for a bleeding disorder. Children who merit a high index of suspicion for a bleeding disorder need diagnostic tests beyond a complete blood count (CBC), platelet count, and prothrombin time (PT) measurement.

In most instances epistaxis is unilateral and is caused by local irritation or trauma. Bilateral epistaxis, in contrast, may be due to a bleeding disorder, a posterior source of bleeding, or severe craniofacial trauma. Gradual-onset bleeding often results from overuse of medications such as aspirin or ibuprofen in an older child or from slowly growing tumors. In contrast, sudden-onset bleeding usually is due to trauma or nose picking. Intermittent bleeding may be caused by changes in the weather, allergies, or low humidification of inspired air. It also can be associated with menses.

The location of the bleeding may be useful in determining the cause and the treatment. An anterior bleed, which can be viewed with a nasal speculum, can be treated by simple compression. In contrast, a posterior bleed can be visualized only if the anatomy of the nose is normal and adequate premedication and special instruments are used. A high nasal bleed may represent a fracture involving the nasoethmoid complex and orbit. Recurrent epistaxis may occur in a patient who has a minor bleeding disorder or in one who suffers from chronic irritation of the nasal mucosa.

ASSOCIATED SIGNS AND SYMPTOMS

Although epistaxis is a dramatic symptom, it usually is not the only one related to the nose. Other symptoms can be useful in arriving at a diagnosis. For example, a child who has a nasal obstruction and epistaxis may have a foreign body or a polyp in the nose. Obstruction also can be caused by a deviated septum, which may predispose the patient to local dryness and cracking of the mucosa. If the nasal obstruction is chronic and related to lower airway symptoms, the child may have perennial allergic rhinitis associated with asthma.

It is important to know if the patient has had facial pain or headaches. Facial pain may be present with sinusitis or an enlarging mucocele of one of the sinuses. It also can be caused by a tumor involving the nose, the sinuses, or the base of the skull, which may bleed intermittently. Headaches associated with epistaxis in infants can be caused by an encephalocele or meningocele.

Children who have trauma-induced epistaxis should be tested for visual acuity because injury to the nose or ethmoid sinuses may disrupt the lamina papyracea and injure the eye, resulting in retroorbital bleeding, orbital fractures, and damage to the eye muscles. The cribriform plate also can be fractured, which can result in meningitis, anosmia (lack of smell), or chronic leakage of cerebrospinal fluid (CSF) through the nose.

Occasionally the only symptom noticed by the parents of a child who has chronic mild epistaxis is unexplained melena. This is due to the child swallowing blood from the pos-

Table 127-1 Blood Supply of the Nose

Vessel	Location
Internal carotid artery	
Ophthalmic artery	
Anterior ethmoid	Anterosuperior septum, anterior lateral wall
Posterior ethmoid	Posterior septum, posterior lateral wall
External carotid artery	
Internal maxillary artery	
Sphenopalatine branch	Posterior septum, posterior lateral wall
Nasopalatine branch	Posterior septum, floor of the nose
Descending palatine branch	Posterior lateral wall
Pharyngeal branch	Nasopharyngeal roof
Facial artery	
Superior labial branch	Tip of septum, nasal alar

terior nares. Similarly, hematemesis can result from epistaxis when the child swallows blood.[10]

All children who have epistaxis should have their vital signs monitored closely. Hypotension and syncope-like episodes can occur if the blood loss is significant. Some children who have had chronic nasal bleeding may tolerate a surprisingly low hematocrit. Younger children and infants tolerate blood loss less well than do older children; a blood transfusion may be required in severe cases.

CIRCUMSTANCES

One of the most useful observations the physician can make is whether other members of the family have bleeding disorders or problems with epistaxis. Although episodes of epistaxis are relatively rare in the general population, they are common in patients who have coagulation disorders. Beran and Petruson[3] studied habitual nose bleeders (primarily in adults) and found that 27% had bleeding disorders, such as factor V, VII, or X deficiencies. Kiley and colleagues[13] found a 30% incidence of such disorders in a similar group of children. Families of children who have chronic bleeding may have hereditary hemorrhagic telangiectasia syndrome (Osler-Weber-Rendu disease). This is an autosomal dominant disease associated with increased fragility of small blood vessels. McCaffrey and colleagues[14] reported that 70% of patients who have this disease have a positive family history for epistaxis.

If a child has epistaxis associated with trauma, it is important to determine the type of injury that occurred. Blunt trauma with a heavy instrument to the nose may point to other facial fractures. A bicycle fall may suggest an "accordion" injury to the nose and a potential septal hematoma, which would require immediate incision and drainage. Recurrent trauma that results in epistaxis may suggest child abuse. It has been estimated that 30% of physically abused children have some form of facial trauma.[1]

CAUSES OF EPISTAXIS IN CHILDREN

Local

1. *Trauma:* nose picking, surgery (septoplasty, turbinectomy), blunt impact (fist or instrument), foreign body, child abuse, sports, auto accident
2. *Infection:* viral, bacterial, fungal, parasitic
3. *Chronic irritation:* allergies, recurrent colds, dry environment, chronic sniffers, smoking, cocaine abuse, ciliary dysfunction, chemicals, ingestion of a caustic substance
4. *Structural abnormality:* deviated septum, vomer spur, septal perforation
5. *Drugs:* topical sprays (phenylephrine, aerosol steroids), drying agents (decongestants, antihistamines)
6. *Neoplasms:* polyps, hemangiomas, rhabdomyosarcomas, angiofibromas

Systemic

1. *Bleeding diseases:* von Willebrand, coagulation factor deficiencies, vitamin deficiencies, Osler-Weber-Rendu, idiopathic thrombocytopenia, disseminated intravascular coagulation
2. *Infections:* rheumatic fever, diphtheria, malaria, measles
3. *Neoplasms:* leukemia, lymphoma
4. *Granulomas:* Wegener, midline reticulosis, tuberculosis, sarcoidosis
5. *Medications:* antiinflammatories (aspirin, ibuprofen), anticoagulants (warfarin), steroids
6. *Cancer treatment:* chemotherapy (methotrexate), radiotherapy
7. *Hormonal influences:* menses, birth control pills, pregnancy
8. *Cardiovascular disease:* hypertension, arteriosclerosis
9. *Barometric pressure changes:* scuba diving, air flight, elevator rides
10. *Miscellaneous:* liver disease, renal dysfunction, aplastic anemia, sepsis

DIFFERENTIAL DIAGNOSIS

The easiest way to conceptualize the many causes of epistaxis is to categorize them according to either local or systemic causes (see the box above). Local causes include trauma, surgery, infection, medications, or tumors. Systemic causes may be divided into bleeding disorders, other major diseases (e.g., leukemia, renal dysfunction, and hypertension), and cancer therapy (radiotherapy or chemotherapy).

Most nasal injuries in children occur at home or during sporting events. Bleeding occurs because the nasal septum is abraded. Intranasal hematomas, abscesses, and lacerations can be overlooked unless the physician carefully inspects for them. Failure to recognize an infection or a blood clot lodged in this area may result in pressure necrosis of the nasal septum and eventual external and internal nasal deformities.[18] Major facial fractures also can manifest in this way; thus a complete examination of the facial structures with the use of roentgenograms should be performed when this diagnosis is considered.

Occasionally epistaxis may occur after surgery. Postoperative bleeding from the tonsils and adenoids can mimic epistaxis. Septal surgery, rhinoplasty, and turbinectomies also can lead to postoperative bleeding among adolescents. Whenever a child undergoes nasotracheal intubation, the nasal mucosa may be torn, which can lead to bleeding.

Chronic nasal irritation as a result of infection, allergies, or drugs can cause epistaxis. Local mucosal cellulitis and failure of the mucociliary lining of the nose to function properly after an infection may cause the Little area to become dry and cracked. Children who have chronic rhinorrhea may rub their noses frequently, thereby irritating the septum significantly. Chronic irritation also can occur from overuse of topical antiallergic sprays (e.g., cromolyn sulfate and dexamethasone). Schwartz and colleagues[20] have reported that 27% of adolescents who snorted cocaine routinely complained of recurrent epistaxis. Cocaine causes local infection, chronic necrosis of the mucosa and septum, and foreign body reactions and destroys nasal ciliary function.

A variety of nasal masses can cause bloody rhinorrhea in children. Hemangiomas, which are among the most common benign tumors of the nose during childhood, can cause epistaxis. Juvenile angiofibromas should be considered in adolescent boys who have unilateral spontaneous epistaxis and a nasopharyngeal mass. Neel and colleagues[16] have reported that 73% of boys who had this diagnosis had epistaxis. Angiofibromas can be differentiated from benign choanoantral polyps by computed tomography (CT) scanning using a contrast medium. Blind biopsies of the nasopharynx should be avoided because of the risk of life-threatening epistaxis. The most common benign growths of the nose—antral choanal polyps—and the most common malignant lesions—rhabdomyosarcomas—usually are not associated with epistaxis.[19]

Excessive nasal bleeding may be caused by a variety of acquired or inherited bleeding disorders. Aspirin can cause a relative platelet dysfunction that results in a prolonged bleeding time. Deficiencies of vitamins C and K also can predispose a child to epistaxis because of blood vessel changes and coagulopathies, respectively. Thrombocytopenia can occur after use of sulfasoxazole, chloroquine, carbamazepine, estrogens, and thiazide diuretics. Ingesting toxic substances and eating certain foods such as beans can lead to thrombocytopenia. Viral illnesses may cause idiopathic thrombocytopenic purpura. The most common inherited bleeding disorders that cause epistaxis in children are von Willebrand disease and factor XI deficiency (hemophilia C). Less common disorders are factor VIII deficiency (hemophilia A) and factor IX deficiency (hemophilia B, or Christmas disease).[15]

Severe epistaxis is a common feature of Osler-Weber-Rendu disease (hereditary hemorrhagic telangiectasia). More than 81% of a series of patients from the Mayo Clinic who had this disease had epistaxis. The disease usually occurs with bleeding, skin telangiectasias, and a family history of the condition. McCaffrey and colleagues[14] reported that these symptoms can appear in childhood but usually do not begin until after age 15. Epistaxis is caused by defects in the walls of small mucosal vessels.

Epistaxis may occur in immunocompromised children. Leukemia and lymphomas that involve the bone marrow can lead to thrombocytopenia and concomitant bleeding. In addition, the chemotherapeutic agents used to treat these malignant diseases (e.g., methotrexate and cyclophosphamide) can cause thrombocytopenia. Radiotherapy often causes cracking, irritation in the nasal mucosa, and bleeding.

As noted, epistaxis has many causes. The patient's age and the circumstances that surround the onset of bleeding are important clues to the diagnosis. In neonates the most common cause is birth trauma, especially if forceps are used. Frequently the bleeding is caused by deflection of the nasal septum, which can be manipulated gently back into position or left as is if no deformity results. In childhood, simple nose picking or blunt trauma are the most common causes. In early adolescence, boys have a higher incidence of nasal tumors, such as angiofibromas, than do girls. Pubescent girls may have occasional bleeding during their menses.

MANAGEMENT

The basic approach to treatment of children who have epistaxis should incorporate the "two Cs"—calmness and compression. The patient should be reassured during the history-taking and the assessment of his or her general condition and the amount of blood loss. Most bleeding can be stopped by having the child sit upright and gently squeezing the anterior nose for 5 minutes. Blood pressure and other vital signs should be taken. Blood tests and roentgenograms should be performed only if the bleeding cannot be stopped with simple pressure or anterior or posterior nasal packing. The first few minutes should be used to stem the bleeding while assessing its cause.

Once the initial bleeding has slowed, the nose should be examined more carefully with a nasal speculum and headlight. A simple solution of phenylephrine (¼%, ½%) can be sprayed into the nose for local vasoconstriction to control further bleeding and to help clear any clots that may have formed. A 1% epinephrine solution with or without lidocaine can be used for the same purpose if required. Nose blowing should be avoided even though the nose will feel quite congested. Bleeding sites in the Little area can be cauterized electrically or with silver nitrate sticks. If either form of cautery is used, the septum should be covered with a petroleum jelly–based antibiotic ointment to provide a moist environment for optimum healing. Care should be taken to clean any excess silver nitrate from the anterior nares because it will discolor the skin and may frighten the child and family.

If these simple measures fail to control the bleeding, the next step is placing bilateral anterior nasal packing, using a ½-inch gauze covered with petroleum jelly. Although this is not pleasant for the child, it is a highly effective way to stop anterior nasal bleeding. Bilateral packing is recommended to provide the greatest compression of the anterior septum. When packing is used, antibiotics should be given to prevent sinusitis. The packing usually is left in place for 3 days.

Prepackaged surgical or Avitene-containing gauze can be used as additional hemostatic agents if bleeding persists. Another type of preformed packing, Mercel (Mercel Corp.), is a compressed sponge that expands when wet, exerting pressure on the nasal lining. This sponge comes in many sizes, can be cut down to fit a child's nose, and is easily placed, especially when the child is agitated. Its use is limited by its tendency to adhere to the nasal lining; it must be used with antibiotics to prevent staphylococcal toxic shock and should be removed within 48 hours.[23] All of these agents may be the treatment of choice for patients in whom standard nasal packing might promote more bleeding by destroying the lining of the nose. This group of children includes those undergoing renal dialysis and those who are severely immunocompromised.

Recurrent anterior nasal bleeding or posterior bleeding can be controlled with placement of either posterior or nasopharyngeal balloons. Posterior packs are made from gauze pads inserted through the mouth into the nasopharynx and secured by ties through the nose. Whenever they are used, an anterior pack also is placed. Unfortunately, these standard packs may cause a drop in oxygenation and discomfort for the patient.[7] The balloon catheters are easier to position. Small Foley catheters can be used and filled with methylene blue–stained saline. The methylene blue indicates that the Foley balloon has burst accidently. Cook and colleagues[8] reported that use of balloons reduced the average hospital stay from 12.5 to 5.6 days.

Severe bleeding that does not respond to packing should prompt the physician to consider a different diagnosis and perhaps use more invasive therapeutic procedures. The use of tests for bleeding disorders, including determination of bleeding time, prothrombin time, partial thromboplastin time, and platelet count, as well as other hematological studies, should be based on the family history. Roentgenographic studies should be reviewed for mass lesions, bone erosion, and other bony abnormalities. Angiographic examination of the internal and external carotid arteries should be considered.

Nasal endoscopy may enhance the physician's examination of the nose. Fiberoptic and rigid endoscopes are routine instruments in the office of most otolaryngologists. In an older child or adolescent who has posterior bleeding, rigid endoscopy combined with intranasal suction cautery may help control difficult bleeding.[5,17] The advantage of this technique is that bleeding can be controlled under direct visualization. The limitations are the absence of appropriate-size pediatric instruments in most otolaryngologists' offices and the difficulty obtaining the patient's cooperation.

Embolization with nonresorbable (usually plaster), spherical pellets can be used if a discrete bleeding source or a vascular tumor is discovered. Embolization is a useful procedure with hereditary hemorrhagic telangiectasia, juvenile angiofibromas, hemangiomas, vascular metastatic lesions, arteriovenous malformations, and traumatic arterial tears.[6,9] The failure rate for embolization for difficult bleeding has been reported to be less than 5%, compared with reports of a 14% failure rate for artery ligation and up to 25% failure for anterior nasal packing.[21,22]

Persistent posterior nasal bleeding from the sphenopalatine artery sometimes requires ligation of the internal maxillary artery.[15] This type of bleeding after trauma, which may be due to a tear of the anterior ethmoid artery, requires surgical ligation for control. Children may be more prone to traumatic tears of the anterior ethmoid artery because of immature bony development of the face and congenital dehiscences around the artery.

Although the goals of epistaxis management are to stop the bleeding and to determine its cause, the care of the patient often continues after the bleeding stops. Blood replacement or iron supplements may be required, and humidifying medications such as saline nasal sprays and petroleum jelly–based ointments often are needed to promote healing and subsequent adequate nasal mucociliary function. Children who have had severe epistaxis should be reexamined frequently to determine if further therapy is necessary. Recurrence of epistaxis can be prevented only if its many causes are considered and appropriate preventive measures are instituted.

REFERENCES

1. Becker DB, Needleman H, Kotelchuck M: Child abuse: orofacial trauma and its recognition by dentists, *J Am Dent Assoc* 97:24, 1978.
2. Behrman RE, Vaughan VC III: *Nelson's textbook of pediatrics,* ed 12, 1983, WB Saunders.
3. Beran M, Petruson B: Changes in the nasal mucosa of habitual nose-bleeders, *Acta Otolaryngol (Stockh)* 102:308, 1986.
4. Beran M, Stigendal L, Petruson B: Haemostatic disorders in habitual nose-bleeders, *J Laryngol Otol* 101:1020, 1987.
5. Bingham B, Dingle AF: Endoscopic management of severe epistaxis, *J Otolaryngol* 20:442, 1991.
6. Breda SD et al: Embolization in the treatment of epistaxis after failure of internal maxillary artery ligation, *Laryngoscope* 99:809, 1989.
7. Cassisi NJ, Biller HF, Ogura JH: Changes in arterial oxygen tension and pulmonary mechanics with the use of posterior packing in epistaxis: a preliminary report, *Laryngoscope* 81:1261, 1971.
8. Cook PR, Renner G, Williams F: A comparison of nasal balloons and posterior gauze packs for posterior epistaxis, *Ear Nose Throat J* 64:79, 1985.
9. Davis KR: Embolization of epistaxis and juvenile nasopharyngeal angiofibromas, *Am J Roentgenol* 148:209, 1987.
10. Hutchison SMW, Finlayson NDC: Epistaxis as a cause of hematemesis and melena, *J Clin Gastroenterol* 9:283, 1987.
11. Juselius H: Epistaxis—a clinical study of 1,724 patients, *J Laryngol Otol* 88:317, 1974.
12. Katsanis E et al: Prevalence and significance of mild bleeding disorders in children with recurrent epistaxis, *J Pediatr* 113:73, 1988.
13. Kiley V, Stuart JJ, Johnson CA: Coagulation studies in children with isolated recurrent epistaxis, *J Pediatr* 100:579, 1982.
14. McCaffrey TV, Kern EB, Lake CF: Management of epistaxis in hereditary hemorrhagic telangiectasia, *Arch Otolaryngol* 103:627, 1977.
15. McDonald TJ, Pearson BW: Follow-up on maxillary artery ligation for epistaxis, *Arch Otolaryngol* 106:635, 1980.
16. Neel HB III et al: Juvenile angiofibroma: review of 120 cases, *Am J Surg* 126:547, 1973.
17. O'Leary-Stickney K, Makielski K, Weymuller EA Jr: Rigid endoscopy for the control of epistaxis, *Arch Otolaryngol Head Neck Surg* 118:966, 1992.
18. Olsen KD, Carpenter RJ, Kern EB: Nasal septal injury in children, diagnosis and management, *Arch Otolaryngol* 106:317, 1980.
19. Schramm VL: Inflammatory and neoplastic masses of the nose and paranasal sinus in children, *Laryngoscope* 89:1887, 1979.
20. Schwartz RH et al: Nasal symptoms associated with cocaine abuse during adolescence, *Arch Otolaryngol* 115:63, 1989.
21. Wang L, Vogel DH: Posterior epistaxis: comparison of treatment, *Otolaryngol Head Neck Surg* 89:1001, 1981.
22. Welsh LW et al: Role of angiography in the management of refractory epistaxis, *Ann Otol Rhinol Laryngol* 99:69, 1990.
23. Wurman LH et al: The management of epistaxis, *Am J Otolaryngol* 13:193, 1992.

SUGGESTED READINGS

Guarisco JL, Graham HD III: Epistaxis in children: causes, diagnosis and treatment, *Ear Nose Throat J* 68:522, 1989.

McDonald TJ: Nosebleed in children: background and techniques to stop the flow, *Postgrad Med* 81:217, 1987.

128 Extremity Pain

Michael G. Burke

Extremity pain is a common complaint in primary care pediatric practice. Up to 15% of school-age children report a history of occasional limb pain,[3] and 4.5% have reported that their normal activities had been interrupted for longer than 3 months because of limb pain.[6] Pain in an extremity accounted for 7% of office visits to pediatricians.[4] Fortunately, most of these visits involve pain that occurs because of minor trauma. Occasionally, however, limb pain is the presenting complaint of a systemic illness, a neoplasm, an infectious process, a nutritional derangement, or a specific orthopedic disease. The challenge for the practitioner is to determine when the pain is significant without exposing the child to excessive diagnostic studies and without delaying treatment or referral. For the most part, this determination is based on the history and physical examination.

HISTORY

Both the patient's and the parents' description of the extremity pain may help in determining the cause. Pain described as aching or cramping is likely to have a muscular origin. Bone pain often is described as deep, and nerve pain as burning, tingling, or numbness. The location of the pain, although usually helpful, may be deceiving because referred pain is common in children. Migrating extremity pain is less likely to occur secondary to trauma and is more typical of systemic illness such as leukemia, acute rheumatic fever, disseminated gonorrhea, and arthralgia or arthritis associated with inflammatory bowel disease. The mode of onset, variability, duration, and frequency of pain also help in diagnosing its cause. Activities associated with worsening or relief of pain also can lead to a diagnosis. Likewise, color change associated with extremity pain may indicate inflammation (faint red), infection (intense red), or autonomic dysfunction (pallor, cyanosis, and erythema). Stiffness not associated with trauma should prompt concern about a rheumatological process.

A history specific to trauma associated with extremity pain can be quite helpful. Trauma accompanied by an audible "pop" or "snap" is more likely to result in a sprain or fracture. Mild trauma that leads to a fracture might indicate some previous defect in the bone, as with a pathological fracture. As always, if the physical findings of trauma are greater than would be expected from the history, physical abuse must be considered.

The child's general health history is needed to complete the picture of extremity pain. For example, the differential diagnosis changes with age. Toxic synovitis of the hip is a common diagnosis in a child under age 10; a slipped capital femoral epiphysis is more likely in an adolescent.

As a screen for systemic disease, all systems should be reviewed. Particular attention should be paid to a history of fever, recent weight loss, sweats, rashes, and gastrointestinal symptoms. A history of recent medications is important and might reveal a serum sickness–like illness (particularly associated with cefaclor). Even a short course of systemic steroids can cause aseptic necrosis of the hip or can result in demineralization of bone and the pain associated with osteoporosis. Immunizations, particularly for rubella, may cause joint or extremity pain, and a history of exposure to viral illness might explain myalgia or arthralgia. Specifically, the prodrome of hepatitis B can cause significant arthralgia.

The patient's family history may reveal a tendency toward autoimmune disease or recent exposure to infectious diseases. The family history particularly is helpful in identifying hemoglobinopathies. A family history of sickle cell anemia in a 6- to 24-month-old child whose hands and feet are painfully swollen may lead to the diagnosis of hand-foot syndrome and previously undiagnosed sickle cell disease. A sickle cell pain crisis always must be considered in a black child or one of Mediterranean origin who has a painful extremity. HLA-B27 is associated with Reiter syndrome or ankylosing spondylitis and has been described in association with peripheral enthesitis (inflammation of tendons, ligaments, or fascia at their attachments to bone).[5] Joint hypermobility syndrome and fibromyalgia also can be familial.

Occasionally, extremity pain is a symptom of a functional disorder and can serve as an entry to the physician's office for the child or parent who has a hidden agenda. The history may be either quite dramatic or highly understated. Pain in a nonanatomical distribution or that disturbs unpleasant but not pleasant activities (waxing on school days and waning on weekends) should raise suspicion of a functional disorder. Eliciting a history of recent events at home, recent school performance, and other social history therefore can be essential.

PHYSICAL EXAMINATION

It is worthwhile to do a brief general physical examination, even if the history points to extremity pain from minor local trauma. Abnormalities in blood pressure, heart rate, or growth pattern can reveal an endocrine cause. An elevated resting heart rate is associated with rheumatic fever. Pallor, fever, lymphadenopathy, or organomegaly may be clues to systemic disease. A rash, particularly, may be helpful. Dermatomyositis occurs with muscle pain and proximal weakness associated with a vasculitic rash on the extensor surfaces of knuckles, knees, and elbows (Gottron papules). Palpable purpura and extremity pain are associated with Schönlein-Henoch purpura. A photosensitive rash in a child who has limb pain might point to systemic lupus erythematosus (SLE), dermatomyositis, or parvovirus infection. Nail pitting is associated with psoriasis, a rare cause of extremity pain.

A thorough eye examination can help diagnose Kawasaki

disease and juvenile rheumatoid arthritis (JRA), each of which may cause extremity pain. A complete physical examination can reveal generalized joint laxity and hyperextensibility, differentiating benign hypermobility syndrome from a focal ligament injury. In benign hypermobility syndrome, the joint laxity allows chronic hyperextension, which can cause pain, often located in the popliteal fossa. The pain often is worse in the evening and can be relieved by exercise that tightens the joint. This syndrome, particularly, is common in gymnasts and dancers.

Claudication is a rare cause of extremity pain in children. However, in popliteal artery entrapment syndrome, vascular calf pain that radiates to the foot is associated with an anomalous popliteal artery or anomalous placement of the gastrocnemius muscle.[1] The pain begins with activity, sometimes more with walking than with running. This syndrome is suggested if normal pedal pulses are lost with simultaneous knee extension and foot plantar flexion.

Because referred pain is common in children, the physical examination should include areas proximal and distal to the site of the complaint. A slipped capital femoral epiphysis and Legg-Calvé-Perthes disease, both of which affect the hip, can manifest as knee or lateral thigh pain, whereas an abscess of the psoas muscle may cause hip pain. Some abdominal processes and diskitis also may cause extremity pain.

Examination of a painful extremity should include assessment of peripheral vascular status, muscle strength, and skeletal and joint integrity. Peripheral vascular status is assessed by palpating the pulses and determining the capillary refill time distal to the pain. Skin color and warmth, whether there is pain upon palpation, and the extent of passive and active range of motion should be ascertained. Point tenderness over a bone raises suspicion of a fracture. Point tenderness in the absence of a clear history of trauma may indicate osteomyelitis. It is helpful to compare the opposite limb when assessing swelling, muscle wasting, or joint mobility. Observing the patient's gait or use of the painful limb when he or she is unaware helps in diagnosing a functional process. In evaluating strength, it is important to remember that isolated distal weakness is likely to be of neurological origin, whereas proximal weakness most likely is due to a muscular disease. Finally, with chronic extremity pain, serial examinations of the patient over the course of weeks can be the key to diagnosis.

LABORATORY AND ROENTGENOGRAPHIC EVALUATION

Laboratory studies are unnecessary for most extremity pain. However, if the history and physical examination do not lead to a definitive diagnosis, if they raise suspicion of a systemic or an infectious disease, or if the pain persists longer than anticipated, screening laboratory tests are in order. A basic evaluation should include a complete blood count (CBC), a sedimentation rate, and a sickle cell preparation or hemoglobin electrophoresis when indicated. Rheumatological studies should be considered if the aforementioned diseases are suspected or if the pain becomes chronic. An elevated sedimentation rate raises suspicion of an infectious or inflammatory disorder, or occasionally of a neoplastic one. A C-reactive protein or an alkaline phosphatase test also can be done. A CBC may reveal anemia or may suggest an infectious disease. With leukemia the white blood cell (WBC) count varies, but immature forms or worrisome thrombocytopenia may be present in the differential WBC count. A creatine phosphokinase (CPK) determination occasionally is indicated if muscular pain is suspected.

Radiological studies often are unnecessary in evaluating limb pain. The tendency to obtain numerous radiographs is reinforced, however, because traumatic injury that ordinarily would cause only a sprain in an adult is more likely to result in a greenstick or buckle fracture in a child. Rivara and colleagues[7] have proposed criteria for obtaining roentgenograms with extremity pain that occurs after trauma. By retrospectively analyzing 189 children who had 209 extremity injuries, they concluded that the presence of point tenderness and/or gross deformity in an upper extremity injury identified 81% of children who had fractures. Their absence predicted 82% who did not have fractures. For lower extremity injuries, the presence of a gross deformity and/or pain on motion of the leg identified 97% of fractures. Absence of both indicators correctly ruled out a fracture in 97% of cases. This study speaks for reducing the number of roentgenograms obtained when evaluating extremity pain. However, posttraumatic pain that fails to resolve as expected should be evaluated radiographically, regardless of whether the aforementioned criteria are met.

When there is no clear history of trauma, roentgenograms can help identify bony tumors, pathological fractures, some metabolic defects, and a number of orthopedic conditions. The timing of the roentgenogram depends on the pediatrician's degree of concern, as established by the history and physical examination.

A bone scan is a useful diagnostic tool in evaluating limb pain, and one should be obtained when a stress fracture or osteomyelitis is suspected. Bone scans are more sensitive than plain roentgenograms for establishing these diagnoses.

DIFFERENTIAL DIAGNOSIS

The differential diagnosis of extremity pain is extremely broad (see the box on p. 942). However, most limb pain is benign, requires no intervention, and is self-limited. Characteristic patterns of pain and associated signs and symptoms signal the presence of certain diseases and conditions. A discussion of some of these disorders follows.

Growing Pains

"Growing pains" are a time-honored pediatric disorder. They are intermittent, deep extremity pains that affect the lower more often than the upper extremities. The pain nearly always is bilateral, rarely involves the joints, and almost universally is worse at night, resolving completely in the morning. Despite their name, growing pains do not occur most frequently during periods of rapid growth. Instead, their onset is described at 3 to 5 or 8 to 12 years of age. Most growing pains resolve in 12 to 24 months; however, they may persist into adolescence.

The cause of growing pains remains unclear. A previous emphasis on a psychological cause recently has given way to an emphasis on an overuse type of injury. Apparent worsening of the pain during times of increased activity and re-

EXTREMITY PAIN IN CHILDHOOD: A DIFFERENTIAL DIAGNOSIS

Allergy/collagen-vascular origin

Dermatomyositis
Familial Mediterranean fever
Inflammatory bowel disease
Juvenile rheumatoid arthritis
Mixed connective tissue disease
Polyarteritis nodosa
Rheumatic fever
Schönlein-Henoch purpura
Scleroderma
Serum sickness
Systemic lupus erythematosus

Congenital origin

Caffey disease
Hemophilia
Mucolipidosis
Mucopolysaccharidosis
Popliteal artery entrapment syndrome
Sickle cell anemia/thalassemia

Endocrine origin

Hypercortisolism
Hyperparathyroidism
Hypothyroidism

Idiopathic origin

Fibromyalgia
Growing pains
Sarcoidosis

Infectious origin

- Bacterial
  - Arthralgia/myalgia associated with streptococcal infection
  - Diskitis
  - Gonorrhea
  - Osteomyelitis
  - Pyogenic myositis
  - Septic arthritis
- Enteric disease
- Histoplasmosis
- Immunization reaction
- Kawasaki disease
- Lyme disease
- Meningococcal disease
- Syphilis: periostitis
- Trichinosis
- Tuberculosis
- Viral
  - Myalgia/arthralgia
  - Myositis
  - Toxic synovitis

Metabolic origin

Carnitine palmitoyl transferase deficiency
Fabry disease
McArdle syndrome
Phosphofructokinase deficiency

Neoplastic origin

- Histiocytosis X
- Leukemia
- Lymphoma
- Neuroblastoma
- Tumors of bone
  - Chondrosarcoma
  - Ewing sarcoma
  - Osteoblastoma (benign)
  - Osteogenic sarcoma
  - Osteoid osteoma (benign)
- Tumors of soft tissue
  - Fibrosarcoma
  - Rhabdomyosarcoma
  - Synovial cell sarcoma
- Tumors of the spinal cord

Nutritional origin

Gout
Hypercholesterolemia
Hypervitaminosis A
Osteoporosis
Rickets (vitamin D)
Scurvy (vitamin C)

Orthopedic origin

Chondromalacia patellae
Freiberg disease
Inflexible flat feet/tarsal coalition
Köhler disease
Legg-Calvé-Perthes disease
Osgood-Schlatter disease
Osteochondritis dissecans
Osteogenesis imperfecta
Pathological fracture
Sever disease
Slipped capital femoral epiphysis

Psychosocial origin

Behavior disorders
Psychogenic pain
Reflex neurovascular dystrophy
School phobia

Trauma/overuse

Carpal tunnel syndrome
Cervical disk syndrome
Compartment syndrome
Fracture
Hypermobility syndrome
Myohematoma
Myositis ossificans
Physical abuse
Shin splint
Sprain
Stress fracture
Subluxed radial head
Thoracic outlet syndrome

Modified from Bowyer SL, Hollister JR: *Pediatr Clin North Am* 31:5, 1984.

lief through use of heat and massage seem to support a physical cause. However, headache and abdominal pain—often associated with emotional illnesses—also have accompanied growing pains.

The diagnosis of growing pains is significant for its lack of associated physical signs. Thus any abnormal finding on physical examination should provoke a search for another cause. Similarly, roentgenograms and the results of screening laboratory tests should prove normal. Treatment involves heat, massage, and analgesics.

Sprains

A sprain is a physical disruption of a ligament. This is a less common occurrence in children than in adults because a child's open epiphyseal plate or plastic bony cortex tends to give way more easily than does ligament. Therefore, Salter fractures and buckle fractures should be considered when the history indicates a sprain and physical examination reveals tenderness on palpation or pain on stretching of the ligament. Joint stability also should be assessed. Sprains can be graded according to the degree of associated ligament disruption. A mild, microscopic tear that results in no laxity of the involved joint is a grade I sprain. Grade II sprains involve macroscopic but incomplete ligament tears. Joint laxity is greater, but there is less than a 5 mm movement differential between the strained and the contralateral joint. Grade III sprains result in more than 5 mm of increased mobility of the affected joint compared with the contralateral one. Grade I sprains can be treated by the primary practitioner, using icing and wrapping of the involved joint to minimize swelling. Early range of motion exercises should be encouraged, with a gradual return to activity. The return of pain indicates too rapid a return to a given level of activity. Grade II and grade III sprains generally should be referred to an orthopedist for immobilization and consideration of surgical repair of torn ligaments.

Overuse Syndromes

Overuse injuries have become more common as physical fitness has become popular nationwide. Localized, gradually increasing, persistent extremity pain that worsens with weight bearing, exercise, and activity but that diminishes with rest can indicate a stress fracture. *Stress fractures* are rare in children under age 12. They most commonly affect the second metatarsal, the proximal tibia, or the fibula. Although a roentgenogram may show normal findings, a bone scan can help establish the diagnosis. Treatment consists mostly of rest and treatment with nonsteroidal antiinflammatory agents. Casting or splinting occasionally is necessary.

Little League elbow is an overuse injury caused by the repetitive motion of pitching a baseball; this motion compresses the radial aspect of the elbow and stretches the ulnar aspect. The result is painful inflammation of the epicondyles. The range of joint motion also may be diminished. Fragments of bone splintered into the joint may cause the joint to "catch" or "lock." Treatment consists of resting the arm by avoiding the repetitive movement. A change in pitching technique may reduce recurrences. To prevent this problem, some Little League systems limit the number of innings a youngster may pitch in one game.

Shin splints also are caused by overuse. The term originally referred to pain along the posteromedial aspect of the tibia as a result of irritation at the origin of the posterior tibial muscle. Shin splints now refer to any of a series of painful overuse syndromes of the lower portion of the leg, including irritation of the posterior or anterior tibial muscle, inflammation of the interosseous membrane located between the tibia and fibula, and both anterior and posterior compartment syndromes. All can cause pain in the lower extremities. The condition, which is exacerbated by running and jumping, occurs most commonly at the beginning of a training season. Although the pain occurs initially after activity, it may occur during or before activity as the syndrome progresses. On examination, there may be tenderness over the posteromedial aspect of the tibia, at the site of origin of the posterior tibia, or over the anterior tibia. Treatment involves rest, application of ice, and antiinflammatory drugs. For runners, training on a softer surface or with better quality running shoes may help.

Subluxation of the Radial Head

Nursemaids' elbow is a common injury in toddlers. The injury usually follows sudden, forceful traction of the hand or forearm. The traction pulls the immature radial head briefly from the cuff formed by the annular ligament. Release of the force allows the radius to trap the ligament against the capitellum. A patient who can talk usually indicates that the pain is in the elbow or, occasionally, the wrist. More often the child refuses to use the extremity and holds the arm with the elbow flexed, the forearm close to the chest, and the hand in pronation. The diagnosis usually is made by history alone. Although roentgenograms are not helpful, occasionally they are obtained to rule out a fracture if the history is unclear or if attempts to reduce the subluxation are unsuccessful. The practitioner can reduce the subluxation by using one hand to supinate the patient's forearm quickly while simultaneously exerting traction on the forearm and using the thumb of the other hand to create pressure over the patient's radial head. This latter maneuver is accomplished simultaneously with pronation of the patient's forearm; it is completed by placing the elbow through full extension and flexion while maintaining pressure over the radial head. Normal use of the extremity usually returns within 30 minutes. The rapid recovery is dramatic and rewarding to the parents and the physician. A prompt return to normal may not occur if the subluxation has been present for some time because of swelling of the ligament. In such instances the affected arm should be placed in a simple sling and positioned across the upper portion of the abdomen for 12 to 24 hours. Referral to an orthopedist rarely is required.

Slipped Capital Femoral Epiphysis

A slipped capital femoral epiphysis is caused by a sudden or gradual dislocation of the head of the femur from its neck and shaft at the level of the upper epiphyseal plate. The characteristic pain occurs in the affected hip or the medial aspect of the ipsilateral knee. The displacement may be sudden, in which case the pain usually is severe and associated with inability to bear weight. Gradual displacement is associated with slowly increasing, dull pain. This condition typically affects sedentary, obese adolescent boys. The physical examination may reveal diminished abduction and internal rotation of the hip. The diagnosis is made roentgenographically. Management involves surgical placement of a pin through the femoral head and the epiphysis to prevent further slippage. Avascular necrosis of the femoral head is a common complication, even with early recognition and treatment.

Toxic Synovitis

Toxic synovitis, a self-limited inflammation of the hip joint, commonly occurs in children under age 2. The cause is unknown, but inasmuch as it often occurs within 2 weeks after an upper respiratory infection, a viral inflammatory process is suspected. It usually occurs in a toddler who refuses to walk because of apparent pain in the hip. The hip is held in flexion, abduction, and external rotation. Findings may include a slight elevation in the WBC count and the sedimentation rate—a frustrating development for the practitioner, who hopes to rule out septic arthritis, a concern that may lead to consultation with an orthopedist. Treatment consists of bed rest, usually for fewer than 4 days. In rare cases avascular necrosis of the femoral head may be a late complication.

Osteochondrosis

Osteochondrosis includes a group of disorders in which degeneration or aseptic necrosis of bone and overlying cartilage occurs at an ossification center and is followed by recalcification. The disorders vary in name and presentation according to their locations.

Legg-Calvé-Perthes disease, or osteochondrosis of the femoral head, results from compromise of the tenuous vascular supply to the area. The condition may be idiopathic or may result from a slipped capital femoral epiphysis, trauma, steroid use, sickle cell crisis, or congenital dislocation of the hip. Toxic synovitis also is associated with subsequent Legg-Calvé-Perthes disease, but again this is rare. After compromise of the vascular supply, the bone underlying the articular surface of the head of the femur becomes necrotic. Collapse of the necrotic bone flattens the femoral head and causes a poor fit with the acetabulum, even after new bone is formed. The pain associated with Legg-Calvé-Perthes disease, which results from necrosis of the involved bone, frequently is referred to the medial aspect of the ipsilateral knee. A limp may be the presenting complaint. Often an early diagnosis eludes the practitioner because roentgenographic findings may be normal or show only swelling of the joint's capsule. A bone scan may demonstrate diminished blood flow to the femoral head compared with the contralateral hip. Later, radiographs may show areas of bone resorption, irregular widening of the epiphysis, or dense new bone formation. The goal of therapy is to prevent flattening of the femoral head by allowing it to undergo new bone formation. This is accomplished by keeping the hip abducted so that the head of the femur is held well inside the rounded portion of the acetabulum. Either bracing or an osteotomy may accomplish this goal; both require referral to an orthopedic surgeon.

Two similar processes can affect the knee joint. *Osteochondritis dissecans* involves degeneration of bone and cartilage at the articular surface of the knee, particularly at the lateral aspect of the medial condyle of the femur. Knee pain and crepitus, caused by loose bone and cartilage fragments in the joint, can result. *Chondromalacia patellae* occurs because of a painful softening or breakdown of the inner surface of the patella. The pain is localized to the knee and increases with activities that require prolonged knee bending and even with prolonged sitting. The pain is described as grinding. It sometimes can be elicited by applying pressure over the patella. Crepitus sometimes can be felt by moving the patella from side to side over the knee joint. Treatment usually is limited to relieving pain and reassuring the patient that in time the condition will resolve. Exercise to strengthen the medial quadriceps muscles may promote better alignment of the patella with the knee and thereby diminish the pain. In severe cases, the patella may have to be realigned surgically. Osteochondrosis of the growth plate of the calcaneus, *Sever disease,* can produce heel pain that worsens with activity. This usually mild process requires only padding of the heel to relieve the pain. Avascular necrosis and osteochondrosis of the tarsal navicular *(Köhler disease)* and of the head of the second metatarsal *(Freiberg disease)* can cause foot pain. Treatment usually requires only pain medication and rest.

Osgood-Schlatter disease is a painful degeneration of the tibial tubercle at the site of insertion of the quadriceps ligament. It is characterized by painful swelling of the anterior aspect of the tibial tubercle. Usually it occurs during adolescence. The degree of swelling may be alarming, and the area is tender to palpation. Pain is exacerbated by activity that involves increased use of the quadriceps muscles. The process is self-limited and resolves toward the end of adolescence when the epiphysis at the insertion site closes and the bone becomes stronger than the inserted ligament. Until it resolves, the condition is treated with rest and analgesics. In rare cases casting or surgical attachment of the quadriceps ligament is required.

Osteomyelitis

Osteomyelitis is a local infection of bone, usually involving one of the long bones. The highest incidence is in children 3 to 12 years of age. Although infection often occurs by hematogenous seeding, it can be caused by direct entry after local trauma. In both children and adults the most commonly isolated organism is *Staphylococcus aureus*. However, *Haemophilus influenzae* type b, *Salmonella* species, and group A streptococci all can infect the bone. Group B streptococcus is more likely the cause of infection in newborns. Although osteomyelitis caused by *Salmonella* organisms tends to occur more often in children who have sickle cell anemia than in other children, *S. aureus* is the most common etiological agent, even in this group. In trauma from a puncture wound to the foot, especially through a sneaker, *Pseudomonas aeruginosa* must be considered. In addition, tuberculous osteomyelitis still occurs and may become more common with the resurgence of tuberculosis.

Osteomyelitis can manifest as extremity pain alone or extremity pain with signs of a systemic infectious disease (fever, irritability, septic appearance). In the absence of systemic signs, it often is difficult to distinguish between osteomyelitis and a traumatic cause of the pain. It may take 2 weeks or longer for roentgenographic evidence of osteomyelitis to develop. A bone scan usually, but not always, is diagnostic. In rare cases a reduction in perfusion caused by pressure from the exudative process may result in false negative scans. In addition, the WBC count and sedimentation rate often are elevated in osteomyelitis. The effectiveness of treatment can be monitored by following the sedimentation rate serially.

Management involves collecting culture specimens from the blood, the overlying cellulitis, and the bone itself to determine the causative organism, followed by initiation of antibiotic therapy, which is continued for as long as 6 weeks. A tuberculin skin test is recommended, especially in high-risk groups.

Neoplasms

A neoplasm rarely is the cause of limb pain; however, the possibility of its presence is a common concern in cases of severe limb pain, inasmuch as pain is a symptom in benign and malignant bone tumors and systemic malignancies.

Osteoid osteoma is a benign bone tumor that occurs most often in adolescents. It usually involves the femur or tibia and occurs unilaterally. Pain, the presenting complaint, initially is dull and increases in intensity to deep and "boring." The pain is more intense at night and with weight bearing. Roentgenographic findings of sclerotic bone around a lucent center are diagnostic of this condition; sometimes tomograms are required for confirmation. Surgical excision is curative.

Systemic neoplasms in which extremity pain occurs include leukemia and metastatic neuroblastoma. One third of children who have acute lymphocytic leukemia have bone pain at the time of diagnosis, and in one fourth, joint or bone pain is a significant presenting complaint.[2] Unrelenting, increasing pain that worsens at night or with rest and that is not relieved by analgesics, heat, or massage may indicate the presence of a metastatic bone tumor. Systemic signs (weight loss, pallor, lymphadenopathy, hepatosplenomegaly, or fever) may accompany the pain. In leukemia, examination of the extremity may reveal strikingly little to account for the degree of pain. Radiographic studies of the extremities may show lucent "leukemic lines" in the subepiphyseal area.

Primary malignant tumors of bone may cause severe unilateral pain, with swelling and tenderness at the site. This supports the use of radiographic studies when unilateral limb pain is not explained adequately by a history of trauma and when pain from trauma does not resolve as expected. The peak incidence of both osteogenic sarcoma and the less common Ewing sarcoma occurs in late childhood and during adolescence. The roentgenogram in osteogenic sarcoma may reveal a tumor in the metaphysis with the presence of both radiolucent and radiopaque areas. The characteristic "sunburst" results from extension of calcification into the overlying soft tissue. Although periosteal elevation may be present, it is not diagnostic of the disease.

REFERENCES

1. Cummings JR et al: The popliteal artery entrapment syndrome in children, *J Pediatr Orthop* 12:539, 1992.
2. Leventhal BG: Neoplasms and neoplasm-like structures. In Behrman RE, Vaughan VC, editors: *Nelson's textbook of pediatrics,* ed 14, Philadelphia, 1992, WB Saunders.
3. Naish JM, Apley J: "Growing pains": a critical study of nonarthritic limb pains in children, *Arch Dis Child* 26:134, 1951.
4. National Center for Health Statistics: Viral and health statistics: patient's reasons for visiting physicians—National Ambulatory Medical Care Survey, US, 1977-1978, DHHS Pub No Pt82-1717, Hyattsville, Md, 1981.
5. Olivieri I, Pasero G: Long-standing isolated juvenile onset HLA-B27–associated peripheral enthesitis, *J Rheumatol* 19:164, 1992.
6. Oster J, Nielsen A: Growing pains: a clinical investigation of a school population, *Acta Paediatr Scand* 61:329, 1972.
7. Rivara FP, Parish RA, Mueller BA: Extremity injuries in children: predictive value of clinical findings, *Pediatrics* 78:803, 1986.

SUGGESTED READINGS

Cawkwell GD, Passo MH: Pursuing the source of musculoskeletal pain, *Contemp Pediatr* 11:72, 1994.

Sherry D: Limb pain in childhood, *Pediatr Rev* 12:39, 1990.

Szer IS: Are those limb pains "growing" pains? *Contemp Pediatr* 6:143, 1989.

Tunnessen WW Jr: *Signs and symptoms in pediatrics,* ed 2, Philadelphia, 1988, JB Lippincott.

129 Facial Dysmorphism

Marvin E. Miller

The face is the region of the body that reveals our identity to others. Although each person has two eyes, two ears, a nose, a mouth, a chin, and a head, it is the subtle uniqueness of these features in their form and their relationship to each other that marks each of us as a distinct and identifiable individual. Only monozygotic twins can have apparently identical faces, and even among them one finds facial differences that readily distinguish one from the other.

The face can appear dysmorphic or unusual if any facial part is abnormal in form or function or if a spatial relationship between or among these parts is abnormal.[1]

Physicians and other health care providers should be sensitive in the use of terminology to describe an individual who has a dysmorphic face. The terms "funny looking kid," "FLK," or "funny looking face" add little to the understanding of the situation and may arouse justified parental indignation. In discussing dysmorphic features with parents or describing them in written or verbal communication with colleagues, the physician should be objective in an evaluation that establishes a diagnosis and avoids an insensitive and derogatory approach to the patient. A dysmorphic face may be quite appropriate in relation to the family's physiognomy, or it may indicate a particular syndrome. Thus it is not surprising to find epicanthal folds and a flat nasal bridge in an Oriental child; if these are found in a Caucasian child, however, the physician should be suspicious of Down syndrome and look for other features that suggest this diagnosis. The child with a large head who also has a parent with a large head does not prompt as much concern as the child with a large head whose parents have normal-size heads. Thus it is crucial to evaluate dysmorphic facial features in light of the child's genetic background.

If the child or baby looks like one of the parents or bears a strong resemblance to the baby pictures of one of the parents, then the features obviously are familial. An autosomal dominant condition, such as Waardenburg syndrome, could explain dysmorphism and parental similarity. However, if there is no parental or familial resemblance (especially with other problems in development or growth or other body symptoms), the physician should consider further evaluation.

Facial morphogenesis is primarily determined by genetic information from multiple gene loci. Recently the molecular characterization of several genetic disorders, each associated with characteristic facial dysmorphism, has provided some clues as to which specific genes are part of the process that determines the facial features of an individual.[5] These genetic loci include the PAX 3 gene (Waardenburg syndrome type 1), the gene for fibroblast growth factor receptor 2 (several craniosynostosis syndomes including Pfeiffer syndrome, Crouzon syndrome, Apert syndrome, and Jackson-Weiss syndrome), and the Treacle gene (Treacher Collins syndrome). Many more genes involved in facial morphogenesis will probably be characterized in the near future.

MECHANISMS OF DYSMORPHOGENESIS

There are four general causes of facial dysmorphogenesis: deformation, disruption, primary malformation of the face, and central nervous system (CNS) malformations that cause secondary facial dysmorphism (anatomical and neuromuscular dysfunction).

Deformations

Deformations are structural abnormalities of newborns involving the musculoskeletal system that arise from intrauterine constraint.[2] Any situation that compromises the intrauterine space can cause a deformation, such as primigravida pregnancy, nonvertex presentation, multiple births, small mother, large baby, oligohydramnios, and structural uterine abnormality. Deformations are common and occur in 2% of all newborns. Common facial deformations include plagiocephaly (asymmetry of the head); asymmetry of the mandible, nose, ears, or chin; and micrognathia. The natural history of facial deformation almost always is benign, with restoration of the affected tissue to normal form and function within weeks after birth.

Disruptions

A disruption is the breakdown of previously normal fetal tissue.[3] The most common example is amniotic bands, which are estimated to occur in 1 in 2000 pregnancies. Although they originally were thought to affect limbs primarily, it now is clear that bands can attach to any part of the craniofacial region, causing a vast spectrum of structural defects of varying severity. This diagnosis should be considered in any newborn who has bizarre external craniofacial features. Evaluation of the placenta can be helpful in confirming this diagnosis if strands of amnion can be demonstrated or if they are found attached to the affected tissues.

Malformations

Facial. A malformation is a structural defect resulting from an intrinsic abnormality in the cells of the affected tissue.[3] Malformations have a number of potential causes, including genetic disorders (chromosomes and single genes), drugs, intrauterine infections, metabolic derangements, and hyperthermia. Malformations can involve almost any part of the face; examples of these are given in Table 129-1.

Central Nervous System. Malformations of the brain can cause facial dysmorphogenesis in two ways. First, the facial anatomy is partly directed by the growth of the forebrain. Any situation that grossly alters the normal development of the brain can alter facial development anatomically. An example

Table 129-1 Examples of Causes of Facial Malformation

Cause	Example	Facial dysmorphism
Genetic		
Chromosomal	Cri-du-chat syndrome (5p−)	Micrognathia, ocular hypertelorism
Autosomal dominant	Treacher Collins syndrome	Dysplastic ears, maxillary hypoplasia
Autosomal recessive	Hurler syndrome	Corneal clouding, coarse facies
Intrauterine infection	Congenital rubella	Cataracts
Drug induced	Fetal alcohol syndrome	Smooth philtrum, small eyes
Metabolic	Congenital hypothyroidism	Coarse facies; large, protruding tongue

of this is holoprosencephaly. When the forebrain fails to separate into the right and left ventricles, secondary midfacial abnormalities may occur. Another example is the upward slanting palpebral fissures in Down syndrome, which probably occurs secondary to forebrain underdevelopment. Second, neuromuscular dysfunction of the face resulting from a primary malformation of the brain can cause facial dysmorphism. Whenever a primary CNS malformation exists, neuromuscular control of a number of facial functions can be abnormal. These abnormal conditions include ptosis, nystagmus, strabismus, and lop ears. Prominent lateral palatal ridges that result from a deficit of tongue thrust into the palate are a sign of intrauterine CNS dysfunction.

EVALUATION OF THE INDIVIDUAL WHO HAS FACIAL DYSMORPHISM

1. Describe the dysmorphic facial features
2. Describe any other dysmorphic somatic features
3. Define the growth of the individual in weight, length, and head circumference
4. Define the development of the individual
5. Review the gestational and perinatal history
6. Review the family history
7. Consider laboratory tests
8. Determine if the features fit a recognizable syndrome
9. Discuss the findings with the family

EVALUATION OF THE INDIVIDUAL WHO HAS FACIAL DYSMORPHISM

Evaluation of the baby or child who has a dysmorphic face is summarized in the box on the right and is aimed at establishing an etiological diagnosis. The physician should follow these steps:

1. *Describe the dysmorphic facial features.* The first task is to describe in objective terms why the face appears unusual. Rather than stating that the distance between the eyes appears increased or the ears appear small, the physician should measure these parameters and compare them with known standards.[2]
2. *Describe any other dysmorphic somatic features.* A thorough physical examination should be performed to determine if associated somatic abnormalities are present. Hearing and vision should be evaluated, and fundoscopic examination should be performed. The cranial sutures should be palpated to evaluate for possible craniostenosis, which can cause facial dysmorphism.
3. *Define the growth of the individual in weight, length, and head circumference.* Data should be obtained and "plotted" to assess how the individual is growing in these parameters. The growth curves should be interpreted in light of the parental growth curves. Growth excess or, more often, growth deficiency can be seen as a part of malformation syndromes involving facial dysmorphism; for example, individuals who have cerebral gigantism (Sotos syndrome), who have very characteristic facies, are macrocephalic and are very tall in childhood. Individuals who have any of the three common autosomal trisomies (trisomy 13, 18, or 21) all show postnatal growth deficiency.
4. *Define the development of the individual.* From the patient's history and the physician's examination and testing, the individual's development should be assessed. It is important to know of any developmental delay because it may indicate CNS dysfunction. However, psychosocial deprivation and chronic otitis media, two correctable situations, can cause developmental delay.
5. *Review the gestational and perinatal history.* The gestational history should be reviewed for maternal drug exposure, viral illness, fever, and alcohol consumption. Positive findings may suggest an environmental cause of a malformation. The history also should include factors that might predispose the patient to deformations, such as breech delivery, oligohydramnios, multiple births, or maternal structural uterine anomaly.
6. *Review the family history.* The importance of taking a good family history has already been mentioned; this information may suggest a genetic basis for the condition.[4] Some autosomal recessive disorders are found almost exclusively in certain ethnic groups. Ellis–van Creveld syndrome, a rare ectodermal dysplasia, has a high incidence in the Amish population. The offspring of parents who are related to each other, particularly if they are first-degree relatives (i.e., father-daughter, mother-son, brother-sister), are at greater risk for having autosomal recessive disorders. Incestuous matings probably are more common than thought, and the couple is at relatively high risk for dysmorphic offspring. An *incestuous mating* should be considered in any dysmorphic newborn of a very young mother and no reputed father. A dysmorphic individual born to an older mother may suggest an autosomal trisomy and when born to an older father may suggest an autosomal dominant disorder caused by a fresh mutation.
7. *Consider laboratory tests.* If the dysmorphic features and history suggest a primary CNS problem, brain imaging

should be considered. If several systems are involved, chromosomes should be analyzed. Other laboratory tests and imaging studies of other organ systems should be performed when warranted. Magnetic resonance imaging (MRI), computed tomography (CT) scanning, and ultrasonography are extremely valuable imaging techniques that can be used selectively after consultation with a radiologist to evaluate internal structures.
8. *Determine if the features fit a known condition or syndrome* after all the information has been gathered.*
9. *Discuss the findings with the family.*

SUMMARY

The physician who is confronted with a patient who has dysmorphic facial features must decide whether the patient or family will benefit from a thorough evaluation or referral. The most important task initially is *to determine whether the features are consistent with the individual's genetic background* or whether they represent an abnormal phenotype. Through systematical gathering of information, the physician should attempt to establish an etiological diagnosis and then convey the implications to the appropriate family members.

**Smith's Recognizable Patterns of Human Malformation* is the most valuable resource for this purpose. It also is helpful in determining if a particular condition has a genetical basis.

REFERENCES

1. Aase JM: *Diagnostic dysmorphology,* New York, 1990, Plenum.
2. Graham JM: *Smith's recognizable patterns of human malformation,* ed 4, Philadelphia, 1988, WB Saunders.
3. Jones KL: *Smith's recognizable patterns of human malformation,* ed 4, Philadelphia, 1988, WB Saunders.
4. McKusick VA: *Mendelian inheritance in man,* ed 10, Baltimore, 1992, Johns Hopkins University Press.
5. Winter RM: What's in a face, *Nat Genet* 12:124, 1996.

130 Failure To Thrive

Lewis A. Barness

Failure to thrive is a convenient label applied to children who are behind their age peers in physical growth or development. The term is used most often to refer to infants under 2 years of age. However, it is equally applicable to older children or to those of any age whose mental development is deficient. This discussion is adapted largely to infants who are below the third percentile for height or weight, or both.

Children most often fail to thrive because they don't get enough to eat. Psychosocial difficulties may be the underlying cause, although specific physical defects may be a primary cause or may create psychosocial problems secondarily. If a psychosocial cause is suspected, an investigation is warranted, as it is for children who are victims of parenting problems or more obvious types of neglect.

NORMAL GROWTH FACTORS

The ultimate growth of a normal child is determined most closely by inheritance, but other factors can alter this pattern. One external factor that affects growth is malnutrition. Nutritional deprivation in utero may result in permanent growth retardation; the effects of nutritional deprivation later in life may cause permanent mental and physical retardation or may be reversible, depending on the age at which deprivation occurred, its duration, and the type of rehabilitation used. Nutritional deprivation that results in retardation may be caused by lack of calories, lack of protein, or lack of any one of the specific nutrients, such as a vitamin or mineral.

Malnutrition occurs in children whose families do not feed them for psychological or economic reasons or because of ignorance of how, how often, or what to feed.[1,2,8] However, malnutrition also occurs in children who have organic defects that produce excess waste and abnormal metabolism[3] or inanition that reduces the ability to eat.

Hormones are necessary for normal growth. Pituitary growth hormone induces skeletal muscle, hepatic, and renal protein synthesis.[9] Insulin affects carbohydrate metabolism and stimulates amino acid transport, protein synthesis, and cell division. Thyroid hormone influences the rate of cell division and cell size. Androgens and estrogens increase the rate of cartilage cell division but accelerate maturation and calcification of the epiphyses even faster; thus, with an excess of these hormones, immediate growth is rapid but the growing period is shortened. Glucocorticoids inhibit cell division. All other known hormones affect growth in some way. All acute or chronic diseases can slow growth as a result of increased catabolism of tissue, increased caloric demands, increased waste, or defective metabolism.

EVALUATION

It is essential that children who fail to thrive be evaluated systematically to conserve time and resources and provide remedial measures as quickly as possible. A history, physical examination, and laboratory tests are done, as they are for other children, but care should be directed to certain areas. In cases that have strong psychosocial features, nonroutine laboratory tests may not be indicated.

HISTORY

Birth Weight and Gestational Age

The birth weight in relation to the gestational age may indicate intrauterine growth retardation, causes of which include intrauterine infection, placental insufficiency, chromosomal anomalies, and some of the dwarfing syndromes. Many of these children are born with a smaller-than-normal complement of cells and can never grow normally. The shorter small-for-gestational-age (SGA) babies born at term are more likely to catch up than the longer babies. The former are voracious eaters and usually catch up in the first 6 to 9 months.

Sequential Growth Record

It is important to know if a child has always been of low height or weight for age or if growth slowed at some specified time. The latter circumstance points to a disease or phenomenon that occurred near the time of the change in growth rate.

Family History

The heights of parents and grandparents and the heights and weights of siblings may indicate a genetic growth aberration or some factor common to several family members.

Feeding

A careful 1-day feeding history often is revealing. Caloric intake should be estimated. Well-motivated parents may restrict the intake of fats and calories to prevent obesity or atherosclerosis, but when such a regimen is applied rigidly or at an early age, growth failure results.[7] A history of massive intake with no growth usually indicates that the informant is fabricating or ignorant of the intake, although excessive losses cannot be excluded. A history of pica should be noted.

Stools

Excessive stool losses may be the cause of lack of gain and growth.

System Review

Disease in any system can slow or stop weight and height gain.

Social History

The importance of an adequate social history cannot be overestimated. Family interest and time spent with the child, the degree of caring for the child, and realistic concern can be

Table 130-1 Suggested Blood Studies and Diagnoses Indicated by Abnormal Results

Blood study	Diagnoses
Hemoglobin, smear	Iron deficiency and other anemias, hematological disorders, some hemoglobinopathies
Sodium, potassium, chlorine, blood urea nitrogen	Renal diseases, adrenal disorders, dehydration
Calcium, phosphate, phosphatase	Rickets, thyroid and parathyroid insufficiency or excess
Serum glutamate oxaloacetate transaminase (SGOT), prothrombin	Liver diseases, hepatitis, cirrhosis
Albumin	Chronic malnutrition, protein-losing enteropathy
Fasting blood glucose	Diabetes mellitus, adrenal disorders, glycogen storage disease, hypoglycemia syndromes, pituitary insufficiency or excess
Uric acid	Hyperuricemia
Thyroxine, triiodothyronine (T_4, T_3) resin uptake	Thyroid insufficiency or excess
Growth hormone	Pituitary disease
Alpha-1-antitrypsin	Alpha-1-antitrypsin deficiency
Erythrocyte sedimentation rate	Collagen disorders; infections

estimated. Parents may be frustrated when their children do not eat as much as the parents think they should. If a conflict then develops, feeding may be inhibited. Parents can be depressed for many reasons, and this feeling may be transmitted to their young children, who may then refuse to eat adequately. Economic status and the availability of resources also should be determined.[1,6]

PHYSICAL EXAMINATION

A careful physical examination can lead to detection of disease in body systems, any one of which can be a cause of failure to thrive. Determining the sitting height as a fraction of the total height helps to distinguish specific types of growth failure. Blood pressure measurement should not be forgotten as a screening test for acute or chronic renal disease.

Accurate height and weight measurements are essential. Some parents complain that their children are not growing properly. If the history and physical examination are within normal limits and the child falls within the lower percentiles of the growth charts for height and weight, the physician's explanation of normal growth patterns may reassure the parents and child. Some parents who themselves are short may expect excessive growth of their normal children. An explanation of genetic factors and normal growth rates can lead to realistic expectations of growth without excessive investigation.

In a young child, head circumference is a valuable clue to diagnosis. With caloric deprivation, weight is lost first, linear growth then slows, and finally, the head circumference no longer increases. A head circumference below normal for age indicates either severe malnutrition or primary failure of the skull or brain to develop.

LABORATORY TESTS

Because many children who fail to thrive have inadequate nutritional or emotional support, early admission to a hospital may prevent their rapid deterioration. Laboratory studies should be minimized at this phase so that the child will not fear the hospital environment.

Tests that should be done include a peripheral blood examination (which may suggest iron deficiency anemia, a hemoglobinopathy, or a hematological disorder) and a tuberculin test (which can detect an otherwise unexpected infection). Urinalysis includes determination of the pH, which when high in the presence of acidosis suggests renal tubular acidosis. A low specific gravity may indicate diabetes insipidus. The presence of acetone or glucose may indicate dehydration, poisoning (e.g., lead), or diabetes mellitus. Cellular elements are present with renal inflammatory disease, poisoning, or febrile states. Reducing substances other than glucose should be determined because inborn metabolic errors such as galactosemia can be detected by the presence of a reducing substance in the absence of glucose. Ferric chloride is positive in a host of poisonings and also is a screening test for aminoaciduria.

If the child's problem is failure to gain weight, careful note should be made of the height, weight, and head circumference. The child should then be fed; if he or she gains rapidly, the diagnosis of inadequate feeding is suggested, and careful instruction and discussion with the family are required along with frequent supportive follow-up visits. If the child fails to gain within 3 days, further laboratory studies may reveal a specific cause.

The stool should be examined and its appearance noted; examination should include staining for fat, ova, and parasites. An excessive number of or bulky stools point to a major enteropathy, although parenteral infections also may be responsible for chronic diarrhea. Testing the stool water with a urine dip stick will reveal the pH and the presence of glucose and protein. Demonstration of alpha-1-antiprotease in the stool provides a quantitative estimate of stool protein levels. Excessive fat may indicate a malabsorption syndrome, excess protein, or a protein-losing enteropathy, and a stool pH below 5.5 may be the first indication of a disaccharidase deficiency. Some parasites (e.g., *Giardia*) may cause malabsorption syndromes.

A sweat test is performed to determine the likelihood of pancreatic insufficiency; in short girls, a buccal smear or chromosomal analysis is performed to determine genetic sex and the presence of gonadal insufficiency.

Other blood tests, including blood chemistries, should be performed (Table 130-1). These tests may result in a specific diagnosis or may indicate involvement of a specific organ or system, after which more definitive tests for that organ or system can be performed.

Table 130-2 Comparison of Chronological Age (CA), Height Age (HA), and Bone Age (BA)

Relationship of CA, HA, and BA	Suggested diagnoses
HA < BA; BA = CA	Genetic short stature, chondrodystrophies, trisomy 21, gonadal dysgenesis (XO), trisomy 13, Cockayne syndrome, leprechaunism, Seckel syndrome, intrauterine infection, maternal drugs, storage diseases
HA = BA; BA < CA	Normal variant, constitutional delay, familial trait, mild malnutrition, metabolic or other chronic illness
BA < HA; BA < CA	If marked, hypothyroidism; if moderate, hypopituitarism or malnutrition

Skull, chest, and long bone roentgenograms should be obtained and should include views to determine bone age. Skull films may indicate asymmetry from previous injuries or specific abnormalities; abnormal calcifications suggest intracranial bleeding or intrauterine infections. Chest abnormalities may indicate chronic diseases, such as tuberculosis, cystic fibrosis, or antiprotease deficiency. Long bone roentgenograms help diagnose acute or chronic infection or metabolic and hereditary bone diseases. Bone age should be compared with height and chronological age (Table 130-2).

Other studies that may be suggested include immunoelectrophoresis and special immunological studies in children who have frequent infections; chromosome studies in those who have a peculiar appearance or a conglomeration of abnormalities; 17-ketosteroids and other biochemical studies for adrenal or gonadal diseases; radiological and endoscopic gastrointestinal studies for those who have enteropathies; radiological kidney studies for those who have renal or adrenal diseases or abdominal masses; electrocardiograms in those who have heart abnormalities; and electroencephalograms in those who have seizure disorders. Human growth hormone should not be given to short children who are not growth hormone deficient, even though it initially can increase their height.

Another complaint of failure to thrive occurs in children who approach the age of puberty without having developed secondary sex characteristics. At this time, several other considerations may lead to a definitive diagnosis. The most common cause of delayed adolescence is constitutional delay, including that arising from malnutrition, which requires reassurance of the patient and family. In these cases the characteristics of prepubertal development are normal and proceed as listed in the box above. Male genital development should begin by age 14 and should be complete by age 19. Female sex development should begin by age 10, and menarche should occur within 5 years. If the developmental order is abnormal or if the delay extends beyond these limits, further investigation is required (see Chapter 165, Sexual Developmental Alterations).

ORDER OF ADOLESCENT DEVELOPMENT

Male

Enlargement of testes
Pubic hair
Axillary hair
Facial hair

Female

Growth acceleration
Breast development
Pubic hair
Menarche
Axillary hair

MANAGEMENT

If a specific cause of failure to thrive is determined, it should be treated as an entity. In most children this is related to inadequate food intake. Depending on the type of clinic population served, in some series as few as half and in others as many as 90% of children who were seen because of failure to thrive finally were found to be growing poorly or not at all because of inadequate intake (see the box on the right). In most series the cause of inadequate intake was almost equally divided among economic, educational, or psychological inadequacy.[4,5]

CAUSES OF FAILURE TO THRIVE*

Improper feeding—50%-90%

Economic—10%-40%[2,4,5,10]
Education—10%-40%[2,4,5,10]
Psychological—30%-40%[2,4,5,10]
Intolerance—<5%[4,5,10]

Other causes—10%-50%

Hypothyroidism
Cystic fibrosis
Subdural hematoma
Glycogen storage disease
Celiac disease
Methylmalonic acidemia
Maple syrup urine disease
Mental retardation, unspecified
Urinary tract disease
Diencephalic syndrome
Brain tumors
Chronic liver disease
Congenital heart disease
Ulcerative colitis

*Compendium from various sources. Some obvious causes are missing because the complaint is not failure to thrive but rather is related to the diagnosis.

Realimentation in a marasmic child may be accompanied by no weight gain for as long as 6 weeks, presumably because of shifting of water between intracellular and extracellular spaces. During the phase of rapid weight gain, the liver may enlarge from fat accumulation, and signs of increased intracranial pressure may occur. These usually are temporary and require no treatment. If, however, refeeding is begun after even a short period of inadequate intake, diarrhea may occur. The child may have developed lactase deficiency during the period of low intake of lactose and must be given lactose in small quantities or not at all. He or she may have developed gastrointestinal motility abnormalities, so slow increases in feeding are necessary. After the diagnosis has been made and the treatment begun, frequent visits serve to determine the adequacy of treatment and also the adequacy and completeness of the diagnosis. Regardless of the child's age at the beginning of treatment, some catching up of growth will occur. The more severe, the earlier, and the longer the insult, the less likely the child is to attain his or her genetic potential. Nonetheless, treatment efforts should be persistent. If treatment is not maintained after it is begun, the previous inadequate growth and development pattern likely will recur.

PROGNOSIS

In managing the child whose failure to thrive is nonorganic, the parents should be involved early in both investigation and treatment. A nonthreatening, nonrecriminatory attitude should be fostered as the interaction between the child and parents is observed. A few suggestions or instructions may suffice, but follow-up by a social worker in the home to give continual support usually is helpful. Mental stimulation of the child is necessary.

For children whose failure to thrive is severe, the prognosis for future growth and development may be poor for as many as half of those diagnosed before age 5. The correspondence of statistical outcome between children who fail to thrive and those who have suffered other forms of abuse is striking.

REFERENCES

1. Baertt JM, Adrianzen B, Graham GG: Growth of previously well-nourished infants in poor homes, *Am J Dis Child* 130:33, 1976.
2. Barness LA: Failure to thrive, *Dallas Med J* 58:325, 1972.
3. Barness LA, Morrow G: Clinical clues to diagnosis of metabolic disorders, *Clin Pediatr* 9:605, 1970.
4. Berwick DM: Nonorganic failure to thrive, *Pediatr Rev* 1:265, 1980.
5. Hannaway PJ: Failure to thrive: a study of 100 infants and children, *Clin Pediatr* 9:96, 1970.
6. Klaus MH, Leger T, Trause MA: *Maternal attachment and mothering disorders,* ed 2, Skillman, NJ, 1982, Johnson & Johnson.
7. Lifshitz F, Moses N: Growth failure: a complication of dietary treatment of hypercholesterolemia, *Am J Dis Child* 143:537, 1989.
8. Mitchell WG, Gorrell RW, Greenberg RA: Failure-to-thrive: a study in a primary care setting: epidemiology and follow-up, *Pediatrics* 65:971, 1980.
9. Root AW, Bongiovanni AM, Eberlein WA: Diagnosis and management of growth retardation with special reference to the problem of hypopituitarism, *J Pediatr* 78:737, 1971.
10. Sills RH: Failure to thrive: the role of clinical and laboratory evaluation, *Am J Dis Child* 132:967, 1978.

SUGGESTED READINGS

Frank DA, Silva M, Needleman R: Failure to thrive: mystery, myth and method, *Contemp Pediatr* 10:114, 1993.

Smith DW, Simons ER: Rational diagnostic evaluation of the child with mental deficiency, *Am J Dis Child* 129:1285, 1975.

131 Fatigue and Weakness

Arnold T. Sigler

The signs and symptoms of fatigue and weakness are among those a pediatrician will encounter most often; yet the terms *fatigue* and *weakness* are neither indexed nor discussed in most current pediatric textbooks. Also, these terms are confused and misused by both physicians and patients. Adolescents and children often use other terms to describe their perceptions of somatic weakness and fatigue. Furthermore, pediatric texts have failed to stress that specific complaints, rather than diseases, are what bring most patients to the physician. Fatigue, in fact, is very different from true body weakness. Therefore it is important to define the two terms carefully, even though the definitions must be modified for each age group.

Weakness refers to a decrease in strength either of a part of the body or of the whole body. The definition of true weakness can be met only by demonstration of abnormal neurological or muscular functions, by means of history, by physical examination, or by laboratory techniques. Practically speaking, a history of weakness, on further questioning, will reveal hypotonia in infants and, in older children, trouble running or keeping up in gym class, clumsiness, or lack of agility.

Fatigue may be a normal result of bodily or mental overwork—a feeling of weariness or lassitude, with increasing discomfort and decreasing efficiency, which may have a biochemical basis. The temporary fatigue of long-distance running, cramming for examinations, or food or sleep deprivation are examples of normal fatigue. In these instances, the amount of fatigue, even when prolonged, usually is appropriate for the amount of physical or mental exertion.

On the other hand, fatigue may be a pathological state. The lassitude associated with somatic illness, often with definable physical or laboratory abnormalities, is well known. In contrast, fatigue also may be described as an emotional condition characterized by a state of weariness, boredom, lassitude, and lack of energy and initiative, resulting in the absence of a sense of well-being.

Parents who report that their infant is weak or "floppy" almost always are describing a neuromuscular problem. The term *fatigue* rarely is pertinent or appropriate for a very small child.

Older children, too, complain only infrequently of "feeling fatigued." Remarkably, even with chronic organic diseases, fatigue itself is not expressed verbally by the child. Rather, it is the concerned parent who usually observes and reports that the child appears fatigued. Parents commonly say such things as "He has no energy," "She lies around all the time," "She seems bored and droopy," "He's sleeping a lot of the time," "She has no pep," "He drags around," or "I can't get her to do a thing." On questioning, younger children occasionally express a sense of lassitude and fatigue to a physician. Much of the difficulty in the middle years of childhood (before adolescence), however, is the child's inability to put into words what he or she feels. Fatigue therefore usually is exhibited in terms of a child's physical activity and performance in school, sports, and other organized activities.

Chronic complaints of fatigue are encountered most often in adolescents. It is among the adolescent's most common presentations in pediatric practice and one that usually arouses excessive concern in parents. The normal swings in adolescent moods, from excessive exuberance to fatigue, usually are of more concern to parents and teachers than to the patient; thus the parent most often is the complainant. Often the adolescent may disagree vehemently with the parents' view and not share their concern. Adolescents, however, also initiate visits to the pediatrician because they themselves feel fatigue. Parents may be unable or may refuse to recognize the adolescent's symptoms.

FATIGUE ASSOCIATED WITH MEDICAL ILLNESS

The younger the child, the more likely that the expressed or observed fatigue has a pathological cause. The pediatrician often is astounded by the lack of symptoms, such as fatigue, in younger children who have a profound medical illness. Similarly, minor illnesses are more likely to precipitate prolonged fatigue in adolescents compared with younger children. The box on p. 954 lists disorders associated with prolonged fatigue most likely to be encountered by the pediatrician. Needless to say, any acute illness or trauma may be accompanied by fatigue, but usually only prolonged fatigue is noteworthy.

The most common problem associated with fatigue in children is recurrent or chronic infection. Otitis media, sinusitis, and tonsillitis of a recurrent and often smoldering nature often are overlooked for their systemic effects, among which may be prominent fatigue. *Mycoplasma* pneumonia, often low grade and without fever, produces progressive fatigue. In addition, prolonged viral and parasitic illnesses (e.g., infectious mononucleosis, hepatitis, cytomegalovirus infection, and toxoplasmosis) commonly manifest with fatigue, especially in adolescents.

The terms *chronic infectious mononucleosis* and *chronic fatigue syndrome* have become popular with both physicians and the media. This attention has led to occasional misuse of those terms and also, undoubtedly, to mild mass hysteria among young adults and adolescents who now are convinced that they suffer from one of these disorders. Most adults and many infants and children have been infected with the Epstein-Barr (EB) virus. The clinical manifestations in proved cases are extremely variable: some patients remain symptom free, whereas clinical, hematological, and serological findings support the diagnosis of infectious mononucleosis in others. The symptoms of infectious mononucleosis usu-

DISORDERS COMMONLY ASSOCIATED WITH PROLONGED FATIGUE

- Severe anemia
- Hypothyroidism
- Chronic upper respiratory tract infections
  - Otitis media and sinusitis
  - Tonsillitis
- *Mycoplasma* and other viral pneumonias
- Infectious mononucleosis
- Hepatitis
- Chronic asthma
- Chronic allergies
- Rheumatoid arthritis
- Rheumatic fever
- Lupus erythematosus
- Diabetes mellitus
- Disseminated malignancy
- Inflammatory bowel disease
- AIDS
- Immunological disorders
- Drug abuse, including alcoholism
- Cyanotic heart disease
- Chronic pulmonary disease
- Chronic renal failure
- Depression
- Severe obesity

ally resolve in several weeks, but an occasional patient may have an atypical or a more prolonged course in which the initial clinical findings either persist or are intermittent over a period of months or, in rare cases, years. These unusual but documented cases of chronic infectious mononucleosis typically include complaints of chronic fatigue.

Another much smaller group of patients has now been described as having a serious, sometimes lethal, illness associated with EB virus infection. These patients usually do not manifest the classic findings of infectious mononucleosis; very often their conditions are proved to be either acquired or genetically determined immunological abnormalities. Fatigue frequently manifests as part of allergic rhinitis in children and adolescents. Often mistakenly considered insignificant, upper respiratory tract allergies may cause impressive fatigue, as well as irritability and mild depression.

Of the common endocrine disorders, only hypothyroidism is likely to be associated with fatigue. Certainly the hypothyroid child whose rate of growth has fallen off may manifest increasing fatigue and lassitude, at first subtle, as the only symptoms. Thyrotoxicosis, in contrast, is uncommon in young children but occasionally manifests with isolated fatigue in adolescents.

Although any metabolic disorder can cause fatigue, only diabetes mellitus occurs with enough frequency to merit consideration here. Fatigue almost always accompanies the initial or uncontrolled diabetic state.

Collagen-vascular diseases, especially rheumatoid arthritis and other rheumatoid-like disorders, appear frequently in pediatric practice. Many of these disorders are difficult to diagnose precisely and often eventually are self-limited, but many children have significant fatigue, out of proportion to the musculoskeletal complaints. Lyme arthritis is one example of this circumstance.

Always unpredictable and often secretive, inflammatory bowel disease may arouse concern initially with unexplained fatigue and a loss of sense of well-being. Although eventually accompanied by fever, abdominal symptoms, or abnormal stools, this disorder can continue for months with fatigue as the only major symptom.

Congenital cyanotic heart disease and chronic advanced pulmonary disease, as seen with cystic fibrosis, commonly are associated with marked fatigue; in these cases, however, the underlying disease usually is readily evident before the fatigue becomes severe. In atypical circumstances the pediatrician occasionally may see an older child for the first time who has severe fatigue caused by a previously undiagnosed hypoxic disorder.

Overall, the condition most often suspected as a cause of fatigue in both children and adults is anemia—and, most often, incorrectly so. Although fatigue often is ascribed to mild or moderate anemia, from whatever source, symptoms usually are not seen in children until the hemoglobin level falls to 6 or 7 g/dl; if red cell levels fall gradually, even lower hemoglobin levels may ensue without clinically evident symptoms. Irritability and attention problems may be present with mild to moderate iron deficiency anemia, but fatigue usually is not. Younger children, especially, seem to tolerate incredibly low hemoglobin levels with no symptoms at all.

Malignancy, particularly leukemia or lymphoma, occasionally develops insidiously, with fatigue as the major symptom. Although always feared, these diseases are seen infrequently in pediatric office practice.

Of more current importance in older children and adolescents are alcoholism and drug abuse—causes of chronic fatigue that easily are overlooked.

FATIGUE ASSOCIATED WITH EMOTIONAL FACTORS

Most children and adolescents who come to the pediatrician with unexplained chronic fatigue are found to have an emotionally related disorder. Before adolescence the complaint usually centers on the parents' concern about a child's reduced activity level. A younger child will have been noted to prefer sedentary activities—to "lie around the house a lot," appear tired, lack energy, and shrink from social contacts. These traits may have been long standing, but a comment from grandparents or a teacher may arouse acute anxiety precipitating the first visit to the pediatrician.

At this point the family often is convinced that the child has a serious organic disease. Further evaluation, however, usually reveals that the child is performing at a very satisfactory level, but not up to the family's excessive expectations. The child may be withdrawing because of failure to compete with an exceptional sibling or because of real or imagined failure in school. In other cases a child may feel a lack of well-being because of parental discord. Similarly, lack of parental involvement with a child may lead to lassitude and boredom. Therefore stress and anxiety in these children usually result in either hyperactivity or withdrawal, and the more common withdrawal reaction may exhibit itself as chronic fatigue.

These observations do not mean that most children do not go through transient periods of lassitude or fatigue, but such instances are brief and usually self-limited. At the opposite extreme is the child whose chronic fatigue is a sign of true psychiatric depression. Here, as in the adolescent, the more protracted and severe the periods of withdrawal, the more likely that depression and fatigue are caused by a pathological process. By far the most common and familiar patient for protracted fatigue is the adolescent. The pediatrician can expect to see a generous number who characteristically appear each spring complaining of fatigue or lassitude, lacking energy, and being mildly depressed. This disorder usually appears during periods of greatest school-related stress—before examination time. It is "spring fever." Although the patient may have a real fever, usually secondary to infection (e.g., infectious mononucleosis or influenza), the problem usually is emotionally based. All the uncertainties of late adolescence, including identity and sexual crises, may create a "spring fever" during *any* season, with fatigue often the dominant complaint.

Often the adolescent collapses with fatigue after intense and exuberant activity involving schoolwork, extracurricular activity, sports, or social events. These individuals also may be short on sleep and may have "borderline" eating habits and an additional variety of hypochondriacal symptoms. "Burnout" and fatigue are particularly common in overachieving high school and college students during late adolescence. The emotional reaction actually may be precipitated by a physical illness, particularly an infection. Most of these patients have normal findings on physical examinations and routine laboratory tests.

CHRONIC FATIGUE SYNDROME (see also Chapter 192)

Since 1985 adolescents, adults, and occasionally children have been described as having a disorder commonly referred to as *chronic fatigue syndrome* (CFS). This syndrome most commonly involves persistent or relapsing severe fatigue, fever, headache, sore throat, tender lymphadenitis, nausea or vomiting, myalgia, arthralgia, and abdominal pain. Neurocognitive complaints, such as an inability to concentrate, sleep disturbances, episodical confusion and memory problems, depression, anxiety, and irritability, also are especially common in CSF.

The neurocognitive complaints are the most difficult to evaluate and assess in CFS because of the extreme difference in emotional perception from person to person. Furthermore, careful physical examinations by experienced physicians often fail to document any physical abnormalities, and extensive laboratory evaluations usually produce normal results. In addition, much of the difficulty surrounding both the diagnosis and the search for a cause of CFS is attributable to confusion about the use of the terms *chronic fatigue* and *chronic fatigue syndrome*. Consequently, the Centers for Disease Control and Prevention (CDC) has formulated strict criteria for the case definition of chronic fatigue syndrome. Unfortunately, these criteria were based mainly on observations of adult populations and may not be completely pertinent to children and adolescents.

Nevertheless, the CDC criteria for CFS stipulate that the debilitating fatigue must last at least 6 months, and they exclude patients who have either a current or preexisting chronic psychiatric disorder such as depression. However, because depression and anxiety are so commonly reported in CFS, strict adherence to this definition may falsely exclude some patients who have CFS or may exclude some who have reactive depression secondary to their chronic physical fatigue.

Chronic fatigue syndrome quickly became a popular diagnosis. Initially the syndrome was attributed to infection with the EB virus, although very few patients had documented physical findings or hematological abnormalities consistent with the diagnosis of infectious mononucleosis. In addition, most had no serological evidence of active EB virus infection. Recently, however, a better understanding of the natural course of EB virus antibody activity in healthy individuals months and years after an initial illness with infectious mononucleosis indicates that healthy patients who had mononucleosis years earlier could not be differentiated from fatigued patients who currently had the disease.

Nevertheless, some adolescent patients reported in series of patients who have chronic fatigue also had evidence of IgM antibodies to the EB virus. These antibodies subsequently cleared, and the patients appeared to recover physically but continued to have debilitating fatigue. These patients are examples of chronic fatigue caused by EB virus mononucleosis and clearly not by CFS. Additional diagnostic confusion arises from the common occurrence of depression after mononucleosis and other viral illnesses such as influenza A.

Attempts to implicate many other viruses as the etiological agent in CFS have been inconsistent and nonconclusive. Although various immunological deviations have been reported, such as mild elevations in circulating immune complexes, IgG subclass deficiencies, hypergammaglobulinemia, and low or absent antibodies to EB virus nuclear antigens associated with latency, none of these abnormalities has been specific to CFS. However, the common association of cognitive and psychological abnormalities in CFS also has led to speculation and further investigation into the role of the central nervous system in the causation of chronic fatigue.

Recently a few studies have attempted to link some patients who have chronic fatigue syndrome to so-called neurally mediated hypotension (neurocardiogenic syncope), which is detected by upright tilting of the patient, who soon develops hypotension (postural hypotension). Some patients had improvement in their chronic fatigue when treated with an increase in salt intake plus a variety of drugs used to regulate blood pressure. However, neurally mediated hypotension with or without syncopy is common, especially in early adolescence and usually not in association with chronic disease. Further testing of patients who have both emotional disorders and those recovered from infectious diseases—but *not* chronically fatigued—needs to be carried out before any specific etiological relationship is established.

Historically, epidemics of chronic fatigue syndrome, or

neurasthenia have surfaced episodically since 1750. The term *myalgic encephalomyelitis* still is used in the United Kingdom to describe an illness similar to CFS. Brucellosis and Asian influenza, both prevalent in the 1950s, also were implicated as possible causes of CFS. More recently, chronic yeast infections have been blamed, as well as infection with the herpes 6 virus. However, none of these associations has been proven scientifically.

Additional research is necessary to determine whether CFS in adolescents is depression, a unique psychosomatic illness, or an infectious/immunological disorder that produces depression.

Currently, however, the evidence strongly suggests that CFS is not one disease but rather is associated with a variety of disease processes, both physical and emotional. Similarly, CFS that meets the CDC diagnostic criteria appears to be a very uncommon disorder in the experience of physicians caring for both children and adolescents. In contrast, prolonged fatigue associated with a clear-cut emotional disorder is very common in adolescents and older teenagers.

DIFFERENTIAL DIAGNOSIS AND EVALUATION

Although it may first appear that the patient who is chronically fatigued has an insignificant problem, great care must be taken to rule out underlying medical illness and also to return the child and parents to a state of well-being. The physician must remember that either the child or the parents are worried about the child's fatigue. Because family members may disagree about the significance of the symptoms, adequate time and concern are needed to evaluate the history. The symptoms of chronic fatigue cannot be dismissed casually over the telephone or with a quick office check.

Inasmuch as most patients who come to the physician complaining of fatigue have an emotionally based problem, a careful history, with information from both child and parents (taken separately when appropriate), often limits the differential diagnosis initially. Discrepancies between the child's and the parents' observations soon become evident, and the diagnosis of emotionally related fatigue emerges in most cases on the basis of the history alone. Happily, the information derived from a long-standing physician-patient relationship contributes enormously to increased ease during the evaluation. Although fatigue may be the only presenting symptom, further questioning almost always uncovers other symptoms of somatic disease. Chronic fatigue alone, in the absence of other physical symptoms, usually is emotionally based. Other supporting complaints are somnolence, depression, anxiety, boredom, and decreased activity. Furthermore, the patient's affect may be inappropriate. Often, emotional stress or some disruption in the patient's life also is part of the history.

A careful physical examination should be performed. A normal examination, patiently performed, may be the only treatment necessary, working miracles to reassure the often fearful child or parent. The child's affect and appearance usually are revealing. The impression that the child "looks well" invariably proves to be an accurate measure of the child's health. Because in younger children the parent describes the child's fatigue, the physician and parent often agree simultaneously that the child "appears healthy"—again making the presence of organic disease unlikely. The condition of the adolescent, in contrast, may be more difficult to interpret. Although the physical examination may be benign, the adolescent may appear slovenly, uncommunicative, depressed, and unable to express his or her feelings; thus at first the adolescent sometimes appears to be physically ill.

In all age groups a search should be made for sites of chronic latent infection, adenopathy, enlargement or tenderness of the liver and spleen, and abdominal masses. Careful palpation for an enlarged or tender thyroid gland is essential. Mild scleral icterus and petechiae are easy to overlook. Similarly, a patient's pallor (a common finding, especially after long winters indoors) may evade even the most experienced pediatrician. On the other hand, the congested facies of the chronically allergic or infected child, clubbing, and cyanosis are obvious.

A limited, well-selected group of laboratory tests should be performed on most patients who are chronically fatigued. These results will reassure the family, the patient, and the pediatrician and usually erase any lingering doubt about the diagnosis. Furthermore, normal physical examination findings plus a normal laboratory evaluation may provide all the therapy necessary for recovery.

The laboratory evaluation initially should include a complete blood count (CBC) with red cell indexes, thyroid and liver function tests, a throat culture, and a stool examination for blood. The cold agglutinin test often is valuable, as is a simple initial screening test for a *Mycoplasma* infection. Roentgenograms rarely are necessary and should be discouraged. Critical evaluation of data collected from the history, physical examination, and laboratory tests should enable the pediatrician to detect quickly any organic causes of fatigue. Prolonged fever, however low grade, always must be viewed as significant and may suggest infection, inflammatory disease, or malignancy. Pallor points to the possibility of anemia or hypothyroidism. Cervical adenopathy, even a single enlarged node, in the absence of other findings can be a clue to the diagnosis of infectious mononucleosis. In fact, every pediatrician begins to look for patients who have infectious mononucleosis in the autumn and early winter of each year. However, infectious mononucleosis is a protean illness, and the results of the physical examination sometimes are normal. Children and adolescents who have infectious mononucleosis may have no fever or signs of toxicity but may manifest major fatigue.

Furthermore, results of the heterophil antibody test for infectious mononucleosis may be negative in many young children and infants and in about 10% of older children and adolescents who have the disease. The reliability of EB virus antibody testing has improved to the point where the diagnosis of acute, active infectious mononucleosis can be confirmed. During the evaluation of chronic fatigue, EB virus antibody titers usually can differentiate long-past infection from recent and active infection, thus eliminating EB virus infection and infectious mononucleosis as causes for the fatigue and permitting a search for other likely neuropsychiatric causes. Toxoplasmosis and cytomegalovirus (CMV) infections may mimic mononucleosis closely and manifest with significant fatigue but with only minimal cervical adenopathy and fever. Positive results of a fluorescent antibody test for toxoplasmosis or CMV with negative results of a heterophil antibody test will confirm the diagnosis. Similarly, fatigued children may have hepatitis and may be anicteric (or only slightly icteric), with little or no hepatic tenderness or enlargement. Commonly, other routine but slightly prolonged viral infections, especially during convalescence, can precipitate a prolonged fatigue syndrome accompanied by depression.

The diagnosis of chronic fatigue syndrome should be restricted to patients who meet rigid criteria, including the new onset of persistent or relapsing fatigue in patients having no history of such fatigue and the exclusion of other clinical conditions that might produce similar symptoms. In addition, two of the following three physical criteria should be documented on at least two occasions in a 1-month interval: (1) low-grade fever, (2) nonexudative pharyngitis, and (3) palpable or tender postcervical or axillary lymph nodes (less than 2 cm in diameter). Furthermore, symptoms must include several of the following: muscle weakness, muscle discomfort, headaches, migratory arthralgia, neuropsychological complaints, and sleep disturbances. After other medical conditions are excluded, some older children and adolescents may meet these criteria for diagnosis. Certainly these patients should not be labeled with a diagnosis of chronic infectious mononucleosis syndrome or chronic EB virus infection, which recently has become a "quick fix" diagnosis for patients who are chronically fatigued.

Children who have a collagen-vascular disease have fatigue but little else at first. Mild articular or periarticular inflammation easily may be missed by the physician. The emphasis must be on a careful examination and the observation of subtle or minimal physical findings, inasmuch as children usually do not manifest fulminant findings initially. Children who have inflammatory bowel disease, arthritis, or an arthritis-like illness and some patients who have a malignancy—monocytic leukemia, in particular—may have especially prolonged symptoms, including fatigue, without any physical findings whatsoever.

An enlarged, tender thyroid gland and fatigue may indicate thyroiditis with emerging hypothyroidism. However, the thyroid often is palpable and full in healthy adolescents. In any event, chronic fatigue from thyroid disease usually can be ruled out quickly with a thyroxine (T_4) test. Some patients who have hypothyroidism also demonstrate mild to moderate anemia, and those who have active thyroiditis may have an elevated sedimentation rate. To be acceptable as an explanation for fatigue, the diagnosis of pure anemia requires marked reduction of hemoglobin. Red cell indexes and a reticulocyte count will characterize the anemia and the probable cause. Anemia accompanied by thrombocytopenia, however, suggests leukemia or aplastic anemia. The white cell count may be normal in infectious mononucleosis or hepatitis, but lymphocytosis with atypical lymphocytes most likely will be present. The heterophil antibody screening test ("mono test") is diagnostic in most such circumstances.

The erythrocyte sedimentation rate is the most valuable screening test for inflammatory diseases of all varieties. A normal sedimentation rate almost always rules out collagen-vascular disease, inflammatory bowel disease, chronic smoldering infections, and disseminated malignancies. An elevated sedimentation rate requires further investigation. A routine urinalysis almost always reveals diabetes, and most patients who have chronic renal failure have urinary abnormalities as well as significant anemia. In these cases the subsequent measurement of blood glucose in diabetes and of creatinine or blood urea nitrogen in renal disease can confirm these diagnoses.

MANAGEMENT

Inasmuch as significant organic disease is ruled out in most patients, further management requires meaningful communication between the pediatrician, the patient, and the parents. In younger children, one must put the variability in performance and behavior of normal children into perspective. Again, appropriate parental expectations must be emphasized. In addition, the child's and the family's daily schedule should be reviewed. A chaotic life-style that is frantic with poorly structured activity and inadequate sleep patterns often is revealed. Occasionally, true psychiatric depression is discovered, which calls for referral to a psychiatrist.

Older children and adolescents benefit from personal, warm attention. The value of a continuous relationship with one physician becomes self-evident. An understanding, thorough session with the patient's own pediatrician usually "streamlines" the evaluation and eliminates the need for excessive testing. Conversation after the physical examination should attempt to (1) reassure the child or adolescent about his or her basic health, (2) reiterate the common and "normal" occurrence of fatigue, (3) examine the daily routine and stresses on the patient, and (4) suggest modifications of the patient's life-style and approaches to life's situations. It is a time for respectful give-and-take. It is the pediatrician's responsibility to attempt to establish the probable cause of the fatigue before the patient is referred to a specialist. If emotional fatigue is suspected, the adolescent in particular must be comfortable with the conclusion that organic diseases have been ruled out. The patient then must be made aware of the emotional underlay for the fatigue, and if psychiatric referral is needed, the reasons must be made clear; otherwise the fatigue, like any psychosomatic symptom, may continue and worsen. A knowledgeable pediatrician therefore will be reassuring but firm in approaching the child or adolescent who has the potential need for further evaluation and referral. Fortunately, such a referral usually is not necessary.

SUGGESTED READINGS

Bou-Holaigah I et al: The relationship between neurally mediated hypotension and the chronic fatigue syndrome, *JAMA* 274:961,1995.

Carter BD et al: Case control study of chronic fatigue in pediatric patients, *Pediatrics* 95:179, 1995.

Cassidy J: *Textbook of pediatric rheumatology,* New York, 1990, Churchill Livingstone.

Dale JK, Straus SE: The chronic fatigue syndrome: considerations relevant to children and adolescents, *Adv Pediatr Infect Dis* 7:63, 1992.

Hofmann A: *Adolescent medicine,* ed 2, Menlo Park, Calif, 1989, Addison-Wesley.

Holmes GP, Kaplan JE, Gantz NM: Chronic fatigue syndrome: a working case definition, *Ann Intern Med* 108:3087, 1988.

Kaplan S: *Clinical pediatric and adolescent endocrinology,* ed 2, Philadelphia, 1990, WB Saunders.

Katz BZ, Andiman WA: Chronic fatigue syndrome, *J Pediatr* 113:944, 1988.

Klein GL et al: The allergic irritability syndrome, *Ann Allergy* 55:22, 1985.

MacBryde CM, Blacklow RS: *Signs and symptoms,* ed 5, Philadelphia, 1970, JB Lippincott.

Malmquist CP: *Handbook of adolescence,* New York, 1978, Jason Aronson.

Nathan DG, Oski FA: *Hematology of infancy and childhood,* ed 3, Philadelphia, 1987, WB Saunders.

Sigler A: Chronic fatigue syndrome: fact or fiction, *Contemp Pediatr* 7:22, 1990.

Smith MS, et al: Chronic fatigue in adolescents, *Pediatrics* 88:195, 1991.

Wilson A et al: The treatment of chronic fatigue syndrome: science and speculation, *Am J Med* 96:544, 1994.

132 Fever

Élise W. van der Jagt

For centuries fever in both human beings and animals has been associated with illness. Today, as many as 30% of all patients seen by pediatricians have fever as their principal complaint, making it one of the most common reasons children are taken to a physician. The multitude of telephone calls about fever received day and night by pediatricians makes it obvious that the proper evaluation and management of fever is a basic and necessary skill for physicians and nurse practitioners.

Even though clinicians have dealt with this common clinical sign for decades, its mechanism, meaning, and management have remained sufficiently unclear and controversial that research on these matters continues. Although advances in neurochemistry and neurophysiology have improved our understanding of the pathophysiology of fever, clinical investigators continue to search for practical knowledge that will enhance the care of the febrile patient. Availability of such information can simplify the challenging role of the physician, who must evaluate the patient quickly and effectively, arrive at a diagnosis, institute appropriate therapy, and both educate and support the parents and child during the entire process. The extent to which health care providers accomplish these goals depends on their knowledge of the mechanisms of disease, the various clinical manifestations of disease, and their awareness of the social context in which the disease occurs.

DEFINITION

The word *fever* is derived from the Latin *fovere* (to warm) and commonly means an elevation of body temperature. Although this general definition is acceptable in common parlance, fever is described more accurately as a *disorder* of thermoregulation. It must be differentiated from hyperthermia, an elevated body temperature resulting from conditions that overwhelm the normal process of thermoregulation.

The thermoregulatory center resides in the preoptic nuclei of the anterior hypothalamus. These nuclei consist of warm- and cold-sensitive neurons that respond both to the temperature of the blood coursing near them and to stimuli received from peripheral thermal sensors, particularly those in the skin. By regulating peripheral thermoregulatory control mechanisms in response to these stimuli (e.g., sweating, vasoconstriction), the hypothalamic thermostat maintains core body temperature at about 37° C (98.6° F), the so-called set-point of the hypothalamus.

Excessive body heat generated during strenuous exercise, from excessive coverings, or from high environmental temperatures normally is dissipated by peripheral thermoregulation to maintain core body temperature at 37° C. If peripheral thermoregulation is unable to accomplish this task, heat will be retained and hyperthermia will occur. In the case of fever, however, the thermostat itself has been "reset" at a higher set-point, causing core body temperature to be maintained at a higher level.

The primary substance responsible for elevating the set-point has been known since 1948. It originally was named *endogenous pyrogen* and was believed to originate from leukocytes. Evidently, however, endogenous pyrogen is not the only leukocyte product that can induce fever; others, including interferon and tumor necrosis factor (cachectin), also can do so. As additional products of macrophages exhibiting properties almost identical to endogenous pyrogen have been described, they have been grouped and called interleukin-1 (IL-1). Subsequent research with the use of in vitro lymphocyte assays and recombinant IL-1 has shown that IL-1 is a low-molecular-weight cytoplasmic protein contained within bone marrow–derived phagocytes (predominantly macrophages and monocytes but also neutrophils and eosinophils) and is released when these phagocytes are active at inflammatory sites. As might be expected, multiple disease processes may precipitate the release of IL-1, including infections, antigen-antibody mediated reactions, and tumors. After its release, this intriguing substance appears not only to stimulate the production of prostaglandins (primarily prostaglandin E_2), prostacyclins, and thromboxanes (all arachidonic acid metabolites) that directly elevate the set-point of the hypothalamic thermostat (resulting in fever), but also to cause T cell proliferation and an increase in B cell–derived antibodies. Thus IL-1 would seem to have a role in immune regulation as well. Although other substances, such as serotonin, norepinephrine, and cyclic adenosine monophosphate (cyclic AMP), also have been implicated in fever production, their precise relationship to IL-1 has yet to be defined.

In addition to knowing the pathophysiology of fever, knowing the range of normal body temperature also is important. Ever since 1850, when the use of the thermometer first was recommended to measure body temperature,[25] normal core body temperature measured rectally has been found to range between 97° and 100° F (36.1° and 37.8° C), although on rare occasions it may be as low as 95.5° F (35.3° C) or as high as 101° F (38.3° C). Of note is that the "normal temperature" of 98.6° F was derived from Wunderlich's study[24] of over 1 million *axillary* temperatures taken in adults. This may have no relevance for children not only because adults were studied but also because axillary and rectal (core) temperatures have been shown to correlate poorly. Young children appear to have higher core body temperatures than adults, with temperatures slightly greater than 37.8° C occurring frequently in those younger than 2 years of age. Most recently, a study by Herzog and Coyne[8] suggested that the upper limits of normal for a rectal temperature is 38.0° C for infants less than 1 month old, 38.1° C in 1-month-olds, and 38.2° C in 2-month-olds. In this study, 6.2% of infants (well babies) had a rectal temperature of 38.0° C. Lowest temperatures occur from 2 to 6 AM and highest ones from 5 to 7 PM, a diurnal variation that persists even during a febrile illness. Because of the range of normal body temperatures, knowing a child's usual body temperature occasionally can be useful so that an abnormal elevation can be recognized more easily. The extent to which body temperature is elevated from normal may help determine the presence and significance of fever. This especially may be true in a young infant, in whom even a mild fever may be associated with serious disease. Although the variability and range of normal temperatures in children have made it difficult to define fever precisely and consistently, a recent consensus panel of experts[2] has recommended that the lower limit of fever be defined as a **rectal** temperature of 38° C (100.4° F).

MEASUREMENT

Inasmuch as accurate measurement of body temperature is relied on extensively to determine the presence of fever, every physician should ensure that patients and parents are knowledgeable about the techniques for temperature measurement, as well as its rationale. Ideally this discussion should be held at the time of the child's birth, just before hospital discharge.

The traditional locations for measurement of temperature are the rectum, the mouth, and the axilla. Glass thermometers with mercury or alcohol-filled bulbs commonly are used at home, although most physicians' offices and hospitals now use electronic thermometers that have digital readouts and disposable sheaths to reduce the spread of communicable disease. Attempts to measure temperature at home by use of a liquid crystal temperature strip applied to the forehead or sensor-containing pacifiers have not been successful uniformly and are not sufficiently reliable. A more recent advance in temperature measurement is the development of a device that is inserted into the outer part of the ear canal and measures thermal infrared energy emitted from the tympanic membrane. Because the tympanic membrane's blood supply is common with that going to the hypothalamus, core body temperature can be measured. This method is not uncomfortable, takes only 1 second, and has correlated well with pulmonary artery ($r = 0.98$) and rectal ($r = 0.90$) temperatures in adults.

A number of studies have demonstrated that acceptable correlations of tympanic membrane temperatures with rectal temperatures also exist in children.[4,23] However, in children who are very young (less than 3 months) or exceptionally active (toddlers), correlation with rectal temperatures has not been found to be as good, particularly if the child is febrile.[21] Caution is advised, therefore, in using this technique in the very young infant. In addition, environmental temperature (either hot or cold) has been shown to affect tympanic temperatures significantly,[26] something that is not true of rectal temperatures. Nevertheless, in the older infant or child and in the child for whom a rectal temperature is contraindicated (e.g., a neutropenic child), the advent of a tympanic thermometer has made the process of temperature-taking more pleasant, more reliable, more efficient, and more acceptable to parents.

Because the rectal temperature generally reflects core body temperature best, this location is preferred unless a specific contraindication to minor rectal trauma exists. After the procedure is explained to the parent and, as appropriate, to the child, a well-lubricated glass thermometer or a sheathed electronic thermometer should be inserted 3 to 7 cm into the anal canal. If care is taken that the thermometer stays in the anal canal, peak temperature will be reached in 2 to 3 minutes by using a glass thermometer or in about 30 seconds by using an electronic thermometer.

Taking temperatures orally should not be attempted until the child is older than 5 to 6 years and is cooperative. After the thermometer has been placed under the tongue for a minimum of 1 minute, a temperature reading will be obtained that is about 0.5° C less than the rectal temperature. Because hot and cold foods may alter the oral temperature by as much as 1° to 2° C, they should be avoided for an hour before measurement.

Axillary temperature measurements have been recommended in the very young infant because of a concern that rectal temperature measurement in infants might result in rectal perforation. However, very few cases of rectal perforation have been reported (11 cases reported in the world literature over the past 30 years), and all have occurred in neonates, in the hospital, and in the first few days of life. Thus little risk and no advantages are associated with taking an axillary temperature after the first few days of life. Moreover, although axillary temperatures have been shown to correlate well with rectal temperatures in preterm infants under radiant warmers,[16] they correlate poorly in older infants and children.[17,18] Several recent studies have demonstrated that as much as 3° C difference can exist between the axillary and rectal temperature. In addition, although a mean difference of up to 1.8° C between axillary and rectal temperatures has been demonstrated in group studies, this cannot be used as a standard number to convert axillary to rectal temperatures because of significant individual patient variability. For all these reasons, axillary temperature measurements should be avoided if possible. If neither oral nor rectal temperatures can be measured, a tympanic temperature reading would be preferable.

ASSOCIATED SIGNS AND SYMPTOMS

Donaldson[7] has noted the behavior of humans and animals to be remarkably similar when fever is present. After IL-1 has elevated the set-point in the hypothalamus, patients, as much as they are able, attempt to adjust the environment to keep their body at this higher temperature. Young children usually seek close contact with a warm person (generally a parent), wish to be covered by a blanket, sit near a warm stove or register, and refuse cold liquids or foods. Although children may be quite comfortable at this elevated body temperature, they interact less with others, have a decreased ability to concentrate, substitute quieter activities for energetic ones, and become less communicative except to indicate discomfort and distress. This "adaptive withdrawal" often is accompanied by loss of appetite and complaints of headache.

Such a combination of behavioral symptoms is a familiar indicator of illness to most parents and usually results in the "hand on the forehead" maneuver, followed by measurement of the temperature. Unfortunately, parents may not recognize the onset of fever in the younger child because the alterations in behavior are fewer and more subtle. In a small infant, irritability and anorexia may be the sole evidence of fever and disease. If a parent is not familiar with these subtle cues, recognition of serious illness may be significantly delayed.

In addition to the behavioral changes that may accompany fever, the general physical examination may reveal a pronounced hypermetabolic state. The child may have flushed cheeks and an unusual glitter in the eyes and may be either sleepy and lethargic or exceptionally alert and excited (particularly 5- to 10-year-olds). With rare exception the pulse is elevated by about 10 to 15 beats per degree centigrade of fever, and the respiratory rate is increased. (If the pulse rate is less than expected from the degree of fever, typhoid fever, tularemia, mycoplasmal infection, or factitious fever should be considered.) The skin may feel very hot and dry ("burning up with fever"), although the distal extremities may be cold and pale (vasoconstricted), obscuring a very high core body temperature. Most children are not particularly uncomfortable, but some may shiver or sweat, mechanisms by which the body increases or decreases temperature. Sweating may be so excessive that significant dehydration may occur, particularly if the intake of fluids has been poor. Thus a dry mouth and lips may result not only from rapid mouth breathing but also from dehydration. Finally, increased irritability of the central nervous system may occur, reflected in a febrile seizure.

The aforementioned signs and symptoms may be less obvious in a small infant. Shivering does not occur in the first few months of life, and diaphoresis is seen less frequently than in the older child. Because irritability and pallor may be the only suggestions of illness, careful attention should be given to the child if the parent mentions these signs.

PRESENTATION

How a febrile child comes to the attention of a physician or nurse practitioner determines the urgency and type of management initiated. Probably the most dramatic and frightening manifestation of fever in a child is the sudden occurrence of a seizure. Usually lasting less than 15 minutes and occurring within 24 hours of the onset of fever, a generalized tonic or tonic-clonic seizure may begin without warning. Most parents are not aware that a fever was present and then feel guilty for not having noted it. The pediatrician may be called after the seizure has taken place and often is first alerted when the child already has been transported to the local emergency room. There the child may be postictal and have a temperature of 102° to 104° F (39° to 40° C). A careful assessment of the patient is indicated because a seizure may be the first sign of meningitis or encephalitis.

Although some have recommended that every patient who has a first febrile seizure automatically have a lumbar puncture, most authorities recommend that diagnostic evaluations be individualized. Reexamination of the child after defervescence and after resolution of the convulsive episode may be helpful in determining whether an examination of the cerebrospinal fluid is needed. However, in children younger than 24 months and especially under 18 months of age, it probably is prudent to perform the lumbar puncture because the telltale signs of meningitis (meningismus, Kernig sign, and Brudzinski sign) may be absent. More commonly, the patient first is seen when the fever has been present for longer than 24 hours and is associated either with nonspecific symptoms, such as those mentioned before, or with symptoms referable to a particular organ system. Inasmuch as many of the evaluations of the febrile child take place over the telephone (the first contact with the clinician), the physician must be able to take a pertinent history. Of particular significance are the age of the patient (the younger the child, the more careful the evaluation), associated signs and symptoms, exposure to illness in the family or community, history of recent immunization, and a history of any recurrent infections (e.g., urinary tract infections, streptococcal infections, or otitis media). The time of year should be considered because certain viral diseases are more prevalent at different times of the year. Respiratory syncytial virus and influenza virus are more common during the winter. Parainfluenzae infections (most common cause of croup) are more common during the spring and, especially, the fall. Enteroviruses typically are present primarily during the summer. In addition, questions should be asked about the duration and the height of the fever. A low-grade fever that has been present for many days usually does not need to be evaluated as urgently as a temperature of 106° F (41° C) that has been present for a few hours. The former is likely to indicate either a chronic or benign illness, whereas the latter has a greater risk of being an acute, perhaps serious, disease.

A visit or telephone call for minimal fever and little evidence of disease should prompt a careful assessment of the psychosocial factors that may be contributing to parental concern. Is the main concern about something else—the "hidden agenda"? What knowledge about fever and disease does the caregiver have? Has there been a previous traumatic experience with disease? Could this be a "vulnerable child"? Is this a dysfunctional family in which minor illness either cannot be dealt with or is used as a means to meet other needs? These questions and others may clarify the situation.

DIFFERENTIAL DIAGNOSIS

Innumerable conditions may cause fever, but an extensive discussion about each condition is beyond the scope of this chapter. However, to classify conditions associated with fever into broad categories is useful: (1) infections, (2) collagen-vascular diseases, (3) neoplasia, (4) metabolic diseases (e.g., hyperthyroidism), (5) chronic inflammatory diseases, (6) hematological diseases (e.g., sickle cell disease, transfusion reaction), (7) drug fever and immunization reactions, (8) poisoning (e.g., aspirin, atropine), (9) central nervous system abnormalities, and (10) factitious fever. In addition, dehydration, activity, and heat exposure all can cause an elevation in temperature (hyperthermia).

Although any disease in these categories may cause fever at any age, some diseases are more likely to occur at some ages than at others. Collagen-vascular disease and inflammatory bowel disease, for example, are unusual in infants but become progressively more frequent with increasing age. Similarly, febrile immunization reactions are much more common during the first year of life, the time during which immunizations usually are administered.

Infections account for the majority of fevers in all age

groups, primarily affecting the respiratory and gastrointestinal tracts. Most of these infections have a viral origin (e.g., enterovirus, influenza virus, parainfluenza virus, respiratory syncytial virus, adenovirus, rhinovirus, rotavirus) and generally are self-limited. Knowledge of the seasonality of these viruses promotes correct and efficient diagnoses. In addition, knowledge of the typical physical findings in these infections and their course may help distinguish them from bacterial disease. For example, high fever, irritability, cervical adenopathy, and painful vesicles on the gums and tongue are characteristic of herpes gingivostomatitis. Failure to examine the tongue and gums may result in an unnecessary septic workup in search of a possible bacterial infection. On the other hand, assuming that a high fever in a 2-month-old child is due to roseola (exanthem subitum) would be erroneous because this infection (human herpesvirus 6) usually does not occur at that early an age. Failure to evaluate the fever further might result in missing a serious bacterial infection. Although viral infections may cause significant morbidity and mortality, the more aggressive course and serious outcomes of bacterial infections make early diagnosis especially important, particularly because effective antibiotic treatment usually is available. Bacterial infections may be especially devastating in younger children, who are relatively immunocompromised because of their immature immune system. What remains as a localized infection in the older child may be disseminated rapidly to other soft tissues in the infant and toddler, particularly the blood (bacteremia), the lungs (pneumonia), the meninges (meningitis), the bones (osteomyelitis), and the joints (arthritis). Because these infections may be fatal if not recognized, the physician must be equipped to differentiate bacterial infections from the more benign viral infections.

The younger the child, the more difficult it is to recognize bacterial infection. Complaints cannot be verbalized, and physical signs and symptoms are more subtle and easily missed unless a high index of suspicion is maintained. Of particular concern is the difficulty in diagnosing bacterial disease in children who have no obvious focus of infection. For this reason, many attempts have been made during the last 15 years to identify children in whom fever portends a high likelihood of a serious bacterial infection.[22] Children between birth and 36 months of age have been of special interest because fever is most common in this age group and they may be difficult to assess, particularly during the first 6 months of life. Efforts have focused on three areas: (1) data from the history and physical examination,[9,15] (2) laboratory data,[13] and (3) response to antipyretics.[1] Of the three areas, the response to antipyretics has been shown most clearly *not* to be helpful in distinguishing between patients who have a serious bacterial infection and those who have a more benign viral infection.[1] Children who have a serious infection respond to antipyretics no differently than those whose illness is less significant. In fact, some children who have viral illnesses do not defervesce as well. With respect to the other areas, many studies now have been performed attempting to delineate the precise combination of clinical or laboratory variables that might identify the febrile child at risk for serious disease. Specifically, recommendations have been made for the initial management of febrile infants and children who do not have an obvious source of infection.[2]

Fever during the first 4 days of life has been associated with a high incidence of bacterial disease.[24] A temperature above 37° C (98.6° F) occurs in 1% of all newborns; of these children, 10% have a bacterial infection caused primarily by group B streptococcal or gram-negative enteric pathogens.

Although febrile (≥38.0° C) infants younger than 3 months of age were previously believed to have a higher incidence of bacteremia, more recent studies suggest that the incidence is similar to that of older infants and children. The presence of bacterial disease ranges between 8% and 15% and that of bacteremia between 3% and 4%.[2] In fact, neither age, sex, height of fever, nor apparent degree of toxicity has been a reliable predictor of bacteremia or serious bacterial infection.[3,14] Instead, several studies now have identified a combination of clinical and laboratory criteria that can be used to recognize infants who are at low risk for having a bacterial infection (low-risk criteria). The infants must satisfy all of the following conditions: previously healthy, no clinical signs of toxicity, no focal bacterial infection on physical examination (except otitis media), WBC 5000 to 15,000 with <1500 bands, and normal urinalysis (<5 WBC/hpf) or gram-stained smear <5 WBC/hpf in stool if diarrhea is present.[6] Infants who in the first 3 months of life satisfy these criteria have only a 1.4% probability of having a serious bacterial infection, a 1.1% probability of having bacteremia, and a 0.5% probability of having meningitis.

Because it is especially difficult to determine whether an infant less than 3 months of age is at a low or high risk for bacterial disease solely on the basis of the degree of fever (septicemia has occurred in infants who have even low grade fevers[19]), an evaluation should be prompt and thorough in all such infants who have a fever of ≥38° C, paying particular attention to obtaining the data necessary for classifying the child as at low or high risk. Such a comprehensive evaluation should include a thorough physical examination, total and differential white blood cell count, urinalysis,[11] examination of the cerebrospinal fluid, and cultures of the blood, urine, and spinal fluid. A urine culture is especially important because a urinary tract infection is the most common bacterial infection observed in this age group, even in the absence of pyuria.[5,12] Because urinary tract infections have been shown to occur more often in uncircumcised males, this physical characteristic should be noted.

In infants and children between 3 months and 3 years of age who have a fever ≥39° C that has no obvious source, the risk of bacteremia ranges from 3% to 11% (mean, 4.3%). Below this temperature, an associated bacteremia is much less common. *Streptococcus pneumoniae* (pneumococcus) and *Hemophilus influenzae* are the bacteria implicated most commonly in bacteremia and are associated with tissue invasion in 5% of cases of the former and in almost all cases of the latter. Fortunately, the advent of the *Hemophilus influenzae* type B vaccine (HIB) has diminished greatly the likelihood of developing a serious infection because of this organism. *Hemophilus influenzae* meningitis and epiglottitis have become very uncommon since the vaccine has become widely available. On the basis of many studies performed over the last decade, several recommendations can facilitate the identification of children between 3 months and 3 years of age who have a fever ≥39° that has no obvious focus of infection but who are most at risk for a serious bacterial infection.[2] After a thorough history is taken, including queries about illness of a similar nature in other family members, the child should be assessed clinically and the degree of toxicity should be determined. If the child shows signs of toxicity (lethargy, noninteractiveness, perfusion problems, and the like), hospitalization should be considered along with further diagnostic tests to assess for sepsis. If the child does not appear toxic, a white blood cell count should be obtained, and if this is >15,000, blood samples should be obtained for culture. (Children who have a WBC >15,000 are five times as likely to be bacteremic than those who have a WBC <15,000). Practically, obtaining the white cell count and blood samples at the same time is easiest, sending the blood samples for culture only if the white blood cell count warrants it. A urine culture is recommended for male infants under 6 months of age and female infants under 2 years because 5% to 8% of children in this age group who have an undifferentiated fever have a urinary tract infection.[10] A urinalysis is not adequate by itself as a screening device to determine which child should have a urine culture because 20% of children who have a urinary tract infection have a normal urinalysis, including a negative test for urinary nitrites or leukocyte esterase. A chest radiograph is necessary only if any clinical symptoms or signs suggest pneumonia (e.g., tachypnea, dyspnea, and the like).[9]

Once the infant or child who has an undifferentiated fever has been evaluated, a plan of management similar to the one developed recently by a consensus panel of experts (derived from a meta-analysis of 85 published studies on this subject) should be instituted[2] (see Figs. 132-1 and 132-2).

Children older than 3 years of age are more likely to have

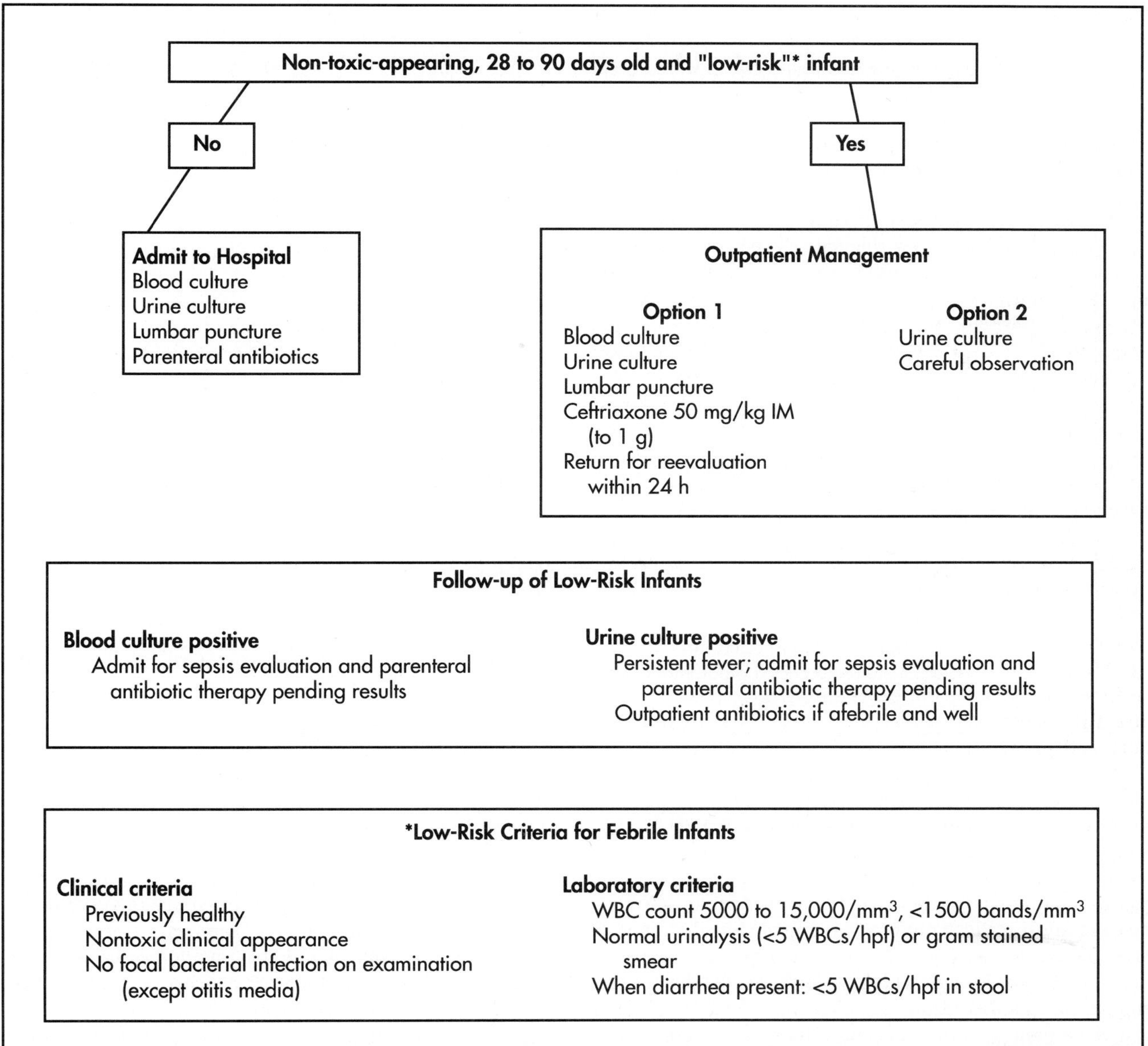

FIG. 132-1 Algorithm for the management of a previously healthy infant 0 to 90 days of age with fever without source ≥38.0° C.

(From Baraff LJ et al: *Pediatrics* 92:1, 1993.)

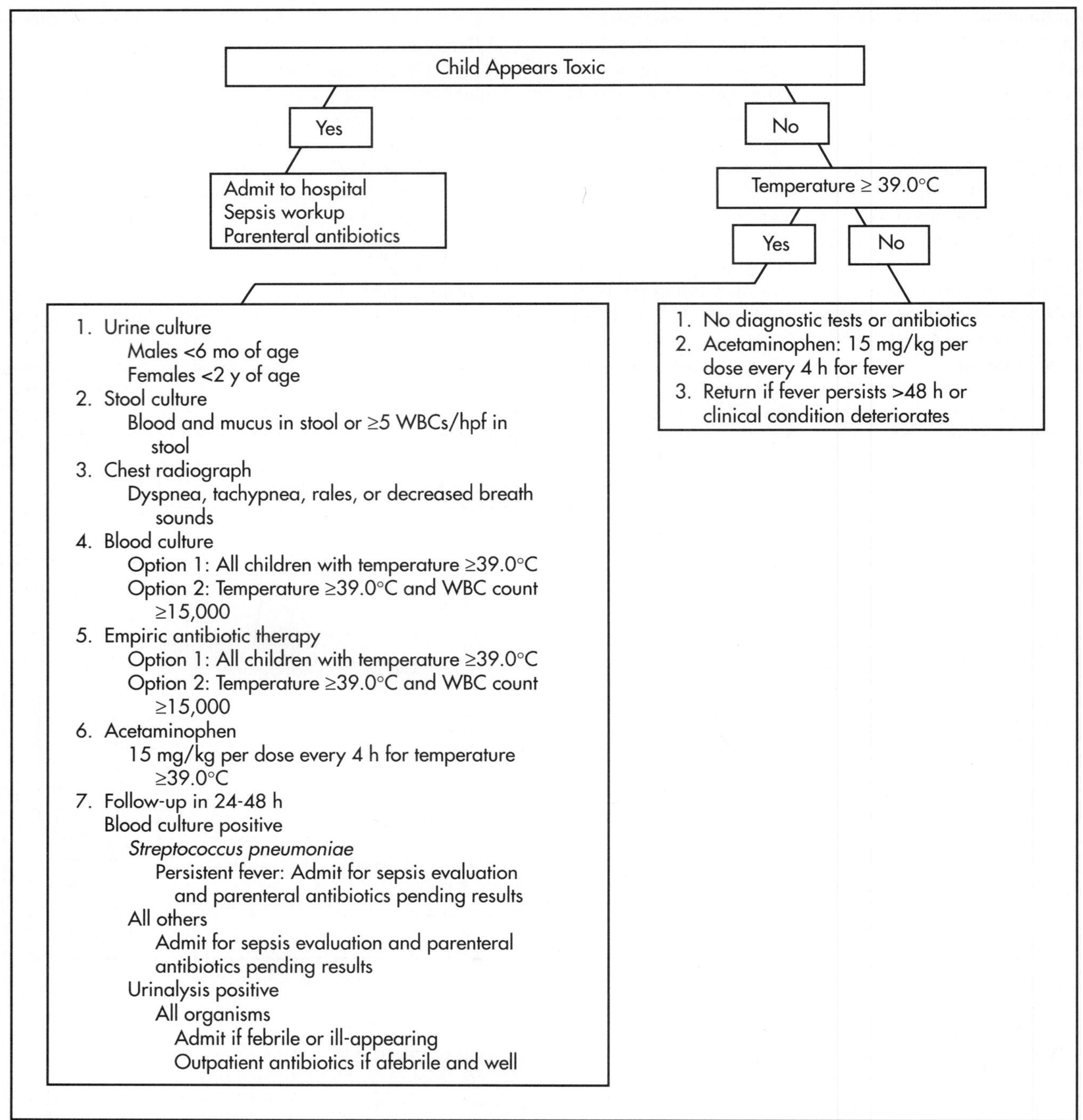

FIG. 132-2 Algorithm for the management of a previously healthy child 91 days to 36 months of age with fever without source.

(From Baraff LJ et al: *Pediatrics* 92:1, 1993.)

signs and symptoms suggestive of a recognizable illness. If they have nonspecific symptoms, an urgent consultation with the physician probably is unnecessary; however, regardless of age, all febrile children who have such localized signs and symptoms as swollen joints, meningismus, labored respirations, chest pain, dysuria, petechiae, alteration of consciousness, and severe abdominal pain should be seen immediately.

Although many children who have fever do not have obvious signs and symptoms pointing to a clear cause, a careful physical examination may reveal important clues to its origin. Because the majority of infections involve the respiratory tract, this area must be examined carefully. In all instances the tympanic membranes should be examined for otitis media, the pharynx for streptococcal or viral pharyngitis, the nose for the nasal discharge of sinusitis or a viral upper respiratory tract infection, and the lungs for evidence of pneumonia or bronchiolitis. Conjunctivitis may be a clue to adenovirus infection, conjunctivitis-otitis syndrome, or even Kawasaki disease.

The skin is no less important and may demonstrate typical

viral exanthems, such as those associated with rubella, roseola, or chickenpox, or it may show the erythema marginatum of rheumatic fever or the rose spots of typhoid fever.

Generalized lymphadenopathy often occurs with viral illnesses, such as infectious mononucleosis, hepatitis, or cytomegalovirus infection, but it also may be a clue to the diagnosis of leukemia or lymphoma. Localized enlargement of lymph nodes should prompt a search for a skin infection or for a tumor. Isolated cervical lymphadenopathy may be associated with tuberculosis infection or cat-scratch disease.

The musculoskeletal system must be examined with care. Localized bone tenderness may suggest osteomyelitis, and a restricted range of motion in a warm joint may suggest arthritis. The latter finding may occur in many different diseases, but a careful examination of the heart is always indicated to detect the carditis of rheumatic fever or infective endocarditis. The spine should be palpated for any evidence of diskitis, and any costovertebral angle tenderness should prompt an examination of the urine for evidence of a urinary tract infection or pyelonephritis.

Factitious fever is a final consideration; it is an uncommon but nevertheless real entity, even in children. Children as young as 8 years of age have been known to increase the thermometer reading artificially by rubbing the mercury thermometer bulb on the sheets or by exposing it to warm liquids. Clues on physical examination include a pulse that is not correlated with the temperature elevation, inability to document fever when it is measured rectally, and an absence of sweating during defervescence. Investigation of psychosocial disturbances within the family usually is necessary.

MANAGEMENT

During the last decade a large body of evidence has accumulated that appears to support the positive role fever plays as a part of the host defenses. Increased leukocyte mobility, increased leukocyte bactericidal activity, enhanced interferon effect, and decreased available trace metals (notably iron) for pathogenic bacteria are just a few of the ways in which fever improves the body's ability to fight infection. The inability of animals to mount a febrile response to infection has been demonstrated to be highly associated with increased mortality.

Provided that an appropriate evaluation has been undertaken and that specific therapy has been instituted for the underlying disease, the physician should question whether the best interest of the patient is served by eliminating fever through environmental and pharmacological manipulations. Three factors need to be considered in answering this question: (1) the complication rate associated with fever, (2) the ability of the patient to handle the increased metabolic demands of the fever, and (3) the comfort of the patient.

Complications in children who have a temperature below 105.8° F (41° C) are unusual unless the fever is associated with febrile status epilepticus or heatstroke. Of febrile seizures, 1% to 2% last longer than 15 minutes; if they continue beyond 60 minutes, they may be associated with severe brain damage (probably resulting from hypoxia). Heatstroke is uncommon in childhood and usually is associated with a temperature higher than 107.6° F (42° C), coma, and anhidrosis; it has a mortality rate of 80%. In both these instances body temperature obviously should be decreased. Children who have a seizure disorder may have an exacerbation of their seizures in the presence of fever and therefore may benefit from antipyretic management.

The child who has limited cardiopulmonary reserve, as might occur in congenital heart disease, cardiac infections, cystic fibrosis, or asthma, should be kept as normothermic as possible in spite of some of the benefits of fever in fighting disease. The high metabolic demand induced by fever otherwise may result in irreversible decompensation and death.

Although many children exhibit no discomfort until the temperature is higher than 102° to 104° F (39° to 40° C), discomfort at lower temperatures may be treated with antipyretic therapy. If the child is comfortable, no treatment is necessary up to a temperature of 105.8° F (41° C), except for the administration of additional fluids to prevent dehydration. A complete discussion of antipyretic therapy is provided in Chapter 25, Management of Fever.

Finally, the physician should provide sound education to parents about fever—its definition and meaning, its benefits and disadvantages, when to be concerned about it as an indicator of serious disease, its initial home management, including proper dosing with antipyretics, and when to contact the physician. Such education has been shown to improve home management and to enhance parental confidence in caring for their febrile child.[20]

SUMMARY

Although fever can be a frightening symptom that may be associated with serious illness, its treatment is much less crucial than the evaluation and treatment of the illness causing the fever. Health care professionals are responsible for educating parents about the proper management of their febrile child, emphasizing their role in the observation for symptoms that are more likely to be associated with serious disease. Fever is but one symptom that should be evaluated in the total context of the care of the patient.

REFERENCES

1. Baker RC et al: Severity of disease correlated with fever reduction in febrile infants, *Pediatrics* 83:1016, 1989.
2. Baraff LJ et al: Practice guideline for the management of infants and children 0 to 36 months of age with fever without source, *Pediatrics* 92:1, 1993.
3. Berkowitz CD et al: Fever in infants less than two months of age: spectrum of disease and predictors of outcome, *Pediatr Emerg Care* 1:128, 1985.
4. Chamberlain JM et al: Comparison of a tympanic thermometer to rectal and oral thermometers in a pediatric emergency department, *Clin Pediatr* 30(suppl):24, 1991.
5. Crain EF, Gershel JC: Urinary tract infection in febrile infants younger than 8 weeks of age, *Pediatrics* 86:363, 1990.
6. Dagan R et al: Identification of infants unlikely to have serious bacterial infection although hospitalized for suspected sepsis, *J Pediatr* 107:855, 1985.
7. Donaldson JF: Therapy of acute fever: a comparative approach, *Hosp Pract* 16:125, 1981.
8. Herzog LW, Coyne JL: What is fever? Normal temperature in infants less than 3 months old, *Clin Pediatr* 32:142, 1993.

9. Heulitt MJ et al: Febrile infants less than 3 months old: value of chest radiography, *Radiology* 167:135, 1988.
10. Hoberman A et al: Prevalence of urinary infection in febrile infants, *J Pediatr* 123:17, 1993.
11. Hoberman A et al: Pyuria and bacteriuria in urine specimens obtained by catheter from young children with fever, *J Pediatr* 124:513, 1994.
12. Krober MS et al: Bacterial and viral pathogens causing fever in infants less than 3 months old, *Am J Dis Child* 139:889, 1985.
13. McCarthy PL: Controversies in pediatrics: what tests are indicated for the child under two with fever, *Pediatr Rev* 1:51, 1979.
14. McCarthy PL, Dolan T: The serious implications of high fever in infants during their first three months, *Clin Pediatr* 15:794, 1976.
15. McCarthy PL et al: Observation scales to identify serious illness in febrile children, *Pediatrics* 70:802, 1982.
16. Moen JE et al: Axillary vs rectal temperatures in preterm infants under radiant warmers, *J Obstet Gynecol Neonatal Nurs* 16:348, 1987.
17. Morley CJ et al: Axillary and rectal temperature measurements in infants, *Arch Dis Child* 67:122, 1992.
18. Ogren JM: The inaccuracy of axillary temperatures measured with an electronic thermometer, *Am J Dis Child* 144:110, 1990.
19. Roberts KB, Borzy MS: Fever in the first eight weeks of life, *Johns Hopkins Med J* 141:9, 1977.
20. Robinson JS et al: The impact of fever health education on clinic utilization, *Am J Dis Child* 143:698, 1989.
21. Selfridge J, Shea SS: The accuracy of the tympanic membrane thermometer in detecting fever in infants aged 3 months and younger in the emergency department setting, *J Emerg Nurs* 19:127, 1993.
22. Teele DW, Marshall R, Klein JO: Unsuspected bacteremia in young children, *Pediatr Clin North Am* 26:773, 1979.
23. Terndrup TE, Milewski, A: The performance of two tympanic thermometers in a pediatric emergency department, *Clin Pediatr* 30(suppl):18, 1991.
24. Voora S et al: Fever in full-term newborns in the first four days of life, *Pediatrics* 69 (suppl):40, 1982.
25. Wunderlich C: *Das Verhalten der Eigenwarme in Krankenheiten,* Leipzig, Germany, 1868, Otto Wigard.
26. Zener WJ, Terndrup TE: The impact of moderate ambient temperature variance on the relationship between oral, rectal, and tympanic membrane temperatures, *Clin Pediatr* 30 (suppl):61, 1991.

SUGGESTED READINGS

Bonadio WA: Evaluation and management of serious bacterial infections in the febrile young infant, *Pediatr Infect Dis J* 9:905, 1990.

Cone TE: Diagnosis and treatment: children with fevers, *Pediatrics* 43:290, 1969.

Dagan R et al: Epidemiology and laboratory diagnosis of infection with viral and bacterial pathogens in infants hospitalized for suspected sepsis, *J Pediatr* 115:351, 1989.

Dinarello CA, Cannon JG, Wolff SM: New concepts on the pathogenesis of fever, *Rev Infect Dis* 10:168, 1988.

Jaffe DM et al: Antibiotic administration to treat possible occult bacteremia in febrile children, *N Engl J Med* 317:1175, 1987.

Kluger MJ: Fever, *Pediatrics* 66:720, 1980.

Kramer MS, Naimark L, Leduc DG: Parental fever phobia and its correlates, *Pediatrics* 75:1110, 1985.

Schmitt BD: Fever phobia, *Am J Dis Child* 134:176, 1980.

133 Fever of Unknown Origin

Élise W. van der Jagt

One of the more frustrating symptoms for the clinician to evaluate is that of a fever that has no discernible cause. Because fever suggests disease, the inability to identify its cause strikes at one of the physician's *raisons d'etre* and may undermine any credibility he or she previously has established with the patient and family. The longer the fever persists, the more concern is raised by the family and the more plentiful the demands made on the physician. A fever that is of only a few days' duration and that is not associated with any localizing signs or symptoms frequently does not even come to a physician's attention unless the child appears quite ill. Fever that continues beyond 5 to 7 days, however, usually alarms parents sufficiently to prompt a medical consultation. This discussion focuses on these more prolonged fevers and their evaluation.

DEFINITION

The classic definition for a fever of unknown origin (FUO) was proposed by Petersdorf and Beeson[7] in 1961 to be a fever (1) that is higher than 38.3° C (101° F) on several occasions, (2) that is present for more than 3 weeks, and (3) whose cause still is unexplained after 1 week of evaluation in the hospital. This definition, based on a study of adult patients, has not been accepted completely by most pediatricians, who would prefer not to delay evaluation for 3 weeks. More commonly, therefore, an FUO in children has been defined as a rectal temperature greater than 38.3° C, lasting for at least 2 weeks, whose cause has not been elicited by simple diagnostic tests, including a thorough history and physical examination.[3] Some would add that 1 of the 2 weeks of fever should be documented in the hospital.

Careful documentation of fever is necessary before labeling a child with a diagnosis of FUO. A thorough explanation of the range of normal core body temperature for age, with its diurnal variation, may help in excluding patients who truly are not febrile but who instead have a high normal body temperature. The physician should instruct the parents in the technique of taking a rectal temperature and define a day of fever as a 24-hour period in which a temperature greater than 38.3° C occurs at least once. All medications taken, the various activities participated in, and the environmental temperature during this time should be recorded, since each may affect body temperature. However, although much importance has been attached to fever patterns in the past (i.e., remittent, intermittent, sustained), detailing them is not necessary because they rarely are diagnostic of a specific disease.[6]

Careful documentation of fever will help to exclude what Kleiman[5] has called a pseudo-FUO. Children who have a pseudo-FUO do not have a true fever if their body temperature is measured accurately and consistently (at times this needs to be done under hospital supervision), but do exhibit a definite constellation of findings that is recognizable and, many times, diagnostic (see the box above). In addition to the inability to document fever and in the face of a completely normal physical examination, the parents may tell of a previous serious illness and their concerns about its recurrence or lasting effect ("vulnerable child syndrome"). Their child may have missed an excessive amount of school considering the general degree of illness described; however, school absence often is prompted by the presence of fatigue, abdominal pain, and headache in the morning—symptoms that are conspicuously absent during the rest of the day. Finally, a sequence of minor illnesses may have occurred, mimicking a single, continuous illness. Only careful questioning and record keeping will clarify this so that one can provide a reassuring explanation to the parents.

CHARACTERISTICS OF THE CHILD WHO HAS PSEUDO-FUO

1. Absence of documented, persistent fever
2. Lack of objective, abnormal physical findings
3. History of significant or near-fatal illness
4. Parental fear of malignant or crippling disease
5. Frequent environmental exposure to illness
6. Absence of persistent weight loss
7. Normal erythrocyte sedimentation rate and platelet count
8. Large number of missed school days because of subjective morning complaints
9. Discordance of fever and pulse rate
10. Medical or paramedical family background
11. Majority have, singly or in sequence, mild self-limited diseases, behavioral problems, parents who have misconceptions concerning health and disease, or families under stress

From Kleiman MB: *Pediatr Clin North Am* 29:201, 1982.

DIFFERENTIAL DIAGNOSIS

The box on p. 968 lists the causes of FUO in children. The causes are subdivided into four categories: infectious diseases, collagen-vascular diseases, malignancies, and miscellaneous. This list clearly shows that the majority of FUOs eventually are found to be caused by common pediatric illnesses that are either self-limited or treatable.

An infectious illness is the most common cause for an FUO in children, making up as many as 60% of the reported cases; the second most common cause is collagen-vascular disease, making up about 20% of the cases. Children under 6 years

CAUSES OF FEVER OF UNKNOWN ORIGIN IN CHILDREN

Infectious diseases

Bacterial
- Brucellosis
- Bacterial endocarditis
- Leptospirosis
- Liver abscess
- Mastoiditis (chronic)
- Osteomyelitis
- Pelvic abscess
- Perinephric abscess
- Pyelonephritis
- Salmonellosis
- Sinusitis
- Subdiaphragmatic abscess
- Tuberculosis
- Tularemia

Viral
- Cytomegalovirus
- Hepatitis viruses
- Epstein-Barr virus (infectious mononucleosis)

Chlamydial
- Lymphogranuloma venereum
- Psittacosis

Rickettsial
- Q fever
- Rocky Mountain spotted fever

Fungal
- Blastomycosis (nonpulmonary)
- Histoplasmosis (disseminated)

Infectious diseases—cont'd

Parasitic
- Malaria
- Toxoplasmosis
- Visceral larva migrans

Unclassified
- Sarcoidosis

Collagen-vascular diseases

Juvenile rheumatoid arthritis
Polyarteritis nodosa
Systemic lupus erythematosus

Malignancies

Hodgkin disease
Leukemia-lymphoma
Neuroblastoma

Miscellaneous

Central diabetes insipidus
Drug fever
Ectodermal dysplasia
Factitious fever
Familial dysautonomia
Granulomatous colitis
Infantile cortical hyperostosis
Nephrogenic diabetes insipidus
Pancreatitis
Periodic fever
Serum sickness
Thyrotoxicosis
Ulcerative colitis

From Feigin RD, Cherry JD: *Textbook of pediatric infectious diseases,* ed 2, Philadelphia, 1987, WB Saunders.

Table 133-1 Diagnosis of Prolonged Fever, Children's Hospital Medical Center, Boston[8]

	Infection						
Age	"Viral"	Nonviral	Collagen	Malignancy	Miscellaneous	No diagnosis	Totals
<6 yr	14 (27%)	20 (38%)	4 (8%)	4 (8%)	7 (13%)	3 (6%)	52
>6 yr	7 (15%)	11 (23%)	16 (33%)	2 (4%)	3 (6%)	9 (19%)	48
TOTALS	21	31	20	6	10	12	100

of age are more likely to have an FUO resulting from an in fection, whereas collagen-vascular diseases are found much more frequently in children older than 6 years (Table 133-1).

Although the majority of infections that manifest themselves as an FUO are an atypical or incomplete manifestation of a common infectious disease, unusual infections should be considered. The appearance during the 1980s and subsequent increased incidence of human immunodeficiency virus (HIV) infection, with its associated acquired immunodeficiency syndrome (AIDS), should encourage the pediatrician to consider this diagnosis and assess the child carefully for the presence of known risk factors (parental intravenous drug abuse, parental promiscuity, parental sexual contact with individuals who may be HIV positive, an HIV-positive mother, hemophilia requiring transfusion of blood products) and characteristic physical signs and symptoms. Fever alone is not usually the sole manifestation of HIV infection. However, HIV infection should be considered and the appropriate laboratory tests performed if the fever has been present for more than 2 months *and* is associated with one or more of the following: failure to thrive or a weight loss of more than 10% from baseline, hepatomegaly, splenomegaly, generalized lymphadenopathy (lymph nodes measuring at least 0.5 cm in two or more sites, with bilateral lymph nodes counting as one site), parotitis, and diarrhea that is either persistent or recurrent.[2]

Of the collagen-vascular diseases, juvenile rheumatoid arthritis is the most common. Fever is associated almost 100% of the time with systemic onset juvenile rheumatoid arthritis, frequently preceding the joint manifestations by weeks or months. The typical double quotidian fever (two fever spikes in 24 hours with a normal temperature in between) is a helpful clue to this diagnosis. Other inflammatory diseases that should be considered are lupus erythematosus and regional enteritis. The latter is more common among children over 6 years of age.

Malignancy, the most anxiety-producing diagnosis, is present in only a small percentage of patients in most studies (1.5% to 6%). This is in contrast to adults who have an FUO, of whom up to 31% are found to have a neoplastic process. Most common in children is leukemia, although solid tumors such as lymphoma, hypernephroma, and hepatoma all have been described. The exact reason for fever in these diseases is unclear but may be related to endogenous pyrogen produced by the neoplastic cells.

As can be seen from the box on p. 968, a large spectrum of miscellaneous diseases can cause fevers. In as many as 25% of patients who have prolonged fevers, however, a true diagnosis never is obtained. (In one recent study, no diagnosis was ever found in 67% of the children.) These are the genuine FUOs. The majority of these patients appear to do well, and the fever eventually disappears after months or even years.

EVALUATION

Whether the child has a true FUO or a pseudo-FUO cannot be determined without a thorough and precise history and physical examination, with the physician paying close attention to behavioral, social, and environmental factors. Information regarding travel, animal exposure, frequency of exposure to other persons who have common febrile illnesses, previous illness, hospitalizations, drug treatments, family history of disease, and the precise course of the manifested symptoms must be obtained methodically and efficiently. Meticulous documentation of dates especially is important.

For children over 11 to 12 years of age, a separate interview is indicated to obtain the child's perspective on the illness and to elicit information that may be difficult to express in the presence of parents. School, peer relationships, family functioning, and sexual identity and activity all should be explored.

Once a complete history has been taken, a full physical examination must be performed. Rectal temperature, respiratory rate, heart rate, and blood pressure measurements should not be forgotten. Any discrepancy between heart rate and temperature should suggest factitious fever. A careful examination of the respiratory tract is indicated. Inspection of the pharynx for hyperemia and exudate and the tympanic membranes for chronic otitis media, transillumination of the sinuses for sinusitis, a search for a purulent nasal discharge, and auscultation of the chest for localized wheezing all are important. In the older child, an examination of the teeth to exclude caries and periodontal disease must be included. A new cardiac murmur may be a clue to rheumatic fever or infective endocarditis. Lymphadenopathy, especially if generalized, may suggest a viral infection, such as infectious mononucleosis, cytomegalovirus infection, toxoplasmosis, or HIV infection. Joints must be examined meticulously for swelling, restricted range of motion, and tenderness. Skin rashes may suggest a viral disease or a collagen-vascular disease such as juvenile rheumatoid arthritis. The absence of sweating and the presence of a smooth tongue are consistent with familial dysautonomia, a rare genetic disorder of thermoregulation. Finally, a rectal examination with a sample of stool for a stool guaiac test is imperative, because pararectal lymphadenopathy suggests a pelvic infection, and a positive stool guaiac result might be consistent with inflammatory bowel disease.

If the history and physical examination disclose no specific findings, simple diagnostic tests are indicated. Routine blood counts and urinalysis have not been shown to be of major benefit, although no one advocates their elimination from the workup. A PPD (tuberculin skin test) should be placed to detect tuberculosis, although anergy may occur in active tuberculosis infection. Negative blood, urine, and throat cultures exclude infections of these areas.

Probably the most useful laboratory tests are the erythrocyte sedimentation rate (ESR) and the albumin/globulin ratio. If the ESR is over 30 or the albumin/globulin ratio is reversed, a high probability of serious disease exists—particularly a collagen-vascular disease or a malignancy—and further evaluation should be pursued vigorously.

How the evaluation then should proceed is variable and clearly should be individualized. Because infectious causes are the most common, it is reasonable to pursue special serological tests for such diseases as hepatitis A and B, Epstein-Barr virus infection (infectious mononucleosis), toxoplasmosis, and cytomegalovirus infection. Radioactive gallium scans may be useful in detecting occult abscesses and infections, although this scan has been found to be much less useful in children than in adults.[1] Total body computed tomography scans may help delineate tumors, although, if the abdomen is of primary concern, an abdominal ultrasound will detect significant abnormalities as well.[9] Radiological studies of the sinuses, the gastrointestinal tract, and the chest all may be appropriate in certain individuals. A bone marrow examination occasionally may help in the diagnosis of tuberculosis, leukemia, metastatic cancer, or fungal infections but should be considered only in those children who either have a clinical or laboratory suggestion of malignancy or who are immunocompromised.[4] Finally, if the child is not deteriorating visibly, a period of observation may be necessary until new findings appear that can give more direction.

If the ESR and the albumin/globulin ratio are normal, little can be gained from any of the previously mentioned tests. Observation and periodic evaluation are all that are required while remaining alert for the occurrence of new symptoms or signs that might lead the investigation in a specific direction.

SUMMARY

The evaluation of the child who has an FUO must be individualized to accommodate the history, the physical examination, and the particular social environment in which the child and family live. An intensive examination of all these factors is the physician's responsibility and is the first stage of managing the patient. Whether hospitalization is part of this approach depends ultimately on the amount of parental anxiety, the necessity to document fever, and the performance of diagnostic tests that cannot be done on an outpatient basis.

REFERENCES

1. Buonomo C, Treves ST: Gallium scanning in children with fever of unknown origin, *Pediatr Radiol* 23:307, 1993.
2. Centers for Disease Control: Classification system for human immunodeficiency virus (HIV) infection in children under 13 years of age, *MMWR* 36:225, 1987.
3. Feigin RD, Shearer WT: Fever of unknown origin in children, *Curr Probl Pediatr* 6:1, 1976.
4. Hayani A, Mahoney DH, Fernbach DJ: Role of bone marrow examination in the child with prolonged fever, *J Pediatr* 116:919, 1990.
5. Kleiman MB: The complaint of persistent fever, *Pediatr Clin North Am* 29:201, 1982.
6. Musher DM et al: Fever patterns: their lack of clinical significance, *Arch Intern Med* 139:1225, 1979.
7. Petersdorf RG, Beeson PB: Fever of unexplained origin: report on 100 cases, *Medicine* 40:1, 1961.
8. Pizzo PA, Lovejoy FH, Smith DH: Prolonged fever in children: review of 100 cases, *Pediatrics* 55:468, 1975.
9. Steele RW et al: Usefulness of scanning procedures for diagnosis of fever of unknown origin in children, *J Pediatr* 119:526, 1991.

SUGGESTED READING

Lohr JA, Hendley JO: Prolonged fever of unknown origin: a record of experiences with 54 childhood patients, *Clin Pediatr* 16:768, 1977.

134 Foot and Leg Problems

Robert A. Hoekelman

Pediatricians and family practitioners often have to make judgments concerning actual or presumed problems of the feet and legs in infants and children. The frequency and natural history of these problems is such that referral to orthopedic consultants is not always appropriate. In most instances the problems presented require no treatment, others can be managed easily without consultations, and only a few require the services of an orthopedist.

The *ped* in pediatrics and orthopedics is derived from the Greek word *paidios,* meaning child, not from the Latin *pedalis* or French *ped,* meaning foot. Therefore pediatrics is the medicine (Greek *iatrike*) of the child, and orthopedics is the straightening or correction (Greek *orthos*) of deformities in children. Orthopedics has expanded its scope well beyond this initial thrust; nevertheless, the orthopedist and the pediatrician are concerned with many problems involving the feet of children.

SHOES

Anatomy of the Shoe

Because some foot problems in childhood are treated with corrective shoes, understanding the anatomy of the shoe is necessary. The *last* is the wooden or metal form on which a shoe is constructed. Shoes for regular use are built on a straight last; shoes designed to deviate the forefoot outward are built on an out-flare last; those designed to deviate the forefoot inward are built on an in-flare last. Actually, most of the shoes sold for general use in the United States have an adducted forefoot last rather than a truly straight last.

The *sole* is that part of the shoe that covers the ventral surface of the foot. It consists of the *outsole,* usually made of firm leather or rubber that comes in contact with the surface on which the shoe is placed, and the *insole,* made of soft leather or synthetic material that comes in contact with the plantar surface of the foot. The *heel,* also made of leather, rubber, or synthetic material, elevates the rear portion of the shoe. It usually is absent in the shoes of infants and toddlers. It may be low and flat (common sense), somewhat higher (military), or more elevated and tapered (Cuban or high). The Thomas heel is of medium height and has a forward medial extension.

The *shank* of the shoe is that part of the sole between the forwardmost edge of the heel and ball of the foot. A narrow flat piece of steel sometimes is placed between the inner and outer soles to prevent flexion of the shank of the shoe. The *counter* of the shoe is placed above the heel between the outsole and insole and provides a shelf for the rear portion of the foot. It usually is made of firm leather and may be extended forward on the medial aspect of the shoe to provide added support to the instep. The *upper* or top of the shoe may be made of leather or a variety of other materials. The upper of low shoes (Oxfords) rises to a point below the malleoli; the upper of high shoes extends above the malleoli. The *vamp* is the part of the upper attached to the sole.

Functions of Shoes

The physician often is asked by parents *when* their child should begin wearing shoes and *what* kind of shoe should be worn. In answering these questions, the reasons for wearing shoes must be borne in mind. The shoe has two functions, the most important of which is protection of the feet from trauma and extreme temperatures. Protection implies comfort; therefore the shoe must fit properly to avoid discomfort to the foot. The second function of the shoe is to provide style. Older children often will sacrifice comfort for style despite parental or medical advice to the contrary.

Support to the foot and ankle is *not* a function of the shoe except when a pathological condition is present. Low shoes that have soft uppers are worn by athletes in all sports that place the feet and ankles under severe strain. Ski boots are worn not to support the foot and ankle but to make them "one with the ski," to ensure response to movements originating in the knee and lower leg. High shoes usually are worn by babies and toddlers not to provide support to the foot and ankle but to make it more difficult for the child to remove the shoes.

Style is the only reason for a baby to wear shoes at all until he or she begins walking outdoors or is taken out in cold weather. Some babies may gain a certain degree of stability from hard-sole shoes when beginning to stand, but this has not been shown to enhance learning to walk. Properly fitting shoes that have firm soles and soft uppers should be recommended initially and subsequently. They need not be expensive. Sneakers are perfectly adequate for summer wear and for winter indoor wear.

Fitting Shoes

Determining the proper fitting of shoes involves no great science. The counter should hug the heel snugly, the length should allow ¾ inch between the tip of the great toe and the front end of the upper, and the width should allow ¼ inch between the edge of the fifth toe and the lateral edge of the upper when the foot is pushed medially within the shoe. These measurements should be made with the child standing and should apply only to the time the shoes are newly acquired. There is no reason why shoes in good condition cannot be handed down from one child to another.

The frequency with which shoes should be changed depends on the rate of growth of the feet, the quality of the shoes, and the degree of their use. Parents usually are able to tell when shoes become too small (or rather, feet become too large) without professional advice. The toes will be felt to press against the front end of the upper, and getting the

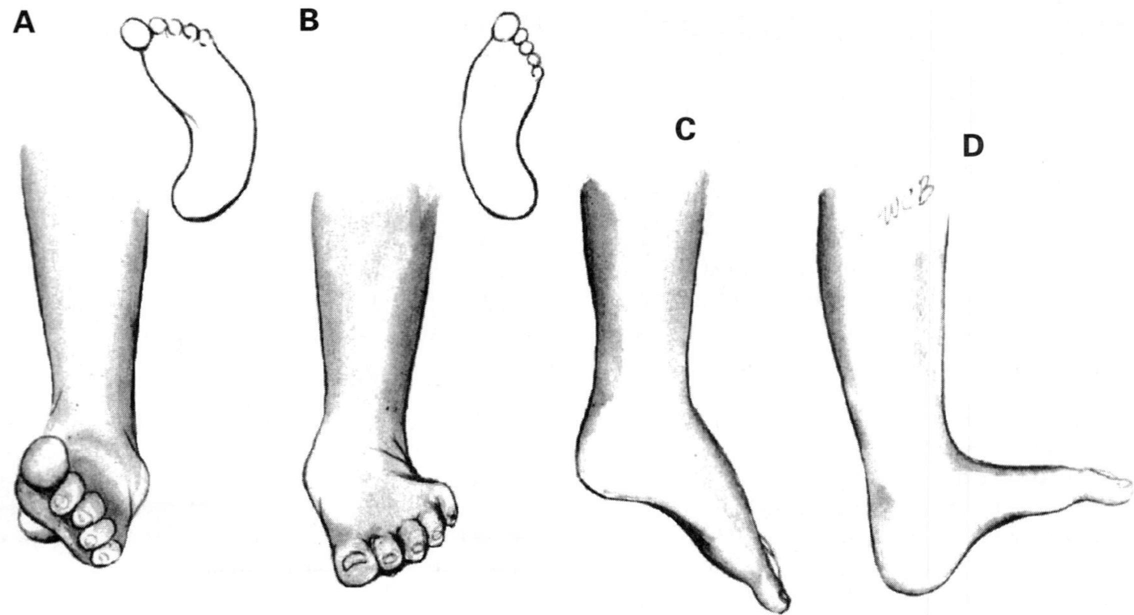

FIG. 134-1 Positional deformities of the foot and ankle. **A,** Varus. **B,** Valgus. **C,** Equinus. **D,** Calcaneus.
(From Tachdjian MO: *Pediatric orthopedics,* 2 vols, Philadelphia, 1977, WB Saunders.)

shoes on or having the child keep them on will be increasingly difficult.

Lightweight cotton, nylon, or wool socks that adjust to the length and width of the foot present no problem in the attainment of maximal foot comfort for children of all ages.

ORTHOPEDIC TERMINOLOGY

Certain terms are used by practitioners to describe positional variations of the lower extremities and often are used in the nomenclature of specific orthopedic conditions.

In general, the joint that is primarily involved in the condition constitutes the first word; the subsequent word or words relate to the positioning of the extremity in relation to the midline of the body. For example, *coxa vara* is a condition of the hip (coxa) that results in a deviation of the leg toward the midline (varus position).

The following orthopedic terms have special reference to abnormalities of the feet (Fig. 134-1):

Talipes—congenital deformities of the foot that, if untreated, result in walking on the ankle (talus)
Pes—acquired deformity of the foot
Inversion—foot twisted inward on its long axis
Eversion—foot twisted outward on its long axis
Adduction—deviation toward the midline of the body
Abduction—deviation away from the midline of the body
Varus—heel and forefoot inverted; forefoot adducted
Valgus—heel and forefoot everted; forefoot abducted
Equinus—foot plantar flexed, placing the toes below the level of the heel
Calcaneus—foot dorsiflexed, placing the heel below the level of the toes
Planus—medial longitudinal arch of the foot flattened
Cavus—medial longitudinal arch of the foot elevated

CLINICAL CONDITIONS

A variety of positional deformities of the legs and feet are encountered by physicians who provide primary care for children from birth through adolescence. The distinction between a pathological and functional cause must be made. The former should be referred to an orthopedist for treatment. When a pathological deformity of the legs or feet is diagnosed, the physician should look for other congenital anomalies, especially those involving the skeletal system. Most functional deformities of the legs and feet are self-correcting in time without treatment. This must be considered in weighing the results of any treatment prescribed. Unfortunately, studies of those conditions, analyzing treated versus untreated paired control patients, have not been performed, so clinicians are left to their own or others' anecdotal experiences in making therapeutic decisions.

Clubfoot

The term *clubfoot* denotes a pathological deformity that causes the leg and its appended foot to resemble a clubbing instrument. Two varieties occur. The more severe is *talipes equinovarus,* in which the heel and forefoot are inverted, the forefoot is adducted, and the entire foot is plantar flexed. Figure 134-2 shows bilateral clubfoot in a newborn; Figure 134-3 shows an untreated right clubfoot. The other, *talipes calcaneovalgus,* is characterized by eversion of the heel and forefoot, abduction of the forefoot, and dorsiflexion of the entire foot (Fig. 134-4). Both forms occur in about 1 of every 200 live births, are bilateral in 50% of the cases, and affect boys almost twice as frequently as girls. When present, associated neurological, muscular, or other skeletal anomalies should be sought.

Often in the newborn period, functional deformities of the feet secondary to in utero positioning will mimic both var-

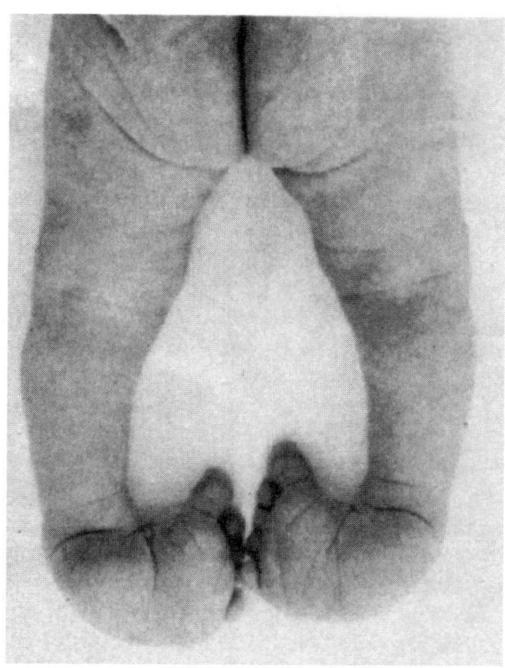

FIG. 134-2 Bilateral talipes equinovarus in a newborn infant.

(From Tachdjian MO: *Pediatric orthopedics,* ed 2, 4 vols, Philadelphia, 1990, WB Saunders.)

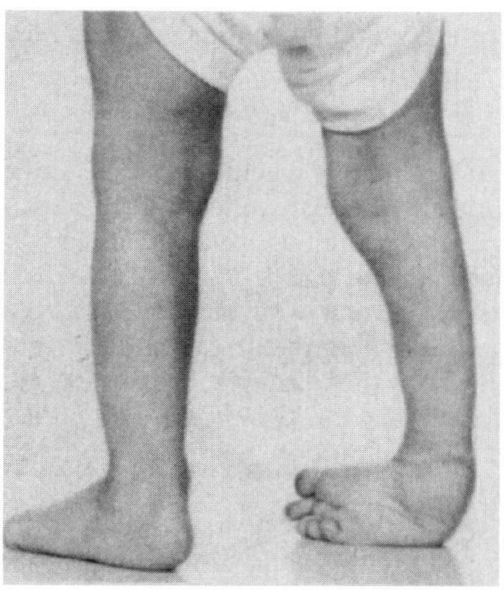

FIG. 134-3 Untreated talipes equinovarus in a 3-year-old child.

(From Tachdjian MO: *Pediatric orthopedics,* ed 2, 4 vols, Philadelphia, 1990, WB Saunders.)

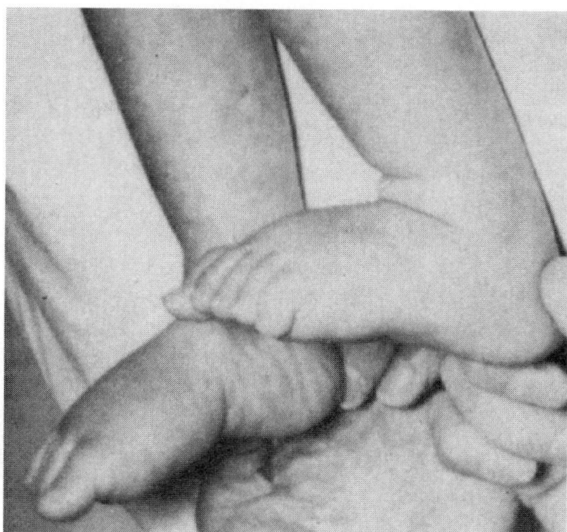

FIG. 134-4 Bilateral talipes calcaneovalgus. The left foot is held dorsiflexed and the right plantar flexed to show the range of ankle movement.

(From Sharrard WJW: *Paediatric orthopaedics and fractures,* ed 2, Oxford, 1979, Blackwell Scientific.)

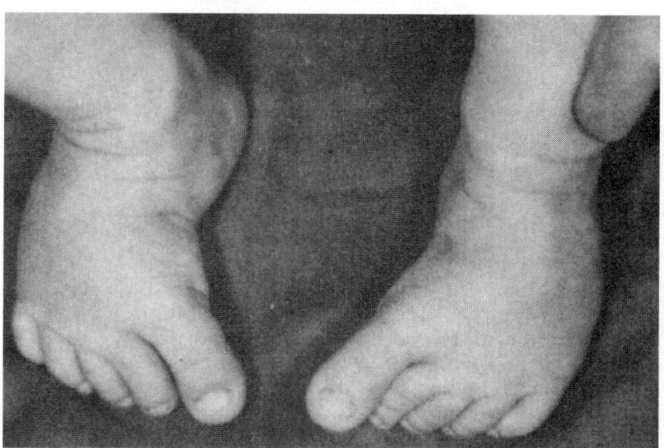

FIG. 134-5 Bilateral talipes varus. The entire foot is twisted inward on its longitudinal axis, and the forefoot is adducted.

(From Tachdjian MO: *Pediatric orthopedics,* ed 2, 4 vols, Philadelphia, 1990, WB Saunders.)

ieties of clubfoot. These can be differentiated readily in that the functionally deformed foot can be brought easily to a neutral position and overcorrected. This is not possible when pathological deformities are present, and an orthopedic consultation should be sought immediately. Treatment with casting usually is required for initial correction. In severe cases, tenotomies, muscle transplants, and arthrodeses are necessary when the child is older. Functional deformities are self-correcting and require no treatment.

Metatarsus Varus

Much confusion surrounds the incidence and management of metatarsus varus because three deformities are characterized by adduction of the forefoot: talipes varus (Fig. 134-5) in which the entire foot is inverted and the forefoot is adducted, metatarsus varus (Fig. 134-6) in which the forefoot is inverted and adducted while the hind foot and heel are in the normal position, and metatarsus adductus (Fig. 134-7) in which the only finding is adduction of the metatarsals at the tarsometatarsal joints. The combined incidence of these three forefoot adductive deformities is in the neighborhood of 1 per 100 live births (the most frequent musculoskeletal congenital malformation), with metatarsus adductus being the most common and talipes varus the least common.

Talipes varus and metatarsus varus have been considered lesser degrees of clubfoot and are fixed deformities of the foot that require early treatment. The medial border of the foot is concave with a widening of the space between the first and second toes and a high medial longitudinal arch. The

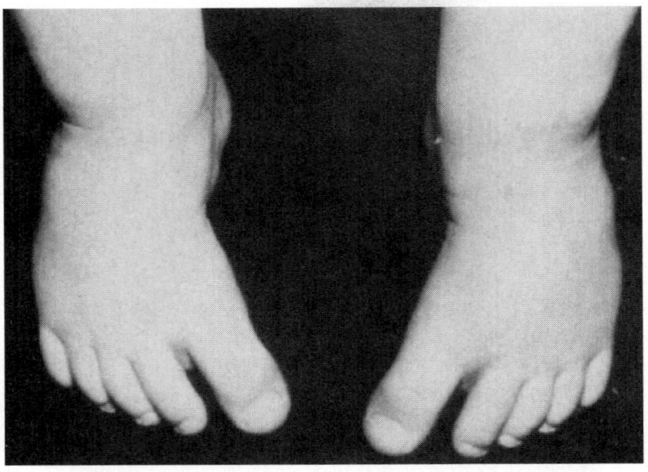

FIG. 134-6 Bilateral metatarsus varus. The forefoot is inverted and adducted, the great toe is widely separated from the second toe, and the lateral border of the foot is convex. The hindfoot is in a neutral position.

(From Sharrard WJW: *Paediatric orthopaedics and fractures,* ed 2, Oxford, 1979, Blackwell Scientific.)

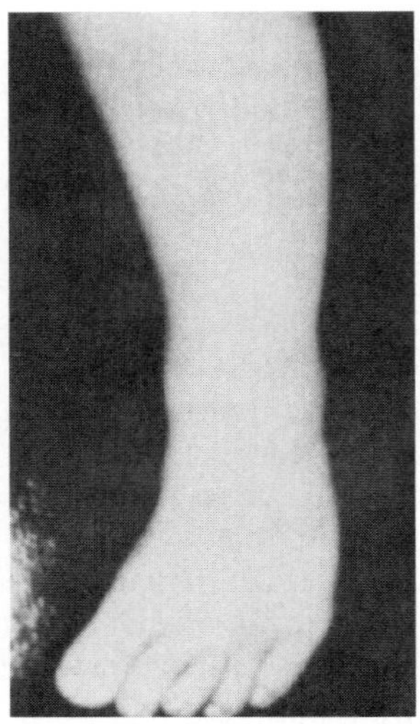

FIG. 134-7 Metatarsus adductus. The forefoot is adducted but not inverted.

(From Ferguson AB: *Orthopedic surgery in infancy and childhood,* ed 4, Baltimore, 1981, Williams & Wilkins.)

lateral border of the foot is convex, and the base of the fifth metatarsal bone is prominent. Treatment consists of serial casting. Abduction stretching exercises and out-flare-last shoes may be used as an adjunct to cast treatment but should not be relied on as the only therapy.

Metatarsus adductus, a functional deformity, can be distinguished from the two fixed forefoot deformities by observing lateral movement of the infant's forefoot in response to stimulation of the sole. This condition requires no treatment because it corrects spontaneously, usually during the first year. Primary care physicians see metatarsus adductus frequently and observe its resolution without treatment, whereas orthopedists are more likely to see talipes varus and metatarsus through referrals, sometimes unfortunately in late infancy when treatment results are less satisfactory.

Pronation

Almost all children develop some degree of pronation during the early stages of weight-bearing. Pronation is characterized by an outward rolling of the foot with eversion of the heel and eversion and abduction of the forefoot. The Achilles tendon is seen to curve inward, and the medial longitudinal arch of the foot, observed without weight-bearing, disappears on standing. These changes occur because a wide-based stance is assumed for balance (accentuated by bulky diapers), causing the weight to be borne on the medial aspect of the feet (Fig. 134-8). Laxity of the ligaments supporting the feet contributes to pronation. Flexible foot, relaxed foot, fatfoot, and flatfoot also are used to describe this condition, leading to considerable confusion in terminology.

Pronation is transient in most children, usually disappears before 2½ years of age, and requires no treatment. In those in whom it persists, treatment is not necessary unless symptoms occur. These include aching of the feet and legs, muscle cramps in the calves at night, easy fatigability, and reluctance to participate in strenuous activity. Symptoms result from the strain caused by the child's continual attempt to shift weight-bearing laterally toward the center of the foot, bringing about some degree of toeing-in. Persistent pronation without symptoms occurs in some children who may have a family history of pronation and often demonstrates hyperextensibility of other joints, including the knees, elbows, wrists, and thumbs.

When symptoms do occur, they may be alleviated by use of corrective shoes that have a long medial counter and a Thomas heel. Support to the medial longitudinal arch with a flexible felt, rubber, or leather pad placed beneath the inner sole may help. Wedges ⅛- to 3⁄16-inch thick applied to the medial aspect of the heel and the lateral aspect of the sole of the shoe sometimes are helpful. Steel arch supports placed within the shoe rarely are required, and foot exercises are of no value. Treatment with these simple measures usually brings relief of symptoms but may need to be continued for several years until the muscles and ligaments that support the foot mature sufficiently.

Planovalgus

Certain congenital anomalies involving the bones of the foot produce flattening of the medial longitudinal arch and eversion of the forefoot. These include vertical talus, accessory tarsonavicular, and fusion of one or more of the tarsal bones (tarsal coalition). The first two conditions usually can be detected in the newborn by the presence of a bony prominence on the medial and plantar aspects of the foot, with limitation of plantar flexion and inversion of the forefoot. Surgical correction should be accomplished early in infancy.

Tarsal conditions usually are not detected until late childhood or adolescence, when they produce pain with walking and inability to invert the foot. The foot is held in a pronated position with eversion of the forefoot. The peroneal tendons stand out prominently when attempts are made to invert the foot. This condition, commonly called spastic flatfoot, is not related etiologically to simple pronation. Treatment in most cases is symptomatic with orthopedic shoes. Surgical correction, usually performed in adulthood, is necessary in only about 10% of cases.

The incidence of pes planovalgus is unknown. Vertical talus and accessory tarsonavicular are very rare. Tarsal coali-

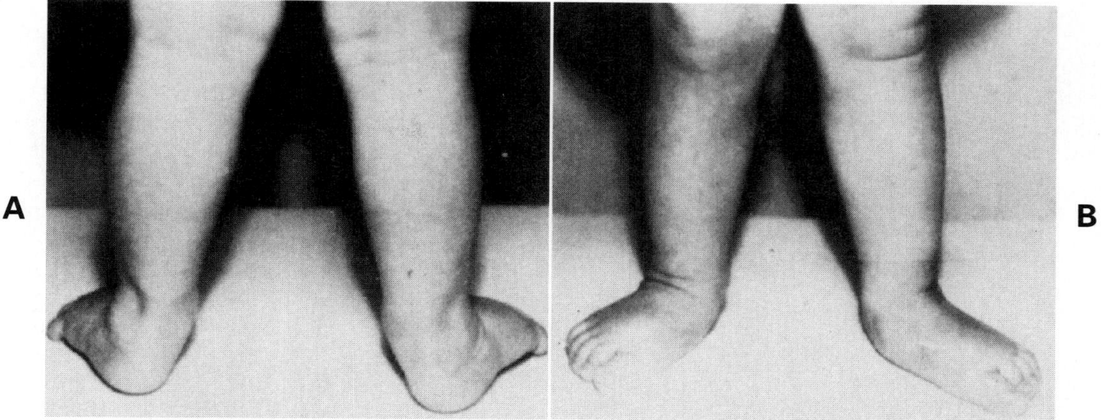

FIG. 134-8 Pronation. **A,** Viewed from behind, the hindfoot is everted. **B,** Viewed from in front, the forefoot is everted and abducted.

(From Sharrard WJW: *Paediatric orthopaedics and fractures,* ed 2, Oxford, 1979, Blackwell Scientific.)

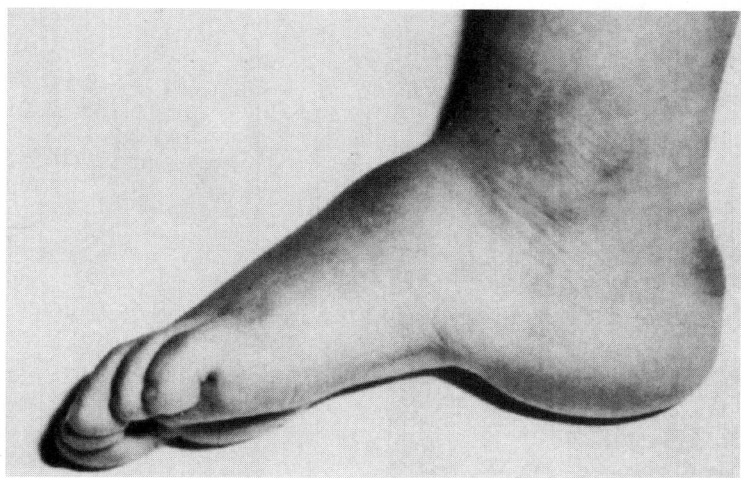

FIG. 134-9 Pes cavus, viewed from the outer side. There is abnormal height of the medial and lateral longitudinal arch.

(From Sharrard WJW: *Paediatric orthopaedics and fractures,* ed 2, Oxford, 1979, Blackwell Scientific.)

tions probably occur in 1% of the population and usually are hereditary.

Pes Cavus

Pes cavus is manifested by an equinus deformity of the forefoot in relation to the hindfoot, producing a high medial longitudinal arch (Fig. 134-9). It is referred to as *clawfoot* when associated with flexion deformities of the toes. The primary pathological condition is neuromuscular rather than bony, with weakness or paralysis of the intrinsic muscles of the foot and its dorsiflexors, leading to the deformity over time. It therefore is not seen at birth and usually does not manifest clinically until late childhood or adulthood, depending on the underlying neuromuscular disease.

Pes cavus is seen in muscular dystrophy, peripheral neuropathies, and disease of the spinal cord, brainstem, and cerebral cortex. Cerebral palsy, meningomyelocele, poliomyelitis, Charcot-Marie-Tooth disease, and Friedreich ataxia are examples of conditions of neurological origin that produce pes cavus as a late manifestation. Because of the variety of conditions in which pes cavus is seen and its variability as a manifestation of some of these, its incidence in the general population is not known. A family history of pes cavus should be sought because many of the conditions producing this deformity are inherited. Early treatment includes exercises designed to strengthen the affected muscles and application of metatarsal pads to the innersoles of the shoes or metatarsal bars to the outersoles. Surgical correction of the fixed deformities, including plantar fasciotomy, tendon transplants, osteotomies, and arthrodeses, may be required later.

Toe-Walking

Walking on the toes or the ball of the foot is a variation of normal gait for many children as they begin to walk. This usually progresses to a toe-heel gait and eventually to the normal heel-toe gait pattern within 3 to 6 months. Reassurance to parents is all that is required.

A congenitally short tendocalcaneus causes persistent toe-walking even though the child can toe-heel and heel-toe walk. These latter gaits are awkward and are less comfortable for the child until he or she is 6 to 8 years of age, when toe-walking disappears. No treatment is required.

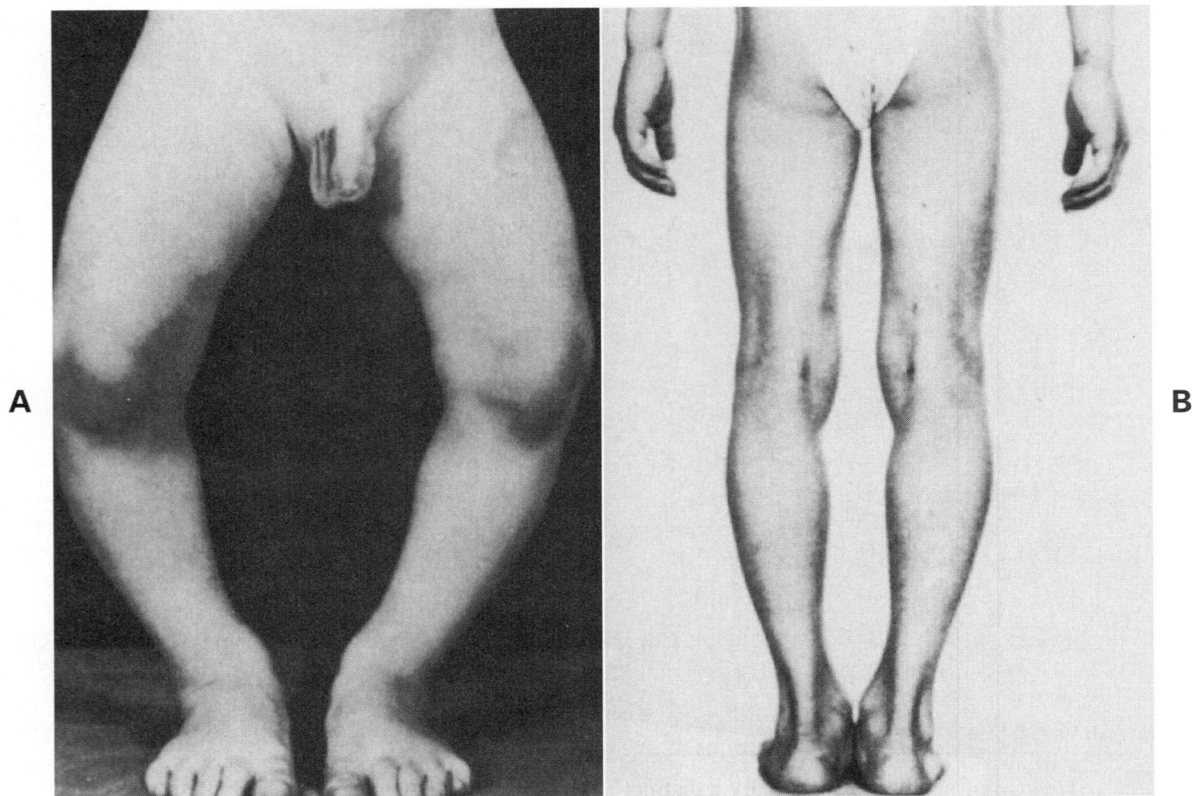

FIG. 134-10 **A,** Extreme physiological bowing of the legs at age 18 months. **B,** Spontaneous resolution over time (age 7 years).

(From Sharrard WJW: *Paediatric orthopaedics and fractures,* Oxford, 1971, Blackwell Scientific.)

As with pes cavus, certain rare muscular, peripheral, spinal, and central neurological diseases should be ruled out when toe-walking persists beyond 2 years of age.

Bowed Legs and Knocked Knees

From birth until 18 months of age a distinct bowing of the lower extremities is normal. This is followed by a transitional period over the next year or so during which a knocked knee pattern assumes prominence. This persists until later childhood or early adolescence when a balancing and straightening occur spontaneously. Physicians must be aware of this normal developmental pattern to avoid unnecessary treatment of mild to moderate degrees of bowed legs and knocked knees. However, marked degrees of these conditions require investigation to rule out underlying disease that can result in permanent deformity.

Bowing of the legs (genu varum), when extreme or unilateral, requires roentgenographic examination to exclude rickets, dyschondroplasia, osteogenesis imperfecta, osteochondritis (Blount disease), or injury to the medial proximal epiphysis of the tibia. Extreme degrees of physiological bowing of the legs may occur in the young child and resolve over time without treatment (Fig. 134-10).

Knocking of the knees (genu valgum) often is associated with pronation and is more apt to be marked in the child who is overweight. The degrees of knocked knee can be gauged by measuring the distance between the medial malleoli when the child is standing with the knees approximated (Fig. 134-11). Injury to the lateral proximal tibial epiphysis can cause

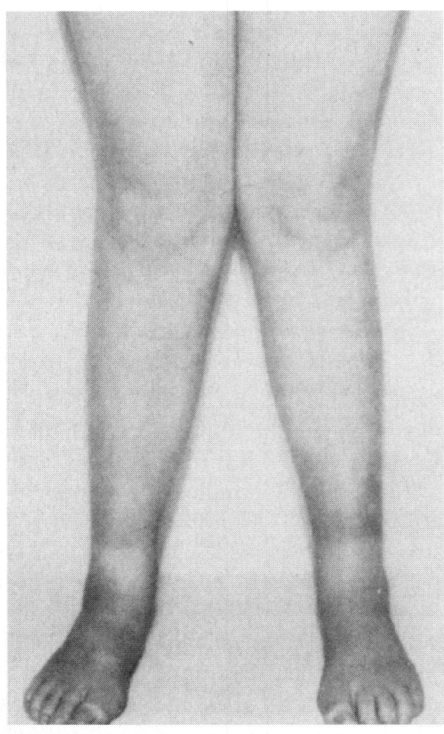

FIG. 134-11 Marked degree of physiological genu valgum. At age 11 years the distance between the medial malleoli measured 4 inches.

(From Sharrard WJW: *Paediatric orthopaedics and fractures,* ed 2, Oxford, 1979, Blackwell Scientific.)

unilateral genu valgum (Fig. 134-12). As with extreme bowing, underlying generalized diseases of the bone can cause marked bilateral genu valgum.

Treatment of severe bowing or knocking of the knees caused by underlying disease is determined by the nature of the condition and may include wedge osteotomy or epiphyseal stapling.

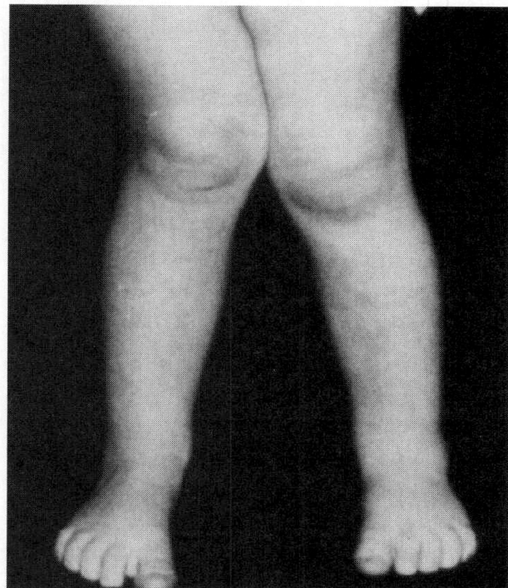

FIG. 134-12 Unilateral genu valgum caused by previous injury to the lateral aspect of the right proximal tibial epiphysis.
(From Sharrard WJW: *Paediatric orthopaedics and fractures*, ed 2, Oxford, 1979, Blackwell Scientific.)

Toeing-In and Toeing-Out

Toeing-in (pigeon toe) and toeing-out (slew foot) are frequently seen at all ages and are caused by a variety of conditions affecting the feet, ankles, legs, knees, and hips. Toeing-in is more common than toeing-out and is more likely to be caused by benign conditions. Protective or compensatory shifting of the body weight to the middle or outside of the foot in pronation and knocked knee, both normal developmental stages, is the most common cause of toeing-in and corrects itself in time. Developmental bowing of the legs, also self-correcting, may lead to temporary toeing-in. Talipes equinovarus and metatarsus varus are associated with toeing-in, whereas toeing-out is seen with calcaneovalgus and pes planovalgus. Spasticity of the internal rotator muscles of the hip, as seen in cerebral palsy, produces toeing-in; flaccid paralysis of these muscles results in toeing-out. Anterior and posterior maldirections of the acetabulum produce toeing-in and toeing-out, respectively. The remaining causes of both are related to internal or external torsion of the tibia and femur. In general, if in cases of toeing-in the child's patellae are noted to be rotated inward while walking, the underlying problem is above the knee; if they face straight forward, the underlying problem is below the knee.

Tibial Torsion. During fetal life the tibia is rotated inward on its longitudinal axis relative to the transverse axes of the knee and ankle joints. At birth, it reaches a neutral position

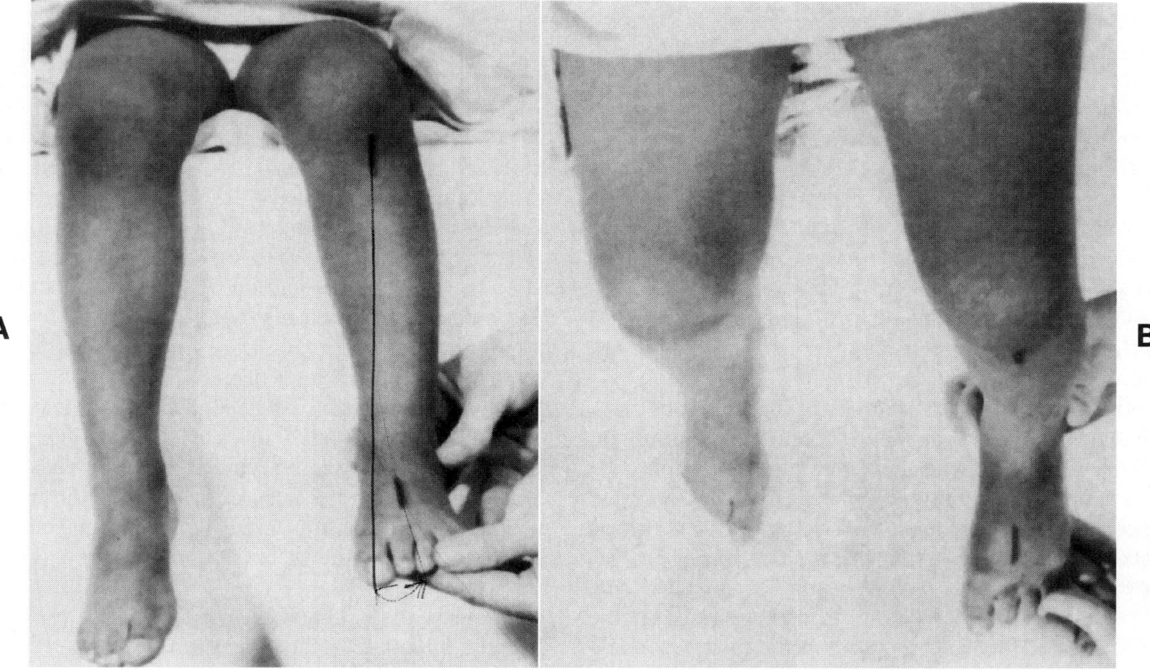

FIG. 134-13 Testing for tibial torsion. **A,** The patient is seated on the examining table with the knees flexed at 90 degrees and the legs hanging over the edge. A mark is drawn along the longitudinal axis of the tibia through the proximal tibial tubercle. Another mark is drawn over the second metatarsal bisecting the foot. The two marks are then aligned. **B,** With the left hand holding the foot in this neutral position, the thumb of the right hand is placed over the lateral malleolus and the forefinger over the medial malleolus. The angle at which an imaginary line joining the malleoli intersects the longitudinal axis will approximate the degree of internal or external tibial torsion.
(From Tachdjian MO: *Pediatric orthopedics*, ed 2, 4 vols, Philadelphia, 1990, WB Saunders.)

and thereafter gradually rotates outward, reaching 20 degrees of lateral torsion by the time walking is fully established and 23 degrees by adulthood. The degree of internal and external tibial torsion can be determined by observing the relative position of the medial and lateral malleoli while the child is sitting on the edge of a table or chair with legs dangling, the patellae facing forward, and the feet in their relaxed position (Fig. 134-13). The medial malleolus is placed posterior to the lateral malleolus in internal tibial torsion and anterior to it in external torsion.

The degree of torsion can be measured exactly either radiographically or with special instruments but is not required in most cases. The incidence of internal tibial torsion is 12% at birth. This gradually diminishes to near zero at 2 years of age. External tibial torsion develops in most babies shortly after birth and is almost universal by age 2 years. Pathological degrees of internal and external tibial torsion are found only in association with deformities of the feet, ankles, knees, and hips or as a result of improperly applied casts, braces, or Denis Browne splints. Treatment of primary internal tibial torsion is not required in most cases. Occasionally, if a child trips on his or her feet and falls frequently or if parents are unduly concerned over toeing-in, passive stretching exercises (externally rotating the foot at the ankle), corrective shoes (Thomas heel, longitudinal arch pad, inner-heel and outsole wedges), or application of torque heels may be prescribed. Denis Browne splints should not be used without orthopedic consultation because they may create abnormal stress on the hip joint. Derotation osteotomy of the tibia rarely is required and then almost always when tibial torsion is associated with other orthopedic anomalies of the lower extremity.

Femoral Torsion. The proximal portion of the femur rotates on its longitudinal axis in relation to the transverse plane of the knee when the femoral neck is twisted anteriorly (anteversion) or posteriorly (retroversion) in relation to the femoral condyles. Anteversion produces "kissing knees," toeing-in, and a clumsy gait (Fig. 134-14). With the patella in neutral position, the greater trochanter of the femur lies posterior to the lateral, longitudinal midthigh line. External rotation is decreased and internal rotation of the hip in extension is increased (normally 35 to 45 degrees for both). External rotation of the hip in flexion is normal, however. The findings in retroversion are the opposite of those found in anteversion of the femoral neck.

In utero and postnatal positioning of the legs and hips produces stresses that bring about these rotational deformities of the femoral neck. The true incidence of anteversion and retroversion is not known, but the former is much more common and occurs twice as frequently in girls as in boys. Most femoral torsion deformities correct themselves by 7 years of age. If they do not, an orthopedist should be consulted because the persistence of these deformities may lead to degenerative arthritis of the hip joint. Orthopedic treatment consists of the use of a bivalve lower-trunk and leg cast during sleeping hours or in rare cases a derotation osteotomy of the middle or lower femoral shaft. A simple measure that can be employed by the primary care physician early on for parental concern over toeing-in is to have the child learn to sit in the tailor, modified lotus, or Indian-style sitting position. The use of Denis Browne splints is contraindicated, and corrective shoes are of no value.

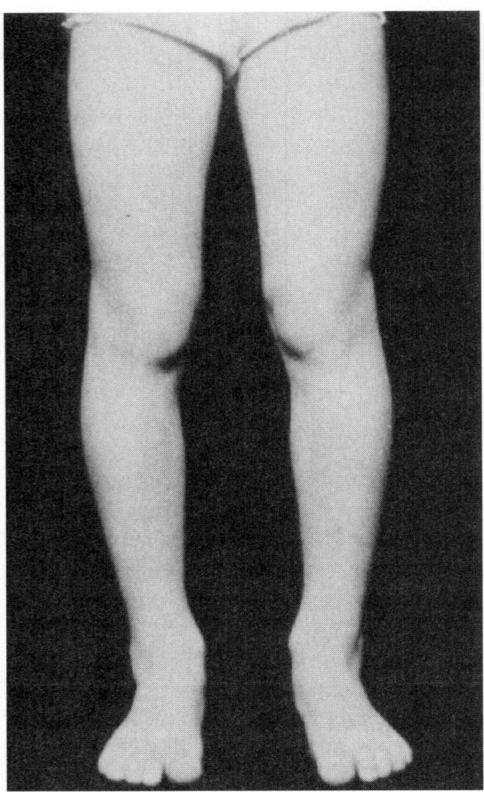

FIG. 134-14 Anteversion of the femoral neck or medial femoral torsion.

(From Sharrard WJW: *Paediatric orthopaedics and fractures,* ed 2, Oxford, 1979, Blackwell Scientific.)

Positions Leading to Toeing-In and Toeing-Out. Infants and children often assume certain positions during sleep or while sitting for long periods (watching television) that lead to positional deformities of the femur, tibia, or feet.

Sleeping in the prone, knee-chest position with the legs internally rotated may lead to anteversion of the femoral neck, internal tibial torsion, and varus of the forefoot; having the legs externally rotated may lead to valgus of the feet; and having the legs in a neutral position may lead to equinus of the feet and toe-walking. Sleeping in the prone position with the legs extended and rotated inward may lead to anteversion of the femoral neck, internal tibial torsion, and varus of the forefoot; having them rotated outward may lead to retroversion of the femoral neck and valgus of the feet. Sleeping in the frog-leg position prone or supine may lead to retroversion of the femoral neck and valgus and abduction of the feet.

Sitting in the reversed tailor position (on one's feet) with the feet internally rotated may produce anteversion of the femoral neck, internal tibial torsion, and varus of the forefoot; having the feet rotated externally may produce anteversion of the femoral neck and valgus of the feet.

When these sleeping or sitting positions are noted to occur in conjunction with the positional deformities listed, and when they raise concern, some effort can be made to change the positional sleeping or sitting habit. Success, however, is not often attained.

Although toeing-in or toeing-out may reflect a variety of underlying orthopedic diseases, no evidence suggests that toeing-in or toeing-out of developmental origin will lead to any functional disabilities if left uncorrected.

SUGGESTED READINGS

Bleck EE: The shoeing of children: show or science? *Dev Med Child Neurol* 15:188, 1971.

Heinrich SD, Sharp CH: Lower extremity torsional deformities in children: a prospective comparison of two treatment modalities, *Orthopedics* 14:655, 1991.

Kling TF, Hensinger RN: Angular and torsional deformities of the lower limbs in children, *Clin Orthop* 176:136, 1983.

Staheli LT et al: Lower-extremity rotational problems in children, *J Bone Joint Surg* 67:39, 1985.

Tachdjian MO: *Pediatric orthopedics,* ed 2, 4 vols, Philadelphia, 1990, WB Saunders.

135 Gastrointestinal Hemorrhage

David M. Steinhorn and Wallace F. Berman

Bleeding from the gastrointestinal (GI) tract in children requires prompt evaluation and appropriate treatment. The potential severity of this problem often is underestimated, thereby putting some children at even greater risk for life-threatening hemorrhage. A thorough assessment is made possible by taking into consideration basic pediatric principles. The age of the child, the history, and the associated findings, such as vomiting, pain, bruisability, and medication use by the patient or, if nursing, by the mother, will help direct the physician's subsequent workup. Although earlier literature suggested that a cause for GI bleeding could not be found in many cases, a diagnosis now can be determined in the majority of cases. This advance in diagnostic ability stems from increasing skill with and widespread use of flexible fiberoptic endoscopy in small children.

AGE AT PRESENTATION

Newborn

Gastrointestinal bleeding in newborns usually appears as rectal bleeding or blood suctioned from the infant's stomach during routine immediate postnatal care. There often is no readily discernible lesion, the cause may remain obscure, and the bleeding may cease spontaneously and permanently. In the first 24 hours the infant should be evaluated for maternal blood swallowed during delivery. The Apt test, which detects reduced fetal hemoglobin, can be performed easily by mixing 1 part bright red stool or vomitus with 5 to 10 parts water and then centrifuging the mixture; 1 ml of 0.2 N NaOH is added to the supernatant. A pink color developing in 2 to 5 minutes indicates fetal hemoglobin; adult hemoglobin produces a brown color.

Premature and newborn infants who have *upper GI bleeding* and low Apgar scores are at increased risk for developing gastric ulceration and erosions. In young infants who have *blood in the stool* one must consider anorectal fissures, enteric infections, and congenital or acquired hemorrhagic disorders. Maternal aspirin ingestion within 1 week of delivery, promethazine use during delivery, or maternal use of phenytoin or phenobarbital, all of which lower vitamin K–dependent clotting factors, may be associated with altered platelet function or coagulopathy. The loss of large quantities of blood suggests an intrinsic structural lesion of the GI tract, such as duplication, an enteric cyst, erosive mucosal lesions, Meckel diverticulum, volvulus, hemangioma, or enterocolitis. Bleeding associated with a hemangioma or Meckel diverticulum usually is not associated with pain. Hemorrhage secondary to volvulus tends to occur with abdominal pain, a mass, or distention; however, these findings may be difficult to appreciate in the neonate. Occasionally a colitic picture can be seen with cow milk protein allergy and in allergy to the mother's breast milk. Elimination of the offending protein is curative.

Infants

Among infants up to 1 year of age, a number of other lesions in addition to most of those already mentioned for the neonate must be considered. Children in this age group are introduced to a wide variety of foods. Food sensitivities, most frequently cow milk and soy protein allergy, can produce a fulminant enterocolitis. This reaction can be seen even in breast-fed infants when the offending agent is consumed by the mother. Children who have food sensitivities that produce colitis usually have varying degrees of iron deficiency anemia from chronic blood loss. Immunodeficiency states also are associated with potentially severe enterocolitis.

As infants become mobile, with improved hand-to-mouth ability, their proximity to small objects on the floor makes a significant risk. Other causes of GI bleeding tend to be similar to those in older children. Juvenile polyps usually are first noted in this age group. They usually are evidenced by painless bright red blood passed through the rectum. Rectal bleeding associated with abdominal pain can be a sign of intussusception.

Children and Adolescents

In children and adolescents, esophageal varices, peptic ulcer disease, and gastritis must be considered, as well as many of the structural lesions described previously. *Varices at this age can result* from the cavernous transformation of the extrahepatic portion of the portal vein, leading to portal hypertension; this has been associated with umbilical vessel catheterization, omphalitis, or neonatal conditions associated with hypoxia, prolonged jaundice, or sepsis. Intrahepatic causes of cirrhosis, leading to portal hypertension that may first manifest during childhood or adolescence, include Wilson disease *(after age 6 years),* alpha-l-antitrypsin deficiency, or other forms of chronic liver disease—either metabolic, infectious, or anatomical. These latter diseases also may be associated with coagulopathies and thrombocytopenia secondary to the hypersplenism that usually accompanies them.

In acute variceal bleeding the portal system may be acutely decompressed, emptying an otherwise palpable spleen. If the cause of the portal hypertension is extrahepatic, the bleeding may be remarkably well tolerated in contrast to those patients who have cirrhotic liver disease in whom rapid hepatic decompensation may occur. Variceal bleeding may be induced following routine aspirin use, upper respiratory tract illnesses, excessive physical exertion, or the ingestion of rough, bulky foods.

The true incidence of peptic ulcer disease in the general pediatric population is unknown. The reasons for this gap in our knowledge come from the difficulty in separating causes of upper GI bleeding—that is, "pill" gastritis, stress ulceration, or acid-peptic disease—as well as from the extremely variable occurrence of symptoms that differ according to age group. The classic history of epigastric pain that worsens with an empty stomach and improves with eating is more typical in the adolescent but may be absent in the younger child. Peptic ulcers may be evidenced by acute bleeding or as a chronic anemia secondary to ongoing blood losses.

Polypoid lesions of the GI tract may produce painless rectal bleeding as a result of local irritation and usually represent simple, solitary, juvenile polyps of the colon. This bleeding may be seen either as minor streaking on the stools or, less frequently, as frank, bright red blood. Of these polyps, 70% are located within 25 cm of the anus and are readily removed by using a snare-cautery technique. If bleeding is not a problem, many of these polyps will autoamputate if left alone. Polyps not easily reached by this method usually can be removed by using a fiberoptic colonoscope and snare technique after appropriate patient preparation. Adenomatous polyps may present with rectal bleeding as early as infancy. They are managed differently from juvenile polyps. *Juvenile polyps are benign inflammatory excrescences that do not cause later complications. Adenomas, on the other hand, are premalignant tumors.*

Many parents are extremely concerned and anxious over the possibility that their child's rectal bleeding represents a malignancy. Colonic carcinoma is extremely rare in children, occurring predominantly in older children who have long-standing ulcerative colitis or familial polyposis syndromes. The Peutz-Jeghers syndrome consists of diffuse polyps of the GI tract that may twist on their stalks and infarct. It is associated with melanotic spots of the oral mucosa and skin. Gardner syndrome is a genetic disorder of intestinal polyposis (adenomatous), with bony and soft tissue tumors. This disease can become malignant as early as the early teenage years.

Hemangiomas and other vascular lesions, such as hereditary hemorrhagic telangiectasia (Rendu-Osler-Weber syndrome), must be considered in the evaluation of painless rectal bleeding. Its most common form is the larger cavernous hemangioma, either polypoid or diffuse, extending several centimeters through the submucosa of the small or large intestine. The large bowel, specifically the rectum, is the area usually involved in the diffuse type. Cutaneous vascular malformations often are present but may require scrupulous searching to detect. Selective arteriography or digital subtraction angiography may aid in demonstrating the abnormal vessels if they are not visible on direct inspection. The clinician must determine whether the patient has, indeed, bled and whether the discolored vomitus or stools truly represent the presence of blood. This task may be accomplished easily and rapidly by confirming the presence of blood by using the Hematest, Hemoccult (guaiac), or Gastroccult test. Some false positive and negative results have occurred with these tests; however, the ability to determine the presence of blood accurately in most cases mandates their use in evaluating suspected GI bleeding.

GENERAL APPROACH TO PATIENTS WHO HAVE GASTROINTESTINAL BLEEDING

In evaluating a patient who has GI blood loss, the physician should keep two goals in mind: first, the severity of the blood loss must be quickly assessed (see following section) to institute appropriate resuscitative measures; second, the physician must consider the most likely causes so that the problems requiring immediate surgery can be separated from those requiring medical management and evaluation. Thus the workup is based on clinical appearance, age, history, and the physician's familiarity with the patient and on the family's reliability and compliance. A list of lesions commonly associated with GI bleeding is provided in the box below. These include lesions with upper gastrointestinal (UGI) bleeding and those with rectal bleeding, since blood is a potent cathartic and reduces transit time.

If during the initial assessment the physician determines that the degree of blood loss is neither enormous nor life threatening, a more leisurely diagnostic approach is suitable. In infants and small children, particular attention should be paid to a history of chronic or familial diseases, allergies, medications the child or nursing mother is receiving, diet, recent behavior pattern, and growth pattern, particularly to recent weight loss or failure to thrive. The sequence of diag-

CAUSES OF GASTROINTESTINAL HEMORRHAGE

Infants under 1 year of age

Manifesting as upper gastrointestinal bleeding
- Swallowed maternal blood
- Gastritis, acid-peptic disease
- Stress ulceration
- Mallory-Weiss syndrome
- Vascular malformations

Manifesting as lower gastrointestinal bleeding
- Anal fissure or trauma
- Gastroenteritis
  - Enteric infections
  - Enterocolitis
- Intussusception
- Coagulation disorders
- Congenital malformations
  - Malrotation
  - Intestinal duplications, Meckel diverticulum
- Food allergies

Children over 1 year of age

Manifesting as upper gastrointestinal bleeding
- Stress ulcers
- Gastritis, acid-peptic disease
- Esophageal varices
- Esophagitis
- Mallory-Weiss syndrome
- Swallowed blood from nasopharynx

Manifesting as lower gastrointestinal bleeding
- Anal fissures
- Polyps
- Gastroenteritis, enteric infections
- Intussusception
- Inflammatory bowel disease
- Congenital malformations
  - Malrotation or volvulus
  - Intestinal duplication
  - Meckel diverticulum
- Henoch-Schönlein purpura

nostic studies should be designed to determine whether the blood most likely is coming from a site proximal or distal to the ligament of Treitz. From that point, the physician concentrates either on looking for upper GI lesions by using endoscopy, a UGI series, or angiography or on examining the lower tract through bacterial cultures, proctoscopy or colonoscopy, barium contrast studies, labeled red cell studies, or a Meckel scan (Fig. 135-1).

For a child having acute massive GI bleeding, the approach must be the same as in any other emergency. The physician must approach the patient with an efficient, rational plan in mind that will allow him or her to obtain the pertinent histological information, perform a brief but adequate examination, stabilize the patient clinically, arrive at a working diagnosis, and institute appropriate therapy or consultations. As soon as possible, cardiovascular status should be evaluated by measuring blood pressure, pulse, capillary refill time, and respiratory rate. Skin turgor and the color of the mucous membranes also should be noted.

If signs of shock are present (e.g., orthostasis or frank hypotension, tachycardia, poorly perfused extremities, pale mucous membranes, or altered mental status), a large-bore intravenous catheter should be placed. If any intravenous line cannot be placed in a patient who evidences hypotension and hypovolemia or if one of sufficient size cannot be placed to administer 20 ml/kg of crystalloid fluid in less than 30 minutes, then one should consider inserting an intraosseous needle for fluid resuscitation and administering any necessary medications. This technique may be lifesaving and carries an extremely low risk of complications.[1]

In addition, 20 ml/kg of lactated Ringer solution, Hetastarch, normal saline, or plasma should be given rapidly to reexpand the vascular volume. This dose may be repeated once if needed. Additional fluid should be given as needed to make up for equilibration of these solutions with the extravascular space. Red cells should be given as soon as possible, while watching for signs of circulatory overload. Next, an appropriately sized nasogastric (NG) tube, preferably of the vented sump type, should be placed to help determine the source and estimate the volume of ongoing blood loss. This tube should be left in place and attached either to low-pressure continuous suction, if vented, or to intermittent suction, if nonvented. The only instances in which an NG tube may be frought with problems are in patients who have documented varices in whom NG placement may aggravate bleeding. Nonetheless, even in these cases an NG tube may be required to quantitate blood loss adequately.

The presence of blood in the stomach, either fresh or acidified (coffee ground appearance), suggests that the bleeding is occurring proximal to the ligament of Treitz. If the pylorus is closed, bleeding may not be evident from the appearance of the NG tube aspirate. Therefore duodenal bleeding may be evidenced by bloody stools rather than by bloody vomitus. Lower GI bleeding is characterized on the basis of the stool's appearance as hematochezia (bright red bloody stools), blood-streaked stools, melena (black, tarry stools), or currant-jelly stools. Hematochezia usually indicates massive upper GI or colonic bleeding. Blood streaking often is associated with disease involving the rectum or the perianal region. Melenic- to maroon-colored stools may be seen with small bowel or proximal colonic bleeding. The presence of currant-jelly stools usually is ominous, suggesting impending infarction of bowel with the sloughing of necrotic mucosa; in these cases one also may see signs similar to those associated with an acute surgical abdomen.

With this basic information in hand, the physician can proceed to a more complete history of the present illness. Pertinent points include the presence of pain, vomiting, diarrhea, or fainting. A history of chronic or predisposing illnesses (e.g., liver disease, bleeding disorders, or familial GI disor-

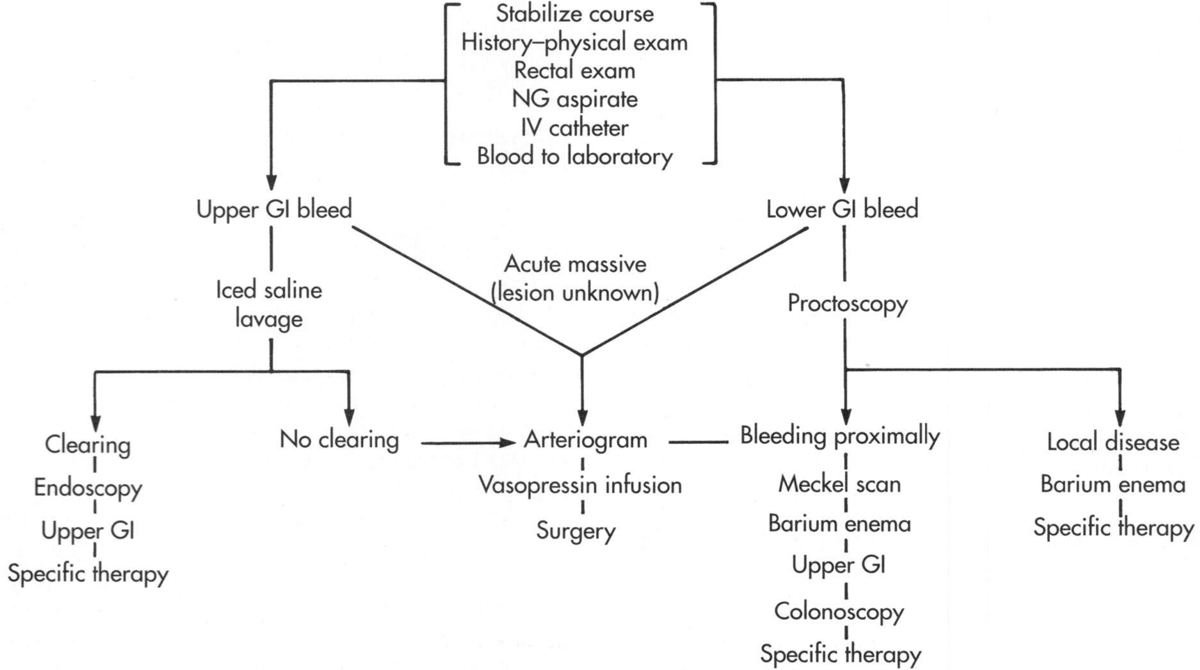

FIG. 135-1 Management of gastrointestinal hemorrhage.

ders) must be sought. The pediatrician should inquire as to all medications and substances taken by the child before or during the episode, particularly emphasizing salicylates, iron, alcohol, or caustic agents such as household cleaning products.

A complete neonatal history, including complications such as hypoxia, umbilical vessel catheterization, prolonged jaundice, and omphalitis, must be obtained. Prior surgery, trauma, and chronic illnesses must be asked about directly. To expedite the treatment of unstable patients, the physical examination should be performed while taking the history and initiating therapy. Pulse rate, respirations, and postural blood pressure measurements should be recorded. Of particular importance in any patient who is bleeding is the presence of petechiae, ecchymoses, or blood in the nares, throat, or urine. The physician also must look for signs of chronic liver disease, such as the presence of telangiectasias, jaundice, hepatosplenomegaly, and a prominent abdominal venous pattern. With lower GI bleeding a careful rectal examination should be performed, paying special attention to (1) the perianal region, observing for skin tags, abscesses, fissures, bleeding points or, much less commonly, hemorrhoids; (2) the character of the stool; and (3) the presence of occult blood. It also is necessary to palpate for polyps and pelvic masses during the rectal examination.

Having completed all the above, which in practice usually takes less than an hour, controlling the bleeding and determining the specific diagnosis become the next orders of business. If the nasogastric aspirate contains blood or if the patient has hematemesis, iced saline irrigation may be instituted in an attempt to decrease mucosal blood flow and thereby stop profuse bleeding. Although the efficacy of lavage in decreasing and controlling upper bleeding has not been demonstrated conclusively, it allows easier assessment of the rate of bleeding and helps in removing clotted blood. Iced saline is instilled through an NG tube and is withdrawn after 5 minutes, while signs of blood in the aspirate return are watched for. The procedure is repeated until the aspirate return is clear or no diminution occurs in the blood content of the aspirate return for 30 to 45 minutes.

If the bleeding ceases, gastroduodenoscopy should be performed to demonstrate the bleeding source and to determine the type of lesion present. Upper endoscopy can establish the diagnosis in 75% to 90% of patients. If the bleeding is massive and cannot be controlled with iced saline lavage, adequate visualization is not likely to be achieved with the fiberoptic endoscope. If the bleeding is not immediately life threatening, arteriography can be considered, which may demonstrate bleeding that occurs at a rate of 0.5 ml/minute or more. *Endoscopy and arteriography can be therapeutic as well as diagnostic.*

Of greater sensitivity and reduced invasiveness is the use of a sulfur-colloid isotopic study, which can demonstrate active bleeding at rates as low as 0.1 ml/minute. This method demonstrates active bleeding by using a tracer with a very short half-life. In small infants a large uptake of the isotope by the liver may mask the right upper quadrant. An additional isotopic method of determining the bleeding site consists of injecting the patient with technetium-99-pertechnetate-labeled red blood cells. These labeled cells may remain in the circulation for more than a day and allow repeated imaging to locate the site of intermittent bleeding.

If the lesion is one of mucosal erosion or inflammation, antacid therapy with or without the concomitant use of a H_2-blocker should be instituted. If the bleeding source is found to be a variceal bleeding, the cause of these lesions must be considered, with appropriate treatment of the underlying cause. Liver or portal venous disease should be sought. Clotting factors and platelets should be replaced as indicated.

Variceal bleeding requires special mention because of the myriad settings in which varices may be seen. Although the treatment of variceal bleeding continues to evolve, it may be divided into those therapies that can be instituted in most emergency facilities and those that require a pediatric endoscopist skilled at sclerotherapy. Of the former therapies, balloon tamponade and vasopressin therapy are most common. Although Blakemore tubes are available in pediatric sizes, their use has been associated with an unacceptably high incidence of airway problems and even esophageal rupture. Vasopressin may be used as a mesenteric vasoconstrictor to reduce portal blood flow and thus decrease variceal pressure. Initially, 0.3 U/kg of vasopressin is diluted in 2 ml/kg of 5% dextrose and given over 20 minutes, preferably through a central or intraosseous line. A continuous infusion of vasopressin 0.15 to 0.35 U/m^2/minute may be continued for 12 hours after bleeding stops; the dose then is tapered gradually. Extreme care must be taken to avoid malignant hypertension in patients receiving vasopressin infusions, and arterial pressure must be monitored continuously.

Endoscopic sclerotherapy, which controls variceal bleeding caused by a variety of underlying disease, has taken its place in recent years as a valuable treatment option for children. The number and magnitude of complications are exceedingly small, with a low incidence of rebleeding when performed for esophageal varices. This technique is somewhat more effective when used for varices associated with extrahepatic portal hypertension rather than those associated with primary liver disease. A major drawback to this technique is the frequent need for general anesthesia and endotracheal intubation when initially performed on small children and the need for a facility skilled at managing small children who are critically ill. For many patients, however, sclerotherapy offers a relatively less invasive means for controlling variceal bleeding than more risky portal shunting procedures.

The workup for lower GI bleeding differs in several aspects from that of upper GI bleeding. The abdomen and perianal and rectal region are carefully examined. Stool must be analyzed for the presence of blood, ova and parasites, and enteric pathogens. If diarrhea is present, the stool should be examined microscopically for polymorphonuclear leukocytes and mucus, both of which are evidence of bacterial infection. Proctosigmoidoscopy, which can be performed in even the smallest infants, should follow in an attempt to discover the presence of fissures, polyps, or mucosal disease. One must look for signs of mucosal friability and edema. The presence of blood coming from above the reach of the proctosigmoidoscope indicates the need to proceed with other diagnostic studies. Depending on the circumstances, these may include (1) an upright and supine view of the abdomen, looking in particular for signs of obstruction or for calcifications; (2) a radionuclide scan, using pentagastrin to enhance uptake in search of a Meckel diverticulum; (3) a sulfur-colloid isotopic scan; (4) arteriography; and (5) an isotope-labeled red blood cell infusion (usually reserved for cases of intermittent bleeding). If the rate of bleeding does not permit the delay necessary to perform these studies, vasopressin may be administered perenterally in an attempt to control the bleeding and to stabilize the patient.

An air contrast barium enema to identify mucosal lesions and an upper GI series with small bowel follow-through should be the last studies performed because they make the further use of arteriography, isotope scans, and endoscopy impossible for several days thereafter. In those cases in which the gut is compromised vascularly, or the rate of bleeding is excessive and uncontrollable by more conservative methods, prompt surgical intervention is required. Fortunately, however, most acute episodes of GI bleeding can be controlled relatively easily by using conservative measures; in those patients who require surgical intervention, it can be handled electively at a later time.

REFERENCE

1. Rossetti VA et al: Intraosseous infusions: an alternative route of pediatric intravascular access, *Ann Emerg Med* 14:885, 1985.

SUGGESTED READINGS

Alavi A, Ring EJ: Localization of gastrointestinal bleeding: superiority of ^{99m}Tc sulfur colloid compared with angiography, *Am J Radiol* 137:741, 1981.

Caulfield M et al: Upper gastrointestinal tract endoscopy in the pediatric patient, *J Pediatr* 115:339, 1989.

Donovan TJ, Ward M, Shepherd RW: Evaluation of endoscopic sclerotherapy of esophageal varices in children, *J Pediatr Gastroenterol Nutr* 5:696, 1986.

Fox VL et al: Endoscopic ligation of esophageal varices in children, *J Pediatr Gastroenterol Nutr* 20:2, 1995.

Goenka AS et al: Therapeutic upper gastrointestinal endoscopy in children: an audit of 443 procedures and literature review, *J Gastroenterol Hepatol* 8:44, 1993.

Hyams JS, Leichtner AM, Schwartz AN: Recent advances in diagnosis and treatment of gastrointestinal hemorrhage in infants and children, *J Pediatr* 106:1, 1985.

Kelly DA: Do H_2 receptor antagonists have a therapeutic role in childhood? *J Pediatr Gastroenterol Nutr* 19:270, 1994.

McKusick KA et al: ^{99m}Tc red blood cells for detection of gastrointestinal bleeding: experience with 80 patients, *Am J Radiol* 137:1113, 1981.

Steffen RM et al: Colonoscopy in the pediatric patient, *J Pediatr* 115:507, 1989.

Teach SJ, Fleisher GR: Rectal bleeding in the pediatric emergency department, *Ann Emerg Med* 23:1252, 1994.

136 Headache

Henry M. Seidel

Headache—quite literally, a pain in the head—is a common presenting complaint in childhood, increasing in frequency as the child becomes more verbal and better able to be explicit about aches and pains. We cannot, of course, accurately appreciate its frequency in the very young. Eventually, virtually every one experiences a headache—probably humanity's most commonly experienced pain—usually, for the first time, at some point during childhood or adolescence. It is a complaint that elicits empathy easily.

Occasionally, serious concern and frustration also accompany this complaint. The physician does not want to overlook the relatively infrequent causes that require lifesaving therapeutic interventions. Parents and many older children and adolescents who have headaches often worry about a major disease, particularly a brain tumor. Because of the several categories of headache (migraine, "abdominal" migraine, tension, and "cluster"), each with imprecise starting and end points, diagnosis and management can be difficult (see the box on p. 986).

Nonetheless, most headaches during childhood are transient, bearable, and associated with the general wear and tear of life—from the nonthreatening viral and upper respiratory tract infection to the results of stress-producing experiences of day-to-day living. The older the child, the more likely the latter. However, if an acute episode persists or the intensity of the complaint accelerates, be aware of the possibility of an organic cause for the complaint, particularly if any localizing findings are evident after the history has been taken and the physical examination performed.

MECHANISM OF HEADACHE

Headache may have both extracranial and intracranial origins. An extracranial cause is most common, not surprising in that almost all extracranial structures are pain sensitive. Thus headache frequently is associated with dilation and distention of the extracranial vessels or with spasmodic contracture of the scalp and neck musculature. Infections or other diseases in any of the extracranial structures of the head—eyes, teeth, sinuses, and ears—can cause headache and usually are identifiable readily with localized findings. However, this is not always so; extracranial causes may not be made immediately evident by localized signs.

Not all intracranial structures are pain sensitive. Those that are include cranial nerves V, VII, IX, and X; cervical nerves I through III; and the venous sinuses and some of their branches. Most of the rest of the intracranial structures—skull, substance of the brain, and most of the meninges—are not pain sensitive. However, the "traction" produced by a mass of any sort, the pulls and displacements of the venous sinuses and their branches, and inflammation from any cause can and do influence those cranial and cervical nerves that are pain sensitive. However, the exact mechanism by which pain results is not known, particularly when no identifiable anatomical displacements are evident.

CONCOMITANT SIGNS AND SYMPTOMS

Meningismus and fever, for example, may accompany headache and, when present, increase concern for an acute, treatable condition. Meningitis is an obvious first thought. However, other major conditions may produce a severe headache along with meningismus: retropharyngeal abscess, superior longitudinal sinus thrombosis, and subarachnoid hemorrhage, as well as typhoid fever and pneumonia. And, of course, the common infecting bacteria or viruses may not always be the cause of meningitis or meningoencephalitis. Other agents (e.g., cryptococci) also must be considered.

HISTORY AND PHYSICAL EXAMINATION

The history and physical examination are, as usual, the bedrock of diagnosis. They often will quickly help to rule out many diagnoses that may require extensive investigation and therapeutic intervention. Actually, while taking the history, the pediatrician can begin to eliminate (or include) many concerns—for example, by an immediate look to observe the movement of the eyes (for evidence of cranial nerve VI palsy, frequently the first manifestation of intracranial pressure) or an initial question directed to the associated complaint of vomiting (whether it is accompanied by nausea, which usually is not the case with increased intracranial pressure).

Occasionally the acute circumstance for which treatment is sought requires great speed to reach even a tentative diagnosis. The patient's physical condition and level of consciousness may direct the diagnostic search. Certainly, the following accompanying complaints and findings suggest organic causes and therefore a less leisurely approach:

- Fever
- Meningismus
- Trauma (even if obscure or distant in time)
- Seizures
- Severe hypertension
- Confusion
- Diminished awareness
- Petechiae and ecchymoses
- Lethargy
- Vomiting, with or without nausea, with or without headache, if otherwise unexplained
- Intense irritability
- Great specificity in description of headache
- History of pica
- Changes in gait, personality, behavior

PARTIAL LIST OF CAUSES OF HEADACHES

Intracranial masses (sharply localized or diffuse)

Intracranial tumor, benign or malignant
Brain cyst
Subdural hematoma
Central nervous system leukemia
Acute onset of hydrocephalus for any reason caused by obstruction within the ventricular system

Vascular causes

Migraine
- Classic
- With ophthalmoplegia or hemiplegia
- Basilar artery
- Complicated by tension
- With ornithine transcarbamoylase deficiency

Arteriovenous malformation
Venous sinus engorgement
Hypertension
Cranial arteritis
Intracranial aneurysm
Subarachnoid hemorrhage
Vascular occlusion
- With congenital heart disease
- With sickle cell disease

Vascular dilation secondary to fever, hypoxia, hypercapnia, or severe anemia

Specific focal disease

Inflammation, new growth, foreign body, or other injury of:
- Eye
- Ear
- Nose
- Throat
- Teeth
- Sinuses
- Cervical spine

Emotional causes

Conversion reactions
Daily stress, psychogenic causes, familial patterning
Depression

Infections

Meningitis or encephalitis
- Bacterial
- Viral

Sinusitis (less frequent in the younger child, who has poorly developed sinuses)
Otitis media
Mastoiditis
Retropharyngeal abscess
Brain abscess
Cervical adenitis
Systemic infection

Neural causes

Epileptic equivalent
Trigeminal neuralgia
Glossopharyngeal neuralgia
Excessive auditory, visual, or gustatory sensory stimuli
Seizures (postictal)

Trauma

Lumbar puncture (with subsequent decreased intracranial pressure)
Head injury
- Concussion
- Subdural hematoma
- Subarachnoid hemorrhage

Other posttraumatic events

Noxious stimuli

"Gas leak" syndrome
Alcohol
Lead
Oral contraceptives
Other drugs (e.g., steroid withdrawal)

Other causes

Allergy
Hyperaldosteronism
Hypoglycemia
Occipital neuralgia with malformation at C1 and C2
Pseudotumor cerebri (with otitis media, use of vitamin A, tetracyclines, steroids)
Renal disease
Unknown origin

Similarly, the headaches characterized by one or more of the following suggest an organic cause:

- Initial, dramatic episode
- Sudden onset
- Progressive severity and frequency over a short period (a history of several months tends to argue against the organic)
- Intense pain upon awakening
- A dramatic description (e.g., "jackhammer in the head")
- Occurrence in the morning; subsidence after arising, particularly after vomiting
- Precipitation by the Valsalva maneuver, cough, sneeze, strain (particularly if headache is of short duration—a few minutes to 30 minutes)

A sharply defined, acute onset is worrisome, and the age of the child is a prime consideration—the younger the child, the greater the risk. Also, the precision of the complaint suggests a more life-compromising diagnosis. Even the young child (usually by 3 to 4 years of age) can point a finger very accurately. A frontal location of the headache suggests frontal or ethmoid sinusitis, cerebral tumors, a migraine, and problems with the eyes; an occipital or suboccipital location suggests a cerebellar tumor, occipital neuralgia, sphenoid sinusitis, or tension. The more severe the complaint, the more likely an organic cause. However, children under 8 to 10 years of age usually do not have recurrent headache due to sinusitis nor, in general, do those who have so-called "eyestrain" due to refractive errors.

Some characteristics of headache particularly suggest increased intracranial pressure. These include those that wake the patient from sleep or occur in the morning and that are accompanied by vomiting free of nausea; those related to a change in position from prone to supine and from either of those to the erect position; and those related to physical activity, coughing, sneezing, and straining. Increased intracranial pressure does not provide a warning, a prodrome like that of scotomata (visual "fireworks"), pallor, and abdominal pain that may precede a migraine headache. The headache that wakes the patient from sleep and that does not respond to aspirin, acetaminophen, or other over-the-counter drugs often may have a more serious cause. The simple, transient episode generally responds most readily. In addition, pica, particularly in the younger child, suggests lead encephalopathy; the description of "throbbing" suggests hypertension. A clear history of trauma always requires particular attention.

These considerations underscore the need for a careful history and sharp dissection of the often intermingled psychosocial and organic variables. Clearly, the family history is important. Children who have migraine headaches tend to have parents who have them. Care should be taken, however: children under stress are apt to mimic their parents' behavior. Beyond that, the description of the headache, its frequency, duration, and location, and the report of prodromata are all very important. Clues to stress and tension may reside in the events that precede the headache, such as the experience and thoughts of the patient, the time of day, and the day of the week. Understanding all the experiences of the child, both at home and at school can help—the nature of relations with family, teachers, and friends, reading and television habits, eating patterns, environmental noise, sleep habits, and any recent change in bowel and urination patterns. Even the presence of a gas stove in the home is important because it may be leaking. The search, then, must be for hints of organic cause and for evidence of emotional stress and tension.

A "concept" of the child emerges from this inquiry. The depiction of behavioral patterns, past coping mechanisms, any recent behavioral change, hints of any change in the flow of normal development, and diminished school performance all help characterize the child. Is the child shy or compulsive, too sensitive to the needs of others, obsessively neat—in all, a possible "worrywart?" These traits may facilitate a migraine or the so-called tension headache. Certainly, the physician should look for evidence of depression, since headache may be the prime complaint of the chronically depressed child.

The physical examination must be precise and include a careful neurological evaluation and a conscientious attempt at ophthalmoscopy, a visual field check, an evaluation of ocular muscle balance and convergence, palpation and auscultation of the skull and mastoid and of the optic globes, palpation and transillumination of the sinuses, a careful check of the teeth, ears, and throat, a blood pressure reading, and a urinalysis. Eye drops may be used to improve the visualization of the fundus, but only after a description of the pupils and their reactions to light and accommodation are carefully recorded. Rarely, then, are laboratory and imaging examinations necessary.

INTERPRETING INFORMATION

Characterization of the headache is most important. Two major groups exist: those having an apparent first acute episode in the absence of a significant prior complaint and those suggesting chronicity and recurrence. This latter group bestows the advantage of hindsight in determining the patterns. However, the acute episode may be the first of many; the boundary can be obscure, at least at the start. A tendency to the diffuse and nondescript suggests tension or a more "distant" cause—an association, perhaps, with anemia, fever, some infectious process, or hypoglycemia. It is worth repeating that youth and specificity—the younger the child and the more specific the headache—increase the likelihood of an organic disorder. But make haste cautiously; time usually allows for a careful approach to differentiate the organic from the benign.

The trap to avoid is relying too greatly on a mechanical and unthinking use of the laboratory and other diagnostic aids, that is, the workup. Most headaches should be diagnosed and managed successfully without the skull roentgenographic series, computed tomography (CT) scan, magnetic resonance imaging (MRI), lumbar puncture, or arteriogram; most patients are helped by a conscientious history and physical examination, a meticulous explanation, and a ready and willing ear. It is the ability to listen wisely and to respond constructively that will do most for the patient who has a rather diffuse, chronic, or recurrent headache—that and, perhaps, a little acetaminophen.

Headache, more than most complaints, tends to force the physician's behavior to extremes—on the one hand, intervening forthrightly for major problems; on the other, responding gently in a conscientious attempt at understanding the patient's sometimes submerged feelings and needs. The physician must reject mechanistic diagnostic intervention unless the situation clearly calls for it.

DIFFERENTIAL DIAGNOSIS

Given a precise history and physical examination, resorting to the laboratory becomes necessary if there is a genuine indication of *infection* or *increased intracranial pressure* from whatever source. The choice of studies at the start is relatively simple. The suspicion of infection suggests the need for a complete blood count and, quite often, a lumbar puncture and blood culture. The lumbar puncture should be approached with care and only after verification that no papilledema or other evidence of increased intracranial pressure exists. A urinalysis is easy to obtain and certainly is indicated in the presence of hypertension. Auscultation for a cranial bruit may detect an aneurysm or other vascular deformity.

Although skull and sinus films can be helpful, a need for the CT scan, sonography, MRI, or radioactive isotope brain scans may arise, particularly if the history does not suggest a clearly definable diagnosis or when there are focal findings. If so, consultation is indicated with the neurologist and the "imagists," who can help decide on the most effective and least invasive of the various imaging techniques. Arteriography, still used occasionally, should be avoided if at all possible because it increases morbidity and the risk of hemiplegia.

The electroencephalogram (EEG), of itself relatively benign (save for its cost and impressive, intimidating trappings), is of questionable help. Its findings, for example, often are abnormal in patients who have migraine and often normal in those who have epilepsy. It sometimes is helpful in localizing an intracranial lesion, but it is not nearly as specific as the imaging techniques. The EEG therefore is not the first line in the study of acute problems.

At this point, the individual problem often becomes sufficiently clear that an appropriate therapeutic intervention is evident. Infection can be defined further by appropriate cultures and treated with antibiotics, surgical drainage, or both; expanding lesions and any trauma and bleeding mandate neurosurgical consultation. Fortunately, the diagnosis of pseudotumor cerebri sometimes can be made.

However, once the history and physical examination are complete, the pediatrician still may be confronted with a complaint that seems nonspecific and difficult to clarify. For example, some helpful information indicating a behavioral change may become evident, as well as information eliminating the possibility of organic disease; sometimes the organic and the functional components are concurrent. If migraine is present about 75% of the time in a family history, the physician should turn the evaluation in that direction. In this circumstance other factors are helpful. Migraine, quite common in childhood, usually begins during the early school years, from 5 or 6 to about 9 years of age. However, it is not uncommon in the younger child. There often has been a history of cyclic vomiting or car sickness. These headaches, usually unilateral, tend to predominate in females after puberty and sometimes are accompanied, particularly in "classic" migraine, by prodromal periods that may include sensory, motor, or visual auras, scotomas, abdominal pain, nausea and vomiting, irritability, and paresthesias; prodromes, however, are reported less commonly in children than in adults. At times, retroorbital pain occurs, usually on one side.

The physician should ask about odd visual phenomena—gaping "holes," dots, lines, and "stars." The older child should be asked to draw the scotoma. The often associated gastrointestinal complaint can be severe, and the occasional transient neurological finding of aphasia, hemiplegia, or ophthalmoplegia can be very disturbing. This complicates matters and leads to more extensive testing, particularly to the use of the CT scan or MRI and to the investigation of a urea-cycle abnormality (ornithine transcarbamoylase deficiency), believed by some to be a cause of migraine.

A migraine headache lacks consistency in that it may occur on either side of the head and may vary in frequency. It often may begin during periods of emotional stress, intense use of the eyes (reading, television), menstruation, use of oral contraceptives, or exposure to loud sound (rock music played at high volume); it may occur when menses have been missed or chocolate and cheeses have been eaten. A period of sleep following the headache often terminates the episode.

A variant of the "classic" migraine is "common" migraine, in which the abdominal pain, nausea and vomiting, aura, and other prodromata are unusual but family history of the symptoms and relief with sleep are similarly typical. Notably, the headache accompanying "common" migraine tends to be somewhat less dramatic. Some effort has been made to relate the incidence of all forms of migraine to family income, but this at best is an uncertain differential diagnostic point.

Tension headaches, sometimes called muscle contraction headaches, usually follow periods of stress and may last for days or weeks; they are dull (not pulsating) and usually bilateral. They may be correlated with behavioral change and, particularly, with difficult relations with family, friends, or teachers. These undercurrents and any suspicion of them should have been explored during the history and should prompt the interviewer to go beyond initial denials. An effort must be made to gain a clear understanding of those feelings and attitudes that may provoke anger, hostility, or anxiety. The history also may reveal a disruption of sleep patterns, particularly difficulty in falling asleep.

Such headaches usually begin at about 8 to 12 or 13 years of age and usually in females, particularly those who are overweight. The description of a tension headache is more fuzzy than that of migraine (although it may be compulsively precise), and it often is said to involve the entire head or the occiput. No prodromal period akin to that of migraine occurs and, generally, no conclusion of the episode by a period of sleep takes place; neither are reports of aura, nausea and vomiting, or visual changes common. Finally, these headaches do not have associated objective findings, such as an abnormal EEG.

The depressed child often may have a severe headache that lasts for days or longer. Acute anger and subsequent guilt may underlie the depression. Although no particular behavioral pattern suggests either migraine or tension headache, these children frequently have a demeanor that sharpens the intensity of concerns common to all people—for example, sensitivity to criticism and meeting new people, worry about grades, and precision in doing homework. Such children may seem to be compulsive and to worry very much if they do not meet the personal demands they place on themselves.

Occipital neuralgia, often suggested by tenderness over the cervical spinous processes, usually occurs first during adolescence. A roentgenogram may reveal subluxation or narrowing at the level of the first and second cervical vertebrae. No prodrome occurs, nor does cessation of the pain with sleep.

Finally, vascular headaches, often called "cluster" headaches, begin to occur in older teenagers, predominantly in males. When they do occur in females, there is no association with menses. They usually are unilateral and accompanied by ipsilateral tearing of the eye. They are recurrent and tend to occur in clusters, often at night, each one lasting for perhaps an hour and then disappearing. Thus they are briefer and perhaps more frequent than migraine. They are not accompanied by vomiting or nausea.

Headache manifestations, then, are age related. The organic lesion is not confined to any age, yet headache in the very young suggests organicity. Thereafter, a sequence of diagnostic possibilities emerges: migraine during the early school years, tension headaches just before the onset of puberty, occipital neuralgia during adolescence, and finally, the vascular headache of the older teenager. It should be emphasized that the patient who has an already recognized headache disorder may, as time goes by, report a different sort of headache. Always respect the possibility of a new and superimposed problem.

MANAGEMENT

The symptomatic management of headache is less difficult when there is a specific cause requiring a specific management. The therapeutic task is less certain in the chronic circumstance when the headache is described less precisely and its true chronicity, severity, and recurrence often are obscured by fuzzy verbiage. The child most often involved is older than 6 or 7 years, and the circumstances almost invariably suggest at least some emotional basis. The desire, then, is to be more specific in getting at the cause, invoking at times the psychologist or psychiatrist, and to use drugs sparingly. In fact, the very process of meticulous evaluation and sympathetic response sometimes is enough to break the cycle of complaint, particularly with the older child and adolescent.

Parents, properly advised, are central to the management. They can be effective in supervising the maintenance of the expected schedule—that is, attendance at school—and helpful in arranging a compassionate yet disciplined approach when headaches occur at school. Given the age of the patient, they can keep or help to keep a headache record, noting the time of occurrence, the characteristics, and the relationship to events of the time. The patient, of course, is central to all of this and should be expected to be a full participant in age-appropriate ways.

Although the cautious use of drugs has much to recommend it, do not be too cautious. A limited list of agents is helpful (Table 136-1). Headaches that are not severe, not particularly frequent, and not prolonged are best managed with acetaminophen rather than aspirin or nonsteroidal antiinflammatory drugs, with their greater risk of side effects. Usually, the response is not dose related, and an increase in the amount or frequency of the dosage is *not* justified when the headache persists. In addition, a period of rest and sleep (if that is achievable) is synergistic. A migraine headache, particularly, responds to sleep. Although the chronic use of sedatives as an additional management "crutch" should be avoided, the use of short-term daily phenobarbital or phenytoin in anticonvulsant doses may help.

The next steps are guided by the diagnostic conclusion and the age of the child. Some children will persist in experiencing an intense and frequently recurrent headache (one or two times a month) and may, if they have migraine or cluster headaches, require ergot. The primary care pediatrician must then consider consulting with a neurologist or a physician whose specific concern is the treatment of headache. The use of ergot derivatives to treat acute migraine is uncommon in pediatric practice, and they certainly should not be used in the prepubertal child or in any young person in whom gastrointestinal symptoms predominate. If they are used, they should be given in the prodromatal phase so that the subsequent headache might be prevented. In addition, the cluster headache often is managed more effectively by potentiating the effect of ergot with methysergide. However, the potential toxic effect of methysergide (retroperitoneal fibrosis and fibrotic syndromes) suggests the need for great caution.

Therefore the pediatrician's relative unfamiliarity with these drugs and occasional inadequate understanding of their toxicity in the young (e.g., ergot will intensify an abdominal complaint) require the direction of a consultant more experienced in their use. If the clinical picture includes significant depression, amitriptyline can be prescribed. This, too, requires the advice of a consultant, preferably a psychiatrist.

Eliminating certain foods thought to be associated with migraine, such as chocolate, citrus fruits, red wines, and some beans may be relatively easy, but first try to establish some relation between the use of these foods and the occurrence

Table 136-1 Drug Dosage for Relief of Headache

Drug	Dose	Comments
Acetaminophen	<1 yr: 60 mg q4-6h PO 1-3 yr: 60-120 mg q4-6h PO 3-6 yr: 120-180 mg q4-6h PO 6-12 yr: 240 mg q4-6h PO >12 yr: 325-650 mg q4-6h PO Alternative: 5-10 mg/kg q4-6h Maximum adult dosage: 4 g/day	
Amitriptyline	1-2 mg/kg/day: ⅓ in morning, ⅔ at bedtime	Prescribe only after consultation
Codeine phosphate	0.5-1 mg/kg PO or SC stat; repeat q4-6h Maximum dosage: 3 mg/kg/day	May be habit forming
Cyproheptadine	0.25-0.5 mg/kg/day, divided, q6-8h PO Maximum total dose: 0.5 mg/kg/day	use with caution in asthma because of atropine-like effects; contraindicated in neonates
Diazepam	0.1-0.8 mg/kg/day, divided, q6-8h PO	
Ergot	<12 yr: no more than 4 mg per episode; preferably 2 mg sublingually	Prescribe only after consultation
Phenobarbital	2-4 mg/kg/dose PO, IM, or PR; repeat prn q8h	
Propranolol	<35 kg: 10-20 mg PO tid >35 kg: 20-40 mg PO tid	May cause hypotension, nausea and vomiting, and bradycardia; contraindicated in asthma and heart block; caution advised in presence of obstructive pulmonary, renal, or liver disease

of migrainous episodes. After all, abstinence from some foods can more often lead to problems than help and in any event can be difficult to enforce in children. Suggested preventive or prophylactic medications for migraine—propranolol and cyproheptadine hydrochloride (Periactin)—should be used with caution. Propranolol *is not* to be used once an attack has begun, and its value compared with a placebo is not certain. Periactin's sedative and appetite-stimulant properties make it less desirable.

Tension headache is apt not to respond to acetaminophen, particularly if the underlying circumstance goes beyond the usual wear and tear of living and involves a more deep-seated problem, intense anxiety, or depression and particularly if these contributors have been present for some time. In fact, the failure to respond to simple medication strongly suggests a tension headache. The temptation to intervene with tranquilizers should be resisted in spite of an occasional reason to offer one. However, a frequent need for its use in a particular patient should suggest intense underlying factors that must, if possible, be discovered. Given this, sometimes with the help of a psychologist or psychiatrist, the pediatrician may be more secure in the use of diazepam or, in the instance of a child who is chronically depressed, amitriptyline. Such a serious and persistent problem, however, requires psychiatric intervention. Biofeedback and relaxation techniques can help if supervised by an experienced person, but only when the child is old enough and motivated enough to use them consistently.

There are occasional patients who have a headache so severe and persistent that there is a temptation to use narcotics or an intramuscular sedative. In this event the diagnosis must be secure because an as yet unrecognized organic cause may exist, requiring a specific intervention. The primary pediatrician should seek consultation at this point. Severity, whether defined by intensity of the episodes, their frequency, or the persistence of an individual episode, often requires this. The failure of relatively simple medication to provide relief also suggests consultation before riskier drugs are tried. In any event, the long-term outlook for children who have nonorganic headaches generally is good, although adolescents who have tension headaches often may suffer them into and throughout adulthood.

SUGGESTED READINGS

Barlow CF: *Headaches and migraine in childhood,* Philadelphia, 1984, JB Lippincott.

Basbaum AI, Fields HL: Endogenous pain control mechanisms: review and hypothesis, *Ann Neurol* 4:451, 1979.

Elser JM: Easing the pain of childhood headaches, *Contemp Pediatr* 8:108, 1991.

Fenichel G: Migraine in children, *Neurol Clin* 3:77, 1985.

Johnson K, editor: *The Harriet Lane handbook,* ed 13, St Louis, 1994, Mosby.

Prensky AL: Differentiating and treating pediatric headaches, *Contemp Pediatr* 1:12, 1984.

Singer HS, Rowe S: Chronic recurrent headaches in children, *Pediatr Ann* 21:369, 1992.

Sullivan JF: Diagnostic imperatives in neurology. In Proger S, Barza M, editors: *Diagnostic imperatives,* New York, 1981, Thieme-Stratton.

Welch KMA: Drug therapy of migraine, *N Engl J Med* 329:1476, 1993.

137 Hearing Loss

Michael H. Weiss, Patricia M. Chute, and Simon C. Parisier

The early identification and remediation of hearing loss among children is highly desirable so that these individuals may develop normal communication skills. The incidence of congenital hearing loss is approximately 1 per 600 live births. About 50% of these cases are attributable to a genetic disorder, the great majority of which are autosomal recessive.

Acquired hearing loss in childhood is extremely common.[2] More than 75% of children have at least one episode of otitis media, with concomitant conductive hearing loss. Many of these cases readily resolve over time with antibiotic treatment, but others go on to chronic effusion, which causes hearing loss that requires intervention. Chronic otitis media, cholesteatoma, and otosclerosis are other causes of acquired conductive hearing loss in the pediatric population.

DEFINITION AND CHARACTERISTICS OF HEARING LOSS

Hearing loss is defined and quantified according to the hearing thresholds measured (i.e., the softest tone heard by the subject at a given frequency) during the performance of pure tone audiometric testing. Zero decibels (0 dB) is the reference standard set by testing a cohort of normal young adults. Normal hearing ranges between 0 and 25 dB, mild impairment from 26 to 40 dB, moderate from 41 to 55 dB, moderately severe from 56 to 70 dB, severe from 71 to 90 dB, and profound being 91 dB and above.[18] The degree of hearing loss determines the type of treatment required.

ASSOCIATED SIGNS AND SYMPTOMS

The evaluation of hearing loss in an infant or child starts with the history. A family history of congenital hearing loss places all subsequent children at high risk. Prenatal or perinatal infection such as rubella or cytomegalovirus is significant. Birth trauma and anoxia also are important to note. Medications, such as aminoglycosides, may cause ototoxicity. In the older child, behavior or personality changes may signify hearing loss. A history of frequent ear infections or other nonspecific signs and symptoms (e.g., fever, irritability, or gastrointestinal upset) may accompany otological abnormalities. Vestibular problems may well accompany hearing impairment; thus a history of dizziness or imbalance should be sought. All prior medical problems should be reviewed, as these may shed light on the cause of the hearing loss.

The physical examination includes careful examination of the entire head and neck to note the presence of any anomalies. Examination of the ear will disclose abnormalities of the external ear and reveal a middle ear infection or effusion. While examining the patient, the pediatrician should note his or her responsiveness to auditory and verbal cues.

ASSESSMENT OF AUDITORY AND MIDDLE EAR FUNCTION

Older children are tested with a standard battery of audiometric tests that includes pure tone tests of air and bone conduction. The child signals the tester whenever he or she hears a tone, and a graph of the hearing thresholds at a variety of test frequencies is generated.[19] Speech reception and discrimination testing, as well as tympanometry, also are performed.[10]

Unfortunately, one cannot test infants and very young children this straightforwardly, but several tests have been devised to determine hearing thresholds in young subjects. A common form of behavioral testing uses sound generators and observation of the auropalpebral reflex, the startle reflex, and arousal. However, these behavioral testing techniques provide estimates of hearing acuity only for the better hearing ear.[17] The most recent development in evaluating young children is otoacoustic emissions (OAE).[5] The emission, also called the "cochlear echo," is spontaneous in some individuals but can be evoked reliably by clicks or tones. Through the insertion into the ear canal of a probe that contains small microphones, the cochlear response to a variety of stimuli can be measured. Although the sensitivity of this test decreases once the stimulus intensity reaches 30 to 40 dB, it has been shown to be an excellent method of screening hearing in newborns.[15] This test is being used in conjunction with the more traditional electrophysiological test known as the auditory brainstem response (ABR).

ABR uses the measurement of electrical potentials generated within the brainstem in response to monaural acoustic stimuli. Electrodes are placed on the scalp, and a computer is used to record responses to many auditory clicks. Hearing thresholds for each ear may be generated separately with this method. ABR results should be considered in conjunction with behavioral testing to obtain a total picture of the infant's capabilities.[3]

At 2 years of age, the hearing of 70% of children can be evaluated by play audiometry. With this technique, children are conditioned behaviorally to respond to sounds during play. A skilled tester can elicit responses to threshold-level stimuli, and the percentage of children who can be evaluated by play audiometry rises to 96% by 3 years of age.[17] In addition to pure tone testing, speech discrimination can also be estimated by a variety of picture identification tests. Such tests require the child to point to the correct picture in response to an auditory cue. Thus it is possible to assess a young child's hearing ability for pure tones and speech accurately.[10,19]

Because one of the most common causes of hearing loss in young children is otitis media, an assessment of middle ear function is necessary for this group. Tympanometry is the measurement of the acoustic impedance of the ear as a function of ear canal pressure. It is helpful in identifying abnormalities of the middle ear, particularly problems characterized by high impedance (middle ear effusions).[11,16]

The acoustic reflex also has been employed as a diagnostic measurement. In the demonstration of the acoustic reflex, the impedance meter measures the sudden change in ear canal sound pressure caused by the decrease in compliance of the middle ear system as the stapedius muscle contracts in response to an auditory stimulus. The threshold for the acoustic reflex has been employed to estimate the level of hearing loss in young children.[4] The absence of an acoustic reflex often is noted in conductive hearing loss. An absent or abnormal acoustic reflex is a common finding in the presence of retrocochlear abnormalities.

DIFFERENTIAL DIAGNOSIS

After complete testing, hearing loss may be characterized as conductive, mixed, or sensorineural. Conductive losses are those that involve the external or middle ear or both. These losses may be congenital (as in the cases of anomalies of the external or middle ear such as congenital atresia) or acquired. Sensorineural hearing loss implies damage to the cochlea or the acoustic nerve[14] (part of cranial nerve VIII). Such losses may be congenital or acquired. A subset of sensorineural hearing loss is retrocochlear hearing loss, which implies dysfunction of the acoustic nerve or the brainstem, usually secondary to neoplasm. Retrocochlear abnormalities are rare in children. Mixed hearing loss is a combination of conductive and sensorineural hearing loss.

Central auditory dysfunction is characterized by hearing loss in combination with one or more of the following: deficits in foreground-background discrimination, poor auditory attention, limitations in memory and retrieval, and delays in receptive language development. Finally, there is functional hearing loss. This hearing loss is pretended, exaggerated, or hysterical. It is a diagnosis of exclusion and must be made with caution but has been noted unequivocally in several studies.[8]

With the newer techniques available to test newborns, one can diagnose hearing loss very early in life. Although the cost initially might appear to be large, the overall cost to society when hearing losses are missed is much greater. Current recommendations are that all infants admitted to the neonatal intensive care unit be screened, as well as other infants considered to be at high risk because of family history or associated syndromal anomalies (see Chapter 20, Nine, Auditory Screening). In addition, any child recovering from meningitis must have audiometric testing. Ideally, all children should be screened in the first 3 months of life. Few institutions employ this practice, but screening all neonates by using the techniques of OAE and ABR in combination is feasible. A recent NIH Consensus Panel strongly recommended this approach.[7]

A radiological workup consisting of a high-resolution noncontrast computed tomography (CT) scan of the temporal bones often is helpful in cases of documented hearing loss. Several anomalies of the inner ear, notably Mondini dysplasia, can be diagnosed definitively in this way. Computed tomography is an important adjunct in the workup of aural atresia to define the anatomy of the middle and inner ear, thus determining suitability for surgical correction of the hearing loss. Individuals who have congenital sensorineural hearing loss must be examined carefully for associated anomalies of the head and neck, integument, and internal organs. More than 60 genetic syndromes have been characterized, including Usher, Alport, Pendred, Waardenburg, and many other eponymic syndromes.[6,14] Other cases are caused by prenatal or perinatal insult, such as low birth weight, infection, or anoxia. Appropriate blood serological samples are tested, and a CT of the temporal bone is ordered.

A substantial number of cases of congenital sensorineural hearing loss will not yield an obvious diagnosis following this workup. Many of these probably occur genetically, although this is difficult to prove.

Acquired sensorineural hearing loss may be caused by ototoxicity, meningitis, labyrinthitis, temporal bone trauma, a perilymph fistula, and acoustic trauma.[14]

Conductive hearing loss usually is caused by otitis media or middle ear effusion. Chronic otitis media, cholesteatoma, otosclerosis, and ossicular fixation or discontinuity are less frequent causes.

PSYCHOSOCIAL CONSIDERATIONS

Any degree of hearing loss during a child's early life can impair that child's development of language and communication skills. In the case of a child who has a severe or profound hearing loss, this effect is most pronounced. Early identification of such children therefore is imperative because it enables the child to be rehabilitated. Amplification through the use of hearing aids often can provide some useful hearing. The special educational needs of the child who has a hearing impairment may be addressed early, allowing for maximal benefit. For a child whose severe impairment remains unidentified for the first 2 or 3 years of life, a severe handicap in all areas of interpersonal communication is the usual result. Such an individual has been understimulated during a crucial phase of language development, and making up for that lost opportunity is extremely difficult.

Milder degrees of hearing loss also may induce significant hardship because children who have hearing losses in the 20 to 50 dB range do not follow conversations fully and may miss instructions from teachers. Such children may be thought of as inattentive, antisocial, or unintelligent. Following treatment of such hearing losses, one often sees remarkable improvement in school performance and personality.[10]

MANAGEMENT

Mild and moderate conductive hearing losses caused by middle ear infections are treated with antibiotics. Middle ear effusion frequently is seen after an acute infection, but such effusions often resolve spontaneously. When an effusion lasts several months, or if the tympanic membrane is severely retracted with marked hearing loss, surgical intervention may be indicated. Myringotomy and insertion of drainage tubes usually is performed, along with adenoidectomy if concomitant nasopharyngeal obstruction is evident (see Chapter 266, Tonsillectomy and Adenoidectomy for discussion of the indications for adenoidectomy).

Severe and profound hearing losses require an intensive rehabilitative and educational program.[1] Hearing aid technology has advanced in recent years with miniaturization and improved acoustic characteristics. The child should be fitted with an appropriate device early in life. Frequency modulated (FM) assistive listening devices are excellent adjuncts in the classroom and home. With such a device the individual who has a hearing impairment has an FM receiver and earphone, and the speaker has a microphone. The effects of background noise are reduced substantially with the use of such a device. The range of the device can extend up to several hundred feet. Speech reading and auditory training help to maximize communication skills. Children who are successful in oral communication have been increasingly successful with "mainstreaming" into a regular classroom. When oral communication is less successful, a manual mode of communication (e.g., sign language) is introduced. For profoundly deaf children who do not benefit from conventional hearing aids, the use of vibrotactile aids may improve communication performance.[9,13] Cochlear implants have emerged as a new and exciting modality in the treatment of children who have a profound hearing impairment.[12] Data on the use of cochlear implants indicate that children fitted at an earlier age perform better than do children fitted with implants after sustaining long durations of deafness.[18]

The key to proper treatment of children who have hearing impairment is early identification and intervention. Today's technology makes it possible to diagnose hearing loss in infants and children of any age and thus to treat and rehabilitate these individuals at the earliest possible time.

REFERENCES

1. Erber N: *Auditory training,* Washington, DC, 1982, AG Bell Association for the Deaf.
2. Ginsberg IA, White TP: Otologic disorders and examination. In Katz J, editor: *Handbook of clinical audiology,* ed 4, Baltimore, 1985, Williams & Wilkins.
3. Hecox K, Galambos R: Brainstem auditory-evoked responses in human infants and adults, *Arch Otolaryngol* 99:30, 1974.
4. Jerger S: Studies in impedance audiometry. II. Children less than 6 years old, *Arch Otolaryngol* 99:1, 1974.
5. Kemp DT: Stimulated acoustic emissions from the human auditory system, *J Acoust Soc Am* 64:1386, 1978.
6. Konigsmark BW, Gorlin TJ: *Genetic and metabolic deafness,* Philadelphia, 1976, WB Saunders.
7. Matz GJ et al: Early identification of hearing impairment in infants and young children, *NIH Consensus Statement* Mar 1-3; 11:1, 1993.
8. McCanna D, DeLapa G: A clinical study of 27 children exhibiting functional hearing loss, *Language Speech Hearing Services in Schools* 12:26, 1981.
9. Miyamoto RT et al: Comparison of sensory aids in deaf children, *Ann Otol Rhinol Laryngol* 99(suppl 142):2, 1989.
10. Northern JL, Downs MP: *Hearing loss in children,* Baltimore, 1978, Williams & Wilkins.
11. Paradise JL, Smith C, Bluestone CD: Tympanometric detection of middle ear effusion in infants and young children, *Pediatrics* 58:198, 1976.
12. Parisier SC, Chute P, Hellman S: The use of cochlear implants for profound hearing loss, *Surgical Rounds* 12:15, 1989.
13. Pickett J, MacFarland W: Auditory implants and tactile aids for the profoundly deaf, *J Speech Hear Res* 28:134, 1985.
14. Schuknecht HF: *Pathology of the ear,* ed 2, Cambridge, Mass, 1993, Harvard University Press.
15. Smurzynski J et al: Distortion-product and click-evoked otoacoustic emissions of preterm and full-term infants, *Ear Hear* 14:258, 1993.
16. Terkildsen K, Thomsen K: The influence of pressure variations on the impedance of the human eardrum, *J Laryngol Otol* 73:409, 1959.
17. Thompson G, Weber B: Responses of infants and young children to behavior observation audiometry, *J Speech Hear Disord* 39:140, 1974.
18. Tyler R: Speech perception by children. In Tyler R, editor: *Cochlear implants: audiological foundations,* San Diego, 1993, Singular Publishing.
19. Yantis P: Pure tone air conduction testing. In Katz J, editor: *Handbook of clinical audiology,* ed 4, Baltimore, 1994, Williams & Wilkins.

138 Heart Murmurs

Edward B. Clark

The normal murmur that most children develop sometime during childhood must be distinguished from a pathological murmur indicating a structural heart defect. Yet not all patients who have heart disease have a murmur; cyanotic patients who have pulmonary atresia and healthy looking children who have coarctation of the aorta may have no murmur. Thus the cardiac examination includes what one sees and feels, in addition to what one hears.

INSPECTION

Much can be learned from careful observation. Asymmetry of the chest often reflects long-standing enlargement of the heart. Retraction of the suprasternal notch and grooving of the lower rib cage may be caused by vigorous pulling of the diaphragm in an infant who has stiff lungs from pulmonary overcirculation.

PALPATION

Palpation adds to the examination. Thrills felt over the heart or neck vessels reflect high-velocity blood flow. The cardiac thrust or heave correlates with ventricular enlargement. A palpable pulmonary artery signifies pulmonary hypertension. The peripheral pulses should be palpated simultaneously. A strong brachial pulse and weak femoral pulse suggest the diagnosis of coarctation of the aorta. A water-hammer pulse may be the clue to aortic insufficiency or another cardiac lesion associated with a wide pulse pressure. The plateau pulse of aortic stenosis can be easily recognized. An enlarged liver correlates with vascular engorgement.

AUSCULTATION

The heart sounds relate to the hemodynamic events of the cardiac cycle. The first heart sound is generated by closure of the tricuspid and mitral valves. The second heart sound is produced by closure of the semilunar valves and is particularly important for diagnosis. The first component of the second heart sound (S_2A) is caused by aortic valve closure and the second component by pulmonary valve closure (S_2P). The intensity of S_2A and S_2P and their relationship to each other and to respiration provide information about the pressure at which the valves close and about blood flow across the valves. Other sounds such as systolic click of a bicuspid semilunar valve, an opening snap of the mitral valve, diastolic gallop, friction rub, and bruits over intercostal arteries or an arteriovenous fistula help make an accurate cardiac diagnosis.

TYPES OF HEART MURMURS (Fig. 138-1)

A heart murmur is caused by turbulent blood flow. The timing, intensity, and location of heart murmurs define the anatomical cause of the turbulent flow. A thrill is palpable when the murmur is a grade 4 or more in intensity in the grading system of 1 to 6.

An *ejection murmur* reflects turbulence as blood flows in increased volume through a narrowed orifice or normal semilunar valve. Murmurs arising in the pulmonary outflow tract are best heard in the left second intercostal space. Those arising in the aortic outflow tract radiate to the right second intercostal space.

A *pansystolic murmur* denotes turbulent blood flow during the isovolemic phase of contraction. Ventricular septal defect (VSD), mitral insufficiency, and tricuspid insufficiency cause such a murmur. The location of maximal intensity distinguishes the murmur of a ventricular septal defect from that of mitral insufficiency. The VSD murmur is heard best along the left lower sternal border and radiates to the right. A mitral insufficiency murmur is heard best at the apex and radiates to the left axilla. The murmur of tricuspid insufficiency is maximal at the fourth left interspace and varies with respiration.

A *continuous systolic and diastolic murmur* arises from turbulent flow across a patent ductus arteriosus or another direct connection between a high- and low-pressure system such as a pulmonary arteriovenous fistula.

An *early diastolic murmur* begins with the second heart sound and is caused by insufficiency of the aortic or pulmonary valve. A high-pitched murmur indicates aortic insufficiency; a low-pitched, soft murmur indicates pulmonary regurgitation.

A *middiastolic murmur* heard at the apex is caused by excessive blood flow across the mitral or tricuspid valve. This murmur is heard with large left-to-right shunts such as an atrial septal defect, a ventricular septal defect, or a patent ductus arteriosus.

ASSOCIATED HEART SOUNDS

The *second heart sound* is particularly important in the diagnosis of congenital heart defects. Normally this sound is split, with the aortic component preceding the pulmonary component. The two elements separate on inspiration and fuse on expiration. The louder the pulmonary component and the narrower the splitting, the greater the pulmonary artery pressure. Conversely, delay and diminution of the pulmonary component signify increasingly severe pulmonary stenosis. A wide and fixed split second heart sound occurs with mild pulmonary stenosis and with increased right heart ejection volume, as in the left-to-right shunt of an atrial septal defect.

An *early systolic ejection click* denotes a bicuspid aortic or pulmonary valve. Clicks also can be heard from a dilated aorta or pulmonary artery. A *midsystolic click* and a late systolic murmur at the apex characterizes the mitral valve prolapse.

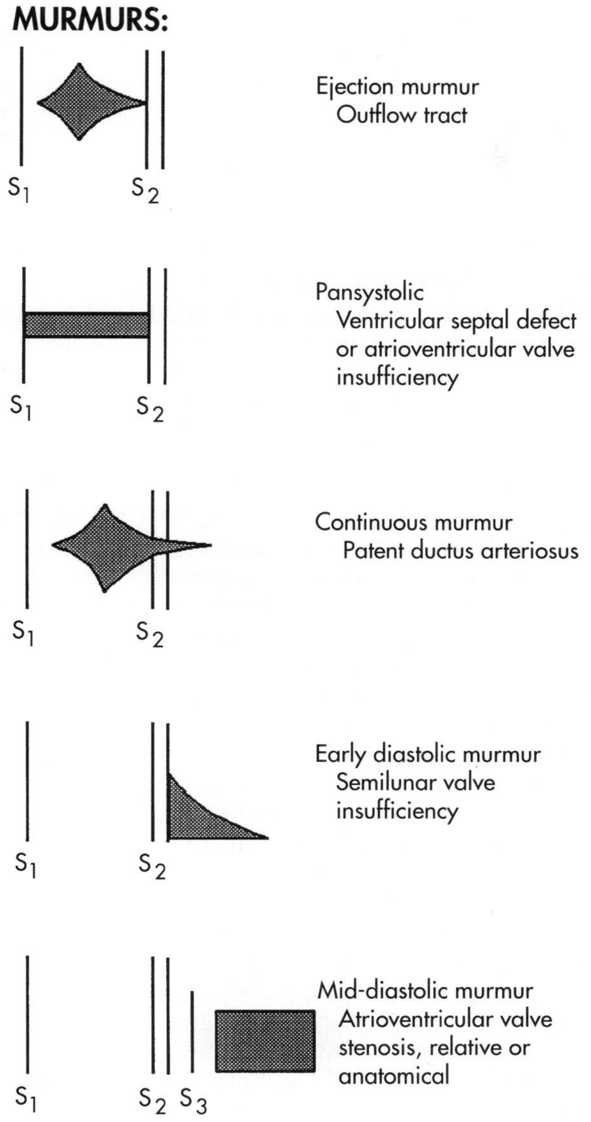

MURMURS:

FIG. 138-1 Diagram of the five most common types of cardiac murmurs: ejection murmur, pansystolic murmur, continuous murmur, early murmur, and middiastolic murmur. The shaded areas show the timing and intensity of the cardiac murmur in relation to the first (S_1) and second (S_2) heart sounds; the third heart sound exhibits a gallop rhythm (see text for further description).

An intermittent *third heart sound* at the apex is heard in many normal children; a *fourth heart sound,* however, often is pathological. The S_3 and S_4 gallops reflect blood flow into a stiff ventricle and are often associated with heart failure.

DIFFERENTIAL DIAGNOSIS: NORMAL MURMUR

Most heart murmurs arise from turbulent blood flow in a normal heart. Four common kinds of normal murmurs are distinguishable:

1. *Still murmur:* A short, vibratory, grade 1 or grade 2 ejection murmur heard over the precordium; it is the most common innocent murmur. A Still murmur is noted in at least 50% of normal, healthy children by 3 or 4 years of age.
2. *Venous hum:* A continuous murmur heard above the clavicle when the patient is upright. The murmur disappears when the patient is supine or when the head is turned and the external jugular vein is compressed.
3. *Pulmonary souffle:* A soft, midsystolic murmur heard in the second left interspace (pulmonary area). This murmur is heard in high cardiac output states such as fever, anemia, or hyperthyroidism.
4. *Benign peripheral pulmonary murmur:* An ejection murmur heard in the left second intercostal space that radiates to both axilla. Frequently heard in infants and small children, it represents blood flow turbulence at the branch point of the main and right and left pulmonary arteries.

MANAGEMENT

The only management needed in a child who has a normal heart murmur is complete reassurance. A child who has an organic murmur merits evaluation by a pediatric cardiologist.

SUGGESTED READINGS

Emmanouilides GC et al: *Heart disease in infants, children and adolescents,* ed 5, Baltimore, 1994, Williams & Wilkins.

Neill CA, Clark EB, Clark CI: *The heart of a child,* Baltimore, 1992, Johns Hopkins University Press.

Park MK: *Pediatric cardiology for practitioners,* ed 2, Chicago, 1988, Mosby.

139 Hematuria

Edward J. Ruley

The diagnostic approach to hematuria in pediatric patients is quite different from the strategy employed for adults. Having an organized plan of investigation is important if one is to determine the diagnosis most cost effectively while subjecting the child to the fewest invasive and uncomfortable procedures.

It is helpful to consider the occurrence of hematuria in several clinical settings: (1) macroscopic or gross hematuria, (2) spots of blood found on the underclothing or diapers, with an otherwise clear urine, and (3) microhematuria found by chemical or direct microscopy in an otherwise grossly normal urine. The presence of symptoms, either localized to the urinary tract or more generalized, is variable in each of these circumstances. The most likely causes of the hematuria in these clinical scenarios are different; therefore the clinical approach to the diagnosis of each also differs.

GROSS HEMATURIA

Incidence

Gross hematuria is a relatively uncommon urinary symptom, the occurrence of which varies according to the population being studied. In a report of more than 128,000 consecutive patients visiting an emergency clinic in a large city in the northeastern United States, the incidence of "red urine" as the chief complaint was 1.4 per 1000 visits. When other causes of a red urine were eliminated, the incidence of true gross hematuria was 1.3 per 1000 visits.[3]

Etiology

Urinary tract infection (either bacterial or viral) is the most common cause of gross hematuria in children, accounting for approximately half the cases. Irritation or ulceration of the perineum or urethral meatus is the next most common cause, constituting about 20% of the cases. Trauma is the third most common etiology. When relatively minor trauma results in gross hematuria, the clinician should be alerted to the possibility of an undiagnosed dilated urinary system. Such dilated structures may be fluid-filled cysts associated with various types of congenital cystic kidney diseases or a urine-filled renal pelvis and ureter caused by obstructive uropathy. These dilated systems are much more susceptible to gross bleeding after minor direct or indirect trauma than is the normal urinary system. Urinary stones as well as hypercalciuria without lithiasis have been recognized as important causes of gross hematuria in children. In one study significant hypercalciuria was found in 64% of the children who had gross hematuria.[2] Although coagulopathy has always been included among causes of gross hematuria, it is very uncommon. In contrast, gross hematuria is not uncommon in patients who have sickle cell trait or sickle cell disease. Glomerulonephritis usually accounts for fewer than 10% of patients who have gross hematuria, although the incidence varies considerably depending on whether there is a nephritogenic strain of *Streptococcus* in the community. Even with a complete and thoughtful approach, a specific cause cannot be proved in 10% to 20% of children.

History

It is important to ascertain a description of the color, clarity, and pattern of the gross hematuria. Pink or red urine most often indicates bladder or urethral bleeding; greenish or brown urine is seen most commonly in upper tract or renal parenchymal bleeding. An opaque or cloudy specimen usually results from the presence of blood cells in the urine, whether they originate from the upper or lower urinary tract. In contrast, a urine that is discolored but clear in character usually indicates the presence of pigmenturia (hemoglobinuria or myoglobinuria). Gross hematuria that occurs sequentially in each voiding, even though it may differ in the degree of discoloration, usually is consistent with infection or the presence of upper tract (parenchymal) disease. Gross hematuria that occurs interspersed with normal-appearing urine is most consistent with hypercalciuria and lithiasis. The presence of symptoms, either generalized or localized to the urinary tract, is important in determining the most likely cause. Generalized symptoms such as fever, abdominal pain, arthralgia, arthritis, and rash imply that the gross hematuria is part of a more extensive illness. In contrast, urinary frequency, urgency, and dysuria would lead one to consider the lower urinary system and the bladder outlet as the site of the pathology. The past medical history, in particular previous diagnoses, prior episodes of gross hematuria, recent or concurrent illness, as well as the events surrounding the onset of gross hematuria, are important. Certain diagnoses such as sickle cell disease, hypercalciuria, or IgA nephropathy are characterized by recurrent episodes of gross hematuria. The occurrence of antecedent or concurrent upper respiratory tract infections may favor a particular type of glomerulonephritis as the etiology (see Chapter 232, Nephritis). Prior voiding habits such as the frequency and style of voiding can be important clues to the etiology. It has been noted that young boys may squeeze or compress the penis in an attempt to thwart an urge to micturate when it is experienced at a time when they do not want to interrupt their play or activities. Other boys may have the habit of bending their penis over the elastic in their underpants when voiding, causing a sharp bend in the urethra. Both of these practices may lead to urethral irritation and produce gross or microscopic bleeding. In girls it is important to consider menarche as being misinterpreted as an episode of gross hematuria. Finally, a history of other family members who have gross hematuria, urinary stones, hearing loss, sickle cell disease, or coagulopathies can be pertinent.

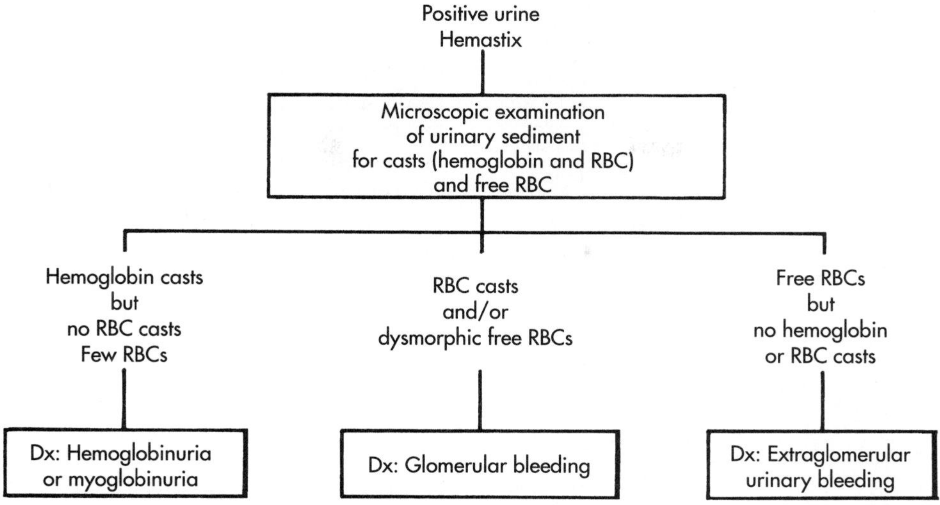

FIG. 139-1 A clinical algorithm for microhematuria in children.

Physical Findings

A comprehensive general physical examination is appropriate for children who have gross hematuria. Specifically, blood pressure measurement, abdominal examination, and direct visualization of the penile meatus or the female introitus, including the urethral meatus, is important.

Laboratory Findings

Obviously the most important laboratory test is the urinalysis. The centrifuged sediment of a freshly voided urine specimen should be examined very carefully under the microscope, giving attention to the presence and morphology of any erythrocytes, as well as to the presence of any cellular casts (Fig. 139-1). Should there be only relatively homogeneous pigmented casts without significant numbers of erythrocytes, one should suspect hemoglobinuria or myoglobinuria as the cause of the discolored urine. The dip-and-read strips for blood react to both hemoglobin and myoglobin. Some causes of hemoglobinuria and myoglobinuria are given in the box on the right. These situations are relatively uncommon in pediatric patients.

When erythrocytes are present, scrutiny of their appearance helps to determine their origin.[1] Red blood cells that originate from the urinary structures outside the nephrons look like normal peripheral-circulating erythrocytes on a blood smear. They will be eumorphic, that is, of uniform size and shape. Also, no casts will be seen. In contrast, erythrocytes originating from the kidney parenchyma are dysmorphic; that is, they vary in size and have irregular outlines, with blebs of cytoplasm appearing to bud from the cell surface (Fig. 139-2). The dysmorphic appearance of the erythrocytes may be the result of cell damage during extrusion through the glomerular basement membrane, the effect of osmotic forces during the cell's passage down the tubule, or some other as yet undefined factor. In addition to dysmorphic erythrocytes, a variety of casts containing erythrocytes, leukocytes, or tubular cells, as well as casts that appear coarsely and finely granular or hyaline, may be present (see Fig. 139-1). Regardless, dysmorphic erythrocytes and erythrocyte casts originate only from diseases in the kidney parenchyma; nowhere in the urinary system from the calyx to the meatus are there conditions that can create dysmorphic erythrocytes or casts. However, there are certain situations in which kidney insult can cause some overlap. One of the most obvious is trauma, in which bleeding can come from the kidney parenchyma and the urinary system at the same time. In this circumstance both dysmorphic and eumorphic erythrocytes, as well as erythrocyte casts, may be present in the same specimen.

Proteinuria also can be found in urine specimens in which there is gross hematuria. However, the dip-and-read test for protein is inaccurate in the presence of gross hematuria because of the effect on interpretation of color change. Therefore another method of protein quantitation, such as sulfosalicylic acid precipitation, must be used to assess proteinuria. In urine specimens that are isotonic or hypertonic, gross hematuria can result in modest amounts of protein being detectable. In urine specimens that are hypotonic, the degree

CAUSES OF HEMOGLOBINURIA AND MYOGLOBINURIA

Hemoglobinuria

Hemolytic anemia (e.g., glucose-6-phosphate dehydrogenase [G6PD] deficiency, Coombs'-positive hemolytic anemia)
Mismatched blood transfusions
Intravascular coagulation (e.g., disseminated intravascular coagulation [DIC], hemolytic-uremic syndrome)
Infections (e.g., sepsis, malaria)
Freshwater near-drowning
Mechanical erythrocyte damage (e.g., artificial heart valves, cardiopulmonary bypass)

Myoglobinuria

Muscle injury (e.g., crush injuries, electrical burns)
Myositis
Rhabdomyolysis

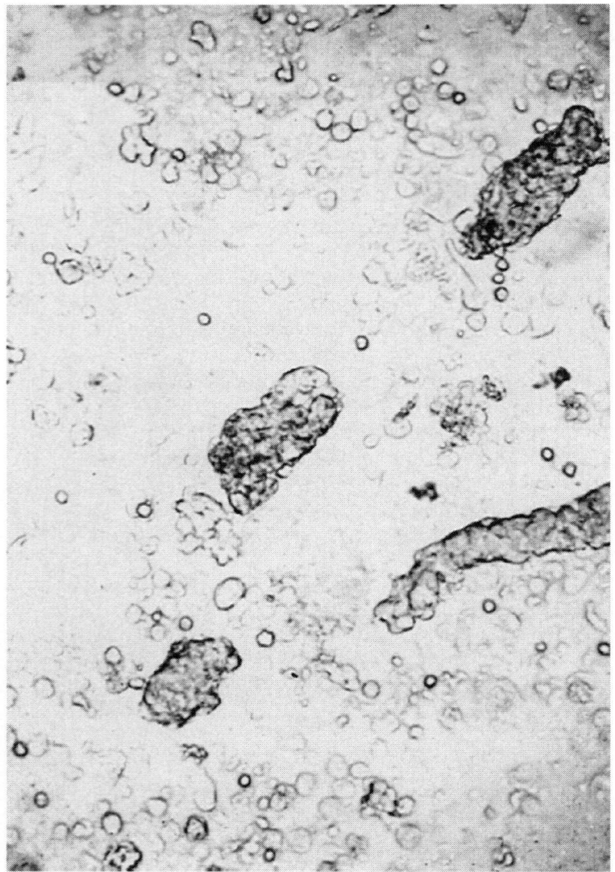

FIG. 139-2 Unstained urine sediment showing a red blood cell cast and dysmorphic red blood cells (×100).

of proteinuria can be marked. Studies have shown that the protein in this latter circumstance originates from the hemoglobin released from the lysed erythrocytes. Microhematuria does not result in any significant proteinuria,[5] therefore proteinuria in the presence of microhematuria needs to be investigated as an additional harbinger of significant renal disease.

Because urinary tract infection is so common, a urine culture is indicated in all instances of gross hematuria. To investigate hypercalciuria, calcium and creatinine quantitation should be determined on a random urine specimen. If the calcium-creatinine ratio is above 0.21, a 24-hour specimen should be obtained to determine the calcium excretion.[2,4] Imaging of the kidneys and the urinary system by ultrasound also is indicated to investigate kidney size and the character of the kidney parenchyma and to screen for dilated collecting systems. Gross hematuria is one instance in which cystoscopy may be indicated to look for sites of bleeding within the bladder or to determine from which kidney the blood is originating. Obviously such direct visualization is indicated for selected cases only and must be done when the patient is actively bleeding to be of value. Further investigation and the institution of treatment depend on the working diagnosis as suggested by recent, past, and family histories and the results of the preliminary tests. In contrast to adults, in children tumors of the urinary system are very uncommon causes of gross hematuria.

Blood on Underclothing

The discovery of dried spots of blood on diapers or underclothing can be very distressing for parents. The urine usually is normal in appearance and actually may dilute the appearance of the blood spots. This most often is seen in male infants who are otherwise well. The most common cause of this finding is irritation of the urethra, particularly at the meatus. These infants usually pass a normal urine, but at the end of urination a drop or two of blood seeps out the meatus, creating a discolored spot in a wet diaper. This can be diagnosed by direct observation of the penis and associated with an otherwise normal physical examination. More invasive tests are not indicated. The application of petroleum jelly and leaving the infant undiapered for a short period is all that is needed to resolve the problem.

MICROHEMATURIA

Incidence

Microhematuria occurs much more frequently than gross hematuria in the pediatric population, with a prevalence of 0.05% to 2.0%, depending on the definition of significant hematuria (see Chapter 20, Eight, Use of Urinalysis and the Urine Culture in Screening). Although the definition of significant microhematuria differs among studies, many investigators consider more than 10 erythrocytes per high-power field in the sediment of a centrifuged aliquot of freshly voided urine to be pathological.

Etiology

Many of the causes of gross hematuria also may cause microhematuria, although infection does so less commonly. Microscopic hematuria in the asymptomatic child usually is discovered during a routine well-child examination. This frequent clinical problem requires a thoughtful, systematical approach. The same algorithm given for macroscopic hematuria (see Fig. 139-1) can be applied to the child who has microhematuria.

History and Physical Findings

The same questions should be asked and a similar physical examination performed in the child who has microhematuria as that outlined for the child who has gross hematuria. Not uncommonly the history is completely noncontributory, and the physical examination is unrevealing.

Laboratory Findings

As with gross hematuria, the carefully done urinalysis becomes the crucial first test for the child who has microhematuria. Pigmenturia should be considered, although significant hemoglobin or myoglobin filtration more often causes macroscopic urine discoloration. When true hematuria exists, the morphology of the erythrocytes and the presence of casts assume the same significance as in gross hematuria. Differentiation of the causes of glomerular bleeding often requires hospitalization and more extensive testing (see Chapter 232, Nephritis). Should the urine contain only eumorphic erythrocytes and be free of casts, extraglomerular bleeding is most likely. Some causes are listed in the box on p. 999. Random and 24-hour urine specimens should be collected for calcium-creatinine ratios and calcium excretion determination. Spe-

CAUSES OF EXTRAGLOMERULAR HEMATURIA

Infection (e.g., cystitis, urethritis, balinitis)
Hypercalciuria (e.g., absorptive hypercalcuria, renal tubular hypercalciuria)
Trauma (e.g., vehicular accidents, falls, child abuse)
Urinary lithiasis (e.g., hypercalcuria, cysteinuria)
Malformations (e.g., cystic kidney diseases, posterior urethral valves, ureteropelvic junction obstruction)
Hemoglobinopathy (e.g., sickle cell disease, thalassemia)
Drugs (e.g., antibiotics, cytoxan)
Bleeding diathesis (e.g., von Willebrand disease, hemophilia)
Instrumentation (e.g., suprapubic aspiration, urinary catheterization, cystoscopy, self-stimulation)
Tumors (e.g., Wilms tumor, rhabdomyosarcoma, bladder papilloma)

cific treatment regimens depend on the cause of the microhematuria.

REFERENCES

1. Birch DF et al: Urinary erythrocyte morphology in the diagnosis of glomerular hematuria, *Clin Nephrol* 20:78, 1983.
2. Garcia CD, Miller MLT, Stapleton FB: Natural history of hematuria associated with hypercalciuria in children, *Am J Dis Child* 145:1204, 1991.
3. Ingelfinger JR, Davis AE, Grupe WE: Frequency and etiology of gross hematuria in a general pediatric setting, *Pediatrics* 59:557, 1977.
4. Stapleton FB et al: Hypercalciuria in children with hematuria, *N Engl J Med* 310:1345, 1984.
5. Tapp DC, Copley JB: Effect of red blood cell lysis on protein quantitation in hematuric states, *Am J Nephrol* 8:190, 1988.

SUGGESTED READINGS

Lieu TA, Grasmeder HM, Kaplan BS: An approach to the evaluation and treatment of microscopic hematuria, *Pediatr Clin North Am* 38:579, 1991.
Norman ME: An office approach to hematuria and proteinuria, *Pediatr Clin North Am* 34:545, 1987.

140 Hemoptysis

Beryl J. Rosenstein

Hemoptysis, defined as the expectoration of blood or blood-tinged sputum that originates from the tracheobronchial tree or pulmonary parenchyma, is a potentially life-threatening but unusual occurrence in the pediatric age group. Over a 10-year period at a large pediatric referral center, hemoptysis was diagnosed in only 40 children.[17] In seven of these children, hemoptysis was the sole presenting manifestation; in the remaining patients hemoptysis often was associated with fever and cough. The amount of bleeding usually was small; only two children had blood loss in excess of 200 ml. Because hemoptysis often is a sign of significant underlying disease and may be life threatening, patients who have this condition deserve rapid and complete evaluation. If hemoptysis occurs as something more than blood-tinged sputum or mild bleeding, the evaluation best is carried out in a hospital in collaboration with a pediatric pulmonologist and endoscopist.

CHARACTERISTICS AND ORIGIN

The majority of children brought to medical attention because of "spitting up blood" have an identifiable source of bleeding outside the lower respiratory tract—usually epistaxis, gingivitis, pharyngeal ulceration, or trauma to the oropharynx. At times it may be difficult to differentiate hemoptysis from hematemesis.[12,16] With hematemesis the blood is dark red or brownish, may contain food particles, and has an acid pH; bleeding usually is preceded by nausea or accompanied by retching. With hemoptysis the blood usually is bright red and frothy, may be mixed with sputum, has an alkaline pH, and microscopically may contain hemosiderin-laden macrophages; such bleeding may be preceded by a gurgling noise in the large airways and usually is accompanied by coughing. Older patients who have bleeding in the lung may describe a vague sensation that enables them to localize the site of the bleeding.

It sometimes is difficult to determine the origin of bleeding when the child is both coughing and vomiting. In infants, swallowed blood originating in the lungs may be vomited in the absence of coughing. Therefore the possibility that the respiratory tract is the source of the bleeding should be considered in children whose hematemesis is unexplained, particularly if the chest roentgenogram shows abnormalities. Children under 6 years of age rarely expectorate sputum; in this age group, the presence of hemoptysis may not be apparent unless the amount of bleeding is large. Children who have a hard, forceful cough may produce sputum that has small streaks of blood on the surface but is not mixed with blood. This finding may occur in association with respiratory tract infections and usually is of little clinical significance.

The treatment of hemoptysis is by management of the underlying disorder, making a correct etiological diagnosis mandatory. Hemoptysis is a relatively common occurrence in adults. The leading causes are chronic bronchitis/bronchiectasis, lung cancer, and tuberculosis.[16] However, almost any disease that affects the respiratory tract can result in hemoptysis. The number of disorders associated with hemoptysis is not as large in children as in adults but is still extensive (see the box on p. 1001). The most common cause is infection, followed by foreign body aspiration.[17] Many of the underlying conditions occur infrequently and may be difficult to diagnose.

EVALUATION

Evaluation of the patient who has hemoptysis should begin with a detailed history and physical examination. The history should be elicited as to underlying illnesses, fever, cough, sputum production, stridor, wheezing, dyspnea, joint pain, weight loss, menstrual history, family illnesses, recent trauma, prior episodes of bleeding, choking episodes, medication use, substance abuse, exposure to toxins, and travel to areas endemic for parasitic infestations and mycobacterial disease. Any history of travel especially is pertinent because of the large-scale immigration from southeast Asia to the United States. Some patients who have hemoptysis, however, otherwise will be asymptomatic and have an entirely negative history.

When confronted with a child who is presumed to have hemoptysis, it first must be determined if the blood originated from the lungs or lower airways or from the mouth, upper airway, or gastrointestinal tract. Careful examination of the nasopharynx and oral cavity for bleeding sites is essential. Nasopharyngoscopy and laryngoscopy may be helpful. Pertinent physical findings include saddle-nose deformity, bruits, thrills, unequal chest wall movement and air entry, abnormal breath sounds (especially localized wheezing, heard with bronchial lesions and foreign bodies), pleural rub, heart murmur, hypertension, digital clubbing, lymphadenopathy, hepatosplenomegaly, hemangiomas, telangiectases, neuropathies, deep vein thrombosis, and evidence of trauma to the head, neck, or chest.

Roentgenographic Evaluation

If the source of bleeding is not apparent on the basis of the history and physical examination, a chest roentgenogram is the next step in the evaluation.[1] The presence of an infiltrate suggests a parenchymal source for the bleeding, whereas a normal chest roentgenogram suggests an airway source. The most common abnormalities found on chest roentgenograms are atelectasis, areas of parenchymal consolidation, and interstitial infiltrates. Other helpful findings include localized air trapping, pulmonary nodules, hilar adenopathy, pleural effusion, pneumothorax, cardiomegaly, and foreign bodies.

CAUSES OF HEMOPTYSIS IN CHILDREN

Infection

Bacterial
- Bronchitis
- Lung abscess
- Necrotizing pneumonia
- Tuberculosis
- Bronchiectasis
- Immune deficiency
- Cystic fibrosis
- Ciliary dyskinesia

Fungal
- Actinomycosis
- Aspergillosis
- Coccidioidomycosis
- Histoplasmosis

Parasitic
- Echinococcosis (hydatid disease)
- Paragonimiasis
- Strongyloidiasis

Foreign bodies

Congenital defects

Cardiovascular
- Congenital heart defects
- Absent pulmonary artery
- Arteriovenous malformation
- Hemangiomatous malformation
- Telangiectasia (Rendu-Osler-Weber syndrome)

Other
- Pulmonary sequestration
- Bronchogenic cyst
- Intrathoracic enteric cyst

Vasculitis

Periarteritis nodosa

Autoimmune disorders

Wegener granulomatosis
Pulmonary hemosiderosis
Milk allergy
Goodpasture syndrome
Collagen-vascular disease

Trauma

Compression or crush injury
Iatrogenic
- Postsurgical
- Diagnostic lung puncture
- Transbronchial biopsy

Inhalation of toxins

Neoplastic conditions

Endobronchial metastases
Primary lung tumors
- Benign (hamartoma, neurogenic tumors)
- Malignant (bronchial adenoma, bronchogenic carcinoma, pulmonary blastoma)

Endometriosis

Drug induced

Propylthiouracil

Pulmonary embolism

Hemoglobinopathy with pulmonary infarct

Factitious

Ring shadows and parallel lines represent thick-walled bronchi and suggest bronchiectasis. One third of children who have hemoptysis have normal initial roentgenograms; however, a pulmonary source for the bleeding eventually is identified in half of those patients whose chest roentgenograms are negative.[17]

Inspiratory and expiratory roentgenograms help detect any partially obstructing endobronchial foreign body. The lung on the side of the foreign body demonstrates air trapping on expiration relative to the normal side. On a decubitus view the side that does not deflate normally in the dependent position is the side that has air trapping. With complete obstruction secondary to a foreign body, obstructive atelectasis or pneumonia occurs. High kilovoltage roentgenograms can help to visualize the upper airway and define mass lesions better. Fluoroscopy or computed tomography can be used to (1) confirm questionable parenchymal lesions on plain roentgenogram; (2) localize an identified lesion or mass on a chest roentgenogram to lung parenchyma, pleura, chest wall, mediastinum, or vascular structures; or (3) identify and localize a suspected bronchial foreign body causing air trapping when findings are equivocal or not apparent on chest roentgenogram. An esophagram may help to localize a mass to the middle mediastinum. Based on the results of the roentgenographic evaluation, the diagnostic workup may require additional laboratory and imaging procedures.

Laboratory Evaluation

A variety of laboratory tests may be helpful, including a complete blood count and indices, eosinophil count, erythrocyte sedimentation rate, urinalysis, arterial blood gas measurements, skin tests for *Mycobacterium, Aspergillus,* and *Echinococcus,* clotting studies, sputum cytology, and cultures for bacteria, fungi, and mycobacteria. Gastric aspirates can be examined for ova, parasites, and hemosiderin-laden macrophages (hemosiderosis) and cultured for mycobacteria. Other helpful procedures include measurement of sweat electrolyte concentration (cystic fibrosis), milk precipitins in serum (milk allergy, hemosiderosis), and antinuclear antibody, lupus erythematosus (LE) cell preparation, and rheumatoid factor (collagen-vascular disease). In patients who have hemoptysis and renal involvement (Goodpasture syndrome, collagen-vascular disease, and Wegener disease), renal function studies, measurement of antiglomerular basement membrane antibody, and renal biopsy may be needed for a definitive diagnosis.

Diagnostic Imaging

Computed tomography (CT) may detect parenchymal infiltrates or foreign bodies unrecognized roentgenographically and usually is the procedure of choice to define further the anatomy of an abnormality found on chest roentgenogram.[1,16] Computed tomography can outline the extent of a mass and localize it properly to the anterior, middle, or posterior mediastinum, lung parenchyma, pleura, chest wall, or spine. The trachea and major proximal bronchi are well defined. Computed tomography is good for the detection of cystic bronchiectasis, broncholithiasis, and endobronchial obstruction secondary to adenoma or a blood clot. The use of intravenous contrast identifies vascular structures and can determine if a suspected mass is vascular in nature. The internal characteristics of a mass also can be identified; calcification, hemorrhage, and fat can be differentiated by their relative densities. Computed tomography also may be useful in guiding diagnostic procedures.

Magnetic resonance imaging (MRI) gives superior soft tissue contrast resolution and is useful in the evaluation of the mediastinum and hila, but has not been as useful in the evaluation of pulmonary parenchymal abnormalities.[1] Because vessels can be distinguished from other mediastinal structures without the use of vascular contrast, this technique often can be used to demonstrate arteriovenous malformations and congenital anomalies of the pulmonary arteries.

Conventional or *digital subtraction pulmonary angiography* is useful for the evaluation of congenital malformations of the lungs and abnormalities of pulmonary vessels—that is, arteriovenous malformations, pulmonary embolus, and congenital anomalies of the pulmonary vessels—and can be used to define the blood supply to a pulmonary sequestration. It is the most accurate method for locating the source of arterial bleeding in the lungs and is necessary when planning embolization therapy.

Ventilation-perfusion scanning is helpful in evaluating regional lung perfusion and ventilation, particularly when planning surgical excision of a pulmonary lesion. This procedure can detect a decrease in pulmonary blood flow—that is, pulmonary artery agenesis or hypoplasia, and pulmonary embolus. The hallmark of a pulmonary embolus is ventilation without perfusion (V/Q mismatch). A *radionuclide scan* using technetium sulfur colloid or radiolabeled red blood cells can be used to identify bleeding sites (even with bleeding rates as low as 0.1 ml/minute)[4] or ectopic gastric mucosa.

Endoscopy

If the source of hemoptysis still is not apparent after laboratory and roentgenographic evaluation or if bleeding recurs or is substantial, endoscopy is indicated.[14,16] A bleeding site is localized best when bronchoscopy is performed during bleeding. The availability of the flexible fiberoptic bronchoscope has been a great advance. Compared with the rigid bronchoscope, this instrument has increased maneuverability and is tolerated more readily and for longer periods. The fiberoptic bronchoscope usually can be passed transnasally with the use of sedation rather than general anesthesia. It can be used to visualize subsegmental airways that are beyond the reach of the rigid bronchoscope. There still is a role, however, for the rigid bronchoscope; it is better for removing foreign bodies and for maintaining a secure airway while providing adequate suctioning in those patients whose bleeding is massive.

Bronchoscopy is particularly useful to detect foreign bodies and to diagnose infection and endobronchial lesions. Material can be obtained for cultures, stains, and cytology. Bronchial brushings can be obtained and transbronchial biopsy performed. Old blood can be removed by saline lavage of segmental bronchi; the airway then can be reexamined. The need for bronchography virtually has been eliminated by the availability of CT and high kilovoltage roentgenography. In rare cases it may be indicated as an adjunct to fiberoptic bronchoscopy to define type, site, and extent of bronchiectasis or to identify a congenital abnormality of the bronchus. It also may be used to differentiate an extrinsic from an intrinsic defect in the airway.

DIFFERENTIAL DIAGNOSIS

Among 40 children who had hemoptysis who were seen at a pediatric referral center, bleeding was caused by infection in 16 cases and by an aspirated foreign body in 6.[17] The remaining cases were associated with a variety of other disorders. In some cases, such as those associated with cystic fibrosis, congenital heart disease, or bleeding secondary to surgical procedures, diagnosis of the underlying disorder usually is well established at the time of hemoptysis. In most cases, however, the underlying diagnosis is not apparent immediately. In general, it is rare for children who have pulmonary neoplasms or bleeding disorders to have hemoptysis. The diagnoses of bronchial wall neoplasms, mediastinal tumors, and arteriovenous malformations should be considered in young children whose airway bleeding is massive. Most aspirated foreign bodies occur in children under 4 years of age. Worldwide, echinococcosis and paragonimiasis probably are the most common causes of hemoptysis in childhood. This is not so, however, for hemoptysis occurring in North America.

Foreign Bodies

In children who have hemoptysis it always is important to be aware of the possibility of foreign body aspiration, even in the absence of a suggestive history.[11,13] Although most cases of an aspirated foreign body involve children younger than 4 years of age, teenagers who have retained aspirated foreign bodies may have hemoptysis.[11] The major complication of foreign body aspiration is bronchial obstruction, which may result in atelectasis, abscess formation, pneumonia, and bronchiectasis. Hemoptysis is secondary to the extensive neovascularization that may occur in the bronchiectatic portion of the lung.

In many patients the initial choking episode either is not observed or not remembered, and there may be a long latent period between the episode of aspiration and the appearance of symptoms.[13] The likelihood that an aspirated foreign body is the cause of hemoptysis is increased if the episode of hemoptysis is accompanied by pronounced coughing, localized wheezing, and locally diminished or absent breath sounds.

On examination there may be localized rales or wheezes or both, but some patients' examinations are normal. Patients commonly have recurrent infiltrates or clear a focal infiltrate incompletely. The chest roentgenogram may be normal (20% of cases) or may show localized air trapping, atelectasis, or signs of unresolved pneumonia. A radiopaque object is seen in approximately 15% of cases. Fluoroscopy may reveal unequal aeration, asymmetrical diaphragmatic movement, or a mediastinal shift. Inspiratory and expiratory roentgenograms may help to demonstrate localized air trapping. Foreign bodies also may be identified by CT. However, normal roentgenographic findings do not eliminate the need for bronchoscopy, at which time the diagnosis usually is confirmed. A flexible fiberoptic bronchoscope may be used for diagnosis, but a rigid bronchoscope is more useful for removal of foreign bodies. Because there may be more than one foreign body, it is important to examine both sides during bronchoscopy.

Hemosiderosis

Idiopathic pulmonary hemosiderosis (IPH) is an unusual and often baffling cause of hemoptysis in children.[2,8] It is a disorder of unknown cause characterized by recurrent episodes of diffuse intraalveolar hemorrhage. Although familial cases have been reported, the inheritance pattern is not clear.[2] Patients usually manifest the disorder during infancy and early childhood by having hemoptysis, respiratory distress (cough, dyspnea, wheezing), diffuse parenchymal infiltrates, and iron deficiency anemia. It is one of the few conditions in which refractory iron deficiency anemia occurs without an obvious bleeding site.

Hemosiderosis may occur as a primary condition or in association with glomerulonephritis (Goodpasture syndrome), collagen-vascular disease, IgA deficiency, and, in rare cases, cow milk protein allergy. The diagnosis of pulmonary hemosiderosis is suggested by the clinical picture along with the finding of iron-laden macrophages in bronchial or gastric washings and confirmed by the demonstration of these macrophages in open lung biopsy material. Nuclear scanning of the lungs after radiolabeled red blood cells have been injected can confirm that lung infiltrates are secondary to intrapulmonary hemorrhage. Patients who have hemosiderosis should have (1) an immunological evaluation (collagen-vascular disease), (2) renal function studies, including renal biopsy and measurement of antiglomerular basement membrane antibody (Goodpasture syndrome), and (3) measurement of circulating precipitins to constituents of cow milk (milk allergy).

Treatment depends on associated disorders. In patients who have cow milk allergy, all dairy products should be eliminated from the diet. Patients who have Goodpasture syndrome and collagen-vascular disease are treated with immunosuppressive agents. Patients who have persistent pulmonary infiltrates may benefit from an iron-chelating agent such as deferoxamine (Desferal). General supportive treatment consists of oxygen, bronchodilators, iron replacement, and transfusions as necessary. Corticosteroids often are used, but there are no data to support their efficacy.

Infections

Hemoptysis can occur with a variety of pulmonary infections, including necrotizing pneumonia, tuberculosis, aspergillosis, coccidioidomycosis, actinomycosis, histoplasmosis, and parasitic infestations. Worldwide, echinococcosis and paragonimiasis probably are the most common causes of hemoptysis in children. Bronchiectasis may be seen after lower respiratory tract infections (measles, adenovirus, tuberculosis), after foreign body aspiration, with allergic bronchopulmonary aspergillosis, and with genetic disorders such as cystic fibrosis, ciliary dyskinesia, immunodeficiencies, and alpha-1-antitrypsin deficiency. About 5% of patients who have bronchiectasis have significant hemoptysis.[9] This diagnosis should be considered when hemoptysis occurs in conjunction with pulmonary infiltrates, cough, purulent sputum, and localized abnormal breath sounds. Plain roentgenography, CT, and ventilation-perfusion scans may aid in the diagnosis. Bronchoscopy may help to confirm the diagnosis and to obtain material for stains and culture. In the child who has a suspected infection, serological studies, cultures, and skin testing all may aid in arriving at a specific etiology. In some cases needle aspiration of a lesion or open lung biopsy is necessary.

Cystic Fibrosis

In patients who have cystic fibrosis and bronchiectasis/chronic suppurative pseudomonas bronchitis, there are dilation, increased tortuosity, and hyperplasia of the bronchial arteries.[18] Anastomoses develop between the bronchial and pulmonary circulations in the walls of larger bronchi in chronically infected segments of lung. The right upper lobe is the most common site of bleeding. Secondary to exacerbations of pulmonary infection, there may be erosion of bronchial arteries and episodes of moderate to massive hemoptysis. Although episodes may subside spontaneously, recurrences are common. Bronchoscopy can be performed to help localize the bleeding site, but may not be successful if bleeding has stopped or when massive bleeding prevents adequate visualization of the airways. Identification of a hypervascular area of lung by arteriography also may help to localize the bleeding site.

Conservative treatment consists of bed rest, sedation, temporary withholding of chest physiotherapy, and intravenous antibiotics. Blood losses should be replaced and vitamin K administered if the prothrombin time is prolonged. Percutaneous bronchial artery embolization now is accepted as the standard procedure for treating episodes of hemoptysis in patients who have cystic fibrosis.[18]

Indications for embolotherapy include either massive acute bleeding (300 ml over 24 hours) or chronic bleeding (75 to 100 ml per day) recurring over weeks or months. With this technique immediate cessation of bleeding can be achieved in greater than 90% of patients. On long-term follow-up one can expect recurrent episodes of minor bleeding in 70% of patients and major rebleeding in 30%. Recurrent hemoptysis may occur secondary to recanalization of vessels, aberrant vessels, or collateral flow. In rare cases, as in an unstable patient who has cystic fibrosis and massive hemoptysis, pulmonary resection may be indicated.[10]

Miscellaneous

A number of unusual causes of hemoptysis need to be considered in pediatric patients, including pulmonary embolus, neoplasms (pulmonary blastoma, hamartoma, bronchial adenoma), congenital defects (arteriovenous malformation, sequestration, hemangiomatous malformation, intrathoracic gastrogenic cyst, hereditary hemorrhagic telangiectasia), and cardiovascular lesions (Eisenmenger complex, severe pulmonic stenosis, extreme hypoplasia, or unilateral absence of a pulmonary artery).[6]

Thyrotoxic adolescents *may* develop a clinical picture of purpura, nephritis, severe anemia, and hemoptysis (secondary to pulmonary cavitation) during treatment with propylthiouracil.[3]

In rare cases recurrent episodes of hemoptysis may occur coincident with the onset of menses in patients who have bronchopulmonary endometriosis.[5,7] The chest roentgenogram usually is normal or it shows only nonspecific changes. Bronchopulmonary endometriosis is a clinical diagnosis based on the association of unexplained hemoptysis coincident with menses, but the bleeding site can be localized through CT at the time of bleeding.[5] Angiography is not helpful.[7]

Factitious bleeding is one of the most baffling of all causes of hemoptysis in children.[15] This represents a form of Munchausen syndrome by proxy in which blood other than the patient's is presented as evidence of hemoptysis. Innovative detective work may be needed in such cases, including video monitoring and blood typing from the patient and caretakers.

MANAGEMENT

Management of the patient who has hemoptysis depends almost entirely on the underlying cause and extent of bleeding.[16] Once the underlying cause is found, treatment is directed at the source. In children whose bleeding is massive (more than 8 ml/kg/24 hours), an aggressive approach is mandatory. Arterial blood gases should be monitored. Once the airway is established, vigorous suctioning may be necessary. Supplemental oxygen, transfusions, and mechanical ventilation may be required. Bronchoscopy, useful both diagnostically and therapeutically, can localize the bleeding site, protect and maintain the airway, and prevent asphyxiation. In cases in which bleeding is active, the open ventilating bronchoscope is preferable. It allows for simultaneous ventilation and inspection of the airway and is better than the flexible bronchoscope for suctioning and clearing the airway. Lavage with iced saline solution, topical application of a vasoconstrictor, or laser coagulation may be helpful. Control of massive bleeding may require endoscopic tamponade with a balloon catheter, embolization of involved arteries, or thoracotomy with a direct surgical approach to the source of bleeding.

REFERENCES

1. Ablin DS, Newell JD: Diagnostic imaging for evaluation of the pediatric chest, *Clin Chest Med* 8:641, 1987.
2. Beckerman RG, Taussig LM, Pinnas JL: Familial idiopathic pulmonary hemosiderosis, *Am J Dis Child* 133:609, 1979.
3. Cassorla FG et al: Vasculitis, pulmonary cavitation, and anemia during antithyroid drug therapy, *Am J Dis Child* 137:118, 1983.
4. Coel MN, Druger G: Radionuclide detection of the site of hemoptysis, *Chest* 81:242, 1982.
5. Elliot DL, Barker AF, Dison L: Catamenial hemoptysis: new methods of diagnosis and therapy, *Chest* 87:687, 1985.
6. Haroutunian LM, Neill CA: Pulmonary complications of congenital heart disease: hemoptysis, *Am Heart J* 84:540, 1972.
7. Katoh O et al: Utility of angiograms in patients with catamenial hemoptysis, *Chest* 98:1296, 1990.
8. Levy J, Kolski GB, Scanlin TF: Hemoptysis and anemia in a 3-year-old boy, *Ann Allergy* 55:439, 1985.
9. Lewiston NJ: Bronchiectasis in childhood, *Pediatr Clin North Am* 31:865, 1984.
10. Marmon L et al: Pulmonary resection for complications of cystic fibrosis, *J Pediatr Surg* 18:811, 1983.
11. Pattison CW, Leaming AJ, Townsend ER: Hidden foreign body as a cause of recurrent hemoptysis in a teenage girl, *Ann Thorac Surg* 45:330, 1988.
12. Putnam JS, Tellis CJ: Hemoptysis, *Prim Care* 5:67, 1978.
13. Pyman C: Inhaled foreign bodies in childhood, *Med J Aust* 1:62, 1971.
14. Selecky PA: Evaluation of hemoptysis through the bronchoscope, *Chest* 73:741, 1978.
15. Shafer N, Shafer R: Factitious diseases, including Munchausen's syndrome, *NY State J Med* 80:594, 1980.
16. Thompson AB, Teschler H, Rennard SI: Pathogenesis, evaluation, and therapy for massive hemoptysis, *Clin Chest Med* 13:69, 1992.
17. Tom LWC, Weisman RA, Handler SD: Hemoptysis in children, *Ann Otolaryngol* 89:419, 1980.
18. Tonkin ILD et al: Bronchial arteriography and embolotherapy for hemoptysis in patients with cystic fibrosis, *Cardiovasc Intervent Radiol* 14:241, 1991.

141 Hepatomegaly

Kenneth Kenigsberg

Hepatomegaly, or enlargement of the liver, in children presents predominantly in four forms—neonatal, neoplastic, metabolic/genetic, and infectious/inflammatory.

Enlargement of the liver must be differentiated from displacement of the liver. Tension pneumothorax, congenital adenomatous malformation, congenital diaphragmatic hernia, and thoracic tumors all may occupy space in the right hemithorax, pushing the liver down and making it appear enlarged. The upper level of the child's or infant's liver should be placed by percussion at about the fifth intercostal space in the mid-axillary line. The normal liver is palpable less than 4 cm from the costal margin in infants and less than 2 cm in children. Radiographs may give a false impression of enlargement. Scans, computed tomography (CT) and magnetic resonance imaging (MRI) are more reliable.

NEONATAL PERIOD

Before the widespread use of immune globulin (Rhogam) in 1968 to prevent erythroblastosis fetalis, about 1% of pregnancies were sensitized to the rH antigen. It was common to see hepatomegaly in the infants who survived to delivery. Today, erythroblastosis fetalis caused by rH sensitization is almost never seen. However, occasionally ABO or other blood group sensitization may be severe. In these rare cases hepatic hematopoiesis may be so great as to cause liver enlargement in the newborn. If, in addition, there is congestive heart failure due to hemolytic anemia, the liver enlargement will become even more pronounced.

Other causes of congestive heart failure also may result in hepatomegaly. Indeed, enlargement of the liver in a newborn is one of the earliest manifestations of heart failure.[12] The leading causes of congestive failure with resultant hepatomegaly are aortic atresia, transposition of the great vessels, coarctation of the aorta, and patent ductus arteriosis. Heart failure also may be produced by idiopathic paroxysmal tachycardia. In these infants peripheral edema rarely is seen, and the initial signs usually are tachypnea and hepatomegaly.

Although two thirds of liver tumors in children are malignant, almost all that present as hepatomegaly in the first month of life are benign.[5,7,14] Although their names—capillary hemangioma, cavernous hemangioma, and hemangioendothelioma—sound quite innocuous, the outcome in these cases may be far from "benign." Because of the extremely vascular and friable nature of these tumors, they may cause death in the neonatal period from the intraperitoneal bleeding precipitated by delivery. Lethal bleeding into the peritoneum also can be caused by ill-advised percutaneous needle biopsy of these masses. The bleeding also may be systemic and life-threatening because of platelet trapping (Kasabach-Merritt syndrome). The initial liver enlargement may be increased quickly by congestion if the vascularity is so great as to cause cardiac failure secondary to high cardiac output.

A rare cause of hepatic enlargement in the newborn infant, and one requiring immediate and intense care, is subcapsular hemorrhage.[6] In earlier days the child predisposed to subcapsular hemorrhage and rapid blood loss was the very large infant. Today this is more common in premature infants. Along with the rapidly enlarging liver and abdominal distention are signs of acute blood loss, including tachycardia, tachypnea, and cardiac failure. The rapid postpartum bleeding of a child must be differentiated from intraventricular hemorrhage and from hemorrhage involving the adrenals.

Neoplasms

Another group of benign tumors may present during infancy (though rarely in the neonatal period) or later in life. Unlike the vascular tumors of the newborn, they do not constitute a risk to life. These are mesenchymal hamartomas,[13] which are seen predominantly in males, and focal nodular hyperplasia, which occurs primarily in females.[10,17] Both occur in the absence of liver disease and usually present as abdominal enlargement or a palpable lump in the region of the liver.

The malignant tumors presenting as a liver mass primarily are hepatoblastomas and hepatocellular carcinoma.[3,15] Hepatoblastoma usually is seen before 5 years of age and may present as an asymptomatic mass, although anorexia and weight loss are common.

Hepatocellular carcinoma occurs in older children and rarely presents with only a liver mass; most commonly there are jaundice, pain, and weight loss.[11]

Metabolic/Genetic Diseases

Metabolic/genetic diseases cause enlargement of the liver because of abnormal storage of some metabolite in the liver. The type of material storage is the result of an enzyme deficiency that, in turn, is determined by a genetic abnormality, usually an autosomal recessive one. Thus in glycogen storage disease the liver is swollen with glycogen as well as with fat, in Gaucher disease with glucosylceramide, and in mucopolysaccharidosis with heparin and dermatin sulfates.[11] Any of the storage diseases may present from infancy onward with a smoothly enlarged liver.

Inflammatory Diseases/Inflammation

Viral hepatitis of any type may involve liver enlargement as part of the evolution of the disease. Usually this occurs after the child has developed jaundice.

Two types of liver inflammation may present as liver enlargement, however, before other manifestations of liver disease. Hepatomegaly and focal cirrhosis develop in about 18% of patients who have cystic fibrosis.[2] The incidence of this complication in cystic fibrosis patients who have meconium ileus is three times higher than in those cystic fibrosis patients who have no meconium ileus.

Presumably the pathophysiology that causes meconium ileus is the same as that causing cirrhosis and hepatomegaly. The defective chloride secretion in the bowel, leading to thickened meconium and obstruction, also occurs in the biliary tract, causing bile duct plugging and cirrhosis (see Chapter 36, Cystic Fibrosis).

Sclerosing cholangitis is another condition that may give rise to hepatomegaly before other signs of hepatic disease.[4] In children this disease usually is associated with chronic inflammatory bowel disease, immune deficiency, or histocytosis X. Occasionally, however, it develops in the absence of any other apparent disease. The final pathology of sclerosing cholangitis resembles inflammation, but the etiology is unknown.

The etiology of liver abscess, on the other hand, is well known.[9,16] The most common cause of liver abscess among infants is an umbilical vein catheter. Infection starts at the skin, spreads up along the umbilical vein, up the portal vein, and into the liver, where it causes an abscess. Neonatal intraabdominal operations such as those for biliary atresia or necrotizing enterocolitis may cause abscess in the infant by direct spread or transmission along the vascular or biliary tracts. In older children the abscess frequently is preceded by a staphylococcal infection elsewhere in the body. Frequently the child has chronic granulomatous disease. As in the infant, the older child's hepatic abscess may be caused by intraabdominal surgery, particularly appendectomy.

Diagnosis

In the neonate it may be vital to establish a prompt diagnosis because hepatomegaly may be the harbinger of a lethal condition. The newborn who has hepatomegaly and tachycardia, a murmur, or decreased femoral pulses requires rapid cardiac evaluation, including echocardiography and electrocardiography. The child who has a vascular tumor may have a hemangioma elsewhere, which suggests the nature of the liver tumor. Frequently a flow murmur can be heard over the vascular tumor. A radioisotope scan and CT scans are useful for defining the nature of the mass. Perhaps the easiest and most definitive test is an arteriogram carried out through the umbilical artery (Fig. 141-1). If the newborn child has splenomegaly and anemia as well as hepatomegaly, with or without jaundice, the possibility of isoimmunization is very strong. A direct and indirect Coombs test should establish the diagnosis. In the extremely uncommon instance of the infant who has hepatomegaly as a result of bleeding under the capsule of the liver, the clinical signs primarily are those of hypovolemia. Sonography or a CT scan may suggest the diagnosis, and a peritoneal tap may be confirmatory if blood is found.

The important question in diagnosing neoplasms is whether the tumor is benign or malignant. Children who have benign liver tumors such as mesenchymal hamartomas or focal nodular hyperplasia may not have any symptoms. However, children who have hepatoblastoma may seem similarly unaffected. Frequently the children who have hepatoblastoma will have elevated levels of alphafetoprotein, which is a significant diagnostic clue. Children who have hepatocellular carcinoma rarely are entirely well. Usually they have signs

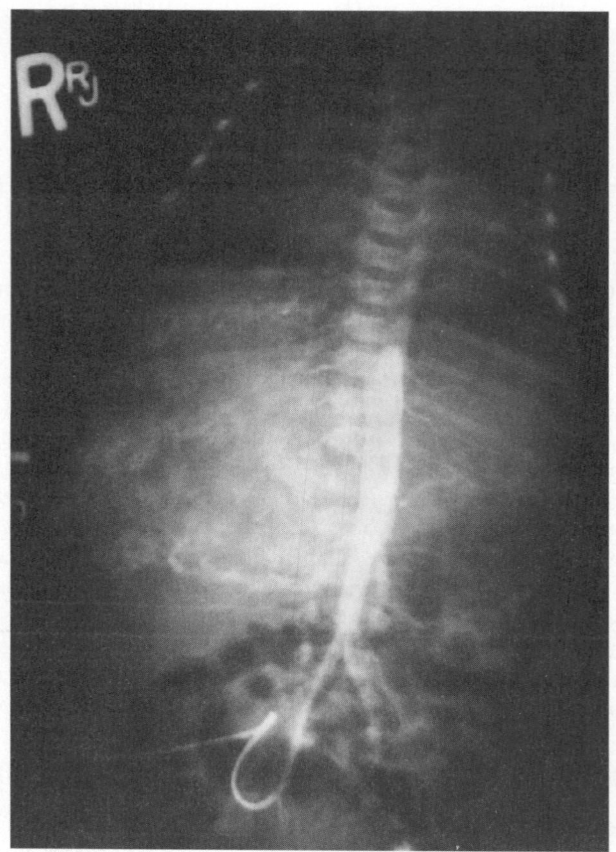

FIG. 141-1 Hepatic arteriogram in a newborn child via umbilical artery. A vascular tumor occupies most of the liver.

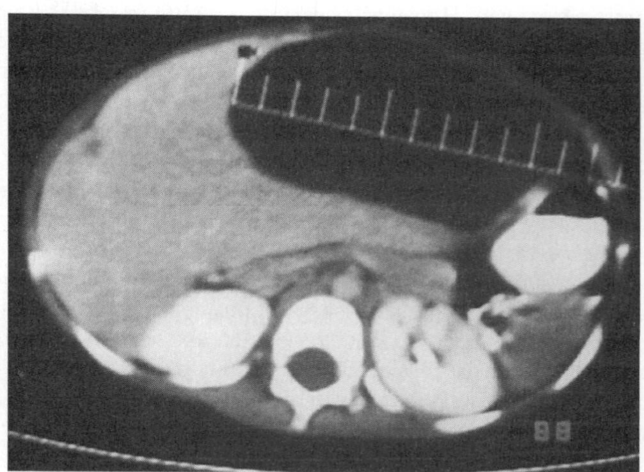

FIG. 141-2 CT scan of the liver showing a large hamartoma.

of liver disease, with altered liver function tests. A CT scan is the modality most useful for defining these liver tumors (Fig. 141-2). Ultimately, angiography and an open biopsy may be necessary for diagnosis.

Metabolic/genetic hepatomegalies frequently are diagnosed on the basis of clinical signs and symptoms. Infants who have galactosemia, for instance, present with vomiting and lethargy in the first few days of life after they have been fed milk. Infants who have glycogen storage have enlarged livers at birth but may have hypoglycemia as their first clinical sign. To define the specific type of glycogen storage disease, it may be necessary to carry out a liver biopsy for histological and biochemical study. Infants who have a neuropathic form of Gaucher disease can be diagnosed via a marrow biopsy and demonstration of the typical Gaucher cells. Children who have mucopolysaccharidosis usually are diagnosed within the first year of life because of their characteristic physical presentation and facies. Their growth is retarded, and they have thick lips, an enlarged tongue, and profuse hair growth on the forehead.

The diagnosis of focal biliary cirrhosis should be suspected in any patient who has cystic fibrosis, an altered liver function, and an enlarged nodular liver. The diagnosis can be confirmed by sonography, radioisotope scanning, or biopsy.[2] The definitive diagnosis of sclerosing cholangitis is made by cholangiogram. Liver abscess can be defined well by CT scan, radioisotope scanning, or sonography. The final diagnosis can be made by percutaneous aspiration of the abscess.

Treatment

For the treatment of the neonatal liver enlargements, a balance between immediate intervention and cautious delay is necessary. In the infant who has subcapsular hepatic hemorrhage, immediate transfusion may be lifesaving; surgical intervention rarely is necessary. Similarly, the survival of the child may hinge on whether the liver-enlarging tachycardia or aortic stenosis is dealt with promptly by medical or surgical means. The child who has an exsanguinating hemangioma will die unless the tumor is treated very vigorously. Currently the common method of dealing with this tumor and preventing the direct bleeding or the bleeding secondary to platelet trapping is by embolizing the tumor and giving large doses of steroids. A recent treatment that has some promise is the use of alpha-interferon.[8]

However, if the patient is not bleeding and if the hemangioma does not represent an immediate threat to the life of the infant, the better treatment may be watchful procrastination. The child shown in Figure 141-1, in spite of the enormous size and vascularity of the tumor, had almost no residua of the tumor at 18 months of age, despite no treatment whatsoever.

The treatment of the malignant tumors of the liver—hepatoblastoma and hepatocellular carcinoma—remain primarily excisional. A number of chemotherapeutic agents are helpful in reducing the size of inoperable tumors to excisional size. They also have been used, occasionally successfully, in destroying residual tumor after resection. If mesenchymal hamartoma or focal nodular hyperplasia can be diagnosed definitively, an operation may not be necessary. In treating the focal cirrhosis of cystic fibrosis, it has been suggested that choleretics are useful in preventing further liver disease. The only treatment available for sclerosing cholangitis is liver transplantation.

The treatment of the metabolic-genetic diseases involves dealing with the metabolic effect of the enzymatic deficiency. Galactosemia, for instance, is treated entirely successfully by total avoidance of any galactose-containing carbohydrate. Glycogen storage disease is treated quite satisfactorily by giving small feedings of complex carbohydrates and nighttime feeds. There is no treatment for mucopolysaccharidosis. However, in regard to Gaucher disease a new and experimental treatment involves the use of a synthesized enzyme, Ceredase. However, the cost of this medication for a single patient for a single year is about $150,000. Although the cost of the treatment is prohibitive at the present time, the biochemical victory of having synthesized this enzyme truly is uplifting.

REFERENCES

1. Clift DAL, Campbell PE et al: Primary liver tumours in children in Victoria: incidence and pathology, *Pediatr Surg Int* 3:382, 1988.
2. Colombo C et al: Analysis of risk factors for the development of liver disease associated with cystic fibrosis, *J Pediatr* 124:393, 1994.
3. Davidson PM et al: Liver tumours in children, *Pediatr Surg Int* 3:377, 1988.
4. Debray D et al: Sclerosing cholangitis in children, *J Pediatr* 124:49, 1994.
5. Ein SH, Stephens CA: Benign liver tumors and cysts in childhood, *J Pediatr Surg* 9:847, 1974.
6. French CE, Waldstein G: Subcapsular hemorrhage of the liver in the newborn, *Pediatrics* 69:204, 1982.
7. Graivier L, Votteler TP, Dorman GW: Hepatic hemangiomas in newborn infants, *J Pediatr Surg* 2:299, 1967.
8. Hatley RM et al: Successful management of an infant with a giant hemangioma of the retroperitoneum and Kasabach-Merritt syndrome with α-interferon, *J Pediatr Surg* 28:1356, 1993.
9. Larsen LR, Raffensperger J: Liver abscess, *J Pediatr Surg* 14:329, 1979.
10. Luks FI et al: Benign liver tumors in children: a 25-year experience, *J Pediatr Surg* 26:1326, 1991.
11. Mowat AP: *Liver disorders in childhood,* ed 2, Stoneham, Mass, 1987, Butterworth Publishers.
12. Schaffer AJ, Avery ME: *Diseases of the newborn,* ed 3, Philadelphia, 1971, WB Saunders.
13. Stocker JT, Ishak KG: Mesenchymal hamartoma of the liver: report of 30 cases and review of the literature, *Pediatr Pathol* 1:245, 1983.
14. Tawes RL, Nelson JA, Hyde GA: Hepatic hemangioma: successful resection in a neonate, *Surgery* 70:782, 1971.
15. Walker WA et al: *Pediatric gastrointestinal disease—pathophysiology, diagnosis and management,* vol 1, Philadelphia, 1991, BC Decker.
16. Wyllie R, Hyams JS: *Pediatric gastrointestinal disease,* Philadelphia, 1993, WB Saunders.
17. Yandza T, Valayer J: Benign tumors of the liver in children: analysis of a series of 20 cases, *J Pediatr Surg* 21:419, 1986.

142 High Blood Pressure in Infants, Children, and Adolescents

Edward B. Clark

Blood pressure, the dynamic force driving blood flow through the body, varies greatly during each day. Transient increases in blood pressure are essential in meeting the metabolic demands of the body, but a sustained increase in blood pressure can lead to premature vascular changes in the heart, brain, and kidneys. Most physicians suspect that the seeds of adult-onset hypertensive disease are sown during childhood. Therefore abnormalities in blood pressure are of great interest to all who care for children. Although the highest levels of blood pressure in a child likely correlate with essential hypertension as an adult, data on the long-term outcome in children are only now becoming available.[6] Lauer found that 45% of young adults who have high blood pressure had had childhood high blood pressure recorded on at least one measurement; he concluded that although in an individual child there is variable predictability of adult blood pressure, on a population basis early childhood blood pressure elevations are predictive of risk for future high blood pressure.[6] This important, ongoing study and others confirm that regular measurement of blood pressure in childhood is an essential part of good primary pediatric care.

DEFINITION

High blood pressure is a level of systolic or diastolic blood pressure at which there is an unacceptable risk for cardiovascular complications for that individual. Setting that level is difficult because there are no long-term studies relating blood pressure beginning in childhood to vascular disease arising during adult life. Thus the current definition is statistical and closely correlated with age, gender, physical activity, body size, and sexual maturity.

Primary (essential) hypertension occurs without identifiable pathological cause and is likely related to genetic factors. Secondary hypertension is caused by chronic vascular, renal, or neuroendocrine causes.

DIAGNOSIS

Most children who have high blood pressure do not have symptoms. Therefore recognition requires regular measurements of blood pressure during normal growth and development. The current recommendation is for infants and children to have their blood pressure checked beginning at 3 years of age and annually thereafter. All symptomatic children, including those evaluated in emergency rooms, hospitals, or critical care units, and high-risk or premature infants should have their blood pressure measured routinely (Fig. 142-1).

Blood pressure must be measured in a quiet, resting infant or child, because the normative data were gathered under these conditions. The blood pressure cuff must cover more than two thirds of the upper arm, the bladder positioned over the brachial artery, and the sensor (Doppler crystal, oscillometer, or stethoscope) placed over the artery.

Systolic blood pressure is the first sound (phase 1 Korotkoff) as the cuff is deflated; diastolic blood pressure is either the muffling (phase IV Korotkoff) or disappearance (phase V Korotkoff) of the sounds. The most frequent "cause" of elevated blood pressure is an improperly taken measurement.

According to the standard blood pressure tables for age, gender, and weight, *normal blood pressure* is a systolic and diastolic pressure less than the 90th percentile; *high normal blood pressure* is the average of three or more systolic and/or diastolic pressure measurements from the 90th percentile to the 95th percentile; and *high blood pressure* is the average of three or more systolic and/or diastolic pressures greater than the 95th percentile. Note that a child who is taller or heavier for age will have a higher blood pressure than a child of average size. (See Figs. 142-2, 142-3, and 142-4 for gender-, age-, and weight-corrected systolic and diastolic blood pressures.)

Severe symptomatic high blood pressure (hypertensive crisis) includes evidence of cardiovascular or cerebrovascular malfunction.

DIAGNOSTIC EVALUATION

Patients who have normal blood pressure on a single reading require continued annual surveillance. Those who have high normal blood pressure on three consecutive measurements separated by at least 3 days should have three extremity blood pressures (right arm, left arm, and a leg) taken to rule out coarctation of the aorta, urinalysis and a quantitative urine culture to rule out chronic urinary tract infection, counseling for dietary salt and weight reduction where appropriate, and more frequent surveillance.

Children who have high blood pressure should be evaluated for a possible treatable cause of secondary hypertension. The evaluation includes the tests listed in Table 142-1. The younger the child and the higher the blood pressure, the more likely it is that renal or renovascular disease or other cause of secondary hypertension is present. Children who have symptomatic severe high blood pressure fitting the criteria for hypertensive crisis should have aggressive treatment to reduce blood pressure to safer levels (see Chapter 284, Hypertensive Emergencies) and a thorough diagnostic evaluation to determine the underlying cause (Table 142-2).

Children who have high normal blood pressure and most

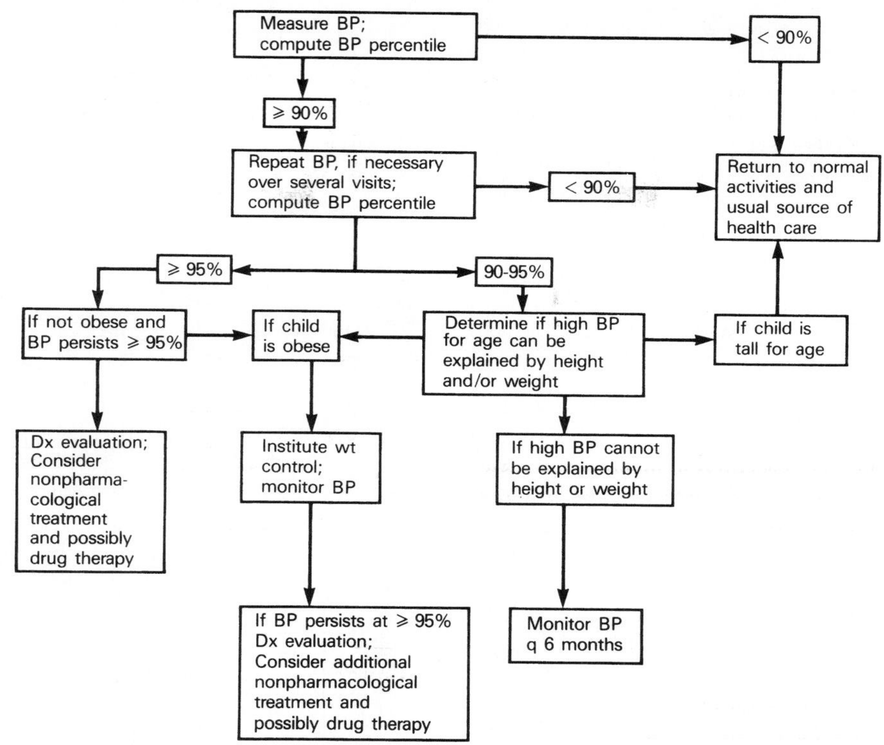

FIG. 142-1 Algorithm for identifying children with high blood pressure.

(From Task Force on Blood Pressure Control in Children: *Pediatrics* 79:1, 1987; courtesy Dr. Michael J. Horan.)

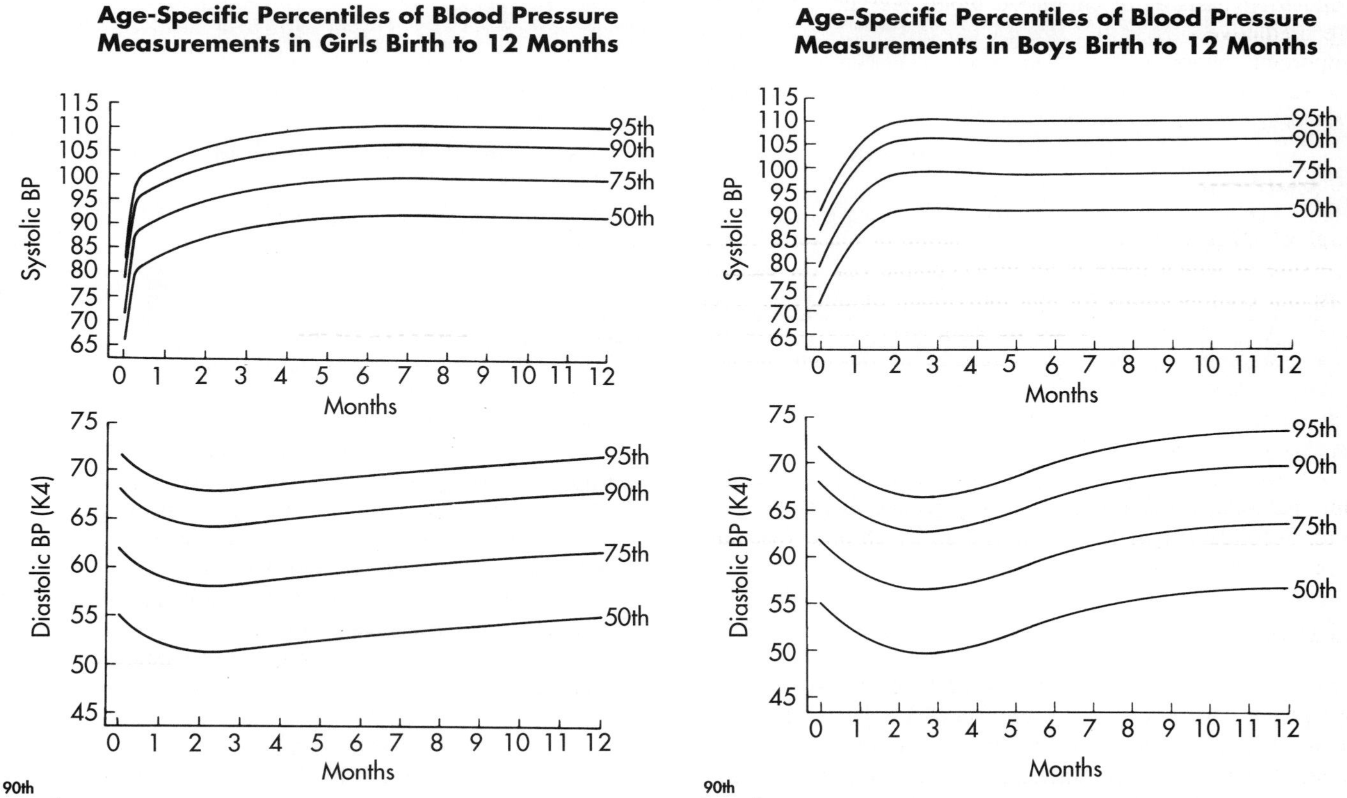

Age-Specific Percentiles of Blood Pressure Measurements in Girls Birth to 12 Months

Systolic BP: 115 110 105 100 95 90 85 80 75 70 65; 95th, 90th, 75th, 50th; Months 0 1 2 3 4 5 6 7 8 9 10 11 12

Diastolic BP (K4): 75 70 65 60 55 50 45; 95th, 90th, 75th, 50th; Months 0 1 2 3 4 5 6 7 8 9 10 11 12

90th Percentile													
Systolic BP	76	98	101	104	105	106	106	106	106	106	106	105	105
Diastolic BP	68	65	64	64	65	65	66	66	66	67	67	67	67
Height CM	54	55	56	58	61	63	66	68	70	72	74	75	77
Weight KG	4	4	4	5	5	6	7	8	9	9	10	10	11

Age-Specific Percentiles of Blood Pressure Measurements in Boys Birth to 12 Months

Systolic BP: 115 110 105 100 95 90 85 80 75 70 65; 95th, 90th, 75th, 50th; Months 0 1 2 3 4 5 6 7 8 9 10 11 12

Diastolic BP (K4): 75 70 65 60 55 50 45; 95th, 90th, 75th, 50th; Months 0 1 2 3 4 5 6 7 8 9 10 11 12

90th Percentile													
Systolic BP	87	101	106	106	105	105	105	105	105	105	105	105	105
Diastolic BP	68	65	63	63	63	65	66	67	68	68	69	69	69
Height CM	51	59	63	66	68	70	72	73	74	76	77	78	80
Weight KG	4	4	5	5	6	7	8	9	9	10	10	11	11

FIG. 142-2 Age-, gender-, height-, and weight-specific percentiles of systolic and diastolic blood pressure for birth to 12 months of age.

(From Task Force on Blood Pressure Control in Children: *Pediatrics* 79:1, 1987; courtesy Dr. Michael J. Horan.)

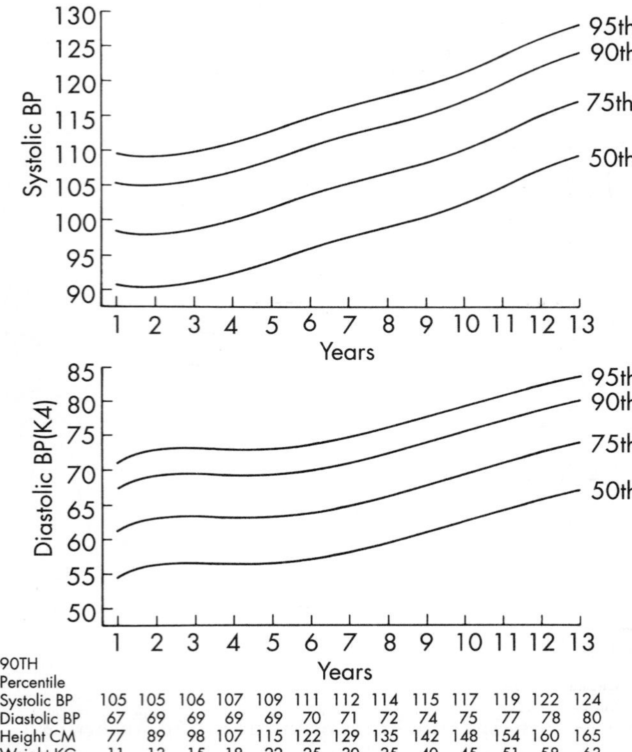

90TH Percentile													
Systolic BP	105	105	106	107	109	111	112	114	115	117	119	122	124
Diastolic BP	67	69	69	69	69	70	71	72	74	75	77	78	80
Height CM	77	89	98	107	115	122	129	135	142	148	154	160	165
Weight KG	11	13	15	18	22	25	30	35	40	45	51	58	63

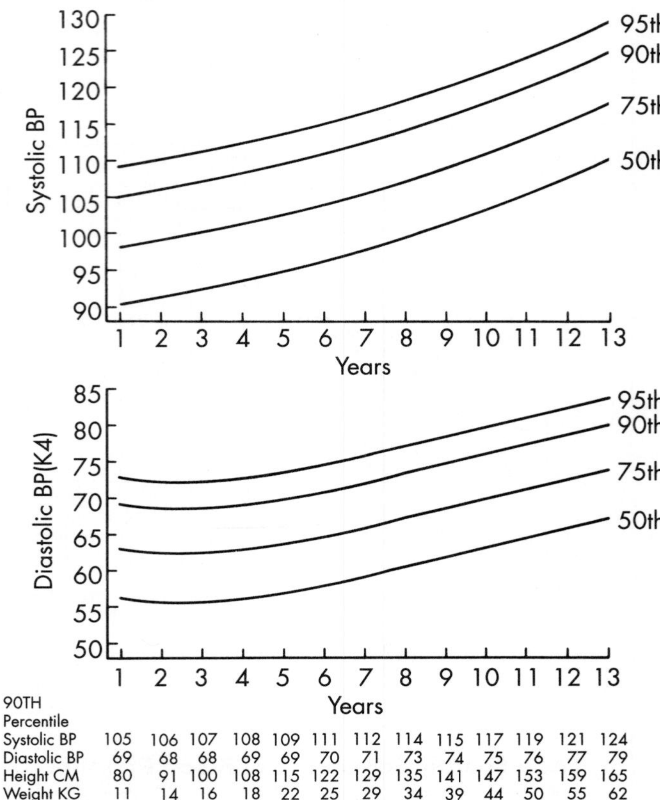

90TH Percentile													
Systolic BP	105	106	107	108	109	111	112	114	115	117	119	121	124
Diastolic BP	69	68	68	69	69	70	71	73	74	75	76	77	79
Height CM	80	91	100	108	115	122	129	135	141	147	153	159	165
Weight KG	11	14	16	18	22	25	29	34	39	44	50	55	62

FIG. 142-3 Age-, gender-, height-, and weight-specific percentiles of systolic and diastolic blood pressure for 1 to 13 years of age.

(From Task Force on Blood Pressure Control in Children: *Pediatrics* 79:1, 1987; courtesy Dr. Michael J. Horan.)

Table 142-1 A Diagnostic Strategy in the Evaluation of High Blood Pressure

Item	Action
Exclude drugs or prior illness	Conduct history, physical examination
Exclude coarctation of the aorta	Measure blood pressure in all extremities
Identify renal causes	Auscultate for abdominal bruits; perform urinalysis; obtain urine culture; measure electrolytes and blood urea nitrogen
Assess for end organ changes	Obtain echocardiogram for evidence of left ventricular hypertrophy; perform ophthalmoscopy
Assess vascular disease risk factors	Obtain family history; perform lipid screen, including high-density lipoproteins and triglycerides
Assess general health	Conduct history and physical examination; obtain complete blood count

children who have high blood pressure can be evaluated and cared for in the primary physician's office or clinic.[3,7] Children or adolescents who have severe hypertension or a perplexing presentation should be referred to a consultant with expertise in the diagnosis and management of pediatric patients. A summary of the approach to such severe and complex cases was published recently.[1]

Table 142-2 Commonest Causes by Age Group of Chronic Sustained Hypertension

Age group	Cause
Newborn	Renal artery thrombosis Renal artery stenosis Congenital renal malformations Coarctation of the aorta Bronchopulmonary dysplasia
Infancy to 6 years	Renal parenchymal disease Coarctation of the aorta Renal artery stenosis
6 to 10 years	Renal artery stenosis Renal parenchymal disease Primary hypertension
Adolescence	Primary hypertension Renal parenchymal disease

ASSOCIATED SIGNS AND SYMPTOMS

Symptoms are rare in children who have high blood pressure; when present, they are usually associated with either sudden acute or chronic severe elevation in blood pressure. Table 142-3 lists the most common causes of the chronic

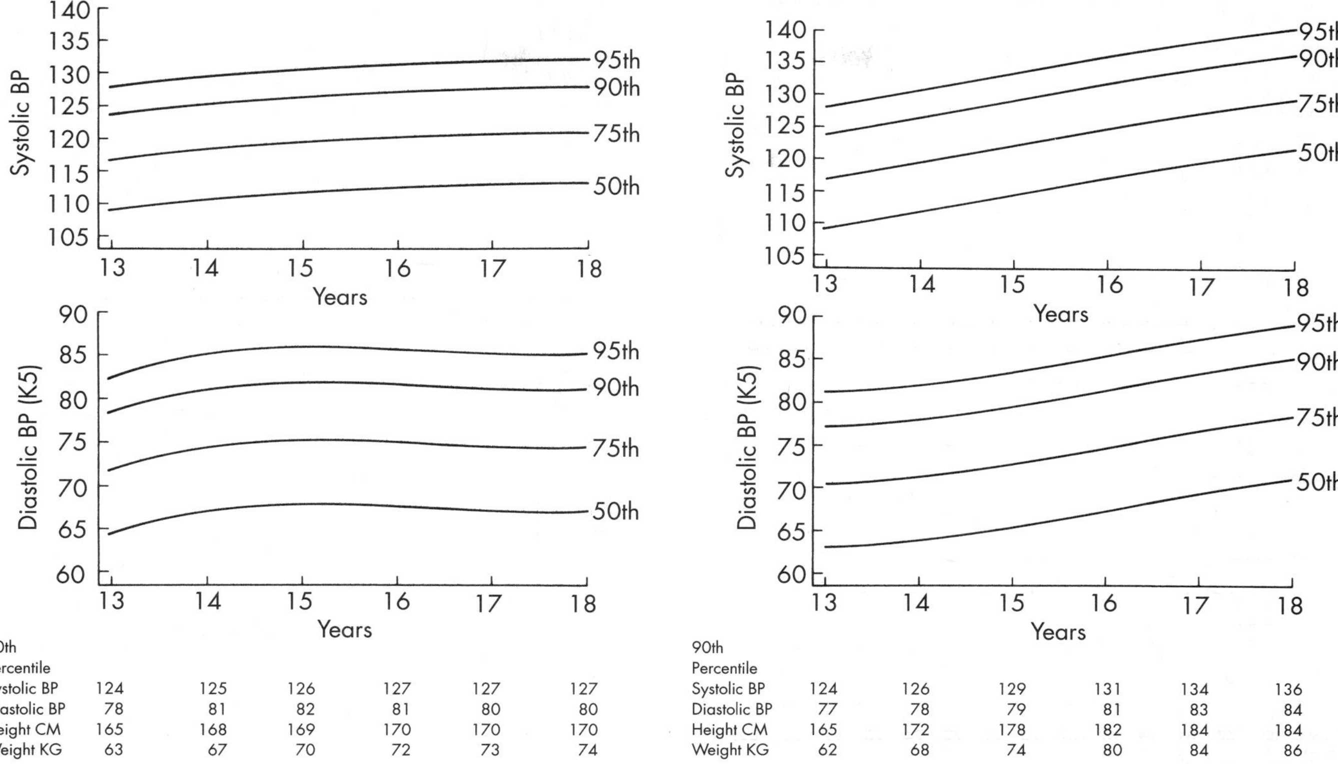

Girls:

90th Percentile						
Systolic BP	124	125	126	127	127	127
Diastolic BP	78	81	82	81	80	80
Height CM	165	168	169	170	170	170
Weight KG	63	67	70	72	73	74

Boys:

90th Percentile						
Systolic BP	124	126	129	131	134	136
Diastolic BP	77	78	79	81	83	84
Height CM	165	172	178	182	184	184
Weight KG	62	68	74	80	84	86

FIG. 142-4 Age-, gender-, height-, and weight-specific percentiles of systolic and diastolic blood pressure for 13 to 18 years of age.

(From Task Force on Blood Pressure Control in Children: *Pediatrics* 79:1, 1987; courtesy Dr. Michael J. Horan.)

Table 142-3 Causes of Secondary Hypertension

Cause	Mechanism
Renal	Renal parenchymal disease
	Glomerulonephritis
	Chronic pyelonephritis
	Polycystic kidney
	Connective tissue disease
	Hydronephrosis
	Renal tumors
Cardiac	Coarctation of the aorta
Adrenal	Cortical
	Mineralocorticoid secreting tumors
	Adrenogenital syndrome
	Medullary
	Pheochromocytoma
Neurogenic	Increased intracranial pressure from a variety of pathological causes
Drug induced	Oral contraceptives
	Amphetamines
	Sympathomimetic amines
	Cocaine, phencyclidine (PCP), illicit drugs, licorice

type. The cardiovascular complications of congestive heart failure and pulmonary edema often are associated with left ventricular hypertrophy (determined on the electrocardiogram) and/or an increase in myocardial mass measured from the echocardiogram. Cerebrovascular complications include persistent headache, blurred vision, coma, convulsions, or, in rare cases, stroke. Retinal vascular changes are evidence of chronic severe hypertension.

ETIOLOGY OF HIGH BLOOD PRESSURE

The dynamic control of blood pressure occurs through a complex feedback mechanism regulating cardiac output, vascular resistance, and blood volume.[4] A number of pathophysiological defects are recognized as causes of *secondary hypertension* (see Table 142-2). In childhood, renal and renovascular disorders are among the most frequent and important causes.

*Primary (*or *essential) hypertension* has as yet no clearly defined pathophysiological mechanism or mechanisms but probably has a strong genetic component. This concept is supported by studies showing that high blood pressure tends to aggregate in families. Studies in experimental animals, together with human studies of blood pressure in twins, of erythrocyte sodium-lithium transport, and of familial patterns of blood pressure response to stress all demonstrate the importance of genetic factors in control of blood pressure.[2]

Table 142-4 Antihypertensive Medications*

	Dose	Times/day	Route
Diuretics			
Hydrochlorothiazide (Hydrodiuril, Esidrix)	1-2 mg/kg	2	Oral
Chlorthalidone (Hygroton)	0.5-2 mg/kg	1	Oral
Furosemide (Lasix)	0.5-2 mg/kg	2	Oral, intravenous (IV)
Spironolactone (Aldactone)	1-2 mg/kg	2	Oral
Triamterene (Dyrenium)	1-2 mg/kg	2	Oral
Adrenergic inhibitors			
Beta-adrenergic antagonists			
Metoprolol (Lopressor)	1-4 mg/kg	2	Oral
Atenolol (Tenormin)	1-2 mg/kg	1	Oral
Propranolol (Inderal)	1-3 mg/kg	3	Oral
Central adrenergic inhibitors			
Methyldopa (Aldomet)	5-10 mg/kg	2	Oral
Clonidine (Catapres)	0.05-0.40 mg	2	Oral
Guanabenz (Wytensin)	0.03-0.08 mg	2	Oral
Alpha-adrenergic antagonist			
Prazosin hydrochloride (Minipress)	0.5-7 mg	3	Oral
Vasodilators			
Hydralazine (Apresoline)	1-5 mg/kg	2 or 3	Oral, intramuscular, IV (drip)
Minoxidil (Loniten)	0.1-1.0 mg/kg	2	Oral
Diazoxide (Hyperstat)†	3-5 mg/kg/dose		IV (bolus)
Nitroprusside (Nipride)†	1-8 μg/kg/minute		IV (drip)
Angiotensin-converting enzyme inhibitor			
Captopril			
≤6 mo of age	0.05-0.5 mg/kg	3	Oral
≥6 mo of age	0.5-2 mg/kg	3	Oral

Adapted from Task Force on Blood Pressure Control in Children: *Pediatrics* 79:1, 1987; courtesy Dr. Michael J. Horan.
*Not to exceed usual adult dosage with all drugs.
†Primary use is in hypertensive emergencies.

Identification of children at risk for primary hypertension is important because elevated blood pressure is one of the risk factors for stroke, myocardial infarction, congestive heart failure, and renal failure in adults.

PSYCHOSOCIAL CONSIDERATIONS

Although it is important to detect children who have high blood pressure, it is equally important to avoid erroneous identification of a child as "hypertensive." The dangers of a false positive diagnosis include labeling within the family and at school, limiting participation in sports, creating an obstacle to obtaining life and health insurance, losing employment opportunities, and risking the potentially harmful side effects of treatment.

Rigorous diagnosis and care of the severely hypertensive child is essential. Careful evaluation and management of the child who has normal high blood pressure is judicious.

MANAGEMENT

The treatment of high blood pressure depends on the cause and the degree of elevation. Acute symptomatic severe elevation in blood pressure requires immediate evaluation and treatment. Other forms of secondary hypertension frequently require direct intervention such as surgery for coarctation of the aorta or pharmacological management for children who have chronic renal disease.

The management of high normal or high blood pressure without an identifiable cause is more difficult. The current recommendation is for conservative therapy: weight reduction if obese, exercise, moderate salt restriction (to around 2500 mg of sodium per day), and avoidance of tobacco, particularly cigarette smoking. There is unanimity on the benefits of dynamic exercise; because isometric forms of exercise such as wrestling and weight lifting may lead to elevated blood pressure, these activities are questioned more often. The present consensus is that supervised, graduated isometric exercise is not harmful and may be beneficial.

Weight reduction is particularly important, especially since tracking data from childhood to adulthood indicate that obesity in a child is most predictive of obesity and hence high blood pressure in an adult. Therefore strategies designed to prevent the acquisition of excess weight during adolescence may be useful in preventing adult hypertension.[5]

There is a small role for drug treatment, because the natu-

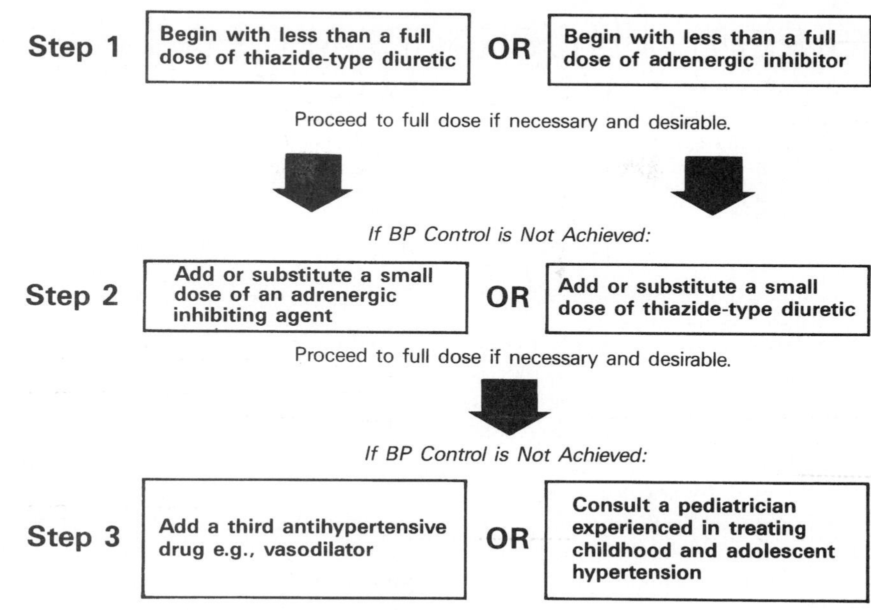
Step 1
Begin with less than a full dose of thiazide-type diuretic
OR
Begin with less than a full dose of adrenergic inhibitor
Proceed to full dose if necessary and desirable.
If BP Control is Not Achieved:
Step 2
Add or substitute a small dose of an adrenergic inhibiting agent
OR
Add or substitute a small dose of thiazide-type diuretic
Proceed to full dose if necessary and desirable.
If BP Control is Not Achieved:
Step 3
Add a third antihypertensive drug e.g., vasodilator
OR
Consult a pediatrician experienced in treating childhood and adolescent hypertension

FIG. 142-5 Stepped-care approach to antihypertensive drug therapy (reproduced from Fig. 142-1).
(From Task Force on Blood Pressure Control in Children: *Pediatrics* 79:1, 1987; courtesy Dr. Michael J. Horan.)

ral history of blood pressure elevation is obscure, the side effects of lifelong drug treatment are undefined, and the risk of target organ disease is unknown. When pharmacological therapy is necessary, a stepped-care approach traditionally has been used by the pediatrician (Fig. 142-5). Step 1 usually is a thiazide diuretic or adrenergic inhibitor at less than a full dose; step 2 is the addition of a second drug gradually increased to full dose; step 3 is the addition of a third drug, usually in consultation with a physician skilled in treating children and adolescents who have more refractory forms of high blood pressure. Table 142-4 provides a list of antihypertensive medications and their doses. Once blood pressure returns to the normal range, discontinuing medication is more often feasible and desirable in the young than in older subjects who already have fixed arterial wall changes.

REFERENCES

1. Balfe JW et al: Hypertension in childhood. In Barness LA, editor: *Advances in pediatrics,* Chicago, 1989, Mosby.
2. Burns TL, Lauer RM: Blood pressure in children. In Pierpont MEM, Moller JH, editors: *Genetics of cardiovascular disease,* Boston, 1986, Martinius Nijhoff.
3. Gifford RW et al: Office evaluation of hypertension: special report—a statement for health professionals by a writing group of the Council for High Blood Pressure Research, American Heart Association, *Hypertension* 13:283, 1989.
4. Guyton AC: The kidney in blood pressure control and hypertension. In Holliday MA, Barratt TM, Vernier RL, editors: *Pediatric nephrology,* ed 2, Baltimore, 1987, Williams & Wilkins.
5. Lauer RM et al: Factors related to tracking of blood pressure in children, *Hypertension* 6:307, 1984.
6. Lauer RM, Clarke WR: Childhood risk factors for adult high blood pressure: the Muscatine study, *Pediatrics* 84:633, 1989.
7. National Heart, Lung and Blood Institute Task Force on Blood Pressure Control in Children: Report of the Second Task Force on Blood Pressure Control in Children in 1987, *Pediatrics* 79:1, 1987.

SUGGESTED READINGS

Emmanouilides GC et al: *Heart disease in infants, children and adolescents,* ed 5, Baltimore, 1994, Williams & Wilkins.
Neill CA, Clark EB, Clark CI: *The heart of a child,* Baltimore, 1992, Johns Hopkins University Press.

143 Hirsutism, Hypertrichosis, and Precocious Sexual Hair Development

Cynthia H. Cole

Both hirsutism and hypertrichosis technically imply excessive hair growth. When a patient with an excess of hair is seen, one must decide if it is a normal variant or pathological. An increase in body hair in areas under sex hormone control increases the likelihood of an endocrine origin. The areas of the body primarily influenced by sex hormone levels are the face, chest, axilla, abdomen, and pubic region. There is little chance of an endocrine cause if the disproportionate hair growth is in or limited to body areas not primarily under sex hormone control. These areas include the extremities, the eyebrows, and the scalp. Human hair can be classified into two types: vellus and terminal hair. Vellus hair is soft, unmedullated, less pigmented, and shorter in contrast to terminal hair, which is coarser, longer, medullated, and pigmented. Transformation of sexual hair from vellus to terminal is caused by androgen stimulation. Nonsexual hair is unresponsive to androgen stimulation and will not change from its original type.

DEFINITIONS

Hypertrichosis

Hypertrichosis is excessive growth of nonsexual hair and is associated with normal androgen metabolism. This excessive body hair is in normal distribution for the patient's race, age, and sex. The quantity of total body hair varies considerably among normal individuals and is influenced by race and genetics. Females of Mediterranean origin have more hair than do those of Scandinavian origin, and Caucasians have more than Asians. Therefore the quantity of hair, as opposed to its distribution and type, is of little diagnostic significance.

Disproportionate hair growth also may be a feature of various congenital syndromes, including congenital hypertrichosis lanuginosa, generalized lipodystrophy, fetal hydantoin syndrome, mucopolysaccharidoses, trisomy 18, leprechaunism, and de Lange syndrome, among other disorders of infancy and childhood. In each of these, excessive body hair should be considered in context with other features of the specific syndromes.

Hirsutism and Precocious Sexual Hair Development

Hirsutism is excessive growth of androgen-dependent sexual hair in females, which primarily involves pubic, axillary, facial, chest, and abdominal hair. This excessive, coarse, terminal hair in a female is distributed in a male sexual pattern. It most often is associated with increased production of total or free androgen. When an overproduction of androgens cannot be demonstrated, the cause of hirsutism may be related to increased "sensitivity" of the hair follicle to normal levels of androgen. Hirsutism is but one manifestation of virilization and refers to the development of a "male" hair growth pattern in a female.

Pubic hair usually starts growing after the child is 13 years of age. Development of sexual hair in boys younger than 9 years of age or in girls younger than 8 years of age deserves further evaluation. Disorders that result in premature development of sexual hair in prepubertal children include premature adrenarche, precocious puberty, virilizing congenital adrenal hyperplasia (classical, cryptic), Cushing syndrome, and tumors of the adrenal glands, ovaries or testicles, or central nervous system (CNS). Exogenous administration of androgens also may cause premature or excessive sexual hair development.

Evaluation of a child who has premature sexual hair development should include a complete history and physical examination, observing for or inquiring about (1) a history of obesity, of an unusual growth spurt, or of electrolyte problems, (2) a family history of infant deaths or of ambiguous genitalia, and (3) the rapidity of onset and progression of symptoms and their duration and severity. It is important to look for the advancement of other secondary sexual characteristics or for signs of virilization. Evidence of virilization in prepubertal boys or girls includes advanced genital growth (clitoris, penis, testicles), accelerated muscle development, and growth of facial, chest, abdominal and thigh hair in addition to pubic and axillary hair, a deepened voice, and acne. Hirsutism and virilization in any prepubertal child or in girls of any age are the result of increased androgen stimulation; the source of these signs must be sought.

The endogenous sources of excess androgen production include the adrenal glands, the ovaries and testicles, the enhanced peripheral conversion of androgenic precursors to potent androgens, and hypothalamopituitary dysfunction.[3,6-9,12] Hyperandrogenism in some pubescent or postpubescent girls may result from increased androgen production by both the adrenal glands and the ovaries. Potential exogenous sources of androgens should be evaluated.

DIFFERENTIAL DIAGNOSIS

Adrenal Causes of Hirsutism

Premature Adrenarche. *Premature adrenarche* (PA) is defined as the precocious growth of pubic hair in the absence of other signs of precocious puberty (under 8 years of age in girls and under 9 years of age in boys); it occurs more commonly in girls than in boys. It also is common in large children and in children who have CNS disorders. Axillary hair, oily skin, and acne also may be observed. Height and bone age usually are slightly accelerated. Pubertal development appears to ensue normally or slightly earlier than usual in children who have premature adrenarche.

In many patients who have premature adrenarche the mean androgen concentrations and their metabolites are similar to those in pubertal children. Therefore dehydroepiandrosterone (DHEA), DHEA-sulfate (DHEA-S), testosterone, androstenedione, and urinary 17-ketosteroids are elevated for the age of the child who has PA but are normal for those at midpuberty. In these patients it has been assumed that PA was caused by a precocious maturation of the adrenal zona reticularis. Patients who have normal androgen concentrations are assumed to have an increased sensitivity to adrenal androgens.

Recently it was demonstrated that some individuals who have PA have enzyme defects in steroidogenesis and exaggerated responses to adrenocorticotropic hormone (ACTH) stimulation. Some of the abnormal hormonal responses resembled late-onset 21-hydroxylase deficiency or heterozygosity for classic adrenal hyperplasia, and others evidenced 3-beta-hydroxysteroid dehydrogenase deficiency.[9,10,13,16]

The differential diagnosis for children who have PA should include idiopathic PA, PA with enzyme deficiencies, isosexual precocious puberty presenting with pubic hair, and gonadotropin-producing tumors.

Evaluation of a child who has PA should include a complete history and physical examination; an abdominal ultrasound may be needed. Hormonal evaluation of androgens, cortisol, precursor steroids [DHEA, DHEA-S, testosterone, androstenedione, dehydrotestosterone (DHT), 17-OH progesterone (17-OHP), 17-OH pregnenolone (D5-17OHP), desoxycorticosterone (DOC)], luteinizing hormone–releasing hormone (LH–RH) stimulation, ACTH stimulation, and dexamethasone suppression tests also may be required.

For patients who have PA periodic follow-up every 3 to 6 months is important to determine growth velocity, bone age, and evidence of precocious development of other secondary sexual characteristics. Repeat hormonal evaluation may be considered if precocious puberty or an androgen-producing tumor still is in the differential diagnosis.

Congenital Virilizing Adrenal Hyperplasia. Congenital virilizing adrenal hyperplasia (CVAH) may not be accompanied by hirsutism, virilization, cortisol deficiency, or electrolyte disturbance for varying periods of time (sometimes years), depending on the degree of enzyme deficiency present. Several enzyme deficiencies have been identified. The most common adrenal enzyme deficiency associated with CVAH is that of 21-hydroxylase, whereas 11-beta-hydroxylase deficiency occurs in a small percentage (5%) of CVAH cases and may be associated with hypertension.[1] In both types of CVAH, urinary excretion of 17-ketosteroids and pregnanetriol usually is increased.

Depending on the degree of enzyme block, urinary levels of 17-hydroxycorticosteroids (17-OHCS) may be normal or decreased with 21-hydroxylase deficiency, whereas these levels may be increased in 11-beta-hydroxylase deficiency. Urinary metabolites of tetrahydric derivatives of compound S and deoxycorticosterone usually are increased in patients who have 11-beta-hydroxylase deficiency.

Twenty-four hour urine specimens are difficult to collect in some children and, even if properly collected, may yield equivocal results. Plasma hormone determinations of 17-hydroxyprogesterone, DHEAS, and 11-beta-hydroxyandrostenedione are elevated in 21-hydroxylase deficiency. Diagnosis usually is based on an 8 AM 17-hydroxyprogesterone level followed by ACTH stimulation tests.[17] There are two classic forms of 21-hydroxylase deficiency, salt-wasting and simple virilizing, which tend to appear early in life. The nonclassic variants of congenital adrenal hyperplasia (CAH) can be classified as late-onset symptomatic CAH and cryptic-asymptomatic CAH. The late onset variants of CAH result from specific mutations in the gene encoding adrenal 21-hydroxylase. Late-onset CAH appears around peripubertal and postpubertal periods with manifestations of hirsutism, menstrual abnormalities, acne, clitoromegaly, and infertility. Although late-onset CAH has been associated most often with 21-hydroxylase deficiency, it also has been described with 3-beta-hydroxysteroid and 11-beta-hydroxylase deficiencies.[4,5,10,12-15,17] Determining levels of 11-deoxycortisol, cortisol, and 17-alpha-OH-progesterone during ACTH stimulation test may detect 11-beta-hydroxylase deficiency.

Partial 3-beta-hydroxysteroid deficiency results in elevated DHEA following ACTH stimulation. 17-beta-hydroxysteroid oxidoreductase deficiency results in elevated and rostendione levels.

Treatment of CVAH consists of hydrocortisone replacement (15 to 30 mg/m^2/day). The dosage may vary, depending on the severity of the enzyme deficiency and the presence of stress factors. Mineralocorticoid replacement (e.g., deoxycorticosterone acetate) is required for patients who have the salt-wasting features of CVAH.

Virilizing Adrenal Tumors. A virilizing adrenal tumor (VAT) is uncommon in childhood. When such tumors do occur, they usually appear in early childhood and affect females more often than males. VATs may be associated with other congenital anomalies (e.g., hemihypertrophy), other nonadrenal tumors, and Beckwith-Wiedemann syndrome.[2,8,13]

The clinical features of VAT include rapid linear growth and advanced bone maturation. In boys the development of the penis, scrotum, and pubic hair is advanced, but the testicles usually remain small. In girls pubic hair grows and the clitoris enlarges. Some degree of breast development is not uncommon in patients who have virilizing adrenal tumors, which also have an associated increased estrogen production. Acne, greasy hair, adult body odor, deepening voice, masculine habitus, and hypertension may be other features of VAT. Rapidly growing carcinomas may develop with abdominal pain, weight loss, fever, or abdominal mass. VATs often are associated with excess glucocorticoid secretion; therefore features of Cushing syndrome, or glucocorticoid excess, also may be apparent.

Virilizing adrenal tumors produce excessive androgens, primarily DHEA and DHEA-S, although a few may produce testosterone primarily. Serum DHEA levels usually are higher than 20 ng/ml, and serum DHEA-S levels usually are higher than 9000 ng/ml. Depending on the amount of androgen produced by the tumor, 24-hour urinary 17-ketosteroids are significantly increased. Dexamethasone suppression studies usually do not suppress androgen production, but exceptions occur occasionally.[2,8] In addition, some VATs demonstrate heterogeneous steroid production with deficiencies or enhancement in specific enzyme systems. The hormonal secretion pattern of VAT may change with time, therapy, or both.[8]

Computed tomography (CT) provides more reliable imaging, particularly of small adrenal tumors.

The prognosis is related largely to completeness of surgical removal and the presence or absence of metastases. If the VAT is associated with excess glucocorticoid production, postoperative management may require glucocorticoid support because of the possibility of contralateral adrenal gland suppression. Postoperative follow-up also requires long-term hormonal surveillance for years. Malignant VATs do not respond well to radiation or chemotherapy.

Cushing Syndrome. Cushing syndrome, which results from abnormally high levels of cortisol, usually manifests with a characteristic pattern of truncal and facial obesity, buffalo hump, striae, and hypertension. Virilization caused by excess adrenal androgen production may result in hirsutism, acne, deepened voice, and clitoral or penile enlargement. Linear growth is impaired or arrested.

Among infants and young children, adrenocortical tumors (carcinoma, adenoma, and nodular hyperplasia) most often are the cause of Cushing syndrome. Bilateral adrenal hyperplasia, caused by pituitary microadenomas or basophilic adenomas (Cushing disease), is the most common cause of Cushing syndrome in older children. Extrapituitary ACTH-producing tumors are rare in children.[2,13,17]

Cushing syndrome must be ruled out in any female who has cystic ovaries, obesity, hirsutism, hypertension, and diabetes mellitus. The cystic ovaries in Cushing syndrome may be the result of chronic anovulation with ovarian androgen overproduction and increased peripheral estrogen production.[12]

Laboratory evaluation of Cushing syndrome usually reveals hypercortisolism with loss of the circadian rhythm of cortisol production. Urinary 17-hydroxycorticosteroid and free cortisol levels are elevated. Plasma ACTH levels and the response to dexamethasone suppression will vary, depending on the syndrome's etiology. Lack of cortisol suppression by prolonged (7 to 10 days) dexamethasone administration is presumptive evidence of a tumor. A low or undetectable baseline level of ACTH eliminates Cushing disease as a cause. CT scanning is helpful in localizing adrenal tumors.[2,13]

Treatment of Cushing syndrome depends on the cause, but involves either surgery to remove an adrenal or other tumor or bilateral adrenalectomy. Patients who have Cushing disease may require pituitary irradiation or transsphenoidal surgery for selective removal of pituitary microadenomas. Adrenocortical carcinoma is highly malignant and frequently has metastasized by the time of presentation.

Gondal Causes of Hirsutism

Polycystic Ovarian Disease (PCOD). Polycystic ovarian disease is a disorder of androgen excess diagnosed frequently in postpubertal females who have manifestations of hirsutism, menstrual disorders (including anovulation), obesity, and cystic ovaries. Hirsutism in PCOD may be mild to severe; virilization is not usual with this disease. A number of other endocrine disorders (e.g., CAH, Cushing disease, androgen-secreting neoplasm, hypothyroidism, hyperprolactinemia, and ovarian hyperthecosis) may have similar components in their clinical presentations and must be differentiated from PCOD. Also, PCOD may accompany these endocrine disorders. Galactorrhea, acanthosis nigricans, and insulin receptor defects may be seen in PCOD.[1,9,11-14,17] PCOD appears to have a genetic basis. However, the pathophysiology of polycystic ovarian syndrome is not understood entirely, in part because of the heterogeneity of clinical and biochemical features of the disorder among affected women. The aberrant ovarian steroidogenesis and follicular maturation are related to dysfunctional feedback within the hypothalamopituitary-ovarian-adrenal axis. Hyperandrogenism is one feature of this syndrome. Excessive androgen production from the adrenal gland and the ovary has been documented, as has increased peripheral conversion of androgen precursors to testosterone and dehydrotestosterone, the two most potent androgens. The luteinizing hormone/follicle-stimulating hormone ratio is increased because of increased LH secretion and low or normal FSH secretion. Urinary 17-ketosteroid excretion and total serum testosterone levels are not always abnormal in these patients. Free serum testosterone and 5-alpha-androstane-3-alpha, 17-beta-diol glucuronide (3-alpha-diol G) levels correlate well with hirsutism, but neither of these assays is available routinely to the clinician. Other serum androgens whose levels may be elevated are serum testosterone, DHEA, DHEA-S, and androstenedione. An abdominal sonogram is useful in documenting polycystic ovaries. No one test can diagnose PCOD definitively. Even after a baseline LH, FSH, and androgen evaluation, a dexamethasone suppression test, and corticotropin or GNRH stimulation tests, there may be overlap and confusion as to ovarian versus adrenal causes of hyperandrogenism.[11,13,17]

Treatment of polycystic ovarian syndrome may include suppression of ovarian function using combination estrogen-progestin oral contraceptives to decrease LH secretion and therefore ovarian androgen production. Adrenal suppression has been used in patients in whom the excess androgens appear to originate from the adrenal gland or from a mixed adrenal-ovarian source. Weight reduction should be incorporated in the treatment program of obese women who have PCOD. Other agents that have antiandrogen effects (e.g., cyproterone acetate, clomiphene citrate, spironolactone, cimetidine, and bromocriptine) have been used in specific circumstances to treat PCOD.[12,17] The eventual decrease in hirsutism is variable, depending on the duration of hirsutism before treatment and the levels of androgens present during treatment.[7,11]

Androgen-Secreting Tumors of the Ovaries. Androgen-secreting tumors of the ovaries, such as Sertoli-Leydig cell tumors, hilus cell tumors, lipid cell tumors, and cystic teratomas, are exceedingly rare but need to be considered in girls who have hirsutism, virilization, and markedly elevated serum testosterone levels.[6]

The most frequent manifestations are abdominal pain and abdominal mass. Torsion occurs more frequently in young females than in older ones and in those who have benign rather than malignant tumors. The clinical features reflect the predominant hormone secretion pattern: estrogens, androgens, or both. Virilizing tumors are much less frequent than feminizing tumors. In young children who have virilizing tumors, the presenting signs and symptoms include precocious development of sexual hair, clitoromegaly, acne, deepened voice, and accelerated growth and bone age. Adolescent girls and young women have abrupt menstrual abnormalities, breast atrophy, hirsutism, clitoromegaly, and male-type muscle development.

Laboratory evaluation of virilizing ovarian tumors reveals marked elevation of plasma testosterone and DHT; CT scans may help to identify small tumors.

The differential diagnostic process includes ruling out the two main adrenal disorders causing masculinization in childhood (VAT and CAH) by assessing plasma DHEA, DHEA-S, and 17-OHP. In both VAT and CAH, urinary 17-ketosteroids and ketogenic steroids are elevated. Differentiating between a small virilizing ovarian tumor and a small virilizing adrenal tumor may require selective venous catheterization of ovarian and adrenal veins for hormonal sampling. Adrenal tumors should be strongly suspected in the presence of marked elevation of DHEA-S (over 2000 μg/dl). Polycystic ovarian disease (PCOD) also must be considered in the differential diagnosis, although patients who have PCOD usually do not experience the abrupt onset of virilization and menstrual abnormalities seen with virilizing ovarian tumors.

Optimum surgical and medical management of ovarian tumors depends on the type of tumor.

Ovarian Hyperthecosis. Ovarian hyperthecosis manifests with signs of androgen excess (severe hirsutism, mild clitoromegaly, obesity, temporal balding, and oligomenorrhea). The androgen excess (testosterone, androstenedione) is ovarian in origin. Histologically the ovaries are characterized by theca interna hyperplasia. The ovaries usually are not cystic and may be of normal size. LH and FSH levels can be normal. Diabetes mellitus and hypertension may be associated clinical problems. The diagnosis of hyperthecosis is made by wedge biopsy of the ovary.[12,13]

Gonadal Dysgenesis. Hyperandrogenism may be seen in patients who have Turner syndrome who have some component of Y chromosome (Turner mosaic with XY or H-Y antigen positive). A remnant of testicular tissue is found, which should be removed.[13]

Peripheral Causes of Hirsutism

Idiopathic Hirsutism. Idiopathic hirsutism (IH) by definition has normal total circulating androgen levels and is not associated with other signs of excess androgen secretion (e.g., virilization). This condition may reflect different sensitivity to circulating androgens or increased 5-alpha-reductase activity in the skin of hirsute patients. Elevated free testosterone (T) and metabolites of T and DHT have been demonstrated in some women who have IH. Even if basal androgen levels are normal, there is other evidence that pituitary or adrenal response may be abnormal to CRF or ACTH stimulation tests. Dynamic testing demonstrates that some cases of IH really have ovarian or adrenal androgen production response for hirsutism.[9] Ethnic differences do exist with respect to the frequency of IH diagnosis (it is more common among women of Mediterranean background). The diagnosis is made by exclusion of other hyperandrogen disorders. Treatment of IH has included agents that have antiandrogenic effects such as diethylstilbestrol (DES), medroxyprogesterone, cimetidine, spironolactone, and cyproterone acetate.[9]

HAIR-AN. HAIR-AN syndrome consists of *h*irsutism, *a*ndrogen excess, *i*nsulin *r*esistance, and *a*canthosis *n*igricans. Recently, mutations in the insulin receptor gene have been found that correlate with abnormal insulin receptors, compensatory hyperinsulinemia, and hyperandrogenism. Insulin-induced hyperandrogenism is not understood. Some cases have been associated with PCOD and androgen-producing ovarian tumors.[1,13,17]

Precocious Puberty

Precocious puberty (PP) should not be confused with hirsutism per se. It includes premature isosexual development of secondary sexual characteristics and advanced sexual hair growth. Precocity in sexual development is defined as premature sexual development in boys under 9 years of age and in girls under 8 years of age.[7]

True PP is caused by a disorder of premature maturation of the hypothalamohypophyseal complex, resulting in increased gonadotropin secretion and gonadal maturation. In boys the increased secretion of testosterone produces a hyperandrogenic state. In girls the increased secretion of estradiol produces a hyperestrogenic state. Precocious puberty occurs less frequently in boys than in girls, with idiopathic PP more common in girls; CNS lesions are distributed evenly between the sexes.

The clinical course is variable in tempo, although the clinical symptoms are those of normal puberty but occurring at an abnormally early age. The evolution of secondary sexual characteristics may be slow or fast. The more rapid evolution frequently is associated with CNS lesions. Linear growth velocity and bone age maturation are accelerated, leading to premature epiphyseal closure and, ultimately, short stature. Bone age is consistent with the child's pubertal stage.

Hormonal changes may be similar to those observed in normal puberty. Episodic, pulsatile secretion of gonadotropins occurs as in normal puberty but is of lesser amplitude than expected in normal children for the comparable stage of pubertal development. Gonadotropin levels, although usually elevated for the age of the patient, also may overlap with normal levels for the patient's age. Thus, according to the stage of puberty, levels of testosterone, luteinizing hormone (LH), and follicle-stimulating hormone (FSH) usually are higher than normal for age in boys. Estradiol, LH, and FSH levels usually are elevated for age in girls, although estrogen levels may fluctuate widely.[7]

Idiopathic precocious puberty is a diagnosis of exclusion and may be familial in origin. Sexual precocity also may occur after various CNS injuries (e.g., trauma, meningitis, sarcoidosis, toxoplasmosis, hydrocephalus). Septooptic dysplasia, McCune-Albright syndrome, and neurofibromatosis are other disorders in which precocious puberty is a component. Magnetic resonance imaging has enhanced the ability to diagnose CNS tumors (e.g., hamartomas) associated with true PP. True PP must be differentiated from false PP. False PP occurs when secondary sexual characteristics develop without maturation of the gonads and when serum gonadotropin levels are normal. False PP usually is caused by an abnormality of the gonads (e.g., tumors) or of the adrenal cortex. In boys false PP may result from congenital virilizing adrenal hyperplasia, a virilizing adrenal tumor, or a virilizing gonadal tumor.[3] False PP in girls rarely is caused by an estrogen-secreting tumor of the adrenal gland or of the ovaries; it more commonly is a result of exogenous estrogen administration.

MANAGEMENT

When a prepubertal child develops sexual hair prematurely, or when a postpubertal female has hirsutism, it is imperative to perform a careful clinical and biochemical evaluation to distinguish between pathologically significant and pathologically insignificant causes. This provides the basis for a rational therapeutic regimen.

Regardless of the pathophysiological basis and whether the condition is deemed to be hirsutism or hypertrichosis, there may be some particular advantage to removing the existing excess hair, specifically, positive cosmetic and emotional effects. The pediatrician will encounter cases in which the presence of excess hair can be managed appropriately by physical removal. This may be accomplished by bleaching (6% hydrogen peroxide solution), shaving, plucking, or using depilatory agents (sulfides of alkali metals, thioglycolate-containing agents). Electrolysis, if performed properly, also is effective and safe. Because commercial electrolysis is unlicensed in many states, one should choose an electrologist carefully. The use of glucocorticoids and oral contraceptives decreases the rate of new hair growth but has no effect on existing hair.

REFERENCES

1. Barbieri RL: Some genetic syndromes associated with hyperandrogenism, *Contemp Ob/Gyn* 39:35, 1994.
2. Behrman RE, Vaughn VC, Nelson WE, editors: *Nelson textbook of pediatrics,* ed 13, Philadelphia, 1987, WB Saunders.
3. Berthelsen JG et al: Testicular tumors in infancy and childhood. In Forest MG, editor: *Androgens in childhood pediatric and adolescent endocrinology,* vol 19, Basel, Switzerland, 1989, S Karger AG.
4. Eldar-Geva T et al: Secondary biosynthetic defects in women with late-onset congenital adrenal hyperplasia, *N Engl J Med* 323:855, 1990.
5. Ehrmann DA, Rosenfield RL: Hirsutism—beyond the steroidogenic block, *N Engl J Med* 323:909, 1990.
6. Forest MG: Ovarian tumors in infancy, childhood, and adolescence. In Forest MG, editor: *Androgens in childhood pediatric and adolescent endocrinology,* vol 19, Basel, Switzerland, 1989, S Karger AG.
7. Francois R, dePerett E, Forest MG: Precocious puberty in boys. In Forest MG, editor: *Androgens in childhood pediatric and adolescent endocrinology,* vol 19, Basel, Switzerland, 1989, S Karger AG.
8. Grant DB: Virilizing adrenal tumors. In Forest MG, editor: *Androgens in childhood pediatric and adolescent endocrinology,* vol 19, Basel, Switzerland, 1989, S Karger AG.
9. Korth-Schutz S: Precocious adrenarche. In Forest MG, editor: *Androgens in childhood pediatric and adolescent endocrinology,* vol 19, Basel, Switzerland, 1989, S Karger AG.
10. Pang S et al: Late-onset adrenal steroid 3β-hydroxysteroid dehydrogenase deficiency: a cause of hirsutism in pubertal and post-pubertal women, *J Clin Endocrinol Metab* 60:428, 1985.
11. Rodin A et al: Hyperandrogenism in polycystic ovary syndrome, *N Engl J Med* 330:460, 1994.
12. St Louis Y, Levy R, Saenger P: Hyperandrogenism in females: hirsutism and acne. In Forest MG, editor: *Androgens in childhood pediatric and adolescent endocrinology,* vol 19, Basel, Switzerland, 1989, S Karger AG.
13. Sanfilippo JS: Hyperandrogenemia: clinical perspectives. In Sanfilippo JS, Finkelstein JW, Styne DM, editors: *Adolescent medicine: state of the Art reviews, medical and gynecologic endocrinology,* vol 5, no 1, Philadelphia, 1994, Hanley & Belfus.
14. Sielgel SF et al: ACTH stimulation tests and plasma dehydroepiandrosterone sulfate levels in women with hirsutism, *N Engl J Med* 323:849, 1990.
15. Sperling LC, Heimer WL: Androgen biology as a basis for the diagnosis and treatment of androgenic disorders in women. II, *J Am Acad Dermatol* 28:901, 1993.
16. Temeck JW et al: Genetic defects of steroidogenesis in premature pubarche, *J Clin Endocrinol Metab* 64:609, 1987.
17. Winter JSD: Hyperandrogenism in female adolescents. In Nathan DG, Oski F, editors: *Current opinion in pediatrics,* vol 5, no 4, Philadelphia, 1993, Current Science.

144 Hoarseness

Susan E. Levitzky

Hoarseness, a symptom of voice dysfunction, is a change in voice quality often described as harsh, grating, rough, noisy, or raspy. Hoarseness should not be confused with (1) stridor, which is a high-pitched whistling sound, (2) the muffled "hot potato mouth" speech of persons who have supraglottic lesions, or (3) the weak "breathy" speech of persons who have neuromuscular disorders. The main significance of hoarseness is that some process has affected the structure or function of the vocal cords. This may be an early sign of local disease or a manifestation of a systemic illness. This chapter highlights the common causes of hoarseness in newborns, infants, children, and adolescents.

According to voice surveys conducted among elementary school children, the prevalence of chronic hoarseness ranges from 5% to more than 20%.[39] Statistics reflecting the incidence of acute hoarseness are not available because data from outpatient surveys have focused on general diagnostic categories rather than on specific symptoms and diagnoses.

HISTORY

When evaluating a child who is hoarse, it is essential to obtain a thorough history from the parents. In hoarseness of sudden onset, an inflammatory process should be considered. In acute laryngitis, symptoms of rhinorrhea, cough, and sore throat often precede the hoarseness. Occasionally a history of foreign body aspiration or direct laryngeal trauma may explain acute hoarseness. Gradually progressive or persistent hoarseness implies a more insidious and chronic disease process. Information should be gleaned regarding age of onset, excessive use of the voice, associated allergies, chronic chest congestion with recurrent pneumonias (gastroesophageal reflux), sluggishness associated with any decrease in the yearly rate of height increase (hypothyroidism), chronic postnasal drip, recent tuberculosis intradermal test conversion, underlying systemic disease, and change of hoarseness with change in position (mobile lesion). Thus a thorough review of systems is indicated to uncover any conditions that may be responsible for or associated with persistent hoarseness.

PHYSICAL EXAMINATION

A complete physical examination should be performed to detect any unsuspected disease. One especially should observe for any signs of increased respiratory effort (stridor, drooling, nasal flaring, retractions, tachypnea, or use of accessory muscles). If any of these is present, the child should be evaluated promptly by a qualified, experienced physician for potentially life-threatening airway obstruction (see Chapters 169, Stridor, and 271, Airway Obstruction). If stridor is not present, the physician may proceed with the examination, noting any of the following: neck masses (hemangiomas, lymphangiomas), local adenopathy, tracheal shift, thyromegaly or thyroid nodule, pale boggy nasal mucosa (allergies), chest congestion (gastroesophageal reflux), cardiac murmurs or enlargement, cutaneous hemangiomas, café-au-lait spots, pallor, rash, joint swelling, or splenomegaly. With clues from the history and physical examination, the physician must decide what further investigation is indicated.

FURTHER INVESTIGATION

Direct laryngoscopy by a skilled endoscopist has become the mainstay in diagnosing laryngeal disease.[1,4] Categories of hoarseness meriting direct laryngoscopy include (1) congenital hoarseness, (2) possible foreign body in the larynx, (3) progressive, unremitting hoarseness of unknown cause, (4) hoarseness of unknown cause with stridor, and (5) acquired hoarseness persisting for longer than 2 to 3 weeks.[37] Other diagnostic modalities complement but do not replace laryngoscopy. True lateral and anteroposterior roentgenographic views of the soft tissues of the neck, computed tomography (CT) scans, and magnetic resonance imaging (MRI) studies may reveal vocal cord immobility, cysts, foreign bodies, or masses. A chest roentgenogram may demonstrate a mediastinal mass. Fiberscopic stroboscopic videolaryngoscopy, a procedure described recently for documenting laryngeal images and voice simultaneously, can be very useful for clinical diagnosis.[40] Another recently developed quantitative method for evaluating vocal cord dysfunction is a valuable adjunct in following perturbation (the degree of hoarseness of the voice).[28] This procedure is simple, brief, highly accurate, and cost effective.

CAUSES OF HOARSENESS

Newborns

Lifesaving measures increasingly are successful in treating premature and newborn infants who are in respiratory distress, but reports on resultant laryngeal injuries also have increased. Following intubation an infant may sustain arytenoid cartilage dislocation, ulceration, or edema of the vocal cords. Unilateral vocal cord palsy may result from birth trauma, with stretching of the neck and the recurrent laryngeal nerve during a breech delivery.

Congenital anomalies causing hoarseness include the following[10]:

1. *Laryngeal web,* a persistent membrane of tissue usually located at the anterior commissure between the true vocal cords. The thickness and extent of the web are variable and determine the mode of therapy. Webs have been associated with cardiac defects, most often with ventricular septal defects.

2. *Laryngeal cysts and laryngoceles,* cysts arising from the laryngeal ventricle and containing either fluid or air. A hoarse cry eventually leads to stridor, especially when air cysts are present. Lateral neck roentgenograms show a supraglottic mass, which may disappear when the child is quiet. The endoscopist must be prepared to deal with complete airway obstruction, because laryngeal edema or hemorrhage into the cyst may occur during endoscopy.
3. *Laryngeal fissure or cleft,* a rare anomaly characterized by an incomplete closure of the posterior larynx. This vertical slit often extends below the vocal cords causing a tracheoesophageal fistula in 20% of cases. Feeding-associated respiratory distress usually overshadows the voice disorder.
4. *Laryngeal hemangiomas,* rare causes of hoarseness in newborns. In 50% of cases skin hemangiomas also are present. Symptoms worsen with crying or with an intercurrent upper respiratory tract infection. Most of these hemangiomas regress spontaneously, but if airway compromise develops, surgical laser and/or steroid therapy may avert a tracheostomy.

Infants who have Down syndrome have a harsh, flat, low-pitched cry. Infants who have Cornelia de Lange syndrome have a coarse, growling cry. The cry of babies who have untreated hypothyroidism has a hoarse, "gravelly" quality resulting from myxedematous infiltration of the vocal cords. Rarer causes of hoarseness with onset in the newborn period include Farber lipogranulomatosis,[7] lipoid proteinosis of Urbach and Wiethe,[29] pachyonychia congenita,[6] Weaver syndrome,[35] and laryngoonychocutaneous syndrome.[31] Hypocalcemic tetany may cause laryngospasm with accompanying hoarseness and stridor.

Infants, Children, and Adolescents

Infectious Inflammatory Causes. By far the majority of cases of acute hoarseness in childhood are related to respiratory tract infections, especially those caused by adenoviruses 4 and 7, influenza A, and parainfluenza I. Acute laryngitis and acute laryngotracheobronchitis (infectious croup) result in vocal cord inflammation. Children who have postnasal drip associated with the common cold, sinus disease, or adenoiditis are hoarse as a result of bathing of the vocal cords with purulent material. Impaired nasal respiration during a cold leads to mouthbreathing and drying of the vocal cord mucosa, with resultant hoarseness on arising in the morning. Children who have spasmodic croup have recurrent episodes of laryngeal obstruction and wake up at night with a harsh voice and inspiratory stridor. Children who have epiglottitis are *not* hoarse, and cough is *not* a prominent symptom. As the epiglottis swells, the voice becomes *muffled* and drooling sets in. Laryngeal diphtheria should be considered in the differential diagnosis of progressive hoarseness. With lapses in immunization practices and the ongoing influx of refugees into the United States, sporadic outbreaks still occur. Laryngeal diphtheria usually develops as a downward extension of the tonsillar-pharyngeal membrane. Sudden death from laryngeal obstruction also may occur. Other causes of hoarseness in this age group are laryngeal candidiasis or tuberculosis,[36,38] especially in the immunocompromised host. Febrile immunocompromised or neutropenic children who are hoarse should have laryngoscopy promptly so that fungal involvement can be ruled out.[12,16] Cytomegalovirus (CMV) infection of the laryngeal nerve has resulted in hoarseness in adults who have AIDS[33] and should be considered in immunocompromised children who have CMV infection who also develop vocal cord paralysis. Hoarseness secondary to left recurrent laryngeal nerve palsy can develop during the healing stage of fibrosing tuberculous mediastinitis and may be permanent.[32] The recent upsurge in maternal and congenital syphilis requires physicians to consider this infection in the evaluation of a hoarse infant.[23]

Noninfectious Inflammatory Disease. Gastroesophageal reflux may result in hoarseness secondary to acid or chemical laryngitis.[2,19,26,27,34] Thickened feedings, 30-degree prone upright positioning, antacids, and histamine H_2 receptor antagonists usually control the reflux, and eventually a normal voice returns. In allergic laryngeal disease, children whose respiratory allergies and rhinosinusitis are documented develop vocal cord edema and inflammation and the hoarseness that accompanies these changes.[3] Occasionally, patients using inhaled steroids for asthma control may develop secondary dysphonia. Discontinuation of this route of treatment or the addition of a volumetric spacer device for administration leads to resolution.[17]

Inhalation of a caustic or hot gas or ingestion of salicylic acid may lead to vocal cord edema and hoarseness in susceptible individuals.[18] Cricoarytenoid arthritis, sometimes associated with juvenile rheumatoid arthritis, can cause painful hoarseness.

Traumatic Causes. The most common cause of chronic hoarseness in school-age children is the development of vocal cord nodules. The nodules usually occur bilaterally and are whitish protuberances on the free margin of the true vocal cords, located at the junction of their anterior and middle thirds, which is the area of maximum vibration. Nodule formation is attributed to submucosal hemorrhages caused by screaming or shouting. The hemorrhages then are organized into fibrous nodules or polyps. Speech therapy may resolve the nodules and alleviate the hoarseness. Surgical removal of the nodules usually is not indicated, but in specific situations, such as when the hoarseness has lasted for several years without improvement, with worsening, or with psychological sequelae, vocal nodule microsurgical removal should be considered.[5]

Acute hoarseness may follow endotracheal intubation, aspiration of a foreign body, or fracture of the larynx. Laryngographic investigation of postoperative hoarseness may be helpful.[20]

Tumors. Juvenile laryngeal papillomatosis is the most common benign laryngeal tumor that occurs during childhood. Such papillomas usually present with hoarseness in children between 2 and 7 years of age, but they may occur in newborns. The tumor consists of wartlike proliferations of stratified squamous epithelium arising in the glottic region, but occasionally it spreads to involve the trachea, the bronchi, and rarely the lung parenchyma. Caused by human papilloma viruses, this tumor may involute spontaneously during puberty.[13,15] Carbon dioxide laser excision has been very successful in maintaining a patent airway and preserving vocal cord function.[24] Leukocyte interferon administration and ribavirin treatment have shown promise in inducing remission.[21,22] Osteochondroma of the cervical spine has resulted in hoarseness caused by edema, erythema, and deviation of the larynx; surgical excision is curative.[30]

Laryngeal granular cell tumor is an uncommon benign tumor usually seen in adults. However, this tumor should be considered in a hoarse child who has a vocal cord tumor or a subglottic mass. Local excision performed endoscopically usually is curative.[9]

Rhabdomyosarcoma of the larynx is a rare but highly malignant tumor that presents with painful hoarseness. Combined partial laryngectomy, radiotherapy, and chemotherapy have effected high cure rates.[11]

Miscellaneous Causes. Miscellaneous causes of hoarseness during childhood and adolescence include sarcoidosis, which may cause supraglottic granulomas and compression of the left recurrent laryngeal nerve by enlarged lymph nodes; laryngeal neurofibromatosis, amyloidosis, or lipid proteinosis; and vocal cord paralysis secondary to central nervous system malfunction, such as the Arnold-Chiari malformation. In cardiovocal syndrome vocal cord paralysis results from impingement on the left recurrent laryngeal nerve by an enlarged pulmonary artery or an enlarged left atrium.[8]

Relapsing polychondritis is a rare autoimmune-related disorder that has an insidious onset of hoarseness, airway narrowing, and nonspecific systemic complaints. Its management includes steroids and immunosuppressive agents; tracheostomy to maintain an airway is required in some cases.[25]

Other causes of hoarseness that occur during adolescence include abusive, vigorous, loud singing and yelling (without vocal cord nodule formation), pubertal voice changes, laryngeal trauma complications of car and motorcycle accidents, smoking, myasthenia gravis, multiple sclerosis, and functional dysphonia (whispering syndrome in girls and falsetto voice in boys).[14]

RESTORING AND PRESERVING NORMAL PHONATION

Speaking in a pleasant-sounding voice is especially important for older children and adolescents because peers are very cognizant and often intolerant of deviations from the norm. Once the cause of a child's or adolescent's hoarseness is determined, every attempt should be made to restore and preserve vocal function. Voice therapy with a speech pathologist is useful for children who have functional hoarseness as well as for those who have organic hoarseness.

REFERENCES

1. Autier C, Grimfeld A: Endoscopy of the respiratory tract. In Gerbeaux J, Couvreur J, Tournier G, editors: *Pediatric respiratory disease,* New York, 1982, John Wiley & Sons.
2. Bain W et al: Head and neck manifestations of gastroesophageal reflux, *Laryngoscope* 93:175, 1983.
3. Baker BM, Baker CD, Le T: Vocal quality articulation and audiological characteristics of children and young adults with diagnosed allergies, *Ann Otol Rhinol Laryngol* 91:277, 1982.
4. Benjamin B: A new pediatric microlaryngoscope, *Ann Otol Rhinol Laryngol* 93:468, 1984.
5. Benjamin B, Groxson G: Vocal nodules in children, *Ann Otol Rhinol Laryngol* 96:530, 1987.
6. Benjamin B, Parsons DS, Molloy HF: Pachyonychia congenita with laryngeal involvement, *Int J Pediatr Otorhinolaryngol* 13:205, 1987.
7. Burck U et al: A case of lipogranulomatosis Farber: some clinical and ultrastructural aspects, *Eur J Pediatr* 143:203, 1985.
8. Condon LM et al: Cardiovocal syndrome in infancy, *Pediatrics* 75:22, 1985.
9. Conley SF, Milbrath MM, Beste DJ: Pediatric laryngeal granular cell tumor, *J Otolaryngol* 21:450, 1992.
10. Cotton RT, Richardson MA: Congenital laryngeal anomalies, *Otolaryngol Clin North Am* 14:203, 1981.
11. DeGroot TR, Frazer JP, Wood BP: Combination therapy for laryngeal rhabdomyosarcoma, *Am J Otolaryngol* 1:456, 1980.
12. Dole M et al: Hoarseness in children with neutropenia, *J Pediatr* 113:782, 1988.
13. Doyle DJ et al: Recurrent respiratory papillomatosis: juvenile vs adult forms, *Laryngoscope* 104:523, 1994.
14. Froese AP, Sims P: Functional dysphonia in adolescence: two case reports, *Can J Psychol* 32:389, 1987.
15. Hartley C et al: Recurrent respiratory papillomatosis—the Manchester experience 1974-1992, *J Laryngol Otol* 108:226, 1994.
16. Hass A et al: Hoarseness in immunocompromised children: association with invasive fungal infection, *J Pediatr* 111:731, 1987.
17. Henry RL: Inhaled cortiocosteroid agents and dysphonia, *Med J Aust* 147:365, 1987.
18. Hillerdal G, Lindholm H: Laryngeal edema as the only symptom of hypersensitivity to salicylic acid and other substances, *J Laryngol Otol* 98:547, 1984.
19. Katz P: Ambulatory esophageal and hypopharyngeal pH monitoring in patients with hoarseness, *Am J Gastroenterol* 85:38, 1990.
20. Lesser T, Williams G: Laryngographic investigation of postoperative hoarseness, *Clin Otolaryngol* 13:37, 1988.
21. McCabe BF, Clark KF: Interferon and laryngeal papillomatosis, *Ann Otol Rhinol Laryngol* 92:2, 1983.
22. Morrison GA, Kotecha B, Evans JN: Ribavirin treatment for juvenile respiratory papillomatosis, *J Laryngol Otol* 105:423, 1993.
23. Murphy FK, Patamasucon P: Congenital syphilis. In Holmes KK et al, editors: *Sexually transmitted diseases,* New York, 1990, McGraw-Hill.
24. Ossoff RH, Toriumi DM, Duncavage JA: The use of the laser in head and neck surgery, *Adv Otolaryngol Head Neck Surg* 1:220, 1987.
25. Prasid S, Grundfast KW, Lipnick R: Airway obstruction in an adolescent with relapsing polychondritis, *Otolaryngol Head Neck Surg* 103:113, 1990.
26. Putnam PE, Orenstein SR: Hoarseness in a child with gastroesophageal reflux, *Acta Paediatr* 81:635, 1992.
27. Richter JE: Hoarseness and gastroesophageal reflux: what is the relationship? *Gastroenterology* 98:1717, 1990.
28. Rontal E et al: Quantitative and objective evaluation of vocal cord function, *Ann Otol Rhinol Laryngol* 92:421, 1983.
29. Savage MM, Crockett DM, McCabe BF: Lipoid proteinosis of the larynx: a cause of voice change in the infant and young child, *Int J Pediatr Otorhinolaryngol* 15:33, 1988.
30. Scher N, Panje WR: Osteochondroma presenting as a neck mass, *Laryngoscope* 98:550, 1988.
31. Shabbir G, Hassan M, Kazmi A: Laryngo-onycho-cutaneous syndrome—a study of 22 cases, *Biomedica* 2:15, 1986.
32. Shah P, Ramakantan R: Hoarseness of the voice due to recurrent laryngeal nerve palsy in tuberculous mediastinitis, *Arch Otolaryngol Head Neck Surg* 116:108, 1990.
33. Small PM et al: Cytomegalovirus infection of the laryngeal nerve presenting as hoarseness in patients with acquired immunodeficiency syndrome, *Am J Med* 86:108, 1989.
34. Sutphen JL: Pediatric gastroesophageal reflux disease, *Gastroenterol Clin North Am* 19:617, 1990.
35. Teebi AS et al: A new autosomal recessive disorder resembling Weaver syndrome, *Am J Med Genet* 33:479, 1989.
36. Varteresian-Karanfil L et al: Pulmonary infection and cavity formation

caused by *Mycobacterium tuberculosis* in a child with AIDS, *N Engl J Med* 319:1018, 1988.

37. Vaughan CW: When to refer the hoarse patient, *Hosp Pract* 24:21, 1989.
38. Vyravanathan S: Hoarseness in tuberculosis, *J Laryngol Otol* 97:523, 1983.
39. Wilson DK: *Voice problems of children,* Baltimore, 1979, Williams & Wilkins.
40. Yanagisawa E, Yanagisawa K: Stroboscopic videolaryngoscopy: a comparison of fiberscopic and telescopic documentation, *Ann Otol Rhinol Laryngol* 102:255, 1993.

SUGGESTED READINGS

Aronson A: *Clinical voice disorders: an interdisciplinary approach,* New York, 1980, Thieme-Stratton.

Bluestone, CD, Stool SE: *Pediatric otolaryngology,* Philadelphia, 1990, WB Saunders.

Tucker HM: *The larynx,* New York, 1993, Thieme.

145 Hyperhidrosis

Nancy K. Barnett

Hyperhidrosis, or sweating more than normal, occurs commonly in childhood. The child or the family usually expresses concern because the sweating is either odiferous or so intense that it interferes with hand or foot functions, (e.g., holding a pencil). Axillary hyperhidrosis usually becomes more of a problem in adolescence because of the odor associated with bacterial degradation of apocrine sweat—the apocrine glands being stimulated at puberty by androgenic hormones. However, palmar and plantar hyperhidrosis secondary to eccrine sweat production may occur at any age.

Palmoplantar hyperhidrosis is thought to be stimulated by anxiety, whereas axillary hyperhidrosis probably is stimulated by both heat and emotion. It is postulated that emotions and the temperature of the blood perfusing the hypothalamus stimulate the secretion of the hormones that regulate the autonomic nervous system's control of perspiration.[1]

Excessive sweating that is not chronic or limited to the palms, soles, and axillae may indicate a systemic disorder, such as infection, lymphoma, thyrotoxicosis, Riley-Day syndrome, hypoglycemia, drug withdrawal, or pheochromocytoma. These disorders must be diagnosed and evaluated only in the face of *generalized* increased perspiring.

Systemic anticholinergic agents will control hyperhidrosis, but the side effects of cholinergic blockage preclude their long-term use. The application of aluminum salts (Drysol) every other day probably is the most effective treatment for palmar sweating. Plantar hyperhidrosis also responds to aluminum salts, and one can use absorbent powders (e.g., Zeasorb) more easily here than on the palms. The patient should be allowed to go barefoot whenever possible. For bromhidrosis (malodorous hyperhidrosis) of the soles, cleansing frequently with drying deodorant soaps and applying topical antibiotics (erythromycin, tetracycline, or clindamycin) may help.

Axillary hyperhidrosis is troublesome because in the face of continual sweating, it is difficult to maintain an effective antiperspirant in contact with the axillary skin. One approach consists of applying a saturated solution of aluminum chlorohydroxide in absolute ethanol or isopropyl alcohol to the axillary vault at night under occlusion. For individuals who have axillary hyperhidrosis and bromhidrosis, frequent clothing changes may be necessary, as well as the use of topical antibiotics and deodorant powders. In extreme cases, when these measures fail and the patient is desperate for relief, local axillary skin can be excised with reasonable expectation of success. Because of its attendant complications, ganglion sympathectomy cannot be recommended for most patients who have axillary hyperhidrosis.[2,3]

REFERENCES

1. Cage GW, Shwachman H, Sato K: Hyperhidrosis. In Fitzpatrick TB et al, editors: *Dermatology in general medicine,* New York, 1979, McGraw-Hill.
2. Hurwitz S: *Clinical pediatric dermatology,* Philadelphia, 1981, WB Saunders.
3. Shelley WB, Hurley HJ: Studies on topical antiperspirant control of axillary hyperhidrosis, *Acta Derm Venereol (Stockh)* 55:241, 1975.

146 Hypotonia

Cynthia H. Cole

Infants who have hypotonia ("floppy" infants) are born with sufficient frequency to require the pediatrician to have some experience in their initial assessment and eventual management. Often the extensive list of potential causes of hypotonia may be narrowed based on the history, perinatal events, and physical examination. Even in cases in which a careful history and physical examination yield limited or confounding information, the cause of hypotonia may be clarified through diagnostic studies (e.g., muscle biopsies, muscle chemistry analysis, electromyography, nerve conduction studies, or nerve biopsy). Tracking the course and evolution of manifestations may contribute to the final diagnosis. The following discussion approaches the topic of hypotonia from the perspective of the clinical presentation (with emphasis on the "anatomical" localization of dysfunction) and laboratory evaluation. In addition, a brief profile of various disorders is provided.

CLINICAL EVALUATION OF HYPOTONIA

Hypotonia is a dysfunction of the motor system and should be suspected in any infant who assumes unusual postures, has decreased resistance to passive movements, and demonstrates relative immobility. Hypotonic infants may have excessive range of joint mobility or joint contractures caused by immobility in utero (e.g., arthrogryposis multiplex congenita). Some hypotonic infants may have additional problems such as difficulty sucking and swallowing, reduced respiratory excursion, which leads to frequent respiratory infections, and delays in attaining motor milestones.

The history and family evaluation often are relevant to specific disorders. The pregnancy history may be significant for polyhydramnios (secondary to dysfunctional fetal swallowing) and decreased fetal movement. The perinatal history may reveal intrauterine exposure of the baby to magnesium, obstetrical analgesia or anesthesia, or evidence of obstetrical trauma. Family history and examination of the parents may be positive for a specific motor disorder (e.g., myasthenia gravis or myotonic dystrophy).

Physical evaluation of the hypotonic infant requires an orderly approach. Consideration of the effects of the major contributors of the motor system is critical for "localization" of the dysfunction. The major levels and components of the motor system include (1) central or "above the lower motor" neuron, (2) the lower motor neuron (anterior horn cells of spinal cord), (3) the peripheral or cranial nerve level, (4) the myoneural junction, and (5) the muscle itself. Motor dysfunction at any level results in hypotonia.[1,4,8] The first goal is to determine if the hypotonia is central (i.e., above the lower motor neuron) or peripheral (at or below the lower motor neuron). Peripheral hypotonia is associated with *significant* weakness; central hypotonia is *not* associated with *significant* weakness.

Thus it is important from a localization perspective to assess whether *significant* muscle weakness accompanies hypotonia.[3,7,9] This assessment may be difficult. Significant weakness is not present if an infant can move spontaneously and withdraw an extremity or raise it against gravity. Hypotonia often is associated with some degree of weakness, so *complete* absence of weakness is unusual. Therefore the evaluation should distinguish whether *significant* muscle weakness is or is not associated with the hypotonia.

Additional evaluation of mental status, response to deep tendon reflexes and sensory stimuli, sucking, swallowing, respiratory distress, facial movements, ophthalmoplegia, gesticulations, and joint contractures help to localize the category of hypotonia.

Hypotonia without Significant Weakness

If significant muscle weakness does *not* accompany hypotonia, then the etiology of the baby's "floppiness" is *central* and involves pathology of the cerebral cortex, the corticospinal-corticobulbar and other spinal tracts; involves the basal ganglia or the cerebellum; or is caused by a systemic disorder (e.g., connective tissue disorders, endocrinopathies, genetic or syndromal disorders, or metabolic disorders) that can affect motor function. The majority of hypotonic infants have a "central" CNS disorder or systemic illness that explains the "floppy baby" presentation. Specific features characteristic of "central" motor disorders include preservation of the deep tendon reflexes and the presence of additional signs of CNS involvement (e.g., lethargy, failure to track visually, altered mental status, seizures). Arthrogryposis, or joint contractures, secondary to prolonged, severe in utero inactivity, may be apparent. A narrow arched palate may result from decreased fetal thrusting.

The differential diagnosis of central hypotonia is diverse and includes such entities as hypoxic-ischemic encephalopathy (HIE), intracranial hemorrhage or infection, neurodegenerative disorders, developmental anomalies of the CNS and spinal cord, and CNS or spinal cord trauma. Systemic disorders, as noted above, should be considered as well. Therefore the diagnostic evaluation will be guided by the history and clues derived from the patient's presentation. Hypoxic-ischemic encephalopathy, the most common cause of hypotonia in the neonatal period, usually is apparent based on the perinatal history and the neonatal examination. It is important to consider whether HIE is the *primary* cause of hypotonia or whether HIE is a *secondary* complication of respiratory failure and accompanying hypotonia of some other cause.

Hypotonia with Significant Weakness

Hypotonia with weakness is caused by (1) disorders of the lower motor neuron, (2) peripheral neuropathies, (3) disorders of the neuromuscular junction, and (4) disorders of the muscle itself.

Disorders of the lower motor neuron involve the anterior horn cells of the spinal cord and are characterized by hypotonia, muscle weakness, and eventually areflexia. These features are observed in the presence of an alert infant whose sensory and sphincter function is intact. Fasciculations may be visualized or detected on an electromyogram (EMG). Werdnig-Hoffmann disease, glycogen storage disease type II (Pompe disease), and anterior horn cell neurogenic arthrogryposis multiplex congenita are examples of lower motor neuron disorders. Each of these has specific features that may distinguish them from each other. Werdnig-Hoffmann disease typically follows a deteriorating course, in contrast to the nonprogressive course of most cases of neurogenic arthrogryposis multiplex congenita. Pompe disease may be distinguished from the other lower motor neuron disorders by the presence of cardiac failure, hepatomegaly, and glycogen in muscle, tongue, and anterior horn cells.

Peripheral neuropathies seldom are diagnosed in the neonatal period but manifest signs similar to those of lower motor neuron disorders, such as hypotonia, weakness, and hypoactive or absent reflexes. In addition, sensory deficits may be elicited in some peripheral neuropathies. Elevation of cerebrospinal fluid (CSF) protein and reduction of nerve conduction velocities are features of polyneuropathies. The diagnosis of peripheral neuropathy may be established with a nerve biopsy. A muscle biopsy shows a denervation pattern of group atrophy, and the EMG reveals fasciculations. Hypomyelinating neuropathies are rare disorders that present with severe generalized hypotonia.[6] Charcot-Marie-Tooth disease is a peripheral neuropathy seen in infants; Guillain-Barré syndrome and infectious and toxic polyneuritis may occur at any age.[6]

Disorders of the neuromuscular junction (presynaptic and postsynaptic defects) share common features of hypotonia and weakness. However, they are distinguished by differences in onset and evolution, patterns of hypotonia and weakness, characteristic EMG findings, and pathogenesis. Deep tendon reflexes and muscle biopsy results are normal. Examples of myoneural junction disorders include neonatal transient myasthenia gravis and congenital myasthenia gravis syndromes (postsynaptic defects) and infantile botulism (presynaptic defect). Dysfunction of the myoneural junction also may be induced by hypermagnesemia and aminoglycoside antibiotic therapy. (Infantile botulism [presynaptic defect] presents relatively acutely with feeding difficulties, constipation, and severe hypotonia at 2 to 4 months of age.) Disorders of the neuromuscular junction are important to recognize because supportive and anticholinesterase therapeutic interventions are available. The myasthenia gravis disorders that affect neonates and older infants are profiled clinically below.

Disorders of the muscle share nonspecific features of hypotonia, weakness, and depressed deep tendon reflexes. The EMG may reveal a characteristic but nondiagnostic pattern. Muscle enzymes are variably elevated, depending on the particular myopathy. A muscle disorder often is diagnosed based on the particular myopathic pattern shown on the muscle biopsy.

Additional Neurological Evaluation. Assessment of specific neurological features may help to determine the cause of hypotonia. Altered or depressed mental status or seizures suggest that the hypotonia is "central" in origin. Neuroimaging EEG may be informative. The pattern and distribution of significant weakness (if present) vary among disorders. Disease of the peripheral nerve is characterized by weakness that often is greater in the distal than in the proximal limbs, whereas the opposite is true for myopathies and variably true for lower motor neuron disorders. The facial muscles may be involved more prominently in disorders of the myoneural junction compared with a late or variable involvement in disorders of the anterior horn cell or in myopathies.

Deep tendon reflexes are normal in "central" and myoneural junction disorders, depressed in peripheral neuropathies and myopathies, and eventually absent in anterior horn cell disease.

Evaluation of the sensory level may differentiate transection of the spinal cord from anterior horn cell disease. Diminished touch and vibratory perception may be found in some peripheral neuropathies. Cranial nerve function may be abnormal in myasthenia gravis, ocular dystrophies, myotubular myopathy, and Möbius syndrome. Additional information that influences clinical evaluation of the hypotonic infant includes the age of the patient at the onset of signs and symptoms and the clinical course (nonprogressive or progressive).

DIAGNOSTIC STUDIES

The initial diagnosis of a hypotonic patient may be sufficiently clear from a thorough history and physical examination alone. Laboratory evaluation for systemic or CNS infection, drug effect, biochemical or metabolic abnormality, karyotype analysis, and neuroimaging should be considered. This occurs more commonly in the group of disorders in which hypotonia is present without weakness. Floppiness resulting from hypotonia associated with weakness usually requires further diagnostic studies. Patterns of abnormality determined by EMG, nerve conduction studies (NCS), and muscle biopsies can help to localize the site of pathology and facilitate definitive diagnosis. However, whether and when these adjunctive tests should be obtained requires careful consideration because appropriate timing affects how informative the result may be.

Muscle Enzyme Levels

Serum levels of creatinine phosphokinase (CPK), creatine kinase (CK), serum glutamic-oxaloacetic transaminase (SGOT), serum glutamic pyruvic transaminase (SGPT), aldolase, and lactic acid dehydrogenase (LDH) help to identify only a few muscle disorders. These levels are increased moderately in Duchenne and Becker muscular dystrophies and less so in the facioscapulohumeral and limb-girdle dystrophies. CPK levels may be increased slightly in spinal muscular atrophy and in many congenital myopathies; CPK levels also are increased during the first few days of life and remain elevated for 4 to 6 weeks. Some infants who have primary muscle disease or denervating disease have variably elevated levels of CK although a normal CK before 6 weeks of age does not rule out a muscular dystrophy. Thus it may not be helpful to measure muscle enzyme levels in the initial evaluation of infants and young children who have hypotonia.

Muscle Biopsy

A muscle biopsy is essential in diagnosing a disorder in which weakness is associated with hypotonia. It must be kept in mind that muscle biopsies may be nonspecific or nondiagnostic in newborns and that biopsy results may change with time. A biopsy in 3 to 6 months time may be necessary to make a diagnosis. It is important that an individual assessing the biopsy specimen of a newborn be expert in the pathological conditions associated with that age and, specifically, with neonatal muscle biopsies. Various histological patterns—denervation, myopathy, and inflammation—may shed light on the diagnosis. Proliferation of adipose and connective tissue is common in muscular dystrophy, neurogenic atrophies, and other myopathies. Characteristic morphological, histochemical, and electron-microscopic markers are essential in the diagnosis of congenital myopathies because these disorders often have similar clinical presentations.

Electrodiagnostic Studies

Electromyography and nerve conduction studies, both sensory and motor, may help to distinguish among myopathies, neuromuscular junction disorders, and denervation myopathy. Although electrodiagnostic studies are useful, both tests have limitations. Electromyograms may be unreliable and difficult to interpret in the newborn period, and the results may change with time. An EMG performed on a muscle at rest in which fasciculations and sharp waves are present may indicate denervation, but these may be seen in the distal muscles of normal infants. Disorders of the CNS demonstrate normal EMGs, with the exception of spinal cord defects, where denervation is confined to a specific level or segmental distribution. An abnormal EMG may direct attention to specific diseases. If an EMG suggests myopathy, sufficient sampling of muscles helps to define the most affected site whose contralateral homologue would optimize biopsy information. However, an EMG may be normal in some congenital and metabolic myopathies.[6] Nerve conduction studies may be difficult to interpret in small children. Slow conduction velocities may be seen in peripheral neuropathies, and repetitive stimulation is useful in diagnosing myasthenia gravis. EMG and NCS should be performed and interpreted by someone skilled in neonatal EMG and NCS. The results should be considered within the clinical context of the patient. The individual interpreting the results should be familiar with normal maturation of neuromuscular function and the spectrum of diseases encountered in neonates or infants.

Ultrasound Imaging

Ultrasound imaging recently has been used to differentiate neuromuscular from nonneuromuscular disorders.[4,5] The ultrasonic pattern of Werdnig-Hoffmann disease is heterogeneously hyperechoic and distinctly different from myopathic images obtained of Duchenne muscular dystrophy and polymyositis. Muscle sonogram also may be useful in locating muscles most appropriate for biopsy or electrodiagnostic testing because all muscles may not be affected uniformly.

COMMON DISORDERS OF THE HYPOTONIC INFANT

When all data have been gathered from the available sources a definitive diagnosis often is possible. The most frequent diagnoses encompass relatively few conditions; it therefore is useful to highlight these more common causes of hypotonia.

Disorders of Hypotonia Without Associated Weakness

Disorders of the Central Nervous System. Disorders of the CNS commonly are associated with hypotonia and delayed motor milestones. Mental retardation may be present, along with global developmental delay. In the majority of patients who have nonspecific mental retardation, no diagnosis or clinical disorder can be recognized. However, in some (Down syndrome and other genetic syndromes) the clinical features may be sufficient to define a specific disorder. If a child demonstrates loss of acquired developmental milestones, a degenerative CNS disorder resulting from various storage diseases must be considered and investigated. Hypotonia associated with CNS disorders varies in degree and subsequent course. Hypotonic cerebral palsy has features of athetosis and ataxia with or without increased deep tendon reflexes (DTRs), in addition to hypotonia. Various metabolic disorders (aminoacidopathies, organic acidemias, mucopolysaccharidoses, and lipidoses) may manifest with hypotonia, failure to thrive, and other nonspecific symptoms. Acidosis, hypoglycemia, and hyperbilirubinemia may be found with chemical screening tests. The ferric chloride test is a useful metabolic urine screen for some aminoacidopathies. However, specific analysis of blood and urine for amino acids, organic acids, or urinary sulfates (keratan, dermatan, haparan) should be requested if clinical judgment suggests one of these metabolic disorders. Cultured fibroblasts also are used to diagnose the specific enzyme deficiency in mucopolysaccharidoses. Lipidoses (Tay-Sachs disease, metachromatic leukodystrophy, Krabbe leukodystrophy) are disorders of lipid metabolism and are characterized by progressive mental retardation, hypotonia, and possible diminished nerve conduction velocity. Eventually, muscle biopsy may reveal degenerative changes. Cerebral trauma, hemorrhage, or anoxic insult will produce varying degrees and durations of hypotonia.

Connective Tissue Disorders. Connective tissue disorders may be associated with lax joints, hypotonia, and delayed motor milestones. Ehlers-Danlos syndrome also exhibits hyperelasticity of the skin. Marfan syndrome is characterized by hypotonia, delayed motor milestones, increased joint laxity, tall stature, dislocated lenses, and vascular lesions. Osteogenesis imperfecta varies in presentation depending on the specific form of this disorder's spectrum. Hypotonia, blue sclerae, multiple fractures, and delayed motor milestones are classic features. Congenital laxity of ligaments has no other clinical features in addition to increased joint laxity. Mucopolysaccharidoses may manifest with hypotonia and delayed motor and intellectual milestones. The diagnosis usually is based on characteristic facial and clinical features and is confirmed by appropriate biochemical screening of acid mucopolysaccharides in urine and by cell cultures of lymphocytes and fibroblasts.

Endocrine Disorders. Hypothyroidism, hypopituitarism, and Cushing syndrome may be associated with hypotonia. Clinical features and biochemical analyses of serum electrolytes, glucose, and various hormones usually reveal the specific disorder.

Metabolic Disorders. Many of the previously mentioned disorders are metabolically based. Infantile hypercalcemia and renal tubular acidosis may have associated hypotonia and failure to thrive; serum and urine chemistry analyses are necessary to establish the diagnosis.

Miscellaneous Disorders. It is not practical to discuss here all the possible causes of hypotonia without associated weakness. However, a few deserve mention. Prader-Willi syndrome manifests in the newborn with extreme floppiness, feeding difficulties, weak cry, sticky saliva, genital hypoplasia, and cryptorchidism. The characteristic facies of this disorder may not be prominent and therefore may be overlooked. Obesity begins around 2 to 3 years of age in association with hyperphagia. Short stature and mental retardation are two additional features. Prader-Willi syndrome may be diagnosed by clinical criteria and molecular genetic techniques, looking for deletions of chromosome 15q11-13 region.[2] Nutritional disorders (e.g., celiac disease and rickets) may exhibit hypotonia associated with malnourishment and failure to thrive. Some infants defy diagnosis and exhibit hypotonia as an isolated feature, with no other demonstrable disorder. In these instances the hypotonia may improve with time.

Disorders That Produce Significant Weakness and Incidental Hypotonia

Spinal Muscular Atrophy Syndromes. Spinal muscular atrophy syndromes are a group of heritable degenerative diseases caused by degeneration of the nuclei of the motor cranial nerves and anterior horn cells of the spinal cord. The denervation leads to muscular atrophy. The acute form of spinal muscular atrophy (Werdnig-Hoffmann disease) is autosomal recessive and the most definable cause of severely hypotonic, floppy infants.[8] Weakness may have its onset in utero, be apparent in the neonatal period in one third of the cases, or apparent in more than half the cases in the first 3 months of life. Other forms of spinal muscular atrophy may not have their onset until after a few months or even after 5 to 10 years of age. Although these disorders usually progress quite rapidly, with many infants dying before 3 years of age, it is difficult to predict the clinical course. These infants characteristically have few spontaneous movements and appear floppy, with poor head, trunk, and extremity control. Breathing is abdominal with little chest movement. The alert facial expression is in striking contrast to the general paralysis. Weakness of bulbar musculature is manifested as impaired sucking and weak cry. Fasciculations may be seen in the tongue of some patients. The deep tendon reflexes usually are diminished or lost early in the course of the disease. Infants do respond to painful stimuli. Muscle enzyme levels usually are normal, except that CPK levels may be mildly elevated. Biopsy shows a classic denervation pattern: large groups of uniformly atrophic muscle fibers interspersed with single or groups of normal or enlarged fibers. Electromyography reveals a denervation pattern. Supportive treatment is all one can offer. Most of these infants develop complications of contractures and osteoporosis (resulting from immobilization) and are prone to the morbidity of repeated respiratory infections and aspiration pneumonia. Less severe forms of spinal muscular atrophy may manifest with delay in motor milestones, hypotonia, and muscle weakness. In early- or late-onset forms proximal muscles always are affected more than distal muscles. Inheritance is of the autosomal recessive type.

Myasthenia Gravis. Different forms of myasthenia gravis may appear during the neonatal period. These forms are broadly categorized as (1) neonatal transient myasthenia gravis and (2) congenital myasthenia syndromes. Each of these disorders manifests with hypotonia and muscle weakness. Both respond to anticholinesterase therapy and display decremental response to repetitive motor nerve stimulation.

Neonatal transient myasthenia gravis is the most common of these disorders. It is an immune-mediated process that occurs in 10% to 15% of infants born to mothers who have myasthenia gravis, presumably as a result of passive transfer of antiacetylcholine receptor antibody across the placenta. No correlation exists between the severity of neuromuscular dysfunction of the newborn and the degree or duration of maternal myasthenia gravis. The occurrence of one affected child increases the risk that future siblings will be symptomatic. Symptoms of feeding difficulties, weak cry, and respiratory problems may evolve rapidly during the first 24 to 72 hours of life. Generalized hypotonia is apparent in approximately 50% of affected infants. Deep tendon reflexes generally are normal. Although facial diplegia is frequently observed, ophthalmoplegia and ptosis are seen infrequently in neonatal transient myasthenia gravis, in contrast to the prominent ocular involvement in congenital myasthenia gravis syndromes. The diagnosis may be confirmed by evidence of the myasthenic phenomena in response to repetitive motor nerve stimulation and by a positive response to anticholinesterase medication (e.g., neostigmine 0.1 mg/kg intramuscularly). Symptoms may last from 2 to 8 weeks. Patients who have marginal motor deficits should receive electrophysiological therapy to minimize the risk of serious deterioration and morbidity.

Congenital myasthenia gravis syndromes occur in infants of normal mothers, have a rare tendency to occur in siblings, and demonstrate a variety of defects in the neuromuscular junction. A true genetic basis for all congenital myasthenia syndromes is not established. "Congenital myasthenia," the most common of these syndromes, has its onset in the first weeks of life, and is characterized by prominent ptosis and evolving ophthalmoplegia. In general, hypotonia and weakness are not pronounced. However, fluctuating facial diplegia and a weak suck and cry are common. The course is persistent and mild. All features of the disorder, except for ophthalmoplegia, respond to anticholinesterase therapy.

Electrophysiological studies and treatment are as for neonatal transient myasthenia gravis except that therapy is required for life. "Familial infantile myasthenia" syndrome may be dramatically apparent at birth with apnea, respiratory distress, feeding problems, facial diplegia, less pronounced ptosis, and no ophthalmoplegia. The course is episodic and has natural remissions and relapses. Diagnosis and treatment are as for the other myasthenia gravis syndromes.

Congenital Myotonic Dystrophy. Classic myotonic dystrophy primarily is a disease of early childhood. It is an autosomal dominant inherited disease.[1,4,8] The congenital form of myotonic dystrophy manifests with general hypotonia (often profound), difficulty in sucking and swallowing, and varying degrees of respiratory difficulties (which may necessitate assisted ventilation), associated skeletal deformities (e.g., scoliosis, talipes equinovarus), arthrogryposis of lower extremities, facial diplegia (open, triangular-shaped mouth and open eyes), and diminished or absent reflexes. Abdominal distention and ileus may result from smooth muscle involvement. Mental retardation is another common feature that may manifest subsequently.

The clinical course of congenital myotonic dystrophy is one of gradual improvement in muscle tone over several weeks, so the infant may be weaned from assisted ventilation and fed from a bottle. Patients subsequently develop the clinical and electromyographical features characteristic of classic myotonic dystrophy.

The explanation for the congenital form of myotonic dystrophy is the presence of an unidentified maternal intrauterine factor that affects babies who have inherited the dominant gene for myotonic dystrophy. The congenital form is not seen in infants who have not inherited the dominant gene and are born to affected mothers.

The pregnancy history frequently is remarkable for evidence of decreased fetal movement and polyhydramnios, presumably resulting from the inability of the fetus to swallow.

The diagnosis is based on the infant's clinical features and confirmation of myotonic dystrophy in the mother by examination and electromyography.

Congenital Muscular Dystrophy

Congenital muscular dystrophy represents a group of poorly defined muscle disorders that may or may not have CNS involvement along with diffuse hypotonia and weakness. Congenital muscular dystrophy is not a distinct disease with specific histological findings. Other features of congenital muscular dystrophy at birth include weakness of face, neck, and limbs (proximal more than distal); presence of arthrogryposis multiplex congenita; and swallowing and respiratory problems. The progression of the clinical course varies. Three forms of congenital muscular dystrophy associated with CNS involvement differ neuropathologically. The serum CPK is elevated, and electromyography reveals a myopathic pattern. CT scan of the brain is useful in identifying gyral abnormalities and cerebral hypodensity, and muscle biopsy reveals a dystrophic process that may vary in severity in terms of muscle replacement by adipose tissue and connective tissue proliferation. Inheritance is consistent with an autosomal recessive pattern. Duchenne muscular dystrophy (a common, sex-linked recessive muscle disease of childhood) is not symptomatic in the neonatal period, but can have a presumptive neonatal diagnosis based on elevated CPK and a positive family history. Gene therapy research for Duchenne muscular dystrophy is in progress.[10]

Congenital Myopathies. Congenital myopathies include a number of entities that manifest with hypotonia from the neonatal period through infancy. Weakness may be proximal or diffuse and can range from mild to severe. Because it can be diagnosed only by muscle biopsy with detailed histochemical and electron microscopic studies, the names of congenital myopathies have been based on the results of these studies. They include those that have (1) *structural abnormalities*—central core disease, nemaline rod myopathy, minicore disease, myotubular myopathy, mitochondrial myopathies, nonspecific congenital myopathies, congenital fiber-type disproportion, and congenital type 1 fiber predominance; and (2) *metabolic abnormalities*—glycogen storage diseases (types II, III, IV, V, and VII with variable degrees of muscular, cardiac, and hepatic involvement, depending on the specific enzyme deficiency); and abnormal lipid metabolism (carnitine deficiency, carnitine palmitoyl transferase deficiency, and periodic paralysis).

CONCLUSION

Often the underlying cause of hypotonia in the neonate is diagnosed accurately through a systematic approach and use of information from investigative procedures that complement one another. Appropriate diagnosis is important for specific treatment (e.g., myasthenia gravis syndromes), prognosis, planning supportive treatment, and genetic counseling.

REFERENCES

1. Brzustowicz LM et al: Genetic mapping of chronic childhood-onset spinal muscular atrophy to chromosome 5q11.2-13.3, *Nature* 344:540, 1990.
2. Donaldson MDC et al: The Prader-Willi syndrome, *Arch Dis Child* 70:58, 1994.
3. Dubowitz V: *The floppy infant,* Philadelphia, 1980, JB Lippincott.
4. Fischer AQ: The use of ultrasound in evaluating neurologic diseases of childhood, *Neurol Clin* 8:759, 1990.
5. Heckmatt JZ, Leeman S, Dubowitz V: Ultrasound imaging in the diagnosis of muscle disease, *J Pediatr* 101:656, 1982.
6. Jones HR: EMG evaluation of the floppy infant: differential diagnosis and technical aspects, *Muscle Nerve* 13:338, 1990.
7. Menkes JH: Diseases of the motor unit. In Avery ME, Taeusch HW, editors: *Diseases of the newborn,* Philadelphia, 1984, WB Saunders.
8. Miller VS, Delgado M, Iannaccone ST: Neonatal hypotonia, *Semin Neurol* 13:73, 1993.
9. Volpe JJ: *Neurology of the newborn,* ed 2, Philadelphia, 1987, WB Saunders.
10. Wolff JA: Gene therapy for neuromuscular disorders, *Pediatr Res* 35:155A, 1994.

SUGGESTED READINGS

Clairezux AE, Lake BD: Muscle disorders in the floppy child. In Rosenberg HS, Bolande RP, editors: *Perspectives in pediatric pathology,* vol 4, Chicago, 1978, Mosby.

Dubowitz V: *Muscle disorders in childhood,* Philadelphia, 1978, WB Saunders.

Low NL: Spinal muscular atrophy syndromes, *Pediatr Ann* 6:35, 1977.

Paine RS: The future of the "floppy infant": a follow-up of 133 patients, *Dev Med Child Neurol* 5:115, 1963.

Sarnat HB: Diagnostic value of the muscle biopsy in the neonatal period, *Am J Dis Child* 132:782, 1978.

Slater GE, Swaiman KF: Muscular dystrophies of childhood, *Pediatr Ann* 6:50, 1977.

Spiro AJ: Approach to diagnosis in the child with muscle weakness, *Pediatr Ann* 6:11, 1977.

147 Irritability

C. Jean Ogborn

Irritability as a presenting complaint is a common and vexing problem in the pediatric age group. Although experienced clinicians can recognize irritability in a child, agreeing on a concise definition is difficult. *Webster's Ninth New Collegiate Dictionary* defines irritability as "abnormal or excessive excitability of an organ or body part." In the context of pediatrics irritability is an alteration in sensorium that evokes negative behaviors outside the range of normal for the child, including overreaction or inappropriate reaction to normal stimuli.

At the root of the symptom of irritability is the lack of something vital (e.g., oxygen, glucose) and/or the presence of something noxious (e.g., pain, toxins). Irritability may have different causes and manifestations in infants, children, and adolescents. An infant or preverbal child will be unable to offer information about his or her complaint, whereas some older children and adolescents may offer verbal clues to the disease process. In addition, an infant or child who is irritable and has other symptoms generally will have a different underlying disorder than one who has irritability as a sole presenting complaint. An organized approach to the differential diagnosis is essential to minimizing unnecessary testing while making the correct diagnosis.

ACUTE IRRITABILITY

Categories of conditions that can cause acute irritability include infections, trauma, toxins or drugs, metabolic derangements, hypoxic/ischemic events, allergies, and inflammatory processes, among others. Acute irritability may be associated with life-threatening illnesses and physical findings, requiring urgent intervention. A parent who seeks care for an infant who is "fussier than usual" may present with a child who is in shock, in respiratory distress, or having a seizure. The child must be stabilized before a search for the cause begins. Some life-threatening conditions that may cause acute irritability are listed in the box on p. 1030.

If the child does not have an immediately life-threatening condition, a careful history and physical examination are the first steps in the evaluation of irritability and, in many cases, will reveal the cause of the symptom. Many common infectious, traumatic, toxic, allergic, and inflammatory conditions can be diagnosed by history and physical examination alone. Laboratory or radiological procedures may confirm a clinical suspicion. Some conditions associated with acute irritability but generally without life-threatening presentations are listed in the box on p. 1030. Common and some unusual causes of acute irritability are discussed below.

Infections

Meningitis often is suspected when the complaint is irritability in the presence of fever. Lumbar puncture followed by spinal fluid analysis often settles the issue quickly. Encephalitis also must be considered when the infant or child is irritable and has fever without another apparent focus or fever that is associated with hallucinations, seizures, or rash. Spinal fluid pleocytosis and focal findings on MRI or EEG may be suggestive, and viral cultures may yield a pathogen. Treatment mostly is supportive, with parenteral acyclovir for proven or suspected herpes simplex encephalitis.

Urosepsis, *E. coli* sepsis, or group B streptococcal sepsis in a neonate or young infant may present with irritability, fever, and a toxic or shocky appearance. Urinary tract infections in preverbal or nonverbal children may cause fever and irritability without the expressed specific complaints of dysuria or flank pain. Examination of the urine for blood, leukocytes, nitrites, and bacteria is necessary to establish the diagnosis.

Myocarditis and pericarditis with poor cardiac output can present with fever and irritability as the most prominent signs. The presence of tachypnea, tachycardia, and cough may mislead the examiner toward a diagnosis of pneumonia. Chest radiography may or may not show cardiomegaly or pulmonary edema in early stages of these disorders. The findings of hepatomegaly, poor capillary refill, or tachycardia out of proportion to the fever may be clues to the presence of these underrecognized and sometimes deadly causes of heart failure. An echocardiogram and electrocardiogram are useful in making the diagnosis.

Kawasaki disease is thought to result from an infectious process leading to a toxin-mediated generalized vasculitis.[15] Early in its course, fever and extreme irritability may be the most pronounced signs. Conjunctival, dermal, and mucosal vasculitis are responsible for the red eyes, rash, and stomatitis that occur in typical cases. No definitive diagnostic tests exist, but an elevated erythrocyte sedimentation rate (ESR), sterile pyuria, toxic granulations of the neutrophils, and uveitis on slit lamp examination, in conjunction with fever, rash and lymphadenitis, all combine to make the diagnosis. Although not immediately life threatening, recognition of this disorder and treatment with intravenous immunoglobulin within the first 10 days of illness are critical to decreasing the likelihood of coronary artery vasculitis and the formation of an aneurysm.[16,21]

Musculoskeletal infections such as osteomyelitis, diskitis, and septic arthritis may cause fever with pain and irritability. A careful history and physical may yield these diagnoses, or the suspicion of them, but skeletal infectious processes may be nearly indistinguishable from inflammatory or malignant processes, or even behavioral reactions in young infants. Diagnosis may require serial examinations and tests. Plain films of bones and joints may be unrevealing, and further evaluations including ESR, C-reactive protein, complete blood count, blood cultures, bone scan, bone biopsy, and joint aspiration may be necessary.

SOME LIFE-THREATENING CAUSES OF ACUTE IRRITABILITY

Infections

Meningitis
Encephalitis
Myocarditis
Pericarditis
Kawasaki disease*

Trauma

Shaken baby syndrome
Child abuse
Cerebral edema
Acute blood loss

Hypoxia/ischemia

Stroke
Myocardial infarction
Respiratory failure
Carbon monoxide poisoning
Methemoglobinemia
Pulmonary embolism

Metabolic

Hypoglycemia
Hyponatremia
Hypernatremia
Hypocalcemia
Hypercalcemia
Acidosis
Hyperammonemia
Pheochromocytoma
Thyrotoxicosis

Toxins/drugs

Heavy metal intoxication
Chemical exposure
Medication toxicity
Drugs of abuse

Miscellaneous

Heat illness
Malignancy*

*May be life threatening but may not present with emergent symptoms.

SOME CAUSES OF ACUTE IRRITABILITY

Infections

Otitis media and externa
Urinary tract infection
Stomatitis
Dental caries and abscess
Balanitis
Gastroenteritis
Sinusitis
Measles
Osteomyelitis
Septic hip

Trauma

Fractures and dislocations
Corneal abrasions
Anal fissures
Foreign body (eye, ear, nose, skin)
Sunburn
Bites and stings

Toxins/drugs

Medication toxicity and side effects
Substance abuse or withdrawal
Chemical or drug exposure

Allergies

Food and environmental
Contact dermatitis
Eczema

Inflammations

Juvenile rheumatoid arthritis
Toxic synovitis
Inflammatory bowel disease

Miscellaneous

Teething
Colic
Constipation
Hunger
Hyperthermia or hypothermia
Dactylitis and vasoocclusive crisis
Hernia
Diaper rash
Constrictive or abrasive clothing and shoes
Altitude sickness
Phimosis
Torsion of the testis or the ovary
Insect bites or stings

Trauma

In general, irritability will not be the most salient finding in a child who has sustained life-threatening trauma. Important exceptions to this generalization are the shaken baby syndrome, the battered child syndrome, and massive occult blood loss. Infants and very young children who have been shaken may suffer retinal hemorrhages and detachment, subdural or subarachnoid hemorrhages, and cerebral edema.[5] Irritability without an obvious source may be the only external sign of these life-threatening situations. A child who is battered repeatedly (and ultimately at high risk for loss of life) may have occult fractures or intraabdominal contusions and yet evidence very few outward findings except irritability. The clinician should consider carefully the issue of child abuse or neglect in the case of unexplained irritability or irritability resulting from fracture or dislocation, especially in very young or nonambulatory children.[1,5,12]

The pressure of the lap belt of a restraint system in a motor vehicle crash or other blunt abdominal trauma can lead to intraabdominal bleeding from a laceration of the liver, spleen, or bowel wall and the resultant irritability that occurs from hypoperfusion and pain.

Many traumatic causes of irritability that are not life threatening may be apparent on initial physical examination and include fractures or dislocations, anal fissures, corneal abrasions, sunburn, and foreign bodies (including insects) in the eye, nose, or ear or under the skin.

Hypoxic/Ischemic Events

Carbon monoxide poisoning and methemoglobinemia each cause irritability by producing hypoxia. The history and arterial measurement of carboxyhemoglobin or methemoglobin are diagnostic. A cherry red (carboxyhemoglobin) or chocolate brown (methemoglobin) appearance of arterial blood are immediate clues. Pulmonary embolism can cause irritability by inducing sudden hypoxia, and respiratory failure from any cause may be associated with irritability progressing to lethargy.

Altitude sickness from relative hypoxia may cause acute irritability in infants and children, as it may in adults.[2] Reactions to changes in altitude vary among individuals and are difficult to predict. Altitude sickness must be considered in a child from a lower altitude who recently has arrived in the mountains.

Cerebral ischemia from thrombosis or a hemorrhagic stroke may have irritability as a component. Myocardial ischemia is not common in children but can present with irritability. Children who have had Kawasaki disease or have certain congenital heart defects are at risk for thrombosis, arrhythmia, ischemia, and infarction. Vasoocclusive crisis in a child who has sickle cell anemia is an ischemic cause of pain and irritability. With any ischemic insult, older children and adolescents may be able to describe pain, but younger children and infants simply may be irritable.

Metabolic Derangements

Hypoglycemia, hyponatremia or hypernatremia, hypocalcemia or hypercalcemia, hyperammonemia, and acidosis all can cause irritability. In a child who appears toxic and irritable, a quick check of electrolytes may indicate sodium, glucose, calcium, and acid-base abnormalities. Dehydration, hyponatremia, hypernatremia, and acidosis all can result from common gastrointestinal illnesses in infants and young children. Hypoglycemia can result from many causes, including starvation. Infants who are underfed acutely or chronically (e.g., have marasmus or kwashiorkor) may be quite irritable. Older children and adolescents also may exhibit an irritable response to the relative hypoglycemia that occurs if regular meals are delayed. Obtaining ammonia levels is not often part of an initial screening in a child, but the clinician should consider checking it in children who have encephalopathy or evidence of liver disease along with their irritability, all of which could indicate Reye syndrome or congenital enzyme deficiencies.[23] Detection of a metabolic derangement is far simpler than determining the precise cause, and detailed discussion is left to the chapters on metabolic diseases.

Toxins and Drugs

Life-threatening intoxications may result from heavy metals such as lead and mercury,[9] drugs of abuse such as cocaine and alcohol, envenomations by scorpions and snakes, overdoses of or idiosyncratic reactions to medications, and contact with agricultural, industrial, or household chemicals. Careful questioning about recent use of lawn chemicals, pesticides, and cleaning products may be the only clues to these as a cause of irritability because many of these chemicals will not be detected by standard toxicology screenings of blood and urine. Prescribed or over-the-counter medications such as theophylline, beta-agonists, antiepileptics, decongestants, antihistamines, antitussives, and various "cold preparations" may cause irritability even when used as directed, and certainly when overused. Cocaine,[20] alcohol, PCP,[24] inhalants, and other drugs of abuse are known to cause irritability. Infants and children may be exposed to these substances by passive means transplacentally,[17] by ingestion of breast milk,[6] by inhalation, or they may accidentally ingest alcohol or cigarettes and other substances left within reach. A positive history may be difficult to elicit, and a toxicology screen may be helpful. Substance use or withdrawal should be considered in the differential diagnosis when any adolescent presents with irritability. Rarely, intentional poisoning may be the cause of a child's distress.[25]

Allergies

Allergies are a controversial cause of irritability, but one that more and more parents and clinicians recognize. Food allergies, environmental allergies, contact allergies, and severe eczema may result in irritability. Bizarre behavior, temper tantrums, and outbursts of rage reportedly have been caused in some children by allergic responses to foods and environmental allergens.[13,22]

Miscellaneous

Increased intracranial pressure from a brain tumor may present with acute irritability and altered behavior without preceding symptoms such as headache or loss of coordination. Many clinicians remember at least one child who presented with complaints of irritability and intermittent fever and in whom leukemia with bone pain was diagnosed. Malignancies of all sorts may have a component of irritability among their symptoms and must be considered carefully in the child when no other diagnosis is forthcoming.

Heat illness, heat stroke, and malignant hyperthermia all are life-threatening alterations in the body's homeostatic mechanism that may present with irritability. Thyrotoxicosis and pheochromocytoma also may have irritability as a symptom.

Irritability in infants has been attributed to a variety of causes of pain or discomfort that may become obvious during the evaluation, including teething, colic, constipation, diaper rash, hernia, hair wrapped around a digit or penis, prolapsed rectum or urethra, phimosis, testicular torsion, dacty-

SOME CAUSES OF CHRONIC/RECURRENT IRRITABILITY

Psychosocial/psychiatric

Abuse and neglect*
Temperament mismatch
Family discord
Maternal depression
Substance abuse or withdrawal*
Depression*
Psychosis*
Autism

Toxins/drugs

Lead poisoning*
Mercury poisoning*
Hypervitaminosis A
Medication effects

Neurological

Seizures
Migraine
Tumors*
Degenerative diseases*
Postconcussion syndrome

Metabolic/genetic

Urea cycle defects*
Storage diseases*
Fetal alcohol syndrome
Phenylketonuria
Acute intermittent porphyria
Dietary deficit

Miscellaneous

Colic
Vision or hearing impairment
Glaucoma
Reflux esophagitis
Kwashiorkor/marasmus*
Idiopathic hypercalciuria
Pseudotumor cerebri
Hormone effects

*Potentially life threatening.

litis, insect and spider bites or stings, constrictive clothing, and inappropriate clothing leading to hyperthermia or hypothermia. Ovarian torsion is fairly uncommon but can cause pain and irritability in a child and can be difficult to diagnose. An ultrasound examination can be helpful in this regard.

CHRONIC OR RECURRENT IRRITABILITY

Chronic or recurrent irritability in a child challenges both the parents'[11] and the clinician's skills. Psychosocial causes may head the list, but toxic, neurological, metabolic, and miscellaneous causes must be considered and are shown in the box above.

Psychosocial/Psychiatric Disorders

Irritability as a chronic feature of a child's behavior may indicate significant problems with his or her familial relationships and ability to master the environment. Infants may be irritable because of maternal/infant temperament mismatches, maternal depression,[26] or stress within the family surrounding the addition of the new child to the family. Abuse and neglect of a child at any age may provoke irritable behavior or outbursts. An older child or adolescent who has a psychiatric problem such as depression, psychosis, autism, or posttraumatic stress disorder may be described as irritable by parents and others. The investigation and treatment of irritability in these situations may require a multidisciplinary and long-term approach.

Toxins and Drugs

As discussed earlier any medication or drug of abuse may cause irritable behavior in some individuals in some circumstances. Hypervitaminosis A, pseudotumor cerebri,[14] and transient intracranial hypertension of infancy[18] can cause chronic recurrent irritability resulting from elevations in intracranial pressure. Use of steroids among adolescents who are trying to "bulk up" for sports is known to cause irritability and aggression.[3]

Neurological Disorders

Degenerative diseases, brain tumors, migraine headaches, seizures, and postconcussion syndrome are neurological causes for cyclical, chronic, or recurrent irritability among older children and adolescents. Postconcussion or post–head trauma syndrome is particularly distressing to families because the head injury may have occurred months or years before and even might have been minor, yet the irritability and behavior changes may be major and persistent.[7,10]

Metabolic/Genetic Diseases

Urea cycle defects,[23] storage diseases, congenital drug or alcohol syndromes, phenylketonuria, vitamin B_{12} deficit, and acute intermittent porphyria are a few significant disorders that must be considered in the recurrently irritable child.

Miscellaneous

A wide variety of chronic disorders have irritability as a prominent or sole component. Colic is one well-known but little understood disorder that is characterized by recurrent bouts of irritability and crying. Other causes in infants or young children include vision or hearing impairment, glaucoma, reflux esophagitis, and idiopathic hypercalciuria.[8] Hormonal effects associated with adolescence in both males and females can cause moodiness and irritability.[4,19]

CONCLUSION

Irritability has a variety of causes and can be indicative of life-threatening or relatively trivial or transient disorders. A careful history and physical examination most often can determine the cause. In puzzling cases serial examinations and staged laboratory investigations may be necessary. Treatment of irritability depends on its cause.

REFERENCES

1. AAP Committee on Child Abuse and Neglect: Shaken baby syndrome: inflicted cerebral trauma, *Pediatrics* 92:872, 1993.
2. Bahrke MS, Shukitt-Hale B: Effects of altitude on mood, behavior and cognitive functioning: a review *Sports Med* 16:97, 1993.
3. Bahrke MS et al: Psychological moods and subjectively perceived behavioral and somatic changes accompanying anabolic-androgenic steroid use, *Am J Sports Med* 20:717, 1992.
4. Buchanan CM, Eccles JS, Becker JB: Are adolescents the victims of raging hormones: evidence for activational effects of hormones on moods and behavior at adolescence, *Psychol Bull* 111:62, 1992.
5. Caffey J: On the theory and practice of shaking infants, *Am J Dis Child* 124:161, 1972.
6. Chasnoff IJ, Lewis DE, Squires L: Cocaine intoxication in a breast-fed infant, *Pediatrics* 80:836, 1987.
7. Evans RW: The postconcussion syndrome and the sequelae of mild head injury, *Neurol Clin* 10:815, 1992.
8. Fivush B: Irritability and dysuria in infants with idiopathic hypercalciuria, *Pediatr Nephrol* 4:262, 1990.
9. Florentine MJ, Sanfilippo DJ: Elemental mercury poisoning (clinical conference), *Clin Pharmacol* 10:213, 1991.
10. Goldstein J: Posttraumatic headache and the postconcussions syndrome, *Med Clin North Am* 75:641, 1991.
11. Keefe MR, Froese-Fretz A: Living with an irritable infant: maternal perspectives, *Am J Child Nurs* 16:255, 1991.
12. Kempe CH et al: The battered-child syndrome, *JAMA* 181:17, 1962.
13. Klein GL et al: The allergic irritability syndrome: four case reports and a position statement from the Neuroallergy Committee of the American College of Allergy, *Ann Allerg* 55:22, 1985.
14. Lessell S: Pediatric pseudotumor cerebri (idiopathic intracranial hypertension), *Surv Ophthalmol* 37:155, 1992.
15. Leung DYM et al: Toxic shock syndrome toxin-secreting *Staphylococcus aureus* in Kawasaki syndrome, *Lancet* 342:1385, 1993.
16. Levy M, Koren G: Atypical Kawasaki disease: analysis of clinical presentation and diagnostic clues, *Pediatr Infect Dis J* 9:122, 1990.
17. Levy M, Spino M: Neonatal withdrawal syndrome: associated drugs and pharmacologic management, *Pharmacotherapy* 13:202, 1993.
18. Mann NP, McLellan NJ, Cartlidge PH: Transient intracranial hypertension of infancy, *Arch Dis Child* 63:966, 1988.
19. Mortola JF: Issues in the diagnosis and research of premenstrual syndrome, *Clin Obstet Gynecol* 35:587, 1992.
20. Mott SH, Packer RJ, Soldin SJ: Neurologic manifestations of cocaine exposure in childhood, *Pediatrics* 93:557, 1994.
21. Nadel S, Levin M: Kawasaki disease, *Curr Sci* 5:29, 1993.
22. Price CE, Rona RJ, Chinn S: Associations of excessive irritability with common illnesses and food intolerance, *Paediatr Perinat Epidemiol* 4:156, 1990.
23. Rowe PC, Newman SL, Brusilow SW: Natural history of symptomatic partial ornithine transcarbamylase deficiency, *N Engl J Med* 314:541, 1986.
24. Schwartz RH, Einhorn A: PCP intoxication in seven young children, *Pediatr Emerg Care* 2:238, 1986.
25. Woolf AD et al: Intentional infantile ethylene glycol poisoning presenting as an inherited metabolic disorder, *J Pediatr* 120:421, 1992.
26. Zuckerman B et al: Maternal depressive symptoms during pregnancy, and newborn irritability, *J Dev Behav Pediatr* 11:190, 1990.

148 Jaundice

Joel M. Andres and Mary Pat Francisco

Jaundice, a yellow discoloration of skin and mucous membranes, is the most common presenting manifestation of liver dysfunction in infants and children. This important physical finding is a direct indicator of hyperbilirubinemia, or excessive unconjugated and/or conjugated bilirubin in blood and tissues. The spectrum of conditions associated with jaundice ranges from physiological immaturity of bilirubin metabolism in the neonate to life-threatening disruption of liver function in the adolescent who is using illicit drugs. Jaundice always prompts concern and anxiety in the physician, parents, and older child; it is a clinical sign that demands evaluation.

EVALUATION OF THE PATIENT

History

The history is important in determining the patient's age at the onset of the illness, in defining the chronicity of the hepatic dysfunction, and in understanding the clinical manifestations, especially jaundice and hepatomegaly. Inquiry may point to prolonged abdominal distention suggestive of longstanding hepatomegaly, splenomegaly, or ascites. Other manifestations of chronic liver disease are easy bleeding or bruising and peripheral edema. The occurrence of jaundice, dark urine, and acholic stools may help date the onset of illness; also, jaundice usually appears in a cephalad to caudad progression. Pruritus and skin excoriations suggest prolonged cholestasis. The historical assessment also should include questions about maternal illness during pregnancy, exposure to sick individuals, blood products, or hepatotoxins, or recent surgery involving anesthesia. Because inheritable metabolic disease is a more common cause of liver dysfunction in the infant than in the older child or adult, a careful family history is essential and should include information about early childhood deaths, pulmonary problems, and neurological or liver disease.

Clinical Assessment

The infant liver, a large organ relative to body size during the first 2 years of life, normally is palpable about 2 cm below the right costal margin[84] and should not be felt to the left of the midline. Knowledge of vertical liver span for normal children may provide a guideline for estimating liver size in children under age 2; a liver span greater than 7 cm should be considered an indication for further evaluation.[86] Changes in structures adjacent to the liver can influence apparent liver size; for example, gas in the hepatic flexure of the colon may obscure hepatic dullness, and hyperinflation of the lungs, with subsequent depression of the diaphragm, may displace the liver downward, making it easier to palpate.

The consistency and character of the liver's surface may help determine the nature of the underlying liver disorder. The liver's edge normally is sharp, but soft and nontender. A large liver that develops secondary to congestive heart failure has a rounded, smooth edge and a firm consistency; a cirrhotic liver is hard and has an irregular surface and edge. Auscultation over the liver area is valuable for detecting increased hepatic arterial blood flow (bruit) caused by primary liver tumors, metastatic disease of the liver, hepatic hemangiomas, or arteriovenous fistulas. A complete abdominal evaluation of an infant who has jaundice or is suspected of having hepatomegaly should include palpation of the spleen. In normal infants under age 2, the spleen can be palpated 1 to 2 cm below the left costal margin; under most circumstances this organ should not be felt in normal children over age 2. Splenomegaly suggests portal hypertension, especially in a child who has a prominent abdominal venous pattern, peripheral edema, and ascites. Splenic enlargement may be the first manifestation of previously undiagnosed progressive liver disease because it is not always associated with jaundice. Table 148-1 presents the clinical manifestations of liver dysfunction with associated differential diagnostic considerations for infants and children.

JAUNDICE IN THE NEONATE AND YOUNG INFANT

In this chapter, jaundice in the neonate and young infant (see the box on p. 1035 for differential diagnosis for this age group) is considered separately from jaundice in the older infant and child (see the box on p. 1036 for differential diagnosis) for two reasons: (1) the infant liver mounts a unique response to injury (i.e., active fibroblastic proliferation, Kupffer cell hyperplasia, and formation of multinucleated giant cells); (2) unconjugated hyperbilirubinemia is common in early life and relatively uncommon after the neonatal period.

Unconjugated Hyperbilirubinemia

Unconjugated bilirubin in neonates is hazardous because of the potential for deposition of free bilirubin in neuronal tissues, with associated brain damage (kernicterus), especially in premature infants. Also, more subtle central nervous system (CNS) abnormalities can occur in infants, although a critical level of serum unconjugated bilirubin (at which only physiological changes rather than brain cell injury occur) has not yet been identified clearly. A total bilirubin of 14 mg/dl or higher may be associated with a significant risk of deafness in high-risk preterm infants whose birth weight is 1500 g or less.[15] Others have suggested that moderate hyperbilirubinemia (10 to 20 mg/dl) in full-term infants affects adjoining areas of the brainstem, including both the auditory pathway and the cry production pathways.[82]

A persistent unconjugated hyperbilirubinemia suggests excessive production of bilirubin, an inherited or acquired block

DIFFERENTIAL DIAGNOSIS OF JAUNDICE IN THE NEONATE AND YOUNG INFANT

Unconjugated hyperbilirubinemia* (noncholestatic jaundice)

Overproduction of bilirubin

Sepsis
Rh/ABO incompatibility
Hematoma (birth trauma)
Drugs (e.g., vitamin K)
Polycythemia
- Maternal-fetal or twin-to-twin transfusion
- Delayed clamping of umbilical cord

Erythrocyte defects (e.g., congenital spherocytosis)
Hemoglobinopathies
Physiological jaundice

Impaired transport of bilirubin

Hypoxia, acidosis
Drugs (e.g., sulfonamides, aminosalicylic acid [ASA])
Serum free fatty acids
- Breast milk
- Fat emulsions

Hypoalbuminemia of prematurity

Impaired hepatic uptake of bilirubin

Decreased sinusoidal perfusion (e.g., diminished venous flow after birth)
Gilbert syndrome
Physiological jaundice

Impaired conjugation of bilirubin

Breast milk jaundice
Drugs (e.g., chloramphenicol)
Hypoglycemia
Hypothyroidism
High intestinal obstruction
Glucuronyl transferase deficiency (types I and II)
Physiologic jaundice

Enterohepatic circulation of bilirubin

Delayed passage of meconium
- Low intestinal obstruction
- Cystic fibrosis

Diminished intestinal motility
Physiological jaundice
- Negligible intestinal bacterial flora
- Presence of intestinal beta-glucuronidase

Conjugated hyperbilirubinemia* (cholestatic jaundice)

Acquired cholestatic jaundice

Sepsis
Other infections
- Bacterial
- Congenital (TORCH)
- Viral (e.g., hepatitis A, B, or C; HIV)
- Parasitic (e.g., toxoplasmosis)

Chemical liver injury (e.g., drugs)
Total parenteral nutrition (TPN)

Idiopathic cholestatic jaundice

Hepatocellular cholestatic jaundice
- Neonatal hepatitis

Ductal cholestatic jaundice
- Biliary atresia
- Biliary hypoplasia
- Paucity of intrahepatic bile ducts
- Choledochal cyst

Inherited cholestatic jaundice

Familial cholestatic syndromes (e.g., benign recurrent cholestasis)
Metabolic cholestasis
- Galactosemia
- Hereditary fructose intolerance
- Hereditary tyrosinemia
- Cystic fibrosis
- Alpha-1-antitrypsin deficiency
- Glycogen storage disease
- Inborn errors of bile acid metabolism

Other storage disease
- Niemann-Pick disease
- Gaucher disease

"Noncholestatic" syndromes
- Dubin-Johnson syndrome
- Rotor syndrome

*When this is the predominant form of bilirubin, the following diagnoses should be considered.

in bilirubin transport, uptake, or conjugation, or abnormal enterohepatic circulation of bilirubin. More than one mechanism may be involved at any time during the course of an illness. Normally, bilirubin metabolism commences with the breakdown of hemoglobin and subsequent conversion of heme (by the enzyme heme oxygenase) to biliverdin, which then is reduced to bilirubin. Unconjugated bilirubin binds to albumin, is transported to the hepatocyte, and then is taken up across the hepatocyte-plasma membrane. Cytoplasmic proteins help transport bilirubin to the smooth endoplasmic reticulum for conjugation. Only bilirubin glucuronide conjugates are secreted at the bile canaliculus into bile and subsequently to the small intestine. Because unconjugated bilirubin is not secreted into bile, urobilinogen does not appear in the intestine or subsequently in the urine.

Sepsis, one of the important treatable problems associated with *bilirubin overproduction,* causes a hyperbilirubinemia that is a consequence of rapid hemolysis. Severe infection eventually causes a more prominent conjugated hyperbilirubinemia because of the bacterial or viral hepatocellular damage. The jaundice associated with hemolytic states such as erythroblastosis occurs during the first 36 hours of life; the

DIFFERENTIAL DIAGNOSIS OF JAUNDICE IN THE OLDER INFANT AND CHILD

Unconjugated hyperbilirubinemia* (noncholestatic jaundice)

Overproduction of bilirubin

Hemoglobinopathies (e.g., sickle cell disease)
Erythrocyte defects (e.g., congenital spherocytosis)

Impaired uptake of bilirubin

Gilbert syndrome

Impaired conjugation of bilirubin

Glucuronyl transferase deficiency (types I and II)

Conjugated hyperbilirubinemia* (cholestatic jaundice)

Acquired cholestatic jaundice

Sepsis
Other infections
- Bacterial (e.g., syphilis, leptospirosis)
- Viral (e.g., hepatitis A, B, C, D, and E; HIV, Epstein-Barr virus)
- Parasitic (e.g., toxoplasmosis)

Chemical liver injury
- Drugs (e.g., valproic acid, erythromycin, sulfonamides, isoniazid, methyldopa)
- Total parenteral nutrition (TPN)

Idiopathic cholestatic jaundice

Autoimmune hepatitis
Sclerosing cholangitis

Inherited cholestatic jaundice

Wilson disease
Cystic fibrosis
Alpha-1-antitrypsin deficiency

*When this is the predominant form of bilirubin, the following diagnoses should be considered.

Table 148-1 Manifestations of Liver Dysfunction

No jaundice		Jaundice		
Generalized hepatomegaly	**Asymmetrical hepatomegaly**	**Generalized hepatomegaly**	**Apparent hepatomegaly**	**No hepatomegaly**
"Benign" hepatomegaly	Tumors	Unconjugated hyperbilirubinemia (hemolytic)	Choledochal cyst	Unconjugated hyperbilirubinemia (nonhemolytic)
Congestive hepatomegaly	Trauma	Bile duct abnormalities		
Malnutrition		Infections		
Metabolic liver disease (storage)		Metabolic liver disease (with cell necrosis)		
Infiltrative liver disease (cellular)		Chemical (e.g., drug) injury		
With splenomegaly		With splenomegaly	With cholestasis	
Metabolic liver disease	All conditions except chemical injury	All conditions except hemolytic disease		
Infiltrative liver disease				

From Andres JM, Mathis RK, Walker WA: *J Pediatr* 90:686, 1977.

risk of kernicterus is high if the infant develops early severe anemia and splenomegaly. Blood group typing and a direct Coombs test will establish the diagnosis of Rh incompatibility. Late hyporegenerative anemia occurs in some of these infants.[31] In a patient who has ABO incompatibility, numerous spherocytes may be noted in the blood smear, which can be obtained in addition to the appropriate blood group typing of infant and mother. A hematoma or polycythemia can lead to hemolysis because of the increased red blood cell (RBC) mass. Certain drugs administered during pregnancy or to the infant after birth may increase the risk of significant unconjugated hyperbilirubinemia. Vitamin K, for example, may cause hemolysis by acting as an oxidizing agent. Congenital erythrocyte defects such as spherocytosis cause chronic hyperbilirubinemia in infancy. The diagnosis is suspected when maternal agglutination antibodies are not demonstrated, especially if there is a family history of splenomegaly or hemolysis.

Most cases of neonatal unconjugated hyperbilirubinemia occur secondary to physiological jaundice, a transient, benign condition. This common form of jaundice has no single cause; it results from the interaction of many complex factors and is noted in approximately 15% of normal newborn infants. Overproduction of bilirubin occurs in these children because catabolism of fetal hemoglobin is increased and RBC survival is shortened.

Other newborn developmental factors include delayed conjugation of bilirubin that occurs secondary to immaturity of the glucuronyl transferase enzyme, poor hepatocellular transport of bilirubin because of a decrease in cytoplasmic transport proteins, and increased intestinal reabsorption of unconjugated bilirubin. For a full-term infant the serum bilirubin concentration rarely exceeds 10 mg/dl; jaundice occurs on the second or third day after birth and usually disappears by the fifth to eighth day of life. Bilirubin levels may increase to 12 mg/dl by the fifth to seventh day of life in a premature infant, returning to normal by the fourteenth day. Physiological jaundice is of no clinical significance unless additional factors such as prematurity, acidosis, or hemolysis also are present. Odell[48] has outlined four criteria to help distinguish physiological jaundice from pathological jaundice; these criteria should prompt careful diagnostic evaluation: (1) jaundice before 36 hours of age, (2) serum total bilirubin concentration above 12 mg/dl, (3) jaundice that persists beyond the eighth day of life, and (4) a conjugated bilirubin level above 1.5 mg/dl.

Numerous other conditions can cause unconjugated hyperbilirubinemia in the neonate. Drugs such as aspirin and sulfonamides can lead to *impaired transport of bilirubin* as a result of displacement of the bilirubin molecule from albumin-binding sites. Other albumin-binding sites also can be blocked by free fatty acids, known to be in high concentration in breast milk and the main metabolic product of intravenous lipid (e.g., Intralipid or Liposyn).[2,50] Various cephalosporins[59] and sodium fusidate[8] also increase the risk of bilirubin encephalopathy by altering bilirubin-albumin binding. Although the precise mechanism of action is not known, benzyl alcohol, a bacteriostatic agent used to flush intravascular catheters, has been associated with the development of kernicterus in infants.[28] Other changes in care may have contributed to the findings in this latter group of patients (many also had intraventricular hemorrhages), but drug interference with bilirubin-albumin binding was suspected. Bilirubin displacement from albumin is amplified in the neonate who is hypoxic and acidotic, especially in a premature infant who has hypoalbuminemia.

Impaired hepatic uptake of bilirubin occurs in Gilbert syndrome, a common familial condition that usually is diagnosed in the second decade of life and in sick neonates who have diminished hepatic sinusoidal blood flow or persistent patency of the ductus venosus. Although alteration of bilirubin-albumin binding probably is the main defect, breast milk jaundice may occur because of the hormone pregnanediol in the mother's milk.[20] This hormone is capable of inhibiting glucuronyl transferase activity, which leads to *impaired conjugation of bilirubin*. Clinical jaundice occurs in about 1% of breast-fed infants, usually between the sixth and eighth days of life in a normal-appearing, thriving child. The serum concentration of unconjugated bilirubin rarely exceeds 20 mg/dl; this level recedes after breast-feeding is discontinued, and the jaundice usually does not recur if breast-feeding is reinstituted after 2 or 3 days.[33] Even if breast-feeding is continued, the serum bilirubin usually declines over a period of 2 to 3 months. Kernicterus has never been reported with this common form of jaundice; however, a brief discontinuance of breast milk always should be considered because of the small potential for subtle neurological dysfunction after prolonged exposure to unconjugated bilirubin. This should be done before the child is subjected to a detailed diagnostic evaluation.

The possibility of drug-induced jaundice again should be emphasized; for example, chloramphenicol and novobiocin can diminish bilirubin conjugation by competing for glucuronyl transferase. Hypoglycemia also may exacerbate jaundice in young infants because glucose is a required substrate for synthesis of the bilirubin-glucuronide conjugate. Prolonged elevation of unconjugated bilirubin is seen in congenital hypothyroidism, presumably because of delay in maturation of the bilirubin-conjugating enzyme.[35] This is a treatable disease; therefore it is critical to obtain thyroid function studies in all children who have indirect hyperbilirubinemia. Some infants who have intestinal obstruction (e.g., pyloric stenosis or duodenal atresia) develop unconjugated hyperbilirubinemia. The mechanism for jaundice in this circumstance is not known, but some evidence suggests diminished glucuronyl transferase activity in these infants, who improve rapidly after the anatomical problem is corrected surgically.

A rare familial cause of unconjugated hyperbilirubinemia is glucuronyl transferase deficiency.[4] Two forms have been described, depending on the patient's clinical response to phenobarbital. Type I, Crigler-Najjar syndrome, is a severe, rare autosomal recessive disease in which no glucuronyl transferase enzyme can be demonstrated. Nonhemolytic jaundice develops in the first hours of life, and early signs of kernicterus often are present. Phototherapy is required, and exchange transfusion often is necessary. As the child becomes older, phototherapy is less effective. Plasmapheresis can then be tried, but patients usually require liver transplantation; phenobarbital therapy is ineffective. The type II deficiency is autosomal dominant. These infants have reduced levels of glucuronyl transferase enzyme, and the action of the enzyme is enhanced by phenobarbital. Serum bilirubin levels may decline dramatically with the use of phenobarbital, which is required for the individual's entire life. Lower intestinal obstruction syndromes and clinical conditions that lead to decreased intestinal motility promote increased enterohepatic circulation of unconjugated bilirubin. Elevated serum bilirubin can occur, especially in the early days of life when the intestinal lumen sequesters bilirubin-rich meconium together with deconjugating glucuronidase enzyme.

Conjugated Hyperbilirubinemia

Immature secretory mechanisms, damage to the hepatocyte canalicular membrane, or an anatomical abnormality of bile ducts can cause conjugated hyperbilirubinemia. This always is a pathological condition, and it usually is associated with hepatocellular disease. The conjugated molecule is not known to be harmful to body tissues, including the central nervous system, but a serum conjugated bilirubin level above 1.5 mg/dl always should be considered abnormal and a development that occurs secondary to hepatic injury.

Hepatic excretion of organic anions such as bilirubin depends in part on the movement of bile acid and water across the canalicular membrane. Jaundice usually is associated closely with a reduction in bile flow, or cholestasis—hence the term *cholestatic jaundice*. Various acquired, idiopathic, and inherited conditions that cause neonatal cholestatic jaundice are discussed briefly in this section (see the box on p. 1035).[39]

Hepatocellular cholestatic jaundice includes neonatal hepatitis and is the diagnosis given for most infants who have conjugated hyperbilirubinemia in the early months of life. Symptoms usually occur in the first 2 weeks after birth, and the typical presentation is that of an unwell, jaundiced infant who has hepatomegaly. The main differential diagnostic consideration is ductal cholestatic jaundice, especially biliary atresia—that is, determining whether the jaundice occurs secondary to a surgical or a nonsurgical problem. An evaluation to determine the type of hyperbilirubinemia and to establish an early diagnosis of a treatable disease always should be considered immediately. Studies that should be done include total and direct serum bilirubin determinations, a hemoglobin count, Coombs test, blood glucose test, serum amino acid determinations (e.g., for tyrosine), and serological tests for toxoplasmosis, syphilis, hepatitis B virus (HBV) (especially anti-HBc), and human immunodeficiency virus (HIV). HIV infection is slowly beginning to emerge as an important problem affecting the liver in neonates and young infants. Clinical symptoms of HIV perinatal infection can develop as early as 1 month of age; however, the median interval from birth to the emergence of symptoms is 8 months. The commonest early manifestations of HIV infection in infants are poor growth, interstitial pneumonitis, and hepatosplenomegaly. However, the overall spectrum of liver disease and pathological features among neonates and young infants is unknown, and jaundice is not common. Cholestatic jaundice and hepatitis occurred in seven infants as the first manifestation of their perinatally acquired disease.[53] No specific etiological agent was identified as the cause of the cholestasis. Six of the seven infants died within 12 weeks of the onset of hepatitis, mainly because of complications of *Pneumocystis carinii* pneumonia and cytomegalovirus infection. Only one infant died as a consequence of liver failure.

Other important tests include urine testing for non-glucose-reducing substances and organic acids (to eliminate galactosemia and hereditary fructose intolerance), blood cultures, and urine cultures. The syndrome of cholestatic jaundice in association with urinary tract infection is not uncommon, especially among neonates and infants under 2 months of age. The liver histology may suggest the cause of the infant's problem, but failure to diagnose hepatocellular cholestasis specifically necessitates studies to determine patency of the biliary tree such as hepatobiliary scintigraphy (e.g., *d*i*is*opropyl *i*mino*d*iacetic *a*cid [DISIDA]), duodenal intubation for bile, and percutaneous liver biopsy. Factors related to an unfavorable prognosis are prolonged jaundice and cholestasis, early appearance of portal fibrosis, and coexistence of systemic disease.[11] Approximately 30% of infants who have hepatocellular cholestatic jaundice develop progressive liver failure, another 30% survive the early months of illness but have chronic disease (including cirrhosis), and the remainder recover completely. The overall outlook for these patients has improved because of the success of liver transplantation.

Children who have cholestatic jaundice who die have significantly more liver histological abnormalities, including prominent periportal inflammation and fibrosis and diffuse giant cell transformation.[73] *Ductal cholestatic jaundice* includes diagnoses such as biliary atresia, sclerosing cholangitis, biliary hypoplasia, and choledochal cyst. Infants who have biliary atresia usually appear well until jaundice persists beyond the first week after birth. About 20% of infants who have biliary atresia have other congenital anomalies, mainly cardiovascular, gastrointestinal, or splenic malformations.[67] Although the theory is controversial, *Reovirus* (type 3) has been implicated as an important etiological agent for hepatobiliary disease in infants.[43] This virus has been localized in biliary remnants in the inflamed porta hepatis.[44] Jaundice increases with time, and the liver becomes hard and firm as cirrhosis progresses over the first months of life.

In the past the prognosis for infants who had biliary atresia correlated best for those who had expert surgical treatment performed by operating teams skilled in biliary microsurgery[10]; however, the long-term outcome for these children now is related more strongly to the skill of the liver transplantation surgeon. In some Japanese surgery units, bile drainage is reported in almost 90% of patients; in North America, the overall success rate of Kasai portoenterostomy is less satisfactory,[56] but this procedure always should be done before transplantation is considered except for infants seen after 120 days of life, in whom the transplantation procedure may be considered primary therapy.[16] The Kasai operation restores bile flow in about 80% of children operated on before 60 days of life. Despite this success, fewer than 20% of patients with biliary atresia who have no jaundice generally survive for long periods.[42] Most of these patients have portal hypertension and abnormal liver function. Postoperative cholangitis often leads to deteriorating liver function, which continues to be a major problem despite surgical technological advances; it occurs in more than half of successful portoenterostomies before the age of 1 year but is unusual after age 2.[22] Liver transplantation is the only chance of survival for many patients who have this form of end-stage liver disease.[80]

Sclerosing cholangitis of neonatal onset may be confused with biliary atresia. The former is a cholestatic syndrome associated with abnormal intrahepatic bile ducts and increased serum levels of gamma-glutamyl transpeptidase. Infants who have hypoplasia of bile ducts and antitrypsin deficiency also have high serum levels of this transpeptidase enzyme, which may be considered an index of bile duct damage.[36]

Biliary hypoplasia is noted in infants who have acute infections of the liver, various familial cholestatic syndromes such as arteriohepatic dysplasia (Alagille syndrome),[1,14] and the more common metabolic cholestatic syndrome, alpha-1-antitrypsin deficiency.[64] The clinical course of infants who have biliary hypoplasia varies; overall survival is much longer than for children who have biliary atresia, but some patients require liver transplantation.[79] Clinical recognition of a jaundiced child who has a choledochal cyst depends on the size of the cyst and whether biliary obstruction occurs.[65] Ultrasonographic scans can improve the preoperative diagnosis of this problem, which can be resolved surgically before progressive biliary obstruction and cirrhosis occur. Identifying the gallbladder by using ultrasound and noting a change in its size after oral feeding aids in the differential diagnosis of the ductal versus hepatocellular problem.[27] For example, infants who have biliary atresia may have a small gallbladder that is not affected by oral feeding. Further, ultrasound-guided percutaneous cholecystocholangiography may help differentiate extrahepatic from intrahepatic causes of cholestatic jaundice in infancy.[77]

Just as rare as the *familial cholestasis* syndromes are the *metabolic hepatocellular* problems (except for cystic fibrosis and alpha-1-antitrypsin deficiency); nevertheless, they are important to diagnose because of the potential for effective treatment. Specifically, infants who have galactosemia, fructose intolerance, and tyrosinemia have similar clinical manifestations, usually within days to weeks after birth. Marked jaundice, hepatosplenomegaly, bleeding, and failure to thrive usually are prominent. However, infants who have galactosemia may have less apparent findings; after several months they may develop cataracts, cirrhosis, and psychomotor retardation. Similarly, the tyrosinemic infant may escape the acute phase of illness and be discovered months later to have cirrhosis, rickets, and renal disease; these patients have a high incidence of hepatoma in later childhood.[85] A jaundiced child who has cataracts and psychomotor retardation might very well have galactosemia, whereas jaundice associated with a history of vomiting, distaste for sweet foods, and fructosuria more likely would result from fructose intolerance. Each of these metabolic disorders also may cause renal dysfunction manifested by aminoaciduria, glycosuria, and phosphaturia (Fanconi syndrome). Their definitive diagnosis depends on specific tolerance tests and the measurement of enzyme activity in red blood cells (galactosemia), liver, or kidney (fructose intolerance) and of serum metabolic products (succinylacetone in tyrosinemia). Analyzing the urine for non-glucose-reducing sugars, organic acids, and amino acids is appropriate for initial screening. The long-term prognosis for all of these metabolic diseases depends on early introduction of dietary restrictions.

Jaundice is unusual in children who have glycogen storage disease[41] except for types III and IV. Hepatocellular dysfunction is more prominent in infants who have type IV glycogenosis; jaundice occurs in the first months of life and usually is followed by cirrhosis and death before age 2. Persistent jaundice is unusual in infants who have cystic fibrosis, but it may occur when the disease is associated with increased enterohepatic circulation of bilirubin (meconium ileus), drug hypersensitivity, parenteral alimentation, or common duct inflammation secondary to inspissation of biliary secretions. Alpha-1-antitrypsin deficiency,[64] a genetic defect of glycoprotein metabolism, is the most common metabolic disorder associated with liver disease among infants. The usual presentation is that of cholestasis with associated jaundice and hepatomegaly. The diagnosis is suspected if a diminished or absent alpha-1-globulin peak is observed in the serum protein electrophoretic pattern. The diagnosis is confirmed by a low serum alpha-1-antitrypsin level and protease inhibitor (Pi) typing. No specific treatment is available, but infants at risk must be identified and proper genetic counseling provided to the family. Liver transplantation has been performed in older children who have end-stage liver disease caused by antitrypsin deficiency.[24] The prognosis varies considerably. Despite the persistence of mild hepatocellular dysfunction, clinical improvement may occur in infants a few months after birth. Biliary cirrhosis and portal hypertension eventually develop in some older children.

In rare cases an infant who has cholestatic jaundice will be discovered to have a primary metabolic defect in bile acid synthesis,[9,63] a disorder that affects transformations in the bile acid steroid nucleus. These rare but important inborn errors of metabolism have the potential for successful diagnosis (urine and serum analysis for the presence of bile acids and bile precursors) and treatment (chenodeoxycholic or ursodeoxycholic acid). Other rare, difficult to treat entities include children who have hepatitis and autoimmune hemolytic anemia, neonatal hemochromatosis,[30] and syncytial giant cell hepatitis that occurs secondary to paramyxovirus infection.[54]

Inherited storage diseases (e.g., Niemann-Pick and Gaucher disease) usually cause hepatosplenomegaly in infants, but jaundice is unusual. These diseases are exceedingly rare and should not be considered in the initial evaluation of children who have cholestatic jaundice.

Dubin-Johnson syndrome[3] is another type of familial jaundice that probably has an autosomal recessive mode of inheritance. It is considered a benign condition, but the child has a reduced capacity to secrete several organic anions, especially conjugated bilirubin, sulfobromophthalein (SBP), rose bengal, and cholecystographic dye. Interestingly, excretion of bile acids is normal; therefore the term *noncholestatic jaundice* is applicable and the extrahepatic biliary tree always is patent. Recurrent episodes of jaundice, which can be precipitated by infection, may begin in infancy and can be misdiagnosed as acute hepatitis because of the abrupt onset of illness. There often is a family history of jaundice and vague upper abdominal pain in older children. Routine tests of liver function produce normal results except for an increase in total bilirubin (usually below 15 mg/dl) with predominance of conjugated bilirubin. Grossly, the liver appears black owing to accumulation of melanin-like pigment in lysosomes. Rotor syndrome is similar to (or may be a variant of) Dubin-Johnson syndrome except that pigmentation of hepatocytes has not been demonstrated and secretion of cholecystographic dye is normal. Recognition of these benign "noncholestatic" jaundice syndromes may obviate the need for diagnostic tests.

JAUNDICE IN THE OLDER INFANT AND CHILD

Unconjugated Hyperbilirubinemia

Unconjugated hyperbilirubinemia in 1- to 2-year-old infants (after maturation of the blood-brain barrier) and in older children usually is of no pathological significance. It is uncommon in an older child who does not have an underlying hemolytic disease such as sickle cell disease or spherocytosis. Gilbert syndrome[55] is a common familial syndrome of autosomal dominant inheritance that may occur secondary to an abnormality of bilirubin uptake at the hepatocyte sinusoidal membrane. Mild fluctuating jaundice can be noted during early infancy, but the syndrome usually is not diagnosed until the second decade of life. Fatigue and caloric deprivation accentuate the jaundice. The mechanism is not understood, but it may be related to increased production of bilirubin after fasting. Abdominal pain, malaise, and other vague symptoms usually accompany the jaundice. The criteria for diagnosing Gilbert syndrome are a serum unconjugated bilirubin level above 1.5 mg/dl but below 6 mg/dl, lack of other demonstrable abnormalities of liver function, absence of overt hemolysis, and no evidence of liver disease on examination except for jaundice. The main differential diagnostic considerations are glucuronyl transferase deficiency (type II) and mild hemolytic syndromes. No treatment is necessary for Gilbert syndrome except resumption of an adequate caloric intake. This is a benign condition but one important to recognize so that unnecessary diagnostic investigations are avoided.

Conjugated Hyperbilirubinemia

Acute viral hepatitis is the most common cause of jaundice in older infants and children. Hepatitis A virus (HAV) often is the etiological agent, but most of these children do not have jaundice or significant liver dysfunction. Fulminant hepatitis may occur, however, and is associated with a high mortality.[19] Hepatitis B virus (HBV) produces a similar symptom complex of nausea, vomiting, and anorexia that often precedes the jaundice. In children, liver disease that occurs secondary to HBV may be mild, but persistent jaundice and hepatocellular dysfunction with eventual occurrence of chronic hepatitis can occur. Antigenemia and clinical disease occur often in infants born to mothers who have acute hepatitis during the latter part of pregnancy or early in the postpartum period.[62] Another mode of transmission is contact with the HBV-positive mother during infancy, including ingestion of contaminated breast milk.[7] From a worldwide perspective, perinatal and postnatal transmission of HBV is an extremely important public health problem. For example, before an extensive, controlled HBV vaccine trial in Senegal, striking evidence of the endemicity of HBV infection was found; 12% of blood donors were HB_sAg positive, and 80% of 6- and 7-year-olds had at least one serum marker of past or present HBV infection.[40] In areas where HBV is endemic, the relative risk of hepatocellular carcinoma is much higher in carriers than in noncarriers.

Routine HBV screening of all pregnant women is essential. If the woman proves to be positive, the newborn should receive hepatitis B immunoglobulin (HBIG) for passive immunity and begin the recombinant vaccine series immediately at birth. In the United States and other developed countries, adolescent users of parenterally administered illicit drugs may develop acute HBV liver disease. The HBV vaccine now is available for patients at risk of developing this serious infection.[71,75]

Although there is no specific treatment for hepatitis B disease, alpha-interferon now is being used in children. The results of large multicenter adult trials[52] are encouraging, but further studies are necessary to evaluate the degree and duration of resolution of HBV infections after use of interferon.

Hepatitis C virus (HCV), formerly known as non-A, non-B hepatitis virus, recently was discovered to be an important pathogen in children.[5,6] The significance of this virus in infant cholestatic jaundice is not clear, but it is known that HCV probably transmits vertically.[49,76] Further, infants born to HCV-positive mothers coinfected with HIV have a higher vertical transmission rate.[76] It also is known that anti-HCV antibodies can be detected, although infrequently, in infants who have jaundice, abnormal liver function, and biopsy-proven hepatitis. HCV is transmitted to older infants and children through transfusion of infected blood; this virus probably is responsible for most cases identified as posttransfusion hepatitis. Acute and chronic infection with HCV usually is milder and anicteric compared with HBV infections; however, persistent HCV infection leads to chronic liver disease in 25% to 50% of patients. For example, 24% of multiply transfused leukemic children in long-term remission were discovered by anti-HCV reactivity to have a persistently polyphasic pattern of elevated serum transaminase and abnormal liver histology, such as chronic active hepatitis.[34] In general, anti-HCV antibodies persist in patients who have chronic disease. The mean interval from onset of hepatitis to detection of anti-HCV antibodies may be 15 weeks but can be much longer. HCV is detected much more rapidly by polymerase chain reaction (PCR) technology, but this still is a research tool not yet generally available for clinical practice.[47] Detection of HCV-RNA by reverse transcription PCR is the best means of confirming the diagnosis,[32] although recombinant immunoblot assay (RIBA) now is readily available and also confirms the presence of infection. Treatment of HCV is problematical, and clinical trials using alpha-interferon are just commencing in children. In adults, half of patients who have persistent HCV infection respond to interferon with normalization of transaminase and improvement in liver histology.[12] Unfortunately, half of these patients relapse after therapy is discontinued.

Hepatitis D virus (HDV) is diagnosed as a concurrent infection in patients who have acute and chronic HBV hepatitis. Transmission of HDV (delta agent) from mother to infant has been reported.[87] This RNA virus requires HBV for replication. The severity of HBV infection is greatly increased by the presence of HDV. Testing for anti-HDV antibodies is recommended for any patient who is HBV positive. No therapy is available to treat this viral infection, which is not common in the United States.

Hepatitis E virus (HEV) may be the most common cause of acute sporadic hepatitis among children living in some developing countries.[25,26] Its fecal-oral or waterborne transmission is similar to that of HAV infection. Hepatitis E infection has not been documented to occur in Western countries; it is endemic to Southeast Asia and India and should be suspected in travelers returning from these areas of the world. Clinical manifestations of HEV resemble those of HAV except that the attack rates are highest among adolescents and young adults. Fulminant hepatitis may occur in outbreaks of HEV disease, especially in young pregnant women. This infection is confirmed by a Western blot assay for anti-HEV IgM.[26]

Chronic active hepatitis was discovered in older infants and children who had clinical and immunological characteristics of acquired immunodeficiency syndrome (AIDS).[17] Epstein-Barr virus (EBV) infection may have been the cause of the hepatic inflammation in these AIDS patients as a consequence of a generalized immune disturbance. Another report documented hepatic opportunistic infections caused by *Cryptosporidium* organisms and *Mycobacterium avium-intracellulare,* as well as small epithelioid granulomas on liver histology.[51] In general, liver histopathology in pediatric patients shares some features with that in adults. However, granulomas are less common in children, whereas young patients who have interstitial pneumonitis are more likely to have evidence of hepatic lymphoplasmocytic infiltrates.[29] In adults with AIDS, macrocytosis and nonspecific portal inflammation are the most common histological abnormalities.

Sporadic cases of jaundice in childhood may be noted with other infections, such as infectious mononucleosis. Jaundice occurs in only a small percentage of children infected with EBV, despite hepatic involvement in most patients. This diagnosis should be suspected in an adolescent who has acute pharyngitis and splenomegaly with or without hepatomegaly. A large number of children under age 4 also acquire this disease and are prone to develop pneumonia during their acute course.[74]

Cholecystitis is a rare problem in children; acute disease usually develops among adolescent girls, who often experience jaundice, right upper quadrant pain, vomiting, and fever. Gallbladder ultrasonography will suggest the correct diagnosis and identify the presence of gallstones, which most often are seen in children who have hemolysis. Gallstones also are seen in pregnant adolescents, in patients receiving parenteral nutrition or ceftriaxone therapy, in patients with cystic fibrosis, and in some children who have cirrhosis.[57,58] Laparoscopic cholecystectomy is the treatment of choice for most children who have cholelithiasis.[81] Cholangiography may be important to exclude the presence of stones in the common bile duct, especially in a patient with hemolytic disease who is acutely ill with fever and abdominal pain. For children who have evidence of common duct stones, especially those who have undergone cholecystectomy previously, endoscopic sphincterotomy is the treatment of choice.[23] Hemolytic anemia may be the mode of presentation for Wilson disease in children over age 5. Individuals who have this important, treatable disease have jaundice during the early hepatic stage of illness, when the liver is becoming saturated with copper. A careful evaluation should be done to detect Kayser-Fleischer rings and subtle neurological dysfunction.

Chronic active hepatitis probably is rare in infants under age 2. In more than 25% of these children, the illness begins as acute hepatitis with jaundice, and the severity, course, and prognosis vary considerably. An immunological form of chronic active liver disease (autoimmune hepatitis) occurs primarily in young girls. The extrahepatic autoimmune manifestations they develop are skin rash, arthritis, and hemolytic anemia. This inflammatory liver disease often is associated with high serum titers of anti-liver-kidney microsome (anti-LKM) antibody, and it is a potentially fatal disease for which immunosuppressive treatment must be started early.[37] Exposure to drugs such as isoniazid and methyldopa occasionally leads to liver dysfunction and a histological abnormality indistinguishable from chronic active hepatitis. The appearance of jaundice may be delayed for months after institution of isoniazid therapy, and the severity of the liver dysfunction correlates with continued use of the drug.[70] Children who have immunodeficiency syndromes and increased serum gamma-glutamyl transferase activity may have sclerosing cholangitis.[13] This chronic cholestatic disease also is associated with chronic inflammatory bowel disease, histiocytosis X, congenital psoriasis, and cholestatic jaundice of the neonate. Cholangiography reveals abnormal intrahepatic bile ducts in all these children. The prognosis is poor, but liver transplantation should be considered except in those who have severe immunodeficiency disorders.

The anticonvulsant agent valproic acid also causes cholestatic jaundice with diffuse hepatocellular injury.[72] The mechanism for hepatic damage is uncertain; concurrent administration of valproic acid with other anticonvulsants should be monitored carefully. Other common drugs (e.g., erythromycin estolate and sulfonamides) can cause jaundice with either a hepatitis-like or cholestatic pattern. Hepatotoxic reactions occur in children who have tuberculosis and are treated with isoniazid combined with rifampin; jaundice occurs more rapidly if the dose of isoniazid exceeds 10 mg/kg/day.[78] Jaundice occurs in children, especially infants, who are receiving total parenteral nutrition (TPN). The precise mechanism is unknown, but the problem may be related to amino acid imbalance and a subsequent decrease in bile acid synthesis or to inadequate secretin stimulation of bile flow in a child who has minimal oral alimentation. Clinical characteristics associated with the development of TPN-associated jaundice include low birth weight, duration of TPN administration, interval before enteral feeding is initiated, sepsis, central venous catheter infection, and the number of surgical procedures performed.[21,45]

MANAGEMENT

Unconjugated Hyperbilirubinemia

Excellent general reviews are available in the literature on the treatment of newborns with unconjugated hyperbilirubinemia.[38] An extensive discussion of such treatment can be found in Chapter 47, Common Neonatal Illnesses. Intravenous infusion of albumin, especially before exchange transfusion, increases the potential binding sites for the unconjugated molecule. A double-volume exchange transfusion is indicated infrequently except for hemolytic disease when the serum indirect bilirubin concentration exceeds 20 mg/dl in full-term neonates or 10 mg/dl in ill premature infants or in any child who experiences a rapid rise (more than 0.5 mg/dl/hour) in serum bilirubin. Phototherapy is more efficacious than exchange transfusion for nonhemolytic jaundice and may help prevent a rapid increase in serum bilirubin. However, its effectiveness in terms of preventing brain injury is unknown and, as noted earlier, it should not be instituted before any underlying pathological condition is excluded. This form of therapy never is considered routine and should be reserved for premature infants or term infants who have high serum bilirubin concentrations, as well as for the rare patient who has type I glucuronyl transferase deficiency who requires continuous therapy. Specific guidelines for initiating phototherapy include treatment if the bilirubin level exceeds 15 mg/dl at any time of life in the full-term infant, at 12 hours of age in neonates weighing less than 1500 g at birth, and when the serum bilirubin rises to 10 mg/dl in infants weighing 1500 to 2000 g at birth. Phototherapy probably induces increased biliary excretion of photoisomers of bilirubin after the molecule in exposed skin reacts photochemically.[18] Potential side effects are well recognized, including an increase in insensible water loss, retinal damage, unusual bronzing of the skin,[18] and even alteration of intracellular deoxyribonucleic acid (DNA). When the hyperbilirubinemia is refractory to conventional phototherapy, treatment with high-dose intravenous gamma globulin may be useful in some patients who have isoimmune hemolytic disease.[60]

The effectiveness of agar in treating neonates who have jaundice is uncertain, but it may be associated with reduced peak serum bilirubin levels by binding bilirubin in the gut. Recently a new treatment with tin (Sn)-protoporphyrin has been proposed for infants who have unconjugated hyperbilirubinemia. This synthetic metalloporphyrin is a competitive enzyme inhibitor (of heme oxygenase) that blocks the degradation of heme to the bile pigment, biliverdin. The excess heme is not converted to bilirubin; instead, it is excreted in bile. This synthetic compound may prove useful, especially if it helps lessen dependence on phototherapy and exchange transfusion.

Phenobarbital is used to treat unconjugated hyperbilirubinemia in older infants who have type II glucuronyl transferase deficiency. In this situation, continuous use of phenobarbital is necessary in the early weeks of life when the risk of kernicterus is greatest. Children who have Crigler-Najjar syndrome do not respond to phenobarbital. An exchange transfusion is the only effective early therapy to reduce toxic serum bilirubin levels in these patients, but curative treatment has been reported with home phototherapy, followed by orthotopic liver transplantation at an early age.[66]

Collaborative perinatal projects have examined the association between neonatal bilirubin levels and subsequent neurodevelopmental outcome in terms of intelligence quotient (IQ), neurological examination, and sensorineural hearing loss. In general, by 6 to 8 years of age, neonatal bilirubin levels seem to have little effect on IQ, neurological abnormalities, or hearing loss. Higher bilirubin levels are associated with minor motor abnormalities.[46,61] Infants born prematurely did not fare as well in that the percentage of children who had minor and major handicaps increased consistently as the bilirubin concentration increased.[83]

Conjugated Hyperbilirubinemia

It is not necessary to treat the jaundice of patients who have conjugated hyperbilirubinemia because the conjugated molecule is nontoxic. Therapy is aimed at optimizing nutrition and controlling pruritus. Using choleretic agents (e.g., phenobarbital, cholestyramine, and ursodeoxycholic acid) may increase bile flow effectively, which in turn lowers the level of total serum bilirubin. Fat-soluble vitamins also are essential in these children who have cholestatic liver disease.

Vitamin K is given in a starting dose of 2.5 to 5 mg every day or every other day. The dose is monitored by following the coagulation studies, especially prothrombin time. Excessive vitamin K can cause hemolysis. Vitamin D is administered as the 25-hydroxy vitamin D. Serum calcium levels are monitored carefully because vitamin D intoxication leads to hypercalcemia, which is responsible for CNS depression, ectopic calcification, and nephrolithiasis.

A water-miscible preparation of vitamin A is given in a dose of 5000 to 25,000 IU/day. Vitamin A deficiency can cause xerophthalmia, keratomalacia, night blindness, and pigmentary retinopathy. Manifestations of vitamin A toxicity include hepatotoxicity and pseudotumor cerebri. Serum vitamin A and retinal ester levels should be followed.

Vitamin E supplementation is indicated in all infants and young children who have cholestatic jaundice. For vitamin E–deficient patients (who have hyperreflexia, areflexia, ptosis, mild truncal ataxia, or hypotonia),[68] 50 IU/kg/day of vitamin E or standard alpha-tocopherol acetate suspension should be administered. Tocopherol polyethylene glycol-1000 succinate (TPGS) is a water-soluble ester of vitamin E (Liqui-E, Nutr-E-Sol) that is more effective in maintaining vitamin E sufficiency.[69] The dose of vitamin E is modified according to serum concentrations and the ratio of serum vitamin E to total serum lipid concentration (normally above 0.8 mg : 1 g).

REFERENCES

1. Alagille D, Odievre M, Gautier M: Hepatic ductular hypoplasia associated with characteristic facies, vertebral malformations, retarded physical, mental, sexual development, and cardiac murmur, *J Pediatr* 86:63, 1975.
2. Andrew G, Chan G, Schiff D: Lipid metabolism in the neonate. II. The effect of Intralipid on bilirubin binding in vitro and in vivo, *J Pediatr* 88:279, 1976.
3. Arias IM: Inheritable and congenital hyperbilirubinemia: models for the study of drug metabolism, *N Engl J Med* 285:1416, 1971.
4. Arias IM et al: Chronic nonhemolytic unconjugated hyperbilirubinemia with glucuronyl transferase deficiency: clinical, biochemical, pharmacologic, and genetic evidence for heterogeneity, *Am J Med* 47:395, 1969.
5. Blanchett VS et al: Hepatitis C virus infection in children with hemophilia A and B, *Blood* 78:285, 1991.
6. Bortolotti F et al: Cryptogenic chronic liver disease and hepatitis C virus infection in children, *J Hepatol* 15:73, 1992.
7. Boxall EH et al: Hepatitis B surface antigen in breast milk, *Lancet* 2:1007, 1974.
8. Brodersen R: Fusidic acid binding to serum albumin and interaction with binding of bilirubin, *Acta Paediatr Scand* 78:874, 1985.
9. Buchmann MS, et al: Lack of 3B-hydroxy-C27-steroid dehydrogenase/isomerase in fibroblasts from a child with urinary excretion of 3B-hydroxy bile acids, *J Clin Invest* 12:2034, 1990.
10. Danks DM: Biliary atresia: lessons from Japan, *Lancet* 1:219, 1981.
11. Danks DM et al: Prognosis of babies with neonatal hepatitis, *Arch Dis Child* 52:368, 1977.
12. Davis GL et al: Treatment of chronic hepatitis C with recombinant interferon-alpha: a multicenter randomized controlled trial, *N Engl J Med* 321:1501, 1989.
13. Debray D et al: Sclerosing cholangitis in children, *J Pediatr* 124:49, 1994.
14. Deprettere A, Portmann B, Mowat AP: Syndromatic paucity of the intrahepatic bile ducts: diagnostic difficulty; severe morbidity throughout early childhood, *J Pediatr Gastroenterol Nutr* 6:865, 1987.
15. DeVries LS, Lary S, Dubowitz LMS: Relationship of serum bilirubin levels to ototoxicity and deafness in high-risk low-birth-weight infants, *Pediatrics* 76:351, 1985.
16. Dorney SF et al: Outcome of surgery for biliary atresia, *Aust NZ J Surg* 59:855, 1989.
17. Duffy LF et al: Hepatitis in children with acquired immune deficiency syndrome: histopathologic and immunocytologic features, *Gastroenterology* 90:173, 1986.
18. Ennever JF, Knox I, Speck WT: Differences in bilirubin isomer composition in infants treated with green and white light phototherapy, *J Pediatr* 109:119, 1986.
19. Friedland IR et al: Fulminant hepatitis in children: report of 12 cases, *Ann Trop Paediatr* 11:207, 1991.
20. Gartner LM, Arias IM: Studies of prolonged neonatal jaundice in the breast-fed infant, *J Pediatr* 68:54, 1966.
21. Ginn-Pease ME, Pantolos D, King DR: TPN-associated hyperbilirubinemia: a common problem in newborn surgical patients, *J Pediatr Surg* 20:436, 1985.
22. Gottrand F et al: Late cholangitis after successful surgical repair of biliary atresia, *Am J Dis Child* 145:213, 1991.
23. Guelrud M et al: ERCP and endoscopic sphincterotomy in infants and children with jaundice due to common bile duct stones, *Gastrointest Endosc* 38:450, 1992.

24. Hood JM et al: Liver transplantation for advanced liver disease with alpha-1-antitrypsin deficiency, *N Engl J Med* 302:272, 1980.
25. Hyams KC et al: Acute sporadic hepatitis E in children living in Cairo, Egypt, *J Med Virol* 37:274, 1992.
26. Hyams KC et al: Acute sporadic hepatitis E in Sudanese children: analysis based on a new Western blot assay, *J Infect Dis* 165:1001, 1992.
27. Ikeda S, Sera Y, Akagi M: Serial ultrasonic examination to differentiate biliary atresia from neonatal hepatitis: special reference to changes in size of the gallbladder, *Eur J Pediatr* 148:396, 1989.
28. Jardine DS, Rogers K: Relationship of benzyl alcohol to kernicterus, intraventricular hemorrhage, and mortality in preterm infants, *Pediatrics* 83:153, 1989.
29. Jonas MM et al: Histopathologic features of the liver in pediatric acquired immune deficiency syndrome, *J Pediatr Gastroenterol Nutr* 9:73, 1989.
30. Knisely AS et al: Neonatal hemochromatosis, *Birth Defects* 23:75, 1987.
31. Koenig JM et al: Late hyporegenerative anemia in Rh hemolytic disease, *J Pediatr* 115:315, 1989.
32. Lau JYN et al: Significance of antibody to the host cellular gene–derived epitope GOR in chronic hepatitis C virus infection, *J Hepatol* 17:253, 1993.
33. Lascari AD: "Early" breast-feeding jaundice: clinical significance, *J Pediatr* 108:156, 1986.
34. Locasciulli A et al: Hepatitis C virus infection and chronic liver disease in children with leukemia in long-term remission, *Blood* 78:1619, 1991.
35. MacGillivray MH, Crawford JD, Robey JS: Congenital hypothyroidism and prolonged neonatal hyperbilirubinemia, *Pediatrics* 40:283, 1967.
36. Maggiore G et al: Diagnostic value of serum gamma-glutamyl transpeptidase activity in liver disease in children, *J Pediatr Gastroenterol Nutr* 12:21, 1991.
37. Maggiore G et al: Liver disease associated with anti-liver-kidney microsome antibody in children, *J Pediatr* 108:399, 1986.
38. Maisels MJ: Jaundice in the newborn, *Pediatr Rev* 3:305, 1982.
39. Mathis RK, Andres JM, Walker WA: Liver disease in infants. II. Hepatic disease states, *J Pediatr* 90:864, 1977.
40. Maupas P et al: Efficacy of hepatitis B vaccine in prevention of early HB_sAg carrier state in children: controlled trial in an endemic area (Senegal), *Lancet* 1:289, 1981.
41. McAdams AJ, Hug G, Bove BE: Glycogen storage disease, types I to X: criteria for morphologic diagnosis, *Hum Pathol* 5:463, 1974.
42. Miyano T et al: Current concept of the treatment of biliary atresia, *World J Surg* 17:332, 1993.
43. Morecki R et al: Biliary atresia and *Reovirus* type 3 infection, *N Engl J Med* 307:481, 1982.
44. Morecki R et al: Detection of *Reovirus* type 3 in the porta hepatis of an infant with extrahepatic biliary atresia: ultrastructural and immunocytochemical study, *Hepatology* 4:1137, 1984.
45. Moss RL, Das JB, Raffensperger JG: Total parenteral nutrition–associated cholestasis: clinical and histopathologic correlation, *J Pediatr Surg* 28:1270, 1993.
46. Newman TB, Klebanoff MD: Neonatal hyperbilirubinemia and long-term outcome: another look at the Collaborative Perinatal Project, *Pediatrics* 92:651, 1993.
47. Novati R et al: Mother-to-child transmission of hepatitis C virus detected by polymerase chain reaction, *J Infect Dis* 165:720, 1992.
48. Odell GB: Neonatal jaundice. In Popper H, Schaffner F, editors: *Progress in liver disease,* New York, 1976, Grune & Stratton.
49. Ohto H et al: Vertical Transmission of Hepatitis C Virus Collaborative Study Group: transmission of hepatitis C virus from mothers to their infants, *N Engl J Med* 330:744, 1994.
50. Ostrea EM et al: Influence of free fatty acids and glucose infusion on serum bilirubin and bilirubin binding to albumin: clinical implications, *J Pediatr* 102:426, 1983.
51. Patrick CC et al: A patient with leukemia in remission and acute abdominal pain, *J Pediatr* 111:624, 1987.
52. Perrillo RP et al: A randomized, controlled trial of interferon-alpha-2b alone and after prednisone withdrawal for the treatment of chronic hepatitis B, *N Engl J Med* 323:295, 1990.
53. Persaud D et al: Cholestatic hepatitis in children infected with the human immunodeficiency virus, *Pediatr Infect Dis J* 12:492, 1993.
54. Phillips MJ et al: Sporadic hepatitis with distinctive pathologic features, a severe clinical course, and paramyxoviral features, *N Engl J Med* 324:455, 1991.
55. Powell LW: Clinical aspects of unconjugated hyperbilirubinemia, *Semin Hematol* 9:91, 1972.
56. Psacharapoulos HT et al: Extrahepatic biliary atresia: preoperative assessment and surgical results in 47 consecutive cases, *Arch Dis Child* 55:351, 1980.
57. Reif S, Sloven DG, Lebenthal E: Gallstones in children: characterization by age, etiology, and outcome, *Am J Dis Child* 145:105, 1991.
58. Riccabona M et al: Ceftriaxone-induced cholelithiasis: a harmless side-effect? *Klin Padiatr* 205:421, 1993.
59. Robertson A, Fink S, Karp W: Effect of cephalosporins on bilirubin-albumin binding, *J Pediatr* 114:291, 1988.
60. Sato K et al: High-dose intravenous gamma globulin therapy for neonatal immune hemolytic jaundice due to blood group incompatibility, *Acta Paediatr Scand* 80:163, 1991.
61. Scheidt PC et al: Intelligence at six years in relation to neonatal bilirubin levels: follow-up of the National Institute of Child Health and Human Development Clinical Trial of Phototherapy, *Pediatrics* 87:797, 1991.
62. Schweitzer IL: Vertical transmission of the hepatitis B surface antigen, *Am J Med Sci* 270:287, 1975.
63. Setchel KDR et al: 3-Oxosteroid 5B-reductase deficiency described in identical twins with neonatal hepatitis: a new inborn error in bile acid synthesis, *J Clin Invest* 82:2135, 1988.
64. Sharp HL: The current status of alpha-1-antitrypsin, a protease inhibitor, in gastrointestinal disease, *Gastroenterology* 70:621, 1976.
65. Sherman P et al: Choledochal cysts: heterogeneity of clinical presentation, *J Pediatr Gastroenterol Nutr* 5:867, 1986.
66. Shevell MI et al: Crigler-Najjar syndrome type I: treatment by home phototherapy followed by orthotopic hepatic transplantation, *J Pediatr* 110:429, 1987.
67. Silveira TR et al: Congenital structural abnormalities in biliary atresia: evidence for etiopathogenic heterogeneity and therapeutic implications, *Acta Paediatr Scand* 80:1192, 1991.
68. Sokol RJ et al: Frequency and clinical progression of the vitamin E deficiency neurologic disorder in children with prolonged neonatal cholestasis, *Am J Dis Child* 139:1211, 1985.
69. Sokol RJ et al: Treatment of vitamin E deficiency during chronic childhood cholestasis with oral d-alpha-tocopheryl polyethylene glycol 1000 succinate (TPGS); *Gastroenterology* 93:975, 1987.
70. Stein MT, Liang D: Clinical hepatotoxicity of isoniazid in children, *Pediatrics* 64:499, 1979.
71. Stevens CE et al: Yeast-recombinant hepatitis B vaccine: efficacy with hepatitis B immune globulin in prevention of perinatal hepatitis B virus transmission, *JAMA* 257:2612, 1987.
72. Suchy FJ et al: Acute hepatic failure associated with the use of sodium valproate, *N Engl J Med* 300:962, 1979.
73. Suita S et al: Fate of infants with neonatal hepatitis: pediatric surgeons' dilemma, *J Pediatr Surg* 27:696, 1992.
74. Sumaya CV, Ench Y: Epstein-Barr virus infectious mononucleosis in children. I. Clinical and general laboratory findings, *Pediatrics* 75:1003, 1985.
75. Szmuness W et al: Hepatitis B vaccine: demonstrations of efficacy in a controlled clinical trial in a high-risk population in the United States, *N Engl J Med* 303:833, 1980.
76. Thaler MM et al: Vertical transmission of hepatitis C virus, *Lancet* 338:17, 1991.
77. Treem WR et al: Ultrasound-guided percutaneous cholecystocholangiography for early differentiation of cholestatic liver disease in infants, *J Pediatr Gastroenterol Nutr* 7:347, 1988.
78. Tsagaropoulou-Stinga H et al: Hepatotoxic reactions in children with severe tuberculosis treated with isoniazid-rifampin, *Pediatr Infect Dis J* 4:270, 1985.
79. Tzakis AG et al: Liver transplantation for Alagille's syndrome, *Arch Surg* 128:337, 1993.

80. Vacanti JP et al: The therapy of biliary atresia combining the Kasai portenterostomy with liver transplantation: a single center experience, *J Pediatr Surg* 25:149, 1990.
81. Vinograd I et al: Laparoscopic cholecystectomy: treatment of choice for cholelithiasis in children, *World J Surg* 17:263, 1993.
82. Vohr BR et al: Abnormal brainstem function (brainstem auditory evoked response) correlates with acoustic cry features in term infants with hyperbilirubinemia, *J Pediatr* 115:303, 1989.
83. Vohr BR: New approaches to assessing the risks of hyperbilirubinemia, *Clin Perinatol* 17:293, 1990.
84. Walker WA, Mathis RK: Hepatomegaly: an approach to the differential diagnosis, *Pediatr Clin North Am* 22:929, 1975.
85. Weinberg AG, Mize CE, Worthan HG: The occurrence of hepatoma in the chronic form of hereditary tyrosinemia, *J Pediatr* 88:434, 1976.
86. Younoszai MK, Mueller S: Clinical assessment of liver size in normal children, *Clin Pediatr* 14:378, 1975.
87. Zanetti AR, Ferroni P, Magliano EM: Perinatal transmission of the hepatitis B virus and the HBV-associated delta agent from mothers to offspring in northern Italy, *J Med Virol* 9:139, 1982.

SUGGESTED READINGS

Barrera JM et al: Incidence of non-A, non-B hepatitis after screening blood donors for antibodies to hepatitis C virus and surrogate markers, *Ann Intern Med* 115:596, 1991.

Krugman S: Viral hepatitis: A, B, C, D and E infection, *Pediatr Rev* 13:204, 1992.

Newman TB, Maisels MJ: Evaluation and treatment of jaundice in the term newborn: a kinder, gentler approach, *Pediatrics* 89:809, 1992.

Nowicki MJ, Balisteri WF: Hepatitis A to E: building up the alphabet, *Contemp Pediatr* 9:23, 1992.

Ramirez RO, Sokol RJ: Medical management of cholestasis. In Suchy FJ, editor: *Liver disease in children,* St Louis, 1994, Mosby.

Suchy FJ: Approach to the infant with cholestasis. In Suchy FJ, editor: *Liver disease in children,* St Louis, 1994, Mosby.

149 Joint Pain

David M. Siegel and John Baum

Pediatricians and others who provide primary health care to children often are faced with clinical situations involving musculoskeletal aches and pains; within this group of symptoms is the subset of joint pain. In fact, 1 of every 6 to 10 pediatric outpatient visits includes a musculoskeletal complaint.[1] Discomfort in a joint can result from a wide variety of diagnostic entities that must be sorted out to allow appropriate evaluation and management. Using a systematical approach to patients who have pain and swelling in one or more joints helps the clinician arrive at an accurate diagnosis and course of therapy.

ARTHRALGIA VERSUS ARTHRITIS

As always, a careful, thorough history is indispensable in initially approaching a child who has joint pain; the physical examination then can substantiate or alleviate suspicions raised during the interview. It is essential to distinguish between arthralgia and arthritis. Joint pain, or *arthralgia,* is the subjective experience of pain referable to a bony articulation. In a young child this sensation of pain might be inferred from the patient's refusal to move a particular extremity or joint, but the term *arthralgia* refers only to *discomfort* in a joint. On the other hand, the term *arthritis* (as suggested by the *-itis* suffix) should be used only when the joint can be shown to be inflamed, as evidenced by the classic signs of inflammation: redness, warmth, swelling, tenderness, and pain with motion. In the joint this kind of inflammation can be accompanied by loss of motion. Thus all that is arthralgia is not arthritis—an invaluable distinction in the differential diagnosis of joint pain.

With these definitions in mind, what would be the characteristics of children who have joint pain, and what information must be elicited through the interview and physical examination? Before enumerating specific entities, it is helpful to discuss general characteristics of clinical presentations.

The onset of joint pain can be rather sudden or quite indolent (over days or weeks). In cases of sudden onset, an associated history of a fall or direct blow to the joint immediately suggests a traumatic etiology, whereas the presence of fever points to an infectious process such as septic arthritis or a systemic inflammatory disease such as juvenile arthritis. Often the complaint expressed to the physician is loss of motion in a joint, with or without obvious swelling. Further clues are provided by the time of day the stiffness occurs and its duration. A child who has juvenile arthritis typically complains of joint stiffness on arising in the morning, which may last from half an hour to several hours and may be relieved by gradual exercise. On the other hand, a patient who has hypermobility syndrome or some other mechanical, noninflammatory condition associated with joint pain usually gives a history of pain and stiffness occurring at the end of a vigorous day. Besides fever, other distinguishing signs can include rash, mucous membrane involvement, lymph node inflammation or enlargement, or the presence of some recognizable chronic diseases that can involve the joints.

DIFFERENTIAL DIAGNOSIS AND MANAGEMENT

A useful format for beginning a discussion of the differential diagnosis of joint pain is the division between rheumatic and nonrheumatic diseases. Juvenile arthritis, sometimes called Still disease,[8] is a classic rheumatic disease of childhood involving the joints. It typically peaks in children 1½ to 2 years of age, although onset can occur through late adolescence. The clinical presentation can be limited to a few (four or fewer), usually large joints (pauciarticular disease), or a greater number of joints, both large and small, might be involved (polyarticular disease). There also is a systemic and at times initially fulminant form of juvenile arthritis known as systemic-onset disease that is marked by high spiking fevers, a typical salmon-pink, maculopapular, evanescent rash, lymph node and spleen enlargement, anemia, and general malaise. These more systemic findings often precede the onset of any joint involvement, although arthritis must be present for at least 6 consecutive weeks to establish the diagnosis of the other two subgroups of juvenile arthritis (pauciarticular and polyarticular). The clinician may glean only a history of ill-defined arthralgias and stiffness, whereas on physical examination he or she may find contractures of the elbows, knees, and wrists or limitation of cervical motion, all of which provide evidence of previous episodes of active inflammation in these joints. Although not a common disease, juvenile arthritis has a prevalence of 0.1 to 1 child per 1000 children worldwide.[2]

The diagnosis can be reinforced by laboratory studies, including the erythrocyte sedimentation rate (ESR), the C-reactive protein, and a complete blood count (CBC), as well as by more specialized studies such as the antinuclear antibody test (the result most commonly is positive in girls who have pauciarticular disease), rheumatoid factor titer (RF factor is present in only a small subset of children who have polyarticular juvenile arthritis), serum immunoglobulin levels, and others.

Management focuses on subduing inflammation and preserving the normal range of joint motion. Salicylate therapy remains a mainstay, beginning with a daily dosage of 80 to 100 mg/kg of body weight in divided doses. Other (more expensive) nonsteroidal antiinflammatory drugs (NSAIDs) increasingly are useful when the disorder does not respond adequately to the maximum tolerated salicylate dose. More rheumatologists now advocate NSAID therapy from the outset.[10] The enteric-coated form of aspirin is particularly useful because it achieves a more gradual rise and fall in blood concentrations while protecting the gastric mucosal lining. Long-acting agents, including gold, hydroxychloroquine, D-penicillamine, and especially methotrexate, have their place in persistent cases, whereas systemic steroid therapy is used only when these other modalities have failed. Surgery is used mostly in joint reconstruction or prosthetic replacement as a means of dealing with sequelae of synovial inflammation and destruction (see Chapter 224, Juvenile Arthritis).

Acute rheumatic fever (ARF) is another classic rheumatic disease of childhood. Although not the scourge that it once was, the incidence of ARF is increasing, and its inclusion in the differential diagnosis of arthritis and arthralgia remains important. The characteristics of the disease are described at length in Chapter 252; suffice it to say that the arthritis usually involves large joints such as the knees and typically is migratory, with the joints being quite tender to palpation. Although signs of marked inflammation commonly are present, arthralgia alone can be seen.

Ankylosing spondylitis, which can involve large joints of the lower extremities during childhood and early adolescence, is typified in late adolescence by involvement of the sacroiliac joint (which can be seen on roentgenograms) and by pain elicited on palpation over the joint. In adulthood further axial involvement occurs; the classic "bamboo spine" develops, with its diffuse vertebral fusions and often severe limitation of back motion. The HLA-B27 transplantation antigen is seen in 90% of patients who have ankylosing spondylitis, although the converse is not true (only 20% of those born with HLA-B27 develop arthritis). Treatment with one of the nonaspirin NSAIDs usually is more successful.

Reiter syndrome, a triad of urethritis, conjunctivitis, and arthritis, can be seen in adolescents and children. In children it often starts with enteritis. It is more common in boys, and making the diagnosis depends on ruling out infectious causes of the inflammation. The arthritis occurs predominantly in large joints; again, there is a strong association with the HLA-B27 locus in these patients (about 60%). The disorder is treated with antiinflammatory drugs. Most children recover within a few months, although some follow a more chronic and relapsing course, occasionally progressing to ankylosing spondylitis.

Also showing a predisposition for larger joints is an arthritis sometimes seen with psoriasis: either the characteristic involvement of the skin is present, or there is at least a history of psoriatic skin disease.

Systemic lupus erythematosus (SLE) can cause chronic joint pain. Seen most commonly in girls, SLE is a true multisystem disease that can involve almost every organ in the body; the joints, however, may merely be stiff and painful, or they may show frank signs of inflammation. This disorder, then, would be within the differential diagnosis of joint pain or arthritis in an adolescent girl. Dermatomyositis and polymyositis also can cause inflamed joints in addition to muscle and skin involvement. Other rheumatic diseases that can affect children and cause joint involvement are scleroderma, mixed connective tissue disease, and mucocutaneous lymph node syndrome (Kawasaki disease; see Chapter 225). Each of these entities has its own distinguishing features, as seen on physical examination and in laboratory findings.

Unlike most of the rheumatic diseases that cause joint pain and tend to be chronic (having waxing and waning courses), many of the nonrheumatic diseases are acute in onset and short in duration, given appropriate therapy. Foremost among this group, and representing something of a medical emergency, is *acute bacterial infection* of the joint, or septic arthritis (see Chapter 257). The usual presentation is one of a child complaining of a painful joint (rapid onset), usually accompanied by fever. The joint itself is red, warm, swollen, and exquisitely tender to palpation or with movement. This clinical situation demands immediate arthrocentesis for diagnosis and therapy. Analysis of the fluid for appearance (opaque), viscosity (usually low), mucin clot (friable), cell count (more than 100,000 WBC/mm^3 with 80% polymorphonuclear cells), glucose (usually low, much less than serum), and protein (high) helps to establish the diagnosis. Most important, a portion of the fluid must be gram stained to check for bacterial organisms. Cultures can direct definitive antimicrobial therapy. In the absence of direct (traumatic) inoculation of the joint, a child under approximately age 4 is at high risk for *Haemophilus influenzae* infection (seeding from a bacteremia), whereas in an older child *Staphylococcus aureus* and *Streptococcus* organisms are more likely to be the offending organism. Blood cultures also may yield growth of the organism. The incidence of *H. influenzae* infection is expected to drop with regular immunization of children.

Systemic bacterial infections, notably those caused by *Neisseria gonorrhoeae* and *Neisseria meningitidis,* also can produce arthritis, although the organism usually is not isolated from the joint in these cases. After joint aspiration and establishment of at least a strong suspicion of a purulent arthritis, the child should be hospitalized and appropriate intravenous antibiotic therapy started. Prompt, aggressive therapy usually effects recovery without sequelae, although some foci, such as the hip joint, can remain persistent problems. Because of the tenuous blood supply to the femoral capital epiphysis (as it courses intracapsularly via the ligamentum teres), purulent arthritis of the hip can lead to chronic problems despite timely intervention.[5]

In addition to bacteria, other infectious organisms can cause joint disease. Viruses, including rubella, mumps, chickenpox, and adenovirus, as well as the Epstein-Barr virus (in infectious mononucleosis), all can affect synovial tissue. Manifestations of the *viral syndrome* (rash, fever, mucous membrane involvement) usually precede joint involvement. Infectious hepatitis, on the other hand, can cause arthritis before overt hepatic involvement. Rubella immunization also is associated with arthralgia and arthritis in as many as 3% of children who receive the vaccine—rarely, if ever, with any sequelae.[6] Other infections that can involve the joints include brucellosis, leptospirosis, tularemia, Rocky Mountain spotted fever, and rat-bite fever. Mycobacteria can cause arthritis, as can various fungal agents, particularly in immunocompromised individuals.

Ixodes dammini, a newly identified offender, is a tick that harbors the spirochete *Borrelia burgdorferi*. This tick is carried by a number of mammals. The infection and arthritis produce the syndrome of *Lyme disease*. First described in Old Lyme, Connecticut, the syndrome is characterized by an initial tick bite that often (but not always) causes a large circular spreading erythematous lesion known as erythema chronicum migrans. Meningoencephalitis, neuritis, and carditis also may occur. The arthritis manifests later in the course as recurrent attacks of inflammation of the large joints (85% of cases involve the knee), with each recurrence usually lasting no more than a week or two. Occasionally symptoms may persist for several months, and chronic persistent arthritis of the knee has been reported in rare instances. A short course of high-dose penicillin therapy seems to shorten the course of the rash and perhaps attenuate the arthritis, and salicylate or other NSAID therapy relieves the symptoms[9] (see Chapter 225, Lyme Disease).

Congenital syphilis (see Chapter 258, Sexually Transmitted Diseases) can be seen in the infant as painful bony lesions and refusal to move the involved limb (Parrot pseudoparalysis), along with other associated stigmata. In adolescence, an individual born with this syndrome can develop bilateral knee effusions known as Clutton joints.

Osteomyelitis is another acute infection of the bone. However, when one of the long bones is involved adjacent to a joint (such as the distal femur and knee), the patient may describe pain in the joint, and a sterile effusion may even be present.[5] In some rare instances, particularly in younger patients, the bacterial infection directly invades the joint space.

Diskitis is another infection that can cause joint pain. This disorder manifests low-grade fever, back pain, and tenderness over the spinous process contiguous to the involved disk space. *S. aureus* has been isolated from the blood and disk space in some instances, but often there is no culture-proven cause. The presentation can involve sensory and motor complications that occur secondary to nerve root impingement, and an epidural abscess must be considered in the differential diagnosis.

Noninfectious origins of arthralgia and arthritis abound. Large joint involvement is the most common extraintestinal manifestation of inflammatory bowel disease. This can involve pain alone or inflammation as well; we have seen the joint complaints precede the appearance of bowel disease. The activity of the bowel disease may or may not correlate with joint flare-ups. Sarcoidosis can include arthritis, as can the unrelated diseases of polyarteritis nodosa and Marfan disease. In the group of vasculitic disorders, Henoch-Schönlein purpura is a disease of childhood evidenced by fever, abdominal pain (with or without melena), purpuric lesions of the buttocks and lower extremities, and warm, swollen, painful, tender joints (usually large joints such as the knees and ankles). Hematological diseases that have articular manifestations include hemophilia and sickle cell disease. In the latter disorder, the physician must consider the hand-foot syndrome type of vasoocclusive crisis in a child between 1 and 4 years of age. Although primary gout is exceedingly rare in children, hyperuricemia and subsequent joint disease can be seen in those who have leukemia (with chemotherapy producing sudden lysis of cells), hemolytic anemia, glycogen storage disease, and Lesch-Nyhan syndrome. In Lesch-Nyhan syndrome, a sex-linked, recessive, genetic, inborn metabolic error results in overproduction of uric acid. Polyarthritis and limb pains can be seen in children following traumatic pancreatitis. Infantile cortical hyperostosis (Caffey disease), which occurs in infants under 6 months of age, involves fever, irritability, an increased ESR, and tender swellings of facial, trunk, and limb bones, with associated arthralgia. Toxic synovitis of the hip also can cause arthralgia (see Chapter 128, Extremity Pain).

A fascinating condition seen primarily in children and adolescents that can induce arthralgia without arthritis is *hypermobility syndrome*. Children with this disorder have increased joint laxity, and with vigorous activity, especially that requiring extremes of joint flexion and extension, they can experience significant arthralgia. The diagnosis is made by physical examination and observation of at least three of the following five signs: (1) hyperflexion of the wrist, bringing the thumb in contact with the volar surface of the forearm, (2) hyperextension of the fingers to parallel with the forearm, (3) hyperextension of the elbow to at least −10 degrees, (4) hyperextension of the knee to at least −10 degrees, and (5) hyperflexion of the back such that the palms can be placed flat on the ground with the feet together and without flexing the knees. All laboratory and radiological studies are normal. The syndrome is treated with NSAIDs and reassurance.

In *chondromalacia patellae,* or *patellofemoral pain syndrome,* the child has knee pain that usually is related to activity, especially descending stairs. The problem is a roughening of the underside of the patella, with resultant pain as the patella moves in the patellofemoral groove. Exercises directed toward strengthening the quadriceps femoris and adductor muscles can produce marked improvement. Analgesic medication can be used as an adjunct to the physical therapy.

"Growing pains" are an actual discomfort in the lower limbs and joints (often worse at night) that children experience during a phase of rapid linear growth. A bedtime dose of enteric-coated aspirin or NSAID can help alleviate this pain until it resolves spontaneously with the slowing of growth.

Physical abuse must be strongly considered whenever signs of trauma are evident, and accidents that represent neglect on the part of parents or guardians need to be recognized and pursued. Any suspicious history or circumstance demands complete investigation.

There are many other orthopedic reasons for arthralgia and arthritis; these are discussed elsewhere in this text.

Management of Psychological Aspects

Having arrived at a diagnosis and plan of therapy, the practitioner also must offer management for the psychological aspects of joint disease. In children afflicted with an ongoing joint problem, all the issues of chronic pediatric disease also must be addressed. The child may not be able to keep up with peers in physical activity and also may be faced with making numerous health care visits. Many clinicians feel that not only does the disease create stress in these patients, but also stress in their environment can exacerbate the disease, as may occur in children who have juvenile arthritis. A child faced with hospitalization for an acute problem, such as septic arthritis, is exposed to all the complications of being taken out of his or her family and school environment, as well as those dealing with an institutional setting. Any child who has ongoing joint disease, even those who have a mild disability, should be provided with the expertise and services of a social worker or counselor experienced with this population of patients. Family resources (both emotional and financial) need to be assessed and support provided when needed. Discussion groups composed of these children and their families can be very beneficial because they offer an opportunity to compare experiences and coping mechanisms. Attention to the physical dimension alone does not provide adequate care in these diseases. A functionally minor disability can cause major problems of body image and feelings of lack of independence, which must be dealt with appropriately.[3,4] As with other chronic physical disorders of childhood, long-term psychosocial sequelae also may develop.[7]

REFERENCES

1. Cassidy JT, Petty RE: An introduction to the study of the rheumatic diseases of children. In Cassidy JT, Petty RE, editors: *Textbook of pediatric rheumatology,* ed 3, Philadelphia, WB Saunders.
2. Gewanter HL, Roghmann KJ, Baum J: The prevalence of juvenile arthritis, *Arthritis Rheum* 26:599, 1983.
3. Lowit IM: Social and psychological consequences of chronic illness in children, *Dev Med Child Neurol* 15:75, 1973.
4. McAnarney ER et al: Psychological problems of children with chronic juvenile arthritis, *Pediatrics* 53:523, 1974.
5. Petty RE: Septic arthritis and osteomyelitis in children, *Curr Opin Rheumatol* 2:616, 1990.
6. Phillips P: Viral arthritis in children, *Arthritis Rheum* 20(suppl 2):584, 1977.
7. Pless IB et al: Long-term psychosocial sequelae of chronic physical disorders in childhood, *Pediatrics* 91:1131, 1993.
8. Siegel DM, Baum J: Juvenile arthritis, *Prim Care* 20:883, 1993.
9. Steere AC et al: The spirochetal etiology of Lyme disease, *N Engl J Med* 308:733, 1983.
10. Stiehm ER: Nonsteroidal anti-inflammatory drugs in pediatric patients, *Am J Dis Child* 142:1281, 1988.

150 Limp

Alain Joffe

A limp in a child is *never* normal. It suggests that weight bearing on one extremity either is painful or is difficult because of pelvic or thigh muscle weakness. The causes of limp are legion; they can be as obvious as a foreign body embedded in the foot or shoe or as subtle as appendicitis or diskitis.[5]

CAUSES AND CHARACTERISTICS

Table 150-1 lists the causes of limp in children and adolescents.[3] Although the list is formidable, most of the causes usually can be excluded by obtaining a complete history and performing a comprehensive physical examination.

Some of the causes listed in Table 150-1 are likely to be associated with systemic signs and symptoms. Tumors, neoplastic disease, and infections might reasonably be expected to produce constitutional symptoms such as fever, anorexia, weight loss, malaise, and fatigue. Diseases such as infectious myositis, Rocky Mountain spotted fever, dermatomyositis, Gaucher disease, or leukemia, which involve more than one muscle or bone group, likely will cause pain at more than one site, although the pain may be most severe in a lower extremity.

The child's age also is helpful in determining the cause of a limp. Anatomical causes of a limp, such as congenital coxa vara or congenital dislocation of the hip, become manifest shortly after an infant begins to walk. Occult trauma (toddler fracture) always should be considered as a cause of a limp in small children, who cannot report that a significant fall occurred.[10] Legg-Calvé-Perthes disease occurs most often in children 4 to 10 years of age, whereas slipped femoral capital epiphysis and Osgood-Schlatter disease are most common among adolescents.

Whether the limp is associated with pain can help to exclude certain causes.[1] Severe pain is associated with fractures, dislocations, severe trauma, or infections of bones or joints. The various osteochondroses generally cause only moderate pain. A very mild pain in the knee or medial aspect of the thigh above the knee is consistent with slipped femoral capital epiphysis, whereas such pain in the groin or lateral hip is associated with Legg-Calvé-Perthes disease. Pain is likely to be absent if the cause of the limp is solely muscle weakness (as in muscular dystrophy) or a discrepancy in leg length. The practitioner always should keep in mind that pain in a child often is referred distally, so pain in the knee or lower thigh may be caused by a pathological process in the hip, and pain in the hip may indicate pelvic, vertebral, or spinal cord problems.

HISTORY

The physician needs to ask about the onset of the limp and its antecedents. A history of trauma may be helpful, but parents often focus on an insignificant event in an effort to determine the cause of the limp; conversely, a seemingly trivial past trauma may cause a significant injury. If the nature of the injury does not seem to correlate with the clinical illness, child abuse should be suspected. Details of the injury (e.g., whether it was a flexion or a hyperextension injury) may help pinpoint the anatomical structures involved. If the associated symptoms are recurrent, a chronic illness such as juvenile rheumatoid arthritis may be the cause of the limp. Adolescent girls who receive a rubella vaccination often develop a transient but painful arthritis 1 to 2 weeks after vaccination. In a young boy who has a swollen, painful knee, a family history of bleeding problems suggests a hemarthrosis as the cause of the limp. A history of a previous flulike illness followed by a large, erythematous skin lesion with central clearing suggests the possibility of Lyme arthritis[11] (see Chapter 228).

Athletic individuals are prone to a variety of injuries. Stress fractures caused by overuse, patellofemoral malalignment syndrome (chondromalacia patellae), and Osgood-Schlatter disease are more common among runners than nonrunners.[7,9] A sudden increase in the amount or duration of exercise (e.g., suddenly increasing a jogging regimen from 1 mile to 3 miles) frequently is associated with injury.[2]

PHYSICAL EXAMINATION

If there is any indication that a systemic illness may be causing the limp, a complete physical examination should be done, including height, weight, and body temperature measurements. Obese boys are more likely to develop slipped femoral capital epiphysis. If systemic signs are lacking, most of the physical examination should be directed toward the affected limb. Some useful information also may be gathered by watching the patient walk. For example, a child who has a painful knee might be expected to walk with the leg outstretched so as to minimize any flexion of the painful joint, whereas one who has an inflammatory condition affecting the spine likely would hold his or her trunk rigid.[8]

The skin should be inspected carefully for redness, warmth, bruises, or puncture wounds. It is logical to assume that any such findings indicate a process involving the underlying subcutaneous tissue, muscle, or bone. For example, osteomyelitis of the distal metaphysis of the femur produces redness and tenderness in the skin overlying that area of bone.

Each joint should be examined systematically for range of motion, both active and passive, and for redness, swelling, or warmth. If there is any question about whether swelling is present, the examiner can measure the same area on the opposite extremity. Pain with active but not passive motion suggests a muscle or tendon problem. Examination of the knee should include attention to the patella because some causes of knee pain and limp are related to problems in the patella or its ligaments.

Table 150-1 Causes of Limp

Causes	Infants and toddlers	Children	Adolescents
Foreign bodies in foot	+*	+	+
Trauma to bone, periosteum, muscle, or ligaments	+	+	+
Bone, joint, or muscle infections			
Osteomyelitis	++	++	+
Septic arthritis	++	++	+
Myositis	−	+	+
Rocky Mountain spotted fever	−	+	+
Lyme arthritis	+	++	++
Neoplastic diseases			
Leukemia	−	++	+
Tumors of bone (e.g., Ewing sarcoma, osteogenic sarcoma)	−	+	+
Metastatic diseases	−	+	+
Bone or cartilage diseases			
Osteochondroses (e.g., Legg-Calvé-Perthes disease, Osgood-Schlatter disease)	−	++	+
Slipped femoral capital epiphysis	−	+	++
Neuromuscular disorders			
Spinal cord tumor	−	+	+
Muscle weakness	−	+	+
Muscular dystrophy	−	+	+
Systemic diseases			
Juvenile rheumatoid arthritis	+	++	+
Autoimmune diseases	+	+	+
Rheumatic fever	−	+	+
Scurvy	+	−	−
Hyperparathyroidism	−	+	++
Crohn disease	−	+	+
Gaucher disease	+	−	−
Pancreatitis	−	+	++
Hematological diseases			
Sickle cell anemia	+	+	+
Hemophilia	+	+	+
Congenital deformities			
Dislocated hip	+	−	−
Leg length discrepancies	++	+	+
Otto pelvis	−	−	+
Miscellaneous causes			
Appendicitis	+	+	+
Inguinal adenopathy	+	+	+
Toxic synovitis	−	+	−
Drug-induced causes			
Steroids	+	+	+
Vitamin A poisoning	+	+	+
Rubella vaccination	−	+	++

Modified from Green M: *Pediatric diagnosis,* ed 3, Philadelphia, 1980, WB Saunders.

*−, Not likely to cause limp in this age group; +, causes limp in this age group; ++, more likely to cause limp in this age group.

Unless the site of the pain is evident from a simple examination, it also is worthwhile to palpate the entire extremity anteriorly and posteriorly from the lower spine to the toes. Again, pinpoint tenderness suggests a process involving the structures at that point. If the hip or upper thigh appears to be involved, the lower spine, paraspinal areas, abdomen, and inguinal area also should be examined. A rectal examination may help confirm a diagnosis of appendicitis or some other pelvic pathological condition.

If examination of the extremity is equivocal or if some kind of congenital anatomical process or neurological disease is suspected, other physical signs may be present. Discrepancy in leg length can be detected by measuring both legs from the anterior iliac crest to the ipsilateral medial malleolus. Performing the Ortolani maneuver to check for dislocated hips still can be useful in an ambulatory toddler. Asymmetry in deep tendon reflexes or alterations in sensation suggest a pathological condition of the spinal cord; difficulty raising the leg against mild resistance suggests muscle weakness.

LABORATORY DIAGNOSIS AND MANAGEMENT

If the cause of the limp is obvious from the history and physical examination, treatment should be directed toward it.

Causes such as bruises or muscle sprains generally can be managed with mild analgesics, heat, and rest until the injury heals. If a slipped femoral capital epiphysis or some of the osteochondroses cause the limp, combined management with an orthopedist may be necessary. Infectious causes such as osteomyelitis or septic arthritis may require drainage in addition to obtaining appropriate cultures and instituting antibiotic therapy.

Often, however, a clear cause may not be obvious. The complete blood count (CBC) and erythrocyte sedimentation rate (ESR) or C-reactive protein (CRP) may be helpful in this context as markers of systemic illness or infection. A normal ESR or CRP generally is inconsistent with a systemic disease or an inflammatory process, although in some diseases (e.g., osteomyelitis) the ESR can be normal. An elevated value strongly suggests local inflammation or a systemic disease.

When the physical findings are ambiguous, consultation with a radiologist can be extremely helpful.[6] Some fractures are difficult to detect with routine anteroposterior and lateral views of the affected part. Specialized (oblique) views often are required, and these views can best be selected if the pediatrician and radiologist review the clinical symptoms jointly. Views of both limbs occasionally may be necessary. An inexperienced examiner often can miss early and subtle signs of a problem, such as periosteal elevation or changes in the fat pads surrounding the joints.

In certain situations, such as osteomyelitis or various types of stress fractures, plain roentgenograms are normal in the early phases of the disease.

Radionuclide scans often are positive earlier on.[4] Computed tomography (CT) scans and magnetic resonance imaging (MRI) also may be of use in studying various anatomical sites; ultrasonography is particularly useful for detecting swelling or fluid in and around joints such as the knee or hip.

If the initial history does not suggest a systemic illness or infection, if the physical examination is essentially normal, and if radiological investigation (if it seems necessary) fails to reveal an abnormality, a short period of observation, perhaps 1 to 2 weeks, is appropriate. Then the history and physical examination should be repeated if the limp persists. A repeat ESR or CRP and radiological examination likely will establish a diagnosis at that time. If the picture remains confusing, consultation with an orthopedist or perhaps a neurologist is warranted.

REFERENCES

1. Chung SMK: Identifying the cause of acute limp in childhood, *Clin Pediatr* 13:769, 1974.
2. Garrick JG: Knee problems in adolescents, *Pediatr Rev* 4:235, 1983.
3. Green M: *Pediatric diagnosis,* ed 3, Philadelphia, 1980, WB Saunders.
4. Hensinger RN: Limp, *Pediatr Clin North Am* 24:723, 1977.
5. Illingworth CM: 128 limping children with no fracture, sprain, or obvious cause, *Clin Pediatr* 17:139, 1978.
6. Kaye JJ: Roentgenographic evaluation of children with acute onset of a limp, *Pediatr Ann* 5:11, 1976.
7. Keller EK: Patellar management syndrome in runners, *Nurs Pract* 8:27, 1983.
8. MacEwen GD, Dehne R: The limping child, *Pediatr Rev* 12:268, 1991.
9. Newell SG, Bramwell ST: Overuse injuries to the knee in runners, *Physician Sports Med* 12:81, 1984.
10. Singer J, Towbin R: Occult fractures in the production of gait disturbance in childhood, *Pediatrics* 64:192, 1979.
11. Steere AC, Schoen RT, Taylor E: The clinical evolution of Lyme arthritis, *Ann Intern Med* 107:725, 1987.

SUGGESTED READINGS

Cankwell GD, Passo MH: Pursuing the source of musculoskeletal pain, *Contemp Pediatr* 11:72, 1994.

Eichenfield AH et al: Childhood Lyme arthritis: experience in an endemic area, *J Pediatr* 109:753, 1986.

Henrickson M, Passo MH: Recognizing patterns in chronic limb pain, *Contemp Pediatr* 11:33, 1994.

151 Loss of Appetite

Martin H. Ulshen

Loss of appetite (anorexia) is a common symptom in pediatric practice. Acute illness in childhood often is associated with transient loss of appetite. Prolonged loss of appetite associated with poor weight gain or loss of weight usually signifies a serious chronic illness, either organic or psychogenic.

The mechanisms that regulate hunger and satiety are complex and still poorly understood.[2,4,6] Hypothalamic control of the appetite may be influenced by anticipation of a pleasurable meal, visual and taste sensations, ambient temperature, and changes in blood levels of glucose or other nutrients, as well as by limbic signals from higher central nervous system regions. Satiety appears to be initiated through the vagus nerve by gastric distention, by cholecystokinin release from the intestine after ingestion of food and from endogenous stores in the central nervous system, and by other possible humoral influences, such as glucagon and endorphins. Each individual may have a set point for body fat content, and deviations from this level may cause alterations in diet intake. Because no hypothesis appears to explain the mechanism of appetite control fully, it seems most likely that this function is influenced simultaneously by several stimuli. Certain physical characteristics of food (e.g., appearance, aroma, and bulk) undoubtedly contribute to the generation of appetite. Cytokines may be important in the appetite suppression that occurs with acute and chronic diseases. Beta-interleukin-1 and tumor necrosis factor-a, for example, both have been shown to act directly on the hypothalamus, which mediates appetite.

In considering anorexia, the physician first must separate complaints based on unrealistic parental dietary expectations from justified parental concern over a child's diminished nutritional intake. This usually is not difficult because children in the former situation thrive and gain weight appropriately. Although significant gastrointestinal disease commonly leads to poor appetite, anorexia may be the result of disease distant from the bowel. In the newborn period, poor oral intake by an infant developmentally capable of feeding may be the only indication of a major disorder, such as sepsis, meningitis, urinary tract infection, congenital viral infection, a gastrointestinal anomaly, central nervous system disease, renal failure, or a metabolic disorder.

During infancy, a wide spectrum of causes can account for inadequate caloric intake that has no obvious cause. An acute infectious disease is a common cause of transient anorexia in infants. If there is no obvious explanation for poor feeding, the practitioner always should consider the possibility of an oral disease such as thrush, gastroesophageal reflux, or a neurological disease. Emotional deprivation is a common cause of failure to thrive; a careful social history is essential to the evaluation. Early observation of parent-infant interaction in the hospital, including feeding techniques, may be appropriate. An infant who has not received oral feedings for a prolonged period because of medical problems (e.g., esophageal disease or short bowel syndrome) may not be interested when feedings are introduced by mouth. The mother and infant may require training (typically provided by a physical or speech therapist) and gradual advancement of an oral diet.

A state of chronically inadequate caloric intake can be established objectively by computing the total calories ingested (most of which come from formula) and comparing this with the estimated caloric requirements for weight. This is more difficult with breast-fed infants, although intake may be established by weighing the infant before and after feedings. If the nursing infant has a reduced intake, the physician must establish whether maternal milk production is inadequate or the infant is too weak or uninterested to nurse.

In older children and adolescents, an adequate evaluation of nutritional intake requires careful calorie counts. If the possibility of malabsorption is a concern, calories may be counted in conjunction with a 72-hour stool fat collection. It is important at the outset to separate children who have poor appetites from children who do not eat for fear of worsening their symptoms. Children who have abdominal pain resulting from chronic inflammatory bowel disease or chronic constipation may not eat because this increases their pain. Similarly, children who have chronic diarrhea may eat less if doing so seems to lead to improved stools. These patients actually may not have anorexia, and treatment aimed at improving the other symptoms may result in a rapid improvement in appetite.

The box on p. 1053 presents a list of causes of loss of appetite applicable to both infants and children. Generally, the best approach to anorexia is to treat the underlying condition.

Enlisting the help of a dietitian to plan diets can be useful for maximizing nutritional intake in older children. Nutritional supplements may be indicated (e.g., high-calorie milk shakes, Carnation Instant Breakfast, Ensure, and Sustacal). Other nonspecific treatments include a trial of cyproheptadine, which, although controversial, has been shown in a number of studies to stimulate appetite. In some disorders (e.g., congenital heart disease), a nasogastric or nasoduodenal infusion of nutrients may be necessary to promote growth.[10] Parenteral nutrition may be indicated in very specific situations; however, both expertise with this modality and close supervision are required. Caretakers need special training if parenteral nutrition is to be provided at home.[9] Refeeding after severe malnutrition requires careful consideration of potential cardiac and metabolic complications.[8]

REFERENCES

1. Bernstein IL, Sigmundi RA: Tumor anorexia: a learned food aversion? *Science* 209:416, 1980.
2. Brobeck JR: Nature of satiety signals, *Am J Clin Nutr* 28:806, 1975.

CAUSES OF LOSS OF APPETITE IN INFANTS AND CHILDREN

Organic disease

- Infectious (acute or chronic)
- Neurological
  - Congenital degenerative disease
  - Hypothalamic lesion
  - Increased intracranial pressure (including a brain tumor)
  - Swallowing disorders (neuromuscular)
- Gastrointestinal
  - Oral lesions (e.g., thrush or herpes simplex)
  - Gastroesophageal reflux[3]
  - Obstruction (especially with gastric or intestinal distention)
  - Inflammatory bowel disease
  - Celiac disease
  - Constipation
- Cardiac
  - Congestive heart failure (especially associated with cyanotic lesions)
- Metabolic
  - Renal failure and/or renal tubule acidosis
  - Liver failure
  - Congenital metabolic disease
  - Lead poisoning
- Nutritional
  - Marasmus
  - Iron deficiency
  - Zinc deficiency
- Fever
  - Rheumatoid arthritis
  - Rheumatic fever
- Drugs
  - Morphine
  - Digitalis
  - Antimetabolites
  - Methylphenidate
  - Amphetamines
- Miscellaneous
  - Prolonged restriction of oral feedings, beginning in the neonatal period
  - Systemic lupus erythematosus
  - Tumor[1]

Psychological factors

- Anxiety, fear, depression, mania (limbic influence on the hypothalamus)[5]
- Avoidance of symptoms associated with meals (abdominal pain, diarrhea, bloating, urgency, dumping syndrome)
- Anorexia nervosa (see Chapter 98)
- Excessive weight loss and food aversion in athletes, simulating anorexia nervosa[7,11]

3. Dellert SF et al: Feeding resistance and gastroesophageal reflux in infancy, *J Pediatr Gastroenterol Nutr* 17:66, 1993.
4. Plata-Salaman CR: Regulation of hunger and satiety in man, *Dig Dis Sci* 9:253, 1991.
5. Pugliese MT et al: Fear of obesity: a cause of short stature and delayed puberty, *N Engl J Med* 309:513, 1983.
6. Robinson PH et al: Gastric control of food intake, *J Psychosom Res* 32:593, 1988.
7. Smith NJ: Excessive weight loss and food aversion in athletes simulating anorexia nervosa, *Pediatrics* 66:139, 1980.
8. Solomon SM, Kirby DF: The refeeding syndrome: a review, *J Parenter Enteral Nutr* 14:90, 1990.
9. Strobel CT, Byrne WJ, Fonkalsrud EW: Home parenteral nutrition: results in 34 pediatric patients, *Ann Surg* 188:394, 1978.
10. Vanderhoff JA et al: Continuous enteral feedings: an important adjunct to the management of complex congenital heart disease, *Am J Dis Child* 136:825, 1982.
11. Yates A, Leehey K, Shisslak CM: Running: an analogue of anorexia? *N Engl J Med* 308:251, 1983.

152 Lymphadenopathy

George B. Segel and Caroline Breese Hall

Lymphadenopathy, or enlargement of the lymph nodes, is a common problem in childhood. Lymphadenopathy may be defined as any lymph node enlargement; all lymph nodes that are palpable technically are considered to be enlarged. However, nodes in the cervical chain and occipital areas drain regions commonly infected in childhood and often are mildly enlarged (less than 1 cm in diameter) in children who otherwise are normal.

The clinically relevant problems in assessing lymphadenopathy are (1) whether any lymph node or lymph node aggregate or chain is abnormal and requires further assessment, (2) if abnormal, whether the nodes are benign, primarily inflammatory, or malignant, and (3) the appropriate evaluation, diagnosis, and management.

CHARACTERISTICS OF LYMPH NODE ENLARGEMENT

Components of the Lymphatic System

The lymphatic system includes not only lymph nodes but also the spleen, thymus, tonsils, Waldeyer ring, and Peyer patches in the intestine, as well as the appendix. Potentially palpable lymph node groups and their drainage areas are shown in Table 152-1, which may serve as a guide to palpation of these superficial nodes.

Lymph Node Features

Abnormalities of the palpable lymph nodes are assessed by noting the node's size, location, mobility, inflammatory reaction, and consistency. Small nodes (less than 1 cm) are found often in the cervical chain and the femoral and inguinal areas. Likewise, nodes less than 0.5 cm may be palpated in the occipital, postauricular (mastoid), and axillary chains (see Table 152-1). In the submental or submaxillary regions, intraoral or facial infections may enlarge the nodes to over 1 cm. It is unusual, however, to find lymph nodes of any size in the supraclavicular or epitrochlear areas. Thus the same size lymph node observed in two different regions may have markedly different implications. For example, a 1 cm node in the cervical region is very likely to be benign, whereas a 1 cm supraclavicular node requires a biopsy because it is unlikely to result from superficial inflammatory disease and may reflect intrathoracic or intraabdominal malignancy.

Fluctuance and signs of inflammation surrounding a group of enlarged lymph nodes are helpful in reaching a diagnosis, particularly if an infectious source is present distal to the node area. These findings strongly suggest an infectious etiology (Table 152-2), usually requiring systemic antibiotic therapy. If no inflammation is found, the consistency and mobility of the nodes may heighten suspicion of underlying malignancy. Hard, fixed nodes are seen more often in adults who have metastatic carcinoma. The nodes of Hodgkin disease and lymphoma are more matted than hard, although nodes associated with neuroblastoma, rhabdomyosarcoma, and other childhood malignancies may mimic the findings in adults.

DIFFERENTIAL DIAGNOSIS

The major differential diagnostic categories for enlarged lymph nodes include infectious (inflammatory) and neoplastic diseases. Table 152-2 provides a summary of the common and not so common conditions associated with lymphadenopathy for newborns, infants, children, and adolescents, since the relative occurrence varies with age. The classification of these conditions is somewhat arbitrary and not all-inclusive but does reflect the diagnostic likelihood within a given age group.

Infections

Infectious problems may be localized or systemic. If localized, the primary site of infection draining to the involved lymph node area should be identified.

The common pyogenic bacteria, atypical mycobacteria, anaerobic bacteria, and cat scratch are most likely to cause localized adenopathy. Generalized adenopathy or regional adenopathy associated with adenopathy elsewhere is more likely to be caused by infections from viruses, spirochetes, or sometimes *Toxoplasma. Mycobacterium tuberculosis* may produce localized or multiple sites of adenitis. Fungal infections, such as histoplasmosis, occasionally may cause generalized lymphadenopathy, but most fungal infections, if associated with adenopathy at all, produce regional enlargement.

Neoplastic Diseases

Primary neoplastic diseases are the other major consideration in both localized and generalized adenopathy. Included in this category are lymphomas, leukemia, histiocytosis, and metastases from solid tumors such as neuroblastoma, Wilms tumor, Ewing sarcoma, and rhabdomyosarcoma.

Immunological and Inflammatory Diseases

Generalized lymphadenopathy also may be associated with chronic inflammatory conditions, such as collagen-vascular diseases and sarcoidosis, with reactions to certain drugs, such as phenytoin and isoniazid, or serum sickness. Such divergent causes as hyperthyroidism and Addison disease also must be included in the differential diagnosis of generalized adenopathy.

ASSESSMENT

History, Physical Examination, and Chest Roentgenogram

The history and physical examination may reveal a source of a localized infection, such as a dental abscess, mastoiditis, scalp infection, insect bite, or cat scratch. Alternatively,

Table 152-1 Palpable Lymph Nodes and Lymphatic Drainage

Node area	Area of drainage
Occipital	Posterior scalp, neck
Mastoid	Mastoid area
Submental	Apex of tongue and lower lip
Submaxillary	Tongue, buccal cavity, lips, and cheek
Cervical	Cranium, neck, and oropharynx
Axillary	Greater part of arm, shoulder, superficial anterior and lateral thoracic and upper abdominal wall
Supraclavicular	Right: Inferior neck and mediastinum Left: Inferior neck, mediastinum, and upper abdomen
Epitrochlear	Hand, forearm, and elbow
Inguinal	Leg and genitalia
Femoral	Leg
Popliteal	Posterior leg and knee

systemic diseases such as infectious mononucleosis, juvenile rheumatoid arthritis (JRA), infection with the human immunodeficiency virus (HIV), and others may be suggested by other characteristic historical and physical findings. The physical examination should include all the palpable nodes listed in Table 152-1. Furthermore, assessment of enlarged lymph nodes without an obvious inflammatory explanation requires a chest roentgenogram to determine whether enlarged mediastinal or hilar nodes are present. The chest roentgenogram is the study most commonly omitted in the evaluation of patients who have lymphadenopathy and are referred to our center. Mediastinal or hilar adenopathy would preclude "trials of antibiotics," with the attendant delay in performing a diagnostic biopsy.

Imaging

The abdominal lymph nodes, including retroperitoneal, periportal, and celiac nodes, as well as the nodes of the splenic hilum, are more difficult to evaluate without more sophisticated imaging techniques. The spleen, which is primarily lymphoid tissue, may be enlarged in infectious, immunological, collagen-vascular, and neoplastic disorders and may be delineated by ultrasound or computed tomography (CT) examination. Abdominal and pelvic lymph nodes may be visualized by ultrasonography or may require techniques such as CT and magnetic resonance imaging (MRI). In some special circumstances lymphangiograms are used to define the iliac and periaortic nodes for the staging of Hodgkin disease.

Complete Blood Count

A number of other studies may be useful in the assessment of lymphadenopathy. The complete blood count (CBC) may reveal the reactive lymphocytes of infectious mononucleosis or a granulocytosis with a "shift to the left," suggesting systemic bacterial infection. Any cytopenia (e.g., anemia, granulocytopenia, or thrombocytopenia) would be a "red flag" that a hematological malignancy, such as leukemia or lymphoma, or metastatic disease involving the bone marrow, such as neuroblastoma, may underlie the lymphadenopathy. The finding of nucleated erythrocytes and immature granulocytes ("leukoerythroblastic blood picture") on the peripheral blood film is an ominous sign suggesting bone marrow "irritation"; this is seen in metastatic diseases such as neuroblastoma and rhabdomyosarcoma and with immunological vasculitis.

Infectious Evaluation

The diagnostic workup of potential infectious lymphadenopathy is diverse and depends on the history, the patient's age, the location of the nodes, and the signs of inflammation accompanying the adenopathy, as previously noted. For acute, inflamed, and localized adenopathy, an infectious etiological diagnosis is achieved most frequently by obtaining material for culture and histological or pathological examination. In children who have acute cervical adenitis, needle aspiration of an acutely inflamed, sometimes fluctuant node demonstrates the infecting organism in two thirds or more of cases. The aspirated material should be cultured aerobically and anaerobically and for fungi and mycobacteria. Histochemical evaluation should include a gram and acid-fast stain. In certain cases a biopsy may be required, and this may be evaluated by additional special stains, such as the Warthin-Starry silver stain for cat-scratch disease. Intradermal skin tests should be applied when mycobacterial infection is suspected. Although a skin test exists for cat-scratch disease, the antigen is neither standardized nor available commercially. However, serological tests for *Bartonella henselae,* the major agent of cat scratch disease, have been developed and are available commercially. Specific serological or antigen detection tests also are available for syphilis, toxoplasmosis, brucellosis, tularemia, fungi, and some viral infections such as Epstein-Barr virus, HIV, cytomegalovirus, and herpes simplex virus (HSV). Viral cultures are appropriate for the last two and for the common respiratory viruses, such as the adenoviruses and enteroviruses. The erythrocyte sedimentation rate may be useful in assessing underlying inflammation, but it is not unique to infectious diseases because it may be elevated in immunological and neoplastic diseases as well.

After initial evaluation by history, physical examination, chest roentgenogram, and preliminary laboratory studies, the clinician may not yet have an obvious explanation for the node enlargement. If a bacterial source for localized adenopathy (e.g., pharyngitis and cervical nodes) is suggested, a limited course of 7 to 10 days of antibiotic therapy may be tried. However, if the nodes have not regressed significantly, prompt further evaluation is necessary. At this time a chest roentgenogram should be obtained, if it has not already been done, and even in the absence of mediastinal or hilar adenopathy, significantly enlarged, unexplained lymph nodes should be biopsied promptly to permit institution of appropriate therapy.

Biopsy

Biopsy of significant adenopathy should be performed early if no evidence suggests an infection or other etiology, and particularly if mediastinal or hilar nodes are enlarged. The biopsy should encompass the central mass of the enlarged nodes to avoid a misdiagnosis of reactive inflammation in adjacent nodes. This is particularly common in Hodgkin disease, in which an adjacent smaller lymph node may be more

Table 152-2 Etiology of Lymphadenopathy

Differential diagnosis	Newborn	Infant	Child	Adolescent
Infections				
Bacterial	Group B streptococci			
Pyogenic		Streptococci/staphylococci, and other gram positive and gram negative organisms		
			Cat-scratch fever →	→
			Typhoid fever →	→
			Tularemia →	→
Spirochetal	Syphilis →	→		Syphilis
				Anaerobes
				Vincent angina
Granulomatous		Mycobacteria →	→	→
		Atypical mycobacteria →	→	→
Viral			Rubella →	→
			Rubeola →	→
			Varicella →	→
		→	→	→HHV6 syndrome
		Adenovirus →	→	→
		Enterovirus →	→	→
			Epstein-Barr virus (EBV) →	→
			Cytomegalovirus (CMV) →	→
			Herpes simplex virus (HSV) (stomatitis, pharyngitis, or skin infection) →	→
		Human immunodeficiency virus (HIV) →	→	→
Protozoan	Toxoplasmosis →	→	→	→
Fungal		Histoplasmosis →	→	→
		Other fungi (rare cases) →	→	→
Rickettsial			Rocky Mountain spotted fever →	→
Chlamydial				Lymphogranuloma
Parasitic			Toxocara →	→
			Myiasis →	→
Neoplastic				
Endogenous		Leukemia →	→	→
		Lymphoma →	→	→
		Histiocytosis →	→	→
			Hodgkin disease →	→
Exogenous (Metastatic)		Neuroblastoma →	→	→
		Wilms tumor →	→	→
			Ewing sarcoma →	→
			Rhabdomyosarcoma	
Immunological		Juvenile rheumatoid arthritis (JRA) →	→	→
			Systemic lupus erythematosus (SLE) →	→
		Serum sickness →	→	→
			Sarcoidosis →	→
Other				
(Reactive)		Kawasaki disease →	→	
			Hemoglobinopathies →	→
			Hemophilia →	→
			Phenytoin →	→
			Addison disease →	→
			Hyperthyroidism →	→
	Chronic granulomatous disease (CGD) →	→	→	→
	Agammaglobulinemia →	→	→	→

accessible and technically easier to biopsy but may not demonstrate the presence of Reed-Sternberg cells.

It is critical that the biopsy be performed at a medical center specializing in the care of children so that all of the appropriate touch preparations, cultures, special cytochemical or immunological stains, and biochemical or cytogenetic studies are obtained. The pathology of Hodgkin disease, lymphoma, and other similar round cell tumors may be difficult to establish and requires the assessment of a pediatric pathologist who has experience in these diseases. The biopsy diagnosis obviously is critical for subsequent management, which may involve treatment with radiation or chemotherapy, or both.

TREATMENT

Infectious Diseases

Therapy of lymphadenitis depends on determining its etiology or judging the most likely cause. Acute adenitis, particularly of the cervical area in young children, frequently is associated with infection from group A beta-hemolytic streptococci or *Staphylococcus aureus*. The latter is particularly likely in adenitis that progresses to fluctuance. In the neonate and rarely in older children, group B streptococci may cause localized adenitis with or without cellulitis. In children beyond the neonatal period who have acute localized adenitis, primarily cervical, antibiotic therapy should be directed at group A streptococci with an antibiotic that covers penicillinase-producing strains of *S. aureus*. For most patients, oral therapy with drugs such as dicloxacillin or cloxacillin is adequate. The broader spectrum oral agents (e.g., Augmentin) and especially first and second generation oral cephalosporins also may be used.

The usual course of therapy is 10 to 14 days, but therapy should be continued for at least 5 days after the signs of acute inflammation have subsided. For patients who have suppurative adenitis from these organisms, drainage is not only diagnostic (by culturing the exudate obtained), but also therapeutic. A few patients may not respond to oral therapy, even with a drug to which the organism is known to be sensitive. Parenteral antibiotic therapy then is required.

If an anaerobic infection is suspected, therapy depends in part on the location of the adenitis and the type of organism. Most anaerobic infections of the cervical and submental area are associated with mouth flora, most of which are sensitive to penicillin. Occasionally, however, such infections require alternative therapy such as clindamycin.

Both *M. tuberculosis* and atypical mycobacteria may cause adenitis, with the latter being more frequent in children. Differentiating the two may be difficult but is important because many strains of atypical mycobacteria are resistant to the usual antitubercular chemotherapy, and excisional biopsy may be required. If tubercular infection is suspected, appropriate therapy for *M. tuberculosis* (e.g., isoniazid and rifampin) should be initiated while awaiting identification and sensitivities of the organism. Adenitis suspected to be tubercular should not be incised or drained.

Cat-scratch adenitis usually is self-limited. The recent discovery of *Bartonella* spp., especially *B. henselae* as the prime cause of cat scratch disease has raised the potential for specific antibiotic therapy. However, treatment with antibiotics should be reserved for the severely ill because reports of controlled trials showing efficacy are not yet available. If nodes become markedly enlarged, tender, and fluctuant, aspiration may help relieve symptoms; incision and drainage, however, should be avoided.

For the unusual case of severe primary HSV infection with localized adenitis, treatment with oral acyclovir has been tried, but no data are available indicating its efficacy.

Neoplastic Disease

The treatment of neoplastic diseases today is oriented toward cure in most instances. The effectiveness of treatment for lymphocytic and myelocytic leukemia, lymphomas, and Wilms and other tumors has improved markedly in the past 2 decades. The specific treatment of childhood cancer often involves combinations of chemotherapy, radiation therapy, and surgery, which depend on the individual diagnosis and are beyond the scope of this presentation (see Chapter 190, Cancers in Childhood). However, prompt, accurate diagnosis is essential for institution of specific treatment and optimum care of these patients.

SUGGESTED READINGS

Filston HC: Common lumps and bumps of the head and neck in infants and children, *Pediatr Ann* 18:180, 1989.

Freidig EE et al: Clinical-histologic-microbiologic analysis of 419 lymph node biopsy specimens, *Rev Infect Dis* 8:322, 1986.

Knight PJ, Mulne AF, Vassy LE: When is lymph node biopsy indicated in children with enlarged peripheral nodes? *Pediatrics* 69:391, 1982.

Lake AM, Oski FA: Peripheral lymphadenopathy in childhood, *Am J Dis Child* 132:357, 1978.

Starke JR: Nontuberculous mycobacterial infections in children, *Adv Pediatr Infect Dis* 7:123, 1992.

153 Malocclusion

Lindsey K. Grossman

The incidence of malocclusion in school-age children and adolescents may be as high as 90% or more, according to some reports. In evaluating such statistics, however, one first must consider the definition involved, because in the field of orthodontics any deviation from absolutely ideal tooth alignment is considered malocclusion, although at most probably only 10% to 15% of these can be viewed as handicapping.[11] Indeed, the 1963 to 1965 National Health Survey, which examined 7400 children 6 to 11 years of age, found 14.2% to have severe or very severe malocclusion.[5] This national survey of malocclusion has not been repeated to date; however, there is no reason to believe that the incidence has changed during the past 3 decades.

A major problem hindering objective evaluation of orthodontic treatment is the lack of a universally acceptable classification system. The Treatment Priority Index, which was used in the National Health Survey, is a quantitative measure of severity, but because of its complexity has not been adopted widely. The commonly used Angle classification system effectively expresses qualitative but not quantitative differences in dental occlusion; hence it is not helpful in determining the need for referral or in evaluating the treatment outcome.[4] It therefore is difficult to determine objectively which patients require orthodontic correction or to compare the results of various treatments.

The etiology of malocclusion involves a number of factors, with both heredity and environment playing a role.[7] Significant evidence links nasal obstruction, especially when caused by enlarged tonsils or adenoids, with the development of a high arched palate and posterior crossbite.[8]

Significantly abnormal dental occlusion has been said to predispose individuals to many risks.[2,8,10] Caries, periodontal disease, increased susceptibility to trauma or root resorption, and disturbances of physiological functioning, including muscular dysfunction, speech defects, and masticatory disturbances, have been linked to malocclusion, although the data supporting such outcomes are either scanty or conflicting.[6] Temporomandibular joint (TMJ) dysfunction increasingly has been cited as a possible cause of headache and other symptoms in adolescents and school-age children. Some studies show an amazingly high incidence of signs referable to the temporomandibular joint but usually without symptoms of TMJ dysfunction. Signs such as joint sound or condyle position do not correlate well with symptomatic TMJ dysfunction requiring treatment, especially in children. Furthermore there is no convincing evidence that orthodontic therapy either promotes or prevents the development of temporomandibular symptoms.[13]

Most patients seek orthodontic treatment because of malocclusion's effect on their appearance. In our society, the individual's own sense of attractiveness can influence behavior and ultimate success in life. However, there is no direct evidence that treating dental irregularities affects these outcomes positively.

The pacifier, as well as thumb- and finger-sucking habits,[9] play a role in malocclusion problems. Most children develop such habits during infancy, and by 4 or 5 years of age most have stopped the practice; however, as many as 5.9% of children may continue into school age.[3] If sucking continues into the periods of mixed and permanent dentition, the potential for developing malocclusion is greater, although a specific causal relationship may not always hold. Often, abnormal bites revert to normal after the habit is dropped. Anterior open bite, overjet, crossbites, and other malocclusions have been reported in association with oral habits, although other children who have such habits may show no abnormalities. Thumb-sucking may be preferable to finger-sucking because fewer physical stresses are exerted on the teeth. A pacifier probably has the least deleterious effects. Most studies show that use of a pacifier stops earlier than thumb- or finger-sucking.

In the assessment of occlusion, both the maxillary and mandibular arches should be observed with the mouth open to determine if the teeth are crowded or have excess space between them.[11] Crowding almost always increases over time, whereas excess space either improves or worsens. Excess space, especially between the upper lateral incisors and canines and the lower canines and first deciduous molars, is the norm in young children who have primary dentition and allows room for the eruption of the larger, permanent teeth.

Occlusion of the posterior teeth is assessed with the teeth set in the biting position. The tongue should not be visible between the upper and lower teeth; the presence of such a space, albeit very small, or the contrasting problem of a deep bite (lower incisors biting on palatal gingiva) nearly always requires treatment. The maxillary teeth should overlap their mandibular partners slightly in the lateral plane and be placed slightly anterior (approximately one-half tooth) to them. The degree of malalignment at this point will determine the need for referral.

Anterior dentition problems, readily apparent when the patient smiles, are the source of many orthodontic referrals. Open bites with space visible between the upper and lower arches, as well as deep bites, are difficult problems to treat, whereas overbite ("buck teeth") or anterior crossbite often can be corrected easily. Occasionally, one or more of the permanent teeth, often incisors, erupt before the corresponding primary teeth have been shed, giving the child a double row of teeth and causing much parental concern. Extraction rarely is necessary, since the primary teeth almost always are shed by age 8. Normal tongue movements usually ensure correct final placement of the permanent teeth.

Few data link maloccluded primary dentition with maloccluded permanent teeth. However, the presence of anterior crossbite, wherein the upper lateral incisors erupt behind the lower ones or the upper posterior teeth erupt medial to the lower ones, may interfere with ultimate maxillary growth and tooth position. The absence of normal spacing in primary dentition almost always leads to severe crowding of the permanent teeth. Children who have conditions should be referred to an orthodontist early.[10,12] Probably the most important influence that pediatricians have in promoting good dental occlusion is their advice concerning primary dentition. Congenital absence or loss of one or more of the primary teeth to decay or trauma can seriously affect the spacing required for normal occlusion of the permanent teeth. Thus a dental referral is advisable if any primary tooth fails to erupt or is prematurely lost.[9]

In general, however, the decision to refer a child or young adolescent for orthodontic treatment may be difficult; there are few objective referral guidelines.[1] Treatment nearly always results in an improved, although not necessarily a flawless, appearance; nevertheless, the pediatrician should assess the patient's and family's expectations as well as their willingness to comply with the discomfort and cost of treatment before arranging for referral.

REFERENCES

1. Currier GF: Fundamentals of orthodontics with criteria for referral, *Pediatr Ann* 14:117, 1985.
2. Helm S: Etiology and treatment need of malocclusion, *J Can Dent Assoc* 45:673, 1979.
3. Gellin ME: Digital sucking and tongue thrusting in children, *Dent Clin North Am* 22:603, 1978.
4. Jago JD: The epidemiology of dental occlusion: a critical appraisal, *J Public Health Dent* 34:80, 1974.
5. Kelly JE, Sanchez M, VanKirk LE: An assessment of the occlusion of teeth of children 6-11 years. *NHS* Series 11, No 130, US Department of Health, Education and Welfare Publications (PHS) 74-1612, 1973.
6. McLain JB, Profitt WR: Oral health status in the United States: prevalence of malocclusion, *J Dent Educ* 49:386, 1985.
7. Proffit WR: On the aetiology of malocclusion, *Br J Orthod* 13:1, 1986.
8. Richter HJ: Obstruction of the pediatric upper airway, *Ear Nose Throat J* 66:209, 1987.
9. Schneider PE, Peterson J: Oral habits: considerations in management, *Pediatr Clin North Am* 29:523, 1982.
10. Shaw WC, Addy M, Ray C: Dental and social effects of malocclusion and effectiveness of orthodontic treatment: a review, *Commun Dent Oral Epidemiol* 8:36, 1980.
11. Smith RJ: Development of occlusion and malocclusion, *Pediatr Clin North Am* 29:475, 1982.
12. Sweeney EA: Pediatric dentistry, *Curr Probl Pediatr* 11:1, 1980.
13. Tallents RN, Catania J, Dommers E: Temporomandibular joint findings in pediatric populations and young adults: a critical review, *Angle Orthod* 61:7, 1991.

154 Nervousness

Richard M. Sarles and Henry M. Seidel

Some chief complaints occasion a sinking feeling in a busy physician, especially when he or she first hears them in the middle of a busy afternoon in the office. The nature of such complaints implies that the physician and patient are about to embark on an often murky and abstract search for the root of an evanescent symptom or problem. One such complaint is nervousness, whether it is voiced by an older child or an adolescent or by a parent about a child. For example, the mother who describes her 12-year-old as "nervous all the time," to which the patient responds vaguely, "I don't know, maybe I just feel funny."

Such moments call for discipline on the part of the physician. They remind us that this may be a circumstance in which an inarticulate patient literally is shouting for help. It is the kind of complaint with which patients may signal that they are among those most in need of help. The physician must look beyond the chief complaint to the "iatrotropic," the "doctor-seeking," stimulus: Why is this patient here having this complaint? What does it mean?

Finding the answer will take time, perhaps a great deal of time. The approach, however, is clear. A good history and physical examination are needed. The circumstance is not life threatening; everything does not have to be done immediately. Indeed, some of the effort may be delayed until a time when the physician can schedule more time and is more at ease and less stressed. Certainly the abstraction of the term *nervousness* and the difficulty in defining it more precisely underscore the need and the necessary care.

What accompanies the nervousness—anorexia, restlessness at night, sluggishness, overactivity? A physical problem is implied but quite often is not at the root. Nervousness, for example, often is part of the constellation of complaints in a variety of endocrine disorders (hyperthyroidism, hypoglycemia, Addison disease) and in dermatitis, pinworm infestation, and allergy. Caffeine ingestion (colas and coffee) and abuse of a variety of drugs also can cause "nervousness." Mitral valve prolapse and paroxysmal auricular tachycardia are cardiac diseases that can create symptoms of nervousness. Clearly, a careful history and thorough physical examination can be productive.

The physician also should consider the possibility of an attention deficit disorder with or without hyperactivity, as well as a variety of anxiety disorders including separation anxieties and school phobia and somatization of depression. Many more serious problems, such as autism, childhood psychoses, obsessive-compulsive and manic-depressive disorders, panic attacks, and Tourette syndrome, all can be verbalized as nervousness as the parents or patient try to define perceptions and feelings. However, such problems rarely are defined as nervousness alone; the history and physical examination quickly can uncover a host of concomitant findings.

It is after a conscientious biopsychosocial search has been made and when little if anything more has been discovered that the chief complaint of nervousness becomes ever more difficult to approach. Time, caring, and sensitive understanding of the patient's needs are required. Unfortunately, little help is available in the literature. Nervousness usually is not defined or described in textbooks and is not listed in the American Psychiatric Association's *Diagnostic and Statistical Manual of Mental Disorders* (DSM-IV) or in any standard psychiatric textbook, and a discussion of its implications generally is not included in most medical school curricula.

How, then, is the practitioner to conceptualize, diagnose, and treat nervousness, nervous stomach, or other disorders that occur as symptoms without any readily discernible underlying pathophysiology? First, of course, comes the careful search; then come the devotion of time, the "listening ear," the sensitive exploration, and if necessary, referral to a colleague who has expertise in emotional disorders of childhood and adolescence to attempt to unravel the sometimes intricate psychosocial puzzle.

By this time the physician may know that the patient has no physical disorder; however, emotional tension, restlessness, agitation, fearful apprehension, acute uneasiness, undue excitability, or excessive irritability is evident. These manifestations, quite real and requiring care, may require individual attention to the child or work with the family in a group; indeed, the approaches may be as infinite as the variety of complaints. A physician who is unprepared or unwilling to provide this degree of time and effort should refer the patient in order to ease the morbidity inevitably associated with these complaints.

155 Nonconvulsive Periodic Disorders

Sarah M. Roddy

A variety of paroxysmal nonepileptic disorders occur in children. These disorders have a wide range of clinical features that mimic seizures, and it is important to distinguish them from seizures so that the child is not treated with anticonvulsants inappropriately. A careful history often is all that is needed to make the diagnosis, although a few patients may require a more extensive evaluation. Some of the more common paroxysmal nonepileptic disorders are reviewed here.

BREATH-HOLDING SPELLS

Breath-holding spells, or infantile syncope, occur in approximately 5% of children.[13] Most children who have breath-holding spells begin having episodes between 6 and 18 months of age, although some may begin in the first few weeks of life. The frequency of episodes ranges from once a year to several times daily. The history of the episode and the surrounding events are the most important part of the evaluation of a child who has such spells. Because the familial incidence of breath-holding spells is high, the parents should be questioned about episodes in other family members.

Two types of breath-holding spells occur. The cyanotic type is more common and usually is precipitated by frustration or anger. The child cries vigorously and then holds his or her breath in expiration. This apnea is followed by cyanosis with opisthotonic posturing and loss of consciousness. Recovery usually is quick, with return of respiration and consciousness within 1 minute. Evaluation of children who have severe cyanotic breath-holding spells has shown an underlying autonomic system dysregulation that may contribute to the pathophysiology of the episodes.[7] Pallid breath-holding episodes usually are provoked by sudden fright or minor injuries, especially falling and hitting the occiput. The child gasps or cries briefly and then abruptly becomes quiet, loses consciousness, has pallor, and becomes limp. The child then may develop clonic jerks. Pallid breath-holding spells are a vasovagal phenomenon. The precipitating event induces a vagally mediated asystole with a secondary cerebral ischemia. Ocular compression during simultaneous electroencephalographic and electrocardiographic tracing in children who have pallid breath-holding spells has shown asystole with flattening of the electroencephalogram without electrical seizure activity.[13,17] The clonic jerks are caused by cerebral hypoxia rather than by epileptiform discharges from the brain.

The prognosis for children who have either type of breath holding is excellent; most outgrow the episodes by school age. Children who have pallid breath-holding spells later may develop syncope.[13] Treatment is directed mainly at reassuring the family of the benign nature of the episodes. It is important to emphasize that the episodes are not seizures and that they do not lead to mental retardation or epilepsy. Because cyanotic episodes often are precipitated by temper tantrums, anger, and frustration, advice about behavior management may be helpful. Anemia has been described as a contributing factor in breath-holding spells, and treating it may reduce the incidence of the episodes.[13] Atropine is effective for pallid breath-holding episodes, but its use rarely is warranted. Anticonvulsants should not be used because they are not effective in the treatment of either type of breath-holding spell.

SYNCOPE

Syncope (or fainting) is an acute and transient loss of consciousness caused by reduced cerebral perfusion. These episodes are relatively common in teenagers. Postural hypotension, which may occur after a sudden change from a sitting or reclining position to a standing position, can precipitate an episode. Emotional upset, fright, or overheating also are common provoking stimuli. Cardiac disorders, including arrhythmias, aortic stenosis, and severe cyanotic heart disease, may cause syncope by reducing cardiac output. In rare cases, episodes of syncope have been reported with swallowing, coughing, urinating, and defecating.[6,14,19]

Patients have presyncopal symptoms that may include light-headedness, anxiety, sweating, nausea, generalized numbness, and visual changes described as constriction or darkening of vision. Observers notice marked pallor and clammy skin. These symptoms are followed by loss of consciousness and slumping to the floor. Once the patient is recumbent and cerebral perfusion is restored, consciousness returns within a few seconds. If the patient is held with his or her head above the body and cerebral perfusion is not restored, clonic movements may occur. As with the pallid breath-holding spells, these movements occur secondary to cerebral ischemia rather than to epileptiform discharges from the brain. Patients are not disoriented or confused after an episode of syncope, although they may be tired.

The history is very important in diagnosing syncope, and it should include a description of the event by the patient and an observer. Laboratory evaluation seldom is needed, but if atypical features are involved, such as absence of a precipitating factor or confusion after the episode, an electroencephalogram or a cardiac evaluation, including Holter monitoring, may be necessary. Evaluation with tilt table testing has been recommended for children who have unexplained syncope.[16] Treatment consists of teaching the patient and family about managing an episode. Because patients have presyncopal symptoms, they should be instructed to sit or lie down as soon as the symptoms begin, thereby preventing progression to loss of consciousness. If the patient does lose consciousness, the family should place him or her in a recumbent position with the head lower than the body. Parents often pick up a child who has fainted; they should be cautioned against doing this because they could prolong the period of unconsciousness (see Chapter 170, Syncope, for a more detailed discussion of syncope and its causes.)

BENIGN PAROXYSMAL VERTIGO

Benign paroxysmal vertigo of childhood is a disorder characterized by brief attacks of vertigo. Symptoms usually appear within the first 3 or 4 years of life, although they may begin later. Episodes are characterized by abrupt onset, with the child appearing fearful and unable to maintain normal posture and gait. The child may seek support and clutch the parent or abruptly sit down or fall. In severe cases the child may be limp and incapable of using his or her extremities. Pallor and diaphoresis usually are apparent, and vomiting and nystagmus occur in some cases. Typically an episode lasts less than 30 seconds, in rare cases, a few minutes. A brief period of postural instability may follow the episode, but within a few minutes the child is back to normal and playing. Consciousness is not altered during the episode, nor does the child feel sleepy after it. The frequency of episodes varies from as many as several weekly to as few as one every 4 months. Audiograms are normal, but caloric testing, which is difficult to perform in young children, is abnormal, demonstrating reduction of vestibular sensitivity.[3,12] Radiographic studies of the temporal bone and electroencephalographic recordings also are normal. Included in the differential diagnosis of vertigo in childhood are brainstem lesions, posterior fossa tumors, and epilepsy. Usually the history and physical examination differentiate benign paroxysmal vertigo from these more serious disorders. In most cases no treatment is necessary, and anticonvulsants are not effective. Antihistamines such as dimenhydrinate have been used in some patients who have frequent episodes, with an apparent reduction in the number of episodes. Because the frequency of attacks varies, it is difficult to assess the effect of therapy accurately. Attacks of vertigo usually stop spontaneously over a period of a few years. Some children who had had benign paroxysmal vertigo later developed migraine headaches[9] (see Chapter 121, Dizziness and Vertigo).

SHUDDERING ATTACKS

Shuddering or shivering episodes are a benign movement disorder that probably occurs in many children at one time or another. The episodes are brief and characterized by paroxysmal rapid tremors primarily involving the head and arms. Some episodes may involve flexion of the head, elbow, trunk, and knees, with adduction of the elbows and knees.[18] Consciousness is not altered during the episodes. The frequency varies, with some children having more than 100 episodes daily. Emotional factors, including excitement, fear, anger, and frustration, may precipitate episodes. Shuddering episodes may start as early as a few months of age or not until later in childhood. Usually the number of episodes gradually declines. The pathophysiology of the episodes is unclear, although it has been postulated that the attacks are an expression of an essential tremor.[18] Electroencephalographic monitoring has shown that the episodes are not epileptiform in nature.[10] Usually no treatment is necessary. If episodes are severe and interfere with activities, treatment with propranolol may be helpful[2]; anticonvulsants are ineffective and should not be used.

BENIGN NEONATAL SLEEP MYOCLONUS

Sudden brief jerks of the extremities are normal in children and adults when falling asleep. Sleep-related myoclonus in neonates is called *benign neonatal sleep myoclonus*. The myoclonic jerks begin in the first month of life, often within the first day of life. The myoclonus is present only during sleep and may be present in both quiet and active sleep states. The jerking movements may start in one extremity and then progress to involve the other extremities, or they may begin bilaterally. They occur every 2 to 3 seconds for several minutes, although they have been reported to last up to 90 minutes.[5] The neonates develop normally and have no neurological deficit. Electroencephalographic results are normal, with no epileptiform discharges associated with the myoclonus.[15] The major differential diagnosis of neonatal sleep myoclonus is a seizure disorder. A history of episodes only during sleep and a normal electroencephalogram help to differentiate this benign disorder from seizures. The myoclonus usually diminishes gradually during the first 6 months of life. No treatment is necessary.

NIGHT TERRORS

Night terrors are a sleep disorder with some features that mimic partial complex seizures. They occur in up to 6% of children, with a peak incidence in late preschool and early school-age children.[8] There often is a family history of night terrors or sleep disorders. The episodes usually occur during the first 2 hours after falling asleep. The child sits up in bed abruptly and screams or talks unintelligibly. If the child's eyes are open, he or she has a glazed look. During the episode the child appears to be hallucinating and does not respond to the parents. Tachycardia and diaphoresis result from the response of the sympathetic nervous system. In some cases the child may sleepwalk. A night terror usually lasts about 10 minutes, with the child relaxing and abruptly falling back to sleep. Upon awakening the child does not remember the episode. Night terrors are caused by a rapid partial arousal from deep, slow-wave sleep.

Electroencephalography does not show seizure activity during the episodes. It is important to differentiate night terrors from nightmares, which occur during rapid eye movement (REM) sleep and are associated with easy arousal and recall of the content, or at least the occurrence, of the nightmare. Night terrors usually occur less often as the child gets older, although episodes may continue into adolescence and adulthood. The nature of the episodes should be explained to the parents. Although parents tend to try to wake and reassure the child, they should be told that the child is not aware of their presence, and attempts to awaken him or her are not helpful. Usually no medication is indicated, but if episodes are frequent or severe, diazepam is the drug of choice.[1]

NARCOLEPSY

Narcolepsy is a sleep-wake disorder characterized by excessive and inappropriate periods of sleep during the day. The daytime sleepiness interrupts activities and does not diminish in response to adequate amounts of sleep at night. Naps may last from a few minutes to longer than 1 hour. In addition to the excessive daytime sleep, patients often have cataplexy, sleep paralysis, and hypnagogic hallucinations. Cataplexy is a transient partial or complete loss of tone, often triggered by an emotional reaction such as laughter or fright. The individual does not lose consciousness. Sleep paralysis occurs as the patient falls asleep or awakens and is characterized by the inability to move or speak. Hypnagogic hallucinations occur while falling asleep, can be auditory or visual, and may be very frightening to a child. The prevalence of narcolepsy is 0.04% to 0.09% in the entire population, but it increases to 50% with a family history of the disorder.[11] Onset usually occurs in the second decade, although it has been reported in children as young as age 3. Sleep studies in patients who have narcolepsy show that sleep occurs within 15 minutes of sleep onset; in normal subjects, 90 minutes of non-REM sleep precede the first REM period.[20] Narcolepsy and the presence of the HLA-DR2 antigen are strongly associated.[4] HLA typing and sleep studies are important in diagnosing narcolepsy. Included in the differential diagnosis of excessive daytime sleepiness are chronic illness, sleep apnea, hypothyroidism, depression, and seizures.

Narcolepsy is a lifelong condition, but central nervous system stimulants such as methylphenidate help reduce the frequency of naps. Tricyclic medications such as imipramine are used to treat cataplexy and the other associated symptoms.

REFERENCES

1. Anders TF, Weinstein P: Sleep and its disorders in infants and children: a review, *Pediatrics* 50:312, 1972.
2. Barron TF, Younkin DP: Propranolol therapy for shuddering attacks, *Neurology* 42:258, 1992.
3. Basser LS: Benign paroxysmal vertigo of childhood (a variety of vestibular neuronitis), *Brain* 87:41, 1964.
4. Billiard M, Seignalet J: Extraordinary association between HLA-DR2 and narcolepsy, *Lancet* 1:226, 1985.
5. Blennow G: Benign infantile nocturnal myoclonus, *Acta Paediatr Scand* 74:505, 1985.
6. DiMaria AA Jr, Westmoreland BF, Sharbrough FW: EEG in cough syncope, *Neurology* 34:371, 1984.
7. DiMario FJ Jr, Burleson JA: Autonomic nervous system function in severe breath holding spells, *Pediatr Neurol* 9:268, 1993.
8. DiMario FJ Jr, Emery S III: The natural history of night terrors, *Clin Pediatr* 26:505, 1987.
9. Fenichel GM: Migraine as a cause of benign paroxysmal vertigo of childhood, *J Pediatr* 71:114, 1967.
10. Holmes GL, Russman BS: Shuddering attacks: evaluation using electroencephalographic frequency modulation radiotelemetry and videotape monitoring, *Am J Dis Child* 140:72, 1985.
11. Kessler S, Guilleminault C, Dement WC: A family study of 50 REM narcoleptics, *Acta Neurol Scand* 50:503, 1974.
12. Koenigsberger MR et al: Benign paroxysmal vertigo of childhood, *Neurology* 20:1108, 1970.
13. Lombroso CT, Lerman P: Breathholding spells (cyanotic and pallid infantile syncope), *Pediatrics* 39:563, 1967.
14. Proudfit WL, Forteza ME: Micturition syncope, *N Engl J Med* 260:328, 1959.
15. Resnick TJ et al: Benign neonatal sleep myoclonus: relationship to sleep states, *Arch Neurol* 43:266, 1986.
16. Samoil D et al: Head-upright tilt table testing in children with unexplained syncope, *Pediatrics* 92:426, 1993.
17. Stephenson JBP: Reflex anoxic seizures ("white breath-holding"): nonepileptic vagal attacks, *Arch Dis Child* 53:193, 1978.
18. Vanasse M, Bedard P, Andermann F: Shuddering attacks in children: an early clinical manifestation of essential tremor, *Neurology* 26:1027, 1976.
19. Woody RC, Kiel EA: Swallowing syncope in a child, *Pediatrics* 78:507, 1986.
20. Young D et al: Narcolepsy in a pediatric population, *Am J Dis Child* 142:210, 1988.

156 Odor (Unusual Urine and Body)

Modena E. H. Wilson

An unusual or offensive odor may be the presenting or even the only complaint. Odor may provide a diagnostic clue when other symptoms have prompted a visit to the pediatrician, or it may confirm a suspected diagnosis. An unusual odor may be noticed first by the child, family members, others who have contact with the child, or the examiner. Each of these situations suggests a set of possibilities that may overlap.

UNUSUAL ODOR AS THE CHIEF COMPLAINT

When an unusual body odor is the chief complaint, relevant questions include: When was the odor first noticed? What does it smell like to the patient or parents? Does it seem to come from any particular piece of clothing? Does bathing modify it, and if so, for how long? What other symptoms have been noted? Is there any reason to suspect that the child might have an object lodged in a body orifice? Is there drainage from any orifice or skin lesion? Is the child using any medications, either taken by mouth or applied topically? How has the odor affected the child and family?

ODOR AS A CLUE TO DIAGNOSIS

When a particular infection, metabolic defect, or ingestion is suspected for reasons other than odor, the practitioner may inquire about or note the presence or absence of an odor that often is associated with that condition to clarify the clinical situation.[11,14,19]

Any unexpected odor the physician detects during the history-taking or physical examination requires explanation. For example, the lingering odor of feces or urine on a child who should have attained continence may prompt consideration of encopresis or enuresis.

If a patient reports an unusual odor (especially intermittently) but it is never detected by others, the possibility of temporal lobe epilepsy should be entertained. On the other hand, if the practitioner notices an offensive body odor but the patient or parent does not, anosmia in either the child or the parent should be considered.

ODOR AND THE PHYSICAL EXAMINATION

In assessing an odor, the examiner should (1) note the character of the odor, (2) determine the patient's age (and stage of pubertal development), (3) check for any other signs or symptoms during a complete examination with the child unclothed, and (4) localize the odor to a particular body site.

In a medical examination, the sense the physician uses least is the sense of smell. Satisfactory methods of classifying, quantifying, or even describing odors have been lacking. Gas-liquid chromatography now allows more precise identification of odors. Historically and practically, odors have been compared with others for which we have common experience, and their strength is characterized either by the distance from which the odor is obvious or by such adjectives as "strong" or "faint." Also, individuals differ in their ability to detect at least some odors.

CAUSES OF UNUSUAL ODOR

An array of odors can be associated with the human body and with personal effects, such as clothing, and subtle differences in odor can be found among people as well. Therefore the first task may be to decide whether a particular odor truly is peculiar and whether it emanates from the body. The odor may be simply a normal body odor that drew attention because of its intensity or because the complainant is unusually sensitive to or concerned about it.

Normal Body Odor

Normal body odors derive from secretions of the sweat and apocrine glands, vagina, cervix, and respiratory tract and from urine, feces, breath, and flatus.[11] Odor may be modified by the action of normal or abnormal microbial flora. *Halitosis* is offensive breath and *bromhidrosis* is fetid perspiration.

In Western culture people often minimize body odors by frequently changing their clothing, bathing, and using deodorants or antiperspirants, mouthwashes, douches, or scents applied to the skin. If one of these artificial odors is too strong, the practitioner may wonder what the patient is trying to hide. On the other hand, if a patient does not practice these customs, the physician may detect an odor that he or she finds offensive and then must decide if the patient's failure to comply with these social expectations is either precipitating or precipitated by psychosocial stress.

Body odor changes with puberty, and a characteristic adult odor may prompt a child (or the child's parents) to seek medical attention. Axillary odor, which varies in intensity from person to person, often is the strongest odor associated with adolescents and adults.[11] Its pungency results from the action of aerobic diphtheroids on apocrine secretions. Axillary hair appears to retain or spread odor.[10]

Vaginal Odor

The odor of postpubertal vaginal secretions varies among individuals and with the menstrual cycle. Vulvar secretions, vaginal wall transudates, exfoliated cells, cervical mucus, fluids from the endometrium and uterine tubes, and metabolic products of the vaginal microflora all contribute.[8] Some characterize the resulting odor as unpleasant, even in the absence of vaginitis. Odor during menses usually is rated as the most offensive.[8] Some individuals may be concerned about these normal odors. The "rotten fish" smell of the vaginal discharge associated with bacterial vaginosis is caused by trimethylamine.[1]

Mouth Odor

The odor of a healthy mouth is assumed to be inoffensive in childhood; however, "bad breath" is not uncommon, even in an otherwise well child. Halitosis in the absence of disease is thought to be caused at least partly by volatile sulfur compounds, which are formed when the oral flora metabolize compounds containing amino acids that are found in the saliva or adhering to the teeth, tongue, or gums. Halitosis is exacerbated by infrequent eating and drinking, which ordinarily have a flushing action. Halitosis also accompanies a variety of childhood respiratory tract and gastrointestinal in-

Table 156-1 Abnormalities of Metabolism Associated with Unusual Odor

Disease	Description of odor	Clinical features	Metabolic defect
Phenylketonuria	Musty, like a mouse, horse, wolf, or barn	Vomiting, progressive mental retardation and microcephaly, eczema, decreasing pigmentation, seizures, spasticity	Phenylalanine hydroxylase
Maple syrup urine disease	Maple syrup, burnt sugar, malt, caramel	Feeding difficulty, irregular respiration beginning in first week, marked acidosis, seizures, coma leading to death in first 1-2 years of life Intermittent form without mental retardation but with episodes of ataxia and lethargy that may progress to coma Other variants, including thiamine, respond to treatment	Branched chain decarboxylase
Oasthouse urine disease (methionine malabsorption syndrome)	Yeast, dried celery, malt, hops, beer	Diarrhea, mental retardation, spasticity, attacks of hyperpnea, fever, edema	Kidney and intestinal transport of methionine, branched chain amino acids, tyrosine, and phenylalanine
Odor of sweaty feet syndrome 1 (isovalericacidemia)	Sweaty feet, cheese	Recurrent bouts of acidosis, vomiting, dehydration, coma, mild to moderate mental retardation, aversion to protein foods	Isovaleryl CoA dehydrogenase
Odor of sweaty feet syndrome 2 (*N*-butyric and *N*-hexanoic acidemia; may be same as odor of sweaty feet syndrome 1)	Sweaty feet	Poor feeding, weakness and lethargy developing in first week of life with acidosis, dehydration, seizures, and death in early months of life from bone marrow depression	Green acyldehydrogenase
Odor of cat urine syndrome (beta-methylcrotonylglycinuria)	Cat urine	Neurological symptoms resembling Werdnig-Hoffmann disease, failure to thrive, ketoacidosis Biotin-responsive form	Multiple carboxylase deficiency
Fish odor syndrome 1	Dead fish	Stigmata of Turner syndrome, neutropenia, recurrent infections, anemia, splenomegaly	Unknown
Fish odor syndrome 2 (trimethylaminuria)	Dead or rotting fish, rancid butter, boiled cabbage	Normal development; has been induced in two premature infants by oral choline	Trimethylamine oxidase
Rancid butter syndrome	Rancid butter, boiled cabbage, decaying fish	Poor feeding, irritability, progressive neurological deterioration with coma and seizures, death caused by infection in first 3 months	Unknown; hypermethioninemia, hypertyrosinemia, and generalized aminoaciduria present; may be a form of acute tyrosinosis

Data from Mace JW et al: *Clin Pediatr* 15:57, 1976; Hayden GF: *Postgrad Med* 67:110, 1980.

Table 156-2 Inhalations, Poisonings, and Ingestions Associated with Recognizable Odors

Odor	Site	Substance implicated
Fruity, like acetone or decomposing apples	Breath	Lacquer, chloroform, salicylates
Fruity, alcohol	Breath	Alcohol, phenol
Fruity, pearlike, acrid	Breath	Chloral hydrate, paraldehyde
Wintergreen	Breath	Methyl salicylate
Severe bad breath	Breath	Amphetamines
Bitter almond	Breath	Cyanide (chokecherry, apricot pits), jetberry bush
Burned rope	Breath	Marijuana
Camphor	Breath	Naphthalene (mothballs)
Coal gas	Breath	Coal gas (associated with odorless but toxic carbon monoxide)
Disinfectant	Breath	Phenol, creosote
Garlic	Breath	Phosphorus, arsenic, tellurium, parathion, malathion
Metallic	Breath	Iodine
	Stool	Arsenic
	Vomitus	Arsenic, phosphorus
Shoe polish	Breath	Nitrobenzene
Stale tobacco	Breath	Nicotine
Hydrocarbon	Breath, vomitus	Hydrocarbons
Violets	Urine, vomitus	Turpentine
Medicinal	Urine	Penicillins
Sulfides or amines	Skin	War gases

Data from Hayden GF: *Postgrad Med* 67:110, 1980; McMillan JA, Nieburg PI, Oski FA: Diseases and poisonings associated with unusual breath odor. In *The whole pediatrician catalog*, Philadelphia, 1977, WB Saunders; Goldfrank L, Kirstein R: *Hosp Phys* 3:12, 1976; Smith M, Smith LG, Levinson B: *Lancet* 2:1452, 1982.

fections. Persistent halitosis should prompt a search for dental or gingival disease or a nasal foreign body. In some cases halitosis may reflect lung disease or gastroesophageal reflux.

Simple oral hygiene can modify mouth odor for about 3 hours. Brushing the teeth and the dorsoposterior surface of the tongue and then rinsing with water or a mouthwash supposedly reduces both the concentrations of volatile sulfur compounds and the offensive odor.[18,21]

Foot Odor

Several types of localized dermatitis including eczema, tinea pedis infection (athlete's foot), and pitted keratolysis have been associated with increased foot odor. Little is known about the causes of excessive foot odor that occurs despite the seeming absence of skin lesions. One group of investigators found that cultures of particularly smelly feet, compared with those from other feet, had higher bacterial counts, especially of organisms that produce lipid- and protein-degrading exoenzymes.[13] Moisture may promote the growth of such bacteria.

Metabolic Abnormalities

Certain metabolic defects are associated with an unusual odor of the urine,[2] sweat, and other body fluids because of accumulation of odoriferous metabolic precursors or byproducts. These disorders (listed in Table 156-1), although infrequently the cause of odor, are the pediatric conditions most commonly linked to diagnosis by odor.[3,4,12] They should be suspected if an infant has an unusual body odor, especially if the he or she is doing poorly or is ketotic. Recognizing the odor in a compatible clinical situation may lead to early diagnosis and therapy, which may prevent progressive brain damage or death. A specialist in metabolic disease should be consulted and an appropriate diet instituted while blood and urine amino acid analyses are completed.

Foreign Bodies

Retention of a foreign body in an orifice may lead to a fetid or foul smell with or without drainage or to generalized body odor, apparently because odoriferous substances are absorbed and secreted in sweat.[5] Nasal foreign bodies are the most common.[9,16] Vaginal tampons or diaphragms that have not been removed also may promote odor. All orifices must be inspected.

Inhalation, Poisoning, and Ingestion

When inhalation or ingestion of a toxic substance is suspected, odor may provide a clue to the substance involved. Table 156-2 lists some common associations. When puzzled, the practitioner should consult a poison control center.

Penicillin and cephalosporins give the urine a "medicinal" or musty smell. Topical benzoyl peroxide has been implicated in at least one case of persistent body odor.[15] Thiourea compounds give the breath a sweet smell, resembling that of decaying vegetables.[20] Newborns have smelled spicy when their mothers ate particular curries before labor.[6]

Other Diseases

Odor may suggest either the presence of an infection or the type of infection (Table 156-3), or it may confirm an acquired but noninfectious medical condition (Table 156-4).[7]

SUMMARY

Odor is imprecise. It is not surprising that, with many other diagnostic aids at hand, today's practitioners have minimized olfactory cues.[7] However, odor should not be neglected; it may be the patient's chief concern and, more important, it may be the most specific early indication of a diagnosis, thereby guiding the choice of diagnostic tools and prompt initiation of therapy.

Table 156-3 Odor As a Clue to Infection

Odor	Infection
Foul, putrid breath or sputum	Lung abscess, empyema (especially anaerobic), bronchiectasis, fetid bronchitis
Severe halitosis	Trench mouth, tonsillitis, gingivitis
Ammoniacal urine	Urinary tract infection with urea-splitting bacteria
Musty or grapelike, especially in a patient with burns or wounds	*Pseudomonas* skin infection
Fetid sweat	Intranasal foreign body
Rancid stool	Shigellosis
Fishy vaginal discharge	Bacterial vaginosis
Foul vaginal discharge	Vaginal foreign body
Pus that smells like feces or overripe cheese	Proteolytic bacteria
Foul cerumen	*Pseudomonas* infection
Putrid smell from skin	Scurvy
Sweetish odor from mouth	Diphtheria
Butcher shop	Yellow fever
Beer odor in peritoneal dialysate	*Candida* infection[22]
Mousy	*Proteus* infection
Rotten apples	*Clostridium* gas gangrene
Stale beer	Scrofula
Fresh-baked brown bread	Typhoid fever
Alcohol smell to cerebrospinal fluid	*Cryptococcus* meningitis
Malodorous newborn	Amnionitis

Data from Hayden GF: *Postgrad Med J* 67:110, 1980; Smith M, Smith LG, Levinson B: *Lancet* 2:1452, 1982; Schiffman SS: *N Engl J Med* 308:1337, 1983.

Table 156-4 Some Other Diseases Associated with Specific Odors

Disease	Odor
Diabetic ketoacidosis, starvation	Ketones are present in the breath and smell fruity, like acetone or decomposing apples
Uremia	Fishy smell to urine caused by dimethylamine and trimethylamine Ammoniacal smell to the breath caused by ammonia
Acute tubular necrosis	Urine smells like stale water[17]
Hepatic failure	Breath smells like musty fish, raw liver, feces, or newly mown clover; caused by mercaptans and/or dimethyl sulfide
Intestinal obstruction, esophageal diverticulum	Breath smells feculent, foul
Schizophrenia	Sweat smells unpleasant, pungent, heavy; caused by trans-3-methyl-2-hexanoic acid
Skin diseases with protein breakdown	Skin smells foul, unpleasant
Intestinal obstruction, peritonitis	Vomitus smells like feces
Malabsorption	Stool smells foul
Portacaval shunt, portal vein thrombosis	Breath smells sweet

Data from Hayden GF: *Postgrad Med J* 67:110, 1980; McMillan JA, Nieburg PI, Oski FA: Diseases and poisonings associated with unusual breath odor. In *The whole pediatrician catalog*, Philadelphia, 1977, WB Saunders; Smith M, Smith LG, Levinson B: *Lancet* 2:1452, 1982.

REFERENCES

1. Brand JM, Galask RP: Trimethylamine: the substance mainly responsible for the fishy odor often associated with bacterial vaginosis, *Obstet Gynecol* 68:682, 1986.
2. Burke DG et al: Profiles of urinary valatiles from metabolic disorders characterized by unusual odors, *Clin Chem* 29:1834, 1983.
3. Chen H, Aiello F: Trimethylaminuria in a girl with Prader-Willi syndrome and del(15)(q11q13), *Am J Med Genet* 45:335, 1993.
4. Cone TE: Diagnosis and treatment: some diseases, syndromes, and conditions associated with an unusual odor, *Pediatrics* 41:993, 1968.
5. Feinstein RJ: Nasal foreign bodies and bromhidrosis (comment), *JAMA* 242:1031, 1979.
6. Hauser GJ et al: Peculiar odors in newborns and maternal prenatal ingestion of spicy food, *Eur J Pediatr* 144:403, 1985.
7. Hayden GF: Olfactory diagnosis in medicine, *Postgrad Med J* 67:110, 1980.
8. Huggins GR, Preti G: Vaginal odors and secretions, *Clin Obstet Gynecol* 24:355, 1981.
9. Katz HP et al: Unusual presentation of nasal foreign bodies in children, *JAMA* 241:1496, 1979.
10. Leyden JJ et al: The microbiology of the human axilla and its relationships to axillary odor, *J Invest Dermatol* 77:413, 1981.
11. Liddell K: Smell as a diagnostic marker, *Postgrad Med J* 52:136, 1976.
12. Mace JW et al: The child with an unusual odor, *Clin Pediatr* 15:57, 1976.
13. Marshall J, Holland KT, Gribbon EM: A comparative study of the cutaneous microflora of normal feet with low and high levels of odor, *J Appl Bacteriol* 65:61, 1988.
14. McMillan JA, Neiburg PI, Oski FA: Diseases and poisonings associated with unusual breath odor. In *The whole pediatrician catalog*, Philadelphia, 1977, WB Saunders.
15. Molberg P: Body odor from topical benzoyl peroxide, *N Engl J Med* 304:1366, 1981 (letter).
16. Moriarty RA: Nasal foreign body presenting as an unusual odor, *Am J Dis Child* 132:97, 1978.

17. Najarian JS: The diagnostic importance of the odor of urine, *N Engl J Med* 303:1128, 1980 (letter).
18. Schmidt NF, Tarbet WJ: The effect of oral rinses on organoleptic mouth odor ratings and levels of volatile sulfur compounds, *Oral Surg* 45:876, 1978.
19. Smith M, Smith LG, Levinson B: The use of smell in differential diagnosis, *Lancet* 2:1452, 1982.
20. Stewart WK, Fleming LW: Use your nose, *Lancet* 1(8321):1983 (letter).
21. Tonzetich J, Ng SK: Reduction of malodor by oral cleansing procedures, *J Oral Surg* 42:172, 1976.
22. Turney JH: Use your nose, *Lancet* 1(8321):426, 1983 (letter).

157 Petechiae and Purpura

Reggie E. Duerst

Although patency of the body's vascular system is required to ensure continued delivery of nutrients and oxygen to the tissues, immediate steps must be taken to limit any blood loss if the integrity of a blood vessel is disrupted. In primary hemostasis, platelets adhere to the injured endothelium or subendothelium, and a thrombus begins to form. Defects in primary hemostasis are manifested by minute, 1 to 2 mm hemorrhagic spots called *petechiae* after capillary injury. *Purpuric lesions* represent a confluence of petechiae or extravasated blood from a larger vessel; *ecchymoses* result if the extravasated blood extends along a fascial plane.

Many disorders cause the formation of petechiae or purpura or both. Although the underlying etiology may be benign, serious life-threatening illnesses also must be considered such as meningococcemia, disseminated intravascular coagulopathy (DIC), and purpura fulminans. Immediate action must be taken to halt progression of these life-threatening diseases. Also, intracranial hemorrhage must be considered in any child being evaluated for changes in consciousness who also has petechiae or purpuric lesions.

The differential diagnosis of disorders leading to development of petechiae or purpura includes many other serious, potentially life-threatening syndromes or diseases. The pathophysiology of these disorders, although varied, ultimately leads to defective primary hemostasis. These disorders can be manifestations of (1) a decrease in the number of platelets, (2) platelet dysfunction, or (3) defective vessels. An approach for evaluating a patient who has petechiae or purpura (or both) is presented in the box on p. 1070.

The rapidity of onset of the purpura and associated signs of systemic illness provide clues that help the physician initially assess the gravity of the illness. A well-appearing child who has petechiae isolated to a well-circumscribed location may have self-inflicted them by suction (factitious petechiae). A lethargic, febrile patient who has had a rapid onset of diffuse petechiae needs immediate management of sepsis and DIC. As noted above, the distribution of purpuric lesions also may help the examiner make a diagnosis. Involvement of the buttocks and lower extremities is classic for Henoch-Schönlein purpura; prominence of purpura around hair follicles is characteristic of scurvy. Localization of petechiae to the head and neck may result from increased transmural pressure transmitted to vessels after a prolonged Valsalva maneuver (e.g., cough, weight lifting). Well-circumscribed lesions also may result from trauma, and child abuse must be considered.

NORMAL HEMOSTASIS

The pathophysiological mechanisms underlying formation of petechiae are associated with different steps in primary hemostasis. Following vascular injury, the subendothelium is exposed, and the blood elements are no longer confined within the vessel. Primary hemostasis (Fig. 157-1) is initiated when von Willebrand factor is released from endothelial cells and adheres to the exposed collagen matrix; von Willebrand factor, in turn, binds to platelets via the platelet surface glycoprotein Ib(gpIb). Next, the platelets that have adhered to the subendothelium release their granule contents. Additional platelets aggregate in response to adenosine diphosphate (ADP) released from the granules. Synthesis and release of thromboxane A_2 (TxA_2) by the platelets result in vasoconstriction and further enhancement of platelet plug formation.

Secondary hemostatic mechanisms include activation of factor X at the platelet membrane surface, prothrombin conversion to thrombin, and thrombin-catalyzed polymerization of fibrin. Thrombin also provides positive feedback for primary hemostasis by stimulating platelets to release ADP and synthesize TxA_2. Finally, the clot is stabilized by cross-linking of fibrin strands, a reaction catalyzed by activated factor XIII.

After the damaged endothelium has been repaired, the clot that was formed needs to be degraded so that normal blood flow may resume. Plasminogen (which is incorporated into the fibrin clot as it is produced) is converted to the proteolytic enzyme plasmin by the action of plasminogen activators (e.g., tissue plasminogen activator and urokinase). Plasmin cleaves fibrin, forming fibrin degradation products (or fibrin split products) and causing clot dissolution. Thus hemostasis—formation and degradation of a clot—is an ongoing "homeostatic" process designed to maintain vascular integrity and thereby blood flow.

THROMBOCYTOPENIA

Thrombocytopenia is the most common cause of bleeding. Regulation of platelet production and maintenance of the normal platelet count (150,000 to 400,000/μL) is poorly understood. If platelet function is normal, abnormal bleeding usually will not occur unless the platelet count is below 100,000/μL. Declines in the platelet count may result from hypoproduction, enhanced destruction, maldistribution, or dilution (e.g., a patient who is hemorrhaging and receiving insufficient platelet replacement). If the decrease in the platelet count is caused by excessive platelet destruction despite greatly increased production, symptomatic bleeding often does not develop until the platelet count falls below 20,000/μL. This suggests that the newly produced platelets may have enhanced coagulant function.

Hypoproductive Thrombocytopenia

Inadequate production of platelets can be divided into congenital and acquired conditions. One such congenital disor-

EVALUATION OF PETECHIAE AND PURPURA

1. History and physical examination

Duration/speed of onset
"Sick versus well"
Distribution of lesions

2. Low platelet count (<150,000)

a. Blood smear

Verify low platelet count
Look for *microangiopathic changes*
- Kasabach-Merritt syndrome
- DIC/purpura fulminans
- Hemolytic uremic syndrome (HUS)
- Thrombotic thrombocytopenic purpura (TTP)
- Liver disease

b. PT, aPTT (±FDP, fibrinogen)

Abnormal
As above plus:
- Histiocytosis X
- Familial erythrophagocytic lymphohistiocytosis (FEL)

Normal
See below

c. Bone marrow examination

Decreased megakaryocytes
Aplasia, congenital
- Thrombocytopenia with absent radii (TAR) syndrome
- Fanconi anemia
- Bernard-Soulier syndrome
- Wiskott-Aldrich syndrome
- Metabolic disorders

Aplasia, acquired
- Idiopathic
- Nutritional (iron, vitamin B_{12}, folate)
- Drug, chemical, toxin, radiation
- Rubella, other "TORCH"

Infiltration
- Leukemia, lymphoma
- Neuroblastoma or other metastatic solid tumor
- Storage disease

Normal or increased megakaryocytes
Immune destruction
- Immune thrombocytopenic purpura (ITP) (acute and chronic)
- Alloimmune thrombocytopenia
- Posttransfusion purpura
- Drugs
- HIV/AIDS

Other
- Histiocytosis X
- Virally associated hematophagocytic syndrome (VAHS)
- FEL
- Intravascular prosthesis
- May-Hegglin anomaly
- Hypersplenism with sequestration

3. Normal platelet count (>150,000)

Platelet dysfunction, congenital

Glanzmann thrombasthenia
Bernard-Soulier syndrome
Wiskott-Aldrich syndrome
Storage pool defect

Platelet dysfunction, acquired

Aspirin or aspirinlike drugs
Liver disease
Uremia
Paraproteinemia (dysgammaglobulinemia, cystic fibrosis)

Von Willebrand disease

Vascular defect, congenital

Ehlers-Danlos syndrome
Osler-Weber-Rendu syndrome

Vascular defect, acquired

Trauma (lacerations, abuse)
Lacerations
Abuse
Factitious
Vasculitis
- Drugs
- Infection (bacterial, viral, rickettsial)
- Henoch-Schönlein purpura

Senile purpura
Steroid purpura
Scurvy

der is thrombocytopenia with absent radii (TAR) syndrome. Infants who have TAR syndrome are recognized readily by their upper extremity deformities. The platelet count is in the 15,000 to 30,000/μL range, and megakaryocytes are reduced or absent in the bone marrow. Platelet production improves gradually after the first year of life. Congenital amegakaryocytic thrombocytopenia also is present in Fanconi anemia. Patients who have Bernard-Soulier syndrome also may be mildly thrombocytopenic secondary to hypoproduction (the functional defect in the platelets in these individuals is related more significantly to bleeding; see below). May-Hegglin anomaly (giant platelets and Döhle bodies in the leukocytes) rarely is associated with thrombocytopenia and bleeding. Wiskott-Aldrich syndrome (WAS) is an X-linked recessive disorder characterized by immunodeficiency, platelet dysfunction, and thrombocytopenia. The combination of thrombocytopenia and platelet dysfunction places the patient at great risk for hemorrhage. Treatment of these disorders is supportive—avoiding aspirin or aspirinlike drugs and using protective head gear, plus administration of the antifibrinolytic agent epsilon-aminocaproic acid (EACA) and, if necessary, platelet transfusions.

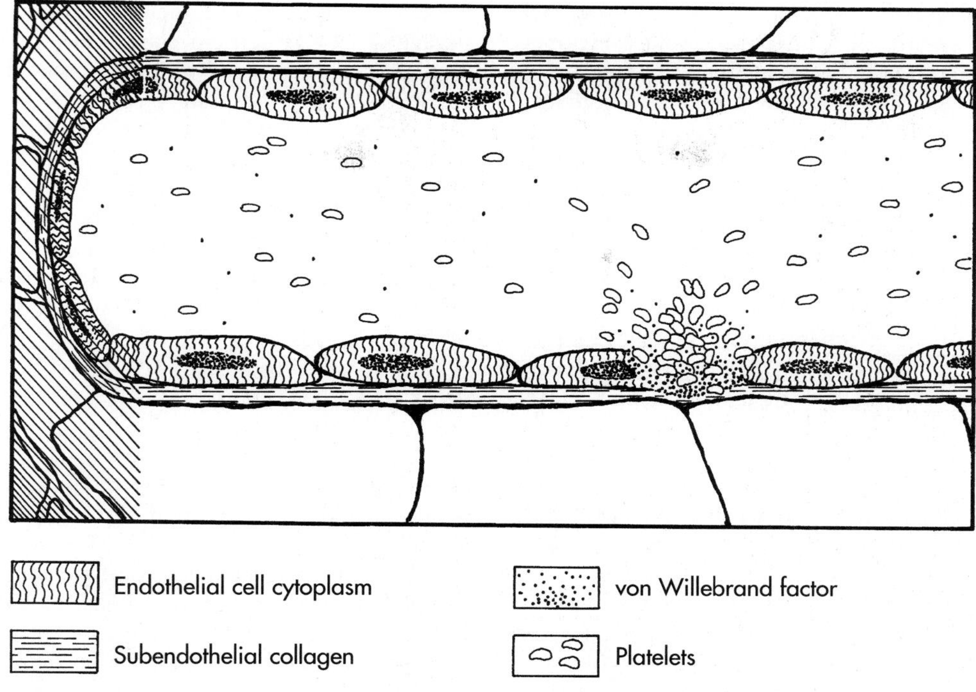

FIG. 157-1 In primary hemostasis, platelets adhere to subendothelial collagen coated with von Willebrand factor. Platelet aggregation ensues, and a platelet "plug" forms.

Marrow aplasia also results in hypoproductive thrombocytopenia. Marrow aplasia that develops after exposure to drugs or other toxic chemicals may be temporary and may resolve when the causative agent is withdrawn. Immunosuppressive therapy, bone marrow transplantation, or both may be required for patients who have severe aplastic anemia. Extensive infiltration of bone marrow in patients who have leukemia, lymphoma, or a metastatic solid tumor prevents normal platelet production. Infectious agents also may cause ineffective thrombocytopoiesis and thrombocytopenia.

Destructive Thrombocytopenia

Acute idiopathic thrombocytopenic purpura (ITP) is the most frequent cause of severe thrombocytopenia and bleeding in childhood. ITP usually is a temporary disorder, and 80% to 90% of children recover completely within 1 year of diagnosis. The incidence of life-threatening hemorrhage or intracranial bleeding is less than 0.1% to 1%, and it is greatest at the onset of the disease. Chronic ITP or other diseases associated with immune dysfunction (e.g., lupus erythematosus, Evan syndrome) develop in 10% to 20% of patients who manifest acute ITP. Thrombocytopenia is a result of increased removal of platelets from the circulation by monocyte-macrophage cells of the reticuloendothelial (RE) cell system. Adherence to the platelet surface of specific antiplatelet autoantibody or immune complexes leads to phagocytosis of the platelets by the RE cells. Bone marrow should be examined to exclude an infiltrative process. Treatment with corticosteroids or high doses of intravenous immunoglobulin appears to shorten the initial period of severe thrombocytopenia but has not been shown to affect the long-term prognosis for this generally self-limited disorder.

Neonatal alloimmune thrombocytopenia develops when maternal antibody is made to a paternal platelet antigen (not expressed on maternal platelets) inherited by the infant. $P1^{A1}$ is a platelet antigen expressed on 98% of the population's platelets; thus approximately 1% of women are at risk of developing anti-$P1^{A1}$ antibody during pregnancy. Antibody to the $P1^{A1}$ antigen also has been implicated in posttransfusion purpura. In this condition severe thrombocytopenia and mucocutaneous bleeding develop 5 to 8 days after a blood product transfusion. It occurs most commonly in women who have been sensitized previously to $P1^{A1}$-positive platelets. Drugs that act as a hapten with platelet surface antigens to form an immunogenic moiety can cause an immune thrombocytopenia. Platelet destruction continues as long as the drug-platelet neoantigen is present. Quinidine, cimetidine, and trimethoprim-sulfamethoxazole have been shown to cause thrombocytopenia by this mechanism.

Destruction of platelets resulting from nonimmunological platelet injury occurs in children who have hemolytic uremic syndrome (HUS) and adults who have thrombotic thrombocytopenic purpura (TTP). These disorders are both associated with microangiopathic hemolytic anemia, endothelial cell injury, and platelet consumption. HUS affects the renal glomerular capillaries primarily, but other organs, including the brain, may be involved. Thrombocytopenia of Kasabach-Merritt syndrome results from platelet consumption in a giant hemangioma. Intravascular prostheses also may cause significant platelet destruction.

Several disorders associated with RE cell proliferation also result in platelet consumption that is not antibody mediated. Patients who have histiocytosis X, virally associated hematophagocytic syndrome (VAHS), and familial erythrophagocytic lymphohistiocytosis (FEL) can develop thrombocytopenia as a result of excessive phagocytosis of platelets by abnormal histiocytic cells. If these disease processes are active, splenomegaly often is present, and the spleen is a major site of platelet destruction. Sequestration of platelets in an enlarged spleen (regardless of cause) also causes a reduction in measured circulating platelet concentration. However, bleeding symptoms are uncommon because the platelet count is not reduced severely.

DEFECTIVE PLATELET FUNCTION

Defects in platelet function can be subdivided by the step in primary hemostasis (platelet adhesion, release, and aggregation) at which the defect is expressed. Adherence of platelets to the exposed subendothelium is mediated by von Willebrand factor. Von Willebrand factor is a glycoprotein of 240,000 molecular weight subunits synthesized primarily by endothelial cells. It is "complexed" with factor VIII and circulates as multimers of the basic subunit. Larger multimers are more active in promoting coagulation than are monomers or small oligomers. Von Willebrand disease (vWD) is a heterogeneous disorder involving von Willebrand factor that has three major subtypes; type I accounts for 75% of patients with the disease. Patients may have (1) reduced synthesis of vWF, (2) synthesis of defective vWF, or (3) disordered assembly of the vWF complexes. The inheritance of most forms of vWD follows autosomal dominant transmission. The prevalence of the disease is estimated to be as high as 1 per 100 individuals. The activated partial thromboplastin time and bleeding time generally are prolonged. Factor VIII activity is normal, but ristocetin cofactor activity is reduced. Treatment of active bleeding or prophylaxis before elective surgery involves infusion of desmopressin acetate (DDAVP) or cryoprecipitate. DDAVP is effective for most forms of vWD and acts by stimulating endothelial cell release of vWF. Cryoprecipitate provides an exogenous source of factor VIII-vWF and secondarily stimulates further production and release of vWF. However, cryoprecipitate can be associated with transmission of bloodborne viral infections. DDAVP is the current treatment of choice (subtype IIb of vWD is the exception). Bernard-Soulier syndrome also is characterized by a defect in platelet adhesion. Platelet binding to vWF is diminished because of lack of the vWF ligand, gpIb, on the platelet membrane. Platelet transfusion is necessary to correct this disorder, but refractoriness to later transfusions because of development of antibody to platelet gpIb mandates that transfusion be withheld unless absolutely necessary.

Glanzmann thrombasthenia is caused by congenital deficiency or absence of platelet surface antigen glycoprotein IIb/IIIa. This deficiency results in defective binding of platelets to fibrinogen and a decrease in platelet aggregation after activation. Platelet transfusion can be lifesaving, but its use should be minimized to prevent antibody formation. Deficiency of alpha-granules in the platelets of patients who have gray platelet syndrome (named for the platelet appearance on routine blood smears) results in a decrease of coagulation factors available for release after aggregation. Several heterogeneous deficiencies in dense granules, collectively called *storage pool defects,* result in defective platelet release of ADP and serotonin. This defect also is associated with Wiskott-Aldrich syndrome, Chédiak-Steinbrinck-Higashi syndrome, and Hermansky-Pudlak syndrome. Other diseases associated with defects in platelet granule release include disorders of platelet arachidonic acid metabolism and type 1 glycogen storage disease (glucose-6-phosphatase deficiency). The latter disorder is associated with decreased ADP release during episodes of hypoglycemia.

Acquired platelet dysfunction is characteristic of uremia. Retention of metabolites otherwise cleared by the kidneys appears to be causative, and significant bleeding may occur as a result. DDAVP is very useful for prophylaxis against bleeding if a uremic patient requires a surgical procedure. Liver disease and myeloproliferative and lymphoproliferative disorders also have been associated with acquired platelet dysfunction.

VASCULAR DEFECTS

Congenital Defects

A consequence of several congenital vascular disorders is a predisposition to the development of purpuric lesions. The telangiectasia of Osler-Weber-Rendu syndrome is a consequence of vascular anomalies that include a thin endothelial lining. The thrombocytopenia of Kasabach-Merritt syndrome is a result of consumption within the cavernous arteriovenous malformation. Patients who have congenital connective tissue disorders that result in defective collagen or elastin can exhibit "vascular purpura." These disorders include osteogenesis imperfecta, Ehlers-Danlos syndrome, Marfan syndrome, and pseudoexanthoma elasticum.

Acquired Defects

Acquired vascular conditions can be manifested by petechiae or purpura. Vasculitis develops in response to drugs, toxins, or a host of infectious organisms (e.g., meningococcus, yellow fever virus, and rickettsiae). In response to endotoxin (or other mediators of inflammation), interleukin-1 and tumor necrosis factor are produced by endothelial cells. These cytokines, in turn, bring about endothelial cell changes that impair primary hemostasis, and petechiae or purpura result. Similarly, systemic lupus erythematosus, rheumatoid arthritis, or other collagen-vascular diseases can display purpura resulting from vasculitis. Henoch-Schönlein purpura is a syndrome of widespread acute vasculitis that may cause a rash (vasculitis in the skin) and arthralgia (vasculitis in the joints). Vasculitis in the gastrointestinal tract may cause abdominal pain, bowel wall edema, partial obstruction, and intussusception. Renal complications (proteinuria, hypertension, renal failure) are possible. Late renal sequelae are confined to patients who have renal involvement during the acute illness.

Vitamin C is required for normal collagen synthesis. Patients who have scurvy may develop purpuric lesions as a result of the abnormal collagen in the subendothelium. Prominence of bleeding at the base of hair follicles is characteristic of scurvy. Senile purpura (purpura of the elderly) is another manifestation of abnormal collagen in the subendothelium. Dysproteinemias and conditions that result in elevated gamma globulinemia (including cystic fibrosis) have been shown to promote formation of petechiae or purpura.

SUGGESTED READINGS

Beardsley DS: Platelet abnormalities in infancy and childhood. In Nathan DG, Oski FA, editors: *Hematology of infancy and childhood,* Philadelphia, 1993, WB Saunders.

Beutler E et al, editors: *Williams' hematology,* 1995, New York, McGraw-Hill.

Bowie EJW, Owen CA: Primary vascular disorders. In Colman RW et al, editors: *Hemostasis and thrombosis: basic principles and clinical practice,* 1994, Philadelphia, JB Lippincott.

Handin RI: Physiology of coagulation: the platelet. In Nathan DG, Oski FA, editors: *Hematology of infancy and childhood,* Philadelphia, 1987, WB Saunders.

Hawiger J, Handin RI: Physiology of hemostasis: cellular aspects. In Nathan DG, Oski FA, editors: *Hematology of infancy and childhood,* Philadelphia, 1993, WB Saunders.

Hoffman R et al, editors: *Hematology: basic principles and practice,* New York, 1991, Churchill Livingstone.

Stuart MJ, Kelton JG: The platelet: quantitative and qualitative abnormalities. In Nathan DG, Oski FA, editors: *Hematology of infancy and childhood,* Philadelphia, 1987, WB Saunders.

158 Polyuria

Samuel M. Libber and Leslie P. Plotnick

Polyuria, or excessive urinary volume, is a symptom common to a large number of pediatric disorders. It may be defined clinically as urine production of more than 900 ml/m^2/day or functionally as an inappropriately high urine output relative to circulating volume and osmolarity.[12] It often is associated with frequent urination, nocturia, or enuresis. Sometimes the pediatrician is called on to evaluate this symptom without knowing the exact daily urinary volume; in such situations a detailed history of fluid intake and urinary habits may help delineate the primary symptom.

A normal homeostatic response to polyuria is increased thirst; with subsequent liquid intake, then, water balance remains intact. In an older child the parent may perceive this symptom as more prominent than the polyuria. However, in infants who have polyuria and are unable to maintain free access to fluids, negative water balance results, and weight loss, dehydration, and electrolyte disturbances often occur. When chronic or recurrent electrolyte disturbances plague the infant, growth failure and central nervous system (CNS) injury may result.

DIFFERENTIAL DIAGNOSIS

In reaching a diagnosis in a patient who has polyuria, the clinician must bear in mind a general overview of the systems that may cause this symptom, as indicated in the box on p. 1075. A CNS or pituitary lesion may reduce vasopressin secretion; a renal defect may limit the kidney's ability to respond to vasopressin; an excessive fluid intake may be the primary cause of polyuria; or excretion of an osmotically active urine may effect a large volume loss.

Central or neurogenic diabetes insipidus is a condition in which secretion of vasopressin by the posterior lobe of the pituitary gland is limited. Consequently, a dilute urine of large volume is passed, and the crucial function of water conservation in times of volume depletion is lost. In rare cases there may be a familial idiopathic vasopressin deficiency, inherited generally as an autosomal dominant trait but occasionally in an X-linked recessive pattern.[4] More commonly, however, cases are sporadic; in these cases a search for a specific underlying organic lesion and concomitant anterior pituitary dysfunction is necessary.[2] Injury to the CNS, whether traumatic or surgical, may be associated with a decline in the production or release of vasopressin. Likewise, thrombosis or hemorrhage involving the hypothalamus or pituitary gland may result in vasopressin deficiency. Abnormalities in vasopressin secretion may accompany CNS infections. Just as the syndrome of inappropriate antidiuretic hormone (SIADH) may accompany meningitis in the acute states, clinical diabetes insipidus may supervene as a chronic sequela to CNS infections.[16]

Congenital intracranial defects (such as septooptic dysplasia, holoprosencephaly, and encephalocele) also have been associated with diabetes insipidus. Brain tumors (craniopharyngioma, glioma, dysgerminoma, and metastatic tumor) are the most common causes of central diabetes insipidus. In addition, patients who have any of a variety of systemic illnesses (histiocytosis, syphilis, tuberculosis, sarcoidosis, and Guillain-Barré syndrome) have developed vasopressin deficiency.

An unusual association between diabetes mellitus, diabetes insipidus, optic atrophy, and hearing loss (Wolfram syndrome) has been described.[7] A review by Greger and colleagues[6] suggests that, in recent years, fewer cases have been diagnosed as idiopathic and a higher proportion has been diagnosed as occurring secondary to CNS infection or intracranial birth defects. Also, autoantibodies to hypothalamic vasopressin cells have been detected in some children previously thought to have idiopathic diabetes insipidus. Interestingly, about half of patients with histiocytosis also have vasopressin cell antibodies.[17] The practitioner must search diligently for an organic lesion because an underlying lesion may not be evident at the initial evaluation.

In some situations polyuria is a consequence rather than a cause of excessive fluid intake. Primary polydipsia, or compulsive water drinking, is a rare cause of polyuria in childhood.[11] It occurs most often in older children or adults who have emotional disturbances; about 80% of cases are believed to occur in girls and women. The ailment has a gradual onset, unlike the more abrupt onset typical of central diabetes insipidus. Although some believe this disorder is caused by a primary psychiatric disturbance, a recent study of adult psychiatric patients who have polydipsia and hyponatremia showed evidence of a defect in water excretion, osmoregulation of water intake, and vasopressin secretion.[5]

Water intoxication is another cause of polyuria, seen in increasing numbers over the past 20 years.[9] It is particularly common in infants living in impoverished circumstances in which caretakers feed diluted formula or water when formula supplies are exhausted. Life-threatening hyponatremia may ensue unless such infants are treated promptly.

Renal disorders may be associated with polyuria because of an inability of the renal tubule to concentrate urine despite normal circulating levels of vasopressin. This may be a congenital or an acquired abnormality. In hereditary nephrogenic diabetes insipidus, renal tubular cells lack the ability to respond to vasopressin because of a defect in vasopressin V_2 receptors in the distal convoluted tubule and collecting duct.[15] This is an X-linked, recessive disorder in which polyuria, fever, failure to thrive, and hypernatremic dehydration occur in early infancy. Older children and adults may be able to adjust their oral fluid intake to maintain constant serum osmolality, but infants do not have this ability. The condition can be associated with damage to the CNS or even death if

DIFFERENTIAL DIAGNOSIS OF POLYURIA IN CHILDHOOD

- I. Neurogenic vasopressin deficiency
  - A. Idiopathic
    1. Familial
    2. Sporadic
  - B. Organic
    1. Posttraumatic
    2. Vascular event
    3. After infection
    4. CNS tumor
    5. Systemic infiltrative diseases (histiocytosis, syphilis, tuberculosis, sarcoidosis)
    6. Guillain-Barré syndrome
    7. Congenital intracranial defect
    8. Autoimmune disorders
- II. Excessive fluid intake
  - A. Primary polydipsia
  - B. Water intoxication
- III. Renal vasopressin insensitivity
  - A. Congenital
    1. Hereditary nephrogenic diabetes insipidus
    2. Other renal tubular defects (cystinosis, distal renal tubular acidosis, Bartter syndrome)
    3. Structural defect
  - B. Acquired
    1. Postinfectious
    2. Postobstructive
    3. Drug induced
    4. Associated with systemic disease (sickle cell disease, sarcoidosis, amyloidosis)
    5. Metabolic (hypercalcemia, hypokalemia)
- IV. Osmotic diuresis
  - A. Diet induced
  - B. Drug induced
  - C. Insulin-dependent diabetes mellitus
  - D. Non-insulin-dependent diabetes mellitus
  - E. Renal glycosuria

the infant develops recurrent hypernatremic dehydration. Thus prompt recognition and treatment are needed to prevent such sequelae.

Besides the hereditary form of nephrogenic diabetes insipidus, the clinician must consider other renal tubular defects in which vasopressin resistance has been observed. Patients who have cystinosis, distal renal tubular acidosis, and Bartter syndrome may have a clinical picture of polyuria.

In addition to this functional tubular impairment, congenital structural abnormalities that can cause polyuria also may occur. In medullary cystic disease and oligomeganephronia, a condition in which the renal tubules are abnormally large and reduced in number, the architecture of the kidney is distorted, resulting in an abnormality in the regulation of renal output. In chronic pyelonephritis or obstructive uropathy, damage to the tubules or a disturbance in the medullary osmotic gradient may result in nephrogenic diabetes insipidus. Drugs such as lithium, demeclocycline, and amphotericin have been known to result in functional vasopressin insensitivity. Likewise, hypercalcemia and hypokalemia each may be associated with a nephropathy in which tubular ability to conserve water is lost. Finally, systemic disorders such as sickle cell disease, sarcoidosis, and amyloidosis may cause renal tubular dysfunction and result in polyuria.

The final major group of disorders that cause polyuria is that in which renal water loss results from an osmotic diuresis. In rare cases this may be diet induced, as in individuals who are tube fed a diet high in protein and sodium. Drugs such as mannitol, urea, and glycerol, as well as radiological contrast agents, may be responsible for this picture. Glycosuria is one of the most frequent findings in children who have acquired polyuria; in these patients, insulin-dependent diabetes mellitus (IDDM) is the most likely explanation (see Chapter 199, Diabetes Mellitus). Polyuria, polydipsia, polyphagia, and weight loss compose the symptom complex seen most commonly in these patients. Non-insulin-dependent diabetes mellitus (NIDDM) is relatively rare in childhood but may occur in an obese child or adolescent. In both situations glycosuria results from diminished carbohydrate utilization, and loss of water and electrolytes ensues. In renal glycosuria, insulin secretion and activity are entirely normal, but the maximum glucose reabsorption rate of renal tubular cells is diminished. As a result, glycosuria occurs without hyperglycemia. When present in the urine in large amounts, glucose acts as an osmotic diuretic and causes polyuria.

EVALUATION

The initial laboratory procedure of highest yield is a urinalysis performed on a "first morning" voided specimen. A high specific gravity (1.020 or higher) generally is found in patients who have osmotic diuresis or in normal individuals, whereas a specific gravity of 1.008 or lower is found in patients who have nephrogenic or central diabetes insipidus. Patients whose renal tubular epithelium has been damaged (e.g., individuals who have sickle cell disease) are more likely to have isosthenuria with specific gravities in the neighborhood of 1.010. Protein, casts, or formed blood elements in the urine likewise would suggest a renal disorder. In patients who have glycosuria, ketonuria would strongly suggest IDDM; if glycosuria without ketonuria is present, one must distinguish further whether the patient has diabetes mellitus or renal glycosuria. A normal serum glucose concentration would point to a diagnosis of renal glycosuria.

Examination of serum electrolytes, glucose, urea nitrogen, phosphate, creatinine, calcium, and osmolality also is indicated, as is evaluation of urinary amino acid excretion. A hyperosmolar state would suggest vasopressin deficiency or insensitivity, provided the serum glucose concentration is normal. A low serum osmolality would suggest either primary polydipsia or water intoxication as the most likely diagnosis. A careful feeding history can help identify infants suffering from water intoxication. Evidence of renal impairment, hypercalcemia, and hypokalemia also will be uncovered in such an examination.

In polyuric individuals who have a low urine specific gravity and no glycosuria, the next step in evaluation is a water deprivation test, the purpose of which is to determine the child's ability to conserve water at times when antidiuresis is necessary for homeostasis. After a 24-hour period of adequate hydration, blood is drawn to determine sodium, osmolality, and urea nitrogen levels and to perform a hematocrit; the urine osmolality and specific gravity are measured, the child is weighed, and his or her intake and output are recorded. The child then is restricted from any food or fluid intake for a 6- to 8-hour period, during which the child's weight, urine output, urine specific gravity, and serum sodium are determined. After the study period, the initial blood tests are repeated, urine osmolality is measured again, and the final weight is recorded. If at any point the child has lost 5% or more of his or her body weight, the test is stopped, once final blood studies are obtained. Because of the possibility of volume depletion, it is recommended that the study be carried out during the day when supervision is optimal. In normal children and in most children who have psychogenic polydipsia, the weight remains constant, the urine specific gravity increases to at least 1.010, the urine volume decreases, and the ratio of urine to plasma osmolality rises to at least 2:1. However, if diuresis continues in the absence of oral intake and if weight loss and hyperosmolarity develop, one should suspect a diagnosis of diabetes insipidus, either central or nephrogenic.

The vasopressin test is the next step in the evaluation of a polyuric patient when the water deprivation test shows a specific gravity of less than 1.015 (Table 158-1). The purpose of this test is to determine whether the excessive urine flow responds to exogenous vasopressin. This test is best done immediately after the water deprivation test. Aqueous vasopressin in a dose of 6 U/m^2 is administered subcutaneously, and the patient is allowed free access to water. Subsequently, intake, output, and urine specific gravity are recorded every 30 to 60 minutes. Normal subjects and patients who have vasopressin deficiency evidence a reduced fluid intake and output and a rise in urine specific gravity to at least 1.015. Urine osmolality, likewise, increases significantly. Individuals who have partial diabetes insipidus demonstrate a modest rise in urine concentration on water deprivation testing (urine osmolality less than 400 mOsm/kg), but the urine becomes concentrated after administration of vasopressin. Patients who have primary polydipsia maintain a constant intake but generally have a reduced urine output and increased urine specific gravity. If no response to vasopressin occurs after 6 hours, the test should be repeated using a dose of 12 U/m^2 subcutaneously. If the patient shows no effect after this double dose, nephrogenic diabetes insipidus probably is the diagnosis.

MANAGEMENT

Patients who show evidence of vasopressin deficiency are best referred to an endocrinologist or neurologist so that the cause of the diabetes insipidus can be determined. Skull roentgenograms, visual field examination, full investigation of other pituitary functions, or magnetic resonance imaging (MRI), or computed tomography (CT) scans of the head likely will be the next steps in evaluation. Patients should be allowed free access to fluids, and their serum and urine osmolality should be monitored closely. In a severely ill patient, aqueous vasopressin (0.1 to 0.2 U/kg) may be given subcutaneously every 4 to 6 hours.

Aqueous vasopressin also may be given by constant intravenous infusion. Reported starting dosages vary from 1.3 to 4.6 mU/kg/hour, and these should be increased or decreased as needed.[1,14] Once the child's condition has stabilized, management consists of desmopressin acetate (DDAVP), a synthetic derivative of vasopressin, instilled intranasally at a dosage of 5 to 20 μg twice daily. Recent studies have shown that DDAVP may be administered effectively and safely either orally[3] or sublingually,[8] although therapeutic doses are larger and more variable than those administered intranasally. Use of thiazide diuretics, chlorpropamide, and clofibrate has met with some success in the management of diabetes insipidus but generally lacks the efficacy of vasopressin derivatives.

In patients who have primary polydipsia, once a neurogenic lesion has been ruled out, medical therapy is not indicated. Psychotherapy, however, may be useful in addressing the emotional problem causing the polydipsia. Water-intoxicated infants require prompt attention to fluid and electrolyte balance, and some whose hyponatremia is severe have required treatment with either isotonic or hypertonic (3%) saline solution. Once the acute sequelae have been treated, preventive efforts should focus on educating caretakers so that feeding techniques may be corrected.

Patients who have structural renal diseases leading to polyuria can be referred to a nephrologist; patients who have nephrogenic diabetes insipidus commonly are seen by an endocrinologist or a nephrologist. They should be allowed free access to fluids; parents of infants who have this disorder need to offer frequent water feedings to allow their infants to maintain osmotic homeostasis. A low-salt diet has been helpful in reducing urine output; thiazide diuretics can further reduce polyuria by reducing the amount of urine delivered to the distal tubule. Indomethacin[13] and amiloride,[10] when given concurrently with a thiazide, each have been found to be effective at reducing urine output.

Osmotic diuresis induced by drugs or diet generally is self-limited. Although renal glycosuria requires no specific therapy, such a diagnosis can be made only when other renal tubular functions are normal. In overweight patients who have NIDDM, weight reduction is paramount. This measure alone usually is sufficient to reverse the carbohydrate intolerance. If glycosuria persists, an endocrinologist may prescribe insulin. In IDDM, patients who have polydipsia and polyuria may be hospitalized to stabilize the abnormal car-

Table 158-1 Interpretation of Vasopressin Test

	Intake	Output	Urine specific gravity
Normal	↓	↓	↑
Psychogenic polydipsia	Unchanged	↓	↑
Central diabetes insipidus	↓	↓	↑
Nephrogenic diabetes insipidus	Unchanged	Unchanged	Unchanged

bohydrate metabolism with exogenous insulin, to correct the electrolyte disturbance, and to educate the patient and family about home management (see Chapter 199).

Management of polyuria, therefore, depends heavily on the underlying diagnosis and must be individualized carefully. In most cases the results are gratifying, but patients often are found to have a chronic disease that requires close, long-term surveillance.

REFERENCES

1. Chanson P et al: Ultralow doses of vasopressin in the management of diabetes insipidus, *Crit Care Med* 15:44, 1987.
2. Czernichow P et al: Diabetes insipidus in children. III. Anterior pituitary dysfunction in idiopathic types, *J Pediatr* 106:41, 1985.
3. Fjellestad-Paulsen A et al: Central diabetes insipidus: oral treatment with dDAVP, *Regul Pept* 45:303, 1993.
4. Forssman H: Two different mutations of the X chromosome causing diabetes insipidus, *Am J Hum Genet* 7:21, 1955.
5. Goldman M, Luchins D, Robertson G: Mechanisms of altered water metabolism in psychotic patients with polydipsia and hyponatremia, *N Engl J Med* 318:397, 1988.
6. Greger N et al: Central diabetes insipidus: 22 years' experience, *Am J Dis Child* 140:551, 1986.
7. Grosse Aldenhovel H, Gallenkamp U, Sulemana C: Juvenile onset diabetes mellitus, central diabetes insipidus, and optic atrophy (Wolfram syndrome): neurological findings and prognostic implications, *Neuropediatrics* 22:103, 1991.
8. Kappy M, Sonderer E: Sublingual administration of desmopressin: effectiveness in an infant with holoprosencephaly and central diabetes insipidus, *Am J Dis Child* 141:84, 1987.
9. Keating J, Schears G, Dodge P: Oral water intoxication in infants: an American epidemic, *Am J Dis Child* 145:985, 1991.
10. Knoers N, Monnens L: Amiloride-hydrochlorothiazide versus indomethacin-hydrochlorothiazide in the treatment of nephrogenic diabetes insipidus, *J Pediatr* 117:499, 1990.
11. Kohn B et al: Hysterical polydipsia (compulsive water drinking) in children, *Am J Dis Child* 130:210, 1976.
12. Leung A, Robson W, Halperin M: Polyuria in childhood, *Clin Pediatr* 30:634, 1991.
13. Libber S, Harrison H, Spector D: Treatment of nephrogenic diabetes insipidus with prostaglandin synthesis inhibitors, *J Pediatr* 108:305, 1986.
14. McDonald J et al: Treatment of the young child with postoperative central diabetes insipidus, *Am J Dis Child* 143:201, 1989.
15. Merendino J et al: A mutation in the vasopressin V2-receptor gene in a kindred with X-linked nephrogenic diabetes insipidus, *N Engl J Med* 328:1538, 1993.
16. Moses AS: Diabetes insipidus and ADH regulation, *Hosp Pract* 12:37, 1977.
17. Scherbaum W: Autoimmune hypothalamic diabetes insipidus ("autoimmune hypothalamitis"), *Prog Brain Res* 93:283, 1992.

159 Proteinuria

Edward J. Ruley

The presence of abnormal amounts of protein in the urine may be asymptomatic or, if severe enough to cause hypoproteinemia, associated with varying degrees of edema. The techniques and pitfalls of detecting proteinuria and determining its prevalence are discussed in Chapter 20, Eight, Use of Urinalysis and the Urine Culture in Screening.

The crucial factors in the consideration of proteinuria are (1) its constancy, (2) its quantitation, and (3) its concurrence with other urinary abnormalities. The first two factors can be determined simultaneously by having the patient collect a 24-hour urine specimen following the instructions shown in the box on p. 1079.

The constancy of proteinuria in relation to posture and activity can be determined if the amount of protein in each voiding during the 24-hour collection is measured by the patient or parent using dip-and-read strips. Because the collection begins and ends with the first void after waking on consecutive days, two urine determinations after the patient has been supine overnight will be available. More information on the effect of activity on proteinuria can be obtained if the patient is instructed to have periods of both vigorous and quiet activity during the waking hours of the 24-hour collection.

The total collection should be assayed for volume, creatinine, and protein content. One can determine whether the 24-hour urine was collected properly by calculating the urinary creatinine excretion (mg/kg/day). Children of normal habitus excrete about 18 mg/kg/day of creatinine, although there is individual variation that is partly determined by age and gender.[1] If the creatinine excretion is near this amount, one can presume that the 24-hour urine specimen was obtained correctly and that the urinary protein quantitation is a good reflection of the degree of proteinuria. Although creatinine excretion may vary between individuals, each person is very consistent in his or her creatinine excretion. Thus, if the urinary creatinine excretion varies in serial collections, one must suspect that the collection methodology has been inconsistent, and the protein quantitations cannot be compared in terms of trends. If the creatinine excretion is not near normal or varies greatly, the urine collection should be repeated after the technique of urine collection has been reviewed with the patient and parents. Normally, children excrete less than 200 mg of protein per square meter, although there may be some variation in quantity between diagnostic laboratories because of different methods of measurement.

The third crucial factor is the concurrence of other urinary abnormalities such as hematuria and cylindruria. The probability that proteinuria represents a more severe pathological state increases when it occurs with other urinary abnormalities. An algorithm for the investigation of proteinuria using the 24-hour urine collection in which each individual specimen has been tested is shown in Fig. 159-1. If all specimens are negative and the total 24-hour protein excretion is normal for the child's size, the previous finding of proteinuria in random urine samples probably was an artifact. Such an occurrence is not unusual in pediatric practice. The two most common causes of artifactual proteinuria are (1) improper urine collection, in that the cleansing solution or an extraneous source of protein (e.g., vaginal discharge) contaminates the specimen, and (2) collection of a specimen from a person who has had a poor fluid intake. In this latter circumstance, the normal amount of excreted protein that usually is below the range of detection by the dip-and-read strips is concentrated to a detectable level. This commonly occurs in handicapped children (e.g., blind or mentally retarded children) who have limited access to water and apparently adjust to a chronic low intake of fluid. Usually a history of poor fluid ingestion and infrequent voiding can be obtained. Despite the positive result on the dip-and-read test, the quantitative protein will be normal. High positive dip-and-read results (3+ and 4+) usually are not caused by poor fluid intake.

If the patient has negative urine protein results after he or she has been supine or inactive but positive results following upright posture or physical activity, a clinical diagnosis of postural, or orthostatic, proteinuria is justified, providing such a postural effect occurs (1) as an isolated urine abnormality, (2) with a quantitative protein excretion that is less than five times the 95th percentile for age, (3) in the absence of symptoms and of a personal or family history of renal disease, and (4) with a normal physical examination and laboratory tests of renal function. Orthostatic proteinuria usually is discovered on routine urinalysis in an asymptomatic adolescent or young adult. The diagnosis of orthostatic proteinuria is a clinical one; therefore renal biopsy and an extensive radiographic investigation are not indicated. When renal biopsies have been performed, they have been normal or have shown only nonspecific changes.[4] Orthostatic proteinuria resolves in early adulthood in half of these patients. Follow-up studies of patients (for as long as 50 years after diagnosis) have revealed no tendency for the urinary abnormality to progress to serious renal disease.[2,3] Even so, the child should have a semiannual reexamination and a repeat 24-hour urine collection with individual specimen testing. Such a follow-up can detect any change in the pattern of proteinuria, which may be a harbinger of an underlying serious renal problem.

If all urinary specimens test positive for protein regardless of position or activity, a significant renal pathological condition is likely. Such pathological proteinuria also is associated more frequently with hematuria or other abnormalities of the urinary sediment. The nephritic range for total 24-hour proteinuria usually is 5 to 10 times normal and often is associated with hypertension, mild edema, and nonspecific generalized symptoms, such as malaise and fatigue. In such pa-

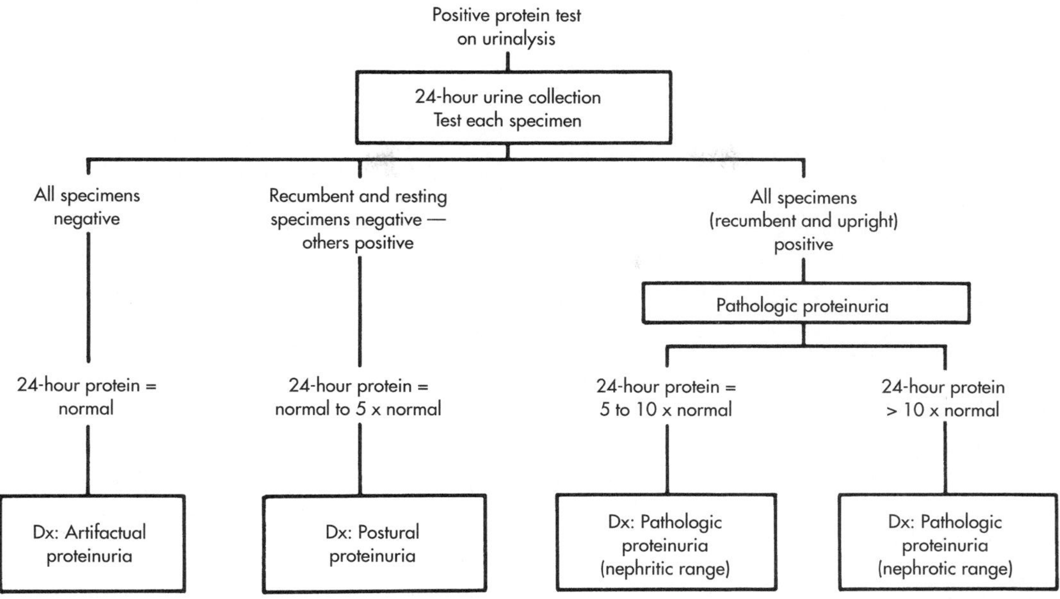

FIG. 159-1 A clinical algorithm for proteinuria in children.

PATIENT INSTRUCTIONS FOR SIMULTANEOUS COLLECTION OF 24-HOUR URINE SPECIMEN AND POSTURAL PROTEIN TEST

This test involves the simultaneous collection of a 24-hour urine specimen (for quantitation of total urinary protein) and the testing of each individual urine specimen for protein. The amount of protein in each urination should be recorded along with the date, time of day, and the activities of the patient since the previous urination. The specific instructions for the patient are as follows:

1. On the day the test begins, urinate immediately after rising (________AM), test for protein, record the results, and then *discard* the urine.
2. Test each subsequent urination, record the result, and add the entire specimen to the 24-hour collection, which should be kept refrigerated. A good intake of fluid is helpful throughout this test.
3. Sometime during the day, exercise (e.g., bike riding, playing ball) so that there is a urine specimen to test after a period of vigorous activity. Test it, record the results, and add it to the collection as you did with the others.
4. During another time of day (evening is best), remain relatively quiet (e.g., doing homework, watching television) so that there is urine to test after a period of rest. Test it and add it to the collection.
5. On the next day, rise at the same time, urinate immediately, test for protein, record the results, and add to the 24-hour collection.
6. Bring this paper with the written urine tests results, the unused protein test strips, and the 24-hour specimen to the office. The patient need not come to the office unless an appointment has been scheduled.

Results

Date	Time	Activity	Urine Protein

tients a complete renal functional examination and imaging of the kidneys are important. Most of these children should be referred to a pediatric nephrologist for more complete evaluation, which usually includes a renal biopsy[5] (see Chapter 232, Nephritis).

Pathological total 24-hour proteinuria over 10 times normal can be labeled as being in the nephrotic range. Hypoproteinemia and hypercholesterolemia often are found concomitantly. These patients usually have edema or other obvious signs and symptoms that bring them to medical attention. A complete evaluation is indicated in these circumstances (see Chapter 233, Nephrotic Syndrome).

REFERENCES

1. Meites S: *Pediatric clinical chemistry,* ed 3, Washington, DC, 1989, AACC Press.
2. Robinson RR: Isolated proteinuria in asymptomatic patients, *Kidney Int* 18:395, 1980.
3. Rytand DA, Spreiter S: Prognosis in postural (orthostatic) proteinuria: forty- to fifty-year follow-up of six patients after diagnosis by Thomas Addis, *N Engl J Med* 305:618, 1981.
4. Sinniah R, Law CH, Pwee HS: Glomerular lesions in patients with asymptomatic persistent and orthostatic proteinuria discovered on routine medical examination, *Clin Nephrol* 7:1, 1977.
5. Yoshikawa N et al: Asymptomatic constant isolated proteinuria in children, *J Pediatr* 119:375, 1991.

SUGGESTED READINGS

Kiel DP, Moskowitz MA: The urinalysis: a critical approach, *Med Clin North Am* 71:607, 1987.

Normal ME: An office approach to hematuria and proteinuria, *Pediatr Clin North Am* 34:545, 1987.

160 Pruritus

Nancy K. Barnett

Pruritus, or itch, is the subjective perception of a cutaneous disturbance that is relieved by scratching or rubbing. It usually is not brought to the pediatrician's attention unless it is generalized, chronic, or associated with an eruption. In such instances, however, it must be treated with great respect because severe itching can be physically incapacitating. In addition, scratching or rubbing the itch can produce extensive disfigurement in the form of linear excoriations or lichenified plaques. The constant scratching can even cause social isolation, for at times the pruritic child is viewed by others as contagious or unclean.

PATHOPHYSIOLOGY

Because it is a subjective sensation, objective evaluation to delineate the pathophysiology of itch has been difficult. However, current thinking implicates a local production of chemomediators that stimulate "itch receptors," thought to be free fine nerve endings at the dermoepidermal junction.[6] The exact mediators and their release triggers are unknown. Histamine and endopeptidases have elicited itch fairly consistently in experimental settings and may be active in human disease. Experimental triggers that have produced itch are physical pressure, heat, and electric shock.

It is believed that the nerve impulses travel along the anterolateral spinothalamic tract to the thalamus, where they are transferred to the sensory cortex via the internal capsule, where they are interpreted as itch.[4,7] This is the same pathway for pain, and some contend that itch is a mild degree of "pain"; however, aspirin alone does not relieve itch.

Certain circumstances alter the interpretation of the degree of pruritus. For example, the itch threshold in and around areas of active dermatitis can be lowered by psychic stress, decreased skin hydration or increased skin temperature, and during the night.[2,3]

CLINICAL MANIFESTATIONS

In children, local cutaneous rather than systemic disease is by far the most common cause of generalized pruritus. The major differential diagnoses of generalized pruritus with skin lesions in children are infestation (scabies, pediculosis, insect bites, and papular urticaria), atopic dermatitis, miliaria, contact dermatitis, and acute urticaria.[7]

Children may itch with cutaneous diseases such as psoriasis, lichen planus, and bullous disease of childhood. These children should be referred to a dermatologist for evaluation and management, as should a pruritic child who otherwise is healthy and does not have bites, eczema, "heat rash," contact dermatitis, or hives. The child who has pruritus, from whatever cause, is at risk for psychological damage, infection secondary to impetiginization, and scarification.

Systemic causes of pruritus in childhood that should be sought in the occasional child who has pruritus but no evident skin lesions are hyperthyroidism, leukemia or lymphoma, chronic renal failure, obstructive biliary disease, and xerosis (generalized dry skin).

EVALUATION AND TREATMENT

All of the common cutaneous diseases associated with generalized pruritus can be diagnosed on the basis of a good history and physical examination. The answers to the following questions may help in diagnosing infestation of one sort or another and direct therapy toward topical steroids, long clothes, and repellents: Are there individual pruritic papules with a central punctum? If so, are they on exposed or nonexposed areas? Does anyone else in the family have similar lesions?

A family history of allergy, asthma, or eczema in a child who has a chronic eczematous dermatitis over extensor surfaces in infancy and flexural areas in childhood suggests atopic dermatitis. Hydration and emollients will reduce the pruritus and should be the mainstay of therapy, although topical steroids, antibiotics, and cool compresses may be required to bring the scratch-itch cycle under control. A tolerable (nonsoporific) dose of an antihistamine may relieve itch, especially if it is given about 1 hour before bedtime, since the itch threshold is lower at night. Hydroxyzine seems to be the most effective agent.[5] Data conflict about the use of nonsedating antihistamines for controlling itch.[1]

Pinpoint crystalline or erythematous papules in areas of occlusion and sweating—that is, miliaria crystallina and miliaria rubra (heat rash)—can be controlled by simple measures such as applying dusting powders, avoiding tight clothing, and reducing exposure to high ambient temperature.

Contact dermatitis usually is readily recognizable because of the linear array of papulovesicular, erythematous lesions and their sharp borders conforming to the shape of the contactant. The use of antihistamines, topical steroids, and compresses is discussed in detail in Chapter 196, Contact Dermatitis.

Acute urticaria that occurs secondary to a drug or other ingestant is indicated by intensely pruritic, erythematous, and edematous plaques and papules. Careful historical and environmental sleuthing may reveal the cause of contact allergic or contact irritant dermatitis, but the cause of 90% of acute urticaria cases remains a mystery. If the patient has not used any new drug or food and if the hives persist despite regular use of antihistamines for several days, it is reasonable to obtain a throat culture and to screen for hepatitis to rule out occult streptococcal and viral hepatitis infections.

To relieve itching and prevent scarring (both mental and physical), the scratch-itch cycle must be broken. Scratching relieves itching only temporarily, perhaps by substituting the perception of pain for that of itch. Itching provokes scratching, and when the scratching stops, the itching returns. To control itching, the following steps can be helpful: keep the patient's fingernails short (to prevent damage from scratching); keep the patient fully clothed except when applying medications; apply emollients frequently, especially after bathing; apply cool compresses to relieve intense pruritus and to remove crusts and debris; apply topical steroids for short periods (less than 10 days) to control inflammation; increase the dosage of antihistamine until the scratching stops or marked drowsiness occurs, and then reduce the dosage to a level that controls the scratching; have the patient avoid stress, heat, and irritants; and see the patient frequently to provide support and, if the child is old enough to understand, to explain why these methods are being used. Topical capsaicin and pramoxine may be indicated in some cases. Referral to the dermatologist generally is indicated in such a circumstance. Ultraviolet B (UVB) light therapy may be very helpful for generalized pruritus such as occurs in biliary cirrhosis or severe chronic atopic dermatitis.

REFERENCES

1. Bernhard JD: Itching: some answers but no panacea, *Dermatol Perspect* 5:1, 1989.
2. Cormia FE: Experimental histamine pruritus, *J Invest Dermatol* 19:21, 1952.
3. Edwards AE et al: Pruritic skin disease, psychological stress, and the itch sensation, *Arch Dermatol* 112:339, 1976.
4. Gilchrest BA: Pruritus: pathogenesis, therapy, and significance in systemic disease states, *Arch Intern Med* 142:101, 1982.
5. Rhoades RB et al: Suppression of histamine-induced pruritus by three antihistamine drugs, *J Allergy Clin Immunol* 55:180, 1975.
6. Shelly WB, Arthur RP: The neurohistology and neurophysiology of the itch sensation in man, *Arch Dermatol* 76:296, 1957.
7. Tonnesen MG: Pruritus. In Fitzpatrick TB et al, editors: *Dermatology in general medicine,* ed 3, New York, 1987, McGraw-Hill.

161 Rash

Nancy K. Barnett

Rash is an ambiguous term used to describe an acute skin eruption that usually is temporary. It does not define any specific lesion. The term also does not convey information about the evolution or progression of a disorder, which are data needed to arrive at a logical differential diagnosis.

Tables 161-1 and 161-2 list descriptions of lesions and contain historical or characteristic information for particular diagnoses. The tables are not valid for "rashes" that have been altered by therapy. They are not all-inclusive but cover the major acute eruptions that the pediatrician will encounter.

Before reviewing the tables, a few points are worth making. Within all of medicine, a careful history is necessary. However, we too often are prone to look at a rash before exploring its past. We must know when it arose, how it progressed, and whether there were accompanying symptoms or signs—for example, an itch or a fever. A sound history includes that of the family. It is easy to ask if someone else in the family is scratching or similarly beset now or in the past.

The most important lesson one pediatrician learned early in his career about evaluating a rash involved light: the rash of scarlet fever became evident when he raised the window shade. The light should be adequate when performing a physical examination; natural lighting is preferred. Be sure your view of the field is unobstructed. Clothing must be shed. Don't limit your look to a rolled-up sleeve or a lifted shirttail. Feel the rash—is it smooth or rough? Once the site has been inspected and palpated, the rash must be described as accurately as possible. What does it look like? (Use a magnifier to discern, for example, a burrow or a pinpoint puncture.) Where is it? Are the lesions discrete or confluent, large or small? Use a tape measure to define the lesions accurately by size. Is it oozing or dry? Excoriated or relatively untouched in appearance? Describe carefully in writing what is seen.

A *macule* is a spot that is set apart from its immediate surroundings by a difference in color. It is a discoloration of the skin that is not elevated above the surface and may be of any color or of many colors. It is small, generally less than 1 cm. Larger areas may be described as patches. *Papules* are small (less than 5 mm in diameter), well-circumscribed solid elevations of the skin. A *nodule,* too, is solid and usually elevated or palpable in the subcutaneous area, but it is larger than a papule. Its solidity, like the papule, enables it to be detected by touch, although its borders are indistinct. A *vesicle* is a small sac that contains liquid. With respect to the skin, it may be described as a circumscribed elevation of the epidermis containing a serous liquid. As the diameter approaches 1 cm, it is more appropriately called a bulla or bleb. A *bulla,* or blister, similarly is an elevation above the level of the skin that is filled with fluid, usually serous. It may have either a quite delicate or tough "roof," depending on the level of the skin in which it appears.

Once one has become familiar with Tables 161-1 and 161-2 and their precepts, it becomes evident that many dermatological diagnoses are not particularly difficult to make. On the other hand, problems of either diagnosis or treatment are sure to arise. Children and adolescents who have eczema, acne, and psoriasis, for example, often will benefit from consultation with a dermatologist.

Regardless, for pediatrician and dermatologist alike, *primum non nocere* (i.e., above all, do no harm) should be the rule. Iatrogenic difficulties from the overuse of drugs such as topical corticosteroids and antibiotics must be avoided. Seldom should adrenal suppression be risked because of continuous steroid use, and we already are too far along in encouraging bacterial readaptations to the environment. Fortunately, some principles of therapy help guide the pediatrician. First, the least amount necessary of the most effective medication should be given by mouth or applied locally. Second, the use of household aids can be convenient and inexpensive; for example, oatmeal can serve as a colloid compress or bath for itching; an emery board will keep the fingernails smooth and short to reduce excoriations from scratching; and tea bags can be used as compresses for odd places (weeping behind the ears). Third, a moistened gauze wrapped twice around atopic areas helps to reduce oozing, to relieve itching, and to potentiate the effect of topical steroids. Fourth, children whose itching is generalized, as in atopic dermatitis, should always be kept fully clothed, using long-sleeved shirts and leotards during the day and pajamas with feet at night. Fifth, emollients, such as Eucerin or Aquaphor lubricate and smooth dry skin and diminish itching, whereas powder or cornstarch, dusted on lightly, is useful on moist or oozing surfaces (particularly between the toes and other intertriginous areas) to prevent maceration. And last, precise instruction is essential; the patient or parent should be asked to repeat the plan for treatment and the steps for its implementation to ensure complete understanding of what is to be done, and written instructions should be sent home with the patient.

SUGGESTED READINGS

Cohen BA: *Atlas of pediatric dermatology,* London, 1993, Wolfe.

Rasmussen JE: Principles of diagnosis. In Schachner LA, Hansen RC, editors: *Pediatric dermatology,* New York, 1988, Churchill Livingstone.

Table 161-1 Descriptions of Lesions

	Number			Pattern						Distribution									Size			Spread			Other characteristics				
Diagnosis or differential diagnosis	Few	Many	TNTC*	Discrete	Confluent	Annular†	Localized	Generalized	Symmetrical	Face/scalp	Palmoplantar	Truncal	Intertriginous	Extremities	Acral	Extensor	Flexor	Mucosae	<1 mm	1-5 mm	>5 mm	Centripetal	Centrifugal	Caudal	Sun exposed	Fever/illness	Pruritus	Scale	Crust
Macule																													
Erythematous																													
Dermatomyositis‡					X					X						X									X			X	
Drug reaction‡			X	X	X			X		X	X	X	X	X	X				X	X	X						X		
Erythema infectiosum					X		X			X		X		X						X	X			X					
Erythema marginatum‡		X				X						X		X							X		X			X			
Erythema multiforme, Stevens-Johnson syndrome	X	X	X	X			X	X	X	X	X	X			X	X		X		X	X	X				X			
Infectious mononucleosis‡					X			X				X		X												X			
Juvenile rheumatoid arthritis‡		X		X	X			X				X		X						X	X					X			
Kawasaki disease‡					X			X		X	X	X		X				X								X			
Rubella			X	X	X			X		X		X		X				X		X						X			
Lyme disease	X	X		X		X	X	X				X									X					X			
Roseola infantum (exanthem subitum)			X	X	X			X				X								X						X			
Rubeola			X	X	X			X		X		X		X				X		X				X		X			
Staphylococcal scalded skin syndrome					X		X	X		X		X	X	X												X			X
Sunburn, phototoxic reaction	X				X		X	X													X				X				
Toxic epidermal necrolysis					X			X		X		X	X	X				X								X			
Toxic shock syndrome					X			X				X						X								X			
Viral exanthem‡			X	X	X			X		X	X	X		X				X		X						X			
Hypopigmented																													
Pityriasis alba	X	X	X	X	X		X	X		X		X		X						X	X							X	
Tinea versicolor‡	X	X	X	X	X		X	X		X		X		X						X	X			X			X	X	
Vitiligo in evolution	X	X		X	X		X	X	X	X	X	X		X	X	X				X	X								
Hyperpigmented																													
Tinea versicolor‡	X	X	X	X	X		X	X		X		X		X						X	X			X			X	X	
Transient neonatal pustular melanosis	X	X	X	X	X			X		X		X	X							X									

Nonblanching (petechiae, purpura)																													
Atypical measles		X	X	X	X			X		X		X		X	X			X	X	X					X	X			
Battered child syndrome‡	X	X		X			X			X		X		X							X								
Leukemia, coagulation defect, ITP	X	X	X	X	X			X		X		X		X				X	X	X									
Rocky Mountain spotted fever‡	X	X	X	X	X			X		X	X	X		X	X		X		X	X		X				X			
Viral exanthem, TORCH infection, drug, hepatitis‡		X	X	X	X			X		X		X		X				X	X	X					X	X			
Papules, nodules																													
Erythematous																													
Atopic dermatitis	X	X	X	X	X		X	X		X		X		X		X	X		X	X	X						X		X
Granuloma annulare	X	X		X		X						X		X	X					X	X								
Insect bites	X	X	X	X			X			X		X	X	X	X					X					X				
Miliaria rubra (heat rash)	X	X	X	X			X			X		X	X						X							X	X		
Scarlet fever			X	X	X				X				X	X	X			X		X	X			X			X		
Seborrheic dermatitis	X	X	X	X	X		X	X		X		X	X							X	X							X	
Tinea corporis	X	X		X		X	X			X		X		X					X	X	X			X					
Hypopigmented																													
Lichen nitidus		X	X	X			X					X		X					X	X									
Lichen striatus, linear lichen planus, epidermal nevus		X	X	X	X		X				X			X							X								
Molluscum contagiosum	X	X	X		X		X			X		X		X					X	X	X								
Violaceous																													
Lichen planus	X	X	X	X	X			X	X			X		X	X			X	X	X	X						X		
Nonblanching																													
Gonococcemia, SBE	X			X			X				X	X		X						X						X			
Henoch-Schönlein purpura§	X	X	X	X	X			X	X					X		X				X	X	X				X			
Letterer-Siwe disease	X	X	X	X	X		X	X		X	X	X	X	X						X	X					X		X	X
Leukemia cutis/lymphoma	X	X	X	X	X			X				X		X					X	X	X					X			
Mastocytosis (urticaria pigmentosa)§	X	X	X	X	X		X	X		X		X		X						X	X						X		
Meningococcemia, sepsis	X	X	X	X	X			X		X	X	X		X				X	X	X						X			
Neuroblastoma, TORCH infection, leukemia	X	X		X				X		X		X		X						X	X					X			

*Too numerous to count.
†Raised border.
‡May be papular in parts.
§May be edematous.

Continued.

Table 161-1 Descriptions of Lesions—cont'd

	Number			Pattern						Distribution									Size			Spread			Other characteristics				
Diagnosis or differential diagnosis	Few	Many	TNTC*	Discrete	Confluent	Annular†	Localized	Generalized	Symmetrical	Face/scalp	Palmoplantar	Truncal	Intertriginous	Extremities	Acral	Extensor	Flexor	Mucosae	<1 mm	1-5 mm	>5 mm	Centripetal	Centrifugal	Caudal	Sun exposed	Fever/illness	Pruritus	Scale	Crust
Vesicles																													
Contact dermatitis	X	X	X	X	X		X	X		X		X	X	X	X				X	X							X		X
Coxsackievirus hand, foot, and mouth disease	X	X		X			X			X					X			X		X						X			
Dyshidrotic eczema (pompholyx)	X	X	X	X	X		X				X				X				X	X							X		
Flea bites	X	X	X	X			X							X	X					X							X		X
Herpes simplex; herpes zoster	X			X	X		X			X		X		X				X	X	X						X	X		X
Miliaria crystallina	X	X	X	X			X	X		X		X	X	X					X						X	X	X		
Tinea pedis	X	X	X	X	X		X				X								X	X							X		X
Varicella		X	X	X				X	X	X	X	X	X	X				X	X	X		X				X	X		X
Bullae																													
Bullous disease of childhood	X	X	X	X	X	X		X		X		X	X	X	X						X						X		X
Bullous impetigo	X	X		X	X		X			X		X	X	X							X						X		X
Pustules																													
Acne neonatorum	X	X		X			X		X	X									X	X									
Candidiasis	X	X	X	X	X		X	X		X	X	X	X	X				X		X						X		X	
Erythema toxicum neonatorum	X	X	X	X	X		X	X		X	X	X		X						X									
Folliculitis	X	X	X	X			X	X				X		X					X	X									
Transient neonatal pustular melanosis	X	X	X	X	X		X			X		X	X							X									
Plaques																													
Acute urticaria	X	X	X	X	X		X	X		X		X		X				X	X	X	X						X		
Nummular eczema	X	X	X	X			X					X		X		X					X						X	X	X
Psoriasis	X	X	X	X	X		X	X	X	X	X	X		X		X				X	X				X		X	X	

*Too numerous to count.
†Raised border.

Table 161-2 Laboratory Studies and Characteristics of Lesions

Diagnosis or differential diagnosis	Laboratory studies	Comments
Macule		
Erythematous		
Sunburn, phototoxic reaction		Look for patterns and sharp edges, e.g., clothing lines after exposure to sun
Rubeola		Koplik spots, preauricular lymph nodes
Drug reaction*	Leukocytosis with eosinophilia	History of drug ingestion
Toxic shock syndrome	Blood, throat, urine, stool, vaginal cultures for *Staphylococcus aureus* or *Streptococcus pyogenes*	Shock, tampon use
Infectious mononucleosis*	Heterophil antibody; atypical lymphs on smear	Generalized adenopathy, splenomegaly; ampicillin use
Kawasaki disease*	Thrombocytosis 3-5 wk after onset	Conjunctival injection, cervical adenopathy
Staphylococcal scalded skin syndrome	*S. aureus* cultured from focus	Tender erythema, positive Nikolsky sign, bullae
Toxic epidermal necrolysis	*S. aureus* cultures negative	Search for new drug use
Erythema multiforme, Stevens-Johnson syndrome	Skin biopsy may aid diagnosis	Central papule or vesicle, iris lesions; may be bullous
Viral exanthem*	Leukocytosis with lymphocytosis	
Rubella	Fourfold rise in antibody titer	Postauricular lymphadenopathy; monarticular arthritis
Roseola infantum (exanthem subitum)	Leukopenia may be present	Eruption appears with resolution of fever; periorbital edema
Erythema infectiosum	Lymphocytosis, eosinophilia	Reticulated pattern may appear for months with stress; arthritis
Erythema marginatum*		Acute rheumatic fever with active carditis; fleeting
Juvenile rheumatoid arthritis*	Rheumatoid factor may be positive	Arthritis; lesions may be papular
Dermatomyositis*	Electromyography, creatinine phosphokinase, aldolase	Muscle weakness; periungual telangiectasia; heliotrope eyelid edema; Gottron papule
Lyme disease	Most nonspecific; may look for antibodies to *Borrelia burgdorferi* (see Chapter 228 on Lyme disease)	Erythema chronicum migrans appearing as enlarging rings after tick bite
Hypopigmented		
Tinea versicolor*	Potassium hydroxide (KOH) smear—short, branched hyphae and spores	Chronic; prevalent if immunosuppressed
Pityriasis alba	Wood light—hypopigmented	
Vitiligo in evolution	Wood light—depigmented if vitiliginous; T_4, TSH to rule out thyroid disorder	Observe for scleroderma, melanoma
Hyperpigmented		
Tinea versicolor*	See above	See above
Transient neonatal pustular melanosis	Pustule gram stain—sterile with polymorphonuclear neutrophils (PMNs)	Pustules; superficial desquamation
Nonblanching (petechiae, purpura)		
Atypical measles		History of killed measles vaccine; pneumonitis; acral petechiae, purpura, vesiculobullous lesions
Viral exanthem, TORCH infection, drug, hepatitis*	Complete blood count (CBC), liver enzymes, viral titers	Drug history
Rocky Mountain spotted fever*	Fluorescent antibody screen; OX-19, OX-2; skin biopsy of fluorescent stain	History of tick bite
Leukemia, coagulation defect, ITP	CBC, PT, PTT, platelet count, bone marrow aspirate and biopsy	
Battered child syndrome*		History incongruous with pattern and/or degree of lesions

*May be papular in parts.

Continued

Table 161-2 Laboratory Studies and Characteristics of Lesions—cont'd

Diagnosis or differential diagnosis	Laboratory studies	Comments
Papules, nodules		
Erythematous		
Miliaria rubra (heat rash)		Prominent in occluded areas
Seborrheic dermatitis		Intertriginous with yellow greasy scale, cradle cap
Atopic dermatitis	IgE level	Family or personal history of allergies, asthma, eczema; flexural in infancy and extensor in childhood
Scarlet fever	Throat culture, ASO titer	Malar flush, circumoral pallor, Pastia lines, desquamation
Insect bites		Check for central punctae
Tinea corporis	KOH smear—long, thin-branched hyphae	
Granuloma annulare		Lack of scale distinguishes from tinea corporis; no epidermal component
Hypopigmented		
Molluscum contagiosum		Pearly papule with central umbilication containing easily expressed white cheesy core
Lichen nitidus		Check penis for grouped lichenoid papules
Lichen striatus, linear lichen planus, epidermal nevus	Skin biopsy	Linear
Violaceous		
Lichen planus		Purple pruritic polygonal papules
Nonblanching		
Meningococcemia, sepsis	Blood, cerebrospinal fluid (CSF) culture; gram-stain lesion	Check conjunctivae for hemorrhage
Gonococcemia, SBE	Blood, throat, cervical, rectal cultures	Check for heart murmur, arthritis, tenosynovitis
Henoch-Schönlein purpura†	Stool guaiac, urinalysis, skin biopsy	Abdominal pain, arthritis; crops of lesions
Mastocytosis (urticaria pigmentosa)†	Skin biopsy—mast cells	Wheal and flare on stroking
Letterer-Siwe disease	Skin biopsy—histiocytes	Distinguish from seborrheic dermatitis
Leukemia cutis/lymphoma	Skin biopsy—atypical leukemic infiltrate	Lymphoma, especially Hodgkin disease, may be pruritic
Neuroblastoma, TORCH infection, leukemia	Skin biopsy	"Blueberry muffin" baby
Vesicles		
Miliaria crystallina		Superficial
Tinea pedis	KOH scraping of vesicle roof—hyphae	
Herpes simplex; herpes zoster	Tzanck preparation—multinucleated giant cells; viral culture to distinguish simplex from zoster	Grouped vesicles on an erythematous base; simplex labialis, progenitalis, whitlow—zoster usually linear and dermatomal
Contact dermatitis	Patch testing	Sharp borders, linear arrays, bizarre patterns, asymmetrical
Varicella		Crops in various stages—macule, papule, vesicle, pustule, and cyst
Coxsackievirus hand, foot, and mouth disease	Throat culture—coxsackievirus A16, 5, and 10	May be recurrent
Flea bites		Treat pet
Bullae		
Bullous disease of childhood	Skin biopsy for hematoxylin and eosin (H&E) stain and immunofluorescence	Refer to dermatologist to rule out bullous pemphigoid and dermatitis herpetiformis
Bullous impetigo	Culture blister fluid for phage group II *S. aureus*	

†May be edematous.

Table 161-2 Laboratory Studies and Characteristics of Lesions—cont'd

Diagnosis or differential diagnosis	Laboratory studies	Comments
Pustules		
Erythema toxicum neonatorum	Wright stain of pustule—eosinophils	Pustule in center on erythematous macule
Transient neonatal pustular melanosis	Gram stain of pustule—sterile with PMNs	Hyperpigmented macules; superficial desquamation
Candidiasis	KOH smear of scale or pustule—budding yeast and pseudohyphae	
Folliculitis	Gram stain—staphylococcal or sterile	Follicular, i.e., hair shaft central in pustule; pseudomonas causes hot tub follicuitus
Plaques		
Psoriasis		Well-demarcated erythematous plaque with adherent scale; check family history, arthritis
Acute urticaria	Eosinophil count, throat culture for streptococci, HB_5AG	Erythematous, edematous plaque, drug history, food history (shellfish)
Nummular eczema		Papules and vesicles grouped into plaques

162 Recurrent Infections

John H. Dossett

The notion of frequently recurring infection implies that the child is having infections with such frequency and severity as to be perceived as having more infections than a generally healthy child should. Such a notion necessarily is related to the parents' concept of normal and of the acceptable number of infections in children. The prevalence of a truly unusual number of serious infections among children actually is quite low; however, children whose parents perceive them as having an unusual number of infections are seen often in pediatric practice—so much so that they make up a major part of the practice of consultants in immunology and infectious disease.

Generally healthy children may be expected to have 6 to 10 separate respiratory virus infections in a year. This especially is true where prolonged exposure to large numbers of children occurs in places such as day care centers, nursery schools, and regular schools. A series of new and unrelated respiratory viral infections interspersed among two or three bacterial complications of respiratory virus infections (e.g., otitis media) will make a child appear to be "sick all the time."

Moreover, many children have frequent recurrences of rhinitis and cough and appear to be infected but actually have respiratory allergy in addition to the usual number of respiratory virus infections, making them appear to be "infected all the time." Other children, commonly labeled as having recurrent infections, are those whose skin is colonized by a virulent strain of *Staphylococcus,* resulting in recurrent episodes of folliculitis or furunculosis.

DEFINITION

Any concise definition of recurrent infection is necessarily arbitrary and very likely to be either too general or too restrictive. Rather than define by some arbitrary criteria whether a child has recurrent infections, the physician more appropriately should determine whether the child generally is well and whether some specific condition can be identified and treated.

Recurrent infection traditionally has been viewed as the hallmark of persons who have deficiencies in host defense, such as hypogammaglobulinemia, leukocyte-killing defects, or thymic hypoplasia syndromes. However, children who have frequent pneumonia secondary to asthma or cystic fibrosis and those who have frequent otitis media are much more prevalent than children who have immunodeficiency syndromes. Children who generally are well despite frequent symptoms of infection usually will be thriving, as manifested by normal growth and development. Their infections usually are less severe and generally are limited to the skin and upper respiratory tract. Most often such children have not been hospitalized or were hospitalized only briefly for uncomplicated illnesses.

DIFFERENTIAL DIAGNOSIS

In sorting out the causes of recurrent infection, the physician first should establish whether the child's infections are usual and associated with generally good health or whether the infections herald some underlying illness that requires a systematic laboratory evaluation. Careful history-taking is of utmost importance in that it provides the information with which one decides whether to pursue laboratory evaluation (see the box on p. 1091). It also will determine the direction of the laboratory investigation to be undertaken, if one is indicated.

The Generally Well Child

Because the parents of generally well children (*category A* in the box, p. 1091) usually have concluded already that their child is "sick all the time," recording the actual dates and duration of each episode becomes necessary. Most often this demonstrates significant intervals during which the child is well. Moreover, specific episodes of illness frequently can be related temporally to similar illness in other family members. In general, those *children whose recurrent infections are limited to the upper respiratory tract, who have intervals of distinct wellness, and who are growing normally do not need a laboratory evaluation of possible immunodeficiency syndromes.* Children who have frequent recurrences of otitis media may need chronic prophylaxis throughout the respiratory virus season, namely, November to April (see Chapter 240, Otitis Media and Otitis Externa). However, unless they have other manifestations of chronic illness, they do not merit an extensive laboratory evaluation.

The important diagnosis of *general wellness* should be an early *primary diagnosis* based on a detailed history, growth records, physical examination, and chest roentgenogram, rather than a delayed diagnosis of exclusion, which one stumbles upon after multiple normal laboratory test results. An astute and sympathetic physician can reassure parents that their child generally is well, even when there have been multiple episodes of respiratory infection or otitis media.

The Generally Unwell Child

When the detailed history (including family history), physical examination, and chest roentgenogram suggest that the child is not generally well (*category B* in the preceding box), the best investigation is that which follows the clues. Clearly, the signs and symptoms listed in category B are not very specific. Most of them may be found in dozens of specific diseases that are associated with recurrent infections. In fact, chronic or recurrent respiratory tract infections are seen in almost every disease that predisposes to recurrent infection. Because of the tremendous overlap in clinical manifestations, one must play the odds as well as follow the clues. Although all the diseases discussed below may seem very similar, *asthma and cystic fibrosis are much more common*

EVALUATION OF CHILDREN WHO HAVE RECURRENT INFECTIONS

Category A: generally well child*

1. Normal growth and development
2. Usual illness with common viruses
3. Infections usually of skin and upper respiratory tract, such as furunculosis, otitis media, and rhinitis
4. Infection usually with common pathogens such as respiratory viruses, *Staphylococcus,* and *Streptococcus*
5. Periods of complete wellness
6. Chest roentgenogram usually normal
7. Palpable lymph nodes and normal-to-enlarged tonsils

Category B: child who has specific signs and symptoms that may indicate immunodeficiency or another chronic illness†

1. Failure to thrive
2. Severe disease with common viruses such as chickenpox and measles
3. More than one *serious infection,* such as meningitis, pneumonia, bone and joint infection, or bacteremia
4. May be infected with organisms that usually are of low virulence in the normal host (e.g., *Serratia, Klebsiella, Pseudomonas, Proteus*)
5. Few periods when child is completely well
6. Chest roentgenogram usually abnormal
7. Physical signs such as the following:
   a. Rales or wheezing
   b. Chronic eczema and alopecia
   c. Small tonsils and nonpalpable lymph nodes
   d. Chronic blepharitis
   e. Opacified sinuses
   f. Clubbing of fingers
   g. Nasal polyps
   h. Chronic mucopurulent nasal or postnasal drainage
8. Chronic diarrhea or stools characteristic of malabsorption
9. Frequent fever

*Children in this category usually need to have their acute infections (e.g., otitis media) treated and their *parents reassured* that generally they are well. Drawing specific attention to each of the items of information that caused them to be put in this category is very comforting to most parents.
†Any one of the items in this category may indicate a need for systematic laboratory evaluation that is specifically designed to *follow the clues.* It is painful, expensive, and reckless to try to rule out every possibility in the differential diagnosis with a "laboratory shotgun" approach.

than are agammaglobulinemia or alpha-1-antitrypsin deficiency.

In the decade of the 1990s, infants and children who have human immunodeficiency virus (HIV) infection and acquired immunodeficiency syndrome (AIDS) have become increasingly prevalent among those who have chronic and recurrent infections. HIV infection should be in the differential diagnosis of every child who has manifestations in category B.

Recurrent Pneumonia or Abnormal Chest Roentgenogram. The box on the right lists chronic diseases that may be associated with recurrent pneumonia. *The most common cause of recurrent lower respiratory tract infection is respiratory allergy.* This diagnosis is easy to make when the child has obvious, frequent asthma attacks; however, many children who have bronchospastic disease have never had severe wheezing, and one depends on the family history or a history of mild, exercise-induced wheezing to find a clue. Careful questioning usually elicits a history of wheezing. Review of all medical records may reveal that another physician has heard wheezing on auscultation or a previous roentgenogram has shown air trapping. The diagnosis usually is supported by an elevated serum IgE level, and the recurrent infections are controlled by the administration of adrenergics.

HIV infection and AIDS are seen primarily among children born to women who are drug users, who are sexual partners of drug users, or who have multiple sexual partners. Even so, HIV testing should be done on any child who has only

CHRONIC DISEASES ASSOCIATED WITH RECURRENT PNEUMONIA

1. Asthma
   a. Overt wheezing
   b. Subacute bronchospasm with atelectasis
2. Aspiration
   a. Tracheoesophageal fistula
   b. Gastroesophageal reflux
3. Cystic fibrosis
4. Alpha-1-antitrypsin deficiency
5. Immunodeficiency syndromes
   a. HIV infection
   b. Hypogammaglobulinemia
   c. Leukocyte defects
   d. Complement deficiencies
   e. Cellular immunodeficiency
6. Immotile cilia syndrome
7. Bronchopulmonary dysplasia of prematurity
8. Anatomical malformations
9. Bronchiectasis resulting from pneumonia of measles, *Bordetella pertussis,* or *H. influenzae*

IMMUNODEFICIENCY SYNDROMES

Humoral-mediated immunodeficiency
Antibody deficiency syndromes

Transient hypogammaglobulinemia of infancy
X-linked infantile hypogammaglobulinemia
Common variable immunodeficiency or acquired hypogammaglobulinemia
Isolated IgA deficiency
Isolated IgM deficiency
Antibody deficiency with normal immunoglobulins
Miscellaneous dysgammaglobulinemias

Leukocyte deficiency syndromes

Decreased number of leukocytes
- Marrow toxicity
- Immune injury to marrow
- Myelothisic suppression of marrow
- Familial hypoplasia

Defective leukocyte function
- Chronic granulomatous disease
- Chédiak-Higashi disease
- Lazy leukocyte syndrome

Humoral-mediated immunodeficiency—cont'd
Complement deficiency syndromes

Isolated C3 deficiency
Isolated C5 deficiency
C2 and C4 deficiencies

Cell-mediated immunodeficiency

Congenital thymic hypoplasia (DiGeorge syndrome)
Chronic mucocutaneous candidiasis

Mixed B and T cell immunodeficiency

HIV infection
Severe combined immunodeficiency
Wiskott-Aldrich syndrome
Immunodeficiency with ataxia-telangiectasia
Immunodeficiency with thymoma
Immunodeficiency with short-limbed dwarfism
Cellular immune deficiency with abnormal immunoglobulin synthesis (Nezelof syndrome)

the slightest indication because many mothers who have HIV infection do not know that they are infected. Just as in a previous era when tuberculosis was a major scourge, a sick infant commonly is the first clue that the family harbors HIV (see Chapter 180, Acquired Immunodeficiency Syndrome (AIDS) and Human Immunodeficiency Virus (HIV) Infection).

Aspiration pneumonia is seen primarily in children who have some form of neurological impairment. Neurologically, children who aspirate chronically are similar to those alcoholics who vomit and aspirate while drunk—that is, who temporarily are impaired neurologically. Although *gastroesophageal reflux* is quite common, aspiration rarely occurs without accompanying neurological impairment. Babies who have congenital *tracheoesophageal fistulas* usually start having recurrent pneumonia very early in life and typically cough with feeding.

Cystic fibrosis may be mild or severe and may involve primarily the respiratory tract or the gastrointestinal tract. It is more common than most of the other causes of recurrent pneumonia; consequently, the sweat chloride test should be done early and on minimal provocation.

Alpha-1-antitrypsin deficiency most often is associated with hepatic cirrhosis; however, it sometimes is associated with emphysema and chronic lung disease.

All of the *immunodeficiency syndromes* (hypogammaglobulinemia, leukocyte defects, complement deficiencies, and cellular immunodeficiencies) are likely to result in recurrent pneumonia. In fact, of all the possible sites for infection in the immune-deficient host, the respiratory tract is the most common.

Immotile cilia syndrome manifests commonly as sinusitis, bronchiectasis, and situs inversus (Kartagener syndrome). Children so affected have a heritable (autosomal recessive) defect of the myofibrils that are responsible for mucociliary motion. The diagnosis is made by nasal biopsy. Motility is assessed by light microscopy and structural abnormalities by electron microscopy.

Bronchopulmonary dysplasia is a form of chronic lung disease often seen in children who have had intensive respiratory support in the neonatal period. The cause is not determined; however, most such children were born prematurely having hyaline membrane disease requiring oxygen therapy and mechanical ventilation. In the first 2 or so years of life they often manifest severe respiratory distress when infected with common respiratory viruses.

Anatomical malformations, such as congenital anomalies of the bronchial tree and anomalous blood supply to one or more segments of lung (e.g., sequestered lobe), may result in recurrent pneumonia. *Mediastinal tumors* or *enlarged lymph nodes* may compress a bronchus, resulting in atelectasis or recurrent pneumonia. *Foreign bodies* within the bronchial tree usually result in recurrent pneumonia.

Some infectious agents can cause such severe damage to the bronchi that children may recover from an acute infection only to be left with *chronic bronchiectasis.* This is seen most often following infections with measles virus, *B. pertussis,* or *H. influenzae* type b.

Recurrent Skin Infections. Recurrent furuncles occur quite commonly and are a source of significant discomfort and embarrassment. They are rarely, however, a manifestation of subnormal host defenses. Most often such patients simply are colonized with especially virulent strains of staphylococci that cause recurrent infection of the skin and subcutaneous tissues. Such patients do not need laboratory evaluation; they require only a short course of antistaphylococcal antibiotics and daily baths with a povidone-iodine scrub soap for 2 to 3 weeks.

In rare cases, children who have immunodeficiency diseases may have recurrent and chronic skin infections; however, they are associated with other manifestations, such as chronic eczema, alopecia, growth failure, short limbs, and fungal infections of the nails.

Recurrent Otitis Media. Many young children have multiple episodes of otitis media. These usually are children who had their first episode in the first year of life and who eventually may have three to six episodes per year. Most of these children do not have immunodeficiency diseases; rather, abnormal middle ear mucosa and eustachian tube dysfunction generally cause their frequent recurrences. Although otitis media is a major problem among children who have allergies and immunodeficiency, other clues to these diseases should surface before one embarks on a laboratory evaluation. Most children who have recurrent otitis media are served best by being prescribed sulfisoxazole prophylactically through the respiratory virus season.

Multiple Pyogenic Infections. Children who have multiple pyogenic infections, and especially those pyogenic infections caused by bacteria that usually are of low virulence, are more likely to have one of the (rare) immunodeficiency syndromes. The normally functioning host defense system of humoral-mediated immunity requires adequate quantities of normal opsonic antibodies, normal granulocytes, and normal complement components. Deficiencies of opsonic antibodies include the various forms of hypogammaglobulinemia and dysgammaglobulinemia. Granulocyte deficiencies include the various forms of agranulocytosis, intracellular killing defects (chronic granulomatous disease), and the granulocyte migration defects (lazy leukocyte syndrome). Chronic and recurrent infections have been associated with deficiencies of several components of the complement system. Except for deficiencies of IgA and transient hypogammaglobulinemia of infancy, these immunodeficiency syndromes are rare; most of them are listed in the box on p. 1092.

Children who have deficiencies in the system of cell-mediated immunity are likely to have serious infections with viruses and fungi as well as with bacterial disease. The more serious forms are seen at an early age and are likely to be fatal.

To detail the unique characteristics of each immunodeficiency syndrome listed in the preceding box is beyond the scope of this text. However, children who have the signs and symptoms found in category B of the box on p. 1091 may need to be evaluated for immunodeficiency. Screening tests that are readily available are listed in the box above. Whether these tests do or do not establish a presumptive diagnosis, the child will be served best by referral to an immunology or infectious disease consultant who has access to specialized tests for pursuing the diagnosis, who has experience with these rare diseases, and who can provide a diagnosis, genetic counseling, and long-term care for a chronic illness.

LABORATORY SCREENING TESTS FOR IMMUNODEFICIENCY SYNDROMES

1. Antibody deficiency syndromes
   a. Immunoglobulin levels (normal level is age related)
   b. Isohemagglutinin titers
   c. Specific antibody titers (i.e., polio and tetanus)
   d. HIV antibody
2. Leukocyte deficiency syndromes
   a. Granulocyte count (should have 1500 or more granulocytes)
   b. Stained peripheral smear (look at granule size)
   c. Nitroblue tetrazolium (NBT) test
3. Complement deficiency syndromes
   a. Total hemolytic complement
   b. C3 level (radial diffusion kits available)
4. T cell deficiency syndromes
   a. Chest roentgenogram for thymus shadow
   b. Skin test using *Candida* organisms, mumps, SK-SO, and tetanus toxoid
   c. Total lymphocyte count (should have 1500 or more)
   d. HIV antibody

SUGGESTED READINGS

Insel RA: The child with recurrent infections. In Ziai M, editor: *Bedside pediatrics,* Boston, 1983, Little, Brown.

Insel R: Disorders of lymphocyte function. In Hoffman R et al, editors: *Hematology: basic principles and practice,* New York, 1991, Churchill Livingstone.

Johnston RB Jr: Recurrent bacterial infections in children, *N Engl J Med* 310:1237, 1984.

Rubin BK: The evaluation of the child with recurrent chest infections, *Pediatr Infect Dis J* 4:88, 1985.

Stiehm ER, editor: *Immunologic disorders in infants and children,* ed 4 Philadelphia, 1996, WB Saunders.

163 The Red Eye

James W. McManaway III and Carl A. Frankel

The red eye has hyperemia of the bulbar conjunctiva, which occurs with inflammation of the conjunctiva, cornea, episclera, sclera, or anterior uvea. The differential diagnosis of the red eye in childhood includes (1) conjunctivitis, (2) nasolacrimal duct obstruction, (3) keratitis, (4) iritis, and (5) glaucoma. "Pink eye" is a lay term that refers to conjunctivitis.

CONJUNCTIVITIS

Conjunctivitis means inflammation of the conjunctiva, which is characterized by conjunctival hyperemia and discharge that varies from clear to purulent. Because of the close association of the conjunctiva with the eyelids and cornea, many forms of conjunctivitis involve the eyelid and cornea as well. The causes of conjunctivitis in children include (1) allergens, (2) bacteria, (3) viruses, (4) chlamydia, (5) toxins, (6) immunological reactions, and (7) ophthalmia neonatorum. Although most types of conjunctivitis do not present an acute risk to the eye, conjunctivitis should be evaluated promptly so that appropriate intervention can be instituted.

Allergic Conjunctivitis

Allergic conjunctivitis is a noninfectious form of conjunctivitis characterized by itching, conjunctival chemosis (edema), and conjunctival hyperemia. Frequently, tearing also is present. The condition may be unilateral or bilateral and may be asymptomatic. The six types of allergic conjunctivitis are (1) seasonal allergic rhinoconjunctivitis, (2) vernal keratoconjunctivitis, (3) giant papillary conjunctivitis, (4) contact allergic dermatoconjunctivitis, (5) atopic keratoconjunctivitis, and (6) phlyctenular keratoconjunctivitis.[3]

Seasonal Allergic Rhinoconjunctivitis. Seasonal allergic rhinoconjunctivitis, also called hay fever conjunctivitis, is the most common form of allergic conjunctivitis. It is an IgE-mediated immediate hypersensitivity reaction to airborne allergens. During times of high pollen counts, patients have red, itchy, tearing eyes. Minimal ocular signs are present besides conjunctival redness, although patients occasionally may show eyelid edema or increased skin pigmentation called "allergic shiners." Treatment includes avoidance of known allergens and use of artificial tears as necessary. Children who have more severe symptoms can be treated with topical mast cell stabilizers such as lodoxamide tromethamine (Alomide) or cromolyn sodium (Crolom). Children 12 years of age and older can be treated with the topical antihistamine levocabastine hydrochloride (Livostin) or the topical nonsteroidal antiinflammatory agent ketorolac tromethamine (Acular); the safety and efficacy of these drugs have not yet been established in younger children.

Vernal Keratoconjunctivitis. Vernal keratoconjunctivitis is a rare form of allergic conjunctivitis characterized by severe ocular itching, ropy mucus discharge that can be pulled like a string from the conjunctival surface, and giant papillae on the upper tarsal conjunctiva (Fig. 163-1). Gelatinous nodules at the corneoscleral limbus are more common in dark-skinned races. Corneal complications such as limbal neovascularization, central epithelial keratitis, and corneal "shield" ulcer may occur. As the name implies, the allergy is much worse in the spring and early summer. Patients often develop symptoms first between age 10 and 13 years and may be symptomatic each spring for the next 10 or so years. Because of the severity of the symptoms, the frequent need for topical corticosteroids to control symptoms, and the risks of cataracts, glaucoma, and herpes simplex keratitis associated with long-term topical steroid use, these patients should be referred to an ophthalmologist for management. Typical management includes topical corticosteroids, topical mast cell stabilizers such as cromolyn sodium (Crolom) or lodoxamide tromethamine (Alomide), and topical and systemic antihistamines.

Giant Papillary Conjunctivitis. Giant papillary conjunctivitis (GPC) nearly always is associated with contact lens wear and has been reported among patients wearing hard, rigid gas-permeable, and soft contact lenses. Patients initially have conjunctival hyperemia, mucus accumulation, increased awareness of the contact lens, and itching upon removal of the lens. End-stage GPC is characterized by the presence of giant papillae on the upper tarsal conjunctiva, copious mucus production, and contact lens intolerance. GPC is felt to be an allergic reaction to antigen (degraded mucus) coating the contact lens as well as a reaction to mechanical trauma by the lens. These patients should be referred to the eye care professional who dispensed the contact lenses for treatment. Treatment options include stopping contact lens wear, better contact lens hygiene, use of a different contact lens type, and topical cromolyn sodium.

Contact Allergic Conjunctivitis. Contact allergic conjunctivitis is characterized by itching, watery discharge, conjunctival edema, and hyperemia associated with redness and edema of the periorbital skin. Possible sources include topical ophthalmic medications, contact lens solution preservatives, and cosmetics. Environmental sources such as soap or detergents are common; because of the higher incidence of right-handed individuals, the right eye is affected more commonly. A careful history including a list of all medications placed on or near the eyes helps to establish the diagnosis. Treatment consists of withdrawal of all ocular medications and solutions, good hand washing, attempts to discourage hand-eye contact, and use of topical and systemic antihistamines in more bothersome cases. Steroid lotions or ointments can be used for skin lesions but should be used with care to prevent secondary atrophy of the eyelid skin.

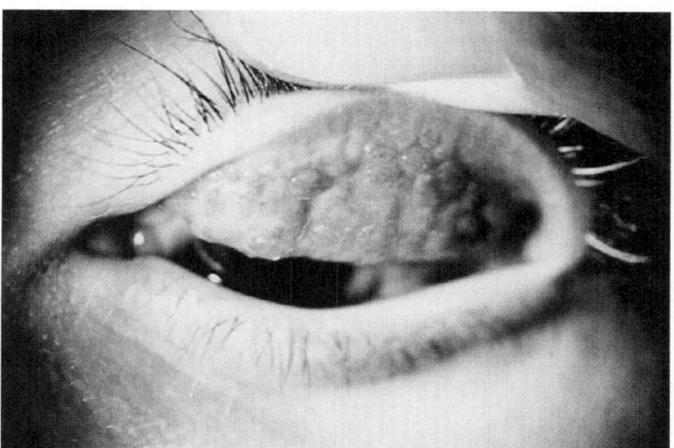

FIG. 163-1 Vernal conjunctivitis with giant papillae on the upper tarsal conjunctiva.

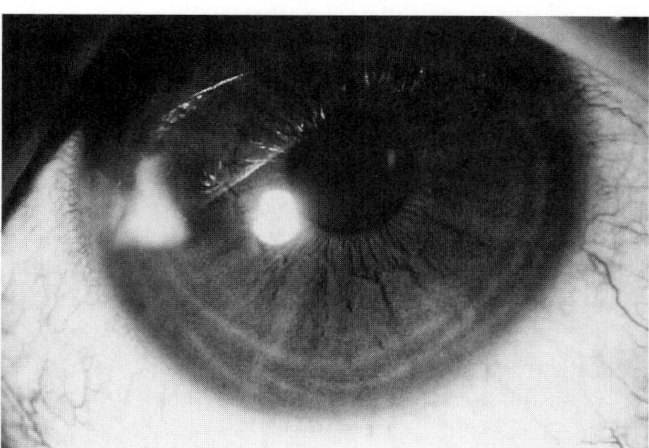

FIG. 163-2 Phlyctenular keratoconjunctivitis with corneal scarring and trailing "leash" of conjunctival vessels.

Atopic Keratoconjunctivitis. Atopic keratoconjunctivitis is a vision-threatening disease that occurs in 25% to 40% of atopic individuals. It occurs most frequently in males around 20 years of age. Patients have extreme itching, copious discharge of mucus, conjunctival hyperemia, and redness, scaling, and maceration of the eyelids and periorbital skin. Conjunctival papillae develop on the upper and the *lower* tarsal conjunctiva; the location of the papillae and the older age of these patients differentiate atopic from vernal keratoconjunctivitis. The eyelid appearance and discharge of mucus distinguish atopic keratoconjunctivitis from seasonal allergic rhinoconjunctivitis. Corneal complications include epithelial keratitis, chronic epithelial defects that can become infected secondarily, and corneal scarring and vascularization. Teenagers who have atopic keratoconjunctivitis are at risk of developing cataracts. Patients who have atopic keratoconjunctivitis should be referred to an ophthalmologist. Management includes short courses of topical corticosteroids, topical cromolyn sodium, oral antihistamines, eyelid hygiene to treat associated blepharitis, and steroid ointments to the eyelid skin.

Phlyctenular Keratoconjunctivitis. Phlyctenular keratoconjunctivitis is characterized by a heavily vascularized, whitish yellow, elevated lesion, usually located near the limbus. Left untreated, the conjunctival phlyctenule advances into the cornea with a trailing leash of vessels (Fig. 163-2). In developing nations, tuberculosis is the most common association; however, in industrialized nations an allergic reaction to the *Staphylococcus* exotoxin is the suspected cause. Treatment with topical steroids is extremely efficacious but should be performed under the care of an ophthalmologist.

Bacterial Conjunctivitis

Patients who have bacterial conjunctivitis often experience tearing, photophobia, and foreign body sensation. The conjunctiva has moderate to severe hyperemia; the conjunctival discharge may be watery to serous initially but becomes mucopurulent with a green to yellow color. The discharge may be mild or so copious that the eyelids may be pasted shut. Eyelid edema and erythema may be worrisome. Typical causative agents include strains of *Staphylococcus, Streptococcus, Pneumococcus,* and *Haemophilus influenzae;* strains of *Pseudomonas, Klebsiella,* and *Neisseria* are encountered less frequently.

Neisseria gonorrhoeae causes a hyperacute conjunctivitis with copious purulent discharge and severe eyelid edema. The examiner should wear eye protection because infected secretions can be expelled forcibly upon attempts to open the swollen eyelids. Gonococcal conjunctivitis is a medical emergency because the organism can invade intact corneal epithelium, resulting in corneal ulceration or perforation with resultant bacterial endophthalmitis. An ophthalmologist should be consulted immediately.

Bacterial conjunctivitis generally is diagnosed on clinical grounds alone. Because most bacterial conjunctivitis responds readily to topical antibiotics, cultures and sensitivity determinations usually are not necessary unless *Pseudomonas, Neisseria,* or another particularly virulent organism is suspected. Treatment with ophthalmic solutions is easier than with ophthalmic ointments, and the response frequently is dramatic. Sodium sulfacetamide (10% solution) is useful in most cases, although polymyxin B sulfate-trimethoprim sulfate solution (Polytrim) has a broader spectrum and is well tolerated. Because of the small volume of the conjunctival cul-de-sac, only one drop is needed. Gentamycin and tobramycin should be reserved for suspected gram negative bacterial conjunctivitis and for cases in which culture and sensitivity results justify their use. Treatment should be continued for 24 to 48 hours after the conjunctival hyperemia and purulence have subsided.

Gonococcal conjunctivitis should be treated with a single intramuscular dose of ceftriaxone (1 g or 50 mg/kg in patients weighing less than 20 kg).[2] If keratitis is present, saline lavage and topical erythromycin ointment four times daily should be added. The patients also should be evaluated for chlamydial conjunctivitis and other sexually transmitted diseases such as syphilis and AIDS.

Viral Conjunctivitis

Three major causes of viral conjunctivitis exist: adenovirus, herpes simplex virus, and varicella-zoster virus. Adenoviral infections are the most common and have two types, epi-

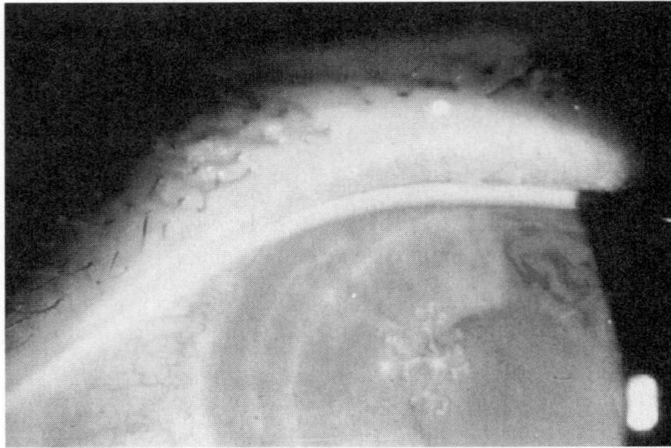

FIG. 163-3 Typical herpes simplex virus dendrites stained with fluorescein and viewed with a cobalt blue light.

demic keratoconjunctivitis and pharyngoconjunctival fever. Epidemic keratoconjunctivitis (EKC) is caused by adenovirus types 8, 19A, and 37. Transmission occurs through respiratory tract to eye and finger to eye pathways, as well as by contaminated swimming pools. Affected patients have moderate conjunctival hyperemia, watery discharge, photophobia, and a tender preauricular node. Treatment consists of artificial tears to lubricate the eyes and isolation of the patient to prevent further outbreaks. Some patients develop inflammatory membranes and keratitis; these should be treated with topical steroid drops by an ophthalmologist. Pharyngoconjunctival fever is caused by adenovirus types 3, 4, and 7. These patients have similar ocular signs but also have pharyngitis, fever, and malaise.

Herpes Simplex Virus. Herpes simplex virus can cause a host of ocular problems and is associated with disseminated encephalitis in infants. A primary herpetic ocular infection typically manifests as a unilateral conjunctivitis with watery discharge and photophobia several days to 2 weeks following close personal contact. Patients frequently have eyelid vesicles and a tender preauricular node. Some patients have an epithelial keratitis, which may be punctate, or may show a classical dendrite (Fig. 163-3) after application of fluorescein dye when the eye is viewed with a cobalt blue light source. The initial infection is self-limited, but the virus remains latent in the cornea and trigeminal ganglion and can recur. The recurrences are characterized by corneal involvement and lead to corneal scarring, vascularization, and decreased vision. Amblyopia is a common problem in young children who have recurrent herpes simplex keratitis. Children who have conjunctivitis and lid vesicles or corneal staining with fluorescein dye should be referred to an ophthalmologist for further evaluation.

Varicella-Zoster Virus. Immunocompromised children may have reactivation of a previous varicella infection in the distribution of the ophthalmic division of the trigeminal nerve; this is called herpes zoster ophthalmicus (Fig. 163-4). Affected patients can have conjunctivitis, keratitis, uveitis, glaucoma, optic neuritis, and other cranial nerve palsies. The diagnosis is easy when the characteristic skin changes are present, but these do not always precede the ocular signs. Patients who have herpes zoster ophthalmicus should be evaluated by an ophthalmologist immediately.

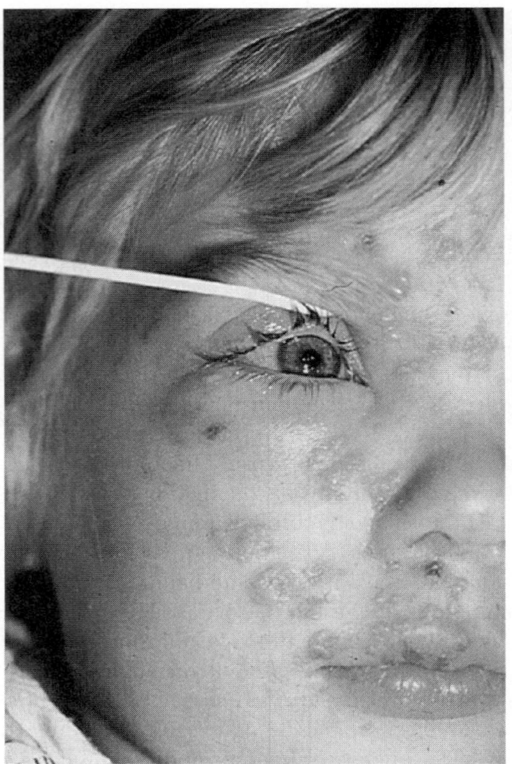

FIG. 163-4 Herpes zoster ophthalmicus in a child.

Chlamydial Conjunctivitis

Chlamydial conjunctivitis is an acute, mucopurulent conjunctivitis often seen in the adolescent population and accompanies sexual promiscuity. Transmission usually is by autoinoculation from genital secretions, although spread through unchlorinated swimming pools occurs rarely. Typically the conjunctivitis begins 4 to 12 days after contact with a new sexual partner. Infected patients have conjunctival hyperemia, tearing, photophobia, mucopurulent discharge, eyelid edema, and a painless preauricular node. The diagnosis is made most readily using direct immunofluorescent antibody testing of conjunctival scrapings. Topical therapy alone is ineffective; it must be combined with systemic antibiotics such as erythromycin (250 mg orally four times daily for 3 weeks). Untreated patients may have a chronic conjunctivitis for up to 18 months. Sexual contacts also must be treated to prevent continued spread to or reinfection from sexual partners.

Toxic Conjunctivitis

Toxic conjunctivitis occurs as a direct (not allergic) effect of some ocular medications and a host of foreign substances that can be splashed, sprayed, aerosolized, or rubbed onto the eye. Toxic conjunctivitis occurs immediately to several hours after contact by the offending substance. Contact allergy generally requires about 2 days for symptoms to develop. Treatment of toxic conjunctivitis includes ocular irrigation and methods to avoid future exposure. Ocular chemical injuries are discussed in Chapter 237, Ocular Trauma.

Immunological Conjunctivitis

Erythema multiforme is an acute systemic disorder thought to be an acute hypersensitivity reaction that occurs after exposure to infectious agents, drugs, or certain foods. Some patients develop a mild skin rash that resolves after several days. Other patients have severe skin and mucous membrane disease with conjunctival involvement; this form is known as Stevens-Johnson syndrome. Patients who have Stevens-Johnson syndrome develop a mucopurulent conjunctivitis that may progress to conjunctival necrosis. The conjunctival damage leads to complications including adhesions between the tarsal and bulbar conjunctiva (symblepharon), eyelid margin changes with inturned lashes (entropion with trichiasis), and a chronic dry eye syndrome due to loss of normal conjunctival function. These problems can lead to corneal scarring and permanent visual loss.

Patients who have Stevens-Johnson syndrome require admission to the hospital and systemic steroids to control the immune complex–mediated vasculitis. Ocular management includes topical ocular steroids and antibiotics to reduce conjunctival inflammation and prevent secondary infection. Conjunctival adhesions must be lysed daily with a glass rod under topical anesthesia. After the acute conjunctivitis resolves, these patients require artificial tears and careful observation for the development of vision-threatening corneal complications.

Ophthalmia Neonatorum

Ophthalmia neonatorum is defined as conjunctivitis occurring in the first month of life. The causes can be (1) chemical, (2) chlamydial, (3) bacterial, and (4) viral. The most common cause of ophthalmia neonatorum is a chemical conjunctivitis from the 1% silver nitrate drops given as prophylaxis for gonococcal or chlamydial conjunctivitis. This conjunctivitis usually is characterized by conjunctival hyperemia, mild lid edema, and scanty discharge. Chemical conjunctivitis usually resolves over 24 to 48 hours without sequelae. Because of the chemical conjunctivitis caused by silver nitrate drops, many hospitals use erythromycin ophthalmic ointment, which also prevents most cases of chlamydial ophthalmia neonatorum.

The most common infectious cause of ophthalmia neonatorum is inclusion conjunctivitis caused by *Chlamydia trachomatis*. Inclusion conjunctivitis usually is characterized by a mucoid or mucopurulent discharge and mild lid edema with conjunctival hyperemia. Bacterial ophthalmia neonatorum usually is caused by *Neisseria, Staphylococcus, Pneumococcus,* or *H. influenzae* organisms. The bacterial conjunctivitis is characterized by a moderate or profuse purulent discharge with significant conjunctival hyperemia (Fig. 163-5); eyelid edema also may be severe. Viral ophthalmia neonatorum caused by herpes simplex virus (Fig. 163-3) also must be considered. Viral ophthalmia neonatorum has mild conjunctival hyperemia with a serous discharge, although the cornea may be hazy if a simultaneous keratitis is present.

Diagnosis is determined by direct immunofluorescent antibody testing for *Chlamydia* organisms and by culture for bacteria and herpes simplex virus. Conjunctival scraping and plating at the bedside recovers the organism superiorly compared with the use of a cotton applicator sent to the microbiology laboratory. Treatment is organism specific, with systemic therapy reserved for herpes simplex virus, *Chlamydia*, or *Neisseria* infections.

As a guide, gram positive organisms usually are well treated with sodium sulfacetamide 10% solution every 4 hours. *Haemophilus* species should be treated with topical polymyxin B sulfate-trimethoprim sulfate solution (Polytrim). Gentamycin or tobramycin should be reserved for gram negative organisms. Inclusion conjunctivitis should be treated with topical and systemic erythromycin (10 mg/kg four times a day) for at least 3 weeks. Herpes simplex keratoconjunctivitis is treated best with idoxuridine (Herplex) or trifluridine (Viroptic) solution topically, under the direction of an ophthalmologist, with appropriate systemic antiviral agents. *Neisseria gonorrhoeae* ophthalmia neonatorum is treated with a single dose of intramuscular ceftriaxone (50 mg/kg).[2] The parents and any sexual partners of either also need to be treated in cases of gonococcal and chlamydial ophthalmia neonatorum.

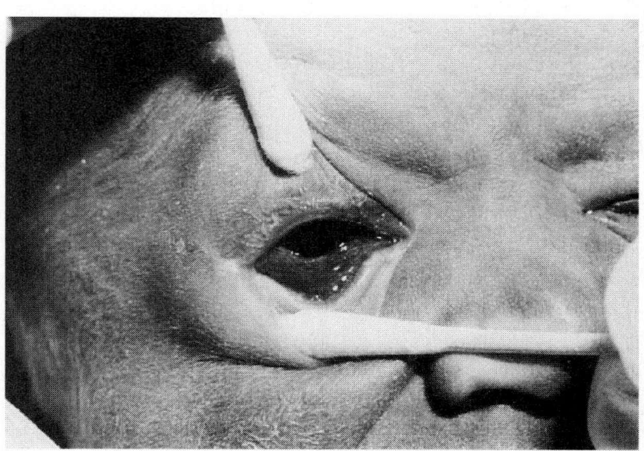

FIG. 163-5 Early bacterial ophthalmia neonatorum that was treated successfully with topical antibiotics.

In the past, the causative agent of ophthalmia neonatorum was predicted based on the time of onset of the conjunctivitis; however, because of the risk of a misdiagnosis, nothing substitutes for appropriate diagnostic evaluation to determine the exact cause. Additionally, the presence of any corneal findings or any uncertainty should prompt consultation with an ophthalmologist.

NASOLACRIMAL DUCT OBSTRUCTION

Nasolacrimal duct obstruction may be present in as many as 6% to 7% of healthy full-term infants (Fig. 163-6). Fortunately, this common condition resolves spontaneously in about 90% of infants by 12 months of age. Occasionally, dacryocystitis (infection in the nasolacrimal sac) (Fig. 163-7) may occur and can progress to preseptal or orbital cellulitis. Treatment of nasolacrimal duct obstruction is varied; ophthalmological opinion is split between early nasolacrimal duct probing and conservative management via nasolacrimal sac massage and topical antibiotics when purulence is present. Nasolacrimal sac massage is performed with five strokes from just beneath the medial aspect of the brow in a downward direction just nasal to the medial canthus and terminating about ¼ inch to ½ inch below the level of the medial canthus. The use solely of downward strokes serves to raise the pressure in the nasolacrimal sac in an attempt to overcome the obstruction usually found at the distal nasolacrimal duct. The success rate with conservative treatment is about 90% by 1 year of age, although nasolacrimal duct probing

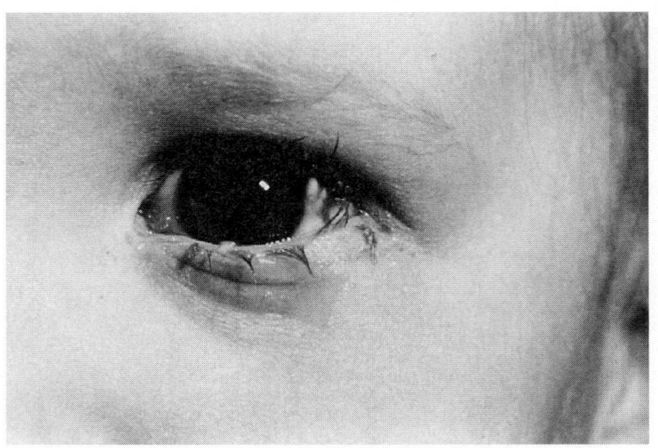

FIG. 163-6 Congenital nasolacrimal duct obstruction. Note the significant discharge, usually accompanied by epiphora. In the absence of conjunctival hyperemia, antibiotic therapy is not indicated and treatment is with nasolacrimal sac massage.

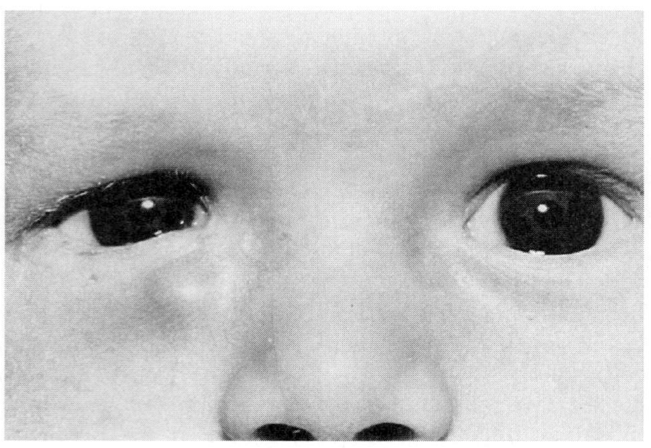

FIG. 163-7 Acute dacryocystitis secondary to nasolacrimal duct obstruction where massage was not performed. Pressure on the tear sac led to mucopurulent reflux from the superior and inferior puncta. Resolution of the dacryocystitis was complete with topical and systemic antibiotics, and nasolacrimal sac massage was successful at overcoming the obstruction.

often is performed early to deal with parental unhappiness with the chronic tearing and accumulation of mucus in the conjunctival sac.[4] Referral to an ophthalmologist is indicated by 6 months of age if the condition persists or earlier if the purulent discharge cannot be controlled by topical antibiotic eye drops.

KERATITIS

Inflammation of the cornea (keratitis) indicates significant ocular disease that needs urgent attention from an ophthalmologist. Because the cornea is relatively avascular, keratitis usually is associated with perilimbal conjunctival hyperemia (ciliary flush), which may simulate conjunctivitis. If the corneal epithelium is damaged, the pain can be quite intense. Otherwise, a mild to moderate foreign body sensation, blepharospasm, and significant tearing are present. Under normal conditions the cornea has a bright luster; however,

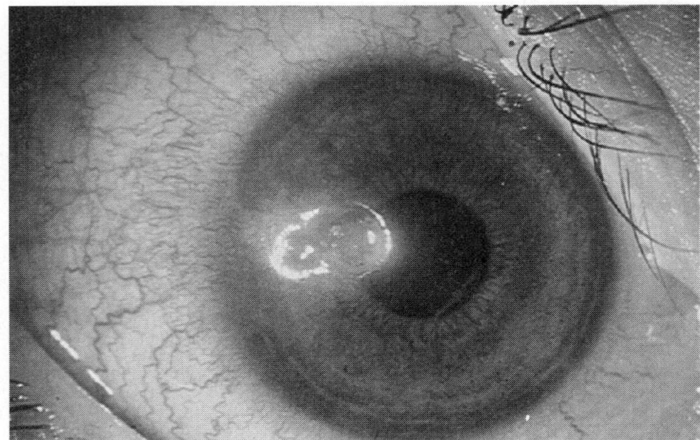

FIG. 163-8 Neurotrophic keratitis in a child who has neurofibromatosis and decreased corneal sensation of the right eye.

when keratitis is present, the cornea often is hazy with a dull corneal light reflex on direct illumination with a penlight. Important forms of keratitis include (1) trauma, such as a corneal abrasion or chemical injury; (2) exposure, such as in patients who have decreased corneal sensation (Fig. 163-8) or a facial nerve palsy; (3) infectious, such as in patients who have bacterial, viral, fungal, or parasitic infections of the cornea; and (4) interstitial, such as in patients who have congenital syphilis who develop symptoms between 5 and 15 years of age. Fluorescein staining can help distinguish herpes simplex virus keratitis from other forms by the characteristic dendrites.

IRITIS

Iritis is an inflammation of the anterior uvea (iris or ciliary body) and can indicate a severe, vision-threatening condition or even the initial manifestation of systemic disease. As in keratitis, the primary symptom frequently is a ciliary flush or generalized conjunctival hyperemia. Blepharospasm, reactive ptosis, photophobia, epiphora, and pupillary miosis (secondary to spasm of the constrictor muscle) are common. Iritis may be either unilateral or bilateral, and the more posterior layers of the eye also may be involved. Untreated iritis can result in glaucoma, cataracts, posterior synechiae (adhesions between the iris and the lens), and blindness. Because of the conjunctival hyperemia and epiphora, a diagnosis of conjunctivitis often is entertained first, and treatment with a topical antibiotic is instituted; however, the lack of a rapid clinical response soon should prompt suspicion. Chronic treatment with an antibiotic may allow the posterior synechiae to become quite advanced (Fig. 163-9); thus any patient who has presumed conjunctivitis that does not readily respond should be referred to an ophthalmologist to rule out iritis. If iritis is diagnosed, systemic disease should be ruled out. Patients who have pauciarticular, antinuclear antibody positive juvenile rheumatoid arthritis can have significant iridocyclitis without the typical conjunctival hyperemia; these patients must be examined by an ophthalmologist via a slit-lamp biomicroscope at the time of diagnosis and every 3 months thereafter for several years.[1] Iritis is treated with mydriatic and cycloplegic agents to reduce the ciliary spasm

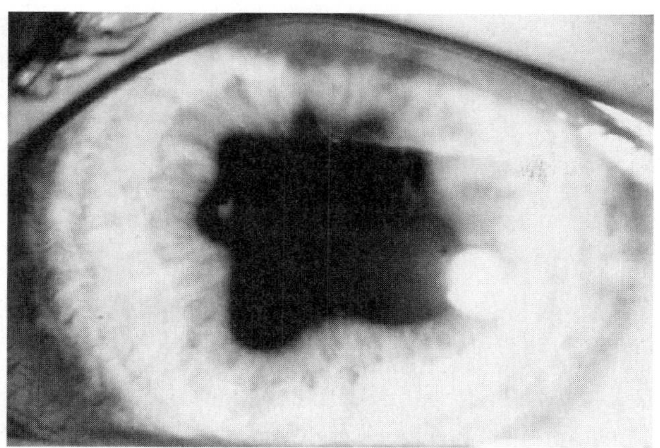

FIG. 163-9 Chronic anterior uveitis treated for 5 months as a chronic "conjunctivitis." Note the irregular pupil caused by posterior synechiae.

and topical steroid agents (under the care of an ophthalmologist) to reduce inflammation and lessen the risk of posterior synechiae.

GLAUCOMA

Infantile or congenital glaucoma usually is diagnosed readily by the presence of corneal enlargement. However, this rare condition sometimes is mistaken for conjunctivitis or nasolacrimal duct obstruction. The symptomatic constellation of tearing, photophobia, fussiness, and failure to thrive with signs of corneal enlargement (buphthalmos) and cloudiness should prompt urgent referral to an ophthalmologist so that the intraocular pressure can be managed (usually by surgery) to minimize loss of vision.

REFERENCES

1. American Academy of Pediatrics Section on Rheumatology and Section on Ophthalmology: Guidelines for ophthalmologic examinations in children with juvenile rheumatoid arthritis, *Pediatrics* 92:295, 1993.
2. Haimovici R, Roussel TJ: Treatment of gonococcal conjunctivitis with single-dose intramuscular ceftriaxone, *Am J Ophthalmol* 107:511, 1989.
3. Jackson WB: Differentiating conjunctivitis of diverse origins, *Surv Ophthalmol* 38(suppl):91, 1993.
4. Kushner BJ: Congenital nasolacrimal system obstruction, *Arch Ophthalmol* 100:597, 1982.

SUGGESTED READINGS

Beauchamp GR, Meisler DM: Disorders of the conjunctiva. In Nelson LB, Calhoun JH, Harley RD, editors: *Pediatric ophthalmology,* ed 3, Philadelphia, 1991, WB Saunders.

Calhoun JH: Disorders of the lacrimal apparatus in infancy and childhood. In Nelson LB, Calhoun JH, Harley RD, editors: *Pediatric ophthalmology,* ed 3, Philadelphia, 1991, WB Saunders.

Day S: Lacrimal system. In Taylor D, editor: *Pediatric ophthalmology,* Boston, 1990, Blackwell Scientific.

Day S: Uveal tract. In Taylor D, editor: *Pediatric ophthalmology,* Boston, 1990, Blackwell Scientific Publications.

Friedlaender MH: Conjunctivitis of allergic origin: clinical presentation and differential diagnosis, *Surv Ophthalmol* 38(suppl):105, 1993.

Giles CL: Uveitis in children. In Nelson LB, Calhoun JH, Harley RD, editors: *Pediatric ophthalmology,* ed 3, Philadelphia, 1991, WB Saunders.

Good W, Hoyt C: Corneal abnormalities in childhood. In Taylor D, editor: *Pediatric ophthalmology,* Boston, 1990, Blackwell Scientific.

Hoyt C, Lambert S: Childhood glaucoma. In Taylor D, editor: *Pediatric ophthalmology,* Boston, 1990, Blackwell Scientific.

Jackson WB: Differentiating conjunctivitis of diverse origins, *Surv Ophthalmol* 38(suppl):91, 1993.

Laibson PR, Waring GO: Diseases of the cornea. In Nelson LB, Calhoun JH, Harley RD, editors: *Pediatric ophthalmology,* ed 3, Philadelphia, 1991, WB Saunders.

Lambert S, Hoyt C: Ophthalmia neonatorum. In Taylor D, editor: *Pediatric ophthalmology,* Boston, 1990, Blackwell Scientific.

Taylor D: External eye diseases. In Taylor D, editor: *Pediatric ophthalmology,* Boston, 1990, Blackwell Scientific.

Walton DS: Glaucoma in infants in children. In Nelson LB, Calhoun JH, Harley RD, editors: *Pediatric ophthalmology,* ed 3, Philadelphia, 1991, WB Saunders.

164 Scrotal Swelling

Mark F. Bellinger

The nature of the scrotal contents makes the differential diagnosis of scrotal swelling challenging. Swelling may be acute or chronic, congenital or infectious, traumatic or neoplastic. The source of the swelling may be the scrotal wall, the testis, its adnexa, or the cord structures (see the box on p. 1101). Differential diagnosis requires an appreciation of both anatomy and embryology of the scrotal contents.

The testis develops in the retroperitoneal space at the level of the internal inguinal ring. Descent through the inguinal canal occurs late in the third trimester of gestation and is complete within the first year of life.[1] As the testis descends, the spermatic cord becomes elongated so that the testis hangs on a pedicle containing its neurovascular supply and the vas deferens (Fig. 164-1). The tongue of peritoneum, which elongates to follow the testis into the scrotum (the processus vaginalis), forms a serous lubricating surface over most of the testis. The neck of the processus vaginalis normally pinches off during development, isolating the tunica vaginalis from the peritoneal cavity (Fig. 164-2, *A;* see Fig. 164-4). The posterior testis and epididymis, excluded from the processus vaginalis, normally are attached to the scrotal wall, making torsion of the cord impossible. The testis and epididymis frequently exhibit small appendages (appendix testis and epididymis) that are developmental remnants of embryonic ductal systems (Fig. 164-3). The testis and its adnexal structures are contained within the scrotum, a sac of smooth muscle capable of considerable contraction, whose rugated skin bears hair and sebaceous glands.

EVALUATION OF THE CHILD WHO HAS SCROTAL SWELLING

Determining both the onset and duration of scrotal swelling is important. A history of urinary symptoms, urethral instrumentation, urological anomalies, or urological surgery can indicate a predisposition to urinary infection and epididymitis. Because of the embryonic origin of the testis, pain from scrotal disease may be referred to the lower abdomen; conversely, pain of renal origin may be referred to the scrotal skin. Therefore all children who have abdominal or scrotal complaints must have a complete abdominal and genital examination. Genital examination may be anxiety provoking and embarrassing, especially for teenagers. Younger boys generally are more comfortable having their parents present; teenage boys may prefer to be alone with a male physician. Examining the patient in both the upright and supine positions may facilitate differential diagnosis. Inspection of the scrotum is important and may help to determine whether the process is unilateral or bilateral. With painful unilateral lesions the patient may be put at ease by examination of the normal hemiscrotum first. Palpation may distinguish lesions of the scrotal wall from those of the spermatic cord. Testicular masses must be differentiated from adnexal or paratesticular spermatic cord lesions. Transillumination may help to differentiate cystic from solid lesions.

In certain clinical settings, laboratory testing may influence differential diagnosis. The urinalysis and white blood cell count (WBC) may be abnormal in infectious processes. Scrotal ultrasound may provide information about the nature of mass lesions. Color Doppler ultrasound[15] and nuclear scans[8,14] aid in evaluating blood flow to the testis in acute scrotal conditions and are most helpful in ruling out torsion of the spermatic cord. In addition, color flow Doppler may assist differential diagnosis by displaying intrascrotal anatomy.

NEONATAL INTRASCROTAL MASSES

In the newborn infant, a firm upper scrotal mass most likely is the result of an extravaginal torsion of the spermatic cord that has occurred before birth. Salvage of these testes is almost unheard of, and surgery is not indicated in most cases.[4] However, if a mass develops acutely after birth, prompt surgical exploration is appropriate. The role of prophylactic contralateral testicular fixation remains the subject of debate.[3] Testicular *tumors* in neonates are rare. *Hydroceles* are common, frequently imparting a bluish translucency to the scrotal skin; moreover, hydroceles transilluminate easily. The testis is normal, but may be difficult to palpate if the hydrocele is tense. Infantile hydroceles usually resolve spontaneously over a period of months.

ACUTE, PAINFUL SCROTAL SWELLING

The acute onset of scrotal pain is a *pediatric urological emergency.* Any process causing acute inflammation may produce massive scrotal swelling and exquisite pain rapidly, making differential diagnosis difficult.

Torsion of the Spermatic Cord

Torsion of the spermatic cord is the most important diagnosis to exclude when acute scrotal swelling occurs. Because the testis hangs at the end of a narrow vascular pedicle, ischemic necrosis occurs quickly in the absence of collateral blood supply. Salvage of endocrine function requires detorsion within 4 to 8 hours, and oligospermia or aspermia may result after only short periods of ischemia.[2] Torsion may occur at any age but is most common between 6 and 12 years. Severe unilateral scrotal pain of sudden onset is most commonly encountered. Frequently, a history of episodes of acute scrotal pain can be elicited (intermittent torsion with spontaneous detorsion). Vomiting is common, but fever is unusual. Although torsion may be triggered by trauma or athletic activity, many boys are awakened from sleep by pain. Inspec-

CAUSES OF SCROTAL SWELLING

Acute, painful scrotal swelling

- Torsion of spermatic cord
- Torsion of appendix, testis, epididymis
- Acute epididymitis, orchitis
- Mumps orchitis
- Henoch-Schönlein purpura
- Trauma
- Insect bite
- Thrombosis of spermatic vein
- Fat necrosis
- Hernia
- Folliculitis
- Dermatitis

Acute, painless scrotal swelling

- Tumor
- Idiopathic scrotal edema
- Hydrocele
- Henoch-Schönlein purpura
- Hernia

Chronic scrotal swelling

- Hydrocele
- Hernia
- Varicocele
- Spermatocele
- Sebaceous cyst
- Tumor

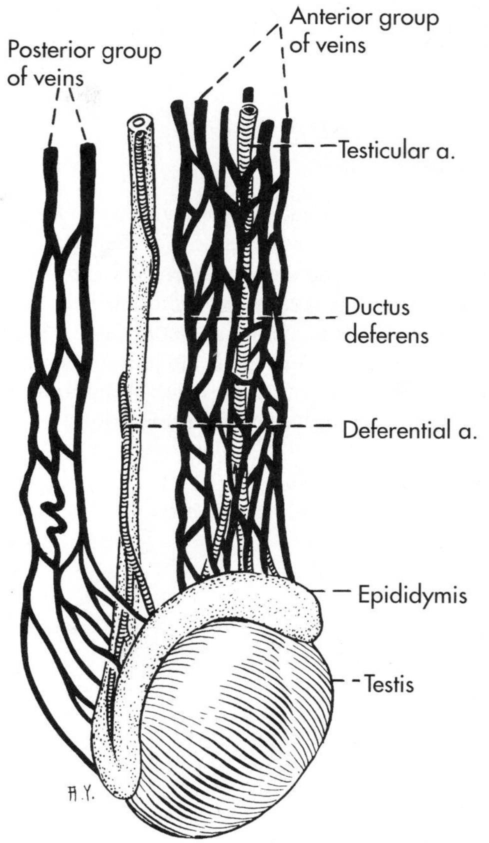

FIG. 164-1 Structure of the spermatic cord.
(From Hollinshead WH, Rosse C: *Textbook of anatomy*, New York, ed 4, 1985, Harper & Row.)

tion of the scrotum may reveal an immobile testis located high in the scrotum. This is the result of shortening of the cord as it twists (up to 720 degrees). The contralateral testis should be examined for a transverse axis, presumptive evidence of abnormal fixation ("bell-clapper" deformity) (see Fig. 164-2, *B*). The cremasteric reflex may be absent in the presence of cord torsion but can be elicited in all other causes of acute scrotal swelling.[18] Scrotal skin over the involved testis may be reddened and taut with loss of normal rugations. Transillumination usually is absent, although an acute, tense hydrocele may form. The scrotum is acutely tender, often making adequate examination difficult. Laboratory examination may reveal a slightly elevated white blood cell count and normal urinalysis.

Torsion of Testicular or Epididymal Appendages

Torsion of testicular or epididymal appendages (see Fig. 164-3) may produce acute scrotal pain whose onset is indistinguishable from that of torsion of the cord. The peak age of presentation is approximately 10 years.[22] Soon after torsion, examination is relatively normal with the exception of exquisite tenderness localized at the anterosuperior surface of the testis, where the twisted appendage may be palpable as a tender mass. The black, necrotic appendage may be visible through the skin of light-skinned children, appearing as a "blue dot."[7] Testicular mobility is normal. When this en-

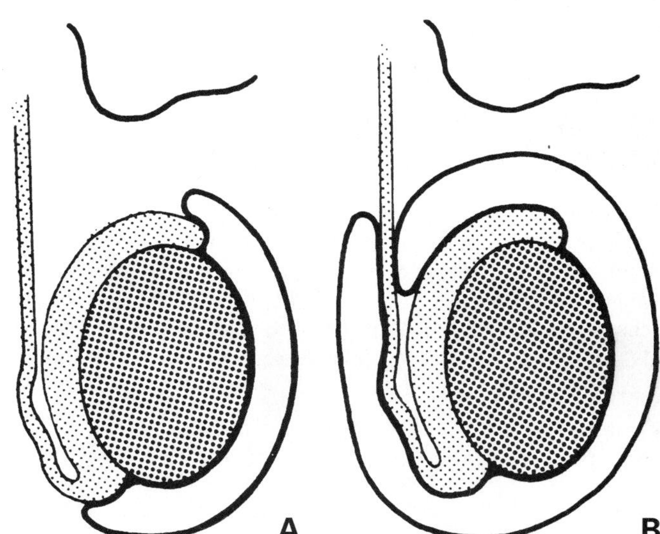

FIG. 164-2 ***A,*** Normal configuration of the tunica vaginalis. ***B,*** Bell-clapper configuration of the tunica vaginalis.
(From Gonzalez R: *J Urol* 116:673, 1976.)

tity is encountered at a later age, skin fixation, reactive hydrocele, and massive scrotal edema make it indistinguishable from torsion of the spermatic cord. Radionuclide scan or color flow Doppler examination will reveal normal or increased blood flow to the testis.[8,14,15]

Acute Epididymitis

Acute epididymitis is relatively uncommon in younger children and may indicate the presence of congenital or acquired lower urinary tract anomalies (ectopic ureter, urethral valves, urethral stricture). All young boys should have radiological investigation, including renal ultrasound and contrast voiding cystourethrography after the acute episode has resolved.[21] A history of sexual activity, dysuria, or urethral discharge should be sought in the older child and adolescent. The onset of pain and swelling usually is less acute than seen with torsion, but the two may be difficult to distinguish on the basis of history alone. Pain and swelling usually are accompanied by fever, usually 102° F (38.9° C) or greater. Dysuria may be present and may antedate other symptoms. Early examination may reveal a normal testis with posterior epididymal tenderness. Later, the epididymis and testis swell into a globular mass as scrotal swelling obliterates all landmarks. The cremasteric reflex usually is present.[18] Passive elevation of the testis may relieve pain (Prehn sign). Rectal examination may indicate prostatic tenderness or result in the expression of a urethral discharge, which should be examined microscopically and cultured for gonorrheal or other organisms. Urinalysis may reveal infection, but results of the microscopic examination and culture are not infrequently normal in adolescents who have epididymitis. The white blood cell count usually is elevated.

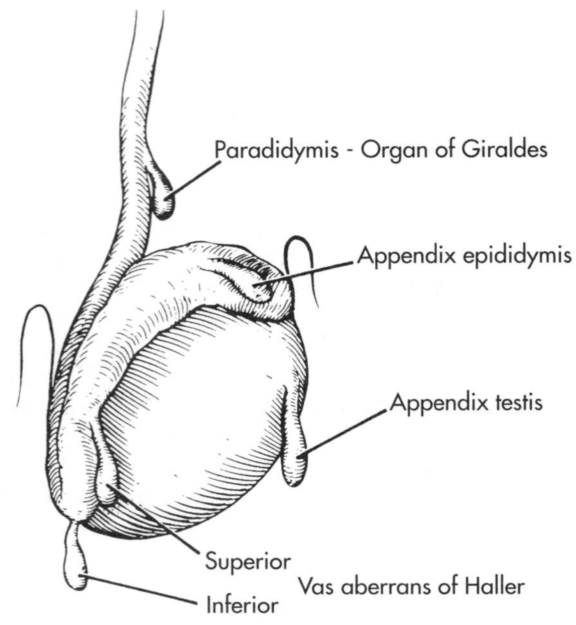

FIG. 164-3 Testicular appendages.
(From Cromie WJ: *Urol Clin North Am* 5:237, 1978.)

MANAGEMENT OF ACUTE CONDITIONS OF THE SCROTUM

Management of acute conditions of the scrotum should be based on the concept that all cases represent torsion of the spermatic cord until proved otherwise. Hence, urological consultation should be obtained while the patient is prepared for immediate surgery. If torsion of the cord cannot be ruled out definitively, scrotal exploration must be undertaken immediately.[5] Manual detorsion of the testis frequently is possible, resulting in immediate relief of pain and resolution of physical findings as blood flow is restored to the testis.[11] Although manual detorsion can provide evidence of blood flow to the testis, surgical exploration is mandatory to confirm complete detorsion of the cord, to fixate the testis, and to perform contralateral testicular fixation, since the opposite testis invariably has the same abnormal anatomy and thus is at risk for asynchronous torsion. If a testis is found to be even marginally viable, it usually is left in situ, although recent evidence of possible immunological damage to the contralateral testis has rendered this practice controversial.[17] If torsion of the spermatic cord seems to be an unlikely diagnosis, confirma-

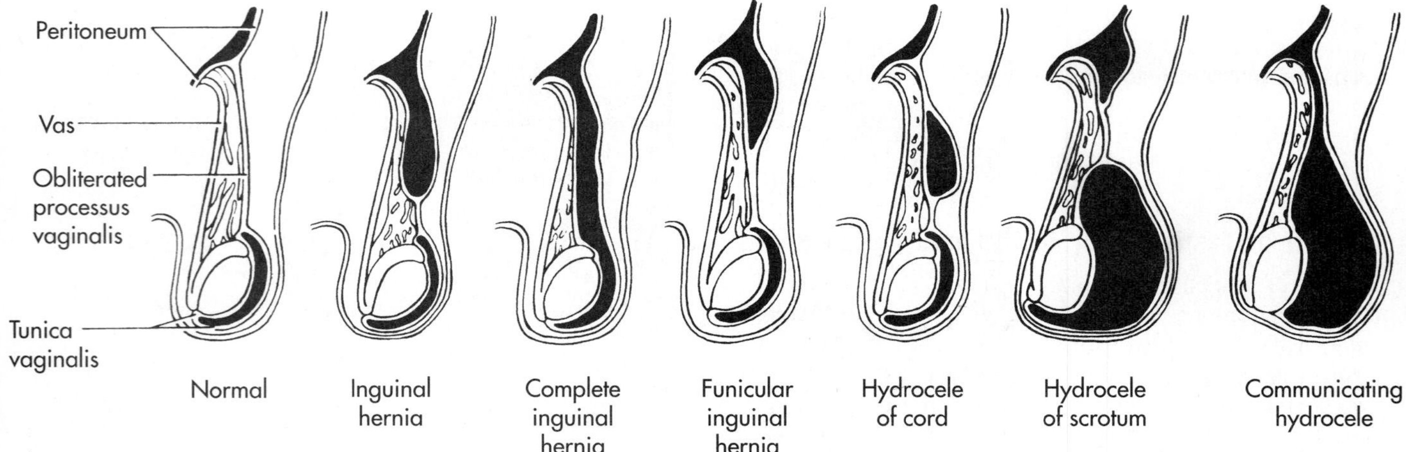

FIG. 164-4 Abnormalities of the processus vaginalis.
(From Woolley MM: Inguinal hernia. In Ravitch MM et al, editors: *Pediatric surgery,* vol 2, ed 3, Chicago, 1979, Mosby.)

tion should be made by either nuclear scan[8,14] or color flow Doppler ultrasound.[15] Bedside Doppler examination, originally considered to be a reliable indicator of testicular blood flow, has proved to be unreliable and should no longer be employed in the differential diagnosis.

Torsion of a testicular or epididymal appendage may be treated conservatively when the diagnosis is certain, but many children undergo excision of the infarcted appendix because the diagnosis is uncertain or pain is severe or persistent.

If epididymitis is diagnosed, cultures should be taken, scrotal elevation instituted, and antibiotic therapy begun. Severe cases may require hospitalization and parenteral antibiotics. Follow-up radiological examination should be performed.[21]

Rare Causes of Acute, Painful Scrotal Swelling

Acute, painful scrotal swelling may be caused by mumps orchitis,[19] Henoch-Schönlein purpura,[23] insect bites, or scrotal trauma. *Mumps orchitis* occurs commonly in adolescence but is rare in younger boys.[19] Acute orchitis or epididymitis usually occurs within a week after parotitis and rarely occurs in isolation. Clinical findings are typical of orchitis, and treatment is symptomatic. Infertility following bilateral disease may occur secondary to testicular atrophy, but this is quite unusual.

Henoch-Schönlein purpura may involve the scrotal wall, producing various degrees of erythema and edema, and may involve the testis and epididymis, producing acute pain of sufficient intensity to mimic testicular torsion.[23] Although some form of scrotal involvement may be seen in as many as 15% to 38% of cases, severe acute scrotal disease is uncommon. Testicular torsion coincident with purpura has been reported, so surgical exploration is warranted if the diagnosis is in doubt. Nuclear or color flow Doppler scans may be extremely valuable in determining the presence of testicular torsion.[8,14,15]

Insect bites and allergic dermatitis may cause edema of the scrotal wall; examination should reveal a normal spermatic cord and testis. Scrotal trauma may result in hematoma of the scrotal wall, a hematocele, or testicular rupture. Scrotal ultrasound may provide valuable information. If massive swelling makes diagnosis impossible, exploration is necessary.

Painless Scrotal Swelling

Painless scrotal swelling may be acute or chronic. Scrotal masses discovered on routine examination may have been present for an unknown period of time. Painless swelling may originate in the scrotal wall, testis, adnexal, or cord structures.

Idiopathic scrotal edema is a self-limited process of unknown origin that causes acute erythema, edema, and perhaps mild tenderness of the scrotal wall.[9] The process usually involves the entire scrotum, although the testis and cord are normal. It may occur at any age from 18 months to 14 years. The process resolves spontaneously, although diphenhydramine has appeared to hasten resolution. Edema or lymphedema from any origin also may cause scrotal wall swelling, as may various other soft tissue processes.[6,12]

Painless swelling of the testis should be regarded as a *tumor* until proved otherwise. Most tumors occur after age 15 years, but a small peak in incidence occurs at 2 years.[13] Tumors are firm, painless masses that may give a sensation of heaviness in the testis; they do not transilluminate. The mass cannot be delineated from the substance of the testis. Because solid lesions of the epididymis are rare and invariably benign, firm lesions in the sulcus between the testis and the epididymis should be considered testicular in origin until proved otherwise. Testicular tumors require prompt inguinal exploration and orchiectomy. Preoperatively a chest roentgenogram and serum markers (alpha-fetoprotein, beta-human chorionic gonadotropin) should be obtained.

The most common cause of painless scrotal swelling in infants is a *hydrocele,* a collection of serous fluid within the tunica vaginalis surrounding the testis (see Fig. 164-4). These cystic swellings may impart a bluish tinge to the scrotum, especially when tense. They exhibit transillumination, and it usually is possible to palpate a normal testis within the hydrocele. Infantile hydroceles resolve spontaneously within several months. Communicating hydroceles vacillate in size. A reliable history of a flat scrotum in the morning with a gradual increase in fluid during the day is diagnostic because a hydrocele may not be grossly apparent at the time of office examination.

Examination may reveal a variable amount of fluid or a "silk glove" sign in the groin, as the surfaces of the tunica vaginalis glide over each other. Communicating hydroceles rarely resolve, and because of the potential for herniation of abdominal structures, elective repair is indicated.[20] Boys under 2 years of age should have a bilateral exploration because of the high incidence of a contralateral patent processus vaginalis. Adolescents who have communicating hydroceles frequently are found to have omental hernias. A hydrocele associated with an inguinal mass is likely a *hernia.* If the mass cannot be reduced or if vomiting or signs of intestinal obstruction occur, emergency surgery is indicated.

Painless masses of the epididymis occur with some frequency. Epididymal solid tumors are very rare and invariably are benign.[16] Cystic lesions of the epididymis *(spermatocele, epididymal cyst)* often are found in teenagers. These transilluminate, are nontender, and can be separated from the testis by examination. No surgical intervention is indicated unless discomfort arises, since postoperative epididymal scarring may obstruct ductal structures and result in infertility. Swellings of the spermatic cord are not uncommon in childhood. Solid, painless lesions should be pursued aggressively because spermatic cord and paratesticular sarcomas are not rare. Cystic lesions that transilluminate may represent encysted hydroceles of the cord, many of which are associated with a patent processus vaginalis (see Fig. 164-4).

Varicoceles are found in older boys and adolescents. These dilated veins of the pampiniform plexus commonly are asymptomatic and usually occur on the left side. The veins may collapse when the patient is sitting or supine. The left-sided predominance suggests origin from increased pressure in the left gonadal vein, which has no valves and enters the renal vein at a right angle. Acute onset of a varicocele, or a right-sided varicocele in a younger child, may represent acute venous obstruction from a retroperitoneal tumor. Abdominal sonography is indicated in these cases. Recent data indicate that diminished testicular volume may result from noxious effects of a varicocele, thought perhaps to be due to increased scrotal temperature. Although a subject of some debate and much uncertainty, indications for varicocele ablation include pain, ipsilateral testicular growth failure, and abnormal semen analysis. Varicocele ablation can be achieved by surgical, laparoscopic, or radiological means.[10]

Physical examination of a boy who has acute scrotal swelling should rule out *folliculitis, sebaceous cyst, local trauma* (e.g., zipper injury), and other miscellaneous local scrotal wall processes as etiological factors.

REFERENCES

1. Arey LB: *Developmental anatomy,* ed 7, Philadelphia, 1965, WB Saunders.
2. Bartsch G et al: Testicular torsion: late results with special regard to fertility and endocrine function, *J Urol* 124:375, 1980.
3. Blyth B, editor: Neonatal testicular torsion, *Dialogues in Pediatric Urology* 14:1, 1991.
4. Brandt MT et al: Prenatal testicular torsion: principles of management, *J Urol* 147:670, 1992.
5. Cass AS, Cass BP, Veeraraghhavan K: Immediate exploration of the unilateral acute scrotum in young male subjects, *J Urol* 124:829, 1980.
6. Coolsaet B, Weinberg R: Thrombosis of the spermatic vein in children, *J Urol* 124:290, 1980.
7. Dresner ML: Torsed appendage: diagnosis and management—blue dot sign, *Urology* 1:63, 1973.
8. Falkowski WS, Firlit CF: Testicular torsion: the role of radioisotopic scanning, *J Urol* 124:886, 1980.
9. Kaplan GW: Acute idiopathic scrotal edema, *J Pediatr Surg* 12:647, 1977.
10. Kass EJ, editor: Options for adolescent varicocele, *Dialogues in Pediatric Urology* 13:1, 1990.
11. Kiesling VJ et al: Spermatic cord block and manual reduction: primary treatment for spermatic cord torsion, *J Urol* 132:921, 1984.
12. Koster LH, Antoon SH: Fat necrosis in the scrotum, *J Urol* 123:599, 1980.
13. Kramer SA, Kelalis PP: Pediatric surgical oncology. In Gillenwater JA et al, editors: *Adult and pediatric urology,* ed 2, St Louis, 1991, Mosby.
14. Mendel JB et al: Testicular torsion in children: scintigraphic assessment, *Pediatr Radiol* 15:110, 1985.
15. Meza MP et al: Color flow imaging in children with clinically suspected testicular torsion, *Pediatr Radiol* 22:370, 1992.
16. Mostofi FK, Price EB: Tumors of the male genital system. In *Atlas of tumor pathology,* Series 2, Fasc 8, Washington, DC, 1973, Armed Forces Institute of Pathology.
17. Nagler HM, White RD: The effect of testicular torsion on the contralateral testis, *J Urol* 128:1343, 1982.
18. Rabinowitz R: The importance of the cremasteric reflex in acute scrotal swelling in children, *J Urol* 132:89, 1984.
19. Riggs S, Sandford JP: Viral orchitis, *N Engl J Med* 266:990, 1962.
20. Rowe MI, Lloyd DA: Inguinal hernia. In Welch KJ et al, editors: *Pediatric surgery,* ed 4, Chicago, 1986, Mosby.
21. Siegel A, Snyder H, Duckett JW: Epididymitis in infants and boys: underlying urogenital anomalies and efficacy of imaging modalities, *J Urol* 138:1100, 1987.
22. Skoglund RW, McRoberts JW, Ragde H: Torsion of the testicular appendages: presentation of 43 new cases and a collective review, *J Urol* 104:598, 1970.
23. Turkish VJ et al: Scrotal swelling in the Schönlein-Henoch syndrome, *J Urol* 115:317, 1976.

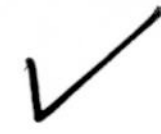

165 Sexual Developmental Alterations

Leslie P. Plotnick and Robert K. Kritzler

Disorders of pubertal development constitute one of the most frequent referrals to pediatric endocrinology clinics. In many cases no endocrine problem is found. Frequently, a costly referral can be avoided by a careful evaluation, including family history, and a few simple laboratory procedures.

At puberty a series of complex hormonal changes takes place. The hypothalamus secretes pulses of gonadotropin-releasing hormone (GnRH), which stimulates pituitary gonadotropin production of luteinizing hormone (LH) and follicle-stimulating hormone (FSH). Concomitantly, the previously very sensitive hypothalamic-pituitary-gonadal feedback loop becomes less sensitive to the negative effect of gonadal steroids; thus gonadotropin levels increase. This results in the secretion of greater amounts of androgens or estrogens, depending on the sex of the child, leading to the physical changes of puberty. There also is an increase in secretion of adrenal androgens. The mechanism that triggers the maturation of the adrenal cortex at puberty remains poorly understood.

In girls, breast development usually is the first sign of puberty, with the mean age of onset at about 10½ years and a standard deviation of 2½ years. This is followed in about 6 months by the appearance of pubic hair. Menarche follows the onset of breast development by about 2 years. A growth spurt accompanies the changes, usually peaking before menarche. The range of normal variation, however, is quite wide. In boys, testicular enlargement and scrotal thinning are the first signs of puberty, with a mean age of onset at about 11½ years and a standard deviation of 2 years; this is followed in about 6 months by pubic hair growth and some penile enlargement. Approximately 2 years after the first changes, axillary hair and then facial hair appear. The male growth spurt peaks about 2 years after that of the female. As with girls, the normal range is wide.

The time of puberty is one of profound change, both physical and psychological. Problems of sexual identity, body image, adolescent independence, and peer acceptance are frequent. When pubertal development is precocious or delayed, many of these problems are compounded.

DELAYED DEVELOPMENT

Few matters are of greater concern to the adolescent than remaining short in stature or sexually underdeveloped. Delayed development demands the immediate attention of the practitioner.

Puberty is considered delayed in girls who have no breast development by 13 years of age or in boys who have no testicular enlargement at 14 years of age. In girls a delay of more than 5 years from onset of puberty to menarche also is cause for concern. Similarly, maturation arrest in boys warrants evaluation. Delayed puberty is more common in boys than in girls.

Constitutional delay, a slow maturation with appropriate hormonal levels, accounts for the majority of all cases of delayed pubertal development. This problem is identified much more frequently in boys, perhaps because of general societal and peer group reaction to short and sexually underdeveloped boys. It frequently is familial. Often, early signs of puberty are found on careful examination, which permits the physician to reassure the child and the parents. Chronic systemic diseases that can lead to delayed puberty may be difficult to differentiate from constitutional delay as a cause for the difficulty; these diseases are listed in the box on p. 1106.

The remainder of the differential diagnosis of delayed development relates to failure at either the hypothalamic-pituitary level, shown by low serum gonadotropins *(hypogonadotropic hypogonadism),* or at the gonadal level, shown by elevated gonadotropins *(hypergonadotropic hypogonadism).* Either of these conditions may result from genetic disorders or acquired illnesses (see the box on p. 1106). The workup of the patient is directed toward identifying the specific cause.

Treatment should be directed, when possible, toward the cause of the delayed development. If sex steroid secretion is deficient, due to either gonadal failure or gonadotropin deficiency, treatment centers are replacing the appropriate sex steroid. In constitutional delay, waiting is the best course. In males, however, a short course of injectable testosterone may be indicated if the delayed development is affecting the boy's psychological well-being. In girls, cosmetic treatment, such as the use of a padded bra, is very helpful. Estrogen therapy is necessary only occasionally. In patients who have GnRH or gonadotropin deficiency, fertility may be induced with GnRH or gonadotropin therapy. In any case, strong psychological support must be provided to the adolescent and sometimes to the family. If the problem is difficult diagnostically or if hormonal therapy is desired, referral should be made to an endocrinologist.

PRECOCIOUS DEVELOPMENT

Precocious puberty is the appearance of secondary sexual characteristics before 8 years of age in girls and 9 years in boys. It may be isosexual (appropriate for phenotype) or heterosexual (appropriate for opposite sex phenotype). Precocious puberty is much more common in girls than in boys. In girls, idiopathic precocious puberty is the single most common diagnosis, but precocious puberty in boys is more likely (more than 50% of cases) to be secondary to organic causes.

Isosexual Precocious Puberty

Stimulation of the hypothalamic-pituitary axis, with gonadotropin secretion and resultant sex steroid secretion, is termed *central precocious puberty.* Sex steroid secretion independent of pituitary gonadotropin secretion may be termed *peripheral*

CAUSES OF DELAYED PUBERTY

I. Constitutional delay
II. Deficiency of GnRH secretion by the hypothalamus
  A. Genetic
    1. Isolated deficiency
    2. Kallmann syndrome
    3. Laurence-Moon-Bardet-Biedl syndrome
    4. Prader-Willi syndrome
  B. Acquired
    1. Infection
    2. Neoplasm
    3. Infiltrative disease
    4. Trauma
III. Deficiency of gonadotropin secretion by the pituitary
  A. Genetic
    1. Panhypopituitarism
    2. Isolated deficiency
    3. Fertile eunuch (normal FSH, low LH)
  B. Acquired
    1. Infection
    2. Neoplasm
    3. Trauma
IV. Gonadal disorders
  A. Genetic
    1. Turner syndrome (45, X or structural X abnormalities or mosaicism)
    2. Klinefelter syndrome (47, XXY abnormality)
    3. Noonan syndrome
    4. Syndromes of complete androgen insensitivity (no sexual hair)
    5. Del Castillo syndrome (Sertoli cells only)
    6. Pure gonadal dysgenesis
    7. Myotonic dystrophy
  B. Acquired
    1. Infections
      a. Gonorrhea (male)
      b. Virus (usually mumps)
      c. Tuberculosis (male)
    2. Radiotherapy or chemotherapy
    3. Mechanical causes
      a. Torsion
      b. Surgery
      c. "Vanishing testes"
    4. Autoimmune
V. Adrenal and gonadal steroid enzyme deficiencies
VI. Chronic systemic diseases
  A. Congenital heart disease
  B. Chronic pulmonary disease
  C. Inflammatory bowel disease
  D. Chronic renal failure and renal tubular acidosis
  E. Hypothyroidism
  F. Poorly controlled diabetes mellitus
  G. Sickle cell anemia
  H. Collagen-vascular disease
  I. Anorexia nervosa

CAUSES OF ISOSEXUAL PRECOCIOUS PUBERTY

I. Central (with pituitary gonadotropin secretion)
  A. Idiopathic
  B. Central nervous system abnormalities
    1. Congenital anomalies (hydrocephalus)
    2. Tumors (hypothalamic, pineal, other)
    3. Hamartoma
    4. Postinflammatory condition
    5. Trauma
    6. Syndromes
      a. Neurofibromatosis
      b. Tuberous sclerosis
  C. Hypothyroidism (severe)
II. Pseudoprecocious puberty
  A. Exogenous sex steroids
  B. Gonadal tumors or cysts
  C. Adrenal hyperplasia or tumor
  D. Ectopic gonadotropin-secreting tumors (chorioepithelioma, hepatoblastoma, teratoma)
  E. Familial Leydig cell hyperplasia
  F. McCune-Albright syndrome

or *pseudoprecocious puberty*. The box above lists the causes of these two conditions.

The diagnosis of precocious puberty is based on the physical examination and laboratory evidence of sex steroid secretion. Measurement of serum gonadotropin levels before and after an injection of GnRH usually allows classification of the condition as either central or pseudoprecocious puberty. In central precocious puberty, further workup centers on a search for the cause of the gonadotropin secretion. The diagnosis of idiopathic central precocious puberty can be made only after a search for a pathological cause is negative. In pseudoprecocious puberty, one must search for the source of sex steroid, remembering that exogenous sources (e.g., contraceptive pills in girls) are easily available. In males physical examination of the testes is particularly useful in the differential diagnosis. If both testes are of pubertal size, then clearly the patient has gonadotropin-stimulated precocious puberty; if one testis is enlarged, a testicular tumor probably is present; if both testes are small, the androgens are either exogenous or of adrenal origin.

Treatment of the isosexual precocity centers on removal of the underlying cause. The treatment of idiopathic central precocious puberty is with GnRH analogs. GnRH analogs produce sustained levels of GnRH, which lead to pituitary desensitization and a reduction in gonadotropin secretion to prepubertal levels. Several GnRH analogs are available in intramuscular (depot), subcutaneous, and intranasal forms. In all cases, psychological support is important. In general, evaluation and treatment of precocious puberty is a matter for a pediatric endocrinologist.

Variations of Puberty

Two entities not requiring treatment are isolated premature breast development (thelarche) and isolated premature development of sexual hair (adrenarche). *Premature thelarche*

CAUSES OF HETEROSEXUAL PRECOCIOUS PUBERTY

I. Female
  A. Congenital adrenal hyperplasia
  B. Androgen-secreting tumors
    1. Adrenal
    2. Ovarian
    3. Teratoma
  C. Exogenous androgens
II. Male
  A. Estrogen-producing tumors
    1. Adrenal
    2. Teratoma
    3. Hepatoma
    4. Testicular
  B. Exogenous estrogens
  C. Increased peripheral conversion of androgens to estrogens

typically occurs in girls between 6 months and 2 years of age. Breast development usually is moderate, often regresses, and is seen without other signs of precocious puberty. Specifically, estrogen or gonadotropic levels do not increase significantly, and statural and skeletal maturation accelerate only mildly, if at all. Premature thelarche does not progress to complete precocious puberty.

Premature adrenarche usually occurs between 5 and 8 years of age. The development of sexual hair frequently is accompanied by a mild growth spurt (with slight bone age advancement) and signs of increased adrenal androgen (slightly elevated urinary 17-ketosteroids and increased levels of plasma dehydroepiandrosterone and its sulfate); in girls there are no signs of increased estrogen secretion. An abnormal androgen source such as a tumor or adrenal hyperplasia must be excluded.

In both premature thelarche and premature adrenarche, careful follow-up is necessary because the early stages of complete sexual precocity may appear similarly.

Heterosexual Precocious Puberty

Heterosexual precocious puberty is uncommon. The box above lists its causes. Exogenous sex steroids (including creams) must be considered. The diagnostic workup must center on the search for a sex steroid–producing tumor. These patients should be referred to a pediatric endocrinologist. Treatment is aimed at removal of the sex hormone source (exogenous or tumor) or suppression with glucocorticoid replacement therapy (congenital adrenal hyperplasia).

SUMMARY

In most cases of delayed or precocious sexual development, a careful history and physical examination and a few basic laboratory tests identify those patients likely to have a pathological cause requiring referral to a pediatric endocrinologist. In all cases physical care, as well as psychological care and support, is extremely important particularly in cases in which medical therapy is only partially satisfactory.

SUGGESTED READINGS

Blizzard PM, Rogol AD: Variations and disorders of pubertal development. In Kappy MS et al, editors: *Wilkins diagnosis and treatment of endocrine disorders in childhood and adolescence,* ed 4, Springfield, Ill, 1994, Charles C Thomas.

Clemons RD, Kappy MS et al: Long-term effectiveness of depot GnRH analogue in the treatment of children with central precocious puberty, *Am J Dis Child* 147:653, 1993.

Kappy MS, Stuart T, Perelman A: Efficacy of leuprolide therapy in children with central precocious puberty, *Am J Dis Child* 142:1061, 1988.

Kelch RP, Beitins IZ: Adolescent sexual development. In Kappy MS et al, editors: *Wilkins the diagnosis and treatment of endocrine disorders in childhood and adolescence,* ed 4, Springfield, Ill, 1994, Charles C Thomas.

Kulin HE, Reiter EO: Managing the patient with a delay in pubertal development, *The Endocrinologist* 2:231, 1992.

Lee PA, Page JG: Effects of leuprolide in the treatment of central precocious puberty, *J Pediatr* 114:321, 1989.

Parker KL, Lee PA: Depot leuprolide acetate for treatment of precocious puberty, *J Clin Endocrinol Metab* 69:689, 1989.

Rosenfield RL: The ovary and female sexual maturation. In Kaplan SA, editor: *Clinical pediatric endocrinology,* Philadelphia, 1990, WB Saunders.

Saenger P, Reiter EO: Premature adrenarche: a normal variant of puberty? *J Clin Endocrinol Metab* 74:236, 1992.

Styne D: The testes: disorders of sexual differentiation and puberty. In Kaplan SA, editor: *Clinical pediatric endocrinology,* Philadelphia, 1990, WB Saunders.

Tanner JM: Growth and endocrinology of the adolescent. In Gardner LI, editor: *Endocrine and genetic diseases of childhood and adolescence,* Philadelphia, 1975, WB Saunders.

Wheeler MD, Styne DM: The treatment of precocious puberty, *Endocrinol Metab Clin North Am* 20:183, 1991.

Wilson DM, Rosenfeld RG: Treatment of short stature and delayed adolescence, *Pediatr Clin North Am* 34:865, 1987.

166 Splenomegaly

Allen Eskenazi

The spleen has intrigued physicians for centuries. Pliny the Elder associated it with mirth and laughter, and Galen described it as an organ full of mystery. Over the years the immunological and hematological roles of the spleen have been defined more precisely. Understanding the role of the spleen in health and disease permits the clinician to evaluate rationally the child or adolescent who has an enlarged spleen.

The spleen is fixed in the left upper quadrant of the abdomen by the splenorenal and phrenosplenic ligaments. Congenital or acquired abnormalities of the support structure can result in *splenic ptosis* and thus allow palpation of a spleen that actually is normal in size. An estimated 5% to 10% of normal infants have a palpable spleen tip, whereas a palpable spleen in an adult almost always is pathological.

A useful framework for evaluating the child who has splenomegaly is to consider the four major physiological functions of the spleen: immunological, phagocytic, hemodynamic, and hematopoietic. First, the spleen is the major lymphoid organ in the body. It is the primary site of B lymphocyte activity related to antibody production, and it is an important reservoir of T lymphocytes and natural killer cells, the mediators of cellular immune responses. Second, the spleen serves a major role in the removal of abnormal and senescent blood cells, as well as of circulating particulates. Third, the vasculature of the spleen plays an important role in the regulation of portal blood flow. Finally, the spleen is an important site of hematopoiesis in children and adults who have pathological conditions and of extramedullary hematopoiesis in the fetus.

Splenomegaly is a prominent or associated feature in numerous disease states (see the box on the right). Splenomegaly caused by recurrent viral infections often is seen in young infants. The degree of splenic enlargement is relatively small and should resolve within a short period of time. A greater degree of splenic enlargement occurs specifically in infectious mononucleosis (Epstein-Barr virus), cytomegalovirus, and human immunodeficiency virus infections. Chronic bacterial infections (such as subacute bacterial endocarditis, syphilis, and tuberculosis) may be associated with splenomegaly. Acute overwhelming bacterial infections with pneumococcus or meningococcus also may result in splenic enlargement. In many areas of the world the spleen may harbor a large burden of protozoan-infected cells.

Inherited and acquired hemolytic anemias generally result in splenomegaly because of either increased phagocytic activity by the reticuloendothelial network (membranopathies, hemoglobinopathies, autoimmune hemolysis) or the development of extramedullary hematopoiesis (thalassemia major). Splenic sequestration of blood is a common, acute event in children who have sickle cell anemia, resulting in pallor, irritability, tachypnea, tachycardia, and variable degrees of splenic enlargement. Recognition of splenic sequestration is imperative because hypotension and shock can develop rapidly as a result of accumulation of blood in the spleen.

Infiltrative diseases of the spleen require prompt evaluation. The spleen rarely is the site of metastatic solid tumors but often is infiltrated by leukemias and lymphomas. Nonmalignant infiltration is seen in lipidosis and mucopolysac-

SOME CAUSES OF SPLENOMEGALY

Infections

Viral: Epstein-Barr, cytomegalovirus, human immunodeficiency virus
Bacterial: acute bacterial infections, subacute bacterial endocarditis, congenital syphilis, tuberculosis
Protozoal: malaria, toxoplasmosis
Fungal: candidiasis, histoplasmosis, coccidioidomycosis

Hematological disorders

Hemolytic anemias—congenital and acquired
- Red cell membrane defects: hereditary spherocytosis, hereditary elliptocytosis
- Red cell hemoglobin defects: sickle cell disease and related syndromes, thalassemia
- Red cell enzyme defects: pyruvate kinase deficiency and others
- Autoimmune hemolytic anemia

Extramedullary hematopoiesis
- Thalassemia major, osteopetrosis, myelofibrosis

Infiltrative disorders

Leukemias
Lymphomas
Lipidoses
Mucopolysaccharidosis
Histiocytosis X

Congestive splenomegaly

Chronic congestive heart failure
Portal hypertension secondary to hepatic cirrhosis

Inflammatory diseases

Systemic lupus erythematosus (SLE)
Rheumatoid arthritis (Still disease)
Serum sickness
Sarcoidosis
Immune thrombocytopenias and neutropenias

Primary splenic disorders

Cysts
Hemangiomas and lymphangiomas
Subcapsular hemorrhage

charidosis, as well as in histiocytosis X. Autoimmune disorders (e.g., systemic lupus erythematosus and rheumatoid arthritis) and alloimmune disorders (serum sickness) may lead to expansion within the spleen of its lymphoid elements, as well as the phagocytic elements that remove antibody-coated cells and proteins. These conditions often mimic other infiltrative processes and may result in hypersplenism.

EVALUATION

Splenomegaly is diagnosed by physical examination and only rarely requires confirmation by radiographic, ultrasonographic, or radionuclide imaging. These studies, which may be useful in the evaluation of the child who has lymphoma, are not indicated in the routine evaluation of splenomegaly. A careful history, including family history, and physical examination permit the clinician to narrow the differential diagnosis to a few entities. A complete blood cell count, a reticulocyte count, and careful evaluation of the peripheral blood smear are extremely useful studies in the majority of patients who have splenomegaly. The results of these simple diagnostic procedures help dictate further diagnostic procedures such as hemoglobin electrophoresis, bone marrow aspiration, or lymph node biopsy.

HYPERSPLENISM

Hypersplenism is not a specific disease entity. The term refers to the condition in which the spleen removes excessive numbers of normal circulating blood cells, resulting in one or more cytopenias. The affected blood element(s) are formed in the bone marrow to compensate for their accelerated destruction in the spleen. Splenectomy will correct the cytopenia(s). Establishing the cause of the hypersplenism is vital, however, inasmuch as other therapeutic modalities may correct the hypersplenism and thus obviate the need for splenectomy.

SUGGESTED READINGS

Crosby WH: The spleen. In Wintrobe MM, editor: *Blood, pure and eloquent,* New York, 1980, McGraw-Hill.

Pearson H: The spleen and disturbances of splenic function. In Nathan D, Oski F, editors: *Hematology of infancy and childhood,* Philadelphia, 1993, WB Saunders.

167 Strabismus

James W. McManaway III and Carl A. Frankel

INTRODUCTION

Strabismus is the general term for any misalignment of the eye. The misalignment can be present under binocular conditions, in which case it is a *manifest strabismus (tropia),* or under monocular conditions, in which case it is a *latent strabismus (phoria).* Many persons have a small phoria, which is of no clinical significance; these latent deviations usually are found on routine ophthalmological examination. Tropias (manifest deviations) are present under binocular conditions, either intermittently or constantly, and may be alternating or unilateral. Alternating tropias imply equal or near-equal visual acuities, whereas monocular tropias may indicate reduced vision (amblyopia) (Fig. 167-1).

Strabismus occurs in approximately 3% of the population and, while familial tendencies have been well documented, no clear-cut genetic mode of inheritance has been demonstrated. The direction of deviation of one eye with respect to the fixating eye names the deviation. An inward deviation is called an *esotropia,* an outward deviation an *exotropia.* A vertical deviation is referred to as a *hypertropia* or *hypotropia,* depending on whether the deviating (nonfixating) eye is higher or lower, respectively, than the fixating eye. Torsional deviations are named for *incyclotorsion* or *excyclotorsion* of the 12 o'clock position to the eye and usually are associated with an abnormality in superior oblique muscle or inferior oblique muscle function with a secondary vertical strabismus; these conditions usually are referred to as *cyclovertical strabismus.*

Congenital or infantile strabismus deviations acquired before maturation of the visual system (between the ages of 7 and 9 years for most children) are not associated with diplopia due to suppression. *Suppression* is the adaptation to strabismus that inhibits the image at the deviating eye from reaching consciousness. In an alternating strabismus, alternating suppression is evidence for normal monocular visual development in both eyes and abnormal binocular visual development. However, in a youngster who has monocular strabismus, visual development in the fixating eye is expected to proceed normally, whereas binocular visual development and monocular visual development in the nonfixating eye can be expected to be impaired. This impairment in monocular visual development leads to amblyopia (poor vision, or "lazy eye"), which requires patching of the fixating eye to restore normal vision in the nonfixating eye. After the visual acuities have been equalized, surgery may be indicated to correct the ocular misalignment.

Because one eye is the fixating eye, *bilateral strabismus* is a misnomer. *If both eyes appear deviated when the patient is facing an examiner, visual inattention or visual impairment is suggested* and further evaluation is indicated to assess the function of the visual system. This assessment can be in the form of the visual evoked potential (VEP) or visual evoked response (VER), electroretinogram (ERG), or forced preferential looking (FPL). The first three are electrophysiological tests that require surface electrodes; the latter requires some demonstrable visual interest for the child.

Acquired strabismus, whether esotropia, exotropia, or a cyclovertical deviation, should prompt concern as to the exact cause, because of the long-term implications for the patient. Poor vision may be the cause, as strabismus caused by retinoblastoma (the most common intraocular tumor of children with an incidence of 1:12,000 to 14,000 live births) is the second most common presenting sign (after leukocoria). Head trauma, either accidental or deliberate, can cause third, fourth, or sixth cranial nerve palsies that may result in an acute acquired strabismus. Because of other diagnostic considerations, any patient who has an acquired strabismus should be referred to an ophthalmologist for evaluation and intervention as needed, including that necessary to restore the integrity of binocular vision.

In a newborn infant, inattention or somnolence is the most common cause of variable ocular alignment. During periods of full wakefulness, the ocular alignment usually is normal. Even in normal infants, however, an intermittent esotropia or exotropia may be noted. This usually represents central nervous system immaturity and typically resolves during the first 2 to 3 months of life. *In any infant in whom strabismus persists beyond 10 to 12 weeks, evaluation by an ophthalmologist is indicated,* earlier if other signs of developmental delay are present or if the strabismus is constant.

DETECTION OF STRABISMUS

The Corneal Light Reflection Test

The simplest method to determine the presence of strabismus is the corneal light reflection test (Hirschberg method). In this test a penlight is directed at the cornea, and the observer notes the position of the corneal reflection with respect to the center of the pupil. If the light reflex is deviated toward the nose, an exotropia may be present; an esotropia should be suspected when the light reflex is deviated toward the lateral side of the visual axis. Although this method is used as a rapid screening test, the high incidence of false positive findings results in unneeded referrals. On the other hand, the presence of a false negative result may give a false sense of security (Fig. 167-2).

The Cover-Uncover Test

A more sensitive test for the presence of a strabismus is the cover-uncover test. To perform this test the examiner uses some bright, pleasant object to attract the youngster's attention and then covers one eye with a hand, finger, or occluder. The examiner should watch the other eye carefully for a refixation movement, which indicates the presence of a hetero-

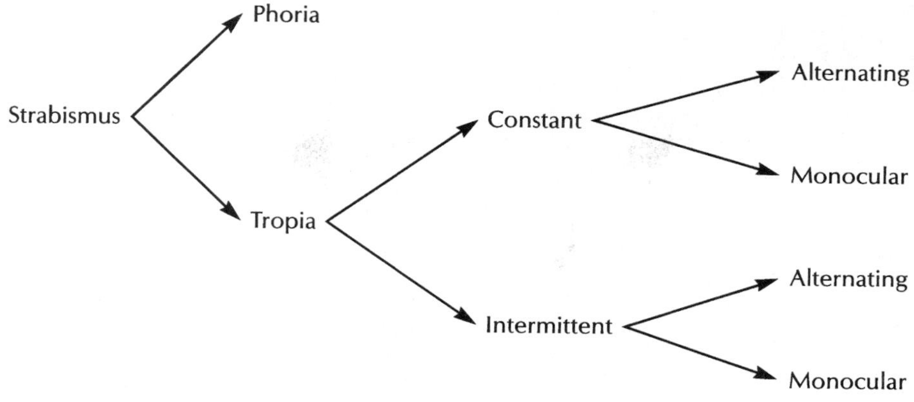

FIG. 167-1 Classification of strabismus.

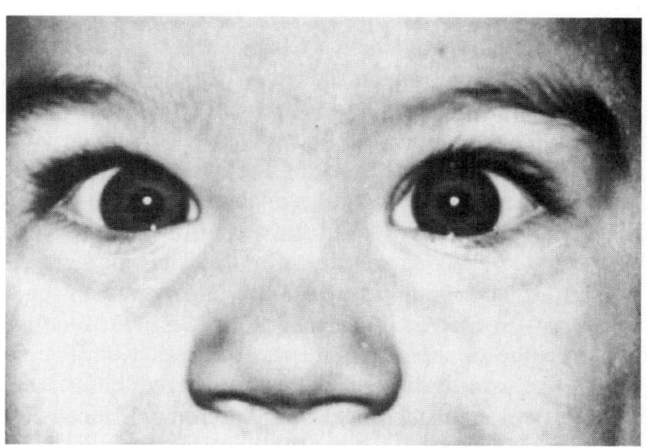

FIG. 167-2 Pseudostrabismus. This child's eyes, in fact, are aligned perfectly, even though the right eye appears "crossed" (esotropic). Epicanthal skin folds produce this illusion, which here is enhanced by the face being turned slightly toward the side. Notice that the corneal light reflections are quite symmetric.

tropia. The examiner then removes the cover and covers the other eye after 1 to 2 seconds, again watching for a refixation movement. Each eye must be tested several times, and the cover should be removed briefly before the next eye is covered. *The presence of a shift of one eye while covering the fellow eye is evidence of a strabismus* and should prompt referral for further evaluation and intervention as indicated.

PSEUDOESOTROPIA

A common misconception among the lay public is that children may outgrow "crossed" eyes by the time they are 2 to 3 years of age. Unfortunately, this is not so. What children do tend to outgrow is the pseudoesotropia that is caused by the prominent epicanthal folds and broad, flat nasal bridge present in most infants. This condition creates an illusion of esotropia because of the decrease in the amount of nasal conjunctiva visible to the observer (see Fig. 167-2). Because the nasal cornea tends to "dip" under the epicanthal fold on adduction, the parent frequently reports that the eyes are crossed more with right or left gaze and with near viewing (where convergence accentuates the illusion).

ESOTROPIA

The most common type of strabismus is esotropia, which is characterized by a nasal deviation of the nonfixating eye (Fig. 167-3). In patients in whom the visual function is equal, alternate fixation may be present, giving rise to an alternating (*not* bilateral) deviation, whereas a monocular deviation is present in those in whom visual function is better in one eye. The corneal light reflection test will show the light to be centered in the pupil of the fixating eye, with the deviating eye showing the light reflection to be toward the temporal side of the center of the pupil. Because of variation in the location of the visual axis with respect to the center of the pupil, a small deviation may be either accentuated or, of greater concern, minimized. In fact, deviations of up to 7 degrees (15 prism diopters) may be missed. Thus the cover-uncover test is more reliable in the detection of a deviation.

Congenital Esotropia

Congenital esotropia is defined as having its onset within the first 6 months of life. Because the deviation may not be present at birth, a more accurate term is *infantile esotropia.* Infantile esotropia is characterized by a large angle of deviation and, at least initially, by equal visual function and cross fixation. Cross fixation is that condition in which a patient prefers to look to the left with the already deviating right eye and to the right with the already deviating left eye. Because of cross fixation, a unilateral or even bilateral sixth cranial nerve palsy may be diagnosed. Normal abduction of each eye may be demonstrated by occluding one eye and using rotational testing or observing following eye movements of the unpatched eye.

In an attempt to normalize the ocular alignment, early surgical intervention is indicated in youngsters who have congenital esotropia. Current medical opinion recommends surgical intervention between 6 and 18 months (possibly up to 24 months) in an effort to obtain more stable binocular vision than might be possible if the surgery were performed later. Prerequisites for early surgical intervention include stable ocular deviation, treatment of amblyopia (poor vision), and minimal risk for undergoing general anesthesia.

Less common conditions in which an esotropia is present include the congenital abducens nerve palsy (very rare) and Duane syndrome, which typically affects the left eye. Duane

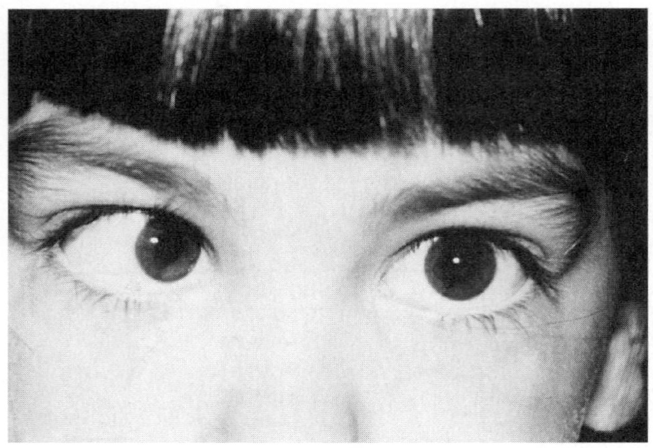

FIG. 167-3 Note the nasal deviation of the right eye with the corneal light reflection temporally displaced on the right eye and centered in the left pupil, indicating an esotropia.

syndrome is distinguished from a true sixth nerve palsy by narrowing of the palpebral fissure with retraction of the globe on adduction as a result of contraction of the medial rectus muscle and inappropriate simultaneous contraction of the lateral rectus muscle of the same eye.

Acquired Esotropia

Any esotropia first detected beyond 6 months of age is classified as acquired; although it may represent a late-onset form of infantile esotropia, it requires careful diagnostic evaluation. Visual function needs to be assessed because *unilateral visual loss in the first several years of life typically results in an acquired esotropia.*

Accommodative Esotropia. This type of acquired esotropia typically has its onset in patients between 2 and 3 years of age. The history is that of an intermittent esotropia that becomes more frequent in its occurrence and is of increasing duration. The condition is based on the accommodation reflex. For an emmetrope (person who has no refractive error) to focus at near objects, a synkinetic near reflex must occur. *The three components of this synkinetic near reflex include accommodation* (the alteration in the shape of the lens to make it a more powerful refracting element), *accommodative convergence* (nasal movement of the eyes so that the visual axes may be directed to the near object of regard), and *pupillary miosis* (irrelevant to this discussion). In accommodative esotropia, one of two scenarios typically is encountered and depends on the relationship between accommodation (A) and accommodative convergence (AC)—the AC/A ratio.

NORMAL AC/A RATIO. When the deviation (esotropia) of a patient who has a normal AC/A ratio is measured and found to be the same for both near and distant targets, a normal relationship between accommodation and accommodative convergence is defined. A hyperopic (farsighted) patient is not able to view distant objects clearly when the lens is in its normal, relaxed state (the usual state for distant viewing). To focus, the patient increases the refractive power of the eye by forced accommodation for distant viewing. Accommodative convergence ensues because of the synkinetic near reflex, and esotropia results (Fig. 167-4, *A*). Spectacle correction of the refractive error obviates the need for the accommodation reflex during distant viewing (with its secondary accommodative convergence) and promotes normal ocular alignment while spectacles are worn (Fig. 167-4, *B*).

HIGH AC/A RATIO. Patients who have a high AC/A ratio have excessive convergence for each unit of accommodation generated and have an esotropia that is larger at near than at distance. Those patients who have no refractive error may have nearly straight eyes at distance but develop an esotropia at near because their normal accommodative effort results in excessive convergence. Hyperopic patients will have an esotropia at distance that becomes larger at near because of the additional accommodation required at near.

These patients are treated with bifocal spectacles containing their distance refractive correction in the upper segment and a stronger correction for near in the lower segment to relieve the need for accommodation at both distance and at near. An alternative treatment is the use of topical ophthalmic anticholinesterase agents such as isoflurophate or echothiophate iodide to facilitate accommodation (less effort needed) and thus reduce the excessive convergence. Unfortunately, these agents have ocular and systemic side effects, so they are used most commonly for short periods in the summer so that the child will not have esotropia at the swimming pool when glasses are not worn. Patients who have esotropia at distance looking through the upper segment of the glasses or with esotropia at near looking through the lower segment of the glasses often are candidates for surgical correction of their strabismus. Fortunately, many children have their esotropia controlled with bifocal glasses. Because the AC/A ratio typically begins to normalize by about 8 years of age, the bifocals eventually can be discontinued.

Paralytic Esotropia. An esotropia secondary to paralytic causes (abducens nerve palsy) is characterized by a deviation that varies with the direction of gaze and depends on whether the patient is fixating with the affected or the unaffected eye. When the patient looks in the direction of the affected side, the deviation is increased (horizontal incomitance). For example, in a patient who has left abducens nerve palsy, the esotropia will increase in left gaze and decrease in right gaze in relation to the primary (straight ahead) gaze position. Additionally, the deviation accompanying fixation by the unaffected eye (primary deviation) is less than that obtained with fixation by the affected eye (secondary deviation), unless the paralytic strabismus is long-standing, in which case the secondary deviation may approximate the primary deviation. An acquired abducens palsy is a nonlocalizing sign; it may reflect any cause of increased intracranial pressure or may be the benign sixth nerve palsy of childhood.[1,2] An appropriate evaluation to rule out the causes of increased intracranial pressure should be undertaken.

PSEUDOEXOTROPIA

Illusory exotropia occurs much less frequently than illusory esotropia. Because of the strikingly prominent appearance of pseudoexotropia, referral is made much more frequently and at a much earlier age, but the cover-uncover test reveals no refixation movement on covering either eye.

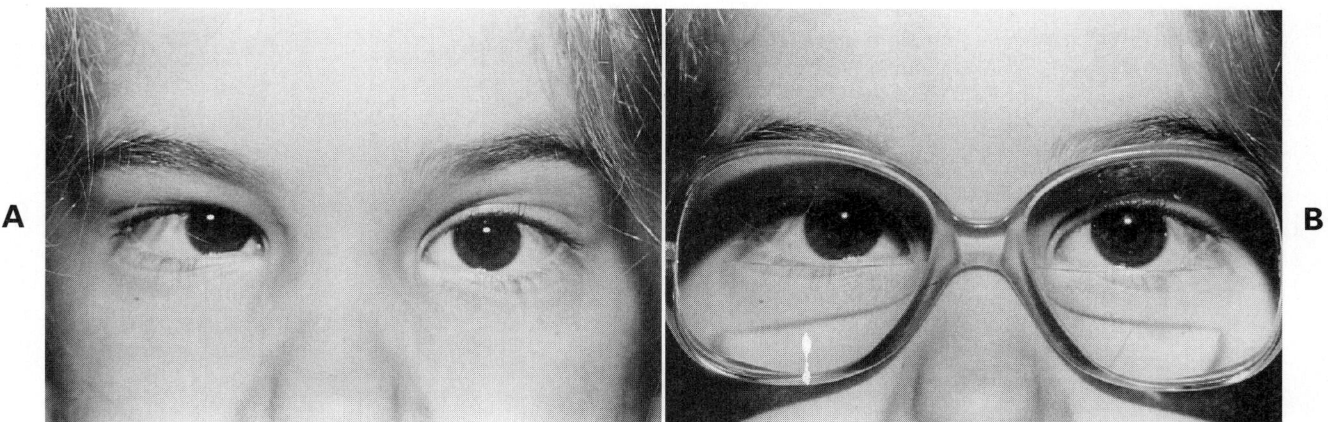

FIG. 167-4 **A,** Esotropia in a patient who has accommodative esotropia. **B,** Same patient, now having straight eyes upon refractive correction. Note the small increase in pupil size because of the reversal of accommodative miosis upon correction.

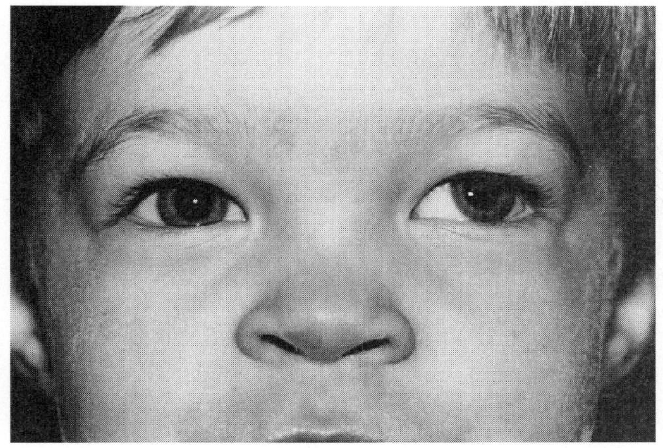

FIG. 167-5 Divergent strabismus of the left eye, defining an exotropia.

EXOTROPIA

Exotropia, or divergent strabismus (Fig. 167-5), occurs less frequently than does esotropia. As with esotropia, the deviation may be congenital or acquired and alternating or monocular. In addition, the exotropia may be constant or intermittent. Careful analysis of all these factors determines the treatment to be selected by the ophthalmologist.

Congenital Exotropia

Congenital exotropia is defined as having its onset in the first 6 months of life and is called, more appropriately, *infantile exotropia*. Infantile exotropia occurs much less frequently than infantile esotropia but similarly is characterized by a large angle of deviation and normal refractive error (mild hyperopia). Pseudoadduction deficit may be present, but full adduction usually is demonstrable on occlusion of one eye and then the other. As with infantile esotropia, early surgery is indicated to improve ocular alignment and binocular vision that is more stable than that obtained with later surgery (in those over 2 years of age).

Acquired Exotropia

Any exotropia that has its onset after 6 months of age is an acquired exotropia. Visual function must be assessed because the strabismus secondary to visual loss from a retinoblastoma is more likely to be an exotropia than an esotropia.

Intermittent Exotropia. This is the most common type of exotropia seen in children and typically has its initial onset at about 2 to 3 years of age. Late-onset intermittent exotropias typically are diagnosed beyond 3 years of age, although these are perhaps atypical only in the age at which they are first noted. During periods when the eyes are well aligned, binocular vision may be developing normally and the presence of binocular vision can help determine when, or if, surgical intervention is indicated. If binocular vision is deteriorating or if the frequency and duration of the deviation are increasing, surgical intervention is justified.

Convergence Insufficiency. A subset of intermittent exotropia, convergence insufficiency is characterized by complaints of eyestrain, fatigue, blurred vision, diplopia, and headache. As a result of the nature of the fusion mechanism, orthoptic exercises for symptomatic convergence insufficiency have a high rate of success as measured by relief of patient symptoms. Orthoptic exercises should not be confused with "vision training," which is of dubious value.

Divergence Excess. This is characterized by an exotropia that is larger at distant fixation than at near. The exotropia sometimes is noted only when a distant object is viewed. Surgical intervention is directed at the distance deviation, and a postoperative overcorrection (esotropia) for near fixation may occur.

Consecutive Exotropia. This deviation may occur spontaneously in previously esotropic patients who have poor vision of one eye, but generally follows surgical correction of an esotropia in patients who have poor fusional ability or unrecognized accommodative esotropia. Surgical intervention frequently is indicated in an attempt to obtain normal ocular alignment.

Paralytic Exotropia. Paralytic exodeviations, which usually are seen with acute third cranial nerve palsies, are character-

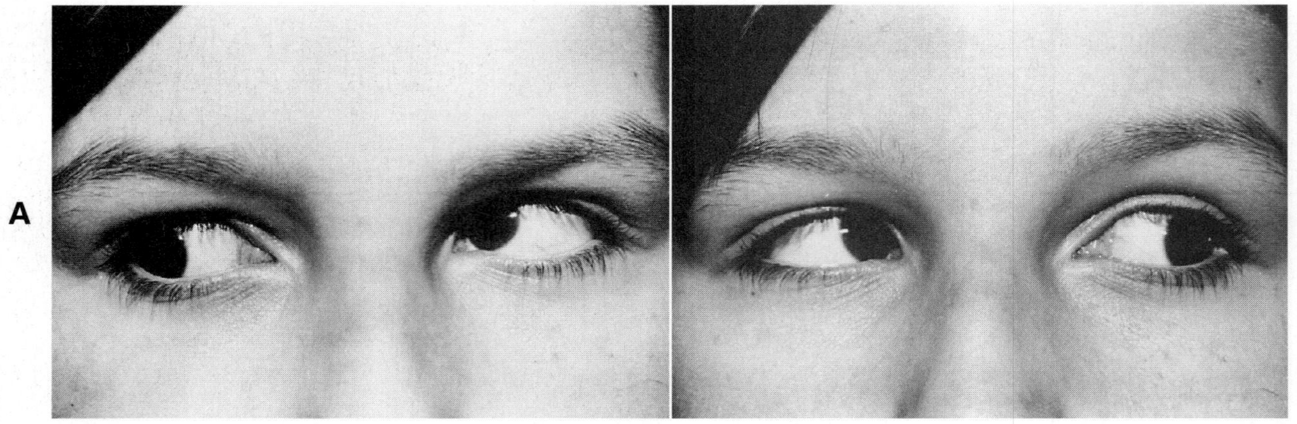

FIG. 167-6 **A,** Left hypertropia on right gaze characteristic of a left superior oblique muscle palsy. **B,** Right hypertropia on left gaze characteristic of a right superior oblique muscle palsy. This is the same patient shown in **A,** implying bilateral superior oblique muscle palsies.

ized by pupillary mydriasis, ptosis, an exotropia, and a hypotropia. Head trauma is the most frequent cause, and neuroradiological imaging (computed tomography and magnetic resonance imaging) usually is indicated. Because of the ptosis, diplopia is not a complaint; thus complete evaluation can be obtained during the wait to see if spontaneous improvement occurs. Special care should be taken in young children because of the possibility of deprivation amblyopia resulting from the ptotic lid.

VERTICAL AND CYCLOVERTICAL DEVIATIONS

Four muscles in each eye contribute to vertical and torsional eye movements: the superior and inferior rectus muscles and the superior and inferior oblique muscles. The two rectus muscles are concerned primarily with vertical eye movement, with secondary actions of incyclotorsion for the superior rectus muscle and excyclotorsion for the inferior rectus muscle. Conversely, the two oblique muscles are concerned primarily with torsional movements: the superior oblique for incyclotorsion and the inferior oblique for excyclotorsion. Secondary actions of the oblique muscles are depression and elevation for the superior and inferior oblique muscles, respectively. As a result of this arrangement, the two elevators (superior rectus and inferior oblique) have opposite torsional actions (incyclotorsion and excyclotorsion, respectively), whereas the two depressors (inferior rectus and superior oblique) also have opposite torsional actions (excyclotorsion and incyclotorsion, respectively). Thus *an imbalance in any one of the four muscles of either eye can result in a significant cyclovertical strabismus.*

Superior Oblique Muscle Palsy

The superior oblique muscle is innervated by the trochlear nerve (fourth cranial nerve), and superior oblique muscle palsies are the most commonly undiagnosed forms of strabismus. Although head trauma is a frequent cause of superior oblique muscle palsy, most of these palsies are congenital and bilateral. In a youngster who has bilateral superior oblique muscle palsy, fusion is not possible (because of the bilateral excyclotorsion), and the head position typically is normal,

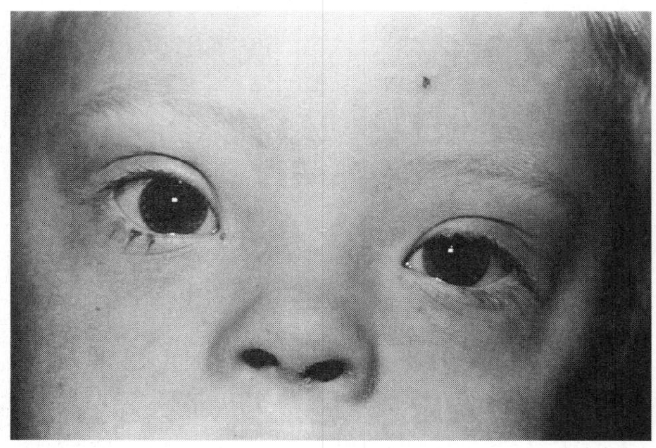

FIG. 167-7 Left head tilt in a patient who has a unilateral right superior oblique muscle palsy. Fusion was present, indicating binocular vision.

giving no clue to the existence of a problem. On right gaze, however, a left hypertropia typically is present because of the relatively unopposed action of the left inferior oblique muscle (Fig. 167-6, *A*). Similarly, on left gaze a right hypertropia usually occurs as a result of the action of the right inferior oblique muscle (Fig. 167-6, *B*). In addition, in down gaze a large esotropia is typical, resulting from an absence of the abduction function of both superior oblique muscles.

In unilateral superior oblique muscle palsies, the unopposed excyclotorsion action of the inferior oblique muscle causes the affected eye to rotate outward. In an attempt to obtain and maintain fusion, a head tilt toward the opposite side from the palsied muscle results in normal ocular alignment, and fusion may be normal (Fig. 167-7). When the patient's head is straightened, the torsional action of the synergistic incycloductor (superior rectus muscle) results in an upward drift (hypertropia) of the affected eye, which is exaggerated by tilting of the head to the side opposite the naturally occurring head tilt. For example, a patient who has a right superior oblique muscle palsy usually will have a left head tilt to overcome the excyclotorsion of the right eye. On forced right head tilt, a large right hypertropia typically becomes obvious. Any patient who has torticollis should be evaluated for the presence of ocular torticollis, inasmuch as patients unwittingly may be subjected to such unnecessary treatments as physical therapy and braces for presumed nonocular torticollis. If any doubt exists about a possible superior oblique muscle palsy, the patient should be referred to a pediatric ophthalmologist for further evaluation.

Dissociated Vertical Deviations

Dissociated vertical deviations (DVDs), also termed *alternating hyperphorias* or *double dissociated hyperphorias,* typically are seen in patients who have infantile esotropia, even if strabismus surgery has been successful in obtaining normal horizontal ocular alignment. DVDs are characterized by an alternating upward deviation of first one eye and then the other on alternate cover testing. Occasionally, excycloduction may be noted with a lateral deviation of the eye on its upward movement. The exact cause of DVD is unknown, but both superior rectus and inferior oblique muscle dysfunctions have been implicated. In most patients the deviation is only a clinical curiosity; unless spontaneously present, surgery rarely is indicated. When surgery is indicated, even for unilateral DVDs, bilateral superior rectus muscle recessions usually are performed to prevent the "unmasking" of a bilateral DVD.

Miscellaneous Vertical and Cyclovertical Deviations

Other deviations that may be seen in the pediatrician's office include generalized or isolated congenital fibrosis syndromes, inferior oblique muscle palsies, dysthyroid orbitopathy, double elevator palsies, third nerve palsies, Brown syndrome, double depressor palsies, or inferior rectus muscle restriction or fibrosis secondary to orbital floor fractures. These entities all are unusual, the descriptions of which can be found in any text on pediatric ophthalmology or strabismus.

REFERENCES

1. Knox RL, Clark DB, Schuster FF: Benign VI nerve palsies in children, *Pediatrics* 40:560, 1967.
2. Werner DB, Savino PJ, Schatz NJ: Benign recurrent 6th nerve palsies in children, *Arch Ophthalmol* 101:607, 1983.

SUGGESTED READINGS

Ernest JT, Costenbader FD: Lateral rectus muscle palsy, *Am J Ophthalmol* 65:721, 1968.

Harley RD: Paralytic strabismus in children, *Ophthalmol* 87:24, 1980.

Khawam E, Scott AB, Jampolsky A: Acquired superior oblique palsy, *Arch Ophthalmol* 88:761, 1967.

Kodsi SR, Younge BR: Acquired oculomotor, trochlear, and abducent cranial nerve palsies in pediatric patients, *Am J Ophthalmol* 114:568, 1992.

Nelson LB et al: Congenital esotropia, *Surv Ophthalmol* 31:363, 1987.

Nelson LB: Strabismus disorders. In: Nelson LB, Calhoun JH, Harley RD, editors: *Pediatric ophthalmology* ed 3, Philadelphia, 1991, WB Saunders.

Rubin SE, Wagner RS: Ocular torticollis, *Surv Ophthalmol* 30:366, 1986.

von Noorden GK: Cyclovertical deviations. In *Binocular vision and ocular motility: theory and management of strabismus,* ed 4, St. Louis, 1990, Mosby.

von Noorden GK: Esodeviations. In *Binocular vision and ocular motility: theory and management of strabismus,* ed 4, St. Louis, 1990, Mosby.

von Noorden GK: Exodeviations. In *Binocular vision and ocular motility: theory and management of strabismus,* ed 4, St. Louis, 1990, Mosby.

von Noorden GK: Paralytic Strabismus. In *Binocular vision and ocular motility: theory and management of strabismus,* ed 4, St. Louis, 1990, Mosby.

von Noorden GK: Special forms of strabismus. In *Binocular vision and ocular motility: theory and management of strabismus,* ed 4, St. Louis, 1990, Mosby.

168 Strange Behavior

Lois T. Flaherty

Strange behavior is a relatively unusual presenting problem, but one that may be indicative of serious psychopathology. In a large national survey using the Child Behavior Checklist, Achenbach[1] found that parents endorsed the item "strange behavior" for only 15% of girls and 18% of boys who had received mental health services; among children who had not received mental health services, only 1% to 2% were identified by their parents to exhibit strange behavior. Thus this item was a relatively strong discriminator between clinically and nonclinically identified youngsters but was a relatively infrequent problem even among those enrolled in mental health clinics.[1]

Although not a precise term, *strange* usually is the word used to describe behavior that (1) is socially inappropriate, that is, does not conform to that expected in a given situation, and (2) is not understandable in its context. The boy at nursery school, for example, who suddenly, with no apparent provocation, bites or kicks the child standing next to him will be seen as "strange." The young adolescent girl who goes to school garishly made up (by standards of her age mates), in a misguided attempt to beautify herself, certainly will be considered "weird" by her peers. The school-age child who, evidently misinterpreting a friendly "hello" across the backyard fence, shouts back "shut up!" will have a reputation as being odd, to say the least.

Another way of understanding the labeling of behavior as strange is that it reflects a sense of confusion on the part of the observer, which in turn is related to something about the child that does not make sense. The human organism, probably from fetal life onward, is engaged in a constant struggle to impose organization and structure on sensory inputs—in other words, to give meaning to experience. The process by which this occurs involves classification, integration, and storage of information received through sensory channels. Infants and young children are assisted in this process by their parents, with whom they become involved very early in complicated communication processes and who act as modulators of sensory inputs. Defects in children's cerebral integrative functioning, their sensory apparatus, their ability to communicate, or the care they receive can result in impairment of this process by which the child gradually makes sense of his or her world. As a result the child, to some degree, experiences fragmentation, disorganization, and chaos, which he or she continues to struggle to overcome. From an early age, this child will have difficulty coping with most, if not all, of the major developmental tasks that must be mastered by all children if they are to grow into emotional maturity. The behavior of such a child, reflective of the child's own confusion, appears strange and confusing to others.

These children are considered to have *pervasive developmental disorders.* [2] Although experts in the field disagree over the use of this term, it refers to a category of disorders that are characterized by severe impairment in social interaction, communication, and thinking; it includes disorders that in the past were termed *autism, childhood psychosis, atypical development,* and *borderline states.* Once considered to be the result primarily of faulty parenting, these disorders now are recognized to involve serious deficits in neurobiological functioning, which in turn interferes with many aspects of social, emotional, and cognitive development. No specific locus of abnormality has been found in the brain, and possibly, similar clinical manifestations could result from different kinds of central nervous system abnormalities. Children who have pervasive developmental disorders frequently have "soft" neurological signs, and abnormal findings on computed tomography (CT) scans have been found in some.

Fortunately, the number of such children is small. Although the prevalence of severe emotional disturbance among children in the general population has been estimated to be 2% to 5%, the majority of them are neither autistic nor psychotic. Various epidemiological studies consistently have placed the prevalence of autism at about 4:10,000[3]; the prevalence of other pervasive developmental disorders is not as easy to pinpoint because diagnosis is less reliable, but it probably is similar. For comparison, the prevalence of schizophrenia, an illness that affects adults predominantly, is about 1% of the population.

STRANGE BEHAVIOR IN YOUNG CHILDREN

Autism

Of all "strange" children, those who are autistic probably are the most strange. The syndrome of early infantile autism originally was described by Kanner[5] in 1943 on the basis of his experience with 11 cases; this description still stands as a model of careful clinical observation.

The most striking feature of autistic children is the disturbance in their ability to relate to others. They often appear aloof and uninterested in people, preferring inanimate objects. They may avoid eye contact. A concomitant deficit is in communication, both verbal and nonverbal. Some do not acquire speech at all, and those who do tend not to use it to communicate. A variety of speech and language abnormalities have been described, the most common of which are echolalia (rote repetition of what is heard) and pronominal reversal (the use of "you" for "I," for example). Another major deficit is the inability to think flexibly and imaginatively, thought to be related to a basic deficit in conceptualization. This commonly is manifested in a lack of imaginative play. An autistic child may stack blocks repetitively but not *build* anything. Autistic children frequently display poor coordination and motor abnormalities, such as hand flapping, twirling, or head banging, although these are not diagnostic because they occur in other conditions. About 60% have concomitant mental retardation. Autism is three to four times as common in boys as in girls. A variety of metabolic, genetic, and infectious conditions that result in central nervous system damage or dysfunction have been found in association with autism. These have included maternal rubella, untreated phenylketonuria, tuberous sclerosis, perinatal anoxia, encephalitis, infantile spasms, and fragile X syndrome. It now is recognized that in addition to "classic autism," a spectrum of disorders falls within this diagnostic category, and autistic children vary considerably in their functioning.

Recent research has supported the notion that autism is a spectrum of disorders that may have multiple causes. In its most typical form, it includes abnormal verbal and nonverbal communication, aloofness, impaired social skills, and sensory disturbances. Subgroups have been described who are moderately to severely retarded, as well as those who are higher functioning, overactive, and aggressive. Of particular interest is another subgroup who is socially and linguistically impaired and has restricted interests. The latter group tends to have family members who have learning disabilities. The degree of social impairment tends to be related to IQ. A combination of a higher IQ, together with a lack of empathy, overactivity, and impulsiveness, produces a tendency for these children to be quick to strike out at others to meet self-directed needs, with the result that they appear violent and aggressive and can be difficult to manage. The finding of birth complications, such as being limp or needing resuscitation, is consistent among the most retarded group, whereas a family history of learning problems is least prevalent in this group.[3]

Current treatment of autism and related disorders primarily involves special educational approaches; supportive counseling to families is extremely important.[8] Psychotropic medications sometimes are helpful in controlling aggressive behavior and improving learning, but their usefulness is fairly limited (see Chapter 88, Psychosis, for further discussion of infantile autism).

OTHER PERVASIVE DEVELOPMENTAL DISORDERS

Many of the children who often are described as strange have disorders that are more difficult to diagnose. Unlike the autistic child, who usually shows developmental abnormalities in infancy, their development in the neonatal period and infancy may be described as normal. Somewhere between the second and third year of life they undergo what apparently is a dramatic change, and their developmental progression ceases. They not only fail to acquire new functions but also may lose those previously acquired, such as language or bowel and bladder control. These children may develop some of the features of autistic children, such as engaging in isolated, repetitive play, avoiding eye contact, and being obsessively preoccupied with sameness. They lack self-control and frequently have uncontrolled outbursts of aggressive behavior toward others, as well as severe temper tantrums. Unlike autistic children, these children are extremely attached to their parents—they cling and are overly dependent. They are extremely prone to anxiety and often may not be able to tolerate any separation from their parents, or they may fly into a panic over the appearance of strangers, darkness, or loud noises. Thus, although these children have a better ability than autistic children to form attachments, they have not been able to master the basic developmental tasks of early childhood. Instead of striving for independence like the normal toddler, they fear it. They have been described as resembling toddlers whose parents are perpetually out of the room.[4]

All children regress at times, and most children have fears, temper tantrums, and displays of aggression. What is different about these children is the intensity and prevalence of their disturbed behavior. Their aggression toward another child, for example, involves more than the occasional shove, slap, or bite, and it may be seriously hurtful. Rather than simply having one fear, they have many, and the fears are only part of the whole spectrum of disturbed behavior.

Many of these children are grossly confused about reality and lack a concept of themselves as distinct from others, often confusing their own thoughts with those of others. They may believe, for instance, that they are about to be attacked by another child, when in reality their *own* anger toward the other is the problem. They tend to be totally preoccupied with trying to protect themselves from what they perceive to be menacing forces all around them, which in reality are their own uncontrolled fantasies and feelings. One child, for example, when asked to draw a person, drew a large stomach, reflecting a preoccupation with eating and being eaten.

Others of this group are in better touch with reality but have only a limited ability to control their own thoughts, feelings, and behavior; they readily become overwhelmed. Typically, children in this group tend to improve with appropriate handling and become dramatically worse with adverse changes in the environment. Placement in a special therapeutic nursery school, for example, may result in a marked improvement in the child's functioning, whereas parental separation may have disastrous effects.

For the severely emotionally disturbed child, a variety of mental health and educational approaches are involved in management. These may range from outpatient psychiatric treatment to inpatient or residential treatment in special facilities. Often special school placement in a class for emotionally handicapped children is also required. Pediatricians can help families of such children by familiarizing themselves with the resources available in their area and assisting families in finding needed services, as well as supporting and encouraging families to help them persevere in an often discouraging task.

The use of psychotropic medications, including the major tranquilizers, has been of some help in decreasing the extreme anxiety and out-of-control behavior of these youngsters, but they should be prescribed for children only by someone who has extensive experience with their use, usually a child psychiatrist.

The diagnosis of childhood schizophrenia and whether it should be considered one of the pervasive developmental disorders is controversial.[6] The diagnosis can be problematical, particularly in young children, whose intellectual functioning is not yet sophisticated enough for them to form organized delusions and paranoid thinking, although they show the disorganized thought processes and severe impairment in functioning that are characteristic of the adult forms of this disorder, and they may hallucinate. Similar to the adult form, the onset in some cases is gradual and insidious and in other cases acute. The older the child the more likely the disorder is to resemble schizophrenia in adults (see Chapter 88, Psychosis).

OTHER CONDITIONS THAT MAY BE ASSOCIATED WITH STRANGE BEHAVIOR

Many other conditions may be associated with strange behavior in children and will occur far more commonly in pediatric practice than those already discussed. These include the following:

1. Organic brain syndromes, including degenerative neurological disorders, psychomotor disturbances, and petit mal epilepsy
2. Mental retardation
3. Sensory deficits (e.g., deafness and blindness)
4. Speech and language disorders
5. Learning disabilities
6. Child abuse and neglect
7. Underlying chronic illness characterized by failure to thrive (e.g., celiac syndrome and cystic fibrosis)

In addition to the organic conditions previously noted to be associated with autism, various degenerative neurological disorders can manifest clinically as pervasive developmental disorders. Psychomotor seizures and the staring spells of children who have petit mal epilepsy may be mistaken for signs of emotional disorder.

Metabolic disorders often are associated with behavioral disturbances and developmental delays; these children should be screened for inborn errors of metabolism. Occasionally, children found to have celiac disease have autistic features; however, what seems to be emotional withdrawal actually is caused by severe cachexia.

Mentally retarded children frequently manifest behavioral disturbances. Often what is described as strange simply is behavior that is inappropriate for the child's chronological age, although it is not necessarily so when one considers mental age—for example, playing with feces by a 6-year-old child who has a mental age of 2 years. On the other hand, the prevalence of behavior disorders and emotional disturbances (including psychoses and autism) is greater among this population than among children of normal intelligence. Many of the children who meet all the criteria for autism also are retarded. If one understands both psychoses and mental retardation as developmental disturbances involving delays in cognitive functioning, it is possible to see that they may coexist within the same child.

Congenitally deaf or blind children may show autistic features as a result of their sensory deficits, which hamper communication and reduce stimulation.

Impairment in the child's ability to communicate, associated with hearing or visual impairment or speech and language disorders, inevitably will cause some difficulty in responding to normal social situations. The more severe the child's sensory or language deficit, the more bizarre his or her behavior may seem.

Increasingly it has been recognized that learning-disabled children frequently have difficulty understanding and responding to social cues because of their problems in processing information. Therefore their behavior in social situations may be inappropriate. Although these children are not as impaired as those who have pervasive developmental disorders, they often are notably handicapped socially. An interesting type of learning disability, termed nonverbal learning disability (NVLD), thought to be related to right hemisphere brain dysfunction, has been described. Individuals who have this syndrome have higher verbal than nonverbal abilities and deficits in social nonverbal communication and visual perception. They have difficulty handling novel situations and thus often appear strange and awkward—"autistic-like." They often are good readers but lack commensurate comprehension.[7] A relationship between this syndrome and attention deficit/hyperactivity disorder has been postulated. Its relationship to autism is not clear.

Children who have been the victims of neglect or abuse may show autistic or psychotic-like behavior. These children usually improve, often dramatically, on removal from their homes and placement in a good residential treatment facility or foster home. In some cases, several months to a year may be necessary before change is noticed. Their deficits result from failure of their environment to provide the necessary stimulation and nurturance, rather than from any intrinsic deficits in the child. These children can be understood best as reacting to extreme degrees of psychological stress (see Chapter 56, Child Abuse and Neglect).

The emotionally disturbed parent may have a distorted view of his or her child and describe the child as strange. In extreme cases this may involve misinterpreting normal child behavior as deviant. A psychotic parent, for example, may see a child as "possessed by the devil." Abusive parents typically ascribe malevolent meanings to their children's actions. For example, an infant's fussiness may be interpreted as "meanness" or a toddler's hyperactivity as being "out to get" the parent. In both cases the parent is attributing something to the child that is, in fact, an anxious preoccupation of the parent's own mind.

STRANGE BEHAVIOR IN ADOLESCENTS

Psychotic disorders, including schizophrenia and manic-depressive disorder, may appear for the first time during adolescence and can be manifested by changes in behavior and appearance. Adolescents' strange behavior mainly may be in the eye of the beholder; in the assessment of adolescents, in particular, one may encounter dress and hair styles that appear strange. These are the adolescent's way of establishing an identity distinct from that of his parents as well as from his childhood identity. Teenage fads in dress and hairstyles offer a relatively superficial and symbolic way of taking a stand against the adult world, allowing the teenager to continue to hold the more essential values, such as succeeding in school. Indeed, families of healthy adolescents are more likely to argue about these things than they are about whether the teenager works at getting good grades or plans to attend college. Adolescents who truly are disturbed often appear bizarre to their peers as well as to adults. To distinguish psychotic disorders from other severe kinds of psychopathology in adolescence is difficult because disturbed adolescents often are uncommunicative. Disturbed adolescents can be differentiated from normal adolescents, however.

EVALUATION OF THE CHILD WHO EXHIBITS STRANGE BEHAVIOR

Although what identifies a child's behavior as strange usually is its failure to conform to social expectations, together with its confusing nature, the evaluation of strange behavior involves an assessment of the child's developmental status and overall level of functioning.

The first task of the pediatrician is to ascertain the accuracy of the description given of the child. Although the parents' description may be exaggerated, one should never dismiss it without attempting to verify it through collateral sources of information. If the child is in a school or day care program or otherwise comes in contact with adults outside the home, this task is simplified. The first step should be to inquire about the setting in which the behavior occurs, the usual reactions of those around the child, and the child's responses to these. As a rule, the more disturbed the child, the more ubiquitous the behavior. One should keep in mind that unless the child clearly is autistic or psychotic, observations made in the clinic or office can be misleading. The child who has violent temper tantrums at home and is described as socially isolated and withdrawn is unlikely to have a tantrum in the pediatrician's office, and his or her poor capacity for social interaction may not be obvious, given a situation that engenders anxiety and reticence in normal children; in some cases, abnormalities in psychological functioning will be apparent only in evaluations by specialists.

The reactions of the child's age mates are a particularly sensitive barometer. Adults may be willing to overlook minor degrees of social ineptness among children, but other children are not. The child who is even a bit strange frequently will be physically avoided by other children in nursery school and later on often will be labeled as weird and treated as a social outcast by school-age peers, so harsh are the standards of child society. Adolescents who are borderline or psychotic often appear bizarre to their peers as well, so learning from the school how the patient appears to function with peers provides important diagnostic information.

The evaluation of the child who exhibits strange behavior is outlined in Table 168-1. It should address each of the essential components of the process by which children make sense of their environment. Referral to a special diagnostic clinic within a medical school is one way to facilitate the evaluation, which often necessitates involving several specialists. Another approach is for the pediatrician to refer the child for psychiatric evaluation and psychological testing and, on the basis of these evaluations, determine whether an additional speech and language evaluation is in order (see Chapters 13, The Art of Consultation, and 93, Consultation and Referral for Behavioral and Developmental Problems).

Evaluation of the *sensory apparatus* includes testing hearing and vision. The *capacity to store, classify, and integrate information* can be assessed through various tests of cognitive functioning. The standard intelligence tests, such as the WISC-R and Stanford-Binet, are helpful, as are more specialized tests designed to identify difficulties with auditory or visual processing (see Chapter 20, Screening). The *ability to communicate* is evaluated through a speech and language assessment. The *caregiving environment* is assessed on the basis of information obtained from parents and others as part of the *developmental and social history,* as well as by direct observation of the caregivers and their interactions with the child. Finally, the *psychiatric interview with the child* includes careful observations of the child's behavior, thinking patterns, capacity for relationships, and methods of coping with stress. The synthesis of all available information about the child and family then can be used to arrive at an integrated view of the child's functioning and an assessment of the degree and nature of the psychopathological condition present. To promote this synthesis, the pediatrician should meet with the other specialists who have evaluated the child.

In addition to recognizing that emotional disturbance in parents may lead to misperceptions of normal child behavior, the pediatrician should be equally aware that the disturbed child has a major and often devastating impact on the family's functioning; what may appear to be distortions in the parent-child relationship may in reality be the result of the parents' reaction to the child's emotional disturbance. Autistic and psychotic children, in particular, place an extraordinary burden on families. Typically, families are confused and frustrated in their attempts to manage the child. Focusing only on the parents' apparent psychopathological condition can blind one to the extent of an emotional disturbance in the child.

Table 168-1 Evaluation of the Child Who Exhibits Strange Behavior

Diagnostic procedure	Entity identified	Primary specialist involved
Developmental history	Developmental delays	Pediatrician
Complete psychosocial history	Problem with child's social and emotional adjustment, family functioning, parent-child relationship	Pediatrician
Physical examination	Growth failure secondary to underlying chronic illness	Pediatrician
Hearing and vision screening	Hearing or visual deficits	Pediatrician
Urinary metabolic screening	Inborn errors of metabolism	Pediatrician
Psychiatric evaluation	Psychiatric disorder	Child psychiatrist
Neurological evaluation	Degenerative conditions, brain lesions	Pediatric neurologist
Psychological testing	Abnormalities of cognitive functioning	Child psychologist
Speech and language evaluation	Speech and language disorders	Speech and language specialist

During the overall physical examination, the pediatrician always should do a neurological examination, including an assessment for "soft" neurological signs. If a pervasive developmental disorder is suspected, urinary metabolic screening should be undertaken. Because of the likelihood of Rett syndrome, chromosomal studies are indicated in girls who show features of autism. Although abnormal findings on a CT scan and an electroencephalogram (EEG) have been found among children who have pervasive developmental disorders, they are not diagnostic and should be obtained only if a degenerative neurological disorder or space-occupying lesion is suspected.

TREATMENT

Treatment obviously needs to be determined by the physician's understanding of the type of disorder involved. In the various kinds of developmental disorders, and in those resulting from sensory or cognitive impairments, treatment is aimed at maximizing functioning and teaching skills that will enable the child to be as self-sufficient as possible. These children's needs are complex and require multipronged treatment that includes special education, help in language development, and emotional support for themselves and their parents.[8] Most children who are autistic or have other pervasive developmental disorders are able to be managed at home with appropriate special educational placement and family support. A comprehensive school program that emphasizes structure and behavioral methods is important, and a very high level of individual attention often is necessary. As the child progresses through adolescence, training in skills that will allow for as much independent functioning as possible should be emphasized. Used judiciously, drug treatment can help in some cases to reduce dangerous or extremely bothersome behaviors, such as self-injurious behavior, aggression toward others, or extreme temper tantrums.[2] The drugs used most commonly are the neuroleptic agents, such as haloperidol or thioridazine. These drugs, which possibly have serious side effects such as tardive dyskinesia, may impair the child's ability to learn; they should be used cautiously and prescribed only by a physician experienced in their use. Newer antipsychotic drugs, such as clozapine and risperidone, that offer the promise of improved efficacy and fewer side effects have been shown to be effective in adults, but experience with them in children and adolescents is limited.

Psychotherapy can help learning disabled children who suffer social handicaps by giving them a better understanding of their handicaps and helping them to develop compensatory strategies.

The importance of emotional support and guidance for parents cannot be overemphasized. The pediatrician is likely to be the professional who has the most long-term relationship with the child and family and is in an excellent position to provide such support. The pediatrician can interpret the findings and recommendations of other specialists to the parents and guide them in the difficult and often frustrating task of obtaining necessary services for their child. In recent years, support and advocacy groups for parents of mentally ill children have developed; such groups also can be extremely helpful.

Awareness of any distorted parental perceptions should lead the pediatrician to intervene immediately to prevent the pathological influences from affecting the child irreparably. The pediatrician's task, after listening carefully, is to empathize with how difficult things must be for this parent and gently, but directly, suggest that it would be helpful to have someone to talk to in more depth about these problems. If one simply attempts to convince the parent that nothing is wrong with the child, one almost guarantees that the parent will continue in his or her belief and seek confirmation of his or her opinions elsewhere.

OUTCOME

Outcome in the pervasive developmental disorders is variable, which should not be surprising given the heterogeneity of these disorders. Outcome has been studied most in autism, which also is the entity of the group most clearly defined. Outcomes have been reported that range from good to very good (5% to 18%), fair (16% to 27%), and poor (60% to 75%). Children who have higher intellectual functioning tend to do better; outcome is poor if they fail to develop speech by the age of 6 years. Unfortunately, no long-term controlled studies reveal the impact of various kinds of interventions. In general, children who have pervasive developmental disorders require intensive supportive services throughout childhood and adolescence and into adulthood. Although children who function at a higher level than most and some children who have otherwise pervasive developmental disorders may attain economic self-sufficiency, the majority do not.

The outcome of schizophrenia in adolescence can best be described as bimodal, with an equal distribution of good and poor outcomes. Outcome is predicted by several features, including premorbid functioning, presence of schizophrenic relatives, and others.

SUMMARY

Strange behavior may be the manifestation of a variety of different entities, ranging from severe psychiatric disorders to behavioral responses to abuse and neglect. Strange behavior resulting from so many causes underscores the importance of understanding the context in which the behavior occurs, the social environment of the child, and the child's own thoughts and feelings. A careful and comprehensive evaluation is necessary in all cases. Treatment, likewise, needs to be comprehensive and address the complex needs of the child and the family.

REFERENCES

1. Achenbach TM: *Manual for the child behavior checklist: 4-18 and 1991 profile*, Burlington, Vt, 1991, University of Vermont Dept of Psychiatry.
2. American Psychiatric Association: *Diagnostic and statistical manual of mental disorders*, ed 4, Washington, DC, 1994, The Association.
3. Eaves LC, Ho HH, Eaves DM: Subtypes of autism by cluster analysis, *J Autism Dev Disord* 24:3, 1994.
4. Frijling-Schreuder ECM: Borderline states in children, *Psychoanal Study Child* 24:307, 1969.
5. Kanner L: Autistic disturbances of affective contact, *Nerv Child* 2:217, 1943.

6. Kestenbaum CJ, Canino IA, Pleak RR: Schizophrenic disorders of childhood and adolescence. In Tasman A, Hales RE, Frances AJ, editors: *American Psychiatric Press review of psychiatry,* vol 8, Washington, DC, 1989, American Psychiatric Press.
7. Semrud-Clikeman M, Hynd G: Right hemisphere dysfunction in nonverbal learning disabilities: social, academic and adaptive functioning in adults and children, *Psychol Bull* 107:196, 1990.
8. Volkmar FR: Autism and the pervasive developmental disorders. In Lewis M, editor: *Child and adolescent psychiatry: a comprehensive textbook,* Baltimore, 1991, Williams & Wilkins.

SUGGESTED READINGS

Cohen DJ: Child and adolescent mental health: neurobiological and social knowledge and their application for children and families, *Bull N Y Acad Med* 65:381, 1989.

169 Stridor

Morton E. Salomon

Stridor is a high pitched crowing respiratory noise caused by partial obstruction of the large airways at the level of the pharynx, larynx, or trachea. Stridor commonly is heard on inspiration, but may be heard on expiration or on both inspiration and expiration *(biphasic stridor),* if the obstructive lesion is more distal.[8,9,12]

Stridor must be differentiated from *stertor,* a noisy heavy snoring-type breathing heard during inspiration as a result of obstruction at the level of the nose, nasopharynx, or oropharynx. One also must distinguish stridor and stertor from wheezing. *Wheezing* is a high pitched musical whistling sound generally associated with prolongation of exhalation.[12]

Although stridor can be a manifestation of a benign, static, and self-limited condition, it also can herald a rapidly progressive deterioration in ventilation leading to complete airway obstruction. Therefore a patient who has stridor requires prompt attention so that the degree of airway compromise can be assessed and its etiology determined.

PATHOPHYSIOLOGY

Stridor is produced by turbulence of air flow in the large airways. During inspiration, pressure gradients in the extrathoracic airway favor narrowing of the lumen because intraluminal pressure becomes slightly lower than atmospheric pressure. During expiration intraluminal pressure is greater than extraluminal pressure and the airway dilates. More distally, in the intrathoracic airway the situation reverses itself and the airway tends to narrow during exhalation.[9]

These transmural gradients normally are not significant clinically. However, the airways of infants and young children are narrow in diameter and have a soft cartilaginous superstructure. Therefore the pediatric airway can experience air flow turbulence even with small degrees of edema, inflammation, mucus accumulation, or anatomical protuberances; for this reason stridor is a common pediatric phenomenon.

APPROACH TO DIAGNOSIS

As the boxes on pages 1123 and 1124 demonstrate, numerous diagnostic entities cause stertor and stridor. How one approaches the diagnostic evaluation depends on the condition of the child at presentation. With the patient who has severe airway compromise, characterized by retractions, nasal flaring, diminished air entry, pallor or cyanosis, and change of mental status, airway maintenance takes precedence over diagnostic evaluation. Attention is directed toward controlling the airway, ventilating the patient, and relieving obstruction. Under these circumstances most diagnostic maneuvers, including blood drawing, could compromise the integrity of the airway even further and should be postponed. On the other hand, in the uncompromised child whose obstruction does not seem life threatening, one can proceed with an orderly, thorough diagnostic investigation on an outpatient basis. But even in this situation diagnosis must be prompt, since some pathological entities—for example, hemangiomas or papillomas—can progress to obstruction rapidly. (For a more detailed discussion of the management of acute airway obstruction, see Chapter 271, Airway Obstruction.)

For the child who has a single episode of acute stridor the diagnosis might be obvious, and evaluation can stop with a history and physical examination. But for the patient who has congenital or continuous or frequently recurrent stridor, a more thorough investigation is warranted. In these situations one follows the history and physical examination by radiographic studies—both plain films and specialized procedures—and fiberoptic laryngoscopy and, possibly, bronchoscopy.

History

In evaluating stridor two aspects of the patient's history are key to the diagnosis: age of onset and chronicity. Stridor, as well as other manifestations of airway problems that present postnatally, usually indicates the presence of a congenital anatomical abnormality of the upper airway. Symptomatology within hours of birth most likely is caused by choanal atresia, bilateral vocal cord paralysis, or a large laryngeal web or cyst. On the other hand, stridor that presents at several days to weeks of life usually is caused by laryngomalacia, an external vascular compression of the trachea (a ring or sling), or a subglottic hemangioma. Subglottic stenosis—either congenital or acquired—often will not be evident until the infant develops his or her first respiratory illness, and thus usually is diagnosed as viral croup.

Acute Stridor. Stridor that has been present for only a few hours to a few days is significantly more common than chronic stridor in the pediatric practice, and the cause often is readily apparent. A single episode of acute stridor usually is caused by an infectious process. It is estimated that 80% of all cases of stridor are caused by an airway infection. When one looks at these infectious episodes, laryngotracheobronchitis (viral croup) accounts for approximately 90% of all airway infections in the infant and child.[9] In addition to laryngotracheobronchitis (LTB), one also must consider supraglottitis (epiglottitis), bacterial tracheitis, and retropharyngeal abscess. The only fairly common *noninfectious* cause of acute stridor is foreign body of the airway or the esophagus. Of course the practitioner must be aware that recurrent episodes of crouplike illnesses might mean that the child has an underlying anatomical abnormality of the airway such as subglottic stenosis or hemangioma.[12]

Chronic Stridor. Stridor present for weeks to months or frequently recurrent episodes of stridor is a less common prob-

CAUSES OF ACUTE STRIDOR IN PEDIATRIC PATIENTS

Infectious

Laryngotracheobronchitis (croup)
Epiglottitis
Bacterial tracheitis
Retropharyngeal abscess
Peritonsillar abscess
Severe adenotonsillitis (infectious mononucleosis)
Ludwig angina
Diphtheria
Membraneous croup

Immune-mediated

Anaphylaxis
Angioneurotic edema

Trauma

Foreign body (in larynx, trachea, or esophagus)
Laryngeal fracture
Cricoarytenoid dislocation
Hematoma
Caustic ingestion
Thermal/inhalation injury

Metabolic

Hypocalcemia (vocal cord tetany)
Biotinidase deficiency

lem in pediatric practice and presents a diagnostic challenge because the possibilities are much more numerous and less obvious (see the box on p. 1124). Chronic or recurrent stridor generally indicates a fixed anatomical obstruction. In the young child this usually is congenital, but in the older child one must consider acquired conditions as well.

The perinatal history is another aspect of the patient's history that is useful in the evaluation of stridor. Children who have congenital airway problems frequently will have a perinatal history of polyhydramniosis. A history of birth trauma or difficult delivery might suggest vocal cord paralysis, and a history of neonatal intubation and ventilation raises the possibility of acquired subglottic stenosis.[7]

Physical Examination

Once the degree of respiratory distress has been assessed and the airway stabilized (if necessary), the physical examination should focus on the quality of the stridorous sound. Low pitched snoring sounds on inspiration (stertor) generally denote obstruction in the nose or nasopharynx. A harsh high pitched stridor generally will point to a lesion in the supraglottic area. Inspiratory stridor is produced mostly by obstruction above the level of the glottis. Biphasic stridor usually connotes obstruction at the glottic or subglottic level. Exclusively expiratory stridor generally points to a lesion in the intrathoracic trachea.

When examining the patient it also is important to note the quality of the voice and cry. Hoarseness, aphonia, or a weak cry generally indicates a problem at the glottic level, either a glottic web or vocal cord paralysis.[1] Progressive hoarseness suggests an expanding lesion in the larynx such as a laryngeal papillomatosis or another form of neoplasm. A barking cough generally points to pathology in the subglottic and tracheal area. Pronounced drooling associated with stridor characteristically is associated with obstruction and inflammation in the oropharyngeal area and suggests epiglottitis or retropharyngeal abscess. Stridor that increases with agitation or crying probably stems from floppy airway structures and classically is associated with laryngomalacia. The position of the patient also should be noted. An infant whose stridor diminishes while in the prone position is likely to have laryngomalacia. In contrast the child who holds his or her neck in the hyperextended position might have a mass in the retropharyngeal region or an aberrant artery in the mediastinum.[1,12] Finally, stridor that increases with drinking and eating suggests a tracheal esophageal connection such as a laryngotracheal-esophageal cleft or a tracheoesophageal fistula.

The practitioner should look for evidence of trauma to the body that would suggest an injury to the larynx or neck. Cutaneous hemangiomas would raise a suspicion of a hemangioma in the larynx. Craniofacial dysmorphia should prompt the examiner to look for micrognathia and glossoptosis. Tongue size should be noted and the oropharynx gently examined for enlarged tonsils, a retropharyngeal bulge, and an enlarged epiglottis. Any child who has both stridor and concomitant meningomyelocele or hydrocephalus should be assumed to have bilateral vocal cord paralysis unless proven otherwise.[8]

Associated Signs

The simultaneous occurrence of acute stridor and wheezing in a patient presents a diagnostic challenge frequently encountered by the clinician. Undoubtedly, any patient who has stridor and wheezes may have two pathological processes occurring together, such as croup and bronchiolitis or croup and asthma. But in one unscientifically sampled hospital-based series of 25 patients presenting with both symptoms, fewer than one third of the patients fit into this dual-diagnosis category. The other two thirds had a single problem accounting for both symptoms. The two largest groups were infants who had congenital lesions of the trachea (e.g., vascular ring) and children who had foreign bodies in the esophagus or airway.[11] These authors suggest that the history was not always reliable in these cases and that a physical examination could not distinguish between patients who had single lesions and those who had dual pathology. They did point out, however, that a thorough history and physical examination supplemented by plain radiography of neck and chest established the correct diagnosis in more than 75% of the patients.[11]

Radiography

Although the patient's history, physical examination, and associated findings may suggest the location of the obstruction and even the specific anatomical diagnosis, generally radiographic, and sometimes even endoscopic studies, are necessary for confirmation. A plain radiograph of the chest and the neck, coupled with fluoroscopy or a barium esophagram, can pinpoint the cause of chronic stridor in more than half of cases.[6]

A chest radiograph should be taken in all newborns who

CAUSES OF CHRONIC/FREQUENTLY RECURRENT STRIDOR IN PEDIATRIC PATIENTS

Nasal cavity

Bilateral choanal atresia
Anterior encephalocele
Polyps
Neoplasms
Dermoid cysts

Oropharynx/nasopharynx

Craniofacial dysmorphia (micrognathia and glossoptosis; e.g., Pierre Robin and Treacher Collins syndromes)
Macroglossia (e.g., Beckwith syndrome, congenital hypothyroidism, glycogen storage disease, lingual thyroid)
Hyperplasia of the tonsils and adenoids
Thyroglossal duct cyst
Cystic hygroma

Supraglottic area

Laryngomalacia
Cysts of vallecular, epiglottis, arytenoids
Laryngeal web
Papillomatosis

Glottic and subglottic area

Vocal cord paralysis
Psychogenic stridor (paradoxical vocal cord motion)
Glottic and subglottic webs
Subglottic stenosis (congenital and acquired)
Subglottic hemangioma

Trachea

Tracheal stenosis
Tracheomalacia
Vascular rings and slings
Enlarged thyroid
Spasmodic croup

Esophagus

Esophageal atresia
Tracheal-esophageal fistula
Laryngotracheal-esophageal cleft
Gastroesophageal reflux
Achalasia

Mediastinal masses

Bronchogenic cysts
Ectopic thymus
Neoplasm
Enlarged lymph nodes

have stridor and in all older children in whom the cause of stridor is not evident immediately. Plain radiographs of the chest can reveal a mediastinal mass, external tracheal compression, or a right-sided aorta, which suggests the presence of a vascular ring.[8] One also might visualize a foreign body or infer its presence because of asymmetrical air trapping.

Anterior-posterior (AP) and lateral views of the neck can elucidate anatomical obstruction when done with the correct technique and *when the clinical situation is not critical.* The films should be taken with high-energy (high KV) exposure to emphasize soft tissue detail. The lateral view is best performed with the head slightly extended in order to view the retropharyngeal space more accurately and to avoid overinterpretation.[8,13] The AP view allows viewing of the subglottic and tracheal area and is particularly helpful in making the diagnosis of subglottic stenosis, subglottic hemangioma, and tracheal stenosis. The lateral view allows assessment of the adenoids and tonsils, the epiglottis, and the retropharyngeal profile. However, it should be noted that radiographs are not always indicated in acute stridor cases. An AP view of the neck is unnecessary to confirm the diagnosis of croup (see Chapter 273). And for the patient with epiglottitis (see Chapter 280), roentgenographic studies can be dangerous and are generally contraindicated when the diagnosis seems fairly certain.[8]

Making the diagnosis of a foreign body in the airway or esophagus is easily confirmed when that object is radiopaque. However, in the majority of cases more subtle signs are needed. In addition to unilateral air trapping seen on a regular chest radiograph, one frequently relies on forced expiratory films to establish the diagnosis. Because young children cannot perform this maneuver, one of the best approaches to the diagnosis of nonopaque foreign bodies is bilateral cross-table decubitus films of the chest. In this examination one would expect, under normal circumstances, the dependent side to have increased vascular markings. However, when the side containing a foreign body is placed in the dependent position, vascular markings are not enhanced because of the hyperinflation on that side.

Fluoroscopic evaluation of the airway also plays a role in diagnosis. It provides a dynamic view of the airway during both phases of respiration. Thus fluoroscopy can be used to confirm the diagnosis of subglottic stenosis (when suggested by an AP view of the neck) and can reveal other fixed lesions. It is particularly useful in diagnosing tracheomalacia. Fluoroscopy of the chest might reveal air trapping during exhalation, further confirming the diagnosis of bronchial foreign body.

Another radiographic study that is useful in the evaluation of airway obstruction is the barium esophogram. Although this study would not be done routinely, it is indicated if one suspects a non-radiopaque foreign body in the esophagus, a tracheoesophageal fistula, or a laryngotracheal-esophageal cleft. In the latter two instances barium can be seen being aspirated into the trachea from the esophagus. Vascular compressions are also revealed by the esophagram because they are likely to indent the esophagus as well as the trachea.[8] Computerized tomography (CT) and magnetic resonance imaging (MRI) are not routinely used in the evaluation of stridor and airway obstruction; however, they have their place in specific instances. Computerized tomography is useful for defining masses in the neck and mediastinum, whereas MRI is particularly useful in delineating vascular anomalies. In some instances MRI has obviated the need for angiography before surgical repair of aberrant vascular structures.[8,13]

Endoscopy

Whereas history, physical examination, plain radiographs of the chest and neck, and barium esophogram will define the cause of stridor in many cases—especially cases of acute stridor—endoscopy with a flexible fiberoptic laryngoscope or a rigid bronchoscope is required to reach a definitive diagnosis in most patients who have chronic/recurrent stridor.

Flexible fiberoptic laryngoscopy is a simple, safe, and well-tolerated procedure. Although some older children, especially those who are cooperative, can be examined by the heated mirror technique of indirect visualization, most are best examined using a fiberoptic scope. This scope can visualize the airway anatomy from the nasal vestibule to the glottic opening. It can be done with the patient—even an infant—in a sitting position, awake, with local topical anesthesia and little or no sedation. The technique is enhanced by a video display and recording of the examination. The flexible endoscope is introduced through both nostrils so that the nasal cavities can be examined for atresia, masses, polyps, and foreign bodies. The scope is then advanced to the nasopharynx where the adenoids, tonsils, and base of the tongue are visualized. The supraglottic area is examined next, looking for hemangiomas and other masses, webs, and evidence of laryngomalacia. Finally the examiner assesses vocal cord dynamics, noting abnormal movement or anatomical irregularities. On occasion the flexible endoscope reveals significant lesions below the vocal cords, in the subglottic area, although this area is better examined with roentgenograms and a rigid bronchoscope.[8,13]

More often than not, flexible laryngoscopy establishes the diagnosis in the evaluation of chronic stridor. However, in select cases a diagnosis cannot be determined definitively without rigid endoscopy of the esophagus and the airway below the glottis. Rigid endoscopy is the definitive procedure in airway evaluation. Not only does it allow for visualization, it also helps therapeutically. With a rigid endoscope one can biopsy lesions, drain abscesses and cysts, remove polyps, remove foreign bodies, and perform laser surgery.[13] In one study of chronic stridor 12% of patients had two or more airway lesions. Of those patients with two lesions, the majority of the lesions were below the vocal cords. Therefore one can argue that patients who have severe airway symptomatology or cyanosis should be evaluated for multiple lesions, even if one diagnosis is made by laryngoscopy.[3] The practitioner should be aware that rigid endoscopy involves general anesthesia and must be done in the operating room.

SPECIFIC DIAGNOSTIC ENTITIES

A discussion of each of the stridor-producing diagnostic entities listed in the boxes on pages 1123 and 1124 and their management is beyond the reach of this chapter. For an in-depth discussion of the management of severe acute airway obstruction, the reader is referred to Chapter 271, Airway Obstruction. The most important causes of acute airway obstruction are described in Chapters 273, Croup, 280, Epiglottitis, and 204, Foreign Bodies of the Ear, Nose, Airway, and Esophagus. Craniofacial abnormalities are discussed in Chapter 193, Cleft Lip and Cleft Palate, and other airway-obstructing abnormalities in Chapters 198, Cystic and Solid Masses of the Face and Neck, and 216, Hyperthyroidism.

Table 169-1 Etiology of Chronic Stridor in Children

Diagnosis	Frequency (%)
Laryngomalacia	45
Acquired subglottic stenosis	17
Congenital subglottic stenosis	13
Subglottic hemangioma	10
External vascular compression of trachea	6
Tracheomalacia	5
Vocal cord paralysis	3
All other diagnoses	1

Based on retrospective review of 60 hospitalized patients.[3]

One hospital-based series retrospectively reviewed 60 pediatric cases of patients admitted for chronic stridor; the most common etiologies in this series are listed in Table 169-1.[3] As this table indicates laryngomalacia is far and away the most common cause of congenital stridor in children and, along with tracheomalacia, makes up almost half of all cases of chronic stridor. Acquired and congenital subglottic stenosis occur with almost equal frequency and constitute another 30% of cases. Other common causes of chronic/recurrent stridor include subglottic hemangiomas, external vascular rings and slings, and vocal cord paralysis. The anatomy and physiology of each of these entities, as well as their diagnosis and management, are discussed briefly below. Some attention also will be directed to psychogenic stridor. Although this condition is not nearly as common as other causes of stridor, the practitioner caring for adolescent patients should be aware of it.

Laryngomalacia and Tracheomalacia

Laryngomalacia, also known as *congenital laryngeal stridor,* is the most common cause of chronic stridor in children and the most common congenital anomaly of the larynx.[8,9,13] The problem arises from a weakness in the cartilaginous support of the laryngeal structures. As a result of this anatomical immaturity the epiglottis, aryepiglottic folds, and arytenoid cartilage collapse over the glottic opening, causing inspiratory stridor. Sixty percent of patients who have laryngomalacia demonstrate symptoms within the first week of life; almost all cases are apparent by the fifth week of life. However, most authors have described "outlying" cases that are not diagnosed in infancy and do not come to recognition until childhood or adolescence.[3,10] These late-presenting cases often are associated with additional abnormalities of the respiratory tract and, in some cases, probably are acquired rather than congenital.[10] In the typical congenital case the infant's stridor is exacerbated by upper respiratory tract infection and by agitation and crying, but is relieved by prone positioning.

The prevailing understanding of laryngomalacia is that it is a benign self-limited entity that requires no intervention, generally resolves by the time the infant is 18 months old, and has no long-term sequelae. [3] Although this is true in the majority of cases, 10% to 22% of infants who have laryngomalacia will develop life-threatening respiratory compromise that requires some sort of airway intervention.[3,5,9] These patients also will have feeding difficulties and failure to thrive secondary to their airway problems. This "sicker" subset of patients will go on to require intubation during respiratory tract infections and, in many cases, tracheostomy. With or without airway intervention the laryngomalacia ultimately will resolve when the larynx matures and the cartilaginous structures become firmer. In 17% of cases symptomology will persist beyond the infant's 18-month birthday. In some congenital cases the stridor will persist up to the child's fifth birthday.[3]

The simplest and most direct way to diagnose laryngomalacia is by flexible fiberoptic laryngoscopy. It also can be diagnosed by fluoroscopy, where the examiner notes inspiratory collapse of the laryngeal structure. However, many patients—up to 68% in one series—who have laryngomalacia will have additional abnormalities of their respiratory tract. The two most common anatomical abnormalities associated with laryngomalacia are subglottic stenosis and tracheal compression by an anomalous innominate artery.[9,10] Patients with additional airway lesions are the ones most likely to have severe airway obstruction and to require medical or surgical intervention. Therefore it is sometimes necessary to go beyond flexible laryngoscopy in the evaluation of laryngomalacia and undertake bronchoscopy of the airway, especially in patients with significant obstruction.

Most patients who have laryngomalacia will not require medical intervention. For those patients who have severe airway collapse, a tracheostomy is performed. More recently, a procedure in which the aryepiglottic folds are trimmed down endoscopically has been described; this allows some patients to have their symptoms relieved without a tracheostomy.[5]

Tracheomalacia similarly is caused by floppy cartilaginous support of the trachea. Patients who have tracheomalacia typically have biphasic stridor caused by inspiratory collapse of the extrathoracic trachea and expiratory collapse of the intrathoracic trachea. Although the pathophysiology of tracheomalacia is similar to that of laryngomalacia, the two entities usually occur independently and only rarely coexist in the same patient.[1] Like laryngomalacia, tracheomalacia often can be a benign self-resolving condition that disappears in a child between 12 and 18 months of age as the cartilage becomes firmer. However, some patients who have this entity also have severe airway compromise and require surgical intervention. Diagnosis is made by fluoroscopy or more definitively by flexible or rigid endoscopy of the trachea. Those patients who have severe and unremitting airway obstruction require tracheostomy or placement of a tracheal stint to prevent collapse.[1]

Subglottic Stenosis

Subglottic stenosis is a narrowing of the larynx at the level of the cricoid cartilage, usually 2 to 3 mm below the glottic opening.[3] It can be caused by a congenital malformation or it can be acquired as a result of prolonged or especially traumatic neonatal intubation. Acquired subglottic stenosis is slightly more common than the congenital variety, but congenital stenosis often is more severe.[1]

Subglottic stenosis usually is not diagnosed until the patient is several months old. Frequently the patient will be asymptomatic until the airway is challenged by a respiratory tract infection. At this time the patient will develop respiratory distress, barking cough, and biphasic stridor and will be diagnosed as having croup. Subglottic stenosis is suspected when the croup fails to resolve or the patient develops recurrent episodes of stridor.

The diagnosis of subglottic stenosis is initially made by a high KV AP view of the neck that shows the characteristic "steeple" sign of subglottic narrowing. However, this is the same radiologic finding seen in croup (see Fig. 273-3). If the clinical course of the patient suggests a fixed lesion, the diagnosis is made definitively by bronchoscopy.

If the patient does not develop critical airway obstruction during any bout of inflammation, the child eventually will outgrow the condition as the larynx enlarges and the obstruction becomes relatively less consequential. However, some patients who have subglottic stenosis will require an emergency tracheostomy during an acute episode of inflammation and obstruction. For patients who have severe obstruction and can escape emergency tracheostomy, an anterior cricoid split can be done to widen the airway diameter. This procedure, which usually requires 10 to 14 days in the hospital, is performed so that a tracheostomy can be avoided.[13]

Subglottic Hemangioma

Congenital cavernous hemangiomas of the airway always are located in the subglottic area. Like other congenital hemangiomas airway hemangiomas grow rapidly in the first several months of life, and the patient generally becomes symptomatic at the age of 3 to 6 months. Symptoms include biphasic stridor, respiratory distress, and in more severe cases, feeding difficulties. Fifty percent of patients who have subglottic hemangiomas also have cutaneous hemangiomas, which provides a valuable clue to the diagnosis.[1,9]

The diagnosis is suggested by a lateral roentgenogram of the neck. One can often visualize larger hemangiomas by direct laryngoscopy, as they can been seen protruding below the glottic opening. However, a definitive diagnosis is made by rigid bronchoscopy, where a compressible lesion, located asymmetrically on one side of the subglottic area and covered by normal mucosa, is visualized. Biopsy is not necessary for confirmation.[1,9]

Like other hemangiomas, subglottic hemangiomas begin to regress spontaneously after the first year of life. For the patient who does not develop life-threatening airway obstruction, it therefore is possible to wait for remission; a tracheostomy is necessary in more severe cases.[13]

Vascular Rings and Slings

The trachea and/or esophagus can be compressed externally by persistent aberrant segments of the embryonic aortic arch. Although many people have anomalous vessels in their mediastinum and are asymptomatic, vascular anomalies account for 1% to 6% of all cases of congenital stridor.[3,9]

A vascular *ring* is created when the trachea and or esophagus is encircled tightly by aberrant vascular structures. The most common vascular ring is created by a double aortic arch. Rings also can arise from a right-sided aortic arch and left-sided ductus arteriosus or an anomalous right subclavian artery arising from a left aortic arch.[1,9] A vascular *sling* is created by the anterior compression of the trachea by a nonencircling anomalous vessel. Slings generally are created by anomalous innominate arteries or pulmonary arteries.[9]

The superior mediastinum of the infant is more crowded than that of a larger person and the trachea is softer; therefore the infant is most prone to respiratory symptoms from anomalous vessels. Symptoms, when present, usually begin in the neonatal period. Biphasic stridor is common and is present in 95% of symptomatic patients. Other symptoms might include feeding problems secondary to esophageal compression, expiratory wheezing, and opisthotonic posturing to relieve the tracheal compression. If left untreated these patients are prone to recurrent episodes of croup and recurrent lung infections.[1]

When suspected, diagnostic workup of a vascular compression starts with a chest radiograph to detect a right-sided aorta. A barium esophagram will reveal external compression of the esophagus and is diagnostic in 95% of cases.[2] The diagnosis is confirmed by rigid bronchoscopy, where one sees a pulsatile external indentation on the trachea. If surgery is contemplated, precise mapping of the vascular anatomy is required. Vascular anatomy is defined best by an arteriogram. However, this highly invasive procedure ultimately might be replaced by MRI.

As the trachea firms and the mediastinum enlarges, becoming less crowded, the patient who has a vascular anomaly will become less symptomatic. Tracheostomy is contraindicated in patients who have vascular anomalies. Therefore intubation is used to secure the airway. However, cardiovascular surgery is indicated for patients who have severe airway obstruction, recurrent pneumonia, or recurrent lung atelectasis. If surgical repair is undertaken early, one can expect the trachea to achieve normal configuration with growth.

Vocal Cord Paralysis

Vocal cord paralysis (VCP) can be congenital or acquired, unilateral or bilateral, benign or urgently life threatening. The paralyzed cord generally is frozen in adduction owing to paralysis of the vocal cord abductors. Unilateral VCP generally is caused by a peripheral injury to the recurrent laryngeal nerve (RLN). The RLN injury usually is caused by a cardiovascular abnormality such as an enlarged left atrium or a dilated pulmonary artery. However, RLN dysfunction also can be caused by masses in the neck or mediastinum, traction on the neck at time of delivery, or surgery on the neck, chest, or mediastinum.[1,9]

Bilateral vocal cord paralysis sometimes can be caused by bilateral RLN impingement, but more likely is due to CNS pathology. A pediatrician sees bilateral VCP most frequently in patients who have Arnold-Chiari type II malformations. Patients who have this neural tube defect will manifest stridor alone or stridor in association with dysphagia and apnea. In this setting VCP heralds the onset of brainstem compression, which must be neurosurgically alleviated or death is certain. Brain tumors, and any other cause of increased intracranial pressure, can cause caudad displacement of the brainstem and traction on the vagal nerve before it exits the skull. Vocal cord paralysis and its associated symptoms can be the first manifestation of this intracranial pathology.[12]

The patient who has VCP generally will have stridor, continuous respiratory distress, difficulty with feeding, and a weak or absent cry. Patients who have unilateral VCP, however, often have minimal respiratory distress and normal phonation.[8,9,13]

The diagnosis of VCP is made by direct fiberoptic laryngoscopy with the patient unanesthetized. The endoscopist will observe the absence of vocal cord motion during inspiration and phonation. Once the diagnosis of vocal cord paralysis is made, it is necessary to do a chest roentgenogram and barium swallow to rule out mediastinal and cardiovascular anomalies. If the paralysis is bilateral, a head CT must be performed urgently to rule out intracranial pathology. Management of the patient with vocal cord paralysis depends on the etiology and severity. Patients with bilateral VCP need a tracheostomy to preserve their airway unless they have intracranial pathology that can be immediately addressed. If the vocal cord paralysis is not reversed within 24 hours it generally becomes irreversible.[9] Unilateral VCP rarely requires tracheostomy and can be treated more temperately.

Psychogenic Stridor

The practitioner treating adolescent patients should be aware of the rare but instructive condition known as psychogenic or "functional" stridor. This condition can be seen in adolescents and adults, males and females, but occurs most often among adolescent females. In most cases it represents a true conversion reaction (see Chapter 96, Conversion Reactions in Adolescents).

A person whose stridor is psychogenic often will present having intermittent and recurrent bouts of stridor. They typically show little anxiety about their symptoms and maintain normal oxygen saturation levels. However, sometimes their stridor is so convincing that they will be intubated repeatedly.

Diagnosis generally is made at laryngoscopy. With the patient awake, the vocal cords are noted to have normal anatomy and mobility. However, there is paradoxical adduction of the false and true cords during inspiration, with normal motion or abduction on expiration.[4] These laryngoscopy findings have led some to call this condition *paradoxical vocal cord motion*.[11]

Psychogenic stridor must be diagnosed by laryngoscopy. If suspected and confirmed early, it can save the patient many unnecessary diagnostic procedures and interventions. Effective treatment can be provided by psychotherapy, which allows the patient to recognize the underlying depression and the symbolic import of their stridor.[4,11]

REFERENCES

1. Bellet PS: Stertor and stridor. In *The diagnostic approach to common symptoms and signs in infants, children and adolescents,* Philadelphia, 1989, Lea & Febiger.
2. Chun K et al: Diagnosis and management of congenital vascular rings: a 22-year experience, *Ann Thoracic Surg* 53:597, 1992.
3. Friedman EM et al: Chronic pediatric stridor: etiology and outcome, *Laryngoscope* 100:277, 1990.
4. Geist R: Diagnosis and management of psychogenic stridor caused by a conversion reaction, *Pediatrics* 86:315, 1990.

5. Jani P et al: Surgical treatment of laryngomalacia, *J Laryngol Otol* 105:1040, 1991.
6. John SD, Swischuk LE: Stridor and upper airway obstruction in infants and children, *Radiographics* 12:625, 1992.
7. Kilham H et al: Severe upper airway obstruction, *Pediatr Clin North Am* 34:1, 1987.
8. Letourneau MA et al: Respiratory disorders. In Barkin RM, editor: *Pediatric emergency medicine,* St Louis, 1992, Mosby.
9. Maze A, Bloch E: Stridor in pediatric patients, *Anesthesiology* 50:132, 1979.
10. Nussbaum E, Maggi JC: Laryngomalacia in children, *Chest* 98:942, 1990.
11. Poole SR et al: The child with simultaneous stridor and wheezing, *Pediatr Emerg Care* 6:33, 1990.
12. Ross DA, Ward PH: Central vocal cord paralysis and paresis presenting as laryngeal stridor in children, *Laryngoscope* 100:10, 1990.
13. Tunkel DE, Zalzal GH: Stridor in infants and children; ambulatory evaluation and operative diagnosis, *Clin Pediatr* 31:48, 1992.

170 Syncope

Diane L. McDonald

Syncope (fainting) is defined as a rapid, transient, complete loss of consciousness and postural tone as a result of cerebral ischemia, hypoxia, or hypoglycemia. In the pediatric population it usually occurs among older children and adolescents. In a study by Pratt and Fleisher,[2] half of the patients examined in the pediatric emergency room for fainting were diagnosed as having vasovagal syncope. Other diagnoses included orthostatic hypotension (20%), atypical seizure (7.5%), migraine (5%), and minor head trauma (5%).

Although syncope often is a benign occurrence, an effort must be made to rule out serious causes. A thorough history and physical examination must be performed, with added attention to the patient's cardiac and neurological status. If the cause of the syncopal event is cardiac, the child may be at risk for an arrhythmia or even sudden death. In addition, a child who is lethargic or unconscious is not one who has simple syncope and needs to be evaluated for an underlying disorder of the central nervous system. Therefore a child in whom cardiac disease is suspected or one who manifests impairment of consciousness after the initial event requires immediate attention and intervention.

Any available witness should be interviewed to obtain a full description of the event. Issues to be noted include the premorbid state of the child, circumstances surrounding the episode, the onset and duration of the loss of consciousness, any associated body movements, and the quality of the recovery period. Inquiry should include the circumstances precipitating the event. For example, with vasovagal syncope the child is often standing in a warm, stuffy room and is hungry, tired, or frightened. The prodrome of a seizure may consist of an aura, whereas a cardiac event often is without warning or is induced by exercise.

It is helpful to attempt to determine if the child was completely unconscious or if there was some degree of responsiveness, suggesting hysteria or malingering. A truly unconscious person will not respond if the eyelashes are lightly brushed; a hysterical person will respond, albeit often with just a mild flickering of the lids. Seizurelike movements are important; however, generalized tonic-clonic movements may be seen in all forms of syncope because of cerebral anoxia or hypoglycemia.

The duration of the episode should be estimated. In general, the conscious state is regained quickly in the case of vasovagal syncope (a few seconds to 1 or 2 minutes), whereas a seizure may last longer and the postictal state may be characterized by prolonged confusion and fatigue.

The medical history, like the history of the event, may provide significant clues to the likely cause. A history of congenital heart disease, seizure disorder, or endocrine abnormalities such as diabetes may be important. Recurrent syncopal episodes are unusual and may require more extensive testing, for example, Holter (cardiac) monitoring, echocardiographic examination, electrophysiological studies, or an electroencephalogram to uncover occult cardiac or neurological disease.

The family history may be helpful. Seizure disorders and cardiac disease leading to syncope, such as Marfan syndrome, idiopathic hypertrophic subaortic stenosis, and prolonged QT syndrome, may be inherited. Breath-holding spells also have been noted to occur more frequently in those who have such a family history.

As can be inferred from the disorder-specific descriptions that follow, particular importance should be paid during the physical examination to the cardiorespiratory systems. Murmurs, gallops, and irregular rhythms may suggest that the syncopal event is of cardiac origin. Wheezing, rales, and evidence of hypoxia suggest cardiac or respiratory disease. Attention also should be directed to the gastrointestinal tract for signs of hemorrhage or hypovolemia.

DIFFERENTIAL DIAGNOSIS

Syncope can be categorized by its various causes (see the box on p. 1130).

Neurocardiogenic Syncope

A fainting episode in which the child has been standing or sitting for a prolonged period in an uncomfortable environment suggests *vasovagal or vasodepressor syncope.* A noxious event that causes fear, pain, or anxiety also may precipitate the faint. The child may feel dizzy, weak, or nauseated and appear cold and clammy. A rapid drop in blood pressure associated with vagally stimulated bradycardia may lead to the loss of consciousness. The exact mechanism is unknown; however, it is known that the normal response to standing is a decrease in venous return to the heart. The ensuing message of hypotension to the brain results in an increase in sympathetic outflow and a consequent increase in heart rate, an increase in diastolic blood pressure, and no change in systolic blood pressure. It is believed that when patients who have vasodepressor syncope have a sudden decrease in venous return to the heart, the heart responds by increasing the force of ventricular contraction. This may send a paradoxical message of hypertension to the brain that results in decreased sympathetic output. The result is bradycardia and hypotension.[4] This response usually is short-lived and, depending on the degree of cerebral hypoperfusion, may end with tonic-clonic movements. The patient usually awakens to full consciousness within a short time.

Cyanotic breath-holding spells usually begin around the age of 6 months and end by age 6 years. Clinically the child is upset, frightened, or hurt, begins to cry, gasps, and then becomes apneic and cyanotic. Stiffening of the body and a loss of consciousness soon may follow. The pathophysiologi-

DIFFERENTIAL DIAGNOSIS OF SYNCOPE

Neurocardiogenic

- Vasovagal/vasodepressor episodes
- Breath-holding spells
  - Cyanotic
  - Pallid infantile syncope

Psychophysiological

- Hyperventilation
- Hysteria/conversion reaction

Neurological factors

- Generalized tonic-clonic seizure
- Atonic seizures
- Complex partial seizures
- Migraine
- Trauma/concussion
- Narcolepsy

Cardiac

- Structural abnormalities
  - Aortic stenosis
  - Idiopathic hypertrophic subaortic stenosis
  - Left atrial myxoma
  - Tetralogy of Fallot
  - Pulmonic stenosis
  - Primary pulmonary hypertension
- Arrhythmia
  - Bradycardia
    - Sick sinus syndrome
    - Atrioventricular block
  - Ventricular tachycardia/fibrillation
    - Myocarditis/pericarditis
    - Intoxication/medication
    - Congenital heart disease
    - Postoperative cardiac surgery
    - Prolonged QT syndrome
    - Ischemic heart disease
  - Supraventricular tachycardia
    - Wolff-Parkinson-White syndrome
    - Caffeine/stress

Orthostatic

- Hypovolemia
- Postural hypotension
- Medications

Metabolic

- Hypoglycemia
- Anemia

Miscellaneous

- Cough
- Swallowing
- Micturition
- Pregnancy

cal basis is unclear, but it may be that crying during expiration causes increased intrathoracic pressure, which in turn leads to low cardiac output. Hypoxia combined with decreased cerebral blood flow leads to the loss of consciousness. The event is brief, and afterward the child becomes fully conscious. A pallid type of breath-holding spell *(pallid infantile syncope)* is less common, although it can occur in the same age range as does the cyanotic spell and likewise may begin with pain or crying. The mechanism differs: the child suddenly becomes pale and limp and loses consciousness. The pathophysiological basis is increased vagal tone, which causes an apparent asystole. The event ordinarily lasts only seconds to minutes, and the child awakens to full consciousness.[1] (see Chapter 155, Nonconvulsive Periodic Disorders).

Psychophysiological Syncope

Hyperventilation may occur as a response to anxiety or pain. For instance, the child may hyperventilate in anticipation of venipuncture or as a reaction to fright. Rapid, short breaths cause hypocapnia and a resultant cerebral vasoconstriction and hypoperfusion. The individual experiences a feeling of lightheadedness along with numbness and tingling of the hands and feet; loss of consciousness is brief and recovery rapid.

A *conversion reaction* transforms an unacceptable unconscious desire into a physical complaint. In the older child or adolescent the conversion reaction may take the form of hysterical fainting. The child often is sitting or recumbent or may exaggerate a fall from a standing position to avoid injury. The child usually responds quickly to a mildly painful stimulus, and the physical examination reveals nothing extraordinary.

Neurological Syncope

Generalized tonic-clonic movements can occur with all forms of syncope, so the diagnosis of seizure disorder as a specific underlying cause for syncope may be difficult. Intercurrent fever or a history of seizures, head trauma, or adverse perinatal events may be helpful leads; frequently there is a family history of epilepsy.

The *generalized tonic-clonic* or *grand mal seizure* is characterized by a rather sudden onset of complete unconsciousness with stiffening of the body and rolling back of the eyes. After a tonic phase, clonic movements of the extremities may occur. Although the duration is variable, it usually lasts longer than a simple fainting spell. Incontinence is common, and the postictal recovery period is characterized by prolonged confusion and weakness.

Some *complex partial seizures* can resemble fainting episodes. Partial seizures may begin with an aura, which the child may describe as an uncomfortable feeling or an unusual visual or olfactory sensation. During the seizure the child may be unresponsive and lose postural tone. The complex partial seizure is characterized by semipurposeful yet involuntary action, for example, picking at clothing. In the postictal period the child is tired and returns to full consciousness slowly.

A *basilar artery migraine* may manifest as a syncopal event believed to result from impaired blood flow to the brainstem during the vasoconstrictive phase of migraine. After the initial spasm the affected artery dilates and a classic or common migraine occurs. A family history of migraine may help in making this diagnosis.

It is not uncommon to lose consciousness for a short time after relatively minor *head trauma* (concussion). Other symptoms such as vomiting, headache, and amnesia also may occur. Abnormal findings on neurological examination, clear drainage from the nose or ears, bleeding from the ears, a Battle sign, or a prolonged period of altered consciousness should alert the physician to the possibility of serious injury such as a subdural hematoma, basilar skull fracture, or cerebral contusion; such injuries require intervention.

Cardiac Syncope

Cardiac syncope is rare in childhood; however, when it occurs, it may be life threatening. Cardiac disease can cause syncope in a number of ways. Structural heart disease may obstruct blood flow from the left ventricle, with consequent hypoperfusion, or may shunt blood flow from right to left, leading to hypoxia. A person who has a diseased or stressed myocardium from hypoxia, myocarditis, toxic drug ingestion, or a congenital heart lesion is at risk for a sudden arrhythmia. Arrhythmias, by decreasing either the cardiac stroke volume or the heart rate, can lead to a reduced cardiac output and cerebral hypoperfusion.

Structural lesions such as *aortic stenosis* and *idiopathic hypertrophic subaortic stenosis* (IHSS) can cause dizziness or fainting after exercise. On auscultation a systolic murmur may be heard at the right sternal border. The murmur of IHSS is accentuated by a Valsalva maneuver, and the electrocardiogram shows signs of left ventricular enlargement. Children who have cyanotic congenital heart disease, in particular *tetralogy of Fallot,* may have spells of cyanosis that occasionally lead to unconsciousness. These episodes, called "tet spells," are caused by a sudden decrease in pulmonary blood flow and the shunting of deoxygenated blood from right to left through the ventricular septal defect and thence the aorta.

Bradycardia, as seen with *sick sinus syndrome,* is associated with periods of extreme sinus slowing or arrest and may require a pacemaker. Tachycardia, as with *ventricular tachycardia* and *ventricular fibrillation,* is most serious and usually is the result of severe underlying cardiac disease. *Ventricular fibrillation* also may be seen with the *prolonged QT syndrome.* The etiology of this disease is unclear; it may involve an imbalance of sympathetic cardiac innervation. Two inherited diseases characterized by a prolonged QT interval are notable. The *Jervell and Lange-Nielsen syndrome* is autosomal recessive and associated with deafness; the *Romano-Ward syndrome* occurs with normal hearing and an autosomal dominant pattern of inheritance. Sinus rates of 200 to 300 per minute are possible with *supraventricular tachycardia (SVT),* which can be associated with *Wolff-Parkinson-White syndrome.* In this circumstance an accessory pathway, the bundle of Kent, bypasses the atrioventricular node and speeds conduction from the atria to the ventricles. Stress, coffee, and drugs (e.g., amphetamines) also can cause an attack.[3]

Orthostatic Syncope

Hypovolemia from dehydration or acute blood loss can lead to *orthostatic hypotension* and syncope. Medications (e.g., diuretics, antihypertensives, and antidepressants) also can cause orthostatic blood pressure changes. In addition, *postural hypotension* can occur from rising quickly, prolonged standing, or prolonged bed rest.

Metabolic Syncope

Syncope caused by *hypoglycemia* is encountered most frequently in the young patient who has insulin-dependent diabetes. Better control, with appropriate insulin dosing and an understanding of the warning signs of hypoglycemia, may prevent further episodes. Chronic *anemia* can lead to fatigue, weakness, or a syncopal attack. A thorough search for the source of blood loss is required, and a blood transfusion may be necessary.

Miscellaneous Causes of Syncope

Cough-induced syncope has been described in patients who have the paroxysms of pertussis, laryngeal spasm, laryngeal nerve irritation, and asthma. Rarely in childhood, syncope is associated with micturition or strenuous swallowing.

Pregnancy always should be considered when a female of childbearing age faints. Pregnancy-associated fainting results from increased estrogen and progesterone levels that cause decreased peripheral vascular resistance and hypotension.

PSYCHOSOCIAL CONSIDERATIONS

The majority of benign vasovagal fainting episodes occur in places outside the home. Perhaps at school or church, for example, the child is forced to sit or stand for long periods of time but at home is more free to move about and alter body position. Thus a "faint" at home or while exercising may suggest a more serious cause, including cardiac syncope.

Atypical syncopal episodes, hysteria, or pseudoseizures may reflect "acting-out" behavior and should prompt evaluation for evidence of physical, verbal, or sexual abuse. Effort should be made to determine whether the family is subject to unusual stress, for example, marital conflict, divorce, or recent death.

MANAGEMENT

The physical examination of the syncopal patient begins with assessment of neurological status. A child who arrives unconscious or with depressed consciousness has not had a simple fainting episode and requires immediate care. If the child is alert, a careful physical examination should be performed with special attention to the cardiovascular system. The examiner should listen for murmurs, extra heart sounds, and an unusual rhythm or rate. A simple workup for a first-time fainting episode may include an electrocardiogram and determination of hematocrit, electrolyte, and glucose levels. Vital signs should be taken while the patient is upright and supine (see the box on p. 1132). The electrocardiogram should be evaluated for rhythm disturbances, chamber hyper-

WORKUP FOR THE FIRST EPISODE OF SYNCOPE

History
Physical examination
Vital signs, including orthostatic blood pressure and pulse
Electrocardiogram
Glucose level
Electrolyte levels
Hematocrit measurement
Consider:
- Pregnancy test
- Toxicology screen

Table 170-1 Relating History to Etiological Factors

History	Possible causes
Prolonged seizure activity or postictal state	Seizure disorder
Precipitation by crying	Breath-holding spell
Precipitation by cough, swallow, or urination	Cough, swallow, micturition syncope
Precipitation by exercise or a sudden onset of syncope	Cardiac syncope
Head trauma	Concussion
Precipitation by noxious event or environmental stress	Vasovagal syncope
Inconsistent findings or incomplete unconsciousness	Hysteria or malingering

trophy, abnormal voltage, and a prolonged QT segment. If an abnormality is found on cardiac examination or electrocardiogram, monitoring and cardiology consultation most often are mandated. A patient who has recurrent syncopal episodes should be evaluated for occult cardiac disease. A referral to a cardiologist for Holter monitoring, an echocardiogram, stress testing, or an electrophysiological study is indicated. Abnormalities such as a low hematocrit or blood glucose level are rare but, if present, require a vigorous search for the cause. If postprandial hypoglycemia is suspected, a glucose tolerance test may help in making the diagnosis. Children who have symptoms of obvious dehydration or abnormal orthostatic vital signs require rehydration therapy.

Frequently the results of the physical examination are normal and no abnormality is found in the initial laboratory workup. As is so often the case, the history becomes most important in establishing a cause (Table 170-1). A seizure disorder can be particularly difficult to diagnose because seizurelike activity can occur with all forms of syncope, and the electroencephalogram often does not reveal significant findings. Therefore a high index of suspicion and consultation with a neurologist may be needed.

Most other causes of syncope are benign. Reassurance and common-sense management are required. A child who has vasovagal syncope should be placed supine before venipuncture. Children who hyperventilate need to learn its relationship to fainting; attention should be paid to the reasons for hyperventilation. Breath-holding spells are best treated by educating the parents and by emphasizing the harmless nature of the spells. In severe instances a neurology consultation is warranted.

The diagnosis of hysteria or malingering may be difficult. Hospitalization for observation and a psychiatric referral may be indicated. Finally, pregnancy always should be considered in the evaluation of postpubertal female who has syncope. If there is any possibility of pregnancy or if the date of the last menstrual period is unknown, a urine or serum pregnancy test should be instituted.

Recurrent Syncope

In the past, recurrent idiopathic syncope has been a diagnosis of exclusion. Recently, head-upright tilt-table testing has become a means of provoking vasodepressor syncope in susceptible children and adults, after other more serious causes have been ruled out. Patients are placed supine on a table that has a footboard. The table then is tilted up between 60 to 80 degrees for 30 to 60 minutes. Patients are monitored closely for a syncopal episode. Some centers use low-dose intravenous isoproterenol infusions to increase the sensitivity of the test, which ranges from 30% to 80% depending on the laboratory.

Therapy includes avoiding precipitating factors, educating the patient to lie down when symptoms occur, and pharmacological treatment. Fluorocortisone, beta-adrenergic blocking agents, and transdermal scopolamine have been effective in some individuals.[4]

REFERENCES

1. Holmes GL: Breath-holding attacks in children, *Postgrad Med* 84:191, 1988.
2. Pratt JL, Fleisher GR: Syncope in children and adolescents, *Pediatr Emerg Care* B5:80, 1989.
3. Ruckman RN: Cardiac causes of syncope, *Pediatr Rev* 9:101, 1987.
4. Samiol D et al: Head-upright tilt-table testing in children with unexplained syncope, *Pediatrics* 92:426, 1993.

SUGGESTED READINGS

Anderson RH et al: *Pediatric cardiology,* Edinburgh, 1986, Churchill Livingstone.

Castor W, Skarin R, Roscelli JD: Orthostatic heart rate and arterial blood pressure changes in normovolemic children, *Pediatr Emerg Care* 1:123, 1985.

DiMario F et al: Pallid breath-holding spells, *Clin Pediatr* 29:17, 1990.

Driscoll DJ, Edwards WD: Sudden unexpected death in children and adolescents, *Am Coll Cardiol* 5:6 (suppl): 118B, 1985.

Farmer TW: *Pediatric neurology,* Philadelphia, 1983, Harper & Row.

Katz RM: Cough syncope in children with asthma, *Pediatrics* 77:48, 1970.

Woody RC, Kiel EA: Swallowing syncope in a child, *Pediatrics* 78:507, 1986.

171 Tics

John S. Werry

DEFINITION AND CLASSIFICATION

Tics are recurring, nonrhythmic, sudden, rapid, stereotyped, involuntary movements or vocalizations.[3] The muscles affected mostly are those of the head, neck, and respiratory system. Tics may be motor or vocal and simple or complex in form. The commonest simple motor tics are eyeblinking, neck-twisting, shoulder-shrugging, and grimacing; coughing, throat-clearing, sniffing, grunting, and hiccuping are the usual simple vocal tics. Complex motor tics include facial gestures, grooming of the head or hair, touching, jumping, stomping on or sniffing objects, and echokinesis (automatic imitation of another person's movements). Complex vocal tics include palilalia (repeating one's own words), echolalia (repeating the words of others), and coprolalia (uttering obscenities). Tics are exacerbated by emotion, disappear in sleep, and can be controlled to some degree, but not completely, with treatment. These characteristics are not as helpful in differential diagnosis as might be supposed because they also characterize many neurological movement disorders. Although children generally report that they are unaware of their tics, premonitory urges may occur especially in severe cases and as the child gets older.[6,7]

Motor tics are distinguishable easily from chorea (with which they often are confused) by their centripetal location, fixed repetitive form, and normal muscle tone and from most other neurologically based abnormal movements by their rapidity, fixity, and normal muscle tone. They are distinguished from self-stimulating behaviors, such as rocking, by their later onset, more restricted localization and complexity, involuntary nature, and lack of apparent pleasure associated with the movement (see Chapter 89, Self-Stimulating Behaviors). However, distinguishing these from complex motor tics may be difficult. Vocal tics often are mistaken for otolaryngological or respiratory symptoms, but other essential diagnostic characteristics of such disorders are absent.

The fourth edition of the American Psychiatric Association's *Diagnostic and Statistical Manual of Mental Disorders* (DSM-IV) describes four rather arbitrary subtypes of tic disorder: transient (duration longer than 4 weeks but less than 1 year), chronic (longer than 1 year), Tourette disorder (at least 1 year duration with less than a 3-month remission; severe, multiple tics including vocal tics but not necessarily contemporaneously), and tic disorder not otherwise specified (NOS), in which criteria of minimum duration of 4 weeks or frequency of many times a day and most every day, are not met.[3] It is not known whether these four disorders simply are more or less severe instances of the same disorder[8]; most of the recent research has been restricted to Tourette disorder. However, pedigree studies regarding Tourette disorder suggest that they probably are related somewhat.[6]

FREQUENCY

Tics can begin as early as age 2 years. Peak prevalence is between 10 and 12 years (2 to 3 years earlier for Tourette disorder), after which tics decline rapidly.[3,9] At peak they may affect from 5% to 24% of children, depending on the criteria used for diagnosis. Higher figures probably include many cases of tic disorder NOS that are short-lived and inconspicuous, because this is the commonest kind of tic disorder. Boys are affected more often than girls, especially in severe cases; the ratio is as high as three to one.[3]

ETIOLOGY

The cause of tics is unknown, but it is the focus of intensive and fascinating biobehavioral research[5-7] that shows the boundaries between psychiatry and neurology to be ill defined and increasingly obsolete. In a small number of cases tics reflect or portend a neurological disorder.[9] Such tics are likely to be much more persistent and to be accompanied by signs of the causative disorder.

Some of the factors that have been shown to be associated with tics and thus may give clues to the cause follow.[3,6,9]

1. *Developmental stage*. That tics are common in middle childhood and disappear soon after points to maturational factors in the neuromuscular apparatus mirrored in the high frequency of all spontaneous movements (such as choreiform movements) at this age.
2. *Gender*. The preponderance of boys affected also supports the motor developmental view because boys are more active motorically than girls at all ages but especially in middle childhood.[9] There is evidence that androgens may mediate this vulnerability because postnatal exposure to such hormones may elicit Tourette syndrome.[6]
3. *Prenatal, perinatal, and postnatal insults*. There is some association between tics and the same group of factors that has been proposed repeatedly for hyperactivity; as in that condition, however, this association is weak, because it has appeared only in epidemiological studies.[6,9] Nevertheless, recent studies suggest that prenatal and perinatal factors (including maternal vomiting and stress during pregnancy, fetal nutrition, and exposure to androgens) may be of more significance in Tourette syndrome.[6] Apart from drugs (see below) and a few neurological disorders, thermal stress is the only other established physical insult.[6]
4. *Psychological factors*. Anxiety is associated with tics, in that it makes existing tics worse and may precipitate them in some cases; furthermore children who have anxiety disorders or overanxious personalities are overrepresented in clinical cases.[9] Little is known, however,

about the psychological status of most children who have tics, for they rarely are seen in clinics.

5. *Psychiatric disorders.* The reason for separating psychiatric disorders from psychological factors is because some psychiatric disorders, especially those more severe, are biogenic or require a biological vulnerability to develop. Family pedigree and clinical studies of tics and occurrence of stimulant-induced tics in hyperactivity show that there is a strong relationship, most marked in Tourette syndrome, between tics and attention deficit/hyperactivity disorder (AD/HD)[3,5,6] (see Chapter 69, Attention Deficit/Hyperactivity Disorder). There also is some relationship between tics and obsessive-compulsive disorder because symptomatology (e.g., premonitory urges, intrusive thoughts, and compulsive actions), putative anatomical locus (cortico/striato/thalamic circuits), hypothesized pathophysiology (rogue reverberating microcircuits), and family pedigrees all show elements in common.[6]
6. *Genetic factors.* There is evidence to suggest that tics are, in some cases, a genetic disorder.[6,7,10] This is most true of Tourette disorder, in which the gene seems to act as an autosomal dominant one. However, the gene seems to be of variable expression in that most relatives have much more mild and transient forms of tic disorder. This suggests that in addition to genes, protective and risk factors must also exist. Penetrance increases if obsessive compulsive disorder is accepted as an alternative expression of the gene; indeed, a majority of patients who have Tourette disorder develop obsessive-compulsive symptoms if the disorder persists into adulthood.[6] Although there is an association between tics and AD/HD, it is by no means clear that this is another expression of the tic/Tourette gene.[6]
7. *Drugs.* Amphetamine and other dopaminergic drugs induce stereotypies in rats and occasionally can produce tics and other abnormal movements in children. Stimulants given for hyperactivity may precipitate tics or Tourette disorder in vulnerable children,[5] though some believe that this merely reflects the common association of the two disorders.[8] However, it is prudent not to give stimulants to hyperactive children if there is any history of tics or Tourette disorder.[5] Also, stimulants aggravate tics and therefore should not be given if tics are present. If tics emerge subsequently, the stimulants should be stopped and other medications such as antidepressants or clonidine substituted.[5,8] Drugs of abuse, especially cocaine and other stimulants, are capable of producing tics. Neuroleptic drugs also can produce tics/Tourette disorder as an analog of tardive dyskinesia[2] presumptively caused by hypersensitivity of dopamine receptors following chronic blockade. This is yet one more reason for caution in using these drugs.

It seems reasonable to posit that in most cases tics appear spontaneously during middle childhood as exaggerations of spontaneous movements, normal at that stage of development. In others, they are catalyzed by states of increased motor activity or excitability such as in AD/HD or anxiety disorders or the use or abuse of dopaminergic drugs interacting with neuromuscular developmental status. In some cases, notably Tourette disorder, tics probably are the result of an as yet unestablished abnormality of the neuromotor system of genetic origin or rarely some other neurological disorder. As with any other motor behavior, however, tics may be influenced by learning or conditioning, which may serve to prolong or shorten their course.

Tics should never be assumed to indicate a psychiatric disorder unless they are associated with other signs or symptoms of such a disorder that affect other areas of function beyond the motor system. Also, although tics can be controlled to some degree for variable periods in public situations (e.g., a pediatrician's office), this does not mean that the child can or should be expected to control them most of the time. Such control requires considerable emotional energy from the child and can be sustained only for limited periods. As soon as the child relaxes, is distracted, or lets up concentration in the least, the tics will reappear.

TREATMENT

The vast majority of tics in children will be mild, short-lived, and flit from one muscle group to another. As in so much of medicine, the best treatment for most tics is masterly inactivity coupled with authoritative information to child and parents about the condition.[9] Clearly, any unreasonable and avoidable stress on the child should be reduced; however, tics should not be a sign to treat the child as though she or he is necessarily overstressed or anxious. First, that presumes a cause that may not be present; second, if it is so, some stress is not only an inexorable part of life but also is one of the ways children learn how to cope. AD/HD or obsessive-compulsive disorder or drug abuse also may be present and require attention. Other kinds of medication such as stimulants, neuroleptics, androgenic steroids, or any drug that interferes with dopamine such as metoclopramide or antiemetics should be borne in mind because their removal may be the required treatment.

Once a tic has been present and unchanged in form or site for more than a year, treatment may be considered—but only if the tic is conspicuous, disabling, or distressing to the child. Treatments shown to be effective include the following, discussed below.

1. *Behavioral methods.*[4,9] These are the only methods that are truly curative. However, they usually are not completely successful, although some improvement can be expected, even in Tourette disorder.[4] There is a variety of such techniques (e.g., massed practice, habit reversal, and avoidance learning); all, however, are specialized and best carried out by a psychologist who is used to working with children because the procedures are difficult and children are passively resistant.
2. *Anxiety-reducing procedures.*[9] These include relaxation training, biofeedback, psychotherapy, and where possible, general adjustment of the child's life-style. Unlike behavioral methods, however, none of these is of proven value in tics. Neither should these procedures be considered specific; rather, they are ancillary and holistic in meeting therapeutic objectives.
3. *Acceptance.* In the overwhelming majority of cases the best management is explaining to parents, teachers, and peers that the tics are a physical disability, that the child cannot help them, and that acceptance of both child and

tics is the kindest, safest, and simplest way to deal with them. Criticizing and belittling the child are likely to make tics worse and prolong their course.[6]

4. *Pharmacotherapy.* Only physicians thoroughly familiar with the drugs indicated and experienced in their use should undertake pharmacotherapy, and only after reading one of the specialized publications on the topic.[5,8] Because of the risks involved and the lack of any truly curative value, drugs should be used only when tics are seriously disabling. This is most likely to be in Tourette disorder or in chronic severe tics. Medication should not be given simply for superficial reasons except for brief periods during special socially embarrassing circumstances. Even then it is important to ensure that dramatic and distressing side effects such as dystonic reactions will not ensue or that the embarrassment will be far greater than that from the tics.

The mainstays of pharmacotherapy are the dopamine-blocking neuroleptic drugs. Their utility stems from the fact that whatever their cause, tics are executed through the basal ganglia and appear to reflect a relative overactivity in the dopaminergic nigrostriatal systems that inhibit cholinergic basal ganglion systems. These latter regulate movement through the twin mechanisms of increased tone and synchronization seen in exaggeration in parkinsonian states; dopamine has the opposite effect—that is, it produces unregulated or spontaneous movements seen in chorea or occasionally with dopamine agonists such as dextroamphetamine or L-dopa.

Any one of the neuroleptics may be used,[8] although haloperidol and pimozide (for no apparently valid reasons) in doses starting at 0.5 mg and increasing slowly up to 3 mg/day seem to be preferred.[5] Pimozide has a reputation for cardiotoxicity in doses in excess of 0.2 mg/kg.[5,8] Even these relatively low doses may produce acute dystonic reactions, sedation, parkinsonism, the highly uncomfortable and usually overlooked akathisia (restless legs), and in the long term, tardive dyskinesias.[2] In some cases initial effects wear off, subsequent doses needed may be quite high, and the risk of side effects rises accordingly. Although neuroleptics often are effective to some degree, their action is symptomatic rather than curative. A number of lawsuits in the United States have been successful against physicians for tardive dyskinesias, and it is necessary that this and other risks involved be discussed fully and that informed consent be obtained. A second opinion, by a specialist who has obtained knowledge of tics/Tourette disorder before neuroleptic pharmacotherapy is undertaken, offers the physician added protection.

If neuroleptics are unsuccessful or, more commonly, create unacceptable side effects, clonidine may be tried in doses of 50 μg/day and slowly raised, if needed, over several weeks to 150 to 300 μg/day after preliminary EKG and blood work has been done.[5,8]

Although it may seem logical to use anxiolytic drugs in the management of tic disorders, these thoroughly undesirable drugs[8] should be used only in unusual instances in children. They affect the highest functions of the brain, including learning, can make children irritable and lead to dependence, and withdrawal symptoms[1] may make children more irritable.[8] The muscle relaxant properties of the benzodiazepines are insignificant clinically, so they cannot be defended on that basis either.[1,8]

In summary, tics should be treated pharmacotherapeutically only as a last resort and by a physician skilled in the use of the drugs concerned. Such treatment should be considered and discussed carefully, closely monitored, and undertaken only with knowledge and consideration of the risks and disadvantages involved.

REFERRAL TO MENTAL HEALTH SPECIALISTS

Criteria for referring children who have tics to a mental health specialist are: (1) tics associated with *additional* evidence of psychiatric disorder, such as overanxiety, AD/HD, or obsessive-compulsive disorder; (2) chronic or recurrent tics that seem to have a clear relationship to stress and when there is reason to believe that mental health procedures may be helpful; (3) chronic, disabling, or discomforting tics for which differential diagnosis or treatment is indicated; or (4) when the primary physician knows little about tics and feels the need of expert opinion.

In general, the preferred mental health specialist is a well-trained child and adolescent psychiatrist—one who has a broad biopsychosocial perspective, including a good grasp of neuropsychiatry and pharmacotherapy but a "light" prescribing hand and a capacity to work closely with behavioral psychologists. This kind of child psychiatrist most likely will be alert to the possibilities of the rare neurologically induced tics and will order any appropriate neuroimaging and neurological consultations.

PROGNOSIS

Most tics last only a few weeks, although they may flit from one muscle group to another or change their form at irregular intervals.[8] Even chronic tics are likely to disappear in adolescence, although the longer a tic has been present and unchanged in form or site, the less likely it will be to disappear. Because the prevalence drops sharply after age 13 years, a tic that persists after that age is more likely to become chronic. Tourette disorder may be a lifelong condition, but better recognition of the disorder shows that most cases generally will improve somewhat and even abate in late adolescence or adulthood.[3,6] Behavioral methods of treatment can influence the course of tics, but there is no evidence that any other treatment affects prognosis as opposed to suppressing symptoms.

Children who have tics and especially Tourette disorder can suffer secondary problems of self-image when adult criticism and peer rejection ensue.[6] Occasionally, severe complex motor tics result in injury or self-mutilation.[3] Finally, obsessive-compulsive disorder may develop during adolescence or late in Tourette disorder.[6]

REFERENCES

1. American Psychiatric Association: *Benzodiazepine dependence, toxicity and abuse,* Washington, DC, 1990, The Association.
2. American Psychiatric Association: *Tardive dyskinesia: a task force report,* Washington, DC, 1992, The Association.
3. American Psychiatric Association: *Diagnostic and statistical manual of mental disorders (DSM-IV),* ed 4, Washington, DC, 1994, American Psychiatric Press.
4. Azrin NH, Peterson AL: Behavior therapy for Tourette's syndrome and

tic disorders. In Cohen DJ, Leckman JF, Bruun RD, editors: *Tourette's syndrome: clinical understanding and treatment,* New York, 1988, John Wiley & Sons.
5. Cohen DJ et al: Pharmacotherapy of Tourette's syndrome and associated disorders, *Psychiatr Clin North Am* 15:109, 1992.
6. Cohen DJ, Leckman JF: Developmental psychopathology and neurobiology of Tourette's syndrome: advances in treatment and research, *J Am Acad Child Adolesc Psychiatry* 33:2, 1994.
7. Leckman JF et al: Premonitory urges in Tourette's syndrome, *Am J Psychiatry* 150:98, 1993.
8. Werry JS, Aman MG: *A practitioner's guide to psychoactive drugs for children and adolescents,* New York, 1994, Plenum.
9. Werry JS: Physical illness, symptoms and allied disorders. In Quay HC, Werry JS, editors: *Psychopathological disorders of childhood,* ed 3, New York, 1986, John Wiley & Sons.
10. Zausmer DM, Dewey ME: Tics and heredity: a study of the relatives of child tiqueurs, *Br J Psychiatry* 150:628, 1987.

SUGGESTED READING

Cohen DJ, Leckman JF, Bruun RD, editors: *Tourette's syndrome: clinical understanding and treatment,* New York, 1988, John Wiley & Sons.

172 Torticollis

Beryl J. Rosenstein

Torticollis, or wryneck, refers to abnormal positioning (tilt) of the head and neck. It is a physical finding, not a diagnosis, and an accurate cause must be determined before appropriate treatment can be initiated. It is found in association with many childhood illnesses and, depending on the age of the patient, has a wide spectrum of underlying etiological factors (see the box on p. 1138).[21] In evaluating the patient who has torticollis, it is important to inquire as to maternal obstetrical history, recent surgery, head and neck infections, trauma, family history of torticollis, drug ingestion, and presence of associated findings such as pain, fever, vomiting, ataxia, ocular abnormalities, and abnormal posturing.[21] The examination should focus on the head, neck, and nervous system to look for evidence of localized infection, neck masses, sternocleidomastoid (SCM) muscle abnormalities, cervical vertebrae tenderness, eye abnormalities, and neurological deficit.

DIAGNOSIS

Neonates

When a head tilt is recognized in the early neonatal period, the usual cause is *congenital muscular torticollis*.[2,3,6,11,21] This disorder occurs in 0.4% of live births and affects males more often than females. It is characterized by tilting of the head to the involved side and turning of the face to the opposite side, in association with unilateral fibrotic contracture of the SCM muscle. The head cannot be moved passively into a normal position. Torticollis may be noted at birth and almost always is obvious by 2 to 4 weeks of age. A firm, nontender, discrete fusiform mass ("tumor") 1 to 3 cm in diameter may be palpable in the body of the muscle. The mass contains fibrous tissue and does not represent a resolving hematoma. It may increase gradually in size over the first month, but then it regresses; by 4 to 6 months it usually no longer is palpable. By this time only contracture and fibrotic thickening of the involved muscle will be obvious. The cause is not known, but it is postulated to result from trauma to the soft tissues of the neck during delivery, an intrauterine positional deformity, ischemia secondary to venous occlusion, or a sequela of an intrauterine or perinatal compartment syndrome.[3] The family history will be positive for muscular torticollis in 10% of cases.[20] Associated musculoskeletal disorders such as talipes equinovarus, metatarsus adductus, and hip dysplasia occur in up to 20% of cases.[2,3,9]

Other causes of congenital torticollis include anomalies of the atlas, odontoid, or atlantoaxial articulation; abnormal skin webs or folds *(pterygium colli);* lesions such as cystic hygroma and branchial cleft cyst in the region of the SCM muscle; vertebral dislocation; and fusion abnormalities associated with cervical hemivertebrae, as seen in Klippel-Feil syndrome or Sprengel deformity.[6,7] Ultrasound examination of the neck may help to identify cystic lesions in the neck. When a mass is *not* palpable within the SCM muscle, cervical spine roentgenograms should be obtained. Rarely the SCM muscle may be absent unilaterally, in which case the head tilt is away from and the chin is rotated toward the side of the absent muscle, compared with the positions associated with muscular torticollis.

Infants

After the newborn period infants may have abnormal tone and posturing of the head, neck, and upper portion of the trunk in association with gastroesophageal reflux, esophagitis, and hiatus hernia *(Sandifer syndrome)*.[1,13,21] Posturing, which can take the form of torticollis, opisthotonos, or dystonia, has been attributed to an attempt by the infant to decrease the pain of esophagitis. There may be other manifestations of reflux, including vomiting after feeding, gastrointestinal bleeding, dysphagia, episodes of apnea, recurrent cough, wheezing, pulmonary infiltrates, and failure to thrive. It needs to be emphasized that esophagitis secondary to reflux can occur in the absence of vomiting. Intermittent occurrence and alternating direction of the torticollis, in association with normal SCM muscles and normal cervical spine roentgenographic findings, strongly suggest gastroesophageal reflux/esophagitis as the underlying cause of the torticollis. In an infant with obvious regurgitation a trial of medical management should be considered. If an infant has severe symptoms or is refractory to medical management, esophageal pH probe monitoring and endoscopy should be carried out.

Benign paroxysmal torticollis of infancy is a puzzling disorder of unknown etiology characterized by recurring attacks of head tilt and often accompanied by vomiting, pallor, ataxia, and behavior changes.[4,5] Although usually no specific precipitating factors occur, a familial pattern may exist. The cardinal feature is the periodicity of the attacks; between attacks the infant appears normal. Onset is within the first year of life. Attacks typically last from several hours to several days and usually cease before age 5 years. Apart from the head tilt and ataxia, results of physical and neurological examinations are normal, as are laboratory tests. Other disorders that need to be considered in the differential diagnosis include recurrent cervical dislocation, posterior fossa tumor, seizure disorder, and gastroesophageal reflux. An electroencephalogram, cervical spine films, esophageal pH probe monitoring, barium swallow, cervical computed tomography (CT) scans, and magnetic resonance imaging (MRI) may help in the diagnostic evaluation. Suggested causes of benign paroxysmal torticollis include episodic vasospasm, migraine, and paroxysmal dysfunction of central vestibular structures. Clinical features of benign paroxysmal vertigo or infantile migraine develop in some patients. Although there is no specific therapy, it is important to recognize this entity and to reassure the family that its course is benign and its prognosis usually good.

Torticollis may occur secondary to ocular abnormalities, including strabismus, paresis of the extraocular muscles, nystagmus, and refractive errors.[21]

Older Children

Acquired torticollis in older children may be secondary to a variety of disorders, as outlined in the box below. Some of these conditions can be managed adequately by the pediatric practitioner; however, patients who have cervical spine injuries or neurological signs are best evaluated in conjunction with neurology and orthopedic consultants.

Most cases of acquired torticollis seen by the pediatric practitioner are related to ligamentous or muscular injuries of the cervical soft tissues.[6] The onset is sudden and usually follows strenuous activity, a minor injury, or a sudden change in position. The head is fixed in a tilted position, and the affected muscle often has spasms and is tender. Fever and manifestations of systemic illness are absent; laboratory and roentgenographic studies usually are not indicated.

Sudden onset of difficulty in rotating the head to one side, often after mild trauma or an upper respiratory tract infection and accompanied by torticollis and muscle spasm, may occur as a result of rotational subluxation of the atlas (C1) on the axis (C2) or of C2 on C3. This seldom is accompanied by neurological signs or symptoms. The diagnosis usually is confirmed by cervical spine roentgenograms but may require a CT scan of the neck.

Children who have bone dysplasia, Morquio syndrome, and spondyloepiphyseal dysplasia have a high incidence of C1-C2 instability with accompanying torticollis.[7] Atlantoaxial instability secondary to laxity of the transverse ligaments occurs in 15% of patients who have Down syndrome.[15] Although the vast majority are asymptomatic, some cases manifest torticollis, neck discomfort, and/or neurological deficits secondary to spinal cord compression. These patients are at risk for developing progressive neurological impairment and apnea, especially following trauma or surgical and rehabilitative procedures.[12] All patients who have Down syndrome should have their cervical spine evaluated roentgenographically.

Spasmodic torticollis can occur as an idiosyncratic dystonic reaction to a variety of drugs, including the phenothiazines, methylphenidate, metoclopramide, and haloperidol.[21] There may be other extrapyramidal manifestations, such as opisthotonos and trismus, sometimes in association with spasmodic conjugate deviations of the eyes *(oculogyric crisis)*. Torticollis may occur as a result of cervical adenitis in children whose tonsils and pharynx are infected and who have a retropharyngeal abscess. With a retropharyngeal abscess there also is drooling, sore throat, dysphagia, noisy and difficult mouth breathing, fever, and leukocytosis. The diagnosis can be made by direct finger palpation of a fluctuant mass on the posterior pharyngeal wall or by a roentgenogram of the lateral neck. Following surgical procedures to the head and neck, children may develop torticollis, pain, and diminished neck movement 4 to 7 days after surgery.[17,21] This may result from reflex irritation of neck muscles, localized infection, or rotational subluxation of C1 on C2. Children who have bacterial meningitis may develop torticollis, probably secondary to irritation of the spinal nerve roots supplying the sternomastoid.[10] There also have been reports of epidemic torticollis of acute onset, presumed to be of viral origin.[14]

Torticollis also may occur secondary to *spontaneous calcification of a cervical disk.*[19] Other symptoms include muscle spasm, localized pain, and low-grade fever. Although the cause is unknown, onset may be related to trauma or to an upper respiratory tract infection. Roentgenograms show fluffy calcification of the nucleus pulposus. Treatment consists of analgesics and a soft cervical collar. Symptoms may last from a few days to several months; the calcification may disappear after 2 to 3 months or may be permanent.

Osteomyelitis of a cervical vertebra should be suspected in a child who has torticollis accompanied by an unexplained low-grade fever.[22] Leukocytosis may be present, the erythrocyte sedimentation rate may be elevated, and often there is a history of mild trauma. Because of a low index of suspicion, the diagnosis often is delayed until the appearance of neurological signs. Cervical spine roentgenograms demonstrate bone destruction, but bone scans may help to establish an early diagnosis before destruction is detectable.

Torticollis accompanied by motor weakness, muscle atrophy, and fasciculations suggests a spinal cord tumor.[22] There may be neck pain and stiffness, back pain, nerve root pain, impaired gait, and sensory disturbances. Nystagmus may be

CAUSES OF ACQUIRED TORTICOLLIS

Trauma

Injury to cervical musculature (spastic torticollis)
Subluxation (atlantooccipital, atlas-axis [C1-C2], or C2-C3)
Intervertebral disk calcification

Infection

Cervical adenitis
Retropharyngeal abscess
Osteomyelitis of cervical vertebrae
Acute epidemic torticollis

Neurological causes

Ventricular shunt malfunction
Dystonic drug reactions (oculogyric crisis)
Tumors (posterior fossa, intraspinal, or extradural)
Syringomyelia
Wilson disease
Dystonia musculorum deformans

Other causes

Hiatal hernia with gastroesophageal reflux (Sandifer syndrome)
Benign paroxysmal torticollis of infancy
Vertebral abnormalities
- Atlantoaxial instability (nontraumatic dislocation)
- Bone dysplasia
- Eosinophilic granuloma

Strabismus (ocular torticollis)
Nystagmus
Hysteria
Psychogenic
Soft tissue tumors of the neck
Rheumatoid arthritis

present in patients who have high cervical cord tumors. Cervical spine roentgenograms may show gross bone destruction, erosion of spinal pedicles or vertebral bodies, and widening of the interpediculate spaces. The diagnosis usually is confirmed by CT scan or MRI. Torticollis accompanied by headache, vomiting, nystagmus, or cranial nerve signs suggests a posterior fossa tumor with herniation.

For reasons unknown, intermittent torticollis may occur because of blockage of a ventriculovenous or ventriculoperitoneal shunt. Revision of the shunt is followed by resolution of the torticollis. Torticollis also may result from formation of a subcutaneous fibrous cord along the length of a ventriculoperitoneal shunt tract.[16]

MANAGEMENT

In infants who have congenital muscular torticollis, the prognosis for a good cosmetic and functional outcome depends on the severity of the deformity and the age at which treatment is started.[2,11,21] All infants, including those who have moderate-to-severe deformities and tumors in the SCM muscle, should be prescribed a trial of medical management consisting of passive stretching exercises to the involved muscle and positioning in which the most interesting aspects of the child's surroundings are placed opposite the side of the contracted muscle.[2,11] This therapy almost always is successful in infants who have mild-to-moderate deformities for which treatment is started before 1 year of age. Surgery is indicated if torticollis persists beyond 1 year of age, if there is a residual craniofacial deformity (plagiocephaly), or if there is >30% loss of range of motion.[18] Surgical management consists of an open bipolar tenotomy of the involved muscle, followed by neck traction, a soft cervical collar, and passive and active range-of-motion exercises. After successful medical or surgical therapy, however, potential sequelae include mild residual craniofacial asymmetry, intermittent head tilt, decreased range of neck motion, asymmetrical motor development, and rarely, scoliosis. [2] Residual head and neck positioning problems may be caused by rotational subluxation of C1 on C2.[18]

The medical management recommended for gastroesophageal reflux consists of using thickened feedings, a histamine-2 (H_2) blocker, and drugs such as bethanechol and metoclopramide to enhance gastric emptying. Patients who do not respond to medical therapy should have endoscopy and esophageal biopsy; some may require surgical correction (fundoplication).

Treatment of acquired torticollis as a result of ligamentous and muscular injuries consists of local heat, analgesics, and a soft cervical collar; symptoms usually resolve completely in 7 to 10 days. If rotational subluxation of the atlas occurs, analgesics and light cervical traction followed by the wearing of a cervical collar usually are sufficient; cervical fusion rarely is required. Patients who have anomalies of the occipitocervical junction or of the cervical spine often require surgical stabilization by fusion of the cervical spine.[6-8]

Patients who have Down syndrome and atlantoaxial instability require careful neurological follow-up and should be counseled to restrict participation in activities that involve potential trauma to the head and neck.[15] In symptomatic patients, cervical stabilization is indicated to prevent progressive neurological impairment. Patients who have acute onset of neck pain, torticollis, or neurological deficit require immediate immobilization of the neck followed by cervical roentgenograms and CT scans or MRI. Prophylactic stabilization in asymptomatic patients who have Down syndrome is not indicated.

Drug-induced spasmodic torticollis may be treated by discontinuing the offending drug and slowly administering diphenhydramine intravenously at a dose of 1 to 2 mg/kg. If cervical adenitis and abscess are the causative conditions, treatment consists of surgical drainage and appropriate antibiotics. In patients whose torticollis is secondary to an ocular abnormality, treatment of the eye problem leads to resolution of the torticollis.

REFERENCES

1. Bray PF et al: Childhood gastroesophageal reflux, *JAMA* 237:1342, 1977.
2. Binder H et al: Congenital muscular torticollis: results of conservative management with long-term follow-up in 85 cases, *Arch Phys Med Rehabil* 68:222, 1987.
3. Davids JR et al: Congenital muscular torticollis: sequela of intrauterine or perinatal compartment syndrome, *J Pediatr Orthop* 13:141, 1993.
4. Deonna T, Martin D: Benign paroxysmal torticollis in infancy, *Arch Dis Child* 56:956, 1981.
5. Hanokoglu A, Somekh E, Fried D: Benign paroxysmal torticollis in infancy, *Clin Pediatr* 23:272, 1984.
6. Hensinger RN: Orthopedic problems of the shoulder and neck, *Pediatr Clin North Am* 33:1495, 1986.
7. Hensinger RN, MacEwen GD: Congenital anomalies of the spine. In Rothman RH, Simeone FA, editors: *The spine,* ed 2, Philadelphia, 1982, WB Saunders.
8. Holmes JC, Hall JE: Fusion for instability and potential instability of the cervical spine in children and adolescents, *Orthop Clin North Am* 9:923, 1978.
9. Hummer CD Jr, MacEwen GD: The coexistence of torticollis and congenital dysplasia of the hip, *J Bone Joint Surg (Am)* 54:1255, 1972.
10. McIntosh D et al: Torticollis and bacterial meningitis, *Pediatr Inf Dis* 12:160, 1993.
11. Morrison DL, MacEwen GD: Congenital muscular torticollis: observations regarding clinical findings, associated conditions and results of treatment, *J Pediatr Orthop* 2:500, 1982.
12. Msall ME et al: Symptomatic atlantoaxial instability associated with medical and rehabilitative procedures in children with Down syndrome, *Pediatrics* 85:447, 1990.
13. Murphy WJ, Gellis SS: Torticollis with hiatus hernia in infancy, *Am J Dis Child* 131:564, 1977.
14. Neng T et al: Acute infectious torticollis, *Neurology* 33:1344, 1983.
15. Peuschel SM, Scola FH, Pezzullo C: A longitudinal study of atlanto-dens relationships in asymptomatic individuals with Down syndrome, *Pediatrics* 89:1194, 1992.
16. Robb JE, Southgate GW: An unusual case of torticollis, *J Pediatr Orthop* 6:469, 1986.
17. Singer JI: Evaluation of the patient with neck complaints following tonsillectomy or adenoidectomy, *Pediatr Emerg Care* 8:276, 1992.
18. Slate RK et al: Cervical spine subluxation associated with congenital muscular torticollis and craniofacial asymmetry, *Plast Reconstr Surg* 91:1187, 1993.
19. Sonnabend DH, Taylor TKF, Chapman GK: Intervertebral disc calcification syndromes in children, *J Bone Joint Surg (Br)* 64:25, 1982.
20. Thompson F, McManus S, Colville J: Familial congenital muscular torticollis: case report and review of the literature, *Clin Orthop* 202:193, 1986.
21. Tom LWC et al: Torticollis in children, *Otolaryngol Head Neck Surg* 105:1, 1991.
22. Visudhiphan P et al: Torticollis as the presenting sign in cervical spine infection and tumor, *Clin Pediatr* 21:71, 1982.

173 Vaginal Bleeding

Alain Joffe

As with other symptoms referable to the female genital tract, physician assessment of vaginal bleeding depends largely on the pubertal status of the patient. In prepubertal girls, vaginal bleeding probably reflects a localized problem in the vagina or uterus; in pubertal females, the differential diagnosis includes disorders affecting the hypothalamic-pituitary-ovarian axis and complications of pregnancy, as well as local causes. In both cases, however, a careful history and physical examination will provide important clues to the diagnosis.

PREPUBERTAL GIRLS

In the neonatal period a decrease in circulating maternal estrogen, which diffuses across the placenta, results in a physiological discharge that can be either blood-tinged or frankly bloody.[5] No treatment, except reassurance, is necessary, and the discharge usually disappears within 10 days after birth.

A number of factors can result in vaginal bleeding in the prepubertal child, including vulvovaginal infections, excoriations secondary to pruritus, foreign bodies, sexual abuse, trauma, tumors (including condyloma), and coagulopathies.

Coagulopathies

A history of exposure to diethylstilbestrol (DES) in utero raises the possibility of a vaginal carcinoma; the patient should be examined carefully by an experienced gynecologist. If there is any suggestion of sexual abuse, such as bruises, lacerations, or other signs of trauma, careful, nonthreatening questioning of the child or caretaker may reveal whether further referral (to the appropriate social agencies) is necessary. If there is concern about sexual abuse, cultures for *Neisseria gonorrhoeae* and *Chlamydia trachomatis* should be obtained.

Nighttime pruritus may indicate a pinworm infestation. The Scotch tape slide test, to look for pinworm eggs, can help to establish *Enterobius vermicularis* infestation. The review of systems that indicates the presence of petechiae or considerable numbers of bruises on physical examination suggests a bleeding tendency. If so, platelet counts and clotting studies are indicated. A history of foreign bodies elsewhere suggests that a foreign body in the vagina is the cause of the bleeding. The physician also should make sure that the bleeding *is* vaginal in origin, since a prolapsed urethra can mimic vaginal bleeding.

If excoriations, redness, or a rash in the perineal area is noted, vaginitis is a distinct possibility. If there is discharge and microscopic examination demonstrates large numbers of white blood cells, vaginitis is certain. Concern about sexual abuse should prompt cultures for *N. gonorrhoeae* and *C. trachomatis*. Other bacterial cultures may be necessary; for example, a history of diarrhea in the weeks preceding suggests vaginitis caused by *Shigella* organisms.

Vaginal bleeding caused by vulvitis or foreign bodies will respond to removal of the foreign body and proper perineal hygiene. Occasionally, systemic antibiotics may be necessary. Foreign bodies often can be washed out with a flexible red Robinson catheter—sharp objects should be removed carefully, under direct visualization; referral to a gynecologist may be required if the patient is uncooperative.

Bleeding that does not subside within 10 days should be evaluated by a gynecologist. The entire foreign body may not have been removed, or a tumor, not readily visualized by a primary care provider, may be the actual cause of the bleeding.

PUBERTAL FEMALES

Evaluation

Abnormal vaginal bleeding in pubertal females can indicate a variety of disorders. Evaluation of this symptom depends on the nature of the problem: is she bleeding between normal periods, or have her regular menses become more frequent or heavier? It also is possible that a teenager whose prior menses have been regular will begin to have infrequent but heavy menstrual bleeding. In general, normal periods are 28 days apart (measured from the first day of one period to the first day of the next) with a range of 21 to 35 days and should not last more than 5 days.[4] Thus some teenagers will have only 2 weeks without bleeding between menses. How much bleeding is too much is difficult to quantify objectively. An increase from previous baseline menses is suggestive; Huffman et al.[7] recommend that a flow requiring use of more than 6 pads or 10 tampons in a 24-hour period is excessive.

The causes of abnormal bleeding in this age group are summarized in the box on p. 1141. Although "dysfunctional uterine bleeding" (DUB) secondary to an immaturity of the hypothalamic-pituitary-ovarian axis with resultant anovulatory cycles most likely is the cause, this diagnosis requires a careful search for and exclusion of many other causes. Nonetheless, it is worth noting that menstrual irregularity is frequent in the year following menarche: in one study of 5000 adolescents, 43% had irregular menses in the first year and 20% still had irregular periods 5 years after menarche.[4,12]

Most of the causes indicated in the box can be ruled out by history and physical examination. Certain key aspects of the history may be difficult to obtain: a young woman may hesitate to reveal that she has engaged in sexual intercourse or that she has been sexually abused. It is extremely unlikely that today's patient will have been exposed to DES in utero, but the question still is worth asking. If the teenager describes a discharge that is foul smelling and bloody, a foreign body or retained tampon is likely; however, necrotic tumors can

POSSIBLE CAUSES OF ABNORMAL UTERINE BLEEDING

Pregnancy complications

Spontaneous abortion
Ectopic pregnancy
Retained gestational products
Trophoblastic disease

Coagulation disorders

von Willebrand disease
Idiopathic thrombocytopenia
Other causes of thrombocytopenia
Glanzmann disease
Leukemia

Systemic disease

Renal failure
Hepatic failure
Malignancy

Pathology of the reproductive tract
Vagina

Vaginitis
Trauma
Foreign body
Congenital anomaly (septum)
Neoplasia

Cervix

Cervicitis, erosion
Cervical polyp
Neoplasia

Uterus

Endometritis
Endometrial polyp
Submucosal leiomyoma
Arteriovenous malformation
Congenital anomaly
Neoplasia

Pelvis

Endometriosis

Endocrine disorders
Hypothalamus/pituitary

Immature hypothalamic-pituitary-ovarian axis
Hyperprolactinemia
Anorexia nervosa, malnutrition
Excessive exercise

Ovary

Polycystic ovary syndrome
Luteal phase abnormality
Premature ovarian failure
Neoplasia (hormone secreting)

Adrenal

Congenital adrenal hyperplasia
Cushing disease
Adrenal insufficiency
Neoplasm

Thyroid

Hypothyroidism
Hyperthyroidism

Iatrogenic

Hormonal medications
Anticoagulants
Neuroleptics
Intrauterine contraceptive device

From Namnoun AB, Carpenter SEK: *Adolescent Medicine: State of the Art Reviews* 5:162, 1994.

result in similar bleeding patterns. Pruritus or dysuria suggests vaginitis as the cause of the bleeding. Bleeding between periods is common during the first two or three cycles of oral contraceptive use and generally does not require any additional therapy. Young women who have levonorgestrel implants (Norplant) or who receive depot medroxyprogesterone acetate (Depo-Provera) injections often have frequent and irregular periods of excess bleeding. Occasionally, women may have a small amount of bleeding or spotting after sexual intercourse, and some will have spotting around the time they ovulate.

Normal findings on physical examination, including pelvic and bimanual rectoabdominal examinations, help to rule out many of the causes listed in the box. Vulvar or vaginal bruising or lacerations suggest the probability of sexual abuse. Lack of adnexal or cervical motion tenderness generally excludes pelvic inflammatory disease. If the ovaries are of normal size, ovarian tumors or cysts are unlikely sources of the bleeding. A minimally enlarged uterus, consistent with early pregnancy, may not be noted by an inexperienced examiner. Measurement of human chorionic gonadotropin (HCG) level in urine or serum (if ectopic pregnancy is under consideration) will help to include or exclude diagnoses such as a missed or an incomplete abortion or an ectopic pregnancy.[9] Complications of pregnancy (e.g., ectopic pregnancy or incomplete abortion) are more likely if there is a history of one or two missed periods, if the prior menstrual period was lighter than normal, if other symptoms of pregnancy are present (breast tenderness or nausea), or if the bleeding is accompanied by crampy lower abdominal pain. A history of "passing tissue" or tissue in the vaginal canal also is suggestive. Although a blood dyscrasia (e.g., thrombocytopenia or von Willebrand disease) occasionally can present with heavy vaginal bleeding and should be excluded, this condition is often, but not always, accompanied by cutaneous manifestations of easily provoked bleeding.

Pelvic tuberculosis is extremely rarely seen in most practices, but a negative intradermal purified protein derivative

(PPD) result is simple to document for a teenager from a high-risk environment. A complete blood count with indices, red cell distribution width, and reticulocyte count also should be obtained inasmuch as iron deficiency anemia can cause increased uterine bleeding. Determining whether the anemia, if found, is responsible for or secondary to the heavy bleeding can be difficult; consultation may be necessary to sort this out. Alternatively, if the bleeding is not heavy and the patient is not severely anemic, a short trial of iron therapy may be instituted and the bleeding followed to see if it persists.

Endometrial polyps or submucous leiomyomas are distinctly unusual in women younger than 20 years of age. They cannot be felt by the examiner on the usual pelvic examination. If the patient has an intractably heavy flow, the presence of one of these entities should be considered. Curettage may be necessary, or an ultrasound examination of the uterus may suggest their presence.[6,7] In either case, referral to a gynecologist for appropriate therapy is necessary.

Normal menstrual function requires that the hypothalamic-pituitary-ovarian axis be intact and functioning properly. When this occurs, the following sequence of events transpires. Follicle-stimulating hormone (FSH) causes maturation of ovarian follicles, which produce estrogen. Rising levels of estrogen stimulate the endometrial lining of the uterus to proliferate and, at the same time, induce a midcycle surge of luteinizing hormone (LH) that causes the primary follicle to release an ovum, after which LH and FSH levels fall. The remnants of the follicle (termed *corpus luteum*) now produce progesterone, which converts the proliferative endometrium to a secretory phase. At the end of a normal cycle the corpus luteum involutes, and both estrogen and progesterone levels fall. The endometrial lining is now shed, and bleeding occurs.

In adolescents, especially young adolescents, the hypothalamic-pituitary-ovarian axis is relatively immature and highly sensitive to disturbance by a number of endogenous and exogenous factors, and this perturbation leads to irregular bleeding. Among young adolescents (but in some older ones as well) the axis has not yet matured, and most cycles are anovulatory.[2] Thus the endometrium proliferates under estrogen stimulation from the maturing follicle, but the midcycle LH surge is absent, ovulation does not occur, and the progesterone-secreting corpus luteum never forms. Toward the end of the cycle, estrogen levels fall and bleeding occurs. Influenced by estrogen only, endometrial shedding is incomplete and irregular, accounting for the excessive bleeding of anovulatory cycles. Alternatively, fluctuating estrogen levels during an anovulatory cycle result in estrogen withdrawal bleeding.

Most teenagers who seek evaluation for genital bleeding will have "dysfunctional uterine bleeding"; in one series 74% did so.[3] Nonetheless it is important to search for other causes that affect the integrity of the hypothalamic-pituitary-ovarian axis and therefore can mimic DUB. Because any significant stress in a teenager's life can affect the axis, a general assessment of her well-being is valuable. Fluctuations in weight, particularly if rapid and significant, also can affect menstrual function. Questions about dietary habits (including fad or crash diets), concerns about body image, and exercise patterns should be part of the physician's evaluation. Symptoms of the other endocrine disorders listed in the box (e.g., cold intolerance, polyuria, headache, and increased facial hair) should also be sought.

The physical examination should include measurement of height, weight, and blood pressure as well as careful palpation of the thyroid gland. Visual field and funduscopic examinations are necessary to help rule out a prolactinoma. Increased facial hair would be consistent with polycystic ovaries or an adrenal tumor. Striae suggest Cushing disease; enlargement of the clitoris would be consistent with an androgen-secreting tumor or congenital adrenal hyperplasia.

For most cases relatively few laboratory tests are needed. A urinalysis, pregnancy test, and complete blood count should be obtained. If suggested by the history or physical examination or if hormonal therapy is contemplated, thyroid function tests (TSH), a prolactin level, and LH, FSH, and coagulation tests should be requested.[8] An LH:FSH ratio greater than 3:1 is highly suggestive of polycystic ovary syndrome but is not a sensitive indicator. Any evidence of hyperandrogenism necessitates measurement of testosterone, dehydroepiandrosterone and its sulfate, and 17-OH progesterone.

MANAGEMENT

If a specific cause for the bleeding is discovered, treatment should be directed at ameliorating this condition. As the aforementioned series indicates, a specific cause is not found in most instances, and the clinician must manage the bleeding without knowing the precise cause. Whether and how to treat is a matter of judgment; some physicians may feel comfortable using hormonal therapy, whereas others may prefer the guidance of a more experienced clinician.

Mild cases of bleeding that do not result in anemia and that do not upset the patient and her parents greatly can be managed expectantly with no immediate, specific therapy. Those who have mild anemia (hemoglobin value 11 to 12) should receive iron supplementation. Some will have the problem resolved within three or four cycles.[1]

Hormonal therapy is indicated in those teenagers with moderate bleeding—that is, enough to cause a small decrease in the hemoglobin level or to cause bleeding for 7 to 10 days per cycle. Teenagers who have menses every 1 to 3 weeks also need treatment. Although there are differences, most authorities recommend combined estrogen-progestin therapy.[4] Emans and Goldstein[5] recommend birth control pills, medroxyprogesterone (Provera) or norethindrone (Norlutate) as initial therapy; medroxyprogesterone should be given (10 mg once or twice daily) for 10 days beginning 14 days after the onset of the last period or at the time of the visit. This pattern of beginning the medication 14 days after the onset of menstrual flow can be continued for 3 to 6 months. Norethindrone (10 mg/day) also can be given using the same schedule. For the sexually active teenager, oral contraceptive pills abate the bleeding as well as protect against pregnancy.

A 2 to 3 g drop in hemoglobin associated with heavy or prolonged bleeding requires more aggressive therapy. Emans and Goldstein[5] suggest using an oral contraceptive such as Ovral, Lo/Ovral, or Ortho-Novum (Norinyl). They argue that Ovral particularly is useful because it contains 50 μg of estrogen as well as a potent progestin. The patient begins by taking a pill twice daily for 3 to 4 days until the bleeding stops, and then once daily until a total of 21 days of therapy have elapsed. Oral contraceptive pills then can be continued monthly if contraception is needed, or medroxyprogesterone (Provera) can be given for 2 weeks on a monthly basis to counteract unopposed estrogen stimulation of the uterus.

Should these methods fail or the hemoglobin level fall below 9 g, gynecological or adolescent medicine consultation should be sought; clotting studies should be obtained and hospitalization should be considered. Blood transfusion and endometrial curettage may be necessary. Even if these measures succeed in controlling the vaginal bleeding, these adolescents require long-term follow-up because an appreciable number of them will continue to have menstrual abnormalities and will be at increased risk for difficulties in conceiving. Persistent anovulation also may lead to endometrial hyperplasia and carcinoma in later life. In these cases joint management by the pediatrician and a gynecologist is optimal.[1,10,11]

REFERENCES

1. Altchek A: Dysfunctional menstrual disorders in adolescence, *Clin Obstet Gynecol* 14:975, 1971.
2. Askel S, Jones GS: Etiology and treatment of dysfunctional uterine bleeding, *Obstet Gynecol* 44:1, 1974.
3. Claessens CE, Lowell CA: Dysfunctional uterine bleeding in the adolescent, *Pediatr Clin North Am* 28:369, 1981.
4. Coupey SM, Ahlstrom P: Common menstrual disorders, *Pediatr Clin North Am* 36:551, 1989.
5. Emans SJH, Goldstein DP: *Pediatric and adolescent gynecology,* ed 3, Boston, 1990, Little, Brown.
6. Gailey TA, McDonough PG: Atypical uterine bleeding, *Pediatr Ann* 40:66, 1975.
7. Huffman JW, Dewhurst CJ, Capraro VJ: *The gynecology of childhood and adolescence,* ed 2, Philadelphia, 1981, WB Saunders.
8. Litt I: Menstrual problems during adolescence, *Pediatr Rev* 7:203, 1983.
9. Little HM: Managing incomplete abortion, *Am Fam Physician* 9:137, 1974.
10. Southam AL: Disorders of menstruation, *Clin Obstet Gynecol* 9:779, 1966.
11. Southam AL, Richart RM: The prognosis for adolescents with menstrual abnormalities, *Am J Obstet Gynecol* 94:637, 1966.
12. Vaughn TC: Dysfunctional uterine bleeding in the adolescent, *Semin Reprod Endocrinol* 2:359, 1984.

174 Vaginal Discharge

Alain Joffe

Vaginal discharge is a common complaint that confronts the pediatrician. Not all vaginal discharges, however, represent disease; some are physiologically normal, and the physician need only reassure the patient and her parents. To a large extent the age of the patient and her pubertal status also determine the cause of the discharge.

NEWBORN PERIOD

In utero the vaginal epithelium of the neonate is stimulated by maternal hormones that diffuse across the placenta into fetal circulation. After delivery these hormone levels fall rapidly, and the parents may note a thick, grayish white or mucoid discharge from the neonate's vagina. Often the discharge is blood tinged or even grossly bloody.[8] No treatment is needed, and the discharge usually resolves by 10 days of age.

PREPUBERTAL GIRLS

The genital area of prepubertal girls is more susceptible to infection than that of older, pubertal girls. The labial folds are smaller, and there is a relatively short distance between the vagina and the rectum in comparison with adolescents and adults. Low levels of circulating estrogen render the vaginal mucosa relatively thin and more susceptible to irritation or infection. The alkaline pH of the vaginal secretions affords a more hospitable environment to bacteria. As such, together with poor perineal hygiene, fecal flora can establish themselves more easily in the genital area[1,3] (see the box on p. 1145 for causes of vaginal discharge in prepubertal girls).

Evaluation

When evaluating a premenarcheal girl with vaginal discharge, the physician should inquire about her hygiene. Wiping from the rectum toward the vagina brings intestinal flora to the vaginal introitus. Use of chemicals such as bubble baths or deodorants or of strong detergents to launder underwear can irritate the vulva and vagina. Occlusive nylon or rayon underwear provides a moist environment for potential pathogens, and the material itself can be an irritant. Although accounting for less than 5% of vaginal discharges, foreign bodies (e.g., toilet paper, coins, and small toys) should be considered and inquiries made regarding the possibility that the girl may have placed some foreign body in her vagina.[5]

The parents should be asked about recent or concomitant illness. Vaginal discharge is associated with streptococcal infection (e.g., scarlet fever) and with *Shigella* infection occurring coincident with or after an episode of diarrhea.[4] Rectal infestations with *Enterobius vermicularis* (pinworms) also can lead to vaginitis if the eggs are deposited around or in the vagina. A history of nocturnal itching accompanying vaginal discharge suggests this diagnosis.

Many organisms, especially *Neisseria gonorrhoeae,* that are sexually transmitted are known to cause vaginal infections in prepubertal girls; thus the possibility of sexual abuse always should be considered in the evaluation. It is not known whether these organisms occasionally can be transmitted in other than a sexual manner.

The mother of the child also should be asked whether the daughter was exposed to diethylstilbestrol (DES) in utero. An affirmative response requires thorough evaluation by a gynecologist because of the possibility of vaginal carcinoma.

The physical examination should include the entire genital and rectal area. The condition of the vulva, urethral opening, and vaginal introitus should be noted. Infections in prepubertal girls usually involve the vulva and outer vagina as opposed to only the vagina. Bruises, lacerations, or scrapes in the genital area raise high suspicions of some form of sexual abuse. Excoriations around the rectum or vagina suggest itching caused by pinworms. A rash that spares skin folds is consistent with an irritative cause; one that is predominantly within the skin folds suggests candidiasis.

Use of a veterinary otoscope and speculum will allow for examination of the outer portions of the vagina without causing undue discomfort to the girl.[2] If a foreign body is suspected (because of a thick, yellowish, foul-smelling discharge) but not visualized, irrigating the vagina with a red Robinson catheter and tepid saline solution often will flush out bits of toilet paper or small objects.

If sufficient vaginal discharge is present, several drops of the secretion should be placed on three glass slides. If the discharge is scant, a saline-moistened cotton swab can be introduced into the vagina and the material so obtained placed on the glass slides. Several drops of normal saline solution should be added to one slide. Several drops of 10% potassium hydroxide should be added to the second slide and then gently heated to dissolve epithelial cells. A gram stain of the material on the third slide also should be made. All slides should be examined as indicated in Table 174-1. A gram stain that shows gram negative intracellular diplococci strongly suggests a gonococcal infection, and appropriate cultures should be obtained. A piece of Scotch tape applied to the rectal area and examined microscopically may reveal the typical eggs of *E. vermicularis* infection.

Management

If the history or physical examination suggests an "irritative" origin, parents should discontinue the offending agent and have the patient wear cotton underpants. Sitz baths will provide temporary relief until natural healing takes place. Removal of a foreign body will result in rapid improvement and cessation of the discharge. Pinworm infestations should be treated in the usual manner[7] (see Chapter 246). Infections caused by poor personal hygiene will respond to the general

CAUSES OF VAGINAL DISCHARGE IN PREPUBERTAL GIRLS

- Irritative (bubble baths, sand)
- Poor perineal hygiene
- Foreign body
- Associated systemic illness (group A streptococci, chickenpox)
- Infections
  - *Escherichia coli* with foreign body
  - *Shigella* organisms
  - *Yersinia* organisms
- Infections (consider sexual abuse)
  - *Chlamydia trachomatis*
  - *Neisseria gonorrhoeae*
  - *Trichomonas vaginalis*
- Tumor (rare)

measures just listed, coupled with instructions about proper perineal hygiene. If the discharge is associated with another infection (such as scarlet fever or *Shigella* organisms), it will disappear as the underlying infection is treated.

When the organism causing the vaginal discharge is found to be sexually transmitted, a more comprehensive evaluation and treatment are required (see Chapters 65, Sexual Abuse of Children, and 258, Sexually Transmitted Diseases). Antibiotic treatment adjusted to the girl's weight should be prescribed and a report that includes a comprehensive evaluation of the social situation of the patient should be sent to the appropriate agencies.

PUBERTAL AND POSTPUBERTAL ADOLESCENTS

With the onset of puberty, circulating estrogen and progesterone levels rise, stimulating vaginal mucus production and an increase in the turnover of vaginal epithelial cells. Bartholin and sebaceous glands also are stimulated. Generally the clear mucoid discharge that results will not cause problems. The amount of secretion, however, can increase with sexual excitement, as well as midway through a normal menstrual cycle. It is particularly prominent at the onset of puberty (physiological leukorrhea). Examination of a wet preparation will reveal vaginal epithelial cells only. The high protein content of this discharge, absorbed onto underwear, causes yellow staining when the underwear is laundered. Traditionally, occlusive nylon or rayon underpants have been alleged to cause a nonspecific vaginal discharge; recent research, however, suggests that such an association may be spurious.[4]

A wide variety of organisms normally are found in the vagina.[6] These organisms, especially the lactobacilli, help to maintain the normal acidic pH of the vagina, which resists infection. Except for *Candida* organisms, virtually all the organisms that cause vaginitis and vaginal discharge in this age group are sexually transmitted. If the patient denies sexual activity, sexual abuse should be considered. If the patient is sexually active, her partner should be treated simultaneously, especially if the infection is caused by *Neisseria gonorrhoeae, Chlamydia trachomatis,* or *Trichomonas vaginalis;* otherwise the infection is likely to recur. The presence of a foreign body (e.g., a retained tampon or condom) also should be considered. Because many teenagers fear admitting to sexual activity, a negative response should not rule out consideration of a sexually transmitted organism as the cause of the discharge. As with prepubertal girls, teenagers or their mothers should be queried about the possibility of DES exposure in utero. Those who have been so exposed should be referred to a gynecologist.

Table 174-1 lists the organisms and conditions responsible for producing vaginal infections or vaginal discharge in pubertal young women. Although the characteristics of each type of infection are said to be typical, the discharge observed on examination does not always fit these classic presentations. The laboratory methods outlined in Table 174-1 therefore are of considerable diagnostic utility. However, they are not 100% sensitive: *Trichomonas vaginalis* may not be noted during microscopic examination of vaginal fluid even though a subsequent Pap smear will show evidence of this infection. Regardless of the type of discharge noted, appropriate screening tests for *N. gonorrhoeae* and *C. trachomatis* should be obtained if the patient reports a new sexual partner or has not been screened in the last 6 to 12 months.

Bacterial vaginosis is a syndrome resulting from replacement of lactobacilli by high concentrations of a variety of anaerobic organisms. It generally is not considered a sexually transmitted infection. However, many of the organisms recovered from women who have bacterial vaginosis are also recovered from women who have pelvic inflammatory disease. Therefore prompt treatment of this cause of symptomatic vaginal discharge is essential; if found in women who have no symptoms, it does not need to be treated. Treatment of sex partners generally is not indicated.

Occasionally, herpesvirus infections of the vulvovaginal area and/or cervix are associated with vaginal discharge. Typically there is pain or a burning sensation in the genital area. The vulva is reddened, and groups of small vesicles are noted on the vulva, in the vagina, or on the cervix. If the vesicles rupture, the examiner sees only small ulcerations. Inguinal adenopathy is present, as are fever and systemic signs such as malaise if this is a first attack (see Chapter 214, Herpes Infections).

Approximately 50% of women will have recurrent episodes, usually milder than the first. Oral acyclovir has been approved for treatment of genital herpes infections. Women with herpes should have an annual Pap smear.

If the discharge does not appear to fit any of the causes described earlier and if cultures are negative for *N. gonorrhoeae* and *C. trachomatis,* a trial of sitz baths and vinegar douches (15 ml white vinegar in 1 quart of water taken twice daily for 1 week) is warranted.

A teenager who has a persistent discharge unresponsive to therapy may not actually be complying with the therapy or may have become reinfected by an untreated partner. If the physician believes that neither is the case, referral to a physician specializing in adolescent medicine or a gynecologist should be made to ensure a more thorough evaluation.

Candidal infections can be especially difficult to treat and may recur. Factors that predispose to candidiasis include oral contraceptive or broad-spectrum antibiotic use and diabetes mellitus.[6] Treatment with one of the medications listed in

Table 174-1 Major Causes of Vaginal Infections in Pubertal Girls

Agent	Discharge	Odor; pH	Dysuria; pruritus	Other clues	Diagnosis	Treatment
Candida albicans	Thick, white, curdlike, "cheesy"	None usually; pH 4.5 (obtained from midvagina with nitrazine paper)	Dysuria frequent; pruritus (4+)	Vulva affected; association with use of oral contraceptives and tetracycline	Hyphae on potassium hydroxide examination	A variety of effective treatment regimens are available for candidiasis. The author recommends the following because they are of brief duration or because they are available without prescription. All treatments usually are administered at bedtime: butoconazole 2% cream 5 g intravaginally for 3 days; clotrimazole (OTC) 100 mg vaginal tablet, two tablets once daily for 3 days; miconazole 2% cream (OTC) 5 g intravaginally for 7 days; miconazole 200 mg vaginal suppository, one suppository for 3 days; miconazole 100 mg vaginal suppository (OTC), one suppository for 7 days; terconazole 0.8% cream 5 g intravaginally for 3 days.
Trichomonas vaginalis	Frothy; yellow-green or gray	Foul-smelling; pH 5.2-5.5	Dysuria frequent; pruritus	Low abdominal pain; "strawberry" cervix; punctate vaginal hemorrhages	Motile trichomonads on wet preparation; avoid drying specimen. PAP smear may indicate trichomonads	Metronidazole 2 g orally in a single dose. Alternatively this medication can be given as 500 mg bid for 7 days. Partners of the patient must be treated. Some strains of *T. vaginalis* have diminished susceptibility to metronidazole. If failure occurs with either of the indicated regimens (and reinfection is not a possibility), the patient should be treated with 500 mg bid for 7 days. Repeated failures should be treated with 2 g qd for 3 to 5 days. The patient should be told to avoid alcohol until 24 hours after completion of therapy.
Neisseria gonorrhoeae	Purulent, but usually not prominent	None usually; pH <6.0	Occasional dysuria; not usually pruritic	Partner has discharge or dysuria	Gram negative intracellular diplococci suggestive; confirm with culture	Cefixime 400 mg orally in a single dose (see Chapter 258, Sexually Transmitted Diseases)
Bacterial vaginosis (formerly *Gardnerella vaginalis*)	Gray or clear, not curdlike*	Fishlike and foul; increased when mixed with potassium hydroxide*; pH 5.0-5.5*	No dysuria; slight pruritus	Probably occurs in association with other anaerobic organisms	Clue cells on wet preparation (bacteria-coated epithelial cells)*	Metronidazole 500 mg orally bid for 7 days has a cure rate of approximately 95%. An alternative regimen, 2 g of metronidazole as a single dose, has a cure rate of approximately 84%. Other alternative regimens include clindamycin cream, metronidazole gel, and clindamycin tablets. However, experience with these regimens is limited.
Chlamydia trachomatis	Purulent	None usual; pH > 4.5	Dysuria often; no pruritus	Partner has discharge or dysuria	Purulent material in endocervix, >10 WBCs per field (oil immersion). Endocervix is friable	Azithromycin 1 g orally *or* doxycycline 100 mg orally bid for 7 days (see Chapter 258, Sexually Transmitted Diseases)

Data from Amsel R et al: *Am J Med* 74:14, 1983; Brunham RC et al: *N Engl J Med* 311:1, 1984; and Rein MF, Chapel TA: *Clin Obstet Gynecol* 18:73, 1975.
*Must have three of these four criteria to make diagnosis.

Table 174-1 for a full 30 days (including during menstruation) may be necessary. Alternatively, 1% gentian violet applied to the vagina and cervix every other day for 2 weeks can be tried. Male sex partners also may need treatment.

REFERENCES

1. Capraro VJ, Gallego MB: Vulvovaginitis in children, *Pediatr Ann* 3:74, 1974.
2. Emans EJH, Goldstein DP: *Pediatric and adolescent gynecology,* ed 3, Boston, 1990, Little, Brown.
3. Hammerschlag MR et al: Microbiology of the vagina in children: normal and potentially pathogenic organisms, *Pediatrics* 62:57, 1978.
4. Paradise JE et al: Vulvovaginitis in premenarcheal girls: clinical features and diagnostic evaluation, *Pediatrics* 70:193, 1982.
5. Paradise JE, Willis ED: Probability of vaginal foreign body in girls with genital complaints, *Am J Dis Child* 139:472, 1985.
6. Rosenfeld WR, Clark J: Vulvovaginitis and cervicitis, *Pediatr Clin North Am* 36:489, 1989.
7. Schneider GT, Geary WL: Vaginitis in adolescent girls, *Clin Obstet Gynecol* 14:1057, 1971.
8. Singleton AF: Vaginal discharge in children and adolescents, *Clin Pediatr* 19:799, 1980.

SUGGESTED READINGS

Centers for Disease Control and Prevention: Sexually transmitted diseases treatment guidelines, *MMWR* 42(RR-14):67, 1993.

Shafer MB: Sexually transmitted diseases in adolescents: prevention, diagnosis, and treatment in pediatric practice, *Adolescent Health Update* 6:2, 1994.

175 Visual Problems

James W. McManaway III

Detection of visual problems in children may be difficult for several reasons: (1) children usually do not complain of monocular or mild bilateral visual loss, and even those who have significant bilateral visual loss may navigate familiar surroundings without notable difficulty; (2) vision-threatening ocular disease may have subtle ocular signs; (3) measurement of visual acuity in preverbal children requires special techniques; and (4) children who have monocular visual loss tend to peek around the occluder to escape detection (Fig. 175-1). Nonetheless, the primary care pediatrician must use accurate screening techniques to ensure the ocular health of children.

THE VISION SCREENING EXAMINATION

A basic but effective pediatric vision screening examination consists of three steps: (1) measurement of visual acuity in each eye, (2) assessment of ocular alignment, and (3) assessment of the fundus red reflex. All newborns' red reflex should be assessed in the nursery, and children should have this vision screening examination at 2, 4, and 6 years of age. Children passing all three steps are unlikely to have vision-threatening ocular problems.

Measurement of Visual Acuity

The method of visual acuity measurement (Table 175-1) depends largely on the age and level of cooperation of the child. The simplest of these tests is to look for a fixation preference by alternately covering one eye. The normal response is to maintain fixation with the uncovered eye. A child who consistently objects to covering one eye and has no objection to covering the other eye is said to have a fixation preference for one eye (Fig. 175-2). The methods used to measure visual acuity in young children do not yield a numerical measurement; *what is important is that both eyes show the same response.* Children often perform better if the test is practiced at near and under binocular conditions before one eye is completely covered with an eye patch or an occluder. When performing a "fixes and follows" acuity test, be sure not to provide audible clues—a blind child can track with eye movements a subtle sound all over the examination room!

Children more than 2 to 3 months of age should follow the examiner's face for several seconds with each eye. Children 6 to 12 months of age should follow a brightly colored toy (Fig. 175-3). A very useful and well-accepted method is the localization of small candy beads in the examiner's hand; children 12 to 30 months of age should sweep at or grasp a 1-mm bead at 13 inches using each eye. The examiner should extend both hands so as to force the child to choose the hand holding the candy (Fig. 175-4). Older children can be tested by using the picture chart, "E" game, or letters in the usual fashion at a 20-foot testing distance. Children who have significant differences in visual acuity between their two eyes (two Snellen lines difference) or who have abnormal acuity in both eyes (20/50 or worse for a 3-year-old, 20/40 or worse for a 5-year-old) should be referred to an ophthalmologist.

Assessment of Ocular Alignment

Strabismus in children may be associated with amblyopia due to suppression of the deviating eye or with vision- or life-threatening ocular disease such as cataracts, retinoblastoma, or congenital ocular malformations. Thus detection of strabismus is a key part of the vision-screening examination. Two major methods to detect strabismus exist—the corneal light reflex test and the alternate cover test.

The *corneal light reflex test* shows centration of the corneal reflection of a lighted toy in both pupils of a child who has normal ocular alignment. Temporal displacement of the reflex occurs in esotropia, and nasal displacement occurs in exotropia (Fig. 175-5). Any decentration is abnormal, but this test yields both false positive and false negative results because the visual axis may not coincide with the center of the pupil. A much superior test is the *cover-uncover test.* The examiner covers one of the child's eyes with a finger or occluder and looks for a refixation movement by the other eye. Both eyes must be tested, but the cover should not be moved from eye to eye; instead, the cover is used to cover one eye and then is removed. A few seconds later, the other eye is tested similarly. A refixation demonstrates the presence of strabismus (Fig. 175-6); an outward refixation means esotropia, and an inward refixation means exotropia. Further details of the testing methods can be found in Chapter 167, Strabismus. Any refixation is abnormal and should be referred for further evaluation.

Assessment of the Fundus Red Reflex

A normal fundus red reflex rules out any opacity of the ocular tissues that could cause amblyopia; it also rules out an intraocular tumor or coloboma involving the posterior retina. This test is performed with a direct ophthalmoscope in a semidark room (Fig. 175-7). With the ophthalmoscope on the zero power setting, the examiner should sit 3 to 5 feet from the child and direct the ophthalmoscope beam on the child's face. When looking through the ophthalmoscope, the examiner immediately will see a bright orange-red reflection from the fundus through the patient's pupils. Asymmetry, dimness, or whiteness of the reflex is abnormal and should be evaluated immediately by an ophthalmologist.

REFRACTIVE ERRORS

Refractive errors are the most common cause of decreased visual acuity in children. Four major types of refractive errors exist: (1) myopia, (2) hyperopia, (3) astigmatism, and

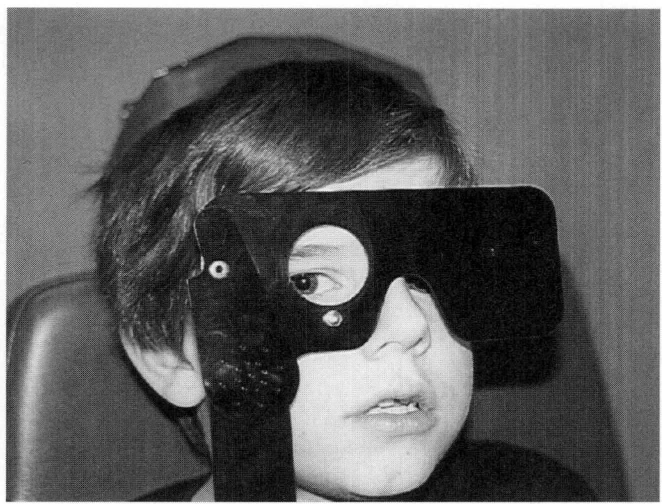

FIG. 175-1 This child is peeking around the occluder to use his left eye instead of the amblyopic right eye to see the visual acuity chart. This subtle behavior results in false negative visual acuity testing and a delay in the diagnosis and treatment of his amblyopia.

Table 175-1 Visual Acuity Measurement in Children

Method	Age of child
Fixes and follows examiner's face	3-6 months
Fixes and follows toy	6-12 months
Localizes candy beads	12-30 months
Picture chart	30-60 months
"E" game	5-6 years
Snellen letter chart	6+ years

(4) anisometropia. A detailed discussion of ophthalmic optics is beyond the scope of this chapter, but a few basic points will be set forth.

Myopia

Myopia (nearsightedness) exists when the refractive power of the eye is too strong for the length of the eye. Images from distant objects are focused in front of the retina and are blurred, but images from near objects are seen clearly. Myopia is the most common cause of decreased distance acuity in children. Mild myopia does not have to be corrected until the child reaches school age, but high myopia, as seen in many infants born prematurely, should be corrected by 9 to 12 months of age.

Hyperopia

Hyperopia (farsightedness) exists when the refractive power of the eye is too weak for the length of the eye. Without accommodation (focusing of the crystalline lens of the eye for near vision), images from distant objects are focused "behind" the retina and are somewhat blurred, and images from near objects are focused farther "behind" the retina and are more blurred. Children have a tremendous amplitude of accommodation, and hyperopic children can easily accommodate somewhat to see distant objects clearly and can accommodate more to see near objects clearly. Some children who have uncorrected hyperopia have eyestrain from constant accommodation, and others develop accommodative esotropia because excessive accommodation is linked to excessive convergence through the near reflex.

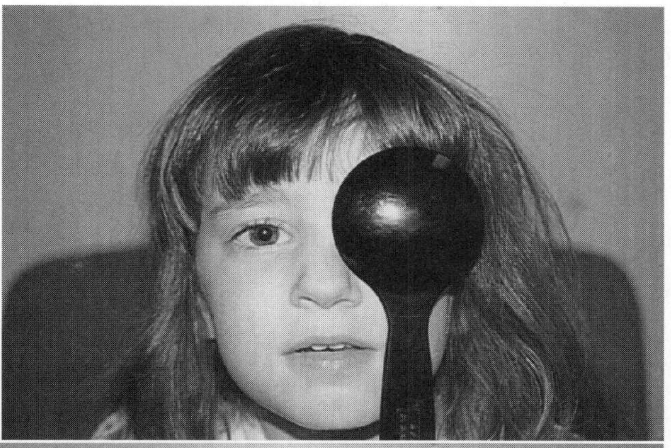

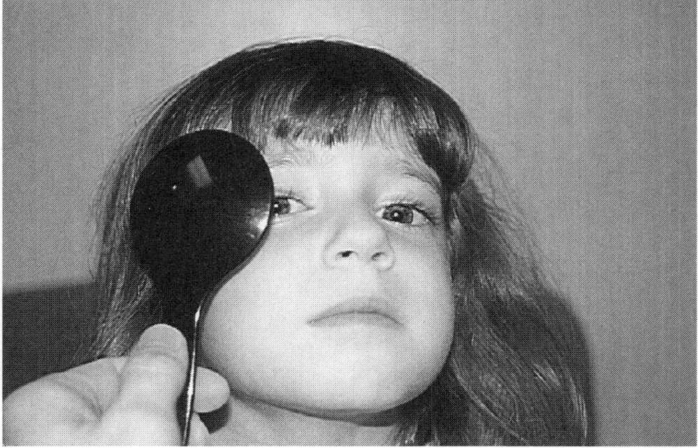

FIG. 175-2 **A,** This child happily fixes with her right eye and does not object if the left eye is covered. **B,** When the right eye is covered she moves her head away and tries to remove the cover, demonstrating a fixation preference for the right eye and amblyopia of the left eye.

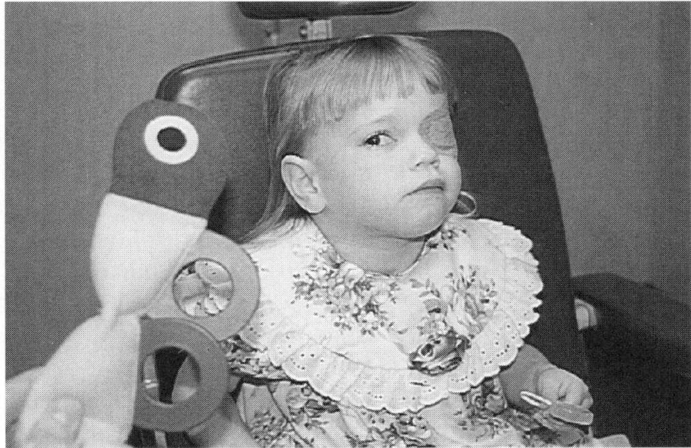

FIG. 175-3 This child follows the brightly colored toy easily with each eye.

Astigmatism

Astigmatism occurs when the refractive power of the eye is different in the horizontal than the vertical meridian of the eye. This generally occurs when the corneal curvature is

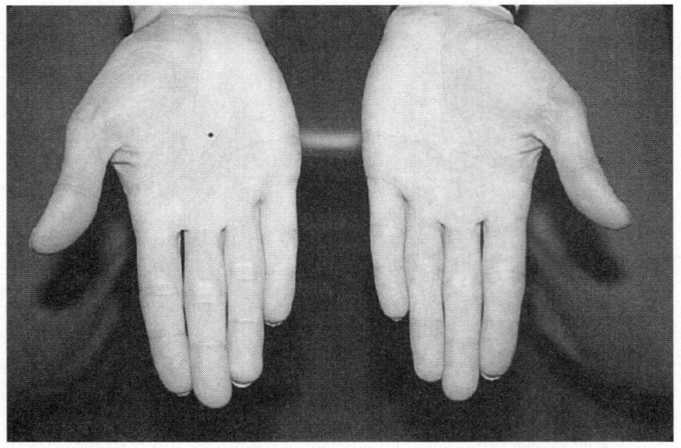

FIG. 175-4 Technique of visual acuity testing using a 1-mm candy bead in one hand while presenting both hands.

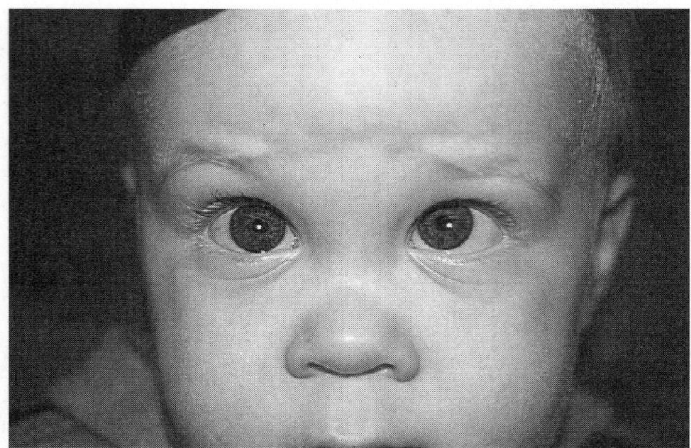

FIG. 175-5 The corneal light reflex test in a child who has esotropia.

steeper in one meridian than in the other. A descriptive exaggeration is that the cornea is shaped more like a football than a basketball. This causes a point object to be focused into a vertical line image in front of the retina and into a horizontal line image behind the retina. This lack of a point focus earns this condition the name *astigmatism* (without a point). Astigmatism causes both distant and near objects to be blurred.

Anisometropia

Anisometropia occurs when the refractive power between the two eyes is significantly different. One eye could be hyperopic and the other myopic, or one eye could have more hyperopia, myopia, or astigmatism than the other. Anisometropia is a common cause of amblyopia because the eye that has the larger refractive error has a constantly blurred image and does not have normal visual development.

FUNCTIONAL VISUAL LOSS

Functional (psychogenic) visual loss is a common cause of unilaterally or bilaterally decreased visual acuity. This occurs most commonly in the pediatric clinic because the child is fearful of upcoming injections or painful procedures. Another

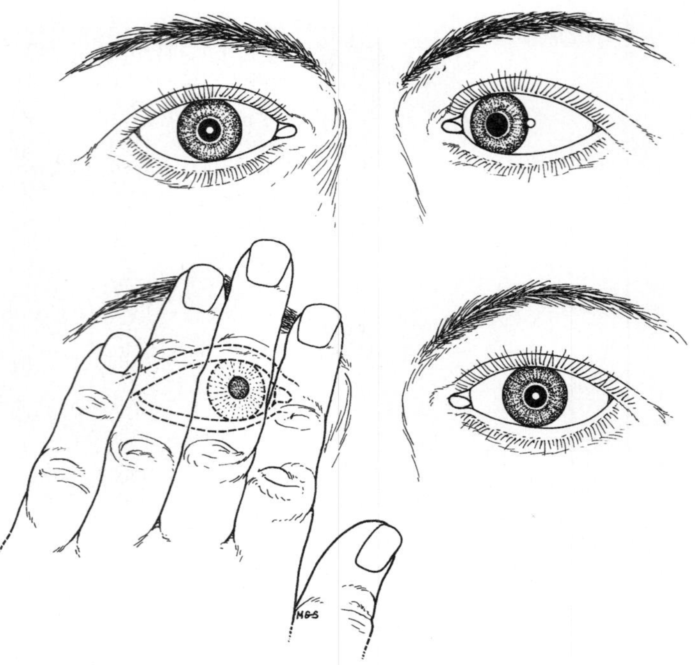

FIG. 175-6 The cover-uncover test demonstrating a temporal ocular refixation in a child who has esotropia.

common cause is the desire to obtain glasses because a classmate or sibling has them. A pair of medium-size spectacle frames that have plano (no power) lenses can be made by a local optician and will establish the diagnosis quickly in the child who wants to obtain glasses. Some children will continue to show abnormal visual acuity despite encouragement and retesting with plano lenses; these children should be referred to an ophthalmologist to rule out amblyopia, refractive errors, or ocular disease.

AMBLYOPIA

Amblyopia is a decrease in visual acuity in one or both eyes, with no apparent abnormality on physical examination. It is a very important cause of permanent visual loss and affects 5% of the United States population; the incidence of amblyopia may be much higher in economically deprived children or those who were born premature. Detection of amblyopia in young children is important for two reasons: (1) amblyopia can be treated successfully only in young children, and (2) life-threatening disorders (retinoblastoma) may present as amblyopia. Because the results of amblyopia treatment are much better in young children, the National Children's Eye Care Foundation aims to eliminate permanent visual loss caused by amblyopia through *effective vision screening of all children before they reach 3 years of age.*

Five types of amblyopia exist: (1) deprivation, (2) strabismic, (3) anisometropic, (4) occlusion, and (5) ametropic. *Deprivation* amblyopia occurs when the visual axis is blocked and a clear image cannot reach the retina. Typical causes include severe congenital or acquired ptosis, congenital cataract, and opacities of the vitreous body. Amblyopia often adds to the visual loss already caused by cataracts or other opacities of the ocular media. Bilateral deprivation am-

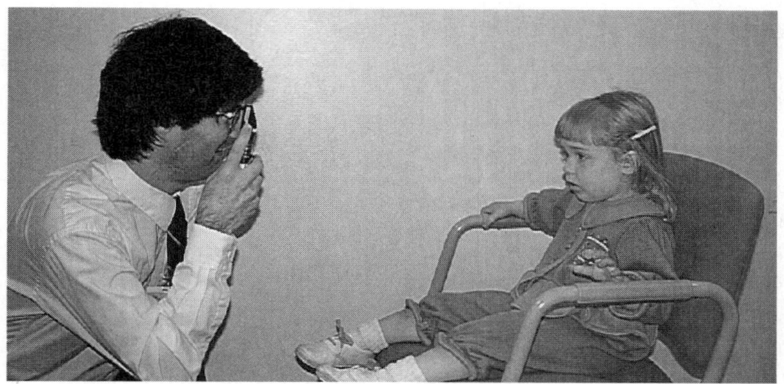

FIG. 175-7 The technique of assessing the fundus red reflex.

blyopia is possible in children who have bilateral occlusion of the visual axis. *Strabismic* amblyopia occurs when the same eye constantly is deviated; the brain ignores the image from the deviating eye and amblyopia results. *Anisometropic* amblyopia occurs when a significant difference in refractive power exists between the two eyes. The brain ignores the blurred image from the eye that has the larger refractive error and amblyopia results. *Occlusion* amblyopia is a subtype of deprivation amblyopia that occurs when the better-seeing eye is patched excessively in an attempt to improve the visual acuity of the amblyopic eye. The poorer-seeing eye becomes the better-seeing eye and vice versa. Frequent follow-up visits during patching therapy prevent this complication. *Bilateral ametropic* amblyopia occurs when both eyes have a large and equal refractive error, typically hyperopic astigmatism. Neither eye sees well at distance or at near, and bilateral amblyopia occurs.

OCULAR AND NEUROLOGICAL DISORDERS CAUSING VISUAL LOSS

Disorders causing visual loss can be categorized into (1) opacities of the optical media, (2) retinal disease and detachment, (3) optic nerve disorders, and (4) disorders of the visual pathways and the cerebral cortex. Common examples of each category will be provided, but summarizing the field of pediatric ophthalmology is beyond the scope of this chapter.

Opacities of the optical media can occur in the cornea, lens, and vitreous body. Corneal opacities can be caused by congenital anomalies, glaucoma, herpetic or bacterial keratitis, metabolic disease, corneal dystrophies, and trauma. Any opacity of the crystalline lens is called a cataract, which can be congenital, traumatic, or caused by other ocular or metabolic disorders. Common examples of vitreous opacities include a congenital anomaly called *persistent hyperplastic primary vitreous* and one called *vitreous hemorrhage* that is caused by child abuse or bleeding abnormalities.

Many retinal diseases can cause visual loss in children. Common examples include cicatricial changes from retinopathy of prematurity, congenital retinal infections (TORCH), metabolic storage diseases, and retinal dystrophies. Retinal detachment in children is rare, but can occur congenitally or in association with retinopathy of prematurity or trauma to the eye. Optic nerve disorders include congenital anomalies of the optic disk, optic nerve hypoplasia, optic atrophy, and optic neuritis. Optic nerve hypoplasia is a very important cause of visual loss because of a common association with midline CNS defects and a pituitary insufficiency called *De-Morsier syndrome*.

Disorders of the visual pathways posterior to the optic chiasm usually cause loss of visual field instead of an overall loss of visual acuity. Patients who have infarcts of both occipital lobes following prolonged hypotension or anoxia will have severe loss of overall visual acuity and of visual fields; this condition is called *cortical blindness*. Some infants will have delayed myelination of the visual pathways or the visual cortex and will demonstrate profound visual inattention during the first several months of life; this condition is called *delayed visual maturation*. This usually resolves by 6 months of age in otherwise healthy infants, but may take longer in infants who have other developmental delays caused by delay of myelination throughout the CNS. Migraine is a disorder of the visual pathways that may cause transient visual loss in children as the scintillating scotoma expands from a small spot near the fixation point to a large area covering nearly half of the visual field of each eye. This scintillating scotoma may not be associated with a headache, and the child may not be able to explain the visual phenomenon sufficiently for the examiner to consider migraine as the diagnosis. A carefully directed history may allow the child to explain the visual symptoms.

SUGGESTED READINGS

Berson FG: *Basic ophthalmology for medical students and primary care residents,* San Francisco, 1993, American Academy of Ophthalmology.

Nelson LB, Calhoun JH, Harley RD: *Pediatric ophthalmology,* ed 3, Philadelphia, 1991, WB Saunders.

Taylor D: *Pediatric ophthalmology,* Boston, 1990, Blackwell Scientific.

176 Vomiting

Martin H. Ulshen

Vomiting is a ubiquitous symptom of acute and chronic illness in childhood. This highly coordinated, active process must be distinguished from regurgitation, which is free reflux of gastric contents into the esophagus and mouth through an incompetent lower esophageal sphincter. Vomiting is a coordinated event usually preceded by nausea in association with increased salivation, gastric atony, and reflux of duodenal contents into the stomach. This phase may not be apparent in infants. Retching (coordinated contraction of abdominal and intercostal muscles as well as the diaphragm, with simultaneous closure of the glottis) immediately precedes the actual vomiting. Increased intragastric pressure from contraction of the abdominal wall musculature, lowering of the diaphragm, and pyloric contraction are associated with elevation and relaxation of the cardia, and vomiting occurs. The total process of vomiting is coordinated in the medullary vomiting center. This center may be influenced directly by visceral afferent stimuli or indirectly through the chemoreceptor trigger zone. The latter region is the site of action of many of the drugs that cause nausea and vomiting, including apomorphine and digitalis, as well as the site of initiation of motion sickness. Higher CNS centers may also influence the medullary vomiting center.

Recent understanding of the role of neurotransmitters as mediators of the initiation of vomiting has led to a range of new antiemetics. The area postrema, which is a major lower brainstem center for coordination of drug-induced vomiting, is rich in enkephalins, 5-hydroxytryptamine (HT) receptors, and dopamine receptors. Enkephalins and 5-HT both stimulate release of dopamine. Dopamine and 5-HT antagonists have been successful in the treatment of chemotherapy-induced nausea and vomiting. Antihistamines and anticholinergics prevent motion sickness by acting at H_1 and muscarinic cholinergic receptors, respectively, in the nucleus ambiguus in the lower brainstem and the lateral vestibular nucleus in the mid-pons.[1]

CAUSES AND DIFFERENTIAL DIAGNOSIS

The box on p. 1153 lists the most frequent causes of emesis in infants and children. In infancy, *regurgitation,* or spitting up, is very common and most often is a developmental event called *chalasia,* which has no sequelae and gradually resolves. Pathological *gastroesophageal reflux,* however, can be associated with severe complications (esophagitis with anemia secondary to blood loss, esophageal stricture, aspiration pneumonia, or failure to thrive). *Bilious vomiting* (especially associated with the first vomitus) usually occurs only with serious disease. In patients of any age it usually suggests gastrointestinal tract obstruction below the ampulla of Vater (in the second portion of the duodenum), although in newborns bilious vomiting also commonly is associated with necrotizing enterocolitis. In older children who vomit persistently, reflux of bile from the duodenum into the stomach may lead to bilious vomiting without gastrointestinal tract obstruction. Projectile vomiting commonly occurs with *pyloric stenosis.* When this condition persists, however, gastric atony may eliminate the projectile character. A *succussion splash* may be present, as in other causes of gastric outlet obstruction. Vomiting associated with increased intracranial pressure may be projectile and may take place in the absence of nausea or retching.

Persistent vomiting in a newborn or young infant who has no evidence of infection usually suggests a congenital gastrointestinal anomaly, inborn error of metabolism, or CNS abnormality such as hydrocephalus or subdural effusion. If the history and physical examination results do not suggest a cause, it is best to evaluate all three possibilities simultaneously. When the sudden onset of bilious vomiting, especially within the first few days of life, develops in a previously well newborn, one must consider a *malrotation* with secondary *midgut volvulus.* A plain film of the abdomen may show a paucity of gas distal to the upper small intestine; however, the plain film may not be helpful. If a midgut volvulus is suspected, an upper gastrointestinal roentgenographic series should be done at once with the controlled introduction of barium through a nasogastric tube after gastric aspiration. The lack of complete correlation of developmental rotation of the cecum with that of the duodenum makes a barium enema investigation of cecal position a less reliable study in evaluating a patient for malrotation. Midgut volvulus is a surgical emergency requiring early diagnosis and surgical intervention. In a sick newborn the diagnosis of *necrotizing enterocolitis* always must be considered in the event of bilious vomiting, especially with blood in the stool. Beyond the first week of life, but within the first 2 months, *pyloric stenosis* is the most common cause of persistent vomiting (but not regurgitation). In the older infant or child the entire spectrum of causes of vomiting listed in the box should be considered. It is interesting that patients who have *celiac disease* occasionally may have minimal or no diarrhea but prominent vomiting. When an older child manifests acute vomiting and somnolence, one always should consider drug overdose (especially aspirin toxicity), meningoencephalitis, and Reye syndrome in the differential diagnosis. Persistent or recurrent vomiting without other symptoms may be the major manifestation of an emotional disorder in childhood. Therefore a careful psychosocial history is an important part of the evaluation.

Cyclic Vomiting

Cyclic vomiting is characterized by repeated episodes of vomiting, sometimes occurring in clusters and sometimes associated with abdominal pain.[6] Uncontrollable vomiting and

CAUSES OF EMESIS (ARRANGED BY USUAL AGE OF EARLIEST OCCURRENCE)

Infancy

Gastrointestinal tract

Congenital
- Regurgitation—chalasia, gastroesophageal reflux
- Atresia—stenosis (tracheoesophageal fistula, prepyloric diaphragm, intestinal atresia)
- Duplication
- Volvulus (errors in rotation and fixation, Meckel diverticulum)
- Congenital bands
- Hirschsprung disease
- Meconium ileus (cystic fibrosis), meconium plug

Acquired

- Acute infectious gastroenteritis, food poisoning (staphylococcal, clostridial)
- Pyloric stenosis
- Gastritis, duodenitis
- Intussusception
- Incarcerated hernia—inguinal, internal secondary to old adhesions
- Cow milk protein intolerance, food allergy, eosinophilic gastroenteritis
- Disaccharidase deficiency
- Celiac disease—presents after introduction of gluten in diet, inherited risk
- Adynamic ileus—the mediator for many nongastrointestinal causes
- Neonatal necrotizing enterocolitis
- Chronic granulomatous disease with gastric outlet obstruction

Nongastrointestinal tract

- Infectious—otitis, urinary tract infection, pneumonia, upper respiratory tract infection, sepsis, meningitis
- Metabolic—aminoaciduria and organic aciduria, galactosemia, fructosemia, adrenogenital syndrome, renal tubular acidosis, diabetic ketoacidosis, Reye syndrome
- Central nervous system—trauma, tumor, infection, diencephalic syndrome, rumination, autonomic responses (pain, shock)
- Medications—anticholinergics, aspirin, alcohol, idiosyncratic reaction (e.g., codeine)

Childhood (additional causes)

Gastrointestinal tract

- Peptic ulcer—vomiting is a common presentation in children younger than 6 years old[2]
- Trauma—duodenal hematoma, traumatic pancreatitis, perforated bowel
- Pancreatitis—mumps, trauma, cystic fibrosis, hyperparathyroidism, hyperlipidemia, organic acidemias
- Crohn disease
- Idiopathic intestinal pseudoobstruction
- Superior mesenteric artery syndrome[7]

Nongastrointestinal tract

- Central nervous system—cyclic vomiting, migraine, anorexia nervosa, bulimia

retching are typical of an attack, but between episodes patients are well. Recently, low-dose erythromycin has been noted to treat some of these children successfully.[10]

Recurrent, episodic vomiting can be the major symptom of abdominal migraine or epilepsy. Abdominal migraine is characterized by the paroxysmal onset of repetitious attacks often relieved with sleep. A strong family history of migraine usually is present. Headache typical of migraine may occur with episodes. Propranolol is highly effective as prophylactic treatment for abdominal migraine, and its success helps to confirm the diagnosis. A careful history of the sequence of events and electroencephalographic evaluation are useful in the consideration of abdominal epilepsy. Anticonvulsants can be tried when this condition is suspected.

EVALUATION

Evaluation of the gastrointestinal tract usually includes an upper gastrointestinal contrast roentgenographic study. *Endoscopy* is feasible in all children, even newborns, if performed by an experienced examiner using a pediatric instrument.[4,9] Esophageal pH monitoring, esophageal biopsies, and gastroesophageal scintiscan all are useful in establishing a diagnosis of gastroesophageal reflux.[8,11] Ultrasound is helpful in diagnosing atypical pyloric stenosis, as is endoscopy. If brain tumor is a consideration in an infant, an MRI is more sensitive than a CT of the head.

TREATMENT

The most significant complications of vomiting include aspiration pneumonia, hemorrhage from a tear at the gastroesophageal junction *(Mallory-Weiss syndrome),* rupture of the esophagus (rare in children), and dehydration and electrolyte imbalance associated with persistent vomiting. Acute intercurrent vomiting *without serious underlying disease or significant dehydration* should be treated by administering clear liquids by mouth (e.g., in acute gastroenteritis or otitis media). It usually is advisable to start with a period of 4 to 6 hours without oral intake and then begin with frequent small quantities of clear liquids (1 teaspoonful to tablespoonful every 15 to 20 minutes for infants) and gradually increase the volume and extension of the period between oral fluids. Clear liquids may include Jell-O water (packet of gelatin to 1 quart of water), Kool-Aid, or flat cola or ginger ale. Carbonated beverages may increase vomiting. Fluids of high osmolality, long-chain triglycerides, and anticholinergic drugs all tend to slow gastric emptying and should be avoided.

Antiemetic drugs should be avoided in infants, although they may at times be useful in older children. The drug used most commonly for acute symptoms is promethazine (Phenergan). In the controlled studies that have been carried out, trimethobenzamide (Tigan) appears to have been less effective.[3] Rectal suppositories probably are preferable to oral drugs because nausea is associated with gastric atony and unpredictable absorption. Dopamine-receptor antagonists (such as metoclopramide) are effective for chemotherapy-induced vomiting, although 5-hydroxytryptamine$_3$ receptor antagonists (ondansetron) appear to have even greater efficacy without the risks of dystonic reactions associated with metoclopramide.[1] Histamine (H_1) receptor antagonists (including diphenhydramine, dimenhydrinate, meclizine, and promethazine) and muscarinic cholinergic receptor antagonists (e.g., scopolamine) prevent motion sickness.[1] Metoclopramide, cisapride, and erythromycin can help to treat poor gastric emptying without mechanical obstruction. Experience with cisapride in children is limited.

Patients should be monitored for signs of dehydration. For certain patients (e.g., those who have severe psychomotor retardation), a nasoduodenal infusion may circumvent the problem. Significant vomiting that requires intravenous fluid therapy usually is associated with hypochloremic alkalosis with secondary hypokalemia. Intravenous fluids should repair the deficits (see Chapter 28, Fluid Therapy).

Management of gastroesophageal reflux must be individualized. The extent of treatment depends on the volume of emesis and the presence of any of the complications of reflux (esophagitis with or without esophageal stricture or intractable anemia, failure to thrive, or respiratory manifestations). Medical management includes thickening feedings with cereal (a standard concentration is 1 tablespoonful of cereal for each ounce of formula). The efficacy of placing an infant in a supine or lateral, head-elevated position for sleep is questionable, although elevating the head of the bed remains standard therapy for older children and adults.[5] Older children also should avoid snacks or liquids after dinner and agents that exacerbate esophagitis (alcohol, caffeine, and smoking). Medications also can be used in an attempt to improve lower esophageal function and gastric emptying (e.g., metoclopramide or cisapride) and to decrease exposure of the esophageal mucosa to acid (antacids and histamine blockers). A slurry of sucralfate (a cytoprotective agent) four times a day has been used occasionally as well. When a child has severe gastroesophageal reflux, medical management may be unsatisfactory. In this case antireflux surgery (fundoplication) should be considered. In this group of children the results of surgery generally are good when performed by an experienced surgeon, and the benefits can be long lasting. In children who have psychomotor retardation and gastroesophageal reflux, antireflux surgery may not eliminate respiratory symptoms inasmuch as other factors such as swallowing dysfunction may contribute to these findings. Among all children undergoing a Nissen fundoplication, the risk of a postoperative complication that requires further surgery may be as high as 10% and underscores the need for careful patient selection for this operation.

REFERENCES

1. Allan SG: Antiemetics, *Gastroenterol Clin North Am* 21:597, 1992.
2. Deckelbaum RJ et al: Peptic ulcer disease: a clinical study in 73 children, *Can Med Assoc J* 111:225, 1974.
3. Ginsburg CM, Clahsen J: Evaluation of trimethobenzamine hydrochloride (Tigan) suppositories for treatment of nausea and vomiting in children, *J Pediatr* 96:767, 1980.
4. Hargrove CB, Ulshen MH, Shub MD: Upper gastrointestinal endoscopy in infants: diagnostic usefulness and safety, *Pediatrics* 74:828, 1984.
5. Orenstein SR: Prone positioning in infant gastroesophageal reflux: is elevation of the head worth the trouble? *J Pediatr* 117:184, 1990.
6. Reinhart JB, Evans SL, McFadden DL: Cyclic vomiting in children: seen through the psychiatrist's eye, *Pediatrics* 59:371, 1977.
7. Shandling B: The so-called superior mesenteric artery syndrome, *Am J Dis Child* 130:1371, 1976.
8. Shub MD et al: Esophagitis: a frequent consequence of gastroesophageal reflux in infancy, *J Pediatr* 107:881, 1985.
9. Ulshen MH: Unique aspects of gastrointestinal procedures for pediatric patients. In Drossman DA, editor: *Manual of gastroenterologic procedures,* ed 3, New York, 1993, Raven Press.
10. Vanderhoof JA et al: Treatment of cyclic vomiting in childhood with erythromycin, *J Pediatr Gastroenterol Nutr* 17:387, 1993.
11. Winter HS et al: Intraepithelial eosinophils: a new diagnostic criterion for reflux esophagitis, *Gastroenterology* 83:818, 1982.

177 Weight Loss

Carole A. Stashwick

The documentation of weight loss in an infant, child, or adolescent is an uncommon but highly significant event. A child's weight should be measured at each visit and plotted on standard growth charts in the medical record. Weight loss, as the chief complaint or as an incidental finding, should be evaluated and followed carefully. Illingworth[8] ranks the symptom "loss of weight" as 1 of 13 that may signal a serious problem in the child.

Parents may have the impression that a child has lost weight on the basis of a decrease in appetite or a change in the fit of clothing. Subjective impressions of weight loss always should be verified objectively before an evaluation is undertaken. True weight loss, however, sometimes may be difficult to differentiate from factitious weight loss, even when weights are documented in the medical record. A survey of child health clinics by the Centers for Disease Control and Prevention[12] revealed that specific errors in weighing children occurred at frequencies ranging from 5% to 20% of all children weighed. Errors were caused by faulty equipment and by poor technique—for example, weighing with the clothes on.

NEWBORNS AND YOUNG INFANTS

The normal full-term newborn who is breast-fed is likely to lose about 6% (±3%) of weight during the first 3 days of life, and at least 7% of infants will lose more than 10% of their birth weight.[10,11] A loss of more than 12% of birth weight in the few days after birth is uncommon and is cause for an investigation to ensure that the infant is well, that adequate intake is being provided, and that fluid losses from vomitus, urine, or stool are not excessive.[10] It generally is believed that the infant who is breast-fed should have regained the lost weight and thus be at or above birth weight by 2 weeks of age.[11]

The most common reason for the breast-fed infant to have lost more weight than expected or to have failed to regain the lost weight by age 2 weeks is inadequate intake at the breast, not because of "insufficient milk" or milk that is not sufficiently "rich." Inadequate weight gain occurs because of infrequent or short feedings, failure of the let-down reflex, or improper positioning of the infant for an effective suck.[15] The infant will appear well, although perhaps slim, and may or may not act hungry. A number of case reports have documented passivity and infrequent demands to be fed in some infants who are starving at the breast.[7,15]

The breast-feeding mother should be observed during a feeding, if possible, and specific evidence of a let-down or oxytocin reflex should be sought (uterine cramps, milk dripping or spraying from the opposite breast, a pins-and-needles sensation in the breast at the beginning of each nursing, and loud swallowing or occasional choking by the baby at the beginning of the feeding). The mother's motivation to breast-feed and her positive or negative feelings about the experience should be discussed; encouragement and support should be given for continuation of the nursing; and specific suggestions should be made for the mother to rest, to nurse frequently (every 2 to 3 hours in the day) to build up the milk supply, and to arrange relaxed, pleasant, and unhurried nursings. Formula or other fluids should not be recommended unless there are serious concerns about the infant's well-being. It is inappropriate for the physician prematurely to recommend discontinuing the nursing.[15] Demonstration of an appropriate weight gain in the following few days (120 to 200 g or more each week) is evidence that the infant is well and confirms the diagnosis of initial underfeeding. Infants who demonstrate failure to thrive while breast-feeding require more intensive nutritional rehabilitation while still preserving breast-feeding.[15]

The formula-fed infant rarely loses more than 5% of birth weight in the first few days inasmuch as complete nutrition is available beginning a few hours after birth.[10] Because it is unusual for a bottle-fed infant to weigh less than birth weight at the age of 2 weeks, such an infant should be evaluated carefully. An error in feeding caused by maternal inexperience or ignorance is the usual explanation, but a careful search for an organic problem, as well as an evaluation of the family's functioning, support mechanisms, and adjustment to the new infant, is indicated. Rarely the newborn will lose weight as a result of (1) inadequate intake for other reasons, such as infection, congenital heart disease, metabolic abnormality, somnolence from maternal medications or substance abuse, or poor suck resulting from a craniofacial or CNS abnormality, or (2) excessive fluid loss, such as vomiting associated with congenital gastrointestinal malformations (duodenal atresia, annular pancreas, volvulus), diarrhea, or polyuria (diabetes insipidus, renal disease) (see the box on p. 1156).

OLDER INFANTS, PRESCHOOLERS, AND SCHOOLCHILDREN

The infant may lose weight because of excessive vomiting, as in pyloric stenosis or severe gastroesophageal reflux. Tumors of the CNS in infancy may manifest with vomiting, anorexia, and cachexia.

The most common reason for weight loss in older infants and toddlers is fluid loss as a result of fever, vomiting, and diarrhea. The loss of weight may amount to 5% or more of premorbid body weight and usually is reversed with a few hours of oral or intravenous fluid replacement.

Weight loss also is a frequent concomitant of any severe febrile illness, such as pneumonia, pyelonephritis, septic arthritis, osteomyelitis, or meningitis, as well as less severe ill-

DIFFERENTIAL DIAGNOSIS OF WEIGHT LOSS BY AGE GROUP

Newborns

- Difficulties in establishing breast-feeding
- Inappropriate choice of formula or dilution
- Inadequate intake
  - Infection
  - Metabolic abnormality
  - Craniofacial abnormalities
  - CNS dysfunction
  - Somnolence from maternal medications/substance abuse
  - Congenital heart disease
  - Maternal depression/inexperience/lack of knowledge
- Excessive losses
  - Vomiting because of gastrointestinal malformations (duodenal atresia, others)
  - Polyuria (diabetes insipidus, renal disease)
  - Diarrhea

Infants, preschoolers, and school-age children

- Excessive losses
  - Pyloric stenosis
  - Gastroesophageal reflux
  - CNS tumors
  - Vomiting
  - Diarrhea
  - Fever and infection
  - Diabetes mellitus
  - Excessive activity
- Inadequate intake
  - Fever and infection
  - Tuberculosis
  - Surgery
  - Medication effect (loss of appetite)
  - Malignancy
  - Congenital heart disease
- Poor utilization
  - Malabsorption syndromes
  - Inflammatory bowel disease
- Immunodeficiency disorders, especially HIV infection
- Psychosocial dysfunction
  - Neglect; nonorganic failure to thrive
  - Parental depression
  - Childhood depression
  - Rumination
  - Childhood eating disorder

Adolescents

- "Dieting" behavior
- Adolescent eating disorders
  - Anorexia nervosa
  - Bulimia nervosa
  - Other eating disorder
- Psychiatric affective disorders, especially depression
- Malignancy
- Inflammatory bowel disease
- Diabetes mellitus
- Hyperthyroidism
- Tuberculosis

nesses such as stomatitis and pharyngitis. Resolution of the infection often is followed by a period of "catch-up" growth and weight gain. Surgical procedures commonly result in a temporary loss of weight.

Weight loss also may be caused by poor utilization of ingested foodstuffs. Cystic fibrosis, the most common disease in which malabsorption occurs in childhood, may appear in infancy as poor weight gain or actual weight loss. Malabsorption, weight loss, and constipation may occur in the child who has Hirschsprung disease. Children who have chronic diarrhea or severe immunodeficiency also may have weight loss. An infant or child who loses weight should be evaluated carefully for infection caused by the human immunodeficiency virus.[14]

Although emotional reasons often are the basis for an infant's or child's failure to thrive, actual weight loss is much less common than a slowdown or cessation of weight gain and linear growth. Psychosocial dysfunction (poor parent-child interaction, infant or childhood depression, rumination) that results in a child's weight loss requires a prompt and thorough evaluation.[5] Eating disorders have been described in prepubertal children as young as 7 years.[4]

The young child who has new-onset juvenile diabetes mellitus commonly loses weight (often 10% or more of body weight) despite polyphagia and polydipsia. Hyperthyroidism in childhood may manifest as weight loss. Children who have inflammatory bowel disease usually demonstrate poor weight gain or actual weight loss.

A diagnosis of tuberculosis should be considered in every child who has lost weight, particularly in those who have night sweats or cough. Malignancies, such as lymphoma, also may cause loss of weight with few other symptoms initially.

ADOLESCENTS

Planned dieting is widespread among adolescent girls and is the most common cause of weight loss in adolescents. Dieting must be distinguished carefully from an eating disorder, such as anorexia nervosa, which may affect as many as 1% to 2% of adolescent women in the United States, or bulimia nervosa, which may affect 1% to 5% or more.[6] Anorexia nervosa should be suspected when the adolescent is unwilling or unable to maintain body weight over a minimally normal weight for age and height and when attitudes and behaviors about eating or body image are distorted.[1] The anorectic adolescent may experience amenorrhea associated with emaciation and overactivity and may demonstrate clinical signs of malnutrition (hypothyroidism, bradycardia, hypothermia, growth of lanugo-like hair on the body and extremities).[6,9] Nutritional rehabilitation and psychiatric counseling are indicated (see Chapter 98, Anorexia and Bulimia Nervosa).

Bulimia nervosa is an eating disorder that to some degree overlaps to anorexia nervosa. Adolescents who have bulimia indulge in binge eating, followed by self-induced vomiting, self-starvation, overactivity, or the use of cathartics or diuretics to reduce weight.[1] These behaviors are practiced in secret, and the adolescent often denies them. An elevated serum bicarbonate or hypokalemia may provide evidence of chronic vomiting. The patient often is depressed and self-deprecating and may seek medical aid when the eating-vomiting pattern becomes compulsive and out of the patient's control. Psychiatric evaluation and counseling are indicated.[6,9]

Although severe degrees of weight loss during adolescence often can be ascribed to eating disorders, weight loss in adolescence also may result from other psychiatric disturbances, especially affective disorders; CNS tumors, particularly those of the hypothalamus, sella turcica, or other midline areas; or gastrointestinal problems, such as undiagnosed inflammatory bowel disease or other syndromes of malabsorption. Diabetes mellitus may manifest during adolescence with significant weight loss. Tuberculosis always should be considered and ruled out when an adolescent patient reports weight loss. Malignancies, particularly lymphoma, may present as weight loss.

INITIAL EVALUATION OF A COMPLAINT OF WEIGHT LOSS

The following should be included in the initial evaluation (Table 177-1):

1. A careful *history* and *physical examination,* with special attention to dietary intake, family functioning, and the patient's emotional well-being. The growth chart should be reviewed and updated.
2. A *complete blood cell count (CBC)* and *erythrocyte sedimentation rate (ESR).* The CBC screens for oncological factors and provides an overview of the nutritional state. The ESR may be elevated in collagen-vascular diseases, chronic infections, certain malignancies, and inflammatory bowel disease; it may be abnormally low in anorexia nervosa.[2]
3. *Serum electrolyte* and *kidney function* tests to evaluate dehydration, to reveal evidence of pernicious or self-induced vomiting, and to rule out renal or adrenal disease.
4. *Serum protein and albumin levels* to assess liver function, to determine whether the weight loss represents malnutrition, and to rule out protein malabsorption. Reversal of the albumin/globulin ratio is seen often in collagen-vasular diseases and malignancies.[13]
5. *Tuberculosis skin test.*
6. *Stool for occult blood* and *tests of malabsorption* to diagnose gastroenteritis, inflammatory bowel disease, and the various causes of malabsorption. The *serum carotene* level may be low in infancy and in malabsorptive conditions but often is elevated in anorexia nervosa.[2]
7. *Urinalysis and urine culture* to rule out diabetes mellitus, diabetes insipidus, dehydration, urinary tract infection, and renal disease. The urine pH may be high (≥8) in adolescents who have eating disorders, particularly when vomiting occurs.[3]

Table 177-1 Laboratory Studies Helpful in Weight Loss

Suggested studies	Suggested diagnoses
Complete blood count, smear	Anemia Infection Nutritional deficiencies Malabsorptive syndromes Malignancy
Erythrocyte sedimentation rate (ESR)	Collagen-vascular disease Infection Inflammatory bowel disease Malignancy Anorexia nervosa (very low ESR)
Serum electrolytes, kidney function tests	Dehydration Vomiting, self-induced or pernicious Renal dysfunction Adrenal disorders Metabolic disorder (with acidosis) Collagen-vascular disease
Serum protein and albumin levels	Liver dysfunction Malignancy Malnutrition Protein malabsorption Protein-losing enteropathy
Tuberculosis skin test	Tuberculosis
Stool for occult blood	Gastroenteritis Inflammatory bowel disease Enteropathies
Serum carotene; specific tests of malabsorption	Malabsorption syndromes Cystic fibrosis Anorexia nervosa (high carotene)
Urinalysis, including specific gravity; urine culture	Diabetes mellitus Diabetes insipidus Dehydration Urinary tract infection Renal disease Adolescent eating disorder (high pH)

REFERENCES

1. American Psychiatric Association: *Diagnostic and statistical manual of mental disorders*, ed 4, Washington, DC, 1994, The Association.
2. Anyan WR: Changes in erythrocyte sedimentation rate and fibrinogen during anorexia nervosa, *J Pediatr* 85:525, 1974.
3. Arden MR et al: Alkaline urine is associated with eating disorders, *Am J Dis Child* 145:28, 1991.
4. Atkins DM, Silber TJ: Clinical spectrum of anorexia nervosa in children, *J Dev Behav Pediatr* 14:211, 1993.
5. Bithoney WG et al: Failure to thrive/growth deficiency, *Pediatr Rev* 13:453, 1992.
6. Fisher M et al: Eating disorders in adolescents: a background paper, *J Adolesc Health* 16:420, 1995.
7. Gilmore HE, Rowland TW: Critical malnutrition in breast-fed infants, *Am J Dis Child* 132:885, 1978.
8. Illingworth RS: *Common symptoms of disease in children,* ed 9, Oxford, 1988, Blackwell Scientific.

9. Kreipe RE: Eating disorders among children and adolescents, *Pediatr Rev* 16:370, 1995.
10. Lawrence RA: *Breastfeeding: a guide for the medical profession,* ed 4, St Louis, 1994, Mosby.
11. Maisels MJ, Gifford K: Breast-feeding, weight loss and jaundice, *J Pediatr* 102:117, 1983.
12. *Nutrition surveillance,* Atlanta, Sept 1975, p 10, Centers for Disease Control.
13. Pizzo PA, Lovejoy FH, Smith DH: Prolonged fever in children: review of 100 cases, *Pediatrics* 55:468, 1975.
14. Rand TH, Meyers A: Role of the general pediatrician in the management of human immunodeficiency virus infection in children, *Pediatr Rev* 14:371, 1994.
15. Stashwick C: When a breastfed infant isn't gaining weight, *Contemp Pediatr* 10:116, 1993.

178 Wheezing

Thomas A. Hazinski

The term *wheezing* is often used by parents and children to refer to any noise made during breathing; to avoid ambiguity, however, the term should be used precisely to describe a high-pitched sound heard with a stethoscope during the terminal phases of exhalation. Wheezes also may be heard without the use of a stethoscope, usually in patients who have chronic asthma, acute foreign body inhalation, or psychogenic asthma.

Wheezing usually implies obstruction of the distal airway, but a wheezelike sound also can be produced by patients who have peribronchial edema (e.g., congestive heart failure) and disorders of the proximal or middle airway. The presence or absence of wheezing correlates poorly with the degree of impairment in pulmonary function. As shown in Tables 178-1 and 178-2, the differential diagnosis of wheezing is extensive, so if one approaches the wheezing patient with only asthma in mind, life-threatening but correctable disorders may be missed.

Lower airway obstruction usually causes wheezing only during exhalation, because of dynamic changes in airway caliber during spontaneous breathing. During inhalation, normal airways (or even narrowed or unstable airways) inside the thorax are expanded by the inspiratory decrease in pleural pressure (as the pressure in the airway becomes positive with respect to pleural pressure). In contrast, narrowed or poorly supported intrathoracic airways will narrow further during exhalation, when intrathoracic pressure begins to exceed the pressure inside the airway lumen. Although small airway closure can thus occur at the end of exhalation, in the normal lung this is counterbalanced by the alveolar walls, which act as springs to hold the small airways open at low lung volumes. In addition, at low flow rates (e.g., as respiratory muscle fatigue in the wheezing child develops), a wheeze may not be generated, despite the presence of severe obstruction. In these patients the appearance of wheezes actually may indicate a beneficial response to therapy as flow rates improve and airways open.

In addition to wheezing, another useful sign of airway obstruction is a prolongation of the expiratory time. During a normal breath the ratio of inspiratory time to expiratory time is approximately 1 : 1. During airway obstruction, however, expiratory airflow resistance increases, and this ratio approaches 1 : 2. Indeed, in some wheezing patients who have acute tachypnea, the next inhalation actually may occur before complete exhalation has occurred, thus eliminating the pause between breaths and producing a progressive increase in end-expiratory lung volume, termed *dynamic hyperinflation.*

DIFFERENTIAL DIAGNOSIS OF WHEEZING

Among the anatomical causes of wheezing, large airway "floppiness" is common in infancy and is termed *tracheomalacia.* Most of these infants have had inspiratory *stridor* as a major sign since birth, but wheezing may occur if the lack of airway rigidity is limited to the bronchi. Wheezing develops as the abnormal airway is opened on inspiration but dynamically narrows on expiration, with airflow occurring through the distorted areas. A coarse, low-pitched expiratory sound is generated.

Fixed lesions of the trachea or bronchi may not cause wheezing, inasmuch as the degree of obstruction is not influenced by the respiratory cycle. These lesions, however, may cause or be associated with softening of the adjacent airway wall sufficient to cause wheezing occasionally. Two examples are a completely circular *tracheal stenosis* or a *vascular ring;* these lesions encircle the airway and essentially are unyielding. Many of these patients have residual tracheomalacia after surgical correction.

In patients who have *acute infections* and *asthma,* wheezing is generalized on auscultation, whereas localized wheezing may indicate the presence of a discrete obstruction *(mucus, foreign body,* or *tumor).* Tumors or granulomata may be found in the lumen of the airway, but most lung tumors in children occur outside the lumen and compress the airway to produce obstruction with focal hyperinflation or atelectasis.

Patients who have *emphysema* or *interstitial inflammation* may wheeze because damaged alveolar walls cannot act as springs to hold the small airways open. The wheezing of patients who have *bronchopulmonary dysplasia* or *cystic fibrosis* may be intermittent and asymmetrical because the wheezing is caused by a combination of mucous obstruction, inflammation, loss of airway tone, and bronchial hyperreactivity.

Most of the causes of wheezing in the lower airway are acquired. Infection is the most common cause of acute wheezing, with viral agents being implicated the most frequently. The smaller airways most often are affected by *respiratory syncytial virus* (RSV) or *parainfluenza,* but tracheal involvement, as in viral tracheobronchitis *(croup)* and *bacterial tracheitis,* may occur. These infections, especially in infants, lead to coarse expiratory wheezes. Bacterial tracheitis can involve the large airway, creating such limited airflow that fine wheezing develops, which leads to its confusion with severe asthma.

Tables 178-1 and 178-2 summarize the causes of wheezing.

EVALUATION OF THE WHEEZING CHILD

Physical signs to be recorded are the expiratory time, respiration rate, and the degree to which accessory respiratory muscles are used. Anteroposterior and lateral chest radiographs provide the key laboratory procedure for diagnosis of the wheezing patient, because they allow identification of fo-

Table 178-1 Causes of Diffuse Wheezing

Location	Pathological or anatomical cause	Clinical diagnosis	Type of wheeze generated
Trachea	Loss of airway wall rigidity	Laryngotracheomalacia	Generalized, coarse
	Airway inflammation	Tracheobronchitis, bacterial tracheitis	Generalized, coarse to fine
Bronchi	Less airway wall rigidity	Bronchomalacia	Localized, fine
	Foreign body	Aspirated foreign body	Localized, fine
	Inflammation and mucous obstruction	Bronchiectasis	Localized, fine, bubbly
	Extrinsic compression	Mediastinal tumor or nodes	Localized, coarse
	Airway and elastic tissue destruction	Emphysema	Generalized, fine
	Inflammation	Bronchitis	Generalized, fine
Bronchioles	Inflammation and mucous obstruction	Bronchiolitis	Unusual—generalized, fine, but occasionally localized with mucous obstruction
	Airway wall edema, smooth muscle hypertrophy	Asthma	Same as for bronchiolitis
	Peribronchial edema	Congestive heart failure	Diffuse, fine
	Peribronchial hemorrhage	Hemosiderosis	Focal or diffuse, fine

Table 178-2 Differential Diagnosis of Diffuse Wheezing as a Function of Age

Age group	Acute	Chronic or recurrent
Infants	Infection (bronchiolitis), including tuberculosis and opportunistic infection in immunosuppressed patients Congestive heart failure Asthma	Tracheomalacia Cystic fibrosis Tracheoesophageal malformations Vascular ring Tracheal stenosis Congenital lobar emphysema Diaphragmatic hernia Bronchopulmonary dysplasia Gastroesophageal reflux Aspiration pneumonitis Extrinsic compression of airway by tumors (e.g., neuroblastoma) Visceral larva migrans Histiocytosis Hemosiderosis Asthma
Children and adolescents	Infection Foreign body Asthma	Foreign body Asthma Allergic bronchopulmonary aspergillosis Cystic fibrosis Ciliary dysmotility syndromes Tumors, lymph nodes Alpha-1-antitrypsin deficiency Sarcoidosis Vocal cord dysfunction Psychogenic causes

cal lesions. The clinician should remember that 50% of patients ultimately found to have a foreign body have no history of choking or cough. When a foreign body is suspected, additional radiographs should be obtained to demonstrate asymmetrical and sustained hyperinflation.

Asthma should not be diagnosed in an infant or child during the first episode of wheezing until a pattern of recurrent wheezing responsive to bronchodilator therapy is documented. In infants the differential diagnosis of acute wheezing should include usual or unusual infections, a foreign body, and congenital malformations. Viral and bacterial infections may cause transient bronchial hyperreactivity, and wheezing with respiratory infections can develop in patients who have bronchial hyperreactivity. For this reason patients who have respiratory infections often may respond to bronchodilator therapy.

SUGGESTED READINGS

Benjamin B: Tracheomalacia in infants and children, *Ann Otol Rhinol Laryngol* 93:438, 1984.

Gilbert EF, Opitz JM: Malformations and genetic disorders of the respiratory tract. In Stocker JT, editor: *Pediatric pulmonary disease,* New York, 1989, Hemisphere.

Hillman BC: Evaluation of the wheezing infant, *Allergy Proc* 15:1, 1994.

Kraemer R, Abeischer CC, Shoni MH: The "wheezy infant": diagnosis, epidemiology, and management, *Agents Actions* 40:13, 1993.

O'Connell MA, Sklarew PR, Goodman DL: Spectrum of presentation of paradoxical vocal cord motion in ambulatory patients, *Ann Allergy Immunol* 74:341, 1995.

Sporik R: Early childhood wheezing, *Curr Opin Pediatr* 6:650, 1994.

PART EIGHT

Specific Clinical Problems

179 Acne

Donald P. Lookingbill

Acne is so prevalent in young adults that some consider it a physiological event. However, this perspective does not take into account the impact of acne on the patient, and it may preclude therapeutic intervention. This chapter addresses acne as a treatable disease that deserves medical attention.

ETIOLOGY

Hormones

Acne is a disease of the pilosebaceous unit.[1,14,18] Androgens stimulate the sebaceous glands, which enlarge and increase their production of sebum. Before puberty the responsible androgens are of adrenal origin.[10] With puberty, gonadal androgens further stimulate the sebaceous glands. In most studies to date, patients with acne have not had abnormal levels of circulating testosterone; therefore tissue androgen metabolism may be the more important factor in the pathogenesis of acne.[9] One of the major organs for androgen metabolism is the skin, where the enzyme 5-alpha-reductase metabolizes testosterone to dihydrotestosterone, which has much more potent activity at the tissue level. Some evidence suggests that 5-alpha-reductase is more active in the skin of acne patients. This would be expected to increase androgenic stimulation of the sebaceous glands, ultimately causing acne. Increased sebaceous gland activity is necessary for acne to develop, yet alone it is insufficient to cause disease. Additional factors are needed.

Follicular Obstruction

If sebum is allowed to drain freely to the surface, the surface skin becomes oily, but acne does not develop. Acne can develop only if the outlet of the follicular canal is obstructed, which occurs when adherent, keratinized cells within the canal accumulate and form an impaction that blocks the flow of sebum (Fig. 179-1). Production of keratinized cells within the lining of the follicular canal is normal, but accumulation and subsequent impaction are not. This follicular obstruction, which also may be influenced by androgens, is a prerequisite for the development of acne.

Bacteria

Sebum and keratinous debris accumulate proximal to the follicular outlet obstruction. This provides an attractive environment for the growth of anaerobic bacteria, particularly *Propionibacterium acnes,* that play a role in the pathogenesis of inflammatory acne.[17] Several factors may be involved in causing the inflammation. One theory suggests that the lipase enzymes elaborated by *P. acnes* hydrolyze sebaceous lipids, releasing free fatty acids, which then cause irritation when the follicle ruptures. *P. acnes* also produces chemotactic factors that may attract inflammatory cells directly to a sebaceous follicle. Some evidence indicates that complement-mediated inflammation is directed against *P. acnes* itself. Whatever the mechanism of inflammation, there is little question of the therapeutic benefit of antibiotics.

The pathogenic events involved in the development of acne, then, include (1) androgenic stimulation of sebaceous glands, which increases sebum production, (2) keratinous impaction in the pilosebaceous canal, causing outlet obstruction, (3) accumulation of sebaceous and keratinous debris behind the obstruction, and (4) proliferation of *P. acnes,* which alters this milieu in such a way as to contribute to the rupture of the dilated pilosebaceous unit, resulting in extravasation of its contents into the surrounding dermis and inflammatory acne lesions.

CLINICAL FINDINGS

The disease process may begin at a surprisingly young age. In a recent study of premenarchal girls, 78% were found to have some acne.[10] The same investigators found acne to be present in 100% of adolescent boys.[11] Although the severity of the disease increases during adolescence, acne by no means is confined to these years. It is not uncommon for acne activity to continue into the third and fourth decades of life, much to the consternation of the afflicted patient.

The pathogenic mechanisms previously described result in the following types of clinical lesions: noninflamed open and closed comedones and inflammatory papules, pustules, nodules, and cysts.

The acne found in prepubertal children is predominantly noninflammatory and so may easily be overlooked. The open comedo (blackhead) and closed comedo (whitehead) are lesions caused purely by obstruction of the pilosebaceous canal; there is no accompanying inflammation.

Inflammatory acne is rare in young children and should raise the suspicion of a possible hyperandrogenic condition, such as that associated with congenital adrenal hyperplasia or even a rare androgen-secreting tumor. Girls should be examined for virilization, and boys and girls should be checked for precocious puberty. Screening blood studies should include serum levels of testosterone, dehydroepiandrosterone sulfate (DHEA-S), and 17-hydroxyprogesterone.

Not surprisingly, acne lesions have a predilection for skin rich in sebaceous glands. Accordingly, the face is the prevailing site, although acne also is often found on the chest and back. The lower portions of the trunk, buttocks, and thighs are involved much less commonly, and the distal extremities are always spared.

DIFFERENTIAL DIAGNOSIS

It rarely is difficult to diagnose acne; usually the condition can be diagnosed from "across the room," although, as men-

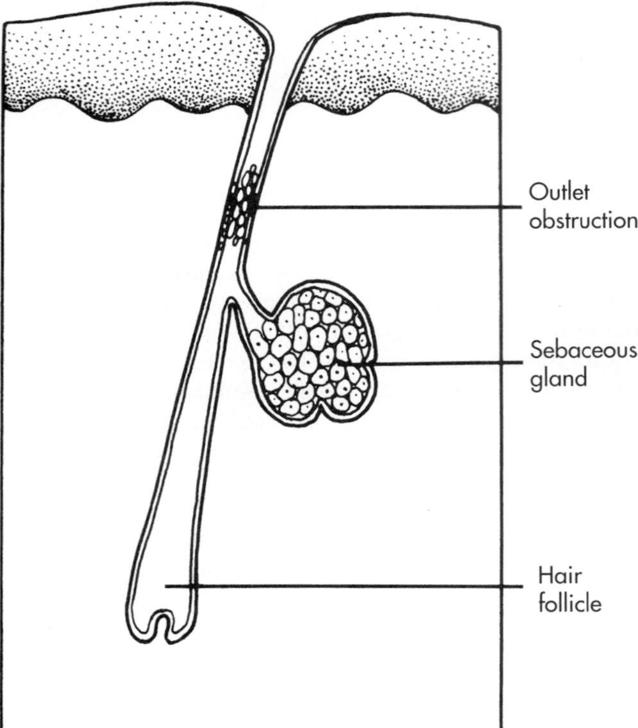

FIG. 179-1 Obstruction of the pilosebaceous unit in acne.

tioned, the comedonal lesions may require closer inspection (Fig. 179-2). Occasionally acne may be confused with flat warts, milia, or adenoma sebaceum, and acne variants may occur.

Flat Warts

Small, flesh-colored warts may be confused clinically with closed comedones. The question usually can be resolved with very close inspection—a flat wart has a sharp right-angled edge and a finely roughened surface, whereas a closed comedo has a dome shape and a smooth surface. Flat warts also vary in size; closed comedones are uniformly small.

Milia

Milia are small epidermal inclusion cysts that sometimes also are confused with comedones and occasionally with inflammatory pustules, especially in infants who have neonatal acne.

Adenoma Sebaceum

A misnamed disorder (the lesions actually are angiofibromas), adenoma sebaceum is one of the skin manifestations in tuberous sclerosis. Clinically the lesions appear as pink papules, which occasionally are confused with the lesions of acne. Adenoma sebaceum should be suspected if the papules are (1) clustered primarily in the center of the face, (2) persistent, and (3) resistent to acne therapy.

Acne Rosacea[14]

Acne rosacea is an acneiform eruption that can be distinguished from acne by a background blush of erythema and

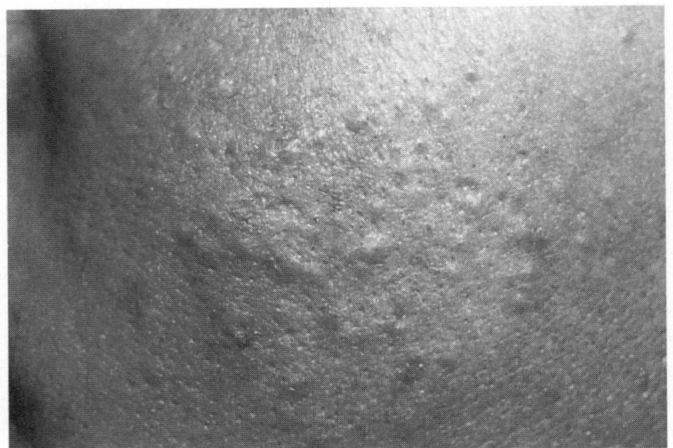

FIG. 179-2 Closed comedones (whiteheads) appear as dome-shaped, flesh-colored papules, which often are overlooked.

telangiectasia and by the absence of comedones. Also, rosacea most often occurs in middle-aged adults.

Steroid Acne[4]

Both systemic and topical steroids can induce acne. Acne from systemic steroids usually appears as numerous small, uniform-size papules and pustules with a predilection for the upper trunk. The condition involutes slowly and spontaneously after the steroids are discontinued.

Gram Negative Folliculitis

Gram negative organisms occasionally can produce a pustular folliculitis in patients being treated for acne with systemic antibiotics. This condition should be suspected in any patient whose disease flares up during therapy, especially if the flare-up is manifested by numerous pustules. A bacterial culture with antibiotic sensitivity studies should be done so that the diagnosis can be confirmed and the antibiotic therapy changed.

PSYCHOSOCIAL CONSIDERATIONS

Acne can be a devastating disease. In an ironic quirk of timing, it occurs at a time of life when personal appearance is of prime concern and self-consciousness is at its peak. Some young people appear to be more affected psychologically by acne than others, but no one is comfortable with it.[5,6] Patients who have severe cystic acne may even be socially ostracized. Regardless of the acne's severity, the condition is important to the patient seeking help and deserves serious attention. Patients are not impressed with soothing advice that trivializes their disease and reassures them that they eventually will "outgrow it." Fortunately, an alternative to this advice is possible—medical therapy is available that can produce effective, gratifying results.

MANAGEMENT

Three methods of treatment have proved effective for acne: topical comedolytic agents,[12] topical and systemic antibiotics,[3] and systemic retinoids.[8,13] The most traditional, yet still effective, treatment regimen comprises comedolytics and antibiotics.

Comedolytics

Topical *retinoic acid* (Retin-A) and *benzoyl peroxide* both help disimpact the keratinous plug in the follicular canal. They are most helpful in treating superficial acne lesions, that is, comedones and superficial papules and pustules.[14] Of the two agents, retinoic acid has a somewhat more active effect on comedones,[16] but benzoyl peroxide preparations also exert an antibacterial effect. When both agents are used, the patient should be instructed to apply the retinoic acid at bedtime and the benzoyl peroxide each morning. Both Retin-A and benzoyl peroxide are available in a variety of preparations. The "strength" of a given preparation reflects its irritancy and probably also its efficacy. Benzoyl peroxide gels are marketed in concentrations of 2.5%, 5%, and 10%. For Retin-A, the strength of the preparation depends both on the concentration of the drug and the nature of the vehicle in which it is contained (Table 179-1). Patients initially are prescribed the mildest preparations, and the potency is increased at subsequent visits if necessary.

Skin irritation, which usually becomes less of a problem with continued use, is the major side effect of the comedolytics. Also, about 1% of patients develop a true allergic contact dermatitis to benzoyl peroxide, which requires permanent discontinuation of this agent. Because topical retinoic acid may make the skin more susceptible to the effects of sunlight, patients should be instructed to avoid excessive exposure to the sun and to use sunscreens if they need to be exposed to the sun for prolonged periods.

Antibiotics

Antibiotics are indicated for patients who have inflammatory acne lesions. Topical agents such as tetracycline, erythromycin, and clindamycin have been formulated for commercial use. However, if a patient already is using the two topical comedolytics mentioned earlier, the addition of a third topical agent becomes confusing. Therefore systemic antibiotics are preferred for most patients. *Tetracycline is the drug of choice* because of its proved efficacy, its relatively low cost, and its low incidence of side effects, even when given over a long period. However, because of dental staining, tetracycline should not be used in patients under age 9. Food, particularly dairy products, interferes with the absorption of tetracycline, and so it needs to be taken on an empty stomach. The most convenient times are on awakening in the morning and on retiring at night. For the occasional patient who does not respond adequately to tetracycline, erythromycin may be used as an alternative. Doxycycline and minocycline also may be substituted, but doxycycline is more likely to cause photosensitivity, and minocycline is very expensive.

Systemic Retinoids

The systemic retinoid 13-*cis*-retinoic acid (isotretinoin, or Accutane) became commercially available in September 1982 for use in the treatment of *severe cystic acne*.[8] This drug reduces follicular keratinization, sebum production, and intrafollicular bacterial counts. The net result of these (and possibly other) effects is a dramatic improvement in acne. The therapeutic effect usually takes several months to begin and often is sustained long after the recommended 20-week course of therapy is discontinued. Unfortunately, side effects are common. Almost all patients experience mucocutaneous

Table 179-1 Retin-A Preparations

	Mildest	Mild	Moderate	Strongest
Cream	0.025%	0.05%	0.1%	
Gel		0.01%	0.025%	
Solution				0.05%

reactions (cheilitis, conjunctivitis, and dry mucous membranes of the mouth and nose), and extracutaneous complications also occur. For example, systemic retinoids can elevate plasma lipid levels and cause asymptomatic vertebral hyperostoses.[2] Most important is the drug's teratogenicity. Exposure to isotretinoin in pregnancy has been associated with a 25-fold increased risk of major fetal malformation.[7] Thus it is *mandatory* that female patients exercise strict birth control while taking this drug. As mentioned before, isotretinoin is recommended only for those who have severe cystic and/or scarring acne, a minority of acne patients.

Patient Compliance

Patient compliance is the single most important aspect of successful acne treatment. Without patient compliance, even the most effective medications are doomed to failure. To maximize compliance the physician must take time at the initial visit to explain in detail the use of each medication, as well as the effects and side effects to be expected. To reinforce these instructions it is helpful to give the patient printed instructions, an example of which is shown in the box on p. 1168. Medications are used only twice daily. If this activity is linked to an established daily routine, such as brushing the teeth, it, too, can become habitual. Given careful, specific instructions, most patients who have acne are exceptionally compliant and, given time, obtain good results for their efforts. In this regard, the "it takes time" concept needs to be emphasized to all patients; otherwise they may become prematurely, and inappropriately, discouraged. The acne instruction sheet also can be used to answer several other questions, often unasked, that acne patients or their parents frequently have. The most common of these pertain to diet, cleanliness, cosmetics, and picking at the lesions.

Diet. Although some evidence indicates that the usual American diet may have adverse effects on acne,[15] specific foods have not been implicated. For the vast majority of patients, it is useful to remember Dr. A.M. Kligman's admonition,[14] "The disease is enough of a curse without gustatory deprivations." For most, a sensible diet is all that is suggested.

Cleanliness. The question of cleanliness is pondered more by parents than by patients. To help maintain peace at home it is useful to dispel the notion that acne is a function of poor hygiene. It is not. In general, acne cleaning agents need not be recommended, since most irritate the skin, unnecessarily compounding the irritation caused by the recommended topical comedolytics.

Cosmetics. Because cosmetics have been implicated as possibly contributing to the acne process, it is preferable not to use them. If cosmetics are used, they should be water based and used sparingly.

Picking. In many patients who have acne, much of the skin damage is self-inflicted. Although the temptation to squeeze

ACNE INSTRUCTION SHEET

Topical medications: benzoyl peroxide and retinoic acid

A. Action
   1. Both help open up clogged pores.
   2. Benzoyl peroxide also helps kill bacteria in the pores.
B. Method of use (apply to *all* affected areas)
   1. Apply retinoic acid at bedtime.
   2. *Do not* use acne scrub cleaners.
   3. Apply benzoyl peroxide in the morning.
C. Possible problems
   1. May make the condition look worse rather than better after several weeks ("bringing acne to surface").
   2. May cause irritation (e.g., redness, dryness, and tenderness). If too much irritation does occur, use every other night until the skin becomes accustomed to it. If irritation is severe, stop medication and schedule a return visit.

Tetracycline

A. Action—helps kill bacteria; particularly useful for deep and inflamed lesions.
B. Method of use—needs to be taken on an *empty* stomach. Therefore take it as soon as you get out of bed in the morning (wait ½ hour before eating breakfast) and at bedtime, at least 1 hour after taking any evening snack.
C. Potential side effects
   1. Uncommon; most patients have no trouble.
   2. May upset your stomach and cause nausea and/or diarrhea.
   3. Occasionally causes a yeast vaginitis, particularly if you are taking birth control pills.
   4. Should not be taken if you are pregnant or trying to get pregnant.

General

A. Diet—for most patients, foods have no effect on acne. If you notice that a certain food aggravates the condition, simply avoid that food. Otherwise, no restrictions are necessary.
B. Washing—acne cannot be washed off. Wash your face with regular soap two to three times and bathe or shower daily.
C. Results from medicines—*it takes time,* usually several months, to begin to see benefits. At a return visit in 2 months, some improvement should be present, but it is unlikely that the acne will be cleared. The medications and their dosage will be altered at that time, depending on the response.
D. Conscientious and *regular* use of the medications is essential. They will not do any good if not used regularly.
E. Cosmetics—they may aggravate your acne. If you must use them, do so sparingly and use only those which are water based.
F. No picking!

a fresh pustule can be overwhelming, the practice must be discouraged. Picking, probing, and squeezing cause more tissue damage and sometimes produce scars. For some acne patients, picking may become so obsessive that excoriations are the only lesions seen.

COMPLICATIONS

The major complications of acne are its psychosocial ramifications.[5,6] In addition to the cosmetic liability of active lesions, permanent scars compound and perpetuate the problem in some unfortunate patients, mainly those who have inflammatory lesions. Established scars are difficult to treat. Many patients have been disappointed with the results of *dermabrasion.* Bovine *collagen injections* have been used in some patients, producing short-term improvement, but repeated injections often are necessary, and the long-term results are not yet known. Because scars are prevented more easily than treated, the emphasis in acne is on early, aggressive medical therapy such as that outlined earlier.

PROGNOSIS

With proper treatment the prognosis for acne is good, if not excellent. Patients should understand that most therapies control rather than cure the disease and that improvement does not occur overnight. However, improvement does occur, usually within 2 months of starting therapy, and it is at this time that the first revisit is best scheduled. At that visit the acne regimen can be adjusted as necessary. For example, the potency of the comedolytics can be increased (or reduced) and the dosage of the antibiotic altered, depending on the initial response. Continued improvement is to be expected with continuation of therapy. For many patients the dose of systemic antibiotics can be reduced gradually and eliminated after a number of months, but most patients require prolonged maintenance therapy (often over years) with topical agents and, in some cases, continued antibiotic therapy.[3]

Historically, cystic acne has been the most difficult to treat, but isotretinoin has become a powerful tool for dealing with this disastrous disease. This drug has the potential to effect prolonged remissions, sometimes lasting for years after a single course of therapy. However, as was previously discussed, isotretinoin has serious side effects, and its use is reserved for patients who have severe cystic and/or scarring acne that does not respond to standard treatment.

REFERENCES

1. Cunliffe WF: *Acne,* Chicago, 1989, Mosby.
2. Ellis CN et al: Long-term radiographic follow-up after isotretinoin therapy, *J Am Acad Dermatol* 18:1252, 1988.
3. Hughes BR et al: Strategy of acne therapy with long-term antibiotics, *Br J Dermatol* 121:623, 1989.
4. Hurwitz RM: Steroid acne, *J Am Acad Dermatol* 21:1179, 1989.
5. Koo JYM, Smith LL: Psychologic aspects of acne, *Pediatr Dermatol* 8:185, 1991.

6. Krowchuk DP et al: The psychosocial effects of acne on adolescents, *Pediatr Dermatol* 8:332, 1991.
7. Lammer EJ et al: Retinoic acid embryopathy, *N Engl J Med* 313:837, 1985.
8. Layton AM, Cunliffe WJ: Guidelines for optimal use of isotretinoin in acne, *J Am Acad Dermatol* 27:S2, 1992.
9. Lookingbill DP et al: Tissue production of androgens in women with acne, *J Am Acad Dermatol* 12:481, 1985.
10. Lucky AW et al: Acne vulgaris in premenarchal girls: an early sign of puberty associated with rising levels of dehydroepiandrosterone, *Arch Dermatol* 130:308, 1994.
11. Lucky AW et al: Acne vulgaris in early adolescent boys, *Arch Dermatol* 127:210, 1991.
12. Melski JW, Arndt KA: Topical therapy for acne, *N Engl J Med* 302:503, 1980.
13. Peck GL et al: Prolonged remissions of cystic and conglobate acne with 13-*cis*-retinoic acid, *N Engl J Med* 300:329, 1979.
14. Plewig G, Kligman AM: *Acne and rosacea,* ed 2, New York, 1993, Springer-Verlag.
15. Rosenberg EW: Acne diet reconsidered, *Arch Dermatol* 117:193, 1981.
16. Thomas JR, Doyle AR: The therapeutic uses of topical vitamin A acid, *J Am Acad Dermatol* 4:505, 1981.
17. Webster GF: Inflammatory acne, *Int J Dermatol* 29:313, 1990.
18. Winston MH, Shalita AR: Acne vulgaris: pathogenesis and treatment, *Pediatr Clin North Am* 38:889, 1991.

180 Acquired Immunodeficiency Syndrome (AIDS) and Human Immunodeficiency Virus (HIV) Infection

John H. Dossett

Acquired immunodeficiency syndrome (AIDS) is a moderately advanced stage of infection with the human immunodeficiency virus (HIV). AIDS appears to be a relatively new infectious disease that has burgeoned into a devastating worldwide pandemic since the late 1970s. The designation *AIDS* is a descriptive term that was applied to a new clinical syndrome when it was first recognized in 1980. The term was used as an epidemiological tool to study this new syndrome. The infectious agent was identified in 1983, and since then, the designation *AIDS,* however well-entrenched, has no longer been a useful concept. Although HIV infection eventually causes an immune deficiency syndrome in most patients, it has many other clinical manifestations that are not related to immune deficiency.

The rapid spread of HIV since 1980 has resulted in tens of thousands of infected infants and children. Moreover, the huge number of infected adults in their childbearing years has threatened to produce an ever-increasing number of infected infants and children. Early in the epidemic, the Centers for Disease Control and Prevention (CDC) recognized that the designation *pediatric AIDS* was confusing. A system for classifying pediatric HIV infection (see the box on p. 1171) was established and has been used very effectively for describing the manifestations and clinical course of HIV infection in infants and children.

Children who fulfill the CDC case definition of HIV infection may be classified according to the presence or absence of clinical signs and symptoms and subclassified according to the status of their immune function and clinical findings. *Class P-0* includes indeterminate infection in children who have antibody to HIV, indicating exposure to an infected mother, but in whom the diagnosis of HIV infection has not yet been confirmed. *Class P-1* includes patients who have documented infection with HIV but who have no clinical signs or symptoms. The subclassifications of this group rely on immunological testing, which should include quantitative immunoglobulin determination, a complete blood cell count with differential, and T lymphocyte subset quantitation. *Class P-2* includes children who have symptoms of longer than 2 months' duration, such as the nonspecific findings of *subclass A,* which include fever, failure to thrive, generalized lymphadenopathy, hepatomegaly, splenomegaly, parotitis, and diarrhea. The lymphoid interstitial pneumonitis noted in *subclass C* is based either on histological confirmation or on chronic pneumonitis of at least 2 months' duration that is confirmed with a chest roentgenogram.

This classification system is based on current knowledge and diagnostic abilities. The criteria may need to be revised as diagnostic techniques are refined further and become available generally.

EPIDEMIOLOGY

HIV infection is primarily a disease transmitted both heterosexually and homosexually. It also is transmitted easily through transfusions of blood or blood products and by needles contaminated with blood. Most children are infected through longitudinal transmission from mother to child, either transplacentally, perinatally, or, in rare cases, through breast milk. Early in the HIV epidemic many children were infected through blood or platelet transfusions and infusions of antihemophiliac factors; however, effective tests and screening of blood were introduced in 1985, and virtually all pediatric infections are now longitudinal infections. Adolescents are an exception in that most of their infections are acquired, just like those of adults, through unsafe sexual practices or intravenous (IV) drug use. The rising rate of HIV infection among children parallels and reflects the rising rate of infection in women of childbearing age. Such women increasingly are infected through heterosexual transmission rather than IV drug use. However, they commonly have a drug use connection in that many are the sexual partners of men who are IV drug users.

Approximately one third of infants born to infected mothers are infected with HIV. In children who have transfusion-acquired HIV infection, the latency period from time of infection to development of symptoms approximates the latency period of adults, 5 to 7 years. However, in longitudinally transmitted HIV infection, the latency period is much shorter; the average age of onset of clinical symptoms is closer to 8 or 9 months. The range of latency in longitudinally acquired disease is wide. Some infants manifest symptoms shortly after birth, and others are not sufficiently symptomatic for parents to seek medical attention until the infant is 2 to 3 years old. All races and socioeconomic groups are vulnerable to HIV infection, but it is far more prevalent among those who are poor, Hispanic, or African-American. This is true for adults and children.

Although symptomatic HIV infection is not common among adolescents, it is clear that a large number of adolescents are being infected because clinical symptoms are prevalent in individuals between 21 and 29 years of age. Many of these cases reflect infection during adolescence in that the latency period from time of infection to onset of symptoms commonly is 5 to 7 years.

SUMMARY OF THE CLASSIFICATION OF HIV INFECTION IN CHILDREN YOUNGER THAN 13 YEARS OF AGE

Class P-0.

Indeterminate infection

Class P-1.

Asymptomatic infection

Subclass A.

Normal immune function

Subclass B.

Abnormal immune function

Subclass C.

Immune function not tested

Class P-2.

Symptomatic infection

Subclass A.

Nonspecific findings

Subclass B.

Progressive neurological disease

Subclass C.

Lymphoid interstitial pneumonitis

Subclass D.

Secondary infectious diseases
Category D-1. Specified secondary infectious diseases listed in the CDC surveillance definition for AIDS
Category D-2. Recurrent serious bacterial infections
Category D-3. Other specified secondary infectious diseases

Subclass E.

Secondary cancers
Category E-1. Specified secondary cancers listed in the CDC surveillance definition for AIDS
Category E-2. Other cancers possibly secondary to HIV infection

Subclass F.

Other diseases possibly due to HIV infection

PATHOPHYSIOLOGY

HIV is a member of the lentivirus family. Currently, two serotypes of HIV (HIV-1 and HIV-2) have been identified; however, the great majority of patient isolates are HIV-1.

HIV predominantly infects cells that have a CD4 receptor (most commonly the T_4 lymphocyte). However, studies have shown that other cell surface moieties also may be important for entry of the virus. The virus consists of (1) an outer lipid envelope that has an external surface antigen (gp 120) and an anchoring segment (gp 41), (2) a cylindrical core referred to as P_{24}, and (3) genomic RNA, consisting of polymerase genes, structural genes, and functional genes.

The polymerase enables the transcription of the viral RNA genome into a DNA copy that eventually becomes integrated into the host cell chromosomal DNA. In this form, replication of the virus may be suspended for varying periods (up to 8 years), during which the individual may be relatively well and less infectious. On the other hand, the virus may reproduce actively, leading to cytopathic effects characterized by syncytium formation, degeneration, and lysis. The infected cells may be stimulated to reproduce the virus by a variety of factors, such as interaction of the infected cell with other agents such as cytomegalovirus (CMV) or herpes simplex virus (HSV). It is during this period of active replication that clinical symptoms, as well as increased infectivity, may be marked.

Inasmuch as the T_4 cells are particularly susceptible to HIV, this cell group, normally responsible for destruction of viruses, undergoes dramatic qualitative and quantitative change; this is the basis for the immunological abnormalities and profound immunodeficiency, with subsequent clinical consequences, seen in HIV infection.

Although HIV primarily infects the lymphoid cells, ultimately causing immunodeficiency, it also clearly infects other tissues, producing devastating consequences that are independent of the immunodeficiency syndrome. Most specifically, HIV infects the brain, producing an encephalopathy that is out of proportion to the immunodeficiency.

CLINICAL ILLNESS

The most important factor in diagnosing pediatric HIV infection is *a high clinical index of suspicion*. With this in mind, meticulous attention to details in the history and the physical examination will alert the clinician, allowing early confirmation. Because most HIV infection in children is acquired perinatally, the disease affects younger children predominantly. In more than half of cases the diagnosis can be made within the first year of life, and in most of the others it can be made by age 3. Generally, the time between infection and the onset of symptoms is shorter among children who acquire the infection longitudinally than among those who are infected through blood transfusion.

HIV infection is a chronic infection that causes chronic disease. Within weeks after infection, many individuals have an acute mononucleosis-like syndrome associated with fever, sore throat, lymphadenopathy, splenomegaly, and a sense of being unwell. This usually resolves within 1 to 2 weeks, and the patients most often return to their previous state of health. They remain asymptomatic for a variable period, which may last for several years. When the asymptomatic period is over, they begin to develop manifestations of immune deficiency and other illnesses (discussed later).

Children who have longitudinally acquired infection can be divided into two distinctly different subsets. In one group, the illness remains quiescent well through the first 2 to 3 years of life; then the children begin to manifest symptoms of HIV infection. In the other group, intrauterine growth may be retarded, and major manifestations of HIV infection may appear within the first 8 to 9 months of life. Many of the patients in this second group develop lymphadenopathy, hepatosplenomegaly, and failure to thrive in the first months of life. Others develop encephalopathy by 7 or 8 months of age and have either progressive deterioration of the central nervous system (CNS) or static encephalopathy.

It generally is believed that these two courses reflect developmental maturity at the time of infection. As with other intrauterine viral infections (e.g., congenital rubella and CMV infections), infants infected early in gestation commonly have profoundly severe clinical manifestations. In contrast, the children in the other subset are thought to be infected intrapartum or immediately postpartum. These children have a more mature immune system that can handle the virus better, and they develop clinical manifestations later in life.

History

A thorough pediatric history begins with a careful review of the antenatal history. It is clear that the presence of any one of a number of risk factors in women of childbearing age significantly increases the risk of HIV infection. These factors include IV drug use, multiple sexual partners, blood transfusions before the year 1985, or sexual partners who have known risk factors (known infection with HIV, bisexual practices, history of IV drug use, hemophilia, or blood transfusions before 1985) (see the box on the right, top).

The important clinical clues that suggest HIV infection in infants and children are prematurity and low birth weight, recurrent oral thrush, failure to thrive, recurrent fevers, chronic diarrhea, recurrent infections, opportunistic infections, blood transfusions, and sexual abuse (see the box on the right, center).

The adolescent history, as always, needs to address the issues of IV drug abuse and approach the details of sexual practices carefully and sensitively. This information must include not only participation in any sexual activity but also the number of partners, homosexual or bisexual encounters, and the use of contraceptive methods (especially the consistent use of condoms) (see the box on the right, bottom). Tattooing also may be a risk factor for HIV infection.

THE ANTENATAL HISTORY: HIV RISK FACTORS IN WOMEN OF CHILDBEARING AGE

Intravenous drug use
Multiple sexual partners
Blood transfusions before 1985
A sexual partner with any of the following characteristics:
- Known infection with HIV
- Bisexual practices
- History of IV drug use
- Hemophilia
- Blood transfusions before 1985

THE HISTORY: NEONATAL AND EARLY CHILDHOOD

Prematurity
Low birth weight
Recurrent oral thrush
Failure to thrive
Recurrent fevers
Chronic diarrhea
Recurrent infections
Opportunistic infections
Blood transfusions
Sexual abuse

THE HISTORY: ADOLESCENTS

IV drug abuse
Tattoos
Sexual practices
- Number of partners
- Homosexual preference
- Bisexual preference
- Contraceptive methods

Clinical Signs

After a careful history is obtained, attention should be paid to the details of the examination. The clinical manifestations of HIV infection are numerous and are addressed here systematically.

Nonspecific Findings. These include failure to thrive, recurrent or intermittent fevers, a diminished level of activity, and myalgia. Involvement of the lymphoid system is common, and generalized lymphadenopathy may be the only presenting clinical sign. Although lymphadenopathy is generally a common finding in the pediatric age group, the presence of more than two lymph nodes larger than 1 cm in diameter in two noncontiguous sites and particularly the presence of axillary adenopathy are important indicators of HIV infection.

Pulmonary Findings. Pulmonary disease is responsible for much of the morbidity and mortality among pediatric patients. Lymphoid interstitial pneumonitis (LIP) is common. It manifests clinically with tachypnea and progressive respiratory distress and often progresses to profound hypoxia. Radiographically, peribronchiolar lymphonodular aggregates and interstitial infiltrates are characteristic (Fig. 180-1). Biopsy, which may be required to distinguish this disorder from *Pneumocystis carinii* pneumonia (PCP), classically shows interstitial and peribronchial infiltration by lymphocytes and plasma cells. Recurrent bacterial pneumonias are common in children who have HIV infection. Of the opportunistic pulmonary infections, PCP is the most important pathogen, occurring in more than half of children who have HIV infection. Clinically it manifests with fever, tachypnea, and sometimes hypoxia. Radiographically it is characterized by a diffuse reticular pattern and pulmonary infiltration. Biopsy sometimes may be necessary to distinguish among LIP, PCP, and other opportunistic infections such as CMV and fungi.

Gastrointestinal Findings. The most common gastrointestinal manifestation is chronic or recurrent diarrhea. This may be secretory diarrhea, resulting from primary HIV involvement of the gastrointestinal tract. Alternatively the diarrhea may be caused by secondary agents such as enteroviruses, salmonella, or shigella; *Campylobacter, Cryptosporidium,* or

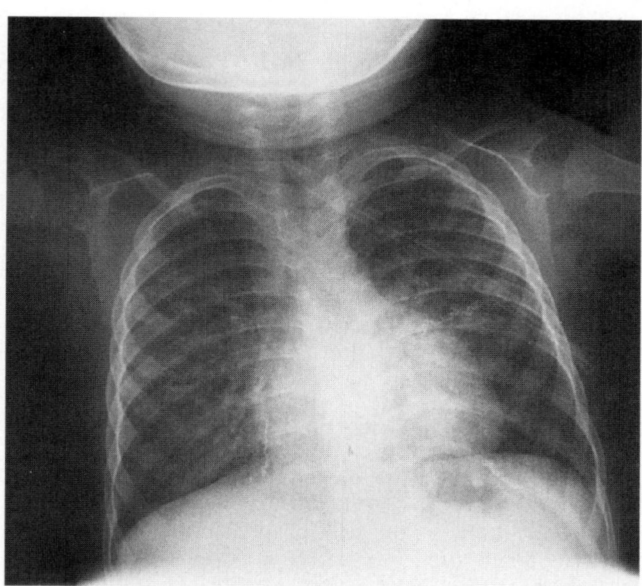

FIG. 180-1 Chest roentgenogram of a child with lymphoid interstitial pneumonitis (LIP). The infiltrates are diffuse, interstitial, and bilateral and have been described as reticulonodular.

Candida organisms; CMV or HSV; or *Giardia lamblia, Mycobacterium avium, Isospora belli,* or *Clostridium difficile.* Direct invasion of the bowel by some strains of HIV (e.g., invasion of the enterochromaffin cells that produce hormones responsible for bowel motility and digestion) may induce malabsorption and chronic secretory diarrhea. Infected macrophages in the stroma may be an indirect source of toxic cytokines that contribute to the secretory diarrhea.

Other gastrointestinal manifestations include parotitis, oral thrush, and esophagitis caused by *Candida,* CMV, or HSV organisms. Hepatitis, manifested by elevated transaminase levels, commonly is seen without serological evidence of hepatotropic virus infection. Biopsy may show nodular lymphoid aggregates in the portal triads, hepatocellular and bile duct damage, sinusoidal cell hyperplasia, endothelialitis, and changes that suggest chronic active hepatitis. Both HIV and CMV are possible infective causes. Pancreatitis also has been reported in the pediatric age group.

Neurological Findings. The prevalence of CNS manifestations of HIV disease among children has been reported to be as high as 90%. The clinical presentation varies and includes an encephalopathy characterized by delayed neurological development or loss of developmental milestones. Seizures may occur but are not typical. The physical examination may reveal extrapyramidal tract signs, paresis, peripheral neuropathy, ataxia, and pseudobulbar palsy. The encephalopathy seen in HIV infection almost always is due to the presence of HIV in the central nervous system. Secondary CNS infection, CNS lymphoma, and microvascular accidents are less common among children. Neuroradiological studies may show cerebral atrophy, white matter abnormalities, and basal ganglia calcification. Spinal fluid may show pleocytosis and an elevated protein; however, the cerebrospinal fluid (CSF) often is normal. Electroencephalograms may show normal findings or diffuse background slowing.

COMMON BACTERIAL PATHOGENS IN HIV

Streptococcus pneumoniae
Haemophilus influenzae
Streptococcus pyogenes
Salmonella spp.
Staphylococcus aureus
Escherichia coli
Pseudomonas spp.

Pathological findings include reduced brain weight consistent with atrophy, as well as microscopic calcifications in the walls of blood vessels. Multinucleated giant cells may be associated with inflammatory cell infiltrates. The inflammatory cells (microglia, mononuclear cells, lymphocytes, and plasma cells) may be found throughout the gray and white matter but are most prominent in the brainstem and basal ganglia.

Cardiovascular Findings. Cardiomyopathy with congestive heart failure has been seen in a number of children. Arteriopathy, characterized by vasculitis that progresses to fibrosis of the intima and media, has been reported.

Renal Findings. Children who have HIV infection may have renal disease that commonly manifests as proteinuria. The pathologic condition is most consistent with focal glomerulosclerosis or mesangial hyperplasia.

Dermatological Findings. An eczematoid rash commonly is found early in HIV infection. Infective causes of rashes may include candidiasis, herpetic gingivostomatitis, CMV, herpetic whitlow, chronic varicella eruptions, herpes zoster, molluscum contagiosum, condyloma acuminatum, impetigo, and cellulitis. Kaposi sarcoma is exceedingly rare in children.

Ophthalmological Findings. These may include a perivasculitis of the retinal vessels for which no infectious agent has yet been found. Opportunistic ocular infections include CMV retinitis, *Toxoplasma* retinitis, and fungal infections.

Hematological Findings. Thrombocytopenia has been reported in 10% to 20% of cases. It usually is an immune thrombocytopenia, although nonimmune thrombocytopenia is seen. Leukopenia, neutropenia, and anemia (including hemolytic anemia) are common hematological manifestations.

Infectious Findings. Recurrent bacterial and viral infections are the common initial markers that lead the practitioner to suspect HIV infection. Much like children who have congenital hypogammaglobulinemia syndromes, children who have HIV infection frequently have infections with common pyogenic bacteria. These may be relatively mild infections (e.g., pyoderma, recurrent otitis media, sinusitis, and other respiratory tract infections) or more serious bacterial infections (e.g., pneumonia, bacteremia, meningitis, cellulitis, and empyema). The bacteria usually responsible for these infections are listed in the box above.

Children who have HIV infection are deficient in cell-mediated immunity. This lack is reflected in their frequent viral, fungal, and protozoal infections. Although PCP (protozoan) is by far the most often seen, other opportunistic infections also are common (see the box on p. 1174). Children are particularly vulnerable to herpes viruses (CMV, Epstein-Barr virus, herpes simplex virus, and varicella-zoster virus).

OPPORTUNISTIC INFECTIONS IN CHILDREN WITH HIV

Pneumocystosis
Candidiasis (of the mouth, esophagus, trachea, bronchi, or lungs)
Cryptococcosis
Cryptosporidiosis
Cytomegalovirus infection
Persistent herpes simplex infection
Histoplasmosis
Isosporiasis
Toxoplasmosis
Mycobacteria infections
Herpes viruses (CMV, HSV, Epstein-Barr virus, varicella-zoster virus)

Infection with the measles virus may result in fatal disease, especially in those children who have a nutritional deficiency. Oral thrush is extremely common. Less commonly, *Candida albicans* causes extensive local invasion or severe systemic disease.

LABORATORY DIAGNOSIS

The clinical manifestations of HIV infection are protean and overlap with those of many other infectious diseases. Moreover, the implications of the diagnosis are of such medical and social significance that *reliable laboratory diagnosis is essential.* Culture of HIV from blood or other tissues is the gold standard; however, this method is prohibitively expensive and not readily available. Because HIV culturing generally is not available, the diagnosis depends on less direct methods of detecting the virus (antigen and antibody).

Methods of Detecting Antibody

Enzyme-Linked Immunosorbent Assay (ELISA). The ELISA is used widely to screen for HIV antibodies. Because it was developed initially for blood donor screening, it is more sensitive (95% to 99%) than specific. Its other advantages include reproducibility, rapid availability, and low cost. Inasmuch as there is a small risk of false positive results, *all positive ELISA reactions must be confirmed* by more specific tests such as the Western blot test.

Western Blot Test. This test identifies antibodies to specific antigens (such as the P_{24} antigen) by electrophoretically running the antigen through gel against the patient's sera and identifying specific bands. Standards have been published that allow test results to be identified as positive, negative, or indeterminate. Sera from individuals recently infected and from those who have advanced disease may produce an indeterminate pattern.

Crucial principles that bear on the interpretation of the tests for detecting antibodies include the following:

1. Maternal antibodies cross the placenta and may be detectable in an infant (infected or not) for approximately 15 months. That is, all babies born to seropositive women have detectable antibodies, regardless of whether they are infected. Approximately 30% of these infants eventually will have confirmed HIV infection.
2. Approximately 75% of seropositive infants who ultimately are found to be uninfected become antibody free by 1 year of age. However, a single negative result on an antibody test does not confirm that the infant is not infected. Absence of antibody may reflect an inability of the humoral system to respond to antigen or a phase of viral replication that results in binding of the limited amount of circulating antibody. Some infants under 6 months of age who have very severe disease produce no antibody at all.
3. Children older than 15 months of age who have a consistently positive result for HIV antibody are presumed to be infected with the virus.

Methods of Detecting the Virus

Culture. Culturing plasma and peripheral monocytes is an excellent means of diagnosing HIV infection; however, because of the expense and lack of availability this technique is not frequently used.

Antigen

1. Antigen capture immunoassay, which relies on viral replication for detection of HIV antigen (most important is the P_{24} [core] protein), depends on the quantity of virus present at the time of testing. Therefore P_{24} antigen can be detected most readily early in the course of infection (before or early during antibody production) and very late (when the humoral defense mechanisms may be overwhelmed). The absence of easily detectable P_{24} antigen in the blood does not indicate absence of infection. Persistence or recurrence of antigen in the blood of patients who have symptomatic disease may be an ominous sign, often heralding clinical deterioration.
2. The indirect fluorescent antibody (IFA) and immunohistochemical techniques are additional tests that may be used to detect viral antigen.

Polymerase Chain Reaction. The polymerase chain reaction is a new technique in which proviral sequences of HIV within host DNA are amplified, making small amounts of virus much easier to detect. This procedure may prove to be an important diagnostic tool in confirming the diagnosis in young infants.

Supplementary Laboratory Investigations

The aforementioned serological tests plus other studies that are listed in the box on p. 1175 may confirm the diagnosis. Immunological dysfunction is a hallmark. The affinity that HIV has for the lymphocyte explains many of the cellular and humoral abnormalities that are found. Lymphocytes infected with HIV may be killed, resulting in lymphocyte depletion (and reversal of the T_4/T_8 ratio). The function of infected cells that are not killed is altered, resulting in deregulation of the immune system. These functional derangements include depressed responsiveness to certain mitogens and absence of cutaneous-delayed hypersensitivity responses, such as to *Candida* and mumps antigens. The B lymphocytes also are affected, and despite the frequent occurrence of hypergammaglobulinemia, specific responses to antigenic stimulation are impaired. The hypergammaglobulinemia most often includes elevations of IgM and IgG and often precedes an obvious T cell defect. Increased circulating immune com-

POSSIBLE LABORATORY FINDINGS IN PEDIATRIC PATIENTS INFECTED WITH HIV

Immunological

- B cell abnormalities
  Hypergammaglobulinemia
  Increased circulating immune complexes
- T cell abnormalities
  Quantitative: reversed T_4/T_8 ratio
  Qualitative

Hematological

- Lymphopenia
- Neutropenia
- Anemia
- Thrombocytopenia

Hepatic

- Elevated transaminase levels

Pancreatic

- Elevated serum amylase

Renal

- Proteinuria
- Azotemia

plexes also have been reported. The abnormalities of the B lymphocytes help explain the increased risk of autoimmune diseases.

The immunological markers may help distinguish seropositive infants who are infected from those who are not. By 3 to 8 months of age, HIV-infected children show significantly higher IgG, IgM, and IgA levels and significantly lower T_4, T_8, and T_4/T_8 ratios than do children who have maternal antibodies but who are not infected. As early as the first month of life, infected infants also may have an elevated beta$_2$-macroglobulin compared with infants who are not infected.

Other laboratory abnormalities might include lymphopenia, neutropenia, thrombocytopenia, and anemia.

TREATMENT: PRINCIPLES AND PRACTICE

Providing care for pediatric and adolescent patients who have HIV disease requires a multidisciplinary approach with at least as much emphasis on psychosocial problems and methods of preventing further spread of the disease as on the specifics of medical management. Because most children who have HIV disease acquired the infection perinatally, appropriate counseling of adolescents and seropositive mothers is critical to the effort to prevent further transmission by this route. Thus physicians need to become comfortable with inquiring into the details of patients' sexual practices, sexual history, and use of contraceptives and drugs.

Social Aspects

Many pediatric patients who have HIV infection (more specifically, those who have transplacentally acquired disease) may be members of families that are unable to care for them. This may result from simultaneous complications of HIV disease in one or both parents, financial or social difficulties, and sometimes the paralyzing effects of drug addiction. Thus an enormous need exists for individuals who are willing to provide comprehensive care outside the hospital. The HIV epidemic has brought forward many compassionate heroes who have adopted these children and others who have become foster parents, providing long-term and respite care in their homes.

Parents and alternate caregivers often face a tremendous lack of support and often are alienated from the community (e.g., day care, school, religious groups, and family gatherings). This is due to ignorance and unfounded fear regarding the transmission and communicability of this disease. *One of the most important functions of the pediatrician is to become an advocate for the patient—one who will help the community understand that there is no reason why a child infected with HIV should be denied full participation in the school and social environment.*

Physicians commonly are asked to advise those in schools, churches, and day care centers about the risks of HIV transmission in these settings. We are reassured by the observation that HIV has not spread in the families of infected individuals except in situations in which people are sharing needles with or are sexually active with the index case. Good hand washing and appropriate disposal of debris should apply to *all* hospital and day care settings, regardless of whether HIV is a factor. Thus no specific precautions are required for those known to have HIV infection.

Care of Infants Born to HIV-Positive Mothers and Mothers Who Have Risk Factors for HIV

As already mentioned, all babies born to seropositive mothers have HIV antibodies. Seropositivity in infants or toddlers may represent passive acquisition of maternal antibody or active HIV infection. An algorithm for determining which of the infants are infected and which have only passively acquired antibodies is shown in Figure 180-2.

Because HIV can be transferred in breast milk, *infants born to seropositive mothers should not be breast-fed;* it is one of the few situations in which the risk outweighs the benefit. In countries where malnutrition and diarrhea are major causes of infant mortality, breast-feeding may be preferable to formula feeding.

Care of HIV-Infected Women

A large multicenter study has demonstrated clearly that the incidence of perinatal transmission is remarkably reduced by administration of zidovudine (AZT) to HIV-infected pregnant women. In this study the women were given AZT from the second trimester until delivery. In the intrapartum period they were given AZT intravenously to ensure that therapeutic concentrations of AZT were maintained through this critical period. The infants were given oral AZT for the first 6 weeks of life. Using this protocol, the transmission of HIV from mother to infant was reduced from 26% to 8%.

Immunizations

The observation that children who have other immunodeficiency syndromes sometimes have serious or fatal complica-

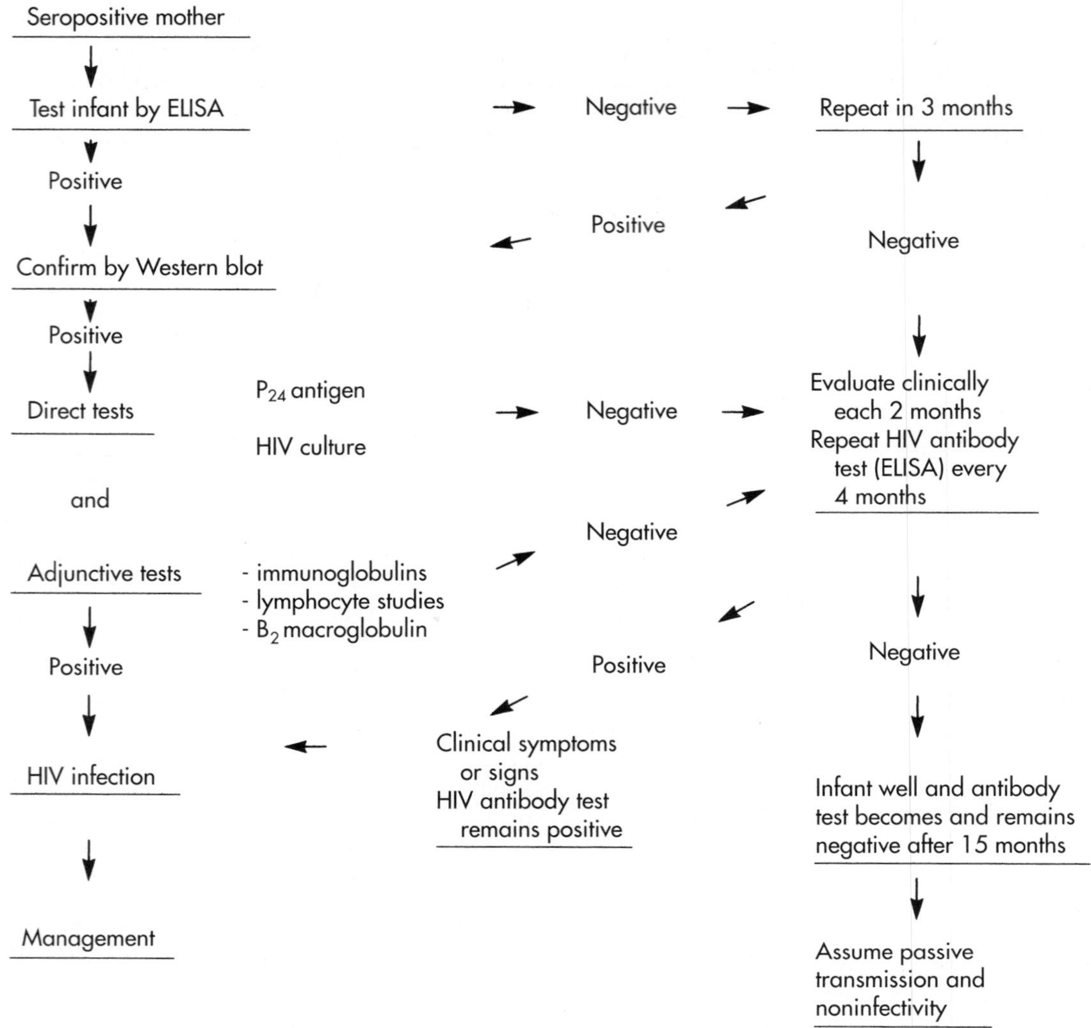

FIG. 180-2 Algorithm for determining whether an infant has HIV infection or only passively acquired antibodies.

(From Dossett JH: Perinatal HIV infection. In Nelson NM: *Current therapy in neonatal-perinatal medicine,* ed 2, Toronto, 1989, BC Decker.)

tions from live virus vaccinations has raised concern about immunization of children who have HIV infection. Initially it was recommended that the measles-mumps-rubella (MMR) vaccine not be given to children who have HIV symptoms. This recommendation has been changed because of reports of serious and fatal measles in HIV-infected children and because there have been no reports of adverse effects in the children who received this vaccine. In the event of contact with measles, even children who have received MMR should receive immunoglobulin because their response to the vaccine may have been suboptimal. Inactivated polio vaccine rather than oral attenuated poliovirus vaccine should be given to HIV-infected patients and also to their household contacts. All HIV-infected children should receive the diphtheria-pertussis-tetanus (DPT) vaccine, as well as a *Haemophilus influenzae* type b (Hib) conjugate vaccine, according to the usual schedule. Moreover, these children should be given pneumococcal vaccine and influenza virus vaccine even though immunocompromised children may have an attenuated response to them.

Varicella vaccine has been licensed for general use in children. Although experience with this vaccine in HIV-infected children is limited, it seems appropriate to immunize with varicella vaccine shortly after the infant is 1 year old. Based on experience with other attenuated virus vaccines (polio, measles, rubella, mumps), it is expected to be safe and to provide protection against serious varicella disease as the child becomes progressively more immunocompromised. Severely immunocompromised children who have not had chickenpox should be given varicella-zoster immunoglobulin after exposure to chickenpox or herpes zoster infection.

Nutritional Support

In severely ill children who have HIV infection, especially those who have intractable diarrhea, chronic intravenous alimentation may become essential. Home nursing often can ac-

Table 180-1 Pathogens in HIV-Infected Children

Organism	Syndrome	Method of diagnosis	Treatment	Comments
Pneumocystis carinii	Pneumonia	Pneumocysts seen on special stains of respiratory specimen or tissue	TMP-SMX (20 mg/kg TMP component/day IV or PO) or pentamidine isethionate (4 mg/kg/day IV or IM)	Toxic effects of therapy are common; treat for 21 days, relapses are common, prophylaxis may be beneficial
Toxoplasma gondii	Brain abscess	Brain scans; biopsy	Sulfadiazine and pyrimethamine (PO)	Toxic effects of therapy are common; use folinic acid; lifelong therapy is required to prevent relapse
Cryptosporidium sp.	Gastroenteritis	Stool examination (special procedure); biopsy	Best therapy is not known; supportive	Chronic infection
Candida sp.	Thrush, esophagitis	Wet mount or gram stain of lesions (thrush); esophagoscopy and biopsy (esophagus)	Clotrimazole, ketoconazole, fluconazole, amphotericin B	Relapses are common; consider maintenance
Cryptococcus sp.	Meningitis, fungemia, pneumonia	Cryptococcal antigen tests on blood, CSF; culture of blood, respiratory specimen, CSF; India ink test on CSF	Amphotericin B	Flucytosine can be used if tolerated; chronic suppressive therapy is required to prevent relapse
Cytomegalovirus	Chorioretinitis, pneumonitis, hepatitis, colitis, esophagitis, encephalitis, disseminated (including adrenals)	Ophthalmological examination (retinitis); tissue biopsy; culture (urine, sputum, buffy coat)	Gancyclovir	Relapses occur after therapy; suppressive regimen is required; isolation of virus does not alone provide diagnosis
Herpes simplex virus	Stomatitis, perianal infection	Tzanck preparation; culture	Acyclovir (750 mg/m^2/day IV, can treat PO)	Recurrences are frequent; chronic suppressive therapy may be needed
Varicella zoster virus	Primary varicella, local or disseminated zoster	Tzanck preparation; culture	Acyclovir (1500 mg/m^2/day IV)	Chronic or relapsing zoster lesions occur; indications for and effectiveness of oral therapy are not clear
Mycobacterium avium/intracellulare	Disseminated infection (blood, bone marrow, liver, spleen, GI tract, nodes)	Acid-fast blood culture; acid-fast stain or culture of tissue or fluid specimen	Clarithromycin	Drugs used have included ansamycin, clofazimine, ethambutol, amikacin, rifampin, isoniazid, and ethionamide, but their efficacy has not been documented

Modified from Falloon J et al: *J Pediatr* 114:17, 1989.
TMP-SMX, Trimethoprim-sulfamethoxazole.

commodate this procedure, so that the patient does not have to be hospitalized.

Treatment of Infectious Complications

Fever is a major manifestation of HIV infection. The fever may be a direct effect of HIV, or it may herald a secondary infection stemming from HIV-induced immunodeficiency. Some individuals who have acute HIV infection have an infectious mononucleosis-like illness characterized by fever, lethargy, and lymphadenopathy. This acute illness typically is mild and usually resolves completely within 1 or 2 weeks. Months to years later fever and lymphadenopathy may recur for which no specific infectious agent is found. It is believed that such fever is a primary manifestation of HIV. As has been mentioned, progressive immunodeficiency eventually develops. Consequently, fever in these children frequently may be caused by secondary infection with bacteria (often pyogenic), protozoa, fungi, or viruses. Such infections require appropriate antimicrobial therapy. Because of their antibody deficiency, these children also may need supplementation with intravenous immunoglobulin (IVIG). Moreover, monthly infusions of IVIG seem to reduce the frequency and severity of recurrent infections. Controlled studies in progress will determine the effectiveness of maintenance IVIG. Opportunistic infections with PCP, CMV, HSV, *Candida* organisms, and other agents are common. If these infections are to be treated appropriately, the definitive diagnosis must be pursued diligently. This requires aggressive tissue collections and thorough collaboration among the clinician, the pathologist, and the microbiologist. Table 180-1 summarizes some of the important organisms and requirements for their diagnosis and treatment.

Pneumocystis carinii Pneumonia Prophylaxis

Children who have HIV infection are at great risk of developing PCP. This risk is reduced remarkably if trimethoprim-sulfamethoxazole (TMP-SMX) is administered 3 days a week. Such prophylaxis also reduces the incidence of infection with some pyogenic bacteria.

Lymphoid Interstitial Pneumonitis

LIP is believed to be a primary manifestation of HIV rather than a secondary infection. Exacerbations and remissions are characteristic, making assessment and treatment difficult. Periodic monitoring of oxygen saturation is useful for detecting subtle progression of the disease. Supplemental oxygen therapy may make children more comfortable, and they adapt well to long-term administration at home.

Antiretroviral Therapy

Clinical trials to assess the efficacy and safety of antiretroviral drugs in children are in progress. The best studied drug is AZT, which prolongs the interval between infection and the development of symptoms. It also prolongs the life of individuals who already have symptoms. It does not eradicate HIV and consequently does not cure the disease. Although there are many potential sites for interrupting viral replication, most antiretroviral agents under investigation focus on inhibition of reverse transcriptase. Zidovudine (3^1-acido-3^1-deoxythymidine) is a nucleoside analog that is incorporated into viral DNA where it is believed to inhibit reverse transcriptase and possibly result in chain termination. This drug, which can be administered orally, penetrates the central nervous system. Because it inhibits viral replication but has no effect on latent virus, therapy probably will need to be continued indefinitely. AZT's toxicity is related both to the dose and the duration of therapy. Toxic effects include anemia, neutropenia, thrombocytopenia, headaches, nausea, myalgia, insomnia, and neurological side effects. Current dosages range from 120 mg/m^2/dose to 180 mg/m^2/dose (orally).

Recent clinical trials have shown that AZT in combination with dideoxyinosine (ddI) is superior to either one given alone. Clinical trials of the new protease inhibitors are in progress.

Vaccines

Numerous barriers block the development of an effective vaccine, including the genetic diversity of HIV, the lack of a good animal model, the appropriate reluctance to experiment with attenuated strains, the lack of evidence that humoral immunity is protective, and the absence of a controllable study population. Clinical trials of a recombinant HIV envelope vaccine are in progress.

PROGNOSIS

The spectrum of illness caused by HIV infection among children ranges from fully developed HIV-associated immunodeficiency in the first 6 months of life to perinatally acquired infection in children still clinically well at 10 years of age. For perinatally acquired disease, the mean incubation period is estimated to be 7 to 9 months. The range, however, extends to a decade or more. The mean incubation period of transfusion-acquired HIV disease is estimated to be 17 months. These incubation periods may be biased by patients who have early symptoms of disease because the patients included were identified by clinical illness rather than by prospective surveillance of seropositivity.

SUMMARY

Children constitute a rapidly growing group of patients who have confirmed HIV infection. Pediatricians need to become familiar with the wide spectrum of clinical manifestations and the subtleties encountered in diagnosing HIV infection. Surely the principles of clinical care will evolve rapidly over the next 2 decades; however, the need for social and educational intervention to prevent HIV infection is immediate and compelling.

We abide in the hope that a preventive vaccine or a cure will be found; however, we must continue emphasizing that responsible sexual behavior and avoiding intravenous drug use will prevent the further spread of this incurable disease.

SUGGESTED READING

Pizzo PA, Wilfert CM, editors: *Pediatric AIDS: the challenge of HIV infection in infants, children, and adolescents,* Baltimore, 1994, Williams & Wilkins.

181 Allergic Rhinitis

Kenneth C. Schuberth

Allergic rhinitis is the most common clinical expression of atopic hypersensitivity. It occurs in as many as 15% of the general population and may exist alone or in combination with asthma or eczema. In children it is unusual before age 3 but increases in frequency thereafter, especially at puberty.[8] The most easily recognizable form is the typical "seasonal" spring-fall pattern, often referred to as hay fever or pollenosis. Year-round, "perennial" allergic rhinitis triggered by household inhaled allergens is more common but often less dramatic and more difficult to diagnose.

ETIOLOGY

The tendency to develop allergic rhinitis clearly is inherited.[8] When a child who has a genetic predisposition to allergy is exposed to a strong allergic stimulus, antigen-specific IgE molecules are produced, which bind to submucosal mast cells in the respiratory tract epithelium. Once the individual has been sensitized in this way, reexposure to the allergen causes an immediate type I hypersensitivity reaction, in which cross-linking of cell surface IgE molecules triggers the rapid release of mast cell mediators (e.g., histamine, prostaglandins, and leukotrienes), as well as the slower synthesis of cell interactive compounds, called cytokines.[5] Histamine causes immediate local vasodilation, mucosal edema, and increased production of mucus. Cytokines summon cells to the area, accounting for the slower "late-phase reaction" and causing inflammation and destruction of the mucosal surface that progresses to chronic nasal obstruction.

The severity of the symptoms varies tremendously and depends both on the individual's level of sensitivity and the intensity of the antigen exposure.

The allergens responsible most often include the following:

1. *Pollens.* Wind-borne pollens from trees and grasses in the spring and from weeds, especially ragweed, in the fall cause well-defined seasonal symptoms, but variation is tremendous according to location. Most flower pollens are insect borne and rarely cause problems.
2. *Molds.* In cold climates, outdoor molds produce spores beginning in the early spring and peaking in late fall. In warm climates without frost, molds can grow year-round.
3. *Animal dander.* Scales from the skin of house pets such as dogs and cats can produce severe intermittent as well as perennial symptoms.
4. *Dust mites.* These ubiquitous, microscopic insects are the major allergen in house dust. Mites prosper in warm, moist, indoor environments and colonize in pillows, mattresses, and carpets. They are the major cause of perennial rhinitis.[2]

CLINICAL FEATURES

The triad of nasal congestion, sneezing, and rhinorrhea is characteristic of allergic rhinitis.[2] Younger children usually have perennial symptoms, whereas pollen sensitivity becomes more common after age 6. In the acute, seasonal pollen-related variety, the symptoms may be quite intense and often include an itchy palate and throat, headaches, and itchy, tearing eyes. The patient often can identify the specific allergen responsible. Perennial sufferers may have more nonspecific problems such as frequent "colds," recurrent otitis media, nasal speech, mouth breathing, snoring during sleep, fatigue, malaise, and poor school performance. Epistaxis is common. The rhinorrhea usually is clear unless the child has a superimposed infection. Many children perform the "allergic salute," a maneuver in which they sniff and sweep the palm of their hand upward across the nose in an attempt to open their nasal passages or to relieve nasal itching.

The physical examination usually reveals striking features. The nasal mucosa is pale, bluish, and boggy, with a clear serous discharge. The nasal turbinates are enlarged, sometimes enough to obstruct the airway almost completely. Children who have perennial problems often have the typical "allergic facies," consisting of (1) "allergic shiners"—dark discoloration beneath both eyes, (2) "Dennie lines"—extra wrinkles below the lower eyelids, and (3) mouth breathing. The tonsils and adenoids often are enlarged, and there may be evidence of middle ear effusion. Nasal polyps are uncommon in childhood allergic rhinitis.

COMPLICATIONS

Early in life children who have allergic rhinitis may suffer from an increased incidence of respiratory infections, acute otitis media, and eustachian tube dysfunction, leading to more chronic serous otitis media. Many authors have suggested an association between allergy and chronic serous otitis media, although this is only one of many risk factors. Adenoidal enlargement, nasal speech, and abnormal facial development from chronic mouth breathing occasionally develop in these patients.[6] Acute and chronic sinusitis are common, probably the result of reduced ciliary clearance and obstruction of sinus ostia. Asthma appears to be a concomitant development in atopic individuals and not a complication of untreated allergic rhinitis. There is no good evidence that immunotherapy for allergic rhinitis prevents the subsequent development of asthma.

LABORATORY FINDINGS

The nasal smear for eosinophils is a simple office procedure that can help confirm the clinical diagnosis.[4] The patient blows his or her nose into a plastic or wax paper wrap, and the secretions are spread onto a glass slide and left to dry overnight. The slide then is prepared with Hansel stain. A cotton swab may be used to obtain secretions if the patient cannot blow. If more than 10% of the cells seen on the smear are eosinophils, an ongoing allergic process is probable. Strongly positive results are most likely during heavy exposure to the allergen. Concurrent nasal infection may obscure the results, and eosinophils may be absent during the "off season."

Blood eosinophilia occasionally is found (more than 5% eosinophils on the differential white blood count or more than 250/mm^3 on the proportionate total white blood cell count). An elevated total serum IgE suggests atopy, but many patients who have uncomplicated allergic rhinitis have a normal serum IgE.

Skin tests and radioallergosorbent tests (RAST) can detect antigen-specific IgE and identify individual allergens in patients who need aggressive management. Skin tests always should be performed by a physician trained in allergy, and they should be interpreted in the light of the clinical history. Compared with skin testing, screening with RAST has the disadvantages of higher cost and lower sensitivity.

In some patients impedance audiometry may help to document eustachian tube dysfunction. Sinusitis, diagnosed on a roentgenogram, is common, especially among older children, and pulmonary function testing occasionally demonstrates reversible obstructive airway disease.

DIFFERENTIAL DIAGNOSIS

Usually there is very little difficulty making the clinical diagnosis of seasonal allergic rhinitis on the basis of the family history, clinical presentation, physical examination, and a knowledge of local pollens. On the other hand, children who have nonspecific perennial problems often pose a difficult diagnostic challenge. Two other conditions often confused with allergic rhinitis are recurrent upper respiratory tract infections and vasomotor rhinitis. Recurrent viral and/or bacterial infections can be differentiated from allergies by their intermittent course, a history of contagion, the presence of fever, purulent nasal discharge, red, inflamed nasal mucosa, and the absence of eosinophils on a nasal smear. The family history for allergy is negative, and the serum IgE is normal.

Vasomotor rhinitis is an ill-defined condition that begins in early childhood. It is characterized by hyperreactivity of the nasal mucous membranes to a wide variety of irritant stimuli.[2] The most prominent symptom usually is perennial nasal obstruction that does not respond to environmental controls and/or medications. There is no family history of allergy, the nasal smear and skin test results are negative, the serum IgE is normal, and no eye signs or other atopic manifestations are present. Treatment is based on the symptoms.

A third variant of perennial rhinitis, eosinophilic nonallergic rhinitis, recently was described. In this disorder, which affects adolescents and adults, the nasal smear results are positive for eosinophils, but the serum IgE is normal, and the skin test results are negative.[3]

Other, less common conditions that may mimic allergic rhinitis are presence of a nasal foreign body, choanal atresia, congenital syphilis, enlarged adenoids, rhinitis medicamentosa, cystic fibrosis, and nasopharyngeal tumors.

TREATMENT

Management of allergic rhinitis incorporates the information from a careful history and physical examination into a stepwise program consisting initially of avoiding the allergen and treatment with medication. If the symptoms are perennial, do not respond to medication, or worsen each year, an allergist should be consulted; he or she can confirm the diagnosis, identify specific allergens, and possibly prescribe immunotherapy.

Measures to avoid the allergen are the first priority and are easier for small children confined to the home. Particular attention should be directed to the child's room or other settings where he or she spends a lot of time. The first steps are to reduce dust mite exposure with miteproof encasings of mattresses and pillows, remove animals, and eliminate indoor mold. Children allergic to pollen can be helped dramatically by closing windows and using a room air conditioner. Forced air heating and cooling systems can be improved by adding humidifiers and air filters.

Antihistamines are the mainstay of pharmacological treatment for allergic rhinitis.[7] They inhibit the histamine effect by preventing histamine from binding to H_1-receptors and are most effective in treating sneezing, rhinorrhea, and nasal itching. Antihistamines are divided into several large classic and nonsedating groups. Three examples of classic antihistamines commonly used are:

Class I: ethanolamines (diphenhydramine [Benadryl])

Class II: ethylenediamines (tripelennamine [Pyribenzamine])

Class III: alkylamines (chlorpheniramine [Chlortrimeton]

These medications are most effective when given before exposure to the allergen and often must be used in doses larger than those recommended on the packages. Many are available in long-acting form, which allows twice-daily dosing. Their usefulness sometimes is limited by their sedative side effects or by the development of tachyphylaxis, which can be averted by switching to an antihistamine in another class.

Newer, nonsedative antihistamines such as terfenadine (Seldane), astemizole (Hismanal), and loratidine (Claritin) provide an alternative for older children who are unable to tolerate the sedative side effects of traditional antihistamines.[5] These drugs also have long half-lives, which allow once- or twice-a-day dosing.

Alpha-adrenergic agents such as pseudoephedrine and phenylephrine cause vasoconstriction of the small blood vessels in the nose. They are helpful, either alone or in combination with antihistamines, when nasal congestion is a major symptom. Most of the over-the-counter oral cold preparations contain a combination of adrenergic and antihistamine compounds. Side effects that limit their usefulness include nervousness and tachycardia. Nasal sprays may provide transient relief, which usually is followed after several days by rebound congestion. Because prolonged use of nasal sprays has led to worsening of symptoms, a condition known as rhinitis medicamentosa, their use should be discouraged.

Antiinflammatory nasal sprays also can be helpful.[9] Nasal cromolyn sodium (Nasalcrom) is an extremely safe drug similar in potency to oral antihistamines without the side effects. It must be used preventively before and during seasons or before periodic exposure. Its usefulness is limited somewhat by the need to use it four to six times a day. Nasal topical steroids are the most effective drug, but with children, these usually are saved for those whose allergy is not controlled by avoidance, antihistamines, or nasal cromolyn. The potent antiinflammatory effect of nasal topical steroids reduces swelling and obstruction over 3 to 5 days, with a peak effect by 2 weeks. They are most useful when used preventively but will work well in the midst of illness. Available preparations include beclomethasone, flunisolide, triamcinolone, and budesonide. Side effects are minimal, with occasional epistaxis but no systemic steroid toxicity. Finally, short courses of oral steroids (e.g., prednisone) should be reserved for severe intransigent cases that do not respond to other therapies.

If the patient's allergy does not respond to the avoidance steps mentioned previously or to medication, he or she should be referred to an allergist for skin testing to identify specific allergens. If the clinical history and skin test results correlate, immunotherapy becomes a logical part of treatment.[1] Usually a 3- to 5-year course of regular injections is necessary. This regimen is most effective in the treatment of seasonal pollenosis, but it also is beneficial for dust mite and cat dander allergy. As treatment progresses, patients can expect a gradual decline in symptoms and reduced reliance on medication. Because of the risk of local and generalized reactions to the material injected and because of the inconvenience and expense associated with weekly injections, it is essential that immunotherapy be used selectively.

PROGNOSIS

Allergic rhinitis, like other allergic disorders, is an illness that waxes and wanes over time. Most children tend to improve with time, although very few (probably fewer than 10%) lose their sensitivity completely. Remission of symptoms may result from changes in environment, avoidance programs, and immunotherapy. It is important to counsel patients that allergic symptoms can be controlled but not eliminated entirely and that the success of any treatment depends on an understanding of the causes of symptoms and compliance with the prescribed regimen.

REFERENCES

1. Creticos PS: Immunotherapy with allergens, *JAMA* 268:2834, 1992.
2. Meltzer EO, Schatz M, Zeiger RS: Allergic and nonallergic rhinitis. In Middleton E Jr et al, editors: *Allergy: principles and practice,* ed 3, St Louis, 1988, Mosby.
3. Mullarkey MF: Eosinophilic nonallergic rhinitis, *J Allergy Clin Immunol* 82:941, 1988.
4. Mullarkey MF, Hill JS, Webb DR: Allergic and nonallergic rhinitis: their characterization with attention to the meaning of nasal eosinophilia, *J Allergy Clin Immunol* 65:122, 1980.
5. Naclerio RM: Allergic rhinitis, *N Engl J Med* 325:860, 1991.
6. Shapiro GG, Shapiro P: Facial characteristics of children who breathe through the mouth, *Pediatrics* 73:662, 1984.
7. Simons FER: Allergic rhinitis: recent advances, *Pediatr Clin North Am* 35:1053, 1988.
8. Smith JM: Epidemiology of asthma, allergic rhinitis, and atopic dermatitis. In Middleton E Jr et al, editors: *Allergy: principles and practice,* ed 3, St Louis, 1988, Mosby.
9. Welsh PW et al: Efficacy of beclomethasone nasal solution, flunisolide, and cromolyn in relieving symptoms of ragweed allergy, *Mayo Clin Proc* 62:125, 1987.

182 Animal Bites

Neil E. Herendeen and Peter G. Szilagyi

It is estimated that more than 2 million people a year across the United States are bitten by animals.[7] Dog bites account for more than 90% of these injuries, and cat bites cause most of the remainder. Although wild animal bites are rare, they potentially are more serious, given their risk of rabies and other infection. Half of all animal bites are trivial, requiring no medical treatment; only 10% are severe enough to require suturing, and only 2% result in hospitalization. Bite wounds account for an estimated 1% of pediatric visits to an emergency department. Children sustain the greatest number of animal bites (the peak age group is 5 to 14 years), with half of all school-age children reporting an animal bite at some point in their life. With dog bites, adults primarily are bitten on an extremity; children, however, are bitten on the head and neck 75% of the time.[13] Boys are twice as likely to be bitten by a dog, whereas girls receive twice as many cat bites.[3,7] Not surprisingly, the vast majority of the animals live in the victim's neighborhood (75%) or home (15%); in most instances the bites are provoked by humans. With the recent trend among many urban families of buying guard dogs, including pit bulls, the incidence of dog bites is likely to rise, and pediatricians should be familiar with preventive strategies and management of these injuries.[2]

The major morbidity from animal bites results from direct trauma and infection. Although dog bites are more likely to cause lacerations or avulsions, these open wounds can be debrided and cleaned to prevent infection. Puncture wounds, however, which usually do not require suturing, can result in deep tissue infections.[2,6,10]

MICROBIOLOGY

As shown in Table 182-1, the risk of infection varies according to several factors. Hand wounds are most likely to become infected, partly because of the type of wound (most frequently a puncture wound), the relatively poor vascular supply, and the vulnerability of the closed spaces of the hand. As previously noted, puncture wounds, often made by cat or human bites, are more likely to become infected than are lacerations. If more than 24 hours has elapsed before medical attention is sought, the risk of infection is increased substantially. Cat and human bites pose a greater risk of infection than dog bites, partly because these bites more often cause puncture wounds and dog bites frequently cause open lacerations.

Most bacteria associated with bite wounds are common organisms that reside in the animal's oral cavity. In addition, bacteria on the victim's skin may contribute to infection. Most infections involve several pathogens,[8] often both aerobes and anaerobes. *Pasteurella multocida,* a gram negative, facultative anaerobe found in the mouths of most dogs and cats, is highly associated with cat bite infections (up to 80%) and to a lesser extent with dog bite infections (12% to 50%). Although the exact prevalence of other pathogenic bacteria isolated from infected animal bites varies across studies, gram negative aerobes (e.g., *Pseudomonas, Klebsiella,* and *Enterobacter* spp.) are found more often than other organisms sometimes seen, which include gram positive aerobes (e.g., staphylococci and streptococci) and anaerobes (e.g., *Bacteroides, Fusobacterium,* and *Peptococcus* spp.).[1-3,6-10]

Another group of gram negative bacteria, classified by the Centers for Disease Control and Prevention (CDC) as alphanumeric organisms, frequently has been isolated from dog bite wounds. Interestingly, human bites rarely are infected by *P. multocida* but often are associated with gram positive organisms, gram negative anaerobes, or *Eikenella corrodens,* a genus almost unique to human bites that in rare cases is found in cat bites.

CLINICAL DIAGNOSIS

Important historical points include the length of time since injury, the type of animal (including domestic or wild), the animal's present location and health, and the prior wound management. The physical examination entails a careful musculoskeletal and neurological examination to determine if underlying structures were damaged and a thorough inspection of the wound for signs of infection. Special attention must be given to bites on the hand because, particularly in deep puncture wounds, superficial signs of infection (redness, swelling, purulent drainage) may be absent. Finally, the clinician should be aware that deep infections of tendons or bones and systemic infections can occur if animal bites go untreated. The time of the infection's onset may be a clue to *P. multocida* infection. Cellulitis from this organism generally develops rapidly, within hours of the animal bite, whereas systemic signs (fever, lymphangitis) usually are absent.[9] A cellulitis that develops gradually, over days, more likely is due to gram positive cocci or other pathogenic bacteria.

A gram stain of a wound specimen is not useful because findings do not correlate with culture results. Cultures of clinically infected animal bite wounds are reported to have "no growth" in as many as one third of cases; conversely, cultures of clinically noninfected bite wounds grow a wide spectrum of oral flora bacteria in the same proportion of cases.[11] Moreover, such cultures do not predict the likelihood of subsequent infection, nor do results correlate with culture findings when clinical infection becomes apparent. However, cultures of clinically infected wounds may help to ensure that the causative bacteria are sensitive to the antibiotic used.

The clinician should remember that cat-scratch disease is a relatively common complication of cat bites and, less commonly, of bites by other animals. This disease often begins

Table 182-1 Risk Factors for Infection in Animal Bites

Risk factor	Infection rates
Location of bite[6]	Hand (18%-36%) > arm or leg (12%-16%) > face (5%-11%)
Type of wound[2,6,10]	Puncture with laceration (17%-26%) > laceration alone (9%-12%)
Interval between bite and medical care	If >24 hr, risk of infection is higher
Type of animal	Cat bites (40%-50%) Dog bites (10%-30%) Human bites (13%-40%)[8]

with the development of a red, painless papule at the site of a recent scratch or bite; within weeks, a tender, enlarged, regional lymph node appears, usually associated with fever, malaise, and other systemic symptoms. This self-limited illness, caused by a gram negative bacillus, is diagnosed clinically because the cat-scratch skin test reagent used to substantiate the clinical diagnosis is not licensed and therefore not available for use in most clinical settings. The role of antibiotics in the treatment of this disease is not clear; however, because the disease is self-limited, their use is seldom indicated. Large, tender, fluctuant lymph nodes may require aspiration or incision and drainage.

Animal bites from nondomestic animals require careful attention. Although most pediatricians will never treat a child who has rabies, they will evaluate children who may have been exposed to it. With the increasing spread of rabies among nondomestic animals, the number of people exposed to rabies and requiring vaccination is increasing dramatically. A full postexposure series can cost $2000 or more and requires five visits to the doctor in a single month. Knowing whom and when to treat requires an understanding of rabies transmission and epidemiology. The animals most often involved are rats, mice, skunks, raccoons, foxes, cattle, bats, and a variety of others.[12] In the United States, in all cases of rabies resulting from a dog or cat bite, the infected animal has been noted to become ill during the standard 10-day confinement and observation period; thus location, confinement, and observation of the animal are important.

In cases involving wild animal bites, consultation with the local health department is helpful in determining the risk of rabies in a specific animal for a particular geographical region. In general, bats and wild skunks, foxes, raccoons, and other carnivores are considered rabid until proved otherwise by laboratory tests[12]; in the interum, or if the animal cannot be found, treatment with human rabies immunoglobulin (HRIG) plus human diploid cell vaccine (HDCV) is recommended.

A variety of rare diseases have been described after wild animal bites; consultation with the local health department may help in establishing the diagnosis and managing treatment. Rat bite fever, a systemic illness caused by *Streptobacillus moniliformis* or *Spirillum minus,* is one such example. The *Red Book* (published by the American Academy of Pediatrics' Committee on Infectious Diseases) contains comprehensive, up-to-date descriptions of unusual diseases transmitted by various domestic and wild animals.

Table 182-2 Rabies Vaccination Guidelines

Animal	Management
Wild carnivores	Begin HRIG and HDCV. Submit animal's head for testing.
Healthy domestic dogs and cats	Quarantine animal; treat only if animal develops symptoms.
Stray or sick dogs and cats	Submit animal's head for testing. Delay treatment until test results are known unless clinical likelihood of rabies is high. If animal is unavailable, complete full series of HRIG and HDCV.
Rodents, rabbits	Unlikely to be rabid (except woodchucks). Treat only if animal acted strangely and cannot be tested.

Data from Schmidt MJ et al: *Contemp Pediatr* 10:36, 1993.

MANAGEMENT

The initial step in treating animal bites is meticulous wound care. This involves gently cleaning the wound with soap and water and vigorously irrigating with saline solution. Saline irrigation of the wound with a syringe and a 19-gauge needle generates increased pressure that facilitates cleansing of the wound and reduces the risk of infection.[5] Devitalized tissue should be debrided. Puncture wounds should be cleaned, but irrigation is ineffective and may result in further damage to underlying structures. Elevation and immobilization are important for significant extremity injuries. The child's immunization status should be assessed and tetanus prophylaxis given if indicated. Primary closure of lacerations caused by animal (or human) bites is controversial.[5,6] Clearly, infected wounds should not be closed. The consensus is that most noninfected lacerations can be sutured, after meticulous cleansing and irrigation, for cosmetic purposes or for hemostasis, without increasing the risk of infection. Hand wounds may be an exception[5,10] because of the great likelihood of infection and the risk of serious complications from deep, closed space infections; in these cases suturing is recommended only for large wounds.

Radiological studies may be necessary for deep puncture wounds to determine if the periosteum has been penetrated. These include studies of the calvaria of small children who sustain bites to the head. The use of prophylactic antibiotics in noninfected animal bite wounds is controversial.[4-6,10] It is prudent to treat prophylactically (for 5 to 7 days) bites that have a high likelihood of infection, including (1) puncture wounds (particularly from cat bites), (2) human bites, and (3) bites of the hands and face. If infected, bite wounds brought to medical attention after 24 hours should be treated with antibiotics. The choice of antibiotics depends on culture results or, if cultures are not available, on the likely pathogens. Although penicillin is active against *P. multocida* and many oral flora, the addition of a penicillinase-resistant antibiotic provides more effective coverage. Amoxicillin/clavulanic acid (Augmentin) is an excellent choice for empirical treatment of bites from all animals. As mentioned, administration of rabies prophylaxis depends on the type of animal and the prevalence of rabies in the community (see Table 182-2).

ANTICIPATORY GUIDANCE

Although pets provide hours of delight and companionship for children, education about responsible care of a pet is important. Preschool-age children should not be left alone with a pet, and they should be advised never to tease animals, approach strange animals, or play with pets that are eating.[10] Families who have children should be advised not to buy wild animals or dogs bred for aggressiveness. Finally, vaccinations for pets and routine visits to a veterinarian should be encouraged (see Chapter 23, Injury Prevention, for a more detailed discussion of animal safety rules for children).

REFERENCES

1. Aghababian RV, Conte JE Jr: Mammalian bite wounds, *Ann Emerg Med* 9:79, 1980.
2. Baker MD: Bites and scratches: when pets fight back, *Contemp Pediatr* 6:76, 1989.
3. Berzon PR: The animal bite epidemic in Baltimore, Maryland: review and update, *Am J Public Health* 68:593, 1978.
4. Boenning DA, Fleisher GR, Campos JM: Dog bites in children: epidemiology, microbiology, and penicillin prophylactic therapy, *Am J Emerg Med* 1:17, 1983.
5. Callaham ML: Treatment of common dog bites: infection risk factors, *J Am Coll Emerg Med* 7:83, 1978.
6. Callaham M: Prophylactic antibiotics in common dog bite wounds: a controlled study, *Ann Emerg Med* 9:410, 1980.
7. Kizer KW: Epidemiologic and clinical aspects of animal bite injuries, *J Am Coll Emerg Physicians* 8:134, 1979.
8. Lindsey D et al: Natural course of the human bite wound: incidence of infection and complications in 434 bites and 803 lacerations in the same group of patients, *J Trauma* 27:45, 1987.
9. Lucas GL, Bartlett DH: *Pasteurella multocida* infection in the hand, *Plast Reconstr Surg* 67:49, 1981.
10. Marcy SM: Management of pediatric infectious diseases in office practice: infections due to dog and cat bites (special series), *Pediatr Infect Dis J* 1:351, 1982.
11. Ordog GJ: The bacteriology of dog bite wounds on initial presentation, *Ann Emerg Med* 15:1324, 1986.
12. Peter G et al: *Report of the Committee on Infectious Diseases (Red Book),* Elk Grove, Ill, 1988, American Academy of Pediatrics.
13. Rosekrans JA: Animal bites: a summertime hazard, *Contemp Pediatr* 10:23, 1993.
14. Schmidt MJ, Olson JG, Krebs JW: Rabies goes wild, *Contemp Pediatr* 10:36, 1993.

183 Anuria/Oliguria

Edward J. Ruley

Anuria, the failure to excrete any urine, or *oliguria,* the failure to excrete at least the minimal amount of urine that would be considered normal—defined as less than 500 ml/1.73 m/BSA (body surface area) in children or less than 0.5 ml/kg/hr in infants—may be a physiological or a pathological phenomenon. In a water-deprived child the kidney tubules reabsorb most of the glomerular filtrate to maintain the body's water content. In an extreme case this physiological response may result in oliguria or anuria. Conversely, a large number of acute renal insults or chronic kidney diseases can reduce glomerular filtration by damaging the kidney parenchyma, thereby producing anuria or oliguria. In clinical practice, oliguria occurs more often than anuria. An organized approach to the child who has anuria or oliguria begins with a careful physical examination (Fig. 183-1). If the urinary bladder or one or both kidneys are palpable and enlarged, urine is being formed but for some reason is not being emptied from the urinary tract. In contrast, if the urinary bladder and kidneys are not palpable, the patient's state of hydration must be considered in assessing why urine apparently is not being formed. The systematical approach to these physical findings follows the algorithm shown in Fig. 183-1.

ACUTE URINARY RETENTION

One of the more common clinical circumstances of anuria in pediatric practice is acute urinary retention. In this situation a distended, often painful urinary bladder can be palpated or percussed just above the symphysis pubis, sometimes extending as high as the umbilicus. Such a circumstance often occurs when the child's regular schedule is interrupted and the child feels that circumstances are not convenient or familiar enough to allow micturition. The child then consciously overrides the urge to micturate, and the urinary bladder becomes progressively more distended. Eventually the child feels considerable lower abdominal pressure and pain but cannot void voluntarily because overdistention has exceeded the muscular compliance of the bladder, and an organized contraction coordinated with relaxation of the internal sphincter cannot be achieved. Simple catheterization to empty the bladder usually relieves the symptoms and restores the compliance of the bladder musculature. Urinary retention is unlikely to recur, and indwelling bladder catheterization is not indicated. If retention does recur, the practitioner should consider the possibility of a functional or anatomical bladder outlet obstruction, although this is rare.

URINARY OBSTRUCTION

Chronic partial urinary obstruction usually causes polyuria rather than anuria or oliguria. Polyuria occurs in this circumstance because obstruction first affects the medullary functions of the kidney, specifically the ability to resorb sodium and water. Chronic partial obstruction can be complicated by an acute complete obstruction that can cause anuria. Occasionally, severe chronic obstruction may so damage the kidney parenchyma that oliguria may develop.

Visualizing the urinary system through ultrasound or computed tomography (CT) scans or excretory urography will confirm the diagnosis of obstruction and provide some indication of the site and degree of blockage. Urological consultation is important in developing a plan for further evaluation and treatment of these children.

DEHYDRATION

If a patient has no abdominal masses, the next step is to assess the state of hydration by clinical examination (see Fig. 183-1). With significant dehydration, oliguria or anuria caused by poor perfusion (functional renal failure mediated by a physiological antidiuretic hormone response) must be differentiated from oliguria or anuria caused by established parenchymal renal failure. This is accomplished by assessing the quality of urine remaining in the bladder and then determining the volume and quality of urine produced in response to prompt rehydration. To maximize the value of these studies, the child should be catheterized during rehydration. Catheterization allows the residual urine to be quantified and renal function to be characterized as to sodium and water resorption capabilities (see Table 291-1). If the residual urine, however small the volume, demonstrates maximal water and sodium resorption (i.e., a high osmolality or specific gravity and a low urinary sodium concentration), and if urine production during rehydration increases promptly, it may be presumed that the patient's oliguria or anuria was a physiological response to dehydration. This should not recur, provided that hydration is maintained.

If urine production does not increase on rehydration or if oliguria or anuria has occurred with near-normal hydration, the patient most likely has severe parenchymal renal failure. This usually is the result of an extensive parenchymal disease, such as acute tubular necrosis, or of a sudden renovascular catastrophe, such as renal cortical necrosis.

A third possibility is a partial response to rehydration, in which urine output increases but remains suboptimal. Such a patient most likely has partial parenchymal renal failure oliguria (see Chapter 291, Acute Renal Failure).

Prompt differentiation of functional (prerenal) failure from parenchymal renal failure is extremely important. Significant parenchymal renal failure may result if functional renal failure goes untreated, as in a dehydrated patient who does not undergo prompt rehydration. Diagnostic evaluation and management of a child who has severe renal failure are discussed in Chapter 291.

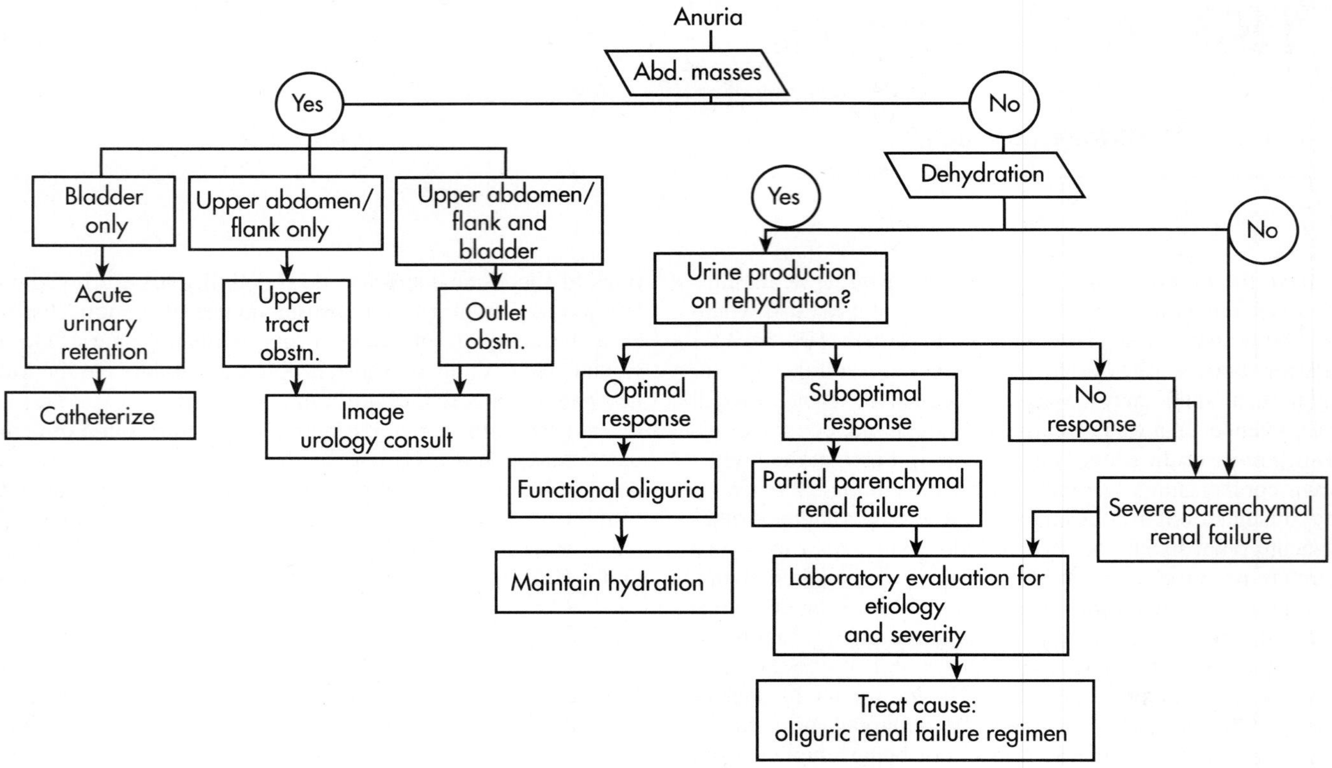

FIG. 183-1 Algorithm of the physical examination of a child with anuria.

NEWBORNS

Anuria or oliguria in a newborn may be caused by bilateral renal agenesis or some other major congenital urological anomaly. Often a maternal history of oligohydramnios reflects a deficient production of fetal urine, a major source of amniotic fluid. An adequate volume of amniotic fluid is important in normal fetal development because it promotes lung maturation and acts as a cushion for the fetus. Clues to a major urinary anomaly include a maternal history of small uterine size for gestational age, scanty passage of amniotic fluid at delivery, and positional somatic abnormalities discovered on examination of the newborn. Prenatal fetal sonographic examination may confirm the oligohydramnios and/or demonstrate renal structural abnormalities. Such information is important in parental counseling and in deciding on the optimal delivery date. At birth the results of the child's blood chemistry tests are normal because the mother maintains the neonate's biochemical status in utero. Biochemical abnormalities attributable to renal failure usually become evident gradually over the first several weeks of life. Pneumothoraces develop in most children who have severe renal damage or bilateral renal agenesis, and in the latter case the child dies of pulmonary immaturity rather than renal failure.

A pediatric nephrologist who has experience with renal failure in newborns should be involved in determining treatment options and in counseling the parents early in the course, prenatally if possible. With the advent of newer dialysis techniques and renal transplantation in small infants, the outlook is not as bleak as before, providing the infant can survive the pulmonary problems so common in the first month of life.

SUGGESTED READINGS

Anand SK, Northway JD, Crussi FG: Acute renal failure in newborn infants, *J Pediatr* 92:985, 1978.

Giangiacomo J: Unilateral renal agenesis presenting as anuria, *J Urol* 116:790, 1976.

Koff SA: Clues to neonatal gentourinary problems, *Postgrad Med* 62:93, 1977.

Olavarria F et al: Renal function in full-term newborns following neonatal asphyxia: a prospective study, *Clin Pediatr* 26:334, 1987.

Shapiro SR, Stratton ML, Adelman AD: Anuria in infants and children, *J Urol* 120:227, 1978.

184 Appendicitis

R. Scott Strahlman

Although appendicitis is a surgical emergency, the pediatrician has a crucial role in its initial diagnosis and management and often is the first to suspect appendicitis and to contact the surgical team. The pediatrician's high index of suspicion can be the driving force that leads to an appropriate, timely appendectomy. Prompt diagnosis and preoperative management help to reduce the high morbidity associated with a perforated appendix.

Appendicitis is the most common cause of an acute surgical condition of the abdomen in childhood. The exact incidence is unknown, but appendicitis is rare in early childhood and becomes more common after age 10. Boys and girls are affected equally before puberty, but after age 15 twice as many boys are affected as girls. An increased incidence in the spring and autumn months also has been observed. In addition, appendicitis is more common in children who have a family history of appendicitis.[4] Whether this tendency is genetic or diet related is unclear because the risk of appendicitis may be reduced with a high-fiber diet.[5]

ETIOLOGY AND PATHOPHYSIOLOGY

Appendicitis always is initiated by obstruction of the appendiceal lumen, usually by a fecalith or by lymphoid hyperplasia. In rare cases a parasite, tumor, or foreign body may obstruct the lumen. Inspissated secretions of cystic fibrosis also may obstruct the appendiceal lumen (thus, although rarely, cystic fibrosis may manifest as appendicitis).[16] As secretions accumulate within the obstructed appendix, the walls become distended. Continued distention causes ischemia and necrosis of the appendix, leading to irritation of the surrounding peritoneum.

Clinically the initial distention of the appendiceal wall is manifested by a dull, steady periumbilical pain. After 4 to 6 hours this pain often shifts to the right lower quadrant as local peritoneal inflammation develops. Without surgical intervention the appendix eventually may rupture, causing peritonitis. The incidence of rupture increases dramatically 24 to 36 hours after the onset of abdominal pain. Delaying surgery more than 36 hours results in at least a 65% incidence of perforation.[3] Organisms cultured in perforated appendicitis have included both aerobic and anaerobic bacteria.[19] The most common aerobic bacteria are *Escherichia coli* and *Klebsiella* and *Proteus* organisms. Common anaerobes include *Bacteroides* and *Clostridium* species.

INITIAL ASSESSMENT

History

A thorough history is invaluable in differentiating appendicitis from other disorders. An important component of that history is pain. The onset of symptoms often is heralded by a dull, steady periumbilical pain. The pain more often is thought to be caused by acute appendicitis if it awakens the patient from sleep. Anorexia is a consistent finding. One or two episodes of vomiting may follow, but essentially never precede, the pain. After 4 to 6 hours the pain commonly migrates to the right lower quadrant. Given the many variations in the location of an appendix, however, the location of abdominal pain in appendicitis may vary. Usually, bowel habits do not change. The child may have a low-grade fever, but the temperature rarely is above 100.3° F (37.9° C). If the clinical picture suggests but does not convince the physician that appendicitis is the problem, it is best to watch the progression of signs and symptoms carefully over several hours. Because an appendix rarely perforates within 24 hours of the onset of pain, a period of observation can safely differentiate a potential surgical condition from a nonsurgical one.

Physical Examination

As always, a gentle, nonthreatening approach is most effective during the physical examination. The physician should look for peritoneal signs such as pain upon walking or coughing. If the patient can jump up on the examining table, he or she usually does not have appendicitis. Patients may be most comfortable lying supine with their legs flexed. Abdominal tenderness always is present and often is greatest at McBurney's point (two thirds of the distance from the umbilicus to the anterosuperior iliac spine). Rebound tenderness of the abdomen (particularly that which is referred to the right lower quadrant) is common, as is hyperesthesia of the skin overlying the painful area. Bowel sounds may be diminished or hyperactive. A rectal examination is essential and may reveal right-sided tenderness. Examination of the lungs is important to rule out a right lower lobe pneumonia that may generate referred pain to the right lower quadrant of the abdomen. A pelvic examination is indicated in any adolescent girl who has abdominal pain to rule out gynecological conditions.

Laboratory Tests

The only essential laboratory studies are a blood count and urinalysis. The white blood cell count most often is in the range of 10,000 to 20,000/mm^3, with a slight increase in the number of neutrophils, particularly younger forms. The erythrocyte sedimentation rate usually is normal. Urinalysis is performed to rule out urinary tract infection or diabetic ketoacidosis as causes of the abdominal pain.

If the diagnosis is in doubt, abdominal roentgenograms occasionally are helpful. Radiographic features that suggest appendicitis include a calcified appendicolith or an air-filled appendix, although the absence of abnormalities does not rule out the diagnosis. Ultrasonography,[18] barium enema,[10] CT scanning,[1] and even technetium scanning[12] have helped to delineate appendicitis in cases that are not clear-cut.

The typical progression of signs and symptoms in appendicitis may be summarized as follows: abdominal pain, followed by nausea, vomiting, and localization of the pain to the right lower quadrant. Low-grade fever, tenderness on rectal examination, and a mild leukocytosis often accompany these symptoms.

DIFFERENTIAL DIAGNOSIS

The differential diagnosis of appendicitis, which is the same as the differential diagnosis of acute abdominal pain, is extensive (see the box below). Gastroenteritis can be differentiated from appendicitis on the basis of a benign abdominal examination in the former condition. Vomiting and diarrhea usually occur before the onset of pain, not afterward, as in appendicitis. Constipation often can appear to be appendicitis. However, this pain usually is diffuse, not localized to the right lower quadrant, and the patient often has a history of constipation. An abdominal flat plate roentgenogram can help in the diagnosis, and a small Fleet enema often is both diagnostic and therapeutic.

An appropriate initial evaluation can rule out the following nonsurgical conditions in a patient who has abdominal pain: urinary tract infection, diabetic ketoacidosis, sickle cell crisis, right lower lobe pneumonia with referred pain, nephrotic syndrome with primary peritonitis, and inflammatory bowel disease. Gynecological disorders can be ruled out on the basis of the history and a pelvic examination; pelvic inflammatory disease, ovarian torsion, ectopic pregnancy, dysmenorrhea, and mittelschmerz all can mimic appendicitis.

Unusual conditions such as Henoch-Schönlein purpura and hemolytic-uremic syndrome may be indistinguishable from appendicitis.[9] Even Rocky Mountain spotted fever can mimic appendicitis.[8] Surgical emergencies that mimic appendicitis (see the box below) can be ruled out only in the operating room.

DIFFERENTIAL DIAGNOSIS OF APPENDICITIS

- Common conditions
  - Gastroenteritis
  - Constipation
- Medical problems
  - Urinary tract infection
  - Diabetic ketoacidosis
  - Sickle cell crisis
  - Right lower lobe pneumonia
  - Primary peritonitis
  - Inflammatory bowel disease
- Gynecological problems
  - Pelvic inflammatory disease
  - Ovarian torsion
  - Ruptured ectopic pregnancy
  - Dysmenorrhea
  - Mittelschmerz
- Unusual conditions
  - Henoch-Schönlein purpura
  - Hemolytic-uremic syndrome
  - Rocky Mountain spotted fever
- Surgical emergencies
  - Meckel diverticulitis
  - Intestinal adhesions
  - Intussusception
  - Necrotizing enterocolitis

NEONATAL APPENDICITIS

Appendicitis in the first 2 years of life is rare, accounting for fewer than 2% of all childhood cases.[11] The mortality is high, however, and approaches 100% in cases with perforation.[13] Therefore appendicitis must be considered in any infant suspected of having abdominal pain. The presenting symptoms consist of vomiting and fever, and the baby may appear to be colicky. Physical examination shows abdominal distention with diffuse tenderness. Abdominal roentgenograms can be diagnostically helpful in a neonate by showing an appendicolith, free peritoneal fluid, bowel wall edema, or free air. With a high index of suspicion, surgery must be performed immediately to prevent perforation, with its high mortality.

MANAGEMENT

Once the diagnosis is made, the patient must be prepared for immediate surgery. Nothing is given by mouth, and a nasogastric tube is inserted and placed on low suction. Intravenous hydration is started (e.g., 10 ml/kg/hr of lactated Ringer), and fever may be controlled with acetaminophen given by rectum. Broad-spectrum antibiotics (e.g., ampicillin, gentamicin, and clindamycin, or a cephalosporin) are administered before surgery. Antibiotics have been shown to reduce morbidity even in nonperforated cases.[6] An appendectomy is performed as soon as the patient's condition has been stabilized. Many institutions are gaining experience with laparoscopic appendectomy[14] (see Chapter 32, Minimally Invasive Surgery).

For patients who have symptoms for 5 days or longer and a palpable mass consistent with an appendiceal abscess, many surgeons prefer nonsurgical management initially.[17] The patient is treated with broad-spectrum antibiotics and, barring interim complications, returns in 4 to 6 weeks for an elective appendectomy. This approach lowers the incidence of peritonitis and the associated complications precipitated by surgical manipulation during the acute inflammatory stages of the disease.

PROGNOSIS

For uncomplicated appendicitis treated with prompt surgical repair, the mortality is less that 1%, and there is essentially no long-term morbidity. The average hospital stay is about 4 days.[2] A ruptured appendix increases the risk of mortality only slightly (with most of the increase occurring in the neonatal age group) but extends the average hospital stay to about 10 days. Complications that increase morbidity include peritonitis, postoperative abscesses, and prolonged ileus. In women, infertility is a possible long-term complication of a ruptured appendix.[15]

The incidence of perforated appendicitis is about 35%, a disconcertingly high figure.[7] A higher index of suspicion on the part of pediatricians and the general public may lead to earlier diagnosis of the condition and reduce the incidence of appendiceal perforation and its morbid complications.

REFERENCES

1. Balthazar EJ et al: Appendicitis: prospective evaluation with high-resolution CT, *Radiology* 180:21, 1991.
2. Berry J, Malt R: Appendicitis near its centenary, *Ann Surg* 200:567, 1984.
3. Brender JD et al: Childhood appendicitis: factors associated with perforation, *Pediatrics* 76:2, 1985.
4. Brender JD et al: Is childhood appendicitis familial? *Am J Dis Child* 139:338, 1985.
5. Brender JD et al: Fiber intake and childhood appendicitis, *Am J Public Health* 75:399, 1985.
6. Busuttil RW et al: Effect of prophylactic antibiotics in acute nonperforated appendicitis, *Ann Surg* 194:502, 1981.
7. Cooperman M: Complications of appendectomy, *Surg Clin North Am* 63:1233, 1983.
8. Davis AE, Bradford WD: Abdominal pain resembling acute appendicitis in Rocky Mountain spotted fever, *JAMA* 247:2811, 1982.
9. Edmonson MB, Chesney RW: Hemolytic-uremic syndrome confused with acute appendicitis, *Arch Surg* 113:754, 1978.
10. Garcia C et al: Appendicitis in children: accuracy of the barium enema, *Am J Dis Child* 141:1309, 1987.
11. Grosfeld JL, Weinberger M, Clatworthy HW: Acute appendicitis in the first two years of life, *J Pediatr Surg* 8:285, 1973.
12. Henneman PL et al: Evaluation of children with possible appendicitis using technetium 99m leukocyte scan, *Pediatrics* 85:838, 1990.
13. Kwong MS, Dinner M: Neonatal appendicitis masquerading as necrotizing enterocolitis, *J Pediatr* 96:917, 1980.
14. Miller JP: Laparoscopic appendectomy, *Pediatr Ann* 22:664, 1993.
15. Mueller BA et al: Appendectomy and the risk of tubal infertility, *N Engl J Med* 315:1506, 1986.
16. Oestreich AE, Adelstein EH: Appendicitis as the presenting complaint in cystic fibrosis, *J Pediatr Surg* 17:191, 1982.
17. Powers RJ et al: Alternate approach to the management of acute perforating appendicitis in children, *Surg Gynecol Obstet* 152:473, 1981.
18. Sivit CJ et al: Appendicitis: usefulness of US in diagnosis in a pediatric population, *Radiology* 185:549, 1992.
19. Stone HH: Bacterial flora of appendicitis in children, *J Pediatr Surg* 11:37, 1976.

SUGGESTED READINGS

Ballantine TV: Appendicitis (review), *Surg Clin North Am* 61:1117, 1981.

King DR et al: Antibiotic management of complicated appendicitis, *J Pediatr Surg* 18:945, 1983.

Ravitch MM: Appendicitis (review), *Pediatrics* 70:414, 1982.

Shaul WL: Clues to the early diagnosis of neonatal appendicitis, *J Pediatr* 98:473, 1981.

Siler W, editor: *Cope's early diagnosis of the acute abdomen,* New York, 1983, Oxford University Press.

185 Asthma

Philip Fireman

Asthma can best be defined as a recurrent, reversible obstructive lung disease caused by hyperreactive airways. The obstruction of the hyperreactive airways results from bronchial smooth muscle contraction, increased secretion of mucus, and edema with inflammation. Both large and small airways can be involved to a variable degree and are hyperresponsive to a variety of environmental stimuli. Symptoms and signs usually are episodical because of reversible airway obstruction that can improve either spontaneously or as the result of therapy. Although it can occur at any age, *asthma usually has its onset within the first 5 years of life*. It is among the leading causes of both acute and chronic illness in children.[5] It is estimated that 5% to 10% of children have asthma at some time during childhood.[2] In a recent survey conducted at Children's Hospital of Pittsburgh, asthma accounted for 10% of medical emergency room visits and 10% of medical hospitalizations. According to a U.S. Public Health Service survey, asthma is the most common cause of school absenteeism and chronic illness in children under age 17.[8] Before adolescence boys are affected more often than girls (3:1), but the male preponderance does not persist past adolescence. The clinical spectrum of asthma is that of an illness that begins early in life, tends to improve during midchildhood and adolescence, but continues on into adulthood in some patients.[4,10] One matter of concern is the increase in hospital admissions and mortality during the past decade.[1] Asthma therefore is particularly important to pediatricians and to all physicians interested in the care of childhood respiratory illnesses.

ETIOLOGY AND PATHOGENESIS

The pathogenesis of asthma is only partly understood; it is a multifactorial, familial respiratory illness that involves allergic and other immunological, infectious, biochemical, autonomic nervous, and psychological factors to a varying degree in different individuals. Thus an affected individual may develop respiratory symptoms after exposure to a variety of environmental stimuli, such as specific inhalant antigens, infectious agents, cold air, tobacco smoke, aerosolized chemicals, inert dusts, strong aromas, and the hyperventilation that can be associated with exercise, laughing, or crying. These environmental factors trigger the release or generation of certain mediators of inflammation, such as histamine, leukotrienes, prostaglandins, and other agents, that can induce smooth muscle contractions, mucus gland secretion, and inflammatory edema to provoke symptoms. An increase in plasma histamine has been reported during acute asthma in children.[9]

The fundamental abnormality, however, appears to be a genetically influenced hyperreactivity of the airways. Specifically, it has been proposed that the basic abnormality in asthma is that of a defect in beta-adrenergic responsiveness, either with or without increased cholinergic activity of the airways.[11] Inhalation challenge with methacholine or histamine to provoke airway obstruction has been developed as a diagnostic provocative test in individuals who have asthma, but it is not suitable as a test for children under age 6. Recent studies have confirmed the impression of many pediatricians that *a history of bronchiolitis or croup is a risk factor for the development of asthma;* approximately 33% to 50% of children who have had more than one episode of bronchiolitis or croup during early life subsequently demonstrate bronchial hyperreactivity.[3] It is interesting that one third of these patients' first-degree relatives also have airway hyperreactivity, which suggests a genetic predisposition. A relation between allergy and asthma also exists whenever specific antigen (allergen) inhalation challenge is documented as provoking signs and symptoms of asthma in the hypersensitive (allergic) host. An increase in serum immunoglobulin E (IgE) has been documented in both familial and epidemiological studies of asthma patients.[1] In fact, specific allergen sensitization has been reported in 70% to 80% of children who have asthma.

CLINICAL MANIFESTATIONS

Asthma in infants and children varies markedly among patients and sometimes even in the same patient. The illness may manifest in several clinical patterns. The National Institutes of Health (NIH) has set guidelines for asthma management, and these classify the disease as mild, moderate, or severe (Table 185-1).[6] Patients may have occasional acute episodic episodes of symptoms that can vary from mild (requiring only minimal medication) to severe, life-threatening attacks of status asthmaticus, which demands hospitalization and treatment in an intensive care unit. Other children may have episodes every several months, yet appear to be well and symptom free between episodes. Still others may have chronic or daily symptoms that interfere in some way with their life-style and have superimposed on this a number of acute episodes that can be severe but may vary in duration from several hours to days. Finally, a small number of patients (probably fewer than 1% of all asthmatic individuals) have severe daily symptoms that require several medications and careful clinical monitoring. Studies indicate that *the most severely affected children* experience the onset of wheezing during the first year of life and have *a family history of asthma or other allergic* disease, especially atopic dermatitis (infantile eczema).

Many pediatricians hesitate to diagnose asthma in infants because of the difficulty involved in documenting the signs and symptoms of reversible obstructive airway disease. Yet in most children who subsequently are diagnosed as having asthma, suggestive signs appear during the first year or two

Table 185-1 Estimation of Severity of Acute Exacerbations of Asthma in Children

Sign/symptom	Mild	Moderate	Severe
Respiratory rate	Normal to <1 standard deviation (SD) from the norm for age	Normal to <2 SD for age	Normal to >2 SD for age
Alertness	Normal	Normal	May be diminished
Dyspnea*	Absent or mild; speaks in complete sentences	Moderate; speaks in phrases or partial sentences	Severe; speaks only in single words or short phrases
Pulsus paradoxus	<10 mm Hg	10-20 mm Hg	20-40 mm Hg
Use of accessory muscles	No intercostal use to mild retractions	Moderate intercostal retraction with tracheosternal retractions; use of sternocleidomastoid muscles	Severe intercostal retractions, tracheosternal retractions with nasal flaring
Color	Good	Pale	Possibly cyanotic
Auscultation	End-expiratory wheeze only	Wheezes during entire expiration and inspiration	Breath sounds nearly inaudible
Oxygen saturation	>95%	90%-95%	<90%
Pco_2	<35 mm Hg	35-40 mm Hg	>40 mm Hg
PEFR	70%-90% predicted or personal best	50%-70% predicted or personal best	<50% predicted or personal best

Adapted from the National Heart, Lung, and Blood Institute: National Asthma Education Program: Guidelines for the Diagnosis and Management of Asthma, NIH Consensus Report No 91-3042, National Institutes of Health, Bethesda, Md, 1991.

Note: Within each category, the presence of several, but not necessarily all, parameters indicates the general classification of the exacerbation.

*Parents' or physician's impression of the degree of breathlessness.

Pco_2, Carbon dioxide pressure; *PEFR*, peak expiratory flow rate.

of life, usually associated with a viral respiratory infection that induces cough and "wheezy," labored respirations. The mechanism of this virus-induced wheezing has been shown to involve virus-specific IgE antibody and increased release of histamine into the secretions of young children infected with respiratory syncytial virus.[13] The infectious agents involved during the preschool years are primarily the respiratory syncytial virus, with fewer episodes associated with parainfluenza virus; rhinovirus and influenza viruses are more significant among older children and adults.[4] Mycoplasma infections can promote asthma symptoms in children of school age, especially adolescents. Bacterial infections are rarely associated with acute exacerbations of asthma except as secondary invaders or as a cause of an associated sinusitis. There is no correlation between the severity of allergic rhinitis or atopic dermatitis and the severity of asthma.

An acute episode of asthma may begin with rhinorrhea and fever, then rapidly progress to cough, audible wheeze, and dyspnea. Many pediatricians label these viral respiratory illnesses "asthmatic bronchitis," "wheezy bronchitis," or "wheezy cold," but this reluctance or actual failure to recognize the underlying reactive airway disease may delay institution of appropriate management. Between infections an infant may be relatively free of respiratory symptoms, but cough can persist for longer than the usual 7 to 10 days.

Between the ages of 3 and 5 years, the typical asthmatic child begins to have some episodes without apparent infection. Acute symptoms may commence abruptly and range from paroxysms of cough to severe dyspnea. Symptoms may be seasonal or perennial and can be precipitated by exercise, infection, allergens (e.g., pollens, dust mites, animal products, and organic dusts), tobacco smoke, fumes, odors, laughter, or other stimuli. In rare instances foods can provoke an asthma attack. *Allergic rhinitis, seasonal or perennial, often is evident in children whose asthma has an allergic basis.* Between episodes the patient may be free of symptoms or may have latent reactive airway obstruction provoked by forced expiration (elicited by the astute clinician as compression expiratory rhonchi during chest auscultation). *A chronic cough in children or adults may be the only manifestation of airway hyperreactivity.* Sputum production is minimal in children, who usually swallow excess bronchial secretions.

During an acute episode of asthma the patient appears anxious and dyspneic. The pediatrician will recognize the characteristic prolonged expiratory phase of respiration, the raised clavicles, and subcostal retractions. If the asthma has been long-standing, the child may have a distended or barrel-chest appearance caused by air-trapping. Auscultation of the chest may reveal the characteristic high-pitched musical expiratory rhonchi (wheeze), but both inspiratory and expiratory coarse rhonchi also can be heard. Lack of breath sounds or rhonchi in a dyspneic, asthmatic child should suggest poor air exchange and potential respiratory failure, requiring immediate therapy and close observation in the office, emergency room, or hospital.

LABORATORY FINDINGS

Laboratory studies of pulmonary function in mild cases of asthma during remission may well show no abnormalities. A chest roentgenogram shows hyperinflation during acute attacks, with persistent hyperinflation changes in the more severe and chronic states. Atelectasis, particularly in the right middle lobe, is a common finding on chest radiography during acute episodes and should not be misconstrued as pneumonia. Pulmonary function testing may be a valuable adjunct in assessing the degree of pulmonary impairment in children over age 6, especially when performed both before and after treatment with an aerosolized sympathomimetic bronchodilator. Long-term management of the chronic asthmatic child may include home monitoring of pulmonary function (e.g., with the mini-Wright peak flow meter). Pulmonary testing after exercise can be helpful in assessing an asthmatic child who is involved in athletic activities. Monitoring patients by means of pulse oximetry during an acute asthma attack is a valuable adjunct, as is determining arterial blood gas and pH values in the intensive management of a child who has severe acute asthma or status asthmaticus.

All children suspected of allergic (immune-mediated) asthma should be evaluated. Skin testing usually is preferred over serological IgE antibody testing, because of its greater sensitivity and lower cost. Serum immunoglobulins, especially total serum IgE, often are elevated but nonspecifically. Unconventional allergy tests, including the controversial cytotoxic, sublingual neutralization, and titration techniques, should be avoided until their sensitivity and specificity have been established in controlled studies. Eosinophilia in sputum and blood is a common finding in asthmatic individuals, but sputum bacterial cultures generally are not helpful.

DIFFERENTIAL DIAGNOSIS

During the first few years of life, other conditions that can cause partial airway obstruction and provoke recurrent cough and wheezing must be considered. As already indicated, *bronchiolitis* and asthma are often difficult to differentiate in infants under 1 year of age. *Cystic fibrosis* may cause symptoms that mimic asthma, even in the absence of growth failure. Thus a sweat test is warranted in children with recurrent wheezing. *Congenital anomalies* of the respiratory, cardiovascular, and gastrointestinal tracts may obstruct the airway and produce symptoms that warrant appropriate radiological studies, especially during the first 2 years of life. Aspiration of a *foreign body* usually causes a sudden onset of symptoms, but if the acute event is not appreciated at the time of aspiration, it may result in chronic or recurrent wheezing. *Gastroesophageal reflux* may be associated with subtle aspiration that causes respiratory symptoms, including wheezing, during infancy and childhood. On occasion an *immunodeficiency* may be associated with repeated respiratory infections accompanied by wheezing. IgG subclass deficiency should be considered in children who have recurrent infections and asthma.[7] Yet the child who has recurrent episodes of coughing and wheezing, after appropriate study, most often is shown to have asthma.

TREATMENT

The goals of therapy for asthma are to reverse symptoms and, of course, to prevent their development. To achieve both these goals, the clinician must classify the asthma as mild, moderate, or severe and, following NIH guidelines (see Table 185-1), institute appropriate incremental pharmacological therapy along with suitable measures of environmental control to reduce or eliminate specific and nonspecific factors that provoke symptoms.[6] The pharmacotherapy of children who have asthma comprises two classes of medications, bronchodilators and antiinflammatory agents (Table 185-2). The sympathomimetics and theophyllines are specific bronchodilators, whereas antiinflammatory cromolyn, nedocromil, and steroids do not act directly on the airway smooth muscle and provide clinical improvement only over hours or days. The efficacy of these medications can be additive, and they may be used simultaneously. Unfortunately, multiple-drug treatment regimens are potentially confusing, not only to the patient but also to the pediatrician.

To simplify the use of appropriate pharmacotherapy, Figure 185-1 presents a step-up or step-down flowchart of drug treatment based on the clinical patterns of asthma described above.[6,12] Efficient reversal of symptoms requires a prompt-acting bronchodilator; thus sympathomimetics are the drugs of choice for the acute, occasional asthma attack. *Theophylline* does not appear to be effective during acute attacks. Several of these agents, along with their formulations and appropriate dosages, are listed in Table 185-2. Severe acute symptoms may require administration of *subcutaneous epinephrine* or a *sympathomimetic aerosol*, the latter often seeming to be a faster and safer treatment route. Home use of metered-dose inhalers demands proper instruction and has the potential for overuse and abuse by some children, particularly adolescents. A sympathomimetic aerosol generated by an air compressor can be used for the child under age 6 who cannot use the metered-dose inhalers properly, and spacers and holding chambers have been devised, which may help facilitate metered-dose inhaler therapy. Mild acute symptoms may be controlled with oral sympathomimetic agents. *If symptoms cannot be managed with one of the sympathomimetics, an antiinflammatory drug should be added to the regimen.* If symptoms are severe or unresponsive, hospitalization is indicated. *As an alternative to hospitalization for a known asthmatic child, administration of a short course of oral steroids may be warranted.* Prednisone in a dosage of 2 mg/kg/24 hr (up to a maximum daily dose of 60 mg) can be given in several divided doses for 3 to 5 days; it then can be stopped or tapered as clinically indicated over several days.

Cromolyn can be effective for preventing asthma attacks in a patient who has recurrent or daily wheezing. It should be used as a prophylactic agent, however, and not as an acute bronchodilator for ongoing established episodes of asthma. *Cromolyn and nedocromil* are available as a metered dose that is used four times a day. For children under age 6, a liquid form of cromolyn is available for inhalation via a nebulizer with compressed air. If cromolyn therapy proves beneficial, certain children may be maintained on as few as two or three inhalations per day, and it may even be possible then to reduce or stop administration of bronchodilators.

Intermittent corticosteroid therapy with prednisone may be necessary in certain children who have chronic or severe asthma that has failed to respond to the other drugs. Judicious use of prednisone in dosages of 1 to 2 mg/kg/24 hr for several days, followed by rapid tapering of the dose over 1 week, may prevent frequent hospitalization of a child who has severe chronic asthma. An alternative to *oral corticosteroids* is prophylactic use of a *topical metered-dose steroid* (beclomethasone, triamcinolone, or flunisolide) aerosolized by inhaler. The usual pediatric dose (two inhalations three or four times daily) produces minimal side effects, other than a rare instance of oral candidiasis. Metered-dose flunisolide, triamcinolone, or beclomethasone also can be delivered via a spacer or holding chamber to children under age 6. At this time, however, a corticosteroid solution is not yet available for aerosol use via an air compressor.

Table 185-2 Medications Used To Treat Children Who Have Asthma

Drug	Formulation/administration	Dose/duration
Bronchodilators		
Sympathomimetics		
Epinephrine		
Epinephirine	1:1000 solution SQ	0.01 ml/kg up to 0.33 ml
Sus-Phrine*	1:200 suspension, SQ	0.005 ml/kg up to 0.25 ml
Albuterol		
Proventil*	Metered aerosol	90 μg/puff
Ventolin*	Tablet: 2, 4 mg	0.1 mg/kg tid
	Syrup: 2 mg/5 ml	0.1 mg/kg tid
	Aerosol solution: 1%	0.5 ml/2.5 ml saline
Metaproterenol		
Alupent*	Aerosol solution: 5%	0.25 ml/2.5 ml saline
Metaprel*	Metered aerosol	650 μg/puff
	Syrup: 10 mg/5 ml	0.5 mg/kg tid
	Tablet: 10, 20 mg	0.5 mg/kg tid
Terbutaline		
Brethine*	Solution SQ	0.25 ml/dose
Bricanyl*	Tablet: 2.5, 5 mg	0.075 mg/kg tid
Theophyllines (the normal dosage [12-16 mg/kg/24 hr] must be individualized)		
Theo-Dur Sprinkle*	Capsule: 50, 75, 125 mg	q8-12h (long duration)
Theo-Dur*	Tablet: 100, 200, 300 mg	q8-12h (long duration)
Slo-Phyllin*	Gyrocap: 60, 125, 200 mg	q8-12h (long duration)
Slo-Bid*	Gyrocap: 100, 200, 300 mg	q8-12h (long duration)
Antiinflammatory drugs		
Cromolyn	Aerosol solution: 2 μg/2 ml	20 g qid
	Metered aerosol	2 puffs qid
Nedocromil	Metered aerosol	2 puffs qid
Inhaled corticosteroids		
Beclomethasone (Vanceril,* Beclovent*)	Metered aerosol	44 mg/puff
Triamcinolone (Azmacort*)	Metered aerosol	100 mg/puff
Flunisolide (AeroBid*)	Metered aerosol	250 mg/puff

*Trade name.

Severely affected children may require alternate-day steroids, which should be tapered to the smallest dose (given as a single morning dose) that controls symptoms. Long-term daily use of oral corticosteroid should be avoided in children at all costs because of the severe impairment of growth and development caused by daily corticosteroids.

The child who has episodic (recurrent) asthma may benefit from regular maintenance therapy with a *sustained-release theophylline,* as may the child who has chronic daily wheezing. It must be remembered, however, that there is substantial intersubject variation in theophylline metabolism. The preschool and primary school-age child, for instance, metabolizes theophylline faster than does the adolescent or infant. Other factors that can alter theophylline metabolism include liver disease, viral infection, nicotine (from cigarette smoking), and other drugs. Ingestion of sustained-release theophylline with meals can alter its pharmacokinetics and should be avoided. It usually is best to begin with a modest dose (12 to 16 mg/kg/24 hr) and then cautiously increase it weekly if wheezing persists. Chronically ill children who are to be treated with daily maintenance theophylline probably should have their serum theophylline concentration measured a week after therapy is begun and thereafter at approximately 6- to 12-month intervals. Still, it may be sufficient to monitor the serum theophylline level only in children who do not respond to the usual recommended dose or who have adverse symptoms while receiving the usual dosage. Although the therapeutic range for serum theophylline is 10 to 20 μg/ml, it probably is best not to exceed 16 μg/ml in most children. Several reliable sustained-release theophylline products are available. The bead-filled capsules may be particularly useful for a young child who is unable to swallow a capsule or tablet but who can swallow the beads mixed into or sprinkled on food. Another adjunct therapy for chronic asthma is the anticholinergic ipratropium (Atrovent), which is available as a metered-dose inhaler and a solution for nebulization.

Other aspects of therapy should not be overlooked in planning a comprehensive treatment program. Passive inhalation of cigarette smoke or other respiratory irritants can provoke hyperreactivity in the airways of an asthmatic person. Thus appropriate *environmental control measures* should be pursued to prevent exposure to known irritants. Appropriate play and exercise are necessary for all children. Should exercise provoke asthma, prophylactic inhalation of an aerosolized bronchodilator may allow active play and can be especially useful for children engaged in competitive sports.

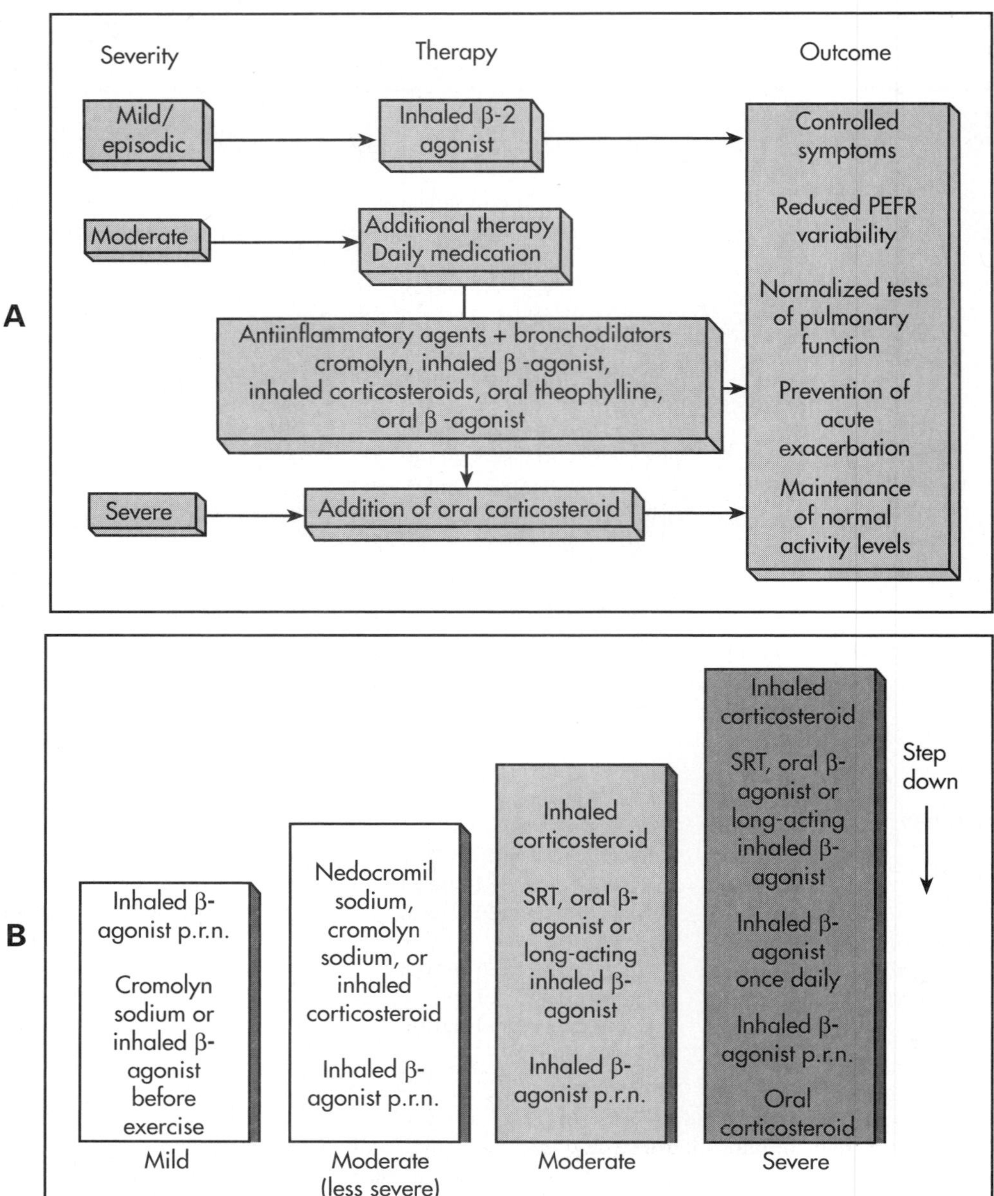

FIG. 185-1 Stepwise approach to the pharmacological treatment of asthma as proposed by the National Heart, Lung, and Blood Institute[6] **(A)** and the International Consensus Report[12] **(B)**. *PEFR*, Peak expiratory flow rate; *SRT*, sustained-release theophylline.

In certain children, allergic asthma is seasonal. If the offending allergens (which are not easily avoided) are identified, a trial of hyposensitization by injection with the specific allergen may be considered. The stresses, both emotional and financial, on the family of a child who has chronic asthma create an environment conducive to psychological problems. Attention to these potential behavioral problems should lessen the anxiety associated with asthma and improve compliance with the total therapeutic program.

PROGNOSIS

In general, the prognosis for a child who has asthma is good. Yet long-term studies of asthmatic patients show abnormal airway hyperreactivity even among those who have been symptom free for years. Many children whose asthma is intermittent tend to improve during adolescence, with symptoms developing only during viral respiratory infections or strenuous exercise. Of those who have persistent daily wheezing during childhood, however, fewer than 20% become asthma free during adolescence. Thus persistent daily bronchospasm may indicate an unfavorable prognosis, and appropriate therapy should be pursued aggressively so that the child who has asthma can have a normal life-style, including regular school attendance, uninterrupted rest at night, appropriate recreation, and enjoyment of sports.

REFERENCES

1. Burrows B et al: Association of asthma with serum IgE levels and skin-test reactivity to allergens, *N Engl J Med* 320:271, 1989.
2. Gergen PV, Mulladly DI, Evans R: National survey of prevalence of asthma among children in US: 1976-1980, *Pediatrics* 81:11, 1988.
3. Gurwitz D, Mindorff C, Levinson H: Increased incidence of bronchial reactivity in children with a history of bronchiolitis, *J Pediatr* 98:551, 1981.
4. Martin AJ et al: Natural history of asthma from childhood to adult, *Br Med J* 280:1397, 1980.
5. McIntosh K et al: The association of viral respiratory infections with wheezing in young asthmatic patients, *J Pediatr* 82:578, 1973.
6. National Heart, Lung, and Blood Institute: National Asthma Education Program: Guidelines for the Diagnosis and Management of Asthma, NIH Consensus Report No 91-3042, National Institutes of Health, Bethesda, Md, 1991.
7. Page R et al: Asthma and selective IgG subclass deficiency: improvement of asthma following IgG replacement therapy, *J Pediatr* 112:127, 1988.
8. Schiffer CG, Hunt EP: Illness among children: data from the National Health Survey, US Public Health Service Pub No 2074, Washington, DC, 1970, US Government Printing Office.
9. Skoner DP et al: Plasma elevations of histamine and a prostaglandin metabolite in asthma, *Am Rev Respir Dis* 137:1004, 1988.
10. Smith JM: The changing prevalence of asthma in schoolchildren, *Clin Allergy* 1:51, 1971.
11. Szentiavanyi A: The beta-adrenergic theory of atopic abnormality in bronchial asthma, *J Allergy* 42:203, 1968.
12. US Department of Health and Human Services: International Consensus Report on Diagnosis and Management of Asthma, Public Health Service, National Institutes of Health, Bethesda, Md, 1992.
13. Welliver RC et al: The development of respiratory syncytial virus–specific IgE and release of histamine in nasopharyngeal secretion after infection, *N Engl J Med* 305:841, 1981.

186 Atopic Dermatitis

Ana M. Duarte and Lawrence A. Schachner

Atopic dermatitis is a multifactorial, chronic skin disorder common in children. It sometimes is called *eczema,* which is a general term used to describe a condition of redness, scaling, vesicles, and crusting. Eczematous eruptions include atopic dermatitis, seborrheic dermatitis, contact dermatitis, and dermatophyte infection. This chapter focuses on atopic dermatitis.

EPIDEMIOLOGY

Atopic dermatitis (AD) is predominantly a disease of infancy and childhood. In 60% of affected individuals, the onset occurs in the first year of life; 85% have symptoms by age 5.[12] Studies indicate an increasing prevalence in developed countries, with as many as 10% to 20% of the general population having atopic disease. In the United States the prevalence of AD increased from 3% in the 1960s to 10% in the 1980s.[8,15] AD affects all races, but it is particularly common in Caucasians and Asians.[13] Males and females are affected equally.[14] As many as 50% of children who have acquired immunodeficiency syndrome (AIDS) also have atopic dermatitis.

GENETICS

Atopic dermatitis appears to be inherited in a polygenic pattern. If one parent is affected, there is a 60% chance the child will have AD; if both parents are affected, the likelihood increases to 80%. If neither parent has the disorder, the child has a 19% chance of having AD.[7,9]

CLINICAL FEATURES

AD is characterized by three distinct stages—infantile, childhood, and adult forms. The patient may manifest *acute dermatitis* (Fig. 186-1), which is characterized by severe pruritus, redness, vesicles, and exudation, or may have a *subacute* pattern (Fig. 186-2), with pruritus, redness, and scaling. Over time the lesions show the changes of *chronic dermatitis,* marked by excoriations, lichenification (thickened skin and deeper skin lines), and postinflammatory hypopigmentation or hyperpigmentation (Fig. 186-3).

The *infantile stage* begins at about 3 months of age and lasts through the first 2 years of life. The eruption begins on the cheeks and extensor surfaces of the arms and legs. The hair is dry, and the scalp often is scaly. The dermatitis usually is a more acute form.

The *childhood stage* begins at about age 3 and lasts through puberty. The areas most often affected are the antecubital and popliteal areas, the neck, and the flexures of the wrists and ankles (Fig. 186-4). Clinically these patients in this stage display a more subacute and chronic dermatitis.

The *adult stage,* which lasts from puberty onward, is an extension of the childhood stage. The clinical signs include diffuse involvement of the body, central facial pallor, xerosis, and lichenification.

Associated Clinical Manifestations

Dennie-Morgan folds (infraorbital folds) and *atopic shiners* (infraorbital darkening) (Fig. 186-5, *A*), as well as *hyperlinear palms* (Fig. 186-5, *B*) and *soles,* frequently are seen in patients who have AD.

Twenty percent of patients with AD have *ichthyosis vulgaris,* marked by areas of scaling, on the lower extremities. *Keratosis pilaris* (KP), characterized by follicular keratotic papules, affects predominantly the lateral surfaces of the upper or lower extremities, although the face also may be involved (Fig. 186-6).

Lichen spinulosus, marked by annular, grouped follicular keratotic papules, may occur on the trunk and extremities (Fig. 186-7). *Pityriasis alba,* a condition of ill-defined mildly scaling hypopigmented patches, occurs primarily on the face, although other areas often are involved (Fig. 186-8).

Cataracts (anterior or posterior subcapsular form), *keratoconjunctivitis,* and *keratoconus* also are seen in AD patients. Periodic ophthalmological examinations are recommended.

Juvenile plantar dermatosis (Fig. 186-9), which manifests as redness, scaling, and painful fissuring of the plantar surfaces of the feet, often is worse in atopic individuals. Treatment involves applying a moderate-potency topical corticosteroid (e.g., Kenalog) to the fissured areas for 7 days, followed by a low-potency corticosteroid in combination with a topical antibiotic (e.g., Silvadene). If the condition fails to improve, a dermatologist should be consulted.

Nummular eczema, a condition marked by coin-shaped, scaling, red lesions, also is seen in association with AD (Fig. 186-10). The treatment is the same as that for AD (see Management in this chapter).

DIAGNOSIS

The criteria for diagnosing atopic dermatitis were defined by Hanifin and Lobitz.[5] These criteria are presented in the box on p. 1197.

PATHOGENESIS

Atopic dermatitis is characterized by two basic immune abnormalities: an increase in immunoglobulin E (IgE) and a decrease in T suppressor cells. Also, production of gamma-interferon (INF-gamma) and interleukin-4 (IL-4), which play reciprocal roles in regulating IgE production, is abnormal. Production of INF-gamma is inadequate, and production of

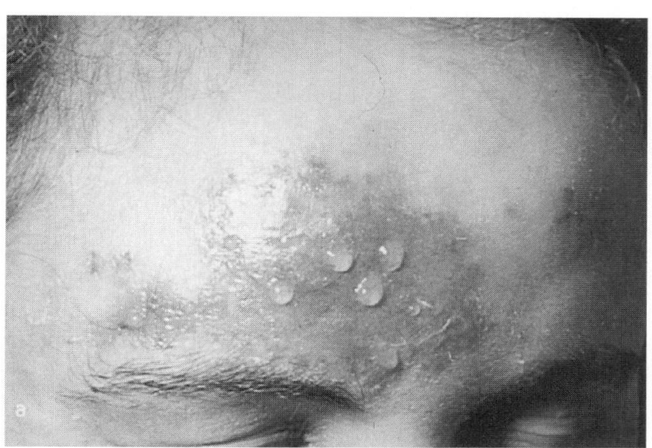

FIG. 186-1 Acute dermatitis characterized by redness and vesiculation.

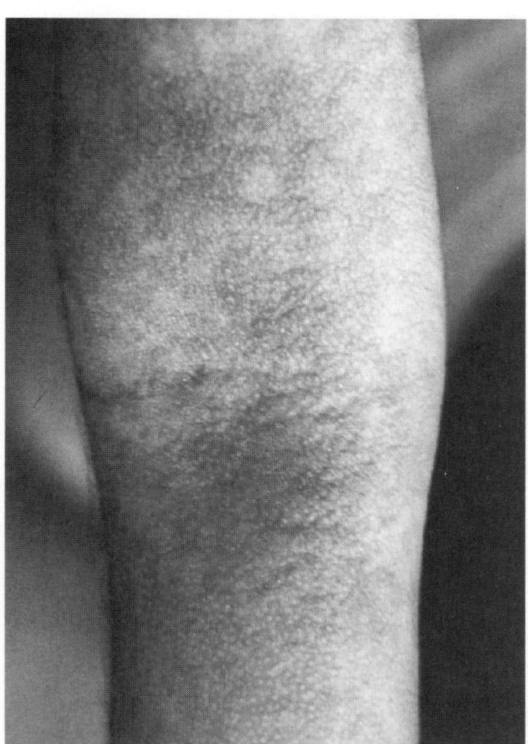

FIG. 186-2 Subactute dermatitis of the antecubital region. The skin is pink and dry and shows mild scaling.

IL-4 is excessive.[17] These disturbances effect IgE-mediated activation of mast cells and mononuclear cells, which includes the release of histamine and other pharmacologically active mediators, resulting in the clinical manifestations of AD.

DIFFERENTIAL DIAGNOSIS

The differential diagnosis of AD includes disorders characterized by an eczematous eruption. These include seborrheic dermatitis, contact dermatitis (allergic and irritant forms), and

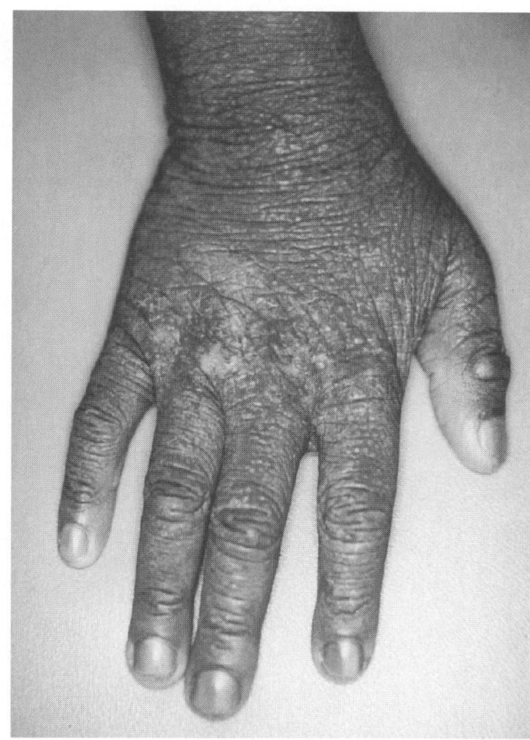

FIG. 186-3 Chronic dermatitis. The skin is dry and hyperpigmented, and the skin markings are accentuated.

CRITERIA FOR THE DIAGNOSIS OF ATOPIC DERMATITIS

Major criteria (all three must be present)

1. Pruritus
2. Typical morphology and distribution
   a. Facial and extensor involvement during infancy and early childhood
   b. Flexural lichenification and linearity by adolescence
3. Chronic or recurring dermatitis

Minor criteria (two or more must be present)

1. Personal or family history of atopy (e.g., asthma, allergic rhinoconjunctivitis, atopic dermatitis)
2. Immediate skin test reactivity
3. White dermatographism and/or delayed blanch to cholinergic agents
4. Anterior subcapsular cataracts

Associated conditions (four or more must be present)

1. Xerosis/ichthyosis/hyperlinear palms
2. Pityriasis alba
3. Keratosis pilaris
4. Facial pallor/infraorbital darkening
5. Dennie-Morgan fold
6. Elevated serum IgE
7. Keratoconus
8. Nonspecific hand dermatitis
9. Recurring cutaneous infections

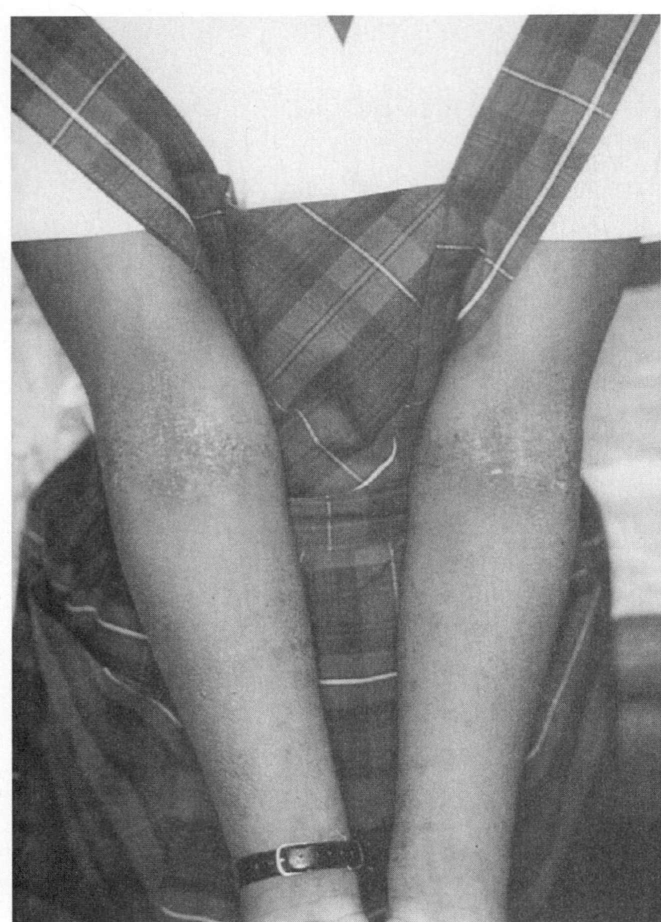

FIG. 186-4 Atopic dermatitis, childhood stage. Note the flexural distribution of the eruption.

dermatophyte infection, as well as other immunological and metabolic disorders.

Seborrheic dermatitis is a disease of unknown cause that affects infants and some adolescents. It usually manifests in the neonatal period and consists of asymptomatic, greasy, yellow, scaling plaques. When these occur on the scalp, the condition is called *cradle cap*. Areas typically affected include the flexural creases, the axillae, the retroauricular area, and the neck. Seborrheic dermatitis may occur with AD (see Chapter 255).

Contact dermatitis may be a primary irritant reaction, resulting from application of an irritating substance, or the result of true allergic sensitization (a type 4 delayed hypersensitivity reaction). The most common causes of allergic contact dermatitis are poison ivy, nickel, and rubber. The lesions, which may be acute, subacute, or chronic, occur on exposed sites in the distribution of the contactant (Fig. 186-11). A careful history and patch testing can help determine the cause.

Dermatophyte infection (Fig. 186-12), which is characterized by red, scaling, annular plaques on the trunk and interdigital maceration and scaling of the feet, may be confused with nummular eczema and juvenile plantar dermatosis. A potassium hydroxide preparation will identify the septate hyphae.

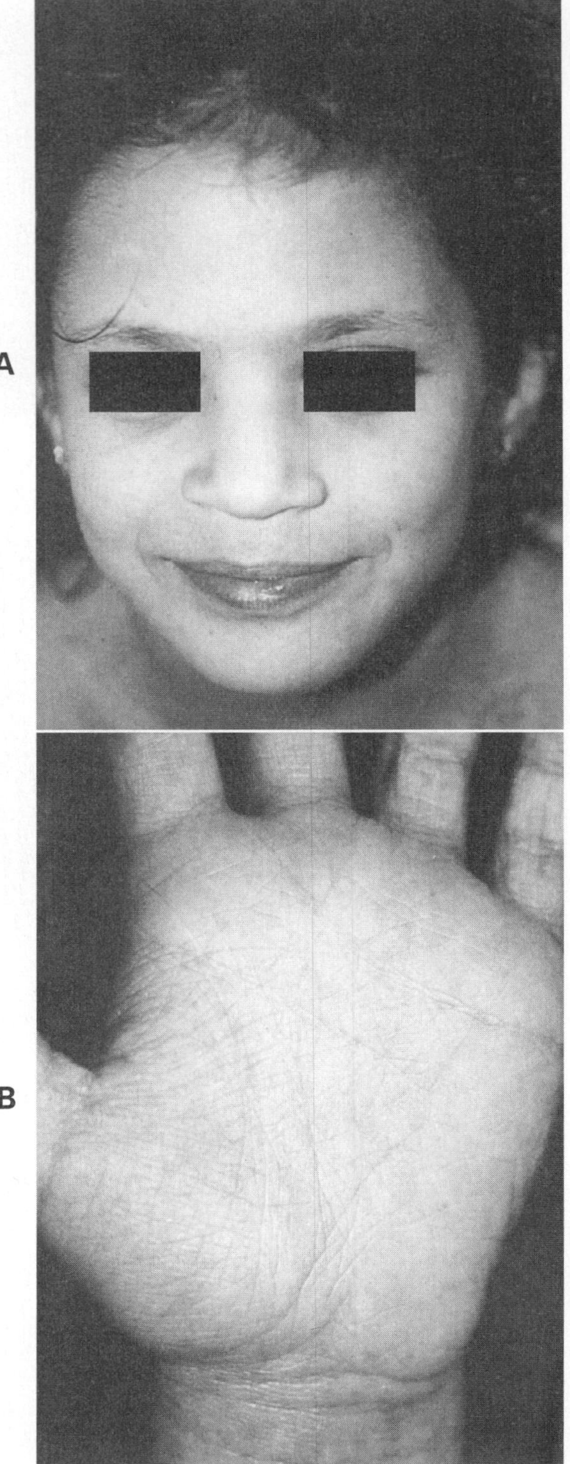

FIG. 186-5 **A,** Infraorbital folds (Dennie-Morgan folds) and atopic shiners. **B,** Hyperlinear palms.

A detailed discussion of other disorders that may produce eczematous lesions is beyond the scope of this chapter. Some of these diseases are Wiskott-Aldrich syndrome, Leiner disease, histiocytosis X, ataxia telangiectasia, ahistidinemia, agammaglobulinemia, Hartnup disease, Hurler syndrome, and phenylketonuria.

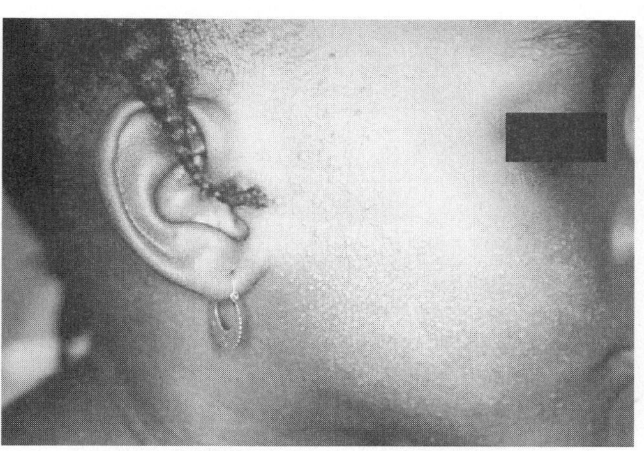

FIG. 186-6 Keratosis pilaris.

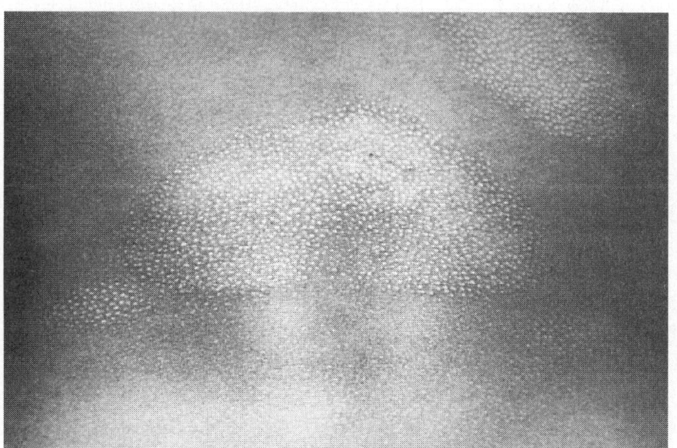

FIG. 186-7 Lichen spinulosus.

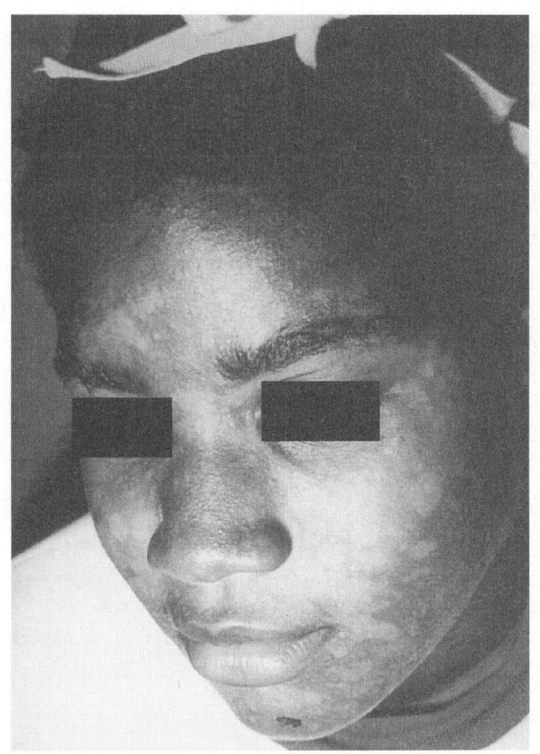

FIG. 186-8 Pityriasis alba.

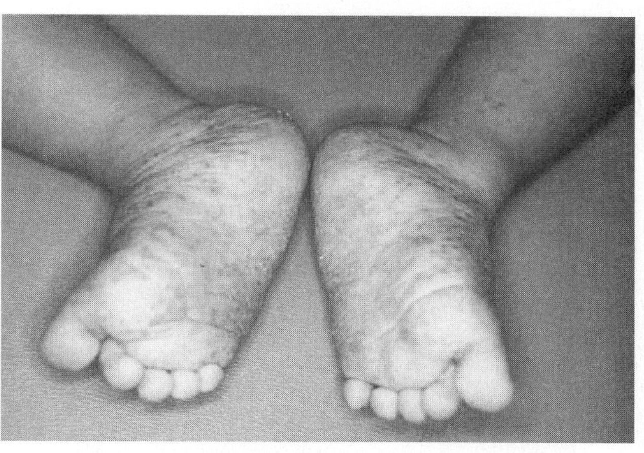

FIG. 186-9 Juvenile plantar dermatosis.

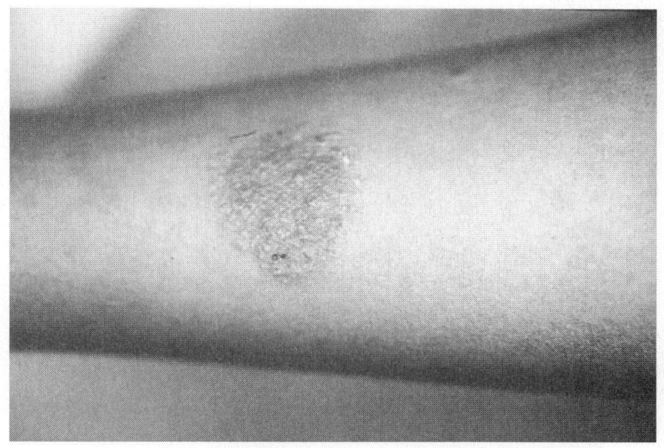

FIG. 186-10 Nummular eczema.

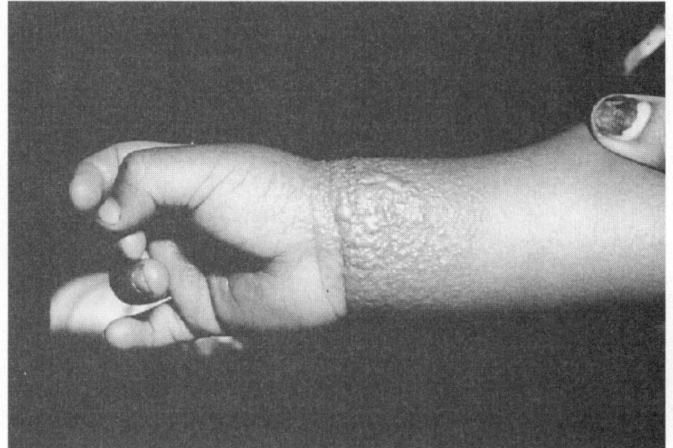

FIG. 186-11 Contact dermatitis caused by poison ivy. (Courtesy of Dr. Harvey Blank.)

COMPLICATIONS OF ATOPIC DERMATITIS

Cutaneous Infection

Staphylococcal Infections (Impetigo). Many patients who have AD have significant colonization with *Staphylococcus aureus* and may easily develop a secondary infection, known as impetigo (Fig. 186-13), in areas of dermatitis. This infec-

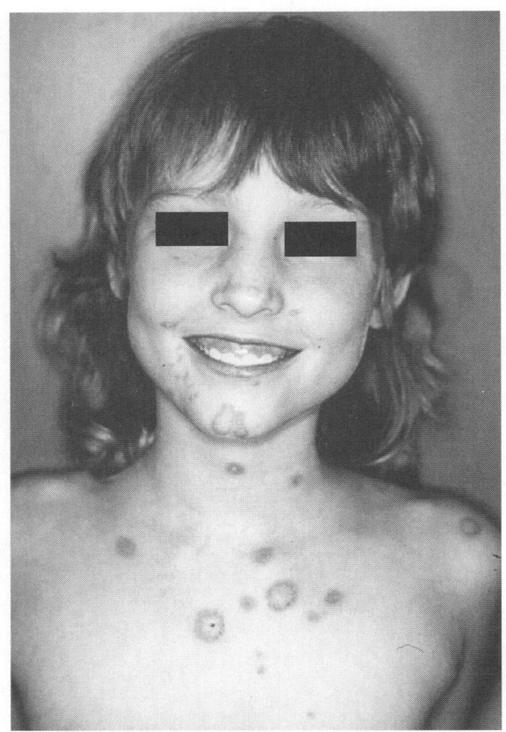

FIG. 186-12 Dermatophyte infection.

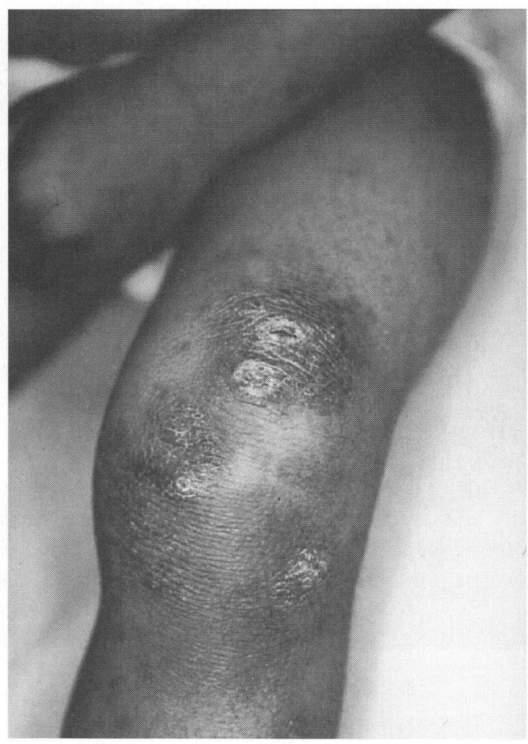

FIG. 186-13 Impetigo.

tion usually responds well to topical or oral antibiotics. However, an *S. aureus* superinfection may be widespread and serious. Such patients may have generalized exfoliative erythroderma, which requires hospitalization for aggressive skin care and systemic antibiotics.

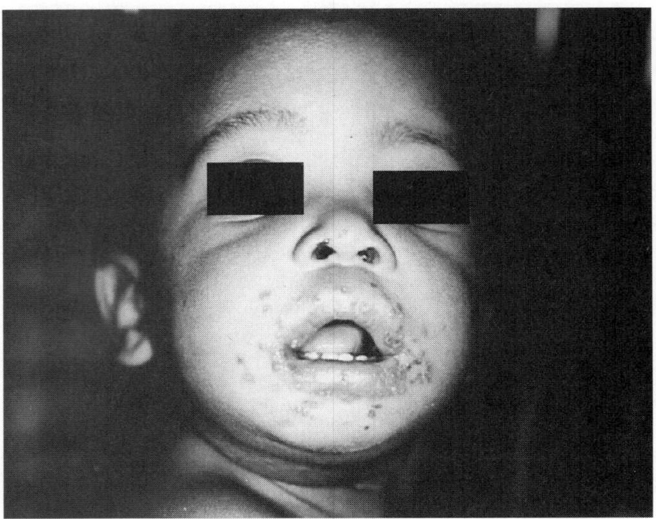

FIG. 186-14 Eczema herpeticum.

Herpes Simplex Infections. Eczema herpeticum (Fig. 186-14), also known as Kaposi varicelliform eruption, is a widespread herpes simplex virus or varicella virus infection of the skin that occurs in patients who have AD. The eruption may be serious, especially in very young or immunodeficient patients. The morbidity and mortality rates are greater than those for superinfection with *S. aureus*. Patients with eczema herpeticum may require treatment with acyclovir.

Human Papillomavirus. Verruca vulgaris (warts) also may occur more commonly in AD patients. Various types of treatment can be used, including topical vesicants (e.g., Duofilm or Cantharone). Some cases may require more aggressive treatment, such as immunomodulaters (e.g., interferon), cryotherapy, or ablation with a carbon dioxide laser.

Molluscum Contagiosum. Molluscum contagiosum is a cutaneous, self-limited viral infection caused by the pox virus It is thought to be more common in patients with AD, who may have widespread eruptions. Treatment is optional. In extensive cases, manual expression, cryotherapy, or topical Cantharone may be helpful.

Short Stature

In children who have severe atopic dermatitis (i.e., involvement of more than half of the body surface area), linear growth may be diminished.[10] Also, elimination diets and long-term treatment with corticosteroids may further retard growth.[10] The release of growth hormone may be impaired in some children with AD who show growth retardation.[3]

MANAGEMENT

Treatment of AD is directed primarily at relieving inflammation, dryness, and pruritus, treating superinfection by *S. aureus*, and managing associated conditions. *If the condition does not respond to the following measures, the patient should be referred to a dermatologist.*

Inflammation

Inflammation is best treated with corticosteroids. A cream should be used for acute dermatitis (weeping, red lesions).

For chronic dermatitis, in which dryness and lichenification predominate, an ointment base is more therapeutic.

Low-potency steroids (e.g., 1% hydrocortisone ointment or cream) can be used on the face and groin twice a day as needed. *Strong, halogenated steroids should not be used for the face, axillae, or groin.* A midpotency corticosteroid (e.g., 0.1% triamcinolone acetonide cream or ointment) may be applied to lesions on the extremities or trunk as needed twice a day. Systemic corticosteroids are used only in rare cases because of the many undesirable side effects and the rebound flare-ups that occur when the drug is discontinued. As a last resort, prednisone may be given at 1 mg/kg daily for 4 days and then tapered slowly over the next 2 weeks.

Some patients may respond to a modified Goeckerman regimen, which involves applying tar to the affected area and then exposing it to ultraviolet light (using sunlight or a light box). This treatment is used in addition to the course of topical corticosteroids described above.

Dryness

Dryness can be alleviated by having the patient take lukewarm baths instead of showers, which are more drying. The bath should last only about 5 minutes, and a mild soap, such as unscented Dove, Cetaphyl, or Lowila, should be used. The patient should be patted dry (not rubbed) with a towel, and immediately an oil-based emollient (e.g., Vaseline) should be applied to unaffected skin and the appropriate corticosteroid to areas of dermatitis. This effectively seals in moisture.

Pruritus

Pruritus can be relieved with oral antihistamines such as hydroxyzine or diphenhydramine, especially at bedtime, so that the child sleeps more peacefully. Behavior modification (e.g., teaching the child to rub rather than scratch and having him or her wear mittens to bed) will lessen the itch-scratch cycle. Keeping the child's nails cut short is essential because it helps to reduce skin damage and the incidence of superinfection.

Staphylococcal Superinfection

A staphylococcal superinfection may manifest as a flare-up in the patient's dermatitis. Local infections are treated with topical antibiotics, and oral medications are used for more extensive involvement. Cultures of skin and nares samples may help identify appropriate antibiotic sensitivities, as well as a nasal carrier state (in which case Bactroban applied three times a day may eradicate the bacterium).

Associated Manifestations

Ichthyosis vulgaris can be treated with keratolytics (e.g., LacHydrin) in combination with emollients. Treatment for *keratosis pilaris* and *lichen spinulosus* involves topical isotretinoin, keratolytics, and emollients. *Pityriasis alba* may improve if treated with low-potency topical steroids, emollients, and sunscreen. As mentioned before, juvenile plantar dermatosis may respond to a short course of a moderate-potency corticosteroid (e.g., Kenalog) followed by a low-potency corticosteroid in combination with a topical antibiotic (e.g., Silvadene cream).

A range of controversial treatments using Chinese plant extracts has been found therapeutic compared with a placebo in many AD patients.[16] No short-term toxicity has been found; however, long-term, well-controlled studies are needed. The medications are available in pills, tablets, or liquid.

Immunomodulators, such as cyclosporine, INF-gamma, thymopentin, and PUVA (psoralen and ultraviolet A light), which may play a therapeutic role in recalcitrant cases of AD, are not widely used because of their significant side effects.

Dietary Management

Dietary management of patients who have AD remains controversial. However, for patients whose food allergy has been identified (peanuts, milk, and eggs account for 80% of adverse reactions in patients with AD), eliminating these allergens has been shown to improve the dermatitis. The major drawback is the potential for nutritional and psychological hazards with an elimination diet. Prophylactic avoidance of food allergens, both for infants (i.e., breast-feeding exclusively for the first 6 months) and for lactating mothers who have a strong family history of atopy, may be helpful in some cases of AD.[6,18] Measuring the level of beta-lactoglobulin and soya protein antibody in affected children may help predict the response to an exclusionary diet.[2]

Oral sodium cromoglycate is useful in treating children who have AD that is aggravated by food hypersensitivities when the food or foods have high nutritional value or are very common in the diet and therefore cannot be eliminated easily.[1]

Environmental Control

Measures to control *house dust mites* may improve AD in patients with this allergy. Such measures include encasing pillows and mattresses in plastic liners, eliminating plants, stuffed animals, drapes, and carpeting from the home, dusting frequently, and using acaricides (mite killers). Determining IgG antibody titers against Der P1 Ag (the major allergenic component of house dust mite extract) may predict which children will benefit from these control measures.[2]

The patient's environment should be kept cool, and 100% cotton clothing is recommended (wool should be avoided).

PSYCHOSOCIAL CONSIDERATIONS

Atopic dermatitis is a chronic condition that very often is physically and psychologically distressing to both the patient and the family. Children who have a moderate to severe form of the disease often are irritable, restless, aggressive, and manipulative. Stress reduction and relaxation in the form of massage therapy is under investigation and may be an important therapeutic adjunct. Behavior modification (i.e., teaching the child not to scratch) is important to relieving the itch-scratch cycle. In some cases referral for professional family and individual counseling may be appropriate.

The child's activities, including sports, should be as mainstream as possible. If the child enjoys swimming, a thin barrier of petroleum jelly should be applied to the skin before the child enters the pool. He or she should shower quickly upon getting out and then reapply the petrolatum to counteract the drying, irritating effects of chlorine.

PROGNOSIS

Atopic dermatitis tends to resolve with age. Studies have shown clearing rates up to 40% of patients.[11] Those who have the most severe AD, as well as those who have food allergies, are more likely to have persistent cutaneous disease and respiratory involvement.[4,11]

REFERENCES

1. Businco L, Cantani A: Oral sodium cromoglycate in the management of atopic dermatitis in children, *Allergy Proc* 12:333, 1991.
2. Casimir GJ et al: Atopic dermatitis: role of food and house dust mite allergens, *Pediatrics* 92:252, 1993.
3. David TJ, Ferguson AP, Newton RW: Nocturnal growth hormone release in children with short stature and atopic dermatitis, *Acta Derm Venereol* 71:229, 1991.
4. Guillet G, Guillet MH: Natural history of sensitization in atopic dermatitis: a 3-year follow-up in 250 children: food allergy and high risk of respiratory symptoms, *Arch Dermatol* 128:187, 1992.
5. Hanifin JM, Lobitz WC: Newer concepts of atopic dermatology, *Arch Dermatol* 113:663, 1977.
6. Kajosaari M, Saarinen UM: Prophylaxis of atopic disease by six months total solid food elimination, *Acta Paediatr Scand* 27:411, 1983.
7. Kaufman HS, Frick OL: The development of allergy in infants of allergic parents: a prospective study concerning the role of heredity, *Ann Allergy* 38:339, 1983.
8. Larsson PA, Liden S: Prevalence of skin diseases among adolescents 12-16 years of age, *Acta Derm Venerol* 160:415, 1980.
9. Luoma R, Koivikko A, Viander M: Development of asthma, allergic rhinitis, and atopic dermatitis by age five years, *Allergy* 38:339, 1983.
10. Massarano AA et al: Growth in atopic eczema, *Arch Dis Child* 68:677, 1993.
11. Musgrive K, Morgan JK: Infantile eczema, *Br J Dermatol* 95:365, 1976.
12. Rajka G: Clinical aspects. In Rajka G, editor: *Essential aspects of atopic dermatitis,* Berlin, 1989, Springer-Verlag.
13. Rajka G: Some aetiological data on atopic dermatitis. Paper presented at the Second International Symposium on Atopic Dermatitis, Norway, 1984.
14. Schachner L, Ling NS, Press S: A statistical analysis of a pediatric dermatology clinic, *Pediatr Dermatol* 2:157, 1983.
15. Schultz-Larsen F: Atopic dermatitis: etiological studies based on a twin population, thesis, Copenhagen, 1985, Legeforeningens.
16. Sheehan MP, Atherton DJ: A controlled trial of traditional Chinese medicinal plants in widespread nonexudative atopic dermatitis, *Br J Dermatol* 126:179, 1992.
17. Tang M, Kemp A, Varigos G: IL-4 and interferon-gamma production in children with atopic disease, *Clin Exp Immunol* 92:120, 1993.
18. Zeiger RS et al: Effect of combined maternal and infant food allergen avoidance on development of atopy in early infancy: a randomized study, *J Allergy Clin Immunol* 84:72, 1989.

ditions in warm, humid environments. In contrast to staphylococcal impetigo, the streptococcal skin lesions occur most commonly on the lower extremities, where they usually are preceded by trauma such as a scratch or insect bite. Family members also may be affected.

Physical Findings

The early lesion is a pustule (hence the term *pyo*derma) with surrounding erythema, but the more advanced lesion of ecthyma is seen more often. At first glance this looks like a thick, usually brown crust surrounded by erythema. When the crust is removed, an actual ulcer is revealed (Fig. 187-3) (in contrast to the superficial erosion underlying the crust of a staphylococcal lesion). Also in contrast to staphylococcal impetigo, regional adenopathy often is present with streptococcal pyoderma.

Laboratory Studies

A culture sample taken from the base of the denuded ulcer grows group A beta-hemolytic streptococci. *S. aureus* occasionally is recovered concomitantly, in which case it is thought to be a secondary invader. Because some strains of group A streptococci are nephritogenic, screening for renal complications may be done by obtaining a urinalysis 2 to 3 weeks after the onset of infection.

Differential Diagnosis

Ecthyma gangrenosa is an uncommon but serious manifestation of *Pseudomonas* septicemia. Clinical features that help to differentiate this lesion from streptococcal ecthyma are (1) the location (usually inguinal or axillary folds), (2) the lesion's appearance (a deeper ulcer covered with a tightly adherent, black [gangrenous] crust), and (3) the host (a seriously ill, usually immunocompromised patient who manifests other signs of sepsis).

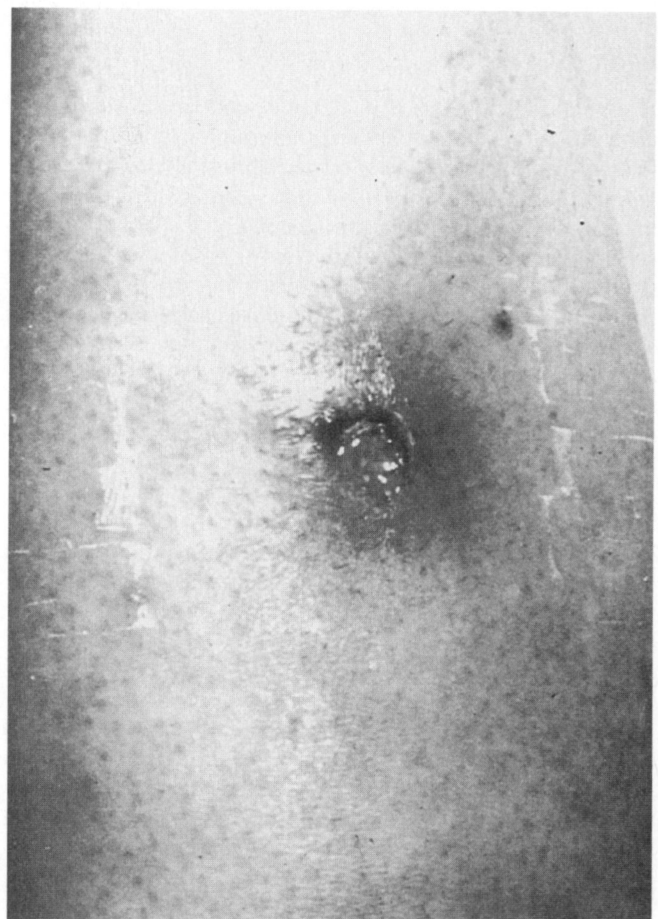

FIG. 187-3 Streptococcal pyoderma (ecthyma). After the crust is removed, the depth of this ulcerative lesion can be appreciated. The surrounding erythema and the location on the lower leg also are typical of this streptococcal lesion.

Management

Streptococcal pyoderma is treated with antibiotics, although the most appropriate route of administration still is a matter of debate. Some evidence indicates that applying topical antibiotics to scratches and insect bites reduces the incidence of subsequent pyoderma[3]; thus topical antibiotics may be advocated prophylactically for traumatic skin lesions.[12] Although topical mupirocin has proved effective for impetigo caused by group A streptococci, systemic antibiotics still are recommended for streptococcal infections, particularly if the infection is extensive. Injectable benzathine penicillin G is effective, but a 7- to 10-day course of oral penicillin or erythromycin often is used with compliant patients. Penicillin treatment occasionally fails, presumably because of the persistence of coexisting penicillinase-producing *S. aureus* organisms.

Complications

Complications are uncommon, although both local and systemic problems can result from streptococcal pyoderma. *Cellulitis* may develop if the infection extends into larger and deeper areas of skin and subcutaneous tissue. Some strains of group A streptococci produce the toxin responsible for scarlet fever; in fact, streptococcal pyoderma was the most common cause of scarlet fever in one series. But the potential immunological sequelae from streptococcal infections is the complication of most concern.

Acute rheumatic fever does *not* follow streptococcal infection of the skin, but *glomerulonephritis* may. It is caused by only a few nephritogenic serotypes of pyoderma-inducing streptococci. The usual period from onset of infection to development of the glomerulonephritis is 18 to 21 days. Even though treating streptococcal pyoderma has not been proved to prevent this nephritic complication, treatment nonetheless is recommended. Systemic antibiotic therapy clears the skin infection and helps to reduce the spread of streptococcal infection to the patient's playmates and family.

Prognosis

The aforementioned complications are uncommon, and in most patients the lesions heal uneventfully. Because they are deeper, streptococcal lesions often take longer than staphylococcal lesions to heal; however, bacteriological cures usually are accomplished within a week. If a prompt response is not achieved, a secondary infection from a penicillinase-producing staphylococcal strain should be considered, particularly if penicillin was used for treatment. Erythromycin-resistant strains of group A streptococci also may be encountered.

FOLLICULITIS

Etiology

Bacterial folliculitis is a moderately common disorder that primarily affects older children and young adults. It is an infection of the hair follicles, caused almost exclusively by *S. aureus*. In rare cases the infection is caused by gram negative organisms; this occurs occasionally in patients whose acne is being treated with antibiotics.[10] Also, with the recent popularity of hot tubs and whirlpools, some of which become contaminated, *Pseudomonas aeruginosa* has been identified as the cause of an uncommon and unusual type of folliculitis *(hot tub dermatitis),* which causes pruritic papules and pustules on the trunk and proximal extremities. In the usual case, however, *S. aureus* is the responsible pathogen, and it is this type of infection that is discussed.

History

Staphylococcal folliculitis appears most commonly as a chronic, smoldering eruption unaccompanied by symptoms, although occasionally a patient notices mild discomfort or pruritus.

Physical Findings

The lesions in staphylococcal folliculitis usually are located on the buttocks and upper portion of the thighs, over which individual small papules and pustules are scattered. The key to the diagnosis is that, on close inspection, hairs can be seen growing out of the very center of many of the lesions.

Laboratory Studies

In the typical case, culturing usually is not necessary. If, however, the presentation is atypical and laboratory confirmation is desired, the contents of a fresh pustule should be cultured.

Differential Diagnosis

Clinically, folliculitis caused by gram negative organisms differs from staphylococcal folliculitis in its distribution, with lesions occurring primarily on the face and shoulder. Hot tub folliculitis usually appears on the lower trunk.

Keratosis pilaris is another common follicular disorder that manifests as tiny, rough, scaling papules on the back of the upper parts of the arms, the buttocks, and the thighs. Although the distribution may be similar to that of staphylococcal folliculitis, the appearance of the lesions is not. In keratosis pilaris the lesions are smaller, more numerous, and scaling, but not pustular.

Management

The usual mild case of staphylococcal folliculitis can be managed by having the patient use an antiseptic cleanser (e.g., chlorhexidine) daily or every other day for at least several weeks. For more extensive involvement, a 7- to 10-day course of systemic antibiotics is suggested (e.g., erythromycin or dicloxacillin) in addition to the topical regimen.

Complications and Prognosis

In rare cases the follicular infection extends more deeply, producing a furuncle. Most patients respond to the treatment outlined above. If not, a bacterial culture should be done to rule out infection by gram negative organisms. Some patients are plagued with recurrences, for which a more prolonged course of antibiotic therapy is recommended.

FURUNCLES AND ABSCESSES

Etiology

Furuncles and abscesses are forms of skin infection (pus-filled nodules or boils) that usually follow folliculitis. *S. aureus* almost always is the responsible organism. Bacteria also may be inoculated into the skin and underlying soft tissue by traumatic injury, including surgery. Gram negative and anaerobic organisms also can be causes.[2,13] In children, anaerobic organisms commonly are isolated from abscesses in the perirectal area, hand, fingers, and nail beds.

History

A history of trauma may be elicited but often is not, especially with furuncles. Immunodeficiency states and diabetes may predispose certain patients to bacterial skin infections, but the typical patient who has a furuncle or abscess has no underlying medical disease.

Physical Findings

Furuncles and abscesses are fluctuant masses filled with pus. They often begin as hard, tender, red nodules and become more fluctuant and painful with time. Abscesses tend to be larger and deeper than furuncles, but sometimes the two lesions may be difficult to differentiate clinically.

Laboratory Studies

A Gram stain of the pustular material may provide a clue to the bacterial cause, but for precise identification, cultures are required. If anaerobic cultures are desired, material ideally is collected by aspirating the pus, sealing the syringe, and promptly delivering it to the laboratory. If insufficient material is available to aspirate, swab culturettes can be used for anaerobic as well as aerobic cultures. Blood culture results rarely are positive and are not indicated unless the patient shows signs of sepsis.

Management

Incision and drainage remain the mainstay of therapy. This results in complete healing in most cases, even in patients not treated with systemic antibiotics.[13] Systemic antibiotics may result in involution of early lesions, thereby halting their progression and averting the need for incision and drainage. Erythromycin or dicloxacillin is the antibiotic of choice. Culture results from abscesses may help in the ultimate selection of the appropriate antibiotic.

Complications

Recurrent furunculosis sometimes prompts a search for an underlying immunodeficiency—a search that almost always goes unrewarded. However, many such patients harbor *S. aureus* in a sequestered mucocutaneous site, the most common of which is the nose. The application of an antibiotic ointment (e.g., Bacitracin) to the external nares twice daily may decrease this bacterial colonization and thereby prevent furuncles from recurring. This should be accompanied by an every-other-day total body scrub with an antiseptic cleansing agent, such as chlorhexidine.

In rare cases a staphylococcal abscess may be the focus of toxin production, resulting in staphylococcal *scalded skin syndrome* (most commonly seen in infants and neonates) or *toxic shock syndrome*.

Prognosis

Untreated lesions often rupture and drain spontaneously. After either surgical or spontaneous drainage, uneventful healing is the rule. Larger lesions may leave scars.

CELLULITIS

Etiology

Cellulitis is a deep, locally diffuse infection of the skin with systemic manifestations and life-threatening potential.[8] It usually involves the face, an extremity, or the perianal area.[15] On an extremity the bacteria presumably have been externally inoculated into the deep dermal tissue, although the portal of entry often is not detectable clinically. A hematogenous or lymphangitic source also is possible and may explain the development of cellulitis in some cases in which the underlying skin is unbroken. In children under age 3, facial cellulitis often is associated with otitis media, *Haemophilus influenzae* type b usually being the responsible organism. *S. aureus* and group A streptococci more commonly are responsible for cellulitis of the extremities. Group A streptococci cause perianal cellulitis. In rare cases other aerobic and anaerobic bacterial organisms, as well as deep fungal agents such as *Cryptococcus neoformans,* can cause cellulitis. These infections occur in immunosuppressed individuals.

History

Children who have cellulitis often feel and look ill. Fever frequently is present and may precede the clinical skin signs. Patients may complain of pain in the affected area. There may be symptoms of an accompanying otitis media in buccal cellulitis. Patients who have perianal cellulitis often have pain with defecation. However, patients who have this disorder usually are not systemically ill; thus the disease may persist for weeks or months before it is correctly diagnosed.

Physical Findings

Fever at the time of presentation is common. The area of involved skin shows the classic signs of inflammation: redness, swelling, heat, and tenderness. *H. influenzae* facial cellulitis has a violaceous hue, and this type of cellulitis often is associated with otitis media and sometimes meningitis, with or without meningismus.

Laboratory Studies

Leukocytosis is a common finding. Cultures are required to identify the responsible pathogen, and samples should be obtained from the skin, the blood, and, with facial cellulitis, the cerebrospinal fluid (CSF). Middle ear aspirates also may reveal significant findings in patients who have otitis media. Skin aspirates from the leading edge of the lesion sometimes help in isolating pathogens when other cultures are negative.[8,17] This procedure is performed by preparing the skin with an antiseptic, introducing an 18- or 21-gauge needle into the deep dermis, and aspirating material. If no material is obtained (which usually is the case), 0.5 to 1 ml of nonbacteriostatic saline is injected and then aspirated. All aspirates should be Gram stained as well as cultured.

Differential Diagnosis

Erysipelas sometimes is considered separately from cellulitis. Classic erysipelas has more sharply demarcated borders than does cellulitis and may be caused more commonly by group A streptococci. However, the distinction between these two entities often is more semantic than real, inasmuch as the diagnosis and therapeutic considerations are the same.

A severe, local, confluent *contact dermatitis* sometimes may be confused with cellulitis in that both may show marked erythema of the skin. The important differences are that with contact dermatitis, the patient complains of itch rather than pain, the skin usually is not tender, and the patient is not febrile. The presence of vesicles also favors contact dermatitis, although vesicles and bullae sometimes may occur in erysipelas as the condition evolves.

Perianal cellulitis may be misdiagnosed as candidiasis or a diaper dermatitis. Pain and tenderness of the involved skin suggests bacterial infection, and a swab culture often confirms it.

Erythema of the cheeks occurs characteristically in *erythema infectiosum,* in which a "slapped cheek" appearance is noted. Important diagnostic differences between erythema infectiosum and cellulitis are that in the former, the involvement is bilateral, the site usually is not very tender, and the patient does not appear toxic, although he or she may be mildly febrile.

Management

Systemic antibiotics are the mainstay of therapy. Mild cases of cellulitis on an extremity may be treated with an oral antibiotic, warm soaks, and outpatient follow-up in several days. Inasmuch as cellulitis of the extremity most often is caused by gram positive organisms, erythromycin, dicloxacillin, or cephalexin is an appropriate drug to use. More seriously ill patients in whom sepsis is suspected, as well as most patients who have facial cellulitis, should be hospitalized for parenteral antibiotic therapy. Because facial cellulitis most commonly is caused by *H. influenzae* type b organisms, antibiotics must be selected accordingly. Intravenous therapy with a third-generation cephalosporin (e.g., ceftriaxone) is recommended.[18]

Complications

H. influenzae type b facial cellulitis often is accompanied by otitis media and less commonly by meningitis. Bacterial sepsis often accompanies cellulitis, however, and was present in 86% of one series of pediatric cases. Local abscesses and osteomyelitis are rare sequelae. Although cellulitis once was a serious, life-threatening disease, antibiotics have reduced the fatality rate to nearly zero in otherwise healthy patients.

Prognosis

With appropriate antibiotic therapy, fever usually resolves within 24 hours. If it does not, a change in antibiotic therapy should be considered, optimally guided by early culture results. The skin reaction resolves more slowly than does the fever, sometimes taking a week or longer to subside completely—the outcome to be expected in most patients.

REFERENCES

1. Barton LL, Friedman AD: Impetigo: a reassessment of etiology and therapy, *Pediatr Dermatol* 4:185, 1987.
2. Brook I, Finegold SM: Aerobic and anaerobic bacteriology of cutaneous abscesses in children, *Pediatrics* 67:891, 1981.
3. Coskey RJ, Coskey LA: Diagnosis and treatment of impetigo, *J Am Acad Dermatol* 17:62, 1987.
4. Dajani AS, Ferrieri P, Wannamaker LW: Natural history of impetigo. II. Etiologic agents and bacterial interactions, *J Clin Invest* 51:2863, 1972.
5. Demidovich CW et al: Impetigo: current etiology and comparison of penicillin, erythromycin, and cephalexin therapies, *Am J Dis Child* 144:1313, 1990.
6. Dillon HC: Impetigo contagiosa: suppurative and nonsuppurative complications. I. Clinical, bacteriologic, and epidemiologic characteristics of impetigo, *Am J Dis Child* 115:530, 1968.
7. Ferrieri P et al: Natural history of impetigo. I. Site sequence of acquisition and familial patterns of spread of cutaneous streptococci, *J Clin Invest* 51:2851, 1972.
8. Fleisher G, Ludwig S, Campos J: Cellulitis: bacterial etiology, clinical features, and laboratory findings, *J Pediatr* 97:591, 1980.
9. Hayden GF: Skin diseases encountered in a pediatric clinic, *Am J Dis Child* 139:36, 1985.
10. Leyden JJ et al: *Pseudomonas aeruginosa* gram-negative folliculitis, *Arch Dermatol* 115:1203, 1979.
11. Lookingbill DP: Impetigo, *Pediatr Rev* 7:177, 1985.
12. Maddox JS, Dillon HC: The natural history of streptococcal skin infection: prevention with topical antibiotics, *J Am Acad Dermatol* 13:207, 1985.
13. Meislin HW et al: Cutaneous abscesses: anaerobic and aerobic bacteriology and outpatient management, *Ann Intern Med* 87:145, 1977.
14. Mertz PM et al: Topical mupirocin treatment of impetigo is equal to oral erythromycin therapy, *Arch Dermatol* 125:1069, 1989.
15. Rehder PA, Eliezer ET, Lane AT: Perianal cellulitis: cutaneous group A streptococcal disease, *Arch Dermatol* 124:702, 1988.
16. Tunnessen WW: Practical aspects of bacterial skin infections in children, *Pediatr Dermatol* 2:255, 1985.
17. Uman SJ, Kunin CM: Needle aspiration in the diagnosis of soft tissue infections, *Arch Intern Med* 135:959, 1975.
18. Wortman PD: Bacterial infections of the skin, *Curr Probl Dermatol* 6:193, 1993.

188 Brain Tumors

Jerome Y. Yager and Robert C. Vannucci

Primary brain tumors, the most common type of solid tumor in childhood, are second only to leukemia as a cause of death from malignancy in children.[4,24] Advances in the fields of neuroradiology, neurosurgery, and cancer chemotherapy have improved the identification, management, and survival of affected children. Accordingly, pediatricians and primary care physicians have become involved in the long-term management of children who have central nervous system (CNS) tumors, thereby increasing their need to keep abreast of current trends in cancer diagnosis and treatment.

EPIDEMIOLOGY

The incidence of primary childhood brain tumors has not changed significantly over the years, remaining at 2.2 to 2.4 per 100,000 population at risk per year.[21,25] This figure equates to between 1200 and 1500 new cases identified each year. No significant gender or ethnic differences in incidence are evident among pediatric patients.[25]

Both the incidence and histopathological typing of brain tumors in children vary with age. In the first year, supratentorial tumors—those of the cerebral hemispheres and the diencephalon—predominate. Thereafter infratentorial tumors—those involving the brainstem and the cerebellum—are more prevalent. The highest incidence of tumors occurs between 5 and 9 years of age; these predominantly are astrocytic, with a smaller proportion being medulloblastomas. A slightly lesser number of tumors occurs between birth and 4 years of age; these, unfortunately, tend to be both clinically and histologically more malignant than those that occur at an older age. Histopathological types and their respective locations are shown in the box on p. 1210. Astrocytomas (both in the cerebral hemisphere and the cerebellum) represent 48%, medulloblastomas 23%, brainstem glioma 9%, ependymomas 8% (both supratentorial and infratentorial), and craniopharyngomas between 6% and 10% of all CNS tumors of childhood. Oligodendrogliomas, optic nerve gliomas, choroid plexus papillomas, and pineal gland tumors each make up 2% or less.

Primitive neuroectodermal tumors make up a group of poorly differentiated cerebral malignancies whose classification has yet to be clarified. Because they are of primitive neuroectodermal origin, several investigators include medulloblastomas among them. The tumors arise in either supratentorial or infratentorial regions of the brain, favor the younger age group, and are rapidly progressive in their growth.

PATHOGENESIS

The cause of the majority of primary brain tumors in childhood remains unknown. Recent work in the field of molecular biology, however, has brought us closer to an understanding of tumor pathogenesis in general.

Chromosomal abnormalities, manifested as deletions, translocations, and duplications, have long been known to exist in a variety of tumors, including brain tumors.[2,20,21] Highly malignant tumors appear to show extensive heterogeneity in DNA content. Benign tumors, on the other hand, display a more homogeneous cellular karyotype. Extensive evidence also exists, at least in laboratory animals, for a role of both RNA and DNA viruses in the induction of primary intracranial neoplasms.

The mechanism by which either viruses or chromosomal aberrations lead to tumor induction and propagation likely involves oncogenes, a group of genes involved in cell growth and differentiation.[22] Activation of these oncogenes releases the cell from its normal growth constraints and allows malignant transformation to occur. One theory proposes that viral genes integrate into host DNA and allow expression of the cellular oncogene; a second proposes that structural chromosomal abnormalities predispose a cell to oncogene enhancement.[20]

Several genetic syndromes are associated with an increased risk of CNS tumors; two of the most common are neurofibromatosis (NF) and tuberous sclerosis (TS). Both syndromes exhibit autosomal dominant modes of inheritance with high rates of spontaneous gene mutation. Peripheral neurofibromatosis (NF-I) and central neurofibromatosis (NF-II) have been linked to loci on chromosomes 17 and 22, respectively.[23] The relative risk of benign or malignant CNS neoplasms in NF-I is four times that in the general population,[24] and optic gliomas occur in as many as 15% of affected individuals.[7] A similar rate (15%) has been quoted for the occurrence of giant cell astrocytomas in patients who have TS.[14] The vast majority of these tumors are supratentorial gliomas. Whether an association exists between malignant transformation and the genetic abnormalities of these conditions is as yet unknown. Several investigators have suggested a role for neuronal growth factors as a possible cause of oncogenesis in patients who have NF-I.[19]

Other mechanisms that likely play a role in the development of childhood CNS tumors include prior radiation[15] and exposure to environmental toxins.[26] Some tumors, often appearing in the first year of life, are congenital in the sense that they arise from embryonic rests (e.g., craniopharyngioma) or result from errors in development (e.g., epidermal and dermoid cysts, hamartomas, and colloid cysts). A strong association exists between primary CNS lymphoma and acquired immunodeficiency syndrome.[16]

CLINICAL MANIFESTATIONS

The diagnosis of brain tumor in a child is based on clinical suspicion, a thorough history, and a detailed neurological examination. Signs and symptoms may be subtle and depend

PRIMARY BRAIN TUMORS OF CHILDHOOD

Supratentorial (cerebral hemisphere)

Astrocytoma
Oligodendroglioma
Ependymoma
Choroid plexus papilloma
Meningioma

Midline (diencephalon)

Craniopharyngioma
Pinealoma
Optic nerve glioma

Infratentorial (brainstem and cerebellum)

Astrocytoma (cerebellum)
Medulloblastoma (cerebellum)
Glioma (brainstem)
Ependymoma

Other

Primitive neuroectodermal tumors

on the age of the child and location of the tumor and its biological aggressiveness.

Although brain tumors lack pathognomonic features, several general concepts should be kept in mind. Intracranial mass lesions produce symptoms as a result of indirect effects caused by an increase in intracranial pressure (ICP) or of direct effects arising from the displacement or destruction of surrounding tissue. The duration of symptoms before diagnosis is affected by tumor site and growth characteristics. *Symptoms typically are progressive rather than intermittent.* Malignant, rapidly growing lesions have a more explosive manifestation than benign and slow-growing lesions.

In addition to tissue displacement within a fixed cranial volume, elevated ICP is caused by obstruction of cerebrospinal fluid (CSF) flow and secondary hydrocephalus or more rarely by increased CSF production. *Symptoms appear insidiously;* a change in personality, deterioration in school performance, headache, nausea, vomiting, and lethargy are the most common presenting complaints. Rarely, acute ventricular obstruction leads rapidly to coma.

The *signs of increased ICP* may be subtle. Young infants and children, whose cranial sutures have not yet fused, are able to tolerate a relatively greater expansion of the intracranial contents than are older children and adults. Compensatory head growth and ultimate macrocephaly are presenting features and may be accompanied by (1) failure to thrive from anorexia, (2) lethargy, or (3) irritability. Funduscopic examination may reveal *papilledema.* If increased ICP is longstanding, *optic atrophy* can occur with associated visual loss and nystagmus. Pressure on the sensitive abducens cranial nerve VI causes lateral gaze impairment, resulting in *diplopia.*

Signs and symptoms of intracranial hypertension are common among children who have brain tumors, inasmuch as the majority of such mass lesions lie in the midline of the posterior fossa and cause ventricular obstruction. Such neoplasms include cerebellar astrocytomas, medulloblastomas, ependymomas, and pineal gland tumors. Choroid plexus papillomas, although rare, cause increased ICP by excessive production of CSF.

Direct symptom-producing effects of a brain tumor vary according to their site of origin. Supratentorial lesions within a cerebral hemisphere lead to headache, unilateral muscle weakness *(hemiparesis),* visual disturbance, or unilateral sensory loss. *Headaches* may not be localized, but their presence should arouse suspicion, particularly if they worsen while lying down or coughing, sneezing, or straining. Headaches that awaken a child in the early morning hours also are of concern.

Seizures occur rarely as an initial manifestation of brain tumors in children. When present, they typically are focal and tend to be refractory to anticonvulsant medication before definitive therapy. The electroencephalogram shows persistent focal slowing. The tumors usually are benign and slow growing.[1]

Craniopharyngiomas and hypothalamic germinomas, both midline diencephalic tumors, manifest with headache, *endocrine dysfunction* (growth failure, precocious puberty, diabetes insipidus, hypothyroidism), and *visual disturbance.* The accompanying symptoms of abnormal visual fields and hormonal imbalance strongly suggest the presence of a midline supratentorial mass. Infratentorial tumors are associated with increased ICP, usually secondary to hydrocephalus, and brainstem or *cerebellar dysfunction,* including truncal and limb ataxia, long-tract signs (spasticity and hyperreflexia), and cranial nerve deficits.

The differential diagnosis of intracranial tumors includes less common space-occupying lesions and other causes of increased ICP, such as (1) arteriovenous malformation, (2) subdural hematoma, effusion, or empyema, (3) abscess, (4) infarction, and (5) hemorrhage. Pseudotumor cerebri, especially in adolescents, is a common cause of increased ICP without clinical evidence of a mass lesion. Classic hemiplegic migraine or Todd paralysis after a focal seizure may mimic the signs of an intracerebral mass lesion. The residual signs for migraine or a prior seizure, however, are transient and usually resolve within 24 hours. Occasionally, venous sinus thrombosis manifests with signs of increased ICP.

DIAGNOSIS

The advent of computed tomography (CT) and magnetic resonance imaging (MRI) has revolutionized the diagnosis and subsequent management of CNS tumors. *Initial evaluation should include both an unenhanced and enhanced CT scan.* A noncontrast CT scan affords the opportunity to determine (1) tumor density in comparison with surrounding tissue, (2) the existence of hydrocephalus, and (3) the presence of calcifications or hemorrhage, which may suggest certain tumor types or their aggressiveness. Contrast enhancement delineates tumor margins from surrounding edema and differentiates neoplasms from suspected vascular malformations. Although CT scanning has shown a greater than 90% sensitivity, relevant limitations exist in the assessment of pediatric tumors. In particular, poor resolution of posterior fossa structures (brainstem and cerebellum) hinders the evaluation of more than 55% of childhood tumors.[11]

Where available, *MRI is now supplanting CT as the imaging procedure of choice.* Greater resolution, the ability to image in more than one plane, and the lack of artifact produced by the surrounding skull make MRI particularly suitable for assessment of posterior fossa structures. MRI has been reported to provide more information than does the CT scan in up to 50% of patients and has proved its superiority for the early detection of neoplasms and determining the limits of their extension.[17] Disadvantages include the inability of MRI to detect calcification and to distinguish tumor from surrounding edema, although contrast enhancement with gadolinium (a paramagnetic contrast agent) can obviate this limitation.[3] MRI requires a much longer scanning time—thus the need for prolonged sedation or even anesthesia, which potentially is hazardous in children who have increased ICP. *MRI and CT scans currently are complementary;* both provide important information regarding tumor location, type, and degree of invasiveness.

Once the diagnosis of an intracranial mass is confirmed, further information is required to delineate histological typing and extent of spread. Angiography, less often required with the advent of MRI scanning, can help differentiate certain lesions from arteriovenous malformations.

Approximately 50% of medulloblastomas have developed seeding along the subarachnoid pathways by the time of diagnosis.[11] CT myelographic examination detects CSF dissemination most accurately and generally is performed as part of the initial assessment of posterior fossa tumors. *Caution must be exercised in performing lumbar punctures* in patients who have brain tumors, particularly of the posterior fossa, because of the risk of brainstem herniation. For the most part such procedures are accomplished postoperatively after decompression of the intracranial contents.

Determination of CSF cytology, although historically of interest in early tissue diagnosis, is of little value in the initial investigation of brain tumors. Although cells frequently are present postoperatively in the CSF, whether they are the result of preoperative seeding or intraoperative shedding is uncertain. Therefore *cytological examination of CSF rarely is helpful in tumor staging or histological diagnosis.* Several *biochemical tumor markers* have been shown to be of assistance in the early diagnosis and progression of CNS tumor recurrences. The polyamines, specifically putrescine, are accurate markers for the recurrence of medulloblastomas, whereas CSF alpha-fetoprotein and beta–human chorionic gonadotropin are good indicators of germ cell tumor activity.[8,11]

MANAGEMENT

In the past 10 years substantial gains have accrued in the management of childhood brain tumors through the availability of microsurgical techniques, refined modes of radiation therapy, and chemotherapeutic agents that cross the blood-brain barrier.

Stabilization of the child's neurological condition through the use of *osmotic agents* and *corticosteroids* to reduce surrounding brain edema and early *CSF shunting* for hydrocephalus is the first step toward comprehensive treatment planning. Histological diagnosis has been aided by the advent of *stereotaxic biopsy* for most tumors regardless of location, including certain brainstem gliomas.[10] *Complete excision* and cure are possible for several localized CNS tumors, including choroid plexus papilloma, craniopharyngioma, and cystic cerebellar astrocytoma. Survival generally is aided by a *"debulking" procedure, followed by radiation or chemotherapy, or both.* Operative mortality has been reduced in most centers to less than 5%. Refinement in the use of *microoperative techniques, laser surgery,* and *interstitial radiation* with stereotaxic implantation has improved outcome further, with diminished morbidity.[13]

Most childhood brain tumors that cannot be excised totally will benefit from a combination of surgical debulking and radiation therapy. Medulloblastomas in particular have a high incidence of CSF and meningeal seeding by the time of diagnosis, and affected children should receive craniospinal radiation. Recent reports have suggested prolonged survival of children who have brainstem gliomas after the use of *hyperfractionated radiation therapy.*[9,13]

Substantial evidence now exists that chemotherapy plays a vital role in the treatment of primary childhood CNS tumors. The Children's Cancer Study Group (CCSG) has reported an improved *5-year survival rate of 42% among patients who have high-grade astrocytomas treated with combined radiation/chemotherapy* as compared with survival rates of only 10% among patients treated with radiation alone. Unfortunately, similar results as yet have not been forthcoming for medulloblastomas or brainstem gliomas.[12]

A regimen of eight chemotherapeutic drugs administered in 1 day has shown encouraging preliminary results among children who have newly diagnosed brain tumors, including medulloblastomas and malignant astrocytomas. The rationale for this regimen relates to CNS malignant tumors displaying histological heterogeneity. This *cellular diversification enables a greater degree of drug resistance* to single-drug therapy, whereas multiple drugs attack a tumor by a variety of mechanisms, thereby increasing the likelihood of sensitivity. Studies are in progress to evaluate the effectiveness of "8-in-1" therapy on highly malignant astrocytomas and medulloblastomas.

PROGNOSIS

Prognosis for brain tumors depends on tumor type, size, and location. Overall, 5-year survival rates approach or exceed 50% for all age groups and tumor types.[4] Less virulent cerebellar and supratentorial astrocytomas have excellent long-term survival rates of 70% to 100%. Survival of patients who have medulloblastoma has been reported variously at 40% to 75%. The poorest prognosis occurs in children who have brainstem gliomas, and the survival rate has remained stable at just under 20%. *For all tumor types, survival generally is poorest in affected children younger than 2 years of age.*

The treatment of brain tumors carries with it significant morbidity. Acute effects of radiation and chemotherapy are well known. Bone marrow suppression brings the risk of infection and bleeding diathesis. Cranial radiation is accompanied by hair loss, which though temporary, can be psychologically distressing, particularly for adolescents.

As improvements in therapy lengthen survival, long-term adverse effects of treatment play a greater role. Delayed effects of radiation include progressive demyelination and radiation necrosis. The latter can be misdiagnosed as tumor recurrence. Recent studies have documented a slow decline in intelligence quotients over years among children receiving radiation and chemotherapy.[5] At higher risk are those treated at a young age.[14]

Growth hormone deficiency and subsequent growth deceleration occur frequently among children who receive cranial radiation. Replacement of multiple hormones is required for patients who have been treated for craniopharyngiomas by surgery with or without radiation therapy.[6,18]

FUTURE PROSPECTS

Prospects for improved treatment modalities of childhood brain tumors continue with advances in our understanding of the molecular biology of tumors, sophistication of diagnostic techniques, and the advent of microsurgical procedures and chemotherapeutic programs. The care of children who have brain tumors involves a greater number of physicians as long-term survival and neurological morbidity continue to improve. Therefore management requires an ongoing, multidisciplinary approach with participation by specialists in oncology, neurosurgery, neurology, primary care, social work, psychology, and rehabilitative services.

REFERENCES

1. Blume WT, Girvin JP, Kaufman JCE: Childhood brain tumors presenting as chronic uncontrolled focal seizure disorders, *Ann Neurol* 12:538, 1982.
2. Cusimano MD: An update on the cellular and molecular biology of brain tumors, *Can J Neurol Sci* 16:22, 1989.
3. Dickman CP et al: Unenhanced and gadolinium-DTPA-enhanced MR imaging in postoperative evaluation in pediatric brain tumors, *J Neurosurg* 71:49, 1989.
4. Duffner PK et al: Survival of children with brain tumors: SEER program 1973-1980, *Neurology* 36:597, 1986.
5. Duffner PK, Cohen ME, Parker MS: Prospective intellectual testing in children with brain tumors, *Ann Neurol* 23:575, 1988.
6. Duffner PK et al: Long-term effects of cranial irradiation on endocrine function in children with brain tumors: a prospective study, *Cancer* 56:2189, 1985.
7. Dunn DW: Neurofibromatosis in childhood. In Lockhart JD, editor: *Current problems in pediatrics,* vol 17, Chicago, 1987, Mosby.
8. Edwards MSB, Davis RL, Laurent JP: Tumor markers and cytologic features of cerebrospinal fluid, *Cancer* 56:1773, 1985.
9. Edwards MSB, Prados M: Current management of brain stem glioma, *Pediatr Neurosci* 13:309, 1987.
10. Epstein F, McClearly EL: Intrinsic brain stem tumors of childhood: surgical indications, *J Neurosurg* 64:11, 1986.
11. Finlay JL, Goins SC: Brain tumors in children. I. Advances in diagnosis, *Am J Pediatr Hematol Oncol* 9:246, 1987.
12. Finlay JL, Goins SC: Brain tumors in children. III. Advances in chemotherapy, *Am J Pediatr Hematol Oncol* 9:264, 1987.
13. Finlay JL, Uteg R, Giese WL: Brain tumors in children. II. Advances in neurosurgery and radiation oncology, *Am J Pediatr Hematol Oncol* 9:256, 1987.
14. Kingsley DPE, Kendall BE, Fitz CR: Tuberous sclerosis: a clinicoradiological evaluation of 110 cases with particular reference to atypical presentation, *Neuroradiology* 28:38, 1986.
15. Leviton A: Principles of epidemiology. In Cohen ME, Duffner PL, editors: *Brain tumors in children: principles of diagnosis and treatment,* New York, 1984, Raven Press.
16. List AF, Greco A, Vogler LB: Lymphoproliferative disease in immunocompromised hosts: the role of Epstein-Barr viruses, *J Clin Oncol* 5:1673, 1987.
17. Packer RJ, Batnitzky S, Cohen ME: Magnetic resonance imaging in the evaluation of intracranial tumors of childhood, *Cancer* 56:1767, 1985.
18. Rappaport R, Brauner R: Growth and endocrine disorders secondary to cranial irradiation, *Pediatr Res* 25:561, 1989.
19. Riopelle RJ, Riccardi VM: Neuronal growth factors from tumors of von Recklinghausen neurofibromatosis, *Can J Neurol Sci* 14:141, 1987.
20. Schmidek HH: The molecular genetics of nervous system tumors, *J Neurosurg* 16:1, 1987.
21. Schoenberg BS et al: The epidemiology of primary intracranial neoplasms of childhood: a population study, *Mayo Clin Proc* 51:51, 1976.
22. Shapiro JR: Biology of gliomas: heterogeneity, oncogenes, growth factors, *Semin Oncol* 13:4, 1986.
23. Sorensen SA, Mulvihill JJ, Nielsen A: Long-term follow-up of von Recklinghausen neurofibromatosis survival and malignant neoplasms, *N Engl J Med* 314:1010, 1986.
24. Tomita T, Mclone DG: Brain tumor during the first twenty-four months of life, *Neurosurgery* 17:913, 1985.
25. Young JL et al: Cancer incidence, survival and mortality for children younger than age 15 years, *Cancer* 58:598, 1986.
26. Zeller WJ et al: Experimental chemical production of brain tumors, *Ann NY Acad Sci* 281:250, 1982.

SUGGESTED READINGS

Cohen ME, Duffner PK: *Brain tumors in children: principles of diagnosis and treatment, ed 2,* New York, 1994, International Review of Child Neurology Series, Raven Press.

Cohen ME, Duffner PK: Tumors of the brain and spinal cord including leukemic involvement. In Swaiman KF, editor: *Pediatric neurology: principles and practices, ed 2,* St Louis, 1994, Mosby.

Kadota RP et al: Brain tumors in children, *J Pediatr* 114:511, 1989.

189 Bronchiolitis

Caroline Breese Hall and William J. Hall

Bronchiolitis is an acute infectious respiratory illness of children that usually occurs in the first 2 years of life. The hallmarks of the clinical picture are wheezing and hyperaeration, commonly associated with tachypnea, respiratory distress, and retractions of the chest.

Although the clinical picture of bronchiolitis has been described since the beginning of this century, bronchiolitis was not recognized as a separate entity until Engle and Newns[8] gave it its sovereignty by designating the distinctive infantile disease as *bronchiolitis*.

ETIOLOGY

Viruses and occasionally *Mycoplasma pneumoniae* now are recognized as the causes of bronchiolitis.* As shown in Fig. 189-1, respiratory syncytial virus is by far the most frequently isolated agent, with the parainfluenza viruses being the next most common agents.[9,16] In Henderson and colleagues' study[16] of bronchiolitis occurring among children in a private pediatric practice, respiratory syncytial virus, parainfluenza viruses types 1 and 3, adenoviruses, rhinoviruses, and *M. pneumoniae* accounted for 87% of the isolates from children of all ages. Respiratory syncytial virus accounted for 44% of the isolates from children in the first 2 years of life, with parainfluenza type 1, parainfluenza type 3, and adenoviruses each accounting for about 13%. In two group practices in Rochester, New York, respiratory syncytial virus was isolated from 55% and parainfluenza type 3 from 11% of cases of bronchiolitis. If only hospitalized cases of bronchiolitis are examined, the contribution of respiratory syncytial virus is much higher.[11,33] In the Newcastle-upon-Tyne studies, respiratory syncytial virus was isolated from 74% of hospitalized bronchiolitis patients.[11]

EPIDEMIOLOGY

The seasonal pattern of bronchiolitis reflects the activities of its viral agents, particularly respiratory syncytial virus.[1,10,13] Because respiratory syncytial virus is causative in the majority of cases, bronchiolitis peaks during the winter to spring months when respiratory syncytial virus is epidemic in the community. As shown in Fig. 189-2, in Monroe County, New York, the greatest number of cases are reported during the yearly January to February peak of respiratory syncytial virus activity. Lesser peaks are seen during the fall when parainfluenza virus type 1 has been present in the community and during the spring period of parainfluenza virus type 3 activity. Cases of bronchiolitis commonly are designated as epidemic or sporadic bronchiolitis, which essentially means cases that are or are not associated with respiratory syncytial virus.

*References 1, 5, 6, 9, 10, 13, 16.

The incidence of bronchiolitis varies according to the age and definition of the syndrome. Over 80% of bronchiolitis cases occur during the first year of life.* The peak attack rate occurs between 2 and 10 months of age and is relatively uncommon during the first weeks of life. The highest reported incidence is from Denny and colleagues' long-term studies[6] in Chapel Hill, North Carolina, in which 115 cases per 100 children up to 6 months of age were detected per year. Because these children in a day care center were examined at regular intervals, and the diagnosis of bronchiolitis did not have to include tachypnea or air-trapping, the mildest cases were included. In subsequent Chapel Hill studies of ambulatory children, the incidence was 11 cases per 100 children per year for both the first and second 6 months of life.[5,16] In both of these studies the incidence fell rapidly during the second year of life to 32 cases per 100 children per year in the day care center and to 6 cases per 100 children per year in the private practice. In hospitalized cases the incidence is highest during the first 6 months of life and in the study by Foy et al.[10] was found to be 6 per 1000 children per year. The attack rate in boys generally is 1½ times greater than that in girls among both outpatients and hospitalized patients.[1,5,13]

PATHOPHYSIOLOGY

Host, environmental, and immunological factors have appeared to play a role in the development and severity of bronchiolitis. The risk of bronchiolitis appears to be increased in children who come from poorer socioeconomic areas, crowded and polluted surroundings, who have more siblings attending day care, and who have not been breast fed.[2,17,32,33,35] Children who have a genetic predisposition to hyperreactive airways appear more likely to manifest their initial respiratory viral infections as bronchiolitis, especially those of respiratory syncytial virus and the parainfluenza viruses, although the role of atopy, genetics, and an allergic family background is unclear.[2,17,21,27,35] Immunological mechanisms, however, have been suggested in the pathogenesis of bronchiolitis.[17,25,30,31] An enhanced responsiveness to viral antigens and allergens in infants who have bronchiolitis has been suggested as resulting in release of lymphokines, inflammation, and hyperreactivity of the airways. Increased production of specific IgE antibody and histamine release in the secretions of infected infants have been associated with the presence, duration, and severity of wheezing.[30,31]

Paramount in the pathogenesis of bronchiolitis is the age of the child and the specific viral agents, particularly respiratory syncytial virus and parainfluenza virus type 3, which infect children early in life and are capable of infecting the

*References 1, 5, 6, 9, 13, 16, 33.

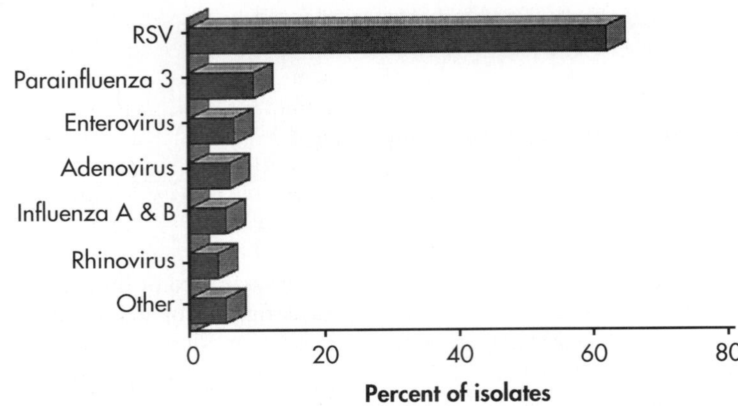

FIG. 189-1 Viral origin of bronchiolitis from patients in pediatric practices participating in an ongoing community surveillance program in Monroe County, New York, 1976-1992. *RSV*, Respiratory syncytial virus.

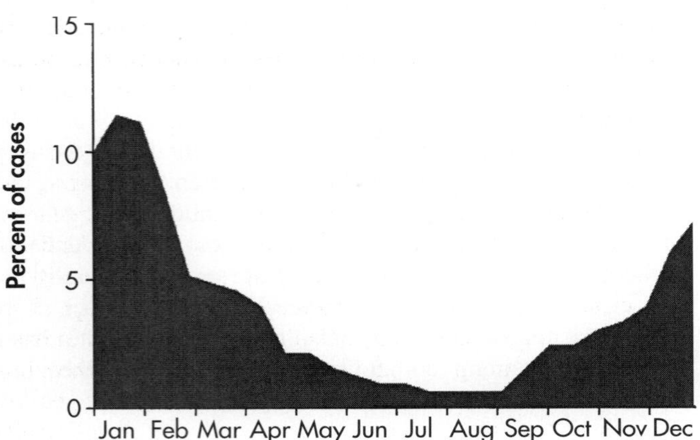

FIG. 189-2 Seasonal occurrence of bronchiolitis cases obtained over an 18-year period from a community surveillance program in Monroe County, New York.

lower respiratory tract in a high proportion of young infants. As important in this young age group as gender are anatomical and physiological factors, such as the small diameter of the peripheral airways, the poor collateral ventilation, and the relatively increased number of mucus-secreting glands.[32] Furthermore, males appear to have greater muscle tone of the airways and increased risk of hyperresponsiveness.[17,18,20]

Initially the viral agent usually causes infection of the upper respiratory tract and subsequently spreads to affect the medium and small bronchi and bronchioles. The virus characteristically causes inflammation and necrosis of the respiratory epithelium.[32,33] Histologically, peribronchiolar infiltration and proliferation, mostly of mononuclear cells, are observed. The bronchiolar epithelium subsequently becomes necrotic and sloughs. In most cases of bronchiolitis, spread of the inflammation beyond the peribronchiolar area is slight, with little involvement of the surrounding alveoli. The inflammation of the small bronchi and bronchioles, nevertheless, is generalized, but with areas varying in severity. The small diameter of the lumen makes the infant particularly vulnerable to this obstruction caused by the developing edema and exudate. Peripheral to the sites of partial obstruction, air becomes trapped by a process similar to a "ball valve" mechanism. During inspiration the negative intrapleural pressure allows air to flow past the site of partial obstruction. On expiration, however, the positive pressure decreases the lumen's size, causing an increase in the degree of obstruction. The lung becomes hyperinflated. Expiration, in particular, becomes difficult and prolonged. If the inflammation progresses, complete obstruction occurs. When the trapped air becomes absorbed, multiple areas of focal atelectasis result.

Two important physiological sequelae occur from these pathological processes. First, the resistance to airflow markedly increases.[33] This leads to dyspnea and an increased respiratory rate and lower tidal volume. Thus the volume of air reaching the gas-exchanging alveoli diminishes with each breath, and proportionately more air ventilates only "dead space." This eventually may elevate the arterial Pco_2. The second sequela resulting from the small-airway obstruction is the marked change in the distribution of ventilation within the lung. The low ratio of ventilation compared with the perfusion of the lung results in arterial hypoxemia. Almost all infants hospitalized with bronchiolitis have some degree of hypoxemia, which commonly is appreciable and protracted.[14,33] Despite clinical improvement the hypoxemia may persist for weeks, reflecting the relatively slow resolution of the inflammation and atelectasis.

CLINICAL FEATURES

Bronchiolitis usually is heralded by the signs of a common cold. Rhinorrhea, nasal congestion, a slight fever, and cough may develop over a prodromal period of 1 to 7 days. As bronchiolitis develops, the cough may become more prominent, and an increased respiratory rate, pulse rate, and tachypnea appear. Fever commonly is present during the prodromal period but usually is not high; by the time bronchiolitis has developed, less than half of the children are febrile.

Physical examination of the infant who has bronchiolitis often is striking. Tachypnea is a constant finding, often accompanied by tachycardia; the respiratory rate usually is 45 to 80 breaths per minute. The infant may appear lethargic and distressed with circumoral cyanosis. The increased work of breathing is evidenced by flaring of the nasal alae and grunting. Retractions of the chest wall in the subcostal, intercostal, and suprasternal areas and use of the accessory muscles of respiration are notable.

Physical examination of the baby's chest verifies the hyperinflation resulting from the trapping of air peripheral to the small airway obstruction. The diameter of the chest appears increased, and the percussion note has a hyperresonant ring. The liver and spleen may become easily palpable from the downward placement of the overinflated lungs. Expiration usually, but not always, is prolonged and may be difficult to detect in a small baby who has a rapid respiratory rate. The flow of air also is obstructed on inspiration but to a lesser extent. Auscultation usually reveals the diagnostic hallmark of wheezing. The degree of wheezing and the fine moist rales commonly heard on inspiration may vary from hour to hour. A decrease in the auscultatory findings with increasing respiratory distress may indicate progressive obstruction to the flow of air in the small airways and impending respiratory failure. As this stage of respiratory acidosis becomes manifest, the respirations become shallow and ineffective, as if the effort to breathe becomes too great for the infant.

Associated findings that may complicate the infant's course include otitis media (in about 10% to 30% of infants) and dehydration. Babies who have bronchiolitis are prone to dehydration because of paroxysms of coughing that trigger vomiting and because of a decreased fluid intake resulting from their respiratory distress and lethargy. In addition, tachypnea and fever may increase fluid requirements.

Most infants who have bronchiolitis improve appreciably within several days, and the cough and other signs resolve gradually thereafter over 1 to 2 weeks. For some infants the entire course is one of slow, gradual improvement. Most children who worsen and require hospitalization will do so within the first 3 or 4 days.

In most infants the white blood cell count and differential count are within normal limits. However, in the more severely affected and hypoxemic infant the white blood cell count may be elevated, and the differential count may demonstrate a shift to the left. In these more distressed infants, determination of the blood gas tensions is helpful.[14] The degree of hypoxemia is extremely difficult to judge clinically, and cyanosis may not be apparent in the face of moderate degrees of hypoxemia.

The chest roentgenogram in infants who have bronchiolitis may appear relatively benign, and the severity of illness generally cannot be correlated with the roentgenographic findings. Hyperinflation is the most frequent finding. An increased anteroposterior diameter of the chest on a lateral film and flat or depressed diaphragms may be present. Increased bronchovascular markings are common, appearing as abnormal streaks or linear densities radiating out from the hila. Scattered small areas of atelectasis and interstitial infiltrates of varying intensity and distribution also may be seen. Differentiation of these areas of atelectasis from those of pneumonic infiltration often is not possible.

DIAGNOSIS

Bronchiolitis usually is diagnosed on the characteristic clinical and epidemiological features; a specific cause may be diagnosed by viral isolation or antigen detection in the nasopharyngeal secretions. Most of the respiratory viruses causing bronchiolitis are identifiable in cell culture within 3 to 7 days. A variety of rapid viral diagnostic techniques, such as immunofluorescence and enzyme-linked immunoassays, are now available to identify RSV and a number of other viral respiratory pathogens in the respiratory secretions within hours.[7] Antibody determinations on acute and convalescent sera in the young infant rarely are helpful because of the time required to obtain a convalescent serum, the presence of passive maternal antibody, and the diminished antibody response of young infants to RSV and other viral respiratory agents.

DIFFERENTIAL DIAGNOSIS

Asthma is the major consideration in the differential diagnosis of bronchiolitis. Often in a single episode it is not possible to differentiate these two entities; indeed, the two may be combined.[17] A great proportion of wheezing episodes occurring in an atopic child may arise from viral infections. In asthmatic children 1 to 5 years of age, McIntosh and colleagues[23] found 42% of the episodes of wheezing to be associated with a viral infection and respiratory syncytial virus to be the agent isolated most frequently.

Respiratory syncytial virus has an unexplained propensity for producing wheezing in infants. Therefore children who first wheeze during an epidemic of respiratory syncytial viral infections may be less likely to have an atopic predisposition than do children who develop sporadic bronchiolitis at other times of the year. The role of atopy also is apt to be greater in a child older than 18 months and in one who has a family history of allergy and previous episodes of wheezing.

Another diagnostic consideration is gastric esophageal reflux, which in the infant may produce a picture clinically identical to that of bronchiolitis. Aspiration of a foreign body also may result in wheezing and respiratory distress. Wheezing also may occur in congestive heart failure and in cystic fibrosis.

TREATMENT

Management of most infants who have bronchiolitis consists mainly of supportive care, including adequate hydration and antipyretics, if necessary. In the hospitalized child the mainstay of care is supportive, ensuring adequate oxygenation and hydration. In infants who have RSV bronchiolitis with more severe disease and in those who have underlying conditions predisposing them to more complicated disease, aerosolized ribavirin may be used.[4,15,24] This drug is administered by small-particle aerosol via an oxyhood, tent, or ventilator to the infant intermittently or continuously for up to 8 to 20 hours per day, usually for 2 to 5 days. The duration of treatment should be guided by the infant's clinical improvement rather than by a set number of days. Infants in controlled studies treated with ribavirin have been shown to have diminished production in their secretions of specific IgE antibody and leukotrienes associated with inflammation and wheezing.[12,26]

The use of bronchodilators in bronchiolitis remains controversial. In young infants inflammation from the viral infection often is the prime cause of the impedance to air flow, rather than airway hyperresponsiveness, although this may aggravate the obstruction. Studies evaluating bronchodilators in bronchiolitis have produced conflicting results. A carefully monitored trial of aerosolized or parenteral bronchodilators has been recommended by some for hospitalized infants, especially for those over a year of age.[19,28] The use of steroids in bronchiolitis has been studied and found to be of no benefit.[29,34] On this basis the Committee on Drugs of the American Academy of Pediatrics advises against the use of steroids in those who have bronchiolitis. Antibiotics should not be used to treat bronchiolitis because bacteria have no role in its origin. Secondary bacterial infection rarely is observed after bronchiolitis, and unless such is documented, antibiotics should not be used.

COMPLICATIONS AND PROGNOSIS

The prognosis for normal infants who have bronchiolitis is good; mortality is less than 1%. In certain children who have underlying diseases such as cardiopulmonary disease, bronchiolitis may be accompanied by increased morbidity and mortality.

Pneumonia so commonly coexists with the clinical manifestations of bronchiolitis that the diseases may be considered a continuum, particularly in respiratory syncytial viral infection. Bacterial pneumonia is an uncommon complication.

Apnea may complicate the course of approximately 20% of infants hospitalized with respiratory syncytial viral infection.[3] Apnea is most likely to occur in the youngest infants and in premature infants.

Infants who have bronchiolitis appear to be at risk for recurrent episodes of wheezing and long-term pulmonary function abnormalities.[17,27,32,33] However, in one study of ambulatory children who had a history of relatively mild bronchiolitis, follow-up examination did not show an increased incidence of abnormal pulmonary function.[22] In those infants who had recurrent wheezing and lower respiratory tract disease, the number of episodes tended to be most frequent in the first 1 to 2 years after hospitalization for bronchiolitis and subsequently diminished in frequency.[17]

REFERENCES

1. Brandt CD et al: Epidemiology of respiratory syncytial virus infection in Washington, DC. III. Composite analysis of eleven consecutive yearly outbreaks, *Am J Epidemiol* 98:355, 1973.
2. Carlsen KH et al: Acute bronchiolitis: predisposing factors and characterization of infants at risk, *Pediatr Pulmonol* 3:153, 1987.
3. Church NR et al: Respiratory syncytial virus related apnea in infants: demographics and outcome, *Am J Dis Child* 138:247, 1984.
4. Committee on Infectious Diseases: Use of ribavirin in the treatment of respiratory syncytial virus infection, *Pediatrics* 92:501, 1993.
5. Denny FW, Clyde WA: Acute lower respiratory tract infections in nonhospitalized children, *J Pediatr* 108:635, 1986.
6. Denny FW et al: Infectious agents of importance in airways and parenchymal diseases in infants and children with particular emphasis on bronchiolitis, *Pediatr Res* 11:234, 1977.
7. Drew LW: Direct detection of viruses, *Pan American Group for Rapid Viral Diagnosis* 18:1, 1992.
8. Engle S, Newns GH: Proliferative mural bronchiolitis, *Arch Dis Child* 15:219, 1940.
9. Everard ML, Milner AD: The respiratory syncytial virus and its role in acute bronchiolitis. *Eur J Pediatr* 151:638, 1992.
10. Foy HM et al: Incidence and etiology of pneumonia, croup and bronchiolitis in preschool children belonging to a prepaid medical care group over a four year period, *Am J Epidemiol* 97:80, 1973.
11. Gardner PS: How etiologic, pathologic, and clinical diagnoses can be made in a correlated fashion, *Pediatr Res* 11:254, 1977.
12. Garofalo R, Welliver RC, Ogra PL: Modulation of leukotriene (LT) release with ribavirin during infection with respiratory syncytial virus (RSV), *Pediatr Res* 25:163A, 1989.
13. Glezen WP, Denny FW: Epidemiology of acute lower respiratory disease in children, *N Engl J Med* 288:498, 1973.
14. Hall CB, Hall WJ, Speers DM: Clinical and physiologic manifestations of bronchiolitis and pneumonia, *Am J Dis Child* 133:798, 1979.
15. Hall CB et al: Aerosolized ribavirin treatment of infants with respiratory syncytial viral infection: a randomized double blind study, *N Engl J Med* 308:1443, 1983.
16. Henderson FW et al: The etiologic and epidemiologic spectrum of bronchiolitis in pediatric practice, *J Pediatr* 95:183, 1979.
17. Landau LI: Bronchiolitis and asthma: are they related? *Thorax* 49:293, 1994.
18. Landau LI et al: Gender related differences in airway tone in children, *Pediatr Pulmonol* 16:31, 1993.
19. Mahesh VK, Taussig LM: When an infant wheezes: clues to the differential diagnosis, *J Respir Dis* 11:739, 1990.
20. Martinez FD et al: Diminished lung function as a predisposing factor for wheezing respiratory illness in infants, *N Engl J Med* 319:1112, 1988.
21. Martinez FD et al: Initial airway function is a risk factor for recurrent wheezing respiratory illnesses during the first three years of life, *Am Rev Respir Dis* 143:312, 1991.
22. McConnochie KM et al: Normal pulmonary function measurements and airway reactivity in childhood after mild bronchiolitis, *J Pediatr* 107:54, 1985.
23. McIntosh K et al: The association of viral and bacterial respiratory infections with exacerbations of wheezing in young asthmatic children, *J Pediatr* 82:578, 1973.
24. Rodriguez WJ et al: Aerosolized ribavirin in the treatment of patients with respiratory syncytial virus disease, *Pediatr Infect Dis J* 6:159, 1987.
25. Ronchetti R et al: Enhanced allergic sensitization related to parental smoking, *Arch Dis Child* 67:496, 1992.
26. Rosner IK et al: Effect of ribavirin therapy on respiratory syncytial virus-specific IgE and IgA responses after infection, *J Infect Dis* 155:1043, 1987.
27. Sims DG et al: Atopy does not predispose to RSV bronchiolitis or postbronchiolitic wheezing, *BMJ* 282:2086, 1981.
28. Soto ME et al: Bronchodilator response during acute viral bronchiolitis in infancy, *Pediatr Pulmonol* 1:85, 1985.
29. Stecenko AA: Treatment of viral bronchiolitis: do steroids make sense? *Contemp Pediatr* 4:121, 1987.
30. Welliver RC et al: The development of respiratory syncytial virus-specific IgE and the release of histamine in nasopharyngeal secretions after infection, *N Engl J Med* 305:841, 1981.
31. Welliver RC et al: Parainfluenza virus bronchiolitis: epidemiology and pathogenesis, *Am J Dis Child* 140:34, 1986.
32. Wohl MEB: Bronchiolitis, *Pediatr Ann* 15:307, 1986.
33. Wohl MEB: Bronchiolitis. In Chernick V, Kendig EL Jr, editors: *Kendig's disorders of the respiratory tract in children,* ed 5, Philadelphia, 1990, WB Saunders.
34. Yaffe SJ et al: Should steroids be used in treating bronchiolitis? *Pediatrics* 46:640, 1970.
35. Young S et al: The influence of a family history of asthma and parental smoking on airway responsiveness in early infancy, *N Engl J Med* 324:1168, 1991.

190 Cancers in Childhood

Cindy L. Schwartz

Advances in the treatment of solid tumors of childhood during the past 20 years have ensured the long-term survival of at least two thirds of children who have these diagnoses. The pediatrician who initially discovers a solid tumor may not, and need not, know the best treatment available. However, early referral of such a child to the appropriate specialist, a pediatric oncologist, significantly affects the likelihood and the quality of survival. Many common childhood tumors are unique in the pediatric age range. For all solid tumors in children, therapies must be designed to minimize effects on growth and development. Appropriate use of the therapeutic modalities—surgery, chemotherapy, and radiation—provides maximum efficacy and minimal toxicity of therapy.

The child and his or her family should be encouraged to plan for the future. Educational and developmental needs must be addressed by the pediatric team—generalist and specialist together. Such a team also is best able to address the needs of the child, the parents, and the siblings if treatment is not successful. Fortunately, most children are cured and return to the pediatrician for many years of general pediatric care.

The following solid tumors seen in the pediatric population are described herein: Wilms tumor, neuroblastoma, rhabdomyosarcoma, germ cell tumors and teratomas, retinoblastoma, Ewing sarcoma, osteogenic sarcoma, Hodgkin disease, and non-Hodgkin lymphomas. The role of the pediatrician in the care of these children also is examined.

WILMS TUMOR

Wilms tumor, or nephroblastoma, is a malignant renal tumor of childhood that occurs at an annual rate of 7.6 per 1 million children in the United States. It is the second most common abdominal tumor of childhood.[20] Patients usually are between 2 and 5 years of age, and the incidence of bilateral disease is increased in younger patients. Wilms tumor rarely occurs in teenagers and adults.

The chemosensitivity and radiosensitivity of this tumor, in conjunction with the ability to resect most nonmetastatic tumors, have allowed a multidisciplinary approach to be highly successful. Wilms tumor has become the model for treatment of childhood cancer. The National Wilms' Tumor Study (NWTS) has evaluated over the past 2 decades successive therapeutic regimens with the goal of increasing the cure rate and decreasing the toxicity of therapy. The cooperative group approach has made possible the gathering of more data than could have been obtained at single institutions. The findings, such as the superiority of multiagent chemotherapy and the importance of tumor histology, are relevant for many tumors.

Etiology

Wilms tumor has occurred in siblings, cousins, and parent-child pairs, particularly in association with specific congenital anomalies and bilateral disease.[90] Although it has been proposed that 40% of patients who have Wilms tumor may have had a genetic predisposition to the disease, a much lower incidence of Wilms tumor in patients who have affected relatives has been reported (approximately 1%).[12]

Anomalies are commonly reported in patients who have Wilms tumor; most involve the genitourinary tract.[12] Hemihypertrophy is second in frequency, sometimes noted as a component of the Beckwith-Wiedemann syndrome (excessive growth of many body organs). Of children who have the sporadic form of congenital aniridia, 33% have Wilms tumor. WAGR syndrome is the association of Wilms tumor–aniridia, genitourinary abnormalities, and mental retardation. Drash syndrome represents the association of Wilms tumor with male pseudohermaphroditism and diffuse glomerular disease.[34] Neurofibromatosis occurs with increased frequency in patients who have Wilms tumor.

Clinical Manifestations

Wilms tumor in children usually manifests as a painless mass discovered by a relative, often during bathing.[20] The mass usually is firm, occasionally lobulated, and confined to one side of the abdomen. Rapid abdominal enlargement, anemia, and hypertension (perhaps because of a sudden subcapsular hemorrhage) occasionally occur at the time of presentation. Hypertension, malaise, abdominal pain, and hematuria each occur in 20% to 30% of patients. Hypertension has been attributed to hyperreninemia.

Table 190-1 presents the differential diagnosis of abdominal and pelvic tumors of childhood that may mimic Wilms tumor.

Evaluation

The evaluation of a patient with presumed Wilms tumor begins with a history and physical examination. Particular attention should be paid to the associated congenital anomalies and the family history. Laboratory studies should include a complete blood cell count, urinalysis, and liver function testing. Bleeding within the tumor may cause anemia.[100] An erythropoietin-secreting Wilms tumor may cause polycythemia. Hypercalcemia occurs in patients who have congenital mesoblastic nephroma or a rhabdoid tumor.

A plain radiograph of the abdomen should be obtained. Calcification, if noted in a Wilms tumor, usually is quite coarse, unlike the fine, stippled pattern commonly seen in neuroblastoma. A chest film may reveal pulmonary metastases. An abdominal computed tomography (CT) scan with contrast or intravenous pyelographic examination may reveal an intrarenal mass displacing and distorting the collecting system of the involved kidney. Ultrasonographic examination is particularly helpful in evaluating the renal vein, vena cava, and the right side of the heart for tumor spread. Liver metastases may be diagnosed either by ultrasound or by CT scan.

Table 190-1 Differential Diagnosis of Abdominal and Pelvic Tumors in Infants and Children

Tumor*	Age	Clinical signs	Laboratory findings
Wilms	Preschool	Unilateral flank mass, aniridia, hemihypertrophy	Hematuria
Neuroblastoma	Preschool	GI/GU obstruction, raccoon eyes, myoclonus-opsoclonus, diarrhea, skin nodules (infants)	Increased VMA; increased HVA; increased ferritin; stippled calcification in mass
Non-Hodgkin lymphoma	>1 yr	Intussusception in >2-year-old	Increased urate
Rhabdomyosarcoma	All	GI/GU obstruction, sarcoma botryoides, vaginal bleeding, paratesticular mass	
Germ cell/teratoma	Preschool, teens	Girls: abdominal pain, vaginal bleeding Boys: testicular mass, new onset "hydrocele" Sacrococcygeal mass/dimple	Increased HCG; increased AFP
Hepatoblastoma	Birth-3 yr	Large, firm liver	Increased AFP
Hepatoma	School age, teens	Large, firm liver; hepatitis B, cirrhosis	Increased AFP

AFP, Alpha-fetoprotein; *GI,* gastrointestinal; *GU,* genitourinary; *HCG,* human chorionic gonadotropin; *HVA,* homovanillic acid; *VMA,* vanillylmandelic acid.
*Other causes: constipation, splenomegaly, hydronephrosis, kidney cyst, and full bladder.

A CT scan of the chest to detect small pulmonary metastases should be performed before surgery inasmuch as postoperative atelectasis can otherwise interfere with the evaluation. Bone scans are indicated in patients who have the variant known as clear cell sarcoma, which often spreads to bone.

At the time of surgery the tumor is staged as follows[41]:

1. Stage I: Tumor is limited to the kidney and is completely excised.
2. Stage II: Tumor extends beyond the kidney but is completely resected.
3. Stage III: Residual nonhematogenously spread tumor is confined to the abdomen, such as lymph node involvement, peritoneal contamination before or during surgery, peritoneal implants, residual tumor postoperatively, or incomplete resection caused by local infiltration.
4. Stage IV: Tumor metastasizes hematogenously to areas such as lung, liver, bone, or brain.
5. Stage V: Bilateral renal involvement is found at diagnosis.

Management

In the United States the initial therapeutic approach is a complete resection by nephrectomy. This requires careful and gentle surgical techniques to prevent tumor spillage. The large transabdominal incision facilitates exploration and excision. The entire ureter is removed, lymph nodes are sampled, and the contralateral kidney and abdominal cavity are examined for evidence of disease. For bilateral disease, chemotherapy is recommended after bilateral biopsy. "Second-look" excision of residual disease may be accomplished by partial nephrectomies when possible.[67,129] Alternatively, nephrectomy of the more involved side, with partial nephrectomy on the opposite side, may be preferred.

Actinomycin D and vincristine were noted to be effective agents in the mid-1960s. The initial NWTS-I study revealed that radiation therapy in combination with a single agent (actinomycin D or vincristine) provided approximately 55% relapse-free survival in patients whose disease was localized. An 81% relapse-free survival was found when both agents were administered in conjunction with radiation.[21] The two drugs have since been the mainstay of chemotherapy for Wilms tumor. Patients who have low-stage disease now are treated with these two agents without the use of radiotherapy.[21,22] For those with high-stage disease, doxorubicin is added to actinomycin D, vincristine, and radiation therapy.[22] The NWTS-IV evaluated shorter duration, dose-intensified regimens. Results of this study are being evaluated.

Radiation therapy is initiated within 70 days of surgery to prevent local and regional recurrences in patients who have stage II unfavorable histology and who have stages III and IV disease, as well as those who have the clear cell variant. Lower radiation doses (10 to 20 Gy) and irradiation of the entire width of the vertebrae adjacent to the renal bed have decreased the severity—but not entirely prevented the development—of scoliosis.[122] Peritoneal seeding or a major tumor rupture necessitates radiation of the entire abdomen. Thoracic radiation is used for pulmonary metastasis.

Prognosis

The prognosis of patients who have Wilms tumor is determined by the histopathology of the tumor. In the NWTS-I, 50% of 26 patients who had unfavorable histological findings died, compared with 6.9% of 376 patients who had favorable histological findings.[6] These findings have been confirmed in succeeding protocols. More intensive regimens are being studied for those patients who have stages II to IV disease and unfavorable histological findings.

The prognosis also depends on the stage of disease at diagnosis. Most relapses occur within 2 years of diagnosis. Two-year relapse-free survival for stages I and II disease that has favorable histological findings is approximately 91%. For stage III disease, relapse-free survival at 2 years is approximately 76%. The 2-year relapse-free survival rate is 69% for patients who have stage IV disease or unfavorable histological findings (stages II to IV).[23]

Follow-up

While patients are receiving therapy, they are monitored for disease recurrence at the primary site and in the lungs. Such monitoring continues until approximately 3 years after diagnosis or until age 5 years, whichever occurs later.

Long-term survival is likely in patients who have Wilms

tumor. Virtually all have had a nephrectomy and should be discouraged from engaging in contact sports. A kidney guard can be recommended for particularly active children, if only to serve as a reminder of the need for caution.

Scoliosis was a major problem for early survivors treated with moderate-dose radiation (30 to 40 Gy), particularly if the adjacent vertebrae were not included in the field. The scoliosis is less severe in patients treated more recently. Close observation of patients who received irradiation, particularly during the pubertal growth spurt, remains necessary. Prevention of obesity will minimize the asymmetry associated with a decreased quantity of adipose tissue in the radiation field.

Although fertility is preserved in most patients who have Wilms tumor, the average size of infants born to female survivors of irradiation is smaller than that of normal women.[75] Continued follow-up of these offspring is necessary to evaluate the genetic factors involved in the occurrence of Wilms tumor.

NEUROBLASTOMA

Neuroblastoma arises from the fetal neural cells that normally develop into the sympathetic nervous system. It is a tumor that provides insight into the biological processes of malignancy. Tumors in infants may regress spontaneously or mature to benign ganglioneuromas, whereas patients older than 1 year who have disseminated disease rarely are cured in spite of aggressive use of active agents. Neuroblastoma is the most common malignancy of infants, accounting for over half of infantile cancers.[45] Two thirds of patients who have neuroblastoma are younger than 5 years. Approximately 8.5 white children and 7.4 black children per million in the United States are afflicted with neuroblastoma each year.[131] This accounts for 7% of all children diagnosed as having cancer and 15% of childhood cancer mortality.

Etiology

The high incidence of neuroblastoma in early infancy suggests that its development may be related to abnormal maturation of fetal neural crest cells. The finding of microscopic nodules of adrenal neuroblastoma in infants younger than 3 months of age who have died of unrelated causes suggests that spontaneous maturation or regression occurs in many children.[7]

Families have been reported in which neuroblastoma occurred in multiple siblings or occasionally in multiple generations.[16,95] Some have proposed that 20% to 25% of neuroblastomas occur in patients who have a prezygotic germinal mutation.[69] Neuroblastoma also has been reported to occur with an increased incidence in patients who have fetal hydantoin syndrome, von Recklinghausen disease, Beckwith-Wiedemann syndrome, and Hirschsprung disease.

Clinical Manifestations

Neuroblastoma may arise anywhere along the sympathetic nervous system chain, including the adrenal gland (40%), the paraspinal regions of the abdomen (25%), the thorax (15%), the neck (5%), and the pelvis at the organ of Zuckerkandl (5%). The presenting features depend to a large extent on the location of the tumor. A large, firm, irregular abdominal mass that may cross the midline often is the first sign of disease. Disturbances of bowel or bladder function may be due to compression by a pelvic mass. Thoracic masses may cause a persistent cough or respiratory distress and are diagnosed by a chest film. Cervical masses often are diagnosed initially as lymphadenitis, but they do not respond to antibiotic therapy. Horner syndrome or heterochromia iridis suggests the possibility of neuroblastoma.

Neuroblastomas that arise in the paravertebral ganglia tend to grow into the intervertebral foramina, forming a dumbbell-shaped mass. Paralysis, weakness of an extremity, or incontinence may result from spinal cord compression by the intraspinal component. This is an oncological emergency that requires surgical decompression, radiation, or chemotherapy to prevent permanent paraplegia.

Many children who have neuroblastoma have metastatic disease at the time of diagnosis. The symptoms then usually are related to the metastatic tumor rather than to the primary tumor. Infants may have metastatic hepatic involvement. Rapid liver enlargement can cause marked abdominal distention followed by respiratory compromise. Bluish skin nodules, which may release catecholamines if palpated, sometimes are noted in infants who have neuroblastoma. An erythematous cutaneous flush occurs, lasting for 2 to 3 minutes, and is followed by blanching because of vasoconstriction.[56]

Older children who have neuroblastoma often have infiltration of the bone marrow with tumor causing pancytopenia. Bone involvement may produce pain, with or without palpable bone masses. Lytic bone lesions are found most often in the skull, orbit, or proximal long bones. A raccoonlike appearance caused by proptosis and eyelid ecchymosis has been described in those who have orbital involvement. Intracranial disease usually is due to meningeal metastases.[70] In infants this may manifest as separation of cranial sutures. Intracerebral lesions are extremely rare.

Secretory products of the tumor may be the cause of the presenting features. Vasoactive intestinal polypeptide (VIP) has been found in 7% to 9% of children who have neural crest tumors, most frequently ganglioneuromas or ganglioneuroblastomas.[109] Intractable diarrhea is caused by this hormone.

An unusual symptom of neuroblastoma is the syndrome of opsoclonus-myoclonus.[11] These patients have acute cerebellar ataxia and rapid, dancing-eye movements. Although these patients often have localized disease and usually are cured, residual neurological dysfunction, including residual ataxia and mental retardation, is common. The etiology of this syndrome is unclear. An autoimmune factor, perhaps an antibody directed against neuroblastoma that cross-reacts with the cerebellar cell antigen, may be causative.

Tables 190-1 to 190-3 present the differential diagnosis of abdominal, pelvic, head, neck, and mediastinal tumors that may mimic neuroblastoma.

Evaluation

Evaluation of a patient who has neuroblastoma requires radiological examination of the area of primary disease, as well as of areas to which neuroblastoma spreads. In addition to the chest film, a CT scan of the abdomen, pelvis, and chest should be performed. For those patients who have cervical masses, the CT scan should include this area. Because paravertebral lesions may extend into the intervertebral foramina, any patient who has such a lesion should be evaluated by use of myelography or magnetic resonance imaging. A skel-

Table 190-2 Differential Diagnosis of Head and Neck Tumors in Infants and Children

Tumor*	Age	Clinical signs	Laboratory findings
Non-Hodgkin lymphoma	>1 yr	Lymphadenopathy—NR to antibiotics; immunodeficiency; EBV (in Africa)	Increased urate
Hodgkin disease	>10 yr	Lymphadenopathy—NR to antibiotics; weight loss, night sweats, fever, pruritus	Increased ESR
Rhabdomyosarcoma	All	Orbital mass; hoarseness; persistent otitis, sinusitis	
Neuroblastoma	Preschool	Heterochromia iridis, Horner syndrome, myoclonus-opsoclonus, raccoon eyes, skin nodules (infants)	Increased HVA in urine; increased VMA in urine; calcification
Retinoblastoma	Preschool	Cat's eye reflex, strabismus, family history	Calcification

EBV, Epstein-Barr virus; *ESR,* sedimentation rate; *HVA,* homovanillic acid; *NR,* no response; *VMA,* vanillylmandelic acid.
*Other causes: infectious lymphadenopathy, histiocytosis, Caffey disease, acquired immunodeficiency syndrome.

Table 190-3 Differential Diagnosis of Mediastinal Tumors in Infants and Children

Tumor*	Age	Clinical signs	Laboratory findings
Non-Hodgkin lymphoma	All	Cough, respiratory distress, anterior mediastinal mass, immunodeficiency syndrome	Increased urate; malignant effusion
Hodgkin disease	>10 yr	Middle mediastinum lymphadenopathy—NR to antibiotics; weight loss, night sweats, fever, pruritus	Increased ESR; increased copper
Neuroblastoma	Preschool	Posterior mediastinum; heterochromia iridis, myoclonus-opsoclonus, raccoon eyes, skin nodules (infants)	Increased HVA; increased VMA; calcification
Thymoma	>10 yr	Anterior mediastinum, myasthenia gravis, red cell aplasia, hypogammaglobulinemia	
Germ cell/teratoma	All	Anterior mediastinum (rarely, posterior mediastinum), cough, wheeze, dyspnea	Increased AFP; increased HCG

AFP, Alpha-fetoprotein; *ESR,* sedimentation rate; *HCG,* human chorionic gonadotropin; *HVA,* homovanillic acid; *VMA,* *vanillylmandelic acid.
*Other causes: infection, bronchogenic cysts, aneurysms, lipoid tumors, thoracic meningocele.

etal survey and a bone scan should be performed to detect bony lesions.[66] Radiographs are useful for the detection of small lytic lesions at the end of bones; the bone scan helps find lesions of the skull and tubular bones. A bone marrow biopsy specimen should be obtained in all patients because the marrow is a common site of metastatic involvement. The liver should be examined by contrast CT scan or liver-spleen scan in all patients, and biopsy specimens should be obtained in those who have abdominal disease.

Neuroblastoma must be diagnosed by histological examination after biopsy. In patients who have localized disease, the biopsy specimen must be obtained from the primary tumor. For those who have metastatic disease, neuroblastoma cells can be identified in the primary tumor or in areas of metastases, including the bone, bone marrow, or liver. Neuroblastoma comprises small round cells with scant cytoplasm that must be differentiated from other small cell tumors of childhood, including lymphoma, leukemia, Ewing sarcoma, and retinoblastoma. Neuroblastoma cells often are densely packed and separated by thin fibrils or bundles. Necrosis and calcification may be seen. The small round cells often form clusters surrounded by pink neurofibrillary material called *rosettes*. With increasing maturation, more fibrillary material is present, and ganglionic differentiation may be seen. Cytoplasmic structures consisting of neurofibrils, neurotubules, and neurosecretory granules that contain catecholamines may be noted.[80] Secretion of catecholamines from the granules results in elevated levels of vanillylmandelic acid (VMA) and homovanillic acid (HVA) in 24-hour urine samples or in elevated VMA:creatinine or HVA:creatinine ratios in "spot" urine samples.[48,71] These findings can be used to confirm the diagnosis of neuroblastoma in patients who have a small round cell infiltrate in the bone marrow. In addition, elevated urinary catecholamine levels can be used to monitor the response to therapy.

Amplification of the N-*myc* oncogene is an intrinsic biological property of some neuroblastomas, which has been associated with poor prognosis regardless of clinical stage (although most commonly seen in patients who have advanced disease).[110] Conversely, tumors that have hyperdiploid neuroblastoma (ONA index >1) are sensitive to chemotherapy, resulting in good prognosis; specimens should be analyzed for their biological features.[78]

Management

Neuroblastoma is sensitive to both chemotherapy and radiation therapy. For those whose disease is localized, however, surgical therapy alone may suffice. Complete removal of the tumor offers the best chance of cure. Residual tumor in patients who have stages I and II disease may regress spontaneously. Because patients who have advanced disease have disease that cannot be completely resected, only a diagnostic biopsy is required initially. Tumor recurrence in such patients often is at the site of the primary tumor. Thus surgical reduction after initial cytoreductive therapy may affect the likelihood of cure.

Chemotherapy is the major modality of therapy in neuroblastoma. Complete and partial responses have been found with the following agents: cyclophosphamide (59%), doxorubicin (41%), cisplatin (46%), epipodophyllotoxin (30%), vincristine (24%), and dacarbazine (DTIC) (14%).[14] Cyclophosphamide and vincristine individually or in combination have been used to treat localized neuroblastoma. For patients who have advanced stage disease, cyclophosphamide, ifosfamide, doxorubicin, cisplatin, carboplatin, and etoposide are used in various combinations. Long-term survival for patients who have Evans stage III neuroblastoma has improved in recent years, but survival with conventional therapy remains inadequate for patients (older than 1 year of age) who have stage IV disease or undesirable biological features (e.g., N-*myc* amplification). More intensive regimens that use high-dose cisplatin and other newer agents are being investigated. A recent study questions the need for any chemotherapy in young children who do not have any adverse prognostic features.

Intensive regimens are at the limits of bone marrow tolerance. Total body irradiation and higher doses of chemotherapy may increase the likelihood of long-term survival but require a bone marrow transplantation to restore hematopoiesis. Autologous transplantation using the patient's own bone marrow is preferred to allogeneic transplantation (using another person's bone marrow, e.g., a sibling's), which is limited to human leukocyte antigen (HLA)-matched donors and carries the risk of graft-versus-host disease. Techniques to eliminate ("purge") residual tumor cells from autologous marrow are in clinical use.[51] A number of long-term survivors of stage IV neuroblastoma have been reported after bone marrow transplantation.[5]

Neuroblastoma is a radiation-sensitive tumor. In early-stage disease, surgery alone or surgery with a small amount of chemotherapy may obviate the need for radiation therapy. Patients whose disease is advanced may receive radiation therapy to make residual disease surgically resectable or less likely to recur. Emergent situations, such as a large mediastinal mass resulting in respiratory compromise or a dumbbell lesion protruding into the intervertebral foramen that causes cord compression, frequently are treated with radiation. Radiation also is a component of the preparative regimen used before bone marrow transplantation for the treatment of stage IV neuroblastoma. In the terminal stage of neuroblastoma, bone pain or compression of organs such as the trachea, bowel, or urinary tract may require palliative radiation therapy.

Prognosis

Age and stage of disease appear to be the most important predictors of survival. Patients who are younger than 1 year of age do markedly better than those who are older than 2 years. Older studies report 2-year survival rates of 80%, 60%, 13%, 7%, and 75% for patients who have Evans stages I, II, III, IV, and IVS neuroblastoma, respectively. Patients who have IVS neuroblastoma have a small primary lesion in addition to metastatic disease (other than bone involvement). Most are less than 1 year of age. The review of patients treated with more intensive approaches during the decade 1970 to 1980 found survival rates of 100%, 93%, 81%, 23%, and 90% for Evans stage I, II, III, IV, IVS disease.[103] From 2 to 12 years had elapsed since these patients' diagnosis, with a mean follow-up of 46 months for all patients (66 months for surviving patients). Thus intensive multiagent chemotherapy appears to result in improved cure rates. The use of biological features (N-*myc,* DNA index) to determine "risk groups" for treatment purposes may allow further tailoring of therapy (minimizing treatment for good prognosis; intensifying treatment for high risk groups).

Follow-up

Although late recurrences have been reported, most tumors recur while patients are receiving therapy or shortly afterward. Close follow-up with physical examination and radiological studies should continue for 2 years after completion of therapy. Urinary catecholamine levels may be useful in the surveillance of those who had elevated values at diagnosis. The patient should be monitored for late toxicities (e.g., of cyclophosphamide, doxorubicin, and cisplatin).

RETINOBLASTOMA

Retinoblastoma is a congenital malignant tumor of the retina that occurs once in 18,000 live births.[28] Retinoblastoma develops in approximately 200 children in the United States annually, 20% to 30% of whom have bilateral disease. The disorder is diagnosed in 80% before age 4 years, with the median age of diagnosis being 2 years. Patients who have bilateral disease appear to have an inherited form of this tumor that manifests at an earlier age. Most patients who have unilateral disease have a sporadic form of the tumor.

This tumor is the model for understanding the role of genetics in the development of malignancy. The pediatrician plays an important role in detecting this disorder initially and in providing support to the family, who may carry a genetic predisposition to this malignancy.

Etiology

Knudson[68] has proposed that two independent mutations must occur in a single retinal cell for retinoblastoma to develop. The initial mutation may occur in a germinal cell (inheritable form) or in the somatic retinal cell itself (sporadic form). Those patients who have an abnormality in the germinal cell have one mutation in each retinal cell. A second mutation is relatively likely to occur, causing retinoblastoma (often multiple, bilateral tumors). If the initial mutation arises in a retinal cell, it must be followed by a second mutation in the same cell for the sporadic form of retinoblastoma to arise. The likelihood of two such events is low; hence single, unilateral tumors develop. Because the germinal cell is not involved, the mutation is not inherited.

Clearly, a patient who has a family history of retinoblastoma or bilateral retinoblastoma has a germinal mutation—thus the hereditary form of the disease. The germinal mutation also may have arisen in an affected parent or in one who had an undiagnosed retinal lesion. Parents are recommended to have an ophthalmological examination. If the first child of "normal" parents has unilateral retinoblastoma, their second child has a 1% risk of being affected. In some families, recombinant DNA techniques may aid in determining which relatives are predisposed to retinoblastoma.[130] All families should be sent for genetic counseling.

Clinical Manifestations

Patients who have a family history of retinoblastoma currently are screened by examination under anesthesia every 2 to 3 months during early childhood. These patients therefore are diagnosed before the occurrence of any clinical symptoms. Pediatricians and parents usually detect the abnormality in children who have the sporadic form of disease, because young children rarely complain of unilaterally decreased vision. Leukocoria, or cat's eye reflex, describes a whiteness detected in the pupillary area caused by a large retrolental mass. It is the most commonly encountered sign of retinoblastoma.[111] If a normal red reflex is not present in a young child, it should be investigated. The second most common presenting feature is strabismus. Although this is common in childhood because of abnormalities of ocular muscle strength, it rarely arises suddenly in a child who has had normal extraocular movements. Rarely, pain in the eye may occur as a result of glaucoma. New-onset strabismus or an abnormal red reflex requires prompt ophthalmological evaluation.

The differential diagnosis of retinoblastoma includes Coats disease, retrolental fibroplasia, toxoplasmosis, *Toxocara canis,* persistent hyperplastic primary vitreous, and severe uveitis.[111] In one review, 25% of patients had nonneoplastic disorders at the time of enucleation.[86] Of the patients who had retinoblastomas, 14% have been found to have had a significant delay from the time of onset of symptoms to diagnosis.[114] Newer methodologies, including ultrasonic examinations and MRI, may help differentiate retinoblastoma from other diseases of the eye. Patients in whom retinoblastoma is a possibility should be referred to an ophthalmologist who has a working relationship with radiation and pediatric oncologists and is experienced in the diagnosis and initial evaluation of these patients.

Evaluation

Examination under anesthesia, after pupillary dilation, is necessary to evaluate fully the retina in a young child. Ultrasonographic examination is useful to evaluate the mass, particularly if the fundal examination is obscured by hemorrhage or retinal detachment.[115] Calcification in retinoblastoma may be apparent on roentgenogram, ultrasound examination, or CT scanning. The CT scan is useful to demonstrate the extent of intraocular disease and to detect possible extraocular extension. MRI can help to evaluate the tumor's involvement with the optic nerve, the subarachnoid, and the brain.

This is not a tumor in which biopsy is a feasible method of diagnosis. Patients who have the hereditable form do not need a tissue diagnosis. In most cases of unilateral disease, enucleation is necessary to establish the diagnosis and to treat the tumor. For high-risk patients, bone marrow and cerebrospinal fluid specimens are obtained for evidence of dissemination. The extent of local disease (extension beyond the globe or optic nerve infiltration) is assessed at the time of enucleation.

Management

Treatment for retinoblastoma is individualized on the basis of the extent of disease and the possibility for the preservation of vision.[64] Treatment modalities available include enucleation, cryotherapy, photocoagulation, and radiotherapy. Most patients who have unilateral sporadic disease have large lesions and visual compromise. They usually require enucleation; cryotherapy and photocoagulation are used for small lesions, most commonly in those who have hereditary bilateral disease. These approaches prevent the need for bilateral enucleation. Radiation therapy is used for those who have massive bilateral disease. If vision can be preserved in one eye by photocoagulation or cryotherapy, but not in the other, then a unilateral enucleation may be performed. Studies are ongoing to assess the role of chemotherapy as initial treatment of bilateral retinoblastoma. It is hoped that such an approach will reduce the need for enucleation, preserve vision, and minimize the number of patients who will require radiotherapy.

Chemotherapy rarely is used for unilateral intraocular retinoblastoma. Triethylenemelamine given by intracarotid artery injection in combination with radiotherapy is not clearly superior to radiotherapy alone.[15] The role of adjuvant chemotherapy in those who have larger amounts of intraocular disease is not well defined. Combinations of agents such as cyclophosphamide, doxorubicin, vincristine, cisplatin, and epipodophyllotoxins have been used with some evidence of success in patients who have advanced or recurrent disease.[98] Bone marrow transplantation for the treatment of recurrent disease has been reported.[36]

Prognosis

Survival of patients who have retinoblastoma is excellent; 90% have no recurrence of their tumor.[15] Unfortunately, those who have hereditary retinoblastoma have a high incidence of second malignancy. Approximately 50% occur within the radiation field; osteogenic sarcoma or other sarcomas particularly are common. Approximately one third of such patients have a second malignancy within 15 years. By 30 years, two thirds will have a second malignancy.[3,50]

Follow-up

Patients who have been treated for retinoblastoma will need close follow-up for evidence of recurrence and for second malignancies. Most recurrences manifest within 3 years of diagnosis. Examinations under anesthesia should be performed every 2 to 3 months during the first year, every 3 to 4 months during the second year, and every 6 months thereafter until age 6 years. Patients who have bilateral or familial disease are at great risk of second malignancies and thus should seek medical care promptly for unexplained masses, pain, or other symptoms. These patients experience a number of long-term complications. After enucleation a prosthesis is necessary. In young children the orbit will not grow normally after enucleation or radiation. Although bilateral radiation prevents asymmetry, cataract development is likely. Retinal vascular injury also may occur. Growth and pubertal development should be followed after high-dose orbital irradiation because the pituitary gland or hypothalamus might be affected.

RHABDOMYOSARCOMA

Rhabdomyosarcoma is an aggressive tumor arising from embryonal mesenchyme that can differentiate into skeletal muscle. It can arise almost anywhere in the body and disseminates early in the course of disease. Before the advent of chemotherapy, cure required extirpative surgery of localized disease and then radiotherapy. The rapid progress, with survival rates increasing from less than 20% in the 1960s to 70% currently, has been due to the multidisciplinary cooperative group approach of the Intergroup Rhabdomyosarcoma Study (IRS) teams.[88]

Rhabdomyosarcoma is the most common pediatric soft tissue sarcoma, accounting for 4% to 8% of childhood malignancies and 5% to 15% of childhood solid tumors.[131] It occurs in 4.5 per million white and 1.3 per million black children in the United States; 38% of children are younger than 5 years of age, 47% are 5 to 14 years of age, and 15% are older than 15 years.[88]

Etiology

The cause of this tumor is unknown. It has occurred in association with neurofibromatosis, in families who have a history of multiple tumors, and in patients who have congenital abnormalities of the central nervous system, the heart, the gastrointestinal tract, and the urinary tract.[107]

Clinical Manifestations

Rhabdomyosarcoma manifests as a painless mass that has poorly defined margins.[31] One common site is the orbit, in which swelling, proptosis, discoloration, and limitation of extraocular motion occur. Patients who have a tumor of the head and neck may have hoarseness, polyps, obstruction, difficulty swallowing, decreased hearing acuity, persistent otitis, sinusitis, parotitis, or cranial nerve palsies. In parameningeal sites, penetration to the brain may cause headache, vomiting, or diplopia. Retroperitoneal tumor may manifest as a mass or as gastrointestinal discomfort because of partial obstruction. Vaginal bleeding, pelvic or perineal masses, hematuria, urinary frequency, and urinary retention suggest genitourinary tract involvement. A hydrocele, incarcerated hernia, testicular torsion, or testicular mass may be an indication of paratesticular rhabdomyosarcoma.

Evaluation

The initial evaluation should include a complete blood cell count, liver and renal function tests, and a urinalysis. Roentgenograms, CT scans, and in some instances (e.g., genitourinary tract) ultrasound examination of the involved and adjacent areas should be performed. For those who have a parameningeal tumor, the spinal fluid should be examined for cellular evidence of meningeal disease. The skull should be examined for erosion into its base. A head CT and dental films may be helpful. A barium enema, voiding cystourethrogram, and cystoscopic and pelvic examinations (sometimes under anesthesia) may be necessary for patients who have genitourinary tract involvement. At times an arteriogram or inferior vena cavagram is performed to assess operability of the tumor. If spinal cord symptoms are present, a myelogram or MRI of the spinal cord is necessary. Biopsy of the lesion establishes the diagnosis and should be performed before extensive resection. The bone, bone marrow, and liver must be evaluated for evidence of metastasis before any major surgical resections are attempted. The current Integroup Rhabdomyosarcoma Study (IRS) determines chemotherapy by preoperative extent and site of disease (stage) and radiotherapy by residual disease postoperatively (clinical group).

Management

Rhabdomyosarcoma is a tumor that requires a multitherapeutic approach, including chemotherapy, surgery, and radiation. Aggressive surgical approaches have become less essential as chemotherapy and radiation therapy have become more efficacious.

The initial surgical procedure should be a diagnostic biopsy. When possible a wide resection of the primary tumor, including surrounding normal tissue, is preferable if excessive morbidity can be avoided.[89] Extensive en bloc lymph node dissection is no longer indicated; however, biopsy for staging purposes is indicated for large regional nodes. At times, second-look surgery is appropriate after chemotherapy or radiotherapy to assess therapeutic responses.

Chemotherapeutic regimens used in the treatment of rhabdomyosarcoma include vincristine, actinomycin D, cyclophosphamide, ifosfamide, and etoposide.[88] Patients who have localized paratesticular tumors and orbital tumors can be treated with vincristine and actinomycin D alone. Patients who have more advanced disease also receive cyclophosphamide, ifosfamide, doxorubicin, and etoposide.

Rhabdomyosarcoma is an infiltrative disease, and radiation portals should include the entire extent of tumor volume. Although high doses of radiation (60 to 65 Gy) control local residual disease excellently, substantial late morbidity results.[119] Unfortunately, lower doses of radiation result in an increased recurrence rate. New methodologies using lower total doses of radiation administered twice daily are being evaluated to determine if disease can be controlled while late toxicities are decreased.[84]

Prognosis

The likelihood of survival for patients who have rhabdomyosarcoma is determined by the site and the stage of disease.[73] The prognosis is particularly good for patients who have orbital tumors and localized tumors that can be resected fully (90% to 95% long-term survivors). Extremity lesions are particularly difficult to treat, perhaps because many are of the alveolar subtype and tend to metastasize. Treatment of genitourinary primary tumors has improved markedly in recent years with the use of extensive chemotherapy. Pelvic exenteration and other morbid surgeries can now be avoided in most patients. The recent use of cranial radiation and intrathecal chemotherapy in patients who have parameningeal lesions has prevented meningeal involvement and has improved survival markedly.[101] Eighty percent of recurrences occur within 2 years of treatment. Local relapse is most common, although distant spread to the lungs, central nervous system, lymph nodes, bone, liver, bone marrow, and soft tissues does occur. Patients who have metastatic disease at diagnosis (20%) continue to have a low likelihood of survival.[106] Bone marrow transplantation or the use of new agents may offer hope to these patients.

Follow-up

Patients who have rhabdomyosarcoma should receive close follow-up for evidence of recurrent disease for approximately 3 years from the time of diagnosis. Later recurrences may even occur thereafter. Most of these patients have been treated with high-dose radiotherapy; thus bone films of the area should be obtained periodically. Patients who have orbital tumors often have significant cosmetic effects as a result of the radiation therapy. Those who have orbital parameningeal lesions have received radiation to the sinuses, hypothalamus, and pituitary gland. Sinusitis is a common complaint. Hormonal levels (e.g., gonadotrophins and growth hormone) may need monitoring. The patient also should be monitored for any potential late effects of chemotherapeutic agents (e.g., cyclophosphamide and doxorubicin) (Table 190-4).

GERM CELL TUMORS AND TERATOMAS

Germ cell tumors are growths arising from primordial germ cells; they account for 3% of tumors in children.[131] The sacrococcygeal teratoma (named from the Greek *teras,* or monster) is benign in 80% of patients. It occurs in 1 per 35,000 live births, more commonly in girls than in boys (2 to 4:1); 60% of childhood germ cell tumors originate in other sites, including the gonads, mediastinum, intracranial region, and retroperitoneum.

Etiology

Germ cells appear in the yolk sac endoderm, migrate around the hind gut to the genital ridge on the posterior abdominal wall of the embryo, and congregate, becoming part of the developing gonad. A slightly aberrant path of migration may account for the occurrence of extragonadal germ cell tumors along the dorsal wall of the embryo in midline sites (sacrococcygeal, retroperitoneal, mediastinal, and pineal regions).[4] Children who have sacrococcygeal teratomas have an approximately 15% incidence of associated anomalies (e.g., imperforate anus and rectal stenosis).[53] An association with a family history of twinning resulted in early theories suggesting that teratomas were abortive attempts at the development of twins. Of interest, the common sites of teratomas—the brain, mediastinum, abdomen, and sacrococcygeal region—are all sites of twin attachment. Although most germ cell tumors arise in "normal" individuals, a genetic tendency for abnormal germ cell development may exist in some families. These tumors have been reported to develop in siblings, twins, and subsequent generations. Gonadal dysgenesis has been associated with dysgerminoma or gonadoblastoma.[55]

The type of germ cell tumor that forms is determined by the subsequent development of the germ cell.[120] Those that

Table 190-4 Long-Term Side Effects of Chemotherapy

Drug	Potential organ damage	Evaluation
Anthracyclines, e.g., doxorubicin	Cardiac: myocardial damage, congestive failure, arrhythmias	*Cardiac* History: Exercise intolerance, palpitations; ECG (QTc interval); echocardiogram (shortening fraction q3-5 yr); Holter monitor; exercise ECG; exercise nuclear angiography
Bleomycin	Lungs: fibrosis, impaired diffusion capacity, exacerbated by increased oxygen (e.g., anesthesia)	*Pulmonary* History: Shortness of breath, dyspnea on exertion, cough. Chest film and pulmonary function tests (with diffusion capacity) q3-5 yr
Cyclophosphamide, ifosfamide	Gonadal damage: infertility, sterility, early menopause	*Gonadal* History: Menses, question of fertility; LH/FSH/testosterone or estradiol during pubertal development, or if a problem with fertility/amenorrhea exists; semen analysis (prn childbearing)
	Bladder: hemorrhagic cystitis	Urinalysis—annually
	Marrow: secondary AML	CBC—annually
Lomustine (CCNU) Carmustine (BCNU)	Gonadal, lungs	Pulmonary, gonadal evaluation (as above)
Cisplatin	Kidney: decreased glomerular filtration rate Ears: hearing loss (high frequency)	Serum creatinine q1-3 yr Creatinine clearance q3-5 yr Audiogram q3-5 yr
Methotrexate	Liver dysfunction CNS: learning impairment (high intravenous dose)	Liver function tests q1-3 yr
6-Mercaptopurine (6-MP), 6-thioguanine, actinomycin D	Liver dysfunction	Liver function tests q1-3 yr

AML, Acute myeloblastic anemia; *CBC,* complete blood cell count; *ECG,* electrocardiogram; *FSH,* follicle-stimulating hormone; *LH,* luteinizing hormone; *prn,* as required.

maintain their total potentiality become embryonal sarcomas. The development of extraembryonic structures results in the formation of choriocarcinomas (placental tumors) or endodermal sinus tumors (yolk sac tumors). Seminomas or dysgerminomas arise when the gonads differentiate. Teratomas form as a result of embryonal differentiation into ectoderm, mesoderm, and endoderm.

Clinical Manifestations

The clinical manifestations of a germ cell tumor depend on the tumor's location. Sacrococcygeal tumors occur as a mass between the anus and the coccyx.[127] An abnormality of the overlying skin may be noted. An intrapelvic tumor may be associated with an external tumor or may be the only evidence of disease, noted by the onset of urinary or rectal obstruction. The incidence of intradural tumor extension is 3% to 5%. Maternal polyhydramnios may be associated with infantile sacrococcygeal teratomas.

Ovarian tumors[83] in infants manifest as abdominal masses. Older girls have symptoms of abdominal pain, nausea, vomiting, constipation, or urinary tract obstruction, with palpable masses noted in 50%. Torsion or hemorrhage within the tumor may be responsible for acute abdominal pain; 5% of such children have bilateral tumors. Vaginal germ cell tumors in preschool girls (younger than 3 years old) may cause bloody vaginal discharge.

Testicular tumors[39] most often manifest as symptom-free scrotal masses, sometimes with a coexisting hydrocele. Torsion of the tumor in an undescended testis may result in acute abdominal pain. Testicular malignancy is 20 to 40 times more common in boys who have undescended testes. Because the ipsilateral or contralateral testis may be affected, an intrinsic testicular defect is likely.

Retroperitoneal teratomas that occur in children younger than age 2 years usually are symptom-free abdominal masses. In older children, anorexia, vomiting, or abdominal pain may be noted. Intradural extensions also may occur, and gastric and hepatic tumors have been reported.

The symptoms of patients who have germ cell tumors of the anterior mediastinum include coughing, wheezing, dyspnea, and chest pain.[72] Newborns may require immediate intubation for respiratory distress caused by mediastinal, cervical, or oropharyngeal germ cell tumors. Intrapericardial tumors can cause heart failure and cardiac tamponade. In the fetus that has an oropharyngeal mass, the inability to swallow can cause maternal polyhydramnios. Cranial tumors (80% in the pineal region) cause hydrocephalus and increased intercranial pressure in infants. Teenagers have headaches, lethargy, vomiting, visual disturbance, diabetes insipidus, and seizures.

The differential diagnosis of children who have germ cell tumors depends on the location of the primary tumor. For those who have sacrococcygeal masses, meningocele is the most frequent alternative diagnosis. Abdominal or pelvic masses may be due to neuroblastoma, Wilms tumor, rhabdomyosarcoma, or lymphomas. Nonmalignant disorders such as hydronephrosis, benign ovarian cysts, constipation, and splenomegaly must be considered. Anterior mediastinal tumors include T cell lymphoma or thymoma. The differential diagnosis for an intrascrotal mass includes testicular torsion, epididymitis, and testicular infarction. (See Tables 190-1 and 190-3 for details of the differential diagnosis of germ cell tumors.)

Evaluation

As in any ill child, evaluation includes a careful physical examination. For those patients who have sacrococcygeal mass or abdominal pain, particular attention should be given to the abdominal and rectal examination. A pelvic examination (performed under anesthesia in young girls) will be necessary if an ovarian or a vaginal tumor is suspected.

Careful evaluation by CT or ultrasound examination, or both, is essential. A CT scan of benign germ cell tumors often will reveal calcifications. A teratoma frequently shows cystic and solid components on ultrasound examination. A chest CT scan and bone scan should be performed to detect pulmonary and bony metastases.

Malignant germ cell tumors that have evidence of extraembryonic differentiation often produce proteins elaborated by the corresponding normal embryonic structure. Serum levels of these markers, alpha-fetoprotein (AFP) and beta–human chorionic gonadotropin (B-HCG), should be assayed before surgery. AFP is found in germ cell tumors that have endodermal sinus tumor histology. The evaluation of AFP levels must account for their elevation during fetal development; they do not fall to normal levels until the child is approximately 9 months of age.[123] B-HCG, a glycoprotein normally produced by specialized placental cells, is present in increased quantity in patients who have choriocarcinomas and who have hydatidiform moles and during pregnancy. Detection of AFP or B-HCG improves the ability to follow the disease status. The rate of disappearance after resection reflects the adequacy of the tumor removal. With response to chemotherapy the levels of these proteins fall. A significant rise in these levels suggests disease recurrence.

Management

Germ cell tumors may have components of teratoma, endodermal sinus tumor, embryonal carcinoma, choriocarcinoma, seminoma, or dysgerminoma. Teratomas are classified as mature, immature, or teratoma with malignant components. Mature teratomas (well-differentiated tissues) and immature teratomas (embryonic-appearing neuroglial elements and mature elements) most commonly are found in infants. Malignant evolution may occur years after removal of an apparently benign tumor, particularly in the sacrococcygeal area. For this reason, complete excision of the coccyx often is recommended, and careful follow-up is necessary.

In the past, malignant teratomas, embryonal carcinomas, endodermal sinus tumors, and choriocarcinomas were fatal almost uniformly. Complete surgical resection rarely was attained and was only infrequently curative. Only embryonal carcinoma of the infant testis could be cured by radical orchiectomy. In the 1960s, however, the efficacy of chemotherapy for gestational choriocarcinomas and testicular germ cell tumors was demonstrated.[76] Methotrexate was noted to be effective in gestational choriocarcinoma. Ovarian tumors responded to vincristine, actinomycin D, and cyclophosphamide. In the 1970s, additional agents such as vinblastine and cisplatin were found to have significant single-agent response in testicular germ cell tumors of young men. The combination of these two agents with bleomycin produces a 70% complete remission rate and a 55% long-term disease-free survival for patients who have advanced testicular carcinoma.[35]

Prognosis

The regimens already described have been effective in children; 79 children who had malignant germ cell tumors, 39% of whom had widely disseminated metastases at diagnosis, were treated with these agents.[1] Of these, 45% remained free of disease 4 years after diagnosis. Newer agents such as ifosfamide and etoposide, as well as higher doses of cisplatin, are now being incorporated into the treatment regimens. It is hoped that these additions will increase the percentage of cured patients.

The prognosis for a teratoma depends on its degree of maturity. Patients who have a mature teratoma do best. Age also is important: sacrococcygeal teratomas usually are benign in children younger than 2 months of age, but thereafter the likelihood of malignant evolution increases rapidly. This may be the reason that intrapelvic teratomas that are not detected early often are found to be malignant. Mediastinal teratomas behave benignly in children and young teenagers; in older patients they are more aggressive. Cervical and intracranial teratomas in infants usually are benign, whereas those in adolescents and adults often are malignant.

Follow-up

The response of malignant germ cell tumors to chemotherapy is very encouraging. These patients, however, may relapse late in the course of the disease, as many as 10 years from the time of diagnosis. For this reason, close follow-up care is essential, including frequent physical examinations, use of ultrasound, and chest films. Late brain metastases also have been described. Salvage therapy may prolong survival or even provide a cure. Late effects of the chemotherapeutic agent administered (e.g., bleomycin, cisplatin, doxorubicin) should be monitored (see Table 190-4).

EWING SARCOMA

Ewing sarcoma is a malignant nonosseous tumor that usually arises in bone but also may occur in soft tissues. It accounts for 3% of childhood cancers and is the most common bone tumor in children younger than 10 years of age.[131] In the second decade of life it is second in incidence only to osteogenic sarcoma. The peak incidence is between the ages of 11 and 17 years, with a range of 5 months to 60 years of age. Ewing sarcoma is extremely rare in children younger than 5 years of age, as well as in black and Asian persons.

Etiology

Ewing sarcoma is a primitive small round cell tumor. The cell of origin may be derived from primitive mesenchymal cells.[30] A possible neural origin of Ewing sarcoma is suggested by the finding of a chromosomal abnormality involving a reciprocal translocation of chromosomes 11 and 22 [t(11,22)] in tumor tissue that is identical to that of peripheral neuroepithelioma.[128] No evidence suggests hereditary transmission of Ewing sarcoma, nor has it been associated with known congenital syndromes or constitutional karyotypic abnormalities.

Clinical Manifestations

Patients who have Ewing sarcoma most commonly consult the clinician for pain.[38] Swelling also may be seen. Symptoms often begin insidiously, several months before diagnosis, and initially are attributed to trauma. At the time of diagnosis a mass is palpable in 60% of patients, resulting from the propensity of this tumor to break through the bony cortex and involve the surrounding tissue.[91] The primary lesion most often is found in the femur (22%), the fibula or tibula (21%), or the pelvis (22%).[25] The ribs and vertebrae are other common sites of origin. Demonstrable metastatic lesions are present in 14% to 35% of patients, occurring in the lungs, bones, lymph nodes, and bone marrow.[125] Central nervous system involvement is not common.

The differential diagnosis includes osteogenic sarcoma, osteomyelitis, benign bone tumors, and bone cysts. Other tumors that occasionally involve the bone and have a similar histological pattern of small round cells include lymphoma, leukemia, neuroblastoma, and rhabdomyosarcoma (Table 190-5).

Evaluation

A roentgenogram should be obtained in a patient who has a mass overlying bone or bone pain that is not characteristic of trauma (by lack of history or duration of symptoms). Radiographs of a bone that has Ewing sarcoma often show a

Table 190-5 Differential Diagnosis of Malignant Tumors Involving the Extremities

Tumor*	Age	Clinical signs	Laboratory findings
Ewing sarcoma	≥5 yr	Pain, swelling; GU/skeletal anomaly; weight loss, fever; malaise (metabolic)	"Onion skin" on roentgenogram
Osteogenic sarcoma	Teens	Pain, swelling; familial retinoblastoma; prior radiation to bone; Paget disease	Codman triangle (cortical elevation, new bone formation); "sunburst" ossification of soft tissue; soft tissue mass; elevated alkaline phosphatase level
Lymphoma	All	Pain	
Fibrosarcoma	Infants, teens	Painless mass; prior radiation; plastic implant	
Rhabdomyosarcoma	All	Mass	
Synovial sarcoma	Teens	Mass	Calcification (40%)

*Other causes: trauma, bone cysts, osteomyelitis.

destructive lesion in the diaphysis. An onion-skin appearance arises from periosteal elevation and subperiosteal new bone formation associated with tumor extension through the cortex. A mottled pattern may be seen as a result of bone destruction, sclerosis, and cystic formation. An associated soft tissue mass occurs in more than 50% of patients who have primary tumors of long bones. In addition to a plain roentgenogram of the involved bone, a CT scan and perhaps MRI may help to determine the extent of the primary lesion.

Radionuclide bone scanning detects primary and metastatic lesions, but it is not particularly useful in determining the extent of the primary disease. However, it may aid in following the response to therapy. A chest film and a CT scan of the chest are necessary to determine whether pulmonary lesions are present. The possibility of bone marrow involvement should be evaluated by marrow biopsy. Cerebrospinal fluid should be examined in patients who have parameningeal tumors.

A biopsy of the lesion is necessary to establish the diagnosis. If possible, diagnostic tissue should be obtained from soft tissue rather than cortical bone to reduce the potential for pathological fracture. Ewing sarcoma is characterized by a pattern of monomorphic sheets of small tumors made up of round cells with hyperchromatic nuclei and relatively little cytoplasm.[38] Schiff stains of the cells show positivity, but this finding is not specific for Ewing sarcoma, which remains a diagnosis of exclusion, depending on the absence of characteristics specific for other small round cell tumors.

Ewing sarcoma has no staging system; tumors are classified and treated as being either localized or metastatic.

Management

Approximately 75% of patients who have Ewing sarcoma apparently have localized disease. Localized therapies alone, however, are unlikely to be curative because of the presence of micrometastases. Chemotherapy has made it possible to cure the majority of patients who have Ewing sarcoma, and it assists in the treatment of local disease by reducing the need for radical surgery or high-dose, large-volume irradiation.

The choice of radiation or surgery for local control is based on the likelihood of preserving function. Functionally expendable bones should be removed. Aggressive surgical procedures (amputation or radical limb-sparing excisions) are being used more commonly now than in the last decade. However, radiotherapy remains the standard form of local control except when growth impairment by radiotherapy is likely or in the presence of severe pathological fractures. Local control is attained after radiotherapy in 90% of patients who have distal extremity lesions, 75% who have proximal extremity lesions, and 65% who have central lesions.[121] Radiation therapy also may be helpful after subtotal resection of the primary tumor or for treatment of pulmonary or osseous metastases.

Ewing sarcoma is extremely chemosensitive. Active agents, including vincristine, doxorubicin, cyclophosphamide, and actinomycin D (i.e., VACA) have been used in the most efficacious regimens. Etoposide and ifosfamide, in combination, elicited good therapeutic responses in many patients whose disease had relapsed. A recent study has shown improved survival for patients treated with etoposide and ifosfamide in addition to the standard VACA regimen.[52]

Dose intensity of the more active agents (cyclophosphamide and doxorubicin) has played a major role in improving disease-free survival.[103] However, the outcome remains extremely poor for patients who have bone metastases or bone marrow involvement. Further dose intensification is being investigated in new studies. Pulmonary metastases often can be treated effectively with intensive chemotherapy regimens and radiation therapy.

Prognosis

Before the use of multiagent chemotherapy, 85% of children who had Ewing sarcoma died within 2 years of diagnosis.[40] Five-year, disease-free survival is now 55% to 70%, influenced by the extent and location of disease.[64,97] Approximately 80% of patients who have small, distal extremity Ewing sarcoma tumors survive, compared with only 30% of those who have large, central extremity lesions, perhaps because of the difficulties in delivering adequate amounts of radiation therapy. Factors associated with poor prognosis include extensive soft tissue masses, large primary tumors, and high serum levels of lactate dehydrogenase.[37,42,91]

Follow-up

Patients who have Ewing sarcoma require close follow-up for evidence of recurrent disease for approximately 3 years from the time of diagnosis, although recurrences may occur later. Particular attention should be paid to the irradiated field of long-term survivors, because second malignancies may arise (Table 190-6). Bone films should be obtained periodically. Patients who have lower extremity lesions whose growth is incomplete should be monitored for evidence of leg length discrepancies, which may need to be treated by arresting the growth in the opposite limb. Monitoring for potential late effects of specific chemotherapeutic agents administered (e.g., cyclophosphamide and doxorubicin) is important (see Table 190-4).

OSTEOGENIC SARCOMA

Osteogenic sarcoma is the most common bone tumor encountered in the first 3 decades of life; approximately 2000 to 3000 patients are diagnosed per year in the United States.[24,60] Seven teenagers per million are diagnosed annually with osteogenic sarcoma, with a male to female ratio of approximately 1.5 : 1. The peak incidence occurs at age 14.5 for boys and 13.5 for girls, corresponding to the age of their growth spurts. Taller children appear to be at increased risk.[44]

Etiology

The hallmark of osteogenic sarcoma is the production of osteoid or mature bone by proliferating malignant spindle cell sarcoma. The high incidence of this tumor in adolescents who are undergoing rapid skeletal growth, as well as individuals who have Paget disease of the bone, suggests that increased bone growth may play a role in the induction of the malignancy.[57] Although patients often report a history of trauma before the diagnosis, injuries most likely allow the recognition of an already proliferating tumor.

Patients at increased risk of osteogenic sarcoma include those who have received irradiation to the bone, usually for the treatment of malignancy.[112] Whether radiographs are

Table 190-6 Long-Term Side Effects of Radiation

Irradiated area*	Risks	Monitoring
Cranium and nasopharynx	Cataracts	Physical examination
	Growth: impaired	Growth charts (bone age, growth hormone)
	Central nervous system: learning impairment	Monitoring of school function; neuropsychological evaluation
	Dentition: abnormal formation	Dental evaluation
	Thyroid: overt or compensated hypothyroidism	Free T_4/TSH levels
	High dose (>2500 Gy)	
	Hypothalamic dysfunction (decreased growth hormone; decreased gonadotropin, hyperprolactinemia)	Growth; pubertal, menstrual, and fertility history (growth hormone, LH, testosterone, estrogen, prolactin levels)
	Hearing (especially with cisplatin)	Audiogram
Neck and mandible	Hypoplasia of bone/soft tissues	Examination of area
	Dentition: abnormal formation, abnormal salivary function	Dental evaluation
	Thyroid: hypothyroidism	Free T_4, TSH
Thorax	Hypoplasia (includes impaired chest wall growth)	Examination of area
	Thyroid: hypothyroidism	Free T_4, TSH levels
	Lungs: fibrosis, decreased capacity	History, pulmonary function tests, chest film q3-5 yr
	Cardiac: pericardial and valvular thickening; possibility of early myocardial infarction	History, ECG, echocardiogram q3-5 yr
	Breasts: impaired growth, possibility of increased malignancy	Breast self-examination, early mammograms
Abdomen/pelvis	Hypoplasia (including scoliosis)	Examination of area, x-ray film of spine during puberty
	Liver (if in field)	Liver function tests
	Kidneys (if in field)	Serum creatinine, urinalysis—protein, (24-hour collection for creatinine, protein)
	Gonads (if in field)	Pubertal, menstrual, and fertility history, LH, FSH, estradiol or testosterone levels during puberty and if fertility is doubtful, semen analysis
	Gastrointestinal tract	Nutritional history
Extremities	Hypoplasia	Examination of area

ECG, Electrocardiogram; *FSH,* follicle-stimulating hormone; *LH,* luteinizing hormone; *T_4,* thyroxine; *TSH,* thyroid-stimulating hormone.
*All: Consider roentgenograms of bones every 5 to 10 years after ≥35 Gy radiation (risk of secondary malignancy). Examine skin for abnormal pigmented nevi (risk of second malignancy).

causative or whether these patients who have already had one tumor are at a higher than normal risk for a spontaneous, second primary malignancy is unclear. For example, patients who have hereditary retinoblastoma and a constitutive deletion in chromosome 13 have an increased incidence of osteogenic sarcoma; however, only half the sarcomas occur within the radiation field.[2] Thus the abnormality in chromosome 13 itself may predispose to osteogenic sarcoma. Osteogenic sarcoma has been described in sisters with a constitutional translocation between chromosomes 13 and 14.[47]

Clinical Manifestations

The presenting symptom of virtually all patients is pain. Palpable masses, swelling, and limited motion are common signs. Weight loss and other systemic symptoms such as anorexia rarely are seen; if these symptoms are present, overt metastatic disease is likely. A few patients have fractures. Cough, chest pain, or dyspnea may be seen in those who have extensive pulmonary metastases at the time of diagnosis, although most patients who have such metastases are symptom free. The metaphyses of bones are common sites of osteogenic sarcoma origin. The lower extremities are involved most frequently, with 60% of tumors occurring around the knee (40% in the distal femur and 20% in the proximal tibia).[124] Three quarters of osteogenic sarcomas occur in the bone of the upper and lower extremities. The sacrum, jaw, and phalanges are involved less commonly. Patients who have Paget disease of the bone or those who have had radiation therapy in the area of the orbit may have osteogenic sarcoma of the skull bones.

The presenting symptom, bone pain, is ubiquitous. It most commonly is due to trauma. Prolonged symptoms, or a history inconsistent with trauma, suggest the need for further evaluation. Bone abnormalities that may be confused with osteogenic sarcoma include benign cysts, Ewing sarcoma, lymphoma, or tumor metastases. (See Table 190-5 for the differential diagnosis of osteogenic sarcoma involving the extremities.)

Evaluation

Roentgenograms of the involved bone show bony destruction with periosteal new bone formation. A “sunburst” appearance is characteristic, a result of the eruption of tumor through the cortex with subsequent formation of new bone. Soft tissue swelling often is noted. Adequate biopsy and histological examination are necessary to establish the diagnosis of osteogenic sarcoma.

Osteoid found within a sarcomatous tumor is the characteristic histological pattern. Osteogenic sarcoma in the child or adolescent usually is a high-grade tumor characterized by osteoblasts that demonstrate pleomorphism and bizarre mitoses. Necrosis, fibrosis, and calcification may be noted. This classic form usually arises from the medullary cavity. A less aggressive form of osteogenic sarcoma arises in the paraosteal area of the bone and tends to spread along the shaft of the bone without invading the cortex. Periosteal, intracortical, and extraskeletal osteogenic sarcomas also have been described.

Baseline lactic dehydrogenase and alkaline phosphatase levels should be obtained. The extent of the primary lesion is defined further by the use of CT or MRI scanning. Arteriographic examination may be necessary in patients considered for limb salvage procedures, in which the vascular and neurological integrity of the limb must be ensured. Metastatic disease in the lung should be sought by the use of CT scanning. Bone scans can be helpful both for outlining the primary tumor and for detecting multiple primary lesions and metastasis.

Management

The traditional therapy of osteogenic sarcoma has been amputation of the affected limb. The natural history of disease in such patients is notable for the rapid appearance of pulmonary metastases 6 to 12 months after diagnosis.[24] Five years from the diagnosis, only 10% to 20% of patients are alive. High-dose radiotherapy is even less effective than amputation.[117] In the early 1970s, favorable responses to high-dose methotrexate with leucovorin and to doxorubicin were noted.[19,59,60] Patients treated with these agents had markedly improved survival rates (40% to 50%) compared with historical control subjects (treated with amputation alone).[19,59] Unfortunately, a report of 50% survival after surgery alone suggested that the improved outcome was a result of improved surgical techniques rather than the chemotherapy.[118] Adjuvant chemotherapy therefore was not recommended by many physicians until the 1980s, when a controlled randomized study confirmed that adjuvant chemotherapy improves disease-free survival of patients who have osteogenic sarcoma.[77] Adjuvant chemotherapy regimens now being recommended use high doses of methotrexate, doxorubicin, and cisplatin. The role of ifosfamide in osteosarcoma is being investigated.

The availability of effective chemotherapy has made limb-sparing or subamputative therapies possible for many patients who have osteogenic sarcoma.[85] The portion of bone involved with tumor is removed and replaced by an artificial prosthesis or a bone graft. This procedure can be performed only if the vascular and neurological integrity of the limb is not compromised. Preoperative chemotherapy may reduce the size of the mass so as to make such surgery possible. In many protocols the efficacy of the chemotherapy used initially is evaluated on the basis of the biological response to therapy.[105] The subsequent chemotherapeutic regimen may be modified. For those who have lower extremity tumors, limb-salvage procedures are limited to patients who have achieved most of their growth potential. For patients who have lesions of the humerus, any preservation of hand function will improve the patient's life-style significantly.

For patients in whom pulmonary metastases develop, surgical resection of these nodules may result in long-term survival.[87,92] A similar approach has been used in patients who have metastatic pulmonary disease at the time of diagnosis, with long-term survival of 20% to 40%.

Prognosis

Two randomized studies have confirmed the role of adjuvant chemotherapy in improving the long-term disease-free survival of patients who have nonmetastatic osteogenic sarcoma. Approximately 65% to 75% overall disease-free survival can be achieved.[77,104] The initial biological response to chemotherapy appears to have prognostic significance, although it is unclear whether subsequent tailoring of therapy achieves a better result than aggressive, early chemotherapy for all patients. The advantage of preoperative chemotherapy compared with immediate surgical excision also is unclear. Preoperative chemotherapy, however, allows for the possibility of limb-salvage procedures by decreasing tumor size, as well as by allowing time for a prosthesis to be made.

Prognostic factors in this disorder are related to the site of the tumor (patients who have distal tumors do better than those who have proximal or central-axis tumors) and the patient's age (prognosis improves with increased age).

Follow-up

Adjuvant chemotherapy has resulted in an increased number of long-term survivors of osteogenic sarcoma. Virtually all these patients will have undergone either amputation or limb-salvage procedures. It is hoped that at some time, less disabling therapies will be feasible. Most of these patients, however, maintain a relatively normal life-style, including participation in a variety of sports. Their long-term, follow-up care to detect recurrent disease includes (1) chest films and alkaline phosphatase determinations performed semiannually for 5 years and annually until 10 years from the time of diagnosis, (2) orthopedic evaluations to consider necessary adjustments in prostheses, and (3) monitoring for the late effects of chemotherapeutic agents used (e.g., doxorubicin, cisplatin, bleomycin, ifosfamide, and cyclophosphamide).

NON-HODGKIN LYMPHOMAS

Non-Hodgkin lymphoma (NHL) of childhood comprises a heterogeneous group of malignancies arising from lymphocytes and lymphoid precursors. The migratory nature of these cells is reflected by the variable sites at which the tumors occur and to which they spread. Recognition of the systemic nature of disease, even in those patients who have only locally detectable disease, has resulted in a marked improvement in survival rates in recent years. Childhood NHL is markedly different from adult NHL both in the immunohistopathological types that occur and in the better survival rates noted in children.

Lymphomas account for 10% of childhood cancer[131]; 60% are NHLs. The incidence of NHL is low in children younger than 5 years and then increases steadily throughout life. It occurs more commonly in males than in females (2 to 3:1). The frequency of NHL itself and of its various subtypes varies markedly in different geographical regions.[81] NHLs of childhood have a high growth rate, approaching 100% in some cases, and short doubling-in-size times (as few as 12 hours). They have a high frequency of dissemination, particularly to the bone marrow and central nervous system. Although the distinction between lymphoma and leukemia is defined by <25% versus >25% marrow blasts, respectively, the distinguishing biological parameters are not clear. Lymphoid malignancies involving immature thymocytes more frequently occur as leukemia, whereas more mature thymocytes are associated with lymphomatous manifestations.[8]

Etiology

Childhood NHL arises from lymphoid precursors in the marrow and thymus. Burkitt and non-Burkitt small, nonclefted cell lymphomas and most large cell lymphomas are B cell phenotypes, usually manifesting surface immunoglobulin and B cell–specific antigens. Lymphoblastic lymphomas almost invariably express the enzyme terminal deoxynucleotidyl (TdT), as well as T cell markers.[8] Specific chromosomal aberrations have been described in Burkitt lymphoma.[9,132]

Different breakpoints of chromosomal translocations may be seen in the Burkitt lymphoma of equatorial Africa, which usually harbors Epstein-Barr virus (EBV), compared with the North American variety, which does so only rarely.[96] The presence of EBV in lymphoma specimens suggests that viral infection may play a role in the development of NHL. Immunodeficiency states also are associated with the development of lymphomas, usually of the B cell immunoblastic or large cell variety.[43] A defect of T cell regulation that permits the expansion of EBV-affected clones of B cells has been hypothesized to result in lymphomas, particularly in immunologically abnormal hosts. Lymphomas occur with increased frequency in children receiving immunosuppressive therapy for renal, cardiac, or bone marrow allografts.

A number of specific, nonrandom chromosomal abnormalities have been reported in lymphoblastic lymphoma and large cell lymphomas. The variation in subtypes described suggests that these tumors may be more heterogeneous than Burkitt lymphoma.

Clinical Manifestations

Localized lymphadenopathy is a common presentation of NHL. Common areas of involvement are supradiaphragmatic, particularly the cervical, axillary, and mediastinal areas, or Waldeyer ring.[93] The histological pattern of supradiaphragmatic disease often is lymphoblastic. Dissemination to the bone marrow, the central nervous system, or the gonads is common. Patients who have mediastinal masses frequently have a history of cough and, occasionally, acute respiratory distress. Unless careful attention is paid to the state of the airway, obstruction can occur during evaluation, even in patients who have minimal symptoms, particularly with the administration of sedation. The obstruction may involve the lower airway, beyond the reach of an endotracheal tube, resulting in an inability to ventilate the lungs effectively.

An abdominal mass that may involve the iliocecal region, mesentery, ovaries, or retroperitoneum is seen in 30% to 40% of patients.[93] Such tumors often are of B cell origin. Extranodal sites of involvement include the tonsils, lungs, bone, testicles, and soft tissue.

Patients whose disease is localized often feel well. Those who have disseminated disease experience weight loss and malaise, as well as symptoms referable to the primary site of the disease.

The differential diagnosis of cervical adenopathy includes a variety of infectious and inflammatory processes. Malignant processes that cause enlarged cervical nodes include Hodgkin disease, neuroblastoma, leukemia, nasopharyngeal carcinoma, rhabdomyosarcoma, and thyroid carcinoma. Anterior mediastinal masses may be due to T cell leukemia or thymoma. Abdominal masses may be due to constipation, splenomegaly, Wilms tumor, rhabdomyosarcoma, or neuroblastoma. Lymphoma is a rare type of bone tumor. (Tables 190-1 to 190-3 provide differential diagnostic aids in evaluating patients who have NHL.)

Evaluation

The diagnosis of NHL should be established by surgical biopsy; removal of the most suspicious node is recommended. Frozen sections and needle biopsies are to be discouraged to ensure proper diagnosis. Although the primary diagnosis is based on histological findings, immunophenotyping and enzyme studies (TdT) can be helpful. If possible, cytogenetics studies should be performed. A sufficient number of malignant cells may be present in patients who have bone marrow involvement or pleural effusions to establish the diagnosis. In this instance a lymph node biopsy may not be necessary. Biopsy may be contraindicated for patients who have large mediastinal masses with imminent airway obstruction unless endotracheal intubation will ensure airway patency. If the distal end of the endotracheal tube lies proximal to the mass, localized radiation to the mediastinum may be necessary before the diagnostic specimen is obtained. Alternative sites for obtaining diagnostic specimens then must be considered.

All patients should receive a complete blood cell count and platelet and reticulocyte counts. Serum electrolyte, uric acid, calcium, and phosphorus levels and renal and liver function tests should be obtained. A low serum alkaline phosphatase level predicts a good outcome. A lumbar puncture should be obtained with cytocentrifugation of cerebral spinal fluid to detect meningeal involvement. Imaging studies should include a chest film and a CT scan of the chest and abdomen in all patients. Bone scans and gallium scans can be helpful in selected patients.

A variety of staging systems are used for lymphomas.[81] The most common, the Ann Arbor system used for Hodgkin disease, is not of prognostic significance in pediatric NHL because of noncontinuous patterns of spread. The National Cancer Institute staging system is used primarily for Burkitt lymphoma. The St. Jude system, applicable to most forms of NHL, is devised to reflect the prognostic significance of involvement in various areas of the body.

Management

The majority of patients who have NHL have disseminated disease at the time of diagnosis. Even those who have clinically localized disease rarely are curable with localized surgical or irradiation therapy alone. The choice of chemotherapeutic regimens is based on the clinical stage and the immunohistological tumor subtype.

Lymph node biopsy usually is required for diagnosis and characterization of NHL. Removal of the tumor is indicated only for those patients who have Burkitt lymphoma whose tumor can be removed en masse (90%) with minimal morbidity.[82] In general, major surgical procedures should be avoided because subsequent healing time may delay initiation of chemotherapy, the most essential component of treatment.

The high incidence of micrometastatic disease at the time of diagnosis necessitates that all children who have NHL receive chemotherapy. Many agents are active in lymphomas. Optimal treatment regimens differ for patients who have lymphoblastic lymphoma compared with those who have nonlymphoblastic lymphoma. A study comparing two lymphoma regimens showed that the histological class of lymphoma predicted the efficacy of the regimens. For those with lymphoblastic lymphoma, the LSA2L2 regimen, which uses pairs of agents in rapid succession, was the most effective. For patients who had nonlymphoblastic lymphoma, the more effective regimen included cyclophosphamide, vincristine, prednisone, methotrexate, and doxorubicin.[63] Agents such as cytosine arabinoside, etoposide, and ifosfamide are successfully replacing some of the more toxic or less effective agents used in these regimens.

Local measures of control rarely are essential in the treatment of childhood NHL. Lymphomas are radiosensitive, but the use of radiation therapy does not improve disease-free survival in patients whose disease is advanced. Unnecessary morbidity may be added. Radiotherapy is helpful in the treatment of emergent situations such as airway compromise or spinal cord compression and for treating overt meningeal involvement. Radiation therapy also plays a role in the treatment of patients who do not achieve a complete remission after standard chemotherapy. After relapse, radiotherapy is used as part of consolidation therapy before bone marrow transplantation. For terminally ill patients, radiation provides effective palliation for localized pain.

Prognosis

The prognosis is excellent for most children who have NHL. Although histological findings are not of great prognostic significance for outcome, they provide the basis for choice of therapeutic regimen. Clinical staging is of particular relevance because it is determined by a combination of the tumor burden, disease extent, and primary location. New intensive chemotherapy or bone marrow transplantation regimens should improve the likelihood of survival in patients whose prognosis is poor.

Follow-up

Patients who have NHL who are disease free 2 years from the time of diagnosis usually are cured. During this initial period they should be monitored on the basis of complete blood cell counts, chest films, and evaluation of the primary site of disease. The follow-up of long-term survivors of childhood lymphomas should reflect the types of therapy (e.g., cyclophosphamide, doxorubicin, methotrexate) administered (see Table 190-4).

HODGKIN DISEASE

Hodgkin disease is a malignancy of the lymphoreticular system characterized by multinucleated giant cells, known as Reed-Sternberg cells, interspersed in an infiltration of normal-appearing cellular elements (lymphocytes, macrophages, histiocytes, plasma cells, and eosinophils).[102] The Reed-Sternberg cells appear to be the mitotically active malignant cell of Hodgkin disease. Controversy exists as to the normal counterpart from which these cells derive.

In the more developed nations the incidence of Hodgkin disease exhibits two age peaks, one in young adults (15 to 30 years of age) and one in late adulthood.[54,113] In developing nations the early peak occurs in preadolescence. Hodgkin disease is extremely rare before the age of 5 years. A male predominance is present throughout the preadolescent age range; thereafter the incidence is approximately equal in males and females. Hodgkin disease in older teenagers and young adults is most common in Caucasian persons.

Etiology

The role of environment or genetics in the acquisition of Hodgkin disease is suggested by national and racial differences in the epidemiological features of the disease. First-degree relatives of patients who have Hodgkin disease have an increased risk of acquiring the disease,[54] possibly because of genetic susceptibility or similar exposures (viral, environmental).

High serum titers to EBV in some patients who have Hodgkin disease may reflect a causative role for the virus.[94] Alternatively, patients may have an inappropriate immune response to this virus. The incidence of Hodgkin disease is known to be increased in patients who have certain underlying immunodeficiency diseases (e.g., ataxia-telangiectasia and acquired immunodeficiency syndrome).[46,58]

Clinical Manifestations[74]

The most common presenting feature of Hodgkin disease is painless enlargement of the lower cervical lymph nodes. Approximately half of the patients who have this manifestation also have mediastinal disease. The classic pattern of spread is from the cervical lymph nodes to the mediastinum and then into the spleen and abdominal lymph nodes. Spread via the thoracic duct may result in disease of the right side of the neck and of the abdomen, without mediastinal involvement. Axillary or inguinal adenopathy or extranodal primary sites (e.g., bone) are seen occasionally. Pleural involvement occurs in approximately 10% of patients. Renal, skin, or nervous system involvement is less common. Constitutional symptoms related to Hodgkin disease occur in approximately one third of patients at the time of diagnosis. The symptoms that predict a poor prognosis ("B" disease) are fever (oral temperature >38° C), weight loss (>10% of body weight within 6 months), and drenching night sweats. Absence of these symptoms provides a better prognosis ("A" disease).

Hematological abnormalities may be present in Hodgkin disease (usually in advanced stages), even in the absence of bone marrow involvement. Hemolytic disease or the anemia of chronic disease associated with impaired mobilization of iron storage may occur. Neutrophilia in the absence of infection occurs in approximately 50% of the patients. Thrombocytopenia caused by immunologically mediated platelet destruction also is seen.

Lymphadenopathy occurs in children for a variety of reasons. Infection with bacteria, viruses, tuberculosis, atypical mycobacteria, and toxoplasmosis may cause lymphadenopathy. Malignancies that can be considered in the differential diagnosis include non-Hodgkin lymphoma, nasopharyngeal carcinoma, soft tissue sarcoma, or in a younger child, neuroblastoma. Histiocytosis and other inflammatory processes also present similarly. A chest film, a complete blood cell count, and a sedimentation rate should be obtained in any patient who has lymphadenopathy that is atypical for infection. Persistent lymphadenopathy, even after a transient "response" to antibiotic therapy, requires biopsy. (Tables 190-2 and 190-3 provide differential diagnostic aids in evaluating patients who have Hodgkin disease.)

Evaluation

Evaluation of the child who has Hodgkin disease should begin with a careful history and physical examination. Particular attention should be paid to "B" disease symptoms. Lymphatic areas to be evaluated include Waldeyer ring and the cervical, supraclavicular, axillary, and inguinal lymph nodes. The sizes of the nodes found should be recorded carefully, and it should be noted whether they are tender. In addition, a careful abdominal examination should be performed, particularly to evaluate liver and splenic size. Retroperitoneal lymph nodes are not palpable. The blood cell counts may show anemia (caused by hemolysis or chronic disease), neutropenia, or thrombocytopenia. Elevation of the sedimentation rate and the serum copper level occurs in some patients and may be useful for following response to therapy. Serum hepatic alkaline phosphatase isoenzyme levels also may be elevated.

Radiographic evaluation of a patient with a possible diagnosis of Hodgkin disease includes a chest film and CT scans of the chest and abdomen. Bipedal lymphangiography can be used to detect pelvic and paraaortic lymph nodes in institutions in which radiologists commonly perform such tests. Gallium scanning also detects Hodgkin disease and can be useful in detecting disease in obscure sites. Although bone involvement is rare, a bone scan should be considered in patients who have advanced disease, particularly those who have bone pain or an elevated serum alkaline phosphatase level.

Laparotomy with splenectomy is the only precise way to define the subdiaphragmatic extent of Hodgkin disease.[49] Biopsy specimens of even normal-appearing lymph nodes should be obtained in each of the following areas: splenic hilar, celiac portal hepatic, mesenteric, paraaortic, and iliac regions. In addition, any suspicious lesions should be removed. Evaluation of other organs includes a careful examination of the spleen, with sectioning at intervals of 1 mm to 3 mm to detect small nodules. Wedge biopsies of the liver are necessary because needle biopsies are unlikely to detect focal lesions. A bone marrow biopsy must be obtained either before or coincidentally with laparotomy. Although bone marrow involvement is not common, the detection of Hodgkin disease in the marrow would be consistent with stage IV disease, obviating the need for a staging laparotomy.

The importance of defining subdiaphragmatic involvement is most clear when radiation therapy is the primary therapeutic modality. A staging laparotomy with splenectomy allows limited fields to be irradiated, thus preventing the morbidity associated with total nodal irradiation. When chemotherapy is used, the benefits of staging laparotomy with splenectomy are lower. The current trend is to perform laparotomies in those settings in which exact staging of disease extent would facilitate reduction of radiotherapy or chemotherapy.

Unfortunately, overwhelming bacteremia with polysaccharide-encapsulated organisms occurs in 10% of patients after splenectomy, with a mortality of 50% in these patients.[105] The risk is greatest for young children who previously have not been exposed to these pathogens. All patients who have undergone splenectomy will require presurgical vaccination against pneumococci, *Haemophilus influenzae* type b, and *Neisseria meningitidis*. Prophylactic antibiotics also are recommended throughout their lives.

The extent of disease spread usually is classified by the Ann Arbor staging system by means of either the clinical stage (CS) or the pathological stage (PS).[13] PS implies that the most extensive degree of involvement has been confirmed pathologically. The stages are as follows:

Stage I—involvement of one lymphatic region only
Stage II—involvement of two or more lymphatic regions on the same side of the diaphragm
Stage III—involvement on both sides of the diaphragm, including nodal regions and/or the spleen
Stage IV—involvement of extranodal organs such as lungs, liver, bone marrow, kidneys, bone, or skin, in addition to lymph nodes

Direct extranodal extension to adjacent tissue is denoted by the subscript E. Stage III disease is subdivided by the degree of abdominal involvement. Stage III_1 involves nodes of the upper portion of the abdomen alone (celiac portal nodes and/or spleen). Stage III_2 involves paraaortic nodes as well; stage III_3 additionally involves iliac nodes.

Four subtypes of Hodgkin disease are described by review of pathological specimens. [79] The nodular sclerosing type (NS) is most common in childhood. Collagenous bands divide the lymphoid tissues into nodules, and a "lacunar variant" of the Reed-Sternberg cell is seen. Lymphocyte-predominant Hodgkin disease is characterized by destruction of the lymph node architecture with the cellular proliferation of benign-appearing lymphocytes. Reed-Sternberg cells rarely are found in the absence of fibrosis. In mixed cellularity Hodgkin disease, lymph node architecture is not preserved. Approximately 10 Reed-Sternberg cells are seen per high power field, often with interstitial fibrosis; necrosis is not pronounced. Lymphocyte-depleted Hodgkin disease is characterized by the presence of fibrosis, necrosis, and abnormal cells (but only a rare lymphocyte).

Management

Hodgkin disease responds to radiation or to chemotherapy. Protocols using radiation therapy alone, chemotherapy alone, or both forms of therapy all have been successful, at least in some groups of patients. Choosing an appropriate therapeutic plan necessitates assessing the risk of disease recurrence and the potential for long-term effects in a particular patient.

Contiguous spread of Hodgkin disease via lymphoid organs allows for success with radiation therapy alone.[65] Full-dose radiation therapy (35 to 45 Gy) is used most frequently in the treatment of patients who have stages I, II, and III_1 disease. The involved fields, and one field beyond the area of proved disease, are treated. Those patients who have large mediastinal masses (more than one third the thoracic diameter) also require chemotherapy for optimal results. Skeletal and soft tissue growth, particularly in the neck and clavicular areas, are severely compromised when these doses of radiation are used. Cardiac and pulmonary complications occur as well. Children who have not achieved full adult size at the time of diagnosis will have significant skeletal deformity if full-dose irradiation is used to the neck and mediastinum. Low-dose radiation (20 to 25 Gy) to involved fields, in conjunction with chemotherapy, is being used for most younger children.[33]

Hodgkin disease responds to a number of single chemotherapeutic agents, but rarely are lasting, complete remissions achieved in this manner. Combination chemotherapy, with active agents that have differing mechanisms of action and nonoverlapping toxicities, is used. The original combination that proved to be successful in the treatment of Hodgkin disease was MOPP (mechlorethamine, Oncovin [vincristine], procarbazine, and prednisone).[29] Cyclophosphamide or a nitrosuria may be substituted for mechlorethamine, or vinblastine for vincristine. Full doses of drugs should be used in as short a period as possible. In 1974, 10 years after the initial discovery of MOPP, another combination regimen ABVD (Adriamycin [doxorubicin], bleomycin, vinblastine, and dacarbazine) was devised for the treatment of patients whose disease had relapsed.[10] The efficacy of this combination has resulted in combined ABVD/MOPP regimens. Chemotherapeutic regimens have been used successfully alone or in combination with radiation for all stages of disease.

Combined therapies (chemotherapy and radiation together) are used (1) to improve cure rates in patients whose prognosis is poor and (2) to reduce the dose of radiotherapy administered to children who have low-stage disease so that skeletal development will proceed more normally. Chemotherapy has side effects as well, including infertility after MOPP chemotherapy, cardiotoxic effects of the doxorubicin of ABVD, and pulmonary toxicity caused by bleomycin.[26,108] Secondary leukemias have been described, particularly after the combination of MOPP and radiation.[17] Second-generation treatment protocols are being devised to decrease the number of courses, to eliminate particularly toxic components of therapy (i.e., bleomycin), and to substitute less toxic agents. In choosing an appropriate regimen for a given patient, the following must be considered: (1) the age of the patient (likely effects on the developing organism), (2) the extent of disease present (how much therapy is necessary), and (3) symptoms that might predict a poor prognosis. Because so many regimens currently appear equivalent in terms of outcome, an experimental protocol should be used (if one is available) to help delineate the best treatment for patients in the future, while ensuring appropriate treatment for those under study.

Prognosis[74]

Radiation therapy alone may cure up to 70% of patients who have stage I or IIA Hodgkin disease. The success of this approach varies significantly among institutions. When three to six courses of MOPP are added to radiotherapy, the 5-year disease-free survival rate increases to approximately 90% at all institutions.

Patients who have stage IIB or IIIA disease are treated in a variety of fashions, including chemotherapy alone, extended field irradiation, or a combination of the two. Many oncologists use full-dose radiation for fully grown patients. Relapse will occur in approximately 50% of these patients after such treatment. The subsequent use of chemotherapy will enable half of those who relapse after radiation therapy to be cured of the disease.[116,126] Combined modality therapy often is used for younger patients or for those in whom a poor prognosis is indicated (e.g., large mediastinal mass).

Patients who have stage IIIB or IV disease are treated with multiagent chemotherapy, with or without radiation, to areas of bulk disease. Results of recent studies suggest that approximately 50% to 75% of patients will remain disease free 5 years later. In some patients who experience relapse, improvement can be effected with bone marrow transplantation.

Follow-up

Patients who have Hodgkin disease should be monitored for evidence of recurrent disease for as long as 10 to 15 years after the original diagnosis. Useful tests for prolonged follow-up include complete blood cell count, sedimentation rate, and chest film.

After high-dose radiotherapy to the neck and mediastinum, soft tissue and bone growth abnormalities include shortening of clavicles and underdevelopment of the soft tissues of the neck. Sitting height decreases after radiation to the axial skeleton in proportion to the growth potential remaining at the time of radiation.[99] In prepubertal girls, breast development may be impaired. The incidence of breast cancer may be increased after irradiation.[62] Serial mammography examinations beginning at an early age (approximately 25 years) may be appropriate.

Overt hypothyroidism (low thyroxine) occurs in approximately 5% to 10% of patients who have undergone irradiation, whereas compensated hypothyroidism (elevated thyroid-stimulating hormone) occurs in 50% to 90% of such patients.[18] Thyroid function should be assessed for at least 15 years. Thyroid replacement therapy is recommended when the thyroid-stimulating hormone level is elevated.

Patients who receive mediastinal irradiation may have pulmonary fibrosis with variable abnormalities detected by pulmonary function testing.[32] Late cardiac abnormalities include pericardial thickening and, occasionally, valvular dysfunction. Early myocardial infarctions have been reported. These toxicities may be exacerbated by the use of bleomycin and anthracyclines.

Fertility in women is affected by the use of radiation and chemotherapy. Pelvic irradiation of a woman causes infertility unless oophoropexy (moving ovaries to the midline) is performed. After oophoropexy, all teenage girls treated with radiation alone and 88% of those treated with combined modality therapy maintained normal menses.[32] Older women (older than 30 years of age) experience ovarian failure more frequently than do younger women after treatment with MOPP. All should be advised of the possibility of early menopause. A menstrual history should be elicited at each visit.

Testes are more severely affected by cytotoxic therapies than are ovaries. Fortunately, the radiation fields used in Hodgkin disease spare the gonads in male patients. Six courses of MOPP chemotherapy, however, result in universal male sterility. Approximately 50% of patients treated with three courses of MOPP are sterile.[27] ABVD causes less impairment of spermatogenesis. Men interested in fathering a child may benefit from the monitoring of gonadotropin levels and from semen analysis. Recovery has been documented in previously sterile men.

Acute nonlymphocytic leukemia occurs at the rate of approximately 1% per year for the first 10 years after treatment with MOPP and radiotherapy.[17] Thereafter the risk appears to decrease. The incidence is lower with single modality therapy or after ABVD and radiation. Solid tumors, particularly breast cancer, thyroid cancer, bone tumors, and NHL, may occur after Hodgkin disease.

Patients who have Hodgkin disease remain at risk for overwhelming infections secondary to splenectomy.[106] Patients who have a high fever should be hospitalized and treated empirically with antibiotics for the potential of sepsis caused by polysaccharide-encapsulated organisms.

GENERAL ONCOLOGICAL CARE

Referral to a Pediatric Oncologist

Fortunately, children who have malignancies represent a very small proportion of patients in a general pediatrics practice. The treatment of such patients is specialized and changes rapidly each year. Proper care of such patients begins with referral to a pediatric oncologist, even if the initial procedure is surgical. For many tumors, appropriate baseline studies must be obtained before surgical procedures are begun. For example, AFP and B-HCG levels fall rapidly after removal of the germ cell tumor, as do catecholamine levels after removal of a neuroblastoma. Delayed assays for such markers may result in the inability to recognize an important indicator of recurrent disease in a given patient. The chest CT scan should be performed before surgical procedures because perioperative atelectasis may impair the ability to detect metastatic disease in the pulmonary parenchyma.

The tumors of childhood behave differently from those of adults, even when histologically identical. In addition, children tolerate radiation and chemotherapy differently than do adults. Therefore all children should receive the care of a pediatric oncologist. Services available for children and their families at pediatric referral hospitals often ease the pain of being diagnosed with a life-threatening disease. Pediatric social workers, child life workers, and nurses experienced in dealing with children and adolescents who have cancer are available. For patients living at a distance from a center, it often is possible to initiate therapy at a referral center and administer most of the treatments and evaluations closer to the patient's home. At times, a local oncologist can assist in administering chemotherapy to children living at a distance from a center, but such oncologists should not be relied on to choose a therapeutic regimen or to evaluate major problems that may arise.

A number of oncological emergencies exist that general pediatricians must recognize. Cord compression may result from neuroblastoma, Ewing sarcoma, lymphoma, or any other tumor that invades the spinal canal. Such patients experience incontinence, loss of reflexes in the lower extremities, or decreased ability to use the lower extremities. Rectal spincter tone may be decreased. Rapid institution of therapy may reverse such findings, markedly changing the long-term functioning of the patient. Thus recognition of such findings should prompt immediate referral to a pediatric oncologist who, in conjunction with a neurosurgeon or radiation therapist, will be able to deliver emergent therapy.

Patients whose bone marrow has been infiltrated by leukemia, Ewing sarcoma, neuroblastoma, or lymphoma may have pancytopenia and thus be at risk of infection from neutropenia, bleeding caused by thrombocytopenia, and congestive failure as a result of anemia. Rapid lysis of cells (tumor lysis syndrome) because of the high cell turnover rate of the tumor itself (as is seen in Burkitt lymphoma) or to cytotoxic therapy is characterized by elevated uric acid (risk of urate nephropathy), hyperkalemia, hypocalcemia, and hyperphosphatemia. Medical management includes allopurinol, urinary alkalinization, and binders of potassium and phosphate. Dialysis may be necessary. If delayed arrival to the medical center is anticipated, allopurinol should be started by a referring physician when a tumor that has a large cell burden (e.g., leukemia, Burkitt lymphoma, and marrow involvement with either neuroblastoma, Ewing sarcoma, or rhabdomyosarcoma) is suspected.

Role of the Pediatrician During Therapy

The most prominent toxicity that results from chemotherapy is myelosuppression. Infections in neutropenic patients can rapidly result in septic shock, particularly if gram negative organisms are involved. Primary physicians who follow up these children can help by recognizing the risk of fever and referring the patient immediately to the pediatric oncologist. If the center is at a distance, the pediatrician becomes the frontline caretaker, obtaining proper culture specimens and initiating antibiotics (usually an aminoglycoside and semisynthetic penicillin or a fourth generation cephalosporin). In such circumstances the primary pediatrician should discuss aspects of care with the pediatric oncologist to ensure that all appropriate measures are performed. Many patients receiving intensive chemotherapy have indwelling central venous catheters that increase the risk for septicemia with gram positive organisms. These patients, even in the absence of neutropenia, should have blood cultures performed and the administration of antibiotics considered if fever develops. Any person who is febrile and who has undergone a splenectomy should be given antibiotics empirically to treat polysaccharide-encapsulated organisms.

In the absence of splenectomy and a central line, pediatric treatment of patients whose blood cell counts are normal usually is similar to that of the typical child. The primary pediatrician can be of great assistance in seeing such children for common pediatric complaints, including skin rashes, earaches, and respiratory and gastrointestinal infections inasmuch as these children appear to handle such infections without undue difficulty. Varicella, however, is a major threat to all immunocompromised patients (because dissemination of disease is likely even in the absence of neutropenia). Before the availability of acyclovir, significant morbidity and mortality occurred in such patients. Immunocompromised children who are exposed by a sibling or a close playmate should receive varicella-zoster immunoglobulin within 4 days of the exposure. Should chickenpox occur, the patient should be admitted for treatment for 5 to 7 days with acyclovir. Chemotherapy usually is withheld during treatment of varicella.

Children who are receiving treatment for a malignancy should continue to see their primary pediatrician for well-child visits. This is in anticipation of their ultimate successful treatment and cure. Immunizations are delayed until 1 year after therapy is terminated, because live vaccines may cause disease, and inactivated vaccines rarely result in a normal immune response. The pediatrician should remain involved in continuing developmental issues that at times are exacerbated by the treatment of a malignancy. With the current success rates in treating children who have cancer, pediatricians should anticipate the return of these children to their practice for most of their care. Maintenance of a relationship with the patient and family is essential.

Care of Long-Term Survivors

Patients treated for childhood malignancy have, for the most part, received a number of extremely toxic agents, the long-term implications of which are incompletely known. Studies of a therapy's late toxicities are just beginning. Children should continue to return at least annually to the treating institution or to a similar institution elsewhere to be monitored for potential side effects and to be informed of problems occurring in patients treated similarly. Toxicities of radiation to particular areas (see Table 187-6) and of currently used chemotherapeutic agents (see Table 187-4) are listed, and recommended follow-up studies are described. The pediatrician should ensure that his or her patients are being screened appropriately.

Multidisciplinary clinics, which evaluate all survivors for potential late effects, are being formed in some hospitals. Subclinical evidence of cardiac damage after anthracycline administration and of pulmonary toxicity (decreased diffusing capacity) after bleomycin administration is found in some survivors, but whether the damage will be progressive is not clear. The long-term effects on renal function and hearing are not yet known. Fertility has been impaired in some patients who received alkylating therapies, but the incidence of dysfunction is lower than in adults treated similarly. Radiation to the gonads also causes infertility. Affected women need hormone replacement for feminization and to prevent the osteoporosis associated with estrogen depletion. Testosterone levels in treated males usually remain in the normal range, but they should be monitored.

Endocrine dysfunction after radiation may involve the thyroid, hypothalamus, and pituitary. Studies of the mechanism of impairment may help in treating other affected patients more effectively. Thyroid radiation often causes compensated (increased TSH, normal T_4) or overt (increased TSH, decreased T_4) hypothyroidism and should be treated with thyroid hormone.

Secondary malignancies are reported in long-term survivors. Mutagenic agents such as mechlorethamine and cyclophosphamide, and possibly etoposide and radiation therapy, play a role. A genetic predisposition to malignancy exists for those who have certain disorders (e.g., bilateral retinoblastoma).

The psychosocial effects of childhood cancer also differ from patient to patient. Some were so young when they received treatment that they do not remember the ordeal, whereas others had to forsake normal childhood experiences because of their illness. Some have no physical deficits, and others have permanent deformities (amputations, scoliosis, hair loss, scars). Although memories and physical handicaps may linger, survivors usually are cured of their cancer. They are emotionally intact people who are able to live and work normally within the mainstream. Unfortunately, certain workplaces and insurance companies continue to discriminate on the basis of a history of cancer. Because each tumor and treatment regimen is different, businesses and agencies must be educated to accept those who are cured and are likely to have a normal future.

Pediatricians must be advocates for these successfully treated persons. Past medical conditions that will not interfere with future health should not be a barrier to success; however, we must remain aware of potential late effects of therapy. Screening for toxicities will allow for interventions that can maintain health.

REFERENCES

1. Ablin AR et al: Malignant germ cell tumors in childhood: an outcome analysis, *Proc Am Soc Clin Oncol* 5:213, 1986.
2. Abramson DH, Ellsworth R, Zimmerman L: Nonocular cancer in retinoblastoma survivors, *Trans Am Acad Ophthalmol Otolaryngol* 81:454, 1976.
3. Abramson DH et al: Retinoblastoma: survival, age at detection and comparison 1914-1958, 1958-1983, *J Pediatr Ophthalmol Strabismus* 22:246, 1985.
4. Ashley DJB, Path FRC: Origin of teratomas, *Cancer* 32:390, 1973.
5. August CS et al: Treatment of advanced neuroblastoma with supralethal chemotherapy, radiation, and allogeneic or autologous marrow reconstitution, *J Clin Oncol* 2:609, 1984.
6. Beckwith JB, Palmer NF: Histopathology and prognosis of Wilms' tumor, *Cancer* 41:1937, 1978.
7. Beckwith JB, Perrin EV: In situ neuroblastoma: a contribution to the natural history of neural crest tumors, *Am J Pathol* 43:1089, 1963.
8. Bernard A et al: Cell surface characterization of malignant T cells from lymphoblastic lymphoma using monoclonal antibodies: evidence for a phenotypic difference between malignant T cells from patients with acute lymphoblastic leukemia and lymphoblastic lymphoma, *Blood* 57:1105, 1981.
9. Bernheim A, Berger R, Lenoir G: Cytogenetic studies on African Burkitt's lymphoma cell lines: t(8,14), t(2,8) and t(8,22) translocation, *Cancer Genet Cytogenet* 3:307, 1981.
10. Bonadonna G et al: Combination chemotherapy of Hodgkin's disease with adriamycin, bleomycin, vinblastine, and imidazole carboxamide versus MOPP, *Cancer* 36:252, 1975.
11. Bray PF et al: The coincidence of neuroblastoma and acute cerebellar encephalopathy, *J Pediatr* 76:983, 1969.
12. Breslow NE, Beckwith JB: Epidemiological features of Wilms' tumor:

results of the national Wilms' tumor study, *J Natl Cancer Inst* 68:429, 1982.

13. Carbone PP et al: Report of the Committee on Hodgkin's Disease Staging Classification, *Cancer Res* 31:1860, 1971.
14. Carli M et al: Therapeutic efficacy of single drugs for childhood neuroblastoma: a review. In Raybaud C et al, editors: *Pediatric oncology,* Amsterdam, 1982, Excerpta Medica.
15. Cassady JR et al: Radiation therapy in retinoblastoma, *Radiology* 93:405, 1969.
16. Chatten J, Voorhees ML: Familial neuroblastoma, *N Engl J Med* 277:1230, 1967.
17. Coleman CN: Secondary malignancy after treatment of Hodgkin's disease: an evolving picture, *J Clin Oncol* 4:821, 1986.
18. Constine LS et al: Thyroid dysfunction after radiotherapy in children with Hodgkin's disease, *Cancer* 53:878, 1984.
19. Cortes EP et al: Amputation and adriamycin in primary osteosarcoma, *N Engl J Med* 291:998, 1974.
20. D'Angio GJ: Wilms' tumor and neuroblastoma in children, *Pediatr Rev* 6:16, 1984.
21. D'Angio GJ et al: The treatment of Wilms' tumor: results of national Wilms' tumor study, *Cancer* 38:633, 1976.
22. D'Angio GJ et al: The treatment of Wilms' tumor: results of the second national Wilms' tumor study, *Cancer* 47:2302, 1981.
23. D'Angio GJ et al: Results of the third national Wilms' tumor study (NWTS-3): a preliminary report, *Am Assoc Cancer Res* 25:183, 1984.
24. Dahlin CD, Coventry MB: Osteosarcoma: a study of 600 cases, *J Bone Joint Surg (Am)* 49:101, 1967.
25. Dahlin DC, Coventry MB, Scanlon PW: Ewing's sarcoma: a critical analysis of 165 cases, *J Bone Joint Surg (Am)* 43:185, 1961.
26. Damewood MD, Grochow LB: Prospects for fertility after chemotherapy or radiation for neoplastic disease, *Fertil Steril* 45:443, 1986.
27. deCunha MF et al: Recovery of spermatogenesis after treatment for Hodgkin's disease: limiting dose of MOPP chemotherapy, *J Clin Oncol* 2:571, 1984.
28. Devesa SS: The incidence of retinoblastoma, *Am J Ophthalmol* 80:263, 1975.
29. DeVita VT Jr, Serpick A, Carbone PP: Combination chemotherapy in the treatment of advanced Hodgkin's disease, *Ann Intern Med* 73:881, 1970.
30. Dickman P, Liotta L, Triche T: Ewing's sarcoma: characterization in established cultures and evidence of its histogenesis, *Lab Invest* 47:375, 1982.
31. Donaldson SS: Rhabdomyosarcoma. In Carter S, Glatstein E, Livingston RB, editors: *Principles of cancer treatment,* New York, 1982, McGraw-Hill.
32. Donaldson SS, Kaplan HS: Complications of treatment of Hodgkin's disease in children, *Cancer Treat Rep* 66:977, 1982.
33. Donaldson SS, Link MP: Combined modality treatment with low-dose radiation and MOPP chemotherapy for children with Hodgkin's disease, *J Clin Oncol* 5:742, 1987.
34. Drash A et al: A syndrome of pseudohermaphrodism, Wilms' tumor, hypertension, and degenerative renal disease, *J Pediatr* 76:585, 1970.
35. Einhorn LG, Donahue JP: Combination chemotherapy in disseminated testicular cancer, *Semin Oncol* 6:87, 1979.
36. Ekert H et al: Experience with high dose multiagent chemotherapy and autologous bone marrow rescue in the treatment of twenty-two children with advanced tumors, *Aust Paediatr J* 20:195, 1984.
37. Evans R et al: Local recurrence, rate and sites of metastases, and time to relapse as a function of treatment regimen, size of primary and surgical history in 62 patients presenting with non-metastatic Ewing's sarcoma of the pelvic bones, *Int J Radiat Oncol Biol Phys* 11:129, 1885.
38. Ewing J: Diffuse endothelioma of bone, *Proc NY Pathol Soc* 21:17, 1921.
39. Exelby PR: Testicular cancer in children, *Cancer* 45:1803, 1980.
40. Falk S, Albert M: The clinical and roentgen aspects of Ewing's sarcoma, *Am J Med Sci* 54:44, 1965.
41. Farewell VT et al: Retrospective validation of a new staging system for Wilms' tumor, *Cancer Clin Trials* 4:167, 1981.
42. Farley F et al: Lactose dehydrogenase as a tumor marker for recurrent disease in Ewing's sarcoma, *Cancer* 59:1245, 1987.
43. Filipovitch A et al: Lymphomas in persons with naturally occurring immunodeficiency disorders. In Magrath I, O'Connor G, Ramot B, editors: *Pathogenesis of leukemias and lymphomas: environmental influences,* New York, 1984, Raven Press.
44. Frauman JF: Stature and malignant tumors of bone in childhood and adolescence, *Cancer* 20:967, 1967.
45. Gale G et al: Cancer in neonates: the experience at the Children's Hospital of Philadelphia, *Pediatrics* 70:409, 1982.
46. Gatti RA, Good RA: Occurrence of malignancy in immunodeficiency disease: a literature review, *Cancer* 28:89, 1971.
47. Gilman PA et al: Familial osteosarcoma associated with 13;14 chromosomal rearrangement, *Cancer Genet Cytogenet* 17:123, 1985.
48. Gitlow SE et al: Diagnosis of neuroblastoma by qualitative and quantitative determination of catecholamine metabolites in urine, *Cancer* 25:1377, 1970.
49. Glatstein E et al: The value of laparotomy and splenectomy in the staging of Hodgkin's disease, *Cancer* 24:709, 1969.
50. Grabowski EF, Abramson DH: Intraocular and extraocular retinoblastoma, *Hematol Oncol Clin North Am* 1:721, 1987.
51. Graham-Pole J et al: High dose chemotherapy supported by marrow infusion for advanced neuroblastoma: a Pediatric Oncology Group study; *J Clin Oncol* 9:152, 1991.
52. Grier H et al: Improved outcome in non-metastic Ewing's sarcoma (EWS) and PNET of bone with the addition of ifosfamide (I) and etoposide (E) to vincristine (V), Adriamycin (Ad) and Actinomycin (A), *Proc ASCO* 13:421, 1994.
53. Grosfeld JL et al: Benign and malignant teratomas in children: analysis of 85 patients, *Surgery* 80:297, 1976.
54. Grufferman SL, Delzell E: Epidemiology of Hodgkin's disease, *Epidemiol Rev* 6:76, 1984.
55. Hart WR, Burkons DM: Germ cell neoplasms arising in gonadoblastomas, *Cancer* 43:669, 1979.
56. Hawthorne HC et al: Blanching subcutaneous nodules in neonatal neuroblastoma, *J Pediatr* 77:297, 1970.
57. Hems G: An etiology of bone cancer, and some other cancers, in the young, *Br J Cancer* 24:208, 1970.
58. Ioachim HL, Cooper MC, Hellman GC: Lymphomas in men at high risk for acquired immune deficiency syndrome (AIDS): a study of 21 cases, *Cancer* 56:2831, 1985.
59. Jaffe N: Recent advance in the chemotherapy of metastatic osteogenic sarcoma, *Cancer* 30:1627, 1972.
60. Jaffe N: Malignant bone tumors, *Pediatr Ann* 4:10, 1975.
61. Jaffe N et al: Adjuvant methotrexate and citrovorum-factor treatment of osteogenic sarcoma, *N Engl J Med* 291:994, 1974.
62. Janjan NA et al: Mammary carcinoma developing after radiotherapy and chemotherapy for Hodgkin's disease, *Cancer* 61:252, 1988.
63. Jenkin R et al: The treatment of localized non-Hodgkin's lymphoma in children: a report from the Children's Cancer Study Group, *J Clin Oncol* 2:88, 1984.
64. Jurgens H et al: Multidisciplinary treatment of primary Ewing's sarcoma of bone: a 6-year experience of a European Cooperative Trial, *Cancer* 61:23, 1988.
65. Kaplan HS: *Hodgkin's disease,* ed 2, Cambridge, 1980, Harvard University Press.
66. Kauffman RA et al: False negative bone scans in neuroblastoma metastatic to the ends of long bones, *Am J Roentgenol* 130:131, 1978.
67. Kay R, Tank E: The current management of bilateral Wilms' tumor, *J Urol* 135:983, 1986.
68. Knudson AG: Mutation and cancer: statistical study of retinoblastoma, *Proc Natl Acad Sci USA* 68:820, 1971.
69. Knudson AG, Strong LC: Mutation and cancer: neuroblastoma and pheochromocytoma, *Am J Hum Genet* 24:514, 1972.
70. Koizumi JH, Dal Canto MC: Retroperitoneal neuroblastoma metastatic to brain: report of a case and review of the literature, *Child's Brain* 7:267, 1980.
71. LaBrosse EH: Biochemical diagnosis of neuroblastoma: use of a urine spot test, *Proc Am Assoc Cancer Res* 9:39, 1968.
72. Lack EE, Weinstein HJ, Welch KJ: Mediastinal germ cell tumors in childhood: a clinical and pathologic study of 21 cases, *J Thorac Cardiovasc Surg* 89:826, 1985.

73. Lawrence W et al: Prognostic significance of staging factors of the UICC staging system in childhood RMS: a report from the Intergroup Rhabdomyosarcoma Study (IRS-II), *J Clin Oncol* 5:46, 1987.
74. Leventhal BG, Donaldson SS: Hodgkin's disease. In Pizzo PA, Poplack DG, editors: *Principles and practice of pediatric oncology,* Philadelphia, 1989, JB Lippincott.
75. Li FP et al: Adverse pregnancy outcome after radiotherapy for childhood Wilms' tumor, *Proc ASCO* 5:202, 1986.
76. Li MC, Hertz R, Spencer DB: Effect of methotrexate on choriocarcinoma and chorioadenoma, *Proc Soc Exp Biol Med* 96:361, 1956.
77. Link MP et al: The effect of adjuvant chemotherapy on release-free survival in patients with osteosarcoma of the extremity, *N Engl J Med* 314:1600, 1986.
78. Look AT et al: Cellular DNA content as a predictor of response to chemotherapy in infants with unresectable neuroblastoma, *N Engl J Med* 311:231, 1984.
79. Lukes RJ, Butler JJ: The pathology and nomenclature of Hodgkin's disease, *Cancer Res* 26:1063, 1966.
80. Mackay B et al: Diagnosis of neuroblastoma by electron microscopy of bone marrow aspirates, *Pediatrics* 56:1045, 1975.
81. Magrath IT: Malignant non-Hodgkin's lymphomas. In Pizzo PA, Poplack DG, editors: *Principles and practice of pediatric oncology,* Philadelphia, 1988, JB Lippincott.
82. Magrath IT et al: Surgical reduction of tumor bulk in management of abdominal Burkitt's lymphoma, *BMJ* 2:308, 1974.
83. Mahour GH, Woolley GH, Landing BH: Ovarian tumors in children: a 33 year experience, *Am J Surg* 63:367, 1976.
84. Mandell L et al: Preliminary results of alternating combination chemotherapy (CT) and hyperfractionated radiotherapy (HART) in advanced rhabdomyosarcoma (RMS), *Int J Radiat Oncol Biol Phys* 15:197, 1988.
85. Marcove RC, Rosen G: En bloc resections for osteogenic sarcoma, *Cancer* 45:3040, 1980.
86. Margo CE, Zimmerman LE: Retinoblastoma: the accuracy of clinical diagnosis in children treated by enucleation, *J Pediatr Ophthalmol Strabismus* 20:227, 1983.
87. Martini N et al: Multiple pulmonary resections in the treatment of osteogenic sarcoma, *Ann Thorac Surg* 12:271, 1971.
88. Maurer H, Beltangody M, Gehan E: The Intergroup Rhabdomyosarcoma Study-1: a final report, *Cancer* 611:209, 1988.
89. Maurer H et al: Rhabdomyosarcoma in childhood and adolescence, *Curr Probl Cancer* 2:3, 1977.
90. Meadows AT, Lichtenfield JL, Koop CE: Wilms' tumor in three children of a woman with congenital hemihypertrophy, *N Engl J Med* 291:23, 1974.
91. Mendenhall C et al: The prognostic significance of soft tissue extension in Ewing's sarcoma, *Cancer* 51:913, 1983.
92. Meyer WH et al: Thoracotomy for pulmonary metastatic osteosarcoma, *Cancer* 59:374, 1987.
93. Murphy SB: Classification, staging, and end results of treatment of childhood non-Hodgkin's lymphomas: dissimilarities from lymphomas in adults, *Semin Oncol* 1:332, 1980.
94. Nonoyama M et al: Epstein-Barr virus DNA in Hodgkin's disease, American Burkitt's lymphoma and other human tumors, *Cancer Res* 34:1228, 1974.
95. Pegelow GH et al: Familial neuroblastoma, *J Pediatr* 87:763, 1975.
96. Pellici PG et al: Chromosomal breakpoints and structural alterations of the c-myc locus differ in endemic sporadic forms of Burkitt lymphoma, *Proc Natl Acad Sci USA* 83:2984, 1986.
97. Perez CA et al: Radiation therapy in the multimodal management of Ewing's sarcoma of bone: report of the Intergroup Ewing's Study, *Natl Cancer Inst Monogr* 56:262, 1981.
98. Pratt CB, Crom DB, Howarth C: The use of chemotherapy for extraocular retinoblastoma, *Med Pediatr Oncol* 13:330, 1985.
99. Probert JC, Parker BR, Kaplan HS: Growth retardation in children after megavoltage irradiation of the spine, *Cancer* 32:634, 1973.
100. Ramsey NKC et al: Acute hemorrhage into Wilms' tumor, *J Pediatr* 91:763, 1977.
101. Raney R et al: Improved prognosis with intensive treatment of children with cranial soft tissue sarcomas arising in nonorbital parameningeal sites: a report from the Intergroup Rhabdomyosarcoma Study, *Cancer* 59:147, 1987.
102. Reed DM: On the pathological changes in Hodgkin's disease, with especial reference to its relation to tuberculosis, *Johns Hopkins Hosp Rep* 10:133, 1902.
103. Rosen G et al: Ewing's sarcoma: ten year experience with adjuvant chemotherapy, *Cancer* 47:2204, 1981.
104. Rosen G et al: Preoperative chemotherapy for osteogenic sarcoma, *Cancer* 49:1221, 1982.
105. Rosenstock JG, D'Angio GJ, Kiesewetter WB: The incidence of complications following staging laparotomy for Hodgkin's disease in children, *Am J Roentgenol* 120:531, 1974.
106. Ruymann F et al: Bone marrow metastases at diagnosis in children and adolescents with RMS, a report from the Intergroup Rhabdomyosarcoma Study, *Cancer* 53:368, 1984.
107. Ruymann F et al: Congenital anomalies associated with RMS: an autopsy study of 115 cases—a report from the Intergroup Rhabdomyosarcoma Study Committee, *Med Pediatr Oncol* 16:33, 1988.
108. Santoro A et al: Long-term results of combined chemotherapy-radiotherapy approach in Hodgkin's disease: superiority of ABVD plus radiotherapy versus MOPP plus radiotherapy, *J Clin Oncol* 5:27, 1987.
109. Scheibel E et al: Vasoactive intestinal polypeptide (VIP) in children with neural crest tumors, *Acta Paediatr Scand* 71:721, 1982.
110. Seeger RC et al: Association of multiple copies of the N-mcy oncogene with rapid progression of neuroblastomas, *N Engl J Med* 313:111, 1985.
111. Shields JA: *Diagnosis and management of intraocular tumors,* St Louis, 1983, Mosby.
112. Sim F et al: Postradiation sarcoma of bone, *J Bone Joint Surg* 54A:1479, 1972.
113. Spitz MR et al: Ethnic patterns of Hodgkin's disease incidence among children and adolescents in the United States, 1973-1982,*J Natl Cancer Inst* 76:235, 1986.
114. Stafford WR, Yanoff M, Parnell B: Retinoblastoma initially misdiagnosed as primary ocular inflammations, *Arch Ophthalmol* 82:771, 1969.
115. Sterns JK, Coleman DJ, Ellsworth RM: The ultrasonographic characteristics of retinoblastoma, *Am J Ophthalmol* 78:606, 1974.
116. Sullivan MP et al: Intergroup Hodgkin's disease in children study of stages I and II: a preliminary report, *Cancer Treat Rep* 66:937, 1982.
117. Sweetnam R, Knowelden, Jedden H: Bone sarcoma: treatment by irradiation, amputation, or a combination of the two, *BMJ* 2:363, 1971.
118. Taylor WF et al: Trends and variability in survival from osteosarcoma, *Mayo Clin Proc* 53:695, 1978.
119. Tefft M et al: Acute and late effects on normal tissues following chemo- and radiotherapy for childhood RMS and Ewing's sarcoma, *Cancer* 37:1201, 1986.
120. Teilum G: Special tumors of ovary and testis and related neoplasms. In Levine AS, editor: *Cancer in the young,* New York, 1982, Masson Publishing USA.
121. Tepper J et al: Local control of Ewing's sarcoma of bone with radiotherapy and combination chemotherapy, *Cancer* 46:1969, 1983.
122. Thomas PRM et al: Late effects of treatment for Wilms' tumor, *Int J Radiat Oncol Biol Phys* 9:651, 1983.
123. Tsuchida Y et al: Evaluation of alpha-fetoprotein in early infancy, *Pediatr Surg* 13:155, 1978.
124. Uribe-Botero G et al: Primary osteosarcoma of bone: a clinicopathologic investigation of 243 cases with necropsy studies in 54, *Am J Clin Pathol* 67:427, 1977.
125. Vietti TJ et al: Multimodal therapy in metastatic Ewing's sarcoma: an intergroup study, *Natl Cancer Inst Monogr* 56:279, 1981.
126. Vinciguerra V et al: Alternating cycles of combination chemotherapy for patients with recurrent Hodgkin's disease following radiotherapy: a prospectively randomized study by the Cancer and Leukemia Group B, *J Clin Oncol* 4:838, 1986.
127. Whalen T et al: Sacrococcygeal teratomas in infants and children, *Am J Surg* 150:373, 1985.
128. Whang-Peng J et al: Chromosome translocation in peripheral neuroepithelioma, *N Engl J Med* 311:584, 1984.

129. White JJ et al: Conservatively aggressive management with bilateral Wilms' tumors, *J Pediatr Surg* 11:859, 1976.
130. Wiggs J et al: Prediction of the risk of hereditary retinoblastoma using DNA polymorphisms within the retinoblastoma gene, *N Engl J Med* 318:151, 1988.
131. Young JL et al: Cancer incidence, survival and mortality for children younger than age 15 years, *Cancer* 58:598, 1986.
132. Zech L et al: Characteristic chromosomal abnormalities in biopsies and lymphoid-cell lines from patients with Burkitt and non-Burkitt lymphomas, *Int J Cancer* 17:47, 1976.

191 Chickenpox

Evan G. Pattishall III

Chickenpox (varicella) is a common childhood viral disease characterized by a pruritic vesicular rash that appears in crops. It is highly contagious and has been regarded as a relatively benign disease, inasmuch as symptoms usually are mild and complications rare in healthy children. However, because of the increasing population of patients who are immunosuppressed or receiving therapy for malignancies, the educational impact of the disease through days lost from school, the financial impact of days lost from the work force by parents, and the developing possibility of prevention through immunization, the disease is now of greater concern.[43]

The *chicken* part of chickenpox is believed to derive from its likeness to the chickpea *Cicer areitinum,* or from the French for chickpea, *pois chiche.*[17,26] The word *varicella* is derived from a disease that is similar in appearance but is much more severe: variola (smallpox). Traditionally, *chickenpox* has been used to refer to the disease and *varicella* or *varicella-zoster virus* to refer to the virus.

ETIOLOGY

Chickenpox is caused by the varicella-zoster virus, a DNA virus and member of the herpesvirus family, along with the herpes simplex virus, cytomegalovirus, and Epstein-Barr virus. It has been established that the same virus causes both chickenpox and herpes zoster, the latter being a reactivation (after a latent phase) of the initial varicella infection.[17] Varicella-zoster virus can be isolated from the vesicles of both chickenpox and herpes zoster. It also has been isolated from blood and tissue during an infection but has proved more difficult to isolate from respiratory secretions. The virus is highly labile, losing its infectivity quickly in the external environment. Inactivation also can be accomplished by heat and trypsin. There is only one serotype of varicella-zoster virus, but different virus strains have been identified by means of restriction endonuclease patterns of DNA.[28]

TRANSMISSION

Chickenpox is one of the most contagious viral infections to cause disease in humans and is only slightly less contagious than measles and smallpox. Infection is thought to be spread by respiratory secretions as airborne particles from patients who can transmit infection before onset of the rash.[16] Virus has not been isolated from these secretions, however. Contact with the vesicular fluid of chickenpox or herpes zoster also will result in the transmission of chickenpox infection. Indirect contact (fomite transmission) probably is rare because of the lability of the varicella-zoster virus.

Varicella-zoster virus can cross the placenta during the first and early second trimester of pregnancy to produce a congenital varicella syndrome.[1,13,18,35] Maternal infection during the late third trimester of pregnancy similarly may result in transplacentally acquired varicella in the newborn.[31,39] Transplacentally acquired antibody to herpes zoster virus is partially protective to the newborn, but chickenpox has occurred in young infants born to immune mothers.

EPIDEMIOLOGY

Humans are the only known reservoir, or natural host, of the varicella-zoster virus. Transmission in the majority of cases is by droplet or by direct contact. The communicability period is considered to last from 1 or 2 days before the onset of the rash until 5 days after the onset of the rash or until all vesicles have crusted. Most vesicles have lost virus particles after 5 days. The incubation period is between 10 and 21 days, with an average of 14 to 15 days. With household exposure, clinical disease will develop in approximately 90% of susceptible contacts after one incubation period.[21,38]

Chickenpox, mainly a disease of childhood, has its maximum incidence at 6 years of age; 80% to 90% of children have been infected by 9 to 10 years of age.[17,30,37] Recently in England and Wales the incidence has changed, with the infection found most commonly in the neonate to 4-year age group.[24] Approximately 3 million cases occur each year in the United States. The disease occurs throughout the year, but most cases occur during the winter and spring months. There are epidemic occurrences every 2 to 3 years and are worldwide in distribution, but children in tropical climates have a lower rate of infection, so a greater number of susceptible persons remain uninfected among older age groups in the tropics than in temperate climates.

Subclinical infections with serological conversion rarely occur. Second clinical infections have been reported but are also rare.[16] Death rates from chickenpox are estimated to be 2 per 100,000 for children, 50 per 100,000 for adults, 7000 per 100,000 for immunocompromised patients, and 31,000 per 100,000 for neonates.[21]

PATHOGENESIS

Varicella infection is transmitted by droplet or airborne spread, with entrance into the susceptible individual through the respiratory tract. The virus migrates to the regional lymph nodes, where primary replication occurs. Approximately 4 to 6 days later a primary viremia spreads the virus to internal organs, where secondary replication occurs. This is followed by a secondary viremia, which spreads the organism to the skin and is followed by clinical chickenpox. Viremia has been documented in blood-borne monocytes after exposure but before onset of the rash or symptoms.[48] The appearance of the rash in crops probably is the result of an intermittent secondary viremia.[19]

The rash at first is macular and then progresses to a papular lesion that contains a minute vacuole. Fluid accumulates in the vacuole, causing a vesicle to appear on a reddened base to produce the classic "dewdrop on a rose petal" lesion. Multinucleated giant cells can be identified in the base and on the edges of the vesicle along with eosinophilic type A intranuclear inclusions. As the rash resolves, the vesicle becomes cloudy and fills with fibrinous fluid and leukocytes. A crust develops that may remain attached for 1 to 2 weeks.

When a vesicle occurs on mucous membranes, its roof sloughs to leave a shallow ulcer. There is evidence that interferon, produced by the polymorphonuclear cells in the lesion, may contribute to resolution of the disease.[46]

CLINICAL MANIFESTATIONS

Normal Children

Chickenpox usually begins with either no prodrome or only a slight malaise and low-grade fever. This is followed in a few hours to days by a macular rash, usually on the scalp, neck, or upper portion of the trunk. The macules progress to a papular, vesicular, pruritic rash usually within 12 to 24 hours. Vesicles appear in crops, with a new crop occurring every 1 to 2 days over the next 2 to 5 days, resulting in two to four crops during the illness. The vesicles turn to pustules and then crust. The case usually runs its course in 5 to 10 days. At the height of the disease lesions in all phases from early vesicles to crusts can be seen. Fever varies from none to 102° F (38.9°C) at the onset of the disease and may continue until vesicles cease to appear. The rash spreads centrifugally and involves all areas of the skin in severe cases. Vesicles are pruritic, and excoriations frequently are seen. Lesions occur more frequently in areas of irritation, dermatitis, or skinfolds. Occasionally the skin rash will appear as a macular rash in the diaper area or on the trunk and remain for a day or two before becoming vesicular, making early diagnosis more difficult. Vesicles may occur on the mucous membranes of the mouth, conjunctiva, esophagus, trachea, rectum, or vagina. Generally little scarring occurs, unless the lesions become superinfected or are continually traumatized. Areas where pox have occurred may, however, remain hypopigmented or hyperpigmented months after the rash has resolved. Occasionally lesions are bullous, as a variant of the disease itself, but these more often are caused by a staphylococcal superinfection. White blood cell counts and other laboratory test results usually are normal.

Older Children and Adults

Chickenpox in older children and adults usually is more severe than in younger age groups, with a prodrome that may include irritability, listlessness, headaches, chills, anorexia, and myalgias. Fever usually is present and is higher and more prolonged than in the young child. The rash, too, tends to be more severe. The risk of complications is 9 to 25 times greater; for example, varicella pneumonia has been observed to occur in 15% to 50% of older patients.[29]

Immunocompromised Children

Immunocompromised children usually have the most severe symptoms and are at greatest risk of death from chickenpox infection, with the exception of the neonate. "Progressive varicella" can be seen in children who are immunocompromised naturally or are being treated by immunosuppression for malignancies.[46] It manifests by a more severe prodrome followed by dissemination of the varicella-zoster virus. This occurs in 30% of cases in which spread to the lungs, liver, pancreas, or CNS can be identified. Even if progressive varicella does not develop, these patients still have higher fevers and more prolonged vesicular eruption than does the nonimmunocompromised child. Vesicles may be larger and hemorrhagic. All complications of chickenpox are increased in this population, with varicella pneumonia being the most common cause of death. Children receiving steroid therapy for disease other than cancer also are at risk for more severe involvement and complications.

Congenital and Neonatal Varicella

Infants born to mothers who contract chickenpox during the first trimester of pregnancy have a 2% to 17% risk of having congenital varicella. This syndrome includes one or more of the following defects: low birth weight, cicatricial skin lesions, a hypotrophic limb, eye abnormalities, brain damage, and mental retardation.[1,13,20,35]

When mothers have clinical chickenpox immediately before delivery, there is a 24% infection rate among their infants. If the onset of maternal rash is earlier than 5 days preceding delivery or if the onset of rash in the infant occurs at less than 4 days of age, there seems to be little risk of death. This reprieve probably is attributable at least in part to maternally transferred immunity. If, on the other hand, the maternal rash emerges within 4 days of delivery or if the newborn rash begins at 5 to 10 days of age, there is an associated 21% to 31% mortality.[31,35,39] The risk is uncertain for infants who are nursing when the mother contracts chickenpox.

COMPLICATIONS

Secondary Bacterial Infection

Secondary bacterial infection is the most common complication of chickenpox. Infection usually is by group A streptococci or *Staphylococcus aureus* and can lead to all the complications associated with these organisms, including scarlet fever, nephritis, cellulitis, abscess, gangrene, pneumonia, conjunctivitis, sepsis, and erysipelas. Bullous lesions caused by *S. aureus* may begin on the second or third day of the rash and manifest as bullous impetigo.[7,17]

Reye Syndrome

The association of Reye syndrome and chickenpox has been publicized and may cause parental concern. Approximately 16% to 28% of cases of Reye syndrome are preceded by varicella infection. It is less common, however, for Reye syndrome to follow varicella than to occur after influenza A or B infection. The age distributions of chickenpox-associated Reye syndrome and chickenpox itself are similar, being most common in 5- to 9-year-olds, followed by 10- to 14-year-olds and then 1- to 4-year-olds. Because of the suggested association between Reye syndrome and aspirin, it is recommended that aspirin be avoided in the treatment of chickenpox.

Neurological Complications

Nervous system complications include cerebral encephalitis—the most common—followed by cerebellar encephalitis, aseptic meningitis, myelitis, and peripheral neuropathy.[23] In a more recent study cerebellar complications were more common than cerebral infections, occurring in 1 in 4000 cases of chickenpox.[20] The onset of symptoms has been reported 4 days preceding until 3 weeks after the appearance of the rash. Symptoms are those that normally would be associated with encephalitis, meningitis, myelitis, or peripheral neuropathy. A toxic encephalopathy caused by diphenhydramine toxicity has been reported, which may mimic neurological complications.[12]

Pneumonia

Varicella pneumonia occurs most often among adults and immunocompromised children.[29] It is one of the more common causes of death. In children it occurs in 1 per 10,000 cases of chickenpox, but in adults it may be present in 30% to 50% of cases of varicella. Manifestations range from a lack of clinical symptoms with abnormal findings on the chest roentgenogram to symptoms that include rales, tachypnea, hemoptysis, chest pain, cyanosis, and respiratory failure.

Hematological Complications

Febrile purpura, malignant chickenpox with purpura, postinfectious purpura, purpura fulminans, and Henoch-Schönlein purpura all have been described as occurring with varicella infections.[8] Onset occurs from 3 to 5 days to 2 to 3 weeks after the chickenpox rash appears.

Hepatitis

Hepatitis has been reported during chickenpox infections and is marked by the onset of abdominal pain, vomiting, and continued fever on the second to fourth day after the rash appears.[11] Liver function tests become abnormal but return to normal with resolution of the abdominal symptoms. No progression to Reye syndrome occurs, and the blood ammonia level is normal. One study of 39 children who had uncomplicated chickenpox found 47% to have a mildly increased level of AST (SGOT) and 29% to have markedly increased AST levels.[36] Whether this condition actually is hepatitis or early Reye syndrome still is not clear.

Zoster

Zoster is the reactivation of the varicella-zoster virus that has remained dormant after clinical chickenpox.[17] It is believed that the virus resides in the dorsal nerve ganglia and is reactivated by periods of decreased host immunity or other unknown stimuli. During reactivation the rash covers the dermatome that corresponds to the infected nerve root. Disseminated zoster, however, also can occur. Zoster has been described in all age groups, including in infancy after prenatal exposure to varicella virus resulting from maternal chickenpox. Children who have varicella infections at younger ages, especially when the infection occurs before the child is 1 year of age, have an increased incidence of zoster later in life.[3]

Other Complications

Appendicitis, myocarditis, arthritis, nephritis, orchitis, splenic hemorrhage and rupture, conjunctivitis, necrotizing fasciitis, pancreatitis, pericarditis, optic neuritis, and parotitis have been reported, but rarely.[7,17]

DIAGNOSIS

Chickenpox usually is diagnosed on a clinical basis. There may be a history of exposure. White blood cell counts usually are normal. A Tzanck smear (scraping of the base of a vesicle and staining with Giemsa or Wright stain) will be positive for multinucleated giant cells in varicella-zoster virus infections.[41,42] Herpes simplex types 1 and 2 also produce a positive Tzanck smear.[34] Electron microscopy and viral cultures can be used to demonstrate virus in the vesicular fluid. Viral antigen has been identified in vesicular fluid by countercurrent immunoelectrophoresis. Polymerase chain reaction (PCR) tests have been demonstrated to be superior to viral culture in identification of varicella virus from vesicles.[32] Viral titers during acute and convalescent stages can document a recent infection if acute titers are obtained early in the illness (preferably day 1 or 2) and higher titers are noted during convalescence 2 to 6 weeks later.

DIFFERENTIAL DIAGNOSIS

Smallpox (variola) historically has been the most important disease to be differentiated from chickenpox. This can easily be done with a Tzanck smear or other of the aforementioned laboratory tests, but it has not been necessary since the eradication of smallpox.

Vaccinia (cowpox) will produce a vesicular rash resulting from exposure to infected livestock or, in former years, from direct contact with a smallpox vaccination.

Disseminated *herpes simplex* can resemble the chickenpox rash, but the history and progression of the disease usually differentiate these two entities. Such a situation is more confusing in newborns because disseminated herpes is rare in normal children; a Tzanck smear will be positive in both diseases.[34,41,42] *Rickettsial pox* can resemble chickenpox, but its vesicles are deeper and occur at the same stage of development, and there is a more severe prodrome.

Viral exanthems, especially *coxsackievirus* and *echovirus,* can produce vesicular exanthems that usually do not crust and that follow a distinctly different course. The Tzanck smear is negative in these infections. Lesions of *Stevens-Johnson syndrome* can resemble chickenpox, but the two diseases follow different clinical courses and the rashes develop differently. A Tzanck smear will be negative. *Contact dermatitis* may produce a rash similar to that of chickenpox (including pruritus) but has a different distribution and evolution.

Insect bites and scabies occasionally cause confusion if they are vesicular. *Bullous impetigo* (especially staphylococcal skin infection) may produce bullae that resemble chickenpox.

TREATMENT

Treatment of symptoms with acetaminophen for control of fever and relief of prodromal symptoms, along with measures to control pruritus, usually are sufficient. However, treatment of children with acetaminophen has been associated with a prolongation of the illness.[9] Pruritus can be controlled with antihistamine (diphenhydramine), calamine lotion, or Cetaphil lotion (containing cetyl alcohol, stearyl alcohol, sodium lauryl sulfate, propylene glycol, butylparaben, methylparaben, propylparaben, and purified water), and with 0.25% menthol lotion. Diphenhydramine, applied topically in lotions and administered orally, has been associated with encephalopathy in patients who have chickenpox.[12,40,44]

Despite the popular belief that bathing is contraindicated, patients should be encouraged to take daily baths to help prevent bacterial superinfection. Adding baking soda to a warm (not hot) bath helps to relieve the pruritus. Children's nails should be cut and kept clean, and scratching should be discouraged. Occasionally gloves or socks on the hands are required to prevent opening of lesions by scratching. If superinfection is present, it is usually a result of group-A streptococci or *S. aureus*. This may be treated topically with bacitracin ointment or systemically with an appropriate antibiotic. The Centers for Disease Control and Prevention recommend avoiding aspirin in the treatment of chickenpox until its suspected association with Reye syndrome is further defined. Physicians caring for patients who are taking aspirin on a chronic basis for juvenile rheumatoid arthritis or other diseases will need to consider the risks versus the benefits of this therapy on an individual basis if these patients develop chickenpox.

Treatment with adenine arabinoside, acyclovir, transfer factor, and interferon has been attempted in immunosuppressed patients or patients who have progressive chickenpox.[6,46] Acyclovir and adenine arabinoside have been effective in varicella therapy. The choice of therapy, however, must be individualized by a consideration of the patient's age, weight, and other concurrent conditions or diseases.[2,15,45]

Acyclovir has been shown to be effective in the treatment of varicella infections in normal children and adolescents. When instituted within 24 hours of the onset of rash, treatment has resulted in a reduction in duration of illness, number of cutaneous lesions, fever, and systemic symptoms.[4,5,10] Antibody titers 1 year later were equal in the treated and untreated patients.[10] In one study treatment of the index case with acyclovir did not change the transmission rate to other susceptible household contacts.[4] Routine use of acyclovir for varicella infection in normal children and adolescents continues to be controversial in the pediatric literature.

Occasionally pruritus is so severe that sedation of a patient is considered. If done, this procedure should be regarded with extreme caution because of possible "masking" of CNS complications or Reye syndrome.

Hospitalization should be avoided whenever possible because hospital epidemics can occur even when the strictest isolation procedures are followed. These generally have spread by infection of staff members who were thought to be immune or by airborne spread of the virus through ventilation systems. When unavoidable, hospitalization requires strict isolation. *Hospitalization on an adult ward* with no immunosuppressed patients may lessen the chances of spread in hospitals where effective strict isolation is not available.[14]

PREVENTION

Isolation of the patient to prevent subsequent exposure is the easiest means of prevention. This is not always effective, however, inasmuch as the disease is contagious 1 to 2 days before the appearance of the rash.

When indicated, passive prevention may be attempted by administering varicella-zoster immunoglobulin (VZIG) within 72 to 96 hours of a known or suspected exposure.[18,21,27,47] With VZIG administration, disease usually will be prevented in normal children and less severe in adults and immunocompromised patients. Guidelines for the administration of VZIG are outlined in the February 24, 1984, issue of *Morbidity and Mortality Weekly Report*.[21] The use of interferon and transfer factor in prevention is experimental.[46]

A live virus vaccine has been developed and tested successfully both in immunosuppressed and in normal children.[22,25,33] The varicella vaccine has been licensed for use in the United States and has been shown to be effective in preventing infection in most recipients.[25] It is recommended for administration to children 1 year and older who are susceptible to varicella infection. When incomplete immunity is conveyed after vaccine administration, the disease is reduced in severity and duration. Varicella vaccine is an attenuated live vaccine; therefore its use in immunocompromised persons needs to be individualized.

REFERENCES

1. Alkalay A, Pomerance JJ, Rimoin DL: Fetal varicella syndrome, *J Pediatr* 111:320, 1987.
2. Arvin AM: Oral therapy with acyclovir in infants and children, *Pediatr Infect Dis J* 6:56, 1987.
3. Baba K et al: Increased incidence of herpes zoster in normal children infected with varicella zoster virus during infancy: community-based follow-up study, *J Pediatr* 108:372, 1986.
4. Balfour HH Jr et al: Acyclovir treatment of varicella in otherwise healthy children, *J Pediatr* 116:633, 1990.
5. Balfour HH Jr et al: Acyclovir treatment of varicella in otherwise healthy adolescents, *J Pediatr* 120:627, 1992.
6. Bean B, Balfour HH: Varicella-zoster infection: advances in prevention and treatment, *Minn Med* 66:623, 1983.
7. Bullowa J, Wishile SM: Complications of varicella, *Am J Dis Child* 49:923, 1935.
8. Charkes ND: Purpuric chickenpox: report of a case, review of the literature and classification by clinical features, *Ann Intern Med* 54:745, 1961.
9. Doran T et al: Acetaminophen: more harm than good for chickenpox? *J Pediatr* 114:1045, 1989.
10. Dunkle LM et al: A controlled trial of acyclovir for chickenpox in normal children, *N Engl J Med* 325:1539, 1991.
11. Ey J, Smith S, Fulginiti V: Varicella hepatitis without neurologic symptoms or findings, *Pediatrics* 67:285, 1981.
12. Filloux F: Toxic encephalopathy caused by topically applied diphenhydramine, *J Pediatr* 108:1018, 1986.
13. Fuccillo D: Congenital varicella, *Teratology* 15:329, 1977.
14. Gardner P, Breton S, Charles D: Hospital isolation and precaution guidelines, *Pediatrics* 53:663, 1974.
15. Gershon AA: Live attenuated varicella vaccine, *J Pediatr* 10:154, 1987.
16. Gershon AA et al: Clinical reinfection with varicella-zoster virus, *J Infect Dis* 149:137, 1984.
17. Gordon JE: Chickenpox: an epidemiological review, *Am J Med Sci* 244:362, 1962.
18. Greenspoon J: Fetal varicella syndrome, *J Pediatr* 223:505, 1988 (letter).
19. Grose C: Variation on a theme by Fenner: the pathogenesis of chickenpox, *Pediatrics* 68:735, 1981.
20. Guess HA et al: Population-based studies of varicella complications, *Pediatrics* 78:723, 1986.

21. Immunization Practices Advisory Committee: Varicella-zoster immunoglobulin for the prevention of chickenpox, *MMWR* 33:84, 1984.
22. Johnson CE et al: Live attenuated varicella vaccine in healthy 12- to 24-month-old children, *Pediatrics* 81:512, 1988.
23. Johnson R, Milbourn P: Central nervous system manifestations of chickenpox, *Can Med Assoc J* 102:831, 1970.
24. Joseph CA, Noah ND: Epidemiology of chickenpox in England and Wales, 1967-85, *Br Med J (Clin Res)* 296:673, 1988.
25. Krause PR, Klinman DM: Efficacy, immunogenicity, safety, and use of live attenuated chickenpox vaccine, *J Pediatr* 127:518, 1995.
26. Lerman SC: Why is chickenpox called chickenpox? *Clin Pediatr* 20:111, 1981.
27. Lipton SV, Brunell PA: Management of varicella exposure in a neonatal intensive care unit, *JAMA* 26:1782, 1989.
28. Martin JH: Restriction endonuclease analysis of varicella-zoster vaccine virus and wild-type DNAs, *J Med Virol* 9:69, 1982.
29. Mermelstein R, Freiveich A: Varicella pneumonia, *Ann Intern Med* 55:456, 1961.
30. Muench R et al: Seroepidemiology of varicella, *J Infect Dis* 153:153, 1986.
31. Myers J: Congenital varicella in term infants: risks reconsidered, *J Infect Dis* 129:215, 1974.
32. Nahass GT et al: Comparison of Tzanck smear, viral culture, and DNA diagnostic methods in detection of herpes simplex and varicella-zoster infections, *JAMA* 268:2541, 1992.
33. Ndumbe PM, Cradock-Watson J, Levinsky RJ: Natural and artificial immunity to varicella zoster virus, *J Med Virol* 25:171, 1988.
34. Oranje AP et al: Diagnostic value of Tzanck smear in herpetic and nonherpetic vesicular and bullous skin disorders in pediatric practice, *Acta Derm Venereol (Stockh)* 66:127, 1986.
35. Paryani SG, Arvin AM: Intrauterine infection with varicella-zoster virus after maternal varicella, *N Engl J Med* 314:1542, 1986.
36. Pitel PA et al: Subclinical hepatic changes in varicella infection, *Pediatrics* 65:631, 1980.
37. Preblud S, D'Angelo L: Chickenpox in the United States 1972-1977, *J Infect Dis* 140:257, 1979.
38. Ross AH: Modification of chickenpox in family contacts by administration of gamma globulin, *N Engl J Med* 267:369, 1962.
39. Rubin L et al: Disseminated varicella in a neonate: implications for immunoprophylaxis of neonates postnatally exposed to varicella, *Pediatr Infect Dis* 5:100, 1986.
40. Schunk JE, Svendsen D: Diphenhydramine toxicity from combined oral and topical use, *Am J Dis Child* 142:1020, 1988 (letter).
41. Solomon AR: The Tzanck smear: viable and valuable in the diagnosis of herpes simplex, zoster and varicella, *Int J Dermatol* 25:169, 1986.
42. Solomon AR, Rasmussen JE, Weiss JS: A comparison of the Tzanck smear and viral isolation in varicella and herpes zoster, *Arch Dermatol* 122:282, 1986.
43. Sullivan-Bolyai JZ et al: Impact of chickenpox on households of healthy children, *Pediatr Infect Dis J* 6:33, 1987.
44. Tomlinson G, Helfaer M, Wiedermann BL: Diphenhydramine toxicity mimicking varicella encephalitis, *Pediatr Infect Dis J* 6:220, 1987.
45. Vilde JL: Comparative trial of acyclovir and vidarabine in disseminated varicella-zoster virus infections in immunocompromised patients, *J Med Virol* 20:127, 1986.
46. Weller T: Varicella and herpes zoster, *N Engl J Med* 309:1362, 1984.
47. Wurzel CL, Rubin LG, Krilov LR: Varicella zoster immunoglobulin after postnatal exposure to varicella: survey of experts, *Pediatr Infect Dis J* 6:466, 1987.
48. Yoshizo A et al: Viremia is present in incubation period in nonimmunocompromised children with varicella, *J Pediatr* 106:69, 1985.

SUGGESTED READINGS

Krause PR, Klinman DM: Efficacy, immunogenicity, safety and use of attenuated chickenpox vaccine, *J Pediatr* 127:518, 1995.

Straus SE et al: NIH conference. Varicella-zoster virus infections: biology, natural history, treatment and prevention (published erratum appears in *Ann Intern Med* 109:438, 1988).

192 Chronic Fatigue Syndrome

Leonard R. Krilov and Stanford B. Friedman

Chronic fatigue syndrome (CFS) has been used to describe an illness characterized by prolonged periods of debilitating fatigue for which no definitive cause has been determined. Although the U.S. Centers for Disease Control and Prevention has created a working definition of CFS for study purposes,[2] CFS nevertheless is not a well-defined clinical entity. No specific etiological agent(s) and no characteristic pathophysiological model have been identified for CFS. Debate centers on the contributions of infectious, immunological, and psychological factors to the clinical manifestations of CFS. It is likely that all these factors interact to produce CFS, albeit to differing degrees in each individual.

Historically a variety of syndromes that appear similar to CFS have been described.[9] These include chronic infectious mononucleosis, total allergy syndrome, chronic candidiasis, hypoglycemia, neurasthenia, myalgic encephalomyelitis, postviral syndrome, and fibromyalgia. All these diagnoses are characterized by signs and symptoms similar to those of CFS, as well as the inability to develop a definitive diagnostic test or confirm a definitive causative agent. Cases of CFS have been reported to occur both sporadically and epidemically.

The majority of reported cases of CFS have occurred in white women—a median age of 35 to 40 years and from upper socioeconomic groups, although adolescents who have the diagnosis also have been described.[5,8] Minorities, the indigent, and those living in developing countries are strikingly underrepresented in reports of CFS. Whether this observation reflects a bias in patient selection or predisposing factors for development of CFS remains to be determined.

CLINICAL MANIFESTATIONS

The primary manifestation of CFS is severe fatigue greater than 6 months in duration that limits the individual to activity less than 50% of the premorbid level of function. Associated symptoms frequently include sore throat, low-grade fever (oral temperatures of 37.5° to 38.6° C), painful lymph nodes, unexplained generalized weakness, myalgias and/or arthralgias, prolonged fatigue after exercise, headaches, difficulty concentrating or memory loss, and sleep disturbances (hypersomnia or insomnia). The majority of patients describe a sudden onset of the syndrome with an initial mononucleosis or flulike illness, although in some cases a more gradual onset is related. Many patients also describe a history of atopy and/or multiple allergies.

The initial history should include questions about the nature and duration of symptoms, as well as possible exposures to or contacts with ill persons that might suggest an alternative diagnosis. Personal and social history to assess family dynamics, prior level of functioning, response to illness, and family history of psychiatric illness may be helpful.

The physical examination may reveal abnormalities including (1) mild inflammation of the pharynx, (2) cervical or axillary lymphadenopathy, and/or (3) low-grade temperature elevation in up to 50% of cases. However, the primary goal of the physical examination is to eliminate other causes for the patient's symptoms. Significantly elevated temperatures, enlarged lymph nodes (>2 cm), weight loss of more than 10% of body mass without dieting, or focal neurological abnormalities should suggest an alternative diagnosis. The differential diagnoses of illnesses associated with extensive fatigue are listed in the box on p. 1245.

PSYCHOLOGICAL FACTORS

Clinicians and investigators have noted a relationship of CFS to depressive symptoms, frank depression, and a family history of depression.[3] Conceptually, depression may be both part of the etiology of CFS *and* a secondary reaction to having CFS. We have been impressed with the family dynamics of adolescents who have CFS.[6] School avoidance behaviors related to high expectations for academic performance compared with the teenager's abilities have been noted frequently. In many families we also have noted overprotection and overindulgence of the child, often associated with difficulty in mother-teen separation. A recent analysis of adolescents who have CFS compared with age-matched adolescent survivors of childhood cancer and a healthy control group showed that the CFS group had higher scores on measures of somatic complaints, depression, internalizing symptoms, and feeling different from others.[6]

The manifestations of CFS can be considered in this framework as a conversion reaction in which an infection or other stressor serves as a model for persistent symptoms that offer the individual a mechanism by which to maintain an overprotective environment or to avoid going to school (see Chapter 96, Conversion Reactions in Adolescents).

LABORATORY DIAGNOSIS

There are no specific laboratory tests by which to diagnose CFS. As with the physical examination the primary aim of laboratory evaluations is to eliminate other conditions that may be responsible for the patient's symptoms. A suggested battery of screening tests might include a complete blood count and differential; measurement of the erythrocyte sedimentation rate (ESR), serum electrolytes, creatinine, BUN, and glucose; liver function tests; thyroid function tests; tuberculin skin test with controls; measurement of alkaline phosphatase, antinuclear antibodies (ANA), rheumatoid factor, and HIV antibody; and chest and sinus radiographs. Additional tests (e.g., Lyme serology, viral serologies) may be indicated based on history and physical examination findings. Although potential immunological abnormalities, including

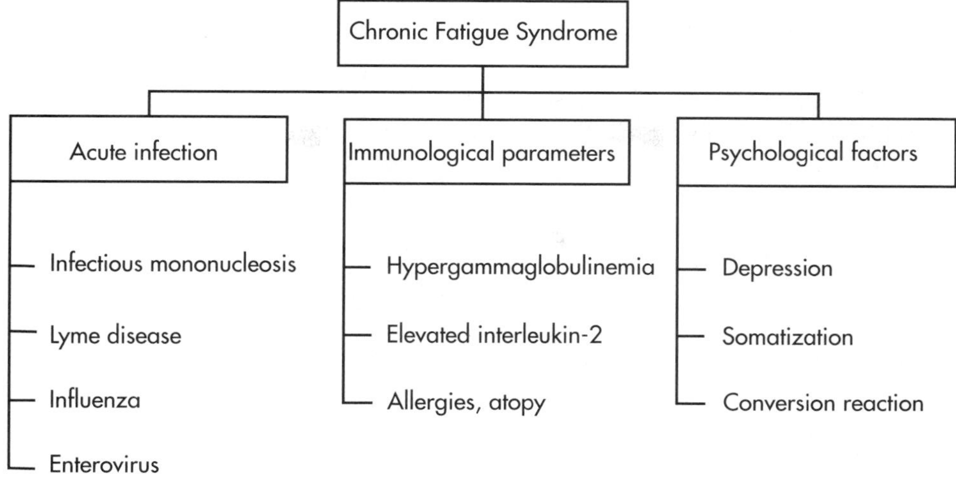

FIG. 192-1 Pathogenesis of chronic fatigue syndrome.

DIFFERENTIAL DIAGNOSIS OF A PATIENT WHO IS CHRONICALLY FATIGUED

- Malignancy
- Autoimmune disease
- Localized infection (e.g., sinusitis, occult abscess)
- Chronic or subacute infection (e.g., Lyme disease, endocarditis, tuberculosis)
- HIV infection
- Fungal disease (e.g., Candidiasis, histoplasmosis, coccidioidomycosis, blastomycosis)
- Parasitic disease (e.g., toxoplasmosis, giardiasis)
- Chronic inflammatory disease (e.g., sarcoidosis, Wegener granulomatosis)
- Endocrine disease (e.g., hypothyroidism, Addison disease, diabetes)
- Neuromuscular disease (e.g., myasthenia gravis, multiple sclerosis)
- Drug dependency
- Side effects of chronic medications or other toxic agents (e.g., chemical solvent, heavy metal, pesticide)
- Psychiatric disorder

altered lymphocyte subsets, qualitative defects in natural killer cell activity, hypo- or hypergammaglobulinemia, elevated titers to herpes viruses (e.g., EBV, HHV-6), abnormal lymphokine levels, and decreased lymphocyte proliferation responses, have been described in patients who have CFS, they have not been observed consistently in different groups of patients.[1] Additionally the magnitude of immunological abnormalities detected in patients who have CFS has been small compared with classic immunodeficiencies; the degree of immune aberrations does not correlate with the severity of symptoms, and opportunistic infections do not occur in CFS.

Although of uncertain significance, increased white matter on T2 MRI scans suggestive of possible infiltration of the perivascular spaces, focal demyelination, or disease of the small blood vessels of the cerebral white matter has been reported in a number of CFS patients.[7]

PROPOSED MODEL OF PATHOGENESIS

Exact definition of a case of CFS is difficult in that there are few objective findings in these individuals and their most severe symptoms are difficult to quantify. To date no specific infectious cause for CFS has been defined, and it seems unlikely that a single infectious agent is responsible. It seems reasonable to suggest that it is the interaction of multiple factors, as depicted in Figure 192-1, that results in the development of CFS. The relative importance of each of the factors probably varies from individual to individual.

THERAPY

No specific therapy for the CFS has been proven to be effective. However, management strategies aimed at alleviating the patient's symptoms may help. An approach to the management of CFS is outlined in the box on p. 1246. The primary goals of this treatment are to provide symptomatic relief for depression, sleep disorders, musculoskeletal pains; offer emotional support with involvement of a social worker, psychologist, or psychiatrist, as needed; identify and eliminate "secondary gain" from continuing to contribute to the illness; and to devise programs with the patient to increase school (or work) attendance and exercise capability gradually. Periodic physical examinations for possible other conditions also are important. Family therapy often helps the parents manage these issues and addresses the role of family dynamics in the evolution of a patient's symptoms. A team approach with coordination of services to avoid "doctor shopping" and fad therapy is critical to the successful management of the patient who has CFS.

Some of the unproved fad therapies described are megavitamin treatment, immune modifiers (e.g., Ampligen, thymic extract, interleukin-2), magnesium sulfate, liver extract injections, anti-candida diets, colonic irrigation, and removal of dental fillings. Immunoglobulin injections have been reported to be beneficial in one study of CFS patients,[4] although two subsequent studies failed to confirm this observation.

MANAGEMENT OF PEDIATRIC PATIENTS WHO ARE CHRONICALLY FATIGUED

Confirm the diagnosis of CFS and acknowledge the symptoms as real
Explain and explore the potential relationship to psychological symptoms
Stress a coordinated approach; minimize doctor shopping, unnecessary testing, and unconventional therapies
Use stress-coping skills: modify life-styles, decrease stress, develop a realistic schedule including working with school (gradual return to classes, home tutoring, neuropsychometric testing), and develop a graduated exercise program
Use cognitive-behavioral approaches: pay attention to sleep patterns and nutrition; increase activity gradually
Provide psychological support: individual therapy, family therapy, decrease secondary gain
Maintain follow-up: monitor physical symptoms and psychological issues; provide ongoing guidance and continued reassurance

PROGNOSIS AND FUTURE PROSPECTS

Despite the vagaries associated with the diagnosis of CFS and differences in each case, long-term follow up suggests that most individuals report improvement or resolution of symptoms over a 2- to 3-year period. Few patients report progressive symptoms, although symptoms may wax and wane in severity. With better definition of the nature of the neurological and immunological alterations in CFS, additional therapeutic approaches may become available.

REFERENCES

1. Barker E et al: Immunologic abnormalities associated with chronic fatigue syndrome, *Clin Infect Dis* 18 (suppl 1):136, 1994.
2. Holmes GP et al: Chronic fatigue syndrome: a working case definition, *Ann Intern Med* 108:387, 1988.
3. Katon WJ et al: Psychiatric assessment of patients with chronic fatigue and those with rheumatoid arthritis, *J Gen Intern Med* 6:278, 1991.
4. Lloyd A et al: A double-blind, placebo-controlled trial of intravenous immunoglobulin therapy in patients with chronic fatigue syndrome, *Am J Med* 89:561, 1990.
5. Marshall GS et al: Chronic fatigue in children: clinical features of Epstein-Barr virus and human herpes virus 6 serology and long-term follow-up, *Pediatr Infect Dis J* 10:287, 1991.
6. Pelcoviz D et al: Psychosocial correlates of chronic fatigue syndrome in adolescence, *J Dev Behav Pediatr* 16:333, 1995.
7. Schwartz RB: Neuroradiologic features. In Dawson DM, Sabin TD, editors: *Chronic fatigue syndrome,* Boston, 1993, Little, Brown.
8. Smith MS et al: Chronic fatigue in adolescents, *Pediatrics* 88:195, 1991.
9. Straus SE: History of chronic fatigue syndrome, *Rev Infect Dis* 13 (suppl 1):2, 1991.

SUGGESTED READINGS

Dawson DM, Sabin TD, editors: *Chronic fatigue syndrome,* Boston, 1993, Little, Brown.
Klonoff DC: Chronic fatigue syndrome, *Clin Infect Dis* 15:812, 1992.
Levine PH, editor: Chronic fatigue syndrome: current concepts, *Clin Infect Dis* 18(suppl 1):1, 1994.

193 Cleft Lip and Cleft Palate

Archie S. Golden

The complex problems associated with cleft lip and cleft palate require that the primary care pediatrician coordinate management, family support, and a variety of medical needs over the years. The goal is a good psychosocial outcome, as well as a satisfactory anatomical result. Cleft lip or cleft palate, or both, occurs in approximately 1 in 750 births. Cleft lip with or without cleft palate is most frequent in native Americans and least so in African-Americans. Cleft palate alone has similar frequency in all groups. Isolated cleft lip is more common in girls; cleft lip *and* cleft palate more so in boys.

ETIOLOGY AND PATHOGENESIS

The pathogenesis of this malformation is related to hereditary and environmental factors and their interactions. Clefts of the face have been described as a component of more than 250 syndromes. Cleft palate, in particular, occurs more frequently as a constituent of certain syndromes. Because many of these syndromes exhibit single-gene inheritance, their recognition is important so that genetic counseling can be provided. Although a specific environmental cause rarely is identified, several substances are known to increase the risk of this birth defect. Among these are alcohol, some tranquilizers, and a few anticonvulsant medications; one third of all infants who have fetal alcohol syndrome have a cleft. Amniotic bands and maternal phenylketonuria also may play a role. Because these deformities may have ramifications far beyond the oral cavity, affected children often present a continuing, complex diagnostic and treatment challenge to a wide range of professionals.

CLINICAL EVALUATION

History

A full family and gestational history is necessary, with particular attention to the maternal use of alcohol, medications, and drugs. A family tree is helpful in identifying those family members who have had clefts, other congenital anomalies and syndromes, mental retardation, odd speech and dental problems, and parental consanguinity. A physical examination of parents and other relatives can confirm the clues provided in the history.

Physical Examination

All infants must have an examination of their gums, the hard and soft palates, the uvula, and the throat, including palpation in all areas. The degree of clefting will vary. A cleft lip may manifest as a small notch in the vermilion border or a complete separation extending into the nose. Clefts may be unilateral or bilateral. Isolated cleft palate occurs in the midline and can vary from minimal involvement of the uvula to extension through the soft and hard palates. Associated lip and palatal clefts can involve the soft or hard palate on one or both sides, thereby exposing one side of the nasal cavity, or both. A complete examination is necessary to uncover the existence of possible associated anomalies in a variety of described syndromes. Prognosis varies with the particular constellation of findings.

COMPLICATIONS

Giving birth to a baby who has a facial defect can be emotionally traumatic for parents. The emotions experienced are varied and may include shock, anger, confusion, guilt, anxiety, and sadness. Because most parents are unprepared for the birth of a child who has a cleft and are not familiar with the defect, the manner in which the physician first presents the infant and the defect to the parents is of utmost importance. The knowledge, reassurance, and counseling that the primary physician can provide at such a critical time may do much to alleviate the uncertainties and anxieties of the parents. Parents should be encouraged to express their feelings openly and should be reassured that these feelings are normal. The physician should listen attentively and help the parents to understand the importance of their role in the baby's habilitation. Also, the physician should emphasize his or her intent to support the family after the infant is discharged from the hospital. The parents also should be advised that the treatment may take several years and include many types of management. Of paramount importance to the parents is knowing the degree of risk that the cleft will recur in subsequent children. Predictions can be made for individual families by using tables that provide risk data for almost every pedigree; consultation with a geneticist should be sought.

Feeding

The most immediate need in the newborn period and during early infancy is adequate nutrition.[1] The infant born having a cleft lip only usually has little or no difficulty feeding; however, those who have a cleft palate with or without a cleft lip may have some difficulty. One of the major causes of difficulty in feeding is the inability to generate effective oral suction.

Breast-feeding should be encouraged and can be accomplished with most infants who have a cleft lip. When breast-feeding the infant is not possible or not desired, a variety of feeding techniques can be effective. The position of the infant while feeding is important. Holding the infant in an upright or semiupright position generally works best and keeps food from coming out through the nose. This also decreases the probability of formula entering the eustachian tubes and causing ear problems. Because these babies often swallow an excessive amount of air, the feeding period may be prolonged and a great deal of energy used in obtaining a marginal amount of nourishment. The use of a soft nipple with an enlarged crisscross cut often works well. Alternatively, a Haberman nipple, a Brecht feeder, or medicine dropper can be tried. Milk should be directed to the inside of the cheek, rather than into the throat. If choking on liquids is a problem, rice cereal may be used as a thickener.

The most important factor in feeding an infant who has a cleft lip or palate is patience. Smaller but more frequent feedings may help to avoid tiring the infant and frustrating the parents. Parents should be encouraged to be creative, determining what works best for their particular infant. Gavage feedings or gastrostomy rarely are needed. It is important that another person (or persons) knows how to feed the infant to enable the mother or other primary caretaker to obtain some respite.

Speech and Language

A hypernasal tone to the voice is the most common speech defect associated with clefts, particularly of the palate. Functioning of the palatal and pharyngeal muscles is impaired. The development of expressive language and speech may be retarded in children who have a cleft palate, and their articulation is less advanced than that of children who do not have such a defect. An associated hearing defect may play an important role in delayed or abnormal speech development. Because problems may persist even after successful anatomical closure, early referral to a speech therapist should be considered.

Dental and Orthodontic Problems

Irregularities in the upper anterior dental arch associated with cleft lip may result in supernumerary incisors, rotation and malformation of the lateral incisors, or malocclusions. When there is a cleft of both lip and palate, the dental deformities may be greater, involving the canine teeth and the molars. Children who have these problems tend to have more cavities, thus requiring meticulous oral hygiene and constant dental care. Orthodontic treatment usually is necessary.

Middle Ear Disease and Hearing Loss

Recurrent otitis media and hearing loss are almost universal complications of cleft palate. A key factor in the cause of secretory otitis in patients who have a cleft palate is eustachian tube dysfunction. Although middle ear disease is almost universal in these patients, the hearing loss that often accompanies recurrent disease usually can be avoided by close supervision that results in early recognition and treatment of middle ear infections. Educating the parents in the recognition of the signs and symptoms of middle ear disease is important and can aid the physician tremendously. The likelihood of otitis media decreases after palate repair, but an increased incidence may continue, as compared with unaffected children. Antibiotic prophylaxis should be prescribed readily for these infants and children; referral to an otolaryngologist for possible surgical correction of the cleft, tympanostomy tubes, and adenoidectomy is common; careful audiological follow-up clearly is necessary.

Upper Airway Problems

Occasional apneic episodes have been described in children who have a cleft palate, especially in those who have the Pierre Robin malformation.

Psychological Problems

Without question the presence of such a visible defect adds to the burden of childrearing and increases the stress experienced by the child and the parents. However, psychological disorders common to these children have not been found. It is most important that the primary physician, as well as others involved in the medical management, remain sensitive to the emotional needs of these children throughout the total process of rehabilitation. The stability of the family, available support, existing emotional problems and those arising from the condition, the possibility of the child being unwanted, and ethnic and cultural beliefs that might affect parental attitudes toward the baby should be explored. Economic status is important because children who have clefts require long-term medical care and rehabilitation, which is considerably expensive.

Because of our mobile society, pediatricians may "inherit" children who have clefts at varying states of repair and rehabilitation. The practical matters of anatomical revisions must be addressed, as well as the psychosocial needs of older children and adolescents and peer and family relationships.

SURGICAL CORRECTION

A cleft lip usually is repaired in early infancy. Traditionally most surgeons prefer to wait until the child reaches a body weight of 10 to 12 pounds. However, in an otherwise healthy infant in whom no complications of general anesthesia are expected, the cleft lip may be repaired at birth or at 3 months of age, depending on the preference of the surgeon.

Speech development is of primary consideration in palate repair. The purpose of the operation is to close the palate anatomically and to minimize maxillary growth retardation accompanied by associated dental alveolar deformities. Eighteen months generally is accepted as the latest age for surgical repair of a cleft palate because frequent speech usually develops soon thereafter; six months of age is preferable. If the operation is delayed until 2 years of age or older, the child is more likely to have speech problems. Revisions of the primary procedure may be necessary by 5 or 6 years of age and further plastic surgery and rhinoplasty at 11 to 14 years.

LONG-TERM CARE: THE CLEFT LIP AND PALATE TEAM

Although the pediatrician must assume the responsibility for the child's overall health management and for parental counseling and guidance, referral to an interdisciplinary cleft lip and cleft palate team is essential. There are at least 215 such groups in the United States today, varying in size from some 20 members in major academic centers to 3 in community-based programs; a plastic surgeon, a dentist or pedodontist, and a speech pathologist are the core of the team. In addition, university-based teams often include an otolaryngologist, a geneticist, a psychologist, a public health nurse, a social worker, a vocational and rehabilitation counselor, an orthodontist, and a prosthodontist. A well-functioning team is cost effective in that it allows a comprehensive group of specialists to evaluate and manage a patient through a minimum of closely coordinated visits over time, thus limiting time lost from school by the patients and from work by the parents.

Clearly the specialization of team members mandates the pediatrician's coordinating effort. This need may continue for decades. The anatomical problems associated with clefts may emerge any time in a patient's life, and the rehabilitative process may be prolonged.

REFERENCE

1. Clarren S. Anderson B, Wolf L: Feeding infants with cleft lip, cleft palate, or cleft lip and palate, *Cleft Palate J* 24:244, 1987.

SUGGESTED READINGS

Kaufman, FL: Managing the cleft lip and palate patient, *Pediatr Clin North Am* 38:1127, 1991.

Moller KT, Starr CD, Johnson SA: *A parent's guide to cleft lip and palate,* Minneapolis, 1989, University of Minnesota Press.

Pashley NRT, Krause CJ: Cleft lip, cleft palate and other fusion disorders. In *Symposium on congenital disorders: otolaryngologic clinics of North America,* Philadelphia, 1981, WB Saunders.

Rood SR, Stool SE: Current concepts of the etiology, diagnosis and management of cleft palate related otopathologic disease. In Caldarelli DD, editor: Craniofacial anomalies, *Otolaryngol Clin North Am* 14:865, 1981.

Suslak L, Desposito F: Infants with cleft lip/cleft palate, *Pediatr Rev* 9:331, 1988.

Tier WC, editor: Symposium on cleft lip and cleft palate, *Clin Plast Surg* 12:533, 1985.

194 The Common Cold

Philip E. Thuma

Colds are viral infections of the upper respiratory tract, with involvement of the mucosal surfaces that are lined with respiratory epithelium. Thus nasal passages, sinuses, eustachian tubes, middle ears, conjunctiva, and the nasopharynx potentially are affected with the symptoms of the common cold. The distribution of this illness is worldwide—adults and children of all ethnic and geographical groups may become afflicted. Colds are most common in children during the preschool years, who average three to eight colds per year, which is about half the number expected in adults. Those attending day care centers or exposed to other school-age children tend to have the higher number of annual colds.

Colds always have tended to occur more frequently during the cooler months in temperate climates, probably leading to the popular myth that exposure to cold weather leads to a cold. Fortunately the common cold has been extensively researched in the last 3 to 4 decades, allowing us to have a more scientific understanding of this age-old malady. In fact, the incidence of colds peaks in early fall, followed by a peak in late January and another in early April in the northern hemisphere. Studies have shown that exposure to a cold environment neither causes a cold nor decreases immunity that potentially may allow a viral infection to begin. It does appear clear, however, that colds are more frequent in crowded situations, and evidence suggests that the infection begins most commonly after self-inoculation of a virus onto one's own nasal or conjunctival mucosa.[5] Because the viruses of infected individuals are shed in large amounts in nasal secretions, they can be spread easily by way of fingers and hands to objects such as clothing or environmental surfaces, from where fingers of other children can acquire them and then self-inoculate their respiratory tract by picking their nose or rubbing their eyes. Other epidemiological data suggest that colds and other respiratory tract infections may be more common in those exposed to passive tobacco smoke or other indoor air pollution. It also has been shown that some adults are more prone to develop cold symptoms during periods of emotional stress; whether these data can be reproduced in other populations or in children is not known.[11] Interestingly, not all those infected with cold viruses develop symptoms,[10] which has led to a better understanding of the variable attack rates based on symptomatology only.

ETIOLOGY

Over 100 different infectious agents may cause cold symptoms, with rhinoviruses, small RNA viruses of the picornavirus family, being implicated most frequently. In addition to many rhinovirus serotypes, other viruses and a few nonviral organisms are associated with the common cold (Table 194-1) whereas respiratory syncytial virus and parainfluenza viruses most commonly cause a croupy cough and bronchiolitis in infants, they are more likely to cause a cold in older children and adults. Adenoviruses and enteroviruses tend to cause other symptoms in addition to those of a common cold, including pharyngitis and gastrointestinal problems.

CLINICAL PRESENTATION

Once a cold-causing virus is introduced into the host's respiratory tract, assuming there is no immunity to that particular serotype, a local infection usually begins after a variable incubation period, depending on the specific virus. However, not all people developing a viral respiratory tract infection (defined as evidence of viral shedding and an increase in antibody titers) develop symptoms of a cold. In one study, only 75% of experimentally infected adults who shed rhinovirus type 2 and developed antibody titers with a greater than fourfold rise actually developed symptoms.[3] Others have found that the symptoms of a cold are related primarily to the host's production of kinins in response to the viral infection,[7] resulting in increased vascular permeability and the symptomatology associated with a common cold.

Younger infants may begin their illness with a fever; older children, however, usually are afebrile, with the earliest symptoms being a stuffy nose and watery nasal discharge, followed in a few days by sneezing. Generalized symptoms such as headache and malaise are uncommon in a rhinovirus infection, although they are seen in adenoviral and other viral infections. Infants tend to be irritable, have changes in feeding and sleep patterns, and sometimes develop mild diarrhea. By the third or fourth day of the illness a dry cough may be present, and the nasal discharge usually becomes more purulent. Although such purulence has been interpreted in the past as indicating a secondary bacterial infection (such as sinusitis) or the shedding of damaged epithelial cells, little evidence is available to support that impression. Rather, recent studies on adults who had colds documented that, whereas 87% had evidence on CT scan of sinus abnormalities during the illness, 79% of those studied again after 2 weeks resolved spontaneously despite no treatment with antibiotics.[4] In addition, examination of purulent secretions has not shown increased aerobic bacterial growth or sloughing of nasal epithelial cells,[12] and biopsies in volunteers only demonstrate loss of cilia and ciliated cells.[8]

The symptoms of a cold generally last about a week, with an occasional child having mild rhinorrhea and a dry cough for 2 to 3 weeks. The cilia necessary for proper function of the respiratory epithelium may take as many as 3 weeks to return to their normal state,[8] thus delaying the return to a state of no respiratory tract symptoms.

DIFFERENTIAL DIAGNOSIS

There are no routine confirmatory tests to diagnose the common cold because viral cultures are expensive and generally

Table 194-1 Infectious Agents Associated with the Common Cold

Category	Agents
Common viruses that usually cause the common cold	Rhinovirus, parainfluenza viruses, respiratory syncytial virus, coronaviruses
Common infectious agents that occasionally cause illness with symptoms of the common cold	Adenoviruses, enteroviruses, influenza viruses, reoviruses, *Mycoplasma pneumoniae*
Unusual causes of common cold–like illness	*Coccidioides immitis, Histoplasma capsulatum, Bordetella pertussis, Chlamydia psittaci, Coxiela burnetti*

From Cherry JD: The common cold. In Feigin RD, Cherry JD, editors: *Textbook of pediatric infectious diseases,* ed 2, Philadelphia, 1987, WB Saunders.

unnecessary, so the diagnosis must be made on clinical grounds. However, the most common concern is that an underlying bacterial infection (such as a sinus or ear infection) is being missed or improperly treated. In most cases, if a cold follows its expected course of causing the usual symptoms for 5 to 7 days, a concurrent sinus or ear infection is unlikely. What is well known is that when the symptoms of a cold are prolonged a secondary infection may be present, especially if fever persists or is prominent or if ear pain or a productive cough develops. Thus a good ear and lung examination is essential in all children in whom a cold has persisted for longer than expected. The routine use of radiographs or CT scans to diagnose sinusitis in these individuals is controversial, because the radiological finding of opacification of the sinuses does not correlate with clinical sinusitis in older individuals.[1]

Persistent nasal symptoms also can be caused by an allergy, and it is not uncommon for allergies to be diagnosed initially as a cold and only later to be recognized as being seasonal or associated with nasal eosinophilia. Another consideration is that cold symptoms associated with significant pharyngitis, rashes, or other systemic symptoms usually are caused by a virus other than those causing the common cold.

One also must be aware that in children under 2 years of age, a persistent purulent nasal discharge has been seen in individuals infected with beta-hemolytic streptococci, although this usually is associated with mild excoriations around the nares. Unilateral nasal discharge also must be evaluated carefully to rule out a foreign body in the nose. Finally, irritation and swelling of the nasal passages from inhalation of drugs such as cocaine or the chronic use of medicated nasal sprays should be considered in the differential diagnosis of the older child who has cold symptoms.

MANAGEMENT

Although the various remedies available for the common cold constitute a significant portion of any pharmacy's shelf space, all of them constitute symptomatic rather than curative treatment. In the pediatric population most of the remedies give only marginal symptomatic relief and, in many cases, are potentially harmful. Most pediatricians advise against using any of these cold remedies in infants and, at most, suggest saline nose drops with the use of a bulb syringe to aspirate secretions, and a cool-mist vaporizer to humidify the air.[2] The malaise and fever sometimes associated with a cold can be treated with acetaminophen or ibuprofen; aspirin should be avoided because of its association with Reye syndrome. Recent data suggest that ibuprofen theoretically may be more beneficial during a cold than acetaminophen because it appears to lead to a shorter period of viral shedding and a better neutralizing antibody response than when acetaminophen is used.[3]

Studies conducted on preschoolers have not demonstrated a beneficial effect of the decongestants, antihistamines, or their combinations that are readily available in multiple colors and flavors.[6,9] In older children and adolescents an oral decongestant such as pseudoephedrine hydrochloride either alone or with an antihistamine such as chlorpheniramine maleate provides symptomatic relief with a very low possibility of side effects. The regular use of nasal spray or drops containing vasoconstrictors such as oxymetazoline hydrochloride should not be encouraged because of the high incidence of rebound nasal congestion after only a few days of their use.

Many parents will ask about the advisability of giving vitamin C during a cold, as well as request that the physician prescribe antibiotics; both these practices have little validity and should be discouraged.

COMPLICATIONS

The vast majority of colds resolve on their own without the help of the doctor or any medication. When a secondary fever occurs or symptoms continue longer than expected, a complication such as otitis media or sinusitis should be suspected. It appears that a cold can contribute to eustachian tube dysfunction, especially in younger children, resulting in an otitis media. A fever, headache, and unilateral purulent nasal discharge may herald a secondary bacterial sinusitis, although this is probably diagnosed much more frequently than it really occurs. In rare occasions a lower respiratory tract infection develops and can progress into a pneumonia manifested by cough, tachypnea, and usually fever and can be confirmed by a chest radiograph.

REFERENCES

1. Cooke LD, Hadley DM: MRI of the paranasal sinuses: incidental abnormalities and their relationship to symptoms, *J Laryngol Otol* 105:278, 1991.
2. Gadomski A, Horton L: The need for rational therapeutics in the use of cough and cold medicine in infants, *Pediatrics* 89:774, 1992.
3. Graham NM et al: Adverse effects of aspirin, acetaminophen, and ibuprofen on immune function, viral shedding, and clinical status in rhinovirus-infected volunteers, *J Infect Dis* 162:1277, 1990.
4. Gwaltney JM Jr et al: Computed tomographic study of the common cold, *N Engl J Med* 330:25, 1994.
5. Hendley JO, Wenzel RP, Gwaltney JM: Transmission of rhinovirus colds by self-inoculation, *N Engl J Med* 288:1361, 1973.
6. Hutton N et al: Effectiveness of an antihistamine-decongestant combination for young children with the common cold: a randomized, controlled clinical trial, *J Pediatr* 118:125, 1991.
7. Proud D et al: Kinins are generated in nasal secretions during natural rhinovirus colds, *J Infect Dis* 161:120, 1990.

8. Rautiainen M et al: Ultrastructural changes in human nasal cilia caused by the common cold and recovery of ciliated epithelium, *Ann Otol Rhinol Laryngol* 101:982, 1992.
9. Smith MB, Feldman W: Over-the-counter cold medications: a critical review of clinical trials between 1950 and 1991, *JAMA* 269:2258, 1993.
10. Sperber SJ et al: Effects of naproxen on experimental rhinovirus colds: a randomized, double-blind, controlled trial, *Ann Intern Med* 117:37, 1992.
11. Stone AA et al: Development of common cold symptoms following experimental rhinovirus infection is related to prior stressful life events, *Behav Med* 18:115, 1992.
12. Winther B, Kawana R, Saito H: Fireside conference 11: common cold, *Rhinol Suppl* 14:228, 1992.

195 Congenital Heart Disease

Edward B. Clark

Most children will have a heart murmur noted on examination sometime during infancy or early childhood. The challenge to the pediatrician is to identify the children who require cardiac care. This chapter is a review of the most common congenital cardiac defects.

EPIDEMIOLOGY

Congenital cardiovascular malformations remain a major public health problem in the United States and other industrialized nations. Eight of every 1000 liveborn infants have a congenital cardiovascular malformation. For some the defect is of little clinical significance; for others surgical palliation and repair permits a longer life. In spite of dramatic advances in treatment over the last 50 years, cardiac defects account for a large proportion of infant mortality. In addition, many survivors of surgery are not cured but have an ongoing morbidity and mortality from their heart defect.

ETIOLOGY AND PATHOGENESIS

The etiology of most congenital heart defects is as yet undefined. Many defects are probably the result of single or multiple gene abnormalities, others arise as the consequence of genetic and environmental interaction, and some are chance occurrences in the complex process of cardiovascular development. Of the 2600 infants studied in the Baltimore-Washington Infant Study of Congenital Cardiovascular Malformations, 12% of the cases were associated with chromosomal abnormalities, 8% with multiple congenital malformations, and 80% with isolated cardiac defects.

Abnormalities in cardiovascular development are responsible for a broad spectrum of heart diseases, yet we know relatively little about the process that brings about the shape and function of the heart. The heart begins as a muscle-wrapped tube and becomes a complex four-chambered pump through growth and morphogenesis. Most congenital cardiovascular malformations have their origins during primary morphogenesis in the first 8 weeks after conception; a few defects may arise during later secondary morphogenesis of the heart. Risk factors for congenital cardiovascular malformations include maternal illnesses such as diabetes mellitus and systemic lupus erythematosus. The known cardiac teratogens include rubella, thalidomide, retinoic acid, and alcohol.

CLINICAL PRESENTATION

Children who have a congenital heart defect are recognized because of a heart murmur, cyanosis, congestive heart failure, or an arrhythmia. The differential diagnosis of congenital heart defects requires the integration of the history, symptoms, and findings on physical examination, chest roentgenogram, electrocardiography, and two-dimensional Doppler echocardiography. Serious congenital heart disease appears most frequently in infancy, but can be diagnosed prenatally by fetal echocardiography. Less severe cardiac abnormalities are identified during early childhood. Mild defects may be identified in adulthood or go unrecognized.

LABORATORY STUDIES

Chest Roentgenogram

The chest roentgenogram shows the size of the heart and the amount of pulmonary blood flow. With normal pulmonary blood flow, the heart occupies 50% of the cardiothoracic dimension, and the pulmonary vessels decrease in size from the hilar area through two thirds of the chest. The heart and pulmonary vessels are large and the vascular markings are visible in the peripheral one third of the lung fields because of increased pulmonary blood flow. Abnormal size, shape, or location of specific chambers and vessels can be determined from the chest roentgenogram.

Electrocardiogram

The electrocardiogram (ECG) shows cardiac rhythm and myocardial mass. A normal newborn's ECG has right ventricular dominance that gradually shifts to left ventricular dominance as the child grows and the left ventricular forces increase.

Echocardiography

Echocardiography and Doppler measurement of blood velocity give precise information and should be used, as should most laboratory data, as an adjunct to careful clinical evaluation of the patient and not as a prediagnostic screening tool.

SPECIFIC DEFECTS

Right-to-Left Shunts

Right-to-left shunts are characterized by cyanosis secondary to decreased pulmonary blood flow. In many defects having a right-to-left shunt, pulmonary blood flow depends on a patent ductus arteriosus. As the ductus closes in the first hours to days after birth, the infant becomes progressively cyanotic. If these early signs are ignored, the progressive cyanosis leads to hypoxemia, metabolic acidosis, and death; therefore aggressive initial evaluation and stabilization is essential.

Tetralogy of Fallot (Fig. 195-1, A)

Tetralogy of Fallot is characterized by pulmonary outflow tract obstruction, a ventricular septal defect, an overriding aorta, and right ventricular hypertrophy. Infants who have tetralogy of Fallot manifest symptoms in the first days to

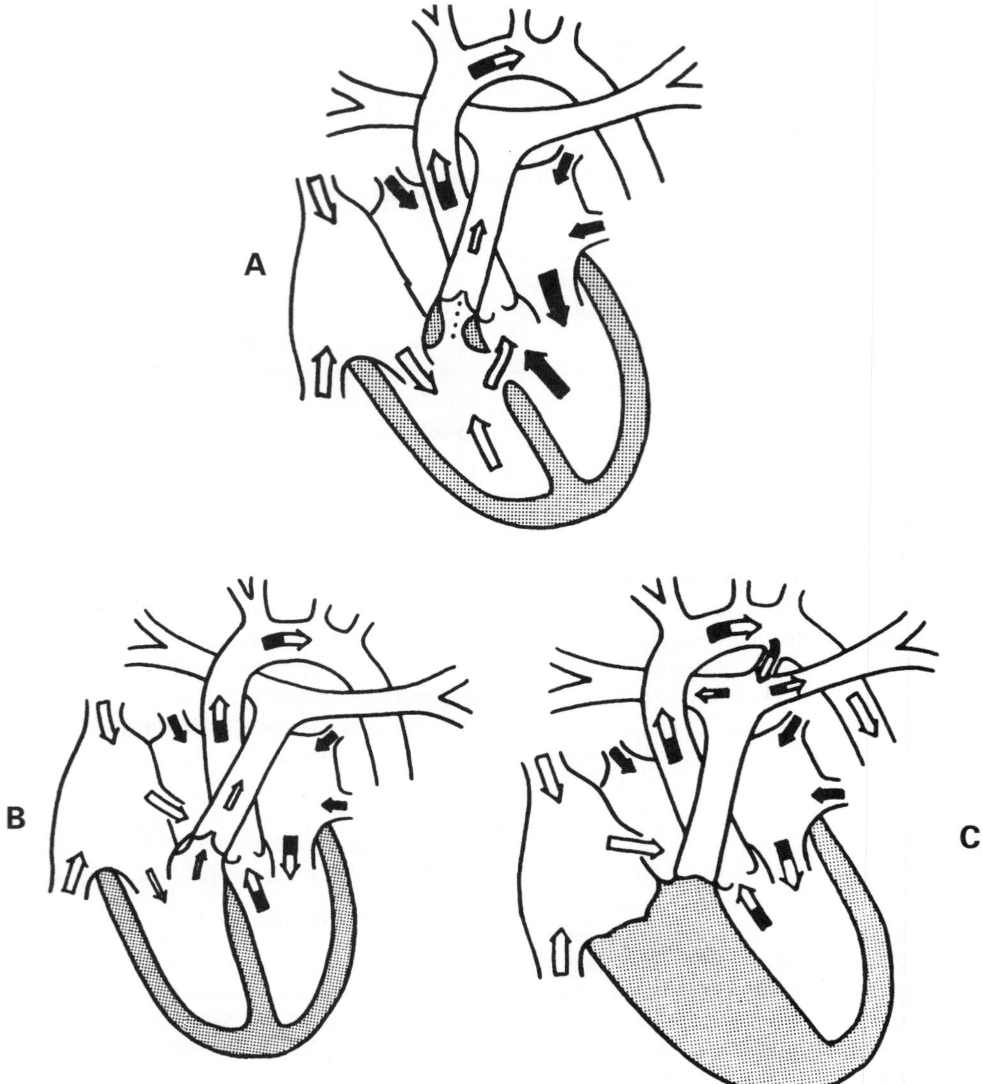

FIG. 195-1 Right-to-left shunts. **A,** Tetralogy of Fallot. **B,** Pulmonary atresia. **C,** Tricuspid atresia. Closed arrows indicate saturated blood; open arrows indicate desaturated blood. (See text for details.)

(From Clark EB: Heart disease. In Paxson CL Jr, editor: *Van Leeuwan's newborn medicine,* ed 2, St Louis, 1979, Mosby.)

months of life and initially may have the auscultatory findings of a simple ventricular septal defect. However, as the infundibular obstruction increases, the cardiac murmur changes to reflect pulmonary stenosis. Symptoms consist initially of intermittent cyanotic spells that progress to persistent cyanosis. The ECG shows right axis deviation and right ventricular hypertrophy. The chest roentgenogram shows a heart that is normal in size with normal to slightly decreased pulmonary blood flow. The echocardiogram defines an intracristal ventricular septal defect, an overriding aorta, and infundibular and pulmonary valve stenosis. For infants who have hypercyanotic spells, the knee-chest position increases systemic resistance and decreases the right-to-left shunt. Some infants respond to propranolol, which decreases infundibular obstruction. Surgical management is either a primary repair of the intracardiac defects or, in cases that have a complex pulmonary artery anomaly, a systemic-to-pulmonary shunt.

Pulmonary Valve Atresia and Critical Stenosis (Fig. 195-1, *B*)

Neonates who have pulmonary valve atresia manifest cyanosis in the first hours or days of life as the ductus arteriosus closes and pulmonary blood flow decreases. Physical findings often include a soft murmur of the patent ductus arteriosus. The ECG shows variable right ventricular forces, and the chest roentgenogram shows a heart that is normal in size and decreased pulmonary blood flow. The diagnosis is established by echocardiography, which defines atresia or critical stenosis of the pulmonary valve. The ventricular anatomy can be that of a single ventricle, two ventricles having a large ventricular septal defect, or a hypoplastic right ventricular cavity having an intact ventricular septum. An infant initially is stabilized with the use of prostaglandin E_1 to maintain ductal patency. Surgical treatment includes a systemic-to-pulmonary artery shunt to increase pulmonary blood flow. Many children eventually undergo surgical repair to reconstruct the pulmonary outflow tract.

Tricuspid Atresia (Fig. 195-1, *C*)

Infants who have tricuspid atresia manifest cyanosis and a heart murmur in the neonatal period. The chest roentgenogram shows a heart that is normal in size that has an enlarged right atrium and decreased pulmonary blood flow. The ECG shows left-axis deviation, a predominant P wave, and absent right ventricular forces. Echocardiography defines atresia of the tricuspid valve and often a slitlike right ventricle and ventricular septal defect. Initial management includes the use of prostaglandins to maintain ductal patency, followed by a surgical shunt. Many children who have tricuspid atresia undergo a Fontan procedure to separate systemic and pulmonary circuits by direct connection of the right atrium to the pulmonary artery.

Ebstein Malformation of the Tricuspid Valve

In Ebstein malformation the septal and anterior tricuspid valve leaflets are displaced into the right ventricle, often obstructing the pulmonary outflow tract. The clinical presentation varies. In the severe form an infant may have severe cyanosis because the valve leaflet obstructs the right ventricular outflow tract. In the mild form a child may have only trivial tricuspid insufficiency. Diagnostic studies include an ECG that shows left-axis deviation, a prominent P wave, and preexcitation (Wolff-Parkinson-White syndrome) (see Chapter 115, Cardiac Arrythmias). Children who have Ebstein malformation are predisposed to supraventricular tachycardia. In severe cases the chest roentgenogram shows massive cardiomegaly and decreased pulmonary blood flow. Echocardiography defines the displacement of the tricuspid valve leaflets and a right-to-left shunt at the atrial level. Infants may require prolonged respiratory support until pulmonary vascular resistance decreases. Some children require chronic antiarrhythmic therapy because of their supraventricular tachycardia. Older patients may require surgical closure of an atrial septal defect and plication of the tricuspid valve.

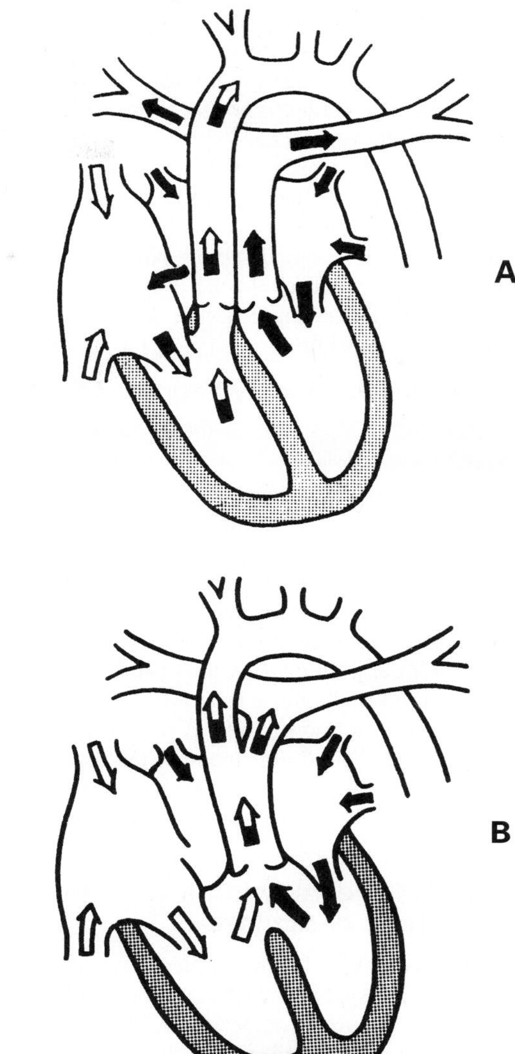

FIG. 195-2 Admixture lesions. **A,** Transposition of the great arteries. **B,** Truncus arteriosus communis. Closed arrows indicate saturated blood; open arrows indicate desaturated blood. (See text for details.)

(From Clark EB: Heart disease. In Paxson CL Jr, editor: *Van Leeuwan's newborn medicine,* ed 2, St Louis, 1979, Mosby.)

Admixture Lesions

Admixture lesions are characterized by increased pulmonary blood flow but have mixing of systemic and pulmonary venous return at the cardiac or great artery level. Cyanosis varies depending on the relative amount of pulmonary blood flow.

Transposition of the Great Arteries (Fig. 195-2, *A*)

In transposition of the great arteries the aorta arises from the right ventricle and the pulmonary artery from the left ventricle. Infants who have this defect are profoundly cyanotic in the first few hours or days of life. The clinical examination reveals a soft systolic ejection murmur and profound cyanosis. The chest roentgenogram and ECG usually are normal. Echocardiography defines the origin of the great arteries. Management includes the use of prostaglandins to maintain ductal patency and palliation by atrial septostomy to allow for the mixing of saturated and desaturated blood at the atrial level. Surgical repair is either an arterial switch during the first week of life or an atrial baffle (Mustard procedure) before 6 months of age.

Truncus Arteriosus Communis (Fig. 195-2, *B*)

In truncus arteriosus communis the septation of the embryonic outflow tract into the aorta and pulmonary artery is incomplete. Infants who have truncus arteriosus communis have mild cyanosis and congestive heart failure in the first days or weeks of life. Characteristics of the physical examination include a hyperactive precordium, bounding pulses, an ejection click from the truncal valve, and a systolic ejection murmur. The ECG shows a normal axis along with right or biventricular hypertrophy, and the chest roentgenogram shows cardiomegaly and increased pulmonary blood flow. The right and left pulmonary arteries arise from a higher position than normal. Echocardiography demonstrates a ventricular septal defect, with the truncal root and pulmonary arteries arising distal to the truncal valve. Aortic arch anomalies occur in most cases. Cardiac catheterization and angiography may be needed to define the defect completely. Initial management includes control of congestive heart failure. Definitive management is surgical repair with placement of a conduit from the right ventricle to the pulmonary artery and closure of the ventricular septal defect so that the truncus arises from the left ventricle.

Total Anomalous Pulmonary Venous Return

Children who have total anomalous pulmonary venous return usually manifest mild cyanosis and congestive heart failure as neonates. The characteristics include a hyperdynamic precordium, a soft systolic ejection murmur, and a widely fixed, split, second heart sound. This defect can be difficult to diagnose by noninvasive studies alone. Neither chest roentgenogram nor the ECG provides specific information. Echocardiography can be problematic because of the difficulty in identifying individual pulmonary veins. Cardiac catheterization often is required to diagnose total anomalous pulmonary venous return and to define the site of the common pulmonary vein connection. Initial management includes treatment for congestive heart failure and ventilatory support. Surgery involves the anastomosis of the common pulmonary vein to the left atrium.

Hypoplastic Left Heart Syndrome: Aortic Atresia with Mitral Atresia or Stenosis

Neonates who have hypoplastic left heart syndrome, aortic atresia, and mitral atresia have abrupt onset of shock and cyanosis within a few hours or days of life. Clinical findings include pallor, a hyperdynamic precordium, weak or absent pulses, and congestive heart failure. The echocardiogram shows a diminutive left ventricle, an ascending aorta less than 6 mm in diameter, and retrograde blood flow to the coronary arteries. The infant depends on the patent ductus arteriosus for systemic blood flow. Aortic atresia with mitral atresia usually is a lethal lesion because death follows closure of the ductus arteriosus. Heart transplantation or surgical palliation (Norwood procedure) is being performed experimentally in some institutions.

Left-to-Right Shunts

Left-to-right shunt defects have increased pulmonary blood flow through a defect at the atrial, ventricular, or great artery level.

Atrial Septal Defect (Fig. 195-3, *A*)

Most children who have atrial septal defects have a cardiac murmur. Clinical characteristics include a hyperdynamic precordium, a fixed, split, second heart sound, and a pulmonary ejection murmur. The ECG shows right-axis deviation and volume-overload right ventricular hypertrophy. The chest roentgenogram shows mild cardiomegaly and increased pulmonary blood flow. The echocardiogram shows a defect in the midportion of the secundum atrial septum and a dilated right ventricle having paradoxical septal motion. The child who has an atrial septal defect should have the defect closed before he or she enters school. Closure techniques include direct surgical repair or closure with an umbrella-like device that is positioned with a cardiac catheter.

Ventricular Septal Defect (Fig. 195-3, *B*)

The clinical presentation of a ventricular septal defect varies. The murmur of small defects may be heard in the first few days of life, but large defects may be silent and lead to congestive heart failure at 6 to 8 weeks of age. The physical examination reveals a harsh, pansystolic murmur heard along the left lower sternal border that radiates to the right. Muscular ventricular septal defects may generate a short pansystolic murmur. Noninvasive study results also vary. Although the ECG may be normal with small defects, children who have large septal defects evidence biventricular hypertrophy. Similarly, the chest roentgenogram shows an enlarged heart only if the left-to-right shunt is large. Echocardiography often shows the location and size of the defect and is important in assessing the prognosis. Small defects are likely to close spontaneously, and even perimembranous defects of moderate size have a greater than 50% chance of closing spontaneously. Large symptomatic ventricular septal defects are closed surgically to reduce the risk of pulmonary vascular obstructive disease.

Patent Ductus Arteriosus (Fig. 195-3, *C*)

Infants who have patent ductus arteriosus present variably. Premature infants have congestive heart failure; term infants may develop heart failure at 2 to 3 weeks of age when pulmonary vascular resistance drops; older children may be asymptomatic. The physical findings also vary with age. Premature infants often have no murmur but do have bounding pulses and a hyperdynamic precordium. Full-term infants and older children usually have a continuous murmur heard best in the left second intercostal space. The ECG shows left ventricular hypertrophy, and the chest roentgenogram shows normal to increased pulmonary vascularity and an increase in left atrial and left ventricular size. Echocardiography defines retrograde turbulent blood flow in the main pulmonary artery. Management is surgical closure of the patent ductus. Large defects are closed to prevent pulmonary vascular obstructive disease; small defects are ligated to reduce the risk of bacterial endocarditis.

Atrioventricular Canal Defects

Atrioventricular canal defects make up a spectrum of abnormalities, including complete atrioventricular canal, ostium primum atrial septal defect with mitral valve cleft, and inflow-type ventricular septal defect. These defects frequently are found in children who have Down syndrome. Clinical findings include a hyperdynamic precordium and the murmurs of increased pulmonary flow and AV valve insufficiency. The ECG shows a characteristic counterclockwise superior axis in the frontal plane and ventricular hypertrophy. The chest roentgenogram shows cardiomegaly and increased pulmonary blood flow. Echocardiography defines defects in the atrial and ventricular septa and the abnormal position of the atrioventricular valves. Initial management is directed to-

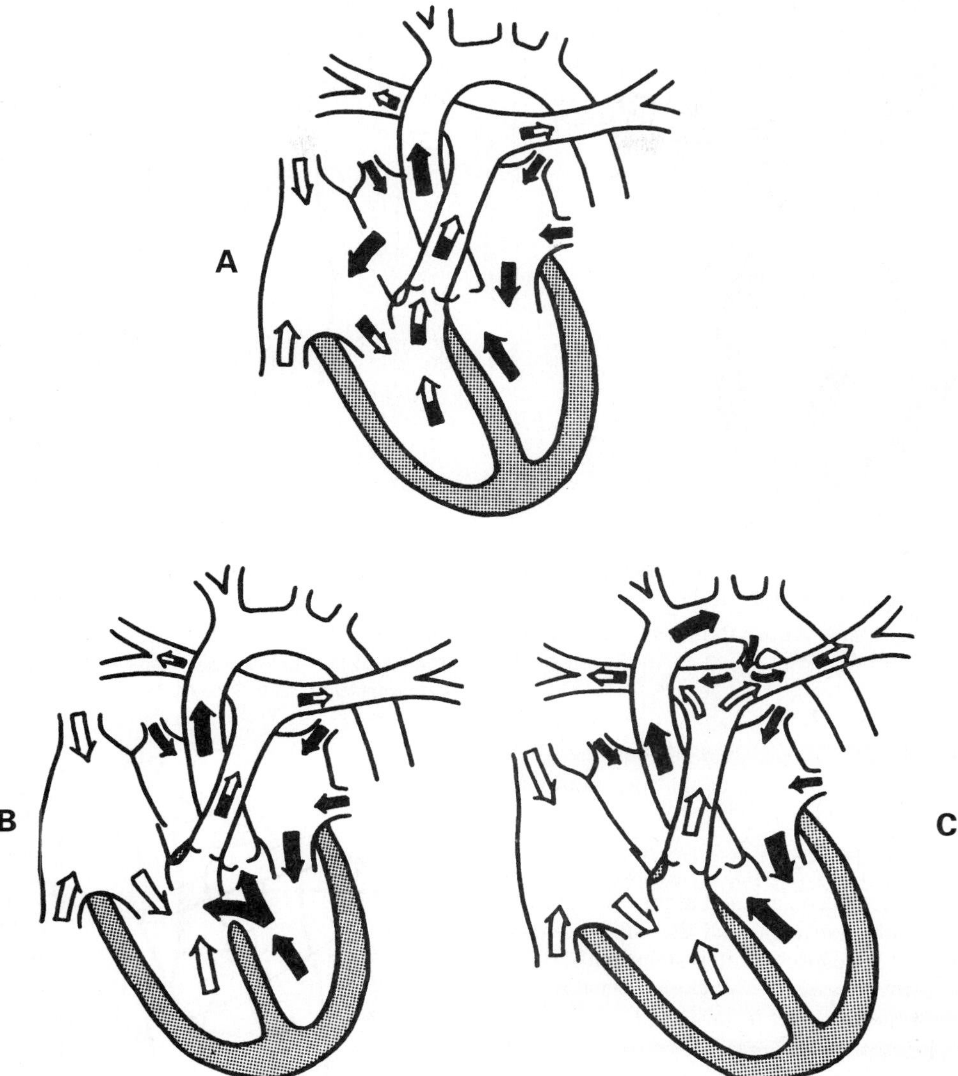

FIG. 195-3 Left-to-right shunt. **A,** Atrial septal defect. **B,** Ventricular septal defect. **C,** Patent ductus arteriosus. Closed arrows indicate saturated blood; open arrows indicate desaturated blood. (See text for details.)

(From Clark EB: Heart disease. In Paxson CL Jr, editor: *Van Leeuwan's newborn medicine,* ed 2, St Louis, 1979, Mosby.)

ward control of congestive heart failure. Most children require surgical repair to protect the pulmonary vascular bed from high blood pressure-flow damage. Children who have Down syndrome are at particular risk for irreversible pulmonary vascular obstructive disease as early as 6 months of age and thus require early surgical repair.

Obstructive Cardiac Defects

Obstructive cardiac defects are characterized by outflow tract obstruction.

Pulmonary Stenosis (Fig. 195-4)

The pulmonary outflow tract can be obstructed at the infundibulum, the pulmonary valve, the supravalvular area, and the peripheral levels. Pulmonary valve stenosis is the most frequent obstruction. Presentation of pulmonary valve stenosis depends on the severity of the outflow tract obstruction. Mild pulmonary valve stenosis often is found as an incidental condition of little or no clinical significance. Critical valve stenosis can manifest in infancy with profound heart failure and a right-to-left atrial level shunt. Clinical examination reveals a systolic ejection click followed by a systolic ejection murmur heard best in the left second intercostal space. The ECG is normal in mild pulmonary valve stenosis and shows increasing right ventricular forces that parallel the increase in the right ventricular myocardial mass. The chest roentgenogram shows a prominent main pulmonary artery, reflecting poststenotic dilation. Echocardiography defines the site of obstruction, and Doppler determination of blood velocity estimates the pressure gradient from the right ventricle to the pulmonary artery. The child who has mild pulmonary valve stenosis requires no treatment. Moderate to severe pulmonary

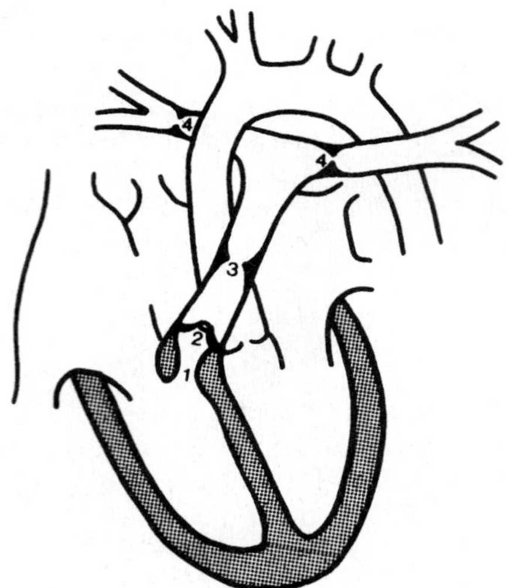

FIG. 195-4 Sites of obstruction to blood flow in right ventricular outflow tract. *1,* Infundibulum; *2,* pulmonary valve; *3,* supravalvular; *4,* peripheral. (See text for details.)

(From Clark EB: Heart disease. In Paxson CL Jr, editor: ***Van Leeuwan's newborn medicine,*** ed 2, St Louis, 1979, Mosby.)

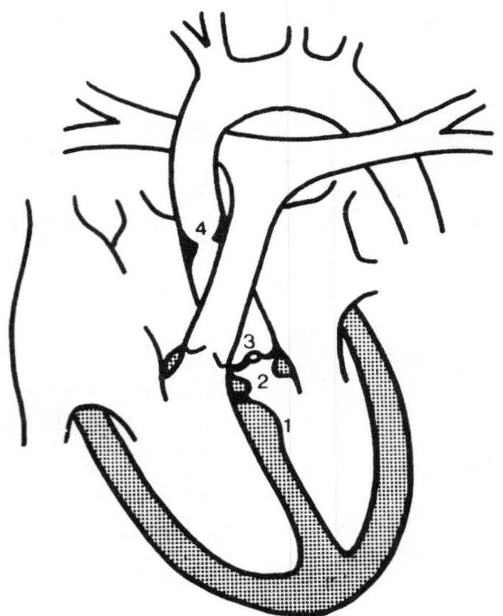

FIG. 195-5 Sites of obstruction to blood flow in left ventricular outflow tract. *1,* Ventricular septum; *2,* subaortic valve membrane; *3,* aortic valve; *4,* supravalvular. (See text for details.)

(From Clark EB: Heart disease. In Paxson CL Jr, editor: ***Van Leeuwan's newborn medicine,*** ed 2, St Louis, 1979, Mosby.)

valve stenosis can be reduced by transvenous balloon valvuloplasty. Critical valve stenosis or a dysplastic pulmonary valve may require surgical repair.

Aortic Stenosis (Fig. 195-5)

The aortic outflow tract can be obstructed at the left ventricular outflow tract, the subvalve area, and the supravalve region, but the most frequent cause is valve stenosis. The presentation of aortic valve stenosis varies from a benign click and murmur heard on auscultation to profound heart failure associated with critical obstruction of the aortic outflow tract. On physical examination there is a systolic ejection click followed by a systolic ejection murmur heard maximally in the right second intercostal space. The ECG shows left-axis deviation and left ventricular hypertrophy; the chest roentgenogram may show mild dilation of the ascending aorta. Echocardiography defines the stenotic aortic valve and an increase in ventricular wall mass. The Doppler measure of blood velocity estimates the pressure gradient across the stenotic valve. Long-term management is more complex for aortic valve stenosis. A nonobstructive bicuspid aortic valve can progress to severe stenosis; thus all children must be monitored into adulthood for progression of the disease. Relief of the pressure gradient is achieved by balloon valvuloplasty in some patients, but surgical valvulotomy or valve replacement often is necessary.

Coarctation of the Aorta (Fig. 195-6)

Children who have coarctation of the aorta present variably. Neonates can have cardiovascular collapse, whereas absent femoral pulses may be the only sign of disease in older children. The cardiac examination typically reveals a systolic ejection murmur that arises from a bicuspid aortic valve and murmurs from the enlarged collateral blood vessels that bypass the site of coarctation. The femoral pulses are decreased or absent, and blood pressure in the legs is less than in the

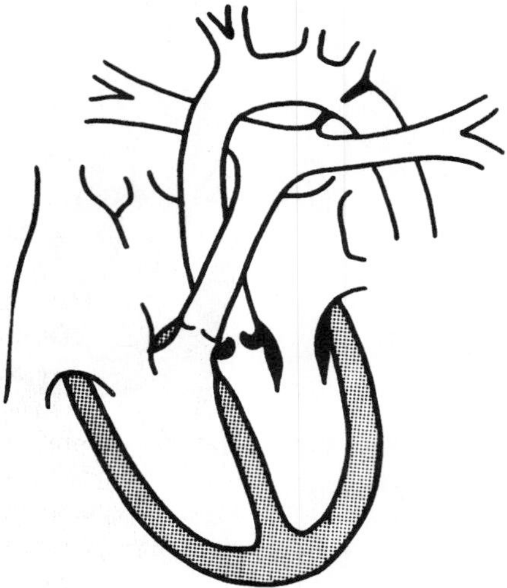

FIG. 195-6 Coarctation of the aorta and associated abnormalities of the mitral and aortic valves. (See text for details.)

(From Clark EB: Heart disease. In Paxson CL Jr, editor: ***Van Leeuwan's newborn medicine,*** ed 2, St Louis, 1979, Mosby.)

arms. The ECG shows right ventricular hypertrophy, reflecting the increased work of the right ventricle during fetal life. The chest roentgenogram usually is normal, but older children may have an aortic indentation at the coarctation site and rib erosion caused by collateral intercostal blood vessels. Echocardiography defines aortic valve abnormalities and aortic arch dimensions, and Doppler velocity estimates the pressure gradient across the coarctation site. Neonates who have critical coarctation and heart failure can be managed by prostaglandin infusion to reopen the ductus arteriosus, thereby reducing the obstruction. The timing for surgical repair depends on the severity of symptoms and the level of the systemic blood pressure. Repair should be accomplished before 5 years of age to reduce the long-term complications of systemic hypertension.

MYOCARDIAL DISEASE

Cardiomyopathy is a primary congenital abnormality of the ventricular muscle that occurs as a sporadic or genetic defect. Cardiomyopathies are classified as either hypertrophic or dilated; each requires thorough evaluation.

Hypertrophic cardiomyopathy usually manifests in children who are asymptomatic and identified either because of a family history of the disease or the discovery of a cardiac murmur. In some adolescents hypertrophic cardiomyopathy may be recognized only after sudden death. Physical examination often is unremarkable. However, in severe forms of cardiomyopathy, there is outflow tract obstruction that produces a long systolic ejection murmur. The ECG often shows bizarre ventricular voltages and an abnormal axis. The chest roentgenogram usually is normal. Echocardiography defines a marked ventricular myocardial thickening and obstruction of the left ventricular outflow tract during late systole. There is no definitive treatment. Some patients are treated with beta blockers or calcium channel blocking agents in an attempt to reduce the obstruction. The prognosis varies. Sudden death can occur and probably is related to primary arrhythmias.

Children who have cardiomyopathy can present in severe congestive heart failure with a dilated and poorly contractile ventricle. The etiology often is undefined, although a viral illness sequela or an undefined metabolic abnormality is often suspected. Physical examination findings include congestive heart failure with a prominent gallop rhythm and hepatosplenomegaly. The ECG often is normal or shows diffuse low-voltage and nonspecific T wave changes. The chest roentgenogram shows cardiomegaly. Echocardiography defines a dilated, poorly contractile ventricle. Management is directed toward pharmacological support of the failing myocardium with inotropic agents, diuretics, and afterload reduction (see Appendix A, Pediatric Basic and Advanced Life Support). The prognosis is uncertain, and some patients eventually are considered for heart transplantation.

SUMMARY

The primary care physician is responsible for recognizing the wide spectrum of congenital heart defects. Along with the pediatric heart team, the primary care physician focuses on supporting the child and family and being an advocate for the child in the community.

SUGGESTED READINGS

Clark EB: Congenital cardiovascular defects in infants with Down syndrome, *Pediatr Rev* 11:99, 1989.

Emmanouilides GC et al, editors: *Heart disease in infants, children and adolescents, including the fetus and young adult,* ed 5, Baltimore, 1994, Williams & Wilkins.

Freedom R, Bensen LN, Smallhorn JF, editors: *Neonatal heart disease,* New York, 1992, Springer Verlag.

Neill CA, Clark EB, Clark CI: *The heart of a child,* Baltimore, 1992, Johns Hopkins University Press.

196 Contact Dermatitis

Nancy K. Barnett

When considering the diagnosis of contact dermatitis, the medical provider should distinguish between *contact irritant dermatitis* and *contact allergic dermatitis*. Contact irritant dermatitis is a nonallergic reaction of the skin to direct contact by an irritant. Contact allergic dermatitis is a delayed hypersensitivity phenomenon that requires immunological sensitization to a contact allergen to become manifest.[4]

Contact irritant dermatitis in childhood is most common in infancy when the skin is thinner. Contact allergic dermatitis is eight times more common in allergy-prone adults than in children, possibly because a mature immune system, as well as prolonged exposure to contact allergens, is required for it to occur. Contact allergic dermatitis is rare in infancy, less rare in childhood, and approaches adult incidence figures by age 8 years.[2]

The diagnosis of contact dermatitis should be entertained when an eruption (1) is limited to exposed contact surfaces, (2) shows sharp delimitation (i.e., at contactant borders and in linear arrays), or (3) reveals bizarre asymmetrical distributions. A good history should provide clues to the offending allergen; if not, a well-kept diary may be helpful.

CONTACT IRRITANT DERMATITIS

There are a variety of common childhood irritants, including soaps, perfumed baby lotions and oils, feces, saliva, food, and detergents. The eruptions vary in severity according to the duration of contact, the strength of the irritant, and the age of the patient. Confluent papular erythema confined to the pattern of contact is the usual manifestation. This will respond readily to the regular (three times a day) application of a topical steroid cream of medium strength over 5 to 7 days. Low-potency steroids should be used on the face whenever possible. With particularly noxious or potent irritants, an acute dermatitis with erythematous vesiculation, weeping, and crusting may occur. Applying compresses (tepid water, saline, or Burow solution) four times daily to the weeping areas for 5 minutes before applying the steroid will help dry the involved areas and remove serous debris. If secondary impetiginization has occurred, then appropriate antibiotic therapy based on Gram stain and culture results should be instituted.

Diaper Dermatitis

Diaper dermatitis is the most frequent contact irritant dermatitis in infancy (see Chapter 200, Diaper Rash). The usual irritant is urine or feces that has been in contact with the skin too long as a result of infrequent diaper changes or occlusion by plastic pants. Occasionally, detergents used to wash cloth diapers or synthetic components of paper diapers or wipes are direct skin irritants. The dermatitis usually is a confluent macular or papular erythema confined to the areas of contact, with sparing of the inguinal folds. However, contact irritants in oils or lotions applied to the diaper area usually will involve the skin folds. If the irritation is severe, the skin may macerate and erode, leading to oozing and crusting.

In diaper dermatitis the most important aspect of treatment is to dry the involved area (with aeration and powder) while preventing further contact with the irritant. Also helpful at times is the use of a low-potency antiinflammatory steroid cream three times a day, alternating its application with that of an anticandidal cream such as nystatin or clotrimazole two times a day. If the dermatitis persists for more than 3 days (the area usually becomes colonized with *Candida albicans*), the patient probably has a candidal superinfection, which can be recognized as a beefy red dermatitis with frequent satellite papules and pustules; a potassium hydroxide (KOH) preparation of skin scrapings may be positive for pseudohyphae or budding yeast.[5]

Other Irritants

In older children soaps and detergents are frequent irritants. The dermatitis often is limited to those areas of tight contact with clothing (e.g., wrists, axillae, waistbands), where detergent often accumulates. Soaps may be general irritants and cause the most severe eruptions on the face and hands. Bubble bath solutions often are a cause of perivaginal dermatitis and vaginitis in young girls. Woolens and formaldehyde resins (flame retardants) in clothing also can cause severe irritant dermatitis. In soap or detergent dermatitis, use of the suspected inciting agent should be discontinued. All new clothes should be washed and rinsed twice before initial wearing.

CONTACT ALLERGIC DERMATITIS

In contact allergic dermatitis, it is postulated that the contact allergen penetrates the epidermis as a hapten, which binds to a carrier protein and thus travels via the lymph system to the lymph node, where antigen processing occurs in macrophages. T lymphocytes with specific antigen recognition properties presumably proliferate and return in the bloodstream to the skin, where they are available for rapid (6 to 18 hours) antigen recognition and reaction on subsequent contact rechallenges. The time required for sensitization varies with the strength of the allergen—it takes weeks or months in the case of weak allergens and less than a week for strong ones. On recognition of and reaction to the contact allergen, the T lymphocytes are assumed to release inflammatory mediators, which cause an acute erythematous papulovesicular eruption confined to the areas of allergen contact. The treatment is the same as that outlined above for acute contact irritant dermatitis. For intense pruritus, liberal use of oral antihistamines, cool compresses, cool baths, and soothing lotions (e.g., calamine) may be indicated. If the area of involvement is extensive or involves the face or genitals, a course of oral prednisone may be warranted in otherwise healthy children, beginning with 1 mg/kg/day (maximum 30 to 40 mg) and tapering the dose over 2 to 3 weeks to avoid a rebound resurgence of the dermatitis when the drug is discontinued.

Rhus Dermatitis

The most frequent contact allergic dermatitis seen in children is rhus dermatitis, caused by poison ivy, oak, and sumac. The contact allergen is pentadecylcatechol, an ingredient of the oleoresin urushiol. The characteristic pruritic, vesicular red eruption conforming to the typical contact distribution (i.e., on exposed surfaces and in linear patterns where leaves and branches touch the skin) is not always present. The oleoresin can persist on animal fur, clothing, or furniture for months as long as it is not destroyed by heat and can continue to be a contactant, sometimes at unusual sites. The burning of rhus leaves can create an airborne contact dermatitis that may be confluent and extensive over exposed sites. Ragweed pollen dermatitis, another airborne contact dermatitis, may be confused with rhus dermatitis in autumn.

To manage this type of dermatitis effectively, the patient and the family must be educated about the appearance of the *Rhus* plants and how the oleoresin is spread. Specifically they should be told to wash all garments (including shoes, packs, and purses) and themselves after possible exposure to the oleoresin to decrease potential ongoing contact. The transfer of vesicle fluid during scratching does *not* cause the dermatitis to spread.

Other Common Allergens

Nickel sensitivity, a frequent cause of contact dermatitis, may be seen following ear piercing when nickel studs are placed in the newly formed earring holes.[3] Other common objects to which children may be exposed and that can cause nickel dermatitis include zippers, watch bands, toys, coins, metal underwear snaps, and the like.[3] Adolescents and children also may suffer dermatitis from allergens such as parabens, lanolin, and paraphenylenediamine contained in nail polish, hair dyes, perfumes, deodorants, sunscreens, and other cosmetics. Neomycin and ethylenediamine, present in certain topical preparations, also may cause contact allergic dermatitis.

SHOE CONTACT DERMATITIS

Shoe contact dermatitis may be either of the irritant or allergic type. The diagnosis usually is suggested by the presence of a bilateral, symmetrical dermatitis involving the dorsum of the toes and feet, with relative sparing of the web spaces. The dermatitis may range in appearance from a chronic eczema with mild confluent erythema and postinflammatory hyperpigmentation of lichenified plaques to an acute papulovesicular eruption with oozing and crusting. Various shoe compounds are irritants or sensitizers; the most common is rubber, but also implicated are dyes and adhesives. Weston et al.[6] found a positive patch test in 8 of 19 children who had dorsal foot dermatitis. Patients who have shoe contact dermatitis should wear loose-fitting, open shoes and go barefoot whenever possible. Plantar hyperhidrosis (see Chapter 145, Hyperhidrosis) frequently accompanies shoe contact dermatitis and should be managed with frequent changes of socks and the application of absorbent powder and aluminum chloride (Drysol). Acute dermatitis will respond to topical steroids, antipruritic agents, and compresses (see above), but the inciting irritant or sensitizer must be avoided to prevent recurrences. In Weston's study,[6] all who avoided the allergen remained disease free at the 2-year follow-up. To determine if the patient is allergic to a shoe component, he or she should be referred to a center where patch testing is performed routinely. Patch testing can be done with a standard shoe patch test tray or parts of the suspected offending shoes. If a shoe allergy is identified, nonallergenic footwear should be recommended.

PATCH TESTING

Patch testing, the process by which dilute quantities of suspected allergens are applied to the skin, should be performed by trained personnel. This can be used to identify many contact allergens, but its results are only significant if there has been exposure to the allergen in question or to a similar compound and if exposure to the identified allergen causes a dermatitis. Care must be taken not to perform the test when active dermatitis is present. Patch test results are of questionable value in young children. Reliable plant allergens for patch testing are not available routinely.[1]

REFERENCES

1. Adams RM: Patch testing—a recapitulation, *J Am Acad Dermatol* 5:629, 1981.
2. Fisher AA: Contact dermatitis in childhood. In *Contact dermatitis,* ed 3, New York, 1986, Lea & Febiger.
3. Fisher AA: Nickel dermatitis in children, *Cutis* 47:19, 1991.
4. Hurwitz S: *Clinical pediatric dermatology,* Philadelphia, 1981, WB Saunders.
5. Weston WL: *Practical pediatric dermatology,* ed 2, Boston, 1985, Little, Brown.
6. Weston JA, Hawkins K, Weston WL: Foot dermatitis in children, *Pediatrics* 72:824, 1983.

197 Contagious Exanthematous Diseases

John H. Dossett

The literal translation of *exanthem* is *to bloom* or *to break out*. Thus parents are quite accurate when they say that "my child 'broke out' in a rash." Exanthem refers to an eruption or rash that usually is associated with fever and generally implies that the eruption is infectious in origin. These eruptions are extremely common in children and present the clinician with a major challenge in differential diagnosis, inasmuch as many illnesses manifest by rashes (exanthems) that can look very similar. Consequently the clinical manifestations other than the rash itself often must be explored to distinguish one disease from another. These would include the incubation period, prodromal signs, the age of the patient, immunization history, contact history, distribution and progression of the rash, evidence of other organ involvement, and pathognomonic signs, such as enanthem, peeling, or Koplik spots.

Confusion is compounded further by the knowledge that these rashes may be caused by viruses, bacteria, rickettsia, mycoplasma, and fungi. Moreover, certain allergic and immune complex diseases such as childhood arthritis can mimic the infectious exanthems.

It is not sufficient to conclude that the child who has moderate fever and rash has a "viral exanthem" and forget about it. For example, if rubella or erythema infectiosum (human parvovirus) is included in the differential diagnoses, one needs to investigate recent and potential exposures of the sick child to pregnant women, in that fetal infection with these viruses may be devastating. Diseases that might respond to specific therapy require special consideration. These include the exanthem of *Mycoplasma pneumoniae* infection, which will respond to erythromycin, or the exanthem of *Rickettsia rickettsii* (Rocky Mountain spotted fever), which most desperately necessitates early treatment with tetracycline or chloramphenicol. The rash of streptococcal or staphylococcal scarlet fever (scarlatina) needs specific identification so that it can be treated appropriately, and scarlatina must be differentiated from Kawasaki disease so that the latter receives careful monitoring and specific treatment. Some of the differentiating characteristics of these eruptions are found in Table 197-1 and in Tables 161-1 and 161-2 (see also Chapter 191 for a discussion of chickenpox).

ENTEROVIRAL EXANTHEMS

Inasmuch as rubeola (measles) and rubella have been controlled largely by the administration of effective vaccines, enteroviral infections are now the most common cause of exanthems in children. Many serotypes of echoviruses and coxsackieviruses are associated with rashes; often these are generalized maculopapular rashes with discrete lesions much like those of rubella. They may appear very much like roseola, with an initial 2 to 3 days of fever followed by the eruption. Generally, though, the prodromal fever is much lower than that of roseola.

Although maculopapular rashes predominate, vesicular lesions have been observed in coxsackievirus A5, A9, and A16 infections. Hand-foot-mouth disease commonly is seen with coxsackievirus A16 infection and is manifested by vesicles on the palms and soles and ulcers in the mouth.

Enteroviral exanthems typically occur in the late summer and early fall and are associated with epidemics of aseptic meningitis. These infections are presented in more detail in Chapter 230.

EXANTHEM SUBITUM (ROSEOLA)

On the basis of its clinical course and epidemiology, roseola long has been presumed to be an infectious illness. In 1988 a newly discovered virus called human herpesvirus–6 (HHV-6) was shown to be the infectious agent.[2] Moreover, this virus has been isolated from infants who have had roseola without a rash—a condition experienced pediatricians have long suspected.[1] Roseola is characterized by 3 or 4 days of high fever (104° to 105°FF [40° to 40.6°C]), followed by abrupt resolution ("lysis") of the fever and the eruption of a pink maculopapular rash that begins on the neck and then spreads to the trunk and extremities, usually sparing the face. The lesions are discrete and last only for 1 or 2 days.

The child usually has no other manifestation of illness and does not appear as ill ("toxic") as the severity of the fever might imply.

Roseola occurs year round and is limited to children between the ages of 6 months and 3 years.

Complications are limited to febrile seizures, which may be precipitated by the rapid rise in body temperature. Most children who have seizures associated with roseola show normal findings on spinal tap and have an excellent prognosis.

There is no specific treatment for roseola, but affected children can be made more comfortable by controlling their fever (see Chapter 254 for a more complete discussion of this disease).

ERYTHEMA INFECTIOSUM (FIFTH DISEASE)

As the name implies, erythema infectiosum is a contagious disease, as manifested by its epidemic occurrence. The infectious agent was identified in 1984 as human parvovirus (HPV). Susceptible persons are infected by droplets via the respiratory tract; in epidemics the attack rate is high.

The diagnosis depends exclusively on the clinical presentation, which is one of rash *without* fever or other systemic signs. The rash first erupts as a bright red erythema of the cheeks and forehead with circumoral pallor. This slapped-cheek appearance is the result of many large maculopapular lesions that coalesce to form a confluent red rash. These confluent lesions are hot to the touch and commonly palpable, but they are nontender.

Table 197-1 Differentiating Common Childhood Exanthems

Disease	Character of rash	Prodrome	Pathognomonic signs	Helpful signs
Enterovirus infection	Maculopapular; generalized to most of body; discrete	May have 3-4 days of mild fever before rash, or rash may appear with constitutional signs	Herpangina, hand-foot-mouth syndrome	Aseptic meningitis, pharyngitis, petechiae with some coxsackievirus strains; occurs in summer and early fall
Exanthem subitum (roseola)	Maculopapular and discrete; begins on trunk and spreads to face and limbs	3-4 days of high fever and irritability with no other signs	None	Dramatic drop in fever simultaneous with onset of rash
Erythema infectiosum (fifth disease)	Red and flushed cheeks with circumoral pallor; maculopapular rash on extremities (lacelike)	None	Slapped-cheek appearance in otherwise healthy child	Possible recurrence of eruption with irritation of skin by heat, cold, or pressure
Rubella (German measles)	Pink, maculopapular, discrete; begins on face and spreads to trunk and extremities	Commonly none; adolescents may have 1-3 days of low-grade fever and malaise	None	Tender postauricular and suboccipital lymph nodes; possibly arthralgia in adolescents
Mumps	Maculopapular, discrete, concentrated on trunk; may have urticaria	1-2 days of fever, headache, and malaise	None	Diffuse swelling of parotid glands, with pain and tenderness; aseptic meningitis; orchitis or pancreatitis; erythema of the Stensen duct
Infectious mononucleosis	Macular or maculopapular and discrete; when associated with ampicillin administration, is confluent (morbilliform) and more intense	2-4 days of fever, pharyngitis, malaise	None	Exudative pharyngitis, lymphadenopathy, splenomegaly, atypical lymphocytes on peripheral smear
Mycoplasma pneumonia	Maculopapular on trunk and extremities in 10% of cases; common spectrum of urticaria, erythema multiforme, and vesicular/bullous lesions	3-5 days of progressive fever, headache, malaise, and cough	None	Pneumonia, cold agglutinins may be elevated
Rubeola (measles)	Red to brown macular rash that spreads from face and neck to trunk and extremities; confluent (morbilliform), particularly on face; fades after 6-7 days with temporary staining of skin	3-4 days of high fever, conjunctivitis, cough, and coryza	Koplik spots	Always an associated conjunctivitis and cough
Atypical measles	Rash may be maculopapular, purpuric, petechial, or vesicular; prominent at wrists and ankles	2-3 days of fever, headache, and cough	None	History of killed measles vaccine, myalgia, pneumonia
Scarlet fever	Erythematous papular eruption sometimes associated with generalized erythema; concentrated on trunk and proximal extremities; feels like fine sandpaper	Occurs within 1-4 days of onset of focal infection	None	Focal infections such as pharyngitis, vaginitis, cellulitis, erythema of palms and soles; strawberry tongue; desquamation in recovery phase
Kawasaki disease	Rash ranges from maculopapular to scarlatina form to urticaria; marked erythema of palms and soles	1-3 days of fever and irritability	None	Conjunctivitis, tender lymphadenopathy, strawberry tongue, meatitis, diarrhea, meningitis, prolonged fever, late desquamation, arthritis in recovery phase

After a single day a maculopapular rash next appears on the proximal extremities. This then gradually spreads to the trunk and distal extremities, leaving a lacelike appearance as it clears. This stage lasts 2 to 4 days. In a third stage the rash may reappear transiently when the skin is traumatized by pressure, sunlight, or extremes of hot and cold.

RUBELLA

Our grandmothers knew rubella as "German measles" or "3-day measles." These names served to distinguish the disease from rubeola ("hard measles" or "10-day measles"). The virus was cultivated first in 1962; its clinical spectrum was documented thoroughly in the 1965 epidemic.

The typical clinical illness is mild and brief. In most children the rash is itself the first sign of infection. It typically is a pink, maculopapular eruption beginning on the face and spreading downward to the trunk and extremities. The lesions remain discrete and pink, the appearance of which contrasts with the raised, confluent, and deep red lesions of rubeola. The facial rash clears as the extremity rash erupts, and all are cleared by the third to the fifth day.

Fever is very mild, ranging between 99° and 101° F (37.2° and 38.3° C). Lymphadenopathy frequently is impressive, the nodes most commonly involved being those in the posterior auricular and suboccipital chains. They usually are tender at the onset of rash, but the tenderness resolves rapidly over 2 to 3 days. Although lymphadenopathy is an important sign of rubella infection, it is not pathognomonic, in that other viral infections also cause enlargement of these same nodes. Some children who have rubella have tiny reddish spots on the soft palate. These lesions, however, themselves are not distinguishable from those of scarlet fever or rubeola. The incubation period is 2 to 3 weeks, with a peak at 16 to 18 days.

Of all the childhood exanthems, it is most important to pursue objective confirmation of suspected rubella because the risk of spread to susceptible pregnant women has potential for such devastating consequences.

The rubella virus usually can be grown from the pharynx within 5 days of the onset of the rash. Serological diagnosis is made by demonstrating an antibody titer rise between acute and convalescent sera. Hemagglutination-inhibition (HI) antibody titers are readily available, and a fourfold rise after 2 weeks indicates recent infection.

Complications of rubella are rare in children, but a transient arthritis develops in approximately 15% of adolescents and young adults. The arthritis rarely becomes chronic.

The major serious complications of rubella virus result from fetal infection. If a pregnant woman is infected in the first trimester of gestation, there is a very high probability that the fetus will become infected, with involvement of virtually every organ in the body.

INFECTIOUS MONONUCLEOSIS

The exanthem of Epstein-Barr virus (EBV) mononucleosis occurs in approximately 15% of children who have infectious mononucleosis who are not treated with ampicillin. The rash is pink to red and macular or maculopapular. The lesions are discrete and have no specific distinguishing characteristic, so it most often is diagnosed on the basis of other signs of infectious mononucleosis and confirmed by the peripheral blood smear and serological tests.

The *administration of ampicillin* to persons who have infectious mononucleosis results in approximately 50% of them developing a much more intense rash. This ampicillin-associated rash is deep red and confluent, giving it a morbilliform appearance. This iatrogenic exanthem resolves spontaneously within a week, but its significance extends beyond its mere presence. First, such patients commonly are identified as "allergic to penicillin." Second, administration of ampicillin to a person who has infectious mononucleosis indicates that an incorrect diagnosis of antibiotic-treatable disease was made. This happens most often when rash and exudative pharyngitis are observed, a careful examination for generalized lymphadenopathy and splenomegaly is neglected, and a diagnosis of streptococcal or staphylococcal disease is concluded. The full spectrum of EBV infection is discussed in Chapter 221.

MEASLES (RUBEOLA)

Measles clearly is the most serious of the childhood exanthems because of the morbidity of the acute infection and its potential for producing permanent sequelae. The virus is highly contagious, and typical clinical disease begins after an incubation period of 10 to 11 days. The prodromal illness is manifested by increasing fever, cough, conjunctivitis, and coryza. By the fourth day the fever commonly is high (104° F [40° C]) and the rash erupts—typically a deep red macular rash that begins on the face and neck and spreads down the trunk and extremities. The lesions on the face and upper portion of the trunk soon become confluent to produce the characteristic morbilliform rash. By the sixth day the fever subsides and the rash begins to fade; as it fades, it leaves a faint brown stain in the skin and a fine desquamation ensues.

The *enanthem* of measles is pathognomonic. *Koplik spots* begin approximately 2 days before the rash erupts and increase in number until the first or second day of the exanthem. They are tiny bluish white spots on an erythematous base and cluster adjacent to the molars on the buccal mucosa.

The combination of Koplik spots, fever, cough, conjunctivitis, and morbilliform rash is sufficient to make a firm clinical diagnosis of measles. Although the children usually are very ill, they recover rapidly after the eighth or ninth day and most often are back to normal in a few days.

Measles virus induces inflammation throughout the respiratory tract, so respiratory complications are common; these include otitis media, pneumonia, and croup. The otitis media is treated as any acute otitis media. The pneumonia may be either a primary measles pneumonia or a superimposed bacterial pneumonia. All children who have measles need daily examination of the chest and observation for tachypnea. Development of clinical pneumonia is indication for a chest roentgenogram, white blood cell count, blood culture, sputum examination, and treatment with antibiotics because of the probability of bacterial infection.

Acute encephalitis is the major complication of measles infection. It occurs in approximately 1 per 1000 cases and commonly results in death or permanent neurological sequelae.

It manifests by headache, vomiting, drowsiness, personality changes, seizures, and coma. In most cases the cerebrospinal fluid reveals pleocytosis and elevated protein levels. Some of these children have only a mild disease and recover in a few days, but others may have a fulminant course.

Prevention of measles is discussed in Chapter 17, Immunizations.

Atypical Measles

In recent years some children who had been immunized with inactivated measles vaccine have had an atypical presentation of wild measles virus infection. Typically such children have had 2 to 3 days of fever and headache, followed by a rash erupting on the wrists and ankles. The rashes have varied from maculopapular to purpuric to petechial or vesicular. There has been marked myalgia, with swelling of the hands and feet; pneumonia is common.

The constitutional symptoms and the distribution of the rash may be confused easily with Rocky Mountain spotted fever. Elicitation of a history of having received killed measles vaccine obviously is crucial to the diagnosis.

MYCOPLASMA PNEUMONIA

Although cutaneous signs are not major manifestations of mycoplasmal infections, they occur with sufficient frequency to justify attention. A maculopapular eruption may appear on the trunk and extremities of 10% to 15% of persons infected with *Mycoplasma pneumoniae.* It is even more common for these infections to be associated with allergic-type eruptions that display a spectrum of cutaneous lesions ranging from urticaria and erythema multiforme to vesicles or bullae. Such patients frequently have had a prodromal illness of fever, headache, malaise, and cough. The pneumonia may escape physical diagnosis, only to crop up on the chest roentgenogram as an "incidental," accidental finding. Such a combination of symptoms is indication for treatment with erythromycin, whether or not one has access to laboratory confirmation.

MUMPS

An exanthem will develop in fewer than 10% of persons infected with mumps virus, but when a rash does occur, the lesions are maculopapular, pale pink, discrete, and concentrated on the trunk. The virus more typically involves the salivary glands, the testicles (after puberty), the pancreas, and the meninges. After an incubation period of 16 to 18 days, clinical mumps develops in approximately 60% of infected persons. The remaining 40% have inapparent infections, without salivary gland swelling.

The typical illness begins with 1 or 2 days of anorexia, headache, and mild to moderate fever. This is followed by complaints of discomfort when chewing and pain around the ear. There usually is a diffuse but noticeable enlargement and tenderness of the parotid gland, which can be distinguished from lymph node enlargement in that it extends anterior to the ear and below the ramus of the mandible posteriorly to the mastoid bone, usually obliterating the angle of the jaw. Lymph nodes are more discrete and generally submandibular in location. Accompanying the parotitis one commonly sees erythema around the opening of the Stensen duct. The fever usually lasts 2 to 5 days. Rarely, only one parotid gland is involved, or the submandibular salivary glands rather than the parotids will be swollen.

Meningoencephalitis is estimated to occur in 10% of all cases of mumps and is characterized by headache, nausea, vomiting, and mild nuchal rigidity. It may occur before, during, or after the parotitis phase of the disease. It follows a course similar to the aseptic meningitis that is caused by other viruses, and it usually has no sequelae. Some cerebrospinal fluid pleocytosis is present in most cases of mumps without clinical evidence of meningeal irritation.

Orchitis is uncommon in children, but unilateral involvement of the testes and epididymis is observed in approximately 25% of males who are infected with mumps virus *after* puberty. Patients who have orchitis usually are quite ill; however, the incidence of sterility in males who experience mumps orchitis is no greater than in those who do not.

The pancreas and other exocrine glands rarely are involved.

Late neurological complications include nerve deafness and a very rare postinfectious encephalitis.

SCARLET FEVER

The rash of scarlet fever (scarlatina) is caused by a circulating erythrotoxin that is produced by certain strains of streptococci and staphylococci. This rash is characterized by a fine papular eruption on an erythematous base. Often there is a generalized erythema of the skin, including even those areas that are not yet involved with the papular rash. The eruption of scarlet fever is concentrated on the trunk and proximal extremities. It feels rough to the touch like fine sandpaper. The rash commonly is associated with prominent erythema of the lips, soles, and palms. Transverse red streaks (Pastia lines) sometimes are present, usually in the antecubital spaces. Desquamation of involved skin typically occurs in the recovery phase. On the tongue one can observe prominent papillae on a very red base, giving a "strawberry tongue" appearance.

If streptococci are the source of the erythrogenic toxin, the pharynx is the usual site of focal infection. Other focal infections, however (such as vaginitis or cellulitis) also may be found. When staphylococci are the source of erythrogenic toxin, the infective focus usually is some site other than the pharynx; infected surgical or traumatic wounds have been common sites. Toxic shock syndrome (associated with staphylococcal vaginitis from tampon use) is a cause of scarlet fever rash.

The treatment of scarlet fever is directed toward eradication of the focal infection. Streptococcal infections are treated with penicillin or erythromycin, whereas staphylococcal infections are treated with erythromycin or dicloxacillin. If systemic illness is severe, the patient should be hospitalized to receive parenteral antibiotics and general supportive care.

The eruption that needs to be differentiated most carefully from scarlet fever is *Kawasaki disease.* Its cutaneous manifestations overlap remarkably with those of scarlet fever, but it usually can be distinguished by the additional signs of conjunctivitis, cracking of the lips, very tender lymphadenopathy, meatitis, and diarrhea. These children are profoundly irritable, and their fever persists for more than a week in most cases. Just as in scarlet fever, however, they have erythema of the palms and soles with striking desquamation during the second and third weeks of the disease. Kawasaki disease is presented in more detail in Chapter 225.

REFERENCES

1. Suga S et al: Human herpesvirus–6 infection (exanthem subitum) without rash, *Pediatrics* 83:1003, 1989.
2. Yamaniski K et al: Identification of human herpesvirus–6 as a causal agent for exanthem subitum, *Lancet* 1:1065, 1988.

SUGGESTED READING

Feigin RD, Cherry JD: Viral infections. In Feigin RD, Cherry JD, editors: *Textbook of pediatric infectious diseases,* ed 3, vol 2, Philadelphia, 1992, WB Saunders.

198 Cystic and Solid Masses of the Face and Neck

Neil E. Herendeen and Peter G. Szilagyi

The differential diagnosis of a neck mass is broad, ranging from common inflammatory lymph nodes and cysts to rare neoplasms. Therefore an orderly approach to the workup and management of a neck mass is needed. The most practical approach involves differentiating the anatomical location of the mass into lateral neck masses versus midline neck masses and determining the exact anatomical position of the mass.[9] It is helpful to localize a lateral neck mass further into either the anterior cervical triangle (anterior to the sternocleidomastoid muscle) or the posterior cervical triangle.

ETIOLOGY

Masses in the neck can be classified into two broad categories: cystic lesions and solid masses.[2] Cystic lesions are either congenital cysts or vascular malformations; however, traumatic hematomas and abscesses may appear to be cystic. Solid neck masses usually are inflammatory lymph nodes or, rarely, neoplastic lesions. In general, a careful history and physical examination will lead the clinician to the correct diagnosis. Carefully chosen laboratory tests or radiological studies then may confirm the diagnosis.

In evaluating neck masses it is important to be familiar with key anatomical structures of the neck. Because most neck masses encountered by pediatricians are lymph nodes and not cysts, it is crucial to understand the location of the different groups of lymph nodes within the anterior and posterior anatomical triangles of the neck. Figure 198-1 shows the location of the major groups of lymph nodes (in *solid circles*), the sternocleidomastoid muscle, and the typical locations of the congenital cysts *(open circles)* encountered most frequently.

HISTORY

It is important to determine whether the neck mass was observed at birth, whether it has increased or decreased in size, whether it has changed color, and whether the lesion has drained or opened. Knowing the age of onset may help because lymph nodes rarely appear at birth, whereas many congenital cysts are noted in the newborn period. Some congenital cysts, however, may not be noted until childhood or beyond and are detected only when they become infected.

The history of pain or tenderness is important. Congenital cysts are nontender unless they become infected. Inflamed lymph nodes are quite tender and painful. Pain during eating suggests parotid gland involvement.

PHYSICAL EXAMINATION

The first step in the physical examination is to determine whether abnormalities exist in other parts of the body, such as other cysts, lymphadenopathy, hepatosplenomegaly, skin lesions, or signs of infection. The exact anatomical location of the neck mass must be determined, and the clinician should note whether the mass is in the typical location of a lymph node (See Fig. 198-1). The consistency, color, and firmness of the mass should be noted, as well as the presence of tenderness. The size of the mass also should be measured.

Midline masses usually are related to a thyroid abnormality. Those that move with swallowing or with tongue protrusion suggest a thyroglossal duct cyst, inasmuch as these lesions may be tethered to the foramen cecum by the thyroglossal duct remnant. A mass along the anterior edge of the sternocleidomastoid muscle that moves with swallowing or that has a sinus opening to the surface of the overlying skin is likely to be a branchial cleft cyst. Both cysts and benign lymph nodes are freely mobile, whereas malignant lesions are more likely to be fixed to underlying structures.

Rapidly growing, painless neck masses are worrisome because they might be neoplastic. Additional signs associated with a neoplastic process include fixation of the mass to subcutaneous tissue, firm consistency, size of greater than 3 cm, and presence of constitutional symptoms. Neck masses in the posterior cervical triangle are more likely to be malignant than are masses anterior to the sternocleidomastoid muscle.

TYPES OF CONGENITAL CYSTS

Thyroglossal duct cysts account for more than 70% of congenital cysts of the neck, branchial cleft cysts for more than 20%, and vascular malformations and other lesions for 4% to 5%.[4]

Thyroglossal duct cysts result from failure of the embryological thyroglossal duct to degenerate during the fifth week of gestation, leaving a fistula, sinus tract, or cyst at the midline of the neck just below the hyoid bone.[3] Thyroglossal duct cysts are not often detected at birth but usually are noted first after the age of 2 years; they may first manifest as an inflamed, tender mass. When not infected they are smooth, firm, mobile, and nontender and move upward with tongue protrusion or with swallowing. The differential diagnosis includes sebaceous cysts, epidermal cysts, submandibular lymph nodes, and lipomas. Unless normal thyroid tissue is palpable, it is important to confirm the presence of the thyroid gland by ultrasonography or technetium scan, because what may appear to be a thyroglossal duct cyst actually may be an ectopic thyroid gland, and its removal would leave the

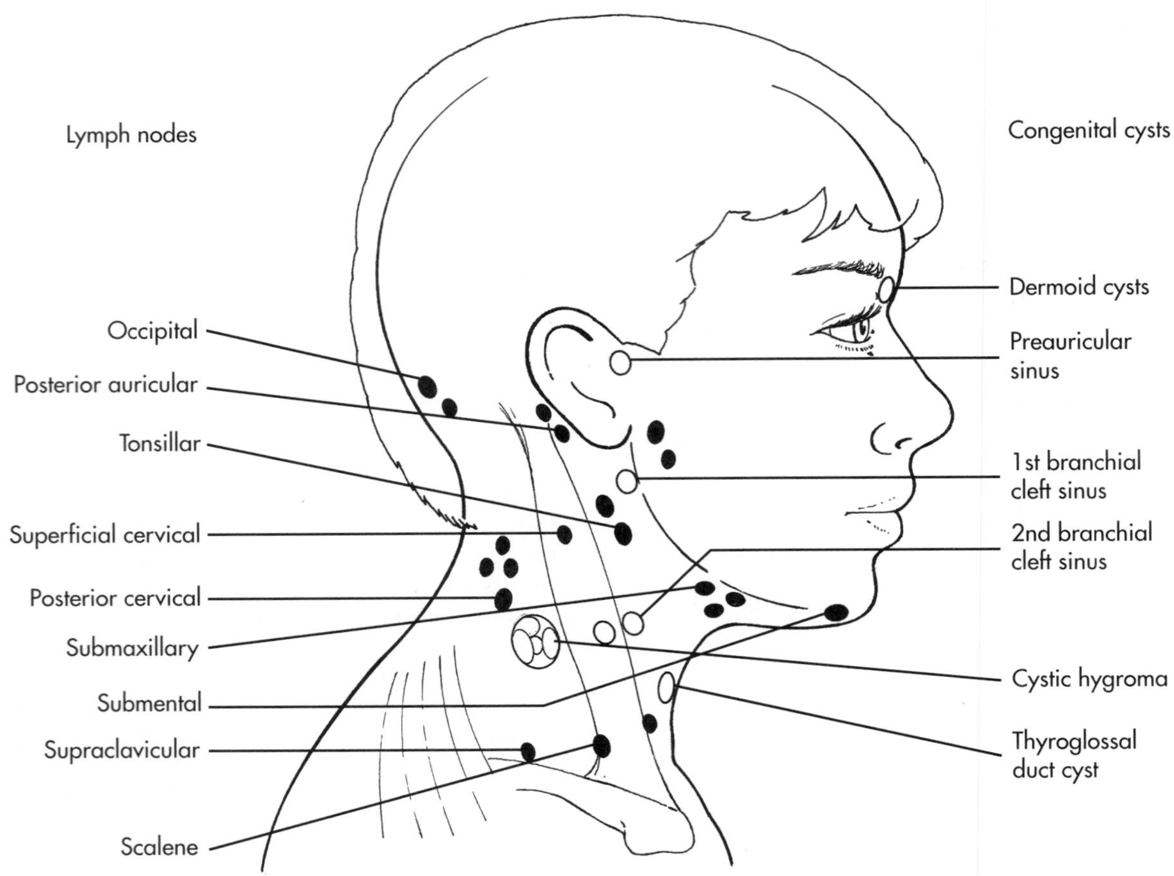

FIG. 198-1 Common locations for cystic and solid masses of the face and neck.

child dependent on thyroid hormone supplementation throughout life.[8] Because the likelihood of infection is high, thyroglossal duct cysts should be removed surgically.

Branchial cleft cysts are congenital remnants of the lateral four branchial pouches and clefts, which, interestingly, correspond to embryological gill slits in fish.[1] The vast majority of branchial cleft cysts arise from the second cleft or pharyngeal pouch. They appear as a small dimple or opening anterior to the middle portion of the sternocleidomastoid muscle. The cyst is nontender, firm, and mobile and is located just under the skin. A small sinus, which occasionally drains fluid to the surface of the overlying skin, may be present, and a long fistulous tract may extend from it to the tonsil bed.[3,5] Branchial cleft cysts without sinuses often are unnoticed until later childhood when they become infected. Infected cysts can easily be confused with lymphadenitis. Other lesions included in the differential diagnosis are sternocleidomastoid muscle masses associated with torticollis, small cystic hygromas, epidermoid cysts, neurofibromas, lipomas, and an ectopic thyroid gland. Treatment involves surgical removal of the cyst and fistula.

Cystic hygromas are congenital, avascular masses derived from congenital obstruction of lymphatic vessels. They generally are multilocular, fluid-filled, soft, compressible, painless masses located in the posterior triangle just behind the sternocleidomastoid muscle and in the supraclavicular fossa. They usually can be transilluminated. These masses may grow rapidly because of accumulation of lymph and can reach an enormous size, compressing important structures and obstructing the airway.[4] Although the diagnosis usually is obvious on physical examination, smaller cystic hygromas may resemble hemangiomas or other cysts. Ultrasonographic examination will reveal fluid and multiple cystic components, confirming the diagnosis. Because spontaneous regression is rare and the risk of compression of vital upper airway structures is high, surgical removal is indicated. Often multiple procedures are necessary to remove large lesions in their entirety. Cystic hygromas occur infrequently in the axilla, on the trunk, or on the extremities; in older children, when they occur within the subcutaneous tissues they may be mistaken for a lipoma or a hemangioma.[1]

Cavernous hemangiomas are vascular lesions within the subcutaneous tissues that may appear in any part of the body and may be difficult to differentiate from congenital cysts. They often are noted in the newborn period and enlarge (sometimes very rapidly) during the first year of life. Cavernous hemangiomas are less firm, more diffuse, and more easily compressible than are cystic masses (except for cystic hygromas). Unlike cystic hygromas, cavernous hemangiomas do not transilluminate, and their size may increase with crying or straining. Often the skin overlying these vascular lesions is bluish; cavernous hemangiomas frequently begin to increase in size during the first few months of life but usually regress spontaneously by school age.[9] Thus surgery is indicated only for masses that compress vital structures or that cause severe cosmetic disfigurement.

Epidermoid cysts are relatively common masses that may arise from an embryological or fusional defect. They usually are located at midline on the face, most often at the level of the eyebrows. These small cysts feel doughy and smooth and contain sebaceous material and sometimes even hair, cartilage, or bone. One third are present at birth; the remaining two thirds appear by school age.[5] Because these cysts may become infected and may form deep tracts, surgical excision is indicated.

Preauricular cysts and sinuses are the most common anomalies arising from an embryological fusion failure of precursor tissues that develop into the external ear. The sinuses are pinhole-size pits usually located anterior to the helix (see Fig. 198-1), and they may contain a short sinus tract.[3] Preauricular cysts often are bilateral. These sinuses and cysts are inherited in an autosomal dominant manner, with incomplete penetrance and are found more commonly in African-Americans than in Caucasians. They are a far more common cause of preauricular lesions than are first branchial cleft cysts, which are located in the same area.[5] Because they may become infected, elective surgical removal is a preferred treatment. Hearing deficits may be associated with these lesions, but their prevalence is unknown.

Other congenital masses occur rarely in the head and neck; the aforementioned lesions account for the vast majority of congenital masses. The major challenge in the differential diagnosis involves (1) differentiating congenital masses from lymph nodes and (2) determining the type of congenital lesion.

SOLID NECK MASSES

Cervical lymph nodes frequently are palpable in normal children and can be distinguished by their location (see Fig. 198-1), size, shape, consistency, and mobility. Enlarged cervical lymph nodes (>1 cm) should be defined further by their association with surrounding nodes or generalized adenopathy, the presence of an infection of the head or pharynx, and localized signs of inflammation and erythema. Cervical adenitis typically presents in a child who has a fever and a swollen, tender, erythematous mass. *Staphylococcus aureus* and *Streptococcus pyogenes* account for 80% of acute unilateral cervical adenitis and usually respond to oral antibiotics such as a semisynthetic penicillin or cephalosporin. Lymph node aspiration usually is reserved for those patients who do not respond to the initial course of therapy. Incision and drainage is an option for those masses that turn fluctuant. Some of the various causes of cervical lymphadenopathy include viral infections of the upper respiratory tract, bacterial infections, HIV infection, Kawasaki syndrome, and certain systemic disorders (lupus, juvenile rheumatoid arthritis, sarcoidosis, histoplamosis). Chronic inflammation of the lymph nodes can be seen with infections like cat scratch disease (see Chapter 182, Animal Bites), atypical mycobacterium, and toxoplasmosis.

Malignant tumors often are found as a single mass in the posterior triangle or as multiple or matted masses crossing into both the anterior and posterior triangles. Over 25% of children who have malignancies have a tumor of the head or neck.[9] The most common neck malignancies include Hodgkin disease, lymphosarcoma, rhabdomyosarcoma, fibrosarcoma, thyroid tumors, and neuroblastoma.

MANAGEMENT

As already discussed, all congenital cysts and masses should be followed up closely by the pediatrician. Acute infections must be treated with systemic antibiotics. Patients who have thyroglossal duct cysts, branchial cleft cysts, cystic hygromas, and epidermal cysts should be referred to a surgeon experienced at excision of these congenital lesions. Elective surgery before a bout of infection is preferable because excision of an entire sinus tract, fistula, or embryological connection is more difficult after an infection. Many pediatricians and surgeons prefer to delay surgery until the child is beyond infancy and will tolerate the procedure better. For patients who have thyroglossal duct cysts, a pediatrician or surgeon should confirm the presence of normal thyroid tissue by ultrasonographic examination or a technetium scan. Hemangiomas can be observed without referral unless they begin to impinge on vital structures.

For those children who have enlarged cervical lymph nodes and evidence of infection, the antibiotic therapy should improve the condition within 7 days; the condition should resolve completely over the next few weeks. If the adenopathy is persistent, with no inflammation, and has any worrisome characteristics (size >3 cm, not mobile, associated with systemic symptoms, in an abnormal location), the child should be evaluated further and followed up until the enlarged node has resolved.[6,7,9]

REFERENCES

1. Feins NR, Raffensperger JG: Cystic hygromas, lymphangioma and lymphedema. In Raffensperger JG, editor: *Swenson's pediatric surgery,* ed 5, Norwalk, Conn, 1990, Appleton & Lange.
2. Friedberg J: Clinical diagnosis of neck lumps: a practical guide, *Pediatr Ann* 17:620, 1988.
3. Friedberg J: Pharyngeal cleft sinuses and cysts, and other benign neck lesions, *Pediatr Clin North Am* 36:1451, 1989.
4. Gray SW, Skandalakis JE: *Embryology for surgeons,* Philadelphia, 1972, WB Saunders.
5. Hogan D, Wilkinson RD, Williams A: Congenital anomalies of the head and neck, *Int J Dermatol* 19:479, 1980.
6. Knight PJ, Reiner CB: Superficial lumps in children: what, when and why? *Pediatrics* 72:147, 1983.
7. May M: Neck masses in children: diagnosis and treatment, *Ear Nose Throat J* 57:12, 1978.
8. Raffensperger JG: Congenital cysts and sinuses of the neck. In Raffensperger JG, editor: *Swenson's pediatric surgery,* ed 5, Norwalk, Conn, 1990, Appleton & Lange.
9. Zitelli BJ: Evaluating the child with a neck mass, *Contemp Pediatr* 7:90, 1990.

199 Diabetes Mellitus

Robert E. Greenberg

DEFINITIONS AND FREQUENCY

Diabetes mellitus refers to a number of related disorders, all characterized by impaired glucose tolerance associated with a deficiency in either insulin secretion or its metabolic effect. Although disordered glucose homeostasis is the most striking and well-recognized characteristic of diabetes, many other metabolic abnormalities occur, affecting amino acid, protein, and lipid metabolism. The current classification, depicted in Table 199-1, emphasizes the distinction between insulin-dependent and non-insulin-dependent forms of diabetes, IDDM and NIDDM, as well as the heterogeneity of factors that may underlie hyperglycemia.

The prevalence of type I IDDM varies strikingly among various populations, with the highest rate in Northern Europeans (1 in 300 to 500 18-year-olds) and much lower rates in African and Asian children. The incidence in Northern Europeans approximates 10 per 100,000, with the peak incidence between 11 and 14 years of age. There is some suggestion that type I IDDM is less common in those groups in which the prevalence of type II diabetes appears to be markedly increasing (Native Americans, Polynesians, and Africans). The disease can affect adults at any age.

HETEROGENEITY

Recognition of the heterogeneity within diabetes was a critical step in understanding the separate nature of IDDM and NIDDM. This demonstration of heterogeneity has been based on family, twin, hormonal, immunological, and genetic studies. Family studies indicate that type I and type II diabetes segregate in an unrelated fashion. Studies of twins have set forth the difference between the two clinical syndromes: only 50% or fewer of monozygotic twins demonstrate concordance for type I diabetes, whereas 100% of twins show concordance for type II diabetes. Hormonal studies have demonstrated deficient insulin secretion as the primary event in type I diabetes. In type II diabetes, both insulin deficiency and resistance to the action of insulin are demonstrable, with the latter considered to be the primary event.[5] An altered immune response is associated with IDDM in that most type I diabetic patients have autoantibodies against several pancreatic antigens demonstrable in their sera at the time of clinical diagnosis. Finally, HLA association studies have continued to reveal the striking association between specific alleles in the major histocompatibility locus with type I but not type II diabetes. More than 90% of Caucasian patients bear the serologically defined tissue specifications HLA-DR1, HLA-DR3, or HLA-DR4. If the fifty-seventh amino acid on the DQB chain is aspartic acid, occurrence of diabetes is low; a noncharged amino acid at the same site raises the risk.[4] During the middle years of life, distinguishing between type I and type II diabetes mellitus may be difficult, requiring use of hormonal and immunological data in addition to demonstrating alterations in carbohydrate metabolism. Further, both forms of diabetes may exhibit common aspects of their natural history, especially because the vascular and neuropathic complications partly are a consequence of similar disturbances in metabolic regulation.[12]

ETIOLOGICAL MECHANISMS IN TYPE I DIABETES MELLITUS (IDDM)

Genetic and Environmental Interplay

The striking fact that fewer than 50% of identical twins show concordance for type I diabetes strongly suggests that an interplay between genetic and other biological mechanisms must occur to produce disease.[10] Available data indicate that *type I diabetes is the ultimate result of autoimmune (self-directed) mechanisms.* Evidence for this includes (1) the presence of infiltration of the pancreatic islets by lymphocytes and macrophages in newly diagnosed patients, (2) islet cell–reactive antibodies and T cell clones in the sera of patients at the time of clinical onset, and (3) an increased frequency of non–islet cell specific autoimmunity in affected individuals or their family members. Of importance is the observation that autoantibodies may be demonstrated long before aberrant carbohydrate tolerance can be detected in both humans and experimental animal models. Further, a marked increase in the incidence of autoantibodies is seen in genetically predisposed, but healthy first-degree relatives of persons who have type I diabetes. The initiating environmental events for such autoimmune islet cell destruction remain unknown. Recently, evidence has accumulated suggesting that this immune defect may be triggered, in at least some children, by exposure to a protein in cow milk, and that antibodies to cow milk proteins also recognize antigens on the pancreatic beta cell membrane (the phenomenon of molecular mimicry).[9]

History

The classic presentation is that of a child who demonstrates the clinical consequences of reduced glucose utilization (polyphagia, weight loss) and hyperglycemia (polyuria, polydipsia). It still is common for the physician to be confronted with a child in whom the early clinical signs were unappreciated, leading to the classic clinical picture of diabetic ketoacidosis (vomiting, Kussmaul respirations, altered state of consciousness). Diabetic ketoacidosis is discussed in detail in Chapter 275. The coexistence of abdominal pain in a child who has diabetic ketoacidosis is extremely common and remains the leading cause of confusion in making the initial diagnosis. Although preexisting infections may be present (as in any child), no convincing evidence exists that newly diagnosed patients with type I diabetes are more susceptible to significant infections. Although the majority of affected children have type I diabetes, the occurrence of NIDDM is ap-

Table 199-1 Classification of Diabetes Mellitus

Current terminology	Older terminology
Insulin-dependent diabetes mellitus (type I)	Juvenile, growth onset, insulin-sensitive, labile, or ketosis-prone diabetes
Non-insulin-dependent diabetes mellitus (type II)	Maturity onset, insulin-resistant, or ketosis-resistant diabetes
Impaired glucose tolerance	Chemical, latent or borderline, or asymptomatic diabetes
Potential abnormality of glucose tolerance	Prediabetes
Gestational diabetes	Gestational diabetes

preciable. In this circumstance the clinical signs of diabetes usually are more subtle, and ketoacidosis rarely occurs.

Decreased glucose utilization (leading to hyperglycemia) may be found in any severely ill young child, especially in those who have reduced blood volume and peripheral hypoperfusion. Hyperglycemia in these circumstances is neither diagnostic nor predictive of IDDM.

Physical Examination

The findings on physical examination are determined by the duration and severity of insulin deficiency. If decreased glucose utilization has been present for weeks or months, poor weight gain will be an almost universal finding. If glucose utilization has been severely impaired, dehydration, respiratory compensation for metabolic acidosis, and altered consciousness will be the primary findings.

Laboratory Findings

Laboratory confirmation of carbohydrate intolerance requires the demonstration of hyperglycemia either when fasting or after food intake. Because of significant individual variations in the renal threshold for glucose reabsorption, *glucosuria alone is not diagnostic*. Elevation in the amount of glycosylated hemoglobin confirms persistent or chronic hyperglycemia. Depending on the severity and duration of insulin deficiency, the laboratory findings of diabetic ketoacidosis—reduced plasma bicarbonate, reduced blood pH, increased anion gap, and hyperlipemia (increased cholesterol and/or triglycerides)—may be present. Hyperkalemia often accompanies significant metabolic acidosis; hypokalemia in untreated diabetic ketoacidosis usually signifies a massive depletion of total body potassium. Hyponatremia may be partly artifactual because of the altered water distribution produced either by hyperglycemia or by the water displacement in plasma produced by severe hyperlipemia.

Rapid bedside diagnosis and management of diabetes are facilitated by use of glucometers for the determination of blood glucose and serial dilution of plasma for determination of ketone bodies (Acetest).

Differential Diagnosis

Glucose intolerance can result from a number of different conditions: (1) decreased insulin secretion (type I diabetes), (2) defects in the binding of insulin to receptors (altered affinity or numbers of receptors, antireceptor blocking antibodies), (3) defects in the glucose transport system, such as a reduced affinity and number or mobility of glucose transporters, (4) increased secretion of counterregulatory hormones (catecholamines, corticosteroids, growth hormones), and (5) postreceptor defects in insulin action (genetic or nongenetic). A useful path through such confusion is to determine whether the glucose intolerance coexists with a reduced or an increased level of insulin secretion (plasma insulin or C-peptide, determined by radioimmunoassay), as measured during a standard oral glucose tolerance test. If insulin levels are increased, the differential diagnosis of insulin-resistant states may be made more confidently.

Another form of diabetes, namely *maturity-onset diabetes of youth (MODY),* is a genetic disease that has an autosomal dominant pattern of inheritance. It appears to result from defects in the gene coding for the enzyme glucokinase. When the activity of this enzyme in pancreatic beta cells is reduced, the ability of the B cell to respond accurately to changes in blood glucose concentration by altering insulin secretion is blunted. Accordingly, hyperglycemia may occur with suboptimal increases in insulin secretion.[11]

Management

Natural History. When the diagnosis of diabetes mellitus is first made, insulin requirements may be high (>1 unit of insulin/kg/day). It should be noted, however, that the young child may be exquisitely sensitive to exogenous insulin, especially when the diabetes is diagnosed before the onset of ketoacidosis. Soon after initial stabilization, a respite may occur wherein requirements for exogenous insulin may fall or even vanish as endogenous insulin secretion resumes (documented by increased plasma C-peptide levels). This "honeymoon" period may last for weeks or even months with longer periods following intensive intravenous insulin therapy at initial diagnosis; after this phase, insulin requirements are determined primarily by body weight, hormonal changes during puberty, and psychological factors.

The clinical course of the child who has diabetes is determined primarily by levels of understanding and the acceptance of the disease, psychological adjustment, family interactions, and stability of life-style. These factors are more significant determinants of metabolic control and frequency of hospitalization and illness than are the strictly biological factors affecting the action of insulin.

The progression of the natural history of type I diabetes depends on the attack rate and severity of occurrence of the vascular and neuropathic complications. The significance of these long-term complications is made dramatically evident by the fact that renal failure caused by diabetes is the most prevalent diagnosis among adults beginning hemodialysis or undergoing transplantation and that blindness is 25 times more common in individuals who have type I diabetes than in the nondiabetic population.

Importance of Metabolic Control. The entire design and implementation of strategies to manage insulin-dependent diabetes effectively are determined by the relation between its metabolic control and the histopathological events noted during its course. Studies during the last decade have provided strong evidence to support the view that microangiopathy and neuropathy have their origin in the metabolic defects associated with insulin deficiency and resistance to insulin

EVIDENCE THAT MICROANGIOPATHY IS A CONSEQUENCE OF ABERRANT METABOLIC CONTROL

Genetic issues

Microangiopathy does not occur in monozygotic twins in the absence of clinical diabetes.

Secondary diabetes (i.e., hemochromatosis and pancreatic resection) is accompanied by microangiopathy.

Animal studies

Experimental diabetes is associated with vascular lesions in proportion to the severity of metabolic disturbance.

Vascular lesions can be prevented or reversed by intensive insulin treatment or pancreatic transplantation.

The injured kidney of a diabetic animal may improve when transplanted into a nondiabetic recipient.

Human studies

Histological changes are not present at the onset of clinical symptoms in type I diabetes.

A normal kidney develops microangiopathic lesions when transplanted into a diabetic person.

Pathological changes are related to the duration and severity of metabolic derangement.

Effective metabolic control of diabetes limits the rate of progression of microangiopathy.

action. This evidence is summarized briefly in the box above. In addition, the results of the Diabetes Control and Complications Trial have been published recently, summarizing the results of a multicenter randomized clinical trial designed to compare intensive with conventional diabetes therapy with regard to the development and progression of the early vascular and neurological complications of type I diabetes mellitus.[6] This very significant study demonstrated that intensive therapy "effectively delays the onset and slows the progression of diabetic retinopathy, nephropathy, and neuropathy in patients with IDDM." These observations have sharply heightened the mandate to assist children and youth who have type I diabetes in establishing glucoregulation as close to the normal range as possible without producing severe and recurrent hypoglycemia. This mandate represents a significant departure from previous pediatric practice, wherein adequate control was defined simply as normal physical and emotional growth and development in the absence of significant hypoglycemia or ketoacidosis. The practical questions now focus on the best methods to effect such a demanding level of metabolic control.

Monitoring. Short-term glycemia glucosuria will occur only when the concentration of glucose in blood exceeds the renal threshold for glucose reabsorption (the tubular maximum [Tm] for glucose). Inasmuch as the Tm for glucose normally approximates 180 mg/dl (with wide variations), glucosuria usually cannot occur without significant preceding hyperglycemia, nor does the absence of glucosuria ensure the absence of moderate hyperglycemia or distinguish normoglycemia from hypoglycemia. If metabolic balance is to be brought under more rigorous control, the glucose concentration of blood, rather than of urine, must be measured precisely. Hence, monitoring the blood glucose level has become the modern cornerstone of diabetes management. Assuming use of proper technique, the self-monitoring of blood glucose has many potential consequences for the patient: (1) it may stimulate interest and motivation in self-control of the disease; (2) it documents the precise nature of metabolic problems; (3) it reinforces learning behavior by demonstrating that metabolic control is possible; (4) it reinforces the acceptance of responsibility; and (5) it teaches through personal experience. Lack of compliance, however, may be associated with inaccurate and invalid blood glucose data, as has long been recognized to be the case in home monitoring of the urinary glucose level.

Daily monitoring can easily become an unthinking routine, especially if the data are not used to alter management. When daily monitoring at multiple times is beyond the current capability of a child or family, the following approach has been shown to lead to improved control:

1. Determine the blood glucose level before each meal and before bedtime during 3 days of every week (M, W, Sat or T, Th, Sun).
2. Determine the blood glucose level whenever symptoms suggest hypoglycemia or hyperglycemia.
3. Determine the blood glucose level whenever clinical situations arise that often are associated with hyperglycemia (infections, injuries, emotional distress).
4. Analyze available data weekly in terms of average blood glucose at each time of sampling.
5. Determine urine ketone levels whenever the blood glucose level is elevated markedly, or the child/youth is symptomatic.

By using the weekly blood glucose record to adjust insulin dosage systematically, exercise pattern or dietary intake not only improves diabetic control, but convinces patients that blood glucose measurements are used to make their lives better, rather than being a mandate from either parents or physicians. Further, this approach provides an incentive for regularity and places responsibility for documenting and interpreting metabolic control with the patient or parent, depending on the age of the child.[1]

LONG-TERM GLYCEMIA. When foods are heated or stored in the presence of reducing sugars for long periods of time, a brown color results, which is produced by a direct reaction between the free amino groups of proteins and the reducing sugars (this is the Schiff reaction of nonenzymatic glycosylation). Because some minor hemoglobin electrophoretic variants were glycosylated, such variants might be a consequence of nonenzymatic glycosylation, just as in the browning of foods. The detection of elevated levels of the principal glycosylated hemoglobin variant Hb A_{1c} among diabetic patients supported this proposal. The rate and extent of the nonenzymatic glycosylation of any protein in vivo depend in part on the concentration of protein and sugar, on the turnover rate of the protein, and on accessibility of sugar to the protein. Thus if a protein has a rapid turnover rate it cannot become significantly glycosylated, regardless of the concentration of blood glucose. Similarly, if the concentration of blood glucose is significantly elevated only for a small fraction of time, the extent of protein glycosylation will be minimal even if the specific protein has a very slow rate of turnover. The measurement of glycosylated hemoglobin provides a sort of integrated assessment of the mean blood glucose concentration over the preceding 1 to 2 months. Measurement of fructosamine is a reflection of glycated serum proteins (one half the half-life of hemoglobin).

More than simply providing a handy index of long-term glycemia, nonenzymatic glycosylation may have far greater implications in diabetes; many proteins may exhibit significant changes in their functional properties after glycosylation and thus be responsible for some of the tissue-specific consequences of the diabetic state.[3]

MONITORING COMPLICATIONS. Careful monitoring of blood pressure is an important part of monitoring procedures. Monitoring quantitative urinary albumin excretion also appears to be significant because microalbuminuria exhibits a relationship to the development of significant nephropathy. Yearly monitoring of thyroid function and blood cholesterol/triglyceride levels is recommended. Beginning approximately 5 years after clinical onset of type I diabetes, complete ophthalmological examination and urinalysis must become regular components of ongoing management.

Patient and Family Education. Critical to the successful management of insulin-dependent diabetes is the extent to which the patient and family are kept informed. The physician who can convey the message that "freedom from diabetes" can be achieved only by mastery of both practical and theoretical aspects of the disease has a much greater chance of achieving optimal diabetic control. Several principles underlie the education of the diabetic family:

1. A natural period of shock and grieving accompanies a new diagnosis of diabetes, during which the family is not easily capable of assimilating extensive information.
2. Education about diabetes must be organized into discrete modules (digestible bites) of information (see the box above).
3. Opportunity for self-study, using instructional aids, must be provided.
4. Educational outcome criteria need to be developed and incorporated into the patient's ongoing record.
5. Education must be directed initially toward the more practical procedures of blood glucose monitoring and insulin administration.
6. Education must be an ongoing, continuous part of patient-physician interaction and management.[3]
7. Problem-solving situations to enhance education are most effective when two approaches are used: (a) analyzing and interpreting the data derived from the patient's own monitoring program, and (b) creating "problem cases" that require the child/youth and the parent(s) both to understand the issues and to formulate approaches to management.

Diet. Of overriding importance to helping children and their families manage diabetes is the concept of diet regularity. When an individual has lost the capacity to modulate the amount of insulin secreted from moment to moment in response to varying stimuli (glucose or amino acids), it becomes essential to keep constant from day to day the magnitude of the substrate load to be metabolized. Fortunately the average child in a stable family has a uniform pattern of nutrient intake, but when that nutrient intake becomes the prime focus of parental attentions, mealtime can become a focus for family anxiety. Soon, regularity in intake is replaced by marked irregularity and variation.

In addition to regularity in the timing and quantity of food intake, several other principles are important:

1. The diet should be adequate nutritionally, just as for the nondiabetic person.
2. The diet prescribed should be within the bounds of cultural patterns and individual preferences and also should be based, whenever possible, on the family's usual pattern of eating.
3. Caloric and protein intake should be sufficient for optimal growth without obesity.
4. Caloric intake in the morning should be proportionally less than at other meals. The "dawn phenomenon" refers to that period between approximately 5 and 9 AM when insulin requirements increase in the absence of antecedent hypoglycemia for both diabetic and nondiabetic individuals.[8]
5. Exchange diets, based on individual dietary assessment, may be used as an educational tool for establishing and maintaining a pattern of regularity in nutrient intake. However, the blood glucose response to various food that contain isocaloric amounts of total carbohydrate varies widely; thus the basic premise that underlies the older "exchange lists" actually may not be valid.
6. Readily available pure carbohydrate (e.g., candy) makes interpretation of blood glucose patterns difficult and

TOPICS FOR PATIENT AND FAMILY EDUCATION

1. Nature of diabetes
   a. Blood glucose regulation
   b. Role of insulin
   c. Significance of hyperglycemia and ketonuria
2. Monitoring
   a. Short term
      (1) Home blood glucose determination
      (2) Urine testing
   b. Long term: glycosylated protein levels
3. Insulin therapy
   a. Types of insulin
   b. Methods of injection
4. Dietary management
   a. Importance of regularity
   b. Exchange lists
5. Effect of environment
   a. Emotional factors
   b. Exercise
6. Special problems and emergencies
   a. Ketoacidosis
   b. Insulin reactions
   c. Illness
7. Informing family, friends, and school personnel about diabetes
8. Resources for diabetics
   a. Peer or family groups
   b. Organizations
   c. Camps

thereby reduces the effectiveness of a self-monitoring program.

Insulin Administration. All mammalian insulin is of a similar structure and contains 51 amino acids in two polypeptide chains (A and B). Pork insulin is closer in structure to human insulin than is beef. Allergic reactions to insulin, usually lipodystrophy or IgE-mediated local or systemic reactions, may be stimulated either by the beef or the pork insulin itself or by additives, preservatives, and contaminants. Use of recombinant DNA technology has enabled the synthesis of human insulin, which theoretically should not be immunogenic. Beyond an avoidance of allergic manifestations or antibody-mediated insulin resistance, however, human insulin offers only theoretical advantages over beef or pork insulin.

The proper use of insulin in the management of diabetes is restricted by the following considerations.

1. The normal pattern of insulin secretion is one of rapid changes (pulses, almost) in response to substrate stimuli, with a subsequent rapid decline in insulin levels. No current system of insulin administration, including the newer extracorporeal and implanted pumps, can mimic the rapidly changing secretory patterns found in the nondiabetic individual.
2. Fifty percent of endogenous insulin, secreted into the portal vein, is extracted by the liver in a single passage, but when insulin is given parenterally (except by intraperitoneal administration), the liver is bypassed. Thus the hepatic extraction rate for exogenously administered insulin theoretically can be only half the physiological secretory rate without producing peripheral hyperinsulinemia; at physiological peripheral blood insulin levels the portal vein concentration remains only half that seen in the nondiabetic person.

Practical aspects of insulin administration include the following.

1. Insulin absorption from sites of injection is highly variable from day to day, from site to site, and from one individual to another. Furthermore, insulin absorption is more rapid from a site of injection in which vasodilation by exercise has occurred.
2. After administration of either intermediate- or long-acting forms of insulin, a relation between the dose administered and the blood insulin level observed can be demonstrated *only* by measuring the total area under the curve of blood insulin concentrations obtained over a period of 24 to 36 hours, that is, no single time after injection can be selected to measure "peak" levels. Thus intermediate- and long-acting insulins cannot be used effectively where changing levels in circulating insulin are needed to handle sudden changes in substrate load (e.g., after meals).
3. Accordingly, it generally is advisable to give insulin under the following guidelines: (a) in the "established" diabetic (i.e., beyond the honeymoon period) less than 1 U/kg/day of insulin should be given; (b) the usual division of insulin should approximately two thirds of the total before breakfast and one third before the evening meal; and (c) approximately half of the morning insulin should be given as short-acting insulin, whereas increasing ratios of intermediate-acting insulin to regular insulin are given before the evening meal. In some instances additional short-acting insulin may have to be given before the noon meal if further optimal metabolic control is to be achieved. The intermediate-acting evening insulin may be given separately before bedtime to reduce the likelihood of hypoglycemia during sleep.[2,13]

Physical Activity. Regular physical activity is an important part of diabetic management, not only as an effective means to facilitate glucose utilization but also as an integral component of a life-style designed to minimize the risk of large vessel disease. Because the physical activity of children often is sporadic and unpredictable, it is wiser to ask the child to take extra calories than to attempt to alter insulin administration in anticipation of exercise, which can improve glucose utilization sufficiently to produce a relative insulin overdose.

Psychological Considerations. Like any chronic illness, diabetes presents new problems that may affect the child who has diabetes and his or her family. Many normal developmental tasks may be more difficult and less spontaneous for both child and parents. The family's ability to lead a normal life may be compromised by ignorance of the principles of good control or by unnecessary rigidities that impose excessive restrictions on life-style. An adolescent with diabetes may use the disease and the quality control it requires as a weapon against his or her parents; the parents in turn may use the disease as a mechanism to restrain the adolescent's establishment of appropriate independence from them.

The intimate relation that exists between the emotional state and the metabolic control of diabetes is well recognized. Numerous studies have demonstrated that emotional disturbances lead to compromised rates of glucose utilization, presumably through increased secretion of counterregulatory hormones. Conversely, emotional well-being of a patient who has diabetes can be affected by primary disturbances in metabolic control.

Uninformed responses to the child's disease by the extended family, friends, and school personnel can magnify his or her emotional distress. Careful attention therefore must be paid to informing and educating such well-meaning contacts so that the child's living opportunities are not restricted unnecessarily.

With careful attention to family dynamics, effort should be focused on improving the family's interactions, facilitating the communication of individual and group needs, and allowing both the child and family the opportunity to express the fears, concerns, and frustrations generated by the predictable problems every family with a child who has diabetes faces.

As the child grows older, the effect of microangiopathic and neuropathic complications on the emotional state becomes pronounced. Yet many patients remain able to maintain the balance necessary between the demands and excitement of their normal lives and the insistent constraints imposed by their disease.

FUTURE DEVELOPMENTS

Attempts to reduce the impact of type I diabetes reflect three primary approaches: (1) preventing the development of diabetes, (2) improving the physiological delivery of insulin, and (3) understanding the biological basis for the complications of diabetes, with the assumption that pharmacological tools will become available to impede the natural history of diabetes.

Prevention

The demonstration that immunotherapy at the time of clinical onset can delay the rate of beta cell destruction has set the stage for multiple approaches toward either primary prevention or treatment of subclinical disease in high-risk individuals. Primary prevention may be the consequence of restricting access of infants to cow milk proteins, if it is validated that such exposure leads to autoimmune destruction of the beta cells. Clinical research protocols are addressing several approaches to early treatment of subclinical disease: (1) nicotinamide in relatives who have increased levels of islet cell antibodies, (2) parenteral insulin trial in autoantibody-positive family members who already have exhibited loss of the first phase of insulin response to an intravenous glucose challenge, (3) oral insulin in a larger population, (4) different immunotherapy programs directed toward minimizing side effects.[3]

Improving the Physiological Delivery of Insulin

Insulin Delivery Systems. "Open loop" devices for chronic subcutaneous insulin infusions can provide normal metabolic control in certain patients, but they require a higher order of individual responsibility and compliance; such devices also are associated with complications (infection, erratic absorption, ketoacidosis). Therefore the "brittle" and often unmotivated child who has diabetes usually is not a good candidate for use of these open loop devices.

"Closed loop" infusion devices (where insulin is delivered in response to the blood glucose level) will require the preceding development of a reliable and implantable glucose sensor before such a system can be used.

Beta Cell Transplantation. Islet cell or intact pancreas transplantation has been successful; however, ongoing immunosuppression is required to maintain graft acceptance. Attempts to alter the antigenicity of donor cells before transplantation so far have been only partially successful. Modification of the donor tissue is the necessary approach, rather than attempts to inhibit rejection of the graft by the recipient.

Understanding the Biological Basis of Diabetic Complications

If the biochemical mechanisms that underlie diabetic complications were completely understood, specific therapies might be formulated that could forestall or prevent pathophysiological sequelae. For instance, nonenzymatic glycosylation of proteins leads to increased protein cross-linking, a process that can be impeded chemically. Further, in chronic hyperglycemia, shunting of glucose through the sorbitol or polyol pathway increases (leading to increased tissue concentrations of sorbitol), and this process can be impeded by inhibitors of the enzyme aldose reductase. Impaired synthesis of heparin proteoglycan may cause increased permeability of the vascular endothelium to macromolecules, a mechanism that also may be subject to chemical modification. These putative mechanisms exemplify exciting possibilities concerning chemical prevention of the pathological consequences of diabetes.

COMPLICATIONS

Insulin Resistance

The most common form of insulin resistance is that produced by excessive insulin administration (e.g., the Somogyi phenomenon). When poor metabolic control of the disease is attended by insulin dosages exceeding 1 U/kg/day, concern should be raised about excessive insulin administration; a stepwise reduction in insulin dose eventually will lead to improved control. Insulin resistance also may accompany use of the same site for repetitive injections. Sequestration of insulin at injection sites is an additional problem that appears more commonly during puberty. Antibody-mediated insulin resistance (commonly diagnosed but rarely present) may respond to human insulin. Further dissection of rare instances of insulin resistance requires sophisticated study of insulin-binding and postreceptor phenomena.[7] The child who has so-called brittle type I diabetes in reality most often is the child for whom family disruption and emotional factors lead to irregularity in diet, activity, and insulin administration, along with the metabolic consequences of emotional distress. Physiological insulin resistance can occur during puberty, when insulin requirements may increase to 2 U/kg/day.

Hypoglycemia

Coma or convulsions as a result of hypoglycemia are common complications of diabetes management that affect up to one third of children who have diabetes. Hypoglycemia occurs in the presence of unanticipated exercise, diminished food intake, or excessive insulin administration. The loss of glucagon and epinephrine secretion as a counterregulatory factor during the natural history of type I diabetes may be significant.[4]

Organ-Specific Complications

The major goals in diabetic management are the facilitation of normal physical and emotional growth and development, as well as postponement or actual prevention of the microangiopathic and neuropathic complications of the disease. Signs of microangiopathy are observed readily in many children within 5 to 10 years after the clinical onset of diabetes, although the actual clinical consequences are seen only rarely in childhood. Individuals caring for children who have insulin-dependent diabetes therefore constantly must recall the consequences of the disease in later life and the resulting overriding importance of establishing and maintaining optimal metabolic control.

REFERENCES

1. Blohme B: Home blood glucose monitoring—the key to good control, *Acta Med Scand (Suppl)* 671:29, 1983.
2. Bolli GB, Gerich JE: The "dawn phenomenon"—a common occurrence in both non-insulin-dependent and insulin-dependent diabetes mellitus, *N Engl J Med* 310:746, 1984.
3. Brownlee M: Glycation products and the pathogenesis of diabetic complications, *Diabetes Care* 15:1835, 1992.
4. Daneman D et al: Severe hypoglycemia in children with insulin-

dependent diabetes mellitus: frequency and predisposing factors, *J Pediatr* 115:681, 1989.
5. DeFronzo RA, Bonadonna RC, Ferrannini E: Pathogenesis of NIDDM: a balanced overview, *Diabetes Care* 15:318, 1992.
6. The Diabetes Control and Complications Trial Research Group: The effect of intensive treatment of diabetes on the development and progression of long-term complications in insulin-dependent diabetes mellitus, *N Engl J Med* 329:977, 1993.
7. Flier JS: Syndromes of insulin resistance: from patient to gene and back again, *Diabetes* 41:1207, 1992.
8. Gale EAM, Bingley PJ: Can we prevent IDDM? *Diabetes Care* 17:339, 1994.
9. Gerstein HC: Cow's milk exposure and type I diabetes mellitus, *Diabetes Care* 17:13, 1994.
10. Maclaren NK: How, when, and why to predict IDDM, *Diabetes* 37:1591, 1988.
11. Mueckler M: Glucokinase, glucose sensing, and diabetes, *Proc Natl Acad Sci USA* 90:784, 1993.
12. Ostman J: Can adequate control of diabetes prevent the development of vascular complications? *Acta Med Scand (Suppl)* 671:5, 1983.
13. Santiago JV: Insulin therapy in the last decade: a pediatric perspective, *Diabetes Care* 16:143, 1993.

200 Diaper Rash

Gregory S. Liptak

Diaper rash is the most common skin disorder of infants and toddlers. For example, a survey of suburban infants revealed that 25% had some diaper dermatitis; 4% of the sample had a rash that was classified as severe.[9] The greatest frequency occurs in infants between 9 and 12 months of age.[1] Diaper rash is not a single disorder but represents the reaction of the skin to a host of factors, both local and systemic, and on occasion may result from serious illness.

ETIOLOGY

Four factors have been associated with the occurrence of diaper rash: (1) wetness of skin (2) elevated pH level of skin (3) fecal enzymes, and (4) microorganisms.[2,5,18] Wet skin has been shown experimentally to have greater friction and higher permeability. In one study infants whose diapers had been changed eight or more times during the day (and presumably were dryer) had less rash than those whose diapers were changed less often.[7] Diapers made with water-absorbent gel material (usually cross-linked sodium polyacrylates) have been shown to keep skin drier and decrease the occurrence of diaper rash.[4,12,16]

The normal pH concentration of the skin is between 4.5 and 5.5. Elevated pH levels increase irritation and have been associated with more severe diaper rash. When urine and stool mix on an infant's skin, urease from the stool breaks down urea in the urine, increasing the pH. Although ammonia, which once was believed to be the primary irritant causing diaper rash,[14] may play a role in increasing the pH level it no longer is considered to be the major factor.

Normal stool contains enzymes such as proteases and lipases that inflame skin and increase permeability to substances such as bile salts, which worsen the inflammation. Infants who have more frequent bowel movements, such as those who have gastroenteritis or who are taking antibiotics, have a higher prevalence of diaper dermatitis.[4] Infants who are breast-fed have lower levels of enzymes in their stools, lower urinary pH, and a lower occurrence of diaper rash.

The most important microorganism found on the skin of infants who have diaper rash is *Candida albicans*.[5] This yeast, which produces a protease that penetrates the skin, can (1) cause a primary infection, (2) be a secondary invader in systemic conditions such as seborrheic dermatitis, and (3) be found in many infants who have nonspecific diaper rash. Even a small number of *Candida* organisms can cause significant infection. The use of oral or parenteral antibiotics can increase the number of *Candida* organisms on the skin (as well as the frequency of stools) and contribute to the occurrence of diaper rash.[8] *Staphylococcus aureus* also has been isolated as a secondary invader of systemic illness, such as atopic dermatitis; however, it does not appear to be a common primary pathogen in other forms of diaper rash.[13]

PATHOLOGY

A few histopathological studies of diaper rash have been described; however, most of these have dealt with unusual or chronic cases. The more common diaper rashes are believed to manifest nonspecific inflammatory changes.

HISTORY

Historical factors that may help determine the factors contributing to diaper rash include duration of the rash; associated symptoms (e.g., diarrhea); type of diaper; frequency of changing; method of laundering (if cloth diapers are used); use of watertight coverings, such as plastic (rubber) pants; past illness (especially dermatological, allergic, infectious); medication use (e.g., antibiotics), including the therapy for the rash; exposure to contagious disease (e.g., scabies, varicella); the presence of systemic symptoms; and a family history of illness (e.g., psoriasis, allergy).

PHYSICAL EXAMINATION

Although diaper rashes can be classified by presentation (appearance and location), this approach should be viewed with caution because one agent (e.g., *C. albicans*) can lead to different presentations, and a single presentation may be caused by many agents (acting either alone or in concert).

Three common distribution patterns for diaper rash occur. *Chafing* (irritative or ammoniacal) dermatitis (Fig. 200-1) is an erythematous desquamative rash involving the convex surfaces that touch the diaper and spare the inguinal folds. There is mild erythema with or without papules. The skin has a shiny, glazed appearance. This rash is associated with the irritants mentioned previously. Prolonged contact with water (uncontaminated urine) probably facilitates the production of all diaper rashes, especially those in this category. Meatitis (urethritis) may be seen in boys who have this type of diaper rash. Diaper rashes that have persisted for more than 72 hours usually are found to have significant *Candida* involvement.

Atopic dermatitis may have the same distribution as chafing as do zinc deficiency, Kawasaki disease, and Wiskott-Aldrich syndrome. The eczematoid appearance with lichenification (thickening), pruritus, and the occurrence of the atopic dermatitis elsewhere on the child should help substantiate this diagnosis. Diaper rash caused by atopic dermatitis is uncommon in children younger than 6 months.

The second pattern of diaper dermatitis involves skinfolds and spares convex surfaces (Fig. 200-2). Rashes involving the perianal area only are common in the neonatal period and may be the result of irritation from diarrhea (and are especially common in children whose diarrhea is secondary to disaccharidase deficiency). They also may be caused by infection with *C. albicans*.

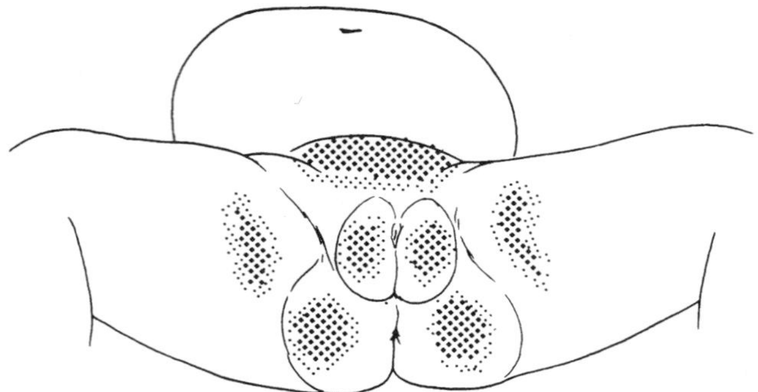

FIG. 200-1 Irritative pattern of diaper dermatitis.

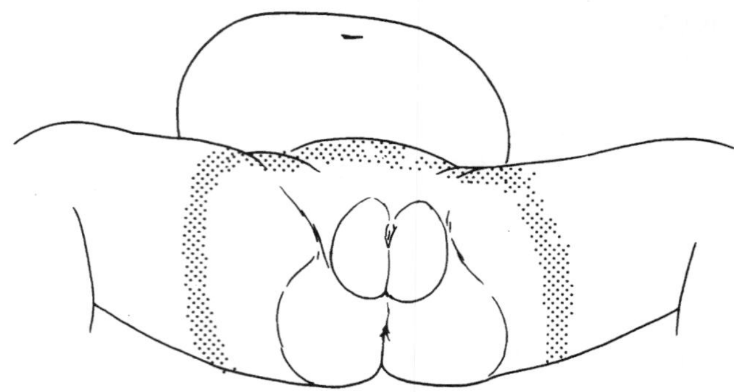

FIG. 200-3 Constrictive pattern of diaper dermatitis.

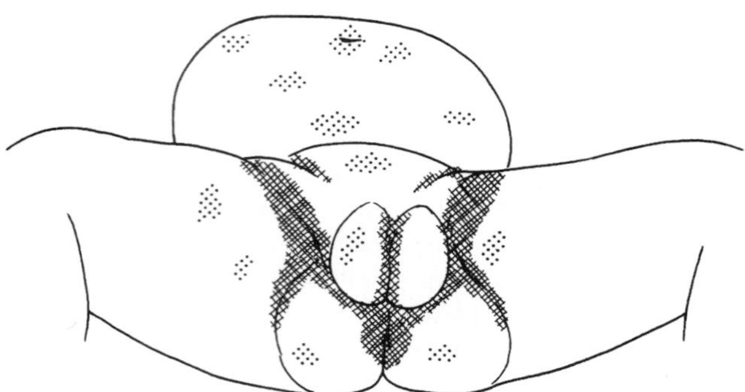

FIG. 200-2 Intertriginous pattern of diaper dermatitis.

Moist, macerated symmetrical eruptions in the skinfolds and creases (Fig. 200-2) may result from seborrhea or *intertrigo,* an ill-defined entity. Both commonly are infected secondarily by *C. albicans,* especially when satellite lesions are present. The classic primary candidal (monilial) diaper rash has this pattern with bright red confluent lesions, often with raised borders, and occasionally with pustular-vesicular satellite lesions on the trunk and legs. Other areas, such as the folds of the neck, the postauricular area, and the oral mucosa (thrush), may be involved. Dermatitis caused by *Candida* organisms usually is painful and tender. Letterer-Siwe disease (histiocytosis) may have the same skin rash distribution as seborrhea or *Candida* infections but is more papular and more likely to be ulcerated. It also fails to respond to conventional therapy; the child may have constitutional symptoms such as malaise and abnormal physical findings such as hepatosplenomegaly. *Seborrheic dermatitis,* which also has been termed *psoriaform napkin dermatitis,* is characterized by beefy red confluent erythema with scaling involving the entire diaper area; however, the intertriginous areas are involved more prominently. The rash looks worse than it appears to feel to the child. Some of these infants have a family history of psoriasis; true psoriasis will develop in approximately 3% as they get older.

The third major distribution pattern of diaper dermatitis is shown in Figure 200-3. Erythema in this distribution has been termed *tide mark dermatitis* and is believed to be related to frequent cycles of wetting and drying. Irritation from diapers that are too tight (constrictive) and that may have an elastic band also can lead to a similar rash.

Diaper rashes that do not fit any of these patterns—for example, from herpes simplex virus infection, also occur. In one study the less a rash looked like the one shown in Figure 198-1, the more likely it was to be associated with *Candida* organisms.[4] Diaper dermatitis from any cause can become secondarily infected with *Staphylococcus* or *Streptococcus* organisms, leading to impetigo or bullous impetigo.

DIFFERENTIAL DIAGNOSIS

Systemic conditions such as seborrhea, atopic dermatitis, primary herpes simplex infection, psoriasis, varicella, miliaria, and scabies may begin or occur with greater intensity in the diaper area.[10] Such predilection for the diaper area probably represents the Koebner (isomorphic) response in which the skin lesions of a systemic illness concentrate on areas previously injured by other factors, for example, friction.[9] Table 200-1 lists some of the less common causes of diaper rash.

In addition to the aforementioned conditions, histiocytosis (Letterer-Siwe disease), acrodermatitis enteropathica,[15] congenital syphilis, granuloma gluteale infantum,[3] and Wiskott-Aldrich syndrome may lead to rashes that are prominent in the diaper area. Kawasaki syndrome may manifest as a red, desquamating perineal eruption, often during the first week after onset of the syndrome[6] (see Chapter 225). Serious illness always must be considered in the child who has an atypical or a severe rash, as well as in the child who fails to respond to customary therapy. For instance, the child who has severe "seborrhea" may have histiocytosis; fulminant atopic dermatitis may be the result of Wiskott-Aldrich syndrome; and severe, persistent, and recurrent infections with *Candida* organisms may (albeit rarely) result from immunodeficiency, including infection with human immunodeficiency virus (HIV) or diabetes mellitus. Children who are immunosuppressed from HIV infection or neoplasia (or its treatment) may have diaper rash from organisms such as herpes simplex or cytomegalovirus. If an immunosuppressed child has a serious or unresponsive diaper rash, aggressive pursuit of an etiological agent, including skin biopsy, should be considered.[17] The physician should suspect child (including sexual) abuse or neglect in the child who has lesions in the diaper area (especially burns) that are inconsistent with the history provided.

LABORATORY FINDINGS

Laboratory tests generally are not indicated for most diaper rashes. Those that may be helpful in identifying the cause of

Table 200-1 Less Common Conditions Associated with Diaper Rash

Conditions	Comments
Infectious or presumed infectious	
Herpes simplex virus	Vesicular; may be associated with immunosuppression
Cytomegalovirus	Usually associated with immunosuppression
Kawasaki disease	Desquamating rash associated with fever
Syphilis	May have other manifestations of secondary syphilis
Trychophyton	Extremely uncommon; annular scaly patches
Neoplastic	
Histiocytosis (Letterer-Siwe)	Resembles seborrhea plus reddish brown papules
Nutritional and metabolic	
Zinc deficiency (acrodermatitis enteropathica)	Mimics monilial rash; vesicular eruptions elsewhere
Presumed iatrogenic	
Granuloma gluteale infantum	May be secondary to use of halogenated steroid creams
Genetic	
Wiskott-Aldrich	Thrombocytopenia and recurrent infections in boys

a diaper rash include a potassium hydroxide preparation and a fungal culture of skin scrapings for *Candida* organisms, a bacterial culture for *Staphylococcus* organisms, a mineral oil slide preparation for scabies, a serum zinc level (to rule out acrodermatitis enteropathica), serological tests for syphilis, and roentgenograms of the skull and long bones for evidence of child abuse. Laboratory studies for atopic dermatitis, Wiskott-Aldrich syndrome, and histiocytosis are discussed elsewhere in this text. Rarely a skin biopsy may be useful in cases in which the diaper rash is atypical or unresponsive to therapy.

MANAGEMENT

Because most diaper rashes, whatever the cause, are worsened by prolonged contact with wet or soiled diapers, the initial step in their management should be to keep the skin free of such diapers as much as possible. However, because total abstinence from diapers is impractical, most clinicians recommend that during therapy the diapers be changed frequently (at least eight times a day, using diapers with absorbent gel material) and kept off as much as possible and that plastic pants that retain water not be used.

Most systemic conditions such as scabies, atopic dermatitis, and varicella can be managed for the diaper area as they are for other parts of the skin. Seborrheic dermatitis, however, is an exception. Because it so often is infected secondarily with *Candida* organisms, measures to treat the yeast must be undertaken as well. For this and other diaper rashes in which *Candida* organisms are present, topical miconazole, clotrimazole, haloprogin, nystatin, or ketoconazole should be applied. Miconazole has the advantage of requiring only twice-daily applications, is less irritating than nystatin, and probably is more effective. It also is more expensive. Gentian violet also is effective but is extremely messy. The simultaneous use of 1% hydrocortisone usually hastens healing. Steroids more potent than 1% hydrocortisone should never be used in the diaper area because diapers form an occlusive dressing. Their chronic use may lead to granuloma gluteale infantum (a rash characterized by purple granulomatous nodules),[3] skin atrophy, telangiectasis, striae, irritation, and systemically, Cushing syndrome. The effectiveness of oral nystatin in the therapy of candidal diaper rash is uncertain. In a controlled study Dixon et al.[4] found that oral nystatin did not decrease the recurrence of candidal diaper rash significantly.

For irritative diaper rashes, changing diapers frequently and washing the skin with plain water and allowing it to dry between diaper changes usually are the only interventions needed. The use of diapers with absorbent gel materials has been shown to decrease wetness in the diaper area and may hasten the disappearance of a diaper dermatitis.[12] Scrubbing the rash or diaper area should be discouraged; a soft cloth with water should provide sufficient cleansing in most cases. A barrier ointment that contains zinc oxide or vitamins A and D may help to protect the skin from further irritation. Rinsing cloth diapers in methylbenzethonium chloride (Diaperene), a bacteriostatic agent, or in a vinegar solution (1 ounce in a gallon of water) has been shown to reduce recurrences.[7] Agents to acidify the urine (cranberry juice, vitamin C), cornstarch, and ointments that contain vitamins A and D are widely used; however, there is no experimental evidence that they are effective. Eliminating fabric softeners and changing detergents may be effective in some cases, but this approach also is undocumented scientifically. In cases of significant inflammation, 1% hydrocortisone may promote healing. The meatitis that occurs in this form of rash may be treated with topical antibiotics to prevent stricture by use of an ophthalmic solution applied by partially inserting the tip of the dispensing bottle into the urethra every 4 to 6 hours.

Many more children have been harmed by well-intended diaper rash therapies than have ever been harmed by the rash itself. Boric acid, mercury compounds, and pentachlorophenol used in the treatment and prevention of irritative diaper rash have led to illness and death in infants.[9] Talcum powder never should be used because inhalation of a large quantity can produce serious, even fatal, pulmonary damage. The dangers of topical steroids already have been mentioned. Hair dryers should never be recommended as a means to dry the skin in the diaper area; perineal burns may result. Products containing iodochlorhydroxyquin, such as Vioform, should never be used because they may lead to optic atrophy and neuropathy. Prudent use of therapeutic agents is necessary to avoid harm. The use of commercial diaper wipes, which contain an emollient and cleansing agent, is on the increase; their role with regard to diaper dermatitis is uncertain.

PREVENTION

If there were no diapers, there would be no diaper rashes. Because the complete elimination of diapers is unacceptable, alternatives to keep the skin dry, such as changing as soon as the diaper becomes wet or soiled and avoiding plastic pants, have been recommended.

Whether the type of diaper used affects the occurrence of diaper rash is controversial. Most recent studies have shown that diapers that contain absorbent gel are associated with the lowest incidence of diaper rash.[4,11,12,16] Although plastic diapers that contain absorbent gel material have been shown to decrease the occurrence of diaper rash and to contain stool and urine better, an important factor for decreasing the spread of disease in sites such as day care centers, attention also should be paid to the effect of plastic diapers on the environment. It is estimated that commercial nonbiodegradable diapers make up 1% to 2% of landfills. The cost of their disposal, which is borne by all citizens, should be considered when recommending their use. On the other hand, washing cloth diapers (and soiled clothes and bed linens) requires water and energy as well as human labor.[19] Parents who usually use cloth diapers may consider using commercial diapers that contain absorbent gel materials when their children are at increased risk for developing diaper rash, such as when they are taking antibiotics or have gastroenteritis. Commercial diapers also are convenient during travel away from home.

Breast-feeding and frequent diaper changes have been associated with a lower occurrence of diaper rash; both should be recommended. The physician should be certain that other recommendations do not harm the child.

REFERENCES

1. Benjamin L: Clinical correlates with diaper dermatitis, *Pediatrician* 14:21, 1987.
2. Berg RW, Buckingham KW, Stewart RL: Etiologic factors in diaper dermatitis: the role of urine, *Pediatr Dermatol* 3:102, 1986.
3. Bluestein J, Furner BB, Phillips SD: Granuloma gluteale infantum: case report and review of the literature, *Pediatr Dermatol* 7:196, 1990.
4. Campbell RL et al: Effects of diaper types on diaper dermatitis associated with diarrhea and antibiotic use of children in day-care centers, *Pediatr Dermatol* 5:83, 1988.
5. Dixon PN, Warin RP, English MP: Alimentary *Candida albicans* and napkin rashes, *Br J Dermatol* 86:458, 1972.
6. Friter BS, Lucky AW: The perineal eruption of Kawasaki syndrome, *Arch Dermatol* 124:1805, 1988.
7. Grant WW, Street L, Fearnow RG: Diaper rashes in infancy: studies on the effects of various methods of laundering, *Clin Pediatr* 12:714, 1973.
8. Honig PJ et al: Amoxicillin and diaper dermatitis, *J Am Acad Dermatol* 19:275, 1988.
9. Jacobs AH: Eruptions in the diaper area, *Pediatr Clin North Am* 25:209, 1978.
10. Jenson HB, Shapiro ED: Primary herpes simplex virus infection of a diaper rash, *Pediatr Infect Dis J* 6:1136, 1987.
11. Jordan WE et al: Diaper dermatitis: frequency and severity among a general infant population, *Pediatr Dermatol* 3:198, 1986.
12. Lane AT, Rehder PA, Helm K: Evaluations of diapers containing absorbing gelling material with conventional diapers in newborn infants, *Am J Dis Child* 144:315, 1990.
13. Leyden JJ, Klingman AM: The role of microorganisms in diaper dermatitis, *Arch Dermatol* 114:56, 1978.
14. Leyden JJ et al: Urinary ammonia and ammonia-producing microorganisms in infants with and without diaper dermatitis, *Arch Dermatol* 113:1678, 1977.
15. Munro CS, Lazaro C, Lawrence CM: Symptomatic zinc deficiency in breast-fed premature infants, *Br J Dermatol* 121:773, 1989.
16. Seymour JL et al: Clinical effects of diaper types on the skin of normal infants and infants with ectopic dermatitis, *J Am Acad Dermatol* 17:988, 1987.
17. Thiboutot DM et al: Cytomegalovirus diaper dermatitis, *Arch Dermatol* 127:396, 398, 1991.
18. Weston WL, Lane AT, Weston JA: Diaper dermatitis: current concepts, *Pediatrics* 66:532, 1980.
19. Wong DL et al: Diapering choices: a critical review of the issues, *Pediatr Nurs* 18:41, 1992.

201 Down Syndrome: Managing the Child and Family

Paul T. Rogers

The pediatrician is a source of education and support, as well as medical care, for the family of a child born having Down syndrome (DS). The physician's role is critical if the family is to adapt to the child's special needs. However, it may be frustrating at times to meet this responsibility. Often it is difficult to locate current information about the special health problems of a child who has DS. In addition, coordinating care with medical subspecialists and early child education specialists often can be time consuming. This chapter provides the pediatrician with a guide to the special needs of these families and children. It also discusses interventions that can identify and remediate many disorders that prevent a child from reaching his or her full potential.

DS occurs in about 1 in every 1250 births,[6] a decline from the incidence of 1 in 700 births just a decade ago.[30] The specific reason for this decline is not clear. The incidence of DS is closely related to advanced age of the mother, and the number of infants with DS born to women over age 35 increases dramatically.[17]

Recent advances have improved noninvasive techniques for identifying a fetus that has DS. Previously, measurement of the maternal serum alpha-fetoprotein (MSAFP) level was offered to pregnant women under age 35 because low levels of MSAFP are associated with DS.[1] Diminished levels of other maternal serum factors, unconjugated estriol, and human chorionic gonadotropin (hCG) also are associated with Down syndrome.[1] For pregnant women under age 35, the serum screening usually is completed by using a combination of MSAFP, estriol, and hCG. In pregnant women over age 35, amniocentesis or chorionic villous sampling (CVS) is offered instead of MSAFP. In the future, prenatal testing will be offered primarily to high-risk women almost entirely through noninvasive methods.[21]

ETIOLOGY

An abnormality in chromosome replication leads to DS. The abnormality, known as nondisjunction, results from a fault in chromosome replication during meiosis. During normal replication, the process of disjunction reduces the number of chromosomes in the sperm and ova from 46 to 23. At fertilization, the egg and sperm unite, giving the developing fetus the full number of 46 chromosomes in 23 pairs. Nondisjunction is the improper division of the 46 chromosomes in the cell, resulting in 24 chromosomes in the sperm or egg. At fertilization, 24 chromosome pairs, usually in the egg, unite with 23 pairs of chromosomes in the sperm, resulting in a total of 47 chromosomes. Recent DNA testing has shown that nondisjunction takes place in the egg 96% of the time. The extra chromosome in the karyotype results in three chromosomes (the extra chromosome plus the normal pair), which is designated *trisomy.*

About 90% of the time the extra chromosome is located in the 21 group. A small group of patients have a mixture of cell types (mosaicism), some cells with 46 chromosomes and some with 47. *Translocation* refers to a chromosome rearrangement in which the extra chromosome attaches to yet another chromosome. One of the chromosomes from the 21 group attaches very often to one in the 14 group. This results in a normal number of 46 chromosomes in 23 pairs, but the karyotype shows the abnormal attachment. Both translocation and mosaicism produce the clinical picture of DS. Translocation is especially significant because it can be inherited.

Every newborn who has DS requires chromosome testing. This information forms the basis of genetic counseling for the parents regarding the risk of recurrence. Because DS can recur, it is important to have a chromosome analysis done to complement a detailed family history. With this information, the family can better make a decision about future pregnancies.

Down syndrome, in effect, is a gene overdosage disease.[2] A DS-specific segment on a normal 21 chromosome produces excess proteins. The overproduction results in an imbalance of the biochemical pathways, which causes the physical characteristics of DS. Recent chromosome mapping shows that the DS-specific region is located around D21S55 in 21q22.2-22.3.[8]

PREVENTIVE MANAGEMENT

Preventive management refers to early detection and correction of medical problems seen in children who have DS. Children who have this disorder require the usual preventive intervention and anticipatory guidance given to other children, but the special problems of children with DS require close evaluation and monitoring. The most common types of problems include the following:

1. Ophthalmological: strabismus, myopia, and cataracts
2. Otological: chronic otitis media, conductive hearing loss
3. Cardiac: congenital heart disease (CHD)
4. Endocrine: hypothyroidism
5. Gastrointestinal: constipation, failure to thrive
6. Neurological: congenital malformation, seizures

Careful examination and testing should be done at critical ages to detect these common problems and correct them if possible.

Occasionally a woman who has learned that she is carrying a fetus with DS will contact a pediatrician with questions

COMMON FEATURES OF DOWN SYNDROME

May or may not be present:

Head
- Brachycephaly (flat occiput)

Dermatoglyphics
- Increased ulnar loops
- Single flexion crease on fifth finger
- Four-finger sign (simian crease): transverse palmar lines

Eyes
- Brushfield spots (speckling of the iris)
- Inner epicanthal folds
- Upward slanting palpebral fissures (mongolian characteristic)

Face
- Flat appearing
- Low nasal bridge
- Small ears with small or no earlobes

Fingers and toes
- Brachydactyly (short hands and fingers)
- Wide-spaced first and second toes

Heart (commonly congenital defects)
- Endocardial cushion defects
- Ventricular septal defects

Hips and pelvis
- Dysplasia

Neck
- Short
- Superabundant skin at nape

Neuromuscular system
- Absent or diminished Moro reflex
- Muscular hypotonia
- Joint hyperflexibility

Tongue
- Macroglossia
- Excessive protrusion

Potential for:

Increased incidence of leukemia
Increased susceptibility to infection
Increased incidence of duodenal atresia

about the challenges of raising a child with this disorder. A good source for information, in addition to the physician's discussion, is the National Down Syndrome Congress (1-800-232-6372). Besides information, this organization provides the names of other parents who have a child with DS.

DIAGNOSIS

The birth of a child who has DS presents an abundance of clinical and family management issues. The first critical task is making an accurate diagnosis. This often can be done at the bedside by means of a careful examination. When eight of the many characteristics commonly associated with DS are present (see the box above), the diagnosis is relatively simple.[14] However, when the diagnosis is based on one or two findings, errors can occur. For example, 50% of children with DS have the four-finger sign (formerly called a *simian crease*), but so do 15% of normal children. Small ears also are characteristic, but not diagnostic, of Down syndrome.

Many pediatricians are reluctant to share the diagnosis of DS with the parents unless it is confirmed in the laboratory by chromosomal karyotyping. Physicians delay the diagnosis until it is definitive so as to avoid giving the family the wrong diagnosis. However, in an informal survey (Patterson B., personal communication), families reported that they would like the physician to share the information with them as soon as the diagnosis of DS is suspected (see the box above). The pediatrician must decide which approach is best for the individual situation.

SUGGESTIONS FOR INFORMING THE PARENTS

1. Talk to both parents in a quiet place
2. Report the diagnostic information in a hopeful fashion
3. Allow time for the parents to respond
4. Give the parents current information to read
5. Give the parents the number of the local Down syndrome support group.
6. Discuss future expectations briefly
7. Allow the parents time to express their feelings and ask questions

MANAGEMENT

Newborn to 2 Months of Age (see the box on p. 1283)

After the diagnosis is made, the child is observed for signs of gastrointestinal malformations (vomiting, weight loss, and absence of stools), cardiac malformations (cyanosis, murmur, and irregular heart rate), and cataracts (absent red reflex). Laboratory testing includes chromosomal karyotyping, thyroid screening, and a complete blood count (CBC). Thyroid screening is particularly important because children who have DS have a higher incidence of congenital hypothyroidism.[11] Occasionally a DS child has leukocytosis, suggesting congenital leukemia. This usually benign condition is called *leukemoid reaction* (transient myeloproliferative disease), but careful follow-up is needed.[31] Hearing screening is suggested because 15% of children who have DS may have congenital hearing loss. In addition, an ophthalmological consultation should be arranged for any abnormalities (e.g., lens opacities) seen on the eye examination. A pediatric cardiologist should evaluate the baby for cardiac disease. A genetic consultant can help educate the family about prenatal detection and the risk of recurrence.

Once the diagnosis is made, the physician must inform the family fully; the approach must be gentle and hopeful. Some suggestions in this regard include the following:

1. Inform both parents together. Do this in a quiet place where the physician and parents will not be interrupted.

MANAGING THE NEWBORN

History

1. Evaluate the feeding pattern
2. Evaluate the stooling pattern

Physical examination

1. Perform a general physical examination and a neurological examination
2. Check for signs of CHD
3. Examine the eyes for congenital cataracts

Laboratory tests

1. Chromosomal karyotyping
2. Thyroid screening

Consultation

1. Cardiological examination
2. Genetic counseling

2. Provide current information to the family in a hopeful fashion.
3. Allow time for the parents to respond.
4. Provide written information about DS. Parents find it useful to have something to read after their discussion with the physician. Most information over 5 years old should be considered outdated.
5. Provide the name and number of a local DS support group. The National Down Syndrome Congress (1-800-232-6372) will provide the names of local support groups, as well as educational information for the physician and family.
6. Discuss future expectations briefly. Also discuss the potential medical problems, but point out that many children who have DS are healthy and participate in most of the usual childhood activities. Point out that the average life span of those who have DS now is 55 years. Discuss the plan to identify and manage medical problems.
7. Allow the family time to voice concerns and raise questions. Parents need time to express feelings of anger, guilt, or depression.
8. Arrange for a follow-up meeting with the family to give them time to begin adjusting to the new information and to formulate questions. Offer to meet extended family members, as well as the parents, to answer questions.

Most families accept a child born with DS. Some have greater initial difficulty and require more extended counseling. In rare cases a family will not be able to accept a child with DS. In this event, adoption should be discussed. There often are families waiting to adopt children who have DS. The Down Syndrome Adoption Exchange (914-428-1236) can be called for more information.

In this time of abbreviated hospital stays, the physician should arrange a visit with the parents and child 1 to 2 weeks after discharge. This provides time for further discussion with the family as well as for a follow-up medical assessment.

In the first few weeks of the infant's life, the physician may be asked questions about the following:

MANAGING THE INFANT: AGES 2 TO 12 MONTHS

Health Concerns

History

1. Evaluate the parents' concerns
2. Determine the incidence of otitis media and upper respiratory tract infection
3. Assess the infant's nutritional intake

Perform or refer the patient for the following tests and examinations:

Physical examination

1. Plot growth on a DS growth chart
2. General physical examination and neurological examination

Laboratory tests

1. Thyroid screening

Consultation

1. Cardiological examination
2. Ophthalmological examination
3. Audiological screening

Psychosocial concerns

Habilitation

1. Refer the parents to an infant education program
2. Continue educating the family about Down syndrome

1. *Oral motor problems.* Anatomical and neuromotor problems often result in a poor suck and frequent spitting. Mild feeding problems usually resolve in 2 to 3 weeks. However, some measures can help simplify feeding. The parents should be instructed to (1) make sure the child is fully awake when fed at night, (2) clear mucus from the baby's nose and mouth before feeding so that breathing will be easier during feeding, and (3) support the infant's chin during feeding.

   The pediatrician should follow the baby's weight and caloric intake carefully. If feeding problems are particularly severe or do not resolve with these interventions, referral to an oral motor (swallowing) specialist should be considered.
2. *Breast-feeding problems.* Most babies who have DS breast-feed successfully. If breast-feeding appears to be going poorly, the pediatrician should arrange a visit to review the baby's weight gain and the mother's breast-feeding technique. After a medical examination, particularly severe problems should be referred to a lactation specialist.
3. *Constipation.* If an infant has constipation that does not respond to dietary changes and stool softeners, evaluation for Hirschsprung disease should be considered.

Infants 2 to 12 Months of Age (see the box above)

In many cases families with a child who has DS need to see the pediatrician frequently for medical care and education. Often it is difficult to find the extra time in a busy office, where most visits may be for routine checkups or acute care. How does the physician find time for extended discussion? Following are a few suggestions:

1. Set aside a period each week, perhaps half a day, for consultation and family education. Keep this time free of acute care office visits.
2. Consider the contribution of a nurse practitioner (e.g., to help meet the extra educational and health care needs of the children and family).
3. Use a problem-oriented approach to the office chart. At the start, set up the medical record with special sections for:
   a. Problems
   b. Procedures (date, site, and result of all special medical procedures completed)
   c. Consultants involved in the child's care (with emergency numbers)
   d. An updated, one-page medical summary to be used for emergency admissions and consultations
   e. A flow chart of significant laboratory data and medications
4. Provide special check-out instructions for "covering" or "on-call" physicians, especially if they are outside the office and not familiar with the patient.

Medical care for infants in this age group who have DS involves particular diagnostic and consultative procedures (e.g., physical and occupational therapy and speech assessment) to detect both routine and potentially serious medical disorders. It is important to remember that the first year of life holds the highest probability of death for children who have DS.[3] Cardiac malformations cause 60% of the deaths that occur during the first 12 months.[4]

During office visits for periodic health assessments, the physician should ask about the baby's feeding sessions and the caloric intake. He or she also should discuss enrollment in an early education program.

On the physical examination, the pediatrician should check carefully for signs of cardiac and neurological disorders. Because frequent episodes of otitis media and upper respiratory tract infection are common in this age group, the tympanic membranes should be inspected. Hearing screening should be repeated if the newborn testing was equivocal or if signs of recurrent middle ear effusion are seen. The ophthalmological examination needs to be repeated at 9 months of age. A repeat cardiac consultation is indicated even in the absence of a murmur. Occasionally a congenital heart lesion is missed in the newborn period and manifests without typical cardiac findings at 6 to 9 months of age. Children who have DS *and* CHD have a greater tendency to develop early pulmonary hypertension compared with other children who have the same heart lesions.[7] All this underscores the need for early referral to a pediatric cardiologist.

The pediatrician can identify failure to thrive by plotting and following the infant's weight and height on the DS growth chart.[9] Further extensive evaluation may be indicated for pulmonary, cardiac, and gastrointestinal malformations. Recently, celiac disease has been added to the list of disorders that present with failure to thrive.[16]

Thyroid screening should be repeated at the end of the first year. Because clinical signs of hypothyroidism often are subtle, routine screening is suggested. Hypothyroidism occurs 28 times more often in infants who have DS than in the general population.[11]

Extra time should be arranged at office visits to allow families to talk about how they are adjusting to their child. The practitioner should review with them the information about DS provided earlier. The family also should be informed about Supplemental Security Income (SSI) and other government programs that help families financially with the extra costs of raising a child who has special needs.

Parents of infants who have DS often ask questions about the following issues:

1. *Tongue protrusion.* The factors that produce tongue protrusion include macroglossia, a small oral cavity, and mouth breathing.[2] Behavior management techniques can be used to manage tongue protrusion. Partial glossectomy should be considered when the macroglossia violates the airway.[27]
2. *Controversial therapies.* Some families contemplate controversial therapies as a means of obtaining a magical cure for their child. For example, facial plastic surgery techniques available include tongue resection to improve speech and silicone implants to correct micrognathia. Experts still are not sure if tongue resection improves speech,[22,23] and complications have been reported from facial surgery.[24,25] The pediatrician should try to educate families about the risks as well as the benefits of any surgical procedures. Preparations high in vitamins and minerals initially seemed to result in increased intelligence scores.[15] However, because no studies to date have replicated these results and side effects from megavitamin regimens have been reported,[5] unproven megavitamin and mineral therapies should be avoided. Routine nutritional screening should be done at the health assessment visit and vitamins prescribed when suggested by standard criteria.

Child 1 to 12 Years of Age (see the box on p. 1285)

Children who have DS need an annual health assessment. At these office visits, the pediatrician should ask about respiratory infections, constipation, and hearing problems. The practitioner also should ask about sleep problems to determine if the child has any symptoms of sleep apnea (e.g., snoring or difficulty breathing during sleep). Excessive drowsiness during the day also may be a symptom of sleep apnea.

The physician also should ask about behavior problems. Many children who have DS have unique personalities and do not fit the stereotype of being placid or compliant, and many parents may not volunteer information about obstinance or noncompliance. When there seems to be a behavior disorder, a careful history should be obtained, and the parents should be asked about changes in the environment or their expectations. A complete physical examination should be done, as well as laboratory tests, if warranted, to identify medical problems that may lead to behavior disorders. A trial of behavior management should be initiated for mild problems, and the diagnoses of pervasive developmental disability or physical abuse should be considered for serious behavior disorders. For severe behavior problems or persistent mild to moderate problems that have no medical cause, the child should be referred to a behavior specialist.

MANAGING THE CHILD: AGES 1 TO 12 YEARS

Health concerns

History

1. Assess any parental concerns about the child's behavior and school program
2. Ask if the child has shown any symptoms of a vision or hearing disorder

Perform or refer the patient for the following tests and examinations:

Physical examination

1. General physical examination plus a careful neurological examination
2. Height and weight plotted on a DS growth chart

Laboratory tests

1. Thyroid screening—each year
2. Hearing screening
3. Consider a cervical spine roentgenogram

Consultation

1. Eye examination—every 2 years
2. Hearing test—every 2 years
3. Roentgenogram of the cervical spine
4. Dental examination—twice a year

Psychosocial concerns

Habilitation

1. Discuss respite and long-term care plans with family
2. Review the child's education program

The pediatrician needs to review the current individual educational plan (IEP) to make sure that appropriate developmental testing has been completed and that the parents have had an opportunity to provide information in the IEP process. School problems may come to the physician's attention more often as children who have DS are placed in mainstreamed or regular classes.

School learning problems require further evaluation. The history should be reviewed carefully to ensure that the parents' and teachers' expectations are appropriate for the child's developmental age. A careful physical examination should be done to identify medical problems that can affect learning and behavior. For example, the ears should be examined for impacted cerumen that can cause a moderate hearing loss. An eye examination should be done to detect cataracts.[12] Vision screening should be done yearly or more often if indicated.

The physical examination must include plotting of appropriate measurements on the DS growth chart. It also includes a careful neurological search because atlantoaxial subluxation presents special problems in children who have DS. Atlantoaxial instability, which occurs in about 15% of children who have DS, refers to excess mobility of the atlantoaxial joint without neurological complications.[26] A roentgenogram of the cervical spine in flexion reveals an atlantoodontoid interval greater than 5 mm. Atlantoaxial subluxation, however, refers to backward movement of the odontoid process of the axis compressing the spinal cord, resulting in the signs and symptoms of cord compression, which may include neck pain, head tilt, progressive weakness, and loss of bladder or bowel control. Neurological examination reveals long tract signs such as increased deep tendon reflexes in the lower extremities, a positive Babinski sign, and ankle clonus. This indicates a neurosurgical emergency and requires immediate referral and treatment. Although atlantoaxial subluxation occurs in only 1.5% of children who have DS, it is a life-threatening complication.

Unfortunately, the natural history of atlantoaxial instability and subluxation still is understood poorly. It is not clear if one set of cervical spine roentgenograms is necessary or if these films need to be repeated. In addition, cervical spine roentgenograms may be unreliable in identifying all children at risk.[28] Until further information is available about the natural history of atlantoaxial subluxation, the diagnosis depends on a neurological examination plus neurophysiological and imaging studies.[25] Given this incomplete understanding, the following are some general guidelines for the pediatrician:

1. A cervical roentgenogram should be taken at 3 and 12 years of age to identify children who have atlantoaxial instability. The child also should have a yearly neurological examination to identify long tract signs. The child also should have a careful examination before participating in school sports or Special Olympics. The roentgenograms should be read by an experienced radiologist. If the child has a normal neurological examination and the roentgenograms are normal, he or she may participate in all sports. The films should be repeated in adolescence.
2. If the roentgenograms are read as abnormal (the atlantoodontoid distance is greater than 5 mm) and the neurological examination is normal, the child should be followed up closely on a yearly basis with repeated neurological examinations. It also is prudent for the child to avoid certain sports that place the neck in extreme extension (e.g., tumbling, gymnastics, and diving). The child also would need careful monitoring during intubation for induction of anesthesia if surgery is necessary.
3. If the roentgenograms are normal but the neurological examination is abnormal, the child should be referred to an experienced neurosurgeon or orthopedic physician. Further diagnostic testing may be suggested, such as a computed tomography (CT) scan of the cervical spine.

The studies suggested for children 1 to 12 years of age include annual thyroid, vision, and hearing screening.

General habilitation includes monitoring of exercise and recreational activities, good daily care of the teeth, and a dental examination twice a year beginning at the first birthday. Obesity often becomes a problem at about age 2. The pediatrician should ask about the child's snacks and the amount of time he or she spends watching television. The family should be asked again if they have checked into eligibility for SSI and Medicaid benefits. Parents also should investigate trust and guardian arrangements. The Association for Retarded Citizens (ARC) helps guide parents through these financial and custody arrangements. The local ARC chapter or the national office can be contacted for further information.

Parents of school-age children who have DS ask about the following issues most frequently:

1. *Obesity.* The cause of obesity in DS is multifactorial. Children who have greater hypotonia and shorter stature and those at preschool age and in adolescence are at greater risk. A preventive approach includes monitoring the child's diet, promoting regular exercise, and screening yearly for hypothyroidism.
2. *Hyperactivity.* Because children who have DS often attend regular schools for their education, hyperactivity comes to the physician's attention more frequently. A careful assessment should be done to identify some of the medical problems (e.g., mild to moderate hearing loss due to middle ear effusion) associated with inattention in children who have DS. After obtaining a careful history that includes information from the child's teacher, the physician should perform a complete physical and neurological examination and evaluate the child's vision and hearing. Thyroid testing should be considered when clinically suggested to rule out hyperthyroidism.[19] Behavior management techniques and classroom adaptations should be tried before resorting to medications.

Adolescence (see the box below)

Adolescence is a special challenge for any family. The physical, emotional, and educational needs in adolescents who have DS, however, require a special approach from the pediatrician. During the annual health assessment visit, the pediatrician should discuss with the family their child's infections, educational program, behavior problems, and prevocational experience and training.

The general physical examination should include plotting the child's height and weight to monitor for obesity. The need for a careful neurological examination for long tract signs persists at this age.

A gynecological examination should be done by at least 17 years of age. Because it often is not tolerated well by the adolescent, the pediatrician should consider referral to a specialist who has had experience evaluating women who have developmental disabilities. Often the examination can be done less invasively with pelvic ultrasound, which requires an examiner who has appropriate experience with the procedure.

Routine examination and consultation includes thyroid screening, a cervical spine roentgenogram at 12 and 18 years of age, and vision and hearing screening. The higher risk for periodontal disease among children who have DS is a major reason for dental examination twice a year.

Although many adolescents who have DS receive some formal education about sexuality in school, it is important to make sure that it is complete and to discuss this with the family. Although young men who have DS usually are sterile, a small number of girls and women have given birth to children. When a young woman who has DS does become pregnant, the father usually is a close relative.[29] Families need to know about birth control options and routine procedures for safeguarding their adolescent. If the primary care physician is not experienced in answering these questions, referral to a community specialist should be considered.

Adolescents who have DS also need education about smoking and drug abuse. If at all possible, they should have well-balanced diets, continue regular exercise, and be involved in appropriate social activities. When appropriate, they also should have opportunities for prevocational experiences such as doing volunteer work at a library or other

MANAGING THE ADOLESCENT

Health concerns

History

1. Answer the parents' questions
2. Ask about any education or behavioral problems
3. Make sure the patient is up to date on his or her immunizations

Perform or refer the patient for the following tests and examinations:

Physical examination

1. General physical examination
2. Obesity
3. Gynecological examination
4. Neurological examination

Laboratory tests

1. Thyroid screening

Consultation

1. Eye examination—every 2 years
2. Hearing test—every 2 years
3. Roentgenogram of the cervical spine
4. Dental examination—twice a year

Psychosocial concerns

Habilitation

1. Check to see whether the patient is obtaining vocational training
2. Have the patient continue speech therapy

Family concerns

1. Ask about community living plans for the patient
2. Discuss enrolling the patient in Medicaid and Supplemental Security Income (SSI) if he or she is eligible
3. Discuss the issue of sexuality, including preventing pregnancy
4. Help the parents teach their child to avoid smoking and drug abuse

facility that can provide adequate supervision. The school curriculum should make the transition to planning for a life vocation. Psychoeducational testing often is helpful in this regard to determine the individual's aptitudes, as well as his or her interest in community jobs.

Disruptive behavior, as well as anxiety disorders, may arise in adolescence.[20] A good mental status examination is helpful as part of the routine health assessment. When completing a mental status examination on an individual whose verbal skills are limited, it is necessary to talk with the family and teachers about any changes or regression in self-care skills. Often the family will report important information about withdrawal or loss of interest in recreational activities. Some emotional disorders manifest with excessive anger, frustration, or aggressive behaviors. Other signs of a possible disorder include self-injurious behavior (hitting or biting oneself), crying spells, or refusal to participate in self-care activities.

When the physician is evaluating a patient who has a sudden increase in behavior problems, it is important to look for underlying medical problems. For example, changes in vision or hearing may result in withdrawal or temper tantrums. Hypothyroidism can cause lethargy and lack of interest in activities. In rare cases, Alzheimer disease may appear in adolescence. When skills have been lost, it is important to document this with psychological testing that includes an assessment of self-care skills. Referral to a neurologist is suggested if this loss of skills is documented and initial assessment shows no signs of a correctable problem.

The pediatrician needs to discuss with the family a long-term plan for the adolescent's living arrangements. Most communities have a spectrum of community living facilities that range from small, heavily supervised group homes to apartments that have minimal supervision. Families need to arrange this early on because often there is a waiting list for placement in a community facility. The family should visit and discuss the options 2 or 3 years before they anticipate needing this arrangement.

Most families have questions about their adolescents with regard to the following issues:

1. *Sexuality.* There usually are many questions about a teenager's sexuality, but families often do not ask the pediatrician about them. For example, many parents wonder about the sexual interests of their children and the level at which they experience sexual feelings. They do not know how to deal with masturbation or questions about wanting to have a baby. Management of menstrual hygiene also presents problems. The school may provide sexuality education for adolescents. Referral to community resources should be considered for parents who have these additional questions if the pediatrician's expertise or the school curriculum needs to be complemented.
2. There may be inquiries about sterilization procedures for both young men and young women. In most states it is difficult to perform sterilization procedures because of the difficulty in obtaining consent. The pediatrician should counsel the family as well as the adolescent about preventing conception. Additional sources of counseling are available for families and professionals.[10]

Young Adult (see the box below)

Often, pediatricians continue to follow up adolescents into the early adult years to maintain continuity of care. Families often are attached to the physician and ask about continuing care; this discussion can center on aspects of preventive medical care for the young adult. The special interventions are an adjunct to the routine health assessment.

MANAGING THE YOUNG ADULT

Health concerns

History

1. Evaluate the family's concerns
2. Ask about symptoms of dementia and mental disorders

Perform or refer the patient for the following tests and examinations:

Physical examination

1. Gynecological examination and Pap smear
2. Testicular and breast examination
3. Neurological examination

Laboratory tests

1. Thyroid screening

Consultation

1. Cardiological examination and echocardiogram—to check for mitral valve prolapse
2. Eye examination—every 2 years
3. Hearing test—every 2 years
4. Dental examination—twice a year
5. Cervical spine examination—at age 30

Psychosocial concerns

Habilitation

1. Inquire about the patient's exercise and recreational activities
2. Urge the patient and family to continue with vocational and adult education programs to allow better job placement
3. When appropriate, check to see whether the patient has registered to vote and (for young men) has registered with the Selective Service Commission

Family issues

1. Remind the family to update their estate planning and wills
2. Evaluate the patient for community living if he or she is not already in this type of setting
3. Check on patient's eligibility for Medicaid and Supplemental Security Income (SSI)

ORGANIZATIONS PROVIDING PARENT EDUCATION AND SUPPORT

United States

National Down Syndrome Society
666 Broadway
New York, NY 10012
Telephone: 1-212-460-9330 **or** 1-800-221-4602

National Down Syndrome Congress
1800 Dempster St.
Park Ridge, IL 60068-1146
Telephone: 1-312-823-7550 **or** 1-800-232-6372

Down Syndrome Adoption Exchange
56 Midchester Ave.
White Plains, NY 10606
Telephone: 1-914-428-1236

Association for Retarded Citizens
P.O. Box 6109
Arlington, TX 76011
Telephone: 1-817-261-6003

Canada

The Canadian Down Syndrome Society
#303 501 18th Avenue, S.W.
Calgary, Alberta
Canada T2T 0C7
Telephone: 1-403-235-0746

National Institute on Mental Retardation
Kinsmen NIMR Building
York University Campus
4700 Keele St.
Downview, Ontario
Canada M3J 1P3
Telephone: 1-416-661-9611

Mexico

Asociacion Mexicana de Sindrome de Down A.C.
Boulevard de la Luz 232
Jardines del Pedragal
01900 Mexico, D.F.
Telephone: 1-525-652-4200

Down Association of Monterrey A.C.
20 De Noviembre Sur 846
Monterrey, N.L., Mexico

Adults who have DS require an annual health assessment. At this assessment, the physician should seek out symptoms of dementia such as loss of adaptive skills, diminished memory, personality changes, and confusion. Screening for hypothyroidism or problems with vision or hearing should continue. The parents should be asked about family or community living arrangements.

The general physical examination includes a gynecological and breast examination in women and testicular examination in men. The neurological assessment must include testing for long tract signs. Thyroid, vision, and hearing screening should continue, and the patient should be referred to a neurologist and/or a psychiatrist if symptoms of dementia, behavior problems, or depression arise. The dental examination continues at twice a year. Because about half of adults who have DS develop mitral valve prolapse, an echocardiogram needs to be done when clinical findings suggest it.[13] A Pap smear is necessary annually for sexually active women; in addition, a baseline mammogram is appropriate at age 35, with follow-up based on the physical examination and family history. Immunizations should be reviewed and kept current. Hepatitis B and pneumococcal vaccines should be considered for adults at special risk.

The young adult should be enrolled in a vocational training program to enhance his or her skills for either a community job or workshop placement. The program also should include some basic educational activities for continued improvement in skills.

Again, the physician should discuss with the family future living arrangements if the adult continues to live at home. Plans for guardianship and will or trust plans should be reviewed. The young adult also should be referred for registration with the Selective Service Commission and for voter registration. Health education, especially about drug and alcohol abuse, smoking, and sex, should continue.

Parents of adults who have DS usually have a compelling question: what will happen to their child after the parents' death? Most adults will need various levels of supervision because they are not independent economically. The family should be counseled to seek community resources for information about community living options. The state office of disabilities can provide information about social insurance and medical benefits available for adults with DS. A booklet published by ARC provides further information for the family.[18] The names and addresses of organizations providing parent education and support in the United States, Canada, and Mexico are listed in the box on the left.

REFERENCES

1. American Academy of Pediatrics, Committee on Genetics: Prenatal genetic diagnosis for pediatricians, *Pediatrics* 93:1010, 1994.
2. Anneren G, Edman B: Down syndrome: a gene dosage disease caused by trisomy of genes within a small segment of the long arm of chromosome 21, exemplified by the study of effects from the superoxide-dismutase type 1 (SOD-1) gene, *APMIS* 40:71, 1993.
3. Baird P, Sadovnick A: Life expectancy in Down syndrome, *J Pediatr* 110:849, 1987.
4. Bell JA, Pearn JH, Firman D: Childhood deaths in Down syndrome: survival curves and causes of death from a total population study in Queensland, Australia, 1976 to 1985, *J Med Genet* 26:764, 1989.
5. Bidder RT et al: The effects of multivitamins and minerals on children with Down syndrome, *Dev Med Child Neurol* 31:532, 1989.
6. Centers for Disease Control: Congenital malformation surveillance report: January 1981-December 1983, September 1985, US Department of Health and Human Services.
7. Chi TPL, Krovetz LJ: The pulmonary vascular bed in children with Down syndrome, *J Pediatr* 86:533, 1975.
8. Crete N et al: Mapping the Down syndrome chromosomal abnormality, *Clin Pediatr* 5:4, 1966.
9. Cronk C et al: Growth charts for children with Down syndrome: 1 month to 18 years of age, *Pediatrics* 18:102, 1988.
10. Edwards JP, Elkins TE: *Just between us: a social sexual training guide for parents and professionals who have concerns for persons with retardation,* Portland, Ore, 1988, Ednick Communications.

11. Fort P et al: Abnormalities of thyroid function in infants with Down syndrome, *J Pediatr* 104:545, 1984.
12. Gaynon MW, Schimek RA: Down's syndrome: a ten-year study, *Ann Ophthalmol* 9:1493, 1977.
13. Goldhar S, Brown WD, St John M: High frequency of mitral valve prolapse and aortic regurgitation among asymptomatic adults with Down syndrome, *JAMA* 258:1793, 1987.
14. Hall B: Mongolism in newborn infants: an examination of the criteria for recognition and some speculation on the pathogenic activity of the chromosomal abnormality, *Clin Pediatr* 5:4, 1966.
15. Harrell RR et al: Can nutritional supplements help mentally retarded children? An exploratory study, *Proc Natl Acad Sci USA* 78:574, 1981.
16. Hilhorst MI et al: Down syndrome and coeliac disease: five new cases with a review of the literature, *Eur J Pediatr* 152:884, 1993.
17. Hook EB, Fabia JJ: Frequency of Down syndrome by single-year maternal age interval: results of a Massachusetts study, *Teratology* 223, 1978.
18. "How to Provide for Their Future," Association for Retarded Citizens, National Headquarters, PO Box 6109, Arlington, TX 76011.
19. Lambyah PA, Cheah JS: Hyperthyroidism and Down syndrome, *Ann Acad Med Singapore* 22:603, 1993.
20. Myers BA, Pueschel SM: Psychiatric disorders in persons with Down syndrome, *J Nerv Ment Dis* 179:609, 1991.
21. Nicolini U: Prenatal diagnosis and fetal therapy, *Curr Opin Obstet Gynecol* 5:50, 1993.
22. Olbrisch RR: Plastic surgical management of children with Down's syndrome: indications and results, *Br J Plast Surg* 35:195, 1982.
23. Parson CL, Lacono TA, Rozner L: Effect of tongue reduction on articulation in children with Down syndrome, *Am J Ment Deficiency* 91:328, 1987.
24. Peled IJ et al: Mandibular resorption from silicone chin implants in children, *J Oral Maxillofac Surg* 44:346, 1986.
25. Pueschel SM et al: Atlantoaxial instability in Down syndrome: roentgenographics, neurologic, and somatosensory evoked potential studies, *J Pediatr* 110:515, 1987.
26. Pueschel SM, Scola FH: Epidemiologic, radiographic and clinical studies of atlantoaxial instability in individuals with Down syndrome, *Pediatrics* 80:555, 1987.
27. Purdy AH, Deitz JC, Harris SR: Efficacy of two treatment approaches to reduce the tongue protrusion of children with Down syndrome, *Dev Med Child Neurol* 29:469, 1987.
28. Selby KA et al: Clinical predictions and radiological reliability in atlantoaxial subluxation in Down's syndrome, *Arch Dis Child* 66:876, 1991.
29. Sheridan R et al: Fertility in a male with trisomy, *J Med Genet* 26:294, 1989.
30. Smith GF, Berg JM: *Down's anomaly,* Edinburgh, 1976, Churchill Livingstone.
31. Wong KY et al: Transient myeloproliferative disease disorder and acute nonlymphoblastic leukemia in Down syndrome, *J Pediatr* 112:18, 1988.

SUGGESTED READINGS

Lou IT, McCoy EE: *Down syndrome: advances in medical care,* New York, 1992, Wiley-Liss.

Rogers RT, Coleman M: *Medical care in Down syndrome,* New York, 1992, Marcel Dekker.

202 Drug Eruptions

Donald P. Lookingbill

The clinical expression of drug eruptions varies considerably. Because systemically administered drugs can cause almost any kind of rash, the practitioner should remember a general principle of dermatological diagnosis: "For any rash, think of drugs." The types of skin reactions caused by drugs include morbilliform eruptions, urticaria, erythema multiforme, erythema nodosum, vasculitis, photosensitivity reactions, acneform eruptions, alopecia, blistering disorders, fixed drug eruptions, lichenoid reactions, and drug-induced lupus erythematosus.[2,3] Tables in Fitzpatrick and coworkers' general dermatology text[2] conveniently list the drugs most commonly responsible for each of these different types of eruptions. This chapter deals only with the three types of eruptions most commonly seen in children; in order of decreasing incidence they are morbilliform eruptions, urticaria, and erythema multiforme.

MORBILLIFORM ERUPTIONS

Etiology

Morbilliform eruptions, also known as *exanthematous* or *maculopapular* eruptions, are the most common cutaneous expression of a drug reaction. Although a variety of drugs can cause this reaction, the drugs that most often cause morbilliform or urticarial eruptions are listed in Table 202-1.

History

A drug-induced morbilliform eruption usually does not have an immediate onset; rather, it begins within several days of initiation of the drug. The onset sometimes is delayed up to a week but seldom longer. Because no laboratory tests can identify the responsible drug, heavy reliance is placed on the history. Patients receiving more than one drug obviously present a problem. In trying to select a single drug from a list of many, the two variables to consider are (1) the temporal relationship between the drug and the rash and (2) the likelihood that a given drug can cause a drug eruption. For the latter factor, incidence data such as those in Table 202-1 are used.[1] Itching usually is present but is not helpful as a diagnostic marker. Fever is rare.

Physical Findings

The eruption is generalized and comprises brightly erythematous macules and papules that tend to be confluent in large areas. It usually starts proximally and proceeds distally, with the legs the last to be involved and also the last to clear. Drug fever has been well described, but most drug eruptions are not accompanied by an elevation in body temperature.

Laboratory Studies

Laboratory tests usually are not helpful. A peripheral blood eosinophilia sometimes is present and may heighten the suspicion for a drug reaction, but no laboratory tests can incriminate a specific drug.

Differential Diagnosis

For a generalized erythematous, "maculopapular" eruption, the major differential diagnosis is (1) a drug reaction, (2) a viral exanthem, or (3) a toxic erythema.

As the name *morbilliform* (measles like) suggests, a viral exanthem and a drug eruption can be indistinguishable clinically. Often a drug eruption is much more erythematous and more confluent, but not always. Other clinical information can help, including a drug history and the presence or absence of other viral signs and symptoms. Eosinophilia favors a drug etiology. Acute and convalescent serological tests can be obtained for some viral infections to provide a retrospective diagnosis. In most cases, however, a presumptive diagnosis is made on the basis of the combined clinical data.

Examples of toxic erythema are scarlet fever, staphylococcal-induced scarlatiniform eruptions, and possibly Kawasaki disease. Features that help to distinguish these toxic erythemas from drug eruptions include a sandpaper-like roughened texture of the rash, mucous membrane involvement (scarlet fever and Kawasaki disease), fever, a focus of infection, and lymphadenopathy. Postinflammatory desquamation from the skin of the hands and feet often follows the rash of toxic erythema, but this is not specific. Drug eruptions and even viral exanthems also can involve the hands and feet, and if the inflammation has been sufficiently intense, desquamation follows.

Management

When an offending agent is identified, it should be discontinued. If a patient is taking several drugs and it is not possible to be certain of the culprit, the number of drugs administered should be reduced to an absolute minimum and, whenever possible, any remaining possible offenders should be changed to alternative agents.

Therapy otherwise is directed toward the symptoms, with antihistamines used most commonly for the pruritus. Topical agents usually are confined to moisturizing lotions, which are most helpful during the later, desquamative phase of the reaction. Topical steroids are of little value, and systemic steroids rarely are required.

Complications

The complications primarily are cutaneous. When large areas of skin are inflamed, body heat increases and water is lost. If the patient already is seriously ill, this could be a problem; for most patients, however, it is not.

Guessing wrong and continuing an offending agent in the face of a drug eruption can result in two main consequences: cutaneous and renal. The cutaneous risk is that of progres-

Table 202-1 Allergic Skin Reactions to Drugs

Drug	Reaction rate (reactions per 100 recipients)
Amoxicillin	5.1
Trimethoprim-sulfamethoxazole	3.4
Ampicillin	3.3
Blood	2.2
Cephalosporins	2.1
Semisynthetic penicillins	2.1
Erythromycin	2.0
Penicillin G	1.9
Allopurinol	0.8
Barbiturates	0.4
Diazepam	0.04

Data from Bigby M et al: *JAMA* 256:3358, 1986.

sive worsening of the rash, possibly resulting in toxic epidermal necrolysis, a serious problem. Fortunately, this is rare. In fact, in some cases a drug eruption clears even when the offending agent is continued. Of course, it is not desirable to continue the drug if an alternative is available. The renal risk is that of allergic interstitial nephritis, an uncommon development that usually is associated with penicillins and celphalosporins and only rarely with other drugs.

Course

Drug eruptions clear with time after the responsible agent is discontinued. It is important to realize that it usually takes 1 to 2 weeks for the condition to clear completely and that the eruption actually may worsen for several days after the offending drug has been stopped. If a responsible drug has been identified, the patient should be advised about the allergy and the medical record should be clearly labeled to that effect.

URTICARIA (HIVES)[5,6,8]

Etiology

Drug-induced hives can be mediated immunologically by either (1) immediate IgE reactions, usually within hours, or (2) delayed immune complexes that result in serum sickness–like reactions after 7 to 10 days. The immediate reactions are more common.

History

A precise cause usually is not found among patients who have hives. When it is, it is determined from the history. The drug history is the most important but the most difficult to obtain, at least among outpatients. Because many patients and their parents tend to consider over-the-counter (OTC) medications unimportant, it often is helpful to ask about specific medications to help jog their memories. Aspirin is particularly important, inasmuch as salicylates cause hives in some patients and aggravate them in as many as one third of all patients who have urticaria, regardless of its cause. Whenever a drug is suspected, the physician must be aggressive and persistent in eliciting a medication history. Otherwise, some drugs invariably are overlooked.

A history of associated symptoms also may be important. Itching nearly always is present. A history of an obstructed airway or other anaphylactic symptoms suggests a more serious problem. Fever and arthralgia often accompany hives in serum sickness reactions, for which the two most common causes are drugs and viral hepatitis.

Physical Findings

Hives are skin lesions that are more easily recognized than described. They appear as edematous plaques, often with pale centers and red borders. They frequently assume geographical shapes and sometimes are confluent. The lesions may be scattered but usually are generalized. By definition an individual hive is transient, lasting less than 24 hours, although new hives may develop continuously. In serum sickness reactions, lymphadenopathy, in addition to fever and arthralgia, may be present.

Laboratory Studies

Drug-induced hives may be accompanied by an eosinophilia. To evaluate for hepatitis, it is appropriate to obtain liver function tests in patients who have hives and fever. In patients who have no fever, however, laboratory tests rarely are helpful in eliciting a cause, and they are of no help in implicating a specific drug.

Differential Diagnosis

The differential diagnosis of urticaria may be approached in two ways: (1) from the causes of hives per se and (2) from consideration of the cause of lesions sometimes mistaken as hives. As already mentioned, the cause of hives most often cannot be determined. When a cause is found, it usually is drug related. Other causes include infection, physical modalities (e.g., cold, pressure, or sunlight), emotions and, albeit rarely, foods.

Lesions sometimes mistaken for hives include those seen in erythema multiforme and juvenile rheumatoid arthritis (JRA). The lesions in erythema multiforme are discussed later. The individual lesions in JRA behave like hives in that they are transient but differ in size (only 2 to 3 mm), color (typically salmon), and timing (usually appearing with fever spikes).

Management

Any suspected medication, including aspirin, should be discontinued. Symptomatic therapy usually is achieved with antihistamines given on a regular rather than an as-needed schedule. Hydroxyzine is the preferred agent, administered in a dosage of 10 to 25 mg four times a day.

Complications

In rare cases acute urticaria can be accompanied by anaphylactic reactions that require more immediate therapy; usually, however, hives are more a nuisance than a morbid threat.

Course

Drug-induced hives usually clear within several days after the responsible medication is discontinued. As with any drug reaction, if a specific agent has been identified, the patient must be alerted to avoid that drug in the future. Because most hives are IgE mediated, rechallenge with the responsible drug is more likely to result in an anaphylactic response than is rechallenge in a patient who had a previous morbilliform eruption.

ERYTHEMA MULTIFORME[4,7]

Etiology

Erythema multiforme has been ascribed to innumerable causes, which are poorly substantiated except for two: (1) drugs and (2) infection, the latter primarily from *Mycoplasma pneumoniae* and recurrent herpes simplex. Circulating immune complexes have been detected in patients who have erythema multiforme, a finding consistent with the concept that this distinctive cutaneous disorder is an immunological reaction.

History

Sulfonamides, penicillins, barbiturates, and hydantoin have been the drugs implicated most commonly in erythema multiforme; however, a history for all drugs should be elicited. Recurrent herpes simplex infection is the most common cause of recurrent erythema multiforme. The herpetic lesion usually precedes the erythema multiforme by a few days to a week or more. Because, for the more extended intervals, the herpetic lesions may have healed by the time the patient comes for treatment, the history is important. In about half of all cases, a cause cannot be identified. In some patients a febrile prodrome precedes the cutaneous eruption by 1 to 14 days.

Physical Findings

As the name suggests, erythema multiforme is characterized by a variety of lesions, including erythematous plaques, blisters, and iris, or *target* lesions. Hives sometimes are confused with target lesions. The difference is that a hive has only two zones of color: a central pale area surrounded by an erythematous halo. The criteria for a target lesion require three zones: a central dark area or blister, surrounded by a pale zone, surrounded by a peripheral rim of erythema. True target lesions are diagnostic for erythema multiforme. They are seen more often on the palms and soles but may occur anywhere. Typically, erythema multiforme is a strikingly symmetrical eruption that favors the extremities. The disorder can range from mild to severe. In the severe form *(Stevens-Johnson syndrome),* the skin lesions are more extensive and mucous membrane involvement usually is severe as well.

Laboratory Studies

A chest roentgenogram is appropriate to screen for pulmonary involvement, including that caused by *Mycoplasma* infection, which can be confirmed further by acute and convalescent cold agglutinin titers. For herpes simplex disease, if the responsible vesicular lesion is still present, its fluid can be examined for multinucleated giant cells (Tzanck preparation) or cultured for herpesvirus. Laboratory evaluation usually is not helpful in drug-induced cases of erythema multiforme.

A complete blood cell count (CBC) and urinalysis are recommended because erythema multiforme occasionally is accompanied by leukocytosis and (although rarely) by renal involvement.

When the diagnosis is in doubt, a skin biopsy can be helpful. Erythema multiforme blisters are subepidermal.

Differential Diagnosis

The skin reactions most commonly considered in the differential diagnosis are urticaria, viral exanthems, vasculitis, staphylococcal scalded skin syndrome, and other blistering eruptions. The difference in appearance between a target lesion and a hive already has been discussed. In addition, individual hives last less than 24 hours, whereas the lesions in erythema multiforme persist much longer. Viral exanthems usually are monomorphous and tend to be less red, more confluent, and more centrally distributed than the lesions of erythema multiforme. Purpura is the distinguishing feature of vasculitic lesions. The skin in scalded skin syndrome is diffusely red and strips off easily (Nikolsky sign). In the rare case when erythema multiforme involves the whole skin surface (toxic epidermal necrolysis), a skin biopsy helps distinguish it from staphylococcal scalded skin syndrome. In erythema multiforme, the split in the skin is subepidermal, whereas in scalded skin syndrome, it is intraepidermal. Other blistering disorders that might be confused with erythema multiforme are rare in children.

Management

There is no convincing evidence that medical therapy favorably alters the course of erythema multiforme. Treating a precipitating infection seems appropriate, and erythromycin is recommended for *M. pneumoniae* infections, even though there is no proof that this alters the course of the skin reaction.

The use of systemic steroids is more controversial. They have been used frequently in Stevens-Johnson syndrome, but without documented benefit. In fact, Rasmussen's retrospective study[7] found that children who had Stevens-Johnson syndrome treated with systemic steroids required a longer hospital stay and had more complications (e.g., infection and gastrointestinal bleeding) than did untreated patients. Nevertheless, prednisone given systemically in doses ranging from 40 to 80 mg/m^2 still is sometimes used for patients who have severe erythema multiforme. Clearly, a prospective study is needed to determine whether this is helpful or harmful. Although the value of corticosteroid therapy may be unproved, supportive measures are important. These are aimed mainly at (1) restoring and maintaining hydration, (2) preventing secondary infection, and (3) relieving pain. Patients who have severe oral involvement may be unable to drink and thus may require intravenous fluids. When skin involvement is extensive, transcutaneous fluid loss increases and replacement volumes must be adjusted accordingly. Local therapy with antiseptics and dressings may help to prevent secondary infection, and patients who have severe involvement may require treatments similar to those for burn patients. Systemic analgesics are used for pain. Topical anesthetics may be used intraorally to provide temporary relief for patients who have painful mouth lesions. Viscous lidocaine is one such agent, but dyclonine liquid is easier to use, and its anesthetic effects last longer.

Complications

The major complication of erythema multiforme, which occasionally results in death, is worsening of the mucocutaneous involvement. The entire skin surface can become involved with the blistering process, a condition often called *toxic epidermal necrolysis*. Mucous membrane involvement can restrict oral intake, resulting in dehydration. Conjunctivitis can produce residual ophthalmic complications, of which *keratitis sicca* is the most common, occurring in about 15% of patients who have Stevens-Johnson syndrome. Internal organs are affected less often; pulmonary involvement is reported occasionally and renal involvement in rare cases.

Course

Patients who have mild forms of erythema multiforme usually recover uneventfully within 2 to 3 weeks. The course of the disease is longer (4 to 6 weeks) in patients who have severe involvement, and death occasionally occurs from Stevens-Johnson syndrome, with reported rates ranging up to 15%. Erythema multiforme recurs in 10% to 20% of patients and is particularly common in those in whom the disease is precipitated by recurrent herpes simplex infection.

REFERENCES

1. Bigby M et al: Drug-induced cutaneous reactions: a report from the Boston Collaborative Drug Surveillance Program on 15,438 consecutive inpatients, 1975 to 1982, *JAMA* 256:3358, 1986.
2. Blacker KL, Stern RS, Wintroub BU: Cutaneous reactions to drugs. In Fitzpatrick TB et al, editors: *Dermatology in general medicine,* ed 4, New York, 1993, McGraw-Hill.
3. Dunagin WG, Millikan LE: Drug eruptions, *Med Clin North Am* 64:983, 1982.
4. Huff JC, Weston WL, Tonnessen MG: Erythema multiforme: a critical review of characteristics, diagnostic criteria, and causes, *J Am Acad Dermatol* 8:767, 1983.
5. Jorizzo JL, editor: Symposium on urticaria and the reactive inflammatory vascular dermatoses, *Dermatol Clin* 3:1, 1985.
6. Monroe EW: Urticaria: an updated review, *Int J Dermatol* 20:32, 1981.
7. Rasmussen JE: Erythema multiforme in children: response to treatment with systemic corticosteroids, *Br J Dermatol* 95:181, 1976.
8. Wintroub BU, Stern RS: Cutaneous drug eruptions: pathogenesis and clinical classification, *J Am Acad Dermatol* 13:167, 1985.

203 Enterovirus Infections

Jerri Ann Jenista

Enteroviruses affect the practice of every pediatrician. The best known serotypes are the polioviruses, but the other enterovirus serotypes also cause widespread disease. A knowledge of these viruses can save both the practitioner and the patient considerable anxiety and can reduce diagnostic and therapeutic expenses.

CLASSIFICATION

Enteroviruses are Picornaviridae, small ribonucleic acid (RNA) viruses. They are classified into three groups: polioviruses, coxsackieviruses, and enteric cytopathogenic human orphan viruses (echoviruses). The paralytic disease of poliovirus was known in ancient Egypt and was described clinically in 1789 in England. There are three polio serotypes.

Coxsackieviruses, named for the town in New York state where the first recognized patients lived, are divided into groups A and B, depending on the characteristic pathological changes induced in suckling mice; 23 and 6 serotypes, respectively, have been described.

Echoviruses initially were thought not to cause disease but now have been associated with nearly all the enterovirus syndromes. More than 30 types are known.

All newly identified enterovirus serotypes are designated simply as "enterovirus" followed by a number, beginning with 68. Recent dramatic gains in our understanding of enterovirus genetics have resulted in the reclassification of several echoviruses and the hepatitis A virus (formerly enterovirus 72) into nonenteroviral categories.[11]

EPIDEMIOLOGY

The epidemiology of enterovirus infection is complicated by host, virus, and environmental factors. In the United States alone, approximately 10 million cases of symptomatic enterovirus infection occur every year. Since up to 90% of infections are silent clinically and reinfection is common, clearly a large percentage of the population must encounter enteroviruses each year.

Environment

In temperate climates, enterovirus infections show a distinct seasonality, occurring from June through October in the Northern Hemisphere. In tropical regions, however, infection is noted throughout the year, with an increased incidence during rainy periods. Crowding, poor sanitation, and lower socioeconomic conditions also contribute to a higher incidence of infection.

Host

Age correlates inversely with the severity of clinical disease, probably because an individual becomes immune to an increasing number of serotypes over several seasons. With certain enteroviral serotypes, neonates may develop fatal sepsis rapidly, whereas most older children and adults have mild or no symptoms. Some enteroviral syndromes (e.g., poliomyelitis, acute hemorrhagic conjunctivitis, or myocarditis) may be severe at any age. Males seem to suffer both more infections and more disease than do females.

Individuals who have humoral immunodeficiencies may suffer chronic, debilitating infection with enteroviruses. Except for poliovirus, enteroviral infection does not seem to pose a particular threat to individuals who have malignancy or acquired immunodeficiency syndrome (AIDS) or those who are transplant recipients, although there are occasional reports of severe or fatal disease in these groups.

Virus

Most enteroviral syndromes are not serotype specific; that is, several different types may produce the same clinical disease. For example, the coxsackieviruses first were recognized in children who had classic paralytic disease without evidence of poliovirus infection. Conversely, a single serotype may produce varying clinical syndromes in different seasons and communities and even in different individuals infected at the same time and place.

Although outbreaks of illness associated with a single serotype often are reported, the far more common pattern is endemic infection caused by several enterovirus types. The predominant circulating serotypes may vary yearly, by locality, and even within the same year. The pattern of clinical syndromes seen also tends to change over the enterovirus season. A typical sequence might be herpangina in June, nonspecific febrile exanthem in midsummer, and aseptic meningitis by early fall. Pandemic illness is unusual but not unknown. A modern example is the worldwide spread of acute hemorrhagic conjunctivitis caused by coxsackievirus A24 and enterovirus 70, which started in 1969 and affected millions of people.

Transmission and Incubation

Human beings are the only known reservoir for enteroviruses in nature. These viruses nearly always are transmitted by the fecal-oral route, although infections transmitted by food, water, blood, and perinatally occasionally have been reported. Nosocomial transmission has resulted in a number of severe nursery epidemics. In the special case of acute hemorrhagic conjunctivitis, the disease is spread by hand-to-eye contact.

The incubation period for enterovirus infection ordinarily is 3 to 5 days but may range from 2 to 20 days. The period of contagion probably is greatest several days before and immediately after the onset of symptoms; however, it may be prolonged. Because infection is so commonly asymptomatic and because virus excretion in the feces can persist for weeks after a person has recovered from the illness, it often is impossible to identify a patient's contact by history alone. Scrupulous hand washing may reduce the spread of enterovirus infection but is unlikely to control it completely, given the large pool of asymptomatic "shedders" usually present. Reinfection is common and usually clinically inapparent.

PATHOGENESIS

Over the past decade, the technological advances in molecular biology have produced a wealth of new information and have confirmed many long-held theories about the pathogenesis of enterovirus infection. For example, the development of monoclonal antibody systems has allowed researchers to isolate and clone poliovirus receptor sites on human cells.[11] As long suspected, these receptors are different from those for echoviruses. Antibodies directed against the poliovirus receptors block infection by any of the three serotypes of poliovirus but not infection by echoviruses or closely related nonenteroviruses. These and many other data are the first steps toward understanding the specificity of enteroviruses for primates and the tissue tropism of certain serotypes. The ultimate result of these studies may be an all-enterovirus vaccine.

Enterovirus infection is initiated by viral replication in the lymphoid tissue of the oropharynx and gut. This phase occurs over 1 to 3 days and is symptom free. A *minor viremia* follows, with spread of virions to the reticuloendothelial system at 3 to 5 days. At this point the patient is contagious, although symptoms of disease are not yet apparent. In a subclinical infection the process is halted at this point by host defenses. A subsequent *major viremia* results in viral dissemination to secondary organs such as the skin, heart, liver, pancreas, adrenal glands, and central nervous system (CNS). This phase most often is recognized clinically as a nonspecific febrile illness, or the "minor illness" of poliomyelitis. In a very small percentage of cases, viral replication continues, producing the various clinical syndromes of enterovirus infection such as poliomyelitis, herpangina, or pleurodynia. We do not know why serotypes have a tropism for certain tissues, such as poliovirus for the neurons of the brain and spinal cord.

Antibody production may be detectable as early as 1 day after exposure to an enterovirus; both serum and secretory forms are induced. Although some cross-reaction occurs among antibodies to different serotypes, protection against disease is not complete. Thus a person who has suffered paralytic disease with one serotype of poliovirus may still be susceptible to a second episode with another serotype. Enterovirus antibody also is found in human milk; it may prevent enterovirus infection or may interfere with successful immunization with oral (live) poliovirus vaccine in the newborn period.

CLINICAL SYNDROMES

Large-scale epidemiological studies of poliovirus infection indicate that probably more than 90% of enterovirus infections are inapparent. When symptoms do occur, a variety of host factors (e.g., age, genetic background, and antibody status) and viral factors (e.g., strain virulence and inoculating dose of virions) determines the clinical disease present. Although nearly all the protean syndromes associated with enteroviruses have been noted with serotypes from each group, certain diseases are associated more frequently with specific groups (Table 203-1). For example, coxsackievirus A virus is the likely etiological agent of an outbreak of herpangina.

Enteroviruses and the Febrile Infant

Any of the enteroviruses may cause a mild nonspecific febrile illness that lasts 2 to 5 days. Such seasonal infections account for the late summer and early fall peak of office visits noted in community surveillance studies of pediatric febrile illnesses.

Nonpolio enteroviruses are the major cause of hospitalization in febrile infants under 3 months of age. In prospective studies in Rochester, New York, enterovirus infection resulted in hospitalization in 2% of infants in the first month of life and accounted for 82% of admissions for "suspected sepsis." In other studies, enterovirus infection accounted for 33% of year-round admissions and 65% of summer-fall admissions for acute febrile illness in young infants.[8]

The most common presenting symptoms of nonspecific enteroviral illness are fever, irritability, lethargy, and poor feeding. Diarrhea, vomiting, or upper respiratory tract symptoms may or may not be present but are not severe enough to be the cause of the admission. Concomitant aseptic meningitis in infants is common and is not predicted by clinical symptoms.[7] The illness occasionally takes a biphasic course. A relapse of fever associated with irritability within a day or two sometimes results in a second hospital admission for the same illness.

Respiratory Tract Disease

Nonexudative pharyngitis with or without lymphadenopathy is common and probably is the major cause of summertime sore throat. In a few cases this illness may be the first manifestation of more severe disease that appears after an apparent recovery period of 1 to 3 days. Other respiratory syndromes (e.g., bronchitis, croup, or pneumonia) listed in Table 203-1 are less common and generally are mild. Herpangina is a disease commonly diagnosed in a young child who has fever and sore throat or pain on swallowing. An enanthem may be noted early, but it soon is succeeded by small vesicles and then by ulcers on the tonsils, pharynx, and soft palate. Occasionally the lesions are firm, tiny white nodules; the illness then is called *lymphonodular pharyngitis*. Herpangina is differentiated from herpes simplex stomatitis by the former's milder fever, primarily posterior oropharyngeal involvement, and epidemic seasonal occurrence.

The coxsackievirus B serotypes often are implicated in epidemic pleurodynia, or Bornholm disease.[12] Fever with severe pain in the intercostal and abdominal muscles occurring in spasms lasting minutes to hours are characteristic. The succeeding episodes are milder than the first but may occur days and sometimes even months later. In rare cases the symptoms are severe enough to prompt an exploratory laparotomy.

Enanthem and Exanthem Diseases

Hand-foot-mouth syndrome occurs in toddlers and school-age children. The hallmark signs are relatively painless vesicles on a red base, occasionally grouped, that appear on the buccal mucosa and tongue and on the palms and soles.

Table 203-1 Etiological Groups Most Often Implicated in Clinical Diseases Associated with Enteroviruses

	Poliovirus	Coxsackievirus A	Coxsackievirus B	Echovirus	Enterovirus
Asymptomatic infection	X	X	X	X	X
Nonspecific febrile illness	X	X	X	X	X
Common cold		X			
Pharyngitis	X	X	X	X	X
Herpangina		X			
Parotitis			X		
Croup			X	X	
Bronchitis, bronchiolitis			X	X	
Pneumonia			X	X	
Pleurodynia			X		
Myocarditis, pericarditis			X		
Gastrointestinal symptoms	X	X	X	X	X
Hepatitis			X	X	
Pancreatitis			X		
Diabetes mellitus			X		
Orchitis			X		
Hand-foot-mouth disease		X			X
Exanthem		X	X	X	X
Conjunctivitis		X			X
Aseptic meningitis	X	X	X	X	X
Paralysis, encephalitis	X		X	X	X
Chronic meningoencephalitis				X	
Generalized neonatal disease			X	X	

From Amstey MS, editor: *Virus infections in pregnancy,* New York, 1984, Grune & Stratton.

In rare cases the rash may spread to the extremities and buttocks. Patients usually have a low-grade fever and a sore throat and recover within a week.

A variety of exanthems may be the sole or major manifestation of enterovirus infection. Epidemics are reported with the classic macular blanching rubella-like rash, the so-called Boston exanthem, which begins on the face and trunk and spreads to the extremities. It is distinguished from rubella by the lack of posterior auricular and suboccipital adenopathy. Unusual enterovirus rashes may be maculopapular, vesicular, roseola-like, urticarial, or petechial. When such exanthems occur in conjunction with other enterovirus syndromes, such as aseptic meningitis, the illness may be mistaken for a more serious disease, such as meningococcal meningitis.

Gastrointestinal Diseases

Despite the virus group name and the fecal-oral transmission of enteroviruses, enteric disease is not a prominent clinical syndrome. Gastrointestinal symptoms of nausea, vomiting, abdominal pain, constipation, diarrhea, or peritonitis occasionally are seen but almost always with other signs of systemic enterovirus infection, such as aseptic meningitis. Hepatitis or pancreatitis usually is part of a generalized enterovirus syndrome.

Anecdotal cases of juvenile diabetes mellitus have been related to coxsackievirus B.

Acute Hemorrhagic Conjunctivitis

Acute hemorrhagic conjunctivitis is an epidemic disease marked by the sudden onset of severe eye pain, photophobia, tearing, and dramatic subconjunctival hemorrhage and swelling. Recovery occurs in a week to 10 days. The illness most often is observed in middle-age individuals, but epidemics in schools have been noted. Neurological sequelae may be seen in adults, and improvement may take several months. A worldwide pandemic of this disease began in 1969 with waves of disease in Asia and Africa. The disease reached the continental United States only in the early 1980s and has been confined mostly to the southeastern states.

Aseptic Meningitis and Encephalitis

Enterovirus infection is the major cause of aseptic meningitis in countries that immunize against mumps. The classic disease manifests in a school-age child who has a headache, nuchal rigidity, fever, and often photophobia, pharyngitis, or a rash. Cerebrospinal fluid (CSF) analysis shows a moderate pleocytosis with a predominance of lymphocytes, normal glucose levels, and slightly increased protein levels. Occasionally, meningitis (as documented by isolation of the virus) is present with minimal or no pleocytosis, especially in a very young infant.[7]

Diagnostic dilemmas are not uncommon when such an illness occurs in an infant under 1 year of age, in sporadic cases, during a course of antibiotic therapy, or with atypical associated findings such as a petechial rash or encephalitis. Spinal fluid obtained early in the course often has a predominant polymorphonuclear cell type; cell counts over 1000/mm^3 have been reported. In some patients a second spinal tap after a 12-hour observation period may clarify the diagnosis.[9,18] The results of virus identification techniques may reduce the length of the course of antibiotics and hospitalization significantly.[6]

The course of enterovirus-associated meningitis usually is mild, although complications (e.g., the syndrome of inappropriate secretion of antidiuretic hormone [SIADH]) occasionally are seen.[5] Most patients recover within 2 weeks; in rare cases relapses occur. Early information suggested that as many as 10% of survivors of aseptic meningitis that occurred before 3 months of age suffered long-term neurological sequelae, especially speech and language delays.[17,20] However, recent prospective outcome studies indicate no such identifiable long-term sequelae.[14] Older children apparently recover completely.

Paralytic Disease

Paralytic disease with wild-type poliovirus has been eradicated in the Western Hemisphere. Virtually all cases of poliomyelitis acquired in the United States are associated with vaccine virus strains and occur in young adults or in immunodeficient individuals. Cases of wild-type disease are encountered in unimmunized individuals who travel to endemic regions of the world and in some religious groups who do not accept immunization. Infection with other enterovirus serotypes may also result in paralysis. Nonpolio enterovirus paralysis actually may be more common in the United States than classic poliovirus-associated disease.[10] Asymmetrical weakness and/or paralysis without sensory loss differentiates this illness from Guillain-Barré syndrome. Life-threatening disease usually involves paralysis of the primary and accessory respiratory muscles or bulbar poliomyelitis of the respiratory center. Treatment is entirely supportive; recovery of muscle function may continue for several months.

In the 1980s a new syndrome of progressive weakness and fatigue was recognized in long-term survivors of paralytic poliomyelitis. This "postpolio syndrome" is seen decades after the initial infection. Apparently the previously affected muscles suffer denervation as overburdened motor neurons eventually "wear out." The long-term outcome of this syndrome is unknown.

Perinatal Infection

Enterovirus infection in neonates may occur as any of the syndromes seen in older children.[1] However, premature infants and newborns born without specific passively acquired maternal antibody may suffer a fulminant, rapidly fatal disease. This generalized neonatal infection begins as a syndrome of fever, lethargy, and poor feeding indistinguishable from early bacterial sepsis. Progression is swift, with multiorgan involvement, including hepatitis, pancreatitis, myocarditis, and encephalitis. Mortality is high in the disseminated forms of infection. The virus in neonates most often is transmitted from mother to infant at or near the time of delivery; however, nursery outbreaks with fatal cases have been reported. There is some evidence that maternal enterovirus infection may affect the fetus, but no consistent teratogenic pattern has been recognized. Epidemiological evidence suggests that maternal exposure to certain enteroviruses during pregnancy may increase the risk of subsequent juvenile diabetes mellitus in the offspring.

Other Diseases

Unusual enterovirus syndromes include encephalitis, often occurring in severely ill neonates, and the chronic meningoencephalitis of patients who have hypogammaglobulinemia. Myocarditis and pericarditis occur with a high mortality as part of the generalized disease of newborns. Fewer than 50% of older children and adults who have myocarditis die; recovery may be complete, but severe sequelae have been reported. Orchitis occasionally occurs in postpubertal patients in association with coxsackievirus B infection.

LABORATORY DIAGNOSIS

Interpretation of Laboratory Results

When obtaining specimens for enterovirus identification, the clinician must keep in mind the concept of "permissive" versus "nonpermissive" sites. Permissive sites (e.g., the nasopharynx and feces) are those in which enteroviruses may persist for weeks to months after infection. Identification of an enterovirus from a permissive site may be completely unrelated to the illness under investigation.

Nonpermissive sites are those from which virus is identified only during periods of disease. Shedding of virus in these sites usually is brief. Thus finding an enterovirus in blood, spinal fluid, or a skin vesicle is strong evidence that the virus is related to the concurrent clinical illness.

Because almost all enterovirus serotypes can produce any enterovirus syndrome and because no disease is associated uniquely with any enterovirus serotype, an enterovirus usually need not be identified beyond its actual presence. Enterovirus presence from a nonpermissive site is sufficient to diagnose the etiology of the illness in question. In rare cases both enteroviral and bacterial pathogens may be present in blood or spinal fluid. Invariably, the symptoms associated with the bacterial agent are more severe and dictate the clinical management.

Identification of an enterovirus from a permissive site specimen, especially feces, is more problematical. Vague, nonspecific symptoms or highly unusual or rare syndromes may be completely unrelated to the finding of an enterovirus shed in the GI tract. Many disease associations with enteroviruses probably are explained by such incidental enterovirus identification. Classic enterovirus disease during a known epidemic season is interpreted more easily; isolating an enterovirus from the stool of an infant who has fever and CSF pleocytosis in the summer, without any other pathogen isolated, is presumptive evidence of enteroviral meningitis.

Special caution must be used in interpreting enterovirus identification from infants in the first few months of life. Vaccine strains of poliovirus may persist in the stool for several weeks and may be transmitted to household members and caregivers. Fortunately, laboratories usually are able to identify an enterovirus as "vaccine related" versus "non-polio" quite rapidly. Vaccine polioviruses are not found in nonpermissive sites such as CSF or serum.

Virus Isolation

Except for most of the coxsackievirus A group, enteroviruses are isolated readily in cell cultures. A presumptive positive culture can be noted as early as 18 hours but more typically requires 2 to 5 days. Specific identification of an individual serotype takes somewhat longer. Suckling mouse inoculation, an expensive and difficult procedure, is the only available method of isolating most of the coxsackievirus A group serotypes.

Viruses may be isolated from throat swabs, feces, CSF,

blood or serum, skin vesicles, and tissues obtained at autopsy. Specimens from several sites increase the diagnostic yield because it is not always possible to predict the pathological stage of infection and thus the most likely source of the virus. As virology diagnostic laboratories become more available, efforts to isolate a virus may prove cost effective in cases of more severe illness, such as aseptic meningitis. Positive identification of an etiological agent may eliminate the need for further diagnostic tests, reduce the need for antibiotics, shorten the hospital stay, and improve prognostic accuracy.[16,19]

Rapid Virus Identification

Currently, the only rapid diagnostic technique with clinical promise is the polymerase chain reaction (PCR). The test cannot be performed directly on clinical specimens, and the process must be standardized within individual laboratories, which limits its usefulness in routine virology. However, in areas where the test is available, an enterovirus can be identified from a specimen such as CSF in as short a time as 5 hours.[3]

In a clinical trial of PCR on cerebrospinal fluid during a community outbreak of enteroviral meningitis, PCR identified 141 cases of enteroviral infection in 257 specimens within 24 hours.[15] Viral culture identified only 112 positive specimens, with a mean reporting time of 6.8 days. In a study of 20 neonates suspected of having sepsis, PCR was more sensitive than viral culture when serum and urine specimens obtained on the day of presentation were used and was 100% specific for enteroviral infection.[3]

Molecular Genetic Analysis

The genomes of the polioviruses and several of the echoviruses have been sequenced and cloned. These and other advances in genetic analysis have allowed researchers to examine precisely viral strains isolated during epidemics. Thus the epidemic of paralytic poliomyelitis in Finland in 1984 and 1985 was discovered to be caused by a typical wild-type poliovirus strain, not a new mutant, as had been suspected.[11] Ten cases of paralysis and widespread minor infection occurred in this highly immunized population because of an inadequate response to one of the inactivated vaccine components. The epidemic was terminated quickly by mass administration of a live oral polio vaccine.

Investigations such as this may allow better vaccines to be engineered to accomplish the World Health Organization's goal of eradicating polio worldwide by the year 2000.

Serological Diagnosis

It is not practical to obtain serum for analysis of enterovirus antibody titers because of the numerous serotypes and the complexity of the procedure. When the clinical or pathological picture strongly suggests one enterovirus group or a limited number of serotypes (i.e., myocarditis probably related to coxsackievirus B), measuring neutralizing antibody titers may be feasible.

In situations in which it might be desirable to prove the cause of an epidemic or a particularly unusual case (e.g., in paralytic disease related to a strain of poliovirus vaccine), serum-neutralizing antibody titers in acute and convalescent samples may be useful. Unfortunately, because antibody production occurs early, titers already may be high during the acute phase of clinical illness, thus obscuring the diagnosis. Assays to detect enterovirus serotype-specific IgM in serum are not available commercially.

PREVENTION

Attenuated or killed poliovirus vaccines are the only preventive enterovirus preparations currently available. An enhanced-potency inactivated poliovirus vaccine is available in the United States. This formulation should be used to immunize immunocompromised individuals and/or their household contacts. This is particularly important as infection with HIV becomes widespread; some households may have several severely immunodeficient members. Details of vaccination schedules for partly immunized or immunodeficient patients are available from the Centers for Disease Control and Prevention.[4]

In the prevaccine years, 0.2 ml/kg of pooled immune serum globulin given intramuscularly prevented or ameliorated poliovirus infection. In view of the severity of the disease in neonates, such injections might be indicated in nursery epidemics and for infants of mothers who develop a probable enterovirus disease within a few days of delivery. A single recent reported trial of intravenous immune globulin in neonates who had clinical disease did not show any benefit.[2]

A number of antiviral drugs and strategies to combat enteroviruses are under investigation, but none of them are nearing widespread clinical trials.[13]

REFERENCES

1. Abzug MJ: Perinatal enterovirus infections. In Rotbart HA, editor: *Human enterovirus infections,* Washington, DC, 1995, The American Society for Microbiology.
2. Abzug MJ et al: Neonatal enterovirus infection: virology, serology, and effect of intravenous immune globulin, *Clin Infect Dis* 20:1201, 1995.
3. Abzug MJ et al: Diagnosis of neonatal enterovirus infection by polymerase chain reaction, *J Pediatr* 126:447, 1995.
4. Centers for Disease Control: Poliomyelitis prevention: enhanced-potency inactivated poliomyelitis vaccine: supplementary statement, *MMWR* 36:795, 1987.
5. Chemtob S, Reece ER, Mills EL: Syndrome of inappropriate secretion of antidiuretic hormone in enteroviral meningitis, *Am J Dis Child* 139:292, 1985.
6. Chonmaitree T, Menegus MA, Powell KR: The clinical relevance of "CSF viral cultures": a two-year experience with aseptic meningitis in Rochester, New York, *JAMA* 247:1843, 1982.
7. Dagan R, Jenista JA, Menegus MA: Association of clinical presentation, laboratory findings, and virus serotypes with the presence of meningitis in hospitalized infants with enterovirus infection, *J Pediatr* 113:975, 1988.
8. Dagan R et al: Nonpolio enteroviruses and the febrile infant. In Rotbart HA, editor: *Human enterovirus infections,* Washington, DC, 1995, The American Society for Microbiology.
9. Harrison SA, Risser WL: Repeat lumbar puncture in the differential diagnosis of meningitis, *Pediatr Infect Dis J* 7:143, 1988.
10. Hayward JC et al: Outbreak of poliomyelitis-like paralysis associated with enterovirus 71, *Pediatr Infect Dis J* 8:611, 1989.
11. Hellen CUT et al: Enterovirus genetics. In Rotbart HA, editor: *Human enterovirus infections,* Washington, DC, 1995, The American Society for Microbiology.
12. Ikeda RM et al: Pleurodynia among football players at a high school: an outbreak associated with coxsackievirus B1, *JAMA* 270:2205, 1993.
13. O'Connell J et al: Development of antiviral agents for picornavirus in-

fections. In Rotbart HA, editor: *Human enterovirus infections,* Washington, DC, 1995, The American Society for Microbiology.

14. Rorabaugh ML et al: Aseptic meningitis in infants younger than 2 years of age: acute illness and neurologic complications, *Pediatrics* 92:206, 1993.
15. Sawyer MH et al: Diagnosis of enteroviral central nervous system infection by polymerase chain reaction during a large community outbreak, *Pediatr Infect Dis J* 13:177, 1994.
16. Schlesinger Y et al: Enteroviral meningitis in infancy: potential role for polymerase chain reaction in patient management, *Pediatrics* 94:157, 1994.
17. Sells CJ, Carpenter RL, Ray CG: Sequelae of central nervous system enterovirus infections, *N Engl J Med* 293:1, 1975.
18. Singer JI et al: Management of central nervous system infections during an epidemic of enteroviral aseptic meningitis, *J Pediatr* 96:559, 1980.
19. Wildin S, Chonmaitree T: The importance of the virology laboratory in the diagnosis and management of viral meningitis, *Am J Dis Child* 141:454, 1987.
20. Wilfert CM et al: Longitudinal assessment of children with enteroviral meningitis during the first three months of life, *Pediatrics* 67:811, 1981.

SUGGESTED READING

Rotbart HA, editor: *Human enterovirus infections,* Washington, DC, 1995, American Society for Microbiology.

204 Foreign Bodies of the Ear, Nose, Airway, and Esophagus

Jay N. Dolitsky and Robert F. Ward

Foreign bodies of the ear, nose, and upper aerodigestive tract are a common problem among children, particularly those under age 5. The scope of the problem was underscored first by National Safety Council statistics in 1969, which showed that more children died at home from accidental foreign body ingestion or aspiration than from any other cause.[1] In 1992 *foreign body aspiration and asphyxiation was the fourth leading cause of accidental death in the home among children under age 5*, and it still is a major problem.[2] The severity of the problem depends on several factors, including the site, composition, and duration of residence of the foreign body. Similarly the clinical presentation and management of these objects are related to those factors.

Removal of a foreign body usually is not an emergency, unless the airway is compromised, and it should be attempted only after the physician has as many factors as possible under control, including appropriate sedation or anesthesia, proper instrumentation and illumination and, most important, ability. If these elements are lacking, the problem probably will be aggravated by attempts to remove the foreign body, and the child's well-being may be jeopardized.

FOREIGN BODIES OF THE EAR

Earrings can become embedded in the auricle when a chronic infection of the pierced site is followed by overgrowth of granulation tissue. The use of the spring-loaded gun to pierce ears has resulted in numerous cases of embedded earrings as well.[5] Foreign bodies of the external auditory canal are found most commonly among children between 2 and 4 years of age. Curiosity, boredom, and imitation of others often are predisposing factors. Accidental entry of a foreign object through placement in the external auditory canal, either by the child or a companion, can occur during play. Insects also can find their way into the ear canal without any assistance. Das[6] reviewed 233 cases of foreign bodies in the ear and nose and found that the most consistent etiological factor was chronic irritation or inflammation of these orifices. Thus children who have chronic external otitis are more likely to place objects in their ear canals.

Clinical Presentation

Depending on the depth of the foreign object within the external auditory canal, the nature and composition of the object, and its duration in the canal, a wide spectrum of findings can be seen. Usually there is no history of placing an object in the ear canal because most children are reluctant to admit to this activity for fear of punishment.

Nonreactive substances, such as plastic, that are not completely obstructing the canal and not abutting the tympanic membrane may not cause symptoms. Insects tend to incite local irritation, causing discomfort, erythema, and occasionally, drainage. Vegetable matter also may cause local inflammation, which often leads to local pain and itching. Objects that touch the tympanic membrane cause pain, particularly with movement of the drum, as when swallowing. If the entire canal is obstructed, hearing most likely will be decreased.

There have been several reports concerning button-size alkaline batteries as foreign bodies of the ear canal.[4,17,19] These objects may leak battery acid, causing a severe local tissue reaction or destruction with pain, swelling, and discharge. This relatively new type of foreign body should be handled expeditiously to prevent serious injury to the canal, tympanic membrane, or middle ear.

When a small foreign body is suspected from the history but cannot be visualized on examination, it may be lodged anteriorly in the tympanic sulcus. Instillation of water to fill the medial half of the external canal may act as a concave lens, thereby allowing visualization of the tympanic sulcus.[16]

Management

Nonreactive foreign bodies that do not occlude the external canal completely or impinge on the tympanic membrane do not present an emergency. These can be removed with a variety of instruments; the most useful will depend on the shape and composition of the object. Often a 6 or 8 mm Frazier tip suction, an alligator forceps, or a right-angle hook can be used to retrieve the object. The hook is used by passing it beyond the object, hooking it from behind, and pulling it out gently. Gentle irrigation also may be used on nonvegetable substances; vegetable matter tends to swell when water is applied, making it more difficult to remove.

When the tympanic membrane cannot be visualized or if there is evidence of inflammation or injury to the external canal, the foreign body should be removed immediately. This is particularly important with an alkaline battery because tympanic membrane perforations have been reported within only 8 hours of entry.[4] Magnets may be helpful for removing metallic objects such as batteries or metal beads.[12]

Insects should be killed before removal by instilling either mineral oil or 4% Xylocaine into the external canal. Extraction with suction or alligator forceps may then be undertaken.

After any foreign body is removed, the external canal and tympanic membrane should be inspected carefully and thoroughly. Aqueous-based acidic ear drops or ophthalmic drops should be used for 5 to 7 days if the external canal appears injured or inflamed. The affected ear should be protected from water until it has healed completely.

In older children who are cooperative, a local anesthetic injected with a small-gauge needle into the skin lining the external canal may allow complete removal of the foreign body and subsequent examination. In younger children or in those who are uncooperative, general anesthesia may be necessary and certainly is preferable to traumatic removal in a child who is unable to cooperate or who cannot be restrained adequately.

Complications

Complications can be caused by the foreign body itself or by traumatic removal. Laceration and inflammation of the external canal usually is not serious and resolves with instillation of liquid analgesics and antibiotics. Perforations of the tympanic membrane require careful inspection to ensure that a flap of the membrane has not folded into the middle ear, which can lead to a permanent perforation or the development of a cholesteatoma. Likewise, when the drum is not intact, the middle ear space can become contaminated and otitis media can develop.

If it is not possible to remove a foreign object from the ear canal safely or if the tympanic membrane may have been injured by either the foreign body or its removal, the patient should be seen by an otolaryngologist.

FOREIGN BODIES IN THE NOSE

The predicaments that lead to foreign objects in the nasal cavity are quite similar to those of the ear. Boredom, curiosity, and acts of imitation may lead a child to place an object in his or her nose. These objects typically are soft, such as tissues, erasers, clay, or pieces of a toy. Occasionally a foreign object enters the nose accidentally while the child is attempting to sniff or smell it. In Das' study, chronic rhinitis was found to be the most common underlying factor in children placing objects in the nose.[6]

Clinical Presentation

Children usually will not confess to having placed something in the nose. The most common finding with this problem is *unilateral nasal discharge,* which usually is foul smelling. In fact, a unilateral nasal discharge in a young child should be considered evidence of a foreign body until proven otherwise. Occasionally, epistaxis is the presenting symptom.[23] If possible, the anterior nasal cavities should be examined with a nasal speculum and suction. The key to any evaluation is powerful illumination. Roentgenograms may be helpful if the object is radiopaque or has become calcified. An incidental finding of a nasal foreign body on a routine dental roentgenogram has been reported.[11] U.S. toy manufacturers are required by law to make toy parts radiopaque, a regulation that proves quite valuable when a physician is looking for foreign objects in the nasal cavity or in any part of the upper aerodigestive tract. However, toys and toy parts manufactured outside the United States do not have to conform to this regulation.

Management

Nasal foreign bodies should be removed as quickly as possible, particularly in the case of an alkaline battery, which can cause severe local inflammation.[4,9] Young children tend to detest any nasal instrumentation, and removal of a nasal foreign body requires some degree of cooperation. Thus sedation or general anesthesia usually is advised. Topical application of an epinephrine-like decongestant, (e.g., Neosynephrine, Afrin) in conjunction with removal of secretions by a small suction tip helps in visualizing the foreign object, particularly one lodged in the middle or posterior nasal cavity. Use of an endoscope is recommended to visualize this region.[23] A foreign body that has been allowed to remain in the nose for a long time may become calcified and form what is known as a rhinolith. Removing rhinoliths often is difficult and bloody. Various methods of foreign body removal have been described that can be attempted in the office, including using pepper to induce a sneeze while the uninvolved nostril is occluded or blowing in the child's mouth while the contralateral nostril is held shut. We do not recommend these methods. Another method of removal involves using a Fogarty or a small Foley catheter.[10,15] The catheter is placed beyond the foreign body into the posterior portion of the nasal cavity or nasopharynx and then inflated with 2 to 3 ml of saline solution. The catheter then is drawn gently forward and out of the nose, expelling the object. The danger with this technique is that the foreign object may be dislodged by pushing it posteriorly into the nasopharynx, which may lead to aspiration of the object.

Soft, friable objects usually can be removed with a Frazier tip suction. If the foreign body is rigid, it may be removed by using a nasal bayonet or Hartman or alligator forceps. After removal, local inflammation manifested by bloody or purulent oozing may be controlled with saline nose drops and an antibacterial ointment such as bacitracin or mupirocin (Bactroban).

Complications

Complications of nasal foreign bodies usually are limited to local inflammation and irritation. Occasionally, local scars may form, with the development of a scar band, or synechia. These can be prevented by placing a splint made of Gelfilm or Silastic over the raw, exposed area. Obstruction of a sinus ostium by a foreign object may lead to the development of sinusitis. This typically manifests as pain and tenderness over the affected sinus, or clouding and an air-fluid level on x ray. Treatment includes oral antibiotics and nasal decongestant drops.

The differential diagnosis of foreign bodies in the nose includes suppurative rhinitis, adenoiditis, sinusitis, and nasal or nasopharyngeal tumors. Nasal polyps also may manifest as a unilateral nasal discharge, and in a young child, the diagnosis of cystic fibrosis must be ruled out.

FOREIGN BODIES OF THE AIRWAY

A statistic mentioned earlier bears repeating: only a few years ago, foreign body aspiration and asphyxiation was the fourth leading cause of accidental death in the home among children under age 5.[2] It accounts for approximately 9% of all home accidental deaths of children in this age group.[2] The incidence declines rapidly among those over age 5, until age 65, when it increases again to an even higher percentage. Overall the incidence of death from foreign body aspiration has declined significantly during the past 2 decades.[2] This probably is the result of increased parental awareness of the risks of leaving small objects within the reach of young children. Consumer education and awareness have been important in diminishing this potential hazard. Also, the development of lifesaving techniques, such as the Heimlich maneuver, that can be performed by people who are not medical personnel accounts for a higher survival rate.

With regard to foreign body impaction, the airway can be divided into three segments: the larynx, the trachea, and the bronchial tree. Lima[13] reviewed all airway foreign body admissions to his pediatric hospital from 1980 through 1987. Of the 91 cases, 11 involved a foreign body lodged in the larynx. Of these 11 patients, 5 died and 3 suffered anoxic encephalopathy. It is apparent that although most foreign bodies pass through the larynx, the outcome is grave when one does not.

Etiology

The causes of foreign body impaction in the airway are many. As with foreign bodies of other head and neck orifices, curiosity or boredom may lead a young child to put foreign objects in his or her mouth. Infants in particular are known to explore their world with their oral sense and will attempt to place almost anything they can handle into their mouths. A startle may cause inadvertent ingestion or aspiration. Lack of complete dentition, as well as lack of attention to chewing, allows large food particles to enter the posterior pharynx. Incomplete development of mouth and tongue coordination in young children also may account for a greater incidence of foreign body ingestion or aspiration. Reichert[18] reports that a positive association has been noted between the occurrence of upper respiratory tract infections and foreign body aspiration. He postulates that the need for continuous mouth breathing when a child suffers a cold interrupts a smooth breathing-swallowing pattern, leading to an increase in aspiration.

Clinical Presentation

A history of foreign body ingestion or aspiration may or may not be obtained, depending on the patient's age or condition and whether the suspected incident was witnessed. Classically, when a foreign object initially is aspirated into the respiratory tract, it produces a choking, gagging, coughing, or wheezing episode. This may be followed by an asymptomatic interval during which there is little to suggest the presence of a foreign body. At this point the parents and physician often are lulled into a false sense of security.

Depending on the site of the foreign body in the airway, a patient may manifest a spectrum of findings, ranging from an almost complete lack of symptoms to signs of complete airway obstruction.

Laryngeal foreign bodies are likely to produce the most acute and dramatic presentation. Large objects that completely obstruct the airway may result in stridor, high-pitched wheezing, cough, dysphonia, or worse—aphonia and cyanosis. Children who have smaller, partly obstructing objects that allow adequate air exchange have cough, stridor, hoarseness, pain, or discomfort.

Tracheal foreign bodies usually are associated with cough and some degree of stridor or wheezing and may produce an audible "slap" as the object moves from the carina to the glottis with respiration. Bronchial foreign bodies usually cause wheezing or coughing if they are partly obstructing; this often is misdiagnosed as asthma. With complete obstruction of a bronchus, an initial asymptomatic period is followed by a postobstructive pneumonitis or bronchiectasis.[14] Sharp objects such as pins or tacks may cause pain or hemoptysis.

If aspiration of a foreign body into the upper airway is suspected, plain roentgenography may help. For objects suspected to be lodged in the laryngeal inlet, high-kilovolt, anteroposterior (AP) and lateral roentgenograms of the upper trachea or esophageal inlet should be obtained if the patient's condition permits. Bronchial foreign bodies may be suggested by some form of dynamic roentgen ray study, such as inspiratory-expiratory roentgenograms, lateral decubitus films, or videofluoroscopy. These studies can demonstrate air-trapping in the affected lung.

Management

Foreign bodies that completely obstruct the laryngeal inlet create a life-threatening emergency and should be expelled immediately using the Heimlich maneuver (abdominal thrusts). For infants under 1 year of age, the American Academy of Pediatrics recommends five back blows in the head-down position followed by five chest thrusts in the supine position, in place of the Heimlich maneuver[3] (see Appendix A, Pediatric Basic and Advanced Life Support). *Blind finger sweeps are dangerous and should be avoided.*[3] If the foreign body cannot be expelled, a large-bore needle or angiocatheter (14 gauge) should be inserted into the cricothyroid space to allow some degree of ventilation until the patient can be taken to the operating room for removal of the object. Alternately, if skilled personnel are present, an emergency tracheotomy may be necessary. Partly obstructing laryngeal foreign bodies should be treated in a way that prevents total obstruction of the airway; therefore *back blows and abdominal thrusts should not be used in these cases.*

Tracheal and bronchial foreign bodies should be removed by a physician specifically trained for the task, which usually requires controlled endoscopic removal in the operating room. This usually is not an emergency; therefore adequate preparations can be made.

Complications

Abdominal and chest thrusts may damage intraabdominal contents (e.g., liver, spleen) and ribs respectively. Therefore these techniques should be used only in cases of complete airway obstruction that otherwise would cause certain death. Conversion of a partial airway obstruction to a complete obstruction can best be avoided by having skilled personnel retrieve the foreign body. According to Wolach,[22] pneumonia was the most common complication in 127 cases of foreign body aspiration.

A bronchial foreign body that remains in place for an extended period may cause air-trapping and irreversible bronchiectatic changes distal to the obstruction.

Prolonged or difficult instrumentation of the airway during removal of a foreign body can lead to laryngeal edema or injury, with obstructive symptoms. This may require a period of intubation after surgery. As an alternative, postoperative edema sometimes can be avoided by using steroids during and after surgery.

FOREIGN BODIES INVOLVING THE ESOPHAGUS

More than half of the foreign bodies in children involve the esophagus, with the highest incidence in children 14 months to 6 years of age.[21] Younger children are inquisitive and tend to explore objects orally. The objects then are intentionally swallowed or accidentally ingested as the result of a startle. In the United States, coins are the most common foreign body to lodge in the esophagus.[20]

The esophagus has four physiological areas of narrowing: the cricopharyngeal sphincter, the aortic arch, the region of the left main bronchus, and the gastroesophageal sphincter. These correspond to the four most common sites of foreign body obstruction. The cricopharyngeus is the most common, the arch of the aortic region the most dangerous.

Clinical Presentation

The history of foreign body ingestion often is not obtained, and most foreign bodies pass through the normal esophagus undetected. Those that do not pass freely initially stimulate the larynx and cause gagging and coughing. Subsequent symptoms depend on the size, composition, and nature of the foreign body. With young children, poor feeding or refusal to eat or drink, as well as increased salivation, are typical. When the esophagus is completely or almost completely obstructed, choking and vomiting occur. The duration of obstruction can affect the clinical presentation: The longer a foreign object is present, the greater the tissue reaction and local inflammation. Thus, in the later stages, patients can have pain on swallowing, fever, and leukocytosis.

When a foreign body is suspected, posteroanterior (PA) and lateral chest roentgenograms, in addition to neck films, are diagnostic if the object is radiopaque, such as a coin. Contrast studies can be used when an esophageal foreign body that does not show on routine roentgenograms is strongly suspected.

Management

An esophageal foreign body does not usually require emergency measures, but it should be removed as soon as possible after proper evaluation and preparation.[8] Often children will have eaten recently, and generally it is recommended that an appropriate period pass before they are given general anesthesia. If the foreign body is corrosive, such as an alkaline button battery, it should be removed as soon as possible to prevent severe inflammation and potential perforation of the esophageal wall.[7]

Endoscopic removal under anesthesia by a trained expert remains the method of choice because of the safety provided. This technique allows for direct visualization of the esophagus, its mucosa, and the foreign body. Removal with a flexible endoscope also is possible without general anesthesia.

Nonendoscopic techniques for removing an esophageal foreign body (i.e., with a Foley or Fogarty catheter) have been described.[10] The child is sedated and brought to the fluoroscopy suite. While the child is in a steep Trendelenburg position, the catheter is placed beyond the foreign object and the balloon on the catheter is inflated and withdrawn. This technique can lead to aspiration and airway obstruction and generally is not recommended.

Complications

Perforation of the esophagus can result from the endoscopic procedure or may be caused by the foreign body itself, especially if it is sharp or caustic. Endoscopic removal is particularly dangerous with objects lodged at the level of the aortic arch. If an esophageal tear is suspected, contrast roentgenography usually will confirm or negate the suspicion.

Foreign bodies that have been in the esophagus for long periods can cause a stricture to develop. In these cases also, a contrast study should be performed to aid in the diagnosis.

REFERENCES

1. Accident facts, National Safety Council, Chicago, 1969.
2. Accident facts, National Safety Council, Chicago, 1992.
3. American Academy of Pediatrics Committee on Pediatric Emergency Medicine: First aid for the choking child, *Pediatrics* 92:477, 1993.
4. Capo JM, Lucente FE: Alkaline battery foreign bodies of the ear and nose, *Arch Otolaryngol Head Neck Surg* 112:562, 1986.
5. Cohen HA et al: Embedded earrings, *Cutis* 53:82, 1994.
6. Das SK: Etiological evaluation of foreign bodies in the ear and nose, *J Laryngol Otol* 98:989, 1984.
7. Derkay CS et al: Retrieving foreign bodies from upper aerodigestive tracts of children, *AORN J* 60:53, 1994.
8. Giordano A et al: Current management of esophageal foreign bodies, *Arch Otol* 107:249, 1981.
9. Gomes CC et al: Button battery as a foreign body in the nasal cavities: special aspects, *Rhinology* 32:98, 1994.
10. Henry LN, Chamberlain JW: Removal of foreign bodies from the esophagus and nose with the use of a Foley catheter, *Surgery* 71:918, 1972.
11. Kittle PE et al: Incidental finding of an intranasal foreign body discovered on routine dental examination, *Pediatr Dent* 13:49, 1991.
12. Landry GL, Edmanson MB: Attractive method for battery removal, *JAMA* 256:3351, 1986 (letter).
13. Lima JA: Laryngeal foreign bodies in children: a persistent life-threatening problem, *Laryngoscope* 99:415, 1989.
14. Mears AJ, England RM: Dissolving foreign bodies in the trachea and bronchus, *Thorax* 30:461, 1975.
15. Nandapalan V, McIlwain JC: Removal of nasal foreign bodies with a Fogarty biliary balloon catheter, *J Laryngol Otol* 108:758, 1994.
16. Peltola TJ, Scarento R: Water used to visualize and remove hidden foreign bodies from the external ear canal, *J Laryngol Otol* 106:157, 1992.
17. Rachlin LS: Assault with battery, *N Engl J Med* 311:921, 1984 (letter).
18. Reichert TJ: Foreign bodies of the larynx, trachea, and bronchi. In Bluestone CD, Stool SE, editors: *Pediatric otolaryngology,* ed 2, Philadelphia, 1990, WB Saunders.
19. Skinner DW, Chiu P: The hazards of "button-sized" batteries as foreign bodies in the nose and ear, *J Laryngol Otol* 100:1315, 1986.
20. Turtz MG, Stool SE: Foreign bodies of the pharynx and esophagus. In Bluestone CD, Stool SE, editors: *Pediatric otolaryngology,* ed 2, Philadelphia, 1990, WB Saunders.
21. Witt WJ: The role of rigid endoscopy in foreign body management, *Ear Nose Throat J* 64:70, 1985.
22. Wolach B et al: Aspirated foreign bodies in the respiratory tract of children: eleven years experience with 127 patients, *Int J Pediatr Otorhinolaryngol* 30:1, 1994.
23. Yanagisawa E, Citardi MJ: Endoscopic view of a foreign body in the nose, *Ear Nose Throat J* 74:8, 1995.

205 Fractures and Dislocations

R. Scott Strahlman

At first glance the reader may feel that this chapter is unnecessary—that fractures and dislocations are a topic more appropriately discussed by orthopedic surgeons in an orthopedic textbook. The truth, however, is that pediatricians see scores of fractures and dislocations each year. Whether a particular injury is managed conservatively by the pediatrician or referred to an orthopedic specialist is up to the individual primary care provider; regardless, a familiarity with proper management and triage is essential. This chapter covers the pathophysiology, clinical assessment, and classification of fractures and dislocations, as well as some of the more common conditions encountered in primary care.

ETIOLOGY AND PATHOPHYSIOLOGY

A *fracture* is defined as a break or crack in a bone. The fracture may occur directly at the site of injury or indirectly when the break occurs at a site different from the applied force. *Stress fractures* result from recurrent trauma to a bone and often occur in athletes (e.g., long-bone fractures in distance runners). *Pathological fractures* can occur without trauma when a bone is weakened, as with osteogenesis imperfecta or a tumor.

A *dislocation* is defined as a malposition of bone ends that normally appose one another within a joint. Dislocations are far less common in children than are fractures because a child's ligaments are quite strong; with an injury, it is more likely that a bone will break or a growth plate will separate than that a ligament will tear.

Certain broad generalizations can be made about the pathophysiology of childhood fractures.[1] First, fractures in children heal more quickly than in adults. For example, a fractured clavicle in a 4-year-old may heal in as little as 3 weeks! Second, the remodeling that occurs in the healing of pediatric fractures often corrects residual bony deformities. Third, children's bones are resilient; they bend instead of break, or they break on one side only (a greenstick fracture). Fourth, a phenomenon called *overgrowth* occurs in pediatric long-bone fractures. Overgrowth is an accelerated growth rate of bony fragments during healing. Long-bone fractures therefore must be corrected with overriding of the broken ends to prevent length discrepancies with the uninjured side. Finally, the growth plate must be protected in children's fractures because a growth plate injury can result in the loss of growth potential.

INITIAL ASSESSMENT

Whenever a fracture or dislocation is suspected, an accurate history is essential. Historical details may provide clues about the *mechanism* of injury. The practitioner should find out how, where, and when the injury occurred and where any pain is located. Does the parent or child report any loss of function in the affected limb? Is there a previous or recurrent history of trauma?

A complete physical examination, including taking the vital signs, should be performed; a neurovascular assessment also is important. The examiner should look carefully for any unnatural or deformed position of joints or limbs. Pain upon palpation or attempted movement may be a clue. Swelling and discoloration may be seen. Crepitus sometimes can be elicited at a fracture site.

Radiography is a mainstay in the diagnosis of fractures and dislocations. Roentgenograms from two angles are indicated to delineate subtle fractures. It sometimes is helpful to include the joint above and below the injury to rule out a dislocation; often it is necessary to get a film of the unaffected side for a comparison view. Stress fractures often are not seen on roentgenograms. If a stress fracture is suspected, a radionuclide bone scan may be indicated.[5] Occasionally, when injury to the growth plate is a concern, newer imaging techniques such as computed tomography (CT) or magnetic resonance imaging (MRI) scanning can be useful.[2]

CLASSIFICATION

Fractures are characterized in various ways to give the orthopedic surgeon information. This information in turn aids in the formulation of a management plan and prognosis for the fracture. Fractures may be classified according to the clinical appearance. A *closed fracture* has no break in the skin. With an *open,* or *compound, fracture,* a bone fragment is exposed to the air, increasing the risk of infection or injury to adjacent nerves and blood vessels. A *hidden fracture* causes slight pain and swelling but no obvious bone deformity. Roentgenograms are necessary to confirm the diagnosis. An *obvious fracture* or dislocation is an easily seen injury, even with a cursory examination. Immediate medical attention is necessary.

Fractures also are classified according to their radiographic appearance. Breaks in the bone may be described as *transverse, oblique,* or *spiral.* A fracture is *comminuted* when the bone has three or more fragments. With an *impacted fracture* the bone ends are compressed into each other.

Probably the most important classification system for fractures is the Salter-Harris system of describing injury to the growth plate (Fig. 205-1). Growth or epiphyseal plate injuries occur *only* in childhood. They must be treated with care to protect a bone's growth potential. Approximately 15% of all childhood fractures involve the growth plate.[6] In a Salter I fracture, the epiphysis is separated from the metaphysis without a true break in the bone. Roentgenograms often are normal, and the diagnosis is made on the basis of the clinical picture: tenderness over the area of the growth plate.

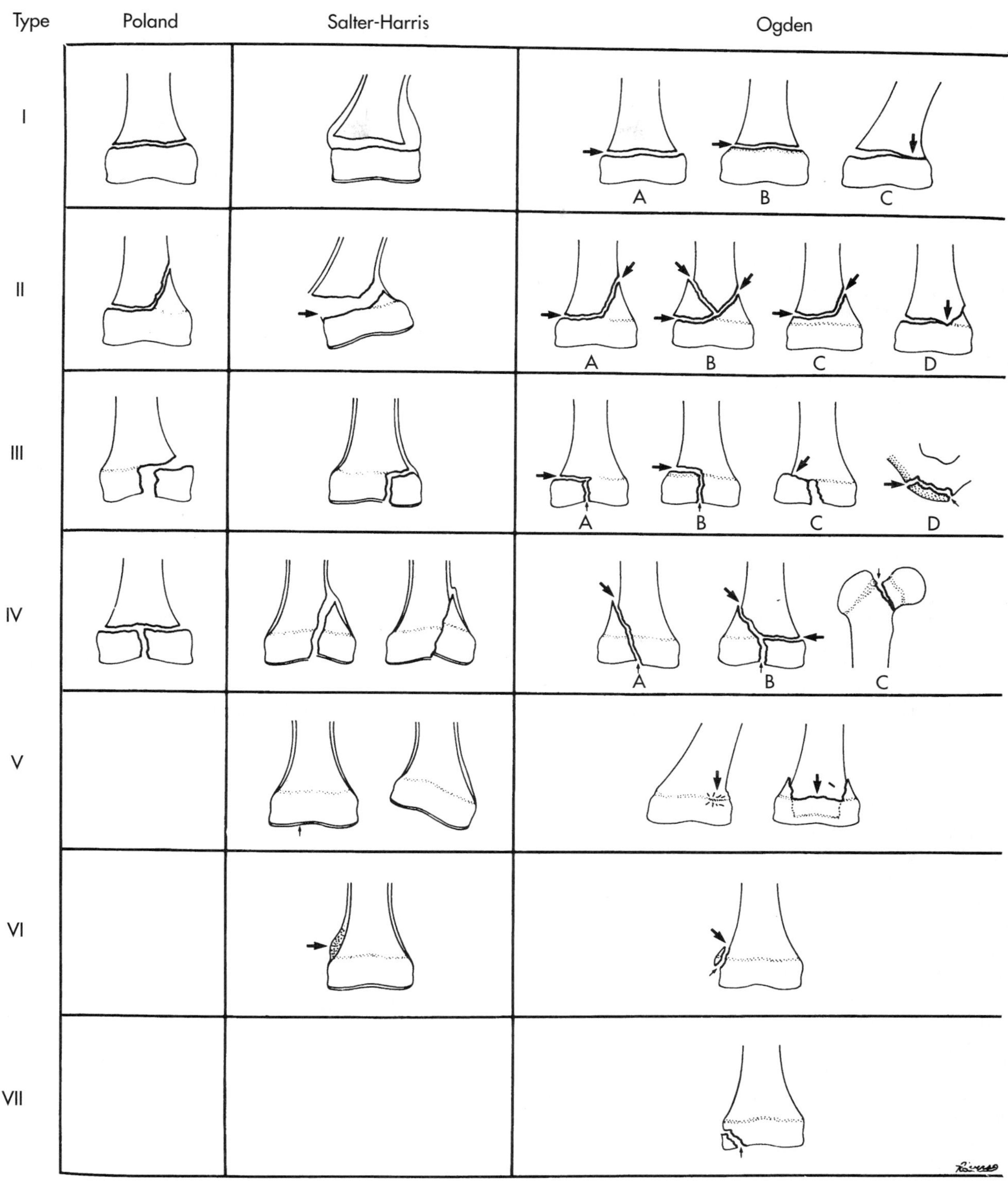

FIG. 205-1 Salter-Harris classification of growth plate injuries.
(From Canale ST, Beaty JH: *Operative pediatric orthopaedics,* St Louis, 1990, Mosby.)

Growth usually is not disturbed. The treatment is immobilization by cast for approximately 3 weeks. The most common growth plate fracture is the type II fracture, in which a fragment of metaphyseal bone separates from the epiphysis. Closed reduction of the fracture usually is possible, and with proper casting, growth is not disturbed.

A Salter III fracture involves a *partial* growth plate injury through the epiphysis. Open repair of the fracture in the operating room is indicated to align articular surfaces and preserve joint function. When a fracture goes *across* the growth plate, injuring both the epiphysis and the metaphysis, it is called a Salter IV fracture. The fracture must be perfectly realigned to protect growth potential.

In a Salter V fracture, the growth plate is compressed. The

prognosis for preserving growth is poor in this case because of a *crush* injury to the growth plate.

Fracture types VI and VII sometimes are not included in the Salter-Harris classification system. These are chip fractures that do not cause any direct injury to the growth plate.

MANAGEMENT

Fractures and dislocations should be splinted and immobilized immediately. For most fractures and dislocations, consultation with an orthopedic specialist is then necessary. Most pediatric fractures respond to closed reduction by the orthopedist. If the growth plate is affected, however, open reduction is performed. Close pediatric and orthopedic follow-up always are important. A child in a cast should be comfortable; if pain is persistent, the child needs reevaluation and possibly recasting.

COMMONLY ENCOUNTERED FRACTURES AND DISLOCATIONS

Fractured Clavicle

A "broken collarbone" is the most common fracture in children. It can occur at any time during childhood as a result of trauma. This fracture often occurs at birth when there is a difficult vaginal delivery. The incidence can be as high as 3.5% in babies delivered vaginally.[3] Physical findings include decreased arm motion on the affected side, crepitus, and swelling at the fracture site. A roentgenogram or ultrasound study may be needed to confirm the diagnosis.[4] If the condition is asymptomatic, no treatment is needed; indeed, the diagnosis often is made after the fact when a callus at the fracture site is noted at a well-baby clinic visit. If the fracture causes pain or reduced arm movement, splinting of the clavicle for 2 to 3 weeks is indicated. In older children treatment requires splinting for 3 to 4 weeks in a figure-eight bandage or a shoulder extension harness. Most of the fracture's healing and realignment are spontaneous.

Congenital Hip Dislocation

Congenital hip dislocation is present from birth but is not always detected in the newborn. For this reason children under 1 year of age should be examined for hip dislocation at every routine visit. The disorder may occur secondary to abnormal intrauterine positioning, and it is more common in infants delivered by breech and by cesarean section.

Roentgenograms are of limited value in the diagnosis of congenital hip dislocation. Therefore the physical examination is of utmost importance. The Ortolani test is used to detect a dislocated hip. With the baby on his or her back, the hips and knees are flexed and the knees brought together. The examiner then places a hand on each of the baby's knees, with each middle finger over the greater trochanter and each thumb over the medial thigh. With gentle abduction of the knees, the dislocated femoral head will slip back into the acetabulum; an audible or palpable "clunk" results. The Barlow test is essentially the reverse of the Ortolani test; the femoral head can be felt slipping out of the acetabulum when the knees are brought back together. An examiner may feel unusual laxity of the hip by pushing up and down on the thigh when the hips are flexed and adducted. If the diagnosis is in doubt, an ultrasound study often will confirm or rule it out. Treatment requires referral to an orthopedist for a harness or casting. Notably, a hip "click" (without a "clunk" and without any movement of the femoral head) does not indicate a hip dislocation.

Nursemaid Elbow

"Nursemaid elbow" is a common dislocation in pediatrics. A transient subluxation of the proximal radial head, it is caused by inadvertent pulling or "yanking" of a child's arm, often by a parent or caretaker. The condition usually occurs in children between 1 and 4 years of age. The child refuses to move the arm and keeps it flexed and pronated. Roentgenograms rarely are necessary; the history and characteristic posture of the child's arm confirm the diagnosis. The treatment, easily performed by the pediatrician, requires rapid, forceful supination of the forearm while placing pressure over the proximal radial head. Symptoms usually resolve within 30 minutes. The condition sometimes is recurrent, in which case great care must be taken when holding hands with the affected child.

Child Abuse

Unfortunately, fractures and dislocations are all too commonly suggestive of child abuse (see Chapter 56, Child Abuse and Neglect). Child abuse may be suspected when there is an unexplained fracture or an inconsistency between the history and the physical findings in a childhood injury. There may be an unusually long delay between the time of injury and the time that medical attention is sought. Multiple bruises may be noted on physical examination. If abuse is suspected, a radiographic bone survey should be done. Silent fractures, or multiple fractures in varying stages of healing, may be seen.

When child abuse is suspected, the child should be hospitalized for protection as well as appropriate orthopedic care. Child protective services and social services should be involved. Pediatric care providers are morally and legally responsible for detecting child abuse and reporting all suspected cases.

TODDLER'S FRACTURE

Radiologists refer to a spiral fracture of the tibia as a "toddler's fracture" when the fracture occurs in a child under age 6. Torsion of the foot creates a spiral break in the tibia. The trauma to the leg often is minor or unwitnessed, so there frequently is no history of trauma. Symptoms can be minimal; the child may be brought for medical attention only because of reluctance to bear weight on the affected leg. The physical examination is significant for tenderness over the affected area of the tibia. A diagnosis can be made with anteroposterior and lateral roentgenograms of the tibia-fibula, but the fracture sometimes is not evident on a roentgenogram for a few days. The physician therefore should not hesitate to repeat films on a child who has an unexplained limp that is not resolving spontaneously. Treatment requires immobilization in a cast for 3 to 4 weeks.

Because the signs and symptoms of a "toddler's fracture" can be subtle, the examiner should have a high index of suspicion in a child who has a limp or fails to bear weight. Because the cause of the fracture often is unexplained, child abuse sometimes is a consideration. However, an isolated spiral fracture of the tibia usually does *not* imply child abuse in a younger child.

REFERENCES

1. Chung SMK: *Handbook of pediatric orthopedics,* New York, 1986, Van Nostrand Reinhold.
2. Jaramillo D et al: MR imaging of fractures of the growth plate, *Am J Radiol* 155:1261, 1990.
3. Joseph PR, Rosenfeld W: Clavicular fractures in neonates, *Am J Dis Child* 144:165, 1990.
4. Katz R et al: Fracture of the clavicle in the newborn: an ultrasound diagnosis, *J Ultrasound Med* 7:21, 1988.
5. Rosen PR, Micheli LJ, Treves S: Early scintigraphic diagnosis of bone stress and fractures in athletic adolescents, *Pediatrics* 70:11, 1982.
6. Salter RB, Harris WR: Injuries involving the epiphyseal plate, *J Bone Joint Surg* 45a:591, 1963.

SUGGESTED READINGS

Conrad EU, Rang MC: Fractures and sprains, *Pediatr Clin North Am* 33:1523, 1986.

Mayer TA: *Emergency management of pediatric trauma,* Philadelphia, 1985, WB Saunders.

Sherk HH et al: Congenital dislocation of the hip: a review, *Clin Pediatr* 20:513, 1981.

Tachdjian MO: *Pediatric orthopedics,* ed 2, Philadelphia, 1990, WB Saunders.

206 Gastrointestinal Allergy

Aubrey J. Katz

Food allergy is a common but often unsubstantiated diagnosis in pediatric practice. Adverse reactions to foods are a feature of many gastrointestinal (GI) diseases; however, although food intolerance is caused by allergy in some patients, many other causes should be considered, such as malabsorption, lactose deficiency, toxic effects of contaminants and additives, and psychological factors.

The GI tract contains lymphoid tissue capable of mounting an immunological response to protect against the penetration of antigens across the epithelium. Lymphocytes and plasma cells are present in Peyer patches and the lamina propria of the small and large intestine; IgA-containing plasma cells account for only 2%. The aberrations in immunological mechanisms that trigger GI allergic reactions are unknown.

Allergic disorders of the GI tract can be subdivided into two general groups: specific allergens and eosinophilic (allergic) gastroenteritis.[4] Removing specific allergens from the diet ameliorates symptoms, which are exacerbated with reintroduction of the allergen. Cow milk protein allergy and soy protein allergy are defined the best. Eosinophilic (allergic) gastroenteritis exists when two or more food sensitivities are present. Usually, several food sensitivities are identified.

COW MILK PROTEIN ALLERGY

The incidence of cow milk allergy is estimated to vary between 0.5% and 7% of all infants under the age of 6 months.[2] Beta-lactoglobulin appears to be the most antigenic component of cow milk, but some babies also may be sensitive to casein or whey protein. The symptoms and signs are listed in the box on p. 1309. GI symptoms predominate in a large number of patients. In other patients, anaphylaxis or pulmonary symptoms occur.[4] The GI manifestations depend on the site of predominant inflammation in the gastrointestinal tract. Esophagitis manifests as recurrent vomiting; gastritis manifests as vomiting, irritability or pain, and occult GI bleeding; enteritis manifests as diarrhea, malabsorption, or protein-losing enteropathy[5]; and colitis manifests as rectal bleeding, with blood or mucus in the stool.

Antral gastritis is a common finding in these patients, with increased eosinophils and inflammatory cells in the antrum. Duodenal biopsy reveals patchy changes ranging from normal mucosa to "flat gut" lesions (see Chapter 209, Gluten-Sensitive Enteropathy [Celiac Sprue]). Esophagitis was described recently, and the biopsies are identical to those for esophagitis associated with gastroesophageal reflux disease. Colitis is common in these patients who have blood or mucus in the stool. Allergy is the most common cause of rectal bleeding among infants under 6 months of age.

SOY PROTEIN ALLERGY OR SENSITIVITY

Thirty percent to 50 percent of infants are allergic to milk protein or allergic to soy protein[1]; however, soy protein allergy may occur without a concomitant sensitivity to milk protein. The clinical features of soy protein allergy are similar to those of milk protein allergy in that gastritis, enteritis, and colitis occur.

ALLERGY VIA THE BREAST MILK

The term "breast milk colitis" is a misnomer. It is apparent that infants who are breast-fed may develop the same symptoms as patients who are formula-fed, manifesting either colitis or evidence of esophagitis, gastritis, or enteritis—the commonest appears to be colitis.[7] These patients often show significant irritability as a manifestation of their symptoms, with either occult blood or obvious rectal bleeding.

Treatment in this instance involves persuading the mothers to avoid dairy products, but only about 20% of infants respond to this measure alone. It then becomes extremely difficult sometimes to prevent many of the breast-feeding mothers to start eliminating many other foods from their diet, resulting in significant maternal weight loss. It is important to emphasize to mothers that by far most infants who show sensitivity to foods the mother is eating do not have a severe disease. Therefore breast-feeding can be continued unless the symptoms are significant. Sometimes using a hypoallergenic formula may be worth a trial to see if the baby's symptoms disappear.

CLINICAL FEATURES OF A SPECIFIC FOOD SENSITIVITY

In most cases of either milk or soy sensitivity, the infant may have peripheral eosinophilia initially or, interestingly enough, the eosinophilia may occur once the allergen has been removed from the diet.

IgE determinations and radioallergosorbent tests (RASTs) to detect these specific milk and soy proteins usually are negative, suggesting that the immunological mechanism occurs by means of an IgG rather than an IgE mechanism. A significant number of these patients also appear to have a concomitant transient hypogammaglobulinemia, and it appears that the sensitivity to either milk or soy or other specific allergens disappears once the immunoglobulin levels, particularly IgG, return to normal. The findings of an elevated IgE or positive RAST result with these foods at this age in most cases would suggest perhaps long-term rather than self-limited sensitivity.

The hallmark of gastrointestinal biopsies in these patients is the increased number of eosinophils. It has been reported that over 20 eosinophils per high-power field on rectal bi-

COW MILK ALLERGY

Systemic signs
- Anaphylaxis
- Iron deficiency anemia (secondary to GI blood loss)
- Rhinitis
- Wheezing
- Pulmonary hemosiderosis
- Nasopharyngeal obstruction leading to cor pulmonale
- Peripheral eosinophilia

Gastrointestinal manifestations
- Vomiting
- Diarrhea/malabsorption/protein-losing enteropathy
- Colic
- Gastrointestinal bleeding
- Failure to thrive

EOSINOPHILIC (ALLERGIC) GASTROENTERITIS

Peripheral eosinophilia (common to all three types of disease)

Mucosal disease
- Protein-losing enteropathy leading to hypoalbuminemia and hypogammaglobulinemia
- Growth failure
- Iron deficiency anemia secondary to occult gastrointestinal blood loss
- Systemic allergy

Submucosal disease
- May have features of mucosal disease
- Pyloric obstruction

Serosal disease: eosinophilic ascites

opsy is indicative enough of an allergic etiology for colitis.[9] It must be remembered, however, that any inflammatory lesions of the GI tract appear to attract eosinophils.

TREATMENT

Once the infant either is suspected of having or has been diagnosed with a specific formula sensitivity, he or she should be placed initially on a hypoallergenic formula, which usually take the form of casein hydrolysate formulas. Commercial preparations include Alimentum, Nutramigen or Pregestimil. In view of their expense, however, many practitioners place their patients on a trial of a whey formula (commercially available, such as GoodStart), because a fair number of patients appear to tolerate whey.

It appears most practical to choose a casein hydrolysate formula for the first 6 to 8 weeks, then to try to switch to the whey formula, and perhaps 4 to 6 months later, to try the infant again on a soy formula. The sensitivity usually lasts from about 2 to 12 months, so this usually is a period of trial-and-error.

EOSINOPHILIC (ALLERGIC) GASTROENTERITIS

Eosinophilic (or allergic) gastroenteritis is a condition characterized by peripheral eosinophilia and infiltration of the GI tract with eosinophils.[10] Hypereosinophilic syndromes, which are characterized by infiltration of many organs with eosinophils, are not included in this category. Three types of disease manifestation are described, depending on the site of GI involvement: (1) mucosal disease manifests as protein-losing enteropathy, malabsorption, and GI blood loss; (2) submucosal disease usually manifests with pyloric obstruction; and (3) serosal disease manifests with eosinophilic ascites. The latter two types are less common in children.

Etiology

The presence of peripheral eosinophilia, systemic allergy, and elevated IgE levels, plus a therapeutic response to steroids, indicates an allergic basis for this disease in some patients.

Pathology

The small intestine reveals lesions, patchy in distribution, ranging from areas of normal mucosa to a flat villus lesion.[8] Eosinophilic infiltration may be mild or marked. Gastric abnormalities, found more commonly in the antrum, have been described as being consistent in the mucosal form of the disease. The stomach shows evidence of gastritis, with destruction and regeneration of gastric glands and surface epithelium. Eosinophilic infiltration usually is marked. Esophagitis with significant eosinophilic infiltration is a common finding in these patients. Preliminary data indicate that biopsies in these cases are identical to those for patients who have reflux esophagitis.

Clinical Features

Peripheral eosinophilia is common to all three types of disease. The mucosal form has many of the features listed in the box above, whereas pyloric obstructive disease, especially serosal disease, commonly does not have all these features. Whether these are variants of a similar disease process or distinctly different conditions remains to be solved. Pyloric obstructive disease manifests with vomiting and serosal disease with ascites. Numerous eosinophils are present in the ascitic fluid. Growth failure is a prominent feature of mucosal disease in childhood; diarrhea often is not a feature. These patients usually have evidence of systemic allergy, especially asthma. Thus this syndrome often is missed at initial presentation. Iron deficiency anemia that occurs secondary to GI blood loss is another consistent feature, together with protein-losing enteropathy.

Diagnosis

Diagnosis is based on the clinical features and laboratory findings described above. A biopsy of the small intestine reveals both normal mucosa (with or without eosinophilic infiltration) and a flat villus lesion. A gastric antral biopsy appears to be of diagnostic value in the mucosal form of the disease and usually is positive, revealing evidence of gastritis with marked eosinophilic infiltration.[6]

Treatment

Eliminating these allergens, which are found to be highly positive in affected patients, from the diet may alleviate most of the symptoms.[8] In many cases corticosteroid therapy may be required intermittently. Pyloric obstructive disease may require surgery.

Prognosis

Extensive follow-up studies are lacking, but the evidence indicates that eosinophilic gastroenteritis is a lifelong condition with remissions and exacerbations, often requiring careful dietary manipulation and intermittent steroid therapy. Preliminary data also suggest that younger adolescents go through a phase in which they are much better able to tolerate foods to which they previously were sensitive.

CONCLUSION

GI food sensitivity can be divided into two types: that involving a specific allergen (a self-limited condition usually found in patients under 1 year of age) and that characterized by eosinophilic or allergic gastroenteritis with multiple food sensitivities (a more permanent condition usually associated with a positive RAST result and elevated IgE). However, the biopsy findings in both types are similar.

REFERENCES

1. Ament ME, Rubin CF: Soy protein: another cause of the flat intestinal lesion, *Gastroenterology* 62:227, 1972.
2. Gryboski JD: Gastrointestinal milk allergy in infants, *Pediatrics* 40:354, 1967.
3. Katz AJ, Goldman H, Grand RJ: Gastric mucosal biopsy in eosinophilic (allergic) gastroenteritis, *Gastroenterology* 73:705, 1977.
4. Katz AJ et al: Milk-sensitive and eosinophilic gastroenteropathy: similar clinical features with contrasting mechanisms and clinical course, *J Allergy Clin Immunol* 74:72, 1984.
5. Kuitenen P et al: Malabsorption syndrome with cow's milk intolerance, *Arch Dis Child* 50:351, 1975.
6. Lake AM: The polymorph in red is no lady, *J Pediatr Gastroenterol Nutr* 19:4, 1994.
7. Lake AM, Whittington PF, Hamilton SR: Dietary protein–induced colitis in breast-fed infants, *J Pediatr* 101:96, 1982.
8. Leinbach GE, Rubin CE: Eosinophilic gastroenteritis: a simple reaction to food allergens? *Gastroenterology* 59:874, 1970.
9. Machida HM et al: Allergic colitis in infancy: clinical and pathologic aspects, *J Pediatr Gastroenterol Nutr* 19:22, 1994.
10. Waldmann TA et al: Allergic gastroenteropathy, *N Engl J Med* 276:761, 1967.

207 Gastrointestinal Obstruction

David L. Dudgeon

Gastrointestinal obstruction (GIO) during infancy, childhood, and adolescence is relatively uncommon but always is a diagnostic challenge. Obstructions that occur distal to the pylorus are surgical emergencies, and the younger the patient, the more ominous the probable cause and the more urgent the required therapy. Therefore the pediatrician continually must be alert for a GIO to facilitate early diagnosis and thus prevent tragedy.

HISTORY

The symptoms and signs of a GIO (Table 207-1) vary considerably but involve the following, either singly or in combination: vomiting, pain, abdominal distention (see Chapter 109), a change in bowel habits, fever, abdominal tenderness, and a palpable abdominal mass.

Vomiting is a ubiquitous symptom seen far more often without a GIO in this age group. However, it frequently can be a sign of obstruction, particularly when marked by certain characteristics.

A small amount of nonbilious, nonprojectile vomitus in an infant is unlikely to indicate a GIO; it commonly denotes a benign, self-limited form of regurgitation or gastroesophageal reflux (chalasia). However, this picture in the newborn can be associated with an esophageal obstruction (atresia).[2] An esophageal block encountered during attempts to pass a transoral soft catheter into the stomach denotes esophageal atresia. Respiratory distress can be associated with this anomaly, caused by pharyngeal aspiration of retained saliva, secondary gastric aspiration, or the development of acute gastric distention as the result of the commonly associated tracheoesophageal fistula distal to the atresia.[2] Esophageal atresia and the rare entity of pediatric gastric volvulus are uncommon and are the only two neonatal conditions in which a congenital or early acquired esophageal obstruction is likely to be encountered. Acute gastric volvulus, rather than esophageal atresia, often is accompanied by severe pain and can be associated with signs of shock. Nonbilious vomiting can be produced by the rare anomaly of a complete or incomplete gastric antral web.[16]

The more dramatic, projectile, nonbilious vomiting of early infancy is associated with the semiurgent condition of congenital hypertrophic pyloric stenosis.[18] Bilious vomiting, usually nonprojectile, is a more ominous problem and denotes a GIO below the level of the ampulla of Vater. Concern arises because of the possibility of an associated condition, intestinal nonrotation with a complicating volvulus, which can produce an intestinal block and necrotic intestine.[9,20] Although a premature infant who has an immature pyloric sphincter can have bilious regurgitation without obstruction, related to an underlying septic process, the threat of intestinal vascular compromise caused by an underlying volvulus mandates immediate radiological examination for diagnosis, usually an upper GI contrast study. Other causes of bilious vomiting in the neonate and infant include duodenal, jejunal, and ileal atresias,[10] duodenal stenosis that occurs secondary to an annular pancreas or Ladd bands (colonic peritoneal bands crossing the duodenum),[24] meconium ileus, colonic atresia, congenital aganglionosis of the colon (Hirschsprung disease),[7] and imperforate anus.[6] An infant or older toddler who has bilious vomiting can have a GIO caused by an incarcerated hernia or an intussusception.[17] The etiology of bilious vomiting in an adolescent can include incarcerated hernias, postoperative adhesions, and meconium ileus equivalent associated with cystic fibrosis,[14] acute inflammation (appendicitis[3] and pelvic inflammatory disease), and chronic inflammation (regional ileitis and ulcerative colitis).

Vomitus containing minimal amounts of blood can be seen in infants who have congenital hypertrophic pyloric stenosis.[18] In rare cases hematemesis with larger amounts of blood is associated with a GIO, as in the uncommon occurrence of an acute peptic ulcer obstruction of a newborn or, more frequently, in an older, chronically stressed infant or child.

Abdominal pain, detectable only as irreconcilable crying or irritability in an infant, usually accompanies a GIO. It is likely to be "crampy" or intermittent and results in flexion of the legs to the abdomen and crying interspersed with periods of no apparent or obviously decreased levels of distress. This is best exemplified by the toddler who has an intussusception.[17] A complete or chronic partial obstruction of the intestine acutely produces intermittent abdominal pain, which in a matter of hours becomes constant and is caused by the resultant intestinal distention or peritoneal inflammation, or both.

Obstipation in a newborn is a significant finding. Full-term, otherwise healthy infants pass normal meconium spontaneously within the first 24 hours of life. With premature infants, those small for gestational age,[8] and infants of diabetic mothers,[15] there frequently is a delay of up to 72 hours before the initial stool. Likewise, a pregnancy complicated by maternal drug abuse (narcotics such as morphine), drug therapy (e.g., magnesium sulfate for toxemia),[19] or neonatal stress (hypoxemia or sepsis) also can delay the initial bowel movement.

Atresias of the upper GI tract do not cause obstipation routinely; however, the meconium passed by these patients usually is sparse and lighter in color and may be hard and dry. The differential diagnosis of newborn obstipation includes meconium ileus (usually with underlying cystic fibrosis), meconium plug syndrome (30% are associated with congenital aganglionosis of the colon),[13] congenital aganglionosis of the colon, imperforate anus, and in rare cases, rectal atresia. Strictures that occur secondary to previous episodes of neo-

Table 207-1 Pediatric Gastrointestinal Obstruction: Clinical Findings

	Findings						
Etiology	**Vomiting**	**Pain**	**Stool pattern**	**Distention**	**Bowel sounds**	**Tenderness**	**Masses**
Esophageal atresia	Nonbilious (saliva)	No	Normal meconium	No	Absent to normal	No	No
Gastric obstruction	Nonbilious (curdled formula)	Severe with gastric volvulus; none with antral web	Normal meconium	Epigastric	Absent to normal	Severe with volvulus	No
Hypertrophic pyloric stenosis	Nonbilious, projectile	No	Constipation (dehydration)	Epigastric	Hyperactive (epigastric)	No	Yes ("olive")
Duodenal obstruction	Bilious	Minimal	Small meconium stool	Epigastric	Absent to normal	No	No
Volvulus	Bilious	Severe	Hematochezia	Epigastric to generalized	Hyperactive	Yes (severe)	No
Jejunoileal atresia	Bilious	No	Small, hard, light-colored meconium stool	Generalized	Variable	No	No
Intussusception	Bilious	Yes (crampy)	Currant jelly stool	Generalized	Hyperactive	Yes	Yes ("sausage shaped")
Meconium ileus	Bilious	No	Obstipation	Generalized	Variable	No	Yes ("doughy beads")
Meconium plug	Bilious	No	Obstipation	Generalized	Variable	No	No
Congenital aganglionosis	Bilious	No	Obstipation, constipation, and intermittent diarrhea	Generalized	Hyperactive	No	Palpable stool
Obstipation of prematurity	Bilious	No	Obstipation	Generalized	Hyperactive	No	No
Incarcerated inguinal hernia	Bilious	Yes	Diarrhea or constipation	Generalized	Hyperactive	Yes	Inguinal or scrotal
Imperforate anus	Bilious	No	Obstipation	Generalized	Hyperactive	No	No

natal necrotizing enterocolitis or previous intestinal surgery, as well as extrinsic compression of the GI tract caused by congenital cysts, inflammatory masses, and/or malignancies, produce obstipation or constipation in an older infant or child.

In pediatric patients, particularly neonates and infants, diarrhea or alternating diarrhea and constipation can occur as a sign of a functional GIO or as a partial or intermittently complete GIO. Congenital colonic aganglionosis or the more critical problem of an intussusception or intermittent volvulus also can produce this picture (the latter two conditions frequently manifest with hematochezia or melena).

Hematochezia or grossly blood stool in association with GIO symptoms indicates intestinal vascular compromise. It occurs most commonly in patients who have an intussusception or volvulus.[17,20] This so-called currant jelly stool results from the admixture of blood and mucus and is a sign of superficial mucosal sloughing, but it also can accompany a full-thickness necrosis of the bowel wall. Occasionally, darker (mahogany to black), melena-type stools resulting from a more proximal bleeding site are noted, with the same potential dire etiology.

PHYSICAL EXAMINATION

The physical examination of the abdomen includes evaluation for distention, which is likely to be prominent if the obstruction is distal to the duodenum (see Table 207-1). Gastric obstruction caused by a congenital antral web, hypertrophic pyloric stenosis, or duodenal atresia produces only mild to moderate epigastric distention, whereas distal intestinal atresias or other forms of lower GIO produce generalized distention. The presence or absence of abdominal distention does not aid in the diagnosis of a potential underlying midgut volvulus because the obstruction may be at the level of the duodenum, with few air- and fluid-distended bowel loops present.

Abdominal auscultation should be performed before any manipulation of the patient. In larger patients an effort should be made to listen to all the abdominal quadrants. High-pitched, "tinkling" bowel sounds heard in "rushes" are diagnostic of a complete GIO. However, the bowel sounds often are normal early in obstruction, becoming diminished to absent late in obstruction or in the case of a GIO produced by an inflammatory process.

If the abdomen is moderately to grossly distended, a mild amount of tenderness or discomfort is to be expected with palpation, because pressure applied to gas- or fluid-filled loops causes pain. However, marked tenderness, especially accompanied by rebound or referred tenderness, clearly indicates an accompanying peritoneal inflammation. This inflammation (or peritonitis) in the face of a GIO means ischemia of the bowel wall with possible necrosis and demands immediate surgical evaluation and treatment.

The presence of multiple, "doughy," compressible, mobile, nontender abdominal masses in a newborn who has a GIO is associated with meconium ileus.[11] A tender, palpable, immobile mass most likely is an area of cellulitis or abscess related to visceral perforation, that is, necrotizing enterocolitis in infants or appendicitis and inflammatory bowel disease in children and adolescents. A nontender, extremely mobile mass that produces GIO symptoms is found with congenital intestinal duplication cysts or mesenteric cysts. Malignancies in the intestinal tract are rare and usually do not produce intestinal obstruction, but lymphomas may do so in older patients. When they cause GIO, intestinal or mesenteric lymphomas in patients over age 4 commonly are manifested as an intussusception.

An incarcerated inguinal hernia is an important cause of GIO in the pediatric age group. Detecting an inguinal hernia in an uncooperative, chubby infant is difficult and requires considerable patience and effort. Sedation with a tranquilizer, with or without an added narcotic analgesic, may be helpful. These medications must be used very cautiously to avoid excessive sedation, since vomiting and aspiration can occur. If possible, the hernia should be reduced gently and then repaired later when the effects of the GIO have subsided. If the hernia is reduced but left unrepaired, repeat incarcerations are likely, with the potential consequences of strangulation and necrosis of the bowel.

Often a rectal examination can clarify the cause of a GIO. In an infant who is suspected of having an incarcerated inguinal hernia, the clinician often can palpate the peritoneal side of the internal inguinal ring transanally and identify an exiting intraperitoneal structure. The rectal examination can be equally important in the diagnosis of any suspected colonic or distal GIO. Previously unsuspected perirectal or presacral pelvic masses (e.g., hydrometrocolpos, appendicial inflammatory mass, or a presacral teratoma) can be identified in this manner. Abnormal stool (as in the patient who has meconium plug syndrome) or blood found in association with an intussusception or accompanying inflammatory bowel disease can be detected during a rectal examination. In rare cases an intraluminal rectal mass can be palpated, such as with a low-lying intussusception.

TREATMENT

Medical Management

A pediatric patient who has a GIO requires gastric decompression to avoid continued bowel distention, vomiting, and possibly aspiration. Intravenous fluid therapy is required immediately to replace the "third space" (i.e., intraluminal and intraperitoneal) fluid loss. When replacing the fluid deficit, it must be remembered that luminal GIO losses are high in electrolyte content, requiring administration of higher-than-maintenance concentrations of sodium, chloride, and potassium. Therefore solutions such as lactated Ringer solution are needed to provide appropriate replacement. A urinalysis, with catheterization if necessary, as well as a complete blood count (CBC) and blood chemistry studies, is mandatory. Because almost all pediatric patients who have a GIO require emergency or semiemergency surgery, they must be well prepared for anesthesia and the surgical procedure. This requires correcting fluid, electrolyte, hematological, and metabolic imbalances beforehand. Such corrective measures should begin before extensive diagnostic ultrasound scans or radiological studies are begun.

Table 207-2 lists roentgenographic diagnostic studies required for a patient who has a GIO and the expected findings; these studies are dictated by the results of the history and physical examination. However, a plain roentgenogram of the abdomen is obtained in all patients suspected of hav-

Table 207-2 Common Causes of Pediatric Gastrointestinal Obstruction: Roentgenographic Findings

	Findings				
Etiology	**Dilated area**	**Air or fluid levels**	**Calcium deposits**	**Noncalcium opacities**	**Further studies that may be indicated**
Esophageal atresia	Esophagus and stomach	Yes (gastric)	No	No	Esophageal air instillation
Gastric obstruction	Stomach	Yes	No	No	Gastric barium instillation*
Hypertrophic pyloric stenosis	Stomach	Yes	No	No	Ultrasonography
Duodenal obstruction	Stomach, duodenum (double bubble)	Yes	No	No	None
Volvulus	Variable	Variable	No	No	Upper GI series or barium enema
Jejunoileal atresia	Stomach and small intestine	Yes	Yes (with prenatal perforation)	No	Barium enema to rule out nonrotation
Intussusception	Stomach and small intestine	Variable	No	Yes (soft tissue densities)	Ultrasonography and/or barium enema†
Meconium ileus	Stomach and small intestine	No	Yes (meconium peritonitis)	Yes (ground-glass appearance)	Water-soluble contrast enema†
Meconium plug	Stomach to colon	Yes	No	No	Barium enema‡
Congenital aganglionosis	Stomach to colon	Yes	No	No	Barium enema
Obstipation of prematurity (short left colon syndrome)	Stomach to colon	Yes	No	No	Barium enema‡
Incarcerated inguinal hernia	Stomach and small intestine	Yes	No	No	None
Imperforate anus	Stomach to colon	Yes	No	No	Complete evaluation of genitourinary tract

*Should be performed cautiously to avoid aspiration.
†Should be performed cautiously to avoid bowel perforation.
‡May be therapeutic and diagnostic.

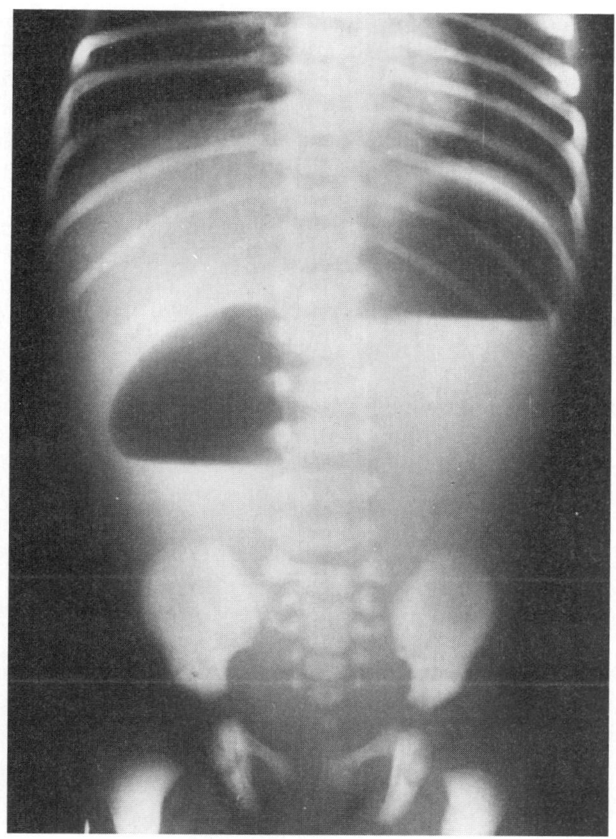

FIG. 207-1 Duodenal atresia. An upright roentgenogram of a 4-day-old girl with persistent vomiting since birth. The double-bubble sign is classic, showing the large gastric fluid-filled air bubble on the right and the similar duodenal bubble on the left.
(From Micro X-ray Recorder, Inc, Chicago.)

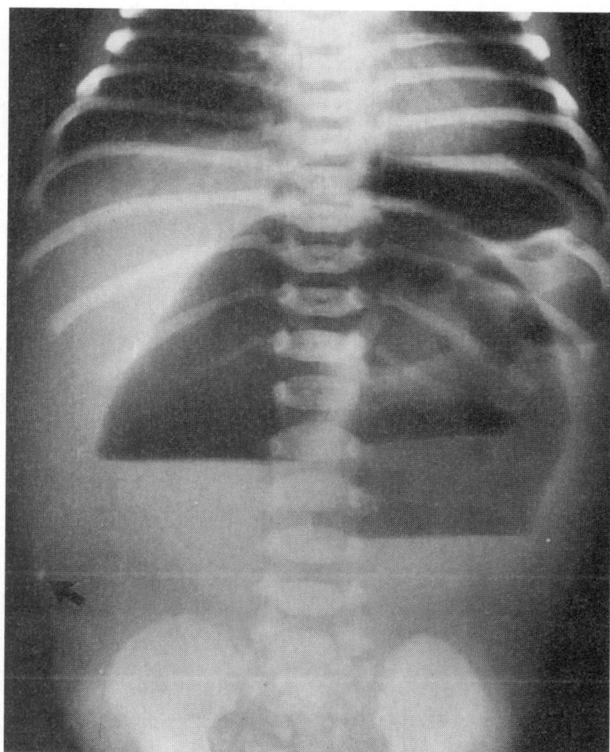

FIG. 207-2 Ileal atresia with meconium peritonitis. An upright roentgenogram of a 36-hour-old girl with persistent vomiting since birth. The numerous dilated loops of small bowel with fluid levels indicate atresia of the ileum; the calcification *(arrow)* is diagnostic of meconium peritonitis caused by prenatal rupture of the small bowel.
(From Micro X-ray Recorder, Inc, Chicago.)

ing a GIO. In a newborn infant, air localized to the stomach and duodenum (double-bubble sign) is diagnostic of a duodenal obstruction[24] (Fig. 207-1). If no distal intestinal intraluminal air is seen, the GIO usually is caused by an atresia; however, if even a small amount of air is found distally, the diagnosis of a malrotation with possible volvulus must be suspected. Use of an upper GI series to determine the relationship between the duodenum and the jejunum and the ligament of Treitz or a barium enema to ascertain cecal position is necessary to rule out a malrotation or nonrotation of the intestine.[20] The presence of even a large number of air-filled loops on the plain roentgenographic study does not eliminate the need for a contrast study, because a volvulus still is possible. Visualization by barium enema of an "unused," small-caliber distal colon (microcolon) in a normal position makes the diagnosis of intestinal atresia or meconium ileus more likely than an acute volvulus.

Calcifications seen on the abdominal roentgenogram in a neonate who has a GIO are evidence of an intrauterine intestinal perforation (meconium peritonitis), which often is associated with intestinal atresia. The calcifications may be small, single, or multiple scattered throughout the entire peritoneal cavity or maybe seen to outline the peritoneal cavity (Fig. 207-2). Cystic fibrosis may or may not be associated with such a presentation.

Infants suspected of having hypertrophic pyloric stenosis usually do not require an upper GI series to confirm the diagnosis. The classic history and the presence of characteristic upper abdominal peristaltic waves and a palpable, olive-size mass in the mid to right upper quadrant are diagnostic; roentgenographic confirmation is needless, costly, and potentially hazardous. The hazard results from the routinely ineffective preoperative efforts to lavage the residual barium from a dilated obstructed stomach. This makes subsequent induction of a general anesthetic hazardous because of possible barium aspiration. An experienced pediatrician or surgeon will be successful in palpating the olive in approximately 80% to 90% of the patients. Diagnostic ultrasound scans can produce a diagnosis in most difficult cases in which there is no palpable mass.[21,23] Contrast studies rarely are required (see Chapter 250, Pyloric Stenosis).

An unusual presentation of nonbilious vomiting, absence of a clinically palpable olive, a normal abdominal ultrasound examination, and a "normal" upper GI contrast study is possible. This sequence of events may lead to prolonged delay in diagnosing an underlying partial gastric antral web. This can be clarified by using esophageal gastric duodenoscopy to identify and possibly divide the web. If the web cannot be treated safely by endoscopy, open gastric antroplasty is effective.[16]

Often an abdominal roentgenogram of a GIO that occurs in association with suspected cystic fibrosis (meconium il-

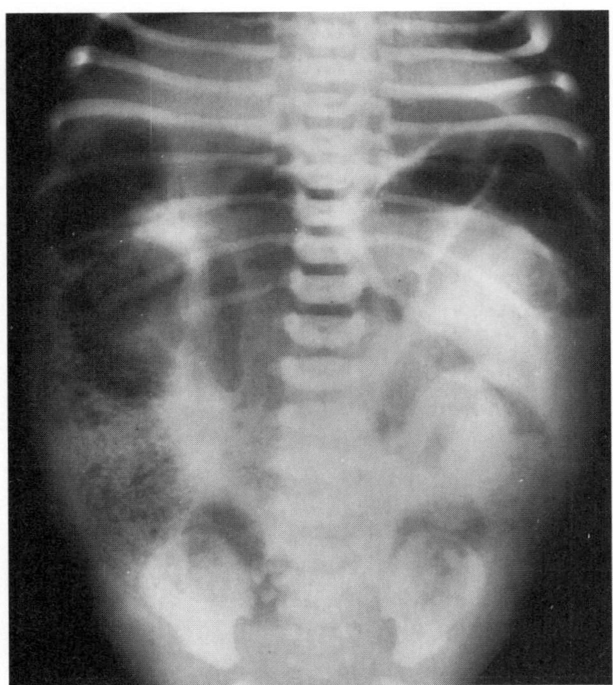

FIG. 207-3 Meconium ileus. An upright roentgenogram of a 2-day-old boy with abdominal distention since birth. The loops of distended bowel of varying size without fluid levels are filled with meconium shadows (radiolucent soap bubbles).

(From Micro X-ray Recorder, Inc, Chicago.)

eus) has a peculiar hazy pattern described as a "ground-glass" or "soap bubble" appearance (Fig. 207-3). This is caused by the abnormal meconium mixed with air that is inspissated in the bowel lumen. Occasionally this hard, dense, abnormal stool, palpable as multiple abdominal masses, appears on the roentgenogram as a chain of radiolucencies, or a "string of beads" sign.[11,13] Meconium ileus, like ileal atresia, is associated with a complete GIO; however, air-fluid levels are rare in meconium ileus. Meconium ileus and meconium plug syndrome are two neonatal GIO conditions that can be diagnosed and frequently can be treated with a contrast enema. A neonate who is suspected of having meconium ileus, who has no evidence of perforation, and who is well hydrated can be given a water-soluble contrast enema cautiously by an experienced radiologist. This identifies the inspissated meconium, localized to the distal ileum, and may free it from the bowel wall for spontaneous expulsion. This technique is somewhat limited in application and duration, with subsequent surgical therapy required in as many as half of the patients. Uncomplicated meconium plug syndrome, a lower GIO lesion infrequently associated with cystic fibrosis but occasionally associated with congenital aganglionosis, also is diagnosed and successfully treated with a barium enema.[1,13] Unlike meconium ileus, the abnormal meconium in meconium plug syndrome is localized to the distal colon. Contrast enemas in either syndrome are contraindicated when there is intestinal vascular compromise or perforation, that is, peritonitis, free intraperitoneal air, or intraperitoneal calcification.

Older infants and toddlers suspected of having a GIO produced by an intussusception can be diagnosed and often successfully treated with a barium enema.[17] The importance of an experienced radiologist for this maneuver cannot be overemphasized. The study is performed with a limited pressure (3-foot) barium column. The intussusception is slowly reduced by the hydrostatic pressure generated by this barium solution. Because of the potential hazard of a barium perforation, the study should never be performed without a surgical team standing by. The procedure, which can be used in about 75% of patients, successfully reduces the intussusception in 35% to 50% of cases.[17,25] The patient always is observed for 12 to 24 hours in the hospital after successful barium reduction. More recently the use of air enema reduction of the intussusception has become available. This consists of air insufflation of the rectum and colon by using an inline pressure-limiting valve and maintaining fluoroscopic or sonographic observation to ensure that the reduction is under control. The advantages of this technique are (1) elimination of barium, with the threat of severe chemical peritonitis it can cause if a perforation inadvertently occurs, and (2) possibly an improved mechanical advantage by using air reduction.[4,5,12]

Surgical Management

The type of surgical procedure performed and the patient's postoperative course and prognosis (Table 207-3) depend on the types of lesion causing the GIO.

ESOPHAGEAL OBSTRUCTION

Esophageal atresia with associated tracheoesophageal fistula (TEF) constitutes an emergency requiring either primary repair or a staged procedure using an initial gastrostomy for gastric decompression and prevention of aspiration. Subsequent definitive repair, including a division of the fistula and anastomosis of the esophageal ends, is carried out after treatment of any existing underlying pneumonic process. Occasionally the gastrostomy and definitive repair are performed simultaneously, or in selected patients the esophageal repair is performed without a gastrostomy. Complications of the definitive procedure include esophageal leaks, infection, and strictures. Anomalies, particularly of the cardiovascular system, are associated problems in as many as half of these cases.[2] Patients who have uncomplicated atresia and TEF have a low morbidity and negligible mortality. Associated cardiovascular anomalies and low birth weight lead to a mortality as high as 70%. Late complications of atresia and TEF include congenital hypertrophic pyloric stenosis and chronic gastroesophageal reflux with hyperactive airway symptoms.

GASTRIC OBSTRUCTIONS

Gastric volvulus usually is an acute problem that requires an immediate surgical gastropexy to prevent ischemia and necrosis. If no gastric necrosis is found, recovery usually is uneventful. Gastric necrosis with secondary peritonitis results in high morbidity and mortality. A gastric antral web is difficult to diagnose and often requires repeated diagnostic studies, but it is not a critical problem. Surgical therapy consists of simple incision of the web and performance of a modified pyloroplasty, resulting in minimal postoperative complications.[22] Hypertrophic pyloric stenosis is a semiurgent surgical problem, with surgical therapy following adequate cor-

Table 207-3 Common Causes of Pediatric Gastrointestinal Obstruction: Surgery and Prognosis

Etiology	Surgical procedure	Complications	Prognosis
Esophageal atresia	Divide tracheoesophageal fistula, perform primary esophageal anastomosis, with or without gastrostomy	Aspiration, leaking anastomosis, stricture	Depends on associated anomalies; with no cardiac anomaly, ≥95% survival
Gastric volvulus	Gastropexy, gastrostomy, with or without resection	Sepsis, leaking anastomosis	With no necrosis, very good; with necrosis, high mortality
Antral web	Gastrotomy, divide web, modified pyloroplasty	Leaking gastrotomy or pyloroplasty	Good
Hypertrophic pyloric stenosis	Pyloromyotomy	Incomplete procedure, mucosal leak	Good
Volvulus	Detorsion of mesentery, divide Ladd bands, and intestinal resection (if necrosis is present)	Leaking anastomosis, sepsis, short-gut syndrome	With no necrosis, good; with necrosis, guarded
Jejunal atresia	Resection and anastomosis	Strictures, leaking anastomosis, poor gut motility	Isolated anomaly, good; associated with cystic fibrosis, poor
Intussusception	Reduction with or without resection	Ischemic bowel, leaking anastomosis, recurrence	With no necrosis, good; with necrosis, potential short-gut syndrome
Meconium ileus	Intestinal cleansing through enterotomy, possible resection	Sepsis, malnutrition	Immediately after surgery, good; long term, poor
Obstipation of prematurity	Colostomy only for severe cases	Sepsis	Good
Congenital aganglionosis	Colostomy, delayed pull-through procedure	Sepsis, incontinence	Good
Incarcerated inguinal hernia	Reduction, possible intestinal resection	Sepsis	Good to guarded
Imperforate anus	Colostomy, delayed pull-through procedure	Sepsis, incontinence	High defects, guarded; low defects, good

rection of the accompanying dehydration and hypochloremic alkalosis. The procedure is a muscle-splitting pyloromyotomy, leaving the mucosa intact. Acute complications are unusual, with the patient resuming postoperative feedings without sequelae within 8 to 24 hours. Chronic complications such as a stricture related to intraoperative mucosal perforations and adhesions are rare.

DUODENAL OBSTRUCTIONS

Duodenal atresia, stenosis, and annular pancreas constitute semiurgent problems as long as they are not accompanied by an associated volvulus. Surgical therapy consists of bypassing the obstructed area by means of a duodenoduodenostomy, a duodenojejunostomy, or a gastrojejunostomy.[24] Moderate feeding problems necessitating a longer hospitalization may be encountered, particularly when a gastrojejunostomy is performed. The prognosis is good; however, with associated congenital cardiac problems, mortality can be as high as 50%. The growth and development of patients who have uncomplicated duodenal obstructions are normal.

JEJUNAL AND ILEAL OBSTRUCTIONS

Jejunal and ileal atresia also are semiurgent conditions unless they are associated with a volvulus. Surgical treatment involves excision of the atretic bowel and primary anastomosis of the dilated proximal and the narrowed distal segment of bowel.[10] When multiple atretic segments of bowel are present, the overall intestinal length and therefore the absorptive surface may be reduced significantly. Total parenteral nutrition commonly is required after surgery. Overall survival and prognosis are good unless the atresia is complicated by cystic fibrosis or the remaining small intestine is too short for adequate absorption.

Nonrotation with a complicating volvulus is the most critical diagnosis in any pediatric patient suspected of having a GIO. The twisted bowel mesentery may lead to ischemia and bowel necrosis within 4 to 6 hours after the onset of symptoms. Untreated volvulus has a high acute mortality rate because of associated metabolic imbalances and sepsis. After successful surgical resection of the involved necrotic bowel, high long-term morbidity can be expected. The entire embryonically derived midgut may have to be resected, leading to reduced intestinal absorption of nutrients and the so-called short-gut syndrome. Thus early diagnosis, rapid correction of fluid and electrolyte imbalances, and surgical reduction of the mesenteric torsion with or without resection of potentially necrotic gut are imperative.[20] Proximal and distal segments of involved intestine that appear ischemic but may be viable should be retained and abdominal enterostomas created or a second-look operation performed in 24 hours rather than performing extensive intestinal resections initially. Postoperative complications include marked fluid and electrolyte disturbances, local and systemic infections, and malnutrition. Long-term parenteral nutrition, dietary adjustments, and repeated surgical procedures should be expected. Survival with reasonable quality of life can be expected if the remaining viable small bowel is 30 cm or longer. Survival is improved when the ileocecal valve remains intact. Long-term hospitalization or prolonged nutritional support through total parenteral nutrition is common.

As noted previously, meconium ileus may respond to water-soluble contrast enemas; however, evidence of an accompanying intestinal perforation or failure of a carefully managed water-soluble contrast enema necessitates surgical therapy.[11] The underlying disease (cystic fibrosis), which almost certainly is present, complicates the postoperative respiratory and nutritional picture. Administration of cleansing solutions by means of an enterotomy usually frees the intestinal lumen of the inspissated material. Associated atretic or necrotic intestinal segments are excised, and primary anastomoses are performed. Enterostomas are created for postoperative lavage of massively impacted meconium or in instances where the viability of the remaining bowel segments is marginal. Surgical survival is good; however, the morbidity is high, and the ultimate prognosis is related to the severity of the other manifestations of the accompanying cystic fibrosis.

COLONIC AND RECTAL OBSTRUCTION

An intussusception uncomplicated by a lead point (i.e., a Meckel diverticulum, a polyp, or a malignancy) can be successfully reduced hydrostatically or by air in more than half of appropriately selected patients.[17] Recurrences after air/hydrostatic reduction range from 5% to 7%. Surgical intervention is required if there is evidence of compromised bowel, such as a free perforation or peritoneal irritation, and in failures of air/hydrostatic reduction. Most patients who have intussusceptions that are reduced intraoperatively do well postoperatively and experience a 2% to 4% recurrence rate. Bowel resection is required when an intraoperatively diagnosed lead point is present or an ischemic complication is found. Early diagnosis and treatment of intussusception results in reduced morbidity and mortality.

Congenital aganglionosis of the colon (Fig. 207-4), or Hirschsprung disease, in infancy can be lethal if complicated by enterocolitis. Hirschsprung disease seldom produces total GIO, which, when present, must be treated as an emergency. The initial diagnosis is made on the basis of clinical suspicion because it cannot be verified by noninvasive diagnostic procedures. A barium enema often is helpful in diagnosing Hirschsprung disease in older children, but either a rectal mucosal or full-thickness rectal wall biopsy specimen is required to confirm the diagnosis in infants. Surgical therapy includes creating a colostomy by using a segment of proximal ganglionic colon. This is followed in 6 months to 1 year by excision of the affected segment of aganglionic colon and anastomosis of the normally innervated (ganglionic) bowel to the anus (pull-through procedure).[7] Infant morbidity and mortality rates are high when the disease is accompanied by a complicating enterocolitis; however, patients who have no such complications usually do well, with good anal continence, growth, and development after these procedures.

Colonic dysfunction of prematurity or short left colon syndrome (SLCS) produces a functional mechanical obstruction that mimics Hirschsprung disease. SLCS can be related to extreme prematurity, maternal diabetes, prenatal maternal

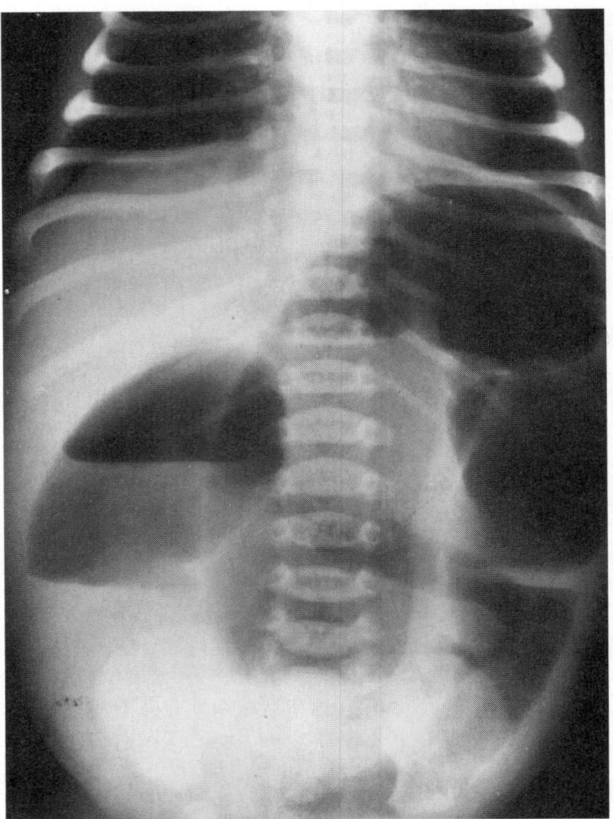

FIG. 207-4 Aganglionic megacolon (Hirschsprung disease). An upright roentgenogram of a 2-day-old boy with a distended abdomen and failure to pass anything by rectum shows extreme distention of the colon with several fluid levels.

(From Micro X-ray Recorder, Inc, Chicago.)

medications for eclampsia (magnesium sulfate), hyperthyroidism, or maternal narcotic use. SLCS is a rule-out diagnosis of exclusion because its barium contrast appearance resembles Hirschsprung disease. Surgically, a temporary colostomy is indicated only for failure to respond to careful, small-volume, saline enema therapy or the presence of signs of peritonitis or intestinal perforation.[15] The prognosis for uncomplicated cases is excellent.

Rectal atresia and imperforate anus require diagnosis and initial therapy (a colostomy) within 24 hours. Definitive therapy, which includes a pull-through procedure and anoplasty, is performed when the infant is approximately 1 year old.[6] If the lesion is not associated with any other congenital anomalies, survival is good. Anomalies should be looked for, particularly those of the genitourinary tract (rectovaginal and rectovesicle fistulas, lower urinary tract obstructions with megacystis, hydroureter, and hydronephrosis). Future stool continence is related directly to the severity of the deformity, which is determined by the degree of normal embryological descent of the colon through the levator muscle. High lesions, or a colon descent limited to a position above the levator muscle, results in stool continence in approximately 50% to 60% of patients after definitive surgery. Low lesions, in which the colon has descended below the levator muscle, result in a stool continence rate of at least 80% after definitive repair.

REFERENCES

1. Ellis DG, Clatworthy WH Jr: The meconium plug syndrome revisited, *J Pediatr Surg* 1:54, 1966.
2. Holder TM, Ashcraft KW: Esophageal atresia and tracheoesophageal fistula: collective review, *Ann Thorac Surg* 9:445, 1970.
3. Janik JS, Firor HV: Pediatric appendicitis: a 20-year study of 1640 children at Cook County (Illinois) Hospital, *Arch Surg* 114:717, 1979.
4. Jinzhe Z, Yenxia W, Linchi W: Rectal inflation reduction of intussusception in infants, *J Pediatr Surg* 21:30, 1986.
5. Katz M et al: Gas enema for the reduction of intussusception: relationship between clinical signs and symptoms and outcome, *Am J Roentgenol* 160:363, 1993.
6. Kiesewetter WB et al: Imperforate anus, *Arch Surg* 111:518, 1976.
7. Kleinhaus S et al: Hirschsprung's disease: a survey of the members of the surgical section of the American Academy of Pediatrics, *J Pediatr Surg* 14:588, 1979.
8. LeQuesne GW, Reilly BJ: Functional immaturity of the large bowel in the newborn infant, *Radiol Clin North Am* 13:331, 1975.
9. Lilien LD et al: Green vomiting in the first 72 hours in normal infants, *Am J Dis Child* 140:662, 1986.
10. Louw JH: Resection and end to end anastomosis in the management of atresia and stenosis of the small bowel, *Surgery* 62:940, 1967.
11. Mabogunjc OA, Wang CI, Mahour GH: Improved survival of neonates with meconium ileus, *Arch Surg* 117:37, 1982.
12. Menor F, et al: Effectiveness of pneumatic reduction of ileocolic intussusception in children, *Gastrointest Radiol* 17:339, 1992.
13. Olsen MM et al: The spectrum of meconium disease in infancy, *J Pediatr Surg* 17:479, 1982.
14. Penketh AR et al: Cystic fibrosis in adolescents and adults, *Thorax* 42:526, 1987.
15. Philippart AI, Reed JO, Georgeson KE: Neonatal small left colon syndrome: intramural not intraluminal obstruction, *J Pediatr Surg* 10:733, 1975.
16. Rodin D, Schwartz S, Dudgeon DL: Antral mucosal diaphragm, *Gastrointest Endosc* 24:33, 1977.
17. Rosenkrantz JG et al: Intussusception in the 1970s: indications for operation, *J Pediatr Surg* 12:367, 1977.
18. Scharli A, Sieber WK, Kiesewetter WB: Hypertrophic pyloric stenosis at the Children's Hospital of Pittsburgh from 1912 to 1967: a critical review of current problems, *J Pediatr Surg* 40:108, 1969.
19. Sokal MM et al: Neonatal hypermagnesemia and the meconium plug syndrome, *N Engl J Med* 286:733, 1975.
20. Steward DR, Colodny AL, Daggett WC: Malrotation of the bowel in infants and children: a 15-year review, *Surgery* 79:716, 1976.
21. Studen RJ, LeQuesne GW, Little KE: The improved ultrasound diagnosis of hypertrophic pyloric stenosis, *Pediatr Radiol* 16:200, 1986.
22. Tunell WP, Smith EI: Antral web in infancy, *J Pediatr Surg* 15:152, 1980.
23. Weiskittel DA, Leary DL, Blane CE: Ultrasound diagnosis of evolving pyloric stenosis, *Gastrointest Radiol* 14:22, 1989.
24. Wesley JR, Majour GH: Congenital intrinsic duodenal obstruction: a 25-year review, *Surgery* 82:716, 1977.
25. West KW et al: Intussusception: Current management in infants and children, *Surgery* 102:704, 1987.

208 Giardiasis

Craig M. Wilson and Donald A. Goldmann

ETIOLOGY

A *Giardia*-like organism was described and associated with gastrointestinal symptoms by Dutch microscopist Anton van Leeuwenhoek in 1681,[7] but only in the past 30 years has the true pathogenicity of this flagellate protozoan been recognized. It now is clear that *Giardia lamblia* is one of the most common intestinal parasites in the United States and the world,[1,18] and it has attained a certain notoriety as a result of diarrhea epidemics at fashionable ski resorts, in day care centers, in major metropolitan areas, among campers, and among international tourists. Nonetheless, the prevalence of giardiasis in children is not widely appreciated, and the diagnosis is easily missed by physicians who do not maintain a high index of suspicion.[19]

G. lamblia is an extracellular parasite that has no intermediate development outside of the intestinal lumen. This unicellular protozoan exists in two forms: a motile, flagellated trophozoite that causes disease and a dormant cyst that transmits infection. The trophozoite is 12 to 15 μm long and has four pairs of flagella and two prominent nuclei (Fig. 208-1). It lacks many eukaryotic subcellular structures, including mitochondria, Golgi apparatus, or a well-developed endoplasmic reticulum, and has a ribosomal RNA structure suggestive of a very primitive organism.[10,26] A large sucking disk, which the parasite uses to attach to the intestinal mucosa, occupies most of the flat ventral surface. Attachment is regulated by contractile proteins, including actin and myosin, which alter the structure of the disk. It is not clear how the organism evades degradation in the intestinal lumen. The motile trophozoites divide by longitudinal binary fission in the upper small bowel and then encyst as they pass into the colon. Trophozoites usually are seen only in the stool when diarrhea is present. Cysts, the more common form seen in stool specimens, are 9 to 12 μm long. Recently formed cysts have two nuclei; mature cysts have four.

EPIDEMIOLOGY

Studies in human volunteers have demonstrated the high infectivity of *G. lamblia* cysts. Although one cyst rarely was infectious, infection occurred in virtually all volunteers receiving 100 to 1 million cysts orally and in 36% of those exposed to 10 to 25 cysts.[20]

G. lamblia is one of the most commonly identified pathogens in waterborne diarrheal disease in the United States, where the organism is holoendemic.[3,18] A number of large common-source outbreaks have been traced to contaminated drinking water. Epidemiological studies have attributed these epidemics to cross-contamination of municipal drinking water supplies with sewage, defective or deficient filtration facilities, and reliance on chlorination as the principal method of water disinfection.[10,24] In mountainous regions, where the prevalence of disease appears to be higher,[4] use of surface water for drinking is the principal problem. It has been suggested that indigenous animal hosts, especially beavers, are responsible for contaminating mountain streams and reservoirs.[9] However, true zoonotic infection has not been proven.[27] As suggested by the occurrence of epidemic giardiasis despite chlorination of municipal water supplies, routine chlorination may not be adequate for killing *G. lamblia*.[23] The level of chlorine necessary to kill cysts depends on many other factors, including pH, contact time, turbidity, and temperature.[16] Thus an adequate water purification system for clearing *G. lamblia* should include filtration, sedimentation, and flocculation systems. Halogen-based, small-quantity disinfection methods are also affected by water clarity and temperature.[15]

Because cysts may be shed in abundance in the stool, it is not surprising that *G. lamblia* may be transmitted by the fecal-oral route. This undoubtedly is the main route of spread in families, in institutions, in day care centers, and among homosexuals. With intensive exposure to stool, as in day care centers caring for infants in diapers, giardiasis quickly may become hyperendemic.[2,22] Although food-borne giardiasis is a theoretical hazard, only four such outbreaks have been reported; in all four the implicated food probably was contaminated during preparation.

PATHOGENESIS

Although many mechanisms have been postulated for the diarrhea and malabsorption caused by *G. lamblia,* how this parasite causes disease remains a mystery. It seems likely that the process is multifactorial, with the severity of symptoms depending on the degree of focal small bowel injury. Infection is associated with injury to the mucosal brush border, with disruption of disaccharidase activity and transport mechanisms.[13] There is a basal membrane and intraepithelial inflammatory cell infiltrate[28] and evidence of an increased enterocyte turnover in the murine model.[11] In either case, less efficient villus function would be expected. In the extreme, the microvilli atrophy, resulting in the severe malabsorptive diarrhea that is a major complication of giardiasis.[13] Recent studies suggest that parasite-induced prostaglandin E_2 production plays a role in the pathophysiology of this infection.[25] Also, evidence indicates that some *Giardia* strains produce more severe symptoms in humans,[17] and differences in phenotype and genotype have been correlated with virulence in experimental models of infection.

Host defense mechanisms appear to be relatively inefficient, given the small number of organisms required to initiate infection and the frequency of relapse and reinfection. However, intraluminal secretory antibody response, nonspecific inflammatory responses at the level of the mucosa, and

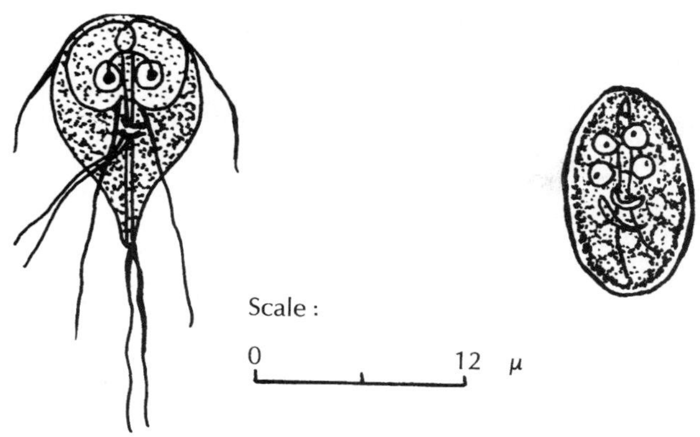

FIG. 208-1 *Giardia* organisms. The trophozoite *(left)* is 12 to 15 μm long and has four pairs of flagella. This form is not commonly seen in stools. Cysts *(right)* are 9 to 12 μm long and may have two to four nuclei.

antibody-dependent cell-mediated cytotoxicity (ADCC) appear to be important in limiting the severity of disease.[25] The role of antibody and ADCC in containing giardiasis is supported by the increased incidence and severity of disease in patients who have immunoglobulin deficiencies. Underlying IgA deficiency and both X-linked and common variable hypogammaglobulinemia have been associated with more severe or prolonged infection.

G. lamblia should be considered in the workup of diarrhea or malabsorption in patients who have human immunodeficiency (HIV) infection. The role and extent of *G. lamblia* infections in children who have HIV infection have not been established. Of course, diarrhea in patients who have acquired immunodeficiency syndrome (AIDS) often is multifactorial, and treatment of documented giardiasis may not result in clinical improvement if other pathogens still are present (see Chapter 180).

CLINICAL MANIFESTATIONS

Based on experimental studies and point-source outbreak observational data, the incubation period of giardiasis is 7 to 14 days.[20] Most patients infected by *G. lamblia* probably remain asymptomatic, although they do shed cysts in their feces and probably are infectious.[12,20] Children are more likely than adults to have symptomatic disease.

The principal symptoms of giardiasis are gastrointestinal. Diarrhea, abdominal cramps, and nausea are reported most often.[23] Vomiting, malodorous stools, flatulence, bloating, anorexia, and even constipation are noted less frequently. Because the colon and rectum are not involved, tenesmus should suggest another diagnosis. Blood almost never is found in the stool, and the presence of mucus is unusual. Gastrointestinal symptoms generally last 7 to 10 days, although a more protracted course is common. Because of the disaccharidase deficiency that accompanies severe infections, some patients complain of milk intolerance, which may last for weeks.

Constitutional symptoms are not prominent in giardiasis, but up to 25% of patients experience fatigue, headache, or a low-grade fever.[23] Extraintestinal syndromes, such as urticaria, erythema multiforme, and arthralgia, have occurred in very rare cases in association with giardiasis.

Some patients, particularly children, develop chronic diarrhea, frank malabsorption, weight loss, malnutrition, and growth retardation. Thus giardiasis must be considered in the differential diagnosis of failure to thrive. Occasionally giardiasis may be misdiagnosed as sprue, food allergy, or psychogenic abdominal pain, and its protean clinical manifestations may mimic a wide variety of gastrointestinal disturbances. Malabsorption leading to an iron deficiency anemia also has been reported with *G. lamblia*.[6]

The physical examination generally is unremarkable unless secondary malnutrition has developed.

LABORATORY EVALUATION[14]

The diagnosis often escapes a physician who performs a casual laboratory evaluation. Unfortunately, eosinophilia, one of the hallmarks of parasitic helminth infections, generally is absent in giardiasis, supporting the observation that *G. lamblia* rarely is invasive beyond the intestinal mucosa.

Careful examination of the stool is of paramount importance in diagnosing giardiasis. Initially, fresh stool suspended in saline or 1% potassium iodide should be examined microscopically. Trophozoites are detected more readily in fresh, diarrheal specimens. The yield of cyst detection can be increased if the stool is concentrated by either the formyl-ether or zinc sulfate methods. Trichrome-stained, polyvinyl alcohol–fixed specimens also are useful for detecting trophozoites or cysts. At least three stool specimens obtained on separate days should be examined, particularly if diarrhea is not present, because cysts can be passed intermittently.

Traditional diagnostic techniques are relatively labor intensive, cumbersome, and slow. Recently the focus has been directed toward developing techniques for detecting *Giardia* antigens directly in stool specimens. Currently at least three kits are available for detecting *Giardia* antigens in fecal material: Pro SpecT/Giardia, Alexon Inc., Mountain View, Calif; Giardia Direct Detection System, Trend Scientific Inc., St. Paul, Minn; and GIARDEIA, Antibodies Inc., Davis, Calif. Overall, these tests compare well with standard microscopic procedures and in some cases are more sensitive. In some clinical centers this methodology has replaced microscopic stool examination. The disadvantage is that the tests are singularly specific for *Giardia* and do not rule out other parasitic infestations that often are in the same diagnostic differential as giardiasis.

A few patients require additional measures to detect the pathogen. Examining the duodenal contents provides the optimum yield in these patients. This can be done either by direct duodenal aspiration or by using the Entero-Test.[21] In rare patients with chronic symptoms in whom the diagnosis must be excluded, the small bowel should be biopsied. Several sections of the biopsy specimen stained with Giemsa may have to be examined to find the parasite; *Giardia* organisms are detected more easily in Giemsa-stained mucosal impression smears.

Serological tests are valuable in epidemiological studies but are of little use diagnostically. Upper gastrointestinal roentgenograms may reveal mild dilation of the small bowel, edema of the mucosa, segmentation of barium, and either increased or decreased transit times; however, these changes are nonspecific. The sedimentation rate is normal, and as noted above, there is no eosinophilia. There may be biochemical evidence of malabsorption, including disaccharidase deficiency, abnormal absorption of D-xylose and fat, and a deficiency of folic acid.

THERAPY[9]

Most authorities agree that giardiasis should be treated when recognized, even if the patient is asymptomatic, because carriers of the parasite are potential transmitters of disease and may have subclinical malabsorption. However, physicians may elect not to treat some patients, particularly if reexposure to *G. lamblia* seems unavoidable. Treatment should be approached cautiously because none of the available drug regimens are universally effective or free of toxicity.

Furazolidone (Furoxone) has the distinct advantages of having a pleasant taste and being available in a pediatric suspension. Side effects, which have been minimal in children, include mild GI distress, hypersensitivity reactions, hemolysis in individuals who have glucose-6-phosphate dehydrogenase (G6PD) deficiency, brown discoloration of the urine, and disulfiram-like reactions (optic neuritis, peripheral neuritis, and/or polyneuritis). The efficacy in children has been as high as 92%, which is comparable if not superior to cure rates seen with alternative agents.[5] The dosage is 6 mg/kg/day (maximum dosage, 400 mg/day) given orally in four divided doses for 7 to 10 days.

Metronidazole (Flagyl) has been widely used to treat giardiasis in adults because it is well tolerated (except for the mild metallic aftertaste), has a very low incidence of serious side effects, and has an acceptable cure rate. However, the U.S. Food and Drug Administration (FDA) has not approved metronidazole for treating giardiasis in children. This agent has received considerable adverse publicity because studies have shown that it is carcinogenic in laboratory animals and mutagenic in bacteria. The relevance of these studies to humans has been questioned; no data suggest carcinogenicity in humans. The dosage of metronidazole is 250 mg three times a day for 5 days in children weighing more than 27 kg and 15 mg/kg/day in smaller children. The drug is not available as a suspension.

Relapse is possible after using any of these regimens. If this occurs, retreatment with the same agent or an alternative drug often is successful. There is no well-documented evidence for actual drug resistance in *Giardia*. Quinacrine, a previously recommended therapy for giardiasis, no longer is manufactured. Albendazole (400 mg/day for 5 days) recently was reported to be as effective as metronidazole in a study in children 5 to 10 years of age.[12] This may be an alternative therapy when the drug becomes more widely available in the United States. Tinidazole, a nitroimidazole similar to metronidazole, is used extensively outside the United States to treat giardiasis in a single-dose regimen. This drug is not marketed in the United States. Paromomycin has been used to treat giardiasis in pregnancy, but data regarding its efficacy are limited.

PREVENTION

Because giardiasis is so prevalent, total prevention of transmission is virtually impossible. When the disease is known to be present in a household, institution, or day care center, good hand washing is essential to limit spread by the fecal-oral route. Personal hygiene is especially important when infants in diapers are affected. In day care centers that have infants in diapers, eradication is difficult unless all *Giardia* excretors are treated, whether symptomatic or not. Because parasitological examinations of the stool are expensive and diagnosis often is delayed because cysts are not always found in a single specimen, all infants in the center may need to be treated to terminate the outbreak.

As noted above, prevention of waterborne giardiasis is contingent on adequate water purification, including filtration, sedimentation, and flocculation in addition to chlorination. Tourists in endemic areas should avoid drinking tap water. Campers should not rely on chlorination tablets, which are ineffective against *Giardia* cysts. Iodination, boiling for at least 10 minutes (particularly at high altitudes), or filtration (pore size under 3 μm) are satisfactory means for preparing drinking water free of *G. lamblia*.

REFERENCES

1. Beaver PC, Jung RF, Cupp EW: *Clinical parasitology,* ed 9, Philadelphia, 1984, Lea & Febiger.
2. Black RE et al: Giardiasis in day care centers: evidence of person-to-person transmission, *Pediatrics* 60:468, 1977.
3. Centers for Disease Control: Intestinal surveillance: United States, 1976, *MMWR* 27:167, 1978.
4. Centers for Disease Control: Waterborne giardiasis: California, Colorado, Oregon, and Pennsylvania, *MMWR* 29:121, 1980.
5. Craft JC, Murphy T, Nelson JD: Furazolidone and quinacrine: a comparative study of therapy for giardiasis in children, *Am J Dis Child* 135:164, 1981.
6. DeVizia B et al: Iron malabsorption in giardiasis, *J Pediatr* 107:75, 1985.
7. Dobell C: The discovery of the intestinal protozoa of man, *Proc R Soc Med Section Hist Med* 13:1, 1920.
8. Drugs for parasitic infections, *Med Lett Drugs Ther* 35:111, 1993.
9. Dykes AC et al: Municipal waterborne giardiasis: an epidemiologic investigation: beavers implicated as a possible reservoir, *Ann Intern Med* 87:426, 1980.
10. Erlandsen SL, Meyer EA, editors: *Giardia and giardiasis: biology, pathogenesis, and epidemiology,* New York, 1984, Plenum.
11. Gillon J, Thamery AL, Ferguson A: Features of small intestine pathology (epithelial cell kinetics, intraepithelial lymphocytes, disaccharidases) in primary *Giardia muris* infection, *Gut* 23:498, 1982.
12. Hall A, Nahar Q: Albendazole as a treatment for infections with *Giardia duodenalis* in children in Bangladesh, *Trans R Soc Trop Med Hyg* 87:84, 1993.
13. Hartong WA, Gourley WK, Arvanitakas C: Giardiasis: clinical spectrum and functional structural abnormalities of the small intestinal mucosa, *Gastroenterology* 77:61, 1979.
14. Isaac-Renton JL: Laboratory diagnosis of giardiasis, *Clin Lab Med* 11:811, 1991.
15. Jarrol EL, Bingham AK, Meyer EA: *Giardia* cyst destruction: effectiveness of six small-quantity water disinfection methods, *Am J Trop Med Hyg* 29:8, 1980.
16. Jarroll EL, Bingham AK, Meyer EA: Effect of chlorine on *Giardia lamblia* cyst viability, *Appl Environ Microbiol* 41:483, 1981.
17. Nash TE et al: Experimental infections with *Giardia lamblia, J Infect Dis* 156:974, 1987.
18. Nelson JD: Etiology and epidemiology of diarrheal disease in the United States, *Am J Med* 78:76, 1985.
19. Pickering LK, Engelkirk PG: *Giardia lamblia, Pediatr Clin North Am* 35:565, 1988.
20. Rendtorff RC: The experimental transmission of human intestinal protozoan parasites. II. *Giardia lamblia* cysts given in capsules, *Am J Trop Med Hyg* 59:209, 1954.
21. Rosenthal P, Liebman WM: Comparative study of stool examinations,

duodenal aspiration, and pediatric Entero-Test for giardiasis in children, *J Pediatr* 96:278, 1980.
22. Sealy DP, Schuman SH: Endemic giardiasis and day care, *Pediatrics* 72:154, 1983.
23. Shaw PK et al: A community outbreak of giardiasis with evidence of transmission by a municipal water supply, *Ann Intern Med* 87:426, 1977.
24. Smith PD: *Giardia lamblia.* In Walzer PD, Genta RM, editors: *Parasitic infections in the compromised host,* New York, 1989, Marcel Dekker.
25. Smith PD: Pathophysiology and immunology of giardiasis, *Annu Rev Med* 36:295, 1985.
26. Sogin ML et al: Phylogenetic meaning of the kingdom concept: an unusual ribosomal RNA from *G. lamblia, Science* 243:75, 1989.
27. Thompson RCA, Reynoldson JA: *Giardia* and giardiasis, *Adv Parasitol* 32:71, 1993.
28. Wright SG, Tomkins AM: Quantitative histology in giardiasis, *J Clin Pathol* 31:712, 1978.

209 Gluten-Sensitive Enteropathy (Celiac Sprue)

Aubrey J. Katz

Gluten-sensitive enteropathy (GSE), also called celiac sprue, is a condition characterized by clinical features of malabsorption and pathological changes in the jejunal mucosa, both of which improve when gluten is removed from the diet and recur when it is reintroduced. After cystic fibrosis, celiac sprue is the second most common cause of malabsorption in childhood.

HISTORY

The classic clinical description of celiac disease was given by Samuel Gee in 1888. In 1950 Dicke noted the association between the ingestion of gluten and celiac disease. During World War II, when grain products in Holland were in short supply, the incidence of gluten-sensitive enteropathy was reduced markedly, and children who had the disease improved. After the war, when cereal grain became plentiful, the incidence of GSE rapidly returned to the prewar level. In 1954 Paulley, studying surgical biopsy material, provided the first accurate description of the intestinal lesion in patients who have gluten-sensitive enteropathy. It was not until 1968 that Rubin and coworkers discovered that adult nontropical sprue and celiac disease in childhood were the same disease.

PATHOLOGY

Gluten-sensitive enteropathy primarily affects the mucosa of the small intestine.[5] The submucosa, muscularis, and serosa are not involved. The mucosal lesion of the small intestine in GSE varies in both severity and extent, the lesion in the jejunum being generally more severe than that in the ileum. This variability may explain the differences in the degree of malabsorption seen in some patients. Those in whom more intestinal area is involved presumably have a greater degree of malabsorption. This difference in the distribution of the lesion suggests that the proximal intestine has greater exposure to undigested gluten than the distal intestine because there is no greater sensitivity to gluten in the proximal than in the distal mucosa. Among patients who have active GSE, surface epithelial cell damage occurs, and the migration of cells from crypt to villus region is increased. Compensatory crypt hypertrophy occurs, with a marked increase in mitotic activity, and gradual villus flattening develops (Figs. 209-1 and 209-2). The surface epithelial cells demonstrate a loss of the basal nuclei polarity and become more cuboidal. Numerous intraepithelial lymphocytes are noted, and the lamina propria shows a marked increase in plasma cells (T cells) and lymphocytes. It should be emphasized at this stage that this flat villus lesion is not pathognomonic of GSE because it may be seen in many other diseases. With the introduction of the flexible endoscope rather than blind suction biopsy, investigators have found nonspecific gastritis in some patients who have celiac disease, suggesting that perhaps there may be some gastric sensitivity.

PATHOGENESIS

GSE is a genetic disease; the exact mode of inheritance, however, remains unknown. In 1972 Falchuk and coworkers observed the association between histocompatibility antigen HLA-B8 and GSE: 80% of patients had HLA-B8, whereas only 22% of the normal population carried this antigen. A similar incidence of HLA-B8 is observed in patients with dermatitis herpetiformis, a skin disorder characterized by vesicular eruptions and a gluten-sensitive intestinal lesion.[2]

The exact mechanism by which gluten damages the mucosa of the small intestine remains unknown. Two contrasting mechanisms have been proposed: (1) GSE results from the lack of a specific enzyme, perhaps a dipeptidase, which results in accumulation of toxic gluten peptides (evidence for this hypothesis is lacking); and (2) gluten toxicity is mediated through immunology aberrations associated with the generically determined cell-surface markers discussed above.[7] Various immunological abnormalities have been described in GSE: (1) elevated levels of serum IgA and diminished levels of serum IgM are abnormalities that are reversed by a gluten-free diet; (2) intestinal mucosal immunoglobin synthesis, notably IgA and IgM, is increased markedly in patients who have active GSE and returns to normal when remission occurs, and 50% of the elevated IgA is associated with specific antigluten antibody; (3) patients who have active GSE respond to treatment with corticosteroids; and (4) in vitro peripheral lymphocyte transformation in response to gluten has been described in GSE patients.

INCIDENCE AND AGE OF ONSET

The precise incidence of gluten-sensitive enteropathy is unknown because a large number of patients have asymptomatic disease. The disorder is more common in certain European countries than in the United States. This may relate to a larger intake of gluten by people in Europe or to the way in which wheat is refined in the United States. The incidence of GSE in the United States is estimated to be 1 case per 3000 people. In certain parts of Ireland, it is as high as 1 in 300. In pediatric patients the average age at the time of diagnosis appears to be between 9 and 18 months, occurring earlier in infants who are fed cereal at an earlier age. The incidence declines markedly after age 2, and it is uncommon to have a newly diagnosed case of GSE in a teenager. For unknown reasons, clinical but not histological remission seems to occur during the teenage years. There is a resurgence of clinically manifest disease in adult life, when GSE may be precipitated by infectious diarrhea, other illnesses, or surgical procedures such as gastrectomy. These patients pre-

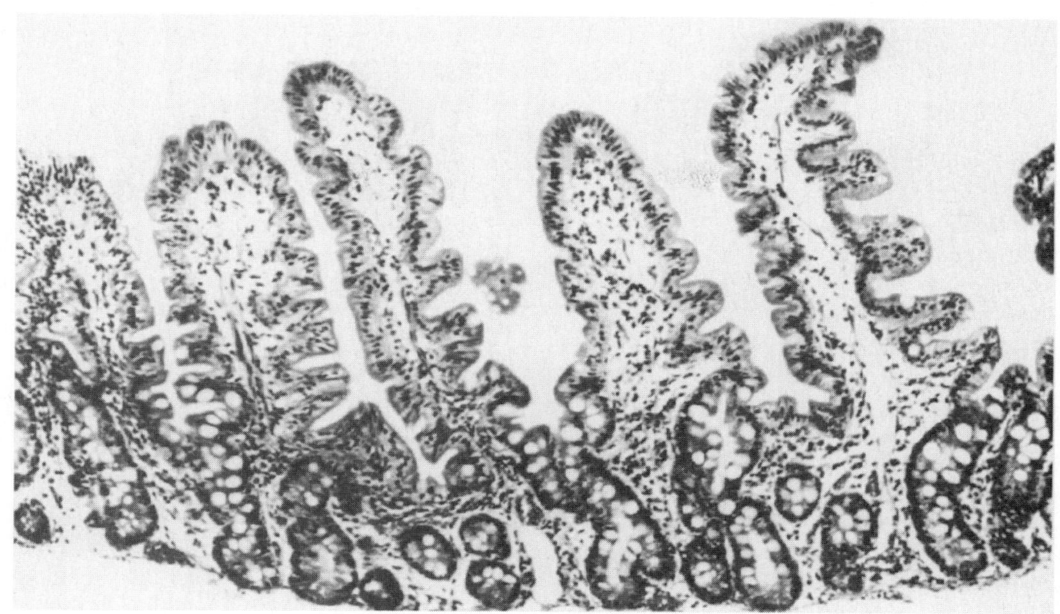

FIG. 209-1 Normal jejunal mucosa. Villi are tall, crypts are relatively short, and the crypt:villus ratio is approximately 1:4. Epithelial cells are columnar, and their nuclei are basally oriented. Some lymphocytes and plasma cells are found in the lamina propria. (×160).

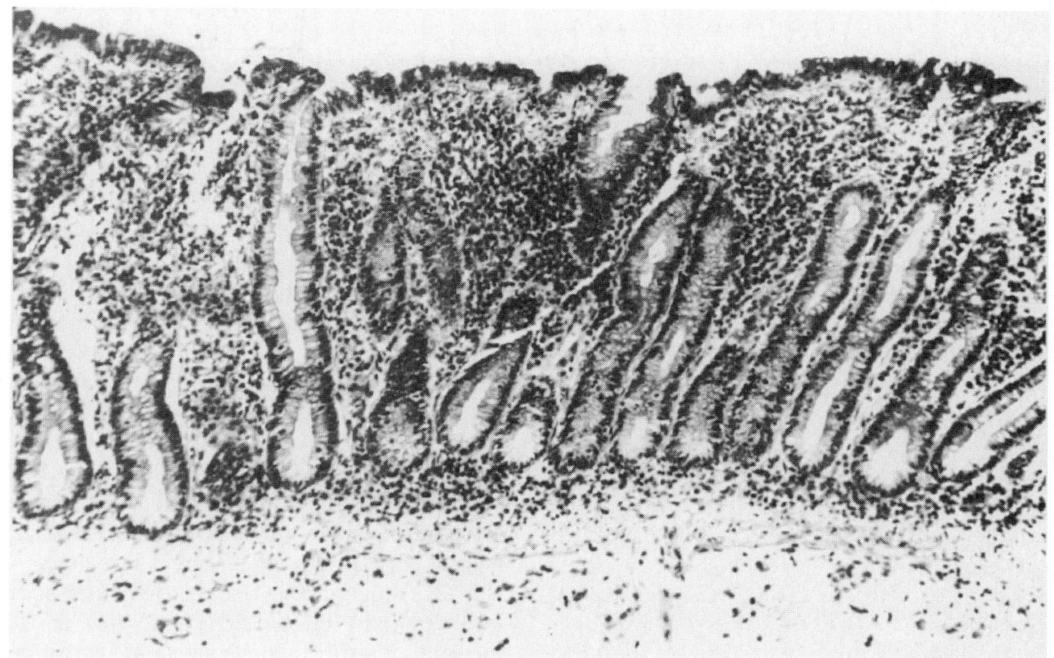

FIG. 209-2 Jejunal mucosa in gluten-sensitive enteropathy (celiac sprue). The mucosa is flat, villi are absent, and crypts are deep. Epithelial cells are cuboidal, and nuclei are not basally oriented. There are increased numbers of mitoses in the crypts. Inflammatory cells, especially plasma cells and lymphocytes, are markedly increased. (×160).

sumably have had the abnormal histological condition since infancy.

CLINICAL FEATURES

A patient who has an advanced case of GSE typically is an irritable, anorectic child who has chronic diarrhea, failure to thrive, a potbelly, and muscle wasting, especially of the buttocks and proximal limbs.[4] These children usually are easy to diagnose (Fig. 209-3). It is extremely important to realize that many patients manifest the disorder atypically (e.g., steatorrhea may be absent). Atypical features of patients who have GSE are listed in the box on p. 1326. These presentations usually are related to selective malabsorption of vari-

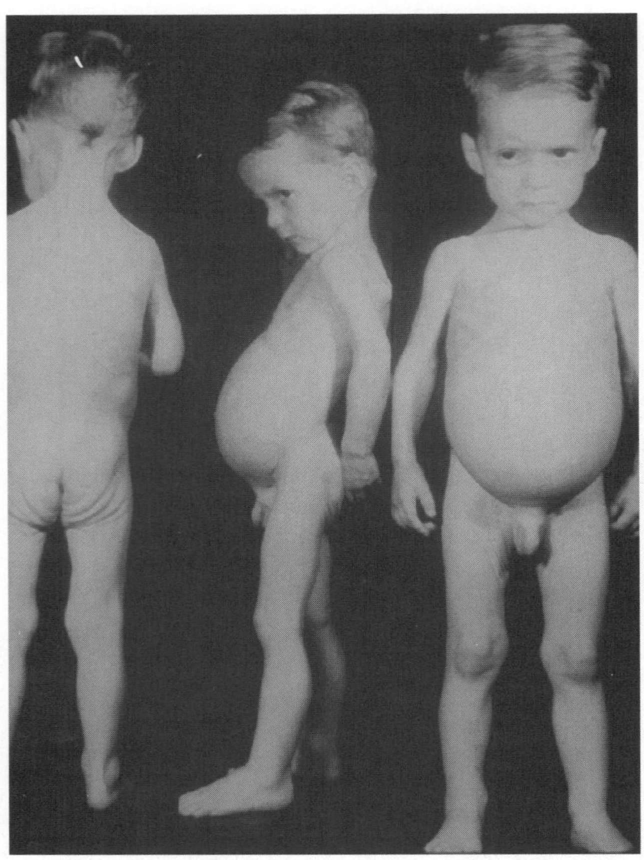

FIG. 209-3 Classic "celiac" profile. Note potbelly, thin buttocks, and proximal muscle wasting.

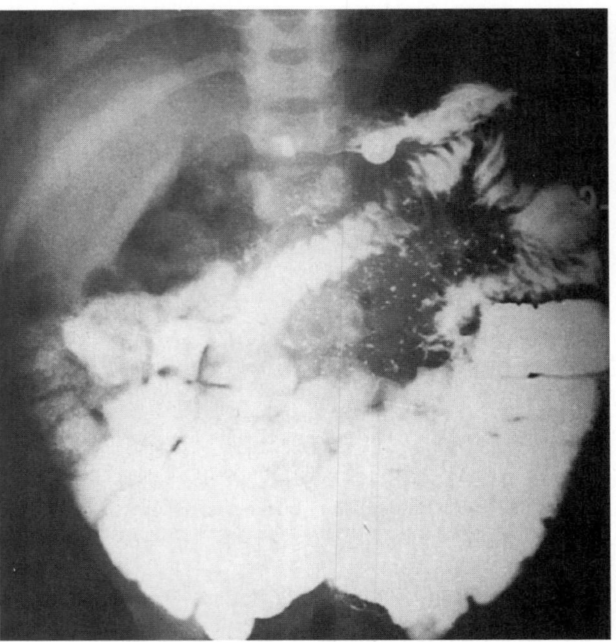

FIG. 209-4 The small bowel follow-through of this child with growth failure shows mild dilation of loops of small bowel, some dilution of barium distally, and mild flocculation. His duodenal biopsy revealed typical celiac sprue, and he responded to a gluten-free diet.

ATYPICAL PRESENTATIONS OF GLUTEN-SENSITIVE ENTEROPATHY

- Growth failure (without GI symptoms)
- Anemia
  - Iron deficiency
  - Folate deficiency
  - Vitamin B_{12} deficiency (rare)
- Rickets, osteoporosis, pathological features
- Bleeding disorders
- Edema
- Constipation
- Vomiting
- Recurrent abdominal pain

ous nutrients. Thus it is not unusual for some patients to have rickets, osteoporosis with bone pain, or pathological fractures. Also seen are bleeding disorders secondary to vitamin K deficiency, iron deficiency anemia, and megaloblastic anemia usually secondary to folate deficiency; deficiency of vitamin B_{12} is rare and usually indicates severe disease that extends to the terminal ileum. Constipation, rectal prolapse, clubbing of the fingernails, edema, and vomiting also have been described as presenting features. Gluten-sensitive enteropathy should always be considered in patients with specific nutritional defects who fail to respond to appropriate replacement therapy.

DIAGNOSIS

Laboratory Findings

Before GSE is diagnosed in childhood, a sweat test should be performed to exclude cystic fibrosis, the most common cause of malabsorption in childhood. A number of reports have described the coexistence of these two disorders. Tests are discussed in detail in Chapter 120, Diarrhea and Steatorrhea.

Anemia is very common in gluten-sensitive enteropathy and usually occurs secondary to iron, folate, or vitamin B_{12} malabsorption. Hypoprothrombinemia may occur secondary to vitamin K malabsorption. Because protein-losing enteropathy may occur in GSE, serum albumin and globulins should be measured. Electrolyte disturbances, especially hypokalemia, are common; calcium, phosphorus, and alkaline phosphatase levels may be abnormal in patients who have rickets. The radiographic findings in gluten-sensitive enteropathy, which are nonspecific (Fig. 209-4), include distention of the small intestine and segmentation of barium as a result of hypersecretion of intestinal fluid.

Intestinal Biopsy

Biopsy of the small intestine is the definitive method of establishing the diagnosis of GSE. Previously, blind biopsies were performed with either the Crosby capsule or the Quinton-Rubin pediatric suction tube; currently, fiberoptic endoscopy routinely is used to obtain biopsy specimens to establish this diagnosis. Various studies have indicated that adequate tissue can be obtained with this technique. In addition, endoscopy allows endoscopic visualization of the duodenum. Scalloping of the small intestinal valvulae of Kerckring[1] has been described as pathognomonic for GSE on endoscopy (Fig. 209-5). In young infants this appearance may

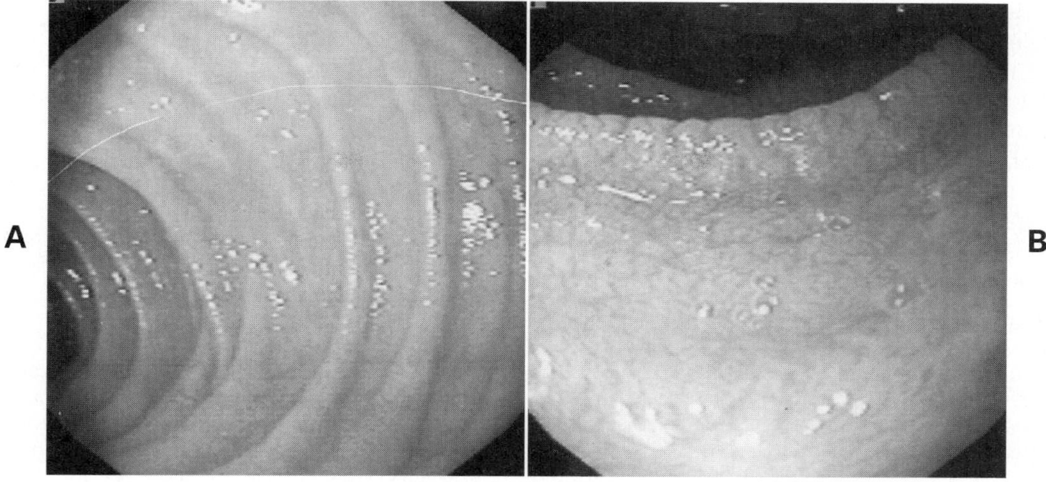

FIG. 209-5 Endoscopic study shows scalloping of the small intestinal valvulae of Kerckring, a pathognomonic finding for GSE.

not be visualized as easily, but edema of the duodenal mucosa appears to be more common.

Differential Diagnosis of Flat Villus Lesion

In children under 18 months of age flat villus lesion can have many causes besides GSE. Many GI insults can damage surface epithelial cells, resulting in increased epithelial cell turnover, crypt hypertrophy, abnormal surface epithelial cells, and eventual villus flattening. Other causes of the flat villus lesion are listed in the box to the right. Thus, for a definitive diagnosis of gluten-sensitive enteropathy, the following criteria must be met: (1) demonstration of clinical malabsorption and abnormal intestinal lesion, (2) clinical and histological response to gluten withdrawal, and (3) subsequent gluten challenge that may exacerbate clinical symptoms but always produces abnormal intestinal histology. Because the diagnosis of gluten-sensitive enteropathy means lifelong gluten restriction and, in an untreated patient, perhaps an increased risk for development of GI cancer in late adulthood, it is essential that this diagnosis be made with assurance.

COMMON CAUSES OF THE FLAT VILLUS LESION

- Food sensitivity
  - GSE
  - Cow milk protein allergy
  - Soy protein allergy
  - Eosinophilic gastroenteritis
- Infections
  - Viral (rotavirus)
  - Bacterial *(Escherichia coli)*
  - Parasitic *(Giardia lamblia)*
  - Fungal *(Candida albicans)*
- Malnutrition (kwashiorkor, not marasmus)
- Tropical sprue
- Immunodeficiency disorders (most notably AIDS)
- Familial enteropathy
- Rarer causes
  - Lymphoma
  - Crohn disease
  - Whipple disease

Serological Markers in Celiac Sprue

Serological markers have emerged as a diagnostic tool and screening test for GSE.[3] These markers include antiendomysial, antigliadin, and antireticulin antibodies. Antiendomysial antibodies (IgA) have demonstrated the most sensitivity and specificity for the diagnosis of GSE compared with other antibodies at this time. Antigliadin IgA antibodies appear to be specific and sensitive as well; however, antigliadin IgG antibodies are not very sensitive and have a high false positive rate. If the diagnosis of GSE is suspected, antiendomysial and antigliadin (IgA) antibodies should be sought. If they are found, the patient needs a small bowel biopsy for definitive diagnosis; if they are not found but the patient still appears to have the classic features or features suggestive of GSE, a small bowel biopsy should be done. About 10% of patients who have GSE may *not* have markers.

Serological Markers in Family Screening

As has been mentioned, many patients who have celiac disease remain asymptomatic. The disease is genetic; about 20% of family members may well have it without being aware of it. Instead of performing biopsies on all these patients, serological markers can be sought, particularly antiendomysial and antigliadin (IgA) antibodies. Parents and siblings should have marker studies performed.[8] If these are positive, then small bowel biopsies should be performed.

TREATMENT

The treatment of gluten-sensitive enteropathy is complete withdrawal of gluten from the diet. Various gluten-free diets and recipes are available[6,9]; this information should be given to all patients and parents. It is important to realize that it may take a number of weeks for symptoms to disappear completely after the gluten is withdrawn. Subjective improvement, however, occurs within the first few days. In children, apathy usually is the first symptom to be alleviated, followed by progressive improvement in muscle tone, abdominal distention, and diarrhea. Disaccharidase activity is markedly depressed in untreated cases, and a lactose-free diet is advocated during the initial 4 to 6 weeks of therapy to alleviate the diarrhea. Lactose is gradually reintroduced, provided there is no concurrent infection, severe electrolyte imbalance, dehydration, or shock (so-called celiac crisis). Replacement iron, folic acid, vitamin K, vitamin D, and calcium should be given when appropriate.

REFERENCES

1. Brocci E et al: Endoscopic demonstration of duodenal folds in the diagnosis of celiac disease, *N Engl J Med* 319:741, 1988.
2. Caffrey C et al: HLA-DP and celiac disease: family and population studies, *Gut* 31:663, 1990.
3. Calabuig M et al: Serological markers and celiac disease: a new diagnostic approach? *J Pediatr Gastroenterol Nutr* 10:435, 1990.
4. Hamilton JR, Lynch JJ, Reilly BJ: Active celiac disease in childhood, *Q J Med* 38;135, 1969.
5. Katz AJ, Falchuk ZM: Current concepts in gluten-sensitive enteropathy, *Pediatr Clin North Am* 22:767, 1975.
6. Sheedy CB, Keifeiz N: *Cooking for your celiac child,* New York, 1969, Dial Press.
7. Strober W et al: The pathogenesis of gluten-sensitive enteropathy, *Ann Intern Med* 83:242, 1975.
8. Unsworth DJ, Brown DL: Serological screening suggests that adult coeliac disease is underdiagnosed in the UK and increases the incidence by up to 12%, *Gut* 35:61, 1994.
9. Wood MN: *Gourmet food on a wheat-free diet,* Springfield, Ill, 1967, Charles C Thomas.

SUGGESTED READINGS

Alper CA et al: Extended major histocompatibility complex haplotypes in patients with gluten-sensitive enteropathy, *J Clin Invest* 79:251, 1987.

Misra S, Ament ME: Diagnosis of coeliac sprue in 1994, *Gastroenterol Clin North Am* 24:133, 1995.

Visakorpi JK, Maki M: Changing clinical features of coeliac disease, *Acta Paediatr Suppl* 83:10, 1994.

210 Hemolytic-Uremic Syndrome

Glenn H. Bock

Hemolytic-uremic syndrome (HUS) is defined as the triad of acute microangiopathic hemolytic anemia, thrombocytopenia, and acute renal insufficiency or failure. The syndromic nature of HUS must be emphasized. The disease manifestations undoubtedly occur as a common pathway resulting from a variety of initiating causes (see the box on p. 1330). In North America and western Europe, epidemic, diarrhea-associated HUS is the most common form. Atypical HUS (also known as sporadic or nondiarrhea-associated HUS) occurs less frequently in children and is classified according to the suspected underlying primary cause.

The clinical manifestations of HUS may be difficult to distinguish from those of thrombotic thrombocytopenic purpura (TTP), particularly at the time of a first episode. Classically, the kidney has been considered the primary target organ in HUS, whereas the presence of more generalized disease, particularly inclusive of the central nervous system, has been considered more characteristic of TTP. However, clinical manifestations overlap broadly.

FREQUENCY

Childhood HUS occurs worldwide, although its incidence varies among countries. Sites of epidemic outbreaks include Argentina, the United States, western Europe, South Africa, and the Indian subcontinent. Typically the illness affects infants and young children of all races and both genders, with the majority of diarrhea-associated cases occurring in the summer months. Even in nonepidemic areas, cases commonly cluster. Although the frequency varies, typical childhood HUS is one of the most common causes of acute renal failure among pediatric patients. Atypical HUS is more common in older children and adults, although diarrhea-associated HUS is being recognized increasingly frequently in this population. The occurrence of atypical HUS tends to be sporadic without geographical or seasonal characteristics.

ETIOLOGY

The initiating events in HUS leading to the clinical manifestations of the syndrome are incompletely established. Nonetheless, most forms of the disease appear to require endothelial cell injury with consequent platelet adhesion and aggregation, resulting in potentially reversible microvascular thrombosis. The diarrheal form of HUS in children is associated most commonly with colonic infection by an *Escherichia coli* (most commonly *E. coli* subtype 0157:H7) capable of producing a Shiga-like verocytotoxin. Currently verocytotoxin is suspected to be the provocative agent for more than 75% of the postdiarrheal cases of HUS. This toxin has many characteristics in common with Shiga toxin produced by *Shigella dysenteriae,* an infectious agent known to cause HUS in underdeveloped countries. Other infectious organisms that do not produce verocytotoxin (e.g., pneumococci, clostridia, and some viruses) also have been associated with HUS. These organisms have in common the production of neuraminidase, an enzyme that can damage platelet, erythrocyte, and endothelial cell membranes. Other atypical forms of HUS may be caused by disturbances of prostacyclin regulation of platelet aggregation, by differences of host resistance to the binding of aggregate materials to endothelial cell surfaces, or from the use of certain medications (e.g., mitomycin and cyclosporine). Those patients who have inherent biochemical or endocrinological disturbances may have recurrent episodes of HUS or demonstrate familial occurrences.

HISTORY

The child who has typical HUS usually experiences a 3- to 10-day prodrome of bloody or watery diarrhea often associated with cramping abdominal pain. Nausea, vomiting, and fever variably are present but not usually prominent features. Extreme pallor and malaise, when reported, usually occur suddenly at a time when the gastrointestinal illness has appeared to have stabilized or improved. Although the renal injury begins with the onset of the hemolytic microangiopathy, signs or symptoms attributable to acute renal failure may take several days to develop.

Extrarenal involvement in HUS often is seen (see the box on p. 1330). In fact, with the general availability of dialysis, extrarenal disease in HUS is the major determinant of early mortality and a significant factor in long-term sequelae. Gastrointestinal manifestations may include bleeding, intussusception, abdominal distention, or rectal prolapse. Gangrene of the colon and intestinal perforation have occurred. Central nervous system abnormalities such as somnolence, irritability, seizures, stroke, or chronic sequelae may occur; such symptoms now are recognized to be much more common than was appreciated when the syndrome was first described. In atypical HUS a prodrome usually is absent or consists of an upper respiratory tract infection. The manifestations at the onset of HUS are similar, except that gastrointestinal complaints are less common.

PHYSICAL FINDINGS

Children who have HUS usually appear acutely ill with pallor, petechiae, and/or purpura. They often are irritable or drowsy and may have any degree of hypertension. Those who have the typical childhood variety may have a distended, tympanitic abdomen with diffuse tenderness. Hepatomegaly frequently is present. The presence of congestive heart failure and pulmonary or peripheral edema results from the oliguria and the consequent intravascular volume overload complicated by the rapidly developing anemia.

LABORATORY FINDINGS

The most striking laboratory findings are the often-profound Coombs-negative anemia, the presence of fragmented erythrocytes on the blood smear, and the thrombocytopenia. Leukocytosis often is present, and more severe degrees have been purported to be a negative prognostic finding. The urinalysis usually demonstrates proteinuria, microscopic or macroscopic hematuria, cylindruria, and pyuria. Laboratory abnormalities resulting from renal dysfunction, including azotemia, hyperkalemia, hyperphosphatemia, and metabolic acidosis, are variable in their degree depending on the magnitude and duration of the renal disease and the degree of red cell hemolysis. The biochemical derangements, especially of potassium, may be life threatening and require emergent treatment to prevent potentially fatal cardiac arrhythmias. Furthermore, the child who has suspected HUS should have some form of electrocardiac monitoring until the initial laboratory data are obtained.

DIFFERENTIAL DIAGNOSIS

The features of HUS are not specific and also may occur in disseminated intravascular coagulation (DIC), overwhelming sepsis, malignant hypertension, and some instances of vasculitis. Although the microangiopathic features of DIC and HUS are similar, coagulation pathway studies most often are normal in HUS. As mentioned, TTP, which occurs more commonly in adults, may share many of the pathophysiological features of HUS. The diagnosis of atypical (sporadic) HUS mandates an evaluation for a noninfectious underlying cause.

CAUSES OF HEMOLYTIC-UREMIC SYNDROME

Infection-related

E. Coli
Shigella
Neuraminidase-producing organisms
Human immunodeficiency virus

Sporadic

Familial
Pregnancy
Transplantation
Malignant hypertension
Drugs
Tumors
Collagen vascular disease

TREATMENT

Management of the oliguric acute renal failure, hypertension, anemia, and central nervous system disturbances are the most common initial therapeutic considerations in patients who have HUS. Prevention of fluid overload (which often provokes significant worsening of hypertension), correction of electrolyte imbalances, and control of uremia is achieved by careful medical management and, if necessary, dialysis. Details of the medical approach to acute renal failure are given in Chapter 291, Acute Renal Failure. Prompt implementation of dialysis is considered an important aspect of care in these patients because a great deal of the morbidity of HUS in earlier reports resulted from complications of fluid overload, hypertension, and electrolyte imbalance. In addition, dialysis permits the modulation of fluid balance in order to allow for infusions of hyperalimentation solutions, erythrocytes, or other necessary preparations. To avoid rapid changes of intravascular volume, where possible, blood cells should be transfused in small quantities as needed to keep the hematocrit around 25%. Platelet transfusions seldom are required in patients who have HUS and should be restricted to children who have active bleeding or those whose platelet counts are below 50,000/mm^3 and who require invasive procedures. Seizures should be treated aggressively and conventionally (allowing for medication dosage adjustments for dialysis and the degree of renal failure); comatose children may require elective ventilation to protect the airway. The common symptom of irritability cannot be treated but resolves gradually.

Attempts to modify the course of HUS by treatment with corticosteroids or anticoagulants have not proved effective. Some success has been reported using several modalities, including drugs that impair platelet aggregation (aspirin, dipyridamole), plasma infusion, plasma exchange, and prostacyclin infusion. The potential benefits of these treatments seem to occur primarily in the atypical forms of HUS. However, few controlled studies assess the actual benefit of these interventions adequately. In contrast, plasma infusion has been suggested to be contraindicated in patients who have neuraminidase-associated HUS, because it may worsen the hemolysis. The complexities of acute renal failure manage-

EXTRARENAL MANIFESTATIONS OF TYPICAL DIARRHEA-ASSOCIATED HUS

Common	Uncommon
Gastrointestinal	Pulmonary hemorrhage
Central nervous system	Myocardial ischemia/infarction
Hepatitis	Retinal hemorrhage
Pancreatitis	Skin necrosis
	Rhabdomyolysis
	Parotitis

ment and the rapidly changing concepts in dialysis and treatment for HUS make early consultation with a pediatric nephrologist an important aspect to individualizing patient management.

PROGNOSIS

Over 80% of children who have typical childhood HUS recover without renal or CNS sequelae. More than 10% may have some degree of persistent renal insufficiency or hypertension. Aggressive management of the renal failure and hypertension has a positive effect on survival during the acute phase of the disease. Severe CNS involvement during the early phase of the disease should raise concerns about possible long-term CNS sequelae. Children who have atypical HUS are at increased risk for permanently impaired renal function. Patients who have recurrent or familial forms of HUS also are at increased risk for progressive deterioration of renal function and often ultimately require dialysis or renal transplantation.

SUGGESTED READINGS

Loirat C et al: Hemolytic-uremic syndrome: an analysis of the natural history and prognostic features, *Acta Paediatr Scand* 73:505, 1984.

Moake JL: Haemolytic-uraemic syndrome: basic science, *Lancet* 343:393, 1994.

Neild GH: Haemolytic-uraemic syndrome in practice, *Lancet* 343:398, 1994.

Remuzzi G: HUS and TTP: variable expression of a single entity, *Kidney Int* 32:292, 1987.

Siegler RL: Spectrum of extrarenal involvement in postdiarrheal hemolytic-uremic syndrome, *J Pediatr* 125:511, 1994.

211 Hemophilia and Other Hereditary Bleeding Disorders

Eva G. Radel

Hemostasis requires adhesion of platelets to an injured vascular endothelium, aggregation of additional platelets with formation of a platelet plug, activation of coagulation factors resulting in the coagulation "cascade," and finally, formation of a fibrin clot that interacts with the platelet aggregate to form a stable hemostatic seal. The coagulation factors exist in the blood mostly as precursors that become activated to become enzymes or cofactors and, in turn, activate other factors. Also involved are anticoagulants, fibrinolysins, and inhibitors, and all form a very complex, delicate, autoregulated system. Abnormalities of platelet function also may exist congenitally but will not be discussed herein.

EVALUATION TO DETECT ABNORMALITIES OF HEMOSTASIS

The most useful screening tests to study the hemostatic and coagulation mechanisms are the activated partial thromboplastin time (APTT), the prothrombin time (PT), and the bleeding time. The PT alone is not adequate for screening children for coagulation disorders because it misses the most common congenital deficiencies. Falsely prolonged clotting tests may result from an insufficient amount of blood in the test tube or difficulty accessing the vein. The tests are sensitive to clotting factor levels <30% to 40% of normal. A prolonged APTT or PT must be followed up by the performance of individual clotting factor assays. The "normal" activity (100%) of a clotting factor is defined arbitrarily as 1 unit/ml of plasma, and the normal range of activity for different factors is from about 50% to 200%. The bleeding time can be measured with one of several commercially available disposable templates.

HEMOPHILIA A AND B

Although factors VIII and IX act in different ways in the coagulation cascade, their sex-linked inheritance and the clinical manifestations of their deficiencies are identical. The incidence of hemophilia is about 1 in 5000 males, 85% being hemophilia A (classical hemophilia, congenital factor VIII deficiency) and 15% hemophilia B (Christmas disease, congenital factor IX deficiency). A positive family history is present in about two thirds of cases.

Diagnosis

The diagnosis can be suspected on the basis of the family and personal history, and laboratory tests will identify the deficiency. Severe hemophilia accounts for 80% of cases of classical hemophilia and is defined by a factor VIII or IX level of <1% to 2%. Levels above 5% to 10% are associated with mild disease and intermediate levels with moderate disease. Severe disease is manifested by hemarthroses and hematoma formation with minimal or no trauma. Mild disease results in bleeding only with trauma. Many different DNA abnormalities have been found in patients who have hemophilia. If the genetic defect in a family has been identified, prenatal diagnosis can be done, but if it has not, only the sex of the fetus can be determined.

Bleeding Manifestations

Hemarthrosis. Recurrent bleeding into joints is the major clinical problem for patients who have severe hemophilia. The knees, ankles, and elbows are involved most frequently. Many patients have one particular "target" joint where recurrent episodes occur and where chronic changes are most likely to occur. Synovial thickening and vascular friability may develop, resulting in increased susceptibility to bleeding and a vicious cycle. Synovitis accompanied by chronic effusion often occurs and may progress to joint destruction. With prompt adequate treatment of bleeding episodes, the incidence of these complications is much less.

Hemarthrosis must be treated as soon as pain or limping *begins*. Watchful waiting is not appropriate for the child who has hemophilia. Synovitis may be managed via administration of short courses of steroids and factor VIII or IX prophylactically. Synovectomy (open or arthroscopic) may be effective if medical management fails.

Soft Tissue Bleeding. Superficial hematomas, unless very large, often do not require treatment. However, bleeding into muscles may result in nerve damage or muscle fibrosis and contractures; such bleeding may be difficult to diagnose because swelling often is minimal. Bleeding into the iliopsoas may cause femoral nerve damage, and it must be considered whenever pain occurs in the hip or groin; limping and flexion of the hip often are the only positive findings. Sonography or a CT scan may help in the diagnosis. Bleeding into the thigh may cause accumulation of a large amount of blood without much external change and may result in significant anemia.

Life-Threatening Bleeding. *Intracranial bleeding* can occur after trauma but also appears to occur spontaneously. All but the most minor head injury must be considered to be significant and treated promptly. *Airway compromise* must be considered a potential threat with any hematoma of the neck or the submental or sublingual areas, as well as the retropharyngeal or parapharyngeal regions; a severe sore throat or dysphagia also suggests bleeding. *Retroperitoneal bleeding* may be quite massive before it can be detected and must be considered when abdominal or groin pain is present. In all of these situations, a CT scan or MRI may be helpful in evaluating the patient.

Mouth Bleeding. The lip, tongue, and frenulum are areas of frequent trauma in young children. Factor replacement should be accompanied by the use of epsilon amino caproic acid (EACA, Amicar) to prevent fibrinolysis of the clot.

Hematuria. Hematuria must be evaluated with noninvasive procedures as in the normal individual. It usually resolves spontaneously with or without factor replacement. Steroid therapy is controversial. EACA should be avoided because it can result in obstruction of the renal pelvis by clot.

Acquired Immunodeficiency Syndrome (AIDS) and Other Viral Infections

Up to 90% of the cases of severe hemophilia in the United States contracted HIV infection in the late 1970s and early 1980s. The production of clotting factor concentrates from large donor pools in the era before the virus was identified and the need for frequent treatment of hemophilia with these concentrates resulted in massive exposure. Chronic liver disease also has been a major problem, presumably most often caused by hepatitis C and sometimes by hepatitis B virus infection. Currently, both donor testing and several methods to inactivate viruses in the production process make the concentrates safe with regard to HIV. Hepatitis B and C also appear to have been largely eliminated.

General Principles of Treatment

Ideal management of the patient who has hemophilia is in a comprehensive center where all the needs of the patient can be met, including medical, orthopedic, physical rehabilitation, dental, and psychosocial help. All elective surgical procedures *must* be done in a center that has experienced personnel, immediate availability of factor assays, and a ready supply of clotting concentrates and should be preceded by factor inhibitor testing. Nerve blocks must be avoided. A patient who has a severe injury or life-threatening bleeding should be given an immediate dose of the appropriate factor to raise its level to 100% and then should be transferred to an appropriate center.

Any significant injury must be treated promptly, even without apparent evidence of active bleeding, because bleeding often is delayed. A small superficial laceration, if not bleeding or in need of cleaning, may be managed with a simple pressure dressing, but if soaking of the wound or suturing is necessary, factor *must* be administered *before* such management. Casts never should be applied unless factor has been administered and is continued for several days, and the involved area watched closely for evidence of pain or nerve compression. Treatment must be given before *all* surgical procedures, arterial punctures, and spinal taps.

Pain management should use acetaminophen whenever possible. Codeine and other oral narcotics can be given if necessary. Aspirin must be avoided, but nonacetylated salicylates (choline magnesium trisalicylate) can be used, and nonsteroidal antiinflammatory agents such as ibuprofen can be given cautiously.

Factor Replacement

Products available for the treatment of coagulation disorders are described in Chapter 29, Blood Products and Their Uses. Whole plasma can raise factor VIII levels to only 40% and factor IX to 20% because of the large volume and protein load required. Early in the AIDS epidemic it was recommended that plasma or cryoprecipitate be given when possible, rather than concentrates made from large donor pools. The safety of current concentrates makes them the preferred mode of treatment in most situations. Recombinant factor VIII has become available recently, appears to be safe and effective in early tests, and is expected to be entirely free of viral contamination.

Factor IX is available in the form of prothrombin complex, as well as in a purified form. Recombinant factor IX is not yet available. Mild bleeding requiring a single treatment can be managed with the complex, but if repeated doses are needed over several days, or for patients who have liver disease, the more purified factor should be used because of the danger of thrombosis or disseminated intravascular coagulation from activated factors in the complex. The cost of the products increases with the degree of purification. The advantages of the more purified preparations for HIV-negative patients are not yet clear, although their use has been shown to result in a slower decrease of CD4 cells in HIV-positive patients.

The desired levels of factor VIII or IX for managing different clinical problems and the expected dose responses are shown in Table 211-1. Preassayed concentrates are available in vials containing different doses. Whole vials to (or slightly above) the calculated desired dose should be given.

Health Care Maintenance

Routine immunizations, which must include hepatitis B, should be given subcutaneously with a 25-gauge needle, and pressure should be maintained for 5 to 10 minutes. Intramuscular injections should be avoided. Routine dental evaluation, prophylaxis, and hygiene should be begun by 3 years of age. The most difficult part of managing the child who has hemophilia is to find the proper blend of caution and allowing for independence. Family education about the disease is essential, and support groups are beneficial. Psychosocial problems must be a major concern in managing patients and families. Not only do they have to live with a very serious chronic illness, associated with frequent pain and limitation of normal activities, but the impact of AIDS on this population has been devastating and in many cases has eroded trust in medical caretakers.

Home Care

If a child has reasonably "good" venous access and the family dynamics allow for it, parents can be taught to administer treatment to children as young as 3 years, and 9- or 10-year-olds may be taught to self-administer factor. This allows for much earlier treatment of bleeding episodes, provides the satisfaction of self-sufficiency, and prevents some of the frustrations of having to get to a treatment center or emergency room. Venous access devices have been used.

Mild Hemophilia

The patient who has mild hemophilia is more likely than the severe hemophiliac to get inadequate treatment of bleeding episodes because neither the family nor the physicians may be aware of the need for treatment. Severe injuries require

Table 211-1 Treatment of Bleeding Episodes in Hemophilia

Type of bleeding	Desired level FVIII or FIX*	Duration of treatment	Ancillary treatment
Hematoma, simple	20%-40%	Usually X1	
Hemarthrosis Mild muscle hematoma	30%-40%	Administer as soon as symptoms begin; repeat daily, if severe, until better	Administer prednisone for severe or recurrent joint episodes (0.5-1 mg/kg/day for 3 days); aspirate joint after treatment if swelling is marked
Mouth bleeding Epistaxis Dental extractions	80%-100%	X1	Start EACA 75-100 mg/kg q6h for 3 to 7 days (until clot is gone)
Severe muscle hematoma	50%-100%	3-7 days	
GI bleeding	100%	3-7 days	
Hematuria	? (factor may not be needed)	3-7 days	Bed rest; hydration; prednisone 2 mg/kg/day; do *not* use EACA
Life-threatening CNS Airway obstruction Retroperitoneal Surgery	100%; do not allow to drop to <50%†	7-14 days	Monitor factor levels

**FVIII:* 1 U/kg increases plasma level by 2%; half-life 10 to 12 hours. *FIX:* 1 U/kg increases level by 1%; half-life 20 to 24 hours. Slightly lower levels of FIX than of FVIII are effective.

†Initial dose 50 U/kg FVIII, 80 to 100 U/kg FIX; repeat half the dose in 8 to 12 hours for FVIII, in 18 to 24 hours for FIX; or give continuous infusion of 3 to 4 U/kg/hour after the initial bolus.

EACA, Epsilon amino caproic acid (Amicar)

management like that of the severe hemophiliac, although smaller doses of factor may suffice to attain the desired factor levels. Desmopressin (DDAVP) is a vasopressin analog that results in release of factor VIII from the endothelial cells where it is produced. Administration of 0.3 μg/kg IV over 20 to 30 minutes usually results in a threefold increase of factor VIII in about 1 hour, which may be maintained for about 24 hours. It can be repeated in 24 hours, but tachyphylaxis may occur. Desmopressin is ineffective in factor IX deficiency. Overhydration must be avoided, since water retention and hyponatremia may occur with desmopressin therapy. A concentrated intranasal preparation is available and has been used in children 6 years and older. A stimulation test with response assessment should be performed in each patient with both the IV and the nasal preparations.

Inhibitors

About 10% to 15% of patients who have hemophilia develop antibodies to factor VIII, usually early in their treatment. Such patients should be managed only by experienced practitioners; this includes the use of very large doses of factor VIII, prothrombin complex, activated prothrombin complex, porcine factor VIII, recombinant factor VIIa (not yet available in the United States), and induction of immune tolerance.

Prophylaxis and Gene Therapy

Prophylactic treatment given three times weekly or every other day has been advocated to prevent hemarthrosis and joint damage and to normalize the life of the hemophiliac. It is hoped that gene therapy will allow these conditions to be cured in the not too distant future.

VON WILLEBRAND DISEASE

Von Willebrand disease (VWD) is the most common hereditary coagulation disorder, with estimates of an incidence as high as 1% of the population. Von Willebrand factor (VWF) is the carrying protein for factor VIII and exists in a series of different-sized multimers of smaller subunits. Decreased VWF is associated with a corresponding decrease of factor VIII activity. The inheritance usually is autosomal dominant with variable penetrance, but autosomal recessive variants occur. In addition to bleeding after surgery and trauma, the major manifestation of VWD is mucosal bleeding, most frequently manifesting as epistaxis. Menorrhagia and, less commonly, gastrointestinal bleeding also may occur. Hemarthrosis without trauma is not seen.

Several components of the VWF-factor VIII complex and function can be determined: factor VIII function, VWF function, VWF antigen, and the pattern of multimers. VWF antigen is normal in classical hemophilia. Many variants of VWD exist. The most common is type I, in which all components are similarly reduced and the multimer pattern is normal. Type II has a decrease or absence of the larger multimers; type IIB exhibits increased binding to platelets. Type III represents very severe deficiency with very low or absent levels of all components.

The bleeding time is the most useful screening test, being prolonged in most patients, and most cases are associated with decreased levels of factor VIII. However, all of the studies may be variable, both from patient to patient and also in the same patient from time to time; if results are normal, studies should be repeated if the index of suspicion is high. The differential diagnosis of a prolonged bleeding time includes thrombocytopenia and congenital or acquired disorders of platelet function.

Most patients who have type I VWD will respond to DDAVP as in mild hemophilia A, and this can be used for most bleeding episodes. Patients who have type IIA and type III VWD do not respond to DDAVP, and it is contraindicated in type IIB disease because it may cause platelet aggregation and DIC. Patients who have severe bleeding or those who do not respond to DDAVP must be treated with fresh frozen plasma (FFP), cryoprecipitate, or Humate P (see Chapter 29, Blood Products and Their Uses). Mild epistaxis often can be controlled with EACA.

OTHER COAGULATION DEFECTS

The other coagulant deficiencies are inherited as autosomal recessives, with the exception of factor XI, which can exist in both heterozygous and homozygous forms. Deficiencies of factors II, VII, and X can be treated with prothrombin complex, and factor XIII is concentrated in cryoprecipitate. Concentrates of factors VII and X are available for compassionate use. Other deficiencies require fresh frozen plasma. The latter also should be used for patients who are bleeding but whose deficiency has not yet been identified. Factor XIII deficiency cannot be detected with the usual screening tests; a normal screening workup in a patient who has a significant bleeding history should be followed with a clot solubility test. The contact factors prekallikrein, high molecular weight kininogen, and factor XII are necessary to initiate clotting in vitro, but their absence is not associated with clinical bleeding.

SUGGESTED READINGS

Aledort LM, editor: Factor VIII inhibitor treatment: strategies for the continuing challenge, *Semin Hematol* 31(suppl 4):1, 1994.

Bray GL et al: A multicenter study of recombinant factor VIII (recombinate): safety, efficacy, and inhibitor risk in previously untreated patients with hemophilia A, *Blood* 83:2428, 1994.

Gomperts ED, de Biasi R, De Vreker R: The impact of clotting factor concentrates on the immune system in individuals with hemophilia, *Transfus Med Rev* 6:44, 1992.

Logan LJ: Treatment of von Willebrand's disease, *Hematol Oncol Clin North Am* 6:1079, 1992.

Lusher JM, Warrier I: Hemophilia A, *Hematol Oncol Clin North Am* 6:1021, 1992.

Nilsson IM: Prophylactic treatment of severe hemophilia A and B can prevent joint disability, *Semin Hematol* 31(suppl 2):5, 1994.

Pfaff JA, Geninatti M: Hemophilia, *Emerg Med Clin North Am* 11:337, 1993.

Roberts HR, Eberts ME: Current management of hemophilia B, *Hematol Oncol Clin North Am* 7:1269, 1993.

Triantafyllou SJ et al: Open and arthroscopic synovectomy in hemophilic arthropathy of the knee, *Clin Orthop* 283:196, 1992.

212 Henoch-Schönlein Purpura

Glenn H. Bock

Henoch-Schönlein purpura (also called HSP, anaphylactoid purpura, or allergic purpura) is a diffuse necrotizing vasculitis, of which the main manifestations are rash, arthritis, gastrointestinal symptoms, and renal abnormalities.

FREQUENCY

A recent study from northern Europe estimated the incidence of HSP to be 13.5 cases per 100,000 child population per year.[4] This likely underestimates the actual incidence of HSP because this estimate was derived from hospital admission data, thereby likely omitting patients who had milder symptoms. Although HSP may occur at virtually any age and has been reported in infants as young as 6 months, its peak incidence occurs in the 4- to 7-year age range. A slight male to female predominance exists, and the disease most commonly is reported in Caucasian, Native American, and Japanese children. In the Northern Hemisphere most cases occur between November and January.

ETIOLOGY

The cause of HSP is unknown; although it is presumed to have an immune pathogenesis. Although the majority of patients have an upper respiratory tract infection preceding the onset of this syndrome, no consistent infectious agent has been identified. The incidence of streptococcal infections is no greater in children who have HSP than in those of the same age who do not have disease. Some cases of HSP have been associated with food allergies, certain medications, bee stings, or prior bacterial infections, but definitive proof of the relationship is lacking. Recent attempts to understand the pathogenesis have focused on abnormalities in IgA production and clearance. These studies are inconclusive and, at times, contradictory.

HISTORY

Approximately 65% to 75% of the patients have a history of an upper respiratory tract illness 1 to 3 weeks before the onset of the HSP symptoms.[1,4] A prodrome of malaise and low-grade fever may occur in half of these patients. The most common initial feature of HSP is a petechial rash that gradually becomes purpuric. Virtually all patients who have HSP contract a rash. Arthritis, the second most common clinical feature, occurs in 60% to 80% of patients and may be the initial symptom in as many as 25%. Nonmigratory pain and swelling of the knee and ankle joints occur most frequently, and involvement of upper extremity joints (elbows, wrists, fingers) also is seen commonly.

Approximately 50% of the patients have gastrointestinal complaints that may include colicky abdominal pain, melena, vomiting, or bloody diarrhea. These abdominal complaints may be severe enough to suggest an acute abdominal emergency. Although many of these complaints do not require surgical intervention, intussusception is a well-recognized complication of HSP that must be considered. Presumably this complication results from bowel wall edema forming a "lead point" that promotes the infolding of the bowel on itself. In about 20% of patients, the gastrointestinal symptoms may precede the rash and arthritis.

A broad spectrum of renal involvement is found in 20% to 70% of patients who have HSP.[2,4] This may range from microscopic hematuria with or without mild to moderate proteinuria to fully manifested glomerulonephritis or nephrotic syndrome. If urine sediments are examined repeatedly in all HSP patients, nearly 80% will demonstrate some evidence of renal involvement during the course of their illness. In the hospitalized population study mentioned above, 20% had renal abnormalities. Of these, 45% had coexisting hematuria and proteinuria, 2% had isolated microhematuria, 18% had coexisting nephritis and nephrotic syndrome, and the remaining 15% had nephritis only.[4] The renal manifestations usually coincide with or follow the rash; they rarely precede it. Renal involvement tends to be more severe in patients who have recurrent purpura or gastrointestinal complaints. Usually the renal abnormality manifests within 4 weeks of the onset of the joint or gastrointestinal symptoms, although nephritis has been reported to precede these manifestations in some patients and to occur as late as 2 years afterward in other patients.

The neurological and pulmonary involvement that may occur in patients who have HSP tends to be rather mild and of little clinical significance. Significant neurological complaints or respiratory compromise should suggest other forms of systemic vasculitis. Testicular and scrotal complaints also may be present in HSP. Pain, tenderness, and swelling of one or both testicles or the scrotum with scrotal bruising may occur. Because these findings may overshadow or precede other symptoms, careful assessment of the testicle is necessary to avoid unnecessary surgery for suspected testicular torsion.

PHYSICAL FINDINGS

The typical rash begins with symmetrical erythematous macules that usually start over the malleoli of the ankle but often spread to involve the dorsal aspect of the legs, the buttocks, and the ulnar aspect of the arm. The trunk, face, palms, and soles usually are spared. Characteristically the rash evolves rapidly to dusky red maculopapules that coalesce to form ecchymoses within 12 to 24 hours. By 2 weeks the rash becomes purple-brown and then gradually fades. Atypically the rash may not be present initially or may be more urticarial or erythematous in character, posing a diagnostic dilemma.

The arthritis as described above usually is characterized by painful and swollen joints; erythema, warmth, or palpable tenderness usually are absent. Abdominal findings may include distention, direct or rebound tenderness, and abnormal bowel sounds. Physical signs of renal involvement usually are absent early in the illness but may develop later.

LABORATORY FINDINGS

No specific diagnostic laboratory findings identify HSP. The platelet counts and bleeding and clotting times are normal. Neutrophilic leukocytosis may be present, and the sedimentation rate often is elevated. Approximately 50% of patients have a transient elevation in their serum IgA level. Urinalysis reveals that some combination of erythrocyturia, proteinuria, leukocyturia, and cylindruria accompanies renal involvement. Laboratory evidence often reveals renal insufficiency, and anemia may be prominent. Some individuals have the typical biochemical abnormalities of nephrotic syndrome, including hypoproteinemia, massive proteinuria, and hypercholesterolemia. Usually the serum complement levels are normal.

DIFFERENTIAL DIAGNOSIS

HSP is a clinical diagnosis based on the characteristic rash and the other typical clinical findings. Similar rashes associated with renal abnormalities may occur in association with poststreptococcal glomerulonephritis and systemic lupus erythematosus. The serum complement levels usually are decreased in these latter two conditions. Other forms of vasculitis such as polyarteritis nodosa and Wegener granulomatosis may be particularly difficult to distinguish from HSP. Although IgG-IgA nephritis (Berger disease) is thought to be the monosymptomatic variant of HSP, it is unlikely to be confused with HSP because of the absence of other organ involvement in the former. The biopsy appearances, however, are indistinguishable. Purpura also may be seen in HUS, thrombocytopenia, and sepsis, whereas the arthritis must be differentiated from juvenile rheumatoid arthritis and acute rheumatic fever. Other causes of an "acute abdomen" such as peptic ulcer, volvulus, and acute appendicitis must be differentiated from the gastrointestinal complaints of HSP.

TREATMENT

The general therapeutic measures for HSP mostly are supportive. Corticosteroids and immunosuppressive medications have been used by many in attempts to modify the clinical course of HSP. These studies usually were not well controlled; thus no consensus on treatment has been established.

Corticosteroids have been used most commonly in the setting of severe or prolonged gastrointestinal, renal, and at times, joint involvement. While a short course of oral steroid treatment is thought by many to ameliorate the gastrointestinal symptoms, assessing benefit in the treatment of the renal involvement is difficult because the majority of the patients have good long-term outcomes regardless of treatment. Nonetheless, the more severe, exudative forms of nephritis associated with HSP (proved by biopsy or clinicolaboratory evaluation) also often are treated empirically with steroids in an attempt to modulate the inflammatory component of the disease. Formulation of a diagnostic and therapeutic plan for the child in whom severe renal involvement is suspected is done best in consultation with a pediatric nephrologist, particularly when nephrotic or nephritic syndromes or azotemia are present.

PROGNOSIS

The rash of HSP resolves without scarring or pigmentary changes, and no permanent deformities result from even the most severe arthritis.

The most important determinant of long-term morbidity and mortality of HSP is the degree, type, and persistence of the renal involvement. Even so, the majority of patients recover completely. In one long-term study, all of the children who had either isolated microhematuria or hematuria associated with proteinuria had normal urinalyses and renal function on follow-up 8 years later.[4] Of those who had either nephritis or combined nephritic and nephrotic manifestations, fewer than 1% had died of renal complications, and only 2% had continued renal abnormalities. However, other studies of long-term outcome have shown that as many as 10% to 15% of HSP patients who had renal involvement have chronic sequelae, including hypertension and renal failure. These differences may be explained by the reports of worse outcomes emanating from nephrology referral institutions, in which the patient population is biased toward those who have more severe renal involvement. Clinically patients who have both nephrotic syndrome and hematuria, especially if associated with hypertension or renal insufficiency, have the greatest likelihood of progressing to chronic renal failure. Clinicopathological studies of renal biopsy findings in HSP patients also have shown histological correlates to poorer outcomes.[6] Generally, a poor prognosis with progression to renal failure has been associated with (1) the onset of HSP nephritis in the child older than 6 years of age, (2) the presence of the nephrotic syndrome, and (3) the presence of crescent formation in the glomeruli. A renal biopsy can help establish the diagnosis and improve prognostic assessment.

REFERENCES

1. Allen DM, Diamond LK, Howell DA: Anaphylactoid purpura in children, *Am J Dis Child* 99:853, 1960.
2. Austin HA III, Balow JE: Henoch-Schönlein nephritis: prognostic features and challenge of therapy, *Am J Kidney Dis* 2:512, 1983.
3. Goldstein AR et al: Long-term follow-up of childhood Henoch-Schönlein nephritis, *Lancet* 339:280, 1992.
4. Stewart M et al: Long term renal prognosis of Henoch Schönlein purpura in an unselected childhood population, *Eur J Pediatr* 147:113, 1988.
5. Waldo FB: Is Henoch-Schönlein purpura the systemic form of IgA nephropathy? *Am J Kidney Dis* 12:373, 1988.
6. Yoshikawa N, White RHR, Cameron AH: Prognostic significance of the glomerular changes in Henoch-Schönlein nephritis, *Clin Nephrol* 16:223, 1981.

SUGGESTED READINGS

Austin HA, Balow JE: Henoch-Schönlein nephritis: prognostic features and the challenge of therapy, *Am J Kidney Dis* 2:512, 1983.

Robson WLM, Leung AKC: Henoch-Schönlein purpura, *Adv Pediatr* 41:163, 1994.

Steward M et al: Long-term renal prognosis of Henoch-Schönlein purpura in an unselected childhood population, *Eur J Pediatr* 147:113, 1988.

Waldo BF: Is Henoch-Schönlein purpura the systemic form of IgA nephropathy? *Am J Kidney Dis* 12:373, 1988.

213 Hepatitis

Jay A. Perman and Kathleen B. Schwarz

Approximately 60,000 cases of viral hepatitis are reported annually to the Centers for Disease Control and Prevention. Not included in these figures are numerous unrecognized anicteric cases, especially in the pediatric population, in whom the anicteric/icteric case ratio is thought to approach 10:1. In addition, an unknown number of subclinical cases must occur, as evidenced by the presence of antibody to hepatitis A in more than 30% of the adult U.S. population and the prevalence of hepatitis B antigen-positive persons identified by bloodbank screening. Two causative agents of non-A, non-B hepatitis have been recognized: hepatitis C, which causes most cases of transfusion-associated cases of hepatitis,[12] and hepatitis E, which causes epidemic (enterically transmitted) non-A, non-B hepatitis.[8] Thus acute viral hepatitis continues as a major infectious disease. Although generally a self-limited illness in children, virus A (infectious hepatitis, short incubation period) and particularly virus B (serum hepatitis, long incubation period) and hepatitis C may be associated with significant morbidity and death. In addition, chronic hepatitis, a potential complication of acute viral hepatitis, is being recognized with increasing frequency in children.

ACUTE HEPATITIS

Virus A[13]

Transmission of hepatitis A is predominantly by the fecal-oral route, although saliva and urine are potentially important vehicles, particularly among siblings. Contaminated shellfish, polluted water, and travel to endemic areas also have been identified in the acquisition of type A infection.

Viruslike particles capable of causing hepatitis A infection in primates have been demonstrated by immune electron microscopy in the stools of patients ill with hepatitis A. Antigen can be detected in the stool (as well as in serum and possibly in urine) as early as 2 to 3 weeks before acute illness and as much as 1 week after the onset of illness; recovery in the stool decreases as jaundice becomes evident. Aggregation of the 27 nm diameter viral particles present in stool can be achieved by adding serum containing hepatitis A antibody. This antibody is recoverable in patients' serum after antigen no longer is found in the stool. Hepatitis A antibody is present at least 10 years after infection and probably confers lifelong immunity to virus A. It now is possible to grow hepatitis A in cell culture. An inactivated vaccine, not yet available in the United States, has been shown to be safe and immunogenic in healthy children[19] (see also Chapter 203, Enterovirus Infections).

Virus B[7]

Hepatitis virus B (HBV) consists of a surface antigen (HB_sAg), a core antigen (HB_cAg), an e antigen (HB_eAg), and DNA with DNA polymerase. Although previously thought to be transmitted only parenterally, hence the designation *serum hepatitis,* it now is accepted that virus B can be transmitted orally. Antigen may be present in saliva and other secretions. Blood-sucking insects also have been incriminated in transmission of the virus, as has ingestion of contaminated shellfish.

Hepatitis B in the Neonate. The neonate delivered of an HB_sAg-positive mother or a mother who has had hepatitis B during pregnancy represents a unique problem. Transmission is more likely if the mother is HB_eAg antigen-positive and appears highly unlikely if maternal antibody to HB_eAg is present. The risk of infection to the infant appears to be markedly increased (80%) if the mother has had clinical hepatitis in the third trimester of pregnancy. The route of infection may be transplacental by the swallowing of blood at the time of delivery or by close contact postpartum. Evidence for acquisition of antigen after birth is based on conversion from antigen negativity to positivity postpartum. Data linking breast-feeding to the acquisition of antigenicity are equivocal, but HB_sAg-positive mothers whose infants have received immunoprophylaxis may breast feed without risk of transmitting HBV to the infant. Infants born to an HB_sAg-positive mother or a mother who has had hepatitis B during pregnancy should be given 0.5 ml of hepatitis B immune globulin (HBIG) intramuscularly immediately after birth and 0.5 ml of hepatitis B vaccine intramuscularly within the first week of life and again 1 and 6 months later.

New recommendations may be forthcoming. A preliminary study of neonates born to mothers who were both HB_sAg-positive and HB_eAg-positive demonstrated that administration of recombinant hepatitis B vaccine to infants at birth, 1, and 2 months of age without concomitant immune globulin resulted in a very high protective efficacy rate against the chronic carrier state[16] and was very safe.[18]

The long-term effects of acquiring antigenicity in infancy include hepatoma. Infants acquiring antigen have a recognized tendency to become chronic carriers and to have features of persistent hepatitis on biopsy. However, infants of carrier mothers have been reported in whom acute fulminant hepatitis occurs in the first 6 months of life.

Hepatitis Delta Virus. Hepatitis delta virus replicates in the liver and is associated with a protein, the hepatitis delta antigen (HDAg), which can be found in both the liver and the serum of individuals who have the disease. The virus is unique in that it is defective and requires a coat of Hb_sAg to replicate effectively. The characteristic clinical feature is that it increases the severity of hepatitis B virus infection.

Virus C[5]

Hepatitis C virus (HCV), which was recognized in 1989, is a 30 to 50 nm RNA virus present in serum of infected individuals.[12] Preliminary studies have shown HCV to cause the majority of cases of posttransfusion hepatitis and 50% to 60% of cases of sporadic non-A, non-B hepatitis.

A whole series of diagnostic tests has been developed. The first-generation enzyme-linked immunoassay (ELISA) for antibody to HCV (C100-3) had relatively poor sensitivity and specificity. Second generation ELISAs are highly sensitive and specific, as is the recombinant immunoblot assay (RIBA) for which the RIBA II test is thought to be best; however, neither of these tests, which now are available commercially, become positive until weeks after exposure to the virus.[1] In contrast, the highly sensitive polymerase chain reaction assay becomes positive within days after exposure to the virus.

Virus E[8]

Hepatitis E virus (HEV), a 27 to 34 nm RNA virus, is the cause of "epidemic" or "enterically transmitted" hepatitis, an illness that has been described in outbreaks in India, Pakistan, Nepal, Russia, China, Algeria, central Africa, Peru, and Mexico. Only imported cases have been identified in the United States. The illness usually occurs in areas where the water supply is contaminated by feces; viruslike particles in stool specimens can be agglutinated by serum from convalescent patients. Serology is diagnostic.

Clinical Features

The clinical features of acute types A, B, and C viral hepatitis in children are reviewed in Table 213-1. Type A is heralded by an abrupt onset associated with fever, malaise, anorexia, nausea, vomiting, and upper abdominal discomfort. Darkening of the urine and enlargement and tenderness of the liver follow. Shortly thereafter, clinical jaundice becomes apparent. The bilirubin level increases in both direct and indirect fractions but generally does not exceed a total of 15 mg/dl. Aminotransferase elevation generally does not exceed 3 weeks in duration. In general, the clinical and laboratory abnormalities do not persist beyond 4 weeks. The disease rarely is fulminant.

Hepatitis B occurs more often in the adolescent than in the younger age group. It generally occurs sporadically in contrast to type A, which may occur in epidemics. Occasionally a history of exposure to blood or blood products may be obtained. The onset usually is insidious. Extrahepatic manifestations such as skin rash and arthralgia are common and may be prodromal. In fact, hepatitis B should be kept in mind in the differential diagnosis of serum sickness–like illness. The duration of illness usually is 4 to 6 weeks, generally somewhat longer than in type A. Aminotransferase elevation usually peaks approximately 1 month after the onset of illness. Although more than 90% of children recover without sequelae, fulminant hepatitis is seen more frequently than in type A. Type C hepatitis cannot be distinguished rigorously on clinical grounds from type B hepatitis. However, two characteristic clinical features are (1) fluctuation in the serum concentration of the aminotranferases and (2) progression to chronicity (50% to 80% of patients). Type E hepatitis is similar clinically to hepatitis A. Cholestasis may be more common than with hepatitis A, and elevation of serum aminotransferases is modest. The most unusual clinical feature of the illness is high mortality in pregnant women (approximately 10%). The disease does not progress to chronicity, cirrhosis, or a carrier state.

Table 213-1 Acute Viral Hepatitis

Characteristics	Virus A	Virus B	Virus C
Age distribution	Children and young adults	All age groups	All age groups
Route of infection	Predominantly fecal-oral	Parenteral-oral	Parenteral-oral
Incubation period (days)	15-40	50-180	20-90
Onset	Acute	Insidious	Insidious
Duration of clinical illness	Weeks	Weeks to months	Weeks to months
Virus present			
Feces	Late incubation, acute	May be present	Absent
Blood	Late incubation, acute	Late incubation, acute, may persist for months to years	Present chronically
Clinical features			
Fever	High, common early	Moderate, less common	Moderate, less common
Nausea and vomiting	Common	Less common	Less common
Anorexia	Severe	Mild to moderate	Mild to moderate
Arthralgia or arthritis	Rare	Common	?
Rash or urticaria	Rare	Common	?
Laboratory findings			
Aminotransferase elevation	1-3 wk	Months	Fluctuates for months
Bilirubin elevation	Weeks	May be months	Unusual
HB_sAg	Absent	Present	Absent
Severity	Usually mild	Often severe	Usually mild
Progression to chronic hepatitis	Rare	More common	High chronicity rate
Immunity	Homologous, lifelong (?)	Homologous, lifelong (?)	?
Prevention	Immune serum globulin	Hyperimmune globulin; vaccine	Screen donor blood

Modified from Krugman S, Katz SL: *Infectious diseases of children*, ed 8, St Louis, 1985, Mosby; and deBelle RC, Lester R: *Pediatr Clin North Am* 22:948, 1975.

Fulminant hepatitis, which can occur with any of the viruses enumerated previously, is heralded by the following laboratory aberrations[17]:

1. Prolonged prothrombin time (>4 seconds over control), unresponsive to large doses of vitamin K
2. Marked elevation of serum bilirubin (>20 mg/dl)
3. Leukocytosis (>12,500)
4. Hypoglycemia

Fulminant disease may occur in two forms: massive hepatic necrosis or submassive hepatic necrosis. Known as acute yellow atrophy, massive hepatic necrosis rarely is associated with survival; the patient dies within 10 days of onset of illness unless a liver transplant is performed. Submassive hepatic necrosis, often extensive, may lead to death within 3 weeks after the onset of illness or progress to chronic liver disease; a small number of patients recover completely. A characteristic form of "bridging" necrosis—that is, necrosis that extends from one portal area to another—has been described in patients who have submassive hepatic necrosis.

Diagnosis

The various types of viral hepatitis often can be discriminated on the basis of their clinical and epidemiological characteristics, although distinction may be difficult in sporadic cases. Sensitive radioimmunoassay techniques are available for detection of antibody to hepatitis A (antihepatitis A). The presence of IgM class antihepatitis A coinciding with clinical symptoms confirms the diagnosis of acute hepatitis A. The IgM response is followed rapidly by the development of IgG antihepatitis A, which persists for years.

The presence of HB_sAg remains the principal means of diagnosing hepatitis B. The ELISA and RIBA II tests for HCV usually become positive several weeks after the acute illness. A fluorescence test for hepatitis E antigen is in hepatocyte cytoplasm; this test has been modified for assay of anti-HEV in the serum of affected patients. However, this assay is not available widely.[11]

If the history, clinical features, and serological tests leave the diagnosis in doubt, other causes, both viral and nonviral, must be ruled out. Clinical features may help discriminate among other infectious causes—for example, Epstein-Barr virus or leptospirosis. Additional agents associated with inflammation of the liver include cytomegalovirus, toxoplasmosis, herpes simplex, echovirus, coxsackievirus, measles, and adenovirus; in children who have acquired immunodeficiency syndrome (AIDS), *Mycobacterium avium intracellulare* should be considered. Noninfectious causes include hepatotoxic drugs, as well as metabolic liver disease such as alpha-1-antitrypsin deficiency, Wilson disease, cystic fibrosis, and hepatic involvement in inflammatory bowel disease. In newborns who have cholestasis, idiopathic giant cell hepatitis is found more frequently than is hepatitis secondary to a specific causative agent.

The decision to biopsy a liver should depend on the duration of illness and whether the patient conforms to the clinical course of acute viral hepatitis. If the history, clinical features, or laboratory values (persistence in elevation of gamma globulin) suggest chronicity (3 to 6 months), a biopsy should be performed. Similarly, if Wilson disease is suspected, a definitive diagnosis generally can be made by determining the liver copper, which is elevated, and serum ceruloplasmin, which is decreased. Wilson disease always must be considered in the differential diagnosis of pediatric liver disease, especially because Kayser-Fleischer rings and neurological findings may be absent and the ceruloplasmin may be normal in juvenile Wilson disease.[20]

Therapy and Prevention

Hospitalization generally is unnecessary for the patient who has acute viral hepatitis. However, the infant and young child should be hospitalized and observed closely because of the rapidity with which hepatic failure can ensue in this age group. Regardless of age, if evidence of impending hepatic failure is present, the child must be hospitalized and appropriate measures begun. Although protein restriction coupled with high carbohydrate intake is important in hepatic failure, no benefit of a particular diet has been demonstrated with respect to course and prognosis for the child who has an uncomplicated case of viral hepatitis. Similarly, restriction of activity does not appear to affect the course or outcome, although the child who has hepatitis will desire increased rest.

Because recovery of virus A in the patient's stool decreases rapidly after the onset of jaundice, return to school at this point, provided the child feels well, does not appear to present an undue risk of infection to others. However, if the child appears noticeably jaundiced, his or her feelings regarding that appearance, as well as the concern of others toward contact, may necessitate staying home from school until the jaundice is reduced.

Although household contacts of the patient who has hepatitis A likely already are infected by the time of diagnosis, the physician still should stress scrupulous hand washing and the use of disposable eating utensils in the patient's home until jaundice clears. Pooled immune serum globulin is of documented benefit in suppressing the clinical symptoms of hepatitis A. Household contacts should receive 0.02 to 0.04 ml/kg of body weight intramuscularly as soon as possible after exposure. Newborn infants of infected mothers do not need special care if the mother is not jaundiced. Neither withholding of breast-feeding nor immunoglobulin is recommended unless the mother is jaundiced. Children traveling to endemic areas also should be immunized prophylactically.[10] The American Academy of Pediatrics has made detailed recommendations for control of HAV in day care centers.[2]

The possibility for preventing hepatitis B has been improved dramatically by introduction of safe, effective recombinant vaccines[9] and by the recommendation by the American Academy of Pediatrics that all healthy newborn infants should be immunized. Detailed recommendations regarding doses and preexposure and postexposure prophylaxis are provided in Tables 213-2 to 213-4. Alpha-interferon is the only antiviral agent available commercially that is recommended for HBV, and its efficacy may be limited to about only 25% of those infected. Studies are under way to test this efficacy in children who have HBV.[5]

The most important strategy for controlling hepatitis C is screening donor blood for anti-HCV because preliminary studies have shown that most cases of transfusion-acquired hepatitis C originate from transfusion of donor blood that was anti-HCV positive. Perinatal transmission of HCV is rare in the absence of HIV infection, but withholding of breast-feeding is probably indicated. The efficacy of alpha-

Table 213-2 Recommended Dosages of Hepatitis B Vaccines*

	Vaccine†,‡			
	Recombivax HB§		Energix-B,‖,¶	
	dose: μg	(ml)	dose: μg	(ml)
Infants of HBsAg-negative mothers and children <11 y	2.5	(0.5)#	10	(0.5)
Infants of HBsAg-positive mothers (HBIG [0.5 mL] should also be given)	5	(0.5)** (1.0)#	10	(0.5)
Children and adolescents 11-19 y	5	(0.5)**	20	(1.0)
Adults ≥20 y	10	(1.0)**	20	(1.0)
Dialysis patients and other immunosuppressed adults	40	(1.0)††	40	(2.0)‡‡

*Heptavax B (available from Merck & Co), a plasma-derived vaccine, is also licensed but no longer produced in the United States.
†Vaccines should be stored at 2° C to 8° C. Freezing destroys effectiveness.
‡Both vaccines are administered in a three-dose schedule.
§Available from Merck & Co.
‖The Food and Drug Administration has approved this vaccine for use in an optional four-dose schedule at 0, 1, 2, and 12 mo.
¶Available from SmithKline Beecham.
#Pediatric formulation.
**Adult formulation.
††Special formulation for dialysis patients.
‡‡Two 1.0-ml doses given at one site in a four-dose schedule at 0, 1, 2, and 6-12 mo.

Table 213-3 Persons Who Should Receive Hepatitis B Immunization

All Infants—Infants of HB_sAg-positive mothers require postexposure immunoprophylaxis with HBIG and vaccine.
Infants and children at risk of acquisition of HBV by person-to-person (horizontal) transmission should be immunized by 6-9 mo of age.
Adolescents*—Special efforts should be made to vaccinate those adolescents in the categories of high risk for hepatitis B virus (HBV) infection.
Users of intravenous drugs.
Sexually active heterosexual persons with more than one sex partner in the previous 6 mo or with a sexually transmitted disease.
Sexually active homosexual or bisexual males.
Health care workers at risk of exposure to blood or body fluids.
Residents and staff of institutions for developmentally disabled persons.
Staff of nonresidential child care and school programs for developmentally disabled persons if attended by a known HBV carrier.
Hemodialysis patients.
Patients with bleeding disorders who receive certain blood products.
Household contacts and sexual partners of HBV carriers.
Members of households with adoptees from countries where HBV infection is endemic who are HB_sAg positive.
International travelers who will live for more than 6 mo in an area of high HBV endemicity and who otherwise will be at risk.
Inmates of long-term correctional facilities.

*Implementation can be initiated before children reach adolescence.

interferon in the treatment of adults who have HCV is similar to results with HBV. Trials of this agent are under way in children who have HCV. Prevention of hepatitis E rests on improvement of hygiene in countries where the illness is epidemic.

Table 213-4 Guide to Postexposure Immunoprophylaxis for Hepatitis B Infection

Type of exposure	Immunoprophylaxis
Perinatal	HBIG + vaccination
Sexual—acute infection	HBIG + vaccination
Sexual—chronic carrier	Vaccination
Household contact—chronic carrier	Vaccination
Household contact—acute case with identifiable blood exposure	HBIG + vaccination
Infant (<12 mo)—acute case in primary caregiver	HBIG + vaccination
Accidental—percutaneous/permucosal	HBIG ± vaccination

CHRONIC HEPATITIS

Continuing evidence of hepatic inflammation beyond the period generally expected for resolution of acute viral hepatitis always should suggest chronic hepatitis.[4] However, acute hepatitis may resolve slowly over a period longer than 6 months, and alternatively, evidence of chronicity may be present earlier than 3 months.

Chronic persistent hepatitis and chronic active hepatitis represent the two forms of chronic hepatitis seen in children. Designated also as chronic active liver disease, chronic active hepatitis has many synonyms: chronic aggressive hepatitis, active chronic hepatitis, lupoid hepatitis, autoimmune hepatitis, subacute hepatitis, plasma cell hepatitis, chronic liver disease in young women, and juvenile cirrhosis. As will be seen, these synonyms reflect many of the features of the disease. Not included in the categories of chronic persistent hepatitis and chronic active hepatitis are other entities associated with chronic hepatic inflammation. These include chronic inflammation secondary to drugs (isonicotinic acid hydrazide or isoniazid [INH], alpha-methyldopa, and oxyphenisatin acetate), metabolic diseases (alpha-1-antitrypsin deficiency, Wilson disease, and cystic fibrosis), and fatty liver secondary to obesity.

Type A hepatitis never progresses to chronic liver disease and cirrhosis. By contrast, type B more frequently is associated with chronicity, at least in the adult population; approximately 10% of patients who have acute viral hepatitis type B contract chronic liver disease, many with the benign clinical pattern associated with chronic persistent hepatitis. The hepatitis B carrier state generally is *unassociated with overt disease*. Further, hepatitis B does not appear to be related etiologically to most cases of chronic active hepatitis. As indicated by the presence of HB_sAg, no more than 25% of adult cases of chronic active hepatitis are related to virus B. This figure appears to be considerably lower in children. Because chronic hepatitis B can evolve to hepatocellular carcinoma, some advocate following serial serum alpha-fetoprotein measurements and liver ultrasound examinations in this setting. Type C hepatitis progresses to chronicity in 50% to 80% of infected adults; comparable data are not yet available for children. However, HCV may be as common a cause of hepatocellular carcinoma as is HBV.

Chronic active hepatitis has been associated in the pediatric population with immunopathic diseases such as ulcerative colitis, thyroiditis, and systemic lupus erythematosus. Indeed, immunological mechanisms have been invoked in its pathogenesis. For example, autoantibodies including antinuclear, antimitochondrial, anti-liver, kidney microsomal antibody,[14] and anti-smooth muscle antibodies have been identified in chronic active hepatitis, although their presence may be an epiphenomenon. Similarly, immune complexes have been associated with the extrahepatic manifestations of both acute and chronic active hepatitis, although no definite role in the perpetuation of liver disease has been identified. Altered cell-mediated immunity to HB_sAg also may play a role in pathogenesis.

Genetic factors also may be relevant in the establishment of chronicity. A higher incidence of the histocompatibility antigens HL-A1 and HL-A8 occurs in patients who have HB_sAg-negative chronic active hepatitis. Characteristics of the causative agent also may be important in the establishment of chronicity, as suggested by the association of e antigen with progression to chronic hepatitis.

Chronic Persistent Hepatitis

Although the long-term outcome is unclear, chronic persistent hepatitis often is thought to be a benign disorder. The child generally feels well, although enlargement of the liver is noted occasionally. Aminotransferases usually are elevated, and gamma globulin levels may be normal. Mononuclear infiltration of the portal areas is seen on liver biopsy specimens; minimal inflammation and necrosis and little or no fibrosis are seen within the lobules.

Chronic Active Hepatitis

In contrast, significant clinical, chemical, and histological findings are associated with chronic active hepatitis. Unlike adults, in whom the onset usually is insidious, 50% or more of affected pediatric patients have an acute onset of disease much like that of those who have acute viral hepatitis. Fever, nausea, anorexia, and jaundice are common. An occasional patient may be seriously ill, with evidence of portal hypertension or hepatocellular failure. Approximately two thirds of affected children are girls. A summary of clinical findings in 38 patients reported by Dubois and Silverman[6] reveals the following: jaundice, 87%; hepatomegaly, 79%; splenomegaly, 74%; ascites, 24%; amenorrhea, 18%; acne, 16%; clubbing, 16%; gynecomastia, 5%. Extrahepatic manifestations such as arthralgia, arthritis, and a skin rash are common. Hypergammaglobulinemia is a common laboratory finding, averaging approximately twice the normal level for age. Aminotransferases and the total bilirubin level are elevated to a variable degree. Autoantibodies such as antinuclear antibody frequently are positive. Histologically, portal tracts are infiltrated by lymphocytes and plasma cells. Inflammatory cells often infiltrate the parenchyma, accompanied by necrosis of cells at the periphery of the hepatic lobule—"piecemeal necrosis" or "destruction of the limiting plate." Fibrosis may be seen to a variable degree, or true cirrhosis may be present. Because chronic active hepatitis may progress, cirrhosis, although not seen initially, may appear later.

Liver biopsy is essential for diagnosis when chronic liver disease is suspected, provided it can be diagnosed safely. A needle biopsy is adequate, and the risks are low. An accurate diagnosis is essential because treatment is predicated, at least partially, on the degree of activity seen on biopsy. As emphasized previously, Wilson disease must be ruled out in any child who has hepatitis because of the availability of therapy (penicillamine). Demonstration of a normal serum ceruloplasmin level alone is insufficient to rule out this disorder. Thus a liver biopsy with determination of the hepatic copper level is essential.[15]

Treatment of Chronic Hepatitis

No specific therapy is indicated for chronic persistent hepatitis. Close follow-up of the clinical status and monitoring of liver function and the gamma globulin level are essential for a period of not less than 2 years. If evidence of active inflammation develops, the patient should be reevaluated with a liver biopsy.

By contrast, specific therapy is indicated in patients who have autoimmune chronic active hepatitis.[3] Prednisone alone and in combination with azathioprine helps prolong survival of these patients. Although azathioprine alone appears to be no more effective than a placebo in the treatment of chronic active hepatitis, its use in combination with prednisone allows a smaller dosage of the steroid to be used. Some patients who are refractory to azathioprine and steroids have responded to cyclosporine.[9]

Because steroids are associated with growth retardation and unpleasant side effects, the use of a small steroid dose is critical in the pediatric population. Prednisone is begun in a dosage of 2 mg/kg/day (maximum 60 mg daily). Alternate-day dosages appear to be less effective in achieving remission in chronic active hepatitis but may be of value once clinical and biochemical remission has been achieved. Remission is defined as a lack of clinical symptoms, aminotransferase elevation no more than two times normal, decreasing serum gamma globulin levels, and resolution of the aggressive histological appearance on a liver biopsy specimen.

When evidence of improvement has occurred, the prednisone dosage may be tapered at weekly intervals to a dosage that achieves and maintains clinical and biochemical remission. The patient generally requires between 10 and 20 mg daily. Azathioprine may be added after evidence of improvement, especially if unpleasant steroid side effects are noted. Duration of therapy once remission is achieved is controversial. Generally, once remission is achieved, steroids may be tapered over 6 weeks. A role for alternate-day steroid therapy in maintaining remission has been suggested.[3]

Clinical remission generally occurs within 3 to 6 months, biochemical remission within 6 to 12 months, and histological remission within 12 to 24 months. The patient must be watched at 2- to 4-week intervals for approximately 3 months for evidence of early recurrence of disease. If a recurrence does not manifest within that time, the frequency of observation can be decreased.

At least 80% of children appear to achieve initial remission. Although the adult relapse rate is 50% within 6 months, the rate of relapse tends to be less frequent in children. Because of the paucity of affected children, evaluating the long-term outcome of chronic active hepatitis is difficult. However, most children are likely to have a prolonged clinical remission and perhaps a cure. Those whose disease is severe at the time of diagnosis, as indicated by prolonged prothrombin times and morphological features of extensive necrosis, frequently already have progressed or will progress to cirrhosis. Their prognosis, unfortunately, remains poor.

Liver Transplantation

Liver transplantation has improved the outlook for children who have a wide variety of severe liver diseases, including disease secondary to the viruses discussed in this chapter.

For transplantation in general, 1- to 5-year survival rates in children approach 70% to 80%. Transplantation for liver failure secondary to hepatitis B is complicated by almost 100% recurrence of infection; therefore transplantation for this indication is controversial. Recurrence of hepatitis C following transplantation is in the neighborhood of 90%, but transplantation is recommended because recurrent disease usually is mild. Because successful transplantation for fulminant hepatitis has been achieved in a number of centers, the affected child must be referred to a transplant center as soon as the diagnosis of fulminant hepatitis is established. The prognosis for transplantation in the setting of viral hepatitis undoubtedly will improve with the development of new, more specific antiviral agents.

REFERENCES

1. Akader HH, Balisteri WF: Hepatitis C virus: implications to pediatric practice, *Pediatr Infect Dis J* 12:853, 1993.
2. American Academy of Pediatrics: *Report of the Committee on Infectious Diseases: hepatitis A,* Elk Grove, Ill, 1991, The Academy.
3. Arasu TS et al: Management of chronic aggressive hepatitis in children and adolescents, *J Pediatr* 95:514, 1979.
4. Czaja AJ: Current problems in the diagnosis and management of chronic active hepatitis, *Mayo Clin Proc* 56:311, 1981.
5. Davis GL et al: Treatment of chronic hepatitis C with recombinant interferon alfa: a multicenter randomized controlled trial, *N Engl J Med* 321:101, 1989.
6. Dubois RS, Silverman A: Treatment of chronic active hepatitis in children, *Postgrad Med J* 50:386, 1974.
7. Fulginiti VA, editor: Hepatitis B virus, *Infect Dis Newsl* 1:25, 1982.
8. Gust ID, Purcell RH: Report of a workshop: waterborne non-A, non-B hepatitis, *J Infect Dis* 156:630, 1987.
9. Hyman JS, Ballo M, Leichtner AM: Cyclosporine treatment of autoimmune chronic active hepatitis, *Gastroenterology* 93:890, 1987.
10. Immunization Practices Advisory Committee: Recommendations for protection against viral hepatitis, *MMWR* 34:313, 1985.
11. Krawczynski K: Hepatitis E, *Hepatology* 17:932, 1993.
12. Kuo G-L et al: An assay for circulating antibodies to a major etiologic virus of human non-A, non-B hepatitis, *Science* 244:362, 1989.
13. Lemon SM: Type A viral hepatitis: new developments in an old disease, *N Engl J Med* 313:1059, 1985.
14. Mackay IR: Toward diagnostic criteria for autoimmune hepatitis, *Hepatology* 18:1006, 1993.
15. Perman JA et al: Laboratory measures of copper metabolism in the differentiation of chronic active hepatitis and Wilson disease in children, *J Pediatr* 94:564, 1979.
16. Poovorawan Y et al: Protective efficacy of a recombinant DNA hepatitis B vaccine in neonates of HBe antigen-positive mothers, *JAMA* 261:3278, 1989.
17. Ritt DJ et al: Acute hepatic necrosis with stupor or coma: an analysis of 31 patients, *Medicine* 48:151, 1969.
18. Safety of hepatitis B vaccine confirmed, *FDA Drug Bull* 15:14, 1985.
19. Shou-Dong L et al: Immunogenicity of inactivated hepatitis A vaccine in children, *Gastroenterology* 104:1129, 1993.
20. Werlin SL et al: Diagnostic dilemmas of Wilson's disease: diagnosis and treatment, *Pediatrics* 62:47, 1978.

214 Herpes Infections

Lindsey K. Grossman

Herpesvirus hominis, or herpes simplex virus (HSV), is one of the most common agents infecting humans, and although 85% to 95% of primary infections may be inapparent, the disease in certain circumstances can be fatal. HSV is a deoxyribonucleic acid (DNA) virus having a protein coat. After an incubation period of 2 to 12 days, the primary infection, if apparent, usually is heralded by constitutional symptoms such as malaise, fever, anorexia, and irritability, as well as by the classic herpetic enanthem or exanthem. This is a painful vesicle, usually several millimeters in diameter, on an erythematous base. After healing and recovery from the initial infection, the organism is not rid from the host but rather is presumed to remain in a latent phase in the ganglion cells or nerves innervating the region of localized infection. Various stimuli, including sunlight, fever, physical or emotional trauma, or menses may induce a recurrent infection. Recurrent infection demonstrates a similar vesicular eruption in the same general anatomical area as the primary eruption but without concomitant constitutional symptoms.

Pathologically, HSV is noted for the presence of multinucleated giant cells and eosinophilic intranuclear inclusions seen in tissue scrapings taken from the base of a vesicle and stained with Giemsa (Tzanck preparation), Pap, or hematoxylin-eosin techniques. Herpes infections can be divided definitively into two immunological types that highly correlate with clinical manifestations: *herpesvirus type 1* (HSV-1), which tends to be associated with disease above the waist, and *herpesvirus type 2* (HSV-2), associated with disease below the waist, sexually related transmission, or disease acquired neonatally.

Studies have shown a sharp rise in the prevalence of antibodies to HSV-1 between 1 and 4 years of age and a slower rise of antibody acquisition between 5 and 14 years of age. From adolescence into early adulthood, coincident with the beginning of sexual activity, the presence of antibodies to HSV-2 is increased markedly. Overall, 80% to 100% of adults in lower socioeconomic groups, where crowding probably plays an important epidemiological role, demonstrate antibodies to HSV-1; 40% or more may be positive for HSV-2. Of those of higher socioeconomic circumstances, 10% demonstrate antibodies to HSV-2; 100% of older prostitutes demonstrate such antibodies.

HERPESVIRUS TYPE 1

Transmission of HSV-1 is presumed to be via person-to-person respiratory spread and probably involves close contact, such as kissing an infected person. Transmission can occur whether or not the contact at the time is symptomatic of having an apparent vesicular lesion. The clinical manifestation varies with site of entry, and the clinical diagnosis rarely requires laboratory confirmation.

Acute gingivostomatitis is the most common form of HSV-1 seen in children; the peak incidence is between 1 and 4 years of age. It is characterized by an abrupt onset of fever, irritability, poor feeding, and 1 to 2 days later, by very tender, red, friable mucous membranes surrounding 2- to 3-mm white ulcerations, and severe halitosis. The vesicular stage is seen rarely, but large, tender anterior cervical and submaxillary lymphadenopathy is common. The duration of the illness varies from 5 to 14 days, and the severity ranges from mild to so severe that oral intake becomes negligible and hospitalization for intravenous hydration may be required. The differential diagnosis includes coxsackievirus A herpangina, which results in lesions very similar in appearance to herpes but located in the posterior oral cavity, as contrasted with the anterior clustering of the herpetic lesions.

Herpes labialis (or cold sores) crust and heal without scarring in 7 to 10 days. They may be found on either the upper or lower lip, and recurrence at the same site is extremely common. *Traumatic herpes* is the result of inoculation at the site of local trauma and includes *herpetic whitlow,* an extremely painful syndrome involving herpetic infection of a digit. Although it may resemble a bacterial paronychia, it should not be incised. This condition is common in thumb-suckers who have oral herpes.

Although HSV-1 infections are self-limited usually, certain syndromes are associated with ominous consequences. Ocular herpes can be extremely worrisome and is one of the most common causes of corneal blindness in the United States. The primary infection usually involves *acute keratoconjunctivitis* with intense swelling of the lids but without exudate. Frequently, typical herpetic vesicles are found on the skin surrounding the involved eye. Recurrent disease can be even more severe and may involve superficial or deep epithelial ulceration, stromal damage, or uveitis. Fortunately, treatment is available (see the discussion on treatment), but these children under all circumstances should be referred to an ophthalmologist for care. Indeed, the pediatrician should be aware that devastating results can occur with the use of localized steroid preparations in an unsuspected case of ocular herpes. This underlines the necessity of an ophthalmological consultation before prescribing topical corticosteroids for any use in the eye.

Certain human hosts are at more serious risk for contracting HSV-1 than are others. Individuals who have deficiencies in cell-mediated immunity, those undergoing immunosuppressive therapy for cancer or transplantation, and those who are extremely malnourished may be more likely to show serious disseminated disease. The inoculation of herpes into eczematous skin can result in *eczema herpeticum,* which can vary in severity from mild to fatal. Constitutional symptoms are the rule, and the temperatures of 39.4° to 40.6° C may last for a week or more. Wide areas of skin can become denuded, with enormous fluid, protein, and electrolyte losses, which are potentially life threatening. Secondary bacterial infection may complicate the condition. Recurrences, milder than the primary infection, occur commonly on areas of the skin affected with chronic eczema.

HSV-1 is the most common reported cause of viral *encephalitis* in the United States, with an estimated 250 to 500 cases per year. The disease is characterized by a rapidly progressive encephalopathy culminating in death in 1 to 2 weeks in more than 70% of untreated cases. Most often the infection localizes to a single lobe, and a definitive diagnosis often can be made by a biopsy of that area demonstrating the typical morphological picture of herpes. Treatment now is available (see following discussion) that may improve the prognosis of this disastrous condition.

HERPESVIRUS TYPE 2

As a result of the increase in sexual activity in young adolescents in recent years, pediatricians have been faced with the challenge of diagnosing and treating all types of venereal disease. Genital HSV-2 is of increasing concern to physicians and patients alike because of its symptomatology, lack of cure, and potential for disastrous consequences to the newborn. Clinically, HSV-2 usually is manifested by typical herpetic vesicles on the penile shaft, prepuce, or glans penis in the male and on the labia minora or majora, mons, or nearby skin or within the vagina in the female. Primary infection is accompanied by significant local pain, burning, or paresthesia and constitutional symptoms of fever and malaise, dysuria, and inguinal lymphadenopathy; recurrent bouts are less severe. The 5% to 10% of cases of genital herpes associated with HSV-1 are believed to result from orogenital sex.

Viral culture is the most sensitive method of diagnosis but requires several days, depending on the size of the inoculum, for the definitive answer. When lesions are available for scraping, direct detection methods, including fluorescent antibody and immunoperoxidase assays, give a rapid answer but with lower sensitivity and therefore still require a viral culture for confirmation. Tzanck test and Pap stains are widely available and inexpensive but are not specific for HSV and have low sensitivity. ELISA testing is available commercially but does not distinguish between HSV-1 and HSV-2. Polymerase chain reaction and Western blot are highly specific and sensitive and do discriminate between the HSV-1 and HSV-2 but are not available commercially.

NEONATAL HERPES

Although most neonatal herpes infections are caused by HSV-2, antibodies to HSV-1 are associated in 25% of cases. Transplacental transmission of HSV can occur and may induce spontaneous abortion or, in rare cases, congenital defects in newborns. More often, however, pediatricians are faced with postnatal herpetic disease contracted by the newborn during the second stage of labor while moving through an infected birth canal. Here the incidence is estimated to vary between 1 clinically affected infant per 3000 deliveries in populations of low socioeconomic status to perhaps an overall risk of 1 case to 20,000 deliveries in the United States, or roughly 160 cases per year.[1,6]

The greatest risk of neonatal HSV infection occurs when the mother has contracted primary herpes 2 to 4 weeks before delivery, although the disease may be transmitted to the baby in recurrent cases with or without a clinically detectable herpetic lesion. The pediatrician should note that most newborns infected with HSV at birth are delivered from women who have no history of genital herpes.

When genital herpes occurs during pregnancy, one must worry about the risk of vertical transmission to the infant, especially at the time of delivery. HSV was isolated from 0.35% of nearly 16,000 women not having signs or symptoms suggesting the virus when they were admitted in early labor to a university hospital. Of those having positive HSV cultures, 35% had evidence of a recently acquired, *subclinical* first episode of genital HSV infection and their infants were 10 times more likely to develop the syndrome of neonatal HSV than were those who had an asymptomatic reactivation of HSV.[2]

The NIAID Collaborative Antiviral Study Group[13] classifies cases of neonatal HSV infection into three categories by clinical manifestation. Infants who have *disseminated disease* involving visceral organs with or without central nervous system (CNS) involvement are most likely to die (more than 80% without treatment and 54% with treatment). In disseminated infection, hepatoadrenal necrosis is virtually always found, and microcephaly, hydrocephalus, mental retardation, or seizures occur in many survivors.

A second category of disease includes infants who have *CNS abnormalities* without involvement of viscera. In this group mortality exceeds 50% and morbidity exceeds 90% without antiviral therapy.[14]

A third category includes infants whose *skin, eyes, or mouth* is involved (SEM) but not the CNS or viscera. Infants who have SEM before antiviral drugs became available were not expected to die, and only 20% to 30% were left neurologically impaired; many who appeared to have SEM, however, went on to develop disseminated or CNS involvement and to suffer disastrous consequences. Classically, more than 50% of all neonatal HSV infections manifested as disseminated disease, with only a minority classified as SEM. However, apparently as a result of earlier diagnosis and treatment, 42% now manifest as SEM and 23% as disseminated disease; the remaining 35%, who have CNS disease, has remained fairly stable. Recently an NIAID study documented no deaths with appropriate therapy for SEM disease and 15% and 57% mortality in neonates who had CNS and disseminated HSV infection, respectively.[12]

Previously, stringent prenatal screening programs were recommended to attempt to prevent HSV infection in offspring of women who had recurrent genital herpes. Such programs proved costly, impractical to administer, and medically ineffective. Current guidelines for managing pregnant women who have a history of genital herpes suggest vaginal delivery if no active genital lesions are present at the time of delivery and expeditious cesarean delivery for women who have apparent genital lesions near or at term and who are in labor or who have ruptured membranes. Scalp electrodes should be avoided when the mother has a history of genital HSV infection.

The American Academy of Pediatrics and the American College of Obstetricians and Gynecologists have developed joint guidelines to avoid the less likely possibility of postpartum herpes infection in the baby.[1] These guidelines specify isolation criteria to protect normal babies from their HSV-infected mothers, other infected infants, or infected staff.

TREATMENT

Although no universal cure exists for herpes infection, the prognosis for its many syndromes is improving greatly because of newly introduced therapies. One of the earliest successes was with topical idoxuridine (IDU) in the treatment of ocular herpetic infections. Unfortunately, early trials of systemic IDU and cytosine arabinoside demonstrated little value in the treatment of generalized herpes because of high drug toxicity.

Vidarabine was the first drug shown to decrease mortality and morbidity markedly without significant drug toxicity in neonatal herpes involving the CNS.[15] This effect is most marked when the diagnosis is made early and treatment begun promptly. Studies of vidarabine in older patients who had primary and recurrent genital herpes showed effectiveness only in immunodeficient patients.[14] Although originally found to be effective in the treatment of HSV encephalitis, more recent data show acyclovir to be superior.[11]

Acyclovir clearly is the most effective weapon against HSV currently available. Topical acyclovir (Zovirax) shortens the duration of symptoms and viral shedding by several days in initial or primary genital herpes,[3,4,7] with a lessened effect in cases caused by recurrent disease.[8,9] The oral preparation is even more effective in primary infections and is of some benefit in patients who have recurrent infection, especially if administered early in the course of the recurrence. Clinical trials of chronic suppressive oral acyclovir for patients who have primary genital herpes have shown a dramatic decrease in their recurrence rate.[5,10] Oral acyclovir currently is recommended for use in the treatment of initial cases of genital herpes but only for certain patients who have recurrent genital herpes that is very severe, frequent, or complicated. Acyclovir may be particularly useful in treating as well as preventing herpetic reactivation in immunocompromised patients.[9]

Although morbidity, mortality, and drug side effects are similar to those seen with treatment via vidarabine, acyclovir usually is considered to be the treatment of choice for neonatal HSV infection on the basis of ease of administration.[12,16] Earlier diagnosis coupled with the availability of efficacious therapy has contributed to a decrease in mortality and morbidity for this potentially devastating medical problem. For specific drug doses used in the treatment of HSV infections, see Table 258-1 in Chapter 258, Sexually Transmitted Diseases.

REFERENCES

1. American Academy of Pediatrics and American College of Obstetricians and Gynecologists: *Guidelines for prenatal care,* ed 3, Elk Grove Village, Ill, 1988, American Academy of Pediatrics.
2. Brown ZA et al: Neonatal herpes simplex virus infection in relation to asymptomatic maternal infection at the time of labor, *N Engl J Med* 324:1247, 1991.
3. Bryson YD et al: Treatment of first episodes of genital herpes simplex virus infection with oral acyclovir, *N Engl J Med* 308:916, 1983.
4. Corey L et al: A trial of topical acyclovir in genital herpes simplex virus infections, *N Engl J Med* 306:1313, 1982.
5. Douglas JM et al: A double-blind study of oral acyclovir for suppression of recurrence of genital herpes simplex virus infections, *N Engl J Med* 310:1551, 1984.
6. Hanshaw JB: *Herpesvirus hominis* infections in the fetus and the newborn, *Am J Dis Child* 126:546, 1973.
7. Mertz GJ et al: Double-blind placebo-controlled trial of oral acyclovir in first-episode genital herpes simplex virus infection, *JAMA* 252:1147, 1984.
8. Reichman RC et al: Treatment of recurrent genital herpes simplex infections with oral acyclovir, *JAMA* 251:2103, 1984.
9. Saral R: Management of mucocutaneous herpes simplex virus infections in immunocompromised patients, *Am J Med* 85 (suppl 2A):57, 1988.
10. Straus SE, Takiff HE, Seidlin M: Suppression of frequently recurring genital herpes: a placebo-controlled double-blind trial of acyclovir, *N Engl J Med* 310:1545, 1984.
11. Whitley RJ et al: Vidarabine versus acyclovir therapy in herpes simplex encephalitis, *N Engl J Med* 314:144, 1986.
12. Whitley RJ et al: Predictors of morbidity and mortality in neonates with herpes simplex virus infections, *N Engl J Med* 324:450, 1991.
13. Whitley RJ et al: Changing presentation of herpes simplex virus infection in neonates, *J Infect Dis* 158:109, 1988.
14. Whitley RJ et al: Vidarabine therapy for mucocutaneous herpes simplex virus infection in the immunocompromised host, *J Infect Dis* 149:1, 1984.
15. Whitley RJ et al: Neonatal herpes simplex virus infection: follow-up evaluation of vidarabine therapy, *Pediatrics* 72:778, 1983.
16. Whitley RJ et al: A controlled trial comparing vidarabine with acyclovir in neonatal herpes simplex virus infection, *N Engl J Med* 324:444, 1991.

SUGGESTED READINGS

Carmack MA, Prober CG: Neonatal herpes: vexing dilemmas and reasons for hope, *Curr Opin Pediatr* 5:21, 1993.

Corey L, Spear PG: Infections with herpes simplex viruses, *N Engl J Med* 314:686, 1986.

Dwyer DE, Cunningham AL: Herpes simplex virus infection in pregnancy, *Baillieres Clin Obstet Gynaecol* 7:75, 1993.

Gold D, Corey L: Treatment of herpes simplex infections, *Clin Lab Med* 7:815, 1987.

Koutsky LA et al: Underdiagnosis of genital herpes by current clinical and viral-isolation procedures, *N Engl J Med* 326:1533, 1992.

Whitley RJ: Neonatal herpes simplex virus infections, *Clin Perinatol* 15:903, 1988.

Whitley RJ: Herpes simplex virus infections of the central nervous system, *Drugs* 42:406, 1991.

215 Hydrocephalus

Dennis L. Johnson

Cerebral spinal fluid (CSF) is produced by the choroid plexus, fills the cerebral ventricles, flows out of the ventricles into the basal cisterns of the subarachnoid space, and percolates up and around the brain to be absorbed into the arachnoid granulations along the sagittal sinus. If the flow in this CSF pathway is increased (e.g., by a choroid plexus papilloma) or blocked (e.g., by a medulloblastoma filling and obstructing the fourth ventricle), the volume of CSF increases and dilates the ventricular system.[5] Hydrocephalus is here defined as enlargement of the ventricular system associated with the accumulation of CSF under pressure. Cerebral atrophy also is associated with enlargement of the ventricular system, but in contrast to hydrocephalus, the CSF pressure is not elevated.

Physicians throughout history have recognized the condition, and history is replete with courageous attempts to treat hydrocephalus. Treatment has included external CSF drainage with gold cannulas, skull binding and casting to prevent head enlargement, removal of the choroid plexus to eliminate the source of CSF, and more recently, CSF diversion through ventriculoperitoneal shunts. The history of CSF diversion is a chronicle of surgeons' courage, ingenuity, and frustration in the treatment of a condition that was hopelessly untreatable before the mid 1960s.[4] Hydrocephalus occurs in 3 to 4 of every 1000 live births, and an estimated 100,000 children currently are under treatment in the United States for hydrocephalus.[2]

CLASSIFICATION

Hydrocephalus traditionally has been classified as communicating or noncommunicating. If CSF within the ventricular system does not communicate with the subarachnoid spaces at the base of the brain, the hydrocephalus is *noncommunicating*. Noncommunicating hydrocephalus is characterized by a relatively small fourth ventricle (which may even be distorted by tumor) on computed tomography (CT) or magnetic resonance imaging (MRI) and implies that the flow of CSF is blocked before it enters the fourth ventricle. The fourth ventricle is enlarged in *communicating* hydrocephalus. In the era before CT and MRI, water-soluble dye injected into the ventricles could be retrieved from the subarachnoid space by lumbar puncture in communicating hydrocephalus, but if dye could not be traced from the ventricle to the lumbar subarachnoid space, the hydrocephalus was noncommunicating; whether or not the dye communicated with the subarachnoid space had specific diagnostic and treatment implications.[9] This classification schema is no less relevant in the current management of the child who has hydrocephalus. Communicating hydrocephalus is more likely to compensate with regard to symptoms over time, and shunt malfunction is more insidious. Neonatal posthemorrhagic hydrocephalus associated with prematurity often is communicating and temporarily can be relieved by lumbar puncture. Lumboperitoneal shunts can be done only for the treatment of communicating hydrocephalus. Noncommunicating hydrocephalus usually is very shunt dependent, and shunt failure may be associated with the rapid onset of intracranial hypertension. A lumbar puncture performed in a child who has noncommunicating hydrocephalus may result in life-threatening cerebral herniation. Endoscopic third ventriculostomy, which creates a communication from the third ventricle directly into the subarachnoid space through the lamina terminales, will not be effective if the hydrocephalus already is communicating.

ETIOLOGY

The further classification and cause of hydrocephalus is distinctive for each age group: infancy (birth to 12 months), childhood (1 to 12 years), and adolescence (13 to 18 years).

Infancy

The premature infant usually develops hydrocephalus following intraventricular hemorrhage associated with bleeding from the germinal matrix. The diagnosis is made and the progression of the hydrocephalus can be followed easily by weekly ultrasound examination of the head. If no fourth ventricle is visible on the scan, then the block to the flow of CSF is most likely at the aqueduct of Sylvius. The hydrocephalus is noncommunicating, and lumbar punctures (LPs) will not drain the ventricular system adequately. If, on the other hand, the blood has only *partially* obstructed the basal cisterns or the arachnoid granulations and the fourth ventricle can be identified on imaging studies, hydrocephalus is communicating, and serial LPs will drain the ventricles and avoid a shunt in the majority of cases.

A diagnosis of *congenital hydrocephalus* often is made on routine prenatal ultrasound examination and most commonly is due to aqueductal stenosis, cytomegalic inclusion virus (CMV), or toxoplasmosis. Congenital hydrocephalus can be associated with Dandy-Walker malformation of the cerebellum (dilation of the fourth ventricle associated with absence of the cerebellar vermis), meningomyelocele (MM), or occipital encephalocele. Hydrocephalus may become evident only after surgical repair of MM and occipital encephalocele. In addition, hydrocephalus can occur after meningitis and following severe head injury. In the full-term infant, the diagnosis is suspected on the basis of macrocrania or sequential head circumference measurements, which cross percentiles on normal growth charts. The most common cause of infant macrocrania, however, is constitutional or familial megalocephaly. The differential diagnosis of progressive infant macrocrania also includes subdural hygromas, subdural hematomas, recovery from starvation, Canavan disease, Alexander disease, thickened skull associated with thalassemia and osteopetrosis, lead encephalopathy, and mucopolysaccharidoses. Posterior fossa tumors are not common in infancy. A rare cause of hydrocephalus in infancy is a choroid plexus papilloma or carcinoma that produces an excessive amount of CSF and enlarges the ventricles. Even after the choroid plexus tumor has been removed, hydrocephalus may persist because of postoperative distortion or stenosis of the CSF pathway.

Childhood

The most common cause of hydrocephalus in a child is a posterior fossa tumor, but congenital hydrocephalus caused by aqueductal stenosis also may be discovered late. The hydrocephalus of posterior fossa tumors is associated with obstruction of the fourth ventricle and its outlets into the subarachnoid space. The most common brain tumors in childhood are medulloblastoma, cerebellar astrocytoma, and ependymoma. In a majority of cases the hydrocephalus is relieved by removing the tumor. In childhood, hydrocephalus does not manifest with macrocrania or delayed development, but rather with signs and symptoms of increased intracranial pressure—headaches, vomiting, papilledema, and ataxia.

Adolescence

In adolescence, hydrocephalus often occurs with the same constellation of signs and symptoms as in childhood, but also may manifest more subtly with a change in school performance or athletic ability. Papilledema is seen more reliably in older, more cooperative young people. In adolescence, a brainstem tumor, a pineal cyst, or a pineal region tumor is more commonly the primary cause of new onset hydrocephalus. An MRI is essential to rule out these possibilities definitively.

TREATMENT

In the hands of a pediatric neurosurgeon, the modern treatment of hydrocephalus is straightforward, and the ventriculoperitoneal shunt is the gold standard. Sufficient peritoneal tubing can be coiled in the peritoneal cavity to accommodate axial growth. Based on the experience of the past 2 decades, 1 to 2 revisions of a shunt can be expected every 10 years. If the peritoneal cavity cannot be used, a ventriculoatrial, ventriculopleural, or ventricle-to-gallbladder shunt can be substituted. Communicating hydrocephalus also can be treated with a lumboperitoneal shunt. A variety of methods have been used to divert the CSF internally: third ventriculostomy (opening the third ventricle directly into the subarachnoid space through the lamina terminalis),[3] choroid plexectomy, and Torkildsen shunt (lateral ventricle shunted to cisterna magna). These modes of treating hydrocephalus are effective only if the subarachnoid space is open and CSF can be absorbed. Several shunt valves and options are available to be tailored to the patient's special needs. In general, however, a low-pressure shunt is implanted in the preterm infant who has hydrocephalus associated with intraventricular hemorrhage and in a neonate who has very severe hydrocephalus (head circumference >42 cm). In all other patients, a medium-pressure shunt generally is preferable. In the older child who has hydrocephalus and a very large head, an antisiphon device incorporated into the shunt helps to prevent collapse of the ventricular system and the development of subdural hematomas. Several devices are available to fulfill this purpose and to suit the surgeon's preference.

The medical treatment of hydrocephalus largely has been unsuccessful. Acetazolamide (Diamox) is administered to decrease the output of the choroid plexus but is not always well tolerated, and tachyphylaxis develops rapidly.

PROGNOSIS

An infant treated for hydrocephalus shortly after birth has greater than an 85% chance of survival and 53% probability of having normal intelligence (IQ >80).[8] The thickness of the cerebral mantle and underlying abnormalities of the brain reduce the probability of a normal outcome. Mean head circumference of 42 cm and a cerebral mantle of 1 cm thickness at birth was seen in retarded (IQ <65) survivors. Children who have severe hydrocephalus and no underlying abnormalities can lead normal, productive lives if the hydrocephalus is treated early.[10] With few exceptions, shunts must be maintained for the lifetime of the patient; children don't "outgrow" hydrocephalus.

MANAGEMENT AND COMPLICATIONS

Shunt Malfunction

Continuing management of the shunted hydrocephalic patient can be quite problematic. Shunt malfunction can manifest in a myriad of ways, but generally causes lethargy, vomiting, and headache, which are symptoms of many common childhood illnesses. In the infant, headaches often are supplanted by a full fontanelle and irritability. In a child, shunt malfunction also can cause a change in behavior and decline in school performance. Aggressive and demanding behavior is not uncommon. Parents often relate by phone that the child's "eyes aren't right." Routine inspection of the shunt tract and measurement of the head circumference are important in screening for shunt complications. A slack fontanelle in an infant who is held in an upright position is reliable evidence of good shunt function. When the fontanelle closes, a CT scan should be done to define a baseline ventricular size. Pumping the valve seldom offers useful information and may occlude the ventricular catheter by aspirating choroid plexus or debris into the tip of the catheter. Papilledema may be present. Lateral eye movement may be diminished, and convergence usually disappears. The classic "sun-setting" sign (downward deviation of the eye with the iris "setting" on the "horizon" of the inferior lid margin) is not common but is a sure sign of shunt failure. Blindness occurs rarely. CT usually will show enlargement of the ventricles when compared with the baseline scan, which was done when the fontanelle closed. The primary care physician must be aware, however, that a child who has severe headaches, vomiting, and increased lethargy may still have life-threatening shunt malfunction, even though a CT scan shows normal-size ventricles.[11] If the CT scan shows enlarged ventricles and obliteration of the perimesencephalic cisterns, an emergent shunt revision is in order.[7] In this author's hands, routine annual CT scans and plain radiographs of the shunt have not helped to anticipate shunt failure.

Shunt Infection

Shunt infection complicates 5% of shunt operations. Infection commonly is associated with fever, an elevated white blood cell count, and redness along the shunt tract. The symptoms may be limited to low grade fever, abdominal discomfort, and anorexia. Most shunt infections occur within 3 months of shunt implantation or a shunt revision. Rarely, infection occurs many years later as focal redness and tenderness along the shunt tract. Adequate treatment dictates removal of the old shunt, placement of a temporary ventriculostomy for external CSF drainage, and intravenous (IV) antibiotics.[6] *Staphylococcus epidermidis* (coagulase-negative staph) and *Staphylococcus aureus* (coagulase-positive staph) are the most common infecting organisms, and vancomycin (60 mg/kg/day) is the antibiotic of choice. Intrathecal antibiotics seldom are necessary if adequate serum peak and trough levels of antibiotic are administered. Shunts can extrude through the urethra, anus, or the vagina and must then be presumed to be infected and treated with removal of the shunt and temporary diversion using an external drainage device. Abdominal pseudocysts or localized pockets of CSF may develop with or without infection.

In the child who has hydrocephalus who also contracts an acute abdominal condition, the diagnosis may well be appendicitis. If the appendix has perforated to produce diffuse or localized peritonitis, the shunt catheter should be removed from the abdomen and connected to a drainage-collection bag until all signs of infection have disappeared. Children who have spina bifida who undergo bladder augmentation to expand the capacity of the bladder may perforate the bladder and exhibit an acute abdominal condition. Temporary externalization of the peritoneal catheter is necessary.

Ventriculoatrial Shunts

Ventriculoatrial shunts can be complicated by septicemia, bacterial endocarditis, glomerulonephritis, pulmonary embolus, migration of the atrial catheter into the pulmonary vasculature, cardiac arrhythmias, and cor pulmonale. The complication rate is comparable to that of VP shunts, but complications are more life threatening.

Seizures

Seizures occur in about 30% of shunted patients, usually because of an underlying abnormality of the brain. Recurrent seizures are an uncommon indication of shunt failure.

Slit Ventricle Syndrome

Overdrainage of the ventricular system by a shunt occurs rarely and manifests as the slit ventricle syndrome.[12] Severe headaches exacerbated by activity in an upright posture are relieved at least partially by lying down. The slit ventricle syndrome is associated with nonexistent or very small slit-like ventricles. Many children have slit ventricles on CT scan but are not symptomatic. Symptoms presumably are caused by stiff, noncompliant ventricles that must first expand to push the ventricular wall away from the catheter. The treatment may be as simple as afternoon rest periods (in horizontal position) or may involve changing the valve to one that incorporates an antisiphon device or a variable resistance mechanism.

Subdural Hygromas

Subdural hygromas may occur in the child who is shunted after the fontanelle has closed and the skull has become more fixed in size and shape. Because the skull has expanded to an abnormally large size to accommodate the brain and hydrocephalus, extra space is created when the ventricles decrease in size and the brain reconstitutes itself. The accumulation of CSF in the subdural space usually resolves spontaneously. If the subdural hygroma enlarges and causes symptoms of pressure, a separate subdural-peritoneal shunt may be necessary. This complication can be avoided if an antisiphon device is incorporated into the valve.

Shunt Metastases

The risk of metastasis from shunting children who have primary central nervous system tumors is small and does not justify the insertion of a Millipore filter to screen tumor cells.[1] The filter often clogs and results in shunt failure.

Prophylactic Antibiotics

Prophylactic antibiotics are given by most pediatric neurosurgeons to prevent shunt infection during shunt implantation and revision. This author, however, does not recommend routine prophylaxis for dental work on the child who has a ventriculoperitoneal shunt. Prophylactic antibiotics are recommended for children who have ventriculoatrial shunts or in children who have VP shunts who undergo abdominal procedures that involve manipulating the peritoneal catheter.

WHEN TO REFER

Unremitting headaches with or without vomiting may be sufficient reason for referring the hydrocephalic patient to a pediatric neurosurgeon. If CT shows enlargement of the ventricular system compared with previous studies, then an urgent referral is indicated. However, even if no change is apparent on serial CTs, shunt malfunction still is possible. Intermittent headaches, especially those that occur in the morning and gradually subside during the day, may be associated with shunt malfunction. The classic symptom triad of shunt failure (headaches, vomiting, lethargy) is not always present and must be differentiated from common childhood illnesses.

Progressive macrocrania may be the only sign of shunt malfunction. Seizures are not a common sign of shunt malfunction. Only 4% of shunted children who are seen in an emergency room for seizures go on to have a shunt revision. Unless a seizure is associated with some other sign of shunt malfunction, the patient need not be referred or hospitalized.

WHEN TO HOSPITALIZE

The hydrocephalic patient who cannot be easily aroused should be hospitalized with the presumptive diagnosis of shunt failure. If emergent CT scan shows enlargement of the ventricle compared with previous baseline scans, then an urgent revision should be done. If the basal cisterns on the CT scan are obliterated, then an emergent revision will be necessary because the malfunction is life threatening.

REFERENCES

1. Berger MS et al: The risks of metastases from shunting in children with primary central nervous system tumor, *J Neurosurg* 74:872, 1991.
2. Carey CM, Tullous MW, Walker ML: Hydrocephalus: etiology, pathologic effects, diagnosis, and natural history. In Check WR, editor: *Pediatric neurosurgery,* Philadelphia, 1994, WB Saunders.
3. Cohen AR: Endoscopic ventricular surgery, *Pediatr Neurosurg* 19:127, 1993.
4. Davidoff LM: Treatment of hydrocephalus: historical review and description of a new method, *Arch Surg* 18:1737, 1929.
5. Davson H, Welch K, Segal MB: *Physiology and pathophysiology of cerebrospinal fluid,* Edinburgh, 1987, Churchill Livingstone.
6. James HE et al: Prospective randomized study of therapy in cerebrospinal fluid shunt infection, *Neurosurgery* 7:459, 1980.
7. Johnson DL, McCullough DC, Schwarz S: Perimesencephalic cistern obliteration: a CT sign of life-threatening shunt failure, *J Neurosurg* 64:386, 1986.
8. McCullough DM, Balzer-Martin LA: Current prognosis in overt neonatal hydrocephalus, *J Neurosurg* 57:378, 1982.
9. Milhorat TH: *Hydrocephalus and the cerebrospinal fluid,* Baltimore, 1972, Williams & Wilkins.
10. Piatt JH Jr, Carlson CV: A search for determinants of cerebrospinal fluid shunt survival: retrospective analysis of a 14-year institutional experience, *Pediatr Neurosurg* 19:233, 1993.
11. Sainte-Rose C et al: Mechanical complications in shunts, *Pediatr Neurosurg* 17:2, 1991.
12. Wisoff JH, Epstein FJ: Diagnosis and treatment of the slit ventricle syndrome, *Concepts Pediatr Neurosurg* 11:79, 1991.

216 Hyperthyroidism

Nicholas Jospe

DEFINITION

Hyperthyroidism is the result of excessive activity of the thyroid gland. The clinical manifestation of excessive circulating thyroid hormone is called thyrotoxicosis.

PATHOGENESIS

With a few exceptions, thyrotoxicosis in pediatrics is the result of Graves disease.[3] Graves disease is most frequent in early adolescence, is rare in infancy, and is infrequent in childhood. Affected subjects frequently have a family history of thyroid disorder. The prevalence of Graves disease is six to eight times greater in girls than in boys.

Graves disease, like Hashimoto thyroiditis, is an autoimmune disorder that occurs in subjects who have a genetic predisposition linked to certain HLA haplotypes.[12] Hyperfunction of the thyroid gland in Graves disease is caused by autoantibodies directed against the receptor for TSH.[13] These antibodies, called thyroid receptor antibodies (TRAb), are characterized by an overall predominant stimulatory effect on the thyroid cell. Included among TRAbs are (1) thyroid-stimulating immunoglobulins (TSI) that mimic TSH, (2) TSH-binding inhibitory immunoglobulins (TBII) that can inhibit TSH from binding at its receptor and do not stimulate the thyroid cell, and (3) TSH-blocking antibodies (TbAb). Other antibodies detected in patients who have Graves disease include thyroid growth-stimulating antibodies, which contribute to goiter formation, and antithyroglobulin and antimicrosomal antibodies that also are found in Hashimoto thyroiditis.[13] Graves disease can occur in conjunction with other endocrine autoimmune disease, such as insulin-dependent diabetes mellitus, hypoparathyroidism, and Addison disease, or with other autoimmune diseases such as myasthenia gravis, periodic paralysis, or vitiligo.

CLINICAL FEATURES (Table 216-1)

Early nonspecific findings in Graves disease include changes in behavior such as nervousness, emotional lability, decreased school performance, or deteriorating handwriting, which largely reflect hyperactivity of the sympathetic nervous system. Not infrequently, Graves disease remains undiagnosed for a long time because children can continue their normal activities without complaints overtly suggestive of hyperthyroidism. When cardiovascular signs are more prominent, these include tachycardia, a widened pulse pressure, and an overactive precordium. Neuromuscular signs and symptoms include tremor, a shortened deep tendon relaxation phase, fatigability, and proximal muscle weakness. Though the child has an increased appetite, he or she loses weight more frequently than gains weight and also has frequent and loose bowel movements. Increased perspiration, warmth, heat intolerance, and smoothness of skin appear later. With longstanding disease, tall stature may accompany advanced skeletal maturation in childhood, though curtailment of final height does not occur.

The size of the goiter when first examined is variable, and its presence frequently goes unnoticed. However, the thyroid gland usually is diffuse and enlarged, soft, and nontender and has a clearly delineated border. Examination should include palpation for the presence of a thrill and auscultation for the presence of a bruit. Measurement of the size of the lobes and of the isthmus is essential in following the course of the disease. Eye findings also are variable, although severe ophthalmopathy is far less common in children than in adults. These eye findings include prominence of the eyes (proptosis or exophthalmos), a conspicuous stare (due to lid retraction and a widened palpebral fissure, as shown in Fig. 216-1), and lag of the upper lid upon downward gaze. These eye findings are due to a combination of hyperactivity of the sympathetic system and of mucopolysaccharide accumulation and cellular infiltration of the orbital fat and muscles. In children, mucopolysaccharide accumulation in skin and subcutaneous tissue, such as pretibial myxedema, is infrequent.

LABORATORY DIAGNOSIS

The initial assessment should include measurement of serum free T_4 and total T_4 concentrations and of TSH concentration by using a sensitive radioimmunoassay. The diagnosis of Graves disease rests on demonstrating elevated levels of T_4 and suppression of TSH levels to below the lower limit of detectability. Age appropriate normal values for T_4 *must* be consulted before a diagnosis of hyperthyroidism can be made.[4] Measurement of T_3 may help confirm the diagnosis, although this rarely is necessary. In thyrotoxicosis, the response of TSH to thyroid-releasing hormone (TRH) is blunted severely or absent. The TRH stimulation test is necessary only when Graves disease is suspected but the diagnosis is unclear. In equivocal situations, measurement of TRAbs may help to confirm the diagnosis. In pregnant patients, high levels of TSI are predictive of neonatal Graves disease.

The measurement of thyroid gland uptake of radioiodine (^{123}I) or technetium (^{99m}Tc) is useful only to distinguish painless thyroiditis from Graves disease. Patients who have thyroiditis have a low uptake; patients who have Graves disease have a high uptake. Generally, this study is not necessary.

DIFFERENTIAL DIAGNOSIS

Rarely, children appear thyrotoxic and have laboratory evidence of Hashimoto thyroiditis because of a high titer of TSI among the spectrum of other autoantibodies present in blood.

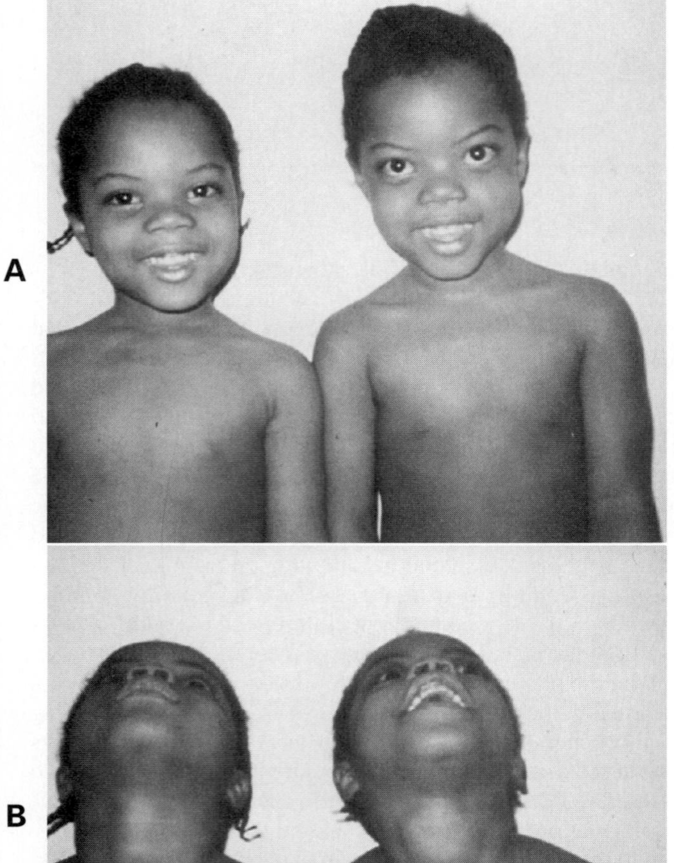

FIG. 216-1 The patient on the right exhibits a widened palpebral fissure and goiter; her twin, on the left, is unaffected.

This condition has been called Hashitoxicosis and may be differentiated from routine Graves disease in that it usually is transient. Other causes of hyperthyroxinemia are rare. These include generalized resistance to thyroid hormone, found in association with attention deficit disorder,[7] factitious hyperthyroidism from excessive administration of thyroid hormone, TSH-secreting pituitary adenomas, and binding-protein changes characterized by normal free T_4 and TSH levels. Finally, hyperthyroidism caused by autonomous thyroid adenomas is rare and can be seen in association with the McCune-Albright syndrome (precocious puberty, café-au-lait pigmentation, and polyostotic fibrous dysplasia).

MANAGEMENT

Antithyroid Medications

The aim of treatment is to reduce thyroid hormone production and block its effect on tissue peripherally. To this end, antithyroid medication consisting of thionamides, either methimazole (Tapazole) or propylthiouracil (PTU), usually are used first.[1,2] They are equally effective in inhibiting thyroid hormone production; however, PTU also blocks the peripheral conversion of T_4 to T_3. The half-life of PTU is 1 to 2 hours, whereas that of methimazole is 6 to 13 hours. Both drugs cross the placenta, although PTU does so less than methimazole and therefore is the preferred drug during pregnancy. Both are present in very small quantities in breast milk, and breast-feeding may be continued. Therapy induces euthyroidism somewhat faster with methimazole than with PTU and from within weeks to a few months, depending on the size of the thyroid gland. Starting doses of PTU range from 5 to 10 mg/kg body weight, with a maximum of 300 mg per day, in three to four divided doses, whereas the dosage of methimazole is approximately 0.5-1 mg/kg, with a maximum of 30 mg per day, in two to three divided doses. Once thyroid hormone secretion is depressed, maintenance doses may be given in two to three daily doses for PTU and one to two for methimazole.

Optimal long-term therapy for Graves disease continues to be the subject of research and some controversy. Some physicians prefer to titrate the dose of antithyroid medication to maintain the patient in a euthyroid state. Others administer antithyroid medication until the patient becomes hypothyroid and supplement thereafter with thyroid hormone. This combined therapy induces maximal suppression of the thyroid gland and appears to increase the likelihood of sustained remission upon discontinuation.[6]

Therapy with antithyroid medication usually is maintained for a minimum of 1 year, during which time monitoring the size of the thyroid gland and following the TRAb levels can be useful, because shrinkage of the thyroid gland and falling TRAb titers predict a greater likelihood of remission after discontinuation of therapy. Thereafter, antithyroid medication can be stopped, and 20% to 40% of patients remain in remission. Continued monitoring of thyroid function tests is indicated to detect any subclinical relapse of Graves disease.

Potential side effects of the thionamides include minor reactions that subside spontaneously, such as a purpuric, papular rash, urticaria, joint pain, stiffness, hair loss, and nausea or headaches and one serious reaction, namely agranulocytosis.[2] Agranulocytosis is an idiosyncratic reaction occurring

Table 216-1 Clinical Signs and Symptoms in Children Who Have Graves Disease

	Prevalence (%)		
Signs and symptoms	Saxena[11]	Mäenpää[8]	Barnes[1]
Goiter	100	100	97
Prominence of eyes	100	69	79
Exophthalmos	77		
Tachycardia	91	41	88
Nervousness	80	74	92
Increased appetite	71		67
Weight loss	67	59	50
Emotional lability	41		40
Heat intolerance	40		25
Frequent stools	16	35	13

in 1:500 to 1:1000 cases, usually within the first few months of therapy after either form of antithyroid medication. White blood cell count monitoring is not useful in anticipating agranulocytosis because its onset is very sudden. Patients thus need to be told about the significance of a sore throat, mouth sores, and fever as potentially heralding agranulocytosis. In addition to supportive treatment, such as antibiotherapy, discontinuation of the thionamide is necessary. Agranulocytosis spontaneously reverses, and resumption with a different thionamide does not usually cause agranulocytosis to recur.[2] Finally, reactions such as drug fever, nephritis, hepatitis, or lupuslike reactions are rare.

In addition to antithyroid medication, adjuvant beta-adrenergic blockade may be accomplished with propranolol, 0.5-2 mg/kg/day to control the sympathetic hyperactivity of severe Graves disease. This form of therapy is necessary only transiently. It may be contraindicated in patients who have cardiac failure, arrhythmias, or asthma.

Iodine has a minor short-term role as adjuvant therapy in patients who develop toxicity to either PTU or methimazole or as adjunctive therapy immediately before thyroidectomy and for treatment of severe thyrotoxicosis. In practice, it seldom is used.

Definitive Therapy

If a relapse of Graves disease occurs upon discontinuation of antithyroid medication, the therapeutic choices include either resumption of antithyroid medication or definitive therapy consisting of radioiodine or surgery. The choice depends on factors that affect the chances of success of each form of therapy, such as compliance, patient preference, and surgical expertise.

Surgery resolves the symptoms faster, but radioiodine is easy to administer, safer, and equally efficacious.[2,5] The potential for surgical complications from injury to adjacent structures (recurrent laryngeal nerve damage and hypoparathyroidism) dictates that referral be made to an experienced surgeon. Permanent hypothyroidism following surgery is frequent.[2] Radioiodine therapy is being used more extensively in the pediatric population, because fears regarding thyroid carcinoma and leukemia and radiation and genetic damage have been alleviated.[5,10] Radioactive iodine concentrates in the thyroid gland and induces cell death over time. Permanent hypothyroidism occurs within a year in 10% to 20% of patients following radioablative therapy. Pregnancy is a contraindication for radioiodine therapy because the iodine crosses the placenta and destroys the fetal thyroid.

PROGNOSIS AND COMPLICATIONS

Unfortunately, no reliable factors predict the natural course of Graves disease in a given patient. The clinical course ranges from progression to overt hypothyroidism on one hand to progression to thyroid storm on the other. Thyroid storm (thyrotoxic crisis) is an exceptional but severe complication.[9] This diagnosis rests on finding uncontrolled hyperthyroidism and is characterized by a constellation of findings including cardiac failure, tachycardia, hyperthermia, and central nervous system abnormalities such as confusion, apathy, or coma. Precipitating factors are stress, such as infection (even relatively minor), and trauma. Therapy must be expeditious and aggressive and include antithyroid medication (as previously described), iodide, beta-blockade, antipyresis, and cardiac medications.

NEONATAL THYROTOXICOSIS

Graves disease, rare in neonates,[4] is due to the transplacental passage of thyroid-directed immunoglobulins from the mother, who may or may not have active autoimmune thyroid disease. In addition, different classes of maternal thyroid antibodies—that is, stimulatory and blocking thyroid antibodies—may disappear at different rates, making the course of neonatal Graves disease difficult to predict. Thus its onset may be immediate or delayed for weeks, and its duration may be brief or prolonged, lasting up to 6 months.[14] Of note, transient neonatal hypothyroxinemia may result from the transfer of maternally derived TBII.

The clinical signs and symptoms of neonatal Graves disease include microcephaly, frontal bossing, tachycardia, hypertension, irritability, failure to thrive, flushing, exophthalmos, and goiter. Vomiting, diarrhea, hepatosplenomegaly, jaundice, and thrombocytopenia also can occur. Cardiac failure and arrhythmias account for a mortality that approaches 25% when the disease is severe and treated inadequately.[4] Long-term complications are severe and include hypothyroidism, premature craniosynostosis, and primarily intellectual developmental defects.

Until the disease resolves spontaneously, usually within 1 to 3 months as the maternal antibodies are degraded, adjunctive therapy may be necessary. The starting dose for methimazole is 0.5-1 mg/kg/day and that of PTU, 5-10 mg/kg/day: these doses can be increased up to 50%. Once thyroid hormone synthesis has been blocked adequately, iodide can be given and has an additive effect. Lugol solution (5% iodine and 10% potassium iodide) is given at a dose of one drop every 8 hours. In severely hyperactive neonates, propranolol, 2 mg/kg/day, and digitalis, for cardiac failure, may be required. Finally, glucocorticoid therapy may be beneficial.

REFERENCES

1. Barnes VH, Blizzard RM: Antithyroid drug therapy for toxic diffuse goiter (Graves' disease): thirty years experience in children and adolescents, *J Pediatr* 91:313, 1977.
2. Cooper SD: Treatment of thyrotoxicosis. In Braverman LE, Utiger RD, editors: *Werner and Ingbar's the thyroid: a fundamental and clinical text,* Philadelphia, 1991, JB Lippincott.
3. Feldmann M et al: Mechanism of Graves thyroiditis: implications for concepts and therapy of autoimmunity, *Int Rev Immunol* 9:91, 1992.
4. Fisher DA: The thyroid. In Kaplan SA, editor: *Clinical pediatric endocrinology,* Philadelphia, 1990, WB Saunders.
5. Hamburger JI: Management of hyperthyroidism in children and adolescents, *J Clin Endocrinol Metab* 60:1019, 1985.
6. Hashizume K et al: Administration of thyroxine in treated Graves' disease: effects on the level of antibodies to thyroid-stimulating hormone receptors and on the risk of recurrence of hyperthyroidism, *N Engl J Med* 324:947, 1991.
7. Hauser P et al: Attention deficit/hyperactivity disorder in people with generalized resistance to thyroid hormone, *N Engl J Med* 328:997, 1993.
8. Mäenpää J, Hiekkala H, Lamberg BA: Childhood hyperthyroidism, *Acta Endocrinol* 51:321, 1966.

9. Roth RN, McAuliffe MJ: Hyperthyroidism and thyroid storm, *Emerg Med Clin North Am* 7:873, 1989.
10. Saenger EL, Thoma GE, Thompkins EA: Incidence of leukemia following treatment of hyperthyroidism: preliminary report of the Cooperative Thyrotoxicosis Therapy Follow-up study, *JAMA* 205:147, 1968.
11. Saxena KM, Crawford JD, Talbot NB: Childhood thyrotoxicosis: a long-term perspective, *BMJ* 2:1153, 1964.
12. Volpe R: Immunoregulation in autoimmune thyroid disease, *N Engl J Med* 316:44, 1987.
13. Volpe R: Graves' disease. In Braverman LE, Utiger RD, editors: *Werner and Ingbar's the thyroid: a fundamental and clinical text,* Philadelphia, 1991, JB Lippincott.
14. Zakarija M, McKenzie JM, Munro DS: Immunoglobulin G inhibitor of thyroid stimulating antibody is a cause of delay in the onset of neonatal Graves' disease, *J Clin Invest* 72:1352, 1983.

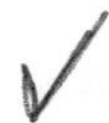

217 Hypospadias, Epispadias, and Cryptorchism

Henry M. Seidel and John P. Gearhart

The male genitalia are much more often a cause of parental preoccupation at the birth of a child than are the female. Untold variables govern this, most of them not readily apparent. The most obvious, of course, is that they are much more accessible. Less concern usually exists about the relationship of the penis to the urinary tract than to sexual function. Still, it is as a part of the urinary tract that it serves its immediate purpose at birth; it must wait until puberty to begin to realize its additional potential.

GENITAL ABNORMALITY

An external genital deformity in the newborn boy usually is obvious immediately—for example, hypospadias, epispadias, injury, swelling, and after careful palpation, undescended testes. To feel both testes is important. Although frequently of somewhat different size in a newborn, they generally are descended in a full-term infant and frequently undescended in the premature infant. One cause of parental distress often is not noted at birth but perhaps several weeks later as the baby gains weight: So much of a suprapubic fat pad can exist that the penis, retracted, may seem to disappear despite its being some 4 cm long. The physician however, must not belittle the concern; the parents should be assured that the condition will correct itself in time. Only rarely does a real problem exist, namely, a micropenis, which suggests a dysmorphic abnormality.

Hypospadias

Among the possible penile abnormalities, hypospadias, which occurs in 8.1 : 1000 newborn boys, still is the most common. In this event, the urethral meatus opens on the ventral surface of the penis, most often between the glans and midshaft of the penis (60%), but it may be located at any point along the shaft or scrotum (25%) or as proximal as the perineum (15%) (Fig. 217-1). The prepuce is incompletely formed, covering only the dorsal surface of the penis. In approximately 10% of cases an associated unilateral or bilateral cryptorchism is present. On rare occasions incomplete scrotal fusion and cryptorchism occurs; this combination suggests the possibility of an intersex anomaly.

The pediatrician must decide when to refer the patient to a pediatric urologist. Obviously the severity of the deformity and the position of the meatus on the undershaft of the penis will greatly influence the decision making regarding surgery. If the hypospadias is mild and situated at or close to the corona, and if relatively little deformity is present, the repair is quite straightforward, accomplished in same-day surgery, and little more than a glorified circumcision. Occasionally a meatal stenosis that can be corrected easily may be associated with the hypospadias at the time of hypospadias repair. Chordee, the downward curving of the penis as a result of abnormal ventral fibrous bands, often is present and is one of the factors that must be addressed at the time of surgical intervention. Currently, most hypospadias defects can be corrected with a single procedure. Although the frequency of an associated anomaly of the upper urinary tract is known to be low, many parents request sonography to be assured that the upper tract is normal. In any event, the pediatric urologist should be consulted immediately, because the judgment concerning the necessity for repair is properly shared with the surgeon.

Even if the hypospadias defect is severe, a single stage repair often will be performed. The decision as to the right time for surgery and the precise approach to use must rest in large part with the pediatric urologist, but usually is performed between 1 and 2 years of age. The pediatrician, however, cannot relinquish responsibility for providing concomitant care; he or she is needed to interpret events and, in a highly charged emotional circumstance, to provide appropriate counseling to parents (and, as the child grows older, to the child). This is especially important when sexual function is threatened and sexual identity worried about. A circumcision should *not* be performed in the presence of hypospadias, however mild. None of the tissue that might be needed for repair should be sacrificed. On occasion, if the hypospadias is severe or accompanied by associated genital anomalies, a referral for endocrine evaluation is indicated. In the presence of hypospadias alone, aside from an infrequent defect in androgen responsiveness, little likelihood exists of significant hormonal disturbance.

Epispadias

Less frequently (1 : 112,000 live male births), the meatus is formed on the dorsum of the penis at various points along the glans and shaft, and on rare occasion so far back as to be beneath the symphysis pubis. The more proximal deformity may be associated with complete incontinence because of involvement of the bladder neck area along with distortion of the normal architecture of the pubic bones. Early consultation with the pediatric urologist is necessary; again, circumcision is to be avoided.

CRYPTORCHISM

Given that the descent of the testes from within the abdomen to the scrotum usually takes place by about week 36 of fetal life, the incidence of cryptorchism (undescended testes) is much higher in the premature infant. Spontaneous descent of the testes after birth, if it is to occur, generally does so

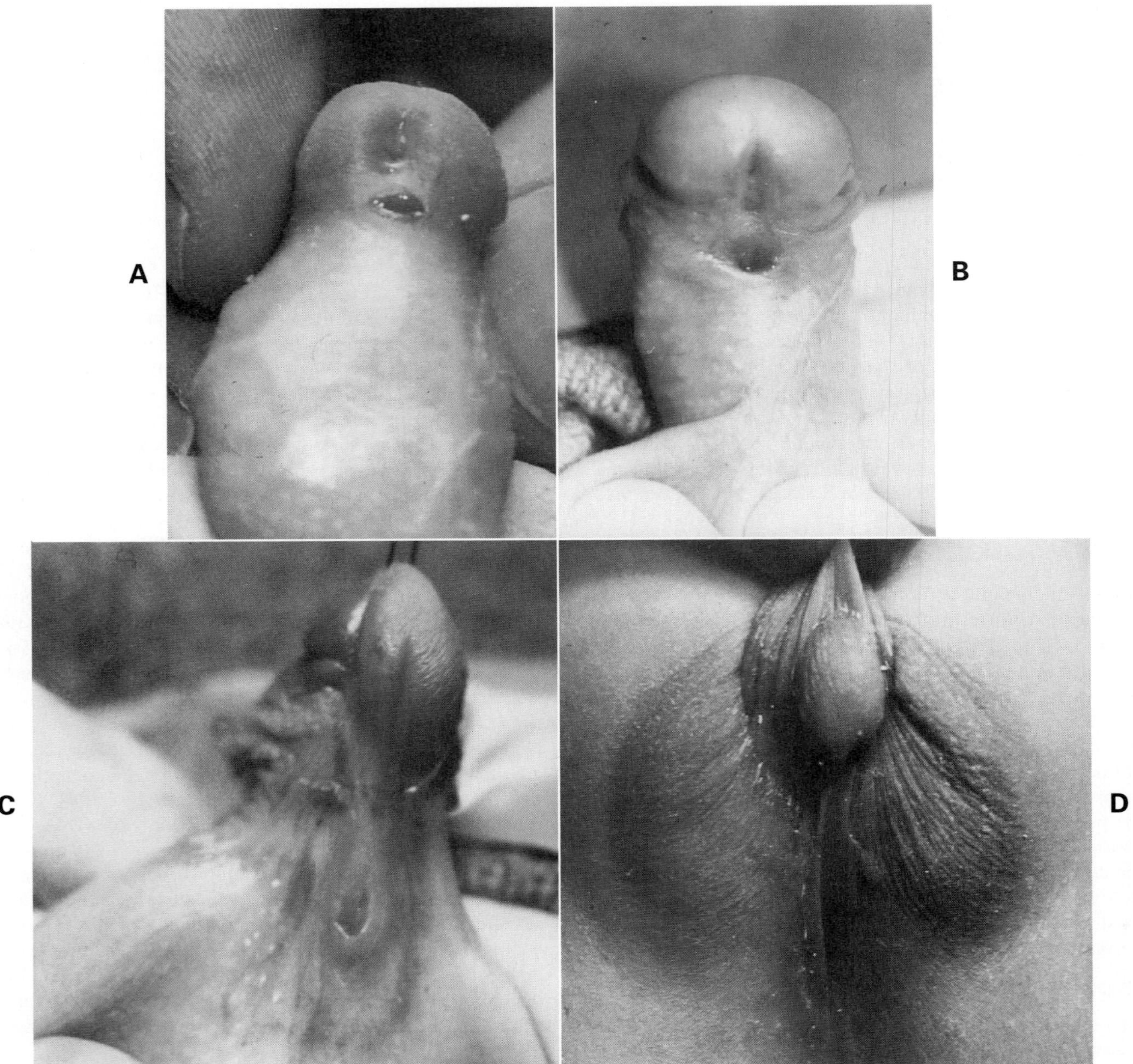

FIG. 217-1 Varieties of hypospadias. **A,** Coronal. **B,** Distal shaft. **C,** Penoscrotal. **D,** Perineal.

well before the end of the first year; if this does not happen by the first birthday, some concern is warranted. This involves the child's potential for childbearing and for sexual function, because with cryptorchism, cellular damage is increasingly likely with each passing year, damage that probably is not reversible after the age of 4 or 5 years. On examination, one must be sure that the testis is truly undescended. Occasionally, an overactive cremasteric reflex may make palpation difficult. Moving the infant or the older child into the tailor position (sitting cross-legged) or a kneeling position can help to overcome this. One must feel from above downward, "milking" the testis from the inguinal canal into the scrotum. The older patient can help this process by coughing or straining. Cold hands and abrupt palpation can invoke the cremasteric reflex. If one or the other of the testes is not felt, one should search beyond the scrotum and the inguinal canal, feeling the femoral triangle and the inner thigh. Many undescended testes are associated with an inguinal hernia and possibly a hydrocele; these masses can make palpation of the testes even more difficult. If the testis is impalpable and a hernia is present, the testis usually lies just inside the internal inguinal ring.

Actually, the testes, if undescended, may have stopped their descent at some point within the inguinal canal or still may be in the abdomen. If a testis has not reached the inguinal canal, the likelihood is greater that it is abnormal; the lower the testis lies in the inguinal canal, the more likely that it is normal. Sonography has proven helpful only with the inguinal undescended testis. Computed tomography (CT) scan exposes the child to radiation, requires sedation, and has many false positive and false negative results. It should be avoided.

A testis that retracts simply because of an overactive cremasteric reflex obviously should not be "repaired." The truly undescended testis needs repair to improve the chance for fertility, provide accessible examination (particularly in the event of malignant change), diminish the possibility of testicular torsion, and prevent the emotional trauma that frequently accompanies the condition.

Given that one or both testes truly are ectopic or "hidden," the management plan raises certain questions: How long should one wait for descent before surgical intervention? Does a "best" time exist emotionally? Is worry about infertility warranted? Can repair help in this regard? If one waits too long, is the child at greater risk for testicular malignancy as an adult?

Certainly no one wants an unnecessary operation. Still, one cannot wait until puberty to see if natural descent occurs. Whenever the location of the testis is uncertain, the potential for natural descent should be explored with a therapeutic trial of human chorionic gonadotropin (HCG), 1500 IU/m^2 body surface area intramuscularly twice a week for 4 weeks. If the testis is to descend, it generally will at this dosage level and duration. Treating with HCG over a longer period has disadvantages; it can hasten the onset of puberty and cause testicular damage and sterility. Surgery is the desirable alternative if the testis does not descend or goes back up after the HCG trial. For those who respond to the administration of HCG, the outlook for full sexual maturity is excellent. If the testes lie within the abdomen and are not palpable in the inguinal canal, HCG will not bring them down into the scrotum but may bring them into the inguinal canal where they are accessible to palpation. However, if a course of HCG (1500 IU/day intramuscularly for 3 days) is given, the functioning of the abdominally placed testes can be determined by detecting a rise in the serum testosterone level on the fourth day.

The optimum age for surgical correction of cryptorchism is between 6 and 12 months of age. Surgical procedures generally are tolerated well in early childhood, and such procedures probably are emotionally advantageous before the child is plunged into the day-to-day demands of school life and the public nakedness that often accompanies physical education classes. If for some reason surgical correction is delayed until adolescence (e.g., delayed diagnosis), a sperm count should be done to reassure the patient and physician regarding fertility or to prepare them for the realities of infertility. Testicular tumors occur with greater frequency in undescended testes. Although bringing the testis down does not diminish the potential of malignancy, it obviously increases the likelihood of detection. Periodic examination is important. Finally, if the patient has an associated inguinal hernia with or without a hydrocele, the hernia, along with orchiopexy, should be repaired immediately. An elective herniorrhaphy is preferable to one done in the face of incarceration and possible strangulation. In any event, cryptorchism should be repaired surgically before 2 years of age, primarily to reduce the risk of infertility.

Surgery may be done on an ambulatory basis when the testis is palpated in the inguinal canal. If it cannot be felt at all, a more extensive surgical procedure with an abdominal incision probably will be necessary unless preliminary laparoscopy reveals the testis to be absent. Either way, a demonstrably *abnormal* testis should be removed and replaced with a prosthesis. As with hypospadias or epispadias, the role of the pediatrician in the care of the patient and his family is obvious. The emotional support necessary when such a vital aspect of human function is threatened is enormous. Preparation for surgery requires full discussion about the child's and the parents' fears and concerns; these discussions should continue following surgery, particularly as the child grows older and begins to reflect on the event.

SUGGESTED READINGS

American Academy of Pediatrics: Timing of elective surgery on the genitalia of male children with particular reference to the risks, benefits, and psychological effects of surgery and anesthesia, *Pediatrics* 97:590, 1996.

Belman AB, Kass AJ: Hypospadias repair in children under one year of age, *J Urol* 128:1273, 1982.

Coloday AH: Undescended testes: is surgery necessary? *N Engl J Med* 314:510, 1986.

Gearhart JP, Jeffs RD: Diagnostic maneuvers in cryptorchidism, *Semin Urol* VI:79, 1988.

Neely EK, Rosenfeld RG: The undescended testicle: when and how to intervene, *Contemp Pediatrics* 7:21, 1990.

Schulze KA, Pfister RR: Evaluating the undescended testis, *Am Fam Physician* 31:133, 1988.

218 Hypothyroidism

Thomas P. Foley, Jr.

Few diseases affect multiple systems so severely as hypothyroidism, yet are associated with so many nonspecific symptoms and signs. Hypothyroidism can occur at any age and affect the fetus as early as the first trimester of pregnancy. Its clinical manifestation during infancy differs markedly from that of childhood and adolescence; for this reason, we must distinguish between congenital and juvenile-acquired hypothyroidism.[6] The clinical distinction of hypothyroidism as a neonate and child is complicated further by the recent recognition of acquired hypothyroidism during the first year of life.[8] As a result of screening programs for the detection of congenital hypothyroidism during the preclinical stage of the disease during the first 2 weeks of life, accurate data on the incidence of congenital hypothyroidism throughout the Western world indicate that approximately 1 infant is affected with congenital hypothyroidism for every 4000 live births.[7] The incidence is greater in iodine-deficient regions. The true incidence of juvenile hypothyroidism is not known. Both congenital hypothyroidism and juvenile hypothyroidism occur as familial or sporadic disease with or without enlargement of the thyroid gland (goiter, thyromegaly) and may progress as either a permanent or a transient disorder.[6]

ETIOLOGY

In most instances the causes of hypothyroidism differ during infancy and childhood[7] (see the box on p. 1359). An occasional patient who has a mild form of congenital hypothyroidism may be missed by newborn screening programs and not exhibit symptoms until childhood. These children usually have either familial goitrous hypothyroidism (dyshormonogenesis)[5] or thyroid dysgenesis with an ectopic thyroid gland located somewhere between the foramen cecum of the tongue and the anterior mediastinum. In most cases of permanent congenital hypothyroidism, the cause is unknown. Approximately 90% of patients have no thyroid tissue (athyreosis), an ectopic thyroid gland, or a hypoplastic thyroid gland found in the normal anterior cervical location.[3] Among infants who have permanent sporadic congenital hypothyroidism, antibody-dependent cell-mediated cytotoxicity (ADCC) was found in 32% of infants and 24% of their mothers.[2] Several inborn errors of thyroid hormone synthesis are inherited as an autosomal recessive trait and usually manifest with thyromegaly on physical examination.[5] In 2% of cases, antibodies that block the TSH receptor and are produced by a mother who has autoimmune thyroid disease cross the placenta and block the function of the fetal thyroid gland.[12] This form of transient hypothyroidism can persist for several weeks or months, and the affected infant requires thyroxine therapy until the antibodies disappear. Other types of transient congenital hypothyroidism may occur when drugs prescribed for the mother, such as propylthiouracil, methimazole, or iodides, cross the placenta to block the fetal thyroid gland. Therefore iodine-containing medications should not be applied to the skin or mucous membranes of neonates for more than a few days because the iodine is absorbed easily and blocks the infant's thyroid gland.

The most common cause of hypothyroidism in children beyond the perinatal period is goitrous or nongoitrous, autoimmune (chronic lymphocytic, Hashimoto) thyroiditis.[13] Rarely, the disease occurs just before the first birthday and progresses rapidly with few symptoms and signs of hypothyroidism.[8] An occasional patient who has hypothalamic or pituitary disease may be seen initially with hypothyroidism. These children usually have other clinical features to suggest an abnormality of the hypothalamus or pituitary.

HISTORY AND PHYSICAL EXAMINATION

Because hypothyroidism can affect most organ systems to varying degrees, it is very important that the clinician consider the diagnosis when the patient has many nonspecific or multisystemic complaints. Furthermore, a family history of thyroid and pituitary disease may disclose important diagnostic information. Many of the symptoms and signs of hypothyroidism are different during infancy compared with childhood.[7,10] These are summarized in the box on p. 1359. During the first month of life, affected infants may have no clinical symptoms or signs of hypothyroidism. Presumably, this occurs either because some transfer of thyroxine occurs in utero from mother to fetus,[16] failure of thyroid gland function (as with ectopic thyroid tissue) is incomplete, or the disease is of short duration, possibly developing during the third trimester of pregnancy.[7] In infants who have no functioning thyroid tissue, clinical symptoms and signs rarely may be present at birth, develop within the first few days of life, or appear as early as the first 2 weeks of life; they certainly are present by 6 weeks of age. The difficulty in diagnosing congenital hypothyroidism is evident when comparing the clinical features of three infants (Fig. 218-1). The infant on the upper left was referred at age 8 months with clinical features very suggestive of hypothyroidism, yet her thyroid studies were normal. The infant on the upper right had documented primary hypothyroidism at 4 weeks of age. Her clinical features at this age were minimal and included only mild periorbital edema, an enlarged posterior fontanelle, decreased stooling, and abdominal distention. The 6-month-old infant pictured at bottom center, in contrast, had severe hypothyroidism.

In addition, the clinical symptoms and signs of older children who have acquired hypothyroidism may be as nonspecific and insidious in their development as those found in infants who have congenital or acquired hypothyroidism.[6] If

CAUSES OF HYPOTHYROIDISM

Congenital hypothyroidism

A. Thyroid dysgenesis
  1. Thyroid aplasia
  2. Thyroid hypoplasia
  3. Ectopic thyroid gland
B. Familial abnormalities of thyroid hormone synthesis and metabolism (familial dyshormonogenesis)
C. Maternal disease
  1. Therapeutic doses of ^{131}I after the eleventh week of gestation
  2. Transplacental autoimmune thyroiditis
  3. Ingestion of goitrogens
D. Endemic goiter and cretinism
E. Hypothalamic-pituitary hypothyroidism
  1. Pituitary agenesis or aplasia
  2. Thyrotropin deficiency: isolated
  3. Hypothalamic hormone deficiency
    a. Isolated thyrotropin deficiency
    b. Multiple tropic hormone deficiencies
    c. Septooptic dysplasia
    d. Anencephaly
  4. Hypothalamic-pituitary lesions

Juvenile hypothyroidism

A. Thyroiditis, autoimmune (Hashimoto)
  1. Atrophic thyroiditis of infancy
  2. Chronic lymphocytic thyroiditis of childhood
  3. Atrophic thyroiditis of childhood and adolescence
  4. Hashimoto thyroiditis (struma lymphomatosa)
B. Congenital thyroid dysgenesis
  1. Ectopic thyroid
  2. Hypoplastic
C. Congenital defects in thyroid hormone synthesis or metabolism
D. Iatrogenic thyroid ablation
  1. Surgical
  2. Radioactive iodine (^{131}I)
E. Ingestion of goitrogens
F. Endemic goiter
G. Hypothalamic-pituitary disease

SYMPTOMS AND SIGNS OF HYPOTHYROIDISM

Congenital hypothyroidism

Facial edema
Large posterior fontanelle (>0.5 cm)
Rectal temperature below 95° F (35° C)
Decreased stooling (less than one stool per day)
Prolonged hyperbilirubinemia (bilirubin above 10 mg/dl after 3 days of age)
Respiratory distress in a term infant
Umbilical hernia
Birth weight above 4000 g
Macroglossia
Bradycardia (pulse below 100 beats/min)
Feeding problems and lethargy
Cutaneous mottling, vasomotor instability
Hoarse cry
Hirsute forehead

Juvenile hypothyroidism

Growth retardation (below 4 cm/yr)
Delayed bone maturation
Delayed dental development and tooth eruption
Onset of puberty: usually delayed; rarely precocious
Myopathy and muscular hypertrophy
Menstrual disorders
Galactorrhea
Increased skin pigmentation
Physical and mental turpor
Pale, gray, cool, mottled, thickened, coarse skin
Constipation
Coarse, dry brittle hair

the disease has been present for more than 6 months, growth deceleration should be evident because normal thyroid hormone secretion is essential for normal linear growth. Hence, most patients who have juvenile hypothyroidism have either thyromegaly or a deceleration of growth and usually are short in stature.[6] Deceleration of linear growth should be identified by the physician who routinely measures the height of the patient; its early recognition will prevent the development of long-standing hypothyroidism and cessation of linear growth. The importance of this easy measurement cannot be overstressed. Frank obesity, however, is an uncommon complaint in children who have hypothyroidism because reduction in physical activity, if it occurs, usually is less than the reduction in caloric intake. On the other hand, children who have advanced hypothyroidism and myxedema usually are chubby and have periorbital edema.

Inspection and palpation of the anterior cervical area will enable the examiner to identify an enlarged thyroid gland, even in the neonate. The easiest method for examining the thyroid gland of an infant is to place the infant prone with the neck extended and feel for the isthmus of the thyroid, just below the hyoid bone. After identifying the isthmus, one should palpate laterally to delineate the lobes, which are very difficult to define in a normal infant. The examination of the

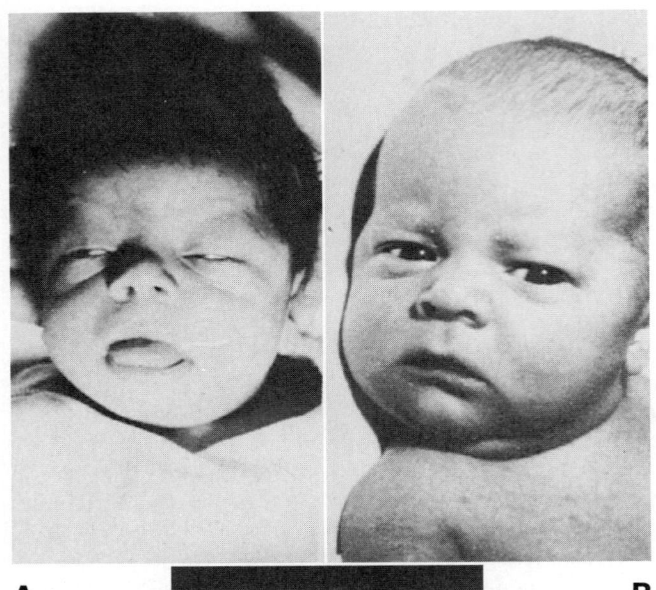

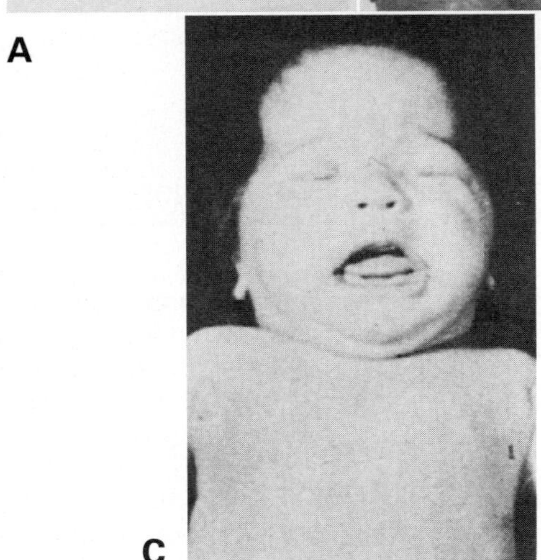

FIG. 218-1 **A,** Normal infant with clinical signs but no clinical symptoms of congenital hypothyroidism. **B,** Affected infant with athyreosis, age 28 days. **C,** Infant at age 6 months with athyreosis and severe congenital hypothyroidism.

(From Foley TP Jr: Sporadic congenital hypothyroidism. In Dussault JH, Walker P, editors: *Congenital hypothyroidism*, New York, 1983, Marcel Dekker.)

thyroid gland in an older child is easier. Having the patient swallow water will facilitate the identification and delineation of both lobes of the thyroid gland as distinct from other adjacent tissue, since the thyroid rises during swallowing.

LABORATORY DATA

Although the clinical laboratory may offer a wide battery of thyroid function tests, rarely are most of these tests necessary for the diagnosis of hypothyroidism. An elevation of the serum thyroid-stimulating hormone (TSH) value is the single most sensitive test for primary hypothyroidism (thyroid gland failure).[6] The combination of a low serum thyroxine (T_4) value and an elevated TSH is diagnostic of primary hypothyroidism, either permanent or transient, at any age, including term and preterm infants.[10] In patients who have hypothalamic or pituitary hypothyroidism, the determination of the T_4 (low) and TSH (not elevated or suppressed, but usually normal) is not adequate for definitive diagnosis because patients who have thyroxine-binding globulin (TBG) deficiency also will have a low T_4 and normal TSH. Hence the free, or unbound, thyroxine (free T_4) and TBG values, as well as specific tests of pituitary function, usually are necessary. The free T_4 determination by direct dialysis is the most accurate method and the least likely to give false positive or negative results from interfering drugs or other substances in serum.[6]

An occasional child or infant who has a coexisting and severe illness, such as idiopathic respiratory distress syndrome, may have the so-called euthyroid sick syndrome (or nonthyroidal illness syndrome) in which the T_4 may be low despite normal TBG levels.[6] The serum triiodothyronine (T_3) value characteristically is low; the TSH value is normal, while the free T_4 and reverse T_3 levels are either in the upper range of normal or are frankly elevated. This problem occurs most frequently in the preterm infant.

Tests other than the serum T_4 and TSH determinations often are not required for children in whom a diagnosis of hypothyroidism is suspected; however, thyroid antibody determinations can be very helpful in finding the cause of infantile or juvenile-acquired hypothyroidism, because the titers of the serum thyroid peroxidase (formerly known as microsomal) or thyroglobulin antibodies usually are elevated in children who have autoimmune thyroiditis.[1,4] Transient congenital hypothyroidism may be caused by TSH receptor–blocking antibodies (TRBAb) acquired from the mother who has autoimmune thyroid disease and primary hypothyroidism.[12] TRBAb levels diagnostically are valuable in these patients and should be measured during pregnancy in mothers receiving thyroxine therapy for primary hypothyroidism from autoimmune thyroiditis.[7] A serum T_3 determination in the infant who has congenital hypothyroidism also may be of prognostic value and often is reassuring for parents if the physician can indicate, on the evidence of a normal T_3 value, that therapy was initiated before chemical hypothyroidism developed.[10] The serum T_3 is not indicated, however, in the diagnostic evaluation of juvenile hypothyroidism.

Radioisotopic studies often are ordered inappropriately. Usually both a thyroid scan and uptake test are not necessary. In infants and children, the isotope ^{131}I-iodine should not be used as a diagnostic test, but a thyroid scan using either ^{123}I-iodine or ^{99m}Tc-technetium is an important test in infants who have abnormal thyroid screening tests for the following reasons:

1. It is the most rapid and definitive diagnostic test on which the initiation of therapy may be decided; the test result can be obtained 2 hours after the dose has been administered.
2. The test will distinguish sporadic disease, such as thyroid dysgenesis, from familial disease (goitrous thyroid dyshormonogenesis), a distinction important for genetic counseling.[7]

The thyroid uptake test using only ^{123}I-iodine should be performed whenever an infant has an enlarged thyroid gland on clinical examination or when the thyroid scan demonstrates an enlarged thyroid gland.

An elevated thyroid uptake in an infant who has a goiter

is very suggestive of an inborn error of thyroid hormone synthesis,[5] although it also may be seen in infants who have an iodine deficiency when living in endemic goiter regions of the world. Radioisotopic studies rarely are needed in older patients who have juvenile hypothyroidism; to exclude the possibility of thyroid carcinoma, the thyroid scan is indicated when a mass is palpated in the thyroid gland of a patient who has normal thyroid function and antibody tests.[4,6] Thyroid uptake studies are indicated when the patient has diffuse thyromegaly and biochemical evidence of hypothyroidism not caused by autoimmune thyroiditis or goitrogen ingestion.[4,6]

Although not essential, the assessment of skeletal maturation can provide additional data regarding the duration of hypothyroidism. A bone age determination consistent with that of a normal newborn would suggest recently acquired, mild congenital hypothyroidism, whereas notation of the absence of ossification centers at the knee in addition to the presence of only the two ossification centers in the foot indicates that the fetus was affected by hypothyroidism during the third trimester of pregnancy.

THERAPY

The treatment of choice for hypothyroidism in infancy and childhood is the daily administration of oral L-thyroxine[6,7,9,15] (Table 218-1). Other thyroid preparations are either more expensive or monitored less reliably for adequacy of dose. The initial dose in a term infant is 50 μg (0.05 mg) of L-thyroxine daily for the first 3 days to 2 weeks and should be started promptly at the initial visit when screening tests are abnormal and serum has been sent for confirmatory tests, or whenever the scan is abnormal.[9] Infants who have hypothalamic or pituitary hypothyroidism should be started on 25 μg/day because their requirements are less and their hypothyroidism mild. At the end of the first and second week, serum T_4 and TSH values should be obtained to determine that the amount of L-thyroxine is adequate but not excessive.[9] In athyreotic infants who have low T_4 values, it is unusual to find that 50 μg/day is inadequate. Often after 1 or 2 weeks, the dose may need to be reduced to 37.5 μg/day and infrequently to 25 μg/day, if (1) clinical symptoms of hyperthyroidism develop or (2) if the serum T_4 value exceeds 16 μg/dl (the normal range for T_4 in the infant is higher than that in older children and adults) and the serum T_3 value exceeds 250 ng/dl. Therapy should be adjusted to maintain the serum T_4 during infancy above 8 μg/dl, preferably between 10 and 12 μg/dl. Within the first 4 weeks of therapy the serum TSH value should decrease into the normal range for age. But in an occasional infant the TSH value will not return to normal even if the thyroxine dose is excessive and causes clinical thyrotoxicosis; these infants may have an abnormality in the feedback set point of TSH secretion.[13] The goal of therapy in this situation should be to maintain normal serum T_4 and T_3 values and clinical euthyroidism. Because excessive thyroxine therapy in infancy may cause cranial synostosis and brain dysfunction, frequent monitoring of serum T_4 and TSH levels at 1- to 3-month intervals during the first year is essential.[7] Additional determinations may be necessary whenever the dose is adjusted.[7] After 2 years of age the need to change the L-thyroxine dose occurs infrequently, so measuring serum T_4 and TSH levels once or twice a year should be adequate. If linear growth and weight gain are progressing satisfactorily, no additional studies are necessary.

Table 218-1 Dose of L-Thyroxine

Age	T_4 dose per day (μg)	T_4 dose/kg/day (μg)
<6 mo	25-50	8-10
6-12 mo	50-75	6-8
1-5 yr	75-100	5-6
6-12 yr	100-125	4-5
>12 yr	100-200	2-3

In contrast to infants who have congenital or acquired hypothyroidism, older children who have hypothyroidism do not share the same degree of urgency in achieving the euthyroid state. Although patients who have had a recent onset of mild hypothyroidism may be started on a full replacement dose of L-thyroxine, children age 3 years and older who have chronic hypothyroidism and clinical symptoms should be started on a low dose (25 μg/day) that gradually is increased every 2 to 4 weeks to the full replacement dose.[4,6]

The rapid correction of the hypothyroid state often can be associated with undesirable behavioral side effects. These children act as though they are thyrotoxic despite biochemical euthyroidism; they often are restless, have a short attention span, and are emotionally labile. These symptoms, in association with the expected hair loss, may lead to inappropriate discontinuance of therapy by the uninformed parent. In such cases a gradual increase in dose seems to minimize these problems in adjustment from the hypothyroid to the euthyroid state. Adequacy of L-thyroxine therapy is monitored by annual serum T_4 and TSH determinations, once the patient is receiving a full replacement dose with normal values. Because patients who have acquired hypothyroidism do not have an abnormality in the feedback control of TSH secretion, an elevated TSH with or without a low T_4 value indicates either inadequate therapy or poor compliance; the latter often is characterized by variable serum T_4 and TSH values. For example, the levels may be normal on one occasion but discordant (normal or elevated T_4 with elevated TSH) on subsequent determinations, despite no change in therapy. In rare cases the medication may not contain the indicated amount of thyroxine. Studies in adults have indicated a reduced absorption of L-thyroxine when administered with meals, especially food containing fiber. Hence it is advisable, particularly in treating infants, that medication be given an hour before the next feeding.

Because an occasional infant receiving treatment merely may have had transient congenital hypothyroidism, therapy should either be reduced to half the dose or discontinued some time after 3 years of age. Serum T_4 and TSH levels then are determined 2 to 4 weeks later and therapy restarted if the TSH is elevated. Radioisotope scan or uptake may be performed while off therapy at this age, if a definitive diagnosis was not obtained at the outset. Temporary cessation or reduction in therapy, however, is not necessary for those patients who have ectopic thyroid dysgenesis or for children who have other causes of hypothyroidism who previously had elevated TSH values after the TSH normalized during initial therapy.

PROGNOSIS

Infants who were treated adequately for congenital hypothyroidism since the first month of age have an excellent prognosis for normal intellectual function and linear growth. However, delays in diagnosis and in the institution of adequate therapy until after 3 months of age usually are associated with an increased risk of mental retardation.[11] In contrast, no permanent intellectual impairment is found among patients who have juvenile hypothyroidism, although adolescents who have chronic hypothyroidism and severe growth retardation may never achieve their full growth potential; often their linear growth response to therapy is not accelerated, and the height percentile achieved as an adult is lower than that predicted by their growth before the development of hypothyroidism.[14]

REFERENCES

1. Bachrach LK, Foley TP Jr: Thyroiditis in children, *Pediatr Rev* 11:184, 1989.
2. Bogner U et al: Cytotoxic antibodies in congenital hypothyroidism, *J Clin Endocrinol Metab* 68:671, 1989.
3. Fisher DA et al: Screening for congenital hypothyroidism: results of screening 1 million North American infants, *J Pediatr* 94:700, 1979.
4. Foley TP Jr: Disorders of the thyroid in children. In Sperling MA, editor: *Clinical pediatric and adolescent endocrinology,* Philadelphia, 1996, WB Saunders.
5. Foley TP Jr: Familial thyroid dyshormonogenesis. In Delange F, Fisher DA, Malvaux P, editors: *Pediatric thyroidology,* Basel, Switzerland, 1985, S Karger.
6. Foley TP Jr, Malvaux P, Blizzard RM: Thyroid disease. In Kappy MS, Blizzard RM, Migeon CJ, editors: *Wilkins the diagnosis and treatment of endocrine disorders in childhood and adolescence,* ed 4, Springfield, Ill, 1994, Charles C Thomas.
7. Foley TP Jr: Congenital hypothyroidism and screening. In Monaco F et al, editors: *Thyroid diseases,* Boca Raton, Fla, 1993, CRC Press.
8. Foley TP Jr et al: Acquired autoimmune mediated infantile hypothyroidism: a pathologic entity distinct from congenital hypothyroidism, *N Engl J Med* 330:466, 1994.
9. Germak JA, Foley TP Jr: Longitudinal assessment of L-thyroxine therapy in congenital hypothyroidism, *J Pediatr* 117:211, 1990.
10. Klein AH et al: Neonatal thyroid function in congenital hypothyroidism, *J Pediatr* 89:545, 1976.
11. Klein AH, Meltzer S, Kenny FM: Improved prognosis in congenital hypothyroidism treated before age three months, *J Pediatr* 81:912, 1972.
12. Matsuura N et al: Familial neonatal transient hypothyroidism due to maternal TSH-binding inhibitor immunoglobulins, *N Engl J Med* 303:738, 1980.
13. Rallison M, Dobyns DM, Keating FR et al: Occurrence and natural history of thyroiditis in children, *J Pediatr* 86:675, 1975.
14. Rivkees SA, Bode HH, Crawford JD: Long-term growth in juvenile acquired hypothyroidism, *N Engl J Med* 318:599, 1988.
15. Sato T et al: Age-related change in pituitary threshold for TSH release during replacement therapy for cretinism, *J Clin Endocrinol Metab* 44:553, 1977.
16. Vulsma T, Gons MH, de Vijlder JJM: Maternal-fetal transfer of thyroxine in congenital hypothyroidism due to a total organification defect or thyroid agenesis, *N Engl J Med* 321:13, 1989.

SUGGESTED READINGS

American Academy of Pediatrics: Newborn screening for congenital hypothyroidism: recommended guidelines, *Pediatrics* 91:1203, 1993.

Vassart G, Dumont JE, Refetoff S: Thyroid disorders. In Scriver CR et al, editors: *The metabolic and molecular bases of inherited disease,* ed 7, vol II, New York, 1995, McGraw-Hill.

Weetman AP, McGregor AM: Autoimmune thyroid disease: further developments in our understanding, *Endocr Rev* 15:788, 1994.

219 Iatrogenic Disease

Cheston M. Berlin, Jr.

Iatrogenic (from the Greek word meaning "produced by the physician") illness is the result of therapy or diagnostic procedures used to manage the health needs of a patient. Few comprehensive studies are available to indicate its prevalence, yet a report in 1981 by Steel et al.[3] found that 36% of 815 patients consecutively admitted to a general medical service had complications during their hospital stay caused by treatment or investigative procedures; 50% of these resulted from drug use.

Pediatric patients are especially vulnerable because of their size, their age, and the use of new therapies that have unknown risk for children. This is an especially significant problem in newborn medicine. Raju[2] surveyed a single pediatric journal and reported that 12.7% of articles published between 1965 and 1976 dealt with iatrogenic problems. Principi et al.[1] surveyed the use of antibiotics in nine pediatric units (765 patients) and found that *nearly one third of the patients received antibiotics on an "irrational" basis* (no proven infection or positive laboratory test). In 75% of the patients the antibiotic choice was not justified by the given clinical condition. This type of therapy invites iatrogenic disease.

The following is a case report of an iatrogenic illness:

Keith was referred by his family physician to an allergist at age 8 years for evaluation of continual nasal sniffing that had been present for years and was attributed to allergies, in part because of a positive family history and because decongestants were ineffective. From age 8 to 10 years he was treated with monthly injections of triamcinolone acetate by the allergist. The parents became concerned at the onset of growth failure during this period. At age 10 he was referred to an endocrinology clinic, where the evaluation revealed his height and weight to be below the 3rd percentile, with essentially no absolute gain since 8 years of age. Also noted in the history was enuresis of many years' duration. The clinic note for that visit describes the patient as "hyperactive, with constant small movements of the body and frequent repetitive sounds from the throat." He was evaluated with the following tests, all of which were normal: insulin-arginine stimulation of growth hormone release, serum thyroxine, skull roentgenograms, bone age, and buccal smear. Conclusions of the endocrine consultation were that the growth failure most likely was caused by the administration of steroids; the family was thus advised to stop the steroids. The patient was referred to a urologist for evaluation of his enuresis and to a pediatrician for evaluation of his hyperactivity.

Keith was first seen by the urologist and hospitalized. He underwent an intravenous program with voiding cystourethrogram, cystoscopy with cystometrogram, and cystourethroscopy. The results of all these studies were normal. The patient was given 25 mg imipramine at bedtime.

The patient was next seen in the pediatrics wing. Tourette syndrome was diagnosed, based on multiple tics and coprolalia. Because of the initial delight of the patient and his family in the efficacy of imipramine in controlling the enuresis, drug therapy for controlling Tourette syndrome was discussed but deferred. Six weeks later, with the patient's resumption of frequent enuresis while still receiving imipramine, this drug was stopped and haloperidol, 1 mg twice daily, was started. There was prompt and considerable diminution of his tics and cessation of coprolalia within 2 days. After 1 week on this dosage the patient experienced acute dystonic posturing of the neck and face, which was reversed by intravenous diphenhydramine, 25 mg. The dose of haloperidol was decreased to 0.5 mg twice daily; there were no further side effects.

The patient remained stable for the next 5 years on this dosage. After the initial diagnosis Keith was placed in a special education class; subsequently, his accomplishments and self-esteem both increased. He also became a rifle marksman. The next year he returned to a regular classroom, and 5 years later he graduated from high school with vocational training. His height was at the 20th percentile, and his weight was at the 50th percentile. At 31 years of age he is fully employed. After 5 years of continuous haloperidol therapy at a dose of 0.5 mg twice daily, the patient now takes the medication at the same dosage two or three times per year for 1 to 2 weeks at a time when he is in stressful situations.

Iatrogenic illness in this patient occurred at several levels and for different reasons. First, he was misdiagnosed as being allergic because of frequent sniffing, a common symptom of Tourette syndrome. Second, he received a potent steroid for this symptom, which stopped his growth; this led to a lengthy, expensive, and negative endocrinology evaluation. Third, he was referred to a specialist for evaluation of a common and usually benign developmental condition: enuresis. He received a lengthy, excessive evaluation that required hospitalization and the administration of an anesthetic agent. Fourth, after the correct diagnosis was made, initial drug therapy caused a severe dystonic drug reaction. And finally, failure to diagnose Tourette syndrome early caused serious educational problems.

ETIOLOGY

Every patient contact is capable of producing iatrogenic disease. Infants under the age of 1 year are especially vulnerable to idiosyncratic central nervous system reactions to drugs (e.g., extrapyramidal reaction to prochlorperazine). The risk varies from virtually zero with the insertion of a tongue depressor (the gag reflex can stimulate the vagus to produce asystole) to 100% with the use of intravenous amphotericin B. The most common but not necessarily the most serious possibilities for iatrogenic disease occur in two broad categories: diagnostic procedures and therapy (Table 219-1).

DATA BASE

Recognition of iatrogenic disorders requires the physician's constant cognizance of the possibility that they may occur. The history and physical examination are most important; laboratory tests may confirm the clinical impression. Many

Table 219-1 Complications That Can Arise from Diagnostic Procedures and Subsequent Therapy

	Complications
Diagnostic procedure	
Physical examination	
Ears	Laceration of auditory canal; perforation of eardrum
Pharynx	Laceration of soft palate and buccal mucosa
Mouth or rectum (with thermometer)	Broken glass (laceration)
Joints	Dislocation
Abdominal examination	Fractured spleen
Laboratory testing	
Throat culture	Gagging; vomiting; aspiration
Venipunctures	Bruising; arterial spasm
Heel sticks	Lacerated heels; infection, osteomyelitis
Roentgenographic procedures	
Position of patient	Dislocation of joints; infiltration of intravenous lines
Use of radiopaque dyes	Allergic reactions
Sedation	Central nervous system (CNS) depression; drug reaction; cardiac arrhythmias
Radiotherapy	Skin erythema; burns; sterility; alopecia
Therapy	
Drug therapy	Drug reaction; drug interaction; errors in type of drug and frequency and route of administration
Fluids and electrolytes	Overhydration or underhydration; incorrect solution; incorrect route; misplacement of intravenous line
Nutrition (including vitamins)	Deficiency states; inadequate knowledge of formula composition; hypervitaminosis
Equipment	
Infant warmers	Burns
Electric hazards	Shocks
Transillumination (fiberoptics)	Burns
Noise (especially in incubators)	Auditory damage; sleep disturbances
Constant light	CNS dysfunction (?); retinal damage (?); hormonal dysfunction (?)
Temperature control	Hypothermia or hyperthermia
Beds: mesh, rails, objects	Choking; falling out
Surgery	Wrong patient operated on; wrong part of body operated on; complication: infection, contracture, scarring, adhesions, fluid and electrolyte imbalance
Cardiopulmonary resuscitation	Fractured ribs, spleen, or liver
Instructions to patient or family	Overly restricted life at home and school; failure to appreciate impact of illness on family's and patient's life; misunderstanding of oral instructions
Immunizations	Local and systemic reactions

iatrogenic disorders are obvious: ocular-gyric crisis from prochlorperazine use; sterile thigh abscesses from diphtheria-tetanus-pertussis (DTP) immunization; and a skin burn from touching an overhead warmer. Others are more subtle: rickets in the rapidly growing premature infant from failure to give sufficient vitamin D; hypernatremia from using boiled skim milk; and thinning skin from long-term use of steroid cream for diaper rash. A careful review of systems coupled with specific questions concerning recent medications or other therapy (by nonphysicians as well as physicians) usually will uncover problem areas.

DIFFERENTIAL DIAGNOSIS

The diagnosis of the condition usually is straightforward, *once considered;* iatrogenic causes of disease are frequently overlooked. A list of a few iatrogenic diseases with alternative causes may be illustrative (Table 219-2).

MANAGEMENT

The management of iatrogenic disease is no different from that of any other condition, except for investigation of the iatrogenic event. The lesson usually learned is that patient-physician communication and the mechanisms of health care delivery have broken down. Some iatrogenic events truly are unavoidable and indeed almost to be expected: limb atrophy after the application of a plaster cast and postoperative scarring in a person known to form keloids. Other iatrogenic events pinpoint serious deficiencies in medical care technology: failure to recheck the position of a decimal point in a digoxin order and inadequate postmarketing drug surveillance. The following are suggestions for preventing (or at least minimizing) iatrogenic illnesses.

1. *Careful explanation to parents and patient upon the institution of any therapy.* Preprinted handouts are helpful in anticipating and recognizing problems—for example, discussion of possible side effects of immuniza-

Table 219-2 Differential Diagnosis of Iatrogenic Diseases

Condition (diagnosis)	Causes
Rickets	No vitamin D supplementation
	Renal disease
	Rapid growth in a premature infant
Seizure	Seizure disorder
	Tap water enemas
	Boiled skim milk
	Fever
Fever of unknown origin	Urinary tract infection
	Phenytoin therapy
Hearing loss	Recurrent otitis media
	Aminoglycoside therapy
	Incubator noise with concomitant aminoglycoside therapy
Short stature	Heredity
	Malnutrition
	Steroid therapy
Loose stools	Enteritis
	Lactose intolerance
	Mineral oil and senna products
Increased intracranial pressure	Meningitis
	Brain tumor
	Vitamin A intoxication
Hair loss	Emotional
	Thallium poisoning
	Vincristine therapy

tion. Patient information brochures on procedures and drug therapy are being developed and used more and more by practitioners and institutions.

2. *Prompt investigation of any iatrogenic event.* Comments such as "Don't worry, this happens frequently," "We see this occasionally," and "Nobody knows" hardly are reassuring to the family. Corrective measures must be instituted immediately.
3. *Continuing education for all health care personnel.* It is the responsibility of the physician to investigate and report suspected links between therapy and unexpected changes in the patient's condition.
4. *Call for help.* This may mean additional consultative opinions from experts within and out of medicine. Electrical engineers can advise on electric current leaks; social workers and teachers can assist in managing a chronically ill child whose medical regimen does not permit normal school attendance.

Iatrogenic disease may be cause for a medicolegal suit by a family. Such a malpractice risk will be considerably minimized if all the above suggestions are followed.

REFERENCES

1. Principi N et al: Control of antibiotic therapy in pediatric patients, *Dev Pharmacol Ther* 3:145, 1981.
2. Raju TNK: The injured neonate of the seventies, *J Pediatr* 91:347, 1977.
3. Steel K et al: Iatrogenic illness on a general medical service at a university hospital, *N Engl J Med* 304:638, 1981.

SUGGESTED READINGS

Koren G, Barzilay Z, Greenwald M: Tenfold errors in administration of drug doses: a neglected iatrogenic disease in pediatrics, *Pediatrics* 77:848, 1986.

Valdes-Dapena M: Iatrogenic disease in the perinatal period, *Pediatr Clin North Am* 36:67, 1989.

220 Idiopathic Thrombocytopenia

Allen Eskenazi and Christopher N. Frantz

APPROACH TO THE THROMBOCYTOPENIC PATIENT

In evaluating the patient who has thrombocytopenia, the physician must determine (1) whether the hemostatic impairment is severe enough to warrant therapy and (2) the cause of the thrombocytopenia. Treatment undertaken without knowledge of the cause of the thrombocytopenia is arbitrary and therefore may be unsuccessful and even harmful.

The most likely cause of thrombocytopenia often may be deduced by performing a careful history and physical examination and analyzing a complete blood count, including the size of the circulating platelets. The history should focus on chronicity of the thrombocytopenia and its manifestations. The family history is helpful but is unlikely to be positive because thrombocytopenia is much more likely to be acquired than congenital. Petechiae are the hallmark of bleeding as a result of a low platelet count or because of platelet dysfunction. Purpura, ecchymosis, and mucosal bleeding, including epistaxis, gastrointestinal hemorrhage, and menorrhagia, commonly are seen, and bleeding from superficial cuts and abrasions usually is prolonged. In contrast, bleeding caused by plasma coagulation defects usually has a single locus (most often in deep tissues such as joints and muscles) and often occurs the day after trauma.

Thrombocytopenia is caused by accelerated destruction, impaired production, or sequestration of platelets in the spleen. Accelerated destruction of platelets is the most common cause of thrombocytopenia in childhood. For a child who appears well except for the presence of easy bleeding, this destruction likely is caused by acute idiopathic thrombocytopenic purpura (discussed below). The platelets in destructive thrombocytopenias usually are large, the hemoglobin level is normal, and the absolute neutrophil count is greater than 1500. In contrast, a febrile, ill-appearing child who has destructive thrombocytopenia is likely to have other manifestations of disseminated intravascular coagulopathy secondary to sepsis.

Thrombocytopenia caused by decreased platelet production almost always is associated with abnormalities of other cell lines, because the most common underlying disorders (e.g., malignancies, aplastic anemia, glycogen storage disorders) involve the entire bone marrow and its ability to sustain normal hematopoiesis. Many of these children are likely to be pale and appear ill, and have hepatosplenomegaly and sometimes bone pain.

Splenic sequestration results in nonspecific removal of platelets as well as white and red blood cells from the circulation (hypersplenism). This can occur secondary to a number of diseases that result in massive splenomegaly (see Chapter 166); a normal-size or only slightly enlarged spleen precludes this diagnosis. Thus the history, physical examination, and CBC usually can direct the clinician toward the likely cause of a patient's thrombocytopenia, resulting in a more rational diagnostic approach and therapeutic intervention.

IDIOPATHIC THROMBOCYTOPENIC PURPURA OF CHILDHOOD

Idiopathic thrombocytopenic purpura (ITP) of childhood is not truly idiopathic; it is caused by the production of autoantibodies that bind to platelets, resulting in their destruction by the reticuloendothelial system, thus leading some to label this disease *immune thrombocytopenic purpura.* The largest subset of children who have ITP also has a well-defined clinical syndrome that may be called *acute ITP of childhood (AITPC).* In other children the ITP may be a manifestation of a more complex underlying disorder that affects the child's long-term prognosis significantly, such as a collagen-vascular disease or hypogammaglobulinemia. Still others may have chronic ITP that has no association with an underlying disorder; chronic ITP is diagnosed when the thrombocytopenia persists for longer than 6 months. Finally 1% to 4% of children who apparently have classic AITPC suffer recurrent episodes of severe thrombocytopenia many months or years after the platelet count initially returns to normal. This disorder is called *recurrent ITP of childhood.*

The annual incidence of new cases of AITPC is 4 per 100,000 children. There is no gender predilection, and the peak onset occurs between 2 and 5 years of age. Typically a previously well child suddenly develops easy bruising and petechiae 1 to 3 weeks following a viral illness. Epistaxis occurs in 20% to 30% of these children, but renal, oral, or gastrointestinal bleeding occurs in fewer than 10%. Except for the presence of bleeding, the physical examination is entirely normal. Splenomegaly rarely is seen in AITPC; the presence of splenomegaly suggests an alternative diagnosis. A very large spleen suggests hypersplenism rather than ITP. In AITPC the platelet count almost always is less than 20,000 at the time of diagnosis. Higher counts should prompt one to entertain alternative diagnoses. Thrombocytopenia is evident on the peripheral blood smear, and the platelets that are present may have bizarre shapes or giant forms or be diffusely increased in size. The red and white blood cells on the smear should be normal; if they are not, other diagnoses should be considered.

The laboratory evaluation of AITPC is quite simple. The complete blood count, including an examination of the blood smear, is usually sufficient in patients who have all the characteristics listed in the box on p. 1367. AITPC typically presents so clearly that a routine bone marrow examination ordinarily is not required. However, it is essential to examine a patient's marrow if an aregenerative thrombocytopenia is suspected or if corticosteroid treatment is contemplated. Because

CRITERIA FOR THE DIAGNOSIS OF ACUTE IDIOPATHIC THROMBOCYTOPENIA OF CHILDHOOD

Platelet count ≤20,000
Normal complete blood count, including the absolute neutrophil count and the examination of red blood cells, white blood cells, and platelet morphology on the blood smear
Age 1 to 9 years
Otherwise patient well
Acute onset (symptomatic <2 weeks)
Preceding viral illness within 1 to 3 weeks
Normal size spleen
No personal history or family history of other possible autoimmune disorders (e.g., hemolytic anemia, nephritis, thyroiditis, collagen-vascular disease, or frequent infections)

DIAGNOSTIC WORKUP FOR ITP

Studies to be performed when a patient who has ITP does not fit all the criteria listed in the box to the left or if apparent AITPC does not resolve within 6 months:
Bone marrow examination
Immunoglobulin levels
Reticulocyte count
Direct and indirect antiglobulin (Coombs) test
Urinalysis
Antinuclear antibody levels
Prothrombin and partial thromboplastin times
Bleeding time
Human immunodeficiency virus antibody

steroid therapy is an integral part of the treatment for acute lymphoblastic leukemia (ALL), steroid treatment of a patient who has evolving ALL but who is presumed to have AITPC not only will delay the diagnosis of ALL, but also will result in the growth of leukemic cells that are resistant to steroids, which would mean a significantly poorer prognosis for the patient. Bone marrow aspiration in patients who have AITPC should reveal a normocellular marrow that has normal erythroid and myeloid maturation. Megakaryocytes are present in normal or increased numbers. Bone marrow examination will not distinguish AITPC from other forms of platelet destruction, including immune-mediated thrombocytopenic disorders other than AITPC. The bleeding time is prolonged and coagulation tests normal in patients who have AITPC, but performing these tests generally is not indicated. The measurement of platelet-associated immunoglobulin is elevated in approximately 85% of children who have ITP, including the majority who have AITPC. Platelet-associated immunoglobulin levels also are elevated in many other thrombocytopenic disorders, so the specificity of this test for AITPC is quite low and rarely helps to establish the diagnosis or prognosis.

Additional diagnostic tests for disorders associated with ITP should be performed in all patients who do not completely meet the criteria for the diagnosis of AITPC as outlined in the box above. This diagnostic workup is summarized in the box above, right. Bone marrow should be examined to document adequate platelet precursors. Immunoglobulin levels should be measured to rule out hypogammaglobulinemia associated with multiple autoimmune phenomena, especially autoimmune hemolytic anemia, ITP, and autoimmune neutropenia. The remaining tests search for evidence of associated autoimmune phenomena, collagen-vascular disease, or coagulopathies. The reticulocyte count is elevated during compensated hemolysis; the Coombs test is positive in most cases of autoimmune hemolytic anemia; urinalysis may reveal evidence of nephritis; the antinuclear antibody may identify patients who have systemic lupus erythematosus. Tests for infection by human immunodeficiency virus (HIV) should be performed because isolated ITP is not an uncommon first manifestation of HIV infection.

PROGNOSIS AND MANAGEMENT

Management of ITP is based on the natural history of the disease and the desire to prevent serious intracranial or gastrointestinal bleeding. The mainstays of therapy are supportive care, corticosteroids, intravenous gammaglobulin (IVIG), and splenectomy, each of which has inherent risks and benefits. The vast majority (>90%) of patients who have AITPC will have complete resolution without therapy and without serious sequelae. However, the clinician is faced with his or her own anxiety as well as parental anxiety in attempting to restrict the activity of young children while awaiting resolution of the thrombocytopenia.

The risk of serious bleeding is greatest in those patients whose platelet counts are <20,000/mm^3. Therapy therefore is aimed at rapidly raising the platelet count above this level. In a recent prospective, randomized trial, patients treated with either prednisone or IVIG had fewer days with platelet counts <20,000/mm^3 than did patients receiving supportive care only. Patients receiving IVIG achieved a platelet count >50,000/mm^3 faster than either of the other two groups.[1] Adverse effects of IVIG include headache, nausea, vomiting, and fever, which are controlled easily by diphenhydramine and acetaminophen. The costs of administering the IVIG (1 g/kg/day for 2 days) are significantly greater than the costs of prednisone. Prednisone generally is administered at a dose of 2 to 4 mg/kg/day for a 2- to 3-week period. The adverse effects of corticosteroids are well known but generally are tolerable for this short duration of therapy. Long-term therapy with corticosteroids should be avoided because of their effects on growth, bone mineralization, and gastric mucosa.

Corticosteroids may have the additional benefit of stabilizing the vascular endothelium in the presence of thrombocytopenia, and this may result in less clinical bleeding at a given platelet count. It again must be emphasized that all patients receiving steroids need to have their bone marrow examined carefully before therapy. Administration of IVIG will not alter the interpretation of a bone marrow examination; therefore it may be used as empirical therapy if a bone marrow examination is not readily obtainable. Treatment with IVIG or steroids does not preclude treatment with the other modality.

There is no role for routine splenectomy in the management of AITPC, but it may be useful in older children who have chronic ITP. Platelet transfusions have a very limited role in the management of AITPC. Because transfused platelets are destroyed immunologically in a fashion similar to that of the endogenous platelets, platelet transfusions will not result in a sustained increase in the patient's platelet count. Platelet transfusions may be useful and should be given to patients experiencing ongoing life-threatening hemorrhage. Defensive management also is important. Restriction of physical activity and avoidance of contact sports and playground activities are indicated. All medications that have antiplatelet activity should be avoided, including ibuprofen, aspirin, antihistamines, phenothiazines, and glycerol guaiacolate. Intramuscular injections should be avoided.

EMERGENCY MANAGEMENT OF BLEEDING

General measures should be directed at the delivery of platelets to the site of hemorrhage. Although the routine use of platelet transfusions in ITP is not indicated, platelet transfusions are useful in an emergency. A bolus infusion of 1 unit/5 kg body weight should be administered immediately because it may exert hemostatic benefit before being cleared by the reticuloendothelial system. Corticosteroids should be administered intravenously (4 mg/kg/day of prednisolone or its equivalent). IVIG also should be administered at the dose described above. If these measures fail to control bleeding, an emergency splenectomy may be indicated. Aminocaproic acid (Amicar), an inhibitor of fibrinolysis, may help to prevent serious rebleeding, especially in mucosal areas.

CHRONIC IDIOPATHIC THROMBOCYTOPENIA PURPURA

Chronic ITP is defined as a platelet count that persists below 100,000 cells/mm^3 for more than 6 months. Approximately 20% of patients who have chronic ITP ultimately will recover spontaneously, but it is not possible to predict in which children this will occur. Chronic ITP in children is similar to ITP in adults and is caused by platelet autoantibodies that bind to specific platelet membrane glycoproteins. The female-to-male ratio for chronic ITP is 3:1. The workup for chronic ITP should include the studies outlined in the box on p. 1367.

Management depends on the overall impact of both platelet count and platelet function on hemostasis in the individual patient. In some patients the antiplatelet antibody also impairs platelet function. A bleeding time is helpful in estimating hemostatic function at a given platelet count. Whereas splenectomy once was the mainstay of treating chronic ITP, other alternatives are available to prevent or postpone splenectomy. IVIG in the doses mentioned above is effective in raising the platelet count temporarily in approximately 80% of children who have chronic ITP, although about 25% of patients eventually become refractory to its effect. In the remainder of patients periodic doses of IVIG are effective long-term therapy and can be given as a single outpatient infusion of 1 g/kg every several weeks. Pulses of high doses of IV methylprednisolone (15 mg/kg/day for 3 days) also have been shown to improve the platelet count in patients who have chronic ITP.[4] Thrombocytopenia in some patients also may be controlled by brief treatment with prednisone (2 mg/kg/day) or low doses of alternate-day prednisone for longer periods of time. This may be useful in postponing splenectomy but is not a desirable long-term option in young children because of long-term side effects. Alternative forms of immunosuppression have been used with some success, but at this point these can be recommended only for highly refractory patients and should be undertaken only after consultation at an experienced clinical center.

Splenectomy effectively raises the platelet count to levels that prevent bleeding in most children who have chronic ITP. There is no definitive test by which one can predict this response. Splenectomy itself appears to be safe in patients who have chronic ITP, and excessive bleeding during surgery is quite rare. During a splenectomy the surgeon must look carefully for an accessory spleen, because residual splenic tissue may result in the relapse of ITP after surgery. The platelet count usually starts to rise in the immediate postoperative period, and platelet counts over 1 million are not unusual. Because there are no reports of thrombosis at these very high levels, antiplatelet agents are not indicated.

Splenectomy should be avoided if at all possible in the younger child because the risk of postsplenectomy sepsis is highest in young children. The risk decreases dramatically with age; by 6 years of age, given proper vaccination and postsplenectomy antibiotic prophylaxis, the incidence of sepsis appears to be quite low. The increased risk of septicemia is limited to encapsulated organisms, pneumococcus, *Hemophilus influenza* type b, and meningococcus. Rapidly overwhelming sepsis almost always is caused by pneumococcus, so penicillin prophylaxis is important and recommended for life by many pediatric hematologists. Pneumococcal vaccinations should be administered at least 2 weeks before splenectomy. The development of fever in children who have had a splenectomy is an indication for prompt evaluation and parenteral administration of a third-generation cephalosporin until blood cultures have been found to be negative.

IMMUNE THROMBOCYTOPENIA IN THE NEONATE

Approximately 10% of infants admitted to neonatal intensive care units have platelet counts $<100,000/mm^3$. The majority of these patients do not have immune thrombocytopenia; instead the thrombocytopenia is secondary to sepsis, congenital infection, asphyxia, or necrotizing enterocolitis. There are, however, two immune causes of neonatal thrombocytopenia that deserve special mention, particularly given the risks associated with future pregnancies.

Maternal ITP may result in the transplacental passage of maternal autoantibodies that may destroy fetal platelets immunologically. Although these infants may become moderately thrombocytopenic (platelet count 20,000 to 50,000/mm^3), significant bleeding in the infant appears to be rare.[2] The thrombocytopenia resolves as the maternally derived antibodies are catabolized. While awaiting resolution one can use IVIG expectantly to support the infant's platelet count.

A more serious situation exists when the mother develops antiplatelet antibodies directed against paternally derived platelet antigens that are present on the infant's platelets. This process, termed *neonatal alloimmune thrombocytopenic purpura (NATP),* is analogous to erythroblastosis fetalis (Rh disease), in which maternal anti-Rh antibodies destroy Rh-positive fetal red blood cells. NATP occurs in approximately 1 in 2000 to 1 in 5000 fetuses and results in severe neonatal thrombocytopenia. The precise incidence of intracranial hemorrhage is unknown, but estimates range between 10% and 30% of affected infants. The severity of thrombocytopenia and intracranial hemorrhage tends to increase with subsequent pregnancies. Postnatal treatment with washed, irradiated maternal platelets as well as with IVIG improve the thrombocytopenia. Identification of NATP is important because antepartum and postpartum neonatal hemorrhages may occur in future pregnancies. Antenatal treatment of the mother with IVIG and perhaps steroids are effective in raising fetal platelet counts[3] and therefore may decrease the incidence of severe injury or death from hemorrhage.

REFERENCES

1. Blanchette VS et al: A prospective, randomized trial of high-dose intravenous immune globulin G therapy, oral prednisone therapy, and no therapy in childhood acute immune thrombocytopenic purpura, *J Pediatr* 123:989, 1993.
2. Burrows RF, Kelton JG: Fetal thrombocytopenia and its relation to maternal thrombocytopenia, *N Engl J Med* 329:1463, 1993.
3. Bussel JB et al: Antenatal treatment of neonatal alloimmune thrombocytopenia, *N Engl J Med* 319:1374, 1988.
4. del Principe D et al: Phase II trial of methylprednisolone pulse therapy in childhood chronic thrombocytopenia, *Acta Haematol* 77:226, 1987.

SUGGESTED READING

Beardsley DS: Platelet abnormalities in infancy and childhood. In Nathan DG, Oski FA, editors: *Hematology of infancy and childhood,* Philadelphia, 1993, WB Saunders.

221 Infectious Mononucleosis and Epstein-Barr Virus Infections

Stephen R. Barone, Leonard R. Krilov, and Ciro V. Sumaya

EPIDEMIOLOGY

Infection with Epstein-Barr virus (EBV), a member of the herpesvirus group, is extremely common but often not apparent clinically. In Africa there is a strong association between infection with EBV and development of Burkitt lymphoma and nasopharyngeal carcinoma; this association, however, has been demonstrated less clearly in Western countries despite the demonstration of serological evidence of past infection by the great majority of children and adolescents. In the United States, interest in EBV infection centers on the typical clinical syndrome—known as *infectious mononucleosis*—that it produces and on its emerging relationship with an increasing number of tumors, noted for the most part in immunocompromised patients.

In childhood, EBV infection usually is inapparent clinically or manifested by a nonspecific, uncomplicated episode of upper respiratory tract infection or pharyngitis.[8] Although EBV antibodies have developed in 70% to 90% of children from low socioeconomic groups by age 5 years, these antibodies occur in only 40% to 50% of those from high socioeconomic groups.[1] Primary infections that do not occur until adolescence and young adulthood are much more likely, for reasons that are unclear, to manifest as infectious mononucleosis. Thus the incidence of infectious mononucleosis is highest among Caucasian high school and college students—approximately 1 in 2500 students.

CLINICAL PRESENTATION

After an incubation period of 2 to 6 weeks (normally 20 to 30 days), signs of classic infectious mononucleosis are seen: fever, sore throat, and lymphadenopathy. This constellation of signs can be preceded by vague symptoms of fatigue, malaise, and anorexia.

Because infectious mononucleosis is the result of a systemic viral infection, virtually every organ system may be involved.[5] Figure 221-1 demonstrates the variety of clinical manifestations compatible with infectious mononucleosis.

The fever usually is not higher than 103° F (39.5° C), but the sore throat, frequently accompanied by exudate and a palatal enanthem, can be excruciating. Lymphadenopathy, perhaps the most striking feature of the illness, can be limited to the cervical nodes but also can be so extensive as to involve virtually all lymph node groups. Posterior cervical adenopathy is noted most frequently. The lymph nodes are not tender, nor do they demonstrate signs of adenitis.

Enlargement of the spleen and possibly the liver, together with posterocervical adenopathy, are the physical signs that usually alert the clinician to the diagnosis of infectious mononucleosis. Some patients who have this illness, however, do not have any palpable splenic enlargement; massive enlargement of the spleen should suggest an alternative diagnosis. Liver enzyme levels are elevated in virtually all patients, but the frequency of jaundice is low.

The severity of illness is extremely variable, and some individuals may have relatively few signs of infection, whereas others will demonstrate virtually all the findings listed in Figure 221-1. In general, the clinical manifestations of the illness last approximately 2 to 3 weeks, with peak involvement during the second week. Eyelid edema has been reported by some observers in about 25% of patients.

DIAGNOSIS AND SEROLOGY

Infectious mononucleosis is diagnosed by the presence of a triad of typical clinical, hematological, and serological findings. In addition to the clinical profile described in the preceding section, minimal hematological features should include a relative lymphocytosis of 50% or more and a relative atypical lymphocyte count of 10% or more of all leukocytes. Other general laboratory findings usually include a decline in the number of granulocytes and platelets.

The heterophil Paul-Bunnell antibody, an IgM antibody produced by humans during infection that reacts with horse, sheep, and beef erythrocytes but not with guinea pig kidney cells, is the cornerstone of laboratory diagnosis. This antibody will be present in only up to 50% of children younger than 4 years of age.[9] Among school-age children and young adults it is detectable 80% to 90% of the time during the second week of clinical illness.[5,9] Occasionally the heterophil response will be brief and minimal or will occur late in the illness and therefore may show negative results at the time of testing. Commercial diagnostic kits, which rely on differential adsorption to detect the heterophil antibody, are readily available and easy to use in a physician's office; they are 96% to 99% sensitive and give a result in 2 minutes.[4] False positive results have been reported in cases of rubella, hepatitis, serum sickness, drug reactions, and systemic lupus erythematosus and through improper use of the kit or inaccurate interpretation of the agglutination reaction. The magnitude of the heterophil antibody titer does not correlate with clinical severity, and repeat testing, once a positive test result is obtained, provides no additional information beyond that gained from clinical assessment of the patient.

If heterophil test results are negative, confirmation of EBV infection should be sought by other serological tests. A variety of antibodies directed against various portions of EBV can be detected by numerous hospital, state health, or commercial laboratories. Patients who have negative heterophil test results will have antibodies against specific components

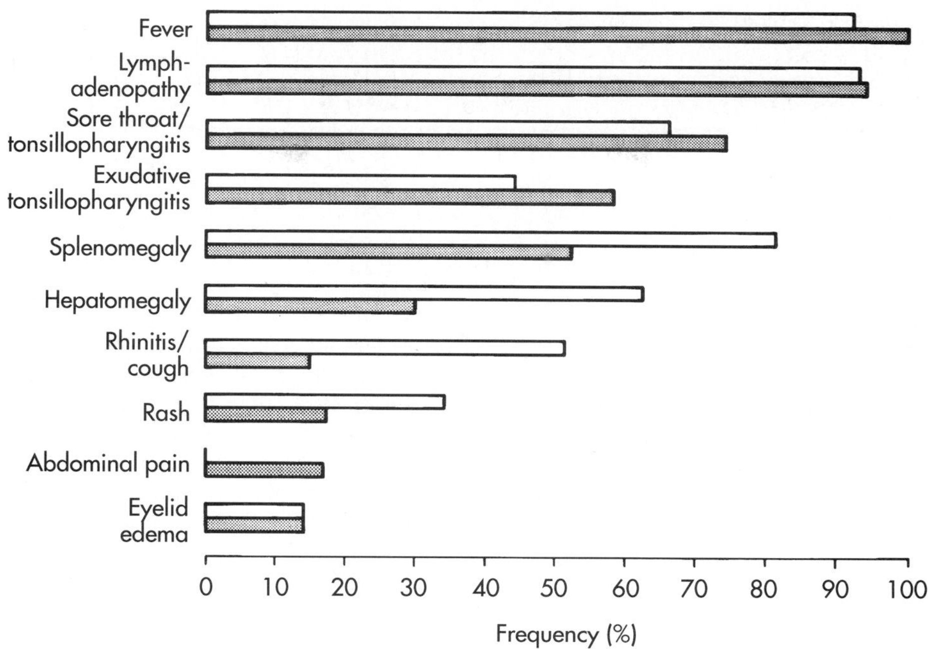

FIG. 221-1 Frequency of clinical findings in two age groups of children with documented Epstein-Barr virus infectious mononucleosis: less than 4 years old *(open bars)* and 4 to 16 years old *(shaded bars).*

(From Sumaya CV, Ench Y: *Pediatrics* 75:1005, 1985.)

of the virus if EBV indeed is the cause of the clinical illness.

Four different antibodies define the EBV serological profile: IgG antibody to the viral capsid antigen (VCA-IgG), IgM antibody to viral capsid antigen (VCA-IgM), and IgG antibody to early antigen (EA). This latter antibody includes two components: diffuse (D) and restricted (R), and IgG antibody to Epstein-Barr nuclear antigen (EBNA). These antibodies usually appear predictably in an individual who acquires a primary EBV infection. The pattern of antibody responses therefore can help the practitioner to date an individual's EBV infection.

In most cases an individual develops a VCA-IgM antibody response in the acute period following an EBV infection. The same is true for the VCA-IgG antibody; however, although IgG antibodies to the VCA persist for life, VCA-IgM tends to disappear in 2 to 3 months. The EA response also peaks at 3 to 4 weeks into the illness and was thought to persist only for several months; therefore it also was considered a good marker for an acute or recent infection. Recent evidence suggests that the EA response may persist for years in some children and may not develop at all in others. Finally, the EBNA antibody response usually appears several weeks to months after a primary infection and therefore is thought to be a marker for a past or convalescent infection. However, even this antibody response has to be interpreted in light of the clinical situation because a number of children develop this response in the acute phase of their infection, yet 10% to 20% of individuals never develop detectable levels of antibody to EBNA. In summary, antibodies in children who acquire an EBV infection typically develop similarly (see Table 221-1); however, not all patients necessarily will follow the same pattern, and clinical judgment remains important in the interpretation of such findings. Additionally, interlaboratory variability in results of EBV antibody testing have been observed, making the reliability of these tests suspect in some cases. If both the heterophil test and specific serologies are negative, other causes for the non-EBV infectious mononucleosis-like illness should be sought.

COMPLICATIONS AND DEATHS

Most persons who have infectious mononucleosis recover uneventfully. Serious complications, however, have resulted from this illness; death occurs in approximately 1 in 3000 cases. The true complication and death rates during this illness are uncertain because many reports do not include strict diagnostic criteria for infectious mononucleosis. The relative frequencies of more common complications associated with this illness, as documented in one large study, are listed in Table 221-2.[4] A number of other complications in virtually every body organ also have been reported with this disease.

Of 20 deaths clearly associated with infectious mononucleosis in one series,[6] 9 were of neurological origin and 3 each were caused by secondary infection or splenic rupture, 2 by hepatic failure, and 1 by probable myocarditis. Because abdominal pain is an infrequent symptom of this illness, its appearance, particularly if severe and in the left upper quadrant, should alert the clinician to the possibility of splenic rupture. Fatal cases of Reye syndrome associated with serological evidence of EBV infection also have been reported.

MANAGEMENT

Because most patients who have infectious mononucleosis recover uneventfully, physicians need do little except establish the diagnosis, explain the nature of the illness, and reassure

Table 221-1 Interpretation of Epstein-Barr Virus Serology

		Epstein-Barr virus antibodies			
	Heterophil antibody	VCA-IgM	VCA-IgG	EA	EBNA
No infection	–	–	–	–	–
Acute infection	+/–	+	+ (>1:320)	+/–	–
Past infection	–	–	+ (1:80-1:160)	+/–	+

Note: Other patterns may occur in an individual patient; the above profile is for a typical individual.

Table 221-2 Complications Present in 113 Children with EBV Infectious Mononucleosis

Complication	No. of children (%)
Respiratory tract	
Pneumonia	6 (5.3)
Severe airway obstruction*	4 (3.5)
Neurological	
Seizures	4 (3.5)
Meningitis/encephalitis	2 (1.8)
Peripheral facial nerve paralysis	1 (0.9)
Guillain-Barré syndrome	1 (0.9)
Hematological	
Thrombocytopenia with hemorrhages	4 (3.5)
Hemolytic anemia	1 (0.9)
Infectious	
Bacteremia	1 (0.9)
Recurrent tonsillopharyngitis	3 (2.7)
Liver	
Jaundice	2 (1.8)
Renal	
Glomerulonephritis	1 (0.9)
Genital	
Orchitis	1 (0.9)
TOTAL	31†

From Sumaya CV, Ench Y: *Pediatrics* 75:1007, 1985.
*Criteria consisted of nasal alar flaring, suprasternal retractions, or stridor.
†Because four children had more than one of these complications, this total is composed of 24 different children, or 21.2% of the study group.

the family. No specific therapy is indicated. Patients should rest to the extent that they feel necessary. As long as the patient can consume adequate amounts of fluids and calories, hospitalization is unnecessary. To minimize the danger of splenic rupture, it seems prudent that ambulatory patients avoid strenuous physical exercise or contact sports until the spleen no longer is palpable. Patients who have late onset of the heterophil antibody response appear to have a prolonged convalescence.

Corticosteroids are of unproved value in treating this illness.[2] They should not be used routinely merely to make the patient feel better. Most clinicians believe that their use is justified in treating severe hemolytic anemia, significant airway obstruction secondary to tonsillar hypertrophy, and thrombocytopenia. However, controlled studies documenting their efficacy in these settings are lacking. Some suggest using them if neurological involvement is significant, but again, proof of efficacy is not available. The antiviral agent acyclovir has good antiviral activity against EBV in vitro, but it has not been shown to be beneficial in a number of clinical trials that involved patients who had infectious mononucleosis. At this time it is not recommended for routine use.

Inasmuch as the pharyngitis of infectious mononucleosis can be indistinguishable from that of true streptococcal pharyngitis, culture specimens of the pharynx should be obtained, and patients who have positive culture findings should be treated accordingly.

A rash, which can be erythematous, petechial, erythema multiforme–like, urticarial, or scarlatiniform, develops in approximately 20% of children who have this illness. However, a rash also develops in 70% to 90% of young adult patients who have this illness and who are treated with ampicillin. In some cases the ampicillin-related rash will appear after the medication has been discontinued. Although the ampicillin effect has not been well demonstrated in young children who have infectious mononucleosis, it is prudent to avoid using this drug under these circumstances.

Infection follows entry of the EBV into the oropharynx, and its recovery from this site can be documented up to 16 months after illness. It appears that EBV establishes latency in the epithelial cells of the oropharynx and that the virus periodically is shed from this site throughout an individual's lifetime. Transmission from one individual to another appears to occur most often through mixing of saliva (thus its description as the "kissing disease"). In the absence of such contact, transfer of infection is unlikely. In a study of families that have a childhood index case of infectious mononucleosis, seroconversion occurred in 34.6% of the susceptible siblings over a period of several months after the acute episode.[10] Even though the rate of transmission of the EBV infection was relatively low and slow, the development of infectious mononucleosis with the eventual primary EBV infection was quite high (55.6%) in these sibling contacts who showed seroconversion.

Secondary infection in typical college settings is even lower. As such, strict isolation of the patient is unnecessary. Instead, separation of drinking and eating utensils (e.g., avoiding drinking from the same glass) is all that is required.

Accounts are increasing (although still rare) of infectious mononucleosis episodes that are quite severe and fatal or else that result in significant long-lasting problems. Most of these patients had some form of immunological abnormality—that is, X-linked lymphoproliferative syndrome, renal transplant recipients, and Chédiak-Higashi syndrome, among others. In contrast, the etiological association initially suspected between EBV, or infectious mononucleosis, and the chronic fatigue syndrome (chronic debilitating illness characterized by extreme fatigue, neuropsychological abnormalities, and a myriad of other problems)[3,7] now appears to be inaccurate. Although many patients who have chronic fatigue syndrome date the onset of their illness to an episode of infectious mononucleosis, virological and clinical studies have confirmed that active EBV infection is not responsible for the patient's illness. The elevated antibody titers to EBV noted in these patients are most likely to be an epiphenomenon related to the subtle immunological disturbances seen in these patients. At present there is no single infectious cause for chronic fatigue syndrome (see Chapter 192, Chronic Fatigue Syndrome).

EPSTEIN-BARR VIRUS–NEGATIVE INFECTIOUS MONONUCLEOSIS

Rubella, hepatitis, toxoplasmosis, cytomegalovirus (CMV), human herpesvirus 6 and adenovirus infections, systemic lupus erythematosus, and drug reactions can have symptoms similar to those of EBV infection. Negative EBV titers and heterophil antibody responses strongly suggest one of these agents as the cause of the illness under consideration. In hepatitis, in which the heterophil test can give a false positive result, liver enzyme levels generally are much more elevated than those seen with infectious mononucleosis. Results of serological tests for hepatitis will be positive, as will rubella titers in rubella infection; CMV can be cultured from urine in those who have infection as the cause of their illness. Illnesses that mimic infectious mononucleosis but lack serological confirmation of EBV infection should be classified as heterophil-negative infectious mononucleosis rather than atypical mononucleosis. The cause of most of these cases is unknown.

EPSTEIN-BARR VIRUS INFECTION AND MALIGNANCY

Lymphocytes that contain the EBV genome can be subdivided indefinitely. The virus remains dormant in human hosts for prolonged periods. These observations, together with the known association of EBV and African Burkitt lymphoma and nasopharyngeal carcinoma, have raised speculation that EBV infection might be oncogenic in the United States as well. Some cases of leukemia occurring shortly after the onset of infectious mononucleosis have been reported, but there is no evidence to support this speculation. Although in the United States the association between EBV and classic Burkitt lymphoma is not as strong as in Africa, a number of lymphomas and lymphoproliferative lesions that contain EBV markers (including markers of viral replication) have been found in American patients. Recent evidence also links EBV with T cell lymphomas and Hodgkin disease. These intriguing findings are the subject of intense investigation.

REFERENCES

1. Andiman WA: The Epstein-Barr virus and EB virus infections in childhood, *J Pediatr* 95:171, 1979.
2. Collins M et al: Role of steroids in the treatment of infectious mononucleosis in the ambulatory college student, *J Am Coll Health Assoc* 33:101, 1984.
3. Jones JF et al: Evidence for active Epstein-Barr virus infections in patients with persistent, unexplained illness: elevated anti-early antigen antibodies, *Ann Intern Med* 102:1, 1985.
4. Karzon DT: Infectious mononucleosis, *Adv Pediatr* 22:231, 1976.
5. Mandell GL, Douglas RG Jr, Bennett JE: *Principles and practice of infectious diseases,* vol 2, New York, 1979, John Wiley & Sons.
6. Penman HG: Fatal infectious mononucleosis: a critical review, *J Clin Pathol* 23:765, 1970.
7. Straus SE et al: Persisting illness and fatigue in adults with evidence of Epstein-Barr virus infection, *Ann Intern Med* 102:7, 1985.
8. Sumaya CV, Ench Y: Epstein-Barr virus infectious mononucleosis in children. I. Clinical and general laboratory findings, *Pediatrics* 75:1003, 1985.
9. Sumaya CV, Ench Y: Epstein-Barr virus infectious mononucleosis in children. II. Heterophil antibody and viral-specific responses, *Pediatrics* 75:1011, 1985.
10. Sumaya CV, Ench Y: Epstein-Barr virus infections in families: the role of children with infectious mononucleosis, *J Infect Dis* 154:842, 1986.

SUGGESTED READINGS

Schuster V, Kreth HW: Epstein-Barr virus infection and associated diseases in children. I. Pathogenesis, epidemiology and clinical aspects, *Eur J Pediatr* 151:718, 1992.

Schuster V, Kreth HW: Epstein-Barr virus infection and associated diseases in children. II. Diagnostic and therapeutic strategies, *Eur J Pediatr* 151:794, 1992.

Straus SE et al: Epstein-Barr virus infections: biology, pathogenesis and management, *Ann Intern Med* 118:1, 1993.

222 Insect Bites and Infestations

Nancy K. Barnett

INSECT BITES

Discrete red pruritic papules and nodules suggest the diagnosis of insect bites. Although mosquitoes are the most common, flies, fleas, gnats, and bedbugs also are potential pests that can cause lesions. The lesions may produce discomfort to the unsensitized individual; the sensitized child, however, can develop aggravating, intensely pruritic wheals or even bullae from bites.

On physical examination a discrete number of erythematous papules and plaques typically are scattered over the body, all in the same stage of development. Some may have central puncta or vesicles; others are capped by a hemorrhagic or serous crust or an excoriation created by scratching. The bites also can be camouflaged by impetiginization or eczematous changes. The reactions usually are found on exposed (not covered by clothing) surfaces. In fact, they often are grouped three in a row and are referred to as "breakfast, lunch, and dinner bites."

Papular urticaria is a common reaction to insect bites. It consists of recurrent crops of urticarial papules on exposed surfaces that may be new or reactivated old bites. Papular urticaria occurs seasonally (particularly in warmer months) in certain hypersensitive individuals. Each lesion can last up to 2 weeks, plaguing the child with itch, and can leave an unsightly postinflammatory pigmentary change. We do not know why one family member may be affected and others not; nevertheless, this bit of history may help to rule out scabies or pediculosis (see below).

Insect bites can be controlled by using repellents and by clothing much of the body. Topical antipruritic agents such as calamine and mentholated lotions sometimes are soothing. Topical corticosteroid creams and oral antihistamines can relieve pruritus temporarily. Persons susceptible to mosquito bites should decrease their use of attractants such as bright clothing and aromatic cosmetics.

Flea bites are suggested by vesiculobullous, pruritic erythematous papules and plaques on the distal extremities and in places where clothes bind. These can be eliminated only by treating the source. The pet should be referred to a veterinarian for flea dipping or dusting, and the house should be treated with a veterinary flea "bomb." Bedbugs must be searched for in old bedding, floorboards, and moldings and be eradicated appropriately with insecticides. A clue to bedbug bites is their appearing in the morning on awakening on areas of the body usually covered by clothing.

INFESTATIONS

Pediculosis

Lice may infest the scalp as pediculosis capitis, the eyelashes as pediculosis palpebrarum, the body as pediculosis corporis, or the pubic area as pediculosis pubis. They are obligate ectoparasites of humans that create pruritic dermatoses by puncturing the skin and injecting inflammatory saliva. Lice can transmit rare rickettsial and bacterial diseases to humans.

Children who are infested with lice sometimes have an itchy scalp, and because lice are spread by close contact and on fomites, the youngsters are referred more often by a concerned school official for evaluation because there is an outbreak of head lice in the classroom. This grayish crawling bug with six legs may be seen in hair, or its eggs (nits) may be found as minute white-gray papules firmly attached to the hair shafts. Family members should be examined, especially if they are symptomatic or if combs, towels, and other personal items are shared. Rarely, pruritic erythematous papules 1 to 2 mm in diameter will be noted about the nape of the neck and the hairline and occasionally on the body; these usually clear after the head lice are eradicated. These lesions presumably are caused by bites of the head louse.

Nits or the insects themselves may be visible on the eyelashes or pubic hair. The sexually active adolescent usually transmits pubic lice. The affected individual should be screened for other sexually transmitted diseases. Pediculosis palpebrarum is most frequent in the toddler who sleeps with his or her parents, and both parents should be examined for pubic lice. The body louse usually is not found on the body; rather, it and its nits may be seen in the seams of clothing or in bedding. Pediculosis corporis should be suspected when extreme generalized pruritus is present. The bites consist of erythematous macules and papules. The lesions often are obscured by the results of scratching: excoriation, impetiginization, eczematization, and pigmentation.

Treatment. The most effective treatment for body lice is the application of 5% permethrin cream (Elimite) topically overnight.[1] A 1% gamma benzene hexachloride (GBH) lotion or shampoo is an alternative. The lotion is used for pediculosis corporis or pubis. It should be applied in a light layer over the entire body surface below the neck, left on for 8 to 12 hours, and then washed off. The optimum length of application has not been established, and shorter periods (e.g., 6 hours) may suffice for young children. For head lice GBH shampoo should be worked through wet hair and allowed to remain for 5 minutes. Then the hair should be shampooed as usual; after rinsing, a fine-toothed comb should be used to remove the nits from the hair shafts. Retreatment may be necessary 1 week after the first application to kill lice that have hatched from viable nits not removed initially.

Nix cream rinse contains 1% permethrin and until recently was probably the most effective agent available for treatment of head lice. A single application usually was sufficient for cure. Resistance of head lice to usual treatments has recently emerged, so repeated treatments with various pediculocides such as permethrin, GBH, and pyrethrins may be required to eradicate head lice. Even the application of Elimite 5% permethrin cream to the hair may be necessary. A vinegar rinse or Step-2 creme rinse (8% formic acid) may be tried to remove stubborn nits.

Pruritus may continue for 1 to 2 weeks after treatments, perhaps because of the continued irritancy of louse antigens or rarely because the topical pediculosides cause a primary irritant dermatitis. Patients should be advised that they might continue to itch so that they do not overtreat themselves by repeatedly applying GBH. Antipruritics and topical steroids will help to control severe pruritus.

Pediculosis palpebrarum can be treated by applying petrolatum to the eyelashes twice a day. Treatment is required for about 1 week, and a moustache comb can be used daily to remove lice and nits from the eyelashes.

The controversy over the use of GBH in younger children largely is unfounded and will be discussed below (see Scabies). Other effective pediculocides are malathion and pyrethrins with piperonyl butoxide. Malathion is available as a 0.5% lotion (Prioderm). Pyrethrins are found in such over-the-counter preparations as A-200 Pyrinate liquid and Rid. It is recommended that clothing, bedding, combs, towels, and other items used by lice-infested persons be washed in hot water or boiled to destroy the insects and their eggs.

Scabies

Infestation with *Sarcoptes scabiei hominis* is common. Scabies is a pruritic dermatosis with various manifestations ranging from a few erythematous papules to diffuse scabies-laden crusts (Norwegian scabies). Because of its varied appearance, scabies must be distinguished from insect bites, atopic dermatitis, impetigo, contact dermatitis, urticaria, secondary syphilis, seborrheic dermatitis, pityriasis rosea, and even Letterer-Siwe disease.[2]

Scabies is spread by close personal contact. All family members and sexual partners of index cases should be examined and treated. Frequently the history will reveal that many people in one household are itching, whereas with papular urticaria, only the patient will be affected. Fomite spread has not been established. However, animal mites can infest humans. Canine scabies is the most common form transferred to humans. It usually lasts for a few weeks because the mite cannot reproduce.

The burrowing of the pregnant female mite into the stratum corneum initiates scabies. She lays ova and defecates in the burrow. Over the next 4 to 6 weeks pruritus develops gradually as the eggs hatch, increasing the mite population. With reinfestation there is a more rapid onset of pruritus, suggesting a hypersensitivity reaction to mite and excreta antigens.

The burrows created by impregnated female mites are helpful in establishing the diagnosis; however, they not always are obvious and often are disguised by excoriations, eczematous reactions, and impetiginization. They should be looked for in the following locations: digital web spaces, the extensor surface of the elbows, and the flexor aspect of the wrists. Once a burrow is found, mineral oil should be applied to it and the burrow should be scraped off with a scalpel blade. Ova, mites, or feces can be found by light microscopy in the removed material.

Burrows are not the only scabious lesions. The papules, pustules, vesicles, and hives that can occur in sarcoptic infestation justify the reputation of scabies being a great masquerader. Therefore, in the face of a gradually worsening pruritus with any of these lesions, the diagnosis of scabies must be considered, particularly if there are close contacts who also are itching. The distribution of lesions can be a clue to the diagnosis. In infants the face, palms, and soles may be involved, with relative sparing of the intertriginous areas, genitals, buttocks, wrists, and extensor surfaces of joints—areas usually involved in adults.

Treatment. The application of 5% permethrin is the treatment of choice for scabies. It should be applied as noted above for lice. An alternative treatment is GBH lotion (e.g., Lindane). Adverse reactions from misuse of or agricultural exposure to 1% GBH lotion have raised concern about possible neurotoxicity from percutaneous absorption. Nevertheless, when used properly, GBH is a safe and effective scabicide, even in infants.[3] It should *not* be applied after a warm bath because absorption might be enhanced. It should be dispensed in limited quantity, sufficient for two applications 1 week apart. Parents may be informed about possible neurotoxic complications to deter overtreatment. Animal data suggest that GBH is fetotoxic but not teratogenic.[3] There are no conclusive studies concerning the use of GBH in pregnant women.

Other treatments for scabies do exist. However, crotamiton 10% (Eurax) is less efficacious than GBH. Precipitated sulfur, 5% or 10% in petrolatum, is a messy and foul-smelling but time-honored therapy. Benzyl benzoate is used widely in developing countries because it is contained in the inexpensive emulsion recommended by the World Health Organization.[4] However, controlled studies need to be conducted on the toxicity and efficacy of these agents.

Despite the absence of documented fomite spread of scabies, most authorities still recommend that clothing, bed linens, and towels be washed in hot water because epidemiological studies have demonstrated a higher rate of spread among families in whom articles such as these are shared.

Certain postscabietic conditions should be noted. Pruritus can continue for weeks despite adequate treatment; retreatment should be undertaken only when mite manifestation is documented. Certain individuals develop reddish purple, discrete nodules up to 2 cm in diameter on surfaces usually covered by clothing, particularly on the genitals. These lesions may persist for months. They are, on biopsy, granulomatous histiocytic or lymphocytic infiltrates. This "nodular scabies" is thought to represent a hypersensitivity reaction because no mites are found. The nodules usually respond to topical applications of steroids or intralesional injections of steroids. Referral to a dermatologist is indicated for treatment of these lesions.

REFERENCES

1. Drugs for parasitic infections, *Med Lett Drugs Ther* 35:111, 1993.
2. Hurwitz S: *Clinical pediatric dermatology,* Philadelphia, 1981, WB Saunders.
3. Rasmussen JE: The problem of lindane, *J Am Acad Dermatol* 5:507, 1981.
4. Schacter B: Treatment of scabies and pediculosis with lindane preparations: an evaluation, *J Am Acad Dermatol* 5:517, 1981.

223 Iron Deficiency Anemia

James Palis

Iron deficiency is the most common cause of anemia in the world and affects all ages. Iron is needed not only for hemoglobin formation and tissue replacement but also for growth. Iron deficiency, as well as other nutritional deficiencies, is most common in early childhood and during adolescence, when growth rates are maximal. Iron deficiency anemia is associated with behavioral and cognitive deficits, which may not improve despite adequate iron therapy; this makes the prevention of iron deficiency an important public health issue.

INCIDENCE

Iron deficiency is surprisingly common, even in Western societies, where nutrition is generally good and the use of iron-fortified foods is widespread. Accurate estimates of iron deficiency are difficult to obtain because the incidence varies depending on the diagnostic criteria used. Several surveys of infants in various urban areas of the United States reveal a prevalence of between 17% and 44%, the highest being among infants of lower socioeconomic status. Adolescent females are affected more commonly than males, with a prevalence as high as 27%.[7]

IRON-CONTAINING COMPOUNDS IN THE BODY

Iron is the most abundant heavy metal in the body. The multiple iron-containing compounds found within the body can be grouped into two major categories—those serving metabolic functions and those involved with iron storage and transport.

The first category includes heme- and non-heme-containing compounds. Heme is composed of a protoporphyrin ring with noncovalently bound iron in the ferrous form (Fe^{++}). The most abundant heme-containing protein in the body is hemoglobin, which transports oxygen from the lungs to the tissues and accounts for more than 60% of total body iron. Myoglobin, which accounts for 10% of total body iron, is a heme protein that provides oxygen for use during muscle contraction. The other major heme proteins, the cytochromes, are found in the mitochondria and are necessary for the oxidative production of cellular energy. There also are several nonheme iron proteins such as the iron-sulfur complexes and flavoproteins. Many of these proteins are found in the mitochondria and also are involved in oxidative metabolism.

The second category of iron compounds is the iron transport and storage molecules. Transferrin is a beta$_1$-globulin capable of binding two atoms of iron in the ferric form (Fe^{+++}). It transports iron from the serosal surface of intestinal epithelium to the bone marrow for the synthesis of hemoglobin. It also plays a major role in the recycling of iron from senescent red blood cells. In adult males approximately 95% of the iron needed for red blood cell production is derived from red blood cell breakdown.[1] Ferritin, an iron storage compound found in all cells of the body, is composed of a hollow protein shell encapsulating iron molecules. Hemosiderin, which also serves to store intracellular iron, is thought to be a partially degraded form of ferritin.

ETIOLOGY AND PATHOPHYSIOLOGY

The four most important factors in the development of iron deficiency in children are (1) the iron endowment at birth, (2) the iron needs during rapid body growth, (3) exogenous iron absorption, and (4) blood loss.

During gestation the fetus is able to extract iron efficiently from the mother independently of maternal iron stores.[9] The ratio of iron content to weight in the human fetus remains constant throughout gestation. The healthy full-term infant has sufficient iron stores to last for 6 months, even if little iron is ingested from the diet. The infant's iron endowment can be compromised by blood loss during the pregnancy or the perinatal period. Common causes of blood loss include third-trimester bleeding, such as abruptio placentae, placenta previa, fetomaternal hemorrhage, and twin-to-twin transfusions.

Because of their lower body weight, premature infants have a smaller absolute amount of body iron compared with full-term infants. Their increased growth requirements after birth coupled with their smaller iron endowment can lead to a rapid depletion of iron stores, resulting in iron deficiency anemia as early as 3 months of age.[4]

Iron is needed not only for many metabolic functions and tissue replacement but also for growth. Growth rates vary with age and are maximal during infancy and adolescence,[10] the same periods associated with the highest frequency of iron deficiency.

Because there are no mechanisms available for the active excretion of iron from the body, iron balance is maintained by regulation of iron absorption. The amount of iron absorbed depends both on the amount and the bioavailability of dietary iron, as well as on regulation of iron absorption by the intestinal mucosa. Most dietary iron occurs in the nonheme form and is much less bioavailable than that in heme proteins. The iron in hemoglobin and myoglobin is particularly bioavailable; up to 30% is directly absorbed by the gastrointestinal tract. Breast milk and cow milk contain small amounts of iron (0.5 to 1 mg/1000 ml). However, 50% of the iron in breast milk is absorbed as compared with only 10% in cow milk. Full-term infants who are exclusively breast-fed for the first 6 to 9 months do not become iron deficient.[7] Nonheme iron absorption is inhibited by bran in cereals, polyphenols in many vegetables, and tannins in tea. The addition of solids to an infant's diet can impair iron absorption significantly and puts the infant at risk for developing iron deficiency. The in-

Table 223-1 Iron Status and Hematological Abnormalities in the Three Stages of Iron Deficiency

	Storage iron depletion	Iron deficient erythropoiesis	Iron deficiency anemia
Storage iron	↓	↓↓	↓↓↓
Erythron iron	Normal	↓	↓↓-↓↓↓
Hemoglobin concentration	Normal	Normal	↓-↓↓↓

Modified from Cecalupo AJ, Cohen HJ: Nutritional anemias. In Grand RJ, Sutphen JL, Dietz WH, editors: *Clinical nutrition: theory and practice,* Boston, 1987, Butterworth.
↓, Decreased.

troduced solids therefore should contain abundant amounts of iron (e.g., iron-fortified cereals).

Blood loss causes iron deficiency in children less frequently than in adults. In infancy and childhood, iron deficiency caused by blood loss most commonly is associated with the ingestion of unprocessed cow milk and with parasitic infections. Hypersensitivity to whole cow milk causes an exudative enteropathy and frequently leads to gastrointestinal blood loss. Other less common causes of blood loss in children include Meckel diverticulum, intestinal duplication, peptic ulcer disease, hemorrhagic telangiectasia, and the chronic use of medications that prolong the bleeding time (e.g., aspirin).

CLINICAL MANIFESTATIONS

The onset and progression of iron deficiency usually is gradual, and most children will not have major symptoms. Iron deficiency in infants and children is associated with generalized weakness, irritability, easy fatigability, headaches, poor feeding, anorexia, pica, and poor weight gain.[7] The physical examination usually is unremarkable except for marked pallor of the mucous membranes and skin. Other less common physical findings associated with iron deficiency anemia include mild hepatosplenomegaly, lymphadenopathy, glossitis, stomatitis, blue sclerae, and koilonychia (spoon-shaped nails).

Many studies have demonstrated an association between iron deficiency anemia and lower scores on tests of mental and motor development, impaired learning, and decreased school achievement.[3,6] These findings may be related to the decreased attention span and increased irritability seen in iron deficient children as compared with nonanemic controls. To what degree iron deficiency is responsible for these clinical findings is not known because iron repletion may not completely correct the behavioral disturbances or the lower developmental, IQ, and achievement scores.[3] More studies are needed to address and clarify these issues.

STAGES OF IRON DEFICIENCY

Iron deficiency occurs when total body iron content is diminished. Iron normally is absorbed only through the gastrointestinal tract. Sites of iron loss include the skin, the gastrointestinal tract, and the urine. Iron also is lost during pregnancy and lactation. When absorption exceeds losses, the iron surplus is stored in the reticuloendothelial system, principally the liver, spleen, and bone marrow. As body iron stores increase, the gastrointestinal absorption of iron decreases so that iron balance is maintained.

Iron is removed from the reticuloendothelial storage pool to compensate for negative iron balance. The development of iron deficiency proceeds through a series of overlapping stages. The first stage of iron deficiency is *storage iron depletion.* During this stage there is no deficit of iron supplied to the erythroid marrow for red cell production. If the negative iron balance continues, the second stage, *iron deficient erythropoiesis,* will occur. During this stage erythroid iron supply is diminished, but the hemoglobin concentration remains in the normal range. If the negative iron balance persists, *iron deficiency anemia* finally develops. This third stage is characterized by a fall in the hemoglobin concentration and a reduction in red blood cell size and hemoglobin content.

DIAGNOSIS

Specific laboratory findings are associated with each of the three stages of iron deficiency. The hematological abnormalities and diagnostic tests characteristic of each stage are reviewed in greater depth below and are summarized in Tables 223-1 and 223-2.

Storage Iron Depletion

During this first stage of iron deficiency, the storage pool of iron in the reticuloendothelial system decreases. This can be detected by a fall in serum ferritin levels or by the absence of stainable iron on a bone marrow sample. No red blood cell changes are present at this time because there is sufficient iron to support normal erythropoiesis.

Serum Ferritin. As seen in Figure 223-1 serum ferritin levels vary with age during infancy and childhood. In healthy individuals serum ferritin levels reflect body iron stores; levels below 12 μg/L indicate iron deficiency. Ferritin is an acute phase reactant. Serum ferritin levels are elevated during infections and inflammatory processes as well as in liver disease. Although low serum ferritin is diagnostic of iron deficiency, an elevated ferritin level associated with inflammation or liver disease does not rule out concomitant iron deficiency.

Bone Marrow Iron. The staining of a normal bone marrow aspirate sample with Prussian blue dye reveals the presence of iron in red blood cell precursors (normoblasts) and serves as a reliable index of body iron stores. In iron deficiency the number of iron granules in normoblasts is decreased and stainable iron in the marrow aspirate is almost completely absent.[2]

Iron Deficient Erythropoiesis

Iron deficient erythropoiesis characterizes the second stage of iron deficiency. The earliest hematological manifestation

Table 223-2 Laboratory Abnormalities in the Three Stages of Iron Deficiency

	Storage iron depletion	Iron-deficient erythropoiesis	Iron deficiency anemia
Bone marrow iron	Absent	Absent	Absent
Ferritin	↓	↓↓	↓↓↓
Red cell distribution width	Normal-↓	↓↓	↓↓↓
Serum iron	Normal	↓-↓↓	↓↓↓
Total iron-binding capacity	Normal	↑	↑↑-↑↑↑
Percent saturation	Normal	↓	↓↓-↓↓↓
Free erythrocyte protoporphyrin	Normal	↑	↑↑-↑↑↑
Red blood cell indices	Normal	Normal	↓-↓↓↓

Modified from Cecalupo AJ, Cohen HJ: Nutritional anemias. In Grand RJ, Sutphen JL, Dietz WH, editors: *Clinical nutrition: theory and practice,* Boston, 1987, Butterworth.
↑, Increased; ↓, decreased.

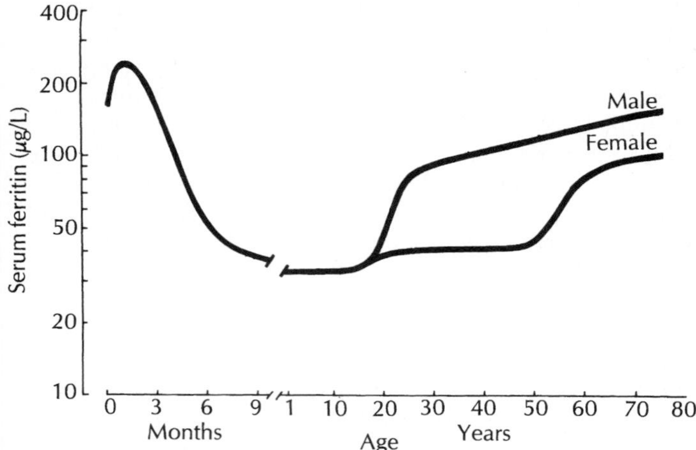

FIG. 223-1 Developmental changes in concentration of serum ferritin.

(From Dallman PR, Simes MA, Stekel A: *Am J Clin Nutrition* 33:107, 1980.)

of iron deficiency is an elevation of the red cell distribution width.[11] The serum iron concentration decreases, and serum transferrin levels rise concomitantly. This leads to an increase in the total iron-binding capacity (TIBC), with a decrease in the percent saturation (iron/TIBC × 100). Because iron is unavailable for incorporation in the protoporphyrin ring, free erythrocyte protoporphyrin (FEP) in both red blood cells and the plasma increases during this stage of iron deficiency. The plasma loses its usual amber color and becomes clear, making inspection of the plasma on a spun hematocrit useful diagnostically.

Iron/TIBC. Serum iron levels normally fluctuate daily, with maximum levels occurring in the morning and minimal levels in the evening. The TIBC varies less than serum iron but is harder to measure accurately.[1] The normal TIBC is 250 to 400 mg/dl, but as serum iron levels decrease, the TIBC increases to 450 mg/dl or more. Iron and TIBC measurements are useful in distinguishing iron deficiency anemia from the anemia of chronic disease. Serum iron levels decrease with both, but the TIBC levels also decrease in chronic disease states. A useful measure of iron deficiency is the percent saturation—the serum iron divided by the TIBC and multiplied by 100. The normal ranges for serum iron and the percent saturation are shown in Table 223-3. In iron deficiency the percent saturation is reduced to less than 16%, at which point

Table 223-3 Means and Standard Errors of Measurement of Serum Iron and Iron Saturation Percentage by Age

Age (years)	Serum iron (μg/dl)	Saturation (%)
½-2	68 ± 3.6	22 ± 1.1
2-6	72 ± 3.4	25 ± 1.2
6-12	73 ± 3.4	25 ± 1.2
18+	92 ± 3.8	30 ± 1.1

Modified from Koerper MA, Dallman PR: *Pediatr Res* 11:473, 1977.

hemoglobin production becomes limited by the lack of iron. The percent saturation is a more sensitive index of iron status than are serum iron measurements alone. Because of the wide variation in serum iron and iron-binding capacity values, these should be tested in conjunction with at least one other test of iron status (e.g., ferritin, FEP) to reach a reliable diagnosis of iron deficiency.

Free Erythrocyte Protoporphyrin (FEP). FEP accumulates in red blood cells when iron is insufficient to combine with protoporphyrin to form heme. FEP levels also are elevated in lead poisoning, infections, inflammatory diseases, and protoporphyria, but not in thalassemia trait. This makes FEP determinations helpful in distinguishing iron deficiency from alpha- or beta-thalassemia trait.

Iron Deficiency Anemia

Anemia characterizes the third stage of iron deficiency. Decreased production of red blood cells in the bone marrow leads to a decrease in hemoglobin levels and the hematocrit. The size of the red blood cells, as measured by the mean corpuscular volume (MCV), and their hemoglobin content, as measured by the mean corpuscular hemoglobin (MCH), begin to decrease as the anemia develops. Thus persistent negative iron balance predictably leads to a microcytic, hypochromic anemia.

Hemoglobin. Percentile curves for hemoglobin values of nonindigent children living at sea level are shown in Figure 223-2. African-American children normally have a hemoglobin concentration 0.3 to 1 g/dl lower than that of Caucasian children. This difference is not explained completely by differences in socioeconomic status or prevalence of iron deficiency.[1] By laboratory definition anemia is a hemoglobin value below the 95th percentile for age and gender.

Unfortunately, capillary blood hemoglobin determinations vary greatly because of dilution by tissue fluids.[8] Venous

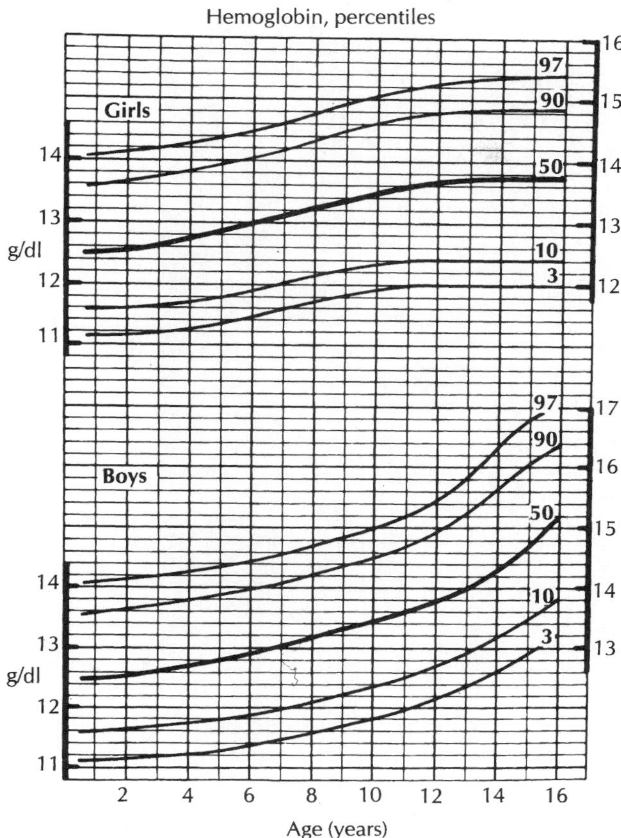

FIG. 223-2 Hemoglobin concentration in infants and children.
(Modified from Dallman PR, Simes MA: *J Pediatr* 94:28, 1979.)

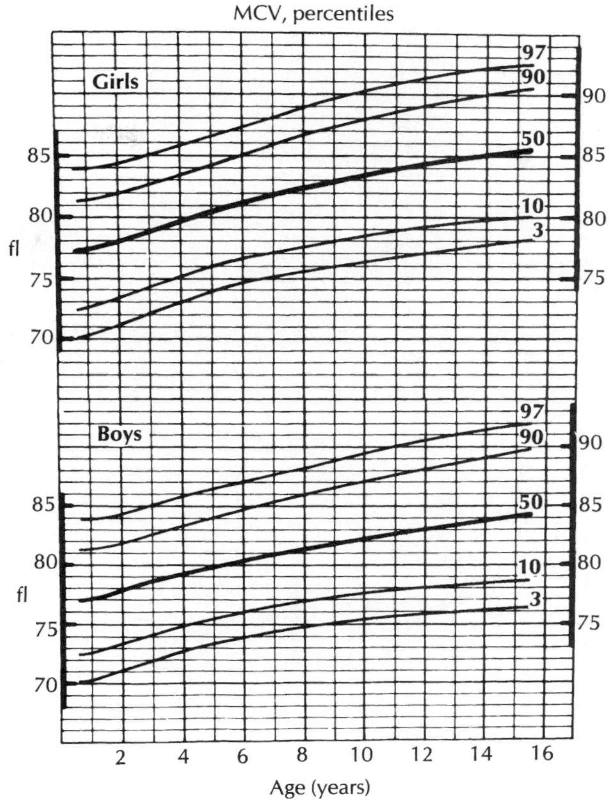

FIG. 223-3 Mean corpuscular volume (MCV) in infants and children.
(Modified from Dallman PR, Simes MA: *J Pediatr* 94:28, 1979.)

blood samples produce more accurate hemoglobin measurements but are more difficult to obtain in infants. These factors limit the usefulness of hemoglobin and hematocrit determinations for the screening of anemia.

RBC Indices. The development of electronic counters has made the use of red blood cell indices widely available for the initial screening of infants and children for iron deficiency. These tests are highly reproducible and less subject to sampling error as compared with hemoglobin determinations because tissue fluid dilution does not affect red blood cell size. Because both the MCV and the MCH normally change during development, it is necessary to consult age-specific reference standards (Fig. 223-3).

Iron deficiency is the most likely diagnosis of anemia characterized by microcytosis and hypochromia. Other causes of anemia with these characteristics include alpha- and beta-thalassemia trait, hemoglobin E disease, and sometimes the anemia of infection and chronic disease. Most other anemias, however, are characterized by a normal or an elevated MCV.

The Mentzer index, defined as the MCV divided by the RBC count in millions, can help to distinguish the anemia of iron deficiency from that of beta-thalassemia trait.[5] In the former the Mentzer index often is greater than 13.5; in the latter it is less than 11.5.

Peripheral Blood Smear. Examination of the blood smear in iron deficiency anemia reveals hypochromic microcytes, poikilocytes, elliptocytes, and target cells (Fig. 223-4). The presence of basophilic stippling suggests associated lead poisoning. Unfortunately, the red blood cell changes seen on the blood smear are not specific for iron deficiency.

The white blood cell count and morphology in iron deficiency anemia usually are normal. Both thrombocytosis and thrombocytopenia occur with iron deficiency. The latter is more common in severe iron deficiency and resolves once iron therapy is instituted.

TREATMENT

Therapeutic Trial of Iron

To confirm the diagnosis of iron deficiency, either additional laboratory tests (ferritin, FEP, Fe/TIBC) or a therapeutic trial of iron can be initiated. Because dietary iron deficiency is by far the most common cause of anemia in an otherwise healthy infant, a 1-month therapeutic trial of iron usually is justified. The treatment of choice is the oral administration of ferrous sulfate. Although other iron salts are available, ferrous sulfate is inexpensive and well tolerated. The dose of oral therapy is 3 to 6 mg/kg/day of elemental iron in three divided doses. About twice as much iron is absorbed on an empty stomach as at mealtime. A response of decreased irritability and increased appetite to oral iron therapy has been noted within 12 to 24 hours. The reticulocyte response peaks at 5 to 10 days after the institution of iron therapy. In an otherwise healthy individual the recovery from anemia is about two thirds complete within 1 month. It is recommended that the hemoglobin be measured again at 1 month

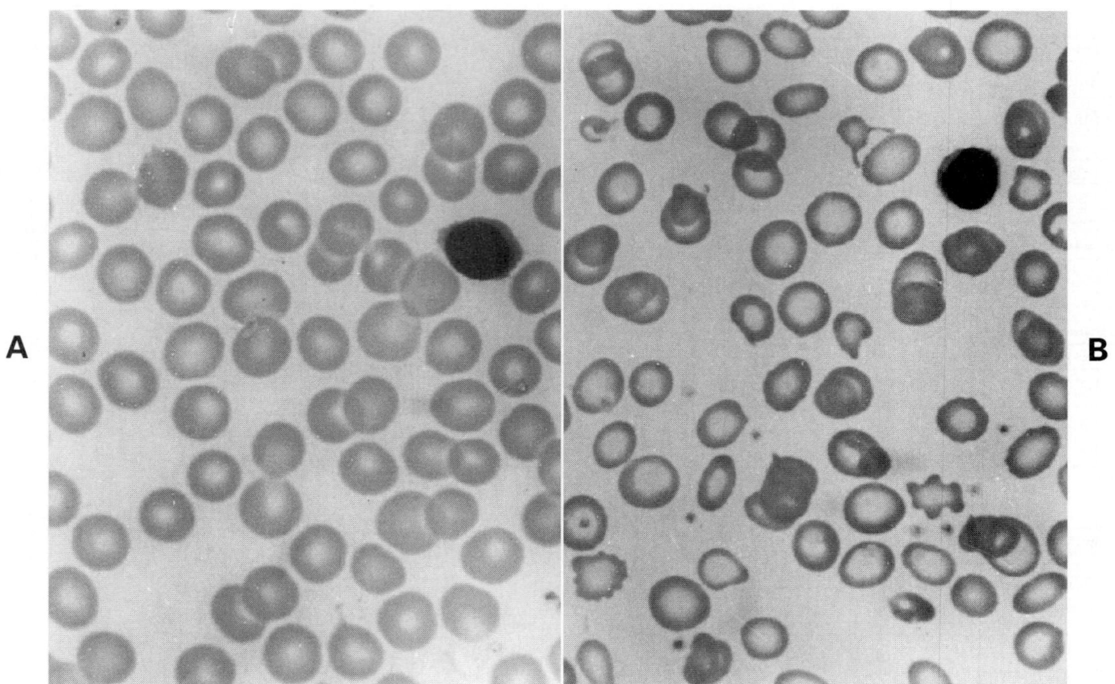

FIG. 223-4 **A,** A normal peripheral blood smear. The size of normocytic red blood cells is similar to the nucleus of a mature lymphocyte. **B,** The peripheral blood smear from an individual with iron deficiency anemia reveals microcytosis, hypochromia, and poikilocytosis.

to check the therapeutic progress as well as to emphasize compliance.

Once the diagnosis of iron deficiency is confirmed either by a response to a therapeutic trial or further laboratory tests, oral therapy at 3 to 6 mg/kg/day should be continued for 2 to 3 months after normal hemoglobin levels have been restored. This allows the repletion of body iron stores. Anemia, microcytosis, and elevated FEP levels are corrected completely with 3 months of treatment. Use of intramuscular or intravenous iron rarely is warranted. Intramuscular injections are painful, and skin discoloration is common. Anaphylactic reactions have occurred with both intramuscular and intravenous injection, and deaths have been reported. Parenteral treatment therefore should be used only when oral therapy is not possible—for example, in patients who have inflammatory bowel disease. A blood transfusion is indicated only when severe anemia leads to congestive heart failure and cardiovascular compromise. If a blood transfusion is warranted clinically, then packed red blood cells should be given slowly or a partial exchange transfusion performed. Vital signs should be monitored carefully.

Failure To Respond to Therapy

When a patient fails to respond to oral iron treatment, the following factors should be considered: (1) noncompliance with oral therapy, (2) inadequate iron dose, (3) persistent or unrecognized blood loss, (4) malabsorption of iron—for example, primary gastrointestinal disease, (5) other diagnoses—for example, alpha- or beta-thalassemia trait and hemoglobin E disease, and (6) poor iron utilization—for example, in chronic inflammation, sideroblastic anemia, lead poisoning, and congenital atransferrinemia.

PREVENTION

Although other important nutritional deficiencies of the past, such as pellagra, scurvy, and rickets, have become rare, iron deficiency remains a current public health problem. Iron deficiency anemia is associated with behavioral and cognitive deficits, some of which may not improve despite adequate iron therapy. Thus prevention of iron deficiency is an important aspect of treatment.

Excessive intake of cow milk during infancy leads to iron deficiency because of the low concentration and poor bioavailability of iron in cow milk. Breast-feeding or the use of milk-based infant formulas supplemented with iron should be encouraged during the first 6 months. The intake of milk thereafter should be limited to less than 1 quart per day. Because the addition of solids to an infant's diet can impair iron absorption significantly, solids should not be started before the infant is 4 months of age. The use of iron-fortified cereals should be encouraged once solids are started. Oral iron supplementation is recommended for preterm infants because they have greater iron needs than do full-term infants. In this instance 2 to 4 mg/kg/day of elemental iron in the form of ferrous sulfate drops should be started when the infant is 2 months of age.

REFERENCES

1. Dallman PR: Iron deficiency and related nutritional anemias. In Nathan DG, Oski FA, editors: *Hematology of infancy and childhood,* ed 3, Philadelphia, 1987, WB Saunders.
2. Krause JR: The bone marrow in nutritional deficiencies, *Hematol Oncol Clin North Am* 2:557, 1988.
3. Lozoff B, Jimenez E, Wolf AW: Long-term developmental outcome of infants with iron deficiency, *N Engl J Med* 325:687, 1991.

4. Lundstrom U, Simes MA, Dallman PR: At what age does iron supplementation become necessary in low birth weight infants? *J Pediatr* 91:878, 1977.
5. Mentzer WG: Differentiation of iron deficiency from thalassemia trait, *Lancet* 1:882, 1973.
6. Oski FA: The non-hematologic manifestations of iron deficiency, *Am J Dis Child* 133:315, 1979.
7. Oski FA, Stockman JA: Anemia due to inadequate iron sources or poor iron utilization, *Pediatr Clin North Am* 27:237, 1980.
8. Reeves JD: Iron deficiency anemia: cost effective screening and management, *Contemp Pediatr* 1:10, 1984.
9. Rio SE et al: Relationship of maternal and infant iron stores as assessed by determination of plasma ferritin, *Pediatrics* 55:694, 1975.
10. Tanner JM, Whitehouse RH, Takaishi M: Standards from birth to maturity for height velocity and weight velocity: British children, *Arch Dis Child* 41:454, 1966.
11. van Zeben et al: Evaluation of microcytosis using serum ferritin and red blood cell distribution width, *Eur J Haematol* 44:105, 1990.

224 Juvenile Arthritis

Harry L. Gewanter

Juvenile arthritis (JA or juvenile rheumatoid arthritis) is an uncommon collection of clinical syndromes with the common feature of chronic childhood arthritis. The diagnosis is applied to any child under 16 years of age who has persistent arthritis of one or more joints lasting for more than 6 weeks in whom all other diseases have been excluded. JA is classified further into three subtypes (systemic-onset, pauciarticular, and polyarticular) based on the clinical course over the first 6 months of illness.[10]

Many American rheumatologists apply the term *juvenile rheumatoid arthritis* only to children who are seropositive for rheumatoid factor. Recent data suggest that many subtypes of pauciarticular and polyarticular JA exist, and it will be a number of years before a universally accepted classification is devised.

Although JA is the most common of the pediatric rheumatic diseases, its true incidence and prevalence are unknown. The peak age of onset is between 2 and 4 years, with a smaller peak later in childhood. There is a general female predominance. The best estimate of prevalence is about 0.5 to 1 case per 1000 children; thus approximately 40,000 to 100,000 children in the United States have JA at any given time.[13]

ETIOLOGY

The exact cause of JA is unknown. Recent data on the frequency of certain subtypes of human leukocyte antigens (HLA) in JA (e.g., HLA-DR5 and DR8 in younger girls who have pauciarticular JA, HLA-DR4 in rheumatoid factor–positive polyarticular JA, and HLA-B27 in older boys who have pauciarticular JA)[16] have led to the concept of a genetic predisposition for the development of an inflammatory arthritis that may be triggered by any of a number of events, such as trauma, infection,[28] or emotional stress.[19]

Other areas of interesting research include investigations of immunological abnormalities involving autoantibodies,[21] cytokines, immunoregulation,[6] and the function of and communication between T and B lymphocytes and antigen-presenting cells.[16] The nature of these interactions and how they result in the development of JA, however, remain to be discovered.

CLINICAL PRESENTATION

Because the diagnosis of JA is based on clinical grounds, the history and physical examination are paramount; no specific diagnostic laboratory tests yet exist. Only by considering all the data on the child's presentation and course is the physician able to diagnose JA.

The presence of arthritis or inflammation within the joint is an absolute criterion for diagnosing JA. Arthritis is defined as being present when there is (1) intraarticular swelling or effusion or (2) when two or more of the following occur: (a) joint pain or tenderness with motion, (b) limitation of joint motion, or (c) increased warmth overlying the joint.[10] Children frequently have arthralgias (pain or tenderness with joint motion), but arthritis is much less common. Other features that may be present in children who have JA include fever, rash, lymphadenopathy, hepatosplenomegaly, polyserositis, rheumatoid nodules, vasculitis, and growth retardation. Younger children rarely complain of joint pain but may instead become irritable, stop walking or using an extremity, or regress in their behavior. Other symptoms include decreased appetite, malaise, inactivity, morning stiffness, night joint pains, or failure to thrive.

Any joint of the body may be involved. The pattern and number of involved joints are important in diagnosing the various subtypes of JA.

SYSTEMIC-ONSET JUVENILE ARTHRITIS

Even though the hallmark of systemic-onset JA is its extraarticular manifestations, the presence of arthritis is necessary to confirm the diagnosis. Affecting about 15% of all children who have JA, systemic-onset JA is slightly more common in males and usually begins at an early age, although it has even been recognized in adults. The systemic features may persist for months and occur or recur independently of the arthritis.

Daily intermittent fevers are frequent components of systemic-onset JA. Rectal temperature recordings may reach 40° C (104° F) to 41° C (106° F), most often in the afternoon, and then return to normal or subnormal levels. An evanescent, salmon-colored rash often accompanies the fevers. The lesions are small macules or papules, frequently with central clearing, and often appear in areas of increased heat (e.g., the axilla); often they can be induced with mild local trauma (Koebner phenomenon).

Enlargement of the lymph nodes, liver, and spleen is frequent and may be of sufficient size to suggest the presence of a malignancy. Polyserositis in the form of pericarditis or pleuritis also is common. The effusions, however, rarely are symptomatic or significant clinically. Although these children frequently complain of myalgias or arthralgias when they are febrile, they may have few symptoms when the fevers resolve. The arthritis may occur at any time, more often is polyarticular involving both large and small joints, and can be quite severe.

The white blood cell count (WBC) can be quite high, with a shift to the left. Most patients are quite anemic. Thrombocytosis is frequent, as are the acute phase reactants (e.g., erythrocyte sedimentation rate [ESR] and C-reactive protein [CRP]). Rheumatoid factor (RF) and antinuclear antibody (ANA) tests usually are negative. Serum immunoglobulin and complement levels usually are normal but may reflect the degree of inflammation. Evidence of a vasculopathy and an intravascular consumption coagulopathy sometimes is found.[33]

The clinical course is extremely variable. Some children have a single systemic episode that lasts weeks to months and have few, if any, joint problems; others have multiple systemic episodes before developing the arthritis, which can be pauciarticular or polyarticular. Poor prognostic signs include the continued presence of systemic features and a platelet count greater than 600,000/mm^3 6 months after onset.[32] At least a third of these children will develop severe and crippling arthritis.

POLYARTICULAR JUVENILE ARTHRITIS

About 30% to 35% of children who have JA have the polyarticular type, which can be subdivided into IgM–rheumatoid factor (RF)-positive (about 10% of the total) and IgM-RF-negative (about 25%) forms. So-called hidden rheumatoid factors have been found in all subgroups, but their significance remains obscure.[26] It is extremely rare to find a significantly positive RF in a child under 7 years of age. Systemic features usually are mild and include low-grade fevers, easy fatigability, and slowing of growth. The growth problems may be local (e.g., micrognathia) or generalized and can occur regardless of whether the child receives corticosteroids. Discrepancies between height and weight are seen and can be significant. For example, children who have polyarticular arthritis may be of low weight for height, whereas children who have systemic onset tend to be average in weight for height.[5] The arthritis most often is chronic and symmetrical and involves five or more joints; any joint of the body, including the temporomandibular joint and the cervical spine, can be affected. Nearly all children have wrist involvement, and small joint involvement of the hands and feet is common. Finally these children may develop a chronic uveitis.[2]

Rheumatoid Factor–Positive Polyarticular Juvenile Arthritis

Patients who have RF-positive polyarticular JA most often are older than 8 to 10 years of age, are more likely to be girls, and are similar clinically to those patients who have adult rheumatoid arthritis. Severe, rapidly progressive, erosive, crippling arthritis, subcutaneous rheumatoid nodules, and rheumatoid vasculitis can develop, just as in adults.

Rheumatoid Factor–Negative Polyarticular Juvenile Arthritis

Children who have RF-negative polyarticular JA usually are younger and overall have a better prognosis than those who are RF-positive. However, even though children who have the RF-negative type typically respond better to therapy and have a lower frequency of severe, early, crippling arthritis than do children who have the RF-positive form, they also may develop many significant problems. Because their arthritis starts earlier, it can lead to significant deformities and problems as a result of the tendency to develop flexion contractures at the involved joints. Compared with adults, hand involvement more often affects the interphalangeal joints than the metacarpophalangeal joints. Ulnar deviation of the fingers is much less common in children compared with adults, whereas flexion contractures, boutonnière (buttonhole) deformities, and radial deviation of the fingers are seen more frequently. Ulnar deviation and subluxation at the wrist may occur. Arthritis of the apophyseal joints of the cervical spine is common and can lead to rapid and significant limitation of extension and rotation. These children are at the highest risk for developing the local and generalized growth problems mentioned above.

Pauciarticular Juvenile Arthritis

Pauciarticular JA involves four or fewer joints, most often the large joints, in an asymmetrical distribution. The pattern and course of joint involvement are as important in distinguishing this form of JA from the others as are the number of joints involved. With a few exceptions, systemic features are infrequent and mild. Nearly half of all children who have JA fall in this subgroup, and they have the best overall prognosis.

At least two, often four and possibly more, subtypes of pauciarticular JA exist.

Early-Onset Pauciarticular Juvenile Arthritis. Early-onset pauciarticular JA (5% to 10% of all patients who have JA) occurs classically in girls under 6 years of age and involves the large joints (knees, ankles, elbows); these girls are at higher risk for developing chronic uveitis.[2,31] Despite the obvious arthritis these children generally function quite well and only rarely complain of pain. Little erosive joint damage typically occurs, even though these children may have ongoing arthritis for many years. Nonetheless, these children are at risk for long-term problems, including leg-length discrepancies and muscle atrophy.[37] Systemic signs and symptoms, except for uveitis, are few. The uveitis rarely is symptomatic until it has progressed to a severe stage and may not occur until years after the onset of the arthritis. It may even occur after the arthritis has resolved. Thus regular ophthalmological examinations, including slit-lamp examinations, should be instituted early, performed every 4 to 6 months, and continued indefinitely. Because the risk of uveitis decreases with time, the interval between examinations can be lengthened after a number of years if no uveitis is present[2] (see Table 224-1).

Few laboratory abnormalities are noted. Although there may be mild WBC and ESR elevations or a low-grade anemia, all these tests may be normal. Most of these children are ANA positive and many are positive for HLA-DR5 and DR8 gene markers.[16]

Late-Onset Pauciarticular Juvenile Arthritis. Late-onset pauciarticular JA typically involves boys over 8 years of age. Their arthritis is more frequently in the lower extremities, involving the knees and ankles but also occasionally the toes (resulting in a dactylitis or "sausage toe"). Complaints and findings of enthesopathies (i.e., inflammation of the attachment of a tendon, ligament, fascia, or capsule to bone) are extremely common in this group and may antedate the joint problems. There often is a family history of arthritis, and many of these children carry the HLA-B27 antigen. These children also seem to be at increased risk for developing spondyloarthropathies later in life, despite there being no evidence of sacroiliac disease initially. For example, some patients will progress to fulfill the criteria for ankylosing spon-

Table 224-1 Frequency of Ophthalmological Visits for Children with Juvenile Rheumatoid Arthritis (JRA) and without Known Iridocyclitis*

JRA subtype at onset	Age of onset	
	<7 y†	≥7 y‡
Pauciarticular		
+ ANA	H§	M
− ANA	M	M
Polyarticular		
+ ANA	H§	M
− ANA	M	M
Systemic	L	L

From The American Academy of Pediatrics Section on Rheumatology's Guidelines for Ophthamologic Examinations in Children with Juvenile Rheumatoid Arthritis, *Pediatrics* 92:295, 1993.

*High risk *(H)* indicates ophthalmological examinations every 3 to 4 months. Medium risk *(M)* indicates ophthalmological examinations every 6 months. Low risk *(L)* indicates ophthalmological examinations every 12 months. *ANA* indicates antinuclear antibody test.

†All patients are considered at low risk 7 years after the onset of their arthritis and should have yearly ophthalmological examinations indefinitely.

‡All patients are considered at low risk 4 years after the onset of their arthritis and should have yearly ophthalmological examinations indefinitely.

§All high-risk patients are considered at medium risk 4 years after the onset of their arthritis.

dylitis or for Reiter syndrome. About 10% will develop an acute iritis; in contrast to the chronic uveitis seen in early-onset pauciarticular JA, this is symptomatic, can be treated early, and usually is self-limited. As with the early-onset group, abnormal laboratory tests are found infrequently.

Other Subtypes of Pauciarticular Juvenile Arthritis. At least two other subtypes of pauciarticular JA might exist. The first lies somewhere between the early-onset and the late-onset subtypes. These children seem to have the best prognosis, are ANA negative, and are at a medium risk for eye or other serious, chronic problems. About 10% to 15% of all children who have JA make up the fourth subtype. They have a pauciarticular onset but evolve into a polyarticular course. These children more often start with three or four joints involved and/or have wrist or small finger joint arthritis.

DIFFERENTIAL DIAGNOSIS

Diseases to be considered in the differential diagnosis of JA are given in the box on p. 1385. The hallmark of JA is its chronicity; frequently, the best diagnostic test is "watchful waiting." Only by meeting the criterion of sustained arthritis for more than 6 weeks and excluding other possible diseases can the physician accurately avoid mislabeling other transient entities as JA.

It is very important to rule out any infectious cause, especially bacterial arthritis. If this is a consideration, arthrocentesis must be performed to establish the diagnosis. *Hemophilus influenzae* type b is the most common organism isolated in children under 2 years, although its incidence is decreasing with increasing immunization rates. *Neisseria gonorrhoeae* is most common in adolescents, whereas various strains of staphylococci may be found at any age. Other infectious agents such as fungi, viruses (including parvovirus, rubella, and hepatitis B), and *Mycoplasma* organisms also must be considered as the cause of arthritis. Lyme disease is a significant cause of childhood arthritis in endemic areas. Osteomyelitis, involving the bone contiguous to a joint, and reactive arthritis from a gastrointestinal (GI) bacterial infection (e.g., *Shigella, Salmonella, Campylobacter,* or *Yersinia* organisms) also may mimic some subgroups of JA. Neoplasms involving the bone, either primary or metastatic (e.g., leukemia, lymphoma, neuroblastoma), can be accompanied by musculoskeletal complaints. Arthritis is uncommon and usually transient, but complaints of pain out of proportion to physical findings and complaints of night pain are common and potentially important clues.

The various osteochondroses and avascular necrosis syndromes, musculoskeletal trauma, chondromalacia patellae, Osgood-Schlatter disease, slipped femoral capital epiphysis, diskitis, psychogenic arthralgias, and nonspecific musculoskeletal aches and pains also can mimic JA in its early stages.

Hemophilia, sickle cell disease, inflammatory bowel disease, the collagen disorders (e.g., Ehlers-Danlos syndrome, Marfan syndrome), familial Mediterranean fever, and sarcoidosis also may be associated with arthritis.

Juvenile ankylosing spondylitis and the other spondyloarthropathies can present as JA at their onset, especially in an older child who is HLA-B27 positive. Acute rheumatic fever, although in decline for many years, now is undergoing a resurgence in many areas.[36] Systemic lupus erythematosus has arthritis as one of its major manifestations but can be differentiated from juvenile arthritis by its other systemic features. Although its gender distribution is equal in younger children, there is female preponderance postpubertally. Dermatomyositis is characterized more typically by inflammatory muscle involvement than by arthritis. Scleroderma occasionally is associated with arthritis but has classic dermatological manifestations.

Children who have various immunodeficiencies can have arthritis, either from their primary problem or secondary to infections. Serum sickness and the various vasculitides, including Kawasaki disease and Henoch-Schönlein purpura, can produce intermittent arthritis. These illnesses are diagnosed by their individual distinguishing features. Finally, a number of conditions may produce significant arthralgias and myalgias and may mimic an arthropathy. The complaints and disability resulting from the hypermobility syndrome[9] and fibromyalgia (fibrositis)[39] can be sufficient to make one believe that an arthritis is present. A reflex sympathetic dystrophy deserves diagnostic consideration in children who have a hot or cold painful extremity that they refuse to move.[8]

MANAGEMENT

It always is necessary to individualize each patient's management in terms of the disease subtype, extent of activity, clinical course to date, and family situation. Although most physicians are accustomed to considering pharmacological therapy of primary importance, it is only one aspect of the treatment of children who have JA. A multidisciplinary team approach is the most effective means to meet the varied needs of a child who has arthritis and of his or her family.

Currently available drug therapy (see the box on p. 1386), although not curative, can suppress the inflammatory activi-

DIFFERENTIAL DIAGNOSIS OF JUVENILE ARTHRITIS

Rheumatic disease of childhood

Acute rheumatic fever
Systemic lupus erythematosus
Juvenile ankylosing spondylitis
Polymyositis and dermatomyositis
Vasculitis
Scleroderma
Psoriatic arthritis
Mixed connective tissue disease and overlap syndromes
Kawasaki disease
Behçet syndrome
Familial Mediterranean fever
Reiter syndrome
Reflex sympathetic dystrophy
Fibromyalgia (fibrositis)

Infectious diseases

Bacterial arthritis
Viral or postviral arthritis
Fungal arthritis
Osteomyelitis
Reactive arthritis

Neoplastic diseases

Leukemia
Lymphoma
Neuroblastoma
Primary bone tumors

Noninflammatory disorders

Trauma
Avascular necrosis syndromes
Osteochondroses
Slipped capital femoral epiphysis
Diskitis
Patellofemoral dysfunction (chondromalacia patellae)
Toxic synovitis of the hip
Overuse syndromes

Genetic or congenital syndromes

Hematological disorders

Sickle cell disease
Hemophilia

Inflammatory bowel disease

Miscellaneous

Growing pains
Psychogenic arthralgias (conversion reactions)
Hypermobility syndrome
Villonodular synovitis
Foreign body arthritis

ties in many children who have JA. Five major categories of drug therapy are available: nonsteroidal antiinflammatory drugs (NSAIDs), slower-acting antirheumatic drugs (SAARDs), corticosteroids, cytotoxic agents, and other therapies (e.g., intravenous immune globulin and plasmapheresis).

Although salicylates constitute the classic NSAID, their use has declined in recent years because of concerns regarding the development of Reye syndrome as well as the emergence of many other agents. Aspirin should be given in divided doses sufficient to achieve a serum salicylate level between 20 and 30 mg/dl; no advantage has been found in increasing the level, and toxicity occurs when this is done. Children weighing under 25 kg usually require dosages of between 80 and 100 mg/kg/day; for those weighing more than 25 kg, the dosage is 2.4 to 4.8 g/day. Enteric-coated aspirin is tolerated better by children who can swallow pills, produces less gastric upset, and delivers adequate serum levels. If a child cannot swallow the tablets or take chewable children's aspirin, both choline salicylate and choline magnesium salicylate are available as liquid preparations. Five to 10 days are needed before steady-state, therapeutic levels are reached, and it may be a few weeks before the full therapeutic benefit occurs. The physician always should be alert for signs of salicylism, including tinnitus, hyperpnea, GI upset, and central nervous system (CNS) alterations. Serum salicylate levels should be obtained if there is any question of lack of effect or if any persistent adverse effects do not resolve with a decrease in dosage. Given the increased risk of Reye syndrome in children taking salicylates,[20] it currently is recommended that these children receive influenza vaccinations and stop their medications if they are exposed to varicella or develop influenza.

Should a child respond inadequately to salicylates or experience adverse effects or if the family or physician is uncomfortable using salicylates because of the risk of Reye syndrome, a number of other NSAIDs are available. All these agents are nearly equivalent in efficacy, toxicity, and mode of action[22]; unfortunately, they also may be more expensive. Individual responses to these agents vary widely; therefore, if a child does not improve with one or two of the NSAIDs, it is reasonable to continue trying others for at least 2 weeks and for up to 2- or 3-month periods to find an efficacious drug.[23] All seem somewhat superior to aspirin for children who have spondyloarthropathies or for older boys who have pauciarticular JA. Naproxen and ibuprofen now are available as liquid preparations that can be quite useful in younger children and in those who have difficulties swallowing pills.

If a child continues to do poorly after 4 to 12 months of treatment with NSAIDs or has aggressive disease, the use of SAARDs should be considered.[30] These include gold, D-penicillamine, hydroxychloroquine, sulfasalazine, and methotrexate. Patients, parents, and physicians should be prepared for at least a 4- to 6-month trial of these drugs.

Three gold preparations now available are for use in the United States: gold sodium thiomalate, aurothioglucose, and auranofin. Gold sodium thiomalate and aurothioglucose are

MEDICATIONS FOR JUVENILE ARTHRITIS

Nonsteroidal antiinflammatory drugs (NSAIDs) currently approved by the FDA for use in children

Salicylates
Indomethacin
Tolmetin sodium
Naproxen
Ibuprofen

Nonsteroidal antiinflammatory drugs (NSAIDs) not yet approved by the FDA for use in children

Diclofenac sodium
Fenoprofen
Flurbiprofen
Ketoprofen
Phenylbutazone
Piroprofen
Piroxicam
Proquazone
Meclofenamate sodium
Sulindac

Slower-acting antirheumatic drugs (SAARDs)

Gold preparations

Gold sodium thiomalate
Aurothioglucose
Auranofin

Hydroxychloroquine

D-Penicillamine
Sulfasalazine
Methotrexate

Corticosteroids

Systemic
Intraarticular

Cytotoxic drugs

Azathioprine
Chlorambucil
Cyclophosphamide
Methotrexate

Other therapies

Pheresis
Intravenous immune globulin
Cyclosporin A

injectable preparations and need to be started on a weekly basis[11]; auranofin is an oral preparation. Careful monitoring for bone marrow, kidney, or skin toxicity is necessary with preinjection WBC and platelet counts, urinalysis, and physical examination. The presence of adverse effects, such as skin rashes, leukopenia, thrombocytopenia, eosinophilia, hematuria, or proteinuria, requires either a dosage adjustment (holding or lowering the dose) or discontinuation of the gold treatment. If the child responds well, the injection interval should be increased as much as possible until it is given on a monthly basis. The dosage for both parenteral preparations is approximately 1 mg/kg/dose to a maximum of 50 mg/dose.

Auranofin is given as a once- or twice-daily dose of 0.1 to 0.2 mg/kg/day. Because it is available as a 3 mg capsule it sometimes is difficult to adjust the dose exactly to the child. In addition to the adverse effects noted above with the injectable gold preparations, it also may cause diarrhea. Although it may not be as efficacious as injectable gold preparations, it also does not cause as many serious adverse effects that require discontinuation. After initial biweekly complete blood and platelet counts and urinalyses are obtained, laboratory studies may be obtained monthly.

D-Penicillamine has been used quite extensively in Europe,[3,29] where it is believed to be as effective as gold; it has the advantage of being an oral preparation. It is given at a dosage of 5 to 10 mg/kg/day. It should be started at 250 mg or less per day and then gradually increased over a 2- to 6-month period to a maximum dosage of 750 mg or 10 mg/kg/day, whichever is lower. Its adverse effects are similar to those of gold therapy, with the addition of occasional GI upset and frequent dysgeusia. The latter signs often resolve with therapy and are not absolute indications for its discontinuation. Other rare adverse effects include Goodpasture syndrome, a lupuslike syndrome, myasthenia gravis, and other autoimmune-induced effects (e.g., hemolytic anemia). Careful monitoring on a schedule similar to that used for gold therapy is necessary.

Antimalarial agents, such as hydroxychloroquine, constitute another therapeutic alternative. Although not as potent as gold or D-penicillamine, these SAARDs have the advantage of producing fewer adverse effects. The dosage for hydroxychloroquine is 5 mg/kg/day given as a single dose. The primary adverse effects that require drug discontinuation are GI upset (e.g., nausea, anorexia, diarrhea), bleaching of the hair, and retinal deposits. Regular ophthalmological examinations every 6 months are necessary to detect the latter effect early; if found, therapy must be stopped.

Sulfasalazine, a drug first synthesized approximately 50 years ago as a specific antirheumatic agent, has seen a resurgence in recent years.[27] It is given at a dosage of approximately 25 mg/kg/day, usually with food or milk. It should not be used in anyone (1) sensitive to sulfa drugs or salicylates, (2) with impaired renal or hepatic function, or (3) with conditions such as glucose-6-phosphate dehydrogenase deficiency. Adverse effects caused by sulfasalazine include rashes, nausea, vomiting, dyspepsia, and a reversible decrease in sperm count. Bone marrow depression occurs in very rare cases. It seems to be as effective as the antimalarials and auranofin and may be superior in patients who are HLA-B27 positive.

A number of international cooperative trials have been conducted comparing the SAARDs to placebos. D-penicillamine and hydroxychloroquine have been found to be variably effective in a number of studies,[12,29] as has auranofin.[14] Many rheumatologists now are reconsidering the use of these agents.

Systemic corticosteroid use in JA should follow these maxims:

1. Only use when other agents have failed or when the child is seriously ill or has progressive severe chronic anterior uveitis unresponsive to local therapy

2. Use as small a dose as possible
3. Try to taper and discontinue their use as soon as possible

Corticosteroids are effective antiinflammatory agents but do not alter the course of the disease, are extremely difficult to discontinue in children who have JA, and their long-term use is associated with many serious adverse effects, the most important being immunosuppression, osteoporosis, and growth retardation. Alternate-day dosing regimens can be tried but are extremely difficult because many children develop problems on the day they do not receive the steroids. Small (1 to 5 mg) daily doses of prednisone that are tapered by 0.5 to 1 mg/day increments every 2 to 3 weeks can be quite effective. High-dose intravenous "pulse" steroid therapy (e.g., intravenous methylprednisolone 30 mg/kg/dose to a maximum of 1 g given over 2 hours daily for 1 to 3 days) can be useful in dire situations but does not seem to be more effective when used as chronic therapy.[25]

Intraarticular steroids can be effective in controlling acute problems associated with an active arthritis but are not a substitute for systemic, ongoing therapy. Children who have a very painful or swollen joint frequently respond to arthrocentesis and instillation of a long-acting steroid preparation (e.g., triamcinolone hexacetonide).[35] One should be careful not to perform this procedure too frequently (more than three or four times per year) and should be sure that concomitant infectious arthritis is not the cause of the acute joint problem.

A variety of cytotoxic agents have been used to treat juvenile arthritis. With the exception of methotrexate, few good long-term studies have been performed to evaluate these agents, and they therefore should be used cautiously in specific, otherwise unresponsive patients. Chlorambucil has been used extensively in Europe, especially in children who have amyloidosis. Azathioprine, although approved for use in adult rheumatoid arthritis, has not been studied as extensively in children. Methotrexate has become a significant addition to the treatment of juvenile arthritis and is among the most effective agents currently used for juvenile arthritis. It has been studied both through a double-blind, controlled trial as well as with extensive clinical use. It is quite effective at a dose of 10 mg/m^2/week as a single-weekly dose.[15] Higher doses (up to 20 mg/m^2/week)[38] and parenteral administration may be effective in recalcitrant cases. At these dosages methotrexate appears to function as an antiinflammatory agent rather than as a cytotoxic drug. Careful monitoring for bone marrow, gastrointestinal, hepatic, and pulmonary toxicity is necessary. Splitting the dose and/or using folinic or folic acid (up to 1 mg daily) may decrease the adverse effects.

A number of other therapies also have been tried for children who have juvenile arthritis. Plasmapheresis and lymphopheresis have not been studied extensively, nor do they seem to be very beneficial. Intravenous immune gamma globulin has been used in children who have systemic-onset juvenile arthritis, with mixed results.[7] Controlled trials will be necessary before this treatment can be recommended.

Pharmacological therapy is only one aspect of the treatment required by children who have JA. Physical therapy and occupational therapy are crucial and important adjuncts to help the child maintain strength and range of motion, to prevent contractures, and to allow the best possible quality of life. All patients should be given a home program of therapy that is reviewed and updated regularly. Heat therapy, such as taking warm baths or using a sleeping bag at night, often helps to minimize morning stiffness. Swimming is an excellent exercise; affected children should be encouraged to swim and to participate in as many other activities as possible. Normal play often is the best therapy available.

The orthopedist's contributions for those whose disease is more extensive range from the application of splints to operative tendon releases and capsulotomies. Some children may require joint resurfacing or joint replacement surgery.[17] Even though most children will not need orthopedic intervention, the orthopedist's perspective is an important part of the management.

In all its forms JA is a chronic illness, and none of the current modes of therapy is curative. Further, JA is one of the few childhood illnesses in which pain is a primary symptom. Different expectations and attitudes therefore are needed when caring for the patient and family. In addition to a caring and understanding physician, a family counselor, social worker, or similar health professional is of particular value in helping the family to cope with and adjust to this chronic illness. Patients, siblings, and parents will experience feelings of denial, guilt, and frustration at the time of the diagnosis and throughout the course of the disease.[4] Siblings frequently find it difficult to cope with the special and extensive treatment the affected child may receive.

Periodic depression and anger are frequent problems, especially in the early stages as the child and family realize that many changes may be necessary in their life-style and dreams. Despite the frequent episodes of family disruption, families often are able to adapt to their child's chronic illness adequately. Poor maternal function, maternal depression, and social isolation are significant risk factors for poor psychosocial outcomes. A sense of control and mastery are important positive factors.[24]

All things being equal, most children who have JA can do well in school; thus all efforts should be made to keep them enrolled. More recent studies of children's school and family adaptations show that children who have JA and their families develop different, albeit generally normal, styles for coping with this chronic illness.[18] Some school adjustments may be necessary, including arranging for different transportation and physical education and allowing the child extra time between classes. Having two sets of books, one for school and one for home, reduces the work of carrying the books to and from school. It may be necessary for the physician or pediatric rheumatology team to advocate on behalf of these children within the school so that they can receive all the necessary services they require.

Although it is important to concentrate on scholastic issues, one must not forget that these children will become adults. Independent living and vocational preparation must begin in childhood to reduce any potential barriers and difficulties. Anticipatory guidance about transitional issues should be provided starting in childhood and early adolescence.

Although children whose disease is severe have a number of obvious problems, the child who has mild disease and a "hidden disability" also may have problems coping, adapting, and trying to accomplish the unrealistic goals set by a society that does not recognize the disability. Finally, it always should be remembered that any chronic illness places a financial burden, both directly and indirectly, on the family—a burden that can add a number of further stresses. Recent estimates for the cost per child who has JA is $8670 per year, with the average family cost being about $1524. Nationally this means that the total cost of juvenile arthritis is approximately $311 million.[1]

COURSE AND PROGNOSIS

Juvenile arthritis rarely is fatal, and in general the long-term prognosis is good, regardless of subtype. Approximately 60% to 75% of children will undergo a remission at some point, and many children will experience permanent remission. Most children who have juvenile arthritis will complete school, be gainfully employed, and raise families, just like their siblings and peers.

Several patterns of disease activity are recognized: (1) persistent active arthritis and destructive arthropathy, (2) active disease, then remission, (3) polycyclic diseases characterized by acute flares of activity followed by temporary remissions, and (4) low-grade continued activity with little if any joint destruction.

Pauciarticular JA has the best prognosis, with 40% to 50% of children undergoing a complete remission, as compared with only 25% to 30% of children who have systemic-onset and polyarticular JA. Children who have IgM-RF or ANA positivity, systemic onset, and certain extraarticular manifestations (e.g., persistent fevers, thrombocytosis, subcutaneous nodules, vasculitis), as well as younger children, usually have a poorer long-term articular outcome. Younger children who have systemic-onset and polyarticular arthritis have a poorer articular prognosis; children who have pauciarticular arthritis and no chronic anterior uveitis have the best prognosis.

Children should be referred to an ophthalmologist at the time of diagnosis. Most clinical uveitis develops within the first 2 years of the diagnosis, but can occur at any time. Therefore ophthalmological examinations should be performed indefinitely. As shown in Table 224-1, The American Academy of Pediatrics recommends that children at high risk (younger children who are ANA positive and who have pauciarticular or polyarticular onset) have eye examinations every 3 to 4 months. These children are at moderate risk after 4 years, and then they should have ophthalmological examinations every 6 months. Children who have systemic-onset JA are at low risk and should have annual eye examinations; all other children initially are at moderate risk. After 4 years all children at moderate risk become low risk; after 7 years, all children are at low risk. Should a child develop uveitis, he or she should be followed as per the ophthalmologist's recommendations; uveitis can become the child's most vexing problem.

The increasing awareness of the pediatric rheumatic diseases, which has resulted in earlier diagnosis and treatment, and the rapid advances in understanding the diseases and their therapies are encouraging signs that the number of children disabled by these illnesses will decrease in the future.

REFERENCES

1. Allaire SH et al: The economic impacts of juvenile rheumatoid arthritis, *J Rheumatol* 19:952, 1992.
2. American Academy of Pediatrics: Guidelines for ophthalmologic examinations in children with juvenile rheumatoid arthritis, *Pediatrics* 92:295, 1993.
3. Ansell BW, Hall MA: Penicillamine in chronic arthritis in childhood, *J Rheumatol* 8:112, 1981.
4. Athreya BH, McCormick MC: Impact of chronic illness on families, *Rheum Dis Clin North Am* 13:123, 1987.
5. Bacon MC et al: Nutritional status and growth in juvenile rheumatoid arthritis, *Semin Arthritis Rheum* 20:97, 1990.
6. Barron KS et al: Abnormalities of immunoregulation in juvenile rheumatoid arthritis, *J Rheumatol* 16:940, 1989.
7. Barron K, Sher M, Silverman E: Intravenous immunoglobulin therapy: magic or black magic? *J Rheumatol* 19(suppl 33):94, 1992.
8. Bernstein BH et al: Reflex neurovascular dystrophy in childhood, *J Pediatr* 93:211, 1978.
9. Biro F, Gewanter HL, Baum J: The hypermobility syndrome, *Pediatrics* 72:701, 1983.
10. Brewer EJ Jr et al: Current and proposed revision of JRA criteria, *Arthritis Rheum* 20:195, 1976.
11. Brewer EJ Jr, Giannini EH, Barkley E: Gold therapy in the management of juvenile rheumatoid arthritis, *Arthritis Rheum* 23:404, 1980.
12. Brewer EJ Jr et al: Penicillamine and hydroxychloroquine in the treatment of severe juvenile rheumatoid arthritis: results of the USA-USSR double-blind placebo controlled study, *N Engl J Med* 314:1269, 1986.
13. Gewanter HL, Roghmann KJ, Baum J: The prevalence of juvenile arthritis, *Arthritis Rheum* 26:599, 1983.
14. Giannini EH, Brewer EJ, Person DA: Auranofin in the treatment of juvenile rheumatoid arthritis, *J Pediatr* 102:138, 1983.
15. Giannini EH et al: Methotrexate in resistant juvenile rheumatoid arthritis, *N Engl J Med* 326:1043, 1992.
16. Grom AA, Giannini EH, Glass DN: Juvenile rheumatoid arthritis and the trimolecular complex (HLA, T cell receptor, and antigen), *Arthritis Rheum* 37:601, 1994.
17. Harris CM, Baum J: Involvement of the hip in juvenile rheumatoid arthritis: a longitudinal study, *J Bone Joint Surg [Am]* 70:821, 1988.
18. Harris JA, Newcomb AF, Gewanter HL: Psychosocial effects of juvenile rheumatic disease, *Arthritis Care Res* 4:123, 1991.
19. Henoch MJ, Batson JW, Baum J: Psychosocial factors in juvenile rheumatoid arthritis, *Arthritis Rheum* 21:229, 1978.
20. Hurwitz ES et al: Public Health Service study of Reye's syndrome and medications, *JAMA* 257:1905, 1987.
21. Lawerence JM et al: Autoantibody studies in juvenile rheumatoid arthritis, *Semin Arthritis Rheum* 22:265, 1993.
22. Levinson JE et al: Comparison of tolmetin sodium and aspirin in the treatment of juvenile rheumatoid arthritis, *J Pediatr* 91:799, 1977.
23. Lovell DJ, Giannini EH, Brewer EJ Jr: Time course of response to nonsteroidal antiinflammatory drugs in juvenile rheumatoid arthritis, *Arthritis Rheum* 27:1433, 1984.
24. Miller JJ III: Psychosocial factors related to rheumatic diseases of childhood, *J Pediatr* 20:1, 1993.
25. Miller JJ: Prolonged use of huge intravenous steroid pulses in the rheumatic disease of children, *Pediatrics* 65:989, 1980.
26. Moore TL et al: Hidden 19S IgM rheumatoid factors, *Semin Arthritis Rheum* 18:72, 1988.
27. Ozgodan H et al: Sulphasalazine in the treatment of juvenile rheumatoid arthritis: a preliminary open trial, *J Rheumatol* 13:124, 1986.
28. Phillips PE: Evidence implicating infectious agents in rheumatoid arthritis and juvenile rheumatoid arthritis, *Clin Exp Rheumatol* 6:87, 1988.
29. Prieur AM et al: Evaluation of D-penicillamine in juvenile chronic arthritis: a double-blind, multicenter study, *Arthritis Rheum* 28:376, 1985.
30. Rosenberg AM: Advanced drug therapy for juvenile rheumatoid arthritis, *J Pediatr* 114:171, 1989.
31. Rosenberg AM: Uveitis associated with juvenile rheumatoid arthritis, *Semin Arthritis Rheum* 16:158, 1987.
32. Schneider R et al: Prognostic indicators of joint destruction in systemic onset juvenile rheumatoid arthritis, *J Pediatr* 120:200, 1992.

33. Silverman ED et al: Consumptive coagulopathy associated with systemic juvenile rheumatoid arthritis, *J Pediatr* 103:872, 1983.
34. Silverman ED et al: Intravenous gamma globulin therapy in systemic juvenile rheumatoid arthritis, *Arthritis Rheum* 33:1015, 1990.
35. Sparling M et al: Radiographic follow-up of joints injected with triamcinolone hexacetamide for the management of childhood arthritis, *Arthritis Rheum* 33:821, 1990.
36. Stollerman GH: The return of rheumatic fever, *Hosp Pract* 23:100, 1988.
37. Vostrejs M, Hollister JR: Muscle atrophy and leg length discrepancies in pauciarticular juvenile rheumatoid arthritis, *Am J Dis Child* 142:343, 1988.
38. Wallace C, Sherry D: Preliminary report of higher dose methotrexate treatment in juvenile rheumatoid arthritis, *J Rheumatol* 19:1604, 1992.
39. Yunus ME, Masi AT: Juvenile primary fibromyalgia syndrome: a clinical study of thirty-three patients and matched normal controls, *Arthritis Rheum* 28:138, 1985.

SUGGESTED READINGS

Ansell BM, Rudge S, Schaller JG: *Color atlas of pediatric rheumatology,* St Louis, 1992, Mosby.

Brewer EJ Jr, Cassidy JT, editors: Rheumatic diseases of childhood, *Rheum Dis Clin North Am* 13:1, 1987.

Cassidy JT, Petty RE: *Textbook of pediatric rheumatology,* ed 3, Philadelphia, 1995, WB Saunders.

Jacobs JL: Pediatric rheumatology for the practitioner, ed 2, New York, 1993, Springer-Verlag.

Lang BA, Shore A: A review of current concepts on the pathogenesis of juvenile rheumatoid arthritis, *J Rheum* 17(suppl 21):1, 1990.

Lovell DJ, White PH, editors: Pediatric rheumatology into the 90s, *J Rheumatol* 19(33):1, 1992.

Miller JJ III: Psychosocial factors related to rheumatic diseases of childhood, *J Pediatr* (20)20:1, 1993.

Miller ML, editor: Pediatric rheumatology, *Pediatr Clin North Am* 42:999, 1995.

225 Kawasaki Disease

Michael E. Pichichero

Kawasaki disease, formerly known as *mucocutaneous lymph node syndrome,* is the main cause of acquired heart disease in children.[3,13,23,24] It was first described in 1967 by a Japanese pediatrician, Tomisaka Kawasaki[14]; in 1974 the first cases of Kawasaki disease were reported in the United States.

Kawasaki disease is an acute, multisystem vasculitis of infancy and early childhood characterized by high fever, rash, conjunctivitis, inflammation of the mucous membranes, erythematous induration of the hands and feet, and cervical adenopathy. Although the symptoms generally are self-limiting, coronary artery aneurysms develop in 15% to 20% of patients. The Centers for Disease Control and Prevention estimates the incidence for children 8 years old or younger in the continental United States to be 2.74 cases per 100,000 in those of Asian or part Asian descent, 1.03 per 100,000 in African-Americans, and 0.43 per 100,000 in Caucasians. The peak age incidence of Kawasaki disease occurs during the second year of life. More than 80% of all cases occur in children under 5 years of age; the disease is quite uncommon beyond 9 years of age. Boys commonly are more affected than girls, with a male/female ratio of nearly 1.5:1. The incidence in siblings of affected persons is 2.1% and of recurrent cases is 3.9%.[12,30,37] More than 50% of sibling cases develop within 10 days after the first case occurs. A recurrent episode of Kawasaki disease may be seen in about 1% of patients months or years after the first episode.[12]

ETIOLOGY

There is no established cause for Kawasaki disease.[6,30] The clinical features suggest a hypersensitivity reaction, exposure to an environmental toxin, or an infectious etiology.[27] Associations have been described between Kawasaki disease and (1) rug shampooing, (2) exposure to a variant strain of *Propionibacterium acnes* infecting mites found in house dust, (3) living near stagnant water (suggesting an arthropod vector or an animal reservoir), and (4) infection with Epstein-Barr virus, human herpesvirus 6, and retroviruses.[22,27,31]

Kawasaki disease is characterized by immunoregulatory abnormalities: a deficiency of suppressor/cytotoxic T cells, increased numbers of activated helper T cells, and increased B cell activation reflected by high levels of spontaneous immunoglobulin synthesis.[1,2] These are immunological features characteristic of diseases that are caused by bacterial toxins acting as "superantigens."[7,11] Staphylococcal toxic shock syndrome, a disease having many similar clinical features to Kawasaki disease, is caused by staphylococcal toxic shock syndrome toxin 1 (TSST-1), which is a superantigen.[7,11] Superantigens stimulate a large fraction of the T cell population; T cell stimulation is mediated by the dual affinity of superantigens for the class II major histocompatibility complex on macrophages/monocytes and for the relatively invariant sequence of the variable beta region (Vβ2) of the T cell receptor. Streptococcal infections have been described in up to 25% of patients who have Kawasaki disease, based on either serological or culture results.[17,28] A new strain of TSST-1-producing *Staphylococcus aureus* has been isolated from the groin, rectum, throat, and axilla in patients who have Kawasaki disease.[19] Taken together, these observations suggest that Kawasaki disease may be caused by *S. aureus* or group A streptococcal toxins acting as superantigens.

PATHOGENESIS

Kawasaki disease is associated with increased production of interleukin-1beta, tumor necrosis factor-alpha, interleukin-6, interleukin-2, and interferon gamma.[21] The production of these cytokines by T cells and monocytes is thought to play an important role in the pathogenesis of vascular endothelial cell injury during acute Kawasaki disease, because these cytokines elicit proinflammatory and prothrombotic responses in endothelial cells. The capacity to activate T cells and monocytes/macrophages markedly is characteristic of staphylococcal enterotoxin and streptococcal erythrogenic toxin superantigens.

The effectiveness of high-dose intravenous gamma globulin infusions in reducing coronary vasculitis (discussed below) might result from prevention of immune complex deposition on blood vessel walls or from a reversal of immunoregulatory abnormalities.[18,35]

CLINICAL MANIFESTATIONS

To make the diagnosis of Kawasaki disease, five of the six major clinical characteristics associated with the condition must be present (see the box on p. 1391), and all other illnesses having similar features must be excluded. Symptoms vary in severity, but greater than 90% of patients fulfill the first five clinical criteria. All the symptoms are not apparent simultaneously, but the timing of their appearance is remarkably constant.

The course of the disease can best be described as triphasic. The acute phase consists of fever, conjunctival hyperemia, oropharyngeal erythema, swelling of the hands and feet, a polymorphous erythematous rash, and cervical lymphadenopathy. Fever, rash, and lymphadenopathy fade after 10 to 12 days of illness, marking the beginning of the subacute phase. The subacute stage is characterized by lip cracking and fissuring, desquamation of skin overlying the tips of the fingers and toes, and the onset of arthralgias (and/or arthritis), thrombocytosis, and cardiac disease. The convalescent stage usually begins about 25 days into the disease process and is characterized by the absence of clinical signs of disease but

DIAGNOSTIC CRITERIA FOR KAWASAKI DISEASE

A. Principal symptoms (At least five of the following six items should be satisfied for diagnosis.)
 1. Fever of unknown cause lasting 5 days or more
 2. Bilateral congestion of ocular conjunctivae
 3. Changes of lips and oral cavity
  a. Dryness, redness, and fissuring of lips
  b. Protuberance of tongue papillae (strawberry tongue)
  c. Diffuse reddening of oral and pharyngeal mucosa
 4. Changes of peripheral extremities
  a. Reddening of palms and soles (initial stage)
  b. Indurative edema (initial stage)
  c. Membranous desquamation from fingertips (convalescent stage)
 5. Polymorphous exanthema of body trunk without vesicles or crusts
 6. Acute nonpurulent swelling of cervical lymph nodes of 1.5 cm or more in diameter

B. Other significant symptoms or findings
 1. Carditis, especially myocarditis or pericarditis
 2. Diarrhea
 3. Arthralgia or arthritis
 4. Proteinuria and increase of leukocytes in urine sediment
 5. Changes in blood tests
  a. Leukocytosis with shift to the left
  b. Slight decrease in erythrocyte and hemoglobin levels
  c. Increased sedimentation rate
  d. Elevated C-reactive protein (CRP)
  e. Increased beta-2-globulin
  f. Thrombocytosis
  g. Negative antistreptolysin titer (ASO)
 6. Changes occasionally observed
  a. Aseptic meningitis
  b. Mild jaundice or slight increase of serum transaminase
  c. Swelling of gallbladder

the persistence of residual inflammation, marked by an elevated erythrocyte sedimentation rate (ESR).

Fever is the most prominent symptom of the acute phase of Kawasaki disease. Temperatures show a high-spiking remittent pattern in the range of 38.4° C to greater than 40° C. Fever persists despite the use of empiric antibiotics, corticosteroids, and standard doses of antipyretics. Fever is present on average for about 12 days, although prolonged courses of up to 5 weeks have been reported; defervescence occurs over 1 to 3 days. Discrete engorgement of the bulbar conjunctivae blood vessels (without associated discharge, exudate, keratitis, chemosis, or pseudomembrane formation) and an anterior uveitis develop shortly after the onset of fever.[34] The cornea, lens, and retina are not involved. Early oropharyngeal signs include dryness and reddening of the lips and of the buccal and pharyngeal mucosa. The absence of aphthous ulceration or hemorrhagic bullae is noticeable. A "strawberry tongue" frequently is present. Later, as the intensity of the erythema subsides, the lips usually become cracked and fissured.

The most characteristic and unique feature of Kawasaki disease relates to changes that occur in the hands and feet. Early on they become diffusely indurated and swollen, and the overlying skin develops a woody firmness suggestive of acute scleroderma. The palms and soles usually become erythematous or take on a purplish hue. There is fusiform swelling of the fingers, which limits the child's ability to grasp objects. The feet are painful to the touch, and many children will refuse to stand or bear weight. Two to three weeks after the onset of illness and after the early signs involving the extremities have disappeared, an unusual desquamation of the skin beginning at the subungual and periungual regions of the fingertips and toe tips is recognizable in nearly all cases (Fig. 225-1). Progression to complete peeling of the palms and soles may occur, but exfoliation generally does not extend to the remainder of the body surface. During the convalescent phase, deep transverse grooves may appear across the fingernails and toenails, presumably as a result of arrested growth during the illness.

A polymorphous erythematous rash appears 1 to 5 days after the onset of fever; it usually begins on the extremities and spreads centripetally. The three most common patterns of rash are maculopapular (morbilliform), erythema multiforme–like with iris lesions, and scarlatiniform. The rash may be coalescent, producing large, irregular, raised plaques, and it may be pruritic. Vesicles, pustules, and bullae are not seen. The rash is not petechial or purpuric. It usually fades within a week but occasionally persists longer or recurs.

Lymphadenopathy typically involves a single cervical node measuring greater than 1.5 cm in diameter. The node usually is not tender or warm and does not become fluctuant. Generalized lymphadenopathy does not occur. The lymph node diminishes in size with defervescence. This finding is the one least often seen of the major criteria; it occurs in only about 60% of patients in most U.S. series (although it is more common in Japan).

In addition to the six major clinical signs, there are other features of Kawasaki disease frequently noted. Sterile pyuria occurs more often than lymphadenopathy in most American cases; 10 to 100 white blood cells (WBCs) per high-power field may be observed on a clean-catch voided specimen. No WBCs will be seen on a bladder aspiration specimen, because the sterile pyuria is caused by urethral ulceration or inflammation. Occasionally a patient will demonstrate trace proteinuria or hematuria.

Irritability, mild meningismus, and lethargy typically are seen in nearly all of these patients, and nearly all probably have aseptic meningitis. When cerebrospinal fluid (CSF) is analyzed, it typically shows 25 to 100 WBCs/mm^3 with normal amounts of glucose and protein. Diarrhea is seen in about 50% of the patients. Passing 5 to 15 stools per day for 2 to 7 days during the acute or subacute phase is common. Stools

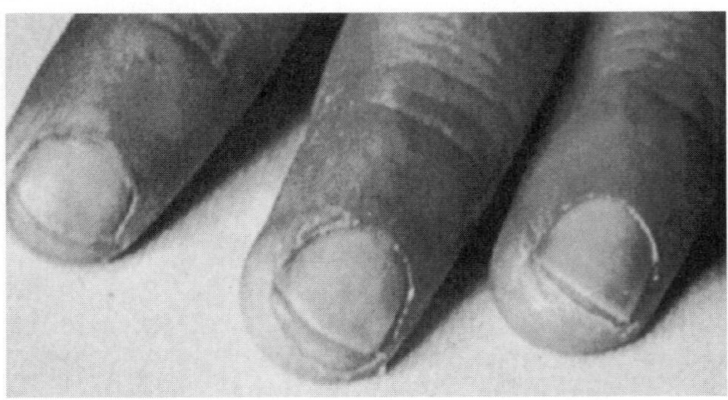

FIG. 225-1 Desquamation of the skin involving the subungual and periungual regions of the fingertips.

From Kawasaki T et al: A new infantile acute febrile mucocutaneous lymph node syndrome (MLNS) prevailing in Japan, Pediatrics 54:273, 1974. Copyright American Academy of Pediatrics, 1974.

do not contain polymorphonuclear cells and are not Hematest positive.

Either arthralgias, arthritis, or both occur in 30% to 40% of the children. Large joints, particularly the knees and ankles, are involved more often. Usually no more than two or three joints will be affected. This symptom occurs 8 to 12 days after the onset of disease. Joint fluid, if analyzed, will reveal findings similar to those of rheumatoid arthritis.

Other findings, such as pneumonia, tympanitis, photophobia, and mild liver dysfunction, are observed somewhat less commonly. Acute hydrops of the gallbladder, jaundice, convulsions, encephalopathy, pancreatitis, orchitis, and pleural effusions are seen rarely but clearly are associated complications of Kawasaki disease.

The most alarming findings of Kawasaki disease are those in the cardiovascular system. Approximately 1% of children who have the disease die, usually as a result of coronary artery aneurysms. During the acute phase, tachycardia and gallop rhythms may appear; however, the most serious manifestations of cardiac involvement occur during the subacute phase. These include serious arrhythmias, congestive heart failure, pericardial effusion, mitral insufficiency, and myocardial ischemia or infarction.

Atypical Kawasaki Disease

Severe or even fatal coronary abnormalities can develop following illnesses that resemble but do not fulfill the classic diagnostic features of Kawasaki disease.* Patients who have "atypical" Kawasaki disease may display prolonged high fever, nonspecific rash, arthralgia or arthritis, fissuring of the lips, nonexudative conjunctivitis, and extreme irritability. Atypical Kawasaki disease can present occasionally with prolonged fever for 5 or more days in the absence of other clinical criteria for the illness. In other patients, unilateral cervical adenopathy refractory to antibiotic therapy is the clue that atypical Kawasaki disease may be present. Atypical Kawasaki disease is likely to present with subtle manifestations in infants less than 6 months of age; this group is at highest risk (50% or greater) for coronary artery lesions if untreated.

*References 4, 5, 8, 9, 15, 20, 29, 33.

LABORATORY FINDINGS

Although there are no pathognomonic laboratory findings in Kawasaki disease, certain laboratory abnormalities frequently are seen and therefore help to establish the diagnosis. In the acute phase of the disease, most patients exhibit an elevated white blood cell (WBC) count with an associated left shift; WBC counts of 15,000 to 20,000/mm^3 are common, and these counts may remain elevated for 1 to 3 weeks. Other laboratory abnormalities in the acute phase usually include an elevated erythrocyte sedimentation rate (ESR) (mean = 55 mm/hr), increased CRP and beta-2-globulin, mild normochromic, normocytic anemia, and slight elevations of the liver enzymes. As previously stated, many patients demonstrate sterile pyuria and cerebrospinal fluid (CSF) pleocytosis. In the second to third week of illness patients characteristically develop significant thrombocytosis, with platelet counts averaging in excess of 700,000/mm^3. Importantly, a number of laboratory studies are negative. Routine cultures of blood, CSF, urine, throat, and lymph node aspirates reveal no growth or normal flora. Serological studies for bacterial and viral agents are negative, including the ASO titer. Antinuclear antibodies and the rheumatoid factor are absent, as are all other autoantibodies.

Sinus tachycardia, nonspecific ST segment and T wave changes, and evidence of mild left ventricular hypertrophy may be seen on an electrocardiogram (ECG) in the acute phase. In the subacute phase myocardial infarction patterns on an ECG may be observed, although infrequently.

A baseline echocardiogram should be performed as soon as the diagnosis of Kawasaki disease is suspected in order to evaluate cardiac function, the presence or absence of pericardial effusion, and the anatomy of the coronary arteries. Coronary artery abnormalities generally are apparent by the third or fourth week of illness. Coronary artery disease rarely, if ever, develops after 6 to 8 weeks, although late-onset valvular disease has been reported.

DIFFERENTIAL DIAGNOSIS

The clinical picture of Kawasaki disease, after all of the major features have become manifest, is not difficult to differentiate from other mucocutaneous syndromes. In the first days of the illness a whole spectrum of acute febrile diseases might be considered. Three to five days after the onset, certain clinical features may be singled out as compatible with other diagnoses—for example, strawberry tongue suggestive of streptococcal infection. However, if all the signs and symptoms are considered carefully, the diagnosis is readily apparent. The clinical features of Kawasaki disease and other mucocutaneous disorders are shown in Table 225-1. Other conditions that share some aspects of Kawasaki disease are ratbite fever, rubella, rubeola, infectious mononucleosis, toxoplasmosis, juvenile rheumatoid arthritis, systemic lupus erythematosus, Behçet syndrome, acrodynia (mercury poisoning), and febrile drug reactions. The similarities between fatal Kawasaki disease and fatal infantile polyarteritis nodosa are striking; pathologically the two diseases cannot be distinguished. The exact relationship between them, however, remains undetermined. At this time one is left with the clear differentiating feature that Kawasaki disease rarely is fatal

Table 225-1 Clinical Features of Kawasaki Disease and Other Mucocutaneous Diseases

	Kawasaki disease	Stevens-Johnson syndrome	Streptococcal scarlet fever	Staphylococcal scarlet fever	Staphylococcal toxic shock syndrome	Leptospirosis
Age (yr)	Usually <5	Usually 3-30	Usually 5-10	Usually 2-8	Usually adolescent	Usually >2
Fever	Prolonged	Prolonged	Variable	Variable	Usually <10 days	Variable
Eyes	Hyperemia of ocular conjunctivae; uveitis	Catarrhal conjunctivitis; chemosis; iritis; uveitis; panophthalmitis	No change	Hyperemia of ocular conjunctivae	Hyperemia of ocular conjunctivae	Hyperemia of ocular conjunctivae; uveitis
Lips	Red, dry, fissured	Erosions; crusted, fissured, bleeding	No change	No change	Red	No change
Oral cavity	Diffuse erythema; "strawberry tongue"	Erythema; bullae, ulcers, pseudomembrane formation	Pharyngitis; palatal petechiae; "strawberry tongue"	Pharyngitis	Erythema; pharyngitis	Pharyngitis
Peripheral extremities	Erythema of palms and soles; indurative edema; periungual, palmar, and plantar desquamation	No change	Periungual desquamation	No change	Swelling of hands and feet; dry gangrene	Gangrene of hands and feet (rare)
Exanthem	Erythematous, polymorphous	Erythematous, polymorphous; iris lesions, vesicles, bullae, crusts	Finely papular erythroderma; Pastia lines; circumoral pallor	Finely papular erythroderma; Pastia lines	Erythroderma	Erythematous, maculopapular, petechial, or purpuric
Cervical lymph nodes	Nonpurulent swelling; unilateral (frequent)	Nonpurulent swelling (occasional)	Nonpurulent or purulent swelling (frequent)	Nonpurulent or purulent swelling (occasional)	No change	Nonpurulent swelling (infrequent)
Other	Meatitis; diarrhea; arthralgia and arthritis; aseptic meningitis; rhinorrhea (uncommon); ECG changes	Malaise; cough, rhinorrhea, pneumonitis; vomiting; arthralgia; recurrent episodes	Malaise; vomiting; headache		Headache; confusion; hypotension; icteric hepatitis; diarrhea; coagulopathy; renal injury	Headache; myalgia; abdominal pain; icteric hepatitis; meningitis

(±1% mortality), whereas infantile polyarteritis nodosa is a pathological diagnosis made at autopsy.

MANAGEMENT

Intravenous immunoglobulin (IVIG) with aspirin is the best available therapy for preventing coronary artery abnormalities in Kawasaki disease and should be administered to all patients diagnosed within the first 10 days of illness.[26,32] Physicians should institute treatment as soon as the diagnosis is established and as early as possible in the course of the illness. Aspirin, given in high doses (80 to 120 mg/kg/day), reduces the length and severity of Kawasaki disease during the acute phase.[16] Aspirin use early in the course of disease also may reduce coronary artery involvement. Salicylate levels should be checked to avoid toxicity. Defervescence apparently is accompanied by improvement in gastrointestinal (GI) absorption of aspirin[16]; therefore dosages should be reduced to 30 to 50 mg/kg/day after fever subsides and until the ESR has returned to normal. Aspirin should be continued throughout the convalescent phase because of its antithrombotic effects at 3 to 5 mg/kg/day until the platelet count has returned to normal. If coronary aneurysms are recognized, salicylates (3 to 5 mg/kg/day) should be continued until careful follow-up echocardiograms demonstrate aneurysm resolution.

High-dose IVIG may prevent coronary artery lesions in Kawasaki disease. A dosage of 400 mg/kg/day for 4 consecutive days has been shown to be effective.[26] A single 2 g/kg dose infused over 10 to 12 hours is at least as effective as the 4-day regimen. The efficacy of IVIG therapy for prevention of coronary lesions when instituted more than 10 days after the onset of illness is not known. However, patients who remain symptomatic beyond the tenth day of illness may still benefit from the effects of IVIG. The decision to administer IVIG later than the tenth day of illness must be individualized. Patients should be monitored carefully during IVIG infusions for signs of anaphylaxis.

Antibiotics are not beneficial. Corticosteroids are contraindicated because some evidence suggests that coronary aneurysms occur more frequently in patients receiving these agents.

RISK FACTORS FOR CORONARY ARTERY ANEURYSMS IN KAWASAKI DISEASE

Risk very increased

Fever lasts longer than 14 days
Biphasic fever pattern*†
Biphasic pattern of skin rash
Maximum WBC count ≥30,000
Maximum ESR (mm/hr) ≥101
Time until normalization of ESR or CRP ≥30 days of illness
Biphasic elevation of ESR or CRP†
Increased Q/R ratio in leads II, III, aV_F >0.3
Symptoms of myocardial infarction

Risk increased

Male sex
Age at onset under 1 year
Hemoglobin ≤10 g/dl† and RBC count ≤3.5 million
Maximum WBC count >26,000
Maximum ESR (mm/hr) >50
Cardiomegaly
Arrhythmia
Recurrence of disease

*Separated by afebrile period of 48 hours or longer.
†Causes other than Kawasaki disease must be ruled out.

COMPLICATIONS

The major complication of Kawasaki disease is the development of coronary artery aneurysms.[3,10,23,24,36] If IVIG is not administered these occur in 15% to 20% of the cases and usually are apparent by echocardiogram during the subacute phase of the illness. Most patients who have aneurysms are asymptomatic; in some cases, however, formation of an aneurysm, particularly giant aneurysms (>8 mm in diameter), is followed by thrombosis or rupture, resulting in a fatal myocardial infarction.

The coronary artery aneurysms seen in Kawasaki disease develop more frequently in boys than in girls, in children less than 1 year of age, in those who have a triphasic fever pattern or prolonged fever (longer than 2 weeks), when a gallop rhythm or other arrhythmia is noted, or when the ESR exceeds 50 mm/hr[10] (see the box above). Cases of atypical Kawasaki disease followed by typical coronary artery involvement have led to the suggestion that an echocardiography examination be undertaken in children who have prolonged unexplainable febrile illnesses associated with subsequent peripheral desquamation.[29]

A rare complication of Kawasaki disease is hydrops of the gallbladder. This occurs in approximately 3% of the cases and is seen most frequently in children who are jaundiced. It becomes evident during the acute phase of the illness and is diagnosed best by ultrasound on recognition of a right upper quadrant abdominal mass. The pathogenesis is unknown. Surgery is not indicated because the problem resolves spontaneously in convalescence.

PROGNOSIS

Kawasaki disease has a .01% mortality, which occurs almost exclusively in children who have giant aneurysms, largely as a result of coronary artery thrombosis, massive myocardial infarction, and cardiogenic shock. Significant morbidity, in the form of coronary artery aneurysms, occurs in 15% to 20% of the cases. Eighty percent of children whose aneurysms are small to moderate in size have complete resolution without apparent sequelae within 5 years.[3,13] The remaining children may experience persisting aneurysms, coronary artery stenosis or obstruction, or aortic regurgitation.[25] Emerging evidence suggests that this latter group of children may be at risk for the subsequent development of significant cardiovascular disease such as coronary arteriosclerosis or persistent aneurysms, placing the patient at risk for sudden death from aneurysm rupture or thrombosis, cardiac arrhythmias, angina, or hypertension.

PSYCHOSOCIAL ASPECTS

Kawasaki disease typically is a self-limited illness without complications, which should be emphasized to the parents. Even if coronary artery aneurysms do develop, these resolve spontaneously in over 50% of the cases in 2 years and 80% in 5 years. Long-term risks still remain undefined, and only as we gain prospective experience with the disease over several more decades will the true incidence of cardiovascular sequelae become evident.

REFERENCES

1. Abe J et al: Selective expansion of T cells expressing T-cell receptor variable regions Vβ2 and Vβ8 in Kawasaki disease, *Proc Natl Acad Sci USA* 89:4066, 1992.
2. Abe J et al: Characterization of T cell repertoire changes in acute Kawasaki disease, *J Exp Med* 177:791, 1993.
3. Akagi T et al: Outcome of coronary artery aneurysms after Kawasaki disease, *J Pediatr* 121:689, 1992.
4. Ammerman SD et al: Diagnostic uncertainty in atypical Kawasaki disease, and a new finding: exudative conjunctivitis, *Pediatr Infect Dis* 4:210, 1985.
5. Avner JR, Shaw KN, Chin AJ: Atypical presentation of Kawasaki disease with early development of giant coronary artery aneurysms, *J Pediatr* 114:605, 1989.
6. Bierman FZ, Gersony WM: Kawasaki disease: clinical perspective, *J Pediatr* 111:789, 1987.
7. Bohach GA et al: Staphylococcal and streptococcal pyrogenic toxins involved in toxic shock syndrome and related illnesses, *Crit Rev Microbiol* 17:251, 1990.
8. Boven K et al: Atypical Kawasaki disease: an often missed diagnosis, *Eur J Pediatr* 151:577, 1992.
9. Cloney DL, Teja K, Lohr JA: Fatal case of atypical Kawasaki syndrome, *Pediatr Infect Dis J* 6:297, 1987.
10. Daniels SR et al: Correlates of coronary artery aneurysm formation in patients with Kawasaki disease, *Am J Dis Child* 141:205, 1987.
11. Drake CG, Kotzin BL: Superantigens: biology, immunology, and potential role in disease, *J Clin Immunol* 12:149, 1992.
12. Fujita Y et al: Kawasaki disease in families, *Pediatrics* 84:666, 1989.
13. Gersony WM: Long-term issues in Kawasaki disease, *J Pediatr* 121:731, 1992.
14. Kawasaki T et al: A new infantile acute febrile mucocutaneous lymph node syndrome (MLNS) prevailing in Japan, *Pediatrics* 54:271, 1974.
15. Kleiman MB, Passo MH: Incomplete Kawasaki disease with facial nerve paralysis and coronary artery involvement, *Pediatr Infect Dis J* 7:301, 1988.
16. Koren G, MacLeod SM: Difficulty in achieving therapeutic serum concentrations of salicylate in Kawasaki disease, *J Pediatr* 105:991, 1984.
17. Lekova ES, Joffe L, Glode MP: Antigenic recognition by intravenous gamma globulin of selected bacteria isolated from throats of patients with Kawasaki syndrome, *Pediatr Infect Dis J* 9:620, 1990.
18. Leung DYM et al: Reversal of lymphocyte activation in vivo in the Kawasaki syndrome by intravenous gamma globulin, *J Clin Invest* 79:468, 1987.
19. Leung DYM et al: Toxic shock syndrome toxin-secreting *Staphylococcus aureus* in Kawasaki syndrome, *Lancet* 342:1385, 1993.
20. Levy M, Koren G: Atypical Kawasaki disease: analysis of clinical presentation and diagnostic clues, *Pediatr Infect Dis J* 9:122, 1990.
21. Lin CY et al: Serial changes of serum interleukin-6, interleukin-8, and tumor necrosis factor alpha among patients with Kawasaki disease, *J Pediatr* 121:924, 1992.
22. Marchette NJ et al: Epstein-Barr virus and other herpesvirus infections in Kawasaki syndrome, *J Infect Dis* 161:680, 1990.
23. Nakamura Y et al: Cardiac sequelae of Kawasaki disease in Japan: statistical analysis, *Pediatrics* 88:1144, 1991.
24. Nakamura Y, Yanagawa H, Kawasaki T: Mortality among children with Kawasaki disease in Japan, *N Engl J Med* 326:1246, 1992.
25. Nakano H et al: High incidence of aortic regurgitation following Kawasaki disease, *J Pediatr* 107:59, 1985.
26. Newberger J et al: The treatment of Kawasaki syndrome with intravenous gamma globulin, *N Engl J Med* 315:341, 1986.
27. Rauch AM: Kawasaki syndrome: review of new epidemiologic and laboratory developments, *Pediatr Infect Dis J* 6:1016, 1987.
28. Rider LG et al: Group A streptococcal infection and Kawasaki syndrome, *Lancet* 337:1100, 1991.
29. Rowley AH et al: Incomplete Kawasaki disease with coronary artery involvement, *J Pediatr* 110:409, 1987.
30. Rowley AH, Gonzalez-Crussi F, Shulman ST: Kawasaki syndrome, *Rev Infect Dis* 10:1, 1988.
31. Rowley A et al: Failure to confirm the presence of a retrovirus in cultured lymphocytes from patients with Kawasaki syndrome, *Pediatr Res* 29:417, 1991.
32. Rowley AH, Shulman ST: Therapy of Kawasaki disease, *Report Pediatr Infect Dis* 3:19, 1993.
33. Schuh S et al: Kawasaki disease with atypical presentation, *Pediatr Infect Dis J* 7:201, 1988.
34. Smith LBH, Newburger JW, Burns JC: Kawasaki syndrome and the eye, *Pediatr Infect Dis J* 8:116, 1989.
35. Takel S, Arora YK, Walker SM: Intravenous immunoglobulin contains specific antibodies inhibitory to activation of T cells by staphylococcal toxin superantigens, *J Clin Invest* 91:602, 1993.
36. Tatara K, Kusakawa S: Long-term prognosis of giant coronary aneurysm in Kawasaki disease: an angiographic study, *J Pediatr* 111:705, 1987.
37. Yanagawa H, Kawasaki T, Shigematsu I: Nationwide survey on Kawasaki disease in Japan, *Pediatrics* 80:58, 1987.

226 Labial Adhesions

Barbara J. Howard

Adhesions of the labia minora, also called *labial fusion, synechia vulvae,* or *agglutination of the labia,* occur commonly in infants and young girls, producing considerable parental concern despite their usual lack of medical significance. What the parents see is a flap of skin formed by the adherence of the labia minora that completely covers all evidence of a vaginal opening. The fear that their daughter may have abnormal sexual anatomy often leads them to ask questions about other problems of the genital area, such as diaper rash, rather than addressing their real concern directly.

The diagnosis of labial adhesions is based entirely on the physical examination. When the labia majora are gently stretched apart, a thin flat membrane of variable length is seen in the midline. This extends from the clitoris to the posterior fourchette in 70% of cases, the rest being cases of partial coverage.[2] There usually is a small opening near the clitoris through which the urine passes. The vaginal introitus is obscured, but one could demonstrate the space beneath the flap by inserting a small probe through the anterior opening and directing it posteriorly beneath the membrane. This, however, is not necessary once the thin line of adherence (or agglutination) between the two nonrugated flat labia minora has been identified.

Labial adhesions very rarely are present at birth, unlike congenital anomalies of the genitals such as vaginal agenesis, familial posterior labial fusion, or the ambiguous genitalia associated with the adrenogenital syndrome with which labial adhesions sometimes are confused. Imperforate hymen also differs in that it is apparent within the vaginal introitus and the labia are normal.

White spots or streaks of the posterior vestibule called *linea vestibularis* are present in 10% to 14% of normal neonates regardless of race, birth weight, or gestational age and are not to be confused with labial adhesions.[11]

Occurrence of the adhesions is ascribed to a combination of inflammation and hypoestrogenization of the labia minora. Commonly the tissue is irritated (usually so mildly as to go unnoticed) through trauma, infection, or poor hygiene, and the medial edges of the labia adhere to each other as they heal. Urine flow may be partially obstructed, resulting in pooling behind the fusion and further irritation, thereby continuing the cycle of inflammation, adhesion, and obstruction. Labial adhesions almost always are found in infants after 2 months of age and at any time up to menarche, irrespective of race. This pattern presumably is caused by the relative immunity to inflammation of epithelium exposed to estrogen, such as that of the newborn under the influence of maternal hormones and that of postmenarcheal girls. One of the rare cases found at birth was associated with infection of the infant in utero.[3] Similarly, adhesions are very rare during the reproductive years in females who have normal ovarian function,[8] although they have been seen as a result of herpes simplex type II infection.[6] Capraro and Greenberg[3] reported the average age at diagnosis to be 2½ years, with 56% of their patients under 2 years of age and 94% under 6 years. Earlier, Huffman reported the highest incidence to be between ages 2 and 6 years.[3] This shift to an earlier age may be the result of a greater awareness of the condition or perhaps a predisposition to inflammation from the occlusion of the plastic diaper covers often used today.

It has been estimated that 10% to 20% of girls have some period of adhesion before 1 year of age.[14] In one series of 93 girls from 3 months to 11 years of age selected for not having been sexually abused, an incidence of 38.9% was found,[4] but 19 of the 35 adhesions were less than 2 mm in length and were detected only because of examination using magnification.[12]

An association has been suggested between labial adhesions and sexual abuse, with two retrospective analyses showing that 3% of children referred for sexual abuse had had adhesions.[2] In another study labial adhesions were the only genital abnormality in 8 of 205 sexually abused girls.[13] Although this is not an increase over the baseline prevalence, because adhesions are thought to be secondary to trauma or infection their presence should alert clinicians at least to examine the child carefully and to ask about caretaking arrangements and express any concerns about inappropriate handling of the child.

Inspection of the vulvae is recommended during each health maintenance physical examination to check hygiene, monitor sexual development, and detect problems.[15,16] This also is important for developing a clinical baseline for normal anatomy. With the apparent increase in sexual abuse of children in whom genital complaints may not be reported, skill in this practice becomes especially important.

Parents may be concerned that the normal self-stimulation of the genitals that starts around 6 months of age and is especially prominent between 18 months and 2½ years of age is damaging to their child. It is helpful to counsel parents routinely about the normality of self-stimulation, particularly when adhesions draw attention to sexual development.[9] An effort must be made to constrain any parental overreaction.

On the other hand, masturbation may be a response to genital irritation from infection or to psychological distress, especially from sexual abuse. These situations should be assessed before providing reassurance about masturbation, particularly if it is persistent or has an acute onset.

Only 20% to 38% of girls who have labial adhesions have any symptoms of dysuria, difficulty voiding, or local discomfort.[3] If there is no evidence of obstruction to voiding, repeated urinary tract infection, discomfort, or excessive parental concern, no treatment beyond explanation is needed. Because adhesions completely resolve spontaneously—50% in 6 months, 90% in 12 months, and 100% in 18 months[10]—

surgical or mechanical lysis not only is unnecessary in the usual case but also is less effective in the long term; it also is potentially painful and can be psychologically traumatic and costly. Should treatment be indicated or urgently desired by the parents in spite of counseling, the topical application of estrogen cream (0.1% or 0.01% dienestrol) is effective in about 90% of cases.[3] Recurrence is rare after this treatment, whereas serious readhesion after mechanical lysis has been noted in 20% to 100% of cases.[1] Separation of the labia is achieved in 90% of cases[5] after 2 weeks of twice-daily estrogen cream treatment with gentle traction of the labia laterally.[7] This should be followed by nightly application of the estrogen cream for 1 to 2 weeks. Treatment is considered to have failed if separation does not occur within 8 weeks.[1] Occasionally a repeat course of treatment is needed.[7] Several more weeks of application of a bland ointment (e.g., petrolatum) after separation has been established is recommended to ensure sustained labial separation.[3] This should be continued for as long as a year in the case of recurrences. The older child can be taught to apply the cream herself with supervision. Reversible vulvar pigmentation or erythema and/or breast tenderness have been reported in up to one third of children managed with topical treatment.[2] However, no serious or lasting complications of treatment have been reported.

If a urinary tract infection is suspected as either a cause of irritation or a complication of outflow obstruction, urinalysis and culture results will dictate the necessary treatment and follow-up. Although labial adhesions are not known to be associated with congenital anomalies, Capraro and Greenberg[3] found 3 of 50 affected girls to have urinary tract anomalies (all were symptomatic). Nevertheless, further specific gynecological or renal evaluation is not needed unless urinary obstruction, persistent urinary tract infection, or vulvar irritation is present, or unless treatment failure is unexplained.

REFERENCES

1. Ariborg A: Topical oestrogen therapy for labial adhesions in children, *Br J Obstet Gynaecol* 82:424, 1975.
2. Berkowitz CD, Elvik SL, Logan MK: Labial fusion in prepubescent girls: a marker for sexual abuse? *Am J Obstet Gynecol* 156:16, 1987.
3. Capraro VJ, Greenberg H: Adhesions of the labia minora: a study of 50 patients, *Obstet Gynecol* 39:65, 1972.
4. Christensen EH, Oster J: Adhesions of labia minora (synechia vulvae) in childhood, *Acta Paediatr Scand* 60:709, 1971.
5. Clair DL, Caldamone AA: Pediatric office procedures, *Urol Clin North Am* 15:15, 1988.
6. DeMarco BJ, Crandall RS, Hreshchyshyn MM: Labial agglutination secondary to a herpes simplex II infection, *Am J Obstet Gynecol* 157:296, 1987.
7. Emans SJH, Goldstein DP: *Pediatric and adolescent gynecology,* ed 2, Boston, 1982, Little, Brown.
8. Goldstein AI, Rajcher WJ: Conglutination of the labia minora in the presence of normal estrogen levels: an exception to the rule, *Am J Obstet Gynecol* 113:845, 1972.
9. Howard BJ: One approach to anticipatory guidance of sexuality for pediatricians. In Charney E, editor: *Pediatric update,* New York, 1981, Elsevier-Dutton.
10. Jenkinson SD, MacKinnon AE: Spontaneous separation of fused labia minora in prepubertal girls, *BMJ* 289:160, 1984.
11. Kellogg ND, Parra JM: Linea vestibularis: a previously undescribed normal genital structure in female neonates, *Pediatrics* 87:926, 1991.
12. McCann J et al: Genital findings in prepubertal girls selected for nonabuse: a descriptive study, *Pediatrics* 86:428, 1990.
13. Muram D: Child sexual abuse—genital tract findings in prepubertal girls. I. The unaided medical examination, *Am J Obstet Gynecol* 160:328, 1989.
14. Parsons L, Sommers SC: *Gynecology,* ed 2, Philadelphia, 1978, WB Saunders.
15. Singleton AF: The vulvar examination of the premenarchal child, *J Natl Med Assoc* 78:203, 1986.
16. Williams TS, Callen JP, Owen LG: Vulvar disorders in the prepubertal female, *Pediatr Ann* 15:588, 1986.

227 Leukemias

Barbara L. Asselin

Even though many pediatricians only infrequently must diagnose a child as having leukemia, they play a crucial role in the treatment of these diseases. As the primary caregiver, the pediatrician is responsible for ensuring that an accurate diagnosis is made quickly, that appropriate emergency measures are initiated when necessary, and that referral to a pediatric cancer center is expedited. Once uniformly fatal diseases, the childhood leukemias now are more appropriately considered treatable and in some cases curable. However, the aggressive treatment protocols that have brought about the therapeutic successes to date also have resulted in significant acute and long-term toxicities. Pediatric subspecialists are vital members of the health care team that implements these complicated, frequently toxic, multiinstitutional clinical trials. The child's pediatrician follows up on his or her patient not only during the acute stage of treatment but also back home during periods of remission and throughout the cure. With the number of long-term survivors of childhood leukemia increasing, the pediatrician, internist, and subspecialists must be knowledgeable about the late sequelae of antileukemic therapy, alert to their emergence, and familiar with appropriate therapeutic interventions.

EPIDEMIOLOGY

Leukemia is the most common form of malignancy seen in children and the second most common cause of death in children between 5 and 14 years of age. Almost one third of cancer cases in children are a form of leukemia (Fig. 227-1). The incidence of all types of acute leukemia has been reported to be 4.2 per 100,000 Caucasian children and 2.4 per 100,000 non-Caucasian children.[82] Each year more than 2000 children under age 15 in the United States are likely to be diagnosed as having acute leukemia.[82] Despite the remarkable gains made in treatment, little has been done that has affected this incidence.[32,58]

As shown in Fig. 227-2, acute lymphoblastic leukemia (ALL) predominates, accounting for 80% of all cases of childhood leukemia.[81] Childhood ALL has a peak incidence at approximately 4 years of age,[48] and it is more common in boys than in girls.[15,24] The observation that acute leukemia is more common in Caucasians than in other races is based primarily on the increased peak incidence of ALL in Caucasian children between 3 and 5 years of age.[16,82] In contrast to ALL, acute nonlymphocytic leukemia (ANLL) in the United States shows no marked age peak.

TYPES OF LEUKEMIA

The leukemia syndromes seen in childhood can be classified as acute, chronic, congenital, and preleukemia. Acute leukemias are characterized by a predominance of immature hematopoietic precursors ("blasts") in the bone marrow (by definition, more than 25% of nucleated cells must be blasts) and a fulminant natural course, resulting in death within months unless effective treatment is instituted. In the chronic leukemias, the mature bone marrow elements hyperproliferate, resulting in a condition of insidious onset of symptoms over months. Even without treatment patients can survive for months to years after diagnosis of these chronic diseases. Congenital leukemia refers to conditions diagnosed in the first 4 weeks of life; they are discussed in more detail at the end of this chapter. The myeloproliferative and myelodysplastic syndromes are characterized by unexplained anemia, neutropenia, or thrombocytopenia and distorted maturation of bone marrow hematopoietic elements. These conditions, commonly referred to as *preleukemia* because of their frequent evolution into acute leukemia, are uncommon among children compared with adults.

The leukemias also are classified according to the predominant cell lines involved. This classification broadly divides the acute leukemias into lymphoblastic (ALL) and nonlymphoblastic forms (ANLL). Acute myelogenous leukemia (AML) is the most common subtype of childhood ANLL, followed by myelomonocytic leukemia (AMML), acute promyelocytic leukemia (APML), monocytic leukemia (AMOL), erythrocytic leukemia, and megakaryocytic leukemia. Very few cases are classified as undifferentiated leukemia (AUL) because of recent technological advances in studies of lineage-specific immunological surface markers and gene rearrangements. The chronic leukemias also can be divided into lymphocytic and myelogenous forms. Among children, chronic myelogenous leukemia (CML) is seen in 3% to 5% of patients diagnosed as having leukemia (see Fig. 227-2). Chronic lymphocytic leukemia (CLL) is extremely rare.

LEUKEMOGENESIS

Normal cell growth is controlled by a complex series of events involving growth factors that are produced by the cell itself, produced by other cells, or produced by cells in other tissues. Leukemia is a disorder of growth and proliferation in which one or more of these growth-regulating events goes awry within a hematopoietic cell.

The exact cause of leukemia is unknown. A number of contributing factors and possible predisposing conditions have been described, including genetic predisposition, immunodeficiency states, viruses, and environmental exposures. Our current understanding of the complicated nature of normal cellular proliferation and differentiation processes suggests that the etiology of leukemia is equally complex, resulting from a series of multifactorial events involving "oncogenes," growth factors, and environmental conditions.

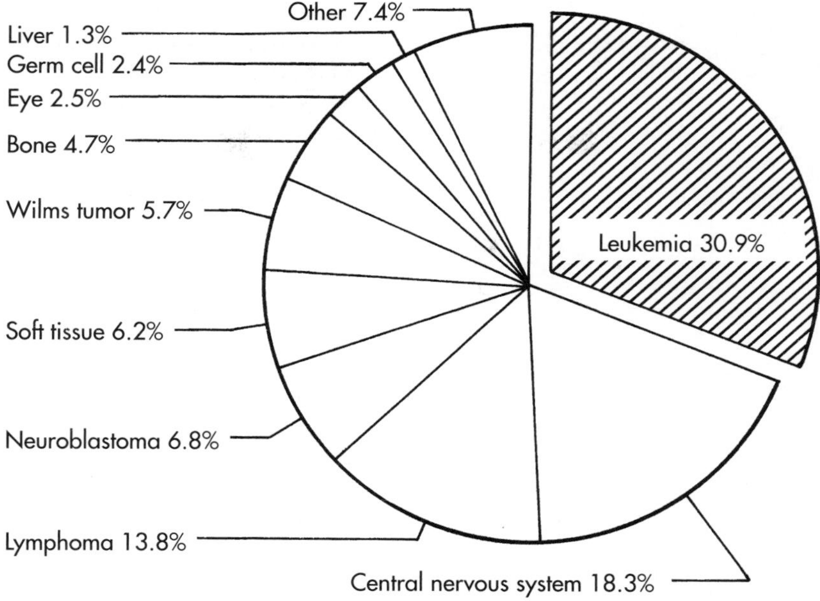

FIG. 227-1 Major forms of cancer in American Caucasian children.

(Modified from Altman AJ, Schwartz AD: *Malignant diseases of infancy, childhood and adolescence,* ed 2, Philadelphia, 1983, WB Saunders.)

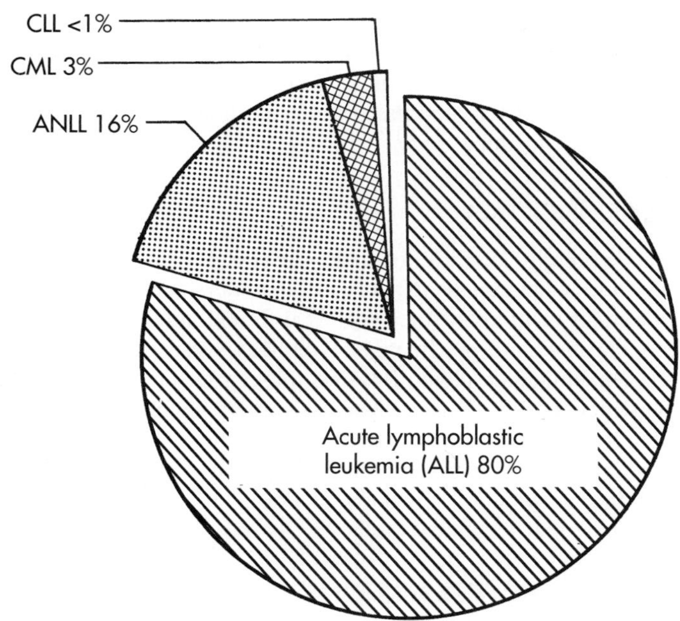

FIG. 227-2 The leukemias of childhood. *ANLL,* Acute nonlymphoid leukemia; *CML,* chronic myelogenous leukemia; *CLL,* chronic lymphatic leukemia.

(From Nathan DG, Oski FA: *Hematology of infancy and childhood,* ed 3, Philadelphia, 1987, WB Saunders.)

Clonal Expansion Theory

It is believed that most cases of leukemia result from a single damaged precursor cell that can self-replicate but that cannot undergo further differentiation. Because these cells do not stop dividing, the burden of leukemic cells increases. The disease apparently is a manifestation of the expansion of a single clone of cells. The clonal origin of leukemia is demonstrated best by studies involving the isoenzymes of glucose-6-phosphate dehydrogenase (G6PD) and by cytogenetics.[19,78,84]

Leukemic Clusters

Numerous reports of "leukemic time-space clusters" have attracted intense epidemiological study. A true leukemic cluster would suggest that a common etiological factor or horizontal transmission of an infectious agent played a role in the development of leukemia. However, the results of intense study suggest that, except for Nagasaki and Hiroshima,[4] the reports of leukemia epidemics can be explained purely by chance.[12,35,56] Inherent in such epidemiological studies is the difficulty of appropriately defining the population at risk and identifying all the potential confounding events that could influence the outcome.

Etiology (see the box on p. 1400)

Familial Predisposition and Genetic Factors. The occurrence of familial leukemia,[20,74] the concordance of leukemia in monozygotic twins,[14] and the increased incidence of leukemia in patients who have certain constitutional chromosomal abnormalities[36,49] are well-documented observations suggesting that genetic factors play an important role in leukemogenesis. It is hypothesized that the preexisting chromosomal defect in patients who have constitutional chromosomal abnormalities makes them more susceptible than normal to extrinsic environmental leukemogenic factors.[30] The common finding of one or more chromosomal abnormalities in the leukemia cells of patients is further evidence of the role genetic events play in the development of leukemia.[79,83]

Patients who have congenital immune deficiency diseases (e.g., Wiskott-Aldrich syndrome, ataxia telangiectasia, and congenital hypogammaglobulinemia) all have an increased risk of developing lymphoid malignancy.[22,49] In addition,

FACTORS ASSOCIATED WITH INCREASED RISK FOR CHILDHOOD LEUKEMIA

Familial predisposition

Twin of a patient with leukemia
Sibling of a patient with leukemia

Genetic factors

Down syndrome
Fanconi anemia
Bloom syndrome
Ataxia telangiectasia
Congenital hypogammaglobulinemia
Wiskott-Aldrich syndrome
Neurofibromatosis
Poland syndrome
Klinefelter syndrome
Schwachman syndrome

Environmental exposure

Viral infection
Ionizing radiation (atomic bomb and nuclear accidents)
Therapeutic radiation (ankylosing spondylitis, thymic enlargement)
Prenatal diagnostic radiation exposure
Certain drugs (benzene, alkylating agents)

Modified from Neglia JP, Robinson LL: *Pediatr Clin North Am* 35:675, 1988.

chronic therapy with immunosuppressive drugs, including long-term use of corticosteroids alone, has been associated with an increased risk of lymphoid malignancy.[57] The increased risk is thought to represent a breakdown in normal host "immune surveillance," allowing proliferation of malignant clones.

Environmental Exposure (see the box above)

Viruses and Leukemias. Certain viruses are known to cause leukemia in animal models,[75] but the relationship of the leukemia that occurs in these species to human leukemia is uncertain. The role of retrovirus in human leukemogenesis recently was demonstrated by the association between human T cell leukemia virus (HTLV-1) and adult T cell leukemia.[5] Epidemiological studies have failed to show a link between exposure to cats or feline leukemia virus and the development of leukemia in humans.[39] Epstein-Barr virus (EBV) infection, which causes infectious mononucleosis in humans, also is associated clearly with the African-type Burkitt lymphoma.[17] Although a link has not yet been demonstrated, EBV infection may be associated with B cell leukemia (i.e., Burkitt lymphoma with bone marrow involvement). The leukemogenic potential in humans of exposure to ionizing radiation is well demonstrated by the following observations: (1) in the 1930s, radiologists had a ninefold greater incidence of leukemia than did physicians and nonradiologists[43]; (2) survivors of the 1945 atomic bomb explosions in Hiroshima and Nagasaki have a 10 to 20 times greater risk of developing leukemia[9]; (3) individuals who have been treated with radiation for ankylosing spondylitis, thymic enlargement, and tinea capitis have a high incidence of leukemia[7]; and (4) children exposed to diagnostic radiation in utero have an increased risk of all childhood cancers.[34]

Controversy persists regarding the diagnostic use of radiation after birth and the development of human leukemia. Diagnostic use of ultrasonography, either before or after birth, has not been associated with an increased risk of childhood leukemia.

Investigations of adult ANLL have provided considerable information about exposure to chemical carcinogens (e.g., solvents and petroleum products) associated with an increased risk of leukemia.[8,76] Partly because of the small number of cases of leukemia among children relative to adults, a link between chemical exposure and childhood leukemia has not been demonstrated. A study completed by the Children's Cancer Study Group suggests that an environmental etiological component may be involved in childhood disease similar to that found in adult cases of ANLL.[63]

A number of studies have shown a link between secondary leukemogenesis and chemotherapy, especially alkylating agents, with or without radiation treatment. For example, acute leukemia (usually AML) has been observed in patients who have Hodgkin disease who received cyclophosphamide or nitrogen mustard as part of therapy, usually with concomitant radiation treatment.[6,55]

Other factors studied for possible association with leukemia include exposure to electromagnetic fields, herbicides and pesticides, and maternal use of alcohol, contraceptives, diethylstilbestrol (DES), or cigarettes. Definitive links between these factors and the risk of childhood leukemia have not been confirmed.[29,52]

CLASSIFICATION

The leukemias of childhood, shown in Fig. 227-2, are actually a very heterogeneous group of disorders that can be subclassified in terms of the level of differentiation (acute versus chronic) and the lineage (lymphoid versus myeloid) of the leukemogenic clone. Because the capacity to distinguish these leukemic cells, or blasts, is important therapeutically and prognostically, various cytological criteria have been established to differentiate them.[2,3,50,67] Newer approaches involving enzymatic,[21] surface marker,[23] cytogenetic,[42,79,83] and gene rearrangement studies[37,61,75] also have been used.

CLINICAL MANIFESTATIONS

Presenting Signs and Symptoms

Leukemia is a process of uncontrolled proliferation of immature hematopoietic cells that results in suppression of normal hematopoiesis and infiltration of extramedullary organs. The common presenting signs and symptoms reflect the degree of bone marrow compromise, the extent and location of leukemic cell infiltration, and the general systemic effects of these processes. In most cases the presenting complaints have been present a few days, a few weeks, or, more rarely, even months. The incidence of presenting complaints among children who have ALL compared with those who have ANLL are shown in Table 227-1.

Fever is the most common feature. In most patients it is caused by the leukemia itself rather than by infection. Pallor,

Table 227-1 Clinical and Laboratory Features in the Diagnosis of Leukemia

Feature	Percentage of all children with ALL*	Percentage of all children with ANLL†
Clinical		
Fever	61	34
Pallor	55	25
Bleeding (i.e., petechiae or purpura)	48	33
Anorexia or weight loss	33	22
Fatigue, malaise	30	19
Bone or joint pain	38	18
Lymphadenopathy	50	14
Hepatosplenomegaly	68	55
Swollen gingivae	—	8
Respiratory symptoms (i.e., sore throat, cough)	—	41
Recurrent infection	—	3
Neurological symptoms	3	10
Laboratory		
Leukocyte count (mm^3)		
<10,000	53	39
10,000-49,000	30	29
>50,000	17	32
Hemoglobin (g/dl)		
<7	43	41
7-11	45	48
>11	12	11
Platelet count (mm^3)		
<20,000	28	15
20,000-99,000	47	67
>100,000	25	18
Coagulopathy	—	17

*Miller DR: *Pediatr Clin North Am* 27:269, 1980.
†Choi SR, Simone JV: *Med Pediatr Oncol* 2:119, 1976.

fatigue, petechiae, purpura, and anorexia often are present. Significant weight loss is rare. Bone pain, lymphadenopathy, hepatomegaly, and splenomegaly are more common with ALL than with ANLL. Young children initially may limp or refuse to walk.

Laboratory Findings

Mild anemia and mild thrombocytopenia are common hematological abnormalities (see Table 227-1). The white blood count (WBC) may be normal, decreased, or increased. Blasts frequently but not always are found in the peripheral blood smear.

Other laboratory studies frequently are abnormal in children newly diagnosed with acute leukemia. In addition to hyperuricemia, serum levels of calcium, potassium, phosphate, and lactic dehydrogenase may be elevated. This constellation of abnormalities often is referred to as "tumor lysis syndrome." The severity of these abnormalities is thought to reflect the total leukemic cell burden and the excessive production and rapid turnover of leukemia cells. These abnormalities are particularly problematical in patients who have high initial WBC and extensive lymphadenopathy and hepatosplenomegaly. Most patients have some extramedullary disease at the time of diagnosis. An anterior mediastinal mass is present in 5% to 10% of patients newly diagnosed with ALL, making a chest roentgenogram crucial in the initial evaluation. Evidence of leukemic infiltration of the periosteum and bone often can be seen on the roentgenogram (including subperiosteal new bone formation, transverse metaphyseal radiolucent bands, osteolytic lesions, diffuse demineralization, and growth arrest lines) even in patients who have no complaints of bone pain.

Special Presentations

Central Nervous System Disease. The most common site of clinically apparent extramedullary leukemia is the central nervous system (CNS); this type is present in as many as 20% of patients at the time of diagnosis. Children who have CNS leukemia most often have increased intracranial pressure (i.e., vomiting, headache, lethargy, and papilledema), occasionally cranial nerve palsies, and, in rare cases, seizures or meningeal signs. Focal signs related to parenchymal involvement include hemiparesis, hemisensory losses, and seizure activity. Children under age 2 and those who have T cell ALL or monoblastic subtypes of ANLL have a higher incidence of CNS leukemia. Generally, cord compression by epidural leukemic infiltrates is rare; it is more common in AML than in ALL.

Chloromas. Chloromas are solid tumor collections of immature myeloid cells that can occur in ANLL patients. These tumors frequently involve periosteal and epidural regions of the head and neck but can occur anywhere on the body. A rare chloroma has been reported to occur months or years before systemic signs of leukemia.

Testicular Leukemia. Although more commonly reported in patients who have ALL, leukemic involvement of the testes in boys who have ANLL has been reported. Testicular leukemia manifests with painless enlargement of one or both testes. Although rarely reported as an initial manifestation of ALL (fewer than 5% of patients) or ANLL, it may be the first identifiable site of the recurrence of leukemia (15% of patients).

T Cell Leukemia. T cell ALL is characterized by several distinctive clinical features. It occurs more often in older boys who have a high WBC and often a mediastinal mass; these patients have a higher incidence of CNS leukemia. They also frequently have massive generalized lymphadenopathy and hepatosplenomegaly. This constellation of bulky infiltration of extramedullary sites historically has been referred to as "lymphomatous presentation" of leukemia.

Specific Clinical Features of ANLL Subtypes. Acute promyelocytic leukemia (M3 subtype) is associated more often with a spontaneous bleeding disorder than are the other variants of ANLL. Bleeding is the result of disseminated intravascular coagulation (DIC) and secondary fibrinolysis triggered by a substance contained within the cytoplasmic granules of the leukemic cells. Acute monoblastic leukemia (M4 and M5 subtypes) occurs at a younger age and is characterized by extensive extramedullary involvement at diagnosis, CNS involvement, leukemia cutis, lymphadenopathy, gingival hypertrophy, chloromas, DIC, an elevated WBC, and an elevated serum muramidase. The M7 morphological subtype of ANLL, or acute megakaryocytic leukemia, is particularly common in children who have Down syndrome. The biopsy specimen usually shows hypocellularity with myelofibrosis.

Preleukemia. Children with this disorder typically have fewer than 25% blasts in the bone marrow, circulating blasts, megaloblastosis, chromosomal abnormalities, and quantitative abnormalities of at least two of the three blood cell lines. These patients may turn out to have juvenile CML, chronic myelomonocytic leukemia, or monosomy 7 syndrome, which can precede the diagnosis of ANLL.

Diagnosis and Differential Diagnosis

The challenge for the physician in diagnosing pediatric leukemias is not that the symptoms are necessarily subtle, but that subtle differences exist between the symptoms of leukemia and those of more common illnesses or infectious conditions seen in children. The box on the right lists the most common malignant and nonmalignant conditions that may masquerade as leukemia. Once suspicion is aroused that a patient may have leukemia, the diagnosis must be confirmed by bone marrow aspiration and the type of leukemia determined. Although leukemic cells may be identified in the peripheral blood of many patients at the time of diagnosis, morphological assessment of these cells may be misleading. Thus examination of the bone marrow is mandatory to diagnose leukemia. Bone marrow aspirate usually provides sufficient material for diagnosis. Occasionally, however, a bone marrow biopsy may be required, particularly in patients who have pancytopenia, in which case bone marrow failure must be excluded.

Normal bone marrow contains fewer than 5% blast cells. By definition, the diagnosis of acute leukemia is confirmed when more than 25% of the nucleated cells in the marrow are blasts; typically, 90% or more of the cells in the bone marrow are blast cells. The presence of 5% to 25% blast cells in the marrow suggests several diagnostic possibilities, including non-Hodgkin lymphoma with leukemic involvement, preleukemia or myelodysplastic syndromes, chronic myelogenous leukemia, or acute monoblastic leukemia, which can manifest primarily with extramedullary disease.

A definitive diagnosis of the specific leukemic cell type is based on review of the morphological appearance of the blast cells, use of histochemical stains (e.g., myeloperoxidase and nonspecific esterases), enzymatic analysis, immunophenotyping, and cytogenetic analysis. These sophisticated techniques are important in establishing the specific leukemic cell type. It is essential therefore that the bone marrow aspiration or biopsy be performed in a center where cellular differentiation techniques are performed routinely. Leukemias must be differentiated from a variety of infectious illnesses. Patients who have these infectious conditions may have fevers, rash, generalized lymphadenopathy, splenomegaly, peripheral blood lymphocytosis and, less frequently, thrombocytopenia or immunohemolytic anemia. Usually these diseases can be differentiated in terms of the morphological appearance of reactive lymphocytes on the peripheral blood smear. Some conditions can be associated with a leukemoid reaction characterized by a reactive leukocytosis (WBC of 50,000 cells/mm^3 or higher) with an orderly progression of immature myeloid cells and occasional nucleated red blood cells (RBCs). Ordinarily, with idiopathic thrombocytopenic purpura, children do not have splenomegaly, anemia, or neutropenia. Juvenile rheumatoid arthritis (JRA) and systemic lupus erythematosus (SLE) may be confused with ALL because of the common complaints of fever, anemia, malaise, and painful, swollen joints. Because there is no reliable, definitive laboratory test for JRA or SLE, bone marrow aspiration may be necessary to exclude leukemia. The absence of lymphadenopathy and hepatosplenomegaly is important in diagnosing aplastic anemia. If the bone marrow aspirate is hypocellular, it should be biopsied. Several pediatric malignancies may show bone marrow involvement, including neuroblastoma, lymphoma, rhabdomyosarcoma, and Ewing sarcoma. Additional laboratory and clinical evaluation may be necessary (e.g., urinary catecholamine determination, radiological imaging) to exclude these malignancies.

DIFFERENTIAL DIAGNOSIS OF CHILDHOOD ACUTE LEUKEMIA

Nonmalignant conditions

- Juvenile rheumatoid arthritis
- Systemic lupus erythematosus
- Infectious mononucleosis
- Idiopathic thrombocytopenic purpura
- Pertussis, parapertussis
- Aplastic anemia
- Acute benign infectious lymphocytosis
- Leukemoid reaction (more common in ANLL)
- Bacterial sepsis with or without coagulopathy (more common in ANLL)
- Osteomyelitis

Malignancies

- Neuroblastoma
- Lymphoma (especially if mediastinal mass, massive adenopathy, and organomegaly are present)
- Retinoblastoma
- Rhabdomyosarcoma
- Ewing sarcoma
- Chronic myelogenous leukemia

Unusual presentations

- Hypereosinophilic syndrome
- Cord compression or cauda equina syndrome
- Eosinophilic granuloma
- Parenchymal brain lesion

TREATMENT

The goal of any antileukemic therapy is to eradicate the invading leukemic cells and their progenitors while preserving the expression of normal blood cell progenitors. Great strides have been made toward this goal, as evaluation, primary combination chemotherapy, bone marrow transplantation, treatment alternatives for patients who relapse, and supportive care have become more sophisticated.

Prognostic Factors

Interest in prognostic factors arose in the late 1970s as therapy became successful in most patients who had ALL.

Pediatric oncologists began looking for common features among groups of patients who did well compared with patients whose disease relapsed. Through retrospective analysis of disease-free survival, certain features present at the time of diagnosis of ALL were identified that were useful in predicting which patients had a good, a fair, or a poor prognosis.

Prognostic factors are useful because they allow physicians to devise "tailored therapy," or therapy that is altered for a patient or group of patients according to the clinical features of the disease and whether it is associated with a higher or lower risk of relapse. If therapy is adequate, the bad prognostic factor no longer predicts a poor outcome, but rather identifies patients who need aggressive therapy. A characteristic identified in a group of patients treated one way may not have the same significance if a different treatment is used. Thus "good risk" patients are treated less aggressively in an attempt to minimize toxicity; "poor risk" patients get more aggressive therapy to better control the disease.

In the treatment of ALL, the initial WBC and the patient's age at diagnosis have been the two most reliable indicators of prognosis, both for the duration of remission and survival.[64] Children who are very young at diagnosis (under 2 years of age) or older (over 10 years of age) have a relatively poor prognosis compared with those in the intermediate age group.[68] The worst prognosis is for infants under 1 year of age. The presence of the Philadelphia chromosome consistently has been associated with a poor outcome among many study groups. Other clinical features that have been correlated with the prognosis include gender, race, degree of organomegaly and lymphadenopathy, presence or absence of a mediastinal mass, cytogenetic features, initial hemoglobin levels, initial platelet count, cell subtype, immunological subtype, immunoglobulin levels at diagnosis, the presence or absence of CNS leukemia at diagnosis, day 14 bone marrow response, and human leukocyte antigen (HLA) type. Because the prognostic importance is not reproducible among different study groups, the value of these variables remains controversial.

Because only recently have more than one third of patients who have ANLL survived long term, prognostic factors in ANLL are defined less clearly than in ALL. A variety of clinical features are being examined as possibly important prognostic factors, including cytogenetic features, day 14 bone marrow response, the presence of Auer rods in affected cells, the blast cells' immune phenotype, in vitro growth characteristics, and in vitro response to chemotherapy. The factors most investigators accept as being associated with an unfavorable outcome are a WBC over 100,000, monoblastic leukemia in infants, monosomy 7 karyotype, and presentation with a preleukemia syndrome.

Death from CML usually occurs within months of the acceleration phase; therefore the major determinant of survival is the duration of the chronic phase. One study found peripheral blood and bone marrow blast counts at presentation to be correlated with survival.[13] The juvenile form of CML is notable for an extremely poor prognosis, with a median survival of less than 9 months from the time of diagnosis.

Acute Management

Initial Evaluation and Referral. Diagnostic evaluation of a child suspected of having leukemia has become more complex, requiring advanced laboratory techniques to perform appropriate cytogenetic, immunological, and biochemical assays. The problems and complications in a child undergoing leukemia therapy often are complex, requiring expert supportive care. A higher death rate has been reported in patients who have ALL and were treated outside of a children's cancer center without a standard protocol.[45] For these reasons and because of the intensity of current regimens, children suspected of having one of the leukemias should be referred for diagnostic testing and treatment to pediatric cancer centers that use cooperative group protocols.

The goal of initial management, often before the diagnosis has been confirmed, is to ensure that the patient does not require urgent medical intervention before transfer to another center. The major clinical problems needing to be addressed by the primary care physician and suggested emergency interventions are listed in the box on p. 1404. Many of these problems can be excluded as emergencies by a careful history, physical examination, and review of the complete blood count (CBC). Very few patients require specific intervention before transfer to a pediatric oncology center. For most patients, initial management involves consultation with a pediatric oncologist, referral to a pediatric oncology center, and admission to the hospital. Admission to the hospital can be helpful in facilitating the child's evaluation and the necessary diagnostic tests, stabilizing the metabolic status, starting chemotherapy, beginning patient and parent education, and building the foundation for long-term relationships between the family and health care providers. A common exception to this is the patient with CML in the chronic phase at diagnosis, who often can be treated as an outpatient if he or she is medically stable.

The primary care physician plays a vital role in ensuring a smooth transition by preparing the child and family for what may lie ahead. This includes apprising them of the facts in a positive manner early on; that is, that this may be a serious illness and that testing is important to determine the problem so that appropriate treatment can be started, emphasizing the need to enlist the help of other pediatric specialists. The primary physician can facilitate the transition by conveying information about previous displays of coping skills by the patient and family to the consulting physician. Follow-up communication between the referring physician, consulting physician, and family is essential in establishing and maintaining a strong patient-family-physician relationship.

Supportive Care

Great strides in supportive care, including transfusion therapy, better infection control, and frequent use of indwelling central venous catheters, have contributed immensely to the reduction in morbidity and mortality. The specific guidelines followed (i.e., choice of antibiotics, indwelling catheter care, isolation procedures, transfusion indications) may vary among institutions, based partly on the previous experience of the institution or investigators.

Blood Product Support. Myelosuppression, with resultant anemia, thrombocytopenia, and neutropenia, often is observed in these patients secondary to leukemia or chemotherapy-induced bone marrow hypoplasia or both. Irradiation of blood products has prevented graft-versus-host disease in patients who have had severe bone marrow depression and immune suppression. Administration of cyto-

APPROACH TO ACUTE MANAGEMENT OF LEUKEMIA

A. Initial evaluation

History—Fatigue, malaise, anorexia, irritability, fever, bone pain, mouth sores

Physical examination—Pallor, petechiae, purpura, fever, lymphadenopathy, hepatosplenomegaly, respiratory distress, neurological abnormalities

Laboratory—Complete blood count with differential and platelet count, abnormal results of one or more cell lines

B. Suspicion of leukemia as a possible diagnosis and potential emergency interventions

Findings	Management
1. Temperature over 100.4° F (38° C), neutrophil count <500; symptoms of infection	Blood culture, antibiotics
2. Bleeding symptoms	Start intravenous unit for access and delivery of a fluid bolus, transfuse platelets, red cells, or plasma
3. Respiratory distress	Chest roentgenogram, oxygen
4. WBC >100,000	Blood urea nitrogen and creatinine, urate, serum potassium, serum calcium, serum phosphate, chest roentgenogram, start intravenous unit for access and delivery of a fluid bolus

C. Refer patient to a pediatric oncology center

Consult with a pediatric oncologist

Arrange for transfer of patient to the pediatric oncology center

Prepare patient and family for what to expect when they get there

megalovirus (CMV)-negative blood products to patients who have had negative CMV antibody titer has decreased the incidence of transfusion-related CMV infection. More sophisticated techniques to test donor blood for evidence of infection such as hepatitis B, non-A, non-B hepatitis, and human immunodeficiency virus (HIV) have reduced but not eradicated transfusion-transmitted infections.

Unless the anemia is rapid in onset (e.g., because of blood loss or hemolysis), RBC transfusion is not necessary until the hematocrit is 25 or less. Platelets generally are transfused when the platelet count falls below 20,000 cells/mm^3; use of "prophylactic" platelet transfusion when platelet counts are higher remains controversial. Indications for platelet transfusion in a patient who has thrombocytopenia, other than absolute platelet count, include fresh bleeding, fever, infection, or anticipated protracted thrombocytopenia as a result of therapy.

Granulocyte transfusions rarely are used. Their value generally is limited to treating patients who have severe neutropenia with proven gram negative sepsis or a perirectal abscess that does not respond to appropriate antibiotics. In addition to the risk of transmission of infection, white blood cell transfusions frequently are associated with the uncomfortable side effects of fever, rigors, and allergic reactions, caused by sensitization to foreign leukocyte proteins.

Infection. Infectious complications are the most common cause of morbidity and mortality in leukemia patients, second only to relapse of leukemia. Leukemia patients who are undergoing combination chemotherapy should be considered immunocompromised hosts. Neutropenia, which can result from chemotherapy-induced bone marrow hypoplasia, contributes to an increased susceptibility to bacterial and fungal infections. In the future, strategies now being tested, including the use of growth factors and recently developed antibiotics, may reduce infectious complications significantly.

Any febrile patient whose absolute neutrophil count (ANC) is below 500 cells/mm^3 must be considered septic.*† Cultures should be obtained promptly, and the patient should be started immediately on intravenous (IV) broad-spectrum antibiotics. Because bowel, respiratory, and skin organisms commonly are identified, antibiotics that cover these gram negative and gram positive bacteria are used. Infections among patients who have fever and neutropenia presumably are bacterial, although specific etiological agents usually are not found. Prophylactic oral antibiotics have not proved useful. *Candida* and *Aspergillus* organisms are the major fungal pathogens reported. Prophylactic oral antifungal agents have not proved effective in preventing invasive disease. Amphotericin B is the treatment of choice for such fungal infections. Thus patients who have neutropenia who remain febrile after 3 to 7 days of treatment with broad-spectrum antibiotics usually are treated empirically with amphotericin B, even before a definitive diagnosis of fungal disease is made.

Viral infections occur frequently in patients who have leukemia, but rarely is specific therapy indicated. Before the routine use of varicella-zoster immunoglobulin and acyclovir, chickenpox often was complicated by pneumonitis, hepatitis, encephalitis, or even death. Acyclovir particularly has contributed to a notable decline in morbidity and mortality from varicella-zoster, herpes zoster, and herpes simplex infections.

Pneumocystis carinii is another organism found to cause severe, often fatal interstitial pneumonitis in children receiving multiagent chemotherapy. Trimethoprim-sulfamethoxazole

*A febrile patient is one whose oral or axillary temperature is over 100.4° F (38° C); the temperature should not be taken rectally in leukemia patients.

†The ANC can be found using this formula: ANC = WBC × (% neutrophils + % bands).

prophylaxis has been shown to reduce the incidence of *P. carinii* infections in the immunocompromised host.

Psychological Aspects. The emotional impact of the diagnosis of cancer is immediate and lifelong for both patient and family; no family member is unaffected. Their lives are changed forever but, it is hoped, not irreparably. For most children leukemia is chronic and life threatening, yet treatable. Attention to the child's and family's adaptation to the phases of diagnosis, treatment, returning to "normal," and eventual survival is essential in truly comprehensive oncological care.

The diagnosis of leukemia is a time of crisis. Feelings of anger, guilt, and loss of control are universal to patients of all ages, their parents, and their siblings. Siblings often are jealous of all the attention the patient receives, which adds to the parents' stress. In the midst of this distress, the child and parents are asked to assimilate vast amounts of information about diagnosis, prognosis, procedures, treatments, side effects, and hospital or clinical routines. Discussions should be gentle, accurate, realistic, hopeful, and, above all, honest.

Several specific techniques can help families with these early adjustments. Repeating information frequently and encouraging any and all questions (they should be written down) are important. Whenever possible, the physician should talk to the parents together to prevent misunderstandings and to avoid making one parent responsible for relaying information and answering questions for the other. Educational materials written in layman's language are helpful supplements to verbal discussions. Information about the child's and the family's previous manner of coping with major events and previous experiences with cancer, serious illness, or death should be obtained from the primary physician and by family interview. Just as with a successful medical outcome, a positive psychosocial outcome depends on early assessment, anticipation, prevention, and intervention for complications.

Regardless of the eventual outcome—good or bad—the treatment course is full of ups and downs, discomforts, uncertainties, and both illness- and non-illness-related stress. The patient and family continue to be challenged by the pressures of day-to-day events such as jobs, school, relocation, marriage, family, finances, and other family illnesses, injury, or death, which may even precede the diagnosis of leukemia. In addition, illness-related stress factors such as separation of family members, frequent traveling, disruption of the normal routine, sleep interruptions, child care arrangements, the high cost of care, and the threat of death take an extreme emotional toll on the child and family.

During the course of therapy there are several times that can be extremely stressful and the need for increased support anticipated. Ironically, getting back to "normal," either at the time of hospital discharge, upon returning to school, or at the completion of therapy, provokes considerable anxiety. Every effort should be made to encourage the child to return to normal social, school, and physical activities as soon as possible. Early communication among family, school, and medical personnel is essential to a smooth reentry into normal routines.

Perhaps more devastating than the initial diagnosis is the news that the disease has recurred, or the realization that all treatments have failed and that the child will die. With a relapse the family must start the treatment process all over again, although with a smaller chance for a successful outcome. More than ever before, they need the support of the health care team to enable them to go on. When a cure is no longer possible, room must always be left for hope. Hope can come from changing the focus toward palliative care, with comfort as the goal. Thus the efforts of the health care team—oncologists, psychosocial workers, family physician, and family—must be redirected toward comfort measures. Physical measures include controlling pain and bleeding without invasive diagnostic or treatment procedures. Frequent reassurance that the child and family will not be left alone are of the utmost importance in providing good, successful palliative care. At this point, perhaps more than ever before, support must be given to staff members, who in turn provide the most support for the child and family.

Chemotherapy

Table 227-2 lists the various chemotherapeutic agents used in treating childhood leukemias and the complications associated with their use. The specific indications for their use are described below in the discussions of therapy for each type of childhood leukemia.

Bone Marrow Transplantation

The role of current bone marrow transplantation (BMT) alternatives for treating leukemia in children is shown in Fig. 227-3. BMT involves initial administration of intensive cytoreductive therapy—usually high-dose chemotherapy with or without total body irradiation—designed to eradicate 100% of the leukemia cells. This therapy is so intense that it also is lethal to normal bone marrow cells. Therefore it must be followed by bone marrow "rescue" with intravenously infused bone marrow from a compatible donor. For an allogeneic bone marrow transplant, the donor is an HLA-matched sibling. Unfortunately, approximately only one third of patients who require transplantation are likely to have an HLA-identical sibling. For this reason, the role of bone marrow transplantation historically has been somewhat limited. With advances in transplantation technology, however, alternatives are being studied, such as autologous donation or transplantation from partially matched related donors (i.e., parents or siblings) or from matched unrelated donors.

Autologous BMT has been curative for small numbers of patients who have had ALL and ANLL. The patient undergoes bone marrow harvest during a time of remission, and the marrow is treated in an attempt to eradicate leukemic cells. The marrow cells then are cryopreserved and infused after completion of the cytoreductive therapy. Posttransplant relapse of leukemia occurs in most patients and is the major reason for failure because posttransplant mortality due to complications is very low. For patients who do not have a matched related donor available or for whom autologous transplantation is not appropriate (e.g., early relapse of ALL, patients who have any form of ANLL, or CML) transplantation is performed at some centers using matched unrelated or partially mismatched donors. To date such procedures have been associated with very poor survival rates secondary to both relapse of leukemia and treatment-related complications. The major limitations of such BMT procedures have been graft rejection and graft-versus-host disease. As progress is

Table 227-2 Use and Complications of Chemotherapeutic Agents in Acute Leukemia

Drug	Route	Common use	Acute toxicity	Delayed toxic effects
Prednisone	PO	Induction and maintenance of ALL	Hyperglycemia, hypertension, emotional lability, increased appetite, fluid retention, weight gain, striae, cushingoid facies, peptic ulcer, diabetes mellitus	Osteoporosis, growth retardation, aseptic necrosis, cataracts, glaucoma, diabetes mellitus
Vincristine	IV	Induction and maintenance of ALL	Alopecia, constipation, paralytic ileus, peripheral neuropathy, jaw pain, SIADH,* danger with extravasation, in rare cases, myelosuppression	Peripheral neuropathy
6-Mercaptopurine	PO, IV	Maintenance of ALL	Alopecia, nausea, vomiting, diarrhea, myelosuppression, hepatic damage, cholestasis	Hepatic disease, cholestasis
Methotrexate	PO, IM, IV	Maintenance of ALL	Nausea, vomiting, mucositis, rash, myelosuppression, hepatic damage, renal toxicity	Hepatic damage, neurotoxicity
Methotrexate and/or cytosine arabinoside	Intrathecal	CNS prophylaxis of ALL and ANLL	Nausea, vomiting, headache, stiff neck, arachnoiditis, seizures	Cortical atrophy, leukoencephalopathy
L-Asparaginase	IM	Induction and consolidation of ALL	Anaphylaxis, nausea, vomiting, fever, chills, hyperglycemia, diabetes, abdominal pain, pancreatitis (increased amylase), CNS depression, coagulation defects with thrombosis or hemorrhage (i.e., stroke), hypoproteinemia, hepatic damage	Pancreatic or hepatic damage, diabetes mellitus
Doxorubicin	IV	Induction and consolidation of ALL	Myelosuppression, alopecia, nausea, vomiting, mucositis, anorexia, hepatic damage, cardiac arrhythmias, red urine, danger with extravasation	Cardiomyopathy, hepatic damage
Daunorubicin	IV	Induction and maintenance of ALL and ANLL	Myelosuppression, alopecia, nausea, vomiting, cardiac arrhythmias, hepatic damage, red urine, danger with extravasation	Cardiomyopathy
Cytosine arabinoside	IV	Induction and maintenance of ANLL Consolidation of high-risk ALL	Myelosuppression, alopecia, nausea, vomiting, diarrhea, mucositis, conjunctivitis, fever, neurotoxicity	Hepatic damage, neurotoxicity
Etoposide/tenoposide	IV	Induction and maintenance of ANLL Consolidation of high-risk ALL	Hypotension, anaphylaxis, myelosuppression, nausea, vomiting, alopecia, mucositis, danger with extravasation	Second malignancy, most commonly ANLL
6-Thioguanine	PO	Induction and maintenance of ANLL	Same as for mercaptopurine but less hepatic toxicity	
Radiation		ALL CNS prophylaxis	Alopecia, nausea, vomiting, skin hypersensitivity, mild myelosuppression	Sleeping syndrome, seizures, leukoencephalopathy, growth retardation

Data compiled from Dorr RT, Fritz WL: *Cancer chemotherapy handbook,* New York, 1980, Elsevier.
**SIADH,* Syndrome of inappropriate secretion of antidiuretic hormone.

made in developing better prophylactic regimens and improved therapeutic strategies for overcoming these limitations, transplantation in the mismatch setting may soon be a more routine and more successful alternative. Another option being explored at some centers is the use of cord blood as a rich source of stem cells for transplantation and hematopoietic reconstitution. For these purposes, cord blood is obtained from the placenta at the time of delivery and cryopreserved. Transplantation with cord blood appears to be particularly advantageous with the mismatched or unrelated donor tech-

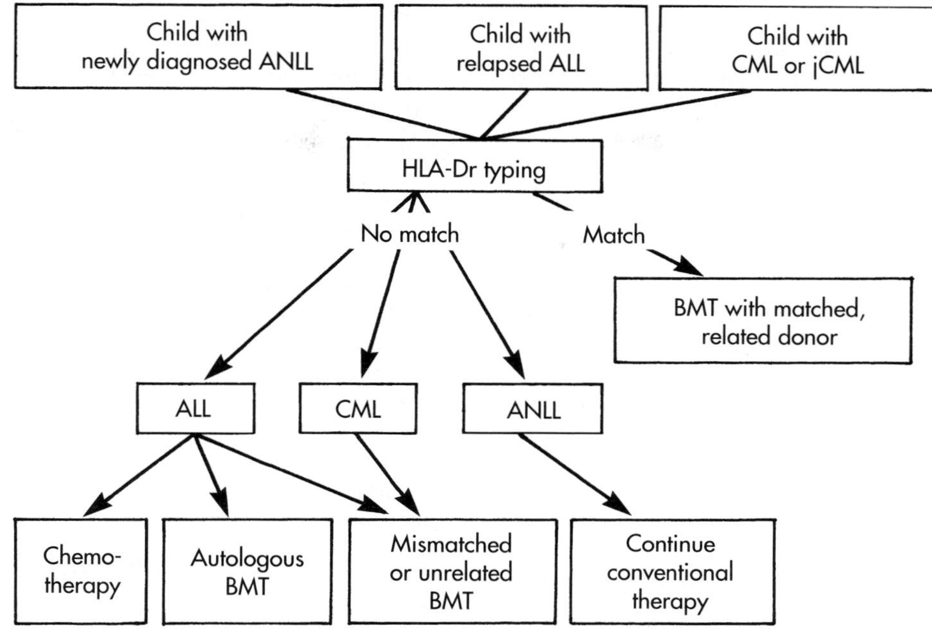

FIG. 227-3 Flow diagram of marrow transplantation for children who have leukemia. (From Trigg ME: *Pediatr Clin North Am* 35:939, 1988.)

nique because the risk of graft-versus-host disease is reduced.

BMT can be associated with significant complications. In addition to the anticipated side effects of the cytoreductive chemotherapy (e.g., nausea, vomiting, mucositis, anorexia, and prolonged bone marrow aplasia), transplantation-related problems may occur such as graft rejection, graft-versus-host disease, and hepatic venoocclusive syndrome. As with all intensive treatment regimens, infections such as bacterial sepsis, invasive fungal disease, CMV interstitial pneumonitis, and *P. carinii* pneumonia (PCP) are significant causes of morbidity and mortality, particularly during the first 6 months after transplantation.

ACUTE LYMPHOBLASTIC LEUKEMIA

Most ALL treatment regimens divide therapy into three phases: induction of remission, CNS prophylaxis and consolidation, and maintenance treatment during remission.

Induction of Remission

The aim of the initial treatment of ALL is induction of remission. Complete remission is defined as the absence of clinical signs and symptoms of disease in the presence of a normal blood count and a normocellular bone marrow with 5% or fewer blasts. However, there is no evidence that the clinical disappearance of leukemic cells from the bone marrow indicates their total eradication.

Although the basic two-drug combination of vincristine and prednisone can induce remission in approximately 85% of children who have ALL, addition of L-asparaginase or an anthracycline improves the remission induction rate to approximately 95% and lengthens the duration of remission.[25,44,69]

Although a period of 4 weeks generally is required to achieve complete remission, in most cases marked regression of symptoms, organomegaly, and peripheral blasts occurs within the first week of treatment. Hospitalization during this time is common. Pancytopenia is seen routinely as a result of leukemia and chemotherapy-induced bone marrow suppression. These patients often are transfusion dependent for red cells and platelets and frequently require antibiotics for empirical treatment of fever with neutropenia.

Central Nervous System Prophylaxis

As soon as bone marrow remission has been achieved, CNS prophylaxis is instituted. The optimum and least toxic prophylaxis has not yet been determined fully. Investigators at St. Jude Children's Research Hospital showed that cranial spinal irradiation could reduce the incidence of CNS relapse to approximately 10%.[1] Because of the excessive myelosuppression and subsequent growth disturbances associated with spinal irradiation, cranial irradiation plus intrathecal methotrexate was adopted universally as the standard form of CNS preventive therapy in the 1970s. In recent years, however, concern has arisen about the apparent adverse effects of this regimen on neurological and intellectual functioning. Reducing the dose of cranial irradiation may be as effective, but it is not clear whether a lower dose is associated with a lower incidence of CNS sequelae. Other approaches studied include triple intrathecal chemotherapy with methotrexate, cytosine arabinoside, and hydrocortisone; intermediate-dose systemic methotrexate, either alone or with concomitant intrathecal methotrexate; intrathecal methotrexate alone; or high-dose systemic methotrexate. For patients at standard risk, cranial irradiation does not appear to be necessary; intrathecal chemotherapy alone appears to offer adequate CNS preventive therapy.

Maintenance Therapy

The rationale for continuing to treat patients in complete continuous remission is based on historical studies in which therapy was discontinued immediately[26] or 6 months after induction of remission.[41] In both studies relapse quickly followed discontinuation of treatment. The backbone of most maintenance regimens includes daily oral doses of 6-mercaptopurine, weekly doses of parenteral methotrexate, postinduction IV doses of vincristine, and oral prednisone at a variety of intervals. These regimens often incorporate anthracyclines, asparaginase, and cytosine arabinoside for high-risk patients. Currently the optimum duration of therapy is unknown. Most centers continue treatment for 2½ to 3 years. For patients who successfully complete a full course of maintenance therapy, the prognosis generally is good. A study from St. Jude Children's Research Hospital demonstrated that approximately 80% of patients who complete therapy remain disease free. Of the 20% who eventually relapse, most do so in the first year of therapy.[27] The risk of relapse after 4 disease-free years is virtually nonexistent.[25]

Relapse Therapy

Most patients who relapse have a grave prognosis. Several factors, such as the duration of first remission, whether relapse occurs during or after completion of therapy, and the site of relapse have been identified—factors that have some predictive value in determining the outcome of subsequent therapy. The most common site of relapse in ALL is the bone marrow. Relapse at any site must be presumed to be associated with systemic reseeding of leukemic cells. Therefore patients who have clinically localized relapses must be treated both locally and systemically with reinduction therapy and reprophylaxis of the CNS. Most patients who have ALL can readily be induced into a second remission; however, these remissions generally last less than 1 year, and long-term remissions are uncommon.

Bone Marrow Transplantation

The current role of BMT in treating ALL is for patients who have relapsed and a select few patients during their first remission (e.g., patients who have the Philadelphia chromosome). For patients who have a bone marrow relapse and are fortunate enough to have an HLA-identical sibling, bone marrow transplantation should be strongly considered. Patients "transplanted" during remission fare better than if the procedure is attempted during relapse, and those transplanted earlier in their disease (i.e., in second remission) do better than those who receive transplantations after several previous relapses.[10,11] Autologous BMT has been curative for some patients. Its exact role in treating relapsed ALL is controversial. Data are conflicting about the benefit in terms of disease-free survival with autologous BMT compared with consolidation chemotherapy. Improved methods of purging the marrow may result in more cures in the future.

ACUTE NONLYMPHOBLASTIC LEUKEMIA

Progress in the treatment of children who have ANLL has not kept pace with advances in the treatment of childhood ALL. As a result of new chemotherapeutic strategies, better supportive care, and improved transplantation technology, overall survival has increased for children who have ANLL, especially for those who have the AML and APML subtypes. In contrast to ALL, the current treatment of ANLL is very intensive for all patients. High WBC, bleeding disorders, chloromas, and symptoms of hyperleukocytosis (see CML below) are much more common findings at diagnosis in ANLL than in ALL.

Induction of Remission

Historically, induction therapy invariably has included cytosine arabinoside (cytarabine) and anthracycline, usually daunorubicin.[70] Approximately 70% to 80% of children achieve complete remission with these two drugs. The duration of severe marrow hypoplasia with peripheral pancytopenia during a typical ANLL induction ranges from 21 to 35 days. The leukemic blasts of almost half of the 20% to 30% of patients who fail to achieve remission are refractory to the standard cytarabine and daunorubicin combination. New treatment alternatives are being studied for this group, including high-dose cytarabine or different drugs (e.g., etoposide, amsacrine, 5-azacytidine).

Central Nervous System Prophylaxis

Without some form of CNS prophylaxis, approximately 10% to 30% of children who have AML have an initial relapse in the central nervous system. Apparently effective CNS prophylaxis regimens consist of intrathecal cytarabine or methotrexate and/or cranial irradiation. High-dose intravenous cytarabine probably also has some activity against CNS leukemia.

Maintenance Therapy

The principles of treatment in ANLL remission are similar to those of ALL, but the strategy differs. Much more intensive treatment appears to be necessary. The consequence of such intense chemotherapy programs is severe myelosuppression and its attendant complications. The need for maintenance therapy beyond the induction-intensification phases remains a controversial issue to be addressed by future studies. There are data to support both conclusions. The answers to questions of optimum duration and drug combinations depend partly on the exact nature and intensity of the therapeutic program used for induction and intensification.

Bone Marrow Transplantation

Allogeneic BMT is the treatment of choice for patients who have ANLL in first remission if a matched related donor is available. Five-year leukemia-free survival is reported to be 60% in children who have AML who are treated by allogeneic transplantation after chemotherapeutic induction of complete remission.[18,72,73] Both leukemia-free survival and overall survival are better than that achieved with chemotherapy alone. The price of BMT in terms of toxicity remains high, with graft-versus-host disease and infection being most problematical. Several groups of children, such as those who have preleukemia syndromes, monosomy 7, and monocytic leukemia, have been identified as being at very high risk for induction failure. For these children who achieve remission and who do not have a histocompatible sibling donor, matched unrelated or partially matched donor transplantation should be the initial approach for consolidation therapy.

It is accepted practice to determine the HLA type of the children and family members when the initial diagnosis of ANLL is made so that therapeutic options can be established and potentially hazardous transfusions from donors or family members can be avoided. Many centers harvest bone marrow on all ANLL patients during the first remission and hold it in reserve for use in the event of relapse. As technology improves, bone marrow transplantation from unrelated or partially mismatched family members will become a more reasonable approach for ANLL patients in second remission.

Relapse Therapy

Approximately 50% of children who have ANLL who have relapsed or were refractory to initial therapy may be induced into a complete remission with one of a number of investigational treatment regimens, such as daunorubicin and cyclocytidine or cytarabine, amasacrine and cyclocytidine, and etoposide and 5-azacytidine.[31,47] The duration of remission has been short for most of these patients. If a second remission is induced, bone marrow transplantation offers the only chance for a cure.

CHRONIC MYELOGENOUS LEUKEMIA

Chronic myelogenous leukemia is rare in children. In childhood the disorder may appear as two distinct clinical syndromes: adult-type CML, which is virtually indistinguishable from that seen in older patients, and juvenile CML, a disease relatively restricted to very young children that has distinct clinical, laboratory, and cytogenetic features.

Adult-Type CML

The adult form of CML is a clonal myeloproliferative disorder involving all of the blood progenitor lineages and at least some of the lymphoid lineages. It is characterized by expansion of the total body granulocyte pool, myeloid hyperplasia of the bone marrow, extramedullary hematopoiesis, and a specific cytogenetic marker, the Philadelphia chromosome.

The natural history of CML is divided into three phases: chronic, accelerated, and blastic. These phases represent the progressive shift in the nature of the disorder, from hyperproliferation, with production of mainly mature blood elements, to production of predominately immature blast cells.

Chronic Phase

The signs and symptoms of CML usually develop insidiously over several months. Patients usually have nonspecific complaints such as fever, night sweats, fatigue, diminished exercise tolerance, weakness, left upper quadrant pain, and early satiation of appetite. Marrow hyperplasia and marrow space expansion may result in bone pain and tenderness. The usual physical findings are pallor, low-grade fever, ecchymoses, sternal tenderness, and hepatosplenomegaly. Neurological abnormalities, visual difficulties, papilledema, retinal hemorrhages, respiratory distress with tachypnea, or priapism may complicate cases involving marked hyperleukocytosis.

Peripheral blood counts typically demonstrate a normochromic, normocytic anemia (mean hematocrit of 25%), marked leukocytosis with "a shift to the left," and thrombocytosis (mean platelet count of 500,000/mm^3). The WBC at diagnosis ranges from approximately 8000 to 800,000 cells/mm^3. The peripheral blood smear is remarkable for (1) increased numbers of myeloid cells at all stages of differentiation, (2) myeloblasts and promyelocytes accounting for fewer than 15% of the total white blood cell differential count, (3) basophilia, and (4) eosinophilia.[66] In the bone marrow, granulocytes at all stages of maturation are seen in increased numbers, although their morphological appearance is normal. The finding of the Philadelphia chromosome in approximately 90% of patients is pathognomonic for CML. The laboratory finding of a decline in leukocyte alkaline phosphatase (LAP) activity is quite helpful diagnostically. LAP activity increases in a number of conditions that can be differentiated, including infection, leukemoid reaction, hematological remission of CML, and a blast crisis of CML. Other common laboratory abnormalities include elevation of serum uric acid and lactate dehydrogenase levels.

Before any specific antileukemic therapy is initiated, the following special management problems and their treatment must be considered: hyperuricemia, hyperkalemia, hyperphosphatemia, priapism, and the neurological, retinal, or pulmonary complications of leukostasis. The goal of treatment in the chronic phase is to provide symptomatic relief by correcting the leukocytosis and organomegaly. The standard approach to chronic-phase CML is single-agent chemotherapy, usually busulfan or hydroxyurea. Hydroxyurea is the drug of choice in children because of its increased margin of hematological safety and its reduced systemic toxicity relative to busulfan. Both drugs must be monitored carefully, and dosages must be adjusted according to the hematological response. Clinical studies of alpha-interferon are underway, and early results suggest that it may be a more effective treatment than busulfan or hydroxyurea.

Conventional therapy rarely produces a true complete remission. Although the CBC may normalize and the organomegaly disappear, the bone marrow continues to show granulocyte hyperplasia and Philadelphia chromosome–positive metaphases. Attempts to ablate the Philadelphia chromosome–positive clone with aggressive multiagent chemotherapy have not succeeded. Therapy does not delay acceleration to blast crisis or prolong survival.

Acceleration Phase

Inevitably, patients develop a more malignant form of their disease. This blast crisis may be heralded by a 3- to 6-month transitional phase referred to as the acceleration phase, or metamorphosis. The clinical features observed in this period include basophilia, new-onset thrombocytosis or thrombocytopenia, leukocytosis refractory to previous therapies, anemia, and splenomegaly. Therapy should be instituted to prevent the complications of this accelerated phase of disease—renewed leukostasis, organomegaly, and hyperproliferation. No therapy short of bone marrow transplantation has been shown to prevent the inevitable development of a blastic phase and death in CML.

Blast Crisis

Acute blastic transformation occurs at a median of about 3 years and is responsible for at least 75% of deaths in CML. Leukostasis and very high WBCs are more common in the blast phase, which is quite refractory to chemotherapy regardless of whether the blastic transformation is myeloblastic or lymphoblastic. Median survival after blastic transformation is only 3 to 6 months. Long-term remissions have been reported in patients who underwent allogeneic bone marrow transplantation while in the accelerated or blastic phase, but the results generally are disappointing.

Bone Marrow Transplantation

Allogeneic BMT is the only curative approach now available for patients who have CML. The disease status at the time of transplantation is the most powerful predictor of disease-free survival. Most centers, therefore, currently recommend allogeneic BMT for any child who has the adult-type CML in the chronic phase who has an HLA-matched donor, preferably within 1 year of diagnosis. Autologous transplantation has been used as a temporizing approach, the objective being to restore the chronic phase. The bone marrow is reconstituted with Philadelphia chromosome–positive cells. Therefore, although the chronic phase may be reestablished and survival prolonged, this technique is unlikely to be curative. Advances in BMT technology have allowed successful unrelated donor transplantation and cure for small numbers of patients who have CML. For the patient who has no HLA-matched sibling, this is the only alternative approach available with curative potential.

Juvenile Chronic Myelogenous Leukemia

Juvenile chronic myelogenous leukemia (JCML) is a myeloproliferative disorder seen mainly in infants and characterized by leukocytosis, splenomegaly, and decreased LAP activity.[33] Despite these clinical similarities to the adult form of CML, JCML clearly is distinguishable with respect to clinical presentation, hematological manifestations, cytogenetic analysis, response to therapy, and prognosis (Table 227-3).

Distinctive clinical features common to JCML at diagnosis include a patient under 2 years of age, persistent respiratory infections (with tachypnea, chronic cough, wheezing), prominent lymphadenopathy, skin rash (eczema, xanthomata, and café-au-lait spots), bleeding, and failure to thrive. In addition to anemia and leukocytosis, frequent laboratory findings are thrombocytopenia, monocytosis, and nucleated RBCs in the peripheral blood. Cytogenetic analysis may be abnormal, but the Philadelphia chromosome is never found.

Most patients who have JCML die secondary to infection. Chemotherapy is of limited value. Patients who have JCML usually do not respond to busulfan or hydroxyurea. Bone marrow transplantation offers the only hope of cure at present and is the treatment of choice for the patient who has a histocompatible sibling.

CONGENITAL LEUKEMIA

Congenital leukemia may be apparent at birth or may develop within the first month of life. Most patients described with this rare disorder had AML, although ALL has been reported

Table 227-3 Differences Between Adult and Juvenile Forms of Chronic Myelogenous Leukemia

Age at onset	Adult form	Juvenile form
Chromosome studies	Philadelphia chromosome–positive Usually over age 2	Philadelphia chromosome–negative Usually under age 2
Physical findings		
Facial rash	Absent	Present
Lymphadenopathy	Occasional	Common with tendency to suppuration
Splenomegaly	Marked	Variable
Hemorrhagic manifestations	Absent	Common
Hematological findings		
WBC at onset	Usually >100,000/mm^3	Usually <100,000/mm^3
Monocytosis of peripheral blood and bone marrow	Absent	Usually present
Thrombocytopenia	Uncommon at onset	Common at onset
Red blood cell abnormalities		
Ineffective erythropoiesis	Absent	Present
I antigen on RBC	Normal	Reduced
Fetal hemoglobin levels	Normal	15%-50%
Normoblasts in peripheral blood	Unusual	Common
Other laboratory findings		
Urinary and serum muramidase	Slightly elevated	Markedly elevated
Immunological abnormalities	None	Strikingly high immunoglobin levels, high incidence of antinuclear antibodies (52%) and anti-IgG antibodies (43%)
Nature of colonies produced in vitro from peripheral blood	Predominantly granulocytic	Predominantly monocytic
Response to busulfan	Uniformly good	Poor
Median survival	2½-3 yr	Less than 9 mo

Modified from Altman AJ, Schwartz AD: *Malignant diseases of infancy, childhood, and adolescence,* Philadelphia, 1983, WB Saunders.

in newborns.[77] The etiology of congenital leukemia is unknown. Leukemia in the neonatal period has been associated with Down syndrome, Turner syndrome, mosaic monosomy 7, and trisomy 9. No cases of congenital leukemia have been reported in infants born to women who had leukemia before or during pregnancy.

The clinical manifestations are similar to those seen with leukemia among older children except that leukemia cutis is more common. These blue-gray skin nodules represent areas of skin infiltration by leukemic cells. Petechiae, purpura, hepatosplenomegaly, and poor feeding are common findings in a newborn who has leukemia. The laboratory findings include thrombocytopenia and hyperleukocytosis.

Congenital leukemia must be differentiated from a number of conditions often found in the neonatal period, including congenital syphilis, intrauterine viral infection (CMV, rubella, toxoplasmosis), neuroblastoma, congenital thrombocytopenic purpura, leukemoid reaction in response to sepsis, hypoxemia, erythroblastosis fetalis, and the transient myeloproliferative syndrome associated with Down syndrome. Myeloproliferative disorders, which are clinically and hematologically indistinguishable from congenital AML, have been reported in newborns who have Down syndrome.[77] These disorders are transient and typically resolve completely within weeks or months of diagnosis without specific antileukemia treatment. No test is available that can distinguish infants who have this transient disorder from those who have true congenital leukemia. Conservative therapy with close monitoring and supportive care as needed is recommended for 6 to 8 weeks to differentiate between these two disorders.

The treatment of congenital leukemia is identical to that for the older child except that cranial irradiation is omitted. The results generally have been disappointing, with many infants dying within a few days to months after diagnosis. A majority of recently reported cases of congenital AML were of the monocytic (M5) subtype. For this group of patients, treatment with etoposide or tenoposide, or both, has been particularly effective.[54]

LATE EFFECTS: THE AGONY OF SUCCESS

The advent of more successful therapy has been accompanied by a growing concern over the physical and psychological well-being of the survivors of these aggressive protocols. Studies of late effects of the leukemias of childhood and their treatment, but particularly of ANLL and CML, are severely limited because of the small numbers that have been studied. The discussion of late effects pertains to studies of survivors of ALL, because there are no similar data about the survivors of ANLL or CML.

Major areas of concern identified among survivors of ALL include second malignancies, CNS damage, endocrine abnormalities with growth failure and reproductive dysfunction, cardiac toxicity, and psychological morbidity. Preliminary results of clinical research suggest that the likelihood and the type and severity of sequelae are at least partly related to (1) the patient's age at the time of diagnosis and institution of treatment, (2) the specific treatment used, and (3) the intensity of treatment. Interpretation of clinical data related to the management of long-term survivors is complicated by uncertainty as to whether a particular problem existed before the diagnosis of cancer, whether the problem is secondary to the treatment or to the life-threatening illness itself, or whether all three scenarios are involved.

Truly successful treatment of childhood cancer must incorporate care of the long-term survivor. This involves not only recognizing the delayed consequences that can emerge after cancer therapy, but also actual follow-up with history, physical examination, and appropriate laboratory testing to monitor the patient's status and provide treatment for any problems identified. Unfortunately for both the patient and the physician, as yet no firm guidelines have been established as to the best method of monitoring cured patients for delayed physical or psychological sequelae. Recommendations for pertinent follow-up must be individualized according to the anticipated problems, based on the patient's disease, therapeutic history, and duration of disease-free, off-therapy survival (see Suggested Readings, Schwartz et al., 1994).

Second Malignancy

The risk of developing a second malignancy after apparently successful treatment of leukemia is estimated to be 3% to 12%.[40,46] Both genetics and treatment have been implicated in this increased risk, which is 20 times greater than that observed in the general population. Most second tumors seen among survivors of childhood ALL are second leukemias or non-Hodgkin lymphomas. Whether these represent a second carcinogenic event or a different manifestation of the primary malignant process is unknown. Brain tumors account for almost one third of secondary solid tumors, and the prognosis is poor.

In follow-up studies of a child who has had ALL, especially if cranial irradiation was used for prophylactic CNS treatment, the head and neck should be inspected carefully because most secondary carcinomas (thyroid, basal cell, parotid gland) have occurred in this region.[59] Biopsy is recommended as soon as possible for any suspicious skin lesions, nodules, or firm, enlarged lymph nodes that do not respond completely to a trial of antibiotic therapy. If seizures, severe headaches, or symptoms of increased intracranial pressure occur in the absence of an obvious clinical explanation, computed tomography (CT) or magnetic resonance imaging (MRI) studies should be done before lumbar puncture to ensure that an intracranial mass is not present.

Central Nervous System Damage

Before the use of effective prophylaxis, the central nervous system was the most common site of first relapse in children who had ALL. Currently, CNS prophylaxis prevents isolated CNS relapse in more than 90% of patients. The functional and structural CNS changes found among long-term survivors of ALL in continuous remission after effective CNS prophylaxis are less common and less severe than among patients who relapse with CNS involvement.

The absolute incidence and natural history of long-term neurological sequelae, including memory and learning problems, among patients treated with intrathecal chemotherapy and cranial irradiation therapy are unknown. Both acute and subacute forms of neurotoxicity have been reported in patients treated with the current methods of CNS prophylaxis.[53] These abnormalities include structural changes, as evidenced by ventricular dilation, calcifications, focal areas of parenchymal hypodensity, and cortical atrophy visible on CT scan. Functional changes, with intellectual deficits, poor memory skills, low IQ scores, and poor school performance, also have been described. Further investigation is required to determine if a correlation exists between these structural and functional CNS changes. Severe permanent neurological sequelae such as a seizure disorder, residual hearing loss, and hemiplegia are observed almost exclusively among children who are cured after one or more CNS relapses.

Endocrine Abnormalities

Endocrine abnormalities involving the hypothalmic-pituitary axis probably occur secondary to cranial irradiation, whereas gonadal dysfunction probably occurs secondary to chemotherapy. Younger age appears to increase the risk for subsequent growth problems and reduce the risk for gonadal dysfunction.

Abnormally low amounts of growth hormone (GH) have been found among children who have had ALL treated with cranial irradiation. Although growth velocities after completion of therapy are not reduced significantly in these children, their final adult height is diminished.[62] Studies are needed to assess the correlations between various treatments, age at diagnosis, GH secretion, pubertal development, and final height attained. The benefits of GH therapy are unknown because results from different investigators are conflicting.[65,80] Follow-up studies of long-term survivors of ALL treated with cranial irradiation demonstrate approximately a 3% to 5% incidence of hypothyroidism and less than a 1% incidence of secondary thyroid malignancies. Palpation of the thyroid, review of hypothyroidism symptoms, and a low threshold for measuring serum triiodothyronine (T_3) and thyroid-stimulating hormone (TSH) should be incorporated into the routine visit of survivors.

Data on infertility and gonadal function in this group are largely unavailable. Studies in this area are complicated by the young age of most patients and the lack of an adequate way of measuring eventual reproductive capabilities. The development of secondary sex characteristics does not necessarily mean that germinal cells are present or functional. Oligospermia related to previous chemotherapy frequently improves with time. Patients who received bilateral testicular irradiation to treat testicular leukemia generally are sterile. Virtually no information is available about the reproductive capabilities of girls. Pubertal progression is more likely to be normal in girls who had leukemia and chemotherapy before the onset of puberty and menarche.

Cardiac Toxicity

The anthracyclines are a vital component of the current antileukemia armamentarium for most patients. The incidence of severe cardiomyopathy has been reduced by limiting the cumulative dose to approximately 350 mg/m^2, monitoring frequently during therapy with electrocardiograms and echocardiograms, and discontinuing the anthracycline if any signs of toxicity are observed (i.e., decreased fractional shorting and arrhythmias). Unfortunately, in most patients the signs and symptoms of cardiac toxicity do not develop until months after the anthracycline treatment has been discontinued. For many patients, congestive heart failure is reversible or at least can be controlled with medication.[28,60] More sensitive diagnostic techniques, such as stress testing and electrophysiological studies, are likely to result in more frequent diagnosis of cardiac abnormalities. Comprehensive follow-up cardiac evaluation with electrocardiograms, echocardiograms, and stress testing is a crucial part of routine checkups for patients treated with anthracycline with or without chest irradiation.

Psychosocial Changes

Because only a few studies have been designed to focus on the psychosocial status of long-term survivors of ALL, information on this subject is limited. Studies of childhood cancer survivors have shown these individuals to have a significantly higher incidence of behavioral and social adjustment problems than normal, including less participation in physical activities, inadequate social relations, poor school performance, frequent somatic complaints, and behavioral maladjustment.[38,51] In particular, children treated for ALL had a greater risk for school-related problems, including the number of grades repeated and special education placement. Psychosocial stressors, which continue to be reported long after therapy for ALL has been completed, include anxiety about potential relapse, financial burdens, rejection for employment or insurance coverage, and rejection for military service. No differences in the frequency of major depressive syndromes, suicide attempts, or hospitalizations for psychiatric reasons have been noted between these patients and their siblings and between them and the general population.[71]

In view of the follow-up information currently available, it is clear that ongoing assessment of neurological functioning, developmental milestones, school and work performance, behavior, and overall quality of life must be an integral part of maintaining health care for the survivor of childhood leukemia.

REFERENCES

1. Aur RJA et al: Central nervous system therapy and combination chemotherapy of childhood lymphocytic leukemia, *Blood* 37:272, 1971.
2. Bennett JM et al: French-American-British (FAB) Cooperative Group proposals for the classification of acute leukemias, *Br J Haematol* 33:451, 1976.
3. Bennett JM et al: Proposed revised criteria for the classification of acute myeloid leukemia, *Ann Intern Med* 103:620, 1985.
4. Bizzozzero OJ Jr, Johnson KG, Ciocco A: Radiation-related leukemia in Hiroshima and Nagasaki, 1946-64: distribution, incidence, appearance in time, *N Engl J Med* 274:1095, 1966.
5. Blattner WA et al: Human T-cell leukemia virus and adult T-cell leukemia, *JAMA* 250:1074, 1983.
6. Blayney DW et al: Decreasing risk of leukemia with prolonged follow-up after chemotherapy and radiotherapy for Hodgkin's disease, *N Engl J Med* 316:710, 1987.
7. Boice JD: Cancer following medical irradiation, *Cancer* 47:1081, 1981.
8. Brandt L, Nilsson PG, Mitelman F: Occupational exposure to petroleum products in men with ANLL, *Br Med J* 1:553, 1978.
9. Brill AB et al: Leukemia in man following ionizing radiation exposure: summary of findings in Hiroshima and Nagasaki, *Ann Intern Med* 56:590, 1962.
10. Brockstein JA et al: Allogeneic BMT after hyperfractionated TBI and cyclophosphamide in children with acute leukemia, *N Engl J Med* 317:1618, 1987.
11. Butturini A et al: Which treatment for childhood acute lymphoblastic leukemia in second remission? *Lancet* 1:429, 1987.
12. Caldwell GG, Heath CW Jr: Case clustering in cancer, *South Med J* 69:1598, 1976.
13. Castro-Malespina H et al: Philadelphia chromosome–positive chronic

myelocytic leukemia in children: survival and prognostic factors, *Cancer* 52:721, 1983.

14. Clarkson BD, Boyse EA: Possible explanation of high concordance for AL in monozygotic twins, *Lancet* 1:699, 1971.
15. Cooke JV: Incidence of acute leukemia in children, *JAMA* 119:547, 1942.
16. Court-Brown WM, Doll R: Leukemia in childhood and young adult life: trends in mortality in relation to aetiology, *Br Med J* 1:981, 1961.
17. De The G et al: Epidemiologic evidence for a causal relationship between Epstein-Barr virus and Burkitt's lymphoma: results of the Ugandar prospective study, *Nature* 272:756, 1978.
18. Dinsmore R et al: Allogeneic bone marrow transplantation for patients with acute nonlymphocytic leukemia, *Blood* 63:649, 1984.
19. Dow LW et al: Evidence for clonal development of childhood acute lymphoblastic leukemia, *Blood* 66:902, 1985.
20. Draper GJ, Heaf MM, Kennier-Wilson LM: Occurrence of childhood cancers among sibs and estimation of familial risks, *J Med Genet* 14:81, 1977.
21. Drexler HG et al: Incidence of TdT positivity in cases of leukemia and lymphoma, *Acta Haematol* 75:12, 1986.
22. Filipovich ATT et al: Immunodeficiency in humans as a risk factor in development of malignancy, *Prev Med* 9:252, 1980.
23. Foon KA, Todd RF III: Immunologic classification of leukemia and lymphoma, *Blood* 68:1, 1986.
24. Fraumeni JF Jr, Wagoner JK: Changing sex differentials in leukemia, *Public Health Rep* 79:1093, 1974.
25. Frei E, Sallan SE: Acute lymphoblastic leukemia: treatment, *Cancer* 42:828, 1978.
26. Freireich EJ et al: The effect of 6-mercaptopurine on the duration of steroid-induced remission in acute leukemia: a model for evaluation of other potentially useful therapy, *Blood* 21:699, 1963.
27. George S et al: A reappraisal of the results of stopping therapy in childhood leukemia, *N Engl J Med* 300:2269, 1979.
28. Gilladoga AC et al: The cardiotoxicity of Adriamycin and daunomycin in children, *Cancer* 37:1070, 1976.
29. Greenberg RS, Schuster JL: Epidemiology of cancer in children, *Epidemiol Rev* 7:22, 1985.
30. Gunz F, Baikie AG: *Leukemia,* ed 3, New York, 1974, Grune & Stratton.
31. Hakami N et al: Combined etoposide and 5-azacytidine in children and adolescents with refractory or relapsed acute nonlymphocytic leukemia: a POG study, *J Clin Oncol* 5:1022, 1987.
32. Hammond DG: The cure of childhood cancers, *Cancer* 58:407, 1986.
33. Hardisty RM, Speed DE, Till M: Granulocytic leukemia in childhood, *Br J Haematol* 10:551, 1964.
34. Harvey EB et al: Prenatal x-ray exposure and childhood cancer in twins, *N Engl J Med* 312:541, 1985.
35. Heath CW, Hasterlik RJ: Leukemia among children in a suburban community, *Am J Med* 34:796, 1963.
36. Hecht F, McCaw BK: Chromosome instability syndromes. In Mulvihill JJ, Miller RW, Fraumeni JF Jr, editors: *Genetics of human cancer,* New York, 1977, Raven Press.
37. Kirsch IR: Molecular biology of the leukemias, *Pediatr Clin North Am* 35:693, 1988.
38. Koocher GP, O'Malley J: *The Damocles syndrome: psychosocial consequences of surviving childhood cancer,* New York, 1981, McGraw-Hill.
39. Krakower JM, Aaronson SA: Seroepidemiologic assessment of feline leukemia virus infection risk for man, *Nature* 273:463, 1978.
40. Li FP, Cassady JR, Jaffe N: Risk of second tumors in survivors of childhood cancer, *Cancer* 35:1230, 1975.
41. Lonsdale D et al: Interrupted versus continued maintenance therapy in childhood acute leukemia, *Cancer* 36:341, 1975.
42. Look AT: The cytogenetics of childhood leukemia: clinical and biologic implications, *Pediatr Clin North Am* 35:723, 1988.
43. March HC: Leukemia in radiologists, *Radiology* 43:275, 1944.
44. Mauer AM: Treatment of acute leukemia in childhood, *Clin Lab Haematol* 7:245, 1978.
45. Meadows AT et al: Survival in childhood acute lymphoblastic leukemia (ALL): the influence of protocol and place of treatment, *Cancer Invest* 1:49, 1983.
46. Mike V, Meadows AT, D'Angio GD: Incidence of second malignant neoplasms in children: results of an international study, *Lancet* 2:1326, 1982.
47. Miller LP et al: Successful reinduction therapy with amsacrine and cyclotidine in children with acute nonlymphoblastic leukemia, *Proc Am Soc Clin Oncol* 3:199, 1984.
48. Miller RW: Ethnic differences in cancer occurrence. In Mulvihill JJ, Miller RW, Fraumeni JF Jr, editors: *Genetics of human cancer,* New York, 1977, Raven Press.
49. Miller RW: Persons with exceptionally high risk of leukemia, *Cancer Res* 27:2420, 1967.
50. Mirro J et al: Acute mixed lineage leukemia: clinicopathologic correlations and prognostic significance, *Blood* 66:1115, 1985.
51. Mulhern RK et al: Social competence and behavioral adjustment of children who are long-term survivors of cancer, *Pediatrics* 83:18, 1989.
52. Neglia JP, Robinson LL: Epidemiology of the childhood acute leukemias, *Pediatr Clin North Am* 35:675, 1988.
53. Ochs J, Mulhern RK: Late effects of antileukemic treatment, *Pediatr Clin North Am* 35:815, 1988.
54. Odom L, Gordon E: Acute monoblastic leukemia in infancy and early childhood: successful treatment with epipodophyllotoxin, *Blood* 64:875, 1984.
55. Pedersen-Bjergaard J, Larsen SO: Incidence of ANLL, preleukemia, and acute myeloproliferative syndrome up to 10 years after treatment of Hodgkin's disease, *N Engl J Med* 307:965, 1982.
56. Pendergrass TW: Epidemiology of ALL, *Semin Oncol* 12:80, 1985.
57. Penn I: Second malignant neoplasms associated with immunosuppression medications, *Cancer* 37:1024, 1976.
58. Pinkel D: Curing of children with leukemia, *Cancer* 59:1683, 1987.
59. Pratt CB et al: Carcinomas in children: clinical and demographic characteristics, *Cancer* 61:1046, 1988.
60. Pratt CB, Ransom JL, Evans WE: Age-related Adriamycin cardiotoxicity in children, *Cancer Treat Rep* 62:1381, 1978.
61. Ribeiro RC et al: Clinical and biologic hallmarks of the Philadelphia chromosome in childhood acute lymphoblastic leukemia, *Blood* 70:948, 1987.
62. Robinson CC et al: Height of children successfully treated for acute lymphoblastic leukemia: a report from the late effects study committee of CCSG, *Med Pediatr Oncol* 13:14, 1985.
63. Robinson LL et al: Environmental exposures as risk factors for childhood ANLL, *Proc Am Assoc Ca Res* 28:249, 1987.
64. Robinson L et al: Assessment of the interrelationship of prognostic factors in childhood acute lymphoblastic leukemia, *Am J Pediatr Hematol Oncol* 2:3, 1980.
65. Romsche et al: Evaluation of human growth hormone treatment in children with cranial irradiation associated short stature, *J Pediatr* 104:177, 1984.
66. Rowe JM, Lichtman MA: Hyperleukocytosis and leukostasis: common features of childhood chronic myelogenous leukemia, *Blood* 63:1230, 1984.
67. Sandberg AA: The chromosomes in human leukemia, *Semin Hematol* 23:201, 1986.
68. Sather HN: Age at diagnosis of childhood acute lymphoblastic leukemia, *Med Pediatr Oncol* 14:166, 1986.
69. Simone JV: Factors that influence haematological remission duration in acute lymphocytic leukemia, *Br J Haematol* 32:465, 1976.
70. Steuber CPPC: Therapy in childhood acute nonlymphocytic leukemia (ANLL): evolution of current concepts of chemotherapy, *Am J Pediatr Hematol Oncol* 3:379, 1981.
71. Teta MJ et al: Psychosocial consequences of childhood and adolescent cancer survival, *J Chronic Dis* 39:751, 1986.
72. Thomas ED et al: Marrow transplantations for the treatment of chronic myelogenous leukemia, *Ann Intern Med* 104:155, 1986.
73. Thomas ED et al: Marrow transplantation for patients with acute lymphoblastic leukemia: a long-term follow-up, *Blood* 62:1139, 1983.
74. Till MM et al: Leukemia in children and their grandparents, *Br J Haematol* 29:575, 1975.
75. Todaro GJ, Huebner RJ: The viral oncogene hypothesis: new evidence, *Proc Natl Acad Sci USA* 69:1009, 1972.
76. Vigliani EC, Forni A: Benzene and leukemia, *Environ Res* 11:122, 1976.
77. Weinstein HJ: Congenital leukemia and the neonatal myeloproliferative

disorders associated with Down's syndrome, *Clin Lab Haematol* 7:147, 1978.

78. Whang-Peng J et al: Cytogenetic studies in acute lymphocytic leukemia: special emphasis on long-term survival, *Med Pediatr Oncol* 2:333, 1976.
79. Williams DL et al: Presence of clonal chromosome abnormalities in virtually all cases of acute lymphoblastic leukemia, *N Engl J Med* 310:640, 1985.
80. Winter RS, Green OC: Irradiation-induced growth hormone deficiency: blunted growth response and accelerated skeletal maturation and growth hormone therapy, *J Pediatr* 106:609, 1985.
81. Young JL Jr, Miller RW: Incidence of malignant tumors in US children, *J Pediatr* 86:254, 1975.
82. Young JL Jr et al: Cancer incidence, survival, and mortality for children under 15 years of age, *Cancer* 58:598, 1986.
83. Yunis JL, Brunning RD: Prognostic significance of chromosomal abnormalities in acute leukemias and myelodysplastic syndromes, *Clin Lab Haematol* 15:597, 1986.
84. Zuelzer WW et al: Long-term cytogenetic studies in acute leukemia of children: the nature of relapse, *Am J Hematol* 1:143, 1976.

SUGGESTED READINGS

Altman AJ, Schwartz AD: *Malignant diseases of infancy, childhood and adolescence,* ed 2, Philadelphia, 1983, WB Saunders.

Green DM: *Long-term complications of therapy for cancer in childhood and adolescence,* Baltimore, 1989, Johns Hopkins University Press.

Halperin EC et al: *Pediatric radiation oncology,* ed 2, New York, 1994, Raven Press.

Nathan DG, Oski FA: *Hematology of infancy and childhood,* ed 4, Philadelphia, 1993, WB Saunders.

Pizzo PA, Poplack DG: *Principles and practice of pediatric oncology,* ed 2 Philadelphia, 1993, JB Lippincott.

Poplack DG: The leukemias, *Pediatr Clin North Am* 35:675, 1988.

Pui CH, Christ WM: Biology and treatment of acute lymphoblastic leukemia, *J Pediatr* 124:491, 1994.

Schwartz CL et al: *Survivors of childhood cancer: assessment and management,* St Louis, 1994, Mosby.

228 Lyme Disease

David M. Siegel

EPIDEMIOLOGY, ETIOLOGY, AND PATHOGENESIS

Lyme borreliosis, or Lyme disease, is a spirochetal infection first observed in a group of children living in and around Lyme, Connecticut, on the eastern shore of the Connecticut River. Although initially these patients mistakenly were diagnosed as having juvenile arthritis, the perceptiveness of two mothers and the follow-up epidemiological work of Steere and others[16] established the infectious etiology and vector of the disease's spread. In their landmark investigation, Steere and colleagues found a total of 15 patients clustered in the area of Lyme, with an overall prevalence of 4.3 cases per 1000 residents. Since then the disease has been reported on all continents except Antarctica and in 48 of the United States. The major clustering of cases in this country has occurred along the eastern seaboard, in the northern Midwest, and in the far West. In the United States, 90% of cases have been reported from Massachusetts, Rhode Island, Connecticut, New York, New Jersey, Wisconsin, and Minnesota. Since 1982, more than 57,000 cases have been reported to the Centers for Disease Control and Prevention (CDC) with a nineteenfold increase in reported cases between 1982 and 1992.[6]

Early study revealed a tick vector as consistent with the pattern of spread of the disease.[14,15,17] Specifically the Lyme disease spirochete is transmitted by *Ixodes* sp. ticks, including *I. scapularis* (previously referred to as *I. dammini*) in the northeastern and midwestern United States,[15] *I. pacificus* in the western United States,[3] *I. ricinus* in Europe,[12] and *I. persulcatus* in Asia.[12] *Ixodes* ticks have a 2-year life cycle; the larval form feeds (on a blood meal) in the late summer and the following spring, and the nymph feeds in early summer. The preferred host at these times is the white-footed mouse, *Peromyscus leucopus*. These mice are able to remain infected with the spirochete without an associated inflammatory response, whereas the spirochete remains in the midgut of the larval tick and later migrates to the salivary glands of the nymph. The adult *I. dammini* prefers the white-tailed deer as a host, although the life cycle of the spirochete does not depend on involvement of the deer.

The actual spirochetal etiology of this multisystem disease was discovered through two pieces of information. First, the skin rash seen in most of these patients was erythema migrans (EM), described in more detail later, which had been recognized in Europe in the 1950s as an eruption of spirochetal origin. This had been established by visualization of spirochetal structures in the lesions of erythema chronicum migrans (EM) and by the subsequent response to penicillin treatment. Second, with this knowledge and with the accumulated epidemiological evidence implicating *I. dammini* as the vector, Burgdorfer et al.[2] began a careful analysis of the digestive tract of the ticks for spirochetes. They isolated previously unrecognized spirochetes later designated *Borrelia burgdorferi*. These organisms were consistently isolated from the blood, skin lesions, and cerebrospinal fluid (CSF) of patients who had Lyme disease, confirming the causation. The infection rate of *I. scapularis* with *B. burgdorferi* in endemic areas is quite high, with spirochetes having been recovered from more than half of the ticks on Shelter Island, N.Y.[1]

CLINICAL MANIFESTATIONS

Because the clinical manifestations of Lyme disease vary with the time that elapses after inoculation by the tick, the infection has been divided into early and late phases. The former is characterized by two stages. Stage 1 of early infection is seen in 60% to 80% of patients and consists of EM, sometimes accompanied by fever, minor constitutional symptoms, and regional lymphadenopathy. The EM rash begins as a red macule or papule (at the site of the tick bite), which expands to form a large annular erythematous patch with a bright red outer border and partial central clearing. In patients who have EM, the rash appears within days of the tick bite and even left untreated fades within 3 to 4 weeks. Specific antibody to *B. burgdorferi* usually is not present at this time. However, the spirochete is cultured more easily from the skin during stage 1 of early infection than at any other time in the illness.

Stage 2 of early infection is marked by dissemination of *B. burgdorferi,* which potentially can involve many organ systems (Table 228-1). The most commonly involved areas, however, are the skin, nervous system, and musculoskeletal system. This is the stage in which patients tend to feel quite ill, with significant malaise and fatigue. Smaller annular skin lesions can appear at sites other than the initial EM eruption. The patient complains of a transient but severe headache and stiff neck, although the CSF usually is normal. Arthritis is not present early in the disease, but patients experience migratory pain in joints, bursae, tendons, muscles, and bones. At this time (3 to 4 weeks after infection) antibody titers to *B. burgdorferi* develop.

As stage 2 disease progresses, meningitis can develop, possibly with subtle signs of encephalitis, including somnolence, poor memory, and mood change. Unilateral or bilateral facial palsy (Bell palsy) and/or a peripheral neuritis, which usually is asymmetrical and accompanied by motor, sensory, or mixed manifestations, develops in 15% to 20% of patients in the United States. Cardiac involvement, which is seen in a smaller group (4% to 8%), is characterized most commonly by varying degrees of atrioventricular block, but it can include myopericarditis or, in rare cases, fatal pancarditis. Complete heart block usually is brief, and only temporary cardiac pacing is needed.[13] Toward the end of stage 2 (6 months after onset of the disease), patients may begin to ex-

Table 228-1 Manifestations of Lyme Disease by Stage*

	Early infection		
System†	Localized (stage 1)	Disseminated (stage 2)	Late infection: persistent (stage 3)
Skin	Erythema chronicum migrans	Secondary annular lesions, malar rash, diffuse erythema or urticaria, evanescent lesions, lymphocytoma	Acrodermatitis chronica atrophicans, localized scleroderma-like lesions
Musculoskeletal system		Migratory pain in joints, tendons, bursae, muscle, bone, brief arthritis attacks, myositis,‡ osteomyelitis,‡ panniculitis‡	Prolonged arthritis attacks, chronic arthritis, peripheral enthesopathy, periostitis or joint subluxations below lesions of acrodermatitis
Neurological system		Meningitis, cranial neuritis, Bell palsy, motor or sensory radiculoneuritis, subtle encephalitis, mononeuritis multiplex, myelitis,‡ chorea,‡ cerebellar ataxia‡	Chronic encephalomyelitis, spastic parapareses, ataxic gait, subtle mental disorders, chronic axonal polyradiculopathy, dementia‡
Lymphatic system	Regional lymphadenopathy	Regional or generalized lymphadenopathy, splenomegaly	
Heart		Atrioventricular nodal block, myopericarditis, pancarditis	
Eyes		Conjunctivitis, iritis,‡ choroiditis,‡ retinal hemorrhage or detachment,‡ panophthalmitis‡	Keratitis
Liver		Mild or recurrent hepatitis	
Respiratory system		Nonexudative sore throat, nonproductive cough, adult respiratory distress syndrome‡	
Kidneys		Microscopic hematuria or proteinuria	
Genitourinary system		Orchitis‡	
Constitutional symptoms	Minor	Severe malaise and fatigue	Fatigue

From Steere AC: *N Engl J Med* 321:586, 1989.
*Classification by stages provides a guideline for the illness's manifestations, but timing and sequence can vary greatly.
†Systems are listed from the most to the least commonly affected.
‡Inclusion of this manifestation is based on one or a few cases.

perience brief attacks of asymmetrical, large joint oligoarthritis, most commonly affecting the knee.

During the latter stages of disease the episodes of arthritis become much more prolonged, with the possibility of chronic arthritis (a year or more of continual inflammation) developing. The arthritis remains confined to one or a few large joints, the knee being the most common site. During this phase patients also may experience neurological complications, including persistent distal paresthesia or radicular pain. Some cases have been reported in which patients who had had classic symptoms of Lyme disease in the past later showed subtle memory deficits, somnolence, or behavioral changes. These patients present a difficult dilemma, although they certainly should be treated for neurological Lyme disease if therapy was not given initially.

CONGENITAL INFECTION

The issue of congenital infection with *B. burgdorferi* is only partly understood. Transplacental transmission of the spirochete has been reported in two infants, who died during the first week of life. Spirochetes were found in the tissue of these infants, but it was not clear that they were etiological in the deaths.[10,18] However, in a study of 463 infants from endemic and nonendemic areas, congenital malformations were not found to be associated with the presence of *B. burgdorferi* antibody in cord blood.[19] Steere[13] has concluded that it is unusual for *B. burgdorferi* to cause an adverse fetal outcome.

SEROLOGICAL TESTING

The major diagnostic tool in evaluating a patient for Lyme disease, outside the history of a summer exposure to a tick bite in an endemic area and development of EM, is detection of antibody to *B. burgdorferi*. Two serological tests currently are available: immunofluorescence assay (IFA), now rarely used, which uses fluorescein-conjugated antihuman immunoglobulins to detect antibodies in patient sera, and enzyme-linked immunosorbent assay (ELISA). Although IFA is relatively sensitive and specific well into stage 1 disease, it is inadequate in detecting antibody early in the illness. In one study, sera obtained from patients who had Lyme disease during the first 3 weeks of their illness showed positivity by IFA

Table 228-2 Treatment Regimens for Lyme Disease

Manifestation	Regimen*
Early infection*	
Adults	Tetracycline, 250 mg orally 4× daily, 10-30 days†
	Doxycycline, 100 mg orally 2× daily, 10-30 days†‡
	Amoxicillin, 500 mg orally 4× daily, 10-30 days†‡
Children (≤8 yr)	Amoxicillin or penicillin V, 250 mg orally 3× daily or 25-50 mg/kg body weight/day in 3 divided doses, 10-30 days
	In case of penicillin allergy:
	Erythromycin, 250 mg orally 3× daily or 30 mg/kg/day in divided doses, 10-30 days‡
Neurological abnormalities (early or late)*	
General	Ceftriaxone, 75-100 mg/kg/day intravenously 1× daily, 14 days§
	Penicillin G, 300,000 U/kg/day intravenously, 6 divided doses daily, 14 days§
	In case of ceftriaxone or penicillin allergy:
	Doxycycline, 100 mg orally 2× daily, 30 days‡
	Chloramphenicol, 250 mg intravenously 4× daily, 14 days‡
Facial palsy alone	Oral antibiotic regimens may be adequate
Cardiac abnormalities	
First-degree atrioventricular block (PR interval <0.3 sec)	Oral antibiotic regimens, as for early infection
High-degree atrioventricular block	Ceftriaxone, 75-100 mg/kg/day intravenously 1× daily, 14 days‡
	Penicillin, 300,000 U/kg/day intravenously, 6 divided doses daily, 14 days‡
Arthritis (intermittent or chronic)†	Doxycycline, 100 mg orally 2× daily, 30 days
	Amoxicillin and probenecid, 500 mg each orally 4× daily, 30 days
	Ceftriaxone, 75-100 mg/kg/day intravenously 1× daily, 14 days
	Penicillin, 300,000 U/kg/day intravenously, 6 divided doses daily, 14 days
Acrodermatitis	Oral antibiotic regimens for 1 mo usually are adequate

Adapted from Steere AC: *N Engl J Med* 321:586, 1989.
*Treatment failures have occurred with all these regimens, and retreatment may be necessary.
†The duration of therapy is based on the clinical response.
‡The antibiotic has not yet been tested systematically for this indication in Lyme disease.
§The appropriate duration of therapy is not yet clear for patients with late neurological abnormalities, and it may be longer than 2 weeks.

in only 38% of cases, whereas patients who had neuritis and arthritis had reactive titers 92% to 100% of the time.[9] ELISA is more sensitive and specific than IFA in diagnosing early Lyme disease, but the deficiency of both tests is their occasional false positive result, which is caused either by the presence of other spirochetal infections in the patient (e.g., syphilis or relapsing fever) or by other confounding patient variables as yet to be defined. Another problem with both IFA and ELISA testing is the lack of standardization and quality controls for these tests in most diagnostic laboratories, which results in poor interlaboratory and intralaboratory agreement.[7,11] Early antibiotic therapy also can blunt antibody production. Given these limitations, most laboratories now consider a titer of 1:256 or higher *in a patient who has compatible clinical symptoms* as sufficient to confirm the diagnosis of Lyme borreliosis.[4] Immunoblotting (Western blot assay) should be used when the physician suspects a falsely positive ELISA. Research into improved serological testing has focused on detecting antigens by using polymerase chain reaction (PCR) techniques. The results of investigations into both CSF and urine concentrations of *Borrelia* DNA suggest their potential diagnostic usefulness, especially in cases of neurological disease.[5,8]

DIFFERENTIAL DIAGNOSIS

In children who have what appears to be Lyme arthritis, the most likely differential diagnosis (as in the first cases of the disease) is pauciarticular juvenile arthritis. Other considerations include aseptic meningitis, Bell palsy or a peripheral neuropathy not caused by *B. burgdorferi,* multiple sclerosis, septic arthritis, acute rheumatic fever, and fibromyalgia syndrome. Such diagnoses are ruled out easily with a history of a tick bite and EM, but many patients who have Lyme disease have no history of these events. Certainly, during the summer in an endemic area, Lyme disease should be considered when consistent symptoms are present.

MANAGEMENT

As a spirochetal infection, Lyme borreliosis can be treated successfully, depending on when in the course of the illness antibiotics are begun. With EM, oral antibiotic therapy is used; tetracycline, doxycycline, penicillin, amoxicillin, or erythromycin (with a penicillin allergy in a child age 8 or younger) shortens the duration of the rash and often prevents later complications. Facial palsy or peripheral neuropathy alone also can be treated with antibiotics given orally, but any other neurological abnormality, such as meningitis or general central nervous system (CNS) symptoms, should be treated with parenteral ceftriaxone, penicillin G, or chloramphenicol. Although first-degree atrioventricular block usually requires only oral therapy, higher grade blocks require parenteral therapy with ceftriaxone or penicillin G. Finally, intermittent or chronic arthritis should be treated with either parenteral or long-term oral therapy. Specific dosages and durations are shown in Table 228-2, as recommended by both Steere[13] and others.

The later antibiotic therapy is instituted, the more likely are complications and persistent problems. Thus a high level of suspicion, followed by prompt diagnosis and treatment, is rewarded with a high likelihood of a mild, short-term illness with a favorable prognosis. Should chronic arthritis persist, the usual management with antiinflammatory medications and physical therapy is required.

REFERENCES

1. Bosler EM et al: Prevalence of the Lyme disease spirochete in populations of white-tailed deer and white-footed mice, *Yale J Biol Med* 57:651, 1984.
2. Burgdorfer W et al: Lyme disease: a tick-borne spirochetosis? *Science* 216:1317, 1982.
3. Burgdorfer W et al: The Western black-legged tick, *Ixodes pacificus:* a vector of *Borrelia burgdorferi, Am J Trop Med Hyg* 34:925, 1985.
4. Eichenfield AH, Athreya BH: Lyme disease: of ticks and titers, *J Pediatr* 114:328, 1989.
5. Huppertz HI, Schmidt H, Karch H: Detection of *Borrelia burgdorferi* by nested polymerase chain reaction in cerebrospinal fluid and urine of children with neuroborreliosis, *Eur J Pediatr* 152:414, 1993.
6. Lyme Disease: United States, 1991-1992, *MMWR* 42:345, 1993.
7. Magnarelli LA: Quality of Lyme disease tests, *JAMA* 262:3464, 1989.
8. Pachner AR, Delaney E: The polymerase chain reaction in the diagnosis of Lyme neuroborreliosis, *Ann Neurol* 34:544, 1993.
9. Russell H et al: Enzyme-linked immunosorbent assay and indirect immunofluorescence assay for Lyme disease, *J Infect Dis* 149:789, 1984.
10. Schlesinger PA et al: Maternal-fetal transmission of the Lyme disease spirochete, *Borrelia burgdorferi, Ann Intern Med* 103:67, 1985.
11. Schwartz BS et al: Antibody testing in Lyme disease: a comparison of results in four laboratories, *JAMA* 262:3431, 1989.
12. Steere AC: Lyme disease, *N Engl J Med* 308:733, 1983.
13. Steere AC: Lyme disease, *N Engl J Med* 321:586, 1989.
14. Steere AC, Broderick TF, Malawista SE: Erythema chronicum migrans and Lyme arthritis: epidemiologic evidence for a tick vector, *Am J Epidemiol* 108:312, 1978.
15. Steere AC, Malawista SE: Cases of Lyme disease in the United States: locations correlated with distribution of *Ixodes dammini, Ann Intern Med* 91:730, 1979.
16. Steere AC et al: Lyme arthritis: an epidemic of oligoarticular arthritis in children and adults in three Connecticut communities, *Arthritis Rheum* 20:7, 1977.
17. Wallis RC et al: Erythema chronicum migrans and Lyme arthritis: field study of ticks, *Am J Epidemiol* 108:322, 1978.
18. Weber K et al: *Borrelia burgdorferi* in a newborn despite oral penicillin for Lyme borreliosis during pregnancy, *Pediatr Infect Dis J* 7:286, 1988.
19. Williams CL et al: Lyme disease during pregnancy: a cord blood serosurvey, *Ann NY Acad Sci* 539:504, 1988.

229 Meatal Ulceration

Mark F. Bellinger

Superficial ulceration of the male urethral meatus (urethritis orificii externi,[2] or Brennemann ulcer[1]) is a common clinical condition seen almost exclusively in circumcised boys; however, it may be seen in uncircumcised boys if the preputial opening is wide enough to expose the meatus and perimeatal skin. Mackenzie[7] reported new meatal ulceration in 20% of boys examined within 5 weeks after neonatal circumcision, but believed that the true incidence was significantly higher, based on historical data of ulcers that had healed by the time of examination.

ETIOLOGY

By approximately 16 weeks' gestation, the prepuce is completely formed, with complete fusion of the epithelium of the glans and prepuce.[5] Normal separation of the prepuce results from a gradual process of keratinization and thickening of these layers.

Desquamation forms smegma, which mechanically separates the two layers, allowing gradual exposure of the now keratinized skin surfaces, which thus are more resistant to the normally harsh environment of the diaper. Preputial separation begins before birth, but in most cases continues well into infancy. Full separation and retraction of the prepuce is found in only 4% of neonates, but 90% have a retractable prepuce by age 3.[3] In contrast, forceful separation of the fused epithelial layers during neonatal circumcision exposes the raw, cherry-red translucent epithelium of the glans and meatus. Trauma to this thin epithelium from diaper contact may result in ulceration.

HISTORY

Although meatal ulceration may be relatively asymptomatic, dysuria is common. Voluntary urinary retention may be caused by severe dysuria during the acute phase of ulceration, whereas involuntary retention may occur secondary to meatal crusting as the lesion heals. Acute crusting or fibrinous adhesion of the meatus may cause a deviated or split urinary stream. Recurrent cycles of ulceration and crusting may lead to scarring, gradual narrowing of the meatus, and a true stenosis with narrowing and upward deviation of the urinary stream.[9]

PHYSICAL FINDINGS

Early ulcers are superficial, clean, and contiguous with the meatus, usually surrounding it. Spreading the lips of the meatus reveals normal urethral mucosa. Meatal ulceration may be seen in conjunction with diaper rash from any cause. When diaper rash is severe, inguinal adenopathy may be present. Meatal ulcers crust quickly, and a cyclical change from ulcer to crust is common as recurrent irritation disturbs the healing process. Crusting transiently may occlude the meatus with a fibrinous exudate, and urinary retention or bladder distention may result. If the crust is rubbed off, bloody spotting may be seen on the diaper. Repeated episodes of ulceration result in a healed but stenotic meatus. Visual examination of the meatus cannot adequately reveal whether significant stenosis is present, but observation of a narrowed stream with upward direction and outpouching of the meatal lips from the force of the stream indicates a urodynamically significant lesion.

DIFFERENTIAL DIAGNOSIS

Glanular trauma may result from circumcision, regardless of whether the Gomco, Plastibell, or freehand technique is used.[4] Older children may suffer glanular trauma during play, and many injuries are caused by falls during bathing. Zipper injuries to the glans are common, and adolescents may suffer trauma during intercourse.

Balanitis (inflammation of the glans) and posthitis (inflammation of the prepuce) are most common in uncircumcised boys. Balanitis xerotica obliterans is a chronic inflammatory process of unknown etiology that may involve a whitish thickening of the glans, prepuce, and distal urethra.[8]

It is important to differentiate cutaneous lesions from urethral lesions that may protrude from the meatus. Urethral malignancies are rare in children, and most benign fibroepitheliomatous polyps originate in the posterior urethra. Venereal diseases are an increasingly common source of genital lesions in adolescents. Condylomata acuminata (venereal warts) may appear on genital skin as small verrucae and may protrude from the urethral meatus as small polypoid masses. Gonorrheal or nonspecific urethritis may cause meatal edema and encrustation. Syphilitic chancre, a painless, indurated ulcer that has sharply demarcated borders, may be found on the penile shaft or glans 3 to 6 weeks after exposure. Herpes progenitalis occurs as perimeatal vesicles on an erythematous base, which may rupture to form a confluent superficial ulcer.[6] Other meatal ulcerations may result from erythema multiforme, contact dermatitis, drug eruptions, and scabies.

TREATMENT

Preventing meatal ulceration in a newly circumcised infant is difficult. Good hygiene, frequent diaper changes and, for babies who wear cloth diapers, proper rinsing of the diapers reduce the risk of ammoniacal dermatitis. On occasion, changing from cloth to disposable diapers or vice versa reduces irritation. Applying a protective ointment (e.g., A and D ointment) to the glans or diaper for a week or two after the circumcision reduces mechanical irritation.

When ulcers are present, local hygiene is important. Simple cleansing with soap and water and applying a protective ointment may suffice. If meatal crusting occurs, cleansing and ointment reduce dysuria. Adherent crusts on the meatus may require mechanical debridement. Diaper rash requires appropriate topical therapy.

Meatal stenosis may occur after repeated episodes of meatitis.[2] The diagnosis should be made by the appearance of the voided urinary stream rather than by the appearance of the urethral meatus. A pinpoint, upward-directed stream with pouting of the meatal lips may indicate the need for meatotomy, which almost always can be performed in the office using local anesthesia. Postoperative care is necessary to prevent recurrent adhesion of the raw meatal edges.

Balanitis xerotica obliterans of the meatus may require meatotomy and topical therapy. Condylomata acuminata may be treated by topical, surgical, or laser therapy. Other genital venereal diseases require specific treatment (see Chapter 258, Sexually Transmitted Diseases).

REFERENCES

1. Brennemann J: The ulcerated meatus in the circumcised child, *Am J Dis Child* 21:38, 1921.
2. Freud P: The ulcerated urethral meatus in male children, *J Pediatr* 31:131, 1947.
3. Gairdner D: The fate of the foreskin: a study of circumcision, *Br Med J* 2:1433, 1949.
4. Gee WF, Ansell JS: Neonatal circumcision: a 10-year overview, with comparison of the Gomco clamp and the Plastibell device, *Pediatrics* 58:824, 1976.
5. Glenister TW: A consideration of the processes involved in the development of the prepuce in man, *Br J Urol* 28:243, 1956.
6. Korting GW: *Practical dermatology of the genital region,* Philadelphia, 1980, WB Saunders.
7. Mackenzie AR: Meatal ulceration following neonatal circumcision, *Obstet Gynecol* 28:221, 1966.
8. McKay DL, Fuqua F, Weinberg AG: Balanitis xerotica obliterans in children, *J Urol* 114:773, 1975.
9. Noe HN, Dale GD: Evaluation of children with meatal stenosis, *J Urol* 114:455, 1975.

230 Meningitis

Keith R. Powell

The meninges of the central nervous system (CNS) include three membranes that support, protect, and nourish the brain and spinal cord. The outermost layer, the dura mater, is a tough, poorly extensive connective tissue layer that sheaths the brain and spinal cord and terminates caudally as the coccygeal ligament. The middle and innermost layers, the arachnoid and the pia mater, respectively, are similar in structure and often are referred to singly as the leptomeninges. The arachnoid and pia are partly separated, leaving a subarachnoid space containing cerebrospinal fluid (CSF). The CSF is formed in the choroid plexuses within the ventricles of the brain, which communicate with the subarachnoid space through the foramina of Magendie and Luschka.

Meningitis, which refers to inflammation of the meninges, often is caused directly or indirectly by an infectious agent. Untreated bacterial meningitis usually is quickly fatal, and because delay in treatment generally increases the chance of death or permanent sequelae, early diagnosis and treatment are essential.

The incidence of bacterial meningitis and the causative organisms are related closely to age. During the first month of life the age-specific incidence is nearly 100 cases per 100,000 live births; it falls to 45 per 100,000 during the second month of life. Until recent years a second peak occurred at 6 to 8 months, with an incidence of nearly 80 per 100,000 infants. This second peak has declined dramatically since 1990, when *Haemophilus influenzae* type b (Hib) conjugate vaccines were approved for use during infancy. As illustrated in Fig. 230-1, between 1980 and 1988 the incidence of *H. influenzae* type b meningitis ranged from 50 to 60 cases per 100,000 children less than 1 year of age. In 1991, 1 year after the licensing of conjugate Hib vaccine for use in infants, the incidence of meningitis fell to 12 cases per 100,000 children less than 1 year of age.[1]

The incidence of aseptic meningitis ranges, in different years, from 1.5 to 4 cases per 100,000 population. The incidence in children actually is much higher because aseptic meningitis is also a disease of the young, with few reported cases occurring in persons over 30 years of age.

The cause of meningitis also changes with age. During the first month of life over two thirds of the cases of neonatal bacterial meningitis are caused by group B streptococci or gram negative enteric organisms, primarily *Escherichia coli* and *Klebsiella* and *Enterobacter* species. In some regions the third most common isolate is *Listeria monocytogenes.* After the first month of life, *Listeria* organisms are found as the cause of meningitis only in debilitated or elderly persons.

BACTERIAL MENINGITIS AFTER THE NEONATAL PERIOD

After the age of 1 month, most cases of bacterial meningitis are caused by *Neisseria meningitidis,* or *Streptococcus pneumoniae* in regions where Hib conjugate vaccines are widely used (Fig. 230-2). A child between 3 and 12 months of age is at greatest risk for acquiring meningitis; after the neonatal period, 90% of meningitis cases occur in children between the ages of 1 month and 5 years. Mortality varies with the pathogen and has been reported to be as high as 26% for *S. pneumoniae,* 10% for *N. meningitidis,* and 6% for Hib.

All three of these pathogens can be isolated from the throat or nasopharynx of healthy individuals. Most studies of microorganism carrier states suggest that children at highest risk for disease also are the most likely to be colonized. During an 18-month period, 71% of the toddlers and 48% of the preschool-age children at a day care center were colonized with *H. influenzae* type b.[23] No invasive *H. influenzae* type b disease occurred. Meningitis usually occurs after bacteremia develops secondary to infection at another site. The site of primary infection might be apparent (e.g., otitis media, sinusitis, pharyngitis, cellulitis, pneumonia, septic arthritis, or osteomyelitis) or may go unrecognized.

Meningitis also can occur after head trauma, particularly with fractures of the paranasal sinuses. The pathogens most often associated with meningitis after trauma are *S. pneumoniae* and *H. influenzae.* Posttraumatic meningitis can recur if CSF leakage persists. Meningitis can occur by direct spread from a congenital dermal sinus that communicates with the central nervous system. Any time meningitis is caused by bacteria that normally reside on the skin or in the gastrointestinal tract, a diligent search of the craniospinal axis should be made.[25] Meningitis can develop after neurosurgery and is not uncommon after procedures done to shunt ventricular fluid. Coagulase-negative staphylococci are the organisms most often associated with shunt infections.

Clinical Manifestations

Children who have bacterial meningitis usually are febrile; however, the absence of fever in a child who has signs of meningeal irritation does not preclude the diagnosis. Inflammation of the meninges can be manifested by irritability, anorexia, headache, nausea, vomiting, confusion, back pain, nuchal rigidity, and photophobia. The signs on physical examination described by Kernig and Brudzinski can be used to demonstrate meningeal inflammation. The Kernig sign is elicited by extending the leg at the knee while the hip is flexed. This maneuver causes pain in the hamstrings of a person who has meningitis. The Brudzinski sign is elicited by flexing the neck of a patient in the supine position and observing involuntary flexing of the hips. In a young infant signs of meningeal inflammation can be minimal, and the signs associated with meningitis in an older child may be absent.[34] In infants, irritability (especially in response to actions that usually are comforting), lethargy, poor feeding, and restlessness often are described. The patient also may have signs of increased intracranial pressure such as a headache or a

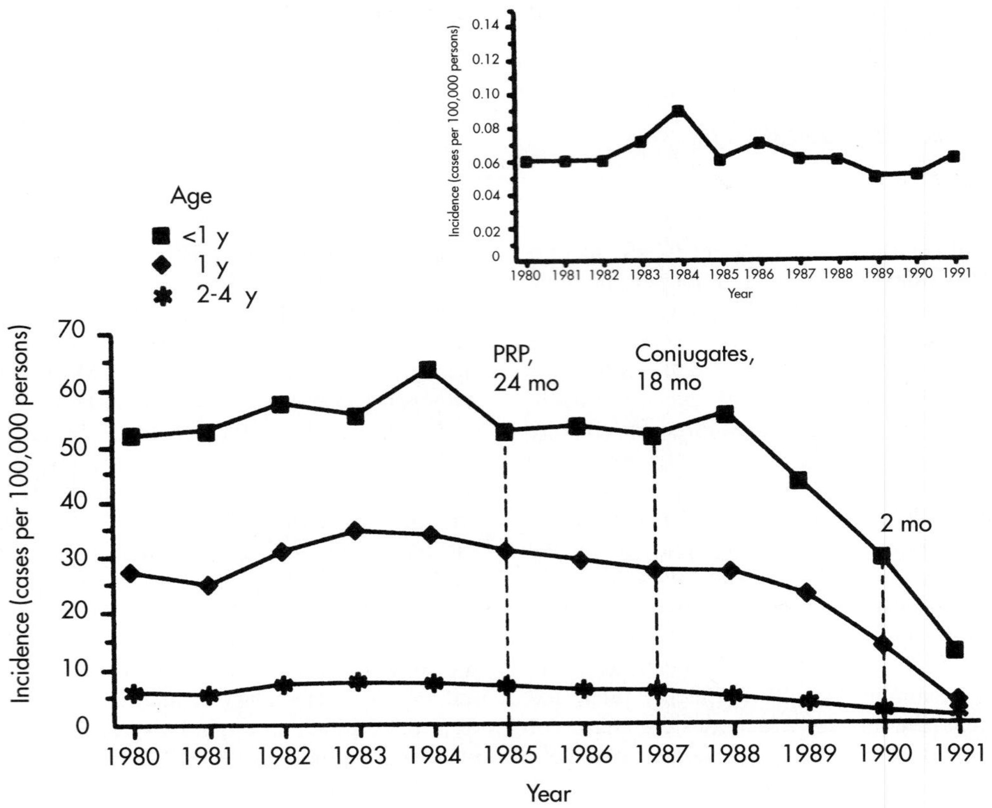

FIG. 230-1 Cases of *Haemophilus influenzae* meningitis, by age, in children under age 5 (according to the National Bacterial Meningitis Reporting System, 1980-1991; 20 continuously reporting states). Licensure dates of polyribosyl ribitol phosphate (PRP) and conjugate vaccines are shown.

(From Adams WG et al: *JAMA* 269:221, 1993.)

bulging fontanelle. However, papilledema is uncommon with bacterial meningitis, and when it is present, other causes should be sought.

Cranial nerve involvement occurs with bacterial meningitis and, although often transient, can be permanent. The auditory nerve often is affected, as manifested by deafness or disturbances of vestibular function. Blindness has been reported but is rare. Children also may have paralysis of extraocular or facial nerves. The degree of CNS derangement observed with bacterial meningitis ranges from irritability to coma. In a prospective series of 124 patients, Feigen[10] found that about 20% of children who had bacterial meningitis were comatose or semicomatose at the time of hospitalization. This occurred more often with *S. pneumoniae* or *N. meningitidis* than with *H. influenzae* type b. Seizures occurred before or within 1 to 2 days after admission in about 30% of patients. Focal neurological signs, present in 14% of the patients, correlated with persistent abnormal neurological examinations 1 year after discharge. Focal signs at the time of admission also correlated with retardation later.

Subdural effusions occur in about 50% of children who have bacterial meningitis but seldom are significant clinically. Therefore, unless focal neurological signs or signs of increased intracranial pressure develop, the presence of such effusions need not be sought through the performance of subdural taps or computed tomography (CT) scans. Infection of subdural effusions is extremely rare.

Arthralgia and myalgia often occur in patients who have meningitis, particularly those who have meningococcemia. Vasculitis can be seen in children who have any type of bacterial meningitis, but petechiae and purpura more commonly are associated with meningococcal disease. Children who have such rashes should be considered in imminent danger of developing septic shock and should be treated accordingly (see Chapter 287, Meningococcemia).

Laboratory Findings

When meningitis is suspected in a patient who does not have papilledema, a lumbar puncture should be performed, the opening pressure measured, and the CSF examined immediately. The clinical situation should influence the amount of data required before a therapeutic decision is made. If the CSF from an ill, febrile child is turbid or purulent, antimicrobial agents should be started and the patient treated for bacterial meningitis before further laboratory results are available. In any case, the CSF should be examined as soon as possible. If the nucleated blood cell count of the CSF is not above 6/mm^3 the only other test likely to be useful in diagnosing bacterial meningitis is a culture of the CSF.[27] If the nucleated blood cell count is 6/mm^3 or above, a Gram stain and differential cell count should be done. The CSF concentrations of total protein and glucose should be determined. If possible, the blood glucose should be measured just before the lumbar puncture so that the CSF to blood glucose

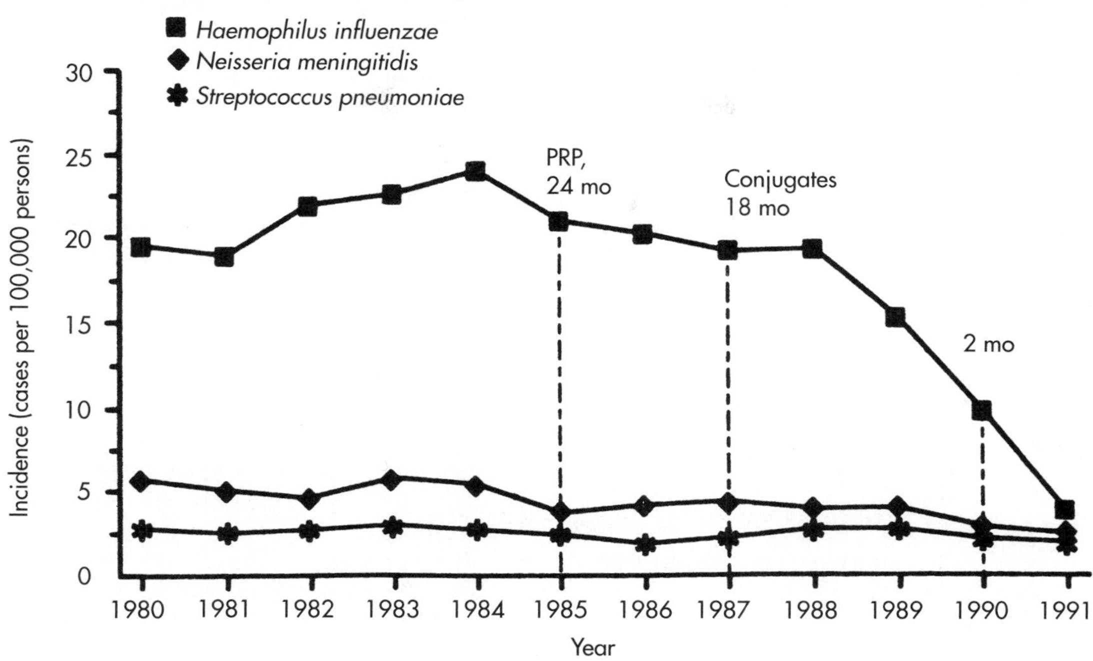

FIG. 230-2 Bacterial meningitis in children under age 5 (according to the National Bacterial Meningitis Reporting System, 1980-1991; 20 continuously reporting states). Licensure dates of polyribosyl ribitol phosphate (PRP) and conjugate vaccines are shown.
(From Adams WG et al: *JAMA* 269:221, 1993.)

Table 230-1 Characteristic Cerebrospinal Fluid Findings in Patients with Meningitis

CSF Findings	Bacterial	Viral	Fungal and tuberculous
Leukocytes			
Usual	>500	<500	<500
Range	0-200,000	0-2000	
Percent polymorphonuclear neutrophils			
Usual	>80%	<50%	<50%
Range	20%-100%	0-100%	
Glucose			
Usual	<40 mg/dl	>40 mg/dl	<40 mg/dl
Range	0-normal	30 mg/dl-normal	
Percent CSF/blood	<30	>50	
Protein			
Usual	>100 mg/dl	<100 mg/dl	>100 mg/dl
Range	Normal-1500 mg/dl	Normal-200 mg/dl	
Stains	Gram stain	—	India ink/acid-fast

ratio can be determined. (The blood glucose is best measured before the lumbar puncture because the stress of the procedure can temporarily elevate the blood glucose.) Characteristic CSF findings are shown in Table 230-1.

The CSF should be cultured on chocolate and blood agar plates and in broth. The etiological agent often can be quickly identified using counterimmunoelectrophoresis (CIE) or agglutination reactions. Soluble capsular antigens can be detected in CSF, serum, and concentrated urine with these methods.

Blood cultures should be obtained for all children suspected of having bacterial meningitis. In one study,[10] blood cultures were positive in 90%, 80%, and 91% of children who had not received antimicrobial agents previously and who had meningitis caused by *H. influenzae*, *S. pneumoniae*, and *N. meningitidis*, respectively. Roentgenograms may help in identifying suspected bone or joint infection. Radionuclide and CT studies have a role in complicated cases of meningitis and may be helpful for decisions on management. However, CT scans should not be obtained routinely because of prolonged or secondary fever when the results of the study are unlikely to affect management.[12]

Differential Diagnosis

Signs and symptoms suggesting meningeal inflammation or increased intracranial pressure can be seen with other infections of the central nervous system as well. The most common cause of meningeal inflammation is viral meningitis, which is discussed later. Meningitis can be caused by *Mycobacterium tuberculosis,* fungi, or parasites. Meningitis or meningoencephalitis also may be present in patients who have Rocky Mountain spotted fever (RMSF), Kawasaki disease, cat-scratch disease, or toxic shock syndrome, and it often is associated with or occurs after mumps, rubeola, rubella, varicella, infectious mononucleosis, roseola, and erythema infectiosum (see the box below). A brain abscess, epidural diseases, embolic diseases (e.g., endocarditis or thrombophlebitis), venous sinus thrombosis, space-occupying lesions, reactions to intrathecal medications, ingestion of toxins, spider bites, pemphigus, and Behçet syndrome can mimic bacterial meningitis. CSF abnormalities similar to those seen with viral meningitis occur with RMSF, Kawasaki disease, toxic shock syndrome, and postinfectious syndromes. However, interpretation of the CSF findings in the context of the clinical manifestations usually differentiates bacterial meningitis from other diseases. Conditions that can simulate a clinical picture of meningitis but that usually have normal CSF findings include pharyngitis, retropharyngeal abscess, cervical adenitis, cervical spine arthritis or osteomyelitis, pyelonephritis, pneumonia, torticollis, tetanus, and oculogyric crisis.[20]

Management

When initially examined, children who have meningitis may appear only mildly ill with fever and irritability, or they may

ETIOLOGICAL AGENTS, FACTORS, AND DISEASES ASSOCIATED WITH ASEPTIC MENINGITIS

Viruses

Enteroviruses (echoviruses, coxsackieviruses A and B, polioviruses, and enteroviruses)
Arboviruses (in the United States: Eastern equine, Western equine, Venezuelan equine, St. Louis, Powassan, California and Colorado tick fever; in other areas of the world, many other arboviruses are important)
Mumps
Herpes simplex type 2
Human immunodeficiency (HIV)
Adenoviruses
Varicella-zoster (VZ)
Epstein-Barr (EB)
Lymphocytic choriomeningitis (LCM)
Encephalomyocarditis (EMC)
Cytomegalovirus (CMV)
Rhinoviruses
Measles
Rubella
Influenza A and B
Parainfluenza
Rotaviruses
Coronaviruses
Variola

Postvaccine reaction

Measles
Vaccinia
Polio
Rabies

Bacteria

Mycobacterium tuberculosis
Pyogenic—partially treated
Leptospira spp. (leptospirosis)
Treponema pallidum (syphilis)
Borrelia spp. (relapsing fever)
Borrelia burgdorferi (Lyme disease)
Nocardia spp. (nocardiosis)

Fungi

Blastomyces dermatitidis
Coccidioides immitis
Cryptococcus neoformans
Histoplasma capsulatum
Candida spp.
Other: *Alternaria* spp., *Aspergillus* spp., *Cephalosporium* spp., *Cladosporium trichoides, Dreschslera hawaiiensis, Paracoccidioides brasiliensis, Petriellidium boydii, Sporotrichum schenckii, Ustilago* spp., *Zygomycete* spp.

Rickettsia

R. rickettsii (Rocky Mountain spotted fever)
R. prowazekii (typhus)

Mycoplasma

M. pneumoniae
M. hominis

Parasites

Angiostrongylus cantonensis (eosinophilic meningitis)
Trichinella spiralis (trichinosis)
Toxoplasma gondii (toxoplasmosis)

Parameningeal infections

Malignancy

Leukemia
CNS tumor

Immune diseases

Behçet syndrome
Lupus erythematosus
Sarcoidosis

Miscellaneous

Kawasaki disease
Toxic shock syndrome
Heavy metal poisoning
Intrathecal injections (e.g., contrast media antibiotics)
Foreign bodies (shunt, reservoir)
Antimicrobial agents

Modified from Cherry JD: Aseptic meningitis and viral meningitis. In Feigen RD, Cherry JD, editors: *Textbook of pediatric infectious disease,* ed 2, Philadelphia, 1987, WB Saunders.

be profoundly ill with an altered state of consciousness and hypotension. The severity of illness at the time of presentation can predict morbidity and should dictate immediate management. The scoring system devised by Herson and Todd[17] and presented in Table 230-2 has been shown to predict morbidity in children who have *H. influenzae* type b meningitis. Children who have a score of 4.5 or higher are significantly more likely to die or to have major sequelae than are children who have lower scores. This scoring system does not predict deafness.[13,17]

Regardless of the patient's Herson-Todd score, acute bacterial meningitis is always a medical emergency, and all infants and children who have an altered state of consciousness should be observed closely and the need for intensive care anticipated.[20]

As soon as bacterial meningitis is diagnosed, intravenous access should be secured and appropriate antimicrobial agents given. The time that it takes for a child who has meningitis to receive antimicrobial therapy after arriving at an emergency department averages 2 to 3 hours.[22,31] The initial laboratory examination should include CSF examination and culture, blood culture, measurement of serum electrolyte concentrations, and measurement of urine specific gravity. If the patient has petechiae or purpura or is in shock, the laboratory tests should include a partial thromboplastin time (PTT), prothrombin time (PT), platelet count, and measurement of fibrin breakdown products. Management of the child who is awake and has stable vital signs consists primarily of administering antimicrobial agents and fluids and careful monitoring for changes in level of consciousness, development of seizures, changes in vital signs, and development of the syndrome of inappropriate secretion of antidiuretic hormone (SIADH).

Other therapies should be considered in more critically ill children (see management of septic shock in Chapter 292). Seizures should be treated with appropriate anticonvulsants, and an open airway that provides good oxygenation should be ensured. Patients who are in profound coma or whose level of consciousness deteriorates while receiving therapy should be evaluated for complications such as a cerebral abscess, obstructive hydrocephalus, or elevated intracranial pressure. A CT scan of the brain is extremely helpful in determining the diagnosis in such cases.

If elevated intracranial pressure is a major concern and treatment has been started or is anticipated, a neurosurgeon should be consulted and an intracranial pressure monitoring device placed. If an intraventricular catheter can be placed, increased intracranial pressure often can be treated by removing CSF. The placement of a pressure transducer affords continuous intracranial monitoring so that mannitol and hyperventilation can be used as necessary to decrease pressure and maintain cerebral perfusion. If a cerebral perfusion pressure (mean arterial blood pressure minus intracranial pressure) of 30 to 40 cm H_2O cannot be maintained, survival is unlikely.[15] Cerebral perfusion pressure increased by 21% within 12 hours of the first dose of dexamethasone in patients who received 0.15 mg/kg per dose given every 6 hours for 4 days compared with a decline of 5% in those who received placebo.[24] Perhaps it is increased cerebral perfusion that accounts for the benefits seen with dexamethasone therapy.[29]

Fluid management and antimicrobial therapy are crucial for all patients who have bacterial meningitis. Traditionally, fluids were restricted to two thirds maintenance in patients who had bacterial meningitis to minimize brain edema and prevent SIADH. A recent study showed that plasma antidiuretic hormone concentrations returned to normal in patients who had bacterial meningitis who received replacement plus maintenance fluids for 24 hours; concentrations remained elevated in patients restricted to two thirds of maintenance requirements.[26] Furthermore, maintenance fluids are necessary to perfuse, oxygenate, and deliver host defenses to the central nervous system, and although SIADH occurs in bacterial meningitis, there is no evidence that fluid restriction *prevents* it. Therefore it is preferable to give full maintenance fluids and monitor the serum sodium concentration. If the serum sodium concentration drops below 125 mEq/L, the test should be repeated as soon as possible. If the serum sodium is still below 125 mEq/L, fluids should be restricted to "keep vein open" until the serum electrolyte concentrations have been corrected.

The use of steroids as adjunctive treatment in patients who have bacterial meningitis has been studied by several groups in the past decade. Recent meta-analyses of these studies concluded that dexamethasone improves the hearing and neurological outcomes of children who have bacterial meningitis.[14,29] Although further studies are needed to confirm these results, the American Academy of Pediatrics Committee on Infectious Diseases recommends that dexamethasone 0.6 mg/kg/day be given for 4 days starting at the time of the first dose of antimicrobial agents to children 6 weeks of age or older who have *H. influenzae* type b meningitis and should be considered for use in infants who have pneumococcal or meningococcal meningitis.[6]

Until recently, all *N. meningitidis*, *H. influenzae* type b, and most *S. pneumoniae* strains were susceptible to very low concentrations of the third-generation cephalosporins ceftriaxone and cefotaxime. Recently there have been numerous reports of infections in infants and children who have resistant strains of pneumococci.[2,32] Some regions have reported that 30% of pneumococcal isolates are resistant to penicillin at some level and that many also are resistant to the third-generation cephalosporins.[4] Therefore in areas where pneumococci are resistant to third-generation cephalosporins, infants and children suspected of having bacterial meningitis should receive vancomycin (10 to 15 mg/kg/dose given every 6 hours) in

Table 230-2 Scoring System for Predicting Morbidity in Haemophilus Influenzae Meningitis

Factor at admission	Points
Severe coma (apnea, nonreactive pupils, no response to pain)	3
Hypothermia (temperature <97.9° F [36.6° C])	2
Seizures (major motor or generalized)	2
Shock (systolic blood pressure <60 mm Hg)	1
Age <12 mo	1
CSF white blood cell count <1000 × 10/L	1
Hemoglobin <110 g/L	1
CSF glucose <1.1 mmol/L	0.5
Symptoms persisting longer than 3 days	0.5

From Gary N et al: *Am J Dis Child* 143:307, 1989.

addition to ceftriaxone (80 mg/kg/dose given once daily) or cefotaxime (50 mg/kg/dose given every 6 hours). Because dexamethasone can decrease the activity of vancomycin, either dexamethasone should not be used or rifampin plus a third-generation cephalosporin should be used. As soon as antimicrobial susceptibility for an isolate is known, vancomycin should be discontinued if the isolate is susceptible to the third-generation cephalosporin. Vancomycin must be used judiciously because it often is the last line of therapy for resistant gram positive pathogens. When vancomycin resistance becomes prevalent, many children will die because of untreatable antibiotic-resistant bacterial infections.

Meningitis caused by *N. meningitidis* usually is treated for 7 days, meningitis caused by *H. influenzae* type b for 7 to 10 days, and that caused by *S. pneumoniae* for 10 days. A 7-day course of antimicrobial therapy for uncomplicated *H. influenzae* type b and *S. pneumoniae* meningitis has been shown to be effective.[18,19] If chloramphenicol is used, serum chloramphenicol concentrations should be monitored when possible, and patients treated with oral chloramphenicol should receive the full course of therapy in the hospital. Although most cases of bacterial meningitis are caused by the three organisms mentioned, other bacteria can cause meningitis; in such cases, antimicrobial therapy must be individualized.

Most therapeutic failures can be related to delayed diagnosis, inadequate therapy with the correct antimicrobial agent, or resistant organisms. A repeat lumbar puncture on completion of therapy does not reflect the adequacy of therapy or predict the likelihood of recurrence and usually is not indicated. However, a delay in sterilizing the CSF beyond 24 to 36 hours has been associated with adverse outcomes; therefore some experts recommend that another lumbar puncture be performed at that time.

Some contacts of patients who have *N. meningitidis* or *H. influenzae* type b meningitis are at increased risk for the disease and therefore should receive prophylaxis. Prophylactic regimens for those at risk for *N. meningitidis* are described in Chapter 287, Meningococcemia. Whether contacts of patients who have *H. influenzae* type b disease should receive prophylaxis remains controversial. The American Academy of Pediatrics recommends that rifampin, 20 mg/kg (600 mg maximum), be given once a day for 4 days to all household contacts, including adults, in households that have at least one contact under age 4. A household contact is anyone who resides with the index patient or a nonresident who has spent 4 or more hours a day with the index patient for 5 of the 7 days before the index patient was hospitalized. Because children younger than 3 years are at risk for a second attack of *H. influenzae* type b disease, some authorities recommend prophylaxis for all household contacts, regardless of age, to prevent recolonization of the index patient. The index patient should receive rifampin either during or at the completion of treatment for meningitis.

Complications

Early in the course of the disease, increased intracranial pressure, septic shock, cardiorespiratory arrest, and disseminated intravascular coagulation (DIC) should be anticipated. Subdural effusions occasionally cause seizures or focal neurological deficits; in such cases the fluid should be removed by subdural taps. Inappropriate secretion of antidiuretic hormone also can complicate bacterial meningitis; therefore the patient should be monitored carefully for this complication, and if it occurs, fluid should be restricted severely. A brain abscess is extremely rare after bacterial meningitis except in neonates who have meningitis caused by *Citrobacter* species.

Sequelae

Although the Herson-Todd scoring system can indicate which children are more likely to have bad outcomes, it is not possible to predict long-term sequelae for an individual child at the time of discharge from the hospital. Some children who apparently are normal subsequently have hearing or learning deficits or develop a seizure disorder. Conversely, some children expected to have a dismal prognosis make remarkable gains. It therefore is important for the practitioner to be optimistic with the family while remaining sensitive to possible sequelae and observing these children closely for attainment of developmental milestones. Hearing should be tested formally before discharge from the hospital because most sensorineural hearing loss can be detected at this time.

PREVENTION

In 1985 a purified capsular polysaccharide vaccine against *H. influenzae* type b was licensed for use in the United States. Subsequently three vaccines made by coupling the capsular polysaccharide to a protein carrier were licensed for use in infants at 2, 4, and 6 months of age (Table 230-3). Wide-

Table 230-3 Haemophilus influenzae Type b Conjugate Vaccines*

Manufacturer	Abbreviation	Trade name	Carrier protein
Connaught Laboratories	PRP-D	ProHIBit	Diphtheria toxoid
Lederle Laboratories	HbOC†	HIBTITER	CRM_{197} (a nontoxic mutant diphtheria toxin)
Merck & Co.	PRP-OMP	PedvaxHIB	OMP (an outer membrane protein complex of *Neisseria meningitidis*)
Pasteur Mérieux Vaccines (distributed by Connaught Laboratories and by SmithKline Beecham)	PRP-T‡	ActHIB OmniHIB	Tetanus toxoid

From Peter G et al, editors: *Report of the Committee on Infectious Diseases,* ed 23, Elk Grove Village, Ill, 1994, The American Academy of Pediatrics.
*PRP-D is recommended by the AAP only for infants 12 months or older. HbOC, PRP-OMP, and PRP-T are recommended for infants beginning at approximately 2 months of age.
†HbOC also is available from Lederle Laboratories as a combination vaccine with DTP (TERAMUNE, referred to here as HbOC-DTP).
‡PRP-T may be reconstituted with DTP manufactured by Connaught Laboratories. Other licensed formulations of DTP have not been approved by the Food and Drug Administration for reconstitution and may not be used for this purpose.

spread use of these vaccines has resulted in the dramatic decline in the incidence of invasive *H. influenzae* type b disease, shown in Figs. 230-1 and 230-2. The meningococcal and pneumococcal vaccines currently available are composed of purified capsular polysaccharides and, like the prototype Hib vaccine, are poor immunogens in infants under age 2. Multivalent pneumococcal conjugate vaccines modeled on the Hib conjugate vaccines have proved to be safe and immunogenic in early trials among children.

Partially Treated Meningitis

Several studies[7,8] have shown that *mean* values for white blood cell (WBC) counts in CSF, the percentage of polymorphonuclear cells, and the level of glucose and protein concentrations in patients who have partially treated bacterial meningitis do not differ from those values in patients not treated previously. However, some patients who have partially treated bacterial meningitis have CSF findings indistinguishable from the classic findings for aseptic meningitis.[7] Unless there is clear evidence of a nonbacterial cause (e.g., isolation of virus from CSF or blood), antibiotics should be administered to partially treated patients for 7 to 10 days at dosages appropriate for bacterial meningitis.

NEONATAL MENINGITIS

Neonatal meningitis merits separate consideration because the incidence is high, the etiological agents are unique, and it often is fatal. The incidence of neonatal meningitis varies with the reporting institute, from 0.2 to 1 case per 1000 live births. The age-specific incidence of bacterial meningitis (estimated from 38 states) reported in 1978 was 96 per 100,000 neonates. Case fatality rates range from 15% to 75%, and in a report from the Neonatal Meningitis Cooperative Study Group the overall case fatality rate was 30%.[21] In general, mortality is lower for full-term infants than for infants of low birth weight (under 2500 g). Early recognition and treatment are critical because the case fatality rate falls to about 5% for neonates who survive the first 24 hours of the disease.[21]

The cause of neonatal meningitis has changed in the past 3 decades, and clinicians should be alert to the possibility of future etiological shifts. During the 1960s most cases were caused by gram negative enteric organisms, primarily *E. coli;* gram positive isolates were likely to be *L. monocytogenes.* During the 1970s group B streptococci entered the scene; currently this organism and *E. coli* account for 60% to 80% of the cases and *L. monocytogenes* for about 5%.[33] Neonatal sepsis and meningitis caused by non–group D alpha-hemolytic streptococci[3] and coagulase-negative staphylococci also have been reported.[16]

The clinical signs associated with neonatal meningitis are nonspecific and therefore not very helpful. Neonates often have apneic episodes or feed poorly, and they can be hyperthermic or hypothermic, irritable or lethargic, and have respiratory distress or diarrhea; only infrequently do they have nuchal rigidity or a bulging fontanelle. The neonate has a limited repertoire of clinical responses to disease or insult; most sick neonates therefore receive a septic workup, including a lumbar puncture, and antimicrobial agents are started pending culture results. The cytology and chemistry of the CSF in neonates have a much broader normal range than in other age groups, especially during the first week of life (Table 230-4). When Sarff and co-workers[28] compared CSF values from high-risk infants who had no meningitis to those who had meningitis, no single test results separated the groups. However, only 1 of 119 infants who had bacterial meningitis had normal CSF on examination.

ANTIMICROBIAL THERAPY

The principles of antimicrobial therapy for neonatal meningitis are the same as for infants and children, but because the organisms are different, the antimicrobial selection must be adjusted. Based on the most common organisms that cause neonatal meningitis, the ideal antimicrobial would be effective against *E. coli* and other enteric organisms as well as against group B streptococci and other gram positive organisms. Two third-generation cephalosporins, cefotaxime and ceftriaxone, are extremely active against the organisms that usually cause neonatal meningitis, with the exception of *L. monocytogenes.* The major difference between these drugs is half-life; cefotaxime has the shortest and ceftriaxone the longest. Data from the Neonatal Meningitis Cooperative Study Group comparing these agents with the combination of ampicillin plus gentamicin or amikacin are not yet available. However, because the drugs are safe, are very active against the common pathogens, and enter the CSF relatively well, one of these agents plus ampicillin should be used to treat documented meningitis. Because some enteric pathogens such as *Pseudomonas aeruginosa* and Enterobacteriaceae readily become resistant to these third-generation cephalosporins, they should not be used empirically for suspected sepsis in neonates. Dosages and characteristics of the antimicrobials used most often to treat neonatal meningitis are listed in Table 230-5. Because ceftriaxone is highly protein bound and can displace unconjugated bilirubin from albumin, it should not be used in premature infants at risk for kernicterus or in term infants who have hyperbilirubinemia.

The role of intraventricular antimicrobial therapy remains controversial; ideally, the newer antimicrobials mentioned

Table 230-4 Representative Cerebrospinal Fluid Findings in High-Risk Neonates Without Meningitis

CSF findings	Full-term neonates—mean (range)	Preterm neonates—mean (range)
White blood cells/mm^3	8.2 (0-32)	9 (0-29)
Polymorphonuclear neutrophils	61.3%	57.2%
Protein (mg/dl)	90 (20-170)	115 (65-150)
Glucose (mg/dl)	52 (34-119)	50 (24-63)
CSF/blood glucose ratio	0.81 (0.44-2.38)	0.74 (0.55-1.05)

Modified from Sarff LD, Platt LH, McCracken GH Jr: *J Pediatr* 88:473, 1976.

Table 230-5 Some Characteristics of Antibiotics Useful or Potentially Useful in the Treatment of Neonatal Meningitis

Drug	Dose (mg/kg/dose) Age 0-7 days	Dose (mg/kg/dose) Age >7 days	Gram positive coverage	Gram negative coverage	Anaerobic coverage	CSF penetration
Ampicillin	50 mg q12h	50 mg q6	Good	Fair	Good	Good
Amikacin	10 mg q12h	10 mg q8	Fair	Good	None	Fair
Gentamicin	2.5 mg q12h	2.5 mg q8h	Fair	Good	None	Fair
Cefotaxime	50 mg q12h	50 mg q8h	Good	Excellent	Good	Good
Ceftriaxone	50 mg q24h	50 mg q24h	Good	Excellent	Good	Excellent
Vancomycin	15 mg q12h	15 mg q8h	Excellent	Poor	None	Fair

Modified from McCracken GM, Nelson JD: *Pediatr Infect Dis J* 1:123, 1982.

will bypass this question. Other therapeutic considerations are the same for neonates as for infants and children who have bacterial meningitis.

PROGNOSIS

The complications of neonatal meningitis, which are similar to those seen among older infants, include hydrocephalus, deafness, and blindness. The case fatality rate is 20% to 50%, and long-term follow-up studies have revealed that about 65% of survivors are normal 3 to 7 years after the illness.[11,21] A brain abscess rarely complicates neonatal meningitis except when the pathogen is *Citrobacter.* For unknown reasons, as many as 80% of neonates who have *Citrobacter* meningitis also have a brain abscess. As with older infants and children, all infants recovering from meningitis should have careful audiology testing and close evaluation for attainment of developmental milestones.

ASEPTIC MENINGITIS

The syndrome of aseptic meningitis consists of a clinical picture of meningitis with CSF pleocytosis and the absence of bacteria on Gram stain or culture. Although aseptic meningitis usually is a viral disease, it is important that treatable causes of this syndrome be considered in the differential diagnosis. The box on p. 1424 lists a wide variety of infectious and noninfectious agents and diseases that have been associated with aseptic meningitis. Nonpolio enteroviruses cause most cases of aseptic meningitis in the United States, but mumps and polio should be considered in endemic areas. Mycobacteria, rickettsiae, fungi, and parasites can be treated, as can parameningeal infections and intoxications. The CSF findings characteristic of aseptic meningitis are shown in Table 230-1.

Clinical Manifestations

Infants and children who have aseptic meningitis often are febrile, irritable, and lethargic. Their temperature usually is 101.3° to 104° F (38.5° to 40° C), rarely higher. Upper respiratory tract symptoms, myalgia, nausea, and vomiting also are commonly present. In general, a child who has viral meningitis does not appear as critically ill as a child who has bacterial meningitis and is less likely to have meningeal signs.[34]

The diagnosis of aseptic meningitis is likely when CSF pleocytosis ranges from 10 to 500 cells, which are predominantly lymphocytes; the CSF protein is mildly elevated at 50 to 150 mg/dl; and the CSF glucose concentration is normal. Early in the course of viral meningitis, polymorphonuclear neutrophils (PMNs) can predominate in the CSF. A transition from a predominance of PMNs to lymphocytes usually occurs rapidly, and a repeat lumbar puncture after 8 to 12 hours may show this transition.

Hypoglycorrhachia (low CSF glucose level) can occur with viral meningitis caused by enteroviruses, mumps, herpes simplex, and Eastern equine encephalitis viruses. Hypoglycorrhachia caused by these viruses tends to result in CSF glucose concentrations that equal about 30% of the simultaneous blood glucose concentration, whereas bacterial meningitis usually results in CSF glucose concentrations of less than 30% of the blood glucose. The CSF glucose concentration also can be low with tuberculous and fungal meningitis.

Many physicians are reluctant to obtain specimens for viral culture because they believe that isolating viruses takes too long to affect patient management. A review of patients who had CSF specimens sent for viral culture showed that of 113 patients who had a discharge diagnosis of aseptic meningitis, 46 had enteroviral meningitis, 2 had tuberculous meningitis, 2 had herpes simplex meningoencephalitis, 1 had leukemic meningitis, and 1 had toxoplasmosis with CNS involvement.[5] It took an average of 3.7 days for CSF cultures to show a typical enterovirus cytopathic effect. The diagnosis of enteroviral meningitis frequently resulted in discontinuation of antimicrobial therapy and early discharge from the hospital. Therefore, when viral meningitis is a possibility, the CSF should be cultured for viruses, as should nasopharyngeal or throat and rectal swab specimens. Although isolation of a virus from a site other than the CSF could be misleading, if taken in the context of other clinical and laboratory findings, a presumptive diagnosis often can be made when a virus is isolated from one or more of these sites. The management of viral meningitis is directed to supportive care. Meningoencephalitis caused by herpes simplex or varicella-zoster viruses should be treated with acyclovir.

Outcome

The outcome of aseptic meningitis relates to both the causative agent and the child's age. Patients who have the most common known cause of viral meningitis, enteroviral meningitis, usually recover completely. However, several groups[9,30,35] have reported low intelligence and delayed speech development after enteroviral meningitis in young infants. In light of these findings, the prognosis for an infant younger than 1 year is somewhat guarded, and the child's development should be monitored carefully.

REFERENCES

1. Adams WG et al: Decline of childhood *Haemophilus influenzae* type b (Hib) disease in the Hib vaccine era, *JAMA* 269:221, 1993.
2. Bradley JS, Connor JD: Ceftriaxone failure in meningitis caused by *Streptococcus pneumoniae* with reduced susceptibility to beta-lactam antibiotics, *Pediatr Infect Dis J* 10:871, 1991.
3. Broughton RA, Krafka R, Baker CJ: Non-group D alpha-hemolytic streptococci: new neonatal pathogens, *J Pediatr* 99:450, 1981.
4. Centers for Disease Control and Prevention: Prevalence of penicillin-resistant *Streptococcus pneumoniae:* Connecticut, 1992-1993, *MMWR* 43:216, 1994.
5. Chonmaitree T, Menegus MA, Powell KR: The clinical relevance of CSF viral culture: a 2-year experience with aseptic meningitis in Rochester, NY, *JAMA* 247:1843, 1982.
6. Committee on Infectious Diseases: Dexamethasone therapy for bacterial meningitis in infants and children. In Peter G et al, editors: *Red Book,* ed 23, Elk Grove Village, Ill, 1994, American Academy of Pediatrics.
7. Converse GM et al: Alterations of cerebrospinal fluid findings by partial treatment of bacterial meningitis, *J Pediatr* 83:220, 1973.
8. Davis SD et al: Partial antibiotic therapy in *Haemophilus influenzae* meningitis: its effect on cerebrospinal fluid abnormalities, *Am J Dis Child* 129:802, 1975.
9. Farmer CJ, Carpenter RL, Ray CG: A follow-up study of 15 cases of neonatal meningoencephalitis due to coxsackievirus B5, *J Pediatr* 87:568, 1975.
10. Feigen RD: Bacterial meningitis beyond the neonatal period. In Feigen RD, Cherry JD, editors: *Textbook of pediatric infectious diseases,* Philadelphia, 1987, WB Saunders.
11. Franco SM, Cornelius VE, Andrews BF: Long-term outcome of neonatal meningitis, *Am J Dis Child* 146:567, 1992.
12. Friedland IR et al: Cranial computed tomographic scans have little impact on management of bacterial meningitis, *Am J Dis Child* 146:1484, 1992.
13. Gary N, Powers N, Todd JK: Clinical identification and comparative prognosis of high-risk patients with *Haemophilus influenzae* meningitis, *Am J Dis Child* 143:307, 1989.
14. Geiman BJ, Smith AL: Dexamethasone and bacterial meningitis: a meta-analysis of randomized controlled trials, *West J Med* 157:27, 1992.
15. Goitein KJ, Tamir I: Cerebral perfusion pressure in central nervous system infections of infancy and childhood, *J Pediatr* 103:40, 1983.
16. Gruskay J et al: Neonatal *Staphylococcus epidermidis* meningitis with unremarkable CSF examination results, *Am J Dis Child* 143:580, 1989.
17. Herson VC, Todd JK: Prediction of morbidity in *Haemophilus influenzae* meningitis, *Pediatrics* 59:35, 1977.
18. Jadavji T et al: Sequelae of acute bacterial meningitis in children treated for seven days, *Pediatrics* 78:21, 1986.
19. Lin TY et al: Seven days of ceftriaxone therapy is as effective as 10 days' treatment for bacterial meningitis, *JAMA* 253:3559, 1985.
20. Lipton JD, Schafermeyer RW: Evolving concepts in pediatric bacterial meningitis. I. Pathophysiology and diagnosis. II. Current management and therapeutic research, *Ann Emerg Med* 22:1602, 1993.
21. McCracken GH Jr: Perinatal bacterial diseases. In Feigen RD, Cherry JD, editors: *Textbook of pediatric infectious diseases,* ed 2, Philadelphia, 1987, WB Saunders.
22. Meadow WL et al: Ought "standard care" be "standard of care"? A study of the time to administration of antibiotics in children with meningitis, *Am J Dis Child* 147:40, 1993.
23. Murphy TV et al: Pharyngeal colonization with *Haemophilus influenzae* type b in children in a day care center without invasive disease, *J Pediatr* 106:712, 1985.
24. Odio CM et al: The beneficial effects of early dexamethasone administration in infants and children with bacterial meningitis, *N Engl J Med* 324:1525, 1991.
25. Powell KR et al: A prospective search for congenital dermal abnormalities of the craniospinal axis, *J Pediatr* 87:744, 1975.
26. Powell KR et al: Normalization of plasma arginine vasopressin concentrations when children with meningitis are given maintenance plus replacement fluid therapy, *J Pediatr* 117:515, 1990.
27. Rodewald LE et al: Relevance of common tests of cerebrospinal fluid in screening for bacterial meningitis, *J Pediatr* 119:363, 1991.
28. Sarff LD, Platt LH, McCracken GH Jr: Cerebrospinal fluid evaluation in neonates: comparison of high-risk infants with and without meningitis, *J Pediatr* 88:473, 1976.
29. Schaad UB et al: Dexamethasone therapy for bacterial meningitis in children, *Lancet* 342:457, 1993.
30. Sells CJ, Carpenter RL, Ray CG: Sequelae of central nervous system enterovirus infections, *N Engl J Med* 293:1, 1975.
31. Talan DA, Zibulewsky J: Relationship of clinical presentation to time to antibiotics for the emergency department management of suspected bacterial meningitis, *Ann Emerg Med* 22:1733, 1993.
32. Tan TQ, Mason EO Jr, Kaplan SL: Systemic infections due to *Streptococcus pneumoniae* relatively resistant to penicillin in a children's hospital: clinical management and outcome, *Pediatrics* 90:928, 1992.
33. Unhanand M et al: Gram-negative enteric bacillary meningitis: a twenty-one-year experience, *J Pediatr* 122:15, 1993.
34. Walsh-Kelly C et al: Clinical predictors of bacterial versus aseptic meningitis in childhood, *Ann Emerg Med* 21:910, 1992.
35. Wilfert CM et al: Longitudinal assessment of children with enteroviral meningitis during the first 3 months of life, *Pediatrics* 67:811, 1981.

231 Meningoencephalitis

Richard S.K. Young

Meningoencephalitis is an infection of the central nervous system and meninges caused by a variety of agents. In children the most common pathogens are viruses, but fungi and parasites also may cause the disorder. Depending on the extent of the infection, the patient may have signs and symptoms of meningitis, encephalitis, or myelitis. By convention, bacterial invasion of the meninges is called *bacterial meningitis* and is considered a disorder distinct from meningoencephalitis.

The actual incidence of infectious meningoencephalitis almost certainly exceeds the nearly 12,000 cases reported each year to the Centers for Disease Control and Prevention (CDC) as aseptic meningitis and encephalitis.[14] However, the difficulty in identifying the specific agent in each suspected case makes statistical accuracy impossible.

ETIOLOGY OF CHILDHOOD MENINGOENCEPHALITIS

The course of meningoencephalitis may vary from aseptic meningitis with a mild clinical presentation to a fulminant encephalitis with paresis, seizures, increased intracranial pressure, and death.[3] Although the initial signs and symptoms produced by viruses often are similar, differences in seasonal occurrence, clinical course, and outcome allow differentiation of some disorders.

Nonpolio enteroviruses, including echovirus and group B coxsackievirus, are responsible for 85% of cases of aseptic meningitis each year.[5] *Enteroviral infection* usually is heralded by the development of malaise and gastroenteritis, more often during the summer months (see Chapter 203, Enterovirus Infections). Progression to meningoencephalitis is uncommon with most enteroviral infections. When meningoencephalitis does occur, it usually is a mild disease. Poliovirus infections have been virtually eliminated through widespread immunization and now occur primarily in immunodeficient children or among small communities of unimmunized children. Echovirus infections commonly begin with a petechial rash; coxsackie infections often start with myalgia and lesions of the palms, soles, and mouth (hand-foot-and-mouth disease). An enterovirus may infect a fetus transplacentally. Eighty-four percent of patients who develop aseptic meningitis are younger than 16 weeks of age.[12]

Herpes simplex virus commonly produces a necrotizing encephalitis, and 50% to 70% of untreated cases are fatal. Herpes simplex encephalitis has a bimodal age distribution, with one third of cases occurring in childhood. Neonatal infection results from passage through an infected birth canal. Mothers of infected infants often have no symptoms of herpes infection during or before gestation, making the diagnosis of a neonatal infection more difficult. Herpes simplex in the neonate may manifest as cutaneous disease, as meningoencephalitis, or as disseminated disease. In all age groups, herpes simplex virus sometimes causes a mild, self-limited meningoencephalitis that resembles the neurological illness caused by the Epstein-Barr virus. Varicella-zoster virus is a herpes virus that causes chickenpox or herpes zoster (shingles).

Arboviral infections caused by *Bunyavirus* species and togavirus are transmitted to humans by arthropods. Arbovirus meningoencephalitis often occurs in epidemics during the summer and early fall. California virus encephalitis should be suspected in any child in a known endemic region who has signs of fever and cerebrocortical dysfunction. The course usually is mild, with a fatality rate of less than 5%. Western equine encephalitis, an arboviral disease primarily of infancy, causes a more severe syndrome. Eastern equine encephalitis has a predilection for infants and young children and usually is fatal. St. Louis encephalitis occurs most often in epidemic form and produces illness in adults more often than in children.

Other viral diseases are transmitted by vectors. The virus that causes Colorado tick fever, a reovirus transmitted by rodent arthropods, produces a denguelike illness in humans. Viral disease transmitted directly to humans from animals includes lymphocytic choriomeningitis (arenavirus), which is transmitted by infected laboratory or domestic rodents, and rabies, which is transmitted by a bite, scratch, or droplet from an infected wild or a unimmunized domestic animal. Recent rabies infections in children have been attributed most often to rabid raccoons, bats, and cats.[2] Rabies characteristically has a long incubation period and invariably ends in a fatal meningoencephalitis. Common childhood viral infections such as rubella, adenovirus, influenza, cytomegalovirus, and Epstein-Barr virus (infectious mononucleosis) occasionally can cause meningoencephalitis.

Meningoencephalitis that occurs in the course of childhood exanthems (measles, mumps, rubella, varicella) may result either from the host's immunological response to the virus or from actual infection of the nervous system. Both varicella and measles viruses cause meningoencephalitis in approximately 1 in 1000 cases and within 4 to 7 days after onset of the rash. The severity of the neurological illness (including irritability, drowsiness, and ataxia) does not appear to be related to the intensity of the systemic illness. Mortality in varicella and measles meningoencephalitis approximates 10%, and as many as half of survivors may have neurological residua. A syndrome of dementia and myoclonic seizures can develop in children of school age many years after measles infection or immunization. This disorder results from a persistent measles infection known as subacute sclerosing panencephalitis (SSPE) (Fig. 231-1). Rubella is a less common cause of meningoencephalitis but can result in a more severe illness than can measles or varicella. In contrast, mumps me-

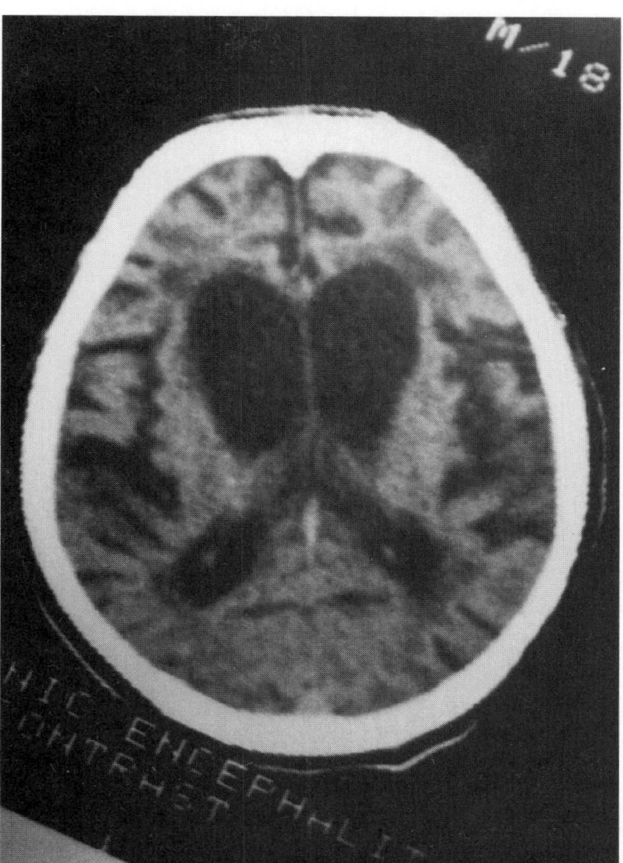

FIG. 231-1 Subacute sclerosing panencephalitis (SSPE). Marked atrophy of both the cerebral cortex and the deep gray nuclei has occurred in this child, who has long-standing SSPE.

ningoencephalitis is a mild illness that generally has a good prognosis. Mumps meningoencephalitis may occur without parotitis within a few weeks of exposure to the virus, or it may occur before the parotitis appears or after it has resolved.

Acquired immunodeficiency syndrome (AIDS), which is caused by a retrovirus known as human immunodeficiency virus (HIV), is noteworthy for meningoencephalitides caused both by HIV and by unusual organisms such as *Toxoplasma gondii* or *Candida albicans* (Figs. 231-2 and 231-3) and Epstein-Barr virus. More than one organism, whether viral or bacterial, can be recovered in immunosuppressed patients who have AIDS.[11]

Nonviral causes of meningoencephalitis include infectious and postinfectious causes and noninfectious conditions associated with cerebrospinal fluid pleocytosis (Table 231-1). These are described more fully by Feigin and Cherry.[6]

SIGNS AND SYMPTOMS

Depending on the extent of the viral infection, the patient may have signs and symptoms of meningitis, encephalitis, or myelitis. A patient who has meningitis characteristically complains of an intense headache, a stiff neck, and photophobia. Physical findings include meningismus with positive Kernig and Brudzinski signs. In encephalitis, a patient who is lethargic, delirious, or hallucinating mistakenly may be diagnosed as being intoxicated or psychotic. A central nervous system infection should be presumed in any child with a fever who has an acute change in mental status.

Encephalitis may reveal focal neurological findings. Herpes simplex encephalitis, for example, classically is heralded by temporal lobe seizures and olfactory hallucinations. Varicella-zoster and other viruses may infect the cerebellum specifically, causing acute ataxia. With myelitis, the viral parenchymal disease causes a symmetrical limb paralysis, transverse sensory symptoms, and bowel and bladder dysfunction.

LABORATORY INVESTIGATIONS

Every attempt should be made to identify and to isolate the offending organism to help determine the prognosis and to document potential epidemic outbreaks. The cerebrospinal fluid (CSF) examination is crucial. Typical CSF alterations among patients who have meningoencephalitis consist of mild pleocytosis, a slight increase in protein level, and no alteration in glucose concentration (Table 231-2); however, the absence of CSF abnormalities does not rule out encephalitis. The sample of CSF should be refrigerated for later virus isolation and determination of viral antibody titers. Red cells in the CSF may indicate hemorrhagic brain necrosis, commonly seen with herpesvirus infections and eastern equine encephalitis. A predominance of mononuclear cells in the CSF is the exception in acute bacterial meningoencephalitis but may be present with syphilis, Lyme disease,[9] listeriosis, or tuberculosis.

Computed tomography (CT) or magnetic resonance imaging (MRI) scans of the brain may demonstrate increased intracranial pressure (ventricular compression) or cerebral cortical enhancement. Temporal lobe enhancement or necrosis may be evidence of herpesvirus infection (Fig. 231-4). Electroencephalographic examination is a useful adjunct in the diagnosis of herpes simplex encephalitis.[8]

Specific identification of viruses requires isolation of the virus by tissue culture. Demonstration of a substantial convalescent antibody rise to a specific virus suggests recent viral infection. Testing the CSF and serum for other organisms may be warranted. A rapid screening test for Epstein-Barr virus (Monospot) is available at most hospitals.

Newborns who have cutaneous vesicles and who are suspected of having herpes simplex meningoencephalitis need not undergo brain biopsy for the diagnosis to be established. Rather, attempts should be made to isolate the virus from the throat, eye, or cutaneous lesions. If herpes simplex meningoencephalitis is suspected in older infants or children, a brain biopsy may be indicated for confirmation.[1] In all other nonherpetic meningoencephalitides, blood, urine, stool, and CSF samples should be obtained to facilitate later confirmation of the virus. Enteroviruses can be isolated relatively easily from throat, stool, and CSF samples. Laboratory diagnosis of mumps meningoencephalitis may be possible within the first week by demonstration of complement-fixing antibodies.

DIFFERENTIAL DIAGNOSIS

Because laboratory tests often only suggest rather than confirm the diagnosis of meningoencephalitis, the clinician must

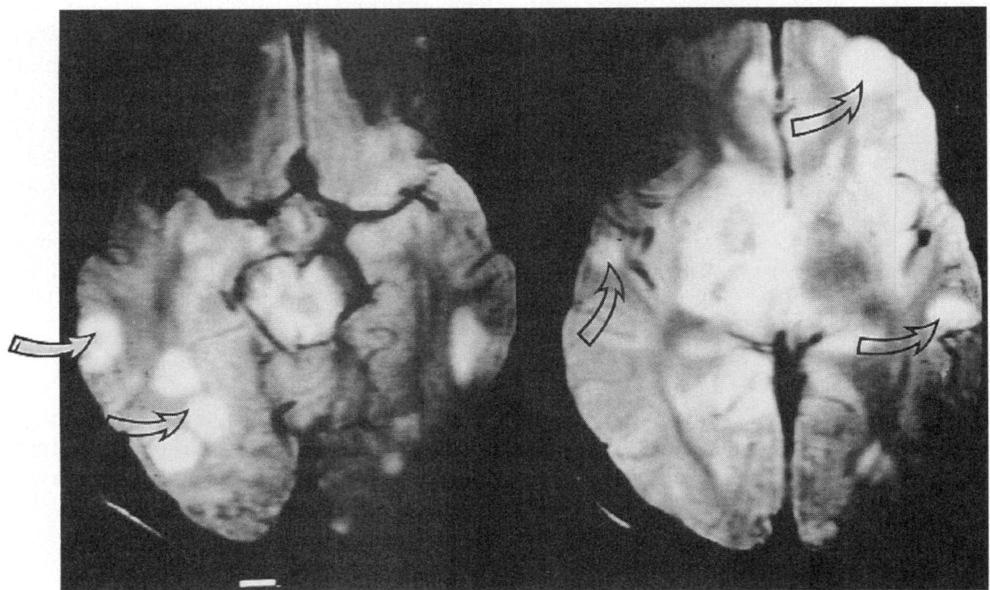

FIG. 231-2 Toxoplasmosis in acquired immunodeficiency syndrome (AIDS). Because patients who have AIDS are immunocompromised, they are at risk for opportunistic infections of the central nervous system. This T2-weighted magnetic resonance image shows several high-intensity lesions caused by ***Toxoplasma gondii*** scattered throughout the frontal, temporal, and parietal lobes *(arrows)*.

(Courtesy of Dr. G. Sze.)

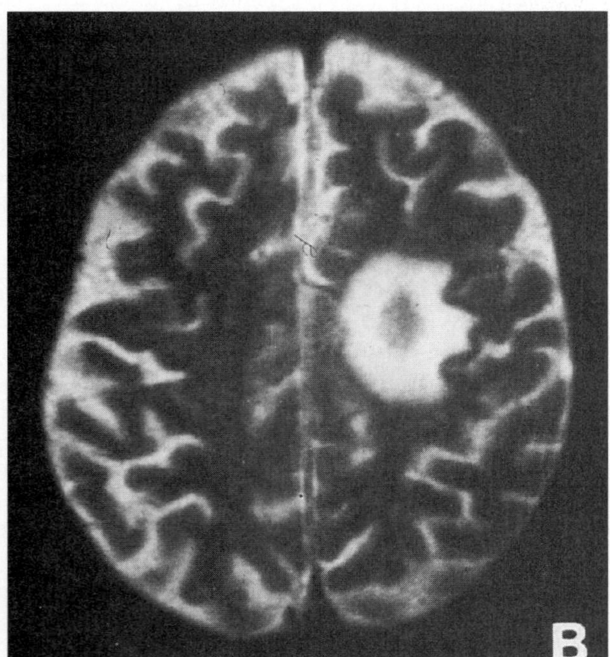

FIG. 231-3 Candidal abscess in AIDS. This T2-weighted magnetic resonance image shows a large left parietal lesion with a mass effect. This lesion is consistent with the diagnosis of toxoplasmosis or lymphoma, but in this patient it proved to be caused by ***Candida albicans***.

(Courtesy of Dr. G. Sze.)

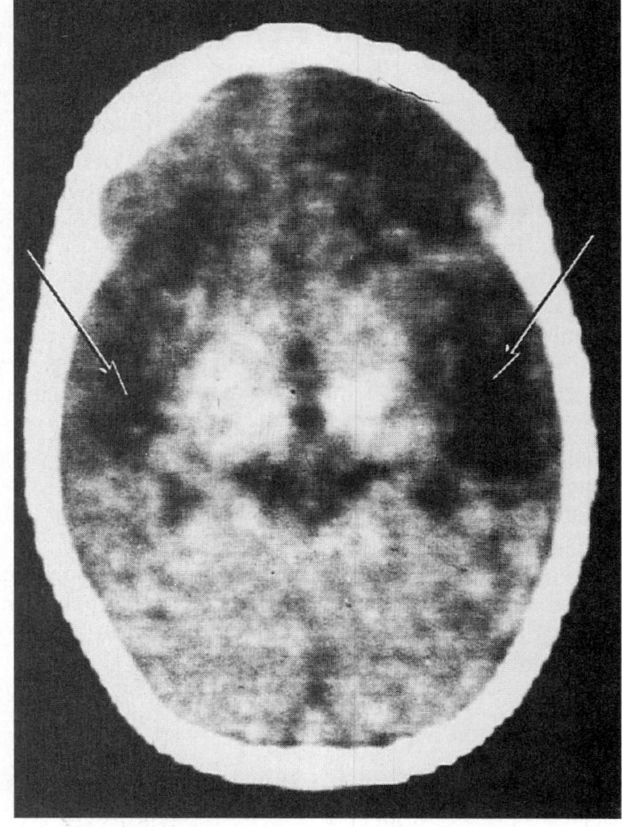

FIG. 231-4 Computed tomography (CT) brain scan of an infant who has herpes simplex encephalitis, showing complete necrosis of the frontotemporal regions *(arrows)*.

Table 231-1 Causes of Meningoencephalitis

Infectious	Postinfectious or unknown	Noninfectious causes of pleocytosis
Viral	Kawasaki syndrome	Intrathecal injections
Enterovirus	Mollaret syndrome	Leukemia
Coxsackievirus	Reye syndrome	Toxins (e.g., lead)
Poliovirus		Trauma
Myxovirus		Lymphoma
Mumps		
Measles		
Influenza		
Rhabdovirus (rabies)		
Arenavirus (lymphocytic choriomeningitis)		
Bunyavirus (California encephalitis)		
Togavirus		
Eastern equine encephalitis		
Western equine encephalitis		
St. Louis encephalitis		
Rubella		
Reovirus (Colorado tick fever)		
Herpesvirus		
Epstein-Barr virus		
Varicella-zoster virus		
Cytomegalovirus		
Adenovirus		
Human immunodeficiency virus		
Nonviral		
Brain or parameningeal bacterial abscess		
Amebae (*Naegleria* and *Acanthamoeba* spp.)		
Brucellosis		
Cat-scratch disease		
Fungi (e.g., *Candida* and *Cryptococcus* spp.)		
Leptospirosis		
Lyme disease *(Borrelia burgdorferi)*		
Lymphogranuloma venereum		
Mycoplasma spp.		
Pertussis		
Rocky Mountain spotted fever		
Syphilis		
Trichinosis		
Tuberculosis		

Table 231-2 Typical Cerebrospinal Fluid Findings in Meningoencephalitis and Bacterial Meningitis

CSF findings	Viral meningoencephalitis	Bacterial meningitis
Leukocytes	Initial predominance of polymorphonuclear neutrophils, followed by shift to mononuclear cells Range: 0-2000/mm^3	Predominantly neutrophils Range: 0-200,000/mm^3
Glucose	>50% of serum concentration	<30% of serum concentration
Protein	Mild to moderate elevation Range: usually <200 mg/dl	Marked elevation Range: usually >150 mg/dl
Gram stain	Negative	Usually reveals bacteria

consider the differential diagnosis carefully. Focal neurological signs often are present. Metabolic encephalopathy resulting from Reye syndrome or from lead, alcohol, or other toxins can be ruled out by appropriate laboratory investigations. The clinical course of a brain abscess usually is slower (Fig. 231-5), and focal findings may be present; a history of sinus infection, bronchiectasis, or congenital heart disease may be elicited. A myelitic form of viral nervous system infection may be mimicked by demyelinating disease or Guillain-Barré syndrome. MRI is superior for ruling out a spinal cord tumor, an arteriovenous malformation, or an infarction.

TREATMENT

Nonspecific treatment of a patient who has meningoencephalitis includes reducing increased intracranial pressure (see

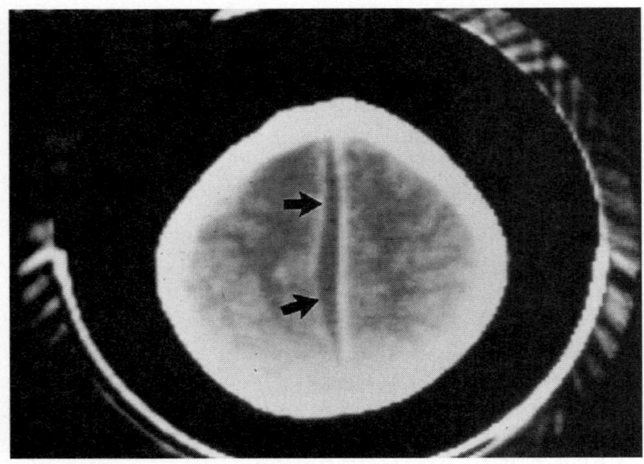

FIG. 231-5 Brain abscess. This MRI scan shows a brain abscess in the temporal lobe. This child had olfactory seizures after repair of his cyanotic heart disease.

Chapter 286), respiratory support, and treating seizures. Maintaining the fluid and electrolyte balance is essential because 64% of infants who have aseptic meningitis develop inappropriate secretion of antidiuretic hormone.[12] Corticosteroids have not proved useful in treating meningoencephalitis and may blunt host defenses.

Specific treatment of acute viral infections of the nervous system is called for with herpes simplex infections. Acyclovir has proved to be superior to vidarabine (ara-A) for parenteral use in herpes infections.[1] Although it is nephrotoxic, acyclovir generally is tolerated by neonates and by children who have renal dysfunction or renal transplants. Other antiviral agents (foscarnet, S-HPMPA) are being developed. Ganciclovir, an antiviral agent similar in structure to acyclovir, has been approved for use in CMV infections.[7] Zidovudine (AZT), an oral preparation, is being administered to symptomatic AIDS patients, although its usefulness is tempered by bone marrow toxicity.[10]

Another drug treatment that may be of benefit is intravenous immunoglobulin, which is known to contain viral antibodies for specific viral infections. These nonspecific immunoglobulin preparations have been used as replacement therapy or as adjuncts to treatment of meningoencephalitis in immunodeficient patients. However, immunoglobulin therapy for overwhelming viral sepsis remains controversial. Alpha-interferon has been used as prophylaxis against CMV and varicella-zoster in immunocompromised children but not as adjunct therapy in meningoencephalitis. Both active and passive postexposure prophylaxis is available for the treatment of rabies.[2]

Prevention is the most cost-effective method of reducing the morbidity and mortality caused by viral meningoencephalitis. Immunization has virtually eliminated poliomyelitis and rubella and has made mumps and measles meningoencephalitis extremely rare. Repeat measles immunizations of older children should reduce the incidence of measles encephalitis and SSPE further. The development of a varicella vaccine holds promise for lowering the morbidity from chickenpox.

PROGNOSIS

The developing nervous system may be more susceptible to viral infection and more likely to sustain serious sequelae. Eastern equine encephalitis, an infectious syndrome seen in children more commonly than in adults, often causes death within 48 hours. Those who survive frequently are severely impaired. Western equine encephalitis is associated with complete recovery in virtually all adults but causes death in 20% of children and a high prevalence of neurological residua among the survivors. Herpes simplex virus commonly produces a destructive encephalitis in neonates, infants, and children (see Fig. 231-4).

Even the more "benign" meningoencephalitides of infancy, such as those caused by enteroviruses, may result in substantial reductions in head circumference, intelligence, and learning ability. California encephalitis, a relatively mild arbovirus infection, causes emotional learning disorders in 15% of affected children.[4,13] Focal epilepsy may be a sequel of a "mild" encephalitis caused by Epstein-Barr virus.

It is essential that every child who has a documented or suspected viral nervous system infection be monitored carefully for auditory, visual, and cognitive aftereffects. Carefully performed prospective, sibling-matched controlled studies have shown that these children are at risk for cerebral cortical dysfunction.

REFERENCES

1. Arvin AA et al: Consensus management of the patient with herpes simplex encephalitis, *Pediatr Infect Dis J* 6:2, 1987.
2. Baevsky RH, Bartfield JM: Human rabies: a review, *Am J Emerg Med* 11:279, 1993.
3. Bell WE, McCormick WF: *Neurologic infections in children,* ed 2, Philadelphia, 1981, WB Saunders.
4. Bergman I: Outcome of children with enteroviral meningitis in the first year, *J Pediatr* 110:705, 1987.
5. Centers for Disease Control: Enteroviral disease in the U.S., 1970-1979, *J Infect Dis* 146:103, 1982.
6. Feigin RD, Cherry JD: *Textbook of pediatric infectious diseases,* ed 2, Philadelphia, 1987, WB Saunders.
7. Ganciclovir, *Med Lett Drugs Ther* 31:79, 1989.
8. Mizrahi EM, Tharp BR: A characteristic EEG pattern in neonatal herpes simplex encephalitis, *Neurology* 32:1215, 1982.
9. Pachner AR, Duray P, Steere AC: CNS manifestations of Lyme disease, *Arch Neurol* 46:790, 1989.
10. Pizzo PA: Therapeutic considerations for children with HIV infection, *AIDS Update* 2:1, 1989.
11. Pizzo PA, Eddy J, Falcon J: AIDS in children, *Am J Med* 85:195, 1988.
12. Rorabaugh ML et al: Aseptic meningitis in infants younger than 2 years of age: acute illness and neurologic complications, *Pediatrics* 92:206, 1993.
13. Sells SJ, Carpenter RL, Ray CG: Sequelae of central nervous system enterovirus infections, *N Engl J Med* 293:1, 1975.
14. Summary of notifiable diseases, U.S., *MMWR,* 1987.

232 Nephritis

Edward J. Ruley

Nephritis is the general term for noninfectious inflammation of the kidney parenchyma. This inflammation may involve primarily the glomerulus (glomerulonephritis), the interstitium (interstitial nephritis), or both. Because glomerulonephritis historically has been the subject of more intense interest, when the term *nephritis* is used, many practitioners think only of glomerular lesions. Even though glomerulonephritis is more common than either interstitial nephritis or combined glomerular and interstitial nephritis in children, the practitioner should have some knowledge of all three disorders.

CLASSIFICATION OF THE GLOMERULOPATHIES

Glomerulopathies previously have been classified according to a variety of schemes, such as the clinical course (e.g., acute, subacute, and chronic glomerulonephritis), the major clinical symptoms (e.g., Ellis types I and II), or some measurable serum abnormality (e.g., normocomplementemic and hypocomplementemic nephritides). All these classifications have proved to be of limited use. An ideal classification system based on cause is not possible because our understanding of the pathogenesis of many types of glomerulonephritis is incomplete. Furthermore, only a limited number of clinical presentations can be caused by a great variety of renal insults. Currently the preferred method of classification is based on glomerular morphological traits.

Understanding morphological classification requires a knowledge of normal renal and glomerular anatomy and of the terms *diffuse, focal, segmental,* and *global.* These terms describe the distribution of disease in the biopsy specimen (a diagram of their use is shown in Fig. 232-1). In glomerulonephritis, diffuse and focal apply to the distribution of disease among the glomeruli present in the biopsy specimen; *diffuse* means that all the glomeruli are involved, and *focal* means that only some glomeruli are involved. Similarly, in interstitial nephritis the inflammation can be diffuse (i.e., general and uniform) or focal (i.e., patchy and irregular).

The terms *segmental* and *global* apply only to glomerular disease, in which they describe the extent of disease involvement in each individual glomerulus; *global* means complete glomerular involvement, and *segmental* means irregular involvement with some loops being normal. Thus glomerular lesions may be described as diffuse and segmental, indicating partial involvement of all the glomeruli in the biopsy specimen, or focal and global, indicating complete involvement of some of the glomeruli, and so on.

One classification scheme based on glomerular morphology is given in the box on p. 1436. In this scheme the category of minimal glomerular lesions includes those that have normal or minimally abnormal glomeruli. The minimal abnormalities usually consist of a mild increase in the amount of mesangium or number of cells (mild hypercellularity). The category of specific glomerular lesions includes more severe lesions characterized by morphological changes attributable to a defined cause. The largest category is that of nonspecific lesions, in which pathological patterns can be defined but the disorder may have more than one cause. Finally, a category of unclassifiable glomerulopathies is included.

The following discussion deals with the common patterns of presentation in an effort to develop a structured way of thinking about the diagnostic possibilities for each clinical problem. It should be recognized that this is only one way of conceptualizing an approach. Furthermore, these clinical patterns are only crude categorizations, and a specific etiology may manifest in a variety of ways. The clinical patterns to be discussed include (1) acute nephritic syndrome, (2) intermittent gross hematuria and proteinuria syndromes, and (3) chronic glomerulonephritis syndromes. In each disease the classification by glomerular involvement is indicated. The disorders of minimal change disease, membranous glomerulopathy, focal glomerular sclerosis, and the nephropathy of chronic bacteremia are discussed in Chapter 233, on nephrotic syndrome, which is their most common pattern of presentation.

ACUTE NEPHRITIC SYNDROME

Acute nephritic syndrome is characterized by hematuria, hypertension, and edema. The hematuria usually is grossly evident, although in some children it may be microscopic only. Red blood cell (RBC) casts and dysmorphic RBCs always are present,[2] although several urine samples may have to be examined to demonstrate them (Fig. 232-2). The edema usually is periorbital and rarely severe. This syndrome is discussed as two clinical presentations: acute nephritic syndrome with no or mild renal failure and acute nephritic syndrome with rapidly progressive renal failure.

Acute Nephritic Syndrome with No or Mild Renal Failure

Acute nephritic syndrome often is the initial symptom in the renal diseases listed in the box on p. 1436.

Acute Poststreptococcal Glomerulonephritis. Acute poststreptococcal glomerulonephritis is a common form of glomerulonephritis in childhood. The true incidence is unknown, inasmuch as only a minority of patients who have this illness have symptoms. Although poststreptococcal nephritis may happen at any age, the peak incidence occurs at age 7, with a slight predominance among boys. It is uncommon before age 3 and in adults.

ETIOLOGY. Poststreptococcal nephritis is the consequence of the host's immune response to a nonrenal infection with group A beta-hemolytic streptococci (GABHS). Not all

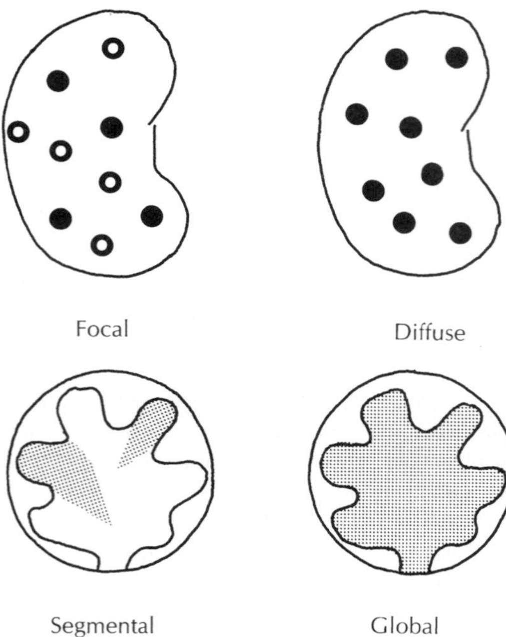

FIG. 232-1 Diagram of the use of the terms *diffuse, focal, segmental,* and *global* in describing glomerular pathological conditions.

MORPHOLOGICAL CLASSIFICATION OF GLOMERULOPATHIES

I. Minimal glomerular lesions (e.g., idiopathic nephrotic syndrome, asymptomatic proteinuria, and asymptomatic hematuria)
II. Specific glomerular lesions (e.g., malarial nephropathy, amyloidosis, diabetic glomerulosclerosis, and thrombotic microangiopathy of hemolytic-uremic syndrome)
III. Nonspecific glomerular lesions
  A. Diffuse glomerular lesions
    1. Nonproliferative (e.g., membranous nephropathy)
    2. Proliferative (e.g., mesangial proliferative glomerulonephritis, membranoproliferative glomerulonephritis, and endocapillary and extracapillary glomerulonephritis with and without crescents)
  B. Focal glomerular lesions
    1. Nonproliferative (e.g., focal glomerulosclerosis)
    2. Proliferative (e.g., focal and segmental proliferative glomerulonephritis
IV. Unclassified glomerular lesions (e.g., Alport syndrome, focal membranoproliferative glomerulonephritis, and lesions too advanced to classify)

Modified from Habib R: Classification of glomerular nephropathies. In Rubin M, Barratt TM, editors: *Pediatric nephrology,* Baltimore, 1975, Williams & Wilkins.

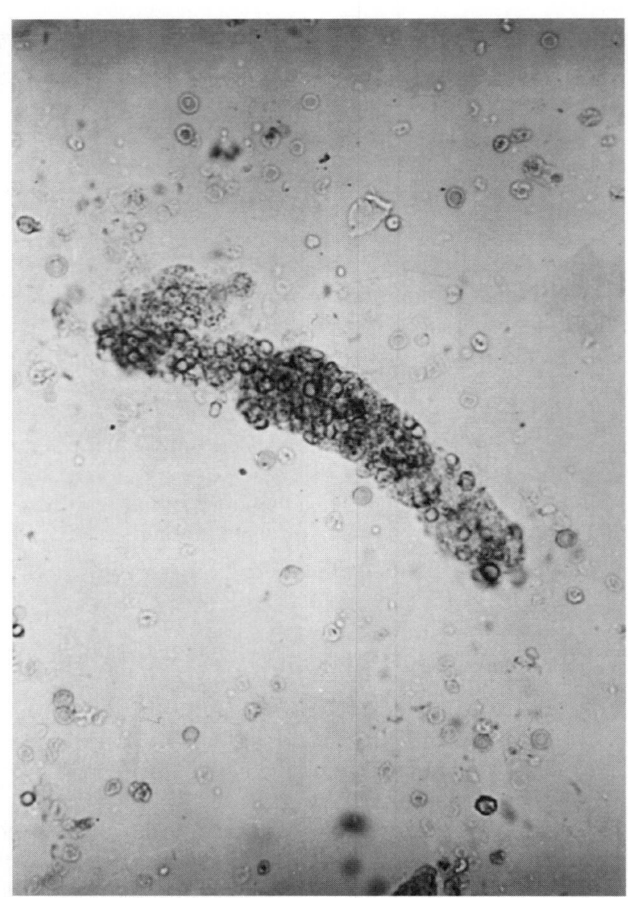

FIG. 232-2 Red blood cell cast—unstained.

DISEASES IN CHILDREN THAT MAY INVOLVE ACUTE NEPHRITIC SYNDROME WITH NO OR MILD RENAL FAILURE

More commonly present

Acute poststreptococcal glomerulonephritis
Henoch-Schönlein purpura with nephritis
Postinfectious (nonstreptococcal) glomerulonephritis
Interstitial glomerulonephritis
Radiation nephritis

Less commonly present

Acute episodes in patients with chronic glomerulonephritis
Hemolytic-uremic syndrome (milder cases)
Membranoproliferative glomerulonephritis (some)
Nephritis of systemic lupus erythematosus (some)

GABHS strains are nephritogenic. Type 12 is the most common nephritogenic strain, whereas types 1, 4, 45, 47, and 55 occur less often. The nephritogenicity of types 3, 6, and 25 is less certain. Recent work has suggested that endostreptocin, a cytoplasmic protein found in large amounts in nephritogenic streptococci, may be the antigen to which the patient reacts.[11] Furthermore, recent evidence suggests that the formation of immune complexes occurs in situ in the kidneys rather than as a passive filtration of preformed immune complexes.[10] Infection with a nephritogenic strain does not guarantee an episode of nephritis, because a variety of incompletely understood factors determines the host response. Renal involvement characteristically manifests 1 to 3 weeks after a pharyngeal or skin infection caused by the nephritogenic streptococci.

PATHOLOGY. Grossly, the kidneys are enlarged and pallid. The typical glomerular morphology is that of diffuse, uniform, cellular proliferation, although it is difficult to determine the type of cell involved. The glomerular tufts are larger than normal, and the capillary lumens are reduced. Polymorphonuclear leukocytes may be present. There is an increase in mesangial matrix, but the basement membranes are normal. On immunofluorescent microscopy examination, deposits of immunoglobulin and complement can be seen. With the use of electron microscopy, electron-dense structures (presumed to be immune deposits) can be seen on the epithelial side of the basement membrane. With healing, the increased cellularity and immune deposits become limited to the mesangial region and then gradually resolve.

CLINICAL PRESENTATION. Most patients who have acute poststreptococcal nephritis have acute nephritic syndrome, with macroscopic hematuria in about half of the cases. Approximately 60% to 70% of the patients have hypertension to some degree. Patients who have severe hypertension may have symptoms of headache, drowsiness, vomiting, personality and visual changes, and convulsions. Although arteriole spasm is common on funduscopic examination, papilledema and hemorrhages are rare, even with severe hypertension. Edema usually is periorbital and rarely severe. Patients may show cardiovascular disturbances similar to those of congestive heart failure. Patients usually have oliguria (urine output less than 240 ml/m^2/day) and, in rare cases, anuria. Anorexia and pain in the abdomen or flank are common, although palpation of the abdomen usually reveals no significant findings. Costovertebral angle tenderness often is present. Although a history of preceding skin or pharyngeal infection supports the diagnosis, such a history cannot be elicited in many cases. Patients rarely have joint symptoms or urinary outlet symptoms, such as urinary frequency, urgency, or dysuria. In rare cases a patient who has convulsions or symptoms of cardiovascular dysfunction as the primary complaint actually has unrecognized poststreptococcal nephritis.

LABORATORY FINDINGS. The urine usually is tea colored and opaque. The specific gravity generally is increased, and hemoglobin can be detected by chemical testing. Any proteinuria that is present usually parallels the degree of hematuria and rarely is the level seen in nephrotic syndrome. Microscopic examination usually reveals erythrocyturia, pyuria, and granular or cellular casts. Because identifiable erythrocyte casts and dysmorphic erythrocytes may or may not be present, serial urine specimens may need to be examined. In rare cases a patient may have a normal urinalysis despite having all other signs of acute glomerulonephritis.

Measurement of the serum complement shows a reduction of C3 in 80% of the patients and C4 in 50%. The erythrocyte sedimentation rate (ESR) usually is elevated. With severe oliguria, azotemia and acidosis may been seen. The plasma volume usually is expanded, causing a decline in serum protein, hemoglobin, and hematocrit levels. Hemolysis, a shortened erythrocyte half-life, and reduced erythrocyte production may contribute to these hematological changes.

Evidence of a preceding streptococcal infection is important to support the diagnosis. The antistreptolysin O (ASO) titer is elevated in 80% of patients, although increases in titer are less common in patients who have skin infection and in those who receive early treatment with antibiotics. If other streptococcal antibodies (antihyaluronidase, antideoxyribonuclease B) are measured, 95% of patients have serological evidence of preceding streptococcal infection. Cultures often are negative for GABHS by the time nephritis develops and are affected particularly by pretreatment with antibiotics.

Roentgenograms of the chest in patients who have hypertension usually reveal a large heart with prominent pulmonary vasculature, pulmonary edema or, in rare cases, hydrothorax.[5] Ultrasound examination usually reveals bilaterally enlarged kidneys.

COURSE. The oliguria and hypertension usually last 4 or 5 days, although in some patients they may last much longer. The onset of diuresis usually heralds resolution of the disease. Gross hematuria resolves within 1 or 2 weeks, although urinary abnormalities may persist for 6 to 12 weeks. Some patients have microscopic hematuria for as long as 2 years and still recover completely. Complement levels should rise gradually to normal by 3 to 6 weeks.

TREATMENT. Acute poststreptococcal glomerulonephritis most often heals spontaneously and is not affected by corticosteroids or immunosuppressive agents. Even so, the practitioner must be aggressive in treating hypertension, oliguria, and the resulting vascular congestion, pulmonary edema, and encephalopathy that occur in the acute phase of the illness because these can be fatal.

Although mild hypertension may resolve spontaneously, more severe degrees of hypertension should be controlled with antihypertensive agents that act quickly. Potent diuretics (furosemide and ethacrynic acid) are logical choices because an expanded vascular volume is theorized to be the determinant of hypertension in acute nephritic syndrome.[5] Diuretics often are ineffective when used in conventional doses. Nifedipine (0.15 to 0.6 mg/kg) can be used sublingually. For small children the approximate amount of drug can be removed from a nifedipine capsule, mixed with 0.5 to 1 ml water, and placed beneath the tongue with a syringe. Diazoxide (2 to 5 mg/kg) injected rapidly intravenously and oral minoxidil (0.1 to 0.2 mg/kg/dose) also can be used. Slower-acting, less potent antihypertensive drugs are not good choices.

Oliguria should be allowed to follow its course of natural resolution and cannot be hastened by administering fluid boluses. Furthermore, excessive fluid administration is contraindicated because it worsens hypertension. The signs of congestive heart failure usually resolve with control of the hypertension. Occasionally a patient develops acute renal failure severe enough to require dialysis.

A 10-day course of antibiotics usually is given to eradicate any remaining GABHS and thus prevent spread of the organism to others. There is no evidence that such treatment affects the course of nephritis in the patient.

Hospitalization for patients who have this disease needs to be determined individually. Although many children who have mild episodes do well as outpatients, the sudden development of hypertension and oliguria may produce life-threatening symptoms quite rapidly. Bed rest may be indicated as a precaution for a patient who has hypertension and may be associated with a decline in the degree of hematuria, but there is no evidence that it affects the healing of the glomerular lesion. Therefore hematuria alone is not an indication for bed rest. After the acute phase, the child may be allowed to resume normal activities gradually. Every child should be followed up regularly until the complement values return to normal. To be certain of the diagnosis, a renal biopsy may be indicated for a child whose clinical or laboratory findings are atypical. Any child whose C3 value does not return to normal within 8 weeks should have a kidney biopsy.

PROGNOSIS. Studies have shown that more than 90% of children who have acute poststreptococcal glomerulonephritis recover from their illness. For most children the critical period is early in the illness, when fatal hypertension or fluid overload presents a danger. Occasionally patients who have severe involvement have some residual damage as evidenced by proteinuria, but in general the kidneys have an outstanding recovery potential in this disease.[3]

Henoch-Schönlein Purpura with Nephritis. This illness may have an acute nephritic onset (see Chapter 212).

Postinfectious (Nonstreptococcal) Glomerulonephritis. A variety of viruses are suspected of causing an acute nephritic syndrome, including varicella, echovirus 10, and coxsackieviruses, as well as the viruses that cause mononucleosis, measles, and mumps. However, significant renal involvement is unusual in infections caused by these viruses. Children who have such involvement have normal complement levels and no serological evidence of recent streptococcal infection. In most cases the acute nephritic syndrome resolves spontaneously and gradually, and renal function returns completely. There is no effective way to differentiate the nonstreptococcal postinfectious glomerulonephritides from the other normocomplementemic nephritides that progress to renal failure except by observing the clinical course.

Other Renal Diseases That May Involve Acute Nephritic Syndrome with No or Mild Renal Failure. Occasionally patients who have undiscovered chronic renal failure suffer a sudden deterioration that may be interpreted as an acute nephritic syndrome (see the box on p. 1436). Evaluation of these patients often reveals evidence of preexisting chronic renal failure, such as osteodystrophy or hyperphosphatemia. Hemolytic-uremic syndrome (see Chapter 210) characteristically occurs as an acute nephritic syndrome. Systemic lupus erythematosus (SLE) may appear to be an acute nephritic syndrome but more often is discovered coincidentally during evaluation of other complaints related to the lupus syndrome. Likewise, membranoproliferative glomerulonephritis or the nephritis of chronic infection initially may manifest acutely with low complement values. However, more often this disease appears as nephrotic syndrome or chronic glomerulonephritis.

Acute Nephritic Syndrome with Rapidly Progressive Renal Failure

This variant of acute nephritic syndrome is characterized by symptoms of acute nephritis associated with relentless progression to renal failure over days or weeks.[9] Although acute interstitial nephritis stemming from pyelonephritis or hypersensitivity may occur in this way, most cases result from glomerular disease, giving rise to the term *rapidly progressive glomerulonephritis* (RPGN). As shown in the box above RPGN can be classified into three categories on the basis of immunopathological findings as seen in kidney biopsies.[4]

CLASSIFICATION OF ACUTE NEPHRITIC SYNDROME WITH RAPIDLY PROGRESSIVE RENAL FAILURE

Immune complex

Postinfectious reaction
- Streptococcal infection
- Visceral abscess
- Other

Collagen-vascular disease
- Systemic lupus erythematosis
- Henoch-Schönlein purpura
- Mixed cryoglobulinemia

Primary renal disease
- IgA nephropathy
- Membranoproliferative glomerulonephritis
- Unknown cases (i.e., idiopathic)

No immune deposit

Unknown cause

Vasculitis
- Polyarteritis
- Wegener granulomatosis
- Hypersensitivity vasculitides

Anti–Glomerular Basement Membrane Antibody

With lung hemorrhage (Goodpasture syndrome)
Without lung hemorrhage
Complicating membranous nephropathy

Modified from Couser WG: *Am J Kidney Dis* 11:449, 1988.

The most common cause of RPGN in pediatric patients is poststreptococcal glomerulonephritis. The diagnosis depends on obtaining a history of a recent sore throat or skin infection and finding reduced serum complement values associated with serological evidence of a recent streptococcal infection. A large proportion of patients who have poststreptococcal RPGN recover spontaneously, provided their course is managed well during the acute phase.

RPGN may be caused by Henoch-Schönlein purpura, although this occurs in children considerably less often than the poststreptococcal and idiopathic (nonstreptococcal) varieties. The multisystem clinical presentation, negative streptococcal serological findings, normal serum complement values, and renal biopsy findings characterize this cause. Some reports suggest that high-dose intravenous corticosteroids, if given early in the course, promote recovery in these patients. Of the primary renal disease group, IgA nephropathy and membranoproliferative glomerulonephritis (types I and II) occur this way in rare cases.

RPGN without immune deposits is much less common among pediatric patients; anti–glomerular basement membrane (GBM) antibody-mediated RPGN is even more rare. Hemolytic-uremic syndrome (HUS) and disseminated intravascular coagulopathy (DIC) must be included in the differential diagnosis, inasmuch as hematuria and rapidly progressive renal failure are common features of their presentations. Hypertension, however, is less common in these two diagnoses. Although the characteristic clinical and laboratory features of these diseases may suggest specific etiological factors, a renal biopsy usually is indicated to make the diagnosis and to determine the extent of the disease.[9]

INTERMITTENT GROSS HEMATURIA AND PROTEINURIA SYNDROMES

The proteinuria in recurrent gross hematuria syndrome is in excess of that expected from bleeding alone. Between episodes, microscopic hematuria and proteinuria often are present, although in some patients the urine is completely normal. The more common illnesses that can cause these syndromes are IgA-IgG nephropathy (nephropathy of Berger), familial (benign) hematuria, hereditary nephritis, and Henoch-Schönlein purpura syndrome.

IgA-IgG Nephropathy

IgA-IgG nephropathy first was described by Berger in 1969 and has been called *Berger disease*. The cause is unknown.

Pathology. The typical lesion is a focal segmental proliferation of mesangial cells, with an increase in mesangial matrix. Immunofluorescent examination reveals mesangial deposits of IgA, IgG, and C3. This lesion is difficult to differentiate morphologically from that of Henoch-Schönlein purpura, which has led to speculation that the former is a partial clinical expression of the latter.

Clinical Presentation. Characteristically, children with Berger disease have a sudden onset of asymptomatic gross hematuria and proteinuria either without intercurrent illness or concomitant with a nonstreptococcal upper respiratory tract infection.[6,8] Hypertension usually is not present. The simultaneous onset of the upper respiratory tract infection and the gross hematuria helps differentiate this disease from acute poststreptococcal glomerulonephritis, in which a delay between infection and hematuria is the rule. The absence of rash, abdominal pain, and arthritis helps differentiate IgA-IgG nephropathy from the nephritis of Henoch-Schönlein purpura nephritis. Atypically, patients who have IgA nephropathy can have nephrotic syndrome or acute renal failure.

Laboratory Findings. IgA-IgG nephropathy is characterized by a lack of abnormal laboratory findings except for the urinalysis. In particular, hypocomplementemia and serological evidence of recent streptococcal infection usually are absent. Azotemia, when it does occur, is a poor prognostic sign. A renal biopsy may be indicated in some patients to confirm the diagnosis and to clarify the prognosis.

Course. The gross hematuria usually resolves spontaneously as the upper respiratory tract infection abates. Many patients continue to have microscopic hematuria and small amounts of proteinuria, although in some the urinalysis findings revert to completely normal. With future intercurrent illness the gross hematuria tends to recur.

Treatment. No treatment has yet proved effective for IgA-IgG nephropathy.

Prognosis. Although the prognosis originally was considered excellent, now it is anticipated that about 10% of pediatric patients progress to renal failure. Progression has been related to the amount of proteinuria and the severity of histological changes found on the kidney biopsy.[1,7]

Familial Hematuria

Familial hematuria is a benign condition inherited as an autosomal dominant trait. Undoubtedly, many of the early reports included patients who had IgA-IgG nephropathy because of the similarities of clinical presentation and because renal biopsy specimens often were not obtained. This condition also has been called *benign recurrent hematuria*.

Etiology. The cause of familial hematuria is not known.

Pathology. Usually light and fluorescent microscopy examinations reveal renal biopsy specimen findings to be normal. Focal or diffuse thinning of the basement membranes often is present on electron microscopy examination.

Clinical Presentation. Most often, children who have familial hematuria have episodes of asymptomatic gross hematuria and minimal to mild proteinuria.

Laboratory Findings. All laboratory test results usually are normal except for the urinalysis. The presence of hematuria in family members suggests this diagnosis. The absence of notable proteinuria, deafness, ocular defects, and renal failure in older family members who have hematuria differentiates this from the hereditary nephritides.

Course. Because recurrent microscopic hematuria with intercurrent infections is common, familial hematuria cannot be differentiated clinically from IgA-IgG nephropathy. Microhematuria usually is present constantly, although it can vary in degree. Proteinuria is never severe and may be present only during episodes of macrohematuria.

Treatment. No treatment is indicated for familial hematuria.

Prognosis. The prognosis is excellent.

Hereditary Nephritis

Hereditary nephritis often manifests as recurrent episodes of hematuria. The best known form is Alport syndrome, in which a hereditary nephritis is associated with neurogenic deafness and (occasionally) ocular abnormalities. Most patients who have the classic form of Alport syndrome inherit it as an autosomal dominant trait. The combination of Alport features and macrothrombocytopenia is known as Epstein syndrome. In addition, some forms of hereditary nephritis are not associated with deafness. Classification of all these hereditary diseases is the subject of molecular genetic study, and their interrelationships should become obvious in the future. A variety of pathological changes have been reported in kidneys obtained from patients who have hereditary nephritis. The most common glomerular alterations include cellular proliferation, focal scarring, focal basement membrane thickening, and periglomerular fibrosis. Often the tubules show varying degrees of atrophy, with mononuclear cell infiltration. So-called foam cells may be seen but are by no means pathognomonic for hereditary nephritis, as originally thought. Immunofluorescent studies of kidney biopsies often are negative, although C3 deposition has been noted in a few cases. Attempts have been made to subclassify familial nephritis by its appearance on electron microscopy examination.

The most common clinical presentation in a child and adolescent is one of recurrent macrohematuria, usually occurring with upper respiratory tract infections or exercise and associated with varying degrees of proteinuria. Microhematuria persists between the episodes of macrohematuria, although its severity also varies. A severe degree of proteinuria usually does not occur until late in the disease, although occasionally it may precede the hematuria, producing nephrotic syndrome when the patient is seen initially. In classic Alport syndrome, high-frequency nerve deafness is more common in boys and usually develops after the onset of renal disease. It is recognized in 75% of these patients before age 15. The hearing impairment may not be noticed at first because the conversational ranges are spared initially. The impairment usually is bilateral but can be asymmetrical. Deafness may skip some generations, only to reappear in later ones and can occur in carriers of the disease who do not have the nephropathy. Detection of a hearing impairment in girls often requires use of audiometry. The ocular abnormalities vary in occurrence and include cataracts, lenticonus, spherophakia (which can produce myopia), nystagmus, and retinitis pigmentosa. In Epstein syndrome, abnormally large platelets associated with defective platelet function have been noted.

Abnormal laboratory findings vary and are nonspecific. Serum complement values usually are normal. A renal biopsy may help to establish the diagnosis in some patients.

The progression of hereditary nephritis to chronic renal failure varies but tends to be the same within a family. The disease generally is more severe in boys, although occasionally a girl progresses to end-stage renal failure. Increasing proteinuria is considered to be evidence of progression. Deafness generally indicates more severe renal involvement and thus a worse prognosis for both genders. Hypertension usually is not prominent. No specific therapy is available. Chronic renal failure is treated in the usual manner, and dialysis and transplantation have been used in some patients. Hearing aids and surgery are of no value for the deafness.

Henoch-Schönlein Purpura Syndrome

Commonly, patients who have Henoch-Schönlein purpura have periodic recurrences of hematuria and proteinuria, often associated with recurrent infections. The presence of a rash and evidence of involvement of other organ systems besides the kidneys help differentiate this syndrome from IgA-IgG nephropathy.

CHRONIC GLOMERULONEPHRITIS SYNDROME

Chronic glomerulonephritis syndrome consists of diminished renal function associated with signs of the detrimental effects of this abnormality on other organ systems. It may be discovered under almost any clinical circumstance, but is found most often as the practitioner investigates nonspecific complaints such as anorexia, intermittent vomiting, and malaise that are found to result from undiagnosed chronic renal failure. The more common disorders are nephritis of SLE, membranoproliferative glomerulonephritis, and "chronic glomerulonephritis." Nonnephritic causes such as renal dysplasia and obstructive uropathies with significant unrecognized parenchymal damage should be considered in the differential diagnosis.

Nephritis of Systemic Lupus Erythematosus

Nephritis of systemic lupus erythematosus is a multisystem disease that occurs mostly in girls (80% to 90%) during their adolescent years. There is an increased familial incidence of the disease.

Etiology. SLE is considered a classic immune complex disease resulting from autoimmunity to endogenous DNA. Both familial predisposition and viral infection have been suggested as important factors.

Pathology. Although the renal disease can vary considerably in presentation, several common patterns have been identified. These include a focal segmental proliferative, a diffuse proliferative, and a membranous lesion. On fluorescent antibody examination, deposition of immunoglobulin and complement components usually is seen. Complement deposition often can be demonstrated even in glomeruli that appear normal on light microscopy examination. Electron microscopy examination often reveals evidence of immune complex deposition, cellular proliferation, and basement membrane thickening. Use of renal biopsies has allowed subcategorization of many of these cases, and attempts are being made to correlate these subcategories with the clinical course.

Clinical Presentation. Although renal involvement in this multisystem disease is common and important as the eventual cause of morbidity and mortality, symptoms of renal involvement usually are not severe enough at the onset to prompt the patient to seek medical attention. More commonly, the patient's complaints relate to skin rash or joint or cardiac involvement. Even if renal disease is not present at the onset, some renal abnormalities develop in most patients as their disease continues. These abnormalities may fit any of the described clinical patterns, including nephrotic syndrome or acute nephritic syndrome.

Laboratory Findings. Serological evidence of SLE can be obtained through a variety of tests that detect DNA antibodies in the patient's serum. These tests include the LE cell test (positive findings in approximately 60% of cases), the fluorescent antinuclear antibody (FANA) test (positive findings in approximately 94% of cases), and the circulating DNA antibody tests (positive findings in more than 95% of cases). None of these tests is specific for SLE.

Serum complement values usually are reduced with acute renal disease and correlate with the activity of the SLE. Other common serological abnormalities include positive test results for rheumatoid factor and false positive test results for syphilis, cryoprecipitable proteins, and Coombs antibodies.

The severity and type of renal involvement (e.g., nephrotic syndrome, chronic renal failure) determine the degree of hypoproteinemia, azotemia, and other manifestations of renal failure. These changes are nonspecific.

Urinalysis usually reveals proteinuria, hematuria, cylindruria, and pyuria. A "telescoped sediment" that consists of every type of element is not pathognomonic of SLE. Changes in urinary sediment are *not* a good indication of disease activity.

Course. The course of SLE varies considerably. Renal manifestations can wax and wane with changes in disease activity, intercurrent illness, and type of therapy.

Treatment. High-dose corticosteroid therapy can reduce the morbidity and mortality from the nephritis of SLE. A renal biopsy should be performed *before* therapy is begun. Treatment usually is associated with varying degrees of steroid-induced side effects that can be as troubling to the patient as the SLE. Other immunosuppressive agents such as intravenous cytoxan are being investigated. The danger of overwhelming sepsis among these immunosuppressed patients is constant. The effectiveness of therapy can be based on changes in serological parameters, blood chemistries, and complement levels. Care of the patient who has lupus is a highly specialized endeavor that requires knowledge of current treatment modalities, the availability of highly specialized tests, and the willingness to deal with a patient who has a chronic, severe, life-threatening illness for which treatment often is disfiguring. These patients are managed best by a team trained in dealing with these aspects.

Prognosis. Childhood SLE has a high incidence of renal involvement, and the survival rate for those who have such involvement is much lower than for those who do not have it. Although nephrotic syndrome generally is associated with a poor prognosis, renal biopsy provides the best means to anticipate the outcome. For this reason it is important to obtain a biopsy specimen early in the course of the illness. Persons who have focal glomerulonephritis rarely progress to renal failure. Diffuse proliferative glomerulonephritis, however, is associated with nephrotic syndrome in more than 50% and hypertension in 33% of the cases; it commonly progresses to renal failure. The membranous lesion also is commonly associated with nephrotic syndrome and may progress to renal failure, although progression usually is slower than with the diffuse proliferative lesion.

Membranoproliferative Glomerulonephritis

Membranoproliferative glomerulonephritis occurs most commonly among older children and young adults, with a slight seasonal predilection for winter. It accounts for 20% to 25% of chronic glomerulonephritis among children. It also has been called chronic hypocomplementemic glomerulonephritis and mesangiocapillary nephritis.

Etiology. The cause of membranoproliferative glomerulonephritis is unknown, and there is no evidence that it is the sequela of streptococcal nephritis.

Pathology. Typically the glomeruli are enlarged and lobulated because of increased mesangial cellularity and matrix. Irregular areas of capillary wall thickening and hyalinization are produced by the presence of nonargyrophilic material. Fluorescent examination usually reveals extensive capillary loop complement deposition (particularly C3) with lesser amounts of IgG and IgM. Several subtypes have been described.

Clinical Presentation. Many children who have membranoproliferative glomerulonephritis initially have nephrotic syndrome or an acute nephritic syndrome, although the disease may be discovered as part of an evaluation of microscopic hematuria. Hypertension and hematuria are common in patients who have nephrotic syndrome. The onset of acute nephritic syndrome cannot be differentiated easily from acute poststreptococcal glomerulonephritis, particularly because both may be associated with hypocomplementemia at the outset. Hypertension may be prominent at the onset in some patients but eventually develops in nearly all patients who progress to renal failure.

Laboratory Findings. Abnormal laboratory findings vary. Renal function often remains normal for a long time. The most typical finding is a persistent reduction in serum C3 with normal C1, C4, and C2. Continual C3 reduction, even after clinical recovery, has been described and is called the *silent phase*. Reduced C3 for longer than 6 to 8 weeks after an acute nephritic syndrome should alert the practitioner to the possibility of membranoproliferative glomerulonephritis. Many patients also have anemia of a severity out of proportion to the degree of azotemia. If renal failure develops later, the patient will have all the usual nonspecific abnormal laboratory findings associated with insufficient renal function. Occasionally C3 levels rise at this time, although they may not completely return to normal.

Course. The course of membranoproliferative glomerulonephritis varies, but half of these patients progress to renal failure by the eleventh year after diagnosis.

Treatment. Currently, no treatment regimens are generally accepted, although a variety of drugs are under investigation. Pediatric nephrology consultation is advised for patients suspected of having this diagnosis (e.g., those who have persistent hypocomplementemia). It is important to provide long-term follow-up care for patients who have this diagnosis because of the documented asymptomatic silent phases and the potential for late renal failure.

Prognosis. The prognosis of membranoproliferative glomerulonephritis is quite variable. Some have suggested that progression to renal failure is slowed if the patient is treated with every-other-day steroids. Furthermore, there is a variable rate of disease recurrence in renal allografts, although such recurrence does not inevitably lead to loss of graft function.

"Chronic Glomerulonephritis"

Chronic glomerulonephritis is a general category for less understood, progressive renal lesions that cause renal failure. Often patients who have severe renal lesions that have progressed so far that the initial process no longer can be recognized are grouped in this category. It is hoped that in the future specific disorders will be recognized and separated from this heterogeneous group.

INTERSTITIAL NEPHRITIS

Inflammation of the interstitium is much less common than glomerular inflammation. The principal manifestations of interstitial inflammation are related to the consequent tubular dysfunction: inability to resorb glucose-producing glucosuria despite normoglycemia, inability to resorb water resulting in urine with a low fixed specific gravity, inability to resorb minerals causing a "salt-losing" syndrome, and inability to resorb bicarbonate and secrete hydrogen ions giving rise to renal tubular acidosis. Hypertension and fluid overload are unusual in these patients, in contrast to children who have isolated glomerulonephritis. Interstitial nephritis may be seen on renal biopsies concomitantly with severe glomerulonephritis when it is the consequence of degeneration of the tubules of the most severely affected glomeruli. This combination has a much more guarded prognosis because the combined glomerular and interstitial involvement reflects the greater severity of the renal disease. In this circumstance the interstitial inflammation tends to heal by fibrosis, thereby damaging segments of the remaining kidney. The finding of glomerulonephritis associated with tubular dysfunction should be evaluated by kidney biopsy.

REFERENCES

1. Berg UB: Long-term follow-up of renal function in IgA nephropathy, *Arch Dis Child* 66:588, 1991.
2. Birch DF et al: Urinary erythrocyte morphology in the diagnosis of glomerular hematuria, *Clin Nephrol* 20:78, 1983.
3. Buzio C et al: Significance of albuminuria in the follow-up of acute poststreptococcal glomerulonephritis, *Clin Nephrol* 41:259, 1994.
4. Couser WG: Rapidly progressive glomerulonephritis: classification, pathogenetic mechanisms, and therapy, *Am J Kidney Dis* 11:449, 1988.
5. Fleisher DS et al: Hemodynamic findings in acute glomerulonephritis, *J Pediatr* 69:1054, 1966.
6. Gallo GH: IgA nephropathy, *Kidney Int* 47:377, 1995.
7. Gallo GR et al: Prognostic pathologic markers in IgA nephropathy, *Am J Kidney Dis* 12:362, 1988.
8. Hogg RJ: IgA nephropathy: clinical features and natural history: a pediatric perspective, *Am J Kidney Dis* 12:358, 1988.
9. Jardim H et al: Crescentic glomerulonephritis in children, *Pediatr Nephrol* 6:231, 1992.
10. Lange K, Seligson G, Cronin W: Evidence for the in situ origin of poststreptococcal glomerulonephritis: glomerular localization of endostreptosin and the clinical significance of the subsequent antibody response, *Clin Nephrol* 19:3, 1983.
11. Lange K et al: A hitherto unknown streptococcal antigen and its probable relation to acute poststreptococcal glomerulonephritis, *Clin Nephrol* 5:207, 1976.

233 Nephrotic Syndrome

Edward J. Ruley

Nephrotic syndrome is characterized by massive proteinuria, hypoproteinemia (particularly hypoalbuminemia), hyperlipidemia, and edema. The incidence of nephrotic syndrome is 1.2 to 2.3 per 100,000 population per year,[9] with the occurrence 15 times more common among children than adults. Two thirds of children who have nephrotic syndrome have the onset between 1 and 5 years of age. In early childhood, nephrotic syndrome develops two to three times more frequently in boys than in girls; by the middle teens, the occurrence is equal in both genders.

ETIOLOGY

Nephrotic syndrome is not an entity but rather a true syndrome in that it can result from diverse causes. Nephrotic syndrome may occur in association with (1) metabolic diseases such as diabetes mellitus and amyloidosis, (2) immune and hypersensitivity diseases such as systemic lupus erythematosus and periarteritis nodosa, (3) nephrotoxin administration such as mercury and trimethadione, (4) allergies resulting from contactants and envenomations, (5) infections such as tuberculosis and malaria, or (6) it can be of undetermined (idiopathic) cause.

In the past the syndrome has been subclassified by a variety of systems in an effort to detect patterns of cause, response to therapy, and prognosis. One of the most definitive classifications was developed by the International Collaborative Study of Kidney Disease in Children on the basis of the findings of renal biopsies.[5,7] In broad terms the pathological appearance of the kidney in nephrotic syndrome has been divided into two groups: those that have moderate to severe morphological abnormalities and those that have mild or no morphological abnormalities. In pediatric patients the former often is part of a defined syndrome (such as systemic lupus erythematosus); therefore the group frequently has been called *secondary nephrotic syndrome*. This group constitutes approximately 10% of childhood cases of nephrotic syndrome. In contrast, biopsy specimens that show no disease or only mild changes often have been equated with the clinical terms *idiopathic nephrotic syndrome of childhood,* NIL (nothing-in-light) disease, or *lipoid nephrosis*. This variety makes up approximately 90% of cases of childhood nephrotic syndrome and is of unknown cause.

PATHOPHYSIOLOGY

The principal pathophysiological abnormality in nephrotic syndrome is an increased permeability of the glomerulus to protein. Whereas the electrochemical properties of the basement membrane of the glomerular capillary usually function as a highly efficient barrier for serum proteins during ultrafiltration of the blood, in nephrotic syndrome a defect in the barrier causes a massive loss of protein. In the nephrotic syndrome characterized by insignificant morphological change, this loss principally is albumin. In contrast, in the instances of nephrotic syndrome associated with notable morphological abnormalities, most of the serum proteins are lost to some degree. The former pattern of protein loss has been termed *selective,* whereas the latter pattern has been termed *nonselective*. Determination of the type of protein loss in the urine has been suggested to be of diagnostic and prognostic value in cases of this syndrome. Recent work also has suggested that tubular reabsorption and catabolism of filtered protein may contribute to the hypoproteinemia.

The liver responds to the low blood protein level by increasing protein synthesis. If the protein loss is mild or moderate, the liver usually can maintain the serum protein at near-normal values. If, however, the loss is greater, the increased synthesis of protein is insufficient and hypoproteinemia ensues. With hypoproteinemia the serum oncotic pressure gradually decreases, allowing fluid to exude from the intravascular space into the intracellular space thereby causing edema. The blood volume often becomes contracted, stimulating the production of aldosterone by the adrenal gland, which acts to increase renal tubular reabsorption of sodium and water. Although such homeostatic response ordinarily would serve to correct the abnormal vascular volume, it is ineffective in nephrotic syndrome because the reduced oncotic pressure allows the fluid to continue to leak from the vascular space. The secondary hyperaldosteronism has been suggested to contribute further to edema formation and the oliguria that is seen commonly in nephrotic syndrome. The pathophysiology of the hyperlipidemia is less clear. Although hyperlipidemia has been suggested to occur secondary to the hypoproteinemia, it has been noted to occur before hypoproteinemia in experimentally induced nephrotic syndrome in animals and to persist even after the resolution of proteinuria in human beings.

CLINICAL FORMS OF NEPHROTIC SYNDROME

Idiopathic Nephrotic Syndrome of Childhood

Idiopathic nephrotic syndrome of childhood (minimal change disease, NIL disease) is the most common variety of nephrotic syndrome in pediatric patients.[4] Although it may occur at any age, 90% of cases of idiopathic nephrotic syndrome occur between the ages of 1 and 5 years, with the peak between 2 and 3 years. The syndrome exhibits a male predominance.

Clinical Presentation. The majority of children have complaints relating to the sudden development of dependent edema (Fig. 233-1). The parents may notice that their child has periorbital edema on rising in the morning, which gradually diminishes with upright activity, only to be followed by

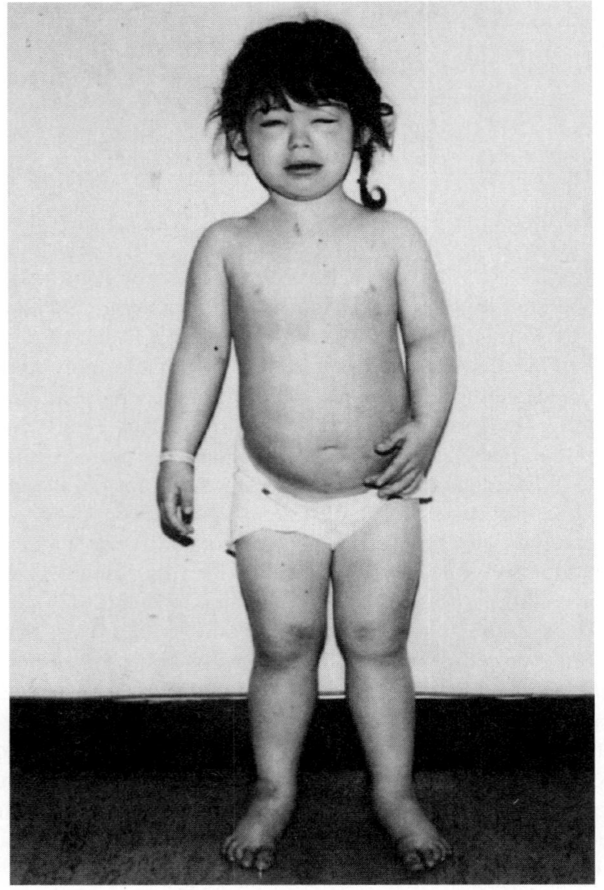

FIG. 233-1 A 2-year-old girl with nephrotic syndrome in relapse.

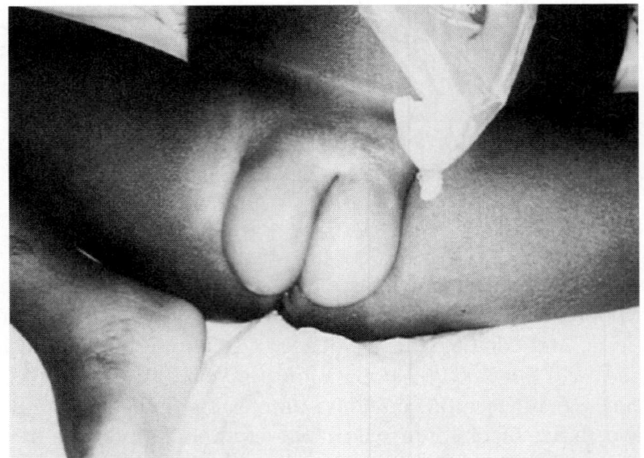

FIG. 233-2 Severe labial edema in a 3-year-old girl with nephrotic syndrome.

ankle and pedal edema later in the day. This ankle edema may manifest as a tight fit of the child's shoes as the day progresses. At first the dependent edema varies in degree from day to day, but gradually it becomes more consistent and severe, so facial or lower extremity edema may be present regardless of the activity and position of the patient. As edema becomes more generalized, ascites and hydrothorax may develop. If the ascites is gradual, it may be noted as an increase in abdominal protuberance, producing the inability to button pants that previously had fit well. Severe ascites often is associated with labial or scrotal edema (Fig. 233-2). Respiratory difficulty in the form of tachypnea, flaring of the ala nasi, or dyspnea may develop as a result of hydrothorax or the pressure of ascites on the diaphragm.

With the development of edema the child may be anorexic, listless, and pale. The appearance is that of a chronically ill, rather than an acutely ill, child. Diarrhea and vomiting are common at this stage, although it is uncertain whether these symptoms are caused by edema of the bowel as has been proposed. Prolonged hypoalbuminemia may result in muscle wasting, malnutrition, and growth failure. Most patients are normotensive, although mild hypertension may occur.

Diagnosis. The urinalysis in idiopathic nephrotic syndrome characteristically contains large amounts of protein and many hyaline and finely granular casts. Microscopic hematuria, which may occur in 33% of patients, almost never is grossly apparent. Cellular casts are seen occasionally. The urine usually is of high specific gravity, and doubly refractile fat bodies may be visualized with polarized light. Quantitative urinary protein determinations often exceed 5 to 10 g/day.

Examination of the serum usually reveals severe hypoproteinemia (serum albumin below 2 g/dl) associated with an increase in triglycerides, high-density lipoproteins, and cholesterol. The hyperlipidemia usually is severe enough to cause the serum to be lactescent on direct examination. This lactescence may interfere with some serum biochemical determinations. The serum calcium level usually is lowered because of the decrease in serum protein. Hyponatremia also may be found. This usually is artifactual inasmuch as sodium is restricted to the aqueous phase of serum, which is relatively diminished in the nephrotic patient as a result of the increase in the nonaqueous phase because of elevated serum lipid levels. Anemia may be present. The serum complement level usually is normal. A diagnosis of idiopathic nephrotic syndrome can be made with 95% certainty on the basis of the clinical impression. Characteristically, these children are between 1 and 10 years of age and have the typical clinical features of the syndrome. They may have either hypertension or hematuria, but not both. Azotemia and hypocomplementemia usually are absent.[7] The presence of selective proteinemia also supports the diagnosis.

Biopsy findings in children who have idiopathic nephrotic syndrome reveal grossly normal glomeruli, although some may have slight mesangial hyperplasia (Fig. 233-3). Typically the biopsy specimen, when examined by immunofluorescent techniques, shows no deposits of immunoglobulin or complement proteins, and examination by electron microscopy reveals only simplification of the foot processes of the epithelial cells. This latter change generally is considered to be a consequence of proteinuria. If clinical and laboratory evidence of idiopathic nephrotic syndrome of childhood is strong, renal biopsy usually is unnecessary. However, biopsy is indicated (1) in children who have both hypertension and hematuria, (2) when hypocomplementemia or nonselective proteinemia is present, or (3) when nephrotic syndrome occurs in an older child or adolescent. Older children and those who fail to respond to a course of corticosteroids are likely

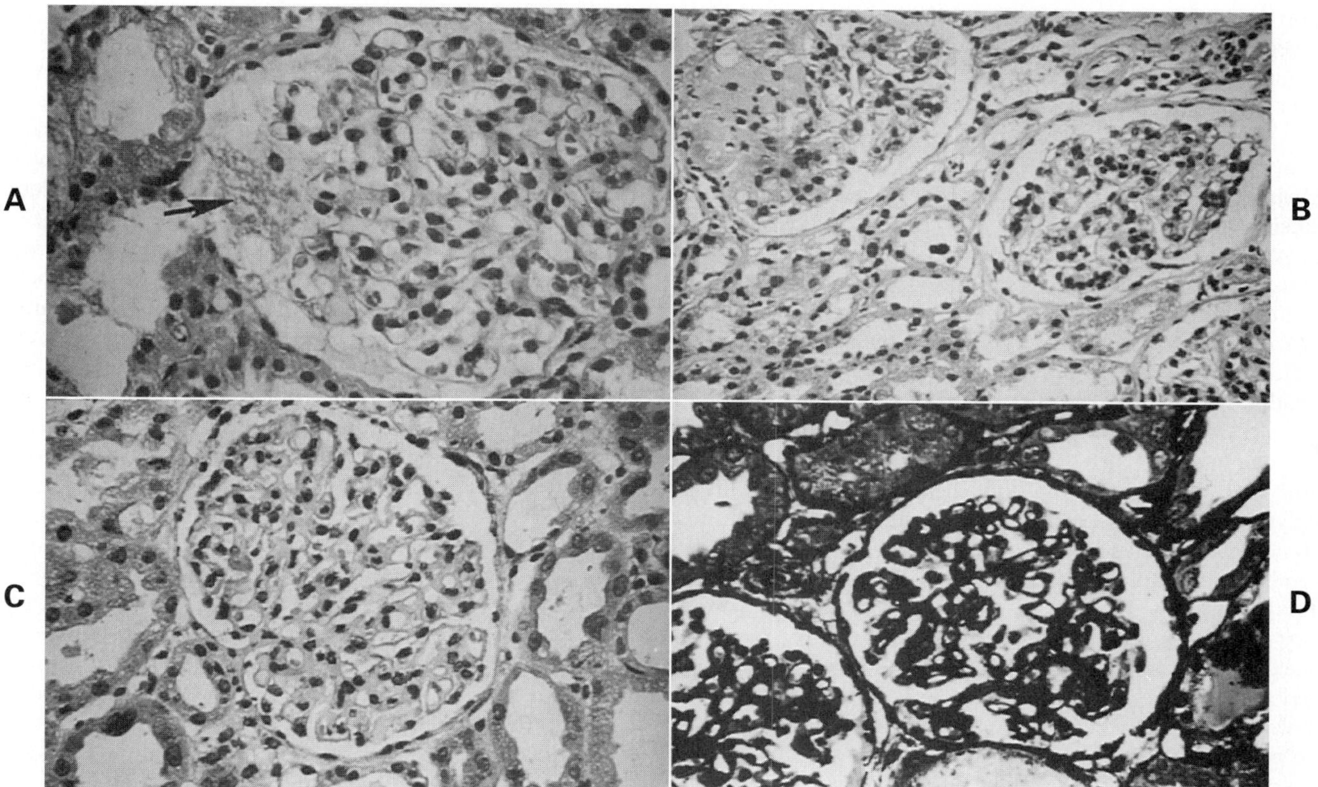

FIG. 233-3 Renal disease in nephrotic syndrome. **A,** Minimal change disease. Arrow indicates proteinaceous material in Bowman space (hematoxylin and eosin stain). **B,** Focal glomerulosclerosis. Note segmental acellular involvement of one glomerulus and virtual sparing of the other (hematoxylin and eosin stain). **C,** Membranous glomerulopathy. Note thickening of basement membranes (hematoxylin and eosin stain). **D,** Membranous glomerulopathy. Thickening of the basement membranes is better seen on silver stain.

to have a renal disease other than idiopathic nephrotic syndrome of childhood.

Occasionally a child will have a complication of nephrotic syndrome such as thromboembolism or infection. The former is related to the propensity to form thrombi in nephrotic syndrome. Furthermore, children who have nephrotic syndrome are particularly susceptible to peritonitis. The presence of fever in any patient who has nephrotic syndrome requires a careful evaluation for sepsis.

Differential Diagnosis. Nephrotic syndrome of any cause needs to be differentiated in general from the hypoproteinemia and edema found in conditions of decreased protein production, such as starvation, liver disease, and protein-losing enteropathy. The absence of notable proteinuria in these diseases differentiates them from nephrotic syndrome.

Idiopathic nephrotic syndrome usually can be differentiated from nephrotic syndrome caused by morphological glomerular disease by the nonselective proteinuria, the tendency for hematuria and hypertension to coexist, and the tendency for onset in older children in the latter condition.[6,7,10] An exception is the child who has a focal sclerosing type of glomerular lesion, who initially may have symptoms similar to those of the child who has idiopathic nephrotic syndrome. These children usually are detected by their incomplete response to corticosteroid treatment.

Treatment. General aspects of treatment include provision for activity, diet, and diuretic therapy. Children kept at bed rest often have a mild spontaneous diuresis with a subsequent fall in weight and decrease in edema. However, because a major complication of nephrotic syndrome of any cause is thromboembolism, the wisdom of inactivity and the attendant increased risk of thrombosis must be considered. Traditionally, a diet high in protein has been prescribed, although it usually has a minimal effect on the serum protein level. Salt limitation usually is unnecessary if the patient is not hypertensive. Salt intake by children usually is not excessive, and severe salt restriction may make the diet unpalatable, thereby defeating the attempt to promote a balanced intake. Restriction of salt to the amount in a "regular" diet with no added salt at the table and the elimination of foods known to be highly salted (e.g., peanuts and potato chips) are all that usually is necessary. Likewise, limitation of fluids also is unnecessary except in the severely hypertensive patient. Marked limitation of fluids in the patient who has hemoconcentration and oliguria may aggravate the hypoperfusion and contribute to the risk of thromboembolism.

Diuretic therapy may be indicated for the patient who has incapacitating edema. However, the response to diuretics usually is less than expected because of the hypoproteinemia in these patients. At best, diuretic therapy can produce only a short-term reduction in the edema. The same is true for intravenous albumin infusion, because the albumin is lost in the urine nearly as rapidly as it is given. A greater effect results from the combined use of albumin (1 g/kg/day intravenously) and diuretics (furosemide, 1 to 2 mg/kg/day orally or intravenously), although the duration of effect is limited. Albumin infusion can be associated with a risk of overexpansion of the vascular space and congestive heart failure. Although such complications are uncommon in nephrotic patients, care always should be exercised in the administration of albumin.

A course of corticosteroids generally is agreed to be capable of inducing a remission in most children who have idiopathic nephrotic syndrome. Prednisone is used most often because of its effectiveness and low cost. Usually the child is begun on a daily dose of 60 mg/m^2 (about 2 mg/kg) given either once daily or in two divided doses, with a maximum daily dose of 60 mg. Such treatment should induce a remission in most patients within 6 to 14 days after starting therapy. Remission usually will be heralded by a rather abrupt diuresis associated with a decrease and then an absence of urinary protein. Recent studies[1,2] have shown that prolonged (6 weeks) daily steroid therapy for the first episode was associated with a more sustained remission than shorter durations (4 weeks) of daily therapy. However, continuing steroids at a high dosage for long periods produces a variety of drug-induced side effects, including increased appetite, weight gain, truncal obesity, moon face, acne, and stria. As with all high-dose continual steroid therapy, serious infections may be masked. At high doses, growth in height is decreased markedly, so prolonged treatment may result in severe stunting. To reduce these side effects, steroids should be changed to an every-other-day schedule after the initial daily regimen. Furthermore, the alternate-day steroids should be discontinued gradually because many patients do well for long periods without steroids. No general agreement exists, however, as to the best method or the rapidity with which to make changes in alternate-day steroid administration.

Patients who respond to corticosteroids are termed *steroid sensitive*. Patients who fail to respond to prednisone after 4 weeks of daily administration are considered to be *steroid resistant*. In other patients a pattern of *steroid dependency* may develop wherein they remain in remission so long as a particular dose of prednisone is given but relapse as soon as the dose is reduced below the "critical level." Other patients respond to the corticosteroid but have *frequent relapses* (defined as more than three relapses within a year while not receiving steroids).

Patients who are steroid resistant, steroid dependent, or frequent relapsers should be referred to a pediatric nephrologist for consideration for renal biopsy and other forms of drug therapy. Effective drug regimens for these children currently are the subject of investigation. Most of the drugs employed have additional side effects about which the parents need to be informed. For a pediatric practitioner to institute a course of therapy with one of these unproved drugs in a sporadic case of nephrotic syndrome is inappropriate.

Infections in children who have nephrotic syndrome should be treated with appropriate antibiotics. *Prophylactic antibiotic therapy is not indicated.* Immunization should be delayed until the child has not relapsed for 6 months to 2 years without steroid therapy.

Prognosis. The overall prognosis for steroid-sensitive nephrotic syndrome is good.[8] Because relapses are the rule, however, parents need to be educated about the natural history of the illness. An occasional relapse should not be portrayed as either a severe setback or a condition to be ignored. Most children remain steroid responsive, and the disease can be controlled with additional courses of therapy. Furthermore, giving the parents some means of testing the urine for protein is helpful, involving them directly in the child's care and allowing them to feel more in control. Finding no proteinuria reassures the parents; thus every change in the physical and emotional state of the child is not viewed as a subtle symptom of a relapse. Furthermore, when relapse does occur, the parents often are able to discover the proteinuria before the development of clinical edema. Prompt reinstitution of corticosteroids often produces a remission before clinical symptoms appear and thereby obviates the need for hospital admission. No advantage is apparent in treating relapse with the prolonged daily prednisone regimen (6 weeks) in terms of subsequent remissions.[2] Therefore relapses should be treated with daily doses of prednisone (60 mg/m^2) until the urine has been protein-free for 3 days. This is followed by 4 weeks of alternate-day therapy at a dose of 40 mg/m^2/day. Nephrotic syndrome is a chronic disease during which patient and parent share a great need for education. Side effects of the disease and the therapy—particularly the corticosteroids—need to be taught. Even in the most uncomplicated case, periodic consultation with a pediatric nephrologist may be helpful. In particular, the use of corticosteroids for this syndrome is constantly changing as various regimens are developed that control the disease effectively with a reduction in side effects. Periodic advice as to the management of these drugs should allow the design of a program that provides the best possible control of the disease with the least treatment side effects, resulting in a child who can lead as normal a life as possible.

Focal Glomerulosclerosis

In a young child, focal glomerulosclerosis can manifest with signs and symptoms identical to those of idiopathic nephrotic syndrome. This illness should be suspected in any nephrotic child who is unresponsive to steroid treatment or who develops steroid resistance, steroid dependence, or frequent relapses after having been steroid sensitive. In addition, azotemia, hematuria, and nonselective proteinuria occur more frequently in these children.[5,7] On the basis of serial biopsy observations, focal glomerulosclerosis has been suggested to be an unfavorable evolution of idiopathic nephrotic syndrome. The diagnosis of focal glomerulosclerosis can be made only by renal biopsy. Typically focal acellular hyalinized areas are in the glomerular segments, although several patterns of disease have been described on the basis of the degree of involvement (Fig. 233-3). The prognosis of this condition generally is poor, with progressive renal failure developing in most patients. Patients who have focal glomerulosclerosis *and* interstitial inflammation tend to have a more rapid rate of deterioration.[3] Definitive drug therapies currently are under investigation. The disease has recurred in some children who have received renal transplants. Because of the complexity in establishing the diagnosis, the probability for development of renal failure, and the uncertainty of beneficial effects with drug therapy, these cases are managed best in consultation with a pediatric nephrologist.

Membranous Nephropathy

Membranous (extramembranous) nephropathy usually has a manifestation similar to that of idiopathic nephrotic syndrome, although it more often affects older children. It, too, is often characterized by steroid resistance. Diagnosis can be made only by renal biopsy, in which the specimen reveals diffuse thickening of the glomerular capillary walls without significant proliferation (see Fig. 233-3). On electron microscopy, subepithelial deposits are found in the capillary loops. As seen by immunofluorescent examination, these deposits usually consist of IgG and C3 and are thought to represent small immune complexes. Although no definite therapy is of proved benefit, the prognosis in children generally is much better than in adults, with spontaneous remission occurring in about 50% of the children. A complete infectious hepatitis serology study should be performed in these children because many are found to be carriers of hepatitis-associated antigens. Controlled trials of various agents currently are under investigation. The disease of these children also is best managed in consultation with a pediatric nephrologist.

REFERENCES

1. Brodehl J: The treatment of minimal change nephrotic syndrome: lessons learned from multicentre cooperative studies, *Eur J Pediatr* 150:380, 1991.
2. Ehrich JHH, Brodehl J: Long versus standard prednisone therapy for initial treatment of idiopathic nephrotic syndrome in children, *Eur J Pediatr* 152:357, 1993.
3. Ellis D et al: Focal glomerulosclerosis in children: correlation of histology with prognosis, *J Pediatr* 93:762, 1978.
4. Grupe WE: Primary nephrotic syndrome in childhood, *Adv Pediatr* 26:163, 1979.
5. Habib R, Kleinknecht C: The primary nephrotic syndrome of childhood: classification and clinicopathologic study of 406 cases. In Sommers SC: *Pathology annual,* East Norwalk, Conn, 1971, Appleton-Century-Crofts.
6. Habib R, Levy M, Gubler MC: Clinicopathologic correlations in the nephrotic syndrome, *Paediatrician* 8:325, 1979.
7. International study of kidney disease in children: nephrotic syndrome in children—prediction of histopathology from clinical and laboratory characteristics at time of diagnosis, *Kidney Int* 31:1368, 1987.
8. Koskimies O et al: Long-term outcome of primary nephrotic syndrome, *Arch Dis Child* 57:544, 1982.
9. Rothenberg MB, Heymann W: The incidence of the nephrotic syndrome in children, *Pediatrics* 19:446, 1957.
10. White RHR, Glasgow EF, Mills RJ: Clinicopathological study of the nephrotic syndrome in childhood, *Lancet* 1:1353, 1970.

SUGGESTED READINGS

Chesney RW, Novello AC: Forms of nephrotic syndrome more likely to progress to renal impairment, *Pediatr Clin North Am* 34:609, 1987.

Kher KK, Sweet M, Makker SP: Nephrotic syndrome in children, *Curr Probl Pediatr* 18:199, 1988.

Strauss J et al: Less commonly recognized features of childhood nephrotic syndrome, *Pediatr Clin North Am* 34:591, 1987.

234 Obesity

Wendi G. Ehrman

Obesity is considered one of the most prevalent nutritional problems among children and adolescents in the United States. Over the past 20 years the prevalence of childhood and adolescent obesity has increased at an alarming rate. Obesity can lead to significant morbidity among youth and has been associated with negative social, economic, and physical outcomes in adulthood. Treatments vary, but few have achieved long-term success in maintaining weight loss.

PREVALENCE

An estimated 25% of the United States population is obese[1] or overweight.[40] Rates of obesity vary by definition and demographical factors but are estimated to be 10% to 30% among children and adolescents.[27,51] Over almost 20 years (1963 to 1980), the prevalence of obesity increased 54% among children 6 to 11 and 39% among adolescents ages 12 to 17.[18]

ETIOLOGY

Overweight is defined as an increase in body weight in relation to height. Obesity is defined as the excess accumulation of body fat relative to lean body mass. Obesity results when energy intake exceeds expenditure and is stored as fat. However, this simplistic explanation fails to address all of the contributing social, cultural, genetic, and environmental factors that can effect accumulation of fat and weight gain.

Obesity often is viewed as a form of overnutrition, supported by evidence that obese children tend to be taller than average, have a larger lean body mass, and have excess body fat.[13,17] Despite these findings, the role of dietary intake in the development of obesity has caused considerable controversy. Although excess caloric intake can lead to increased weight and adipose tissue, studies have indicated that many obese individuals may not eat more than their peers.[24,61] In some children, inactivity and dietary factors such as irregular eating habits and the number of times a child eats per day are associated with childhood obesity.[4]

Infants, children, and adolescents who have low activity levels and energy expenditure may be at higher risk for becoming obese. A study of nonobese infants revealed that those who had lower total daily energy expenditure at 3 months of age went on to become overweight infants at 1 year of age.[44] Overweight adolescent females have been shown to have decreased motor activity in relationship to their nonobese peers.[2] A recent study has shown a highly significant positive relationship between prolonged television viewing time and obesity among children and adolescents.[8]

Despite their decreased activity levels, obese children and adolescents may have energy expenditures equal to those of their nonobese peers. Both activity levels and body weight contribute to energy expenditure. Therefore an obese child would burn more calories than a child of normal weight doing the same activity. When these factors were considered, obese and nonobese children had similar energy expenditure during voluntary activity.[59]

Parental obesity is a well-recognized risk factor for childhood obesity; a direct relationship has been shown between childhood obesity and the degree of overweight or obesity among parents.[16] Studies of adult adoptees show a direct relationship between the body-mass index of biological parents and the weight class of adoptees.[56] In contrast, little or no correlation exists between adoptees and their adoptive parents. Children of normal-weight parents have an estimated 14% risk of obesity compared with a risk of 40% when one parent is obese and 80% if both parents are obese.[34] Studies of twins also suggest a strong genetic contribution to obesity. Body-mass index was shown to be highly correlated among monozygotic and dizygotic twins reared apart.[57] In addition, monozygotic twins show a greater concordance for degree of overweight than dizygotic twins.[55]

Childhood obesity has been associated with other factors such as geographical region, population density, season,[9] and family characteristics such as parental age,[16] marital status, family size,[42] and socioeconomic status (SES). Results of the Ten State Nutrition Survey (1968 to 1970) indicated a "reversal of fatness" for African-American and Caucasian females. Caucasian females were heavier than African-American females up until late adolescence, at which point a reversal in weight categories was seen. This same pattern was seen when low and high socioeconomic groups were compared. Children of all ages from a higher socioeconomic group were heavier than children from lower socioeconomic groups. However, this trend was reversed for females in late adolescence and adulthood.[16] A comprehensive review by Sorbol and Stunkard[53] showed that weight was inversely related to SES for women but not for men or children in developed countries. In developing countries, SES was related positively to weight for women, men, and children.[53]

COMPLICATIONS

Obesity has a major impact on several different aspects of growth. Obese children have increased lean body mass and adipose tissue. Linear growth, bone age, and sexual maturation often are advanced.[13,17] In addition, obese females have earlier menarche than their nonobese peers.[11]

Obesity is associated with a number of cardiovascular risk factors in adults. Factors that predispose individuals to cardiovascular disease are thought to develop during early childhood. Hypertension, hyperlipidemia, and glucose intolerance all are recognized cardiovascular risk factors[28] and have been shown to occur concurrently in adults as well as in obese children and adolescents.[5,52]

Obese adolescents have been found to have blood pressure distributions skewed 1 standard deviation higher than normal. Blood pressures returned within the normal range following weight loss.[45] Cholesterol and triglycerides are related to weight linearly. Data from the National Health and Nutrition Examination Survey demonstrated that the incidence of hypercholesterolemia in a young overweight group was 2.1 times that of a nonoverweight group.[41] In addition, a positive correlation exists between obesity and the risk of non-insulin-dependent diabetes.[41]

Orthopedic problems may result from the stress of excess weight in obese adolescents. Slipped capital femoral epiphysis (SCFE) develops as an abrupt or gradual displacement of the femoral neck from the femoral head through the growth plate. Although a number of factors may contribute to the development of SCFE, more than 50% of the patients are classified as obese, and many are taller than the 90th percentile in height.[3,30] Blount disease, a bowing of the tibia associated with medial osteochondrosis of the proximal epiphysis, also has been associated with obesity in childhood.[10]

Acanthosis nigricans, a skin disorder characterized by a velvety thickening and hyperpigmentation of the neck and axillae, is associated with obesity, hyperinsulinemia, and insulin resistance. Acanthosis nigricans often develops in puberty concurrent with the onset of obesity and may disappear following weight loss.

Menstrual irregularities, predominately anovulatory cycles characterized by dysfunctional uterine bleeding and amenorrhea, have been associated with obesity in adolescent females. Polycystic ovary syndrome is a spectrum of clinical disorders in adolescent females associated with increased androgen production, abnormal gonadotropin secretion and insulin resistance. Obesity is common in adolescents who have polycystic ovary syndrome. In addition, type A HAIR-AN syndrome (a genetic disorder characterized by hyperandrogenism, insulin resistance, and acanthosis nigricans) often is associated with obesity.

Intertrigo, a superficial inflammatory dermatitis, develops in areas of skin subject to friction and maceration. It is seen more frequently among obese children and adolescents because of the overlapping of skin folds.

In adults, obesity is associated with a number of severe pulmonary complications including obesity-hypoventilation syndrome (OHS or Pickwickian syndrome) and obstructive sleep apnea (OSA).[47] Although OHS and OSA have not been documented as well in children, recent evidence indicates that morbidly obese children and adolescents are at risk for hypoventilation and sleep-associated breathing disorders.[33,43]

The most devastating consequence of obesity is believed to be the impact on the psychosocial functioning of the child or adolescent. Overweight children and adolescents reportedly exhibit significant depression,[60] lowered self-esteem,[50] and lower body-esteem.[36] Numerous studies have documented a pervasive "fear of fatness" among adolescent females of all weight categories. This fear can lead to inappropriate eating behaviors and attitudes among the obese and nonobese adolescent female.[38,39] In addition, a recent study showed that women who had been overweight as adolescents were less likely to be married, had lower household incomes, higher poverty levels, and completed fewer years of school than their nonoverweight controls. Men who had been overweight as adolescents also were less likely to be married.[19]

Many obese children and adolescents do not suffer from impaired psychosocial functioning and demonstrate self-esteem equivalent to that of their nonobese peers.[29,58] A number of studies indicate that gender, race, parental perceptions of weight, and socioeconomic status influence self-esteem and body image of obese and nonobese children and adolescents.[7,26,31] Caucasian females of any weight category and females of higher socioeconomic status are more likely to be dissatisfied with their weight and see themselves as heavier than they actually are. Overweight African-Americans are less likely to see themselves as heavy and appear more satisfied with their current weight.

The health care provider should identify and treat those patients who have complications and counsel those at risk for obesity. However, the physical and psychological effects of obesity vary among children and adolescents. Not all obese children and adolescents experience complications as a result of their weight. In fact, many obese children and adolescents are physically and emotionally quite healthy.

DIFFERENTIAL DIAGNOSIS

Obesity is a common feature of several endocrinopathies and a number of syndromes. Primary obesity often is associated with average to above average height and normal to accelerated sexual maturation. Obesity associated with a syndrome or endocrinopathy generally is associated with delayed bone age, short stature, and hypogonadism.

A number of medications can cause obesity. Prolonged use of corticosteroids can lead to cushingoid obesity. Asthmatic patients often experience significant weight gain while receiving chronic oral steroid treatment. Psychotropic medications including lithium, tricyclic antidepressants, and phenothiazines also may cause weight gain.

DIAGNOSIS

Obesity refers to an excess of fat or adipose tissue. Body fat can be estimated by subtracting lean body mass (or fat free mass) from body weight. Methods for estimating lean body mass include underwater weighing to measure body density, measurement of total body water or potassium 40 levels, measurement of total body conductivity, and bioimpedance. In addition, computed tomography (CT) and magnetic resonance imaging (MRI) can define percentages of lean body mass and fat. These procedures are difficult technically and obviously not practical in a clinical setting. As a result, most methods used to estimate obesity do not really measure fat but rely on ratios of body weight to height or on skinfold thicknesses.

The most practical and commonly used methods for estimating obesity in clinical practice involve measurements of weight and height. Tables are available for children and adolescents that allow the practitioner to evaluate weight based on age, gender, and height.[21,22] Ideal body weight is estimated as the 50th percentile weight for the child's age, gender, and height. Obesity often is defined as greater than 120% of ideal body weight. The percent of ideal body weight is calculated by dividing the child's actual weight in kilograms by the child's 50th percentile weight (ideal body weight) and multiplying by 100. Well-trained athletes are an exception; they may have an ideal body weight greater than 120% because of muscle rather than fat mass. In addition, ideal weight may be influenced by factors such as body build, race, and health status.

The body-mass index (BMI) is another useful tool for indirectly estimating obesity in children and adolescents.[48] BMI is defined as weight in kilograms divided by height in meters squared. BMI is calculated easily and is influenced less by the effect of height on weight. BMI is correlated strongly with skinfold thickness,[54] a method of estimating body adiposity in individuals. In addition, BMI values in childhood correlate strongly with values in adulthood.[49] Tables are available to evaluate BMI among children and adolescents by age, race, and sex.[15,23] A BMI of greater than or equal to the 85th percentile has been used as a measure of "overweight" and a BMI greater than or equal to the 95th percentile as a measure of "severe overweight" in adults.[40] These measures are fairly consistent with height/weight criteria from the 1983 Metropolitan Life Insurance tables that are based on morbidity and mortality data. Body mass indexes of 85% and 95% correlate roughly with 20% and 40% above desirable body weight for an adult who has a medium build as described in the 1983 Metropolitan Life Insurance Tables.[37] In children and adolescents, a BMI greater than or equal to the 95th percentile has been suggested as a conservative cutoff point for defining obesity, although studies associating this value with an increased risk of morbidity and mortality have not been clear-cut.[23] BMI can be used for monitoring the development of obesity and changes in BMI for monitoring treatment.

Skinfold calipers have been used to measure subcutaneous fat at various sites (biceps, triceps, subscapular, iliac crest) as an estimate of obesity. Triceps skinfold measurements have been shown to correlate with percentage of weight that is body fat in both children and adults[14,46] but can be limited by lack of experience and technical difficulty. A number of tables are available with distributions based on age, sex, and race.[6,15,40] In general, triceps skinfolds at or above the 85th percentile are accepted as the criterion for obesity.[16,18] All skinfold measurements for males over age 5 correlate well with skinfold measurements for adult males. By contrast, in females, only biceps skinfold measurements are correlated consistently from age 2 years to adulthood.[49]

TREATMENT

Obesity is a complex, chronic problem that provides a significant challenge to practitioners attempting to treat children, adolescents, or adults. The longer the duration of obesity, the poorer the outlook for permanent leanness. An estimated 80% of obese adolescents become obese adults.[32]

Changes in body weight are associated with energy balance. As a result, most weight loss programs combine dietary changes and increased physical activity. In addition, many treatments include behavioral modification, motivational strategies, and environmental changes. More recently, evidence has shown that maternal or family involvement with a weight loss program is associated with increased short-term weight loss and weight loss maintenance over periods of up to 10 years.[12]

Good nutrition needs to be an important part of any weight control program. Fasting and semi-starvation diets are contraindicated in growing children and adolescents because of the potential for growth arrest or retardation. Moreover, these diets are difficult to maintain and do not aid in the development of healthy eating and dietary habits.

Weight goals among young children, should be aimed at slowing excessive weight gain and paralleling the weight curve. Often, investigation into parental feeding practices will reveal opportunities for dietary interventions. Parents should pay attention to an infant's hunger cues and not offer bottles or food to satisfy an infant's need for attention. Feeding environments should be pleasant, supportive, and allow the child to pick and choose from available food. Meals and snacks should be provided regularly and physical activity initiated as early as 1 year of age.

Goals for older children and growing adolescents should focus on slowing the rate of weight gain or maintaining weight throughout linear growth. Treatment should be discussed and developed with the patient. The older child or adolescent can be asked to record all foods consumed as well as the times, places, and circumstances surrounding eating. Examination of the dietary record can be used to identify areas for intervention. Patients can be encouraged to eat regular meals and cut down on the amount of high-fat snack foods such as cakes, candy, and chips. Small, achievable dietary changes that include restriction, elimination, changes in portion size, and changes in dietary composition can be initiated at each visit.

Parents can be encouraged to support their children by providing regular meals and limiting the intake of high-calorie, high-fat foods. In addition, parents and children can be taught to prepare meals in ways that decrease dietary fat and calories, such as trimming fat or boiling and baking instead of frying. Families can be encouraged to help the obese child by consuming the same types of food at meals.

Regular exercise is another important component of any treatment that can improve overall fitness, preserve lean body mass, and improve mental health.[25] Long-term success is achieved best by increasing activities the child or adolescent already enjoys instead of incorporating rigorous exercises and programmed activities that the child or adolescent may not enjoy. Encouraging walking and bicycling instead of vehicular transportation is one way to incorporate exercise into a treatment program. Children and adolescents should be encouraged to use stairs at home, school, or when out shopping. Sedentary activities such as television viewing should be limited and other activities that expend more energy encouraged with friends or family.

Reinforcements should be provided as a means of rewarding weight loss or maintenance and positive behavioral changes. Reinforcement can be given in the form of praise from family, friends, and health care providers and should be offered immediately on performance of a new behavior. Tangible rewards can be negotiated with parents for achievement of weight or behavioral goals. Children and adolescents also can be taught how to reward themselves for positive changes in their life-style and dietary habits.

Commercial programs specially designed for obese or

overweight adolescents are available. One such program, Shapedown, incorporates cognitive, behavioral, and affective techniques to modify diet, exercise, relationships, life-style, communication, and affect. Both long-term and short-term results have been positive.[35] Comprehensive weight loss programs may be ideal for certain patients but may be impossible for others because of location or cost.

Some weight loss treatments (e.g., radical diets, drugs, surgery) generally are not recommended in children and adolescents. Anoretic drugs such as sympathomimetics, diuretics, and hormones have not shown long-term effectiveness, and the potential for stimulant abuse may be high in adolescents.[20] Surgical treatments such as gastroplasty and jejunoileal bypass may lead to life-threatening side effects[1] and should be reserved for the morbidly obese who have serious medical complications.

PREVENTION

Prevention of obesity should start in childhood with the development of healthful eating habits and a positive feeding relationship between parent and child. Regular exercise can be initiated as early as age 1 year, and families should be encouraged to participate in meals and activities together. Children and adolescents who may be predisposed genetically toward obesity should be encouraged to develop or maintain healthy eating and exercise habits and to develop a positive body image. Clinicians can promote these measures by incorporating dietary histories and counseling with each well-infant, child, and adolescent visit.

SUMMARY

Obesity is a common disorder of childhood and adolescence that is associated with long-term complications in adulthood. Although the medical risks for childhood and adolescent obesity are less clear, a large percentage of obese adolescents go on to become obese adults. A number of treatments are available, with the most successful involving a combination of dietary modifications, regular activity, behavior modification, and family involvement. Until completion of linear growth, treatment should focus on weight stabilization rather than on significant weight loss. Although short-term success is seen with a number of commercial and clinical interventions, few have documented long-term success. Health care providers can work to prevent obesity by encouraging healthy eating and exercise habits at an early age and intervening actively when a problem is recognized.

REFERENCES

1. Anderson AE, Soper RT, Scott DH: Gastric bypass for morbid obesity in children and adolescents, *J Pediatr Surg* 15:876, 1989.
2. Bullen BA, Reed RB, Mayer J: Physical activity of obese and non-obese adolescent girls appraised by motion picture sampling, *Am J Clin Nutr* 13:211, 1964.
3. Chung S: Diseases of the developing hip joint, *Pediatr Clin North Am* 24:857, 1977.
4. Crawford PB, Shapiro LR: How obesity develops: a new look at nature and nurture, *Obesity Health* May/June:40, 1991.
5. Criqui MH et al: Clustering of cardiovascular disease risk factors, *Prev Med* 9:525, 1980.
6. Cronk CE, Roch AF: Race- and sex-specific reference data for triceps and subscapular skinfolds and weight/stature, *Am J Clin Nutr* 35:347, 1982.
7. Desmond SH et al: Black and white adolescents' perceptions of their weight, *J Sch Health* 59:353, 1989.
8. Dietz WH, Gortmaker SL: Do we fatten our children at the television set? Obesity and television viewing in children and adolescents, *Pediatrics* 75:807, 1985.
9. Dietz WH, Gortmaker SL: Factors within the physical environment associated with childhood obesity, *Am J Clin Nutr* 39:619, 1984.
10. Dietz WH Jr, Gross WL, Kirkpatrick JA Jr: Blount disease (tibia vara): another skeletal disorder associated with childhood obesity, *J Pediatr* 101:735, 1982.
11. Ellison PT: Skeletal growth, fatness, and menarcheal age: a comparison of two hypotheses, *Hum Biol* 54:269, 1982.
12. Epstein LH et al: Ten-year follow-up of behavioral, family-based treatment for obese children, *JAMA* 264:2519, 1990.
13. Forbes GB: Nutrition and growth, *J Pediatr* 91:40, 1977.
14. Forbes G, Amirhakimi GH: Skinfold thickness and body fat in children, *Hum Biol* 42:401, 1970.
15. Frisancho AR: *Anthropometric standards for the assessment of growth and nutritional status,* Ann Arbor, Mich, 1990, University of Michigan Press.
16. Garn SM, Clark DC: Nutrition, growth, development and maturation: findings from the Ten State Nutrition Survey of 1968-70, *Pediatrics* 56:306, 1975.
17. Garn SM, Clark DC: Trends in fatness and the origins of obesity, *Pediatrics* 57:443, 1976.
18. Gortmaker SL et al: Increasing pediatric obesity in the United States, *Am J Dis Child* 141:535, 1987.
19. Gortmaker SL et al: Social and economic consequences of overweight in adolescence and young adulthood, *N Engl J Med* 329:1008, 1993.
20. Grollman A: Drug therapy of obesity in children, *Pediatr Ann* 4:39, 1975.
21. Hamill PV et al: Physical growth: National Center for Health Statistics percentiles, *Am J Clin Nutr* 32:607, 1979.
22. Hamill PV, Johnston FE, Lemeshaw S: National Center for Health Statistics: height and weight of youths 12-17 years, United States 1966-1970, Vital and Health Statistics, Series 11, No 124, DHEW Pub No (HSM) 73-1606, Washington, DC, 1974, US Government Printing Office.
23. Hammer LD et al: Standardized percentile curves of body-mass index for children and adolescents, *Am J Dis Child* 145:259, 1991.
24. Hampton MC et al: Caloric and nutrient intakes of teen-agers, *J Am Diet Assoc* 50:385, 1967.
25. Hayes D, Ross CE: Body and mind: the effect of exercise, overweight and physical health on psychological well-being, *J Health Soc Behav* 27:387, 1986.
26. Huenemann RL et al: A longitudinal study of gross body composition and body conformation and their association with food and activity in a teen-age population: view of teen-age subjects on body conformation, food, and activity, *Am J Clin Nutr* 18:325, 1966.
27. Huse DM et al: The challenge of obesity in childhood. I. Incidence, prevalence and staging, *Mayo Clin Proc* 57:279, 1982.
28. Kannel WB, McGee D, Gordon T: A general cardiovascular risk profile: the Framingham study, *Am J Cardiol* 38:46, 1976.
29. Kaplan KM, Wadden TA: Childhood obesity and self-esteem, *J Pediatr* 109:367, 1986.
30. Kelsey JL, Acheson DM, Keggi KJ: The body build of patients with slipped capital femoral epiphysis, *Am J Dis Child* 124:276, 1972.
31. Levinson R, Powell B, Steelman LC: Social location, significant others and body image among adolescents, *Soc Psych Q* 49:330, 1986.
32. Lloyd JK, Wolff OH, Whelen WS: Childhood obesity: a long-term study of height and weight, *Br Med J* 2:145, 1961.
33. Mallory GB, Fiser DH, Jackwon R: Sleep-associated breathing disorders in morbidly obese children and adolescents, *J Pediatr* 115:892, 1989.
34. Mayer J: Genetic factors in human obesity, *Ann NY Acad Sci* 131:412, 1965.
35. Mellin LM, Slinkard LA, Irwin CE: Adolescent obesity interven-

tion: validation of the Shapedown program, *J Am Diet Assoc* 87:333, 1987.
36. Mendelson BK, White DR: Development of self-body-esteem in overweight youngsters, *Dev Psych* 21:90, 1985.
37. Metropolitan Life Insurance Company: 1983 Metropolitan height and weight tables, *Stat Bull Metrop Insur Co* 64:2, 1983.
38. Moore Col DC: Body image and eating behavior in adolescent girls, *Am J Dis Child* 142:1114, 1988.
39. Moses N, Banilivy MM, Lifshitz F: Fear of obesity among adolescent girls, *Pediatrics* 83:393, 1989.
40. Najjar MF, Rowland M: Anthropometric reference data and prevalence of overweight, United States, 1976-80. Vital and Health Statistics, Series 11, No 238, DHHS Pub No 87-1688, Washington, DC, 1987, US Government Printing Office.
41. National Institute of Health Consensus Development Panel on the Health Implications of Obesity: Health implications of obesity, *Ann Intern Med* 103:147, 1985.
42. Rawelli GP, Belmont L: Obesity in nineteen-year-old men: family size and birth order associations, *Ann J Epidemiol* 109:66, 1979.
43. Riley DJ, Santiago TV, Edelman NH: Complications of obesity-hypoventilation syndrome in childhood, *Am J Dis Child* 130:671, 1976.
44. Roberts SB et al: Energy expenditure and intake in infants born to lean and overweight mothers, *N Engl J Med* 318:461, 1988.
45. Rocchini AP et al: Blood pressure in obese adolescents: effect of weight loss, *Pediatrics* 82:16, 1988.
46. Roche AF et al: Grading body fatness from limited anthropometric data, *Am J Clin Nutr* 34:2831, 1981.
47. Rochester DF, Enson Y: Current concepts in the pathogenesis of the obesity-hypoventilation syndrome, *Am J Med* 57:402, 1974.
48. Rolland-Cachera MF et al: Adiposity indices in children, *Am J Clin Nutr* 36:178, 1982.
49. Rolland-Cachera MF, Bellisle F, Sempe M: The prediction in boys and girls of the weight/height index and various skinfold measurements in adults: a two-decade follow-up study, *Int J Obes* 13:305, 1989.
50. Sallade J: A comparison of psychological adjustment of obese vs nonobese children, *J Psychosom Res* 17:89, 1973.
51. Shear CL et al: Secular trends of obesity in early life: the Bogalusa Heart Study, *Am J Public Health* 78:75, 1988.
52. Smoak CG et al: Relation of obesity to clustering of cardiovascular disease risk factors in children and young adults: the Bogalusa Heart Study, *Am J Epidemiol* 125:364, 1987.
53. Sorbal J, Stunkard AJ: Socioeconomic status and obesity: a review of the literature, *Psychol Bull* 105:260, 1989.
54. Spyckerelle Y: Adiposity indices and clinical opinion, *Ann Hum Biol* 15:45, 1988.
55. Stunkard AJ, Foch TT, Hrubec Z: A twin study of human obesity, *JAMA* 256:51, 1986.
56. Stunkard AJ et al: An adoption study of human obesity, *N Engl J Med* 314:193, 1986.
57. Stunkard AJ et al: The body-mass index of twins who have been reared apart, *N Engl J Med* 322:1483, 1990.
58. Wadden TA et al: Dissatisfaction with weight and figure in obese girls: discontent but not depression, *Int J Obes* 13:89, 1989.
59. Waxman M, Stunkard AJ: Caloric intake and expenditure of obese boys, *J Pediatr* 96:187, 1980.
60. Werkman SL, Greenberg ES: Personality and interest patterns in obese adolescent girls, *Psychosom Med* 29:72, 1967.
61. Wilkinson PW et al: Energy intake and physical activity in obese children, *Br Med J* 284:756, 1977.

235 Obstructive Uropathy and Vesicoureteral Reflux

Edward J. Ruley

OBSTRUCTIVE UROPATHY

Frequency

The exact frequency of urinary tract obstruction is unknown. An autopsy study suggests that it occurs in 2% to 3.8% of children. More important, it accounts for approximately 20% of renal failure in childhood, and early diagnosis and treatment may delay or prevent the need for dialysis or kidney transplantation later in the child's life.

Etiology

Congenital anomalies account for nearly all of the obstructive lesions of the urinary system. The embryological differentiation of the urinary system is nearly complete by 10 weeks of gestation, at which time the kidneys have migrated to their adult position and urine has begun to form. Aberrations of differentiation during the first 10 weeks may result in structural abnormalities, including the obstructive uropathies, vesicoureteral reflux, and the various forms of cystic dysplasia. Urine first is produced during the second trimester, while nephronogenesis continues until about the 34th week. Kidney mass increases throughout gestation.

Lower Urinary Tract Obstruction. Lower urinary tract obstructive lesions most often are congenital and occur almost exclusively in males because of the length of the urethra and the embryological complexity of its development. *Posterior urethral valves* are the most common obstructive lesions. Abnormal migration of the terminal end of the wolffian ducts is believed to result in the persistence of obliquely oriented ridges along the posterior urethral wall producing a leaflike structure that acts to obstruct urine flow from the bladder. Urethral obstruction usually results in bladder enlargement and muscular hypertrophy as a result of the work involved in forcefully emptying against the obstructive resistance in the urethra. Hypertrophy of the interwoven bladder muscle fibers gives the appearance of a thickened bladder wall, with trabeculation on cystographic examination.

Urethral strictures as a cause of bladder outlet obstruction are uncommon acquired lesions that most often result from urethral trauma such as that induced by instrumentation, a straddle injury, a pelvic fracture, or urethritis, particularly that caused by a sexually transmitted disease. Congenital strictures are very rare. *Bladder outlet obstruction* in the past was a very common urological diagnosis, one made most often in children who had vesicoureteral reflux or recurrent urinary infections. Surgical transurethral resection or bladder neck revision often was performed, usually with little benefit. This disorder is believed to be unusual and limited almost exclusively to boys.

Although *meatal stenosis* in boys and *distal urethral stenosis* in girls were diagnosed commonly in the past as causes of bladder outlet obstruction, the role of these abnormalities in obstructing urine outflow is debated still. From a practical point of view, the visible size of the meatus does not correlate with its calibrated size. Furthermore, in girls urethral diameter correlates inversely with urinary infection, so infection is more common in individuals who have larger urethral lumens.

Phimosis can cause urethral obstruction, although probably not as frequently as once was thought. It may be a developmental anomaly or an acquired condition. *Anterior urethral valves, urethral diverticula,* müllerian *duct cysts,* and *megalourethra* all are rare structural causes of outlet obstruction.

Neurogenic bladder can cause obstructive changes because abnormal innervation may lead to functional obstruction. It may occur as a result of meningomyelocele or other spinal anomalies or with spinal cord injury.

Voiding dysnergia, or *nonneurogenic* bladder, is another functional cause of urinary obstruction. This condition is a form of incorrectly learned behavior associated with voluntary retention of urine and stool. In this circumstance the child constricts the internal sphincter of the bladder rather than relaxing it when voiding, creating a functional obstruction at the bladder neck. This disorder is considered to be psychogenic in origin.

Upper Urinary Tract Obstruction. *Ureteropelvic junction obstruction* is the most common obstructive lesion of the upper urinary system. The ureteric lumen may be constricted either intrinsically from a congenital narrowing of the lumen or extrinsically from pressure of a crossing blood vessel or a fibrous band or adhesion. It occurs in both genders equally, most often on the left side. It is bilateral in 10% of cases. Ureterovesical junction obstruction is the second most common supravesical obstructive site. It is more common among boys than among girls and is unilateral 80% of the time, usually on the left. In this condition the distal ureter usually is aperistaltic, producing functional obstruction and a markedly dilated, tortuous ureter. Occasionally, periureteral diverticula can produce ureteric obstruction by external impingement on the ureter.

Ureteral obstruction also can result from congenital ureteral valves, polyps, a retrocaval position of the ureters, or as a consequence of retroperitoneal fibrosis. All of these are rare among children.

History

The symptoms associated with urinary tract obstruction depend primarily on the degree and the duration of the blockage. In the neonate the severely obstructed urinary system may be dysplastic at birth. In such circumstances a history of oligohydramnios may be a factor, inasmuch as fetal urine makes up most of the amniotic fluid volume. Mild to moderate degrees of obstruction usually are associated with normal amniotic fluid volumes.

In the postnatal period the most common symptoms of children who have lesser degrees of obstruction are related to the occurrence of infection. Urinary tract infection in infants can be associated with nonspecific symptoms and signs such as failure to thrive, diarrhea, vomiting, feeding problems, or recurrent fever. Each infant who has a urinary infection should be examined for urinary tract obstruction. Occasionally an infant or child who has an obstruction comes to medical attention because of a voiding abnormality such as a poor urinary stream or polyuria. Others will have gross hematuria, often occurring after only minor trauma because dilated urinary systems are particularly prone to bleeding even with a slight blow to the abdomen or back. Finally, older children may have been symptom free until later childhood or adolescence when they are found to have azotemia or are referred for the investigation of enuresis or recurrent urinary tract infection.

Physical Findings

An abdominal mass is the most common finding among infants and children who have urinary obstruction. In the neonate, 50% of all abdominal masses are caused by malformations of the urinary system; approximately 65% of these result from obstruction. Upper tract lesions usually result in a unilateral mass, whereas lower tract obstruction often is associated with three masses—the dilated bladder and both hydronephrotic kidneys. In the child who has a significant but undiagnosed obstruction, recurrent infection may result in poor nutrition, which affects physical growth. Such children may be of normal weight and length at birth but grow at a reduced rate, so their weight and height pass through gradually decreasing percentiles on the growth chart during the first year. Obstructive uropathy and undiagnosed urinary tract infection should be included in the differential diagnosis of any child who fails to thrive.

Laboratory Findings

Inasmuch as infection occurs commonly in children who have an obstructed urinary system, a positive urine culture is one of the abnormal laboratory findings encountered most frequently. In addition, isosthenuria or hyposthenuria as a result of damage to the renal medullary concentrating mechanism often is found. Such findings are constant when the obstruction is bilateral but may not be present when the abnormality is unilateral. In addition to obtaining a urine culture, one must measure the urine specific gravity or osmolality in any patient who has an undiagnosed fever. A low specific gravity or osmolality in such a child, particularly if dehydrated, is a clue to urinary tract obstruction, urine infection, or both. Patients who have severe obstruction may have some degree of azotemia. In the neonate this may not be evident at birth because the maternal kidney functions for the fetus. Azotemia often becomes evident during the first week or two. With more severe degrees of renal failure, other abnormalities such as hypocalcemia, hyperphosphatemia, and anemia may occur.

Differential Diagnosis

The widespread use of prenatal ultrasound often alerts the clinician to a potential renal anomaly as early as the beginning of the second trimester. However, even serial prenatal studies cannot differentiate reliably between obstructive lesions and some of the cystic dysplasias (e.g., multicystic dysplasia, polycystic kidney diseases). Definitive differentiation usually must await postnatal imaging studies. Postnatal evaluation should be deferred, if possible, until the newborn is at least 48 hours old so that the transient postnatal period of relative dehydration is past and the diagnostic accuracy of the imaging techniques is greater.

The differential diagnosis of children who have a urinary tract obstruction relies primarily on various imaging techniques. In pediatric patients these usually include abdominal ultrasound, voiding cystourethrography, and radionuclide renal scans. These studies should allow the clinician to determine the site of the obstruction, the effect on renal function, and the potential for surgical correction. Visualizing the lower urinary system directly by cystoscopic examination also may be necessary. Occasionally, intravenous urographic examination is necessary, although its use in pediatrics has declined considerably with the development of newer imaging techniques. Examination by retrograde ureterography is required only under the most special circumstances and should not be part of the routine workup.

Treatment

The initial management of the child who has a newly diagnosed obstruction should be directed toward the aggressive treatment of urinary tract infection and sepsis and the correction of any abnormalities in hydration and blood chemistry values associated with renal failure. Lower tract obstruction may be relieved by catheterization. Early consultation with a urologist skilled in the care of children whose urinary systems are obstructed is crucial. The surgical correction of the obstructing lesion depends on the age and the size of the child, as well as on the site and cause of the obstruction. Definitive surgical treatment such as dilation of urethral strictures, fulguration of urethral valves, or pyeloplasty of ureteropelvic junction obstructions may be possible. Children who have complex anomalies may need several "staged" corrective surgical procedures. Among infants, urinary diversion by vesicostomy or nephrostomy may be the more prudent early approach, with deferral of definitive correction until the child is older and larger. Nonsurgical management by self-catheterization or double voiding often are effective in children who have neurogenic conditions of the bladder who have little to gain from surgical approaches.

Greater use of prenatal ultrasound has changed the medical approach to obstructive uropathy. Before the availability of this tool, only the more severely affected infants and children were detected clinically, and the diagnostic and treatment approaches were relatively aggressive, reflecting the severity of the lesions. It now has become evident that involvement encompasses all gradations, with many of the less severe lesions remaining asymptomatic and nonprogressive or even resolving spontaneously. This has led to a more thoughtful and watchful management of these patients. The advice of a pediatric nephrologist or urologist is valuable in individualizing the approach to these children.

Prognosis

The prognosis of any particular child is related to the degree and duration of the obstructive lesion, as well as to the number of urinary infections that have occurred. Early diagnosis is the most important aspect in minimizing damage. This may be particularly difficult given the nonspecific nature of symptoms of moderate urinary tract obstruction and infection in the infant. The earlier the diagnosis is made, the better the prognosis. Early diagnosis allows prompt treatment of active infection and consideration for surgical correction, thereby preventing future infections through the provision of good urinary drainage and prophylactic antibiotics. In very severe obstruction, because of the severity of the renal damage at the time of diagnosis, even early diagnosis and treatment may not be effective in averting the need for dialysis and transplantation in the future. Prenatal diagnosis of obstruction now provides a means for intervention at birth. Intrauterine corrective surgery has not yet been shown to be practical.

VESICOURETERAL REFLUX

Ureteral reflux is not an obstructive lesion but rather the failure of the normal insertion of the ureter into the bladder to act as a valve to ensure unidirectional urine flow. Vesicoureteral reflux may produce dilatation of the ureter and renal pelvis (often evident on ultrasound) on the involved side. This lesion cannot be diagnosed reliably by prenatal ultrasound because it is difficult to differentiate vesicoureteral reflux from obstructive uropathy. The definitive diagnosis is made postnatally by means of a contrast or nuclear cystogram. In these studies reflux is diagnosed when backflow up the ureter of contrast material or radioisotope is observed after one of these agents has been instilled in the bladder through a urinary catheter.

A grading system based on the contrast cystourethrogram has been developed that classifies reflux as being minimal (grade I) to severe (grade V). In the former the contrast rises no higher than the distal third of the ureter; in the latter the contrast completely fills the urinary collecting system and demonstrates hydronephrosis and loss of significant renal parenchyma. Reflux may be unilateral or bilateral. Although the lower grades of reflux of sterile urine probably do not produce parenchymal damage, evidence suggests that sterile reflux associated with very high intravesicle pressures may damage the renal cortex. In contrast, reflux of almost any degree associated with concomitant infection often produces pyelonephritis, the resolution of which may lead to renal scarring. From 30% to 50% of children who have vesicoureteral reflux have renal parenchymal scarring at the time of clinical presentation. Extensive scarring can cause chronic renal failure or hypertension, or both. As many as 45% of siblings also are found to have vesicoureteral reflux, most of whom are symptom free. Therefore all siblings younger than 5 years old should be screened because they compose the group most susceptible to renal scarring with infection.

Ureteral reflux can be either primary or secondary. Primary reflux can be caused by congenital anomalies at the ureterovesical junction or ectopic insertion of the ureter either alone or as part of a duplicated ureter, or it can be associated with other anomalies such as the so-called *prune belly syndrome*. This syndrome includes bilateral hydroureteronephrosis with reflux, deficient abdominal musculature, and undescended testes.

Secondary ureteral reflux can occur as a result of inflammation at the ureterovesical junction, distal anatomical obstruction (e.g., in urethral valves), or distal functional obstruction, such as a neurogenic bladder. Vesicoureteral reflux associated with inflammation—which occurs, for example, in cystitis—usually is low grade and often resolves with the treatment of the infection. This may take weeks to months, during which time the urinary system is susceptible to reinfection. Such patients should receive prophylactic antibiotics after the initial course of treatment and have routine follow-up urine cultures performed periodically thereafter.

Primary reflux of a lesser degree (grades I through III) usually can be managed medically by low-dose antibiotic prophylaxis. Approximately 60% to 80% of these patients' vesicoureteral reflux resolves on follow-up. Surgical correction more often is necessary for grades IV and V and in the rare patient who has a lower grade of reflux who has "breakthrough" infections despite medical management. Radionuclide cystograms, because of their high level of sensitivity and the low dose of radiation they generate, are particularly useful in follow-up on the resolution or correction of reflux.

SUGGESTED READINGS

Bailey RR et al: Long-term follow-up of infants with gross vesicoureteral reflux, *J Urol* 148:1709, 1992.

Belman AB: A perspective on vesicoureteral reflux, *Urol Clin North Am* 22:139, 1995.

Fine RN: Diagnosis and treatment of fetal urinary tract abnormalities, *J Pediatr* 121:333, 1992.

Hilton S, Kaplan GW: Imaging of common problems in pediatric urology, *Urol Clin North Am* 22:1, 1995.

Johnson CE et al: The accuracy of antenatal ultrasonography in identifying renal abnormalities, *Am J Dis Child* 146:1181, 1992.

King LR: Hydronephrosis: when is obstruction not obstruction? *Urol Clin North Am* 22:31, 1995.

Van den Abbeele A et al: Vesicoureteral reflux in asymptomatic siblings of patients with known reflux: radionuclide cystography, *Pediatrics* 79:147, 1987.

Warshaw BL et al: Prognostic features in infants with obstructive uropathy due to posterior urethral valves, *J Urol* 133:240, 1985.

236 Ocular Foreign Bodies

James W. McManaway III and Carl A. Frankel

Ocular foreign bodies can be classified as (1) surface, in which case they are either nonadherent or only loosely adherent to the corneal or conjunctival epithelium, (2) penetrating, in which case the foreign body goes into but not through the cornea or sclera, or (3) perforating, in which case the foreign body goes through the cornea or sclera and into the globe itself. A foreign body that goes completely through the sclera and rests in the vitreous body causes a perforating wound of the sclera and a penetrating wound of the globe. Although the terminology can be confusing, once it is learned it allows more accurate description of the problem. Careful examination, preferably with magnification, is necessary for all but the most superficial ocular foreign bodies, with referral to an ophthalmologist of all patients who give a history of an injury to the eye via high-velocity objects or in the setting of metal striking metal, for example, while hammering a nail.

SURFACE FOREIGN BODIES

The most likely sources of surface foreign bodies in children are small objects that can be thrown by a child (e.g., dirt, sand, and grass) and small wind-blown particles. Considering the profuse tearing associated with surface foreign bodies, it truly is the exceptional patient who requires medical care for one of these "flying" objects. In fact, even when care is sought after the acute incident, the offending agent often is absent and the cause of the ocular findings usually unknown.

When a patient consults a clinician with the complaint of a foreign body sensation—or when a nonverbal or preverbal patient seeks treatment with a history of pain, photophobia, epiphora, or rubbing of the eye(s)—the initial examination usually is accomplished more easily if a drop of topical ophthalmic anesthetic is instilled in each eye (unless a perforating wound of the cornea or sclera is suspected, in which case no medications should be used); an assessment of visual acuity should then be attempted. Once this is completed, the lids and lashes should be inspected to see if any foreign bodies can be observed and removed. Uncooperative or frightened children may need sedation to allow an adequate examination.

Attention should next be turned to the corneal and conjunctival surfaces to ascertain whether a foreign body can be identified (Fig. 236-1). At this time, magnification, either with a loupe or a slit lamp, is preferred. It may be possible to irrigate or wipe away readily observed foreign bodies with the stretched-out fibers of a cotton applicator. In a cooperative patient sitting quietly by the slit lamp, surface foreign bodies usually can be removed manually with a fine, toothless forceps. Metallic foreign bodies on the corneal surface start to oxidize within several hours; these must be removed and the "rust ring" debrided by an ophthalmologist.

After this procedure, the tarsal conjunctival surfaces should be examined. The clinician usually can pull the lower lid down by placing one finger on the middle aspect of the lid just beneath the lash line and with another, applying gentle traction inferiorly. Again, foreign bodies generally can be irrigated or brushed out and, if adherent, can be removed with a forceps. Attention then should be turned to the upper lid, which should be everted as follows: The lashes should be grasped gently between the thumb and forefinger; with the shaft of a cotton applicator placed at the superior margin of the tarsal plate, the lashes should be pulled out and up to evert the lid onto the cotton applicator (Fig. 236-2, *A*). After the lid is everted, the lashes can be pinned against the superior orbital rim and the cotton applicator removed (Fig. 236-2, *B*). Any foreign bodies that are present usually can be seen and removed readily.

After the foreign body or bodies have been removed, the eye should be checked for a corneal abrasion. This is accomplished best with a minimal amount of sterile fluorescein instilled and the eye examined with a cobalt blue light source, either at the slit lamp or via a penlight with a special filter. Corneal abrasions appear as a green line or patch; multiple fine vertical corneal abrasions that look like ice skate tracks are highly suggestive of a foreign body under the upper eyelid. If an abrasion is present, an antibiotic ointment should be instilled. If the pain was severe before instillation of the anesthetic drops, a sterile eye patch should be taped in place for 6 to 12 hours. Arrangements then should be made for follow-up the next day to ensure that the abrasion has resolved. If it has not, or if significant pain persists, the patient should be referred to an ophthalmologist to be certain that an iritis, which may require more aggressive intervention, has not developed.

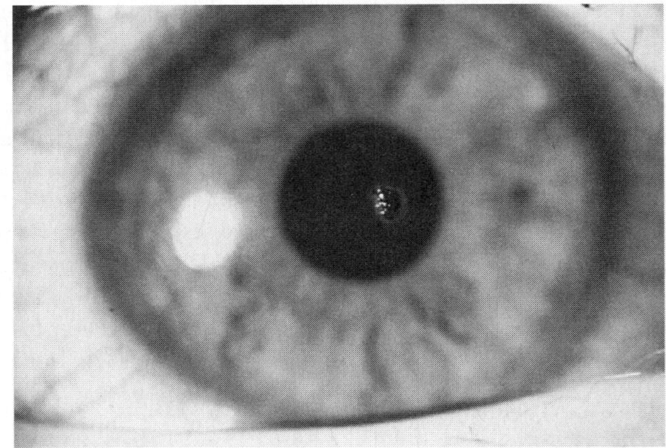

FIG. 236-1 Metallic foreign body on the surface of the cornea. Note the surrounding rust ring, which should be removed to reduce intraocular inflammation from metal breakdown.

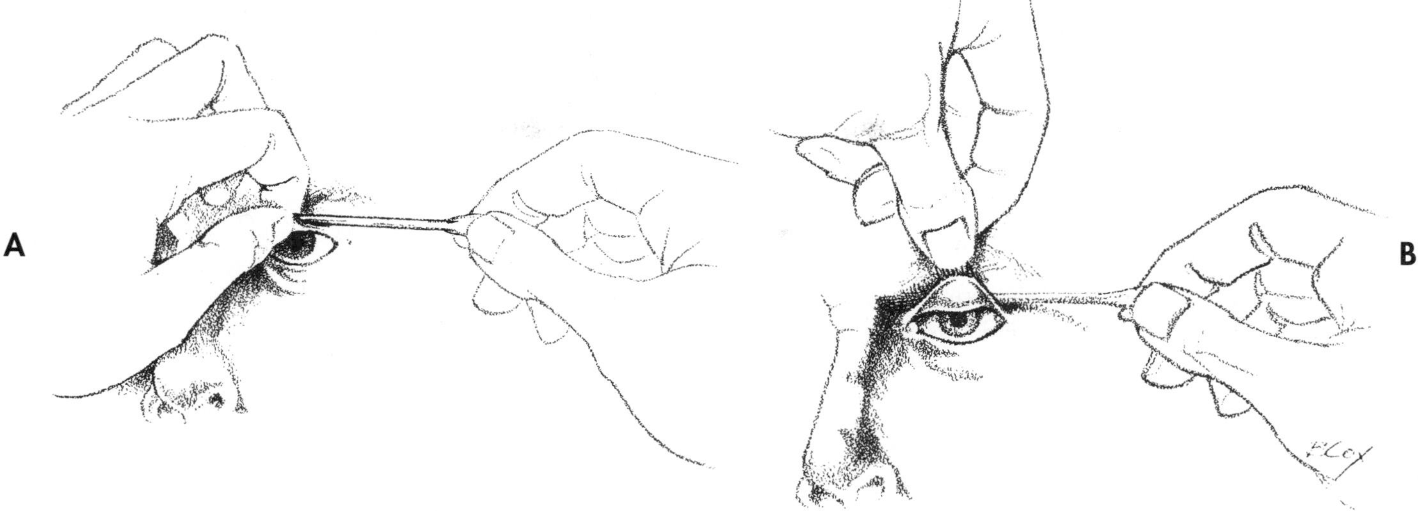

FIG. 236-2 **A,** Demonstration of an easy method for everting a patient's upper eyelid with the lashes and lid being pulled out and up from the globe. **B,** After the eyelid has been everted, the lashes are pinned against the superior orbital rim before removal of the cotton applicator. After the everted lid is examined, the lashes can be pulled inferiorly and released to reposition the lid.

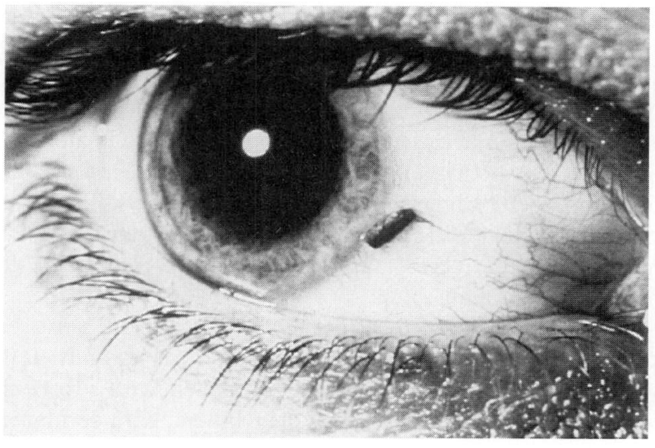

FIG. 236-3 Metallic foreign body that has penetrated the sclera. Care must be taken in determining whether this foreign body has actually perforated the sclera and entered the globe. When in doubt, an ophthalmologist should remove such foreign bodies.

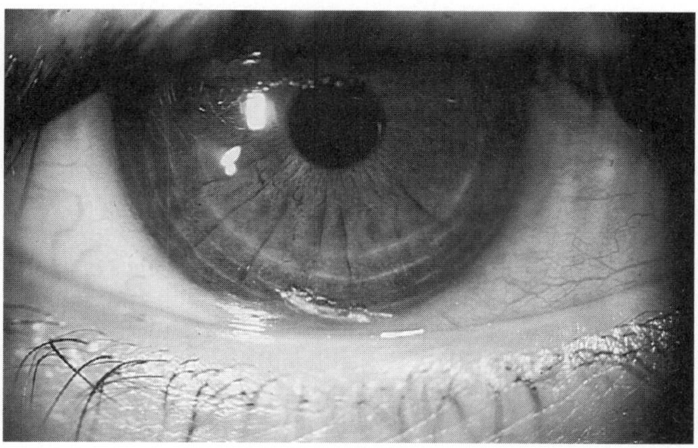

FIG. 236-4 This patient felt pain while hammering a nail. The visual acuity of this eye was 20/20. Note the metallic foreign body that has perforated the cornea and is resting on the inferior iris.

PENETRATING FOREIGN BODIES

When a foreign body is imbedded in the conjunctiva, cornea, or scleral tissue (Fig. 236-3), the examiner must be concerned that it may represent a perforating wound of the cornea or sclera, allowing bacteria to gain access to the intraocular space. In these instances, visual acuity can be surprisingly normal. The examiner, therefore, must maintain a high index of suspicion and have the patient evaluated by an ophthalmologist.

PERFORATING FOREIGN BODIES

Perforating foreign bodies go completely through the cornea or sclera. These high-velocity injuries usually are devastating to ocular integrity and frequently result in severe derangement and permanent visual loss, although initial visual acuity and cursory examination findings may be normal (Fig. 236-4). Visual loss can be minimized in some instances by prompt referral to an ophthalmologist skilled at intervention in corneal, anterior segment, and vitreoretinal trauma.

SUGGESTED READINGS

DeBustros S: Posterior segment intraocular foreign bodies. In Shingleton BJ, Hersh PS, Kenyon KR, editors: *Eye trauma,* St Louis, 1991, Mosby.

Kenyon KR, Wagoner MD: Conjunctival and corneal injuries. In Shingleton BJ, Hersh PS, Kenyon KR, editors: *Eye trauma,* St Louis, 1991, Mosby.

Smiddy WE, Stark WJ: Anterior segment intraocular foreign bodies. In Shingleton BJ, Hersh PS, Kenyon KR, editors: *Eye trauma,* St Louis, 1991, Mosby.

237 Ocular Trauma

James W. McManaway III and Carl A. Frankel

Evaluation of the patient who has ocular trauma requires a thorough knowledge of the anatomy of the eye and orbit and an understanding of the types of injuries that may result from specific types of trauma. Although it is unusual, normal or near-normal visual acuity may be achieved even after a rupture of the globe. As a result, a high index of suspicion must be maintained for each patient who is seen for ocular or orbital trauma. In addition, because many children who have orbital or ocular injuries are in considerable pain and have significant photophobia and fear, the very act of examining or attempting to examine the eye can create greater damage than that produced by the original injury. Uncooperative children who have signs or a history suggestive of significant ocular injury should be examined in the operating room by an ophthalmologist to prevent further ocular injury.

ANATOMICAL CONSIDERATIONS

The orbit is shaped roughly like a quadrilateral pyramid. The orbital roof is formed from the orbital plate of the frontal bone and the lesser wing of the sphenoid bone. The lateral orbital wall is formed by the zygoma and the greater wing of the sphenoid bone. The orbital floor is formed from the maxillary bone, the orbital plate of the zygomatic bone, and a small portion of the palatine bone. The medial orbital wall is formed by the frontal process of the maxilla, the lacrimal bone, the orbital plate of the ethmoid bone, and the body of the sphenoid bone. The orbital rim tends to absorb the impact of most large-object injuries, which may lead to fractures of the orbital bones with preservation of the integrity of the globe itself. Small-object injuries that affect the globe directly tend to cause primary injuries to the globe, with secondary injury to the thinner bones of the orbit, primarily its floor and medial wall. The contour of the object can predispose to penetrating or perforating injuries of the globe.

The globe rests in the orbit, cushioned by orbital fat, and is moved by six extraocular muscles. The lateral rectus muscle is innervated by the abducens (sixth) cranial nerve; the superior oblique muscle is innervated by the trochlear (fourth) cranial nerve. The other four extraocular muscles, the levator muscle of the upper lid, and the iris sphincter muscle are innervated by the oculomotor (third) cranial nerve. Orbital injuries can cause abnormal ocular motility due to cranial nerve palsies, orbital soft tissue scarring, or direct extraocular muscle injury.

The eyelids act to protect the globe from particulate debris and have an important role in maintaining the normal tear film strip over the cornea. Defects in eyelid anatomy or function can cause major problems related to corneal exposure, with subsequent infection or scarring, or both. Injuries to the eyelids can result in unsuspected injuries to the globe, especially when sharp objects lacerate or penetrate the eyelids. Eyelid lacerations that expose the orbital fat pad in the upper lid may injure the levator muscle; improper surgical repair that ignores a levator muscle injury often results in a posttraumatic ptosis. The lacrimal drainage system starts in the medial aspect of each lid and connects to the lacrimal sac via small canaliculi. Lacerations of the medial aspect of an eyelid often result in a canalicular laceration, which must be repaired carefully by an ophthalmologist skilled in this type of surgery.

Between the eyelid fissure lies the exposed surface of the globe—the bulbar conjunctiva and the cornea. These areas commonly are involved when ocular injuries occur. The bulbar conjunctiva covers the sclera from the corneal limbus to the cul-de-sac or fornix; the tarsal conjunctiva then reflects over the inner eyelid surface to the lid margin. The subconjunctival space often fills with blood after ocular injuries; a small amount of blood is spread out into a large area, giving an alarming appearance to the uninitiated. Most subconjunctival hemorrhages are benign, but they also can hide more severe ocular injuries. The clear cornea, approximately 0.5 mm thick, covers the anterior chamber, iris, and lens and provides about 66% of the refractive power of the eye. The sclera forms the wall of the eye and is thinnest (0.3 mm) under the insertions of the rectus muscles. This is a common site for the globe to rupture.

The posterior segment of the eye consists of the posterior sclera, ciliary body, choroid, retina, and vitreous body. Injuries to these areas frequently are associated with severe intraocular hemorrhage and retinal detachment, with permanent visual loss.

EVALUATION

The evaluation of the child who has ocular trauma consists of three steps: (1) recognizing life-threatening nonocular injuries and emergent ocular conditions such as ocular chemical injuries, (2) taking an adequate history to assess the potential risk of injury to the eye, to obtain significant past ocular history, and to identify medical conditions that may complicate the treatment of the injury or administration of general anesthesia, (3) examining the eye in detail ocular examination, which includes visual acuity testing and external, ocular motility, pupil, anterior segment, and fundus examinations.

Occasional patients initially may appear to have only ocular injuries when other severe injuries are present; one example is a patient struck in the eye with a ski-pole tip. The CT scan showed an orbital roof fracture with disruption of the frontal lobe. Ocular alkali injuries can have devastating consequences without immediate and copious ocular irrigation; any patient who has an ocular chemical injury should have irrigation first and be asked detailed questions later! In the evaluation of any child who has ocular injury, a careful history should be obtained, realizing that independent or unsupervised play (coupled with guilt and fear) may make the information obtained unreliable. As many details as possible should be obtained, specifically highlighting the source of injury, which may suggest the nature of potential injuries. Additional history taking should include the date of the last tetanus immunization, prior ocular history (such as amblyopia of the noninjured eye), medications, allergies, and when the patient last had something to eat or drink, in the event surgical intervention is necessary.

After the history has been obtained, with specific regard to symptoms, the examination should proceed in an orderly manner to ensure that nothing is omitted or overlooked. In a child who is old enough to cooperate, beginning with the nontraumatized eye usually will allay anxiety sufficiently to examine the traumatized eye next. When the traumatized eye is tested, care must be taken not to put any pressure on the globe itself.

Visual Acuity Testing

The examination should begin with testing visual acuity. Although normal visual acuity has been reported in patients who have severe injuries, the presence of significantly impaired vision is a sign that the injury is likely to be severe and the services of an ophthalmologist are needed. Children initially may display a poor visual acuity in the injured eye that improves significantly after reassurance and patience. The most objective method available should be used to establish a reliable baseline acuity measurement. The normal eye must be completely covered when the injured eye is being tested.

Preverbal children present a special challenge in measuring visual acuity because they cannot respond to the usual visual acuity tests given to older patients. Fixation on a brightly colored toy or on the examiner's face is very useful; absence of fixation or attempts to move the head to remove the cover over the normal eye indicate poor acuity in the injured eye. Measuring the child's ability to locate small candies in the examiner's hand is well tolerated, but the child should not eat the candy if a trip to the operating room is possible!

Verbal children should have their visual acuity tested with standard picture, E-game, or letter charts. Younger children can "match" the presented picture if they cannot name it. If a child cannot identify the largest picture on the chart (usually 20/200), it should be moved closer until the figure can be identified. If the 20/200 picture is identified at 8 (not 20) feet from the chart, the acuity is recorded as 8/200. If an eye chart is not available, substitutes such as objects, faces, or facial features can be used. The examiner should record details of the objects' size and testing distance so that the data obtained can be compared with subsequent visual acuity measurements.

Patients who have significant ocular injuries still will be unable to read the eye chart even though they are very close to it. Alternative methods of measuring visual acuity under these circumstances include the ability to count fingers (recorded as "counts fingers at X feet"), distinguish the motion of a hand (recorded as "hand motion at X feet"), determine the direction of a light source (recorded as "light perception with projection"), and determine the presence of a light source (recorded as "light perception"). These methods have been listed in order of decreasing visual function.

External Examination

As with the examination of any patient, observation and inspection are important first steps. Key signs to note include edema or ecchymosis of the lids and ocular adnexal structures, asymmetry or discontinuity of the orbital and facial bones, ocular proptosis or enophthalmos, foreign bodies, subconjunctival hemorrhage, laceration(s), and the prolapse of intraocular contents (including iris, ciliary body, vitreous, and retina) through a laceration of the cornea or sclera. If the child is cooperative and no sign of a ruptured globe is present, dried blood should be removed gently to help uncover all injuries present. Significant positive and negative findings should be noted; diagrams of the injuries, including details of the length and depth of lacerations, should be recorded. Photographic documentation of the injuries is very useful.

Ocular Motility

Unless a ruptured globe is suspected, ocular motility should be checked, with attention paid to both ductions (monocular eye movements) and versions (conjugate, binocular eye movements) in all gaze positions, with note made of any abnormalities. The presence of diplopia should be noted, and if possible, the examiner should obtain a description from the patient of the location of the two images with respect to each other.

Pupils

The presence of round pupils should be noted; if a pupil is not round (Fig. 237-1) (oval, teardrop, or pear shaped, for instance), a drawing of the abnormality should be made. Next, the reaction of each pupil to light should be checked, both directly and consensually. When this test is performed, the patient should be instructed to fixate on a distant point so that the accommodation reflex, with its secondary pupillary miosis, does not influence the assessment of pupillary function. The reactivity of the pupils (both direct and consensual) gives important information about both the afferent and efferent limbs of the visual pathway.

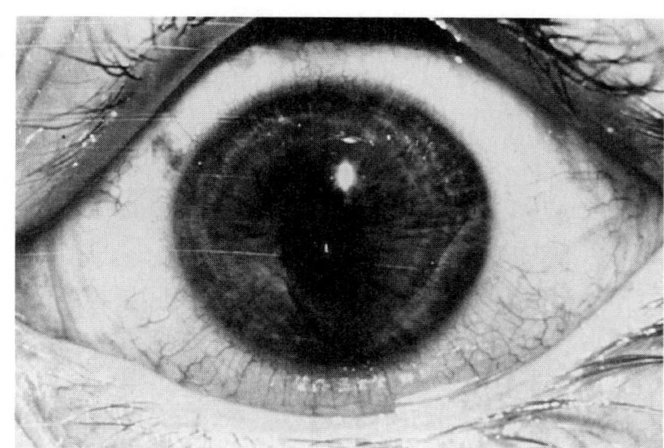

FIG. 237-1 Photograph showing an inverted teardrop-shaped pupil caused by an inferior corneal laceration with the iris drawn to the wound.

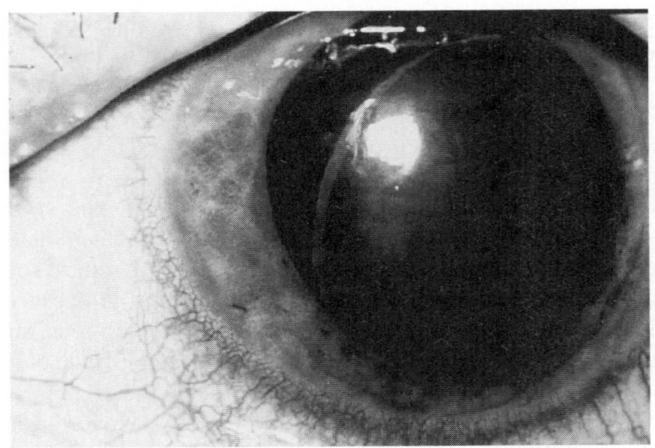

FIG. 237-2 Ocular injury from a fist, with inferior lens subluxation and minimal cataractous changes.

The swinging flashlight test is performed by alternately (i.e., switching eyes every 2 seconds) shining a bright light source into each eye. The normal response is for both pupils to stay constricted. Paradoxical dilation of a pupil when light is illuminating it indicates retinal or optic nerve dysfunction, or both. This is called a *Marcus Gunn pupil* or an afferent pupillary defect. The absence of an afferent pupillary defect on the swinging flashlight test is reassuring confirmation that neither significant optic nerve nor retinal damage has occurred. In the event of posttraumatic iridoplegia, both the direct and consensual reflexes would be diminished because of impairment in the terminal efferent pupillomotor organ—the iris.

Anterior Segment

If a slit lamp is available and if the patient is able, the conjunctiva, cornea, anterior chamber, iris, lens, and red reflex should be examined. Particular attention should be directed to evaluation of (1) the conjunctiva for subconjunctival hemorrhage, conjunctival lacerations, or foreign bodies, (2) the cornea for the presence of epithelial defects (abrasions), lacerations, or foreign bodies, (3) the anterior chamber for depth (shallow or deep) or the presence of red blood cells (hyphema), (4) the lens for the presence of cataracts or dislocation (Fig. 237-2), and (5) the fundus red reflex for subtle lens opacities or abnormalities that might indicate a vitreous hemorrhage or retinal detachment. If a slit lamp is unavailable, if the examiner is not familiar with its use, or if the patient cannot be brought to the slit lamp, the direct ophthalmoscope can be used to examine the anterior segment adequately.

Fundus

A fundus examination always should be attempted unless a ruptured globe is suspected and pressure may have to be placed on the eye to open the lids. In those circumstances, increased pressure on the globe through the eyelids may result in extrusion of intraocular contents, potentially making it impossible to restore the integrity of the visual system. In case of doubt, the examination should be delayed until the arrival of an ophthalmologist.

MANAGEMENT OF SPECIFIC INJURIES

One must keep in mind that just as the orbital relationships comprise a continuum, so too does the extent of orbital and ocular injuries. The result is that when one portion of the orbit or globe is injured, other injuries may be present.

Ecchymosis

Ecchymosis, or bruising, of the periorbital region results in the typical "black" eye. The blunt contusion injury that results in ecchymosis may be either isolated or associated with other orbital or ocular injury. An uncomplicated black eye is treated the same as a contusion anywhere else: cold compresses for the first 24 hours, followed by warm compresses until the swelling subsides, with elevation of the patient's head to help resolve the edema. The patient or parents should be advised that because of gravity, the ecchymosis and edema may appear to spread down the cheek or even to the fellow eye. Although frightening in appearance, this type of spread is not dangerous and resolves spontaneously.

Orbital Hemorrhage

When a contusion injury occurs, ecchymosis of the periorbital region may occur simultaneously with hemorrhage within the orbit itself. Because the orbit is a bony structure open on only one end, an increase in volume of the orbital contents from hemorrhage or edema increases the intraorbital pressure, which can be relieved only with anterior displacement of the globe, resulting in *proptosis*. If the proptosis is severe, compression of the optic nerve or acute glaucoma can permanently impair visual function. If progressive proptosis is noted, emergency lateral canthotomy and possible orbital decompression is indicated. Steroids often are used, but their effectiveness has not been demonstrated. In the absence of signs of optic nerve compromise, treatment consists of ice packs for the first 24 hours, followed by warm compresses, with elevation of the head to reduce edema.

Orbital Fractures

Direct injury to the bony orbit may result in extensive facial and orbital bone fractures and can be associated with significant intracranial and ocular injuries. When a broad concussive force is delivered to the orbit in a manner that rapidly increases the intraorbital pressure, one or more of the thin orbital walls may fracture because of the relative incompressibility of the orbital contents. This condition is called a *blow-out fracture;* the orbital floor is the most common site, with the medial orbital wall the next most common.

Blow-out fractures are seen more commonly in adolescents than in younger children and frequently result from motor vehicle accidents or a blow from a fist; because most people are right-handed, the left orbit is involved more often than the right. The patient frequently complains of diplopia and pain, with clinical signs of proptosis if orbital hemorrhage occurs or enophthalmos if the fracture is large. Movement of the affected eye is limited (typically limitation of upgaze because of inferior rectus muscle entrapment in the fracture), accompanied by eyelid edema and ecchymosis.

The evaluation of a patient who has a suspected blow-out fracture requires the use of orbital computed tomography (CT) scanning to delineate the presence and extent of the fracture accurately. Appropriate positioning of the patient to obtain 1.5 mm slices that slightly overlap is necessary for accurate imaging. Because of the nature of the orbital injury, the possibility of a coexisting injury to the globe must be considered, and an ophthalmologist should evaluate before any other specialist is consulted. The concurrent presence of a ruptured globe and blow-out fracture requires delayed treatment of the fracture until the integrity of the globe is restored.

Blow-out fractures don't have to be treated immediately. Indeed, allowing time for the edema and ecchymosis to diminish may resolve the proptosis and diplopia. Frequently, diplopia is due to a muscle contusion, and the symptoms may resolve over 3 to 4 days. If surgery needs to be undertaken for entrapment of orbital contents, diplopia, or more than 2 mm of enophthalmos, it can be performed safely 5 to 7 days after the injury. Patients who have an orbital blow-out fracture should be managed by, or comanaged with, an ophthalmologist (preferably an ophthalmic plastic surgeon). *Under no circumstances should an orbital blow-out fracture be repaired without prior evaluation by an ophthalmologist.* When surgical intervention is indicated, the goal is to restore the anatomical location of prolapsed orbital contents and to free any restriction of ocular motility. On occasion, an artificial floor needs to be created with the use of implanted material.

Eyelid Lacerations

Although eyelid lacerations and avulsion injuries may occur without significant injury to the globe, ocular injuries must be ruled out before repair of the laceration is attempted; a ruptured globe either missed altogether or not detected until after a lacerated lid has been repaired is indefensible. *An ophthalmologist must be consulted before eyelid repair if any question exists about the presence of ocular injuries.*

Simple lid lacerations that do not involve the eyelid margin, orbicularis muscle, or other structures such as the medial or lateral canthal tendon, the levator palpebrae superioris muscle, or the lacrimal gland and drainage system can be repaired readily with local anesthesia and the use of a size 6-0 nylon suture, which usually is removed 5 to 7 days after injury. In younger children who may not be cooperative for suture removal, 6-0 mild chromic gut should be used instead. If the lid laceration involves deeper orbital structures or if the eyelid margin is involved (Fig. 237-3), an ophthalmologist should be consulted to assess the integrity of the eye and to repair the lacerations. It is not acceptable for a physician to repair the laceration and to notify the ophthalmologist as an afterthought.

Conjunctival Injury

Conjunctival injury typically manifests with only mild to moderate pain because of the relative paucity of a sensory nerve supply. Most conjunctival injuries take the form of subconjunctival hemorrhages (Fig. 237-4), which can be quite frightening but actually are harmless, unless associated with more extensive ocular injuries. No treatment is necessary for isolated subconjunctival hemorrhages, although the patient or parents should be cautioned that a brownish discoloration may result from deposition of hemosiderin. Small isolated conjunctival lacerations do not require intervention, although a thorough ophthalmic examination must be performed to rule out a laceration of the underlying sclera, choroid, or retina.

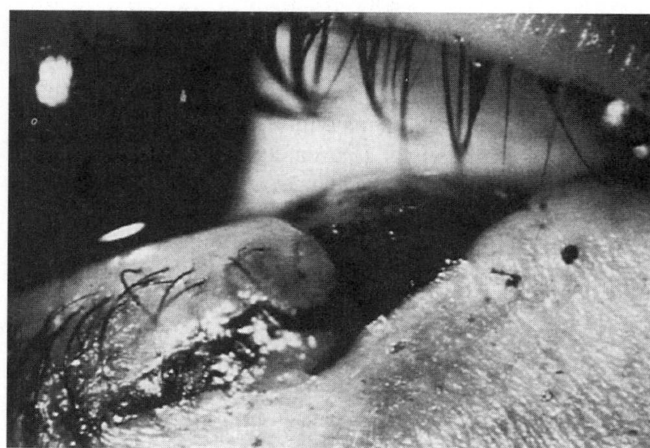

FIG. 237-3 Laceration of the lower lid that was found to involve the inferior canaliculus. Oculoplastic surgical repair was undertaken to restore the function of the inferior tear collection system.

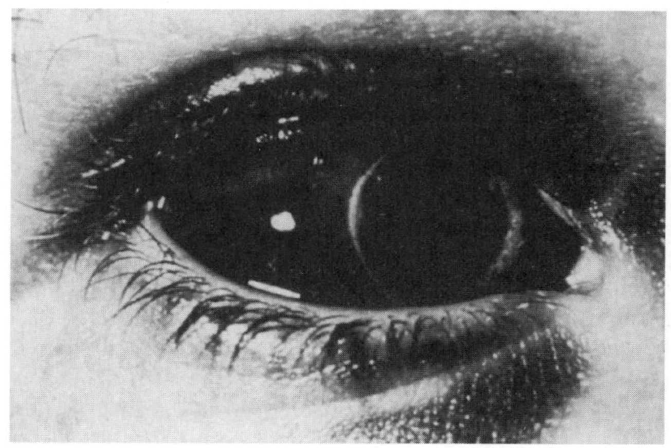

FIG. 237-4 Severe subconjunctival hemorrhage after blunt trauma.

Corneal Injuries

The corneal epithelium is a multilayered structure that rests on a tough basement membrane layer called the Bowman membrane. The corneal epithelium is laced with numerous fine sensory nerve endings, resulting in exquisite pain when the epithelium is disrupted. This epithelial disruption is observed easily with the use of a cobalt blue light after the instillation of sterile fluorescein (Fig. 237-5). Fortunately, most corneal abrasions heal extremely rapidly.

The initial phase of healing is characterized by migration of the remaining corneal epithelial cells over the defect, with subsequent reestablishment of the normal cell-to-cell and cell-to-basement membrane adhesions over a period of several weeks to months. In extensive corneal abrasions in which no corneal epithelium remains, conjunctival cells migrate over the corneal surface and then undergo transdifferentiation eventually to become indistinguishable from normal corneal epithelium.

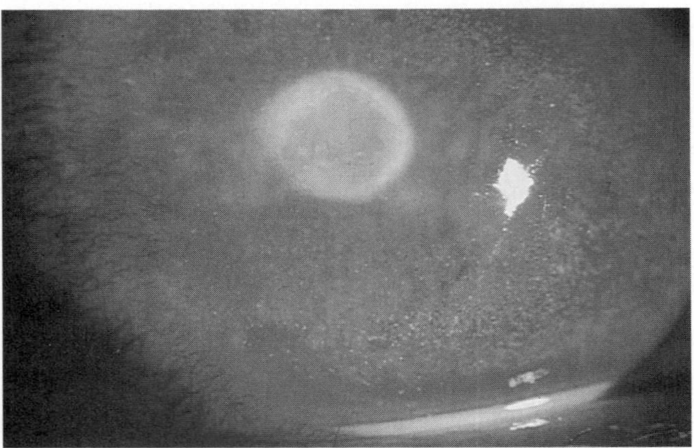

FIG. 237-5 A corneal abrasion revealed by fluorescein dye staining.

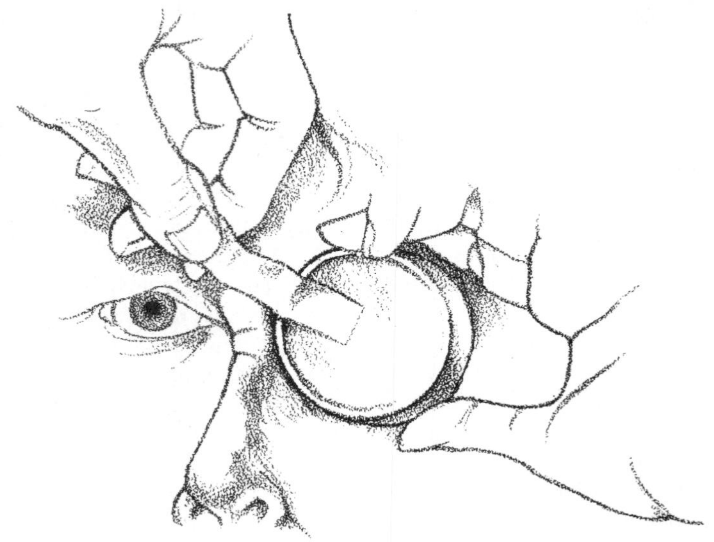

FIG. 237-6 Taping the bottom of a cup to the skin when a shield is not available to protect a suspected open globe from externally applied pressure.

During the healing phase, a tight patch after instillation of an ophthalmic antibiotic ointment may allow the patient to experience only a mild foreign-body sensation, which typically resolves after the epithelial surface of the abraded area has been restored. Typically the period of time that the eye is patched is 12 to 24 hours; in young children the occlusion may be more distressing than the injury itself. Should the abrasion not be healed substantially by 24 hours after injury, referral to an ophthalmologist should be made to rule out infection or other reasons for delayed healing.

Despite the pain that occurs from a corneal abrasion, *under no circumstances should any patient be allowed to use topical anesthetic drops at home*. The topical anesthetic prevents normal epithelial migration and results in a progressively larger abrasion and permanent corneal damage. These agents are to be used only in an acute setting for the diagnosis of ocular disorders or in an attempt to relieve patient discomfort for examination or for brief procedures.

In extremely young children and infants, the plasticity of the visual system should be kept in mind so that occlusion amblyopia (poor vision in the eye under the patch because of visual deprivation) does not ensue. The susceptibility of the development of occlusion amblyopia is inversely proportional to the patient's age. In addition, as a result of impairment of the fusion mechanism, a latent deviation of an eye (typically an esophoria or exophoria—see Chapter 167, Strabismus) may convert to a manifest deviation (either an esotropia or an exotropia, respectively) because of patching of an injured eye for as short a period as 1 to 2 days. Surgical intervention occasionally may be necessary to restore normal ocular alignment.

Corneal lacerations (either full or partial thickness), no matter how well approximated, *require immediate referral to an ophthalmologist*. Patients who have corneal lacerations should have the eye covered with a shield to reduce the likelihood of the intraocular contents prolapsing. If a shield is unavailable, the bottom of a cup can be taped to the skin (Fig. 237-6) to prevent pressure on the globe.

Chemical Injuries

Chemical injuries, from either acid or alkali, are acute emergencies that require immediate, copious irrigation, followed by ocular examination by an ophthalmologist to rule out corneal or other ocular injuries. If the patient complains of pain, instillation of a topical anesthetic will reduce the discomfort from the injury and the irrigation itself. If blepharospasm during attempted irrigation is problem, a lid speculum should be used to keep the eye open; alternatively, an irrigating contact lens can be used. Overirrigation is not a problem, although the use of pH indicator paper can serve to show when the offending solution has been neutralized. Patients who have ocular alkali injuries often have permanent visual loss from corneal scarring, glaucoma, and cataract formation.

Hyphema

In blunt trauma to the globe, the forces transmitted to the intraocular structures by the noncompressible fluid contents of the globe may result in avulsion of the blood vessels at the iris root or the face of the ciliary body. When this happens, grossly visible blood enters the anterior chamber of the eye and a hyphema is formed (Fig. 237-7). When a hyphema occurs, the patient requires the care of an ophthalmologist because of potential associated complications. The purpose of this section is to provide guidelines for initial management.

Although ophthalmologists do not agree universally as to management of the patient who has a traumatic hyphema, many ophthalmologists recommend topical atropine solution, topical prednisolone acetate suspension, a clear plastic shield over the injured eye, and bed rest. The purpose of this management is to prevent rebleeding into the anterior chamber, which is associated with a worse visual prognosis. The atropine stabilizes the pupil to reduce traction on injured iris vessels and paralyzes the ciliary body to reduce discomfort from the associated iritis. Topical prednisolone reduces the associated intraocular inflammation. The shield prevents further injury to the eye, and bed rest reduces fluctuations in the venous pressure transmitted to the eye. Watching television is recommended because the eyes are kept in nearly the same position; reading, however, is contraindicated because of the

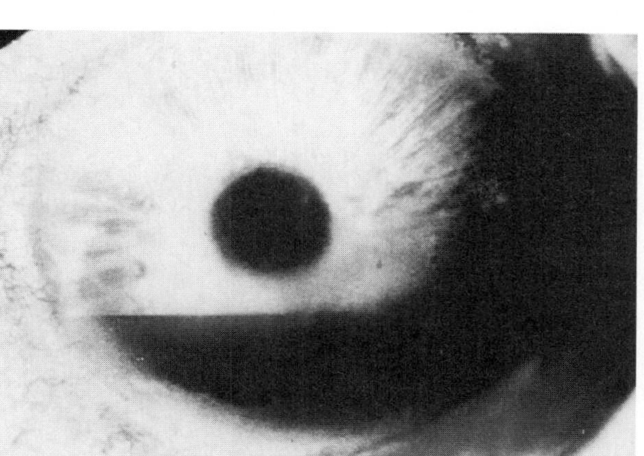

FIG. 237-7 Acute hyphema secondary to blunt ocular injury. Acute glaucoma ensued, which resolved when the hyphema cleared.

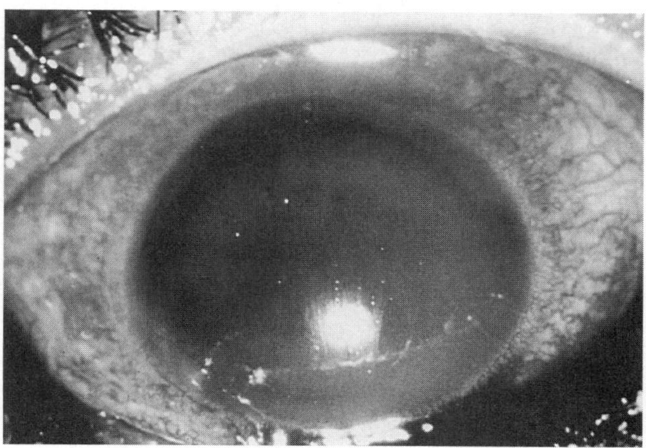

FIG. 237-8 Corneal blood staining following a hyphema in which secondary glaucoma was unable to be controlled.

associated saccadic ocular movements. The preceding treatment can be performed at home if the patient and family are reliable and if the hyphema is small (less than one third of the anterior chamber). If the hyphema is large or if the nature of the child or the social situation warrants it, the child should be hospitalized for 5 to 6 days.

Because of the possibility of rebleeding because of clot resorption, some ophthalmologists hospitalize their patients and administer oral epsilon-aminocaproic acid (Amicar, Lederle) in an attempt to slow clot resorption, although its use is contraindicated in very large hyphemas (greater than 75% of the anterior chamber). If Amicar is used, it is continued through at least the sixth postinjury day, if bleeding has not recurred. Although this agent has been shown to reduce the incidence of rebleeding significantly, hypotension and gastrointestinal side effects, including nausea and vomiting, may prompt some to hold off on its use, except in high-risk situations in which the patient cannot be maintained in a state of quiet.

Children suffering a hyphema are at risk for many ocular complications, including rebleeding, glaucoma, and corneal blood staining (Fig. 237-8) with amblyopia development, as well as the effects of other ocular injuries from the initial trauma, such as iris tears, angle recession, cyclodialysis (an abnormal separation between the ciliary body and sclera), cataract formation, lens subluxation, retinal tears, choroidal rupture (Fig. 237-9), and rupture of the globe. Secondary glaucoma may result from one of two mechanisms. The first is through damage to the filtration angle. The second is caused by obstruction of the filtration angle from the red blood cells; this usually resolves after the blood is absorbed totally. Glaucoma in the presence of a hyphema must be managed carefully to prevent optic nerve damage as well as to prevent corneal blood staining, which can cause severe amblyopia in children under 8 years of age. The glaucoma often is controlled medically, but patients who have uncontrolled glaucoma must have the blood surgically evacuated from the anterior chamber. Patients who have sickle cell anemia or trait are at much higher risk for these complications and need earlier intervention. Any patient who has a hyphema needs daily (and sometimes twice daily) intraocular pressure checks to detect the presence of glaucoma in an attempt to reduce the likelihood of permanent visual loss.

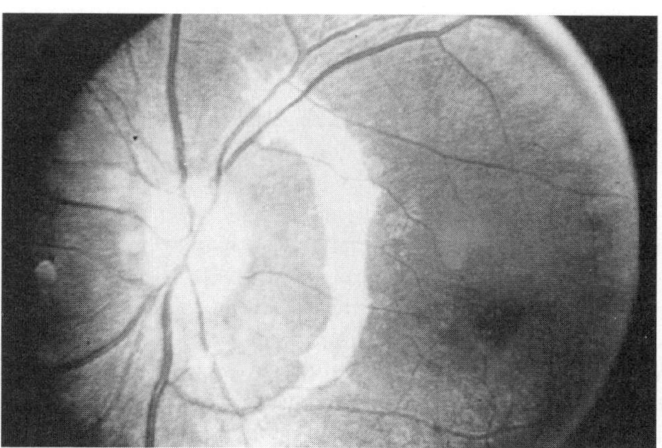

FIG. 237-9 Choroidal rupture resulting from blunt injury to the globe. The overlying retinal vessels are intact, but note the crescent-shaped area caused by absence of choroid overlying the white sclera. The typical location for choroidal and retinal ruptures is between the macula and optic nerve.

Ruptured Globe

Except in the setting of a perforating injury of the cornea or sclera by a small, sharp object or a posterior rupture, patients who have a ruptured globe have several characteristic ocular signs, including poor visual acuity, conjunctival edema, subconjunctival hemorrhage, shallow anterior chamber, and hyphema. Prolapsed intraocular tissue (lens, iris, ciliary body, retina, choroid, or vitreous) may be seen if the rupture occurs at or near the limbus. If a ruptured globe is a possibility, early involvement of an ophthalmologist is essential. In the time before the ophthalmologist's arrival, the patient should be treated as follows:

1. Be kept quiet with sedation and antiemetics as needed
2. Not allowed to lie on the injured side
3. Have a shield placed over the injured eye(s) to reduce the likelihood of further injury
4. Have nothing to eat or drink in anticipation of the need for general anesthesia
5. Have *no* eye drops or ointments instilled until the globe is repaired

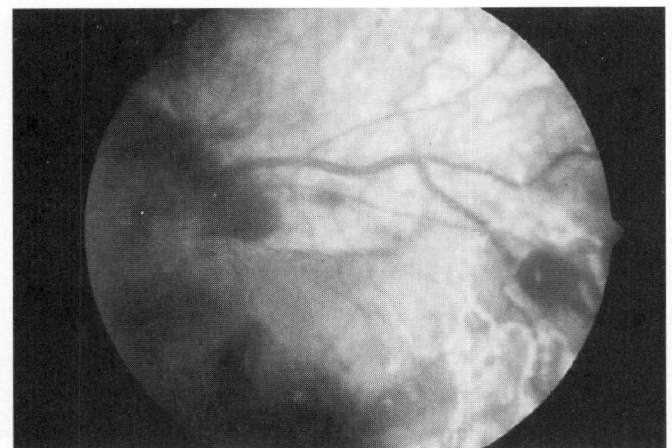

FIG. 237-10 Fundus photograph showing retinal hemorrhages in a victim of shaken baby syndrome.

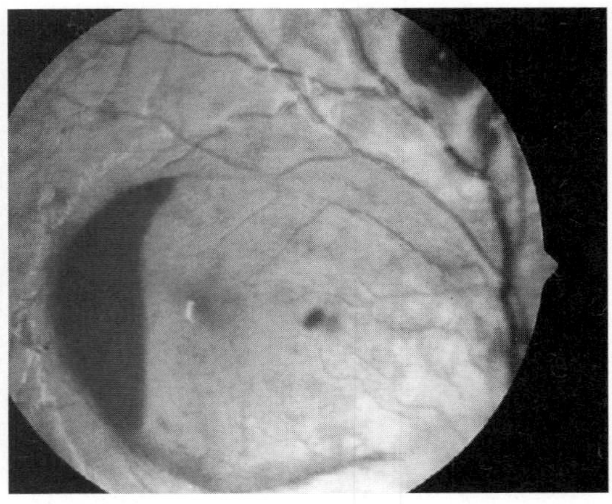

FIG. 237-11 Fundus photograph of the same patient shown in Fig. 235-14 with preretinal hemorrhage. The patient is lying on his side, hence the orientation of the pooled blood.

6. Receive intravenous antibiotics (gentamicin and cefazolin) in an attempt to reduce the likelihood of an endophthalmitis
7. Receive tetanus prophylaxis if it is not up to date

Nonaccidental Trauma (Child Abuse)

The manifestations of child abuse are diverse and can encompass any type of trauma; the explanation of the injury often is either inappropriate or insufficient. Unfortunately the ocular manifestations of child abuse may not be readily observable. Perhaps the most important and most often missed type of child abuse is the *shaken baby syndrome,* characterized by retinal and preretinal hemorrhages (Figs. 237-10 and 237-11), subdural or subarachnoid hemorrhages, and minimal or absent signs of external trauma. A patient who has these signs needs to have a complete systemic evaluation, including evaluation by an ophthalmologist familiar with the ocular manifestations of child abuse. In any case of suspected child abuse, the ophthalmologist should be involved to document and treat any ocular injuries present and to assist in any investigation to locate and prosecute the perpetrator(s). Only through the vigilance of the primary physician and the maintenance of a high index of suspicion may this form of child abuse be diagnosed.

SUMMARY

Most ocular injuries are relatively minor and easily treatable without sequelae. The circumstances surrounding some trauma, however, increase the likelihood of significant ocular or orbital injury. When such significant injury can be ruled out, involvement of the ophthalmologist may not be necessary. However, in any situation in which the primary examiner cannot determine readily the structural integrity of the globe, an ophthalmologist must be consulted.

SUGGESTED READINGS

Agapitos PJ, Noel LP, Clarke WN: Traumatic hyphema in children, *Ophthalmology* 94:1238, 1987.

Hamill MB: Clinical evaluation. In Shingleton BJ, Hersh PS, Kenyon KR, editors: *Eye trauma,* St Louis, 1991, Mosby.

Hersh PS, Shingleton BJ, Kenyon KR: Management of corneoscleral lacerations. In Shingleton BJ, Hersh PS, Kenyon KR, editors: *Eye trauma,* St Louis, 1991, Mosby.

Hoover DL, Smith LEH: Evaluation and management strategies for the pediatric eye trauma patient. In Shingleton BJ, Hersh PS, Kenyon KR, editors: *Eye trauma,* St Louis, 1991, Mosby.

Kenyon KR, Wagoner MD: Conjunctival and corneal injuries. In Shingleton BJ, Hersh PS, Kenyon KR, editors: *Eye trauma,* St Louis, 1991, Mosby.

Kylstra J: Preparation of the eye trauma patient for surgery. In Shingleton BJ, Hersh PS, Kenyon KR, editors: *Eye trauma,* St Louis, 1991, Mosby.

Shingleton BJ, Hersh PS: Traumatic hyphema. In Shingleton BJ, Hersh PS, Kenyon KR, editors: *Eye trauma,* St Louis, 1991, Mosby.

Wagoner MD, Kenyon KR: Chemical injuries. In Shingleton BJ, Hersh PS, Kenyon KR, editors: *Eye trauma,* St Louis, 1991, Mosby.

Weiss RA, McCord CD, Ellsworth RM: Orbital fractures. In Shingleton BJ, Hersh PS, Kenyon KR, editors: *Eye trauma,* St Louis, 1991, Mosby.

238 Osteochondroses

Edward M. Sills

The ossification centers of growing bones may develop irregular mineralization during childhood. Varying degrees of discomfort and dysfunction ensue associated with varying degrees of deformity. In this group of osteochondroses (Table 238-1), the disorders occur in bones preformed in cartilage and ossified from a central nucleus of ossification. Careful study has revealed that the generally assumed causes of interruped blood supply to the affected areas, damage to cartilage, and inflammation likely are inaccurate. The exact causal agents and mechanisms are not known. Excessive endogenous mechanical stress appears to play an important role in each of the disorders, and the degree of deformity and disability depends on the duration and degree of the stress to which the softened fibrous parts are subjected. The disorders that result from these alterations have been referred to as juvenile osteochondroses. Because damage to cartilage is not an instigating factor in these disorders, the root *chondro* is inaccurate. The more commonly involved areas of clinical significance include the femoral head, tibial tuberosity, tibial shaft, tarsal navicular, metatarsal heads, carpal semilunar, and lower thoracic vertebral epiphyses.

FEMORAL HEAD

Two distinctly different affections of the hip joint that occur in childhood involve damage to the femoral head. In Legg-Calvé-Perthes disease, the blood supply to the ossification center of the femoral head is interrupted, resulting in aseptic necrosis of the center. The femoral head, neck, and acetabulum become deformed and, in time, extensively reconstructed. The basis of treatment is to encourage the regaining of a spherical femoral head and to prevent irregular contour, flattening, or mushrooming of the head; shortening and broadening of the neck; and flattening of the vertical wall of the acetabulum. If these occur, osteoarthritis develops at an early age.

In the second common disorder, slipped capital femoral epiphysis, the femoral head begins to slip gradually off the femoral neck, disrupting the epiphyseal cartilage plate. In this disorder, treatment is directed at immediately restoring normal anatomical relationships and preventing further slippage.

Legg-Calvé-Perthes Disease

Legg-Calvé-Perthes disease has its onset in the early school-age years and occurs in boys four times more frequently than in girls. In the vast majority of instances the disorder is unilateral. In those rare instances (less than 10%) when both hip joints are involved, the two joints are involved successively rather than simultaneously.

The earliest sign is an intermittent limp, noticed especially after exertion. This limp may be associated with hip and ipsilateral knee pain. The quadriceps muscles and adjacent thigh soft tissues atrophy, and the hip may develop adduction flexion contracture. The child experiences discomfort in the hip or knee when attempts are made to rotate the hip internally. Associated muscle spasm that anchors the hip to slight external rotation may cause distal thigh or knee tenderness. A roentgenogram taken early in the course of the disease shows widening of the hip joint and, occasionally, metaphyseal demineralization. This "acute phase" generally lasts for a week or two and is followed by the "active phase," which can last for 12 to 40 months, during which time no clinical signs or symptoms are evident; however, the process of reparative revascularization causes an increased radiodensity in the femoral head ossification center (seen on roentgenograms), which is caused by resorption of dead trabecular bone. During this remolding phase, orthopedic care should be directed to maintaining the femoral head abducted and internally rotated in relation to the acetabulum. Use of orthotic devices or surgical approaches can accomplish this goal.

Slipped Capital Femoral Epiphysis

A slipped capital femoral epiphysis causes hip and leg pain in early adolescence, at slightly younger ages in girls than in boys. The gender incidence is nearly equal, with some studies indicating a slight male preponderance. There is a greater prevalence of tall, overweight youngsters among those having this condition than among the general population of young teenagers. About 75% of cases are unilateral, and the left side is involved more often.

Hip pain is the initial complaint, often referred to the thigh or knee in association with a gait that is assumed to protect the hips. In the early "preslipping stage," the pain often commences following a strain or minor injury. A sense of tiredness or mild pain prevails in the hip or knee, accompanied by mild limping or loss of mobility. The "preslipping stage" is succeeded by an "acute slip," with sudden acute pain, pronounced limitation of mobility, and difficulty bearing weight on the affected leg. On examination, the hip is rotated externally, with limited internal rotation and flexion. Earliest roentgenographic abnormalities are seen on a lateral view, with dorsal displacement of the capital epiphysis and widening of the zone of radiolucency between the femoral head and neck. If untreated, further posterior and medial slippage occurs. The hip must be placed in Russell traction and pinned surgically. Manipulation of the hip joint in an attempt at closed reduction may aggravate the slipping and should be avoided. The earlier the slippage is treated and the less the amount of unnecessary manipulation, the greater the likelihood that osteoarthritis can be avoided.

Tibial Tuberosity

Osgood-Schlatter disease results from avulsion of part of the patellar ligament and attached bony and cartilaginous frag-

Table 238-1 Osteochondroses

Site	Peak age of appearance (years)
Upper extremity	
Humeral head	2-8
Humeral capitulum	4-10
Lower ulna	13-20
Carpal navicular	16-24
Carpal semilunar	16-20
Bilateral entire carpus	10-14
Metacarpal heads	9-15
Basal phalanges	8-14
Lower extremity	
Femoral epiphysis slippage	9-16*
Femoral epiphysis	3-12†
Greater trochanter	6-11
Primary patellar center	8-15
Secondary patellar center	8-10
Shaft of tibia	1.5‡ 6-12§
Tibial tubercle	10-15
Distal tibial epiphysis	4
Calcaneal epiphysis	3-18
Astragalus	2-8
Tarsal navicular	3-7
Second metatarsal	8-17
Fifth metatarsal	8-16
Spine and pelvis	
Vertebral epiphysis	13-20
Vertebral disk	Over 16
Vertebral body	
Eosinophilic granuloma (?)	2-11
Symphysis pubis	12-18
Iliac crest	12-19
Ischial apophysis	13-18
Ischiopubic synchondrosis	12-19

*Girls are younger.
†Maximum is 6-8 yr.
‡Infantile form.
§Adolescent form.

ments from the tuberosity. Its incidence is higher in boys, but the age of onset is earlier in girls because ossification of the tibial tuberosity occurs earlier in females. About 25% of cases have bilateral involvement. The child's complaint is that of local pain and tenderness in the region of the knee, particularly the tuberosity. The pain is most severe at the end of active flexion or extension of the knee. If the condition has been present for several months, the tuberosity is enlarged, and one may find a bony prominence on its anterior aspect. The roentgenographic changes vary, depending on the size of the avulsed fragments, cartilage, and bone and on the duration of the condition. The best view is one with the knee rotated inward, giving a tangential view of the tibial tuberosity. One sees soft tissue swelling, an opaque patellar ligament, and a fragmented tuberosity. Treatment is directed at decreasing the stress on the tubercle until the tuberosity fuses with the tibial metaphysis. This bony fusion occurs at about 15 years of age in girls and 17 years in boys. Depending on the degree of pain, strenuous activities involving deep knee bending and jumping may have to be restricted, or casting may be required to immobilize the knee totally. The former approach usually is sufficient.

Tibial Shaft

Infants usually have some leg bowing until 18 months of age, after which time the legs straighten and then progress to a slight degree of knock-knee. Bowing of the legs that persists or progresses beyond 2 years of age should be evaluated. The differential diagnosis lies between tibia vara (Blount disease) and renal or nutritional rickets. In Blount disease, cartilage has failed to transform to bone at the medial aspect of the epiphysis. The metaphysis beneath the epiphyseal ossification center becomes demineralized, and the medial aspect of the proximal tibia fails to grow as rapidly as the lateral aspect, resulting in a bowleg deformity. In rickets, calcification and growth of the epiphyseal cartilage of the long bones are suppressed, their metaphyses become softened, and they flare at both ends with resultant bowing. Appropriate treatment with vitamin D will produce roentgenographic evidence of healing within a few weeks and eventual straightening of the bones. Most children whose Blount disease persists beyond 6 years of age require an osteotomy to correct the bowing.

TARSAL NAVICULAR

Köhler disease of the tarsal navicular bone results from an interruption of the blood supply to the developing navicular bone, causing necrosis of its ossification center. The navicular is in a crucial position in the arch of the foot; thus symptoms can be alarming. The condition is self-limited, and the ossification center becomes revascularized and completely reconstructed. The disorder is seen primarily in boys between 3 and 7 years of age, but predominantly in the younger children.

Pain is localized to the inner aspect of the midtarsal part of the foot. The foot is held in a slight varus position, and the child walks on the outer side of the foot or flat-footedly. The skin over the navicular may be warm, red, and swollen, and palpation of the bone elicits tenderness. Lateral roentgenograms of the feet show a very narrowed, waferlike, irregular navicular ossification center, with increased radiopacity and loss of trabecular markings. The process of revascularization and reconstruction takes from 1 to 3 years. Treatment primarily is directed to reassuring the child and family. Various orthotic pads can be used to absorb weight and pressure forces until the healing occurs. Surgical intervention is to be avoided.

METATARSAL HEADS

Freiberg disease is a condition in which a part of the head of a metatarsal bone undergoes aseptic necrosis and becomes sufficiently weakened to be susceptible to functional trauma (running, jumping), which may cause compressional collapse of the metatarsal head. The second metatarsal bone most often is involved; the third metatarsal bone is the next most likely to be so. Females are affected more often than males.

Pain occurs in the region of the affected metatarsal on walking. Plantar pressure elicits tenderness, as does abrupt release of this pressure. Swelling occurs over the dorsum of the involved metatarsophalangeal joint, plantar flexion becomes limited, and the transverse arch of the involved foot becomes flattened. A callus develops on the plantar surface of the foot, overlying the involved metatarsal head. A deformed, broadened metatarsal head is seen on roentgenogram. High heels should not be worn, and long walks should be avoided until symptoms subside. Symptomatic use of nonsteroidal antiinflammatory agents is recommended.

CARPAL SEMILUNAR

Aseptic necrosis of the lunate bone (Kienböck disease) weakens the bony structure and usually leads to a compression fracture. The lunate bone of the right hand (the usual working hand) is involved more frequently than that of the left, and males are affected more frequently than females.

Pain is experienced on movement of the wrist, and in longstanding cases the pain may be present at rest. Swelling over the dorsum of the wrist and tenderness over the affected bone often are exhibited. The roentgenogram shows a flattened fragmented lunate bone with variations in its radiodensity. The lunate, lying adjacent to the radius, is subjected to great forces and pressures; hence treatment includes wrist immobilization. On occasion, fusion of the lunate with the bones of the wrist that surround it is required for stabilization and relief of pain.

LOWER THORACIC VERTEBRAE

Scheuermann disease is a common cause of kyphosis in teenagers, occurring in about 5% of that population. The lower thoracic vertebrae are affected most often. The pathological condition involves a swelling of the intervertebral disks that exerts pressure on the cartilage plates covering the vertebral bodies; this causes the plates to thin and interferes with endochondral bone formation. The disk spaces become narrowed (more anteriorly than posteriorly), and pressure is exerted on the anterior portions of the contiguous vertebral bodies, which impedes their longitudinal growth and thus leads to kyphosis. An aching pain aggravated by physical exertion is present in the affected portion of the vertebral column. The affected area is tender to palpation. Assuming a stooping position often will cause the pain to increase. Within a year or so, the kyphosis easily is apparent as a round back deformity. In many instances the pain is so minor that the patient's complaint is that of poor posture rather than backache. Roentgenograms reveal narrowing of the anterior disk spaces and defects on the surfaces of adjacent vertebrae. In some children the condition progresses to cause severe deformity and dysfunction; in others the condition stabilizes and the deformity disappears. Treatment is aimed at preventing further deformity, occasionally with the use of casting or bracing. In those rare instances of rapid progression or of persistent, severe pain, spinal fusion is necessary. The majority of youngsters, however, require only careful observation.

SUGGESTED READINGS

Bowen JR, Abrams JS: Legg-Calvé-Perthes disease, *Contemp Orthop* 10:27, 1985.

Riseborough E, Herndon JH: *Scoliosis and other deformities of the axial skeleton,* Boston, 1975, Little, Brown.

Stulberg SD, Cooperman DR, Wallenstein R: The natural history of Legg-Calvé-Perthes disease, *J Bone Joint Surg [Am]* 63:1095, 1981.

Tachdjian M: *Pediatric orthopedics,* ed 2, Philadelphia, 1991, WB Saunders.

239 Osteomyelitis

Edwards P. Schwentker

The vast majority of cases of osteomyelitis are secondary to pyogenic infection. They can result from the direct bacterial contamination of bone, which may occur with an open fracture, during operative procedures, or from direct extension from an adjacent soft tissue infection. Most commonly, however, childhood osteomyelitis is hematogenous in origin.

Hematogenous osteomyelitis may occur at any age, but its incidence is higher in children than in adults. Unless promptly diagnosed and aggressively treated, it may lead to complications resulting in lifelong disability. Because the diagnosis of osteomyelitis may at times be difficult, a high index of suspicion is required.

Pyogenic osteomyelitis initially may manifest either acutely or subacutely. In childhood these two entities are sufficiently distinct to require separate discussion. Chronic osteomyelitis is discussed with acute osteomyelitis, inasmuch as the chronic form of this disease develops from the inadequate treatment of an acute osteomyelitis.

ACUTE OSTEOMYELITIS

Pathogenesis

The pathogenesis and, consequently, the clinical manifestation of acute pyogenic osteomyelitis depend on the anatomy of bone, particularly its pattern of vascular supply. This anatomy is sufficiently different among the infant (birth to 18 months), the older child (18 months to skeletal maturity), and the adult to cause a different form of acute osteomyelitis in each of the three age groups. [9] The concern here is with bone infection only as it occurs during infancy and childhood.

Infancy. In anatomical studies, Trueta[9] demonstrated the presence of vessels that penetrate through the growth plate to connect the metaphysis with the epiphysis. These vessels are seen most commonly before the infant is 6 months of age, but they may be present up to 18 months. When present, infectious spread through the metaphyseal side of the growth plate (physis) into the epiphysis is facilitated by these penetrating vessels. Infection thus is able to damage the growth plate and the epiphysis itself; it also is much more likely to penetrate the adjacent joint. Therefore in infancy *acute osteomyelitis commonly results in an associated septic arthritis.*

As in the older age group, the bone of the metaphysis and the diaphysis also can be destroyed in infancy, with subsequent formation of sequestrum and involucrum. The richness of blood supply and the natural resilience of the young infant provide an enormous capacity for repair. The development of chronic osteomyelitis is less likely in the infant than in the older child, but irreparable damage to the joint surfaces and to growth potential is far more likely.

Childhood. Hematogenous osteomyelitis in childhood (approximately 18 months to skeletal maturity) virtually always arises in the metaphyses of the long bones, gaining entrance to the bone by way of its nutrient vessels. The vasculature on the metaphyseal side of the physis is characterized by vascular loops that extend up into the layer of calcified cartilage of the physis to provide nutritional support for the formation of bone associated with growth. Bacteria within the bloodstream invade the venous side of these vascular loops. It generally is believed that a relatively sluggish blood flow within these venous sinusoids favors bacterial proliferation. Rang,[5] however, points out a relative lack of reticuloendothelial cells in the metaphyses of actively growing long bones, and he postulates that bone defenses against infection are weakest in this area.

Trauma also may play a role. The manifestation of an *acute osteomyelitis frequently is associated with the history of a recent injury* to the affected extremity. Morrissy and Haynes[4] have presented experimental evidence, using an immature rabbit model, to support injury to the physeal plate as a factor in the development of acute hematogenous osteomyelitis. Whatever the cause or combination of causes, *the metaphysis is the predominant site of origin of hematogenous osteomyelitis* in childhood.

In contrast to the situation in infancy, by 18 months of age no direct vascular connections exist between the metaphysis and the epiphysis. The physis becomes a barrier to infection, effectively preventing the spread of infection into the epiphysis.

As bacteria proliferate, local thrombosis occurs, resulting in devascularization of bone. This loss of vascularity further interferes with natural body defenses and prevents the penetration of circulating antibiotics as well. The result is an abscess. Untreated, infection spreads through the haversian system and Volkmann canals, eventually reaching the subperiosteal space. The periosteum then may be elevated by the infection, stripping the periosteal vascular supply from the cortex and causing further bone death.

Rupture through the periosteum at this point may result in a septic arthritis of the adjacent joint if that portion of the metaphysis happens to be intraarticular. This event is most likely in those joints in which the capsule attaches circumferentially well down on the metaphysis of the infected bone. Thus a proximal femoral osteomyelitis may result in septic arthritis of the hip. Similarly, sepsis of the elbow can result from infection of the proximal radius.

If treatment is delayed or inadequate, the infection also may track outward to result in a spontaneously draining sinus. Devascularized bone, the *sequestrum,* becomes a fortress for the bacteria, against which antibiotics and natural body defenses can accomplish little more than to prevent further spread of infection. Meanwhile, the elevated hypervascular periosteum lays down a surrounding wall of new living bone known as the *involucrum.* An inadequately treated or untreated acute osteomyelitis thus becomes a chronic osteomyelitis.

In childhood, unlike infancy, acute osteomyelitis seldom causes growth plate or epiphyseal damage. Growth is unlikely to be retarded and may, in fact, be stimulated, possibly secondarily to the hypervascularity that attends inflammation. Damage to the epiphysis and to the physis can occur, however, when osteomyelitis is complicated by septic arthritis of the adjacent joint.

Clinical Findings

In older infants and children, osteomyelitic infection is most likely to involve a single bone. Fever and sepsis may be prominent, but systemic signs and symptoms usually are mild (or even absent), with the major signs being those localized to the affected part. This is true especially in the infant. Localized tenderness generally is present and often is exquisite. Other local signs may be associated with inflammation, including swelling, redness, and warmth. Characteristically the child is reluctant to move the adjacent joint and, when a lower extremity is involved, may refuse to bear weight. In the young infant the loss of active movement in an extremity may mimic neurological damage, a condition known as pseudoparalysis.

The diagnostic workup should include a complete blood cell count and erythrocyte sedimentation rate, blood cultures, and roentgenograms; however, findings here also may be misleading. The white blood cell count often is normal. An elevation in the sedimentation rate is more sensitive and particularly is useful in monitoring clinical response.

Early in the clinical course, no bony changes are seen roentgenographically, the earliest detectable signs being those of blurred soft tissue planes secondary to edema spreading into fatty tissues. The earliest roentgenographic changes to occur within bone itself are those of bone destruction or lysis, which generally is not apparent until at least 10 days after the onset of symptoms.

The differential diagnosis of acute osteomyelitis includes septic arthritis, acute rheumatic fever, rheumatoid arthritis, leukemia, and cellulitis. The manifestation of septic arthritis may be similar to that of acute osteomyelitis, and especially in the infant, the two entities may coexist. When septic arthritis is present, the urgency for prompt treatment is, if anything, more acute (see Chapter 257). Rheumatoid arthritis and acute rheumatic fever generally exhibit less severity, and tenderness is not localized to the metaphysis of the involved bone as it is with osteomyelitis. Initially, leukemia may mimic or actually be an acute osteomyelitis. The presence of an anemia or a low leukocyte count may be suggestive. Distinguishing between a cellulitis and osteomyelitis may be difficult. In the lower extremities a cellulitis is less likely to interfere with weight bearing. If doubt exists, management should proceed on the assumption that the infection involves the bone.

Radionuclide scanning is not necessary in most cases of acute osteomyelitis, but if signs and symptoms are inconclusive, it may help in establishing the diagnosis. Scanning is far more sensitive than is radiographic examination in the early stages of the disease and is capable of differentiating most cases of soft tissue cellulitis from infection of the bone itself. Scans are most helpful when signs of localization are poor, when multiple sites of involvement are suspected, or for the localization of sites within the axial skeleton. Technetium pyrophosphate scintigraphy is the scanning modality employed most commonly. Technetium scans provide results within 3 to 4 hours and are most helpful when performed with a three-phase protocol to evaluate blood flow, blood pool, and bone uptake.[1]

The use of gallium scans and scans with radionuclide-labeled leukocytes may be even more sensitive and specific; unfortunately these tests require 24 to 48 hours to complete, rendering them of limited usefulness in a situation in which early diagnosis is critical. Of the two techniques, indium-labeled white cell scanning may be the most useful and should be considered when needle aspiration and three-phase technetium scan both show negative results.[1]

Under no circumstances should treatment be delayed to perform a scan when clinical suspicion is high. Both false positive and false negative results with all scanning methods have been reported.[8]

Blood culture results are positive in 40% to 50% of cases of acute osteomyelitis. Needle aspiration of the subperiosteal space and of the metaphysis provides a positive identification of the infecting organism in most cases. In neonates the most common organisms are *Streptococcus pyogenes* (group B), *Staphylococcus aureus,* and enteric bacilli. In the older child *Staphylococcus aureus* is the predominant pathogen; *Streptococcus pneumoniae, Streptococcus pyogenes,* and *Staphylococcus epidermidis* occur less frequently. *Haemophilus influenza* type b rarely causes osteomyelitis without an associated septic arthritis. *Pseudomonas aeruginosa* is becoming more common, particularly in older children who have penetrating trauma or parenteral drug abuse.[7]

High-risk, low-birth-weight infants present a special set of problems with respect to acute osteomyelitis. They often have multiple portals for bacterial entry into the systemic circulation, including infection of other organ systems, indwelling catheters, and heel sticks. They frequently are debilitated; as a result, osteomyelitis often develops at several sites, including the facial bones. Extension of infection from the bone into adjacent joints occurs commonly. *S. pyogenes* (group B) is a frequent offender.

The search for multiple sites of involvement in the neonate would seem to be an ideal application of radionuclide scanning. Unfortunately, false negative results are more common in this age group. Reducing the incidence of false negative scan results in the neonate may be possible with the use of the latest generation of cameras and the application of spot and pinhole views.[1]

Skeletal infections caused by *Candida albicans* may develop in severely debilitated infants and children who have required prolonged antibiotic therapy or hyperalimentation by central venous catheter.

Another special group is composed of patients who have sickle hemoglobinopathies; osteomyelitis occuring in these patients is difficult to differentiate from bony infarction. *Salmonella* spp. are the most common infecting organisms. Osteomyelitis can be differentiated from bone infarction by operative exploration and direct culture of bacteria from the involved bone or by culture of the organisms from the blood.

Because the physical signs are more difficult to interpret when osteomyelitis involves the spine or pelvis, diagnosis becomes more complex. Technetium scans are particularly helpful in making the diagnoses in such cases.

Magnetic resonance (MR) imaging is expensive and often requires patient sedation, but it too is useful in localizing infection beneath the deep tissues surrounding the spine and pelvis. This modality can identify associated epidural abscesses and can guide aspiration. MR imaging also can localize abscesses in the extremities that have been missed by needle aspiration.[3]

Management

Needle aspiration is the single most helpful procedure for diagnosing infections of bones and joints. All children who have suspected osteomyelitis with localized signs should undergo aspiration of the subperiosteum with a large-bore needle; if pus is not encountered, the needle is advanced into the metaphyseal bone. The metaphysis of a long bone can be aspirated quickly without the use of general anesthesia. Aspiration confirms the diagnosis, determines the necessity for operative decompression, and provides a specimen for pathogen identification by culture, as well as material for immediate Gram stain.

Once blood cultures and aspiration have been performed, antibiotics should be given parenterally. In an older child who has no associated septic arthritis and in whom no risk factors for gram negative organisms exist, a penicillinase-resistant penicillin should be sufficient. Neonates should receive the same, plus an aminoglycoside. If reason exists to suspect a pseudomonal infection, the initial treatment should be a carboxypenicillin or acylureidopenicillin combined with an aminoglycoside. Children in whom a salmonella infection is suspected should receive an ampicillin and aminoglycoside combination. In the young child who has osteomyelitis with joint involvement, *H. influenzae* type b may be present, and initial treatment should be a penicillinase-resistant penicillin plus chloramphenicol.[7]

Antibiotics should be adjusted appropriately once cultures and sensitivities are available. Antibiotics should be continued for at least 3 weeks and must be maintained at adequate concentrations in the blood. Oral antibiotics *may* achieve adequate bactericidal titers. Oral antibiotics, however, should be used only if the patient is responding to treatment, the parents are reliable, the antibiotic does not cause a gastrointestinal disturbance that interferes with absorption, and adequate monitored blood levels can be obtained. The erythrocyte sedimentation rate is helpful in monitoring the clinical response and should return to normal values before therapy is discontinued.

Surgical drainage must be undertaken whenever an abscess is detected or suspected. An abscess may be considered as being present whenever a loss of vascularity, and hence viability, has occurred in any part of the skeletal tissues. If a situation exists in which body defenses or antibiotics are ineffective, operative decompression must be used. The aspiration of frank pus is an absolute indication for surgical drainage. Similarly, lytic changes within the bone or periosteal new bone formation, as seen on initial roentgenograms in previously untreated patients, is an indication for operative drainage. On the other hand, in patients already under treatment and responding favorably both clinically and in terms of a falling sedimentation rate, the appearance of radiographic bone changes does not necessarily indicate that an abscess is present, because such changes occur in treated patients as recovery progresses.

A negative aspiration finding is not absolute evidence that operative decompression is not needed. The site of aspiration may have been inaccurate, or pus may be present but too thick to pass through even a large-bore needle. Persistent clinical suspicion or failure of the patient to respond to nonoperative therapy is an indication for MR imaging, or when localizing signs are severe, for immediate operative decompression. The risks of unnecessary surgery in the child who has an acute infection are far less than those of necessary surgery not performed.

SUBACUTE OSTEOMYELITIS

Subacute osteomyelitis in childhood is a clinical entity entirely distinct from acute osteomyelitis. The clinical course is far more benign, both systemically and with respect to the presence of localized signs and symptoms. The sites of subacute osteomyelitis are not restricted to metaphyses but may occur virtually at any site within the bony skeleton. Because of its mild clinical course, the diagnosis of subacute osteomyelitis often is delayed. This entity occurs with a variety of roentgenographic manifestations and frequently is confused with a variety of benign and malignant bone neoplasms.

Pathogenesis

Gledhill[2] has hypothesized that subacute osteomyelitis develops as the result of an altered host-pathogen relation. As in acute osteomyelitis, bacteria appear to gain entrance to the bone through the circulation. After the infection gains a foothold, it is brought under control largely by body defenses and prevented from spreading within the bone. It may be speculated that this situation occurs when bacterial virulence is decreased, either naturally or secondary to antibiotics administered early in the infection. The acute infection also might be aborted by increased host resistance, such as is to be expected within the diaphysis or epiphysis, as compared with the metaphysis. Subacute osteomyelitis may occur in any of these three areas, whereas acute osteomyelitis arises hematogenously almost exclusively in the more susceptible metaphysis.

Whether such an "attenuated" infection occurs because of decreased virulence of the pathogen, increased natural defenses of the host, or a superimposed factor (such as the administration of suboptimal doses of antibiotics), the establishment of the subacute process is characterized by a pathological stand-off between pathogen and host, wherein the infection is contained effectively within a small area of bone. Although the bacteria cannot expand their foothold rapidly, natural body defenses are unable to eradicate the infection completely.

Clinical Findings

Subacute osteomyelitis is of insidious onset. The pain that results is mild to moderate and often intermittent. Little to no functional impairment results, and the systemic signs and symptoms of fever, malaise, anorexia, and weight loss are minimal to nonexistent. The interval between onset of symptoms and diagnosis may be measured in months, whereas the diagnosis of an acute osteomyelitis generally requires no more than a few days.

By the time medical consultation is sought, enough time generally has elapsed since onset of the infection that roentgenograms reveal positive findings. The radiographic appearance may vary considerably and may closely mimic a variety of benign and malignant neoplasms. Roberts and coworkers[6] have proposed an expansion of a system for radiographic classification originally proposed by Gledhill.[2] They describe seven different types of bone lesions, only one of which clearly suggests a subacute osteomyelitis. A lytic defect within the metaphysis surrounded by a dense sclerotic margin suggests the classic form of subacute osteomyelitis, a so-called Brodie abscess. This variety is described as type IB. Type IA is similar in size and location but lacks the sclerotic rim. It most frequently is confused with an eosinophilic granuloma. Type II subacute osteomyelitis is associated with erosion of the metaphyseal cortex, and its appearance may be confused with that of an osteogenic sarcoma. A type III lesion is seen as a localized defect within the cortex of the diaphysis and resembles an osteoid osteoma. The type IV lesion is characterized by onion-skin periosteal reaction and suggests Ewing sarcoma. The type V lesion occurs within the epiphysis and may suggest a chondroblastoma. Finally, the type VI lesion involves a vertebral body, and the roentgenographic appearance is that of erosion or destruction.

The white blood cell count and sedimentation rate in cases of subacute osteomyelitis are likely to be normal or elevated minimally. Blood cultures rarely are positive. Findings on a technetium bone scan may be positive, but if a lesion already is visible on plain roentgenograms, the scan will add little in establishing the diagnosis.

Management

Subacute osteomyelitis can be diagnosed definitively only by isolating an organism on culture of the bone or by histopathological findings consistent with infection. When the lesion involves the long bones of the extremities, curettage generally can be performed easily. Material obtained will establish the diagnosis by culture or histological findings. *S. aureus* is the most commonly isolated pathogen. Operative curettage followed by a course of antibiotic therapy, similar to that used in the treatment of acute osteomyelitis, usually is curative.

When the infection involves a vertebral body, a specimen may be obtained for biopsy with a closed-needle technique. If suspicion of infection is high, treatment may be undertaken with antibiotics and cast immobilization of the spine without resorting to biopsy or aspiration. Again, prognosis for cure is excellent.

REFERENCES

1. Demopulos GA, Bleck EE, McDougall IR: Role of radionuclide imaging in the diagnosis of acute osteomyelitis, *J Pediatr Orthop* 8:558, 1988.
2. Gledhill RB: Subacute osteomyelitis in children, *Clin Orthop* 96:57, 1973.
3. Jaramillo D et al: Osteomyelitis and septic arthritis in children: appropriate use of imaging to guide treatment, *Am J Radiol* 165:399, 1995.
4. Morrissy RT, Haynes DW: Acute hematogenous osteomyelitis: a model with trauma as an etiology, *J Pediatr Orthop* 9:447, 1989.
5. Rang MC: *The growth plate and its disorders*, Baltimore, 1969, Williams & Wilkins.
6. Roberts JM et al: Subacute hematogenous osteomyelitis in children: a retrospective study, *J Pediatr Orthop* 2:249, 1982.
7. Scoles PV, Aronoff SC: Current concepts review: antimicrobial therapy of childhood skeletal infections, *J Bone Joint Surg [Am]* 66:1487, 1984.
8. Sullivan JA, Vasileff T, Leonard JC: An evaluation of nuclear scanning in orthopaedic infection, *J Pediatr Orthop* 1:73, 1981.
9. Trueta J: The three types of acute hematogenous osteomyelitis, *J Bone Joint Surg [Br]* 41:671, 1959.

240 Otitis Media and Otitis Externa

Rickey L. Williams

OTITIS MEDIA

Ear infections most frequently involve the middle ear (otitis media) or outer ear (otitis externa). Otitis media is one of the most common diagnoses made by the practicing pediatrician. The scope of this problem is enormous, especially when one considers the time used in treating this disorder and the costs involved for office visits, medications, and surgery.

Acute Suppurative Otitis Media

Epidemiology. Approximately 75% of children develop at least one episode of otitis media between the ages of 6 and 18 months,[31] and many children suffer numerous bouts of the disease. Younger children are more prone to otitis, especially between 6 and 24 months of age. A second smaller peak occurs between 4 and 7 years of age. Otitis develops more frequently in boys than in girls, and the incidence and prevalence of the disease varies with respect to race. Caucasian children are affected more commonly than African-Americans, and the craniofacial anatomy of Native American and Native Alaskan children is thought to explain in part their high risk for otitis. Clinical data suggest that recurrent acute otitis media is hereditary. This observation is supported by the finding that HLA-A2 antigen is more prevalent in children who have recurrent acute otitis media.[21] Children who have craniofacial abnormalities such as cleft palate also are at especially high risk for contracting acute otitis media, as are those who have Down syndrome.

Children in day care centers are at higher risk than children cared for in homes, presumably because those in day care centers are exposed to more respiratory viral infections.[15] Lower socioeconomic status also is associated with a higher risk for otitis media, as is allergic rhinitis.[12]

The illness occurs most commonly in the winter months in temperate climates, presumably in association with respiratory viral infections. Some children are plagued with numerous bouts of otitis media. Howie and coworkers[18] have found this "otitis-prone" condition to be associated with a first episode of otitis before 6 months of age, especially if *Streptococcus pneumoniae* is the bacterial pathogen.

Pathogenesis. The middle ear cavity normally is filled with air and is sterile. During swallowing, air enters the middle ear through the eustachian tube. When the eustachian tube malfunctions, the middle ear cavity does not ventilate normally, and negative pressure results as the air is absorbed. Fluid effuses into the middle ear, and bacteria from the nasopharynx may be drawn into the cavity, leading to the suppuration found in acute otitis media.[6]

The eustachian tube malfunctions because of obstruction or abnormal mechanical factors. Obstruction can result from inflammation of the tube itself or from hypertrophied nasopharyngeal lymphatic tissue. Viral illnesses and allergies are believed to contribute to eustachian tube obstruction. Mechanical factors that lead to eustachian tube malfunction include diminished patency, poor muscular function, and increased tortuosity.

Microbiology. *S. pneumoniae, nontypeable Haemophilus influenzae,* and *Moraxella catarrhalis* account for most bacterial pathogens isolated from middle ear fluid in older infants and children. Other organisms found less frequently include *Staphylococcus aureus,* group A beta-hemolytic streptococci *(Streptococcus pyogenes),* and various gram negative organisms.

Combinations of organisms can be recovered from middle ear fluid in acute otitis media, and a patient can have one pathogen in one ear and a different pathogen in the other ear. Cultures of the nasopharynx do not correlate well with those of middle ear fluid, although nasopharyngeal carriage of middle ear pathogens increases significantly during respiratory illness. Otitis-prone children tend to carry nontypeable *H. influenzae* at an unusually high rate in the nasopharynx, even during health. This propensity to carry nontypeable *H. influenzae* might explain why nontypeable *H. influenzae* is a major cause of recurrent or chronic otitis media.[11]

In infants during the first few months of life, *S. pneumoniae* and *H. influenzae* are the organisms recovered most often, although the proportion of cases caused by gram negative enteric organisms is higher than in older children, especially if the infant was in an intensive care nursery.

In about one third of the cases in which fluid is obtained for culture, no pathogenic bacteria can be identified, leading to speculation concerning the contribution of anaerobic bacteria or viruses to acute otitis media. Viruses associated with the development of acute otitis media include respiratory syncytial virus, adenovirus, influenza viruses, rhinovirus, parainfluenza viruses, and coronavirus.[1] *Mycoplasma pneumoniae* formerly was thought to cause bullous myringitis, but the data are inconclusive.

Clinical History. In the usual case of acute otitis media, a young child who has had an upper respiratory tract infection for a few days develops fever, becomes irritable, and eats poorly. Other signs and symptoms can include vomiting, diarrhea, vestibular disturbances, a bulging fontanelle, and in older children, complaints of ear pain or hearing loss. Pulling at the ears is an unreliable sign, and it should be noted that fever may be absent in more than one third of children who have bacteriologically proven otitis media.

Diagnosis. Examination of the tympanic membrane by otoscopy is the most common method used by practitioners to diagnose otitis media. The normal tympanic membrane is translucent, and the short process and handle of the malleus are visible through the tympanic membrane. A cone of reflected light is present. The drum moves laterally and medi-

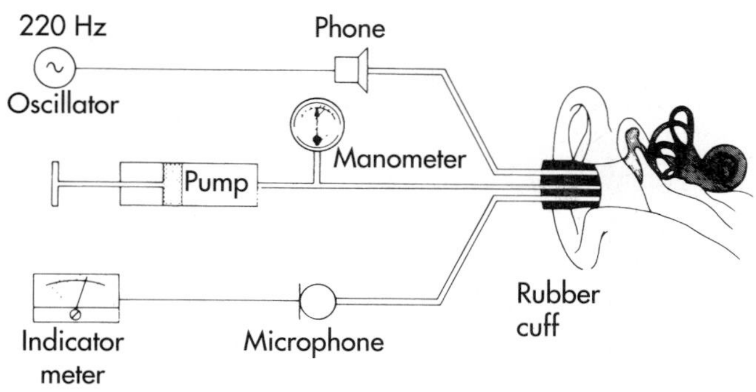

FIG. 240-1 The electroacoustic impedance bridge. (From Paradise JL, Smith CG, Bluestone CD: *Pediatrics* 58:198, 1976.)

ally with negative and positive pressure, respectively, during pneumatic otoscopy.

Pneumatic otoscopy is performed by using a speculum of a size that will ensure an airtight seal in the external auditory canal. Gentle negative pressure followed by gentle positive pressure using a tube that has an attached mouthpiece or rubber bulb allows the examiner to observe motion of the tympanic membrane.

The diagnosis of acute otitis media is based on changes in the tympanic membrane's contour, color, and mobility. A bulging, yellow or red, immobile ear drum in which the bony landmarks and the light reflex are distorted usually is seen in cases of acute otitis media. Redness of the tympanic membrane alone can be caused by crying and is not a reliable sign of acute otitis media.

Tympanometry is being used more frequently as an aid in the diagnosis of otitis media. As described by Paradise,[25] the tympanometer (electroacoustic impedance bridge) gives one an estimate of tympanic membrane compliance (Fig. 240-1).

After an airtight seal is ensured when the probe is placed in the external auditory canal, a tone of constant frequency is emitted into the closed air space. Pressure in the external auditory canal ranging from +200 to −400 mm H_2O then is applied variously by a pump. As the tympanic membrane moves, sound reflected from it is measured with a microphone and displayed on the tympanogram (Fig. 240-2).

A normal tympanogram can be found in the early stages of acute otitis media, so otoscopy also should be performed whenever otitis is suspected. Acoustic reflectometry has been described recently as another possibly helpful adjunct in diagnosing middle ear disease.[35]

Tympanocentesis or myringotomy provides definitive proof of the presence of acute otitis media if fluid is obtained and examined by Gram stain and microbiological culture. These techniques, described in Appendix B, are helpful when dealing with severe illness (especially in infants), otitis that is unresponsive to routine antibiotic treatment, and complications such as mastoiditis and meningitis. Fluid draining into the two external canals after tympanic membrane perforation frequently is contaminated with organisms from the external canal, so culture of this fluid seldom is helpful in assessing the cause of otitis media.

Treatment. Because the microbiological cause of acute otitis media in children usually is not determined, the condition should, under almost all circumstances, be considered of bacterial origin and treated with antibiotics[20,33] (Table 240-1).

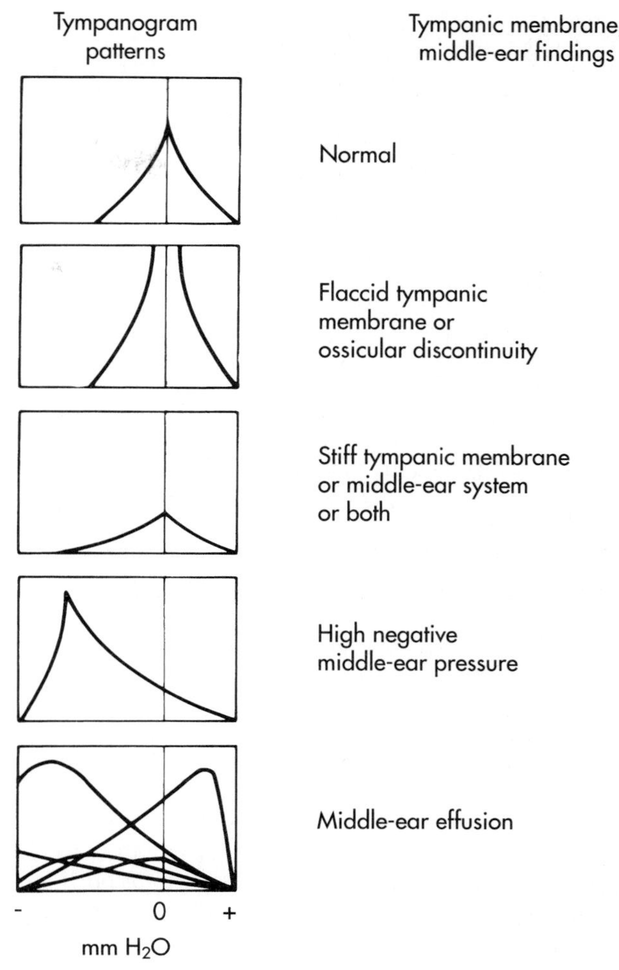

FIG. 240-2 Examples of tympanograms related to tympanic membrane compliance and middle ear pressure (mm H_2O). (From Bluestone CD: *Pediatr Clin North Am* 28:727, 1981.)

Amoxicillin is the treatment of choice for children who are not sensitive to penicillin and who live in regions where the prevalence of beta-lactamase-producing strains of *H. influenzae* and *M. catarrhalis* is low.[5,27] The emergence of penicillin-resistant and multiple drug–resistant *Streptococcus pneumoniae* may force practitioners to choose antibiotics other than amoxicillin as first-line therapy for otitis media.[7] Cefaclor and combinations of erythromycin-sulfisoxazole, amoxicillin-potassium clavulanate, or trimethoprim-sulfamethoxazole also are effective in the treatment of acute otitis media. Trimethoprim-sulfamethoxazole should not be used if infection with group A streptococci is suspected or proven. Cephalosporins are being used more commonly to treat acute otitis media.

The advantages of some of these newer agents include once-daily therapy or even administration of a single intramuscular injection,[14] which should improve treatment compliance, and a broad spectrum of antibacterial activity. Cost considerations preclude use of the cephalosporins as first-line therapy.

Use of antihistamines or decongestants in the treatment of acute otitis media remains controversial; therefore routine use of these drugs is unwarranted. Myringotomy has not been

Table 240-1 Antibiotic Treatment of Acute Otitis Media

Drug	Common trade name(s)	Dose/day (mg/kg)	Dose frequency/day
Amoxicillin	Amoxil, Polymox	20-40	×3
Amoxicillin-potassium clavulanate	Augmentin	40/10	×3
Cefaclor	Ceclor	40	×2
Cefixime	Suprax	8	×1
Cefprozil	Cefzil	15	×2
Cefuroxime axetil	Ceftin	15	×2
Erythromycin-sulfisoxazole	Pediazole	50/150	×4
Loracarbef	Lorabid	30	×2
Trimethoprim-sulfamethoxazole	Bactrim, Septra	8/40	×2

proved to be effective in treating acute otitis media, although it may help relieve the severe pain associated with a bulging eardrum.

The physician should tell parents that their child's symptoms will not resolve immediately with initiation of antibiotic therapy and advise them to give an analgesic such as acetaminophen. Because parents frequently discontinue antibiotics when their child's symptoms improve, they must be advised to continue the antibiotics for a full 10-day course.

For children less than 15 months of age, follow-up office examinations at 2 to 3 weeks are recommended to determine whether the otitis media has resolved. Follow-up also is recommended for children over 15 months of age whose parents feel the infection has not resolved, for children whose symptoms persist, or for children at higher risk for otitis media such as those who have a family history of recurrent otitis.[16]

Persistent Otitis Media. Inadequate resolution of acute otitis media can be attributed to the organism(s) involved, the antibiotic regimen, compliance with medication administration, or a number of other factors. Respiratory virus infection often is present in patients who have acute otitis media unresponsive to initial antimicrobial therapy and may explain the prolongation of symptoms of infection.[2,8] If after 48 hours of antibiotic treatment the child has not improved, Teele and coworkers[38] recommend that tympanocentesis be performed. The antibiotic should be changed, although most recovered organisms prove to be sensitive to the antibiotic prescribed initially. Children who have a history of recurrent otitis media and infection during the winter season more often fail to respond to antibiotic treatment and have a higher risk of developing a persistent middle ear effusion.[3]

Otitis Media with Effusion. Otitis media with effusion, also called nonsuppurative otitis media, secretory otitis media, and glue ear, is a common sequela to acute suppurative otitis media. Persistence of effusion after 10 days of therapy for acute otitis has been demonstrated in about 40% of affected children. The exact incidence and prevalence of this disorder are unknown, although approximately 20% of children who have allergies are said to have nonsuppurative otitis media. Spontaneous resolution occurs in more than 50% of children within 3 months from development of the effusion, and only a small percentage of children experiences otitis media with effusion lasting a year or longer.[36] This condition, caused by eustachian tube malfunction, usually follows an episode of acute otitis media. Negative pressure in the middle ear leads to effusion of fluid into that cavity. Although the effusion formerly was thought to be sterile, bacterial pathogens can be recovered in approximately 33% of cases.

On physical examination, the tympanic membrane appears retracted. An air-fluid level or bubbles of air may be seen behind the tympanic membrane if it is translucent, although it more often is opaque. Mobility of the drum is decreased, and tympanometry frequently reveals high negative pressure in the middle ear cavity.

Otitis media with effusion often is associated with mild to moderate hearing loss, which may lead to delayed language development.[36] A child who has had fluid in both middle ears for a total of 3 months should have a hearing evaluation. Observation or a course of antibiotics as used for acute suppurative otitis media are treatments for children who have effusion that has been present less than 4 to 6 months. Either option can be used for children whose hearing threshold level in the unaffected ear is not reduced by 20 decibels or more.[32,39]

If bilateral effusion has persisted for a total of 3 months and the child has hearing loss, bilateral myringotomy with tube insertion becomes an additional treatment option. Placement of tympanostomy tubes is recommended after a total of 4 to 6 months of bilateral effusion with a bilateral hearing deficit. Antihistamines and decongestants have not proved to be of value in this condition, and steroids are not recommended to treat otitis media with effusion.[4] Tonsillectomy, alone or with adenoidectomy, has not been found effective for treatment of otitis media with effusion (see Chapter 266, Tonsillectomy and Adenoidectomy).

Recurrent Otitis Media. Prophylactic antibiotics are helpful in decreasing recurrences of acute otitis media in children who suffer numerous infections, especially when used during the winter "otitis season."[24] Perrin and coworkers[26] found that giving sulfisoxazole (75 mg/kg/day) every 12 hours decreased recurrences by 81%.

Tympanostomy tube placement is performed frequently, although the controversy over the efficacy of this procedure rages.[23] Immediate improvement in hearing occurs with tube placement and continues until the tube is extruded or removed. Less evidence is available to confirm the efficacy of tympanostomy tubes in preventing recurrences of otitis media. Evidence suggests that tympanostomy tubes should be inserted for recurrent otitis media after failure of medical management with prophylactic antibiotics or in the presence of significant conductive hearing loss.[37]

Care of the Child Who Has Tympanostomy Tubes. Children who have tympanostomy tubes represent a special population for the pediatrician.[19] Problems with these children formerly were dealt with by the otolaryngologist, but recent changes in the health care system have required primary care physicians to care for these problems.

Following tube insertion, visual inspection is used to determine tube patency. Usually the tube can be seen traversing the tympanic membrane. If the tube appears to be occluded with cerumen, blood, or dried pus, reopening the tube can be attempted by instilling an ototopical suspension of neomycin, polymixin B, and hydrocortisone. If this fails, referral should be made to the otolaryngologist.

Water precautions after tympanostomy tube insertion are controversial. Some otolaryngologists recommend strict avoidance of water in the external ear canal, whereas others recommend avoiding water that is likely to be contaminated (bathtubs, lakes).[28]

Otorrhea following tube insertion occurs in up to 30% of children.[9] If the otorrhea is associated with an upper respiratory tract infection, the child should be treated with the same oral antibiotics that are used to treat acute otitis media. Ototopical drops may be used if the otorrhea is persistent or if it is thought to be caused by water contamination. The clinician should prescribe these preparations, surveying closely for potential ototoxicity.[30]

The duration of tube function depends on the type of tube used. In general, tubes should be removed after 2 years to avoid structural complications of the tympanic membrane such as retraction pockets and chronic perforation.

Prevention. No therapy is available to eliminate the occurrence of acute otitis media, although some methods may decrease its frequency. Breast-fed babies suffer fewer episodes of otitis than do bottle-fed babies, especially those bottle fed in a recumbent position.[10] Some postulate that swallowing while lying down allows nasopharyngeal fluid to enter the middle ear, with subsequent infection. Because children exposed to cigarette smoke have more frequent ear infections, parents should be encouraged to avoid having their children around smoke.[17]

Immunization against both the major bacterial pathogens and the viruses associated with acute otitis media is under investigation. Polyvalent pneumococcal polysaccharide vaccines reduce the incidence of pneumococcal otitis media by 50% in children older than 2 years, but the vaccine is not effective in infants, who do not develop antibodies to the polysaccharide vaccines.

Complications. Hearing loss is the most common complication of suppurative and nonsuppurative otitis media. Much concern has been expressed that this hearing loss occurs at the time youngsters are developing language skills, and some postulate that a "critical period" for learning language skills will be missed during the time the child is experiencing hearing loss. Conflicting data exist regarding the impact of recurrent otitis media on speech and language development.[40] The long-term effects of middle ear disease on overall cognitive development have not yet been studied.

Suppurative complications of otitis media such as facial paralysis, subperiosteal abscess, labyrinthitis, meningitis, brain abscess, and mastoiditis are much less common now than before the antibiotic era.[13,22]

OTITIS EXTERNA

Acute otitis externa, or "swimmer's ear," is an infection in the external auditory canal that can be localized or diffuse. Localized infections occur when a hair follicle in the outer third of the canal becomes infected, usually with *S. aureus*. Diffuse infection of the canal follows swimming, aggressive cleaning of the canal, or trauma. *Pseudomonas aeruginosa* is the leading cause of diffuse otitis externa, although other organisms, including fungi, may be the infecting agent.

Clinical Presentation

Patients with otitis externa may present with ear pain, ear swelling, or hearing loss. On physical examination, one finds exquisite tenderness when pressure is placed on the tragus or when the pinna is moved. A furuncle may be seen in localized otitis externa, and moist debris is present on inspection of the ear canal in the diffuse form. The tympanic membrane, if visualized, usually is normal.

Treatment

Treatment of localized infection may require incision and drainage of the furuncle. Diffuse infection is treated by cleaning the debris from the external auditory canal, using suction if possible. A cotton wick may be inserted into the canal to facilitate contact of medication with the skin. Ear drops containing combinations of polymyxin, neomycin, hydrocortisone, and propylene glycol have been found to be effective in combating the infection and decreasing inflammation. Neomycin may cause skin sensitivity in some patients. The patient should lie down with the affected ear upward while the drops are instilled and stay in that position for 5 minutes to allow the drops to penetrate the cotton wick and ear canal. Systemic analgesics often are required to decrease the pain caused by this condition.

Otitis externa may be prevented in persons who have frequent recurrences by instilling 2% acetic acid into the external auditory canal twice daily and after each contact with water.[29] Avoiding swimming and thus keeping the external auditory canal dry also is helpful.

Malignant Otitis Externa

Malignant otitis externa is a more severe form of the illness seen in patients who are susceptible to infections, usually patients who have diabetes mellitus. *P. aeruginosa* is the offending organism in most cases. Infection may extend to the middle and inner ear and to the central nervous system and cause severe sequelae. Computed tomography or radionuclide scanning may be necessary to make the diagnosis. Treatment includes antibiotics administered intravenously and, often, surgical intervention.[34]

REFERENCES

1. Arola M et al: Clinical role of respiratory virus infection in acute otitis media, *Pediatrics* 86:848, 1990.
2. Arola M, Ziegler T, Ruuskanen O: Respiratory virus infection as a cause of prolonged symptoms in acute otitis media, *J Pediatr* 116:697, 1990.
3. Berman S, Roark R: Factors influencing outcome in children treated with antibiotics for acute otitis media, *Pediatr Infect Dis J* 12:20, 1993.
4. Berman S, Roark R, Luckey D: Theoretical cost effectiveness of man-

agement options for children with persisting middle ear effusions, *Pediatrics* 93:353, 1994.
5. Bluestone CD: Modern management of otitis media, *Pediatr Clin North Am* 36:1371, 1989.
6. Bluestone CD, Doyle WJ: Anatomy and physiology of eustachian tube and middle ear related to otitis media, *J Allergy Clin Immunol* 81:997, 1988.
7. Breiman RF et al: Emergence of drug-resistant pneumococcal infections in the United States, *JAMA* 271:1831, 1994.
8. Chonmaitree T et al: Effect of viral respiratory tract infection on outcome of acute otitis media, *J Pediatr* 120:856, 1992.
9. Debruyne F, Degroote M: One-year follow-up after tympanostomy tube insertion for recurrent acute otitis media, *J Otorhinolaryngol Relat Spec* 55:226, 1993.
10. Duncan B et al: Exclusive breast-feeding for at least 4 months protects against otitis media, *Pediatrics* 91:867, 1993.
11. Faden H et al: Nasopharyngeal flora in the first three years of life in normal and otitis-prone children, *Ann Otol Rhinol Laryngol* 100:612, 1991.
12. Fireman P: Otitis media and its relationship to allergy, *Pediatr Clin North Am* 35:1075, 1988.
13. Fliss DM, Leiberman A, Dagan R: Medical sequelae and complications of acute otitis media, *Pediatr Infect Dis J* 13(suppl):34, 1994.
14. Green SM, Rothrock SG: Single-dose intramuscular ceftriaxone for acute otitis media in children, *Pediatrics* 91:23, 1993.
15. Hardy AM, Fowler MG: Child care arrangements and repeated ear infections in young children, *Am J Public Health* 83:1321, 1993.
16. Hathaway TJ et al: Acute otitis media: who needs posttreatment follow-up? *Pediatrics* 94:143, 1994.
17. Hinton AE, Buckley G: Parental smoking and middle ear effusions in children, *J Laryngol Otol* 102:992, 1988.
18. Howie VM: Otitis media, *Pediatr Rev* 14:320, 1993.
19. Isaacson G, Rosenfeld RM: Care of the child with tympanostomy tubes: a visual guide for the pediatrician, *Pediatrics* 93:924, 1994.
20. Kaleida PH et al: Amoxicillin or myringotomy or both for acute otitis media: results of a randomized clinical trial, *Pediatrics* 87:466, 1991.
21. Kalm O et al: HLA frequency in patients with recurrent acute otitis media, *Arch Otolaryngol Head Neck Surg* 117:1296, 1991.
22. Kangsanarak J et al: Extracranial and intracranial complications of suppurative otitis media: report of 102 cases, *J Laryngol Otol* 107:999, 1993.
23. Kleinman LC et al: The medical appropriateness of tympanostomy tubes proposed for children younger than 16 years in the United States, *JAMA* 271:1250, 1994.
24. Paradise JL: Antimicrobial prophylaxis for recurrent acute otitis media, *Ann Otolrhinollaryngol* 155(suppl):33, 1992.
25. Paradise JL: Testing for otitis media: diagnosis *ex machina, N Engl J Med* 296:445, 1977.
26. Perrin JM et al: Sulfisoxazole as chemoprophylaxis for recurrent otitis media: a double-blind crossover study in pediatric practice, *N Engl J Med* 291:664, 1974.
27. Pichichero ME: Assessing the treatment alternatives for acute otitis media, *Pediatr Infect Dis J* 13(suppl):27, 1994.
28. Pringle MB: Grommets, swimming, and otorrhoea—a review, *J Laryngol Otol* 107:190, 1993.
29. Raymond L, Spaur WH, Thalmann ED: Prevention of diver's ear, *Br Med J* 1:48, 1978.
30. Rohn GN, Meyerhoff WL, Wright CG: Ototoxicity of topical agents, *Otolaryngol Clin North Am* 26:747, 1993.
31. Roland PS et al: Otitis media: incidence, duration, and hearing status, *Arch Otolaryngol Head Neck Surg* 115:1049, 1989.
32. Rosenfeld RM, Post JC: Meta-analysis of antibiotics for the treatment of otitis media with effusion, *Otolaryngol Head Neck Surg* 106:378, 1992.
33. Rosenfeld RM et al: Clinical efficacy of antimicrobial drugs for acute otitis media: metaanalysis of 5400 children from thirty-three randomized trials, *J Pediatr* 124:355, 1994.
34. Rubin J, Yu VL, Stool SE: Malignant external otitis in children, *J Pediatr* 113:965, 1988.
35. Schwartz DM, Schwartz RH: Validity of acoustic reflectometry in detecting middle ear effusion, *Pediatrics* 79:739, 1987.
36. Stool SE et al: Clinical practice guideline: otitis media with effusion in young children, AHCPR Pub No 94-0622, July 1994, Rockville, Md, Agency for Health Care Policy and Research, Public Health Service, US Department of Health and Human Services.
37. Teele DW: Strategies to control recurrent acute otitis media in infants and children, *Pediatr Ann* 20:609, 1991.
38. Teele DW, Pelton SI, Klein JO: Bacteriology of acute otitis media unresponsive to initial antimicrobial therapy, *J Pediatr* 98:537, 1981.
39. Williams RL et al: Use of antibiotics in preventing recurrent acute otitis media and in treating otitis media with effusion: a meta-analytic attempt to resolve the brouhaha, *JAMA* 270:1344, 1993.
40. Wright PF et al: Impact of recurrent otitis media on middle ear function, hearing and language, *J Pediatr* 113:581, 1988.

241 Parasitic Infections

Richard Owen Proctor

Parasitism of humans is common. Not all parasites, however, cause disease. Among those that do, light infections frequently are asymptomatic. Recent estimates of prevalence indicate that some progress has been made in controlling selected parasites, locally or regionally. This can occur, however, only when the exposed population is taught the essentials of transmission, and individuals are motivated to change their behavior. A firm governmental commitment to parasite control and dedicated funding also are essential. On a larger scale, many parasites have increased their field in recent years as a result of activities such as the building of dams, new irrigation projects, the clearing of forests, and the construction of housing without adequate sewage and potable water facilities or without adequate protection against insect entry. In areas where civil strife, war, famine, or large refugee populations have complicated social progress, it is difficult for governmental authorities to implement sanitary regulations and environmental control of disease. This is unfortunate because often the economic strength and social cohesion necessary to prevent these disasters stem from just such priorities.

Although many questions remain, researchers are knowledgeable about the general life cycle of the parasites of humans that cause most of the morbidity and mortality. Attempts to control vectors or reservoirs frequently are frustrated by the accompanying toxic effects on other plants or animals, their food chains, and the environment. Therapeutic agents are available against most parasites, but some are dangerously toxic to the patient, and even when a cure rate near 100% with negligible side effects is possible, reinfection may occur quickly and at a high rate. Parasites' development of resistance to antiparasitic drugs, vectors' resistance to chemicals designed to kill them, and immunosuppression caused by HIV infection or therapeutic agents all have expanded the prevalence and lethality of some parasitic diseases (e.g., malaria).

Most people harbor common intestinal parasites with little or no complaint of illness and with small risk of serious sequelae. It therefore is necessary to distinguish between infection and disease. *Infection* occurs when the parasite enters any part of the body, including the integument, and resides, multiplies, or develops there. Some parasites may be unable to develop after entering the human body, but their presence there still constitutes an infection. When the parasite resides on the skin or hair without penetrating the integument or any body orifice, this customarily is referred to as an *infestation*. *Disease* implies some associated host dysfunction that manifests itself by signs or symptoms. When an infection becomes disease, some change has taken place in the delicate balance between maintenance of the host and survival of the parasite. This may stem from changes in the host, agent, or environmental factors.

HOST FACTORS

Multiple host factors may influence the types, numbers, and invasiveness of parasites causing disease in a given person. The epidemiological profile of the patient obtained at interview should thus include age, sex, race, occupation, nutritional and immunological status, and the presence of concurrent infection, chronic noninfectious disease, and medications taken. For example, infection with pinworms or dwarf tapeworms is much more prevalent among children than adults, whereas amebic abscesses are more common in adults than children. Prevalence by gender often is a function of occupation or social custom, as illustrated by the increased rate of infection with *Diphyllobothrium latum* (fish tapeworm) among Jewish women because of sampling the "gefilte fish" before cooking it. Certain races appear to have more natural immunity against infection with a given parasite, such as the relative immunity to malaria seen in some African races. Shepherds in many parts of the world are at greater risk of contracting hydatid disease through handling of their dogs, whose feces disseminate the disease agent. Immunodeficiency already has been noted as a risk factor in parasitic disease.

Aside from genetic predisposition, no other host variable is as fundamental to limiting the invasiveness and duration of parasitic disease as host nutrition. Protein and iron frequently are deficient in the diets of children in tropical countries where the monoculture of coffee, bananas, sugar cane, and similar products has replaced subsistence farming; it is in these settings that polyparasitism of children is most evident.

In advanced industrial societies, parasitism with protozoan and helminthic agents is limited by modern sanitary systems and health education. Immigrants from areas of endemicity can spread the parasites they carry to other areas in which the appropriate vectors, reservoirs, and other host animals are present. Today in the United States it is estimated that hundreds of thousands of recent migrants are carrying parasitic infections, some potentially disabling or lethal. It has been published repeatedly that the snail intermediate hosts of schistosomiasis do not exist in the United States; the presumption that schistosomiasis cannot become a problem here has made us comfortable. However, the rapid transit of military, engineering, and other equipment between countries and the growing international commerce in minerals, timber, and various plants and animals make it inevitable that the vectors and intermediate hosts of this and other parasitic diseases are being introduced and dispersed in the environment. These can become established, of course, only where the thermal, pH, nutrient, moisture, and other essential requirements are also met. Surveillance and enforcement of import laws and customs regulations are essential, as are field surveillance and evaluation of the environment in diagnosed cases. Physicians should consider the potential for transmission of any nonendemic parasitic disease they diagnose. Notification of the appropriate public health authorities may be required.

AGENT FACTORS

Our knowledge of parasitism allows us to assume that a parasite residing in the gastrointestinal (GI) tract attempts to remain as superficial in the bowel wall as is compatible with maintenance of position and feeding. In this way it avoids triggering additional defense systems of the host. When the host's defenses have been compromised by disease, nutritional deficiencies, or therapy with steroids, irradiation, or other immunosuppressants, parasites that normally are not invasive may become so. They then may gain access to the lymphatic system and bloodstream and be transported to distant sites. Parasites that normally enter the deeper tissues of the body as part of their life cycle appear to survive by defeating the body's defenses in a variety of ways, such as rapid transit to their portal of exit from the body, disguising their outer membranes with substances of the host's manufacture, entering cells in which they are equipped to survive, encysting, or repeatedly changing their mantel of antigens to subvert the host's antibody systems. Adaptation is a continuous process, and parasites have much to gain by not injuring their host. However, most parasites do evoke a humoral or cellular response (or both) from the human host. In some cases the hypersensitivity response is the major cause of the pathological condition. Complete, permanent immunity following parasitic infection is not common, probably because the agents are so complex and exhibit such an array of antigens.

ENVIRONMENTAL FACTORS

The spectrum of transmission modalities used by the metazoan parasites of humans is broad but can be covered largely by the following categories: direct, soil dependent, arthropod borne, foodborne, and waterborne.

Direct Transmission

The direct group includes pinworms, dwarf tapeworms, amebas, *Giardia lamblia,* and other parasites that are able to infect humans as soon as they are eliminated by an infected host. Children disseminate such parasites readily among their peers and, to a lesser extent, to adults. Parasites in the direct transmission group often are transmitted in food and water through simple contamination. Superinfections can occur with members of this group through direct reinoculation by way of the fingers—from anus to mouth (i.e., autoinfection).

Soil-dependent Transmission

Simple. Some parasites, such as *Trichuris trichiura, Ascaris lumbricoides,* and the oocyst of *Toxoplasma gondii,* require a period of development outside the body following deposition of feces onto plants or in soil before their embryos become infective for the next host. Only the embryo, still in its case or cyst, is infective. These organisms frequently reach humans on food contaminated by soil or directly with feces on the hands of food handlers. They also may gain entry in contaminated water consumed by the host.

Complex. The embryos of other parasites (e.g., hookworms, *Strongyloides stercoralis*) molt in the soil and give rise to a rhabditiform larvae. When they come into direct contact with skin, these larvae can attach themselves to and penetrate the skin. Humans who go barefoot or recline on soil contaminated by human feces containing these organisms help the parasites to invade a new host and survive.

Arthropod-Borne Transmission

Simple. Parasites in this functional category require a period of metamorphosis in an intermediate arthropod host. Filariasis, malaria, onchocerciasis, leishmaniasis, and the trypanosomiases are examples. In all these examples except Chagas disease (American trypanosomiasis), the parasite is introduced by the insect's bite. In Chagas disease, the insect's feces, which contain the parasite, gain entry to the body, most commonly through the bite wound.

Foodborne Transmission

Apart from food contaminated with soil parasites, this group comprises parasites contained in the flesh of cattle, pigs, fish, snails, crustaceans, or encysted on aquatic plants. Generally the parasite is digested free from its encysted state in the human gut and then undergoes further metamorphosis to complete its cycle. Humans may be either the intermediate or the definitive host. In the latter case the adult parasite with the powers of sexual reproduction are found. *Trichinella spiralis,* the tapeworms, and the endocyst of *T. gondii* are but a few examples.

Waterborne Transmission

Simple. Aside from embryos that contaminate soil and may gain entry to humans through the water they drink, members of this group gain entry because of a water-dependent life cycle. They may be free forms (e.g., schistosome cercariae, amebae, and Giardia), be contained in microscopic copepods (e.g., *Dracunculus medinensis*), or encysted on aquatic plants used as food (e.g., fascioliasis).

DIAGNOSIS AND MANAGEMENT

Diagnosis of a parasitic disease depends on maintaining a strong index of suspicion for a child at higher risk. This category includes children in rural areas, those of lower socioeconomic or educational classes, and those who are undernourished, chronically ill, institutionalized because of mental subnormality, or known to exhibit pica. If a child has visited or lived in an endemic area of parasite transmission anywhere in the world, parasitic diseases should be considered in the differential diagnosis. A systematic and exhaustive attempt to determine the precise species of parasites and the extent of the disease is warranted for those who have significant signs or symptoms and those whose body defenses are known to be compromised. Unlike with many bacterial or viral infections, the physician must obtain more information about polymorphic parasites. This is essential to manage the patient with maximal safety while, when possible, effecting a complete cure.

The following questions should be answered when the diagnosis of a parasite is entertained:

1. What parasites are present?
2. What stages of each parasite are present?
3. What is the site of each stage of each parasite?
4. Do any of the parasites have priority for treatment? (Note: *A. lumbricoides,* if present, must be treated simultaneously with or before other parasites if the treatment for others is likely to cause migration of this roundworm.)
5. Is there any stage of a parasite situated where its death could result in an unacceptable outcome, such as blinding inflammation of the eye?
6. What drug(s) must be used to effect the death of all stages of all the parasites? (Note: For species of malaria that have extraerythrocytic forms, such as *Plasmodium vivax* and *P. ovale,* more than one drug still is needed. Furthermore, drugs that rid the bowel of intraluminal amebiasis may not kill the organism in a liver abscess.)
7. What temporal sequencing of a drug(s) will rid the body of the parasite permanently? (Note: Retreatment is necessary to eliminate parasites such as pinworms or dwarf tapeworms if the drug used does not kill both the adult worm and its eggs.)
8. Is the risk of treating the patient greater than the risk posed by the parasite's presence in the host?

The diagnostician must know the life cycle of a parasite if the history of exposure is to be sought intelligently. Adequate care of the patient and protection for the family and community depend on a knowledge of how the parasite reaches and enters its human host and how soon, how long, and under what conditions the host can transmit the disease to others.

It sometimes is stated that one need not treat light (asymptomatic) infections of *T. trichiura* (whipworm) or hookworm because the worms have a recognized life expectancy and thereby produce a self-limited infection or because reinfection will occur anyway. However, with the newer broad-spectrum therapies, which have a wide margin of therapeutic safety, treatment should be given. The risk is that infection with either of these helminths can lead to serious or fatal outcomes, especially in patients with malnutrition or immunodeficiency. Diseases that have the potential for autoinoculation always should be treated unless specific contraindications exist, such as medication allergy or pregnancy. When a parasite is identified in the patient's stool, blood, or tissue and a parasitism is diagnosed, a warning light must flash for the clinician. Does the parasite adequately explain the findings, or could another disease coexist (e.g., a malignancy, a connective tissue disorder, or an immunodeficiency disorder)? Close follow-up is essential to determine whether the parasite and symptoms have disappeared after therapy. Stool examination and specific serological tests may be helpful.

More than one course of therapy, either with the same drug or another, often is justified. The clinician who lacks experience in treating parasitic infections would be well advised to consult an expert in the field if questions arise.

For discussions of *G. lamblia* and *Enterobius vermicularis* (pinworm) infections, see Chapters 208 and 246, respectively.

AMEBIASIS (*Entamoeba histolytica*)

Epidemiology

Entamoeba histolytica is a cyst-forming protozoan that inhabits the intestinal tract of an estimated 10% of the world's population and accounts for 50,000 to 100,000 deaths a year. *E. histolytica* generally is more prevalent in areas of poor hygiene and inadequate water sanitation and where human waste is used to fertilize food crops.

In the United States fewer than 3000 cases of *E. histolytica* infection were reported during 1992. However, erratic shedding by carriers, the asymptomatic nature of most infections, and incidental cures by amoebicides prescribed for other reasons all have led to underestimation of the prevalence.

The protozoan is transmitted when amebic cysts, shed in the feces of an infected animal, are ingested by another host. Infection also may result from direct inoculation of trophozoites or cysts into injured skin or mucosal surfaces. Ingested trophozoites do not survive the gastric barrier in normal humans. *E. histolytica* cysts are highly resistant to environmental destruction; they survive for months at the temperature of household freezers and may withstand the chlorine concentrations used in city water supplies. However, they are filtered out by modern water purification plants and can be killed by treating drinking water with tetraglycine hydroperiodide (Globaline) or by keeping water at a rolling boil for at least 5 minutes.

Widespread endemicity is the rule in tropical agrarian societies, but pockets of high prevalence occur in temperate industrial societies as well. Clusters in the latter case have been associated with hotels, mental institutions, child care settings, nursing homes, prisons, and male homosexual enclaves. Prevention rests in improved sanitation, health education of target populations, and identification and treatment of hosts who pass cysts in their stools.

Pathogenesis and Life Cycle

The slightly ovoid cysts of *E. histolytica* measure 10 to 20 μm and typically contain four nuclei. They also may contain dark-staining, blunt-ended chromatid bodies, which are refractile. *E. histolytica* has both pathogenic and nonpathogenic strains (zymodemes). These differ in epidemiological as well as pathogenic characteristics. Whether one form can change into the other is in question; they cannot be distinguished microscopically. When a cyst is ingested, the cyst wall is digested in the small intestine, liberating four metacystic trophozoites, each of which divides into two mature trophozoites, measuring up to 25 μm in diameter. These can continue to divide by binary fission. The ameba exhibits unidirectional movement by the extension of clear pseudopodia. The cytoplasm is granular, with recognizable debris of bacteria and red blood cells (RBCs) in some cases. The ameba tends to favor the cecum and rectosigmoid bowel as its habitat. Usually only amebic trophozoites are passed in dysenteric or diarrheal stools. With slow-moving, relatively well-formed stools, trophozoites transform into a precyst and then a smaller, true cyst before passage in the stool. Cysts are infective immediately.

Under certain circumstances that are not yet clear, trophozoites may invade the bowel wall, producing ulcers of varying size, with sharply defined borders and a granular base. Cytolysis of host cells by the ameba follows attachment and probable injection of enzymes through a pore created for this purpose. Phagocytosis of cellular debris by the ameba follows. Only with secondary bacterial infection does much of an inflammatory response occur. Trophozoites can be found in the thin exudate, especially near the ulcer's border. In some patients, especially those who are immunosuppressed, amebae extend into adjacent tissues, even perforating the visceral peritoneum; peritonitis results. Trophozoites also may be disseminated to the liver, lungs, pericardium, and brain through the bloodstream. The presence of a "toxic" hepatitis without evidence of amebae in the liver has led to speculation that products of *E. histolytica* are responsible for this phenomenon. It may precede frank abscess with amebae present, and it clears with successful treatment of the amebiasis. *E. histolytica* cysts do not occur in deep tissues.

Clinical Manifestations

Intestinal Amebiasis. Most infections with *E. histolytica* are asymptomatic, and stool cysts may vanish after treatment with intraluminal amebicides. It is estimated that the bowel wall is invaded in only 10% to 25% of people infected clinically with *E. histolytica*. Clinical illness develops after an incubation period of 1 to 3 weeks and may manifest with acute abdominal pain, cramps, distention, diarrhea or dysentery, fever, toxicity, and lower abdominal tenderness on palpation. Examination also may reveal hepatomegaly. In older children and adults the onset may be more insidious, with intermittent flatulence, watery diarrhea, and constipation plus tenderness in the lower abdomen. Constitutional symptoms may be few. Tenesmus may be pronounced, especially with ulcerations in the rectosigmoid area.

A granulomatous response to *E. histolytica* locally in the bowel may result in constrictions of the bowel, simulating Crohn disease, perforation (in rare cases), or the formation of a large granuloma (ameboma) that may be mistaken for cancer. Amebic granulomas are found most often in the cecum, followed by (in decreasing order) the rectum and anal canal, the transverse colon, and the sigmoid, and then elsewhere.

Extraintestinal Amebiasis. When trophozoites invade the liver, they may cause a hepatic abscess; these are found in the right lobe in 85% to 90% of cases. An abscess may develop within 2 weeks of the initial symptoms or after months of intraluminal infection. Symptoms of abscess formation include pain in the right hypochondrium, fever, weight loss, anorexia, cough, and fatigue. Most patients have a tender, enlarged liver. Bacterial infection occurs more often as the abscess ages. The liver abscess may extend, or rupture into the lung, pleural space, peritoneum, or (particularly from the left lobe) the pericardium. All such events carry a much higher mortality than does an uncomplicated amebic liver abscess, especially if secondary bacterial infection is present. Abscess formation is less common in children than in adults.

Diagnosis

The quickest method of diagnosing acute intraluminal amebic dysentery is to obtain exudate from a colonic ulcer at endoscopy, place it in a drop of normal (1N) saline on a microscope slide, with or without stain (e.g., D'Antoni), and observe it immediately under high power on a light microscope. Kits are available to prepare slides for transfer to an appropriate laboratory. When clinically suspected, *E. histolytica* should not be ruled out until at least three stool specimens taken on separate days have been reported negative by a trusted laboratory. Extraintestinal infections with *E. histolytica* can occur in the absence of intestinal cyst shedding. Serological testing is valuable in cases accompanied by ulcerative bowel lesions and extraintestinal disease. The test results may not be positive in the first week or more of symptoms. The indirect hemagglutination test is positive at 1:256 or higher and is positive in about 90% of cases involving tissue invasion. The counterimmunoelectrophoresis (CIE) test, immunofluorescent assay (IFA), and enzyme immunoassay (EIA) also are used. Cases involving amebic liver abscess almost uniformly test positive. Newer tests, especially those testing for antigen, (e.g., antigen detection enzyme-linked immunosorbent assay [ELISA]) may soon be the standard for diagnosis and monitoring treatment. Ultrasound and computed tomography (CT) scans are valuable in the diagnosis of liver abscess. Needle aspiration under ultrasonographic guidance has been used, largely to rule out bacterial infection; amebae rarely are found. The yellowish proteinaceous fluid is largely free of white blood cells (WBCs). With a large abscess, chest roentgenograms usually demonstrate an elevated diaphragm, with or without pleural effusion and atelectasis. The costophrenic angle may be obliterated. Upper abdominal films may show hepatic enlargement and, if the abscess is in the left lobe, deformation of the stomach shadow.

Treatment

Treatment depends on the anatomical location of the organism, the severity of disease, and coexisting conditions such as pregnancy, secondary bacterial infection, and drug reactions. Table 241-1 shows the current recommendations. Patients who pass cysts in their stools always should be treated because of their role in transmission and the ever-present potential to develop complications such as liver abscess. A drug that is amebicidal in both the intestinal lumen and extraintestinal sites (e.g., metronidazole) must be considered when deep or disseminated infection is a question. An amebic abscess should be aspirated percutaneously when a diagnosis cannot be achieved otherwise, when the patient has not responded to treatment with appropriate therapeutic agents in 3 to 5 days, or when a large abscess, especially of the left lobe, threatens to rupture before it can be controlled with systemic amebic treatment. The abscess should never be drained surgically unless secondary bacterial infection is proven. When surgery is necessary, amebicidal drugs should be given before the procedure.

AMEBIC MENINGOENCEPHALITIS *(Naegleria fowleri, Entamoeba histolytica, and certain species of Acanthamoeba, Leptomyxa, Gephyramoeba, and Balamuthia)*

General

Several known genera of amebae cause central nervous system (CNS) disease. *E. histolytica*, already described, may invade the brain when the agent becomes disseminated, usually when a liver abscess also is present. It causes tissue ne-

Table 241-1 Treatment of Amebiasis

Severity of disease	Drugs	Administration	Total daily dose
Asymptomatic carrier (cyst passer) and mild intraluminal disease	Iodoquinol	3×/day for 20 days (PO)	40 mg/kg/day (max: 2 g)
	OR		
	Diloxanide furoate	3×/day for 10 days (PO)	20-30 mg/kg/day (max: 1500 g)
	OR		
	Paromomycin	3×/day for 7 days (PO)	30 mg/kg/day (max: 1500 g)
Moderate to severe intestinal disease (dysentery)	Metronidazole	3×/day for 10 days (PO)	35-50 mg/kg/day
	(followed by one of the three drugs listed above for asymptomatic carriers)		
Extraintestinal amebiasis or ameboma	Metronidazole	3×/day for 10 days (PO)	35-50 mg/kg/day
	(followed by one of the three drugs listed above for asymptomatic carriers)		
	OR		
	Dehydroemetine	2×/day for 10 days (IM)	1-1.5 mg/kg/day (max: 90 mg)
	PLUS		
	Chloroquine	2×/day for 21 days (PO)	10 mg base/kg/day (max: 300 mg base)

crosis with scant, nonspecific pleocytosis and purulent exudate. Signs of meningeal irritation and hemiplegia may occur before lethargy, seizures, coma, and death. Therapy with metronidazole is indicated, but the fatality rate with cerebral involvement approaches 100%.

More recently, one or more species from the *Naegleria, Acanthamoeba, Leptomyxa, Gephyramoeba,* and *Balamuthia* genera of "free-living" amebae have been identified as a cause of meningoencephalitis. These organisms inhabit fresh and brackish water, sewage, and moist soils. Although acquired as human disease under somewhat different conditions, each nearly always is fatal once the brain is involved. *Naegleria* species seem to predominate in water; *Acanthamoeba* species predominate in moist or wet sediments. Identification requires a knowledge of the taxonomic changes taking place. Zymodemes, no doubt, will be used to bring order to the speciation required for diagnosis. Morphological diagnosis is difficult, even for an expert, and final classification of species still is in question. Currently diagnosis is based on direct observation of trophozoites and cysts in body fluids or tissues, animal inoculation, cell cultures, and the indirect immunofluorescence (IIF) test. Antibodies to *Acanthamoeba* species and, to a lesser extent, *N. fowleri* have been found in normal humans. The implication is that a unique portal of entry or immunodeficiency may result in disease instead of self-limiting infection. The wide distribution of these organisms under conditions that foster human exposure, including the significant resistance of *Acanthamoeba* species to normal concentrations of chlorine in drinking water and swimming pools, supports a concept of human infection without resulting disease.

Naegleria fowleri. *N. fowleri* produces a rapidly fatal disease that mimics acute pyogenic meningitis but fails to respond to antibiotics. The disease is designated primary amebic meningoencephalitis (PAM). Patients give a history of swimming in fresh or brackish water that has a temperature above 86° F (30° C). Some have a history of facial trauma. The clinical course is short, with an incubation period of 3 to 7 days. Headache, nausea, and vomiting are prominent. Evidence of meningeal inflammation, lethargy, coma, and death follow within a few days. The cerebrospinal fluid (CSF) reveals a moderate number of RBCs and WBCs, with polymorphonuclear (PMN) cells predominating. The protein content of the CSF may be elevated and the glucose moderately reduced. *N. fowleri* trophozoites frequently can be found on wet mounts of CSF and can be grown on salt-free, nutrient-free agar that has been inoculated with *E. coli* bacteria. The amebae enter the brain by way of the olfactory nerves, traversing the cribriform plate. At autopsy, lesions have been evident in the olfactory bulbs, posterior fossa, and frontal and temporal lobes. Hemorrhage associated with lesions is more common with *N. fowleri* than with the *Acanthamoeba* species.

Treatment should be started as soon as the history and clinical picture suggest the diagnosis. Despite the nearly 100% fatality rate, treatment with amphotericin B intravenously, intrathecally, and possibly by intraventricular instillation has been recommended. There is some evidence of a synergistic effect when oral rifampin and intraspinal miconazole are administered along with amphotericin B. Survival has been the exception, even with combined therapy.

Acanthamoeba Species. *Acanthamoeba* species cause a subacute to chronic granulomatous disease that generally begins with primary lesions of the skin, pulmonary tract, or eye. This disease is designated granulomatous amebic encephalitis (GAE). When *Acanthamoeba* organisms are atomized in the nasal passages of animals, they cause pulmonary lesions that result in hematogenous spread to the CNS. No history of swimming or other recognizable exposure is elicited consistently. It has been noted, however, that victims of *Acanthamoeba* infection usually are chronically ill, immunosuppressed, or otherwise debilitated (e.g., chronic alcoholics or patients who have malignancies or AIDS or who are taking antibiotics or immunosuppressants).

Symptoms of flulike disease may precede signs of CNS involvement. Headache, fever, nausea, vomiting, hemiparesis, cranial nerve palsies, cerebellar ataxia, and other signs suggesting multifocal brain abscesses may occur. The course of *Acanthamoeba* infection may last weeks or months, but the outcome so far has been uniformly fatal when the brain is invaded. Tissue destruction probably is due to enzymatic action similar to that proposed for intestinal amebiasis. The pathological picture at autopsy is multifocal granulomatous lesions in the brain and leptomeninges. Giant cells, monocytes, and plasma cells can be found. In severely immunosuppressed patients, a granulomatous response may be absent. Both trophozoites and cysts are found in deep tissues. The CSF reveals a pleocytosis with PMN and lymphocytic cells. Elevated protein and normal or reduced glucose levels have been reported. Wet preparations of the CSF should be examined for trophozoites and cysts, even if *Acanthamoeba* is not found in the CSF. It is important to remember that the absence of any species of amebae in the CSF does not rule out an amebic etiology. Acanthamoebic trophozoites found in tissues or cultures are sluggish and may be confused with macrophages, in contrast to the more motile *N. fowleri* ameba, which projects lobopodia rapidly. Sinusitis, otitis media, granulomatous lesions of the skin, lungs, and genitourinary tract, and corneal ulcers all have been attributed to *Acanthamoeba* species. Dissemination to many distant body organs may occur late in the course, when blood vessel walls have been penetrated. The IIF applied to a brain biopsy may help distinguish amebic disease from other causes, but there is much cross-reactivity within the free-living amebae. Treatment of Acanthamoebic encephalitis is unsatisfactory at present. In vitro research with strains taken from fatal cases has shown some drug activity against these pathogens. Paromomycin, 5-fluorocytosine, pentamidine, ketoconazole, polymyxin B, hydroxystilbamidine, amphotericin B, and sulfa drugs all have been suggested or used as therapy.

Surgery for amebic foci in the brain and elsewhere has been tried as a means of halting this highly fatal disease; however, its use must be weighed carefully because of the intrinsic danger of brain surgery where infection is involved and the uncertainty about both the portal and the limiting boundaries of the infection.

All cases of CNS infection from amebae should be treated in a medical setting where neurological, neurosurgical, and infectious disease expertise can be brought to bear on management. Life support systems are essential. Consultation with the Centers for Disease Control and Prevention (CDC) is advisable to make a single repository of experience available to all.

Acanthamoeba species are being reported at an accelerating rate as the cause of keratitis of the cornea, particularly in contact lens wearers. This appears to be due to resistance of *Acanthamoeba* cysts to the disinfection solutions used on contact lenses. Thermal disinfection, on the other hand, seems to be safe. It recently has been suggested that a difference exists in the temperature required for growth. Those that infect the eye may not require as high a temperature for proliferation as those causing encephalitis. Genetic heterogeneity likewise has been proposed. Cures of *Acanthamoeba* keratitis have been reported using propamidine, neomycin in combination with propamidine, ketoconazole, acridine derivatives, and paromomycin.

Prevention

Diving or just swimming in contaminated water, especially heated pools, picking one's nose, or aspirating water into the nose all may be ways of acquiring *N. fowleri*, if not other amebic species. Although the route of transmission for *Acanthamoeba* and other GAE-producing strains is known, it has been suggested that individuals who have a chronic disability or immunodeficiency are at increased risk. This has not been confirmed in all cases. Maintaining a level of 1 ppm free chlorine in swimming pools and sterilizing filters frequently is advisable. Waters known to be high in fecal organisms, warm, or stagnant should be avoided for swimming and bathing. These may need to be posted with warning signs if several cases have resulted from their recreational use. Persons using contact lenses must make sure that only fresh sterile fluids are used to clean lenses and that soiled fingers are not used to handle them.

BABESIOSIS (*Babesia microti, B. divergens, B. bovis, and other species*)

Epidemiology

Babesiosis is caused by a protozoan parasite that infects human erythrocytes much like malaria but possibly without an extraerythrocytic phase. The parasite is transmitted by nymphal ticks of the genus *Ixodes*. In humans the disease initially was believed to be associated only with the postsplenectomy state because the earliest recognized cases occurred in splenectomized humans. Now more than half of cases reported from North America have occurred in individuals who have not undergone splenectomy. Currently, two clinical presentations are recognized. One occurs in splenectomized persons, often of older age, who are infected with the bovine strains of *Babesia*, primarily *B. divergens* and *B. bovis*. These cases have fulminant disease and a high fatality.

The second presentation is that seen with *B. microti*, an organism that commonly infects mice and deer. Humans who have this form, which is found in the United States, have a more benign course. This presentation is found more often in nonsplenectomized persons. More than 100 cases have occurred, clustered in Rhode Island, Massachusetts, Connecticut, Maryland, New York, and Wisconsin. The primary reservoir for *B. microti* is the white-footed mouse, *Peromyscus leucopus*. Transstadial transmission (larva to nymph) maintains the parasite in the *Ixodes* tick-rodent cycle. Babesiosis, which is caused by more than 70 species of *Babesia*, occurs in a wide spectrum of animals. Seroprevalence studies have established the subclinical nature of the infection among humans in most cases. The disease occurs in Mexico, where seroprevalence surveys again demonstrated a silent human prevalence with a few reported overt cases. Babesiosis has been transmitted via transfusion.

Pathogenesis and Life Cycle

The mature protozoan is a small round, oval, or pear-shaped intraerythrocytic parasite. It undergoes asexual division in the red blood cell with periodic release of merozoites, in contrast to the synchronous release of merozoites in *Plasmodium* species. The merozoites attach to and enter other erythrocytes, perpetuating the infection. Lysis of erythrocytes and obstruction of blood vascular channels results in the clinical picture described below. Individuals between 40 and 60 years of age are at greatest risk of manifesting the disease, possibly because of poor splenic defenses (the body depends on the splenic defenses for clearing the circulation of infected

RBCs). Tick larvae that feed on *B. microti*–infected animals in late summer and acquire the parasite pass the infection on to their nymph stage (about 2 mm long). The parasite develops first in the tick gut and then migrates to the salivary glands, where it becomes available for transmission to the human intermediate host. The nymph-stage tick then transmits *B. microti* to humans during its blood meal before molting to the adult tick stage. Accordingly, the disease shows up in humans during late summer or fall. Transmission in newborns has been described, which implies either transplacental or perinatal infection.

Clinical Manifestations

It is believed that many cases of babesiosis occur in the younger-age population but remain controlled and tolerated without clinical illness by the defensive action of a healthy immune system, including the spleen. One of the two reported cases in children (a neonate) was incurred from transfusion. The onset of babesiosis (unlike the infection caused by *Plasmodium falciparum,* with which it often is confused) may be more gradual, owing in part to the nonsynchronous release of merozoites. Intermittent fever (up to 104° F [40° C]), shaking chills, headache, dark urine, sweats, myalgia, arthralgia, nausea, and vomiting are common in symptomatic cases. Numerous other symptoms also have been found, including emotional lability, conjunctival injection, photophobia, sore throat, and nonproductive cough. Mild splenomegaly or hepatomegaly may be present. The illness typically lasts weeks to months and apparently may resolve spontaneously. Recurrences after splenectomy have occurred. In patients without a spleen, fatalities have occurred after as short a period as 1 week of symptoms.

Diagnosis

Giemsa-stained blood smears, inoculation of hamsters, or serological tests (ELISA, IFA) are used to diagnose *B. microti* infection. The ring forms can be distinguished from *Plasmodium* disease (except in early *P. falciparum* infection) by the absence of pigment in *B. microti,* which also may have a large white vacuole in the larger ring forms.

Treatment

Clindamycin alone has proved effective in treating mild cases, although no complete cure has been confirmed. For more severe cases, and probably for all immune-deficient or splenectomized individuals, quinine should be added to the regimen. A regimen of 7 days of clindamycin (20 to 40 mg/kg/day divided into three doses orally) with quinine (25 mg/kg/day divided into three doses orally) appears to clear the blood of *B. microti.*

Prevention

Wearing long sleeves and trousers, tucked in at the boot and waist level, and using diethyltoluamide (Deet) or permethrin repellent are helpful, as is avoiding known areas of high tick infestation during the tick season for that area. However, *Ixodes* ticks are found in urban areas as well as in woods and fields. It is important to inspect the body after outings and to remove promptly any ticks found crawling on the clothing. Hard ticks remain on the body for up to a week or more. A tick should be removed by grasping it with a thin forceps as close to the skin as possible and applying steady, gentle pressure until the tick releases its position. It is essential to examine both the tick and the skin site under magnification to ensure that mouth parts were removed. Applying an antiseptic (isopropyl alcohol) and leaving the wound to air dry is adequate treatment if no secondary infection is obvious.

MALARIA *(Plasmodium falciparum, P. vivax, P. ovale, P. malariae)*

Epidemiology

Despite heroic efforts to eradicate malaria after World War II, the problem has worsened since 1965 because of the ban on the use of DDT as an insecticide, the expanding population in endemic areas, growing resistance to antimalarial drugs, vector resistance to insecticides, and erratic control efforts on the part of governments faced with competing economic goals. Many still believe malaria to be the single greatest infectious scourge in the world today. It is estimated that the current prevalence is at least 800 million people; an estimated 100 million to 300 million new cases occur each year. The annual death toll is put at 1 to 2 million. Malaria is prevalent throughout much of the developing world between the latitudes 40° N and 45° S. It is transmitted from person to person by the bite of the female *Anopheles* mosquito. More than 2 billion people live in areas of transmission, and more than 70 million live births occur annually in those areas. Most of those babies who do not live in major urban areas develop malaria within a few years. Most deaths from malaria occur in children, most of whom live in Africa. There is no suitable test for mass measurement of prevalence or incidence rates among those in endemic areas. However, a crude estimate of prevalence can be obtained by extrapolation from the proportion of 2- to 9-year-olds who have splenomegaly. Likewise, a rough estimate of the incidence of transmission can be obtained from the percentage of randomly selected infants whose blood smears reveal the parasite. Four species of plasmodia infect humans: *P. falciparum, P. vivax, P. malariae,* and *P. ovale*. *P. falciparum* is the most dangerous; *P. vivax* is the most widely distributed; *P. malariae* is the least common and tends to occur in the cooler climates; and *P. ovale* is uncommon and found largely in Africa.

Pathogenesis and Life Cycle

When a female *Anopheles* mosquito feeds on a human who has circulating gametocytes (the sexual stage of malaria), the male microgametes fertilize the female macrogametocytes in the mosquito, and the sporogony phase begins. In 1 to 3 weeks, the infective-stage sporozoites are found in the mosquito's saliva and can enter the bloodstream of a human when he or she is bitten by the infected mosquito. Each sporozoite released into the human circulation travels to and enters a liver parenchymal cell (extraerythrocytic stage), where it divides into as many as 40,000 tiny merozoites. When the cell finally ruptures, these merozoites attach to and enter erythrocytes (erythrocytic stage) by a complex process that causes abnormalities on the RBC surface. Infected cells lose some of their ability to distort during passage through capillaries and become more vulnerable to osmotic change. They have an increased tendency to stick to vascular endothelium. These RBC changes appear to be related to the major symptoms and complication of malaria.

Clinical Manifestations

In childhood malaria, the species of plasmodia in the reservoir population, the seasonality or continuous nature of local transmission, the child's age and nutrition status, and any concomitant illness all influence the nature of the signs and symptoms. A mother who maintains a high rate of natural immunity as a result of repeated exposure passes some protection to the fetus. This passive immunity of the newborn disappears in several months and is followed by several years of high vulnerability unless the infant has received some active immunity through exposure while still protected by maternal antibodies. Malaria in the first several years of life can cause general irritability, periodic fever, vomiting, diarrhea, respiratory symptoms, and poor appetite. The spleen and liver may be enlarged and tender. Drowsiness is common, especially during high fever. An older child may complain of headache, arthralgia, and abdominal pain. Cerebral malaria (usually caused by *P. falciparum*) must be suspected if the patient is lethargic or comatose. About 95% of fatalities are caused by *P. falciparum* infection. Renal failure, cerebral ischemia, countercurrent infection, or severe prostration with cardiovascular collapse are contributory in fatal cases. Because of its release of massive numbers of merozoites from one extraerythrocytic phase and its ability to attack all ages of RBCs, *P. falciparum* may rapidly become fatal in a nonimmune host. Inadequately treated *P. vivax* may recur for several years because it can remain latent in liver cells, with periodic bursts into the circulation. Under favorable conditions *P. malariae* can reappear in the blood periodically for up to 40 years after a single exposure.

Diagnosis

Examination of a Giemsa-stained thick blood smear is the most reliable method of confirming the diagnosis. In *P. falciparum* infection the ring forms (early trophozoites) predominate in peripheral smears, and gametocytes appear later than in other species. Parasitemia rates of over 500,000/mm^3 may be seen in *P. falciparum* infection and constitute a grave sign. In partially treated or immune patients, the parasitemia levels may be low, requiring repeated examination of blood smears. A thick blood smear is used to detect the malarial parasite, although species can be identified by using a thin smear. A trained microscopist can detect as few as 10 to 20 parasites per milliliter of blood. To be useful, a serological test must be simple, quick, and inexpensive and must match that sensitivity. Although specie-specific serological tests are available, they indicate only that infection has occurred at some time. The future use of soluble antigen from the plasma of patients would be useful for diagnosis because it doesn't require circulating infected RBCs, which may be absent in some cases of *P. falciparum* cerebral malaria.

Treatment

No one drug meets all the requirements for prophylaxis and treatment of malaria. The single most important aspect of managing malaria is early recognition and treatment of *P. falciparum* to prevent cerebral malaria and rapid death. Only *P. vivax* and *P. ovale* have potential for recurrent attacks after the initial circulating disease is treated, because these two species continue to release new "crops" of merozoites from infected liver cells. Persons traveling or living in areas of the world where *P. falciparum* is becoming resistant to one or more of the standard remedies must have access to information about what drug(s) still are capable of interrupting the infection. This information often is known only by the local health authorities, but the CDC monitors these developments and may be able to provide the latest reports of drug resistance. When a diagnosis of malaria is entertained but the species is unknown, the patient should be treated for *P. falciparum* immediately and the diagnostic workup continued while the success of treatment is monitored with repeated blood smears. Recurrence of the malaria without continued or repeat exposure can mean drug resistance or the presence of *P. vivax* or *P. ovale*. Chloroquine, quinine, quinidine, and clindamycin have been used successfully and without significant complications to treat pregnant women. However, treating malaria during pregnancy is complex, and the susceptibility of the *Plasmodium* species involved must be considered before subjecting the mother and her fetus to therapy. If the mother is seriously ill, she should be hospitalized and the fetus monitored during therapy. Quinidine must be substituted for quinine when intravenous (IV) treatment is indicated because IV quinine no longer is available in the United States. Both of these drugs may cause hypoglycemia, even if the patient is given IV glucose. Drugs used to manage malaria are listed in Table 241-2. Pay close attention to contraindications and warnings supplied by the manufacturer. Consultation with the CDC is advisable when questions of resistance or adverse reactions arise.*

CHAGAS DISEASE (American Trypanosomiasis)

Epidemiology and Life Cycle

Although estimates vary, as many as 20 million people are infected with *Trypanosoma cruzi,* the agent that causes American trypanosomiasis. Perhaps 2 to 3 million cases accompanied by chronic disease currently exist; another 3 million now infected are expected to progress to chronic disease. Each year 45,000 to 60,000 people die, and about 1 million acquire new infections. It has been estimated that as many as 100,000 immigrants in the United States are carrying the trypanosome. These estimates emphasize the importance of this disease, which is confined to the Western Hemisphere, and should prompt physicians in nonendemic areas to consider it in the differential diagnosis when appropriate. A survey of 500 residents of the Rio Grande valley yielded positive serological results for Chagas disease in 2.4%. The incidence of Chagas disease is approximately equal in males and females, but chronic cardiac disease is greater in males. The acute disease is found more in infants and children, who also evidence the most severe symptoms and the highest mortality. Serological surveys show an increasing prevalence with age, reaching 60% of the population in some villages where the disease is endemic.

*The CDC's Drug Service telephone number in Atlanta, Georgia, is 1-404-639-3356. The CDC's Parasitic Disease telephone number is 1-770-488-7760.

The human disease is incurred most commonly when feces of the reduviid bug containing the metacyclic trypomastigote of Chagas disease are rubbed into the bug's bite wound. The bug is a nocturnal feeder and sucks capillary blood from humans and other vertebrates while they sleep. The bite usually is painless when feeding is intended, but many species of reduviidae can inflict a painful bite that results in protracted healing or, in rare cases, anaphylaxis. The bite wound frequently occurs at the lateral canthus of the eye, the mucocutaneous border of the lip, or other exposed site on the face or upper limbs. Transmission may occur transplacentally, by transfusion, by ingestion or inhalation of reduviid feces, and perhaps by consumption of poorly cooked, infected meat.

Once the metacyclic trypomastigote gains access through the broken skin, mucous membrane, or conjunctiva, it is engulfed by a macrophage. Early in the acute phase, *T. cruzi* is able to survive the killing capability of the macrophage and change into a leishmanial form. This form, the amastigote (without flagellum), divides every 12 hours within a pseudocyst in the host cell's cytoplasm. Some of the amastigotes transform into the blood trypomastigote form before the cell ruptures. The remaining amastigotes disintegrate after cell rupture. Cells may rupture as early as 5 days after being infected. Whether the agent can remain latent in the host cell for any period of time is not known.

When trypomastigotes enter the bug during a vertebrate blood meal, they change into the epimastigote form in the midgut of the bug and multiply actively in this form without apparent harm to the bug. The epimastigotes undergo another metamorphosis to the infective metacyclic trypomastigote before being passed in the bug's feces. More than 90 species of Reduviidae are capable of vectoring Chagas disease. These bugs hide in the cracks and crevices of clay, on wooden or thatch walls and roofs, or on the dirt floors in crude dwellings. The immature forms (instars) of reduviid bugs "kick" dirt onto their own sticky backs to camouflage themselves on the dirt floors of rural houses.

The wild cycle occurs away from human habitats and involves an unknown number of vertebrate species as definitive hosts and reduviid bugs as intermediate hosts. Fowl and amphibians seem to be immune to infection. The paradomestic cycle can involve wild vertebrates that frequent the yards and barns of humans (e.g., opossums, armadillos, rats, bats) as well as domestic pets and farm animals. A domestic cycle may be difficult to distinguish from the paradomestic cycle when the wild animals are as close to the sleeping humans as their pets. The attics and burrows directly under the crawl space beneath many rural farmhouses may harbor any of the wild animals listed in the paradomestic cycle above. Cycles may involve only humans and reduviid bugs.

The adult reduviid bugs lay several dozen to 600 eggs during their relatively short lifespan (210 to 260 days). The eggs hatch in less than a month, and five instars of progressively larger size develop. Transovarial transmission of the flagellate does not occur in the bug's intermediate host and occurs only in perhaps 5% to 10% of human pregnancies when the mother is infected during pregnancy. The three most important vectors are *Triatoma infestans* (found in South America, except for Venezuela), *Rhodnius prolixus* (found in Venezuela), and *Panstrongylus megistus* (found in Brazil). *Triatoma sanguisuga* has been found to be infected frequently in Texas and *T. protracta* in California and Arizona.

Pathogenesis and Immunology

The initial antibody response is polyclonal and fails to protect against the sometimes heavy parasitemia that occurs. Four to six weeks after infection, effective opsonization, phagocytosis, and lysis of the blood trypomastigotes clear the blood of most parasites. After this acute phase, biopsy and autopsy specimens still show amastigotes and an occasional trypomastigote in the untreated host. That, and the finding of a positive xenodiagnosis in as many as 89% of untreated individuals who have a positive result on a complement fixation (CF) test, clearly indicates that the parasite has developed techniques for surviving in the human body despite activation of humoral and cellular immune defenses. In the acute phase, which lasts from a few weeks to 4 months, the trypomastigotes penetrate and parasitize predominantly muscle and neuronal tissues. Some authorities believe that the chronic phase is just the long-term effect of lost muscle and neuronal competency and control over functions. Others believe that the chronic phase results from autoimmune disease. Recent evidence of epitopes (laminin) common to glial cells, cardiac muscle, and perhaps other cells of the host, as well as to the parasite, suggested that the parasite could initiate an autoimmune disease. However, it subsequently was discovered that antilaminin antibodies from chagasic sera recognize a carbohydrate epitope in mouse laminin but not in human laminin, suggesting that they are heterophile antibodies and don't damage human cardiac cells. Fear of this outcome based on research has played a major role in preventing licensing of a vaccine for this disease. However, a 90kD surface glycoprotein isolated from *T. cruzi* is under study for vaccine use and appears to be free of autoimmune potential.

Survival of the trypomastigote has been suggested to be, in part, due to an enzyme of the parasite that can cleave the Fc portion of host IgG antibody from its Fab portion. This could result in removal of the antibody component, which permits effective phagocytosis and lysis, while leaving the antibody receptor site on the parasite covered. Logically this could protect the parasite from further host response. *T. cruzi,* unlike its African trypanosomiasis cousins, cannot multiply in the bloodstream. For the xenodiagnosis test result to be positive decades after initial infection, there are three possibilities: the trypomastigote must be able to reach and infect new cells to keep the cycle going; the pseudocysts in the cells must survive for decades and release trypomastigotes on a schedule that maintains a small but fairly constant parasitemia; or the person must be reinfected. Prospective studies among immigrants to areas where Chagas disease is not transmitted by reduviid bugs could shed light on the third possibility. That, however, would be unconscionable when a relatively effective and safe therapy exists for this potentially fatal disease.

T. cruzi preferentially infects cells of mesenchymal origin (i.e., glial cells, striated and smooth muscle cells, nerve cells, and adipose cells). Different strains of the parasite are said to be neurotropic or myotropic.

Because of the muscle cells' relatively greater capacity for regeneration, damage to these cells results in hypertrophy, hyperplasia, and fibrotic replacement rather than outright per-

Table 241-2 Use of Antimalarial Drugs

Specie	Status of drug resistance in parasite	Prevention of overt disease	Treatment of acute malaria	Eradication of exoerythrocytic stage	Comments
Plasmodium falciparum	Chloroquine resistance suspected **Note:** Many authorities recommend that travelers to areas of known chloroquine-resistant malaria carry three tablets of pyrimethamine/sulfadoxine (Fansidar) to take upon development of a febrile episode. Immediate presentation to competent medical authority is then necessary, since this is considered a temporary suppression of malaria. Suppressive treatment with chloroquine should be continued after use of Fansidar.	Mefloquine (PO) 15-19 kg: ¼ tab/wk 20-30 kg: ½ tab/wk 31-45 kg: ¾ tab/wk >45 kg: 1 tab/wk 1 tab = 250 mg (salt) Begin 1 wk before exposure; continue for 4 wk after exposure **OR** Doxycycline (PO) 2 mg/kg/day in children >8 yr; only up to 100 mg/day for adults Begin 1-2 day before exposure; continue for 4 wk after exposure	*Moderate Cases* Quinine sulfate (PO) 25 mg/kg/day up to 650 mg for adults PO divided tid for 3-7 days (normal saline infusion) **PLUS** Tetracycline (PO) 80 mg/kg/day up to 1 g/day divided qid for 7 days (maximum dose 250 mg qid) **OR** Quinine sulfate (as above) **PLUS** Pyrimethamine 75 mg with sulfadoxine 500 mg (Fansidar) (PO) 5-10 kg: ½ tab 11-20 kg: 1 tab 21-30 kg: 1½ tab 31-45 kg: 2 tab >45 kg: 3 tab *Severe Cases* Quinidine gluconate (IV) in a loading dose of 10 mg/kg delivered over 1-2 hr followed by continuous infusion of 0.02 mg/kg/min continued until parasitemia <1% RBCs or oral medicine is possible; then tetracycline or pyrimethamine/sulfadoxine as above PO.	N/A	Mefloquine should not be used in pregnancy, children <15 kg, heart patients using drugs that affect heart neural conduction, or patients with epilepsy or severe psychiatric disorders. Doxycycline is contraindicated in pregnancy and children <8 yr; may produce photosensitivity. Fansidar contraindicated with known allergy to either component, history of severe skin disease, and in infants < 1 mo. Should be discontinued immediately if rash occurs. Fatal cutaneous reaction can occur. Quinidine should be given in ICU with cardiac monitoring. QT interval >0.6 sec, QRS widening > 25% of baseline, and serum quinidine level >6 µg/ml should prompt decreased infusion or cessation.

P. falciparum	Chloroquine sensitive	Chloroquine phosphate (PO) 5 mg base/kg/wk up to adult dose of 300 mg base/wk Begin 1 wk before exposure and continue 4 wk after exposure If patient is unable to take chloroquine, then substitute mefluoquine or doxycycline as above for chloroquine-resistant *P. falciparum*	Chloroquine phosphate (PO) 10 mg/kg followed in 6 hr by 5 mg/kg then 5 mg/kg/day for 2 additional days (total dose 25 mg/kg up to adult dose of 1000 mg [600 mg base]) followed by 500 mg (300 mg base) in 6 hr. Then 500 mg/day for 2 more days In severe cases it may be necessary to use IV quinidine followed by tetracycline or Fansidar (see above)	N/A	Chloroquine is considered safe in pregnancy.
P. malariae		Chloroquine phosphate (PO) As above for chloroquine-sensitive *P. falciparum*	As above for chloroquine-sensitive *P. falciparum*	N/A	
P. vivax and *P. ovale*		As above for chloroquine-sensitive *P. falciparum* unless resistance to chloroquine is suspected, then substitute with regimen for chloroquine-resistant *P. falciparum*	As above for chloroquine-sensitive *P. falciparum*	Primaquine phosphate 0.3 mg base/kg/day up to adult dose of 15 mg base/day for 14 days to destroy parasites in the exoerythrocytic stage	Primaquine is contraindicated in pregnancy and persons with G6PD deficiency, in whom primaquine may produce severe intravascular hemolysis.

manent loss. Experimental studies indicate that neurons themselves may not be the main neural target of the parasite; rather, it infects Schwann cells, capsular fibroblasts, and satellite cells. When the infected cells rupture, releasing host cell debris and disintegrating amastigotes, an inflammatory response causes ganglionitis. Eosinophils are prominent in these foci. Demyelination occurs, along with axonal shrinkage and disintegration. The chronic form of the disease is seen by many researchers as essentially the result of denervation of muscle and exocrine glands. The composite result is loss of varying degrees of smooth and cardiac muscle power, dilation of hollow viscera, erratic neural control of smooth and cardiac musculature, hypertrophy of glands and hollow viscera, loss of normal peristalsis in the bowel, and hypersecretion from exocrine glands.

Clinical Manifestations

Acute Phase. The course of Chagas disease is divided clinically into an acute, a latent, and a chronic phase. The acute phase usually lasts several weeks to several months. The bloodstream largely is cleared of its high-grade parasitemia at that point, but low-grade parasitemia and tissue damage continue for 10 to 20 years or longer. The damage may be due to direct cell infection or autoimmune or toxic inflammation from the continuous disintegration of cells and release of parasitic antigens.

The usual incubation period is 4 days to 2 weeks after percutaneous infection and 20 to 40 days after transmission by transfusion. When seen by the physician, the disease may be expressed systemically, but this often is preceded by a localized "chagoma," which consists of an erythematous swelling that may be tender and warm to the touch. It is formed by multiplication of the parasite locally and the body's immediate inflammatory response. When this occurs at the lateral canthus of the eye (Romaña sign), it is seen as a unilateral, bipalpebral edema associated with enlargement of the lacrimal gland and conjunctival injection. Regional lymphadenopathy usually can be palpated. With Romaña sign, the preauricular node is palpable.

With dissemination of the parasite in the bloodstream, the patient experiences fever, which often is high (100.4° to 104° F [38° to 40° C]) and may be intermittent or recurring. Evening peaks and two daily peaks have been described. Fever resolves by lysis. It is accompanied by diaphoresis, chills, and myalgia. A transient rash, usually morbilliform, is not uncommon. Edema, which is gelatinous, may be localized to the face or other region of initial infection and to the lower extremities. It can become generalized, especially in fatal cases. Nausea, vomiting, and a persistent diarrhea may be present.

Although less common, cough with mucus, dysphagia, and regurgitation have been seen in acute cases. Pregnant mothers who become infected usually survive, but abortion, stillbirth, and prematurity occur at rates not firmly established. Congenital Chagas disease is believed to occur in up to 10% of cases and carries a high mortality.

Mothers in the latent and chronic phases are at higher risk of death in pregnancy due to cardiac failure.

Some degree of myocarditis probably is present in all cases of symptomatic acute Chagas disease. This usually is mild and may be overshadowed by other aspects of the disease, but it can become severe and is responsible for most deaths in the acute phase.

Signs of acute myocarditis include tachycardia disproportionate to the fever, mild to moderate heart enlargement, mild to moderate cardiomegaly, prolongation of the P-R interval, and T-wave changes. In contrast to the chronic phase, arrhythmias generally are absent. Arrhythmias, cardiac failure, or cardiomegaly are bad prognostic signs.

Although organisms may be found in the CSF occasionally, meningoencephalitis is a rare cause of death. Bronchopneumonia may complicate the management and may be another cause of death in the acute phase.

Latent Phase. Because this phase, by definition, is asymptomatic, little is known about the progress of the disease. Clearly, tissue destruction is occurring, because the chronic phase is heralded by the loss of reserve function and the onset of symptoms. When sought with persistence, the xenodiagnosis in untreated cases is positive in about 90% of patients. Immunosuppression for any reason during this phase can result in renewed parasitemia and active symptomatic disease.

Chronic Phase. The chronic phase manifests most commonly with chagasic heart disease. Complete heart block with Stokes-Adams attacks, high-grade ventricular ectopy, and atrial fibrillation may cause sudden death. Chronic heart failure is the most common cardiac presentation. Because the failure is biventricular, it usually is not accompanied by pulmonary congestion. The heart may become grossly enlarged; weights as high as 800 g have been reported (a normal adult heart weighs 250 to 350 g). Tricuspid and mitral valves may manifest regurgitation. A pathognomonic "apex aneurysm," typically of the left ventricle, is present in many cases. However, rupture of this or other aneurysms is extremely rare. All chambers become enlarged, but the right auricle is notable as the source of pulmonary emboli. Loss of cardiac parasympathetic control, with resultant tachycardia, often is blamed for chronic stress on the heart. Most patients show some electrocardiographic (ECG) changes. PR and QT intervals may be prolonged, and partial or complete atrioventricular (AV) blocks and premature ventricular contractions (PVCs) are common. More than half of all cases develop a right bundle branch block, with an anteriorly directed QRS axis. The QRS complexes often show low voltage. Arrhythmias are a common clinical feature of the chronic phase.

Weakened, fibrotic muscle bundles, loss of autonomic control, hypertrophy, with its attendant potential for ischemia, regurgitation of tricuspid and mitral valves, and thromboembolic phenomena all create a difficult therapeutic challenge.

Another common but less life-threatening problem is that created by loss of autonomic control and/or damage to smooth muscle in the hollow viscera. Köberle[2] places the cause as a "more or less marked diminution of the number of ganglion cells of the myenteric plexuses." This type of clinical pattern may reflect strain differences in *T. cruzi* or an unexplained host factor. It is most prevalent in central Brazil but has been described elsewhere. Megacolon is slightly more common than megaesophagus. Extreme enlargement of the gallbladder, urinary bladder, ureter, and even trachea and bronchi have been reported. Symptoms can be remarkably few in megacolon. Some people go 4 or 5 months without having a bowel movement. The viscus walls are greatly hypertrophied and the lumens grossly enlarged. Fecaloma, volvulus, and rupture accompanied by peritonitis are encountered. In megaesophagus, dysphagia, regurgitation, aspiration, and pneumonia occur. Emaciation, anemia, and general disability are common in advanced cases. Esophageal cancer reportedly is more common in Chagas disease with megaesophagus.

Diagnosis

In the acute phase, the chagoma, protracted fever, and positive results on blood smears usually are sufficient to begin therapy. The CF test becomes positive at about 2 weeks. With experience, it is a highly reliable test for antibodies, although it may cross-react with leishmaniasis and other parasitic diseases. A titer of 1:8 or above is diagnostic. The indirect hemagglutination antibody (IHA) test likewise has problems but commonly is used; a titer of 1:64 or above is diagnostic. The indirect fluorescent antibody test (IFAT) is more sensitive, and field specimens can be processed more easily. It can be used earlier than the IHA. The problem with all of these antibody tests is that the patient may have parasitemia without antibodies early in the acute phase, and thus the tests will yield a false negative. The development of the standard ELISA has greatly improved rapid, reliable testing of blood specimens. Using a combination of recombinant cytoplasmic and flagellar antigens, the direct ELISA has provided a test that may make diagnosis 100% sensitive and 100% specific. Appropriately applied, the test should eliminate the risk of transmitting *T. cruzi* in blood product transfusions. Argentina is using two ELISA test kits, and Brazil is expected to begin using the recombinant direct ELISA imminently. The key to early diagnosis rests with tests for *T. cruzi* antigenemia. The technology is available. Xenodiagnosis may be unnecessary soon, but it has been the most sensitive test when applied by using 40 laboratory-raised, clean reduviid bugs strapped to the arms for 30 minutes. The reduviid bugs then are forced by abdominal pressure to defecate onto a slide that has a drop of normal saline, for direct examination. Alternatively, the bugs are homogenized and studied by use of the IFAT. On the direct slide, the metacyclic trypomastigote can be found in positive cases, but transmission to the laboratory worker is a risk, and *T. rangeli* must be distinguished from *T. cruzi*. *T. rangeli* is about 30 μm and has a very small kinetoplast anterior to the nucleus.

Treatment

Two drugs have shown considerable promise in treating acute-phase Chagas disease. A nitrofuran derivative, nifurtimox (Lampit, Bayer 2502), is available from the CDC in the United States. For children 1 to 10 years old, the dosage is 15 to 20 mg/kg/day, administered orally (PO) and divided into four doses, and given for 90 days. For children 11 to 16 years old, the dosage is 12.5 to 15 mg/kg/day PO, divided into four doses, and given for 90 days. For those over age 17, the dosage is 8 to 10 mg/kg/day PO, divided into four doses, and given for 4 months.

A nitroimidazole derivative, benznidazole (Radinil) still is under investigation and currently not available in the United States. The adult dosage is given as 5 to 7 mg/kg/day for 30 to 120 days.

Although the amastigotes show no evidence of intracellular death when these drugs are used, the xenodiagnosis does revert to negative. Early indications are that antibody titers also decline.

Use of corticosteroids and other immunosuppressives is contraindicated in Chagas disease because they increase parasitemia and symptoms.

Traditional therapy for heart failure is less successful than expected in Chagas disease, probably because of the reduction in cardiac reserve when the patient is first seen and the absolute loss of autonomic neural control that cannot be adequately compensated. Surgery is indicated in the megasyndromes, largely for complications, as previously described.

Prevention

Chagas disease is a preventable tragedy. Adequate housing incorporating concrete slab construction and tight-fitting windows, doors, and ceilings, combined with public education, could eliminate the risk of reduviid feeding on humans. The cost of providing such housing would be immense if it were done everywhere simultaneously. It should be undertaken by communities that cooperate to reduce expenditures for the poor. Identification and early treatment of cases can reduce the human reservoir pool of infection, but this alone is not sufficient. Vector control of the reduviid bugs can make a significant contribution to eliminating the disease in humans. Currently, aerosolization cannisters and insecticide paint are being studied in South America. Spraying the exterior of houses and their entry portals every 6 months with benzene hexachloride has been used with measurable success for many years. For campers and hunters, using mosquito netting on an overhead frame and tucked under the bedding, as well as using insect repellents (e.g., permethrin) may be useful. Use of new, rapid serological tests to screen blood bank donors is essential. Six South American countries already require routine blood bank testing for *T. cruzi* antigen. With the large number of Latin American immigrants already in the United States and Canada, it seems prudent to screen donors and test questionable donors of blood and organs.

LEISHMANIASIS/KALA-AZAR *(Leishmania donovani, L. tropica, L. mexicana, L. braziliensis, L. major, L. aethiopica, L. infantum, L. chagasi)*

Epidemiology

Leishmaniasis is a disease of the skin, mucous membranes, and/or the reticuloendothelial (RE) system, depending on which species of this protozoan parasite has infected the host. Member species of the genus *Leishmania* produce a spectrum of diseases ranging from chronic but self-limiting cutaneous ulcers to the highly fatal kala-azar, in which the parasite invades the body's entire RE system. It is estimated that 12 million people are now infected worldwide, with 1.5 million new cases occurring annually. Three million of those currently infected are believed to be symptomatic and have major economic losses from disabilities. The mortality is near 100% with overt kala-azar. Mortality from other forms is low except for the mucocutaneous form, in which many deaths from secondary bronchopneumonia occur. In 1991, with epidemics of kala-azar in Sudan and India, the worldwide mortality was estimated to be 75,000 lives. Leishmaniasis is increasing due to the living conditions of refugees and the migration of nonimmune populations into endemic areas. The clearing of forests in which the wild parasite life cycle exists has resulted in local or regional epidemics. The agent of leishmaniasis is a spindle-shaped, flagellated protozoan that is injected into the host's skin during feeding by small hematophagus female flies of the genera Phlebotomus, Sergentomyia, and Lutzomyia (sandflies). It survives in the human host as a nonflagellated intracellular parasite that attacks primarily RE cells. People of any race, gender, or age appear to be susceptible, but outdoor occupations and youthful age may increase the exposure and thereby the incidence of the disease. Race appears to play some role in adaptation to the disease. Patients of African descent show greater reactivity to leishmanin skin tests and greater mutilation from the mucocutaneous form of the disease than do South American Indians. People living in endemic zones believe that complete healing results in lifelong immunity. They often have local practitioners inoculate fluid from active lesions onto parts of the body hidden beneath clothing to avoid the social stigma of visible scars, especially in girls. The disease is found in southern Texas and from the Yucatan to southern Brazil, with pockets in central Mexico. It is widespread in both eastern and western Africa and in pockets elsewhere on that continent. It occurs widely around the Mediterranean basin, throughout the Middle East, and in southern Asia. China reports pockets of leishmaniasis.

Phlebotomine flies are small, hairy insects whose wings are held at a 60-degree angle to each other and the body. They are nocturnal feeders, with rare exceptions (*Lutzomyia wellcomei* in Brazil), and weak fliers. Their slow, steady flight can be observed, and they fly only when there is little breeze, hiding the rest of the time in dark, humid crevices with available organic material (e.g., tree hollows, rodent burrows, chinks in walls and rock fences). These sandflies are observed around houses moving in short, "hopping" flights. Many of the females feed on lizards, snakes, and amphibians, as well as on many warm blooded animals. Not all are equally anthropophilic in their feeding habits. Hence, some are better vectors of leishmaniasis in humans. *Phlebotomus papatasi* in the Old World and *P. palpilongis* in Brazil are among the better vectors of kala-azar. In Texas, *Lutzomyia diabolica* is the only phlebotomine vector of leishmaniasis known to feed on humans, and *Leishmania mexicana* is believed to cause local and diffuse cutaneous leishmaniasis and possibly mucucutaneous leishmaniasis in south central Texas.

Pathogenesis and Life Cycle

The flagellated promastigote of leishmaniasis (15 to 26 μm × 2 to 5 μm) divides by binary fission in the midgut of the phlebotomine fly and escapes through the proboscis, which the fly sticks into the human host's skin to suck blood. These promastigotes are rapidly engulfed by macrophages, but until cellular immunity develops some weeks or months later, the macrophages are unable to kill all the parasites. The promastigote transforms into the oval, nonflagellated amastigote form (2 to 6 μm), which divides in the macrophages by binary fission. Upon cell rupture, the amastigotes are taken up by other macrophages and monocytes, and the cycle continues. These collections of parasitized cells evoke a chronic granulomatous response from the host involving lymphocytes, plasma cells, multinucleated giant cells, and histiocytes. Other variations occur, including secondary bacterial infection. The course of the disease appears to be governed by the interplay of factors that promote spread of the disease (interleukins 4 and 10) and those that inhibit it (gamma-interferon). In leishmaniasis-infected mice, Th2 subpopulations of T cells produce the interleukins, whereas Th1 subpopulations produce the interferon (IFN). Fraction 9 of *L. tropica* and *L. braziliensis* have been found to elicit a protective immune response in mice. Fraction 1 increases tumor necrosis factor (TNF), which is associated with increasing severity of disease. *L. chagasi* and *L. infantum* have been recognized to have a subclinical form of infection, which may be important to transmission in the anthroponotic mode (human to human via sandflies). Until more experience is gained, it seems reasonable to assume that any leishmanial species could remain latent and subject to unexpected reactivation in patients infected with the human immunodeficiency virus (HIV).

Killing the intracellular organisms requires activation of macrophages. This appears to require T cell recognition of the antigen and production of a factor (perhaps opsonizing antibody) that prepares the parasite for destruction once it is inside the activated macrophage.

Being able to attribute a specific form of disease (e.g., cutaneous, mucocutaneous, or visceral) to a given species of *Leishmania* now appears to be less certain than previously thought. Finding subclinical cases of all forms, in both the Eastern and the Western Hemispheres, has changed our understanding of the disease. Finding visceral leishmaniasis caused by species previously thought to cause only cutaneous disease *(L. tropica)* also has prompted reexamination of the management and prognosis of cases. Resistance to a given therapy varies with the species being treated. It therefore is increasingly important to identify the species before prescribing a treatment regimen. Polymerase chain reaction (PCR) technology, by providing diagnostic probes, soon may make faster diagnosis possible. Rapid transit between continents and regions is bringing more cases into areas where physicians are not familiar with the complex pathology of leishmaniasis, its diagnosis, and treatment.

The following forms of disease are recognized:

1. *Local cutaneous leishmaniasis (LCL). L. major, L. tropica, L. mexicana, L. aethiopica, L. chagasi, L. infantum,* and the *L. braziliensis* complex all may cause lesions of LCL, although some produce more serious disease as well. This form of leishmaniasis usually begins as a papulonodule at the site of the fly bite. It later ulcerates and may expand and produce satellite lesions before slowly healing over weeks or months. Several lesions may occur simultaneously; most heal without therapy but leave scars and may be disfiguring. These patients have a positive result on a leishmanin skin test, and smears or biopsies from the ulcer's edge reveal the amastigotes. The patients typically have several lesions that may be in different evolving pathological states; that is, papules, nodules, and active and healing ulcers.
2. *Diffuse cutaneous leishmaniasis (DCL). L. aethiopica* and *L. mexicana* have been reported to result in DCL. These patients typically have widespread nodules and plaques without ulceration. Biopsies reveal intracellular and sometimes extracellular amastigotes with large

numbers of amastigote-filled histiocytes. Granuloma formation with multinucleated giant cells and epithelioid cells is uncommon. The skin test result is negative. The cases are difficult to treat, and relapses are common. Conversion of the skin test is believed to be a favorable prognostic sign.

3. *Recurring cutaneous leishmaniasis (RCL).* In these cases the patient's lesion(s) heals and then later recurs. Recurrence usually is seen as ulceration of a nodule at the edge or near a healed ulcer. Healing usually is complete with time if the patient's nutrition and general health are good. Specific therapy generally brings a cure. The skin test result is strongly positive, and amastigotes are few on biopsy. Culture results may be positive or negative.
4. *Mucocutaneous leishmaniasis (MCL).* Classically in *L. braziliensis* (and uncommonly in *L. mexicana, L. aethiopica,* and *L. donovani*), a typical cutaneous ulcer may be the presenting or initial finding. This may expand into a mucosal area, frequently the nasal mucosa. Alternatively, the ulcer heals and a mucosal lesion subsequently is discovered. Metastasis occurs early in the course of the disease but usually is not visible until much later. Although the interval between appearance of the initial skin ulcer and mucosal involvement commonly is several months, years have been reported between the two events. Once mucosal lesions occur, the parasites may mutilate the tissue rapidly, including cartilage and bone. This condition is less easily treated and tends to recur. In many cases the vocal cords, nasopharynx, and hypopharynx are involved. Bronchopneumonia is a common cause of death. The skin test result is positive. Chemotherapy often must be prolonged and given at a higher dosage, bringing with it greater risk from side effects.
5. *Visceral leishmaniasis (kala-azar)*. L. donovani, L. infantum,* and *L. chagasi* can escape from the initial skin wound and invade the entire RE system, producing profound emaciation and almost uniform mortality without chemotherapy. Death often follows countercurrent infection and gastrointestinal (GI) bleeding. The skin and serum test results become positive only after recovery is well established. It is clear now that asymptomatic infection occurs that eventually may resolve or may be reactivated by nutritional deprivation, infection, or other stresses.

Clinical Manifestations

Cutaneous forms of leishmaniasis usually begin with a small, erythematous papule that develops a pinpoint vesicle at its center. This may ooze serous fluid that gradually develops into an open sore with raised, firm, reddened borders and either a crusted or weeping granular center. The ulcer widens in most cases, sometimes reaching 5 cm in diameter. When not infected secondarily, the ulcer is painless. It heals slowly from its center, eventually leaving a depressed and hypopigmented scar. Other nodules and ulcers may occur simultaneously or in sequence. The process may be completed in a few months but often takes a year or more. In chronic cutaneous cases (CCL), the process continues for years with continuous lesions in an active state. If the offending agent is *L. major, L. tropica,* or *L. mexicana,* the lesion may not require treatment. If the location is likely to cause social stigma or disfigurement, treatment can be instituted. If there is evidence of anergy (with DCL), chronicity with spreading occurs, especially to mucosal borders, or if the patient is in a poor nutritional state, immunosuppressed, or has other chronic infectious diseases, treatment should be started.

Visceral leishmaniasis follows an incubation of 2 weeks to 3 months and may begin with fever, anorexia, diaphoresis, fatigue, and weakness. Weight loss with emaciation, especially noticeable in the thorax and shoulders, may be chronic or may follow a more acute course, with death from countercurrent infection within a few weeks. Splenomegaly is a prominent feature, but because of the thick capsule, splenic aspiration rarely has been accompanied by rupture. The fever may develop a twice-daily peak. Adenopathy may be generalized but is not striking.

Diagnosis

Smears of aspirates or scrapings and biopsy material, when stained with Giemsa, may demonstrate the amastigotes in macrophages. Flagellated forms are found in positive tissue cultures on NNN (Novy, Nicolle, and McNeal) medium. The Montenegro (leishmanin) skin test does not yield a positive result until the ulcerative phase and is of little value in diagnosis. It has been useful as a survey tool to establish endemic zones. Recent advances in PCR technology promise to make species-specific diagnosis more available to the practitioner. This will allow the therapy to be tailored to the form of disease expected. Currently the IFA and Dot ELISA tests are used for serological diagnosis.

Treatment

Pentavalent antimonials and amphotericin B have been used as therapy for decades, but a high rate of toxicity has encouraged the development and testing of a number of potentially curative agents. Stibogluconate sodium is the standard drug of choice and is given in a dose of 20 mg/kg/day intravenously or intramuscularly (IM) for 20 to 28 days. It may have to be continued or repeated in refractory cases. Meglumine antimonate may be substituted in a comparable dose schedule.

Amphotericin B has been used at a dose of 0.25 to 1 mg/kg by slow IV infusion on a daily or every-other-day basis for periods up to 8 weeks.

Pentamidine (diamidinophenoxypentane) also has been used as a second-line drug; ketoconazole and allopurinol, local heat, and cryotherapy also have been credited with some success.

Recently, aminosidine, produced by *Streptomyces rimosus* (and virtually identical to paramomycin) was used with considerable success and was well tolerated. However, ototoxicity occurs, resulting in a significantly elevated threshold to frequencies above 2000 Hz, and must be considered a risk, especially if serum titers of aminosidine exceed the recommended dosage. The manufacturer's inserts always should be read before administering any drug. The dose of aminosidine used by Scott and associates[3] was 14 to 16 mg/kg/day ad-

**Kala-azar* is an Indian word that means "black fever," referring to darkening of the skin and the high fever caused by visceral leishmaniasis.

ministered IV in 250 ml of isotonic saline over 90 minutes. This was continued for 21 days or for 1 week after parasitological cure, whichever was longer. Serum assays were conducted on the third day and as needed thereafter. Urea, creatinine, and aspartate transaminase levels, as well as hemoglobin (Hgb) leukocyte and platelet counts, were measured daily, and audiograms were done before and at the conclusion of treatment.

Prevention

Because of the wild parasitical life cycles that perpetuate the disease and cannot be considered eradicable and because of the absence of safe, inexpensive drugs that can attack the intracellular parasite, vaccines are the most viable long-term hope for reducing the human burden of leishmaniasis. Screening domiciles effectively, using insect repellents, and limiting exposure to phlebotomine fly bites from dusk to dawn are important. Early presentation and appropriate treatment can reduce complications. Vaccines combining *L. mexicana* with bacille Calmette-Guérin (BCG) and *L. braziliensis* with BCG are under study. A vaccine made from *L. major* promastigotes is used in the Middle East. The major surface glycoprotein of the promastigote (gp63) and lipophosphoglycans (LPG), which have been shown to enhance the immune response in mice, also are under study.

TOXOPLASMOSIS *(Toxoplasma gondii)*

Epidemiology

Toxoplasma gondii is an obligate intracellular protozoan parasite of the class Sporozoa that can infect most vertebrate animals, including avians and some reptiles. Members of the cat family play host to the entire life span of this organism. Other vertebrates, including humans, become intermediate hosts when they ingest the oocysts shed in the feces of cats. These oocysts, which become infective in 1 to 5 days, can be ingested directly from the soil by pica, nail biting, and thumb sucking. Children are exposed by play in sandboxes to which cats have access or from yard dirt. They can contaminate a gardener's hands and the garden products. Handling cat litter or cats themselves can transfer the oocysts to human hands. Insects such as roaches or filth flies may transfer the oocysts to food mechanically. Transmission also can occur when the tissue cysts are ingested in inadequately cooked meat or are acquired from contaminated transfused blood or transplanted organs; *T. gondii* can be acquired transplacentally if a woman becomes infected during pregnancy.

Serological surveys demonstrate an increasing prevalence of seropositivity with age. Whereas only 5% of children under age 5 are seropositive, as many as 65% of adults over age 40 have been reported to be seropositive. The genders are approximately equal in attack rates. Farm animals and pets show seropositivity rates ranging from about 20% to more than 75% for cats. Interestingly, sheep, which tend to graze grass much shorter than cattle, have a seropositivity rate three times as high as cattle. Tissue cysts also are frequently found in pork (probably because of pigs' diet of swill) and dead carcasses. In its most tragic and costly form, *T. gondii* crosses the placenta and infects the developing fetus. This event, which occurs in an estimated 0.5% of pregnancies in the United States, causes disease in as many as half of infected fetuses, resulting in as many as 450 deaths each year. About 85% of those who survive ultimately have some degree of permanent impairment. Often the congenital infection remains undetected until months or even years later. Seizures, visual acuity problems, or mental retardation can lead to studies that ultimately reveal the diagnosis. Other recognized categories of the disease include acquired and ocular forms and that seen in immunocompromised individuals. This ubiquitous zoonotic parasite may be one of the most common infectious agents in the world, but measures can be taken to limit the damage significantly when the infection is suspected early, or the infection can be prevented altogether.

Pathogenesis and Life Cycle

The asexual cycle in humans begins with ingestion of oocysts from the environment or the ingestion of tissue cysts in uncooked or inadequately cooked meat. The trophozoites are liberated in the GI tract, and epithelial cells are immediately invaded. In these cells the parasite-bearing vacuole protects the parasite from lysis by methods not fully clarified. Trophozoites divide repeatedly by endodyogeny until the cell ruptures and releases more trophozoites. The trophozoites are oval or curved, approximately 3 to 7 μm long, and infective; they may be disseminated via the circulatory and lymphatic vessels. They typically attack the cells of the skeletal muscles, brain, cardiac muscle, lymph nodes, eye, and lung but may infect other organs. A mild initial mononuclear cell response (with some polynuclear cells) is typical, and edema usually is present. In immunocompetent individuals, the dissemination of trophozoites soon diminishes, and both humoral and cellular immunity components become measurable. Oocysts are not shed in the feces of animals other than the cat family. Among other factors, immunity depends, on the extracellular alternate complement pathway, opsonization of the antigen, and subsequent phagocytosis by sensitized mononuclear cells that can then kill the agent. This is made possible by sensitization of the CD4+ T-helper cells, which secrete lymphokinins, notably interleukin-2 (IL-2) and gamma (γ)-interferon (INF-γ). The INF-γ appears to activate the intracellular hydrogen peroxidase killing system of macrophages. However, not all toxoplasma organisms are killed, even in an immunocompetent host. Some trophozoites develop into a tissue cyst that may remain dormant and viable for life or may rupture in response to a change in the host's immune status. Necrosis may occur in the initial infection but usually is limited in an immunocompetent host. Necrosis that occurs secondary to release of trophozoites after a fully active immune response has developed may cause significant impairment, especially in the eye and brain. The inflammatory response in these later lesions involves a granulomatous picture with plasma cells, monocytes, lymphocytes, and sometimes the organisms. Edema and endarteritis are reported.

The cycle of infection in cats begins with ingestion of infected cat "kills" (rats, mice, birds) or inadequately cooked kitchen scraps. Licking its own dirt-contaminated fur might cause infection. The trophozoites released from ingested oocysts or tissue cysts invade the GI epithelial cells and multiply, as in humans, but the sexual stage of trophozoite differentiation into gametocytes occurs in the second generation of multiplication. Their union leads to the oocyst (10 to 12 μm), which is passed in the cat's feces. After an incubation period that varies in length (days to several weeks) and systemic infection, a cat having its first infection passes millions of oocysts in its feces daily for as long as 3 weeks, sometimes longer.

Clinical Manifestations

Congenital Disease. The risk for the fetus depends on when the mother has her first infection with *T. gondii*. The risk of acquiring the infection is less for the first trimester (15% to 20%) and greatest for the last trimester (60% to 65%). However, when infection does occur earlier in gestation, the risk of a serious outcome is much greater because of the expansion of the impact of a few cells destroyed in early development. Some infections in fetuses remain undetected after birth, but such fetuses can show significant impairment later. Others are born with hepatosplenomegaly, hydrocephaly or microcephaly, seizures, neurological deficits, jaundice, rash, chorioretinitis, and anemia. Symptoms and signs of meningoencephalitis may be present. Roentgenograms may show bilateral, scattered punctate calcifications (infection with cytomegalovirus [CMV], conversely, has a pattern of paraventricular calcifications). Obstruction of the aqueduct of Sylvius can result in ventricular enlargement and hydrocephaly. Cerebromalacia can lead to microcephaly and microphthalmia. The CSF may show xanthochromia, increased protein (as high as 2 g/dl in the ventricular fluid), and increased numbers of RBCs and WBCs. The latter predominantly are mononuclear. At autopsy, widespread vasculitis and parenchymal cell necrosis are found, including myocarditis, encephalitis, pneumonitis, and polymyositis. Stillbirths occur, and mortality in the first few months of life is high in live births that demonstrate the classic picture. A third type of congenital clinical picture is the infant who appears normal at birth but proves to have had slowly progressive lesions of the brain or eye that are detected much later. Most survivors develop sequelae, usually serious, involving the brain or eye. *T. gondii* infection in more than one child of a given mother is possible in cases of maternal HIV infection.

Acquired Disease. Infection acquired after birth usually is unreported because the signs and symptoms are similar to those commonly caused by upper respiratory viruses and almost always are self-limiting. When symptomatic, the acquired disease rarely is fatal in immunocompetent patients. The characteristic feature is symmetrical, discrete, usually nontender lymph nodes in the posterior auricular and cervical chains. Generalized lymphadenopathy without suppuration and even splenomegaly may be present. Fever and headache occur with some regularity in the more severe cases, and a nonexudative pharyngitis may occur. Fatigue often is prominent and may last for weeks. Lymphoma and infectious mononucleosis must be considered in the differential diagnosis.

Disease in Immunodeficient Patients. These patients are considered to have reactivated disease, erupting from tissue cysts in their bodies, as a result of their diminished ability to contain the infection. Widely disseminated disease can occur, including meningoencephalitis, pneumonitis, polymyositis, myocarditis, and parenchymal necrosis of other organ systems. However, in immunosuppressed or immunodeficient individuals, the dissemination may be followed by life-threatening disease. Early recognition and treatment can result in full remission, but continued therapy is necessary to prevent relapse. An additional concern is that serodiagnosis may be impossible in these patients, and culture of the organism is required for the delayed diagnosis. For this reason, some advise therapy if infection is suspected at all.

Ocular Disease. *T. gondii* is reported to cause chorioretinitis in 80% of cases of congenital toxoplasmosis; in the great majority, this is bilateral. During the initial infection at any age, chorioretinitis can occur either as the sole finding or with other pathological conditions. In the acquired form it may be unilateral, at least when initially diagnosed. Tissue cysts can rupture at any time and cause additional damage to vision and changes on funduscopic examination. The infection, congenital or acquired, is believed to progress from the brain to its neural extension of vision, the retina. The macula therefore commonly is involved. Viewed through the ophthalmoscope, the active lesion is raised and creamy yellow and has distinct borders, possibly with some satellite lesions. Later the lesion flattens, and the retinal layer atrophies, allowing the whiter sclera to show through. The pigment epithelium migrates to the periphery of the lesions, giving a "rosette" appearance. In some cases the full thickness of the retina, the choroid, and the vitreous itself may be involved. In these cases the vitreous may be cloudy from debris and inflammatory cells. A patient who is old enough may complain of visual disturbances, including increased "floaters." Scotomata may result in the mature lesion. The anterior chamber also may be involved as an extension of retinal infection, resulting in pain, photophobia, and conjunctivitis.

Diagnosis

The clinical picture must be relied on to prompt appropriate serological tests or cultures. The classic triad of congenital toxoplasmosis consists of convulsions, calcifications (intracerebral), and chorioretinitis. However, both congenital and acquired infections may be asymptomatic while painlessly causing damage, especially in the brain and eye. The importance of screening for infection during pregnancy is controversial. Ideally a woman's serological status should be known before she conceives. It may be useful to determine the serological status of any pregnant girl or woman at the initial visit. If the test result is positive, the serum should be tested for IgM antibody, or a second specimen should be obtained 3 weeks later and tested in parallel with the first for a significant titer rise. The CDC recommends EIA as a follow-up test when standard IgG test results are positive in an at-risk host. When serological test results are positive before pregnancy, no further tests are needed unless the woman is immunodeficient. A search for fetal disease clinically and serologically should be made when maternal seroconversion occurs during pregnancy. When this is confirmed in the first or second trimester, therapeutic abortion may be considered. In mothers infected with HIV, repeated fetuses may be infected. If symptoms occur during any pregnancy, tests for active disease should follow. As noted, patients who have immunodeficiency or suppression for any reason should be watched for evidence of fever and lymphadenopathy, tested, and when warranted, treated before the results of tests are available. A neonate who has congenital toxoplasmosis may be seronegative, forcing reliance on clinical grounds or a history of maternal infection for diagnosis. The Feldman dye test has been replaced in most laboratories by the hemaglutination, ELISA, and immunofluorescence tests. Testing for the presence of IgM antibodies by the fluorescent immunoassay (IgM-IFA) method is recommended when standard tests for specific IgG exceed titers of 1:512 in a pregnant woman or the infant. A value of ≥1:16 is considered positive. The CDC can perform the batteries of seroassays using multiple sera to better clarify the meaning of a given positive result. Magnetic resonance imaging (MRI) studies of the head, in the case of brain involvement, are useful, and PCR serological testing of the CSF may help in the diagnosis, particularly when rapid treatment is required because of HIV infection. In acquired disease, serological tests usually yield positive results by at least 2 weeks and peak by at least 2 months. Titers then slowly decline and remain positive for life at a low level. Other diagnostic methods include inoculation of laboratory animals, cell culture of *T. gondii,* and, in rare cases, biopsy from surgical or necropsy specimens.

Treatment

Treatment of acquired toxoplasmosis in an immunocompetent host rarely is necessary. Treatment should be considered when HIV infection or other immunosuppression is a factor, when visual problems are present and progressive, when signs and symptoms become chronic, or when known accidental inoculation occurs in a seronegative host. Currently, combined therapy with pyrimethamine and sulfadiazine is believed to prevent replication of the organism, but it does not inactivate tissue cysts or kill the trophozoites. The pediatric dose of pyrimethamine is 2 mg/kg/day for 3 days, then 1 mg/kg/day to a maximum daily dose of 25 mg given for 4 weeks. Sulfadiazine is given in a dose of 100 to 200 mg/kg/day for 3 to 4 weeks. Adequate hydration should be maintained, and folinic acid, in a daily dose of 5 mg, is given with the pyrimethamine to counteract its inhibition of folate synthesis. The patient should be monitored by means of complete blood counts (CBCs) and platelet counts twice weekly to detect bone marrow suppression. Treating a pregnant woman carries the risk of teratogenic effects on the fetus from pyrimethamine and also from untreated congenital toxoplasmosis; expert consultation is advised. For adult patients with HIV who have *T. gondii* encephalitis, a multicenter study found the following regimen to be necessary: sulfadiazine (1 to 2 g four times daily), pyrimethamine (25 to 50 mg/day), and leucovorin calcium (5 to 10 mg/day) for up to 180 days. Toxicity (especially bone marrow depression) may necessitate treatment cessation in a large percentage of cases, most often between days 14 and 28 of therapy. This was followed by daily therapy for life using pyrimethamine/sulfadiazine. Azithromycin, clindamycin, clarithromycin, and spiramycin have been tried both alone and in combination with pyrimethamine and have had mixed results. The author recommends consultation with a pediatric AIDS treatment group or the CDC, since most trials reported involve adults. Corticosteroids are recommended for active ocular disease in conjunction with the therapy described above. Sulfadiazine is available through the CDC (phone: 1-404-639-3356) and spiramycin through the U.S. Food and Drug Administration (phone: 1-301-594-1012).

Prevention

The ubiquitous nature of *T. gondii* and the ease of its transmission make prevention difficult, especially in children. Those who would benefit most from prevention are women of childbearing age and immunodeficient individuals. Avoiding contact with cats, cat litter, and yard or farm dirt (e.g., no gardening, at least without gloves, and very thorough washing and nail cleaning afterward) is important, as is cooking meat adequately, especially pork and mutton. Holding meat below −4° F (−20° C) until ice crystals form on the outside may reduce or destroy infectivity. Cooking the center of meat to at least 151° F (66° C) kills the infective cysts, but an oven thermometer should be used. All fruit and vegetables should be washed thoroughly; and raw meat and unwashed fruit and vegetables should be handled with impermeable gloves.

TAPEWORM/CYSTICERCOSIS *(Taenia saginata, T. solium)*

Taenia solium (pork tapeworm) and *T. saginata* (beef tapeworm) are acquired by humans when they consume inadequately cooked meat containing the larval form of one of these cestodes. As a definitive host, humans harbor the adult tapeworm in the small intestine. This produces some abdominal discomfort, increased hunger and food consumption, and weight loss. If a human happens to ingest eggs of the pork tapeworm, as by contamination of food or drink with feces from a person harboring the worm, the eggs release larvae that form cysts in the victim's tissues. Both parasites have a worldwide distribution, the actual prevalence varying greatly depending on the number of animals, meat-eating habits, and the amount of human fecal contamination of rangeland. Neither is common in the United States, although both are common in Mexico. Tapeworm disease caused by *Taenia* species can be prevented by cooking all meat adequately; that is, to at least 150° F (65.5° C) measured at the center of the meat with a meat thermometer. Individuals harboring pork tapeworms are dangerous to all contacts, and they should be identified and treated.

Pathogenesis and Life Cycle

The adult worms (strobilae) are segmented and consist of a head (four suckers and a rostellum armed with 22 to 32 hooklets in *T. solium* but no hooklets in *T. saginata*), a neck, and proglottids. Proglottids may be immature, mature, or gravid and contain both male and female reproductive organs and large numbers of eggs. These proglottids eventually drop off, or strings of them may break off the worm and be carried or migrate out of the anus. *T. saginata* proglottids are more muscular, but either may actually crawl after exiting the body. The eggs may leave the proglottid before or after it detaches from the rest of the strobila. They are infective for weeks to months under favorable conditions. They continue their cycle when ingested from plant or soil by the appropriate intermediate host animal. The larvae released from the eggs penetrate the intestinal mucosa, reach the lymphatic or blood vessels, and are carried to all parts of the body, especially muscles and connective tissues. In 2 months or more, they become encysted scolices and remain viable in the muscle for years. The scolix matures fully to a tapeworm when the meat is eaten with the live scolix in it. Both *T. solium* and *T. saginata* gain maturity in the human bowel in about 12 weeks, eventually reaching lengths of 2 to 7 meters and 5 to 15 meters respectively. The eggs of the two species cannot be distinguished microscopically. When a human ingests the pork tapeworm eggs (or possibly when these move retrogradely in the bowel after release from a proglottid), the larvae are digested free from the eggs and enter the circulation. The larvae may attach and encyst anywhere in the body. An increase in size of the cysticercus may produce a significant pathological condition, especially when it occurs in the intracranial space.

Clinical Manifestations

A single tapeworm of either pork or beef origin is likely to be "silent" in an otherwise healthy host. Either can cause abdominal pain or epigastric hunger pains, an increased appetite, weight loss, weakness, and general malaise. Findings elicited less commonly are diarrhea, upper abdominal distention, postprandial vomiting, and in rare cases, intestinal obstruction. Tapeworms have been known to live up to 25 years. Cysticercus infections produce few general symptoms unless large numbers of larvae develop simultaneously. Localized findings are largely a result of the expanding mass and the functions with which it interferes. The most serious threat arises when the cysticercus invades the brain, eye, heart, or spinal cord. Seizures, neurological problems, visual disturbances, headache, and evidence of increased intracranial pressure in a potentially exposed child should raise the suspicion of cysticercus infection.

Diagnosis

Eggs in the stool foretell the presence only of taeniasis. Study of a gravid proglottid for the number of main lateral uterine branches has been used as a means to identify the specie of *Taenia,* but this has been questioned recently. *T. solium* is believed to have 7 to 13 main lateral uterine branches; *T. saginata* is said to have 15 to 20 on each side. Cysticercosis is identified by finding calcified "rice grains" on roentgenograms of any part of the body. A negative series of films does not rule out infection, however, because the calcification usually occurs 5 or more years after initial invasion of larvae. Excision of a cyst provides the opportunity to examine the evaginated scolex (head) of the larva and to look for the typical rostellum and hooklets of *T. solium.* The IHA test has been valuable in the serological diagnosis of difficult cases. Some laboratories also use the indirect fluorescent and CIE tests. The CDC has begun to use an immunoblot test that uses a semipurified extract of *T. solium* cysticerci, which has given a sensitivity of 98% and a specificity of 100%. Diagnosis is possible without multiple cysts being present in the patient.

Treatment

Because of the potential for cysticerci to develop with *T. solium,* this species of tapeworm always should be treated. Routine taeniasis currently is treated with albendazole,* praziquantel,† or niclosamide.† Praziquantel should be taken with a fatty meal to enhance absorption. All three drugs have proved to be effective treatment for taeniasis. In the treatment of neurocysticercosis, it is important to consider the risk of inflammatory reaction upon the death of the worms. Intraocular cysts also are given surgical consideration because of the risk of visual loss from severe inflammation.

Albendazole (15 mg/kg/day in three doses) for 28 days usually is adequate treatment and can be repeated. Dexamethasone may be needed for several days to reduce inflammation, which can be severe, especially if neurological symptoms follow treatment. If seizures occur secondary to neurocysticercosis, anticonvulsive therapy may be required for up to 2 years or longer. The prognosis for intracranial cysticercosis has improved considerably in recent years due to a combined use of CSF shunting, praziquantel, and cyst extirpation. The prognosis for cysts outside the brain parenchyma (in the ventricles, spinal cord area, and subarachnoid space) reportedly is poorer.[1]

*Albendazole is available from SmithKline Beecham, Philadelphia, Pa.

†Praziquantel and niclosamide are available from Miles, Inc. West Haven, Conn.

HYDATID DISEASE *(Echinococcus granulosus, E. multilocularis, E. oligarthrus, and E. vogeli)*

Epidemiology

Echinococcus granulosus is a small tapeworm of canines. The intermediate hosts are herbivorous animals, especially range animals that feed on grass contaminated by canine feces. Humans also serve as intermediate hosts when they become infected through accidental ingestion of the tapeworm eggs. Handling dogs whose fur is contaminated with dog feces is the usual route of egg transmission to humans. Any item contaminated with canine feces may serve as a fomite for transfer to humans. The egg develops into a cystic larval form in the intermediate host. Members of the dog family are reinfested by feeding on dead carcasses or when fed inadequately cooked tripe from infested herbivores. Because human bodies are not available to animals as food, humans are a dead-end host. *E. multilocularis* produces an alveolar larval cyst, but the parasite cannot complete its life cycle in humans and tends to metastasize. Its life cycle occurs largely in wild animals. Both canines and cats are definite hosts because they ingest rodents, which are intermediate hosts. The ecological zone of *E. multilocularis* is the Northern hemisphere. It is found in a pocket of the north central United States, in northern Alaska, and in Canada. In the Eastern hemisphere it is found from central Europe through Siberia, with its southern boundary in northern Iraq and Iran. *E. vogeli* is recognized in Central America and in northern South America. It is a polycystic form of hydatidosis that is transmitted in forests between bush dogs and rodents. Hunting dogs are the primary means of transmission to humans. It also is noted in agoutis and spiny rats, both members of the order Rodentia.

Pathogenesis and Life Cycle

The embryo emerges from the ova in the human duodenum, penetrates a small blood vessel, and is filtered out in the liver (60%), the lung (20%), or by the capillaries of other tissues (20%). The bladderlike cyst (larva) expands at about 1 mm/month until body defenses overwhelm it or its size causes its discovery and treatment. It may manifest as an expanding mass (intracranial) or an inflammatory mass (pulmonary), or it may cause anaphylactic shock if it begins leaking fluid in a hypersensitive person. Secondary bacterial infection has been the cause of leakage or rupture of the cysts. The cyst is filled with fluid but has a germinal layer and a multilayered acellular membrane surrounding the fluid. The germinal layer produces brood capsules that in time collectively contain thousands of tiny protoscolicies (embryos). These eventually break loose and float in the cyst fluid as "hydatid sand." Each protoscolex can develop into either another hydatid cyst or a tapeworm, depending on whether it escapes from the original cyst into the intermediate host's body or is ingested by the definitive host, respectively. In cases of *E. multilocularis,* the boundary of the cyst is poorly demarcated. It rarely produces brood capsules or mature protoscolices. It most commonly is found in the liver and extends its growth to other organs.

Clinical Manifestations

Signs and symptoms of hydatidosis are determined by the number and location of the cysts, as well as by whether they are leaking antigenic fluid or disseminating additional daughter cysts. Cases of hydatid cyst of the brain, heart, lung and liver show very different clinical pictures. *E. multilocularis* often is mistaken for a malignancy or cirrhosis of the liver. It may cause pain, hepatomegaly, bile obstructive disease, or symptoms of metastasis to other organs, especially the lungs and brain. Ascites and secondary bacterial abscess have been reported. Needle aspiration of fluid from massive cysts may be necessary if shortness of breath occurs, but this probably increases the risk of abscess formation. Metastasis to the brain is a grave sign.

Diagnosis

Skillful use of imaging and serological and clinical information are necessary to arrive at the diagnosis. A history of contact with a canine or other carnivore that is in contact with potentially infected herbivores is helpful.

The standard CF test and the Casoni skin test still are used widely. A dose of 0.1 ml Casoni antigen is injected intracutaneously and read at 15 to 20 minutes and at 24 hours. Serum obtained for the CF test, or identification of antigen 5 by immunoelectrophoresis, is proving valuable for diagnosis of the genus, but some cross-reactivity with *T. solium* may occur. Ultimately, identification of the protoscolicies in surgical or autopsy specimens provides definitive proof of the parasitic infection. Needle aspiration usually is not advisable because of the risk of anaphylaxis if fluid leaks from the puncture wound in the cyst. Diagnosis in *E. multilocularis* infection is made by serological tests or a pathological specimen.

Treatment

Albendazole in a dose of 15 mg/kg/day for 28 days, is the drug of choice. When surgical extirpation is needed or when spillage has occurred, praziquantel has been found to be advantageous. Albendazole and percutaneous drainage have been used together successfully in the treatment of hepatic hydatid cyst. Albendazole is given with a fatty meal to enhance absorption. The long-term treatment of *E. multilocularis* with mebendazole appears to result in some amelioration of the disease. Surgical removal, while resulting in long-term cure in a few, often is impossible by the time of diagnosis. The course that any case takes over time is uncertain. Lesions may remain relatively asymptomatic and change little in size for a long period, and then become aggressive and fatal within a short time.

DWARF TAPEWORM *(Hymenolepsis nana)*

Epidemiology

Hymenolepsis nana is a tapeworm of rats and mice. However, it is well adapted to humans and completes its entire life cycle in them, making autoinoculation a problem. Transmission occurs directly from child to child or through contamination of food and drink with human or rodent feces. The parasite is found worldwide, and the prevalence is much higher among children than adults. Children at special risk are those under age 3, those on a protein-deficient diet, immunodepressed children, or those living in a crowded, unhygienic environment infested with rodents. The decreasing prevalence with age reflects a decrease in exposure, but serological studies suggest that previous exposure evokes a measure of resistance against recurrent infestation. The current world prevalence is estimated to be about 50 million cases.

Pathogenesis and Life Cycle

H. nana is the smallest tapeworm infesting humans. It requires no soil or water cycle, and the eggs become infective before leaving the human gut; this allows internal autoinfestation as well as transfer from anus to mouth in the same host. After ingestion of a viable egg, its onchosphere (embryo) is released in the stomach or upper small intestine. The embryo penetrates an intestinal villus and matures into the cysticercoid stage. The larva emerges to attach itself in the small intestine. Maturation to the adult stage is evidenced by the appearance of eggs in the stool several weeks later. The adult worm measures 25 to 40 mm long by 0.5 to 0.7 mm in diameter. The scolex (head and neck) has four suckers and 20 to 30 hooklets arranged in a single crown. The egg is 30 to 40 μm long and is characterized by a wide clear space between the outer membrane and the centrally placed embryo. The embryo contains four to eight polar filaments.

Clinical Manifestations

Although light to moderate infections generally are not associated with patient complaints, a heavily infected child often complains of abdominal pain, headache, and loss of appetite. Diarrhea, abdominal distention, and pallor also may be present in some cases. Diarrhea seldom occurs in patients who have fewer than 15,000 eggs per gram of feces.

Diagnosis

The diagnosis is made by detecting typical worms or eggs in the patient's feces. A moderate eosinophilia is present with heavy infections. Serological tests are of no real value in the diagnosis of *H. nana.*

Treatment

H. nana has been a difficult parasite to eliminate because the drug of choice, niclosamide, was only effective against the adult worm (90% of cases). The eggs released by the adult female hatch while still in the intestine and give rise to new adult worms. This autoinoculation capability and the ineffectiveness of niclosamide in killing the eggs leads to a build up of worms, especially in children whose nutrition is poor or who are immunocompromised. Currently, praziquantel in a single dose of 25 mg/kg provides the best rate of initial cure. A repeat dose still may be necessary. Stools should be checked every 2 weeks for 3 months for eggs. Timing repeat drug therapy at 2 weeks after initial treatment carries the best chance of ridding the patient of the parasite. Close contacts (e.g., family and other closed population) should be treated simultaneously.*

ASCARIASIS/LARGE ROUNDWORM (*Ascaris lumbricoides*)

Epidemiology

Ascaris lumbricoides is the largest roundworm that infects humans. Globally, it is believed to be the most common nematode parasite of humans. It may infect as many as a third of the earth's population. It probably is second only to pinworms in prevalence in the United States. Children are particularly prone to repeated infection because the parasite is contracted by ingestion of the fertile embryonated egg directly from the soil (pica) or by placing dirty fingers or fomites in the mouth. Food or water that is contaminated with human feces is common in parts of the world where human waste is used to fertilize gardens. Although no intermediate host is required, the eggs require a period of embryonation in soil before becoming infective.

Pathogenesis and Life Cycle

Once swallowed, a fertile *Ascaris* egg hatches in the small intestine. The larva penetrates the mucosa, enters a portal venule or the lymphatic system, and is carried to the lungs. Because most of the larvae cannot negotiate the capillary bed, they rupture into the alveoli and migrate up the airways. Upon reaching the epiglottis, they again are swallowed and develop into adults in the small bowel. The larger female commonly reaches 20 to 35 cm in length and 3 to 6 mm in diameter. The male is slightly smaller, and its posterior end curves ventrally. The interval between egg ingestion and the appearance of eggs in the feces is 8 to 10 weeks. The female lays approximately 200,000 eggs a day throughout her 6- to 17-month lifespan. The eggs measure 88 to 95 μm by 44 μm if infertile and 45 to 75 μm by 35 to 50 μm if fertilized. Eggs reaching a favorable soil (i.e., warm, moist, shady clay) develop an infective larva inside the shell that remains viable for many months.

Clinical Manifestations

Most cases of ascariasis are asymptomatic or so mild that medical attention is not sought. The severity of illness is determined in part by the number of infective eggs ingested, the patient's nutritional status, whether other pathological processes are present, the patient's degree of hypersensitivity, and possibly the presence of other helminthic parasites. Two types of uncomplicated clinical presentations are seen. The first occurs concomitant with the migration of the larvae. This is characterized by a dry cough, asthmatic wheezing, mild to severe dyspnea (with or without cyanosis), fever, and auscultatory findings compatible with asthma or bronchopneumonia (Löffler syndrome). Urticaria and, in a few very sensitive children, angioneurotic edema may occur. During this phase the stool may contain no eggs, but peripheral eosinophilia is common, and a chest roentgenogram may reveal patchy central infiltrates or confluent areas of lobar pneumonia or bronchopneumonia. In heavy infections, bronchial secretions increase, and larvae sometimes can be identified in the sputum or gastric secretions. During passage of larvae through the liver, especially in the host who has been exposed previously to ascarids, acute hepatitis may result. Eosinophilic granulomas may develop around larvae that die in the hepatic tissue. In rare cases larvae may pass the pulmonary capillary bed and lodge in other tissues (e.g., the brain), creating a picture compatible with visceral larva migrans. Adult worms may be vomited, may be passed in the stool, or may appear at other body orifices, including the navel of an infant or young child. A small number of adult *Ascaris* worms in the small intestine rarely produces clinical disease, although they unquestionably rob the host of some dietary protein and other nutrients. When only the adult worms are present, the patient suffers little more than periodic cramping abdominal pain with some indigestion, nausea, and vomiting. Headache also has been noted with some regularity in the absence of other detectable causes for it. In rare cases, right upper quadrant tenderness and pain and mild, transient jaundice occur secondary to migration of worms in the biliary tract. Complications are more likely to occur in children because of their smaller visceral lumens and their relatively larger worm burdens. Complications arising from adult *Ascaris* infection include obstruction of the intestine, bile duct, pancreatic duct, and appendix. Unless transient, such obstructions can lead to stasis of the fluid that normally flows through the lumen and the development of secondary infection. Bowel obstruction characteristically is incomplete and may manifest as a soft mass of varying size. Under certain conditions (e.g., high fever, anesthesia, and certain drugs), the worms may migrate indiscriminately through tissue or into the lumens of the ducts, as already noted. This can trigger hemorrhage, tissue inflammation, interruption of organ function, or perforation of a viscus. Infection, such as peritonitis (with or without shock) or liver abscess can follow. Adult worm migration through tissue frequently is attended by allergic phenomena. Infections with 48 or more worms are accompanied by a measurable reduction in fat and protein absorption. During the intestinal phase of ascariasis, eggs usually can be identified in the feces. If no recent migratory activity has taken place, the eosinophilia probably will be absent or nearly so. Abdominal roentgenograms may reveal swirling patterns or air-contrast evidence of the worms. After a barium meal, the worms may be outlined or identified by the examiner seeing barium in the worms' guts.

Diagnosis

During the migratory phase the diagnosis must be suspected and the blood examined for eosinophils. Finding larvae in the sputum is conclusive evidence of the infection, but their absence does not rule out ascariasis. The presence of *Ascaris*

*Praziquantel is available from SmithKline Beecham, Philadelphia, Pa. Niclosamide is available from Miles, Inc. West Haven, Conn.

eggs in the stool confirms the presence of the parasite, but the clinician always must be alert to the coexistence of other causes for the illness, especially in areas endemic for ascariasis. An "all male" or "sterile" female population of worms does not produce eggs in the feces. The presence of a single female worm usually can be detected by examining the stool. Serological tests, although generally not required, may become useful in cases where male worm infection is responsible for biliary tract obstruction and other uncommon expressions of roundworm infection.

Treatment

In the past it was necessary in combined infections to treat *Ascaris* infection first; before, for example, treating hookworm with tetrachlorethylene because the drug sometimes caused *Ascaris* to migrate into ducts or possibly perforate a viscus. With the advent of newer drugs, such as mebendazole and albendazole, this problem appears to have disappeared. Mebendazole in a dosage of 100 mg every morning and evening for 3 days is adequate for both children and adults. A second course should be timed for 3 weeks after the first if the stool examination still reveals eggs. Pyrantel pamoate in a single dose of 11 mg/kg (maximum 1 g) given orally is a reasonable alternative. For children under age 2, the risk of therapy should be weighed before deciding to treat. Mebendazole is not recommended in pregnancy. Children generally should be treated when the problem is discovered, unless a valid contraindication exists, because complications can occur with a single worm. If the history suggests ascariasis, a therapeutic drug trial occasionally is justified. When evidence of ductal (nonbowel) obstruction exists, surgery without prior ascaricide therapy is indicated. Worms that die in bile or pancreatic ducts or in vital tissue pose the risk of a life-threatening illness. If only the bowel is obstructed, a course of medical management generally is warranted. Piperazine citrate suspension (given by nasogastric tube) paralyzes the ascarid muscles, often allowing peristaltic action of the bowel to evacuate the worm or worms. A hospitalized patient can be treated with nasogastric suction and intravenous fluids while being given an effective ascaricidal drug. If this is unsuccessful after 48 hours, surgery is recommended. With a laparotomy, small bowel obstructions usually can be "milked" down into the cecum without opening the bowel itself. The patient then can be treated postoperatively for final removal of the parasites. Entering the bowel should be a last resort. If possible, patients who are likely to harbor *Ascaris* and are going to surgery for any cause should be screened preoperatively.

Prevention

Sanitary disposal of human excreta, reasonable personal hygiene, and avoiding food or water potentially contaminated with human feces constitute the first line of defense against ascariasis. Community-wide treatment, where used, must be repeated every 3 months for several years. Unless basic improvement in sanitation systems and personal hygiene are implemented, the long-term prevalence is unlikely to change. Considering the estimated 20,000 deaths worldwide each year attributed to ascariasis and the cost of medical care and the economic losses from illness, campaigns to control the parasite on a community-by-community basis are worth the effort. Notable examples of reduced prevalence have been reported for approaches that combine education, sanitation, and mass treatment.

TOXOCARIASIS/VISCERAL LARVA MIGRANS (*Toxocara canis, T. cati,* others)

Epidemiology

Toxocara canis (dog ascarid), *Toxocara cati* (cat ascarid), and in rare cases other nonhuman host nematodes are capable of producing a syndrome in humans similar to that produced by larvae of *A. lubricoides* during the migratory phase of its life cycle, but with less predictability. In their natural host, these animal ascarids follow a developmental pattern comparable to that of *Ascaris* organisms in humans, eventually maturing in the bowel and depositing eggs in the feces. Puppies and kittens in the early months of life are infected more heavily and thus disseminate more eggs capriciously into the environment than do older dogs and cats. A sizable percentage of domestic pets are infected and routinely contaminate school grounds, yards, and sandboxes used by children. Small children, especially those in the 1- to 4-year-old age group, are prone to eating dirt and putting soiled hands or toys into their mouths, thus increasing their risk of infection. *Toxocara* eggs become infective 2 to 7 days after being passed in animal feces. Studies of seroprevalence in the United States based on the national Health and Nutrition Examination Survey (HANES) have shown adjusted rates from 4.6% to 7.3% among children ages 1 to 11 years. Because serological tests can yield positive results for years, the infection rates are lower. The higher rates are found in the southern United States and are associated with rural living, increased age of children, number of persons living in the home, lower income, less education, and fewer rooms in the house. The presence of a litter of puppies in the home and the habit of pica in a child also have been correlated with the presence of toxocariasis. It has been estimated that 20% of dogs and 98% of puppies in the United States are infected.

Pathogenesis and Life Cycle

When ingested by a human, the egg hatches and the larva penetrates the upper GI mucosa and either directly begins wandering through the tissues or gets into the circulation and reaches distant organs before breaking out into the parenchymal tissues. The larvae appear to rupture out of the vascular system whenever its size (14 to 20 μm diameter) is too large to negotiate the vessel in which it is traveling. It cannot complete its maturation cycle and so continues to migrate through the tissues until the host encapsulates it. The tissue identified most often as the site of infection is the liver, but involvement of the lungs, kidneys, brain, heart, skeletal muscle, eyes, and other tissues has been reported. At first, only a mild inflammatory response or an eosinophilic abscess forms around the parasite and its tunnel in the tissue. Eventually a granuloma, with eosinophils, lymphocytes, plasma cells, and some giant cells, forms around the larva, and a thick fibrous capsule develops. The larva may remain viable in this state with no significant change for several years. Under certain unknown circumstances, it appears to be capable of breaking out of the capsule to wander again. In time, many of the encapsulated larvae die and become hyalinized. The larva does not mature beyond the second (rhabditiform) stage and measures 350 to 450 μm by 18 to 21 μm *(T. canis)* and 350 to 450 μm by 15 to 17 μm *(T. cati)*. The eggs found in animal feces are spheroid and dark brown and have a rough outer shell surface. They measure 75 to 80 μm *(T. canis)* and 65 to 70 μm *(T. cati)*. In pregnant dogs and cats, transplacental transmission is believed possible.

Clinical Manifestation

The severity of the illness in visceral larva migrans (VLM) is determined in part by the number of fertile viable eggs ingested, the organ system or systems involved, and the host's immunological status. Obviously, several larvae could be encysted in the liver and produce minimal or no symptoms, whereas even a single larva in the eye or brain can be devastating. Infection probably is underdiagnosed. Toxocariasis can manifest in a spectrum of ways, and a high index of suspicion is essential in making the diagnosis.

Asymptomatic Type. Mild constitutional symptoms may be present but apparently do not prompt the person to seek medical attention. Incidental findings of eosinophilia, an enlarged liver, and hypergammaglobulinemia may prompt a search for the diagnosis.

Hepatopulmonary Type. This form primarily involves the liver and lungs but should be distinguished from the migration phase of other nematodes. The child may be mildly to severely ill. Typical findings include episodic fever to 104° F (40° C) with night sweats, hepatomegaly, and pulmonary findings (e.g., wheezing, dyspnea, cough, and patchy pneumonitis or pneumonia). Transient GI disturbances that may recur are anorexia, nausea, vomiting, abdominal pain, and distention. A variety of rashes has been described, but urticaria is the most common. Other common findings include marked leukocytosis with fluctuating eosinophilia (20% to 90%), hypergammaglobulinemia, elevated isohemagglutinins, anemia, a positive test result for blood in the stool, Charcot-Leyden crystals, and eosinophils in the sputum. Chest roentgenograms demonstrate the pulmonary infiltrates. No form of the parasite is found in the sputum or stool.

Generalized Type (VLM). When larvae migrate directly from the intestine or reach the left ventricle, they then may enter virtually any organ system, with subsequent development of corresponding clinical signs and symptoms. These include myalgia, arthralgia, subcutaneous nodules, loss of weight or failure to gain weight, myocarditis, neuritis, and neurological dysfunction, including grand mal or petit mal seizures.

Ocular Type (OLM). This form is found most commonly among individuals over age 4 and is not associated with concomitant systemic manifestations or eosinophilia of any degree. In one series of 245 cases, the average age was 7½ years. Sprent listed 36 species of nematodes responsible for VLM in Australia. The most common cause in the United States probably is *T. canis*. This form manifests as insidious or sudden impairment of vision in one eye. Ophthalmoscopic examination reveals a raised, rounded, or umbilicated granuloma, frequently near the macula. If the larva protrudes into the vitreous, there may be serious inflammation farther anteriorly, carrying with it a high likelihood for impaired vision. This lesion usually is painless and must be distinguished from retinoblastoma. Ophthalmological consultation is advised.

Diagnosis

A syndrome comprising prolonged hypereosinophilia, elevated isohemagglutinins and gammaglobulins, hepatomegaly, intermittent fever, and episodic pulmonary symptoms should suggest the diagnosis. A history of pica, having a pet dog or cat, and poor hygiene are corroborative. The diagnosis is confirmed by finding the causative agent in association with the disease site in biopsy or autopsy specimens. Most experts advocate a liver biopsy (preferably open), although these may be negative even in the presence of the disease. A large number of tissue sections must be viewed, and it must be remembered that the larvae, because of their mobility, may be found away from areas of inflammation. Many serological tests are hindered by cross-reactivity with other nematode infections, especially ascariasis and strongyloidiasis. Negative results on serological tests for *Toxocara* species should cause serious doubt about the diagnosis, except perhaps in ocular cases, in which the serological tests are of less value. An ELISA test for toxocariasis is available, and a positive test result is presumptive. A skin test also is available but cross-reacts with other ascarids.

Treatment

No therapeutic agent has completely destroyed the larvae and controlled symptoms. Great caution must be exercised in treating larvae in tissue because of the potential for damage from hypersensitivity and migration. Diethylcarbamazine, although approved, still is considered investigational by the FDA. It is available as Hetrazan from Lederle Laboratories and from others. It is given in a dosage of 6 mg/kg/day, divided into three doses and continued for 7 to 10 days. Albendazole (400 mg bid for 3 to 5 days) has been reported as a successful cure but is not approved for use in the United States. Mebendazole likewise is believed to be useful in toxocariasis and is relatively safe, but it has not been studied adequately for this disease. It is advisable to consult the CDC.*

TRICHURIASIS/WHIPWORM *(Trichuris trichiura)*

Epidemiology

Trichuris trichiura is an intestinal roundworm that has a fine, hairlike anterior body that becomes thicker posteriorly, giving it the appearance of a whip. Like *A. lumbricoides,* it is acquired through ingestion of the egg after its embryonation in soil. Because of their indiscriminate and repeated play in soil and their thumb-sucking, nailbiting, and pica, children are more prone to become infected and to accumulate heavier worm burdens. The worldwide prevalence of this parasite has been estimated to be 750 million cases. In large surveys of parasites, it often is the nematode found most commonly. Some communities in the United States have shown a prevalence as high as 36% of the population. In the hot, moist tropics, the prevalence may exceed 50% of stools examined. Humans are the only natural host of *T. trichiura* and may pass eggs in their stools for up to 10 years after a single ingestion of eggs.

*Telephone: normal work hours: 1-404-639-3356.

Pathogenesis and Life Cycle

The ova of *T. trichiura* are barrel shaped, have slightly elongated ends containing a mucoid plug, and measure approximately 50 to 22 μm. The outer of the two shells of the egg generally is bile stained. After ingestion and embryonation in the small bowel, migration downward to the large bowel occurs with maturation to the adult worm, which measures 30 to 50 mm long. The adult threads its anterior body into the mucosa of the cecum, ascending colon, or rectosigmoid areas. This elicits no inflammatory response unless competition for nutrients forces deeper burrowing into the mucosa, which triggers infiltration with lymphocytes, plasma cells, and eosinophils down to the muscularis mucosae. This parasite neither causes the degree of blood loss from oozing that hookworms do nor uses blood as a major portion of its diet. However, it can produce significant anemia when 800 or more worms are in residence. One month after ingestion, the fertilized female begins laying about 3000 to 7000 eggs per day. When these fertile eggs are passed into a warm, moist, shady soil, they can become infective as early as 10 days. The average embryonation period in the soil is 21 days.

Clinical Manifestations

Light infections generally go unrecognized. Infections producing 30,000 or more eggs per gram of stool are likely to be accompanied by abdominal pain, headache, pallor, tenesmus, and diarrhea or dysentery. Increased motility and tenesmus, whether caused by physical or chemical irritation, have been blamed for cramping pains, diminished absorption of nutrients, and complications such as volvulus, intussusception, and rectal prolapse. Irritability, lack of concentration, and other emotional problems have been blamed on trichuriasis. Rectal prolapse, presumably secondary to straining when stooling (tenesmus) occurs in about 1% of diagnosed, symptomatic cases. Intense inflammation in the cecum occasionally has led to a symptom complex mimicking appendicitis. In fact, appendicitis has occurred as a result of edema and direct worm obstruction of the appendix. Heavy infection in the presence of chronic debilitation and malnutrition carries a grave prognosis. The invasiveness of both amebiasis and typhoid appears to be enhanced by the presence of *Trichuris* organisms in the same patient. After a single exposure, without treatment, the infection usually subsides in about 3 years. However, it may persist for longer than 9 years.

Diagnosis

The diagnosis must be suspected and the stool examined for the characteristic eggs. The worms may be observed at autopsy, during bowel surgery, or with sigmoidoscopy. When rectal prolapse occurs, the parasite frequently is visible on the mucosa. The stool should be examined in any case of prolapsed rectum. Advanced abdominal tuberculosis, disseminated histoplasmosis, certain malignancies of the abdomen, and severe malnutrition must be excluded. A skin test antigen available from the CDC has been reported to be positive in 93% of proven cases of 1 month's duration or longer. This can be valuable for determining the prevalence of *T. trichiura* infection in a community. Probably the most reliable serological test is the latex flocculation test. Serum from a known case should be used simultaneously for comparing the degree of flocculation present.

Treatment

In the past it often was recommended that light infections not be treated, partly because of the potential toxicity of the drugs used in therapy. With the effectiveness and safety record of mebendazole and now albendazole, treatment should not be withheld except for specific contraindications. Mebendazole is highly effective in a dosage of 100 mg twice daily for 3 days. Albendazole is given in one dose of 400 mg. In heavy infections the dosage may be repeated for 2 or 3 more days. Mebendazole is not recommended in pregnancy.

In severe infections, transfusion and general supportive measures should not be neglected. When a prolapse occurs, the rectum must be inspected for foreign bodies, injury (including perforation), and infarction. When a surgical consultation can be obtained quickly, this is appropriate. A healthy rectum should be returned to the pelvis by using a gloved, lubricated finger while the patient is on his or her knees with the chest flat on the examining table. If the physician is very concerned about possible perforation or infarction of the rectum and the distance from medical care is great, the child should be observed in the hospital for 24 hours. Repeated prolapse has occurred.

HOOKWORM DISEASE/ANCYLOSTOMIASIS
(Ancylostoma duodenale, A. ceylonicum, Necator americanus)

Epidemiology

Necator americanus is the predominant specie of hookworm in the Western hemisphere, southeastern Asia, and sub-Saharan Africa. *Ancylostoma duodenale* infections predominate in the Mediterranean basin, northern India, and northern Asia. Pockets of *A. duodenale* also exist in Central and South America and the Caribbean islands. In the United States the parasite is found in immigrants and travelers. The near-universal use of modern plumbing and the reduction in barefoot children in the United States has reduced the burden of hookworm infection significantly in this country. Still, there are local areas of transmission, mostly asymptomatic, from the mid-Atlantic to the Gulf Coast. *A. ceylonicum* is a hookworm found in southeastern Asia. Humans are found to have only a few worms; therefore, the infections are mild. Hookworm infection constitutes one of the world's more serious economic and health problems. The peak infection rate occurs among men in their teens and twenties. On some coffee plantations, men harvest the beans and women work in the coffee bean processing plant. The barefooted men relieve themselves among the coffee trees and return to harvest more coffee beans at approximately the time the hookworm eggs have hatched into infective larvae. In this manner the bean pickers may become reinfected many times during a single harvest season. The ideal environment for hookworm transmission is slightly sandy, shaded soil that has adequate but not saturated soil moisture. This also is the appropriate environment for coffee bean trees. Children who go barefoot or play on the ground where promiscuous defecation is common may develop large worm burdens. Humans are the only reservoir of infection for *A. duodenale* and *N. americanus*. *A. ceylonicum* has its reservoir in cats and dogs.

Pathogenesis and Life Cycle

When a hookworm egg is deposited on the soil, it hatches in about 24 hours, releasing a rhabditiform larva. Within a week, the third-stage "infective" larva appears. This organism dies in the soil when its stored food supply is exhausted, usually within 6 weeks if conditions otherwise are favorable. The infective larvae have been noted to move upward on plants and stand upright in anticipation of attachment to a passing host. Effective contact with humans can be made when any part of the naked body comes in contact with the soil, even the hands. Only *A. duodenale* is infective when ingested. The larvae not killed by the reaction in the skin enter lymphatic or blood vessels and are carried to the lungs. The larvae eventually migrate upward to the epiglottis and are swallowed. They undergo final development to the adult stage in the small bowel, where they attach to the second or third portion of the jejunum. The worm feeds by grasping a small piece of the intestinal mucosa into its buccal cavity. Cutting blades or teeth mince it, and anticoagulant secretions are introduced until a vessel in the mucosa is ruptured and streams blood into the worm. After the "bite" of mucosa is digested, the worm moves to a new area of mucosa and repeats the meal. The areas abandoned continue to ooze blood or serum for some time. The blood loss per worm is estimated at 0.03 ml/day for *N. americanus* and 0.06 to 0.1 ml/day for *A. duodenale*. Infection with the latter parasite produces greater bowel damage and blood loss. The female lays eggs that are passed in the feces, beginning about 1 to 2 months after skin penetration. The female *N. americanus* is 9 to 11 mm long; the female *A. duodenale* reaches 10 to 13 mm. The eggs are ovoid and contain a two- to eight-segment embryo surrounded by a clear zone. They measure 40 to 60 μm. It is impossible to determine which type of hookworm is present by observing the ova. The female *N. americanus* worm deposits just under 10,000 eggs a day, and *A. duodenale* females deposit 15,000 to 20,000 eggs a day. Without treatment or reinfection, most of the hookworms exit the body within a year, but they have been reported to survive nearly a decade in some cases.

Clinical Manifestations

Hookworm infection must be distinguished from hookworm disease. A single exposure even to moderate numbers of larvae may proceed without notice by the patient except for the skin reaction. During their brief sojourn in the skin, the larvae evoke this reaction, which is characterized by edema, a vesicular, erythematous, or papular rash, and pruritus. Secondary infection may occur, and the name "ground itch" has been given to the visible disorder. Because of further development of the *N. americanus* larvae in the lung, signs and symptoms may be more serious with that species. Pneumonitis, dry cough, and wheezing may occur during the pulmonary phase (1 to 2 weeks after skin penetration). At this time, the larvae are penetrating from pulmonary capillaries into the alveoli and migrating up the bronchial tree. The sputum, especially in *A. duodenale,* may contain larvae and Charcot-Leyden crystals. Once the adult worms begin their ravage of the small bowel, blood loss can be significant. Microcytic, hypochromic anemia, pallor, fatigue, and weakness may be presenting features in moderate cases. Slow blood loss from large worm burdens, coupled with poor diet and reinfection, eventually leads to hypoalbuminemia and cardiac decompensation with shortness of breath, cardiac palpitations, and edema. Reduced activity at work and play are noticeable. GI dysfunction, including diarrhea, anorexia, flatulence, and abdominal aches and pains, add to the patient's anemia, weight loss, and apathy. Although the disease rarely is fatal, it can result in failure to thrive, cardiac failure, acceleration of concominant infections, and increased maternal and fetal morbidity and mortality.

Diagnosis

Diagnosis of hookworm infection rests on identifying the eggs or larvae in the stool specimen. If the specimen is left sitting 24 hours or longer before examination, only larvae may be present. Should this be the case, the larvae must be distinguished from those of *Strongyloides stercoralis*. If more than 20 hookworm eggs are present on a direct 2 mg fecal smear, clinical symptoms can be expected. Potassium iodide saturated with iodine can be used to highlight the eggs in the fecal smear. Concentration techniques are necessary when the number of eggs is small. Blood eosinophilia may be prominent during the tissue migratory phase of larval development, beginning at 2 to 3 weeks after exposure and peaking at 5 to 9 weeks. Untreated disease may result in continued blood eosinophilia for months to years.

Treatment

Both mebendazole and pyrantel pamoate are adequate to treat hookworm infections. Mebendazole is given as 100 mg bid for 3 days and pyrantel pamoate as 11 mg/kg (to a maximum of 1 g) for 3 days. Albendazole also can be given, when available, as a single dose of 400 mg. Children under age 2 have not been studied adequately, and treatment in these cases must be weighed against the risk. Mebendazole is not recommended for pregnant women. Anemia in these patients should be treated as for iron deficiency anemia.

CUTANEOUS LARVAL MIGRANS *(Ancylostoma caninum, A. braziliense, others)*

Epidemiology

"Creeping eruption" commonly is caused by nonhuman hookworm filariform larvae such as *Ancylostoma braziliense, Ancylostoma caninum,* and other species. Because these species only rarely are able to penetrate the skin and reach the GI tract of humans, they wander aimlessly in the skin, producing raised, erythematous, pruritic tracks. They are acquired by children when a child's exposed skin comes into contact with soil or sand contaminated with animal feces containing nonhuman hookworm eggs. The parasite is most prevalent where warm, moist sandy soil with a high humus content is used by dogs and cats to defecate, and subsequently for gardening, a children's playground, or sports field. Beaches also have been the site of transmission. In the United States, the Southeast has the highest incidence.

Pathogenesis and Life Cycle

Although ground itch caused by human hookworm and *Strongyloides* larvae is a form of cutaneous larva migrans (CLM), it differs from the condition caused by nonhuman species in that the latter cannot complete their cycle. The tunneling migrations of these nonhuman hookworms evoke an intense neutrophilic and eosinophilic infiltrate and produce edema and vascular congestion. The tunnel fills with serum. It is believed that the larva advances with the aid of enzymatic action and that the human body elaborates an antibody against the enzyme.

Clinical Manifestations

The serpiginous track through the skin is visualized easily. It is pruritic, often highly so, and has been described as painful by a minority of patients. Localized swelling and rash also may occur. The lesions often are found on the feet, thighs, or buttocks. In some reported series, secondary bacterial infection is present, perhaps enhanced by scratching.

Diagnosis

The diagnosis of "creeping eruption" is made clinically, although the species of larva responsible may remain unknown. The larva is advanced from the reaction that it evokes, and because treatment is successful and the condition is self-limiting, biopsy generally is unwarranted.

Treatment

Topical use of 15% thiabendazole cream applied two or three times a day for 5 days is adequate for cure. Albendazole, given as a single dose of 400 mg, has been used successfully in cases that did not respond to thiabendazole cream. Oral ivermectin has proved very successful and had no side effects in at least one series of patients.

ONCHOCERCIASIS/RIVER BLINDNESS
(Onchocerca volvulus)

Epidemiology

Onchocerca volvulus is a long nematode (females are 23 to 70 cm long and males, 3 to 6 cm). It lives its adult life curled up in an encapsulated nodule with other worms of both sexes in the subcutaneous tissues of humans. Although humans apparently are the only definitive host of *O. volvulus,* the black fly *(Simulium)* transmits it from person to person and serves as the site for intermediate metamorphosis of the parasite. Microfilaria released by the adult female worm move through the human body, particularly the dermis, lymph channels, and eye, producing the characteristic clinical features. These include pruritic skin rashes, blindness, and occasionally elephantiasis, although the elephantiasis seldom is of the magnitude as that produced by lymphatic filariasis. Of the estimated 18 million people who suffer from *O. volvulus* infection 95% are found in tropical Africa. Pockets of disease also are found in Yemen, in northern South America, and in Central America. In some African villages the prevalence of blindness reaches 10%. Although the disease itself is not fatal, those who become blind may become neglected and die prematurely. The economic toll on heavily infected villages is high. In Latin America, the subcutaneous nodules (onchocercomata) typically are found on the head and shoulders; in Africa they are found below the waist, on the trunk, buttocks, and legs. Onchocerciasis may coexist with classic filariasis.

Pathogenesis and Life Cycle

The black fly larvae develop while attached to water plants or rocks in well-aerated, fast-flowing streams, rivers, and irrigation channels. The adult flies are small (1 to 5 mm), tan to black, and have a "hump back" appearance. The wings are broad and irridescent and have a heavier venous pattern toward the anterior edge. These flies are relatively strong fliers, migrating with wind currents in swarms for hundreds of kilometers at times. Only the females feed on blood, but both sexes may use plant juices as a source of energy. Males swarm and the females become fertilized while flying near or through the swarm. Each female lays hundreds of eggs at a time on the water's surface. After the eggs hatch, the larvae attach themselves to plants, rocks, and concrete structures in the water. The pupae also live in the water. The female's life span is just several weeks. Fly bites are made by stylets, and puddle feeding occurs during which microfilariae may be ingested by the fly or infective larvae deposited by the fly. The parasite cycle in the fly is similar to that for other filarids. *Simulium* flies seldom are found inside human domiciles, but they are day feeders and have adequate access to the human host outside. The bite, which is painful, almost certainly is accompanied by the injection of anticoagulants and possibly other substances. The unsheathed microfilariae (210 to 320 μm) taken up in the blood meal from an infected human develop in the fly gut and migrate to the thoracic muscles, from which they can reenter the human, by means of a subsequent bite, as a filariform (infective) larvae (440 to 700 μm). These must be deposited or quickly rubbed into the bite, presumably to infect the definitive human host. Once in the human circulation, they mature over a period of up to 18 or so months. The adult worms coil into a spherical capsule in the subcutaneous areas with several females and a lesser number of males. The long, slender females deposit thousands of microfilariae, which move through the capsule and wander about the body, having an affinity for the dermis and the eye. This behavior probably is controlled genetically to coincide with feeding habits of the vector flies. The damage done to all parts of the eye, the skin, and the lymphatic channels may be a combination of effects from the host immune response, the microfilarial migrations, and possibly substances secreted by one or more stages of the worm.

Clinical Manifestations

The bite of the black fly causes pain, edema, and itching. Secondary bacterial infection may complicate the wound. Symptoms during the maturation of the worms are not acknowledged retrospectively. In less than a year the nodules form and the skin becomes regionally or generally invaded by the microfilariae. Patches of erythematous, edematous skin and pruritus develop, signaling the invasion of microfilariae. The nodules (0.5 to 3 cm) containing the adult worms are painless, spongy or rubbery on palpation, and mobile unless attached to superficially placed bone. If the worms die, fluctuation results. Chronic lichenification occurs, and destruction of the skin's elasticity results in lax, atrophic skin, causing redundancy. "Hanging groin" is seen in chronic cases, especially in Africa. Hernias, hydroceles, and elephantiasis are reported. Leonine facies is seen, especially in patients in the Americas.

Conjunctivitis with photophobia occurs with early invasion of the eye by microfilariae. Death of the microfilariae within the cornea leads to punctate keratitis that proceeds from the limbus toward the central corneum. Over time a pannus forms between Bowman capsule and the epithelium. Proliferation of capillaries and collections of plasma cells and eosinophiles can be seen on pathological specimens. The epithelial layer may show hyperplasia, and melanin is present. Continued infection causes sclerosing keratitis and permanent blindness. This is most common in the savannah type of African onchocerciasis and with long-standing infection. Anterior uveitis can lead to glaucoma. Pupillary dysfunction and posterior synechiae are reported. Damage to the chorioretinal layers of the posterior eye, leading to blindness, is more typical of the African forest type of onchocerciasis.

Diagnosis

Subcutaneous nodules, eye signs, and skin changes are recognized easily by the clinician who sees the disease frequently in endemic areas. Skin snips are obtained by using a sterile hypodermic needle to lift a tiny portion of skin that is shaved off with a Bard-Parker or razor blade. This is placed in a drop of nutrient broth or normal saline and left for several hours before being observed under a light microscope. The unsheathed microfilariae of *O. volvulus* can be identified best with hematoxylin or Giemsa stains.

Treatment

Ivermectin now is the drug of choice for treating onchocerciasis because of its ease of administration and lack of major complications, such as the reactions some patients experience with Hetrazan. One oral dose of ivermectin (150 μg/kg) is sufficient in most cases, but the dose must be repeated every 6 to 12 months if the patient remains in an endemic zone. Ivermectin is available from the CDC Drug Service.*

Prevention

Larvicides and insecticides both have been used. Vector control has been most effective when larvicides are used over large areas for prolonged periods. More recently, mass treatment with the microfilaricide ivermectin has been used. The major obstructions to prevention now are effective host education and reliable distribution and consumption of ivermectin.

TRICHINOSIS (*Trichinella spiralis*)

Trichinella spiralis is a nematode that infests humans, pigs, rats, and a wide variety of other animals globally. Humans contract the disease of trichinosis by ingesting the encysted larvae in inadequately cooked meat. The United States and Europe are the major endemic zones of transmission. Domestic pork is the most common source in these countries, but wild bear, walrus, and boar meats have been the source of infection for humans in Africa and North America. Children rarely are infested and infants virtually never. The incidence of trichinosis in the United States has shown a marked decline, presumably as a result of laws governing the feeding of swine, mandatory slaughterhouse surveillance, food service sanitation, and general public awareness of the causes. Because the parasite is killed by being frozen at 5° F (−15° C) for 21 days, the use of home freezers to store meat also has played an important role in reducing the incidence. The reported incidence in the United States is erratic but with a downward trend; more than 250 cases were reported in 1975 and less than 30 in 1993. However, only 3% of those infected are estimated to develop symptoms resulting in medical diagnosis. The fatality rate in the United States had fallen to less than 1% by the mid-1970s. Evidence for a true decline in prevalence came from a histological study at autopsy of diaphragmatic muscles, for which the *T. spiralis* worm has a predilection. Most cases reported in the United States today are small outbreaks in families or in places where improper meat handling by a food preparer has left the cysts viable. Heating meat to 171° F (77° C) provides a safe margin against trichinosis. Except for the now rare case of cannibalism or consumption of humans by animals, humans are a dead-end host of *T. spiralis*.

Pathogenesis and Life Cycle

Encysted larvae ingested in meat are freed in the acid-pepsin milieu of the stomach and take up residence in the duodenum or upper jejunum. Adult worms appear within 4 to 6 days, and the sexes mate. The males apparently die shortly thereafter, and the females burrow into the columnar cells of the mucosa or remain in the mucoid coating. The females begin depositing larvae at a rate of about 50 per day until they die some weeks later. The fecundity of the mature female has been estimated variously at 1000 to 2000 larvae released before exiting the bowel. The adult females generally are gone from the bowel within 3 weeks. The larvae migrate through the lymphatic and blood vessels before reaching the striated and cardiac muscle bundles where, they are encysted in a host-derived "nurse cell." Within this relatively protected environment the larva molts to its infective form, with a final length of 0.8 to 1 mm. The larvae, so encysted, are believed to remain viable for many years, perhaps decades. Most die within several years. Larvae that fail to reach the muscle bundles before their demise are absorbed by the host. The mature worms in the human bowel are unsegmented and taper from a pointed mouth to maximum diameter in their mid section and then grow smaller again to the posterior tip. The female measures about 3 mm and the male about half the female length. Larvae, released by the female worm in the small bowel, measure about 100 μm. After molting in the nursing cells, they measure about 800 to 1000 μm.

Clinical Manifestations

Most infections are light and produce minor or no symptoms. In heavier infections, three phases may be recognized. Invasion of the upper GI tract by the female worm may occasion anorexia, nausea, vomiting, diarrhea or constipation, and mild fever. These prodromal symptoms develop 2 to 12 days after the contaminated meat is ingested. As early as the end of the second week after ingestion, a high fever, severe myalgia,

*Telephone: normal work hours: 1-404-639-3356.

edema (especially periorbital), and a striking eosinophilia develop. Inflammation in the brain, heart, kidneys, and lungs may cause serious signs related to those organs. Death most commonly is caused by overwhelming larval invasion of the heart, lungs, and/or central nervous system. Heart failure, arrhythmias, pulmonary failure, and seizures, with neurological deficits, must be managed in severe cases.

Diagnosis

The triad of myalgia, eosinophilia (20% to 90%), and periorbital edema, in the presence of fever and a history of eating inadequately cooked meat about 2 to 3 weeks earlier, is presumptive of trichinosis. If others who shared the food are ill with similar symptoms, the diagnosis is strengthened. Available serological tests from state laboratories and the CDC may establish the diagnosis, but only when the disease already has reached the muscle stage. Muscle biopsy may test positive after the larvae reach muscle (second week postingestion), but negative test results do not rule out trichinosis. Fresh specimens of muscle are crushed between two microscope slides and observed for the encysted larvae. If any meat from the suspect meal has been saved, it may be examined for the cysts.

Treatment

Mebendazole recently has been used investigatively for treatment. Because of the potential for toxicity from mass destruction of larvae, the initial dose is 200 to 400 mg/kg given three times daily for 3 days, followed by 400 to 500 mg given tid for 10 days. In patients who have severe symptoms, corticosteroids may be tried, although their benefit has not been confirmed. Analgesics are necessary for heavy infections. Thiabendazole was used earlier but was effective only against the mature worms in the intestinal lumen, and the diagnosis seldom is made before significant release of larvae. The larvae are not susceptible to thiabendazole during their migration or encystment stages.

Prevention

Control of meat-eating animals and their preparation as food for humans, health education, and early diagnosis (to stop further use of contaminated products) have reduced the burden of *T. spiralis* to small numbers in the United States. Vigilance must be continued, however, as evidenced by significant outbreaks seen periodically.

THE FETUS AND MATERNAL PARASITISM

When parasites invade a pregnant woman, the attending physician must consider the effect of both the infection and its treatment on the mother and the fetus. The effects on the fetus may be direct, (e.g. toxoplasmosis) or indirect through damage to the mother (e.g., hookworm anemia). Parasites may cause abortion (e.g., malaria, toxoplasmosis) or the immunosuppression seen in pregnancy may favor invasiveness of existing parasites (e.g., intestinal amebiasis). The placental barrier is remarkably effective in preventing transmission of some parasitic diseases (e.g., malaria, when considering the number of pregnant women and girls with the disease) and fairly ineffective in stopping others (e.g., toxoplasmosis). Some parasites, such as malaria, can occlude the vascular system of the placenta, resulting in compromised blood flow to the fetus. Intrauterine growth retardation and fetal death can result. The buildup of parasites capable of autoinoculation is a special threat to the pregnant woman, because her immune system may be somewhat less competent at this time. *S. stercoralis, H. nana,* and *Enterobius vermicularis* all are capable of autoinoculation. One must weigh the risk of treating a parasitical infection against the risk of the parasite to both mother and fetus. Many intestinal helminths pose minimal risk when their numbers are not excessive during pregnancy. It may be possible, therefore, to postpone treatment until after delivery. Malaria (particularly that caused by *P. falciparum*), invasive amebiasis, trypanosomiasis (both African and American), and visceral leishmaniasis are more dangerous during pregnancy and should be treated if possible. However, many drugs are contraindicated during pregnancy, and these must either be avoided or weighed very carefully against the risk of the parasitical disease. With some drugs, teratogenicity is the problem; with others, carcinogenicity may be of concern. No drug should be used unless the manufacturer's insert has been read to determine the contraindications for pregnant women. If the drug has not received sufficient study, the patient's condition should be sufficiently severe to warrant the uncertain risk of the drug's side effects.

REFERENCES

1. Bandres JC et al: Extraparenchymal neurocysticercosis: report of five cases and review of management, *Clin Infect Dis* 15:799, 1992.
2. Köberle F: Chagas' disease and Chagas' syndromes: the pathology of American trypanosomiasis, *Adv Parasitol* 6:63, 1968.
3. Scott JAG et al: Aminosidine (paromomycin in the treatment of leishmaniasis imported into the United Kingdom, *Trans R Soc Trop Med Hyg* 86:617, 1992.

SUGGESTED READINGS

Abramowicz M: Drugs for parasitic infections, *Med Lett Drugs Ther* 35:111, 1993.

American Academy of Pediatrics: *1994 Red Book: Report of the Committee on Infectious Diseases,* ed 23, Elk Grove Village, Ill, 1994, The Academy.

Benenson AS ed: *Control of communicable diseases manual,* ed 16, Washington, DC, 1995, American Public Health Association.

Connolly KJ, Kvalsvig JD: Infection, nutrition, and cognitive performance, *Parasitology* 107:S187, 1993.

Cook GC: Effect of global warming on the distribution of parasitic and other infectious diseases: a review, *Journal of the Royal Society of Medicine* 85:688, 1992.

Engelhard VH: How cells process antigens, *Sci Am* 271:54, 1994.

Englund PT, Sher A: *The biology of parisitism,* vol 9, New York, 1988, Alan R. Liss.

Feigin RD, Cherry JD, editors: *Textbook of pediatric infectious diseases,* ed 2, Philadelphia. 1987, WB Saunders.

Genta RM: Diarrhea in helminthic infections, *Clin Infect Dis* 16(suppl 2):S122, 1993.

Goldsmith R, Heyneman D: *Tropical medicine and parasitology,* Norwalk, Conn, 1989, Appleton & Lange.

Harwood R, James MT: *Entomology in human and animal health,* ed 7, New York, 1979, Macmillan.

Lambert HP: *Parasitic infection of the central nervous system,* London, 1991, Edward Arnold.

Maddison SE: Serodiagnosis of parasitic diseases, *Clin Microbiol Rev* 4:457, 1991.

Markell E, Voge M, John D: *Medical parasitology,* ed 7, Philadelphia, 1992, WB Saunders.

Muller R, Baker JR: *Medical parasitology,* Philadelphia, 1992, JB Lippincott.

Noble ER et al: *Parasitology: the biology of animal parasites,* ed 6, Philadelphia, 1989, Lea & Febiger.

Santos JI: Nutrition, infection, and immunocompetence, *Diseases of Latin America* 8:243, 1994.

Shulman IA, Appleman MD: Transmission of parasitic and bacterial infections through blood transfusion within the US, *Crit Rev Clin Lab Sci* 28:447, 1991.

Sovoili L, Bundy D, Tomkins A: Intestinal parasitic infections: a soluble public health problem, *Trans R Soc Trop Med Hyg* 86:353, 1992.

Strickland GT: *Hunter's tropical medicine,* ed 6, Philadelphia, 1984, WB Saunders.

Warren KS, Mahmoud AAF: *Trop Geogr Med,* ed 2, New York, 1990, McGraw-Hill.

Weller PF: Eosinophilia in travelers, *Med Clin North Am* 76:1413, 1992.

Wyler DJ, editor: *Modern parasite biology,* New York, 1990, WH Freeman.

Malaria

Cattani J, Davidson D, Engers H: Malaria, *Tropical Disease Research Progress 1991-92* 11:15, 1993.

Groude JRL et al: Imported malaria in the Bronx: review of 51 cases recorded from 1986 to 1991, *Clin Infect Dis* 15:774, 1992.

Hoffman SL: Diagnosis, treatment, and prevention of malaria, *Med Clin North Am* 76:1327, 1992.

Mutabingwa TK: Malaria chemosuppression in pregnancy VI, *Trop Geogr Med* 46:1, 1994.

Subramanian D: Imported malaria in pregnancy: report of four cases and review of management, *Clin Infect Dis* 15:408, 1992.

Voller A, Bidwell DE, Chiodini PL: Evaluation of a malaria antigen ELISA, *Trans R Soc Trop Med Hyg* 88:188, 1994.

Zucker JR, Campbell CC: Malaria: principles of prevention and treatment, *Infect Dis Clin North Am* 7:547, 1993.

Amebic Meningoencephalitis

Duma RJ: Primary amebic meningoencephalitis infection by tree-living amebae. In Lambert HP, editor: *Infections of the central nervous system,* Philadelphia, 1991, BC Decker.

Ferrante A: Immunity to acanthamoeba, *Rev Infect Dis* 13(suppl 5):S403, 1991.

Popek EJ, Neafie RC: Case 4 granulomatous meningoencephalitis due to leptomyxid ameba, *Pediatr Pathol* 12:871, 1992.

Babesiosis

Garnham PCC: Human babesiosis: European aspects, *Trans R Soc Trop Med Hyg* 74:153, 1980.

Gombert ME et al: Human babesiosis: clinical and therapeutic considerations, *JAMA* 248:3005, 1982.

Rowin KS, Tanowitz HB, Wittner M: Therapy of experimental babesiosis, *Ann Intern Med* 97:556, 1982.

Spielman A et al: Ecology of *Ixodes dammini*-borne human babesiosis and Lyme disease, *Annu Rev Entomol* 30:439, 1985.

Wittner M et al: Successful chemotherapy of transfusion babesiosis, *Ann Intern Med* 96:601, 1982.

Chagas Disease

Cimo PL, Luper WE, Scouros MA: Transfusion-associated Chagas' disease in Texas: report of a case, *The Journal of Texas Medicine* 89:48, 1993.

Krieger MA et al: Use of recombinant antigens for the accurate immunodiagnosis of Chagas' disease, *Am J Trop Med Hyg* 46:427, 1992.

Marsden PD: South American trypanosomiasis (Chagas' disease), *International Review of Tropical Medicine* 4:97, 1971.

Moncayo A: Chagas' Disease, *Tropical Disease Research Progress 1991-1992 Report,* 1993, p 67.

Santos-Buch CA: American trypanosomiasis: Chagas' disease, *Int Rev Exp Pathol* 19:63, 1979.

Cryptosporidiosis

Bunyartvej S, Bunyawongwiroj P, Nitiyanant P: Human intestinal sarcosporidiosis: report of six cases, *Am J Trop Med Hyg* 31:36, 1982.

Gellin BG, Soave R: Coccidian infections in AIDS, *Med Clin North Am* 76:205, 1992.

Mehlhorn H: Sarcosporidia (protozoa, sporozoa): life cycle and fine structure, *Adv Parasitol* 16:43, 1972.

Sun T, editor: *Progress in clinical parasitology,* vol 1, New York, 1991, Field & Wood.

Sun T, editor: *Progress in clinical parasitology,* vol 3, New York, 1993, Springer-Verlag.

Hookworm Disease

Gilman RH: Hookworm disease: host-pathogen biology, *Rev Infect Dis,* 4:824, 1982.

Pritchard DI et al: Hookworm *(Necator americanus)* infection and storage iron depletion, *Trans R Soc Trop Med Hyg* 85:235, 1991.

Leishmaniasis

Gustafson TL et al: Human cutaneous leishmaniasis acquired in Texas, *Am J Trop Med Hyg* 34:58, 1985.

Melby PC et al: Cutaneous leishmaniasis: review of 59 cases seen at the National Institutes of Health, *Clin Infect Dis* 15:924, 1992.

Modabber F: Leishmaniasis, *Tropical Disease Research Progress 1991-92 Report,* 1993, p 77.

Pearson RD et al: The immunobiology of leishmaniasis, *Rev Infect Dis* 5:907, 1983.

Scott JAG et al: Aminosidine (paromomycin) in the treatment of leishmaniasis imported into the United Kingdom, *Trans R Soc Trop Med Hyg* 86:617, 1992.

Onchocerciasis

Gibson DW, Heggie C, Connor DH: Clinical and pathologic aspects of onchocerciasis, *Pathol Annu* 15:195, 1980.

Gibson DW, Connor DH: Onchocercal lymphadenitis: clinicopathologic study of 34 patients, *Trans R Soc Trop Med Hyg* 72:137, 1978.

Perez JR: Human onchocerciasis foci and vectors in the American tropics and subtropics, *PAHO Bulletin* 20:381, 1986.

Ramachandran CP: Lymphatic filariasis and onchocerciasis, *Tropical Disease Research Progress 1991-92 Report,* 1993, p 37.

Schistosomiasis

Cook JA, Mecaskey JW: A look ahead in research and control of schistosomiasis, *Rhode Island Medicine* 75:217, 1992.

De Cock KM: Hepatosplenic schistosomiasis: a clinical review, *Gut* 27:734, 1986.

H el Kouni M: Chemotherapy of schistosomiasis, *Rhode Island Medicine* 75:212, 1992.

Jarallah JS et al: Role of primary health care in the control of schistosomiasis, *Trop Geogr Med* 45:297, 1993.

Lucey DR, Maguire JH: Schisotsomiasis, *Infect Dis Clin North Am* 7:635, 1993.

Strickland TG et al: Clinical characteristics and response to therapy in Egyptian children heavily infected with *Schistosoma mansoni, J Infect Dis* 146:20, 1982.

Wiest PM, Olds GR: Clinical schistosomiasis, *Rhode Island Medicine* 75:170, 1992.

Tapeworm

Groll E: Praziquantel for cestode infections in man, *Acta Trop* 37:293, 1980.

Sotelo H, Guerrero V, Rubio F: Neurocysticercosis: a new classification based on active and inactive forms, *Arch Intern Med* 145:442, 1985.

Toxoplasmosis

Kagen LJ, Kimball AC, Christian CL: Serologic evidence of toxoplasmosis among patients with polymyositis, *Am J Med* 56:186, 1974.

MacLeod C, editor: *Parasitic infections in pregnancy and the newborn,* New York, 1988, Oxford Medical Publishing.

McCabe RE et al: Clinical spectrum in 107 cases of toxoplasmic lymphadenopathy, *Rev Infect Dis* 9:754, 1987.

Nussenblatt RB, Belfort R: Ocular toxoplasmosis, *JAMA* 271:304, 1994.

Sun T, editor: *Progress in clinical parasitology,* vol 3, New York, 1993, Springer-Verlag.

Wanke C et al: Toxoplasma encephalitis in patients with acquired immune deficiency syndrome: diagnosis and response therapy, *Am J Trop Med Hyg* 36:509, 1987.

Trichinosis

Compton SJ et al: Trichinosis with ventilatory failure and persistent myocarditis, *Clin Infect Dis* 16:500, 1993.

Ellrodt A et al: Multifocal central nervous system lesions in three patients with trichinosis, *Arch Neurol* 44:432, 1987.

Stehr-Green JK, Schantz PM: Trichinosis in Southeast Asian refugees in the United States, *Am J Public Health* 76:1238, 1986.

242 Pectus Excavatum and Pectus Carinatum

J. Alex Haller, Jr.

Significant chest wall deformities in children may cause physiological, structural, and cosmetic problems that often require surgical correction. If 100 children who have chest wall deformities are referred for surgical evaluation, the most common abnormality is pectus excavatum (funnel chest) (90%); many fewer (about 6%) have pectus carinatum (pigeon or chicken breast) (Figs. 242-1 and 242-2). The remaining chest wall deformities include Poland syndrome,[6] Cantrell syndrome,[4] and Jeune syndrome.[5,11,12] While not thought to be genetic, the exact cause of these chest deformities is unclear. The primary defect in pectus excavatum and pectus carinatum is due to an overgrowth of the length of the anterior costal cartilages. This cartilaginous tissue, for some reason, appears to grow excessively and distorts the entire chest wall, either by holding the sternum posteriorly (pectus excavatum) or by thrusting it anteriorly (pectus carinatum). For pectus excavatum the overgrowth of the ribs occurs in utero; therefore a sunken chest usually is noted at birth or shortly thereafter. Overgrowth in pectus carinatum usually occurs during the pubertal growth spurts; therefore this diagnosis is made most frequently in early adolescence. The cartilage in both conditions appears to be histologically normal.

The surgical repair of both these abnormalities involves removal of the overgrown rib cartilage, which allows the sternum to be repositioned.[8-11] The cartilage then regenerates from the remaining perichondrium. The chest wall is healed solidly and is fully stable after 6 to 8 weeks. Only then can children safely be released to full activity, including contact sports.

A major difficulty in assessing chest wall deformities in children is deciding which of them requires surgical correction. Unfortunately, no absolute criteria prevail. The physician should evaluate each child frequently so as to monitor chest wall growth and development. Sequential evaluations include (1) measurement, with calipers, of the anteroposterior diameter of the chest and (2) determination of any limitation of central thoracic expansion, of abnormalities in posture, and of structural changes in the upper portion of the abdomen.

PECTUS EXCAVATUM

The vast majority of chest wall deformities seen by primary care physicians are some variation of pectus excavatum. If the deformity is severe, it should be repaired in early childhood for three important reasons: (1) chest wall growth and development will be abnormal if correction is not effected; (2) pulmonary and cardiac function will be affected adversely during adolescence, even though this may not be apparent during childhood; and (3) the cosmetic abnormality will be of increasing concern to the patient. A cosmetic concern is not the primary indication for repairing a pectus excavatum deformity because the structural deformity must be significant enough in and of itself to require intervention.

With pectus excavatum a significant structural problem is considered to be present if the depression is greater than 2 cm. Such measurements, however, often are not absolute. By the time a child reaches 5 to 6 years of age, deformities severe enough to cause difficulties usually are obvious. Fortunately, this is early enough to alleviate secondary cosmetic concerns, and the condition can be repaired before any significant psychological problems associated with the deformity occur.

Physiological derangement in breathing and cardiac function can be documented in teenagers and young adults who have severe deformities,[1,2] but such derangements are more difficult to demonstrate in children because of the invasiveness of the evaluative procedures.[3,13] In severe forms of pectus excavatum, the heart is shifted laterally in the left hemithorax, and thoracic compliance is compromised; these changes are reversible, however, if the repair is effected before adolescence. The pectus excavatum deformity should be repaired before the teenage growth spurt if normal growth and development of the chest wall are to be achieved. Thereafter the deformity can be corrected cosmetically to a certain degree, but the basic abnormal chest wall configuration and posture is not altered. The surgeon can employ some plastic surgical procedures to fill the defect with prosthetic material and provide cosmetic correction, but these methods do not correct the physiological and structural aberrations.

Waiting until a child reaches 5 to 6 years of age before performing elective repair of pectus excavatum is important so that the child is more mature emotionally and thus may have a better hospital experience and, to some extent, may participate in the decision for surgical repair of the deformity. Even for young children, alterations in the configuration of the body may affect their perceptions of their body image significantly in later years. Postoperative management of 5- to 6-year-olds is far easier than that of 2- to 3-year-olds, and earlier repair has no technical surgical advantage. Moreover, a 5- to 6-year-old can avoid trauma and rough-house activities better in the postoperative healing period of 6 to 8 weeks than can a young child.

The surgical correction has become standardized in most children's centers.[9,14] The operation essentially is bloodless when electrocoagulation is used, and blood transfusions are not needed. The operation, nevertheless, is *major* because it requires 3 hours of anesthesia followed by considerable discomfort, requiring intravenous sedation and analgesia. Children recover within 48 hours and usually are discharged by the fourth or fifth day after surgery.

Surgery yields excellent results in more than 95% of patients. Long-term results remain good, with a low 1% to 2%

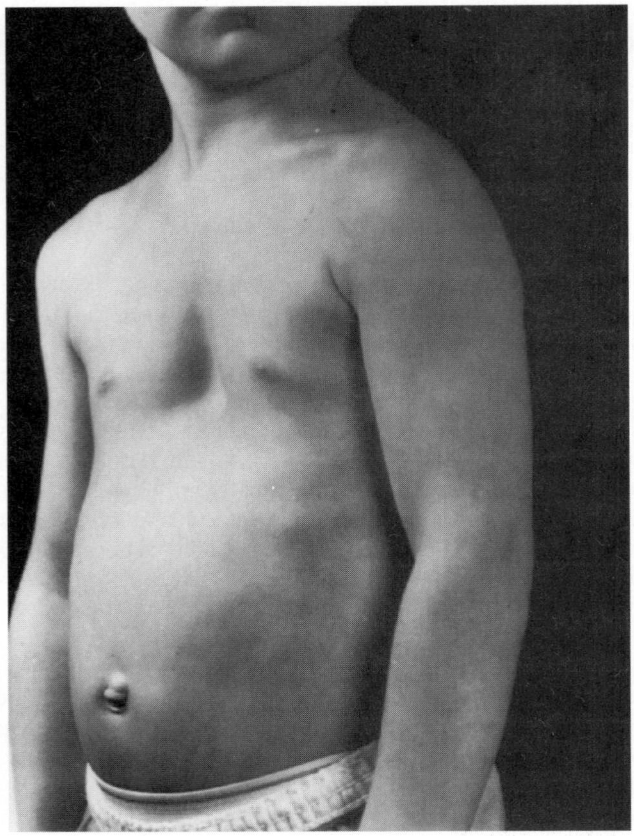

FIG. 242-1 Pectus excavatum.

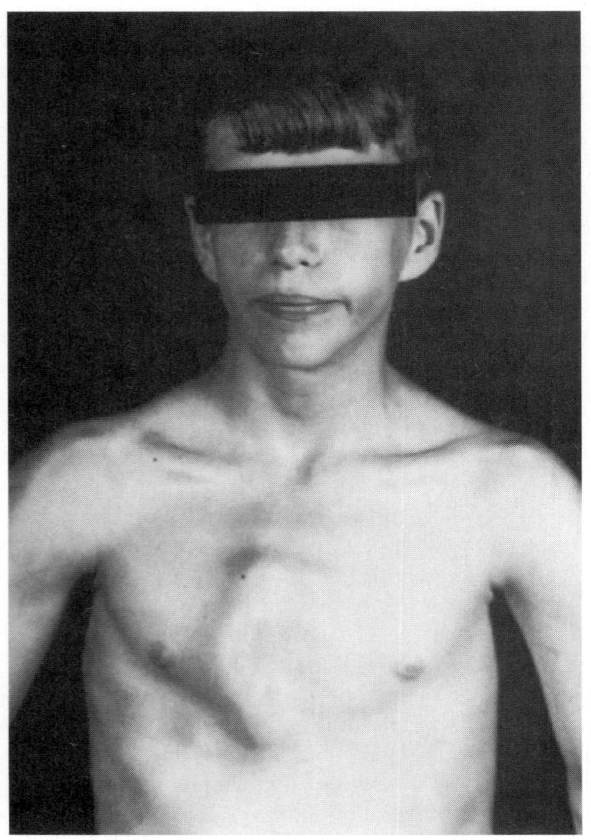

FIG. 242-2 Pectus carinatum.

recurrence rate during adolescence. Complications are extremely uncommon; they include (1) collection of serosanguineous fluid in the substernal and subcutaneous spaces (which is avoided by plastic drains connected to suction), (2) infection (which is avoided by careful sterile technique and prophylactic antibiotics for 48 hours), and (3) bleeding (which is controlled with electrocoagulation). None of these is life threatening. The only postoperative precaution necessary is avoidance of vigorous activities (including contact sports) for 6 to 8 weeks until the cartilages have all regenerated. A postoperative patient may be swimming and jogging in 2 weeks.

PECTUS CARINATUM

Pectus carinatum is much less common than is pectus excavatum, occurring in only 6% of all children who have chest wall deformities. It also appears to result from overgrowth of the involved costal cartilages, which push the sternum into an exaggerated anterior position. Unlike pectus excavatum, which usually is noted in infancy, carinatum deformities occur during rapid pubertal growth. This abnormality is purely cosmetic and does not appear to be associated with any physiological abnormality. Unlike pectus excavatum deformities, recurrence of pectus carinatum is likely after repair in early childhood because of subsequent chest wall growth in which the regenerated cartilage replicates the initial abnormal growth pattern. Therefore surgery should be delayed until the patient is 15 or 16 years old, when maximal growth generally has occurred and the deformity can be corrected with little chance of recurrence. The surgical procedure for the correction of pectus carinatum consists of removing the abnormal costal cartilages and repositioning the sternum posteriorly by means of a transverse osteotomy.[11] Healing occurs within 6 to 8 weeks; the patient then can participate in active contact sports.

REFERENCES

1. Beiser GD et al: Impairment of cardiac function in patients with pectus excavatum, with improvement after operative correction, *N Engl J Med* 287:267, 1972.
2. Bevegard S: Postural circulatory changes at rest and during exercise in patients with funnel chest, with special reference to factors affecting the stroke volume, *Acta Med Scand* 171:695, 1962.
3. Cahill JL, Lees GM, Robertson HT: A summary of preoperative and postoperative cardiorespiratory performance in patients undergoing pectus excavatus and carinatum repair, *J Pediatr Surg* 19:430, 1984.
4. Cantrell JR, Haller JA Jr, Ravitch MM: A syndrome of congenital defects involving the abdominal wall, sternum, diaphragm, pericardium, and heart, *Surg Gynecol Obstet,* 107:602, 1958.
5. Finegold MJ et al: Lung structure in thoracic dystrophy: case reports, *Am J Dis Child* 122:153, 1971.
6. Haller JA Jr et al: Early reconstruction of Poland's syndrome using autologous rib grafts combined with a latissimus muscle flap, *J Pediatr Surg* 19:423, 1984.
7. Haller JA Jr et al: Correction of pectus excavatus without prostheses or splints: objective measurement of severity and management of asymmetrical deformities, *Ann Thorac Surg* 26:78, 1978.
8. Haller JA et al: Evolving management of pectus excavatum based on a single institutional experience of 664 patients, *Ann Surg* 209:578, 1989.
9. Haller JA et al: Operative correction of pectus excavatum: an evolving perspective, *Ann Surg* 184:554, 1976.

10. Haller JA et al: Pectus carinatum: results of surgical therapy, *J Pediatr Surg* 14:228, 1979.
11. Hull D, Barnes ND: Children with small chests, *Arch Dis Child* 47:12, 1972.
12. Jeune M, Beraud C, Carron R: Dystrophic thoracique asphysiante de caractere familial, *Arch Fr Pediatr* 12:886, 1955.
13. Peterson RJ, Young WG, Goodwin JD: Noninvasive assessment of exercise cardiac function before and after pectus excavatus repair, *J Thorac Cardiovasc Surg* 90:215, 1985.
14. Ravitch MM: *Congenital deformities of the chest wall and their operative correction,* Philadelphia, 1977, WB Saunders.

243 Pertussis (Whooping Cough)

Fred J. Heldrich

Few illnesses have a clinical picture as characteristic as pertussis. At the height of the illness, the harsh, persistent cough occurring in paroxysms and ending with an inspiratory whoop and vomiting certainly suggests pertussis as the most probable diagnosis. Although undoubtedly a disease of antiquity, pertussis was first described in 1906 by Bordet and Gengou, who associated it with the *Bordetella pertussis* organism. Although pertussis is one of the communicable diseases of childhood that can be prevented with proper immunization, it nonetheless still occurs, usually in preschool-age children. The reported incidence and the severity of the disease remain highest in patients under 1 year of age. Adolescents and adults who have waning immunity may develop a clinical illness that is not recognized and continue to serve as a reservoir for infecting nonimmunized or partially immunized infants and children.

A well-documented decline in levels of pertussis immunization led to an increased incidence in pertussis in several countries, including the United States,[1,2,12] where the annual incidence rose from 0.82 per 100,000 population in 1982 to 1.74 per 100,000 in 1986.[4] In 1991 the incidence was 1.1 per 100,000, perhaps reflecting an improvement in pertussis immunization efforts.[9] However, unless immunization policies continue to be implemented, outbreaks of pertussis will continue.

ETIOLOGY

B. pertussis, a motile gram negative rod, is the etiological agent in most cases. A special medium (Bordet-Gengou) and special care in obtaining the specimen of this fastidious organism are required to obtain a positive culture. Either coughing directly onto the culture medium or inoculating the medium directly from a nasopharyngeal swab gives the best results. Of the two methods, the nasopharyngeal culture is preferred, especially for younger patients. The direct fluorescent antibody (DFA) test is a more sensitive and rapid diagnostic procedure. It increases the possibility of laboratory confirmation.[1,2,13]

PATHOLOGY

The area involved is the respiratory epithelium, extending from the upper respiratory tract to the trachea, bronchi, and bronchioles. Histologically the organisms are lodged in the cilia of the epithelial cells, with underlying epithelial cell changes consisting of edema and necrosis; also, inflammatory cells infiltrate the interstitial tissues. A mucopurulent exudate, which may cover the respiratory epithelium, can lead to airflow obstruction. Alveolar exudate is thought to be caused by secondary bacterial invasion. The ability of pertussis to elaborate an endotoxin may be responsible for lymphocytic predominance in the peripheral blood count, local tissue damage, and hypoglycemia.

CLINICAL PRESENTATION

Typically the child who has pertussis progresses through three stages, characterized by varying symptoms and clinical severity: the catarrhal stage, the acute stage, and the stage of convalescence. Each stage lasts approximately 2 weeks. The illness may extend longer than the usual 6 weeks, especially the acute stage. In such instances, other causes of persistent cough should be seriously considered and sought.

The incubation period is from 7 to 14 days, with an average of 10 days. The illness is ushered in with symptoms of a "cold"—sneezing, rhinitis, lacrimation, and cough. The cough soon becomes more pronounced than is customary with the usual cold and becomes a dominant feature by the end of the first week. Fever, if present, usually is low grade. Systemic, nonspecific symptoms of malaise and anorexia also are seen.

Unless exposure to pertussis is known, the diagnosis may not be seriously considered until the second week of illness or until the cough has become more persistent and annoying. The cough occurs in bursts or paroxysms and has been described as harsh, dry, irritating, and rapid. It accompanies the expiratory phase of respiration and may be especially prominent at night, disturbing the child's (and the parents') sleep. When these bursts of explosive coughing increase in frequency and are followed by an exaggerated inspiratory effort or "whoop," the acute, or paroxysmal, stage has begun.

When coughing is of this magnitude, the patient also shows signs of respiratory distress. The face becomes suffused and red or cyanotic. Neck veins become more prominent, and the child becomes alarmed and anxious. The face appears swollen, the eyes prominent. The tongue may protrude, and perspiration may be profuse. The child vomits thick, tenacious material and may appear to be "strangling." Facial petechiae, conjunctival hemorrhage, and epistaxis may occur because of the severe coughing episodes. Paroxysms may last 10 to 15 seconds; after these episodes the child frequently is exhausted and obtunded. The frequency of these paroxysmal outbursts may range from several per day to several per hour and may be precipitated by eating or drinking. External stimuli such as smoke, examination of the pharynx, or pressure on the trachea also may precipitate the attack. In younger patients the inspiratory whoops may be absent; however, these patients are at risk for respiratory arrest and may require resuscitation.

After approximately 2 weeks of severe distress (by the fourth week of illness), symptoms begin to abate; the vomiting and whoop clear first. By the sixth week the cough usually has diminished markedly and, barring complications, the patient is well on the way to recovery. After recovery the patient may experience bouts of paroxysmal coughing, with further episodes of respiratory tract infection for the next few months or longer.[7]

Partial immunity provided by inadequate primary immunization or a prolonged interval since immunization, leading to a deficiency in immunological protection, may produce an atypical or attenuated form of illness characterized primarily by a persistent cough.

The physical examination in patients whose pertussis is uncomplicated may reveal, in addition to signs of upper respiratory tract infection, a low-grade fever and, on auscultation of the lungs, rhonchi.

LABORATORY FINDINGS

Success in culturing *B. pertussis* from the nasopharynx is greatest in the prodromal stage of the illness. A cotton swab wrapped on an aluminum wire allows easy access to the nasopharynx. Positive growth of the organism on a Bordet-Gengou plate should occur in 3 days; it can be identified by the use of specific antiserums to produce agglutination. Pertussis may be diagnosed rapidly by the direct fluorescent antibody test (DFA) or by the enzyme-linked immunosorbent assay (ELISA).[2,8] The most distinctive, though nonspecific, finding is a marked leukocytosis, with over 50% of the cells being lymphocytes. When associated with a cough, a total white blood count greater than 20,000 strongly suggests pertussis. The total white count may rise as high as 100,000, with as many as 90% lymphocytes.

Acute and convalescent serums may be compared if there is doubt about the diagnosis and should demonstrate a rise in pertussis antibody titers; this test, however, is most useful for a retrospective assessment of the illness and most often is not necessary. Ten to fourteen days should elapse between the collection of specimens.

COMPLICATIONS

Death from pertussis, although extremely rare today, is most likely to occur in infants. Permanent damage to the lung may lead to bronchiectasis. Bronchopneumonia, usually resulting from secondary invaders, is the most common complication. Although petechiae or purpura, subconjunctival lesions, or epistaxis may occur secondary to the increase in venous pressure associated with the paroxysmal cough, intracranial hemorrhage is a more ominous complication. Another central nervous system complication, an encephalopathy, may occur. Although its exact cause is unknown, some have suggested that it may result from hypoxemia or hypoglycemia. Inguinal hernias and rectal prolapse also have been reported.

DIFFERENTIAL DIAGNOSIS

Conditions to be considered and ruled out by history, physical examination, and appropriate laboratory studies are chlamydial pneumonia, a pertussis-like syndrome caused by other infectious agents, foreign body aspiration, paratracheal lymph node enlargement, and allergic cough. A functional cause also must be considered. Although not an extensive list, these conditions share a common feature—a persistent, irritating cough.

Chlamydial Pneumonia

Frequently found in infants, chlamydial pneumonia is characterized by a dry, staccato-like cough and a chest roentgenogram that reveals pneumonic infiltrates. Patients usually are afebrile. The past history may indicate a chlamydia conjunctivitis perhaps not treated with parenteral antibiotics. Eosinophilia may be noted on the peripheral smear. Chlamydiae can be grown on tissue culture from respiratory tract secretions. A serological study reveals an elevated antibody titer.

Other Infectious Agents

The adenovirus has been associated with a clinical syndrome indistinguishable from pertussis. Other organisms that may produce an illness similar to pertussis include *Mycoplasma pneumoniae, Bordetella parapertussis,* and *Bordetella bronchiseptica*. Marked lymphocytosis usually is not found.

Foreign Body Aspiration

Although a history of aspiration does not always apply, a definite choking episode usually ushers in this condition. Localized changes may appear on the chest roentgenogram secondary to obstruction, or the foreign body may be radiopaque and easily visualized.

Paratracheal Lymph Nodes

If paratracheal lymph nodes are enlarged, diseases such as tuberculosis, histoplasmosis, infectious mononucleosis, or malignancies of the reticuloendothelial system must be considered.

Allergic Cough

In the allergic individual, a persistent, irritating cough may be the earliest manifestation of bronchospasm. A family history of allergy or a history of allergic manifestations in the patient should strengthen the diagnostic suspicion. Upper respiratory tract symptoms, such as clear nasal discharge, sneezing, conjunctivitis, or "allergic shiners," also may be suggestive. Frequently the serum IgE level will be elevated. A therapeutic trial with a bronchodilator will relieve symptoms and thus confirm the diagnosis.

TREATMENT

Supportive care is the mainstay of therapy for the acute phase of pertussis. The patient should be disturbed as little as possible. The paroxysms of coughing, especially in younger patients, may necessitate the removal of secretions via aspiration. Hypoxia, as manifested by cyanosis, may indicate a need for oxygen. Optimum hydration and adequate nutrition usually can be maintained by frequent but small feedings. In infants, intravenous fluid therapy may be required.

Erythromycin, the antibiotic of choice, has been shown to reduce the frequency and severity of coughing and also has been shown to reduce the period during which *B. pertussis* can be recovered from the respiratory tract.[5] In very young infants, periods of apnea may require intubation and assisted ventilation.

While not yet commercially available, intravenous immunoglobulin containing a high level of antitoxin has been given to children who have pertussis and has reduced the severity of illness.[11] Fortunately, a whole cell vaccine is available for active immunization and, when administered at appropriate intervals, affords excellent protection. Routine immunization procedures call for pertussis vaccination—usually combined with diphtheria and tetanus (DPT)—at 2 months, 4 months, and 6 months of age.[10] In the event of a community outbreak, immunization may be started at 2 weeks of age.

Graduates of intensive care nurseries who had chronic pulmonary disease are at great risk of significant morbidity or mortality should they develop pertussis. For these infants, pertussis immunization should be initiated when they are 2 months old, even while in the hospital.[6]

The risk of complications secondary to routine use of pertussis vaccine has recently been reevaluated, and the benefits with proper use of the vaccine greatly outweigh the risks; thus its continued use is warranted.[3]

An acellular pertussis vaccine now is available and recommended for doses four and five of the DPT series for children older than 15 months and younger than 7 years of age. This vaccine reduces side effects and produces effective immunity; however, insufficient data are available to warrant its use in the primary series.[8] Evidence is accumulating that indicates that a pertussis vaccine containing only inactivated pertussis toxoid would be a superior vaccine both to provide immunity and to reduce side effects.[11]

Complications of the disease require specific therapy. Antibiotics should be prescribed for secondary bacterial infections such as pneumonia or otitis media. Bronchial aspiration may be required to relieve segmental atelectasis. Pneumothorax secondary to obstructive emphysema caused by tenacious secretions in the bronchial tree may necessitate the use of closed-tube drainage. Ventilatory assistance may be required for infants who sustain prolonged intervals of apnea and hypoxia. Patients may develop seizures because of tetany precipitated by alkalosis, which is caused by severe vomiting. Correction of blood pH abnormalities is indicated. Direct damage to the central nervous system by anoxia or hemorrhage may occur and requires anticonvulsant medication.

Although the prognosis for those few patients who acquire the infection is good, the proper management is prevention, and this can be accomplished by adhering to recommended immunization schedules.

REFERENCES

1. Broome CV, Fraser DW: Pertussis in the United States, 1979: a look at vaccine efficacy, *J Infect Dis* 144:187, 1981.
2. Centers for Disease Control: Pertussis: Maryland, 1982, *MMWR* 32:297, 1983.
3. Cody CL et al: Nature and rates of adverse reactions associated with DPT and DT immunizations in infants and children, *Pediatrics* 68:650, 1981.
4. Fulginiti VA: The current state of pertussis and pertussis vaccines, *Am J Dis Child* 143:532, 1989.
5. Hoppe JE et al: Comparison of erythromycin estolate and erythromycin ethylsuccinate for treatment of pertussis, *Pediatr Infect Dis J* 11:189, 1992.
6. Koblen BA et al: Response of preterm infants to diphtheria-tetanus-pertussis vaccine, *Pediatr Infect Dis J* 7:704, 1988.
7. Krugman S, Katz SL, editors: Pertussis (whooping cough). In *Infectious diseases of children,* ed 8, St Louis, 1985, Mosby.
8. Mertsola J et al: Serologic diagnosis of pertussis: comparison of enzyme linked immunosorbent assay and bacterial agglutination, *J Infect Dis* 147:252, 1983.
9. Pertussis surveillance—United States, 1989-1991, *MMWR* 42, 1993.
10. *Report of the Committee on Infectious Diseases (Red Book),* ed 21, Evanston, Ill, 1988, American Academy of Pediatrics.
11. Robbins JB et al: Primum non nocere: a pharmacologically inert pertussis toxoid alone should be the next pertussis vaccine, *Pediatr Infect Dis J* 12:795, 1993.
12. Robinson RJ: The whooping cough immunization controversy, *Arch Dis Child* 56:577, 1981.
13. Strebel PM et al: Pertussis in Missouri: evaluation of nasopharyngeal (NP) culture, direct fluorescent antibody (DFA) testing and clinical case definitions in the diagnosis of pertussis, *Clin Inf Dis* 16:276, 1993.

244 Pharyngitis and Tonsillitis

Philip E. Thuma

Acute pharyngitis is one of the diagnoses made most frequently by pediatricians, exceeded only by otitis media and generalized upper respiratory tract infections. The term *pharyngitis* means an infection or inflammation of the throat; when the tonsils are affected the most, the term *tonsillitis* is more appropriate. Pharyngitis may be associated with other inflammatory conditions of the mucous membranes or may be the sole finding in an illness. Generally, a clinical complaint of sore throat indicates some degree of pharyngitis, even though this may not be the main focus of the illness.

ETIOLOGY

While pharyngitis can occur in any age group, it is diagnosed most frequently in children between the ages of 6 and 8 years, when group A beta-hemolytic streptococcal (GABHS) disease is prevalent (Fig. 244-1). In younger children, especially those below the age of 2 years, GABHS is uncommon, and viruses predominate. Data originating from an office practice[3] over 25 years ago demonstrated that 25% to 50% of school-age children who had pharyngitis were culture positive for GABHS; subsequent studies have shown a wide range in the incidence of GABHS. The cause of pharyngitis varies somewhat; depending on the geographical location and season of the year, GABHS, respiratory viruses, or other organisms, such as Mycoplasma, may predominate. In addition to these, many other infectious—as well as some noninfectious— agents have been associated with pharyngitis.

Viruses

Although many practitioners associate pharyngitis and tonsillitis with a bacterial infection, viruses still play a major role in the cause of these illnesses. In fact, whenever pharyngitis is associated with symptoms of nasal congestion and rhinorrhea, viral infection is the most likely cause.[1]

Adenoviruses. At least 12 different types of adenoviruses have been found to cause pharyngitis in children and adolescents, accounting for up to 23% of cases of pharyngitis in some reports.[10] These viruses cause both a nasopharyngitis and a tonsillitis that can be exudative. Outbreaks of a pharyngo-conjunctival fever caused by adenovirus type 3 also have been reported and often are accompanied by a high fever, cough, and myalgias, in addition to pharyngitis and conjunctivitis.

Enteroviruses. Two prominent members of this class of virus, coxsackie A and echovirus, have been shown to cause pharyngitis, often accompanied by respiratory symptoms, commonly in the late summer or early fall. Herpangina is a specific entity caused by coxsackie A, leading to pharyngitis associated with small shallow ulcerated areas on the soft palate and peritonsillar area.

Epstein-Barr Virus. This etiological agent of infectious mononucleosis characteristically causes a rather severe exudative pharyngitis and tonsillitis. In older children this is accompanied by fever, adenopathy, and malaise, as well as splenomegaly in some cases.

Herpes Simplex. Although traditionally believed to cause only "cold sores," this virus can cause a gingivostomatitis and pharyngitis upon initial infection in infants. More recent studies also have documented that it is a not infrequent cause of pharyngitis in adolescents,[9] accounting for 5.7% of pharyngitis in a college-age population.

Other Viruses. Many other viral infections cause a pharyngitis, although it usually is not the primary manifestation of the illness. These include influenza A and B, parainfluenza types 1-4, RSV, polio, cytomegalovirus, reoviruses, measles, rubella, rhinoviruses, and rotavirus.[1]

Bacteria

One of the main considerations in evaluating a child who has pharyngitis and tonsillitis is to determine whether the cause is bacterial, thus requiring specific antibiotic therapy. Group A beta-hemolytic streptococcal infections are the major bacterial cause, but other organisms also should be considered and perhaps sought in certain situations.

Streptococcus Pyogenes. This bacterium causes complete hemolysis when grown on blood agar and hence has been named beta-hemolytic. In addition, it has been subdivided into groups based on the C-substance in the cell wall, and it has been found that most human pathological disease is caused by the A group. GABHS was not fully recognized as a frequent cause of pharyngitis with the possibility of subsequent rheumatic fever until the 1940s. Whereas other groups of streptococcus (B, C, F, and G) have been associated at times with pharyngitis,[2] group A is by far the most frequent bacterial cause, accounting for 35% to 40% of cases (Fig. 244-2). The GABHS can be divided into M and T serotypes, and certain of these have been associated with both the rash of scarlet fever (T4)[11] and the development of rheumatic fever (M3 and M18).[5]

The pharyngitis caused by GABHS characteristically begins after a 2- to 5-day incubation period, usually following exposure to another individual who has the infection. Spread is thought to be by way of respiratory secretions, although fomites, such as shared silverware or household pets, have been shown to be vectors. The ingestion of GABHS-contaminated food also has led to outbreaks of pharyngitis. The illness is heralded by sudden onset of fever, sore throat, and dysphagia, often associated with headache and abdominal pain. Examination of the throat reveals an erythematous pharynx and tonsillar area, often with exudate present. Small petechiae (enanthem) sometimes are seen on the uvula and soft palate. Cervical lymph nodes usually are enlarged and quite tender. These symptoms can last for 4 days and gradually subside, even if no antibiotic therapy is instituted.

Neisseria Gonorrhoea. Pharyngitis in sexually active adolescents or sexually abused children can be caused by gonorrhea acquired from oral sex and should be looked for where appropriate.

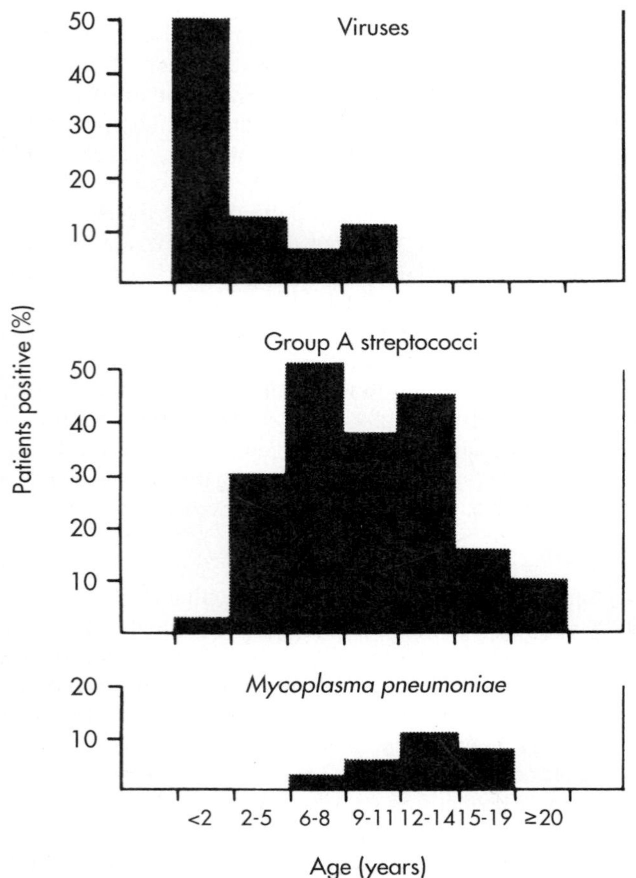

FIG. 244-1 Recovery of microbial agents from persons with pharyngitis, by age.

(From Glezen WP et al: *JAMA* 202:457, 1967.)

***Hemophilus Influenzae* Type B (HIB).** The possible involvement of this organism in pharyngitis and tonsillitis has been controversial, but recent evidence suggests that it may contribute to infection in some children. Fine needle aspiration of tonsils during acute tonsillitis and pathological specimens from tonsillectomy have documented that as many as 20% of tonsils have *HIB* infection.[13,14] However, with HIB immunization of most infants in the United States in recent years, this organism is much less likely to play a role in the pathogenesis of acute tonsillitis and pharyngitis.

Other Bacteria. A century ago, Corynebacterium diphtheria was a frequent and deadly cause of pharyngitis, with a characteristic gray pseudomembranous exudate over the posterior pharynx and tonsils. Fortunately, this now is quite rare in North America, although it still is seen in some developing countries. Various reports have been published of other bacteria causing pharyngitis and tonsillitis, including *Actinomyces, Arcanobacterium* (Corynebacterium) *haemolyticus,*[7] *Chlamydia trachomatis, Yersinia enterocolitica,* and *Francisella tularensis,* the organism that causes tularemia.

Other Causes

Mycoplasma. Two types of mycoplasma have been shown to cause pharyngitis, namely *M. pneumonia* and *M. hominis.* In children, the former causes a mild pharyngitis, often associated with a laryngotracheitis or progressing to a bronchitis or pneumonia. In school-age children, as much as 5% of pharyngitis may be caused by this organism.

Fungi. Candida is an uncommon cause of pharyngitis but certainly can be so in immunocompromised patients or those taking steroids.

Parasites. Toxoplasma gondii is a rare cause of pharyngitis, but the exact incidence of this is unclear.

Kawasaki Disease. This illness of unknown cause manifests mostly in preschool children who have pharyngitis, associated with erythema and fissuring of the lips, as well as with palmar and pedal edema and erythema. An association with staphylococcal toxin has been postulated.[8]

Exposure to Cigarette Smoke. While smoke itself has not been reported to cause pharyngitis or tonsillitis, a recent study has shown a highly significant association between the inci-

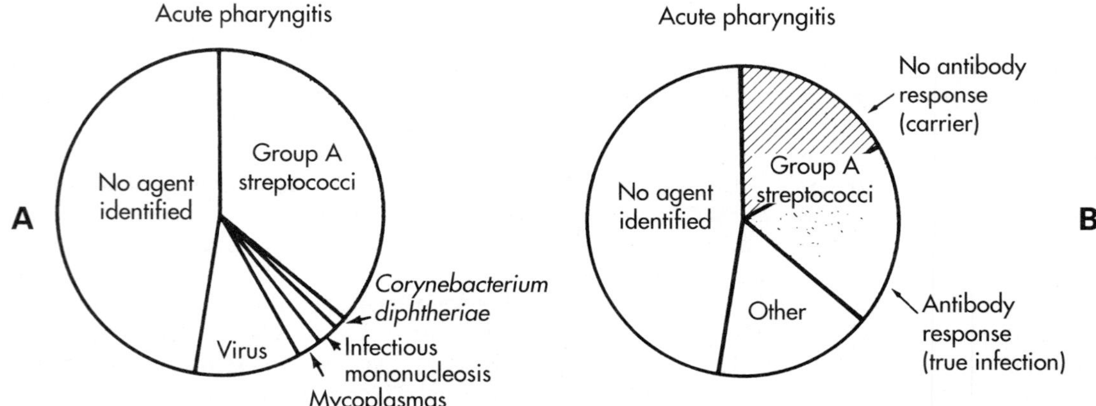

FIG. 244-2 **A,** Proportion of acute pharyngitis associated with various microbial agents. **B,** Proportion of children with clinical pharyngitis who develop a streptococcal antibody response.

(From Wannamaker LW: *Am J Dis Child* 124:353, 1972.)

dence of tonsillectomy in children and parental smoking.[4] These children also had a much higher frequency of attacks of acute tonsillitis compared with those children in a smoke-free environment. Whether this association will be confirmed in other studies remains to be seen, but among children seeking treatment for frequent tonsillitis, a history of parental smoking should be sought. If such a history exists, the physician would be prudent to recommend measures to reduce the child's exposure to cigarette smoke.

DIFFERENTIAL DIAGNOSIS

Because sore throats are so common in pediatric practice, the astute clinician should determine those caused by GABHS because this is the most common reason for needing antibiotic therapy. Unfortunately, multiple studies have been unable to document that so-called strep throats can be recognized on purely clinical grounds. Streptococcal infections should be considered in children over the age of 2 years who have pharyngitis, even if no exudate is present. However, pharyngitis associated with nasal, chest, or "cold" symptoms is much more likely a viral illness.

When a pharyngitis is atypical, either in its duration or its severity, the clinician should suspect infectious mononucleosis or one of the rarer bacterial causes, including those that are sexually transmitted. A peritonsillar abscess or cellulitis also may manifest as a sore throat, but careful examination will reveal swelling extending into the soft palate with deviation of the uvula and a change in the tonal quality of the voice. Allergies may lead to chronic inflammation of the mucous membranes, which could include the pharynx, but this would be infrequent as a sole manifestation. Postnasal drip from a viral respiratory tract infection or allergies has been thought to irritate the posterior pharynx, but this is not well documented.

The one entity in the differential diagnosis not to be missed is epiglottitis, which can be life-threatening. Generally, the child who has epiglottitis has severe throat pain, rapidly becomes ill, having a toxic condition, and experiences respiratory distress accompanied by stridor or a croupy cough. (See Chapter 279, Epiglottitis.)

MANAGEMENT

Laboratory Procedures

Rapid Streptococcal Test and Cultures. The traditional method for determining whether a pharyngitis or tonsillitis was caused by a virus or by GABHS was to take a throat swab and do a culture. Many pediatricians' offices had a candle jar incubator in which many culture plates were placed and bacitracin discs applied daily and read the following morning. Fortunately, with the availability of "rapid strep" tests, this process was made simpler, allowing a result to be obtained in minutes, rather than waiting 1 to 2 days. Unfortunately, with the advent of strict federal guidelines for office laboratories, even the use of these rapid tests requires certification. Despite such encumbrances, most clinicians now perform a rapid strep diagnostic test on all patients whose pharyngitis is suggestive of GABHS.

The various rapid strep tests claim differing levels of specificity and sensitivity. Most all of them (95% to 98%) appear to be rather specific, but their sensitivity can be as low as 70% to 85%, so some cases of GABHS are not detected. For this reason, a positive rapid strep screen generally is thought to be a sufficient indication to treat the patient. However, if it is negative, a culture should be sent. The physician also needs to be aware that some strep carriers in the community (see Fig. 244-2) may well be found to be "strep positive" during a viral illness. Because doing pre- and post-illness titres on every child who presumably has GABHS pharyngitis is impractical, all those who are positive are treated.

Serological Tests. In cases where Epstein-Barr virus (EBV) infection is suspected, a heterophile antibody or specific EBV test can be ordered. One needs to ascertain with the reference laboratory whether an IgG or IgM test is done because a positive heterophile test may confirm only that the child was exposed sometime in his or her life to EBV. Specific IgG and IgM levels of antibody to various components of EBV are available but usually are rather expensive and may take many weeks to get results, making it a less than ideal test to determine the cause of an acute pharyngitis.

Although serological tests exist to determine recent streptococcal infections, they rarely are helpful in evaluating an acute pharyngitis. An antistreptolysin-O titre is used more commonly in diagnosing rheumatic fever, by documenting a recent exposure to streptolysin, with production of antibody.

White Blood Cell Count. The only real value in performing this test is if infectious mononucleosis is suspected. Patients who have an acute EBV infection tend to have a relative lymphocytosis with 10% to 20% atypical lymphocytes. Thus a blood count in a child who has a severe pharyngitis that is culture negative for GABHS may be a helpful diagnostic study, together with a heterophile or specific EBV antibody test.

Treatment

Pharyngitis caused by viruses generally is treated symptomatically with saline gargles, throat lozenges, and analgesics such as acetaminophen. When GABHS has been documented, either by a positive rapid strep test or by culture, antibiotics are indicated primarily to prevent the subsequent development of rheumatic fever. Various antibiotic regimens have been used for GABHS pharyngitis or tonsillitis, but the standard therapy has been a 10-day oral course of potassium penicillin V three or four times a day. Alternatively, intramuscular benzathine penicillin G may be given as a single injection, although these injections often are painful, not only initially but for a few days afterward. Patients allergic to penicillin may be given erythromycin or a first-generation cephalosporin (e.g., cephalexin), again for a full 10 days.

Controversy exists over whether to begin antibiotics for a presumptive GABHS pharyngitis while waiting for culture results. Because rheumatic fever can be prevented even if treatment is started as late as the ninth day of symptoms, the decision to begin therapy immediately rests with the individual physician who knows the circumstances of his or her patients. Although some practitioners believe that early antibiotic treatment will shorten the duration and severity of symptoms, this has not been well documented. What has been shown in a number of studies is that *communicability essentially is eliminated after 24 hours of antibiotic therapy.* Thus it generally is recommended that children not return to school or day care until they have been taking antibiotics for a full 24 hours. Recent data suggest that this rapid elimination of GABHS from the pharynx is more likely when oral or parenteral penicillin is used, rather than erythromycin.[12]

In cases of gonococcal pharyngitis, one intramuscular injection of ceftriaxone is recommended. In young children who have this diagnosis, the possibility of sexual abuse always must be entertained. Other possible bacterial infections are treated with appropriate antibiotics, once the causative organism has been found.

The question of tonsillectomy often is raised by parents after a child has more than one episode of pharyngitis or tonsillitis. Except in documented cases of recurrent, frequent streptococcal infection or the history of the development of a peritonsillar abscess, tonsillectomy is not indicated in children who have recurrent pharyngitis.

COMPLICATIONS

Most cases of pharyngitis present no unusual complications because so many of them are viral and resolve in spite of any therapy. However, the physician must be aware of the possibility of a peritonsillar or retropharyngeal abscess or cellulitis developing and should reexamine the throat of any patient who is not improving. Other suppurative complications also can develop, such as cervical adenitis, otitis media, sinusitis, and pneumonia. In addition, hematogenous spread of an organism is possible and can result in bacteremia, joint, bone, or meningeal infection.

Rheumatic fever (see Chapter 252) is the one complication of streptococcal pharyngitis that can be life threatening, although this occurs some time after the acute throat infection. Although the incidence of rheumatic fever is low in North America, it still occurs and has been seen in increasing numbers at some centers.[6] While acute glomerulonephritis is possible after streptococcal throat infections, it is much more likely after streptococcal skin infections.

REFERENCES

1. Cherry JD: Pharyngitis. In Feigin RD, Cherry JD, editors: *Textbook of pediatric infectious disease,* ed 2, Philadelphia, 1987, WB Saunders.
2. Dudley JP, Sercarz J: Pharyngeal and tonsil infections caused by non–group A streptococcus, *Am J Otol* 12:292, 1991.
3. Glezen WP et al: Group A streptococci, mycoplasmas and viruses associated with acute pharyngitis, *JAMA* 202:455, 1967.
4. Hinton AE et al: Parental cigarette smoking and tonsillectomy in children, *Clin Otolaryngol* 18:178, 1993.
5. Johnson DR, Stevens DL, Kaplan EL: Epidemiologic analysis of group A streptococcal serotypes associated with severe systemic infections, rheumatic fever, or uncomplicated pharyngitis, *J Infect Dis* 166:374, 1992.
6. Kaplan EL: Return of rheumatic fever: consequences, implications, and needs, *J Pediatr* 111:244, 1987.
7. Karpathios T et al: Arcanobacterium haemolyticum in children with presumed streptococcal pharyngotonsillitis or scarlet fever, *J Pediatr* 121:735, 1992.
8. Leung DYM et al: Toxic shock syndrome toxin-secreting staphylococcus aureus in Kawasaki syndrome, *Lancet* 342:1385, 1993.
9. McMillan JA et al: Pharyngitis associated with herpes simplex virus in college students, *Pediatr Infect Dis J* 12:280, 1993.
10. Moffet HL, Seigel AC, Doyle HK: Non-streptococcal pharyngitis, *J Pediatr* 73:51, 1985.
11. Ohga S et al: Outbreaks of group A beta-hemolytic streptococcal pharyngitis in children: correlation of serotype T4 with scarlet fever, *Scand J Infect Dis* 24:599, 1992.
12. Snellman LW et al: Duration of positive throat cultures for group A streptococci after initiation of antibiotic therapy, *Pediatrics* 91:1166, 1993.
13. Stjernquist-Desatnik A, Preller K, Schalen C: High recovery of *Haemophilus influenza* and group A streptococci in recurrent tonsillar infection or hypertrophy as compared with normal tonsils, *J Laryngol Otol* 105:439, 1991.
14. Timon CI, Cafferkey MT, Walsh M: Fine-needle aspiration in recurrent tonsillitis, *Arch Otol Head Neck Surg* 117:653, 1991.

245 Phimosis

Dennis M. Super

Phimosis (derived from the Greek word for muzzling) occurs when the tip of the foreskin becomes scarred (Fig. 245-1). The scarred foreskin loses its suppleness and no longer can be retracted over the glans penis. The incidence of phimosis in uncircumcised males ranges from 2% to 10%. The signs and symptoms of a child who has a scarred, unretractable foreskin are dysuria, hematuria, poor urinary stream, and tenderness of the foreskin. If the tip of the foreskin is severely scarred and if the opening of the foreskin is stenotic, the child's foreskin will "balloon" during urination. If the stenosis progresses, the child develops hydronephrosis and renal failure from the atretic opening of the foreskin.

The actual cause of a scarred, unretractable foreskin is unknown. Some of the proposed theories for the etiology of phimosis are trauma from forcible retraction of the foreskin, irritation from soiled diapers, improperly performed circumcision, congenital anomalies, and recurrent infection of the foreskin.

Not all children who have unretractable foreskins have phimosis. Almost 96% of male neonates have foreskins that cannot be retracted over their glans. These infants do not have phimosis because their foreskins are still supple. The difficulty in retracting the foreskin is caused by adhesions between the foreskin and the glans. These adhesions actually are remnants of the tissue plane that normally bridges the area between the foreskin and the glans. In 90% of these cases the tissue plane will have disappeared sufficiently by age 3 to allow retraction of the foreskin.[2] If these adhesions are lysed prematurely, the foreskin may become scarred and phimotic.

DIFFERENTIAL DIAGNOSIS

Balanoposthitis

Balanoposthitis is an inflammation of the glans (balano) and the foreskin (posthe). This inflammation begins when a few drops of urine remain trapped between the foreskin and glans. Also trapped in this area is a "cheesy" substance called smegma, which is composed of desquamated epithelial cells and the secretions of sebaceous glands. In this intertriginous area the trapped moisture and smegma begin to macerate the delicate surfaces of the glans and the foreskin. If proper foreskin hygiene is not maintained, the moist, macerated skin becomes infected. The foreskin and the glans may be tender, warm, erythematous, edematous, and suppurative. The child may suffer from dysuria and urinary frequency, and he may be febrile. Some of the organisms that can cause this secondary infection are *Staphylococcus aureus,* groups A and D streptococci, coliforms, *Pseudomonas aeruginosa, Candida albicans,* and *Trichomonas vaginalis.*

Children who have recurrent balanoposthitis or who have phimosis secondary to balanoposthitis may have diabetes mellitus. The glucose in a diabetic child's urine enhances the chance for secondary infections in this intertriginous space. In their retrospective review, Cates and coworkers[1] reported that their adult patients who had recent onset of phimosis secondary to balanoposthitis had a tenfold increase in the prevalence of diabetes mellitus over the general population. Almost 20% of these patients previously were undiagnosed diabetics.

Another type of balanoposthitis that may lead to phimosis is balanitis xerotica obliterans. This type of balanoposthitis is a chronic inflammation of the foreskin and glans. It begins as an erythematous lesion and eventually forms a thickened white plaque that may erode into the urethral meatus. These lesions histologically resemble lichen sclerosus et atrophicus, and there is some evidence linking balanitis xerotica obliterans with squamous cell carcinoma of the penis. Balanitis xerotica obliterans was thought to occur only in adults, until Rickwood and coworkers[5] published a prospective review of phimosis in children. In this study they found histological evidence of balanitis xerotica obliterans in 20 of 21 phimotic foreskins. Except for the phimosis, the preoperative physical examination of the glans and the foreskin was normal in all of their patients except one, who had a lesion that may have involved the meatus.

Paraphimosis

Paraphimosis is a condition in which a snugly fitting foreskin or a foreskin that has a partially scarred tip is retracted over the glans and becomes trapped behind it. This incarcerated foreskin begins to obstruct venous return from the tip of the penis, which results in further edema and ischemia. This condition resulted in 0.9% of all childhood admissions per year to the Royal Victoria Infirmary, which serves an area of London in which 88% of the males are uncircumcised.[2] Paraphimosis is a medical emergency because with each passing minute, the amount of edema and the degree of ischemia increase. If the incarcerated foreskin is not released soon, paraphimosis can lead to necrosis of the tip of the penis.

MANAGEMENT

For mild to moderate phimosis, initial management is directed toward preserving the foreskin. Treatment involves topical steroids, lysis of adhesions after inducing anesthesia with an eutectic mixture of lidocaine and prilocaine (EMLA technique), and stretching of the prepuce, with lysis of adhesions using general anesthesia. In one study of boys who had a nonretractable foreskin and ballooning of the foreskin with micturition, the two conditions resolved in 76% of cases (84 of 111) after a 1- to 2-month course of betamethasone valerate (0.5%), which was applied to the tip of the foreskin three

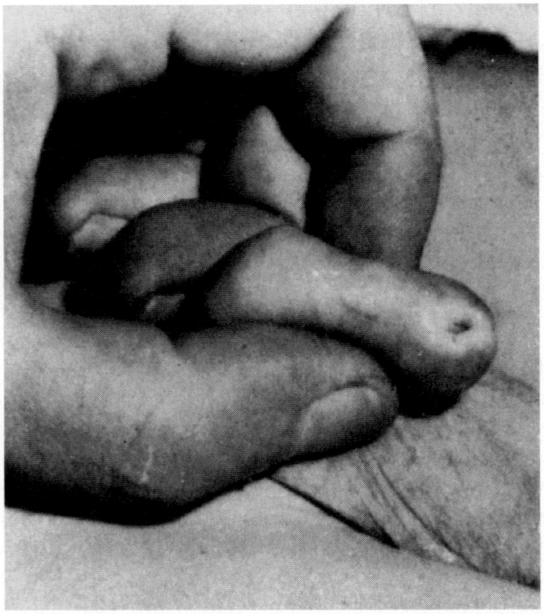

FIG. 245-1 In phimosis, the tip of the foreskin is whitish, scarred, and stenotic.

(From Rickwood AMK et al: *Br J Urol* 52:147, 1980.)

times a day.[7] EMLA lysis of adhesions produced a retractable foreskin in 85% of cases, and stretching of the prepuce was successful in 73% of cases.[4]

If the above regimens fail to produce a retractable foreskin, the child should be circumcised. Circumcision also is the preferred treatment if the phimosis occurs secondary to balanitis xerotica obliterans or if significant renal impairment develops secondary to the phimosis.

In balanoposthitis, a wet mount preparation, a potassium hydroxide (KOH) preparation, and a Gram stain of the exudate may help determine which organism is causing the infection. Because of the association between balanoposthitis and diabetes mellitus, children who have balanoposthitis also should be tested for diabetes mellitus by either a urinalysis or a glucose tolerance test.

The treatment for balanoposthitis consists of elevating the penis and applying warm soaks to the glans. Broad-spectrum systemic antibiotics may be needed if the infection is severe. If the KOH preparation contains hyphae and budding, the treatment also would include topical nystatin for *C. albicans*. The patient should be treated with metronidazole (Flagyl) if the wet mount preparation or urinalysis contains *T. vaginalis*.

Untreated balanoposthitis can cause severe edema, resulting in an ischemic glans. A dorsal slit of the foreskin will reduce this strangulation of the glans. After the edema and ischemia have resolved, the slitted foreskin can be removed (electively) by circumcision. Circumcision also can prevent recurrent episodes of balanoposthitis in children who cannot maintain proper penile hygiene.

The treatment for balanitis xerotica obliterans is circumcision, especially if the patient has phimosis. Penile lesions are removed surgically. If removal of the lesion is impractical, topical or intralesional corticosteroids are used.[5]

In paraphimosis, the patient is given a general anesthetic, and the trapped foreskin is released by applying outward traction on the foreskin while pushing on the glans. Another very successful method is the iced-glove technique. The foreskin is lubricated and anesthetized by applying lidocaine jelly to it for 2 minutes. The foreskin then is retracted, and the glans and shaft are inserted into the thumb of a sealed glove filled with ice water. The entire glove is pushed down the shaft of the penis until it rests on the symphysis pubis. The glove is held in place for about 5 minutes or until the edema is reduced. Finally, the constricting foreskin is slipped over the glans.[3] If these two techniques fail, the foreskin can be anesthetized by using a penile ring block with a local anesthetic, and several punctures (20 to 30) can be made in it with a 25-gauge needle; this may result in seepage of enough transudate to allow reduction of the foreskin.[6] If all of the above techniques fail, a dorsal slit in the foreskin will relieve the strangulation of the tip of the glans. Following reduction of the paraphimosis, the child should be circumcised to prevent recurrence of the paraphimosis.

REFERENCES

1. Cates JL, Finestone A, Bogash M: Phimosis and diabetes mellitus, *J Urol* 110:406, 1973.
2. Gairdner D: The fate of the foreskin: a study of circumcision, *Br Med J* 2:1433, 1949.
3. Houghton GR: The "iced glove" method of treatment of paraphimosis, *Br J Surg* 60:876, 1973.
4. Lafferty DM, MacGregor FB, Scobie WG: Management of foreskin problems, *Arch Dis Child* 66:696, 1991.
5. Rickwood AMK et al: Phimosis in boys, *Br J Urol* 52:147, 1980.
6. Walters TC, Sripathi V: Reduction of paraphimosis, *Br J Urol* 66:660, 1990.
7. Wright JE: The treatment of childhood phimosis with topical steroid, *Aust NZ J Surg* 64:327, 1994.

246 Pinworm Infestations

Donald A. Goldmann and Craig M. Wilson

ETIOLOGY

Pinworm *(Enterobius vermicularis)* infestation is exceptionally common. When looked for carefully, the parasite can be found in at least 30% of children worldwide, and infestation rates may approach 100% in boarding schools and institutions. Good sanitation and advanced socioeconomic status are feeble deterrents to pinworms. Adults often are infested (in one study, 31% of army recruits were found to be infested), and it is not uncommon to find pinworms in all members of a family. The discovery of *Enterobius* eggs in human coprolites from the Hogup and Danger caves in Utah (10,000 BC) proves that the parasite was no stranger to our ancestors.

E. vermicularis is a white, threadlike worm that lives primarily in the cecum and adjacent bowel. The gravid female, which is 1 cm long, migrates to the perianal area to deposit her eggs and dies shortly thereafter. Thus the infestation would be self-limited were it not for reinfestation. Unfortunately, the eggs, which are 50 × 30 μg, oval, flat on one side, and thin shelled, become infestive in about 6 hours. Autoinfestation occurs readily through ingestion of eggs if the host scratches the perianal area or does not wash the hands thoroughly after defecating. Moreover, *Enterobius* eggs are rather hardy and may survive for weeks in dirt, house dust, clothing, and bed sheets, although most die in less than a day. Eggs are easily swept into the air and may cause infestation if inhaled. Pets may carry eggs in their fur. Occasionally, eggs hatch on the perineum, and larvae migrate back into the intestine, where they mature.

In rare cases pinworms invade tissue and cause a granulomatous reaction. Inflammation associated with the parasite has been found in cases of appendicitis, but in such patients it is difficult to be certain whether the acute attack actually was caused by *E. vermicularis*. Pinworms occasionally wander beyond the perianal area, and granulomas containing worms have been an incidental finding in the fallopian tubes, peritoneum, and bladder. It must be stressed, however, that serious problems rarely, if ever, can be blamed directly on the pinworm. Perianal pruritus and recurrent urinary tract infections seem to occur frequently in infested patients, but some studies have questioned whether the parasite causes any symptoms at all.

CLINICAL MANIFESTATIONS

The patient may have perianal pruritus with secondary excoriation and dermatitis. Restlessness and fitful sleep are common complaints. A history of masturbation, enuresis, vaginitis, urinary tract infections, nausea and vomiting, diarrhea, and vague abdominal pain may be elicited, but it seldom is clear that the pinworm is the cause of these problems. As mentioned, it is doubtful whether the pinworm is at the root of any cases of acute appendicitis.

LABORATORY EVALUATION

Occasionally, adult pinworms may be noted near the anus, particularly in the morning. Eggs seldom are found in the patient's feces even if concentration techniques are used. The best way to make a diagnosis is to use the cellophane tape technique. When the child awakens in the morning, the adhesive side of a 2-inch strip of clear cellophane tape should be pressed against the perianal skin. The tape then should be placed on a microscope slide with the adhesive side down and scanned for eggs. Placing a drop of toluene on the slide beneath the tape may make the preparation easier to read. A single test should detect at least 50% of infestations, three tests will detect 90%, and five tests will detect virtually 100%.

PREVENTION AND THERAPY

The zealous physicians who try to eliminate pinworm from their patients are doomed to frustration and failure. The ubiquity and infestivity of the parasite and its persistence in the environment make eradication extremely difficult. Moreover, vigorous pursuit of a permanent cure may provoke needless turmoil and anxiety in the family. When the diagnosis is confirmed in a patient who has symptoms, the following approach seems reasonable.

The entire family should be treated with one of several drug regimens. A single dose of mebendazole (100 mg for all ages) is extremely effective and has virtually no side effects. Pyrantel pamoate, administered as a single dose of 11 mg/kg (maximum 1 g), also is effective; a transient headache and abdominal complaints have been reported. Pyrvinium pamoate, 5 mg/kg (maximum 250 mg) in a single dose, is another alternative; this drug stains clothing and feces red, but it is the least expensive treatment available.

All of these treatments are effective against the adult worms only. Therapy may be repeated in 2 weeks if the infestation is heavy or prolonged, or to eradicate any emerging parasites.

Boiling clothing and bed sheets probably is fruitless. However, some simple, prudent measures can be followed, such as clipping the fingernails (a favorite repository for eggs), washing the hands frequently, and showering daily in the morning. Wearing tight-fitting cotton pants and applying a bland ointment (e.g., petroleum jelly) to the perianal region may limit dispersal of the eggs. The floors in sleeping areas should be cleaned thoroughly, particularly in cases of recurrence.

The most important aspects of treatment, however, are humility on the part of the physician and reassurance of the family.

SUGGESTED READINGS

Drugs for parasitic infections, *Med Lett Drugs Ther* 35:111, 1993.

Pawlowski ZS: Enterobiasis. In Warren KS, Mahmoud AAF, editors: *Tropical and geographic medicine,* New York, 1990, McGraw-Hill.

Russell LJ: The pinworm, *Enterobius vermicularis, Prim Care* 18:13, 1991.

Warren KS, Mahmoud AAF: Algorithms in the diagnosis and management of exotic disease. V. Enterobiasis, *J Infect Dis* 132:229, 1975.

247 Acute Pneumonia

Preston W. Campbell and Thomas A. Hazinski

Acute respiratory infections are the most common illnesses in the pediatric age group. Although pneumonia accounts for only 10% to 15% of all respiratory infections, it causes significant morbidity and mortality among children. This is particularly true during the fall and winter months, when epidemics of parainfluenza, respiratory syncytial virus (RSV), and influenza virus occur. Pneumonia can be distinguished from the more common upper respiratory tract infection by the presence of lower respiratory tract signs (i.e., tachypnea, rales, hypoxemia, and cyanosis) and an associated area of infiltration on the chest roentgenogram. The challenge for the primary care provider is to make the correct diagnosis, to rule out associated serious conditions, and to begin treatment.

ETIOLOGY

The causes of pneumonia in children vary with age and season. A knowledge of which agent is most likely to be the cause in a particular case guides both the diagnostic workup and initial therapy. The maternal genital tract is colonized with group B streptococci and gram negative organisms (e.g., *Escherichia coli* and *Klebsiella pneumoniae*). These organisms are the most common causes of neonatal pneumonia. Other perinatally acquired infections may cause illness later in infancy. For example, perinatally acquired *Chlamydia trachomatis* may cause a characteristic afebrile pneumonitis in children 4 to 11 weeks of age.[1]

Between 2 months and 4 to 5 years of age, viruses constitute the most common cause of pneumonia. RSV is the major cause of pneumonia and bronchiolitis in children, with a peak incidence between 2 and 5 months of age. It occurs in winter and early spring epidemics, with as many as 40% of children becoming infected during their first exposure. Next in importance are the parainfluenza viruses, which cause infection primarily in the fall in slightly older children. Influenza A and B viruses can become the predominant isolate in hospitalized patients during wintertime influenza epidemics. Adenoviruses and rhinoviruses have been associated less frequently with pneumonia. After age 5, viruses become less important as a cause of pneumonia, and *Mycoplasma pneumoniae* replaces them as the most common etiological agent.

Although a potential cause of serious illness, bacterial pneumonia becomes less common after the neonatal period. *Streptococcus pneumoniae* (pneumococcus), *Haemophilus influenzae* type b, and *Staphylococcus aureus* are the usual offending organisms. *S. pneumoniae* is the most common bacterial agent. Use of the *H. influenzae* type b (Hib) vaccine during infancy has reduced the incidence of *H. influenza* pneumonia, but both typical and atypical *H. influenza* infection should still be considered in older or unvaccinated individuals.

Several other infectious agents deserve consideration. Tuberculosis has reemerged as an important pathogen in the last decade. Furthermore, pulmonary mycoses may mimic tuberculosis and are important considerations in endemic regions. Histoplasmosis is endemic to the central United States, and coccidioidomycosis is endemic to the southwestern United States.

It is important to remember that noninfectious diseases also can mimic pneumonia. Gastroesophageal reflux, aspiration, tracheoesophageal fistula with aspiration, asthma associated with atelectasis, hypersensitivity pneumonitis, and pulmonary hemosiderosis are but a few examples. Finally, a number of conditions can mimic pneumonia roentgenographically, such as a prominent thymus, atelectasis, congestive heart failure, and congenital lung malformations.

CLINICAL MANIFESTATIONS

The signs and symptoms of pneumonia vary greatly and depend on the pathogen, the child's age, and his or her ability to mount an immunological response. Although it may not be possible to differentiate clearly between a viral and bacterial pneumonia in an individual case, it is helpful to understand the differences in presentation among the various pathogens.

Viral pneumonia typically begins with upper respiratory tract symptoms of several days' duration, including fever, rhinorrhea, and cough. Respiratory distress usually has a gradual onset. Generalized airway epithelial involvement usually is seen and occurs in the lower respiratory tract as well, accounting for the coarse rhonchi that often are heard along with rales. Wheezing strongly suggests a viral etiology, although *M. pneumoniae* also can trigger wheezing in susceptible individuals. The classic roentgenographic appearance of viral pneumonia is that of a patchy bronchopneumonia. In an infant a perihilar pattern associated with hyperexpansion and atelectasis often is seen. Lobar pneumonia should suggest a bacterial process. Peripheral white blood cell (WBC) counts usually are elevated and not a particularly helpful diagnostic marker, but a significantly elevated count increases the likelihood of a bacterial cause.

Features that suggest *bacterial pneumonia* include acute onset, toxic appearance, productive cough, and chest pain. Lower lobe involvement with diaphragmatic irritation may cause severe referred abdominal pain. Rales often are not heard; instead, the patient has diminished breath sounds over the involved segment, with dullness on percussion and tactile fremitus. In fact, in some cases the only discernible findings may be fever and an increased respiratory rate. Roentgenographic features of consolidation, pleural fluid, pneumatoceles, or abscess indicate a bacterial cause. Finally, associated extrapulmonary bacterial involvement (e.g., meningitis or arthritis) strongly suggests bacterial disease.

In *M. pneumoniae* pneumonia, coryza is unusual. Fever and cough develop first and usually are followed by malaise and headache. Cough is the most persistent symptom and can last 3 to 4 weeks. Rales, pharyngitis, and wheezing, in decreasing order of frequency, are the most common physical signs. The roentgenographic changes vary and often correlate poorly with the clinical status, but most commonly an interstitial pattern is seen.[2] However, other types are possible, such as a lobar pattern, an alveolar pattern, or a combination of these.

The characteristics of chlamydial pneumonia have been well described.[4] The children usually are between 3 and 11 weeks of age and have a persistent staccato cough, rales, and wheezing without fever. Laboratory findings include a mild peripheral eosinophilia and elevated IgM and IgG.

Recurrent pneumonia often presents a challenging dilemma. Some conditions responsible for recurrent pneumonia are listed in the box below.

DIAGNOSIS

Optimal treatment ideally requires precise identification of the offending agent. This may be relatively simple during an RSV epidemic but can prove complex at other times and in patients with underlying chronic disease. The diagnostic workup therefore is tailored to the age of the child, the season, and the nature and severity of the illness.

Although a bacterial cause may be suspected, it may be difficult to make a specific diagnosis because children often are unable to produce an adequate sputum sample. In these cases a blood culture may provide a bacteriologic diagnosis. When available, the sputum should be Gram stained and cultured. On the Gram stain a predominant organism associated with polymorphonuclear leukocytes suggests bacteria as the pathogen. Bacterial antigens can be identified in tissue fluids (i.e., urine or pleural fluid) by use of counterimmunoelectrophoresis, latex agglutination, and enzyme-linked immunosorbent assay (ELISA), even after antibiotics have been started. More invasive approaches, such as flexible bronchoscopy, lung puncture, transtracheal aspiration, or open lung biopsy, may be indicated in the child whose condition is deteriorating, is critically ill, or is immunosuppressed. When tuberculosis is suspected, a purified protein derivative (PPD) test should be used; a positive reaction calls for obtaining a culture specimen.

The ability to diagnose nonbacterial pneumonias rapidly has improved remarkably in recent years. Virologic isolation is available in most major medical centers and public health laboratories. Enzyme-linked immunosorbent assay (ELISA) and fluorescent antibody techniques allow quick diagnosis of infections caused by influenza A virus, parainfluenza viruses, RSV, and *Chlamydia* organisms. Although *M. pneumoniae* can be cultured, the specific diagnosis usually is based on serological conversion. A fourfold rise in antibody titer to *M. pneumoniae* by complement fixation (CF) test is diagnostic. Although false positive results occur, a cold agglutinin titer of 1:32 or higher strongly suggests a mycoplasmal infection. A rapid screening test can be performed for cold agglutinins. Four drops of blood are placed in a tube with sodium citrate or other anticoagulant. The tube is placed in ice water for 30 seconds and then observed for agglutination by rolling the tube on its side. When warmed afterward, the agglutination should resolve. The diagnosis of fungal pneumonia (e.g., histoplasmosis or coccidioidomycosis) is established by isolating the organism from sputum or tissue, or through serological tests.

CAUSES OF RECURRENT PNEUMONIA

Aspiration

Gastroesophageal reflux
Tracheoesophageal fistula
Altered consciousness (i.e., seizures)
Foreign body
Abnormal swallowing reflex

Structural causes

Pulmonary sequestration
Tracheal or bronchial stenosis/web
Extrinsic compression of the airway
  Vascular ring
  Lymph nodes

Immunological deficiency

Acquired: AIDS, chemotherapy, malnutrition
Congenital: humoral, phagocytic

Metabolic causes

Cystic fibrosis
Alpha-1-antitrypsin deficiency

Altered mucociliary clearance

Immotile cilia syndrome

Other

Asthma
Hypersensitivity pneumonitis

TREATMENT

In the neonatal period, antibiotic therapy requires coverage of both gram positive and gram negative organisms. Ampicillin plus an aminoglycoside provides excellent coverage. An afebrile pneumonia in a patient between 4 and 11 weeks of age should be treated with erythromycin.

Amoxicillin is the drug of choice in infants over 3 months and until 5 years of age. An antibiotic with activity against beta-lactamase-producing *Haemophilus* and staphylococci, such as amoxicillin/clavulanic acid (Augmentin), should be used in the sicker child. In children over age 5, when *Haemophilus* is less likely and *Mycoplasma* becomes the most likely agent, the drug of choice is erythromycin. If intravenous antibiotics are needed, a second-generation cephalosporin, nafcillin, or chloramphenicol provides excellent coverage in most cases. When an organism is identified, therapy is guided by that organism's sensitivity pattern.

Treatment of viral pneumonia is primarily supportive. As with all pneumonias, close observation, monitoring of heart rate and oxygen saturation, oxygen supplementation, high humidity, bronchodilators, and chest physiotherapy are used as needed. Specific antiviral therapy is available for RSV (i.e., ribavirin) and influenza A (i.e., amantadine) and should be considered for children who have chronic lung disease or congenital heart disease.

The decision to hospitalize a patient who has pneumonia depends on the severity of the illness, the child's age, the suspected organism, and the adequacy of the home environment. Most older children can be treated at home, but the threshold for admitting a young infant should be low. Certainly, moderately severe respiratory distress, hypoxia, apnea, poor feeding, posttussive emesis, dehydration, deterioration of clinical status despite treatment, or an associated complication such as empyema should prompt hospitalization.

The emergence of penicillin-resistant *S. pneumoniae* is alarming; in some regions, as many as 30% of isolates were penicillin resistant in 1994. Although some of these patients respond to penicillin therapy, intravenous vancomycin is the drug of choice for patients who have severe or unresponsive pneumonia.[3]

Children who have pneumonia should be reevaluated after 2 or 3 weeks. The child who has returned to baseline status needs no further intervention. Repeat chest roentgenograms are indicated for children who have persistent respiratory difficulties, have had previous pulmonary disease, or have had complicated courses. Persistent roentgenographic abnormalities may merely reflect the inherently slow resolution of lung inflammation; thus films should be compared with previous films and interpreted in the context of the clinical course. After an acute pneumonia, the chest roentgenogram may remain abnormal for 4 to 6 weeks.

PROGNOSIS

The complications of bacterial pneumonia include empyema and lung abscess. However, long-term alteration of pulmonary function is rare even when these complications are seen. Death occurs almost exclusively in patients who have underlying conditions. The incidence of long-term complications after viral, bacterial, or mycoplasmal disease is unknown. Significant sequelae have been noted after adenoviral, influenza, and measles pneumonias. These include bronchiectasis, chronic pulmonary fibrosis, and desquamative interstitial pneumonitis. Evidence is accumulating that recurrent viral pulmonary infections in childhood, in association with environmental irritants (i.e., passive smoking), are risk factors for chronic asthma.

REFERENCES

1. Beem M, Saxon E: Respiratory tract colonization and a distinctive pneumonia syndrome in infants infected with *Chlamydia trachomatis, N Engl J Med* 296:306, 1977.
2. Brolin I, Wernstedt L: Radiographic appearance of mycoplasma pneumonia, *Scand J Respir Dis* 59:179, 1978.
3. Friedland IR, McCracken G: Management of infections caused by antibiotic-resistant *Streptococcus pneumoniae,* N Engl J Med 331:377, 1994.
4. Tipple MA, Beem MO, Saxon EM: Clinical characteristics of the afebrile pneumonia associated with *Chlamydia trachomatis* infection in infants less than 6 months of age, *Pediatrics* 63:192, 1979.

SUGGESTED READINGS

Bartlett JG, Mundy LM: Community-acquired pneumonia, *N Engl J Med* 333:1618, 1984.

Campbell PW III: New developments in pediatric pneumonia and empyema, *Curr Opin Pediatr* 7:278, 1995.

Heffner JE et al: Pleural fluid chemical analysis in parapneumonic effusions, *Am J Respir Crit Care Med* 151:1700, 1995.

Peter G: The child with pneumonia: diagnostic and therapeutic considerations, *Pediatr Infect Dis J* 7:453, 1988.

Stark JM: Lung infections in children, *Curr Opin Pediatr* 5:273, 1993.

248 Postoperative Management of the Pediatric Outpatient—Surgical and Anesthetic Aspects

Myron Yaster, Charles N. Paidas, and Lynne G. Maxwell

Over the past 20 years outpatient or "ambulatory" anesthesia and surgery has revolutionized the way surgery and anesthesia is practiced in North America.[16,30] Safe, reliable, inexpensive, and convenient, outpatient surgery is an attractive option for parents, children, their health care providers, and perhaps most important, their insurers. Surgical procedures that routinely required 1 or 2 days of preadmission hospitalization and 1 to 7 days of postsurgical recovery now are performed commonly without any inpatient hospitalization at all. The cost savings are substantial; the average cost of 1 day in an American hospital is more than $1000. Government and private health care insurers are demanding the increasing use of ambulatory surgery services and will pay for fewer and fewer inpatient procedures. Besides cost savings, there are additional advantages. Ambulatory anesthesia and surgery reduces the psychological trauma of hospitalization and family separation, produces fewer nosocomial infections, and hastens recovery.[16,30] In children, examples of surgical procedures that are now performed routinely on an outpatient basis are listed in the box on p. 1526.

Although the incidence of serious postoperative complications in healthy children undergoing ambulatory surgery is relatively low ($<1\%$), some minor postoperative problems occur commonly.[4,30] These common anesthetic and surgical postoperative problems can be classified according to their time of onset into *early* and *late*. Often it is the primary health care provider rather than the surgeon or anesthesiologist who is called on by the family to diagnose and treat these problems.

SELECTION OF PATIENTS

Guidelines to select appropriate procedures and patients for outpatient surgery and anesthesia are evolving continually and are discussed in greater detail in Chapter 8, Preoperative Assessment.[4,12,32] In general the procedure itself should not involve excessive bleeding or entry into a major body cavity. Also, the patient should not require any special postoperative nursing care and must have a responsible adult at home who will be available to provide care until recovery is complete. The patient's physical condition and health also play a role.[12] Anesthesiologists and surgeons often use a short-hand description of a patient's physical status to decide on the suitability of outpatient surgery. This short-hand code, developed by the American Society of Anesthesiologists (ASA), is listed in Table 248-1. Patients undergoing outpatient surgery usually are healthy (ASA physical status 1,2) or have a well-controlled systemic illness (ASA physical status 3). The infant who was born prematurely poses a unique problem because they have a greater risk of developing apnea following general anesthesia.[9,27] It is our practice to either defer surgery until such patients are no longer at risk (institutionally defined; we use 60 postconceptual weeks of age, others use 44, 48, 52 postconceptual weeks of age) or admit these children to the hospital for 12 to 24 hours of cardiorespiratory monitoring following surgery and anesthesia.[10]

EARLY POSTOPERATIVE ANESTHETIC PROBLEMS

The most frequent complications or side effects of general anesthesia are postoperative nausea, retching, and vomiting.[16,17,23] Indeed, this is the most common cause of delayed discharge from the Post Anesthesia Care Unit (PACU, formerly called the Recovery Room) and the most common cause of unanticipated hospitalization following outpatient surgery.[17] The etiology of this side effect is multifactorial. Important factors include predisposition (previous history of perioperative vomiting), the anesthetic drugs or techniques used, the procedure being performed, the skill of the anesthesiologist providing the anesthetic, and motion. Certain surgical procedures such as strabismus surgery, middle ear surgery, orchiopexy, and umbilical hernia repair are associated with a greater than 50% incidence of postoperative vomiting. Similarly the perioperative use of *any* opioid is associated with a very high incidence of postoperative nausea and vomiting, even when less nauseating and less "vomitogenic" general anesthetic drugs such as propofol are used.[25]

The complex act of vomiting involves coordination of the respiratory, gastrointestinal, and abdominal musculature and is controlled by the emetic center. Stimuli from several areas within the central nervous system can affect the emetic center. These include afferents from the pharynx, gastrointestinal tract, and mediastinum, as well as afferents from the higher cortical centers (including the visual center and vestibular portion of the eighth nerve) and the chemoreceptor trigger zone (CTZ) in the area postrema. The area postrema of the brain is rich in dopamine, opioid, and serotonin or 5-hydroxytryptamine (5-HT_3) receptors.[23] Indeed, blockade of these receptors is an important mechanism of action of the antiemetics used most commonly in practice (Fig. 248-1, Table 248-2).

There are several techniques to treat or prevent postoperative nausea and vomiting. These include altering the anesthetic technique (e.g., avoiding the perioperative use of opioids), using antiemetics perioperatively (e.g., droperidol, phe-

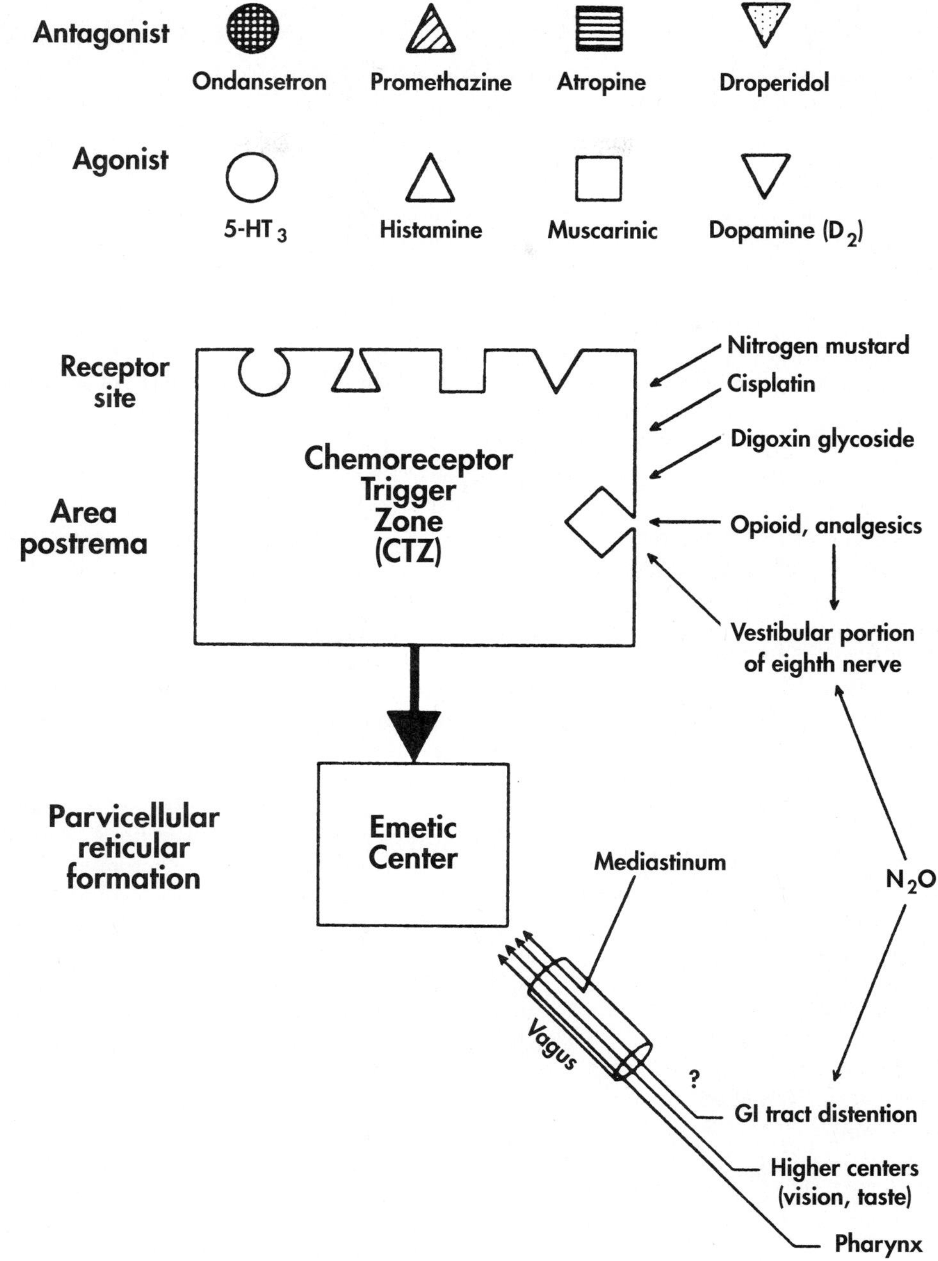

FIG. 248-1 The chemoreceptor trigger zone and the emetic center with the agonist and antagonist sites of action of various anesthetic-related agents and stimuli.
(From Watcha MF, White PF: *Anesthesiology* 77:162, 1992.)

nothiazines, ondansetron, or antihistamines; Tables 248-2 and 248-3), and limiting oral intake postoperatively.[2,23]

Certain anesthetic agents and techniques produce more vomiting than others. The effects of the general anesthetic inhalational agents halothane, enflurane, and nitrous oxide on vomiting are controversial. Some studies report significantly more vomiting when these anesthetics are used; others do not.[14] A new intravenous general anesthetic agent, propofol, produces significantly less vomiting and nausea than other general anesthetic drugs, so long as opioids are not given concomitantly.[24,25] Indeed, the culprit that has been shown to cause nausea and vomiting consistently in virtually every study to date are the opioids. All the opioids used commonly, whether morphine, meperidine, fentanyl, codeine, oxycodone, or hydromorphone, produce nausea and vomiting.[28] Anecdotally, individual patients may find one drug more nauseating than another, and sometimes changing from one drug to another may decrease the amount of nausea and vomiting. Regional anesthetic techniques that use local anesthetics produce less vomiting than general anesthetic techniques.[17,29]

Avoiding opioids perioperatively may solve only part of the puzzle. Obviously, pain control is essential in children who undergo surgery, and opioids are the analgesic drugs used most commonly for this purpose (see below). A new alternative may be the use of ketorolac, a powerful nonsteroidal antiinflammatory drug (NSAID) that is almost as po-

Table 248-1 American Society of Anesthesiologists (ASA) Physical Status Categories

Physical status	Description
1	Healthy patient who has no organic, physiological, biochemical, or psychiatric disturbance
2	Mild-to-moderate systemic disturbance caused either by the condition to be treated surgically or by other pathophysiological processes; examples include hypertension, extreme obesity, mild asthma or diabetes, or extremes of age (neonates)
3	Severe systemic disturbance or disease from whatever cause, even though it may not be possible to define the degree of disability with finality; examples include severe diabetes, congenital heart disease, pulmonary insufficiency (BPD)
4	Severe systemic disease that is life threatening, not always correctable by operation; examples include severely limiting congenital heart disease with evidence of cardiac insufficiency, advanced pulmonary, renal, or hepatic insufficiency
5	A moribund patient who has little chance of survival but is submitted to surgery in desparation; examples include major cerebral trauma with rapidly increasing intracranial pressure, necrotizing enterocolitis with profound shock, and presumptive dead bowel

COMMON OUTPATIENT SURGICAL PROCEDURES BY SPECIALTY

General surgery

Femoral, inguinal, and umbilical herniorrhaphies
Lymph node and other diagnostic biopsies
Central line insertion
Fistulotomy

Genitourinary surgery

Orchiopexy, hydrocele
Circumcision
Hypospadias repair

Otorhinolaryngeal surgery

Myringotomy and tube placement
Adenoidectomy
Tonsillectomy
Bronchoscopy

Ophthalmological surgery

Strabismus
Examination under anesthesia

Orthopedics

Tendon lengthening
Spica changes
Fracture reductions

tent as morphine as an analgesic but does not produce nausea, vomiting, or respiratory depression.[1,11]

Insisting that children drink or ambulate when they are experiencing nausea is as good a recipe for vomiting as any. Many anesthesiologists prefer to keep patients NPO until they are ready and willing to drink and eat, even if this means that the child leaves the hospital while still fasting.[19] In essence the child must say that he or she is thirsty, or better still, hungry, and must specifically ask for something to drink or eat before any food or liquid is offered. Even in the youngest of patients there is little if any risk of dehydration, particularly if intravenous fluid management was administered appropriately perioperatively. In current anesthetic practice virtually all pediatric patients undergoing surgery and anesthesia receive salt- and sugar-containing intravenous fluids in the operating room and PACU. If sufficient fluids to supply maintenance and replacement requirements were given in this period, a postoperative fast would be tolerated readily. Nausea and vomiting that persists beyond 12 to 24 hours is extraordinarily unusual and requires investigation to rule out an alternative pathology. Thus, just as anesthesiologists are abandoning stringent, prolonged preoperative fasts, they increasingly are appreciating their benefits postoperatively.[21] Unfortunately, many institutions continue to require that patients drink and ambulate before they can be discharged from the hospital or same-day care unit. This policy almost certainly contributes to the high incidence of unanticipated admission to the hospital following outpatient surgery—admission that is sought because the patient is vomiting.

The treatment of nausea and vomiting is the same as that for viral gastroenteritis. A "cooling off" period of 2 to 4 hours should be followed by sips of clear sugar- and salt-containing fluids (e.g., oral rehydration solution, Gatorade, etc), each sip being separated by several minutes. Giving fluids or solids prematurely only aggravates the problem. Very rarely, swallowing excessive air in the postoperative period may lead to acute gastric dilation in young children. Recognition of the characteristic distended abdomen and gastric splash, if present, should be followed by nasogastric decompression. Finally, antiemetics can be used either prophylactically or to treat the problem once it develops. The most common antiemetics are those that block receptors within the vomiting center. Four major neurotransmitter systems play a role in mediating the emetic response: dopaminergic, histaminic, cholinergic, and serotonergic. Antiemetic drugs may act at more than one receptor, but they tend to have a more prominent action at one or two receptors[23] (Table 248-2). The antiemetics used most commonly include phenothiazines (chlorpromazine and phenergan), butyrophenones (droperidol, haloperidol), antihistamines (hydroxyzine, diphenhydramine), anticholinergics (scopolamine, atropine), benzamides (metoclopramide), and serotonin antagonists (ondansetron).[2,24] Unfortunately, virtually all these antiemetics produce sedation, which can interfere with rapid return to baseline function. Dosage, site of action, and route of administration of the antiemetics used most commonly are listed in Tables 248-2 and 248-3.

Table 248-2 Receptor Site Affinity of Antiemetic Drugs

Pharmacological group drug	Dopamine	Muscarinic cholinergic	Histamine	Serotonin
Phenothiazines				
Chlorpromazine	++++	++	++++	+
Prochlorperazine	++++			
Butyrophenones				
Droperidol	++++	—	+	+
Haloperidol	++++	—	+	—
Antihistamines				
Promethazine	++	++	++++	—
Diphenhydramine	+	++	++++	—
Benzamides				
Metoclopramide	+++	—	+	++
Anticholinergics				
Scopolamine	+	++++	+	—
Antiserotonin				
Ondansetron	—	—	—	++++

From Watcha MF, White PF: *Anesthesiology* 77:162, 1992.

Table 248-3 Dosage Guidelines For Commonly Used Antiemetics

Pharmacological group (generic)	Brand name	Dosage (mg/kg)	Comments
Phenothiazines			Adverse effects include drowsiness, hypotension, arrhythmias, extrapyramidal symptoms; potentiates effects of opioids, sedatives
Chlorpromazine	Thorazine	IV, PO: 0.5-1 q6-8 hr	
Prochlorperazine	Compazine	PO, PR: 0.1 q6-8 hr (max 10 mg)	
Butyrophenones			Adverse effects include drowsiness, hypotension, arrhythmias, extrapyramidal symptoms; lowers seizure threshold; potentiates effects of opioids, sedatives
Droperidol	Inapsine	IV: 0.01-0.03 q6-8 hr	
Haloperidol	Haldol	IV: 0.01 q8-12 hr	
Antihistamines			Adverse effects include drowsiness, hypotension, arrhythmias; contraindicated in patients taking MAO inhibitors
Promethazine	Phenergan	IV: 0.25-0.5 q6 hr	
Diphenhydramine	Benadryl	0.5-1.0 q4-6 hr (max 50 mg)	
Benzamides			Adverse effects include extrapyramidal symptoms
Metoclopramide	Reglan	IV, PO: 0.05-0.1 q6 hr	
Anticholinergics			Adverse effects include dry mouth, blurred vision, fever, tachycardia, constipation, urinary retention, drowsiness, amnesia
Scopolamine	Hyoscine, transdermal scopolamine	IV, PO: 0.005 q4-6 hr apply behind ear 4 hr before needed; lasts 72 hr	
Antiserotonin			Adverse effects include bronchospasm, tachycardia, headaches, lightheadedness
Ondansetron	Zofran	IV, PO: 0.15 q8hr, (max dose 4 mg)	

Finally, postoperative vomiting may interfere with the resumption of chronic oral medication regimens. With few exceptions (MAO inhibitors, oral hypoglycemics, and diuretics), all chronically administered oral medications should be taken on the morning of surgery.[12] Indeed, the question of whether patients should take oral medications on the morning of surgery has become moot because of the liberalization of preoperative fasting guidelines. That patients are allowed to take their medications preoperatively has reduced greatly the stress of making the decision on when oral medications can be restarted postoperatively. Most chronically administered drugs, such as anticonvulsants, bronchodilators, digitalis, and others, have half-lives of elimination that are long (>12 hours). This means that missing a dose of these drugs for one or two half-lives (12 to 24 hours) will have minimal, if any, effect on blood levels, assuming that therapeutic blood levels existed before surgery began. If vomiting persists beyond 24 hours, parenteral drug administration may be required.

POSTOPERATIVE PAIN MANAGEMENT

The treatment and alleviation of pain is fundamental to medical care.[19] The physician's obligation to manage pain and relieve suffering is a crucial element of our professional commitment to patient care. This is not merely a lofty ideal; effective pain management produces myriad benefits including reduced morbidity and mortality, early mobilization, and more rapid recovery and return to work, school, and play.[19] A detailed discussion of pain management can be found in Chapter 26, Management of Acute Pain in Children.

NONSTEROIDAL ANTIINFLAMMATORY DRUGS (NSAIDS) AND NONOPIOID (OR "WEAKER") ANALGESICS

The weaker or milder analgesics, of which acetaminophen (Tylenol), salicylate (aspirin), and ibuprofen (Motrin) are the classic examples, constitute a heterogenous group of nonsteroidal antiinflammatory drugs (NSAIDs) and nonopioid analgesics.[1] They provide pain relief primarily by blocking peripheral prostaglandin production. These analgesic agents are administered enterally via the oral or, on occasion, the rectal route and are particularly useful for inflammatory, bony, or rheumatic pain. New parenterally administered NSAIDs, such as ketorolac, are now available for use in children in whom the oral or rectal routes of administration are not possible.[11] Unfortunately, regardless of dose, nonopioid analgesics reach a ceiling effect above which pain cannot be relieved by these drugs alone (Table 248-4). Because of this, these weaker analgesics often are administered in combination with other more potent opioids such as codeine or oxycodone.

Aspirin, one of the oldest and most effective nonopioid analgesics, has been abandoned largely in pediatric practice because of its possible role in Reye syndrome, its effects on platelet function, and its gastric irritant properties. A new salicylate product, choline-magnesium trisalicylate (Trilisate), may change our thinking about salicylates both in the postoperative child and in the child who has cancer. Choline-magnesium trisalicylate is a unique aspirin-like compound that does not bind to platelets and therefore has no effect on platelet function.[22] It is a convenient drug to give to children because it is available in both liquid and tablet forms and is administered only twice a day (Table 249-4). The association of salicylates with Reye syndrome will limit its use, even though the risk of developing this syndrome postoperatively is extremely remote.

The nonopioid analgesic used most commonly in pediatric practice remains acetaminophen.[6] Unlike aspirin and the NSAIDs, acetaminophen has minimal, if any, antiinflammatory activity. When administered in normal doses (10 to 15 mg/kg, PO or PR), acetaminophen has very few serious side effects, is an antipyretic, and like all enterally administered NSAIDs, takes about 40 to 60 minutes to provide effective analgesia. Because of this, in our practice we often administer acetaminophen or ibuprofen preoperatively as part of our premedication regimen. Dosage guidelines for the nonopioid analgesics used most commonly are listed in Table 248-4.

OPIOIDS

Morphine is the gold standard for analgesia to which all other opioids are compared. When small doses, 0.1 mg/kg (IV, IM, SQ), are administered to otherwise unmedicated patients who are in pain, analgesia usually occurs without loss of consciousness. Less advantageous side effects of morphine (and all other opioids at equipotent doses) include nausea and vomiting, pruritus (especially around the nose), miosis, constipation, urinary retention, and when administered at high doses, seizures. The most feared complication of morphine and all other opioids is dose-dependent depression of ventilation that is produced primarily by reducing the sensitivity of the brainstem respiratory centers to hypercarbia and hypoxia.

The "unit" dose of intravenously administered morphine is 0.1 mg/kg and is modified based on patient age and disease state. Morphine can be administered orally, making it a useful analgesic in the outpatient setting. Unfortunately only about 20% to 30% of a dose of morphine administered orally

Table 248-4 Dosage Guidelines for Commonly Used Nonsteroidal Antiinflammatory Drugs (NSAIDs)

Generic name	Brand name	Dose (mg/kg) frequency	Maximum adult daily dose (mg)	Comments
Salicylates (aspirin)	Bayer, Bufferin, Anacin, Alka-Seltzer, others	10-15 q 4 hr	4000	Inhibits platelet aggregation, GI irritability, Reye syndrome
Acetaminophen	Tylenol, "aspirin-free," Panadol, Tempra, others	10-15 q 4 hr	4000	Lacks antiinflammatory activity
Ibuprofen	Motrin, Advil, Medipren, others	6-10 q 6-8 hr	2400	Available as an oral suspension
Naproxyn	Naprosyn	5-10 q 12 hr	1000	Available as an oral suspension
Indomethacin	Indocin	0.3-1 q 6 hr	150	Commonly used in NICU to close patent ductus arteriosus
Ketorolac	Toradol	IV or IM: Load 0.5, maintenance 0.2-0.5 q 6 hr	150	May be given orally Adult IM dosing: Load 30 mg, followed by 15-30 mg q 6 hr
Choline-magnesium trisalicylate	Trilisate	8-10 q 8-12 hr	4000	Does not bind to platelets; see Salicylate

reaches the systemic circulation. When converting a patient's intravenous morphine requirements to oral maintenance, the intravenous dose needs to be multiplied 3 to 5 times (Table 248-5). Oral morphine is available as a liquid, tablet, and sustained-release preparation (MS Contin). The liquid is particularly useful in children because it is available in many concentrations (1 to 20 mg/ml).

CODEINE AND OXYCODONE

Codeine and oxycodone (Tylox, Percocet) are mu opioid agonists just like morphine and are the oral opioid analgesics prescribed most frequently in pediatric outpatient surgical practice. Effective when administered either orally or parenterally, these drugs are given most commonly in their oral forms, usually in combination with acetaminophen (Tylox, Percocet). In equipotent doses (Table 248-5), the efficacy of codeine and oxycodone as analgesics and respiratory depressants is similar to that of morphine. In addition, codeine and oxycodone share with morphine and the other opioid agonists common effects on the central nervous system, including sedation, respiratory depression, and stimulation of the chemoreceptor trigger zone (vomiting center) in the brainstem. In our experience codeine is the most nauseating of the orally administered opioids and oxycodone is the least.

Codeine and oxycodone are absorbed from the gastrointestinal tract to a much greater degree than morphine and other opioids. Approximately 60% of a dose of either of these drugs administered orally is absorbed. The analgesic effects occur as early as 20 minutes after ingestion and reach a maximum at 60 to 120 minutes. The plasma half-life of elimination is 2.5 to 3 hours.

Oral codeine and oxycodone almost always are prescribed in combination with acetaminophen. Although conventional pediatric teaching is to prescribe single-agent drugs, this is unwise when prescribing these opioids. As single agents neither codeine nor oxycodone is available as a liquid preparation in most pharmacies. When they are, they are significantly more expensive than the combined forms. Furthermore, acetaminophen potentiates the analgesia produced by these opioids and allows the practitioner to use less opioid and yet achieve satisfactory analgesia. Progressive increases in dose are associated with a similar degree of respiratory depression, delayed gastric emptying, nausea, and constipation as with other opioid drugs. Typically, codeine is prescribed in a dose of 1 mg/kg with a concurrently administered dose of acetaminophen (10 mg/kg). Oxycodone is prescribed in a dose of 0.1 mg/kg with a concurrently administered dose of acetaminophen (10 mg/kg) (Table 248-5).

EMERGENCE PHENOMENA FOLLOWING GENERAL ANESTHESIA

Emergence from general anesthesia in healthy patients often is accompanied by transient symmetrical neurological changes that usually are considered pathological reflexes. These otherwise pathological reflexes include sustained and nonsustained ankle clonus, bilateral hyperreflexia, the Babinski reflex, and decerebrate posturing. These reflexes often can be detected within minutes of discontinuing a general anesthetic and may persists for hours. Why this happens is unknown. However, the discovery of focal neurological deficits in a postoperative patient is never normal and should point to a possible central or peripheral nervous system injury.

Children are prone to disorientation, hallucinations, and at times uncontrollable physical activity during emergence from general anesthesia. This hyperexcitable, hyperactive state sometimes is referred to as *emergence delirium* and occurs most commonly after potent vapor anesthetics (halothane, en-

Table 248-5 Commonly Used Mu Agonist Drugs

Agonist	Equipotent IV dose (mg/kg)	Duration (hr)	Bioavailability (%)	Comments
Morphine	0.1	3-4	20-40	Seizures in newborns and in all patients at high doses Histamine release, vasodilation—avoid in asthmatics and in circulatory compromise MS Contin 8-12 hr duration
Meperidine	1	3-4	40-60	Catastrophic interactions with MAO inhibitors Tachycardia; negative inotrope Metabolite produces seizures; not recommended for chronic use
Methadone	0.1	6-24	70-100	Can be given IV even though the package insert says SQ or IM
Fentanyl	0.001	0.5-1		Bradycardia; minimal hemodynamic alterations Chest wall rigidity (>5 μg/kg rapid IV bolus). R_X naloxone or a succinylcholine, pancuronium
Codeine	1.2	3-4	40-70	PO only Prescribe with acetaminophen
Oxycodone (Tylox, Percocet)	0.05-0.15	3-4	40-60	PO primarily Prescribed with acetaminophen
Hydromorphone (Dilaudid)	0.015-0.02	3-4	40-60	<CNS depression than morphine <Itching and nausea than morphine Can be used in PCA

flurane, isoflurane), ketamine, and high-dose barbiturates have been administered. The most common causes of emergence delirium are pain, sensory deprivation (eye bandages, eye lubricant), residual anesthetic, and awakening in a foreign, "unfriendly" environment—the PACU. Before the child is discharged from the PACU the majority of the disorientation, hyperactivity, excitability, and hallucinatory visual disturbances should be resolved completely. Occasionally, some lingering evidence may persist for several 12 to 24 hours. Thus some children who have undergone general anesthesia and surgery may experience sleep disturbances, nightmares (terrors), and even loss of nighttime bladder control on the night after surgery. Ketamine in particular is associated with sleep disturbances following its administration.[27] Although the incidence of nightmares following ketamine administration is less in children than in adults, it has been reported to occur in 5% to 10% of patients who receive it. Fortunately, regardless of the cause, sleep disturbance is time limited and rarely persists beyond 48 hours after surgery and general anesthesia. If sleep disturbances become overwhelming, they can be treated with oral diazepam (0.02 mg/kg). Usually one dose given at bed time "cures" the problem completely.

INTUBATION-RELATED COMPLICATIONS

Upon awakening from a general anesthetic, many children who have been intubated endotracheally will complain of a sore throat. This discomfort can be alleviated with fruit-flavored popsicles, ice chips, or common throat lozenges once cough, gag, and swallowing reflexes have returned to baseline. Analgesics rarely are required.

Postintubation Croup

Postintubation croup, or postextubation subglottic edema, has been a well-recognized entity since airways were first secured by intubation. Children are more prone to develop croup following intubation than are adults because of differences in their airway anatomy. Children have narrower laryngeal and tracheal lumens, which are obstructed more readily by mucosal edema. Additionally, the narrowest portion of the child's airway is at the level of cricoid cartilage and not at the level of the larynx. This invites internal tracheal injury because an endotracheal tube can pass easily through the vocal cords and become wedged in the subglottic area. Other contributing factors to the development of croup are traumatic or repeated intubations, coughing ("bucking") on the tube, and changing the patient's position after intubation.[7]

The incidence of postintubation croup has been lowered from 6% to 1% of all endotracheally intubated children.[7] This reduction has occurred through the use of sterile, implant-tested endotracheal tubes, the routine intraoperative use of heated, humidified gases, and the use of appropriately sized (air leak pressure of <30 cm H_2O), noncuffed endotracheal tubes. Children who have Down syndrome appear to be particularly likely to develop this problem.

The treatment of postintubation croup is the same as for viral laryngotracheitis. Humidification is effective in most cases. Rarely is nebulized racemic epinephrine therapy necessary. If it is, these patients should not be discharged from the PACU to their homes; rather, they must be admitted to the hospital for overnight observation because of the potential for rebound edema formation. The efficacy of corticosteroids in treating postintubation croup has been controversial.[5] Most anesthesiologists will prescribe dexamethasone, 0.3 to 0.4 mg/kg, for this problem even though there are no controlled, prospective trials to validate its use for this purpose.

Succinylcholine-induced Myalgia

Succinylcholine, a short-acting depolarizing muscle relaxant, frequently is used by many anesthesiologists to facilitate intubation of the trachea. Unfortunately succinylcholine administration in children normally will result in damage to the muscle cell. Myalgia and increased blood levels of creatinine phosphokinase (CPK) and myoglobin are expected "complications" of succinylcholine administration.[8,13] Occasionally, blood myoglobin levels may be high enough to produce myoglobinuria as well. To some degree much of this can be avoided by pretreating the patient with small doses of a nondepolarizing muscle relaxant or calcium. The myalgia is intense and is as debilitating as the myalgia produced by an influenza infection. Treatment is supportive, and the pain usually resolves over several days.

LATE POSTOPERATIVE ANESTHETIC PROBLEMS

Jaundice

The development of hepatic dysfunction (jaundice, abnormal liver enzymes and function) several days to weeks following general anesthesia and surgery has many causes, and arriving at a specific diagnosis may be very difficult. Postoperative hepatic dysfunction may be caused by the surgical procedure, the stress of surgery, ischemia, infection, preexisting but unsuspected liver disease, or drugs. One of the more sensationalized and feared causes is halothane-induced hepatitis. Halothane, a potent vapor general anesthetic, can induce hepatotoxicity in adults and animals by either direct drug injury, by an allergic reaction, or by tissue hypoxia.[15] In adults, 25% of patients exposed to halothane will develop a mild, postoperative increase in serum aminotransferase concentrations that may last for 2 weeks. What, if any, connection this increase in liver enzymes has to do with fulminant halothane-induced hepatitis is unknown. In adults, severe, fulminant halothane-induced hepatitis develops 6 to 11 days after exposure to halothane and has an incidence of between 1:35,000 to 1:200,000 halothane administrations. In the pediatric age group, however, there is no substantiated evidence that halothane-induced hepatitis occurs. Thus if liver dysfunction occurs in a child after surgery, other more likely causes should be sought.

EARLY POSTOPERATIVE SURGICAL PROBLEMS

Fever

Pyrexia (rectal temperature >38.5° C) within 24 hours of surgery and general anesthesia is very common and usually is caused by atelectasis (Table 248-6).[18,31] There are many causes of this postoperative atelectasis. Endotracheal intubation, inhalational general anesthetics, and the use of nonhumidified gases all depress ciliary motion within the tracheal-bronchial tree and thereby interfere with normal pulmonary toileting. When these factors are combined with small tidal volume breathing, somnolence, splinting secondary to pain,

Table 248-6 Common Causes of Postoperative Fever

Site	Etiology	Time	Incidence	Signs and symptoms	Diagnosis	Therapy
Wind	Atelectasis	24-48 hr	Very common	Cough, shortness of breath, retraction	Examination, chest radiograph	Cough, deep breathing, incentive spirometer
Wound	Infection	<24 hr-7 days	Rare	Pain, erythema, induration	Examination, wound cultures	Antibiotics, incise wound
Water (urinary tract)	Urinary tract infection	3-5 days	Very rare	Dysuria, hematuria	Examination, urinalysis, culture	Remove indwelling catheter, +/− antibiotics
Walker	Deep vein thrombosis	>3 days	Extremely rare	Swelling, heaviness of extremities, superficial venous congestion, palpable cord	Examination, duplex Doppler, venogram	Bed rest, elevation, heparin/coumadin, thrombolytics

Table 248-7 Postoperative Wound Infections

Onset (postoperative day)	Usual pathogens	Wound appearance	Other signs
1-3	*Clostridium perfringens*	Brawny, hemorrhagic, cool; occasional gaseous crepitance; putrid "dishwasher" exudate; intense local pain	High standard fever (39° to 40° C); irrational behavior; leukocytosis >15,000/mm^3; occasional jaundice
2-3	Streptococcus	Erythematous, warm, tender; occasionally hemorrhagic with blebs; serous exudate	High spiking fever (39° to 40° C); irrational behavior at times; leukocytosis >15,000 mm^3; rare jaundice
3-5	Staphylococcus	Erythematous, warm, tender; purulent exudate	High spiking fever (38° to 40° C); irrational behavior at times; leukocytosis 12,000 to 20,000/mm^3
>5	Gram negative rod	Erythematous, warm, tender; purulent exudate	Sustained low-grade to moderate fever (38° to 40° C); irrational behavior; leukocytosis 10,000 to 16,000/mm^3
>5	Symbiotic (usually anaerobes plus gram negative rods)	Erythematous, warm, tender; focal necrosis; purulent, putrid exudate	Moderate to high fever (38° to 40° C); leukocytosis >15,000/mm^3; occasional jaundice; variable mentation

and cough suppression caused by pain or opioid analgesics, the result is atelectasis. Early ambulation, deep breathing, and coughing can be extremely helpful in alleviating or preventing this atelectasis and postoperative fever. Indeed, this may be one of the important medical advantages of ambulatory surgery because patients are more likely to be up and about when they are at home rather than in the hospital.

Other causes of postoperative pyrexia are rare. In a retrospective analysis of the postoperative course of 256 febrile children at the Hospital for Sick Children in Toronto, Yeung et al.[31] found that only 4 children had infections that required treatment. All 4 of these children had significant and obvious accompanying signs of infection (local tenderness, crepitance, or erythema at the incision site, tachypnea, cough, dysuria, headache, and the like). Thus most patients who have low-grade postoperative fevers require nothing more than a physical examination to differentiate between a septic and nonseptic process. Extensive (and expensive) diagnostic workups rarely are indicated. Fever in the early postoperative period is so common that it actually can be regarded as a normal response to surgical trauma and general anesthesia in the majority of patients. Other unusual causes of postoperative fever include urinary tract infections, dehydration, infected intravenous access sites, thyroid storm, pheochromocytoma, and malignant hyperthermia. Urinary tract infections usually do not produce symptoms in the immediate postoperative period. Rather, they are a cause of late postoperative fever, usually occurring 3 to 5 days after operation. These children generally are symptomatic and complain of dysuria; infants may have hematuria.

Wound infection as a cause of fever is rare.[18,31] The postoperative day on which a given wound infection becomes apparent and the signs of sepsis produced by the infection vary according to the organism and the concomitant use of antibiotics (Table 248-7). Generally the earlier the onset of wound sepsis, the more destructive and life-threatening the infection. The majority of wound infections do not usually become apparent until the fifth to tenth postoperative day (Table 248-7). Rare exceptions are group A beta-hemolytic streptococci, *Clostridium difficile,* and *C. perfringens.* These organisms produce wound infections that can become apparent within 24 to 48 hours of surgery. Clostridium and streptococcal wound infections are life threatening, and children who have these infections appear acutely toxic. Usually they develop high spiking fevers (39° to 41° C), become irrational, and may even develop jaundice. The surgical incision site is red, warm, and intensely painful on palpation. Additionally, vesicle formation, crepitance surrounding the wound, and an exudate may be present (Table 248-7). Patients who develop this type of wound infection require immediate hospitalization and treatment (see below).

Drainage

A small amount of serosanguineous drainage in the postoperative dressing is normal and should not be a cause for alarm. This is easier said than done; most parents and children are not at all sanguine about the presence of blood in a dressing. Only bleeding that is persistent requires immediate surgical attention. Persistent bleeding is defined as bleeding and bloody ooze that continues for more than 6 to 8 hours after surgery, or a need to change a blood-soaked wound dressing more than twice in the first 6 to 8 hours after surgery. It almost always indicates inadequate hemostasis and usually is caused by a superficial skin arterial bleeding site. Until the bleeding site is investigated surgically and controlled by the operating surgeon, direct digital pressure applied to the wound will slow or stop the flow of blood.

Serosanguineous discharge from the operative site 2 to 3 days after surgery may be caused by a superficial hematoma below the incision site. A hematoma can be recognized by its characteristic ecchymoses and fluctuance. Small hematomas directly below a wound, umbilicus, or scrotum usually drain or resorb spontaneously. A hematoma that progressively expands may require operative exploration so that the clot can be evacuated and any ongoing bleeding controlled. In general, a nonexpanding hematoma usually will resolve within 4 to 6 weeks of surgery. If the wound hematoma is associated with pain, the child should be examined by the operating surgeon.

Serous drainage from a wound may be caused by creation of a large dead space during the operation or by liquification of adipose tissue. Seromas caused by dead space usually drain 4 to 7 days after surgery, whereas liquification of adipose tissue, characterized by yellow drainage, occurs 2 to 3 weeks after surgery.

Regardless of size, both hematomas and seromas are excellent culture media for bacterial organisms and increase the likelihood of wound infection.[18] Both these postoperative problems should be watched closely for and usually are characterized by the triad of pain, wound dehiscence, and persistent drainage.

Urinary Retention

In contrast to adults, urinary retention is rare in the pediatric surgical outpatient. Fisher et al.[3] recently reported that 85 of 92 children (92%) who underwent inguinal canal surgery voided within 8 hours of surgery regardless of intraoperative anesthetic technique or postoperative analgesic regimen. The latter included parenteral and enteral opioids, regional anesthesia (caudal epidural blockade or ilioinguinal-iliohypogastric nerve blocks), or both. This is a significant finding because opioids and regional anesthetics, particularly caudal epidural blockade, can interfere with the neural mechanisms responsible for evacuation of the bladder. Many who argued against the routine use of caudal anesthesia and/or opioids for the treatment of postoperative surgical pain based their opinions on the theoretical risk of urinary retention. Fortunately the data of Fisher et al.[3] will put these concerns to rest.

These data also have important clinical implications in terms of discharge criteria from ambulatory care centers. Many surgeons, anesthesiologists, and ambulatory care administrators have insisted that children void before discharge after undergoing outpatient surgery and anesthesia. Many patients simply cannot void on command, particularly in the very strange setting of a PACU or hospital. In the Fisher study,[3] only 7 of 92 patients (8.5%) required more than 8 hours to void. Eventually all these patients voided at home without the need for any medical intervention.[3] The knowledge that all patients void within 24 hours of surgery and virtually all void spontaneously within 10 hours of surgery strongly suggests that voiding before discharge is unnecessary.

To minimize bladder distention, the child or adolescent should be encouraged to urinate immediately before coming to the operating room and as soon as possible postoperatively. In our practice we do not require patients routinely to void before postoperative discharge from the PACU. Exceptions to this rule include patients who complain of lower abdominal distention and discomfort. Older children and adolescents initially are treated with ambulation; palpation of the lower abdomen is used in infants and toddlers. If these measures do not lead to voiding and amelioration of symptoms, bladder catheterization should be performed. Patients requiring bladder catheterization then should be observed for their ability to urinate voluntarily. If bladder function does not return, the patient should be admitted to the hospital, a specimen of urine sent for urinalysis and culture, and a decision made by the patient's surgeon about reinsertion of a bladder catheter. The need for bladder catheterization is very rare. In our experience, urination following outpatient surgery requires a "less is better" attitude because the more attention one pays to this issue, the more problems one creates.

Scrotal Swelling

Scrotal swelling and concomitant discoloration of the scrotum commonly occurs following inguinal herniorrhaphy and hydrocelectomy. Initially this process can manifest as swelling alone and may progress to bluish discoloration as bleeding and clot lysis occur. The problem usually is the result of bleeding from the cut edge of the peritoneal sac, derived from either a hernia or hydrocele. The swelling and color change should resolve in 4 to 6 weeks. However, if there is fever, erythema, tenderness, and progressive enlargement of the hemiscrotum, an urgent consultation with the patient's surgeon is required. Often this requires reexploration and operative evacuation of the hematoma via a suprainguinal or transscrotal approach.

LATE POSTOPERATIVE SURGICAL PROBLEMS

Infection

Pyrexia (rectal temperature >38.5° C) 48 hours or more after outpatient surgery is unusual and may indicate a serious pulmonary, urinary tract, or wound infection[18,31] (Tables 248-6 and 248-7). It requires evaluation and examination by the patient's pediatrician or surgeon. The wound is examined for signs of inflammation, such as heat, pain, redness, and swelling. If any of these signs or symptoms are present, the operating surgeon should be informed. If the wound appears to be the source of the fever and infection, the wound can be probed with a sterile swab (Q-tip) and a Gram stain and culture obtained. If pus is present, the wound should be opened, copiously irrigated, and debrided. Regardless of the presence of pus, a culture swab always should be sent for Gram stain and culture.

Gram positive infections are the most common causes of wound infection.[18] *Staphylococcus aureus* or *S. epidermidis* wound infections usually are characterized by a milky white, purulent drainage and usually occur 3 to 5 days after surgery (Table 248-7). Staphylococcal infections usually present with high spiking fevers 39 to 40° C and leukocytosis (>12,000 white cells/mm^3). Following Gram stain and culture the patient is treated with a penicillinase-resistant antibiotic such as oxacillin. Enteric encapsulated gram negative organisms such as *E. coli* usually are associated with significant erythema, tenderness, and possibly purulent discharge and usually occur more than 5 days after surgery (Table 248-7). Enteric organisms such as *E. coli* are sensitive to penicillin, cephalosporins, and aminoglycosides.

Patients who develop fevers more than 5 days after surgery may have an anaerobic infection or a mixed infection of anaerobic and gram negative rods. The skin surrounding the wound should be examined closely for the presence of crepitus and vesicle formation, purulent and putrid discharge, and focal necrosis, all of which indicate the development of gas gangrene or necrotizing fascitis. These anaerobic type of infections can be caused by the gram positive cocci *Clostridium perfringens* or the gram negative rod Bacteroides. *C. perfringens* causes exquisite pain, brown discoloration, and a wound that is crepitant to palpation. Gas may be seen in the subcutaneous tissues on roentgenogram. Wound infections caused by bacteroides usually are purulent and malodorous. Both of these anaerobic infections are life threatening and require immediate hospitalization and pediatric surgical intervention.

The treatment of a serious wound infection is straightforward and consists of inpatient hospitalization, opening of the wound along its entire length, drainage, wide debridement of necrotic tissue, high-dose intravenous antibiotics (penicillin, clindamycin, metronidazole, cefotetan), and if available, hyperbaric oxygen therapy. These wounds should not be closed surgically; rather, they should be allowed to close spontaneously with granulation. If only cellulitis is detected, the wound should not be opened, but the patient should be started on intravenous antibiotic therapy. Lymphangitis, manifested by its characteristic red streaks and tender regional adenopathy, also should be treated with intravenous antibiotics in the hospital.

If the surgical incision site does not appear to be responsible for the development of fever, a thorough history and physical examination should be performed. Particular attention should be devoted to the lungs and IV administration sites. As stated previously, atelectasis often follows general anesthesia and surgery. Infected IV insertion sites, phlebitis, or thrombophlebitis, especially in the adolescent female taking birth control pills, also can occur. Additionally, routine causes of pyrexia in children can occur in the postoperative patient and include upper respiratory tract infections, gastroenteritis, and otitis media.

Practical Aspects of the Postsurgical Wound

Wound healing represents a highly dynamic, integrated series of cellular physiological and biochemical events. The morphological events that make up the healing of closed wounds include the following: inflammation, epithelialization, cellular influx, and fibroplasia. The inflammatory phase begins immediately. During its early stages, white cells migrate into the wound and engulf and remove cellular debris and tissue fragments. This phase sets the stage for subsequent events in the healing process.

After dead material is removed the epidermis and dermis immediately adjacent to the wound edge begin to thicken within 24 hours after injury. Within 48 hours the entire wound surface is reepithelialized. This is the critical period during which the wound should be kept dressed and dry. Thus wound dressings are not required after 48 hours. Wound contamination with stool and urine should be cleansed with water or saline and the overlying dressing replaced; detergent soaps and peroxide should be avoided.

Between days two and three, deep to the epithelium there is an influx of fibroblasts into the wound. By the fourth or fifth day the fibroblasts begin to lay down collagen fibers. This continues for several months. However, there is remodeling of collagen that takes place for over 1 year. Practically speaking, by postoperative day four the wound may be washed with warm water and a mild soap (e.g., Ivory, Dove, Neutrogena).

From the surgeon's point of view all the morphological events of wound healing lead to a single important conclusion: wounds become stronger with time. Closing the wound with suture material only serves to hasten the process. Normally, a simple wound will attain 50% of the strength of surrounding uninjured tissue by 28 days. Most wounds are closed by using absorbable suture material, which maintains tensile strength for 60 to 90 days, supplies an appreciable amount of wound strength to allow for the normal healing processes to occur, and does not require suture removal. This allows the child to return to activity at an earlier time. For instance, adolescents who have uncomplicated inguinal hernia repair may return to nonstrenuous activity 7 to 10 days postoperatively; they may return to full activity by 4 to 6 weeks. Whenever possible toddlers are kept off tricycles and bikes for 10 days to 2 weeks. As for the infant, the family should be advised to treat the baby as if no operation was performed (i.e., full bath by the fourth postoperative day and no restrictions for carrying the baby).

Scar Formation

African-Americans and Caucasians of Mediterranean descent are predisposed to forming hypertrophic scars and keloids. Keloids are characterized by massive formation of scar tissue in and deep to skin after any trauma, including surgery. They are different from hypertrophic scars, which tend to resolve with time and as a rule are not associated with prolonged pruritis. Keloids tend to recur after excision. Children have a greater tendency to form and re-form keloids than adults do. A careful family history may be a predictor of this pathological process. An abnormal scar should be observed for a minimum of 6 months postoperatively. If it does not resolve, an attempt to excise the scar should be made, staying within the confines of the lesion to see what response is obtained. If the keloid recurs, it should be reexcised and a mixture of triamcinolone/kenalog 1% should be injected beneath the scar. This mixture will produce some keloid resolution. Overall, the management of the abnormal scar should be determined by the anatomical position of the wound, the age of the patient, and any underlying associated diseases.

Finally, all skin wounds and surgical skin incision sites will scar regardless of the expertise of the surgeon or the use of plastic surgical techniques in closing the skin. Indeed, it is a myth that plastic surgery is "scarless." Further, the scar tissue will permanently pigment (usually it will become red to dark brown or black) when exposed to intense sunlight during the first days to a year of its formation. Thus patients and their families should be advised that when going outdoors and exposing the surgical incision site to the sun, the incision site should be completely covered or be protected with zinc oxide or a sunblock with an SPF of >30 for a year after surgery.

REFERENCES

1. Brooks PM, Day RO: Nonsteroidal antiinflammatory drugs—differences and similarities, *N Engl J Med* 324:1716, 1991.
2. Christensen S, Farrow-Gillespie A, Lerman J: Incidence of emesis and postanesthetic recovery after strabismus surgery in children: a comparison of droperidol and lidocaine, *Anesthesiology* 70:251, 1989.
3. Fisher QA et al: Postoperative voiding interval and duration of analgesia following peripheral or caudal nerve blocks in children, *Anesth Analg* 76:173, 1993.
4. Hannallah RS: Selection of patients for paediatric ambulatory surgery, *Can J Anaesth* 38:887, 1991.
5. Kairys SW, Olmstead EM, O'Connor GT: Steroid treatment of laryngotracheitis: a meta-analysis of the evidence from randomized trials, *Pediatrics* 83:683, 1989.
6. Koch-Weser J: Drug therapy: acetaminophen, *N Engl J Med* 295:1297, 1976.
7. Koka BV, Jeon IS, Andre JM, MacKay I, Smith RM: Postintubation croup in children, *Anesth Analg* 56:501, 1977.
8. Laurence AS: Biochemical changes following suxamethonium: serum myoglobin, potassium and creatinine kinase changes before commencement of surgery, *Anaesthesia* 40:854, 1985.
9. Liu LM et al: Life-threatening apnea in infants recovering from anesthesia, *Anesthesiology* 59:506, 1983.
10. Malviya S, Swartz J, Lerman J: Are all preterm infants younger than 60 weeks postconceptual age at risk for postanesthetic apnea? *Anesthesiology* 78:1076, 1993.
11. Maunuksela EL, Kokki H, Bullingham RE: Comparison of intravenous ketorolac with morphine for postoperative pain in children, *Clin Pharmacol Ther* 52:436, 1992.
12. Maxwell LG, Deshpande JK, Wetzel RC: Preoperative evaluation of children, *Pediatr Clin North Am* 41:93, 1994.
13. McLoughlin C et al: Muscle pains and biochemical changes following suxamethonium administration after six pretreatment regimens, *Anaesthesia* 47:202, 1992.
14. Muir JJ et al: Role of nitrous oxide and other factors in postoperative nausea and vomiting: a randomized and blinded prospective study, *Anesthesiology* 66:513, 1987.
15. Nomura F et al: Halothane hepatotoxicity and reductive metabolism of halothane in acute experimental liver injury in rats, *Anesth Analg* 67:448, 1988.
16. Pasternak LR: Outpatient anesthesia. In Rogers MC et al, editors: *Principles and practice of anesthesiology,* St Louis, 1993, Mosby.
17. Patel RI, Hannallah RS: Anesthetic complications following pediatric ambulatory surgery: a 3-year study, *Anesthesiology* 69:1009, 1988.
18. Pellegrini CA: Postoperative wound infection. In Way LW, editor: *Current surgical diagnosis and treatment,* East Norwalk, Conn, 1991, Appleton & Lange.
19. Schechter N, Berde C, Yaster M: *Pain in infants, children, and adolescents,* Baltimore, 1993, Williams & Wilkins.
20. Schreiner MS et al: Should children drink before discharge from day surgery? *Anesthesiology* 76:528, 1992.
21. Schreiner MS, Triebwasser A, Keon TP: Ingestion of liquids compared with preoperative fasting in pediatric outpatients, *Anesthesiology* 72:593, 1990.
22. Stuart JJ, Pisko EJ: Choline magnesium trisalicylate does not impair platelet aggregation, *Pharmatherapeutica* 2:547, 1981.
23. Watcha MF, White PF: Postoperative nausea and vomiting: its etiology, treatment, and prevention, *Anesthesiology* 77:162, 1992.
24. Watcha MF et al: Effect of propofol on the incidence of postoperative vomiting after strabismus surgery in pediatric outpatients, *Anesthesiology* 75:204, 1991.
25. Weir PM et al: Propofol infusion and the incidence of emesis in pediatric outpatient strabismus surgery, *Anesth Analg* 76:760, 1993.
26. Welborn LG et al: Postoperative apnea in former preterm infants: prospective comparison of spinal and general anesthesia, *Anesthesiology* 72:838, 1990.
27. White PF, Way WL, Trevor AJ: Ketamine—its pharmacology and therapeutic uses, *Anesthesiology* 56:119, 1982.
28. Yaster M, Maxwell LG: Opioid agonists and antagonists. In Schechter NL, Berde CB, Yaster M, editors: *Pain in infants, children, and adolescents,* Baltimore, 1993, Williams & Wilkins.
29. Yaster M, Maxwell LG: Pediatric regional anesthesia, *Anesthesiology* 70:324, 1989.
30. Yaster M et al: The night after surgery: postoperative management of the pediatric outpatient—surgical and anesthetic aspects, *Pediatr Clin North Am* 41:199, 1994.
31. Yeung RS, Buck JR, Filler RM: The significance of fever following operations in children, *J Pediatr Surg* 17:347, 1993.
32. Zuckerberg AL: Perioperative approach to children, *Pediatr Clin North Am* 41:15, 1994.

249 Preseptal and Orbital Cellulitis

James W. McManaway III and Carl A. Frankel

Periorbital infections in children can lead to serious complications, including permanent loss of vision, bacterial meningitis, and death. Although noninfectious disorders can cause eyelid edema and proptosis and can limit ocular motility, bacterial cellulitis always must be ruled out. Noninfectious causes of eyelid edema include trauma, allergic dermatitis (Fig. 249-1), insect stings, sunburn, and systemic diseases, including nephrotic syndrome and congestive heart failure. The differential diagnosis of proptosis in children is outlined in the box on p. 1536.

PRESEPTAL CELLULITIS

A sagittal section through the eyelids reveals an extension of the periorbita (periosteum of the orbit) known as the orbital septum. The orbital septum extends from the orbital rim to the lid margins and provides a natural resistance to the spread of bacteria from the eyelids into the orbit. As defined by the orbital septum, preseptal cellulitis is limited to the eyelids, although in reality there is a continuum between the preseptal and orbital processes.

Preseptal cellulitis (Fig. 249-2) typically occurs with a 12- to 24-hour history of increasing swelling, ptosis, erythema, and edema localized to the eyelids. Occasionally, an insect bite, puncture wound, or area of impetigo may be found to be the origin of this localized infection, but usually no proximate cause is found. The area is warm to the touch and usually nontender. Early on, the patient may be uncomfortable but rarely shows toxicity. These children should have normal visual acuity, normal ocular motility, and no sign of proptosis. Without treatment, preseptal cellulitis progresses rapidly to orbital cellulitis with possible meningitis, cavernous sinus thrombosis, and death.

The management of patients who have preseptal cellulitis consists of ruling out signs of orbital cellulitis, obtaining appropriate cultures, deciding if hospitalization is necessary, starting appropriate oral or intravenous antibiotics, and monitoring for worsening clinical signs. Any patient who has diminished visual acuity, limitation of ocular motility, or evidence of proptosis must have a CT scan of the orbits to rule out orbital cellulitis. Conjunctival and skin cultures may yield the causative agent; blood cultures should be obtained for children who show signs of toxicity. Because toxicity develops so quickly in children under age 3, hospitalization should be considered in this age group, using intravenous antibiotics for treatment. Older patients who develop toxicity or any patient who has signs of *Haemophilus influenzae* preseptal cellulitis should be hospitalized.

The most likely causative organism in preseptal cellulitis depends on the clinical situation.[4] *Staphylococcus aureus* and *Streptococcus pyogenes* are associated with a preexisting skin wound or area of impetigo. These patients initially should be treated with intravenous nafcillin (inpatient) or oral cloxacillin (outpatient).[1] *Haemophilus influenzae* type b and *Pneumococcus* species are associated with a preexisting upper respiratory tract infection. Patients who have purple discoloration of the eyelid often have *H. influenzae* preseptal cellulitis and should be watched especially for worsening clinical signs and for evidence of other sites of *H. influenzae* infection. These patients should be treated initially with intravenous ceftriaxone and later can be converted to oral amoxicillin-clavulanate if this treatment is supported by culture and sensitivity results.[1] Antibiotics should be used for a minimum of 10 days. All patients who have preseptal cellulitis need daily follow-up examinations until significant improvement is noted to ensure that orbital cellulitis is not developing. No clinical sequelae are anticipated when preseptal cellulitis is treated appropriately.

ORBITAL CELLULITIS

Orbital cellulitis usually is a disease of children over 5 years of age and nearly always is due to spread from adjacent sinuses, usually the ethmoid. Rare causes of orbital cellulitis include orbital trauma, complications of retinal detachment, orbital or strabismus surgery, dental infections, or necrosis of an orbital tumor. Children who have orbital cellulitis typically have moderate to severe eyelid edema, ptosis, and proptosis (Fig. 249-3, *A*). When the lid is elevated, the eye shows conjunctival hyperemia and chemosis and typically is deviated in comparison with the fellow eye (Fig. 249-3, *B*). While the patient's lid is elevated, he or she may report diplopia, pain on attempted eye movement, or inability to move the globe; visual acuity may be reduced significantly. When visual acuity is reduced, especially in the presence of an afferent pupillary defect detected by the swinging flashlight test, optic neuritis or optic nerve compression is present, and aggressive management is necessary to prevent permanent visual loss. These patients usually appear acutely ill and almost always have fever and a leukocytosis with a left shift.

The management of patients who have orbital cellulitis includes hospitalization, a CT scan of the head and orbits, blood and conjunctival cultures, appropriate intravenous antibiotics, and ophthalmological and otolaryngological consultation. The purpose of the CT scan is to distinguish exogenous infections (trauma, orbital surgery) from endogenous infections (bacterial sinusitis) and to rule out an orbital abscess, which must be drained surgically. If CT scanning reveals an orbital subperiosteal abscess, a trial of intravenous antibiotics should be given, as reliable correlation has not been shown between orbital subperiosteal abscesses as suspected by CT scanning and the actual clinical findings at the time of surgical drainage.[2,3] A subperiosteal abscess should be drained if the patient's condition worsens despite appropriate antibiotic therapy.

Children who have typical bacterial orbital cellulitis that occurs secondary to sinusitis can be given intravenous nafcillin and chloramphenicol; some physicians prefer intravenous ceftriaxone as a single agent.[1] Patients who have orbital cellulitis that occurs secondary to orbital trauma or surgery should be treated with intravenous nafcillin or tobramycin or both, depending on the Gram stain result of the wound drainage.[1] An ophthalmologist should be consulted to detect and manage potential ophthalmological complications such as corneal exposure, secondary glaucoma, septic retinitis, exudative retinal detachment, central retinal artery occlusion, optic neuritis, and cavernous sinus thrombosis. Otolaryngological consultation should be obtained to manage the sinus disease and to assist in orbital abscess drainage if it becomes necessary. The condition of patients who have orbital cellulitis may worsen for the first 24 hours; thereafter they usually improve dramatically. Intravenous antibiotics should be continued until the patient is afebrile for 24 hours; oral antibiotics then should be substituted. If the patient remains free of fever for 24 hours on an oral antibiotic regimen, discharge from the hospital is reasonable, with oral antibiotics continued so that the patient receives antibiotics for 3 weeks.

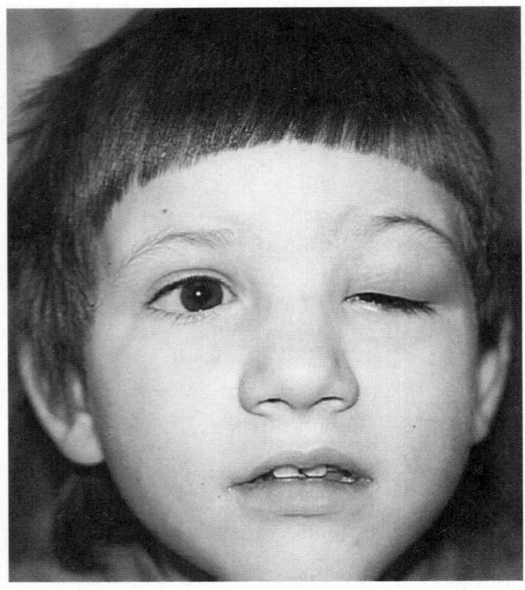

FIG. 249-1 Child who has allergic eyelid edema. The eye beneath the swollen eyelid was quiet and had normal visual acuity and motility. Proptosis was absent.

DIFFERENTIAL DIAGNOSIS OF PROPTOSIS IN CHILDREN

- Capillary hemangioma
- Craniosynostosis
- Dermoid cyst
- Glaucoma (secondary buphthalmos)
- Histiocytosis-X
- Hyperthyroidism
- Idiopathic inflammatory pseudotumor
- Leukemia
- Lymphangioma
- Meningoencephalocele
- Neuroblastoma
- Neurofibroma
- Orbital cellulitis
- Optic nerve glioma
- Rhabdomyosarcoma
- Trauma

A

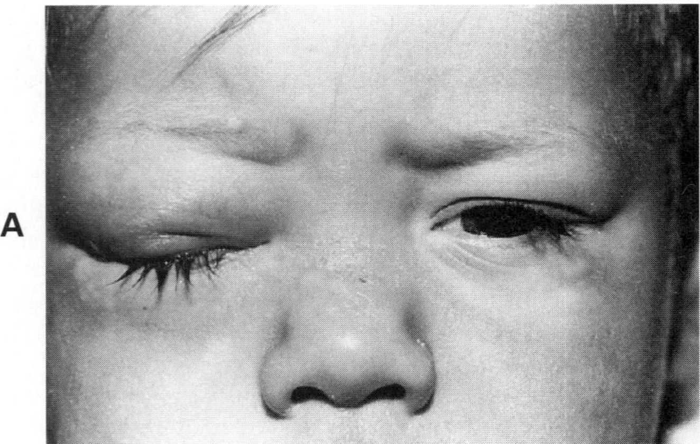

B

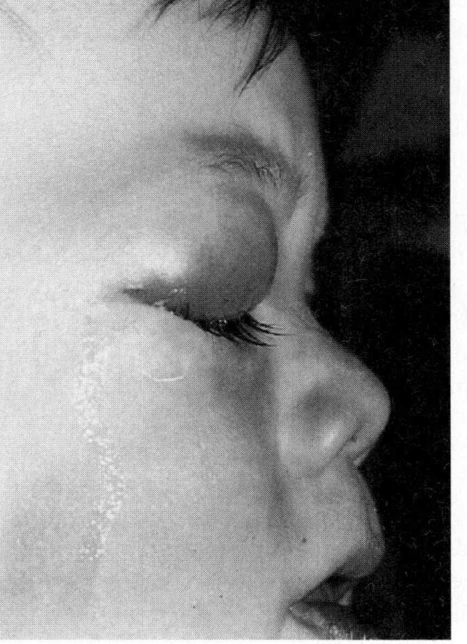

FIG. 249-2 **A,** Frontal view of a patient who has bacterial preseptal cellulitis. When the eyelid was elevated, the eye showed no restriction of motility and produced no pain with movement. Systemic antibiotics readily resolved the condition. **B,** Lateral view of the same patient. Lid edema is significant; however, when the lid was elevated, no evidence of proptosis was noted.

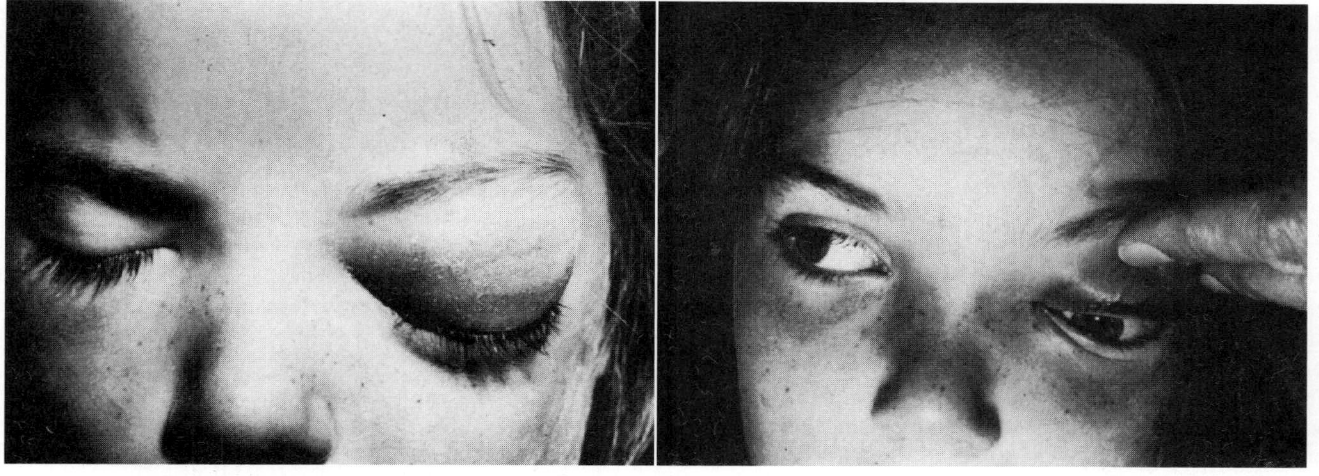

FIG. 249-3 **A,** A girl with severe periorbital inflammatory edema and a suggestion of inferior displacement of the globe. **B,** The same patient; on elevation of the eyelid, proptosis and limited movement of the eye were noted. Patients with this condition also may complain of pain when they attempt to move the affected eye, and their vision may be reduced as a consequence of inflammatory or infectious optic neuritis.

CAVERNOUS SINUS THROMBOSIS

Cavernous sinus thrombosis is a dreaded complication of orbital cellulitis. Because the orbital venous system has no valves, bacteria can leave the orbit via the ophthalmic veins and gain access to the cavernous sinus, leading to thrombosis. Patients who have cavernous sinus thrombosis have the typical signs of orbital cellulitis but are more toxic. Proptosis is marked owing to poor orbital venous drainage; cranial nerves III, IV, V, and VI often are involved. The thrombosis can spread to the contralateral cavernous sinus, giving abnormal ocular motility to the uninvolved eye. The condition should be managed by a neurosurgeon; treatment involves high-dose intravenous antibiotics, anticoagulants and, possibly, systemic steroids.

REFERENCES

1. Jones DB, Steinkuller PG: Microbial preseptal and orbital cellulitis. In Duane TD, Jaeger AJ, editors: *Clinical ophthalmology,* Philadelphia, 1989, JB Lippincott.
2. Rubin SE et al: Medical management of orbital subperiosteal abscess in children, *J Pediatr Ophthalmol Strabismus* 26:21, 1989.
3. Tannenbaum M et al: Medical management of orbital abscess, *Surv Ophthalmol* 30:211, 1985.
4. Weiss A et al: Bacterial periorbital and orbital cellulitis in childhood, *Ophthalmology* 90:195, 1983.

SUGGESTED READINGS

Catalano RA, Smoot CN: Subperiosteal orbital masses in children with orbital cellulitis: time for a reevaluation? *J Pediatr Ophthalmol Strabismus* 27:141, 1990.

Eustis HS et al: Staging of orbital cellulitis in children: computerized tomography characteristics and treatment guidelines, *J Pediatr Ophthalmol Strabismus* 23:246, 1986.

Lessner A, Stern GA: Preseptal and orbital cellulitis, *Infect Dis Clin North Am* 6:933, 1992.

Noel LP, Clarke WN, MacDonald N: Clinical management of orbital cellulitis in children, *Can J Ophthalmol* 25:11, 1990.

Powell KR: Orbital and periorbital cellulitis, *Pediatr Rev* 16:163, 1995.

250 Pyloric Stenosis

Arnold H. Colodny

Pyloric stenosis is one of the more common surgical problems of infancy,[22] and its management delights the pediatric surgeon because surgical treatment is decisive. If the problem goes untreated, the patient's condition will deteriorate. The parents usually are young, inexperienced, and distraught, but the operation is simple and curative and has few complications if the pathophysiology is understood. The mortality has declined steadily from approximately 50% at the turn of the century to well under 1% today.

CLINICAL FEATURES

About 80% of infants who have hypertrophic pyloric stenosis are boys. The firstborn male most often is afflicted. Caucasian infants are affected more than are African-American infants. Fifteen percent of patients are likely to have a family history of the condition. If the mother had pyloric stenosis, the child has a four times greater chance of having pyloric stenosis than if the father had it.[26] Vomiting is the cardinal sign of trouble in most cases. The age of onset varies. The average age is 3 to 4 weeks; in rare cases vomiting from pyloric stenosis has been seen in the newborn period and as late as the fourth month. In the typical case, an infant begins to regurgitate a small amount of formula immediately after some feedings, although he or she continues to gain weight at first. Later the vomiting becomes more frequent and more forceful (i.e., projectile) and eventually occurs after all feedings. The baby continues to be hungry. The vomitus does not contain bile, but if vomiting has occurred for a considerable period, the vomitus may have a brownish discoloration caused by bleeding that occurs secondary to gastritis. Weight loss, dehydration, and metabolic alkalosis are the inevitable results if the vomiting is prolonged, and in neglected cases the infant may develop an extreme degree of nutritional depletion.

The cause of pyloric stenosis is unclear. Various theories have been suggested, such as alterations in gastrin levels,[35] abnormalities of pyloric ganglion cells, changes in breastfeeding practices,[20] changes in infant milk formulas,[48] and neurophysiological alterations.[6] The gastrointestinal (GI) tract harbors several populations of peptide-containing nerve fibers, including the neuropeptides, vasoactive intestinal peptide (VIP), substance P, enkephalin, and gastrin-releasing peptide (GRP). Studies in specimens from patients who have pyloric stenosis have shown a reduction of VIP and enkephalin fibers in their smooth muscle, suggesting that impaired neuronal function may be involved in the pathophysiology of pyloric stenosis.[25]

Congenital hypertrophic pyloric stenosis has been reported in association with malrotation, junctional epidermolysis bullosa,[28] Hirschsprung disease, ovarian cysts, icthyosis,[42] and deletions of the long arm of chromosome 11.[29] An increased incidence has been reported in the children of women who took significant amounts of bendectin in the first trimester of pregnancy.[3,8] However, a dissenting view also has been reported.[27]

DIAGNOSIS

A positive diagnosis is best made by feeling the firm, enlarged pylorus, the so-called olive. This can be done in approximately 90% of the cases, if the baby's abdominal musculature is relaxed, by giving the baby a sugar nipple and holding and elevating the feet with the hand not used for palpation. Emptying the distended stomach with a feeding tube may facilitate the physical examination. The right upper quadrant should be palpated adjacent to the midline because a transverse process of a lumbar vertebra, a piece of fecal material, or the lower pole of the right kidney conceivably could be mistaken for the pyloric mass; with experience, however, there should be no mistaking the typical sensation and movement of the enlarged pylorus while moving the elevated feet, which is like feeling a peanut under a blanket. An infant suspected of having pyloric stenosis but in whom a pyloric tumor is not readily palpable (as often is the case early in the clinical course) is best examined during a sugar water feeding, and infants who have pyloric stenosis usually are eager eaters. Gastric contractions may easily be seen moving across the upper abdomen from left to right, much as a golf ball would appear if it were moved slowly beneath the abdominal wall in the same direction (Fig. 250-1). These contractions increase in size and frequency (working against a hypertrophied, closed pylorus) until projectile vomiting occurs. At this point the pyloric mass is felt most easily, with the patient lying either supine or prone.

It is interesting that in a recent study, even when a palpable pyloric mass was present (85% of cases), most patients (80%) still underwent some unnecessary diagnostic imaging procedure.[11] Such imaging is redundant in the vast majority of infants who have pyloric stenosis and reflects the lack of confidence in the physical findings and too much reliance on technology. Imaging studies should be reserved for infants who vomit persistently and in whom careful and repeated physical examination fails to detect a palpable pyloric mass.[11] Real-time ultrasonography should be the first imaging technique used in vomiting infants who are thought to have pyloric stenosis but who do not have a palpable mass. Several observers[4,40,46] have confirmed Teele's original observation[44] of its value. The thickness and length of the pyloric muscle are measured. If the thickness is greater than 3.7 mm and the length is greater than 17 mm, hypertrophic pyloric stenosis is diagnosed[49] (Fig. 250-2). Postoperative ultrasonography has shown that these values have returned to normal within 6 months.[10] One study showed a return to normal values in 2 to 12 weeks after a successful pyloromyotomy.[30] The

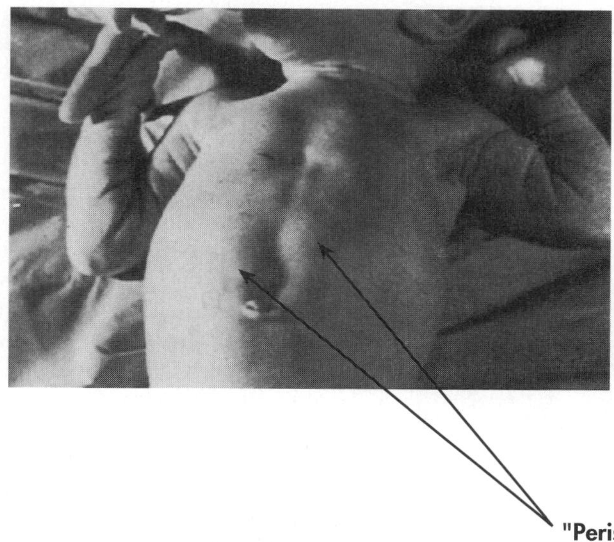

FIG. 250-1 Peristaltic waves seen in the upper abdomen (moving from left to right) in a baby who has pyloric stenosis.

(From Hoekelman RA: The physical examination of infants and children. In Bates B, editor: ***A guide to physical examination and history taking,*** ed 6, Philadelphia, 1995, JB Lippincott.)

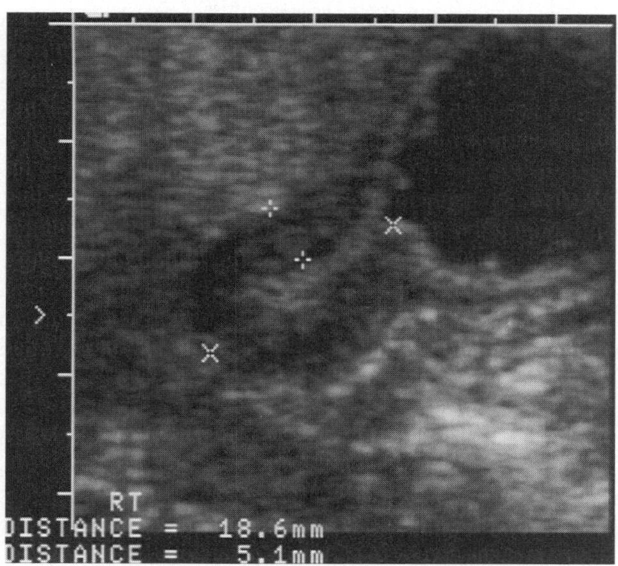

FIG. 250-2 An ultrasound examination of an infant who has hypertrophic pyloric stenosis. Note the increased thickness and length of the pyloric musculature.

overall accuracy of ultrasonography in detecting the presence or absence of pyloric stenosis is 97%.[19,21] In patients initially suspected of having pyloric stenosis who proved to have other congenital GI abnormalities, ultrasonography was able to demonstrate the correct diagnosis (atresia, stenosis, duplications, diaphragms, annular pancreas).[12,33] In addition to associated anomalies of the central nervous system (CNS), the GI tract, and the heart, a possible increase in congenital renal anomalies recently was suggested.[2,9,17] Therefore, when the initial ultrasound scan is performed in an infant suspected of having pyloric stenosis, careful evaluation of the urinary system should be included in the sonogram.

Because some false negative findings occur, a barium swallow and GI series should be done if the ultrasound is negative to ensure that pyloric stenosis is not present and also to seek other lesions that could account for the vomiting.[7,34] The GI series is a less satisfactory method of establishing the diagnosis. When the pyloric mass cannot be felt or the diagnosis cannot be demonstrated on ultrasound examination, roentgenograms with contrast material can rule out alternative diagnoses such as esophageal stenosis, achalasia, chalasia, hiatal hernia, antral spasm, gastric duplication, or pyloric diaphragm. The three criteria for roentgenographic diagnosis of pyloric stenosis are (1) delayed gastric emptying, (2) persistent narrowing, and (3) persistent elongation of the pyloric canal. The double track, or "railroad track," sign is common, consisting of two or more parallel linear streaks of barium extending through the elongated pyloric canal (Fig. 250-3). When a diagnosis of pyloric stenosis cannot be established in a baby who vomits persistently, and who has a normal ultrasound examination and GI series, the possibilities of sepsis, a poor feeding regimen, intracranial disease, renal failure, or adrenal insufficiency should be considered. In these cases it may be crucial to make a prompt diagnosis. Infants who have congenital adrenal hyperplasia who are "salt losers" may be in critical condition and may require immediate therapy. Clues to the correct diagnosis are (1) the baby will be sicker than expected, (2) the genitalia may be abnormal (e.g., an enlarged clitoris and labial fusion in girls [these patients often are mistaken as boys with undescended testicles] or penile enlargement and scrotal hyperpigmentation and hyperrugation in males) and (3) a low serum sodium and a high serum potassium. Otherwise, the infant should be reevaluated in a week or 10 days when the pyloric mass may become palpable or the ultrasound examination or GI series may become diagnostic.[15]

Establishing the diagnosis may be difficult when pyloric stenosis develops after a surgical procedure, as it occasion-

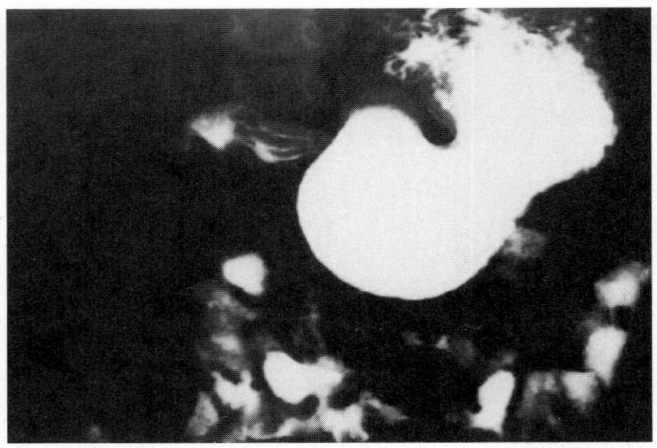

FIG. 250-3 The major features of pyloric stenosis that can be seen on an upper gastrointestinal series include elongation of the pyloric canal, the "railroad track" sign of the compressed pyloric mucosa, and a mass effect on the gastric antrum and duodenal bulb.

ally does in babies who have been operated on for esopha geal atresia.[31] The condition may manifest itself by high residual gastrostomy aspirations or persistent leakage from the gastrostomy site, if the tube has been removed.

COMPLICATIONS

The fluid and electrolyte disturbance in pyloric stenosis is similar to that seen in a patient who has an obstructing duodenal ulcer. Loss of acid gastric juice results in a deficit of sodium, potassium, chloride, and water.[16] Because the gastric juice contains more chloride than sodium, a hypochloremic, hypokalemic alkalosis develops. Potassium shifts out of the cell and sodium into the cell; much of the potassium is lost in the urine and a lesser amount in the vomitus. Although metabolic alkalosis has been regarded as the classic electrolyte derangement, a recent study[45] has shown that a spectrum of derangements may be seen, and variations from this expected pattern are not unusual. The cardinal point to be emphasized in the management of a depleted, alkalotic baby who has pyloric stenosis is that this is not a surgical emergency. Even though this is a form of intestinal obstruction, gangrene and perforation of the stomach do not occur. *No infant should be operated on for pyloric stenosis until the fluid and electrolyte deficits have been corrected.* If infants come to surgery with uncorrected alkalosis, the profound effect of surgical stress on the urinary excretion of sodium may intensify the hypokalemic alkalosis and have disastrous results.

Patients who are mildly to moderately dehydrated usually can be hydrated within 24 hours, using intravenous replacement with a solution of one third saline in 10% glucose; potassium chloride is added at the rate of 40 mEq/liter of solution after urine output has been initiated. The volume replaced depends on the degree of dehydration, the history (intake and degree and duration of vomiting), the physical examination (depression of the fontanelle, skin and tissue turgor, filling of veins, state of the mucous membranes, mental status, type of cry, amount of weight loss, recession of eyes, state of peripheral circulation, type of breathing, and general activity), and the laboratory examination (amount and specific gravity or osmolality of the urine, electrolyte determinations, and hematocrit).

A severely depleted, lethargic infant requires more vigorous therapy. In addition to the electrolyte fluid, plasma may be given rapidly in the amount of 5 ml/kg. If the hematocrit is *very* low after hydration, a small blood transfusion may be indicated (10 to 15 ml/kg). Even though these severely depleted babies may look remarkably better at the end of 24 to 48 hours and their serum electrolytes may be approaching normal, it is wise to continue this therapy for another 24 to 36 hours because their intracellular electrolyte status may not have returned to normal.

Infants who have pyloric stenosis who vomit blood or coffee-ground material are assumed to have severe gastritis. Approximately 8% of patients have hematemesis.[41] They frequently also have significant postoperative vomiting. In these infants it is beneficial to omit oral intake before surgery and for the first 24 hours after surgery. Infants then will tolerate feedings with much less vomiting.

Jaundice is seen in association with pyloric stenosis but recedes rapidly after a satisfactory pyloromyotomy. The hyperbilirubinemia results from indirect, unconjugated bilirubin. As many as 2% of patients have jaundice, with bilirubin in the range of 6 to 12 mg/dl, the indirect fraction ranging from 5 to 10 mg/dl. Bilirubin values return to normal within 7 to 20 days after surgery.[23] The jaundice probably is related to the nutritional deficits and to depression of glucuronyl transferase activity in the liver.

TREATMENT

Preoperative Management

If hematemesis has not occurred and the baby is alert and vigorous, occasional oral feedings of glucose and electrolyte solutions may be given before surgery. Although these babies may not vomit, considerable gastric retention can develop. The stomach must be emptied immediately before the operation; otherwise, vomiting may occur and aspiration may result with induction. Relaxation of the cardia and vomiting also may occur when the stomach is delivered into the incision if it has not been decompressed preoperatively.

Surgery

Surgical management of an infant who has pyloric stenosis usually is straightforward. Bypass procedures were abandoned at the turn of the century when the extramucosal muscle–splitting pyloromyotomy was introduced.[32] This procedure may be performed through the standard right upper quadrant gridiron incision or a transverse rectus incision.[38] Significant wound complications have virtually disappeared. The major intraoperative complication is a duodenal perforation, where the narrowed pyloric lumen changes abruptly to the normal duodenal lumen. Perforation is not catastrophic unless it goes unrecognized. Further complications can be prevented by suture closure of the perforation, omental reinforcement, and maintaining nasogastric suction for 24 to 36 hours.

A second operation for pyloric stenosis is unusual. Because of the abrupt change between the pyloric mass and the duodenum, most surgeons pay great attention to the distal end of the pylorus. In addition to a noticeable color change from white to pink, a distinct ring can be seen at the gastroduodenal juncture. This can be felt by drawing a finger up the soft duodenum onto the firm, rubbery pylorus. The ring will feel broken and the pyloric incision will be eccentric when an adequate pyloromyotomy has been done. The muscle splitting should be carried proximally well onto normal stomach. In most cases requiring a second operation, the pyloromyotomy has been inadequate at the proximal end. Recently, laparoscopic pyloromyotomy has been reported.[1] The advantage of using a laparoscopic approach is not apparent. The open operation is done through a small incision, is simple, is quick, and is as close to a perfect operation as one can be. The laparoscopic approach, although new, is not necessarily better. It adds the real dangers associated with establishing a pneumoperitoneum,[14,18,36,39] requires more expensive instrumentation, takes longer, and increases the cost. A recent report by Alain et al.[1a] on 78 laparoscopic pyloromyotomies had what the authors considered satisfactory results. However, two unrecognized gastric perforations required emergency laparotomies 1 day after the operation. This is a potentially fatal complication if not recognized promptly. This unacceptable complication rate will increase even more if less experienced and less talented laparoscopists than Dr. Alain attempt to equal his results.

Postoperative Management

A significant number of babies may vomit postoperatively; thus it requires discretion to select those who require a second operation. Approximately one third of infants have a day or two of vomiting in the postoperative period. Most of these can be fed, and the vomiting will cease. If vomiting persists, oral feedings should be withheld for 24 to 36 hours and then restarted. If the vomiting recurs, the stomach should be put at complete rest for another day or two by nasogastric suction. Feeding with clear liquids then may be started for 1 to 2 days, followed by dilute formula. If this is retained, full-strength formula may be started. A "chalasia chair" may be helpful. Feedings should be given in small amounts until they are retained without difficulty.

Methylscopolamine nitrate (Skopyl) has been used successfully in the medical treatment of some babies who have mild symptoms of pyloric stenosis and has been tried in patients who have persistent postoperative vomiting.[13] Metoclopramide (Reglan) also may be helpful. If the mother has been breast-feeding, she should be encouraged to continue to do so in the immediate postoperative period; breast milk seems to be tolerated better than commercial formulas.

If vomiting persists despite the above measures, roentgenograms should be obtained. Babies who have pyloric stenosis have a 3% to 12% incidence of other congenital anomalies. Most of these are minor, but distal intestinal obstruction in patients who have pyloric stenosis does occur. The GI series may be difficult to interpret because narrowing and elongation of the pyloric canal usually is persistent in the early postoperative period, even in babies who have no postoperative vomiting. A return to normal pyloric opening time and gastric emptying is the expected response.

A second operation for pyloric stenosis should not be undertaken hastily; the physician should wait 10 days to 2 weeks to make this decision, unless the infant's condition deteriorates. The increased thickness and length of the pyloric muscle may take up to 6 weeks to return to normal after a successful operation.[37]

Hypoglycemia. Reactive hypoglycemia has been recorded in depleted infants who have a wide variety of medical and surgical conditions. This may cause unexpected respiratory arrest and unexplained death. Increases in insulin secretion by constant infusion of glucose can result in severe hypoglycemia if the infusion is stopped suddenly before oral alimentation is adequate. This particularly is likely to happen when the glycogen stores of the liver have been depleted. Liver biopsies performed in babies who have pyloric stenosis and severe postoperative hypoglycemia have revealed depletion of hepatic glycogen stores. Fatalities from postoperative hypoglycemia in babies who have pyloric stenosis have been reported.

Apnea. Babies who have pyloric stenosis may be difficult to anesthetize. After the operation has been completed and anesthesia terminated, apnea may become a problem in the immediate postoperative period in the recovery room. When the painful stimulus of the surgical procedure is no longer present, the level of anesthesia may deepen. Hypoventilation then may proceed to respiratory arrest. Careful attention to respiratory efforts as the baby enters the recovery room is necessary, and stimulation or assisted breathing may be necessary during this period. Administration of naloxone may be helpful.[5]

Long-Term Follow-up. A study of pyloric function revealed an increased rate of gastric emptying and an increase in duodenogastric reflux in some patients who had a pyloromyotomy for pyloric stenosis 5 to 7 years previously.[43] This might account for the increased incidence of peptic ulcer disease and gastritis in some of these patients. A more recent long-term follow-up study has not shown a significant increase in GI difficulties.[47]

CAUSES OF DEATH

The mortality in patients who have pyloric stenosis is well under 1%.[50] Although this is encouraging, the goal is to prevent these deaths altogether. Modern anesthetic management has contributed to these improved results.[24] On review of 754 consecutive patients who had pyloric stenosis, eight causes of death could be identified: (1) delayed diagnosis, (2) inadequate preoperative preparation (rehydration and restoration of a normal electrolyte balance), (3) pulmonary aspiration, (4) unrecognized perforation, (5) hypoglycemia, (6) persistent obstruction, (7) hemorrhage, and (8) the presence of other associated congenital anomalies. The tragedy is that almost all such deaths are avoidable.

REFERENCES

1. Alain JL, Grousseau D, Terrier G: Extramucosal pyloromyotomy by laparoscopy, *J Pediatr Surg* 26:1191, 1991.

1a. Alain JL et al: Extramucosal pyloromyotomy by laparoscopy, *J Laparoscopic Surg* 6(suppl):41, 1996.

2. Angulo JC et al: Congenital mesoblastic nephroma, nephrocalcinosis, and hypertrophic pyloric stenosis, *J Surg Oncol* 48:142, 1991.

3. Aselton P et al: Pyloric stenosis and maternal benedictine exposure, *Am J Epidemiol* 120:251, 1984.

4. Ball TI, Atkinson GB, Gay BB: Ultrasound diagnosis of hypertrophic pyloric stenosis, *Radiology* 147:499, 1983.
5. Beilin B et al: Naloxone reversal of postoperative apnea in a premature infant with pyloric stenosis, *Anesthesiology* 63:317, 1985.
6. Belding HH, Kernohan JW: A morphologic study of the myenteric plexus and musculature of the pylorus with special reference to the changes in hypertrophic pyloric stenosis, *Surg Gynecol Obstet* 97:322, 1953.
7. Bell MJ: Antral diaphragm, *J Pediatr* 90:196, 1977.
8. Benedictine and pyloric stenosis, *FDA Drug Bull* 13:14, 1983.
9. Bidair M, Kalota SJ, Kaplan GW: Infantile hypertrophic pyloric stenosis and hydronephrosis, *J Urol* 150:153, 1993.
10. Bourchier D, Dawson KP, Kennedy JC: Pyloric stenosis: a postoperative ultrasonic study, *Aust Paediatr J* 21:189, 1985.
11. Breaux CW et al: Changing patterns in the diagnosis of hypertrophic pyloric stenosis, *Pediatrics* 81:213, 1988.
12. Chew AL, Friewald JP, Donovan C: Diagnosis of congenital antral web by ultrasound, *Pediatr Radiol* 22:342, 1992.
13. Corner BD: Hypertrophic pyloric stenosis treated with methyl scopolamine nitrate, *Arch Dis Child* 30:377, 1955.
14. Ehrlich RM, Gershman A, Fuchs G: Operative laparoscopy in children, *Soc Ped Urol Newsletter* Feb 28, 1993.
15. Geer LL et al: Evolution of pyloric stenosis in the first week of life, *Pediatr Radiol* 15:205, 1985.
16. Graham JA: Water and electrolyte imbalance in pyloric stenosis, *Gut* 10:1056, 1969.
17. Gupta AK, Berry M: Recessive polycystic kidney disease and congenital hypertrophic pyloric stenosis, *Pediatr Radiol* 21:160, 1991.
18. Kavoussi LR et al: Complications of laparoscopic lymph node dissection, *J Urol* 149:322, 1993.
19. Keller H, Waldmann D, Greiner D: Comparison of preoperative sonography with intraoperative findings in congenital hypertrophic pyloric stenosis, *J Pediatr Surg* 22:950, 1987.
20. Knox EG, Armstrong E, Haynes R: Changing incidence of pyloric stenosis, *Arch Dis Child* 58:582, 1983.
21. Kovalivker M et al: The value of ultrasound in the diagnosis of congenital hypertrophic pyloric stenosis, *Clin Pediatr* 32:281, 1993.
22. Laron Z, Horne LM: The incidence of infantile pyloric stenosis, *Am J Dis Child* 94:151, 1957.
23. Lippert MM: Pyloric stenosis presenting as severe prolonged jaundice, *S Afr Med J* 69:446, 1986.
24. MacDonald NJ et al: Anaesthesia for congenital hypertrophic pyloric stenosis, *Br J Anaesth* 59:672, 1987.
25. Malmfors G, Sundler F: Peptidergic innervation in infantile hypertrophic pyloric stenosis, *J Pediatr Surg* 21:303, 1986.
26. McKeown T, MacMahon B: Infantile hypertrophic pyloric stenosis in parent and child, *Arch Dis Child* 30:497, 1955.
27. Mitchell AA et al: Birth defects in relation to benedictine use in pregnancy, *Am J Obstet Gynecol* 147:737, 1983.
28. Muller H et al: Herlitz syndrome and pyloric obstruction, *Helvetica Paediatrica Acta* 43:457, 1989.
29. O'Hare AE, Grade E, Edmunds AT: Deletion of the long arm of chromosome 11, *Clin Genet* 25:273, 1984.
30. Okorie NM et al: What happens to the pylorus after pyloromyotomy? *Arch Dis Child* 63:1339, 1988.
31. Qvist N et al: Development of infantile hypertrophic pyloric stenosis in patients treated for oesophageal atresia, *Acta Chir Scand* 152:237, 1986.
32. Ramstedt C: Zur operation der angeborenen pylorus-stenose, *Med Klin* 8:1702, 1912.
33. Riebel T, Wurfel A, Gasiorek-Wiens A: Sonography of congenital abnormalities of the gastrointestinal tract, *Ultraschall Med* 12:283, 1991.
34. Rober JM, Bleicher MA: Surgical management of duodenal duplication cyst simulating pyloric stenosis, *Mt Sinai J Med* 51:702, 1984.
35. Rogers JM: Plasma gastrin in congenital hypertonic pyloric stenosis, *Arch Dis Child* 50:467, 1975.
36. Sadeghi-Nejad H, Kavoussi LR, Peters CA: Bowel injury in open technique laparoscopic cannula placement, *Urology* 43:559, 1994.
37. Sauerbrei EE, Paloschi GG: The ultrasonic features of hypertrophic pyloric stenosis with emphasis on the postoperative appearance, *Radiology* 147:503, 1983.
38. Schuster SR, Colodny AH: A useful maneuver to simplify pyloromyotomy for hypertrophic pyloric stenosis, *Surgery* 55:735, 1964.
39. See WA, Cooper CS, Fisher RJ: Predictors of laparoscopic complications after formal training in laparoscopic surgery, *JAMA* 270:2689, 1993.
40. Shkolnik A: Applications of ultrasound in the neonate, *Radiol Clin North Am* 23:141, 1985.
41. Spitz L, Batcup G: Hematemesis in infantile hypertrophic pyloric stenosis, *Br J Surg* 66:827, 1979.
42. Stoll C et al: Hypertrophic pyloric stenosis associated with X-linked ichthyosis in two brothers, *Clin Exp Dermatol* 8:61, 1983.
43. Tam PK et al: Pyloric function 5 to 7 years after Ramstedt's pyloromyotomy, *J Pediatr Surg* 20:236, 1985.
44. Teele RL, Smith EH: Ultrasound in the diagnosis of congenital hypertrophic pyloric stenosis, *N Engl J Med* 296:1149, 1977.
45. Touloukian RJ, Higgins E: The spectrum of serum electrolytes in hypertrophic pyloric stenosis, *J Pediatr Surg* 18:394, 1983.
46. Tunell WP, Wilson DA: Pyloric stenosis: diagnosis by real-time sonography, *J Pediatr Surg* 19:795, 1984.
47. Vilmann P et al: A long-term gastrointestinal follow-up in patients operated on for congenital hypertrophic pyloric stenosis, *Acta Paediatr Scand* 75:156, 1986.
48. Webb AR, Lari J, Dodge JA: Infantile hypertrophic pyloric stenosis: effects of changes in feeding practices, *Arch Dis Child* 58:586, 1983.
49. Wilson DA, Yanhoutte JJ: The reliable sonographic diagnosis of hypertrophic pyloric stenosis, *J Chicago Univ* 12:201, 1984.
50. Zeiden B et al: Recent results of treatment of infantile hypertrophic pyloric stenosis, *Arch Dis Child* 63:1060, 1988.

251 Reye Syndrome

Rebecca Ribovich Matsakis

Reye syndrome, as a distinct clinical and pathological entity, was first reported from Australia by Reye et al.[9] in 1963 when they described a syndrome of encephalopathy and fatty degeneration of the liver. Since then, cases of this syndrome have been reported from all over the world.

The incidence of Reye syndrome in the United States has been decreasing steadily since 1981 and is reported to be less than 0.1 case per 100,000 in populations under 18 years of age.[4] A temporal and geographical association of Reye syndrome with cases of varicella, influenza B, and influenza A has been observed. Reye syndrome has occurred in infants and children of all age groups, and cases have been reported in adults. The highest incidence is in the 5- to 14-year-old age group. There is no sex predilection; 90% of the cases have occurred in whites and 8% in blacks. There have been case reports of recurrent Reye syndrome, familial Reye syndrome, and Reye syndrome following live virus vaccination.

DEFINITION

The case definition for Reye syndrome as established by the Centers for Disease Control and Prevention[3] in 1980 is as follows:

1. Acute noninflammatory encephalopathy with one of the following:
   a. Microvesicular fatty metamorphosis of the liver confirmed by biopsy or autopsy
   b. A serum aspartate aminotransferase (AST), a serum alanine aminotransferase (ALT), or a serum ammonia (NH_3) that is greater than three times normal
2. Cerebrospinal fluid, if obtained, with fewer than eight leukocytes per cubic millimeter
3. No other more reasonable explanation for the neurological or hepatic abnormalities

PATHOLOGY

In Reye syndrome pathological changes have been described in the liver, brain, kidney, heart, pancreas, and skeletal muscle. The liver has a diffuse yellowish appearance caused by lipid accumulation within the cytoplasm of the hepatocytes. Glycogen stains show the diffuse depletion of glycogen. There is no necrosis or inflammatory infiltrates. The mitochondria of the hepatocytes are swollen, and their outer cellular membranes are deformed.

On gross examination the brain is swollen, with flattening of the gyri. Microscopic examination shows cerebral edema. The ultrastructural abnormalities include focal areas of swelling in myelin sheaths and accumulation of edema fluid in glial cells. The brain mitochondria show variable changes, namely matrix distortion and swelling.

Lipid accumulation also has been described in the kidney, the heart, and skeletal muscle. Evidence of mitochondrial injury also has been reported in cardiac and skeletal muscle. Focal necrosis, hemorrhage, and inflammatory changes have been described in the pancreas.

BIOCHEMICAL ABNORMALITIES

Since the original report of Reye syndrome in which elevated serum aminotransferases and hypoglycemia were described, numerous other metabolic abnormalities have been documented. The serum ammonia level is elevated in almost all patients who have Reye syndrome, but this is transient, with levels returning to normal in 24 to 48 hours. Levels greater than 350 μg/dl usually are associated with a less favorable prognosis for survival.

There are various explanations for the hyperammonemia. Reductions in the hepatic activities of ornithine transcarbamoylase and carbamyl phosphate synthetase, which are mitochondrial enzymes of the urea cycle, may explain the hyperammonemia. Also, because of the anorexia and vomiting that occur, the patient is in a catabolic state, which results in an increased release of amino acids from muscle; this too may lead to the hyperammonemia.

The serum aminotransferase levels always are elevated, but the bilirubin is normal or elevated only minimally. Hypoglycemia occurs in about 40% of patients, is seen primarily in children under 4 years of age, and is thought to result from deficient hepatic gluconeogenesis.

Elevated serum lactic acid concentrations frequently are found and may be related to impaired oxidative metabolism of glucose or to accelerated production by extrahepatic tissues such as muscle. Total serum free fatty acids, particularly short-chain fatty acids, are elevated in patients who have Reye syndrome. In some studies clinical improvement has been associated with the clearance of these short-chain fatty acids. Possible explanations for the fatty acidemia include an increased release from adipose tissue secondary to the anorexia and vomiting or a lipolytic response to a virus.

Coincident with the increased free fatty acid concentrations, dicarboxylic acids appear in urine and serum. This finding suggests that mitochondrial beta-oxidation of fatty acids is compromised or overwhelmed by a massive influx of fatty acids. Alternative routes of oxidation then are used.

Other reported abnormalities include elevations in serum amino acids, creatinine phosphokinase, uric acid, blood urea nitrogen (BUN), amylase, and serum osmolality. Transient acute renal failure has been described on occasion.

The prothrombin time is prolonged, but the platelet count usually is normal in patients who have Reye syndrome. Fibrin split products usually are absent from the circulation, and decreased coagulation factors (except for factor VIII) have been observed. Disseminated intravascular coagulation has been described only rarely.

Respiratory alkalosis is present as a result of primary stimulation of the respiratory centers in the brainstem. A mixed metabolic acidosis often is found in addition to the respiratory alkalosis. The hyperthermia that is present early in the disease may be the result of hypothalamic dysfunction.

ETIOLOGY AND PATHOGENESIS

The etiology of Reye syndrome remains unclear, but available evidence suggests a multifactorial cause. Contributing factors may include genetic susceptibility and an exogenous toxin, whether a medication or an environmental agent, which modify the reaction to a viral infection.

An increased incidence of Reye syndrome has been reported during outbreaks of varicella, influenza B, and influenza A. Both influenza A and B infections have been demonstrated serologically in many patients who have Reye syndrome. Adenovirus, coxsackieviruses A and B, echovirus, Epstein-Barr virus, parainfluenza virus, reovirus, rubella virus, rubeola virus, type I poliomyelitis virus, and herpes simplex viruses also have been linked to Reye syndrome.

Much attention has been given to the role of salicylates in the origin of Reye syndrome. Epidemiological studies,[5,7,13,17] including a Public Health Service study,[8] have found a higher rate of salicylate ingestion (by history) in patients who have Reye syndrome as compared with control children who have similar antecedent illnesses. These reports have resulted in the recommendation that the use of salicylates be avoided for children who have varicella infections and during influenza outbreaks. Since the publicity about the association between Reye syndrome and aspirin began in late 1980, much of the decline in its reported incidence has been attributed to the reported decrease in the use of salicylates in treating children who have viral illnesses.[1,2] These epidemiological studies show a strong association between salicylate use and Reye syndrome, although the precise role of salicylates in the pathogenesis of Reye syndrome remains unclear.

Environmental toxins such as aflatoxins and insecticides have been implicated in the etiology of Reye syndrome, but there is little evidence that these toxins play a major role.

The pathogenesis of the encephalopathy in Reye syndrome remains unclear. Some etiological factors that have been suggested are hyperammonemia, lactic acidemia, short-chain fatty acidemia, and direct brain cell mitochondrial damage paralleling that seen in the liver cells.

It also has been suggested that generalized mitochondrial insult and dysfunction are the bases of the metabolic abnormalities found. As noted, there is strong evidence for insult to hepatic mitochondria in terms of both morphological and enzymatic abnormalities. The evidence for a similar primary mitochondrial dysfunction in brain cells is less substantial. As yet, the hypothesis of widespread mitochondrial disease is not well supported.

CLINICAL FEATURES

Patients who have Reye syndrome have a viral prodromal illness usually consisting of an upper respiratory tract infection, gastroenteritis, or varicella. The child appears to be recovering from such illness, but then develops repetitive vomiting. Within 24 to 48 hours the child becomes agitated, combative, disoriented, and behaves irrationally. Periods of lethargy may alternate with the combative behavior. Hyperventilation also may be prominent and is probably a result of primary stimulation of the medullary respiratory centers. Approximately 85% of patients have hepatomegaly, but jaundice is absent. Pancreatitis is found in up to 22% of autopsied cases. The pancreatic involvement can be so severe as to produce hemorrhagic necrosis and death. Seizures can occur at any time during the encephalopathic stages.

The child may begin to recover spontaneously or may deteriorate further into full obtundation. Central nervous system dysfunction progresses from stupor to coma with intact brainstem function, to decorticate or decerebrate posturing, and finally to a flaccid and areflexic state.

Various systems have been devised to stage the severity of the illness in Reye syndrome. The National Institutes of Health Consensus Development Conference on the Diagnosis and Treatment of Reye syndrome held in 1981 generated the revised staging system, shown in Table 251-1. This was done in an attempt to introduce a uniform staging system for use by all treatment centers.

The clinical presentation of Reye syndrome in infants is somewhat different from that previously outlined, so early recognition is more difficult. Following the prodromal illness, vomiting may be minimal or absent. Diarrhea, however, is a frequent occurrence. Seizures also are frequently present, can occur early in the course of the illness, and may be the presenting sign. Respiratory disturbances, such as hyperventila-

Table 251-1 Staging of Reye Syndrome

	I	II	III	IV	V
Level of consciousness	Lethargy; follows verbal commands	Combative/stupor; verbalizes inappropriately	Coma	Coma	Coma
Posture	Normal	Normal	Decorticate	Decerebrate	Flaccid
Response to pain	Purposeful	Purposeful/nonpurposeful	Decorticate	Decerebrate	None
Pupillary reaction	Brisk	Sluggish	Sluggish	Sluggish	None
Oculocephalic reflex (doll's eyes)	Normal	Conjugate deviation	Conjugate deviation	Inconsistent or absent	None

From National Institutes of Health Consensus Development Conference: *JAMA* 246:2442, 1981.

tion and apnea, are prominent and also may occur early in the course of the illness.

DIAGNOSIS

The diagnosis of Reye syndrome should be considered when a history of an antecedent viral illness is followed by vomiting, progressive lethargy, agitation, and obtundation. Early diagnosis is important because prompt treatment may provide a better chance for complete recovery.

Laboratory Tests

Laboratory tests that should be obtained to help establish the diagnosis include serum ammonia, serum aminotransferases, bilirubin, prothrombin time, blood glucose, and urine and blood toxicology screens. A lumbar puncture should not be performed routinely if Reye syndrome is suspected, because of the associated cerebral edema and increased intracranial pressure. If meningitis is suspected, a lumbar puncture should be performed using a small-gauge needle, with removal of as little cerebrospinal fluid as possible to minimize the likelihood of cerebral herniation. A cerebrospinal fluid specimen containing fewer than eight leukocytes per cubic millimeter and normal protein and glucose concentrations, except when there is concomitant hypoglycemia, is consistent with Reye syndrome.

Special Studies and Computed Tomography

A liver biopsy is not essential to diagnose most cases of Reye syndrome because the clinical and laboratory features are typical. However, a liver biopsy to establish the diagnosis firmly should be considered in patients under 1 year of age, in children who have recurrent episodes, in familial cases, in atypical cases that have no antecedent viral infection or vomiting, and when new and potentially dangerous therapeutic regimens are planned.

Computed tomographic (CT) brain scanning is not needed for diagnosing Reye syndrome. A CT scan performed early in the course of the illness will either be normal or show evidence of diffuse brain edema. The electroencephalogram also will be nonspecific and will not help to establish the diagnosis, alter treatment regimens, or determine prognosis.

DIFFERENTIAL DIAGNOSIS

The conditions that should be considered in the differential diagnosis of Reye syndrome are as follows[15]:

1. Infections: meningitis, varicella, hepatitis, encephalitis
2. Toxins: salicylates, methyl bromide, hypoglycin, isopropyl alcohol, aflatoxin, lead, valproic acid
3. Anoxic encephalopathy
4. Inborn metabolic defects: systemic carnitine deficiency, hyperammonemia syndromes, and organic acid disorders.

Meningitis may follow an upper respiratory tract infection and can produce vomiting and lethargy. Aminotransferase elevations may occur in children who have varicella without concomitant Reye syndrome and in hypoxia resulting from a wide variety of causes. Excessive salicylate ingestion can cause vomiting, seizures, obtundation, hyperventilation, hypoglycemia, and abnormal liver function. A serum salicylate level of 25 mg/dl or more suggests salicylism rather than Reye syndrome. Other toxins, such as methyl bromide, hypoglycin, isopropyl alcohol, aflatoxin, lead, and valproic acid may produce disturbances of consciousness and elevation of serum aminotransferase levels.

An increasing number of metabolic disorders have been described that may mimic Reye syndrome, especially in infants and younger children.[6,10,11] These disorders also are associated with vomiting and altered consciousness. The inborn errors of ureagenesis that may mimic Reye syndrome include partial ornithine transcarbamoylase deficiency and partial carbamoyl-phosphate synthase deficiency. Defects of fatty acid metabolism, such as systemic carnitine deficiency and various acetyl-CoA dehydrogenase deficiencies, also can resemble Reye syndrome in presentation. Clinical features that suggest an underlying metabolic disorder include an atypical prodrome with rapid onset, patient age under 2 years, and familial or recurrent episodes of Reye syndrome–like illness.

It has been observed that as the incidence of Reye syndrome declines, an increasing proportion of patients who seem to have its "typical" features may have one of the metabolic disorders that mimic this syndrome.[11] Therefore it has been recommended that investigations to exclude metabolic disorders be considered seriously in all patients suspected of having Reye syndrome.

TREATMENT

Once the diagnosis of Reye syndrome is suspected, the severity of the patient's illness should be staged, using a staging system such as the one shown in Table 251-1. All patients, regardless of their stage of disease, should be hospitalized for careful observation because neurological deterioration can progress rapidly. The primary care physician should arrange for the patient to be transferred to a regional pediatric intensive care unit (PICU) as soon as possible, using a transport team prepared to provide support for all vital functions. Supportive care for patients in stages I and II includes frequent evaluations of neurological status. A 10% dextrose solution containing balanced electrolytes should be administered intravenously at the rate needed to deliver daily maintenance fluid requirements. The use of a high-glucose concentration is designed to decrease lipolysis. Any abnormalities in the serum electrolytes and fluid balance should be corrected.

Children at later stages of the disease require intensive monitoring and aggressive therapy directed toward correction of metabolic abnormalities and reduction of increased intracranial pressure.

Some authorities recommend that fluids be given at two-thirds maintenance; others recommend full maintenance fluid volumes, with adjustments according to electrolyte levels and urinary output. A nasogastric tube and Foley catheter should be inserted so that accurate intake and output can be calculated. An arterial catheter, which permits continuous blood pressure measurement and arterial blood gas sampling, should be placed. Temperature should be maintained at normal levels via a cooling blanket. Endotracheal intubation should be performed and assisted ventilation instituted in comatose patients. Intravenous phenytoin should be used for seizure control. Barbiturates should be avoided because they will alter the patient's level of consciousness and neurological status.

Mannitol (0.25 g/kg, given intravenously over 30 minutes) should be administered in an attempt to reduce cerebral edema, provided that the serum osmolality level is not over 320 mOsm. The use of mannitol requires careful monitoring of the patient's fluid balance.

Neomycin sulfate enemas have been used by some authorities to reduce serum ammonia levels. Vitamin K (5 mg, given intramuscularly) can be administered in an attempt to correct the clotting abnormalities. If a significant amount of bleeding occurs, the administration of fresh-frozen plasma (10 ml/kg) may be helpful.

Arterial blood gases, serum osmolality, glucose, electrolytes, BUN, and hematocrit should be monitored closely. Once the patient is admitted to a PICU, more definitive therapeutic measures can be undertaken. A central venous catheter should be placed to monitor blood volume and cardiac function. In addition, it is recommended that patients receive hypertonic glucose solutions of 15% dextrose; a central line is required for administration of such hypertonic solutions. A pulmonary artery catheter may be required to monitor the pulmonary artery pressure and cardiac output of seriously ill children.

Some centers recommend the use of high-dose glucose and insulin to decrease serum free fatty acid concentrations. Insulin blocks fatty acid release from adipose tissue by inhibiting the enzyme lipoprotein lipase. One unit of insulin per 5 g of glucose is administered intravenously every 4 hours. The insulin dose is adjusted to maintain the serum glucose concentration between 125 and 175 mg/dl. There is no evidence, however, that this therapy improves the clinical course.

Exchange transfusion and peritoneal dialysis have been used to clear the hyperammonemia and to remove "unknown toxins." There is no evidence that the use of these techniques improves outcome either. A double-volume exchange transfusion with fresh blood also has been used to replenish coagulation factor deficiencies.

The most significant adjunct to the management of cerebral edema and increasing intracranial pressure in Reye syndrome has been the development of techniques to monitor intracranial pressure. Most centers recommend that children beyond stage II have an intracranial pressure monitor inserted. Monitoring provides a mechanism to titrate management of the patient and is designed to maintain the intracranial pressure within normal ranges until the illness resolves. The monitoring device can be either an intraventricular cannula or a subarachnoid bolt, and it should be placed after the prothrombin time is brought to normal levels. Intracranial pressure greater than 20 mm Hg should be treated. The cerebral perfusion pressure should be maintained above 50 mm Hg to prevent cerebral ischemia. Cerebral perfusion pressure is equal to the mean arterial pressure minus the intracranial pressure.

The following measures can be undertaken to treat elevated intracranial pressure:

1. Mannitol, 0.25 g/kg/dose, should be administered intravenously. Hyperosmolality is a complication of osmotherapy. Fluid should be replaced to keep the serum osmolality below 310 mOsm, thereby preventing any compromise of renal function.
2. Hyperventilation should be controlled by a mechanical respirator to maintain a P_{CO_2} of 25 to 30 mm Hg. A P_{CO_2} above this leads to increased pressure from vasodilation, and values below this range can be correlated with inadequate cerebral blood flow.
3. Pancuronium bromide, 0.1 to 0.2 mg/kg/dose, should be administered to immobilize the patient.
4. If an intraventricular catheter is used, small amounts of cerebrospinal fluid can be released through the catheter for immediate control of intracranial pressure elevations.
5. Chest physiotherapy, if performed carefully, will remove mucous plugs and decrease intrathoracic pressure, resulting in better control of intracranial pressure.

Corticosteroids have not been shown to be effective in controlling the intracranial pressure.

If the above measures are unsuccessful, high-dose barbiturate therapy may be indicated, although its use remains controversial.[12,16] Varying success rates have been reported with this therapy. Barbiturates are thought to decrease cerebral metabolic demands and cerebral blood flow and thereby control intracranial pressure. This therapy involves the administration of intravenous pentobarbital to maintain a blood level of 30 to 50 μg/dl and is carried out until the intracranial pressure returns to normal. Because possible complications of this therapy include a drop in arterial blood pressure, a change in cardiac output, or unexplained hypoxia, monitoring devices are necessary to measure these indexes accurately.

Some centers have used hypothermia when the above therapeutic measures have failed to control the elevated intracranial pressure.[14] Surface body cooling to a target body temperature of 32° C is achieved with hypothermia blankets. However, this therapy increases the risk of infection because the immune system does not function as well during hypothermia.

A final mode of therapy that has been used for patients who have increased intracranial pressure refractory to all other measures is decompressive craniectomy. Because there are potential risks of infection and bleeding with this therapy, it should be reserved for the most difficult cases.

PROGNOSIS

Early reports indicated that the mortality from Reye syndrome was 80%; this rate has decreased to less than 30%. Some of this decrease may be the result of increased recognition of the illness, especially of mild cases, in addition to greater use of intensive medical support.

Recent studies have attempted to evaluate neurological sequelae in survivors of Reye syndrome. It is estimated that 10% of survivors incur severe brain damage. Several studies suggest that those children who have the most severe illness (as evidenced by the degree and duration of increased intracranial pressure) and those who are under 2 years of age when affected are most likely to suffer sequelae. However, the vast majority of children over 2 years of age who survive Reye syndrome appear to recover completely.

Neuropsychological testing has shown that some children who have recovered from Reye syndrome have difficulty achieving in school and with visual motor integration, sequencing, tactile problem-solving, and concept formation. These more subtle deficits may persist for many months or years. In general, extensive psychological and educational testing of Reye syndrome survivors appears to be unnecessary.

Overprotectiveness of the child by the family should be avoided because this can contribute to behavioral or school problems; family guidance and counseling are essential in this regard.

REFERENCES

1. Arrowsmith JB et al: National patterns of aspirin use and Reye syndrome reporting—United States, 1980 to 1985, *Pediatrics* 79:858, 1987.
2. Barrett MJ et al: Changing epidemiology of Reye syndrome in the United States, *Pediatrics* 77:598, 1986.
3. Centers for Disease Control: Follow-up on Reye syndrome—United States, *MMWR* 29:321, 1980.
4. Centers for Disease Control: Reye syndrome surveillance—United States, 1989, *MMWR* 40:88, 1991.
5. Forsyth BE et al: New epidemiologic evidence confirming that bias does not explain the aspirin/Reye's syndrome association, *JAMA* 261:2517, 1989.
6. Greene CL, Blitzer MG, Shapira E: Inborn errors of metabolism and Reye syndrome: differential diagnosis, *J Pediatr* 113:156, 1988.
7. Halpin TJ et al: Reye's syndrome and medication use, *JAMA* 248:687, 1982.
8. Hurwitz ES et al: Public Health Service study of Reye's syndrome and medications: report of the main study, *JAMA* 257:1905, 1987.
9. Reye RDK, Morgan G, Baral J: Encephalopathy and fatty degeneration of the viscera: a disease entity in childhood, *Lancet* 2:749, 1963.
10. Robinson RO: Differential diagnosis of Reye's syndrome, *Dev Med Child Neurol* 29:110, 1987.
11. Rowe PC, Valle D, Brusilow SW: Inborn errors of metabolism in children referred with Reye's syndrome, *JAMA* 260:3167, 1988.
12. Shaywitz BA, Lister G, Duncan CC: What is the best treatment for Reye's syndrome? *Arch Neurol* 43:730, 1986.
13. Starko KM et al: Reye's syndrome and salicylate use, *Pediatrics* 66:859, 1980.
14. Swedlow DB, Schreiner MS: Management of Reye's syndrome, *Crit Care Clin* 1:285, 1985.
15. Trauner DA: Reye's syndrome, *Curr Probl Pediatr* 12:1, 1982.
16. Trauner DA: What is the best treatment for Reye's syndrome? *Arch Neurol* 43:729, 1986.
17. Waldman RJ et al: Aspirin as a risk factor in Reye's syndrome, *JAMA* 247:3089, 1982.

SUGGESTED READINGS

DeLong GR, Glick TH: Encephalopathy of Reye's syndrome: a review of pathogenetic hypotheses, *Pediatrics* 69:53, 1982.

Heubi JE et al: Reye's syndrome: current concepts, *Hepatology* 7:155, 1987.

Hurwitz ES: Reye's syndrome, *Epidemiol Rev* 11:249, 1989.

Huttenlocker PR, Trauner DA: Reye's syndrome in infancy, *Pediatrics* 62:84, 1978.

National Institutes of Health Consensus Development Conference: Diagnosis and treatment of Reye's syndrome, *JAMA* 246:2441, 1981.

252 Rheumatic Fever

Sylvia P. Griffiths

Acute rheumatic fever is a systemic connective tissue disorder that is clinically manifested by polyarthritis, carditis, or chorea. It would be an illness of little consequence except for its potential for causing inflammatory cardiac valvular involvement and the development of heart disease. The arthritis clears without sequelae of joint dysfunction or deformity, and the chorea leaves no neuromuscular impediment. Although rheumatic fever is a self-limited disease during an acute attack, it has a strong predilection to recur in succeeding years.

Since it has been established that group A beta-hemolytic streptococci play a part in the etiology of rheumatic fever, it has been shown in pediatric populations (as previously demonstrated in military establishments) that the incidence of the first attack of rheumatic fever can be reduced by adequate penicillin treatment of all cases of streptococcal pharyngitis.[10] In contrast to the high incidence of rheumatic fever observed in epidemics of streptococcal pharyngitis (approximately 2% to 3%), the attack rate following sporadic streptococcal upper respiratory tract infection is only about one tenth of that figure. In those who have already had one or more attacks of rheumatic fever, however, the recurrence rate rises to about 15% following subsequent streptococcal infection.[11]

Numerous community primary prevention programs have demonstrated the efficacy of identifying streptococcal infection by performing throat cultures on susceptible children and treating them early. Further, the widespread application of secondary prevention in the form of antistreptococcal prophylaxis programs for patients after their first attack has reduced the recurrence rate and the possible additive effects of repeated bouts of carditis significantly.

Fortunately the severity of acute rheumatic fever in a first attack, as well as the incidence of both initial and recurrent attacks, has declined steadily in the past four decades in the United States and Europe, particularly in communities that have high socioeconomic levels. However, in other parts of the world, such as Asian and other developing countries, rheumatic fever is not uncommon in childhood and may be a fulminating disease, with acute carditis leading to death during a first attack. With the increase in travel by Hispanic families from the Caribbean Islands and South America, as well as refugee population groups from Southeast Asia, rheumatic fever also may be on the rise in certain cities of the United States to which they migrate. A resurgence of rheumatic fever in certain areas of the United States, both urban and suburban, was reported between 1984 and 1988.[5,7,12] Despite the increase in the number of cases the annual incidence at a large teaching medical center may be so small that an intern or resident may not see more than one or two children who have rheumatic fever during his or her 3 years of training in pediatrics.

DIAGNOSIS

Because there are neither pathognomic clinical findings nor specific laboratory tests for rheumatic fever, the designation of this diagnosis must be somewhat arbitrary and empirical. The traditional listing of manifestations into "major" and "minor" criteria, as set forth 50 years ago by Dr. T. Duckett Jones in Boston, was published to offer guidelines for the evaluation and diagnosis of rheumatic fever and rheumatic heart disease.[6] Subsequently they generally were accepted as diagnostic criteria for all ages in the United States and many parts of the world. These guidelines were "modified" (1955) and "revised" (1984) by specifically appointed committees of the American Heart Association. Their most recent review of the Jones criteria, designated as "1992 Update," addresses for the first time the diagnosis of an *initial attack* of acute rheumatic fever.[3] There are five so-called major manifestations that, in order of decreasing frequency today, are polyarthritis, carditis, chorea, erythema marginatum, and subcutaneous nodules. The last two entities involving the skin have been extremely uncommon in the past several decades in the United States.

The category of minor manifestations includes two laboratory findings: (1) elevated acute phase reactants (erythrocyte sedimentation rate and C-reactive protein) and (2) ECG evidence of abnormal prolongation of the PR interval. The clinical observation of fever usually is associated with a temperature under 102° F and may be present early in the course of polyarthritis or carditis. Arthralgia, another minor manifestation, is nonspecific and may affect any joint without objective signs of inflammation.

The tendency to label as rheumatic fever any low-grade febrile illness with arthralgia for which no obvious cause can be found should be strenuously avoided. The distress and anxiety that may lie in the wake of a false diagnosis may be even greater than the possible harm of missed recognition in questionable cases. The institution of effective prophylactic regimens requiring prolonged administration of antistreptococcal agents places a grave responsibility on the physician in diagnosing rheumatic fever. It is advisable to admit a youngster who has arthritis and/or carditis to the hospital for careful observation and appropriate documentation of a poststreptococcal illness. Because of the specificity of Sydenham's chorea with rheumatic fever, hospitalizing a child who has this manifestation should not be mandatory if abnormal neuromuscular activity is mild and unlikely to cause self-inflicted injury.

Age

Rheumatic fever is predominantly a disease of school-age children, with most first attacks occurring between 5 and 15 years of age. It is very uncommon under 5 years of age; when it occurs in this age group it usually is associated with severe carditis and congestive heart failure.

Polyarthritis also is extremely rare in the preschool-age group, where rheumatoid arthritis and other diseases that have joint involvement are statistically much more likely. Chorea also is uncommon in early childhood; most of the cases occur in those over 8 years of age.

Host Susceptibility

The tendency for rheumatic fever to occur in more than one member of a family has long been recognized. The observation is noted even when family members are not concurrently living in the same household; thus environmental influences are not solely responsible. Many investigators have sought to define genetic factors, although none has yet been established clearly.

There is no gender predisposition in the incidence of arthritis or carditis in childhood, although chorea always has been noted to be more common in girls. There are, however, gender differences in the type of valvular lesions that may develop with carditis and ultimately with rheumatic heart disease, with boys having a higher incidence of aortic regurgitation. In young adults, mitral stenosis is more common in women.

STREPTOCOCCAL INFECTION AND LATENT PERIODS

Streptococcal pharyngitis presumptively precedes an attack of rheumatic fever, even though some patients fail to report such a history. Scarlet fever occasionally will be followed by signs of polyarthritis or carditis, but suppurative streptococcal disease, such as skin infection, is not a precursor of rheumatic fever. Throat cultures, however, are of limited value in the workup of patients suspected of having rheumatic fever because the streptococcal infection antedates the common manifestations of polyarthritis and carditis by periods varying from 3 to 8 weeks; only 50% or fewer of patients who have rheumatic fever continue to harbor streptococci during the course of their illness.[11]

The most reliable evidence of a preceding streptococcal infection is obtained by demonstrating an antibody response to one or more of the streptococcal antigens. The most common of these, the antistreptolysin O (ASO) titer, reaches maximal levels 3 to 5 weeks after infection and gradually declines to preinfection levels 6 to 12 months later.[13] The ASO titer is elevated in about 85% of patients who have rheumatic fever. Serological evidence of an antecedent streptococcal infection rises to 95% if other streptococcal antibody tests (including antihyaluronidase, antideoxyribonuclease B, and antistreptokinase) are performed.[11]

The relationship between the times of onset or latent periods of the common manifestations of rheumatic fever and the antecedent streptococcal infection is illustrated in Figure 252-1. As noted, polyarthritis and carditis usually occur 3 to 8 weeks after infection. The streptococcal antibody titer (ASO) peaks before the onset of the clinical symptoms and then declines very gradually. Occasionally, abdominal pain is the conspicuous symptom after a streptococcal infection for which medical or surgical evaluation is sought and may overshadow or precede signs of joint or cardiac involvement. The long latent period of chorea is indicated by the majority of cases beginning 2 months following streptococcal infection, with episodes still developing up to 6 months afterward.

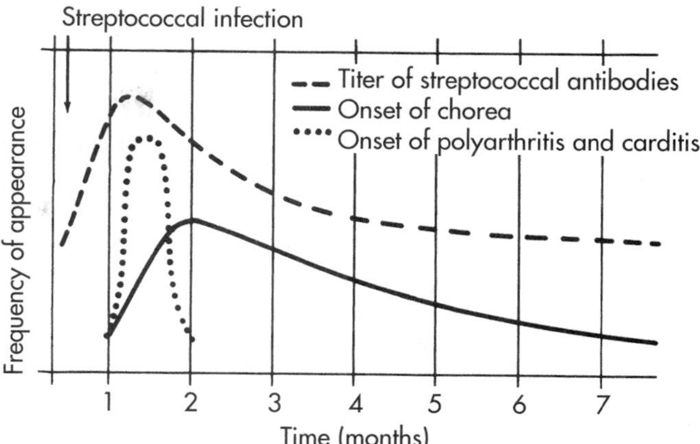

FIG. 252-1 Onset of rheumatic manifestations in relationship to antecedent streptococcal infection and ASO titer.

(Modified from Stollerman GH: *Rheumatic fever and streptococcal infection*, New York, 1975, Grune & Stratton.)

The sequence of the manifestations themselves is noteworthy: polyarthritis, if it is to occur, usually is present before the onset of carditis. Although carditis may occur without any preceding arthritis, if it is to follow the latter, an obvious apical systolic murmur of mitral valvulitis usually occurs within 2 weeks. It frequently is observed, however, that the diastolic murmur of isolated aortic valvulitis takes longer to present itself and may not be heard for 6 to 8 weeks after the joint signs and symptoms appear. Chorea not infrequently develops during the convalescent phase of carditis, though more often than not it has an even longer latent period and appears as an independent manifestation of rheumatic fever long after the initial streptococcal infection. Although chorea and carditis may coexist, chorea and polyarthritis rarely appear concurrently, presumably because of the differences in their latent periods.

MAJOR CLINICAL MANIFESTATIONS

Polyarthritis

This, the most common single manifestation of rheumatic fever, usually involves the large joints of the lower extremities, particularly ankles or knees, and is the cause of the complaint of pain or of some difficulty in walking. Other joints, for example, wrists or elbows, also may be involved in a migratory fashion. An affected joint characteristically is hot and swollen with variable blotchy erythema and may be exquisitely sensitive to touch, as well as painful on motion. Arthralgias, or aching in the joints without objective signs of inflammation, are suggestive of but not specific for rheumatic fever.

Carditis

Involvement of the heart may be expressed as myocarditis, endocarditis (valvulitis), or pericarditis. The characteristic presence of murmurs in rheumatic carditis is caused by endocarditis, secondary to mitral or aortic valvulitis. Implicit in the auscultatory diagnosis of valvulitis is the concurrent existence of myocarditis, which gives a gallop rhythm. Pericarditis typically is diagnosed by distant heart sounds, usually because of the presence of some effusion and a friction rub. Although viral inflammation of the heart by coxsackievirus B or Kawasaki disease may be associated with myocarditis and pericarditis, these entities do not cause valvulitis.

Carditis, clinically diagnosable by the presence of valvulitis with obvious murmurs, arbitrarily may be designated in a first attack of acute rheumatic fever as *mild, moderate,* or *severe.* Such a categorization is useful in the approach to management and expectations in prognosis for developing rheumatic heart disease. Auscultation of the heart and evaluation of murmurs are influenced by fever and tachycardia; therefore the patient should be observed, if possible, after he or she has been given acetaminophen to reduce temperature elevation.

Mild carditis characteristically is defined by the presence of a prominent apical systolic murmur. This usually is of grade 2 to 3 (on a scale of 1 to 6) intensity and occupies all or most of systole. It is consistent with mitral valvulitis; the implication of fixed mitral regurgitation must await a long follow-up period after the acute episode has subsided. Heart size on chest roentgenogram usually is normal.

Moderate carditis designates patients who have (1) both long systolic and prominent mid-diastolic apical murmurs, reflecting a higher degree of mitral valvulitis, (2) a basilar diastolic murmur of aortic valvulitis, or (3) a combination of mitral and aortic valvulitis. An aortic diastolic murmur, which is high pitched and decrescendo in character, usually is heard best with the diaphragm of the stethoscope in the third left intercostal space; in the early stage of aortic regurgitation, the pulse pressure is not widened. A chest roentgenogram may reflect mild cardiac enlargement because of some dilation associated with more extensive myocarditis and valvulitis.

Severe carditis is defined by the presence of either pericarditis or congestive heart failure in addition to mitral or aortic valvulitis. The quality of the heart sounds will be poor either because of pericardial effusion or low cardiac output and associated gallop rhythm. Murmurs may become more intense as cardiac compensation improves. The chest roentgenogram will show obvious cardiomegaly and may reveal pulmonary vascular congestion compatible with left-sided heart failure and pulmonary edema, an appearance sometimes interpreted as "rheumatic pneumonia." Consultation with a pediatric cardiologist would be most desirable for this small group of patients to confirm the diagnosis and to make recommendations for management with cardiotonic (including digitalis and diuretic) and steroid drug therapy.

Two-dimensional echocardiography is invaluable for the documentation of pericardial effusion and its quantitation. However, the interpretation of valvular regurgitation by Doppler ultrasound should not constitute the basis of a diagnosis of carditis without auscultatory evidence of significant mitral or aortic murmurs. Doppler studies in normal subjects quite frequently show some regurgitation across the mitral valve, and in a smaller number, aortic valve regurgitation has been revealed.

Chorea

The clinical picture of Sydenham's chorea includes that of poor neuromuscular coordination, often first detected by a change or sloppiness in handwriting. A wide variety of jerky, involuntary movements may occur during the period of 6 to 8 weeks during which most cases of chorea are active. Neurological testing may give evidence of specific deficiencies, particularly in trunk and upper extremity control of movements. A protective environment is recommended while the process is active. Occasionally, mild sedation with phenobarbital is indicated; the role of other agents, such as clonazepam (Clonopin) or haloperidol (Haldol), for more severe movement disorders has not been established.

When chorea occurs as an isolated manifestation, the patient usually is afebrile, and the sedimentation rate is normal. Because of the long interval following the initiating streptococcal infection, the ASO titer typically is normal or only mildly elevated.

Erythema Marginatum. This is a transient pink rash that has irregular, deeper colored serpiginous borders that may be seen on the smooth glabrous surfaces of the inner aspect of the upper arms and thighs or trunk. Erythema marginatum has been encountered with rheumatic fever infrequently in recent decades, being noted more often in patients with juvenile rheumatoid arthritis.

Subcutaneous Nodules. Subcutaneous nodules characteristically are pea-sized and may be located on the distal digits (fingers and toes), around the elbows or extensor surfaces of other joints, or on the occiput. They usually reflect a long-standing or smoldering illness following severe carditis and persist for several weeks. Currently, subcutaneous nodules rarely are found in children in North America who have rheumatic fever.

MINOR CLINICAL MANIFESTATIONS

Laboratory Findings

Elevated acute-phase reactants, notably the *erythrocyte sedimentation rate,* is an invaluable though nonspecific laboratory sign of inflammation in acute rheumatic fever. Initial values usually range between 60 to 120 mm/hr. It should be noted, however, that in chorea the sedimentation rate is normal because of the long interval, often measured in months, between the antecedent streptococcal infection and its appearance.

Prolongation of the PR interval on the electrocardiogram strongly supports the diagnosis of rheumatic fever. It is an invaluable early clue, most commonly noted while polyarthritis is apparent. If murmurs develop compatible with auscultatory evidence of carditis, the electrocardiogram is characteristically normal.

Delayed atrioventricular (AV) conduction, frequently first-degree heart block with PR interval prolongation, but occasionally second- or third-degree block, may indicate heightened vagal tone, perhaps more pronounced in the rheumatic state than in other acute illnesses.[4] It is not an indicator of carditis or of potential rheumatic heart disease.

MANAGEMENT

The three significant therapeutic approaches include (1) antistreptococcal therapy, (2) antiinflammatory agents, and (3) limitation of activity.

Antistreptococcal Therapy

Intensive antibiotic administration to eradicate group A beta-hemolytic streptococcal infection (even in the absence of a positive throat culture) is the foremost important principle in management, to be immediately followed by a prophylactic program to prevent reinfection. Penicillin is the drug of choice to be prescribed in dosage and duration to maintain therapeutic blood levels for 10 days. Several treatment schedules, which periodically are revised, are outlined by the American Heart Association.[1] The intramuscular administration of the long-acting repository benzathine penicillin G (Bicillin) is the preferred treatment method because it ensures continued treatment for a sufficient length of time. A single injection of 1.2 million units for children 5 to 15 years of age is recommended, to be followed in 10 days by monthly prophylactic injections of 1.2 million units. Alternate methods include (1) oral penicillin, 200,000 or 250,000 units (penicillin G or V), given three or four times a day for a full 10 days, followed by the same dose twice daily thereafter, or (2) a combination of oral and intramuscular penicillin.

In patients sensitive to penicillin, erythromycin may be used for antistreptococcal therapy. The sulfonamide drugs, which are bacteriostatic rather than bactericidal, are not effective for streptococcal eradication, although in rheumatic prophylaxis programs they are helpful in preventing reinfection.

Antiinflammatory Agents

Salicylates are invaluable in the presence of acute, painful arthritis or during the febrile phase of mild or moderate carditis associated with tachycardia. The duration of salicylate therapy in polyarthritis or carditis in childhood is not established and usually ranges from 1 to 8 weeks; the average initial amount prescribed should be approximately 50 to 75 mg/kg/day, given in four divided doses.[8] The administration of steroid hormones, most commonly prednisone (1 mg/kg/day), is indicated for severe carditis manifested by pericarditis or congestive heart failure. In this circumstance (particularly in a first attack), it is projected that the myocarditis, which causes the congestive failure, may be fulminant and life threatening and therefore should be vigorously suppressed. In addition, specific therapeutic measures to control congestive failure may need to be used, namely diuretics and digitalis. The use of a potent diuretic such as furosemide is crucial in the management of pulmonary edema with left ventricular failure. Digitalis (usually in the form of digoxin) should be administered cautiously, remembering that the threshold for toxicity may be lowered because of the presence of inflammatory myocarditis. It may be wise to withhold digitalis for 1 or 2 days until steroid therapy has suppressed myocarditis somewhat. Before steroids are started, the result of the tuberculin test should be determined; if positive, a course of isoniazid should be given concomitantly. Potassium supplementation is advisable to lessen the risk of hypokalemia (from the administration of steroids) predisposing to digitalis intoxication. The duration of steroid therapy frequently may extend upward from 1 to 3 months, with varying schedules of tapering the dosage and possibly adding salicylates. The ultimate development of rheumatic heart disease, following a first attack of rheumatic fever, may be correlated with the severity of the acute carditis. It has been noted in the 10-year follow-up report on the international study of treatment begun in 1951 that approximately 30% of those who had mild carditis and 50% of those who had moderate carditis developed rheumatic heart disease (mitral and/or aortic regurgitation).[9] With severe carditis nearly 75% of the patients may be expected to develop residual heart disease. Any claim of superiority of a given regimen of antiinflammatory agents for rheumatic carditis therefore must be evaluated in terms of altering the expected amount of residual rheumatic heart disease.

Limitation of Activity

The importance and duration of bed rest for optimum management of acute rheumatic fever has not been established: guidelines for bed rest and ambulation in patients who have acute rheumatic fever have been outlined by Markowitz and Gordis.[8] After resolution of painful arthritis, it usually is satisfactory to start ambulation when the sedimentation rate shows a steady decline, even though not to a normal level. Most children who have polyarthritis as their sole major manifestation of rheumatic fever may return to school in 6 weeks.

The period of bed rest recommended for carditis varies according to the estimate of its severity, with the broad range 2 to 12 weeks for mild to moderate cases. For those who have severe carditis, the length of bed rest and restricted activity must be individualized.

EVOLUTION OF RHEUMATIC HEART DISEASE

In the months and years that follow an attack of rheumatic fever, the auscultatory findings frequently change from those heard during the acute episode. For instance, many apical systolic murmurs completely disappear; not infrequently, however, an aortic diastolic murmur may first appear in the follow-up period. "Carditis" having been diagnosed initially does not imply progression to permanent heart damage. When a child is labeled with "history of acute rheumatic fever," the additional appellation of "rheumatic heart disease" must be reevaluated continually.

The majority of children who develop rheumatic heart disease after a single attack of rheumatic fever have mitral regurgitation. The remainder either have mitral and aortic regurgitation or aortic regurgitation alone. The combination of mitral regurgitation and mitral stenosis is uncommon in the United States, and isolated mitral stenosis is rare before early adulthood.

The issue that arises in the follow-up of children who have rheumatic heart disease is the amount of physical activity permitted. In general, those who have mitral regurgitation with normal heart size should be allowed to engage in all sports activities, except perhaps for the most strenuous competitive games or track. Those who have aortic regurgitation or mitral regurgitation with cardiomegaly should have some program restriction. For the very few children or adolescents who have progressive cardiac enlargement, even in the absence of recurrent rheumatic fever, an intensive cardiotonic program with digitalis maintenance should be prescribed. If symptoms of fatigue or exercise intolerance persist in spite of medical management, surgical intervention with valvuloplasty or valve replacement should be considered.

PROPHYLAXIS

The major thrust of prophylaxis in a known rheumatic subject is that of protecting against a recurrence of rheumatic fever through prevention of group A streptococcal infection.

However, among the group that develops rheumatic heart disease with valvular involvement, additional prophylaxis must be given at the time of dental and surgical procedures to protect against bacterial endocarditis.

RECURRENCE OF RHEUMATIC FEVER

One of the most striking characteristics of rheumatic fever is its tendency to recur. Before the introduction of preventive measures, the majority of patients who had an initial attack of rheumatic fever had one or more recurrences. The recurrence rate is highest during the first 3 years following an initial attack; it diminishes with time since the original episode, as well as with the advancing age of the patient.[8]

Continuous antimicrobial prophylaxis should be carried out in all children who have a history of rheumatic fever, including chorea. If by the time of high school graduation or 18 years of age there is no auscultatory evidence of heart disease, prophylaxis may be discontinued. If, however, there is mitral or aortic valvular disease, prophylaxis should be maintained into adulthood.

The method of choice and the most effective protection in reducing the incidence of streptococcal infection and rheumatic recurrence is afforded by an intramuscular injection of long-acting penicillin (benzathine penicillin G, 1.2 million units) every 28 days.[1] If a patient develops a positive throat culture for group A beta-hemolytic streptococci on this schedule, the interval between injections of penicillin should be reduced to 21 days. Acceptance of parenteral therapy is noteworthy in adolescents, when adherence to a program of daily oral medication is difficult if not impossible. Some transient discomfort at the injection site (anterior thigh or buttock) may be relieved by a hot bath and aspirin on the evening of injection.

Alternative methods of secondary prophylaxis include the oral administration of penicillin G (200,000 or 250,000 units, twice a day) or sulfisoxazole (Gantrisin, 0.5 g twice a day). For the exceptional patient who may be sensitive to both penicillin and sulfa, daily prophylaxis with another agent (such as erythromycin) is not essential in the absence of rheumatic heart disease. Successful oral prophylaxis is hard to maintain, and if employed, its value and need for compliance should be reinforced constantly by the pediatrician.

Bacterial Endocarditis

Individuals who have a history of rheumatic fever without evidence of significant murmurs on follow-up examination are not susceptible to bacterial endocarditis because they do not have damaged heart valves. However, those who do have rheumatic heart disease should have specific antimicrobial coverage before dental manipulation or extraction in addition to their regular rheumatic fever prophylaxis. In the case of dental work or oropharyngeal surgery, including tonsillectomy and adenoidectomy, large oral doses of penicillin should be administered to protect the patient from *Streptococcus viridans* bacteremia. The latest recommendation (1990) of the American Heart Association is to give amoxicillin 3 g orally 1 hour before the procedure, then 1.5 g 6 hours after the initial dose.[2] For amoxicillin/penicillin-allergic patients, erythromycin is prescribed. In the event of genitourinary manipulation, appropriate antibiotic coverage should be directed against the enterococci and gram negative organisms.

CONTRACEPTION AND PREGNANCY

The adolescent girl who has rheumatic heart disease should be counseled in regard to contraceptive methods. Prescribing oral medication with a low level of estrogen would be satisfactory, as would be instruction on how to use a diaphragm. An intrauterine device, however, should be avoided because of the risk of bacteremia.

If pregnancy occurs and early termination is sought, therapeutic abortion should be carried out in the hospital and prophylaxis against bacterial endocarditis given, using intravenous antibiotics. Should pregnancy go to term, antibiotics should be employed during delivery to protect against maternal bacteremia. Because of the added cardiovascular burden during pregnancy, obstetrical care throughout pregnancy should be provided, as well as prophylaxis against recurrence of rheumatic fever. Psychosocial support is needed especially for the pregnant teenager with rheumatic heart disease who may face medical complications during pregnancy as well as the added responsibilities of child rearing afterward.

REFERENCES

1. American Heart Association Committee on Rheumatic Fever, Infective Endocarditis and Kawasaki Disease of the Council of Cardiovascular Disease in the Young: Prevention of rheumatic fever, *Circulation* 78:1082, 1988.
2. American Heart Association Committee on Rheumatic Fever, Infective Endocarditis and Kawasaki Disease of the Council of Cardiovascular Disease in the Young: Prevention of bacterial endocarditis, *JAMA* 264:2919, 1990.
3. American Heart Association Committee on Rheumatic Fever, Endocarditis and Kawasaki Disease of the Council of Cardiovascular Disease in the Young: Guidelines for the diagnosis of rheumatic fever: Jones criteria, 1992 update, *JAMA* 268:2069, 1992.
4. Clarke M, Keith JD: Atrioventricular conduction in acute rheumatic fever, *Br Heart J* 34:472, 1972.
5. Griffiths SP, Gersony WM: Acute rheumatic fever in New York City (1969 to 1988): a comparative study of two decades, *J Pediatr* 116:882, 1990.
6. Jones TD: Diagnosis of rheumatic fever, *JAMA* 126:481, 1944.
7. Kaplan EL: Return of rheumatic fever: consequences, implications and needs, *J Pediatr* 111:244, 1987 (editorial).
8. Markowitz M, Gordis L: *Rheumatic fever,* ed 2, Philadelphia, 1972, WB Saunders.
9. Rheumatic Fever Working Party of the Medical Research Council of Great Britain and Subcommittee of Principal Investigators of the American Council on Rheumatic Fever and Rheumatic Heart Disease: Ten-year report of a cooperative clinical trial of ACTH, cortisone, and aspirin, *Circulation* 32:457, 1965.
10. Siegel AC, Johnson EE, Stollerman GH: Controlled studies of streptococcal pharyngitis in a pediatric population, *N Engl J Med* 265:559, 1961.
11. Stollerman GH: *Rheumatic fever and streptococcal infection,* New York, 1975, Grune & Stratton.
12. Veasy LG et al: Resurgence of acute rheumatic fever in the intermountain area of the United States, *N Engl J Med* 316:421, 1987.
13. Wannamaker LW, Ayoub EM: Antibody titers in acute rheumatic fever, *Circulation* 21:598, 1960.

SUGGESTED READING

Ayoub EM: Acute rheumatic fever. In Emmanouilides GC et al, editors: *Moss and Adams' heart disease in infants, children and adolescents,* vol 2, ed 5, Baltimore, 1994, Williams & Wilkins.

253 Rocky Mountain Spotted Fever

Fred J. Heldrich

Rocky Mountain spotted fever (RMSF), an acute infectious disease caused by *Rickettsia rickettsii,* is characterized by the symptoms of fever, headache, myalgia, and distinctive exanthem. The major pathological lesion—a vasculitis—makes RMSF a multisystem disease. Most important, it is a disease that requires a clinical diagnosis and treatment before a confirmatory laboratory diagnosis.

The disease was first reported in patients from the Rocky Mountain region. Today, however, the incidence of the disease is greatest east of the Mississippi River, with the most cases being reported from the southeastern and south central United States. Although the disease occurs predominantly in the United States, it has been reported from other areas in the Western Hemisphere, specifically Canada, Central America, and South America. The reported frequency of the disease has increased slightly over the past several years.

EPIDEMIOLOGY

Ticks serve as a vector for the infectious agent *R. rickettsii.* Transmission to humans occurs when the tick takes a blood meal or when the abraded skin is contaminated by tick feces or a crushed tick, which may occur when ticks are removed. Two specific ticks serve as major carriers: the wood tick, *Dermacentor andersonii,* is the more important vector in the West; the dog tick, *Dermacentor variabilis,* is the usual vector in the East. Ticks, in turn, acquire the rickettsias by feeding on infected wild mammals. In addition, infection of laboratory workers has been reported independent of exposure to ticks.

The seasonal incidence of RMSF—primarily occurring in spring, summer, and fall—is in accordance with the activity of the tick.[5] Dog ticks infected with *R. rickettsii* have been found in urban areas, which suggests this tick's ubiquitous nature and places individuals at risk without travel to endemic areas.[7] In adults, occupational or recreational exposure to ticks increases the risk of infection; however, children are affected with greatest frequency, and boys are affected more often than girls.

Exposure to a tick is not elicited in every case, although a history of removing a tick before the onset of illness is not unusual. The tick bite is painless and leaves no local lesion or regional lymphadenopathy; it is important therefore to question specifically about prior tick removal or activities that increase the risk of exposure (e.g., removal of a tick from a pet dog and camping or picnicking in a high-risk area).

CLINICAL PICTURE

After inoculation with the rickettsias, the incubation period ranges from 3 to 12 days; the usual period is 5 to 7 days. In general, the shortest incubation period is associated with the most serious disease.

In the typical case[4] there is a short prodromal period of 2 to 3 days, with low-grade fever, chills, and muscle aches predominating. Headache also is an early symptom. Younger patients indicate muscle pain and headache by crying. Malaise, anorexia, vomiting, and photophobia also are frequently present. This brief period is followed by accentuation of these symptoms, especially of the fever, which remains elevated, often as high as 40° C or more. The lowest temperatures, although still elevated, are recorded in the mornings. Lethargy and mental obtundation become prominent. Even the severity of symptoms seen at this stage is not diagnostic, and only the history of a tick bite indicates that RMSF is the likely diagnosis.

It is the rash that is most distinctive. It usually appears on the fourth day of fever and begins peripherally on the wrists, ankles, hands, and feet. Initially the lesions are macular, discrete, and erythematous and blanch on pressure. This rash rapidly spreads centrally, involving the arms, legs, axillae, buttocks, trunk, neck, and face. The lesions deepen in color, becoming dusky red and papular to palpation; in several days they are petechial. These petechial lesions may coalesce and form large ecchymotic areas. Before the frank appearance of petechiae, a tourniquet applied when obtaining blood may produce petechial lesions. In severe cases and when treatment is delayed, these ecchymotic areas may ulcerate, and distal regions (e.g., fingers and toes) may become gangrenous. Nonpitting edema, especially notable around the eyes, face, hands, and feet, also occurs frequently.

Tachycardia and an elevated pulse rate are noted early and are proportional to the degree of hyperpyrexia. A sudden increase in pulse rate or fall in blood pressure is ominous and may indicate peripheral circulatory collapse, severe bleeding, or myocardial failure. Photophobia is associated with conjunctival ecchymosis involving both bulbar and palpebral conjunctivae. Petechial hemorrhages also may be seen.

Abdominal pain and vomiting, with generalized abdominal tenderness, may be found[2]; hepatomegaly and splenomegaly may be present. Jaundice usually is not seen, except in the most critically ill patients. Fever, poor fluid intake, and vomiting all contribute to a diminished urinary output. Mild azotemia should respond to rehydration. In addition to the lethargy and obtunded state of consciousness, the patient may exhibit nuchal rigidity. Disorientation and confusion, as well as seizures, may occur. Vasculitis, hemorrhage, or secondary metabolic changes are responsible for these neurological manifestations.[1] When these symptoms occur early in the course of RMSF, they may mask its diagnosis.

DIFFERENTIAL DIAGNOSIS

Illnesses to be considered and differentiated from RMSF include measles, rubeola (atypical), meningococcemia, Henoch-Schönlein purpura, Kawasaki syndrome, idiopathic thrombocytopenic purpura, leukemia, typhus, and infectious mononucleosis. Of these, atypical measles and meningococcemia are confused most frequently; meningococcemia, because of its severe consequences, requires immediate differentiation.

The petechial rash of *meningococcemia* differs from that of RMSF in its distribution, rapid extension, and coalescence of lesions into larger hemorrhagic, purpuric areas. Prostration either is noted on admission or may develop rapidly if untreated. Absence of myalgia and an extremely abrupt onset are helpful differential points. Although the white blood cell count may be elevated, the sickest patients frequently are leukopenic. Meningitis with spinal fluid pleocytosis, low glucose levels, and organisms in the cerebrospinal fluid (identified by Gram stain) also may be found.

Atypical measles has a prodromal period similar in duration to RMSF but differs in that upper respiratory tract symptoms usually are prominent. Atypical measles occurs in patients who have been immunized previously with killed vaccine, and an Arthus response may be noted at the site of prior inoculation. Additionally, joint pain is common in atypical measles, but is not found in RMSF.

Rubeola is characterized by a macular rash (infrequently becoming hemorrhagic), which always begins on the face and neck and is preceded by an exanthem—Koplik spots. The coryza and cough in the prodromal stage of illness are not consistent with RMSF. A history of adequate immunization with rubeola vaccine should help eliminate this possibility.

Henoch-Schönlein purpura may produce a petechial or purpuric rash, frequently concentrated on the lower extremities and buttocks. These cutaneous lesions may be multiform and occur on other parts of the body. Frequently there is an arthralgia with periarticular swelling and accompanying signs and symptoms of upper respiratory tract inflammation, gastroenteritis, or nephritis.

Kawasaki syndrome shares many of the features of RMSF: fever, puffy hands and feet, rash, and conjunctival injection. Usually Kawasaki syndrome is not considered strongly until 5 days of fever and an enlarged cervical node, pharyngeal hyperemia, dry cracked lips, strawberry tongue, and marked irritability tend to set it apart. Although patients who have Kawasaki syndrome do have a rash, it typically does not begin peripherally and spread centrally or become petechial in 1 to 2 days. Leukocyte and erythrocyte sedimentation rates usually are elevated significantly.

Other illnesses that produce petechiae must also be mentioned, even though they lack the distinctive distribution of the rash. Idiopathic thrombocytopenic purpura is seen as a petechial rash in an otherwise healthy patient. Leukemic patients who have fever and petechiae at initial presentation would be expected to be anemic and have lymphadenopathy or hepatosplenomegaly. Patients who have infectious mononucleosis, if they have a petechial eruption, usually have lymphadenopathy, hepatosplenomegaly, and a more gradual onset. *Typhus* is a rickettsial infection to be excluded. Murine typhus produces a milder disease, with a rash that is macular and not petechial. Epidemic typhus may produce a petechial rash that typically begins proximally and extends peripherally, but usually does not involve the palms or soles; history of a tick bite is also absent.

LABORATORY EVALUATION

The diagnosis of RMSF is made clinically, and treatment should be started before laboratory diagnosis is sought. Fluorescent antibody studies of petechial lesions may provide the first positive proof of RMSF, but these studies are not readily available to most clinicians. Appropriate antibiotic therapy started 3 days before biopsy has resulted in negative immunofluorescence. Therefore, when appropriate treatment has been initiated before biopsy, clinical criteria justify a full course of antibiotic therapy.[3]

Complement fixation studies will identify patients who have RMSF, but these do not become positive until the second week of illness or later if early antibiotic therapy has begun. The Weil-Felix reaction, agglutination of *Proteus vulgaris* by the patient's serum, is at best a nonspecific test for RMSF. Again, acute and convalescent serums must be compared, although *Proteus* agglutinins may appear by the end of the first week of illness.

Rickettsias can be isolated from body fluid or tissue specimens when grown in laboratory animals or chick embryos. However, the high rate of disease transmission to laboratory technicians makes such techniques feasible only in laboratories engaged in rickettsia-related research in which all workers are immunized; thus culture identification of rickettsias is not available in most clinical settings.

Leukocyte counts and differential counts usually are within normal limits. Thrombocytopenia is a complication seen in the later stages of the disease. In seriously ill patients, metabolic derangements such as hyponatremia and hypochloremia may occur but are nonspecific findings. Only with the complication of intravascular coagulation will such tests as prothrombin time, partial thromboplastin time, fibrinogen, and fibrin split products become abnormal.

In patients who have neurological symptoms, the cerebrospinal fluid pressure, the number of white and red blood cells, and the level of protein in the cerebrospinal fluid all may be elevated.

COURSE

The disease has a mortality of approximately 5% in recognized cases, but patients have been identified with serological evidence of having had RMSF without clinical detection, suggesting that the disease may occur in a mild or even subclinical form.[6] The importance of abdominal pain mimicking an acute abdominal condition and dominating as an early symptom before the development of or even in the absence of a rash must be emphasized. Rocky Mountain *spotless* fever also has been described.[8] Of great concern is a report suggesting that patients who have "spotless or almost spotless" fever have a significantly higher mortality.[8,9]

It is appropriate to consider RMSF a potentially lethal illness, even though younger patients are likely to be less severely affected. Early diagnosis and prompt therapy lessen disease severity. Under such circumstances death would be extremely unusual; in the majority of patients, early clinical diagnosis and adequate therapy shorten the duration of illness appreciably. Normal temperatures within the first 3 to 4 days may be expected, and patients recover rapidly from other signs of illness (e.g., headache, myalgia, and lethargy). Extension of the rash ceases.[4]

Experience with RMSF before effective therapy indicated that the illness persisted for 2 to 3 weeks and that the overall mortality was 20%. Today, a delay in initiating appropriate therapy will lengthen the duration of illness and increase the likelihood of complications. Although a mortality of approximately 5% still remains, recovery from the illness is accompanied by permanent immunity.

COMPLICATIONS

The major complication of RMSF is disseminated intravascular coagulation. Patients in whom the diagnosis has been delayed are those at greatest risk. This complication may prove lethal or result in local gangrene, with loss of tissue, appendages, or both. Myocardial failure may result from myocarditis and arrhythmias. Edema may be generalized as a result of an increase in capillary permeability secondary to the vasculitis, heart failure, or iatrogenic fluid overload.

Neurological complications, in addition to the lethargy, have already been discussed. Hematuria and anemia also may occur.

TREATMENT

Specific therapy with either chloramphenicol (100 mg/kg/24 hr; maximum 4 g/24 hr) or tetracycline (20 mg/kg/24 hr; maximum 2 g/24 hr; tetracycline should not be used in children under 8 years of age) should be started on the basis of the clinical diagnosis. The intravenous route is indicated for patients moderately or severely ill or for those who are vomiting. Oral medication should be reserved for the mildly ill.

Hospitalization is desirable initially for all patients, both to ensure an adequate differential diagnosis and to ascertain the effect of therapy. Therapy should be continued until the patient has improved and is afebrile for 48 hours.

Supportive therapy includes maintenance of hydration and nutrition by appropriate intravenous fluids, oral feedings if tolerated, or both. Management of disseminated intravascular coagulation remains unsatisfactory, but therapeutic maneuvers such as giving fresh-frozen plasma, transfusing fresh platelets and packed RBCs, and administering vitamin K may be helpful. The use of corticosteroids is believed to be warranted in the most severely ill and toxic patients. Seizures may require the use of anticonvulsant medications.

PREVENTION

The use of vaccine is not indicated except in those individuals at highest risk for exposure. Even then, the availability of effective therapy reduces the need for vaccination. When exposure is likely, ticks should be searched for daily, and for those in tick-infested areas, twice daily. Careful inspection at bath time is an excellent way to discover the presence of ticks. They may be removed by gentle traction with forceps or tweezers, but care must be taken not to crush them.

REFERENCES

1. Bell WE, Lascari AD: Rocky Mountain spotted fever: neurologic symptoms in the acute phase, *Neurology* 20:841, 1970.
2. Davis AE, Bradford WD: Abdominal pain resembling acute appendicitis in Rocky Mountain spotted fever, *JAMA* 247:2811, 1982.
3. Fleisher G, Lennette ET, Honig P: Diagnosis of Rocky Mountain spotted fever by immunofluorescent identification of *Rickettsia rickettsii* in skin biopsy tissue, *J Pediatr* 95:63, 1979.
4. Haynes RE, Sanders DY, Cramblett HG: Rocky Mountain spotted fever in children, *J Pediatr* 76:685, 1970.
5. Lange JV, Walker DH, Wester TB: Documented Rocky Mountain spotted fever in wintertime, *JAMA* 247:2403, 1982.
6. Marx RS et al: Rocky Mountain spotted fever: serological evidence of previous subclinical infection in children, *Am J Dis Child* 136:16, 1982.
7. Salgo MP et al: A focus of Rocky Mountain fever within New York City, *N Engl J Med* 318:1345, 1988.
8. Sexton DJ, Corey GR: Rocky mountain "spotless" and "almost spotless" fever: a wolf in sheep's clothing, *Clin Infect Dis* 15:439, 1992.
9. Westerman EL: Rocky Mountain spotless fever: a dilemma for the clinician, *Arch Intern Med* 142:1106, 1982.

254 Roseola and Related Diseases: HHV-6 and HHV-7 Infections

Jerri Ann Jenista

Roseola is a classic childhood exanthem also known as *roseola infantum, exanthem subitum, 3-day fever, sixth disease,* and *pseudorubella.* Exciting new information has dramatically changed our thinking about this common malady.

Newly discovered viruses, human herpes virus-6 (HHV-6) and human herpes virus-7 (HHV-7), are two of the known causative agents of roseola.[15,16] However, the spectrum of disease associated with these agents is now understood to be far broader than the benign illness of roseola.

ETIOLOGY

HHV-6, formerly called *human B-lymphotrophic virus (HBLV),* and HHV-7 are classified as herpesviruses based on physical and genetic similarities to others of the group: herpes simplex virus-1, herpes simplex virus-2, cytomegalovirus, Epstein-Barr virus, and varicella-zoster virus. HHV-6 and HHV-7 can be distinguished from the other herpesviruses by DNA hybridization or by reactions with virus-specific monoclonal antibodies. HHV-6 exists in two forms, *variant A* and *variant B.*

Sophisticated antigen detection methods demonstrate HHV-6 and HHV-7 in many healthy persons, including those who have virus-specific antibody. HHV-6 has been isolated from saliva, plasma, and many cell lines.[11] HHV-7 is isolated most often from the saliva in healthy persons.[9]

As with other herpesviruses, latent or persistent, asymptomatic viral infection occurs following the primary infection. The site of latency is not clear but may include several sources, including salivary glands, peripheral blood mononuclear cells, kidneys, bronchial glands, and the cerebrospinal fluid (CSF).[5] HHV-6 infection may reactivate during primary HHV-7 infection, acute febrile illnesses, or periods of immunodeficiency. Reactivation characteristics of HHV-7 are unknown.

Both viruses interfere with the function of certain classes of T lymphocytes. There is emerging evidence that HHV-6, and perhaps HHV-7, act as co-factors in the course of human immunodeficiency virus infection. The role of these viruses in lymphoreticular malignancies, chronic fatigue syndrome, and other conditions, such as multiple sclerosis, is under investigation.

EPIDEMIOLOGY

Roseola is so frequent an illness that fully 30% of children will suffer the clinical disease between the ages of 6 months and 2 years.[4] The diagnosis is unusual, however, in children at other ages; rare cases in adults and neonates have been reported. Most cases are sporadic, although family and institutional epidemics occasionally are noted.[13] Cases of roseola are seen year round, with an increased incidence in the late spring.

A child's first episode of roseola is usually caused by HHV-6B, occurring at an average age of 7 months.[3] Primary infection with HHV-7 accounts for about 10% of first and the majority of second cases of roseola. HHV-7 infection occurs somewhat later than HHV-6, at a mean age of about 12 months. Approximately 15% of episodes of roseola cannot be attributed to either HHV-6 or HHV-7.[10]

A prospective study of emergency room visits for acute childhood illness in Rochester, NY, revealed a broader role than previously recognized for HHV-6 infection.[8] Primary HHV-6 infection was documented in nearly 10% of children under age 3 years and in 20% of children between 6 and 12 months of age presenting with an acute febrile illness. HHV-6 infection was the cause of one third of febrile seizures in children under the age of 2 years and resulted in hospitalization of 13% of children following emergency room presentation. Clearly, primary HHV-6 infection is a major cause of morbidity in infancy and early childhood. The contribution of HHV-7 infection to emergency room use, hospitalization, seizures, or physician visits has not been studied.

The incubation periods for HHV-6 and HHV-7 infection are apparently between 5 and 15 days; however, the modes of transmission and the period of communicability are unknown. HHV-6 and HHV-7 can be isolated from the saliva of 70% to 80% of healthy persons over 1 year of age. HHV-6 is isolated most frequently from peripheral blood mononuclear cells. The rate of subclinical disease is high. Most patients have no known exposure.[4] There is indirect evidence of intrauterine or perinatal transmission of at least HHV-6[3]; there are no recognized sequelae attributed to such infection.

Serological surveys show that virtually all full-term infants have passively acquired maternal antibody to both HHV-6 and HHV-7 at birth. The prevalence of antibody falls, reaching a nadir by 6 months of age. By 1 year of age nearly 90% of children have detectable antibody to HHV-6. The prevalence of antibody to HHV-7 also increases with age; 60% of young adolescents have detectable titers. These levels persist unchanged through young adulthood and then decline slightly with age. Prevalence surveys of blood donors show HHV-6 antibody detection rates up to 97%.[17,18]

DISEASE

Roseola

Recognition of roseola is based almost entirely on the observation of a classic clinical course. Interestingly, the signs and symptoms of roseola noted before the discovery of HHV-6 are essentially the same as descriptions of disease proven to be caused by HHV-6 or HHV-7[2,6] (Table 254-1). Typically, a fever as high as 102.2° to 105.8° F (39° to 41° C) suddenly develops in a previously well infant. Except for irritability, the child does not seem as sick as the temperature indicates. Physical findings are sparse and include only painless posterior auricular, suboccipital, or cervical lymphadenopathy accompanied by slight eyelid edema, giving the child a "sleepy-eyed" or "droopy" appearance. Nagayama spots are erythematous macules appearing on the soft palate and near the uvula and are observed regularly after a day or two of illness.[2] Rarely, mild coryza, otitis media, or a bulging fontanelle is observed.

After a 2- to 5-day course the fever resolves dramatically and a rash appears almost simultaneously. With defervescence the child seems to have recovered, despite the rash. The typical exanthem occurs as macular or maculopapular blanching patches surrounded by a lighter halo. The eruption usually begins on the neck and spreads to the trunk and extremities, sparing the face. It fades within 4 hours to 4 days and probably frequently is missed if it is faint or occurs at night.

Clinically inapparent infection certainly occurs. Roseola also may occur in a young infant as an afebrile exanthem or as a nonspecific fever without the characteristic rash.[1,14]

Meningoencephalitis

HHV-6 infection is a major cause of childhood febrile seizures, accounting for up to one third of such incidents in children under the age of 2 years presenting to an emergency room.[8] Complete recovery is the rule. However, there are reports of severe meningoencephalitis with neurological sequelae or death in infants and fatal encephalitis attributed to HHV-6B in adult recipients of bone marrow transplants.

HHV-6 can be isolated from CSF in up to 70% of children during primary infection and in 28% of children who have had past infection.[5] The significance of HHV-6 in relation to recurrent seizures, chronic fatigue, multiple sclerosis, and other neurological conditions is not clear.[11]

Table 254-1 Roseola—Before and After Discovery of HHV-6

Signs and symptoms	1945[6]	1994[2]
Fever	100%	98%
Rash	100%	98%
Pruritis	1.2%	*
Desquamation	10%	0%
Pigmentation	0%	7%
Lymphadenopathy	97.5%	*
Cervical	45%	31%
Erythematous tympanic membranes	92.5%	*
Constipation	40%	*
Upper respiratory tract symptoms	25%	*
Nonspecific prodromal symptoms	*	14%
Diarrhea	15%	68%
Meningismus	5%	*
Bulging fontanelle	*	26%
Convulsions	3.7%	8%
Irritability	92.5%	*
Edematous eyelids	*	30%
Nagayama spots†	87%	65%
Anorexia	80%	*
Abdominal pain	25%	*
Cough	11.2%	50%
Headache	5%	*
Earache	2.5%	*
Aching joints	2.5%	*

*Not reported using this term.

†Erythematous streaks or spots on the soft palate and uvula.

Mononucleosis-like Disease

HHV-6 infection in adults rarely causes a roseola-like illness. Three cases of nonroseola HHV-6 infection in adults were reported in 1988 by Niederman et al.[12] The mild disease lasted several weeks and was associated with slight fatigue, headache, sore throat, and cervical lymphadenopathy. The levels of liver enzymes were elevated transiently. A case of severe mononucleosis-like disease associated with HHV-6 has been reported in an adult recently.

HHV-7 was isolated from a child who had the clinical picture of chronic Epstein-Barr virus infection, characterized by pancytopenia, fever, and hepatosplenomegaly.

Hepatitis

A mild hepatitis associated with HHV-6 infection is recognized in adults and children. A few cases of fulminant and/or fatal hepatitis have been reported, usually with an associated encephalopathy.[11]

Infection in Immunocompromised Patients

HHV-6 infection may reactivate during periods of immunosuppression. A syndrome with fever and rash resembling graft-versus-host disease is recognized in children following bone marrow transplantation. Severe interstitial pneumonitis, disseminated infection, and encephalitis associated with HHV-6 infection have been reported in adult recipients of bone marrow transplants.[7]

The role of HHV-6 in HIV infection is unclear, although there is some evidence to suggest that HHV-6 may potentiate the progression of AIDS. HHV-7 competes with HIV for CD-4 receptors on T cells; theoretically the virus may interfere with the progression of HIV infection.[11]

Other Diseases

HHV-6 has been isolated from patients who have many other conditions. Because HHV-6 is reactivated by many acute illnesses, it is difficult in most cases to attribute causality to the virus. Reported associations include: chronic bone marrow suppression in an immunocompetent adult, idiopathic thrombocytopenic purpura, hemophagocytic syndrome, fatal disseminated disease in an immunocompetent infant, lymphoproliferative disorders, and certain lymphoreticular malignancies.

DIAGNOSIS

In roseola the only helpful laboratory finding is a leukopenia with a nadir count as low as 2000 white blood cells per cubic millimeter by the third day of fever. A relative lymphocytosis or monocytosis is typical. Results of the cerebrospinal fluid examination, urinalysis, and chest roentgenogram are normal. Because roseola is an inconsequential illness, there rarely is any need to confirm the specific diagnosis.

Neither antibody detection methods nor virus isolation techniques are standardized for HHV-6 or HHV-7. These assays are not commercially available. Except in certain situations of infection among immunocompromised hosts, there is no clinical need to confirm infection with HHV-6 or HHV-7 either serologically or virologically.

DIFFERENTIAL DIAGNOSIS

Roseola often is confused with other exanthematous diseases (see Chapter 197, Contagious Exanthematous Diseases). In rubella the rash and fever are concurrent, and enlarged lymph nodes often are tender. Coryza, respiratory symptoms, and Koplik spots distinguish rubeola. Enterovirus exanthems usually occur in epidemics, involve older as well as younger children, and are more common in the late summer and fall. Erythema infectiosum, or fifth disease, affects the school-age child and involves the face most prominently. Scarlet fever has a more confluent rash and is associated with marked pharyngitis. Drug eruptions, especially those resulting from sulfa-containing preparations, are not regularly preceded by fever and tend to be more diffuse.

TREATMENT

Management of roseola is based entirely on symptoms. Acetaminophen is quite effective in controlling the fever. Reassuring the parents that the rash is a sign of recovery often is comforting to them and may prevent unnecessary office visits.

Both HHV-6 and HHV-7 have antiviral agent profiles similar to cytomegalovirus and have little susceptibility to acyclovir. In vitro studies show that either foscarnet or ganciclovir is somewhat effective, but there have been no clinical trials with these drugs. Infection with either of these agents is self-limited in the immunocompetent child. Antiviral therapy is reserved only for life-threatening infection.

OUTCOME

Complications are unusual in the normal child who has roseola. Febrile convulsions are noted in up to 13% of primary HHV-6 infections.[8]

REFERENCES

1. Asano Y et al: Human herpesvirus type 6 infection (exanthem subitum) without fever, *J Pediatrics* 115:264, 1989.
2. Asano Y et al: Clinical features of infants with primary human herpesvirus 6 infection (exanthem subitum, roseola infantum), *Pediatrics* 93:104, 1994.
3. Aubin JT et al: Intrauterine transmission of human herpesvirus 6, *Lancet* 340:482, 1992.
4. Breese BB Jr: Roseola infantum (exanthem subitum), *NY State J Med* 41:1854, 1941.
5. Caserta MT et al: Neuroinvasion and persistence of human herpesvirus 6 in children, *J Infect Dis* 170:1586, 1994.
6. Clemens HH: Exanthem subitum (roseola infantum): report of eighty cases, *J Pediatr* 26:66, 1945.
7. Cone RW et al: Human herpesvirus 6 in lung tissue from patients with pneumonitis after bone marrow transplantation, *N Engl J Med* 329:156, 1993.
8. Hall CB et al: Human herpesvirus-6 infection in children: a prospective study of complications and reactivation, *N Engl J Med* 331:432, 1994.
9. Hidaka Y et al: Frequent isolation of human herpesvirus 7 from saliva samples, *J Med Virol* 40:343, 1993.
10. Hidaka Y et al: Exanthem subitum and human herpesvirus 7 infection, *Pediatr Infect Dis J* 13:1010, 1994.
11. Leach C et al: Human herpesvirus-6: clinical implications of a recently discovered, ubiquitous agent, *J Pediatr* 121:173, 1992.
12. Niederman JC et al: Clinical and serological features of human herpesvirus 6 infection in three adults, *Lancet* 2:817, 1988.
13. Okuno T et al: Outbreak of exanthem subitum in an orphanage, *J Pediatr* 119:759, 1991.
14. Suga A et al: Human herpesvirus 6 infection (exanthem subitum) without rash, *Pediatrics* 83:1003, 1989.
15. Tanaka K et al: Human herpesvirus 7: another causal agent for roseola (exanthem subitum), *J Pediatr* 125:1, 1994.
16. Yamanishi K et al: Identification of human herpesvirus 6 as a causal agent for exanthem subitum, *Lancet* 1:1065, 1988.
17. Yoshikawa T et al: Distribution of antibodies to a causative agent of exanthem subitum (human herpesvirus-6) in healthy individuals, *Pediatrics* 84:675, 1989.
18. Yoshikawa T et al: Seroepidemiology of human herpesvirus 7 in healthy children and adults in Japan, *J Med Virol* 41:319, 1993.

255 Seborrheic Dermatitis

Ana M. Duarte and Lawrence A. Schachner

Seborrheic dermatitis (SD) is a common, usually asymptomatic dermatosis of unknown etiology that is seen primarily in infants, but also in adolescents and adults. It presents in 50% of infants before 5 weeks of age.[1] There is an incidence of 2% to 5% in the general population.[1] Although SD occasionally is seen in infants who have HIV infection, a true increased incidence has not been documented.[4] No evidence suggests a genetic predisposition. Studies have indicated that infants who present with seborrheic dermatitis may be at an increased risk of developing atopic dermatitis and, less often, psoriasis.[3]

CLINICAL FEATURES

Seborrheic dermatitis may present most commonly as a greasy scaly dermatitis, less often as psoriasiform seborrheic dermatitis, and rarely as erythrodermic seborrheic dermatitis.

Seborrheic dermatitis presents in infancy with diffuse red, crusted, and yellow scaling plaques on the vertex of the scalp *(cradle cap)* (Fig. 255-1, *A*). Similar lesions also may be found in the retroauricular creases, the eyebrows, and the nasolabial folds (Fig. 255-1, *B*), as well as in the axillary and inguinal folds, the neck, and the diaper area. The lesions usually are asymptomatic and distributed symmetrically.

The presentation is similar in adolescents. Patients may note a greasy, scaling, pruritic eruption on the scalp. With the exception of inguinal area involvement, the distribution of the lesions is the same as for infants.

HIV-positive children aged 2 to 5 years may manifest SD with lesions similar to those seen in adolescents and adults. This is distinctly unusual in immunocompetent children and appears to be a manifestation of HIV infection.[4]

Psoriasiform seborrheic dermatitis, also known as *sebopsoriasis* or *seborrhiasis,* presents with features of both SD and psoriasis and may represent a bridge between the two conditions. Psoriasiform plaques—that is, annular, red-brown plaques having a silvery scale—may be present among the classical greasy, yellow, scaling lesions of SD (Fig. 255-2). Patients may or may not have "pitted" nails, which are seen with classical psoriasis.

Erythrodermic seborrheic dermatitis is rare and presents with widespread exfoliative erythroderma. (Fig. 255-3). Diffuse desquamation usually begins in the flexures and then spreads. The patient may exhibit signs and symptoms of systemic involvement—that is, fever, chills, lymphadenopathy, peripheral edema, and dehydration. This also may be the presentation of Leiner disease (see Differential Diagnosis).

PATHOGENESIS

The etiology of seborrheic dermatitis remains unknown; several different pathogenic mechanisms are proposed. Based on the distribution of the lesions that involve areas of highest sebaceous gland concentration, an abnormality in the sebaceous gland or an increased sensitivity to circulating maternal or endogenous hormones has been suggested. However, these patients have normal sebaceous secretion and hormonal levels. Recent studies have found that altered essential fatty acids may be important in the pathogenesis of this disorder.[5] In addition, *Pityrosporum ovale* may play a role in the evolution of SD in infant and adult patients.[2]

DIFFERENTIAL DIAGNOSIS

The differential diagnosis of seborrheic dermatitis includes atopic dermatitis, psoriasis, dermatophyte infection, diaper dermatitis, histiocytosis X, and Leiner disease.

Atopic dermatitis usually is distinguished by the presence of extreme pruritus, extensoral distribution in infancy and flexural distribution in older children (tending to spare the scalp and to involve the hands and feet), as well as a family history in 70% of those affected. Seborrheic dermatitis also may occur concomitantly with atopic dermatitis (see Chapter 186).

Psoriasis is a common inherited papulosquamous skin disorder characterized by well-demarcated, annular, thick, red-brown, scaling plaques usually present on the trunk, the extensor areas on the arms, the knees, the elbows, the diaper area, and the scalp (Fig. 255-4), as well as by nail pitting. It usually lacks the specific distribution and the greasy component of SD. However, some cases of SD may overlap with psoriasis and are called *psoriasiform-SD*. Extensive cases of SD become persistent; when there is a positive family history of psoriasis, they should be referred to a dermatologist for biopsy and, potentially, long-term follow-up.

Dermatophyte infection of the scalp *(tinea capitis)* may present with scaling, pruritus, and redness of the scalp. It usually results in alopecia, a distinguishing feature (Fig. 255-5). *Tinea corporis* may be distinguished by its annular configuration. In addition, a potassium hydroxide preparation of the scalp hair roots, or scales from body lesions, will demonstrate septate hyphae.

Diaper dermatitis or *irritant diaper rash (ammoniacal diaper dermatitis)* is characterized by involvement primarily of the convex surfaces by red scaling plaques; the inguinal folds are spared (Fig. 255-6, *A*). In *candidal diaper dermatitis* similar red scaling plaques involve the skin folds, but there also are satellite pustules in areas not covered by the diaper (Fig. 255-6, *B*). Seborrheic dermatitis in the diaper area involves the skin folds; however, there are no satellite lesions.

Histiocytosis X refers to a group of Langerhan cell histiocytoses: Letterer-Siwe disease (diffuse disseminated histiocytosis), Hand-Schüller-Christian disease, and eosinophilic granuloma (chronic multifocal or focal histiocytosis). Letterer-Siwe disease may be confused with seborrheic der-

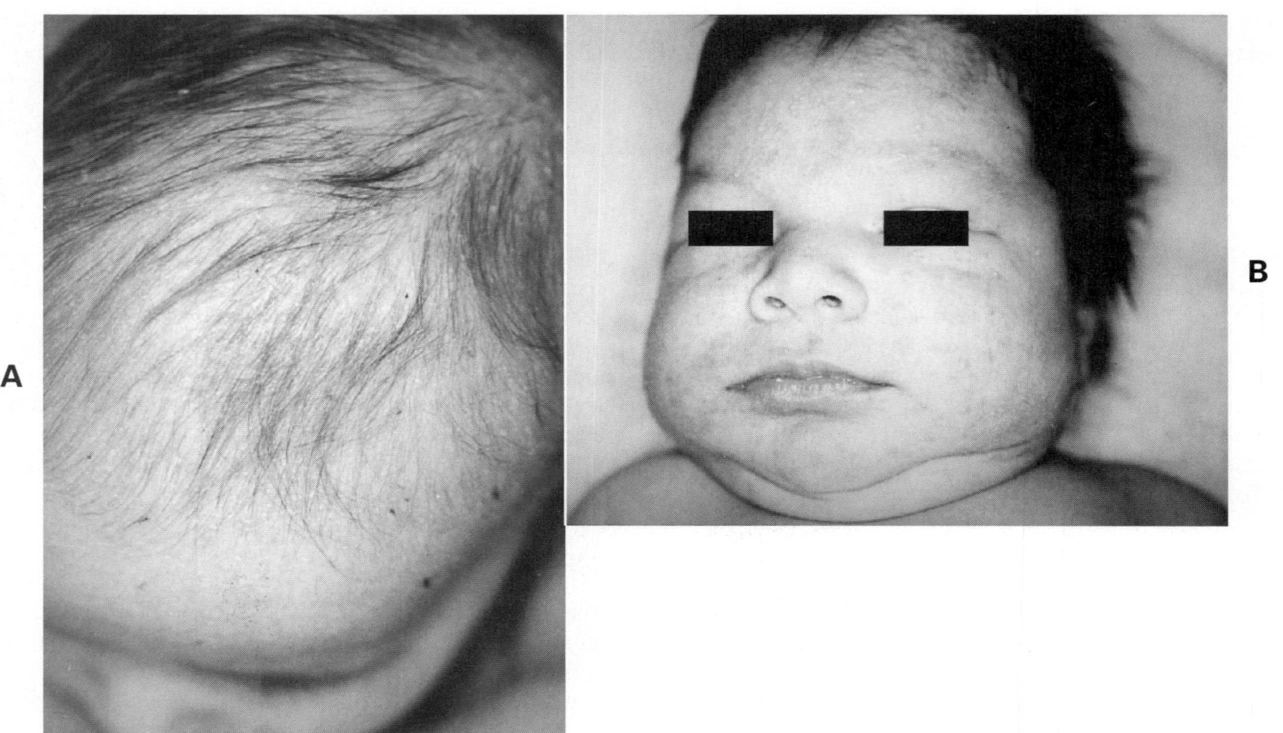

FIG. 255-1 **A,** Cradle cap. **B,** Greasy yellow-red scaling papules.

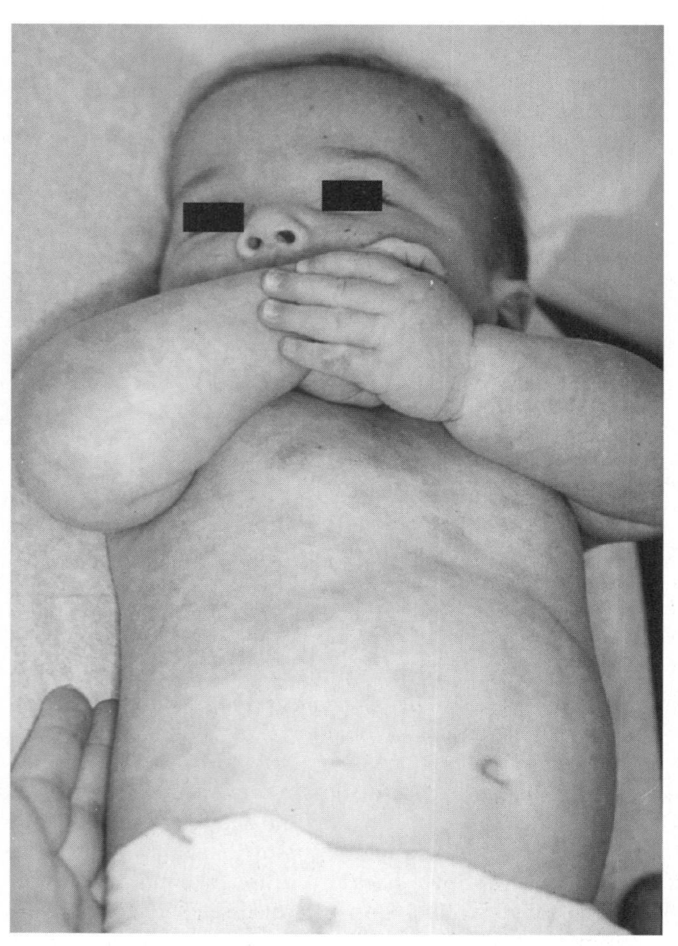

FIG. 255-2 Psoriasiform seborrheic dermatitis.

matitis because its pattern of distribution is similar. However, Letterer-Siwe disease also is characterized by axillary, inguinal, and oral mucosal erosions, purpura and petechiae, and hepatosplenomegaly. A skin biopsy specimen will distinguish the two disorders easily and is recommended in cases of seborrheic dermatitis that are unresponsive to treatment.

Leiner disease, sometimes referred to as *erythrodermic seborrheic dermatitis,* is an inherited immunological disorder characterized by generalized seborrheic dermatitis, persistent diarrhea, failure to thrive, and recurrent gram negative infections caused by C5 and/or C3 dysfunction. The diagnosis is made by demonstrating deficient yeast opsonic activity in the patient's serum.

MANAGEMENT

Therapy for *seborrheic dermatitis (infantile cradle cap)* includes the application to the scalp of a 1% to 2% salicylic acid in liquid or petrolatum form, followed by a keratolytic shampoo (e.g., Sebulex) and a topical low-potency corticosteroid (Synalar solution or Dermasmoothe). The salicylic acid solution or petrolatum should be applied only for 10 minutes and then shampooed out carefully, avoiding the face and particularly the eyes because severe irritant contact dermatitis may occur. The corticosteroid solution should be applied sparingly and left on for several hours. This regimen may be repeated up to twice daily as needed and then tapered. Dramatic improvement occurs usually within a week. Lesions occuring on the face, intertriginous areas, and diaper area may be treated with a low-potency topical corticosteroid cream (1% hydrocortisone cream) twice a day. A midpotency corticosteroid such as 0.1% Kenalog cream may be

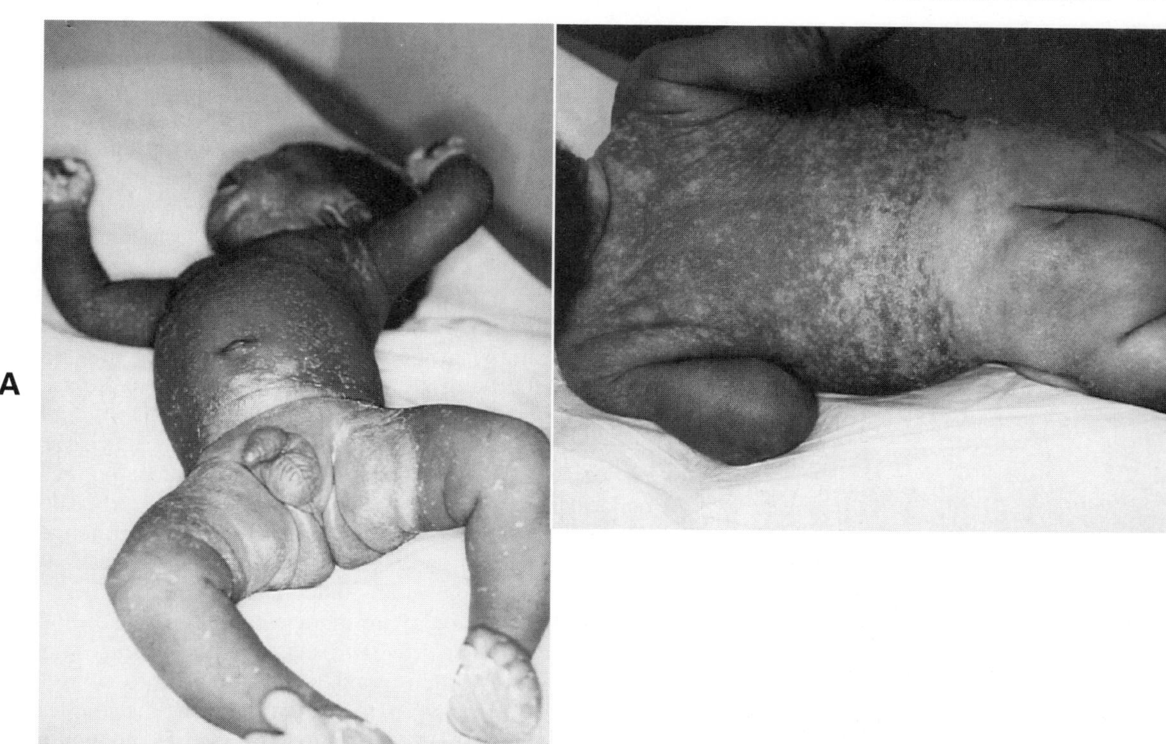

FIG. 255-3 **A** and **B,** Erythrodermic seborrheic dermatitis.

FIG. 255-4 Psoriasis. **A,** Scalp. **B,** Trunk. **C,** Diaper dermatitis.

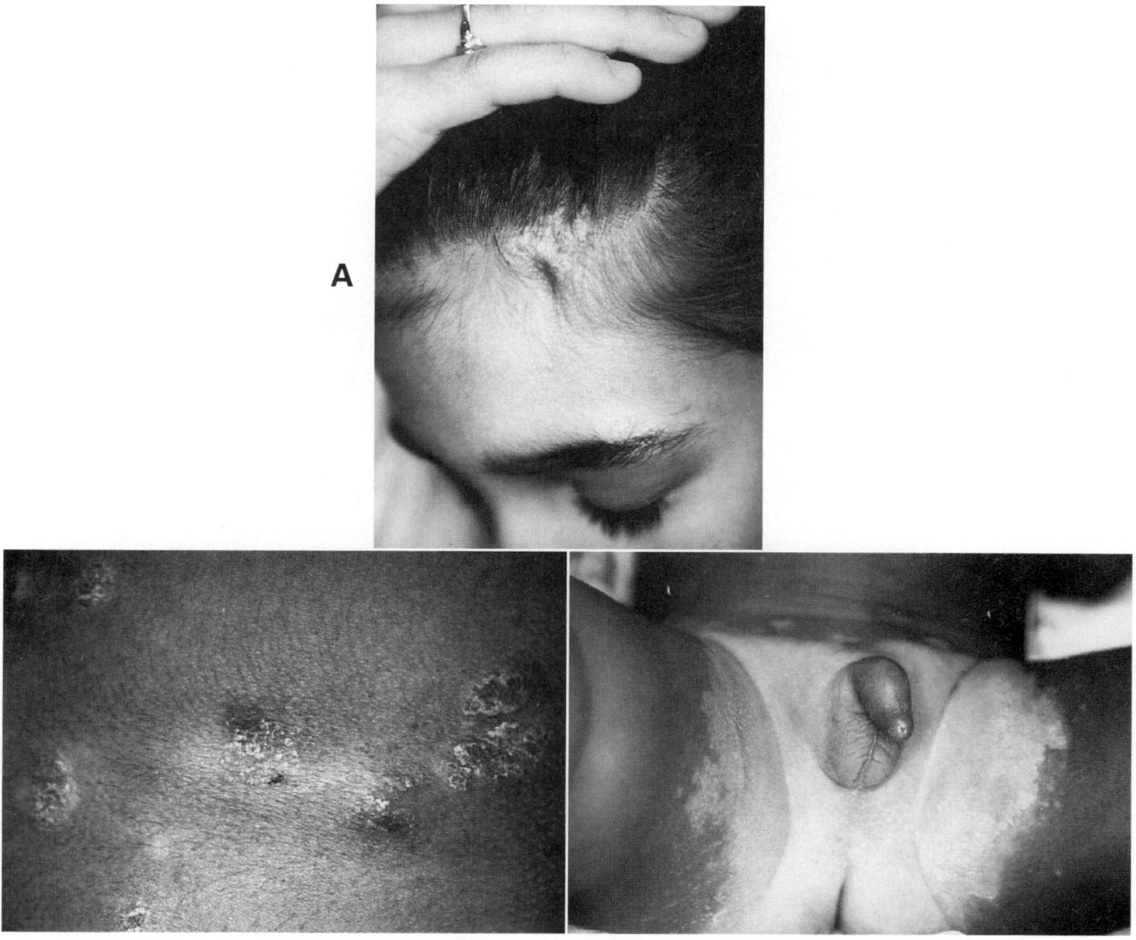

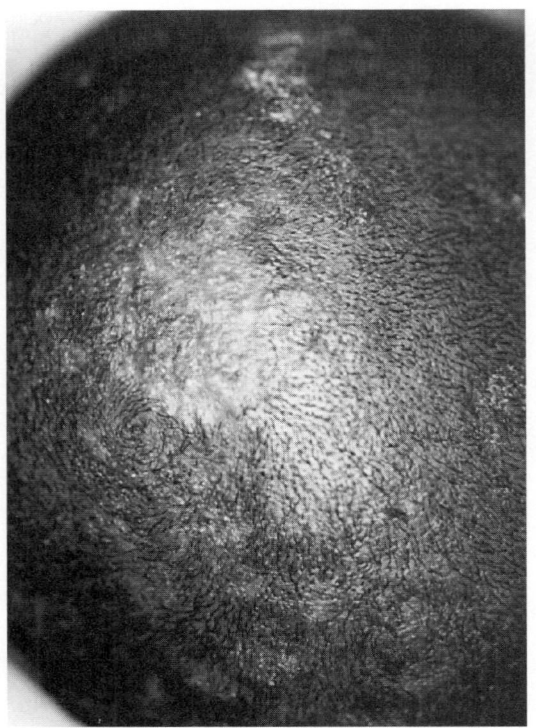

FIG. 255-5 Tinea capitus.

used on the body twice a day. A mid-potency or strong halogenated corticosteroid should not be used on the face, intertriginous areas, and diaper areas. In addition, topical ketoconazole (Nizoral), which has been used to treat adult SD, also has been found to be beneficial in treating infantile SD. Lesions in the diaper and intertriginous areas may become superinfected with *Candida* species and require topical Mycostatin cream twice a day in addition to a topical corticosteroid.

Therapy for *adolescent seborrheic dermatitis* consists of topical corticosteroids and keratolytic shampoos applied to the scalp similar to those described for infants. In addition, topical Nizoral cream and oral ketoconazole may be used in severe cases.

Psoriasiform seborrheic dermatitis of the scalp is treated as described for cradle cap. Psoriasiform lesions on the face and truck respond to treatment with topical corticosteroid ointments and emollients. If lesions persist into childhood, a modified Goeckerman regimen consisting of application of a tar preparation followed by outdoor exposure to sunlight and topical corticosteroids[1] are therapeutic.

Generalized erythrodermic seborrheic dermatitis may require systemic corticosteroids and antibiotics to control superinfection in addition to the antiseborrheic therapies already mentioned. Hospitalization for intravenous antibiotic administration may be required.

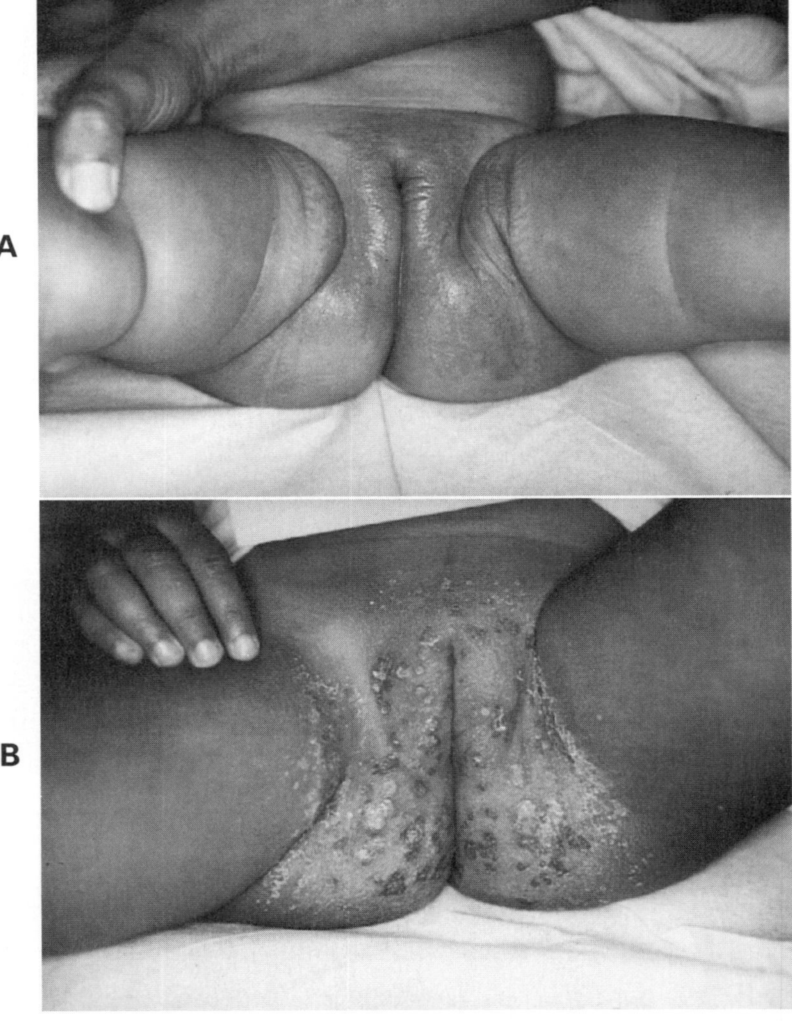

FIG. 255-6 **A,** Irritant diaper dermatitis. **B,** Candidal diaper dermatitis.

PROGNOSIS

The prognosis for infantile seborrheic dermatitis usually is good. Most cases resolve within the first 6 months of life. Adolescent-onset and HIV-related seborrheic dermatitis may be more persistent; however, it usually responds readily to topical therapy. Infants who have seborrheic dermatitis are at an increased risk of developing atopic dermatitis or psoriasis later.

REFERENCES

1. Caputo R: Papulo-squamous disease. In Schachner LA, Hansen R, editors: *Pediatric dermatology,* New York, 1988, Churchill Livingstone.
2. Maldonado RR et al: Pityrosporum ovale in infantile seborrheic dermatitis, *Pediatr Dermatol* 6:16, 1989.
3. Menni SM et al: Infantile seborrheic dermatitis: seven year follow-up and some prognostic criteria, *Pediatr Dermatol* 6:13, 1989.
4. Prose N: HIV infection in children, *J Am Acad Dermatol* 22:1223, 1990.
5. Tollesson A et al: Essential fatty acids in infantile seborrheic dermatitis, *J Am Acad Dermatol* 28:957, 1993.

256 Seizure Disorders

Sarah M. Roddy and Margaret C. McBride

Seizures are caused by abnormal discharges of neurons and may have a wide variety of clinical manifestations. A seizure should be considered a symptom of systemic or central nervous system dysfunction. Management consists not only of controlling seizures, but also of diagnosing any potentially treatable underlying condition. Acute conditions associated with seizures include metabolic disturbances, fever, meningitis, encephalitis, and toxic encephalopathy. The terms *seizure disorder* and *epilepsy* are synonymous and are applied to the condition in which there is a tendency for recurrent, unprovoked seizures. Care of patients who have epilepsy includes managing the psychosocial impact of epilepsy on the child and family.

CLASSIFICATION OF SEIZURES

Classification of seizures (see the box on p. 1565) has provided a means to study seizures that have similar pathophysiology and to determine which medications are effective for which seizure types. Electroencephalographic (EEG) monitoring has aided in the current classification,[6] which is based on characterization of seizure onset and progression. Seizures are either *partial* or *generalized.* Generalized seizures result from involvement of both cerebral hemispheres simultaneously from the onset of the seizure. Types of generalized seizures include absence, myoclonic, atonic, tonic, clonic, and tonic-clonic. Partial seizures are caused by seizure discharges that begin in one hemisphere. Partial seizures are divided further into *simple partial seizures,* in which consciousness is preserved, and *complex partial seizures,* in which consciousness is impaired. Partial seizures of either type may progress to become secondarily generalized.

Epilepsy syndromes also have been defined in terms of a cluster of signs and symptoms, including age of onset, severity, diurnal or nocturnal occurrence, clinical course, associated neurological dysfunction, inheritance, and EEG findings.[5] Generalized epilepsy syndromes include juvenile myoclonic epilepsy, Lennox-Gastaut syndrome, infantile spasms (West syndrome), and childhood absence epilepsy. A common partial epilepsy syndrome is benign partial epilepsy of childhood. Neonatal seizures can be generalized or focal and therefore are considered separately, as are febrile seizures. The accompanying box outlines the classification of the various seizure types and epilepsy syndromes.

Generalized Seizures

Absence Seizures. Absence seizures are generalized, nonconvulsive seizures characterized by interruption of activity, staring, and unresponsiveness; they usually last between 5 and 15 seconds. The episode starts abruptly, without warning, and ends abruptly with resumption of the child's preictal activity. The child may be unaware that the episode occurred. At times, unresponsiveness is accompanied by eyelid fluttering and upward rotation of the eyes and occasionally by mild clonic movements or automatisms such as lip smacking, grimacing, or swallowing. Seizures may occur over 100 times per day and may interfere with the child's learning ability. The age of onset generally is between 4 and 8 years of age; rarely does it occur before 3 years or after 15 years. Girls are affected more commonly than boys. The influence of genetic factors in the etiology of absence seizures is suggested by 15% to 44% of first-degree relatives having a history of absence seizures, paroxysmal EEG abnormalities, or both.[1]

The classic finding on the EEG in patients who have absence seizures is bilaterally synchronous 3-Hz spike-and-wave discharges. Hyperventilation may be used to precipitate the electrical discharge as well as a clinical seizure. Photic stimulation during the EEG also induces the seizure discharge in some patients. Generalized tonic-clonic seizures may occur in some children, especially those who have an onset of absence seizures after 8 years of age. The prognosis for remission is good for children in whom absence is the sole seizure type but less favorable for those who have associated tonic-clonic seizures.

Monotherapy with ethosuximide or valproate usually controls absence seizures effectively. Valproate is the drug of choice if there are associated tonic-clonic seizures. Benzodiazepines also are effective in controlling absence seizures, but their adverse effects on behavior make them second-line therapeutic agents. Phenytoin, phenobarbital, and carbamazepine usually are ineffective for treatment of absence seizures and may exacerbate them.

Myoclonic Seizures. Myoclonic jerks are characterized by brief, sudden muscle contractions that may involve only part of the body or may be generalized. They may occur in clusters, especially during the period of falling asleep or shortly after awakening. There may be no alteration in consciousness associated with the jerks.

Atonic Seizures. Atonic, or astatic, seizures also have been termed *drop attacks.* They are characterized by a sudden decrease in muscle tone, which may result in head nodding or mild flexing of the legs. More significant decreases in muscle tone may cause the patient to slump to the floor. There usually is no detectable alteration in consciousness with these seizures.

Generalized Tonic-Clonic Seizures. Generalized tonic-clonic seizures also are known as *grand mal seizures* and consist of motor manifestations and loss of consciousness. The tonic phase is characterized by a sustained contraction of muscles; as a result the patient falls to the ground, usually in opisthotonus. There usually is extensor posturing with tonic contraction of the diaphragm and intercostal muscles. This halts respirations, which in turn produces cyanosis. The tonic phase lasts less than 1 minute and is followed by the clonic

CLASSIFICATION OF SEIZURES AND EPILEPSY SYNDROMES

Primary generalized
Seizure types

Absence
Myoclonic
Atonic/astatic
Tonic-clonic

Epilepsy syndromes

Infantile spasms (West syndrome)
Lennox-Gastaut syndrome
Childhood absence epilepsy
Juvenile myoclonic epilepsy

Partial
Seizure types

Simple partial
Complex partial
Partial seizures with secondary generalization

Epilepsy syndromes

Benign partial epilepsy of childhood
Epilepsia partialis continua

Unclassified

Neonatal seizures
Febrile seizures
Pseudoseizures

*Data from Commission on Classification and Terminology of the International League Against Epilepsy: Epilepsia 26:268, 1985.

phase, which consists of bilateral and rhythmic jerking. The jerks may be accompanied by expiratory grunts produced by diaphragmatic contractions against a closed glottis. The frequency of the clonic jerks decreases as the seizure progresses, although the intensity actually may increase. The tongue may be bitten, and bowel and bladder incontinence may occur. The clonic activity usually stops after several minutes. The seizure may be followed by vomiting, confusion, and lethargy, with gradual recovery of consciousness over a period of minutes to hours.

Generalized tonic-clonic seizures may be primary generalized or secondary generalized. Primary generalized seizures usually are idiopathic or genetic in origin and are associated with bilaterally synchronous electrical discharges on EEG. Secondary generalized seizures begin as partial seizures but may generalize so rapidly that any suggestion of focal origin is lacking. The EEG may demonstrate a focal discharge that may spread to both hemispheres or may show only bilateral synchronous discharges. History that is helpful in determining that a seizure is secondary generalized is the presence of an aura, head or eye deviation, or focal clonic movement at the onset of the seizure. Neurological examination may reveal subtle focal signs such as a mild hemiparesis or visual field defect. Complete seizure control is less likely in secondary generalized epilepsy than in primary generalized epilepsy.[1] Effective antiepileptic medications for the treatment of generalized tonic-clonic seizures include phenobarbital, phenytoin, primidone, and carbamazepine. Valproate also is an effective anticonvulsant for generalized tonic-clonic seizures with or without focal features.

Infantile Spasms (West Syndrome). Infantile spasms are a unique form of epilepsy, with onset during the first year of life. The seizures are characterized by a sudden contraction of neck, trunk, and extremity muscles. The spasms may be flexor, extensor, or mixed flexor-extensor and last only a few seconds each, but they often occur in clusters of up to 100 individual spasms. A typical episode is characterized by dropping of the head with abduction of the shoulders and flexion of the lower extremities. The infant may cry during or following the spasm. Pallor, flushing, grimacing, laughter, and nystagmus are observed during some episodes. Episodes are common on awakening from sleep, during drowsiness, and with feedings but are rare during sleep. The peak age of infantile spasm onset is between 3 and 7 months,[1] with an estimated incidence of 1 per 4000 to 6000 infants.[10] Males are more likely to be affected than females.

Infantile spasms usually are divided into symptomatic and cryptogenic groups based on the presence of a predisposing etiological factor. Included among symptomatic infantile spasms are infants who have abnormal neurological development before the onset of spasms. Causes include structural abnormalities of the brain, hypoxic-ischemic insults, central nervous system infections or hemorrhages, and inborn errors of metabolism. Children who have tuberous sclerosis account for up to 25% of patients who have infantile spasms.[1] The cryptogenic group includes those patients in whom no etiological factor can be found. Infants in this group tend to be older at the onset of infantile spasms compared with infants in the symptomatic group.

The EEG pattern associated with infantile spasms is known as *hypsarrhythmia* and is characterized by high-voltage slow waves with irregularly interspersed multifocal spike and sharp waves. Hypsarrhythmia may precede the onset of clinical manifestations, or it may occur later or not at all. Over time the hypsarrhythmia usually evolves into other focal or generalized abnormalities; in some cases the EEG may normalize.

Infantile spasms are resistant to treatment with most anticonvulsants. The treatment used most commonly is adrenocorticotropic hormone (ACTH). ACTH in a long-acting form is administered as a single daily intramuscular dose of 20 to 40 IU. Adverse effects of ACTH and steroids are significant and include Cushing syndrome, hypertension, susceptibility to infections, hyperglycemia, gastrointestinal bleeding, and electrolyte disturbance. The benzodiazepines also are effective in controlling infantile spasms. Nitrazepam seems to be more effective than clonazepam or diazepam. Valproic acid also is effective therapy for infantile spasms in some infants.

The prognosis for infants who have infantile spasms remains grave. Even in recently reported series, the average mortality is approximately 20%, with aspiration pneumonia being the most common cause of death.[10] Approximately 80% of survivors are mentally retarded. The spasms usually remit by a few years of age, but 55% to 60% of patients subsequently develop other forms of seizures.[1] The prognosis is more favorable for those infants whose neurological development had been normal before the onset of the spasms.

Lennox-Gastaut Syndrome. Lennox-Gastaut syndrome is a severe epileptic encephalopathy characterized by a variety of primary generalized seizures. Tonic seizures cause sudden, sustained contraction of the muscle groups, at times causing the patient to fall. Atypical absence seizures consist of a brief period of staring and immobility. The onset and recovery of atypical absence seizures are less abrupt than those of typical absence seizures. The episodes may be associated with mild tonic motor manifestations, automatisms, or loss of postural tone. Atonic seizures occur and may be preceded by myoclonic jerks. Tonic-clonic seizures and partial seizures also may occur in patients who have Lennox-Gastaut syndrome.

The majority of these patients begin to have seizures between 3 and 5 years of age,[25] with boys affected slightly more often than girls. Many patients have neurological deficits before the onset of Lennox-Gastaut syndrome, including mental retardation and cerebral palsy, which may be related to hypoxic encephalopathy or other insults to the brain. Patients may have a history of infantile spasms. The EEG typically shows an irregular, high-voltage, slow (2.5 Hz or slower) spike-wave pattern. The discharges are bilaterally synchronous.

The treatment of the seizures associated with Lennox-Gastaut syndrome is disappointing. Valproic acid has been the most successful in treatment of the different seizure types and is the drug of choice. Felbamate as an add-on drug has been shown to reduce the the frequency of atonic and generalized tonic-clonic seizures significantly.[15] The benzodiazepines also have been successful in controlling atonic, myoclonic, and atypical absence seizures. Unfortunately, with increasing doses the frequency of adverse effects also increases. The development of tolerance also is a problem associated with their use. Ethosuximide can help control the atypical absence episodes, and phenytoin can be used for tonic seizures. A ketogenic diet also has been beneficial in seizure control, but because of the nature of the diet, compliance is poor. Generally the goal of treatment is to achieve reasonable seizure control with as few medications as possible in order to minimize adverse effects. Sometimes the seizures typical of Lennox-Gastaut syndrome occur in otherwise normal preschool-age children, associated with normal background and fast polyspike-and-wave changes on EEG. These children have a much better prognosis for seizure control and cognitive development.

Juvenile Myoclonic Epilepsy. Juvenile myoclonic epilepsy is a primary generalized epilepsy with an age of onset of 12 to 18 years. It represents 4% of all epilepsy and is characterized by myoclonic jerks that affect mainly the upper extremities and less commonly the lower extremities. The jerks usually occur shortly after awakening, and patients may complain of clumsiness or difficulty holding objects early in the morning. Approximately 80% of patients have generalized tonic-clonic seizures, and 25% have absence seizures in addition to myoclonic seizures.[9] Myoclonic jerks almost always precede the onset of generalized tonic-clonic seizures by months to years. A teenager who has generalized tonic-clonic seizures should be questioned carefully regarding myoclonic jerks. Both the myoclonic jerks and the tonic-clonic seizures may be precipitated by sleep deprivation, stress, alcohol, and hormonal changes. Patients remain neurologically normal. Juvenile myoclonic epilepsy is genetic; a locus on the short arm of chromosome 6 has been identified. Fifty percent of probands report seizures in first- or second-degree relatives, and EEG changes in relatives are even more prevalent.[7] The ictal EEG typically shows generalized, symmetrical polyspike and waves at 4 to 6 Hz. Photic stimulation precipitates the electrical discharges in some patients. The recommended treatment for juvenile myoclonic epilepsy is valproate. Valproate will control the myoclonic jerks, absence seizures, and generalized tonic-clonic seizures in over 80% of patients. Other anticonvulsants may control certain seizure components of the syndrome, but valproate controls all the seizure components. There is a high rate of seizure recurrence among patients who discontinue valproate. Juvenile myoclonic epilepsy therefore is considered a lifelong condition that requires continuous treatment.

Partial Seizures

Simple Partial Seizures. Simple partial seizures are characterized by seizure activity restricted to one side of the body, with preserved consciousness. The symptoms may be motor, sensory, or cognitive, depending on the location of the neuronal discharge. Motor seizures may be restricted to part of the body, such as the face or a limb, or they may spread to involve the entire side. If the seizure discharge spreads to structures involved in consciousness, the seizure will become a complex partial seizure. The seizure activity also may spread to the opposite side of the brain, causing a generalized seizure. A partial seizure may be followed by Todd paralysis, a weakness of the limbs involved in the seizure. Partial sensory seizures most often are manifested by paresthesias lasting less than 1 to 2 minutes. Seizure discharges from one occipital lobe may cause visual symptoms such as scintillating colored spots or scotomata in the visual field contralateral to the discharge. Seizures with more complex visual hallucinations often progress to complex partial seizures with diminished consciousness. Auditory seizures are manifested by hearing noises and less commonly by having elaborate but usually nonverbal auditory hallucinations such as music.

Although simple partial seizures are caused by focal epileptiform discharges, a focal structural lesion may not be found in 30% to 50% of patients.[10] Causes associated with these seizures include prenatal and perinatal insults, central nervous system malformations, and metabolic disturbances such as hypocalcemia, hypoglycemia, and inborn errors of metabolism. Carbamazepine, phenytoin, and valproic acid are effective drugs in the treatment of simple focal seizures.

Complex Partial Seizures. Complex partial seizures are seizures that originate in a limited area of one cerebral hemisphere and result in impaired consciousness. A complex partial seizure may begin as a simple partial seizure that progresses to impairment of consciousness. The initial portion of a seizure that occurs before consciousness is lost is referred to as the *aura*. The aura may consist of any of a wide variety of symptoms, depending on the location of cortical discharges. There may be auditory, olfactory, or visual illusions or hallucinations. Affective symptoms such as fear or other unpleasant feelings can occur. Anger or rage are extremely rare as a seizure manifestation but may occur during postictal confusion if the patient is restrained.

Déjà vu, the feeling that an experience has occurred before, and *jamais vu,* the feeling that a previously experienced sensation is unfamiliar and strange, have been described. Young children have difficulty describing déjà vu and may say only that there was a "funny feeling" that occurred in the head or stomach. Staring and automatisms, which are involuntary coordinated motor activity, occur when there is clouding of consciousness. Automatisms include simple phenomena such as chewing, lip smacking, swallowing, and hissing and more complicated activities such as picking at clothes, searching, or ambulating. Automatisms usually are followed by postictal amnesia. The child may become tired and go to sleep.

Complex partial seizures must be distinguished from absence seizures, which also are characterized by staring and unresponsiveness. Episodes of absence seizures have an abrupt onset and termination, compared with complex partial seizures, which have a more gradual onset and termination. Absence seizures last less than 30 seconds and are not associated with postictal confusion. Automatisms can occur if absence episodes are prolonged, but they often are just a continuation of motor activity present before the onset of seizure.

The most frequent EEG finding in complex partial seizures is an anterior temporal lobe spike discharge, although some patients will have spike discharges from other areas.[10] Interictal EEGs often are normal. Repeating the EEG increases the likelihood of demonstrating the abnormal discharge. Nasopharyngeal or sphenoidal electrodes rarely add information that is not obtained by scalp recordings that include special temporal placements.

Causes of complex partial seizures include perinatal insults, head trauma, encephalitis, and possibly status epilepticus, all of which may be associated with scarring of the temporal lobe. Indolent tumors such as hamartomas and low-grade gliomas also can cause complex partial seizures and are found in approximately 20% of persons who have intractable partial seizures. Genetic factors play a secondary role in the etiology of complex seizures.[1]

Anticonvulsant drugs used in the treatment of complex partial seizures include carbamazepine, phenytoin, phenobarbital, primidone, and valproate.* Carbamazepine is the drug of choice in children because of its efficacy and relatively mild adverse effects. If seizures are not controlled with carbamazepine, the addition of acetazolamide may result in improved seizure control.[21] Patients who have medically intractable partial seizures should be evaluated at a comprehensive epilepsy center to determine their candidacy for surgical intervention, which results in complete seizure control in 40% to 70% of patients.[13]

Benign Partial Epilepsy of Childhood. Benign partial epilepsy of childhood also is known as *rolandic epilepsy, sylvian seizures,* and *centrotemporal epilepsy.* This epilepsy syndrome is a common type of partial motor epilepsy in childhood. The onset usually is between 5 and 8 years of age. Males more often are affected than females. Genetic factors play a role in the etiology. The seizures typically occur during sleep, although patients occasionally may have an episode during wakefulness. Episodes are characterized by the child awakening with one side of the face twitching. The oropharyngeal muscles are often also involved, causing the child to make unintelligible gurgling sounds. The ipsilateral upper extremity may be involved, but only rarely is the lower extremity involved. In rare cases a seizure episode will become generalized. Consciousness often is retained during the seizure, although the child may not be able to speak. Most seizure episodes last less than 2 minutes. The frequency of seizures is low, with 25% of patients having a single seizure episode and 50% having fewer than five episodes.[1] The typical EEG findings are midtemporal or centrotemporal spike discharges that usually are unilateral, often very frequent, and present in light sleep. Neuroradiological studies show no abnormalities to correlate with the EEG focus. If a child has infrequent episodes, no treatment may be needed. If the episodes frighten the child and a decision is made to initiate treatment, carbamazepine is the drug of choice.[10] Other effective drugs include phenytoin and valproate. The seizure episodes remit when the child is around 9 to 12 years of age, but no later than 17 years. Remission is long lasting, and no developmental or neurological impairment is associated with these seizures.

Epilepsia Partialis Continua. Epilepsia partialis continua is a rare type of seizure in which twitching is continuous and limited to one side of the body. The twitching frequently involves only a few muscles and occurs most often in the hand or foot. Consciousness is preserved, but the seizure activity might weaken the extremity involved. Seizure activity may persist for hours to months. Focal encephalitis and tumor have been associated with this type of seizure. Medical treatment of epilepsia partialis continua generally is unsuccessful, although carbamazepine, phenytoin, and benzodiazepines have been used with varying degrees of success.[10]

Unclassified Seizures

Neonatal Seizures. Seizures are the most common manifestation of neonatal neurological disease and occur in approximately 0.5% of all newborns.[20] The manifestations of seizure activity in neonates differ from those in older children. Volpe[31] has delineated four major seizure types in neonates:

1. *Subtle seizures* occur in both full-term and premature infants and often are overlooked. These seizures consist of eye deviation, blinking, sucking, swimming movements of the arms, pedaling movements of the legs, and apnea. EEG recordings do not always show correlation of electrical seizure discharges with the clinical seizure activity. This has raised the possibility that the seizure discharges arise from regions of the brain that cannot be detected by surface electrodes.
2. *Tonic seizures* are focal or generalized. Focal tonic seizures are characterized by sustained posturing of a limb or asymmetrical posturing of the neck and trunk. There may be accompanying subtle seizure activity such as eye deviation. Generalized tonic seizures are characterized by tonic extension of the limbs. Less commonly, the upper extremities are flexed and the lower extremities are extended. These seizures are more common among premature infants, especially those who have intraventricular hemorrhage.

*Felbamate and gabapentin have been shown to be effective treatment of partial seizures in adults.

3. *Clonic seizures* are categorized as focal or multifocal. Focal clonic seizure activity is characterized by clonic jerking that remains localized. Although focal clonic seizures can result from focal central nervous system lesions such as cerebral infarction, they also can occur with metabolic disturbances. Multifocal clonic seizures are characterized by clonic activity in one extremity that migrates randomly to another area of the body. These seizures occur primarily in full-term infants. The EEG shows multiple areas of sharp activity that discharge independently.
4. *Myoclonic seizures* are flexion jerks of the upper or lower extremities. They may occur singly or in a series of repetitive jerks. Infants with these seizures may later develop infantile spasms. These myoclonic seizures should be differentiated from benign myoclonic jerks that occur during sleep in neonates and are accompanied by a normal EEG.

Jitteriness is a movement in neonates that may be confused with seizure activity. The movement is a tremor that is stimulus sensitive and can be stopped by passively flexing the affected limb. There is no associated eye deviation or other abnormal eye movements. Some investigators advocate identification of neonatal seizures by EEG recording, maintaining that only electrical seizures are *true* seizures and require treatment. However, this remains controversial because identical clinical seizures in the same infant may at times not be associated with electrical seizures.[32] It is clear, however, that electrical seizures may not have clinical correlates; hence, EEG recording should be done for all infants at risk for seizures in order to identify these silent electrical seizures.

ETIOLOGY. There are multiple etiologies of neonatal seizures; however, only a few causes account for most cases. Determining the etiology of neonatal seizures is important because specific treatment may be indicated. The etiology of the seizures also is an important factor influencing prognosis. Some of the most common causes of seizure are described as follows:

1. *Hypoxia-ischemia* is the most common cause of seizure in both premature and full-term infants.[31] These seizures usually begin within the first 24 hours of life and may be very difficult to control. Metabolic disturbances in the infant also may complicate seizure control.
2. *Intracranial hemorrhage* is another cause of seizures in both premature and full-term infants. Intraventricular hemorrhage is seen mainly in premature infants within the first 3 days of life. Generalized tonic seizures may be associated with severe hemorrhage invading the brain parenchyma. Infants who have a primary subarachnoid hemorrhage may not have any clinical symptoms or may develop seizures on the second day of life. These infants often are full-term infants who are normal neurologically except for the seizure. Subdural hemorrhage is associated with trauma and may result in focal seizure activity.
3. *Metabolic disturbances,* especially hypoglycemia and hypocalcemia, also are associated with seizures in neonates. Infants who are small for gestational age and infants of diabetic mothers are at risk for hypoglycemia, and the blood glucose level should be monitored closely. Low-birth-weight infants and infants of diabetic mothers are at risk for hypocalcemic seizures, which occur when calcium levels drop below 7 mg/dl during the first 2 to 3 days of life. Often, infants who have hypocalcemia also have a history of hypoxia, which contributes to the risk of seizure. Hypocalcemic seizures that occur later usually are related to a low calcium and high phosphate intake. Late hypocalcemic seizures are now rare as a result of the development of formula that has an appropriate ratio of calcium and phosphorus supplementation. Other metabolic disturbances less frequently associated with seizures in neonates include hyponatremia, hypernatremia, local anesthetic intoxication, pyridoxine dependence, and disorders of amino acids, organic acids, and the urea cycle.
4. *Infection,* including bacterial and viral intracranial infections, is an important cause of neonatal seizures. The most common bacterial causes are group B beta-streptococcus and *Escherichia coli.* Onset of seizures with meningitis usually is after the first 3 to 4 days of life. Prenatal nonbacterial infections causing neonatal seizures include toxoplasmosis, rubella, herpes simplex virus, coxsackie B virus, and cytomegalovirus.
5. *Malformations of the brain* can cause seizures at any time during the newborn period. The malformations associated most commonly with seizures are those that have cortical dysgenesis such as lissencephaly, pachygyria, and polymicrogyria.[31]

MANAGEMENT. Treatment of neonatal seizures is urgent because repeated seizures may result in brain injury.[31] The following is an approach to the diagnosis and treatment of seizures:

1. Ensure adequate ventilation and perfusion.
2. Obtain blood for glucose, calcium, magnesium, and electrolyte studies. Check a Dextrostix for an immediate determination of glucose.
3. Correct any associated metabolic abnormality.
   A. Hypoglycemia: If glucose is low as shown by Dextrostix (<40 mg/dl), immediately give 10% dextrose intravenously in a dose of 2 ml/kg. Maintain blood glucose levels above 40 mg/dl by continuous intravenous infusion and monitor the levels in both full-term and premature infants.
   B. Hypocalcemia: Correct by administering 5% calcium gluconate solution, 4 ml/kg intravenously at a rate of 1 ml/minute to maintain serum calcium levels above 7 mg/dl while monitoring cardiac rate and rhythm.
   C. Hypomagnesemia: Correct serum magnesium levels to 1 mmol/L with 50% magnesium sulfate solution, 0.2 ml/kg intramuscularly.
4. Continued seizure activity requires administration of anticonvulsants.
   A. Phenobarbital is given in a loading dose of 20 mg/kg intravenously over 10 minutes. Additional doses of 5 mg/kg can be given, up to a total of 40 mg/kg.
   B. Phenytoin is given in a loading dose of 20 mg/kg intravenously while monitoring cardiac rhythm.
   C. Lorazepam can be given in doses of 0.1 mg/kg intravenously for persistent seizures.[8,24] Respiratory status should be monitored.

After seizures are controlled via loading doses of anticonvulsants, infants may be continued on maintenance doses of anticonvulsants. In asphyxiated and premature infants, the half-life of phenobarbital is very prolonged, and doses no higher than 1 to 2 mg/kg/day may be appropriate. There is no consensus as to the duration of treatment for neonatal seizures. The seizure etiology and EEG findings can help to determine the duration of treatment. Infants whose seizures result from a metabolic disturbance or infection may not need to be sent home on anticonvulsants; those who have a central nervous system malformation may need continued treatment. If clinical seizures are no longer present and the EEG does not contain paroxysmal activity, it is reasonable to taper the anticonvulsants.

PROGNOSIS. The prognosis of neonatal seizures relates mainly to the underlying diseases that caused them. Mental retardation and cerebral palsy are more common sequelae than are seizures. Infants who have seizures related to hypoxic-ischemic encephalopathy, hypoglycemia, or bacterial meningitis have a 50% chance of developing normally; those whose seizures result from late-onset hypocalcemia and primary subarachnoid hemorrhage have a greater than 90% chance of developing normally.[31] The interictal EEG is helpful in determining the prognosis. A normal background EEG pattern usually is associated with a good neurological outcome; a markedly abnormal background pattern such as burst-suppression or marked suppression of voltage is associated with a high risk of neurological sequelae.

Febrile Seizures. Febrile seizures are seizures that occur in young children who have fever but no evidence of intracranial infection or acute neurological illness. *Simple febrile seizures* are generalized tonic-clonic convulsions that last less than 15 minutes and do not recur within 24 hours. *Complex febrile seizures* are less common and are focal or prolonged beyond 15 minutes or recur within 24 hours. Febrile seizures occur in children between 3 months and 5 years of age; the median age of occurrence is 18 to 22 months. Approximately 2% to 5% of children will experience a febrile convulsion; boys are more susceptible than girls. Genetic predisposition plays a role in the etiology of febrile seizures, with 60% of patients having a relative who has had at least one seizure.[10]

A febrile seizure may be the first sign that a child is ill. It is not known whether the seizure activity is triggered by the rapid rise of fever or the actual height of the temperature. Febrile seizures can be triggered by any illness that causes fever, most frequently by otitis media and upper respiratory tract infections. There is a high rate of febrile seizures with shigellosis, salmonellosis, and roseola, possibly related to a direct effect they have on the central nervous system or to a neurotoxin they produce.

One third of children who have a febrile seizure will have another one with another febrile illness. The younger the child at the time of the first episode, the greater the risk of recurrence. Approximately 50% of the recurrences occur within 6 months of the initial seizure; 75% occur within 1 year.

Usually seizure activity has stopped by the time the child is evaluated. However, if the seizure continues, lorazepam or diazepam should be administered (see Chapter 293, Status Epilepticus). The temperature should be brought down by using rectal antipyretics, removing blankets and clothing, and sponging. Once seizure activity is controlled, evaluation is directed toward finding the cause of the fever. If the child is under 1 year of age or if the child has not rapidly returned to normal, a lumbar puncture should be strongly considered to evaluate for meningitis.

The EEG generally is not helpful in the evaluation of children who have febrile seizures. EEG tracings recorded within 1 week of the seizure often show posterior slowing. Paroxysmal activity is seen in the EEGs of 35% to 45% of patients who are followed up for several years.[1] These EEG abnormalities do not predict recurrence of febrile seizures or the development of epilepsy.

Treatment of febrile seizures includes family education that addresses the benign nature of the seizures, the use of antipyretics, and first aid for seizures. Administration of oral diazepam (0.33 mg/kg body weight administered every 8 hours during febrile illness) reduces the risk of recurrent febrile seizures.[26] Administration of phenobarbital, however, at the onset of a febrile illness does not prevent seizure activity because therapeutic blood levels are not achieved soon enough. Prophylactic treatment with anticonvulsant agents should be considered if neurological development is abnormal, it is a complex febrile seizure, or the child is under 1 year of age. Administration of phenobarbital in doses that achieve blood levels of 15 μg/ml prevents the recurrence of febrile seizures. Valproate also appears to be effective in prophylaxis; phenytoin and carbamazepine do not prevent recurrences. The adverse effects of anticonvulsant therapy must be weighed against the possible benefits. There is no evidence that prophylactic treatment reduces the risk of subsequent epilepsy.

The risk of subsequent epilepsy in children who have febrile seizures is 2.4%. Factors associated with subsequent development of a febrile partial seizures include focal seizures, prolonged seizures, and repeated episodes of seizures with the same febrile illness. Factors associated with development of a febrile, generalized seizures include more than three febrile seizures, a family history of afebrile seizures, and age over 3 years at the time of the first febrile seizure.[2]

Pseudoseizures. Pseudoseizures are uncommon but must be recognized if inappropriate treatment is to be prevented. They differ from true epileptic seizures in several respects. The movements usually are not clonic but may be quivering or random thrashing movements. There usually is no incontinence, injury, or tongue biting associated with pseudoseizures. Episodes may be dramatic, with screaming and shouting. Episodes also may vary greatly in the same patient. Usually there is no postictal period. Pseudoseizures can occur in early childhood but are more frequent in adolescence, especially in females.[1] Pseudoseizures are most likely to occur in children who have true epileptic seizures. A detailed history and observation of an episode often is all that is needed to diagnose pseudoseizures; EEG monitoring can be used in patients in whom the distinction cannot be made clinically. Once the diagnosis is established, treatment is directed toward the psychosocial issues involved.

APPROACH TO AN INITIAL SEIZURE

The first step in treating the child who has an initial seizure is making the correct diagnosis. The risk of seizure recurrence is important when deciding whether to initiate antiepileptic therapy. Some types of seizures, such as absence, myoclonic, akinetic, and infantile spasms, have a recurrence rate of virtually 100% and usually have recurred by the time the child is seen by the physician. These types of seizures require treatment. However, children who have a generalized tonic-clonic or partial seizure have a recurrence risk of 50% to 60%.[4,18] Factors that increase the risk of recurrence include a partial complex seizure, an abnormal neurological examination, and focal epileptiform abnormalities on the EEG. The best prognosis is in those children who have a generalized seizure, a normal neurological examination, and a nonepileptiform EEG. Many patients who have a single seizure should be observed for recurrence but should not be started on antiepileptic medication. Over 50% of the recurrences occur within 6 months, up to 90% within 1 year. If a second seizure occurs, initiation of antiepileptic medication should be considered because approximately 80% of children who have a second seizure will have more seizures.[4]

Diagnostic Procedures

Laboratory Tests. Laboratory tests usually performed at the time of the initial seizure include measurement of serum electrolytes, calcium, magnesium, and blood glucose. In some cases the history or examination may indicate that a more extensive laboratory evaluation is required.

Electroencephalography. The EEG, which measures the physiological function of the brain, changes throughout childhood, reflecting brain maturation. The EEG is important in the evaluation of a child who has seizures because it helps to define the seizure type. An epileptiform EEG may support the diagnosis of epilepsy, but a normal tracing does not exclude the diagnosis. Other abnormalities such as slowing and background disorganization are much less specific. Repeat tracings increase the likelihood of detecting epileptiform discharges in patients who have seizures. Procedures such as hyperventilation, photic stimulation, and sleep should be used when obtaining EEG recordings. Nasopharyngeal and sphenoidal electrodes may be used to detect mesial temporal discharges, but they rarely add information to that obtainable by special scalp electrode placements. Video EEG monitoring is useful in correlating clinical symptoms with electrical seizure activity and may be useful when clinical manifestations are atypical. Although the EEG provides electrophysiological evidence to support the diagnosis of epilepsy, EEG abnormalities must be interpreted in view of the clinical symptomatology. Some individuals have epileptiform discharges and other EEG abnormalities without ever having a clinical seizure; treatment is not indicated for such individuals.

Neuroimaging Studies. Plain skull roentgenograms can detect calcifications that may be seen in some syndromes, but they rarely help in the evaluation of children who have epilepsy. Computed tomography (CT) and magnetic resonance imaging (MRI) have replaced skull roentgenograms in the evaluation of seizures. CT and MRI scanning detect structural abnormalities; MRI is more sensitive than CT in the detection of low-grade tumors, changes in myelination, and heterotopic gray matter. Neuroimaging studies are not warranted in every child who has epilepsy; however, MRI or CT should be performed in children who have focal neurological abnormalities on examination or have intractable epilepsy. Positron emission tomography (PET) is useful in evaluating metabolic alterations with seizure activity, but the clinical relevance of PET in individual patients is not clear, and its availability is limited.

Lumbar Puncture. The cerebrospinal fluid should be examined in patients in whom meningitis or encephalitis is suspected. In other patients the lumbar puncture rarely is helpful and is not indicated routinely.

TREATMENT WITH ANTIEPILEPTIC MEDICATION

Once the child has had recurrent seizures and antiepileptic medication is indicated, the physician is faced with the decision of which medication to prescribe. Diagnosing seizure type correctly is the critical first step in treatment because some seizure disorders respond to certain medications. In choosing among potentially effective antiepileptic agents, the drug that has the least adverse effects should be selected. The medication is started at a dose that will result in a low therapeutic blood level. The dose should be increased until seizures are controlled or adverse effects become intolerable. If the initial medication is not fully effective, a second medication may be added. Consideration should be given to discontinuing the first medication if seizures are fully controlled with the second medication. It is important to use monotherapy if possible, since polytherapy often does not improve seizure control but may increase toxicity dramatically.

To devise an optimum dosing regimen it is important to consider the pharmacokinetics of the various antiepileptic medications. The dosing frequency is determined by the *half-life,* defined as the time in which the serum level falls to 50% of the initial value. The dosing interval should be no longer than the half-life of the medication, which means that most antiepileptic agents may be administered twice a day and some only once daily.[10] The efficacy of an antiepileptic medication should be evaluated only after five half-lives have elapsed, since this is the period of time required for the medication to reach a steady state. In antiepileptic medications that induce hepatic enzymes (e.g., carbamazepine), the half-life decreases over the first weeks of treatment. If breakthrough seizures occur at times of low (trough) serum drug levels or if toxicity occurs at times of peak serum drug levels, the frequency of dosing should be increased.

Patients requiring higher antiepileptic medication levels usually need more frequent dosing to avoid toxicity.

Serum drug levels can guide the adjusting of doses of antiepileptic medications. A baseline level should be obtained when the patient has been taking an appropriate dose long enough to have stable levels. Other indications for obtaining levels include verification of compliance, breakthrough seizures, and toxic effects. Levels also may be checked when other medications have been added or deleted from the patient's regimen. The timing of the sample in relation to the last dose is important in the interpretation of the levels, especially in drugs with short half-lives.

SPECIFIC ANTIEPILEPTIC MEDICATIONS

Table 256-1 outlines commonly used antiepileptic medications and their properties.

Table 256-1 Common Antiepileptic Medications

Drug	Indications	Half-life (hours)	Usual dose (mg/kg/day)	Therapeutic levels (μg/ml)	Adverse effects
Carbamazepine	Partial, secondary generalized	3-23 (18-55 initially)	5-25 5-10 (monotherapy)	4-12	Allergic rashes, nausea, diplopia, blurry vision, dizziness, hypersensitivity hepatitis, aplastic anemia
Phenytoin	Partial, secondary generalized, primary generalized	7-42 (nonlinear kinetics)	5-7	10-20 (occasionally lower)	Rashes, hirsutism, gingival hyperplasia, coarse features, psychomotor slowing, neuropathy, folate deficiency, myelosuppression, drug-induced lupus
Valproic acid	Primary generalized, absence, myoclonic, akinetic, febrile, infantile spasms, some partial	6-16	10-30 20-50 (infants and in polytherapy)	50-100 (150 if tolerated)	Nausea, tremor, weight gain, hair loss, thrombocytopenia, hepatic failure, pancreatitis
Phenobarbital	Neonatal, febrile, partial, secondary generalized, primary generalized, akinetic	36-120	3-5 (<25 kg) 2-3 (25-50 kg) 1-2 (>50 kg)	10-40	Sedation, inattention, hyperactivity, irritability, cognitive impairment, rare hypersensitivity reactions
Ethosuximide	Absence, myoclonic, akinetic	15-68	15-40	40-100	Nausea, abdominal discomfort, hiccups, drowsiness, behavioral problems, dystonias, myelosuppression, drug-induced lupus
Primidone	Partial, secondary generalized, primary generalized	3-20	5-10 (1-2 initially)	5-12	Sedation, irritability, psychomotor slowing, rare hematological and hypersensitivity reactions
Clonazepam	Absence, primary generalized, infantile spasms	20-36	0.01-0.2	0.01-0.07	Sedation, hyperactivity, inattention, aggressiveness, tolerance, ataxia, withdrawal seizures
Acetazolamide	Absence, myoclonic, akinetic, partial	10-12	10-20	10-14	Diuresis, paresthesias, sedation, CO_2 retention, rashes
Felbamate	Partial (in patients >12 years), Lennox-Gastaut syndrome	20 (in monotherapy)	15-45 (maximum of 3600 mg)	—	Anorexia, weight loss, nausea, insomnia, headache, fatigue, aplastic anemia
Gabapentin	Partial, with or without secondary generalized seizures in patients >12 years	5-7	Total daily dose 900-1800 mg	—	Somnolence, dizziness, ataxia, fatigue
Lamotrigine	Partial, primary generalized, absence, atypical absence, atonic, and myoclonic	7 to 45	5-15 without valproic acid, 1-5 with valproic acid	—	Somnolence, rash, vomiting

Phenobarbital

Phenobarbital is one of the oldest antiepileptic agents still in use. Because of its long half-life, it has the advantage of requiring dosing only once or twice a day. The recommended dose per kilogram decreases as the weight increases. Failure to decrease the per-kilogram dose levels in older children will result in toxic levels. Because phenobarbital is a relatively safe medication in terms of serious toxic effects, monitoring of parameters other than serum levels usually is not necessary. The major disadvantage of phenobarbital is its effect on behavior and cognitive function, including hyperactivity, irritability, and attention deficits. Maintaining serum levels at the minimum level for seizure control may help decrease these adverse effects. Phenobarbital administration will lower the serum levels of carbamazepine and valproate. Administration of valproate will increase phenobarbital levels; therefore phenobarbital doses should be decreased by 25% to 50% to prevent toxicity when prescribed concomitantly with valproate.

Phenytoin

Phenytoin also is among the older antiepileptic medications and has been used widely. Because of its pharmacokinetics, blood levels vary dramatically with small changes in dosage. Therefore changes in dosage should be monitored via serum levels, and only very small dose changes should be made when serum levels are close to or within the therapeutic range. Phenytoin commonly is used for treatment of status epilepticus because intravenous administration results in rapid penetration into the central nervous system. Although phenytoin is an effective antiepileptic agent in generalized tonic-clonic and partial seizures, its adverse effects limit its use. Cosmetic adverse effects include gingival hypertrophy, hirsutism, and coarsening of the facial features. Also of concern are its effects on mood and cognitive function, which include depressed mood, slowed psychomotor functioning, and, in a few, depressed IQ scores.[29] Other adverse effects include folate-deficiency anemia, cerebellar degeneration, and allergic dermatitis. Valproic acid may lower total serum phenytoin, but the free phenytoin level transiently increases and then returns to its original level; thus no adjustment in dosage is necessary. Phenytoin may decrease carbamazepine levels and increase phenobarbital levels.[23]

Carbamazepine

Carbamazepine is widely used because it has relatively few effects on cognitive function. It may also affect behavior positively.[29] The most serious adverse effect associated with carbamazepine has been aplastic anemia. This is extremely rare, occurring at a rate of less than 1 case per 200,000 treatment years.[17] A complete blood count should be obtained before carbamazepine therapy is initiated and should be repeated after 2 to 3 weeks. It is not clear whether further blood counts are useful when the initial counts are normal, but they should be obtained more readily when the child is ill and often are repeated biannually or annually. Neutropenia as low as 3000/mm^3 may occur but does not predict more serious myelosuppression. The dose of carbamazepine may need to be changed during the course of treatment because the drug tends to induce its own metabolic breakdown. Phenobarbital, phenytoin, primidone, and clonazepam decrease carbamazepine serum levels.

Valproic Acid

Valproic acid has a broad spectrum of efficacy and also has the advantage of minimal cognitive adverse effects. Tremor may occur with high serum levels. Other adverse effects include increased appetite, weight gain, transient hair loss, nausea, and vomiting. Fatal hepatotoxicity also has been associated with valproic acid. Most cases occur during the first 3 months of treatment. Those patients at greatest risk for hepatotoxicity are children under 2 years of age who receive valproic acid as part of antiepileptic polytherapy.[11] Successful treatment of valproic acid–associated hepatotoxicity via N-acetylcysteine has recently been reported.[14] Valproic acid should be administered extremely cautiously to patients who have preexisting hepatic dysfunction. Liver function should be monitored in patients taking valproic acid, especially those in the high-risk group. Valproic acid raises the level of phenobarbital; therefore the dose of phenobarbital must be decreased by 33% to 50% if valproic acid is added. Carbamazepine, phenobarbital, and phenytoin decrease valproic acid serum levels.

Ethosuximide

Ethosuximide has a limited spectrum of efficacy; it is used mainly for treating absence seizures and some forms of myoclonic seizures. Behavioral disturbances also can occur in some children, and pancytopenia has been associated with chronic administration. Periodic blood counts therefore may be necessary.[10] Ethosuximide does not interact significantly with other antiepileptic medications.

Primidone

Primidone is not a commonly used antiepileptic agent because it has no specific advantage over other agents. Primidone is metabolized to phenobarbital and phenylethylmalonamide and has many of the same characteristics of phenobarbital, including behavioral and cognitive adverse effects. It may be more sedating than phenobarbital. Because one third of primidone is metabolized to phenobarbital, phenobarbital levels should be monitored. Phenobarbital levels may be 1.3 to 2 times higher than primidone levels. Valproate increases primidone serum levels; phenytoin and carbamazepine increase the phenobarbital to primidone ratio.

Clonazepam

Clonazepam, a benzodiazepine, is not a first-line antiepileptic medication because of its adverse effects. It causes significant behavioral changes, including hyperactivity, decreased attention span, aggressiveness, and restlessness. Because withdrawal of the drug may cause irritability, myoclonus, and increased seizures, it should be withdrawn slowly. Treatment with clonazepam usually is reserved for absence and myoclonic seizures that are refractory to ethosuximide and valproic acid.

Acetazolamide

Acetazolamide is an inhibitor of the enzyme carbonic anhydrase. It is an effective adjunctive therapy for treatment of several types of seizures, although its antiepileptic properties are not well understood. Acetazolamide can be used in combination with valproic acid for treatment of absence, myoclonic, and akinetic seizures. Adding acetazolamide to carbamazepine may improve control of partial seizures.[21] Acetazolamide metabolism is not affected significantly by other medications.

Felbamate

Felbamate is one of the newest antiepileptic medications. It was approved by the FDA in 1993 for treatment of partial seizures in adults and for adjunctive therapy in children who have Lennox-Gastaut syndrome. A placebo-controlled trial of add-on felbamate in patients who have Lennox-Gastaut syndrome demonstrated that felbamate significantly reduced the frequency of atonic and generalized tonic-clonic seizures.[15] The most common side effects of felbamate are anorexia, weight loss, nausea, insomnia, headache, and fatigue. No serious cardiac or hepatic effects have been reported. However, over 20 cases of aplastic anemia among persons taking felbamate have been reported. The true incidence and severity of this problem has not yet been determined. Cases of hepatic toxicity have also been reported. It currently is recommended that felbamate be used only in patients whose epilepsy is so severe that the benefits from its use outweigh the risk of aplastic anemia. Dosage of felbamate is based on weight, with a current maximum recommended total daily dose of 3600 mg. It is not necessary to follow felbamate levels. Felbamate interacts with phenytoin, carbamazepine, and valproate; therefore doses of these medications must be reduced by 25% to 50% when felbamate is added. Felbamate levels are lowered by medications that induce liver enzymes; consequently, felbamate doses may need to be increased.

Gabapentin

Gabapentin is the newest antiepileptic medication. It was approved in 1994 by the FDA for treatment of partial seizures with and without secondary generalization in adults who have epilepsy. Safety and effectiveness in children below the age of 12 years have not been established in this country.

In a multicenter, placebo-controlled, double-blind study among patients refractory to conventional anticonvulsants, gabapentin treatment resulted in a significant reduction in seizure frequency.[3] Gabapentin does not interact with other drugs; consequently, doses of other antiepileptic medications do not have to be adjusted when gabapentin is added. In add-on trials the most common side effects were somnolence, dizziness, ataxia, and fatigue. The effective dose of gabapentin is 900 to 1800 mg/day. Because of its relatively short half-life of 5 to 7 hours, it has to be administered three to four times a day. It is not necessary to monitor levels.

Lamotrigine

Lamotrigine is one of the newest antiepileptic medications. The FDA approved it for treatment of partial seizures in patients over 16 years of age. Studies in this country are ongoing to evaluate its safety and efficacy in children. Studies in other countries in children who have epilepsy reveal that lamotrigine reduced the frequency of both partial and generalized seizures. It was particularly effective in patients with absence, atypical absence, and atonic seizures.[2a] The most common side effects of lamotrigine are somnolence, rash, and vomiting. The rash is usually maculopapular or morbilliform, but a few cases of Stevens-Johnson syndrome have occurred. Comedication with valproic acid increases the incidence of rash. Starting a low dose of lamotrigine in patients who are already being treated with valproic acid and slowly increasing the dose of lamotrigine helps to minimize the risk of rash. Lamotrigine administration has no effect on the metabolism of other antiepileptic drugs; however, phenobarbital, phenytoin, and carbamazepine decrease the half-life of lamotrigine. Valproic acid increases the half-life of lamotrigine by two- or threefold; therefore doses of lamotrigine should be lower when given in combination with valproic acid. Therapeutic plasma concentration has not been established for lamotrigine.

PSYCHOSOCIAL ISSUES

Treatment of the child with a seizure disorder must also address psychosocial issues. Parents and patients may have many fears and need reassurance. The terms *epilepsy* and *seizure disorder* must be explained, and parents need to understand that the diagnosis of epilepsy does not mean that their child has mental retardation or a psychiatric disorder. Guidelines should be given on what to do when a child has a seizure, including positioning on the side and putting nothing in the mouth. Witnessing a seizure can be very frightening. Parents may be afraid that the child is going to die and should be told that death from a seizure is very rare.

Activities of patients with seizures should be restricted as little as possible. A child with a seizure disorder should not swim alone or go bike riding without a helmet. However, these rules apply to all children, whether or not they have epilepsy. Contact sports are permissible when epilepsy is controlled. The decision about climbing up to certain heights should be based on how well the child's seizures are controlled. Older children, who are not supervised when bathing, should be encouraged to take showers rather than baths to minimize the risk of drowning if a seizure occurs. Parents need encouragement to treat the child normally and not be overprotective. The National Epilepsy Foundation and its local chapters can be a valuable resource for families by providing free literature and many other helpful services.

DISCONTINUATION OF ANTIEPILEPTIC MEDICATIONS

After seizures have been controlled for a period of 2 years, consideration should be given to discontinuing antiepileptic medications. Studies have shown that 75% of children who were seizure free for more that 2 years remained seizure free after antiepileptic medications were discontinued.[27] The EEG can be helpful when considering discontinuing antiepileptic medications. If the EEG shows no epileptiform discharges, the prognosis is excellent. However, if the EEG demonstrates spikes or slowing, there is a higher risk of seizure recurrence.[27] The risk of recurrence is not increased if medication is tapered over a period as short as 6 weeks.[28] Long-term follow-up of children after withdrawal of medication has shown that 50% of the recurrences occur within 6 months and 60% to 80% within 2 years.[19]

INTRACTABLE SEIZURES

When seizures continue despite anticonvulsant therapy, it is important to consider three possibilities before deciding that the child's seizures are intractable to anticonvulsant therapy:

1. Seizures may be occurring at times that the child has

lower blood levels of medication because of incomplete compliance or because dosing intervals are too long.
2. The medication may not be appropriate to the child's type of seizures. Primary generalized seizures often will not respond and may even worsen if treated with medications that are indicated for partial or secondary generalized seizures (e.g., carbamazepine).
3. The child's repeated events may represent one of the nonepileptiform paroxysmal disorders rather than an electrical seizure. Pseudoseizures can be especially difficult to differentiate from seizures because they tend to occur in persons who have epilepsy. If a child is having electrical seizures and the seizures continue despite appropriate amounts of the correct medications, the child has intractable seizures.

About 15% of children who have epilepsy have intractable seizures, and about 50% of these may be appropriate candidates for epilepsy surgery. Therefore children who have intractable seizures should be referred to a center that has a multidisciplinary team of professionals including epileptologists, specialized neurosurgeons, neurophysiologists, neuropsychologists, neuroradiologists, psychologists, and family therapists. These professionals can best determine the location of the epileptic zone within the child's brain and the potential morbidity from loss of function in that area or adjacent tissue, can perform the surgery, and can treat the secondary effects of the surgery on the child and his or her family. Although epilepsy surgery can be done at any age, if it is done soon after intractability of seizures has been established, some of the secondary physiological and psychosocial effects of growing up with epilepsy may be prevented, and the child is more likely to be able to live up to his or her potential in adult life.[12,16]

Epilepsy surgery consists either of resecting the epileptic focus, such as a *temporal lobectomy* or a *cortical resection,* or of disconnecting the pathways that may facilitate the spread of epileptic activity within the brain, such as a *corpus callosotomy.*[16] The outcome from temporal lobectomies in appropriately chosen children is as good as in adults—65% become seizure free and another 15% are significantly improved; morbidity is minimal. Hemispherectomies in children who have a congenital hemiparesis and resistant seizures originating in the damaged hemisphere result in control of seizures in 75% of cases and often result in improvement of function because the normal, opposite hemisphere is no longer being interrupted by seizure discharges.[22] A few cases of intractable infantile spasms also may benefit from partial or complete hemispherectomies.[30] The corpus callosotomy is a palliative procedure for individuals who do not qualify for a local resection. It can be quite effective in controlling "drop" attacks and the resultant injuries in children who have multiple seizure types. Results are best in higher-functioning individuals who have localized CNS dysfunction as opposed to diffuse CNS dysfunction.

REFERENCES

1. Aicardi J: *Epilepsy in children,* New York, 1986, Raven Press.
2. Annegers JF et al: Factors prognostic of unprovoked seizures after febrile convulsions, *N Engl J Med* 316:493, 1987.

2a. Besag FMC et al: Lamotrigine for the treatment of epilepsy in childhood, *J Pediatr* 127:991, 1995.

3. Bruni J et al: Efficacy and safety of gabapentin (Neurontin): a multicenter, placebo-controlled, double-blind study, *Neurology* 41(suppl 1):330, 1991.
4. Camfield PR et al: Epilepsy after a first unprovoked seizure in childhood, *Neurology* 35:1657, 1985.
5. Commission on Classification and Terminology of the International League Against Epilepsy: Proposal for classification of epilepsies and epileptic syndromes, *Epilepsia* 26:268, 1985.
6. Commission on Classification and Terminology of the International League Against Epilepsy: Proposal for revised clinical and electroencephalographic classification of epileptic seizures, *Epilepsia* 22:489, 1981.
7. Delgado-Escueta AV et al: Mapping the gene for juvenile myoclonic epilepsy, *Epilepsia* 30(suppl 4):8, 1989.
8. Deshmukh A et al: Lorazepam in the treatment of neonatal seizures, *Am J Dis Child* 140:1042, 1986.
9. Dreifuss FE: Juvenile myoclonic epilepsy: characteristics of a primary generalized epilepsy, *Epilepsia* 30(suppl 4):1, 1989.
10. Dreifuss FE: *Pediatric epileptology: classification and management of seizures in the child,* Boston, 1983, John Wright/PSG.
11. Dreifuss FE et al: Valproic acid hepatic fatalities: a retrospective review, *Neurology* 37:379, 1987.
12. Duchowny MS: The role of surgery in childhood epilepsy, *Int Pediatr* 2:205, 1987.
13. Engel J Jr, editor: *Surgical treatment of the epilepsies,* New York, 1987, Raven Press.
14. Farrell K et al: Successful treatment of valproate hepatotoxicity with N-acetylcysteine, *Epilepsia* 30:700, 1989.
15. The Felbamate Study Group in Lennox-Gastaut Syndrome: Efficacy of felbamate in childhood encephalopathy Lennox-Gastaut syndrome, *N Engl J Med* 328:29, 1993.
16. Goldring S: Pediatric epilepsy surgery, *Epilepsia* 28 (suppl):82, 1987.
17. Hart RG, Easton JD: Carbamazepine and hematological monitoring, *Ann Neurol* 11:309, 1982.
18. Hirtz DG, Ellenberg JH, Nelson KB: The risk of recurrence of nonfebrile seizures in children, *Neurology* 34:634, 1984.
19. Holowach J, Thurston DL, O'Leary J: Prognosis in childhood epilepsy: follow-up study of 148 cases in which therapy had been suspended after prolonged anticonvulsant control, *N Engl J Med* 286:169, 1972.
20. Mellits ED, Holden KR, Freeman JM: Neonatal seizures. II. Multivariate analysis of factors associated with outcome, *Pediatrics* 70:177, 1981.
21. Oles KS et al: Use of acetazolamide as an adjunct to carbamazepine in refractory partial seizures, *Epilepsia* 30:74, 1989.
22. Peacock WJ: The role of hemispherectomy in the treatment of intractable seizures in childhood, *Int Pediatr* 7:291, 1992.
23. Penry JK, editor: *Epilepsy: diagnosis, management, and quality of life,* New York, 1986, Raven Press.
24. Roddy SM, McBride MC, Torres CF: Treatment of neonatal seizures with lorazepam, *Ann Neurol* 22:412, 1987.
25. Roger J, Dravet C, Bureau M: The Lennox-Gastaut syndrome, *Cleve Clin J Med* 56(suppl 1):172, 1989.
26. Rosman NP et al: A controlled trial of diazepam administered during febrile illness to prevent recurrence of febrile seizure, *N Engl J Med* 329:72, 1993.
27. Shinnar S et al: Discontinuing antiepileptic medication in children with epilepsy after two years without seizures, *N Engl J Med* 313:976, 1985.
28. Tennison MB et al: Rate of taper of antiepileptic drugs and the risk of seizure recurrence, *Ann Neurol* 26:439, 1989.
29. Trimble MR, Cull CA: Antiepileptic drugs, cognitive function, and behavior in children, Cleve Clin J Med 56(suppl 1):140, 1989.
30. Uthman BM et al: Outcome for West syndrome following surgical treatment, *Epilepsia* 32:668, 1991.
31. Volpe JJ: *Neurology of the newborn,* ed 3, Philadelphia, 1995, WB Saunders.
32. Weiner SP, Scher MS, Painter MJ: Neonatal seizures: electroclinical disassociation, *Epilepsia* 30:691, 1989.

257 Septic Arthritis

Edwards P. Schwentker

Septic arthritis most commonly involves lower extremity joints and characteristically affects young children and infants. Septic arthritis constitutes a *true clinical emergency* because its complications may include dissolution of articular cartilage, necrosis of the underlying epiphysis, destruction of the adjacent growth plate, and dislocation of the joint itself. Complications can be minimized only by a high index of clinical suspicion, prompt diagnosis, and aggressive treatment.

PATHOGENESIS

Bacteria may reach a joint by any of three routes. Direct introduction may occur through percutaneous puncture, with the needle being either introduced purposely into the joint or wandering from adjacent structures such as from blood vessels during an attempted venipuncture. Second, hematogenous bacterial seeding may occur directly to the membrana synovialis. Finally, septic arthritis may develop from a contiguous metaphyseal osteomyelitis that decompresses into the joint capsule. In young infants, bone infection may extend from the metaphysis into the epiphysis via transepiphyseal vessels and then from the epiphysis directly into the joint. For a more complete discussion of osteomyelitis, the reader is referred to Chapter 239.

With few exceptions, the organisms most commonly responsible for septic arthritis are the same as those in acute osteomyelitis; thus the leading offender is *Staphylococcus aureus*. Particularly in very young children, *Haemophilus influenzae* type b and streptococci of various types are seen. Gonococcal arthritis is fairly rare; when it occurs, however, it often involves several joints. Meningococcal arthritis also can occur and may develop without meningitis or meningococcemia.[3]

The consequences of an established septic arthritis can be severe. Enzymes destructive to both cartilage matrix and collagen are released by leukocytes and synovial cells as part of the inflammatory process. With infections caused by *S. aureus* and some of the gram negative bacteria, the potential for destruction of joint surfaces is increased because these organisms also produce proteolytic enzymes. By raising intraarticular pressure, intracapsular infection may obstruct blood flow, leading to necrosis of the epiphysis and the underlying growth plate. Finally, an untreated joint infection can result in joint instability through destruction of the ligamentous fibers of the capsule. Dislocation of the hip and shoulder particularly are likely.

Considering the possible consequences and, particularly in the young child, the potential for permanent deformity and disability, the need for accurate diagnosis and expeditious treatment of a septic arthritis cannot be exaggerated.

CLINICAL FINDINGS

The source of a hematogenous septic arthritis may be a preexisting infection elsewhere in the body, but frequently none is recognized. As the septic arthritis develops, it generally is accompanied by an acute onset of fever and malaise and marked localized signs and symptoms.[1,4] Swelling, erythema, and tenderness often are prominent but may be hard to detect in a deep joint such as the hip. *The most characteristic finding is pain with joint motion.* When a lower extremity joint is involved, the patient usually refuses to bear weight.

The joint will be held immobile by muscle spasm in a position that maximizes capsular volume, thus minimizing the intraarticular pressure. For the hip, the preferred position is a combination of moderate flexion, abduction, and external rotation; for the knee, gentle flexion; and for the shoulder, adduction against the trunk. It is not at all unusual for a child to appear entirely well and in no distress so long as the affected joint is allowed to remain undisturbed.

The pediatrician should rely most on the physical examination. The only absolutely reliable laboratory tests are Gram stain and culture. White blood cell (WBC) counts may be within normal limits or only mildly elevated. The erythrocyte sedimentation rate is elevated more consistently, but even this test may be unremarkable in the newborn. Blood cultures should be drawn when septic arthritis is suspected because they frequently are positive for the offending organism.

Early in the course of septic arthritis, radiographs are negative for any bone change but frequently demonstrate soft tissue changes, including swelling and edematous infiltration into fatty tissue planes. Radionuclide scanning is not necessary if localizing signs are clear-cut. Scans are contraindicated if they delay appropriate treatment in any way. Scanning may help find or rule out other sites of involvement, particularly in very sick or very young children.

Ultrasonography has proven useful in determining the capsular distention that accompanies septic arthritis of the hip.[6] In the hands of an experienced radiologist, this noninvasive test can exclude the presence of a joint effusion or, if one is present, assist the operator in accurate needle placement during diagnostic aspiration.

Joint aspiration via a large-bore needle is the most important diagnostic maneuver. This generally can be performed in most joints without the use of an anesthetic. An orthopedist should be consulted to aspirate suspected joints, unless the primary care physician is skilled in this procedure. Fluoroscopy or, possibly, ultrasonography should be used to confirm entrance into the relatively inaccessible hip and shoulder joints. A diagnostic aspiration yields fluid with a WBC count exceeding 100,000, with a percentage of polymorphonuclear leukocytes greater than 75%. Lower counts can be found early in the course of a septic arthritis. An effusion with a low WBC count also may be associated with acute osteomyelitis of an adjacent metaphysis, the effusion being sympathetic. In most instances of septic arthritis, the aspiration yields frank pus. In any case, aspirated fluid should be cultured and gram stained.

In septic arthritis, as in osteomyelitis, the neonate presents a unique challenge.[1] Systemic signs may be absent, and laboratory findings may be within normal limits. Nonetheless, localized signs almost always are prominent, particularly pain with motion of the involved joint. The failure of an infant to move an infected joint is a condition known as *pseudoparalysis* and may be seen in a child who otherwise appears completely normal. The clinician may be misled into seeking a neurological deficit, on the assumption that the lack of motion is caused by true muscle paralysis. The pattern of motor dysfunction, however, is usually atypical for a neurological deficit, and almost invariably passive movement of the affected extremity will elicit severe pain, a finding not characteristic of true paralysis. To make the diagnosis of septic arthritis, the pediatrician must suspect infection; *in any infant, failure to move an extremity spontaneously must be considered a result of septic arthritis until proved otherwise.*

MANAGEMENT

Following an expeditious clinical, roentgenographic, and laboratory evaluation, the suspected joint should be aspirated with a large-bore needle. Blood cultures should be obtained. If pus is obtained from the joint, the material should be Gram stained and cultured, and parenteral antibiotics should be begun immediately on the basis of the Gram stain findings. If bacteria are not seen, antibiotic therapy should be instituted empirically while culture results are pending. Neonates should be treated with a penicillinase-resistant penicillin and an aminoglycoside. A penicillinase-resistant penicillin alone is appropriate therapy for a child over 5 years of age. In younger children, coverage for ampicillin-resistant strains of *H. influenzae* should be added. Immunocompromised patients and older patients suspected of parenteral drug abuse should have coverage against enteric gram negative bacilli and *Pseudomonas*. These patients should receive a broad-spectrum penicillin and an aminoglycoside.[5]

Aspiration of a distal extremity joint together with administration of appropriate antibiotics may be sufficient treatment for selected patients.[2] Such patients should have an uncomplicated acute hematogenous septic arthritis of less than 6 days' duration and have no evidence of clinical osteomyelitis, immune deficiency, or other chronic illness. If aspiration and antibiotics fail to provide a prompt clinical response, the involved joint must be drained operatively. Because the hip joint is relatively inaccessible and the capital femoral epiphysis is susceptible to avascular necrosis secondary to increased intraarticular pressure, an infected hip joint should be drained operatively and not treated with aspiration.

Operative drainage unquestionably is more effective than percutaneous aspiration. The findings at the time of arthrotomy often indicate the futility of attempting to eradicate an abscess by needle aspiration, since heavy fibrin deposits frequently are encountered. Such deposits cannot be debrided by needle aspiration. The pediatrician should be quicker to call a surgical colleague when the offending organism is *S. aureus* or a gram negative bacterium that can produce cartilage-damaging enzymes.

Failure to obtain pus from a joint that is otherwise suspected of harboring sepsis must be viewed with skepticism. Fibrin debris or thick pus may prevent aspiration. Exquisite pain with passive joint motion, discretely localized soft tissue swelling and tenderness, and evidence of joint effusion should overrule the negative aspiration and indicate operative exploration. The risks of an unnecessary exploration are minimal compared with the certainty of joint damage that attends a neglected septic arthritis.

Parenteral antibiotics should be continued and adequate blood levels maintained following operative drainage. The choice of antibiotics should be adjusted after the results of cultures are obtained. If methods are available for determining bactericidal activity, substitution of oral medications for parenteral antibiotics may be possible. Oral antibiotics, however, should be used only if the patient is responding to treatment, the parents are reliable, the antibiotic does not cause a gastrointestinal disturbance that interferes with absorption, and blood levels can be monitored adequately. Antibiotic therapy should continue for a minimum of 3 weeks, but treatment should not be discontinued until the clinical response indicates that the condition has been corrected and the erythrocyte sedimentation rate has returned to normal.[3]

Immobilization is the final principle of treating septic arthritis.[4] Splinting should be provided for comfort and rest of the affected distal joints of the upper and lower extremities after drainage, but it need be continued only while swelling, tenderness, and pain with motion persist. Neglected infection of a shoulder or hip may lead to subluxation or frank dislocation; thus these joints should be immobilized long enough for the capsule to restabilize. If diagnosis and treatment are accomplished soon after the onset of the disease, 2 or 3 weeks of immobilization may be adequate. A prolonged infection, particularly of the hip, may require immobilization for 2 to 3 months. The shoulder can be protected adequately with a simple sling and swathe. The hip may be immobilized in a spica cast, or once pain has subsided, protection may be provided by a simple Pavlik harness or any similar device that maintains reduction by centering the hip deeply within the acetabulum. The need for immobilizing a joint should be determined according to the individual's condition, so as to maximize joint stability while avoiding unnecessary stiffness.

REFERENCES

1. Griffin PP, Green WT Sr: Hip joint infections in infants and children, *Orthop Clin North Am* 9:123, 1978.
2. Herndon WA et al: Management of septic arthritis in children, *J Pediatr Orthop* 6:576, 1986.
3. Jackson MA, Nelson JD: Etiology and medical management of acute suppurative bone and joint infections in pediatric patients, *J Pediatr Orthop* 2:313, 1982.
4. Paterson DC: Acute suppurative arthritis in infancy and childhood, *J Bone Joint Surg [Br]* 52:474, 1970.
5. Scoles PV, Aronoff SC: Current concepts review: antimicrobial therapy of childhood skeletal infections, *J Bone Joint Surg [Am]* 66:1487, 1984.
6. Wingstrand H et al: Sonography in septic arthritis of the hip in the child: report of four cases, *J Pediatr Orthop* 7:206, 1987.

258 Sexually Transmitted Diseases

Alain Joffe

For a variety of reasons, teenagers are at high risk for acquiring sexually transmitted diseases (STDs) (see the box on p. 1578). Over the past few decades, rates of sexual activity have increased dramatically among adolescents, especially Caucasian adolescents; hence many more teenagers now are exposed to these infectious agents. Furthermore, by virtue of their cognitive developmental level, many adolescents feel invulnerable and minimize their potential for becoming infected. They may ignore symptoms or believe that as long as they are symptom free, they neither are infected nor infectious.

A large body of evidence now indicates that barrier methods of contraception (diaphragm, condom) when used with a spermicide provide excellent protection against STDs.[14] Although the use of condoms by teenagers has increased over the last decade, many teenagers still do not use them or use them inconsistently. Oral contraceptives, still a popular method of contraception, do not protect against acquisition of STDs, although they may protect against the development of pelvic inflammatory disease (PID) among infected teenagers.

Adolescents have difficulty discussing sexual matters with partners or with parents and so are reluctant to reveal that they are infected or have been treated. They may postpone a visit to a physician because they are embarrassed, fear a lecture, are concerned about the physician maintaining confidentiality, or lack the money or social skills to get to a source of health care.

Some physicians fear treating adolescents who have a sexually transmitted disease, because they are uncertain about an adolescent's capacity to consent to treatment without parental involvement. Currently all 50 states have laws that permit a physician to treat most minors seeking treatment without parental consent or notification. Finally, there may be a physiological basis for adolescent girls being particularly susceptible to infection upon exposure. The transformation zone of the cervix, which is relatively large among pubertal girls, is particularly vulnerable to infection with *Chlamydia trachomatis* and human papillomavirus (Fig. 258-1). Not surprisingly, therefore, current data indicate that adolescents and young adults have higher infection rates than any other age group in the United States. The most recent data from the Centers for Disease Control and Prevention (CDC) for syphilis and gonorrhea are shown in Table 258-1. Reporting of *Chlamydia trachomatis* infections to state and local health departments has only recently become mandatory. Hence accurate data about the extent of this infection are relatively scant. However, several studies have shown that infection rates are highest among sexually active 15- to 19-year olds.

Because *Chlamydia trachomatis* infections are not reportable to state or city health departments, accurate data about the extent of the problem are scant. However, several studies have shown that a greater percentage of 15- to 19-year-olds are infected than are those 20 years or older.

The list of infectious agents having potential to be transmitted sexually is extensive. The box on p. 1579 lists the most common of these. Gonorrhea, chlamydia, herpes, human papillomavirus, and syphilis are discussed in detail in this chapter. The reader is referred to Chapter 214 for further discussion of herpes infections and to Chapter 180 for discussion of human immunodeficiency virus (HIV) infections. Information about the other agents should be sought through the Index.

An alternative way of conceptualizing the spectrum of problems attributable to STDs is to focus on symptoms or diseases rather than on specific agents. More than one STD can produce various signs, symptoms, or syndromes, and many teenagers deny sexual activity for the reasons outlined above. Hence, when an adolescent has a symptom or sign that may be caused by such agents, the physician must proceed with appropriate diagnostic tests or therapy, even though the history may appear to exclude an STD. Most teenagers, however, admit to sexual activity when questioned considerately and given appropriate guarantees about confidentiality. The box on p. 1579 lists a variety of symptoms and clinical entities that frequently are caused by sexually transmitted agents.

SPECIFIC AGENTS

Chlamydia Trachomatis

The obligate, intracellular, chlamydia microorganism causes a wide spectrum of disease and is the most common sexually transmitted bacterial agent in the United States. Of greatest importance is its causative role in urethritis and epididymitis in males and cervicitis and pelvic inflammatory disease in females.[9]

Although data are limited, chlamydia appears to cause 30% to 50% of symptomatic nongonococcal urethritis among adolescent males. Newer detection tests indicate that the proportion may be closer to 70%. Recent data indicate that approximately 10% to 20% of asymptomatic sexually active males will be culture positive for sexually transmitted agents, and almost 75% of them will have chlamydial infection. Males may complain only of mild dysuria, or they may have a scanty, mucoid discharge that is easily ignored. Having the male strip his urethra may produce some discharge if none is apparent. A profuse, purulent discharge should raise the possibility of *Neisseria gonorrhoeae* causing a coinfection or being the single causative agent. Males also may complain of testicular or scrotal pain or both, suggesting that urethral infection has spread to the epididymis.

Because the organism can infect the urethra as well as the cervix, a female may complain of dysuria as the primary

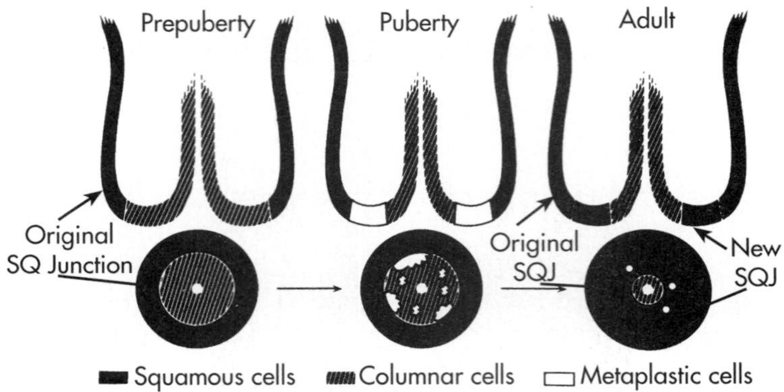

FIG. 258-1 Cervical development. In most prepubertal females, the original squamocolumnar junction is located well onto the ectocervix. During puberty, uncommitted germ cells of the columnar epithelium differentiate into squamous cells during a process called squamous metaplasia. This process begins at the original squamocolumnar junction at various areas and continues caudally. Thus the pubertal cervix is in a transitional state. By adulthood the transformation results in a new squamocolumnar junction, now found near or in the ectocervix.

(From Moscicki B, Shafer MB: *J Adolesc Health Care* 7:505, 1986.)

Table 258-1 Infection Rates per 100,000 Population for Syphilis and Gonorrhea by Age and Gender

Syphilis

1994			
		Total	
Age group	Total	Male	Female
10-14	0.7	0.1	1.2
15-19	13.1	8.6	18.0
20-24	21.5	18.9	24.2
25-29	19.0	17.4	20.6
30-34	16.9	17.4	16.5
35-39	13.8	16.5	11.1
40-44	8.7	11.6	5.8
45-54	5.0	7.6	2.5
55-64	2.4	4.1	0.9
65+	0	1.3	0.1
TOTAL	8.1	8.6	7.6

Gonorrhea

1994			
		Total	
Age group	Total	Male	Female
10-14	50.4	16.6	85.9
15-19	763.4	608.6	926.7
20-24	675.5	715.9	633.5
25-29	312.9	361.1	264.3
30-34	188.4	237.9	135.1
35-39	120.3	174.6	66.6
40-44	69.7	112.6	27.6
45-54	32.7	57.6	9.0
55-64	11.7	22.3	2.2
65+	6.3	9.1	2.7
TOTAL	166.8	182.7	151.7

Data from Division of STD/HIV Prevention: *Sexually transmitted disease surveillance,* 1994, US Department of Health and Human Services, Public Health Service, Atlanta, 1995, Centers for Disease Control and Prevention.

WHY ADOLESCENTS ARE AT RISK FOR STDS

Increased prevalence of sexual activity at earlier ages
Sense of invulnerability ("It can't happen to me.")
Lack of information ("If I don't feel sick, I can't be sick.")
Infrequent use of barrier methods of contraception
Poor communication skills with partners and physicians
Barriers to care (legal obstacles, concerns about confidentiality)
Poor compliance
Physiological changes associated with puberty

manifestation of infection. Hence, *Chlamydia trachomatis* infection should be considered in any adolescent female suspected of having a urinary tract infection. She also may complain of vaginal discharge or, if the infection has spread to the upper genital tract, of low abdominal pain or right upper quadrant pain (Fitz-Hugh-Curtis syndrome). The latter is caused by organisms tracking up the abdominal cavity and causing inflammation of the liver capsule along with adhesions to the diaphragm. Lower abdominal pain suggests the possibility of pelvic inflammatory disease.

As with males, females often are infected asymptomatically. On pelvic examination, however, clues to infection are the presence of mucopurulent discharge from the cervical os ("mucopus"—Fig. 258-2), cervical erythema, and friability.[2] A cervical Gram stain will reveal the presence of 30 or more polymorphonuclear (PMN) white blood cells per oil immersion field in three or more fields. Occasionally, a Papanicolaou (Pap) smear result will reveal the presence of inclusion bodies, suggesting the presence of infection. However, some patients lack signs of infection; given the high prevalence of infection among adolescents and the serious morbidity associated with untreated disease, every sexually active teenager should be screened for chlamydia at least annually. Such an approach becomes cost effective at a prevalence of 7% (when rapid test kits are used) or 14% (when cultures are used).[19]

SEXUALLY TRANSMITTED INFECTIOUS AGENTS

Chlamydia trachomatis
Cytomegalovirus (CMV)
Gardnerella vaginalis (?)
Hepatitis B
Herpes simplex virus (HSV)
Human immunodeficiency virus (HIV)
Human papillomavirus (HPV)
Mycoplasma hominis
Neisseria gonorrhoeae
Treponema pallidum
Trichomonas vaginalis
Ureaplasma urealyticum

SIGNS, SYMPTOMS, AND CLINICAL ENTITIES SUGGESTING SEXUALLY TRANSMITTED DISEASE IN ADOLESCENTS

Males

Dysuria, urethritis
Epididymitis (scrotal pain, swelling)

Female

Mucopurulent cervicitis
Vaginitis
Dysuria
Right upper quadrant pain
Pelvic inflammatory disease (low abdominal pain)

Both

Genital ulcers
Genital warts
Hepatitis B infection
HIV infection
Proctitis
Septic arthritis

Culturing cells for chlamydial infection remains the gold standard for detecting infection, although recent data indicate that polymerase chain reaction (PCR) tests are even more sensitive than culture. PCR is not yet widely available, however. To culture the organism, endocervical or urethral cells must be obtained; the organism cannot be grown from discharge alone. If culture is unavailable or too expensive, the clinician should use whatever rapid diagnostic test is available. Compared with cultures, these tests (excluding PCR) are 70% to 98% sensitive.

Recently, Shafer and colleagues[23] assessed a number of approaches to screening asymptomatic males for chlamydia infection. Use of the "first-part voided" urine technique (see the box above), with positives confirmed by a rapid diagnostic test, gives the best combination of sensitivity, specificity, and cost-effectiveness. To obtain this urine specimen, a nonsterile urine cup is marked at the 15 ml line with a wax pencil, and the male is instructed to collect only the first few drops of urine he produces (up to the line). The urine then is centrifuged and the supernatant poured off. If the sediment contains 10 or more polymorphonuclear nucleocytes per high power field, the test result is considered positive. Alternatively, the unspun urine is tested with a urine dipstick that measures leukocyte esterase activity, with trace or greater reactions considered positive. Either of these positives should be confirmed with enzyme immunoassay (EIA), and samples that are EIA positive should then be confirmed by a direct fluorescent antibody test. Samples positive by all three methods should be treated for *Chlamydia trachomatis* infection.

COLLECTION OF FIRST-PART VOIDED URINALYSIS IN MALES[1,23]

1. Mark a urine collection cup at the 15 ml line.
2. Instruct the patient to *begin* urinating *into* the cup (no skin preparation is necessary).
3. When the urine reaches the 15-ml line *(no more than 15 ml),* the patient should finish voiding into the toilet.
4. To look for white cells, centrifuge urine at 500 g for 10 minutes; decant supernatant. Resuspend sediment in remaining 0.5 ml. Ten white blood cells per high-power field is considered positive for urethritis.
5. Alternately, dip *unspun* urine with leukocyte esterase test strips within 10 minutes of collection. A result of 1+ or higher is positive for urethritis.

Confirmation of these positive urine screens by enzyme EIA coupled with additional confirmation of positive EIA screens by direct fluorescent antibody appears to yield the most clinically effective and cost-effective screening approach. Newer screening techniques that use PCR are likely to be even more effective.

Uncomplicated cervical or urethral chlamydial infection should be treated orally with doxycycline (100 mg bid for 7 days) or azithromycin 1 g as a single dose. Azithromycin is considerably more expensive and has not been evaluated fully in patients 15 years of age or younger. Ofloxacin (for individuals over 17 years), erythromycin, or sulfisoxazole are suitable alternatives (see the box on p. 1581).

As with treatment for any sexually transmitted infection, the patient's abstinence from intercourse is imperative until his or her partner is notified and treated. Complications of chlamydial infection include epididymitis and pelvic inflammatory disease. Long-term complications include Reiter syndrome and the sequelae of pelvic inflammatory disease. Cervical dysplasia also may be a complication of this infection. An untreated, infected woman can pass the infection to her infant through colonization during birth.

Neisseria Gonorrhoeae

Infection with the gonococcus produces a constellation of symptoms very similar to that produced by chlamydia.[10] Approximately 45% of males who have urethral discharge have gonococcal infection. In general, patients who are symptomatic with gonococcal infection tend to have more pronounced symptoms and usually seek health care within a shorter period of time than those infected with chlamydia. However, many patients have no symptoms at all. In large-scale stud-

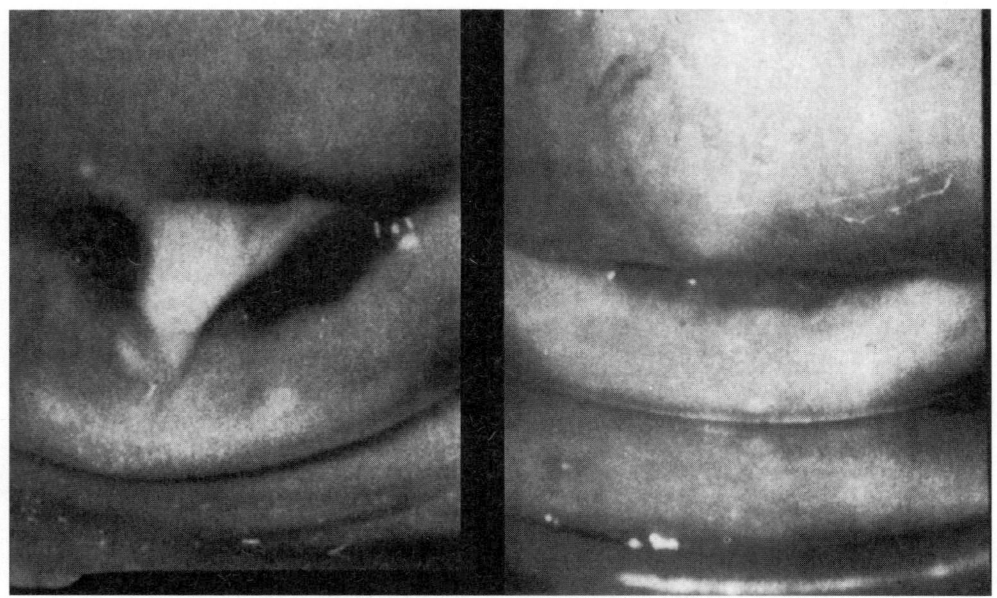

FIG. 258-2 Colpophotograph showing mucopurulent cervicitis before and 2 weeks after treatment with 500 mg of tetracycline four times daily for 7 days. Note disappearance of endocervical exudate after therapy.

(From Brunham RC et al: *N Engl J Med* 311:2, 1984.)

ies, approximately 2% of sexually active males have been shown to be infected with gonorrhea; 70% of these were asymptomatic. The proportion of asymptomatic women with infection is unclear; estimates range from 25% to 80%. The gonococcus can cause pharyngitis and proctitis; females may harbor the organism in the rectum, even though they do not engage in anal intercourse.

The diagnosis of gonococcal infection rests on culture and on the classic Gram stain with gram negative intracellular diplococci. Even under ideal conditions, the organism can be difficult to grow, and each physician should be familiar with the yield from the laboratory he or she uses. In the male, a typical Gram stain from a urethral discharge is diagnostic (Fig. 258-3). For samples taken from females, sorting out gram negative organisms that truly are intracellular versus those that may be overlying the cells is more difficult. However, Wald[24] had shown that when at least eight pairs of such diplococci are seen in at least two PMNs, 96% of cultures are positive. The gonococcus can be grown from urethral or cervical discharge, from swabs of the cervix, urethra, pharynx, or rectum, and in many instances from urine sediment.

Uncomplicated gonococcal infections can be treated with any of the following single dose regimens: 125 mg of ceftriaxone intramuscularly, 400 mg cefixime orally, 500 mg ciprofloxacin orally, or 400 mg ofloxacin orally (see the box on p. 1581). This CDC recommendation is based on the increasing prevalence of beta lactamase–producing organisms. Because of the high likelihood that coinfection with chlamydia is present any treatment for gonorrhea must include an effective regimen for *Chlamydia trachomatis* as well.

Gonorrhea also may produce epididymitis and pelvic inflammatory disease. However, the organism also has the capacity to become bloodborne and can lead to what has been called the arthritis-dermatitis syndrome, or disseminated gonococcal infection (DGI).[17] About 1% to 3% of untreated patients develop DGI. Typically, the patient develops fever (although not always) and may have anorexia or malaise or both. Skin lesions then appear, generally distributed on the extremities (arms more often than legs). These lesions typically are erythematous macules less than 5 mm in diameter; they become pustular and occasionally hemorrhagic or necrotic. They most often are noticed near the small joints of the hands and feet. Such lesions last several days, and at this point, blood cultures are positive in 25% of cases. Accompanying the dermatitis is a tenosynovitis that again tends to occur over the extensor and flexor tendons of the hands and feet.

In general, once the tenosynovitis and dermatitis clear, the patient develops polyarthralgias but usually seeks care only at the point that an oligoarthritis develops. The knee is the joint most commonly infected, followed by the elbow, ankle, and small joints of the hands and feet. Hence, among adolescents, DGI should be considered in the differential diagnosis of septic arthritis. Aspirates of joint fluid reveal the typical changes of a septic arthritis, but cultures usually are negative.

Although the causative organisms usually are exquisitely sensitive to penicillin, patients who have true arthritis should be hospitalized for treatment (see the box on p. 1581). Those who have only skin lesions or who have tenosynovitis may be treated as outpatients if careful follow-up can be ensured; otherwise, inpatient treatment also is justified.

Genital Warts (Human Papillomavirus)

Infections with human papillomavirus (HPV) are the most prevalent sexually transmitted infection in the United States. Such infections have always raised concern because they cause unsightly warts; however, new data suggest that infection with HPV is closely associated with the development of

Text continued on p. 1585.

1993 SEXUALLY TRANSMITTED DISEASES TREATMENT GUIDELINES

Chlamydial infections among adolescents and adults

Recommended regimens

Doxycycline 100 mg orally 2 times a day for 7 days

or

Azithromycin 1 g orally in a single dose

Alternative regimens

Ofloxacin 300 mg orally 2 times a day for 7 days

or

Erythromycin base 500 mg orally 4 times a day for 7 days

or

Erythromycin ethylsuccinate 800 mg orally 4 times a day for 7 days

or

Sulfisoxazole 500 mg orally 4 times a day for 10 days (inferior efficacy to other regimens)

Doxycycline and azithromycin appear similar in efficacy and toxicity; however, the safety and efficacy of azithromycin for persons 15 years of age or younger have not been established. Doxycycline has a longer history of extensive use, safety, efficacy, and the advantage of low cost. Azithromycin has the advantage of single-dose administration. Ofloxacin is similar in efficacy to doxycycline and azithromycin but is more expensive than doxycycline, cannot be used during pregnancy or with persons 17 years of age or younger, and offers no advantage in dosing. Ofloxacin is the only quinolone with proven efficacy against chlamydial infection. Sulfisoxazole is the least desirable treatment because of inferior efficacy.

Gonococcal infections among adolescents and adults

Uncomplicated gonococcal infections

Recommended regimens

Ceftriaxone 125 mg IM in a single dose

or

Cefixime 400 mg orally in a single dose

or

Ciprofloxacin 500 mg orally in a single dose

or

Ofloxacin 400 mg orally in a single dose

plus

A regimen effective against possible coinfection with *C. trachomatis,* such as doxycycline 100 mg orally 2 times a day for 7 days

In clinical trials, these recommended regimens cured more than 95% of anal and genital infections; any of the regimens may be used for uncomplicated anal or genital infection. Published studies indicate that ceftriaxone 125 mg and ciprofloxacin 500 mg can cure 90% or more of pharyngeal infections. *If pharyngeal infection is a concern, one of these two regimens should be used.*

Quinolones are contraindicated for persons 17 years of age or older on the basis of information from animal studies.

Disseminated gonococcal infection

Disseminated gonococcal infection (DGI) results from gonococcal bacteremia, often resulting in petechial or pustular acral skin lesions, asymmetrical arthralgias, tenosynovitis or septic arthritis—and is occasionally complicated by hepatitis and, rarely, by endocarditis or meningitis. Strains of *N. gonorrhoeae* that cause DGI tend to cause little genital inflammation. These strains have become uncommon in the United States during the past decade.

No North American studies of the treatment of DGI have been published recently. The recommendations that follow reflect the opinions of expert consultants.

Treatment

Hospitalization is recommended for initial therapy, especially for patients who cannot be relied on to comply with treatment, for those for whom the diagnosis is uncertain, and for those who have purulent synovial effusions or other complications. Patients should be examined for clinical evidence of endocarditis and meningitis. Patients treated for DGI should be treated presumptively for concurrent *C. trachomatis* infection.

Recommended initial regimen

Ceftriaxone 1 g IM or IV every 24 hours

Alternative initial regimens

Cefotaxime 1 g IV every 8 hours

or

Ceftizoxime 1 g IV every 8 hours

or

For persons allergic to β-lactam drugs:

Spectinomycin 2 g IM every 12 hours

All regimens should be continued for 24 to 48 hours after improvement begins; then therapy may be switched to one of the following regimens to complete a full week of antimicrobial therapy:

Cefixime 400 mg orally 2 times a day

or

Ciprofloxacin 500 mg orally 2 times a day

NOTE: Ciprofloxacin is contraindicated for children, adolescents 17 years of age or younger, and pregnant and lactating women.

Human papillomavirus infection—genital warts

External genital/perianal warts

Cryotherapy with liquid nitrogen or cryoprobe

or

Podofilox 0.5% solution for self-treatment *(genital warts only).* Patients may apply podofilox with a cotton swab to warts twice daily for 3 days, followed by 4 days of no therapy. This cycle may be repeated as necessary for a total of 4 cycles. Total wart area treated should not exceed 10 cm^2, and total volume of podofilox should not exceed 0.5 ml per day. The health-care provider should demonstrate the proper application technique and identify which warts should be treated. If possible, the health-care provider should apply the initial treatment to demonstrate the proper application technique and identify which warts should be treated. *The use of podofilox is contraindicated during pregnancy.*

or

Podophyllin 10% to 25%, in compound tincture of benzoin. To avoid the possibility of problems with systemic absorption and toxicity, some experts recommend that application be limited to ≤0.5 ml or ≤10 cm^2 per session. Thoroughly wash off in 1 to 4 hours. Repeat

Continued.

1993 SEXUALLY TRANSMITTED DISEASES TREATMENT GUIDELINES—cont'd

External genital/perianal warts—cont'd

weekly if necessary. If warts persist after six applications, other therapeutic methods should be considered. *The use of podophyllin is contraindicated during pregnancy.*

or

Trichloroacetic acid (TCA) 80% to 90%. Apply only to warts; powder with talc or sodium bicarbonate (baking soda) to remove unreacted acid. Repeat weekly if necessary. If warts persist after six applications, other therapies should be considered.

or

Electrodesiccation or electrocautery. Electrodesiccation and electrocautery are contraindicated for patients with cardiac pacemakers or for lesions proximal to the anal verge.

Cryotherapy is relatively inexpensive, does not require anesthesia, and does not result in scarring if performed properly. Special equipment is required, and most patients experience moderate pain during and after the procedure. Efficacy during four randomized trials was 63% to 88%, with recurrences among 21% to 39% of patients.

Therapy with 0.5% podofilox solution is relatively inexpensive, simple to use, safe, and is self-applied by patients at home. Unlike podophyllin, podofilox is a pure compound with a stable shelf-life and does not need to be washed off. Most patients experience mild to moderate pain or local irritation after treatment. Heavily keratinized warts may not respond as well as those on moist mucosal surfaces. To apply the podofilox solution safely and effectively, the patient must be able to see and reach the warts easily. Efficacy during five recent randomized trials was 45% to 88%, with recurrences among 33% to 60% of patients.

Podophyllin therapy is relatively inexpensive, simple to use, and safe. Compared with other available therapies, a larger number of treatments may be required. Most patients experience mild to moderate pain or local irritation after treatment. Heavily keratinized warts may not respond as well as those on moist mucosal surfaces. Efficacy in four recent randomized trials was 32% to 79%, with recurrences among 27% to 65% of patients.

Few data on the efficacy of TCA are available. One randomized trial among men demonstrated 81% efficacy and recurrence among 36% of patients; the frequency of adverse reactions was similar to that seen with the use of cryotherapy. One study among women showed efficacy and frequency of patient discomfort to be similar to podophyllin. No data on the efficacy of bichloroacetic acid are available.

Few data on the efficacy of electrodesiccation are available. One randomized trial of electrodesiccation demonstrated an efficacy of 94%, with recurrences among 22% of patients; another randomized trial of diathermocoagulation demonstrated an efficacy of 35%. Local anesthesia is required, and patient discomfort usually is moderate.

Vaginal warts

Cryotherapy with liquid nitrogen. The use of a cryoprobe in the vagina is not recommended because of the risk of vaginal perforation and fistula formation.

or

TCA 80% to 90%. Apply only to warts; powder with talc or sodium bicarbonate (baking soda) to remove unreacted acid. Repeat weekly as necessary. If warts persist after six applications, other therapeutic methods should be considered.

or

Podophyllin 10% to 25% in compound tincture of benzoin. Apply to the treatment area, which must be dry before removing the speculum. Treat ≤ 2 cm^2 per session. Repeat application at weekly intervals. Because of concern about potential systemic absorption, some experts caution against vaginal application of podophyllin. *The use of podophyllin is contraindicated during pregnancy.*

Urethral meatus warts

Cryotherapy with liquid nitrogen

or

Podophyllin 10% to 25% in compound tincture of benzoin. The treatment area must be dry before contact with normal mucosa. Podophyllin must be washed off in 1 to 2 hours. Repeat weekly if necessary. If warts persist after six applications, other therapeutic methods should be considered. *The use of podophyllin is contraindicated during pregnancy.*

Anal warts

Cryotherapy with liquid nitrogen

or

TCA 80% to 90%. Apply only to warts; powder with talc or sodium bicarbonate (baking soda) to remove unreacted acid. Repeat weekly if necessary. If warts persist after six applications, other therapeutic methods should be considered.

or

Surgical removal

NOTE: Management of warts on rectal mucosa should be referred to an expert.

Oral warts

Cryotherapy with liquid nitrogen

or

Electrodesiccation or electrocautery

or

Surgical removal

Genital herpes simplex virus infections

First clinical episode of genital herpes

Recommended regimen

Acyclovir 200 mg orally 5 times a day for 7 to 10 days or until clinical resolution is attained

1993 SEXUALLY TRANSMITTED DISEASES TREATMENT GUIDELINES—cont'd

First clinical episode of herpes proctitis

Recommended regimen

Acyclovir 400 mg orally 5 times a day for 10 days or until clinical resolution is attained

Recurrent episodes

When treatment is instituted during the prodrome or within 2 days of onset of lesions, some patients who have recurrent disease experience limited benefit from therapy. However, since early treatment can seldom be administered, most immunocompetent patients with recurrent disease do not benefit from acyclovir treatment, and it is not generally recommended.

Recommended regimen

Acyclovir 200 mg orally 5 times a day for 5 days

or

Acyclovir 400 mg orally 3 times a day for 5 days

or

Acyclovir 800 mg orally 2 times a day for 5 days

Daily suppressive therapy

Daily suppressive therapy reduces the frequency of HSV recurrences by at least 75% among patients with frequent recurrences (i.e., six or more recurrences per year). Suppressive treatment with oral acyclovir does not totally eliminate symptomatic or asymptomatic viral shedding or the potential for transmission. Safety and efficacy have been documented among persons receiving daily therapy for as long as 5 years. Acyclovir-resistant strains of HSV have been isolated from some persons receiving suppressive therapy, but these strains have not been associated with treatment failure among immunocompetent patients. *After 1 year of continuous suppressive therapy, acyclovir should be discontinued to allow assessment of the patient's rate of recurrent episodes.*

Recommended regimen

Acyclovir 400 mg orally 2 times a day.

Alternative regimen

Acyclovir 200 mg orally 3 to 5 times a day.

The goal of the alternative regimen is to identify for each patient the lowest dose that provides relief from frequently recurring symptoms.

Primary and secondary syphilis

Recommended regimen for adults

Nonallergic patients who have primary or secondary syphilis should be treated with the following regimen:

Benzathine penicillin G, 2.4 million units IM in a single dose

Penicillin allergy

Nonpregnant penicillin-allergic patients who have primary or secondary syphilis should be treated with the following regimen:

Doxycycline 100 mg orally 2 times a day for 2 weeks

or

Tetracycline 500 mg orally 4 times a day for 2 weeks

There is less clinical experience with doxycycline than with tetracycline, but compliance is likely to be better with doxycycline. Therapy for a patient who cannot tolerate either doxycycline or tetracycline should be based on whether the patient's compliance with the therapy regimen and with follow-up examinations can be ensured.

All patients who have syphilis should be tested for HIV. In areas with high HIV prevalence, patients with primary syphilis should be retested for HIV after 3 months.

Follow-up

Treatment failures can occur with any regimen. However, assessing response to treatment often is difficult, and no definitive criteria for cure or failure exist. Serological test titers may decline more slowly among patients with a prior syphilis infection. Patients should be reexamined clinically and serologically at 3 months and again at 6 months.

Patients who have signs or symptoms that persist or recur or who have a sustained fourfold increase in nontreponemal test titer compared with either the baseline titer or to a subsequent result can be considered to have failed treatment or to be reinfected. These patients should be retreated after evaluation for HIV infection. Unless reinfection is likely, lumbar puncture also should be performed.

Failure of nontreponemal test titers to decline fourfold by 3 months after therapy for primary or secondary syphilis identifies persons at risk for treatment failure. Those persons should be evaluated for HIV infection. Optimal management of such patients is unclear if they are HIV negative. At a minimum, these patients should have additional clinical and serological follow-up. If further follow-up cannot be ensured, retreatment is recommended. Some experts recommend CSF examination in such situations.

When patients are retreated, most experts recommend retreatment with three weekly injections of benzathine penicillin G 2.4 million units IM, unless CSF examination indicates that neurosyphilis is present.

Recommended regimen for children

After the newborn period, children diagnosed with syphilis should have a CSF examination to exclude a diagnosis of neurosyphilis, and birth and maternal medical records should be reviewed to assess whether the child has congenital or acquired syphilis (see Congenital Syphilis). Children who have acquired primary or secondary syphilis should be evaluated (including consultation with child-protection services) and treated using the following pediatric regimen:

Benzathine penicillin G, 50,000 units/kg IM, up to the adult dose of 2.4 million units in a single dose

Pelvic inflammatory disease

Therapy regimens for pelvic inflammatory disease (PID) must provide empirical, broad-spectrum coverage of likely pathogens. Antimicrobial coverage should include *N. gonorrhoeae, C. trachomatis*, gram negative facultative bacteria, anaerobes, and streptococci. Although several antimicrobial regimens have proven effective in achieving clinical and microbiological cure in randomized clinical trials with short-term follow-up, few studies have been done to assess and compare elimination of infection of the endometrium and fallopian tubes, or the incidence of long-term complications such as tubal infertility and ectopic pregnancy.

No single therapeutic regimen has been established for persons who have PID. When selecting a treatment regimen, health-care providers should consider availability, cost, patient acceptance, and regional differences in antimicrobial susceptibility of the likely pathogens.

Continued.

1993 SEXUALLY TRANSMITTED DISEASES TREATMENT GUIDELINES—cont'd

Pelvic inflammatory disease—con'd

Many experts recommend that all patients who have PID be hospitalized so that supervised treatment with parenteral antibiotics can be initiated. Hospitalization is especially recommended when the following criteria are met:

- The diagnosis is uncertain, and surgical emergencies such as appendicitis and ectopic pregnancy cannot be excluded
- Pelvic abscess is suspected
- The patient is pregnant
- The patient is an adolescent (among adolescents, compliance with therapy is unpredictable)
- The patient has HIV infection
- Severe illness or nausea and vomiting preclude outpatient management
- The patient is unable to follow or tolerate an outpatient regimen
- The patient has failed to respond clinically to outpatient therapy
- Clinical follow-up within 72 hours of starting antibiotic treatment cannot be arranged

Inpatient treatment

Experts have experience with both of the following regimens. Also, multiple randomized trials demonstrate the efficacy of each regimen.

Regimen A

Cefoxitin 2 g IV every 6 hours or cefotetan 2 g IV every 12 hours

plus

Doxycycline 100 mg IV or orally every 12 hours

NOTE: This regimen should be continued for at least 48 hours after the patient demonstrates substantial clinical improvement, after which doxycycline 100 mg orally 2 times a day should be continued for a total of 14 days. Doxycycline administered orally has bioavailability similar to that of the IV formulation and may be administered if normal gastrointestinal function is present.

Clinical data are limited for other second- or third-generation cephalosporins (e.g., ceftizoxime, cefotaxime, and ceftriaxone), which might replace cefoxitin or cefotetan, although many authorities believe they also are effective therapy for PID. However, they are less active than cefoxitin or cefotetan against anaerobic bacteria.

Regimen B

Clindamycin 900 mg IV every 8 hours

plus

Gentamicin loading dose IV or IM (2 mg/kg of body weight) followed by a maintenance dose (1.5 mg/kg) every 8 hours

NOTE: This regimen should be continued for at least 48 hours after the patient demonstrates substantial clinical improvement, then followed with doxycycline 100 mg orally 2 times a day or clindamycin 450 mg orally 4 times a day to complete a total of 14 days of therapy. When tuboovarian abscess is present, many health-care providers use clindamycin for continued therapy rather than doxycycline because it provides more effective anaerobic coverage. Clindamycin administered intravenously appears to be effective against *C. trachomatis* infection; however, the effectiveness of oral clindamycin against *C. trachomatis* has not been determined.

Alternative inpatient regimens. Limited data support the use of other inpatient regimens, but two regimens have undergone at least one clinical trial and have broad-spectrum coverage. Ampicillin/sulbactam plus doxycycline has good anaerobic coverage and appears to be effective for patients with a tuboovarian abscess. Intravenous ofloxacin has been studied as a single agent. A regimen of ofloxacin plus either clindamycin or metronidazole provides broad-spectrum coverage. Evidence is insufficient to support the use of any single-agent regimen for inpatient treatment of PID.

Outpatient treatment

Clinical trials of outpatient regimens have provided little information regarding intermediate and long-term outcomes. The following regimens provide coverage against the common etiological agents of PID, but evidence from clinical trials supporting their use is limited. The second regimen provides broader coverage against anaerobic organisms but costs substantially more than the other regimen. Patients who do not respond to outpatient therapy within 72 hours should be hospitalized to confirm the diagnosis and to receive parenteral therapy.

Regimen A

Cefoxitin 2 g IM plus probenecid, 1 g orally in a single dose concurrently, or ceftriaxone 250 mg IM or other parenteral third-generation cephalosporin (e.g., ceftizoxime or cefotaxime)

plus

Doxycycline 100 mg orally 2 times a day for 14 days

Regimen B

Ofloxacin 400 mg orally 2 times a day for 14 days

plus

Either clindamycin 450 mg orally 4 times a day, or metronidazole 500 mg orally 2 times a day for 14 days

Clinical trials have demonstrated that the cefoxitin regimen is effective in obtaining short-term clinical response. Fewer data support the use of ceftriaxone or other third-generation cephalosporins, but, based on their similarities to cefoxitin, they also are considered effective. No data exist regarding the use of oral cephalosporins for the treatment of PID.

Ofloxacin is effective against both *N. gonorrhoeae* and *C. trachomatis*. One clinical trial demonstrated the effectiveness of oral ofloxacin in obtaining short-term clinical response with PID. Despite results of this trial, ofloxacin's lack of anaerobic coverage causes some concern; the addition of clindamycin or metronidazole provides this coverage. Clindamycin, but not metronidazole, further enhances the gram positive coverage of the regimen.

Alternative outpatient regimens. Information regarding other outpatient regimens is limited. The combination of amoxicillin/clavulanic acid plus doxycycline was effective in obtaining short-term clinical response in one clinical trial, but many of the patients had to discontinue the regimen because of gastrointestinal symptoms.

Follow-up

Hospitalized patients receiving IV therapy should show substantial clinical improvement (e.g., defervescence, reduction in direct or rebound abdominal tenderness, and reduction in uterine, adnexal, and cervical motion tenderness) within 3 to 5 days of initiation of therapy. Patients who do not demonstrate

1993 SEXUALLY TRANSMITTED DISEASES TREATMENT GUIDELINES—cont'd

Follow-up—cont'd

improvement within this time period usually require further diagnostic workup or surgical intervention, or both.

If the provider elects to prescribe outpatient therapy, follow-up examination should be performed within 72 hours, using the criteria for clinical improvement previously described.

Because of the risk for persistent infection, particularly with *C. trachomatis,* patients should have a microbiological reexamination 7 to 10 days after completing therapy. Some experts also recommend rescreening for *C. trachomatis* and *N. gonorhoeae* 4 to 6 weeks after completing therapy.

Adapted from Centers for Disease Control and Prevention: *MMWR* 42(No. RR-14) 1993.

cervical neoplasia and among adolescent girls represents the most common cause of abnormal Pap smears.[6,18]

More than 50 different types of HPV have been identified: "benign" genital warts usually are caused by types 6 and 11; types 16, 18, 31, 33, and 35 are associated most commonly with squamous intraepithelial neoplasia (SIL) changes on Pap smear. These types have the oncogenic potential to transform normal cells into malignant ones. An individual can be infected with more than one type. Cervical HPV infection has been associated with more than 90% of cervical dysplasia.

As with other STDs, infection rates among adolescents and young adults are quite high—up to 30%. Detection of infection is not always easy. Although 50% to 60% of women who have external warts have cervical infection, only 3% to 6% of those who have cervical disease have external genital warts. Hence, the use of the Pap smear in any sexually active female is extremely important in screening for infection, even among those who have no visible signs of infection.

Males likely constitute a significant reservoir of undetected and untreated HPV infection.[13] In one study, only 21 of 156 male partners of HPV positive women had clinical evidence of warts. However, with use of magnification and acetic acid "soaks" to produce the "acetowhite" changes seen in HPV-infected skin, 77% of males were shown to be infected (Fig. 258-4). All these males were over 20 years of age; virtually no data exist on adolescent males.

Overt warts develop in roughly two thirds of persons having intercourse with an infected individual. Visible warts develop in 6 weeks to 8 months, but the range of the incubation period may be even wider. The typical pedunculated wart with a keratotic and irregular surface usually is easy to recognize, but warts also may be flat and more difficult to detect. Use of a hand-held magnifying glass or even a colposcope is extremely helpful. Among males, warts usually are seen on the shaft, prepuce, frenulum, corona, and glans but also may be present on the skin of the scrotum and the anus (Fig. 258-5). The presence of anal warts often is associated with anal receptive intercourse, but warts in this location have been described in males who deny this type of behavior. Occasionally warts are seen at the urethral opening.

The posterior vaginal introitus, labia minora, and vestibule represent the most common sites of infection among females; again, however, warts can be seen anywhere on the external or internal genitalia. Subclinical disease is most likely to occur on the cervix; the relatively large transformation zone of the maturing adolescent cervix affords a hospitable site of infection for the virus (Fig. 258-6). Extensive disease should raise the possibility of HIV disease.

Evidence continues to accumulate linking the presence of HPV with the development of dysplastic and malignant changes in the cervix. Hence, the role of the routine Pap smear in the care of sexually active teenagers has assumed increased importance. Any patient who has evidence of HPV on Pap smear, usually indicated by the presence of koilocytic changes, should be referred for colposcopic examination, as should any woman who has visible evidence of cervical infection. This is necessary because the physician cannot tell from the Pap smear or from viewing without magnification whether the infected areas contain true neoplastic changes, which require vigorous treatment. If such changes cannot be ruled out by colposcopy alone, biopsy may be necessary. Of untreated cervical infections, 15% to 20% may progress to true malignant changes.

A variety of treatments for genital warts exist (see the box on p. 1581). Each physician who chooses to treat genital warts should determine which technique is most suitable to his or her practice and become familiar with that technique. Regardless of which treatment is chosen, careful follow-up (initially at weekly intervals) is essential to monitor the results and prevent regrowth between too widely spaced treatment intervals.

The benefit of treating subclinical HPV infection is unclear. However, some authorities do recommend the treatment of subclinical cervical disease and localized sites on the penis or scrotum in an attempt to control sexual transmission.

Herpes Genitalis

Herpes simplex viral infections of the male and female genital tract are particularly distressing to patients because of the high likelihood of recurrence after an initial episode.[4] Both herpes simplex type 1 (HSV-1) and type 2 (HSV-2) can cause genital tract disease, although type 2 infections still tend to predominate. Infection rates have increased in the past 2 decades, especially among those 20 years of age or over. Although genital herpes infections were believed at one time to be associated with the development of cervical cancer, current evidence indicates that HSV more likely acts as a cofactor.

Infections with the virus can be classified as primary or nonprimary. Primary infection refers to the first exposure to HSV-1 or HSV-2 in an individual who has had no prior ex-

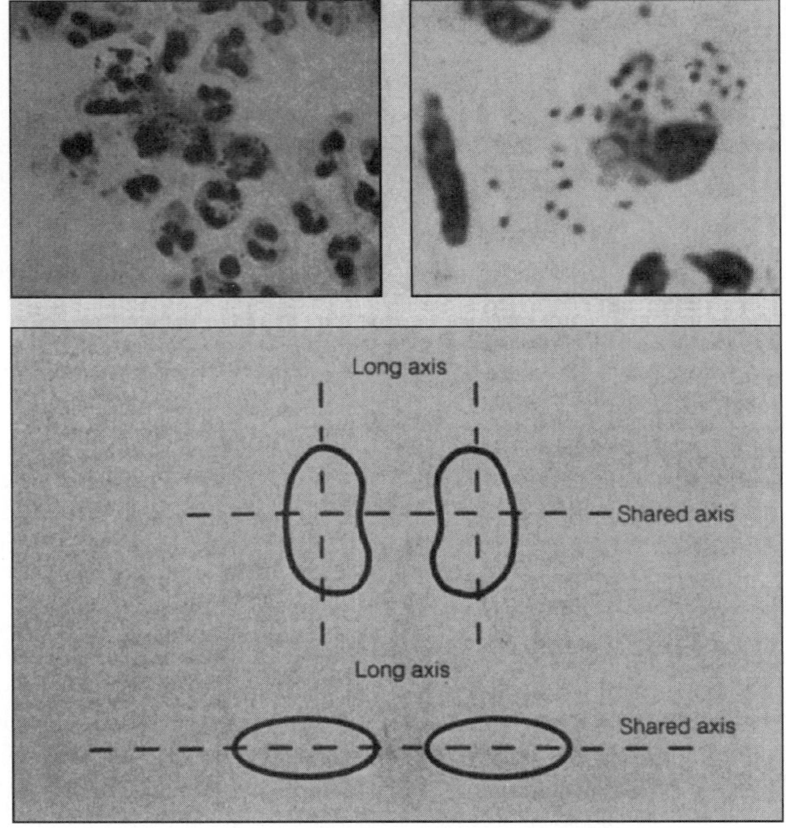

FIG. 258-3 *Neisseria gonorrhoeae* on Gram stains of male urethral smears (×1500 and ×4000 magnification) appear as tiny gram negative diplococci within polymorphonuclear leukocytes (pink-stained nuclei). *Neisseria* organisms are kidney bean shaped, and their long axes are perpendicular to the shared axis, as shown in the diagram.

(From Gilchrist MJR, Rauch JL: *Contemp Pediatr* 4:54, 1987.)

posure to either virus. Nonprimary infection occurs in those who have had prior antibody to either type 1 or type 2 who become infected with the other strain. This type of infection, most commonly occurring in individuals who have existing antibody to type 1 who become infected with type 2, tends to be less symptomatic.

In primary infection, symptoms usually occur within 2 to 20 days after sexual exposure. The patient usually experiences burning or itching at the site of inoculation, followed by erythema and the development of discrete vesicles. Initially the vesicles contain clear fluid, but they rapidly form pustules with an erythematous base. Typically, a patient may have 15 to 30 vesicles, each full of infectious viral particles. Lesions are located on the vulva, cervix, clitoris, or perineum. In males they may occur on the shaft, glans, or prepuce. Infection also can involve the urethra (leading to dysuria or urinary retention). Vesicles also can be seen on the thighs, buttocks, groin, or anus as a result of autoinoculation or anal receptive intercourse.

Because primary infection represents a first exposure to the particular virus type, systemic symptoms such as fever, malaise, and headache are common. About 50% of patients have tender inguinal lymphadenopathy.

After 2 to 4 days, the vesicles break open and coalesce to form wet ulcers. This is usually the time at which patients are seen by physicians. New lesions still may be developing at this point, but within 20 days all the lesions have crusted over and the pain and other symptoms have disappeared. Herpetic lesions heal without scarring.

The diagnosis of herpes genitalis is made most often on clinical grounds. Cultures of intact vesicles generally are positive, as are cultures of the cervix. A Tzanck preparation of a scraping from an ulcer demonstrates the presence of multinucleated giant cells.

Following resolution of the infection, the virus remains latent in the sacral ganglia and may reactivate at any time. This reactivation is referred to as recurrent disease. Recurrences may occur in association with stress, local trauma, fever, or menstruation and tend to be shorter in duration, less symptomatic, and lacking in systemic symptoms. Vesicles usually occur near the initial infection site but tend to be fewer in number. Just before the recurrence, the patient may experience burning or itching at the site of infection. Healing takes from 1 to 2 weeks.

Females whose only site of recurrence involves the cervix may be unaware of the recurrence; during this period they are shedding the virus. About one third of males also may have inapparent recurrences but still are infectious. Hence, unless sex partners reveal their history of infection, many exposures to the virus can occur without an individual being aware that he or she has come into contact with the virus.

The risk of recurrence depends on a number of factors.

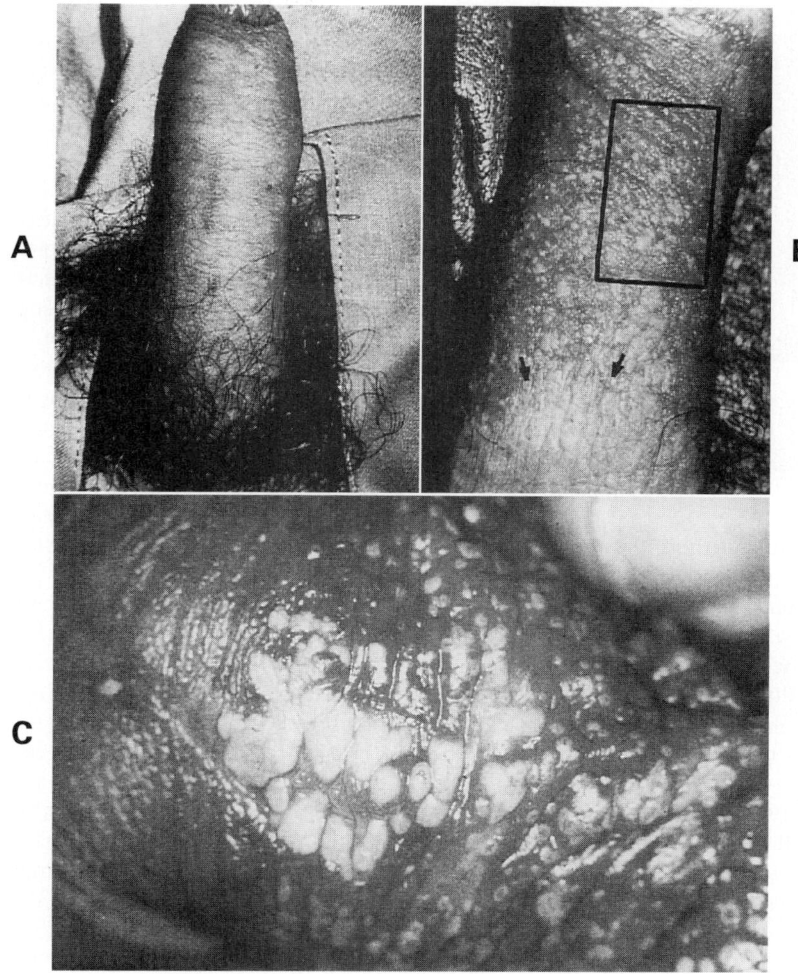

FIG. 258-4 Demonstration of subclinical lesions. **A,** Appearance of penis before acetic acid application. **B,** Penis after 5-minute application of gauze soaked in 5% acetic acid. Note coalescing sheets *(arrows)* and discrete dots of acetowhite staining *(inset)*. **C,** Magnified view of apparent subclinical human papillomavirus infection shown in **B.**

(From Ketelaris PM et al: *J Urol* 140:302, 1988.)

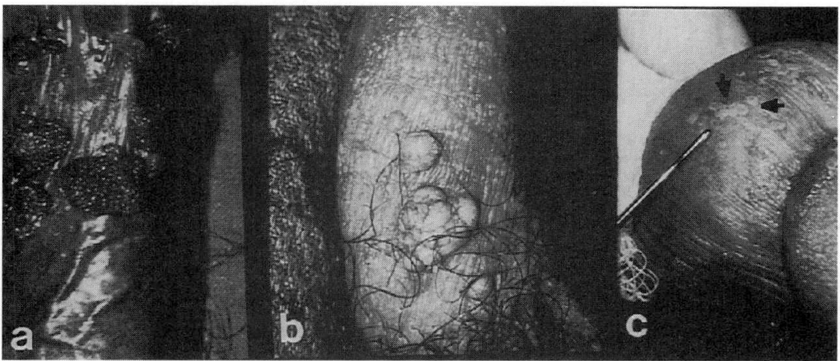

FIG. 258-5 Morphology of macroscopic warts. **A,** Condylomata demonstrated by preputial retraction. **B,** Verrucous wart at penoscrotal junction. **C,** Small, flat warts *(arrows)* on distal third of penis.

(From Ketelaris PM et al: *J Urol* 140:302, 1988.)

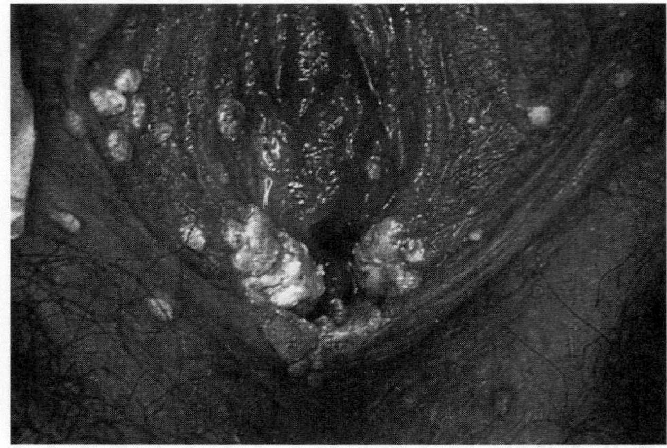

FIG. 258-6 Condyloma accuminatum of the vulva appears as a polypoid mass with a keratotic fissured and irregular surface. (From Moscicki B: *Contemp Pediatr* 6:24, 1989.)

Males are more likely to have recurrent disease, as are those individuals whose infection was caused by HSV-2. In one study, 12 of 14 patients (about 86%) who have HSV-1 infection *did not* have recurrences, compared with only 40% of those who have HSV-2. Once a second episode occurs, the patient is likely to have multiple recurrences.

Development of the antiviral drug acyclovir (Zovirax) has altered the nature of herpes therapy dramatically.[15] Acyclovir tablets (200 mg), taken five times daily for 7 to 10 days, significantly reduces the symptoms associated with primary episodes of genital herpes and decreases both the duration of viral shedding and the time to resolution of lesions (see the box on p. 1582). Some patients who have recurrent disease may derive limited benefit from early initiation of oral acyclovir, and those who have six or more recurrences per year have a 75% reduction in recurrences with daily suppressive therapy (see the box on p. 1583).

Syphilis

Syphilis is on the rise, perhaps because of decreased public health efforts directed toward it in this age of AIDS, and certainly because more women addicted to crack cocaine exchange sex for drugs. Rates of syphilis infection among infants, children, and adolescents peaked in 1991, but the rates in 1993 were still higher in many states than they were in 1989. Pediatricians therefore must remain knowledgeable about the diagnosis, treatment, and prevention of this infection.

The typical chancre of syphilis develops at the site of intimate sexual contact approximately 3 weeks after exposure to an infected individual (range 10 to 90 days).

This lesion, varying from a few millimeters to a few centimeters, is clean-based, painless, and has sharply demarcated, indurated borders. Unilateral, regional lymphadenopathy usually is present. Because the ulcer is painless, its appearance in the vagina or rectum or perhaps in the mouth is likely to go unnoticed. While the ulcer is present, the exudate overlying it is highly infectious.[1] Untreated, the chancre disappears in 2 to 8 weeks.

The rash of secondary syphilis appears 6 weeks to 6 months after the chancre appears in the untreated patient. The rash and the chancre may coexist. Because the spirochetes spread hematogenously from the site of initial infection, constitutional symptoms such as fever, malaise, sore throat, and generalized lymphadenopathy may be present.

The rash typically is papulosquamous but can be macular or pustular. Annular papules can appear on the face, and the rash can resemble impetigo or eczema. Sometimes moist, fissured papules or elevated, thickened papules (condyloma lata) are seen; both are highly infectious. Finally, loss of scalp or eyebrow hair can be associated with secondary syphilis.

At the time the chancre is present, a darkfield examination of the nonbloody exudate should be performed by someone expert in darkfield microscopy. If performed on 3 successive days, the likelihood of obtaining a positive result from an infected individual is extremely high. If the results of all three examinations are negative, the diagnosis of primary syphilis should be reconsidered.

If the darkfield examination is unavailable, a serological test for syphilis should be obtained. A variety of tests for detecting syphilis are available; their relative sensitivities and specificities are outlined in Table 258-2.[5] If the examiner is relatively certain that the chancre is one of primary syphilis, he or she should request the fluorescent treponemal antibody-absorption (FTA-ABS) test, since the sensitivity of the flocculation (VDRL) and rapid plasma reagin (RPR) tests at this point is relatively low. Alternatively a second specimen can be obtained 2 to 4 weeks later.

Recently, Cox and others[4] reviewed the occurrence of syphilis in adolescents: 14% had primary syphilis; 43%, secondary syphilis; 39%, latent syphilis; and 4% were undetermined. A minority of patients had a chancre (14%) or a rash (18%); 47% had no signs or symptoms of the disease. Hence all sexually active adolescents should be screened routinely for syphilis.

The recommended CDC treatment guidelines for primary and secondary syphilis are outlined in the box on p. 1583. Follow-up with repeat serological tests should occur at 3, 6, and 12 months after treatment. Typically, VDRL titers should decline by fourfold at 3 months and eightfold at 6 months. The FTA-ABS test always remains positive. Criteria for reevaluation or retreatment include persistence or recurrence of clinical signs and symptoms, a sustained fourfold or greater rise in titers, or the persistence of a higher than 1:8 titer for more than 1 year after adequate treatment.

Congenital Syphilis

In 1993, 3211 cases of congenital syphilis were reported in children less than 1 year of age. The clinical manifestations of this entirely preventable disease are protean.[12] Infected infants may be identified early in life via routine serological screening or on the basis of various symptoms (early congenital syphilis). Alternatively, some may escape detection and appear after 2 years of age with the sequelae of untreated infection (late congenital syphilis).

Most infected liveborn infants (congenital syphilis is a major cause of stillbirths) are asymptomatic.[11] Common signs of infection include hepatomegaly (with or without splenomegaly or jaundice), nephrotic syndrome (limb edema and proteinuria), eye abnormalities (chorioretinitis, glaucoma, uveitis), generalized nontender lymphadenopathy (especially involving the epitrochlear nodes), anemia or thrombocytope-

Table 258-2 Comparison of Diagnostic Tests for Syphilis

	Sensitivity and Specificity of Serological tests for Syphilis* at Different Stages							
	Percent Sensitivity (Sens.) and Specificity (Spec.)							
	VDRL		RPR		FTA-ABS		MHA-TP	
Stage of syphilis	**Sens.**	**Spec.**	**Sens.**	**Spec.**	**Sens.**	**Spec.**	**Sens.**	**Spec.**
Primary	80 (59-87)	98 (80-99)	86 (81-100)	98 (80-99)	98 (93-100)	98 (84-99)	82 (64-90)	99 (98-100)
Secondary	100 (99-100)	98	100 (99-100)	98	100 (99-100)	98	100 (96-100)	99
Latent	96 (73-100)	98	99	98	100 (96-100)	98	100 (96-100)	99
Late	71	98	73	98	96	98	94	99

From Dans PE: Syphilis. In Barker LR, Burton JR, Zieve PD, editors: *Principles of ambulatory medicine,* ed 2, Baltimore, 1986, Williams & Wilkins.
*The consensus figures for the sensitivity and specificity are for tests done in the Centers for Disease Control Reference Laboratory on samples derived from a well-run STD clinic. The figures in parentheses demonstrate the variability in published reports. Responsible factors include *(a)* study of populations with different prevalences of syphilis and other confounding illnesses, *(b)* variable performance by the laboratory, and *(c)* different clinical criteria for the diagnosis of syphilis.

nia or both, persistent rhinitis (which can be clear, blood tinged, or purulent), and intrauterine growth retardation. Involvement of the central nervous system can mimic bacterial meningitis, although the cerebrospinal fluid (CSF) generally shows a monocytosis with an elevated protein and a normal glucose level.

Skin manifestations also are extremely important. Congenital syphilis always should be suspected when an infant has a persistent diaper rash or an exanthem involving the palms and soles. About 30% to 60% of infected infants have skin lesions, the most common being a large, round, pink macule that turns "coppery" and fades in 1 to 3 months without treatment. The lesions tend to spare the anterior trunk. A fine scale may cover the involved areas. The rash also can be vesiculobullous or, lacking bullae, can manifest as desquamation. Eczematoid, often impetiginized lesions have a predilection for the perineum, for the intertriginous areas, and for the middle third of the face (including the tongue and palate).

Some two thirds of infants also have bony involvement, although in many cases this can be detected only by radiological means. The epiphyses involved most commonly are those of the radius, femur, humerus, and fibula, with infection generally in multiple, symmetrical sites. Bony tenderness can lead to decreased movement of the affected limb and thus a false diagnosis of paralysis secondary to birth trauma (pseudoparalysis of Parrot).

Recently, Dorfman and Glaser[7] reported on seven infants who have congenital syphilis diagnosed between 3 and 14 weeks of age, six of whom were RPR negative at birth. In four cases, the mothers had a negative serological test at delivery; the other three were not tested because of a negative test before delivery. All the infants had hepatomegaly and elevated serum transaminase levels, but other physical findings were inconstant. To ensure complete identification of all infected children, testing of *both* maternal and infant sera is essential.

The box on p. 1590 lists the CDC criteria for surveillance case definition for congenital syphilis. The diagnosis is more difficult in an asymptomatic infant whose treponemal test for syphilis is positive and whose mother also has a positive test. In this case, consultation with an infectious disease specialist may be warranted to differentiate active infection from passive transfer of maternal antibody.

Infants classified as confirmed or presumptive cases of congenital syphilis according to the CDC criteria should be treated for 10 to 14 days with either aqueous crystalline penicillin G (100,000 to 150,000 U/kg/day intravenously every 8 to 12 hours) **or** procaine penicillin G (50,000 U/kg/day intramuscularly once daily).[20] If the infant's mother has not been treated adequately, if it cannot be determined whether the treatment was adequate, or if the infant's mother is HIV antibody positive, a similar regimen should be used. If the mother has been treated adequately, the decision to treat the infant depends on assurances regarding careful follow-up and a normal CSF examination. Under optimum circumstances, no treatment is needed at birth, but serial antibody titers should be obtained at 1, 2, 4, 6, and 12 months. Infants who cannot reliably be followed up but who have normal CSF should receive a single dose of benzathine penicillin (50,000 U/kg intramuscularly).

SYNDROMES ASSOCIATED WITH SEXUALLY TRANSMITTED DISEASES

Pelvic Inflammatory Disease

Pelvic inflammatory disease (PID) refers to infection involving the upper genital tract (uterus, fallopian tubes, ovaries, and pelvis) occurring as a result of undetected or inadequately treated sexually transmitted infections of the lower genital tract (endocervix). In the short term, PID can lead to such problems as a ruptured tuboovarian abscess. In the long run, infertility, chronic pelvic pain, and increased risk for ectopic pregnancy are attributable to this condition, even when the acute episode has been managed appropriately. Among all sexually active females, teenagers under 19 years of age are at greatest risk for contracting this disease; because a major risk factor for developing PID is a prior episode, adolescent girls who experience this illness early in their reproductive life cycle are at great risk for having further significant problems.[22]

Even though this condition is common, the diagnosis of pelvic inflammatory disease is imprecise. Signs and symptoms can be nonspecific, and the only sure method for diagnosis—laparoscopy—is not routinely performed for diagnostic purposes in this country. Hence pediatricians must maintain a high index of suspicion and must obtain a thorough history and perform a careful physical examination to avoid the pitfalls of diagnosis.

SURVEILLANCE CASE DEFINITION FOR CONGENITAL SYPHILIS

For reporting purposes, congenital syphilis includes cases of congenitally acquired syphilis in infants and children, as well as syphilitic stillbirths.

A CONFIRMED CASE of congenital syphilis is an infant in whom *Treponema pallidum* is identified by darkfield microscopy, fluorescent antibody, or other specific stains in specimens from lesions, placenta, umbilical cord, or autopsy material.

A PRESUMPTIVE CASE of congenital syphilis is either of the following:

A. Any infant whose mother had untreated or inadequately treated* syphilis at delivery, regardless of findings in the infant

OR

B. Any infant or child who has a reactive treponemal test for syphilis and any one of the following:
   1. Any evidence of congenital syphilis on physical examination† or
   2. Any evidence of congenital syphilis on long-bone radiograph or
   3. Reactive cerebrospinal fluid VDRL‡ or
   4. Elevated CSF cell count or protein (without other cause)‡ or
   5. Quantitative nontreponemal serological titers that are fourfold higher than the mother's (both drawn at birth) or
   6. Reactive test for FTA-ABS-19S-IgM antibody‡

A SYPHILITIC STILLBIRTH is defined as a fetal death in which the mother had untreated or inadequately treated syphilis at delivery of a fetus after a 20-week gestation or of a fetus weighing more than 500 g.

From Congenital syphilis—New York City, 1986-1988, *MMWR* 38:825, 1989.

*Inadequate treatment consists of any nonpenicillin therapy or penicillin given less than 30 days before delivery.

†Signs in an infant (under 2 years of age) may include hepatosplenomegaly, characteristic skin rash, condyloma lata, snuffles, jaundice (syphilitic hepatitis), pseudoparalysis, or edema (nephrotic syndrome). Stigmata in an older child may include interstitial keratitis, nerve deafness, anterior bowing of shins, frontal bossing, mulberry molars, Hutchinson's teeth, saddle nose, rhagades, or Clutton joints.

‡Distinguishing between congenital and acquired syphilis may be difficult in a seropositive child after infancy. Signs may not be obvious and stigmata may not yet have developed. Abnormal values for CSF VDRL, cell count, and protein, as well as IgM antibodies, may be found in either congenital or acquired syphilis. Findings on long-bone radiographs may help because these would indicate congenital syphilis. The decision may ultimately be based on maternal history and clinical judgment; the possibility of sexual abuse also needs to be considered.

When eliciting the history from a patient who has lower abdominal pain, the physician should keep in mind those factors that place an individual at risk for infection. Hence failure to use barrier methods of contraception, the presence of an intrauterine device (IUD), multiple partners, a recent new partner, or history of other STDs or PID should raise concern. The presence of a new vaginal discharge (or a change in odor, color, or amount), abnormal menstrual bleeding (increased or prolonged or occurring at the wrong time in the cycle), or dyspareunia all suggest PID. Although oral contraceptive pills protect against the development of gonococcal PID, the evidence for protection against *C. trachomatis* PID is uncertain. Oral contraceptive pills actually increase the likelihood of acquisition and persistence of chlamydial infection.

Other symptoms include dysuria, dysmenorrhea (usually more severe than normal), nausea, vomiting, diarrhea, fever, and malaise. Except for dysmenorrhea, these symptoms also can be seen in patients who have diseases of the urinary tract (e.g., pyelonephritis) or gastrointestinal tract (e.g., appendicitis).

Depending on the extent of upper genital tract involvement, physical signs may include pain on cervical movement and endometrial or adnexal tenderness or both. Fever is present in *fewer than* 50% of patients who have documented PID. If the infection has "tracked" up to involve the capsule of the liver, right upper quadrant tenderness also may be elicited. With extensive infection, signs of peritonitis, particularly rebound tenderness, are present. The palpation of an adnexal mass raises the concern of a coexisting tuboovarian abscess. Mucopus visible in the cervical os strongly suggests the presence of infection, but its absence does not rule out the diagnosis. Acute-phase reactants lack the necessary sensitivity and specificity to be routinely helpful in establishing the diagnosis of PID. Although 60% to 80% of patients have an elevated white blood cell count, sedimentation rate, or C-reactive protein, so do many patients who have pyelonephritis or appendicitis.

In an attempt to guide clinicians and minimize the potential for diagnostic confusion, several investigators have suggested diagnostic criteria for infections localized to the female pelvic organs.[8] The criteria for diagnosing of salpingitis are indicated in the box on p. 1591. Despite use of these diagnostic criteria, several studies have indicated substantial false positive and false negative rates in the diagnosis of PID. The physician should take particular note that certain surgical emergency conditions can mimic PID in their manifestation. Hence one should keep in mind the differential diagnosis, as outlined in the box on p. 1591. Because many teenagers at risk for PID are similarly at risk for pregnancy and because ectopic pregnancy can mimic PID, a sensitive urine or serum pregnancy test should be obtained routinely at the time of evaluation. If an adnexal mass is palpated or suspected, an ultrasound should be obtained to determine if a tuboovarian abscess is present. Cultures for *C. trachomatis* and *N. gonorrhoeae* should be obtained routinely.

The hospital admission of any teenager who has PID is recommended by many authorities in an attempt to minimize future sequelae and because teenagers often comply poorly with the lengthy regimens needed for successful treatment. Others argue that if careful follow-up can be ensured, outpatient management can be attempted. The other indications for admission are shown in the box on p. 1592.

Treatment is directed toward eradicating the organism responsible for the infection. Unfortunately, the exact nature of the infection is established with great difficulty. Cultures obtained from the cervix do not necessarily reflect the nature of the tubal infection. Many organisms believed to play a role in PID are difficult to grow; thus studies that did not use state-of-the-art culture techniques may not have identified all relevant organisms. Those studies that have been performed carefully point to the polymicrobial nature of the infection. Both *N. gonorrhoeae* and *C. trachomatis* have been recovered from approximately 25% to 50% of patients. Nongonococcal, nonchlamydial anaerobes (bacteroides and *Peptostreptococcus* spp.), facultative aerobes *(Gardnerella vaginalis, Escherichia coli, Haemophilus influenzae),* and genital tract mycoplasms also have been recovered to varying degrees. Bacterial vaginosis is a likely risk factor for development of PID.

As a result of the uncertainty concerning the nature of the infecting organisms and the lack of controlled treatment and outcome studies, the CDC treatment regimens outlined in the box on p. 1581 reflect empirical therapy based on the assumption that the infection is polymicrobial. The need to use doxycycline as part of therapy underscores the need for obtaining a pregnancy test before treatment. If outpatient therapy is to be attempted, careful follow-up at 48 hours must be ensured, and a mechanism for hospitalizing the patient before that time if symptoms worsen must be in place. Otherwise, admission should occur at the time of diagnosis.

Once therapy is initiated, the patient should improve within 48 hours. Failure to see this improvement should raise concerns about the accuracy of the diagnosis or the presence of complications. The pelvic examination should be repeated in order to look for a tuboovarian abscess if one has not already been detected. Approximately 10% to 20% of patients who have PID develop a tuboovarian abscess; 3% to 15% of these abscesses rupture. If an abscess is detected or if the patient fails to improve, the physician should seek gynecological consultation (or surgical consultation if appendicitis is suspected).

The patient may be discharged from the hospital 48 hours after she demonstrates substantial clinical improvement. Treatment must include a total of 10 days with doxycycline. Follow-up at the end of treatment is important. The patient should be instructed not to have intercourse until her therapy is completed, and her partner must be notified and treated. Because an episode of PID is a major risk factor for development of a second episode, the use of barrier methods of contraception must be stressed to the patient.

Even with optimum diagnosis and treatment, the long-term

SALPINGITIS: CLINICAL CRITERIA FOR DIAGNOSIS

Minimum criteria

Empirical treatment of PID should be instituted on the basis of the presence of all of the following three minimum clinical criteria for pelvic inflammation and in the absence of an established cause other than PID:

- Lower abdominal tenderness
- Adnexal tenderness
- Cervical motion tenderness

Additional criteria

For women who have severe clinical signs, more elaborate diagnostic evaluation is warranted because incorrect diagnosis and management may cause unnecessary morbidity. These additional criteria may be used to increase the specificity of the diagnosis.

Listed below are the *routine* criteria for diagnosing PID:

- Oral temperature >38.3° C
- Abnormal cervical or vaginal discharge
- Elevated erythrocyte sedimentation rate
- Elevated C-reactive protein
- Laboratory documentation of cervical infection with *N. gonorrhoeae* or *C. trachomatis*

From Centers for Disease Control and Prevention: *MMWR* 42(no RR-14):77, 1993.

DIFFERENTIAL DIAGNOSIS OF ACUTE LOWER ABDOMINAL PAIN IN THE ADOLESCENT FEMALE BY ORGAN SYSTEM

Urinary

Cystitis
Pyelonephritis
Urethritis
Other

Gastrointestinal

Appendicitis
Constipation
Diverticulitis
Gastroenteritis
Inflammatory bowel disease
Irritable bowel syndrome
Other

Reproductive

Acute PID
Cervicitis (?)
Dysmenorrhea (primary/secondary)
Ectopic pregnancy
Endometriosis
Endometritis
Mittelschmerz
Ovarian cyst (torsion/rupture)
Pregnancy (intrauterine, ectopic)
Ruptured follicle
Septic abortion
Threatened abortion
Torsion of adnexa
Tuboovarian abscess

From Shafer M, Sweet RL: *Pediatr Clin North Am* 36:513, 1989.

INDICATIONS FOR HOSPITALIZATION OF PATIENTS WHO HAVE PELVIC INFLAMMATORY DISEASE

Many experts recommend that all patients who have PID be hospitalized so that supervised treatment with parenteral antibiotics can be initiated. Hospitalization is especially recommended when the following criteria are met:

- The diagnosis is uncertain, and surgical emergencies such as appendicitis and ectopic pregnancy cannot be excluded
- Pelvic abscess is suspected
- The patient is pregnant
- The patient is an adolescent (among adolescents, compliance with therapy is unpredictable)
- The patient has HIV infection
- Severe illness or nausea and vomiting preclude outpatient management
- The patient is unable to follow or tolerate an outpatient regimen
- The patient has failed to respond clinically to outpatient therapy
- Clinical follow-up within 72 hours of starting antibiotic treatment cannot be arranged

From Centers for Disease Control and Prevention: *MMWR* 42(no 44-14):78, 1993.

morbidity from a single episode of PID is significant. After one episode of PID, 11% of women are infertile; a second episode triples that rate to 34%. Westrom and colleagues[25] have reported a sevenfold to tenfold increase in risk for subsequent ectopic pregnancy following PID. Chronic pelvic pain also is an unfortunate sequela.

Perihepatitis (Fitz-Hugh-Curtis syndrome)

Perihepatis associated with gonococcal salpingitis was described in 1920. Subsequently, Fitz-Hugh described a patient who had "violin string" adhesions between the liver and anterior abdominal wall, and Curtis described localized peritonitis of the liver's anterior surface in a woman who had upper abdominal pain and tenderness who was undergoing laparotomy for suspected gallbladder disease. Since then, it has been well documented that *C. trachomatis* infections can cause a similar picture.

Onset of upper abdominal pain usually follows the onset of lower abdominal pain, but it can precede it. The pain generally is right-sided and can radiate to the shoulder. Fewer than 50% of patients have mildly elevated liver enzymes. Treatment for pelvic inflammatory disease also eliminates the perihepatitis.

Enteric Infections

The syndromes of proctitis, proctocolitis, and enteritis are limited mostly to adolescent males who practice anal receptive intercourse. Symptoms include anorectal pain, tenesmus, constipation, and discharge. Those who have proctocolitis or enteritis will have diarrhea. Patients who have proctitis should be examined with anoscopy and evaluated for *C. trachomatis, N. gonorrhoeae,* and *Treponema pallidum.* Treatment should be with standard doses of cefixime and doxycycline.

Those who have symptoms suggesting proctocolitis or enteritis should receive more extensive evaluation. Such organisms as *Campylobacter jejuni, Shigella* sp., and *Giardia lamblia* can be sexually transmitted.

Vaginitis

As discussed in Chapter 174, Vaginal Discharge, *T. vaginalis,* an important cause of vaginitis among sexually active adolescents, is a sexually transmitted infectious agent. Some evidence suggests that bacterial vaginosis, associated with the overgrowth of *Gardnerella vaginalis,* also is sexually transmitted. Male sex partners of women who have bacterial vaginosis more often have *G. vaginalis* recovered from the urethra than do controls. However, this same organism can be recovered from approximately 15% of females who have never been active sexually. Treatment of male partners does not appear to influence recurrence risks for females who are treated for bacterial vaginosis.

Vaginitis, in and of itself, can be distressing enough to females. However, current concerns about bacterial vaginosis center on its possible role in the pathogenesis of pelvic inflammatory disease. Nongonococcal, nonchlamydial pathogens associated with PID are recovered more often from the endometrium of women who have bacterial vaginosis than from those who do not. Bacterial vaginosis has been related causally to postpartum endometritis. Hence treatment of symptomatic women who have bacterial vaginosis is warranted.

REFERENCES

1. Adger H et al: Screening for *Chlamydia trachomatis* and *Neisseria gonorrhoeae* in adolescent males: value of first-catch urine examination, *Lancet* 2:944, 1984.
2. Brunham RC et al: Mucopurulent cervicitis—the ignored counterpart in women of urethritis in men, *N Engl J Med* 311:1, 1984.
3. Corey L, Spear PG: Infections with herpes simplex viruses. I. and II., *N Engl J Med* 314:686, 749, 1986.
4. Cox J et al: The changing epidemiologic spectrum of syphilis in urban adolescents. Paper presented before the Society for Adolescent Medicine, San Francisco, 1989.
5. Dans PE: Syphilis. In Barker LR, Burton JR, Zieve PD, editors: *Principles of ambulatory medicine,* ed 2, Baltimore, 1986, Williams & Wilkins.
6. Davis AJ, Evans SJ: Human papillomavirus infection in the pediatric and adolescent patient, *J Pediatr* 115:1, 1989.
7. Dorfman DH, Glaser JH: Congenital syphilis presenting in infants after the newborn period, *N Engl J Med* 323:1299, 1990.
8. Hager WD et al: Criteria for diagnosis and grading of salpingitis, *Obstet Gynecol* 61:113, 1983.
9. Hammerschlag MR: Chlamydial infections, *J Pediatr* 114:727, 1989.
10. Hook EW, Holmes KK: Gonococcal infections, *Ann Intern Med* 102:229, 1985.
11. Ikeda MK, Jenson HB: Evaluation and treatment of congenital syphilis, *J Pediatr* 117:843, 1990.
12. Ingall D, Dobson SRM, Musher D: Syphilis. In Remington JS, Klein JO, editors: *Infectious diseases of the fetus and newborn infant,* ed 3, Philadelphia, 1990, WB Saunders.
13. Katelaris PM et al: Human papillomavirus: the untreated male reservoir, *J Urol* 140:300, 1988.
14. Kelaghan J et al: Barrier-method contraceptives and pelvic inflammatory disease, *JAMA* 248:184, 1982.
15. Mertz GJ et al: Double-blind placebo controlled trial of oral acyclovir in first-episode genital herpes simplex virus infection, *JAMA* 252:1147, 1984.

16. Mertz GJ et al: Long-term acyclovir suppression of frequently recurring genital herpes simplex virus infection, *JAMA* 260:201, 1988.
17. Mills J, Brooks GF: Disseminated gonococcal infection. In Holmes KK et al, editors: *Sexually transmitted diseases,* New York, 1984, McGraw-Hill.
18. Mosicki B: HPV infections: an old STD revisited, *Contemp Pediatr* 6:12, 1989.
19. Phillips RS et al: Should tests for *Chlamydia trachomatis* cervical infection be done during routine gynecologic visits? *Ann Intern Med* 107:188, 1987.
20. 1989 Sexually transmitted diseases treatment guidelines, *MMWR* 38(suppl 8):9, 1989.
21. Shafer M et al: Urinary leukocyte esterase screening test for asymptomatic chlamydial and gonococcal infections in males, *JAMA* 262:2562, 1989.
22. Shafer M, Sweet RL: Pelvic inflammatory disease in adolescent females, *Pediatr Clin North Am* 36:513, 1989.
23. Shafer M et al: Evaluation of urine-based screening strategies to detect *Chlamydia trachomatis* among sexually active asymptomatic young males, *JAMA* 270:2065, 1993.
24. Wald ER: Gonorrhea, *Am J Dis Child* 131:1094, 1977.
25. Weström L et al: Incidence, prevalence, and trends of acute pelvic inflammatory disease and its consequences in industrialized countries, *Am J Obstet Gynecol* 66:233, 1985.

SUGGESTED READINGS

Schydlower M, Shafer M: AIDS and other sexually transmitted diseases, *Adolescent Medicine: State of the Art Reviews* 1:409, 1990.

259 Sinusitis

Rickey L. Williams

Infection of the paranasal sinuses in children occurs frequently. Recent estimates suggest that 5% to 10% of upper respiratory tract infections in children are complicated by acute sinusitis.[8] On average, children develop 5 to 10 upper respiratory tract infections yearly, making sinusitis one of the most common problems encountered by the pediatrician.

PATHOPHYSIOLOGY

The paranasal sinuses arise during fetal development as outpouchings beneath the turbinates in the nasopharynx. Only the maxillary and ethmoid sinuses are present at the time of birth, and the sinuses continue to develop and grow until adulthood (Table 259-1). The growth frequently is asymmetrical, and some individuals lack one or more sinuses altogether. Various functions have been ascribed to these sinuses, including warming and humidifying inspired air, trapping inspired particles, secreting mucus, and reducing the weight of the skull.[5]

The lining of the mucosa of the sinuses is similar to that of the nasopharynx, with pseudostratified, ciliated, columnar epithelium interspersed with goblet cells and submucosal glands. The cilia beat toward the ostium of the sinus to expel the mucus and particulate matter contained therein into the nasopharynx.[5]

When the ostia become occluded, the sinus is prone to infection. Sinusitis occurs most frequently after a viral upper respiratory tract infection. The inflammation and edema of the mucous membranes lead to obstruction of the ostium, and the normally sterile sinus cavity is invaded by bacteria. Nasal allergy is another major cause of sinusitis in children. The associated tissue edema, vasodilation, and increased vascular permeability obstruct the ostia of the sinuses, which results in a sinus infection. Other disorders associated with sinusitis in children are listed in the box on p. 1595.

Bacterial pathogens implicated in acute sinusitis are the same as those found in acute otitis media, with *Streptococcus pneumoniae, Moraxella catarrhalis,* and *Haemophilus influenzae* predominating.[7] Anaerobes have been found by Brook[1] to be prevalent in chronic sinusitis, presumably because of the low oxygen content and low pH of fluid retained in the sinus for a long time.

CLINICAL PRESENTATION AND DIAGNOSIS

Children who have either severe or prolonged upper respiratory tract infections are most likely to have sinusitis.[6] Differentiating upper respiratory tract infections or allergic rhinitis from acute sinusitis sometimes is difficult. Most upper respiratory tract infections improve by 5 to 7 days. If symptoms persist without improvement for more than 10 but less than 30 days, a diagnosis of acute sinusitis is made.[9] Cough and nasal discharge are the most common clinical manifestations of acute sinusitis. The cough occurs in the daytime and frequently is worse at night or at any other time when the child is lying supine. The nasal discharge may be clear or purulent. In the infant or young child, fever and irritability following a viral upper respiratory tract infection may be the only manifestations. Malodorous breath, headache, sore throat, a feeling of fullness or pain in the face, and a disturbed sense of smell also suggest the presence of sinusitis.

A less common clinical manifestation of acute sinusitis occurs in children who have severe upper respiratory tract infections. Fever above 39° C, purulent nasal discharge, headache, and eye swelling in a child who has an upper respiratory tract infection suggest the diagnosis of acute sinusitis. Subacute or chronic sinusitis is said to occur if symptoms such as cough and nasal discharge persist more than 30 days.[9]

On physical examination, the nasal mucosa usually is erythematous and swollen, but may be pale and boggy.[8] Mucopurulent material sometimes can be seen draining into the nasopharynx. Palpation of the bones overlying the sinuses may elicit pain.

Transillumination of the maxillary and frontal sinuses is helpful in making the diagnosis of sinusitis in adults and older children; however, the accuracy of transillumination in children younger than 10 years is questionable. A dark room and bright light are used for this technique. To examine the maxillary sinus, the light is placed in the patient's mouth at the center of the hard palate and the lips are closed. Normal sinuses transmit light to the anterior wall of the antrum, giving a "jack-o'-lantern" effect. The frontal sinuses are examined by placing the light below the floor of each sinus. The two sides should be compared, with the examiner keeping in mind that sinus development is asymmetrical in many individuals.[5]

Sinus roentgenograms can help make the diagnosis of sinusitis. When clinical signs and symptoms suggest acute sinusitis and maxillary sinus roentgenograms are abnormal, bacteria is present in a sinus aspirate 75% of the time.[8] With acute inflammation, thickening of the mucous membranes and fluid buildup within the sinus lead to complete or partial opacification, which can be seen roentgenographically. Cysts and polyps also can be seen on sinus roentgenograms.

Computed tomography (CT) imaging of the sinuses is superior to plain radiography, although considerations of cost limit the recommended use of CT to those children whose sinus infections are chronic or complicated. CT has become the primary imaging modality to define anatomical structures before sinus surgery is performed. Currently, the role of magnetic resonance imaging is restricted to the evaluation of complicated sinusitis, intraorbital and intracranial manifestations of aggressive sinusitis, and sinonasal neoplasms.[10]

The diagnosis of sinusitis can be made with certainty only by obtaining a positive culture from sinus aspiration. Nasopharyngeal culture results correlate poorly with sinus culture results. Sinus aspiration and lavage are indicated only in children who fail to respond to conventional antibiotic therapy, in immunosuppressed patients, and in those whose illness is severe or life threatening.

COMPLICATIONS

Complications of sinusitis occur most commonly because of local extension of the disease. Orbital cellulitis is the most common serious complication of sinusitis. The ethmoid sinus is separated from the orbit by the thin *lamina papyracea*. Erosion of this bone leads to invasion of the orbit by bacterial pathogens. Staging of orbital cellulitis is described in Table 259-2. The eyelids appear intensely red and swollen on physical examination. Fever, malaise, and an increased white blood count are present. Orbital pain, proptosis, and limitation of eye movement (ophthlamoplegia) help distinguish this condition from preseptal cellulitis, although computed tomography (CT) scanning may be needed to differentiate the two. Treatment of orbital cellulitis involves parenteral antibiotics; an ophthalmologist and an otolaryngologist should be consulted to determine whether surgical drainage is indicated.[9]

Intracranial infection, most commonly subdural empyema, is the second most common complication of sinusitis. This can occur by direct extension through necrotic bone or by bacterial spread through the venous system. The frontal sinuses are involved most often, making the peak age of incidence of this complication between 10 and 20 years, although it can develop in younger children. Patients have a low-grade fever, malaise, and a frontal headache. Vomiting and a decreased level of consciousness appear as the disease progresses.

In a patient suspected of having an intracranial abscess, CT scanning should be performed. A lumbar puncture should be avoided because of the possibility of brainstem herniation. Treatment in the form of high-dose parenteral antibiotics is required. Neurosurgery is indicated to drain the abscess and to debride necrotic bone. Steroids and hypertonic agents such as mannitol or glycerol are used to control intracranial hypertension.

DISORDERS ASSOCIATED WITH PARANASAL SINUSITIS

1. Anatomical
   a. Nasal malformations
   b. Nasal trauma
   c. Tumors and polyps
   d. Cleft palate
   e. Foreign bodies
   f. Dental infection
   g. Cyanotic congenital heart disease
2. Physiological—barotrauma
3. Abnormalities of local defense mechanisms
   a. Allergy
   b. Cystic fibrosis
   c. Immotile-cilia syndrome and Kartagener syndrome
4. Abnormalities of systemic defense mechanisms—immunodeficiency, primary or secondary

From Shurin PA: *Ann Otol Rhinol Laryngol* 90(suppl 84):72, 1981.

Table 259-1 Sinus Development

Sinus	First appearance	Size (ml) Birth	3 Years	10 Years	14 Years	Age of clinical importance
Maxillary	3 wk of fetal life	0.13	2.5	10.4	11.6	Birth
Ethmoid	6 mo of fetal life	0.06	0.16	2.4	4.8	Birth
Sphenoid	3 mo of fetal life	0.02	0.68	1.8	2.1	5 yr
Frontal	1 yr of life	—	0.08	1.0	3.6	10-12 yr

Modified from Schaeffer JP: *The embryology, development and anatomy of the nose, paranasal sinuses, nasolacrimal passageways and olfactory organ in man,* Philadelphia, 1920, Blakiston.

Table 259-2 Classification of Orbital Cellulitis

Stage	Description
I Inflammatory edema	Inflammatory edema beginning in medial or lateral upper eyelid; usually nontender with only minimal skin changes. No induration, visual impairment, or limitation of extraocular movements.
II Orbital cellulitis	Edema of orbital contents with varying degrees of proptosis, chemosis, limitation of extraocular movement, and visual loss.
III Subperiosteal abscess	Proptosis down and out with signs of orbital cellulitis (usually severe). Abscess beneath the periosteum of the ethmoid, frontal, or maxillary bone (in that order of frequency).
IV Orbital abscess	Abscess within the fat or muscle cone in the posterior orbit. Severe chemosis and proptosis; complete ophthalmoplegia and moderate to severe visual loss present (globe displaced forward or down and out).
V Cavernous sinus thrombosis	Proptosis, globe fixation, severe loss of visual acuity, prostration, signs of meningitis; progresses to proptosis, chemosis, and visual loss in contralateral eye.

From Wald ER et al: *Pediatr Clin North Am* 28:787, 1981; modified from Chandler JR, Langenbrunner DJ, Stevens ER: *Laryngoscope* 80:1414, 1970.

Other less common complications of sinusitis in children include meningitis, osteomyelitis ("Pott puffy tumor"), and cavernous sinus thrombosis.

TREATMENT

Treatment of sinusitis in children involves antimicrobial therapy, symptomatic relief measures, and drainage, if necessary. Antibiotics used in treating sinusitis are the same as those used for acute otitis media (see Table 240-1). Amoxicillin is the drug of choice in those whose sinusitis is uncomplicated in geographic areas where the prevalence of beta-lactamase-producing strains of *H. influenzae* and *M. catarrhalis* is low.[6] Trimethoprim-sulfamethoxazole should not be used if infection with group A streptococci is suspected or proved. Clinical improvement can be expected within 48 to 72 hours. Most patients experience complete resolution of symptoms within 10 days. If the patient's symptoms fail to resolve completely, the patient should be treated until symptom free and then for another 7 days.[9] Decongestants, antihistamines, and saline nose drops have been recommended frequently in an attempt to drain the sinuses, but no proof of the efficacy of these agents exists.[2] In unusually severe cases, parenteral antibiotics such as cefuroxime are required and otolaryngological support is indicated. As with recurrent otitis media, prophylactic low-dose antibiotic regimens to prevent recurrence of acute sinusitis have been recommended, although no scientific studies support this practice.[9] Surgery may be required in cases of medically recalcitrant severe chronic sinusitis in children.[3,4]

REFERENCES

1. Brook I: Bacteriologic features of chronic sinusitis in children, *JAMA* 246:967, 1981.
2. Giebink GS: Childhood sinusitis: pathophysiology, diagnosis and treatment, *Pediatr Infect Dis J* 13(suppl):55, 1994.
3. Lund VJ: Bacterial sinusitis: etiology and management, *Pediatr Infect Dis J* 13(suppl):58, 1994.
4. Parsons DS, Phillips SE: Functional endoscopic surgery in children: a retrospective analysis of results, *Laryngoscope* 103:899, 1993.
5. Rachelefsky GS, Katz RM, Siegel SC: Diseases of paranasal sinuses in children, *Curr Probl Pediatr* 12:1, 1982.
6. Siegel JD: Diagnosis and management of acute sinusitis in children, *Pediatr Infect Dis J* 6:95, 1987.
7. Wald ER: Management of sinusitis in infants and children, *Pediatr Infect Dis J* 7:449, 1988.
8. Wald ER: Sinusitis, *Pediatr Rev* 14:345, 1993.
9. Wald ER: Sinusitis in children, *N Engl J Med* 326:319, 1992.
10. Yousem DM: Imaging of sinonasal inflammatory disease, *Radiology* 188:303, 1993.

260 Spina Bifida

Gregory S. Liptak

Meningomyelocele (myelomeningocele) is a serious and complex congenital malformation, occurring at a rate of 0.4 to 1 case per 1000 live births in the United States.[2,6] The incidence is higher in females, in those of lower socioeconomic status, and in families of English, Irish, or Welsh extraction. The incidence of meningomyelocele (and other neural tube defects) has been declining for the past several decades.

ETIOLOGY

Meningomyelocele belongs to the family of neural tube defects that includes abnormalities of the head (anencephaly, cranial meningocele, encephalocele) and of the spine (spina bifida occulta, meningocele, and meningomyelocele). In spina bifida occulta, the spinal cord and soft tissues are normal, but the vertebral arches are incomplete. In meningocele the spinal cord is normal, but the meninges protrude through abnormal vertebral arches and soft tissue. On rare occasions the meningocele may appear as an anterior mass in the pelvis, abdomen, or thorax. In meningomyelocele, the malformed spinal cord and nerve roots protrude through abnormal vertebral arches and soft tissue. Lipomas or dermoid cysts may accompany the meningomyelocele.

The cause of neural tube defects is unknown, although faulty closure of the neural groove by the twenty-eighth day of gestation seems to be the primary mechanism. The most recent etiological hypothesis is that neural tube defects result from the interaction of many genes (polygenic expression) that can be modified by factors in the fetal (maternal) environment. Assuming an overall incidence of 1 per 1000, the risk for a second affected child from the same parent is 2 or 3 per 100; for a third, it is 10 per 100. An adult who has meningomyelocele has a 2% to 3% chance of having a child who has a neural tube defect—the same risk that exists for the sibling of an affected child.

Environmental factors such as potato blight, organic solvents, aminopterin, valproic acid, and ethanol have been implicated in the origin of neural tube defects; however, maternal malnutrition (especially folic acid deficiency) appears to be the most important variable.[4,25] Meningomyelocele may be seen with certain syndromes, including trisomy 13, trisomy 18, maternal thalidomide and valproate ingestion, and cri du chat syndrome. It also may be associated with cryptorchism, imperforate anus, ventricular septal defect, cleft palate, inguinal hernias, tracheoesophageal fistula, renal anomalies, and diaphragmatic hernia. Most cases, however, are isolated occurrences.

PATHOLOGY

As shown in Figures 260-1 and 260-2, four major malformations account for the findings of meningomyelocele—soft tissue malformation, brain malformation, vertebral body malformation, and spinal cord malformation.

Soft Tissue Malformation

The failure of skin and other soft tissues to close leaves the spinal cord open to infection. The lipomas that occasionally accompany the defect may grow larger, compressing the spinal cord, and may cause progressive neurological symptoms as the child grows. The surgery to cover the cord may itself result in loss of neurological function and may lead to scar tissue that tethers the cord and results in further neurological deterioration as the child grows.

Brain Malformation

Malformation of the brain includes the Arnold-Chiari (type II) deformity, in which the pons and medulla are distorted and elongated and the cerebellar vermis is displaced inferiorly into the spinal canal. This abnormality often is associated with progressive hydrocephalus. Brainstem malformations also may lead to laryngeal nerve palsy and difficulty in swallowing, as well as hypoventilation, apnea, and sudden death. Subtle abnormalities of cranial nerve nuclei may occur in many affected children. Brain malformations also result in the 15% incidence of grand mal seizures experienced by adolescents who have spina bifida.[7]

About 25% of children who have meningomyelocele are born having evidence of hydrocephalus, with an additional 25% to 60% developing such signs within the first year of life.[14] The higher (i.e., the more cephalad) the spinal lesion, the greater the likelihood of hydrocephalus developing. In addition to the usual manifestations of hydrocephalus and complications of shunt placement, strabismus secondary to pressure on the centers that control conjugate gaze occurs in about 50% of children who have hydrocephalus and meningomyelocele. In addition, central precocious puberty develops in many children who have hydrocephalus.

Sudden shunt malfunction in children shunted for hydrocephalus may produce life-threatening elevations of intracranial pressure requiring emergency intervention. Signs and symptoms of acute shunt malfunction include headache, lethargy, irritability, paralysis of upward gaze, sixth cranial nerve palsy, a bulging fontanelle (in infants), and vomiting. Progression to loss of consciousness, abnormal pupillary reflexes, papilledema, deterioration of vital signs, and death may occur rapidly.[14]

Most children who have meningomyelocele have normal overall intelligence quotient (IQ) scores. Yet most of these youngsters have selective cognitive disabilities and score better on verbal than on performance scales. Even those children who have very low performance scores may have surprising verbal fluency, a trait sometimes referred to as the "cocktail party syndrome." Specific cognitive testing often reveals deficiencies of selective visual attention, visual-

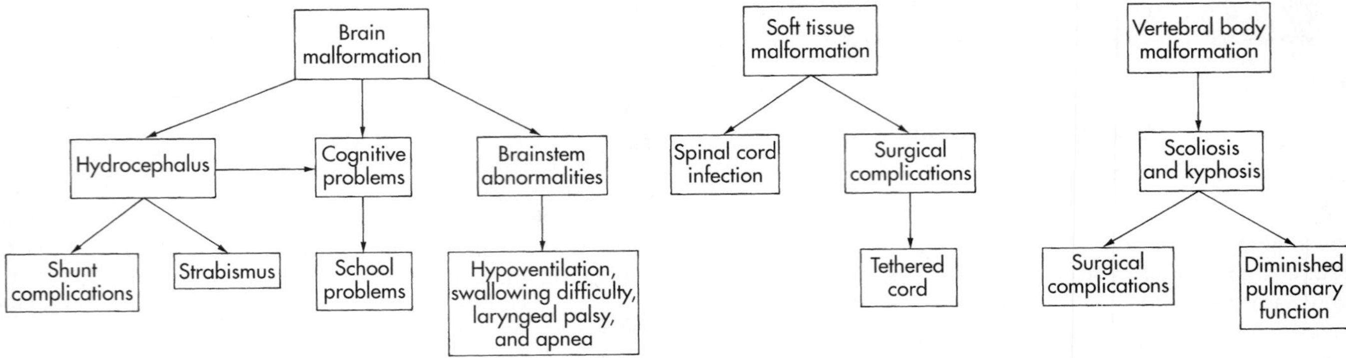

FIG. 260-1 Problems related to meningomyelocele with brain, soft tissue, and vertebral body malformations.

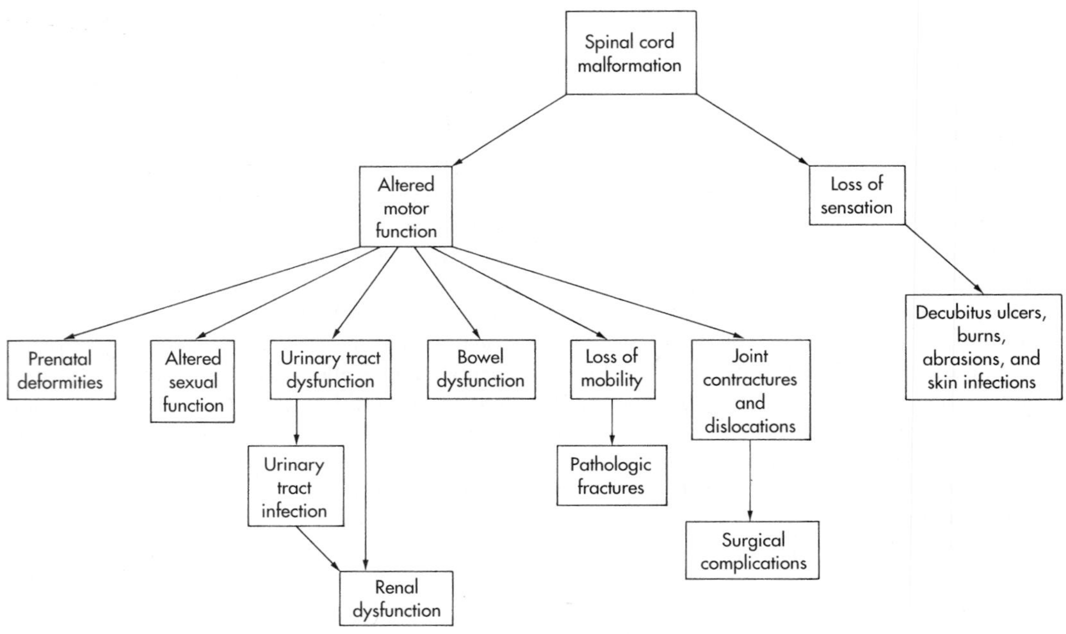

FIG. 260-2 Problems associated with meningomyelocele with spinal cord malformation.

spatial perception, tactile perception, and auditory concentration. Children who have hydrocephalus and higher spinal lesions are more likely to have these deficits. Manifestations seen in school include a short attention span, distractibility, perseveration (the constant repetition of a meaningless word or phrase), and difficulty with subjects requiring visual-motor integration, such as arithmetic.

Vertebral Malformation

Vertebral malformations caused by abnormal segmentation or formation include absent vertebrae, fused vertebrae, hemivertebrae, and butterfly vertebrae. Occasionally, bony or ligamentous spurs lead to diastematomyelia. Of children who have thoracic lesions, 10% are born with kyphosis; by adolescence this rate increases to 33%. Children who have lumbar lesions have a 5% occurrence of kyphosis by adolescence. In addition to cosmetic deformity, severe kyphosis can lead to back pain, pulmonary dysfunction, and recurrent skin ulceration; it also interferes with walking.[20]

The occurrence of scoliosis is related to the level of the lesion, with curves of 30 degrees or more appearing in 81% of adolescents who have thoracic lesions and 23% of those who have lower lumbar lesions. The consequences of scoliosis are similar to those of kyphosis. Lordosis also occurs but is much less common.

Spinal Cord Malformation

Spinal cord malformation results in both loss of sensation and loss of motor function. Loss of sensation leaves these children vulnerable to burns and abrasions. Decubitus ulcers also occur, especially among adolescents and adults who spend large amounts of time in wheelchairs. All three skin lesions are susceptible to infection and may lead to osteomyelitis.

Loss of motor function leads to decreased movement in utero, which may lead to deformities seen at birth, such as clubfoot (talipes equinovarus) and dislocated hip.

Loss of efferent nerve stimuli to the urinary bladder and sphincter results in neurogenic voiding dysfunction in virtually all children who have meningomyelocele. Voiding dysfunction may be classified as (1) failure to store urine or (2) inability to void completely. Failure to store urine may result from a hypotonic urinary outlet or a spastic, hypertonic bladder or both. Inability to void completely may result from spastic urinary sphincter or hypotonic bladder or both. The combination of spastic outlet and hypertonic bladder is especially serious because of the reflux and hydronephrosis that occur frequently with this combination. In addition to incontinence and hydronephrosis, these children have frequent urinary tract infections.[11] These infections lead to fibrosis of the bladder and to chronic renal damage, the most common (spina bifida–related) cause of death in these children beyond the first year of life.[1]

Altered sexual function also occurs, especially in males. Approximately 25% of males who have meningomyelocele are unable to have erections, and of those who can, most have retrograde ejaculation with decreased fertility. Although females have decreased sensation, most can experience orgasm and have normal fertility.

Children who have meningomyelocele usually have fecal incontinence as a result of diminished function of the external rectal sphincter and the levator ani muscles. Most children have intact internal rectal sphincter function, and many have intact rectal sensation. Abnormal migration of neural cells in utero can lead to bowel immotility similar to that seen in Hirschsprung disease.[21] Abnormal rectal function, immobility, and the use of a low-fiber diet because of fear of incontinence may lead to constipation or obstipation with overflow soiling.[15]

Loss of motor function in the lower extremities leads to loss of mobility. The degree of mobility is related closely to the level of the lesion; thus children who have intact quadriceps (L2-4) are much more likely to be ambulatory through adolescence than are those who lack such function.[27] As Table 260-1 illustrates, muscle function around the joints is related directly to the level of the lesion. Contractures and dislocations are more likely to develop in children who have an imbalance of forces around a joint than in those who either have full function or no function. For example, children who have a lesion at the L4-5 level are more likely to develop foot and ankle contractures than are those who have L1-3 or S2-3 lesions. Loss of mobility and innervation also increases the risk for pathological fractures in the lower extremities.

HISTORY

Because meningomyelocele is inherited polygenically, affected newborns may have a family history of neural tube defects or spontaneous abortions (miscarriages). Other historical facts worth noting in the newborn period include length of gestation, type of delivery, complications with and length of labor, maternal nutrition and environmental exposures, current family functioning (including social support and stress), and parental expectations and understanding of the problem. For the older child, information about current and past therapies for neurosurgical, orthopedic, urological, dermatological, and gastrointestinal problems should be obtained. Educational and social functioning at school, relations with peers and with family members, and sexual function and understanding of sexuality should be ascertained. The child's growth, development, mobility, and activities of daily living (personal hygiene, ability to feed oneself, self-help skills) also should be assessed. The onset of new neurological symptoms, such as weakness, change in bowel and bladder function, tripping, and clumsiness, should be sought because these usually indicate treatable conditions such as tethered spinal cord, diastematomyelia, syringomyelia, or ventricular shunt malfunction. Because the prevalence of allergies to latex is high in this population,[28] a history of reactions to products made of latex, such as balloons, bandages, and balls, should be sought.

PHYSICAL EXAMINATION

The backs of *all* children should be examined for pigmented spots, hairy patches, and sinuses that extend into the spine, since these may be signs of occult spinal dysmorphism.[3] These children are at high risk for meningitis and for neurological deterioration secondary to diastematomyelia, lipoma, and tethering of the spinal cord.

Children who have meningomyelocele should have a complete physical examination that emphasizes neurological, orthopedic, and developmental aspects. The *neurological examination* should include motor function (Table 260-1) and sensory level. A rectal examination and assessment of anal wink can assist in the evaluation of lesions at S2-4. Upper extremity strength, including grip, should be assessed because deterioration may indicate syringomyelia. Palpation of the anterior fontanelle, visualization of the eyegrounds via an ophthalmoscope, assessment of the cranial nerves (especially of extraocular movements), and palpation of the shunt valve and tubing may help evaluate shunt functioning.

The orthopedic examination should include an assessment of posture (scoliosis, lordosis, kyphosis) as well as of joint mobility and stability. Erythema and swelling of a joint or bone in an area that lacks sensation represent a fracture until proved otherwise.[20] The skin should be examined for evidence of sores and ulcers in insensate areas.

Formal and informal developmental assessments should be part of the routine examination of these children and should include visual-spatial functioning and verbal, performance, and educational measures, as well as the more standard areas—fine motor, gross motor, language, and social-adaptive skills.

LABORATORY DATA

Laboratory assessments of the newborn should include measurement of length, weight, and head circumference—the latter, daily. Ultrasound or computed tomography (CT) scan or both of the head, roentgenograms of the spine and hips, and a urine culture also should be performed. The kidneys should be examined by ultrasound or intravenous pyelography (IVP) or both. As the child grows, urine and urine cultures should be analyzed routinely, and head circumference, height, and weight should be monitored. Some clinicians recommend substituting arm span for height because growth below the waist is disproportionately slow. A CT scan of the head should be performed routinely to detect asymptomatic ventricular enlargement. The condition of the spine and joints

Table 260-1 Correlation Between Function and Level of Motor Involvement

Functional area—level of lesion	Bowel and bladder function	Toe intrinsics	Foot: Dorsiflexion—inversion	Foot: Plantar flexion—eversion
S2-3	±*	±	+*	±
S1-2	−*	−	+	±
L5-S1	−	−	+	−
L4-5	−	−	±	−
L3-4	−	−	−	−
L2-3	−	−	−	−
L1-2	−	−	−	−

*±, May be present; +, present; −, absent.

should be monitored by roentgenograms. The kidneys should be screened by using routine renal ultrasound (or IVP), voiding cystourethrograms, and urodynamics.

Special studies that may be indicated include (1) grip strength measurement to monitor for syringomyelia, (2) skinfold thickness measurements to evaluate nutritional status, (3) magnetic resonance imaging (MRI)[24] or CT scan of the spine, and (4) injection of radiopaque dye into the shunt and measurement of pressure to evaluate its function. A child who has signs and symptoms suggestive of ventricular shunt malfunction should have a head CT scan and a shunt series (to evaluate the integrity of the tubing) performed.

PSYCHOSOCIAL CONSIDERATIONS

The birth of a child who has meningomyelocele is potentially devastating.[17] Most parents are shocked and begin a journey through a series of phases characteristic of people undergoing a loss (in this case a loss of the expected normal child). These stages include shock, denial, sadness, anger, and guilt, and ultimately, acceptance and equilibrium.[12] In addition to grieving, parents must share in difficult medical decisions. For these reasons parents require support from medical professionals and others. An evaluation of their current levels of social support and the presence of other stressors is critical in helping them through this time. Because most children who have meningomyelocele have multiple medical problems, they require the expenditure of large amounts of money,[5] time, patience, and understanding. Such demands stress parents and can lead to isolation of one from the other. This isolation may be reinforced by a medical system that sees patients during working hours and that is content to deal exclusively with mothers.[10] The stresses also may affect siblings, who may have an increased occurrence of behavioral problems.

Parents may begin mourning but never reach equilibrium, and the clinician may notice manifestations of denial, guilt, or anger. In addition, one spouse may be able to reach equilibrium but be emotionally unavailable to the spouse still struggling with the earlier stages.[12]

The child who has meningomyelocele may have difficulty at home with parents unable to provide affection or set consistent limits. They may have difficulty with peers who see them as "cripples" rather than as children who have disabilities. They may have difficulty performing academically and may lose interest in school because of frequent negative reinforcement. They may have no adult role models. Finally, they may lose self-esteem from frequent visits to clinicians—visits that often are characterized by the identification of new problems without any positive reinforcement of their successes.

MANAGEMENT[14]

The two goals in the management of these patients are (1) to prevent dysfunctions (e.g., physiological and biochemical defects) from becoming disabilities (the functional consequences of the impairment, e.g., "can't walk") and (2) to prevent the disabilities from becoming handicaps (the social disadvantages experienced from the disabilities, e.g., "can't get a job"). Achieving these goals requires comprehensive, coordinated care,[10] as well as routine care such as immunizations and anticipatory guidance.[23]

The newborn and family should be evaluated by a team, usually consisting of a pediatrician, nurse, social worker, neurosurgeon, orthopedist, physical therapist, and urologist. Once the neonate has been examined and given supportive care, central nervous system infection must be prevented. Parenteral antibiotics that provide coverage against gram negative bacilli and *Staphylococcus aureus* organisms should be provided as soon as possible. Surgery to close the open defect may occur within the first 72 hours of life.

Daily measurement of the head circumference and ultrasound or CT scan of the head should be used as guides for ventriculoperitoneal shunt placement to reduce hydrocephalus. No universally accepted criteria exist to determine the need for or the timing of shunt placement. Furosemide (Lasix) and acetazolamide (Diamox) may be administered to transiently delay the insertion of the shunt if the child cannot tolerate surgery.[26]

Deformities such as clubfeet or dislocated hips should be managed with range-of-motion exercises, splinting, and casting. The urological system should be evaluated by urine culture and renal ultrasound or IVP. Baseline roentgenograms of the spine and hips should be taken. Genetic counseling and social support should be provided to the family, and assistance with finances should be a priority. As the child grows, the primary care physician should coordinate the child's care and be his or her advocate.[10] Enhancing environmental stimulation for the maximization of cognitive de-

Knee		Hip			
Extension	Flexion	Flexion	Adduction	Abduction	Extension
+	+	+	+	+	+
+	+	+	+	+	±
+	±	+	+	+	−
+	−	+	+	−	−
+	−	+	+	−	−
±	−	±	±	−	−
−	−	−	−	−	−

velopment should be another goal in the care of these children. In many instances, children may benefit from formal early intervention programs. Opportunities for interactions with people and objects (toys) should be provided. Similarly, the child should be encouraged to develop the best social interaction and self-help skills possible, including the development of independence in hygiene and eating.

According to Bronfenbrenner,[8] learning and development are facilitated by the participation of the developing person in progressively more complex patterns of reciprocal activity with someone with whom that person has developed a strong and enduring emotional attachment and when the balance of power gradually shifts in favor of the developing person.

A child who has a disability has the same psychosocial needs as healthy children, and the clinician should help the family achieve this shifting of power. Although the child's environment should be conducive to learning and exploration, exclusive concern with formal teaching or special programs actually may inhibit those self-directed activities that should be encouraged.

Orthopedic management may include surgery for joint contractures, scoliosis, or kyphosis. To prevent contractures and dislocations, regular passive range-of-motion exercises, splints, body jackets, and casts may be used.[20]

Various exercises and orthoses (braces) may be used to enhance locomotion. The parapodium—a standing brace that allows the child to be in an upright position with hands unencumbered—and reciprocal gait orthosis can be started between 18 and 24 months of age.[16,27] Crutches or walkers that have more standard bracing may be used, and some treatment centers advocate early use of the wheelchair, especially for those children who have quadriceps paralysis. Adaptive equipment such as carts and hand-pedaled tricycles also can enhance the function and self-esteem of these children.

Goals of urological management include prevention of renal damage and attainment of continence.[11] In the past, urinary diversion via ileal loops was performed in most children who had meningomyelocele to achieve these goals. Clean intermittent catheterization, introduced in 1972, is safer, is more acceptable, and results in better renal function than does urinary diversion.[1,19] Vesicotomy may be indicated in the infant who has vesicoureteral reflux or hydronephrosis or both. Most families are able to perform clean intermittent catheterization when the child is 4 to 5 years of age, and many children, even those this young, are able to perform the procedure themselves. Clean intermittent catheterization also has been used in children under 3 years of age and can be helpful in the management of vesicoureteral reflux with or without hydronephrosis or in those who have frequent urinary tract infections.[13] The addition of drugs that relax the detrusor muscle or increase sphincter tone, such as imipramine hydrochloride, oxybutinin chloride, or pseudoephedrine, can enhance continence. For older children in whom catheterization does not provide continence, the use of a surgical procedure such as bladder augmentation plus the creation of a continent stoma with clean intermittent catheterization, may provide continence.[9]

Obtaining regular urine cultures to detect urinary tract infection and administering prophylactic antibiotics in those children who have frequent infections may prevent renal damage. Trimethoprim-sulfamethoxazole, sulfisoxazole, nitrofurantoin, and cephalexin given in less than the therapeutic dosage have been used for prophylaxis.

Bowel continence after 4 years of age and avoidance of severe constipation often is difficult to achieve. However, a high fiber diet, stool softeners, regular toileting, regular stimulants, and biofeedback in those children who have rectal sensation may be used singly or in combination to attain these goals. Regular enemas, using 20 ml/kg of normal saline, have been shown to be effective in many children.[15] A new surgical procedure removes the appendix, opens its distal end, and uses it to create a "fistula" between the colon and the abdominal wall. The fistula allows forward-flowing irrigation of the colon on a regular basis and shows promise for a select group of children and adolescents in whom more conventional constipation-relieving techniques have failed.

Impotence in the male may be managed surgically via penile implants, vacuum pumps, and the injection of prostaglandin. Pregnant women who have meningomyelocele may need to have their babies delivered by cesarean section because of hip contractures. Their intervertebral disks also may become herniated, with neurological sequelae, and therefore they should have frequent neurological evaluations throughout pregnancy.

Because more than 50% of children who have meningomyelocele may have allergies to latex,[28] including anaphylaxis during surgery, contact with products made from latex should be avoided. For example, all surgical procedures should occur in latex-free settings; children who demonstrate latex sensitivity should receive intravenous dexamethasone, diphenhydramine, and ranitidine before any operative procedure. Catheterization should be performed with nonlatex catheters; gloves used during care should be of nonlatex material; toys that contain significant amounts of latex should be avoided, as should products that contact the skin, such as band-aids or ace bandages.

Even though the execution of all these interventions requires tremendous resources and effort, they still may be inadequate in the absence of social changes. To prevent disabilities from becoming handicaps, society's attitudes and practices must be altered. The clinician can advocate for these children by helping remove architectural barriers in the community, which will allow disabled people access to places such as banks, public buildings, transportation, and recreation areas. Altering the attitudes of nondisabled people may be more difficult, but the clinician can help to enable the disabled child and adult to serve as role models in the community—for instance, by encouraging the hiring of disabled workers. Performing all the above tasks requires constant effort and can be achieved only with a multidisciplinary team that is willing to collaborate with the family.

PREVENTION

Periconceptual supplementation of the diets of mothers of children who have neural tube defects has been shown to decrease the recurrence of these defects and may prevent the primary occurrence of such defects as well. The American Academy of Pediatrics recommends that all women of childbearing age receive 0.4 mg of folic acid daily. Mothers of children who have a neural tube defect should receive 4.0 mg folic acid daily.

Open neural tube defects may be diagnosed prenatally by the measuring of alpha-fetoprotein levels in maternal serum between 14 and 16 weeks of gestation, coupled with confirmation of the diagnosis via ultrasound. Amniocentesis is recommended for those who have elevated serum alpha-fetoprotein levels in order to confirm the diagnosis. The prenatal detection of a neural tube defect allows the family to plan rationally, whether or not they elect to continue the pregnancy.[22] If they elect to deliver, the fetus should be monitored for the development of hydrocephalus, which may be treated in utero, and the infant may benefit from cesarean section to avoid trauma to the head and back.[18] Social support should be provided to these families, whatever their decision.

REFERENCES

1. Action Committee on Myelodysplasia, Section on Urology: Current approaches to evaluation and management with meningomyelocele, *Pediatrics* 63:663, 1979.
2. Yen IH et al: The changing epidemiology of neural tube defects, United States, 1968-1989, *Am J Dis Child* 146:857, 1992.
3. Albright AL, Gartner JC, Wiener ES: Lumbar cutaneous hemangiomas as indicators of tethered spinal cords, *Pediatrics* 83:977, 1989.
4. American Academy of Pediatrics Committee on Genetics: Folic acid for the prevention of neural tube defects, *Pediatrics* 92:493, 1993.
5. Anonymous: Economic burden of spina bifida: United States, 1980-1990, *MMWR* 38:264, 1989.
6. Bamforth SJ, Baird PA: Spina bifida and hydrocephalus: a population study over a 35-year period, *Am J Hum Genet* 44:225, 1989.
7. Bartoshesky LE et al: Seizures in children with meningomyelocele, *Am J Dis Child* 139:400, 1985.
8. Bronfenbrenner U: *The ecology of human development,* Cambridge, Mass, 1979, Harvard University Press.
9. Cher ML, Allen TD: Continence in the myelodysplastic patient following enterocystoplasty, *J Urol* 149:1103, 1993.
10. Colgan MT: The child with spina bifida: role of the pediatrician, *Am J Dis Child* 135:854, 1982.
11. Ehrlich O, Brem AS: A prospective comparison of urinary tract infection in patients treated with either clean intermittent catheterization or urinary diversion, *Pediatrics* 70:665, 1982.
12. Irvin NA, Kennell JH, Klaus MH: Caring for the parents of an infant with a congenital malformation. In Klaus MH, Kennell JH, editors: *Parent-infant bonding,* ed 2, St Louis, 1982, Mosby.
13. Lin-Dyken DC et al: Follow-up of clean intermittent catheterization for children with neurogenic bladders, *Urology* 40:525, 1992.
14. Liptak GS et al: The management of children with spinal dysraphism, *J Child Neurol* 3:3, 1988.
15. Liptak GS, Revell GM: Management of bowel dysfunction in children with spinal cord disease or injury using the enema continence catheter, *J Pediatr* 120:190, 1992.
16. Liptak GS et al: Mobility aids in children with high-level meningomyelocele: parapodium versus wheelchair, *Dev Med Child Neurol* 34:787, 1992.
17. McCormick MC, Charney EB, Stemmler MM: Assessing the impact of a child with spina bifida on the family, *Dev Med Child Neurol* 28:53, 1986.
18. McCurdy CM Jr, Seeds JW: Route of delivery of infants with congenital anomalies, *Clin Perinatol* 20:81, 1993.
19. McLorie GA et al: Determinants of hydronephrosis and renal injury in patients with myelomeningocele, *J Urol* 140:1289, 1988.
20. Menelaus MB: *The orthopaedic management of spina bifida cystica,* New York, 1980, Churchill Livingstone.
21. Merkles RG, Solish SB, Scherzer AL: Meningomyelocele and Hirschsprung disease: theoretical and clinical significance, *Pediatrics* 76:299, 1985.
22. Milunsky A: Prenatal detection of neural tube defects. VI. Experience with 20,000 pregnancies, *JAMA* 244:2731, 1980.
23. Raddish M et al: The immunization status of children with spina bifida, *Am J Dis Child* 147:849, 1993.
24. Rindahl MA et al: Magnetic resonance imaging of pediatric dysraphism, *Magn Reson Imaging* 7:217, 1989.
25. Rush D: Periconceptional folate and neural tube defects, *Am J Clin Nutr* 59(suppl 2):511, 1994.
26. Shinnar S et al: Management of hydrocephalus in infancy: use of acetazolamide and furosemide to avoid cerebrospinal fluid shunts, *J Pediatr* 107:31, 1985.
27. Shurtleff DB: Mobility. In Shurtleff DB, editor: *Myelodysplasia and exstrophies: significance, prevention, and treatment,* New York, 1986, Grune & Stratton.
28. Tosi LL et al: Latex allergy in spina bifida patients: prevalence and surgical implications, *J Pediatr Orthop* 13:709, 1993.

261 Spinal Deformities

Edward M. Sills

Back pain in children usually is a sign of an underlying disorder. Postural abnormalities may or may not indicate an underlying disorder, and the challenge to the physician is to determine whether the child's posture is caused by an underlying skeletal deformity or merely is a habit that exaggerates increases or decreases in the normal spinal curves. Abnormal curvatures and protrusions merit careful investigation. The thoracic spine normally has some kyphosis, and the lumbar spine normally has slight lordosis. If either condition is excessive, progressive, or painful, concern is appropriate. Scoliosis, a side-to-side curve, always is abnormal (see the box on p. 1604 for a classification of spinal deformity).

CONGENITAL MALFORMATIONS

The newborn is relaxed when placed prone in the examiner's palm. The infant's back falls into slight flexion, allowing detection of meningomyelocele, congenital scoliosis, kyphosis, or dorsolumbar hyperflexion. Lumbar spinal deformity may be indicated by a hair tuft, dimple, discoloration, or a palpable spina bifida lamina defect.

Congenital scoliosis is the result of asymmetrical growth. It is characterized by a lateral curvature of the spine caused by the asymmetrical structural vertebral deformity. The curve is fixed and inflexible. When located near the middle of the spine, the segments of the spine above and below compensate for it by curving in the opposite direction. The result is a balanced spine and a straight back. Treatment is unnecessary. When, however, the asymmetrical vertebra is at the base of the spine, the compensatory curve that develops above is insufficient, and a curvature progresses as the patient grows. This condition requires surgical correction before adolescence. When the deformity occurs in the cervical spine, a "wryneck" deformity results, and thoracolumbar compensatory curvature severely distorts posture. Unilateral surgical fusions are required to minimize deformity.

Congenital kyphosis is caused by lack of segmentation of vertebral bodies anteriorly or by lack of formation of a vertebral body. Surgical fusion is required to prevent paraplegia.

Other congenital malformations of the spine include the *Klippel-Feil* syndrome, which is characterized by a short neck, limitation of head motion, and a low posterior hairline. Spina bifida often is present in the cervical spine; it is caused by failure of the two lateral halves of the vertebral arch to fuse. Exercises to maintain the neck's functional range of motion are indicated, but surgery is contraindicated because of the danger of injuring the cervical spinal cord. *Spina bifida* can be mild and of no clinical significance (occulta), or it can be severe (vera) with meningeal and neural elements protruding posteriorly. When the protrusion includes bony elements, it may transfix the spinal cord. This transfixing spur is called *diastematomyelia.* These severe forms of spina bifida require prompt neurosurgical correction.

Congenital vertebral anomalies also are seen in several syndromes in which other anomalies may be present. These include the following:

1. Larsen syndrome—vertebral, joint, facial, and palate
2. Waardenburg syndrome—spine and ribs
3. Goldenhar syndrome—oculoauriculovertebral dysplasia
4. Morquio syndrome (mucopolysaccharidosis, type IV)—odontoid dysplasia with atlantoaxial subluxation

ACQUIRED ABNORMALITIES

Scoliosis

Scoliosis can be nonstructural (corrects with side bending) or structural (no improvement with position change). Nonstructural scoliosis results from posture habit, splinting because of pain, muscle spasm, or hysteria. Of the structural forms of scoliosis, the congenital (e.g., absent or fused spinal segments), metabolic (e.g., juvenile osteoporosis), or neuromuscular (e.g., poliomyelitis or cerebral palsy) types are less common than idiopathic scoliosis, which accounts for 75% of all cases. Although most cases are idiopathic, an increased familial risk exists for scoliosis. Idiopathic scoliosis can appear clinically at any age, although the majority of cases begin in adolescence and affect mostly girls, who usually exhibit a right thoracic or right thoracolumbar pattern. The infantile form begins before age 3 years, is predominant in boys, and usually resolves without treatment because of vertebral compensations above and below the area of curve. The juvenile form occurs between ages 6 and 10 years, has no gender predilection, and usually consists of a right thoracic curve. Although some of the mild curves do not progress, the juvenile and adolescent curves tend to rapidly progress during growth spurts.

The condition usually is painless and is discovered on routine physical examinations or at school scoliosis screening programs. When the patient bends forward, prominence of one scapula, of one side of the rib cage, or of the lumbar paraspinous muscles can indicate the site and direction of the scoliosis. An erect anteroposterior spinal roentgenogram determines the degree of curvature and the structure of the vertebrae.

Treatment is undertaken because pulmonary restriction, significant back pain, and cosmetic deformity are the sequelae of unrecognized and untreated scoliosis. Exercises are of no benefit in retarding or reversing the progress of scoliosis. A curvature in excess of 40 degrees requires surgical fusion regardless of the patient's age. Curves between 20 and 40 degrees should not require treatment if skeletal maturation is complete, but they should be braced in the growing

CLASSIFICATION OF SPINAL DEFORMITY

A. Idiopathic
  1. Infantile
  2. Juvenile
  3. Adolescent
B. Neuromuscular
  1. Neuropathic
    a. Upper motor neuron lesion
      (1) Cerebral palsy
      (2) Spinocerebellar degenerations
      (3) Syringomyelia
      (4) Spinal cord tumor
      (5) Spinal cord trauma
    b. Lower motor neuron lesion
      (1) Poliomyelitis
      (2) Other viral myelitis
      (3) Trauma
      (4) Spinal muscular atrophy
      (5) Meningomyelocele (paralytic)
    c. Dysautonomia (Riley-Day)
  2. Myopathic
    a. Arthrogryposis
    b. Muscular dystrophy
    c. Fiber-type disproportion
    d. Congenital hypotonia
    e. Myotonia dystrophica
C. Congenital
  1. Congenital scoliosis
    a. Failure of formation
      (1) Wedge
      (2) Hemivertebra
    b. Failure of segmentation
      (1) Unilateral bar
      (2) Bilateral bar
  2. Congenital kyphosis
    a. Failure of formation
    b. Failure of segmentation
    c. Mixed

C. Congenital—*cont'd*
  3. Congenital lordosis
  4. Associated with neural tissue defect
    a. Meningomyelocele
    b. Meningocele
    c. Spinal dysraphism (diastematomyelia)
D. Neurofibromatosis
E. Mesenchymal
  1. Marfan syndrome
  2. Ehlers-Danlos syndrome
F. Traumatic
  1. Fracture or dislocation
  2. After irradiation
  3. After laminectomy
G. Soft tissue contractures
  1. After thoracoplasty
  2. Burns
H. Osteochondrodystrophies
  1. Achondroplasia
  2. Spondyloepiphyseal dysplasia
  3. Diastrophic dwarfism
  4. Mucopolysaccharidosis
I. Scheuermann disease
J. Infection
K. Tumor
L. Rheumatoid disease
M. Metabolic
  1. Rickets
  2. Juvenile osteoporosis
  3. Osteogenesis imperfecta
N. Lumbosacral anomalies
O. Hysterical
P. Functional
  1. Postural
  2. Secondary to short limb
  3. Secondary to pain

Modified from Scoliosis Research Society.

child. A curve milder than 20 degrees should be observed for possible progression but does not require treatment.

Kyphosis

An acquired dorsal hump can be secondary to a spinal tumor, radiation, infection, or surgery. The most common cause of acquired kyphosis is an osteochondrosis known as Scheuermann disease (see Chapter 238), which occurs in 5% of the population. The most common site is in the lower thoracic vertebrae, but this condition can occur in any site in the vertebral column. The initial event is a bulging of the intervertebral disks in the direction of contiguous vertebral bodies, which exerts pressure against the cartilage plates covering the bodies, causing thinning of the plates. This interferes with endochondral bone formation on the growth surface of the plates, causing gaps that are the basis for the herniation of the disk into the bodies, isolating the apophyseal ossification center from the vertebral body. The disk space narrows, more so anteriorly, causing increased pressure on the anterior portions of contiguous vertebral bodies and impeding their longitudinal growth anteriorly, resulting in attendant kyphosis.

An aching pain aggravated by physical exertion is present in the affected part of the vertebral column. The affected area is tender to palpation. Having the patient assume a stooping position often causes the pain to increase. Once the backache has been present for a year or so, the kyphosis easily is apparent as a round-back deformity. In many instances the pain is so minor that the patient first complains to the physician about pain caused by "poor posture," and then the kyphosis is noted. Roentgenograms reveal a narrowing of the anterior disk space and defects on the surfaces of adjacent vertebrae at sites where the disk tissue has penetrated the bodies. The prolapsed disk tissue, in time, becomes walled off by osseous tissue, forming a bulbous mass of extruded tissue appearing as an area of lucency in the affected body (Schmorl nodule). In some children the deformity can progress to cause severe deformity and dysfunction; in others, the condition stabilizes and the deformity may disappear. Treatment is aimed at preventing further deformity, occasionally by using casting or bracing. In those rare instances of rapid progression or very severe pain, spinal fusion is necessary. The majority of youngsters, however, require careful observation and intervention only if progression of the deformity is noted.

BACK PAIN

Although scoliosis and kyphosis can be painful, usually they are painless postural deformities. The pediatrician should be aware of several painful disorders related to spinal deformity (see also Chapter 114, Back Pain).

Spondylolysis and Spondylolisthesis

Spondylolysis, a defect in the continuity of the pars interarticularis of the posterior portion of L4 or L5, may result in forward slippage of the vertebral body, known as spondylolisthesis. The horizontal slippage usually involves the fifth lumbar vertebral body moving anteriorly in relationship to S1. This deformity, however, can occur anywhere in the vertebral column. Spondylolysis often causes back pain before the spondylolisthesis develops. Trauma, causing disruption of the pars interarticularis, is believed to be the cause of spondylolysis in a genetically susceptible host. The propensity for spondylolysis to become spondylolisthesis with forward slippage is exaggerated during growth spurts.

A flattening of the normal lumbar lordosis with posterior tilting of the pelvis is noted in spondylolysis. An oblique roentgenogram reveals the effect of the pars interventricularis on spondylolysis; a standing lateral roentgenogram demonstrates spondylolisthesis. Activities that hyperextend the lumbar spine should be avoided, and exercises to reduce lumbar lordosis relieve the pain of spondylolysis. Once slippage occurs, surgical spinal fusion is necessary.

Infections

Infections involving the spinal structures are exceedingly rare. Acute pyogenic osteomyelitis and tuberculosis cause bone destruction, initially in the anterior portion of the vertebrae, leading to collapse. Vigorous antibiotic therapy and immobilization are indicated.

Disk space inflammation, or *diskitis,* can appear as a fever of unknown origin accompanied by a limp or low back pain. Narrowing of the disk space is the usual roentgenographic finding. In all cases, blood cultures are indicated. The majority of younger patients do not evidence bacterial infection and require only immobilization. Children older than age 8 years occasionally are found to have a staphylococcal disease. The indications for using antibiotics include positive blood culture results, recurrences of back pain accompanied by systemic signs such as fever, leukocytosis with a "left shift" in the differential white blood cell count, or clinical advancement of disease despite immobilization.

Tumors

Bone tumors occur most commonly in adolescence and usually appear at the end of growth peaks. Of the malignant bone tumors, none primarily involves the spine, although chondrosarcomas and the marrow tumors (leukemias, lymphomas, Ewing tumor, and histiocytic lymphoma) often invade the pelvis early and can cause low back pain in adolescence.

Roentgenograms display bony lesions surrounded by soft tissue mass. Calcification of periosteum lifted away from bone causes a characteristic sunburst appearance.

Of the nonmalignant tumors, the osteogenic group often involves the spine. Both osteoid osteoma and osteoblastoma are reparative rather than infiltrative. Osteoid osteoma occurs in long bones and in the posterior position of the vertebrae; osteoblastoma occurs in the neural arches of the vertebral column. Pain, usually occurring at night, is the common complaint and is relieved quickly by aspirin. On roentgenogram, the examiner sees a hyperostotic lesion surrounding a nidus of sclerotic bone separated by a radiolucent zone. Surgical excision is curative.

SUGGESTED READINGS

Burgos-Vargas R, Petty RE: Juvenile ankylosing spondylitis, *Rheum Dis Clin North Am* 18:123, 1992.

Hensinger RN: Current concept review: spondylolysis and spondylolisthesis in children and adolescents, *J Bone Joint Surg [Am]* 71:1098, 1989.

King HA: Evaluating the child with back pain, *Pediatr Clin North Am* 33:1489, 1986.

Letts M et al: Fractures of the pars interarticularis in adolescent athletes: a clinical-biomedical analysis, *J Pediatr Orthop* 6:40, 1986.

Papanicolaov N et al: Bone scintigraphy and radiography in young athletes with low back pain, *Am J Roentgenol* 145:1039, 1985.

Portenoy RK et al: Back pain in the cancer patient: an algorithm for evaluation and management, *Neurology* 37:134, 1987.

Riseborough E, Herndon JH: *Scoliosis and other deformities: deformities of the axial skeleton,* Boston, 1975, Little, Brown.

Schmorl G: *The human spine in health and disease,* New York, 1959, Grune & Stratton.

Sills EM: What's causing the back pain? *Contemp Pediatr* 5:85, 1988.

Sward L et al: Back pain and radiologic changes in the thoracolumbar spine of athletes, *Spine* 15:124, 1990.

Tachdjian M: *Pediatric orthopedics,* Philadelphia, 1979, WB Saunders.

Williams HJ: Vertebral epiphysitis, *Am J Roentgenol* 90:1236, 1963.

262 Sports Injuries

David E. Hall

More than 5 million young people participate in high school sports each year. According to one study, more than 2% of all visits to pediatric offices are for recreational injuries.[9] Estimates of the frequency of injuries vary widely.

An estimated 10% to 20% of high school athletes sustain an injury that keeps them out of participation for longer than a week.[20] Wrestling and football have the highest significant injury rates per participant in high school, followed by softball, gymnastics, track and field, and soccer. Tennis and swimming produce the fewest injuries.[7] Other sports fall somewhere in between. Frequency of injury, however, is not always the best measure of a sport's risk. The trampoline, for example, accounts for a disproportionately large number of injures that cause paralysis.[6]

Most injuries occur during practice, but competitive events have the highest hourly injury rates.[7] An important determinant of injury is lack of conditioning and recent entry into a sport.[6] The lower extremities are injured the most commonly.[3] Soft tissue injuries, especially sprains and strains, account for the vast majority of injuries and thus may be treated by the primary care physician who has learned basic anatomy and the principles of treatment. Many physicians, unfamiliar with the demands of a particular sport, overtreat and keep the patient out of competition too long. On the other hand, the physician may be pressured by overzealous parents or patients to allow the child to return to activities too soon. Another common mistake is failure to provide appropriate exercises for rehabilitation because many physicians are not familiar with this aspect of care.

Sports medicine is a discipline in itself. This chapter can serve as only an introduction to some of the more common problems. The reader is referred to texts on sports medicine for information on treatment and exercises for rehabilitation.[8,10,19] Sports medicine centers, present in many urban areas, provide consultation and continuing education for interested physicians.

GENERAL PRINCIPLES OF PREVENTION

Pediatricians have become aware that the organization of sports leagues for children—for example, in baseball, football, and soccer—has become so much a part of middle-class American life that, in some ways, it has become the driving force in the experience of many children and adolescents—a force that has thrown the reason for participating in athletics out of context. A potentially marvelous contribution to a child's physical, emotional, and social well-being is distorted by overemphasis, the drive to excel within overorganized, highly structured leagues, the sometimes overzealous participation of parents, and the push to win. Pediatricians can contribute to prevention if they work with the families they serve to provide a context for the participation of children, a context that allows for vigorous effort, enthusiastic participation, and a reawakening, perhaps, of the old Grantland Rice advice that it's how one plays the game that matters, not winning. Given this proper context, the child and the family can anticipate a happier time with less emotional battering and less likelihood of physical injury. This requires the physician to take a sensitive history and subsequently develop insights that can lead to better understanding and therefore to better management.

CLASSIFICATION OF INJURIES

Ligaments connect one bone to another. *Sprains* are injuries to ligaments. *Strains,* on the other hand, are tearing injuries to a muscle or its tendon. Sprains usually are caused by an outside force and are most common in contact sports, whereas strains are dynamic injuries not caused by an outside force. They may be encountered in timed sports such as swimming or running or with overzealous weight lifting. Strains and sprains may be classified as grades 1 through 3 (Table 262-1). Primary care physicians usually can treat grade 1 and most grade 2 injuries.

Most fractures that occur in athletes are not complicated, but many primary care physicians do not feel comfortable treating them and depend on the orthopedist for definitive treatment. Few fractures heal in less than 4 to 6 weeks.

Other types of injuries include *overuse syndromes,* such as tennis elbow, which are associated with excessive or inappropriate use of a body part, often brought about by a recent change in the athlete's activities; *contusions,* which result from a blow to a muscle or bone and result in a painful, swollen area; and *dislocations.* Dislocations may damage surrounding ligaments significantly. Joints having range of motion in few planes (e.g., the knee) are more severely damaged when dislocated than are joints having range of motion in several planes (e.g., the shoulder). Dislocations usually result from an outside force.

DATA BASE

The wise physician obtains a detailed history of the mechanism of injury. Orthopedists use this information, for example, to reduce a fracture or dislocation by reversing the force that led to the injury. Other important information includes the location, character, severity, and radiation of any pain. Was the onset sudden or insidious? What relieves or aggravates the pain? Has the injury occurred before? The sensation or sound of a pop or snap suggests a serious injury. Obtain a brief medical history to rule out illnesses that might complicate treatment. On physical examination, look for any disorders of alignment that may have predisposed the patient to the injury. Note the location of swelling, tenderness, or discoloration. Abnormal bulges in muscle groups may signify a ruptured muscle. Determine the range of motion of the

Table 262-1 Classification of Sprains and Strains

	Sprains	Strains
Grade 1	Minimal tearing of ligament No instability of joint End point present on testing of ligament integrity	Microscopic disruptions of musculotendinous unit No defect on physical examination
Grade 2	Appreciable tearing of ligament (5%-99% of fibers disrupted) with moderate joint instability Testing of instability causes pain End point present on testing of ligament integrity	Some tearing of musculotendinous unit Partial loss of function on examination
Grade 3	Complete tear of ligament with absolute joint instability Testing stability of joint causes little pain No clear end point on testing of ligament integrity	Complete rupture of musculotendinous unit May have little pain after a few minutes but dramatic initial sensation of injury

affected joints and look for instability. Evaluate the integrity of veins and blood vessels.

During the physical examination, keep in mind the possibility of anabolic steroid use. An extensive survey of steroid use in the United States found a prevalence of 6.6% among twelfth grade males.[2] Signs of anabolic steroid use include a sudden flare up of acne, evidence of liver disease such as jaundice, rapid gains in muscle mass and weight, and aggressive behavior. Other effects include decreased spermatogenesis and premature closure of the epiphyses. The doses used by body builders are several times those used for replacement in patients whose puberty is delayed.[12] Steroid use is most common among participants in football, power lifting, shot putting, wrestling, and swimming.

GENERAL PRINCIPLES OF TREATMENT

Much of the disability of soft tissue injuries is increased by soft tissue swelling. Edema, for example, interferes with joint mobility and may keep ligament ends apart, which may cause them to heal with a fibrous scar between the ends, rather than directly together. This makes the ligaments more lax and predisposes to reinjury. Swelling may be minimized by the use of rest, ice, compression, and elevation (RICE), which are the mainstays of initial treatment for virtually all athletic injuries.

Rest is especially important for the first 24 to 72 hours after a significant injury. For lower extremity injuries, crutches should be used to avoid weight bearing.

Randomized studies have demonstrated that athletes return to full activity faster with the use of cryotherapy begun immediately after the injury.[11] The application of ice seems to work by (1) diminishing nerve impulses and conduction velocity, which decreases pain, (2) diminishing muscle spindle firing, which decreases muscle spasm, and (3) inducing vasoconstriction and reducing capillary permeability, which decreases bleeding and edema. In addition, cryotherapy decreases the oxygen demand of the cells by slowing down their rate of metabolism. This minimizes tissue death, which causes cell breakdown and further edema. Continuing cryotherapy beyond 30 minutes, however, can cause a reflex vasodilation.[11]

Ice should be applied for 20 minutes at a time every 2 to 4 waking hours. This is best done by applying a layer of bandage to the skin, preferably wet in order to conduct cold better, then applying the bag of ice, and finally, wrapping it with an elastic or other bandage. The initial layer of cloth reduces the chance of frostbite. Do not apply heat early in the injury; it increases swelling. Do not advise the patient to "run it off." Cryotherapy should be used for at least 24 to 48 hours, but many trainers and sports medicine physicians recommend that it be continued until the swelling has disappeared completely, which may be much later. An alternative way to apply ice is to freeze water in a paper cup, then rub the cup on the injury in a circular motion. As the ice melts, the top portions of the cup are peeled off, and the ice is rubbed on the skin until it becomes bright pink, which usually takes 7 to 10 minutes.[4]

Compression may be applied with an elastic bandage, but this is not very good at filling in sunken areas around bone, where fluid is likely to accumulate. Sometimes, at least initially, the use of gauze pads or disposable diapers is necessary to fill in these spaces under the elastic bandage (see Ankle Sprains below). Once the swelling has stabilized, an elastic stockinet or Tubigrip usually suffices. The injured extremity should be elevated to above the level of the heart whenever possible.

For persistent or severe swelling, contrast baths often are helpful. Fill one container with water warmed to 100° F and the other with ice water. Immerse the injured area in the warm bath 4 minutes, in the cold 1 minute. Repeat four or five times. During the warm bath, the athlete should perform range of motion exercises. These movements seem especially important in reducing swelling during the procedure. Contrast baths usually are performed at least twice a day and continued until the swelling has resolved.

Begin range of motion exercises once swelling is stabilized, usually in 1½ to 2 days. The exercises are carried out through painless range of motion for 5 minutes or so several times a day. Painless motion in physiological planes of motion is not harmful.

Nonsteroidal antiinflammatory medications usually are given for pain.

Rehabilitation is the most neglected aspect of injury treatment, yet it is extremely important to ensure a safe return to activities and to prevent reinjury. Resting the injured part leads to muscle weakness and atrophy. If the physician is not well versed in rehabilitation for specific injuries, referral to a physical therapist is advisable. Most rehabilitation involves gradual strengthening exercises for appropriate muscle groups.

SPECIFIC INJURIES

Ankle Sprains

Between 80% to 90% of ankle sprains are inversion injuries that affect the anterior talofilbular ligament and the calcaneofibular ligament on the lateral ankle (Fig. 262-1). Medial injuries usually involve the deltoid ligament. The interosseous ligament, along with the anterior and posterior tibiofibular ligaments, binds the lower ends of the tibia and fibula together. On examination of the normal foot, the prominence of the fibular malleolus, the talus, and the cuboid on the lateral side can be felt. When the foot is maximally inverted, the calcaneofibular ligament may be felt as a firm band. It usually is possible to determine the injured ligaments by palpation, especially if the physician is fortunate enough to examine the ankle before edema has obscured the findings. Avulsion fractures of the malleoli cause local tenderness over the bone. Pain with compression of the tibia and fibula together suggests a fracture.

Investigators have found that the "Ottowa Ankle Rules"[15] enable clinicians to exclude ankle fractures on clinical grounds without a radiograph. Unfortunately, these rules have been validated for adults only, but for a cooperative teenager they should be useful. According to these rules, a radiograph is indicated if (1) the patient is unable to bear weight within the first hour after the injury or during the visit, or (2) bony tenderness exists at the posterior edge of either malleoli, the base of the fifth metatarsal, or the navicular (this is located on the medial side, a few centimeters anterior and inferior to the malleolus). Concentrating on palpating the posterior edge of the malleoli avoids confusion with ligamentous tenderness. Physicians also must examine the entire distal 6 cm of the fibula carefully to evaluate for spiral fractures. Ability to bear weight is defined as the ability to take four steps without assistance, even in the presence of a limp. This ability has proved to be the most helpful single finding among ankle injury patients when evaluating for fracture.[16]

If a severe ligamentous injury is suspected, the patient should be referred to an orthopedist. Radiographs with stress views are extremely difficult to interpret and are of little value unless the results of the films would alter the management of the ankle sprain. Indeed, regardless of the severity of sprains, they may be treated similarly, thus negating the need for such films. Ice, compression, elevation, and rest with the use of crutches work well to reduce swelling in the beginning. Most physicians do not wrap the ankle properly to reduce swelling. An elastic wrap alone is not sufficient because it puts maximal pressure over the malleoli and leaves the surrounding soft tissues free to swell. To apply pressure over the ligaments, where most swelling occurs, one approach is to cut a disposable diaper in a U shape to fit around the malleolus (with the bottom of the U facing downward); an elastic bandage is then applied over it. If disposable diapers are not available, several pieces of gauze can be used.

Once the swelling and severe pain have subsided, rehabilitative exercises should begin. Before the initial exercises, apply ice as described previously. Have the patient perform range of motion exercises by tracing the capital letters of the alphabet with his or her great toe. If contrast baths are used, perform these exercises during the warm phase. After the exercise, the patient should wear an ankle support or brace. The Air Stirrup* or similar device works wells for this purpose.[17] It allows the patient mobility in an anteroposterior plane but restricts inversion and eversion. It also provides compression to reduce swelling. The patient should begin walking with crutches. He or she should be instructed to use a three-point crutch gait (Fig. 262-2). With this method the patient ambulates with both crutch tips and the injured foot touching the ground simultaneously.[18] The idea is that the patient puts as much weight on the injured foot as is comfortable and does not avoid placing it on the ground. Once the pain on walking is minimal, the patient should walk with only one crutch, on the uninjured side. Once the patient can walk without a limp, he or she may discard the crutch. At this point more rehabilitative exercises should be added. The patient should stop the exercises if he or she experiences pain. The following are useful exercises[18]:

1. *Toe raises.* Spread the feet about 1 foot apart, toeing in. Then rise on the toes as high as possible without pain. Repeat several times with the toes pointed straight ahead, then pointed out.
2. *Resistance press.* Move the foot in all four planes of motion against resistance, holding each position for 10 seconds. For upward resistance, the patient may put the foot under a piece of furniture and press up; for all other directions, he or she may press against a wall. Alternatively, the patient may use surgical tubing, or Theraband (dental dam material, available from dental supply houses) (Fig. 262-3). It also is helpful to perform resistance exercises in inversion and eversion.
3. *Running exercises.* The patient should not be allowed to run until he or she can balance on the toes of the injured foot for at least 20 seconds and hop on the toes at least 10 times without dropping the heel to the ground. Useful running exercises include zig-zags and figure eights. He or she can start with figure eights 20 yards long, gradually reducing the length of the "eight" to about 10 yards. Once the patient can do quick right ankle cuts in both directions, he or she can return to active sports.

Alternatively, the patient may be referred to a physical therapist for rehabilitation. The ankle brace may be worn for weeks to months when exercising or participating in athletics to prevent injury.

Knee Injuries

Knee injuries are the most common pediatric sports injuries and may cause serious lifelong disability. The medial and lateral collateral ligaments stabilize the knee on each side; the anterior and posterior cruciate ligaments provide stability in the anterior and posterior planes.

A precise diagnosis often is difficult in knee injuries, but a detailed history may help. A pop or snap that occurs during deceleration or moving quickly from one direction to another (cutting) often signals an anterior cruciate tear. A rip or tearing sound from a partially bent position often means a patellar dislocation. The tearing sound results from tearing of the patella's supporting structures as it dislocates. A history of locking may be a sign of a loose bony fragment or

*Air Stirrup ankle brace, Aircast Inc., 92 River Road, Summit, NJ 07901; 1-800-526-8785.

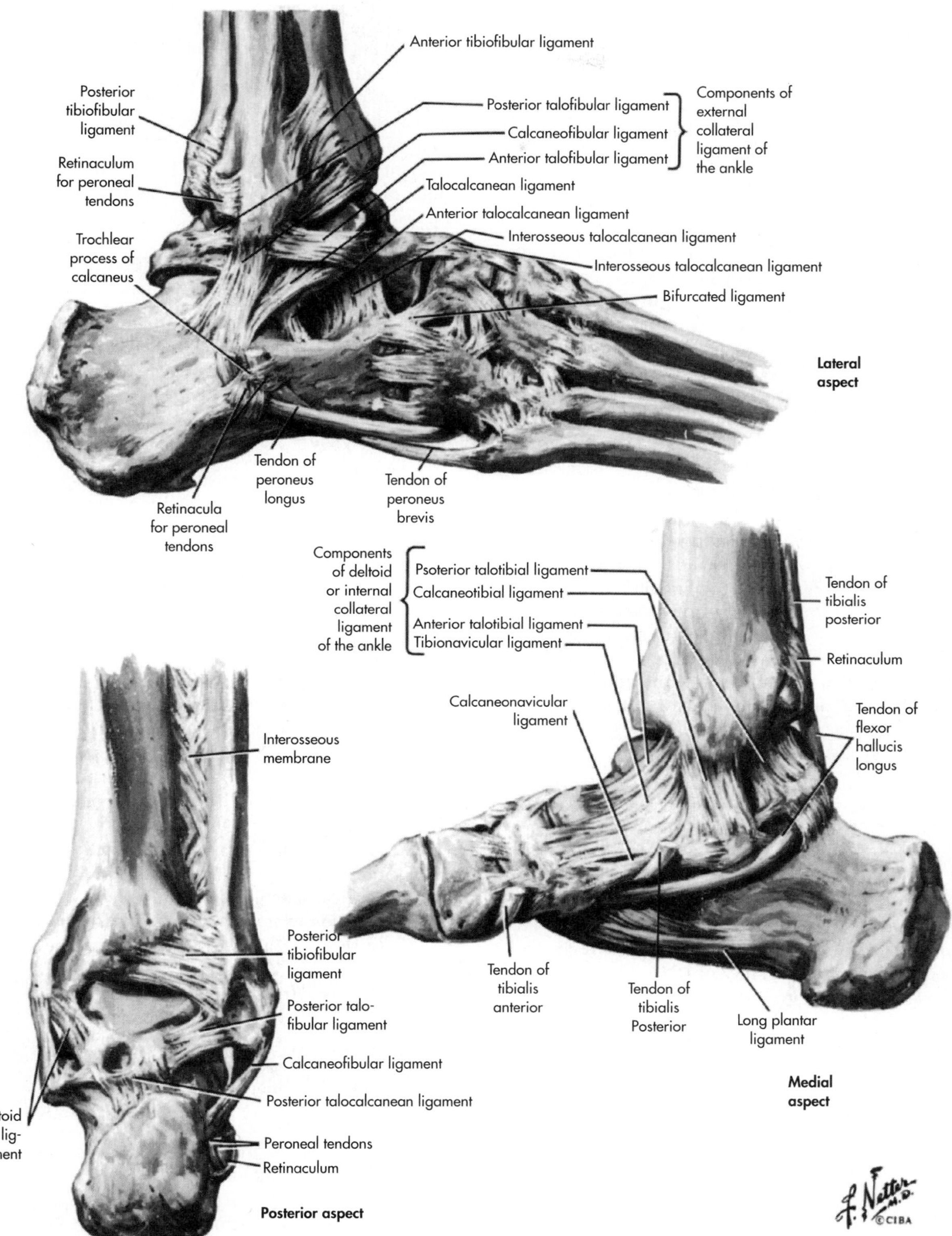

FIG. 262-1 Ligaments of the ankle and foot.

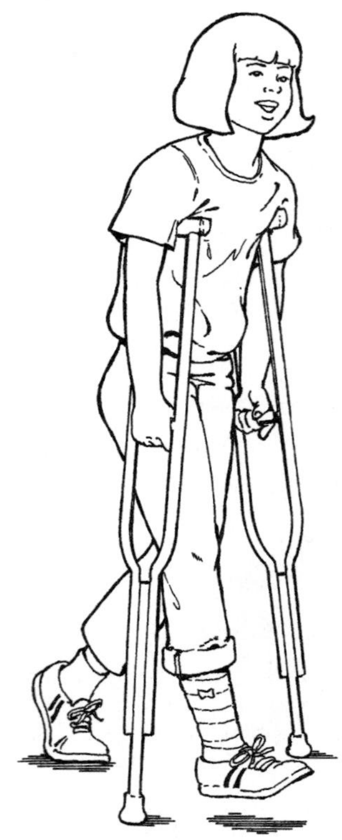

FIG. 262-2 Three-point gait crutch.

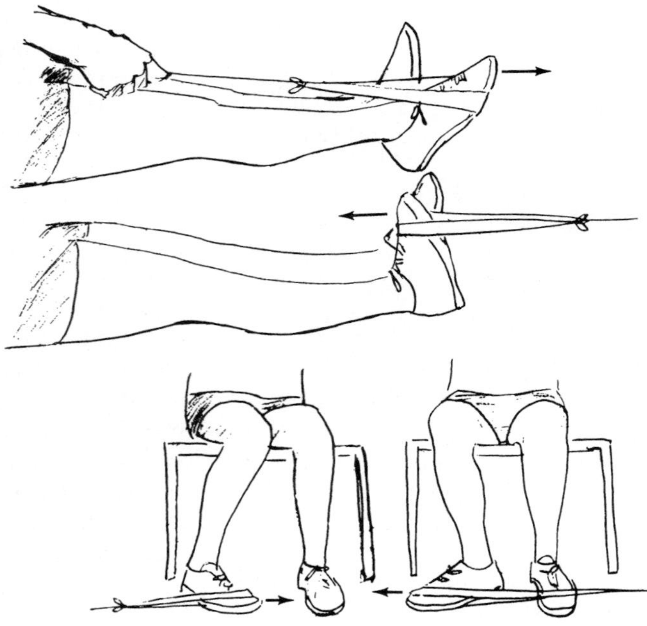

FIG. 262-3 Surgical tubing exercises

torn cartilage in the knee. True locking refers to an inability to extend the knee because something "gets in the way" inside the knee. The sensation appears abruptly and may disappear just as quickly. Patients who have patellofemoral dysfunction also may complain of locking, but they actually are referring to stiffness in the knee after being in one position for a long time. This feeling may go away after a few seconds or minutes and probably is related to muscle spasm.[5] A sensation of looseness in the knee may denote a torn medial collateral ligament. In this situation, a feeling of instability may be more prominent than pain.

Inquiring about the site of initial pain is helpful, for the pain occurs at the site of the injury. Later the discomfort may be more diffuse and less helpful in establishing the diagnosis. Medial collateral ligament injuries cause pain on the medial aspect of the knee. Meniscus tears are tender along the joint line at the tibial plateau. Anterior cruciate tears cause pain on either side of the patellar tendon at the front of the tibial plateau. Dislocation of the patella causes pain along its medial aspect because it dislocates laterally and in doing so tears the soft tissues medially.

An immediate hemarthrosis may indicate an intraarticular fracture or dislocation of the patella. A moderate hemarthrosis occurring over the first 24 hours is a sign of an anterior cruciate ligament tear. A small effusion with swelling over the medial aspect of the knee points to an injury of the medial collateral ligament.[5]

The stability of the anterior cruciate ligament should be determined by using the drawer test (Lachman test). With the patient supine, flex the knee 15 degrees and rotate the leg externally to relax the hamstrings and adductor muscles. Pull the proximal tibia anteriorly and look for (1) excessive motion compared with the opposite extremity and (2) lack of a firm end point to the anterior displacement of the tibia. In all tests of ligament stability, the lack of a firm end point is a sign of a significant tear. To test the posterior cruciate ligament, flex the knee 90 degrees and look for sagging of the tibia posteriorly or for excessive laxity.

To test the collateral ligaments, flex the knee 30 degrees while a valgus stress is applied to test the medial ligaments and then apply a varus stress to test the lateral ligaments. The examiner should place his or her thumb in the joint space while resting the four remaining fingers on the patient's leg above the knee as this test is performed. If the opening of the medial joint is large (more than 1 cm), then the cruciate ligaments also may have been torn.[4] The most common significant knee injury is a sprain of the medial collateral ligament; the most common *severe* injury is a torn anterior cruciate ligament.

These tests are accurate immediately after the injury, but over the next few days the leg may be too painful to test. If a ligament injury is suspected, the patient should be rechecked in 1 to 2 weeks, when pain and muscle spasm have subsided.

Patients who have a dislocation of the patella may show a positive "apprehension test." With the knee flexed 20 degrees to 25 degrees, the patella should be pushed laterally. The patient will be anxious and resist the movement by tensing the quadriceps. This test may be difficult to perform in any patient who has an injured, painful knee. Radiographs may be indicated to rule out osteochondritis dissecans or fractures, but they usually are normal because most knee injuries involve soft tissues. When obtaining radiographs, a tunnel view of the patella should be requested in addition to the usual anteroposterior and lateral views. This view is especially helpful in detecting osteochondritis dissecans.

Patients who have grade 1 collateral ligament strains may be treated by the primary care physician as described under General Principles of Treatment. Patients who have grade 2 or 3 collateral ligament sprains or suspected meniscal or cruciate cartilage injuries are best referred to an orthopedic surgeon.

OVERUSE INJURIES OF THE KNEE

A common condition in the pediatrician's office is the adolescent athlete who has recurrent or chronic knee pain. Treating these patients may be more frustrating than treating acute injuries because the source of the pain is less obvious. The roentgenograms usually are normal, and nothing suggests a medical cause for the condition. No history of trauma may be evident.

Most of these athletes have overuse syndromes of the knee.[8] A careful history usually reveals some change in the patient's activities—the beginning of a new sport or a new activity within that sport. Running or playing sports on a hard surface such as concrete may precipitate problems. Some patients may have conditions that interfere with the mechanical function of the leg, such as ligamentous laxity and excessive valgus of the knee, or foot pronation. Sometimes knee pain follows injuries that do not involve the knee, such as those involving an ankle or hip. The disuse following the injury leads to atrophy of the quadriceps muscles, which causes patellofemoral dysfunction. The most common finding in any of these conditions is loss of tone and muscle mass in the vastus medialis,[5] which is palpable proximal to the knee on the medial side. The vastus medialis ensures proper alignment of the patella in the femoral groove. To examine for this, the patient should sit with legs extended and quadriceps tightened, including the vastus medialis. The quadriceps size and tone then are compared with the quadriceps of the other leg.

The most common overuse syndromes of the knee are patellofemoral syndrome, patellar tendinitis, and Osgood-Schlatter disease. At first the pain occurs only after the athletic activity. As it worsens, the pain begins during or toward the end of the activity.

Patients who have patellofemoral syndrome, often referred to as *chrondromalacia of the patella,* tend to have vague symptoms. The most common site of pain is medial to the patella, but patients may complain of pain anywhere around the patella or behind it or simply of diffuse pain in the knee. They may be unable to point to a specific site of pain. Sometimes the pain is aggravated by walking up and, especially, down stairs or hills. Sometimes sitting with the knees bent for long periods causes pain, as in a car on long trips, in a theater, or in class. Sometimes patients complain of constant anterior knee pain, which is worse after activity.

Patellar tendinitis causes well-localized pain and tenderness at the inferior pole of the patella. It is caused by a partial rupture and inflammation of the tendon where it attaches to the patella. It typically affects athletes in jumping sports such as basketball and volleyball.

Sinding-Larsen-Johansson syndrome is an apophysitis of the patella. It is similar to Osgood-Schlatter disease (see below), but instead affects the inferior patella at the insertion of the patellar tendon. Lateral views of the the patella may show bony abnormalities at this site.

Osgood-Schlatter disease is most common in the early years of puberty. The powerful quadriceps muscle causes avulsion or microscopic disorganization of the tibial tubercle in the area of developing bone. The patient complains of knee pain, which is aggravated by extending the knee against resistance or applying pressure over the tibial tubercle. Occasionally the region of the anterior tibial tubercle swells. Radiological abnormalities do not correlate well with symptoms. Radiographs may be indicated, however, to rule out more serious conditions, such as osteomyelitis, arteriovenous malformation, or osteosarcoma, all of which have been reported to cause symptoms similar to those of Osgood-Schlatter disease.[1] Hip problems such as Legg-Calvé-Perthes disease or slipped capital femoral epiphysis also may cause chronic knee pain.

Treatment of these conditions involves using ice after athletic activities, nonsteroidal antiinflammatory medications, and exercises to strengthen the quadriceps muscle. When the pain is severe, rest from the activities that cause pain (and *only* those activities) is helpful. If walking is painful, crutches may be required for a few days. For patients who have severe pain from patellar tendinitis or Osgood-Schlatter disease, using a Velcro knee immobilizer will rest the knee. A knee immobilizer, however, has the disadvantage of weakening the quadriceps further from disuse and is recommended for only the most severe cases. An Osgood-Schlatter pad that has a hole in the middle and fits around the tender tibial tuberosity prevents repeated painful trauma during sports activities. Sometimes a Neoprene sleeve with a pad placed laterally over the patella is helpful in managing patellofemoral syndrome because it helps keep the patella properly aligned. These devices may be obtained from orthopedic supply companies.* Patients who have excessive pronation of the foot may benefit from cushioned, full-length arch supports, which are available by prescription in many sports-oriented shoe stores. Stretching the quadriceps three times a day or more also is helpful.

Garrick[5] recommends an isometric quadriceps-strengthening program that emphasizes the vastus medialis for patients who have these conditions. These exercises may be performed throughout the day, as often as the patient can think about it, for a total of 20 to 24 times—while waiting for the bus, while in class, or just before meals. To perform these exercises, the athlete should extend the knee and tighten the quadriceps for 5 or 6 seconds, relax it for 2 to 3 seconds, and then repeat the process three times. The patient should palpate the vastus medialis to make sure it tightens during the exercise. The physician should demonstrate this technique in the office. Alternatively, these patients can be referred to a physical therapist to initiate and monitor a rehabilitative program. Sometimes an electrical muscle stimulator is necessary to strengthen the vastus medialis. Most patients improve within 2 to 3 months if they comply with the management plan. Patients who fail to improve require referral to an orthopedic surgeon.

Iliotibial Band Friction Syndrome

Runners often complain of lateral knee pain. Usually this results from inflammation of the iliotibial band where it crosses

*Orthopedic Technology Inc., 14670 Wicks Boulevard, San Leandro, CA 94577. PRO Orthopedic Devices Inc., P.O. Box 1, King of Prussia, PA 19406.

the lateral femoral epicondyle.[13] The iliotibial band is a band of deep fasciae that starts at the iliac crest just posterior to the anterior superior iliac spine, travels down the lateral aspect of the thigh, and inserts on the lateral tibial condyle.

As in many overuse injuries, the pain may occur at first only after running. Later it may develop during the activity. In severe cases the pain may be constant. Some patients complain of lateral hip pain rather than knee pain.

Sometimes the pain may be reproduced with provocative testing.[9] With the patient lying on the uninjured side, ask him or her to abduct the hip and flex the knee 30 degrees. Press down on the lower leg. Attempt to adduct the leg while the patient resists. This may reproduce the pain or increase tenderness at the inflamed site because it puts a varus stress at the knee.

Treatment consists of rest, antiinflammatory medication, ice, and sometimes electrogalvanic stimulation, which may be administered by a physical therapist. Iliotibial band stretching exercises are an important aspect of treatment to prevent recurrences. Patients may have to refrain from running for several weeks.

If the patient has excessive pronation or supination of the foot, appropriate foot orthoses may be helpful. Also, make sure the athlete is not running consistently on one side of the road. The incline built into roads for drainage may lead to a consistent varus stretch on one leg.

OTHER INJURIES

Shin Splint

Shin splint is a poorly defined condition that refers to pain along the medial aspect of the distal two thirds of the tibia. It is an overuse syndrome that may develop in poorly conditioned runners and is associated with running on hard surfaces, with the use of improper shoes, or with excessive foot pronation. At first, patients have pain only while running, but eventually pain is present *after* running as well. Ice, rest, and antiinflammatory medications are effective during the acute state; better shoes, calf stretching, and conditioning should prevent recurrences. The athlete may have to reduce the duration of workouts. Sometimes the use of orthotic devices helps to reduce discomfort. Obtain a radiograph to rule out a stress fracture.

Little League Elbow

Little League elbow is an imprecise term that usually refers to flexor pronator tendinitis, which is an overuse syndrome caused by repetitive valgus stress at the elbow. It is common in young pitchers learning to throw a curve ball. The condition may be less frequent than before, as a result of Little League rules that limit players to pitching no more than six innings per week. It also is important for the growing child to limit pitching practice and to avoid throwing the curve ball. Pain develops first; later tenderness is exhibited over the medial aspect of the elbow. If the pain is severe, contractures and limited range of motion may develop. The mainstay of management is prevention, but in patients who have symptoms, resting the elbow is mandatory.[14] Many patients require flexibility exercises, progressive arm strengthening, and possibly a change in throwing mechanics, arranged in cooperation with an orthopedist and physical therapist.

Stress Fractures

Stress fractures occur most commonly in the fibula and second metatarsal. The onset of pain may be sudden or gradual and without history of direct trauma. Tenderness is present over the fracture site. Radiographs may not show any abnormality until 6 to 8 weeks after the injury. A bone scan will reveal the fracture much sooner. Treatment consists of significantly reducing activity until the patient is pain free for 7 to 10 days. Then, after reexamination, activities may be resumed gradually. Patients who have severe pain may require the application of a cast.

Finger Dislocation

Finger dislocations frequently are reduced immediately after the injury by a trainer or a friend. Because of this, the patient may underestimate the degree of ligamentous damage. Obtaining radiographs is important to rule out avulsion fractures.

Contusions and Hematomas

A contusion to the iliac crest (commonly called a "hip pointer") causes disability out of proportion to the severity of the injury because several muscles are attached to the iliac crest at the injury site and cause pain as they contract during any movement of the hip. In addition to ice, compression, and rest, some patients require crutches. As the patient recovers, stretching and strengthening exercises are helpful.

REFERENCES

1. Adams JE: Injury to the throwing arm: a study of traumatic changes in the elbow joints of boy baseball players, *Calif Med* 102:127, 1964.
2. Buckley WE et al: Estimated prevalence of anabolic steroid use among male high school seniors, *JAMA* 260:3441, 1988.
3. Dehaven KE: Athletic injuries in adolescents, *Pediatr Ann* 7:96, 1978.
4. Dyment PG: Athletic injuries, *Pediatr Rev* 10:291, 1989.
5. Garrick JG: Knee problems in adolescents, *Pediatr Rev* 4:235, 1983.
6. Garrick JG, Requa RK: Girls' sport injuries in high school athletics, *JAMA* 239:2245, 1978.
7. Garrick JG, Requa RK: Injuries in high school sports, *Pediatrics* 61:465, 1978.
8. Garrick JG, Webb DR: *Sports injuries: diagnosis and management,* Philadelphia, 1990, WB Saunders.
9. Goldberg B et al: Children's sports injuries: are they avoidable? *Physicians Sportsmed* 7:93, 1979.
10. Grana WA, Kalenek A, editors: *Clinical sports medicine,* Philadelphia, 1991, WB Saunders.
11. Hocutt JE et al: Cryotherapy in ankle sprains, *Am J Sports Med* 10:316, 1982.
12. Moore WV: Anabolic steroid use in adolescence, *JAMA* 260:3484, 1988.
13. Noble CA: Iliotibial band friction syndrome in runners, *Am J Sports Med* 8:232, 1980.
14. Stanitski CL: Common injuries in preadolescent and adolescent athletes: recommendations for prevention, *Sports Med* 7:32, 1989.
15. Stiell IG et al: Implementation of the Ottawa Ankle Rules, *JAMA* 271:827, 1994.
16. Stiell IG et al: Decision rules for the use of radiography in acute ankle injuries: refinement and prospective validation, *JAMA* 269:1127, 1993.
17. Stover CN: Air Stirrup management of ankle injuries in the athlete, *Am J Sports Med* 2:63, 1983.
18. Stover CN: Functional sprain management of ankle, *Ambulatory Care* 6:25, 1986.
19. Strauss RB, editor: *Sports medicine,* ed 2, Philadelphia, 1991, WB Saunders.
20. Strong WB, Linder CW: Preparticipation health evaluation for competitive sports, *Pediatr Rev* 4:113, 1982.

263 Staphylococcal Toxic Shock Syndrome

Michael E. Pichichero

Staphylococcal toxic shock syndrome (TSS) is a distinct clinical entity characterized by fever, diffuse nonexudative mucous membrane inflammation, vomiting and profuse diarrhea, generalized myalgia, scarlatiniform erythroderma, hypotension, and shock associated with multiple organ failure—renal, myocardial, pulmonary, hepatic, hematological, and central nervous system (CNS).[9]

Staphylococcal toxic shock syndrome is an important consideration in the evaluation of toxic exanthematous diseases in children. It must be distinguished from other serious or potentially life-threatening diseases, including streptococcal toxic shock syndrome, staphylococcal scalded skin syndrome, Stevens-Johnson syndrome, Kawasaki disease, streptococcal scarlet fever, measles, leptospirosis, and drug-related toxic epidermal necrolysis. Staphylococcal TSS occurs most often in menstruating females of childbearing age, particularly in adolescents who use tampons regularly.[2,6] Highly absorbent brands of tampons are especially problematic. The frequency and pattern of tampon use has changed during the past decade with consequent substantial drop in the incidence of staphylococcal TSS.

Currently, 85% of staphylococcal TSS cases occur in females and 15% in males; among cases in females, 55% occur during menses. Nonmenstrual cases of staphylococcal TSS account for approximately 11% of all reported cases and have been associated with use of barrier contraceptives (sponge and diaphragm). Nonsurgical and surgical wounds infected with TSS toxin-producing *Staphylococcus aureus,* staphylococcal empyema, fasciitis, osteomyelitis, sinusitis, peritonsillar abscess, cutaneous and subcutaneous abscess, surgical wound infection, postpartum infection, septic abortion, and bacteremia have all been associated with TSS.[3,5] The overall incidence of staphylococcal TSS is 0.53 cases per 100,000 population, although wide variations exist in different geographical regions; it occurs more often in Caucasians than in non-Caucasians for both menstrual and nonmenstrual cases.[4]

CLINICAL PRESENTATION

Strict criteria for case definition have been established by the Centers for Disease Control and Prevention (see the box on p. 1617. The time sequence of the clinical manifestations of staphylococcal TSS is outlined in Figure 263-1.[2] Patients usually are healthy before the onset of symptoms. Occasionally a prodrome consisting of low-grade fever, malaise, myalgia, or vomiting occurs in the week preceding the beginning of the acute illness. Then the patient abruptly develops a spiking fever of 39° to 41° C, chills, and severe gastrointestinal symptoms consisting of nausea, vomiting, profuse watery, nonbloody diarrhea, and abdominal cramps. Many patients also complain of headache, myalgia, and a sore throat. At this stage of the illness a diagnosis of acute viral gastroenteritis may well be entertained incorrectly and the youngster treated symptomatically. However, over the next 24 to 72 hours additional clinical signs develop suggestive of the diagnosis of staphylococcal TSS. A diffuse, blanching, macular erythroderma (sunburnlike) or scarlatiniform rash erupts. The rash may be faint or evanescent and therefore sometimes is missed or attributed to high fever. The rash is not pruritic but occasionally is petechial. Patients demonstrate bilateral conjunctival hyperemia without discharge and may complain of photophobia. Oropharyngeal inflammation, sometimes with an associated strawberry tongue or buccal ulcerations, also occurs, as does vaginal erythema with minimal clear watery discharge in menstrual cases.

Within 24 to 72 hours of the onset of illness, most patients experience orthostatic dizziness or syncope or both because of orthostatic hypotension. This symptom can manifest abruptly and may be premonitory of the development of hypovolemic shock. The peak of illness in the clinical syndrome occurs on the second or third day and involves multiple organ systems. CNS dysfunction may appear as headache, confusion, disorientation, hallucinations, and complaints of paresthesias of the hands and feet. Some patients have a stiff, tender neck. If a lumbar puncture is performed, normal values for CSF glucose and protein are found, although some patients have up to 100 white blood cells per cubic millimeter, 50% of which may be polymorphonuclear cells. Abdominal musculature tenderness, absent or hypoactive bowel sounds, and radiological evidence of a nonobstructive ileus are common. Azotemia and a diminished creatinine clearance occur as evidence of renal involvement. Oliguria is typical; complete renal shutdown occurs rarely. The musculoskeletal system nearly always is affected. Exquisite muscle tenderness and severe myalgias are common. Arthralgias and joint effusions may be seen. Nonpitting edema over the wrists and ankles and synovitis of the small joints of the hands and feet have been reported to occur in a few patients. Patients may experience shock lung or adult-type respiratory distress syndrome. Hematological involvement includes a progressive normochromic normocytic anemia, thrombocytopenia, and leukocytosis. Arrhythmias or prolonged shock may lead to eventual myocardial failure.

LABORATORY FINDINGS

No laboratory test is available for confirming the diagnosis of staphylococcal TSS. Initial laboratory findings often include a leukocytosis, with a striking increase in the percentage of immature neutrophils, a progressive anemia, and thrombocytopenia. These hematological abnormalities are self-correcting during the convalescent stage. Thrombocytopenia may be accompanied by prolongation of prothrombin

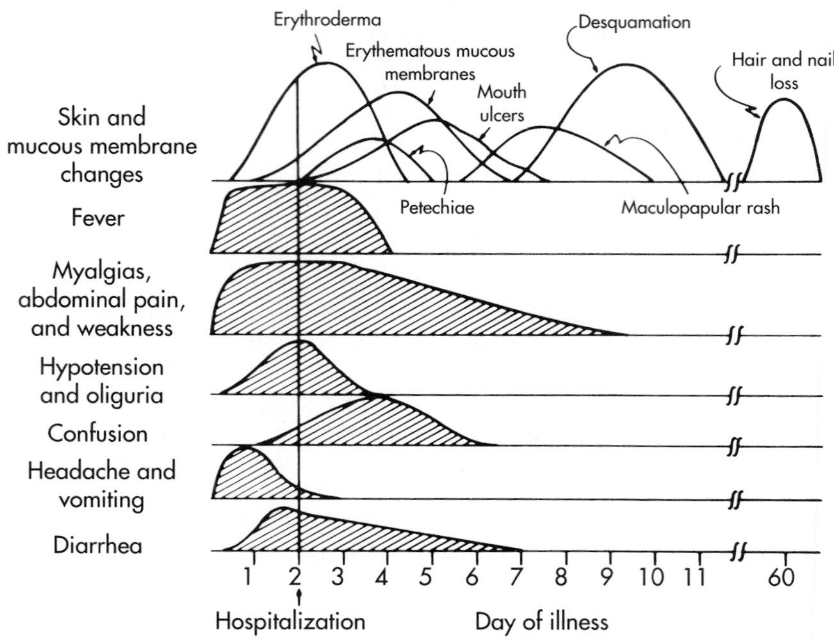

FIG. 263-1 Major systemic, skin, and mucous membrane manifestations of toxic shock syndrome.

(From Chesney PJ et al: *JAMA* 246:743, 1981.)

time and partial thromboplastin time and the appearance of increased fibrin split products. However, neither serious bleeding during the acute phase of illness nor thrombosis resulting from rebound thrombocytosis during recovery has been a significant clinical problem. A majority of patients have hypoproteinemia and hypoalbuminemia, probably as a consequence of increased capillary permeability because of exotoxin-mediated vascular cell membrane change (see section below on etiology). A number of patients also experience metabolic acidosis from inadequate tissue perfusion, and this may be complicated by hyponatremia and hypokalemia as a result of accompanying persistent vomiting and diarrhea. Serum concentrations of calcium may appear dangerously low; however, tetany rarely is seen. The BUN and creatinine usually are elevated early in the illness. Peak abnormal values occur after 5 to 7 days and then return rapidly to normal. However, some patients have required acute hemodialysis or peritoneal dialysis to correct these and other metabolic imbalances. Despite the abnormal renal function, hypophosphatemia typically is present in the first days of illness. The creatinine phosphokinase level often is quite elevated, and occasionally patients experience myoglobinemia. These findings normalize with resolution of the myalgias, usually between the fifth and tenth day of disease. Hepatic enzyme and bilirubin levels typically are elevated initially but tend to revert to normal in convalescence. The relative frequency of these abnormal laboratory findings is presented in Table 263-1.

ETIOLOGY AND PATHOGENESIS

Patients who develop staphylococcal TSS are colonized or infected with specific strains of *S. aureus*. A specific staphylococcal exotoxin known as TSS toxin 1 (TSST-1) has been identified as the most common cause, or a mediator of, the pathophysiological events associated with staphylococcal TSS.[1,8] Apparently, colonization with TSST-1-producing *S. aureus* and concomitant antibody formation is common, whereas the development of staphylococcal TSS is relatively rare. The unique feature in patients who have staphylococcal TSS is that they have sequestered focal sites of *S. aureus* colonization (e.g., the vagina during menstruation with tampon use) or infection (nonmenstrual cases) where growth conditions are established that promote TSST-1 production.[10] TSST-1 is not the only toxin associated with staphylococcal TSS; a few isolates of *S. aureus* from patients who have nonmenstrual TSS do not produce TSST-1. Staphylococcal enterotoxins (A through E) in the appropriate clinical setting (usually nonmenstrual TSS) also may cause the clinical manifestations of TSS. Secondary immune mediators, especially tumor necrosis factor, interleukin-1, and lymphokines released by the host in response to *S. aureus* toxins, appear to play a significant role in the pathogenesis of TSS.[6,7]

MANAGEMENT

The initial steps in management of staphylococcal TSS are outlined in the box on p. 1615. Nearly all patients should be hospitalized, although a few who have a very mild form of the illness may be managed cautiously as outpatients. The first and major resuscitative goal is to administer large volumes of crystalloid (lactated Ringer) or colloid (fresh-frozen plasma or albumin) solutions to restore normal intravascular volume and correct hypotension, since shock is the initial threat to intact survival. Patients may require enormous volumes of fluid (two to four times normal daily maintenance) to maintain tissue perfusion. Adequate treatment of hypotension also may require vasopressor therapy such as dopamine

Table 263-1 Summary of Clinical and Laboratory Data Associated with Staphylococcal TSS

Condition	Relative frequency of occurrence (%)
Clinical	
Fever	100
Temperature >40° C (>104° F)	70
Rash	100
Diffuse erythema	87
Desquamation	90
Myalgia	99
Hypotension (orthostatic hypotension or syncope)	95
Disorientation, irritability, or lethargy	89
Diarrhea	83
Vomiting	82
Sore throat	80
Strawberry tongue	80
Headache	78
Abdominal pain and tenderness	70
Vaginal hyperemia	67
Conjunctivitis	65
Vaginal discharge	42
Stiff neck	36
Arthralgia	15
Joint effusion	12
Adult respiratory distress syndrome	10
Laboratory	
Hematological	
Increased fibrinolytic split products	100
Immature neutrophils	95
Anemia	82
Leukocytosis	76
Prolonged prothrombin time	70
Decreased fibrinogen	68
Thrombocytopenia	64
Prolonged partial thromboplastin time	60
Metabolic	
Hypoproteinemia	95
Hypoalbuminemia	85
Hypocalcemia	83
Hypokalemia	75
Hypophosphatemia	62
Hyponatremia	47
Hepatic	
Elevated hepatic enzymes	67
Hyperbilirubinemia	63
Renal	
Pyuria	100
Increased creatinine	82
Increased BUN	75
Proteinuria	70
Microscopic hematuria	50
Musculoskeletal	
Increased creatinine phosphokinase	75
Metabolic acidosis	75
Myoglobinuria	66

or dobutamine. Much of the administered fluid is sequestered outside the intravascular space, and many patients become markedly edematous. Therefore it frequently is advisable to have a central venous pressure line or a Swan-Ganz catheter to monitor left ventricular end-diastolic pressure to prevent the development of congestive heart failure caused by overvigorous fluid resuscitation. If significant hypotension exists, multiple organ system failure likely is imminent. The management outlined in the box on the right should be pursued while transport to a tertiary care medical facility is arranged. There, continued management largely will be supportive and dictated by the degree of organ dysfunction.

A multidisciplinary approach may well be required to manage the patient who has staphylococcal TSS. The pulmonary specialist may be needed to manage adult-type respiratory distress syndrome or shock lung because endotracheal intubation and ventilatory assistance with positive end-expiratory pressure and high oxygen flow rates may be required. The hematologist may be of assistance in the treatment of DIC. Peritoneal dialysis or hemodialysis may be necessary to manage renal failure or severe electrolyte and acid-base abnormalities; thus a nephrologist may be needed. Ventricular ectopy is common, and refractory ventricular arrhythmias frequently have been a cause of death in severely ill patients.

MANAGEMENT OF STAPHYLOCOCCAL TOXIC SHOCK SYNDROME

1. Consider other possible diagnoses
2. Remove potentially infected foreign bodies (e.g., tampons).
3. Obtain cultures of blood, throat, vagina, nares, rectum, and other appropriate sites
4. Drain and irrigate infected sites
5. Give an intravenous antistaphylococcal beta-lactamase-resistant antimicrobial agent at maximum dosage for weight and age
6. Consider methylprednisolone for severe cases
7. Treat aggressively and monitor for the following:
    - Hypovolemia and inadequate tissue perfusion
    - Adult respiratory distress syndrome
    - Myocardial dysfunction
    - Acute renal failure
    - Cerebral edema
    - Hypocalcemia/hypophosphatemia
    - Metabolic acidosis
    - Disseminated intravascular coagulation
    - Fluid and electrolyte abnormalities

Table 263-2 Differential Diagnosis of Staphylococcal Toxic Shock Syndrome

Disease	Hypotension	Rash	Lips	Oral cavity
Staphylococcal toxic shock syndrome	Yes	Diffuse erythroderma, −Nikolsky sign	Red	Erythematous
Staphylococcal scalded-skin syndrome	No	Erythroderma, bullae, ±Nikolsky sign	—	—
Stevens-Johnson syndrome	No	Erythema multiforme	Bleeding, fissured	Bullous enanthem
Kawasaki disease	No	Polymorphous	Red, fissured	Erythematous, strawberry tongue
Scarlet fever	No	Diffuse erythroderma, circumoral pallor, Pastia lines	—	Strawberry tongue
Measles	No	Morbilliform	—	Koplik spots
Leptospirosis	Sometimes	Erythematous, macular, petechial, purpuric	—	±Pharyngitis
Toxic epidermal necrolysis (drug related)	Sometimes	Painful erythroderma, bullae, +Nikolsky sign	—	—
Streptococcal toxic shock syndrome	Yes	Diffuse erythroderma, maculopapular	Cracked	Erythematous

The cardiac monitoring and management of this aspect of the patient's care can be facilitated by a cardiologist's input.

Because staphylococcal TSS appears to be an exotoxin-mediated disease, the importance of antibiotics could be questioned. However, 1% to 2% of patients who have TSS have an *S. aureus* bacteremia, for which antibiotic therapy would be crucial. Further, it appears that antistaphylococcal antibiotics may reduce the recurrence rate of TSS in girls who have menstrual-related illness. Therefore a 7- to 10-day course of nafcillin (100 to 200 mg/kg/day divided into six equal doses and given intravenously) or other antistaphylococcal antibiotic probably is a prudent part of patient management.

Two somewhat controversial aspects in the management of staphylococcal TSS are the use of corticosteroids and intravenous immunoglobulin (IVIG). Many physicians have elected to use high-dose methylprednisolone (30 mg/kg every 4 hours) during the initial 24 hours of illness on the basis of experimental evidence that steroids may be beneficial in the treatment of shock induced by bacterial toxins. High levels of antibody to TSST-1 have been found in IVIG preparations; animal model studies suggest that administration early in the course of disease can reduce morbidity and mortality of staphylococcal TSS. However, IVIG possibly could diminish the immune response to *S. aureus* toxins, thereby increasing the risk of recurrent episodes. Therefore the risk-benefit ratio of this controversial empirical therapy must be considered carefully in each patient.

DIFFERENTIAL DIAGNOSIS

In some aspects, staphylococcal TSS might be confused with staphylococcal scalded-skin syndrome, Stevens-Johnson syndrome, Kawasaki disease, streptococcal scarlet fever, streptococcal TSS, measles, leptospirosis, or toxic epidermal necrolysis. The differentiating features among these diagnoses are presented in Table 263-2. The strict case definition presented in the box on p. 1617 particularly is useful for epidemiological purposes and serves to exclude patients who have other diseases. However, recent experience suggests that this strict definition may exclude patients who have milder forms of staphylococcal TSS, and this should be kept in mind when confronted with a patient who demonstrates some but not all of the clinical findings of staphylococcal TSS.

PROGNOSIS AND CONVALESCENCE

The majority of patients who have staphylococcal TSS recover within 7 to 10 days. The case fatality rate is 3.3%. Convalescence is characterized by a desquamation of the palms and soles within 1 to 2 weeks after the onset of illness. Some patients also experience hair and nail loss. Prolonged fatigue and weakness for as long as 3 months may occur in the recovery phase.

Staphylococcal TSS can be recurrent in menstruating girls, and multiple recurrences have been reported. The incidence of recurrent staphylococcal TSS may be as high as 28% if antistaphylococcal antibiotics are not employed. The criteria for recurrent disease are less stringent than those required for defining an initial episode. The use of appropriate antistaphylococcal therapy and discontinuation of tampon use reduces the risk of recurrences. An absent or delayed immune response to TSST-1 frequently is associated with susceptibility to recurrent TSS. Physicians who care for adolescent girls having a febrile illness of uncertain cause that occurs during menstruation, is recurrent, or is associated with an exanthem should consider the diagnosis of staphylococcal TSS seriously.

Eyes	Hands and feet	Desquamation	Other findings	Diagnosis
Nonpurulent conjunctivitis	Erythematous, edematous	Hands and feet—can be generalized	Diarrhea, renal, hepatic, CNS, hematological abnormalities	Clinical, culture of *S. aureus* from nasopharynx, vagina, or wound
±Purulent conjunctivitis	Relatively spared or grossly involved	Gross	—	Clinical, culture of *S. aureus* from nasopharynx or wound, skin biopsy
Purulent conjunctivitis	Involved	Involves only individual lesions	Respiratory and GI tract involvement	Clinical, skin biopsy
Nonpurulent conjunctivitis	Erythematous, edematous	Fingertips	Coronary aneurysms, generalized vasculitis	Clinical, no diagnostic test
—	Relatively spared	Fine, flaky	Rheumatic fever, glomerulonephritis	Clinical, culture of group A streptococci from pharynx, serology
Conjunctivitis	Involved	Fine	Respiratory tract involvement	Clinical, serology
Conjunctivitis	Relatively spared	—	CNS, renal, hepatic involvement	Clinical, serology
±Conjunctivitis	±Involved	Gross	—	Clinical, serology
Injected	—	—	Confusion, abdominal pain and vomiting, hyperesthesia	Clinical, culture of group A streptococci

CASE DEFINITION OF STAPHYLOCOCCAL TOXIC SHOCK SYNDROME

Fever: temperature $>38.9°$ C
Rash: diffuse macular erythroderma; desquamation of palms and soles 1 to 2 weeks after onset of illness
Hypotension: systolic blood pressure 90 mm Hg for adults or below 5th percentile by age for children under 16 years of age; orthostatic drop in diastolic blood pressure 15 mm Hg from lying to sitting, or orthostatic syncope
Multisystem involvement—three or more of the following:
- Gastrointestinal: vomiting or diarrhea at onset of illness
- Muscular: severe myalgia or creatinine phosphokinase level at least twice the upper limit of normal for laboratory
- Mucous membrane: vaginal, oropharyngeal, or conjunctival hyperemia
- Renal: blood urea nitrogen (BUN) or creatinine at least twice the upper limit of normal for laboratory or urinary sediment with pyuria (>5 white cells per high-power field) in the absence of urinary tract infection
- Hepatic: total bilirubin, serum glutamic-oxalo-acetic transaminase (SGOT), or serum glutamic-pyruvate transaminase (SGPT) at least twice the upper limit of normal for laboratory
- Hematological: platelets $<100,000/mm^3$
- CNS: disorientation or alterations in consciousness without focal neurological signs when fever and hypotension are absent

Negative results on the following tests, if obtained:
- Blood, throat, cerebrospinal fluid (CSF) cultures
- Rise in antibody titer: Rocky Mountain spotted fever, leptospirosis, and rubeola

REFERENCES

1. Crass BA, Bergdoll MS: Toxin involvement in toxic shock syndrome, *J Infect Dis* 153:918, 1986.
2. Davis JP et al: Toxic-shock syndrome: epidemiological features, recurrence, risk factors, and prevention, *N Engl J Med* 303:1429, 1980.
3. Ferguson MA, Todd JK: Toxic shock syndrome associated with *Staphylococcus aureus* sinusitis in children, *J Infect Dis* 161:953, 1990.
4. Gaventa S et al: Active surveillance for toxic shock syndrome in the United States, 1986, *Rev Infect Dis* 11:28, 1989.
5. Kain KC, Schulzer M, Chow AW: Clinical spectrum of nonmenstrual toxic shock syndrome (TSS): comparison with menstrual TSS by multivariate discriminant analyses, *Clin Infect Dis* 16:100, 1993.
6. Kass EH, Parsonnet J: On the pathogenesis of toxic shock syndrome, *Rev Infect Dis* 9:482, 1987.
7. Resnick SD: Toxic shock syndrome: recent developments in pathogenesis, *J Pediatr* 116:321, 1990.
8. Schlievert PM: TSST-1: structure, function, purification, and detection—role of toxic shock syndrome toxin 1 in toxic shock syndrome: overview, *Rev Infect Dis* 11:107, 1989.
9. Todd J et al: Toxic-shock syndrome associated with phage-group-1 staphylococci, *Lancet* 2:1116, 1978.
10. Todd JK et al: Influence of focal growth conditions on the pathogenesis of toxic shock syndrome, *J Infect Dis* 155:673, 1987.

264 Stomatitis

Julius G. Goepp

Stomatitis (ulceration and inflammation of the mucosa of the oral cavity) is a common problem in children at all ages outside of the neonatal period, with incidence as high as 50% in some populations.[1] Although most cases of stomatitis are mild and self-limited, several types may cause more severe or recurrent disease. Specific treatments generally do not exist, and management usually consists of measures to support comfort and hydration.

ETIOLOGY

Stomatitis in children has numerous causes, including infections (generally viral), trauma, and the effects of cancer chemotherapy. Aphthous stomatitis, which accounts for the largest proportion of cases, has no clear-cut cause.

Infectious Causes

Viral Causes. Several viral classes are capable of causing stomatitis of distinct clinical appearance, whereas others are suspected as causes, but their involvement has not been documented as well.

Herpes Simplex Virus. Herpes simplex virus, type 1 (HSV1), causes acute primary herpetic gingivostomatitis (APHGS) in previously unexposed children. The virus usually is acquired from an individual who has a mouth sore caused by HSV1 or who has a herpetic whitlow of a finger or a toe. Illness begins 5 to 10 days after exposure and is heralded by fever, chills, and a nonspecific "viral syndrome," with subsequent development of a sore throat and cervical adenopathy. Older children may complain of a burning sensation in the mouth. Vesicles develop anywhere on the oral mucosa, primarily in the anterior oropharynx. They may spread to the perioral skin.[1] Anorexia resulting from pain is common and may produce dehydration severe enough to warrant hospitalization.

Recovery from APHGS is spontaneous in 7 to 10 days. About 50% of patients develop at least one episode of "cold sores" subsequently, but APHGS does not recur in immunocompetent children.

Enteroviruses. Milder forms of stomatitis are caused by the enteroviruses, especially coxsackieviruses.[1] Herpangina is caused most commonly by coxsackie A4. In this entity, small vesicles appear posteriorly, especially on the soft palate. Fever in the moderate range is common, as are generalized myalgias and malaise, with diminished oral intake. Dehydration is unusual. Herpangina is seasonal in the United States, being especially prominent in summer. Herpangina usually resolves spontaneously in 3 to 5 days.

Coxsackie A16 infections may produce hand, foot, and mouth disease (HFMD). In this condition, vesicles appearing in the posterior oropharynx may erode to produce small painful ulcers. A characteristic rash, which may be vesicular or appear only as blanching red spots, appears on the palms and soles. Fever is common. HFMD usually resolves in about 1 week.

Bacterial Causes. Acute necrotizing ulcerative gingivitis (ANUG, trench mouth) is caused by fusiform bacilli and spirochetes, which may be part of normal oral flora. The condition is characterized by a rapid progression from gingival redness and pain to ulceration and spontaneous bleeding. Necrotic material accumulates as a pseudomembrane over the gums and is the cause of a characteristic foul breath odor. Children who have ANUG may have fever and malaise and generally do not eat well.

Other bacterial pathogens generally do not cause stomatitis but may play a significant role in superinfection of existing oral ulcers. Oral flora pose a real threat to the immunocompromised patient who may acquire serious systemic bacterial infection when the oral mucosa breaks down.

Noninfectious Causes

Trauma. Minor oral trauma such as cheek-biting or vigorous toothbrushing can cause local oral ulcers that are not recurrent and that resolve spontaneously. Trauma can be significant in the immunocompromised patient and as a precipitant for recurrent aphthous stomatitis (discussed after Chemotherapy).

Chemotherapy. Children undergoing cancer chemotherapy are at high risk of developing mucositis.[2] Its severity depends on the type and duration of chemotherapy, as well as on the state of the oral cavity at the onset of treatment.

Chemotherapeutic drugs are toxic to tissues such as oral mucosa, which normally have high rates of cell turnover. Within 5 days of beginning anticancer treatment, patients may experience thinning of the oral mucosa accompanied by inflammation and pain. Ulceration may follow by day 7, with potential for local and systemic bacterial infection. Routine intraoral trauma may cause or exacerbate local lesions, as can the presence of orthodontic devices.

Aphthous Stomatitis

Aphthous stomatitis (AS) is the most common ulcerative oral disease in children.[1,7] The condition often is recurrent. Terminology in this condition is confusing, in part because the term *aphthae* has been used to describe any undefined oral ulcers. Aphthous stomatitis can occur in isolation or as part of multiorgan disease.[7]

Three categories of AS have been defined on the basis of the size, duration, and tendency of lesions to produce scarring.[1]

"Minor" AS lesions are less than 1 cm in diameter, are round or oval, and appear in groups of one to five. They are yellow-gray in the center and have a red "halo"; they occur mainly on the labial and buccal mucosa and tongue. The recurrence interval is variable and occasionally cyclical. Healing without scarring occurs in 7 to 14 days. About 80% of AS is the "minor" form.

"Major" AS is found in about 10% of cases. Lesions exceed 1 cm in diameter and may occur on any part of the oral mucosa, especially the lips, soft palate, and tonsillar pillars. Lesions may take up to 6 weeks to heal, and submucosal scarring may occur.

"Herpetiform" AS also accounts for about 10% of disease. In spite of the name, "herpetiform" AS does not resemble herpetic stomatitis. Multiple (up to 100) 1 to 2 mm yellow vesicles appear, which may coalesce and produce ulcers. The lesions, which may scar, heal in 7 to 10 days. The anterior mouth, tongue, and floor of the mouth are affected most commonly.

The pathogenesis of AS is unclear for any of the categories. No convincing evidence has been produced for bacterial or viral causes. Strong genetic predisposition appears to exist,[3,5] but specific genetic factors remain unidentified. Minor local trauma is a precipitant[8] but not a cause. Stress and anxiety also are recognized as precipitating factors in susceptible individuals.[6]

Accumulated evidence points to an immunopathological mechanism for AS,[1] but the specific process remains unclear. No good direct evidence for an autoimmune process in response to specific antigens exists.

Stomatitis with an aphthous appearance may occur as part of a number of systemic conditions that should be considered in evaluation. These conditions include various nutritional deficiency states (iron, folate, B_{12}, zinc), as well as blood dyscrasias and inflammatory bowel disease. Cyclic neutropenia is associated with oral ulcers, which recur periodically during neutropenia nadirs. Its cause is unknown. In Behçet disease, aphthous-like ulcers occur in the mouth in conjunction with urethral ulcers and eye findings such as conjunctivitis and uveitis.

DATA BASE

History

When mouth sores are the chief complaint, the history should include the duration, site, and initial appearance of the lesions. Any prior history of stomatitis and pattern of recurrence should be noted. A relationship to oral trauma or to anxiety or stress may be identified. A family history of recurrent stomatitis is helpful in diagnosing aphthous stomatitis. Finally, a general medical history and review of systems may help to identify associated systemic conditions.

Physical Examination

Physical examination, noting the location and size of lesions and any accompanying signs such as fever, adenopathy, and lethargy, often leads to a specific diagnosis. Table 264-1 shows the various features of the most common types of stomatitis.

Laboratory findings usually are not helpful in determining the cause of stomatitis. In rare cases viral titers may be desirable. In recurrent aphthous stomatitis, hematological screening is recommended[1] to exclude iron or folate deficiency. The initial screen should include a complete blood count with red cell indices and hemoglobin. Ferritin, B_{12} level, and serum and red cell folate levels may be needed for further evaluation when anemia is detected.

DIFFERENTIAL DIAGNOSIS

The differential diagnosis of stomatitis in children consists of the entities discussed previously and listed in Table 264-1. Generally, specific diagnosis is not critical, unless symptoms are exceptionally severe or protracted or unless serious systemic disease is suspected.

PSYCHOSOCIAL CONSIDERATIONS

Severe stomatitis resulting in diminished or absent oral intake can be stressful for families. Parents may experience a sense of loss of control and attendant anxiety. Fears of dehydration, while appropriate, may be exaggerated. If a child is reasonably well hydrated, the physician can reassure the parents by pointing that out.

Pain, particularly with APHGS, may be a significant concern. Adequate analgesia is important, and occasionally, hospitalization is indicated for pain control and hydration. The physician should remember that a fussy or irritable child who is refusing to drink is at increased risk for physical abuse when parents become stressed and exhausted.

In APHGS, parents frequently are concerned that the herpetic condition was acquired through venereal contact. Such transmission is rare, and parents should be counseled about the innocent fashion in which the disease usually is transmitted, unless a high index of suspicion exists. In addition, parents should be counseled about the likelihood of recurrence but that the recurrence consists of isolated cold sores, not full-blown stomatitis.

The role of stress in precipitating recurrent AS is well established and should be discussed with parents and older patients.

MANAGEMENT

Primary concerns in management of the child who has any type of stomatitis are comfort and hydration. Supportive therapy alone is sufficient in hand, foot, and mouth disease, herpangina, and mild AS. Pain can be managed with acetaminophen or ibuprofen. Topical relief may be obtained with application, every 4 hours, of occlusive gels such as Oragel or Anbesol, of a 1 : 1 mixture of diphenhydramine and Kaopectate, or in more severe cases, of 2% viscous lidocaine. Systemic toxicity has occurred with the latter, so the dose should be restricted to less than 2 ml, and the parent should be cautioned to keep the bottle away from children.

In addition, APHGS usually may be managed supportively; occasionally, however, pain may be severe enough to warrant parenteral medication. Hydration via intravenous fluids may become necessary. Acyclovir may be helpful if started early enough in the course.

Therapy for trench mouth consists of topical chlorhexidine 0.2% rinses and curettage, which usually are curative. Oral penicillin may be added when systemic signs, such as fever, are present.[4]

Recurrent AS has responded well to treatment via daily

Table 264-1 Features of Stomatitis by Category

Type	Organism	Location in mouth	Appearance of lesion	Time to healing	Associated features	Recurrence
Acute primary herpetic gingivostomatitis	HSV1	Anywhere, especially anterior mucosa	Vesicles on red base	7-10 days	Fever, pain, cervical adenopathy, anorexia, dehydration	As cold sores
Herpangina	Enteroviruses, especially coxsackie A4	Posterior, especially soft palate	Small, gray-white vesicles	3-5 days	Mild pain, fever	None
Hand, foot, and mouth disease	Enteroviruses, especially coxsackie A16	Posterior	Small vesicles erode to small ulcers	7 days	Ulcers painful, papular or vesicular rash on palms and soles, fever common	None
Acute necrotizing ulcerative gingivitis (trench mouth)	Oral spirochetes and fusiform bacilli	Gingiva	Red swelling of gums progressing to ulcers with necrotic, gray pseudomembrane	Variable, depends on treatment	Fever, malaise, foul breath	Possible
Aphthous stomatitis						
Minor	Unknown or none	Tongue, labial, and buccal mucosa	Ulcers <1 cm diameter, round or oral, yellow-gray with red halo	7-14 days	Groups of one to five lesions	Common
Major	Unknown or none	Any part of mucosa, especially lips, soft palate, tonsillar pillars	Ulcers >1 cm diameter, deeper than minor	Up to 6 weeks	Submucosal scarring	Common
Herpetiform	Unknown or none	Any part, especially anterior mouth and tongue	Multiple (up to 100) vesicles 1-2 mm diameter	7-10 days	Vesicles may coalesce to small ulcers	Common

oral washes with triamcinolone acetate 0.1% or 0.2% aqueous solution.[7]

COMPLICATIONS

Complications are unusual in most forms of stomatitis. Scarring is unusual in APHGS and minor AS, but submucosal scarring may occur in major AS and herpetiform AS. In the immunocompromised patient, stomatitis or mucositis may be the site of bacterial invasion, with resulting systemic infection.

PROGNOSIS

Hand, foot, and mouth disease and herpangina rarely recur, although second infections with different viral strains are possible. APHGS does not recur, but up to 50% of patients experience one or more episodes of cold sores. Aphthous stomatitis commonly recurs, exacerbated by trauma and stress, and occasionally occurs cyclically.

WHEN TO HOSPITALIZE

Indications for hospitalization generally are dehydration and refusal of oral fluids or severe pain.

WHEN TO REFER

Most cases of stomatitis may be managed entirely by the primary care provider. Referral to a hematologist or pediatric gastroenterologist may be warranted when nutritional deficiencies or systemic disease are suspected or if laboratory investigations reveal abnormalities not responsive to simple replacement therapy.

REFERENCES

1. Field EA, Brookes V, Tyldesley WR: Recurrent aphthous ulceration in children: a review, *International Journal of Paediatric Dentistry* 2:1, 1992.
2. Hebert AA, Berg JH: Oral mucous membrane diseases of childhood: I. Mucositis and xerostomia. II. Recurrent aphthous stomatitis. III. Herpetic stomatitis, *Semin Dermatol* 11:80, 1992.
3. Miller MF, Ship II, Ram C: Inheritance patterns in recurrent aphthous ulcers, *Oral Surg Oral Med Oral Pathol* 43:886, 1977.
4. Piecuch JF, Topazian RG: Infections of the oral cavity. In Feigin RD, Cherry JD, editors: *Textbook of pediatric infectious diseases,* Philadelphia, 1987, WB Saunders.
5. Ship II: Epidemiologic aspects of recurrent aphthous ulcerations, *Oral Surg Oral Med Oral Pathol* 33:400, 1972.
6. Ship II et al: Recurrent ulcerations and recurrent herpes labialis in a professional student population, *Oral Surg Oral Med Oral Pathol* 13:1191, 1960.
7. Vincent SD, Lily GE: Clinical, historic, and therapeutic features of aphthous stomatitis, *Oral Surg Oral Med Oral Pathol* 74:79, 1992.
8. Wray D, Graykowski EA, Notkins AL: Role of mucosal injury in initiating recurrent aphthous stomatitis, *B M J* 283:1569, 1981.

265 Sudden Infant Death Syndrome

John G. Brooks

Sudden infant death syndrome (SIDS) is the leading cause of death between 1 month and 1 year of age, claiming more than 5000 infant lives each year in the United States. Despite the numerous hypotheses advanced and the extensive research done over the past several decades, the cause of SIDS remains unknown. The loss of a baby to SIDS is devastating for the family, as well as for the health care providers, and it is the pediatrician's responsibility to see that the family receives appropriate support, accurate information about SIDS, and the results of their infant's autopsy.

DEFINITION AND DIAGNOSIS

Sudden infant death syndrome is defined as "the sudden death of an infant under 1 year of age that remains unexplained after a thorough case investigation, including performance of a complete autopsy, examination of the death scene, and review of the clinical history." For clinical purposes the diagnosis of SIDS should not be excluded because of the absence of a death scene investigation, if all other findings point to SIDS. This diagnosis usually is restricted to deaths during the first year of life, although rare deaths have occurred in the second year that have the same clinical picture. Throughout most of this country there are no mandatory autopsy laws for unexpected infant deaths, so pediatricians should do their best to see that an autopsy is performed on any suspected SIDS cases. Because SIDS largely is a diagnosis of exclusion, the autopsy is essential to rule out the 10% to 20% of sudden unexpected infant deaths that are due to other causes such as intracranial hemorrhage, myocarditis, meningitis, and sometimes trauma, which may not be distinguished from SIDS without an autopsy. The autopsy results also are very important for counseling of the bereaved family so that they can be reassured that they had not missed the signs of some potentially treatable disease.

The autopsy characteristic essential for the diagnosis of SIDS is the absence of *any* finding that would constitute an "adequate cause of death," such as myocarditis, significant pneumonia, or intracranial hemorrhage. The most subjective aspect of the diagnosis of SIDS is the determination of what pathological findings constitute an "adequate cause of death." Small amounts of inflammation, in the trachea, for example, or small, isolated foci of pneumonia certainly would not be thought to cause death and therefore are compatible with the diagnosis of SIDS. Some infants who have chronic, stable, underlying diseases such as bronchopulmonary dysplasia (BPD) may die suddenly and unexpectedly, and although their autopsy findings are not normal, no abnormality explains the death. These infants' deaths also can be classified as SIDS.

From the perspective of public health and the clinician, it is more important to understand which infants are at risk of sudden and unexpected death than which autopsy findings constitute an "adequate cause of death." Clinicians should assume that sudden unexpected infant deaths are SIDS until proven otherwise so that family support and counseling can be implemented promptly. Investigating the scene of death and speaking directly with the individuals who found the dead infant are essential aspects of diagnosing SIDS accurately. It is of utmost importance that this search for evidence of environmental risk to, or maltreatment of, the infant be carried out with extraordinary sensitivity to the feelings of the bereaved family. Individuals who conduct death scene investigations of possible SIDS cases must be sensitive and knowledgeable about SIDS, bereavement processes, and child abuse. They must be aware of any of their own biases toward or against any socioeconomic or ethnic groups or child care practices so that such personal biases do not influence the sensitivity, thoroughness, or conclusions of the death scene investigation.

INCIDENCE

The current incidence of SIDS in the United States averages about 1.1 per 1000 live births, but African-American infants probably have a twofold greater incidence than Caucasian infants. In this country, SIDS has a high incidence among Native Americans. In both the United States and England, Asian populations have a lower incidence of SIDS than is found in the general population, and the incidence is lowest among Asians who have immigrated most recently. Nationally, the incidence of SIDS among non-Hispanic Caucasian infants is similar to that among Hispanic infants, despite the significant difference in mean socioeconomic status. There also is a wide variation in the incidence of SIDS in populations outside the United States. SIDS occurs relatively infrequently (fewer than 1 per 1000 live births) in most Scandinavian countries, Japan, Hong Kong, and Israel. Until recently the SIDS rate in New Zealand and Australia was 3 to 4 per 1000 live births, but this diminished significantly over the past few years at the same time that public education campaigns to prevent SIDS were implemented in those two countries. Although some of this variability between populations may be due to differences in reporting procedures and diagnostic criteria, the differences probably are due mostly to other, possibly cultural, diversities. In most countries where accurate SIDS incidence data are available, the incidence has been declining for the past 3 to 7 years. In the United States, the incidence probably has been decreasing since about 1991, but there is a 2-year lag in the availability of accurate national data in this country.

There is a characteristic frequency distribution of age at death of SIDS victims, although the 2- to 4-month peak is significantly less prominent in some recently reported data from Australia and England after their SIDS prevention campaigns. In this country, about 5% of SIDS cases occur in the first month of life, 60% by 3 months of age, 85% by 6 months, and more than 99% in the first year of life. SIDS has been reported to be rare in the first week of life, but this is at least partly because most incidence studies have excluded deaths in the first week of life. In two reported series of autopsies of neonatal deaths, 1% to 10% remain unexplained and may represent SIDS cases. Countries that have low SIDS rates also have low total infant mortality.

POSTMORTEM STUDIES OF SIDS VICTIMS

The diagnosis of SIDS cannot be established without an autopsy. Most states still lack legislation requiring an autopsy and death scene investigation for any sudden unexpected infant death.

Autopsies of such infants should follow standardized, comprehensive protocols. Although nonspecific findings such as vascular congestion, mild pulmonary edema, mild pulmonary inflammation, and an increased number of minor congenital anomalies are common, no diagnostic findings are seen on routine autopsy. The most characteristic finding is the presence of intrathoracic petechiae, which are found on the visceral surfaces of the heart, lungs, and thymus in approximately 80% of SIDS victims. Although intrathoracic petechiae are not unique to SIDS, their localization to the thoracic cavity has led to an unproven hypothesis that they may result from inspiratory efforts against an occluded upper airway.

For the past several decades, studies that used specialized techniques on tissues obtained from SIDS victims and control infants who died suddenly from an explained cause have indicated that some group mean differences exist between the SIDS babies and their controls. These group differences lack sufficient sensitivity or specificity for SIDS to be of any use in establishing the diagnosis. Although there still is some controversy about which "SIDS tissue markers" have been clearly established, those that most generally are accepted include extramedullary hematopoiesis, delayed postnatal resorption of periadrenal brown fat, abnormal pulmonary surfactant, and brainstem gliosis. It is not known whether any of these are related causally to SIDS. Some of these "tissue markers" are compatible with the hypothesis that SIDS deaths are preceded by in utero or postnatal hypoxic insults or both, but these hypotheses remain unproven. Numerous microbiological studies have failed to identify any specific viral or bacterial infection associated with SIDS. Because of methodological shortcomings and conflicting data, it is unclear whether either viral or bacterial infections are more common in SIDS victims than in appropriate controls matched for age and time of year.

EPIDEMIOLOGY

Of the diverse methodologies, disciplines, and approaches to SIDS research, epidemiology has provided the most important and conclusive contributions to an understanding of the disorder. Several clinical, demographic, and environmental characteristics of mothers and infants have been shown to be associated with an increased risk for SIDS. Only those studies that meet minimal criteria for methodological acceptability should be considered. The minimal criteria for an acceptable, epidemiological SIDS study are (1) the study must be population based; (2) the SIDS definition must be clearly stated, acceptable, and consistently adhered to; (3) all SIDS cases must be confirmed by autopsy; and (4) control infants must be appropriately selected. Identification of risk factors for SIDS is important for two reasons: first, true risk factors (in contrast to confounding variables or effect modifiers) should provide clues to the etiology of SIDS; second, these data will serve as the basis for developing a focus for efforts to prevent SIDS.

Maternal risk factors for SIDS that have been reported most consistently include maternal smoking, young maternal age (under age 20), poor prenatal care, and social deprivation. In unadjusted analyses, each of these generally confers a threefold to fourfold increased risk in comparison with mothers who do not have the particular risk factor. Each of these risk factors is still significantly associated with SIDS after socioeconomic status and race have been controlled for. Maternal smoking is one of the strongest and most consistently reported risk factors for SIDS. Both prenatal and postnatal maternal smoking increase the risk for SIDS. The complexity of the relationship between risk factors and SIDS is well illustrated by the synergistic effect of maternal smoking and maternal anemia on SIDS risk.[3] Anemia is not a risk factor for SIDS in nonsmoking mothers; in smoking mothers, however, a maternal hematocrit below 30% is associated with an increased risk of SIDS. There have been several reports of a dose-response effect of maternal smoking, with the risk of SIDS being proportional to the number of cigarettes smoked per day. The effect of maternal smoking on SIDS risk is stronger for infants who die in the first 3 months of life than for older SIDS infants, in contrast to most of the other risk factors that are more highly associated with the risk of SIDS in older infants.

Wintertime is the major environmental risk factor for SIDS, with approximately 65% to 75% of SIDS cases in this country occurring during the 6 winter months. A peak SIDS incidence in the colder months is reported in both the Northern and Southern Hemispheres, although in both Australia and England the seasonal differences in the incidence of SIDS have diminished significantly since the implementation of SIDS prevention campaigns.

Characteristics of infants that confer an increased risk of SIDS include low birth weight, prematurity, small for gestational age, multiple births, male gender, and prone sleeping position. Both prematurity and multiple births remain significantly associated with SIDS after adjustment for birth weight and race. The association of SIDS with low birth weight remains significant after adjusting for smoking, race, and gestational age. Approximately 60% of SIDS babies are boys. In most populations studied, the incidence of SIDS is at least twice as high among infants who usually sleep prone compared with infants who usually sleep on their side or their back.[1] Most of the data supporting this relationship come from studies outside the United States, but there is at least one excellent large U.S. study that indicates that the odds ratio (amount of increased risk conferred by sleeping prone) is about 1.3. After controlling for some confounding variables, such as maternal age, the strength of the association between sleeping prone and SIDS *increased* in the data from the United States and Australia. The incidence of SIDS has declined 50% or more in countries where major public health campaigns have been undertaken to educate families about the risks of infants sleeping prone, which has resulted in dramatic decreases in the prevalence of prone sleeping for infants.[7] This lends further support to the suggestion that sleeping prone truly is associated with an increased risk of SIDS. Relative overheating probably is an "effect modifier" of the risk associated with prone sleeping because overheating is a risk factor for SIDS in prone infants but not in infants who usually do not sleep in a prone position.

Two other factors that probably increase the risk of SIDS are absence of breast-feeding and maternal use of illicit drugs during pregnancy. Although there is a definite relationship between race and the risk of SIDS in this country, this finding most likely is due to confounding effects of other variables, so race probably is not a true risk factor for SIDS. Of all the well-established SIDS risk factors, sleeping prone clearly is the one that can be avoided most simply. Nonetheless, there are several well-documented reports in which the prevalence of risk factors such as low birth weight and having a teenage mother declined, but the SIDS incidence did not change. Despite anecdotal reports to the contrary, SIDS is not associated with diphtheria-pertussis-tetanus (DPT) immunizations. Minor clinical symptoms may be more common in SIDS victims in the 2 weeks before death compared with appropriate controls, but this observation has no clinical role in identifying infants at high risk for SIDS because of the high prevalence of minor clinical symptoms and the low occurrence of SIDS.

PHYSIOLOGY

Despite major efforts to define physiological characteristics that could identify infants at high risk for SIDS prospectively and delineate the mechanism of SIDS death, no clinically useful physiological characteristics have been identified to date. The only data that can illuminate the physiology of the SIDS infant are physiological data that were collected on SIDS infants before they died. Because SIDS is relatively rare, the study of large numbers of normal infants is necessary, and such studies rarely have been carried out. Those who subsequently die of SIDS demonstrate more tachycardia and fewer respiratory pauses than those who do not die of SIDS, but these differences are not sufficiently specific or sensitive to be of any clinical usefulness. There is no evidence that increased respiratory pauses or increased periodic breathing are predictive of SIDS in the general population. In addition, there is no evidence that any abnormalities of cardiac rhythm predict the infant at high risk for SIDS. Several reports of recordings obtained from home monitors while infants were dying of SIDS have demonstrated some bradycardia before the cardiac arrest, but it is not clear in some cases whether any respiratory difficulty preceded the bradycardia.

PROSPECTIVE IDENTIFICATION OF INFANTS AT HIGH RISK FOR SIDS

Efforts to identify infants at high risk for SIDS prospectively generally have focused on three different approaches. First is the *unwarranted* evaluation of 12- to 24-hour recordings of cardiorespiratory activity (pneumogram), based on the assumption that increased amounts of irregularity (pauses, periodicity) identify infants at high risk for SIDS. A second approach, although not appropriate for clinical use, is at least based on a more defensible rationale—the development of scoring systems based on various clinical or demographic characteristics of the infant or the infant's mother.[2] The scoring systems were derived from epidemiological data, but because of high false positive and false negative rates when they were tested prospectively, the scoring systems are not useful clinically. If "high risk" is defined by a score that would identify 20% of the general population as being at high risk, only 50% of the population of SIDS cases would be in the high-risk group. Because there is no proven intervention, use of the scoring systems is not indicated clinically at this time.

Finally, the incidence of SIDS among certain clinically identifiable groups has been noted to be greater than among the general population; this has been the most clinically useful and most widely used method for identifying infants at high risk for SIDS. The clinical groups for which an increased risk has been established most clearly are infants who have experienced apparent life-threatening events (ALTE), prematurely born infants, and subsequent siblings of SIDS victims. The subgroup of ALTE infants who are perceived to have required cardiopulmonary resuscitation for episodes occurring during sleep may have a subsequent mortality of 8% to 10%, and those who have more than one such severe spell (a very small subgroup) may have a risk of subsequently dying as high as 28%.[6] Those who develop a seizure disorder around the time of their ALTE episodes also have a very high risk of subsequently dying. The risk of dying of SIDS for subsequent siblings is 5 to 8 per 1000 live births, which is about three to five times that of the general population.[5] It is unclear whether all this increased risk can be explained by the increased prevalence of adverse risk factors in families that have had one SIDS victim. It is likely, although this has not been established, that in families that have no risk factors for the first SIDS victim, if risk factors still are absent for subsequent pregnancies, the risk of SIDS for that subsequent pregnancy probably is much lower than the risk in the general population. This logic, although not firmly proven, can be useful in counseling many affected families.

It is likely that infants of mothers who use cocaine are at an increased risk for dying of SIDS, but it is difficult to prove that the cocaine is the important risk factor because of the clustering of other adverse characteristics in this same population. Two subgroups of the prematurely born infant group that probably are not at increased risk of SIDS compared with other equally prematurely born infants are those who have a history of apnea of prematurity and those who have bronchopulmonary dysplasia.[4] Although some of these clinical subgroups have quite a high risk of SIDS, as shown in Figure 265-1, they do not account for most SIDS cases. Only about 5% of SIDS victims have been noted to experience apparent life-threatening events, fewer than 1% of SIDS victims are subsequent siblings of SIDS victims, and about 18% of SIDS babies were born prematurely.

ETIOLOGY OF SIDS

Neither the cause of SIDS nor the mechanism of death have been established clearly. The leading hypotheses involve primary respiratory failure due to (1) prolonged central apnea, possibly with impaired arousal, (2) acute hypoventilation due to rebreathing of expired air, as might occur in an infant

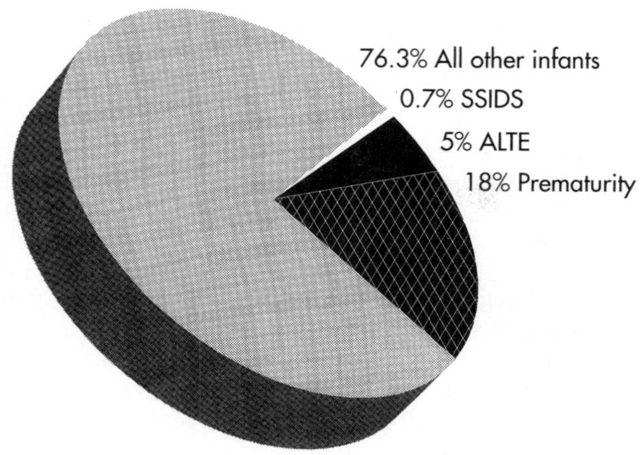

FIG. 265-1 Sources of SIDS cases as a percentage of all SIDS cases.

sleeping prone on soft bedding where a pocket develops around the infant's face, possibly in association with some rebreathing into the soft bedding, or (3) possibly some component of upper airway obstruction. There is little support for a primary cardiac arrhythmia, although neurally mediated bradycardia as the primary event is a possibility. Rare cases of SIDS probably are due to botulism, infanticide, or rare metabolic disorders. There is some evidence that all infants are at increased risk of sudden and unexplained death between 2 and 4 months of age, possibly because of interrelations of developing control systems for arousal and cardiac and respiratory rhythms. This vulnerable period most likely would be explained by dysynchronous, functional development of various components of the central nervous system, resulting in "windows" of particular vulnerability to cardiorespiratory depression, particularly during sleep. Others have proposed that a subgroup of infants is at high risk for SIDS due to some fixed cardiorespiratory vulnerability, which might have resulted from an insult in utero.

SIDS PREVENTION

Over the past 2 decades, three different approaches to preventing SIDS have been promoted. Electronic home cardiorespiratory monitors, usually using thoracic impedance technology, have been used as a preventive intervention with infants from clinically identifiable groups at high risk for SIDS, such as those who have experienced apparent life threatening events. There is no convincing evidence that home monitoring programs have lowered the incidence of SIDS. It is clear that some monitored infants have succumbed despite prompt initiation of effective resuscitation, both at home and in the hospital. In at least half of the reported cases when infants have died despite the prescription of home monitors, the monitor was not being used properly or the resuscitative efforts were not initiated properly.

A second SIDS prevention approach, most widely used in England, has involved increased numbers of home visits by health visitors (community health nurses) to assess the infant and to advise the caregiver about appropriate care practices and available support services and other resources. This intervention has not been evaluated adequately in terms of its ability to lower the incidence of SIDS.

Most recently, in Australia, New Zealand, England, and some Scandinavian countries, national public education campaigns to prevent SIDS have been implemented. These efforts to educate the general public and health professionals by using a variety of media and teaching tools have focused on some combination of encouraging breast-feeding and discouraging maternal smoking, prone positioning for infants, overwrapping or otherwise overheating infants, and using soft bedding for infants. Preliminary assessment of the effects of these campaigns has demonstrated dramatic decreases in the prevalence of prone sleeping among infants, a slight reduction in the prevalence of other targeted risk factors, and a dramatic drop in the incidence of SIDS of approximately 50%. Although it has not been shown clearly that the decrease in the prevalence of sleeping prone is the cause of the decline in the SIDS incidence, these data are encouraging, and a national SIDS prevention "Back to Sleep" campaign now is under way in the United States.

MANAGEMENT AND SUPPORT

The loss of an infant to SIDS is devastating to the family and health care providers. The important role for the physician is to remain informed about SIDS, to ensure that an autopsy is performed in all cases of sudden unexpected infant death, to see that the family is given accurate, appropriate information about SIDS and that opportunities for ongoing support and counseling are readily available and are offered to the family. The family should be provided support for age-appropriate discussions with surviving siblings. The common bereavement reactions of shock, denial, anger, and sadness should be discussed with the family. Current information about SIDS and local counseling and support groups can be obtained through the National SIDS Alliance (1-800-221-SIDS).

REFERENCES

1. American Academy of Pediatrics, Task Force on Infant Positioning and SIDS: Positioning and SIDS, *Pediatrics* 89:1120, 1992.
2. Brooks JG et al: Evaluation of the Oxford and Sheffield SIDS risk prediction scores, *Pediatr Pulmonol* 14:171, 1992.
3. Bulterys MG et al: Chronic fetal hypoxia and sudden infant death syndrome: interaction between maternal smoking and low hematocrit during pregnancy, *Pediatrics* 86:535, 1990.
4. Gray PH et al: Are infants with bronchopulmonary dysplasia at risk for sudden infant death syndrome? *Pediatrics* 93:774, 1994.
5. Guntheroth WG et al: Risk of sudden infant death syndrome in subsequent siblings, *J Pediatr* 116:520, 1990.
6. Oren J et al: Identification of high-risk group for sudden infant death syndrome among infants who were resuscitated for sleep apnea, *Pediatrics* 77:495, 1986.
7. Willinger M et al: Infant sleep position and risk for sudden infant death syndrome: report of meeting held January 13 and 14, 1994, National Institutes of Health, Bethesda, Md, *Pediatrics* 93:814, 1994.

SUGGESTED READINGS

Guntheroth WG: *Crib death: the sudden infant death syndrome,* ed 2, Mt Kisco, New York, 1990, Futura Publishing.

Harper RM et al: *Sudden infant death syndrome: risk factors and basic mechanisms,* New York, 1988, PMA Publishing.

Hunt CE, editor: Apnea and SIDS, *Clin Perinatol* 19:701, 1992.

Kiely M: *Reproductive and perinatal epidemiology,* Boston, 1990, CRC Press.

Valdes-Dapena et al: Histopathology of the sudden infant death syndrome, Washington, DC, 1993, Armed Forces Institute of Pathology.

266 Tonsillectomy and Adenoidectomy

Robert A. Hoekelman

During the twentieth century the most frequently performed operation in children in the United States requiring general anesthesia has been the removal of the tonsils, the adenoids, or both. Tonsillectomy has been more prevalent among adults, whereas adenoidectomy and tonsillectomy and adenoidectomy (T&A) have been more prevalent among children.

The decline in the frequency of these operations is the result of the controversy regarding the indications for performing them that has raged within the medical community for several decades.[3] This is so for two reasons. First, the function of tonsils and adenoids, which constitute the major elements of the Waldeyer ring within the nasopharynx, is not well understood; second, evaluative studies of the worth of T&A have suffered from a host of methodological difficulties and therefore were inconclusive until the 1980s. Consequently, each practitioner had to rely on "clinical judgment and individual experience" in determining the rationale to be used in recommending that a given child be subjected to one of these surgical procedures. Naturally, these approaches vary considerably and form the basis for much of the controversy surrounding the indications for performing these procedures.

INDICATIONS AND RISKS

The indications for T&A that have been advanced seriously by practitioners are listed in the box on p. 1627, beginning with the more generally accepted ones and moving down to those that are more suspect or even capricious. This list probably is incomplete, but it does illustrate the range of indications that have been used from both physician and parental viewpoints to rationalize removal of the tonsils and adenoids. There probably would be little argument given to any surgeon who performed a T&A for the absolute indications listed at the top of the box; however, all those listed below (in some relative order of validity) are controversial and subject to some or serious question.

Of particular note is the recent development of a method to measure the severity of obstructive sleep apnea (OSA)[5] quantitatively and to relate that score to abnormalities in right ventricular function, even before clinical signs of cor pulmonale are present.[14] OSA scores higher than 3.5 are highly predictive of the need for T&A (see the box on p. 1627).

Ultimately the worth of T&A must be measured by weighing the gains it may bring to the patient against the risks involved. In general, the morbidity and mortality from T&A are poorly documented. The mortality has been estimated in the past to be as high as 1 in every 1000 operations[3] and as low as 1 in 27,000 operations.[2] However, under current circumstances of modern anesthetic techniques and high technology and professional competence in monitoring and managing postoperative complications of hemorrhage, shock, and airway obstruction, mortality and severe morbidity following T&A surgery should be extremely rare.

The morbidity rate from T&A, however, is unknown, because no nationwide reporting mechanism is available. In the most recently reported series of T&A surgery performed under the best circumstances, 13 (14%) of 95 patients had surgically related complications. Of these, six required 1 or more extra days of hospitalization. None of the complications was considered serious, and all were managed easily or were self-limited.[6]

Otitis media has been reported to be a frequent sequela of adenoidectomy,[7] but the incidence of otitis media in children who have similar indications for adenoidectomy who did not have surgery was not assessed over the same interval. The incidence and severity of psychological complications are unknown, but asocial and aggressive behavior, excessive dependency, night terrors, and enuresis have been attributed to emotional trauma surrounding hospitalization, separation from parents, anesthesia, and discomfort associated with T&A.

On the other hand, the gains that can be attributed to tonsillectomy, adenoidectomy, or both, although attested to by many parents and physicians, were not demonstrated in adequate, prospective, randomized, controlled studies until the late 1970s and the early 1980s in a study conducted at the Children's Hospital of Pittsburgh.[8] In this study, 95 children severely affected with recurrent throat infections were subjected to tonsillectomy or tonsillectomy with adenoidectomy, whereas 92 children who had similar histories and "matched" with the "tonsillectomized" children (through both randomized and nonrandomized techniques) were not subjected to surgery. During the subsequent 2 years, the surgical group had a significantly lower incidence of throat infection than did the nonsurgical group. On the other hand, many of the children in the nonsurgical group had fewer throat infections during the 2-year follow-up period than previously, and most of these episodes were mild. During the third year of follow-up, the surgical group had fewer throat infections, but these differences overall were not statistically significant.

The criterion for tonsillectomy in the Pittsburgh study[8] was recurrent throat infection (tonsillitis, pharyngitis, or tonsillopharyngitis) characterized by the following:

1. At least three episodes in each of 3 years, or five episodes in each of 2 years, or seven episodes in 1 year
2. Each episode having been characterized by one or more of the following:
   a. Oral temperature 100.9° F (38.3° C) or higher
   b. Enlarged (over 2 cm) or tender anterior cervical lymph nodes
   c. Tonsillar or pharyngeal exudate
   d. Positive culture for group A beta-hemolytic streptococci

INDICATIONS ADVANCED FOR TONSILLECTOMY, ADENOIDECTOMY, OR BOTH

Absolute indications

Alveolar hypoventilation (obstructive sleep apnea) or cor pulmonale, secondary to airway obstruction
Dysphagia
Malignancy (radiotherapy alone preferred in most cases)
Uncontrollable hemorrhage from tonsillar blood vessels
Nasal obstruction causing discomfort in breathing and severe distortion of speech

Controversial indications

Recurrent peritonsillar abscess
Chronic cervical lymphadenitis
Hyponasality, "hot potato" voice, or both
Chronic or recurrent tonsillitis
Chronic or recurrent otitis media
Sensorineural or conductive hearing loss
Chronic mastoiditis
Cholesteatoma
Chronic sinusitis or nasopharyngitis
Diphtheria or streptococcal carrier state
Chronic bronchitis or pneumonia
Mouth breathing, snoring, or both (without obstructive sleep apnea)
Rheumatic fever, when compliance with antistreptococcal prophylaxis cannot be assured
Parental anxiety
Frequent colds with loss of time from school
Adenoidal facies
Allergic respiratory diseases
Chronic cough
Failure to thrive
Poor appetite
Focus of infection
Halitosis
Scarred or cryptic tonsils
Routine procedure

3. Apparently adequate antibiotic therapy having been administered for proven or suspected streptococcal episodes
4. Each episode having been confirmed by examination and its qualifying features described in a clinical record at the time of occurrence

Those who received concurrent adenoidectomy met *one* of the following criteria:

1. Recurrent suppurative or serous otitis media, if myringotomy and insertion of tympanostomy tubes had been performed at least once previously
2. Persistent nasal obstruction
   a. Manifested by stertorous breathing or mouth breathing with or without episodes of obstructive sleep apnea and by hyponasal speech
   b. Accompanied by both clinical and roentgenographic evidence of adenoid hypertrophy
   c. Apparently not caused by allergy

OBSTRUCTIVE SLEEP APNEA SCORE

OSA Score = 1.42D + 1.41A + 0.71S − 3.83
D = Difficulty of breathing during sleep (0 = never, 1 = occasionally, 2 = frequently, and 3 = always)
A = Apnea observed during sleep (0 = No and 1 = yes)
S = Snoring (0 = never, 1 = occasionally, 2 = frequently, and 3 = always)
Scores of >3.5 are highly predictive of the need for T&A
Scores of <−1 rule out OSA
Scores of −1 to 3.4 require polysomography to determine whether OSA requiring T&A exists

3. Chronic sinusitis or nasopharyngitis
   a. Accompanied by both clinical and roentgenographic evidence of adenoid hypertrophy
   b. Apparently not caused by allergy
   c. Persisting despite appropriate antimicrobial and other medical therapy

Although the Pittsburgh study provided evidence of the efficacy of tonsillectomy (with or without adenoidectomy) in reducing the number of throat infections by using these criteria, the efficacy of T&A performed for less stringent criteria (those used for most T&A surgery in the United States) did not prove to reduce the frequency of pharyngitis in a similar Pittsburgh-based study.[10] A nationwide collaborative study on a larger sample representative of all socioeconomic and geographical childhood populations would be needed to determine the absolute criteria for performing T&As that would be acceptable to all, but the difficulties in mounting and conducting such a study reliably have been too formidable to date and probably will never be overcome.

Thus it is likely that the controversy over indications for T&A will continue. Data from the National Center for Health Statistics' National Hospital Discharge Surveys (NHDS) indicate that some overall restraint and discrimination has been exercised in the removal of tonsils and adenoids in recent years. In 1971, 1.019 million tonsillectomies, adenoidectomies, or T&As were performed on inpatients of all ages discharged from hospitals in the United States. This number fell to 584,000 in 1979, to 259,000 in 1987, and to 76,000 in 1992. However, these figures are misleading because in the mid-1980s, changes in reimbursement for these procedures resulted in more being done on ambulatory surgical patients (not included in NHDS) than on hospitalized patients. One study reported that between 1985 and 1988, 60% of these operations occurred in ambulatory surgical centers (ASCs).[12] One must assume that this percentage has risen appreciably since then.

In general, performing these procedures in ASCs is safe unless there are underlying medical conditions (e.g., bleeding disorders, obstructive sleep apnea) that might cause complications. One study found that children under age 3 were more likely to suffer postoperative complications due to airway problems, hemorrhage, and dehydration.[15]

The Pittsburgh group also has investigated the efficacy of adenoidectomy for children at high risk for otitis media who had had tympanostomy tubes placed and had experienced recurrent suppurative or secretory otitis media after the tubes had been removed.[9] Adenoidectomy proved to be beneficial overall during 2 years of follow-up in terms of reducing the number and duration of episodes of otitis media, although many of the adenoidectomized children continued to have recurrent otitis media. The efficacy of adenoidectomy and T&A in reducing episodes of otitis media in children who had not had tympanostomy tubes placed beforehand was not shown to be significant over 3 follow-up years.[11]

The probability of a child receiving T&A surgery may be determined more by parental and physician opinion regarding the worth of T&A than on the basis of the child's health status. Because at least 25% of all visits to pediatricians' offices are for upper respiratory tract infections, including tonsillitis and otitis media, it is not surprising that parental and physician attention frequently is focused on decisions concerning the removal of tonsils and adenoids.

The decision to recommend removal of the tonsils or adenoids should be an individual matter, taking into consideration not only the frequency with which they become infected but also possible relationships to (1) mechanisms of speech, hearing, and swallowing, (2) airway obstruction, and (3) cardiorespiratory function. Many of these relationships, it must be emphasized, are at best hypothetical. Because the worth of T&A, using less stringent criteria than those used in the first Pittsburgh study,[8] has not been demonstrated,[10] conservatism in recommending such surgery is indicated. Under certain circumstances, reasonable alternatives, such as antibiotic prophylaxis or placement of tympanostomy tubes, should be considered.

Although it is not the purpose here to recommend specific indications for T&A, it seems that tonsillectomy or adenoidectomy, or both, should not be performed on any child whose criteria for surgery do not approximate those used in the Pittsburgh studies. In addition, certain indications are considered "urgent," whereas others are considered "reasonable" but in need of verification.

The "urgent" (absolute) indications are so considered because (as in cor pulmonale) surgical intervention is of established value for a serious or life-threatening condition or because surgery, although of uncertain benefit, *may* help prevent worsening of the impairment. They are as follows:

1. Alveolar hypoventilation (obstructive sleep apnea) with or without cor pulmonale and secondary to severe chronic upper airway obstruction (see the box on p. 1627). Depending on the respective size and anatomical relationships of the tonsils and adenoids, this condition may call for either tonsillectomy or adenoidectomy, or both.
2. Tonsillar enlargement sufficient to cause significant difficulty swallowing (tonsillectomy only)
3. Uncontrollable tonsillar bleeding (tonsillectomy only)
4. Tonsillar malignancy (tonsillectomy only)
5. Nasal obstruction caused by hypertrophied adenoids and resulting in manifest discomfort in breathing and severe distortion of speech (adenoidectomy only)

The "reasonable" indications are any *one* of the following:

1. Recurrent peritonsillar abscess
2. Chronic (minimum 6 months) tonsillitis, persisting despite appropriate antimicrobial therapy
3. Muffled, "hot potato" voice if the child is at least 6 years old
4. Chronic (minimum 6 months) enlargement (over 2 cm) or tenderness of anterior cervical lymph nodes, persisting despite appropriate antibiotic therapy

CONTRAINDICATIONS

Removal of the adenoids is contraindicated in children who have hypernasality resulting from velopharyngeal insufficiency. The most common cause of this is complete or incomplete cleft palate. Removal of the adenoids in this circumstance may result in a marked increase in hypernasality. Children who have a cleft palate, repaired or unrepaired, should not be subjected to adenoidectomy without consulting specialists in the management of cleft palate. All children scheduled for adenoidectomy should be examined carefully to rule out a submucous cleft, which involves the palatal muscles but not the overlying mucous membrane. The presence of a bifid uvula, a shortened and widened median raphe of the soft palate, and a palpable V-shaped midline notch (rather than a smooth, rounded curve) at the junction of the hard and soft palate is diagnostic of a submucous cleft (see Fig. 7-26 in Chapter 7). When hypernasality resulting from velopharyngeal insufficiency is suspected, irrespective of the physical findings, consultation with a speech pathologist for palatal function studies should be sought.

Local infection is considered a contraindication to T&A because of the patient's increased risk for anesthetic complications, systemic spread of infection, and hemorrhage during and after surgery. Ordinarily, surgery should be delayed for at least 3 weeks following an acute local infection except in cases in which prolonged antibiotic therapy has been ineffective and when the upper airway is severely obstructed. Some physicians believe that tonsillectomy should be performed immediately as one aspect of the treatment of peritonsillar abscess.[4]

Respiratory allergy is considered by some physicians to be a contraindication for T&A for fear that the surgery may precipitate bronchial asthma. Although such a relationship has not been proven clinically, these physicians advocate at least 6 months of antiallergic treatment for the patient's symptoms before T&A is performed.[1]

ROLE OF THE PRIMARY CARE PHYSICIAN

The pediatrician's responsibility does not end once a decision has been made in favor of T&A. The risks of hospitalization, anesthesia, and the surgery itself, in terms of morbidity and mortality, must be minimized. The pediatrician must assume responsibilities in this regard by choosing a surgeon and anesthesiologist and a hospital that will provide the best expertise and facilities available in the technical performance of the surgery and administration of the anesthesia and by working closely with them in providing the preoperative and postoperative care for the child and the parents.[1] The role of each physician and that of supporting professionals in preparing the child for hospitalization and caring for the patient during hospitalization and follow-up should be discussed and agreed on beforehand so that a coordinated team approach to care can be effected, misunderstanding among the involved professionals and between them and the parents can be avoided, and the experience for the patient and parents can be as pleasant as possible.

Parents and their child should be well informed of the circumstances of the hospitalization and surgery beforehand through preadmission visits to the hospital and age-appropriate literature (see Chapter 24, The Ill Child). A rooming-in arrangement for parents, especially those of younger children, is extremely important in minimizing the potential for psychological trauma. It is particularly important to have one or both parents present just before their child's anesthesia induction and when their child first awakens after surgery in both inpatient and ambulatory settings.

Assessment of the patient for surgery, anesthesia, and risk for complications should be shared by the team of physicians. Under ordinary circumstances, this requires only a careful history and physical examination and coagulation studies. These should include a prothrombin time, a partial thromboplastin time, a bleeding time, a hematocrit or hemoglobin measurement, and a platelet estimate, even in the absence of a positive history of coagulopathy.[2,13] Roentgenographic examination of the chest and prophylaxis against bacteremia are not necessary on a routine basis. Children who have underlying cardiac anomalies, who therefore are at risk for bacterial endocarditis, should receive antibiotic prophylaxis.

Tonsillectomy and adenoidectomy carry the potential of grave risks for each child subjected to them. The physician must consider these and weigh them against the potential benefits to be gained from the operation in reaching a decision to recommend that tonsillectomy, adenoidectomy, or both be performed. If this evaluation is done carefully and conservatively, the benefits of surgery in relation to its costs will be maximized.

REFERENCES

1. Avery AD, Harris LJ: Tonsillectomy, adenoidectomy, and tonsillectomy with adenoidectomy: assessing the quality of care using short-term outcome measures. In *Quality of medical care assessment using outcome measures: eight disease-specific applications,* Santa Monica, Calif, 1976, Rand Corp.
2. Bluestone DC et al: Workshop on tonsillectomy and adenoidectomy, *Ann Otol Rhinol Laryngol* 84 (suppl 19):1, 1975.
3. Bolger WE, Parsons DB, Potempa L: Preoperative hemostatic assessment of the adenotonsillectomy patient, *Otolaryngol Head Neck Surg* 103:396, 1990.
4. Brandow EC Jr: Immediate tonsillectomy for peritonsillar abscess, *Trans Am Acad Ophthalmol Otolaryngol* 77:412, 1973.
5. Browlette R et al: A diagnostic approach to suspected OSA, *J Pediatr* 105:10, 1984.
6. Giebink GS, Thell TE: Tonsillectomy and adenoidectomy practice patterns in Minnesota: a retrospective, multihospital audit, *Minn Med* 63:421, 1980.
7. McKee WJE: A controlled study of the effects of tonsillectomy and adenoidectomy in children, *Br J Prev Soc Med* 17:49, 1963.
8. Paradise JL et al: Efficacy of tonsillectomy for recurrent throat infection in severely affected children: results of parallel randomized and nonrandomized clinical trials, *N Engl J Med* 310:674, 1984.
9. Paradise JL et al: Efficacy of adenoidectomy for recurrent otitis media in children previously treated with tympanostomy tube placement: results of parallel randomized and nonrandomized trials, *JAMA* 263:2066, 1990.
10. Paradise JL et al: Comparative efficacy of tonsillectomy for recurrent throat infection in more vs less severely affected children, *Pediatr Res* 31(part 2):126A, 1992.
11. Paradise JL: Adenoidectomy and adenotonsillectomy (T&A) for recurrent otitis media in children not previously subjected to tympanostomy tube placement. Paper presented at the Sixth International Congress of Pediatric Otolaryngology, Rotterdam, The Netherlands, May 30, 1994.
12. Reiner SA et al: Safety of outpatient tonsillectomy and adenoidectomy, *Otolaryngol Head Neck Surg* 102:161, 1990.
13. Schmidt JL, Yaremchuk KL, Mickelson SA: Abnormal coagulation profiles in tonsillectomy and adenoidectomy patients, *Henry Ford Hosp Med J* 38:33, 1990.
14. Tal A et al: Ventricular dysfunction in children with obstructive sleep apnea (OSA), *Pediatr Pulmonol* 4:139, 1988.
15. Wiatrak BJ, Myer CM III, Andrews TM: Complications of adenoidotonsillectomy in children under 3 years of age, *Am J Otolaryngol* 12:170, 1991.

SUGGESTED READINGS

Bluestone CD: Current indications for tonsillectomy and adenoidectomy, *Ann Otol Rhinol Laryngol* 155(suppl):58, 1992.

Paradise JL: Tonsillectomy and adenoidectomy. In Bluestone CD, Stoll SE, Sheetz MD, editors: *Pediatric otolaryngology,* ed 2, Philadelphia, 1990, WB Saunders.

267 Tuberculosis

Cynthia A. Doerr and Jeffrey R. Starke

Tuberculosis continues to be one of the most important infectious diseases of humans. One third of the world's population is infected with *Mycobacterium tuberculosis*. The World Health Organization (WHO) estimates that 8 million cases of tuberculosis disease and 3 million deaths due to tuberculosis occur annually; 1.3 million cases and 450,000 deaths occur annually in children.[10] In the United States an estimated 15 million people are infected with *M. tuberculosis,* 10% of whom will develop tuberculosis if not properly treated. The tuberculin skin test is the only clinical test available to identify infected individuals. However, the accuracy of this test changes dramatically, depending on the population in which it is used. Although most children in developed countries are at low risk of contracting tuberculosis infection and should not routinely undergo the skin test, some groups in the United States have a high risk of acquiring tuberculosis infection and therefore *should* be tested.

The terminology used to describe the stages of tuberculosis is based on its pathophysiology. The three basic stages are exposure, infection, and disease. Because each of these stages requires different therapy, it is imperative to classify each patient properly. *Exposure* occurs when a child comes in contact with an adult or adolescent who has been confirmed as having or is suspected of having infectious pulmonary tuberculosis. The infectious case (called a source case) typically is a member of the patient's household, although a contagious adult in a school or child care center can be a source of significant exposure. Children who have pulmonary tuberculosis almost never are infectious. The exposed individual has a negative Mantoux skin test reaction (under 5 mm), a normal chest roentgenogram, and no signs or symptoms of tuberculosis disease. If infectious droplet nuclei have been deposited in the lungs of the exposed individual, it may take up to 3 months for a delayed-type hypersensitivity reaction to tuberculin (positive tuberculin skin test result) to develop. Due to the short incubation period of tuberculosis in children age 5 or younger, some of these infected children (as many as 15% in one study[9]) develop severe tuberculosis disease in less than 3 months if left untreated. For this reason, young children who have possible or confirmed exposure should receive chemotherapy for possible infection until 3 months after contact with the source case is broken by physical means, or by instituting antituberculosis chemotherapy for the source case. A second tuberculin skin test then should be done; if the result is negative, the chemotherapy can be discontinued. If the result is positive (5 mm or larger), tuberculosis infection is present and 9 months of chemotherapy should be given.

An individual has tuberculosis *infection* if he or she is harboring *M. tuberculosis* but does not have systemic or local manifestations of tuberculosis disease. The chest roentgenogram usually is normal, but it may show small calcifications and still not be considered indicative of tuberculous disease. In this stage, the Mantoux skin test usually yields a positive result. Approximately 5% to 10% of adults who have untreated tuberculosis infection develop tuberculosis disease during their lifetime, with one half of these cases occurring in the 2 years after the initial infection. Among infected infants, as many as 40% may develop pulmonary, meningeal, or disseminated disease.[8] All children infected with *M. tuberculosis* should receive chemotherapy to prevent disease from developing.

If an infected individual develops clinical manifestations or has an abnormal chest roentgenogram, including hilar or mediastinal adenopathy, he or she has tuberculosis *disease,* commonly referred to as "tuberculosis" (TB). The Mantoux skin test result usually is positive. However, among adults and children who are not infected with the human immunodeficiency virus (HIV), 10% may have a negative result on the Mantoux test[14,15]; among HIV-infected individuals, as many as 50% may have a negative result. Tuberculosis in adults and some adolescents usually occurs when previously dormant *M. tuberculosis* reactivates years or even decades after the initial infection. In contrast, within 1 year, children and most adolescents develop tuberculosis disease as a complication of the initial infection rather than as a reactivation of a previous infection.

Epidemiology

M. tuberculosis is transmitted to children almost exclusively through deposition of infected aerosol droplet nuclei in the alveoli of the lungs. Individuals most likely to be infectious are adults or adolescents who (1) have cavitary pulmonary tuberculosis, (2) cough frequently, and (3) have a positive result with acid-fast staining of sputum. Most children under age 12 who have pulmonary tuberculosis are unable to cough forcefully, rarely produce sputum, have a comparatively low burden of organisms, and therefore rarely are contagious. Because transmission of *M. tuberculosis* usually requires repeated or prolonged (not casual) contact, understanding tuberculosis infection and disease among children necessitates an understanding of contagious pulmonary tuberculosis among adults.

The incidence of tuberculosis in the United States increased by 20% (from 22,201 cases to 26,673 cases) from 1985 to 1992.[2] In the past, tuberculosis disease was diagnosed predominantly in older adults. From 1985 to 1992, however, the median age of those who had tuberculosis disease in the United States dropped, especially among young Hispanic and non-Caucasian adults and children. During the same period the incidence of tuberculosis disease increased 27% (from 7592 cases to 9623 cases annually) among African-Americans and 75% (from 3092 cases to 5397 cases annually) among Hispanics. Although data are fairly com-

CHILDREN AT HIGH RISK FOR TUBERCULOSIS IN THE UNITED STATES

Children who have had contact with adults who are or were:
- Foreign-born persons from countries that have a high prevalence of the disease
- Residents of correctional institutions
- Residents of long-term care facilities
- Homeless
- Users of intravenous and other street drugs
- Poor or medically indigent, especially urban residents
- Infected with HIV
- From families that have a history of tuberculosis

plete for tuberculosis disease because it is reportable in all states, tuberculosis infection in children is reportable in only four states (Indiana, Kentucky, Missouri, and Texas), making true epidemiological patterns of infection among adults and children difficult to determine.

Although the risk of acquiring tuberculosis infection depends mostly on environmental factors—that is, the chance that a child has significant contact with an adult who has contagious pulmonary tuberculosis—the risk of developing tuberculosis disease depends mostly on host-related factors (see the box above). One of the most important risk factors for infection is contact with an HIV-infected adult. These adults are at far greater risk than the general population of developing pulmonary tuberculosis, and they are significantly more likely to harbor a multiply drug-resistant organism.[3] Contact with foreign-born adults, especially those who have immigrated recently, is another risk factor. In 1993, 29.6% of tuberculosis cases in the United States occurred among foreign-born individuals. Adults of Hispanic, Asian, or Pacific Island descent who have immigrated in the past 5 years have a particularly high risk of developing pulmonary tuberculosis and becoming source cases. Certain congregate facilities (e.g., jails, prisons, homeless shelters, nursing homes, and other chronic care facilities) are high-risk settings for *M. tuberculosis* infection and transmission. Finally, the incidence of tuberculosis disease is higher in metropolitan areas; 40% of United States children age 4 or younger who were diagnosed with tuberculosis disease in 1991 lived in cities that had populations greater then 250,000. In general, however, the vast majority of people in the United States and other industrialized countries are at low risk for tuberculosis infection.

Host-related factors help determine which infected individuals develop tuberculosis. Most cases of childhood tuberculosis occur in children under age 5, and these young patients are more likely to develop severe or life-threatening forms of disease. School-age children (5 to 12 years of age) have been called the "favored age" because most of them who are infected do not develop primary tuberculosis disease (although they are more likely to develop reactivation tuberculosis disease as adults than are children who are infected at a younger age). Children who have chronic immunosuppressive medical problems (e.g., malignancy) or who receive medications such as corticosteroids or antineoplastic chemotherapy also are at increased risk of developing tuberculosis disease if infected with *M. tuberculosis*. Infection with HIV appears to be a strong risk factor for the development of tuberculosis disease in children infected with *M. tuberculosis*.[4]

THE TUBERCULIN SKIN TEST

The tuberculin purified protein derivative (PPD) skin test, derived from supernatant extracts of cultures of *M. tuberculosis*, has been in use since 1939. Although nearly 6 decades have passed since the first batch was prepared in Philadelphia, PPD skin testing remains the only clinical test for diagnosing tuberculosis infection.

There are two ways to administer PPD or another antigen, called Old Tuberculin: multiple-puncture devices (MPDs), which typically have metal or plastic prongs coated with dried or liquid antigen, and the Mantoux 5 tuberculin unit intradermal injection, which is considered the gold standard skin test. MPDs should never be used because they have several serious drawbacks.[13] First, the exact dose of antigen introduced into the skin cannot be controlled precisely, so interpretation of the reaction size cannot be standardized. When compared with Mantoux skin tests, MPD reactions vary tremendously with the population studied and sometimes have a high rate of both false positive and false negative results. Another difficulty may be encountered when family members report reactions. Although other medical test results are interpreted nearly universally by medical personnel, parents often are asked to interpret the reaction from an MPD. However, nearly all studies regarding self-interpretation of skin tests indicate that patients and families do not read their tests accurately. Although many self-interpretations of true negative skin test reactions are correct, about half of the true positive skin test reactions are interpreted incorrectly as negative reactions. These false negative interpretations may stem from either an inability to differentiate between positive and negative reactions or a hesitancy to disclose a positive reaction because of fear of social stigma or need for long-term antituberculosis treatment. Finally, because an MPD is not a definitive test, a Mantoux skin test is needed to confirm any suspicious MPD reaction. Unfortunately, if the individual has been sensitized previously by *M. tuberculosis,* a nontuberculous mycobacterial infection, or bacille Calmette-Guérin (BCG) immunization, repetitive stimulation of waned immunological response by serial skin tests may produce a false positive reaction. Using a Mantoux skin test initially eliminates not only the need for a confirmatory skin test but also the potential for this "boosting" phenomenon.

A Mantoux skin test is best administered by anchoring the side of the hand that is holding the syringe against the side of the child's arm and injecting solution containing five tuberculin units of PPD intradermally in a transverse direction (Fig. 267-1). The fluid should make a palpable wheal that is absorbed in a few hours. The reaction size is measured no sooner than 48 hours and preferably at 72 hours. If further induration occurs after 72 hours, the reaction should be considered positive. Erythema, although common, is not considered a positive reaction; only induration, even mild, is palpated, measured, and recorded in millimeters (never as "positive" or "negative").

Neither tuberculosis infection nor disease can be ruled out

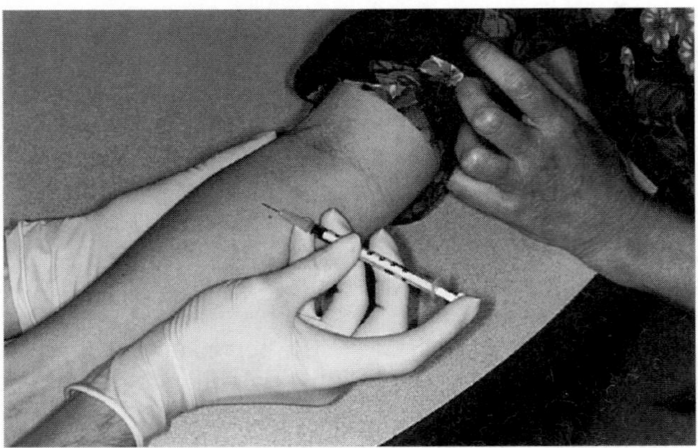

FIG. 267-1 Recommended technique for administering the Mantoux tuberculin skin test.

in a child who has a negative result on a Mantoux tuberculin skin test. A number of factors may reduce responsiveness to tuberculin (see the accompanying box). Overwhelming tuberculosis disease itself may lower tuberculin reactivity in children. Approximately 10% of immunocompetent children who have culture-proven tuberculosis disease have a negative result on the initial Mantoux tuberculin skin test; most of these children develop positive skin test results several months after chemotherapy is started.

Previous immunization with BCG (which is administered routinely in all countries except the United States and The Netherlands) may cause confusion when a Mantoux skin test is interpreted. The BCG vaccines are produced from *M. bovis* organisms that have been passed in serial culture to diminish their virulence. Currently, four principal strains of BCG vaccine, which have widely varying characteristics, are in common use, and immunization schedules vary among countries in the number of immunizations given, the method of administration, and the age at which initial and/or booster doses are administered.[12] Because of these variations, it is difficult to make standard recommendations for interpreting Mantoux skin reactions after BCG immunization. However, it generally has been demonstrated that only 50% of infants who receive a BCG vaccine shortly after birth have a positive result on a tuberculin skin test at 6 to 12 months of age, and virtually all immunized children have a negative result by age 5. Patients who receive a BCG vaccine as an older child or adult are more likely to develop and retain a reaction to a tuberculin skin test than those who are immunized as infants, but by 10 years postvaccination, 80% to 90% of these individuals have little or no reaction to a skin test.[6,7] It is presumed that most recipients of a BCG vaccine will have a PPD reaction below 10 mm after a few months to years. Skin test reactions should be interpreted in the same manner for individuals who have or have not received BCG. Prior BCG immunization is never a contraindication for tuberculin testing.

Although the Mantoux skin test is considered the gold standard, the accuracy of the test depends on proper placement, correct assessment of the reaction's size, and the population being tested. Because *M. tuberculosis* infection in the United States is concentrated mostly in discrete subset populations, most children in the United States are at low risk for tuberculosis infection and disease. Under the best conditions, the sensitivity and specificity of the Mantoux skin test are about 90% (which is very low for a diagnostic test), yielding a high positive predictive value in high-risk populations.[11] However, the predictive value of a positive test result drops dramatically in populations that have a low rate of infection. In other words, most positive Mantoux skin test results in high-risk children are true positives, whereas the vast majority (more than 80%) of "positive" Mantoux skin test reactions in low-risk populations are false positives. Therefore, populations at low risk for tuberculosis infection should not undergo routine testing with the Mantoux skin test.

In 1994 the American Academy of Pediatrics (AAP) with the American Thoracic Society and the Centers for Disease Control and Prevention (CDC) developed guidelines for interpreting Mantoux skin test results based on the patient's clinical, social, and medical history (Table 267-1).[1] This set of guidelines is scientifically valid, but it may be difficult to classify an individual into the proper risk category because of an inability to elicit an accurate medical and social history. A further difficulty is that the risk factors for children depend largely on the risk factors of the adults who care for them. For instance, a child may live with an uncle who recently has been released from a jail that has a population with

FACTORS THAT DIMINISH TUBERCULIN REACTIONS

Host-related factors

Infections
- Viral (rubella, rubeola, varicella, influenza)
- Bacterial (typhoid fever, brucellosis, leprosy, pertussis, overwhelming tuberculosis)
- Fungal (blastomycosis)

Vaccines (live viral)
Chronic renal failure
Malnutrition
Diseases affecting lymphoid organs (leukemia, lymphoma, HIV infection)
Certain drugs (corticosteroids, antineoplastic agents)
Age (newborns and the elderly)
Stress (surgery, burns, mental illness)

Tuberculin-related factors

Improper storage (exposure to light or heat)
Improper dilutions
Chemical denaturation
Contamination
Adsorption to glass or plastic

Administration-related factors

Injection of too little antigen
Delay in administration after antigen is drawn into the syringe
Insufficient interval between injections

Reading-related factors

Inexperienced reader
Conscious or unconscious bias
Error in recording

Table 267-1 Cutoff Size of Reactive Area for Positive Mantoux Tuberculin Reaction

≥5 mm	≥10 mm	≥15 mm
Contacts of infectious cases Abnormal chest roentgenogram HIV-infected and other immunosuppressed patients	Foreign-born people from countries that have a high prevalence Residents of prisons, nursing homes, institutions Low-income populations Users of intravenous street drugs Other medical risk factors Health care workers Locally identified high-risk populations Children in close contact to high-risk adults Infants*	No risk factors

*Infants are not listed as a high-risk group under the guidelines of the American Thoracic Society and the CDC, but they should be included in this category.

a high rate of tuberculosis. A careful history is crucial to classify the child properly. It also may be socially stigmatizing to place students in the same classroom who have identical reactions into different risk categories, since this may create the appearance of cultural, economic, or racial bias. However, if children who have no risk factors for tuberculosis are not tested, the scheme for interpretation is much simplified, and the number of skin tests done and interpreted will be greatly diminished in most pediatric practices or clinics.

DETECTION OF TUBERCULOSIS IN CHILDREN

Infected children are discovered as a result of routine screening, when they develop tuberculosis disease and become symptomatic, or as a result of a health department contact investigation. Routine, periodic screening should be conducted only among children who have risk factors for infection (see the box on p. 1631).

Children most commonly are discovered to have tuberculosis infection or disease through contact investigation of an adult source case. Contact investigations not only have a high yield, but they also find the more recently infected children who are at higher risk of developing primary tuberculosis disease. When a case of suspected contagious pulmonary tuberculosis is reported to the health department, a contact investigation is initiated, ideally within several days of the report. The health department performs a Mantoux skin test on all significant contacts of the index case, beginning with those at highest risk (usually those in the household or immunosuppressed individuals). Individuals who have a Mantoux skin test reaction of 5 mm or larger receive a chest roentgenogram and physical examination to determine if disease is present and then all are placed on proper chemotherapy regardless of the findings. On average, 30% to 50% of household contacts of an infectious adult have a positive Mantoux skin test result, and 1% to 2% already have the disease.[5] About half of childhood tuberculosis cases in the United States are discovered through contact investigation; most of these children are asymptomatic, but significant signs of disease can be seen on the chest roentgenogram.

Any ill child who has signs or symptoms consistent with tuberculosis disease, even in the absence of any identifiable risk factors, should receive a full medical evaluation, including tuberculin skin testing. Specifically, most children who have pneumonia, cervical adenopathy or lymphadenitis, osteomyelitis or chronic arthritis, or meningitis should receive a tuberculin skin test, and their history should be reviewed for tuberculosis exposure if another cause of disease is not readily apparent.

HIV-infected children may benefit from annual Mantoux skin testing. HIV-infected children are more likely to be in contact with HIV-infected adults and have other significant risk factors for tuberculosis infection. Many HIV-infected children have anergy to tuberculin and other antigens, so a negative skin test result should not dissuade the clinician from pursuing a diagnosis of tuberculosis infection or disease in a child who has a significant exposure or signs and symptoms of disease. A difficult situation arises when an anergic, HIV-infected child has significant contact with an adult who has contagious pulmonary tuberculosis. The child should have a careful evaluation for tuberculosis disease. If no disease is found, most experts would treat the child for tuberculosis infection even though its presence cannot be proven.

MANAGEMENT OF CHILDREN WHO HAVE A REACTIVE MANTOUX SKIN TEST

Once a child is found to have a positive tuberculin skin test result, clinical evaluation determines if the child has tuberculosis infection or disease. About 50% of children who have pulmonary tuberculosis are asymptomatic. Infants are much more likely to develop severe respiratory symptoms and extrapulmonary or disseminated disease; older children, particularly adolescents, frequently have fewer clinical manifestations.

The first step in evaluating a child who has a positive result on the Mantoux tuberculin skin test, whether placed for screening or because of a contact investigation, is to obtain a complete history. Specific and nonjudgmental questions must be asked because many families may feel stigmatized by the infection and may be reluctant to disclose possibly embarrassing information about themselves or other family members and friends. It is important to ask every question of every family, regardless of ethnic or social background. The patient or parents should be asked about the immediate family first; then the scope of questions should be widened to include friends, child care, school, or work, and finally social contacts, such as those in a church or other large congregations. Questions must be asked about contacts known to have or to have had tuberculosis infection or disease, whether previously treated or currently receiving therapy; contacts who showed weight loss or were coughing or sick; contacts in nursing homes, jails, prisons, or homeless shelters; and contacts who had immigrated during the past 5 years. The patient's travel history also should be explored. Any history of contacts diagnosed with or treated for tuberculosis disease should be confirmed by the local health department's division of tuberculosis control to determine the extent of the previous contact investigation and treatment. Questions also must be asked about the past and present health of a child who has a positive result on the tuberculin skin test.

After the history is taken, a careful physical examination of the child should be performed because 25% to 35% of tuberculosis disease in children is extrapulmonary. The most common sites are cervical lymph nodes, meninges, pleura, bones, joints, and skin. Often no abnormalities will be discovered. The child should be checked for adenopathy, central nervous system abnormalities, lung involvement, and liver enlargement. All patients also should have high-quality posteroanterior and lateral roentgenographic views of the chest taken to detect any pulmonary involvement. The need for additional testing is determined by the demonstration of any abnormality on the chest roentgenogram or physical examination and by the history.

The most common sites for tuberculosis disease are the lung and perihilar lymph nodes. Small calcified densities in the lung parenchyma or lymph nodes indicate areas of a healed primary complex and are not considered evidence of active disease in the absence of other abnormalities. Perihilar lymph node involvement may be seen as an enlarged silhouette but also may be seen to encircle and compress a mainstem bronchus or to impinge unilaterally on the trachea or mainstem bronchus, causing deviation. Pulmonary disease commonly is manifested as atelectasis, a discrete pulmonary infiltrate, pleural effusion, a miliary pattern (more common in infants) or, in rare cases, cavitary disease in older children and adolescents.

Extrapulmonary sites are involved less commonly but may be associated with significant morbidity or mortality if treated inadequately. The most common extrapulmonary site of involvement is the cervical lymph nodes; surgery rarely is required, and this disease usually is managed effectively by antituberculosis chemotherapy. These lymph nodes may be removed surgically if the diagnosis is in question or if rupture of the node with subsequent scarring is imminent; however, they should never be incised and drained because the surgical incision often is seeded with organisms, resulting in a chronically draining sinus that must be removed surgically. Central nervous system involvement is the second most common form of extrapulmonary disease and is always fatal without proper treatment. Many patients have symptoms of malaise, irritability, and fever for many days or weeks before manifesting cranial nerve abnormalities, hydrocephalus, and basilar meningitis. Other extrapulmonary sites of involvement (e.g., pleura, bone, skin, pericardium, kidney, and gastrointestinal tract) are less common.

An attempt should be made to determine the drug susceptibility pattern of the organism in all cases of suspected or proven tuberculosis infection or disease. If the drug susceptibility results are known for the isolate from the adult source case, it may be presumed that the child's isolate has the same pattern. However, if the source case has not been found for a child who has tuberculosis disease, isolating the organism from the child should be attempted. Children should be evaluated by acid-fast stain and mycobacterial culture of either expectorated sputum (from an adolescent), if it is available, or of early morning aspiration of gastric contents on 3 successive days (from infants and children). Collection of gastric aspirates requires hospitalization because the desired sample is the pooled overnight secretions that have been swallowed and remain in the stomach before the child arises. Decisions about the need for further cultures (urine, cerebrospinal fluid) or histopathological examination of biopsied tissue are dictated by the extent and anatomical location of suspected disease.

Tuberculosis infection and disease are treated with chemotherapy. Commonly used antituberculosis drugs and doses are listed in Table 267-2. Unlike adults, children who take antituberculosis medication experience few side effects. Transient gastrointestinal (GI) distress sometimes is encountered, resulting in vomiting during the first few days of administration. Although rare, the most common serious problem is hepatotoxicity, principally induced by isoniazid (INH) but occasionally associated with rifampin (RIF) or pyrazinamide (PZA). Peripheral neuritis or convulsions caused by inhibition of pyridoxine metabolism in children receiving INH are very rare, and pyridoxine supplementation is not necessary unless the patient has nutritional deficiencies (meat- and milk-deficient diet), is pregnant, or is a breast-fed infant. Discolored secretions are common with RIF administration, which may stain contact lenses permanently. Oral contraceptives may be rendered ineffective by RIF, so an alternative form of birth control should be used while RIF is taken. Reversible optic neuritis is a serious but rare side effect caused by ethambutol (EMB); therefore visual acuity and color discrimination should be monitored monthly in patients receiving this drug. Streptomycin (STM) administration may be associated with ototoxicity and hearing loss. The drug should be avoided as a long-term agent, and hearing should be tested before, during, and after STM therapy. Because hepatotoxicity is rare in children, many tuberculosis experts do not monitor blood chemistries routinely for evidence of abnormalities, but rely instead on early identification of clinical manifestations. Allergic reactions associated with antituberculosis medications, manifested primarily by skin rashes and pruritus, also are rare.

Children who have a positive Mantoux skin test result and no other abnormalities have tuberculosis infection, and treatment with INH for 9 months is considered optimal.[11] Children who have been coinfected by HIV and *M. tuberculosis* should be treated for 12 months. For patients who cannot tolerate INH or who are infected with INH-resistant organisms, RIF for 9 months is a satisfactory alternative. If the adult source case is known to have a multiple drug–resistant isolate of *M. tuberculosis* (INH and RIF resistant), at least two drug therapies based on the susceptibility pattern should be instituted, if possible. It is imperative to search for the adult source case and the drug susceptibility pattern of his or her isolate, if possible, to be sure the correct drugs are given to the child.

Children who have drug-susceptible pulmonary tuberculosis (including hilar or mediastinal adenopathy) may be treated adequately with 6 months of INH and RIF, with the addition of PZA for the first 2 months.[13] If drug resistance is suspected (especially if the adult source case was treated previously for tuberculosis, came from a country or region that has high rates of drug-resistant tuberculosis, or is HIV infected) a fourth drug, usually EMB or STM, should be added to the initial regimen. Extrapulmonary tuberculosis disease may be treated adequately with INH, RIF, and PZA, but longer

Table 267-2 Drugs Used Commonly for the Treatment of Tuberculosis Among Infants, Children, and Adolescents

Drugs	Dosage form	Daily dose (mg/kg/day)	Twice weekly Dose (mg/kg/dose)	Twice weekly Maximum dose	Adverse reactions
Ethambutol	Tablets 100 mg 400 mg	15-25	50	2.5 g	Optic neuritis (reversible), diminished visual acuity, reduced red-green color discrimination, GI disturbance
Isoniazid*	Scored tablets 100 mg 300 mg Syrup 10 mg/ml	10-15	20-30	Daily: 300 mg; twice weekly: 900 mg	Mild hepatic enzyme elevation, hepatitis, peripheral neuritis, hypersensitivity
Pyrazinamide*	Scored tablets 500 mg	20-40	50	2 g	Hepatotoxicity, hyperuricemia
Rifampin*	Capsules 150 mg 300 mg Syrup Formulated in syrup from capsules	10-20	10-20	600 mg	Orange discoloration of secretions/urine, staining of contact lenses, hepatitis, flulike reaction, thrombocytopenia; may render birth control pills ineffective
Streptomycin (intramuscular administration)	Vials 1 g 4 g	20-40	20-40	1 g	Ototoxicity, nephrotoxicity, skin rash

*Rifamate is a capsule containing 150 mg of isoniazid and 300 mg of rifampin. Rifater is a tablet containing 50 mg of isoniazid, 120 mg of rifampin, and 300 mg of pyrazinamide.

courses—6 to 12 months—and the initial addition of EMB or STM (to guard against unknown drug resistance) are indicated for complicated, severe, or central nervous system disease. As with tuberculosis infection, if the adult source case is known to have a multiple drug–resistant *M. tuberculosis* isolate and/or a resistant organism is cultured from a child who has tuberculosis disease, at least four-drug therapy should be instituted, based on the susceptibility pattern. Consultation with an infectious disease specialist or other appropriate specialist is recommended for any case of drug-resistant tuberculosis infection or disease.

The greatest challenge in treating tuberculosis is patient failure to fulfill treatment requirements; this leads to relapse, development of secondary drug resistance, and possible transmission of organisms to others. All patients being treated for tuberculosis disease should have their therapy administered and monitored by a health care worker, usually a member of the health department. This directly observed therapy (DOT) is necessary to monitor for drug side effects and to ensure compliance in taking medications, which essentially eliminates the emergence of secondary drug resistance. Antituberculosis drugs may be given twice weekly under DOT for drug-susceptible tuberculosis infection and for pulmonary and uncomplicated extrapulmonary tuberculosis disease. For these forms of tuberculosis, twice weekly DOT is as effective as daily therapy, has the same or fewer adverse reactions, and is more effective in preventing the emergence of drug resistance.[16]

All household and close contacts under age 5 years of a patient with suspected contagious pulmonary tuberculosis (even if the Mantoux skin test result was nonreactive) should be given INH to prevent disease from occurring rapidly. Some young children, if infected, develop disseminated disease before a tuberculin skin test result becomes apparent. The Mantoux test should be repeated 3 months after contact with the source case has ended. If the second reaction is positive, infection has occurred and the patient should remain on INH and be evaluated for possible tuberculosis disease. If the Mantoux test remains nonreactive, the patient should discontinue INH, provided the source case is undergoing adequate, monitored antituberculosis therapy and his or her sputum tests negative for acid-fast organisms on a smear.

Congenital tuberculosis disease is extremely rare. The more common situation is the newborn in whose family an adult (sometimes the mother) is suspected of having contagious pulmonary tuberculosis. The infant should remain separated from a mother who has a newly recognized reactive tuberculin skin test result until she has had a chest roentgenogram. If the mother has no evidence of pulmonary disease, the infant may safely stay with her. If the mother or any member of the household is suspected of having pulmonary disease but there is no evidence or suspicion of INH-resistant *M. tuberculosis,* the infant should be treated with INH (given daily by the mother or a public health nurse) and a Mantoux skin test should be done 3 months after the mother (or other family member) is no longer contagious. If a member of the household is undergoing treatment for tuberculosis disease, that individual should not have contact with the infant, if possible, unless his or her sputum smear tests negative on acid-fast staining. If the infant and infected family member cannot be separated, the family member must be followed up carefully to ensure compliance with treatment; the infant should be given INH for 3 months, and a Mantoux skin test should be done before therapy is discontinued. If the second tuberculin skin test reaction is positive, infection has occurred, and the infant should continue receiving INH for 9 months and be evaluated for possible tuberculosis disease.

OUTCOME

Children infected with tuberculosis who are treated adequately are nearly universally free of tuberculosis disease upon completion of treatment, and most patients who have uncomplicated pulmonary and extrapulmonary disease have complete resolution of the disease. Patients who have the least favorable prognosis are infants who have severe disseminated disease, children who have tuberculosis meningitis, patients who have multiple drug–resistant tuberculosis disease, and patients who have underlying problems such as immunosuppression (especially HIV infection) or debilitating chronic disorders. Patients should be examined every 4 to 6 weeks during therapy so that their adherence to therapy and any medication side effects may be monitored. Roentgenographic abnormalities should show improvement but may take many months or years to resolve completely. Most children's roentgenograms still show abnormalities after 6 months of therapy, but this does not indicate treatment failure. Patients who have completed medical therapy should be examined within 3 to 6 months to ensure that there is no evidence of recurrent disease.

CONCLUSION

The clinician must be aware of who is at increased risk for tuberculosis and administer and interpret Mantoux skin tests accordingly. Reporting suspected and confirmed cases of tuberculosis disease in adolescents and adults to the health department is essential to prevent source cases from continuing to infect children and other adults. Most important, the physician must institute directly observed therapy whenever possible to ensure complete eradication of infection or disease in the patient. When the patient, the clinician, and the health department interact effectively, nearly all patients with TB recover fully.

REFERENCES

1. American Academy of Pediatrics: Tuberculosis. In Peter G, editor: *1994 Red book: report of the Committee on Infectious Diseases,* ed 23, Elk Grove Village, Ill, 1994, American Academy of Pediatrics.
2. Cantwell MF et al: Epidemiology of tuberculosis in the United States, 1985 through 1992, *JAMA* 272:535, 1994.
3. Frieden TR et al: The emergence of drug-resistant tuberculosis in New York City, *N Engl J Med* 328:521, 1993.
4. Gutman LT et al: Tuberculosis in human immunodeficiency virus–exposed or –infected United States children, *Pediatr Infect Dis J* 13:963, 1994.
5. Hsu KHK: Contact investigation: a practical approach to tuberculosis eradication, *Am J Public Health* 53:1761, 1963.
6. Karalliede S, Katughan LP, Uragoda CG: The tuberculin response of Sri Lankan children after BCG vaccination at birth, *Tubercle* 68:33, 1987.
7. Lifschitz M: The value of the tuberculin skin test as a screening test for tuberculosis among BCG-vaccinated children, *Pediatrics* 36:624, 1965.
8. Miller FSN, Seale RME, Taylor MD: *Tuberculosis in children,* Boston, 1963, Little, Brown.
9. Nolan RC Jr: Childhood tuberculosis in North Carolina: a study of the opportunities for intervention in the transmission of tuberculosis to children, *Am J Public Health* 76:26, 1986.
10. Raviglione MC, Snider DE Jr, Kochi A: Global epidemiology of tuberculosis: morbidity and mortality of a worldwide epidemic, *JAMA* 273:220, 1994.
11. Snider DE Jr: The tuberculin skin test, *Am Rev Respir Dis* 125(suppl):108, 1982.
12. Starke JR, Connelly KK: Bacille Calmette-Guérin vaccine. In Plotkin SA, Mortimer EA Jr, editors: *Vaccines,* ed 2, Philadelphia, 1994, WB Saunders.
13. Starke JR, Jacobs RF, Jereb J: Resurgence of tuberculosis in children, *J Pediatr* 120:839, 1992.
14. Starke JR, Taylor-Watts KT: Tuberculosis in the pediatric population of Houston, Texas, *Pediatrics* 84:28, 1989.
15. Steiner P et al: Persistently negative tuberculin reactions: their presence among children who culture positive for *Mycobacterium tuberculosis, Am J Dis Child* 134:747, 1990.
16. Weis SE et al: The effect of directly observed therapy on the rates of drug resistance and relapse in tuberculosis, *N Engl J Med* 330:1179, 1994.

268 Umbilical Anomalies

Robert W. Marion

It [the umbilicus] is all that remains of the stem that bound us to the parental stalk. It is a reminder that we have been plucked and must sooner or later die. It might be said that when the stem is severed, we cease to live in any true sense. We may be ornamental like roses or useful like cabbages but only for a little while. Our dissolution has begun.[5]

Despite its essential role in the survival of the fetus during prenatal life, the umbilicus, the external vestige of the umbilical cord, frequently is ignored or overlooked by the pediatric primary care provider. However, aberrations in either the formation or the position of this structure can offer helpful clues to an underlying pathological condition in a young child. Major congenital anomalies of the ventral abdominal wall (e.g., omphalocele, gastroschisis, and exstrophies of the bladder and cloaca) are described in detail elsewhere (see Chapter 48, Critical Neonatal Illnesses); this chapter deals with minor anomalies in configuration, placement, and formation of the umbilicus. In addition to the conditions described here, the umbilicus can be the site of both tumors (either vascular or teratomatous neoplasms) and infections (omphalitis).[3]

To understand the etiology and significance of anomalies of the umbilicus, it is necessary to review some basic fundamentals of the embryological development of the umbilical cord.

EMBRYOLOGICAL DEVELOPMENT OF THE UMBILICAL CORD

Appearing within the first 6 weeks of gestation, the umbilical cord is derived from the fusion of three separate embryonic structures: (1) the primitive or primary yolk sac, which contains the allantois and a portion of the vitelline duct, transient structures that ultimately form the central portion of the embryonic gut, the urinary bladder, the urachus, and the umbilical blood vessels (usually two arteries and one vein), (2) the secondary yolk sac, composed of the remainder of the vitelline duct, and (3) the mesenchyme of the connecting body stalk of the embryo, the tissue that produces Wharton jelly, the packing substance that holds the cord together. After fusion is complete, these unified structures become covered by the amnion and ultimately are surrounded by amniotic fluid.[2]

Many of these embryonic structures that form the umbilical cord are transitory, present for only brief periods during embryogenesis. After the seventh week of gestation, the vitelline duct regresses and ultimately becomes completely resorbed. Similarly, the allantois, which is contiguous with the urinary bladder, degenerates, forming a fibrous cord called the urachus, which connects the apex of the bladder with the umbilicus. Anomalies may result when these structures fail to undergo their normal regression, causing them to persist into postnatal life.

ANOMALIES OF THE UMBILICUS

Abnormalities of Position and Morphology

Anatomically the umbilicus usually is situated at a level at the top of the iliac crest ventral to the third or fourth lumbar vertebra.[6] Variations in the position of the umbilicus can result from abnormalities in the way in which the abdominal wall itself formed and, as such, may be a clue to the diagnosis of specific dysmorphic syndromes. For example, as shown in Table 268-1, the umbilicus has been noted to be low set in conditions such as achondroplasia and bladder and cloacal exstrophy[8] and in association with various anomalies of the urinary tract[1]; higher than normal placement of the umbilicus occurs in Robinow syndrome.[8]

Similarly, variations in the appearance of the umbilicus can suggest the presence of a syndrome. In Aarskog syndrome, a disorder that combines abnormalities of the face, digits, and genitalia, the umbilicus is pouting and protuberant, whereas in Robinow syndrome (also known as "fetal face syndrome" because of the striking ocular hypertelorism that occurs in affected individuals), the normal umbilical scar is broad and poorly epithelialized.[8]

Embryonic Umbilical Remnants

As noted above, the umbilical cord is formed from the vitelline duct, which connects the yolk sac to the midgut, the allantois, which ultimately degenerates into the urachus (a structure that forms a connection between the apex of the urinary bladder and the umbilicus), and the umbilical blood vessels. Persistence of these structures can lead to anomalies in the newborn.

Failure of the vitelline duct to completely close and regress by the seventh week of gestation may lead to a Meckel diverticulum (an outpouching of the gut without attachment to the anterior abdominal wall), a vitelline cyst or enterocystoma (a connection between the midgut and umbilicus without communication with either structure), an enteric or vitelline fistula (formed from a communicating connection between the midgut and the umbilicus), or a urachal sinus, cyst, or fistula (resulting from a connection between the bladder and the urachus)[2] (Fig. 268-1). In a child, the presence of these anomalies may be signaled by signs of infection and a lower midline abdominal mass (due to infection of a vitelline cyst), the discharge of feces and urine, which can lead to an erosive dermatitis (from enteric and urachal fistulas), and urinary tract infections (also resulting from urachal fistulas). Further, persistence of a fibrous band of tissue attached to the gut, the result of incomplete involution, may

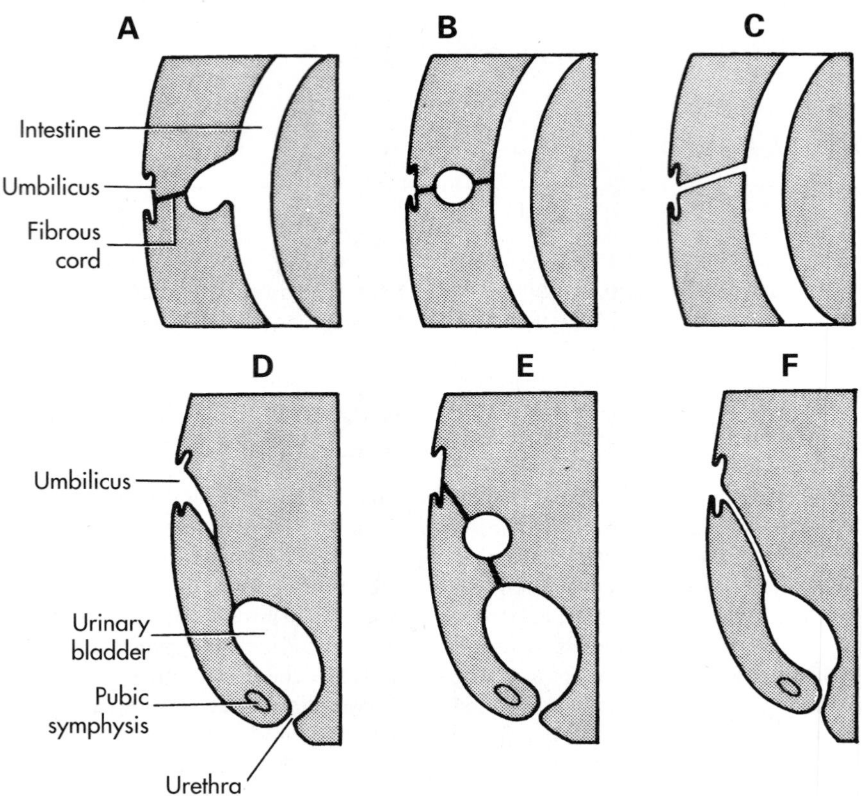

FIG. 268-1 Embryonic umbilical remnants. **A,** Meckel diverticulum. **B,** Enterocystoma. **C,** Enteric (vitelline) fistula. **D,** Urachal sinus. **E,** Urachal cyst. **F,** Urachal fistula.

Table 268-1 Conditions Associated with Abnormalities in Position or Morphology of the Umbilicus

Disorder	Abnormality in position	Abnormality in morphology
Aarskog syndrome	—	Prominent, protruding, pouting
Achondroplasia	Low placement	—
Bladder exstrophy	Low placement	—
Cloacal exstrophy	Low placement	—
Rieger syndrome		Prominent, broad, redundant periumbilical skin
Robinow syndrome	High placement	Broad, poorly epithelialized umbilical scar

Adapted from Curry CJR, Honore L, Boyd E: The ventral wall of the trunk. In Stevenson RE, Hall JG, Goodman RM, editors: *Human malformations and related anomalies,* vol 2, New York, 1993, Oxford University Press.

serve as the lead point for a volvulus or the cause of intestinal obstruction.

Of all these anomalies, Meckel diverticula clearly are the most common. Present in 2.5% of American newborns,[2] they are a well-known cause of clandestine lower intestinal bleeding among children and adults. The bleeding results from the presence of ectopic gastric mucosa within the diverticulum, which leads to ulceration and hemorrhage. Also, because these diverticula, which can occur anywhere from the ileocecal valve to a point 3 feet or more proximal to the valve, resemble a supernumerary vermiform appendix, their presence may be signaled by symptoms and signs similar to those of acute appendicitis.

Embryonic umbilical remnants that are lined with gastric mucosa can be detected by using gastrointestinal (GI) radionuclide scans that use ^{99m}Tc pertechnetate. Sonography or computed tomography (CT) can help delineate vitelline cysts that, after infection, manifest as abdominal masses. A urachal fistula can best be documented by noting methylene blue dye in the urine after it has been instilled at the umbilicus.

The treatment of all internal umbilical cord remnants that are symptomatic is surgical excision and repair.

Umbilical Hernia

Although umbilical hernias often are diagnosed during the first few months of postnatal life, the predisposition to develop such a defect actually occurs during the second trimester of pregnancy, after the midgut (which until then has been developing extraabdominally) returns to the abdominal cavity. Failure to form the normal fascial reinforcements that keep the midgut in place leads to a weakness in the abdominal wall, predisposing the child to the development of a hernia.[6]

Umbilical hernias are so common that, rather than a malformation, they should be considered a variation of normal. The incidence varies widely with race; Evans[7] found that at 6 weeks of age, 32% of African-American infants had umbilical hernias and only 4% of Caucasian infants were affected; at 1 year of age, the prevalence declined to 12% and 2%, respectively. Babies who have a low birth weight also

CONDITIONS ASSOCIATED WITH UMBILICAL HERNIAS

Chromosomal anomalies

Trisomy 13/15
Trisomy 18
Trisomy 21

Metabolic disorders

Hypothyroidism
Mucolipidosis III (pseudo-Hurler syndrome)
Mucopolysaccharidoses
  Type 1 (Hurler syndrome)
  Type 2 (Hunter syndrome)
  Type 4 (Morquio syndrome)

Dysmorphic syndromes

Aarskog syndrome
Beckwith-Wiedemann syndrome
Fetal hydantoin syndrome
Marfan syndrome
Opitz syndrome
Weaver syndrome

From Curry CJR, Honore L, Boyd E: The ventral wall of the trunk. In Stevenson RE, Hall JG, Goodman RM, editors: *Human malformations and related anomalies,* vol 2, New York, 1993, Oxford University Press.

are at markedly increased risk.[7] However, there is no gender predilection in prevalence; boys and girls are affected equally.

Among the vast majority of affected individuals, umbilical hernias are associated with no medical sequelae. One study revealed that incarceration, strangulation, rupture, or skin breakdown occurred in fewer than 5% of 590 children; other studies have revealed even lower rates of complication. Furthermore in most cases the hernia closes spontaneously without any medical intervention.[9] Thus the major indication for surgical treatment of the condition is cosmetic. As such, surgery should be considered only in carefully selected individuals who are older than 5 years of age.

Although most umbilical hernias occur as isolated findings in otherwise normal children, they can be associated with a variety of conditions, many of which are associated with increased abdominal girth or hypotonia. As shown in the box above, these conditions include the common autosomal trisomies, the mucopolysaccharidoses and other inborn errors of metabolism associated with organomegaly, as well as various dysmorphic syndromes, such as Beckwith-Wiedemann syndrome.

Umbilical Granulomas

At birth, the normal umbilical cord contains only the umbilical vessels surrounded by the protective Wharton jelly. Within the first 2 weeks after birth, the umbilical stump normally dries and separates from the abdomen; the region is covered completely by skin in 3 to 4 weeks. Delayed healing with accumulation of excessive amounts of granulation tissue produces an umbilical granuloma—a small, reddened mass. The lesion may be associated with infection at its base or with a foreign body such as talcum, but it recedes rapidly after repeated topical application of silver nitrate. Persistence of a granulomatous-appearing lesion after treatment, the presence of erosive dermatitis at the site, or the egression of gas, feces, or urine from it should suggest persistence of one of the embryonic remnants described above.[4]

Umbilical Polyps

Although they may resemble umbilical granulomas superficially, polyps at the umbilicus actually represent external remnants of the umbilical cord. They may be sinuses of the vitelline duct or of the urachus. Often larger than granulomas, they are bright red and do not respond to treatment with silver nitrate. Diagnosis depends on the histological examination, and the treatment is surgical excision.

REFERENCES

1. Aase JM: Caudal displacement of the umbilicus: implications for diagnosis of genitourinary anomalies, *Proc Greenwood Genet Center* 10:120, 1991.
2. Blackburn W, Cooley NR: The umbilical cord. In Stevenson RE, Hall JG, Goodman RM, editors: *Human malformations and related anomalies,* vol 2, New York, 1993, Oxford University Press.
3. Campbell J et al: Clinical diagnosis of umbilical swellings and discharges in children, *Med J Aust* 145:450, 1986.
4. Cresson SL, Pilling GP: Lesions about the umbilicus in infants and children, *Pediatr Clin North Am* 6:1085, 1959.
5. Cullen TS: *Embryology, anatomy, and disease of the umbilicus together with disease of the urachus,* Philadelphia, 1916, WB Saunders.
6. Curry CJR, Honore L, Boyd E: The ventral wall of the trunk. In Stevenson RE, editor: *Human malformation,* New York, 1994, Oxford University Press.
7. Evans AG: Comparative incidence of umbilical hernias in colored and white infants, *J Natl Med Assoc* 33:158, 1944.
8. Friedman JM: Umbilical dysmorphology, *Clin Genet* 28:343, 1985.
9. Walker SH: The natural history of umbilical hernia, *Clin Pediatr* 6:29, 1967.

269 Urinary Tract Infections

Glenn H. Bock

INCIDENCE

Urinary tract infection (UTI) is the most common nephrological problem encountered in pediatric practice. In newborns, the incidence of UTI has been estimated to be 1.4 to 5 per 1000 live births; boys are affected more than five times as often as girls. Among infants who develop first-time symptomatic UTI during the first year, most cases occur during the first 3 months, and boys account for as many as 75% of cases. Thereafter, and throughout childhood and adolescence, the overwhelming majority of first cases of UTI occur in girls. Although the incidence of UTI in girls during the first decade of life peaks around age 4, the incidence also increases during adolescence, coincident with the onset of sexual activity for many young people. The prevalence of covert (asymptomatic) bacteriuria in preschool girls is 0.8%; in school-age girls it is nearly 2%. After infancy, covert bacteriuria is extremely uncommon in boys.

ETIOLOGY

Both patient-related (host) factors and infection-related (bacterial) factors contribute to the overall risk of UTI. The higher incidence of congenital urinary anomalies in males undoubtedly is a factor in the risk of neonatal UTI in infant boys. However, many affected infant boys have anatomically normal urinary tracts. Insofar as the ratio of sepsis in boys compared with girls is similar to the ratio of UTI, the hematogenous route of urinary infection might also contribute to the gender difference. The incidence of UTI in newborns also appears to be inversely related to gestational age, being greatest in low-birth-weight and premature infants. This has led to speculation that an immature kidney more readily allows the bacteria to pass the renal filtration barrier than does a mature kidney.

In infants and children, most urinary tract infections are "ascending." The high incidence in girls has been attributed to anatomical features of the lower urinary tract, including the short urethra, its proximity to the anus, and its exit within the folds of the vulva. In adolescents it has been demonstrated that during coitus, bacteria are introduced into the urethra, which often becomes inflamed and swollen. This renders the girl susceptible to ascending infection.

A number of other risk factors have been identified that predispose an individual to urinary tract infection. Among the most common are those that result in incomplete urinary drainage and/or stasis in the urinary system. Efficient urinary drainage is an important factor in the resistance to primary and recurring infections. Obstructive urinary lesions that cause poor drainage may be congenital or acquired. The congenital lesions that predispose an individual to urinary tract infections arise when lower urinary tract structures fail to develop normally. Posterior urethral valves and obstruction of the ureteropelvic junction are common findings. Acquired obstructive lesions include urolithiasis, urethral strictures, retroperitoneal fibrosis, and neurogenic bladder. Vesicoureteral reflux is an extremely important factor in urinary tract infections because it is so common and because it plays a role in pyelonephritis and renal scarring. However, although the prevalence of pyelonephritis is high among patients who have reflux and UTI, most infants and young children who have pyelonephritis do *not* have urinary reflux. (Obstructive urinary lesions and vesicoureteral reflux are discussed in Chapter 235, Obstructive Uropathy and Vesicoureteral Reflux.)

Functional disturbances of urinary drainage, such as occur with dysfunctional bladder syndromes, now are recognized as important factors in recurrent UTI. Nonobstructive renal malformations also are associated with an increased incidence of urinary tract infections. These include renal hypoplasia, dysplasia, ectopia, and both autosomal dominant and autosomal recessive polycystic kidney disease. The reason for the increased incidence of infection in these conditions is unknown. A variety of metabolic disorders also have been associated with an increased incidence of urinary tract infections. Although severe malnutrition is of considerable importance worldwide, other disorders associated with an increased incidence of urinary tract infections are hypokalemia, nephrocalcinosis, vitamin A deficiency, diabetes mellitus, and uremia.

Another factor related to urinary tract infection is urethral instrumentation, particularly bladder catheterization. The need for bladder catheterization of hospitalized patients is the primary reason that UTI is the most common nosocomial infection.

Behavioral factors have been purported to contribute to the risk of urinary tract infections, particularly in females. These factors include voluntary deferral of micturition and failure to void promptly after coitus. In addition, certain aspects of hygiene, such as "wiping forward" after bowel movements, chemical irritation of the urethra from soaps and detergents, masturbation, the presence of foreign bodies in the introitus, and infestation of the bowel with *Enterobius* organisms (pinworms) all have been suggested to favor the occurrence and recurrence of UTIs in girls.

Bacterial virulence also is an important determinant in urinary tract infections. Bacteria cause most urinary tract infections, with *Escherichia coli* accounting for 75% to 80% of cases. Recent data suggest that binding sites (pili, or P-fimbriae) are present on the surface of certain uropathogenic *E. coli* organisms, enabling them to combine with receptors on uroepithelial cells; this process is thought to enhance bacterial virulence. Insights into the nature of these and other virulence factors may give rise to new therapeutic approaches to preventing and treating UTI in the future. Less common among the enteric uropathogens are *Enterobacter aerogenes, Enterobacter cloacae,* and the *Klebsiella* and *Proteus* species. Of the nonenteric gram negative pathogens, *Pseudomonas aeruginosa* is the most common. In a sexually active adolescent, gram positive *Staphylococcus saprophyticus* is the most common pathogen after *E. coli.* Infection with *Neisseria gonorrhoeae* should be suspected in boys who have a urethral discharge or purulent balanitis. Urinary outlet symptoms may result from gonococcal vulvovaginitis in girls. Although the presence of gram negative intracellular diplococci in a stain of the discharge strongly suggests gonococcal infection, a culture is necessary to confirm the diagnosis. Other causes of urethritis syndrome (see below) include such sexually transmitted organisms as *Chlamydia trachomatis* and *Ureaplasma urealyticum.*

Viral uropathogens are relatively unimportant except for the adenovirus in acute hemorrhagic cystitis. Fungal infections rarely are significant except in immunodeficient, immunosuppressed, or diabetic patients. Fungal overgrowth, however, may complicate antibiotic treatment of a child who has a normal immune system whose urodynamics are abnormal or who is catheterized. Although protozoan infections are important in many parts of the world, they are rare in the United States. *Mycobacterium tuberculosis* urinary infections may occur in rare cases as part of secondary tuberculosis and should be considered when sterile pyuria is found. The prevalence of tuberculosis currently is increasing, presumably as a result of the rise in infection with the human immunodeficiency virus (HIV).

CLINICAL FINDINGS

History

Urinary tract infections may occur without symptoms, with symptoms that direct attention to the urinary system, or with symptoms that divert the attention to other organ systems. Therefore, in the proper settings, a high degree of suspicion must be maintained by all pediatric practitioners. This concept cannot be overemphasized since, by the time a "first" UTI is diagnosed in a child, renal scars may already be present, indicating an antecedent, previously undetected UTI. Urinary tract infections in newborns and infants usually are associated with manifestations that are nonspecific or are referable to systems other than the urinary tract. Nonspecific symptoms include malaise, anorexia, difficulty in feeding, unexplained jaundice, failure to thrive, fever of inapparent origin, and malnutrition. To confound diagnosis further, newborns and infants who have a urinary tract infection commonly have gastrointestinal (GI) symptoms such as diarrhea or vomiting (sometimes so severe as to mimic hypertrophic pyloric stenosis), as well as neurological symptoms, such as irritability, lethargy, seizures, or hypertonicity. If not absent, specific urinary tract symptoms in this age group are subtle and therefore easily overlooked. They include changes in the caliber and force of the urinary stream, dribbling of urine, or diapers that are constantly wet. In older children, specific urinary tract symptoms are more common; they include dysuria, urinary frequency or urgency, burning on urination, foul-smelling urine, pain in the abdomen, back, or loin, or development of nocturnal enuresis or daytime wetting. Nonetheless, the symptoms of UTI, even in older children, may be quite subtle and only discovered by urine culture. The presence of covert bacteriuria may be associated with recurrent UTI, renal scars, or symptoms of dysfunctional bladder syndromes. It has been noted in untreated patients who have a urinary tract infection that fever and urinary symptoms may resolve after several weeks, even though the infection persists, as can be demonstrated by culture. Investigators have reported that spontaneous cures in such circumstances are uncommon despite resolution of the symptoms.

Physical Findings

Findings in infants who have a urinary tract infection may be normal except for fever and irritability. In addition to specific urinary complaints, an older child may report direct tenderness upon palpation of the abdomen, suprapubic area, or costovertebral angle (CVA). Patients who have a urinary tract obstruction may have palpable abdominal masses, whereas girls with sexually transmitted infections often have a concomitant vulvovaginitis.

Laboratory Findings

Recent data indicate that neither pyuria nor bacteriuria has sufficient degrees of specificity or negative predictive values alone to allow consistent diagnosis of UTI. For this reason, urine cultures are mandatory for appropriate diagnosis of UTI in children. In general, the urine for culture may be collected by the simplest and least painful method.

Proper collection of a clean-caught specimen from a girl requires that a midstream sample be obtained after the vaginal vestibule, vulva, and perineum have been cleansed thoroughly with a nonirritating antiseptic solution. The cleaned area should be rinsed with sterile water or saline and gently wiped dry with a sterile towel before voiding. Care should be taken not to get the cleaning solution into the urine culture. In boys, a midstream urine sample should be obtained after the glans penis has been cleaned with an antiseptic solution, with care taken to retract the foreskin in an uncircumcised individual. Of even greater importance is the handling of the urine after it has been obtained. Cultures should be promptly transported on ice to the laboratory, where they should be "plated out" as soon as possible. Cultured specimens may be accurate after storage for up to 48 hours before plating if kept at 39.2° F (4° C).

Contamination of the urine collection by bacteria from the external genitalia is the most confounding problem in evaluating a positive urine culture result. Bacterial colony counting has been used as a technique to improve the accuracy of cultures. The diagnosis of bacterial urinary tract infection traditionally is based on a colony count of more than 100,000/ml grown from a clean-caught, midstream urine specimen, although recent data suggest that 50,000 colonies/ml may be a more accurate cut off. Colony counts of this magnitude rely on the premise that bacteria thrive in urine at body temperature and multiply significantly in the bladder before voiding occurs. Certain conditions that may produce low colony counts despite significant infection are given in the box on p. 1642. Counts below 50,000 colonies/ml from voided specimens most commonly are due to contaminants. However, certain organisms such as enterococci and *S. saprophyticus* grow slowly and thus may be pathogenic, although the colony counts are less than the usual values.

Consideration of the types of organisms isolated in a

FACTORS THAT CAN CAUSE LOW COLONY COUNTS IN SPITE OF SIGNIFICANT INFECTION

High-volume urine flow
Low urine pH (<5.0) and specific gravity (<1.003)
Recent antimicrobial therapy
Fastidious organisms
Use of inappropriate culture techniques
Bacteriostatic agents in the urine
Complete obstruction of a ureter
Chronic or indolent infection

colony count also is important. Single ("pure") isolates are seen more commonly in actual infections, particularly of the acute variety, whereas multiple species found on culture usually indicate contamination. Multiple isolates, however, are more common in recurrent infections or in cultures taken from sites of urinary diversions.

Suprapubic needle aspiration of the bladder and bladder catheterization are the preferred methods of obtaining urine (1) in the infant or neonate who will not void, (2) when a urine specimen is urgently needed because of the severity of the illness, and (3) to confirm suspected infection in a child whose results on several colony counts are equivocal. Direct bladder aspiration of urine through puncture of aseptically prepared suprapubic skin is safe and reliable (see Appendix B, Special Procedures, for the techniques used for this procedure). Any bacteria grown from urine obtained by this method are significant; thus colony counts are not only *not* necessary but may be misleading, inasmuch as the bacteria obtained by suprapubic tap may not have had sufficient time to multiply to significant numbers in the bladder. Occasionally no urine will be obtained by suprapubic aspiration because the bladder is empty from recent voiding. A repeat attempt at aspiration after a small oral fluid feeding often renders the next attempt more successful. Suprapubic aspiration is contraindicated in patients who tend to bleed. Some patients, particularly neonate boys, may have transient hematuria after suprapubic aspiration, which usually resolves spontaneously. The risk of entering the bowel is minimal if bladder aspiration is performed properly, and even when the bowel has been entered inadvertently, there seems to have been little risk for peritonitis. Catheterization of the bladder can be used for the same indications as suprapubic aspiration. In many ways this is more useful than bladder aspiration because it more likely will produce a specimen for culture.

Using sterile plastic bags attached to a washed perineum is unsatisfactory for collecting urine cultures because the bags are contaminated easily by skin or fecal bacteria. In addition, the time of voiding usually is unknown, and the urine-filled bag may remain attached to the child in a warm environment for a prolonged period. Thus, if the bags are not removed for a colony count soon after voiding, any value of the count is negated.

DIFFERENTIAL DIAGNOSIS

Different sites of infection within the urinary system have "classic" clinical presentations. However, there is a surprising degree of symptom overlap when groups of children who have upper and lower UTI are evaluated. Discussions of the most common ones follow.

Urethritis

Urethritis syndrome (with or without fever) may be sudden or insidious in onset but usually varies somewhat in intensity from day to day. The complaints primarily are related to urinary outlet irritation. The patients, usually girls, void small volumes of urine and have symptoms of frequency, urgency, dysuria, and burning. Occasionally these patients have suprapubic or back pain. Although microscopic hematuria is common, gross hematuria is unusual, and urinary casts are never seen. Fever is uncommon.

Such symptoms usually are attributable to irritation of the vulva. Potential causes of this irritation include poor hygiene, vulvitis, vaginitis, chemical irritation (from soaps or bubble bath), foreign bodies, masturbation, urethral trauma (bicycle seat hematuria), and *Enterobius* infestations. In these circumstances the child has burning on urination because of the urethral or vaginal irritation. This pain causes the child to stop and start the urinary stream, leading to frequent small voidings, hesitancy, and urgency. In boys, such stop-and-start voiding may lead to dilation of the urethra and subsequent microhematuria. Urinalysis may reveal pyuria and bacteriuria as a result of local infection and denudation. Careful examination of the urethral opening is important in making this diagnosis, although urine cultures still are necessary because bacterial infection can cause this syndrome.

Cystitis

In cystitis syndrome the outlet symptoms are more severe, and back and suprapubic pain, as well as fever, are more common. Gross hematuria (without casts) is a common finding. Bacterial infection, particularly with *E. coli,* is the most common cause of this syndrome in girls. An adenovirus infection is a frequent cause of the syndrome in boys, producing dysuria and urinary frequency with terminal hematuria. The urine culture will reveal the offending organisms in the former instance and will be sterile in the latter.

Pyelonephritis

In pyelonephritis syndrome the patient often has generalized symptoms that may include a toxic appearance, high fever, chills, vomiting, diarrhea, and abdominal pain in addition to the urinary outlet symptoms. However, recent studies have shown that in a significant proportion of patients, neither high fever nor CVA tenderness discriminates uncomplicated cystitis from pyelonephritis. Hypertension is seen more often with infection of the renal parenchyma. Urinalysis usually reveals pyuria and bacteria, and occasionally white blood cell (WBC) casts. There may be isosthenuria, which can persist for 8 to 12 weeks after infection because of medullary dysfunction caused by an ascending infection. Urographic evidence of the loss of renal parenchyma, noted in a patient during an episode of pyelonephritis, indicates *previous* kidney infection or congenital structural maldevelopment, inasmuch as such scars take time to form. Blood cultures should be obtained from all patients suspected of having pyelonephritis because bacteremia is common. A renal biopsy in this syndrome, as in all the urinary infection syndromes, is of limited usefulness because of the focal nature of a kidney infection and the nonspecificity of the pathological change.

Radiographic studies are important in the clinical approach to urinary tract infection, both for localizing the infection and for ruling out urinary anomalies. Currently, the most sensitive way to detect pyelonephritis is to perform a ^{99m}Tc dimercaptosuccinic acid (DMSA) renal scan. The scan will show diminished isotope uptake with preserved renal contour in children who have acute parenchymal infection. This imaging test is the current gold standard for diagnosing pyelonephritis.

Imaging also is the most important tool for investigating urinary anomalies. It has been recommended that all children whose first urinary tract infection occurs before age 8 be investigated. The initial test should be a contrast voiding cystourethrogram (VCUG). If this test does not show vesicourethral reflux, a sonogram of the bladder and kidneys often is recommended to rule out structural and developmental disorders associated with UTI. If the results are normal, no further evaluation is necessary. The presence of possible urinary obstruction on renal sonography can be evaluated best by an excretory renal scan such as MAG-3 or ^{99m}Tc diethylenetriaminepentaacetic acid (DTPA). Renal scars caused by previous bouts of pyelonephritis are best detected with the DMSA scan. As mentioned in Chapter 235, if the child being evaluated has vesicoureteral reflux, any siblings under age 5 should be studied because of the high familial incidence of this anomaly.

Recurrent Urinary Tract Infections

Recurrent UTIs are most common in girls. Most often their symptoms are associated with fever, but as mentioned before, they can develop insidiously. When UTIs recur, approximately 50% occur within the first year and 25% occur during the second year. The risk of recurrence within 2 years of the first infection is 80% in Caucasian girls and 60% in African-American girls. The reason for this racial difference is unclear. Infections may recur, particularly in the absence of structural urinary tract abnormalities, in children who have dysfunctional voiding syndromes.

In some children, physical or psychomotor developmental delay may be the only manifestation of the recurrent infection. Urinalysis may reveal abnormal medullary function, as in pyelonephritis syndrome, although in more severe or frequent infections abnormalities of glucose and sodium reabsorption may arise, producing glucosuria and natriuresis. Occasionally there will be evidence of glomerular damage, as reflected by a lowered glomerular filtration rate. The degree of functional impairment has been shown to correlate with the histological severity of the lesion. Similar medullary dysfunction, however, can develop from obstruction without infection. Particular attention should be paid to the possibility of urological abnormalities in the child who has recurrent urinary tract infections. In addition, there is some suggestion that lower urinary tract allergy, *Enterobius* infestation, and poor vaginal hygiene promote recurrent infections.

TREATMENT

The goals of treatment are to eradicate the infection, correct any anatomical or functional abnormalities, and prevent recurrences. Achieving these goals requires the cooperation of the parents and the patient in diagnostic evaluation and treatment.

Before antibiotic therapy is begun, a properly collected, clean-caught urine culture and colony count should be obtained. More accurate culture results are obtained from catheterized or suprapubic aspirate specimens, and these should be sought in infants in whom UTI is suspected. In cases that are symptomatic of acute lower UTI, treatment may begin before culture data are available. Because most first infections are caused by *E. coli,* trimethoprim-sulfamethoxazole, sulfisoxazole, and ampicillin are good drugs of first choice. If the initial culture is sterile, antibiotics can be discontinued and causes other than a bacterial infection should be considered. A second culture should be done 48 to 72 hours after beginning therapy and should be sterile if the choice of antibiotic was correct. The antibiotic can be changed if (1) the initial culture shows an organism unresponsive to the initial antibiotic, (2) the 48-hour culture is not sterile, or (3) the patient has not improved clinically. The antibiotic sensitivities of the initial urine culture are useful in deciding on the best alternative antibiotic. Although various investigators have advised treatment courses of 1 week to 6 weeks, there appears to be little advantage in prolonging initial antibiotic treatment of uncomplicated UTI for longer than 7 to 10 days. Investigation of the efficacy of shorter courses (or single doses) of therapy in children remains controversial. Several recent studies, however, suggest that the efficacy of 3-day courses is similar to that of longer initial treatment regimens. For bacterial urinary tract syndromes thought to be limited to the lower urinary tract, oral antibiotics usually are sufficient. In patients in whom renal parenchymal infection (pyelonephritis syndrome) is suspected or in patients who are vomiting, the antibiotics should be given parenterally. Nitrofurantoin is not a suitable *therapeutic* agent for pyelonephritis because tissue bacteriostatic levels are suboptimal. In addition to the antibiotics, the patient should have a good oral fluid intake (in the absence of vomiting) and void frequently. With a preadolescent girl who has a urinary tract infection, consideration should be given (by history and physical examination) to possible *Enterobius* infestation. Advice also should be given on vaginal and vulvar hygiene and avoiding irritants (e.g., perfumed soaps and bubble bath). Besides the initial and 48-hour urine cultures, follow-up cultures should be obtained within 1 to 2 weeks after treatment is completed. Periodic screening by means of urine cultures should be performed over the subsequent 12 months to identify patients who have covert bacteriuria. The antibiotic sensitivity of the organism should guide the choice of antibiotic in persistent or recurrent urinary tract infections, especially those associated with urinary tract obstruction and instrumentation. The sensitivities of previous infecting organisms may help in selecting an effective antibiotic if reinfection is presumed; the definite choice of an antibiotic again depends on the results of the antibiotic sensitivities of the pretreatment culture. Children who have recurrent urinary tract infections should be given chronic prophylactic therapy. In the absence of urinary reflux and renal scars, prophylaxis can be continued for 6 to 12 months, with several intratreatment urine cultures. The drugs can be discontinued at the end of this period to determine whether the problem of recurrence has resolved. Posttreatment cultures again are necessary to ensure the absence of recurrences in a symptom-free patient.

PSYCHOSOCIAL CONSIDERATIONS

The patient (if old enough to understand) and the parents should be advised of the overall treatment plan (including the follow-up cultures) at the very beginning. This should be done frankly but in a way that should not create undue anxiety. The necessity to complete the full course of antibiotics and the reasons for the long follow-up with cultures should be stressed. In addition, the patients and parents should know that urine cultures should be performed in the event of fevers that have no apparent origin.

REFERRAL

Although usually not needed, a urologist can be helpful in evaluating children who have urinary tract infections, and this specialist should be able to perform a complete urological evaluation of the child with a minimum of psychological stress. Many of the urological abnormalities require surgical procedures, and the primary care physician can expect joint follow-up of such patients. Urological assistance is vital in any child who has a urinary diversion and a history of urinary tract infections. In addition, consultation with specialists in pediatric nephrology and infectious disease often is helpful with a patient who has persistent and/or recurrent infections and in whom urinary tract obstruction has been ruled out or corrected.

SUGGESTED READINGS

Bauchner H et al: Prevalence of bacteriuria in febrile children, *Pediatr Infect Dis J* 6:239, 1987.

Belman B: Urinary imaging in children, *Pediatr Infect Dis J* 8:548, 1989.

Hanson L: Prognostic indicators in childhood urinary infection, *Kidney Int* 21:659, 1982.

Hoberman A et al: Prevalence of urinary tract infection in febrile infants, *J Pediatr* 123:17, 1993.

Majd M et al: Relationship among vesicoureteral reflux, P-fimbriated *Escherichia coli,* and acute pyelonephritis in children with febrile urinary tract infection, *J Pediatr* 119:578, 1991.

Marild S et al: Fever, bacteriuria and concomitant disease in children with urinary tract infection, *Pediatr Infect Dis J* 8:36, 1989.

Zhanel GG et al: Asymptomatic bacteriuria: which patients should be treated? *Arch Intern Med* 150:1389, 1990.

270 Verrucae (Warts)

Donald P. Lookingbill

ETIOLOGY

Warts are virus-induced tumors of the skin.[2,4,5] The wart virus is a human papillomavirus[2,5] (HPV) that infects epidermal cells and causes focal epidermal proliferation, expressed clinically as a verrucous papule.

In recent years, deoxyribonucleic acid (DNA) hybridization analysis has been used to identify different types of human papillomaviruses. To date, more than 60 types have been characterized, and the number continues to grow. Specific DNA types have been associated with certain types of warts. For example, HPV type 1 (HPV-1) is found in plantar warts, HPV-2 in common warts, HPV-3 in flat warts, HPV-6 and HPV-11 in "benign" genital warts, and HPV-16 and HPV-18 in genital warts that have malignant potential (e.g., cervical carcinoma). Thus HPV typing holds promise in helping to identify premalignant warts as well as sources of the transmission of warts.[5,7]

HISTORY

The wart virus presumably is inoculated into the skin from some external source, but neither the source nor the event of inoculation usually is elicitable. Frogs and toads have been unfairly incriminated as carriers.[9] It is reasonable, however, to ask about and search for warts on other areas of the body; for example, patients who have warts on their lips often have them on their fingers. Because warts are transmissible, other family members also may have them.

In young infants, warts (including those in laryngeal and genital locations) are assumed to have been acquired from the mother's vaginal tract during delivery. Genital warts in children raise the possibility of sexual abuse.[3,8] However, several recent studies of anogenital warts in children found no evidence of sexual abuse in most of the subjects.[6,7] Based on HPV typing, anogenital HPV infection in children appears to be acquired most commonly either at birth or by means of nonsexual transmission.[7]

Patients who have systemic defects in self-mediated immunity are more susceptible to warts, which often are recalcitrant to treatment.[1] Also, because cellular immune responses in the skin have been shown to be impaired with atopic dermatitis, these patients, too, have more difficulty with warts and other viral infections of the skin.

PHYSICAL FINDINGS

The clinical appearance of warts varies, depending on the type and the location on the skin. The common wart, or verruca vulgaris, is easily recognized as a superficial, light-colored papule that has a coarse, roughened surface. Warts often are studded with black specks, which many patients call "seeds" but which actually are small, superficial dermal capillaries. Warts sometimes are found in linear array, presumably as a result of autoinoculation through scratching. Not all warts appear as verrucous papules. Variants include flat (planar) warts, plantar warts, periungual warts, and anogenital warts. These are described more fully later in the chapter.

LABORATORY FINDINGS

Warts almost always are diagnosed clinically. If there is doubt, a skin biopsy can provide histological confirmation.

DIFFERENTIAL DIAGNOSIS

The distinctive clinical appearance of the common wart usually presents no problem in diagnosis. *Epidermal nevi,* which are epidermal hamartomas, may be confused with warts, but they usually are softer, more pigmented, more persistent, and much less common. Flat (planar) warts appear as small, flesh-colored papules (Fig. 270-1). When located on the face, they often are confused with the closed *comedones* (whiteheads) seen in acne. On very close inspection, however, flat warts are seen to have sharp borders and a finely verrucous surface, whereas closed comedones are smooth, dome-shaped lesions.

Plantar warts are so named because they appear on the plantar surface of the foot (Fig. 270-2). They often are confused with calluses and corns, although corns are much less common in children than are warts. Large plantar warts often are composed of confluent smaller ones, which form a mosaic wart around which satellite lesions often occur. Additionally, plantar warts differ from corns by having a verrucous surface that interrupts the skin markings and often is punctuated with black specks. Sometimes the two entities can be distinguished only by paring down the surface; wart tissue still has a roughened texture, whereas a corn is smooth. A corn also becomes smaller in diameter as it is pared; a wart does not.

Periungual warts that occur around the nail fold should not pose diagnostic difficulty. Warts under the free edge of the nail, however, can cause the nail plate to separate from the nail bed and may be confused with a *fungal infection.* On close inspection, the verrucous nature of the wart usually can be appreciated.

Anogenital warts (condylomata acuminata) sometimes but not always are acquired by sexual contact.[6-8] They usually can be identified easily as verrucous papules (Fig. 270-3), but sometimes they are small and/or flat and therefore more difficult to see. In this situation the *acetowhitening technique* can aid in the diagnosis. A compress of 5% acetic acid is applied for several minutes to the suspected area, which then is reexamined, under magnification if desired. With this tech-

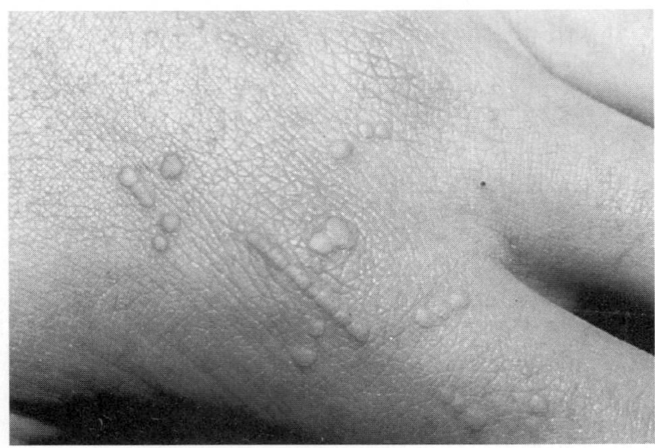

FIG. 270-1 Flat warts. The streaks of warts are due to autoinoculation from scratching. When smaller and located on the face, flat warts may be confused with comedones.

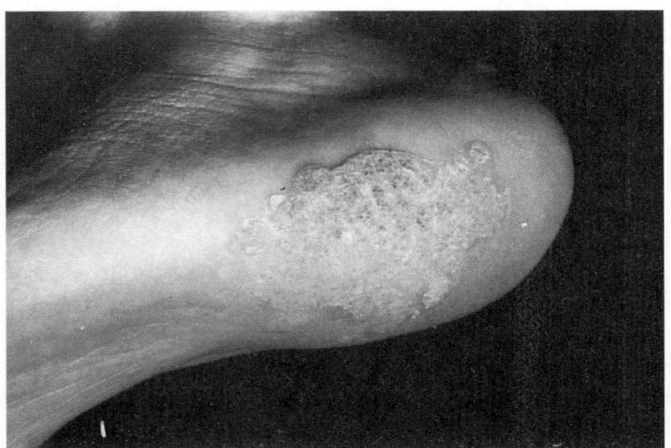

FIG. 270-2 A mosaic plantar wart with a roughened surface punctuated with black specks.

nique, warty tissue turns white and thus is visualized more easily.

Genital warts may be confused with the less common *condylomata lata,* which are skin lesions found in secondary syphilis. In general, *condylomata acuminata* are drier and usually more verrucous than condylomata lata, which are flat and moist. If there is doubt, a serological test for syphilis should settle the issue.

PSYCHOSOCIAL CONSIDERATIONS

Among schoolchildren, warts often are a focus for teasing and insensitive remarks. Consequently, when children ask that their warts be treated, they usually do so because of social pressure. Successful therapy gives patients the opportunity to feel better about themselves and their appearance.

MANAGEMENT

Over the years a wide variety of treatments have been recommended, including some particularly interesting approaches, such as that used by Mark Twain's Tom Sawyer. Therapies such as these probably "worked" because most

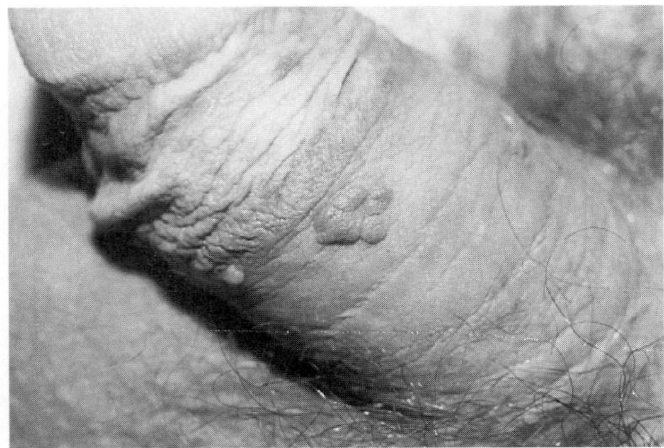

FIG. 270-3 Condylomata acuminata, shown here as verrucous papules on the penis.

warts eventually undergo spontaneous regression. This must be kept in mind when physicians credit their treatment for a successful result. Nonetheless, when a patient requests treatment of a wart, practitioners usually are inclined to oblige. But because a specific antiviral medication for warts has not yet been developed, nonspecific destructive techniques are still relied on as therapy; the following are the most commonly used techniques.

Cryotherapy

Tissue is frozen by applying liquid nitrogen either with a swab or by means of a more sophisticated delivery system. The freezing should extend beyond the wart to include a 1 to 2 mm rim of normal skin. To destroy tissue better, the wart may be refrozen after the initial thaw. The patient must be advised that the frozen area will be sore for several days, that a blister may form, and that it usually takes several weeks for the wart to turn dark and "drop off." This is a favorite office therapy for common warts. For small warts, a single treatment often is successful, but large warts frequently need to be refrozen at about 3-week intervals. Scars may result but are uncommon. The skin also may become hypopigmented. In freezing warts on the fingers, care must be taken not to freeze too deeply, because underlying structures such as digital nerves can be damaged.

Electrodesiccation and Laser Therapy

Electrodesiccation of a wart can be preceded or followed by curettage. One advantage of this technique is that the patient leaves the office without visible evidence of the wart, although the cure rate probably is no higher than with cryotherapy. The disadvantages are that the procedure must be preceded by injection of a local anesthetic, and scarring is more likely. Carbon dioxide laser therapy destroys warts by means of an expensive, "space-age" method, which for most cases provides only a minimal advantage over electrodesiccation.

Acid Therapy

Acid therapy is slower and involves more patient participation, but it is less immediately painful and is least likely to cause scarring. A variety of acids are available for treating warts. A convenient outpatient medication incorporates salicylic acid in a polyacrylic or flexible collodion vehicle (Occlusal-HP and Duofilm). The vehicle dries rapidly to prevent spread of the acid onto surrounding skin. The patient is instructed to put the medication on the wart at bedtime and to cover the area with a bandage. At the end of each week, superficial necrotic tissue should be pared. This usually can be done at home either with a sharp blade or an emery board. Because of its minimal discomfort, this approach is useful with multiple warts and those on very young children. Plantar warts often require a stronger acid, such as a 40% salicylic acid plaster. These can be bought over the counter (Mediplast and Duofilm patch), but the patient needs instruction in application. A piece of plaster the size of the wart is cut, and the adhesive, medicated side is applied to the wart and held in place with the tape. The plaster is changed every 24 hours and the macerated wart pared weekly, as described above. For deeply seeded warts, cryotherapy, following 40% salicylic acid applications and paring, usually provides successful treatment.

Flat warts often are treated successfully with vitamin A acid (Retin A), which probably acts as a "peeling" agent in this situation. Retin A gel or liquid is applied nightly to the entire affected area. Irritation may occur, necessitating less frequent use.

These home acid therapies usually require a minimum of a month of continuous use to be effective. If no progress has been made after several months, other treatments should be considered.

All these treatments are nonspecific, and none is foolproof. Sometimes different modalities are used in sequence. Warts commonly regress spontaneously, although the time required for this varies considerably. In some patients, therapy may only serve to appease the patient while nature takes its course; in others, perhaps the destructive techniques initiate an inflammatory reaction, exposing the wart viral antigen to the body's immune system, which finally rejects the wart. This may explain the phenomenon observed by some, wherein by "treating the mother wart, the baby goes away." In any event, whenever warts are treated, the physician must guard against doing harm by being overzealous. Accordingly, surgical excision usually should be discouraged, and radiotherapy is contraindicated.

COMPLICATIONS

The major complications of warts are those caused by overzealous therapy, resulting in short-term discomfort or long-term scarring. The risk of a wart, which usually is temporary, must be balanced against a scar, which usually is lifelong, may be unsightly, and sometimes is tender, particularly if present on a pressure-bearing surface such as the sole of the foot.

PROGNOSIS

As mentioned before, most warts eventually involute spontaneously, probably through immunological rejection.[1] Because the time required for this varies greatly, it is impossible to predict for an individual patient when this might occur. The goal of therapy, then, is to shorten the time it takes for the wart to disappear. The therapies outlined above result in clearing in most cases, but patients who have resistant, persistent warts will continue to be plagued. It is especially for these patients that more specific therapy is needed.

REFERENCES

1. Adler A, Safai B: Immunity in wart resolution, *J Am Acad Dermatol* 1:305, 1979.
2. Androphy EJ: Human papillomavirus: current concepts, *Arch Dermatol* 125:683, 1989.
3. Bender ME: New concepts of condylomata acuminata in children, *Arch Dermatol* 122:1121, 1986.
4. Birkett DA: Warts and their management, *Practitioner* 226:1251, 1982.
5. Cobb MW: Human papillomavirus infection, *J Am Acad Dermatol* 22:547, 1990.
6. Cohen BA, Honig P, Androphy E: Anogenital warts in children: clinical and virologic evaluation for sexual abuse, *Arch Dermatol* 126:1575, 1990.
7. Obalek S et al: Condylomata acuminata in children: frequent association with human papillomaviruses responsible for cutaneous warts, *J Am Acad Dermatol* 23:205, 1990.
8. Rock B et al: Genital tract papillomavirus infection in children, *Arch Dermatol* 122:1129, 1986.
9. Ross MS: Warts in the medical folklore of Europe, *Int J Dermatol* 18:505, 1979.

PART NINE
Critical Situations

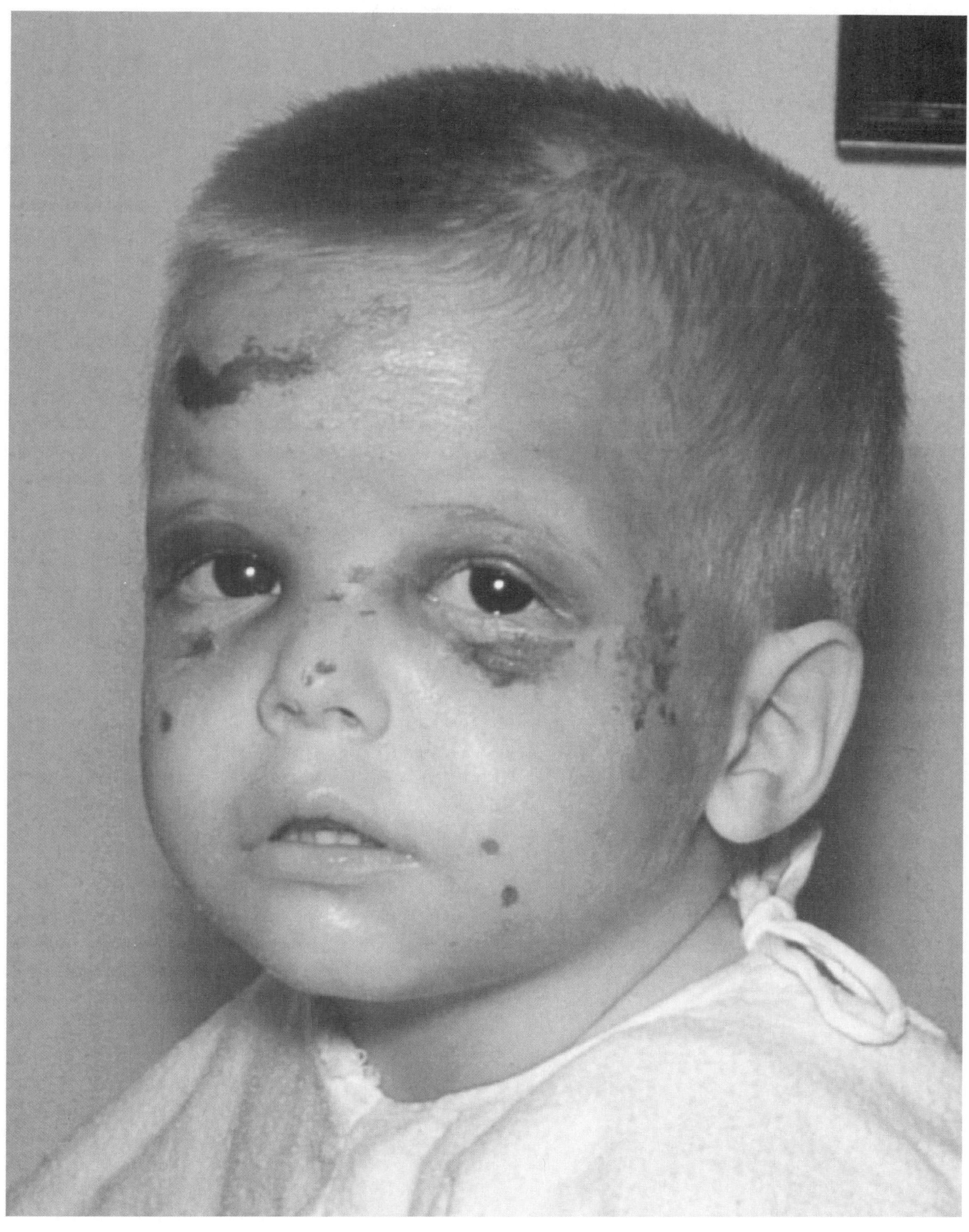

271 Airway Obstruction

Steven E. Lucking

Acute upper airway obstruction presents an immediate threat to life. Because of the fourth-power relationship between airway diameter and airway resistance, the same amount of airway encroachment or edema in millimeters causes a far greater physiological obstruction in a child than in an adult. Inspiratory stridor (a high-pitched sound) is the hallmark of upper airway obstruction. This is not to say, however, that upper airway obstruction cannot occur in the absence of stridor, because profound degrees of obstruction may manifest silently if airflow is nearly absent. When confronted with a child who has acute upper airway obstruction, the practitioner must assess the degree of obstruction quickly and accurately. The possibility of progression to complete airway obstruction with hypoxemia and cardiac arrest must be appreciated.[4] Delaying intervention in a child whose airway is unstable may be costly, but unnecessary instrumentation in a child who has stable upper airway obstruction may precipitate a crisis.

The cause of death in patients who have airway obstruction is progressive hypoxemia and cardiac arrest causing brain damage. Thus the immediate concern when first assessing the child is to provide oxygen and assess the degree of oxygen saturation. A previously healthy infant or child can tolerate significant degrees of hypercapnia without end organ damage. In addition, the degree of hypercapnia can vary over a matter of minutes as a result of factors such as the child's level of agitation, the degree of airway obstruction, the response to palliative therapies, and the onset of fatigue. For these reasons, arterial blood gas (ABG) measurement, which provides an assessment of only one moment in time, generally is not considered sufficiently worthwhile to warrant the amount of distress it causes the child.

HISTORY AND PHYSICAL EXAMINATION

The clinician first should assess the child's level of distress from a distance so as not to agitate the child. One useful approach is to obtain a brief history from the parents or caretaker while merely observing the child. The parents also can be asked to remove the child's clothes to facilitate a quicker assessment of the patient's general appearance. The physician should attempt to obtain as complete an assessment as possible in the least threatening manner because agitation and crying worsen the relative degree of airway obstruction and the attendant work of breathing. After noting all physical signs that do not require direct physical contact with the patient, the examiner should gently approach the child to auscultate the chest and assess the circulation.

The child's appearance gives important clues to the degree of respiratory compromise. The degree of the child's anxiety can be an important clue to the severity of the airway obstruction. Many children who have croup appear quite calm and contented sitting in their parent's arms when not being "threatened" by an examiner. Although these children may have significant stridor, their level of comfort indicates that they are not significantly hypoxic or hypercarbic. Conversely, a child who remains persistently anxious or who has become somnolent to the point of no longer interacting with those around him may be significantly hypoxic or hypercarbic.

Use of accessory muscles indicates the degree of inspiratory effort. Stridor needs to be assessed in the context of the inspiratory breath sounds. Generally, stridor becomes less loud as airway obstruction lessens. However, in extreme cases, stridor may become barely audible as inspiratory flow almost ceases. It is the quality of the inspiratory breath sounds that differentiates improvement (breath sounds clearly heard) from rapid deterioration (breath sounds barely audible) as the reason for diminishing stridor. Respiratory rate has been reasonably well correlated with hypoxemia, but little correlation has been established with hypercapnia.[9] Currently the degree of hypoxemia is easily assessed by pulse oximetry monitoring, which most children tolerate well. In the differential diagnosis of acute infectious upper airway obstruction, the presence of fever, drooling, or cough,[7] a forward-leaning posture, or the appearance of toxicity is useful in leading toward a specific diagnosis and approach to therapy (see Chapters 273, Croup, and 280, Epiglottitis).

A variety of scoring systems have been proposed to aid in assessing the degree of upper airway obstruction. Such systems help focus observation and provide a guide to the effects of therapy (Table 271-1).

DIFFERENTIAL DIAGNOSIS OF AIRWAY OBSTRUCTION

Upper airway obstruction in children can be categorized according to certain features of the presentation and history (see the box on p. 1652 for causes described below).

Early Infancy

Abnormalities of the airway may manifest with airway obstruction and stridor starting early in infancy and occasionally in the immediate newborn period. *Laryngomalacia* is the single most common cause of stridor that begins in early infancy.[10] Most patients have a history of stridor that is audible whenever the child is excited, agitated, or crying, beginning from the first days of life. This is a developmental disorder in that the "floppy" larynx becomes more rigid and less obstructing with time. Endoscopically, the epiglottis is seen to fold over the larynx on inspiration. Another finding is varying degrees of prolapse of the arytenoid cartilages into the center of the larynx on inspiration. These infants typically may have feeding problems, and the stridor often worsens with minor respiratory tract infections. Through continu-

Table 271-1 Scoring System for Assessing the Severity of Upper Airway Obstruction

Sign	Score*
Stridor	
None	0
Inspiratory	1
Inspiratory and expiratory	2
Cough	
None	0
Hoarse cry	1
Bark	2
Retractions and nasal flaring	
None	0
Flaring and suprasternal retractions	1
Flaring plus suprasternal, subcostal, and intercostal retractions	2
Cyanosis	
None	0
In room air	1
In 40% oxygen	2
Inspiratory breath sounds	
Normal	0
Harsh, with wheezing or ronchi	1
Delayed	2

From Downes JJ, Goldberg AI: Airway management, mechanical ventilation, and cardiopulmonary resuscitation. In Scarpelli EM, Auld PAM, Goldman HS, editors: *Pulmonary disease of the fetus, newborn, and child,* Philadelphia, 1978, Lea & Febiger.

*A score of 4 or higher indicates significant airway obstruction.

CAUSES OF AIRWAY OBSTRUCTION

Congenital causes

Craniofacial dysmorphism
Hemangioma
Laryngeal cleft/web
Laryngoceles, cysts
Laryngomalacia
Macroglossia
Tracheal stenosis
Vascular ring
Vocal cord paralysis

Acquired infectious causes

Acute laryngotracheobronchitis
Diphtheria
Epiglottitis
Laryngeal papillomatosis
Membranous croup (bacterial tracheitis)
Mononucleosis
Retropharyngeal abscess
Spasmodic croup

Acquired noninfectious causes

Anaphylaxis
Angioneurotic edema
Foreign body aspiration
Supraglottic hypotonia
Thermal/chemical burn
Trauma
Vocal cord paralysis

ous noninvasive monitoring, it has been demonstrated that infants who have laryngomalacia are more likely than age-matched controls to have transient episodes of hypoxemia and hypercarbia, although none of the episodes was life threatening.[8] Because the disorder improves over time, these infants rarely require an artificial airway.

Unilateral or bilateral *vocal cord paralysis* may occur in otherwise healthy newborns and has been associated with birth trauma. However, vocal cord paralysis also may be associated with other neurological diseases and increased intracranial pressure.[10] In an otherwise healthy child whose vocal cord paralysis is thought to be due to birth trauma, improvement over time is the rule.

Craniofacial dysmorphism (as in Pierre Robin and Treacher Collins syndromes) causes stridor as a result of micrognathia with posterior displacement of the tongue. *Macroglossia* (as in Beckwith-Wiedemann syndrome, congenital hypothyroidism, glycogen storage diseases, Down syndrome, and other conditions) also may cause stridor in the newborn period.

Congenital laryngeal webs and *subglottic stenosis* may cause critical airway obstruction in the immediate newborn period. Some of these children may not be diagnosed correctly at presentation because endotracheal intubation in the newborn period not only provides a lifesaving airway but also temporarily corrects the abnormality. With subsequent scarring, the child may manifest the condition again later in infancy during an upper respiratory tract infection.

Vascular rings and *slings* may cause some degree of airway obstruction in infancy.[10] An infant who has a vascular ring may have persistent wheezing if the obstruction is in the lower trachea near the carina. Conversely the major symptom may be stridor if the obstruction is higher up in the extrathoracic trachea.

Laryngeal clefts are uncommon and may manifest with either stridor or symptoms of recurrent aspiration. Congenital *cysts* and *laryngoceles* also are uncommon causes of stridor in early infancy. Congenital *tracheal stenosis,* a rare disorder, has an extreme form in which the entire trachea may have circumferencial cartilaginous rings much like lobar and segmental bronchi.

Hemangiomas may develop at any level of the airway in infancy, and these may be associated with cutaneous hemangiomas. Corticosteroids (systemic or intralesional) may promote shrinkage, although the hemangiomas generally regress spontaneously after the infant is 1 year old.

Acquired Infectious Causes of Airway Obstruction

The most common cause of acute infectious airway obstruction is viral *laryngotracheobronchitis* (croup). The typical patient is between 3 months and 4 years of age, has had a preceding upper respiratory tract infection, and has a barking cough and loud inspiratory stridor (see Chapter 273, Croup). Membranous croup, also called *bacterial tracheitis,* is becoming the most common cause of acute infectious upper airway obstruction culminating in respiratory failure and requiring referral to a tertiary care pediatric intensive care unit. The consensus is that this condition represents a bacterial superinfection of viral croup.[3] The most common offending agents are *Staphylococcus aureus* and *Moraxella catarrhalis*, although *Streptococcus* and *Haemophilus* organisms have been implicated. The patient initially has a crouplike illness that progresses in severity, with rising fever and increasing toxicity, culminating in respiratory failure, with thick purulent secretions noted upon intubation. This disorder usually is diagnosed at the time of intubation when the child's condition progresses to respiratory failure. Contrary to initial reports, tracheostomy generally is not necessary for treatment, and mortality should be very uncommon in children who have not suffered cardiac arrest before admission to an appropriate intensive care setting. *Acute spasmodic croup* manifests with recurrent nighttime onset of inspiratory stridor and croupy cough. Patients generally are afebrile, and episodes are short-lived.

Retropharyngeal abscess is a relatively rare infectious cause of stridor in children. It usually involves high fever and difficulty swallowing, with airway obstruction to a lesser degree.

Acute epiglottitis has been seen less frequently in the past 5 years, possibly as the reward for the development of effective vaccines. It most commonly is due to infection with *Haemophilus influenzae* type b and may occur at any age, including in adulthood (see Chapter 280, Epiglottitis).

Acute infectious mononucleosis may cause significant upper airway obstruction as a result of tonsillar hypertrophy. This condition rarely leads to respiratory failure, and the airway obstruction generally responds promptly to a short course of corticosteroids. *Laryngeal papillomatosis* may cause persistent stridor in children and adults at any age. Multiple, recurrent, rough-surfaced laryngeal tumors are caused by infection with the human papillomavirus (HPV). Repeated surgical excision generally is required to maintain a patent airway. Most recently, immunological therapy with interferon-alpha has proved beneficial.[6] The condition tends to improve with time, presumably as the child develops immunity to the virus.

Diphtheria is an extremely rare infection in the United States, but it still may occur in unimmunized children.

Other Acquired Causes of Airway Obstruction

Foreign body aspiration may manifest with airway obstruction at almost any level of the pediatric airway.[4] Stridor may be one of the presenting symptoms when a foreign body lodged in the upper esophagus has caused progressive airway obstruction secondary to localized edema that develops over days to weeks. Foreign bodies lodged in the upper airway itself often cause sudden death. Foreign bodies aspirated into the lower airway generally manifest with a combination of wheezing, cough, and infection. Clinical suspicion can be confirmed by appropriate roentgenographic studies. The definitive therapy is removal of the foreign body using rigid bronchoscopy techniques in an operating room, thereby permitting tracheostomy or thoracotomy if either of these becomes necessary.

Thermal or *chemical trauma* of the airway may cause sufficient swelling to precipitate respiratory failure. Flash burns of the face from injudicious use of volatile liquids to start fires commonly causes oropharyngeal and laryngeal edema that may seriously compromise the airway. Empirical use of parenteral corticosteroids is not beneficial for an inhalational injury.[5] Ingestion of corrosive substances likewise may cause sufficient burns of the oropharynx and larynx to require placement of an artificial airway.

External trauma to the head and neck may cause upper airway obstruction by dislocating the laryngeal cartilages or by causing a hematoma or edema.[13] This type of injury is rare in the spectrum of pediatric traumatic injury.

Vocal cord paralysis may occur as a consequence of a variety of serious intracranial injuries. Typical patients have required a tracheostomy, although vocal cord function may improve over ensuing months, allowing decannulation.[1] Children who have suffered brain injuries may have upper airway obstruction secondary to poor supraglottic motor control and hypotonia. The tongue may obstruct the airway, or the pharynx may collapse on inspiration. This can occur as the result of long-standing severe psychomotor retardation or may be acquired as a result of hypoxic, infectious, or traumatic brain injury.

Upper airway swelling can develop suddenly after ingestion of an allergen, an insect sting, or an environmental exposure. This may occur with highly allergic individuals *(anaphylaxis)* or with hereditary *angioneurotic edema,* an extremely rare condition. If an airway can be secured in time, the prognosis is good.

DIAGNOSTIC EVALUATION

With acute, infectious upper airway destruction, diagnostic assessment of the cause of obstruction is urgent, because, depending on the cause, the child's condition may change dramatically in a very short time. Diagnosis is relatively easy when a young child has the classic symptoms of viral croup: upper respiratory tract infection prodrome with subsequent development of stridor, a barking cough, and a mildly elevated temperature.[7] Likewise, an older child who has the classic presenting features of epiglottitis (acute onset of a sore throat, a high fever, a muffled voice, unwillingness to swallow, a toxic, distressed appearance, and rapidly progressive respiratory distress) also presents no special diagnostic dilemma. In practice, however, many children have varying combinations of these features. Indeed, the emergence of membranous laryngotracheobronchitis (bacterial tracheitis) has complicated the diagnosis because this disorder's clinical findings seem to evolve over time from those of more typical croup to those suggestive of epiglottitis.

Considerable controversy still exists over whether roentgenographic neck examinations should be done in a moderately ill child of any age who has acute upper airway obstruction. Although roentgenographic confirmation of the diagnosis of croup may be comforting in some situations, this type of evaluation can be counterproductive. In an uncooperative child who has classic croup, it is not uncommon for a lateral neck roentgenogram (usually an oblique view) to be of such poor quality that it is misinterpreted as showing a swollen epiglottis when evaluated by someone other than an experienced pediatric radiologist. This usually results in an unnecessarily high level of anxiety and referral to a tertiary care pediatric center. The more important scenario, however, is the child who has epiglottitis who develops acute upper airway obstruction and respiratory arrest while being positioned for roentgenographic evaluation, necessitating emergency resuscitation in a suboptimal environment. Finally, membranous laryngotracheobronchitis has no specific roentgenographic features. Because of these considerations, many pediatric institutions forgo routine roentgenographic evaluation of the upper airway if epiglottitis is suspected. Rather, the airway is visualized in the operating room by a pediatric anesthesiologist who has surgical back-up and provisions for emergency tracheostomy if necessary. This approach affords maximal safety for children who have the most dangerous disease, mainly epiglottitis; it also affords an opportunity for early diagnosis and intervention in cases of membranous laryngotracheobronchitis. Some institutions that have not abandoned the use of lateral neck films in cases of suspected epiglottitis now require that an anesthesiologist experienced in managing the pediatric airway accompany the child to the radiology department.

In the case of a neonate who has chronic stable or intermittent stridor and no significant respiratory embarrassment, a number of diagnostic approaches can be taken. A barium swallow or fluoroscopic evaluation of the airway can be helpful in demonstrating a number of congenital lesions. In addition, flexible laryngoscopy and bronchoscopy allow direct diagnostic evaluation and videotaping of airway dynamics. With experienced personnel and appropriate monitoring, this procedure can be done at the bedside.

Blood sampling is a low priority in a child who has an obstructed airway because the crying elicited by this painful procedure increases both the metabolic rate and the inspiratory work of breathing through the obstructed airway. Children who have croup or epiglottitis may have mild hypoxemia in room air, which may be due to atelectasis or early secondary pneumonia. Noninvasive pulse oximetry is a more appropriate way to monitor hypoxemia than intermittent sampling of blood gases. Cultures of blood, purulent tracheal secretions, or the surface of the epiglottis can be obtained, if desired, with the child anesthetized for examination and possible nasotracheal intubation.

MANAGEMENT

Triage

A child who has significant airway obstruction from any cause, as well as any child suspected of having foreign body aspiration or an acute airway injury, should be hospitalized immediately. These children should be placed in a pediatric intensive care unit or in a continuously monitored area in an institution that contains a pediatric intensive care unit to which the child can be transferred immediately should deterioration occur. A child who has mild croup who does not have stridor during quiet breathing need not be hospitalized. A child who has croup who has stridor at rest but who responds well to specific therapies need not be transferred to a pediatric tertiary care center.

A child who has significant airway obstruction should be transported by ambulance and receive oxygen continuously. The child must be accompanied at all times during transport by personnel skilled in airway management. Children suspected of having epiglottitis should not be transported before endotracheal intubation because the medical literature contains numerous reports of cardiorespiratory arrests during transport when the airway has not been secured beforehand. It is a rare circumstance when a community hospital cannot assemble a team for controlled endoscopic examination and nasotracheal intubation in the operating room before transport.

Initial Stabilization

Any child who has significant airway obstruction should be monitored by pulse oximeter and receive supplemental oxygen. Allowing the child or parent to hold the oxygen mask may make this unfamiliar equipment less frightening. The child should be allowed to maintain the position that is most comfortable. Most children who have an obstructed airway prefer to sit up if they are developmentally capable of doing so. If airway obstruction is severe or if controlled examination in the operating room is contemplated, the child should be allowed nothing by mouth.

When acute laryngotracheobronchitis is the most likely diagnosis, aerosolized racemic epinephrine (2.25%, 0.5 ml in 2.5 ml of saline) or L-epinephrine (1%, 0.5 ml in 2.5 ml of saline) in oxygen via face mask generally provides prompt temporary improvement in airflow. Most practitioners hospitalize any child given nebulized epinephrine treatment in an emergency department, regardless of the degree of improvement. However, more recently, some are advocating a prolonged observation period and discharge home if significant airway obstruction does not recur over a number of hours. The most significant toxicity of aerosolized epinephrine in a healthy child is tachycardia, which is well tolerated. Indeed, sometimes the heart rate declines after administration of epinephrine aerosol, coincident with the improvement in airflow. Aerosol treatments may be repeated every 15 to 30 minutes, as necessary, for palliation of upper airway obstruction in croup, provided no signs of toxicity develop.

Most children who have tracheobronchial foreign bodies are not in respiratory distress on arrival because the foreign bodies usually are not located in the proximal airway. In the very rare instance in which the patient is moribund, back blows, chest thrusts, or Heimlich abdominal thrusts may be performed (as appropriate for age) if foreign body aspiration is deemed likely. If these procedures are unsuccessful, direct examination of the airway with a laryngoscope is warranted. If a foreign body is seen to be wedged in the larynx or subglottic space, an emergency crycothyroidotomy may be necessary. If no foreign body is seen, endotracheal intubation should be performed because a foreign body may have migrated to the distal trachea. The only recourse in such circumstances is to push the foreign body forcibly into the right mainstem bronchus and ventilate the left lung. This situation is exceedingly rare.

Definitive Therapy

The definitive therapies for the three most common causes of upper airway obstruction—viral croup, epiglottitis, and membranous laryngotracheobronchitis (bacterial tracheitis)—are very different. Most patients who have croup respond to supportive medical treatment, which includes humidified oxygen, inhalation of epinephrine aerosol, and systemic corticosteroids.[11] It is the unusual patient who has laryngotracheobronchitis who requires an artificial airway. A diminishing response to epinephrine or the development of hyperpyrexia and toxicity may be evidence of bacterial superinfection, heralding the onset of membranous laryngotracheobronchitis (bacterial tracheitis).

Helium has been used to replace nitrogen as the carrier gas for oxygen (Heliox) to reduce the work of breathing in patients who have critical narrowing of the upper or lower airway.[2] Helium concentrations of 60% or greater (i.e., oxygen concentration of 40% or lower) lower the density of inspired gas significantly and reduce airway resistance. Although Heliox temporarily may relieve and palliate airflow obstruction, it is not a specific therapy in itself and cannot be used effectively in children requiring oxygen concentrations above 40%. Heliox should not be used in cases of acute epiglottitis.

Optimal treatment in all cases of acute epiglottitis is securing the child's airway, preferably by nasotracheal intubation. Tracheostomy for treatment of acute epiglottitis is unusual. Inspection and intubation are carried out in the operating room, with the patient undergoing general anesthesia and a pediatric anesthesiologist managing the airway. A surgeon must be present to perform either rigid bronchoscopy or tracheostomy if intubation is not possible. Intubation for epiglottitis generally lasts 18 to 36 hours, until parenteral antibiotics effective against *H. influenzae* have controlled the infection. A second- or third-generation cephalosporin generally is used because of the current emergence of ampicillin-resistant strains. Repeated visualization of the epiglottitis is not necessary for determining the timing of elective extubation.

Most cases of bacterial tracheitis reported to date have required endotracheal intubation to secure an adequate airway. Consequently, most diagnoses are made at the time of intubation. It is not clear whether milder forms of the disease can be treated with appropriate antibiotics and other conservative measures. The usual antibiotic regimen consists of an antistaphylococcal penicillin paired with a second- or third-generation cephalosporin active against *Moraxella* and *Haemophilus* organisms. Generally, extubation is attempted only after thick, purulent secretions have diminished markedly and an air leak is heard on inspiration around the endotracheal tube. The requirement for a air leak is arbitrary because some children have a successful trial of extubation after 5 to 7 days of intubation even without an air leak.

Another scenario encountered in the emergency department involves a child with long-standing, mild upper airway obstruction who has a sudden exacerbation of obstruction. This may be an infant who has mild to moderate laryngomalacia who has increasing difficulty with oropharyngeal secretions arising secondary to a viral infection. Or it may be a child who has poor supraglottic muscle tone as a result of severe psychomotor retardation who has an increase in upper airway obstruction due to a further decrease in mental status secondary to seizures or the effects of medications.

The clinician is guided in responding to the needs of all these children by remembering the "ABCs" of basic life support—*airway, breathing,* and *circulation.*[2] Initial assessment of the child's upper airway function focuses on the degree of airway obstruction and the efficiency of ventilation. The clinician must determine whether the airway is *stable* and patent (which requires no intervention), or *maintainable* (the airway is compromised but can be maintained with basic interventions of oxygen, suctioning, and positioning). The third possibility is that the airway is judged to be *unstable*—this requires immediate placement of an artificial airway to maintain patency. Nasopharyngeal and endotracheal airways are the airway adjuncts of choice to maintain patency of an unstable airway.

Further Care

After a critically impaired airway has been diagnosed and appropriate therapy has been started, the issue of where the child will be cared for must be addressed. A child whose life depends on the patency and stability of an endotracheal tube, nasotracheal tube, or newly created tracheostomy requires the constant attention of nurses, therapists, and physicians experienced in pediatric intensive care. No amount of monitoring equipment can substitute for experienced personnel. Hence, *it is only in dire circumstances that a child should be cared for in an intensive care unit that deals primarily with adults.* The focus of care in a pediatric intensive care unit revolves around vigilant provision of adequate sedation (and paralysis if necessary) to prevent additional trauma to the airway, or even its inadvertent loss. Airways can be kept patent by suctioning and chest physiotherapy. Providing adequate ventilation and lung expansion will prevent parenchymal complications. Attention to other organ system derangements, as well as to the routine needs of a critically ill child, also is essential. When it becomes appropriate to do so, extubation is performed only by personnel experienced in the care of the pediatric airway.

REFERENCES

1. Chaten FC et al: Stridor: intracranial pathology causing postextubation vocal cord paralysis, *Pediatrics* 87:39, 1991.
2. Curtis JL et al: Helium-oxygen gas therapy: use and availability for the emergency treatment of inoperable airway obstruction, *Chest* 90:455, 1986.
3. Donnelly BW, McMillan JA, Weiner LB: Bacterial tracheitis: report of eight new cases and review, *Rev Infect Dis* 12:729, 1990.
4. Downes JJ, Goldberg AI: Airway management, mechanical ventilation, and cardiopulmonary resuscitation. In Scarpelli EM, Auld PAM, Goldman HS, editors: *Pulmonary disease of the fetus, newborn, and child,* Philadelphia, 1978, Lea & Febiger.
5. Herndon DN et al: Treatment of burns in children, *Pediatr Clin North Am* 32:1311, 1985.
6. Leventhal BG et al: Long-term response of recurrent respiratory papillomatosis to treatment with lymphoblastoid interferon-alpha-n1, *N Engl J Med* 325:613, 1991.
7. Mauro RD, Poole SR, Lockhart CH: Differentiation of epiglottitis from laryngotracheitis in the child with stridor, *Am J Dis Child* 142:679, 1988.
8. McCray PB et al: Hypoxia and hypercapnia in infants with mild laryngomalacia, *Am J Dis Child* 142:896, 1988.
9. Newth CJ, Levision H, Bryan AC: The respiratory status of children with croup, *J Pediatr* 81:1068, 1972.
10. Quinn-Bogard AL, Potsic WP: Stridor in the first year of life: the clinical evaluation of the persistent or intermittent noisy breather, *Clin Pediatr* 16:913, 1977.
11. Super DM et al: A prospective, randomized, double-blind study to evaluate the effect of dexamethasone in acute laryngotracheitis, *J Pediatr* 115:323, 1989.
12. *Textbook of pediatric advanced life support,* Elk Grove Village, Ill, 1988, the American Heart Association and the American Academy of Pediatrics.
13. Yarington CT: Trauma involving the air and food passages, *Otolaryngol Clin North Am* 12:321, 1979.

272 Coma

Allen R. Walker

Coma, strictly defined as "a state of unarousable psychologic unresponsiveness in which the subjects lie with eyes closed . . .,"[3] is relatively rare in children and most commonly is caused by blunt trauma to the head. However, the more general syndrome of altered mental status, which includes coma as the most extreme manifestation, is vastly more common and has a more extensive list of possible etiologies.

Alterations in mental status include "clouding of consciousness,"[3] reflecting a primary problem of attentiveness, in which patients seem to be less awake or aware than normal. Delirious patients are out of touch with their environment and may have visual hallucinations. The delirium may be intermittent, alternating with periods of full orientation. Stuporous patients typically seem comatose but can be aroused from their unresponsiveness with strong stimuli, particularly painful ones.

Few studies document the incidence of coma or other alterations of mental status in children[4]; however, it occurs often enough that every primary care physician must have an approach in mind, ready to be called into play quickly. The early management of comatose children can influence the outcome, particularly when the cause is recognized quickly.

ETIOLOGY

Coma and other changes in mental status typically result from processes that involve either both cerebral hemispheres or the brainstem's reticular activating system. Coma may result from direct destruction of brain cells and tissues (trauma, tumor), impairment of function or cell death as a result of insufficient supply of substrate (shock, infarction, hemorrhage, increased intracranial pressure), or impairment of function by endogenous (carbon dioxide) or exogenous (barbiturates) toxins.

Trauma is the most common cause of coma among children; traumatic brain injury caused by child abuse is prominent among infants and young children.[1] The most common nontraumatic cause of coma is intracranial infection, followed by hypoxic-ischemic injury, metabolic causes, and seizures.[4] The list of possible causes of coma is extensive, requiring a logical plan for diagnosis as therapy is initiated.

Plum and Posner[3] have suggested categorizing coma as being due to (1) supratentorial lesions, (2) subtentorial lesions, or (3) diffuse, multifocal, or metabolic causes. Such a classification is useful because it can lead directly to diagnostic and therapeutic considerations early in the management of coma. The box on p. 1657 lists some of the general causes of coma according to this categorization scheme. The boxed material on pp. 1657 and 1658 provides some examples of causes of coma by age group.

Immediate Assessment of Threat to Intact Survival

The "ABC" (airway, breathing, circulation) approach to initial management of emergencies, with the addition of "D" and "E" (disability and exposure), is particularly relevant to coma. Meticulous airway management is the first step in coma therapy, with appropriate respect for the possibility of a cervical spine injury. Not only is appropriate management of the airway a critical step in dealing with threats to intact survival; under some circumstances it also may offer a means of treating increased intracranial pressure by hyperventilation, with resultant hypocapnia and diminished cerebral blood flow.

If there is any suspicion of head trauma, careful in-line immobilization of the cervical spine during airway maneuvers is crucial for protecting the spinal cord.

Comatose children may need help with breathing, either because they are not breathing on their own or because hyperventilation, which produces a modest hypocapnia (P_{CO_2} of 25-35 mm Hg), has been used in managing their increased intracranial pressure. Provision of extra oxygen during resuscitation and initial stabilization has not been shown to be deleterious and may be helpful; ventilation with 100% oxygen should be the rule during the early phases of management.

The goal of maintaining circulation is to provide oxygen and other substrates to the central nervous system (CNS). Clearly, shock must be treated aggressively. Perfusion of the brain to supply oxygen, glucose, and other substrates depends on the difference between mean systemic arterial blood pressure and intracranial pressure; if the systemic arterial pressure is low, cerebral blood flow will be reduced or absent. Fluid restriction has no place in the management of a child in shock, even with a head injury. Restoring circulating intravascular volume, and red blood cell (RBC) mass if necessary, is the critical first step to ensuring adequate perfusion of the central nervous system. Once normal intravascular volume and adequate perfusion have been achieved, fluid administration can be modestly restricted when good evidence of increased intracranial pressure is present.

Arrhythmias rarely are a concern in the management of children in coma, except for bradycardia resulting from increased intracranial pressure and ventricular tachyarrhythmias arising as manifestations of intoxicants (especially tricyclic antidepressants) that can cause coma.

Assessment of *disability* is part of the initial management of coma; this is done by using a coma scale, the best known of which is the Glasgow Coma Scale (GCS). Coma scales offer a reproducible method for assessing neurological disability in a way that can be communicated easily and is useful both for immediate management and for determining the prognosis. A number of coma scales have been developed especially for children[6] because some of the items on the GCS

DIFFERENTIAL DIAGNOSIS OF COMA: GENERAL CAUSES*

Supratentorial causes

Closed head trauma
- Concussion
- Hemorrhage

Hemorrhage/infarction secondary to vascular disease
Neoplasms
- Herniation, obstruction of cerebrospinal fluid, invasion of activating structures

Subdural empyema

Subtentorial causes

Arteriovenous malformation
Basilar migraine
Cerebellar abscess
Cerebrovascular disease
Rupture of vertebrobasilar artery aneurysm
Trauma
- Posterior fossa subdural hematoma

Metabolic causes

Acid-base disorders
Altered temperature regulation
Central nervous system (CNS) infection or inflammation
Dysfunction of non-CNS organs
- Endocrine
- Nonendocrine
- Sepsis

Electrolyte disorders
Failure to provide substrate
- Hypoglycemia
- Hypoxia
- Ischemia

Poisoning

*These causes apply to all pediatric age groups.

DIFFERENTIAL DIAGNOSIS OF COMA: INFANTS

Supratentorial causes

Hydrocephalus
Intraventricular hemorrhage
Subdural empyema
Trauma
- Closed head trauma
- Shaken baby syndrome
- Subdural hematoma

Subtentorial causes

Arteriovenous malformation
Subdural hemorrhage

Metabolic causes

Asphyxiation (child abuse)
Encephalitis
Epilepsy/postictal state
Hypoglycemia
Hyponatremia
Hypothermia
Hypoxia
Inborn errors of metabolism
- Carbohydrate metabolism
- Amino acid metabolism

Intentional poisoning (child abuse)
Intussusception
Meningitis
Sepsis
Shock

are inappropriate; however, none has the widespread acceptability and familiarity of the GCS.

Exposure of the comatose child's whole body permits a search for evidence of trauma, particularly among infants, because even trauma not directed at the head may cause subdural hematomas and coma (shaken baby syndrome[1]). During full body examination, evidence should be sought for other life-threatening diagnoses, such as petechiae/purpura, suggesting sepsis or meningococcemia or an abdominal mass and rectal bleeding, suggesting intussusception.

Diagnosis and treatment must proceed hand-in-hand in the successful management of a child in coma. The initial resuscitation priorities start with a major therapeutic maneuver, that of assuming control of the airway and hyperventilating the child when evidence of increased intracranial pressure is present.

Referral for Care

Many of the conditions that cause coma are within the knowledge and management skills of the general pediatrician. For example, treating diabetic ketoacidosis or meningitis resolves the coma as the underlying disease process improves. Just as clearly, though, some causes of coma require knowledge, skills, and equipment not often within the province of the general pediatrician. Direct measurement of intracranial pressure is one such skill that has assumed increasing importance in the management of traumatic brain injury. Decisions about referral are best made early in the course of management to

DIFFERENTIAL DIAGNOSIS OF COMA: CHILDREN

Supratentorial causes

Arteriovenous malformation
Hydrocephalus
  Malfunction of ventricular shunt
Trauma
Tumor

Subtentorial causes

Arteriovenous malformation
Basilar migraine
Cerebellar abscess
Trauma

Metabolic causes

Acidosis
Altered temperature regulation
Encephalitis
Hepatic failure
Hypertension
  Encephalopathy
Hypoglycemia
Hyponatremia
Hypoxia
Meningitis
Poisoning
Pulmonary disease
  Hypoxia
  Hypercarbia
Renal failure
Seizures/postictal state
Sepsis
Shock
Suicide attempt

DIFFERENTIAL DIAGNOSIS OF COMA: ADOLESCENTS

Supratentorial causes

Arteriovenous malformation
Hemorrhage
Hydrocephalus
  Malfunction of ventricular shunt
Trauma
Tumor

Subtentorial causes

Arteriovenous malformation
Basilar artery migraine

Metabolic causes

Asphyxiation
  Autoerotic
Drug overdose
Encephalitis
Hepatic failure
Hypertension
  Encephalopathy
Hyperthermia
  Heat stroke
Hypothermia
Hypothyroidism
Hypoglycemia
Hypoxia
Meningitis
Occupational exposure to toxins
Poisoning
Pulmonary disease
  Hypoxia
  Hypercarbia
Renal failure
Seizures/postictal state
Sepsis
Shock
Suicide attempt
Vasculitis
  Lupus erythematosus
  Epstein-Barr virus

allow the receiving physician and institution to apply their knowledge and skills to the fullest.

Recognition of local capabilities is crucial to decisions about referral. If 24-hour ventilatory management and one-to-one nursing care are not available, local management of a child in frank coma is not advisable if feasible, safe alternatives are available. The advice of a tertiary care expert should be sought as to the necessity for and timing of referral so that the potential for destabilization during transport is minimized and the child arrives at the most appropriate site—one that is prepared to assume care immediately.

Appropriate transport of a comatose child requires personnel who have the highest level of advanced life-support training, as well as careful decisions about mode of transport (air or ground, high speed or normal speed). Most crucial is maximal stabilization before transport. The more stable the child is before transport, the fewer problems will have to be dealt with under difficult conditions aboard a helicopter or an advanced life-support ambulance. The receiving institution may be able to send a transport team to assist with stabilization and transport.

Common Pitfalls

A number of pitfalls can complicate the management of a child in coma. The most fundamental is underestimating the severity of the symptom. Coma, or any variant of altered mental status, is a fundamental medical emergency, whether it results from head injury, ethanol overdose, status epilepticus, or some other serious cause. Management of the comatose child must include plans to deal with worsening of the condition (e.g., brainstem herniation in the case of trauma, aspiration in the case of a drug overdose, or continued seizures requiring long-term phenobarbital therapy) should that occur.

Concern about increased intracranial pressure may lead to undertreatment of fluid deficits, including frank shock, with disastrous results.

Secondary Needs for General Homeostatic Support

During a short period of coma, most homeostatic needs are met easily by providing intravenous fluids and a neutral thermal environment, in which caloric expenditure for maintaining body temperature is minimal. After 24 to 48 hours, however, nutritional support becomes a major issue, necessitating full parenteral nutrition or enteral nutrition by nasogastric tube or gastrostomy tube.

BRAIN HERNIATION

A critical step in managing coma in children is assessing the risk of herniation of the brain through a bony foramen or its encroachment against a membranous barrier (the falx cerebri or tentorium). There are a number of specific syndromes of herniation, which have been well outlined in classic references.[6] Quick observations should be made repeatedly during management to detect signs of impending herniation. Respiratory pattern and rate, pupillary size, response of the eyes to the doll head maneuver, and the motor system's function at rest and with stimulation all give clues to suggest impending herniation. These signs follow predictable patterns as herniation progresses, with initial changes reflecting reversible lesions and later changes reflecting irreversible lesions resulting from ischemia or hemorrhage.

Respiratory patterns during the early, reversible stages of herniation may appear normal, but more typical are yawns and deep sighs or classic Cheyne-Stokes respirations, with periodic crescendo-decrescendo tachypnea followed by short periods of apnea. As herniation progresses, the respiratory pattern may change to (1) sustained hyperventilation, (2) a pattern indistinguishable from normal breathing, or (3) a slow, irregular pattern.

Coincident with changes in respiratory pattern are changes in pupillary responsiveness. Unilateral pupillary changes are typical of "uncal" herniation, in which midbrain structures are displaced laterally. In "central" (symmetrical) herniation, pupillary changes are bilateral. The earliest pupillary change may be a decrease in the size of the pupils, with limited additional conmtriction in bright light. As herniation continues, becoming progressively irreversible, the pupils become midposition in size, lose their responsiveness to light, and may become unequal. An early sign of uncal herniation is the development of a unilaterally dilated pupil, that initially may be somewhat responsive to light but is progressively less so as the herniation continues.

The doll head maneuver is accomplished by turning the patient's head to one side and then the other (clearly, one must be sure that there is no cervical spine injury before performing this test). In a conscious patient, the eyes normally turn with the head in the direction of the turning. In a comatose patient whose brainstem function is intact, the eyes typically deviate conjugately in the direction opposite that in which the head is turned (doll's eyes are present). Once brainstem function begins to fail, movement of the eyes becomes dysconjugate or totally absent. Should uncal herniation occur, dysconjugate eye movements may be apparent quite early in the herniation sequence.

Motor responses to herniation are assessed both at rest and with stimulation. Early in the course, motor responses may be symmetrical and appropriate, although there may be extensor plantar responses. As central herniation progresses, the child may be motionless at rest and respond to stimulation with stiffened legs and flexed arms (referred to as *decorticate rigidity,*[3] then with extension of both arms and legs *(decerebrate rigidity),* and ultimately *flaccidity.* Motor deterioration during uncal herniation typically is more rapid, often manifesting with decerebrate posturing.

Clearly, herniation is a life-threatening event, so impending herniation must be dealt with aggressively. Immediate intubation and hyperventilation to achieve a Pco_2 in the range of 25 to 30 mm Hg is the initial treatment of choice. Mannitol, an osmotic diuretic, given in a dose of 0.5 to 1 g/kg intravenously, may be helpful. Indiscriminate administration of dexamethasone is controversial, but this drug does appear to be useful in the management of increased intracranial pressure due to brain tumors. It generally is given intravenously in a dose of 1 to 2 mg/kg.

Definitive management of herniation depends on the results of diagnostic studies. Possible etiologies include subdural hematomas in infants, brain tumors in children and adolescents, strokes in children who have underlying vascular anomalies, and malfunctioning ventricular shunts in children who have hydrocephalus. Emergency brain imaging, usually by CT scanning, ordinarily is required after consultation with radiological and neurosurgical specialists to confirm the diagnosis.

INFECTION

If life-threatening herniation syndromes and trauma have been ruled out, intracranial infection is the next most likely cause of the coma.[4] Empirical antibiotic and antiviral treatment may need to be initiated before the infectious etiology is defined clearly. In the presence of signs of increased intracranial pressure or cardiorespiratory instability, lumbar puncture should be deferred.

Treatment of presumed infection should be directed at the most likely etiologies. In young infants, particularly those under 2 months of age, broad-spectrum antibacterial coverage, including an antibiotic active against *Listeria monocytogenes* and an antiviral agent directed against herpes simplex virus are indicated. In older children, broad-spectrum coverage includes drugs with particular effectiveness against *Streptococcus pneumoniae, Neisseria meningitidis,* and *Haemophilus influenzae* type b. Antibiotic therapy should never be delayed because of fear that the results of the lumbar puncture may be affected; eliminating infection is, after all, the point of treatment. If an infectious agent is never recovered but other evidence points to infection, treatment for the most likely organisms should be completed if the child survives the immediate crisis.

ANOXIA/ISCHEMIA

Seshia et al.[4] found that survivors of cardiopulmonary arrest constituted 24% of their series of children with nontraumatic coma. Management of hypoxic-ischemic encephalopathy requires the same knowledge and skills as the management of coma and increased intracranial pressure in general, keeping in mind the overall goal of preventing any further injury to CNS cells that may have the potential to recover after the initial injury. Critical to successful management of children who have suffered hypoxic and/or ischemic brain damage are (1) paying meticulous attention to delivery of oxygen and other nutrients to the CNS, and (2) not overlooking other, potentially treatable causes of coma, particularly metabolic or toxic causes.

SEIZURES

The identification and treatment of seizures that are obvious clinically are discussed in detail in Chapter 256, Seizure Disorders. When stupor or coma is unexplained, the possibility of nonconvulsive seizures should be kept in mind. An EEG may lead to a diagnosis and appropriate therapy.

METABOLIC CAUSES OF COMA

The few metabolic causes of coma are relatively common and vary by age group. Rarer causes are listed in the boxes on pp. 1657 and 1658. In neonates and infants, inborn errors of metabolism must be considered, and measurement of the pH, blood ammonia, and organic and amino acids may be diagnostic. Managing metabolic coma may require avoiding or adding specific substances, and consultation with a metabolic specialist is advised.

In infants, particularly those who are bottle-fed water during the summer months, water intoxication with resultant hyponatremia and seizures is not uncommon. Measuring electrolyte levels confirms the diagnosis, and treatment with isotonic or occasionally hypertonic saline resolves the problem.

Abnormalities of blood sugar, both low and high, are relatively common causes of metabolic coma. Both may be due directly to diabetes and either too much or not enough insulin, respectively. Hypoglycemia also may complicate ethanol ingestion or may be seen as the distinct entity, ketotic hypoglycemia, particularly in toddlers.

Poisonings, intentional (child abuse or suicide) or unintentional, must be considered in the differential diagnosis of coma early in the course. The box above lists some of the common ingestants that can cause coma as part of an overall symptom complex picture; further details on poisoning can be found in Chapter 289, Poisoning.

POISONS ASSOCIATED WITH COMA

Alcohol	Iron
Anesthetics	Lead
Antihistamines	Lithium
Barbiturates	Meprobamate
Benzodiazepines	Monoamine oxidase (MAO) inhibitors
Butyrophenone	Narcotics
Bromide	Organophosphates
Carbamates	Phenothiazines
Carbon monoxide	Salicylates
Clonidine	Sedative-hypnotics
Cyanide	Strychnine
Hydrocarbons	Theophylline
Hypoglycemics (oral and injectable)	Tricyclic antidepressants

From Mandl KD, Lovejoy FH: *Pediatr Rev* 15:151, 1994; and Woolf AD: *Pediatr Rev* 14:411, 1993.

Differential Diagnosis

The boxes on pp. 1657 and 1658 offer a number of specific illnesses and conditions that may cause coma in infants, children, and adolescents, respectively. These lists are not exhaustive, but rather represent common and some of the uncommon etiologies to be considered in the differential diagnosis.

Plum and Posner's classification of coma etiologies into supratentorial, subtentorial, and metabolic is helpful not only in predicting who is likely to be at acute risk of herniation but also in ensuring consideration of the full range of etiologies. Clearly, a child with impending herniation does not require consideration of the metabolic causes of coma; however, the child with undifferentiated coma, particularly an infant, requires consideration of both structural and nonstructural etiologies.

The early steps of differential diagnosis proceed in concert with the early steps of management. Initial observations allow early classification of trauma victims, children who have impending herniation, children who have the petechiae and purpura of meningococcemia, and the like. Early provision of oxygen, along with aggressive fluid resuscitation of those in shock, provides substrate for the brain deprived by poor perfusion. Therapeutic trial of glucose allows identification of some hypoglycemic children; naloxone reverses the CNS depression of opiates. In many instances brain imaging can provide the crucial information to guide the neurosurgeon and the intensive care physician.

Coordination of Multidisciplinary Care

When coma persists over an extended period, the pediatrician plays a central role in the management of the child, either as a direct provider or coordinator of care. Comatose children often are seen by several subspecialty consultants. The general pediatrician can assume the role of advocate for the child, coordinating the efforts of the subspecialists, interpreting their opinions in light of the child's overall condition, and regularly talking with the family. Involving rehabilitation medicine specialists early in the child's course helps ensure the most favorable outcome possible. The pediatrician must know the rehabilitation plans and be sure that acute care interventions in the rehabilitation phase do not interfere with other treatment strategies.

Potential for Organ Donation

Children in coma who ultimately are declared brain dead may be potential organ donors. A responsible organ procurement agency can provide the pediatrician with personnel skilled in discussing donation with families who may in turn see organ donation as allowing some good to come from their loss.

SUMMARY

The primary care pediatrician is crucial to the management of comatose children. Preventing coma by counseling children and parents on injury and poisoning prevention during well-child visits is a daily duty. Evaluating sick and injured children in the office and the emergency department, identifying comatose children early, and rapidly initiating a logical plan for management and diagnosis is a role all primary care pediatricians should be able to assume. Some general pediatricians choose to maintain skills and involvement in the critical care of the comatose child. All can serve as advocates for their comatose patients during the most critical, intensive phases of their care, as well as during rehabilitation.

REFERENCES

1. Committee on Child Abuse and Neglect: Shaken baby syndrome: inflicted cerebral trauma, *Pediatrics* 92:872, 1993.
2. Mandl KD, Lovejoy FH: Common poisonings, *Pediatr Rev* 15:151, 1994.
3. Plum F, Posner JB: *The diagnosis of stupor and coma,* ed 3, Philadelphia, 1980, FA Davis.
4. Seshia SS, Seshia MMK, Sachdeva RK: Coma in childhood, *Dev Med Child Neurol* 19:614, 1977.
5. Woolf AD: Poisoning in children and adolescents, *Pediatr Rev* 14:411, 1993.
6. Yager JY, Johnston B, Seshia SS: Coma scales in pediatric practice, *Am J Dis Child* 144:1088, 1990.

SUGGESTED READINGS

Dietrich AM et al: Head trauma in children with congenital coagulation disorders, *J Pediatr Surg* 29:28, 1994.

Duhaime AC et al: Head injury in very young children: mechanisms, injury types, and ophthalmologic findings in 100 hospitalized patients younger than 2 years of age, *Pediatrics* 90:179, 1992.

Goetting MG, Tiznado-Garcia E, Bakdash TF: Intussusception encephalopathy: an underrecognized cause of coma in children, *Pediatr Neurol* 6:419, 1990.

Levi L et al: Diffuse axonal injury: analysis of 100 patients with radiological signs, *Neurosurgery* 27:429, 1990.

Levin HS et al: Severe head injury in children: experience of the Traumatic Coma Data Bank, *Neurosurgery* 31:435, 1992.

Plum F, Posner JB: *The diagnosis of stupor and coma,* ed 3, Philadelphia, 1980, FA Davis.

Simpson DA et al: Head injuries in infants and young children: the value of the Paediatric Coma Scale: review of literature and report on a study, *Childs Nerv Syst* 7:183, 1990.

273 Croup (Acute Laryngotracheobronchitis)

Caroline Breese Hall and William J. Hall

DEFINITION

Viral croup, or acute laryngotracheobronchitis, is an age-specific syndrome caused by a number of different viral agents. It is characterized by subglottic swelling, respiratory distress, and inspiratory stridor. This syndrome, recognized and respected by physicians for centuries, inherited its name, croup, from the Anglo-Saxon word *Kropan*[4] or from an old Scottish word *roup,* which meant to cry out in a hoarse voice.

Spasmodic croup is a term sometimes used to denote recurrent episodes of croup that affect some children. Allergy or airway hyperreactivity may play a role in predisposing these children to repetitive bouts of croup.

Recent years have seen important advances in our understanding of the etiology, pathophysiology, and treatment of croup, resulting in better management and outcome for these distressed children. An understanding of the physiological abnormalities underlying the child's distress is basic to proper management.

ETIOLOGY

As shown in Table 273-1, a variety of agents may be associated with croup. However, the parainfluenza viruses are the agents identified most frequently as causing this disease, and parainfluenza virus type 1 is the major single agent.[6,10,11,18] In an 11-year study of croup in a private practice in Chapel Hill, North Carolina, the parainfluenza viruses constituted 75% of all the viral isolates obtained from children who had croup; 65% of the parainfluenza viral isolates were parainfluenza virus type 1. Respiratory syncytial virus (RSV), influenza viruses A and B, and *Mycoplasma pneumoniae* were the only other agents isolated with appreciable frequency in this study. Measles (once a major cause of croup) again became a significant cause of severe croup in several large cities most affected by the resurgence of measles during the 1989-1991 upswing of cases in the United States.[9,30]

EPIDEMIOLOGY

Croup occurs primarily in children between 3 months and 3 years of age, with the peak incidence occurring the second year of life. Studies of both hospitalized and ambulatory patients have shown that boys tend to be affected more often than girls.[6,10,11] The incidence of croup varies not only according to age but also by geographical location and season. A prospective study by Hoekelman[15] found that during the first year of life, 1.2% of infants in pediatric practice developed croup. In a prepaid group practice in Seattle, the annual incidence of croup was 7 per 1000 children under age 6.[10] However, between 1 and 2 years of age, this incidence approximately doubled. In the Chapel Hill practice, the attack rate during the second year of life was 4.7 per 100 children per year, and the yearly incidence per 100 children for all ages was 1.82 for boys and 1.27 for girls.

The seasonal flourishes of croup depend on the epidemiological personality of the viral agents (Table 273-1, Fig. 273-1). Parainfluenza virus type 1, the most common cause of croup (Fig. 273-2), has the distinctive pattern of producing epidemics of croup and other associated respiratory illnesses every other year in the autumn.[18] In a continuing surveillance program done in Monroe County, New York, from 1976 to 1992, the parainfluenza viruses overall constituted about 17% of all the viral isolates obtained from outpatients in private practices and for 67% of the isolates from children who had croup.[18] Smaller peaks of croup are associated with outbreaks of influenza, RSV, and parainfluenza virus type 2 and 3.[6,11,18] Cases of croup that occur in the fall most likely are related to the parainfluenza viruses, especially type 1 and to a lesser extent type 2. Winter cases are associated most often with influenza and RSV. In the warmer months of spring and summer, parainfluenza virus type 3 is the agent isolated most often.

Croup in older children (5 years of age or older) has been associated with the influenza viruses or *M. pneumoniae*.[6] RSV tends to cause croup in younger children (in the first year of life) and results more often in prolonged symptoms and hospitalization. The parainfluenza viruses predominately cause croup in toddlers, but they may infect younger and sometimes school-age children.

PATHOPHYSIOLOGY

Infection with one of the viruses usually occurs through person-to-person contact and occasionally through contact with infected secretions. The upper respiratory tract serves as the route of inoculation. The respiratory epithelium offers fertile fields for most of these agents, and viral multiplication occurs easily. Subsequently, the infection spreads farther down the respiratory tract. Involvement of the subglottic tissue appears particularly pronounced. Nevertheless, the infection may extend from the large airways to the alveoli. Inflammation at the subglottic area is especially apt to obstruct airflow seriously because the anatomy of the cricoid and thyroid cartilage make this area both the narrowest and the least distensible part of the larynx. Inflammation, however, commonly affects the conducting airways at all levels. Necrosis of the epithelium is prominent, and the inflammatory exudate and secretions may add to the obstruction.

The age predilection of viral croup can be partly explained by the anatomy of the airway. The subglottic trachea of a young child is relatively smaller and more pliable than that of an older individual. The narrowing that occurs with inspiratory effort therefore may be exaggerated in croup. In ad-

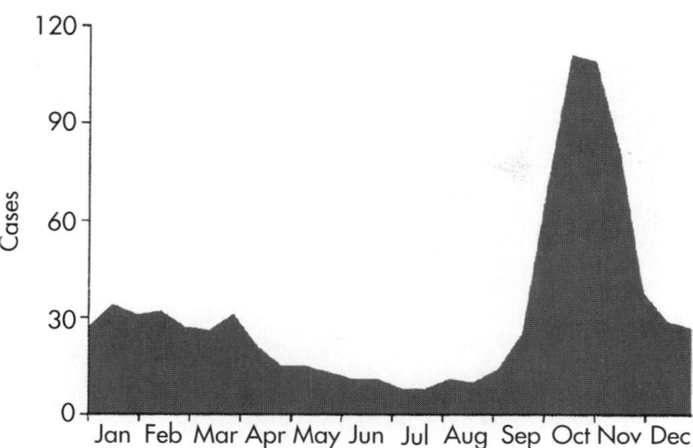

FIG. 273-1 Seasonal occurrence of croup from 1975 to 1992 among patients in pediatric practices that participated in a continuing community surveillance program in Monroe County, New York. Most cases seen in the fall resulted from outbreaks of parainfluenza virus type 1 that occurred in odd-numbered years.

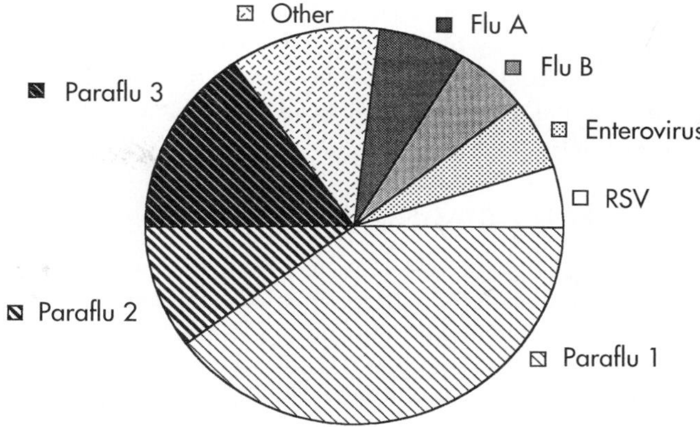

FIG. 273-2 Viral etiology of croup (1975-1992) among patients in pediatric practices that participated in a continuing community surveillance program in Monroe County, New York.

Table 273-1 Causes of Croup

Agent	Epidemiology
Most frequent	
Parainfluenza type 1	Epidemic, fall
Less frequent	
Influenza A	Epidemic, winter
Influenza B	Epidemic, winter
Respiratory syncytial virus	Epidemic, winter-spring
Mycoplasma pneumoniae	Endemic
Parainfluenza type 2	Occasionally epidemic, fall
Parainfluenza type 3	Spring to summer
Uncommon	
Adenoviruses	Endemic
Rhinoviruses	Endemic, fall, spring-summer
Reoviruses	Endemic
Coronaviruses	Epidemic, winter
Herpesvirus hominis	Endemic

dition, obstruction above the subglottic area, such as may occur with nasal congestion, increases the collapsing force, and an increased respiratory rate associated with crying or anxiety may compromise the child's ventilation further.

Other host factors (e.g., genetic and immunological mechanisms), as yet poorly defined, are likely to contribute to the development and severity of croup. Atopy or hyperreactivity of the airways has been suggested as playing a role in spasmodic or recurrent croup by the higher incidence of a family history of allergy and positive skin tests for allergens in such children.[14,20,23,38] Serum IgA levels also have been noted to be lower in these predisposed patients.[39] Abnormalities in the immune response to parainfluenza viral antigens have been observed in children who developed croup when compared with those who had upper respiratory tract illness with parainfluenza virus infection.[35]

CLINICAL FEATURES

Symptoms of an upper respiratory tract infection usually precede the laryngotracheobronchitis. As the infection progresses, the characteristic cough develops. The cough may be spasmodic with a deep "brassy" or "barking" tone. This classic sign therefore has aptly earned the name "seal's bark" and is likened to the notes of a brass bell and even to a crowing cock or a braying ass. Laryngitis with a raspy sounding voice also may develop. Fever commonly is present, particularly with influenza A and parainfluenza viral infections.

These signs herald the usually abrupt onset of the inspiratory stridor. The child may awaken at night with a spasmodic cough and respiratory distress. Although airflow is impeded during both inspiration and expiration, the impediment is most marked on inspiration. Because the subglottic region is outside the pleural cavity, the negative pressures generated on inspiration tend to narrow the passage further, much like sucking on a plugged straw. The child's distress is marked audibly by each stridulous note of inspiration and is accentuated visibly by the retractions of the accessory muscles of the chest wall. The suprasternal, supraclavicular, and substernal retractions particularly are characteristic of the inspiratory obstruction. Further distress may be marked by asynchronous movements of the chest wall and abdomen.

The respiratory rate is increased but usually not more than 50 breaths per minute. This is in contrast to bronchiolitis, in which the picture of respiratory distress may be accompanied by respirations of 80 to 90 breaths per minute. Auscultation of the chest reveals a prolonged inspiration, often accompanied by coarse rales. Wheezes and rhonchi may be heard on expiration. With more severe obstruction, the breath sounds may be diminished. Cyanosis occasionally may be noted, particularly about the lips and nail beds.

The varying intensity of the respiratory distress is characteristic of croup. The child may appear severely compromised and an hour later appear improved, only to worsen over the next hour. Often, for unknown reasons, the symptoms appear to abate on waking in the morning but may worsen again as the day progresses. For most children, the signs of croup extend over 3 or 4 days, but the upper respiratory tract signs and cough may last longer.

In a few children, the respiratory distress may be unremitting or associated with significant pneumonitis and hypoxemia.[27] As the child tires, his or her respirations may become more rapid but also shallow, indicating the need for ventilatory assistance.

DIFFERENTIAL DIAGNOSIS

Viral croup must be differentiated from the two bacterial causes of stridor, bacterial tracheitis and epiglottitis, which without immediate therapy may be fatal. Since the conjugated *Haemophilus influenzae* type b (Hib) vaccines were licensed and incorporated into the routine immunization schedule of young children, epiglottitis has become rare in the United States. The differentiating features of epiglottitis are described in Chapter 280. The rapidly progressive and unrelenting course, the drooling, and the toxicity of epiglottitis tend to distinguish it from croup.

Bacterial tracheitis is the second emergent entity that needs to be differentiated from viral croup.[7,8,22,24] Bacterial tracheitis is an uncommon infection that may affect children of any age, resulting in acute onset of respiratory stridor, high fever, and often copious, purulent secretions. As with epiglottitis, the child may appear toxic, and because the respiratory obstruction progresses rapidly, tracheal intubation is necessary. The pathogens most often involved are *Staphylococcus aureus* and group A beta-hemolytic streptococci. The diagnosis may be confirmed by direct laryngoscopy, which shows the purulent secretions and inflammation in the subglottic area, and sometimes by a lateral neck roentgenogram, which may reveal an area of subglottic narrowing with a shaggy, purulent membrane.

Fortunately, other infectious agents that may mimic croup are now rare. Diphtheria may be excluded by a history of adequate immunizations and by the absence of the characteristic gray pharyngeal or laryngeal diphtheritic membrane. However, there are a number of noninfectious causes of stridor, most of which (e.g., congenital malformations and trauma) can be differentiated by obtaining a good history.[26,32] An aspirated foreign body may cause stridor. Abrupt onset of the stridor, respiratory distress, and lack of preceding respiratory symptoms and fever should suggest this diagnosis. Laryngeal edema caused by an allergic reaction may cause abrupt and severe respiratory distress, occasionally with stridor. The history of the circumstances of the abrupt onset, the lack of previous respiratory signs, and manifestations of an allergic reaction elsewhere should help to differentiate laryngeal edema from other causes of croup.

DIAGNOSIS

Croup usually is diagnosed on the basis of the characteristic clinical findings and a compatible history.[26,32] In cases that are atypical or apt to be confused with other syndromes characterized by stridor, the diagnosis may be aided by a lateral inspiratory and expiratory roentgenogram or by a posteroanterior (PA) roentgenogram of the neck.[5,29,36] The air shadow of the larynx will be seen to narrow like an hourglass in the subglottic region as a result of the characteristic inflammation in this area[29] (Fig. 273-3).

The diagnosis of spasmodic croup has been applied by some to children who have recurrent episodes of croup in which allergic diathesis is believed to play a role.[38] However, the illness in almost all instances still is triggered by a viral infection, and spasmodic croup cannot be differentiated clinically from the usual cases of croup.

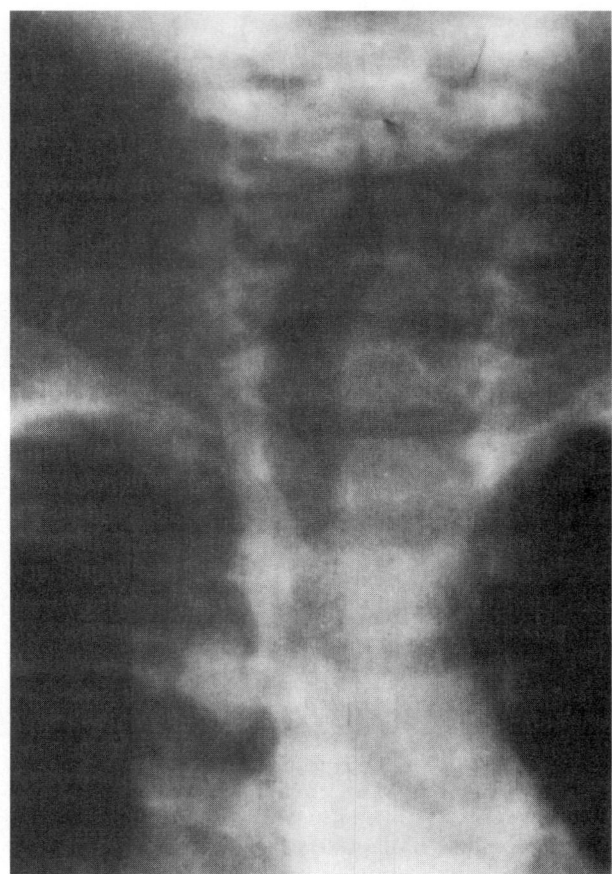

FIG. 273-3 Posteroanterior (PA) roentgenogram of the neck of a child who has viral croup, showing narrowing in the subglottic area.

Laboratory findings are not specific for the diagnosis of acute laryngotracheobronchitis; in fact, they are more helpful in treatment than in diagnosis. The total white blood cell (WBC) and differential counts in children who have croup may be normal or shifted slightly to the left in a more distressed child. Children who have hypoxemia may have an increased proportion of bands in their peripheral count. Most hospitalized children who have acute laryngotracheobronchitis have some degree of hypoxemia.[27] Hypercarbia is unusual except in a severely distressed child.

MANAGEMENT

An understanding of the physiological changes that occur during acute laryngotracheobronchitis is basic to the management of these patients.[1,13,17,21] As depicted in Fig. 273-4, the infecting virus causes inflammation in the subglottic area and lower in the respiratory tract, resulting in two different types of physiological abnormalities. Obstruction in the subglottic area forces the child to increase his or her respiratory effort, causing the respiratory rate to rise. This increased ventilation compensates for the impeded flow of air and results in a

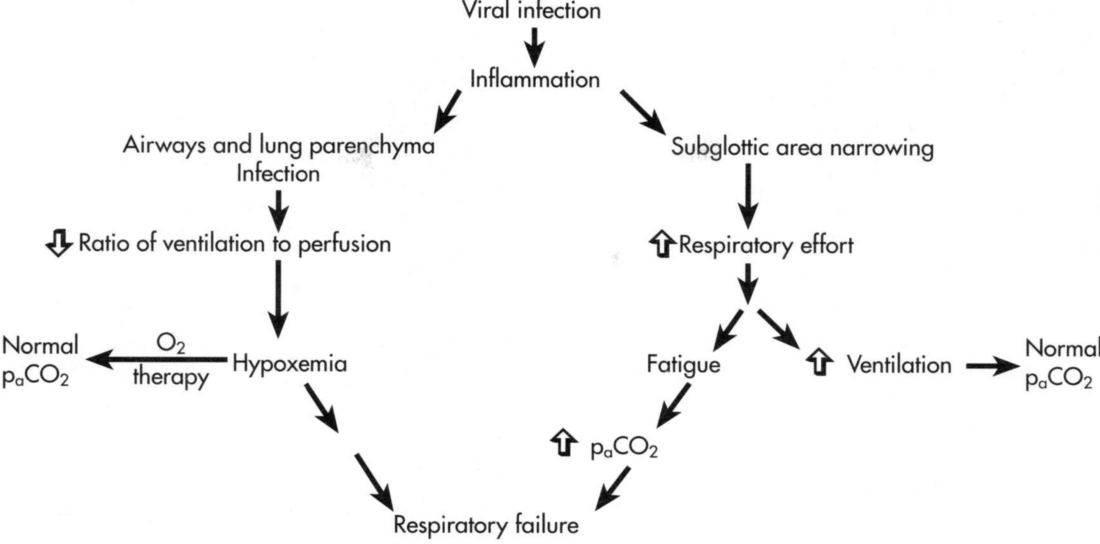

FIG. 273-4 Physiological abnormalities in viral croup.

normal arterial P_{CO_2}. A few children become fatigued from the increased effort of breathing. As their respirations become shallow, the carbon dioxide no longer can be eliminated adequately, and the arterial P_{CO_2} rises.

The inflammation of the airways and lung parenchyma causes concurrent physiological abnormalities that often are not appreciated adequately.[27] Infection of the parenchyma results in an abnormally low ratio of ventilation to perfusion. This produces hypoxemia, seen in more than 80% of hospitalized patients.[27] In contrast to the abnormalities associated with obstruction in the subglottic area, a child who has lower respiratory tract inflammation has little means of compensating. Raising the arterial oxygen saturation requires therapeutic intervention—administration of supplemental oxygen. In a severely distressed child, the hypoxemia contributes to the fatigue. The resulting hypercarbia aggravates the hyoxemia, and respiratory failure may ensue.

The first phase of management is to evaluate which children may be treated at home and which require hospitalization. Severity often is difficult to determine in this fluctuating disease, and no clinical signs are reliably prognostic of a complicated course or of hypoxemia. The severity of the stridor and retractions is better correlated with the degree of subglottic obstruction and the respiratory effort than with hypoxemia. Toxicity, dehydration, and fatigue are indications for hospitalization.

Children who are to be managed at home should be made comfortable to avoid unnecessary anxiety and fatigue. Crying and anxiety tend to make a young child take rapid, short breaths that aggravate the narrowing of the airway and the metabolic need for gas exchange. Fluids should be encouraged, and antipyretics should be given for fever. Despite a cornucopia of cures passed down from generation to generation, few other home therapies have proved beneficial. Because of croup's fluctuating nature, a number of unverified therapeutic modalities may appear to work. Vaporizers and home-devised mist tents, from showers to teakettles, commonly have been tried. However, the water particles produced by these devices are too large to reach the lower respiratory tract and can humidify only the anterior nares and oropharynx. Furthermore, devices that use hot water and steam pose the potential hazard of accidental burns. If the mist is cold, however, it may help to cool the airway, which appears to be beneficial in croup. This might also explain the improvement some children experience when taken out in the cold night air. Cold-dry, cold-mist, and warm-dry air all tend to cool the airway and therefore may be beneficial in croup; this has been supported by animal studies.[37]

In the hospital, the child may be evaluated by the objective criteria of arterial blood gases (ABGs). The degree of hypoxemia may be determined from arterial or capillary blood or by a noninvasive technique such as oximetry. However, laboratory evaluation should be kept to a minimum to avoid upsetting the child further. Humidification in the hospital may be achieved by use of an ultrasonic nebulizer fitted to either a mask or an oxygen tent. This device can produce water particles of a size small enough to reach the bronchioles. The value of such therapy, however, has not been proven. In one small, controlled study, humidification could not be shown to provide any therapeutic benefit for children hospitalized with croup.[3]

Nebulized racemic epinephrine has been shown to be beneficial in children hospitalized with croup.[2,19,31,33] Clinical improvement occurs in most cases in reducing the degree of stridor and retractions, probably as a result of local vasoconstriction from the alpha-adrenergic effect. Such an agent, therefore, may prevent fatigue in a distressed child, but it should be used only with the understanding that (1) amelioration of the clinical signs is transient, and the child may worsen within a couple of hours with rebound mucosal vasodilation and respiratory distress, and (2) the arterial oxygen saturation is not affected.[33] Thus, despite clinical improvement, the degree of hypoxemia remains unchanged.

Use of corticosteroid therapy had been controversial.[2,16,31,34] At least 15 controlled studies using steroids have been published.[2,16,31,34] When subjected to meta-analysis, these randomized trials suggested that for hospitalized children, corticosteroid administration may provide significant clinical improvement when used at a higher dosage—0.3 mg/kg to 0.6 mg/kg of dexamethasone (or its equivalent), given as single dose or up to four doses at 6-hour intervals.[16,31] Antibiotics usually are not indicated for viral croup. Secondary bacterial infection is unusual, and antibiotics should be reserved for such episodes.[28,31]

With these supportive measures, few children require assisted ventilation. General guidelines for determining when a child requires assisted ventilation are (1) progressive carbon dioxide retention, (2) hypoxemia unresponsive to supplemental oxygen administration, and (3) copious secretions that are not mobilized by coughing.

PROGNOSIS

The severity of croup is related partly to the type of infecting virus and partly to unknown host factors. In the great majority of children, croup is a self-limited disease that resolves within a few days. However, several studies have suggested that children who have had croup have a high incidence of bronchial reactivity in subsequent years.[12,23,25,38]

REFERENCES

1. Barker GA: Current management of croup and epiglottitis, *Pediatr Clin North Am* 26:565, 1979.
2. Bass JW, Bruhn FW, Merritt WT: Corticosteroids and racemic epinephrine with IPPB in the treatment of croup, *J Pediatr* 96:173, 1980.
3. Bourchier D, Dawson KP, Fergusson DM: Humidification in viral croup: a controlled trial, *Aust Paediatr J* 20:289, 1984.
4. Cherry JD: Croup. In Kiple KF, editor: *Cambridge History and Geography of Human Disease Project,* Bowling Green, Ohio, 1990, University of Cambridge Press.
5. Currarino G, Williams B: Lateral inspiration and expiration radiographs of the neck in children with laryngotracheitis (croup), *Radiology* 145:365, 1982.
6. Denny FW et al: Croup: an 11-year study in a pediatric practice, *Pediatrics* 71:871, 1983.
7. Donnelly BW, McMillan JA, Weiner LB: Bacterial tracheitis: report of eight new cases and review, *Rev Infect Dis* 12:729, 1990.
8. Dudin AA, Thalji A, Rambaud-Cousson A: Bacterial tracheitis among children hospitalized for severe obstructive dyspnea, *Pediatr Infect Dis J* 9:293, 1990.
9. Fortenberry JD et al: Severe laryngotracheobronchitis complicating measles, *Am J Dis Child* 146:1040, 1992.
10. Foy HM et al: Incidence and etiology of pneumonia, croup, and bronchiolitis in preschool children belonging to a prepaid medical care group over a 4-year period, *Am J Epidemiol* 97:80, 1973.
11. Glezen WP, Denny FW: Epidemiology of acute lower respiratory disease in children, *N Engl J Med* 228:498, 1973.
12. Gurwitz D, Corey M, Levison H: Pulmonary function and bronchial reactivity in children after croup, *Am Rev Respir Dis* 122:95, 1980.
13. Hen J Jr: Current management of upper airway obstruction, *Pediatr Ann* 15:274, 1986.
14. Hide DW, Guyer BM: Recurrent croup, *Arch Dis Child* 60:585, 1985.
15. Hoekelman RA: Infectious illness during the first year of life, *Pediatrics* 59:119, 1977.
16. Kairys SW, Olmstead EM, O'Connor GT: Steroid treatment of laryngotracheitis: a meta-analysis of the evidence from randomized trials, *Pediatrics* 83:683, 1989.
17. Kilham H, Gills J, Benjamin B: Severe upper airway obstruction, *Pediatr Clin North Am* 34:1, 1987.
18. Knott A et al: Parainfluenza viral infections in pediatric outpatients: seasonal patterns and clinical characteristics, *Pediatr Infect Dis J* 13:269, 1994.
19. Kuusela A-L, Vesikari T: A randomized, double-blind, placebo-controlled trial of dexamethasone and racemic epinephrine in the treatment of croup, *Acta Paediatr Scand* 77:99, 1988.
20. Laufer P: The relationship of respiratory allergies to croup, *J Asthma* 23:9, 1986.
21. Lenney W, Milner AD: Treatment of viral croup, *Arch Dis Child* 53:704, 1978.
22. Liston SL et al: Bacterial tracheitis, *Am J Dis Child* 137:764, 1983.
23. Litmanovitch M et al: Relationship between recurrent croup and airway hyperreactivity, *Ann Allergy* 65:239, 1990.
24. Long SS: Bacterial tracheitis, *Report on Pediatric Infectious Diseases* 2:29, 1992.
25. Loughlin G, Taussig LM: Pulmonary function in children with a history of laryngotracheobronchitis, *J Pediatr* 94:365, 1979.
26. McBride JT: Stridor in childhood, *J Fam Pract* 19:782, 1984.
27. Newth CJL, Levison H, Bryan AC: Respiratory status of children with croup, *J Pediatr* 81:1068, 1972.
28. Pianosi P et al: Inappropriate use of antibiotics in croup at three types of hospitals, *Can Med Assoc J* 134:357, 1986.
29. Rapkin RH: The diagnosis of epiglottitis: simplicity and reliability of radiographs of the neck in the differential of the croup syndrome, *J Pediatr* 80:96, 1972.
30. Ross LA et al: Laryngotracheobronchitis as a complication of measles during an urban epidemic, *J Pediatr* 121:511, 1992.
31. Skolnik NS: Treatment of croup, *Am J Dis Child* 143:1045, 1989.
32. Tan HKK, Holinger LD: Tachypnea is often the first sign of respiratory distress: how to evaluate and manage stridor in children, *J Respir Dis* 15:245, 1994.
33. Taussig LM et al: Treatment of laryngotracheobronchitis (croup): use of intermittent positive-pressure breathing and racemic epinephrine, *Am J Dis Child* 129:790, 1975.
34. Tunnessen WW, Reinstein AR: The steroid-croup controversy: an analytic review of methodologic problems, *J Pediatr* 96:751, 1980.
35. Welliver RC, Sun M, Rinaldo D: Defective regulation of immune responses in croup due to parainfluenza virus, *Pediatr Res* 19:716, 1985.
36. Wildin SR, Chonmaitree T, Swischuk LE: Roentgenographic features of common pediatric viral respiratory tract infections, *Am J Dis Child* 142:43, 1988.
37. Wolfsdorf J, Swift DL: An animal model simulating acute infective upper airway obstruction of childhood and its use in the investigation of croup therapy, *Pediatr Res* 12:1062, 1978.
38. Zach M, Erban A, Olinsky A: Croup, recurrent croup, allergy, and airways hyperreactivity, *Arch Dis Child* 56:336, 1981.
39. Zach M, Messner H: Serum IgA in recurrent croup, *Am J Dis Child* 137:184, 1983.

274 Dehydration

Julius G. Goepp

Dehydration resulting from diarrheal illness remains the primary cause of infant and child mortality in the world, accounting for roughly 4 million deaths annually.[7] Although not a leading cause of death in the United States, gastroenteritis and related disorders result in a substantial amount of morbidity and generate significant health care costs. In a recent review, Glass[1] estimated that 16.5 million children less than 5 years of age have at least one episode of diarrhea annually in the United States: 3 million episodes result in a physician visit, and 220,000 hospitalizations occur each year, accounting for about 10% of all pediatric hospitalizations. There are still between 300 and 500 pediatric deaths annually in the United States resulting from dehydration, mainly in the southern states and primarily among African-Americans.

ETIOLOGY

Dehydration in infants and children overwhelmingly is the result of infectious processes. Of these, viral agents are of primary importance in the industrialized countries. Rotavirus and the Norwalk agent account for most cases of viral gastroenteritis in the pediatric population.

Bacterial pathogens also cause significant disease, with the commonest agents being *Salmonella* species, *Shigella sonnei, Campylobacter* species, and *Yersinia enterocolitica.* In addition, in some areas enterotoxigenic strains of *Escherichia coli* produce significant morbidity.

Noninfectious causes of dehydration in children include agents that produce osmotic diarrhea such as laxatives or cathartics containing high concentrations of sugars; obstructive processes in the gastrointestinal tract; and occasionally, vomiting as a sign of elevated intracranial pressure. Although each of these conditions occurs only rarely, they should be borne in mind in the evaluation of the child who is dehydrated and has a history that is not typical for infectious gastroenteritis.

PATHOPHYSIOLOGY OF DEHYDRATION IN GASTROENTERITIS

To make the best-informed decisions about appropriate treatment of dehydration, practitioners should understand the basic principles underlying dehydrating diarrhea and the mechanisms by which rehydration occurs. In this section the mechanisms of diarrheal dehydration and the principles of coupled co-transport on which therapy is based are discussed.

Regardless of which pathogen is involved, diarrhea and fluid loss ultimately result when intestinal fluid secretion exceeds the rate of absorption. In the case of viral agents and cytopathic bacteria such as *Shigella, Salmonella, Campylobacter,* and enteropathogenic strains of *E. coli,* fluid absorption is diminished because absorptive cells at the intestinal villous tip are destroyed, whereas secretory processes that occur at the level of intestinal crypt cells remain unimpaired. On the other hand, toxin-producing bacterial pathogens such as *Vibrio cholerae,* toxigenic *E. coli,* and some strains of *Shigella* cause dramatic increases in fluid secretion from crypt cells by deranging modulation of ion channels in the crypt cell membranes. Intestinal absorptive function is normal in such cases but does not keep pace with secretion, and diarrhea results.

Substantial fluid loss from the gut depletes intravascular volume, resulting in hypoperfusion and poor nutrient and oxygen delivery; ultimately, tissue acidosis develops. Elevated aldosterone levels resulting from hypovolemia lead to renal potassium loss. Eventually circulatory collapse and shock are manifest; irreversible organ damage and death may follow. The chain of events can be interrupted by very rapid repletion of fluids to restore circulating volume, reverse acidosis, and improve perfusion and end-organ function.[4] Traditionally in the United States, volume has been restored directly by intravenous (IV) catheter, and deficits have been replaced rather slowly, over a 24-hour period. There is now growing recognition that even moderate to severe intravascular fluid deficits may be replaced by the enteral (usually oral) route and that better results are obtained with rapid repletion.[4] The balance of this discussion will be devoted primarily to the use of oral rehydration therapy.

ORAL REHYDRATION

Fluid absorption can be promoted by the enteral administration of properly designed fluids, even in the face of ongoing losses. Oral rehydration exploits a normal cellular process known as *co-transport,* in which absorption of a molecule of an organic substrate promotes the absorption of an ion of sodium from the small intestine. With enhanced absorption of sodium, water in turn is absorbed rapidly into the circulation. Intravascular fluid volume can be restored in this fashion rapidly and reliably.

Fluids designed to promote water and electrolyte absorption through the co-transport system in the gut are referred to as *oral rehydration solutions (ORS).* Physiologically appropriate ORS contains 70 to 90 mEq/L sodium and not more than 25 g/L glucose. In addition, ORS typically contains 20 mEq/L potassium and 30 mEq/L base in the form of citrate. It should be noted that almost all juices, soft drinks, and punches contain much higher concentrations of sugars, and almost no sodium, making them inappropriate for use as ORS. In fact, the higher sugar concentrations in these fluids may exacerbate diarrhea by presenting a large osmotic load to the gut.

DATA BASE

In evaluating an infant or child at risk for dehydration, the pathophysiology of the condition should be kept in mind. The interviewer should elicit the duration of symptoms, the frequency and quality of stool (characterized as watery, loose, pasty, or formed), the frequency and approximate volume of emesis, the frequency and volume of urination, and the overall level of activity and appetite displayed by the child. The child who remains active and playful is much less likely to be significantly dehydrated than the child who is fussy, listless, or irritable at home. It is important to bear in mind that infants and younger children may become dehydrated much more rapidly than older children.

The examiner's attention should be directed first to the overall appearance of the child. An alert, interactive, and engageable child is reassuring, whereas somnolence, irritability, and lethargy are of concern. Specific physical findings in dehydration reflect the degree of intravascular volume depletion. Findings suggesting dehydration include a depressed anterior fontanelle, sunken eyes, loss of moisture of the oral mucosa (not dry lips, which may result from mouth-breathing), diminished skin turgor, and delayed capillary refill. To check for the latter, the skin of the thenar eminence is pressed firmly for 1 second and then released. Capillary refill time is the time elapsing before the blanched tissue returns to its normal color. A time longer than 3 seconds is considered indicative of some degree of diminished intravascular volume. Cool extremities and absence of tears do not necessarily denote significant dehydration. Table 274-1 shows a scheme for the assessment of the degree of dehydration as a proportion of total body weight by using physical findings, as well as initial treatment recommendations.

A variety of laboratory studies has been recommended in the past as indicators of the degree of dehydration present in a child. In practice, few such studies are truly necessary in the assessment of the child who has uncomplicated dehydration from gastrointestinal losses. An accurate sense of the severity of dehydration may be formed from physical examination and history. Therapy of dehydration is straightforward and rarely needs to be guided by laboratory studies, which should be reserved for unusual or refractory cases. In such cases measurement of serum sodium, potassium, and bicarbonate levels may be useful, as may determination of the blood urea nitrogen (BUN). It should be noted that ORS can be used to restore both fluid and electrolyte balance in children who have a wide range of initial serum sodium values. By the end of the rehydration period, both hypernatremia and hyponatremia generally have resolved.

MANAGEMENT

The overwhelming majority of dehydrated children can be rehydrated successfully without resorting to parenteral (intravenous or intraosseous) therapy. The combined use of ORS and an appropriate regimen of refeeding is referred to as *oral rehydration therapy (ORT)*.

The first step in ORT is assessment of the degree of dehydration as a proportion of total body weight. Children who have mild dehydration, with thirst as the only presenting sign, are considered to have lost 5% or less of their total body weight. Losses of 6% to 9% of body weight are characterized as moderate dehydration and heralded by sunken eyes, dry mucous membranes, diminished skin turgor, delayed capillary refill time (CRT), and diminution in urine output. Fluid loss of 10% or greater of body weight results in severe dehydration and generally produces signs of shock. Severe dehydration is characterized by marked changes in sensorium (lethargy or irritability), markedly delayed CRT, markedly reduced or absent urine output, tachycardia, and in extreme cases, hypotension. As can be seen from the overlap in descriptors, classifying dehydration is somewhat arbitrary. Therefore fluid replacement calculations are considered to be approximate rather than rigidly accurate.

Table 274-1 Fluid Therapy for Dehydration

Degree of dehydration*	Signs†	Rehydration phase‡ (first 4 hours; repeat until no signs of dehydration remain)	Maintenance phase (until illness resolves)
Mild (6%)	Slightly dry mucous membranes, increased thirst	ORS 60 ml/kg	Breast-feeding, undiluted lactose-free formula, ½-strength cow milk or lactose-containing formula
Moderate (8%)	Sunken eyes, sunken fontanelle, loss of skin turgor, dry mucous membranes, decreased urine output	ORS 80 ml/kg	Same as above
Severe (>10%)	Signs of moderate dehydration plus one or more of the following: rapid thready pulse, hypotension, cyanosis, rapid breathing, delayed capillary refill, markedly reduced or absent urine output, lethargy, coma	IV or IO isotonic fluids (0.9% saline or lactated Ringer), 20 ml/kg; repeat until pulse and state of consciousness return to normal, then 50-100 ml/kg of ORS based on remaining degree of dehydration§	Same as above

*Percent of total body weight lost.
†If no signs of dehydration are present, the rehydration phase may be omitted. Proceed with maintenance therapy and replacement of ongoing losses.
‡In addition to the rehydration amounts shown, replace ongoing stool losses and vomitus with ORS, 10 ml/kg for each diarrheal stool and 5 ml/kg for each episode of vomitus.
§While parenteral access is being sought, nasogastric infusion of ORS may be begun at 30 ml/kg/hr, provided airway protective reflexes remain intact.

Intravenous Rehydration

Patients who present with severe dehydration (shock) should receive initial rehydration fluids parenterally, either intravenously or, when line placement proves difficult, intraosseously. Patients treated parenterally should be given rapid boluses of 0.9% sodium chloride in initial volumes of 20 ml/kg over not more than 20 minutes. Fluid boluses should be repeated until signs of shock begin to disappear. In especially severe cases it is not unusual for patients to require 60 to 100 ml/kg before the restoration of circulating volume is apparent. Even in such cases, however, enteral fluid therapy may begin immediately either by mouth or by nasogastric tube, provided the patient is conscious and that airway protective reflexes are intact.

Oral Rehydration

In the conscious child who has mild or moderate dehydration, fluid replacement always should be initiated orally. Successful ORT depends on proper fluid selection and skilled administration.[2] Simply instructing parents to purchase and feed a child ORS is unlikely to result in success and satisfaction.[3]

Types of ORS. Oral rehydration solutions are most widely available commercially in the industrialized world as premixed liquids. These solutions contain sodium levels varying from 50 to 70 mEq/L. For the mildly dehydrated child, any of these solutions is appropriate. For more significantly dehydrated infants and children, a solution containing 70 to 90 mEq/L of sodium should be chosen. Packets of oral rehydration salts for preparation of a solution containing 90 mEq/L of sodium are available for mixing with 1 liter of water to provide an inexpensive and reliable alternative. These packets always should be distributed with a 1-liter bottle to promote proper mixing. It should again be noted that juices, punches, and other soft drinks are inappropriate solutions for children who have diarrhea because of the high osmotic load they present to the gut. Table 274-2 lists the most commonly available solutions and their compositions. Information on juices and soft drinks is provided for comparison.

Although homemade sugar-salt solutions can be prepared to produce appropriate ORS, the risk of incorrect mixing is high. Such homemade solutions are not recommended when any commercial material is available.

Administration of ORT. In general, ORT can be begun in the office or emergency department immediately after assessment excludes acute abdominal processes and extraintestinal causes of fluid losses (such as intracranial hypertension). Ideally the goal is to replace the entire fluid deficit in the first 4 to 6 hours. A child who is mildly dehydrated is given 60 ml/kg, one who is moderately dehydrated is given 80 ml/kg; severe losses are replaced with 100 ml/kg (including any fluids given parenterally). In addition, 10 ml/kg of ORS for each diarrheal stool and 5 ml/kg for each episode of vomiting should be given.

Fluids are best administered initially by a parent, who is instructed to place into the child's mouth (via a needleless syringe) 1 teaspoon (5 ml)/minute for infants, 10 ml/minute for toddlers, and 15 ml/minute for older children. This steady rate of administration provides 300, 600, and 900 ml/hour, respectively, which generally replaces the calculated deficit within a 4- to 6-hour period. Frequent reassessment of the child and encouragement of the parent is crucial during this period, referred to as the *rehydration phase*. The rehydration phase should be completed in the office or clinic before the child is sent home.

In general, vomiting is not a contraindication to ORT. Even when vomiting occurs, steady fluid replacement is continued orally. Children usually do not discharge their entire stomach contents when they vomit. As dehydration and tissue acidosis are corrected, the frequency and severity of vomiting generally are reduced.

At the end of 4 hours the state of hydration should be reassessed by using the original clinical criteria. If detectable dehydration remains, the rehydration phase should be repeated based on the remaining calculated volume deficit. If rehydration has been completed, the "maintenance phase" is begun. In this phase the parent is instructed to continue to administer ORS in *ad libitum* quantities, but to alternate this fluid with breast milk, formula, or other appropriate feedings. Regular feedings should not be withheld once rehydration is complete. Strong evidence suggests that both volume and duration of diarrhea are reduced when children are fed immediately following rehydration.[5,6]

Table 274-2 Solutions Commonly Used in Children Who Have Diarrhea

Solution	Glucose/CHO (g/L)	Sodium (mEq/L)	Base (mEq/L; citrate or HCO_3)	Potassium (mEq/L)	Osmolality (mmol/L)
Physiologically appropriate solutions					
Pedialyte	25	45	30	20	270
Ricelyte	30*	50	30	25	200
Rehydralyte	25	75	30	20	310
WHO/UNICEF ORS	20	90	30	20	310
Physiologically inappropriate solutions					
Cola	700	2	13	0.1	750
Apple juice	690	3	0	32	730
Gatorade	255	20	3	3	330

*Rice syrup solids.

COMPLICATIONS

Complications of inadequately treated dehydration may be severe, ultimately including full-blown shock and the multiorgan dysfunction syndrome including end-organ damage to the kidneys, liver, and brain, culminating in death. In practice such extreme consequences may be avoided readily by early and aggressive fluid therapy, using the oral or occasionally the intravenous or intraosseous routes. As a rule it is far better to risk overhydration than to be exceptionally cautious with fluid administration. On rare occasions aggressive oral hydration has resulted in mild overhydration, with some transient periorbital puffiness and a 2% to 3% weight gain.[4] These findings generally are self-limited and of no clinical consequence.

Hypokalemia, which results from the losses of total body potassium as a consequence of the increased aldosterone activity in the kidney, is a common occurrence in severe dehydration. As sodium is avidly retained, potassium is lost in urine. Hypokalemia can result in ileus, which may impair fluid and electrolyte absorption from the gut. ORS generally contains 20 mEq/L of potassium chloride; such solutions are capable of restoring potassium balance.

PROGNOSIS

Although diarrheal dehydration is the leading cause of death among children globally, when appropriately treated it carries an excellent prognosis. Rapid restoration of circulating volume coupled with proper dietary management results in maintenance of hydration and earlier resolution of diarrheal symptoms. Parents should be warned, however, that even with ideal therapy, typical episodes of gastroenteritis last 3 to 7 days. Parents and providers must be reassured by the child's state of good hydration. The physician should reinforce the idea that the diarrheal illness itself is of little consequence so long as hydration is maintained and feeding reintroduced in a timely fashion.

WHEN TO HOSPITALIZE

In the industrialized world, otherwise healthy children treated with proper ORT for gastroenteritis and dehydration rarely need to be hospitalized. Most can be rehydrated in the office, clinic, or emergency department and discharged to home for the maintenance phase. Hospitalization should be reserved for the child who has other medical problems (e.g., short-gut and inflammatory bowel disease) or for children whose hydration status cannot be restored or maintained after a 6-hour outpatient treatment period. The expense and occasional adverse consequences of inpatient intravenous therapy warrant keeping dehydrated children who have no other complications out of the hospital.

WHEN TO REFER

Most children in the industrialized world come to medical attention before gastroenteritis results in significant dehydration. Such children almost always can be managed directly from the office or clinic. Children who have moderate or severe dehydration, however, require rehydration under observation, which is not possible in some sites. Such children may be referred to a hospital emergency department for ORT. Emergency department staffs should be trained to initiate and administer ORT and to instruct parents in its use.

SUMMARY

Dehydration resulting from gastroenteritis is a common condition generally managed by ORT on an outpatient basis. Little laboratory evaluation is necessary. Parenteral therapy is reserved for severe or unusual cases. Regardless of route of delivery, fluid should be administered rapidly, with the intent to restore the entire fluid deficit in 4 to 6 hours. Proper dietary management is essential to minimize the severity and duration of symptoms.

REFERENCES

1. Glass RI et al: Estimates of morbidity and mortality rates for diarrheal diseases in American children, *J Pediatr* 118:27, 1991.
2. Goepp J: Oral rehydration. In Henretig FJ, King C, editors: *Textbook of pediatric emergency procedures,* Baltimore, 1994, Williams & Wilkins.
3. Goepp J, Katz S: Oral rehydration therapy: a practice-oriented approach, *Am Fam Physician* 47:843, 1993.
4. Hirschhorn N: The treatment of acute diarrhea in children: an historical and physiological perspective, *Am J Clin Nutr* 33:637, 1980.
5. Santosham M et al: Role of soy-based, lactose-free formula during treatment of acute diarrhea, *Pediatrics* 76:292, 1985.
6. Santosham M et al: Role of a soy-based, lactose-free formula in the outpatient management of diarrhea in infants, *Pediatrics* 87:619, 1991.
7. Snyder JD, Marson MH: The magnitude of the global problem of acute diarrhoeal disease: a review of active surveillance data, *Bull WHO* 60:605, 1982.

275 Diabetic Ketoacidosis

Robert E. Greenberg

Ketoacidosis often may be the initial event leading to the diagnosis of diabetes mellitus. Coexistence of coma is a much less common occurrence because early clinical recognition of the diabetic state has improved and diabetic ketoacidosis thus is often prevented. Yet intercurrent episodes of ketoacidosis remain a frequent occurrence, especially among those diabetic children whose psychosocial and biological factors impose barriers to effective diabetic management or impede the metabolic response to insulin. Although mortality is low, even from coma, meticulous management of diabetic ketoacidosis is required to prevent or detect complications.

DEFINITION

Diabetic ketoacidosis occurs when the rate of endogenous glucose production continues unrestrained, despite the presence of markedly curtailed peripheral glucose utilization. The resultant increase in the breakdown of fat leads to the accumulation of nonesterified fatty acids and, because of the subsequent hepatic conversion of fatty acids to ketone bodies, to the release of hydrogen ion. The combined effects of osmotic diuresis and increased generation of protons lead both to dehydration and to acidosis. If these events are prolonged or severe, stupor, drowsiness, and coma may occur.

ETIOLOGY

Glucose Metabolism

The concentration of glucose in blood is remarkably constant in a normal child, even during periods of fasting. Fasting involves the physiological suppression of insulin secretion, with consequent reduction of peripheral glucose utilization and mobilization of substrate (free or nonesterified fatty acids) from triglyceride stores. The reduction in insulin secretion leads to a marked curtailment of glucose utilization by insulin-sensitive tissues. Glucose utilization is compromised further during fasting by the direct inhibiting effects of both free fatty acids and ketone bodies (Fig. 275-1); it may be impeded still further during severe metabolic acidosis, when the binding of insulin to membrane receptors is impaired.

The reduction in glucose utilization that normally occurs during fasting is necessary to conserve body protein as effectively as possible. Were ongoing glucose utilization not curtailed, increased rates of new glucose formation (*gluconeogenesis*) would be mandatory to replace missing exogenous carbohydrate. However, gluconeogenesis requires precursor amino acids, so the duration of a prolonged fast would be markedly restricted were body protein stores not guarded most zealously.

Gluconeogenesis is not finely modulated in diabetic ketoacidosis but rather persists at a physiologically uncontrolled rate. This lack of control is the complex result of reduced insulin availability, impaired insulin action, increased substrate flow from muscle and adipose tissue, and increased counterregulatory hormones (which accelerate glucose production). Thus, at the very time when glucose utilization is compromised, glucose production is paradoxically increased, with resultant hyperglycemia and consequent osmotic diuresis and dehydration.

Alternate Energy Sources

When the availability of glucose as a substrate for intracellular energy metabolism is reduced, then alternate energy sources must be made available. Hence triglyceride (neutral fat) is broken down into glycerol and fatty acids; the fatty acids release hydrogen ion during their subsequent hepatic conversion to ketone bodies (Fig. 275-2). Ketone bodies accumulate in blood as a consequence both of increased production and of reduced peripheral utilization, because turnover rates for ketone bodies are prolonged in diabetic ketoacidosis (Figs. 275-2 and 275-3).

Role of Counterregulatory Hormones

The action of insulin in diabetic ketoacidosis is resisted for reasons other than the direct effects of acidosis. One such reason is the increased secretion of counterregulatory hormones, a clear example of which is seen in the control of triglyceride breakdown (Fig. 275-4). Insulin inhibits lipolysis, an aspect of its action that is partially independent of its effects on glucose transport. However, catecholamines, cortisol, growth hormone, glucagon, and thyroid hormones all exert—either directly or indirectly—an opposite effect on fat breakdown so as to enhance lipolytic rates, even in the presence of adequate insulin. Activation of counterregulatory hormone secretion, in response to either biological or emotional stimuli, leads to accelerated rates of lipolysis, which in persons who have diabetes impairs metabolic regulation further. Increased secretion of counterregulatory hormones in the presence of relative insulin insufficiency thus compounds the decreased utilization and increased production of glucose and ketone bodies.

INITIAL ASSESSMENT

The severity of acidemia in diabetic ketoacidosis is the summation of increased hydrogen ion generation and reduced hydrogen ion excretion, the latter as a consequence of dehydration. Reversal of this process requires the biological actions of exogenously supplied insulin and replacement of water and electrolytes. The diagnosis of diabetic ketoacidosis usually is not difficult, except when a previously undiagnosed patient is admitted in coma. The antecedent symptoms of nausea and vomiting, thirst and polyuria, weakness, weight loss, and visual disturbances lead most often to a rapid clinical diagnosis.

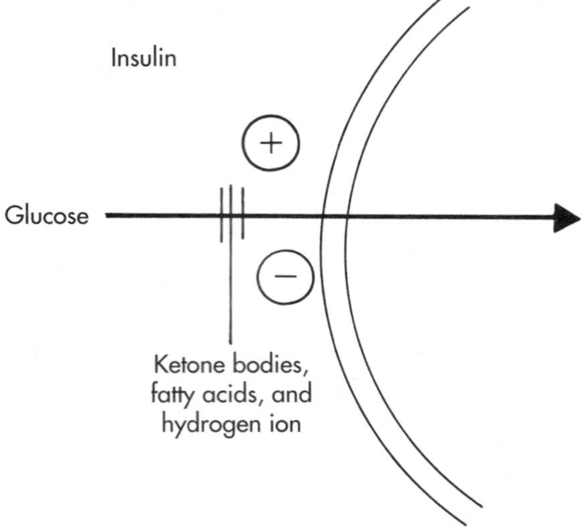

FIG. 275-1 Factors affecting glucose transport across cell membranes. +, Increase; −, decrease.

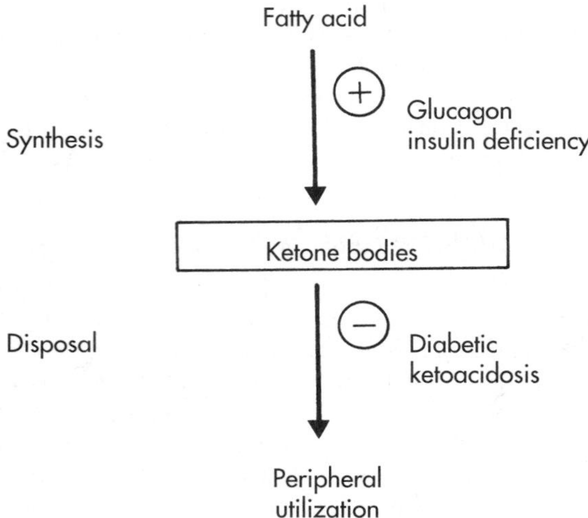

FIG. 275-2 Control of ketone body synthesis and disposal. +, Increase; −, decrease.

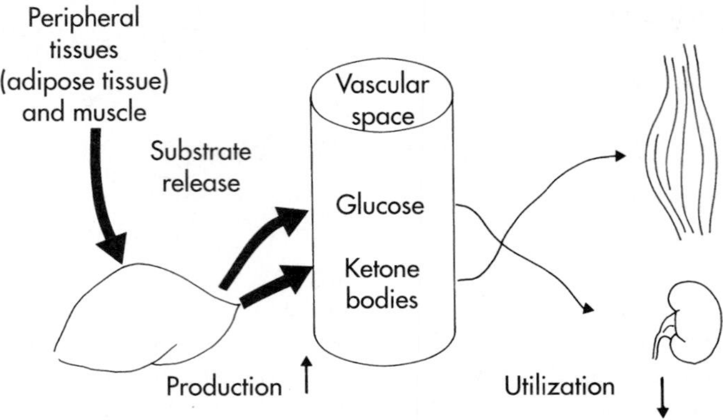

FIG. 275-3 Substrate production and utilization in diabetic ketoacidosis.

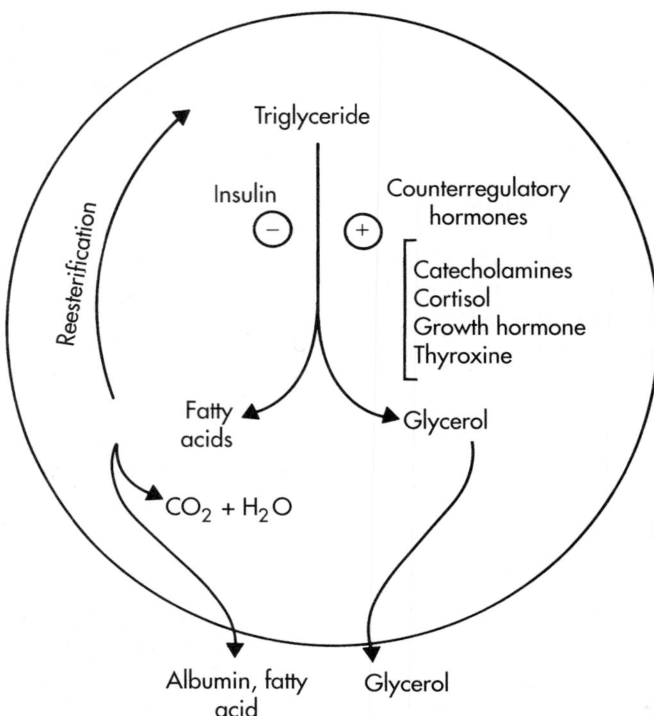

FIG. 275-4 Control of triglyceride breakdown. +, Increase; −, decrease.

In the initial assessment two urgent issues are (1) the evaluation of effective blood volume and (2) the differential diagnosis of coma. Tachycardia, hypotension, and hypothermia all should suggest reduced blood volume; its rapid increase with isotonic saline or colloid is essential. The precise cause of stupor, drowsiness, and coma in a diabetic child may be difficult to document and hence to treat accurately and might well involve hypoglycemia, ketoacidosis, lactic acidosis, or hyperglycemic-hyperosmolar nonketotic coma. Where there is doubt as to the cause of coma, *immediate intravenous administration of glucose (2 to 3 ml/kg of a 50% dextrose solution) may prevent significant neurologic damage;* if hypoglycemia is not present, the amount of glucose given under such a policy is insignificant compared with the total pool of available glucose.

When blood volume is depleted markedly or when ketoacidosis is especially severe, respiratory compensation for metabolic acidosis may not be clinically apparent; that is, the classic Kussmaul respirations of ketoacidosis may become clinically evident only after blood volume has been restored at least partially.

Assessment often is confusing because of the notable frequency of abdominal pain as a symptom of diabetic ketoacidosis. In the comatose patient, gastric atony and dilation may lead to vomiting and aspiration; thus immediate placement of an indwelling gastric tube under constant low suction to remove gastric contents is essential.

TREATMENT

Initial Therapeutic Procedures

The suspected diagnosis of diabetic ketoacidosis is confirmed rapidly by use of methods available in any emergency room that demonstrate elevated glucose and ketone body concentrations in both blood and urine. Blood glucose can be estimated accurately by using glucometers; similarly the severity of ketonemia can be estimated by noting the dilution of serum that still gives a positive test result, with use of crushed or powdered Acetest tablets. Although there are exceptions, it is possible to derive semiquantitative estimates of blood ketone body concentration by multiplying by 0.1 mM the highest dilution still giving a positive test result, to yield a rough estimate of acetoacetate concentration. Because the normal ratio of beta-hydroxybutyrate to acetoacetate is 3:1, multiplying this estimated concentration of acetoacetate by 4 will provide the final estimate for total ketone body concentration. The patient who is dehydrated, has an altered state of consciousness, and has Kussmaul respirations, yet with only a minimal rise in estimated serum ketone body concentration, is the one in whom alternate proton donors must be sought, especially lactic acid. A difficult clinical problem may be presented by the dehydrated, acidemic child who has been given parenteral glucose-containing solutions before blood glucose has been measured; in this setting reduced peripheral perfusion may be associated with impaired glucose utilization to produce "artifactual" (i.e., nondiabetic) hyperglycemia. The correct diagnosis will depend on elicitation of the proper historical evidence to reveal the mechanism producing dehydration.

The severity of blood volume depletion in the child who has diabetic ketoacidosis (blood pH <7.2) can be appreciated from the resultant hormonal changes: serum concentrations of arginine vasopressin, plasma renin activity, aldosterone, and norepinephrine are increased 3-fold to 20-fold, and the concentration of atrial natriuretic peptide is reduced markedly.

After establishing the diagnosis of diabetic ketoacidosis, the physician should center attention quickly on (1) restoring blood volume and (2) initiating a physiological response to insulin. In the presence of significant hyperosmolality (i.e., hyperglycemia), the rapid administration of hypotonic fluids may cause cerebral edema; accordingly, initial intravenous fluids should be isotonic and rapidly administered (10 to 20 ml/kg/hr), even in the absence of evident blood volume depletion, until the results of laboratory tests can clarify the magnitude of hyperglycemia and the severity of acidemia.

Insulin should be administered as quickly as possible and in doses that achieve physiological concentrations of insulin in blood. Low-dose *constant insulin infusion* uses 0.1 unit of regular insulin per kilogram as an initial "push" dose, followed by a similar amount administered over an hour by constant infusion.

Two issues are important to note regarding any form of insulin therapy: (1) the physiological response to insulin must be demonstrated, not assumed, and (2) sensitivity to insulin may change during the course of diabetic ketoacidosis so that a rate of insulin infusion that initially effects stabilization may produce hypoglycemia subsequently. Subcutaneous insulin may be absorbed erratically or poorly by a hypovolemic patient, as compared with intravenous infusion, although insulin administered subcutaneously remains an effective form of therapy.

If clinical evaluation indicates that the blood volume is beginning to be restored and appropriate amounts of insulin are being provided, the question of patient transfer, if necessary, can be decided. A flow sheet should be started, on which the following should be recorded and monitored carefully: the nature and rate of intravenous fluids administered, insulin dosage, urine output, vital signs, and laboratory data.

Subsequent Therapy

During the 6 to 12 hours after initial stabilization, therapeutic concerns should center on the following series of definable problems.

Prevention of Cerebral Edema. The occurrence of cerebral edema is extremely common as a subclinical finding during therapy for diabetic ketoacidosis; clinically evident cerebral edema represents the primary cause of death. Patients at risk for development of cerebral edema include those whose condition has been in prolonged poor control; those who have severe acidemia (blood pH <7.2); those who have normal serum sodium concentrations in the presence of hyperglycemia; and those who have early signs of increased intracranial pressure. Although blood volume depletion initially must be addressed vigorously, the rate of subsequent infusion of hypotonic fluids should not be excessive and must be monitored carefully. A maximum of 4500 ml fluids/M^2/24 hr should guide therapy.

Management of Acidemia. The definitive approach to the management of ketoacidosis is to reduce the generation of increased hydrogen ion (by insulin administration) and to improve the capacity to excrete an acid load (by blood volume expansion). In the presence of severe acidemia (pH <7.0), the irritability of cardiac muscle increases with resultant increased likelihood of cardiac arrhythmias. Because of negative inotropic effects on the heart, cardiac output may fall. When the pH is reduced markedly, the ability of insulin to bind to its membrane receptors is impaired, reducing still further the physiological response to insulin.

Correction of severe acidosis with bicarbonate may thus be necessary before insulin can be effective and, certainly, in instances of aberrant cardiac function. However, use of bicarbonate is not without significant hazard; when it is administered in large amounts, serum bicarbonate rises, raising blood pH values and reducing the stimulus for respiratory compensation so that carbon dioxide accumulates. Because carbon dioxide equilibrates across the blood-brain barrier much more rapidly than does bicarbonate, the intracerebral space may become more acidotic, even as extracellular pH values climb. Further, severe hypokalemia may be precipitated by bicarbonate administration, requiring frequent monitoring and potassium supplementation.

Prevention of Hypoglycemia. The occurrence of significant and even dangerous hypoglycemia during management of diabetic ketoacidosis can be a severe complication. It occurs primarily when glucose is not being provided in the intravenous fluids, excessive amounts of insulin are administered, or the patient's changing sensitivity to insulin is not recognized. Early administration of exogenous glucose and use of the low-dose constant insulin infusion technique minimize the risk of hypoglycemia.

Hyperosmolar nonketotic diabetic coma in childhood is a rare condition; when it does occur, however, the mortality is much higher than in diabetic ketoacidosis. Hyperosmolar nonketotic hyperglycemic coma is defined as a marked increase in blood glucose concentration (usually >800 mg/dl), the absence of ketoacidosis, an altered state of consciousness, and significant dehydration. Thus the initial laboratory studies of severe hyperglycemia without significant ketonemia in a child who has an altered state of consciousness should alert the physician to the presence of this syndrome. A hyperosmolar state also can develop during treatment and is detected by demonstrating marked hyperglycemia and by noting the excessive rate of diuresis in relation to the observed clinical state of hydration and rate of intravenous fluid administration. Because of the rarity of hyperosmolar coma relative to the frequency of therapy-induced hypoglycemia, glucose should be incorporated into intravenous fluids just as soon as it is clear that the blood glucose concentration either is not markedly elevated or is falling during insulin infusion and blood volume expansion.

Replacement of Water and Electrolyte Deficits. The child who has severe diabetic ketoacidosis has marked deficits of water and electrolytes. However, in contrast to other conditions in which dehydration secondary to gastrointestinal losses is the presenting problem, ongoing renal fluid and electrolyte losses in diabetic ketoacidosis may be excessive, as a consequence of osmotic diuresis. When blood glucose values are brought below 200 mg/dl, urinary losses diminish markedly; in that situation excessive urine formation usually is secondary to excessive fluid administration. Because cerebral edema and hypokalemia are the primary reasons for fatality in diabetic ketoacidosis, therapy should be directed primarily toward preventing those complications. Accordingly, full correction of dehydration and resolution of ketonuria need not be accomplished during the initial 24 hours after therapy is initiated, as long as clinical assessment indicates normalization of circulating blood volume and no clinical and/or laboratory evidence of hypokalemia.

Osmotic diuresis produces water losses in excess of electrolyte losses. Thus as soon as blood volume has been expanded and the danger of hyperosmolality assessed, the introduction of hypotonic fluids becomes appropriate. The usual fluid will contain the following approximate contents: Na^+, 30 to 40 mEq/L; K^+, 30 to 40 mEq/L; HCO_3^-, 10 to 20 mEq/L; and Cl^-, 50 to 60 mEq/L. Because prolonged use of chloride ion as the only anion is itself acidifying, the administration of bicarbonate in amounts found in extracellular fluid represents physiological replacement in this case, rather than the use of bicarbonate to combat established acidosis.

Prevention of Hypokalemia. Total body potassium losses may well be excessive in diabetic ketoacidosis and may continue during ongoing osmotic diuresis. Further, the reincorporation of available extracellular potassium into the intracellular space may lead to profound hypokalemia. Adequate amounts of potassium used early in the intravenous fluid program and careful monitoring of both serum potassium and electrocardiographic tracings will minimize the hazard of hypokalemia, the danger of which is greatest during the first 12 hours after the initiation of corrective therapy.

Detection of Lactic Acidosis. Lactic acidosis may occur in several situations in diabetes: (1) lactic acid may accumulate, to some degree, as part of ketoacidosis; (2) it may accumulate during therapy as a complication of tissue hypoxia accompanying severe hypophosphatemia; and (3) lactic acidemia may be a presenting problem in the absence of significant ketonemia. This latter occurrence is much more common in adults, especially in the elderly.

Serum phosphate predictably falls during the management of diabetic ketoacidosis. With significant hypophosphatemia, levels of red blood cell 2,3-diphosphoglycerate also will fall, reducing the ability of hemoglobin to release oxygen. The resultant tissue hypoxia leads to lactic acidosis, which is corrected with phosphate infusions. The presence of lactic acidosis should be suspected whenever the clinical appearance of the child (e.g., Kussmaul respirations) or the measurement of blood pH indicates a degree of acidemia unexplained by the measured or estimated concentration of serum ketone bodies.

The Acetest tablet reflects only acetoacetate, however, and does not detect beta-hydroxybutyrate. On initial examination the patient's degree of ketonemia may be underestimated because the beta-hydroxybutyrate/acetoacetate ratio is increased in diabetic ketoacidosis. Upon correction, the degree of ketonemia may be overestimated inasmuch as the aforementioned ratio will decrease, so a greater proportion of the total ketone bodies will be present as measurable (by Acetest) acetoacetate. Thus the occurrence of a significant anion gap and acidemia in the absence of detectable ketone bodies is an important clue to the presence of other causes for persistent metabolic acidosis.

Treatment of Precipitating Conditions. Diabetic ketoacidosis may be precipitated by other events, including infection. Presence of an underlying infection may be difficult to document because leukocytosis with increased release of nonsegmented leukocytes can occur in diabetic ketoacidosis without infection. Careful observation and repeated physical examination usually clarify coexistent disease and delineate the significance of concurrent abdominal pain.

IATROGENIC DANGERS

The main predisposing factor in iatrogenic complications is the physician's failure to monitor the child as his or her physiological state changes under therapy. Attention to the physiology of the primary problems to be ameliorated and careful observation of the child during the first 6 to 12 hours of treatment should minimize the danger of complications. The most important consideration in evaluating the need to transfer a patient is the availability of competent professionals; the expert who is unavailable cannot help.

CONVALESCENT CARE

Subcutaneous insulin can be initiated after oral intake of fluids and nutrition has become adequate. The principal task then must be to focus on exploring reasons for the occurrence of diabetic ketoacidosis. If the onset of ketoacidosis heralded the initial diagnosis of diabetes mellitus, primary attention must be focused on patient and family education and on helping the family adapt to the new diagnosis of a chronic (and incurable) disease. Where the ketoacidosis represents a recurrent problem in a known diabetic child, primary attention must be focused on determining and resolving the biological and psychosocial factors that led to aberrant metabolic control.

SUGGESTED READINGS

Barrett EJ et al: Insulin resistance in diabetic ketoacidosis, *Diabetes* 31:923, 1982.

Baruh S, Sherman L, Markowitz S: Diabetic ketoacidosis and coma, *Med Clin North Am* 65:117, 1981.

Cahill GF et al: Hormone-fuel interrelationships during fasting, *J Clin Invest* 45:1751, 1966.

Hare JW, Rossini AA: Diabetic comas: the overlap concept, *Hosp Pract* 14:95, 1979.

Harris GD, Fiordalis I, Finberg L: Safe management of diabetic ketoacidemia, *J Pediatr* 113:65, 1988.

Keller V, Bergen W: Prevention of hypophosphatemia by phosphate infusion during treatment of diabetic ketoacidosis and hyperosmolar coma, *Diabetes* 29:87, 1980.

Robinson AM, Williamson DH: Physiological roles of ketone bodies as substrates and signals in mammalian tissues, *Physiol Rev* 60:143, 1980.

Schade DS, Eaton RP: The temporal relationship between endogenously secreted stress hormones and metabolic decompensation in diabetic man, *J Clin Endocrinol Metab* 50:131, 1980.

Schade DS et al: *Diabetic coma,* Albuquerque, 1981, University of New Mexico Press.

Tulassay T et al: Atrial natriuretic peptide and other vasoactive hormones during treatment of severe diabetic ketoacidosis in children, *J Pediatr* 111:329, 1987.

276 Disseminated Intravascular Coagulation

Marilyn J. Manco-Johnson

Disseminated intravascular coagulation (DIC) follows thrombocytopenia as the second most common acquired bleeding disorder in ill children. DIC is a hypercoagulable syndrome in which multiple procoagulant and regulatory proteins as well as platelets are consumed, resulting in a depletion of these factors. Excessive thrombin generation within the circulation either eludes or overwhelms the body's ability to limit and regulate thrombin formation. Fibrin strands that are formed within the microcirculation cause vasoocclusions, which lead to local tissue ischemia and dysfunction. These changes trigger local vascular injury, capillary leak, and the sequelae of shock. The fibrinolytic enzyme, plasmin, is generated. Subsequent fibrin dissolution produces degradation products (fibrin split products, FSP), which inhibit coagulation further by impairing fibrin polymerization and platelet aggregation. Paradoxical concomitant occurrence of hemorrhage and thrombosis is common. DIC can be activated by a large number of triggers including infection, acidosis, trauma, and poor blood flow. Whether blood coagulation normalizes spontaneously depends on effective reversal of the trigger event, adequate clearance of activated proteins by the circulation, and the capacity of the reticuloendothelial system, liver, and bone marrow to compensate with increased production of the elements needed to achieve normal coagulation.

PREVALENCE

At The Children's Hospital, Denver, Colorado, the diagnosis of DIC was made in 36 hospitalized children during 1994, or 0.4% of the 9074 hospital admissions during that year. About half of the diagnoses were made in neonates, with the remainder in older infants, children, and adolescents. This prevalence is typical of a pediatric tertiary care center.

ETIOLOGY

DIC is not a single disease; rather, it is a syndrome that comprises of characteristic clinical and histological findings, which may appear in diverse clinical settings and have in common the excessive activation of the coagulation and fibrinolytic pathways. Coagulation in DIC is activated by exposure of blood to "tissue factor" or to a wide variety of proteolytic enzymes. The box on p. 1677 lists the enormous number of infections and other conditions that have been associated with DIC in infants and children.

DATA BASE

History, Physical Examination, and Laboratory Findings

DIC usually presents in infants and children who are critically ill with hypoxia, acidosis, hypotension, shock or fever and who have multiorgan dysfunction. Patients who have DIC may manifest bleeding primarily in the skin, gastrointestinal tract, central nervous system, and sites where skin and soft tissues have been breached by trauma. Sites of surgery, indwelling central catheters, and skin puncture commonly develop oozing of blood as a first symptom, which responds poorly to pressure or suturing.

Gastrointestinal bleeding may be especially severe among patients who have liver disease, in whom it portends a poor prognosis. Petechiae may be prominent in children who have severe thrombocytopenia.

Capillary leak syndrome is common in DIC. Infants develop peripheral edema, accumulations of fluid in "third spaces," and inadequate intravascular volume. Shock is aggravated by poor cardiac output and peripheral vasoconstriction.

On the peripheral smear a microangiopathic hemolysis may be identified by the presence of schistocytes. Neutropenia and thrombocytopenia are common. Gram negative rods found in smears of the peripheral blood often give the first clue to the presence of bacterial sepsis in the neutropenic neonate.

The laboratory findings of DIC are listed in the box on p. 1678. In acute DIC a severe drop in the platelet count and the fibrinogen level regularly are found, whereas these levels can be normal or even elevated in compensated chronic DIC. Activated partial thromboplastin time (APTT) and thrombin time (TT) are prolonged, both by depletion of coagulation factors and by interference with coagulation by FSP. The prothrombin time (PT) is prolonged moderately in DIC; a PT greater than twice the normal level suggests the possibility of vitamin K deficiency or fulminant liver failure. The reptilase time is normal in the presence of heparin, but is prolonged by a low fibrinogen level or in the presence of FSP.

Plasma markers of thrombin and plasmin activation can be determined. Presence of these markers supports a diagnosis of DIC and excludes a syndrome consisting exclusively of fibrinolysis or end-stage liver disease without DIC. Specific factor assays rarely are necessary. However, levels of factor VII occasionally are helpful, because factor VII has a plasma half-life of only 4 to 6 hours and can be used to assess the short-term synthetic capacity of the liver. In one study low factor V and elevated factor VIII levels were observed in infants who had compensated severe liver disease associated with biliary cirrhosis. Levels of factor VIII and factor V are both decreased in severe DIC.

The box on p. 1678 summarizes the pathophysiological processes that produce DIC. In most cases of DIC, children present with a short history suggestive of rapidly progressive cardiovascular deterioration and features of infection, trauma, and untoward therapy-related or other catastrophic events. Occasionally the onset is insidious, especially with underly-

CAUSES OF DISSEMINATED INTRAVASCULAR COAGULATION

Infections

Gram negative bacteria
- *Neisseria meningitides*
- *Hemophilus influenza*
- *Escherichia coli*
- Pseudomonas sp.
- Enterobacter sp.
- Klebsiella sp.
- *Serratia marcescens*
- Proteus sp.
- Bacteroides sp.
- *Francisella tularemsis*
- *Salmonella typhi*
- *Brucella abortus*
- Selenomonase

Gram positive bacteria
- *Staphylococcus aureus*
- Group A and B beta-hemolytic streptococcus
- *Streptococcus pneumoniae*
- *Streptococcus faecalis*
- *Streptococcus viridans*
- *Clostridium perfringens*
- *Clostridium welchii*
- *Mycobacterium tuberculosis*

Viruses
- Varicella
- Herpes zoster
- Human immunodeficiency virus
- Herpes simplex
- Cytomegalovirus
- Hepatitis B
- Rubella
- Rubeola
- Variola
- Roseola
- Echovirus type 11
- Arbovirus
- Arenavirus

Fungi
- Aspergillus
- Histoplasma
- Candida

Parasites
- *Plasmodium falciparum* (malaria)

Tissue injury

Massive trauma, especially brain and crush injuries
Shock
Asphyxia/acidosis
Ischemia/infarction
Burns
Hyperthermia/hypothermia
Fat embolism
Rhabdomyolysis

Vascular injury

Vascular tumors including giant hemangiomata
Malignant hypertension
Respiratory distress syndrome

Immunological disorders

Collagen vascular diseases
- Systemic lupus erythematosus
- Rheumatoid arthritis
- Wegener granulomatosis
- Inflammatory bowel disease

Antiphospholipid antibodies
- Lupus anticoagulant

Anticardiolipin antibody syndromes
Anaphylaxis
Renal allograph rejection
Hemolytic transfusion reactions

Liver disease

Advanced cirrhosis
Fulminant hepatitis
Reinfusion of ascitic fluid
Reye syndrome

Therapy-related factors

Activated prothrombin complex concentrate infusions
Massive transfusion
Warfarin administration in patients who have severe deficiencies of protein C or protein S
Intravenous lipid infusion

Intrauterine factors

Fetal demise of a twin
Uterine infection
Abruptio placenta
Eclampsia
Acute fatty liver of pregnancy

Malignant neoplasms

Acute leukemia, especially promyelocytic
Lymphoma
Disseminated neuroblastoma
Familial hemophagocytic reticulosis

Other causes

Massive thrombosis, especially stroke
Intravascular hemolysis
- Erythroblastosis fetalis

Snake evenomation
Severe genetic deficiencies of protein C and protein S

From Manco-Johnson MJ: *Int J Pediatr Hematol Oncol* 1:1, 1994.

LABORATORY FINDINGS IN DISSEMINATED INTRAVASCULAR COAGULATION (DIC)

Global screening tests for abnormalities reflecting consumption of coagulation factors and platelets.
- Prolonged activated partial thromboplastin time
- Prolonged prothrombin time
- Prolonged thrombin time and reptilase time
- Prolonged euglobulin lysis time
- Decreased platelet number
- Prolonged bleeding time

Markers of thrombin and plasmin activation. Positive or elevated results are seen in DIC

Thrombin:	F 1.2 (prothrombin fragment 1.2)
	TAT (thrombin antithrombin)
	FPA (fibrinopeptide A)
	Bβ 1-14 (beta fibrinopeptide β)
Plasmin:	Fibrin split products
	Bβ 1-42
Combined:	D-Dimer (plasma fragment of fibrin)
	Bβ 15-42

Specific factor assays. Decreases in all of these proteins reflect consumption of clotting factors in DIC.
- Prothrombin, fibrinogen
- Factor V, factor VIII
- Antithrombin-III, protein C, protein S
- Plasminogen, antiplasmin

From Manco-Johnson MJ: *Int J Pediatr Hematol Oncol* 1:1, 1994.

FACTORS INCLUDED IN THE PATHOPHYSIOLOGY OF DISSEMINATED INTRAVASCULAR COAGULATION

Bleeding diathesis

- Increased fibrinolysis
- Consumption of coagulation factors
- Consumption of platelets
- Interference with platelet aggregation and fibrin polymerization by circulating fibrin split products

Deposition of microthrombi

- Expression of procoagulant surface
- Increased turnover of activated clotting factors
- Consumption of regulatory proteins
- Release of excess fibrinolytic inhibitors
- Release of platelet activating factor

Vascular injury and capillary leak

- Direct toxic effect of endotoxin
- Activation of kinins, complement, and other cytokines
- Neutrophil adhesion and release of elastase and toxic radicals

From Manco-Johnson MJ: *Int J Pediatr Hematol Oncol* 1:1, 1994.

ing malignant or liver disease. *The clinical presentation of DIC predominantly consists of bleeding secondary to systemic fibrinolysis, as well as depletion and dysfunction of coagulation proteins and platelets.* Shock, hypotension, and multiple organ failure usually occur. There may be diffuse thrombosis of small vessels with resulting ischemia of various organs and infarctions, especially in the liver. These abnormalities usually are not apparent on clinical examination; however, infarctions may be prominent when the organs are examined at autopsy. Occasionally infants and children present with thrombosis of large vessels or the presence of gangrene of the extremities. *Frequently a diagnosis of DIC is based on finding a typical pattern of abnormal laboratory tests before clinical signs of this disorder are apparent.* DIC may be acute and fulminant, or it may be chronic and low grade in severity. The clinical picture of DIC is determined both by the intensity and the duration of the disease that triggers the occurrence of intravascular clotting and by the ability of the host to compensate for the associated increase in turnover of coagulation proteins and platelets.

Chemical and cellular pathways that result in DIC are not pathological in and by themselves. Rather, they comprise the normal host response to endothelial injury. Under optimal conditions these processes result in localization of infection and injury; they promote effective bacterial killing and facilitate subsequent tissue repair. The inflammatory response is protective if it is localized and limited.

Endotoxin and Vascular Injury. *Endotoxin initiates the classical alterations resulting in DIC, and it probably causes the majority of cases of DIC in infants and children.* Endotoxin is a lipopolysaccharide produced by certain bacteria, notably gram negative organisms. The lipid moiety of endotoxin promotes cellular adhesion, whereas the polysaccharide component activates complement. After contact with blood cells, most endotoxin that is elaborated within the circulation is carried to the liver, spleen, lungs, and kidneys. These organs are the principal targets of DIC, as shown by histological findings. Endotoxin causes direct toxicity to endothelial cells. This results in structural and metabolic changes, especially to pulmonary endothelial cells, and cell permeability is increased.

Prothrombotic Effects

Endotoxin causes tissue factor to be expressed on the surfaces of endothelial cells, monocytes, and macrophages. Tissue factor itself is an important component of host defense. Complete lack of tissue factor may be incompatible with life, because no living person has been identified with tissue factor deficiency. Expression of tissue factor promotes fibrin formation, both by the activation of factor Xa and through downregulation of thrombomodulin.

Coagulation can be activated by malignancies (especially leukemias), cytokines, hematopoietic growth factors, antigen-antibody complexes, and anaphylatoxin. Furthermore, factor X and other coagulation proteins can be activated in the absence of tissue factor by snake venoms, hemolysis, massive transfusions, burns, and infusions of activated clotting factor concentrates given to children who have hemophilia. Advanced DIC results in excessive release of plasminogen activator inhibitor, especially in the periphery of affected organs, which promotes local organ ischemia and necrosis.

Anticoagulant, Profibrinolytic, and Platelet Inhibitory Effects

Limited coagulation and fibrinolysis not only mobilize protective immune responses but also provide protection from excess coagulation. Tissue plasminogen activator and prostacyclin released from endothelial cells in response to endotoxin promote fibrinolysis and limit platelet aggregation. Degradation products of fibrin and fibrinogen, generated during DIC, inhibit excess fibrin polymerization and platelet aggregation. In this way fibrin and fibrinogen degradation products serve as physiological anticoagulants that promote maintenance of flow in the microcirculation. However, excess fibrinolysis often results in intractable bleeding.

Interleukin-1 and Tumor Necrosis Factor

Both interleukin-1 and tumor necrosis factor are released by endotoxin and cause direct vascular injury. Interleukin-1 causes myriad effects including fever, hypotension, T lymphocyte activation and proliferation, and production of acute phase proteins. Tumor necrosis factor is a very potent mediator of many of the signs of DIC, including shock, massive vascular thrombosis, hemorrhage, adult respiratory distress syndrome, acute renal tubular necrosis, adrenal hemorrhage, and death.

Endotoxin, interleukin-1, and tumor necrosis factor all can cause increased expression of endothelial and leukocyte cell receptors that are important in leukocyte adherence. These receptors include intercellular adherence molecule-1 (ICAM-1), endothelial leukocyte adherence molecule 1 (ELAM-1), and the leukocyte cell surface proteins, LFA-1, MO-1, and p150.

Purpura Fulminans

Purpura fulminans is a clinical syndrome characterized by irregular skin lesions that usually begin on the trunk, the buttocks, and the lower extremities. The lesions at first are flat and red, but they quickly become black and palpable and develop eschars. Diffuse petechiae also are present. Histological examination of the skin shows thrombosis of small blood vessels, together with secondary hemorrhage and necrosis. Thromboses of large vessels can occur, being related to placement of indwelling central venous catheters.

Coagulation studies in purpura fulminans show severe deficiencies in protein C and free protein S. There also is decreased fibrinogen and other evidence of DIC. Neonatal purpura fulminans usually is caused by severe genetic deficiencies of protein C or protein S. A few case reports have described acquired deficiencies from maternal lupus anticoagulants. Severe infections, especially meningococcal sepsis and meningitis, are responsible for purpura fulminans in most older infants and children. In the Waterhouse-Friedrichsen syndrome DIC secondary to meningococcemia is severe, which results in profound shock and adrenal hemorrhage. Recently, purpura fulminans has been described among children who have varicella and acquired autoimmune protein S deficiency. Acquired purpura fulminans is characterized by more peripheral distribution of skin lesions, which can progress to gangrene. Purpura fulminans may also occur upon institution of oral anticoagulation therapy among children who have a genetic deficiency of protein C or protein S, or those who have an anticardiolipin antibody.

PSYCHOSOCIAL CONSIDERATIONS

Rarely, older children and adolescents have presented with multiple purpura lesions caused by self-inflicted trauma that mimics DIC. The diagnosis is suspected because all of the lesions are on skin surfaces accessible to the child's reach. Children who have self-inflicted purpuric lesions require psychiatric evaluation and management.

THERAPY OF DISSEMINATED INTRAVASCULAR COAGULATION

Acute DIC

- Remove trigger (most important)
- Coagulation support
  - Use fresh frozen plasma to maintain PT under 17 seconds (10 ml/kg will raise coagulation factors by 10% to 20%)
  - Use cryoprecipitate to maintain fibrinogen over 100 mg/dl (1 bag/5 kg will raise fibrinogen by 100 mg/dl)
  - Use platelet concentrates to maintain platelet count over 50,000 mm^3 (10 ml/kg will raise platelet count by 75,000 to 100,000 mm^3)
  - Consider use of low-dose heparin therapy
  - Consider replacement of AT-III and protein C

Chronic DIC

- Treat underlying disease
- Administer low-dose heparin to inhibit clotting activation
- Consider replacement of antithrombin-III and protein C
- Consider antifibrinolytic therapy when fibrinogenolysis predominates

From Manco-Johnson MJ: *Int J Pediatr Hematol Oncol* 1:1, 1994.

MANAGEMENT

Therapy of Acute DIC

Therapeutic approaches to DIC are outlined in the box above. The primary treatment of severe acute DIC is to *reverse or eliminate the disease or condition that is triggering the occurrence of intravascular coagulation.* Optimal supportive care via rapid restoration of ventilation and circulation, and administration of appropriate antibiotics, usually is adequate to inhibit the occurrence of consumptive coagulopathy. An abbreviated panel of laboratory screening tests of coagulation, including APTT, PT, fibrinogen level, and platelet count, can be performed on venous, arterial, or capillary samples and should be obtained every 8 to 12 hours. Infants who have respiratory distress syndrome or sepsis complicated by DIC usually will show laboratory and clinical evidence of plasma coagulation improvement within 24 hours of the initiation of therapy. Thrombocytopenia often persists for several days. Worsening of the platelet count during the recovery phase of the illness should trigger a search for a thrombosis or secondary infection. While definitive therapy is being initiated, levels of platelets and clotting factors should be maintained.

There are few studies on replacement of specific factors in infants and children who have consumptive coagulopathy. Antithrombin III concentrate was given to 10 neonates who had sepsis and DIC. In these infants infusions of 40 U/kg/day of human antithrombin III, along with heparin at doses of 200 U/kg/day, raised plasma antithrombin levels by only 8.7%. This small rise probably was related to rapid plasma turnover of antithrombin III. However, 4 infants who had failed to respond to prior therapy with heparin alone showed improved coagulation status within 2 days of being given an infusion of antithrombin. Further study is required before the utility of inhibitor replacement (such as antithrombin) can be assessed in the treatment of DIC.

Therapy of Chronic DIC

Chronic DIC usually presents in children as a low-grade, compensated process with an ongoing disease or triggering condition such as postsurgical cardiomyopathy with poor cardiac output, malignant neoplasms, or inflammatory diseases. Infants and children deficient in antithrombin III, protein C and protein S from developmental immaturity, genetic deficiency, or extreme platelet consumption may require inhibitor replacement in the form of fresh frozen plasma or protein concentrates. Administration of low doses of heparin will help stop consumption of coagulation factors and platelets while awaiting results of definitive therapy.

Purpura Fulminans

Aggressive therapy of the disease or condition precipitating DIC is critical for children who have purpura fulminans. Heparin therapy is controversial. Because some thrombin generation is necessary for protein C activation, high-dose heparin may inhibit endogenous protein C function. In severe cases replacement of protein C via fresh frozen plasma or protein concentrates will help to halt purpuric lesions. With even aggressive therapy, areas of infarction will progress to gangrene and may require amputation, debridement, or skin grafting.

Kasabach-Merritt Syndrome

Infants and children who have giant hemangiomas frequently show laboratory evidence of chronic DIC and may have bleeding complications. Recently several therapeutic approaches have yielded encouraging results. These include use of heparin, steroids, epsilon-aminocaproic acid, recombinant interferon-alpha, cyclophosphamide, surgical excision, pneumatic compression of the hemangioma, and irradiation.

Complications of Therapy

Most children who have acute DIC present with oozing around indwelling vascular catheters and at sites of recent trauma or surgery. Life-threatening intracranial and gastrointestinal hemorrhage can complicate DIC, especially in young infants. Occasionally thrombosis of large vessels develops in an infant or child who has DIC. Anticoagulant doses of heparin may be given safely to patients who have DIC, provided care is taken to minimize the risk of bleeding by maintaining critical levels of platelets, fibrinogen, and clotting proteins, with transfusion of appropriate factors as needed.

Children experiencing chronic DIC (lasting more than 7 days) will begin to suffer the consequences of disseminated microthrombi, causing tissue ischemia with resulting multiorgan failure, acidosis, and deteriorating vital signs.

PROGNOSIS

In general the prognosis of DIC is related to success in treating the underlying disease and reversing the trigger of coagulation activation. In purpura fulminans, infarction of digits and extremities is common, even with initiation of appropriate antibiotics and circulatory support.

HOSPITALIZATION AND SUBSPECIALTY REFERRAL

Most children who have acute DIC require admission to the intensive care unit. If laboratory evidence of DIC does not improve within 24 hours of the initiation of supportive care, referral should be made to a pediatric hematologist. Therapy of any episode of hemorrhage, large vessel thrombosis, or purpura fulminans in a child who has underlying DIC should be managed in consultation with the pediatric hematology service.

SUGGESTED READINGS

Bick RL: Disseminated intravascular coagulation: objective criteria for diagnosis and management, *Med Clin North Am* 78:511, 1994.

Feinstein DI: Diagnosis and management of disseminated intravascular coagulation: the role of heparin therapy, *Blood* 60:284, 1982.

Hathaway WE, Bonnar J: *Hemostatic disorders of the pregnant woman and newborn infant,* New York, 1987, Elsevier.

Mammen EF: Coagulation defects in liver disease, *Med Clin North Am* 78:545, 1994.

Manco-Johnson MJ: Disseminated intravascular coagulation and other hypercoagulable syndromes, *Int J Pediatr Hematol Oncol* 1:1, 1994.

Markwardt F: The development of hirudin as an antithrombotic drug, *Thromb Res* 74:1, 1994.

Martin M: Epidemiology and clinical impact of gram-negative sepsis, *Infect Dis Clin North Am* 5:739, 1991.

Monlar RA et al: Diagnosis and treatment of homozygous protein C deficiency, *J Pediatr* 114:528, 1989.

Sakuragawa N et al: Clinical evaluation of low-molecular weight heparin on disseminated intravascular coagulation: a multi-center cooperative double-blind trial in comparison with heparin, *Thromb Res* 72:475, 1993.

Shimada M et al: Modulation of coagulation and fibrinolysis in hepatic resection: a randomized prospective control study using antithrombin III concentrates, *Thromb Res* 74:105, 1994.

Zenz W et al: Recombinant tissue plasminogen activator treatment in two infants with fulminant meningococcemia, *Pediatrics* 96:144, 1995.

277 Drowning and Near-Drowning

Steven E. Lucking

Drowning is the second leading cause of accidental death among children and adolescents.[5] Motor vehicle injuries remain the leading cause of accidental death in this age group, although rates have declined in the decade ending in 1988. Deaths caused by drowning and other accidents also have shown a decline, whereas the death rates from suicide and homicide have increased.[6] In 1986, 2062 deaths from drowning were reported in children less than or equal to 19 years of age.[5] It also has been estimated that for each drowning fatality in childhood, there are three to four hospital admissions for nonfatal near-drownings.[26] In addition it has been estimated that for each hospital admission, four children are seen in an emergency department for a water-related accident and are released.

The circumstances by which drownings and near-drownings occur vary by age. Bathtub drownings generally occur in children less than 1 year of age who are left in the care of an older sibling and without adult supervision. Children in the 8- to 20-month age range may drown by falling into a pail or other small container of liquid. A strong correlation exists between the incidence of drowning in toddlers and the presence of family swimming pools. Drownings among older children and adolescents may occur as a result of diving accidents. Adolescent and adult drowning incidents often are associated with the use of alcohol. Community education and mandated barriers around private pools may help to decrease the incidence of this clearly preventable source of morbidity and mortality. However, in 1995 children still suffered significant morbidity from near-drowning, even in supervised public pools that have lifeguards on duty.

The oldest and most common definition of drowning is "death from suffocation from submersion in liquid." Additional definitions have been developed over time to reflect certain specific pathophysiological events that may occur. *Near-drowning* most typically defines survival of at least 24 hours after suffocation from submersion in liquid. The term *secondary drowning* usually refers to the development of cardiorespiratory compromise after a variable latent period. The term *dry drowning* is commonly used to reflect that suffocation from submersion in liquid can occur without fluid aspiration into the lung. This phenomenon also is referred to as *drowning or near-drowning without aspiration.* Finally, some have defined *immersion syndrome* as indicating the sudden development of asystole and death upon immersion in cold water; this event probably is mediated vagally.

PATHOPHYSIOLOGY OF DROWNING

The physiological response to submersion is probably quite variable.[17] The classic description of the initial response to submersion includes a period of panic, characterized by vigorous struggling, breath-holding, and automatic swimming. There are a number of eyewitness reports, however, that describe the victim's response as being much more subdued or placid. Children, for instance, are reported to stop playing suddenly and become motionless. Some children will ingest a large amount of water early in the sequence of events. With progressive loss of consciousness, these children may vomit, then aspirate the vomitus with the onset of gasping respirations. As loss of consciousness progresses, airway reflexes eventually are lost and fluid may enter the lungs passively. Conversely, 10% to 20% of autopsy cases of drowning show no fluid aspirated into the lungs. These dry drownings are believed to be caused by laryngospasm occurring early in the sequence of events, preventing aspiration.

Fluid and Electrolyte Shifts

Early interest in the study of drowning in the 1960s focused on fluid and electrolyte abnormalities. Salt water has an osmolarity approximately 3½ to 4 times that of plasma. When aspirated into the lung in sufficient quantities, this hypertonic fluid draws additional fluid into the alveolar space. Intravascular hypovolemia and hemoconcentration result, and the serum concentration of major electrolytes increases. Conversely, fresh water is hypotonic with respect to plasma. Aspiration of sufficient quantities of fresh water will result in intravascular hypervolemia with dilutional hyponatremia as water is absorbed from the lung. Hemodilution and hemolysis may occur in severe cases, leading to hemoglobinuria, acute renal failure, and hyperkalemia. The electrolytic phenomena, which are reported in humans and are easily reproducible in the laboratory, actually are quite uncommon in the clinical setting. In laboratory animals one must instill at least 22 ml/kg into the lung to produce electrolyte changes.[19] It is unusual for nearly drowned humans to aspirate more than 4 ml/kg, and in one study, less than 15% of near-drowning victims aspirated more than 22 ml/kg.[18] Thus significant electrolyte abnormalities are uncommon in patients who survive to reach a medical facility.

Pulmonary Injury

The most important aspect of the fluid aspiration itself is the pulmonary injury that ensues. It has been demonstrated in laboratory animals that fresh water will inactivate pulmonary surfactant on contact whereas salt water will cause surfactant wash-out.[11] Thus the aspiration of sufficient quantities of either fresh or salt water causes loss of functional surfactant, with resultant poor lung compliance. This in turn leads to increased work of breathing, atelectasis, and hypoxemia.

Any child who has a submersion injury may vomit and aspirate during the event. Regardless of the type of liquid in which the submersion occurred, pulmonary aspiration of acid gastric contents may be associated. This can lead to tracheobronchial inflammation with bronchospasm and the development of alveolar capillary injury. Finally, if the patient has suffered a cardiac arrest and has some degree of cardiogenic shock in the aftermath, a secondary pulmonary capillary injury may occur with resultant capillary leak, diffuse edema, and hypoxemia (acute lung injury, adult respiratory distress syndrome [ARDS]).

Neurological Injury

The single most important determinant of morbidity and mortality in near-drowning is the extent of brain injury. Prolonged submersion under water leads to hypoxia and hypercapnia. It is primarily the hypoxemia that leads to myocardial depression and eventual cardiac arrest. During cardiac arrest the entire body is subject to global ischemia and anoxia. Although all organs are affected by global ischemia, the brain tends to be the least forgiving of this insult.

Beginning in the 1980s a considerable amount of interest has focused on the issue of anoxic brain injury and on attempts to improve neurological outcome after global anoxia—an approach called *cerebral resuscitation.*[14]

Within 2 minutes of the onset of anoxia there is loss of substrate for energy production within the cell. This is accompanied by potassium efflux from cells, coupled with the influx of calcium and sodium.[24,25] Following anoxia as much as a 90% reduction in ionic calcium concentration in brain interstitial fluid with toxic accumulation of calcium within neuronal mitochondria has been noted. The enzyme phospholipase A2 is activated by elevated intracellular calcium, resulting in rapid liberation of free fatty acids (predominantly arachidonic acid) from the plasma membrane. Arachidonic acid becomes the substrate for the enzymes cycloxygenase and lipoxygenase, triggering production of prostaglandins, thromboxanes, leukotrienes, and endoperoxides.[2,14,24,25] All these mediators may contribute to neuronal damage through vasoconstriction, by recruitment of platelets and neutrophils after reperfusion, or by other mechanisms as yet undefined.

Endoperoxides also are known to increase the production of toxic oxygen-free radicals. Another source of toxic oxygen-free radicals is the enzyme xanthine oxidase. Under ischemic conditions adenine nucleotides are metabolized to nucleosides and purine bases (adenine and hypoxanthine). When these two compounds are degraded further to xanthine and uric acid by the action of xanthine oxidase in the presence of oxygen during reperfusion, the release of superoxide radical follows. Normally the enzyme xanthine oxidase is in low concentration within the brain. However, during anoxia and in the presence of elevated calcium levels within the cytosol, the enzyme xanthine dehydrogenase undergoes a conformational change to xanthine oxidase. During reperfusion, when oxygen again is presented to the tissues, the production of toxic oxygen-free radicals ensues.[2]

In looking at the circulatory status of the brain as a whole, numerous investigators have described and reproduced the phenomenon of postischemic cerebral hypoperfusion. With reperfusion following global cerebral anoxia, there is a period of transient vasodilation during which blood flow to the brain is as much as two times the baseline level before the anoxic injury. This phase of hyperemia usually lasts 20 to 30 minutes. What follows then is a prolonged period of oligemia with markedly reduced blood flow.[25] In its extreme form this pathophysiological event is referred to as the *no reflow phenomenon.*[1] In these circumstances one can often demonstrate the absence of cerebral blood flow by contrast angiography or radionuclide flow scan and the patient almost always is clinically brain dead.

In recent years research in cerebral resuscitation has focused on ameliorating reperfusion injury by using one or more compounds designed to block some of the pathways in the pathophysiological sequence of events as we understand them.[14,24,25] Drugs such as corticosteroids, barbiturates, and calcium channel blockers show efficacy in certain animal models but have not proved effective in treating humans who have hypoxic brain injury. Presently the use of drugs to block the action of xanthine oxidase (allopurinol),[12] blockers of cyclooxygenase or lypoxygenase and free radical scavengers is being investigated. Although these approaches have been successful in specific animal models, their ability to treat reperfusion injury in humans, when administered sometime after reperfusion has occurred, is questionable.

INITIAL STABILIZATION AT THE SCENE

The factor most crucial to survival after near-drowning is the prompt restoration of ventilation and circulation. In addition to the effects of submersion, the rescuer also must keep in mind that any preexisting condition that can lead to cardiac arrest on land can also do so in the water. All victims of diving-related or unwitnessed submersions must be considered to have suffered a head or cervical spine injury as the cause of their failure to resurface. Beyond these considerations the initial efforts at rescue should follow the procedures of pediatric basic life support, the approach based on the "ABCs" of *airway, breathing,* and *circulation* (see Appendix A). Abdominal thrust (Heimlich maneuver) should not be used routinely in submersion victims because of the risk of vomiting and pulmonary aspiration of gastric contents.[23] Oxygen should be administered to all spontaneously breathing patients regardless of their level of consciousness. Thereafter, immediate transport to the nearest medical facility is crucial.

TREATMENT IN THE HOSPITAL

The management of the nearly drowned child in the hospital must be tailored to the patient's clinical condition. Condition on presentation can vary from the child who, by history, had a serious submersion but who looks essentially well, to the child who presents in cardiorespiratory arrest. One can define reasonably the minimal criteria for a significant submersion to be the presence of cyanosis or the requirement of any form of assisted breathing before spontaneous respirations.

Children who have suffered a significant submersion should be monitored for some time, regardless of how well they look in the emergency department, because lung injury may not be apparent immediately. Numerous reports have demonstrated that the initial chest radiograph may be normal in children who later develop the "secondary drowning" syndrome. Arterial blood gases may be abnormal, even in the presence of a normal chest radiograph, and appear to be a more sensitive indicator of early pulmonary injury. Most would recommend an observation period of 12 to 24 hours for these children, with documentation of a normal respiratory rate and oxygen saturation in room air before discharge.[16]

Guidelines for managing childhood victims of near-drowning who present more severely ill are given below, according to an organ systems approach. This discussion presupposes that basic cardiopulmonary resuscitation has been successful and that spontaneous circulation has been restored, although the child may not be breathing spontaneously.

Central Nervous System

Unfortunately, there are no specific cerebral resuscitation therapies to date that have been shown to be effective in the treatment of hypoxic encephalopathy. Intracranial pressure (ICP) monitoring was practiced widely in the early to mid-1980s in the treatment of comatose children following near-drowning episodes.[9] It was learned that ICP usually is not elevated within the first 72 hours, even in the most severely brain-injured children. Its elevation beyond the 72 hours has been shown to be a marker of the most severe cortical injuries; specific treatment of the increased ICP had no effect on outcome.[22] At present, routine ICP monitoring cannot be recommended in comatose children following near-drowning because it has no therapeutic value for the child and because there are numerous other prognosticators that are noninvasive.

Similarly, we have learned that corticosteroids, barbiturates, and hypothermia have not improved the neurological outcome after near-drowning.[4,20] On the contrary, high-dose barbiturates probably increase the likelihood of cardiopulmonary death, whereas hypothermia actually increases the risk of septicemia.[4] Similarly, the routine use of hyperventilation is of no benefit in the treatment of hypoxic encephalopathy. Because intracranial pressure generally is not elevated in the first 72 hours and cerebral blood flow already is reduced, hyperventilation probably does little more than decrease cardiac output.[22]

The most important therapy for the treatment of hypoxic encephalopathy is an approach that seeks to minimize the possibility of additional neuronal injury following the hypoxic event. The goal therefore is to achieve adequate arterial oxygenation and a systemic blood pressure that is at least within the normal range, if not slightly elevated. Seizures should be treated as they would be with any other neurological condition. Hyperthermia should be treated when it occurs to minimize the metabolic demands placed on the brain and the other organs.

Pulmonary Injury

All children who are breathing spontaneously after a near-drowning initially should receive supplemental oxygen. A common situation facing the clinician in the emergency room is that of a child who required some resuscitation at the scene, usually poolside, and who is now lethargic but is making good respiratory efforts. If his or her oxygen saturation by pulse oximeter is in the high 90s while receiving supplemental oxygen, the child does not need to be intubated immediately. The initial blood gas often will show a mixed metabolic and respiratory acidosis. This also is not an indication for immediate intubation because most of these children will continue to improve. So long as oxygenation and mental status do not deteriorate, the child should continue to be given supplemental oxygen and observed closely because subsequent blood gas levels usually will improve. If one does choose to manage such a patient without intubation, the appropriate setting is the pediatric intensive care unit, where intervention can be undertaken immediately should pulmonary injury worsen. Children in this condition usually are not hypotensive and therefore should not require aggressive fluid infusions. Conversely, if at all possible, the early institution of diuretic therapy will improve their pulmonary condition.

The child who has more severe pulmonary injury is treated as one would treat any other child who has diffuse pulmonary injury and hypoxemic respiratory failure (acute lung injury, ARDS). The same strategies for enhancing oxygenation should be used that are applied to other forms of acute lung injury in children.[21]

The pathophysiology of lung injury caused by near-drowning includes the possibility of significant pulmonary capillary injury. In this situation crystalloid or colloid infusions to increase intravascular volume invariably will increase pulmonary capillary pressure and thus increase the rate of pulmonary edema formation.[27] Early attempts at diuresis should be considered. The pulmonary injury in near-drowning, however, is rarely the determinant of overall morbidity and mortality. It is the rare child who has a good neurological prognosis but dies of the pulmonary injury caused by near-drowning.

Cardiovascular Injury

Some degree of circulatory impairment will be present in the victims of a near-drowning episode affected most seriously. The same pathophysiological events that occur during anoxia and reperfusion in the brain also will occur within the myocardium and may lead to impaired ventricular function after resuscitation. There is no particular reason to believe that children suffer who near-drowning are hypovolemic intravascularly, but invasive monitoring of children following global anoxic injury has demonstrated a vasoconstricted state.[15] Hence it is appropriate that the initial intervention in the hypotensive child be a bolus administration of 20 ml/kg of isotonic crystalloid or colloid solution. If the hemodynamic response to the initial fluid bolus is not impressive, one then should consider the use of inotropic support early in the course, particularly if there is evidence of pulmonary injury. The response to moderate doses of dobutamine is often so impressive that diuresis can be accomplished early. Any child requiring mechanical ventilation for significant cardiopulmonary derangements following a near-drowning should have a multilumen central venous catheter placed. Focus on this procedure, however, should not distract the clinician from attention to the initial priorities of stabilization. The purpose of the catheter is to provide multiple stable sites of vascular access so that vasoactive drug infusion and other therapies may proceed uninterrupted. Central venous pressure monitoring is not itself particularly useful because it does not necessarily reflect events of the left heart and because there is no single optimal range for central venous pressure in the treatment of hypoxemic respiratory failure.

A small subset of nearly drowned children will develop progressive cardiovascular instability with hypotensive shock and metabolic acidosis. This almost invariably occurs in those children who have the most profound global anoxic brain injuries. These events often are heralded by the development of hyperthermia and neutropenia, which may signify the onset of systemic bacterial sepsis.[4] Additional cardiovascular support with fluids, dopamine, or epinephrine may be undertaken, but the prognosis is grim.

Another cardiovascular phenomenon, occasionally displayed in the pediatric patient who has a profound cerebral anoxic injury, is the development within the first 48 hours of marked hypertension and tachycardia. Infants may have blood pressures as high as 180/130 with heart rates greater than 260/min. The rhythm almost invariably is sinus, and the cause is believed to be the unchecked sympathetic outflow from the brainstem cardiovascular center. The phenomenon generally lasts a matter of hours, can be treated with short-acting beta blockers, resolves spontaneously, and almost always indicates a profound neurological injury.

Infection

The infectious complications of near-drowning episodes range from bronchopneumonia to aspiration pneumonia to septicemia. The child who has fever and pulmonary infiltrates should receive antibiotics. Intubated children following near-drownings may develop fever with purulent tracheal secretions. Under these circumstances, regardless of whether there are well-defined parenchymal infiltrates, antibiotic coverage is warranted. The offending organisms include airway flora, gram negative rods, and occasionally *Staphylococcus aureus*. In the children most severely asphyxiated, the scenario of high fever and progressive neutropenia develops. These findings may or may not initially be associated with cardiovascular instability, but often herald the onset of systemic bacterial sepsis. It is not clear whether the neutropenia is entirely caused by the severe global anoxia with migration of neutrophils to anoxic tissue during reperfusion or whether the bacterial invasion produces the neutropenia. These patients may develop a rapidly fulminant cardiopulmonary deterioration. The infecting organisms are the same as those listed above for tracheobronchial infection. The use of induced hypothermia appears to increase the risk of neutropenia with sepsis in nearly drowned children.[4] Anoxic injury seems to diminish in some way the normal barriers to systemic infection, and induced hypothermia only increases the risk.

PROGNOSIS

Numerous attempts have been made to predict outcome after near-drowning. Certain aspects of the history and initial physical examination have been shown to have reasonably good predictive value for outcome. If the child arrives awake or blunted (confused, combative, responsive to voice or pain), chances for a good outcome are quite high. In one study all children who had a Glasgow Coma Scale score greater than 5 had a normal or near-normal outcome.[10] For children who arrive comatose with a Glasgow Coma Scale of 3 or 4, the outcome is mixed. In such patients the presence of spontaneous respirations in the emergency department indicates the potential for a good outcome, whereas the presence of flaccidity with apnea after resuscitation suggests a very poor neurological outcome.[13]

The neurological outcome of children suffering a near-drowning is related to the severity of brain anoxia occurring at the time of submersion. The prognostic information helps the clinician to prepare the parents for the likely outcome because most parents desire some estimate of prognosis at the time of admission.

A child who drowns in cold water may represent an exception to outcome predictions. Cold water (water temperature less than 20° C) rapidly cools the victim, decreasing metabolic rate. Children may cool more rapidly than adults because of a greater relative body surface area. Loss of vasomotor tone occurs in water less than 12° C, further increasing the rate of cooling. The "diving reflex" also may be more prominent in children. This reflex slows heart rate and produces profound redistribution of blood flow so that the heart and brain receive preferential circulation at the expense of the skin, muscle, and gut. Thus rapid cooling with hypothermia and the diving reflex may act to preserve brain function, particularly in small children immersed in very cold water.[16] Intact survival has been reported with up to 40 minutes of submersion in icy water. A recent review of 55 pediatric near-drowning victims examined the variables of core temperature and presence or absence of vital signs upon arrival at an emergency department.[3] All patients who arrived with a detectable pulse, regardless of temperature, survived without neurological sequelae. All patients who had absent vital signs and a temperature greater than 33° C either died or survived in a persistent vegetative state. For the patients who arrived with absent vital signs and hypothermia (temperature less than 33° C), the outcome was mixed. Four of fourteen such patients had intact survival; all four had been submerged under ice or in very cold water. Thus it appears that pediatric near-drowning victims, who present in cardiac arrest but who are profoundly hypothermic, may warrant cardiopulmonary resuscitation throughout the warming phase, provided their hypothermia was secondary to submersion in very cold water. Conversely, presentation of one who is in cardiorespiratory arrest and who has not been rapidly cooled in very cold water at the time of submersion is strongly predictive of poor neurological outcome.

ORGAN DONATION

Organs have varying tolerances to hypoxic injury. It is possible for a pediatric victim of near-drowning who has satisfied criteria for brain death to become a donor for kidneys, heart, liver, corneas, and other tissues. The suitability for organ donation should be explored in every child who meets brain death criteria because the criteria for organ donation continue to be liberalized. When organ donation is possible, the parents or legal guardians should be approached to determine their willingness to make such a gift, once brain death is diagnosed. The making of such a gift can be a comfort to parents in their remembrance of an otherwise terrible sequence of events.

PREVENTION

As a form of accidental injury, drowning and near-drowning ultimately are preventable. Statements from the American Academy of Pediatrics and the Centers for Disease Control have addressed approaches to drowning prevention.[7,8] On the local level it is up to pediatricians, as child safety advocates, both by educating the public and by lobbying public officials, to help to prevent accidental death or disability from submersion injuries in children.

REFERENCES

1. Ames A et al: Cerebral ischemia. II. The no-reflow-phenomenon, *Am J Pathol* 52:437, 1968.
2. Babbs CF: Reperfusion injury of postischemic tissues, *Ann Emerg Med* 17:1148, 1988.
3. Biggart M, Bohn D: Effect of hypothermia and cardiac arrest on outcome of near-drowning accidents in children, *J Pediatr* 117:179, 1990.
4. Bohn D et al: Influence of hypothermia, barbiturate therapy, and intracranial pressure monitoring on morbidity and mortality after near-drowning, *Crit Care Med* 14:529, 1986.
5. Centers for Disease Control: Fatal injuries to children—United States, 1986, *MMWR* 39:442, 1990.
6. Centers for Disease Control: Mortality trends and leading causes of death among adolescents and young adults—United States, 1979-1988, *MMWR* 42:459, 1993.
7. Centers for Disease Control: Setting the national agenda for injury control in the 1990s: home and leisure injury prevention, *MMWR* 41:9, 1992.
8. Committee on Injury and Poison Prevention: Drowning in infants, children and adolescents, American Academy of Pediatrics Committee on Injury and Poison Prevention, *Pediatrics* 92:292, 1993.
9. Conn AW et al: Cerebral salvage in near-drowning following neurological classification by triage, *Can Anaesth Soc J* 27:201, 1980.
10. Dean JM, Kaufman ND: Prognostic indicators in pediatric near-drowning: the Glasgow Coma Scale, *Crit Care Med* 9:536, 1981.
11. Giammona ST, Modell JH: Drowning by total immersion: effects on pulmonary surfactant of distilled water, isotonic saline and sea water, *Am J Dis Child* 114:612, 1967.
12. Itoh T et al: Effect of allopurinol on ischemia and reperfusion-induced cerebral injury in spontaneously hypertensive rats, *Stroke* 17:1284, 1986.
13. Jacobsen W et al: Correlation of spontaneous respiration and neurologic damage in near-drowning, *Crit Care Med* 11:487, 1983.
14. Kirsch JR et al: Current concepts in brain resuscitation, *Arch Intern Med* 146:1413, 1986.
15. Lucking SE, Pollack MM, Fields AI: Shock following generalized hypoxic-ischemic injury in previously healthy infants and children, *J Pediatr* 108:359, 1986.
16. Martin TG: Near-drowning and cold water immersion, *Ann Emerg Med* 13:263, 1984.
17. Modell J: Drowning, *Curr Concepts* 328:253, 1993.
18. Modell JH, Davis JH: Electrolyte changes in human drowning victims, *Anaesthesia* 30:414, 1969.
19. Modell JH, Moya F: Effects of volume of aspirated fluid during chlorinated fresh water drowning, *Anaesthesia* 27:662, 1966.
20. Nussbaum E, Maggi C: Pentobarbital therapy does not improve neurologic outcome in nearly drowned, flaccid-comatose children, *Pediatrics* 81:630, 1988.
21. Royall J, Levin D: Adult respiratory distress syndrome in pediatric patients, *J Pediatr* 112:169, 1988.
22. Sarnaik A et al: Intracranial pressure and cerebral perfusion pressure in near-drowning, *Crit Care Med* 13:224, 1985.
23. Standards and guidelines for cardiopulmonary resuscitation (CPR) and emergency cardiac care (ECC), *JAMA* 255:2905, 1986.
24. Vannucci RC: Experimental biology of cerebral hypoxia-ischemia: relation to perinatal brain damage, *Pediatr Res* 27:317, 1990.
25. White BC et al: Possible role of calcium blockers in cerebral resuscitation: a review of the literature and synthesis for future studies, *Crit Care Med* 11:202, 1983.
26. Wintemute GJ: Childhood drowning and near-drowning in the United States, *Am J Dis Child* 144:663, 1990.
27. Wood L, Prewitt R: Cardiovascular management in acute hypoxemic respiratory failure, *Am J Cardiol* 47:963, 1981.

278 Drug Overdose

Cheston M. Berlin, Jr.

Drug overdose, whether from accidental ingestion, a therapeutic misadventure, or a suicide attempt, is a major problem in pediatric practice. In 1992 1,864,188 case reports of exposure to potentially toxic substances were tabulated by the American Association of Poison Control Centers (AAPCC) National Data Collection System.[4] The participating Poison Control Centers serve a population of 196.7 million; thus the data reported involve approximately 78% of the U.S. population. Children under 6 years of age accounted for 58.6% of case reports; 44.3% occurred in children 2 years of age or younger. Including all reports of children age 12 years or younger, 1.2 million children are exposed yearly to drugs that are potentially able to cause toxicity. These 12 million exposures resulted in 34 deaths, but 15% of total exposures resulted in clinical symptoms.

DEFINITION

Drug overdose or toxicity occurs when a child accidentally ingests or is given (therapeutically or intentionally) an amount of a compound that exceeds the recommended dosage or that causes an idiosyncratic reaction within the recommended dosage.

EPIDEMIOLOGY AND ETIOLOGY

The epidemiology of drug overdose is related to the patient's age, as shown in Table 278-1, which lists the number of exposures and deaths from drugs and other compounds according to patient age. The bimodal frequency of deaths peaks at 5 years or below and again at 15 to 19 years. The former reflects accidental ingestions, the latter, usually suicidal events. For some compounds, aspirin being the prime example, therapeutic misadventure may play a significant role. As Gaudreault et al.[2] have pointed out, most serious salicylate poisonings occur as a result of the therapeutic administration of aspirin. Young children who are febrile or dehydrated are not able to handle antipyretic doses of salicylate effectively. The incidence of therapeutic salicylate poisoning has dropped markedly in recent years because salicylates often are not used in pediatric patients as a result of the concern regarding the relationship between salicylates and Reye syndrome. Preventive measures, such as child-resistant bottle tops, are effective in eliminating acute, single-dose accidental exposures. Iron poisoning is the leading cause of death in children under 6 years of age. Other substances causing deaths are pesticides, antidepressants, hydrocarbons, and alcohols. Chapter 289, Poisoning, provides detailed information on the management of the most common drug ingestions that occur in pediatric practice.

IMMEDIATE ASSESSMENT

An optimum therapeutic response will be achieved if the following steps are taken immediately on encountering the overdosed patient. Detain the person(s) who brought the child to the hospital or office. If initial contact is by telephone, obtain the caller's name and telephone number and then instruct the caller to proceed immediately with the child to the hospital. Be sure to obtain the precise description of the drug thought to have been ingested: name, dose, pharmacy of origin, and prescription number. Instruct the parents to bring the actual container when they come with the patient. Try to determine the amount of drug ingested. This frequently is impossible, and such information, even if obtained, occasionally is misleading. *Assume maximal exposure unless a precise tablet or liquid count is available.*

Initial Procedures for Stabilization and Life Support

Measure the vital signs—temperature, pulse, respirations, blood pressure, pulse oximetry, and continuous electrocardiography. Monitor the sensorium frequently—that is, every 15 minutes for 2 hours until the patient's condition is stable. Changes in frequency and duration of monitoring will depend on the drug, dose, and clinical course.

Assess the adequacy of the airway. Most drug overdoses will not affect the upper airway (larynx, trachea) but will interfere with air exchange by either depressing the central nervous system or paralyzing neuromuscular transmission. Establish an intravenous line. If danger of respiratory depression or ingestion of drugs that alter cardiovascular status exists, consider placing an arterial line. Cleanse the skin if appropriate. Some compounds, such as insecticides, have significant dermal absorption, especially if the skin is inflamed or abraded. If the patient is alert, induce emesis—except in cases of lye, acid, and hydrocarbon ingestion. Save the vomitus for drug analysis.

DIFFERENTIAL DIAGNOSIS

Considerations of other conditions that can mimic the signs and symptoms of drug overdose will depend on the drug ingested. For patients who have alterations in sensorium, head trauma is of prime consideration. Adolescents who have head trauma may have ingested ethanol. Near-drowning victims also may have ingested ethanol. Spontaneous intracranial hemorrhages in the pediatric age group are rare; they usually produce focal neurological signs rather than global depression of consciousness.

Metabolic conditions such as diabetes mellitus, hypoglycemia, and Addisonian crisis may cause clinical states that resemble drug ingestion. Awareness of these possibilities will help narrow down the diagnostic considerations.

Table 278-1 Substances Causing Toxic Exposure (by Patient Age)

Substance	Age (yr)	
	<6	6-17
Pharmaceutical agents	454,689	92,947
Nonpharmaceutical agents (chemicals, plants, gases)	657,044	111,978

	<6 yrs	6-12 yrs	13-19 yrs
Deaths	29	5	58

Data modified from Litovitz TL et al: *Am J Emerg Med* 11:494, 1993.

The most thorny area of all is presented by the patient who has a psychiatric illness, who may develop tremors, hallucinations, or hysterical paralysis. In these patients precise and rapid laboratory analyses are most important in ruling out drug ingestion. If the patient has been receiving psychoactive medications and is having an untoward reaction, management is identical to that discussed in the management section, with special attention directed to the emotional needs of the patient, especially in the recovery phase.

MANAGEMENT

The two factors to consider in deciding location and personnel for management of the patient are (1) expertise of the physician in the management of drug overdose and (2) available hospital support facilities. The latter is of most concern because even the best-trained physician cannot provide care properly in an institution that is inadequately equipped with support staff, equipment, and laboratory facilities. The well-trained pediatrician will not always be able to predict the clinical course of a patient who has "overdosed." Will the patient require charcoal perfusion, renal or peritoneal dialysis, or an exchange transfusion? Is the hospital able to offer pediatric intensive care unit monitoring? Can the hospital provide prolonged ventilation and airway management? Can the nursing staff monitor intracranial and/or intraarterial pressure properly? It is best to decide very early in the clinical course whether special facilities will be needed. It is preferable to transfer a stable patient early than a critically ill child requiring mobile life support later. It is important to maintain frequent and smooth communication with the patient's family. Regardless of the cause of their child's poisoning, these families are in constant need of counseling—especially with regard to any guilt feelings they may be experiencing.

Need for General Homeostatic Support

Thermal monitoring is an important aspect of management in drug overdose. Centrally and peripherally induced hypothermia is a common problem—for example, the hypothermia that occurs with phenothiazine ingestion. Hyperthermia can occur with salicylate and atropine poisoning.

Monitoring fluid balance and electrolyte homeostasis is important. Deficits must be replaced, and the amount of maintenance fluids needed will depend on changes in the vital and physical signs. For example, hyperventilation and increased body temperature require increases beyond normal in the amount of maintenance fluids administered. Continuing losses through vomiting and diarrhea should be replaced as they occur.

Monitoring central venous pressure and arterial pressure to assess vascular volume and tone is important. Evaluate respiratory function with pulse oximetry. Check for an elevation in intracranial pressure to assess the need for treatment of cerebral edema. Consider the need for peritoneal dialysis, hemodialysis, charcoal perfusion, or exchange transfusion to remove the ingested drug.

Nutritional considerations frequently are neglected in patients who require prolonged intensive care. Feeding via a nasogastric tube or with parenteral alimentation should be considered, especially if coma will exceed 3 days.

Diagnostic Procedures

Assays of blood, urine, and gastric contents for barbiturates, antidepressants, phenytoin, iron, digoxin, salicylate, acetaminophen, narcotics, alcohols, cocaine, and propoxyphene must be available. Rapid drug screens should be available; quantitative analyses should follow as quickly as possible.

A flat plate of the abdomen may be required to identify radiopaque tablets (e.g., iron) or foreign bodies. A computed tomography scan of the head should be performed if intracranial hemorrhage is suspected following amphetamine or cocaine ingestion. A chest roentgenogram is needed if narcotic-induced pulmonary edema or aspiration is suspected.

It is important to remember that trauma may have occurred in any poisoned patient, especially the adolescent. One half of adolescent drownings are associated with alcohol use. Because near-drownings often follow diving in which the head and neck may be injured, immobilization of the cervical spine should be accomplished immediately on site.

Definitive Therapy

Specific antidotes exist for some drugs but unfortunately not for most. Thus definitive therapy consists of intensive supportive care and treatment of signs and symptoms as they develop (e.g., hypotension and hypertension, thermal instability, cardiac arrhythmias). The following steps should be taken in treating drug overdosage:

1. Stabilize the patient.
2. Identify the drug ingested and determine the amount ingested.
3. Contact the local poison control center for toxicology data and information regarding the signs and symptoms and clinical course. The "Poisindex" is an excellent comprehensive reference, and the pocket manual by Dreisbach[1] provides essential information that is easy to find.
4. Induce emesis or perform gastric lavage if not contraindicated. Recent work suggests that gastric emptying in the alert patient is not helpful.[3] These authors emphasize the use of activated charcoal and a cathartic.
5. If a specific antidote exists, administer it. It is most helpful to have a table prepared of specific antidotes and their location in the hospital (Table 278-2); the best location is the emergency department. All staff members must know the precise location.
6. Give activated charcoal (1 or 2 g/kg) as a slurry with magnesium sulfate (250 mg/kg).[4] Only a very small number of compounds appear not to be adsorbed to the

Table 278-2 Common Antidotes

Drug	Diagnostic findings requiring treatment	Antidote	Dosage
Acetaminophen	History of ingestion and toxic serum level	N-acetylcysteine	140 mg/kg/dose PO, then 70 mg/kg/dose q 4 hr PO × 17
Anticholinergics Antihistamines Atropine Phenothiazines Tricyclic antidepressants	Supraventricular tachycardia (hemodynamic compromise) Unresponsive ventricular dysrhythmia, seizures, pronounced hallucinations or agitation	Physotigmine	Child: 0.5 mg IV slowly (over 3 min) q 10 min prn (maximum: 2 mg) Adult: 1-2 mg IV slowly q 10 min prn (maximum: 4 mg in 30 min)
Cholinergics	Cholinergic crisis: salivation, lacrimation, urination, defecation, convulsions, fasciculations	Atropine sulfate Physostigmine Insecticides	0.05 mg/kg/dose (usual dose 1-5 mg; test dose for child 0.01 mg/kg) q 4-6 hr IV or more frequently prn
Carbon monoxide	Headache, seizure, coma, dysrhythmias	Oxygen, hyperbaric oxygen	100% oxygen (half-life 40 min); consider hyperbaric chamber
Cyanide	Cyanosis, seizures, cardiopulmonary arrest, coma	Amyl nitrite	Inhale pearl q 60-120 sec
		Sodium nitrite (3%)	0.27 mL (8.7 mg)/kg (adult: 10 ml [300 mg]) IV slowly (Hb ≥10 g/dl)
		Sodium thiosulfate (25%) Also consider hyperbaric oxygen	1.35 mL (325 mg)/kg (adult: 12.5 g) IV slowly (Hb ≥10 g/dl)
Ethylene glycol	Metabolic acidosis, urine Ca^{++} oxalate crystals	Ethanol (100% absolute, 1 ml-790 mg)	1 ml/kg in D5W IV over 15 min, then 0.16 ml (125 mg)/kg/hr IV; maintain ethanol level of 100 mg/dl
Iron	Hypotension, shock, coma, serum iron >350 mg/dl (or greater than iron-binding capacity)	Deferoxamine	Shock or coma: 15 mg/kg/hr IV for 8 hr; if no shock or coma 90 mg/kg/dose IM q 8 hr
Phenothiazines Chlorpromazine Thioridazine	Extrapyramidal dyskinesia, oculogyric crisis	Diphenhydramine (Benadryl)	1-2 mg/kg/dose (maximum: 50 mg/dose) q 6 hr IV, PO
Methanol	Metabolic acidosis, blurred vision; level >20 mg/dl	Ethanol (100% absolute)	1 ml/kg in D5W over 15 min, then 0.16 ml (125 mg)/kg/hr IV
Methemoglobin Nitrate Nitrites Sulfonamide	Cyanosis, methemoglobin level >30%, dyspnea	Methylene blue (1% solution)	1-2 mg (0.1-0.2 ml)/kg/dose IV; repeat in 4 hr if necessary
Narcotics Heroin Codeine Propoxyphene	Respiratory depression, hypotension, coma	Naloxone (Narcan)	0.1 mg/kg up to 0.8 mg initially IV, if no response give 2 mg IV
Organophosphates Malathion Parathion	Cholinergic crisis: salivation, lacrimation, urination, defecation, convulsions, fasciculations	Atropine sulfate	0.05 mg/kg/dose (usual dose 1-5 mg; test dose for child 0.01 mg/kg) q 4-6 hr IV or more frequently prn
		Pralidoxime	After atropine, 20-50 mg/kg/dose (maximum: 2000 mg) IV slowly (<50 mg/min) q 8 hr IV prn × 3

From Barkin RM: *Pediatr Ann* 19:632, 1990.

charcoal (acids, alkali, cyanide, DDT, iron salts, N-methyl carbonate, tolbutamide). Repeated doses of charcoal-magnesium sulfate (every 2 to 4 hours) may be very useful in accelerating clearance of many compounds; this technique is referred to as *gastrointestinal dialysis*.[5] Contraindications to repeated use of oral charcoal include intestinal obstruction, perforation, or poor gastrointestinal motility.

7. Provide supportive care in an intensive or intermediate care unit as appropriate.

8. Meet social service needs as indicated (e.g., drug ingestion by a toddler as a symptom of chaotic family structure or by an adolescent as a symptom of depression or as a suicidal gesture or act).
9. Provide counseling concerning the institution of poison control measures in the home.

Complications

Possible complications of drug overdose are many and varied. Therapy itself can have side effects, such as too rigorous treatment of seizures causing apnea and the need for mechanical ventilation. Many poisoned patients require respirator therapy. Such therapy, especially if prolonged, may lead to complications such as pneumothorax, oxygen toxicity, and airway infections. Nosocomial infections are not uncommon—especially hypostatic pneumonia, urinary tract infection (secondary to catheter placement), or septicemia from vascular catheters. Thrombotic and embolic episodes also can result from vascular catheters.

Permanent central nervous system damage sometimes follows periods of hypoxia or hypoglycemia—usually before therapy is instituted. Topical skin, mucous membrane, and deeper tissue injuries often result from acids, lyes, or corrosives. Specific compounds can cause permanent organ damage (e.g., to the lungs from hydrocarbons, the kidneys from ethylene glycol, the liver from acetaminophen, and the retina from methanol).

Hazards of treatment for drug overdosage include overtreatment, the wrong treatment, an insufficient period of observation, and failure to appreciate drug ingestion as an indication of child neglect or abuse. Especially suspect is the child under age 12 months who is admitted with "accidental ingestion" or the child who has a history of repeated drug ingestions. Overtreatment occurs when errors are made in assessing the amount of drug ingested. A nontoxic ingestion may be vigorously but inappropriately treated with potentially toxic antidotes—for example, using sodium nitrate-sodium thiosulfate for the treatment of cyanide ingestion.

The wrong treatment can occur when a mistake is made in identifying the drug ingested—for example, from a mislabeled prescription vial. An insufficient period of observation can worsen the situation. For example, hepatic necrosis may not occur until day 3 after acetaminophen ingestion, and renal disease may not occur until day 7 to 10.

REFERENCES

1. Dreisbach RH: *Poisoning,* ed 12, Los Altos, Calif, 1987, Lange Medical Publications.
2. Gaudreault P, Temple AR, Lovejoy FH Jr: The relative severity of acute versus chronic salicylate poisoning in children: a clinical comparison, *Pediatrics* 70:566, 1982.
3. Kulig K et al: Management of acutely poisoned patients without gastric emptying, *Ann Emerg Med* 14:562, 1985.
4. Litovitz TL et al: 1992 Annual report of the American Association of Poison Control Centers toxic exposure surveillance system, *Am J Emerg Med* 11:494, 1993.
5. Mofenson HC et al: Gastrointestinal dialysis with activated charcoal and cathartic in the treatment of adolescent intoxications, *Clin Pediatr* 24:678, 1985.

279 Envenomations

Donald Londorf and Sharon Genevieve Humiston

An *envenomation* is the combination of poisonous effects caused by the bite or sting of venomous creatures such as snakes, scorpions, spiders, and insects of the order Hymenoptera (e.g., ants, wasps, bees). Although not uncommon, venomous bites and stings are usually minor in the United States. In 1991 the 73 members of the American Association of Poison Control Centers received a total of 76,941 bite- or sting-related calls. The patient was 17 years of age or younger in 43% of these cases: the vector was a snake in 6.1%, a scorpion in 5.3%, a spider in 20.8%, and a bee, wasp, hornet, or ant in 38.5%. There were no symptoms or only minor ones in more than 90% of the cases for which a final outcome was reported.[30] The clinician must be aware of the venomous species in the area and be prepared to treat envenomations.

HYMENOPTERA

In the United States four families of Hymenoptera are responsible for most insect sting reactions: Apidae (honeybees), Bombidae (bumblebees), Vespoidae (paper wasps, white-faced hornets, yellow hornets, and yellowjackets), and Formicidae (harvester ants and native and imported fire ants).[54] All of these possess venom sacs and stingers that are similar in design.

Bees, wasps, and hornets accounted for 23,224 exposures reported in 1991 to the American Association of Poison Control Centers National Data Collection System. Of these, 11,190 (48%) were in children 17 years of age and younger. Ants and fire ants accounted for 2687 exposures; 1516 (56%) of these were in children less than 17 years of age.[30] These numbers underestimate the problem because most stings are minor in severity and thus are not reported to a poison control center and also because many southern states were not represented fully in this annual report.

Hymenoptera stings can cause local nonallergic and allergic reactions, as well as systemic allergic reactions. Anaphylactic reactions are uncommon. Their prevalence in the general population ranges from 0.15% to 3.9%.[11] Large local cutaneous reactions to stings occur in approximately 2.3% to 18.6% of the general population.[23,35]

Winged Hymenoptera

Characteristics and Distribution. Winged Hymenoptera are found in most areas of the United States. Honeybees usually nest in hollow trees and crevices, whereas bumblebees prefer nesting underground. Wasp nests often can be found under roofs and eaves, hornets prefer to nest in branches and trees, and yellowjackets tend to build their nests in the ground.

Honeybees differ from other Hymenoptera in that they possess a barbed stinger that anchors into the skin. Because of this, bees die from evisceration after they sting. Wasps also have barbed stingers, but they usually are able to withdraw them from the skin and can sting multiple times.[54]

Hymenoptera venoms contain many protein components that account for the various observed reactions. Phospholipase A_2, hyaluronidase, histamine, apam, melittin, mast cell-degranulating peptide, acid phosphatase, norepinephrine, dopamine, and allergen C are the main constituents of honeybee venom. The major vespid allergens are antigen 5 and hyaluronidase, but they also contain histamine, kinins, serotonin, phospholipase A_1 and B, and mastoparans.[54] Cross-reactivity between the apid and vespid venoms is limited, but a significant cross-reactivity exists between the different vespid venoms.[23,29]

The most common areas to be stung are the head, neck, feet, and hands. Stinging is most common during the summer months, and children often are affected.[54] Most patients cannot reliably identify the insect that stung them.

Physical Examination

LOCAL. Types of local reactions to stings are two: nonallergic and allergic. The nonallergic reaction is a direct result of envenomation via mast cell degranulation and the production of a wheal-and-flare response. This produces erythema, swelling, pain, and itching. These symptoms usually subside in a few hours.

Allergic local reactions occur in about 17% of people stung by winged hymenoptera. These consist of erythema and local edema of greater than 10 cm in diameter. These reactions often persist for 48 to 72 hours and may become indurated for a period of up to 5 days.[35,54] Some patients may experience headache, nausea, or malaise with these reactions.

As mentioned previously, a stinger sometimes may be found at the sting site. This usually indicates a honeybee or, in some cases, a yellowjacket sting.

SYSTEMIC. The more common systemic manifestations of an allergic reaction to hymenoptera stings include urticaria, angioedema, wheezing, shortness of breath, stridor, nausea, vomiting, diarrhea, abdominal pain, malaise, dizziness, and anaphylaxis. Dysphagia, dysarthria, hoarseness, weakness, and confusion also have been described. Respiratory and cardiovascular complications are seen in adults more frequently than in children.[35] Fatal anaphylaxis is rare, especially in children.[23]

The risk of developing a systemic reaction appears to be greater with a history of multiple stings or within a few weeks after a previous sting. The risk is higher in patients who have a previous history of anaphylaxis. Their risk of anaphylaxis with subsequent stings is 35% to 60%.[29,35] However, the pattern of reaction is difficult to predict.[23] Atopic patients do not appear to be at greater risk of developing systemic complications, but the severity of their symptoms may be greater than in nonatopic individuals.[35] A history of a large local reaction does not reliably predict progression to systemic complications. The risk of subsequent anaphylaxis after a large local reaction is about 5% to 10%.[23,56]

In rare cases, serum sickness, vasculitis, encephalopathy, neuritis, and renal disease are seen.[32]

Differential Diagnosis. It may be difficult to differentiate between a severe local allergic reaction and cellulitis because the erythema and edema may be very similar in appearance.[56] Other causes of stridor, wheezing, and allergic reaction should be considered if a sting site cannot be identified.

Laboratory Studies. No specific laboratory test is useful in the acute management of hymenoptera stings.

Management. Insect sting sites should be inspected for the presence of a stinger. It is important not to squeeze or grab the free end of the stinger because this may result in further envenomation. It is preferable to use the tip of a 25-gauge needle or the flick of a finger to scrape it off.

Nonallergic local reactions require symptomatic treatment and no further evaluation. Ice may reduce swelling and slow the absorption of venom. Elevation of the affected limb also may decrease the swelling. Local wound cleaning and care usually are all that is required. If local itching is significant, an oral H_1 antihistamine such as diphenhydramine may be useful.

Local allergic reactions require the same kind of wound care as nonallergic reactions. An oral analgesic and an H_1 antagonist may be added for comfort. For very large cutaneous reactions, prednisone (1 mg/kg/day for 3 to 5 days) may be useful. Supportive care is the foundation of the management of systemic reactions, with special attention paid to airway protection and cardiovascular status. Epinephrine is given subcutaneously, intramuscularly, or intravenously depending on the severity of the presentation.* Oxygen, IV fluids, IV diphenhydramine, and steroids should be administered. Children who have severe systemic reactions should be admitted to intensive care for ventilation, pressor support, and monitoring until symptoms improve.

Patients with systemic reactions who respond completely to therapy in the emergency department should be observed for 8 to 12 hours after the sting because of the possibility of a delayed "late-phase" anaphylactic episode. The mechanism of this delayed complication is poorly understood.[29]

At the time of discharge following a systemic reaction, all patients should be given a prescription for a self-administered epinephrine kit. The patient or caretaker should be instructed in the proper use of this kit before discharge from the emergency department. They also should be encouraged to wear a MedicAlert bracelet identifying them as being allergic to insect stings. Patients should be told how to avoid further stings (see the box above).

Children who sustain extracutaneous systemic reactions (other than urticaria) should be referred to an allergist for risk analysis and possible venom immunotherapy.[31,46,54] Immunotherapy with Hymenoptera venom is expensive but it induces complete protection in approximately 80% of subjects allergic to bees and 90% of patients allergic to wasps.

*A 0.01 ml/kg dose of 1 : 1000 aqueous epinephrine solution is injected subcutaneously. The original dose should not exceed 0.3 ml, but it may be repeated in 15 minutes. Alternatively, Sus-phrine (0.005 ml/kg) can be used. It is highly recommended that susceptible individuals carry epinephrine self-administered kits when outdoors. After such a kit is used, medical help should be sought because the drug's duration of action is brief.

HOW TO AVOID INSECT STINGS

- Do not disturb nests or hives—have someone else remove them
- Do not wear perfume, cologne, scented sunscreens, or hairspray when outdoors
- Use footwear when outside
- Avoid picnic areas, garbage sites, orchards, fields of clover, and flowerbeds
- Be extra careful when gardening and cover your hands and body
- Avoid trips outdoors if medical help is not readily available or until maintenance immunotherapy is established
- Do not wear brightly colored clothes or jewelry
- Install screens on windows and doors to prevent insects from entering the home

To ensure long-lasting protection, immunotherapy should be continued for 3 to 5 years. Immediate access to aqueous epinephrine and a thorough understanding of its administration remain important aspects of care for children undergoing immunotherapy until maintenance doses are reached.[31,46] Children who have urticaria are not at an increased risk of having more severe systemic reactions with subsequent stings.[29,35,46]

Skin testing with Hymenoptera venom and a radioallergosorbent test (RAST) are used to assess candidates for immunotherapy. These tests do not distinguish which patient will go on to develop a systemic reaction, and they have no role in the acute management of reactions.

Fire Ants

Characteristics. There are five species of fire ants currently known in the United States: *Solenopsis invicta, Solenopsis richteri, Solenopsis geminata, Solenopsis xyloni,* and *Solenopsis aurea.* The last two species are native to North America and are less aggressive than their imported cousins. The red ant, *Solenopsis invicta,* is native to northern Argentina, Paraguay, and western Brazil; it is the most prevalent of the imported species. *Solenopsis richteri* is black and is native to Argentina and Uruguay. *Solenopsis geminata* appears to have been brought over from the Spanish Carribean Islands.[13]

Fire ants can be red, brown, or black and are approximately 2 to 5 mm long. They live in colonies and build mounds that can measure 10 to 15 inches in height above ground. They are found in meadows, grassy areas, pastures, lawns, and parks. The colonies may extend to 3 to 5 feet below ground and have extensive tunnel systems measuring up to 130 feet in diameter.

Although most of the problems caused by fire ants are related to the imported species, especially *S. invicta* and *S. richteri,* anaphylaxis may occur with any of the mentioned species.[13,44] Imported fire ants (IFA) are aggressive and kill native ants in their area. In infested areas IFA can make up 90% of the ant population.[40] Several authors estimate that between

30% and 60% of the population in infested urban areas is subject to fire ant stings each year.[1,2,13,19,44]

Children are especially vulnerable. Adams and Lofgren[1,2] have noted the highest sting rate (close to 50%) in persons under 20 years of age. Trespassing into the fire ants' territory or disturbing a nest will incite aggressive behavior. However, cases of ants attacking victims indoors are not uncommon.[19,24] Heavy rains appear to increase this occurrence.

Fire ants bite the skin of their victims with their mandibles, then arch their bodies to inject venom through a lancet-shaped stinger located at the distal end of their abdomen. If undisturbed they will continue to sting the victim repeatedly in a circular pattern using their mandibles as a pivot; venom is injected with each sting.[13,20,22,44]

Fire ant venom is mostly composed of alkaloid piperidine compounds and contains very little protein. However, it is this protein moiety that is responsible for the IgE-mediated allergic reactions sometimes encountered with fire ant stings. The alkaloid portion is believed to be responsible for the more common local dermal reactions.[1,13,22,24]

Distribution. *Solenopsis richteri* is found primarily in parts of northwestern Alabama and northeastern Mississippi. *S. invicta* is distributed more widely over the southeastern and south central states—it has been found in Alabama, Arizona, Arkansas, Florida, Georgia, Louisiana, Mississippi, North and South Carolina, Oklahoma, Tennessee, and Texas. Native North American species inhabit similar areas. Imported fire ants also are found in Puerto Rico.

Because imported fire ants have exhibited changes in behavior in their relatively new environment, some authors suggest that these ants ultimately will infest one quarter of the land area of the United States where soil and climactic conditions are favorable, extending along the east coast to Delaware and along the west coast to Washington state.[19,20,44]

Physical Examination: Signs and Symptoms

LOCAL. Stings from imported fire ants frequently occur on children's ankles and feet in the summer. Stings tend to be multiple and cause immediate local burning and itching. Soon after, the area becomes erythematous and raised. This reaction usually subsides after 30 to 60 minutes. The classic finding of small, sterile pustules develops within 24 hours of the sting. Some patients develop a so-called large local reaction, an erythematous, pruritic, warm, indurated area around the sting site. Pustules usually resolve over a period of 3 to 10 days.

Secondary bacterial infections are not uncommon after stings. These are usually minor and localized. However, sepsis may result from superinfected lesions.[19]

SYSTEMIC. Systemic reactions are much less common than cutaneous reactions. Urticaria and angioedema are the most common acute generalized hypersensitivity reactions. Other manifestations include abdominal pain, bronchospasm, laryngeal edema, and hypotension. Hardwick et al.[24] reported a near-fatal envenomation of a neonate who became apneic and asystolic after sustaining over 2000 stings while lying in a playpen in his house. The neonate suffered shock, coma, hemolytic anemia, and coagulopathy. The authors believed these effects were a result of the direct toxicity of the venom.

The incidence of anaphylactic reactions to stings is unknown, but it has been estimated at 0.6% to 1% of stings.[44] Rare neurological complications have been described. These include focal and generalized seizures, loss of consciousness, confusion, blurred vision, drowsiness, wrist drop, and Guillain-Barré syndrome.[20] Death from fire ant stings is rare. In one report, most persons who died were found to have sustained less than five stings.[40]

Laboratory Studies. The diagnosis of fire ant sting is a clinical one; there is no confirmatory test.

Management. Local reactions are treated conservatively with ice and proper wound care. No treatment has been shown to affect the course of the sterile pustules. Topical treatment with antihistamines is not recommended because the patient may become sensitized. A short course of oral steroids or antihistamines has not been shown to make any difference in the clinical course of mild local reactions, but it may be effective for severe local reactions. Anaphylaxis is a life-threatening emergency and is treated with epinephrine, antihistamines, steroids, and supportive care.

Patients who live in fire ant–infested areas and who have had severe hypersensitivity reactions to stings or anaphylaxis should be referred to an allergist for immunotherapy assessment.[21]

Harvester Ants

Harvester ants (genus *Pogonomyrmex*) belong to the Hymenoptera order, subfamily Myrmicinae, which includes the genus *Solenopsis* (fire ants). Over 20 native species inhabit the United States, but only three have been associated with anaphylaxis: *Pogonomyrmex barbatus, P. rugosus,* and *P. maricopa*.[44] Harvester ants occupy a wide geographical area and are found in the southern and western states and in Mexico.

Like fire ants, harvester ants attach to the skin with their mandibles and envenomate their victim through a sting. Their venom differs from fire ant venom in that it contains a much larger fraction of protein constituents; hence it is more like other Hymenoptera venoms.

Unlike imported fire ants, harvester ants do not leave characteristic skin lesions. Their sting resembles that of other insects and may be associated with allergic reactions. Treatment of *Pogonomyrmex* stings is the same as that for fire ants.

ARACHNIDS

Arachnids belong to the phylum Arthropoda, which includes the orders Araneae (spiders) and Scorpionidae (scorpions). Although both of these can inflict envenomations with significant morbidity, fatalities are rare.

Spiders

Most of the 30,000 species of spiders in the world are harmless to humans, but approximately 50 species are of medical importance. In North America *loxosceles* (which includes the brown recluse spider), *latrodectus* (black widow spider), and tarantulas are the species most commonly implicated.

Epidemiology. The true incidence of spider and scorpion bites can only be estimated because of the large number of bites that go unreported. In the 1991 annual report of the American Association of Poison Control Centers National

Data Collection System, 2591 exposures to black widow spiders were reported; 634 (24.5%) of these were in patients less than 17 years of age; 1484 exposures to brown recluse spiders were reported, of which 351 (24%) were in patients less than 17 years of age. Only 66 exposures to tarantulas were reported. No deaths occurred in any of these groups.[30] These numbers clearly are underestimated because several pertinent states were not or not fully represented in this report.

Prevention. Eradicating *loxosceles* and black widow spiders is difficult or impossible. Prevention therefore is focused chiefly on caution in areas inhabited by these spiders.

Spider Venom. Necrotizing venom is produced by many indigenous spiders, including orb weavers, running spiders, jumping spiders, and the commonly implicated brown recluse spider. The latter's venom includes sphingomyelinase D, protease, esterase, and hyaluronidase and is potent enough to kill small animals. Its cytotoxic effects are most pronounced in the destruction of endothelial and red blood cells.[55] It causes liquefaction throughout the dermis and subcutaneous tissue.[48] The extent of the associated destruction may be the result of massive local leukocyte infiltration.

In contrast, black widow spider venom is neurotoxic. It contains proteases and a neurotoxin named alpha-latrotoxin. The latter destabilizes presynaptic receptors, which release neurotransmitters, degenerates motor end plates, and causes cellular calcium influx. The two main peripheral neurotransmitters, acetylcholine and norepinephrine, account for most of the signs and symptoms seen in latrodectism.[4]

Loxosceles

CHARACTERISTICS. The *loxosceles* spiders (including the brown recluse spider) are the most common species implicated in cases of necrotizing skin lesions. They commonly are called *violin* or *fiddleback spiders*. They are hardy and live in dry areas such as wood piles, rodent burrows, vacant buildings, attics, or closets. They are reclusive and nonaggressive, unless disturbed. Their web is irregular and common in appearance.

Loxosceles' body is oval (10 to 15 mm long, 4 mm wide) and light fawn to dark chocolate in color. The leg span is about 25 mm. The most distinguishing feature is the violin-shaped marking on the dorsal aspect of the cephalothorax. The body of this marking is on the cephalothorax, and the neck points toward the abdomen. Another distinguishing feature is the presence of three pairs of eyes instead of the four pairs usually seen in other species.

Bites are usually a result of accidental contact, such as looking through boxes or wood piles, or contact with linens or clothing where the spider has become trapped.

DISTRIBUTION. *Loxosceles* spiders are found throughout the world. Many species are found in the United States, mostly in the south and central areas. Only six of these are known to cause necrotic skin lesions: *Loxosceles reclusa, L. laeta, L. rufescens, L. unicolor, L. arizonica,* and *L. devia.*[3,53]

PHYSICAL EXAMINATION: SIGNS AND SYMPTOMS

Local Manifestations. The bite itself does not cause much discomfort and may go unnoticed. Sometimes a minor stinging or burning sensation may be felt at the site. Erythema, pruritus, pain, and edema typically develop within 2 to 8 hours. These may be followed in the next 24 to 48 hours by the appearance of a blue-gray halo surrounding the erythematous center. Vesicles or bullae containing serous or hemorrhagic fluid soon follow.

Local ischemia and necrosis result in the formation of a black eschar within 7 to 10 days of the bite. This necrotic area may expand slowly in diameter for weeks, especially in fatty areas that have delicate blood supplies such as the abdomen, buttocks, and thighs.[49] The eschar is shed after 2 to 5 weeks and an ulcer remains; the latter may take weeks to months to heal.

Systemic Manifestations. Systemic manifestations of loxoscelism are less common than cutaneous ones. The most common symptoms are fever, chills, and malaise. Symptoms usually occur within 24 hours of the bite and also may include nausea, vomiting, diarrhea, arthralgia, urticaria or maculopapular rash, hemolytic anemia, disseminated intravascular coagulation, jaundice, renal failure, transverse myelitis, seizures, and shock.[3,25]

DIFFERENTIAL DIAGNOSIS. In the absence of a definitive history of spider bites, other diagnostic possibilities must be considered, such as emboli, thrombi, focal vasculitis, envenomation by other insects or reptiles, fat herniation with infarction, pressure sore, pyoderma gangrenosum, poison oak or ivy, cutaneous manifestation of gonorrhea or herpes simplex, diabetic ulcer, purpura fulminans, erythema nodosum, or abusive or self-inflicted trauma.

Other species of spiders have been implicated in the cause of necrotic skin lesions similar to loxosceles. These are *Argiope* (orbweaver spider), *Chiracanthium* (sac spider), *Lycosa* (wolf spider), *Phidippus* (jumping spider), and *Tegenaria agrestis.*[3,50]

LABORATORY STUDIES. No laboratory study can confirm the presence of necrotic arachnidism. Complete blood counts, coagulation profiles, electrolytes, and renal function should be monitored in systemic illness.

MANAGEMENT. Management is controversial because the unpredictable natural course of the wounds makes prospective trials difficult. Serial observations, cleansing, cool compresses, splinting of the affected extremity, and tetanus prophylaxis commonly are recommended wound care measures. Symptomatic relief with antipruritics and analgesics may be useful in some cases.

Different therapies have been proposed, including systemic steroids, antibiotics, antihistamines, dapsone, colchicine, surgical excision, hyperbaric oxygen, and observation. The most suitable therapy in the pediatric population is unclear, but there is general agreement on delaying any surgical repair of skin defects until the necrotic demarcation is discrete and there is no further spread; this takes about 8 weeks.

Black Widow Spider *(Latrodectus)*

CHARACTERISTICS. Although both male and female spiders have venom, only the female has fangs that are powerful enough to bite through skin and envenomate humans. Black widow spiders are among the largest spiders in the world, with a leg span of 40 mm and a body of 1.5 cm. The mature female is black, with a red or orange hourglass-shaped marking on the ventral surface. The immature female may be red, brown, or cream in color, and the hourglass marking may be cream colored or even incomplete.[3]

The web, usually built close to the ground in dimly lit, moist areas, is distinguishable by its irregular pattern. It may be found in barns, outhouses, lumber piles, and sheds where insects are plentiful. Bites usually are a result of the spider being disturbed and acting in self-defense.

DISTRIBUTION. *Latrodectus* spiders are found in both temperate and tropical climates throughout the world. Five species are found in the United States; Alaska is the only state that does not have this genus. The most common spiders implicated in latrodectism are *Latrodectus mactans, L. variolus,* and *L. hesperus.*[12] Envenomations by any of these results in the same clinical syndrome.

PHYSICAL EXAMINATION: SIGNS AND SYMPTOMS

Local. A bite may go unnoticed or may be experienced as a pinprick or burning sensation. Two small punctate lesions may be visible. Within half an hour, pain at the site and in the regional lymph nodes develops. Central pallor at the bite site with surrounding erythema also has been described.[3,12,33] Unlike the bite of *loxosceles,* the black widow bite usually does not induce an impressive inflammatory response.

Systemic. The onset of systemic symptoms frequently is sudden, with crampy, skeletal muscle pains in the legs, abdomen, back, and chest and associated autonomic dysfunction. A review of 163 cases by Clark et al.[12] showed the most frequent systemic signs and symptoms to be generalized abdominal pain or back pain (56%), local or extremity pain (38%), hypertension (29%), diaphoresis (22%), and isolated abdominal (18%) or chest (17%) pains. Nausea and vomiting and tachycardia were present in 11% of patients. Restlessness, salivation, bronchorrhea, priapism, urinary retention, periorbital edema, tremor, and convulsions also may be seen.[3,39] Abdominal rigidity may mimic peritoneal irritation. Respiratory paralysis and heart failure also have been reported.

Patients who do not receive antivenom may have protracted symptoms that last for weeks to months. Symptoms can include fatigue, weakness, paresthesias, generalized aches, diaphoresis, headache, sleeplessness, excessive sweating, impotence, mental status changes, and transient hemiparesis.[33]

LABORATORY STUDIES. No specific laboratory test helps to establish this diagnosis. Leukocytosis and hyperglycemia are common. Creatine phosphokinase may be elevated because of increased muscle activity. Serum calcium is normal.

DIFFERENTIAL DIAGNOSIS. The causes of acute abdominal pain should be part of the differential diagnosis. Of interest is the close resemblance of the autonomic hyperactivity seen after black widow spider bites and that seen in organophosphate poisoning.

MANAGEMENT. The vast majority of black widow spider bites require only cool compresses, elevation of the affected extremity, tetanus status update (if needed), and analgesics. In more severe cases oxygen, cardiac monitoring, and intravenous access are recommended.

Muscle cramps may be relieved with opiates and muscle relaxants. Diazepam, methocarbamol, and calcium gluconate have been used with varying results. Recently the efficacy of 10% calcium gluconate has been questioned by Clark et al.[12] in their retrospective study. Patients who do not receive antivenom gradually will improve over the next 12 to 48 hours. As previously mentioned, some individuals may have protracted symptoms.

Latrodectus antivenom of equine origin is available and neutralizes venom from all related species.[3] Patients should be tested for horse serum hypersensitivity before it is administered. It should be considered in severe envenomations that have evidence of respiratory distress, significant hypertension, and cardiovascular compromise, as well as for pregnant women and for protracted symptoms unresponsive to analgesics and muscle relaxants. Prompt response within an hour of infusion is the rule. The administration of antivenom may decrease length of stay in hospital and prevent lingering neurological complications.[3,33]

Tarantulas (*Mygalomorphs*)

CHARACTERISTICS. Tarantulas, more appropriately called *Mygalomorphs,* are considered primitive forms of true spiders. In the United States the species spends most of the daytime hours in burrows and hunts at night.[53] They are docile, and bites are unusual. Body size varies and can reach up to 10 cm. These spiders possess large vertically oriented fangs that require them to lean back on their hind legs to bite; this is a characteristic defensive posture.

DISTRIBUTION. Over 30 species of tarantulas are found in the tropical and subtropical desert areas of the southwestern United States. Some people keep North American and foreign species as pets.

PHYSICAL EXAMINATION: SIGNS AND SYMPTOMS. Most bites are no more severe than a bee sting and occasionally result in local erythema, swelling, and pain. Nausea and vomiting may occur from the bite. Some species *(Lasiodora, Grammostola, Acanthoscurria,* and *Brachypelma)* are capable of releasing urticaria-producing hairs from their abdomen by rubbing their hind legs on the area. This can result in local histamine release with mild pruritus. However, the itching can last for weeks.[3,53]

MANAGEMENT. Local wound care and tetanus update as required are all that is needed in most cases; antihistamines and oral analgesics may be helpful. Adhesive tape may be useful to remove the urticaria-producing hairs from the skin.

Scorpions

The participating centers of the American Poison Centers National Data Collection System had 1745 pediatric scorpion exposures reported in 1991.[30] Of these exposures, 32% were among patients less than 6 years of age; 68% were in patients less than 17 years old. Although most envenomations are minor, young children, especially those less than 5 years of age, are particularly at risk of complications.[7,8] Morbidity can be significant, but fatalities are rare.

Characteristics. *Centruroides sculpturatus,* also known as *C. exilicauda* or *bark scorpion,* is the only medically relevant species in the United States. It measures 1.3 to 7.5 cm in length and envenomates its victim with a stinger located at the distal end of the tail. The venom is a potent neurotoxin that activates neuronal sodium channels and results in excessive firing of the affected neurons.[7,41]

Stings usually result from accidental contact with a scorpion trapped in linen or clothing or during play outdoors. Fortunately, not all stings result in clinical evidence of envenomation. Although most stings take place in scorpion-endemic areas, scorpions can be accidentally transported to other areas by travellers.

Distribution. Scorpions are found in Arizona and parts of southern California, Nevada, New Mexico, and Texas. *C. sculpturatus,* considered a climbing scorpion, can be sighted on trees, fence posts, and rocks and in cracks and rubbish piles.

Physical Examination: Signs and Symptoms

LOCAL. Pain at the sting site with or without paresthesias is common, especially with species other than *Centruroides.* In mild envenomations this may be the only symptom. Infants may manifest this symptom as unexplained crying.[7] Local erythema and swelling may surround a small puncture wound, but the sting site more often is unidentifiable.

SYSTEMIC. Systemic manifestations of scorpion envenomation can be very dramatic and usually develop within 60 minutes of the sting. They tend to be more common in children less than 10 years of age.[41] Cardiovascular, respiratory, and neurological systems mostly occur.

Cranial nerve dysfunctions such as blurred vision, nystagmus, roving eye movements, hypersalivation, dysphagia, excessive drooling, tongue fasciculations, loss of airway protective reflexes, stridor, slurred speech, and seizures may be seen. Autonomic hyperactivity also may result from the neurotoxin. Tachycardia often is a prominent symptom with or without hypertension or hyperthermia. Paresthesias, apprehension, and restlessness also may be present.

Skeletal muscle findings include twitching or jerking of the extremities, which in some cases may be severe enough to be mistaken for seizure activity; rhabdomyolysis may result from this.[7] Respiratory distress and failure may be encountered in severe cases.[3,41]

Differential Diagnosis. Two factors make it difficult to establish the correct diagnosis. The first is that the sting site may not be identifiable; the second is that the child may not be able to communicate the history of a sting clearly. Seizure disorders, intraabdominal catastrophes, phenothiazine poisoning, and allergic reactions are some of the differential diagnoses. Some children have been misdiagnosed as having asthma in the presence of wheezing and respiratory distress.[41]

Laboratory Studies. Scorpion envenomation is a clinical determination; there is no confirmatory laboratory test. Leukocytosis, CSF pleocytosis, and elevated creatine phosphokinase have been described.[7]

Management. The treatment of scorpion envenomation primarily is supportive, with the use of cold compresses and analgesics for mild symptoms. In severe cases active airway intervention, intravenous access, and sedation may be required. Steroids, antihistamines, and calcium play no role in the management of scorpionism. Gradual resolution of symptoms occurs in 3 to 30 hours.[8,41]

Progression of symptoms is not predictable. A review of cases from Arizona's Regional Poison Management Center revealed that progression to serious symptoms always occurred in less than 5 hours if at all. Numbness, tingling, and pain may persist for 2 weeks.[15] Rimsza et al.[41] found the duration of symptoms to be related inversely to the age of the patient.

Goat serum–derived antivenom to *Centruroides* is available from the Antivenom Production Laboratory of Arizona State University. It is not approved by the FDA. As with other xenobiotic sera, there is a risk of immediate anaphylaxis with its administration and a possibility of delayed serum sickness. Symptoms should resolve fully within 1 to 3 hours after administration. Bond[8] notes that 58% of children 10 years of age or younger who received antivenom developed a rash, hives, or serum sickness within 2 weeks of administration; no acute reactions occurred in 12 patients.

Administration of antivenom is based on the severity of the envenomation and analysis of the risk-benefit ratio. Antivenom therapy may decrease the need for hospitalization, the length of stay, and the number of intensive care procedures the child has to undergo, such as sedation and intubation.[7] Its use should be reserved for severe cases.

SNAKES

The venomous snakes of North America can be divided into two families: Crotalidae and Elapidae. The Crotalidae family gets its name from the Latin for *rattle* and includes rattlesnakes, pygmy rattlesnakes (massasaugas), copperheads, and water moccasins (cottonmouths). As a group these snakes are known as *pit vipers* because of a heat-sensitive pit found behind and below their nostrils. The Elapidae family includes coral snakes as well as the nonindigenous cobras and mambas.

Epidemiology

Type of Snake. In 1991 23.6% of the snakebite-related calls to poison centers referred to nonpoisonous snakes; in 43.2% the type of snake was unknown. Indigenous Crotalidae and Elapidae were the vectors in 24% and less than 1%, respectively. Nonindigenous snakes were the vectors in 8.5%.[30] Fortunately, although all sea snakes are venomous, none inhabits the coastal waters of North America.[45]

Host Factors. Usually the person bitten is a young adult white male. Approximately 40% of bites occur while handling or playing with a snake; 40% of those bitten have a blood alcohol level greater than 0.1%.[51] In one study of rattlesnake bites, only 43% occurred before an encounter with a snake was recognized or while the person was attempting to move away from the snake.[17] The 1975-1980 incidence of snake venom poisoning by state is illustrated in Figure 279-1.[43] More recent data are not available.

Body Area. Most bites are sustained on the upper extremity. A review of inpatient and outpatient cases of snake bite in California reported the following site distribution: 70% finger, 15% hand, 2% arm, 12% leg or foot, and 1% torso.[52] Given the high percentage of bites sustained while the snake was being handled intentionally, these statistics are less surprising than reports of snakebites to the tongue[18] and the glans penis.[14]

Mortality. Between 1975 and 1980 (the most recent years for which data are available) the number of deaths from snakebite in the United States ranged from 9 to 14 per year.[43] Most snakebite deaths are associated with absence of medical care, errors in medical management, or the presence of an underlying medical condition. Once bitten by a snake, children are at increased risk of serious sequelae because of the high venom dose per kilogram of body weight.

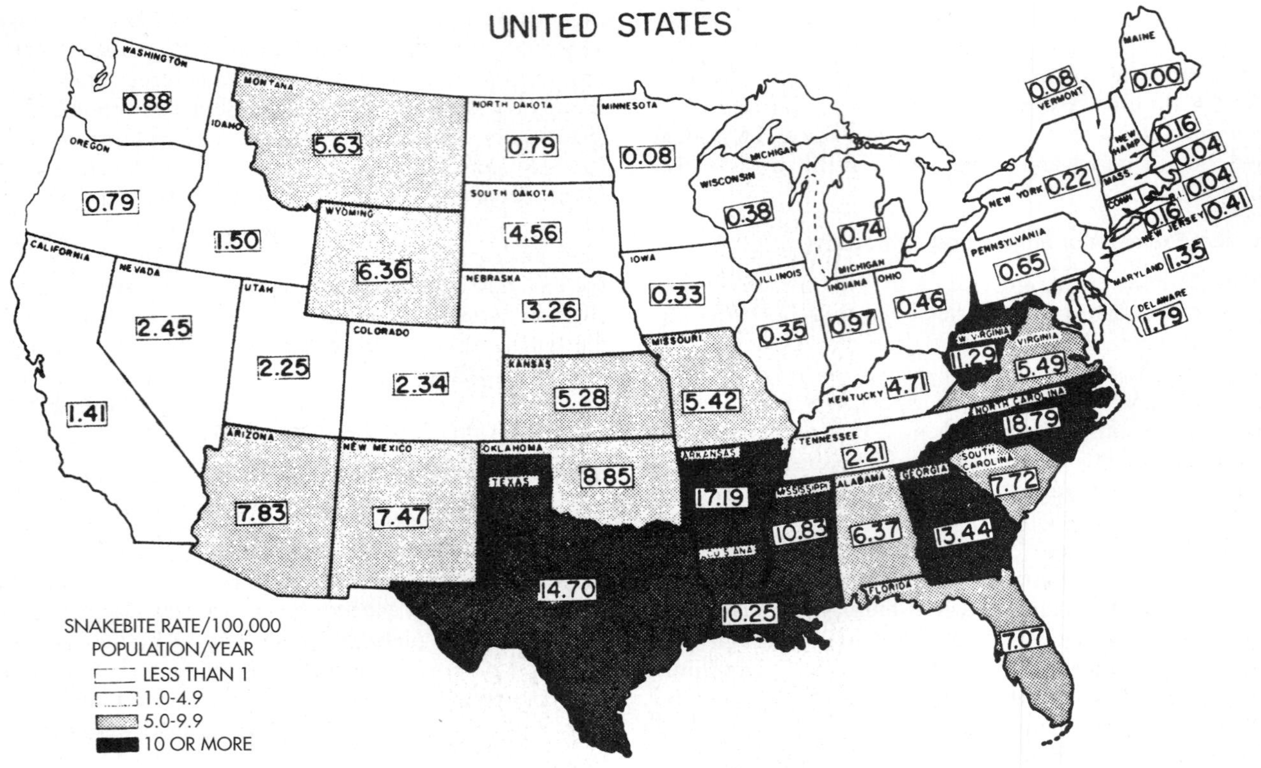

FIG. 279-1 Incidence of snake venom poisoning by state.
(From Russell FE: *Snake venom poisoning,* Philadelphia, 1980, JB Lippincott.)

Prevention

Native Americans used numerous plants, animal tissues, oils, and excrement to prevent snakebites.[43] The box on p. 1697, a summary of more practical suggestions for avoiding snakebites, is based on the epidemiology of these injuries and the nature of snakes.

Snake Venoms

The composition and deadliness of snake venoms vary from species to species. Each venom is a mixture of numerous enzymes (e.g., protease, hyaluronidase, collagenase), polypeptide fractions, and inorganic substances (e.g., sodium, zinc).[43] These substances have two inextricably interwoven chief functions: killing or immobilizing prey and digesting them.

Crotalidae venoms are chiefly, but not exclusively, digestive, causing necrosis of lymphatics, cells, and small blood vessels. The subsequent excessive permeability of blood vessels can lead to tissue edema, adult respiratory distress syndrome (ARDS), shock, and renal failure. Additionally, the venom of pit vipers can cause hemolysis, bleeding diathesis, and disseminated intravascular coagulation. Elapidae venoms, on the other hand, are notoriously neurotoxic, causing paresthesias and paralysis by inhibiting acetylcholine receptors at the neuronal synapse. Some Crotalidae (e.g., the Mojave rattlesnake) also produce a neurotoxic venom.

Pit Vipers

As noted previously, rattlesnakes, copperheads, and water moccasins are members of the pit viper family. Copperheads, which often live in or near cities and suburbs, inflict almost 40% of venomous snake bites in the United States but have a case fatality rate of only 0.01%.[38] Conversely, diamondback rattlesnakes are responsible for only about 10% of venomous snake bites, but 95% of snakebite mortalities.[38] Pit vipers are venomous at birth and as adults can be found in a wide array of sizes that necessarily do not correlate with their deadliness.

Characteristics. Crotalidae are distinguished from coral snakes chiefly by their facial pit. This apparatus is used to locate and estimate the size of prey and predators. The snake can estimate a venom dose in accordance with the size of the prey that is to be immobilized, killed, and digested.[6]

Pit vipers have retractable, hollow fangs that function much like a hypodermic needle. Usually they penetrate to subcutaneous tissue, but large diamondback rattlesnake fangs can reach a depth of 8 to 19 mm.[51] For an envenomation to take place, the pit viper must be venomous at the time of the strike, penetrate the skin, and inject venom during penetration. Approximately 20% to 25% of pit viper bites are "dry," meaning they do not result in envenomation.[28]

Although identifying the type of snake is useful, no time should be lost in getting the victim to medical attention, nor should the rescue party expose themselves to risk while trying to find and identify the snake.

Distribution. The box on p. 1697 lists the indigenous location for North American pit vipers.[6]

First Aid. Commonly accepted guidelines for snakebite first aid are summarized in the box on p. 1698.[6,52] Other forms of first aid are controversial and are discussed here because the physician may see patients less damaged by the snake

SNAKEBITE PREVENTION

1. It is impossible to differentiate poisonous from nonpoisonous snakes without years of experience. Therefore children should not approach, disturb, play with, capture, or kill *any* snake. These practices are dangerous for the human and annoying to the snake.
2. Children should not put their hands or feet in places they cannot see. Children should not put their hands or feet anywhere without first looking.
3. Snakes frequently can be found under rocks, boulders, fallen trees, fences, rubbish piles, and boats that have been left on shore for several hours; in tall grass and heavy underbrush; or sunning themselves on logs, boulders, trees, walls, or cliffs. Extra caution should be used in these areas.
4. The striking distance of a snake is roughly half its length. Children should be taught to keep a good distance from snakes.
5. The striking reflex remains intact for up to an hour after the snake is dead. Therefore, even if one is sure that the snake is dead, it must be examined or transported at the opposite end of a long stick.
6. Rattlesnakes are nocturnal feeders and therefore are active after dark. Never gather firewood after dark. Camp should be set up on open ground; never near wood, rubbish piles, swampy areas, or the entrance of a cave.
7. Children should wear boots when walking in endemic areas.
8. Children should not be allowed to walk alone in an endemic area.
9. Children should not be allowed to swim in waters known to be infested with snakes.
10. Once bitten, everyone present should get away from the snake as quickly as possible. The benefit of identifying the snake is small in comparison to the risk of additional bites.

INDIGENOUS LOCATIONS FOR NORTH AMERICAN PIT VIPERS

Southeast
- Cottonmouths and copperheads
- Eastern diamondback *(C. adamanteus)*
- Timber *(C. horridus)*
- Massasauga pygmy rattlesnakes *(Sistrurus)*

Midwest
- Cottonmouths and copperheads
- Eastern diamondback *(C. adamanteus)*
- Timber *(C. horridus)*
- Prairie *(C.v. viridis)*
- Massasauga pygmy rattlesnakes *(Sistrurus)*

Northeast
- Cottonmouths and copperheads
- Eastern diamondback *(C. adamanteus)*
- Timber *(C. horridus)*
- Massasauga pygmy rattlesnakes *(Sistrurus)*

Northwest
- Great Basin *(C.v. lutosus)*
- Northern Pacific *(C.v. oreganus)*

Southwest
- Western diamondback *(C. atrox)*
- Sidewinder *(C. cerastes)*
- Rock *(C. lepidus)*
- Speckled *(C. mitchelli)*
- Black-tailed *(C. molossus)*
- Twin-spotted *(C. pricei)*
- Red diamond *(C. ruber)*
- Mojave *(C. scutulatus)*
- Tiger *(C. tigris)*
- Prairie *(C.v. viridis)*
- Grand Canyon *(C.v. abyssus)*
- Southern Pacific *(C.v. helleri)*
- Great Basin *(C.v. lutosus)*
- Ridge-nosed *(C. willardi)*

From Banner W: *Curr Probl Pediatr* 18:1, 1988.

than by the field treatment of well-meaning, but untrained (and possibly inebriated) attendants.

Cryotherapy. This form of snakebite treatment was used to constrict blood flow and thus diminish systemic venom absorption. Unfortunately the consequent ischemia is limb threatening. Cryotherapy is contraindicated.

Incision and Suction. The Sawyer extractor, a syringe-type plunger that develops 1 atmosphere of vacuum, has been shown to be beneficial in removing snake venom in both experimental and clinical settings.[9] If this device is not available, incision and suction should be instituted *only if all of the following conditions are met:* (1) the procedure does not delay transport to a medical facility and can be started no more than 30 minutes after the envenomation; (2) the nearest medical care is more than 60 minutes away; and (3) the person performing the procedure is knowledgeable about the method and the underlying anatomy and is prepared to continue suction for 30 to 60 minutes. The single incision should be made through the fang marks, no greater than 3 mm deep, 5 to 6 mm long, and parallel to the axis of the limb. To protect both parties, a clean suction cup rather than the attendant's mouth should be used, if available.[6]

Constricting Bands. Like cryotherapy, use of a tourniquet causes limb-threatening tissue necrosis and is contraindicated. Conversely, wide constricting bands, tight enough to impede lymphatic return but not blood flow, have been found useful according to some studies. Venom spread is not limited to the lymphatic route, and the risk-benefit ratio of this first aid is blurred by the likelihood of a "dry" bite, the relatively benign venom of most North American snakes, and the availability of medical care nearby.

If used at all, the constricting band must be used correctly. A blood pressure cuff should be inflated to 15 to 20 mm Hg 15 to 20 cm proximal to the snakebite, or a wide band may be tied loosely enough to allow two fingers to pass beneath. If swelling occurs, the band should be removed after a more proximal constricting band is placed to prevent the sudden release of venom into the system.[6]

History-Taking. Information elicited in the medical history of known envenomations include the size and species of the

FIRST AID FOR SNAKEBITES

1. Observe the approximate size and characteristics of the snake if this can be done without danger of remaining within the snake's striking range.
2. Move the patient as little as possible.
3. Mark the victim's skin with a pen denoting the area of swelling and the time. Repeat this every 15 minutes.
4. Remove all rings from the victim's fingers.
5. Immobilize the affected limb by splinting as if for a fracture and keep the limb below the level of the heart.
6. Regardless of early symptoms, transport the victim to the nearest medical facility at a safe speed.
7. Avoid the use of ice (tissue damage), aspirin (anticoagulation), alcohol or sedative drugs (vasodilation), or stimulants such as caffeine (acceleration of venom absorption).
8. As soon as possible start basic life support, including volume expansion and Trendelenburg position for hypotensive patients.

snake, the circumstances of the bite (e.g., through clothing, alcohol related), the number of bites and body area affected, first aid methods used, time of bite and transport time, previous snakebite episodes and exposure to horse serum, allergies (e.g., horse serum, antibiotics), and tetanus immunization status.[52]

Physical Examination: Signs and Symptoms

LOCAL. Local signs and symptoms usually include the presence of fang marks as well as pain, edema, ecchymosis, and erythema from 15 minutes to 4 hours after the bite. Fang marks typically have ragged edges but may be obscured by secondary trauma sustained in the flight from the snake or the first aid attempts. Because of the hematoxic effects of pit viper venom, blood may ooze from the puncture sites and hemorrhagic bullae may develop. Muscle necrosis also may become apparent. The absence of any local signs within 30 minutes makes the likelihood of envenomation low; their presence makes 24 hours of observation important.

SYSTEMIC. Hemolysis, consumption coagulopathy, and generalized hemorrhage frequently are present in serious envenomations. The physical examination also should be geared toward detecting signs of ARDS, circulatory collapse, and renal failure. Other findings may include weakness, lightheadedness, diaphoresis, visual disturbances, nausea, vomiting, syncope, and a metallic taste.[10] Paresthesias (of the scalp, face, or extremities), fasciculations, and the formation of bullae have been shown to increase significantly with the severity of the pit viper bite.[52]

Laboratory Studies. Laboratory studies have been found to be of "minor assistance in assessing the severity of (rattlesnake) envenomation."[52] Creatine kinase levels were the only measure to demonstrate a significant difference in severe bites. Prothrombin times, fibrinogen levels, and platelet counts often were altered, and the urinalysis, when performed, was more likely to show hematuria and proteinuria if the bite was considered serious.

Studies often recommended include a complete blood and differential count, red blood cell morphology to evaluate for spherocytosis, and a bleeding screen (prothrombin time, plasma thromboplastin time, fibrinogen levels, fibrin-split products, and platelet count). For severe envenomations electrolytes, blood urea nitrogen, blood type and cross-match, serum bilirubin concentration, arterial blood gas, and urinalysis may also be useful. Enzyme-linked immunoassay (ELISA) and radioimmunoassay (RIA) tests for detection of pit viper venom in wound aspirate, serum, and urine are available.[34]

Supportive Therapy

SHOCK. Because of the increase in membrane permeability, colloid plasma expanders are preferred by many over crystalloids for snakebite victims. Vasopressors may become necessary in the most serious cases.

FLUID AND ELECTROLYTE ABNORMALITIES. Extensive third-space losses may cause fluid and electrolyte imbalances. Intravenous fluids and urine output monitoring become essential under these conditions.

HEMATOLOGICAL COMPLICATIONS. Treatment of thrombocytopenia and anemia (caused by hemolysis) may require multiple transfusions. Disseminated intravascular coagulopathy caused by snakebite does not respond to heparin; antivenin is the drug of choice.

Use of Antivenin. Once venin is bound to the end organ, antivenin has little effect. Therefore, as soon as it is determined that the patient has a serious envenomation, antivenin therapy should be considered. Some reserve its use for large rattlesnakes, water moccasins, or unidentified snakes.[47] Antivenin use should proceed simultaneously with supportive therapy, as shown in the box on p. 1699.

Prevention and Treatment of Serum Sickness. Up to 80% of patients develop serum sickness sometime within 4 weeks after being treated with antivenin, but only 3% require hospitalization for this complication. Oral corticosteroids should be prescribed at the first signs (usually urticaria and pruritus) and should be continued until all symptoms have subsided for 24 hours. The steroid then should be tapered over 72 hours. If necessary, diphenhydramine may be added to control pruritus.

Additional Therapeutic Measures

PAIN CONTROL. Analgesics should not be overlooked in the management of snakebites. Adequate pain control allows rehabilitation to begin as early as possible to prevent contractures.

INFECTION CONTROL. Although snakes have been found to carry a wide variety of bacteria in their mouths (histotoxic clostridia, *Bacteroides,* many gram positive and gram negative aerobes), infection is unlikely in the absence of severe necrosis, and good wound care is believed to be sufficient to prevent secondary infection. Systemic and local changes produced by envenomation and the subsequent vascular damage may be difficult to differentiate from infection. Broad-spectrum antibiotics generally are recommended prophylactically in cases of obvious tissue necrosis.

TETANUS PROPHYLAXIS. *Clostridium tetani* are not part of the mouth flora of snakes. Updating the patient's immunization status is the only necessary intervention.

SURGICAL MEASURES. The debridement of hemorrhagic blebs 3 to 5 days after snakebite is routine if coagulation has

STEPS IN USING ANTIVENIN

1. *Prepare to Manage Anaphylaxis.* Because development of an anaphylactic reaction is unpredictable,[37] all patients receiving antivenin should be monitored and have two intravenous catheters—one for the antivenin and one for emergency drugs and fluids. Intravenous epinephrine, diphenhydramine, and plasma expanders, as well as respiratory support, must be readily available.
2. *Test for Sensitivity to Horse Serum.* Skin testing, detailed on the package insert* of the antivenin, is not reliable.[26] Therefore a negative skin test should not lull one into a sense of false security. However, some physicians have used the antivenin in very serious cases despite a positive skin test. To decrease the risk of an allergic reaction in these cases, give the saline-diluted antivenin slowly with diphenhydramine premedication and a simultaneous infusion of epinephrine.[37]
3. *Start the Infusion.* In the child who weighs over 45 kg the initial dose should be estimated on the basis of the clinical grading system (Table 279-1). Children under this weight usually require *50% more* than this dose. The intravenous antivenin solution infusion should begin at 1 ml/hour and be increased over 30 minutes to a maximum of 150 ml/hour. "One to two vials per hour is appropriate to avoid the risks associated with higher infusion rates."[6]
4. *Repeat Infusion.* If, after the initial infusion, the local signs progress or the systemic signs persist, the initial antivenin dose (usually five vials in children) should be repeated. Although the incidence of serum sickness is proportional to the person's sensitivity and the volume of antivenin received, morbidity and mortality after serious envenomations are related to giving too little hyperimmune serum or giving it too late. Large doses of antivenin may be associated with metabolic acidosis, because each vial contains 0.25% formalin.[5]

*Antivenin polyvalent is hyperimmunized horse serum active against the venom of all species of pit vipers. It is available from Wyeth-Ayerst Laboratories, Box 8299, Philadelphia, PA 19101.

returned to normal. Dermotomy is also routine therapy for fingers if digital swelling compresses the neurovascular bundle. Fasciotomy, however, is very controversial. Although usually unnecessary in cases of indigenous snakebite for which adequate antivenin is given, fasciotomy has a role in cases of dangerously inadequate arterial perfusion caused by elevated intracompartment pressures.[16,42]

Coral Snakes

Coral snakes are the members of the Elapidae family that are indigenous to North America. Although their venom can cause a life-threatening paralysis, coral snakes tend to be small, secretive, and mild-mannered unless provoked. Few bites are reported, and mortality is rare.

Characteristics. The Eastern coral snake often is mistaken for the nonvenomous scarlet king snake because of similar colorful bands encircling the body. The mnemonic "red to yellow, kill a fellow; red to black, venom lack; head of black, step back, Jack!" refers to the color patterns of these snakes. The poisonous black-snouted snake has broad red and black bands separated by narrow yellow ones; the nonpoisonous variety's snout is red, and its broad red bands are separated by narrow yellow ones bounded on each side by black. Despite these distinctions, a large proportion of people bitten by coral snakes thought they were handling a scarlet king snake.[27]

Unlike pit vipers, coral snakes lack facial pits, are diurnal, and have fixed fangs and nearly round pupils. Their bites may produce superficial scratches or definite fang marks. Their retroverted teeth gnaw or chew on their prey and make coral snakes difficult to shake off. Because they must stay attached long enough for their venom to be deposited around their teeth, 50% of coral snake bites are dry.

Distribution. Three types of coral snakes are found in the United States: the Eastern coral snake, the Texas coral snake, and the Arizona or Sonoran coral snake. Their distribution is shown in Figure 279-2. The bite of the Sonoran coral snake produces no more than local pain and a small amount of nausea.

First Aid. Cryotherapy, incision and suction (including the Sawyer extractor), and constricting bands have no proven value in coral snakebites. Russell[43] recommends the following: "No food or drink should be given. If the victim is more than 1 hour's distance from a medical facility, a tourniquet might be placed immediately proximal to the bite area. It should be released for 1 minute every 10 minutes, and it should be left in place until 3 minutes after intravenous antivenin has been started."

Physical Examination: Signs and Symptoms

LOCAL. Erythema and local pain from a coral snake bite are transient or absent. Though 85% of patients will have evident fang marks, envenomations have been reported that were not associated with apparent fang marks on close examination.[36]

SYSTEMIC. Systemic manifestations may be delayed for 12 hours and may appear precipitously. They may include bulbar paralysis with ptosis, dysphagia, dysarthria, excessive salivation, paresthesias, euphoria or apprehension, drowsiness, dizziness, weakness, confusion, nausea, vomiting, diaphoresis, muscle tenderness or fasciculations, and ophthalmoplegias causing visual disturbances. These may be followed by seizures, respiratory paralysis, and pulmonary hemorrhage. It often is unclear which findings are primary and which are secondary to hypoxia.

Laboratory Studies. Coral snake bites do not mandate *routine* laboratory screening.

Supportive Therapy. Elective intubation before impending respiratory paralysis tends to prevent aspiration pneumonia. Elective intubation is recommended if any signs of bulbar paralysis develop.[27]

Use of Antivenin. Russell[43] recommends the use of antivenin effective against Eastern and Texas snake venoms (*Micrurus fulvius;* produced by Wyeth-Ayerst) if a patient definitely has been bitten (five vials) or if any signs or symptoms develop (three vials).[43] These guidelines are based on the judgment that the risks of intravenous hyperimmune horse serum are offset by the potential prevention of respiratory paralysis, which may ensue if therapy is not given early in the disease.

As with pit viper antivenin, skin testing yields many false

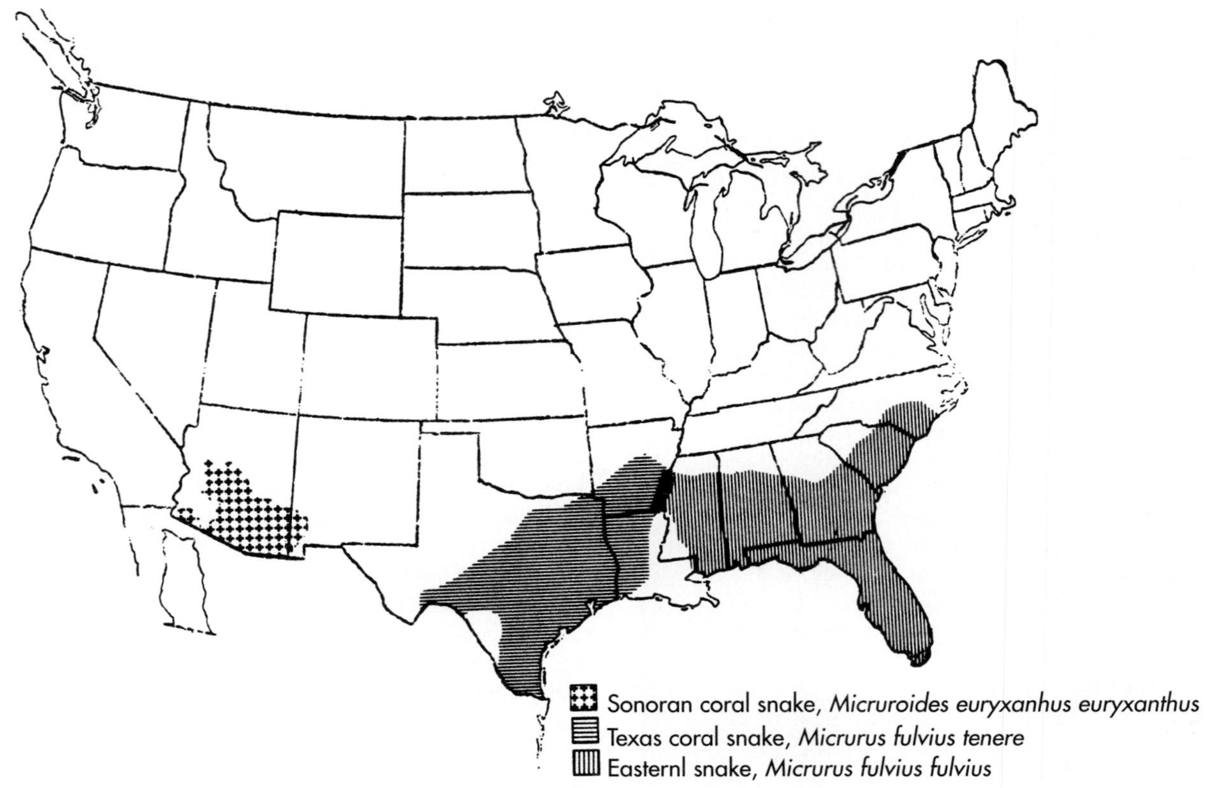

FIG. 279-2 Distribution of coral snakes by type in the United States.
(From Russell FE: *Snake venom poisoning,* Philadelphia, 1980, JB Lippincott.)

Table 279-1 Extent of Envenomation and Dosage of Antivenin

Grade	Signs and symptoms	Initial treatment
No envenomation	Fang marks present; no local or systemic reactions	No antivenin; local care. Tetanus prophylaxis when indicated. Observation in emergency department for at least 4 hours
Mild envenomation	Fang marks present; local swelling but no systemic reaction. Pain may be present or absent	Three to five vials antivenin
Moderate envenomation	Swelling that progresses beyond the site of the bite with systemic reaction or laboratory changes (e.g., fall in hematocrit and fibrinogen levels or platelets or hematuria)	Six to 10 vials antivenin
Severe envenomation	Marked local and systemic reaction. Bleeding diathesis, DIC, shock, or ARDS with marked laboratory changes	15+ vials antivenin

negatives and the same precautions must be taken as outlined above. The diluted vials are put into solution with normal saline—250 ml in children or 125 ml in infants. A starting infusion rate of 1 ml/hour is gradually increased until one or two vials are administered per hour.

Additional Therapeutic Measures. Recommendations for infection and tetanus prophylaxis are the same as for pit viper bites. Additional measures may become necessary if aspiration pneumonia develops. Patients should be aware that muscular weakness may persist for 3 to 6 weeks.

Nonindigenous Snakes

The variety of imported snakes is too great to detail in this text. If an exotic species is suspected, the recommended approach includes local wound care, supportive care, and consultation with experts.*[6]

REFERENCES

1. Adams CT, Lofgren CS: Red imported fire ants (Hymenoptera: formicidae): frequency of sting attacks on residents of Sumter County, Georgia, *J Med Entomol* 18:378, 1981.
2. Adams CT, Lofgren CS: Incidence of stings or bites of the red imported fire ant (Hymenoptera: Formicidae) and other arthropods among patients at Ft. Stewart, Georgia, USA, *J Med Entomol* 19:366, 1982.

*Examples include The Arizona Poison and Drug Information Center (602-626-6016), the Oklahoma Poison Control Center (405-271-5454), and the Bronx Zoo's herpetology section (212-220-5151).

3. Allen C: Arachnid envenomations, *Emerg Med Clin North Am* 10:269, 1992.
4. Atkinson RK, Wright LG: The modes of action of spider toxins on insects and mammals, *Comp Biochem Physiol* 102:339, 1992.
5. Bailey JW: Letter to the editor, *J Trauma* 25:464, 1985.
6. Banner W: Bites and stings in the pediatric patient, *Curr Probl Pediatr* 18:1, 1988.
7. Berg RA, Tarantino MD: Envenomation by the scorpion *Centruroides exilicauda (C. sculpturatus):* severe and unusual manifestations, *Pediatrics* 87:930, 1991.
8. Bond RG: Antivenin administration for *Centruroides* scorpion sting: risks and benefits, *Ann Emerg Med* 21:788, 1992.
9. Bronstein AC et al: Negative pressure suction in suction in field treatment of rattlesnake bite, *Vet Hum Toxicol* 27:297, 1985.
10. Burch JM et al: The treatment of crotalid envenomation without antivenin, *J Trauma* 28:35, 1988.
11. Charpin D et al: Prevalence of allergy to Hymenoptera stings in different samples of the general population, *J Allerg Clin Immunol* 90:331, 1992.
12. Clark RF et al: Clinical presentation and treatment of black widow spider envenomation: a review of 163 cases, *Ann Emerg Med* 21:782, 1992.
13. Cohen PR: Imported fire ant stings: clinical manifestations and treatment, *Pediatr Dermatol* 9:44, 1992.
14. Crane DB, Irwin JS: Rattlesnake bite of glans penis, *Urology* 26:50, 1985.
15. Curry SC et al: Envenomation by the scorpion *Centruroides sculpturatus, J Toxicol Clin Toxicol* 21:417, 1983.
16. Curry SC et al: Noninvasive vascular studies in management of rattlesnake envenomations to extremities, *Ann Emerg Med* 14:1081, 1985.
17. Curry SC et al: The legitimacy of snakebites in central Arizona, *Ann Emerg Med* 18:658, 1989.
18. Danzl DF, Carter GL: "Kiss and yell": a rattlesnake bite to the tongue, *Ann Emerg Med* 17:549, 1988 (letter).
19. deShazo RD, Butcher BT, Banks WA: Reactions to the stings of the imported fire ant, *N Engl J Med* 323:462, 1990.
20. Fox RW, Lockey RF, Bukantz SC: Neurologic sequelae following the imported fire ant sting, *J Allerg Clin Immunol* 70:120, 1982.
21. Freeman TM et al: Imported fire ant immunotherapy: effectiveness of whole body extracts, *J Allerg Clin Immunol* 90:210, 1992.
22. Ginsburg CM: Fire ant envenomation in children, *Pediatrics* 73:689, 1984.
23. Golden DBK: Diagnosis and prevalence of stinging insect allergy, *Clin Rev Allergy* 5:119, 1987.
24. Hardwick WE et al: Near-fatal fire ant envenomation of a newborn, *Pediatrics* 90:622, 1992.
25. Ingber A et al: Morbidity of brown recluse spider bites: clinical picture, treatment and prognosis, *Acta Dermatol Venereol* 71:337, 1991.
26. Jurkovich GJ et al: Complications of crotalidae antivenin therapy, *J Trauma* 28:1032, 1988.
27. Kitchens CS, Van Mierop LHS: Envenomation by the Eastern coral snake *(Micrurus fulvius), JAMA* 258:1615, 1987.
28. Kunkel DB et al: Reptile envenomations, *J Toxicol Clin Toxicol* 21:503, 1983-1984.
29. Li JTC, Yunginger JW: Management of insect sting hypersensitivity, *Mayo Clin Proc* 67:188, 1992.
30. Litovitz TL et al: 1991 Annual Report of the American Association of Poison Control Centers National Data Collection System, *Am J Emerg Med* 10:452, 1992.
31. Lockey RF: Immunotherapy for allergy to insect stings, *N Engl J Med* 323:1627, 1990.
32. Maguire JF, Geha RS: Bee, wasp, and hornet stings, *Pediatr Rev* 8:5, 1986.
33. Miller TA: Latrodectism: bite of the black widow spider, *Am Fam Phys* 45:181, 1992.
34. Minton SA: Present tests for detection of snake venom: clinical applications, *Ann Emerg Med* 16:932, 1987.
35. Muller UR: Epidemiology of insect sting allergy: epidemiology of clinical allergy, *Monogr Allergy* 31:131, 1993.
36. Norris RL, Dart RC: Apparent coral snake envenomation in a patient without visible fang marks, *Am J Emerg Med* 7:402, 1989.
37. Otten EJ, McKimm D: Venomous snakebite in a patient allergic to horse serum, *Ann Emerg Med* 12:624, 1983.
38. Parrish HM, Carr CA: Bites by copperheads *(Agkistrodon contortrix)* in the United States, *JAMA* 201:107, 1967.
39. Rauber A: Black widow spider bites, *J Toxicol Clin Toxicol* 21:473, 1983-1984.
40. Rhoades RB, Stafford CT, James FK: Survey of fatal anaphylactic reactions to imported fire ant stings, *J Allerg Clin Immunol* 84:159, 1989.
41. Rimsza ME, Zimmerman DR, Bergeson PS: Scorpion envenomation, *Pediatrics* 66:298, 1980.
42. Roberts RS, Csemcsitz TA, Heard CW: Upper extremity compartment syndromes following pit viper envenomation, *Clin Orthop* 193:184, 1985.
43. Russell FEL: *Snake venom poisoning,* Philadelphia, 1980, JB Lippincott.
44. Stablein JJ, Lockey RF: Adverse reactions to ant stings, *Clin Rev Allergy* 5:161, 1987.
45. Tu AT: Biotoxicology of sea snake venoms, *Ann Emerg Med* 16:1923, 1987.
46. Valentine MD et al: The value of immunotherapy with venom in children with allergy to insect stings, *N Engl J Med* 323:1601, 1990.
47. Wagner CW, Colladay ES: Crotalid envenomation in children: selective conservative management, *J Pediatr Surg* 24:128, 1989.
48. Wasserman GS: Wound care of spider and snake envenomations, *Ann Emerg Med* 17:1331, 1988.
49. Wasserman GS, Anderson PC: Loxoscelism and necrotic arachnidism, *J Toxicol Clin Toxicol* 21:451, 1983-1984.
50. Willis GA: Loxoscelism in Canada, *CMAJ* July 1988.
51. Wingert WA: Poisoning by animal venoms, *Top Emerg Med* 2:89, 1980.
52. Wingert WA, Chan L: Rattlesnake bites in southern California and rationale for recommended treatment, *West J Med* 148:37, 1988.
53. Wong RC, Hughes SE, Voorhees JJ: Spider bites, *Arch Dermatol* 123:98, 1987.
54. Wright DN, Lockey RF: Local reactions to stinging insects *(Hymenoptera), Allerg Proc* 11:23, 1990.
55. Young VL, Pin P: The brown recluse spider bite, *Ann Plast Surg* 20(5):447, 1988.
56. Zuckerberg AL, Schweich PJ: An arm red and hot: infection or not? *Pediatr Emerg Care* 6(4):275, 1990.

SUGGESTED READINGS

Hutcheson PS, Slavin RG: Lack of preventive measures given to patients with stinging insect anaphylaxis in hospital emergency rooms, *Ann Allergy* 64:306, 1990.

Rees R et al: The diagnosis and treatment of brown recluse spider bites, *Ann Emerg Med* 16:945, 1987.

Valentine MD: Anaphylaxis and stinging insect hypersensitivity, *JAMA* 268:2830, 1992.

280 Epiglottitis

Caroline Breese Hall and William J. Hall

Epiglottitis, or supraglottitis, is an acute infection manifested by progressive, severe respiratory obstruction. Licensure of the conjugated *Haemophilus influenzae* type b vaccines has resulted in a dramatic reduction in epiglottitis cases and changes in the primary ages affected and causative organisms.[6,8,12,24] Nevertheless, epiglottitis remains the same clinically, a potentially fatal disease that requires prompt recognition and treatment.

ETIOLOGY

Before the widespread use of the conjugated *Haemophilus influenzae* type b (Hib) vaccines, epiglottitis was caused almost exclusively by *H. influenzae* type b. *H. influenzae* organisms were discovered by Pfeiffer during the pandemic of influenza in 1890. Believing these to be the cause of influenza, he titled the organism the "influenza bacillus." These gram negative, aerobic bacilli later were designated *H. influenzae*. In clinical specimens these organisms appear pleomorphic, often coccobacillary. Epiglottitis is caused only by the type b organisms, which are distinguished by their capsular polysaccharide. The organisms may be seen to be encapsulated in clinical specimens by stained smears or by the swelling reaction, which produces capsular swelling with type-specific antiserum. On laboratory growth media and broth, the capsules easily may be demonstrated during the first few hours of growth, but with age the morphological traits change.

The effectiveness of the conjugated Hib vaccines has resulted in a significant drop in the proportion of cases caused by *H. influenzae* type b. In Philadelphia from 1979 through 1983, *H. influenzae* type b caused 82% of the cases of epiglottitis and in 1984 through 1989, 75% of cases.[12] (Fig. 280-1) However, from 1990 through 1992 only 25% of cases were identified as being caused by *H. influenzae* type b. Group A beta-hemolytic streptococcus was the only other organism isolated in the Philadelphia study, constituting 4.2% of the total group (six patients); 50% of these cases occurred from 1990 to 1992. In 20% of patients no organism was identified. Other bacteria have been identified occasionally as causing epiglottitis, including pneumococci and *H. parainfluenzae*.[2,4,8,15] Epiglottitis may occur secondary to asymptomatic colonization by these organisms in the upper respiratory tract or, particularly with pneumococci and streptococci, may be secondary to spread from a major nearby focus of infection.

INCIDENCE

The dramatic decline in the incidence of epiglottitis and *H. influenzae* type b infections closely chronicles the history of the Hib vaccines.[5,6] Introduction and use of the Hib conjugate vaccines for children age 18 months in 1988 produced the initial decline in *H. influenzae* disease, reported at 41 cases per 100,000 in 1987 to less than 30 cases per 100,000 reported in 1988.[6] Licensure of the *H. influenzae* type b conjugate vaccines for infants 2 months of age and older in 1990 resulted in a decline to 2 cases per 100,000 in 1993. Of note, however, is that cases of *H. influenzae* type b in patients 5 years of age and older, who would not have received the vaccine, remained essentially stable from 1987 through 1993. The annual incidence of epiglottitis over the 14 years reviewed in Philadelphia was 8.9 cases per 10,000 hospital admissions. Before 1990 the yearly incidence was 10.9 per 10,000 admissions and 1.8 from 1990 through 1992, thus declining by 84%.[12]

Epiglottitis when caused by *H. influenzae* type b, and previous to the current vaccine era, was primarily a disease of children 3 to 7 years of age.* In contrast, other serious disease caused by *H. influenzae* type b, such as meningitis, occurred primarily in infants, whereas viral croup primarily affects children in the second year of life.[23,25] Because other organisms, particularly group A beta-hemolytic streptococci, currently make up a greater proportion of the cases of epiglottitis, a change in the age distribution may be expected. In Philadelphia the median age range of cases of epiglottitis increased from 35.5 months before 1990 to 80.5 months in 1990 through 1992.[12] This reflected the older median age for patients who had group A beta-hemolytic streptococci (117.5 months) compared with that for patients who had *H. influenzae* type b epiglottitis (35 months). Epiglottitis also may occur occasionally during adulthood.[19]

Epiglottitis has had no distinctive seasonal predilection. However, cases from group A beta-hemolytic streptococci would be expected to be more likely to occur during the seasons when group A streptococci infections are more prevalent, which in temperate climates is the winter, usually peaking in February and March.

PATHOGENESIS

The organisms causing epiglotitits commonly reside asymptomatically in the upper respiratory tract or cause other forms of respiratory disease, usually much less severe than epiglottitis. Why certain children should develop epiglottitis is not understood. One hypothesis is that invasion by these organisms colonizing the upper respiratory tract may occur secondary to stress, trauma, or concurrent viral respiratory tract infection. Whether or not the causative organism initially causes clinical signs, such as nasopharyngitis, infection commonly spreads from the upper respiratory tract to involve the

*References 1, 2, 7, 20, 23, 25.

epiglottis, producing marked inflammation and edema. The inflammation is not limited to the epiglottis, however, but involves the surrounding area, the arytenoids, the arytenoepiglottic folds, the vocal cords, and to some extent the subglottic region. The characteristically rapid and pronounced inflammatory response of these structures mechanically obstructs the flow of air. Inspiratory obstruction is particularly pronounced because of the narrowing force generated by the negative intrathoracic pressure. The edematous epiglottis, like a ball valve, is pulled down into the larynx during inspiration and may obstruct the airway completely. In addition, secretions and exudate are formed by the inflammation, which may include the lower tracheobronchial tree as well. The secretions and edema compound the obstruction to the flow of air. The work of breathing increases, and hypoxemia and carbon dioxide retention may result. Thus, even without total occlusion of the airway by the epiglottis, assisted ventilation is likely to be required.[17,22]

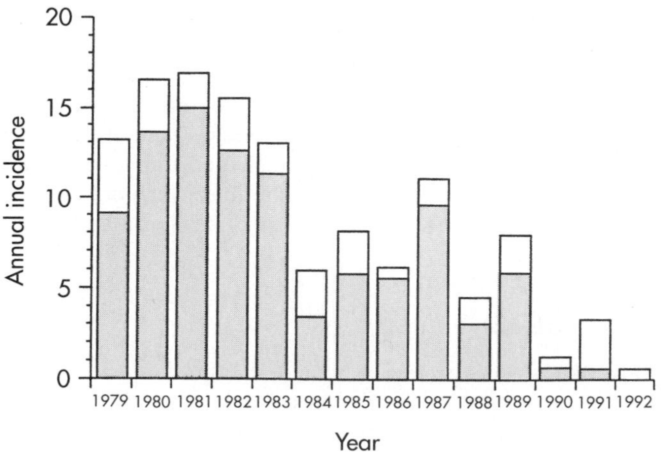

FIG. 280-1 Incidence of epiglottitis. Bars show cases per 10,000 hospital admissions. Solid portion represents cases known to be caused by *Haemophilus influenzae* type b.

(From Gorelick MH, Baker D: *Arch Pediatr Adolesc Med* 148:47, 1994.)

CLINICAL FEATURES

Although the demographics of epiglottitis and the causative organisms have changed in these recent years of vaccine use, the clinical features of epiglottitis remain the same.[12] Hence the clinical manifestations appear related to common pathophysiological processes of the inflamed epiglottis and surrounding structures, whatever the differences in the organisms that initiate the inflammatory response.

Children who have epiglottitis usually have been well previously, although up to 25% may have had some prior upper respiratory tract symptoms that may or may not be related. The hallmarks of epiglottitis are the abrupt onset of severe sore throat, fever, and toxicity in a formerly active child.[1,2,4,25] With fulminant progression, the other classic symptoms and signs occur: dysphagia, drooling, and respiratory distress. Stridor usually develops, but toxicity and respiratory distress may be present initially without overt stridor. Retractions of the chest wall become evident, particularly in the supraclavicular and suprasternal areas, and indicate high airway obstruction. Cough usually is not a prominent part of the picture but may develop as the child tries to clear the increasing secretions. As noted in Table 280-1, the preceding spasmodic, brassy cough and laryngitis

Table 280-1 Characteristic Signs of Epiglottitis Compared with Viral Croup and Bacterial Tracheitis

	Epiglottitis	Viral croup	Bacterial tracheitis
Peak age	3-7 yr	3 mo-3 yr	Any age (mostly ≤12 yr)
History	Previously well	Preceding upper respiratory tract infection common; may have had croup previously	Preceding upper respiratory tract infection common; sometimes viral croup; occasionally previous trauma or manipulation of trachea and upper respiratory tract
Onset	Acute (hours)	Less acute (days)	Acute (hours)
Appearance	Toxic; drooling, dysphagia; sitting forward, mouth open	Less toxic; no drooling	Toxic; respiratory distress and stridor; drooling and sitting forward not characteristic
Cough	Unusual	Very characteristic, spasmodic, "seal's bark"	May be absent or may be present from preceding viral upper respiratory tract infection
Temperature	High (usually 39° C)	Lower (usually <39° C, sometimes none)	High (usually >39° C)
Pharynx	"Beefy" erythema	Normal or slight erythema	Normal or minimal inflammation
White blood cell count and differential	High; left shift	Normal or slight increase; normal or slight left shift	High; left shift
Roentgenogram of neck	"Thumb" sign on lateral view (edematous epiglottis)	Subglottic narrowing on posteroanterior view	Normal epiglottis; subglottic narrowing with membranous tracheal exudate occasionally visible on lateral view

are more characteristic of viral croup. With progression of the epiglottitis, voice changes do occur, however. These may be described more correctly as dysphonia rather than the "scratchy" or "rasping" hoarseness associated with viral laryngotracheobronchitis.

The general appearance of the child who has epiglottitis should suggest the diagnosis. The child who has epiglottitis often appears to have a toxic condition and is in a sitting position, leaning forward with his or her mouth open, tongue protruding, and drooling. The drooling is a particularly characteristic and helpful clinical sign.

Examination of the child reveals a markedly inflamed, "beefy red" pharynx, bathed by copious secretions. Although the "cherry red" epiglottis often may be seen by examination of the pharynx with a tongue depressor, this generally should not be attempted. Fatal occlusion of the airway may result. Inspiratory stridor and expiratory rhonchi may be heard on auscultation, and with progressive obstruction the breath sounds may become diminished.

Bacteremia may occur with development of secondary sites of infection.[20] Most frequent of these are pneumonia, otitis, and cervical lymphadenitis.

DIAGNOSIS

Because of the gravity of epiglottitis, the tentative diagnosis must be made on the basis of the history and clinical manifestation.[2,22] If epiglottitis is suspected, the child should be sent to the hospital immediately, where the diagnosis may be confirmed and trained personnel and equipment are available for establishing an artificial airway.[11,18] Only with these precautions may visualization of the diagnostic epiglottis be attempted.

Roentgenograms of the lateral neck can confirm the diagnosis but usually are unnecessary and unwise for the distressed child who has epiglottitis.[21,22] At all times the child should be accompanied by personnel equipped to handle an airway occlusion. As shown in Fig. 280-2, the characteristic swelling of the epiglottis may be seen as an enlarged, rounded shadow that resembles an adult thumb. This has been called the "thumb sign" by Podgore and Bass[21] and may be compared with the "little finger sign" of the normal epiglottis (Fig. 280-3). The normal epiglottis appears narrower, with the configuration of an adult little finger viewed from the side, as seen in the figure. The total white blood cell count usually is elevated (15,000 to 25,000/mm^3) and often contains a pronounced left shift. Cultures of the upper respiratory tract and blood usually demonstrate the causative pathogen. With *H. influenzae* type b epiglottitis the cultures of blood and secretions almost always are positive. For other organisms, cultures of the respiratory tract secretions may be an unreliable means of definitive etiological diagnosis because the organisms are isolated commonly from the upper respiratory tract without associated disease. Nevertheless, the causative organism is likely to be recovered, along with other organisms, from the respiratory secretions. Such cultures, as a means of diagnosis, therefore usually are sensitive but not specific.

MANAGEMENT

Few illnesses in pediatrics require more swift and careful management.[1] As has been stressed previously, suspicion of the diagnosis of epiglottitis is indication enough to rush the child to the hospital. Once the diagnosis is established, an adequate airway must be maintained. In some intensive care settings, with highly trained personnel in continuous attendance, some children who have early disease have been managed without an artificial airway. In most centers, however, immediate airway intervention is chosen.[2,3,26] With experienced personnel available, nasotracheal intubation is the procedure of choice. Fewer complications occur with this method, and in most patients extubation is possible within 1 to 3 days.

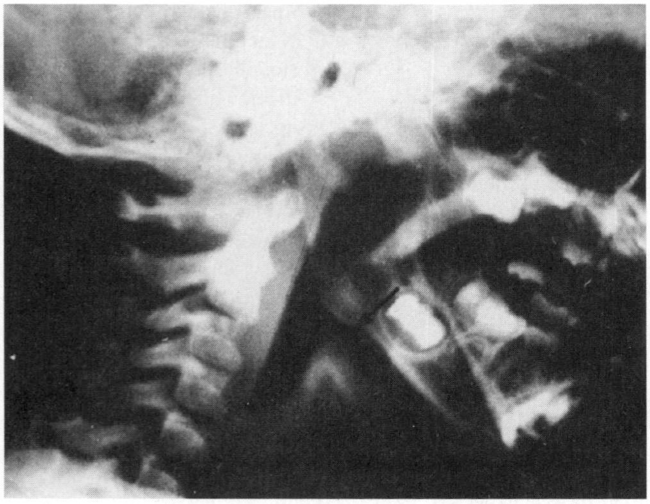

FIG. 280-2 Roentgenogram of lateral neck of a child who has epiglottitis. The arrow points to the shadow of the epiglottitis, which is enlarged and resembles the anteroposterior view of a thumb.

(From Hall CB, Hall WJ: *Update*, 2:665, 1975.)

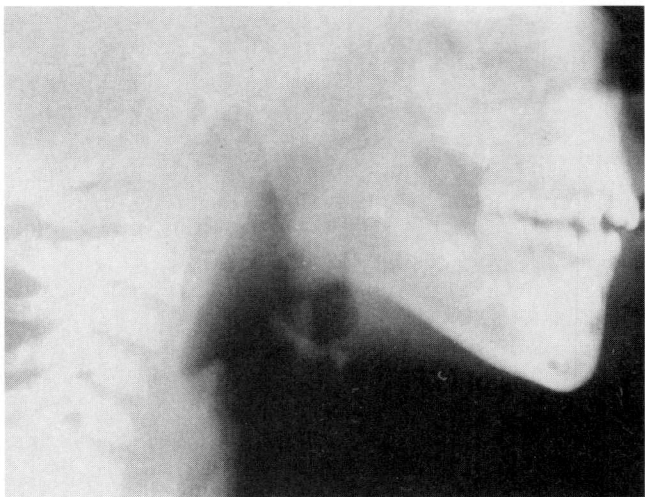

FIG. 280-3 Roentgenogram of lateral neck of a normal child. In contrast to Fig. 280-2, the epiglottis is not enlarged and resembles an adult's fifth finger, viewed laterally.

(From Hall CB, Hall WJ: *Update*, 2:665, 1975.)

Intravenous antibiotic therapy also should be started immediately. Previously, antibiotic therapy has been directed almost exclusively at *H. influenzae* type b. Currently the choice of therapy must be broadened to include not only sensitive and resistant *H. influenzae* type b organisms but also gram positive organisms, particularly *Streptococcus pyogenes* and *S. pneumoniae*. In special circumstances, such as nosocomially acquired infection, antibiotic coverage for *Staphylococci aureus,* gram negative bacilli, and resistant pneumococci may be considered.[9] In most cases a cephalosporin that is stable against the beta-lactamases, such as several third-generation cephalosporins, should be adequate until initial culture results are available. In areas where pneumococci resistant to both penicillins and cephalosporins have been identified, vancomycin may be added until the results of antibiotic sensitivity testing are available.

Supportive care in epiglottitis is of the utmost importance. Direct humidification of the airway and mobilization of the secretions should be maintained. As with any mechanical airway, its position and patency should be monitored carefully. A short course of corticosteroids may help reduce the postintubation edema. Antipyretics may be given during the initial period of high fever. Intravenous fluid should be monitored carefully. The acute onset of the disease means that most of these children are not dehydrated and that only maintenance fluids are necessary.

PROGNOSIS

The outcome in these children often depends on the primary care physician. The clinical acumen of the physician and high index of suspicion suggesting the diagnosis, even over the telephone, will allow the child to reach the hospital rapidly and may prevent an unexpected calamity. The prognosis of epiglottitis is related directly to the speed with which therapy and the precautions against fatal asphyxia are initiated. Once an airway has been established and appropriate antibiotic therapy begun, the clinical response usually is rapid. Progression of the infection usually is controlled in less than 24 hours, and the nasotracheal tube may be removed within the next couple of days.

PREVENTION

Immunization of all children, starting at 2 months of age with the conjugated Hib vaccines, has been the most effective means of preventing *H. influenzae* type b epiglottitis.[12,13] For epiglottitis caused by other organisms, no vaccine or means of prevention is available currently. Conjugated pneumococcal vaccines are being developed for use in young children. Whether such vaccines could affect the occurrence and epidemiological status of epiglottitis, considering the rarity of cases caused by pneumococci, is questionable.

DIFFERENTIAL DIAGNOSIS

The major entities to be distinguished from epiglottitis are viral croup and bacterial tracheitis. The distinguishing features of these diseases are listed in Table 280-1. *Bacterial tracheitis,* in particular, may mimic epiglottitis in its severity and rapid progression and requires equally prompt treatment.[9,10] This unusual entity may affect children of any age. The onset is similar in its acuteness, fever, and toxic condition, but is characterized by respiratory stridor, more severe than that usually observed with viral croup, and the production of copious, purulent sputum. The diagnosis usually is made by direct laryngoscopy, which shows the purulent secretions and an exudate localized to the inflamed subglottic area. The epiglottic and supraglottic structures usually are involved minimally. Roentgenograms of the lateral neck can demonstrate the subglottic narrowing and occasionally even a fibrinous exudate obstructing the airway.[10] The organisms most commonly causing this syndrome are *Staphylococcus aureus* and group A beta-hemolytic streptococci, which usually may be recovered in almost pure culture from the secretions obtained on laryngoscopy.[9,14]

Diphtheria with pharyngolaryngeal involvement may be confused with epiglottitis. However, the slower onset, other signs of diphtheria, and a pharyngeal grayish membrane may help to differentiate the two. Most helpful in the differentiation is the history of inadequate immunizations. Specific diagnosis of diphtheria may be obtained by Gram stained smear and culture of the diphtheritic membrane.

Aspiration of a foreign body should be suspected in a child, usually a toddler, who has a history of acute onset of choking and respiratory distress. Fever is not present early in the course, and the pharynx does not show the "beefy" erythema characteristic of acute bacterial infection. Roentgenograms of the lateral neck will not show the "thumb" sign. Further roentgenographic examination may show the foreign body, if opaque, or endoscopy may be required. In rare cases, thermal injury to the epiglottis has been reported in young children drinking hot beverages, resulting in a clinical picture markedly similar to that of epiglottitis.[16]

REFERENCES

1. Ashcraft CK, Steele RW: Epiglottitis: a pediatric emergency, *J Respir Dis* 9:48, 1988.
2. Bass JW, Steele RW, Weide RA: Acute epiglottitis: a surgical emergency, *JAMA* 229:671, 1974.
3. Battaglia JD, Lockhart CH: Management of acute epiglottitis by nasotracheal intubation, *Am J Dis Child* 129:334, 1975.
4. Berenberg W, Kevy S: Acute epiglottitis in childhood, *N Engl J Med* 258:870, 1958.
5. Black SB et al: Immunization with oligosaccharide conjugate *Haemophilus influenzae* type b (HbOC) vaccine on a large health maintenance organization population: extended follow-up and impact on *Haemophilus influenzae* disease epidemiology, *Pediatr Infect Dis J* 11:610, 1992.
6. Centers for Disease Control: Progress toward elimination of *Haemophilus influenzae* type b disease among infants and children: United States, 1987-1993, *MMWR* 43:144, 1994.
7. Dajani AS, Asmar BI, Thirumoorthi MC: Systemic *Haemophilus influenzae* disease: an overview, *J Pediatr* 94:355, 1979.
8. Daum RS et al: Nosocomial epiglottitis associated with penicillin- and cephalosporin-resistant *Streptococcus pneumoniae* bacteria, *J Clin Microbiol* 32:246, 1994.
9. Davidson S, Yahav BJ, Rubinstein E: Bacterial tracheitis: a true entity? *J Laryngol Otol* 96:173, 1982.
10. Denneny JC, Handler SD: Membranous laryngotracheobronchitis, *Pediatrics* 70:705, 1982.
11. Fulginiti VA: Acute supraglottitis (epiglottitis): to look or not? *Am J Dis Child* 142:597, 1988.
12. Gorelick MH, Baker D: Epiglottitis in children, 1979 through 1992: ef

fects of *Haemophilus influenzae* type b immunization, *Arch Pediatr Adolesc Med* 148:47, 1994.
13. Hoekelman RA: A pediatrician's view: Hib vaccination now! *Pediatr Ann* 19:683, 1990.
14. Jones R, Santos JI, Overall JC Jr: Bacterial tracheitis, *JAMA* 242:721, 1979.
15. Jones RN, Slepack J, Bigelow J: Ampicillin-resistant *Hemophilus paraphrophelus* laryngoepiglottitis, *J Clin Microbiol* 4:405, 1976.
16. Kulick RM et al: Thermal epiglottitis after swallowing hot beverages, *Pediatrics* 81:441, 1988.
17. Margolis CZ, Ingram DL, Meyer JH: Routine tracheotomy in *Haemophilus influenzae* type b epiglottitis, *J Pediatr* 81:1150, 1972.
18. Mauro RD, Poole SR, Lockhart CH: Differentiation of epiglottitis from laryngotracheitis in the child with stridor, *Am J Dis Child* 142:679, 1988.
19. Mayo Smith MF et al: Acute epiglottitis in adults, *N Engl J Med* 314:1133, 1986.
20. Molteni RA: Epiglottitis: incidence of extraepiglottic infection—report on 72 cases and review of the literature, *Pediatrics* 58:526, 1976.
21. Podgore JK, Bass JW: The "thumb sign" and "little finger sign" in acute epiglottitis, *J Pediatr* 88:154, 1976.
22. Rapkin RH: Acute epiglottitis: pitfalls in diagnosis and management, *Clin Pediatr* 10:312, 1971.
23. Robbins JB: *Haemophilus influenzae* type b: disease and immunity in humans, *Ann Intern Med* 78:259, 1973.
24. Schoendorf KC et al: National trends in *Haemophilus influenzae* meningitis mortality and hospitalization among children, 1980 through 1991, *Pediatrics* 93:663, 1994.
25. Todd JK, Bruhn FW: Severe *Haemophilus influenzae* infections, *Am J Dis Child* 129:607, 1975.
26. Weber ML et al: Acute epiglottitis in children: treatment with nasotracheal intubation—report of 14 consecutive cases, *Pediatrics* 57:152, 1976.

281 Esophageal Burns

J. Alex Haller, Jr.

Accidental ingestion of powerful corrosive agents is a much more frequent problem among infants and toddlers than among school-age children and adults. Esophageal burns resulting from ingestion of caustic materials constitute a significant problem, both in immediate management and in subsequent treatment of the serious sequelae of such burns—namely, severe strictures of the esophagus. The ingestion of strong corrosive agents is the most common cause of severe stricture of the midesophagus in infants and young children. Lower esophageal stricture results most commonly from recurrent reflux esophagitis. Although progress has been made in the elimination of dangerous caustic materials from the marketplace, much needs to be done to ensure the packaging of such products in child-safe containers.

The goal of therapy is to minimize esophageal injury and to prevent subsequent strictures that may require complicated and dangerous esophageal substitution operations. The most common form of treatment for caustic injury to the esophagus until 1960 was the Saltzer technique of immediate and continuing esophageal dilation. For more than 2 decades the use of systemic steroids and antibiotics and the avoidance of routine dilation has supplanted the Saltzer technique.[1] Pharmacological treatment decreases inflammation and edema at the burn site and avoids recurrent injury that might result from repeated dilations.

MECHANISMS OF CAUSTIC INJURY

Ingestion of sodium hydroxide is the most common cause of esophageal burns from caustic substances in young children. It is present in toilet bowl, oven, and plumbing cleaners. Recently, liquid cleaners have been added to the list of dangerous agents. Weaker alkaline solutions, such as liquid ammonia, can cause esophageal irritation, but they rarely result in significant tissue damage or strictures. Strong acids are more likely to damage the stomach and small intestine than the esophagus.

Strong alkalis are more common in the child's environment than are strong acids. Clinitest tablets and alkaline disk batteries usually lodge in the esophagus and may lead to esophageal perforation. Oven and drain cleaners usually contain strong alkalis. Bleaches, disinfectants, metal cleansers, and toilet bowl cleansers may be acidic. Household soap, bleaches, and those detergents that are not highly alkaline generally have low toxicity, whereas commercial bleaches may produce caustic burns.[10] Strong alkaline solutions are particularly destructive because they cause *liquefaction necrosis,* which penetrates deeply into the wall of the esophagus and may cause perforation into the mediastinum.[4] The inflammatory reaction that accompanies such burns can cause fibrosis, stricture formation, and mediastinitis. Bacteria can invade the injured tissues and lead to mediastinal abscess and sepsis. Acid burns, on the other hand, produce *coagulation necrosis,* which prevents penetration into the deeper tissues and protects the esophageal wall from further damage.

Animal models of caustic esophageal burns, particularly those in the cat, have demonstrated clearly the pathological changes that occur.[5] In the first week after ingestion of sodium hydroxide, the wall of the esophagus is destroyed to varying degrees, primarily from contact necrosis and secondarily from an intense inflammatory process. The inflammatory reaction extends through the muscle layers and may involve the mediastinum. Over the next week, granulation tissue is formed. By the end of the second to third week, the fibroblasts proliferate, causing early esophageal wall contracture. After 3 to 4 weeks the muscle layer is replaced largely by dense, fibrous tissue, and a pseudoepithelium lines the lumen. Contracture then occurs, leading to severe esophageal stricture. The animals show initial dysphagia, caused by muscle spasm at the injury site and by the intense inflammatory edema. Obstruction of the esophagus may lead to aspiration pneumonia and bacteremia. Antibiotics are used to decrease the risk of pulmonary infection and potential bacterial invasion of the bloodstream through the injured esophageal wall. Steroids significantly diminish the initial inflammation in experimental animals and thereby decrease scar formation.[5,11]

MANAGEMENT

On the basis of animal experiments and clinical experience, a plan of management should include documentation of the caustic agent ingested, identification of the presence and extent of the esophageal burn by means of early direct esophagoscopic examination, immediate institution of steroid and antibiotic therapy, serial evaluation of the esophagus to detect early stricture formation, and immediate and continuing dilation if stricture occurs.[2,3]

HISTORY AND INITIAL PHYSICAL EXAMINATION

Caustic ingestion by infants and young children is either accidental or the result of active (rare) or passive child abuse. The caustic agent is regurgitated immediately; for this reason, gastric lavage is not necessary in the initial management. Usually the caretaker can identify the offending agent. Careful examination of the oral cavity usually reveals areas of edema and superficial burns. Approximately one third of children who have oral burns will have esophageal burns as well. If no oral burn is present but the caustic ingestion is confirmed, a burn of the esophagus, which can occur with or without oral burns, must be assumed until excluded.

ESOPHAGOSCOPIC EXAMINATION

All patients who have oral burns, as well as those in whom caustic ingestion is strongly suspected, should undergo esophagoscopic examination soon after admission to the hospital.[3,5,8] To obviate the danger of perforation during the procedure, the endoscopist should visually examine the oropharynx and upper portion of the esophagus only to the site of the esophageal burn and should not pass the instrument beyond. If an acute esophageal injury is evident, its extent is of no consequence in terms of immediate management, and therapy should be instituted in the hospital. If examination yields negative findings, the patient's care can be managed safely at home.

STEROID THERAPY

Steroid therapy should be instituted within 24 hours because a major inflammatory reaction develops within that period. Steroids must be continued throughout the early phases of injury if the complications associated with the inflammatory reaction are to be prevented. Even in young infants a course of steroid therapy should be given for 3 weeks; with significant burns it should be extended to 4 to 6 weeks. Prospective analyses of long-term outcome in children treated with steroids suggest that very extensive corrosive burns may not respond to steroid therapy.[12]

ANTIBIOTIC THERAPY

Because of the hazards of aspiration pneumonia and mediastinal invasion, especially when steroids are used, prophylactic antibiotic therapy should be instituted. Inasmuch as most of the offending bacteria can be expected to be gram positive organisms, ampicillin is an appropriate drug.

STUDIES OF ESOPHAGEAL FUNCTION

Serial barium swallow studies of the esophagus provide evidence of a developing esophageal stricture. In its presence, steroid therapy should be discontinued and esophageal dilation instituted. Barium swallow studies also help in evaluating the extent of esophageal burn during the healing phase of the injury. Any evidence of difficulties with swallowing after the initial treatment period (3 to 6 weeks) indicates the need for repeated barium swallow studies to identify a late-occurring stricture.

RARE AND SEVERE FORMS OF CAUSTIC INJURY IN INFANTS

With the increased use of strong liquid caustic agents (liquid lye), a severe form of caustic esophageal injury has been reported more frequently. These patients have deep second-degree burns or even full-thickness burns (third degree) and inevitable stricture formation. Reyes and Hill[9] introduced a concept of temporary intraluminal stenting in infants who have such severe burns, and this technique has been extended to older patients with some good results.[7] Reports indicate that a few teenage patients ingested liquid lye to commit suicide. Recent experience suggests that the best survival and long-term rehabilitation of these patients is accomplished if the badly burned esophagus is removed immediately, usually by use of the transhiatal approach, and a cervical esophagostomy is performed.[3,7] Gastric resection also may be necessary. Ultimately, reconstruction must be individualized, including esophageal replacement after 6 to 8 weeks of recovery. Fortunately, these life-threatening caustic injuries are rare in children.

SUMMARY

The immediate establishment of the diagnosis of esophageal injury is mandatory in all infants and young children in whom caustic ingestion is suspected. Early esophagoscopic examination is necessary to document the presence or absence of an acute caustic esophageal burn. Initiation of steroid therapy and antibiotics to decrease the inflammatory response is the only dependable way to prevent late stricture formation. This form of therapy has decreased the incidence of late esophageal stricture significantly. Signs and symptoms of early esophageal stenosis require barium swallow and bougie dilatation.

REFERENCES

1. Buttross S, Bronhard BH: Acute management of alkali ingestion in children: a review, *Tex Med* 77:57, 1981.
2. Cleveland WW et al: The effect of prednisone in the prevention of esophageal stricture following the ingestion of lye, *South Med J* 15:861, 1958.
3. Estrara A et al: Corrosive burns of the esophagus and stomach: a recommendation for an aggressive surgical approach, *Ann Thorac Surg* 41:276, 1986.
4. Haller JA: Caustic burns of the esophagus. In Cameron J, editor: *Current surgical therapy,* ed 3, Toronto, 1989, BC Decker.
5. Haller JA, Bachman K: The comparative effect of current therapy on experimental caustic burns of the esophagus, *Pediatrics* 34:236, 1964.
6. Haller JA et al: Pathophysiology and management of acute corrosive burns of the esophagus: results of treatment in 285 children, *J Pediatr Surg* 6:578, 1971.
7. Meredith JW, Kon ND, Thompson JN: Management of injuries from liquid lye ingestion, *J Trauma* 28:1173, 1988.
8. Mills LJ, Estrera AS, Platt MR: Avoidance of esophageal stricture following severe caustic burns by the use of an intraluminal stent, *Ann Thorac Surg* 28:60, 1979.
9. Reyes HM, Hill JL: Experimental treatment of corrosive esophageal burns, *J Pediatr Surg* 9:317, 1974.
10. Salzer H: Early treatment of corrosive esophagitis, *Klin Wochenschr* 33:307, 1920.
11. Temple AR, Veltri JC: Toxicity of soaps, detergents and caustics. In Rumack BH, Temple AR, editors: *Management of the poisoned patient,* Princeton, NJ, 1977, Science Press.
12. Viscomi GJ, Beekhuis GJ, Whitten CF: Evaluation of early esophagoscopy and corticosteroid therapy in corrosive injury of esophagus, *J Pediatr* 39:356, 1961.

282 Head Injuries

David E. Hall

Head injuries are exceedingly common and a cause for great concern, which leads parents to consult their child's physician more frequently than for other injuries. Of hospitalized patients, about 50% admitted with head injury are under 20 years of age.[15] Boys are injured at least twice as often as girls. Interestingly, left-handed children may be more prone to head injury than right-handed children.[10,22] More than 75% of trauma deaths in children are due to brain injury.[33]

The causes of severe head injury vary with age. In infants, falls and child abuse predominate; in preschool- and school-age children, auto accidents are more common; and in the adolescent years, sports injuries and assault are seen more frequently. For all ages together, falls are the most common cause of head trauma, but auto accidents are the leading cause of serious injury. In most cases the child is a pedestrian. As many as 70% of children hit by an automobile are not supervised by an adult at the time of the accident.[39]

Physicians should be familiar with the initial management of the child who has a severe head injury, but the most common problem faced by the practitioner is distinguishing those patients who require treatment from those who do not. Because these two aspects of care are so different, they are dealt with separately.

INITIAL CARE OF THE SEVERELY INJURED PATIENT

The improved prognosis for survival of the child after a severe head injury compared with an adult,[6,30] plus the potential for organ donation in those patients who are brain dead, dictate that the physician providing emergency care make every effort to resuscitate the child who has a severe head injury.

The level of consciousness is the most important observation in a child who has a head injury. First, determine whether the patient obeys commands, cries, speaks understandably, or opens his or her eyes spontaneously or in response to pain or to speech. If not, do not perform a complete neurological examination; rather, evaluate the airway, breathing, and circulation immediately. The correction of anoxia or poor cerebral perfusion has a far higher priority than detection of an intracranial hematoma.[12,25,38] As Haldane stated in 1919, "Anoxia not only stops the machine but wrecks the machinery."[25] Clear the airway by performing a finger sweep and jaw thrust, but avoid extreme flexion or extension of the neck because the cervical spine also may be injured. Determine the pulse rate and blood pressure and look for signs of shock. Shock is far more common in head injuries than is the Cushing response of hypertension and bradycardia. Examine the chest for signs of a hemothorax and pneumothorax; then check the abdomen for fullness, rigidity, or other signs of a ruptured viscus. The presence of shock almost always means that a serious injury other than to the head exists. Infants are rare exceptions to this rule, because they may lose enough blood intracranially for shock to develop; however, even this is less common than shock from other causes.

Only when certain that the airway, breathing, and circulation are adequate should the examiner proceed to a more detailed neurological evaluation. The Glasgow coma scale (Table 282-1) is convenient for quantitating mental status and is valuable in assessing prognosis and in following the patient's progress later.[5,24,37] It is based on the patient's response in three areas: movement, verbal response, and eye opening.

Evaluate the pupil's response to light. Unilateral dilation of a pupil signifies compression of the ipsilateral third cranial nerve by a herniating temporal lobe or an optic nerve injury. In an unconscious patient the physician must make sure that the tympanic membrane is intact and then test the oculovestibular reflex by elevating the head, neck, and back 30 degrees and injecting 120 ml of ice water into the ear canal. If the eyes develop nystagmus with the fast component away from the side of irrigation, the brainstem is intact from the nucleus of the eighth cranial nerve to the nuclei of the third, fourth, and sixth cranial nerves, which control eye movements. The fifth and seventh cranial nerves should be evaluated by testing the corneal reflexes.

Another method to test brainstem function is to evaluate oculovestibular reflexes with the doll's eye maneuver. Rotate the head briskly to each side. Normally, when the head moves to the right, the eyes move to the left, and vice versa. Loss of doll's eye movements in a comatose patient suggests an injury to the midbrain or pons or very deep coma. Never perform this test until cervical spine trauma has been excluded.

Next, look for bruises, hematomas, or other signs of trauma. Ecchymoses behind the ear (Battle sign) or around the orbits (raccoon sign), cerebrospinal fluid (CSF) rhinorrhea, or bleeding from the ear suggests a basilar skull fracture. Papilledema usually is not present in the acutely injured patient, but retinal hemorrhages may be seen. Computed tomography (CT) scanning and cervical spine films are important for diagnostic purposes but of lower priority than stabilizing the patient.

In addition to ensuring an adequate airway, breathing, and circulation (a large-bore intravenous plastic cannula should be in place), steps to reduce elevated intracranial pressure are important before transferring the patient to a regional center.[12] Excessive stimulation must be avoided. The patient's head, neck, and back should be elevated 30 degrees with the face looking straight ahead to promote venous drainage from the brain. In the absence of shock, fluids should be restricted to two thirds maintenance volumes; 5% dextrose with normal saline solution should be used. The goal is to raise se-

Table 282-1 Glasgow Coma Scale* Modified for Pediatric Patients

Eye-opening response		
Score	> 1 Year	< 1 Year
4	Spontaneous	Spontaneous
3	To verbal command	To shout
2	To pain	To pain
1	None	None

Motor response		
Score	> 1 Year	< 1 Year
6	Obeys commands	Spontaneous response
5	Localizes pain	Localizes pain
4	Withdraws from pain	Withdraws from pain
3	Displays abnormal flexion to pain (decorticate rigidity)	Displays abnormal flexion to pain (decorticate rigidity)
2	Displays abnormal extension to pain (decerebrate rigidity)	Displays abnormal extension to pain (decerebrate rigidity)
1	None	None

Verbal response			
Score	> 5 Years	2 to 5 Years	0-23 Months
5	Is oriented and converses	Uses appropriate words and phrases	Babbles, coos appropriately
4	Conversation is confused	Use inappropriate words	Cries, but is consolable
3	Words are inappropriate	Cries or screams persistently to pain	Cries or screams persistently to pain
2	Sounds are incomprehensible	Grunts or moans to pain	Grunts or moans to pain
1	None	None	None

Adapted from Simon J: Accidental injury and emergency medical services for children. In Behrman RE, editor: *Nelson textbook of pediatrics,* Philadelphia, 1992, WB Saunders.

**Glasgow coma score = sum of best eye opening, motor, and portal response. Range = 3 to 15. Usual definitions of severity of head injury.* Severe = score of < 9; Moderate = score of 9 to 12; Mild = score of 13 to 15.

rum osmolality to about 300 mOsm/kg, but not consistently above 315 mOsm/kg, which may cause renal failure. Hypotonic solutions such as plain 5% dextrose may increase cerebral edema. A decreased P_{CO_2} level lowers cerebral blood volume and thus is very effective in lowering intracranial pressure. Initial bag and mask ventilation with 100% oxygen is effective, but if the patient's condition is deteriorating or if coma is present, an endotracheal tube should be placed. If possible, an anesthesiologist should perform the intubation. The anesthesiologist usually uses thiopental to induce anesthesia, atropine to control secretions and block vagal responses to tube placement, and pancuronium or vercuronium to induce muscle paralysis, along with cricoid pressure to prevent aspiration. These measures help avoid combative behavior and excessive hypercarbia, which further increase intracranial pressure. The usual goal is to maintain P_{CO_2} at 25 to 30 torr.

Evidence of improved outcome with the use of steroids in head trauma is lacking.[17,40] They are useful primarily in increased intracranial pressure caused by a brain tumor or abscess. In a patient whose neurological findings are asymmetrical or whose condition is deteriorating rapidly and one suspects herniation, a mannitol infusion (0.25 to 1 g/kg) may be used. Immediate CT scanning and rapid transfer to the operating room for neurosurgical intervention or to the ICU for increased intracranial pressure management is the current standard in most pediatric trauma centers in this situation.

Computed tomography scanning is the most useful radiological procedure in evaluating the trauma patient. It is faster than magnetic resonance imaging, is less affected by patient motion, and is better for detecting skull fractures. To detect depressed skull fractures on CT scans, ask for bone windows in addition to the usual brain and soft tissue views.

CARE OF THE LESS SEVERELY INJURED PATIENT

Most physicians have little trouble identifying those patients who require intensive care at a regional center. More difficult is making the decision to admit the less severely injured child to the hospital for observation. Information from published studies concerning the indications for such action is scant because most head trauma studies have focused on hospitalized patients only. Evidence to support a decision to hospitalize or not to hospitalize the less severely injured patient therefore is lacking, and each child must be considered individually.

When taking the history, obtain the details of the injury, keeping the possibility of abuse in mind. Children rarely sustain a serious injury when they fall out of bed,[3] so such a history when given as the cause of severe injury is suspect.

Loss of consciousness, seizures, and amnesia of the circumstances surrounding the injury are indicators of more severe head trauma. As mentioned, persistent clouding of consciousness is the most reliable sign of a significant injury. Vomiting and headache are common symptoms after head trauma, and their presence, if not persistent or severe, is not particularly ominous or suggestive of any particular pathological finding.[22] The duration of posttraumatic amnesia (inability to remember ongoing events) repeatedly has been found to correlate with the severity of injury.[39] Diplopia may signify sixth nerve compression caused by increased intracranial pressure.

The physician should check the cranial nerves, use of the extremities, the gait, and coordination and reflexes and look for other injuries or signs of serious injuries such as hemotympanum or CSF rhinorrhea. However, CSF rhinorrhea may *not* be distinguished reliably from garden-variety runny nose with the use of glucose oxidase test sticks.

Much has been written about the overuse of skull roentgenograms; physicians consistently overestimate the frequency of fractures.[20,34] Whether a fracture is present is of less concern than underlying brain injury. The presence of a skull fracture, however, is associated with an increased risk of intracranial abnormalities.[4,11] The risk of a subdural or epidural hematoma is increased two- to threefold in the presence of a skull fracture. However, the absence of a skull fracture does not exclude significant intracranial injury.[18,19]

A depressed skull fracture requires surgical intervention, and a fracture of the parietal bone in the region of the middle meningeal artery may increase the likelihood of an epidural bleed. This is less important in small children because the artery does not lie in a groove on the skull, as in older children and adults.

Skull fractures underlying lacerations are important to detect because they may predispose to meningitis. Basilar skull fractures also increase the risk of meningitis but often do not show up on the radiograph.

Much of the time, the presence of a fracture does not affect treatment or provide prognostic information. With the advent of CT scanning, the isolated skull film has decreased in importance. However, much debate concerns the indications for CT scans in children who have a head injury.[26] Obtaining a CT scan seems prudent when the patient has any degree of obtundation, focal neurological deficits, a history of a high velocity injury, amnesia for the injury, progressive headache, persistent vomiting, serious facial injury, unreliable history of injury, posttraumatic seizure, signs of a basilar skull fracture, or possible skull penetration or is suspected of having been abused.[32] Others would add a Glasgow coma scale of 13 or less or a skull fracture as an indication. Most physicians have lower thresholds for obtaining CT scans in children less than 2 years old.[32,36] Whether a CT scan is indicated is unclear for the patient who has a history of change of consciousness that has resolved. Occasionally, CT scans fail to demonstrate hematomas—usually between 2 to 6 weeks after injury, when the density of the hematoma may equal that of the brain.[16]

Electroencephalograms (EEGs) have little place in the management of acute head trauma. They are neither sensitive nor specific and usually are not available in the emergency room.

Echoencephalography also is of limited diagnostic usefulness in children who have head injuries.

Lumbar punctures are contraindicated unless meningitis is prominent in the differential diagnosis.

Observing the child who has posttraumatic amnesia or loss of consciousness is advisable until the mental status returns to normal. If this does not occur promptly, the child should be admitted to the hospital. Hospitalization also is indicated for patients in whom clear-cut neurological signs, depressed or compound skull fractures, or a suspicion of child abuse or unreliable parents exists. Linear fractures do not mandate admission to the hospital if the child is asymptomatic, but they do require close observation because the force required to fracture a child's skull is significant. A reliable observer at home is required.

One complication of skull fractures in children, albeit rare, is the leptomeningeal cyst, or "growing fracture."[28,42] In this condition a portion of leptomeninges or a porencephalic cyst covered by brain tissue squeezes between the edges of a fracture, especially of those involving the suture line. An enlarging bony defect results, often detectable by palpation. This may resolve with age, but surgical intervention sometimes is necessary.

Some children experience a brief convulsion within minutes after a head injury. Such seizures do not appear to increase the risk of a subsequent seizure disorder. In fact, isolated seizures that occur in the first week probably do not increase the risk of developing seizures later, provided the severity of the injury is taken into account.[2,21] An association, of course, exists between the severity of the injury itself and the development of a subsequent seizure disorder. Seizures that occur after the first week are more likely to recur than are those that occur earlier.[44] Seizures associated with penetrating head injury or intracranial hematomas are more likely to progress to a seizure disorder.[1,27,43] Iron salts and hemoglobin in neural tissue may lead to recurrent seizures by damaging neural cell membranes.[42] An EEG cannot predict which patients will develop a posttraumatic seizure disorder.[23,27] Prophylactic anticonvulsants do not appear to decrease the development of late seizures (those that occur after the first week) or recurrent seizures.[34,44,45] However, phenytoin appears to reduce the development of seizures during the first week. In patients whose intracranial pressure is increased, preventing early seizures is valuable. Therefore many clinicians use phenytoin prophylactically in severe head injury for the first 7 days and then taper it if no seizures develop.[44]

When patients are sent home for observation, the parents should be instructed to watch for drowsiness, vomiting, gait disturbance, or severe headache for the next 2 weeks. Most parents are not reliable observers of pupillary size.

COMPLICATIONS

Even after mild head injuries, children often experience problems such as clinging behavior, irritability, sleep disturbances, hyperactivity, and headaches,[7,13] although how much these symptoms reflect premorbid or concurrent conditions is not certain.[8] Headaches do seem to be more of a problem for mild head injury patients than for "controls" who have other types of injuries.[13] Symptoms are transient and generally resolve within 2 to 8 weeks. Children who have mild traumatic brain injury (Glasgow coma scale 13-15) appear to be indistinguishable from controls at 1 year after injury.[14] Children who have moderate (Glasgow coma scale 9-12) or severe (Glasgow coma scale 3-8) injuries may suffer from multiple physical, cognitive, and psychological difficulties.[31] Costeff et al.[9] investigated 31 children who had severe traumatic brain injury and found that motor skills continued to improve after injury for 3 to 5 years, but cognitive function changed little after 6 to 18 months. Consultation with a psychologist for cognitive testing is helpful in educational planning.[8,29] Patients who have dysarthria may have associated swallowing dysfunction. Anosmia may occur from injury to the olfactory filaments. Basilar skull fractures may be associated with vertigo, tinnitus, and hearing loss.

REFERENCES

1. Alessandro R et al: Computed tomographic scans in post-traumatic epilepsy, *Arch Neurol* 45:42, 1988.
2. Annegers JF et al: Seizures after head trauma: a population study, *Neurology* 30:683, 1980.
3. Bell RS, Loop JW: The utility and futility of radiographic examination for trauma, *N Engl J Med* 284:236, 1971.
4. Bonadio WA, Smith DS, Hillman S: Clinical indicators of intracranial lesion on computed tomographic scan in children with parietal skull fracture, *Am J Dis Child* 143:194, 1989.
5. Braakman R et al: Systemic selection of prognostic features in patients with severe head injury, *Neurosurgery* 6:362, 1980.
6. Bruce DA, Schut L, Bruno LA: Outcome following severe head injuries in children, *J Neurosurg* 48:679, 1978.
7. Casey R, Ludwig S, McCormick MC: Morbidity following minor head trauma in children, *Pediatrics* 78:497, 1986.
8. Chadwick O, Rutter M: Intellectual performance and reading skills after localized head injury in childhood, *J Child Psychol Psychiatry* 22:117, 1981.
9. Costeff H, Groswasser Z, Goldstein R: Long-term follow-up review of 31 children with severe closed head trauma, *J Neurosurg* 73:684, 1990.
10. Craft AW, Shaw DA, Cartlidge NEF: Head injuries in children, *Br Med J* 4:200, 1972.
11. Dacey RG et al: Neurosurgical complications after apparently minor head injury: assessment of risk in a series of 610 patients, *J Neurosurg* 65:203, 1986.
12. Davis RJ, Dean M, Goldberg AL: Head and spinal cord injury. In Rogers MC, editor: *Textbook of pediatric intensive care,* Baltimore, 1987, Williams & Wilkins.
13. Farmer MY et al: Neurobehavioral sequelae of minor head injuries in children, *Pediatr Neurosci* 13:304, 1987.
14. Fay G et al: Mild pediatric traumatic brain injury: a cohort study, *Arch Phys Med Rehabil* 74:895, 1993.
15. Field JH: *Epidemiology of head injuries in England and Wales,* London, 1976, Her Majesty's Stationery Office.
16. French BN, Dublin AB: The value of computerized tomography in the management of 1000 consecutive head injuries, *Surg Neurol* 7:171, 1977.
17. Gudeman SK, Miller JD, Becker DP: Failure of high-dose steroid therapy to influence intracranial pressure in patients with severe head injury, *J Neurosurg* 51:301, 1979.
18. Hahn Y, McLone DG: Risk factors in the outcome of children with minor head injury, *Pediatr Neurosurg* 19:135, 1993.
19. Harwood-Nash DC, Hendrick EB, Hudson AR: The significance of skull fractures in children, *Radiology* 101:151, 1971.
20. Helfer RE, Slovis TL, Black M: Injuries resulting when small children fall out of bed, *Pediatrics* 60:533, 1977.
21. Hendrick EB, Harris L: Post-traumatic epilepsy in children, *J Trauma* 8:547, 1968.
22. Hendrick EB, Harwood-Hash DCF, Hudson AR: Head injuries in children, *Clin Neurosurg* 11:46, 1964.
23. Jennett B: *Epilepsy after non-missile head injuries,* ed 2, London, 1975, William Heinermann.
24. Jennett B, Teasdale G, Braakman R: Predicting outcome in individual patients after severe head injury, *Lancet* 1:1031, 1976.
25. Kalbag RM: Management of head injuries. In Cartilidge NEF, Shaw DA, editors: *Head injury,* London, 1981, WB Saunders.
26. Kaufman B, Dacey R: Acute care management of closed head injury in childhood, *Pediatr Ann* 23:18, 1994.
27. Kollevold T: Immediate and early cerebral seizures after head injuries. IV. *J Oslo City Hosp* 29:35, 1979.
28. Lende RA, Erickson RC: Growing skull fractures of childhood, *J Neurosurg* 19:479, 1961.
29. Levine HS, Bento AL, Grossman RG: *Neurobehavioral consequences of closed head injury,* New York, 1982, Oxford University Press.
30. Luersson T, Klauber M, Marshall L: Outcome from head injury related to patient's age: a longitudinal prospective study of adult and pediatric head injury, *J Neurosurg* 68:409, 1988.
31. Massagli T, Jaffe K: Pediatric traumatic brain injury: prognosis and rehabilitation, *Pediatr Ann* 23:29, 1994.
32. Masters SJ et al: Skull x-ray examinations after head trauma: recommendations by a multidisciplinary panel and validation study, *N Engl J Med* 316:84, 1987.
33. Mayer T et al: Causes of morbidity and mortality in severe pediatric trauma, *JAMA* 245:719, 1981.
34. McQueen JK et al: Low risk of late posttraumatic seizures following severe head injury: implications for clinical trials of prophylaxis, *J Neurol Neurosurg Psychiatry* 46:899, 1983.
35. Phillips LA: A study of the effect of high yield criteria for emergency radiography, Rockville, Md, 1978, HEW publications (FDA) no 78-8009.
36. Pietrzak M, Jagoda A, Brown L: Evaluation of minor head trauma in children younger than 2 years, *Am J Emerg Med* 9:153, 1991.
37. Raimondi AJ, Hirschauer J: Head injury in the infant and toddler, *Childs Brain* 11:12, 1984.
38. Raphaely RC et al: Management of severe pediatric head trauma, *Pediatr Clin North Am* 27:715, 1980.
39. Rutter M et al: A prospective study of children with head injuries, *Psychol Med* 10:633, 1980.
40. Saul TG et al: Steroids in severe head injury: a prospective randomized clinical trial, *J Neurosurg* 54:596, 1981.
41. Simon J: Accidental injury and emergency medical services for children. In Behrman RE, editor: *Nelson textbook of pediatrics,* Philadelphia, 1992, WB Saunders.
42. Taveras JM, Ransohoff J: Leptomeningeal cysts of the brain following trauma with erosion of the skull: a study of seven cases treated by surgery, *J Neurosurg* 10:233, 1953.
43. Willmore L: Post-traumatic epilepsy: cellular mechanisms and implications for treatment, *Epilepsia* 31 (suppl 3):67, 1990.
44. Yablon S: Posttraumatic seizures, *Arch Phys Med Rehabil* 74:983, 1993.
45. Young B et al: Failure of prophylactically administered phenytoin to prevent late posttraumatic seizures, *J Neurosurg* 58:236, 1983.

283 Heart Failure

Bradley B. Keller

The infant or child in heart failure presents a diagnostic and therapeutic challenge to the practitioner. The signs and symptoms of heart failure can occur at any age, even before birth. Heart failure during the first year of life usually occurs as a consequence of congenital or acquired heart disease. Heart failure is the result of specific anatomical, physiological, or metabolic abnormalities, and therapy is directed toward treating the primary cause, as well as toward restoring adequate circulatory function.

DEFINITION

Heart failure is defined as the inability of the heart to meet the circulatory demands of the body. Four factors determine cardiovascular function: heart rate, contractility, preload, and afterload. Thus cardiac pump function depends on both normal filling (diastolic mechanisms) and ejection (systolic mechanisms). If cardiac output decreases below metabolic needs, compensatory mechanisms acutely increase heart rate, sympathetic tone, and circulating blood volume to improve nutrient delivery.

Presenting signs and symptoms depend on the time course and severity of heart failure and reflect circulatory compensatory mechanisms (see the box on p. 1714). Decreased cardiac output produces secondary fluid accumulation in the pulmonary and systemic circulations. The infant heart failure often has a history of diaphoresis, poor feeding, and slow weight gain. Tachypnea and tachycardia are present on examination. Pulmonary vascular congestion results in rales, rhonchi, wheezes, and in premature infants, apnea. Periorbital and peripheral edema reflect systemic venous congestion.

ETIOLOGY

The primary cause of heart failure in most patients can be determined from the physical examination and noninvasive studies (see the box on p. 1714). Heart failure as a result of *pulmonary overcirculation,* which causes pulmonary vascular congestion and pulmonary edema, may result in hypoxemia.

Heart failure can occur as the result of *pump dysfunction* of the right or left ventricle. Passive congestion of the systemic and pulmonary veins results as blood backs up behind the failing ventricle. Cardiac chamber hypoplasia or hypertrophy causes impaired filling and decreases forward output. Primary or secondary tachyarrhythmias reduce ventricular filling and ejection times, further decreasing stroke volume.

Heart failure may be due to pulmonary or systemic *vascular obstruction.* Chronically elevated pulmonary vascular resistance produces right-sided heart failure in some infants who have bronchopulmonary dysplasia. Acute or chronic systemic hypertension likewise can precipitate left-sided heart failure. Pulmonary or aortic valvar stenosis or coarctation of the aorta can cause heart failure.

Heart failure, which can result from intravascular *fluid overload* during renal failure, also can be caused by iatrogenic fluid overload during vigorous intravenous hydration.

INITIAL ASSESSMENT AND STABILIZATION

The diagnosis of heart failure begins with a history and physical examination. Assessment may include use of a chest radiograph, an electrocardiogram, pulse oximetry or arterial blood gas sample, and an echocardiogram. Initial therapy maximizes perfusion to vital organs, which limits organ damage from hypoxia and acidosis (Table 283-1). Volume overload is treated with diuretics, and depressed contractility is treated with digoxin or inotropic agents. The treatment of congestive heart failure with respiratory distress includes intubation and ventilation and prompt intravenous or intraosseous drug delivery.

Therapy for heart failure must be individualized. In patients whose acidosis and circulatory insufficiency is profound, acid-base status must be normalized before inotropic agents can be effective. Prompt management of arrhythmia is essential.

DIAGNOSTIC TESTS AND CARDIOLOGY REFERRAL

Medical management includes the immediate care begun by the pediatrician and the diagnostic and therapeutic plan coordinated by the pediatric cardiologist. To initiate definitive therapy the specific cause of heart failure must be identified soon after patient stabilization. The physical examination is supplemented by means of electrocardiography, echocardiography, and in certain cases, cardiac catheterization to yield a definitive diagnosis. Muscle biopsy and genetic analysis—separately and in conjunction—now are providing definitive diagnoses for several pathogenetic categories of congenital cardiovascular malformations, including several primary diseases of the myocardium.

IATROGENIC DANGERS

Careful attention to drug dosage and delivery is critical in the management of acute heart failure. Monitoring patient response to therapy and reappraising the diagnosis and therapeutic plan continually are essential. Heart failure is the final common pathway of many conditions, and an encouraging early response to therapy is not necessarily predictive of long-term survival.

Table 283-1 Initial Therapy in Heart Failure

Therapy	Route	Dosage	Onset of action
Oxygen	Nasal, endotracheal tube	40%-100%	Immediate
Furosemide	IV, PO	1-2 mg/kg	15-30 min
Digoxin	IV, PO	5-10 μg/kg	5-30 min
Dopamine	IV	5-20 μg/kg/min	Immediate
Dobutamine	IV	5-20 μg/kg/min	Immediate

PRESENTING SYMPTOMS AND SIGNS OF HEART FAILURE

Diaphoresis	Tachypnea
Poor feeding	Tachycardia, gallop rhythm
Failure to thrive	Murmur
Apnea	Rales, rhonchi, wheezes
Peripheral edema	Hepatomegaly

COMMON CAUSES OF HEART FAILURE: DIFFERENTIAL DIAGNOSIS

Pulmonary overcirculation

Ventricular septal defect
Patent ductus arteriosus
Transposition of the great arteries
Truncus arteriosus

Vascular obstruction

Coarctation of the aorta
Aortic valve stenosis
Pulmonary valve stenosis
Pericardial tamponade

Decreased pump function

Hypoplastic ventricle
Cardiomyopathy, carditis
Prolonged tachycardia
Sepsis

Fluid overload

Renal failure
Anemia
Overhydration

SECONDARY NEEDS

Good nutrition with a low-salt, maximum-calorie diet is important. The need to restrict total daily fluid volume is rare; to do so usually limits calories. Small, frequent feedings may be necessary in patients whose tachypnea and fatigue are persistent. The prompt treatment of infections and maintenance of normal body temperature help to limit metabolic requirements.

PLANNING FOR CONVALESCENCE AND REHABILITATION

Home health care, if needed, must be available at discharge. Financial support to help offset uncovered medical expenses can be sought from state and local programs for physically handicapped children. Emotional support for patients and their families is available through social services, family support groups, religious affiliations, and daily interactions with the members of the multidisciplinary care team.

For some children the cause of heart failure is not amenable to medical or surgical management. A long-term medical management plan, which may include cardiac transplantation, should be discussed with the family.

CARDIAC CARE SYSTEM

Care for the infant or child who has an acute, life-threatening illness requires the services of a multidisciplinary team. Management of the acute problem is followed by the careful diagnosis of related disorders, and therapy is directed toward prompt discharge home or to a referring hospital. The referring pediatrician remains an integral part of the child's coordinated care and serves as a resource for following the child's recovery and convalescence. Follow-up with pediatric cardiology appointments supplements routine pediatric care and permits individualizing the patient's care. Home health care may be required to assist in the continued use of diuretics, digoxin, oxygen, and other medications after the acute-management phase of heart failure.

SUGGESTED READINGS

Amidon TM, Parmley WW: Is there a role for positive inotropic agents in congestive heart failure: focus on mortality, *Clin Cardiol* 17:641, 1994.

Dreyer WJ: Congestive heart failure. In Garson A Jr, Bricker JT, McNamara DG, editors: *The science and practice of pediatric cardiology,* ed 1, vol III, Philadelphia, 1990, Lea & Febiger.

Friedman FW, George BL: Treatment of congestive heart failure by altering loading conditions of the heart, *J Pediatr* 106:697, 1985.

Talner NS: Heart failure. In Emmanouilides GC et al, editors: *Moss and Adams' heart disease in infants, children, and adolescents, including the fetus and young adult,* ed 5, Baltimore, 1995, Williams & Wilkins.

284 Hypertensive Emergencies

Glenn H. Bock

Although acute hypertensive emergencies are relatively infrequent in the pediatric population, their full clinical manifestations represent potential life-threatening events demanding prompt identification, evaluation, and treatment. Malignant hypertension most commonly is considered to manifest as some degree of central nervous system dysfunction. However, important end organ insults associated with hypertensive crises, in addition to encephalopathy, may include cardiac failure, renal failure, or vascular endothelial injury and consequent disseminated intravascular coagulation. The timeliness and effectiveness of intervention depend to a great extent on the practitioner's familiarity with the spectrum of potential clinical symptoms and the ability to provide rapid but controlled reduction of blood pressure.

ETIOLOGY

Acute hypertension in children and adolescents almost always is due to an identifiable secondary cause rather than the result of an acute exacerbation of primary hypertension. The probability of secondary hypertension in the pediatric population increases with younger age and the magnitude of the blood pressure elevation. The box on page 1718 lists some of the more common secondary causes that may be associated with acute hypertension in pediatric-age patients. Although the list is not all-inclusive, renal parenchymal diseases, renovascular abnormalities, and coarctation of the aorta compose approximately 93% of the reported secondary causes of hypertension among children. Initial consideration of these three conditions allows the practitioner to focus the hypertensive workup, thereby limiting unnecessary invasive and uncomfortable tests. Important clues to the majority of the remaining diagnoses often can be obtained by history or physical findings. The box on p. 1718 lists some useful initial screening information that can be obtained rapidly during the initial assessment of the acutely hypertensive patient. The more uncommon causes of acute hypertension should be sought only if the initial history and physical examination strongly suggest their presence or after the three most common causes have been ruled out.

HISTORY AND PHYSICAL FINDINGS

Blood pressure may acutely rise to a high level de novo or as a process superimposed on an underlying hypertensive disorder. In either event the clinical manifestations of acute hypertension usually result from neurological or cardiovascular system perturbations, or both, although chronically hypertensive children may be relatively more tolerant of higher pressures. The neurological symptoms are the result of failure of arteriolar blood pressure autoregulation in the brain, with consequent hypertensive encephalopathy. Symptoms of hypertensive encephalopathy include headache, anxiety, restlessness, dizziness, blurred vision, diplopia, nausea, and vomiting. Later, mental confusion, changing levels of consciousness, cranial nerve palsies, and convulsions can occur. Hypertensive encephalopathy should be considered in patients whose convulsions are unexplained. Papilledema and vascular changes in the ocular fundus (Keith-Wagner classification) are much less common in hypertensive children than in adults.

Congestive heart failure can be the predominant manifestation in some patients, particularly neonates and children who have underlying heart disease. Cardiac dysfunction is the net result of a number of factors, including increased peripheral vascular resistance and reduced left ventricular function. Underlying chronic hypertension may contribute to ventricular dysfunction as the result of chronic myocardial hypertrophy. Consideration of the diagnosis of acute hypertension is particularly difficult in neonates and infants, in whom the clinical signs tend to be vague and nonspecific. In these groups, severe hypertension may manifest only as irritability, poor feeding, poor sleeping, restlessness, or vomiting. The diagnosis in these age groups is complicated further by the technical difficulties inherent in accurate blood pressure measurement. A greater awareness by the practitioner is necessary to prevent overlooking this diagnostic possibility.

LABORATORY FINDINGS

The initial basic laboratory tests useful in the evaluation of a pediatric patient who has acute hypertension are a urinalysis (including a carefully performed microscopic examination of the centrifuged urinary sediment), a urine culture, and a study of blood urea nitrogen and creatinine, and of plasma renin and aldosterone. In patients in whom pheochromocytoma is suspected, a plasma or urine catecholamine quantitation or both should be done. If an acquired glomerulonephritis is suspected, serum complement and streptococcal antibody titers should be obtained. Adolescents who have acute hypertension should have urine tests for illicit drug use. Performing thyroid, adrenal, or other endocrine tests is unnecessary unless the patient has multisystem complaints to suggest such diagnoses.

Radiographic imaging studies are very useful in the assessment of possible renal causes of acute hypertension. Renal radionuclide scans (MAG-3 or DTPA) and ultrasound allow noninvasive assessment of kidney number, size, location, relative blood flow, and function. High-quality nuclear and sonographic pediatric studies usually are readily available at most tertiary medical institutions. The kidneys of patients who have acutely acquired glomerulonephritis may be swollen in size and may have abnormal echogenicity. In renal ar-

Table 284-1 Antihypertensive Drugs for Parenteral or Sublingual Administration in Hypertensive Emergencies in Pediatric Patients

Drug	Route	Dosage	Onset	Peak
Sodium nitroprusside*	IV infusion	0.5 μg/kg/min titrated to a maximum of 10 μg/kg/min	Within 30 sec	—
Diazoxide*	IV bolus injection	1-3 mg/kg repeated q5-15 min until BP controlled (minibolus)	1-5 min	1-5 min
Hydralazine	30 min IV infusion or IM	0.15-0.2 mg/kg q6hr	10-20 min	10-90 min
Nifedipine	Sublingual	0.25 mg/kg/dose q4-6hr	10-15 min	60-90 min
Labetalol*	IV infusion	0.5 mg/kg over 2 min. For nonresponse, double dose and repeat every 10 min to a maximum cumulative dose of 5 mg/kg	2-5 min	5-15 min
Phentolamine	IV bolus injection	0.05-0.1 mg/kg	Within 30 sec	2 min

*Manufacturer's warning: safety in children not established.
†*sx,* Symptoms; *Max,* maximum; *BP,* blood pressure; *D/C,* discontinue; D_5W, 5% dextrose in water; *VMA,* vanillylmandelic acid.
‡Vasodilation symptoms include seating, flushing, feelings of warmth, orthostatic hypotension, tachycardia, palpitations, nausea, and vomiting.
§Neurological symptoms include headache, blurred vision, dizziness, and light-headedness.

tery stenosis, the involved kidney often is smaller and has a delay in the blood flow and excretory phases compared with the uninvolved kidney. Currently attracting much interest is radionuclide renal scanning in a patient after a brief course of angiotensin II-converting enzyme inhibitor to diagnose, more sensitively, a critical degree of renal artery stenosis. In this circumstance, the scan done after the converting enzyme inhibitor often shows poorer function on the involved side compared with the function of the same kidney scan done before administering the converting enzyme inhibitor. When these screening tests are abnormal or if the plasma renin value is elevated significantly in the absence of dehydration or any medication that could raise renin directly, a renal angiogram and renal vein renin measurement should be performed. As mentioned in Chapter 235, Obstructive Uropathy and Vesicoureteral Reflux, imaging studies are important in differentiating the various obstructive conditions of the kidney, many of which can produce hypertension. They also are important in the investigation of renal tumors. Physical findings that suggest a coarctation of the aorta should be evaluated by echocardiography, cardiac catheterization, or both.

TREATMENT

Immediate control of blood pressure in a child who has accelerated or malignant hypertension should take precedence over determination of the precise cause. Complicated diagnostic tests, which often require transportation to various departments in the hospital, should be delayed until the practitioner believes that the blood pressure is controlled. Blood pressure control is not the same as blood pressure normalization (see below). Intravenous access should be established immediately in these patients. The general approach to the severely hypertensive child whose airway is compromised or who has convulsive complications for the most part is to use conventional treatment for these problems. The two most important considerations in the initial management of acute hypertension are the chronicity of the blood pressure elevation and the clinical circumstances. The child who has had his or her blood pressure elevated chronically may have minimal hypertensive symptoms but may suffer adverse effects if the blood pressure is suddenly reduced. In contrast, the child who has a true acute blood pressure elevation would be expected to benefit from rapid blood pressure control. Often in an emergency, whether the blood pressure elevation is acute or more chronic is unclear. Therefore the rapid reduction of blood pressure to normal levels generally is not advisable un-

Duration	Adverse effects	Relative contraindications	Comments
Length of infusion	Nausea, vomiting; vasodilation sx†‡; neurological sx§; apprehension, restlessness	Hepatic insufficiency	Solution good for 24 hr; photosensitive (wrap in foil); monitor blood thiocyanate if used longer than 72 hr (D/C for thiocyanate level greater than 10 mg/dl); tachyphylaxis and metabolic acidosis—early cyanide poisoning
Variable; usually <12 hr	Arrhythmias; hyperglycemia; sodium and water retention; vasodilation sx‡; neurological sx§	Thiazide sensitivity; severe tachycardia; diabetes; coarctation	Ineffective in pheochromocytoma; give diuretics to decrease sodium; hyperproteinemia potentiates effects
3-6 hr	Headache; nausea, vomiting; tachycardia, palpitation	Hypersensitivity to hydralazine ("hyperdynamic syndrome")	Undergoes color change in most infusion fluids, which does not indicate loss of potency
Variable; usually 2-3 hr	Headache; palpitations; flushing	Concomitant use of beta-blocking drugs; cimetidine	Dose can be drawn from the 10 mg capsule with a 1 ml syringe and then squirted sublingually
Variable; usually 2-4 hr	Neurological sx†§; bronchospasm; tingling scalp	Jaundice or hepatic dysfunction; pheochromocytoma; asthma; diabetes	Keep supine for 3 hr after administration; ambulate gradually
15-30 min	Tachycardia; arrhythmias; marked hypotension	None	Specific for pheochromocytoma

til a better understanding of the patient's overall condition can be achieved, because rapid normalization may result in acute ischemic organ damage, commonly in kidney and brain tissue. In such cases, the reduction of blood pressure by approximately 25% to 30% usually is well tolerated, regardless of the duration of the elevation. Despite the admonition about diagnostic testing interfering with acute therapeutic intervention, some etiological possibilities should be considered because some medications may be contraindicated in certain conditions. For example, methyldopa should not be used in a child in whom pheochromocytoma is suspected. Severe acute hypertension most often is treated with parenteral therapy so that blood pressure control can be rapid and predictable. Although effective in severe (preencephalopathic) hypertension, some reports suggest that drugs such as nifedipine, hydralazine, and nitroprusside should not be used acutely in hypertensive encephalopathy because these may cause cerebral vasodilatation. Medications that can be titrated to the patient's response are preferred, provided the practitioner has the means to monitor the blood pressure response closely on a continuous basis. Some of the more effective medications for acute blood pressure control are given in Table 284-1. Oral medications should be substituted for parenteral agents as soon as practical. With the determination of cause, the medication that is most specific for the altered pathophysiological condition that is producing hypertension is preferred. In renovascular hypertension, revision or bypass of the renovascular lesion is preferred to long-term medical therapy or nephrectomy. Consultation with a pediatric nephrologist, cardiologist, or vascular surgeon is important in defining a therapeutic plan to serve best the patient's long-term interests.

PROGNOSIS

The immediate prognosis of the child who has acute hypertension depends on the rapidity of recognizing the problem and on blood pressure control. Failure to control blood pressure may result in residual neurological abnormalities such as seizure disorders, cranial nerve palsies, hemiplegia, or blindness. The long-term prognosis depends, for the most part, on the underlying cause. Some causes, such as acute poststreptococcal glomerulonephritis, may resolve spontaneously so that the hypertension eventually remits and does not recur. Other causes, such as hypertension associated with chronic glomerulonephritis, may be controlled via continued medication. Regardless, the longevity of the patient and the subsequent development of end-organ damage, such as hypertensive cardiomyopathy, stroke, and so on, are directly related to the adequacy of long-term blood pressure control.

SUGGESTED READINGS

Bertel O, Conel LD: Treatment of hypertensive emergencies with the calcium channel blocker nifedipine, *Am J Med* 79:31, 1985.

Cressman MD et al: Intravenous labetalol in the management of severe hypertension and hypertensive emergencies, *Am Heart J* 107:980, 1984.

SCREENING ELEMENTS OF THE HISTORY AND PHYSICAL EXAMINATION IN THE ASSESSMENT OF SEVERE HYPERTENSION IN CHILDREN

Present or past medical history of:	Suggests
• Headache, visual disturbance, irritability, abdominal pain (in young child)	Malignant or accelerated hypertension
• Drug use	Drug-induced hypertension
• Umbilical artery catheter	Renovascular hypertension
• Sore throat	Glomerulonephritis
• Recurrent cough, shortness of breath	Preexisting congestive heart failure, pulmonary edema
• Weight loss or gain	Hyperthyroidism, pheochromocytoma, Cushing syndrome, congestive heart failure, renal failure, nephrosis
• Palpitations, flushing, diarrhea	Hyperthyroidism, pheochromocytoma
• Bloody diarrhea	Hemolytic-uremic syndrome
• Purpuric-petechial rash	Vasculitis syndrome
Physical findings of	
• Thin general appearance	Hyperthyroidism, pheochromocytoma
• Obese general appearance (truncal)	Cushing syndrome
• Blood pressure normal or much lower in lower extremity than upper extremity	Aortic coarctation
• Edema	Congestive heart failure, renal failure, nephrosis
• Skin ash-leaf spots	Tuberous sclerosis
café-au-lait spots	Neurofibromatosis
rash	Vasculitis
pyoderma	Glomerulonephritis
• HEENT rounded (moon) facies	Cushing syndrome
proptosis, goiter	Hyperthyroidism
papilledema	Intracranial mass or hemorrhage
• Heart cardiomegaly	Congestive heart failure or long-standing hypertension
murmur	Aortic coarctation
• Abdomen mass involving flank(s)	Tumor (Wilms, neuroblastoma) obstructive uropathy, polycystic kidney disease
bruit	Renal artery stenosis
• Ambiguous genitalia	Virilizing adrenal hyperplasia

Dillon MJ: Investigation and management of hypertension in children, *Pediatr Nephrol* 1:59, 1987.

Evans J et al: Sublingual nifedipine in acute severe hypertension, *Arch Dis Child* 63:975, 1988.

Guignard JP, Gouyon JB, Adelman RD: Arterial hypertension in the newborn infant, *Biol Neonate* 55:77, 1989.

Ruley EJ: Hypertensive emergencies in infants and children. In Ayres SM et al, editors: *Textbook of critical care,* ed 3, Philadelphia, 1995, WB Saunders.

Sigler R, Brewer E: Effect of sublingual or oral nifedipine in the treatment of hypertension, *J Pediatr* 112:811, 1988.

Turner ME: What's new in the antihypertensive armamentarium? *Pediatr Ann* 18:579, 1989.

285 Hypoglycemia

Maurice D. Kogut

Hypoglycemia occurs uncommonly after the first week of life; however, its diagnosis is essential because low blood glucose levels that persist or recur may have catastrophic effects on the brain, particularly in infants. Accordingly, the primary care physician must recognize the clinical symptoms associated with hypoglycemia, document the low blood glucose level, and treat appropriately with glucose. Further, delineating the cause of the hypoglycemia is necessary so that effective continuing treatment can be initiated.

DEFINITION

A child who has a serum or plasma glucose concentration less than 40 mg/dl or a whole blood glucose concentration less than 35 mg/dl, measured by a method specific for glucose, should be investigated and treated for hypoglycemia[14]; those who have plasma glucose concentrations between 40 and 50 mg/dl should be followed up carefully.[14] If hypoglycemia is suspected, the blood glucose level may be approximated quickly by using Dextrostix or Chemstrip bG and later confirmed by an appropriate chemical laboratory test.

CLINICAL MANIFESTATIONS

The clinical findings in hypoglycemia are those caused mainly by cerebral dysfunction and adrenergic discharge. Incoordination of eye movements, strabismus, excessive irritability, motor incoordination, and convulsions may occur after 1 month of age. In the older child, pallor, tachycardia, sweating, limpness, inattention, staring, listlessness, hunger, abdominal pain, ataxia, stupor, coma, and convulsions are frequent findings.

IMMEDIATE MANAGEMENT

In the child in whom hypoglycemia is suspected, a diagnostic blood sample for glucose, insulin, growth hormone (GH), cortisol, ketone bodies, lactic acid, and amino acids must be obtained at the time of hypoglycemia and before the low blood glucose has been corrected.[1,7] This point is absolutely critical because the cause of hypoglycemia cannot be elucidated by measurement of blood glucose alone, and these measurements rapidly provide important information concerning cause. If available blood volume is a limiting factor, judgment must be used in ranking the importance of these tests. At the very least, the blood glucose and insulin levels should be measured. Urinary ketones, as well as specific tests for urinary glucose and nonglucose-reducing substances, also should be determined. If ketones are present, the urine should be tested further for presence of amino and organic acids.

With the exception of those clinical conditions associated with hyperinsulinism (see box on p. 1720), the administration of glucagon has limited therapeutic value in the treatment of hypoglycemia.[7] For diagnostic purposes, however, the administration of glucagon can be useful; a glycemic response to glucagon strongly suggests hyperinsulinism.[7]

Once these essential diagnostic blood samples are obtained, the child should immediately receive an intravenously administered bolus of 10% to 25% glucose to alleviate acute symptoms. Intravenous fluids containing appropriate electrolytes and glucose then should be given at a rate sufficient to maintain plasma or serum glucose levels above 50 mg/dl. The blood glucose level should be monitored every 2 to 4 hours, and the rate of glucose administered should be adjusted accordingly. Urine also is monitored to detect glycosuria, which can produce osmotic diuresis.

Preparation should be made to hospitalize the child to initiate the diagnostic evaluation. During transport to the hospital, personnel experienced in intravenous techniques and Dextrostix or Chemstrip bG determinations must ensure that adequate amounts of glucose are infused continuously. The previously obtained diagnostic blood samples should be sent with the patient to the hospital. The patient who has hypoglycemia should be under the combined care of a pediatric specialist and the child's primary physician.

ETIOLOGY

The blood glucose level is the final balance between hepatic glucose production and peripheral glucose use. An adequate fasting blood glucose concentration depends on sufficient amounts of endogenous nonglucose precursors (e.g., alanine, lactate, and glycerol), effective hepatic enzyme pathways for gluconeogenesis and glycogenolysis, and normal hormonal activities (insulin, growth hormone, cortisol, glucagon, and epinephrine) for the mobilization of substrates and the regulation of these processes.

Many healthy infants and young children, in contrast to adults, cannot maintain normoglycemia during a 24-hour fast.[5,15] The glycogen stores of healthy infants are sufficient only to meet glucose requirements for 8 to 12 hours in the absence of caloric intake,[26] so after 24 to 36 hours of fasting the young child depends totally on gluconeogenesis for glucose production.[21]

Because of diminished protein and fat stores, healthy infants and young children during caloric deprivation may not be able to satisfy the glucose requirements of brain and other tissue and still maintain normal blood glucose levels, because of the limited amounts of these substrates for glucose production. Hence, the physician caring for a child requiring surgery or other procedures accompanied by fasting must prevent hypoglycemia by ensuring that extended fasting is avoided, administering parenteral glucose before and after surgery, and monitoring the blood glucose level.

CAUSES OF HYPOGLYCEMIA IN CHILDHOOD

Hyperinsulinism

Islet cell dysplasia (functional beta-cell secretory disorder)
Islet cell adenoma
Adenomatosis
Beckwith-Wiedemann syndrome

Hereditary defects in carbohydrate metabolism
Glycogen storage diseases

Glucose-6-phosphatase deficiency, types Ia, Ib
Amylo-1,6-glucosidase deficiency, type III
Defects of liver phosphorylase enzyme system

Enzyme deficiencies of gluconeogenesis

Fructose-1,6-diphosphatase (FDPase)
Phosphoenolpyruvate carboxykinase
Pyruvate carboxylase

Other enzyme defects

Galactose-1-phosphate uridyltransferase (galactosemia)
Fructose-1-phosphate aldolase (hereditary fructose intolerance)
Glycogen synthetase

Hereditary defects in amino acid and organic acid metabolism

Maple syrup urine disease
Propionic acidemia
Methylmalonic aciduria
Tyrosinosis
3-Hydroxy-3-methylglutaric aciduria
Glutaric aciduria, type II

Hereditary defects in fat metabolism

Systemic carnitine deficiency
Carnitine palmitoyl transferase deficiency
Long- and medium-chain acyl-CoA dehydrogenase deficiencies

Hormone deficiencies

Congenital hypopituitarism or hypothalamic abnormality
Growth hormone
Cortisol
Adrenocorticotropic hormone (ACTH)
ACTH unresponsiveness
Glucagon
Thyroid hormone
Catecholamine

Ketotic hypoglycemia
Nonpancreatic tumors

Mesenchymal tumors
Epithelial tumors
Hepatoma
Adrenocortical carcinoma
Wilms tumor
Neuroblastoma

Poisoning or toxins

Salicylate
Alcohol
Propranolol
Oral hypoglycemic agents (e.g., sulfonylureas)
Insulin
Unripe ackees (hypoglycin) (Jamaican vomiting sickness)
Pentamidine

Liver disease

Hepatitis, cirrhosis
Reye syndrome

Other causes

Malnutrition
Malabsorption
Chronic diarrhea
Cyanotic congenital heart disease
Postsurgery

Modified from Cornblath MD, Schwartz R: *Disorders of carbohydrate metabolism in infancy,* ed 2, Philadelphia, 1976, WB Saunders. Originally from Kogut MD: Hypoglycemia: pathogenesis, diagnosis, and treatment. In Gluck L et al, editors: *Current problems in pediatrics,* Chicago, 1974, Mosby; and Kogut MD: Neonatal hypoglycemia: a new look. In Moss AJ, editor: *Pediatrics update: review for physicians,* New York, 1980, Elsevier.

CLINICAL APPROACH

Hypoglycemia in the child is not a disease; rather, it reflects failure of one or more factors that regulate the concentration of glucose in the blood. These may be classified as in the box above. Clinical clues enable the physician to plan a logical approach to the diagnostic evaluation of a patient who has hypoglycemia. The age at onset of hypoglycemia is important. The inborn errors of carbohydrate, amino acid, organic acid metabolism, and hormonal deficiencies become apparent during the first 2 years of life.[8] Hyperinsulinism has two peak times of onset: during the first year of life and after age 3 years.[8,17] The most likely cause of hypoglycemia that has its onset after 1 year of age is ketotic hypoglycemia.[8,19] In toddlers, hypoglycemia may result from ingestion of alcohol, aspirin, and other drugs (see the box above). Hypoglycemia is rare after age 5 years.[7]

A history of other affected family members or the occurrence of unexplained infant deaths among close relatives suggests the possibility of one of the inherited metabolic disorders. Some disorders associated with hormonal deficiencies[18] and hyperinsulinism[30] also may be familial. The physician should inquire carefully about the frequency of hypoglycemic episodes, the possibility of drug ingestion, and unfortunately, the malicious administration of drugs.[1,7] The temporal relation of symptoms to food intake is very important in assessing hypoglycemia. In hereditary defects of amino acid and organic acid metabolism, hypoglycemic symptoms may occur shortly after the ingestion of protein.[17] Symptoms that

Table 285-1 Hypoglycemia in Infancy and Childhood

	Inborn metabolic errors of carbohydrate and amino acids	Hormone deficiency	Hyperinsulinism
Family history	+*	Variable	Variable
Hypoglycemia			
Fasting	GSD, fructose-1,6-diphosphatase deficiency	+	+
After lactose	Galactosemia	−	−
After sucrose	Hereditary fructose intolerance	−	−
After protein	Amino acids, organic acids	−	Variable
Hepatomegaly	+	Variable	−
Ketosis	+	Variable	−
Acidosis	+	−	−
Tests	Glucose, glucagon, galactose, fructose tolerance tests; amino acids, gas chromatography	Blood growth hormone, cortisol; stimulation tests	Random blood glucose and immunoreactive insulin; leucine tolerance test
Liver biopsy (enzymes)	Diagnostic for carbohydrate errors (not for galactosemia; use red blood cells)	Not indicated	Not indicated
White blood cells, fibroblasts (enzymes)	Amino acids, organic acids		
Treatment	Specific	Specific	Diazoxide; somatostatin analog; partial excision of the pancreas

Modified from Cornblath MD, Schwartz R: *Disorders of carbohydrate metabolism in infancy,* ed 2, Philadelphia, 1976, WB Saunders. Originally from Kogut MD: Hypoglycemia: pathogenesis, diagnosis and treatment. In Gluck L et al, editors: *Current problems in pediatrics,* Chicago, 1974, Mosby; and Kogut MD: Neonatal hypoglycemia: a new look. In Moss AJ, editor: *Pediatrics update: review for physicians,* New York, 1980, Elsevier.

*+, Present; −, absent; *GSD,* glycogen storage diseases, types I, III, and defects of liver phosphorylase enzyme system.

occur after the ingestion of lactose suggest galactosemia; those after sucrose ingestion suggest hereditary fructose intolerance (HFI).[17] In contrast, fasting hypoglycemia is characteristic of ketotic hypoglycemia, hormonal deficiencies, hyperinsulinism, glycogen storage diseases (GSD), and fructose-1,6-diphosphatase (FDPase) deficiency[17] (Table 285-1).

Metabolic acidosis, ketonemia, or hepatomegaly in association with hypoglycemia strongly suggests the presence of *an inborn error of metabolism* of carbohydrate, amino acid, or organic acid[17] (see Chapter 20, The Recognition of Genetic–Metabolic Diseases by Clinical Diagnosis and Screening). Hypotonia and hyperammonemia also may be present in infants who have defects in organic acid and amino acid metabolism. The presence of nonglucose-reducing substances in the urine may indicate galactosemia or HFI. Nonketotic hypoglycemia in patients who have hepatomegaly, with or without metabolic acidosis, suggests 3-hydroxy-3-methylglutaric aciduria,[25] glutaric aciduria type II,[10] systemic carnitine deficiency,[32] carnitine palmitoyl transferase deficiency,[3] or long- and medium-chain acyl-CoA dehydrogenase deficiencies.[14] In contrast, hepatomegaly, ketonuria, and metabolic acidosis are usually absent in hypoglycemia accompanied by hyperinsulinism.[18] Although ketosis may be present in some hypoglycemic patients who have hypopituitarism[22] and ACTH unresponsiveness,[16] the findings of ketonuria and hypoglycemia without hepatomegaly among small and underweight males after 1 year of age suggest ketotic hypoglycemia.[8,17,19]

Because children who have an inborn error of metabolism may manifest a Reye syndrome–like illness, the physician must be alert to the possibility of an underlying metabolic defect, particularly in young children or in a child who has a recurrence of Reye syndrome–like symptoms.[12,14]

DIFFERENTIAL DIAGNOSIS AND MANAGEMENT OF HYPOGLYCEMIA

Hyperinsulinism

Hyperinsulinism may be caused by any of several abnormalities of the beta cell (see the box on p. 1720) and is the most common cause of persistent or recurrent hypoglycemia in the first year of life.[28] In Beckwith-Wiedemann syndrome (omphalocele, macroglossia, and gigantism), hypoglycemia occurs in 30% to 50% of affected infants, primarily as a result of beta cell hyperplasia.[2] Some of these infants also have hemihypertrophy. An increased incidence of adrenal, liver, and kidney (Wilms) tumors occurs in these patients.

Most children who have hypoglycemia due to persistent hyperinsulinism, previously called *nesidioblastosis* and now *islet cell dysplasia*[14] or *congenital hyperinsulinism*[30] by others, have symptoms beginning during the first year of life. This condition has been described in siblings and is thought to be inherited in an autosomal recessive mode.[30] No definitive hypothesis exists concerning the pathophysiology of this disorder.

Pancreatic islet cell adenomas are uncommon in children. Although hypoglycemia caused by varying histological types of insulinoma may have its onset in the newborn period, symptoms begin after age 4 years in 85% of patients.[8]

Laboratory Investigation. Hyperinsulinism in infants and older children usually is characterized by fasting hypoglycemia, even if of only a few hours' duration,[27] and low fasting plasma levels of beta-hydroxybutyrate (β-OHB) and free fatty acids (FFA).[27] Frequent random simultaneous measurements of blood glucose and insulin levels, particularly before feeding and as hypoglycemia occurs, help identify patients who have hyperinsulinism (Table 285-1). The diagnosis depends on detecting inappropriate insulin secretion by demonstrating insulin levels disproportionately high, relative to blood glucose values, particularly during hypoglycemia.

Abnormalities associated with hyperinsulinism cannot easily be distinguished by available diagnostic tests. Although leucine or tolbutamide may be useful in documenting the presence of hyperinsulinism, their administration is not helpful in delineating its specific cause because many of these patients may respond to these insulin secretogogues with abnormal insulin release.[17,28]

In any child who has intermittent attacks of nonketotic hypoglycemia, the physician should *always* investigate the possibility of malicious or self-administration of insulin or oral sulphonylurea drugs.[9,20,24] Measurement of C-peptide, insulin, and insulin antibodies in blood may identify the patient who has an exogenous source of insulin. In contrast to patients who have endogenous hyperinsulinism, C-peptide levels are suppressed, and insulin antibodies may be present in patients to whom insulin has been administered[20,24]; although plasma insulin and C-peptide levels may be misleading in children who have received oral hypoglycemic agents, the drug itself may be detected in the child's blood or urine.[24]

Management. Acute hypoglycemic episodes must be treated promptly and adequately with intravenously administered glucose. The rate of glucose administration required to maintain normal blood glucose levels among hyperinsulinemic infants often can exceed 12 to 14 mg/kg/min.

Further management of the patient depends on the age at onset of disease. In the infant, the response to diazoxide is of great diagnostic and therapeutic value. Diazoxide raises blood glucose levels primarily by suppressing pancreatic insulin secretion.[23] In patients in whom diazoxide results in restoration of normal glucose levels, the drug is continued and the patients are assessed periodically until approximately 5 to 7 years of age.[23] Corticosteroids are of no value. Some patients remain euglycemic without medication by this age. Because hyperglycemia, ketosis, and hyperosmolar nonketotic coma can occur with diazoxide therapy, the parents should be instructed to monitor urinary glucose and ketones.[17]

If hypoglycemia associated with hyperinsulinism persists or recurs despite diazoxide therapy, the diagnosis of insulinoma or islet cell dysplasia must be considered strongly.[18] In these patients, hypoglycemia usually continues or recurs while they are receiving diazoxide.[18] The two disorders cannot be distinguished without surgical inspection. Location of an adenoma has been achieved by selective arteriography of the celiac axis and by ultrasound.[1] However, because islet cell tumors often are so small, it is unlikely that these procedures or computed tomography can detect the presence of tumor preoperatively in most infants and children. Intraoperative ultrasonography, however, may help to identify adenomas in children.[29] Because the prognosis for subsequent normal mental and neurological development has been poor among infants who have hyperinsulinemia and intractable hypoglycemia, surgical exploration of the pancreas without delay is indicated when no response of hyperinsulinism to diazoxide occurs. Finally, the presence of hyperinsulinemic hypoglycemia in an older child who has no previous evidence of hypoglycemia is very suggestive of an islet cell adenoma; thus any trial of medical therapy should be limited.

At surgery, the pancreas should be inspected carefully and palpated for the presence of tumor. Removal of a tumor usually is curative. If no tumor is found, 85% to 90% of the pancreas should be removed but the spleen preserved. A long-acting somatostatin analog that suppressed insulin secretion has been effective in maintaining adequate blood glucose levels in some infants who have persistent hyperinsulinemic hypoglycemia who were not responsive to diazoxide, thereby sparing initial pancreatic surgery.[11,31] It also was helpful in those patients who had recurrent hypoglycemia postoperatively.[31]

Inborn Errors of Metabolism

Carbohydrate Enzyme Defects. Several enzymatic defects of carbohydrate metabolism result in deficiencies of hepatic glucose formation and release.[17] Glucose-6-phosphatase deficiency is the most common, and the symptoms are more severe than in other glycogen storage disease (GSD) types (see the box on p. 1720).[17] Patients who have GSD types Ia and Ib have growth retardation, cherubic facies, protuberant abdomen, a very large smooth liver, enlarged kidneys, normal intelligence, fasting hypoglycemia of only a few hours' duration, ketosis, lacticacidemia, hyperlipidemia, hyperuricemia, and bleeding diathesis. In type Ib the patients also have neutropenia and an increased frequency of infections. Among infants and young children, poor food intake during an illness may result in severe lactic acidosis and hypoglycemia, and death may result if hypoglycemia and hyperlacticacidemia are not treated adequately and promptly with intravenous glucose and sodium bicarbonate.[17] A dramatic advance in treatment has been the introduction of continuous nocturnal glucose-containing gastric feedings.[13] To maintain normal blood glucose levels during the day, frequent feedings, at least every 3 to 4 hours, are essential. Foods rich in fructose and galactose should be avoided. The daily oral administration of an uncooked cornstarch suspension has been beneficial in older children, but not as effective in infants, in maintaining normoglycemia and attaining adequate metabolic control.[6]

Failure to thrive, jaundice, vomiting, susceptibility to infection, hepatomegaly, edema, ascites, a tendency to bleed, cataracts, proteinuria, aminoaciduria, and galactosuria are characteristic features of the lactose-fed infant who has galactosemia.[17] Mental retardation, progressive liver failure, and death may occur unless galactose-containing feedings are eliminated. Symptomatic hypoglycemia is not a common finding and is reversed quickly by intravenous glucose. When the diagnosis of galactosemia is suspected, the patient should be given a galactose-free diet immediately. This diet should be maintained carefully while the physician awaits the results of erythrocyte enzyme studies and should be continued if the diagnosis is confirmed. Clinical manifestations of hereditary fructose intolerance (HFI) develop only after fructose ingestion and include vomiting, profound hypoglycemia, and convulsions.[17] Continued ingestion of fructose is associated with failure to thrive, prolonged vomiting, jaundice, hepatosplenomegaly, hemorrhage, abnormal liver function, fructosuria, defects in proximal renal tubular function (including proteinuria, glucosuria, and aminoaciduria), and in some, hepatic failure and death. The acute episodes of hypoglycemia are reversed promptly by the intravenous administration of glucose. Long-term treatment consists of strict elimination of dietary fructose and of fructose in cough syrups and other drugs.

Patients who have FDPase deficiency may have episodic hyperventilation, fasting hypoglycemia, lactic acidosis, ketosis, hyperuricemia, and hepatomegaly.[17] Refusal to feed and vomiting, often associated with febrile illness, precipitate the attacks. The disorder is life threatening in the neonate and in young children. In contrast to those who have HFI, these patients do not vomit after fructose intake and do not develop an aversion to sweets. Treatment of the acute attack consists of correcting the hypoglycemia and acidosis by intravenous infusion of glucose and sodium bicarbonate. Long-term management should emphasize the avoidance of fasting and the provision of a fructose-free, high-carbohydrate diet.

Laboratory Investigation. A suggested outline for the investigation of hypoglycemia caused by inborn errors of carbohydrate metabolism has been included in Tables 285-1 and 285-2. These studies should be done in a pediatric metabolic center, but only when the child's condition is stable and the blood glucose level is normal. Judgment must be exercised in choosing the proper diagnostic test to delineate the underlying abnormality. An intravenous galactose test is helpful in the differentiation of some hepatic enzyme defects (Table 285-2) but is dangerous and should not be done to diagnose galactosemia. The presence of specific hepatic enzyme deficiencies may be determined by the use of other tolerance tests (Table 285-2). The tolerance tests are done after a variable period of fasting and only with a physician in attendance, who must be prepared to interrupt the test by administering intravenous glucose should symptoms and signs of hypoglycemia occur or should a low blood glucose level be detected. Definitive diagnosis of any of the inherited disorders of carbohydrate metabolism (see the box on p. 1720), except galactosemia, depends on assay of specific hepatic enzyme activities (Table 285-2); galactosemia, on the other hand, may be detected by the absence of galactose-1-phosphate uridyltransferase activity in red blood cells, so liver biopsy is not necessary for its definitive diagnosis.

Amino Acid and Organic Acid Metabolic Defects. Hypoglycemia has been noted in a variety of inborn errors of amino acid and organic acid metabolism (see the box on p. 1720).[17] Although symptoms usually begin in the neonatal period, they may occur later. The infants tend to improve when protein feedings are discontinued and 10% glucose is administered intravenously. Occasionally, peritoneal dialysis or exchange transfusion may be lifesaving. Amino acid analysis and gas chromatography of blood and urine often are helpful in detecting these inborn errors (Table 285-1). Diagnosis and treatment of a specific disorder depend on detection of its characteristic metabolites in blood and urine and on assays of specific enzyme activities in skin fibroblasts or white blood cells.

Hormonal Deficiencies

Hormonal deficiencies are not common causes of hypoglycemia, occurring primarily in those who are deficient in GH or cortisol.

Hypopituitarism. Congenital hypopituitarism, caused either by a hypothalamic abnormality or by aplasia of the anterior pituitary gland, is associated with severe, often fatal, hypoglycemia during the first few days of life.[1,8,18] Occasionally, however, hypoglycemia may appear first later in infancy or childhood. A few patients may have midline deformities, including hypotelorism, abnormality of the frontonasal process, and cleft lip or palate. Septooptic dysplasia (optic nerve

Table 285-2 Differential Diagnosis of Hepatic Enzyme Defects

Blood values	GSD—I	GSD—III	GSD, phosphorylase enzyme system	FDPase	HFI
Fasting					
Glucose	↓*	↓ or nl	↓ or nl	↓	nl
Lactic acid	↑	nl	nl	↑	nl
After glucose†					
Glucose	↑	↑	↑	↑	↑
Lactic acid	↓	↑	↑	↓	↔
After glucagon†					
Glucose	↔	↑‡	↑ or ↔	↑ or ↔§	↑‖
Lactic acid	↑	↔	↔	↓ or ↑	↔
After galactose†					
Glucose	↔	↑	↑	↑	↑
Lactic acid	↑	↑	↑	↔	↔
After fructose†					
Glucose	↔	↑	↑	↓	↓
Lactic acid	↑	↑	↑	↑	↑

*↑, Increased, ↓, decreased; %, no change; *nl*, normal.

†Tolerance tests done after variable fasting period.

‡Two hours after feeding.

§Variable, dependent on duration of fast.

‖No increase in glucose at time of fructose-induced hypoglycemia.

hypoplasia and absence of the septum pellucidum) is present in some patients and may be accompanied by nystagmus. Some patients who have congenital hypopituitarism may have a small penis (microphallus).

The more usual cause of *GH deficiency* is idiopathic hypopituitarism, in which no organic lesions can be delineated. In affected patients there is an increased occurrence of perinatal problems such as breech and forceps deliveries. Symptomatic hypoglycemia occurs in approximately 10% of patients,[4] with onset usually late in infancy or early childhood. Measurement of height and weight is essential for the evaluation of a child in whom GH deficiency is suspected, because these children have significant growth retardation, which may begin within the first 1 to 2 years of life. These children also tend to be pudgy, and affected boys may have small genitalia.

Cortisol Deficiency. Deficient cortisol production may be secondary to Addison disease, congenital adrenal hyperplasia, ACTH deficiency, or ACTH unresponsiveness.[1,8,16,18] Patients who have ACTH unresponsiveness and Addison disease may have abnormal pigmentation.

Laboratory Investigation and Treatment. Laboratory studies should include determination of GH and cortisol in the blood, particularly when the child has hypoglycemia (Table 285-1). Hypoglycemia is an excellent stimulus for GH and cortisol secretions, so low values of either hormone in the presence of hypoglycemia indicate the need for additional studies for cortisol or GH deficiency, which should be done only when the child's condition is stable and the blood glucose level normal. A lack of response to a definitive GH stimulation test must be demonstrated to confirm GH deficiency. Tests designed to elicit the normal hypothalamic-pituitary-adrenal responses and measurement of adrenal metabolites in blood and urine should be done to identify the child who has either ACTH deficiency, ACTH unresponsiveness, or cortisol deficiency. In patients who have suspected hypopituitarism or GH deficiency, magnetic resonance imaging and computed tomography of the brain may be of diagnostic help. Correction of hypoglycemia by intravenous administration of glucose makes up the treatment of acute episodes. Specific treatment depends on identifying the underlying hormonal deficiency. Patients should be encouraged to avoid prolonged fasting.

Ketotic Hypoglycemia

Although ketotic hypoglycemia previously was the most common cause of hypoglycemia after 1 year of age,[8,17,19] for reasons that are not clear, the incidence of this disorder has decreased. Symptoms mimicking those noted in ketotic hypoglycemia have occurred in children who have GH deficiency, ACTH unresponsiveness, FDPase deficiency, glycogen synthetase deficiency, and Reye syndrome. Before a child is classified as having ketotic hypoglycemia, therefore, careful laboratory investigation to consider these and other diseases must be accomplished.

The combination of ketonuria, hypoglycemia, and central nervous system symptoms, which may vary from unresponsiveness, pallor, and vomiting to coma and convulsions, and which often occur in the early morning hours in association with an upper respiratory tract infection or prolonged fast, is quite typical of ketotic hypoglycemia, for which no cause is known.[17] The onset is between 9 months and 5½ years of age, with a peak incidence at 2 years. Hypoglycemic episodes occur at intervals of from a few months to a year or more; they then decrease in frequency and tend to disappear, usually by 7 to 8 years of age.

Although the pathogenesis of hypoglycemia in ketotic hypoglycemia has not been defined, the evidence suggests that it represents an exaggeration of the starvation state.[8] During hypoglycemia, blood insulin levels are appropriately low; blood alanine levels also may be low; GH, glucagon, cortisol, beta-hydroxybutyrate, and free fatty acid levels in the blood are elevated; urinary ketones are present; and blood glucose levels fail to rise after the administration of glucagon.

The physician should document hypoglycemic blood glucose levels at the time of symptoms by obtaining a diagnostic blood sample. After the child has had several days to recover from the acute episode and is eating well, the administration of a provocative low-calorie, high-fat ketogenic diet has been useful in establishing the diagnosis[8,17] if an acute blood sample is unobtainable. The child must be observed carefully for hypoglycemia during the test period.

The acute hypoglycemic attacks are reversed by the intravenous administration of glucose; glucagon usually has no effect. Because the attacks occur infrequently, long-term drug therapy is not indicated. A liberal carbohydrate diet, including a bedtime snack, is recommended. Prolonged overnight fasting, particularly during weekends or holidays and periods of illness, should be avoided. The parents should be encouraged to test their child's urine for ketones each morning and particularly during illness or periods of fasting.

Carbohydrate-containing foods, given promptly when acetonuria develops, usually are successful in aborting attacks.

REFERENCES

1. Aynsley-Green A: Hypoglycemia in infants and children, *Clin Endocrinol Metab* 2:159, 1982.
2. Beckwith JB: Macroglossia, omphalocele, adrenal cytomegaly, gigantism and hyperplastic visceromegaly. In Bergsma D, editor: Malformation syndromes, *Birth Defects* 5:188, 1969.
3. Bougneres PF et al: Fasting hypoglycemia resulting from hepatic carnitine palmitoyl transferase deficiency, *J Pediatr* 98:742, 1981.
4. Brasel JA et al: An evaluation of 75 patients with hypopituitarism beginning in childhood, *Am J Med* 38:484, 1965.
5. Chaussain JL: Glycemic response to 24 hour fast in normal children and children with ketotic hypoglycemia, *J Pediatr* 82:438, 1973.
6. Chen YT, Cornblath M, Sidbury JB: Cornstarch therapy in type I glycogen-storage disease, *N Engl J Med* 310:171, 1984.
7. Cornblath M: Hypoglycemia in infancy and childhood, *Pediatr Ann* 10:356, 1981.
8. Cornblath M, Schwartz R: *Disorders of carbohydrate metabolism in infancy,* ed 2, Philadelphia, 1976, WB Saunders.
9. Dershewitz R et al: Transient hepatomegaly and hypoglycemia: a consequence of malicious insulin administration, *Am J Dis Child* 130:998, 1976.
10. Dusheiko G et al: Recurrent hypoglycemia associated with glutaric aciduria type II in an adult, *N Engl J Med* 301:1405, 1979.
11. Glaser B, Hirsch HJ, Landau H: Persistent hyperinsulinemic hypoglycemia of infancy: long-term octreotide treatment without pancreatectomy, *J Pediatr* 123:644, 1993.
12. Green CL, Blitzer MG, Shapira E: Inborn errors of metabolism and Reye syndrome: differential diagnoses, *J Pediatr* 113:156, 1988.
13. Greene HL et al: Type I glycogen storage disease: five years of management with nocturnal intragastric feeding, *J Pediatr* 96:590, 1980.

14. Haymond MW: Hypoglycemia in infants and children, *Endocrinol Metab Clin North Am* 18:211, 1989.
15. Kaye R et al: The response of blood glucose, ketones, and plasma nonesterified fatty acids to fasting and epinephrine injection in infants and children, *J Pediatr* 54:836, 1961.
16. Kershnar AK, Roe TF, Kogut MD: Adrenocorticotropic hormone unresponsiveness: report of a girl with excessive growth and review of 16 reported cases, *J Pediatr* 80:610, 1972.
17. Kogut MD: Hypoglycemia: pathogenesis, diagnosis and treatment. In Gluck L et al, editors: *Current problems in pediatrics,* vol 4, Chicago, 1974, Mosby.
18. Kogut MD: Neonatal hypoglycemia: a new look. In Moss AJ, editor: *Pediatrics update: review for physicians,* New York, 1980, Elsevier.
19. Kogut MD, Blaskovics M, Donnell GN: Idiopathic hypoglycemia: a study of 26 children, *J Pediatr* 74:853, 1969.
20. Mayefsky JH, Sarnaik AP, Postellon DC: Factitious hypoglycemia, *Pediatrics* 69:804, 1982.
21. Pagliara AS et al: *Hypoglycemia in infancy and childhood,* part 1, *J Pediatr* 82:365, 1973.
22. Roe TF, Kogut MD: Hypopituitarism and ketotic hypoglycemia, *Am J Dis Child* 121:296, 1971.
23. Roe TF, Kogut MD: Idiopathic leucine-sensitive hypoglycemia syndrome: insulin and glucagon responses and effects of diazoxide, *Pediatr Res* 16:1, 1982.
24. Scarlett JA et al: Factitious hypoglycemia: diagnosis by measurement of serum C-peptide immunoreactivity and insulin-binding autobodies, *N Engl J Med* 297:1029, 1977.
25. Schutgens RBH et al: Lethal hypoglycemia in a child with a deficiency of 3-hydroxy-3-methylglutaryl coenzyme A lyase, *J Pediatr* 94:89, 1979.
26. Shelly HJ, Neligan GA: Neonatal hypoglycemia, *Br Med Bull* 22:34, 1966.
27. Stanley CA, Baker L: Hyperinsulinism in infancy: diagnosis by demonstration of abnormal response to fasting hypoglycemia, *Pediatrics* 57:702, 1976.
28. Stanley CA, Baker L: Hyperinsulinism in infants and children: diagnosis and therapy, *Adv Pediatr* 23:315, 1976.
29. TeLander RL, Charboneay JW, Haymond MW: Intraoperative ultrasonography of the pancreas in children, *J Pediatr Surg* 21:262, 1986.
30. Thornton PS et al: Familial and sporadic hyperinsulinism: histopathologic findings and segregation analysis support a single autosomal recessive disorder, *J Pediatr* 119:721, 1991.
31. Thornton PS et al: Short and long-term use of octreotide in the treatment of congenital hyperinsulinism, *J Pediatr* 123:637, 1993.
32. Ware AJ et al: Systemic carnitine deficiency: report of a fatal case with multisystemic manifestations, *J Pediatr* 93:959, 1978.

286 Increased Intracranial Pressure

Todd F. Barron

Increased intracranial pressure (ICP) is a potentially life-threatening problem that can be a neurological/neurosurgical emergency if it occurs acutely. Rapid identification of the cause and expedient management can prevent serious morbidity and possible mortality. Increased ICP has many causes, and symptoms can be acute, subacute, or chronic.

PATHOPHYSIOLOGY

In older children and adults the skull is a closed, rigid space. This container is filled with three compartments—the brain accounting for 80% to 90% of the volume, the circulating cerebrospinal fluid accounting for 5% to 10%, and the circulating blood accounting for the remainder.[3,7] In that the relative volume is fixed, small increases in any one of these compartments result in a compensatory decrease in the other two. If the increase exceeds normal compensatory mechanisms, intracranial pressure rises. Also affecting this is the compliance (stiffness) of the brain, which is altered in various disease states. Because the brain accounts for most of the intracranial volume, changes in brain compliance dampen compensatory mechanisms.[7]

The normal intracranial pressure in older children and adults usually is 15 mm Hg in the recumbent position; in young children it is less.[9] ICP is pulsatile and varies around a baseline; variation is due to cardiac and respiratory activity.[5,7] Transient increases up to 50 mm Hg or higher occur normally with actions that increase intrathoracic pressure or that impede venous return such as coughing, sneezing, and straining. However, with discontinuation of these maneuvers, ICP returns rapidly to baseline.

Under normal conditions, blood flow to the brain is autoregulated, maintaining a constant level of perfusion over a range of blood pressures.[5,7] Any disruption in this makes blood flow pressure passive, which in turn can lead to significant changes in cerebral perfusion with any change in blood pressure. The cerebral perfusion pressure (CPP) is defined as the mean arterial pressure (MAP) minus the ICP.[7] With increasing ICP, the CPP falls, leading to further cerebral compromise—ischemia, swelling, and further increases in ICP. This cycle, if untreated, persists and ultimately causes death.

ETIOLOGY

The causes of increased ICP in children are numerous and can be classified as shown in the box on p. 1727. Cause also affects whether intracranial hypertension is chronic, such as with pseudotumor cerebrii, or acute, as with head trauma, causing cerebral edema or intracerebral hemorrhage. Common causes of increased ICP in children include head trauma, infection, hydrocephalus, and mass lesions. Causes also affect clinical signs and symptoms.

SYMPTOMS AND SIGNS

Symptoms of both acute and chronic ICP are presented in the box on p. 1727. Many of these are the same, demonstrating their somewhat nonspecific nature. The temporal pace of development differs between the two. Acute signs of rapidly increasing ICP are due to displacement of neural tissue through the several dural openings, with subsequent compression and ischemic changes to the cerebral structures. For example, with uncal herniation in association with supratentorial masses, the uncus is displaced through the tentorial opening, leading to compression of the ipsilateral third nerve and displacement of the peduncles and brainstem laterally[6] (Fig. 286-1). Clinically, the patient is in a comatose state and has an ipsilateral pupillary dilatation (third nerve palsy) and ipsilateral hemiparesis. This is the classic "Kernohan notch"; the ipsilateral hemiparesis suggests a lesion in the contralateral hemisphere that is falsely localizing. The pupil reliably localizes the side of the lesion. Downward herniation of the cerebellar tonsils through the foramen magnum leads to compression and vascular compromise of the lower brainstem structures (medulla) (Fig. 286-1). Patients are comatose and exhibit decorticate or decerebrate rigidity and autonomic changes (respiratory and circulatory changes). Classically, the symptoms of a widened pulse pressure, bradycardia, and deep, slow respiration are referred to as "Cushing triad." Clinically, this triad rarely is seen.[6]

DIAGNOSIS

Key to the management of increased ICP is the rapid recognition of the patient who has intracranial hypertension. As with any individual who has neurological complaints, the history and physical/neurological examination are the most important aspects of the initial diagnostic evaluation. These provide the physician information on the pace of illness and therefore allow him or her to discern the need for urgent versus emergent management. If a rapidly evolving process (e.g., impending herniation) is evident, stabilizing the patient is essential before proceeding to definitive diagnosis and therapy.

Performing a lumbar puncture (LP) provides an opportunity to evaluate the intracranial pressure by inserting a spinal needle into the thecal sac, attaching a manometer, and measuring the height of the column of CSF while the patient is in the lateral decubitus position with the legs extended. The normal is between 12 and 18 cm. However, if a mass lesion is suspected, the withdrawal of CSF may precipitate a herniation syndrome; therefore neuroimaging generally is recommended before an LP. The one exception is in children who are suspected of having meningitis, in which case, in general, neuroimaging before performance of an LP is unnecessary.[2] A spinal fluid analysis always should include measurement of glucose and protein and a differential cell

CAUSES OF INCREASED ICP IN CHILDREN

Head trauma

Cerebral edema
Intracerebral hemorrhage
Extracerebral hemorrhage (subdural, epidural)

Vascular causes

Arterial/venous infarctions
Intracerebral hemorrhage
Dural sinus thrombosis
Subarachnoid hemorrhage
Vascular anomalies (vein of Galen malformation, AVMs)

Neoplastic causes

Primary brain tumors
Metastatic (intracerebral, meningeal infiltration)

Hydrocephalus

Congenital or acquired
Communicating or noncommunicating

Pseudotumor cerebrii (benign intracranial hypertension)

CNS infections

Meningitis (bacterial, fungal, mycobacterial)
Encephalitis (focal or diffuse)
Abscess

Metabolic causes

Inborn errors of metabolism (hyperammonemia)
Hepatic encephalopathy
Diabetic ketoacidosis
Renal failure
Reye syndrome
Hypoxic-ischemic encephalopathy
Fluid-electrolyte abnormalities (hyponatremia, hypernatremia)

Structural causes

Craniosynostosis

Status epilepticus

Adapted from Pickard JD, Czosnyka M: *J Neurol Neurosurg Psychiatry* 56:845, 1993.

SYMPTOMS AND SIGNS OF ACUTE AND CHRONIC INCREASED INTRACRANIAL PRESSURE IN CHILDREN

Infants
Acute

Irritability
Poor feeding/emesis
Split sutures (especially lambdoidal)
Bulging fontanelle
Altered mental status
Seizures
Parinaud sign (upgaze paresis)

Chronic

Irritability
Poor feeding/emesis
Increased head circumference
Bulging fontanelle
Split sutures (especially lambdoidal)
Apparent developmental arrest or regression
Parinaud sign

Children
Acute

Severe, acute headache
Seizures
Emesis
Rapidly deteriorating mental status
Decerebrate/decorticate posture
Focal neurological deficits
+/− Papilledema
Pupillary abnormalities
Autonomic dysfunction (Cushing triad)

Chronic

Chronic, progressive headache
Seizures
Early morning emesis
Change in school performance
Altered mental status
Cranial neuropathy (e.g., sixth cranial nerve palsy)
Focal neurological deficits
Papilledema
Visual changes

count. Depending on the clinical situation, other studies can be obtained, including microbial cultures (bacterial, fungal, viral, mycobacterial), special stains, lactate, and cytology.

Neuroimaging

CT or MRI can provide essential information in the diagnosis and management of patients who have increased ICP. While MRI provides better anatomical differentiation, it frequently is unavailable in the emergency setting; therefore CT is performed most often. If a mass lesion is suspected, neuroimaging, regardless of modality, should include contrast enhancement. Both the modalities are effective in evaluating the cause of intracranial hypertension and are done primarily to determine any presence of a mass lesion. The one exception is in the patient suspected of having a subarachnoid hemorrhage, when CT followed by LP remain the mainstays of initial diagnosis. And finally, in infants suspected of having aqueductal stenosis, ultrasonography is a reasonable alternative to CT or MRI (Fig. 286-2). Other neuroimaging studies such as angiography rarely play a role in the initial diagnosis and management of intracranial hypertension.

MANAGEMENT

Rapid recognition and stabilization of the patient suspected of having acutely increased ICP is essential in preventing greater morbidity and mortality. The goal of early management is to lower ICP without compromising cerebral perfu-

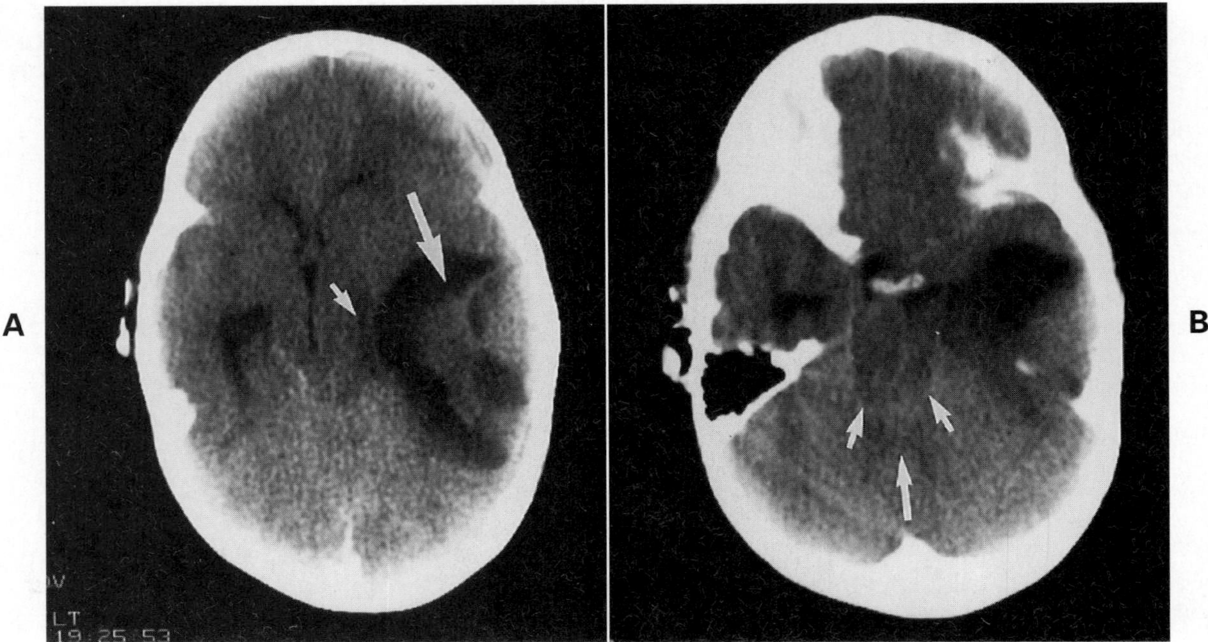

FIG. 286-1 Two sections from a CT scan of a 5-year-old girl who is comatose and has increased intracranial pressure. **A,** Large, cystic left temporal lobe mass *(large arrow)* causing left uncal herniation *(small arrow)* with loss of perimesencephalic cistern and midline shift. **B,** A lower cut demonstrating loss of the fourth ventricle *(large arrow)* and a quadrigeminal cistern *(small arrows),* suggesting downward (tonsillar) herniation.

sion and to identify the cause so that more definitive therapy can be provided, be it medical or neurosurgical. In patients who have evidence of chronically elevated ICP, management usually is directed toward definitive therapy.

As in any emergency situation, the first step in management is to assess the airway, breathing, and circulation (the ABCs). It also is useful to obtain a Dextrostick and, in the case of the trauma patient, to expose the patient so that injuries can be identified rapidly. When acutely increased ICP is suspected, the following initial steps should be applied:

1. Stabilize the airway. In most instances this requires rapid, controlled intubation, taking care to minimize patient Valsalva, which increases ICP further, albeit transiently.
2. Obtain IV access. Use only isotonic solutions, minimizing fluids initially unless circulatory compromise is evident.
3. Measure the vital signs and assess the neurological state rapidly and frequently.
4. Position head at 30 degrees and maintain a midline position.
5. Maintain adequate intravascular volume and blood pressure.
6. Maintain adequate oxygenation.

After these maneuvers, the interventions detailed in the following sections might be attempted.

Hyperventilation

Cerebral blood flow is exquisitely sensitive to CO_2 levels. Low carbon dioxide levels lead to cerebral vasoconstriction, whereas elevated levels lead to dilatation. Early hyperventilation of the patient who has increased ICP leads to a decrease in cerebral blood volume and therefore a decrease in the ICP. This provides the most rapid, effective method of lowering ICP acutely. This effect is transient; therefore other methods must be employed to maintain normal or near-normal ICP. In general, CO_2 should be lowered to the low thirties (mm Hg). Further decreases can lead to a significant decrease in cerebral blood flow, producing ischemia and increasing ICP further. Failure to respond to hyperventilation often is a poor prognostic sign.[8] Evidence suggests that the alkalizing effect of hyperventilation and, therefore, lowered ICP can be maintained through the use of intravenous buffers such as tris hydroxymethyl aminomethane (THAM).[8]

Osmotic Agents and Diuretics

Intravenous osmotic agents (mannitol and glycerol) are unable to permeate the blood-brain barrier and therefore draw fluid from the intracellular brain compartment to the vascular space, thereby reducing ICP and allowing increased cerebral perfusion. In general, mannitol is the drug of choice and is given rapidly in an initial IV bolus of 0.75 to 1 g/kg. Following this initial bolus, additional boluses ranging from 0.25 to 0.5 g/kg should be considered every 3 to 5 hours, depending on the status of the patient. Response to IV mannitol is rapid and occurs usually within 10 to 20 minutes. Serum osmolarity should be maintained in the 295-320 mOsm/l range. Because mannitol is excreted renally, it cannot be given in the face of renal failure, because this provokes potentially life-threatening pulmonary edema. Loop diuretics such as furosemide act to reduce ICP by provoking a diuresis of water and electrolytes, thereby establishing a gradient between the

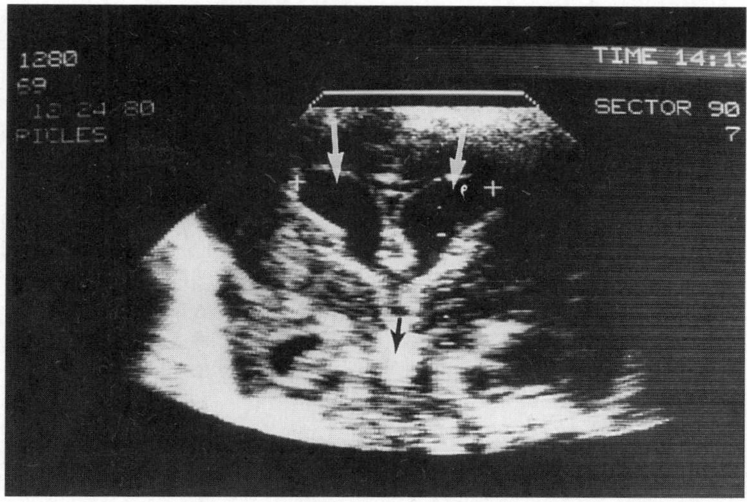

FIG. 286-2 A coronal head ultrasound of a baby born at 30 weeks with a history of an intraventricular hemorrhage now with increasing head circumference. Prominent dilated lateral ventricles *(white arrows)* and a clot-filled third ventricle *(black arrow)* are demonstrated.

intravascular compartment and the brain. They frequently are used in combination with osmotic diuretics but are used alone infrequently. In using any of the aforementioned agents, care must be given to maintain intravascular volume and adequate blood pressure. Electrolytes must be monitored carefully.

Neuromuscular Blockade

Use of agents such as pancuronium and vecuronium can be effective in decreasing ICP by preventing maneuvers that increase intrathoracic pressure such as coughing, straining, or "bucking" the ventilator. The physician must remember that these agents do not provide analgesia or sedation; therefore they should be used in conjunction with analgesic agents and short-acting sedatives.

Temperature Control

Hyperthermia leads to greater cerebral metabolism; therefore measures should be taken to prevent fevers. This generally includes judicious use of antipyretics, cooling blankets, and antibiotics if infection is suspected. Conversely, hypothermia decreases cerebral metabolism and may be advantageous in the management of elevated ICP as long as shivering is prevented and efforts are made to maintain full cardiorespiratory status. Body temperature should be maintained between 30° and 37° C.[5,8]

Seizure Control

Seizure activity, whether clinical or subclinical, places an excessive metabolic demand on already compromised brain tissue. Treatment with antiepileptic drugs is necessary for any patient who is having or is suspected of having seizures, especially if neuromuscular blocking agents are to be used. In general, diazepam (0.1 mg/kg/dose IV) or lorazepam (0.05 to 0.1 mg/kg/dose) are the drugs to be used in treating acute conditions. For more prolonged therapy, either phenytoin or phenobarbital can be used. Phenytoin has the distinct advantage of not depressing mental status, but it needs to be given slowly (5 mg/kg/min or 50 mg/min). If possible, the physician should identify and treat the cause of seizure activity (e.g., fever, drug toxicity, hypoglycemia, electrolyte abnormalities).

Corticosteroids

The use of corticosteroids remains controversial in the management of acutely elevated ICP associated with head trauma, intracerebral hemorrhage, and ischemic stroke.[8] They have clear utility in the management of edema associated with brain tumors and in the management of refractory pseudotumor cerebrii. Their mechanism of action is unknown, but hypotheses include stabilization of the blood-brain barrier, enhancement of brain energy supplies, decrease in tumor growth, reduction of CSF production, and stabilization of cellular membranes.[5,8] In general, dexamethasone is used.

High-Dose Barbiturates

In situations of refractory ICP, treatment with high-dose barbiturates (pentobarbital) can be effective. These agents act to decrease cerebral blood flow and metabolism. Pentobarbital is the agent of choice for prolonged therapy; in general, a loading dose of 3 to 10 mg/kg IV is given, followed by a maintenance infusion of 1 to 2 mg/kg/hr. The dose should be titrated to EEG, with a goal of obtaining a burst-suppression pattern. This therapy should be maintained for 24 hours or more and then tapered. Side effects are frequent and include hypotension, often requiring use of pressors. Which groups of refractory patients benefit from this therapy is not yet certain.[3,5,8]

Intracranial Pressure Monitoring and Removal of CSF

Numerous devices are available for assessing the ICP invasively. These include intraventricular catheters that have the added advantage of allowing drainage of CSF and, therefore, reduction in ICP. The disadvantage of this particular device is the higher risk of infection, seizures, and hemorrhage as compared with the other devices available. Fluid-filled catheter and fiber optic systems can be placed both extradurally and intradurally, allowing relatively accurate assessment of ICP with fewer complications. Measuring cerebral venous oxygenation via a jugular bulb indwelling catheter and noninvasively by transcutaneous, transcranial near infrared spectroscopy can assess ICP and cerebral perfusion indirectly.[3,5,8]

Surgical Decompression

Obviously, in children who have large intracranial masses causing acutely increased ICP, definitive therapy with surgical removal of the mass can be life saving. Surgery also may play a role in decreasing ICP in those patients who have large intracerebral hemorrhages by removing the clot, and in trauma patients who have massive edema and contusion or in patients who have a large cerebral infarction through either craniectomy or decompression of the edematous mass. In the latter two instances, this therapy is performed only after all other measures have failed and increased ICP is refractory.[3,5,8] Effectiveness remains anecdotal.[8]

Future Trends

In the future, cerebral protectants, including free radical scavengers, excitotoxic amino acid antagonists, lazeroids, and NMDA receptor antagonists, may be part of the "cocktail" in the initial emergent management of acutely increased ICP.[5,8]

With respect to patients who exhibit evidence of chronically increased ICP who are neurologically stable, management is directed toward definitive therapy—that is, evacuation of the chronic subdural, appropriate tumor management (surgery or radiation and chemotherapy or both), and treatment with acetazolamide, loop diuretics, steroids, or lumbar drain (in refractory patients) in patients who have benign intracranial hypertension.

OUTCOME

In at least 50% of children who have severe head injuries and in comatose children from other cerebral insults—hypoxia, infections, metabolic disorders—increased ICP is a major complication that affects morbidity and, possibly, ultimate outcome.[1,4] Which variables—intracranial pressure, cerebral perfusion pressure, or initial Glasgow coma score—are helpful in predicting prognosis remains uncertain.[1,4] In any regard, significant morbidity remains for children who have increased ICP. Clearly, in those children who have mass lesions or treatable metabolic disorders, early identification and treatment before a catastrophic increase in ICP occurs will improve outcome.

REFERENCES

1. Barzilay Z et al: Variables affecting outcome from severe brain injury in children, *Intensive Care Med* 14:417, 1988.
2. Haslam RHA: Role of computed tomography in the early management of bacterial meningitis, *J Pediatr* 119:157, 1991.
3. Lehman LB: Intracranial pressure monitoring and treatment: a contemporary view, *Ann Emerg Med* 19:295, 1990.
4. Lieh-Lai MW et al: Limitations of the Glasgow Coma Scale in predicting outcome in children with traumatic brain injury, *J Pediatr* 120:195, 1992.
5. Pickard JD, Czosnyka M: Management of raised intracranial pressure, *J Neurol Neurosurg Psychiatry* 56:845, 1993.
6. Plum F, Posner JB: *The diagnosis of stupor and coma,* ed 3, Philadelphia, 1982, FA Davis.
7. Ropper AH, Rockoff MA: Physiology and clinical aspects of raised intracranial pressure. In Ropper AH, editor: *Neurological and neurosurgical intensive care,* ed 2, New York, 1993, Raven Press.
8. Ropper AH: Treatment of intracranial hypertension. In Ropper AH, editor: *Neurological and neurosurgical intensive care,* ed 2, New York, 1993, Raven Press.
9. Shapiro K, Morris WJ, Teo C: Intracranial hypertension: mechanisms and management. In Cheek WR, editor: *Pediatric neurosurgery,* ed 3, Philadelphia, 1994, WB Saunders.

287 Meningococcemia

Mary T. Caserta

Meningococcemia is a classic example of fulminant bacterial sepsis and is the most dreaded consequence of infection with *Neisseria meningitidis.* Although occult or chronic meningococcemia occasionally is detected, children who have the severe form of the disease can progress from a state of good health to death in hours, regardless of whether meningitis is present.

EPIDEMIOLOGY

N. meningitidis is a gram negative coccus that appears typically in pairs (diplococci) with the adjacent sides flattened. The organism is enclosed by a cell envelope containing outer membrane proteins and a lipopolysaccharide (LPS or endotoxin) and by a polysaccharide capsule. Nine serogroups have been identified on the basis of the antigenic structure of the capsular polysaccharide.[12]

N. meningitidis is found only in the human nasopharynx and is spread from person to person via respiratory droplets or direct contact with secretions. Invasive meningococcal disease is a relatively uncommon event, with most individuals colonized only intermittently with the organism. Approximately 5% to 20% of adults in nonepidemic conditions are colonized. Subgroups, such as military recruits, can have rates as high as 80%, and carriage rates are even higher in household contacts of patients with infection or in noninfected carriers.[6] Colonization with both pathogenic and nonpathogenic *Neisseria,* in addition to other gram negative organisms that have similar capsular polysaccharides, induces the development of natural immunity to *N. meningitidis.* Nonetheless, *N. meningitidis* causes both epidemic and endemic disease worldwide. Since the introduction of an effective vaccine against *Haemophilus influenzae* type B, the meningococcus is the leading cause of meningitis and sepsis in children and young adults in the United States (approximately 2600 cases per year). Data from the Centers for Disease Control and Prevention show that from 1989 to 1991 the overall incidence of meningococcal disease was 1.1 cases per 100,000 people. The highest incidence of disease consistently is found in infants, with a peak attack rate of 26.4 cases per 100,000 population. From 25% to 33% of all cases of meningococcal disease occur in children less than 1 year of age. Almost 50% of all cases of meningococcemia occur in children under age 2 years, when passively acquired maternal antibody concentrations have reached their nadir and substantial numbers of children have not yet acquired protective antibodies following colonization. By age 5 years the incidence reaches adult levels[14] (Fig. 287-1).

Historically, the majority of cases of invasive meningococcal disease in the United States have been caused by serogroup B meningococcus. In the last decade, however, organisms of serogroups B and C have *each* been identified in approximately 45% of cases of meningococcal disease. Despite this relative equality, 69% of disease caused by group C occurred in persons over 2 years of age. Only 37% of disease caused by group B occurred in those children 2 years of age or older, making group B meningococcus more of a threat to the younger age groups. The occurrence of meningococcal infection also varies with the seasons. Winter and spring constitute the peak time of disease in the United States. Several studies have shown an association between meningococcal disease and influenza and other viral respiratory infections, although the exact nature of the interaction is not clear.[7,18]

Sixty percent of cases of invasive meningococcal disease are associated with meningitis; approximately 40% are classified as sepsis without central nervous system involvement. The overall mortality for meningococcal disease is 10% to 15%. Subgroups of patients, such as those who have fulminant meningococcemia, can have fatality rates as high as 50% to 80% despite aggressive intensive care therapy.

DIAGNOSIS AND DIFFERENTIAL DIAGNOSIS

The early recognition of meningococcemia is an important determinant of survival. In a study of 100 children who had meningococcal infections reported by Wong and colleagues,[29] the predominant findings on examination were fever and rash, each noted in 71% of patients. Other important symptoms and signs included irritability or lethargy in just over 50% of the patients; vomiting occurred in approximately 35% of children, and shock was noted in 42 patients. Less common symptoms included delirium, headache, coryza, diarrhea, myalgia, and hypothermia.

The type and duration of the rash provide important information about the course and prognosis of the disease. Early in the infection a tender pink maculopapular rash similar to that seen in rubella, secondary syphilis, or disseminated gonorrhea can appear on any part of the skin. The rash often fades rapidly with treatment, and patients who have this type of manifestation are less likely to have a fulminant course. A generalized petechial rash most prominent on the distal extremities, including the palms and soles, usually is associated with meningococcal disease. Initially the lesions are discrete, 1 to 2 mm in diameter, and found in clusters where clothing puts pressure on the skin.[3] This rash must be differentiated from that seen with Rocky Mountain spotted fever, bacterial endocarditis, and enterovirus infections. Scrapings of petechial lesions reveal the organism approximately 70% of the time.

The most ominous manifestation of meningococcal disease is an ecchymotic or purpuric rash with a centrifugal distribution usually present in cases of fulminant meningococcemia. The differential diagnosis includes Rocky Mountain spotted fever, plague, rubeola, septicemia with other bacteria (Table

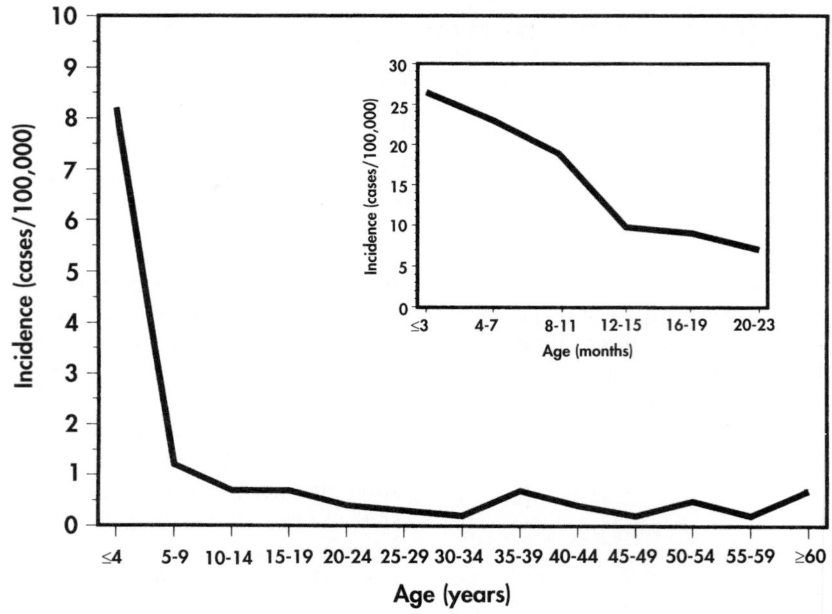

FIG. 287-1 Incidence of meningococcal disease, by age group, in selected areas in the United States, 1989-1991.

(From Jackson LA, Wenger JD: *MMWR* 42:25, 1993.)

287-1), and Henoch-Schönlein purpura. Meningococcemia is the most common cause of purpura. In the classic series by Toews and Bass[26] of 151 patients who had meningococcal infections, 7 of the 16 patients who had ecchymotic or purpuric lesions died; only 4 of the 135 patients who had either maculopapular or petechial lesions, or no rash at all, died. More recent reports also have noted an association between the presence and type of rash with outcome. A review by Tesoro and Selbst[23] published in 1991 demonstrated that mortality in children who had invasive meningococcal disease and a petechial or purpuric rash was 19%, compared with no deaths in those children who had no rash. Similarly, in the aforementioned review of 100 children, patients who had purpura fulminans had a 50% mortality. The case fatality rate is also significantly higher in patients who have petechiae for 12 hours or less. Therefore a febrile child who has purpura or petechiae that have been present for less than 12 hours should be managed as a medical emergency.

MANAGEMENT

An infant or child who has an acute onset of fever and a purpuric or petechial rash requires aggressive monitoring and treatment as soon as possible. If the patient must be transported to a pediatric intensive care unit, blood should be drawn, antibiotics given, and intravenous access secured beforehand. The patient should be attended during transport by a physician prepared to treat shock and respiratory failure. Initial laboratory tests should include a blood culture, a complete blood count and differential, a partial thromboplastin time (PTT), a prothrombin time (PT), measurement of fibrin breakdown products, and serum chemistries. If the patient is stable when first evaluated, a lumbar puncture should also be performed to determine if meningitis is present in order to examine the CSF for organisms, obtain cultures, and assess the prognosis more accurately. If the patient is unstable on initial assessment, the lumbar puncture should be deferred until a later time.

The recommended antibiotic regimen for treatment of meningococcemia is aqueous penicillin G 250,000 to 500,000 units/kg/day in four to six divided doses. No resistance of the meningococcus to penicillin is reported in the United States. However, strains that have decreased susceptibility to penicillin have been reported from several other countries in Europe and Africa. Chloramphenicol, ceftriaxone, and cefotaxime are alternative antibiotics recommended for penicillin-allergic patients or in the rare instance where resistance might be present. Antibiotic therapy generally is continued for 5 afebrile days or 7 days total. Rifampin (10 mg/kg per dose given twice a day for 2 days) is added at the end of the course of penicillin to eliminate carriage of the organism from the nasopharynx.[1,2]

In addition to antibiotic therapy, patients who have meningococcemia often require aggressive supportive therapy in an intensive care setting with invasive monitoring of hemodynamic, neurological, and respiratory function. Mechanical ventilation often is necessary to treat respiratory failure. Maintenance of optimal plasma expansion with intravenous fluids is the first step in stabilizing the circulatory system. Large amounts of fluid may be needed because of the capillary leak associated with endotoxic shock. In addition, multiple transfusions with platelets and fresh frozen plasma may be necessary to correct the coagulopathy associated with meningococcemia. Several studies have demonstrated that myocardial dysfunction precedes shock in adult and pediatric patients who have meningococcal sepsis.[4,17] This phenomenon is believed to be secondary to endotoxemia. The use of inotropic agents aimed at reversing myocardial depression and improving tissue perfusion is recommended on the basis of these observations.

Table 287-1 Infectious Agents Associated with Illnesses in Which Petechial or Purpuric Exanthems, or Both, Occur

Infectious agent	Illness
Varicella-zoster virus	Hemorrhagic chickenpox
Cytomegalovirus	Congenital cytomegalovirus infection
Variola virus	Hemorrhagic smallpox
Coxsackieviruses A4, A9	Fever
Coxsackieviruses B2 to B4	Exanthem and enanthem
Echoviruses 4, 7, 9	
Colorado tick fever virus	Colorado tick fever
Rotavirus	Gastroenteritis
Alphaviruses	Chikungunya fever, o'nyong-nyong fever, Ross River fever, Sindbis fever
Rubella virus	Rubella (German measles)
	Congenital rubella
Respiratory syncytial virus	Bronchiolitis
Measles virus	Hemorrhagic (black) measles
	Atypical measles
Lassa virus	Lassa fever
Marburg virus	Hemorrhagic fever
Rickettsia typhi	Murine typhus
Rickettsia prowazekii	Epidemic typhus
Rickettsia rickettsii and other tickborne rickettsiae	Rocky Mountain spotted fever
Ehrlichia canis	Ehrlichiosis
Mycoplasma pneumoniae	Atypical pneumonia
Streptococcus pyogenes	Scarlet fever; septicemia
Streptococcus pneumoniae	Pneumococcal septicemia
Enterococcal and viridans group streptococci	Endocarditis
Neisseria gonorrhoeae	Gonococcemia
Neisseria meningitidis	Meningococcemia
Moraxella catarrhalis	Sinusitis, otitis media, sepsis
Haemophilus influenzae	*H. influenzae* septicemia
Pseudomonas aeruginosa	Ecthyma gangrenosa
Streptobacillus moniliformis	Rat-bite fever
Yersinia pestis	Septicemic plague (Black Death)
Bartonella henselae	Cat-scratch fever
Treponema pallidum	Congenital syphilis
Borrelia spp.	Relapsing fever
Toxoplasma gondii	Congenital toxoplasmosis
Trichinella spiralis	Trichinosis

Modified from Cherry JD: Cutaneous manifestations of systemic infections. In Feigen RD, Cherry JD, editors: *Textbook of pediatric infectious diseases*, Philadelphia, 1992, WB Saunders.

Supportive measures for severe purpura include treatments aimed at relieving the ischemic complications associated with vasculitis. Case reports have demonstrated the successful use of continuous epidural anesthesia in restoring perfusion of the lower extremities and preventing gangrenous necrosis.[25] The mechanism of action is thought to be vasodilation of partially occluded vessels via sympathetic blockade. If no evidence exists of coagulopathy, an anesthesiologist can perform this type of regional block with an indwelling catheter in the caudal space without an appreciable effect on overall cardiovascular status. The topical administration of nitroglycerin also has been reported to be useful in restoring blood flow to the skin and superficial tissues without notable adverse effects.[13]

Other ancillary treatments evaluated experimentally are aimed at interrupting the disease process pathophysiology via interference with secondary mediators of inflammation induced by the release of endotoxin. These treatments include plasmapheresis, whole blood exchange, or the administration of monoclonal antibodies directed against endotoxin or specific mediators such as tumor necrosis factor. Several studies have shown a correlation between plasma levels of endotoxin or tumor necrosis factor and multiorgan failure or disease severity, making these strategies theoretically attractive.[5,28] Heparin therapy was advocated in the past to treat disseminated intravascular coagulation caused by sepsis, but it has not been found to alter the disease course or the mortality in human or animal studies. Recent reports have associated purpura fulminans induced by sepsis with acquired deficiencies of the natural anticoagulation factors proteins C and S.[19] In a pilot study, Fourrier and colleagues[10] treated five adult patients who had purpura fulminans with concentrates of antithrombin III, a modulator of the clotting cascade and protein C activator; all patients survived without sequelae. This result supports further trials of this type of therapy among patients who have meningococcal sepsis and purpura fulminans. In patients who have meningitis, adjunctive treatment with dexamethasone (0.15 mg/kg per dose every 6 hours for 4 days) to prevent neurological sequelae is supported by limited studies involving small numbers of patients who have meningococcal disease. The use of high-dose steroids in the treatment of adults who have sepsis and shock, caused primarily by gram negative bacteria, has not proved to be of benefit in decreasing either morbidity or mortality. The use of high-dose steroids in children who have meningococcal disease remains controversial.

Numerous investigators have attempted to predict the outcome for individual patients who have meningococcal disease, on the basis of various laboratory and clinical data. In 1966, Stiehm and Damrosch[22] developed a prognostic score whereby patients who had three or more of these findings—the presence of petechiae for less than 12 hours before admission, shock, the absence of meningitis, normal or low white blood cell counts, or normal or low erythrocyte sedimentation rates—had fatality rates of 85% or greater when the score was validated. The Glasgow prognostic score was developed in 1987 and is designed for rapid bedside assessment without the need for multiple laboratory tests.[24] Points are assigned for shock, a skin to rectal temperature differential of greater than 3° C, a pediatric-modified coma scale score of less than 8, absence of meningismus, an extending purpuric rash, deterioration in the hour before scoring, and a base deficit greater than 8. The scale was tested retrospectively on a group of 123 children who had meningococcemia in an effort to predict mortality reliably. A score of 10 or greater had a positive predictive value of 87.5% and a negative predictive value of 100%. In general, these scoring systems are used to determine what patients might benefit from more aggressive or experimental therapies and to help evaluate the usefulness of newer treatments.

COMPLICATIONS

The majority of children who survive meningococcal disease recover completely; 15% to 40% of patients, however, develop a complication of infection that may be categorized broadly as suppurative, neurological, or allergic. The suppurative complications include subdural effusions, subdural empyema, myocarditis, and acute suppurative arthritis. In a retrospective review by Edwards and Baker,[9] suppurative complications were detected in approximately 9% of children. Deafness is the most common neurological sequelae and was noted in 6% of children by Edwards and Baker. Most other series report deafness in 2% to 3% of patients, which is similar to the percentage of survivors who have ischemic complications such as gangrenous necrosis of the extremities or skin. Arthritis and pericarditis are the most common sequelae of meningococcal infection and are reported in 8% to 24% of cases. Both of these complications are thought to be secondary to an allergic phenomenon with immune complex deposition rather than a direct invasion of the heart or joints by the organism. Allergic arthritis and pericarditis are late in onset and more common in adults than in children. The symptoms usually are self-limited. Specific therapy generally is not required; however, drainage of pericardial or joint fluid occasionally is necessary.

Although not a true complication, complement deficiency can be detected in 8% of adults and children who have meningococcal disease. These patients are at high risk for recurrent episodes of invasive infection. In a study limited to pediatric patients, 18% had deficiencies of complement identified by screening for total hemolytic complement during convalescence.[15] Mayatepek and colleagues[16] detected a terminal complement component abnormality in 26.6% of patients who had meningococcal disease caused by the uncommon serotypes Y and W135. Similarly, the rate of deafness in patients infected with uncommon serotypes is increased significantly compared with those who had disease caused by the group B meningococcus (26.6% versus 3.3%). On the basis of this information, screening for complement deficiencies should be considered in any pediatric patient who has meningococcal disease.

DISEASE CONTROL AND PREVENTION

Antimicrobial chemoprophylaxis is an integral component in the control of meningococcal disease. Several studies have demonstrated that household, day care, and preschool contacts of patients who have invasive disease have a rate of infection approximately 100 to 800 times that in the general population.[8] In addition, 50% of secondary cases occur within 5 days of the index case and 70% within 1 week. Rifampin is 90% effective in eliminating carriage of the meningococcus from the nasopharynx. In addition, the recent Centers for Disease Control and Prevention surveillance study did not detect any resistance to rifampin in isolates from disease cases. On the basis of these data, the American Academy of Pediatrics recommends that all household, day care, or preschool contacts or anyone directly exposed to a patient's secretions, be given rifampin within 24 hours of recognition of the primary case.[20] The dosage is 10 mg/kg per dose (maximum adult dose is 600 mg) every 12 hours for 2 days for children over 1 month of age and 5 mg/kg per dose every 12 hours for 2 days for infants less than 1 month of age.

Newer agents being evaluated for use in chemoprophylactic regimens include ceftriaxone and ciprofloxacin. Schwartz and colleagues[21] demonstrated that a single 250 mg dose of intramuscular ceftriaxone was 97% effective at eliminating nasopharyngeal carriage of group A meningococcus. Although ceftriaxone is not recommended for widespread chemoprophylactic use, this regimen has the advantage of being safe for pregnant women. Several studies also have shown that use of ciprofloxacin results in a greater than a 90% meningococcal carrier reduction.[27] Although not approved for children or pregnant women, ciprofloxacin can be used in older adolescents and young adults and has the advantage of being administered as a single oral 500 mg dose.

Another important aspect of disease control and prevention is vaccination. A quadrivalent meningococcal vaccine, composed of purified capsular polysaccharide of meningococcal groups A, C, Y, and W135, is licensed for use in the United States. The dose for adults and children is 0.5 ml administered as a single dose subcutaneously. Routine vaccination is recommended only for those individuals at high risk of contracting meningococcal disease either through travel to highly endemic areas such as sub-Saharan Africa or via altered host defenses such as individuals who have asplenia or complement deficiencies. Vaccination also is a key component of outbreak control and has been used in selected areas in the United States and Canada for this purpose. The immunity induced by vaccination is serogroup specific; therefore no cross-reactive antibody to other serogroups is produced by this vaccine.[11] In general, protective antibody levels are achieved 10 to 14 days after administration, and the vaccine can be given concurrently with other immunizations if necessary. Adverse reactions are mild and infrequent, usually limited to local reactions.

The group A polysaccharide vaccine is safe, immunogenic, and efficacious in protecting against epidemic disease among adults and children as young as 3 months. Although not a major cause of disease in the United States, serogroup A is responsible for the majority of epidemic disease worldwide and for most cases of disease in the meningitis belt of Africa. Group C vaccine is neither immunogenic nor efficacious in children less than 2 years of age. Efficacy is 90% or more in adults, and this vaccine has been very useful in controlling outbreaks in the military. Group Y and W135 vaccines are safe and immunogenic in adults and children over age 2 years. Unfortunately, no vaccine is available for protection from group B meningococcal disease. The group B capsule is not immunogenic in humans and has been found to share cross-reacting antigens with human neural tissue. Attempts to create vaccine by using outer membrane proteins are being investigated but are not available for widespread use.

REFERENCES

1. Abramson JS, Spika JS: Persistence of *Neisseria meningitidis* in the upper respiratory tract after intravenous antibiotic therapy for systemic meningococcal disease, *J Infect Dis* 151:370, 1985.
2. Alvez F et al: Effect of chemoprophylaxis on the meningococcal carrier state after systemic infection, *Pediatr Infect Dis J* 10:700, 1991.
3. Baxter P, Priestley B: Meningococcal rash, *Lancet* 1:1166, 1988.
4. Boucek MM et al: Myocardial dysfunction in children with acute meningococcemia, *J Pediatr* 105:538, 1984.
5. Brandtzaeg P et al: Plasma endotoxin as a predictor of multiple organ failure and death in systemic meningococcal disease, *J Infect Dis* 159:195, 1989.
6. Cartwright KAV, Stuart JM, Robinson PM: Meningococcal carriage in close contacts of cases, *Epidemiol Infect* 106:133, 1991.
7. Cartwright KAV et al: Influenza A and meningococcal disease, *Lancet* 338:554, 1991.
8. De Wals P et al: Meningococcal disease in Belgium: secondary attack rate among household, day-care nursery and pre-elementary school contacts, *J Infect* 3:53, 1981.
9. Edwards MS, Baker CJ: Complications and sequelae of meningococcal infections in children, *J Pediatr* 99:540, 1981.
10. Fourrier F et al: Meningococcemia and purpura fulminans in adults: acute deficiencies of proteins C and S and early treatment with antithrombin III concentrates, *Intensive Care Med* 16:121, 1990.
11. Frasch CE: Vaccines for prevention of meningococcal disease, *Clin Microbiol Rev* 2(suppl):134, 1989.
12. Glode MP, Smith AL: Meningococcal disease. In Feigen RD, Cherry JD, editors: *Textbook of pediatric infectious diseases,* ed 3, Philadelphia, 1992, WB Saunders.
13. Irazuzta J, McManus ML: Use of topically applied nitroglycerin in the treatment of purpura fulminans, *J Pediatr* 117:993, 1990.
14. Jackson LA, Wenger DJ: Laboratory-based surveillance for meningococcal disease in selected areas, United States, 1989-1991, *MMWR* 42:21, 1993.
15. Leggiadro RJ, Winkelstein JA: Prevalence of complement deficiencies in children with systemic meningococcal infections, *Pediatr Infect Dis J* 6:75, 1987.
16. Mayatepek E et al: Deafness, complement deficiencies and immunoglobulin status in patients with meningococcal diseases due to uncommon serogroups, *Pediatr Infect Dis J* 12:808, 1993.
17. Monsalve F et al: Myocardial depression in septic shock caused by meningococcal infection, *Crit Care Med* 12:1021, 1984.
18. Moore PS et al: Respiratory viruses and mycoplasma as cofactors for epidemic group A meningococcal meningitis, *JAMA* 264:1271, 1990.
19. Powars DR et al: Purpura fulminans in meningococcemia: association with acquired deficiencies of proteins C and S, *N Engl J Med* 317:571, 1987.
20. Report of the Committee on Infectious Diseases: Meningococcal infections. In Peter G et al, editors: *1994 Red Book,* ed 23, Elk Grove Village, Ill, 1994, American Academy of Pediatrics.
21. Schwartz B et al: Comparative efficacy of ceftriaxone and rifampicin in eradicating pharyngeal carriage of group A *Neisseria meningitidis, Lancet* 1:1239, 1988.
22. Stiehm ER, Damrosch DS: Factors in the prognosis of meningococcal infection: review of 63 cases with emphasis on recognition and management of the severely ill patient, *J Pediatr* 68:457, 1966.
23. Tesoro LJ, Selbst SM: Factors affecting outcome in meningococcal infections, *Am J Dis Child* 145:218, 1991.
24. Thomson APJ, Sills JA, Hart CA: Validation of the Glasgow meningococcal septicemia prognostic score: a 10-year retrospective survey, *Crit Care Med* 19:26, 1991.
25. Tobias JD et al: Use of continuous caudal block to relieve lower-extremity ischemia caused by vasculitis in a child with meningococcemia, *J Pediatr* 115:1019, 1989.
26. Toews WH, Bass JW: Skin manifestations of meningococcal infection: an immediate indicator of prognosis, *Am J Dis Child* 127:173, 1974.
27. Visakorpi R: Ciprofloxacin in meningococcal carriers, *Scand J Infect Dis Suppl* 60:108, 1989.
28. Waage A, Halstensen A, Espevik T: Association between tumour necrosis factor in serum and fatal outcome in patients with meningococcal disease, *Lancet* 1:355, 1987.
29. Wong VK, Hitchcock W, Mason WH: Meningococcal infections in children: a review of 100 cases, *Pediatr Infect Dis J* 8:224, 1989.

288 Pneumothorax and Pneumomediastinum

David I. Bromberg

Pneumothorax and pneumomediastinum are defined as the presence of air in the potential pleural or mediastinal spaces, respectively. These conditions are relatively rare in pediatrics, having their greatest incidence in the neonatal period. However, in several clinical situations pneumothorax is a serious complication, and failure to recognize its presence could result in serious morbidity. Pneumothorax may play a prominent role (1) in the neonatal period, (2) as a complication of specific respiratory diseases, especially asthma and cystic fibrosis, (3) as a complication of mechanical ventilation, (4) as a result of trauma, and (5) when it occurs spontaneously.

The classic studies of Macklin and Macklin[1] have helped elucidate the mechanism of pneumothorax and pneumomediastinum. When a pressure gradient exists between the alveolus and interstitial tissue (usually as a result of high inspiratory pressures), alveolar rupture may result, with escape of air into the perivascular interstitium. This accumulation of air travels along the vascular ray (seen clinically as pulmonary interstitial emphysema) to the surface of the lung or to the mediastinum and eventually may result in a pneumothorax or pneumomediastinum. The entities, then, of pulmonary interstitial emphysema, pneumothorax, and pneumomediastinum are all expressions of a single pathological process.

The clinical manifestation varies with the extent of disease. Pain almost universally is present. As the size of the pneumothorax increases, tachypnea, dyspnea, and cyanosis may occur. Physical findings also vary from a normal examination to the presence of hyperresonance to percussion, the absence of breath sounds, and a mediastinal shift to the opposite end.

When air enters the pleural space through a ball valve mechanism, a tension pneumothorax is produced. The pneumothorax increases in size, with each inspiration greatly reducing lung volume. Clinical findings include severe and progressive dyspnea and cyanosis and may include shock. This constitutes an emergency in which thoracentesis can be lifesaving.

Pneumothorax has been demonstrated by radiological studies to occur in between 1% and 2% of all newborns. Some of these are undoubtedly related to overaggressive resuscitation, but others have been shown to occur spontaneously. Less than half the total number are symptomatic. The incidence of pneumothorax is much greater in neonates with pulmonary disease, especially hyaline membrane disease, meconium aspiration, and pulmonary hypoplasia. An increased incidence of renal anomalies in association with neonatal pneumothorax and pneumomediastinum has been noted.

Pneumothorax in older children, rather than occurring spontaneously, is seen as a complication of an underlying pulmonary disease or as a result of trauma or mechanical ventilation. Although rare, it has been reported in conjunction with asthma, cystic fibrosis, pneumonia (especially staphylococcal), and tuberculosis. Any entity that pathologically includes interstitial emphysema may potentially progress to include pneumothorax or pneumomediastinum as well. In a study of hospitalized asthmatics, over 5% were found to have pneumomediastinum, with the incidence increasing to greater than 15% in patients over 10 years of age. The therapeutic significance of this is clear, contraindicating the use of positive-pressure breathing in these patients. In thoracic trauma cases, a large percentage of patients have pneumothorax, which usually is apparent. These patients may have tension or "sucking" pneumothoraces and require immediate attention.

In late adolescence and young adulthood, in addition to the causes discussed above, spontaneous pneumothorax becomes a significant entity, occurring predominantly in otherwise healthy males who have no known underlying respiratory disease. These individuals are believed to have a pulmonary or pleural site of structural weakness or abnormality, but this seldom is proved. Activity levels appear to have little correlation with the onset of symptoms that may begin while the patient is at rest. Less than 20% have a recurrence; those who do frequently have the ipsilateral side involved within a year of the initial attack.

The diagnosis of pneumothorax and pneumomediastinum should be entertained seriously in patients who fall into the clinical categories discussed and who manifest sudden onset of sharp chest pain. Confirmation is made by obtaining posteroanterior and lateral chest roentgenograms and demonstrating the presence of free pleural or mediastinal air. Quantification of the pneumothorax also should be attempted. In the neonatal nursery fiberoptic transillumination has proved a valuable adjunctive tool for the rapid bedside diagnosis of pneumomediastinum and pneumothorax.

Iatrogenic causes of pneumothorax also must be considered. Pneumothorax can occur as a complication of tracheostomy, internal jugular puncture, subclavian vein line insertion, and mechanical ventilation. When a patient is given pressurized oxygen, care must be taken to ensure that the system is vented, or a tension pneumothorax could result.

Therapy depends on the size of the lesion, the cause, and the clinical status of the patient. In neonates, most pneumothoraces are managed with the insertion of a thoracostomy tube attached to a water seal. In symptomatic patients who have underlying pulmonary disease, needle aspiration of the pneumothorax is attempted while continuing to direct therapy toward the primary disease. If air reaccumulates in the pleural space, insertion of a thoracostomy tube connected to a water seal is indicated. The therapeutic approach to spontaneous pneumothorax usually is conservative. In the patient who is asymptomatic with a minor pneumothorax, observation alone is sufficient. In the case of larger lesions the physician should perform thoracentesis, removing as much air as possible. In cases of spontaneous pneumothorax without an identifiable cause, the patient and family should be reassured that the initial therapy is curative and that the majority will not recur.

After resolution, no activity reduction is indicated. Pneumomediastinum rarely produces symptoms. When this lesion becomes large enough to produce respiratory or circulatory distress, aspiration under fluoroscopic control is indicated. General supportive care is of the utmost importance in managing both lesions and should include adequate pain control and cough suppression when necessary.

REFERENCE

1. Macklin MI, Macklin CC: Malignant interstitial emphysema of the lungs and mediastinum as an important occult complication in many respiratory diseases and other conditions: an interpretation of the clinical literature in the light of laboratory experiment, *Medicine* 23:281, 1944.

SUGGESTED READINGS

DeVries WC, Wolfe WG: The management of spontaneous pneumothorax and bullous emphysema, *Surg Clin North Am* 60:851, 1980.

Melton LJ, Hepper NGG, Offord KP: Influence of height on the risk of spontaneous pneumothorax, *Mayo Clin Proc* 56:678, 1981.

Peters JI: When to suspect—and how to treat—a pneumothorax, *J Respir Dis* 7:17, 1986.

Pollack MM, Fields AI, Holbrook PR: Pneumothorax and pneumomediastinum during pediatric mechanical ventilation, *Crit Care Med* 7:536, 1979.

289 Poisoning

Robert J. Nolan

EPIDEMIOLOGY

The ingestion of potentially toxic substances usually is accidental in the child under 6 years of age; in the adolescent and the adult, the ingestion of a potentially toxic substance generally is the result of a willful act, although the resulting toxicity may be either intentional (i.e., attempted murder or suicide) or unintentional (e.g., adverse experience with an illicit drug). The incidence of ingestion episodes, the probability of resulting toxicity, and the agents involved are divergent for those two age groups.

Significant morbidity and mortality occur in both age groups as a result of therapeutic misuse of medications. This may be accidental, as in the administration of multiple doses to a child by the two parents, each unaware of the actions of the other, or intentional, excessive dosage administration to achieve an enhanced therapeutic effect (e.g., enhanced antipyresis with aspirin or acetaminophen, enhanced antienuretic effect with imipramine).

The American Association of Poison Control Centers (AAPCC)[6] estimates that more than 2.4 million human poison exposures occur each year in the United States. Nearly 60% of the 1,864,188 exposures voluntarily reported in 1992 were among children under 6 years of age; 90% of these were among children 3 years of age or younger. Many nontoxic or symptomless ingestions are assumed not reported or brought to medical attention. Symptomatic ingestions whose medical management is straightforward also are less likely to be reported by physicians. The morbidity in this high-incidence age group is small; only 20% of reported ingestions among children under 6 years of age result in any symptoms. However, more than 60% of adolescent ingestions are symptomatic. Of the 705 fatalities in all ages reported in 1992, only 29 were among children under 6 years of age. Poisoning deaths in adolescents and adults are not unusual and rarely are accidental; poisoning deaths among children are rare and almost always unintended.

Categories of agents most frequently involved in childhood poisonings are medications (42%), caustics and cleaning agents (11%), cosmetics (12%), plants (9%), hydrocarbons (3%), and insecticides or pesticides (3%). A significant incidence of exposure does not imply resultant toxicity; most ingested cosmetics and plants, for example, are harmless. The major categories of agents responsible for fatal poisoning among children under 6 years of age reported by the AAPCC from 1988 through 1992 are medications (53%), carbon monoxide inhalation (14%), hydrocarbons (11%), insecticides or pesticides (7%), and caustics or cleaning agents (7%). Iron-containing medications, psychotropic agents (including tricyclic antidepressants), and analgesics (salicylates and acetaminophen) in rank order account for almost 70% of the fatal *medication* ingestions among children under 6 years of age.

Over the past 30 years, mortality from accidental poisoning and the agents involved in poisoning episodes have changed significantly. Currently, mortality in the preschool-age child is about 10% of the rate during the mid-1960s. The causes for this decline are not defined adequately but generally are believed to include child-resistant closures (the declining death rate clearly antedated implementation of the Poison Prevention Packaging Act of 1970), increased public awareness of childhood poisoning, improved diagnosis and management of the poisoned child, and a decreased need for certain highly toxic substances (e.g., kerosene, lye) in the home. Aspirin used to be the single substance ingested most frequently by children, but the prevalence of aspirin ingestion has declined both absolutely and as a percentage of total ingestions. Fatalities from salicylates have declined more than tenfold, principally as a result of the legislated use of child-resistant closures and the voluntary restriction (by manufacturers) in packaging quantities for children's aspirin. This trend has accelerated since the early 1980s with declining use of aspirin in children resulting from concerns regarding its association with the onset of Reye syndrome. Childhood ingestions of iron-containing medications and psychotropic agents each account for more than three times as many fatalities as does aspirin.

Normal developmental phenomena, such as oral exploration, increasing mobility, and an insatiable curiosity, play a fundamental role in accidental poisoning in young children. In early childhood boys predominate slightly in accidental ingestions. Females predominate in adolescent ingestions. Family stress, social isolation, poor parenting skills, and maternal depression are among the family variables that predispose to accidental early childhood poisonings. Recidivism is high, with estimates ranging from 10% to 40%. Repetitive poisonings in a child may be the result of disturbed family dynamics resulting from diminished parental vigilance.

Accidental ingestions tend to occur at times of family disorganization, with deviations from normal routines (e.g., household moving, spring cleaning, vacation, or holidays), and during times of family stress (e.g., sickness, death, or divorce). The majority of early childhood ingestions occur in the child's home. The homes of grandparents who have medications of significant toxicity (e.g., cardiovascular medications and psychotropic agents) and a potential lower level of vigilance and "child proofing" also is a common site of ingestions. Ingestions occur most frequently in the kitchen, where cleansing products, polishing fluids, and other poisonous household products commonly are stored beneath the sink or on easily accessible lower cabinet shelves. The bathroom also is a common site for an accidental ingestion; agents involved most commonly are medications and cosmetics. In addition to improper storage of toxic products in easily accessible sites, improper storage of solvents and cleaning agents in drinking glasses, cups, or beverage bottles is a contributing epidemiological factor.

PREVENTION

Injury from the ingestion of toxic substances is best prevented by preventing the unintended, accidental ingestion. Because the child at risk is identified effectively only after the fact (the recidivist), effective prevention is directed toward the environment of all children and in most instances requires parental compliance. It therefore is not surprising that the only preventive measure of proven efficacy is societal intervention through the legislated requirement of child-resistant closures for toxic household products and drugs.

Appropriate selection of products to be stored in a household that has young children, selection of reasonable sites of storage, and prompt, proper disposal of unnecessary toxic materials are facets of the protective parental obligation. The environment may be rendered safer by the use of locked cabinets or boxes for all drugs and for toxic household products. All drugs and household products should be kept in their original containers. Materials no longer required should be discarded in a manner that precludes access by the child, such as flushing them down the toilet. Certain medications can be fatal to an average size toddler when 1 to 2 teaspoons or capsules are ingested. These medications, which include camphor, chloroquine, desipramine, hydroxychloroquine, imipramine, methyl salicylate, and quinine, require special safeguarding.

Advising parents and caretakers of children about these protective measures and alerting parents to the dangers of failing to supervise children during periods of family stress are recommended anticipatory guidance practices. In addition, the physician should provide educational materials in the office, participate in community education programs, limit prescribed drugs to necessary quantities, and instruct parents to use the entire prescribed quantities.

PRINCIPLES OF MANAGEMENT

General Considerations

The pediatrician should be able to deal effectively with the vast majority of acute ingestions. To facilitate this care, specific textbooks on poisonings should be readily available in the office library. Two excellent books are *Clinical Toxicology of Commercial Products* by Gosselin and associates[2] and *Clinical Management of Poisoning and Drug Overdose* by Haddad and Winchester.[4] The POISINDEX system,[8] a poison information software package, is widely available in emergency treatment facilities. The POISINDEX system can be accessed by most office computers.

Prompt removal of the offending agent can obviate the need for future treatment and may ameliorate subsequent developing symptoms. Cleansing from the skin any toxins that can produce a local effect or that can be absorbed cutaneously is accomplished easily in the office. Prompt gastric evacuation, using syrup of ipecac to induce emesis, is possible in the office, as is administration of an adsorbent, such as activated charcoal, or of a demulcent, such as evaporated milk or milk of magnesia. Further definitive treatment of seriously poisoned children is accomplished more easily in the hospital or emergency facility.

The physician should be familiar with and have ready access to community resources that may provide information or practical help with acute poisonings. A hospital emergency room or treatment facility should be readily available for the transfer of patients who are in need of care beyond that available in the office. Poison control centers are a good source of information on poisoning. From 1953 to 1970, local poison control centers were established throughout the United States; improved data retrieval and communication technologies during the 1970s led to regionalization, with a decline in the number of local centers. By 1992 about 75% of the U.S. population was served by regional poison control centers of the AAPCC. These regional centers offer comprehensive information 24 hours a day, toll-free telephone access, and access to a regional treatment facility for patient referral. Protocols for giving advice are used for the initial management of consumer calls.

Pharmacists sometimes can provide information about medications when the name of the medication or the amount dispensed does not appear on the label. Similarly, manufacturers may need to be called to determine the ingredients in a household product. A list of many manufacturers and their addresses can be found in *Clinical Toxicology of Commercial Products*.[2]

Telephone Calls

Most poisoning episodes are handled over the telephone. Typically, the mother calls and usually is anxious, even frantic. The person answering the telephone needs to be calm and firmly directive. Initially the practitioner needs to determine the agent, the amount ingested, and the presence or absence of symptoms. From this information, the risk of toxicity can be determined. This may depend on the relative toxicity of the agent involved or on the amount of the agent ingested. Alternatively, the presence of symptoms may suggest that toxicity is a risk, despite neither the agent nor the amount ingested seeming to be toxic.

If no toxic risk is present, the appropriate response is reassurance. If, however, a toxic risk exists, further data must be collected before advice can be given. The resources available to the caller need to be identified, such as the presence of first-aid drugs in the home (e.g., syrup of ipecac) or the proximity to a pharmacy or to a hospital and whether transportation is readily available. Using this information, the practitioner can recommend appropriate management.

Poisoning and accident prevention should be discussed with the parents within a few days of such a call; experience has shown that addressing prevention at the time of the initial call is less effective than doing so later. A recent accidental ingestion focuses the minds of the parents, providing a valuable opportunity to impart advice on poison prevention.

Approach to the Symptomatic Patient

Diagnosing poisoning in patients who are symptomatic can be difficult when an ingestion has not been observed. Although some poisons produce characteristic signs and symptoms, most do not; they may simulate many acute illnesses seen in pediatrics. The physician always should consider the possibility of poisoning when faced with a puzzling situation in which the diagnosis is not clear. The rapid onset of central nervous system, gastrointestinal, or respiratory symptoms should alert the physician to ask about medications or toxins within the home. Unexplained signs of central nervous system stimulation, such as delirium or convulsions, or of central nervous system depression, such as stupor or coma, should be considered to result from poisoning until proved otherwise. The presence of hyperpnea in a child or a young infant who has a febrile illness may be caused by the overzealous use of salicylates by the parents. A characteristic odor of specific poisons on the breath or in the vomitus sometimes can be discerned.

Therapeutic Modalities

The important principles of management of acute poisonings are (1) elimination of the poison from the body, (2) adsorption and inactivation of the poison, (3) administration of specific antidotes, and (4) provision of supportive measures. A calm and reasoned approach is far more effective than overtreatment with stimulants, depressants, or antidotes. Heroic measures are not needed with most poisoning episodes.

Syrup of ipecac is the most efficacious means of inducing vomiting when an ingestion has occurred. Emesis that can remove up to half of an ingested toxin is most effective within an hour of an ingestion. Syrup of ipecac is available without prescription in 30 ml containers. Contraindications to its use include neurological symptoms (depressed level of consciousness, seizures), caustic ingestions, most hydrocarbon ingestions, and antiemetic ingestions. Infants under 6 months of age have a poorly developed gag reflex and should not receive syrup of ipecac. Close medical observation is required when syrup of ipecac is administered to infants 6 to 9 months of age. The dose of syrup of ipecac is 10 ml for infants and children under 1 year and 15 ml for children; adolescents may receive 30 ml. The dose should be followed by one or two glasses of water and may be repeated if vomiting has not occurred within 20 to 30 minutes. The absence of vomiting after an additional 20 to 30 minutes necessitates gastric lavage. While ipecac-induced emesis has the temporal advantage of immediate home administration, evidence is accumulating that vigorous gastric lavage is more effective in removing the gastric contents.

Gastric lavage clearly is preferable to induced emesis for the patient in whom central nervous system depression is present or possible. In the conscious, alert patient, it has the advantage of being a controlled means of gastric evacuation. It is contraindicated in caustic and most hydrocarbon ingestions. As large a plastic catheter as can be passed into the stomach without trauma should be used, and the stomach should be irrigated with 50 to 200 ml aliquots of isotonic saline until the returns are clear. Tap water should not be used in children because of the danger of producing water intoxication. Before the catheter is withdrawn, it should be either pinched off or the suction maintained to prevent aspiration of material into the lungs.

Activated charcoal is an effective adsorbent for most drugs, including acetaminophen, aspirin, sedative hypnotics, tricyclic antidepressants, stimulants (amphetamines and cocaine), and phenothiazines. It is *ineffective* in alcohol, cyanide, iron, and other heavy metal poisonings. Given as a water slurry (20 to 50 g in children, 50 to 100 g in adolescents), it is effective immediately after ingestion and can be given safely by nonprofessionals. In general, charcoal should be administered as soon as possible, preferably within the first few hours after the ingestion. Repeated administration of activated charcoal every 3 to 4 hours effectively can "trap" a toxin in the luminal space of the gut. Cathartics (sorbitol) may be required because activated charcoal can be constipating. Activated charcoal is contraindicated in caustic ingestions because it is ineffective and will obscure later endoscopic findings; it also should not be used simultaneously with syrup of ipecac because charcoal adsorbs the ipecac, rendering it ineffective. It should be administered after emesis has been induced or lavage completed successfully.

Relatively few effective specific antidotes exist. Oxygen is the specific effective antidote for carbon monoxide poisoning. Naloxone hydrochloride (Narcan) safely and effectively antagonizes the pharmacological effects of natural and synthetic narcotics. Flumazenil improves consciousness in ingestions of benzodiazepine. Specific antibody fragments can reverse the arrhythmias associated with ingestions of digitalis. Ethanol infusion effectively blocks the alcohol dehydrogenase conversion of ethylene glycol or methanol to more toxic metabolites. Pyridoxine reduces isoniazid-induced seizure activity. For the treatment of organophosphate poisoning, pralidoxime (2-PAM) is highly effective if used in conjunction with atropine. N-acetylcysteine is effective when administered early in severe acetaminophen poisoning. Of the chelating agents used to treat heavy metal poisonings, deferoxamine mesylate (Desferal) is specific for iron poisoning; dimercaprol (BAL) combines with arsenic, bismuth, lead, and mercury; and calcium EDTA chelates cadmium, copper, iron, and lead. Methylene blue may be lifesaving in drug-induced methemoglobinemia; sodium thiosulfate and inhalation of amyl nitrate combined with intravenous sodium nitrite (both of which may cause methemoglobinemia) may be lifesaving in cyanide poisoning. Although vitamin K effectively counteracts the anticoagulant properties of coumarin and warfarin, its use rarely is needed because repeated ingestions over a period of days are necessary to produce toxicity.

When poisoning has resulted from an ionizable drug, intracellular and central nervous system drug levels may be reduced and renal excretion increased by therapy directed toward achieving "ion trapping." Ionizable drugs, such as amphetamine, phencyclidine, salicylate, and phenobarbital, cross lipid membranes (the cell wall or blood-brain barrier) only in the nonionized state. Gradients in pH across the membrane "trap" the ionized drug in the milieu, favoring dissociation. A more alkaline pH favors dissociation (and hence, ion trapping) of weakly acidic drugs (e.g., phenobarbital, salicylate); a relatively acidic milieu favors higher concentrations of weakly basic drugs (e.g., amphetamines, phencyclidine). Occasionally in acute salicylism, and almost invariably in chronic salicylism, potassium depletion (with or without hypokalemia) precludes the excretion of an alkaline urine.

Drugs that have a small apparent volume of distribution (V_D less than 1 liter per kg)—that is, most of the drug remains in the blood or extracellular fluid—such as salicylates or amphetamines, can be "cleansed" from the body by hemodialysis, charcoal hemoperfusion, exchange transfusion, or peritoneal dialysis. Drugs that have high degrees of tissue binding and a large V_D, such as digoxin and phenothiazines, are removed poorly by those techniques.

Supportive therapy is the mainstay of treatment in most intoxications. This consists of administering intravenous fluids, supporting respiration, and treating shock, congestive heart failure, cerebral edema, and convulsions.

SALICYLATE POISONING

Salicylism is seen in all age groups, including congenital salicylism caused by maternal ingestion of toxic quantities, accidental ingestion in early childhood, and attempted suicide in adolescence and adulthood. Poisoning also can occur following excessive topical application of oil of wintergreen to denuded skin. Over 50% of hospitalized cases of salicylism result from chronic ingestion associated with therapeutic misuse; 25% of patients who have salicylism have an associated intercurrent infection. Oil of wintergreen (1400 mg methyl salicylate/ml) was the cause of the majority of fatal acute salicylate ingestions in children under 6 years of age reported from 1989 to 1992.

Laboratory Findings

Diagnosis depends on either elicitation of a history of ingestion or recognition of the characteristic clinical findings. A positive urine ferric chloride reaction can confirm salicylate ingestion but not toxic exposure because the test is sensitive to ordinary therapeutic doses. The anion gap usually is elevated. The serum salicylate level confirms the diagnosis. Single acute ingestions of greater than 150 mg/kg generally result in clinical symptoms; acute ingestions greater than 500 mg/kg are potentially fatal. The nomogram introduced by Done[1] (Fig. 289-1) correlates the serum salicylate level with the time since ingestion and is essential to assessment of clinical severity following ingestion of a single dose. The serum salicylate level is of limited value in assessing clinical severity when the drug has been administered repeatedly or ingested chronically. The clinical picture of salicylism is characterized by vomiting, hyperpnea, and dehydration. Salicylism should be considered in the diagnosis of cryptogenic metabolic acidosis, particularly in the 18-month to 4-year age group.

Clinical Findings

The major toxic effects of salicylate are (1) local gastrointestinal irritation, (2) direct stimulation of the central nervous system respiratory center, (3) increased metabolic rate, (4) interference with carbohydrate metabolism through the inhibition of several Krebs cycle enzymes and the uncoupling of oxidative phosphorylation, and (5) interference with normal blood coagulation mechanisms.

The net disturbance in hydrogen ion concentration in salicylism is the product of two simultaneously occurring challenges to acid-base homeostasis. Central nervous system-mediated inappropriate hyperpnea may lead to respiratory alkalosis. Deranged carbohydrate metabolism and dehydration are potent stimuli for metabolic acidosis. In children under 4 years of age, metabolic acidosis generally predominates clinically; in older children and adults, however, the patient frequently has respiratory alkalosis. Profound acidemia among

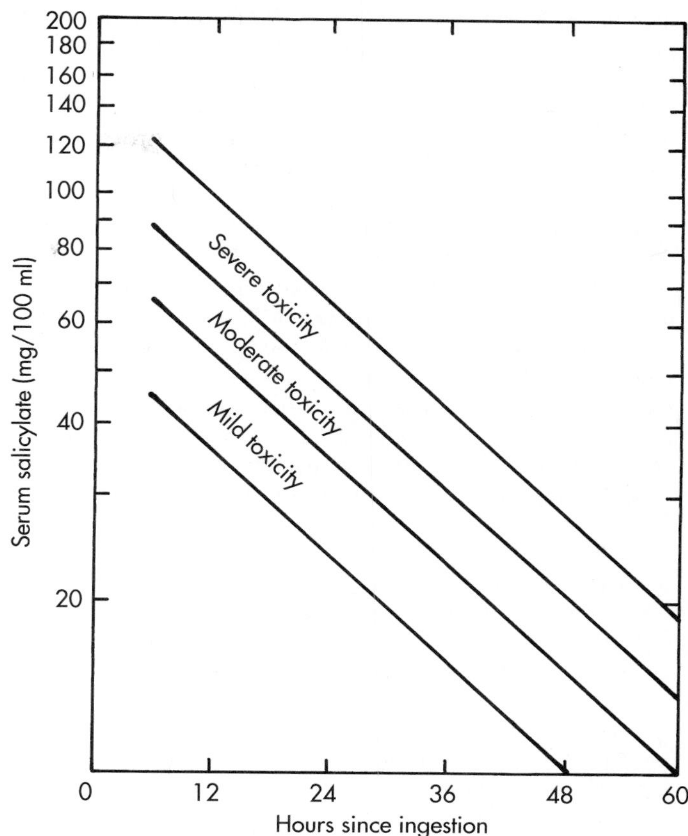

FIG. 289-1 Done nomogram for estimating the severity of poisoning after a single acute salicylate ingestion.
(Adapted from Done AK: *Pediatrics* 26:800, 1960.)

older children and adults heralds a poor prognosis. Hyperthermia, resulting from the increased and disregulated metabolic state, is common.

The clinical findings of hyperglycemia, hyperpnea, polyuria, glucosuria, and ketonuria early in the course of intoxication simulate diabetic ketoacidosis closely. In salicylism, however, blood glucose exceeding 200 mg/dl is unusual. Hypoglycemia may supervene as glycogen stores are depleted. Dehydration causing decreased renal blood flow often results in oliguria later in the course. Hypokalemia is common, and total body stores of potassium often are depleted.

Therapy

Therapy has three objectives: (1) prevention of further salicylate absorption, (2) correction of existent solute and fluid deficits, and (3) reduction of tissue salicylate levels. Further salicylate absorption is prevented by removing salicylate from the gastrointestinal tract through lavage or induced emesis and by binding the medication within the gastrointestinal lumen through the repeated administration of activated charcoal. Gastric emptying should be employed regardless of the time since ingestion.

The initial consideration in fluid therapy is the establishment of an adequate circulating fluid volume. In the presence of shock or impending shock, an isotonic solution should be administered at a rate of 20 ml/kg/hr. This may be continued safely a second hour in the absence of improved tissue perfusion. Blood pressure, pulse, capillary filling, and in extreme circumstances, central venous pressure are effective monitors of adequate volume expansion.

The correction of existent solute and water deficits may require total fluid volumes from 115 ml/kg/24 hr to 250 ml/kg/24 hr. A solution containing 40 to 50 mEq/liter of sodium should be used. A urine volume of 2000 ml/m^2/day and a specific gravity less than 1.010 (300 mmol/liter) are reasonable goals.

Both hypokalemia and hypoglycemia can present life-threatening situations. A minimum of 25 mEq/liter of potassium should be included once adequate renal function has been established; all intravenous fluids should include a minimum of 5 g/dl of glucose; with hypoglycemia or neurological symptomatology, the use of 10 g/dl of glucose should be considered. Correction of acidemia and hypokalemia is essential to the lowering of tissue salicylate levels; the establishment of an alkaline urine dramatically increases urine salicylate excretion. Sufficient bicarbonate should be administered intravenously to raise the urine pH to 8. Although a forced alkaline diuresis is ideal, diuresis in the absence of alkalinization is not effective in eliminating salicylates, and alkalinization of the urine may be difficult to achieve during a rapid diuresis.

Peritoneal dialysis and hemodialysis are effective therapies for serum salicylate values in excess of 100 mg/dl, coma, renal insufficiency, refractory acidosis, or failure of response to conservative therapy.

ACETAMINOPHEN

Ingestion of acetaminophen is a common cause of death among adults and adolescents who have suicidal intent. A widespread lack of appreciation of the toxicity of acetaminophen and the frequent delay in onset of symptoms increase the potential for fatal outcomes in adolescent suicide gestures. Although 70% of the acetaminophen ingestions reported by the AAPCC from 1988 through 1992 occurred in children under 6 years of age, less than 1% of the fatalities reported were in that age range. The majority of fatal ingestions in young children are the result of therapeutic misuse.

More than 90% of an ingested acetaminophen load is inactivated in the liver through conjugation with sulfate or glucuronide. A third hepatic metabolic pathway dependent on cytochrome P-450 detoxifies acetaminophen through conjugation with glutathione. This pathway produces a variety of hepatotoxic metabolites from acetaminophen if the hepatic glutathione reserves are depleted. A diminished toxic state occurs in children under 6 years of age as a result of relatively increased glutathione stores or lessened metabolic detoxification by the P-450 pathway. Comparable toxic doses are five to ten times more likely to be hepatotoxic in the child over 6 years of age.

Clinical Findings and Therapy

During the first 24 hours after ingestion, the child who has toxic plasma levels of acetaminophen may have anorexia, nausea, and vomiting. A latent period follows during which gastrointestinal symptoms resolve concurrent with evolving liver function abnormalities in the untreated individual. The transaminases, bilirubin levels, and prothrombin time peak 2 to 4 days after ingestion; fulminant hepatic failure may intervene. Children who survive the hepatic insult have no clinical or pathological sequelae.

N-acetylcysteine functions as a specific antidote through its substitution for glutathione in the P-450-dependent pathway. The decision to use N-acetylcysteine is based on the plasma acetaminophen level at least 4 hours after ingestion[9] (Fig. 289-2). Individuals at risk for hepatotoxicity should receive therapy. Although maximum benefit is realized if N-acetylcysteine is begun within 8 hours of an ingestion, it is indicated up to 24 hours after an ingestion. Beginning therapy without knowing a plasma level is reasonable if a significant ingestion has occurred (greater than 125 to 150 mg/kg in a child under 6 years of age) and if a level will not be available within the first 8 hours after ingestion. A loading of 140 mg/kg of N-acetylcysteine is given orally, followed by 17 doses of 70 mg/kg at 4-hour intervals. Following an ingestion, the gastric contents should be evacuated;

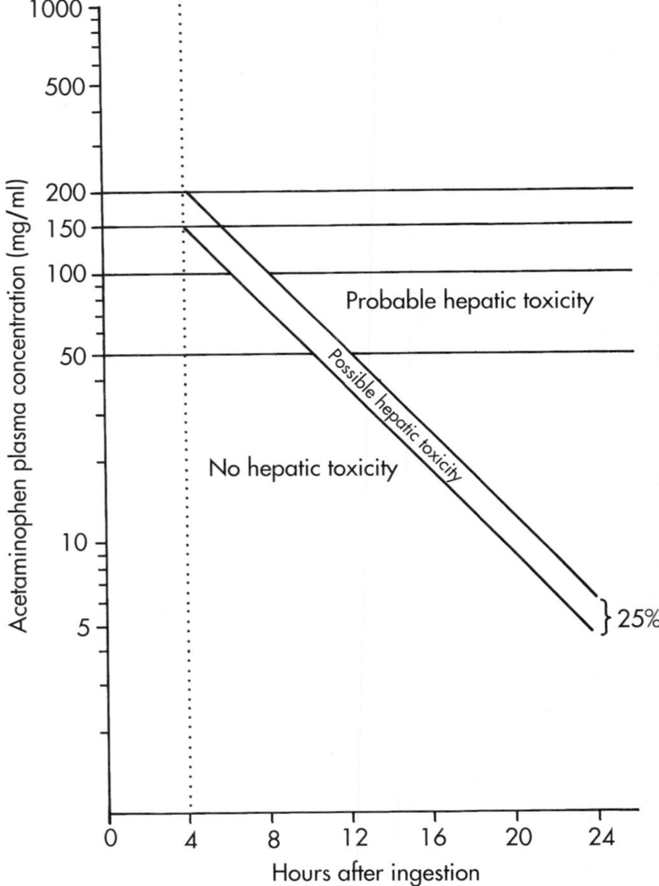

FIG. 289-2 Rumack-Matthew nomogram for estimating the probability of hepatic toxicity after a single acute acetaminophen ingestion. The lower solid diagonal line is placed 25% below the upper solid diagonal line, which divides the "no hepatic toxicity" area. This allows for potential errors in estimating the time after ingestion of the acetaminophen and potential errors in the measurement of acetaminophen plasma levels.

(Adapted from Rumack BH, Matthew H: *Pediatrics* 55:871, 1975.)

catharsis may be considered to remove the drug from the lower gastrointestinal tract. Activated charcoal adsorbs both acetaminophen and N-acetylcysteine. The standard loading dose of 140 mg/kg of N-acetylcysteine generally is sufficient if a single dose of activated charcoal has been given. The emetic quality of N-acetylcysteine may complicate management if an increased loading dose is used. Activated charcoal should be administered if acetaminophen is taken as part of a mixed drug ingestion.

ORGANOPHOSPHATES

Pesticides continue to be a source of serious poisoning among children in both rural and urban settings. The particular substance or the particular chemical group into which it falls must be identified. Standard references are invaluable in this regard.[2]

Organophosphates account for most reported pesticide exposures and most deaths from such exposures. These insecticides, with few exceptions, are highly toxic to humans. Because organophosphates are readily absorbed from the skin, lungs, and gastrointestinal tract, they need not be ingested to cause symptoms of toxicity. Contaminated clothing can lead to symptoms.

Organophosphate insecticides and their metabolic byproducts inhibit acetylcholinesterase. The result is the accumulation of unhydrolyzed acetylcholine. This causes excessive and continued stimulation and then depression of the parasympathetic nervous system, the somatic motor nerves, and the central nervous system.

Clinical Findings

The clinical manifestations of organophosphate poisoning are protean. Stimulation of the autonomic nervous system leads to increased sweating, salivation, and miosis. Bradycardia may develop. Bronchial secretions and bronchial constriction are increased with resultant cough, dyspnea, and cyanosis. Pulmonary edema may occur. Gastrointestinal symptoms include vomiting, abdominal cramps, and intestinal hypermotility. Effects on striated muscle are evidenced by incoordination, tremors, and weakness, then muscle fasciculations followed by paralysis, particularly of the respiratory muscles. Central nervous system manifestations are headache, confusion, anxiety, emotional lability, ataxia, convulsions, coma, and eventual depression of the respiratory and circulatory centers. Hypotension or hypertension may be seen.

Children who are poisoned significantly commonly exhibit pinpoint pupils, excessive respiratory tract secretions, central nervous system excitement or depression, and respiratory arrest. The onset of symptoms may be extremely rapid, and death generally occurs within 24 hours. After sublethal doses, with reversal of inhibition of cholinesterase, the symptoms disappear; the rate of recovery varies with different compounds, from a few hours to several weeks.

Proximal limb paralysis and respiratory muscle compromise can occur in occasional patients after the resolution of cholinergic symptoms, the "intermediate syndrome." These patients require appropriate supportive measures. Organophosphates may cause a delayed (1 to 4 weeks after exposure) polyneuropathy accompanied by ataxia and spasticity.

Diagnosis

Once thought of, the diagnosis of organophosphate poisoning is not difficult to make. The diagnosis should be made on the basis of (1) history of exposure or a reasonable possibility of exposure, (2) the onset of symptoms within 12 hours of exposure, and (3) a clinical picture consistent with this diagnosis. In addition, these insecticides have a disagreeable garliclike odor, and children who have been poisoned may have a garliclike odor on their clothes or breath. This diagnosis can be confirmed by determining depression of serum and red cell cholinesterase levels before therapy is begun. Although serum concentrations (pseudocholinesterase) are measured in most hospitals, many hospitals are not prepared to do the more specific erythrocyte (true cholinesterase) determination. Treatment should be initiated without waiting for laboratory results.

Therapy

Treatment of organophosphate poisoning involves both general measures and specific antidotes. If the skin has been exposed, all clothing should be removed and the skin washed with copious amounts of soap and water. If intoxication has resulted from ingestion, the gastric contents should be emptied. Health care providers should avoid contact with the vomitus or lavage fluid. Activated charcoal adsorbs many of the organophosphates. The oronasopharynx should be cleared of secretions and an airway inserted. Endotracheal intubation and mechanical ventilation may be required to treat respiratory depression. Atropine 0.05 to 0.10 mg/kg should be administered every 10 to 30 minutes until complete atropinization (clearing of excessive oral and pulmonary secretions) and the reversal of cholinergic signs has been achieved. Atropinization should be maintained intermittently for 24 to 48 hours. Atropine blocks the action of acetylcholine without restoring the action of cholinesterase. After atropinization, in moderate to severe intoxication, pralidoxime (Protopam or 2-PAM), a cholinesterase reactivator, 25 to 50 mg/kg (up to 0.5 to 1 g) should be given intravenously in saline solution over 15 to 30 minutes. The dose may be repeated in 1 to 2 hours if muscular weakness does not resolve and every 6 to 8 hours thereafter if symptoms warrant. Pralidoxime does not cross the blood-brain barrier; reversal of central nervous system symptoms depends on atropine therapy. Pralidoxime is of minimal benefit if given more than 36 to 48 hours after exposure.

Atropine should be tapered slowly under close observation and reinstituted if symptoms recur. Observation for a minimum of 24 hours is necessary after the cessation of atropine and pralidoxime therapy. Diazepam can help control the agitation and muscle fasciculations.

PSYCHOACTIVE DRUGS

Sedatives, Hypnotics, and Opiates

Clinical Findings. Central nervous system (CNS) depression (e.g., somnolence, stupor, coma) may constitute the presenting signs for patients whose toxicity results from the ingestion of sedatives, hypnotics, anxiolytics, or opiates. There frequently are no distinguishing clinical features. Occasionally, a constellation of findings may suggest a specific drug class. Hypotension and respiratory depression are seen frequently following ingestion of toxic quantities of barbiturates or a glutethimide; they are observed occasionally with phenothiazine or methaqualone poisoning. Hypothermia usually is associated with the ingestion of barbiturates or a glutethimide. Pulmonary edema frequently complicates the course of poisoning by glutethimide or methaqualone and occasionally is seen with barbiturate poisoning. Seizures, opisthotonos, and torticollis frequently are observed with phenothiazine poisoning; myoclonus, hypertonia, and increased reflexes are associated with methaqualone intoxication. Focal and rapidly changing neurological symptoms and signs are characteristic of glutethimide poisoning. Opiate overdose classically shows respiratory and CNS depression and miosis; pulmonary edema, hypertension, and hypothermia also occur. Cyclic variations in the depth of coma with multiple episodes of abrupt onset of apnea are common with poisoning by these drugs; fixed, dilated pupils with anisocoria also may be seen and do not necessarily indicate a grave prognosis.

Central nervous system depression resulting from the opiates or pentazocine is reversed safely and effectively by the narcotic antagonist naloxone hydrochloride (Narcan). Reversal of central nervous system depression by naloxone also has been reported among patients poisoned by diphenoxylate (Lomotil) and propoxyphene (Darvon). Naloxone has no agonist activity. It is administered intravenously, 0.01 mg/kg; this dose can be repeated safely without fear of increasing respiratory depression, and empirically can be used safely and effectively among patients whose coma is of unknown origin.

Therapy. Supportive care is the mainstay of therapy for patients in coma resulting from poisoning that has not responded to naloxone therapy. Immediate attention is directed to stabilization and maintenance of ventilation and perfusion. Patients in coma require intubation. Atelectasis and aspiration pneumonia frequently are complications of coma from poisoning. Gastric lavage late in the course of ingestion-induced coma is hazardous and of questionable efficacy; it should be undertaken only after a protected airway has been carefully secured. Hypotension resulting from barbiturate ingestion generally is caused by decreased peripheral vascular resistance and hypovolemia and usually responds to plasma volume expansion. The frequency of pulmonary edema as a complication of methaqualone or glutethimide poisoning precludes rapid fluid administration in these poisonings in the absence of careful central venous pressure monitoring. In the profoundly ill, comatose, poisoned patient, a central venous pressure monitor is essential. Analeptic drugs are not indicated in the management of poison-induced coma. Forced diuresis, with alkalinization of the urine to achieve ion trapping, is effective in facilitating clearance of phenobarbital but is of no value in treating poisoning from the short-acting barbiturates and is contraindicated in the management of methaqualone poisoning.

Phencyclidine, Amphetamine, and Cocaine

Poisoning by phencyclidine (PCP) is characterized by aggressive, even assaultive, behavior, which may seriously impede evaluation and therapy of the gravely ill patient. Symptoms and signs may include confusion, irritability, hallucinations, tremor, chest pain, palpitations, hypertension, tachycardia, auditory hyperesthesia, sweating, excessive salivation, anxiety, panic, hyperpyrexia, hyperreflexia, and rhabdomyolysis. Coma and convulsions occur with severe poisoning. Psychotic states (which may persist), nystagmus (horizontal or vertical), increased muscle tone (which may be associated with opisthotonos), and fixed staring are prominent features of PCP intoxication.

Amphetamines and cocaine, although structurally different, are powerful CNS stimulants. Abuse of cocaine, particularly the free-base form, "crack," which can be smoked, has reached epidemic proportions. Cocaine deaths reported to the AAPCC more than doubled since the mid 1980s. Severe morbidity or death may occur from high-dose chronic or "binge" use or may occur after a single exposure. Intoxication results in a sense of enhanced energy, which may progress to violent and bizarre behavior, delirium, seizures, paranoia, agitation, and death. Adverse effects include systemic hypertension, tachycardia and other cardiac arrhythmias, hyperthermia, and respiratory depression. Myocardial infarction, stroke, aortic rupture, and rhabdomyolysis have been reported.

Therapy. Immediate therapy includes careful limitation of sensory stimuli and supportive care. Seizures may be difficult to control. Diazepam is the preferred anticonvulsant. Diazoxide or hydralazine is preferred for the management of hypertension. Additional alpha-adrenergic blocking drugs (phentolamine) may be required. Chlorpromazine, highly useful in the treatment of amphetamine poisoning, is contraindicated in PCP intoxication. Amphetamine and PCP levels in the central nervous system can be reduced and excretion in the urine increased by acidification to achieve ion trapping. Careful monitoring of serum pH, potassium, and ammonia levels is required. In addition, the physician should interrupt the gastroenteric recirculation of PCP by initiating repeated doses of activated charcoal every 3 to 4 hours (independent of the PCP's route of administration).

Tricyclic Antidepressants

The widespread use, accessibility, and toxicity of the tricyclic antidepressants imipramine, amitriptyline, nortriptyline, desipramine, amoxapine, maprotiline, protriptyline, and doxepin make these medications the most common cause of fatal ingestion with prescription drugs in individuals under 17 years old. Tricyclics are used for depression in adults and adolescents; several are used to treat enuresis and hyperkinesis in children. In excess of 95% of the fatal ingestions by adolescents reported by the AAPCC between 1988 and 1992 were suicides. Accidental ingestion and therapeutic misuse predominate in the younger population.

Clinical Findings. Patients have anticholinergic effects, such as dry mouth and skin, mydriasis, urinary retention, delayed gastric emptying and intestinal ileus, and hyperthermia. Tricyclic poisoning should be suspected when hypotension and cardiac arrhythmias or coma are present. Evidence of central nervous system toxicity may include initial excitement that progresses to coma; myoclonus or choreoathetosis, central respiratory depression, and seizures also occur. The primary cause of death in tricyclic overdose is cardiac malfunction; arrhythmias and myocardial depression are common.

Therapy. Initial treatment of tricyclic ingestion is aimed at removing the gastric contents. Lavage rather than emesis is the preferred means of gastric decontamination because of the potential for coma and seizures. The decreased gastric motility secondary to the anticholinergic effects of the ingestion makes gastric decontamination beneficial up to 18 hours after the ingestion. Repeated administration of activated charcoal should follow gastric emptying. All patients should be hospitalized for continuous electrocardiogram monitoring, preferably in an intensive care unit. The pharmacokinetics of tricyclic ingestion are complex. Drug levels should not be used as the sole criterion for therapeutic intervention; initial management should be based on the patient's clinical status. A QRS complex of greater than 100 milliseconds is the most reliable indicator of tricyclic toxicity (occurring in patients who have tricyclic levels greater than 1000 ng/ml) and is correlated strongly with the risk of serious arrhythmias, most commonly ventricular tachycardia degenerating into ventricular fibrillation. Life-threatening arrhythmias usually occur within 24 hours of ingestion but can occur as long as 5 days after ingestion. ECG monitoring should continue for at least 24 hours after the resolution of signs of cardiac toxicity (QRS interval less than 100 milliseconds).

Treatment of intoxication is symptomatic and supportive. The mainstay of treatment is alkalinization to a pH of 7.45 to 7.55 with intravenous sodium bicarbonate, which decreases the risk of arrhythmias, which are potentiated by acidosis. Ventricular tachycardia or fibrillation should be treated with a 1 to 2 mEq/kg sodium bicarbonate bolus as well as appropriate resuscitative measures. Direct ventricular pacing may be necessary. Excessive alkalinization ($pH > 7.6$) is unnecessary and is associated with increased mortality.

Hypotension should be treated with volume expansion. Excessive fluids can result in pulmonary edema because of decreased myocardial contractility. Norepinephrine, dopamine, or dobutamine are recommended as pressor agents if volume therapy is insufficient. Seizures, which may be difficult to control, respond best to diazepam followed by phenytoin.

HOUSEHOLD CLEANING AGENTS AND CAUSTICS

Household disinfectants and cleaning agents (e.g., ammonia and bleach, laundry detergent, automatic dishwater detergent, and oven, drain, and toilet cleaners) contain variable amounts of acidic or alkaline caustics. The severity of damage to the oropharynx, esophagus, and stomach upon ingestion depends on the volume and concentration of the caustic and its duration of contact with the mucosal surfaces. The concentration of the caustic must be determined through history, examination of the container, or consultation with a regional poison control center.

Household bleach (sodium hypochlorite), weak ammonia solutions, and phosphate-based laundry detergents usually don't damage tissue but may irritate the mucosa. Industrial-strength ammonia, bleaches, and detergents brought to the home from the work place constitute a significant hazard. Children on farms who have access to industrial strength liquid alkaline cleaners are a high-risk group. Ecologically sound "low phosphate" detergents containing carbonates and other alkaline agents, such as trisodium phosphate, and dishwater detergents have a high pH and may destroy tissue. Most caustic injuries are caused by ingestion of liquid or particulate alkaline drain or oven cleaners. Recent reductions in the alkali concentration of liquid cleaners to the 8% to 10% range have reduced but not eliminated morbidity. Adolescents and adults who ingest caustics with suicidal intent are more likely to have severe burns than are children who have unintentional exposures.

Clinical Findings

Alkali ingestions generally result in greater tissue destruction than do acid ingestions. The bitter taste and instantaneous burning sensation associated with strong acids limit the volume of the ingestion and prompt immediate expectoration. A greater volume of the relatively tasteless liquid alkaline preparation may be swallowed before the child experiences significant distress. Acid mucosal injury results in a coagulation necrosis, with the formation of a dense eschar that tends to limit tissue penetration. The liquefaction necrosis characteristic of an alkali injury permits deep penetration of the alkali through the mucosa, submucosa, and muscular layers of the upper gastrointestinal tract. Acidic agents generally cause greater damage to the gastric mucosa, particularly the lesser curvature and the prepyloric area; alkaline ingestions result in greater damage to the esophagus. Liquid ingestions often produce circumferential burns; particulate ingestion causes spotty or streaklike burns. The intense inflammatory response may cause acute or subacute viscus perforation or stricture formation 14 to 28 days after the ingestion.

The patient may be in severe distress, with drooling, inability or refusal to swallow, abdominal pain, and violent retching. Air hunger and stridor may result from burns and subsequent edema of the glottic structures. Circumferential or patchy burns or ulcerations of the oral mucosa may be present, with edema of the oral and pharyngeal tissues. Significant ingestions may show minimal symptomatology. Esophageal damage with the potential for stricture formation may occur in the complete absence of oral lesions.

Therapy

Management is supportive and expectant. Induction of emesis is contraindicated. The child should be kept upright to minimize vomiting and reflux. If the child is able to swallow, several ounces of water or milk may be given to dilute the poison. Attempts to neutralize an alkali ingestion with a mild acid such as vinegar are contraindicated because the resulting exothermal reaction will result in further tissue damage. Although serious burns are more likely in symptomatic patients, the initial presenting symptoms are not reliably predictive of esophageal injury; endoscopy should be considered in all patients who have a credible history of caustic ingestion. The efficacy of steroids (prednisolone 2 mg/kg/day) to reduce the inflammatory response and subsequent potential for stricture formation is based on anecdotal and retrospective data; controlled prospective studies have shown no benefit. H_2-blockers may be used to suppress gastric acid production and secondary gastric or esophageal acid injury. Parenteral fluid therapy and antibiotics are used as clinically indicated. Bougienage may be used to prevent or dilate strictures. Long-term morbidity results from esophageal or pyloric strictures and the attempts to maintain patency through chronic dilation or surgical reconstruction.

HYDROCARBONS

Hydrocarbon ingestion is a leading cause of death from poisoning with household products. Hydrocarbons include petroleum distillates such as gasoline, kerosene, mineral seal oil, lighter fluids, paint thinners, and pine oil derivatives such as turpentine. Deaths from hydrocarbon poisoning are the result of pulmonary involvement.

Pulmonary Complications

The pulmonary complications of hydrocarbon ingestions are the result of aspiration into the tracheobronchial tree. With significant ingestions, symptoms usually begin within 30 minutes and often are associated with choking, gagging, and vomiting. Signs of pulmonary involvement include grunting respirations, a persistent nonproductive cough, intercostal retractions, cyanosis, tachypnea, tachycardia, and fever. Rales, rhonchi, or diminished breath sounds may be heard. Frequently the sensorium is depressed, and the odor of the ingested hydrocarbon can be smelled on the breath. A depressed sensorium signifies hypoxemia. Signs and symptoms of respiratory involvement usually peak in the first 24 hours and then regress over the next 2 to 5 days.

Radiographic Findings

The risk of aspiration depends on the chemical and physical properties of the hydrocarbons ingested. Low surface tension allows a hydrocarbon to spread rapidly over the mucosal surfaces, and low viscosity enables deeper penetration of the fluids into the distal airways. Highly volatile hydrocarbons cause acute chemical pneumonitis. Highly viscous, nonvolatile petroleum distillates such as mineral oil, motor oil, most baby oils, and liquid petrolatum are not aspirated as easily and do not cause chemical pneumonitis unless large amounts are aspirated.

Chest roentgenographic changes can be seen as early as 30 minutes after ingestion. Initially multiple, small, mottled densities are seen in the perihilar area and may extend into the midlung field. The mottled densities may become confluent and give a picture of consolidation. Lower airway obstruction with air trapping often is evident. Pleural effusions may develop. Occasionally, pneumatoceles form. Correlation between the chest roentgenographic findings and the clinical symptoms is poor. Whereas approximately 75% of patients who have ingested hydrocarbons exhibit roentgenographic evidence of lung involvement, only 25% to 50% of these have respiratory symptoms.

Therapy

Management of hydrocarbon ingestion is nonspecific, symptomatic, and supportive. Because aspiration is the principal hazard, vomiting should not be induced. Gastric lavage is not recommended. (Hydrocarbons that act as carriers for heavy metals or insecticides, as well as certain halogenated or aromatic hydrocarbons that have systemic toxicity such as carbon tetrachloride or benzene, should be evacuated from the stomach.) Patients who are asymptomatic should be observed for up to 6 hours after ingestion. Patients who have respiratory symptoms warrant hospitalization. Oxygen administration, humidification of inspired air, and intravenous fluids should be instituted. The severely symptomatic patient may require mechanical ventilation with positive end-expiratory pressure. Adrenocorticosteroids have not been effective in preventing or ameliorating pulmonary complications and are not recommended. Leukocytosis and fever are common findings in hydrocarbon aspiration without infection. The use of antimicrobial therapy is not warranted initially. Damage to the pulmonary clearance mechanisms and aspiration of oral flora may cause a secondary bacterial pneumonia requiring antimicrobial therapy.

PLANTS

Because definitive identification of the ingested plant usually is not available, most practitioners find the management of plant ingestions confusing and frustrating. Most plants produce minimal symptoms in the quantities usually ingested. Fatalities are quite rare. In doubtful situations, most physicians prefer to empty the stomach. Activated charcoal adsorbs many plant toxins.

The ingestions reported most commonly involve members of the arum family (dieffenbachia, philodendron, caladium, colocasia). These plants contain needlelike calcium oxalate crystals, which produce intense mucosal irritation. Although treatment at home with a demulcent usually suffices, upper airway obstruction and esophageal erosions occur in rare cases and can be life threatening. Corneal damage may result from contact with the crystals. Oleander and lily of the valley contain cardiac glycosides similar to foxglove's digitalis. Digitalis toxicity has occurred following ingestions of these plants, particularly if they are used in the brewing of "herbal" tea. Digoxin-specific antibody fragments have been used to treat plant ingestion digitalis toxicity.

Jimsonweed (locoweed, angel trumpets) contains belladonna alkaloids that produce anticholinergic symptoms. Therapy with physostigmine may be required but should not be employed for mild symptomatology. Mistletoe berries, Jerusalem cherries, and holly berries represent seasonal hazards and may poison when consumed in quantity; lavage or induced emesis then is indicated. The ingestion of poinsettias usually does not result in symptoms but occasionally is followed by oral or anal irritation or mild gastrointestinal symptoms. Improperly prepared pokeweed (pokeweed salad) produces severe gastrointestinal symptoms and occasionally neurotoxicity. Dangerously poisonous plants, occasionally ingested, include castor bean, precatory bean (jequirity bean, rosary pea), and lantana berry. Ingestion of water hemlock, a highly toxic plant toxin, may result in the rapid onset of seizures and death.

Most toadstools that grow in the yard are not poisonous. Mushroom poisoning is most common with mycetophiles and their families. Because wild mushrooms are difficult to identify accurately, all such ingestions must be considered potentially toxic. Ingestion of *Amanita* species may cause irreversible hepatic failure. Appropriate supportive management should follow gastric decontamination, catharsis, and the administration of activated charcoal.

VITAMINS

The accidental ingestion of modest amounts of the routinely used pediatric multiple vitamins with or without fluoride (not containing iron) does not present a toxic risk. Ingestions of elemental fluoride of 4 to 8 mg/kg of body weight has been associated with nausea, vomiting, diarrhea, and abdominal pain. Fluoride ingestions in excess of 8 mg/kg can cause electrolyte disturbances, particularly hypocalcemia with resultant convulsions, cardiac arrhythmias, and coma. Fatalities have been reported following the ingestion of sodium fluoride insecticides, sodium fluoride tablets, and 4% stannous fluoride solution. The standard toothpaste preparations present minimal risk of acute toxicity.

Toxicity may result from the chronic ingestion of excess quantities of both vitamin A and vitamin D. Excess intake of vitamin D may result in renal damage secondary to nephrocalcinosis, as well as hypercalcemia, bone pain, nausea, and vomiting. Chronic ingestion of excessive vitamin A may result in skin changes, hair loss, cortical thickening of tubular bones, and anorexia.

Acute intoxication with vitamin A results in the abrupt onset of increased intracranial pressure (pseudotumor cerebri). Symptoms include drowsiness, irritability, severe headache, and vomiting. A bulging fontanel may be present in infants. Desquamation, usually beginning around the mouth, may follow over the next few days. Induced emesis or gastric lavage should be considered in patients who have ingested 100,000 units or more of vitamin A.

Toxicity from excessive ingestion of water-soluble vitamins has been reported, usually in association with fad diets or megavitamin "ortho molecular" therapy. Dosages of pyridoxine, vitamin B_6, in excess of 2 g per day, cause peripheral nerve degeneration. Excessive dosages of vitamin C may result in chronic diarrhea and kidney stone formation.

IRON

Ingestion of iron-containing medications, particularly the commonly prescribed maternal prenatal 325 mg ferrous sulfate (65 mg elemental iron) tablets, is a major cause of death among accidental ingestions by toddlers. Lack of widespread public appreciation of the toxicity of iron and the close resemblance of prenatal ferrous sulfate to M & M brand candies contribute to the incidence of this common ingestion. Iron has a direct corrosive effect on the small bowel and gastric mucosa. The lesion is pathologically similar to the coagulation necrosis caused by acid ingestions. Significant ingestions cause severe abdominal pain, diarrhea, vomiting, and gastrointestinal hemorrhage. Shock may ensue as a result of the hemorrhage and attendant coagulopathy; significant hypovolemia can occur secondary to "third spacing" of fluid in the injured bowel in the absence of hemorrhage. Free iron in the circulation causes disregulation of the coagulation cascade. Inhibition of cellular oxidative metabolism and the conversion of ferrous ions to ferric ions in the circulation may intensify the metabolic acidosis. Acute hepatic failure may complicate the course of acute iron poisoning. Scarring and stricture formation, usually at the pylorus, may occur as late as 4 weeks after the ingestion. The asymptomatic or quiescent period traditionally described as occurring after the gastrointestinal symptoms have subsided and before the onset of shock may represent a failure to recognize early signs of hypovolemia.

Therapy

The minimal toxic dose is 20 to 60 mg of elemental iron per kilogram of body weight. Ingestions in this range or greater should be managed with gastric emptying by induced emesis or gastric lavage. A plain roentgenogram of the abdomen is helpful in detecting residual iron tablets. Large concentrations of iron tablets in the stomach or small bowel should be removed by whole bowel irrigation with a polyethylene glycol electrolyte solution (250-500 ml/hr via nasogastric tube). Endoscopic or surgical removal of iron tablet bezoars may be necessary.

Serum iron concentrations in excess of 500 μg/dl, measured 4 to 6 hours post ingestion, are associated with a significant risk of shock; levels under 300 μg/dl often are tolerated. Ingested doses exceeding 60 mg per kilogram of body weight usually are associated with toxic levels. Symptomatic individuals who have levels greater than 300 μg/dl and all individuals with levels greater than 500 μg/dl should receive chelation therapy. An elevated serum total iron binding capacity is not protective and does not diminish the need for chelation therapy in the iron-intoxicated child.

The slow, continuous intravenous infusion of deferoxamine at 15 mg/kg/hr may cause the color of the urine to change to "vin rose" in the intoxicated individual. Lack of a urine color change in severely poisoned children (levels greater than 500 μg/dl), particularly in those in early shock or whose urine output is decreased is not unusual. Because the vin rose color change is unreliable, the duration of chelation therapy is based on the child's clinical status and generally should continue until the serum iron level is below 300 μg/dl. Supportive care with early intensive management of shock through volume therapy is essential.

LEAD

Lead poisoning (plumbism) in the young child is a chronic disease. Although leaded gasoline emissions into the atmosphere constitute the preponderant industrial lead burden on society, the ingestion of lead-based paint chips and paint-soaked plaster and putty remain the most significant source of high-dose lead exposure for young children. Dirt contaminated by automobile emissions along congested urban thoroughfares and household dust from crumbling wall fixtures constitute "intermediate dose" sources of lead for the toddler through repetitive hand-to-mouth contamination.

Toxicity has resulted from a variety of less common exposures. Water and food contamination can result from lead-soldered plumbing systems or containers. Acidic foods and beverages can be contaminated through storage in improperly lead-glazed ceramic ware. Smelter dust, the contaminated work clothing of lead-acid storage battery factory workers, and the burning of discarded battery casings are a hazard. Slow absorption from ingested lead weights, sinkers, and retained bullets or shotgun pellets may result in poisoning. Certain Mexican-American and Asian Indian folk remedies may contain up to 86% lead by weight. The recurrent intentional inhalation of leaded gasoline for recreation by Native Americans has resulted in encephalopathy.

Physiological Effects

Blood lead levels reflect the equilibrium among absorption, excretion, and soft tissue and bone pools. A variable percentage of ingested lead, 5% to 10% in adults and up to 50% in younger children, is absorbed. Iron, zinc, and calcium deficiency and the excessive dietary intake of fat potentiate gastrointestinal lead absorption. Respiratory absorption of lead depends on particle size. Lead is excreted at a relatively limited rate in the urine, bile, and sweat. Ingestion of greater than 5 mg/kg of body weight per day generally results in retention, which results in increased tissue levels and toxic effects on bone marrow, kidneys, and nervous system and deposition of lead in bone (Fig. 289-3).

Lead in soft tissues has serious but reversible effects on hemoglobin production, renal function, and vitamin D metabolism. Lead interferes with the biosynthesis of heme, leading to decreased activity of delta-aminolevuline acid dehydratase, increased erythrocyte protoporphyrin levels, and increased excretion of coproporphyrin in urine. Globin synthesis also is impaired. The effect on the bone marrow is confounded by the frequent coexistence of iron-deficiency anemia. A reversible Fanconi syndrome (hypophosphatemia with hyperphosphaturia, glycosuria, and generalized aminoaciduria), caused by proximal renal tubular damage, may be seen in acute poisoning.

Lead has irreversible effects on the central nervous system. Severe intoxication causes cerebral edema with resultant acute encephalopathy. Capillary permeability is increased with transudation of protein-containing fluid into the brain. Necrosis of vessel walls is present and may be accompanied by petechial hemorrhages. Neurons are damaged irreversibly. Lower-level intoxications result in mild neurological disabilities. High-level intoxication causes peripheral nervous system injury with a motor neuropathy; lower-level ex-

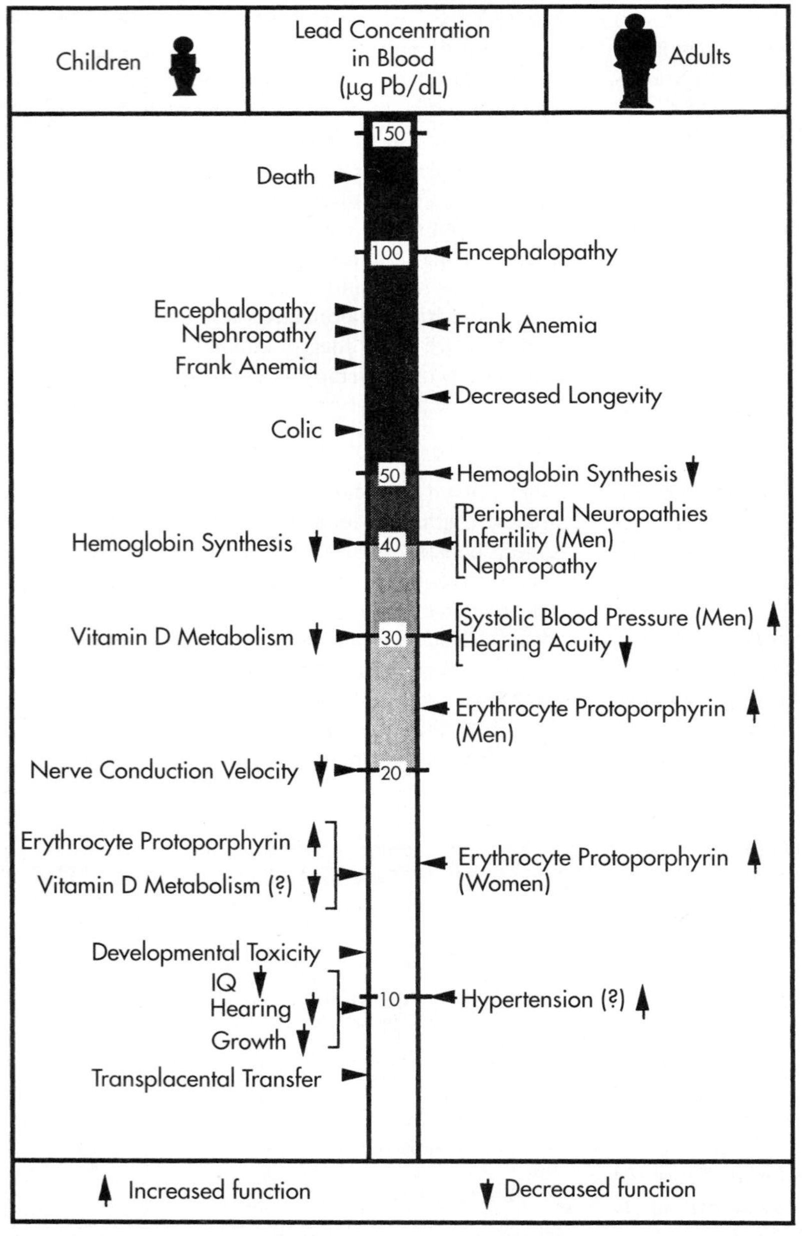

- Effects in children generally occur at lower blood lead levels than in adults.
- The developing nervous system in children can be affected adversely at blood lead levels of less than 10 μg/dL.

FIG. 289-3 Effects of inorganic lead on children and adults—lowest observable adverse effect levels.

(From Agency for Toxic Substances and Disease Registry, U.S. Department of Health and Human Services.)

posure results in an asymptomatic decrease in motor nerve conduction velocity.

Diagnosis and Clinical Findings

The blood lead level reflects the risk of symptomatic lead intoxication and acute encephalopathy. The Centers for Disease Control and Prevention (CDC) revised its guidelines for lead toxicity in 1991 to reflect its position that blood lead levels (PbB) as low as 10 μg/dl result in neurological toxicity (see Chapter 20, Six, Screening for Lead Poisoning, for further discussion of this topic). Blood lead levels are classified into five risk categories: class I ("normal"), PbB under 10 μg/dl; class II, PbB of 10 to 19 μg/dl; class III, PbB of 20 to 44 μg/dl; class IV (high risk), PbB of 45 to 69 μg/dl; and class V (urgent risk), PbB of 70 μg/dl or higher. Risk of neurological damage increases, particularly for class IV and class V individuals, the longer the elevated levels are sustained. Erythrocyte protoporphyrin, as an index of the metabolic effect of lead poisoning, often is elevated in association with lead levels greater than 25 μg/dl. The frequent coexistence of iron deficiency in high-risk populations may account for some of the hematological effects traditionally ascribed to lead intoxication. A minority of iron-sufficient class III, IV, and V individuals will have anemia or microcytosis.

The symptomatology of chronic lead poisoning is protean, nonspecific, and may wax and wane. Initial symptoms may include anorexia, constipation, and bouts of abdominal pain, nausea, and vomiting. Apathy, lethargy, and irritability may be mistaken for a primary behavioral disturbance. Incoordination, ataxia, and loss of recently acquired developmental milestones may occur. The process may abate or may progress to the gross ataxia, persistent vomiting, lethargy, coma, and intractable convulsions characteristic of acute encephalopathy. Absence of papilledema and vital sign changes does not exclude the possibility of cerebral edema in acute encephalopathy. A child may suffer recurrent symptomatic episodes without developing obvious acute encephalopathy. These nonspecific complaints may seem to be explained adequately by a minor intercurrent illness. A lumbar puncture generally is contraindicated because of the risks associated with increased intracranial pressure. Long-term sequelae of encephalopathy include seizure disorders, nonspecific mental retardation, and hyperkinetic behavior disorders. Widespread public recognition of the dangers of lead intoxication, screening programs, the decreased use of leaded gasoline, and the reduction of lead content in household paints have led to a dramatic reduction in the incidence of encephalopathy over the past 30 years.

Neuropsychiatric deficits, distractibility, diminution of IQ scores, and decreased academic achievement are associated with lead levels below 25 μg/dl. Intrauterine exposure to maternal PbB levels greater than 10 μg/dl results in quantifiable and persistent developmental delay. The neurotoxicity of low level lead exposure (PbB levels below 25 μg/dl) has been adequately documented despite the coexistence of confounding variables such as socioeconomic class in exposed populations. The threshold lead level below which adverse biological effect does not occur has yet to be defined.

For further discussion of the public health problem presented by PbB levels between 10 and 25 μg/dl in the general population, see Chapter 20, Six, Screening for Lead Poisoning.

Therapy

Chelation therapy is adjunctive to the most imperative intervention in lead poisoning: separation of the child from the source of lead. Acute encephalopathy is a medical emergency. In addition, because the course of encephalopathy is fulminant and its onset unpredictable, any child who has an elevated PbB, particularly 45 μg/dl or higher, who has symptoms potentially referable to lead should be treated as an emergency. CaEDTA, dimercaptopropanol (BAL), and meso-2, 3-dimercaptosuccinic acid (Succimer) are the three chelating agents used to treat plumbism. Piomelli and Chisholm[7] have extensively described the protocols for inpatient chelation therapy of children who have lead poisoning using CaEDTA and BAL. Consulting such a reference is essential before treating children to appreciate the inherent dangers and precautions for such therapy. Their recommendations are summarized in Table 289-1.

Succimer, an oral chelating agent, has been demonstrated

Table 289-1 Chelation Therapy of Lead Poisoning

Status	Therapy	Comments
Encephalopathy	BAL* 75 mg/m^2 IM every 4 hr for 5 days CaEDTA† 1500 mg/m^2/day IV over 6 hr for 5 days	Give BAL 4 hr before CaEDTA infusion. Treat 5 additional days (after 2-day break) if PbB remains high. Additional cycles may be necessary depending on PbB rebound.
PbB of 70 μg/dl or higher or nonencephalopathic symptomatology	BAL 50 mg/m^2 IM every 4 hr for 3-5 days CaEDTA 1000 mg/m^2 /day IV over 6 yr for 5 days	Give BAL 4 hr before CaEDTA infusion. BAL may be stopped after 3 days if the PbB falls below 50 μg/dl. Additional cycles may be necessary depending on PbB rebound.
PbB of 50 μg/dl or higher under 70 μg/dl PbB of 25 μg/dl or higher under 50 μg/dl	CaEDTA 1000 mg/m^2 /day IV over 6 hr for 5 days	Additional cycles may be necessary depending on PbB rebound.

Adapted from Piomelli S et al: *J Pediatr* 105:527, 1984.

*Medicinal iron should not be given concurrently with BAL therapy.

†Adequate diuresis is essential (IV or oral fluid) to minimize renal toxicity.

‡See text.

to be as effective as CaEDTA in reducing PbB levels in children who had initial levels between 50 and 69 μg/dl.[3] Succimer is as effective in reducing PbB levels in children who have levels between 25 and 45 μg/dl as it is in children whose levels are greater than 45 μg/dl.[5] Chelation therapy with succimer consists of 5 days of 10 mg/kg three times a day followed by 14 days of 10 mg/kg twice a day. Because succimer is an oral agent and can be given on an outpatient basis, this does not relieve the physician of his or her paramount obligation: removal of the child from the lead-contaminated environment. Succimer has a much lower affinity for iron than CaEDTA. Succimer penetrates and effectively mobilizes lead from soft tissues, including the brain.

The symptomatic or encephalopathic child should be hospitalized without oral intake. After cautious parenteral fluid therapy has established an adequate urine output, chelation may begin. Seizures initially may be controlled with diazepam. If plain roentgenograms of the abdomen demonstrate radiopaque flecks, usually in the region of the colon, signifying recent ingestion of foreign matter containing lead, the bowel should be evacuated. Metaphyseal lead lines present on roentgenogram, signifying increased lead storage in bone, are not related to the severity of symptoms. Renal and liver function and PbB levels should be monitored daily. Repeated cycles of chelation may be necessary to reduce the PbB levels to acceptable levels.

The decision to initiate chelation therapy in the clinically asymptomatic child who has an increased lead burden depends on the lead level. Although chelation therapy has never been definitively demonstrated to benefit the asymptomatic child or reverse subtle neurotoxicity, the general consensus is that asymptomatic children who have PbB levels greater than 45 μg/dl should be chelated. The increasing appreciation of the toxic effects of lower lead levels and the availability of an effective oral chelating agent has led many physicians to chelate children whose PbB levels are between 25 and 45 μg/dl. Use of the CaEDTA provocation test (lead mobilization test) to determine which asymptomatic children who have PbB levels below 45 μg/dl should be chelated has been tempered by the potentially undesirable shifts of lead into the soft tissues (brain) during the test. It is hoped that scientifically sound research will be available over the next few years to guide clinicians in their chelation decisions.

Children receiving chelation therapy should not be released from the hospital until lead hazards in their environment are controlled or suitable alternative housing has been arranged. Exposure to aerosolized leaded dust during the deleading of a home containing lead-based paint is particularly hazardous, with the potential for precipitating encephalopathy in the lead-intoxicated child. Children must be excluded from the dwelling until the procedure is complete. Following chelation therapy, children still are at high risk and should have follow-up blood lead determinations at 1- to 2-week intervals until these levels stabilize or show a decline continually for at least 6 months. Thereafter, they should be followed up at 1- to 3-month intervals until 6 years of age or longer. Neurological and psychological conditions should be assessed at the time of diagnosis and in the following years. Effective management of each case of lead poisoning should involve the sustained cooperation of health department personnel, the medical social worker, visiting nurse, and pediatrician.

The systematic screening of high-risk toddlers to detect lead deposits in soft tissue before symptoms occur is essential. Therapy does not prevent neurological sequelae after the onset of encephalopathy.

REFERENCES

1. Done AK: Salicylate intoxication: significance of measurements of salicylate in blood in cases of acute ingestion, *Pediatrics* 26:800, 1960.
2. Gosselin RE et al: *Clinical toxicology of commercial products,* ed 5, Baltimore, 1984, Williams & Wilkins.
3. Graziano JH et al: Controlled study of meso-2,3-dimercaptosuccinic acid for the management of childhood lead intoxication, *J Pediatr* 120:133, 1992.
4. Haddad LM, Winchester JF: *Clinical management of poisoning and drug overdose,* ed 2, Philadelphia, 1990, WB Saunders.
5. Liebelt EL, Shannon M, Graef JW: Efficacy of oral meso-2,3-dimercaptosuccinic acid therapy for low-level childhood plumbism, *J Pediatr* 124:313, 1994.
6. Litovitz TL et al: 1992 annual report of the American Association of Poison Control Centers Toxic Exposure Surveillance System, *Am J Emerg Med* 11:494, 1993.
7. Piomelli S et al: Management of childhood lead poisoning, *J Pediatr* 105:527, 1984.
8. Rumack BH: *POISINDEX information system,* ed 84, Denver, 1994, Micromedex.
9. Rumack BH, Matthew H: Acetaminophen poisoning and toxicity, *Pediatrics* 55:871, 1975.

SUGGESTED READINGS

Anderson KD, Rouse TM, Randolph JG: A controlled trial of corticosteroids in children with corrosive injury of the esophagus, *N Engl J Med* 323:637, 1990.

Bellinger DC, Stiles KM, Needleman HL: Low-level lead exposure, intelligence and academic achievement: a long-term follow-up study, *Pediatrics* 90:855, 1992.

Clark M, Royal J, Seeler R: Interaction of iron deficiency and lead and the hematologic findings in children with severe lead poisoning, *Pediatrics* 81:247, 1988.

Fine JS, Goldfrank LR: Update in medical toxicology, *Pediatr Clin North Am,* 39:1031, 1992.

Gawin FH, Ellinwood EH: Cocaine and other stimulants: actions, abuse, and treatment, *N Engl J Med,* 318:1173, 1988.

Gilman AG, Goodman LS, Gilman A: *Goodman and Gilman's the pharmacological basis of therapeutics,* ed 8, New York, 1990, Pergamon Press.

Gorman RL et al: Initial symptoms as predictors of esophageal injury in alkaline corrosive ingestions, *Am J Emerg Med,* 10:189, 1992.

Haddad LM: Managing tricyclic antidepressant overdose, *Am Fam Physician,* 46:153, 1992.

Lampe KF, McCann MA: *AMA handbook of poisonous and injurious plants,* Chicago, 1985, American Medical Association.

Mortenson ML: Management of acute childhood poisonings caused by selected insecticides and herbicides, *Pediatr Clin North Am* 33:421, 1986.

Peterson RG, Peterson LN: Cleansing the blood: hemodialysis, exchange transfusion, charcoal hemoperfusion, forced diuresis, *Pediatr Clin North Am* 33:675, 1986.

Smilkstein MJ et al: Efficacy of oral N-Acetylcysteine in the treatment of acetaminophen overdose: analysis of the national multicenter study (1976-1985), *N Engl J Med,* 319:1557, 1988.

Spiller HA et al: A prospective evaluation of the effect of activated charcoal before oral N-Acetylcysteine in acetaminophen overdose, *Ann Emerg Med,* 23:519, 1994.

290 Rape

Margarete Parrish, Andrew S. Bernstein, and Marianne E. Felice

Rape is a legal definition, not a medical diagnosis. Hence every state has statutory definitions of sexual assault and rape, and clinicians should be familiar with the statutes in their local jurisdictions. An accurate definition of rape includes three elements: (1) the absence of, or the impossibility of, obtaining consent from the victim, (2) the use of physical force, coercion, threats, punishments, or rewards, and (3) acts of sexual intimacy involving penetration.[11] This definition includes both *statutory rape* (consensual relations between a legal minor and an adult) and *date* or *acquaintance rape* (the victim and the perpetrator know one another socially or professionally). In general, rape refers to sexual intercourse with force or the threat of force or without a person's consent. Rape is not a sexual act, it is an assault acted out sexually.

INCIDENCE

Exact statistics on the incidence and prevalence of rape are unknown because many victims never report the crime. Estimates of unreported rape range from 40% to 90%.[16] About 50% of all rape victims are less than 18 years old, and most are adolescents.[16] Adolescents who engage in high-risk behaviors that impair judgment, such as the use of drugs and alcohol, are at an increased risk for rape.[15] Ninety percent of adolescent rape victims are assaulted by someone they know, and more than 50% of these cases occur on a date.[11] Although most rape victims are female, 5% to 10% of victims are male.[14] About half of all reported rapes in the United States eventually lead to arrests; about two thirds of those arrested are prosecuted, and about half of those prosecuted are found guilty. In other words, for every 100 reported rapes, there are 16 convictions.[16]

TYPES OF RAPES

Types of rape differ based on the relationship of the victim to the assailant. These various types of rapes raise different issues that are important to consider when providing care for the victim.

Known Assailant

In many reported pediatric rape cases the victim knows the assailant, who may be a parent, a stepparent, an adult relative or friend of the family, a neighbor, an acquaintance, or a classmate. The victim-assailant relationship may cause conflicting family loyalties. In these cases victims are less likely to report the rape, thereby contributing to the high estimates of underreporting. Rape victims who know their assailants also are prone to self-doubt and self-blame, and when they do report the rape, their reports may be received with skepticism and disbelief, even by the professionals to whom they turn for help.

Stranger Rape

It is estimated that 15% to 55% of reported rapes are committed by individuals who are not known by the victim.[1] Stranger rape is more likely to entail threats or use of violence and fear of immediate danger and it is associated with a higher incidence of reporting the rape and of subsequent conviction of the assailant.

Date Rape

Estimates of the incidence of date rape are unclear. However, in one survey of middle and high school students nearly 20% of the females and over 10% of the males reported a history of unwanted sexual activity on dates.[8] Surveys of college students indicate that about 25% of female students and 6% of male students report a history of sexual assault that meets the definition of rape while on a date.[13] Almost none of the college students in those surveys reported the sexual assault to authorities. Of the various types of rape, date rape is the least likely to be reported. It is of particular concern to adolescents that the incidence of date rape appears highly correlated with one or both parties having been drinking or using other drugs before the rape. As would be expected, date rapes are more likely to occur on weekends between 10 PM and 1 AM, in automobiles or at the home of the assailant.[1]

The profile of the date rape victim indicates that she frequently is new to an environment (e.g., a newcomer to school or town, or a college freshman), lacks a strong social support system, is not particularly assertive in establishing limits and boundaries with others, and may have been intoxicated at the time of the incident. The date rape perpetrator is believed to be more sexually active than others his age and to have a history of aggressive and/or antisocial behavior toward women. He typically perceives a victim's passivity as permission and denies the element of coercion. He, too, is likely to be intoxicated.[1] Manipulative verbal threats and physically trapping the victim are tactics used commonly by the date rapist.

Long-term issues of trust, self-blame, and vulnerability are important issues for victims of date rape, as in any other form of rape. The date rape victim may not trust her judgment concerning men, and she may blame herself for the rape, erroneously believing that she did not resist clearly or did not resist convincingly enough. She may be ashamed that she ended up in a situation that resulted in rape. It is easy to understand why victims have reservations about reporting date rape. Unfortunately, such secrecy also applies to discussing the incident in general, making catharsis as well as verbal and emotional support from others difficult to obtain.

Gang Rape

Gang rape typically involves a group of young males raping a solitary female victim. This type of rape may be associated with ritualistic behavior as well as displaced rage on the part of the assailants. Issues of sexualized rites of passage apply both to stereotypical adolescent gangs as well as to college fraternities. Victims of college campus gang rapes are more likely to drop out of college following the rape than to pursue legal recourse,[1] thus perpetuating the dynamics of avoiding confrontation with the perpetrators at the long-term expense of the victim.

Male Rape

In this discussion male rape refers to same-sex rape. Although there are sporadic reports of male rape by females, the law is very unclear in this area, and data are practically nonexistent. The area of male rape remains understudied and is far less understood than female rape.

Specific subgroups of young men are at particular risk for sexual abuse: those in institutionalized settings (such as the criminal justice system), street youth (who may engage in prostitution), young male homosexuals (who may be runaways), and youth who have a parental history of physical or sexual abuse (parents who were abused themselves may become abusers as adults).[16] The occurrence of male rape in institutionalized settings often is attributed to displaced heterosexual behavior or undifferentiated sexual orientation, along with aggressive dominance of a weaker partner.[3,10] Male rape outside institutions often occurs through coercion by an individual perceived as an authority figure to the victim.[16]

Issues of loss of control are particularly relevant for the male rape victim, along with subsequent symptoms of depression, anxiety, sleep disturbances, and suicidal ideation. Conflicted sexual identity is common among all male rape victims, whether or not they are homosexual.[10] Male rape victims nearly always perceive the rape as a life-threatening event; this may result in long-term psychological problems.[10] Because of the pervasive reluctance of males to report rape, the preclusion of social support and intervention is a particularly challenging issue in this population.

LEGAL ISSUES

All states have laws that require physicians to report cases involving violent assault, including rape. This is particularly true of minors because rape obviously is a form of sexual and/or physical abuse. Some states require parental notification of a minor's sexual assault, and in those states, this statute overrides issues of confidentiality; most states permit a minor to receive treatment for sexual assault without parental consent. It is essential that all clinicians be familiar with local statutes.

Giving consent for *treatment* of rape is different from giving consent for *collection of evidence*. In most states patients may limit their consent to a confidential report that includes only the patient's name, address, type of crime, and extent of injuries, rather than a full evidentiary examination. The physician must ask the patient for permission to complete a full evidentiary examination and to release the evidence to the police. Many victims are reluctant to give permission because they fear social isolation and possible retribution by the perpetrator. Furthermore, the evidentiary examination may be viewed as another form of assault by the victim.

From a medical-legal perspective the physician must realize that his or her responsibility is limited to the documentation of evidence. It is not the physician's role to determine whether a rape really occurred; that is a court decision. The physician will be of most help to the victim and the authorities by presuming that the victim is telling the truth, being thorough in the evaluation, and keeping accurate medical records.

MEDICAL EVALUATION

Rape is a serious medical and psychological emergency for both the victim and family. The purpose of the initial evaluation is fourfold: treatment of injury and infection; prevention of pregnancy, collection of evidence, and psychological assessment with referral for follow-up counseling.

General Concepts

Many metropolitan areas have treatment centers that have trained interdisciplinary teams available for adolescent and child victims of rape. This probably is the ideal site for the initial evaluation. But rapes also occur to minors in communities where there are no such centers. To minimize the physical and psychological trauma of the evaluation, eliminate the need for repeat evaluations, and maximize the probability of collecting forensic evidence of good quality, this investigation should be performed by the most skilled professional available. The gender of the examiner is less important than the individual's comfort with adolescents and children, skill at conducting the examination, and compassion.

The rape evaluation can be long and tedious, but it should never be rushed. While the youngster is coping with his or her personal outrage and physical and psychological pain, he or she is expected to tolerate and cooperate with uncomfortable procedures that may appear to be similar to the acts of intrusion and aggression experienced previously. Hence it is crucial that the approach to the evaluation be calm and gentle. Rape protocols, if available, are quite helpful and will serve to minimize the chance for error or omission in the evidence collection process. Most jurisdictions have printed standardized forms for the evidence procurement process[17]; *prior* to examining a victim the clinician should become familiar with those forms.

It is important that the clinician not make inappropriate assumptions about the victim based on his or her psychological state. Many victims are in a state of shock or denial immediately after the event. How a patient responds in the emergency room varies and depends on numerous factors, including developmental maturity. It is not uncommon for a 13-year-old child to look older physically, but function cognitively at the level of a preadolescent. The physician should assume that the patient is uncomfortable with the assault and the ongoing rape assessment and attempt to minimize the victim's sense of personal guilt, shame, and anxiety by offering reassurance immediately. Taking a few minutes to empathize with the patient and acknowledge her feelings before proceeding with the evaluation helps both the patient and the physician.

It always is prudent to take a few moments at the beginning of the evaluation to explain the process of the examination and allow for questions. This is particularly true for those rape victims who never had previous sexual relationships or a prior gynecological examination, but it also is helpful for more experienced patients who understandably still may be anxious and fearful of anticipated pain and discomfort. Whenever possible, allow the patient some control over the proceedings; let the patient set the pace of the examination. If the victim becomes severely uncomfortable with the proceedings, stop and allow her to regain composure before continuing with the examination. At no point should a physician continue to examine a child or adolescent against his or her will.

After obtaining consent from the patient, the physician should obtain a detailed and relevant history, followed by a thorough general physical examination and a gentle but complete pelvic examination. It usually is helpful to have a nurse or assistant present during this process, and for small children or very young adolescents it may be helpful to have a parent present *during the examination* if the parent is reassuring rather than openly distraught during the procedure. Some aspects of the evaluation will change depending on the temporal proximity of the evaluation to the alleged event. The following guidelines are recommended for evaluations conducted within 72 hours of the assault. Modifications are necessary if the evaluation is conducted after this time. In some centers the interdisciplinary team obtains the history simultaneously and together so that the victim does not have to repeat his or her story unnecessarily.

History

The history should include the time, date, and location of both the event and the examination. Recalling the event may be emotionally traumatic for the patient, so it sometimes is useful to begin with a relevant medical history, such as a thorough menstrual history including the age of menarche, the date of the last menstrual period, the frequency of menses, sexual activity if relevant, previous pregnancies, miscarriages, and abortions, and the use of contraceptives as well as of feminine hygiene products.

Next, focus on the event itself. Questions should be asked calmly, caringly, sensitively, and patiently. Some of the questions asked may seem invasive and, when taken out of context, inappropriate, but it is important to obtain all relevant information the first time the interview is conducted. Studies show that repeated attempts at obtaining a history are emotionally traumatic, often confusing to the victim, and actually may discredit the victim's testimony. *Use the victim's own words whenever possible*. The medical chart is a legal document and will be subjected to the same scrutiny as any other form of evidence. Do not embellish or offer interpretation; record only the facts.

Ask the victim about the use of intoxicating substances prior to or during the event; ask the victim to describe in detail the location of the event, the appearance of the perpetrator, the type of sexual contact and the positions used, the utilization of force (by both the perpetrator and the victim), the removal of clothing and the manner in which it was removed, what measures if any the patient has taken to cleanse himself or herself (e.g., bathing, douching, changing clothes, urinating, or defecating). Finally, the physician should ask about the presence of clinical symptoms in the musculoskeletal, gastrointestinal, and genitourinary system.

Physical Examination

A complete physical examination from "head to toe" is warranted. Often there is little physical evidence obtained from the genital examination, but an inspection of the entire body may provide the corroborative evidence necessary to convict the perpetrator.

Note the patient's physical appearance, emotional state, and condition of clothing. If the patient presents in the same dress worn at the time of the event, take notes on the condition of the clothing and save each piece in a separate labeled bag. Applying a Wood light to the clothing may illuminate the presence of dried semen. These specimens should be marked for later analysis for the presence of seminal vesicle-specific antigen. Next, conduct a topical survey of the body, documenting any evidence of recent trauma or bruising. The use of photographs may be useful during subsequent litigation.

Pay particular attention to the region of the head and neck. Compression injuries of the neck are fairly common if force is used. This may lead to obstruction of venous return from the head, causing the development of neck bruising and/or petechial hemorrhages in the eyelids and conjunctiva. Examine the inner surface of the lips for evidence of tiny abrasions resulting from forced pressure applied to the mouth by the perpetrator to prevent the victim from screaming. If the patient reports biting the assailant in self-defense, an imprint of the bite plate and a saliva sample should be taken for later comparison.

Examine the breasts for bite marks or bruises. Note the Tanner stage, or sexual maturation state, of the victim (breasts and pubic hair in females; genitalia and pubic hair in males). It is not improbable that by the time a case comes to trial, a child may grow from a Tanner stage 2 to a stage 3 or 4. This significant physical change may bias an uneducated jury inappropriately.

Genital Examination

The Female Patient. The patient should assume the lithotomy position. If the patient seems too anxious and a speculum examination is not required to investigate for a source of undiagnosed internal bleeding, the knee-chest position may be a suitable alternative, particularly for younger adolescents or children. In some cases it may be necessary to perform the pelvic examination with the patient under sedation or, on rare occasions, under general anesthesia.

Begin the examination by inspecting the thighs and perineum for evidence of trauma, bruising, semen, or blood. Appropriate forensic evidence should be taken at this time (see the box on p. 1754). Palpate the inguinal lymph nodes for evidence of ongoing or previous genital infection. Erythema and engorgement of the clitoris is common after intense local stimulation. The effect usually wears off in 1 to 2 hours.

RECOMMENDED PROCEDURES FOR THE COLLECTION OF FORENSIC DATA

Combed and plucked pubic hair
Wet mount of secretions from the vaginal vault
Wet mount and fixed smear for the detection of both motile and dead sperm
Vaginal aspirate for acid phosphatase
Vaginal aspirate for p30 and MH-5 testing
Cervical cultures for both chlamydia and gonorrhea
Rectal cultures for gonorrhea even if sodomy has not occurred
Oral culture for gonorrhea if fellatio occurred
Dried secretions from skin, pubic hair, or clothing for analysis
Blood tests: ABO typing, syphilis, pregnancy test, and HIV test (if patient requests it)

In myths and legends an intact hymen is synonymous with virginity. Hence the patient, and often her parents, may want to know about the structural integrity of the hymen. It is next to impossible, however, to ascertain from a visual inspection of the hymen whether rape has taken place. The presence of hymenal tears is not proof of rape because such tears may be old and the result of nonrape trauma (e.g., forceful use of a tampon). Nevertheless, because of the emphasis placed on this area of the anatomy, careful inspection and documentation of the hymen is required. A saline-moistened cotton swab rolled around the edges of the hymen, the use of an otoscope, or the application of toluidine blue to the hymenal margin may help to locate and identify fresh tears. Many experts use colposcopy for this purpose, but because standards have not been defined clearly and because many evaluation centers do not have access to a colposcope, it still is considered investigational. Measurements of the width of the hymenal opening should be recorded.[7]

Most female adolescents should be able to undergo a speculum examination of the internal genitals, which will allow a clear view of the vaginal walls, fornices, and cervix. Appropriate specimens for culture and forensics should be obtained (see the box above).

After the speculum examination is completed, a vaginal bimanual and rectovaginal examination should be conducted to rule out the presence of trauma. A history of sodomy in both male and female victims indicates the need to conduct a careful anal inspection and digital examination. In addition to looking for evidence of rectal bleeding (hemorrhoids, erythema, engorgement, and constipation if the offense is chronic), particular attention should be paid to the quality of anal sphincter tone.

The Male Patient. The evaluation of the male rape victim is essentially the same as that of the female. A detailed history and physical examination as well as specimens for forensic and laboratory evaluation should be obtained in the same manner as for the female. Particular focus should be placed on the evaluation of the oral cavity, the genitals, and the anus. Specifically, the physician should look for evidence of infection in the mouth or pharynx. The testes, epididymis, vas deferens, penile shaft, foreskin, and glans should be evaluated thoroughly for the presence of infection or trauma. Inguinal lymphadenopathy may indicate the presence of an ongoing infectious process. The physician should check for the presence of external hemorrhoids, rectal fissures, or fistulas. Sphincter tone should be assessed, and a digital evaluation of the internal anal canal, sphincter, and prostate should be performed. The use of an anoscope may be helpful to inspect the internal anal canal visually. A make-shift anoscope can be fabricated by using an empty test tube and flashlight or an otoscope.

Summarizing the Examination

When the physical examination is completed, allow the patient ample time to dress and regain his/her composure before discussing any findings. Most patients will benefit from knowing that their genital anatomy is normal. It also is important to discuss physical findings and treatment options and to confirm plans for follow up.

Forensic and Laboratory Information

The recovery of laboratory and forensic data is probably the most controversial aspect of the evaluation.[17] This is especially true when it comes to the recovery of semen and sperm, yet the finding of male ejaculate is neither predictive nor essential for criminal conviction. In one study physical evidence of rape was found in only 23% of all of the cases that resulted in felony convictions.[5] The newest developments in forensic science have occurred in the laboratory analysis of semen and include quantifiable levels of acid phosphatase in vaginal fluids and the monoclonal antibody test (MH-5 ELISA), specific for seminal vesicle antigen.

Sexually Transmitted Disease

Most patients are concerned about the risk of acquiring a sexually transmitted disease (STD) as a result of the rape. This risk is variable and related directly to the health status of the assailant and the victim, the site of the assault, and the infectivity of the disease in question. Overall, the risk of contracting an STD from a single encounter remains small. Repeat assaults or assaults by more than one assailant obviously increase the risk of infection. Many adolescent victims of rape, however, also engage in high-risk behaviors that put them at increased risk of having a preexisting sexually transmitted disease. The Centers for Disease Control and Prevention recommends the use of prophylactic antibiotics for treatment of potential sexually acquired infections (see Chapter 258, Sexually Transmitted Diseases).

Regardless of the antibiotics given, it must be emphasized to the patient that the incubation time for STDs varies, and it is highly possible that an infection may not be detected or may be missed or treated inadequately at the time of the evaluation examination. Therefore, medical follow up, no matter how discomforting a thought to the patient, is absolutely necessary. After 2 weeks the patient should be reexamined for the presence of an STD. Twelve weeks after the assault, thought should be given to obtaining serological tests for syphilis and HIV infection.

Pregnancy

The incidence of pregnancy after one unprotected mid-cycle exposure is between 1% and 17%.[6] Many adolescents, however, have irregular menstrual cycles; therefore the occurrence of ovulation for any particular cycle may be in question. Also, it has been shown that some perpetrators of sexual crimes are sexually dysfunctional.[10] Nevertheless, if the assault occurred within 48 to 72 hours of the evaluation, a form of postcoital contraception should be offered to the patient *after* a negative pregnancy test has ruled out the presence of an already existing pregnancy[6] (see Chapter 41, Contraception and Abortion). If menses does not occur within 4 weeks of the rape, the patient should return for a repeat evaluation.

PSYCHOLOGICAL ASSESSMENT

The psychosocial and emotional implications of rape in children and adolescents are complex. Three distinct areas must be considered: sexual behavior that is nonconsensual (and possibly premature), the threat of physical danger or violence, and the child's (or adolescent's) loss of control. These three factors are tempered further by the young person's stage of development and the family's response to the rape. For example, a young adolescent who is just beginning to grapple with his or her own sexual feelings and sexuality may feel that he or she deserved to be raped because of having begun to experience sexual feelings. A child who sees her mother respond with tears and wailing to the news that her child was raped may feel guilt not just because of the rape but because of the emotional trauma inflicted on the mother.

How the youngster copes with the rape also is related to how society responds to victims of rape. Unlike most crimes, the crime of rape often is blamed on the victim rather than on the perpetrator, particularly in adolescents. Following no other crime is the victim's prior reputation, appearance, and behavior as subject to scrutiny as in rape. In the case of delinquent adolescents, such behaviors as running away, hitchhiking, and sexual activity are used as justification for the rape, placing further blame on an already troubled young victim.

The Role of Interdisciplinary Care

The evaluation of a rape victim is best conducted by an interdisciplinary care team, usually consisting of a physician, nurse, and social worker. An interdisciplinary approach is beneficial for several reasons, including the ability to provide support to the child and family simultaneously and the ability to serve as a resource for future services. Ideally, a supportive health professional should be available to the child or adolescent as soon as he or she presents to the evaluation site and, if possible, should stay with the young rape victim throughout the evaluation process. This individual is in a position to establish trust and continuity at a time when the rape victim may be afraid to trust anyone. Establishing trust is paramount for the successful provision of future needed services.

Ideally the child should be able to tell the account of the rape once to all the professionals involved. For legal reasons, the parents should not be present during this narrative in case any aspect of the assault involves the family. Also, this enables the child to give his or her version of the events without parental interruption or coaching. However, the family's needs should not be ignored, and another supportive health professional can address the many questions that concerned parents or friends may have.

Immediate Response to Rape by the Victim

Immediate responses to rape vary considerably, ranging from distraught histrionics to near-mute withdrawal. Most victims have intense levels of fear and anxiety. This postrape acute phase also is characterized by varying levels of cognitive disorganization, "shock," and disbelief.[2] As occurs in any crisis, many children and adolescents regress to previous stages of development. An adolescent rape victim who previously was self-assured and appropriately independent may become clinging and dependent on the parent or health professional.

The potential for confusion as well as further trauma on the part of the victim also should be considered. For example, the natural reaction to embrace or try to comfort a rape victim in fact may be unwelcome, if not traumatic, following rape. Many victims, including children and adolescents, may not want to be touched by *any stranger* after the rape, including caring health professionals. Following the trauma of rape, some victims experience psychological symptoms that are both foreign and frightening. For example, a previously articulate individual may have difficulties describing the rape and simply may not be able to speak about the event. Obviously, a minor's cognitive level of development may contribute to this difficulty.

Immediate Response by the Family

Unlike other crime victims, the victim of rape rarely contacts the police immediately. Typically, there is an intermediary (a friend or family member) whom the victim contacts first. That individual's response is crucial in the ensuing medical and legal processes, but most family and friends need guidance to know how best to be supportive to the victim. The disclosure of rape usually is traumatic for the family as well as the victim. Parents may blame themselves inappropriately for the rape. In other instances, parental activities (e.g., neglect) may have contributed to the rape. In either scenario, the issues are highly sensitive and need to be addressed with skill and compassion.

Familial responses to a child's rape range from denial and disbelief to shame and outrage. There is no guarantee that a family is prepared to respond appropriately to a raped child's or adolescent's needs at this time. In some cases, a victim's mother's financial dependence on a perpetrator may confound reactions. During the initial evaluation session health care professionals therefore must spend some time with the family and/or friend of the victim to determine their own psychological response and their ability to be supportive of the victim.

Follow-up Care

After the initial evaluation is completed, arrangements should be made for follow-up care not only for the medical issues discussed previously, but also to assess the victim's ability to cope with the rape and to provide counseling concerning the rape. All rape victims and their families should be seen 1 to 2 weeks after the rape (or sooner) by a mental health professional who is trained to work with children or adolescents and who is knowledgeable about the emotional sequelae to rape.

Rape Trauma Syndrome

The term *rape trauma syndrome* is used to group the constellation of emotional and behavioral symptoms that follow rape. This term encompasses both short- and long-term considerations and addresses both mental and physical reactions. It was introduced first by Burgess and Holstrom[2] to describe the responses of adult women to rape, but it also has been applied to younger rape victims. It is now used as a variation of posttraumatic stress disorder.

There are three phases of response following rape: the acute trauma period, followed by an adaptive period, then a long-term reorganizational period. In the acute phase (days and weeks following the rape), symptoms associated with posttraumatic stress disorder frequently are noted: increased startle response, diminished concentration, sleep disturbances, mood swings, nightmares, and flashbacks. Such symptoms are usually short-lived, but they have been reported to persist in some patients from 1 to 3 years after the rape.[3] During the adaptive phase the child or adolescent is faced with readjustment to a normal life-style. Normal eating and sleeping patterns usually resume (although aversive dreams and nightmares may continue), and the rape victim usually grapples with fear, anxiety, and issues of self-worth. Finally, during the reorganization period survivors face the disruption caused by the rape. They usually question why they were victims and others were not, and they search for explanations to help them understand why the trauma occurred.

Short- and Long-Term Psychological Sequelae

Multiple factors will determine how a child or adolescent responds to the rape, such as level of social support, coping styles and strengths, and developmental and cognitive function. Hence one cannot predict how any given individual will respond to rape. But it does appear that children and adolescents who have been rape victims consistently have lower levels of self-esteem following rape than the general population.[1,3] In addition, sexually traumatized children have been noted to have higher levels of precocious sexualization than nontraumatized children.[9] There may be confusion about what is normal adult sexual behavior, especially in cases in which children were rewarded following inappropriate sexual activities. Some children experience developmental arrests at the time of the trauma; such arrests are not necessarily readily apparent. Although child and adolescent studies are still too scarce to be considered definitive, it appears that the earlier and more traumatic the rape, the greater chance of developmental and functional impairment.[3]

Behavioral concerns frequently associated with childhood and adolescent rape sequelae include school phobias, generalized fearfulness and withdrawal, and especially in adolescents, the onset of truancy. Suicidal ideations are not uncommon, with increased lifetime risks of major depression and suicide attempts being associated with women in the aftermath of rape.[3] For male rape victims the existing research is less clear, but it appears that male sexual trauma in childhood may be associated with sexually abusive behavior toward other boys in adolescence.[10] Obviously, not all children and adolescents who have been raped will have psychiatric sequelae, but all children and adolescents who have been raped should be assessed for these serious sequelae.

MALE PERPETRATORS

Just as adolescent females constitute a large proportion of reported rape victims, adolescent males make up a large proportion of convicted rape assailants: 40% of convicted rapists are 16 to 20 years of age; another 25% are between 20 and 24 years of age.[16]

Perpetrators tend to fall into one of three clusters: those for whom anger is the primary dynamic; those for whom power or conquest is the central issue; and the sadistic, for whom anger and control are in and of themselves erotic.[2] For the *anger-driven rapist,* the act tends to be impulsive, with the intent of hurting, humiliating, and degrading the victim. Physical brutality is common. Rape functions as the outlet for anger, essentially by using sex as a weapon. The *power-oriented rapist* is more likely to engage in premeditated, obsessive, and/or stalking behavior, in which the rape essentially compensates for social and sexual incompetence or inadequacy. Aggression for the power-oriented rapist is less likely to be violent than a means of dominating his prey. Both anger- and power-driven rapists have serious deficits in social skills and the inability to interpret and respond to social cues from others. For the *sadistic rapist,* eroticism and violence are enmeshed; victims typically are subjected to premeditated, deliberate acts of cruelty and dehumanization. The sadistic perpetrator finds gratification in his victim's pain and powerlessness.

Although some rapists are dysfunctional sexually (e.g., suffer from a failure to ejaculate) at the time of the rape,[10] the act of rape rarely is necessary for sexual gratification. Most rapists are sexually active with available, consensual partners outside the rape.[2] Perpetrators usually appear quite ordinary by most standards; most do not have symptoms of major psychiatric illnesses such as psychoses, nor is there a preponderance of mental retardation. However, other conditions such as antisocial, schizoid, paranoid, and narcissistic personality disorders are noted more commonly among convicted rapists than in the general population.[12]

Alcohol and drug use have been associated with the occurrence of rape. Ironically, in the current legal environment alcohol intoxication seems to have the effect of diminishing a perpetrator's sense of responsibility and increasing a victim's culpability. Specifically, victim intoxication consistently is linked with the process of "unfounding" or disproving rape charges. For date rape victims, having been seen drinking with the perpetrator before the attack has serious implications in relation to public, social, and legal responses to the charges.

SUMMARY

Rape is an act of violence that involves a disparity of power between the perpetrator and the victim. Because of its sexual context, rape is easily misinterpreted as erotic and/or sexual behavior, which it is not.

Children and adolescents who have been raped should have sensitive, careful, and thorough evaluations and follow-up assessments. From the time of initial disclosure through eventual legal outcome, many developmental, familial, and social variables can shape the experience for young victims and their families. Long-term adjustment following rape varies considerably, with both developmental and familial factors having considerable impact.

REFERENCES

1. Allison J, Wrightsman LS: *Rape: the misunderstood crime,* Newbury Park, Calif, 1993, Sage.
2. Burgess A, Holstrom L: *Rape: crisis and recovery,* Bowie, Md, 1979, Prentice-Hall.
3. Calhoun K, Atkeson B: *Treatment of rape victims: facilitating psychosocial adjustment,* New York, 1991, Pergamon.
4. Centers for Disease Control (CDC): Sexual assault and STDs, *MMWR* 42:97, 1993.
5. De Jong AR, Rose M: Legal proof of child sexual abuse in the absence of physical evidence, *Pediatrics* 88:506, 1991.
6. Dixon GW et al: Ethinyl estradiol and conjugated estrogens as postcoital contraceptives, *JAMA* 244:1336, 1980.
7. Emans SJH, Woods ER, Allen EN: Hymenal findings in adolescent women: impact of tampon use and consensual sexual activity, *J Pediatrics* 125:153, 1994.
8. Erickson PI, Rapkin AJ: Unwanted sexual experiences among middle and high school youth, *J Adolesc Health* 12:319, 1991.
9. Friedrich W: Behavior problems in sexually abused children. In Wyatt GE, Powell GJ, editors: *Lasting effects of child sexual abuse,* Newbury Park, Calif, 1988, Sage.
10. Groth AN: Male rape: offenders and victims, *Am J Psychiatr* 137:806, 1980.
11. Heger A et al: *Evaluation of the sexually abused child: a medical textbook and photographic atlas,* New York, 1992, Oxford University Press.
12. Knight R, Rosenberg R, Schneider B: Classification of sex offenders: perspectives, methods, and validation. In Burgess AW, editor: *Rape and sexual assault: a research handbook,* New York, 1985, Garland Press.
13. Koss MP, Gidycz CA, Wisniewski N: The scope of rape: incidence and prevalence of sexual aggression and victimization in a national sample of higher education students, *J Consult Clin Psychol* 55:162, 1987.
14. Lacey HB, Roberts R: Sexual assault of men, *Intl J STD AIDS* 2:258, 1991.
15. Nagy S, Adcock AG, Nagy MC: A comparison of risky health behaviors of sexually active, sexually abused, and abstaining adolescents, *Pediatrics* 93:570, 1994.
16. Neinstein LS: *Adolescent health care,* Baltimore, 1991, Urban & Schwarzenberg.
17. Young WW et al: Sexual assault: review of a national model protocol for forensic and medical evaluation, *Obstet Gynecol* 80:878, 1992.

291 Acute Renal Failure

Glenn H. Bock

Acute renal failure (ARF) is a syndrome of sudden diminution or cessation of renal function that can result from various causes. The clinical symptoms and signs result from both the inciting disease process and the altered homeostasis produced by cessation of renal function. Acute renal failure may occur at any age but is less common in children and adolescents than in adults. The exact incidence is unknown because many self-limited episodes may go undetected. This especially is true for the nonoliguric type of ARF.

ETIOLOGY

Acute renal failure may be considered to arise as the result of prerenal, renal (parenchymal), and postrenal causes or a combination thereof. Prerenal causes are those that diminish renal perfusion without producing renal damage. In the pediatric age group hypovolemia is the most common clinical setting in which this occurs. In children the hypovolemia usually results from dehydration associated with abnormal gastrointestinal losses, although it also may occur in shock, which may follow hemorrhage, burns, sepsis, and trauma. Less common causes of prerenal azotemia are those that diminish renal blood flow in the absence of hypovolemia, such as congestive heart failure, renal vascular obstruction from thrombosis or embolism, and increased renal vascular resistance as is seen occasionally following anesthesia or surgery. Although the patient develops oliguria and azotemia as part of this prerenal syndrome, adequate renal tubular function usually persists, as evidenced by the high urinary osmolality and urea concentration and the low urinary sodium concentration as the result of renal water and sodium conservation. Acute renal failure from intrinsic renal damage may result from lesions that involve either the glomeruli, the tubules, or the interstitium. Glomerular damage most commonly results from any of the glomerulonephritides or the microangiopathy of the hemolytic-uremic syndrome. Tubular damage can result from prolonged unrecognized inadequate renal perfusion as may be seen in hypotensive episodes, severe dehydration, sudden hemorrhage, or sepsis. Tubular toxins (e.g., hemoglobin and myoglobin) and various chemicals (e.g., carbon tetrachloride, diethylene glycol, and heavy metals) may cause acute parenchymal renal failure. Drugs can produce renal failure because of either direct toxic effects or hypersensitivity reactions. Acute bacterial infections of the renal interstitium (pyelonephritis) also may result in ARF, particularly in infants. Renal cortical necrosis associated with infection, hemorrhage, or dehydration can produce significant injury to both glomeruli and tubules.

Postrenal causes of acute renal failure are discussed in Chapter 183, Anuria/Oliguria.

History

The type of insult that caused the ARF usually is evident from the patient's history. It is important to note that the volume of urine production is not included in the definition of ARF because a patient may be anuric, oliguric (urine volume <240 ml/m^2/day), or nonoliguric (normal or increased urinary output). Some renal insults, such as various glomerulonephritides and hemolytic-uremic syndrome, frequently are associated with oligoanuric ARF; others, such as aminoglycoside toxicity, more often will cause nonoliguric renal failure. Determination of the type of insult will provide the clinician clues to the expected type of renal failure, the probable duration of renal insufficiency, and the overall prognosis. The history often helps to distinguish between an episode of ARF in an otherwise healthy child and the acute deterioration of a child who has undiagnosed, smoldering chronic renal failure. A preceding history of urinary abnormalities, fatigue, pallor, slowed linear growth, poor school performance, and anorexia extending over a period of time would lead the practitioner to suspect the latter.

Physical Findings

Obviously the child who has oligoanuric acute renal failure will have markedly diminished urine output. Anuria should suggest a catastrophic renovascular event or urinary obstruction. In the child who has anuria or oliguria, fluid retention can produce edema, water intoxication, vascular overload with congestive heart failure, pulmonary edema, and/or hypertension. Fluid overload often is iatrogenic, resulting from attempts to increase urinary output by increasing fluid intake. Early detection of fluid retention is determined best by short-term weight gain on serial measurements. In contrast, acute nonoliguric renal failure may be clinically covert; it usually is suspected only after the laboratory tests reveal azotemia.

Laboratory Findings

The biochemical disturbances that produce the clinical findings in acute renal failure are complex and interrelated. Inherent to the diagnosis of acute renal failure is the accumulation of nitrogenous waste products, as indicated by a rise in blood urea nitrogen and creatinine. If hypotonic fluids have been used in excess to hydrate the patient, dilutional hyponatremia, hypoproteinuria, and anemia may result.

Hyperkalemia may result from the inability of the kidney to excrete potassium and is a potentially life-threatening complication of ARF. It can be especially severe in disease states associated with cellular damage and the consequent release of intracellular potassium. These states include hemolysis, burns, trauma, and infections. Hyperkalemia produces a state of increased neuromuscular excitability, making the heart liable to arrhythmias. However, there are no reliable physical signs of hyperkalemia; diagnosis depends on serum measurement of potassium and electrocardiographic evidence of altered cardiac electric activity. In ARF, metabolic acidosis develops as the result of the kidney's failure to excrete hydrogen ions and reabsorb bicarbonate. Furthermore, any state associated with increased catabolism such as shock, fever, poor caloric intake, or extensive tissue damage may accentuate the degree of acidosis as a result of increased production of organic and inorganic acid radicals. The acidosis promotes further hyperkalemia resulting from movement of intracellular potassium into the extracellular space as the body attempts to accommodate the higher hydrogen ion concentration. Respiratory compensation for an underlying metabolic acidosis may manifest as tachypnea or Kussmaul breathing.

Failure of phosphate excretion can produce phosphate retention. The hypocalcemia associated with hyperphosphatemia may manifest clinically as tremors, tetany, or seizures. Other causes of seizures in acute renal failure include hypertensive encephalopathy, uremia, and water intoxication. It is not unusual for a child to present first with the sudden onset of seizures and other signs of central nervous system dysfunction, only to be found to have acute renal failure.

Children who have nonoliguric acute renal failure do not have the fluid and electrolyte problems seen with anuric or oliguric renal failure. The former usually have a salt-losing type of urine production that blunts the harmful effects of the renal failure.

DIFFERENTIAL DIAGNOSIS

The sine qua non of acute renal failure is the detection of retained nitrogenous waste products in the blood. A recommended clinical approach to the child who has anuria and oliguria is discussed in Chapter 183 and is portrayed in Figure 183-1. All children who have ARF in whom the cause is unclear should undergo renal and bladder ultrasonography.

In considering prerenal and parenchymal renal failure, it first is important to correct any preexisting hypovolemia before evaluating the state of renal function. It is inappropriate to begin provocative tests for renal parenchymal failure while the patient remains significantly dehydrated because the persistent oliguria may merely represent the normal homeostatic response of the kidney to the altered fluid balance.

A variety of tests have been proposed to differentiate prerenal from intrinsic renal failure (Table 291-1). *Urine sodium content* usually is low in prerenal azotemia, reflecting maximal sodium and water reabsorption by the kidney in an attempt to expand the circulating fluid volume. The normal value for urinary sodium concentration varies according to the amount of sodium in the diet. Similarly, despite the drive for sodium conservation in hypovolemic states, variability of urinary sodium concentrations is sufficient in prerenal (functional) and parenchymal renal failure to limit the usefulness of this measurement alone in discriminating between these two conditions. A more reliable test is the fractional excretion of sodium (Table 291-1). In general, tests of renal sodium conservation are not interpretable if the child has received large amounts of sodium intravenously, has been given diuretics, or has the nonoliguric form of ARF. The state of renal water conservation is assessed by the urine osmolality or the ratio of urine osmolality to plasma osmolality. Although the latter is more discriminatory, it may be unreliable in children who have received hypotonic intravenous rehydration, in those who have nonoliguric acute renal failure, and in those who are malnourished.

Finally, the renal response to mannitol or furosemide after a fluid challenge also has been proposed as a means to differentiate prerenal from intrinsic renal disease. Although mannitol (0.5 g/kg intravenously) and furosemide (1 mg/kg intravenously) were evaluated initially as separate challenges, many clinicians combine these agents to decrease the incidence of false negative responses. A good provocative response is the formation of 6 to 10 ml of urine per kilogram over the subsequent 1 to 3 hours. To evaluate the response accurately, the patient should be catheterized. Repetitive doses of mannitol and furosemide in instances of nonresponse may be harmful, with fluid shifts and convulsions being produced by the former and ototoxicity by the latter. Some clinical data also suggest that the infusion of "low-dose" dopamine (3 to 5 μg/kg/min) in conjunction with furosemide early in the course of the ARF may attenuate the severity of the ARF or convert oligoanuric to nonoliguric forms of the injury.

Prompt differentiation of prerenal ARF from the oliguria of renal parenchymal injury is extremely important in view of the effects of further fluid management. If prerenal oliguria is unrecognized, adequate fluids may not be given, leading to the development of intrinsic renal damage as a result of the hypoperfusion. In contrast, if intrinsic renal oliguria already is present but unrecognized, vigorous fluid adminis-

Table 291-1 Clinical Tests to Differentiate Functional from Parenchymal Oliguric Acute Renal Failure (ARF)

Test	Functional ARF	Parenchymal ARF	Discrimination
Sodium conservation			
Urine sodium concentration (UNa)*	<20 mEq/L	>40 mEq/L	Poor
Fractional excretion of sodium (FENa)	<1	>1	Good
$FENa = \frac{UNa/SNa}{UCr/SCr^*} \times 100$			
Water conservation			
Urine osmolality (Uosm)	>500 mosm/L	>350 mosm/L	Poor
Urine serum osmolality ratio (Uosm/Sosm)	>2	<1.1	Fair
Response to diagnostic challenge with IV mannitol and furosemide (see text)	Urine flow increase	No change	Good

**U,* Urine; *Na,* sodium; *Cr,* creatinine.

tration to induce diuresis may lead to clinically significant fluid overload.

TREATMENT

Management of oliguric parenchymal renal failure requires attention to many details. Hyperkalemia is a particular immediate risk to the patient and must be treated immediately when present. The electrocardiographic changes of hyperkalemia often reflect more accurately the state of potassium balance than does the serum potassium measurement.

Peaking of T waves on the ECG generally is considered to be an early sign of potassium-induced disturbances of myoelectrical activity in the heart. However, the rapidity with which this finding may be followed by P-R interval prolongation, QRS complex widening, and tachyarrhythmias is variable and often quite rapid. Various means to lower serum potassium are outlined in Table 291-2. The administration of calcium salts, sodium bicarbonate, glucose, and insulin are immediate measures whose effects, although of short duration, may be lifesaving. These treatments are effective in that they either decrease the sensitivity of the myocardium to the elevated levels of serum potassium or displace potassium from the extracellular space; they do not reduce the increased body burden of potassium. Actual net removal of potassium may be accomplished effectively, but slowly, through the use of enteral potassium-exchange resins (see Table 291-2). Ultimately the child who has potentially life-threatening hyperkalemia may require emergency dialysis so that the serum value can be reduced to a safe level when time is of the essence.

Strict attention must be given to fluid, electrolyte, and caloric intake in these patients to minimize other potentially dangerous homeostatic disturbances and to avoid the development of uremia-enhancing catabolism. If acute renal failure persists, the patient may be given intravenous alimentation, which includes essential amino acids that will provide calories, thereby promoting healing and minimizing uremia.

Children who have nonoliguric acute renal failure generally require less complicated management than those who have oliguric renal failure because strict fluid restrictions are not necessary. In addition, the volume of fluid these children require gives the clinician a means of providing calories, alkalinizing agents, calcium, and other drugs that are required to minimize the biochemical abnormalities of the ARF.

The patient who has any type of acute renal failure is best managed in collaboration with a pediatric nephrologist. With vigorous attention to details of management, dialysis may be unnecessary. However, peritoneal dialysis is useful for disturbances resistant to more conservative measures, regardless of the age of the patient. Hemofiltration, hemofiltration-dialysis, and hemodialysis may be indicated in settings where peritoneal dialysis is inadequate or not feasible. The former two forms of invasive therapy are more suited for use in neonates and smaller infants than is hemodialysis. All these procedures should be performed in collaboration with a pediatric nephrologist who has experience in them.

COMPLICATIONS

The most common complications of acute renal failure in children, beyond the immediate biochemical and fluid problems already mentioned, are infection and gastrointestinal hemorrhage. Infection is more common in patients who have had trauma or surgery and is a factor in as many as two thirds of the deaths occurring in patients who have ARF. The urinary system is the most common site of infection, followed by the bloodstream (septicemia) and the respiratory tract. Although urinary catheterization is an important part of the initial evaluation of the oliguric child, prolonged urinary catheterization predisposes the child to infection. Prophylactic antibiotics in catheterized patients who have ARF also increase the risk of serious urinary infection. Therefore neither prolonged urinary catheterization for monitoring of urine output nor prophylactic antibiotics are recommended as part of routine management of these patients. Meticulous care should be given to all intravenous catheters to decrease the incidence of septicemia.

Table 291-2 Treatment of Hyperkalemia in Pediatric Patients

Agent	Dose	Effect	Remarks
Calcium gluconate (10%)	0.5 ml/kg IV over 2-4 min	Rapid but transient	Monitor ECG for bradycardia during injection; may be repeated but *not likely* to be effective
Sodium bicarbonate (7.5%)	2.5 mEq/kg (approximately 3 ml/kg) IV by slow push	Rapid but transient	Repetition *not* recommended
Glucose (50%)	1 ml/kg IV by slow push	Within 1-2 hr	Attempt to increase blood glucose to 250 mg/dl; may be maintained by infusion of 30% glucose at rate equal to insensible fluid loss
Insulin (regular)	0.1 U/kg IV	Rapid	Give *only* with hypertonic glucose infusion (30%)
Sodium polystyrene sulfonate (Kayexalate)	1 g/kg PO or PR	Hours to days	Side effects: gastric irritation (nausea and vomiting), diarrhea, *or* fecal impaction; PO more effective than PR; enemas should be retained 4-10 hr for effectiveness—removed by cleansing enema; may cause *hypokalemia;* use cautiously in patients who tolerate sodium loads poorly; also chelates Ca^{++} and Mg^{++}

PROGNOSIS

The short-term outcome depends on the physician's ability to recognize acute renal failure and to construct an individualized treatment plan that will minimize the biochemical abnormalities as well as complications. The long-term prognosis depends most on the nature of the underlying condition that produced the renal failure. For example, a patient who has ARF following cardiac surgery has a poor prognosis if the cardiac function remains inadequate, whereas a patient who has renal failure following hemolytic-uremic syndrome generally has a good prognosis.

SUGGESTED READINGS

Baquero A et al: Dopamine and furosemide in oliguric acute renal failure, *Nephron* 37:39, 1984.

Bock GH: Acute renal failure. In Kher KK, Makker SP, editors: *Clinical pediatric nephrology,* New York, 1992, McGraw-Hill.

Dixon BS, Anderson RJ: Nonoliguric acute renal failure, *Am J Kidney Dis* 6:71, 1985.

Ellis EN, Arnold WC: Use of urinary indices in renal failure in the newborn, *Am J Dis Child* 136:615, 1982.

Gaudio KM, Siegel NJ: Pathogenesis and treatment of acute renal failure, *Pediatr Clin North Am* 34:771, 1987.

Schaffer SE, Normal ME: Renal function and renal failure in the newborn, *Clin Perinatol* 16:199, 1989.

Weiss L et al: Continuous arteriovenous hemofiltration in the treatment of 100 critically ill patients with acute renal failure: report on clinical outcome and nutritional aspects, *Clin Nephrol* 31:184, 1989.

292 Shock

Joseph R. Custer and John H. Fugate

The traditional method of writing about and teaching the diagnosis and treatment of shock can be bewildering to a primary care practitioner who rarely encounters critically ill children.[34] However, the practitioner should bear in mind that the cause of the shock state rarely affects treatment, especially in its early stages. Prompt recognition and management of shock minimizes mortality and morbidity, even if transfer to a tertiary care facility is required.[8]

The clinician should recognize that simple principles of therapy are effective despite the various causes of the shock. When treating shock the clinician should be confident in treating the hemodynamic abnormalities first and establishing the etiology later.

Several guidelines are axiomatic:

1. Vascular access must be established immediately.
2. Volume restoration is always the correct first step.
3. Children who require more than two 20 ml/kg fluid boluses usually will require tertiary ICU care.
4. Dopamine is almost uniformly the vasopressor of first choice in pediatric age groups.
5. Sequelae are minimized if hypoxemia is avoided; therefore oxygenation and ventilation must be preserved.
6. Children in septic and cardiogenic shock will require referral for definitive care *after* primary care stabilization.

These few axioms are supported by consideration of pitfalls encountered in the evaluation of children referred to a tertiary unit for definitive care (see the box on p. 1763). All these issues can be addressed easily by the primary care provider.

CLASSIFICATIONS OF SHOCK

Etiology

Historically, shock has been classified by mechanism: hypovolemic, distributive, and cardiogenic. The diagnosis, treatment, and therapy of shock have always fascinated investigators; a textbook chapter published recently cites 320 references![36] Those who provide care for children would do well to simplify the early management of shock states. Shoemaker has commented on the complex literature surrounding the etiology and mechanism of shock and the seemingly paradoxical simplistic approach to treatment:

> The traditional approach is simple, clear, logical, straightforward, readily understandable, and generally accepted by most textbooks and educators. The only problem with this conceptualization is that it is wrong. Real life is not that simple. *Irrespective of the initiating event, the interacting circulatory alterations of flow, volume, and oxygen transport produce characteristic patterns that lead to survival or to circulatory failure, shock, and death.*[34]

The clinician who initially encounters a child in shock must resist the temptation to perform elaborate, complex diagnostic tests before the patient is stabilized. Securing the airway, establishing vascular access, giving fluid volume, and providing 100% oxygen are urgent priorities. Clinical suspicion of the underlying diagnostic process must lead to instant treatment. Once the patient is stabilized, diagnostic tests and evaluation of response to therapy will lead to an expanded appropriate differential diagnosis.

Underscoring the need to treat first and establish etiology later is the observation of common sequential sequences of physiological and hemodynamic patterns in studies that compare children who have either septic or cardiogenic shock. No significant differences in the early or later stages of disease could be found when patients in cardiogenic shock were compared with those in septic shock in terms of cardiac index and oxygen consumption or delivery.[7]

Shock traditionally has been classified as follows:

- *Hypovolemic*
  - Dehydration
  - Gastrointestinal losses
  - Blood loss
  - Excess urine output
    - Diabetes mellitus
    - Diabetes insipidus
  - High-output renal failure
  - "Third space" fluid losses
    - Peritonitis
    - Burns
    - Hypoalbuminemia
  - Mannitol administration
  - Diuretic agent administration
- *Distributive*
  - Septic shock
  - Hypoadrenal states
  - Anaphylaxis
  - Drug overdose
- *Cardiogenic*
  - Pump or inotropic
    - Myocarditis
    - Myocardiopathy
    - Decreased contractility acquired in sepsis syndromes
    - Hypoplastic left heart syndrome
    - Arrhythmia
  - Obstructive
    - Coarctation of the aorta
    - Tamponade caused by excessive pericardial blood, fluid, or air

HYPOVOLEMIC SHOCK

Hypovolemic shock is by far the most common form of shock encountered among children. The most frequent causes include trauma, loss of plasma volume subsequent to burns, gastrointestinal losses, or third space fluid losses.

COMMON PITFALLS NOTED IN A POPULATION OF CHILDREN WHO HAVE SHOCK PRESENTING FOR TERTIARY INTENSIVE CARE

Failure to or delay in obtaining adequate intravenous or intraosseous access
Failure to infuse adequate fluid volume
Failure to document vital signs
Failure to protect the airway
Failure to determine or treat hypoglycemia
Failure to recognize hypoxemia
Failure to recognize occult blood loss
Failure to diagnose an acute abdomen as a source of sepsis

Because shock is defined by hypoperfusion rather than by hypotension, it may be present in a child who maintains a near-normal blood pressure, albeit tachycardic, with poor capillary refill, oliguria, and mental status changes. When the blood pressure finally falls below normal in the already vasoconstricted, traumatized child, the situation becomes even more critical because the child has lost more than 25% of his or her blood volume.

The rate at which an infant loses vascular volume will alter the presentation and observed physical signs. For example, an acute blood or fluid loss of 15% of the blood volume will precipitate all the classic signs of shock: pallor, tachycardia, poor perfusion, and coma. Compared with adults the infant has a much larger extravascular fluid compartment. Thus slow fluid losses over days are compensated for modestly, so clinical signs of shock are blunted. Taken as a whole, however, it will be obvious to the astute clinician that the infant is volume depleted, even if the blood pressure is only modestly, rather than catastrophically, decreased.[14]

Blood Loss

Blood loss resulting from trauma is the most common cause of shock in children, including victims of child abuse.

Gastrointestinal bleeding, which occasionally can be rapid and severe, may be seen with esophageal variceal ulcers, Meckel diverticulum, intussusception, volvulus, or inflammatory bowel disease. Hemolytic uremic syndrome may present with bloody diarrhea, azotemia, and a coagulopathy.

Plasma Loss

Plasma loss regularly is associated with severe burns; the degree of loss is related to the extent and depth of the burn. Continuing losses can be extremely large until eschar is formed, grafting commenced, or artificial skin placed. Peritonitis produces a significant loss of plasma through the peritoneal surface; this loss, being hidden in a "third space," frequently is underestimated.

Electrolyte Loss

Electrolyte loss and imbalance are seen most commonly in pediatric conditions associated with vomiting and diarrhea. Significant electrolyte loss also occurs in paralytic ileus and intestinal obstruction; large volumes of fluid can fill dilated loops of bowel; and continuous suctioning of gastric content can remove significant amounts of fluid and electrolytes. Excessive diuresis from mannitol or furosemide also may produce significant iatrogenic fluid and electrolyte loss. Hyperosmolar agents, as used in radiological diagnostic procedures, can produce an osmotic diuresis.

ADVANCED TRAUMA LIFE SUPPORT CLASSIFICATION OF SHOCK

Class I

15% or less loss of acute blood volume
Blood pressure normal
Age-related pulse increased 10% to 20%
No change in capillary refill

Class II

20% to 25% loss of blood volume
Tachycardia >150 beats/min
Tachypnea 35 to 40 breaths/min
Capillary refill prolonged >3 sec
Systolic blood pressure decreased
Pulse pressure decreased
Orthostatic hypotension
Urine output >1 ml/kg/hr

Class III

30% to 35% blood volume loss
All of the above signs
Urine output <1 ml/kg/hr
Lethargic, clammy skin, and vomiting

Class IV

40% to 50% blood volume loss
Nonpalpable pulses
Obtunded

The advanced trauma life support classification of shock (as shown in the box above) emphasizes the relationship of volume loss to physical signs.[36]

CARDIOGENIC SHOCK

The heart may fail because of primary muscle failure, secondary functional depression, or an obstruction to blood flow. Causes of primary or secondary cardiac pump failure include myocarditis, overwhelming sepsis (bacterial and viral), hypoxemia, myocardial ischemia from inadequate coronary perfusion associated with hypovolemia and hypoxemia, and pericardial tamponade from blood, other fluid, or air.

Cardiac failure is a rare cause of shock in children. The possibility of a cardiac etiology for shock should not delay venous access, and it is safe to administer a fluid bolus of 10 to 20 ml/kg. If the patient develops congestive symptoms—that is, pulmonary edema, an enlarged heart, hepatomegaly—and exhibits clinical signs of poor perfusion, a cardiac etiology should be suspected. An electrocardiogram, echocardiogram, and chest radiograph should be obtained.

Management of cardiogenic shock is complex and requires sophisticated monitoring devices, cardiac catheterization, and technically complex treatment. Consultation with an intensivist or cardiologist is needed, and transport to a tertiary pediatric intensive care facility usually is necessary.[27]

DISTRIBUTIVE SHOCK

The many causes of shock in this classification produce vasodilation and decreased blood flow to some organs, but spare others. As in the other "classes" of shock, early rapid restoration of fluid volume and stabilization of the airway are the foundations of successful therapy.

Causes of distributive shock include sepsis, drug overdose, some poisonings, and anaphylaxis. The hallmark of the clinical presentation is peripheral vasodilation, warm, red skin in the presence of tachycardia, and altered mental status and oliguria, a constellation often referred to as *hyperdynamic shock*.[24] Septic shock may be more common than historical reports would suggest.[16]

The bacterial etiology of septic shock has been altered by vaccination against *Haemophilus influenzae* type B. If sepsis in the (increasingly common) immunocompromised patient is excluded, meningococci and streptococci are the bacterial causes of sepsis encountered most frequently. In a retrospective analysis of 2110 admissions to a pediatric intensive care unit published in 1990, 564 patients had septic shock, one half (268) of whom required inotropic support. In the patients who had positive blood cultures, causes were *Haemophilus influenzae* type b in 41%, *Neisseria meningitidis* in 18%, and *Streptococcus pneumoniae* in 11%.[16] These distributions are not likely today because of the effectiveness of Hib vaccine.

Studies of children who have meningococcemia highlight important issues in the care of those in septic shock.[5,33] Mortality remains high, despite modern advances in critical care.[34] Clinicians who recognize these clinical stigmata in primary care settings should recognize the importance of early stabilization, the need for referral for definitive therapy, and the high mortality despite aggressive intervention.

The development of multisystem organ failure in a group of 100 children who had meningococcemia was predictive of death. Patients in shock, who had a white blood count less than 10,000 cell/mm^3, and who had coagulopathy had extremely high mortality.[2] Multisystem organ failure among patients in septic shock correlates with the development of cardiac depression. The hallmark of this presentation is persistent tachycardia despite restoration of blood volume.[24] When cardiac failure can be controlled with catecholamines and judicious fluid management aided by Swan-Ganz catheters, survival is possible. If aggressive volume replacement and catechol therapy do not correct the plasma volume and cardiac failure occurs, death is likely.[20,30]

Toxic shock syndrome is caused by local infection with toxin-producing strains of bacteria, often *Staphylococci* or *Streptococci*. The condition may affect children of any age and of either gender. Cases have been associated with the use of tampons by menstruating women. Closed-space infections, such as retropharyngeal abscess, and infections involving elaboration of large amounts of toxin may be associated with the syndrome. Clinicians should know that only 50% of cases occur in menstruating females. Any focal staphylococcal infection can produce the syndrome (see Chapter 263, Staphylococcal Toxic Shock Syndrome).

The patients present with a remarkably rapid downhill course. Fever, accompanied by vomiting, diarrhea, headache, and myalgia, proceeds abruptly to cardiovascular collapse. A scarlatiniform exanthem with flexor surface accentuation and palmar-plantar erythema are common cutaneous manifestations. The differential diagnosis includes Kawasaki syndrome, Rocky Mountain spotted fever, rubeola, and erythema multiforme.[31]

OTHER COMMON TYPES OF SHOCK

Hypoxic-Ischemic

The primary cause of cardiac arrest in children is hypoxemia.[18] The type of shock following hypoxemic-ischemic insults, a common occurrence in the pediatric age group, is unique. Cardiac output is reduced, oxygen delivery inadequate, and systemic vascular resistance elevated. The poor perfusion and cool, "clamped down" appearance of the child may be misinterpreted as hypovolemia. In this circumstance aggressive volume infusion can produce symptoms of congestive heart failure. Dopamine, in doses greater than 10 μg/kg/minute, may intensify vasoconstriction and produce tachyarrhythmia.

Hypoadrenal Shock

Many pediatric patients who have increasingly complex chronic disease are cared for in primary settings. Many of these children are treated with steroids; these include patients who have asthma, rheumatic disease, or renal disease and post–organ transplant patients. Patients who may have secondary depression of the adrenal response should be treated with steroids, usually hydrocortisone (Solu-Cortef), in stress doses of 150 mg/m^2.[9]

SEQUELAE OF SHOCK

The molecular biology of shock, especially septic shock, is complex; detailed reviews are available.[36] When oxygen transport to the tissues is reduced and cellular hypoxemia and anaerobic glycolysis occur, the resultant production of lactic acid causes a fall in blood pH and bicarbonate levels. Inflammatory mediators, such as tumor necrosis factor and interleukins, are released. In turn, a cycle of complement activation and endothelial interaction with leukocytes, macrophages, and platelets is initiated, resulting in tissue ischemia and cell death. General metabolic changes during shock include increased glucagon production, decreased insulin response to glucose, and marked protein catabolism. Metabolism of the cell is disrupted, and less adenosine triphosphate (ATP) is available. Cellular changes include the passage of sodium into and potassium out of the cell, as well as intracellular calcium accumulation. Lysozymes are broken down, and the cell finally is destroyed. However, restoration of adequate tissue perfusion may reverse some of these cellular changes.

Several organ systems may be affected by shock. A common form of hypoxemic respiratory failure known as adult respiratory distress syndrome (ARDS) occurs 24 to 48 hours after initial presentation. The child becomes dyspneic and has significant hypoxemia ($Pao_2/Fio_2 \leq 150$). Physical examination reveals rales and tachypnea; a chest roentgenogram reveals "diffuse infiltrates." These changes may be delayed and may appear for the first time 12 to 24 hours after the onset of the dyspnea. The interstitial edema that develops appears to be caused by a capillary leak syndrome. This complication is life threatening, and the patient should be referred to a pediatric ICU. Mechanical ventilation and positive end-expiratory pressure, right heart catheters, high-frequency oscillatory ventilation, or extracorporeal membrane support may be required.[4]

Inadequate perfusion and the presence of inflammatory mediators of the heart affect contractility and may lead to a decrease in cardiac output. Myocardial depression is encountered commonly in septic shock.[23]

Renal failure, especially acute tubular necrosis, is common. Renal failure is suspected when the urine output is less than 0.5 ml/kg/hr, despite adequate restoration of blood volume as evidenced by a central venous pressure greater than 5 cm H_2O. An increase in the blood urea nitrogen and creatinine levels supports this diagnosis. Aggressive use of dialysis and hemofiltration has minimized the morbidity resulting from this complication. Unrecognized renal failure will increase the mortality resulting from shock. Serum levels of drugs in the blood become uncertain. Doses of antibiotics, sedatives, and analgesics must be monitored carefully, following blood levels in serum whenever possible. Fluid therapy must be titrated carefully to insensible fluid loss replacement, otherwise congestive heart failure will result. Anuria complicating shock requires referral or consultation with a nephrologist or intensivist.[17]

The central nervous system is most susceptible to hypoxemia and ischemia. A child may suffer significant neurological impairment while other organs are spared. Early central nervous system signs of shock include delirium, irritability, confusion, and coma. Signs of increased intracranial pressure usually are delayed 24 to 72 hours after a hypoxemic-ischemic insult. The presence of increased intracranial pressure in the acute presentation of shock implies a traumatic or metabolic etiology.[36]

Liver function may become impaired as a result of inadequate perfusion of that organ. Bilirubin and liver enzymes are elevated, and clotting factors may be diminished. In septic shock, liver perfusion may be adequate, but bacteria or toxins may damage hepatic cells. Liver failure is rarely an acute complication.

Adrenal failure is uncommon, but may occur in septicemia. Meningococcemia may result in the lethal complication of Waterhouse-Friderichsen syndrome. The common use of steroid therapy in asthma, other allergic states, and immune suppression therapy has produced a population of patients in whom "stress doses" of steroids need to be administered should such patients be in shock. Such a child exhibits a high cardiac output and low peripheral resistance shock syndrome that is refractory to intravascular volume infusion.

DIAGNOSIS OF SHOCK

History

Appreciating the effects of age and circumstance helps one to arrive at a more precise differential diagnosis, minimize time and expense for extraneous laboratory tests, and determine appropriate consultation.

Age

Newborns less than 6 weeks of age who are in shock merit special attention, and a broader differential diagnosis should be considered than in older children. Early discharge of well babies shortly after birth requires attention to both acquired and congenital or inherited conditions. Algorithmic diagnostic and treatment flow sheets designed for older children have proved too general in the evaluation of this age group. The box above lists the most common diagnoses to consider when approaching infants who are in shock.[28,29]

CAUSES OF SHOCK IN THE YOUNG INFANT

Cardiac

Hypoplastic left heart syndrome
Coarctation of the aorta
Myocarditis
Arrhythmia

Infectious

Bacterial meningitis
Urinary tract sepsis
Herpes (meningitis and sepsis)
Streptococcal sepsis

Metabolic

Hypoglycemia
Inborn errors of metabolism

Traumatic

Child abuse
Occult CNS hemorrhage

Surgical

Bowel obstruction
Occult blood loss

Shock in toddlers usually has a determinable, apparent cause. The clinician should recognize the propensities unique to this age group, especially poisonings, ingestions of medications, inhalation and swallowing of foreign bodies, exposure to day care compatriots, and trauma resulting from falls, playground and household accidents, and child abuse.

The adolescent may not be forthright in volunteering an accurate history. The risk-taking behavior of the teen years should be considered when a differential diagnosis is generated in this age group. Ingestion and poisoning after attempted suicide may not be reported by those available to give a history. Experiments with drugs and alcohol can have catastrophic consequences.

In all age groups history of travel and migration may lead to further etiological clues. Rocky Mountain spotted fever and Lyme disease rarely present with cardiovascular collapse. In a child with recent exposure to pets and who has diarrhea, the possibility of *Salmonella* infection must be considered. Recent ingestion of meat and early onset of central nervous system symptoms with bloody diarrhea imply hemolytic uremic syndrome. Exposure to organophosphates and carbonates should be sought if weakness is part of the presentation.[25]

Physical Diagnosis of Shock

Hypotension and tachycardia are the hallmarks of shock (see the box on p. 1766). In uncomplicated shock, restoration of blood pressure and reduction of heart rate are indicators of

SYMPTOMS AND SIGNS ASSOCIATED WITH SHOCK

Tachycardia
Hypotension
Oliguria
Capillary refill >3 seconds
Tachypnea
Dry mucous membranes
Altered mental status

From Crone RK: *Pediatr Clin North Am* 27:525, 1980.

Table 292-1 Normal Vital Signs

	Heart rate	Blood pressure (S/D)
Neonate	140±40	65±10/40
<1 year	120±30	80±20/50
1-2 years	110±20	90±20/55
2-5 years	90±20	90±20/60
>5 years	80±10	100±20/60

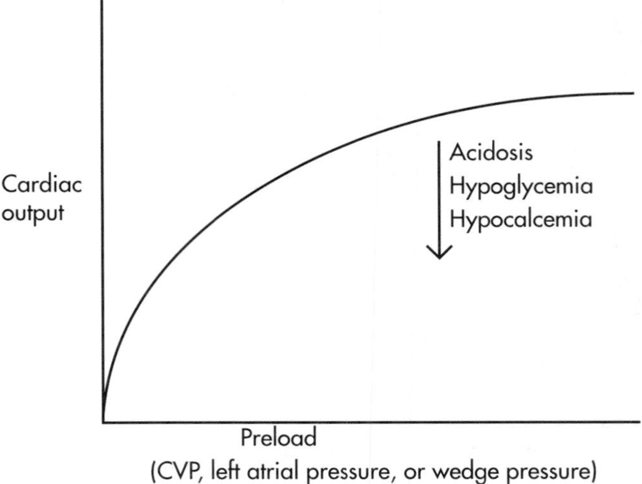

FIG. 292-1 Relationship of stroke volume to preload, determining myocardial contractility (Starling curve). A depressed response may be caused by hypoxemia, acidosis, hypocalcemia, sepsis, or drug toxicity.

therapeutic success. Normal vital signs are seen in Table 292-1.[23,30]

The signs and symptoms of shock are a result of inadequate perfusion, which is a clinical representation of the combined effects of cardiac output and peripheral resistance. Cardiac output is the product of heart rate and stroke volume expressed in liters of blood flow per minute. In older children and adults, hypotension (loss of peripheral vascular tone) is sensed by baroreceptors, which act to increase the heart rate and stroke volume.

In hypovolemia, inadequate blood volume is returned to the ventricles, cardiac muscle fibers are less distended and contract less efficiently, and stroke volume decreases. Contractility of the heart also is depressed by acidosis, hypoxemia, decreased levels of ionized calcium, and hypoglycemia.

Decreased preload is the term used to describe inadequate return of blood to the heart. Preload is measured clinically by determining central venous pressure (CVP).[13] Figure 292-1 demonstrates the interaction of adequate volume status (preload, or CVP) and contractility (cardiac output). In uncomplicated shock, restoration of blood volume alone increases preload and thus restores cardiac output. Acidosis, hypoglycemia, and hypocalcemia decrease cardiac output by reducing preload.

Heart rate is a valuable clinical sign in shock. Infants are not able to increase stroke volume as well as adults; therefore cardiac output in the very young is affected by increasing the heart rate.[13] Thus an infant in shock whose heart rate is 2 standard deviations above normal is attempting to increase cardiac output. The improvement of the infant will correlate with the heart rate decreasing to the normal range. Thus pulse rate is a valuable predictor of success.[8,11,23]

Mental status is a remarkably sensitive and important indicator of degree of illness and response to therapy. Presence of coma or neurological compromise implies significant brain hypoperfusion. Restoration of neurological well-being is the goal of therapy. Shock must be ruled out in children who demonstrate changes in mental status, such as agitation, lethargy, confusion, and coma.[36]

Urine output is usually an accurate indicator of blood volume and perfusion. However, several caveats are important. Many children have multiple caretakers during a typical day, so the frequency and volume of urination may not be recounted accurately. Patients who have high output renal failure or hyperglycemia from diabetes mellitus, patients on diuretics, and children who have received mannitol will have obligatory urine losses that reflect inadequate hydration.

Capillary refill within 3 seconds is not helpful as a single clinical sign, but when interpreted in constellation with heart rate, blood pressure, and mental status, it does help to determine the degree of illness.[3]

TREATMENT

Early volume resuscitation and vasopressor therapy always are indicated in the treatment of shock. One should be conservative in using these treatments only if patients show pulmonary edema, congestive heart failure, or renal failure. In these cases judicious use of fluid and evaluation of response to therapy by measurement of the central venous pressure lead astute clinicians to a diagnosis of shock due to cardiac or renal causes. Rather than fearing fluid overload and thus undertreating the vast majority of patients, one should use the patient's response to fluid administration as a diagnostic test.[26]

Treatment of shock, especially in primary care settings, is based on simple principles of restoring adequate circulating blood volume, thereby achieving adequate delivery of glucose and oxygen to all tissues. Timely documentation of response to each intervention is essential.

Clinicians not involved customarily with critically ill children often worry about which type of fluid and vasopressor is most effective.[38] This concern is unwarranted. The most important therapy, often overlooked or delayed, is the immediate establishment of an intraosseous or large-bore intravenous device; standards of care require this to be placed within minutes of presentation.[22] The second most important priority is giving adequate fluid volume and restoring the circulation. This can be accomplished with commonly available fluids, such as normal saline or lactated Ringer solution with glucose added to maintain adequate blood glucose levels. A reasonable volume is 20 ml/kg with a range of 10 to 30 ml/kg.[11]

Oxygen cannot be delivered to tissues without adequate oxygen intake. One of the urgent priorities in all shock patients is to ensure that the airway is patent. All patients in shock should immediately be given 100% oxygen; oxygenation should be monitored continuously with a pulse oximeter and the values documented in the patient's record. Because a normal oxygen saturation does not reflect adequate oxygen content, the hemoglobin (the carrying vehicle for oxygen) must be at a normal level. Clinicians need to appreciate that a normal oxygen saturation does not imply adequate tissue delivery.[32]

Acidosis is a common sequela of shock. The salutary effects of restoring the pH to greater than 7.25 are crucial: myocardial contractility is enhanced, sensitivity to catecholamines is improved, and potassium is returned to the intracellular space.

Several doses of sodium bicarbonate often are required to improve blood pH to greater than 7.25 and serum bicarbonate levels to greater than 15 mEq/dl. Any remaining base deficit may be corrected by using the following guide: 0.3 × body weight in kilograms × base deficit[19]

Hypocalcemia may accompany shock. Total calcium measurements do not correlate with measurements of the biologically more important ionized calcium.[19] Restoring ionized calcium to normal levels can be an important component of later stages of therapy, as both blood pressure and stroke volume increase.

Clinicians must appreciate the crucial role of hemoglobin, especially when low cardiac output is combined with hypoxemia. Clinicians should also realize that a normal oxygen saturation and "adequate" arterial PO_2 are not accurate reflections of adequate tissue oxygen delivery.[1,21,32]

Blood transfusions are an essential component of shock therapy. If the circulation is compromised and cardiac output falls, oxygen delivery to tissues will be compromised. Oxygen delivery is merely the product of oxygen content and cardiac output. Oxygen content = 1.36 × % saturation × hemoglobin (in grams) and is expressed as milliliters of O_2/100 ml blood. Cardiac output is the product of heart rate and stroke volume expressed as liters of flow per minute (L/m).

In health, O_2 consumption is 25% of O_2 delivery. In shock states, oxygen consumption may increase simultaneously with inadequate cardiac output, leading to inadequate tissue oxygenation. If lung disease is present or hypoventilation occurs, hemoglobin is less than 100% saturated and oxygen delivery is compromised further.[7,25]

Although arguments have been advanced that red blood cell transfusion is an overused resource in routine patient care, adequate oxygen content must be ensured for a patient in shock; transfusion is indicated if anemia is present. For the patient in shock, a hemoglobin of at least 12 gram must be maintained.

As an example, a 3-year-old presents with a lung contusion and splenic hematoma. The hemoglobin is 10, heart rate is 180, systolic blood pressure is 80, and Sao_2 by pulse oximetry is 90%. The patient's level of consciousness waxes and wanes.

Let us consider the oxygen content in this child compared with normal circumstances (SaO_2 100, Hb 13), because O_2 content in ml O_2/100 ml blood = 1.36 × Hb × % saturation, then the patient's O_2 content is 1.36 × 10 × 90 = *12.3 ml of O_2/100 ml* blood, whereas normal O_2 content is 1.36 × 13 × 100 = *17.68 ml O_2/100 ml* blood.

Evidence is ample that our patient's cardiac output is compromised as heart rate is elevated, blood pressure is decreased, and mental status is depressed. Transfusion of red blood cells to reach a hemoglobin of 13 thus increases oxygen content of the blood nearly 50% (from 12.3 to 17.8 ml/100 ml blood).

Preservation of coagulation balance is in the second tier of therapies. In general, unless bleeding is evident, platelet counts of 20,000 to 50,000/mm^3 are tolerated well. Prothrombin time and partial thromboplastin time should be maintained at 1.3 times the normal values. Fresh frozen plasma, administered at 10 ml/kg, is a reasonable method both of repairing volume deficit and replenishing coagulation factor.[10,35]

Glucose replacement is crucial, especially in the very young. Glucose should be maintained at greater than 60 mg/dl in infants and at least at 80 mg/dl in adolescents. Clinicians who use normal saline or lactated Ringer as a volume expander need to remember to provide 10% glucose to these fluids in infants and 5% in other age groups. Rapid serum glucose determinations are available. These values should be monitored and recorded as a "vital sign" whenever blood pressures are measured. Persistent hypoglycemia is an ominous sign in sepsis and may indicate the presence of an inherited metabolic disorder in infants. Calcium may be important in the maintenance of blood measure and cardiac output. Ionized calcium, not the total calcium, should be maintained within the normal range.[19]

VASOPRESSOR DRUGS

The clinician should not be misled or seduced by unneeded complexities when choosing an appropriate vasopressor.[38] In the vast majority of situations that a primary care physician will encounter, knowledge of the effects of dopamine will carry the day. A very basic knowledge of vasopressor physiology is required[37] (see Table 292-2).

Catecholamine drugs commonly used in shock include dopamine, norepinephrine, and dobutamine. Catecholamines are classified by their relative effects on the alpha or beta receptor. The alpha receptor produces vasoconstriction, which accounts for its salutary effect in raising blood pressure. Alpha agonists are not delivered with peripheral intravenous devices because skin and muscle necrosis can result. Intense alpha stimulation can decrease renal blood flow, but this can be offset by the dopaminergic effect of low-dose dopamine.[36]

Beta agonists have type 1 and 2 receptors. Beta 1 receptors stimulate heart rate and cardiac muscle contractility; thus toxicity is reflected in cardiac tachyarrhythmias and ischemia. Beta 2 agonists occur in bronchial and arteriole smooth

Table 292-2 Specific Vasopressor Agents Used to Treat Shock

Agent	Site of action (receptor)	Dose* (μg/kg/min)	Effect
Dopamine	δ	1-3	"Dopaminergic;" renal vasodilation; inotropic
	α>β	5-20	Peripheral vasoconstriction; increased systemic vascular resistance; dysrhythmias
Dobutamine	β_1, β_2	1-20	Inotropic, chronotropic; vasodilation (β_2); lowers systemic vascular resistance; lowers pulmonary vascular resistance; tachycardia and arrhythmia (β_1)
Epinephrine	α>β	0.05-1.0	Inotropic Tachycardia; arrhythmia; decreased renal flow from α effect; increase in myocardial oxygen consumption; intense vasoconstriction
Norepinephrine	α>β	0.005-1.0	Profound vasoconstriction; inotropic; dramatic increase in myocardial oxygen consumption and systemic vascular resistance

*The doses listed are suggested starting ranges. The drugs can be titrated to the desired effect depending on the patient's response.

muscle; thus these muscles relax when stimulated. At low doses (1 to 4 μg/kg/min) dopamine acts at a unique dopaminergic receptor that can enhance or preserve renal blood flow.

A vasoactive drug should be infused continuously with a calibrated infusion pump; continuous heart rate and blood pressure monitoring is required, preferably with an intraarterial catheter and transducer. Vasoactive agents should be infused into a central catheter. Norepinephrine, epinephrine, and dopamine increase blood pressure by vasoconstriction, which decreases microcirculatory flow and, possibly, renal blood flow. These drugs are only adjuncts to volume replacement in hypovolemic shock; blood and fluid replacement is the cardinal therapeutic principle.[12,38]

Dopamine is used frequently to increase cardiac output and augment renal perfusion in the critically ill child. The effects are dose dependent, with renal (dopaminergic, δ) effects seen at the low-dose range (1 to 4 μg/kg/min). At higher doses (>10 μg/kg/min), alpha-adrenergic effects predominate with vasoconstriction and reduced peripheral perfusion.

Dobutamine differs from dopamine because of its enhanced inotropic effect with less chronotropic effect than dopamine; also, it has less effect on systemic vascular resistance. In some circumstances, especially shock induced by hypoxemia-ischemia, dobutamine may be preferred because dopamine may precipitate tachyarrhythmias and increase myocardial oxygen consumption.[18]

Norepinephrine is a valuable agent when dopamine proves futile, as may occur in severe septic shock. Adequate preservation of renal blood flow has been reported when this drug has been used alone or in combination with "renal-dose" dopamine, especially in septic shock, in which peripheral vasodilation is significant.[15]

Steroids are not indicated in shock therapy except when adrenal suppression occurs after corticosteroid treatment. In large prospective human trials, steroids used to treat septic shock have increased mortality and the incidence of secondary infection.[6] Therefore steroids are indicated only in patients suspected of having secondary adrenal suppression from prior steroid use.[9]

In selected situations and in tertiary settings only, the use of vasodilator drugs (nitroprusside, nitroglycerin) may be beneficial in reducing afterload when increased afterload is detrimental to myocardial performance. This therapy optimizes myocardial contractility and improves cardiac output, but requires sophisticated monitoring, including pulmonary arterial oximetry, cardiac output measurement, and pulmonary vascular pressure catheters.[13]

Trials of several new therapies have been unsuccessful and have not affected outcomes for pediatric patients. Extracorporeal membrane oxygenation has not been explored adequately and should be performed only at the few centers capable of supporting this technology.[4] A randomized trial of methylprednisolone demonstrated more complications and no improvement in mortality.[6] Trials of ibuprofen, antibody to endotoxin, and antibody to tumor necrosis factor alpha have not met expectations for improving survival in cases of septic shock.[33]

EVALUATION

Response to therapy is important, simple to assess, and of diagnostic value. Documentation of serial interventions and responses is a standard of care. Pulse, respiratory rate, O_2 saturation, blood pressure, capillary refill, urine output, mental status, and glucose level should be recorded every 15 minutes while the patient remains unstable.

Several laboratory tests help to determine further therapy or appropriate consultation. A persistent anion-gap metabolic acidosis ($[HCO_3^-] < 15$ mEq) may support the diagnosis of renal failure, ketoacidosis, lactic acidemia from sepsis, or poisoning from a salicylate, ethanol, or methanol.

Patients who remain in coma or have a depressed sensorium despite evidence of adequate volume repletion are at high risk for neurological sequelae. An inherited metabolic disorder, hypoglycemia, hepatic failure, azotemia, trauma, and poison ingestion must be considered if normalization of blood pressure does not improve mental status.

If two bolus infusions do not result in an improvement, determination of central venous pressure is invaluable. If the CVP is less than 5 cm H_2O, aggressive volume support and additional pressor therapy should be performed.

If the CVP is greater than 10 cm H_2O and congestive failure, pulmonary edema, and poor perfusion are present, a cardiac etiology should be suspected. An ECG, echocardiogram, and chest radiograph are indicated, and consultation with a pediatric intensive care unit should be obtained.

REFERENCES

1. Akingbola OA et al: Management of severe anemia without transfusion in a pediatric Jehovah's Witness: case report and literature review, *Crit Care Med* 22:524, 1994.
2. Algren JT et al: Predictors of outcome in acute meningococcal infection in children, *Crit Care Med* 21:447, 1993.
3. Barraff LJ: Capillary refill: is it a useful clinical sign? *Pediatrics* 92:723, 1993.
4. Beca J, Butt W: Extracorporeal membrane oxygenation for refractory septic shock in children, *Pediatrics* 93:726, 1994.
5. Bone RC: Let's agree on terminology: definitions of sepsis, *Crit Care Med* 19:973, 1991.
6. Bone RC, Fisher CJ Jr, Clemmer TP: A controlled clinical trial of high-dose methylprednisolone in the treatment of severe sepsis and septic shock, *N Engl J Med* 317:653, 1987.
7. Carcillo JA et al: Sequential physiologic interactions in pediatric cardiogenic and septic shock, *Crit Care Med* 17:12, 1989.
8. Carcillo JA, Davis AL, Zaritsky A: Role of early fluid resuscitation in pediatric septic shock, *JAMA* 266:1242, 1991.
9. Chamberlin P, Meyer WJ III: Management of pituitary-adrenal suppression secondary to corticosteroid therapy, *Pediatrics* 67:245, 1981.
10. Colman RW, Robboy SJ, Minna JD: Disseminated intravascular coagulation: a reappraisal, *Ann Rev Med* 30:359, 1979.
11. Crone RK: Acute circulatory failure in children, *Pediatr Clin North Am* 27:525, 1980.
12. Fisher DG, Schwartz PH, Davis AL: Pharmacokinetics of exogenous epinephrine in critically ill children, *Crit Care Med* 21:111, 1993.
13. Friedman WF, George BL: Treatment of congestive heart failure by altering loading conditions of the heart, *J Pediatr* 106:697, 1985.
14. Friis-Hansen B: Body water compartments in children, *Pediatrics* 28:169, 1961.
15. Hesselvick JF, Bradin B: Low-dose norepinephrine in patients with septic shock and oliguria: effects on afterload, urine flow, and oxygen transport, *Crit Care Med* 17:179, 1989.
16. Jacobs RF et al: Septic shock in children: bacterial etiologies and temporal relationships, *Pediatr Infect Dis J* 9:196, 1990.
17. Lucas CE: The renal response to acute injury and sepsis, *Surg Clin North Am* 56:953, 1976.
18. Lucking SE, Pollack MM, Fields AI: Shock following generalized hypoxic-ischemic injury in previously healthy infants and children, *J Pediatr* 108:359, 1986.
19. Meliones JM, Moler FW, Custer JR: Hemodynamic instability after the initiation of extracorporeal membrane oxygenation: role of ionized calcium, *Crit Care Med* 19:1247, 1991.
20. Mercier JC et al: Hemodynamic patterns of meningococcal shock in children, *Crit Care Med* 16:27, 1988.
21. Mink RB, Pollack M: Effect of blood transfusion on oxygen consumption in pediatric septic shock, *Crit Care Med* 18:1087, 1987.
22. Orlowski JP: Comparison study of intraosseous central intravenous and peripheral intravenous infusions of emergency drugs, *Am J Dis Child* 144:112, 1990.
23. Parker MM et al: Serial cardiovascular variables in survivors and nonsurvivors of human septic shock: heart rate as an early predictor of prognosis, *Crit Care Med* 15:923, 1987.
24. Parrillo JE et al: Septic shock in humans, *Ann Intern Med* 113:227, 1990.
25. Perkin RM: Shock states. In Fuhrman BH, Zimmerman JR, editors: *Pediatric critical care,* St Louis, 1992, Mosby.
26. Perkin RM, Anas NG: Cardiovascular evaluation and support in the critically ill child, *Pediatr Ann* 15:30, 1986.
27. Perkin RM, Levin DL: Shock. In Levin DL, Morris FC, editors: *Essentials of pediatric intensive care,* St Louis, 1990, Quality Medical Publishing.
28. Perkin RM, Levin DL: Shock in the pediatric patient. I. Therapy, *J Pediatr* 101:319, 1982.
29. Perkin RM, Levin DL: Shock in the pediatric patient. II. Therapy, *J Pediatr* 101:613, 1982.
30. Pollack MM, Fields AI, Ruttiman UE: Distributions of cardiopulmonary variables in pediatric survivors and nonsurvivors of septic shock, *Crit Care Med* 13:454, 1985.
31. Resnsick SD: Toxic shock syndrome: recent developments in pathogenesis, *J Pediatr* 116:321, 1990.
32. Rodriguez LR et al: A study of pediatric housestaffs' knowledge of pulse oximetry, *Pediatrics* 93:810, 1994.
33. Saez-Llorens X, McCracken GH Jr: Sepsis syndrome and septic shock in pediatrics: current concepts of terminology, pathophysiology, and management, *J Pediatr* 123:497, 1994.
34. Shoemaker WC: Circulatory mechanisms of shock and their mediators, *Crit Care Med* 15:787, 1987.
35. Sinclair JF: The management of fulminant meningococcal septicaemia in children, *Intensive Care World* 5:89, 1988.
36. Wetzel RC, Tobin JR: Shock. In Rogers M, editor, *Textbook of pediatric intensive care,* ed 2, Baltimore, 1992, Williams & Wilkins.
37. Zaritsky A, Chernow B: Use of catecholamines in pediatrics, *J Pediatr* 105:341, 1984.
38. Zaritsky A, Miles M: Too much pharmacokinetics? *Crit Care Med* 21:1620, 1993.

293 Status Asthmaticus

Colleen L. Cook and Michael D. Dettorre

Asthma represents a significant cause of morbidity and mortality and afflicts 5% to 7% of the pediatric population.[7] In the decade before 1987 hospital admissions for children who had asthma increased by over 4% per year. Paradoxically, however, total pediatric hospitalizations decreased by 4.6% per annum.[6] For the same time period mortality rose by 10% among patients between the ages of 5 and 14 years.[26] Between 1979 and 1983 the percentage of asthma admissions requiring intubation or CPR was 0.11%. Data for 1983 to 1987 reveal an increase in this morbidity to 0.50%.[8]

As defined by NIH guidelines, asthma is a lung disease characterized by airway obstruction, airway inflammation, and increased airway responsiveness to stimuli. Asthma is defined further as a chronic illness with acute exacerbations that either resolve spontaneously or in response to treatment.[15] The diagnosis usually is made based on the clinical symptoms of recurrent episodes of wheezing and coughing. Other symptoms include dyspnea, chest tightness, use of accessory muscles of respiration, and cyanosis.

Status asthmaticus represents episodes of airway obstruction that are refractory to initial conventional treatments and require hospital admission for further therapy. Avoiding repeat exacerbations and treating acute episodes require an understanding of the pathophysiology of asthma so that effective treatments, both medical and educational, can be designed for the child and the family. The ultimate goal is to improve pulmonary function and the quality of life during periods of "wellness."

PATHOPHYSIOLOGY

During severe exacerbations of asthma, the central event is irregular airway narrowing secondary to bronchospasm, mucosal edema, epithelial sloughing, and the formation of mucus plugs. Fiberoptic bronchoscopy has identified the presence of mast cells, eosinophils, activated macrophages, and T lymphocytes in airway secretions. Eosinophils, along with T lymphocytes, are found in the submucosa and epithelium of the airways. Eosinophilic cytokine products and mast cell proteases likely are responsible for epithelial destruction in the airway and the loss of the ability to respond to host-generated bronchodilators, such as nitric oxide.[10]

Histologically, smooth muscle cell hyperplasia and hypertrophy occur, as well as increased collagen deposition in the basement membrane. Additionally, mucosal edema and increased mucous production occur as a result of damage to the airway at the cellular level by cytokines released from recruited inflammatory cells.[10]

Airway smooth muscle constriction produces increased airway resistance, collapse of small airways, and a prolonged expiratory phase of the respiratory cycle, resulting in increased work of breathing, gas trapping, and hyperinflation of lung volumes. Mechanical disadvantages imposed by lung hyperinflation result in diaphragmatic fatigue.[13]

These pathophysiological changes result in ventilation-perfusion (V/Q) mismatch, producing increased physiological deadspace and profound hypoxemia. With severe airway disease, hypercapnia develops and produces a respiratory acidosis.[12]

Patients who have severe obstructive disease create large amounts of negative pleural pressure during the inspiratory phase of respiration. This pleural pressure increases the afterload imposed on the left ventricle. Additionally, increased venous return to the right ventricle shifts the intraventricular septum toward the left ventricle and impedes its filling.[19] Subsequently, these factors combine to diminish cardiac output and oxygen delivery to tissue beds.

Furthermore, children acutely affected by asthma often have poor oral intake and increased insensible fluid loss due to increased ventilatory drive and fever, resulting in the development of a fluid deficit. Subsequently this fluid deficit contributes to increased viscosity of secretions and the development of a metabolic acidosis secondary to hypoperfusion and hypoxemia.

The combination of acute respiratory and metabolic acidosis can produce a sharp decline in intravascular pH. Acidosis results in depressed cardiac contractility, increased pulmonary vascular resistance, and decreased glycolytic pathway activity.[1,20,27] These factors contribute to the spiraling nature of respiratory failure by depressing oxygen delivery to the tissues further, impairing ATP synthesis, and leading to further muscle fatigue and impending cardiorespiratory collapse.

MANAGEMENT OF STATUS ASTHMATICUS

Assessment of Severity

Subjective and objective signs of the magnitude of airflow limitation and respiratory fatigue should be evaluated initially upon patient presentation and frequently during therapy. The respiratory rate and pattern correlate with the severity of the asthmatic attack; tachypnea, tachycardia, expiratory grunting, and accessory muscle use are ominous signs. The use of sternocleidomastoid muscles for movement of the chest wall correlates with peak expiratory flow rates of less than 50%.[4] Dyspnea can be assessed by determining the degree of breathlessness, that is, the inability of the verbal patient to speak without appearing short of breath. Fatigue and lethargy may be signs of hypercapnia; confusion or combativeness are signs of hypoxia.

Some signs, however, may be misleading; for instance, if airway obstruction is severe, wheezing may not be heard and cyanosis may not be apparent until late in the course of the illness. One study has shown that peak expiratory flow rate

(PEFR) decreased by as much as 25% before wheezing was audible.[21]

PEFR is the greatest flow velocity obtained during a forced expiration, starting with fully inflated lungs.[29] PEFR measurement is objective, reproducible, quantitative, inexpensive, and simple to perform. Furthermore, PEFR correlates well with the spirometric value of forced expiratory value at 1 second (FEV_1).[16] *PEFR can be used in the cooperative child older than 5 years.* Measured values of PEFR can be compared with normograms based on height or may be approximated by the following formula:

$$\text{Predicted average PEFR} = (\text{height in inches} - 43) \times 15 + 150$$

Serial measurements of PEFR are used to quantitate the severity of acute airway obstruction and its response to therapy.

Initial laboratory evaluation should include a complete blood count and serum potassium level. If muscle fatigue is present, the levels of serum magnesium and phosphorus should be assessed. Chest radiographs should be reserved for those children thought to be at risk for complications of asthma such as pneumothorax, pneumonia, and atelectasis.

Pulse oximetry (Sao_2) is a good noninvasive monitor of oxygenation and response to therapy. Continuous oximetry should be performed on all patients in status asthmaticus. Measuring arterial blood gases is reserved for patients exhibiting signs of respiratory muscle fatigue or hypoxemia (Fio_2 >60% with Sao_2 <92%) via pulse oximetry.

Therapy for Acute Asthma

Successful treatment of status asthmaticus requires the reversal of the three pathological components of asthma, namely hypoxemia, bronchospasm, and inflammation (Table 293-1). Suboptimal therapy for any single component will result in the propagation of respiratory failure and contribute to the overall morbidity of the disease.

Supportive Care. Dehydration caused by increased insensible fluid loss, poor oral intake, and vomiting is corrected by an initial intravenous bolus of 5 to 10 ml/kg of normal saline. Fluids administered at a volume of 100% to 125% of calculated maintenance requirements will help to improve tissue perfusion, decreasing viscosity of respiratory secretions and replacing fluid deficits. If evidence of hypoperfusion persists, an additional fluid bolus of 5 to 10 ml/kg of normal saline is appropriate. Serial physical examinations to assess the development of pulmonary edema are necessary throughout the acute course of therapy because of the propensity of patients to develop cardiac dysfunction as a result of severe pulmonary disease.

Chest physiotherapy and postural drainage have been performed routinely on asthmatic patients, but the therapeutic benefit of such treatment has been questioned.[2] Further studies are needed to make a definitive statement regarding the benefits of this procedure.

Bacterial and viral infections are known triggers of airway

Table 293-1 Therapy for Acute Asthma

Drug	Mode	Dosage
Antiinflammatory		
Methylprednisolone	Intravenous	2 mg/kg load, then 2 mg/kg/day ÷ q 6 hr
Hydrocortisone	Intravenous	4-8 mg/kg load (max 250 mg), then 8 mg/kg/day ÷ q 6 hr
Beclomethasone dipropionate	Metered dose inhaler	1-2 puffs q 4-6 hrs
Cromolyn sodium	Nebulized (10 mg/ml)	20 mg q 6 hr
Nedocromil sodium	Metered dose inhaler	2 puffs q 6 hr
Adrenergic		
Epinephrine	Subcutaneous (1:1000)	0.01 ml/kg/dose (max 0.5 ml) q 15-20 min × 3
Sus-Phrine	Subcutaneous (1:200)	0.005 ml/kg/dose (max 0.15 ml) q 6 hr
Albuterol	Nebulized (5 mg/ml)	0.05-0.15 mg/kg q 1-3 hr (max 5 mg)
	Intermittent	
	Continuous	0.15-0.3 mg/kg q 1 hr continuously
	Metered dose inhaler	2-4 puffs q 1-3 hr
Terbutaline	Nebulized (11 mg/ml)	0.1-0.3 mg/kg q 2-6 hr (max 11mg)
	Subcutaneous (0.5 mg/ml)	0.01 mg/kg q 20-30 min × 3 (max 0.25 mg)
	Intravenous	0.002 mg/kg load over 5 min, 0.0045 mg/kg/hr
Isoproterenol	Nebulized (5 mg/ml)	0.05-0.1 mg/kg q 2-6 hr (max 2.5 mg)
	Intravenous	0.05 μg/kg/min, then titrate by 0.05-0.1 μg/kg/min q15-30 min (max 1 μg/kg/min)
Theophylline	Intravenous (25 mg/ml)	6 mg/kg load, then <1 yr = 0.65 mg/kg/hr >1 yr = 0.9 mg/kg/hr; modify load if history of recent theophylline dosage, noting that 1 mg/kg = 2 μg/ml serum level
Anticholinergic		
Atropine	Nebulized	0.05 mg/kg
Glycopyrrolate	Nebulized (0.2 mg/ml)	0.4 mg q 4-6 hr
Ipratropium bromide	Nebulized	250-500 μg q 6 hr
	Metered dose inhaler	2-4 puffs q 4-6 hr

responsiveness, but routine use of antibiotics should be withheld, except for those patients exhibiting signs of bacterial infection.

Most patients presenting in status asthmaticus exhibit signs of irritability and agitation because of high levels of endogenous and exogenous catecholamines, hypoxia, and sleep deprivation. The use of sedation in these patients may be of benefit. However, caution is advised because sedation may precipitate respiratory collapse in patients who have a marginal respiratory drive or high levels of pulmonary obstruction. Sedation is best reserved for patients in a monitored setting where endotracheal intubation and mechanical ventilation can be accomplished without delay, if needed.

Oxygen. Humidified oxygen is the first line of treatment in any child who is in respiratory distress. Benefits of oxygen therapy include improved V/Q matching, reduced pulmonary hypertension, and improved oxygen delivery to tissues. Pulse oximetry should be used to assess oxygenation; oxygen saturation should be kept greater than 92%.

Antiinflammatory Agents. Corticosteroids are the most effective drugs for treating airway obstruction caused by inflammation. They are known to improve beta-receptor regulation in the airway, inhibit the activation and influx of inflammatory cells, and interfere with the metabolism of arachadonic acid to prostaglandins and leukotrienes.[15] Oral or parenteral administration appears to be equally potent. In the acutely dyspneic child, parenteral administration is preferred to ensure adequate delivery of the medication. Inhaled corticosteroids have added benefit in that levels are elevated in the airways without concomitant systemic elevation. Side effects of systemic corticosteroids over long-term use include cataracts, osteoporosis, Cushing-like syndrome, myopathy, aseptic necrosis of the femur, and increased weight gain.[15] Inhaled steroids can increase the incidence of oral candidiasis and dysphonia. To minimize the frequency of these side effects, mouthwashes and spacer devices are recommended.[11,15] A recent study showed no increases in cataracts over several years' use of inhaled corticosteroids, but debate remains concerning the effect of inhaled corticosteroids on long-term growth potential.[22,28]

Cromolyn sodium and nedocromil sodium (nonsteroidal antiinflammatory agents) stabilize mast cells and prevent release of mediators of early and late allergen-induced airway hyperresponsiveness and bronchoconstriction.[15] These drugs may have benefit when initiated during the acute phase of illness, but serve better as long-term neutralizers of this chronic disease. If possible, these agents should not be discontinued during an acute flare-up so that their long-range effects can be maintained.

Bronchodilators. The most effective therapies for status asthmaticus are the bronchodilators. These include the beta-agonists, the methylxanthines, and the anticholinergics. Historically, parenterally administered nonselective adrenergic agonists and methylxanthines have been the mainstay of therapy. Recently, however, these agents have been supplanted largely by aerosolized selective beta-adrenergic agonists.

Agents such as albuterol and terbutaline dilate smooth muscle by stimulating $beta_2$-adrenergic receptors. These drugs can be administered either through a nebulizer or a metered-dose inhaler. Delivering a high dose of drug directly to the site of action is thought to be beneficial by producing the desired therapeutic effect while minimizing systemic side effects. However, recent evidence indicates that significant bronchodilatation also may be derived from drug absorbed systemically from the mucosa of the gastrointestinal tract.[18]

Side effects of $beta_2$-agonists include cardiac arrhythmias, tremors, headaches, hypokalemia, and nausea. Overuse of $beta_2$-agonists can result in the development of tachyphylaxis resulting from downregulation of beta receptors.[23] One recent study linked overreliance on $beta_2$-agonists with increasing mortality associated with asthma.[24] Subsequent studies have refuted this conclusion and implied that the increased mortality is caused by the underuse of antiinflammatory agents, as well as to various socioeconomic factors.[3,14]

Patients who have impending respiratory failure because of status asthmaticus can be treated by continuous nebulizations. This has been shown to result in a more rapid improvement in pulmonary function as compared with intermittent therapy.[17] Because systemic and bronchial absorption occurs and is dose related, the likelihood of cardiac side effects (tachycardia, hypertension, hypotension, and ventricular arrhythmia) is increased, and therefore these patients require monitoring in an emergency department or pediatric intensive care unit (PICU). Patients requiring more frequent nebulizations than every 3 hours will require a cardiorespiratory monitor.

The use of subcutaneous epinephrine has diminished as nebulized therapies have become popular, but there remains a subset of patients who have severe bronchospasm who deliver aerosolized medication poorly because of inadequate air movement. These patients may benefit from an initial subcutaneous injection to improve air movement and delivery of aerosolized drug. Subcutaneous epinephrine and Sus-Phrine also are indicated when nebulizations are unavailable or the patient is uncooperative.

Intravenous beta-agonists have been replaced largely by continuous nebulizations. Occasionally patients remain refractory to all therapy and are given a trial of isoproterenol or terbutaline to avoid intubation and mechanical ventilation. All patients receiving intravenous beta-agonists should be admitted to an intensive care unit and have cardiorespiratory and invasive arterial blood pressure monitoring. Side effects of these therapies include cardiac arrhythmias, cardiac ischemia, hypotension, and worsening of V/Q matching.

Theophylline relaxes smooth muscles in airways and strengthens diaphragmatic contraction, but it has a narrow therapeutic window and requires careful drug monitoring and adjustment of dosage with such illness as liver disease, congestive heart failure, fever, and when used with certain drugs such as cimetidine, erythromycin, and other antibiotics. Side effects, including tachycardia, arrhythmia, diuresis, hypokalemia, and hyperglycemia, may occur. Furthermore, theophylline has been found to have no additive benefits when combined with aerosolized $beta_2$-agonists.[5]

Nebulized anticholinergics can be used to block vagal reflex bronchospasm. The sites of action of anticholinergic agents depend on the route of administration. The bronchodilatory effect of intravenously administered anticholinergics occurs in both large and small airways, whereas nebulized formulations act predominantly on the large airways.[9,25] Atropine has lost favor as an agent because of its systemic antimuscarinic effects. Glycopyrrolate has fewer side effects than atropine but continues to induce tachycardia, drying of secretions, and mydriasis. Ipratropium bromide does not have the systemic effects of the other anticholinergic drugs. Clinical trials have found ipratropium bromide to have an additive effect with beta$_2$-agonists in the relief of bronchospasm.[8] Ipratropium bromide has become available recently in nebulizer form.

Unusual and investigational forms of therapy for refractory cases of status asthmaticus are reserved for use in pediatric intensive care units. These therapies include intravenous magnesium sulfate, inhalational anesthetics, calcium channel blockers, extracorporeal membranous oxygenation, and heliox (helium with oxygen). No randomized studies evaluating these modalities in pediatric patients have been published yet, but sporadic case reports have offered hope for severe cases of asthma.

Transfer to Intensive Care Unit

Indications for transfer to an intensive care setting include any patient who has signs of respiratory fatigue, such as somnolence or diminishing respiratory effort, hypoxemia with modest levels of supplemental oxygen (Pao_2 <60 mm Hg in 60% Fio_2), cyanosis, hypercapnea ($Paco_2$ >40), electrocardiographic abnormalities, or air leak (pneumothorax, pneumomediastinum, or pneumoperitoneum). Additionally, any patient who has shown a poor therapeutic response to initial or ongoing treatment should be transferred to a PICU for escalation of therapy. The first-line treatment for these children usually is IV steroids, continuous beta$_2$ nebulizations, plus the addition of nebulized anticholinergics. Patients in severe status will require arterial line placement. With worsening respiratory or neurological status, mechanical ventilation may be required. At this point intravenous adrenergic agonists and/or theophylline usually are added to the treatment regimen.

Status asthmaticus remains a complex problem among pediatric patients. Worsening morbidity and mortality statistics have raised concerns about current therapies. Aggressive management of all patients, including broad use of both antiinflammatory and bronchodilatory agents, is necessary to improve patient outcome. Early intervention, frequent patient observation, and titration of therapies, including transfer of appropriate patients to a pediatric intensive care setting, are needed to reverse these statistical trends.

REFERENCES

1. Anderson MN, Borden JR, Mouritzen CV: Acidosis, catecholamines and cardiovascular dynamics: when does acidosis require correction? *Ann Surg* 166:344, 1967.
2. Asher MI et al: Effects of chest physiotherapy on lung function in children recovering from acute severe asthma, *Pediatr Pulmonol* 9:146, 1990.
3. Chang CC et al: Asthma mortality: another opinion—is it a matter of life and . . . bread? *J Asthma* 30:93, 1993.
4. Commey JO, Levison H: Physical signs in childhood asthma, *Pediatrics* 58:537, 1976.
5. Fanta CH, Rossing TH, McFadden ER: Treatment of acute asthma: is combination therapy with sympathomimetics and methylxanthines indicated? *Am J Med* 80:5, 1986.
6. Gergen PJ, Mullaly DI, Evans R: National survey of prevalence of asthma among children in the United States, 1976-1980, *Pediatrics* 81:1, 1988.
7. Gergen PJ, Weiss KB: Changing patterns of asthma hospitalization among children: 1979 to 1987, *JAMA* 264:1688, 1990.
8. Higgins RM, Stradling JR, Lane DJ: Should ipratropium bromide be added to beta-agonists in treatment of acute severe asthma? *Chest* 94:718, 1988.
9. Holtzman MJ et al: Intravenous versus inhaled atropine for inhibiting bronchoconstrictor responses in dogs, *J Appl Physiol* 54:134, 1983.
10. Howarth PH, Redington AE, Montefort S: Pathophysiology of asthma, *Allergy* 48(suppl 17):50, 1993.
11. Konig P: Inhaled corticosteroids—their present and future role in the management of asthma, *J Allergy Clin Immunol* 82:297, 1988.
12. Leffert F: The management of acute severe asthma, *J Pediatr* 96:1, 1980.
13. Martin JG, Shore S, Engel LA: Effect of continuous positive airway pressure on respiratory mechanics and pattern of breathing in induced asthma, *Am Rev Respir Dis* 126:812, 1982.
14. Mullen M, Mullen B, Carey M: The association between beta-agonist use and death from asthma: a meta-analytic integration of case-control studies, *JAMA* 270:1842, 1993.
15. National Asthma Education Program Expert Panel Report: *Guidelines for the diagnosis and management of asthma,* US Department of Health and Human Services, 1991, Pub No 91-3042.
16. Nowak RM, Pensler MI, Parker DD: Comparison of peak expiratory flow and FEV1: admission criteria for acute bronchial asthma, *Ann Emerg Med* 11:64, 1982.
17. Papo MC, Frank J, Thompson AE: A prospective, randomized study of continuous versus intermittent nebulized albuterol for severe status asthmaticus in children, *Crit Care Med* 21:1479, 1993.
18. Penna AC, Dawson KP: Nebulized salbutamol (albuterol): systemic absorption could be important in achieving bronchodilatation, *J Asthma* 30:105, 1993.
19. Rebuck AS, Read J: Assessment and management of severe asthma, *Am J Med* 51:788, 1971.
20. Roos A, Boron WF: Intracellular pH, *Physiol Rev* 61:296, 1981.
21. Shim CS, Williams H: Relationship of wheezing to the severity of obstruction in asthma, *Arch Intern Med* 143:890, 1983.
22. Simons FE et al: Absence of posterior subcapsular cataracts in young patients treated with inhaled glucocorticoids, *Lancet* 342:776, 1993.
23. Skorodan MS: Beta-adrenergic agonists: a problem, *Chest* 103:1587, 1993.
24. Spitzer WO et al: The use of beta-agonists and the risk of death and near death from asthma, *N Engl J Med* 326:501, 1992.
25. Weiss JW, Mcfadden ER, Ingram RH: Parenteral vs inhaled atropine: density dependence of maximal air flow, *J Appl Physiol* 53:392, 1982.
26. Weiss KB, Wagener DK: Changing patterns of asthma mortality: identifying target populations at high risk, *JAMA* 264:1683, 1990.
27. Wildenthal K et al: Effects of acute lactic acidosis on left ventricular performance, *Am J Physiol* 214:1352, 1968.
28. Wolthers OD, Pederson S: Controlled study of linear growth in asthmatic children during treatment with inhaled glucocorticosteroids, *Pediatrics* 89:839, 1992.
29. Wright BM, McKerrow CB: Wright peak flow meter, *Br Med J* 2:1041, 1959.

SUGGESTED READINGS

Bentur L et al: Controlled trial of nebulized albuterol in children younger than 2 years of age with acute asthma, *Pediatrics* 89:133, 1992.

National Asthma Education Program Expert Panel Report: *Guidelines for the diagnosis and management of asthma,* US Department of Health and Human Services, 1991, Pub No 91-3042.

Portnoy J et al: Continuous nebulization for status asthmaticus, *Ann Allergy* 69:71, 1992.

294 Status Epilepticus

Sarah M. Roddy and Margaret C. McBride

Status epilepticus is defined by the World Health Organization as "a condition characterized by an epileptic seizure that is sufficiently prolonged or repeated at sufficiently brief intervals as to produce an unvarying and enduring epileptic condition."[4] There has been much variability in the interpretation of what constitutes an "unvarying and enduring epileptic condition." The most widely accepted criterion for diagnosis of status epilepticus is any seizure that continues for 30 minutes, or intermittent seizures lasting for 30 minutes or longer in which the person does not regain consciousness between the episodes.

Status epilepticus can be classified in terms of the type of seizure. Generalized convulsive status epilepticus is the form most common and easily recognized type of seizure in children. The seizure activity usually is tonic-clonic or clonic and less often is tonic or myoclonic. In simple partial status epilepticus or epilepsia partialis continua, focal seizure activity is prolonged and restricted to one side of the body without loss of consciousness. Nonconvulsive status epilepticus manifests as a confused, drowsy state in which the patient moves in slow motion. This condition results from continuing or repetitive absence seizures or partial complex seizures.

The annual incidence of status epilepticus in patients who have epilepsy ranges from 1.3% to 16%.[5] Its relative frequency, based on age, is highest in the younger age groups.[3] Infants and children also are much more likely than adults to have status epilepticus as the manifestation of their first seizure. In one study of children who had status epilepticus, 77% had an initial seizure that lasted more than 1 hour.[1] Fever commonly precedes the development of status epilepticus, both in neurologically normal children and in those who have a history of neurological insult before the onset of seizure. Central nervous system infection and electrolyte disturbances are other causes of status epilepticus that require prompt identification and treatment. Poor compliance with antiepileptic therapy is a common precipitating factor of status epilepticus in patients who have epilepsy.

Nonconvulsive status epilepticus and epilepsia partialis continua require prompt treatment, but there is less urgency because these seizures do not alter the body's homeostatic mechanisms to the degree that convulsive status epilepticus does. Convulsive status epilepticus is considered a medical emergency because it is life threatening and sometimes is followed by neurological sequelae. The longer convulsive status epilepticus continues, the more resistant it is to therapy and the greater the incidence of mortality and morbidity. Experimental studies have shown that continued seizure activity for more than 60 minutes results in permanent cell damage, even in ventilated animals whose metabolic parameters are kept in the normal range. Clinical studies in humans have found that the mean duration of convulsive status is 1½ hours in patients who have no neurological sequelae, 10 hours in those who have neurological sequelae, and 13 hours in those who die of convulsive status epilepticus.[2] Mortality from status epilepticus in children has gradually dropped over the past century and currently does not exceed 6%.[6,7] Death attributable to status epilepticus is rare, with most deaths resulting from the illness that precipitated the seizure.[5,6]

The objectives of treating convulsive status epilepticus are to maintain vital functions, identify and correct any precipitating factors, and control seizure activity. A plan for management is outlined in the box on p. 1775. A history should be obtained from an accompanying family member and should include any history of previous seizures, chronic and recent medication use, intercurrent illness, head trauma, and details of the onset of status epilepticus. On physical examination, fever, any evidence of head trauma, increased intracranial pressure, or infection should be noted. A urine toxicology screen is helpful in determining if the seizures were precipitated by drug ingestion. Computed tomography (CT) scanning may be required to rule out an intracranial lesion if the etiology of status epilepticus remains obscure. If the history or physical examination suggests a central nervous system infection, antibiotics should be administered immediately and a lumbar puncture performed as soon as seizure activity has been controlled. Because neurological sequelae of status epilepticus can result from complicating factors such as hypoxia, hypotension, and acidosis, attention should be given immediately to the respiratory and cardiovascular status of the child. If the patient is febrile, reducing body temperature is extremely urgent because of the synergism of fever and status epilepticus in producing brain damage. Fortunately most episodes of status epilepticus are controlled by one or more of the drugs listed in the box.

Once seizure activity is controlled, management should be directed toward preventing recurrence of seizures, including maintenance anticonvulsant therapy. The appropriate duration of therapy following an initial episode of idiopathic status epilepticus is not clear. Recurrence of seizures in this situation may be as low as 25%,[6] and recurrence of status epilepticus only 4%.[8]

TREATMENT OF STATUS EPILEPTICUS

A. Assess cardiovascular function by making sure the airway is clear and the patient is breathing. Provide oxygen or respiratory support as necessary.

B. Establish an intravenous line and obtain blood samples for electrolytes, blood urea nitrogen, calcium, a complete blood count, and anticonvulsant medication levels. A blood Dextrostix test should be performed immediately, and if the glucose is under 60 mg%, then 1 to 2 ml/kg of D25W should be administered.

C. One member of the emergency team should obtain a history while another does a brief physical examination.

D. Administer anticonvulsant drugs in the following order until seizure activity is controlled:

1. Initial therapy
   a. Lorazepam should be the initial anticonvulsant administered intravenously at a dose of 0.1 mg/kg (maximum 4 mg) over 2 minutes; a dose of 0.05 to 0.1 mg/kg may be repeated every 5 minutes if necessary up to a maximum of 0.5 mg/kg, but not over 10 mg in toto.
   b. If lorazepam is not available, diazepam should be administered intravenously at a dose of 0.1 to 0.2 mg/kg (maximum 10 mg) by "pushing" half the dose over 1 minute and the remainder at 1 mg/minute. A dose of 0.1 mg/kg may be repeated in 5 minutes if necessary. Because of diazepam's short duration of anticonvulsant effect, another anticonvulsant such as phenytoin must be administered immediately.
   c. If the patient is known to be receiving phenytoin on a chronic basis, it should be administered as the initial anticonvulsant (see D.2.).
2. If status epilepticus continues, administer phenytoin 15 to 20 mg/kg intravenously up to a total dose of 1000 mg. A quarter of the dose may be administered during the first 2 minutes and then at a rate of 1 to 2 mg/kg/minute (maximum rate of 50 mg/minute). If the patient is known to be receiving phenytoin chronically, 5 to 8 mg/kg of phenytoin may be administered as the initial anticonvulsant. Monitor the heart rate, and slow the rate of phenytoin infusion if bradycardia occurs. If seizure activity continues despite a full loading dose of phenytoin, correct for presumed acidosis with a modest dose of sodium bicarbonate.
3. If status epilepticus continues, administer phenobarbital 15 to 20 mg/kg intravenously up to a total dose of 800 mg. Administer phenobarbital over 15 minutes, monitoring respirations and blood pressure, especially if the patient has been given a benzodiazepine.
4. If status epilepticus persists, administer paraldehyde 0.3 ml/kg mixed with mineral oil (maximum of 5 ml) per rectum.

E. If seizure activity still persists, consult a neurologist to determine the need for other anticonvulsants, general anesthesia, or induction of pentobarbital coma.

REFERENCES

1. Aicardi J, Chevrie JJ: Convulsive status epilepticus in infants and children: a study of 239 cases, *Epilepsia* 11:187, 1970.
2. Delgado-Escueta AV et al: Current concepts in neurology: management of status epilepticus, *N Engl J Med* 306:1337, 1982.
3. Dreifuss FE: *Pediatric epileptology: classification and management of seizures in the child,* Boston, 1983, John Wright/PSG.
4. Gastaut H, editor: *Dictionary of epilepsy. I. Definitions,* Geneva, 1973, World Health Organization.
5. Hauser WA: Status epilepticus: frequency, etiology, and neurological sequelae. In Delgado-Escueta AV et al, editors: *Advances in neurology,* vol 34, New York, 1983, Raven Press.
6. Maytal J et al: Low morbidity and mortality of status epilepticus in children, *Pediatrics* 83:323, 1989.
7. Phillipe SA, Shanahan RT: Etiology and mortality of status epilepticus in children: a recent update, *Arch Neurol* 46:74, 1989.
8. Shinner S et al: Recurrent status epilepticus in children, *Ann Neurol* 31:598, 1992.

295 Thermal Injuries

L.R. Scherer III

The leading cause of death among children between 1 and 15 years of age is traumatic injury. Each year thermal injuries affect an estimated 1 million children in the United States; 10%, or 100,000, require hospitalization.[6] Of these, 3000 die as a result of their injuries, making thermal injuries the third leading cause of traumatic death in children, after motor vehicle accidents and drowning. Permanent disability remains a major complication in the long-term rehabilitation of the pediatric patient.

ETIOLOGY

Most childhood thermal injuries occur in the child's home. Approximately 80% to 90% of these injuries are potentially preventable.[6] The pattern of injury is related to the child's age and gender. During the first 2 years of life, 60% of the injuries are caused by scald burns from hot liquids; they involve boys twice as often as girls,[1] which may be because of the seemingly more active and inquisitive nature of males in this age group. Most scald burns occur when a young child accidentally pulls a pan or pot of hot liquid off the stove or table onto the head, chest, and arms. Occasionally a small child may manage to turn on the hot water in the bathtub, or a parent may carelessly or deliberately place a child in a bathtub of scalding water, causing burns to the arms, buttocks, legs, or feet. Although scald burns more commonly involve only partial-thickness injury, infants and toddlers have skin that is quite thin, and scald burns may result in full-thickness loss.

Because toddlers insist on exploration, the next most common childhood burn results from contact with hot surfaces in the home. These injuries usually involve only the "exploring" surfaces of the extremities.

Flame burn injuries are more common in children over 3 years of age. There is no gender predilection in this age group.[6] Causes include the careless use of matches, space heaters, outdoor fires, and stoves. Governmental restrictions on the manufacture of children's sleepwear have decreased the risk of flame injury in young children, but flammable products still are involved in most flame burn injuries. Because of the intense thermal energy of flame burns, full-thickness injury is more common with major burns; that and the associated inhalation injury increases the mortality in this age group.

PATHOPHYSIOLOGY

During the assessment of the burn patient it is necessary to determine the depth and extent of injury so that a treatment plan can be developed. Classically the depth of a burn has been categorized as first, second, or third degree. A first-degree burn is a superficial burn that involves only the epidermis. First-degree burns are erythematous and painful and do not produce blisters. The most common first-degree burn occurs after overexposure to the sun. Occasionally, first-degree burns are seen secondarily to flashburns from an explosion. First-degree burns should not be included in the estimation of the total extent of a burn wound injury. A second-degree burn, more commonly regarded as a partial-thickness skin loss, is usually erythematous or appears mottled red. The epidermal and dermal injury is evident with blistering, is moist to the touch, and is extremely painful to touch and exposure. A deep partial-thickness burn appears mottled and waxy because of complete injury to the entire epidermis and dermis, with only skin appendages spared, therefore it may look like a full-thickness injury. A full-thickness injury involves the epidermis, dermis, and subcutaneous tissue. These injuries appear dry or waxlike. There are no blisters, and the skin may be white or black. The texture of the skin is hard, dry, and leathery with no elasticity, and coagulated veins are noticeable. These injuries are painless to touch because of complete injury to all appendages.

Injury from partial-thickness and full-thickness burns results in increased capillary permeability and sequestration of large quantities of fluids within the extravascular space. Because of the larger surface area of the infant and child, as well as the thinner skin and subcutaneous tissue, young burn victims tend to lose more fluid and body heat than do adults. These greater evaporative water and body heat losses require the use of larger quantities of fluid for resuscitation and external temperature regulation.

Significant morbidity and mortality occur secondarily to inhalation thermal injuries. The manifestations of these injuries may not be apparent for the first 24 hours. Major injuries to the respiratory tract result from inhaling products of incomplete combustion and toxic fumes and/or direct thermal injury to the upper or lower respiratory tract.

Inhaling products of incomplete combustion or toxic fumes may lead to chemical tracheobronchitis and pneumonia. Carbon monoxide (CO) exposure should always be assumed in children who sustain burns in an enclosed space. Because of the high affinity of CO for hemoglobin (240 times that of oxygen), CO displaces oxygen from the hemoglobin molecule and shifts the dissociation curve to the left. Carbon monoxide dissociates from hemoglobin very slowly; when breathing 100% oxygen, 50% of the patient's CO will dissociate within 40 minutes; it takes 250 minutes for this to happen when one is breathing room air. Therefore the patient who has suspected smoke inhalation should be treated with 100% oxygen.

Direct thermal injury is caused by inhaling heated gases; it rarely causes injury below the vocal cords except when volatile gases or steam are inhaled. Airway injury produces edema and obstruction, mucosal sloughing, bronchorrhea, and pulmonary edema. Early management of inhalation injuries includes endotracheal intubation and administration of 100% oxygen.

HISTORY

A detailed clinical history is extremely important in the evaluation of a burned pediatric patient. This should include when, where, and how the burn occurred and the nature of the burning agent. If the injury occurred within an enclosed environment, a smoke inhalation injury should be suspected and aggressive airway management initiated. Evaluation should include the child's general health, any preexisting medical problems, allergies, and most important, immunization status. Recent infection should be noted, especially the possibility of a streptococcal organism. A careful clinical history helps to determine the depth of the wound, potential associated trauma, particulate or thermal airway injury, and carbon monoxide poisoning.

The diagnosis of child abuse can be obtained from detailed information of the history of the injury. The physician obtaining a history that includes the following should suspect child abuse: (1) an accident that occurs when the child is alone, (2) an injury incurred by a sibling, (3) an unclear or inconsistent history, (4) a previous history of accidental injury, (5) an injury incompatible with the description of the event, (6) a delay in seeking medical attention, and (7) an unstable social environment.[2]

CLINICAL FINDINGS

On initial evaluation all clothing should be removed from the child to stop the burning process and to allow complete assessment of all potential injuries. Airway assessment is particularly important in flame injuries and injuries encountered in an enclosed environment. The child should be assessed for facial burns, singed eyebrows and nasal hairs, carbon deposits in the oropharynx, and carbonaceous sputum, all of which indicate significant airway injury. Early airway management includes endotracheal intubation; delayed intubation may compromise airway management critically because of upper airway edema. Early and rapid assessment for associated injuries is necessary when the child has neurological impairment, a history of trauma, an electrical injury, or evidence of abuse. Unrecognized visceral or long-bone injuries will result in significant morbidity and mortality in the burned child.

At this point a careful, thorough inspection of the burn wounds is necessary. The child should be disrobed completely and all wounds covered with sterile dry linens or towels. Mask, gown, and gloves are worn to inspect the depth and extent of the burn. The burned surface area in children is estimated by using the Lund and Browder chart (Fig. 295-1), because in younger children the surface area of the head is relatively large and the surface area of the lower extremities is small. Estimation of the surface area is required for the management of fluid therapy and for wound care and prognosis. Pitfalls in estimation occur in chemical and electrical injuries, in which extensive tissue damage may manifest few signs of injury to the skin.

OUTPATIENT MANAGEMENT

As stated earlier, approximately 90% of childhood burns can be treated outside the hospital. Minor burns may be classified as partial-thickness burns involving no more than 10% of the body surface or full-thickness burns involving no more than 2% of the body surface (see the box on p. 1779).

Generally these patients can be treated with oral fluids and burn wound care in the emergency room or the pediatrician's office. The wounds should be cleansed with water or saline and a mild antibacterial solution. Blisters should be left intact, as this provides greater comfort and ease of care; however, open blisters should be debrided. Silver sulfadiazine cream is applied to the wound twice daily after cleansing, and dry, sterile, occlusive dressing is applied to the wound. Close observation is required in the initial management of burns, and the child should be seen every 48 hours for evaluation of the depth of the burn and potential complications. Once intact blisters begin to leak or are no longer tense, the blisters should be debrided. Over the past 30 years laboratory and clinical research has found that the maintenance of a moist wound environment facilitates wound healing. The beneficial effects include prevention of tissue dehydration and cell death, accelerated angiogenesis, increased breakdown of dead tissue and fibrin, and accelerated interaction of tissue growth factors and target cells.[5]

As an alternative to the conventional antimicrobial gauze dressing, the burn wound may be covered with an occlusive moisture-retentive dressing such as the semipermeable membrane film or the hydrocolloid occlusive dressing. Clinical research documents a healing rate that is 3 to 4 days faster and involves less pain during and between dressing changes.[5] In the overall care of a minor injury, the child should be managed with oral hydration; pain should be alleviated with acetaminophen or codeine. Most important, the child's tetanus immunization status must be documented and updated, if necessary. Facial burns may be treated with open dressings, applying an antibacterial ointment such as bacitracin, neosporin, or polymyxin B to the partial-thickness burn wound areas three times daily. Partial-thickness burns should reepithelize within 14 to 21 days. Follow-up care calls for monitoring wound healing and patient compliance with the healing regimen, comfort, and early rehabilitation.

PRIMARY CARE HOSPITAL MANAGEMENT

More extensive burns require hospitalization for wound care and intravenous fluid therapy (see the box on p. 1779). Hospital treatment is required in cases of partial-thickness burns involving 10% to 20% of the body surface; full-thickness burns involving 2% to 10% of the body surface; partial-thickness injury to the face, hands, feet, and perineum; questionable burn wound depth and extent; minor chemical burns; inadequate family support; or suspected abuse. In the emergency room the assessment of a child who has a thermal injury involves evaluation of the airway and associated injuries and estimation of the burned area and depth of injury. Intravenous fluid resuscitation is required for severe injuries, and one or two peripheral intravenous lines are required for intravenous fluid therapy. In the approach to fluid management, the Parkland formula may be used in burns involving

Burn Estimate Age vs Area

Area	Birth 1yr.	1-4 yr.	5-9 yr.	10-14 yr.	15 yr.	2°	3°	Total
Head	19	17	13	11	9			
Neck	2	2	2	2	2			
Ant. Trunk	13	13	13	13	13			
Post. Trunk	13	13	13	13	13			
R. Buttock	2 1/2	2 1/2	2 1/2	2 1/2	2 1/2			
L. Buttock	2 1/2	2 1/2	2 1/2	2 1/2	2 1/2			
Genitalia	1	1	1	1	1			
R.U. Arm	4	4	4	4	4			
L.U. Arm	4	4	4	4	4			
R.L. Arm	3	3	3	3	3			
L.L. Arm	3	3	3	3	3			
R. Hand	2 1/2	2 1/2	2 1/2	2 1/2	2 1/2			
L. Hand	2 1/2	2 1/2	2 1/2	2 1/2	2 1/2			
R. Thigh	5 1/2	6 1/2	8	8 1/2	9			
L. Thigh	5 1/2	6 1/2	8	8 1/2	9			
R. Leg	5	5	5 1/2	6	6 1/2			
L. Leg	5	5	5 1/2	6	6 1/2			
R. Foot	3 1/2	3 1/2	3 1/2	3 1/2	3 1/2			
L. Foot	3 1/2	3 1/2	3 1/2	3 1/2	3 1/2			
					Total			

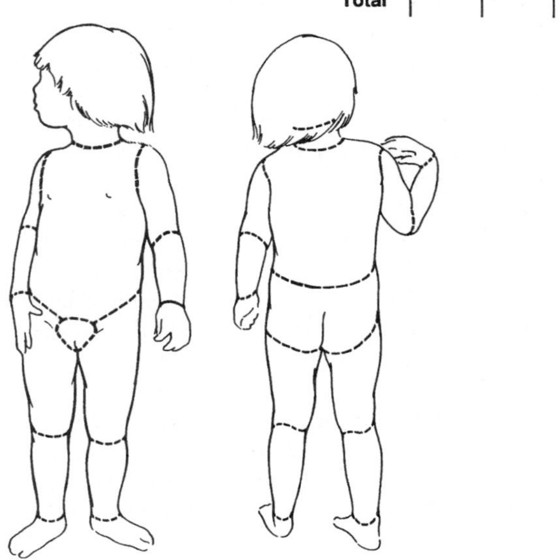

FIG. 295-1 Burn chart for estimating extent of injury. Numbers equal percentage of total body surface.

more than 15% of the body surface. The formula uses 3 ml of lactated Ringer solution per kilogram per percent burn in addition to the child's regular maintenance fluid during the first 24 hours after the burn occurs. Half of the fluid is given over the first 8 hours after injury, and the remaining half is delivered over the following 16 hours. The adequacy of fluid therapy is determined by urinary output, which should be maintained at 1 to 2 ml/kg/hr (measuring output may require the use of a Foley catheter). With extensive burns a central venous pressure line may be required in the management of fluid therapy. Children who have a burn covering 15% or more of the body surface often develop a paralytic ileus, and therefore nasogastric tube decompression often is required. All medications, including antibiotics, analgesics, or sedatives should be given intravenously because perfusion is unpredictable. Initial management of the wound is similar to that of minor wounds except for the extent and potential depth of the wound. Therefore early involvement by the surgical team is required for the overall assessment and management of the burned child.

BURN CENTER MANAGEMENT

Thermal injuries of greatest magnitude—that is, partial-thickness burns involving more than 20% of body surface area; full-thickness burns involving more than 10% of body surface area; full-thickness burns of the face, hands, feet, or perineum; a respiratory tract injury; an associated major injury, or major chemical or electrical burns—require the special facilities and personnel of a regional burn center (see box on p. 1779). A burn center offers specialists involved in the long-term physical, psychological, and social needs of these infants and children.[4,8] These centers have produced remarkable improvements in the morbidity and mortality of those who have major burns. The injured child needs to be care-

TRIAGE CRITERIA FOR THERMAL INJURIES

Outpatient management

Partial-thickness burn <10% body surface area (BSA)
Full-thickness burn <2% BSA

Inpatient management

Primary care hospital
Partial-thickness burn 10%-20% BSA
Full-thickness burn 2%-10% BSA
Partial-thickness burn to face, perineum, hands, or feet
Questionable burn wound depth or extent
Inadequate family support
Suspected abuse

Burn center

Partial-thickness burn >20% BSA
Full-thickness burn >10% BSA
Full-thickness burn to face, perineum, hands, or feet
Respiratory tract injury
Associated major trauma
Significant coexisting illness
Chemical or electrical burns

fully evaluated and adequately resuscitated before being transferred to a burn center. Initial evaluation and resuscitation include early airway stabilization, adequate intravenous access, fluid resuscitation with lactated Ringer solution, tetanus immunization, and covering the burn wounds with sterile, dry linens or towels. To initiate the transfer, early telephone communication between the referring physician and the coordinator of the burn center is important. All pertinent information regarding laboratory evaluation, temperature, pulse, fluids administered, and urinary output should be recorded and a flowchart sent with the patient. Any other information deemed important by either the referring physician or the burn center physician should be sent with the child. At the time of transport, the child must be well prepared and have a secure airway, an established and secure intravenous line, burn dressings, adequate pain relief, and a nasogastric tube and Foley catheter in place.

SPECIAL BURN REQUIREMENTS: ELECTRICAL BURNS

Electrical burns result when a source of electrical power makes contact with a person's body.[6] Electrical burns are frequently more serious than they appear externally. A current passing through the body may destroy muscles, nerves, and blood vessels but spare skin and bone because of their high resistance. Rhabdomyolysis results in myoglobin release, which may cause acute renal failure. As with any serious injury, immediate management of the patient includes attention to the airway and breathing, establishment of intravenous access, electrocardiographic monitoring, and placement of an indwelling urinary catheter. If the urine is cola colored, one must assume myoglobin is present in the urine. Fluid should be administered at a rate to ensure urinary output of at least 3 to 5 ml/kg/hr. If the cola coloration does not clear with increased fluid administration, 500 mg/kg of mannitol should be administered immediately, and 12.5 g of mannitol is added to subsequent liters of fluid to maintain diuresis. Metabolic acidosis should be corrected by maintaining adequate perfusion, and sodium bicarbonate should be used to alkalinize the urine and increase the solubility of myoglobin.

The most common electrical burn in children is sustained by the toddler, when the corner of the mouth is injured by chewing on an electrical cord. Initial management of these injuries involves standard wound care and topical application of an antibiotic ointment. These wounds should be allowed to demarcate, and a plastic surgeon should be involved in their early assessment and management.

COMPLICATIONS

A number of complications may occur in the early management of thermal injuries in children[2]; the most catastrophic occurs when an inhalation injury is not recognized. This results in failure to place a secure airway in a child facing severe respiratory distress. If a child suffers thermal injury within an enclosed space, an inhalation injury must be suspected and early endotracheal intubation performed to secure an airway before respiration is compromised. The second most common complication arises from underestimating the size and depth of a burn, which often occurs in scald burns of young children. Early and repeated methodical examination using a burn chart (Fig. 295-1) helps in estimating the size of the injury. A common unrecognized complication is failure to suspect child abuse. Burns frequently are encountered as part of a spectrum of injuries inflicted on children.

Later complications in the management of children who have moderate to severe burns requiring hospitalization include pneumonia,[4] septic thrombophlebitis,[4] burn wound sepsis,[3] peptic ulcer disease,[7] and behavior disorders.[2] The use of appropriate antibiotic therapy, vigorous pulmonary toilet, and intensive ventilatory support are the mainstays of preventing pulmonary complications in a burn patient.

Potentially lethal infections include suppurative skin lesions or thrombophlebitis when both peripheral and central venous catheters are used. The usual organisms involved are *Staphylococcus aureus, Staphylococcus epidermidis,* or a variety of gram negative bacterial organisms. Burn wound sepsis remains a complication with significant morbidity and mortality; thus prevention is essential. Early aggressive debridement and excision of the wound, use of surveillance quantitative culture, and institution of appropriate topical and systemic antibiotic therapy are the cornerstones of prevention and management of burn wound sepsis. One of the lethal complications in a child who has a burn injury is a gastroduodenal ulcer (curling ulcer). Mortality is higher than 60% for children who suffer more than 60% of blood loss over a 24-hour period from peptic ulcer disease secondary to burns. The prevalence, morbidity, and mortality have diminished with the use of antacids, histamine-antagonist therapy, and early enteral feeding of burn patients. Because of the severe and chronic nature of burns, psychological changes often occur in children: characteristically they regress to earlier stages of development. Behavior changes include hostility and self-destructive behavior. Treatment may require sedation, but usually the members of the burn team need to provide a great deal of understanding and support for the patient and the family. A cheerful environment, an experienced staff of child-life personnel, and a humane approach to the numerous painful procedures are most beneficial.

PROGNOSIS

The morbidity and mortality of thermal injuries have declined in the past 20 years because of advances in fluid therapy, management of pulmonary complications, control of wound infections by topical antibiotic agents, and advances in surgical wound management, nutrition, and regionalization of care.[3,4,8]

The most remarkable areas of improvement involve burn care. The use of topical antibacterial therapy has changed the 50% mortality level expected from 35% of body surface area (BSA) burns to 65% of BSA burns.[4,8] Since the development of early excision and grafting of large BSA burns, several authors have reported an LD_{50} of greater than 90% BSA burn. Other authors argue that aggressive fluid resuscitation, early excision and grafting, and the overall improved management of the burned child have improved the survival rate and the quality of survival.

The early determinants of unnecessary mortality include inadequate volume resuscitation and inappropriate assessment of inhalation injury.[4] Later predictors of mortality include secondary development of renal, cardiovascular, and pulmonary organ failure.

Since the evolution of these new therapies, a child has an excellent prognosis with a burn under 70% BSA, but the morbidity remains high because these children may develop hypertrophic scarring and contractures. Physical and occupational therapy and the use of long-term compressive garments have diminished the morbidity of these wound complications, but further investigation of the prevention of these scars and contractures is required. Ninety percent of children suffering from burns can be treated as outpatients, with the expectation of wound reepithelization within 5 to 14 days. Further investigation and development of therapies for the 10% who require long-term hospitalization, physical therapy, and rehabilitation of their burn wounds is required to decrease the morbidity of their long-term care, which may require 4 to 6 months of hospitalization.

REFERENCES

1. Feldman KW et al: Tap water scald burns in children, *Pediatrics* 62:1, 1978.
2. Harmel RP, Vane DW, King DR: Burn care in children: special consideration, *Clin Plast Surg* 13:95, 1986.
3. Herndon DN et al: A comparison of conservative versus early excision, *Ann Surg* 209:547, 1989.
4. Herndon DN et al: Determinants of mortality in pediatric patients with greater than 70% full-thickness total body surface area thermal injury treated by early total excision and grafting, *J Trauma* 27:208, 1987.
5. Kerstein MD: A symposium: wound infection and occlusion—separating fact from fiction, *Am J Surg* 167:1A, 1994.
6. McLoughlin E, Crawford JD: Burns, *Pediatr Clin North Am* 32:61, 1985.
7. Prasad JK, Thomson PD, Feller I: Gastrointestinal hemorrhage in burn patients, *Burns* 13:194, 1987.
8. Tompkins RG et al: Significant reductions in mortality for children with burn injuries through the use of prompt eschar excision, *Ann Surg* 208:577, 1988.

Appendixes

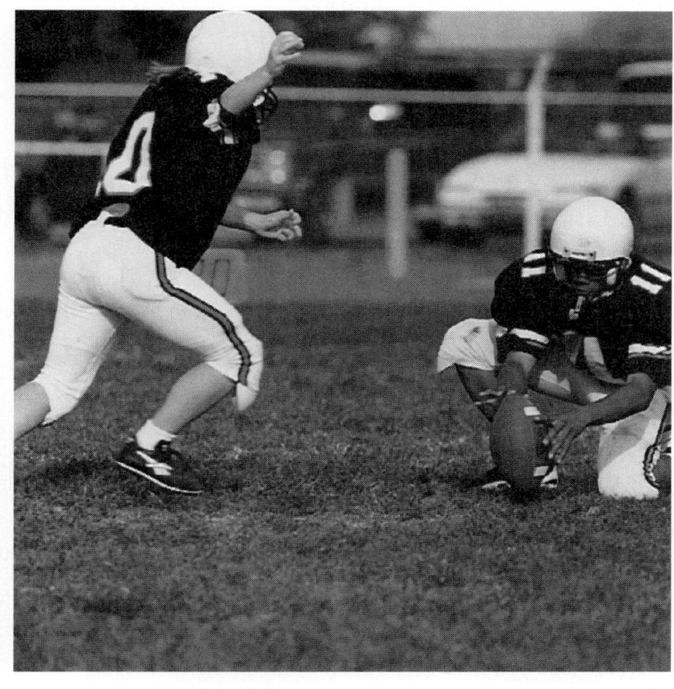

COURTESY NORDMANN PHOTOGRAPHY.

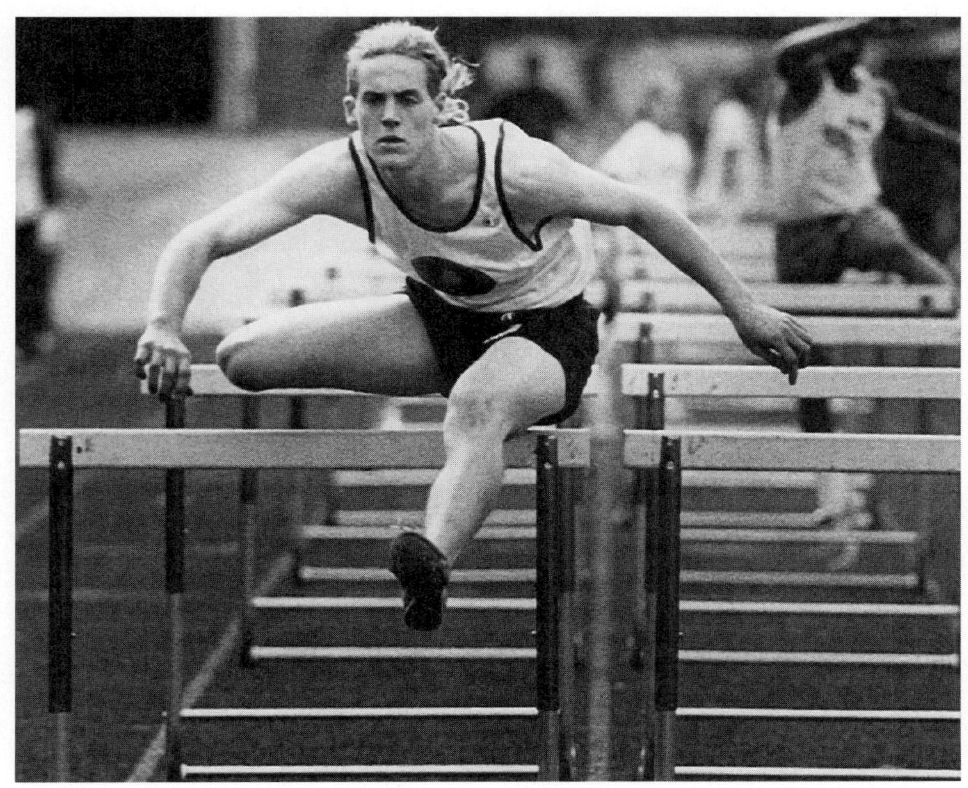

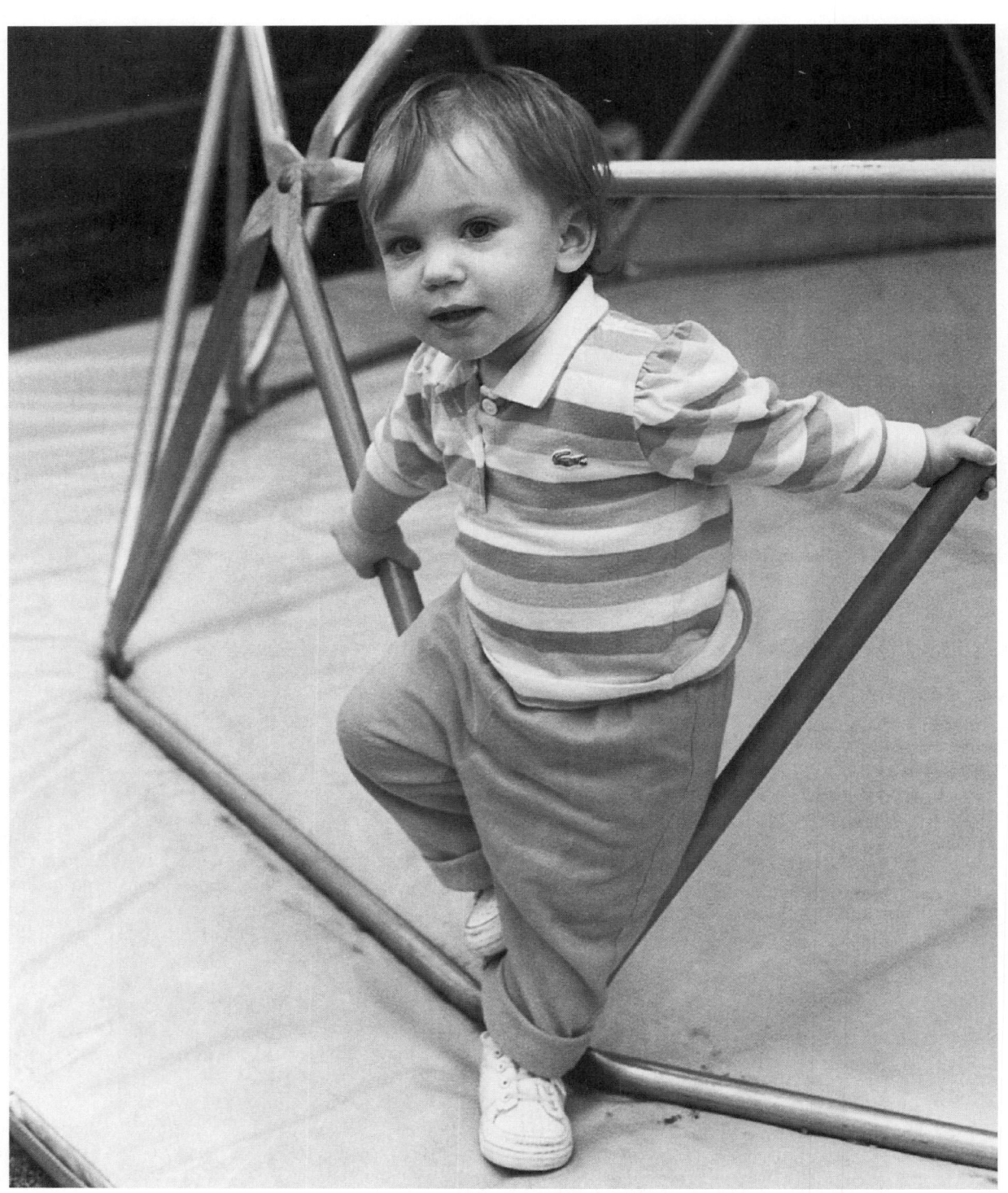

A Pediatric Basic and Advanced Life Support

Howard C. Mofenson and Joseph Greensher

An estimated 40,000 infants under 1 year of age and 16,000 children between 1 and 14 years of age die each year in the United States from all causes. Most deaths in infants under 1 year of age occur before the child is 4 months old.[2]

Pediatric cardiopulmonary arrest occurs biphasically, with the incidence peaking in infants under 1 year of age and in teenagers. During infancy, when most cardiopulmonary arrests occur, the most common causes of death are sudden infant death syndrome (SIDS), respiratory diseases, airway obstruction, submersion, sepsis, and neurological diseases. After 1 year of age, injuries are the most common cause of death.

The mortality of infants under 15 months of age who suffer cardiac arrest outside a hospital is almost 100%.[32] Even inpatient cardiac arrests carry a mortality above 90%, and half of the survivors have major neurological damage.[10]

However, the survival rate approaches 50% after prompt resuscitation in children who have respiratory arrest alone.[34] The amount of time that elapses between arrest and initiation of life-support measures appears to be critical in determining the effectiveness of those measures.

This appendix reviews and updates the guidelines for pediatric basic cardiopulmonary resuscitation and advanced life support. It is not intended as a substitute for participation in the basic and advanced life support courses given by the American Heart Association and the American Academy of Pediatrics. Ideally, basic life support should be integrated into a community effort on education in injury prevention and easy access to emergency medical services.

In the discussion that follows, an infant is defined as 1 year of age or younger, a child as 1 to 8 years of age, and an older child as older than 8 years.

Cardiopulmonary arrest (CPA) is the failure of both effective ventilation and circulation. *Respiratory arrest* is the lack of effective ventilation, as evidenced by absence of breath sounds or air movement or of thoracoabdominal movement. *Cardiac arrest* is the loss of effective circulation, as evidenced by the absence of pulsation in a major artery.

Basic life support is designed to generate perfusion of the vital organs with some oxygenated blood during cardiac arrest. To be successful, it must be coupled with advanced life support measures.

It is important that Emergency Medical Services (EMS) personnel are optimally trained and equipped to care for pediatric emergencies and that hospital emergency departments receiving acutely ill or injured children have transfer agreements with a pediatric tertiary care facility, where advanced pediatric postresuscitative care can be rendered if necessary.

In 1992 the Fifth National Conference on Cardiopulmonary Resuscitation and Emergency Cardiac Care revised the national guidelines for pediatric basic life support, advanced life support, and neonatal resuscitation. These changes were published in *The Journal of the American Medical Association* (JAMA) October 28, 1992.[7,26] The conference based changes in therapeutic interventions on supporting scientific evidence, and each recommendation was assigned to one of the following classes:

Class I: "A therapeutic option that is usually indicated, always acceptable, and is considered useful and effective." Examples are oxygen, endotracheal intubation, and defibrillation.

Class II: "A therapeutic option that is acceptable, but of uncertain efficacy and may be controversial."

Class IIa: "A therapeutic option for which the weight of evidence is in favor of its usefulness and efficacy." An example is a standard dose of epinephrine in ventricular fibrillation.

Class IIb: "A therapeutic option that is not well established by scientific evidence, but may be helpful and probably not harmful." An example is using high-dose epinephrine in adults.

Class III: "A therapeutic option that is inappropriate, is without supporting data, and may be harmful." An example is using sodium bicarbonate in hypoxic lactic acidosis.

The new recommendations also emphasize the importance of following guidelines established by the Occupational Safety and Health Administration (OSHA) to avoid transmitting disease from the victim to the rescuer, and they advocate use of gloves and mechanical ventilation equipment, including resuscitative masks that divert expired air away from the rescuer.

1992 BASIC LIFE SUPPORT CHANGES

1. Children should receive 1 minute of cardiopulmonary resuscitation (CPR) before emergency medical services are begun, because respiratory arrest is the most common cause of cardiac arrest in children and ventricular fibrillation is rare. In adults it is recommended that a lone rescuer begin EMS immediately, before starting CPR.
2. To manage an obstructed airway in infants, a series of five back blows and chest thrusts is recommended (this number makes it easier to remember because it is the same as for cardiac compressions). (The 1986 recommendations specified four back blows and chest thrusts to manage the obstructed airway.)
3. In rescue breathing for adults, it is recommended that the duration of inspiratory filling of the lungs be increased to 1½ to 2 seconds to prevent gastric distention; however, the inspiratory filling time for children is unchanged (1 to 1½ seconds) because children have smaller tidal volumes and higher ventilatory rates.

1992 ADVANCED LIFE SUPPORT CHANGES

1. Epinephrine is to be administered endotracheally in a dose of 0.1 mg/kg (1 : 1000 solution) except in neonates. (The 1986 recommendation for epinephrine administered endotracheally was 0.01 mg/kg [1 : 10,000 solution]) (a class IIb recommendation).[14]
2. Other drugs administered endotracheally are administered in doses two to three times that of the intravenous (IV) route. (The 1986 recommendations for the doses of atropine, lidocaine, and naloxone were the same as for the IV doses.)
3. In asystolic pulseless arrest, the second and subsequent doses of IV and intraosseous epinephrine for unresponsive and pulseless arrest are higher than the initial dose of 0.01 mg/kg (1 : 10,000) and are administered as 0.1 mg/kg (1 : 1000) except in neonates. This is a class IIa recommendation in children because of scientific evidence of better neurological outcome.[23] (The 1986 recommendations were for an initial dose of 0.01 mg/kg [1 : 10,000] of epinephrine, and subsequent doses were the same.)
4. The management of paroxysmal supraventricular tachycardia (SVT), the most common dysarrhythmia to cause circulatory instability in infants, includes a rapid bolus (1 to 3 seconds) of adenosine (0.1 mg/kg) initially in a stable patient and continuous cardiac monitoring. If the initial dose is ineffective, the dose can be doubled. The maximum single dose is 12 mg. In an unstable child, adenosine can be given before 0.5 joules/kg cardioversion, if an IV line is already in place. This is a class I recommendation. (The 1986 recommendations did not include adenosine.)
5. The management of bradycardia no longer includes atropine or isoproterenol. (The 1986 recommendations included atropine in the management of bradycardia.)
6. The management of asystole does not include atropine.
7. Intracardiac administration of emergency drugs is no longer included.
8. It is recommended that pulse oximetry be used in respiratory compromise during stabilization and transport.
9. Use of the Broselow Pediatric Emergency Tape to determine a child's approximate weight by measuring the recumbent length has been validated and can help in calculating drug doses in emergencies. It is suggested that manufacturers print recommended doses on prefilled syringes.
10. The 1992 recommendations advocate a simple protocol for establishing intravascular access quickly. In a child under age 6, an intraosseous line should be established if reliable venous access cannot be achieved within 90 seconds or in three attempts. This technique is not reliable in children over age 6 because the red marrow has been replaced by fat in the long bones. If the intraosseous line cannot be established in 3 to 5 minutes, medications should be given via the endotracheal tube—the least preferred route. An infusion pump is recommended for rapid administration of viscous fluids and large amounts of fluid to overcome the resistance of the emissary veins.

DIFFERENCES BETWEEN CARDIOPULMONARY ARREST IN CHILDREN AND ADULTS

Adults

The cause of cardiopulmonary arrest in adults commonly is an acute cardiac insult, such as myocardial infarction, which leads to a disturbance in cardiac rhythm. It usually occurs in patients whose hearts are damaged already. Ventricular fibrillation is common, and unmonitored defibrillation may be attempted to restore normal cardiac rhythm.

Children

The cause of CPA in children usually is severe hypoxia and acidosis or circulatory collapse, or both. Management focuses on preventing these events with prearrest assessment and anticipatory intervention through respiratory ventilation. Establishing airway patency and adequate ventilation often makes further resuscitative measures unnecessary if the child is not yet in CPA and is experiencing only respiratory arrest or compromise. Because asystole occurs in 90% of pediatric patients who have cardiac arrest, unmonitored defibrillation is not recommended.[2]

• • •

Table A-1 summarizes the distinguishing features of CPA in adults and children.

Children need oxygen more than drugs to correct rhythm disturbances; however, they do require medications for some arrhythmias, such as epinephrine and bicarbonate for asystole, digoxin for supraventricular tachycardia, and lidocaine for ventricular arrhythmias. The anatomical and physiological differences of children, compared with adults, present special problems. For example, in pediatric patients major differences exist in the anatomy of the airways, the airway diameter, the methods used for vascular access, and the choice of medication. A special cart with age-labeled equipment and precalculated drug doses should be available.

Cardiopulmonary arrest in children usually does not occur suddenly. It often can be prevented if respiratory failure and shock are recognized early and treatment is begun promptly.[2,27] Respiratory failure and shock can be recognized within 30 seconds by assessing the "ABCs": *a*irway, *b*reathing, and *c*irculation.

RESPIRATORY FAILURE

Respiratory failure occurs when ventilation and oxygenation become inadequate. Its clinical definition is based on the inability of pulmonary gas exchange to satisfy the body's meta-

Table A-1 Differences Between Adults and Children in Cardiopulmonary Arrest

Feature	Adults	Children
Cause	Myocardial infarction	Hypoxia and acidosis
Cardiac status	Damaged heart	Healthy heart
Arrhythmia	Ventricular fibrillation	Asystole
Defibrillation	Unmonitored	Only monitored
Predominant therapy	Defibrillation	Oxygen

bolic demands for transporting oxygen and eliminating car bon dioxide. Its presence is confirmed by abnormal levels for blood gases (the arterial oxygen [PO_2] and carbon dioxide [Pco_2] pressures and pH), not by physical signs, except for apnea. The presence of or impending respiratory failure is detected by evaluating airway patency and the quality of breathing and by checking for signs of hypoxia and hypercardia (cyanosis, central nervous system depression, and bradycardia).

Airway Patency

The airway is determined clinically to be (1) patent, requiring no intervention, (2) maintainable with noninvasive procedures (e.g., positioning, suctioning, or a bag-valve-mask system), or (3) unmaintainable, requiring invasive procedures (e.g., use of airway adjuncts, endotracheal intubation, cricothyroidotomy, or removal of a foreign body).

Breathing

The effectiveness of breathing and oxygenation is evaluated clinically by analyzing the *respiratory rate,* air entry, respiratory effort, skin and muscosal color, and level of consciousness.

The respiratory rate is classified as apnea, tachypnea, or bradypnea. The rate varies and is nonspecific for age. Tachypnea without respiratory distress may result from attempts to compensate for metabolic acidosis ("quiet tachypnea"). Bradypnea is ominous and may be due to fatigue or CNS depression. Any respiratory rate over 60 breaths/min or under 10 breaths/min is abnormal at any age.

The adequacy of tidal volume (5 to 7 ml/kg) is best assessed by auscultating for breath sounds and *air entry* at the periphery of the lung fields, over the apices and laterally, and by observing excursions of the chest wall. The minute volume equals the tidal volume times the respiratory rate. Minute volume may be low because of breaths that are too shallow or a respiratory rate that is too slow.

Increased *respiratory effort* indicates respiratory distress and represents compensation for inadequate gas exchange. The minute volume is reflected in the work of breathing. The signs of increased respiratory effort are head bobbing, nasal flaring, grunting, stridor, use of the accessory muscles, retractions, seesaw movement of the chest and abdomen, and prolonged expiration. These findings mandate measurement of arterial blood gases (ABGs).

The *skin color* reflects the level of tissue oxygenation. Diminished oxygenation produces an ashen gray or cyanotic color in the skin and mucosa. It is a late sign of hypoxia.

The *level of consciousness* reflects oxygenation and perfusion of the brain. Patients are classified according to their responsiveness (i.e., alert, verbal response, pain response, or unconscious). In infants over 2 months of age, an early sign of diminished cerebral oxygenation and perfusion is failure to recognize his or her parents.

SHOCK (CIRCULATORY FAILURE)

Shock (see also Chapter 292) is a clinical state characterized by failure of the cardiovascular system to perfuse vital organs adequately, resulting in inadequate oxygen delivery. This failure to deliver oxygen and other critical substrates to meet the demand of the tissues and to remove their metabolites results in anaerobic metabolism and accumulation of acids. Shock may occur with normal, increased, or decreased cardiac output and blood pressure. In *compensated shock* the blood pressure is normal. In *decompensated shock* the blood pressure and cardiac output are low.

Shock is classified as either hypovolemic or cardiogenic. *Hypovolemic shock,* or distributive shock, the most common type in pediatric patients, is caused by a loss of vascular space volume as a result of dehydration or blood loss or a loss of vascular tone, such as occurs in sepsis, anaphylaxis, and an acute CNS pathological condition. *Cardiogenic shock* caused by heart failure or arrhythmias is relatively rare among children except in postcardiac arrest patients, in whom it is the primary cause of shock.

Cardiovascular performance can be evaluated by assessing the peripheral pulses, skin perfusion, level of consciousness and heart rate, and later the blood pressure and urinary output.

Pulse

Palpating the peripheral pulse (a reflection of peripheral perfusion) allows the examiner to estimate the stroke volume, heart rate, systemic vascular resistance, and blood pressure. The stroke volume is the volume of blood pumped by each heart beat. The cardiac output is the volume of blood pumped by the heart every minute (heart rate times stroke volume). Organ perfusion is determined by the cardiac output and the peripheral vascular resistance.

Skin Perfusion

The skin is a relatively nonessential organ and loses its perfusion first. This is assessed by capillary refill time, or the time it takes for normal skin color to return after blanching pressure is applied; this should be less than 2 seconds, or less than the time it takes to say "capillary refill." When testing for capillary refill, the extremity used should be elevated above the level of the heart. Poor perfusion also can be identified by mottled skin color, cool hands and feet, and a line of demarcation that separates the warm from the cool skin of an extremity.

Level of Consciousness

Evidence of diminished brain oxygenation and perfusion is discussed under *respiratory failure* above.

Heart Rate

Changes in the heart rate reflect changes in cardiac output but, unfortunately, are nonspecific. Tachycardia is defined as a heart rate above 180 beats per minute (bpm) in patients under age 5; above 160 bpm in patients between 5 and 10 years; and above 100 bpm in patients over age 10. If tachycardia is present, the examiner must distinguish between benign and serious causes. When tachycardia fails to compensate adequately for tissue oxygen needs, hypoxia, hypercapnia, acidosis, and bradycardia develop. Bradycardia in a distressed child is an ominous sign of impending cardiac arrest.

Blood Pressure

The blood pressure is a product of cardiac output times the peripheral vascular resistance. Hypotension is a late and ominous finding in patients who are in shock. The systolic blood pressure should be above 60 mm Hg from birth to 1 month of age and above 70 mm Hg in infants 1 month to 1 year. A formula for determining the lower limit for systolic blood pressure in children over 1 year of age is as follows:

$$70 + (2 \times \text{Age in years})$$

This represents a level that is greater than 2 standard deviations below the mean.

Urinary Output

The normal urinary output is 1 to 2 ml/kg/hr. Although this measure is unavailable to help in the initial evaluation, it is a valuable indicator of kidney perfusion later on. The bladder urine obtained initially should not be used for calculating urinary output.

In respiratory failure the blood is delivered adequately to the body tissues, but the blood delivered is deficient in oxygen. In shock the blood contains adequate oxygen, but it is delivered poorly. Both conditions can lead to hypoxia, hypercapnia, anaerobic metabolism, acidosis, and cardiopulmonary arrest. Table A-2 summarizes the ABCs of cardiorespiratory assessment.

PEDIATRIC BASIC LIFE SUPPORT

In applying pediatric basic life support measures, the priorities of management should be based on clinical assessment. Questionable cases, as well as patients successfully resuscitated in cardiopulmonary arrest, require frequent reassessment by means of ABG determinations and chest roentgenograms.

The patient's condition should be classified as one of the following:

1. *Stable:* requires no intervention but does require continued reassessment
2. *Questionable:* requires very frequent reassessment
3. *Definite respiratory failure or shock:* requires immediate intervention
4. *Cardiopulmonary failure:* requires basic and advanced life support

Table A-2 Summary of Cardiorespiratory Assessment

Respiratory assessment	Cardiovascular assessment
A. Airway patency	C. Circulation
B. Breathing	1. Peripheral pulses
1. Rate	2. Skin perfusion
2. Air entry, breath sounds, chest excursions	3. Level of consciousness
	4. Heart rate
	5. Blood pressure
3. Respiratory effort	6. Urinary output
4. Color	
5. Level of consciousness	

Modified from Chameides L, editor: *Textbook of pediatric advanced life support,* Dallas, 1988, the American Heart Association and the American Academy of Pediatrics.

General Priorities of Management

1. With upper airway obstruction, the child should be allowed to stay with the parents and remain in the selected position of comfort. Feedings are withheld, the normal body temperature is maintained, and the maximum amount of oxygen tolerated is delivered.
2. Respiratory failure requires securing an airway, establishing adequate ventilation, administering maximum supplemental oxygen, instituting cardiorespiratory monitoring and pulse oximetry, and obtaining frequent ABG values and chest roentgenograms.
3. Shock requires delivering maximum supplemental oxygen, establishing vascular access, expanding blood volume, administering appropriate vasopressors (if necessary), obtaining an electrocardiogram (ECG), and instituting cardiorespiratory monitoring and pulse oximetry.
4. Cardiopulmonary failure requires instituting ventilation and oxygenation, establishing cardiorespiratory monitoring and pulse oximetry, gaining vascular access to expand blood volume, and obtaining frequent ABG values and chest roentgenograms.

Basic Airway, Breathing, and Circulation (ABCs) of Cardiopulmonary Resuscitation[1,7,27]

If unconscious, the patient should be placed supine, turned as a unit with firm support to the head and the neck to prevent spinal injury, and placed on a firm, flat surface. The airway should be maintained by using the head-tilt/chin-lift maneuver or, if a neck injury is suspected, by using the jaw-thrust maneuver. If the patient is not breathing, CPR should be performed for 1 minute before help is called. If the patient is conscious and in respiratory distress, the child's position of comfort should be respected, and transport in a properly equipped ambulance should be accomplished without disturbing him or her.

Airway. The *head-tilt* maneuver consists of placing a hand on the forehead and tilting the head backward into a "sniffing" or neutral position. The *chin-tilt* maneuver consists of placing the fingers under the chin and lifting it upward. The neck should not be overextended. The *jaw-thrust* maneuver is accomplished by placing two or three fingers on each side of the lower jaw at the angle and lifting upward with both elbows resting on the surface on which the victim is lying. If the airway is not maintainable with these maneuvers, an oropharyngeal airway or an endotracheal tube should be placed.

Breathing. The patency of the airway must be maintained. The examiner should place his or her ear close to the patient's mouth and nose to listen for breath sounds. The chest should be felt for air movement, and the chest and abdomen observed for movement.

If the patient is not breathing, mouth-to-mouth resuscitation must be instituted: with an infant, this involves tilting the head and sealing the mouth and nose; with a toddler or older patient, the rescuer pinches the nose and seals the mouth. The examiner delivers two slow breaths or puffs (1 to 1½ seconds' duration) after each inhalation, breaking the seal after each puff to allow the patient to exhale. The force and volume of the puff should be sufficient to cause the chest to rise. Using this volume of air and the slow breaths prevents gastric distention in the patient. If air enters the lungs freely and the chest rises, the airway is patent. The most common cause of airway obstruction is improper head positioning; it should be readjusted and mouth-to-mouth breathing repeated. If the chest still does not rise, a foreign body lodged in the upper airway should be suspected, and the recommendations for removing it (given below) should be followed. As soon as possible, the patient should receive ventilation with a bag (with reservoir) and mask attached to oxygen.

Gastric distention with vomiting and aspiration can be minimized in unconscious patients by applying *cricoid pressure* (using one fingertip in infants and the thumb and index finger in children) to occlude the proximal esophagus. The pressure is released once endotracheal intubation is accomplished.

Circulation. Inefficient cardiovascular performance is recognized by the absence of the pulse in a large artery or by bradycardia that does not respond to ventilation and oxygenation. For patients over 1 year of age, the practitioner palpates the carotid artery; for under age 1, the brachial artery is palpated. If the pulse is present but respirations are absent, the head tilt and mouth-to-mouth breathing should be maintained.

Chest Compression. Compression of the chest is performed to effect cardiac compression. Table A-3 summarizes the methods used for chest compression for pediatric patients of varying ages.

The indications for chest compression are asystole, as evidenced by absent pulses, or bradycardia below 60 bpm in a child or 80 bpm in a neonate unresponsive to ventilation and oxygenation.

The patient should be horizontal and supine on a firm surface. With small infants, the palm of the rescuer's hand should support the back.

The site where compression is applied varies with the patient's age.[9,18,21]

In infants, compressions should be applied one fingerbreadth (fb) below the intersection of the internipple line with the sternum; compression should not be applied over the xiphoid. The middle and ring fingers should be used to compress the chest to a depth of ½ to 1 inch (1.3 or 2.5 cm) at a rate above 100/minute. The pressure is released without lifting the fingers off the sternum but allowing it to return to its normal position. Equal time is allotted for each phase (compression and decompression). In applying compressions for a neonate or a small infant, the hands should encircle the thorax, and the thumbs should be placed side by side just below the internipple line over the lower third of the sternum. Chest compressions should then be applied with the thumbs to the same depth and at the same rate as for an older infant.

In children over 1 year of age, the resuscitator places the heel of one hand 2 fb above the sternal notch and uses the pressure generated by his or her arm to compress the sternum 1 to 1½ inches (2.5 to 3.8 cm) at a rate of 80 to 100/minute, taking care to keep the fingers off the ribs. Again, the compression and decompression phases are equal. The compression rate for children over age 8 is also 80 to 100/minute, but the depth of compression is increased to 1½ to 2 inches (3.8 to 5 cm), with the resuscitator using the pressure generated by his or her whole body, applied through clasped hands just above the sternal notch.

The adequacy of the compressions is determined by palpating the pulse during compression. External cardiac compressions must be accompanied by head tilt and ventilations. At the end of every fifth compression, a pause of 1 to 1½ seconds should be made to allow for ventilation (5:1 compression to ventilation ratio). The victim should be assessed after 10 cycles of compressions and ventilations (approximately 1 minute) and every few minutes thereafter. With a single rescuer, the head-tilt maneuver must be performed with each ventilation. As soon as possible ECG monitoring should be instituted and specimens obtained for blood glucose, serum electrolyte, and blood gas analysis.

Relieving Airway obstruction.[2,6,27] The sequence for managing an obstructed airway is as follows:

- I. Conscious patient
  - A. Breathing and coughing → No intervention
  - B. Ineffective cough and increasing stridor with a witnessed or suspected foreign body aspiration
    1. Infant → Back blows and chest thrusts
    2. Child → Heimlich maneuver (abdominal thrusts)
- II. Unconscious, nonbreathing patient
  - A. Nonspontaneous breathing → Head tilt, chin lift, and assisted ventilation
  - B. Assisted ventilation—No chest rise
    1. Reposition head and repeat assisted ventilation
    2. Attempt to relieve obstruction
       - a. Infant: Up to five back blows and chest thrusts
       - b. Child: Up to five Heimlich maneuver abdominal thrusts
    3. Perform tongue-jaw lift, and manually remove a foreign body if one is seen

Infant Back Blows and Chest Thrusts. With the infant straddled over the rescuer's forearm, the head positioned lower than the trunk, and the jaw held open by the rescuer's fingers, up to five back blows are delivered with the heel of the hand between the shoulder blades. If this does not remove the foreign body, the infant should be turned over so that the head, neck, and back are well supported on the rescuer's forearm. Up to five chest thrusts similar to cardiac compressions then are administered.

Table A-3 Methods of Chest Compression

Age	Site	Applicator	Depth	Pressure	Rate/min
Infant (<1 yr)	1 fb below internipple line	Middle and ring fingers	½-1 (1.3-2.5 cm)	Hand	At least 100
Child (1-8 yr)	2 fb above xiphoid	Heel of the hand	1-1½ (2.5-3.8 cm)	Arm	80-100
Child (>8 yr)	2 fb above xiphoid	Both hands clasped	1½-2 in (3.8-5 cm)	Body	80-100

fb, Fingerbreadth.

Table A-4 Summary of Basic Life Support Measures Used in Infants and Children

	Infant (<1 yr)	Child (>1 yr)
Airway		
Head or neck injury	Head tilt/chin lift/jaw thrust	Head tilt/chin lift/jaw thrust
Foreign body obstruction	Back blows/chest thrusts	Heimlich maneuver
Breathing		
Initial	Two breaths at 1-1½ sec	Two breaths at 1-1½ sec
Subsequent	20/min	15/min
Circulation		
Pulse check	Brachial/femoral	Carotid
Compression area	Lower third of sternum	Lower third of sternum
Procedure	Middle and ring fingers	Heel of one hand
Depth	½-1 in	1-1½ in
Rate	At least 100/min	80-100/min
Compression	5:1; pause for ventilation	5:1; pause for ventilation

Modified from Chameides L, editor: *Textbook of pediatric advanced life support,* Dallas, 1988, the American Heart Association and the American Academy of Pediatrics.

The Heimlich Maneuver (Abdominal Thrusts)

1. *Standing patient.* From behind, the thumb of one fisted hand is placed in the midline above the naval and well below the xiphoid. The fist is grasped by the other hand and a quick upward thrust is administered. Each thrust is separate. Up to five thrusts should be completed in an attempt to dislodge and expel the foreign body.
2. *Supine, unconscious patient.* With the child lying supine, the rescuer should kneel at his or her feet. The heel of one hand is placed on the child's abdomen above the navel and well below the xiphoid. The other hand is placed on top of the first and pressed into the abdomen with a quick upward thrust in the *midline.* A series of five thrusts are performed—fewer if the foreign body is expelled.
3. *The tongue maneuver.* This maneuver is used if back blows, chest thrusts, and subdiaphragmatic thrusts fail. The child's mouth is opened, and the tongue and lower jaw are grasped between the rescuer's thumb and index finger and are lifted. This maneuver may relieve airway obstruction even with a foreign body still in place. If a foreign body is seen, it should be removed. Blind sweeps of the throat with the examiner's index finger are contraindicated because they may force a foreign body farther down the airway.

Table A-4 summarizes the basic life support measures used in infants and children.

PEDIATRIC ADVANCED LIFE SUPPORT

When pediatric basic life support measures such as CPR are ineffective in resuscitating and stabilizing affected infants and children, advanced life support measures must be taken immediately. These measures include airway access and management, administration of oxygen, vascular access, administration of fluids and electrolytes, and drug therapy. To implement these measures the physician must be familiar with the ranges of body surface area (BSA), weight, and vital signs for pediatric patients (Table A-5) and the guidelines for use of resuscitation equipment of various sizes, according to the patient's age and weight (Table A-6). Resuscitation of newborns is presented in Chapter 44, One, Peripartum Considerations.

Airway Access and Management

Ventilation can be assisted without placing of an endotracheal tube. The purpose of CPR is to get oxygen into the airway. Oxygen delivery systems include an oropharyngeal airway, a nasal cannula, oxygen hoods and tents, and face shields and masks; however, these methods do not reliably provide oxygen concentrations over 40%. The most effective, noninvasive, assisted ventilation method is the self-inflating bag and mask with a reservoir connected to an oxygen source. Airway patency must be maintained and assessed frequently by observing for adequate symmetrical chest movements, adequate breath sounds, and good color.

Oropharyngeal and Nasopharyngeal Airways. The *oropharyngeal airway* can be used in an unconscious patient to support the tongue. It is not used in conscious patients because it may stimulate vomiting. To estimate the proper size, the flange should be placed at the level of the central incisors and the tip of the appropriate-size airway should reach the angle of the jaw. The tongue should be depressed with a tongue depressor, and the airway should be inserted into the oropharynx in the position of function and rotated into proper position as it approaches the back of the oropharynx. Proper head extension must be maintained.

Conscious patients tolerate a *nasopharyngeal airway* better than an oropharyngeal airway; however, the nasopharyngeal type may injure enlarged adenoidal tissue and cause bleeding in children under age 10.

Suctioning should not last longer than 5 seconds and should be preceded and followed by ventilation with 100% oxygen. The heart rate should be monitored for bradycardia during suctioning.

Endotracheal Airway. Placement of an *endotracheal (ET) tube* should be considered early in the care of an unconscious

Table A-5 Ranges of Body Surface Area, Weight, and Vital Signs for Infants, Children, and Adults

Age	Body surface area (m^2)	Weight (kg)	Pulse*/min	Systolic blood pressure† (mm Hg)	Respiratory rate‡/min
Newborn	0.19	3.5	90-200	60	30-60
1 mo	0.30	4.0	90-180	65	30-60
6 mo	0.38	7.0	90-180	70	24-30
1-2 yr	0.50-0.55	10-12	70-140	72-74	20-24
3-5 yr	0.54-0.68	15-20	60-120	76-80	16-22
6-9 yr	0.68-0.85	20-28	60-120	82-88	14-20
10-12 yr	1.00-1.07	30-38	60-110	90	12-20
12-14 yr	1.07-1.22	38-48	50-100	90	12-20
15-16 yr	1.30-1.60	53-58	50-100	90	12-18
Adult	1.40-1.70	60-70	50-100	90	12-18
Age	**mm Hg**		**Age**	**Tachypnea rate**	**Bradypnea rate**
0-1 mo	<60		<1 yr	>60	<25
1 mo-1 yr	<70		1-5 yr	>40	<15
>1 yr	Formula: 70 + (2 × Age in years)§		>5 yr	>30	<10

*Pulse range includes sound sleep and vigorous crying.
†Systolic blood pressure less than fifth percentile.
‡Respiratory rate >60 or <10/min is abnormal at any age.
§Formula for 50th percentile systolic BP at 2 to 10 yr is 90 + (2 × Age in years); the diastolic BP is two thirds of the systolic BP.

patient because it prevents aspiration, permits suctioning of the trachea and main bronchi, is a route for administering resuscitative medications,[11,12,30] allows for hyperventilation, and permits application of positive end-expiratory pressure (PEEP) when 100% oxygen does not improve oxygenation. Hyperventilation may help reduce increased intracranial pressure and can compensate for metabolic acidosis. PEEP may increase the functional residual capacity of the lungs and improve ventilation and perfusion. If prolonged ventilation is anticipated or if bag-mask and other airway adjuncts cannot accomplish adequate ventilation, an ET tube should be inserted.

The ET tube should be translucent, of uniform diameter (not tapering), and equipped with a standard 15 mm adapter; preferably the tube should have distance markers and an opening on the side wall as well as at the end. Cuffed ET tubes should be used only in children over age 8. An air leak with an uncuffed ET tube should be present when a breath is given at 20 cm H_2O pressure; if it is not, the tube is too large and should be replaced with a smaller one. The internal diameter of the ET tube should equal approximately 16 plus the patient's age in years, divided by 4; after 1 year of age the external diameter of the ET tube used should equal the size of the patient's external nasal orifice or the width of the patient's fifth finger.

Straight-blade laryngoscopes are preferred in children. Before laryngoscopy is begun, the examiner should check the equipment and the light source. Attempts at ET intubation should not exceed 30 seconds, and the heart rate and oxygenation should be monitored during the procedure. Bradycardia below 80 bpm in a neonate or 60 bpm in a child mandates interruption of the procedure and administration of 100% oxygen by face mask and bag. The ET tube should be passed into the trachea to a length that places the distance marker at the level of the vocal chords.

Once intubation has been established, the ET tube should be held securely in position and its position confirmed by (1) observing symmetrical movements of the chest, (2) auscultating the lungs to detect bilateral breath sounds, (3) auscultating over the stomach to ensure that air entry sounds are absent, and (4) looking for condensation in the ET tube during exhalation. An end-tidal carbon dioxide detector allows verification of ET tube placement and displacement during stabilization and transport in the prehospital or hospital setting.

Asymmetrical right-sided breath sounds usually indicate intubation of the right main bronchus. When this occurs, the tube should be withdrawn until breath sounds are heard in both lungs; the ET tube should then be withdrawn another 1 to 2 cm to ensure a midtracheal position. *The final position of the ET tube must be confirmed by chest roentgenogram.*

A properly placed tube but inadequate lung expansion indicates that (1) the tube is too small, (2) a large laryngeal air leak is present (detected by auscultating the neck), (3) the "pop-off" valve on the ventilator bag is not depressed, (4) the bag-valve device leaks, or (5) an insufficiently strong puff was administered.

The tube's position should be verified by noting the distance marked at the lips; it should be secured to the patient's face with benzoin and tape (see Fig. B-20, Appendix B). Its position should be assessed frequently by observing chest wall expansion, listening for bilateral breath sounds, and noting improvement of color and perfusion, obtaining blood gas values, and checking pulse oximeter readings.

Drugs can be administered through the ET tube while vascular access is sought. These drugs are *a*tropine, *n*aloxone, *e*pinephrine, and *l*idocaine (ANEL). Two to three times the usual IV dose (diluted in 1 to 2 ml of 0.9% saline) is administered through a catheter that has been passed beyond the ET tube as deeply as possible into the tracheobronchial tree. The dose of epinephrine, however, should be 10 times the IV dose (0.1 mg/kg of a 1:1000 solution) except in neo-

Table A-6 Pediatric Resuscitation Equipment Guidelines[1]

Age	Weight (kg)	ET tube (mm internal diameter*)	Laryngoscope blade (No.)	Suction catheter (Fr)	Distance from midtrachea to teeth (cm)	Chest tube (Fr)	Venous catheter (gauge)	Foley catheter and nasogastric tube (Fr)
Newborn, premature	<1	2.5	0	5 or 6	8	10-14	22-24	5 fdt
Newborn, full term	3	3.0	1	6	10	12-18	22-24	6 fdt
6 mo	7	3.5	1	8	12	14-20	22-24	8
1 yr	10	4.0	1	8	12	14-24	20-22	10
18 mo	11	4.0	1	8	14	14-24	20-22	10
3 yr	14	4.5	2	8	16	18-26	20-22	10
5 yr	18	5.0	2-3	10	16	20-32	20-22	10-12
8 yr	25	6.0 cuff	2	10	18	28-34	20-22	12
10 yr	34	6.5 cuff	2	10	18	30-38	18-20	12
12 yr	38	6.5-7 cuff	3	10	20	34-38	18-20	12-14
16 yr	55	7.5-8 cuff	3	12	22	34-38	18-20	12-14
Adult		8-8.5 cuff	3	12	22	34-38	18-20	12-14

Cuff, Cuffed endotracheal tube; *ET,* endotracheal; *Fdt,* feeding tube.

*Internal diameter of the ET tube $= \frac{\text{Child's age} + 16}{4}$.

nates.[14] After the drug has been instilled, several positive pressure puffs should be given.[3,11,12,30]

An *esophageal obturator airway* is not recommended for patients under age 16.[2,7]

Cricothyrotomy. In patients under age 8, airway obstruction may occur at the cricoid ring, the narrowest portion of the larynx in this age group. Because the ring is located below the thyrocricoid membrane, cricothyrotomy may not be effective in establishing an airway. In general, this route is *not recommended* in infants and small children.[15]

Airway Emergencies with Endotracheal Tubes. When emergencies occur, the gas delivery system should be disconnected and the patient should receive manual ventilation by means of a resuscitation bag and use of 100% oxygen. Auscultation should be used to determine the tube's position and patency. Problems that may be encountered include (1) loss of oxygen supply to the tube, (2) occlusion or kinking of the tube, or (3) displacement of the tube. If obstruction or displacement is the problem, poor breath sounds, a lack of chest movements, and increased resistance to inflation should be observed. Decreased resistance to inflation occurs when the ET tube has been misplaced into the esophagus. If the ET tube is obstructed, it should be irrigated with 1 ml of saline and suctioned for 3 to 4 seconds. After suctioning, the breath sounds, airway resistance, and adequacy of chest movements should be evaluated. If proper positioning and adequate manual ventilation of the ET tube are ensured, the problem should be assumed to lie with the gas delivery systems, which should be disconnected and manual ventilation instituted. If it is unclear whether the ET tube has been dislodged, its placement can be determined by direct laryngoscopy; sometimes the tube has to be removed and reinserted.

Oxygen Administration

The rational for administering oxygen is that establishing an adequate airway alone cannot reverse the pathophysiology of hypoxemia. Mouth-to-mouth breathing delivers only 16% fractional inspiratory oxygen (Fio_2) and results in an oxygen tension (Pao_2) of only 80 mm Hg. Normally, when one breathes room air, the Pao_2 is 104 mm Hg. Chest compression generates only 25% to 30% of the normal circulation in adults. Oxygen is indicated in any situation in which hypoxia is suspected. Oxygen should be administered even if the Pao_2 is high because a low cardiac output may not deliver sufficient oxygen to the tissues. The oxygen concentration should be 100% (preferably humidified and warmed) to achieve an adequate Pao_2 and tissue saturation. Once the airway has been established, if the respiration is not adequate, oxygen should be administered through an appropriate-size face mask connected to a self-inflating bag with an attached reservoir that delivers 10 to 15 liters of oxygen per minute. When a self-inflating bag is used, the "pop-off" valve should be occluded because the pressures needed to ventilate the lungs may exceed the valve's limit. Administering oxygen through a nasal cannula, a face mask, or a face shield does not provide reliable oxygen concentrations above 40%.[2,7,27]

Vascular Access

In children under age 6, if venous access cannot be established in 90 seconds or after three attempts, the intraosseous fluid access route should be used. For patients over age 6, the lesser saphenous vein or a femoral vein should be accessed.[2]

Infusion pumps or minidrip chambers should be used for infusion therapy. Head and neck vessels should not be used because this interferes with resuscitative measures. Cannulation of central veins should be supervised by experienced operators.

The intraosseous space is a plexus of noncollapsible veins through which any fluid or medication may be infused.[16,24,28,29] Interosseous infusion is recommended for children under age 6 if vascular access cannot be established in 90 seconds or after three percutaneous attempts.[2,27] It is an easily learned technique and quickly accomplished. An 18-gauge short spinal needle with a stylet or a large-bore marrow needle may be used. Intraosseous needles are now available from several commercial distributors. The favorite site is 2 cm below the tibial tuberosity on the medial surface of the tibia. Intraosseous infusions are equivalent to those given intravenously and are preferable to the ET route for administering drugs. (Appendix B, Special Procedures, describes in detail the methods used in intraosseous infusions.)

Resuscitative and Postresuscitative Fluids and Drugs

The purposes of the pharmacological agents used during cardiac arrest and the postresuscitation period are (1) to expand intravascular volume and increase perfusion, (2) to stimulate spontaneous, forceful myocardial contractions, (3) to accelerate the cardiac rate, (4) to correct metabolic acidosis, and (5) to suppress ventricular ectopy. The pharmacological agents used, their indications and doses, and the precautions to apply in using them are discussed below and presented in Table A-7.

Volume Expansion. The types of fluids available for volume expansion include the following:

1. *Crystalloids*—Lactated Ringer or 0.9% saline. Lactated Ringer is preferred because it contains less chloride and does not aggravate acidosis. Because only one fourth of crystalloids remain in the vascular space, four times the deficit is required to restore plasma volume.
2. *Colloids* and *blood products*—albumin, fresh-frozen plasma, human plasma protein fraction (Plasmanate), whole blood or packed red blood cells (RBCs). In general, the patient requires that these products constitute half the amount of the crystalloids given to restore plasma volume.
3. *Glucose*.[2,4,7,25,27] Glucose is not administered in the initial resuscitative fluids unless hypoglycemia exists. In response to stress, the endogenous catecholamines cause glycogenolysis and increase the blood glucose. Excess glucose may be metabolized to lactate and cause an osmotic diuresis.

Small infants and chronically ill children have limited glycogen stores, and hypoxemia-like hypoglycemia may develop. Glucose is a major metabolic substrate for the neonatal myocardium. A rapid blood glucose test should be obtained, and if hypoglycemia exists, glucose should be administered. In children, a $D_{25}W$ solution should be used (dilution of $D_{50}W$ 1 : 1 with sterile water), and in infants, a $D_{10}W$ solution (dilution of $D_{50}W$ 1 : 4 with sterile water). Sufficient amounts should be given to keep the blood glucose level

Table A-7 Drugs Used in Pediatric Advanced Life Support

Drug	Dose	Comments
Adenosine	0.1-0.2 mg/kg (max: 12 mg in a single dose)	Rapid IV bolus
Atropine sulfate	0.02 mg/kg/dose Minimum dose: 0.1 mg Maximum single dose: *Child:* 0.5 mg *Adolescent:* 1 mg	Dose may be repeated once
Bretylium	5 mg/kg; may be increased to 10 mg/kg	Rapid IV bolus
Calcium chloride 10% (100 mg/ml)	20 mg/kg/dose; repeat in 10 min if necessary	Administer slowly Not for cardiac arrest Use for hypocalcemia, hypermagnesemia, and channel blocker Overdose
Dobutamine HCl	2-20 μg/kg/min	Titrate to desired effect
Dopamine HCl	2-20 μg/kg/min	Titrate to desired effect
Epinephrine		
For bradycardia	*IV/IO:* 0.01 mg/kg (0.1 ml/kg) 1:10,000 *ET:* 0.1 mg/kg (0.1 ml/kg) 1:1000	Be aware of preservative administered when large doses are used
For asystole or pulseless arrest	**First dose:** *IV/IO:* 0.01 mg/kg 1:10,000 *ET:* 0.1 mg/kg 1:1000 class IIb* Doses as high as 0.2 mg/kg may be effective **Subsequent doses:** *IV/IO/ET:* 0.1 mg/kg 1:1000 class IIa* Doses as high as 0.2 mg/kg may be effective, class IIa	Be aware of preservative administered when large doses are used Repeat q3-5 min
Epinephrine infusion	*Initial:* 0.1 μg/kg/min Use higher infusion dose with asystole: 20 μg/kg/min	Titrate to desired effect 0.1-1 μg/kg/min Lower dose with effective pulses
Lidocaine	1 mg/kg/dose	
Lidocaine infusion	20-50 μg/kg/min	
Sodium bicarbonate	1 mEq/kg/dose or 0.3 × kg × base deficit Subsequent doses are based on blood gas analysis every 10 min of arrest	Infuse slowly and only if ventilation is adequate Not for cardiac arrest Use for metabolic acidosis

From the Emergency Cardiac Care Committee and Subcommittees of the American Heart Association, *JAMA* 268:2662, 1992.
*Based on classification on supporting scientific evidence.
ET, Endotracheal; *IO,* intraosseous; *IV,* intravenous.

above 100 mg/dl. Repeated hyperosmolar doses have been associated with intracranial hemorrhage in premature infants.

The principle in fluid resuscitation is to administer a bolus of fluid over a period of 10 to 15 minutes and then reevaluate the patient's hydration status. In hypovolemic shock, a 20 ml/kg/dose of crystalloid is administered as soon as vascular access is established. A child who is in hypovolemic shock often requires 40 to 60 ml/kg of fluid in the first hour of resuscitation, occasionally up to 100 to 200 ml/kg in the first few hours. A three-way stopcock attached to a 20 ml or 50 ml syringe may be useful in "pushing" fluids with the aid of the syringe. Subsequently, volume expanders may be needed (e.g., colloid or blood); 20 ml/kg/dose of 5% albumin, 1 g/kg/dose of 25% albumin, or 20 ml/kg/dose of fresh-frozen plasma may be used. Whole blood (20 ml/kg) is administered if hemorrhage has occurred, and packed RBCs (10 ml/kg) are given to a patient who has had chronic blood loss.

Fluid resuscitation should be monitored by reassessing perfusion frequently. Fluid overload is detected by auscultating the chest for signs of pulmonary edema and by noting the size of the heart on a chest roentgenogram. In hypovolemia the heart is normal or small in size; in cardiogenic shock or fluid overload, it usually is enlarged.

Resuscitation Medications.* The resuscitative medications described here are listed in Table A-7, along with their recommended doses and means of administration. The nor-

*References 2, 4, 9, 15, 16, 23, 25, 30.

Table A-8 Normal Values for Arterial Blood (pH, Gases, Oxygen Saturation, Bicarbonate)

Parameter	Unit	Infants and children			Newborn
		Mixed venous	Capillary	Arterial	
pH	units	7.31-7.41	7.35-7.40	7.40-7.45	7.11-7.30
Pco_2	torr	35-40	40-45	35-40	27-40
Po_2	torr	41-51	45-50	80-100	33-75
Sao_2	%	60-80	>70	>90	40-90
HCO_3^-	mEq/L	22-25	22-26	22-26	14-22

Modified from Gordon IB: Reference ranges for laboratory tests. In Behrman RE, Vaughan VC, editors: *Nelson's textbook of pediatrics,* ed 12, Philadelphia, 1983, WB Saunders.

HCO_3^-, Bicarbonate; *Pco_2*, carbon dioxide pressure; *Po_2*, oxygen pressure; *Sao_2*, saturation.

mal values for arterial blood pH, gases, oxygen saturation, and bicarbonate for newborns, infants, and children are shown in Table A-8.

The vagus nerve, through its neurotransmitter acetylcholine, inhibits conduction at the sinoauricular and atrioventricular nodes. The sympathetic nervous system, through its alpha-adrenergic receptors, enhances perfusion by causing vasoconstriction and increased peripheral vascular resistance. Its beta-1-adrenergic receptors increase heart rate, cardiac conductivity, and myocardial contractility, resulting in increased cardiac output. The sympathetic nervous system's beta-2-adrenergic receptors cause vasodilation of skeletal muscle blood vessels and bronchodilation. They do not play a role in cardiopulmonary resuscitation.

Epinephrine. Epinephrine is an endogenous catecholamine that has alpha- and beta-adrenergic receptor properties. In doses used for CPR, it has alpha, beta-1, and beta-2 effects. Its mechanism of action relates to its alpha effect, which increases systemic vascular resistance, leading to increased coronary artery perfusion pressure and increased oxygen delivery to the myocardium. It is indicated in asystole, unstable bradyrhythmias, which constitute 90% of rhythm disturbances in pediatric patients, and ventricular fibrillation (VF), which occurs in only 10% of children who have rhythm disturbances. Epinephrine renders VF more susceptible to conversion by countershock.

Sodium Bicarbonate. Respiratory acidosis is corrected by establishing effective ventilation. By inducing hyperventilation (and thereby reducing the $Paco_2$), respiratory alkalosis results and compensates for any metabolic acidosis that may be present because of poor oxygen delivery. The resultant pH is less acidotic. If acidemia persists despite respiratory compensation and the pH is persistently below 7.20 to 7.25, sodium bicarbonate should be administered to correct the residual metabolic acidosis. Bicarbonate should not be used with inadequate ventilation. The interpretation of blood pH, gases, oxygen saturation, and bicarbonate determinations is complex and can be simplified in terms of determining the acid-base balance and its origins by applying the following "golden rules"[2]:

Rule 1: An acute change in $Paco_2$ of a 10 torr increase or decrease is associated with an increase or decrease of 0.08 units in the pH.

To assess the respiratory component of acidosis: Determine the amount of the measured partial pressure of carbon dioxide in arterial blood ($Paco_2$) that falls below or above 40 torr. Calculate the pH using rule 1. Compare the measured pH with the calculated pH; if they are reasonably close, all acidotic changes are respiratory in origin.

Rule 2: A pH change of 0.15 units is equivalent to (or the result of) a change in bicarbonate (HCO_3^-) of 10 mEq/L from its 20 mEq/L baseline.

To assess the metabolic component: Determine the calculated pH using rule 1 and compare with the measured pH value. If they are not reasonably close, determine the following:

1. If the measured pH is less than the calculated pH (a negative number), the acidosis is metabolic in origin; subtract the measured pH from the calculated pH to determine the base deficit or fixed acid.
2. If the measured pH is greater than calculated (a positive number), metabolic alkalosis is present; subtract the calculated pH from the measured pH to determine the base excess (or negative base excess).

Rule 3: The dose of bicarbonate (mEq) required to correct the metabolic acidosis fully is the base deficit (mEq/L × patient's weight [kg] × 0.3). Usually only half this amount is administered and then the acid-base status is reassessed, which ordinarily indicates that 1 mEq/kg sodium bicarbonate is needed.

If the arrest is observed and brief, bicarbonate usually is not necessary, and in children it may worsen existing respiratory acidosis. Bicarbonate may be required in prolonged arrest (longer than 10 minutes) after initial ventilation and perfusion are established and when the arterial pH remains below 7.2.

Excessive administration of bicarbonate can have adverse effects because it (1) shifts the oxygen dissociation curve to the left and reduces the delivery of oxygen to the tissues, (2) shifts the potassium intracellularly, lowering the serum potassium level, (3) reduces plasma-ionized calcium, (4) lowers the fibrillation threshold, (5) increases the risk of hypernatremia and water overload, (6) increases the risk of hyperosmolality, and (7) may produce paradoxical cerebrospinal fluid (CSF) and intracellular acidosis.[17]

Atropine. Atropine is a parasympatholytic drug by virtue of its competitive antagonism of acetylcholine. It accelerates sinus and atrial pacemaker discharge and atrioventricular conduction. In low doses (less than 0.1 mg) a paradoxical CNS vagal nuclei stimulation may produce atrioventricular node slowing. Higher doses are used in asystole to shorten the response time.

Atropine is indicated to treat hemodynamically unstable bradycardia accompanied by poor perfusion or hypotension and asystole. Bradycardia most often results from hypoxia, and initial treatment should be directed at ventilation, oxygenation, and perfusion.

The vagolytic dose is 0.02 mg/kg with a minimum dose of 0.1 mg. The duration of action is 2 to 4 hours; the pupils remain dilated for 6 hours or longer after injection and thus cannot provide a basis for neurological evaluation of the patient. Repeat doses during asystole can be given every 15 minutes, up to 1 mg in a child and 2 mg in an adolescent.

Calcium Chloride. Calcium has a positive inotropic effect on the heart, but calcium entry into cell cytoplasm is the final common pathway in cell death and may be injurious. *Its use is no longer recommended in cardiac arrest protocols.* The indications for calcium are documented hypocalcemia (total serum calcium below 8.1 mg/dl or ionized calcium below 2.4 mg/dl), hyperkalemia, hypermagnesemia, and calcium channel blocker overdose. Calcium chloride is used in emergency hypocalcemia because it delivers the ionized calcium directly. Calcium always should be injected slowly, concurrently with electrocardiographic and blood pressure monitoring. The injection should be discontinued if bradycardia or hypotension occurs.

Lidocaine. Lidocaine in usual doses has no effect on myocardial contractility, blood pressure, or cardiac conduction. Its action suppresses ectopic foci and reduces automaticity, raises the fibrillation threshold, and inhibits the formation of reentry circuits that lead to ventricular tachycardia and fibrillation. VF occurs in fewer than 10% of pediatric patients in cardiac arrest. If VF is present, a metabolic cause (abnormalities of calcium, potassium, and glucose), hypothermia, and drug intoxication (especially tricyclic antidepressants) should be considered.

The indications for lidocaine administration are (1) ventricular tachycardia, (2) ventricular fibrillation, and (3) frequent (more than 6/min) or potentially serious premature ventricular contractions (couplets, multifocal), particularly if associated with hemodynamic instability. Lidocaine infusion is recommended after successful conversion of ventricular tachycardia or fibrillation.

To ensure adequate plasma concentrations, a bolus of 1 mg/kg should be given when the IV infusion is placed. If the patient is in shock or has liver disease, beginning doses of 1 ml/kg/hr (20 μg/kg/min) should be used to prevent toxicity from impaired lidocaine clearance. The dose for an adolescent is a 50 to 100 mg bolus followed by infusion of 1 to 4 mg/min. The antiarrhythmic effect occurs at a serum concentration of 1 to 5 μg/ml. Concentrations above 6 μg/ml may cause seizures and those above 10 μg/ml, myocardial depression. The practitioner should be prepared to treat bradycardia and hypotension. Lidocaine is contraindicated in severe heart block. Widening of the QRS complex by more than 0.02 seconds or significant ventricular slowing suggests cardiac toxicity. It is important to monitor electrocardiographic activity and plasma lidocaine concentrations because of the erratic pharmacokinetics of lidocaine in patients who have CPA.

Bretylium. Bretylium is a quaternary ammonium compound with postganglionic adrenergic properties and antiarrhythmic activity. It has a biphasic effect. Initially, through norepinephrine release, it increases the blood pressure and heart rate; this is followed by adrenergic blockade of norepinephrine and epinephrine, but cardiac output remains unchanged. Bretylium may raise the fibrillation threshhold and prevent reentry. It is a second-line drug, after lidocaine, and is indicated in refractory ventricular tachycardia or fibrillation. In adults, bretylium improves the susceptibility of a refractory heart to defibrillation, cardioversion, and lidocaine. *It is important to continue CPR for 2 minutes after administering bretylium* to allow for its circulation before attempting defibrillation. The drug's adverse effects are nausea, vomiting, hypotension, and transient hypertension; it may worsen arrhythmias in digitalized patients.

Postresuscitative Medications.* Postresuscitative medications should be administered if the blood pressure or peripheral perfusion remains unstable.

The current teaching is that the following drugs are important in a post-CPA patient:

- With hypotension: epinephrine and norepinephrine
- With normotension but poor cardiac output: dobutamine and epinephrine
- With septic shock accompanied by hypotension: epinephrine and norepinephrine
- With septic shock accompanied by normotension and poor cardiac output: dopamine and dobutamine

Dopamine. Dopamine is an endogenous catecholamine that is an immediate precursor of norepinephrine. *At low doses* (2 to 5 μg/kg/min) it binds to dopamine receptors in splanchnic, coronary, and renal vascular beds, causing vasodilation and increased contractility without affecting the heart rate and blood pressure. *At higher doses* (6 to 20 μg/kg/min) beta-1-adrenergic effects (inotropic and chronotropic) and alpha-adrenergic effects (vasoconstriction) predominate, causing blood pressure to rise as a result of general vasoconstriction and increased cardiac output. At doses *above 20 μg/kg/min,* dopamine produces predominantly vasoconstrictive effects. The indications for its use are hypotension or poor peripheral perfusion in the presence of a stable rhythm and with adequate vascular volume.

A reasonable starting dose of dopamine for a patient in shock is 5 to 10 μg/kg/min. It is not recommended that infusion rates rise above 20 μg/kg/min; if a further inotropic effect is needed, epinephrine and dobutamine should be used. Dopamine may cause tachycardia (which increases myocardial oxygen demands), hypertension, arrhythmias, and extremity ischemia. It should be given in a central vein, if possible. Electrocardiographic activity should be monitored and the skin observed for ischemia; the blood pressure and urinary output also should be monitored closely. Extravasation of dopamine causes tissue necrosis. Table A-9 summarizes the effects of dopamine infusions at various rates.

Dobutamine. Dobutamine is a synthetic catecholamine prepared by manipulation of isoproterenol. It is a direct-acting catecholamine with selective beta-1-adrenergic action and a mild peripheral beta-2 effect (vasodilation), resulting in increased cardiac contractility and heart rate and decreased afterload (systemic resistance); all of this increases the cardiac output. It is less effective in septic shock and in infants under 12 months of age. Its major indication is the treatment of cardiogenic shock. It may cause tachyrhythmias, nausea, vomiting, hypotension, and hypertension.[20]

*References 2, 7, 10, 17, 20, 25, 27, 33.

Table A-9 Effects of the Infusion Rate of Dopamine on the Cardiovascular System

Infusion rate	Cardiac output	Inotropic effect	Vascular resistance	Renal blood flow
2-5 μg/kg/min	0	0	0	+
6-20 μg/kg/min	+ (beta-1)	+ (beta-1)	+/−	+
>20 μg/kg/min	+ (beta-1)	+ (beta-1)	+ (alpha-1)	0

Table A-10 Effects of the Rate of Epinephrine Infusion on the Cardiovascular System

Dose (μg/kg/min)	Chronotropic effect	Inotropic effect	Vasodilation	Vasoconstriction
0.05-0.3	+	+	+	0
0.3-1.5	+	+	0	+

Table A-11 Normal Ranges of Cardiac Function

Age (yr)	Heart rate (beats/min)	PR interval (sec)	QRS complex (sec)
<1	90-180	0.07-0.16	0.03-0.08
1-3	70-140	0.08-0.16	0.04-0.08
4-10	60-120	0.09-0.17	0.04-0.07
>10	55-110	0.09-0.20	0.04-0.08

Modified from Garson A: *Electrocardiogram in infants and children: a systematic approach,* Philadelphia, 1983, Lea & Febiger.

Epinephrine Infusion. Epinephrine is indicated in the treatment of shock with diminished systemic perfusion from any cause. An epinephrine infusion is the treatment of choice and preferable to dopamine in patients with marked circulatory instability. The initial dose is 0.1 μg/kg/min; it can be increased up to 1 μg/kg/min, with the dose titrated to reach the desired effect. Higher infusion rates may be used in asystole. It should be administered through a well-secured peripheral line or, preferably, a central line. The adverse effects of epinephrine infusion are arrhythmias and, at doses exceeding 0.5 μg/kg/min, profound vasoconstriction that compromises skin and extremity blood flow (Table A-10). Epinephrine vasoconstriction reduces renal blood flow but improves renal function through increased cardiac output and tissue perfusion. Extravasation causes tissue necrosis.[33]

EMERGENCY PEDIATRIC CARDIAC RHYTHM DISTURBANCES[4]

Emergency pediatric cardiac rhythm disturbances usually result from hypoxemia and acidosis and rarely cause cardiac arrest; thus ventilation and oxygenation are important in their management. The principle of therapy is to initiate treatment only if the rhythm disturbance compromises the cardiac output or can potentially deteriorate into a lethal rhythm. Electrical therapy includes (1) defibrillation, an untimed depolarization of the myocardium to allow for a spontaneous organized beat, and (2) cardioversion, a timed polarization designed to avoid the vulnerable period in the cardiac cycle.

Table A-11 shows the normal ranges for heart rates, PR intervals, and QRS complexes at various ages; these values are important in interpreting electrocardiograms as part of the assessment and management of cardiac rhythm disturbances.

In children under age 10, a PR interval longer than 0.18 seconds and a QRS complex longer than 0.10 seconds are abnormal. The P wave almost always is upright in lead II; if it is not, or if it is absent, a normal sinus rhythm is not present. An inverted P wave in lead II most commonly is due to incorrect placement of one of the ECG leads. A wide QRS complex may be ventricular in origin or a result of an aberrantly conducted supraventricular beat. However, *a wide QRS complex should always be considered as ventricular tachycardia because of its serious implications* and the relative rarity of aberrant supraventricular tachycardia (SVT) in children.[2,19]

A useful *clinical classification* of emergency arrhythmias in pediatrics would be: (1) rhythms that are too fast (tachyrhythmias) or too slow (bradyrhythmias) associated with hemodynamic instability and reduced cardiac output, (2) rhythms that are disorganized (ventricular fibrillation), or (3) rhythms that are absent altogether (asystole). Other arrhythmias may need evaluation and treatment but usually do not constitute an emergency.[2]

Tachyrhythmias

In infants, *supraventricular tachycardia* usually is associated with a heart rate above 230 bpm; P waves are difficult to find, and the QRS complex is narrow in 98% of cases. If the patient is hemodynamically stable, vagal maneuvers can be tried (e.g., inverting the infant quickly or applying an ice bag to the face). Adenosine, administered intraveneously, is the drug of choice for converting the rhythm to normal. Adenosine is an endogenous nucleoside that causes a temporary block through the atrioventricular node; it is very effective, and side effects are minimal because its half-life is only 10 seconds. Adenosine is given by rapid IV bolus (see Table A-7). If hemodynamic instability and reduced cardiac output are present, synchronized cardioversion (0.5 joules/kg) should be attempted immediately if no IV access is available. If SVT persists, the cardioversion dose should be increased to 2 joules/kg. If it still persists, the diagnosis may be incorrect. Verapamil should not be used to treat SVT in infants or children because cardiovascular collapse has been reported.[2,7,8,22]

Ventricular tachycardia (VT) usually has wide QRS complexes, absent P waves, and T waves that are the opposite in polarity to the QRS complex. VT may degenerate into ventricular fibrillation.

If the patient is hemodynamically unstable and cardiac output is reduced, synchronized cardioversion (0.5 to 1 joules/kg) should be attempted immediately. If a lidocaine bolus can be given without delaying cardioversion, the success of conversion will be greater. If VT recurs, an infusion of lidocaine given after cardioversion will help to maintain the converted rhythm. If this is unsuccessful, cardioversion at a higher voltage (2 joules/kg) should be used. If success still is not achieved, bretylium should be given initially instead of lidocaine, but there are no published data on its usefulness; this is a class IIb recommendation.[7]

Bradycardia

Bradycardia (a heart rate below 80 bpm) requires resuscitation if accompanied by poor perfusion, even if the blood pressure is normal. Epinephrine is the drug of choice. The neonatal dose remains the same (0.01 to 0.03 mg/kg given IV or by endotracheal tube).[7] Atropine is now a class IIb drug if epinephrine is ineffective or bradycardia is caused by atrioventricular (AV) block. Atropine is administered in doses of 0.02 mg/kg, or paradoxical bradycardia may result. Because bradycardia may be caused by hypoxia, atropine should be administered only after adequate oxygenation and ventilation have been established. Isoproterenol is no longer recommended to treat bradycardia (see Fig. A-1).

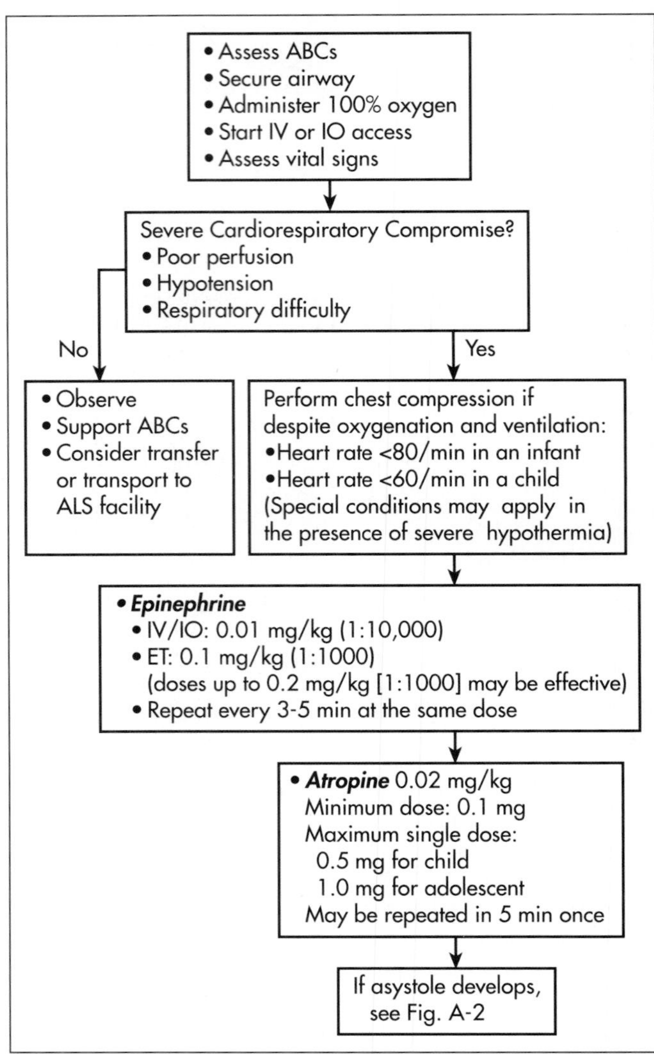

FIG. A-1 Bradycardia decision tree. *ABC,* Airway, breathing, and circulation; *ALS,* advanced life support; *ET,* endotracheal; *IO,* intraosseous; *IV,* intravenous.

(From the Emergency Cardiac Care Committee and Subcommittee of the American Heart Association: *JAMA* 268:2662, 1992.)

Absent or Disorganized Rhythms

Asystole and Pulseless Cardiac Arrest. In making the diagnosis of asystole, it is important to be sure that the clinical picture (no pulse and absent spontaneous respirations) correlates with the electrocardiographic activity that has been monitored. Ventilation, oxygenation, and volume repletion are the standards of treatment. Ventricular arrhythmias rarely occur in children who do not have congenital heart disease; however, the new guidelines endorse prompt defibrillation of pulseless ventricular tachycardia. If an initial dose of 2 joules/kg fails, the dose is doubled and administered twice. If refractory, epinephrine is given, followed by lidocaine and then a rapid infusion of bretylium (5 mg/kg given as the first dose, followed by 10 mg/kg as the second dose). The treatment for asystole and electromechanical dissociation (EMD) is epinephrine. Atropine is no longer recommended (Fig. A-2).

Ventricular fibrillation is characterized by a disorganized series of depolarizations seen on the ECG with no detectible pulse and reduced cardiac output. The ECG pattern is classified as coarse or fine on the basis of the height of the electrical waves.

Cardiopulmonary resuscitative measures should be continued until defibrillation can be applied, using an initial dose of 2 joules/kg. If this is unsuccessful, the dose should be doubled and repeated twice. If this also is unsuccessful, ventilation and correction of any metabolic disturbance (hypoxia, hypoglycemia, severe metabolic acidosis) should be accomplished, followed by a bolus of epinephrine and another attempt at defibrillation. If this, too, fails, a bolus of lidocaine and further defibrillation should be attempted. Finally, if that fails, bretylium should be given initially at a dose of 5 mg/kg and subsequently at doses of 10 mg/kg in place of lidocaine before defibrillation is attempted. Some have recommended lidocaine infusion after cardioversion (see Fig. A-2).

Electromechanical dissociation is characterized by the presence of organized electrical activity with ineffective myocardial contractions, as evidenced by the absence of a pulse. Etiologies include hypoxia, acidosis, volume depletion, tension pneumothorax, and cardiac tamponade. Treatment consists of ventilation, oxygenation, volume repletion, and administration of an epinephrine bolus (see Fig. A-2).

POSTRESUSCITATIVE CARE OF INFANTS AND CHILDREN[2]

Postresuscitative care involves stabilization, frequent assessment, and care during transport to a tertiary care facility, as well as the care rendered in that facility's intensive care unit. Any infant or child who has suffered respiratory or cardiac arrest should be admitted to a pediatric intensive care unit.

Elements of Postresuscitative Care

1. Cardiovascular function should be assessed by determining tissue perfusion clinically and by monitoring urinary

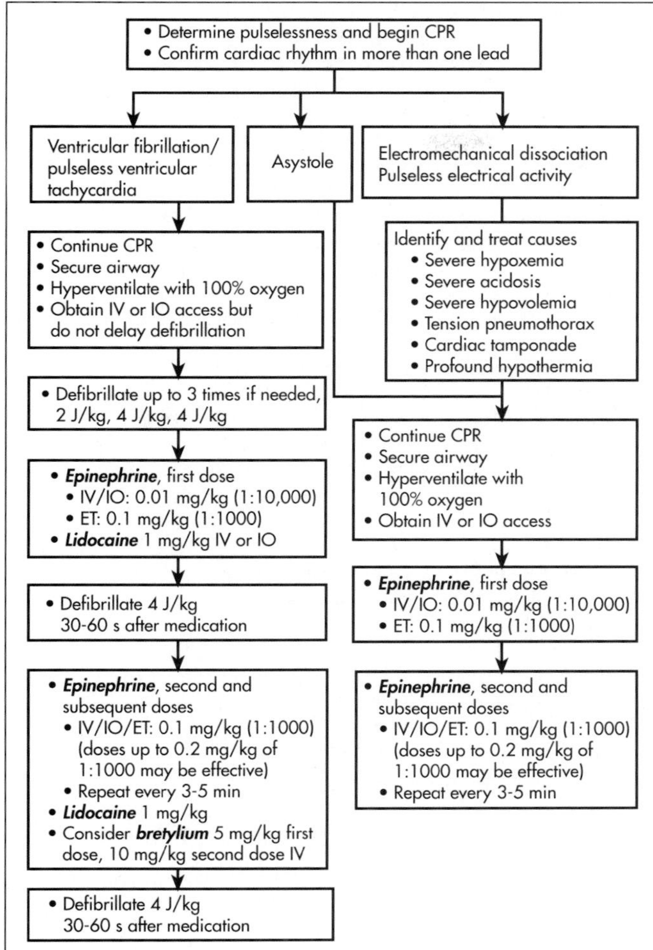

FIG. A-2 Asystole and pulseless arrest decision tree. *CPR,* Cardiopulmonary resuscitation; *ET,* endotracheal; *IO,* intraosseous; *IV,* intravenous.

(From the Emergency Cardiac Care Committee and Subcommittee of the American Heart Association: *JAMA* 268:2662, 1992.)

output, blood pressure, and continuous ECG recordings.
2. Ventilation should be evaluated clinically and by interpretation of ABG levels and pulse oximeter or transcutaneous Po_2 readings.
3. Serial neurological examinations should be performed, with attention given to the level of consciousness and evidence of IIP and seizures.
4. Humidified, warm oxygen at the highest attainable concentration should be administered until ABG levels are available. These levels should be measured after a ventilation system has been in use for at least 15 minutes and before the patient is transported. The hematocrit, serum electrolyte, and blood glucose levels also should be monitored and determined just before transport.
5. Two well-secured functional venous lines should be placed.
6. A nasogastric tube should be connected to gravity drainage to decompress the stomach, especially if positive pressure ventilation has been used.
7. The cause of the cardiopulmonary arrest should be determined and treated.

Transportation to a Regional Pediatric Intensive Care Unit[5]

Agreements, protocols for specific clinical situations, and protocols for transport to the regional pediatric intensive care unit should be prepared in advance by the directors of the Regional Emergency Medical Services for Children (EMS-C) program.

Information Needed for Interhospital Transport

1. The referring hospital's name, physician's name, and telephone numbers
2. The child's name, age, and weight
3. A history of the present illness and significant elements of the past history, including medications present in the home and medications to which the patient may be allergic
4. The current clinical status, including the level of consciousness, heart rate, presence and adequacy of peripheral pulses, capillary refill time, respiratory rate, air entry status, respiratory effort, skin color, body temperature, and blood pressure
5. Laboratory test data, including all roentgenograms and ECG tracings
6. All medications administered, including dosages and times given
7. The number of intravenous lines and fluids administered, including their infusion rates
8. The ventilator settings if the patient is receiving assisted ventilation
9. The availability of parents or their designates for providing consent for treatment

Brain Death[13]

Brain death, the ultimate criterion for removing life-support mechanisms, is defined as (1) irreversible cessation of circulation and respiratory function or (2) irreversible cessation of all brain functions, including those of the brainstem. Caution should be used in reaching the determination of brain death if the patient (1) is under age 5, (2) has hypothermia, (3) nearly drowned, and (4) ingested neuromuscular blocking agents or barbiturates, because early in these circumstance electroencephalographic recordings may be unreliable.*

Do Not Resuscitate (DNR) Orders[31]

The purpose of CPR is to prevent sudden, unexpected death. It may not be indicated in circumstances surrounding a terminal, irreversible illness when death is not unexpected or when prolonged cardiac arrest indicates the futility of such efforts, which are a violation of the right to die with dignity. A DNR order should be written on the patient's order sheet, and the physician should explain in a progress note the rationale for the decision and should identify those who participated in making the decision.

*The determination of brain death is very difficult and must be done precisely. Guidelines for the determination of brain death in children have been drawn up by the Task Force for the Determination of Brain Death in Children (*Arch Neurol* 44:587, 1987).

REFERENCES

1. Bardossi K: Newest guidelines on pediatric CPR and first aid, *Contemp Pediatr* 4:47, 1987.
2. Chameides L, editor: *Textbook of pediatric advanced life support,* Dallas, 1988, the American Heart Association and the American Academy of Pediatrics.
3. Chernow R et al: Epinephrine absorption after endotracheal administration, *Anesth Analg* 63:629, 1984.
4. Committee on Drugs, American Academy of Pediatrics: Emergency drug doses in children, *Pediatrics* 81:462, 1988.
5. Committee on Hospital Care, American Academy of Pediatrics: Guidelines for air and ground transportation of pediatric patients, *Pediatrics* 78:943, 1986.
6. Day RL: Differing opinions on the emergency treatment of choking, *Pediatrics* 71:975, 1983.
7. Emergency Cardiac Care Committee and Subcommittees, American Heart Association: Guidelines for cardiopulmonary resuscitation and emergency cardiac care, *JAMA* 268:2171, 1992.
8. Epstein ML, Kiel EA, Victoria BE: Cardiac decompensation following verapamil therapy in infants with supraventricular tachycardia, *Pediatrics* 75:737, 1985.
9. Finholt DA et al: The heart is under the lower third of the sternum, *Am J Dis Child* 646:649, 1986.
10. Gillis J et al: Results of inpatient pediatric resuscitation, *Crit Care Med* 14:469, 1986.
11. Greenberg MI: Endotracheal drugs: the state of the art, *Ann Emerg Med* 13:789, 1984.
12. Greenberg MI, Roberts RJ: Drugs for the heart by way of the lungs, *Emerg Med* 12:209, 1980.
13. Guidelines for the determination of death: Medical Consultants on the Diagnosis of Death to the President's Commission for the Study of Ethical Problems in Medicine and Biomedical and Behavioral Research Report, *JAMA* 246:2184, 1981.
14. Johnston C: Endotracheal drug delivery, *Pediatr Emerg Care* 8:94, 1992.
15. Mace SE: Cricothyrotomy, *J Emerg Med* 6:309, 1988.
16. Mofenson HC, Caraccio TR: Guidelines for intraosseous infusion, *J Emerg Med* 6:143, 1988.
17. Nieman JT, Rosborough JP: Effects of acidemia and sodium bicarbonate therapy in advanced life support, *Ann Emerg Med* 13:781, 1984.
18. Orlowski J: Optimum position for external cardiac compression in infants and young children, *Ann Emerg Med* 15:667, 1986.
19. Park MK, Guntheroth WG: *How to read pediatric ECGs,* Chicago, 1982, Mosby.
20. Perkin RM et al: Dobutamine: a hemodynamic evaluation in children in shock, *J Pediatr* 100:977, 1982.
21. Phillips GWL, Zideman DA: Relationship of infant heart to sternum: its significance in cardiopulmonary resuscitation, *Lancet* 1:1024, 1986.
22. Radford D: Side effects of verapamil in infants, *Arch Dis Child* 58:465, 1983.
23. Rose JS, Koenig KL: Code blue: what's new? *J Emerg Med* 12:187, 1994.
24. Rosetti VA et al: Intraosseous infusion: an alternate route of pediatric intravascular access, *Ann Emerg Med* 14:885, 1985.
25. Schuman AJ: Pediatric advanced life support: an update and review, *Contemp Pediatr* 6:26, 1989.
26. Schuman AJ: The latest guidelines on pediatric life support, *Contemp Pediatr* 10:25, 1993.
27. Seidel JS, Burkett DL, editors: *Instructor's manual for pediatric advanced life support,* Dallas, 1988, the American Heart Association.
28. Seigler RS, Tecklenburg FW, Shealy R: Prehospital intraosseous infusion by emergency medical services personnel: a prospective study, *Pediatrics* 84:173, 1989.
29. Spivey WH: Intraosseous infusions, *J Pediatr* 111:639, 1987.
30. Stewart RD, Lacovery DC: Administration of endotracheal medication, *Ann Emerg Med* 14:136, 1985.
31. Tomlinson T, Brody H: Ethics and communications in do-not-resuscitate orders, *N Engl J Med* 316:43, 1988.
32. Tsai A, Kallsen G: Epidemiology of pediatric prehospital care, *Ann Emerg Med* 16:284, 1987.
33. Zaritsky A, Chernow B: Use of catecholamines in pediatrics, *J Pediatr* 105:341, 1984.
34. Zaritsky A et al: CPR in children, *Ann Emerg Med* 16:1107, 1987.

B Special Procedures

Joseph R. Custer

The information presented here details the methods by which samples of normal and abnormal body fluids are obtained to enhance diagnosis and treatment of pediatric patients, how therapeutic fluids are introduced parenterally, and how endotracheal intubation can be accomplished in children with respiratory difficulties.

PATIENT PREPARATION

General Approach

The first step in performing any pediatric procedure is to establish an understanding among physician, parents, and child of what is to be done. Failure to do this compromises the physician-patient-parent relationship. The physician who dismisses the parents' and patient's concerns or fears of an impending procedure loses their confidence. Procedures that the physician may consider routine and ordinary have great significance to parents and patients. They have a right to know what will be done and why it will be done.

The information to be gained from the simplest procedure must be explained. The parents and the patient should be informed about the indications for each test and procedure. Parents should be given a reason for their child's inconvenience and discomfort. Reassurance that the physician understands the child and the child's perceptions must be conveyed to the parents.[1]

The spectrum of ages and stages of development of pediatric patients dictates that an adaptive approach be taken by the practitioner. Appreciation of both the child's fears and the parents' reservations requires a calm, empathic, reassuring posture. The newborn, toddler, and older child all present different problems. If one forgets the newborn's individuality in the frustration of repeated attempts at venipuncture, normal protective emotions in the parents may be aroused and the physician-parent relationship may suffer.

The toddler, just beginning to develop a new vocabulary and new emotions, may react to painful procedures submissively or obstinately. The toddler's fear of pain, of being handled by strangers, and of separation from the parents must be respected. A calm, authoritative approach conveys to the child that the adults present are in control.

In older children it is important to appreciate their perception of what will happen. Here the expression "blood test" may conjure up all sorts of mysterious images in the child's mind. A more explicit explanation of what is to be done helps to dispel those mysteries. The older child also responds to contracts of cooperation, such as, "You may cry, but hold your arm still, and we will finish the test quickly," or "You can help by holding very still." One must not violate this contract by denying the child's feelings of pain or discomfort. If the operator sees that the child is terribly upset by a procedure, a few minutes given to reassurance will not be wasted.

Before any procedure is done, a decision as to whether the parents should be in attendance during the procedure needs to be made. It depends on the relative comfort of both the physician and the parents. If their presence causes anxiety for the physician, the success of the procedure may be hampered; on the other hand, children's cooperation may be enhanced by the reassuring presence of their parents. The adolescent at times may feel the presence of parents to be embarrassing.[2]

An "open-door" policy that allows parents to be present when procedures are performed must never represent a demand for demonstration of parenting behavior. Therefore, the wishes of those parents who do not want to be present should be respected. Parents should never be involved in restraining their child or in assisting in the performance of a painful procedure.

Although tradition has kept parents from the bedside and treatment rooms when procedures are performed on their child, this determination should be made on an individual basis.

Restraint and Immobilization

It is necessary to immobilize infants and some children to complete quickly and safely most of the procedures described here. Therefore an assistant always is required to help immobilize the child, to observe the child's cardiorespiratory function during the procedure, and to reassure and comfort the child. In general, parents should not be asked to serve as assistants.

For infants and younger children, the "papoose" board can be used effectively for immobilization. Children up to about age 5 can be immobilized by mummy wrapping, as demonstrated in Figure B-1. The assistant stands at the side or foot of the wrapped child, leans lightly on the trunk, stabilizing the patient's thorax with the elbows, and with the hands fixes the patient's head or free arm for the procedure.

Monitoring During a Procedure

Children are particularly susceptible to hypoxia and ischemia. Safe, efficient performance of a procedure requires sedation. Monitoring of oxygenation, pulse, heart rate, and respiratory rate is mandatory. Patients who receive systemic sedatives and analgesics should be treated as if they were undergoing general anesthesia. The child's recovery from the procedure also should be supervised.[35,36]

The patient's record must show documentation of assessment of risk, doses and timing of drugs administered, vital signs, the intravenous (IV) fluids administered, and the child's recovery from the procedure.[7]

Assessment of Risk

If systemic analgesia or sedation is required, the risks of hypoxemia, hypotension, and hypoventilation must be assessed.

The patient's medical history should be reviewed for al-

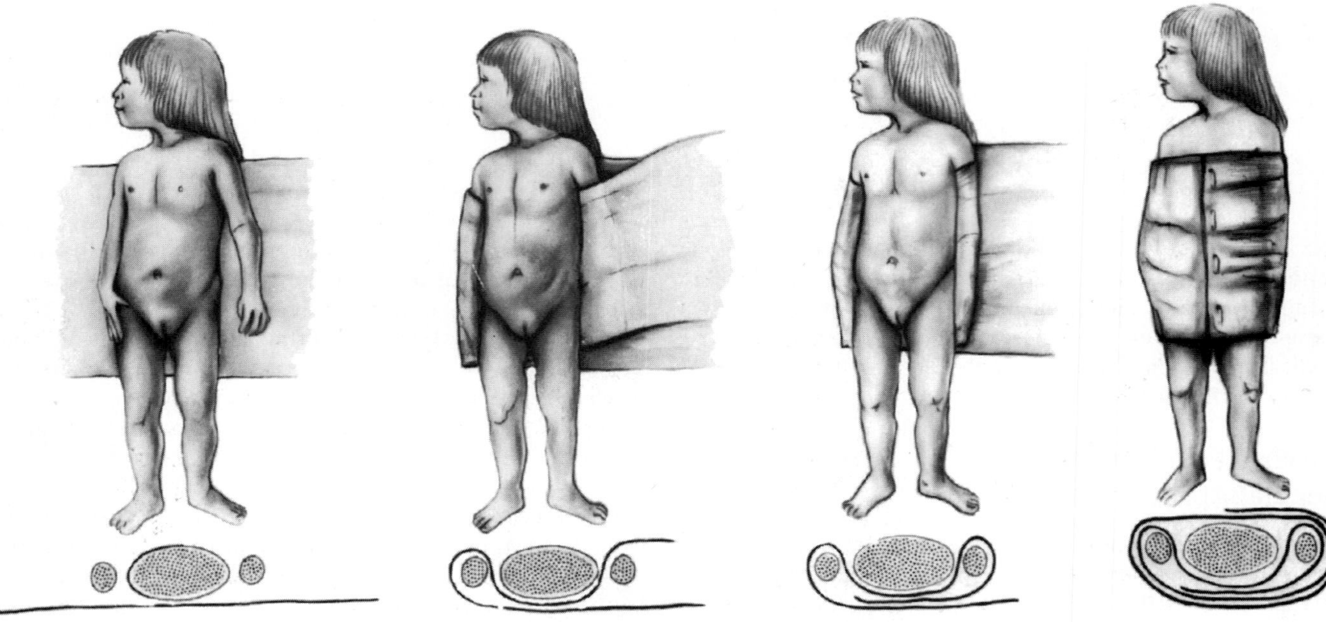

FIG. B-1 Method of mummy-wrapping an infant or child to restrain the upper extremities. The four steps are illustrated with frontal and cross-sectional views. A wider sheet or blanket may be used to restrain the lower extremities.

lergies. The possibility of renal or hepatic disease, which might alter drug pharmacology, should be considered. Pulmonary disease that requires chronic oxygen use places a patient at higher risk for hypoxemia. Patients with cardiac disease require careful monitoring, reduced drug doses, and in some circumstances precautions against bacterial endocarditis. Anemia increases the risk of dysoxia (adequate oxygen saturation but diminished tissue delivery).

Some chronic medications may increase a patient's risk during sedation. Diuretics and antihypertensives may predispose the patient to hypotension. In nonemergency situations requiring systemic sedation or analgesia, the stomach should be empty. An interval of 4 hours since the previous meal usually is sufficient.[35]

Monitoring devices and equipment for procedures should include:

- Pulse oximeter
- Noninvasive blood pressure cuff
- Cardiotachometer
- Respiratory rate monitor
- Resuscitation equipment
- Intubation equipment
- Airway suction equipment
- Flowsheet
- Oxygen delivery equipment
- Antidotes (Flumazenil, Narcan)
- IV access and fluid

The ability to monitor the child's respiratory rate and effort and airway patency continuously is paramount. A common error is to cover the patient's chest and airway with sterile drapes and towels; this deprives the clinician of the most reliable monitor—direct observation. An assistant who is free to circulate during the procedure is invaluable for documenting vital signs, helping to ensure sterility, observing the patient's chest excursion, and monitoring the patency of the airway.

Anesthesia

In general, if the procedure involves only a needle puncture, local anesthesia may be dispensed with, inasmuch as it necessitates additional needle punctures.

Sedation and Analgesia

The primary care clinician can safely administer and monitor sedation in most pediatric patients. Patients who have a chronic disease, especially those who have neuromuscular, pulmonary, cardiac, or renal disease, are difficult to sedate safely. These children also often require several hours of post-sedation observation such as that provided in a recovery room or critical care unit. In elective situations, an intensivist or anesthetist should be consulted when planning sedation.[7,35]

Local anesthesia usually is produced by infiltration of the skin with lidocaine (1% solution, 10 mg/ml). Lidocaine overdose is uncommon but has the serious consequences of hypotension, seizures, and respiratory arrest. The maximum dose of locally infiltrated lidocaine is 5 to 7 mg/kg.

The burning, stinging sensation that accompanies infiltration of a local anesthetic is due to the low pH of lidocaine. These sensations can be oblated by using lidocaine buffered with sodium bicarbonate ($NaHCO_3^-$). Lidocaine is mixed 10:1 by volume with $NaHCO_3^-$ (1 mEq/ml).[34]

Topical anesthetic creams (EMLA) are available. These are applied to the venipuncture site and covered with a patch. However, 20 to 30 minutes of exposure is required. Cost and time should be considered when using these agents. In some extremely anxious children, this technique is helpful when repeated blood sampling is required.[10,12,16]

Deep sedation for invasive procedures may be required.

The risks of sedation include respiratory and central nervous system (CNS) depression, hypotension, and emesis. Therefore patients who are sedated require monitoring of heart rate, respiratory rate and effort, and blood pressure, as well as of noninvasive pulse oximetry. Judgment is required in the choice of sedative dose. Patients who have cardiorespiratory embarrassment need a reduced dose. The best practice is to titrate the dose to the desired effect while adequately monitoring the patient. A key virtue in sedating a child is patience. One should allow adequate time in a quiet, controlled environment, using a calm voice to gain the confidence of the child. A common error is to start a procedure too soon after giving a sedative. When this happens, the child is inadequately sedated, the physician's impatience is tried by the procedure not going well, and consequently, time is wasted.[35]

Deep sedation can be obtained (in patients who are not in danger of respiratory depression) with a lytic "cocktail," composed of meperidine (Demerol), 2 mg/kg (maximum, 50 mg); promethazine (Phenergan), 1 mg/kg; and chlorpromazine (Thorazine), 1 mg/kg. The drugs are mixed in one syringe and administered by deep intramuscular injection. These doses are appropriate for most procedures that produce prolonged discomfort or generate high anxiety, but they should be reduced by 50% for precardiac catheterization sedation of children who have severe cyanotic congenital heart and chronic pulmonary disease.

When one desires cooperation with relatively pain-free procedures, such as immobilization for an echocardiogram or a computed tomographic (CT) scan in infants and toddlers, chloral hydrate is the drug of choice. This drug may be given orally or by rectum in doses of 25 to 75 mg/kg. Side effects include movement disorders, respiratory depression, and vomiting.

Diazepam, a commonly used anxiolytic drug in adults, has an application for older children and adolescents, but its use is hazardous in the young infant. It has a narrow therapeutic index—that is, the difference between the effective dose for sedation and that causing apnea is small. The dose is 0.04 to 0.2 mg/kg given intravenously or 0.2 to 0.8 mg/kg by mouth.

Midazolam is a water-soluble imidazobenzodiazepine with a rapid onset and short duration of action. The drug produces good anxiolytic effect and retrograde amnesia. Experience with neonates and toddlers is inadequate; however, a dose of 0.05 to 0.2 mg/kg given intravenously is well tolerated in older children and adolescents. Respiratory depression is the drug's most serious side effect.[19,25,26,36]

Morphine, 0.1 to 0.2 mg/kg, is commonly used for analgesia in the pediatric population.[1] The drug can be given intravenously, subcutaneously, and intramuscularly. Because the peak effect is delayed for 30 minutes, patience is required for the preprocedure wait. Respiratory depression, hypotension, and bronchospasm secondary to histamine release are complications encountered commonly. Naloxone, 5 to 10 μg/kg given every 5 to 10 minutes, will reverse the hypotension and apnea but must be given repeatedly, inasmuch as its effect is transient.[3]

Fentanyl and ketamine, very useful in specific situations, should be used with the advice of an anesthesiologist or a pediatric intensivist.

SAMPLE COLLECTION

Blood

Capillary Puncture. Blood obtained from the capillary bed of a warm finger can be used for blood gas analysis; blood from the finger, toe, or heel can be used for a wide variety of microdeterminations. After preparation of the skin with alcohol, a firm stab wound is made with a lancet or a No. 11 Bard-Parker blade in the ventrolateral aspect of the terminal phalanx, avoiding the pad and joint. The posterior edge of the heel pad also may be used. Frequent wiping may be needed to prevent clotting and to obtain free flow without squeezing. Local pressure applied with a dry sponge will stop the bleeding after the sample has been obtained.

Venipuncture. Figure B-2 illustrates the location of superficial veins commonly used to obtain blood samples. For infants, the scalp and neck sites provide the easiest access; for older children the veins of the extremities are more accessible, despite the difficulties encountered in restraining movement. The largest superficial veins are those of the cervical and femoral areas, although these should be avoided for routine blood sampling because complications of bloodletting at these sites are more severe than elsewhere. These sites should not be used when bleeding disorders are a factor.

For *venipuncture of the lower arms, lower legs, hands, and feet,* the child is immobilized and the skin is prepared with alcohol. A tourniquet is applied to the extremity (above the point of planned venous puncture) tightly enough to produce venous stasis and distention, yet loosely enough to allow arterial perfusion. This can be demonstrated if there is capillary refilling after blanching created by direct pressure on the extremity distal to the tourniquet. A 20- or 22-gauge needle or "butterfly" infusion needle attached to a syringe may be used. The vein is stabilized by traction on the overlying skin along the axis of the vein. The skin is pierced with the needle bevel up. The needle tip is then advanced subcutaneously, and the vein is entered with a short jab to prevent its rolling away. Negative pressure in the syringe is used to withdraw the amount of blood needed. After the blood is obtained, the tourniquet is released, the needle removed, a dry sponge applied with pressure to the site, and the extremity elevated for a minute or two to prevent bleeding at the puncture site.

For *external jugular venipuncture,* the child is positioned on a table with the head rotated to one side and extended over the edge of the table 45 degrees toward the floor. The assistant, leaning over the mummy-wrapped child, holds the head firmly in this position. Positive intrathoracic pressure created by struggling or crying distends the jugular vein to make it easily located. After preparation of the skin with alcohol, a butterfly needle is attached to a syringe and used to penetrate the skin in a caudal direction where the vein crosses the sternocleidomastoid muscle. The vein is then entered with a separate thrust, and negative pressure is created within the syringe. If a hematoma appears, the procedure should be discontinued at that site. After the sample has been obtained, firm pressure is applied over the venipuncture site for 3 to 5 minutes with the child sitting upright.

Internal jugular venipuncture is a rarely used technique, but this is an accessible site for phlebotomy. This procedure should be reserved as a "last resort" because of the risks of

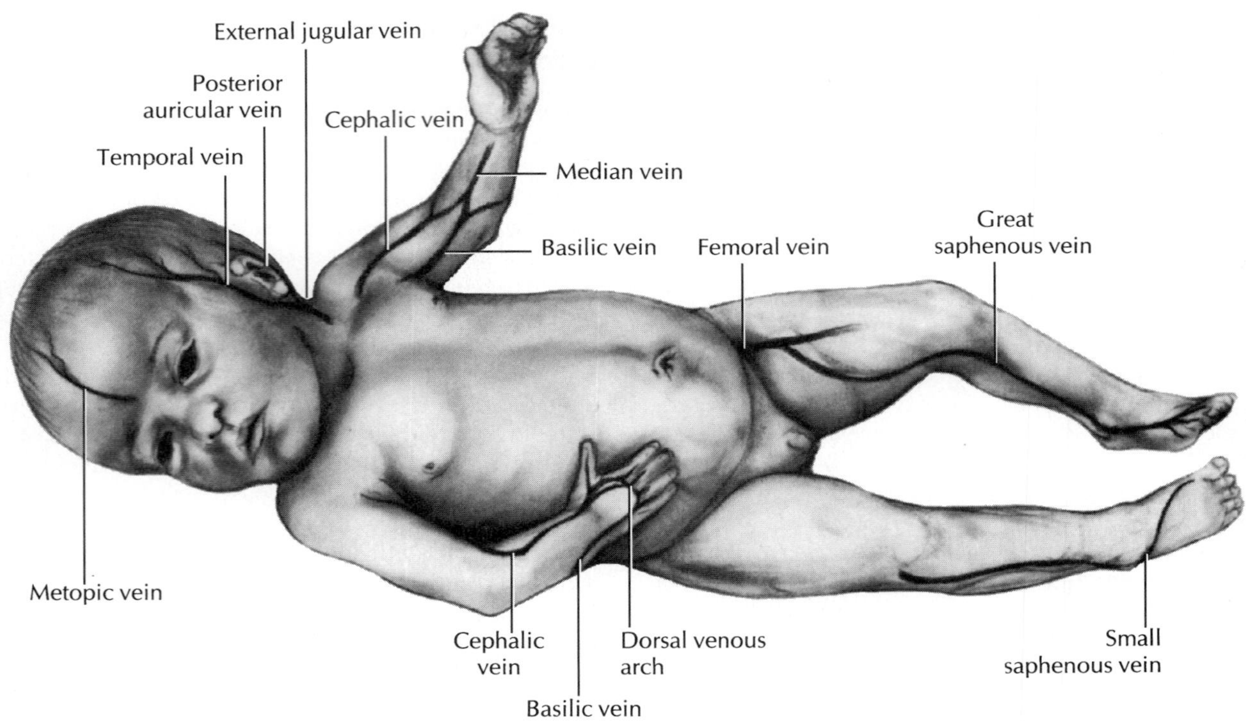

FIG. B-2 Accessible veins for blood sampling and administration of intravenous infusions.

accidental entry into the carotid artery medially and the risk of pneumothorax caused by entering the apex of the lung.

The child is restrained in modest Trendelenburg position, the neck minimally extended at the edge of the table or with the aid of a 2- or 3-inch diameter towel roll at the base of the neck. The child's head is turned 45 degrees away from the proposed side of entry (Fig. B-3).

The internal jugular vein runs lateral to the carotid artery and the trachea. The posterior border of the sternocleidomastoid muscle, as well as its midpoint between the sternal and mastoid insertions, should be identified. A 22-gauge, 1½-inch needle attached to a 10 ml syringe is inserted behind and underneath the posterior border of the muscle at the midpoint, aiming for the ipsilateral nipple. Once the skin is pierced, negative syringe pressure should be maintained continuously so that the blood enters the barrel of the syringe immediately when the vein is entered. Firm pressure should be applied over the site for 3 to 5 minutes after the procedure, with the child sitting upright.

For *puncture of the femoral vein,* the child is placed in the supine position with the leg straight and externally rotated. The assistant holds this position while leaning over the child's trunk from one side. The femoral artery is identified by palpation just distal to the inguinal (Poupart) ligament and medial to the midpoint of the ligament. The femoral vein lies medial and parallel to the artery here (Fig. B-4). The skin is prepared with alcohol, and while the artery is being palpated, the skin is entered 1 to 2 cm distal to the flexion crease of the groin. The needle should be directed medial to the arterial pulsations and cephalad, at a 30-degree angle, while negative pressure is applied to the syringe during insertion and withdrawal. Blood will enter the syringe as soon as the vein is entered. Complications of the procedure, which are caused by faulty needle placement, include septic arthritis of the hip, osteomyelitis of the femur, and femoral arteriospasm (sometimes severe enough to cause gangrene).

Arterial Puncture. Arterial puncture has become a necessary technical skill for physicians who care for critically ill children. Assessment of arterial blood gases (ABGs) is essential in monitoring a variety of cardiopulmonary diseases.

The *right radial artery* is the preferred site for arterial puncture. It is in a consistent anatomical position and is well fixed by surrounding connective tissue. In the newborn, the site has the added advantage of providing preductal arterial blood samples. Other available sites are the brachial and femoral arteries.

Arterial punctures may be hazardous because arterial laceration, spasm, or insufficiency secondary to hematoma may occur.[6] The adequacy of collateral circulation for the radial artery is good, but it may be less so for the femoral and brachial arteries. Septic arthritis of the hip is an infrequent complication of femoral artery puncture. The data from blood gases may be erroneous if venous blood is sampled, if the sample is exposed to air, if the equipment used for analysis is improperly standardized, or if the oxygen concentration to which the patient is exposed during the sampling is not considered or is reported inaccurately.

The wrist is supported in a position of supination and slight dorsiflexion. The artery may be located at the wrist by palpation of the point of maximal pulsation. In newborns it usually is found along the first flexor crease one sixth of the width of the wrist measured from its radial edge (Fig. B-5).

A plastic or glass syringe is rinsed with heparin and emptied. The syringe needs only to be rinsed with heparin; then all the heparin in the solution is ejected. The trace amount of heparin remaining coating the walls is adequate for antico-

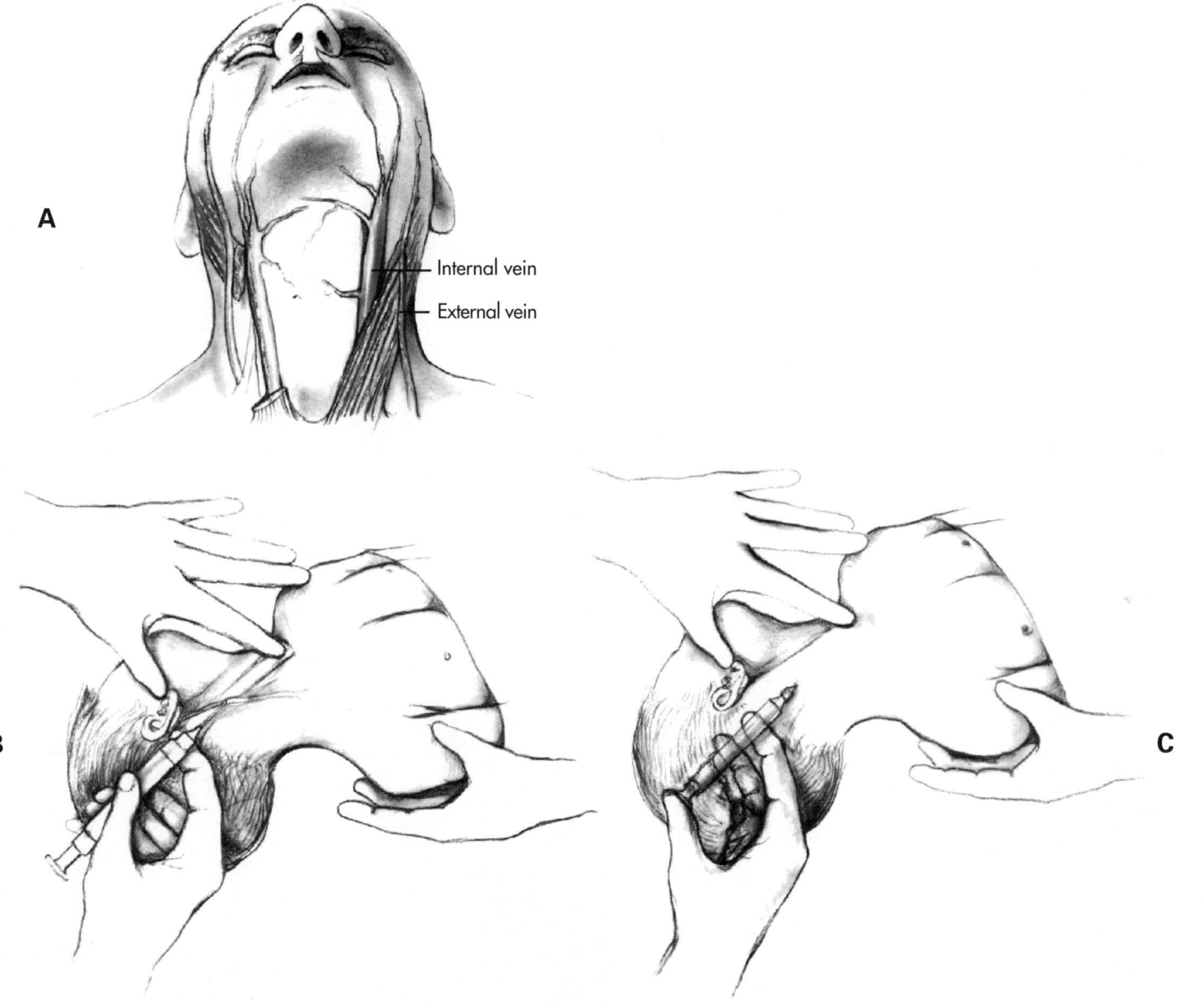

FIG. B-3 Internal jugular venipuncture. **A,** Anatomy of the internal and external jugular veins and their relationship to the sternocleidomastoid muscle. **B,** Positioning of the child, showing the point of the needle overlying the external jugular vein, which must be avoided, and the sternocleidomastoid muscle, beneath which the needle is inserted and thrust toward the suprasternal notch. **C,** Position of the needle and syringe after puncture; with negative pressure on the plunger of the syringe, the barrel should fill quickly with venous blood.

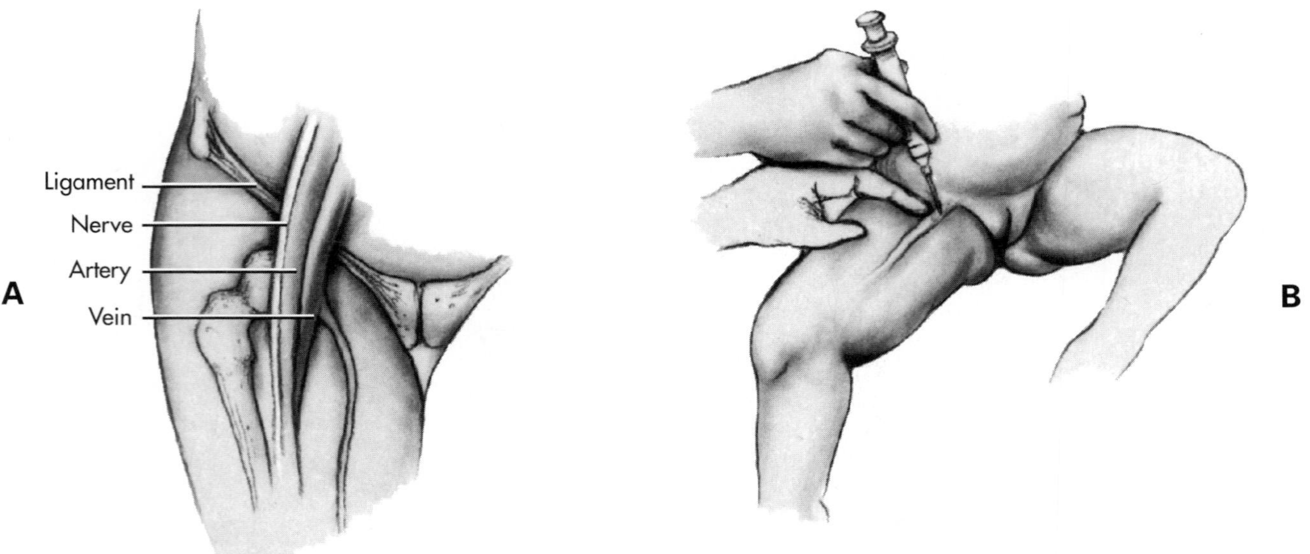

FIG. B-4 Femoral vein or artery puncture. **A,** Anatomical structures. **B,** Position of the patient, with needle poised for piercing the skin, subcutaneous tissue, and femoral vein. The procedure for femoral artery puncture is identical except that the needle is aimed more laterally, directly into the pulsating femoral artery.

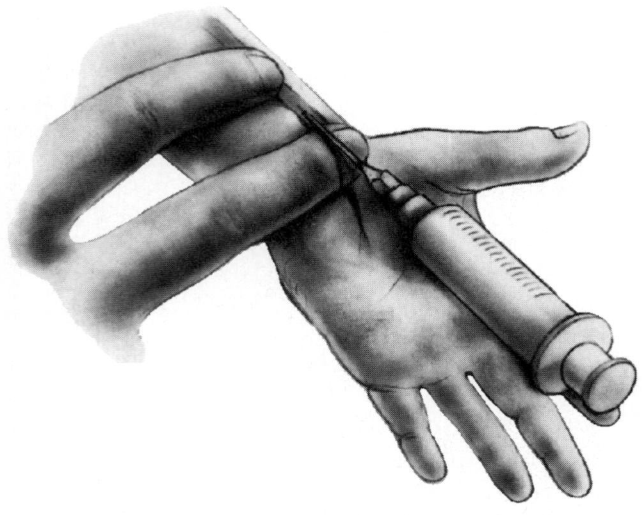

FIG. B-5 Radial artery puncture. The position of the radial artery is determined by palpation; it is fixed with the index and middle fingers while the needle is inserted at a 45-degree angle.

agulation. If heparin solution is left in the syringe, a dilutional acidosis artifact will result.

The size of the needle used varies with the patient's age (25 gauge for newborns and infants to 22 gauge for older children and adolescents). Care must be taken to avoid constricting the artery during restraint. The syringe is held as one would hold a pencil or a dart, and the needle is introduced into the artery at approximately a 45-degree angle. A "flash" of blood spurting into the syringe indicates a successful puncture. Gentle aspiration is required when plastic, disposable syringes are used. A butterfly needle may be used more easily with hard-to-restrain patients; in such cases the syringe is rinsed with heparin, and 0.25 to 0.50 ml of heparin is injected into the butterfly tubing to clear it of air. The butterfly needle, without the syringe attached, then is introduced into the artery as described above. A pulsatile flow of blood into the tubing ensures that arterial puncture has been accomplished. The syringe then is connected to the butterfly tubing, and the sample is collected. The sample should be sealed, placed in ice, and sent to the laboratory for analysis. Direct pressure on the puncture site for a minimum of 5 minutes prevents bleeding and hematoma formation.

The *brachial artery* in the antecubital fossa is a less desirable choice for sampling because collateral circulation is not always adequate and because a vein may be sampled mistakenly. The artery is located by palpation. Either a 22- or 25-gauge needle and syringe or, for infants, a 23- or 25-gauge butterfly needle may be used. The needle should be held at a 45-degree angle and the skin punctured at the point of maximal pulsation. Pressure must be applied to the site of puncture for 5 to 10 minutes after the needle is withdrawn.

The *femoral artery* is the least desirable choice for sampling because the hip joint can be inadvertently entered and contaminated. This area is more apt to be contaminated than are other arterial puncture sites; therefore extra attention to skin preparation is required. The puncture site may be found at the point of maximal pulsation, just inferior to the inguinal ligaments (see Fig. B-4). The femoral nerve is lateral, and the femoral vein medial, to the artery. The artery should be punctured at approximately a 60-degree angle. Gentle aspiration as the needle penetrates the soft tissue aids in detecting a successful puncture. Once the sample has been obtained, careful pressure on the puncture site is necessary for at least 10 minutes.

Cerebrospinal Fluid

The need to perform a lumbar puncture to rule out meningitis and other CNS infections must be weighed against the dangers inherent in performing a lumbar puncture in the pres-

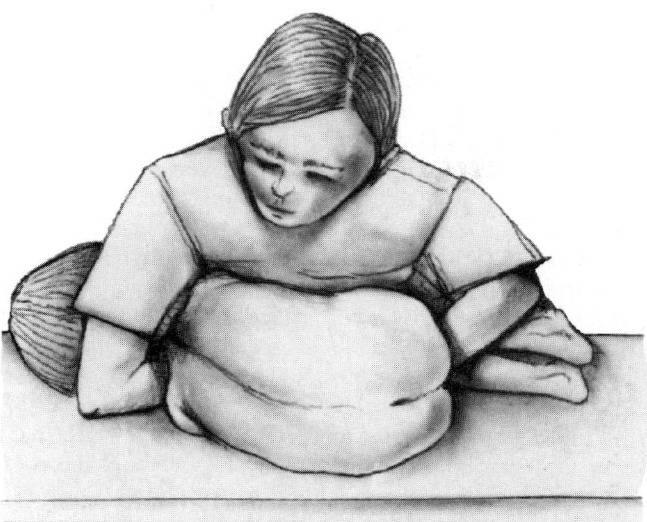

FIG. B-6 Restraining a child during lumbar puncture. The patient's nuchal and popliteal surfaces are in contact with the assistant's antecubital fossae.

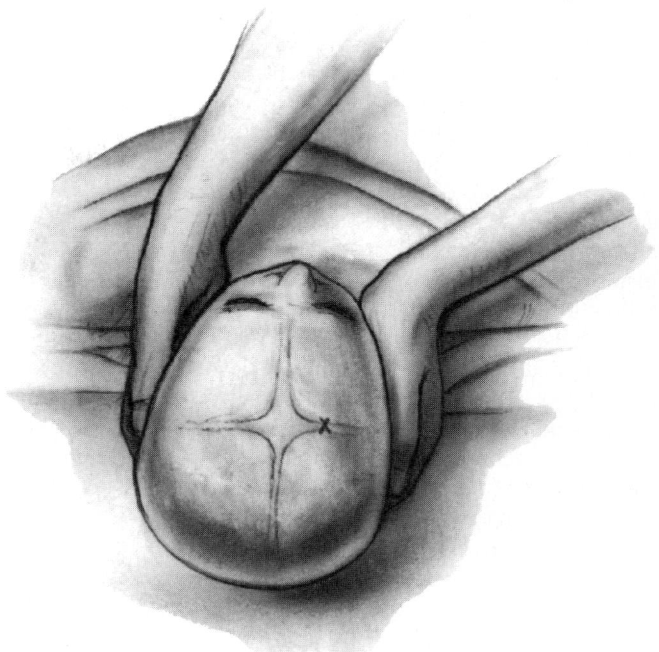

FIG. B-7 Subdural tap. Position of the child for a subdural tap. The subdural needle should be inserted into the coronal suture 1 to 2 cm lateral to the edge of the anterior fontanelle.

ence of a supratentorial space-occupying lesion. Increased intracranial pressure is a relative contraindication to lumbar puncture. Its presence dictates immediate neurosurgical consultation if collection of cerebrospinal fluid (CSF) is judged clinically necessary. If meningitis is suspected, however, antibiotic therapy must not be delayed.

A relative contraindication to lumbar puncture is profound coagulopathy and thrombocytopenia. Again, if bacterial meningitis is suspected, antimicrobial therapy must not be delayed.

The position of the patient during lumbar puncture should be dictated by the mutual comfort of the patient, the assistant, and the operator. Some prefer infants to be held upright; others prefer the lateral recumbent position (Fig. B-6). Use of a local anesthetic is not necessary for infants. Reassurance, an explanation of what is to occur, and a tranquil atmosphere may be as important as a local anesthetic for an older child (see Chapter 27, Hypnosis and Biofeedback Therapy).[20]

The preferred site is the L3-4 interspace. It is located by determining the site at which an imaginary line drawn between the superior edge of the right and left posterior iliac crests crosses the spine. The interspace above and below also may be used. The skin is prepared thoroughly with appropriate antiseptic, the patient is sterilely draped, and sterile gloves are worn.

Care must be taken that the needle enters the intervertebral space in the sagittal plane. This requires several different perspectives of the proposed line of entry with the needle aimed toward the umbilicus.

Once the skin is penetrated, the needle is advanced slowly in the sagittal plane. Although a distinct "pop," or give, may be felt in the older patient when the dura is pierced, this is not the case in the infant. When the physician suspects that the spinal canal has been entered, the stylet is removed and the needle gently rotated to maximize the flow of cerebrospinal fluid through the needle. If no flow is obtained, the stylet is reinserted and the needle is advanced further or withdrawn and redirected. Care must be taken to avoid a "bloody tap," or traumatic tap, caused by pushing the needle into the venous plexus along the anterior wall of the spinal canal. A syringe should *never* be used to enhance the aspiration of cerebrospinal fluid because this creates undue negative pressure and might produce herniation of the brainstem through the foramen magnum.

A stopcock and manometer are attached to the spinal needle to measure the opening and closing pressure of cerebrospinal fluid and, in certain instances, to perform manometric tests. These measures are useless with the struggling child. One milliliter of fluid is collected in each of three sterile test tubes to be used for bacteriological, chemical, and cytological determinations. In the case of a traumatic tap, the red cells in both the first and the third tubes should be counted. A traumatic tap usually gives fewer red cells in the third tube than in the first. Once the fluid is removed, the needle is withdrawn quickly and the puncture site tamponaded briefly. No dressing is required.

Subdural Fluid

The purpose of a subdural tap is to detect a posttraumatic or postinfectious subdural effusion. With closed sutures and ossified fontanelles, neurosurgical assistance should be sought.

The incidence of subdural effusions has declined markedly with the advent of vaccination against *Haemophilus influenzae*. However, the clinician should remain vigilant for this complication. Persistent fever, an increasing head circumference, and transillumination provide clues to the diagnosis.

Figure B-7 illustrates the preferred site of puncture. This is a point in the coronal suture 1 to 2 cm lateral to the anterior fontanelle on an imaginary line drawn posteriorly from the center of the orbit parallel to the sagittal suture.

While the infant is supine, the head should be carefully restrained. The anterior two thirds of the infant's scalp is shaved and cleansed with an appropriate antiseptic. The portion of the unshaved scalp posterior to the planned puncture site should be sterilely draped, and sterile gloves should be used while the procedure is performed.

A short, beveled 19- or 20-gauge lumbar puncture needle or a subdural tap needle is inserted through the skin perpendicular to the scalp and slowly is advanced 2.5 to 5 mm. A hemostat clamped to the shaft of the needle will aid the operator in gauging the depth of insertion and prevent accidental overpenetration. Perforation of the dura usually is recognized by a sudden decrease in resistance and a popping sensation. A few drops of fluid normally are present and flow through the needle when the stylet is removed. Negative pressure applied to the needle with the aid of a syringe should be avoided. The procedure usually is performed on both sides of the head. Current practice in the treatment of subdural effusion is to remove no more than 25 ml of fluid from each subdural space per day. Chronic effusions necessitate daily taps. After removal of the subdural specimen, the needle is withdrawn and a sterile cotton and collodion dressing is applied.

Urine

Urethral Catheterization. To collect a sterile specimen of urine from a child who cannot produce a midstream, clean-catch specimen, or to monitor the urine output continuously, a catheter is inserted into the bladder through the urethra. The child is placed in the supine frog-leg position and prepared with sterile technique, including drapes, gloves, and skin cleansing with benzalkonium chloride. A small (8 Fr) straight or indwelling catheter should be used for a child; for an infant, a No. 5 feeding tube may be used. The catheter or tube should be coated with sterile lubricating jelly. For a female, the labia majora and minora should be widely separated so that the urethral meatus may be identified, cleansed, and entered with the catheter. For a male, the penis is held at a right angle to the abdomen while the catheter is placed in the urethra and is advanced until urine is obtained. If the catheter is to be indwelling, the retaining balloon should be filled with sterile saline or water. The amount of fluid and the site of filling are shown on the catheter itself. When an indwelling catheter is used, it is necessary to establish a closed, sterile urine-collection system.

The catheter should not be forced. Extreme care must be exercised in children who have an acquired or congenital coagulopathy. It is possible to "false pass" a catheter and damage the urethra in both male and female children.

Percutaneous Suprapubic Bladder Aspiration. To obtain sterile urine specimens, a percutaneous suprapubic bladder aspiration is especially useful in infants. Before attempting this procedure, the physician should ensure that the child has not voided for at least 1 hour. An assistant should hold the child in the supine frog-leg position while the operator percusses the bladder above the symphysis pubis and prepares the skin with alcohol. To prevent urination during the procedure, the urethra should be compressed by pressure through the rectum of the female or by direct pressure to the penis of the male. The abdominal wall is entered in the midline 1 to 2 cm above the symphysis pubis with a 22-gauge, 1-inch needle attached to a syringe (Fig. B-8). The needle should be directed slightly cephalad, and negative pressure is maintained in the syringe as it is advanced. Urine entering the barrel of the syringe signals a successful bladder tap.

The procedure may be repeated once if no urine is obtained in the first attempt. If the repeat attempt is unsuccessful, an hour should be allowed to elapse before another attempt is made. When urine is obtained, the needle is withdrawn smoothly, and the entry site is covered with a dry dressing. Complications include transient hematuria and, rarely, perforation of the bowel.

Other Body Cavities

Tympanocentesis. Tympanocentesis is required for bacteriological diagnosis of otitis media in infants and compromised hosts in whom identification of gram negative and

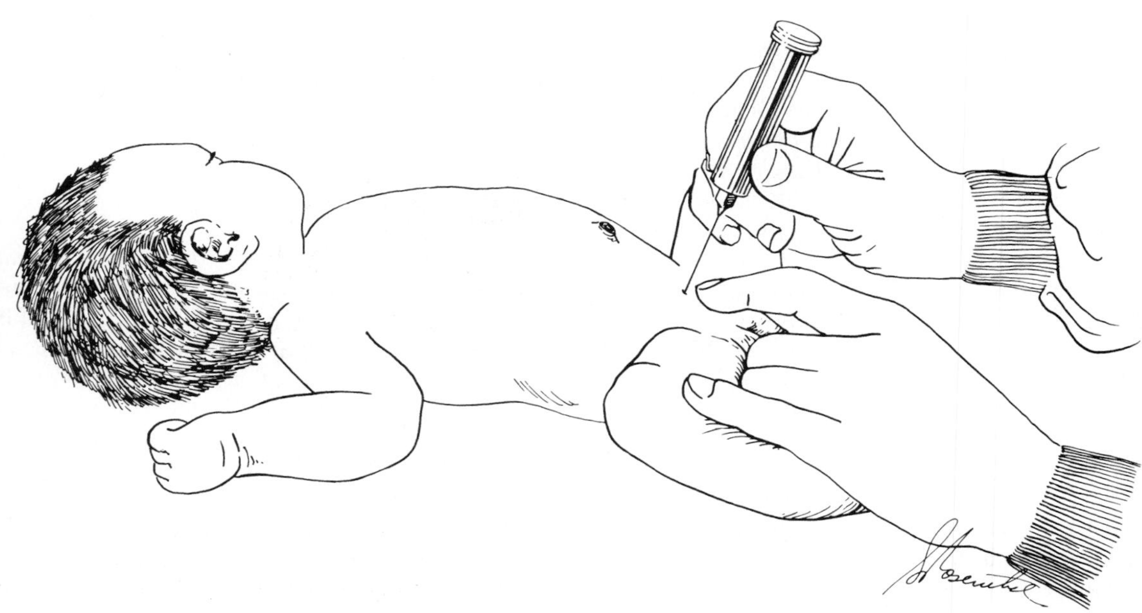

FIG. B-8 Position of an infant before aspiration of urine by suprapubic aspiration. A right-handed physician's left index finger is placed on the symphysis pubis.

other organisms is particularly important. This maneuver also may be therapeutic because it reduces middle-ear pressure. The procedure is contraindicated if the patient has a bleeding disorder.

The child is mummy-wrapped and restrained by the assistant, who should hold the child's head absolutely immobile. The otic canal is cleansed with cotton swabs and alcohol or benzalkonium chloride. After cleansing and before the puncture, specimens should be taken from the ear canal and cultured to identify contaminating organisms.

The tympanic membrane is visualized through the open-ended otoscope. A 3½-inch, 20- or 22-gauge spinal needle with a double bend (Z shape) allows clear visualization of the tip along its axis (Fig. B-9). The needle is connected directly to a tuberculin syringe. The plunger of the syringe is removed, and one end of the length of tubing is placed over the proximal end of the syringe's barrel. The other end of the tubing is placed in the physician's mouth so that controlled negative pressure can be created within the needle-syringe-tubing apparatus. The needle is used to pierce the posteroinferior quadrant of the tympanic membrane, and gentle negative pressure is applied to withdraw middle-ear fluid. A drop should be Gram stained and the remainder cultured appropriately. If there is no visible fluid, the needle should be flushed with 2 to 3 ml of blood culture medium, which may then be Gram stained and cultured.

Abdominal Paracentesis and Peritoneal Dialysis Catheter Placement. The physician who encounters a critically ill child in an emergency department or an inpatient unit can easily obtain access to the child's peritoneal cavity. This might be

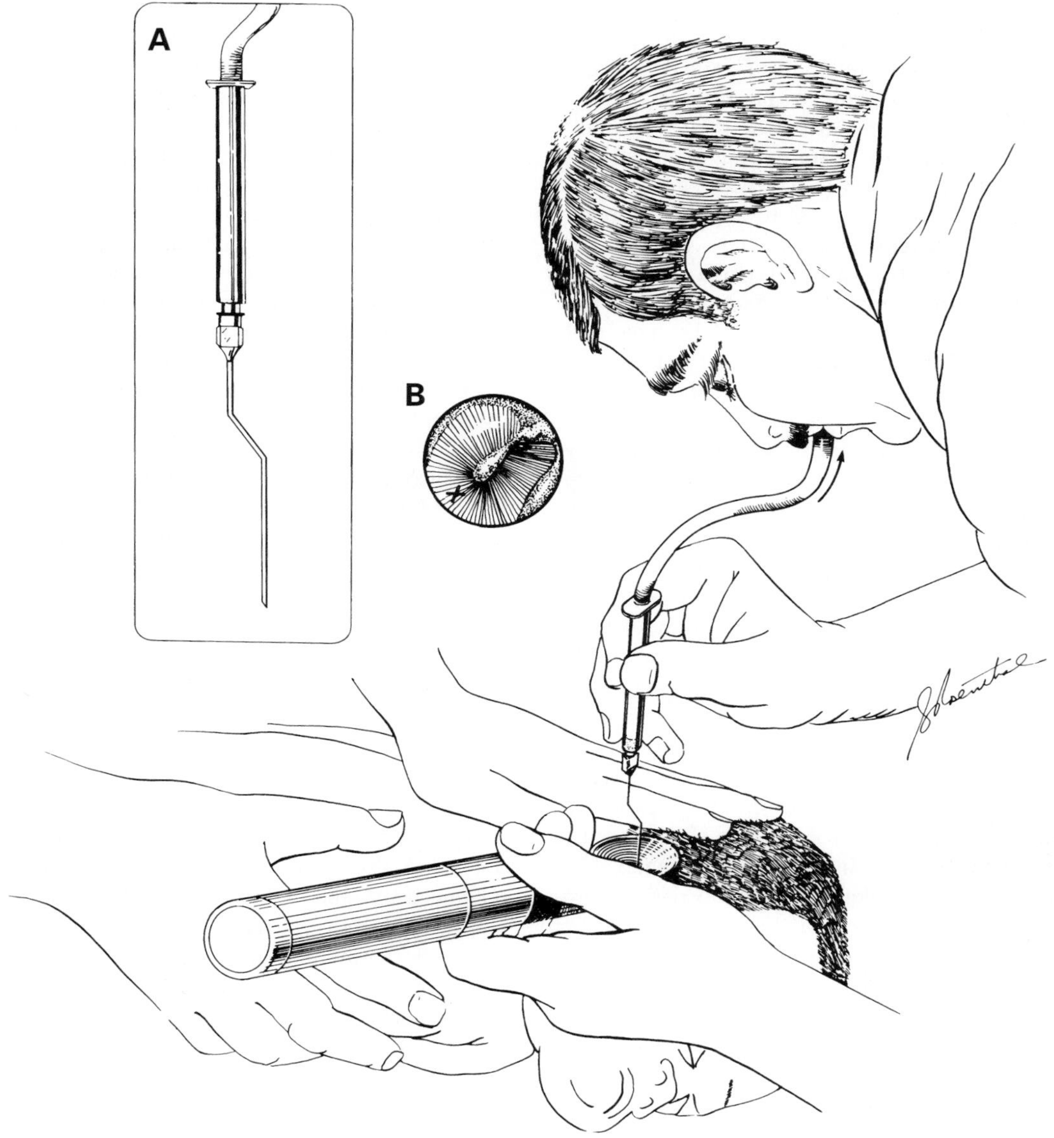

FIG. B-9 Tympanostomy. **A,** A 3-inch, 22-gauge spinal needle that has been shaped to allow direct visualization of the tympanic membrane through the operating otoscope. A tuberculin syringe barrel is attached to the needle, and tubing is attached to the syringe barrel. **B,** The preferred site on the right tympanic membrane for puncture and aspiration of the middle ear. Once the middle ear has been entered, the physician applies negative pressure through the end of the tubing placed in his or her mouth, as illustrated.

done to sample fluid for possible extravasated blood in a trauma victim; to obtain specimens for a white blood cell or differential count, or a Gram stain and culture; to institute peritoneal dialysis for the treatment of renal failure, hyperkalemia, azotemia, or fluid overload; or to remove a dialyzable toxin. Peritoneal dialysis also has been used to control body temperature in severe hypothermia or hyperthermia. Relative contraindications include coagulopathy, distended viscera, and local skin infection. Risks include perforation of bowel and bladder, bleeding, and introduction of infection. The removal of large amounts of ascitic fluid can cause hypotension. The patient should be sedated and placed in appropriate restraints. The abdomen should be prepared with strict aseptic technique. Three sites are available. The first is in the midline, one third of the distance between the umbilicus and the symphysis pubis. The second and third sites are in the right and left lower quadrants, lateral to the rectus muscle sheath and a few centimeters above the inguinal ligament. The bladder should be emptied. The preferred site is in the midline, 2 to 3 cm below the umbilicus. This should be infiltrated with 1% lidocaine. A catheter placed over a guide wire is recommended because the needle used to gain entry to the peritoneum is "protected" from cutting or perforating a viscus by the guide wire.

Peritoneal dialysis catheters are produced by several manufacturers in a variety of lengths and diameters. For paracentesis, lavage, and dialysis, two sizes of guide wire–placed peritoneal dialysis catheters may be used.* The catheters, available in diameters of 9 French (Fr) and 11 Fr, have multifenestrated tips. The catheter is made with the last few centimeters set at approximately a 30-degree angle, which aids placement.

The technique for guide wire–aided placement of a dialysis catheter for lavage or dialysis is simple. A needle, supplied with the manufacturer's "kit," is placed through the abdominal wall. Immediately after the peritoneum is entered, a guide wire of appropriate size is placed through the needle and advanced. The dialysis catheter is advanced over the wire until resistance is encountered. The wire then is removed, and the catheter can be attached to a syringe or intravenous tubing. A purse-string suture placed around the introduction site helps to prevent leakage. To test the system for patency and to document complete return of instilled fluid, an appropriate instillation volume is 20 ml/kg. Care must be taken in the choice of catheter to ensure that all the side holes will be inside the abdominal cavity. A Styrofoam cup can be used to hold the catheter upright over the patient's abdomen. This secures the position of the catheter and improves patient comfort.

Thoracentesis. Thoracentesis is used to remove pleural fluid for diagnosis; the technique also can be used for the emergency relief of tension pneumothorax. The site is determined by roentgenogram and by the findings on physical examination. When fluid is removed from the bases of the lungs, care must be taken that abdominal viscera are not damaged. Anteroposterior, supine, and lateral radiographs should be inspected to determine if the fluid is loculated. Ultrasound examination may help to determine the location of an effusion.

*Cook, Inc., Bloomington, Ind.

The positioning of the patient depends on whether the anterior or posterior aspect of the chest is to be entered. The patient should be sitting and leaning forward, either against the back of a chair while sitting, or against a bed stand when in bed. An infant or a small toddler may be held in a hugging fashion against an assistant's chest.

The needle is inserted in the anterior, middle, or posterior axillary line in the fourth, fifth, or sixth intercostal space. Other sites may be elected as dictated by the location of specific loculated collections of fluid.

A wide site is prepared with an appropriate antiseptic, and local anesthetic is infiltrated with a 25-gauge needle over the body of the rib just below the intended puncture site. The needle is inserted into the skin overlying the rib and then moved over the surface of the rib upward to the interspace, while gentle aspiration is alternated with infiltration of the anesthetic solution so that the subcutaneous tissues and the pleura are anesthetized. The intercostal blood vessels and nerves lie along the inferior margin of each rib and therefore can be avoided by this approach.

The complications of thoracentesis include pneumothorax, hemothorax, and introduction of infection. Laceration of the abdominal viscera through the diaphragm can be avoided by careful selection of the puncture site. An 18- to 22-gauge catheter needle combination, such as is used for venous access, a sterile 50 ml syringe, and a three-way stopcock can be used. The stylet, needle, and catheter are advanced along the previously described tract, with suction applied to the syringe. When the pleura is entered, the plastic cannula is threaded over the needle-stylet and advanced. The three-way stopcock is attached to the syringe and cannula, and fluid is aspirated and placed in appropriate containers for fungal, viral, and bacteriological cultures and Gram staining. Pleural fluid also may be examined for its white blood cell and differential counts, its protein, glucose, and lactate dehydrogenase (LDH) levels, and its cytological characteristics.

An alternative to tube thoracostomy for long-term drainage of effusions is placement of a pigtail catheter by use of a modified Seldinger technique.[9,18] An 8.5 Fr, 15 cm polyurethane tube is placed over a 0.035-inch guide wire.* A kit is supplied that contains the pigtail catheter, an 8 Fr dilator, a needle, a guide wire, and a "Christmas tree" adapter that Luer locks to the catheter and can be firmly attached to large-bore rubber tubing for continuous suction.

The tube is inserted by advancing the needle over the superior margin of a rib, usually T4 to T6, in the midline or anterior axillary line, into the pleural space. A guide wire is advanced through the needle into the pleural cavity. A small stab wound, 2 to 4 mm in diameter, is made at the site where the guide wire enters the skin. An 8 Fr, hard, polyurethane dilator is advanced over the wire. This enlarges the tract to facilitate passage of the catheter. With the wire position fixed, the dilator is withdrawn. The pigtail catheter then is threaded over the wire and advanced into the pleural space; then the wire is withdrawn. The pigtail catheter finally is attached to large-bore rubber tubing with the Christmas tree adapter placed on the appropriate suction device. The pressure in the suction device should be set at 15 to 20 cm H_2O. A chest roentgenogram should be taken to document the catheter's

*Cook, Inc., Bloomington, Ind.

position. The pigtail catheter can be secured to the chest with a small adhesive dressing and/or simply sutured and tied in place. This technique is quick, simple, complication free, and easy to teach; it also is especially valuable to transport and emergency room teams for treatment of pneumothorax.

Pericardiocentesis. Pericardiocentesis is a high-risk procedure. Its dangers must be weighed against the urgency of diagnosing a pericardial effusion or an unchecked cardiac tamponade.

Myocardial injury, laceration of a coronary artery, cardiac arrhythmia, and infection are possible complications of pericardiocentesis. The internal mammary arteries are within 2.5 cm of the sternal border, and they also may be damaged.

The alternate points of entry into the chest are illustrated in Figure B-10. The best site is at the chondroxiphoid angle. The others are in the fourth, fifth, and sixth intercostal spaces, 1 to 2 cm medial to the border of percussable cardiac dullness. A roentgenogram, fluoroscopy, and ultrasound examination also may aid in determining the border of the pericardium.

The patient, who may require sedation, should be supine at approximately a 30-degree angle and carefully restrained. A wide area of the precordium is prepared with an appropriate antiseptic. The chosen site is infiltrated with lidocaine. A 50 ml syringe then is connected to a three-way stopcock and an 18-gauge needle. An electrocardiogram V lead, with an alligator clip, is attached to the needle to detect an injury current should the myocardium or coronary artery be entered.

The needle is directed inward and medially when the intercostal approach is used. When the chondroxiphoid approach is used, the needle is aimed upward and posteriorly.

Gentle negative pressure should be applied to the syringe. The ECG should be monitored constantly and the needle withdrawn if an injury current is detected. The fluid should be aspirated slowly. The needle then is withdrawn, and a simple sterile dressing is applied over the puncture site.

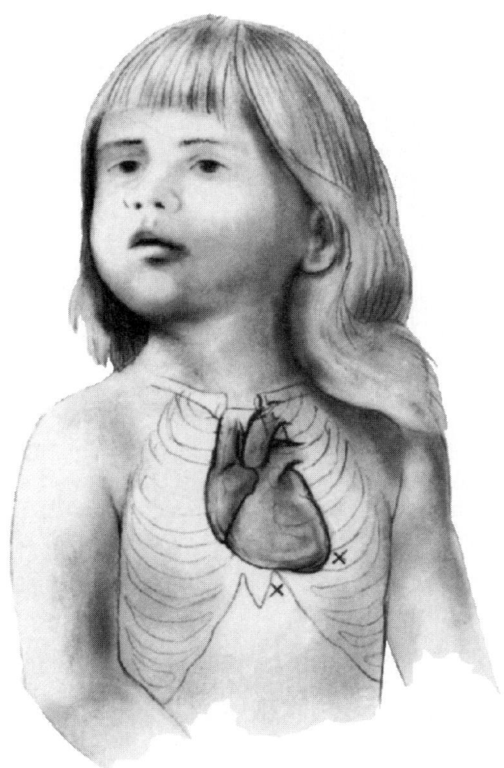

FIG. B-10 Pericardiocentesis. Two sites for aspiration of the pericardial sac are shown. These vary with the extent of the effusion, as determined by examination, contrast study, and/or echocardiography.

Bone Marrow Aspiration. Bone marrow samples aid in the diagnosis of leukemia, metastatic disease, and several of the "storage" diseases, such as the lipidoses. Culture of the bone marrow occasionally is indicated in cases of suspected sepsis. Bone marrow aspiration has few risks; infection is the greatest. It usually is performed safely in those who have thrombocytopenia.

The preferred site is the posterior iliac crest because it is easy to locate, the patient can be easily restrained for its performance, and the site contains active marrow in patients of all ages. Other sites include the tibia, femur, sternum, spinous vertebral process, and anterior iliac crest. The tibia is most useful in children under 18 months of age. The femur also is a useful site in this age group, but overlying muscle tissue makes the procedure more difficult. The sternum is the least safe site for children. The spinous vertebral process requires exceptional restraint of the patient and in general is a technically difficult site to use.

The needle used is a commercially available bone marrow needle and obturator.

The technique for using the posterior iliac crest is described here. The child is restrained in the prone position with a blanket roll or pillow placed under the hips. Use of sedation is effective. The site is scrubbed broadly with antiseptic. The iliac crest is palpable as a bony prominence lateral to the midline above the level of the gluteal cleft.

The site of aspiration is located approximately 1 cm below the lip of the crest. The overlying skin and subcutaneous tissues are infiltrated with local anesthetic down to the periosteum. The aspiration needle with its obturator is then pushed through the skin, angled toward the patient's head, and advanced to the periosteum. A steady, screwdriver-like rotation of the needle with applied pressure forces the needle into the marrow. A decrease in resistance may be felt as the bone's cortex is perforated. The obturator is removed, and a 20 ml sterile syringe is attached to its hub. Firm, quickly applied negative pressure will cause a few drops of blood to spurt into the syringe. Negative pressure should be terminated immediately to avoid dilution of the marrow specimen with peripheral blood. Approximately 1 ml of bone marrow should be aspirated. The syringe is carefully removed from the needle, and six to 10 meticulously cleaned slides are smeared. The obturator then is reinserted, the needle removed, and a sterile dressing applied over the puncture site.[17]

EMERGENCY THERAPEUTIC PROCEDURES

Emergency Intravenous Access Protocol

Significant delay commonly is encountered in the establishment of intravenous access in the critically ill child.[24] The small size of the pediatric patient, the stress of the situation, and venous collapse make insertion of a peripheral intravenous device difficult. An algorithmic, protocol approach to the problem of establishing venous access has been suggested.[14] In one series of pediatric resuscitations, more than 10 minutes was required to establish venous access, and in 6% of the subjects no access could be established. In one algorithm suggested for use in cardiopulmonary resuscitation, attempts at peripheral vein insertion would be made for 1½ minutes.[22,23]

Physicians who might encounter critically ill children should consider the development of such venous access protocols and algorithms. These should be tailored to the needs of the institution or site and to those of the practitioner.

Standard of care guidelines demand early use of the intraosseous needle. All clinicians who might encounter children in cardiovascular collapse should familiarize themselves with this quick, simple, and easy to learn technique.

When caring for a child in cardiovascular or respiratory collapse, undue time must not be spent on attempts at placing peripheral or central venous lines. Placement of a central venous catheter should not be attempted by those inexperienced in the technique. Central venous access is not required for cardiopulmonary resuscitation nor in the early, important stages of shock treatment. If venous access cannot be achieved in 3 minutes, an intraosseous device should be placed.[4]

Likewise, even if the practitioner is skilled in the saphenous vein cutdown procedure, it should not be attempted for venous access in an arrest or shock resuscitation. Cutdown may be indicated for chronic venous access after successful resuscitation.[11]

Intraosseous Infusions

Intraosseous infusion is a procedure that should be familiar to all who provide care to children.[28] This easily learned technique can be used for any critically ill child whenever a delay in establishing venous access might compromise the patient. In many situations, obtaining venous access is time-consuming. A surgeon, intensivist, or anesthesiologist must be brought in to establish a central venous catheter by guide wire or to perform a cutdown. These actions can cause needless delay in treatment. The ability to place an intraosseous needle allows even a technically inexperienced person to gain immediate access to the intramedullary venous system, which is continuous with the venous circulation (Fig. B-11). Crystalloid and colloid for fluid resuscitation, blood, plasma, catecholamines (e.g., epinephrine and dopamine), glucose, calcium, and sodium bicarbonate all can be administered by the intraosseous technique.[4,21] Although a standard 18- or 20-gauge spinal needle with stylet and bone marrow biopsy needles are useful in extreme situations, intraosseous needles, manufactured specifically for this purpose, are available and preferable. The proximal and distal tibias are the sites of choice. The iliac crest, sternum, and femur are alternate sites. The anterior medial surface of the proximal tibia or the medial surface of the distal tibia proximal to the medial malleolus is a preferred site (Figs. B-12 and B-13). The epiphysis must be avoided when the proximal tibia is used. The cortex in the midshaft of the tibia is difficult to penetrate, although this sometimes is used in emergencies. In a child over age 6, the thick cortex at the proximal tibia prevents easy use of this site; the distal tibia is recommended in this instance. The site is aseptically prepared. Then the needle is advanced perpendicular to the bone, with firm pressure and rotary motion.

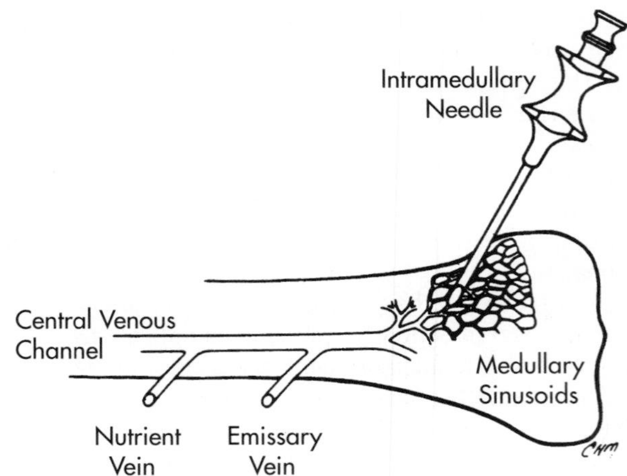

FIG. B-11 The intramedullary venous system demonstrates the position of an intraosseous needle in the medullary sinusoids. Blood may be aspirated from the sinusoids to confirm the position of the needle.

(From Spivey WH: *J Pediatr* 5:111, 1987.)

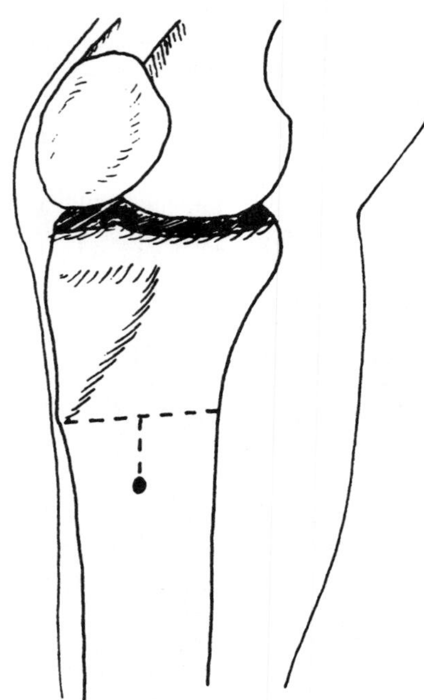

FIG. B-12 Insertion site in the proximal tibia. The tibial tuberosity and medial border of the tibia are palpated. The needle is inserted halfway between these points and 1 or 2 cm distally, pointing away from the joint space and in a caudal direction.

(From Spivey WH: *J Pediatr* 5:111, 1987.)

Entry to the marrow cavity is detected by decreasing resistance. Aspiration with a syringe should produce blood and marrow. To clear the needle, it should be flushed with 3 to 5 ml of sterile saline in a sterile syringe. The device then is connected to standard intravenous tubing. Although the flow rate is slower than that observed in a standard device, it should be steady, with no evidence of extravasation at the site. If the needle dislodges or fluid extravasates, the opposite leg should be used. If large volumes are required, two

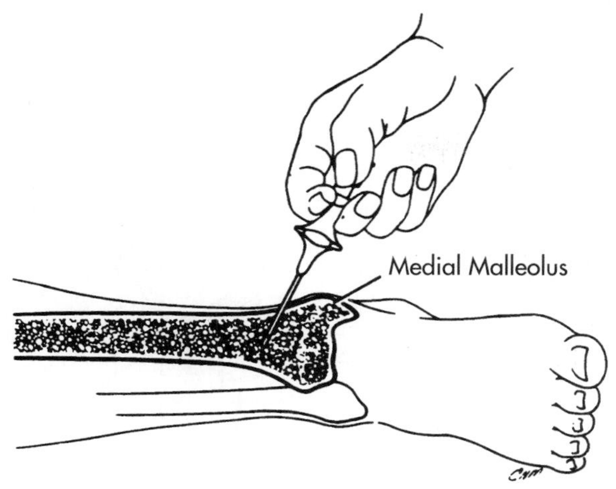

FIG. B-13 The position of an intraosseous needle in the distal tibia. The needle is inserted into the medial surface of the distal tibia at the junction of the malleolus and shaft of the tibia. It is inserted away from the joint space in a cephalad direction.

(From Spivey WH: *J Pediatr* 5:111, 1987.)

devices should be placed. A second device should not be placed on the same leg after removal of the first device, because leakage will occur. Resuscitative drugs should be "flushed" in after 3 to 5 ml of saline have been injected.

INFUSIONS

Percutaneous Intravenous Infusion

Figure B-2 depicts the location of accessible superficial veins suitable for percutaneous intravenous infusions. The veins of the extremities and scalp are commonly used; the latter have no valves and can be punctured in either direction. Skin preparation should be especially meticulous when scalp veins are used because they communicate by means of emissary veins with the dural sinuses.

The child is positioned and immobilized, and the extremity is immobilized further by being taped firmly to a padded board or sandbag. A tourniquet is applied above the vein to be infused, and the skin is cleansed with alcohol. A butterfly 22- or 25-gauge needle or a 20- or 22-gauge intravenous catheter needle (Longdwel or Medicut) filled with saline and attached to the intravenous tubing and solution bottle is used to enter the vein in the direction of venous flow. When the vein is entered, the tourniquet is removed and the blood flow is tested by opening the intravenous tubing to allow the solution to be infused to flow or by gently injecting saline through the needle with a syringe.[32]

If the flow is adequate and there is no extravasation of fluid, a piece of tape is placed over the entry site and the wings of the butterfly needle are taped to the skin. A pad may be used under the hub of the needle to maintain the angle that best allows free flow of fluid. A protective cover is taped over the needle, and the adequacy of the restraints is checked (Fig. B-14). If percutaneous needle catheterization is performed, the vein is entered as described above. When blood is seen in the hub of the needle, it is stabilized and the catheter sleeve is advanced up the vein. The catheter then is stabilized, the needle removed, and the blood flow checked before the catheter hub is taped in position and the intravenous tubing attached.

Cutdown Intravenous Infusion

A *cutdown* intravenous infusion may be required if a vein cannot be entered percutaneously. Generally, these children are chronically ill, and conventional percutaneous catheter placement sites have been exhausted. The useful "life" of a cutdown is less than 5 days. Thus, if chronic access will be a continuing requirement, a chronic indwelling Silastic catheter placed by a surgeon is more appropriate.[11] The catheter is removed by pulling it out through the wound and applying local pressure. The wound sutures should be removed 3 to 4 days after they are placed.

The great saphenous vein is preferred because its position is constant, anterior to the medial malleolus running cephalad, so it may be found even when not visible through the skin. The child is positioned and the limb restrained on a padded board, as for a percutaneous infusion. A tourniquet is applied in the midcalf region, and surgical aseptic technique is observed. Local anesthesia is produced by infiltration of the skin over the site of the incision with 1% lidocaine. A transverse incision, 2 to 3 cm, should be made 1 cm superior and anterior to the medial malleolus, and the skin and superficial fascia should be widely spread. Blunt dissection is used to isolate and identify the vein (Fig. B-15). A curved hemostat is used to scoop the vein off the periosteum and up into the wound. The vein should be freed from connective tissue for 1 to 2 cm along its length by blunt dissection and two No. 000 silk ligatures passed under it. The distal ligature is used to tie off the lower portion of vein and to provide caudal traction on the vein.

An intravenous catheter needle may be used to enter the vein, as described in the section on percutaneous intravenous infusion, or a small nick may be made in the vein and an intravenous cannula threaded cephalad for 2 to 5 cm. The proximal ligature is then firmly tied around the vein and cannula. The wound is closed with fine silk sutures, one of which should be tied around the catheter to anchor it. The wound is dressed with a gauze bandage and cleansed daily.

Heparin Lock

An intravenous catheter needle or a plastic indwelling catheter may be converted to *heparin lock* for intermittent administration of medications or drawing of blood samples. The possible sites are, in order of preference, the great saphenous vein at the ankle, the anterior cubital veins, the external jugular vein, the saphenous vein in the femoral triangle, and the femoral vein.

Heparin in normal saline solution is used to flush and fill the needle and tubing or the catheter. A concentration of 10 units of heparin per milliliter averts heparinization of the patient but still prevents clotting within the needle or catheter; an adapter (which has a rubber diaphragm attached for repeated intermittent injections, infusions, or blood drawing, yet protects the needle or catheter orifice from contamination) is attached to the hub of the indwelling needle or catheter. Prolonged use of any indwelling device carries the risk of local and disseminated infection. Care must be taken to sterilize the adapter port with iodophor solution before each use. When the device is used, 1 to 2 ml of blood should be

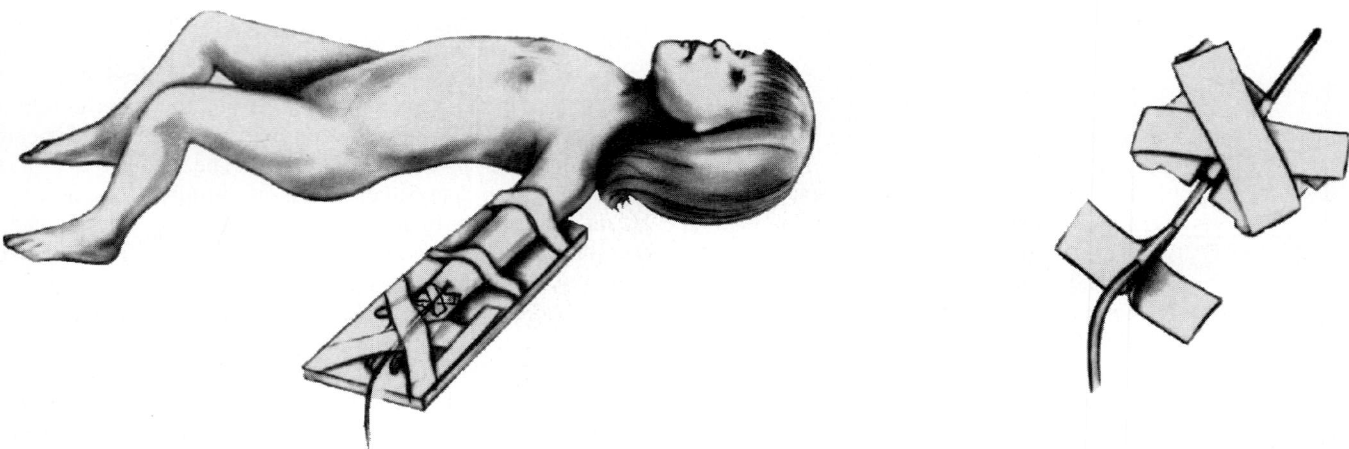

FIG. B-14 Immobilization of the upper extremity for intravenous infusion and a method of securing the needle and tubing with tape.

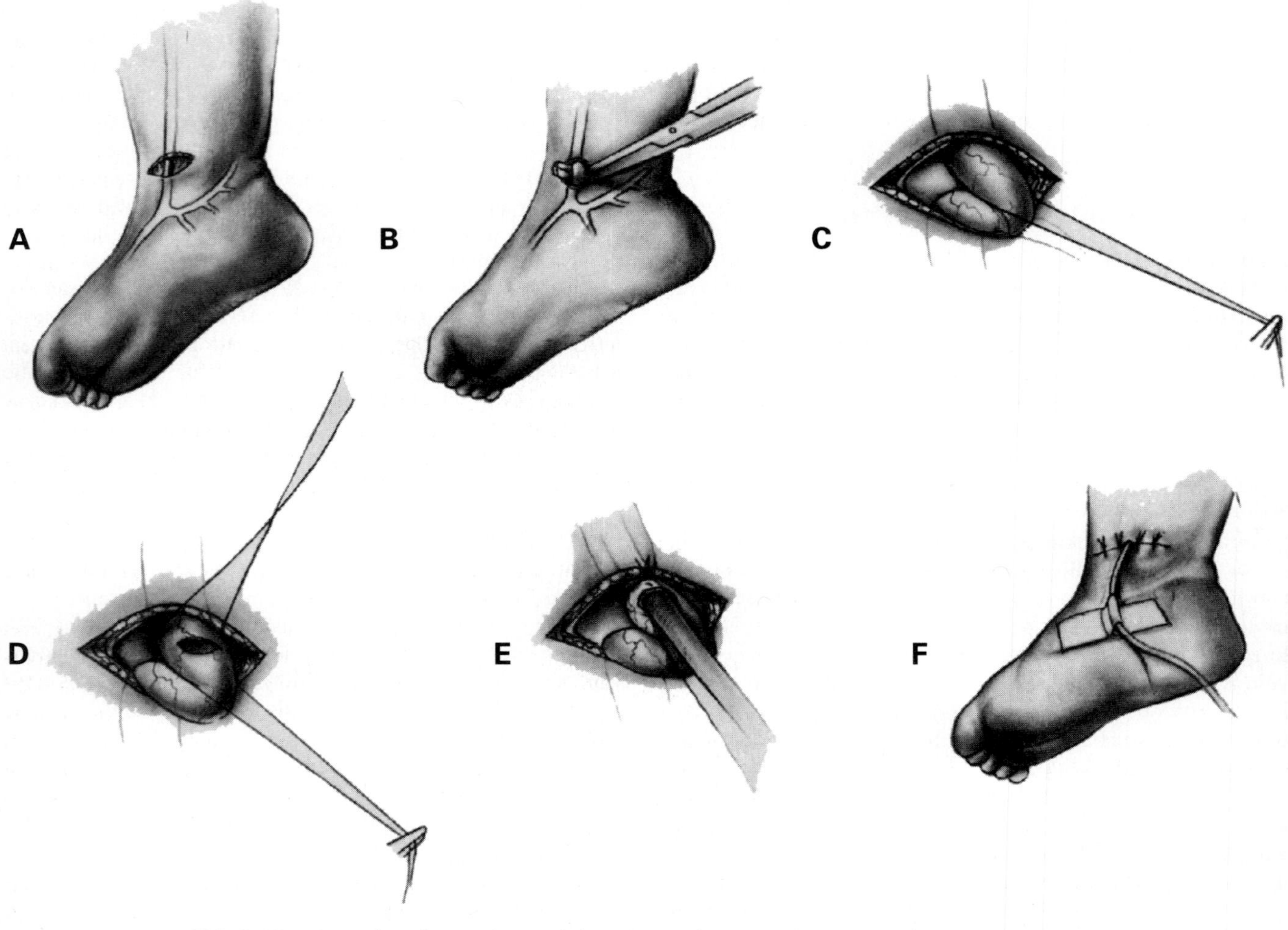

FIG. B-15 Procedure for cutdown of the great saphenous vein. **A,** Site of incision anterior to the medial malleolus. **B,** Elevation of the vein into the wound with a curved clamp. **C,** Application of distal ligature for traction. **D,** Loosely placed proximal ligature and venostomy incision. **E,** Venous catheter tied in place. **F,** Wound sutured and catheter secured.

aspirated before sampling to avoid contamination with heparin and the indwelling fluid. Only the volume of the device should be filled with the heparinized saline. The saline should be changed every 12 hours.

Femoral Venous Cannulation

The femoral vein is a safe, easily accessible vessel for cannulation with a single- or multiple-lumen catheter. The femoral catheter is safe, and with reasonable care it can be used for relatively long-term access as well. Several investigators have reported successful use of femoral venous catheters with minimal infectious complications. In fact, femoral venous catheters compare favorably over other sites in complications from infection.* The consistent anatomy of the area and proximity to the femoral arterial pulse allow the vessel to be easily located, because it lies 1 to 2 cm medial to the artery and 2 to 4 cm below the inguinal ligament. A transcutaneous Doppler device with a hand-held probe and earphones can help locate the artery when the pulse is difficult to palpate.† When the femoral arterial pulse cannot be located because of obesity or hypotension, as is the case in cardiac arrest, the femoral artery easily can be confused with the vein and inadvertently catheterized. In severe cardiorespiratory embarrassment the color of aspirated blood and blood gas tensions may confuse the operator and prevent discrimination of artery from vein.

Placement is simple and easily learned. The patient should be supine and in four-point restraints. The groin area should be widely prepared with an appropriate antiseptic agent. In young children, placement of a Foley catheter in the bladder prevents urine from contaminating the site. The femoral artery is palpated 2 to 4 cm below the inguinal ligament, and the vein is 1 to 2 cm medial to the artery. The skin and immediate subcutaneous tissues are infiltrated with 1% lidocaine. Manufacturer-supplied kits that contain an introducer needle, dilator, guide wire, and catheter are available.‡ The appropriate-size catheter has an outer diameter of 3 to 4 Fr for patients under 1 year of age, 5 to 6 Fr to age 7, and 7 Fr for children 8 years or older. A syringe that contains 2 to 3 ml of heparinized saline is attached to the introducer needle. The needle is introduced at a 30- to 45-degree angle from horizontal and aimed at the umbilicus. Care should be taken to avoid advancing the needle beyond the inguinal ligament because the peritoneum, bowel, and bladder can be perforated. With continuous, gentle aspiration the needle is advanced into the vein. When good blood return is documented, the syringe is removed. The guide wire then is advanced into the vein. There should be minimal resistance to the passage of the wire. If resistance is encountered, the needle and wire must be removed simultaneously to avoid shearing the wire off in the patient's vein. The needle is then withdrawn, leaving the wire in place. An incision, 2 to 4 mm, is made with a scalpel where the guide wire enters the skin. A dilator is threaded over the wire and passed through skin and subcutaneous tissue into the vessel, then withdrawn, again leaving the wire in place. The catheter is threaded over the wire. Care must be taken to ensure that at least 1 to 2 cm of the guide wire extends from the proximal end of the catheter before it is threaded into the vein. Otherwise, the wire can be "lost" in the vessel. Being careful not to change the position of the wire, the practitioner slowly advances the catheter over the wire to the desired distance, then removes the wire. For central venous pressure measurement, the catheter tip should be placed just above the diaphragm. The position should be verified by roentgenogram. The catheter then is sutured in place.

Complications include bleeding, infection, inadequate venous drainage, thrombus formation, and inadvertent penetration of viscera or a vessel wall. These must be weighed against the benefits of obtaining secure, large-bore venous access and the need to determine the central venous pressure.

*References 13, 15, 27, 29, 30, 32.

†Parks Electronics Laboratory, Beaverton, Ore.

‡Cook, Inc., Bloomington, Ind.; Arrow International, Inc., Reading, Pa.

Subclavian Vein Catheter Placement

The subclavian vein is a readily accessible site that provides a secure central conduit for (1) fluid administration (including hypertonic or irritating solutions that cannot be infused into peripheral veins), (2) maintenance of cardiac output by direct infusions of pressor drugs, and (3) central venous pressure monitoring.[33]

The procedure incurs the risk of pneumothorax or accidental penetration of the subclavian artery, with hematoma formation or thrombosis-induced obstruction of venous return. The operator first should be familiar with the use of the Seldinger technique for percutaneous placement of a catheter over a guide wire placed through an introducer needle.

Catheterization kits* provide a guide wire, catheters, and an introducer needle. The following sizes of catheters are used: 3 Fr in infants, 4 Fr in toddlers, 5 Fr in children 4 to 12 years of age, and 7 Fr for adolescents. The right subclavian vein is preferred over the left because of its more direct entry to the superior vena cava and because there is less risk of pneumothorax (the right lung lies lower in the thorax than the left) and injury to the thoracic duct, which lies in the left hemithorax.

The patient is placed in the Trendelenburg position and is restrained. The child's face is turned 90 degrees away from the intended puncture site. A 3-inch thick towel roll is placed along the long axis of the thoracic spine between the shoulder blades.

The area overlying the puncture site is cleansed widely, and drapes are used to provide an aseptic field. Masks, gloves, and gowns are used.

The subclavian vein is cannulated by the infraclavicular approach. The vein lies approximately parallel to the proximal third of the clavicle and is accessed in a triangle bounded by the medial third of the clavicle, the anterior scalene muscle, and the upper surface of the first rib. The subclavian artery runs posterior to the vein behind the anterior scalene muscle. Using a 1½-inch, 22-gauge needle, the skin overlying the puncture site and intended insertion tract is infiltrated with 1% lidocaine.

The introducer needle is placed just medial to the midclavicular line 2 to 3 cm below the inferior border of the clavicle. The needle is aimed toward the midsternal notch and is advanced to the inferior border of the medial portion of the clavicle. A syringe containing a few milliliters of heparinized saline is attached to the introducer needle, and with negative

*Available from Cook, Inc., Bloomington, Ind.

pressure applied to the barrel of the syringe, the needle is advanced deep to the clavicle on a course nearly parallel to its medial portion. Small cephalad adjustments of the target point (approximately 0.25 cm increments) can be made if the vein is not entered immediately.

When the vein has been entered, as evidenced by blood entering the syringe, the hub of the introducer needle is held securely in place by the physician, and the syringe is removed.

Caution must be exercised in a spontaneously breathing patient because air may be introduced into the vein as the patient increases the negative pleural pressure when initiating a breath. Therefore, the patient must be instructed to hold his or her breath, or as with infants and children, the orifice of the needle must be occluded temporarily. The flexible, floppy end of the guide wire now is inserted into the introducer needle and advanced through the bore of the needle into the subclavian vein and beyond into the superior vena cava. A minimum of 3 cm of wire is passed beyond the estimated tip of the needle. A cardiac arrhythmia may signal that the guide wire has been passed too far into the right ventricle, in which case it should be drawn back a bit. The distal end of the wire is held securely, and the introducer needle is removed.

The catheter is flushed with heparin solution and advanced over the guide wire to the desired position in the superior vena cava; care should be taken not to advance the wire simultaneously. The guide wire then is removed, and the proximal end of the catheter is attached to the desired intravenous fluid–administration system or the central venous pressure–monitoring system.

The position of the catheter should be verified roentgenographically. The catheter must be placed so that the distal tip is in the middle third of the superior vena cava. This helps to prevent the complications of vessel or atrium perforation.

Umbilical Vein Catheterization

Catheterization of the umbilical vein is useful in newborns for emergency correction of acidosis, hypoglycemia, and hypotension, in the performance of exchange transfusions, and for the measurement of central venous pressure. The complications of umbilical vein catheterization include sepsis and microembolization from catheter-induced thrombosis. An umbilical venous catheter easily can be misplaced into a branch of the portal venous system, and the injection of hyperosmolar solutions containing substances such as glucose and sodium bicarbonate can lead to portal vein thrombosis and hepatic necrosis. Umbilical vein catheters also have been implicated in cases of necrotizing enterocolitis and spontaneous perforation of the large bowel.[17]

A radiopaque catheter must be used in umbilical vein catheterization to allow verification of its position by roentgenogram. The small premature infant is susceptible to chilling during the catheterization procedure, and use of a radiant warmer, an Isolette, or a heating blanket is necessary. The equipment found on a cutdown tray, with the addition of fine-toothed pickup forceps, is adequate. The catheter size is selected on the basis of the weight of the baby: a 3.5 Fr catheter should be used for infants weighing less than 1500 g and a 5 Fr catheter for those weighing more. Special attention to aseptic techniques, including surgical scrubbing of the operator's hands, antiseptic preparation of the baby's abdomen and umbilical cord, and maintenance of a sterile field, is essential. The physician should be gloved, masked, and gowned as for any surgical procedure.

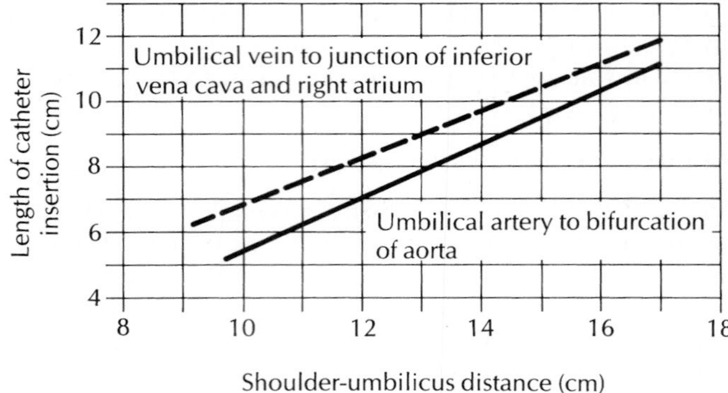

FIG. B-16 Method of determining the optimal length for umbilical catheter insertion.

The length that the catheter is to be inserted should be determined by measuring the distance from the infant's shoulder to the umbilicus by the conversion method shown in Figure B-16. This length ideally places the catheter at the junction of the inferior vena cava and the right atrium. Care must be taken not to cover the infant's chest in such a manner that apnea or malfunction of the heat probes or monitor leads will go undetected. An assistant provides gentle traction to the cord stump while the physician transects the cord with a scalpel 1 to 1.5 cm above the skin. Gauze sponges should be available for tamponade to control oozing of blood from the umbilical vein; the amount of oozing usually is insignificant. The cord stump is inspected to locate the thin-walled umbilical vein and the two thick-walled umbilical arteries. The catheter is attached to a three-way stopcock and a syringe containing heparinized saline solution (1 unit of heparin per milliliter of saline), and the catheter is filled. Minimal traction on the superior edge of the cord stump may be helpful in locating the orifice of the umbilical vein; this is dilated gently with pickup forceps or a small probe, and the catheter is introduced the predetermined distance (Fig. B-17). Resistance occasionally is met at the level of the abdominal wall or at the level of the ductus venosus. Very gentle pressure and partial withdrawal and rotation of the catheter usually overcomes this resistance; force should not be used. The position of the catheter should be verified by roentgenogram except under emergency circumstances.

Care must be taken to avoid iatrogenic blood loss through accidental dislodgment of the catheter. A purse-string suture around the umbilical stump and careful taping of the catheter to the abdominal wall help to avoid this. Antibiotic ointment and a dressing that will show any significant blood loss from the stump should be applied lightly over the umbilicus after successful catheterization. Current practice discourages keeping umbilical vein catheters in place for long periods; however, if neonatal transport requires fixation of the catheter, this can be accomplished with a purse-string suture, a bridge of adhesive tape (Fig. B-17), or umbilical cord tape. Fortunately, these rarely are needed for hemostasis alone. Application of an antibiotic ointment and daily inspection of the

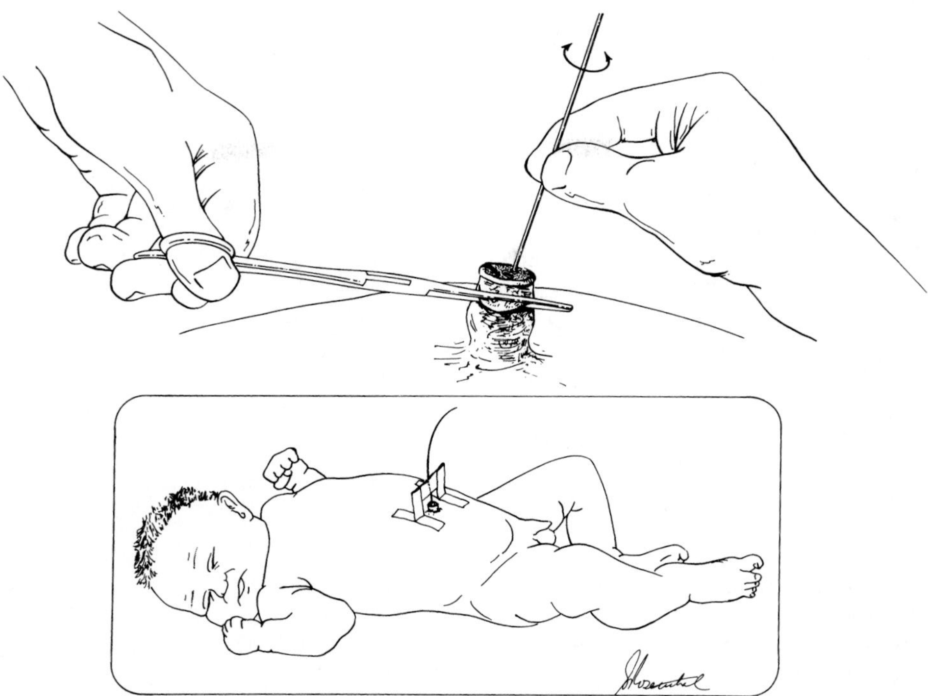

FIG. B-17 Umbilical vessel cannulation. The hemostat is used to grasp the edge of the cord stump, which then is rolled toward the physician to allow visualization and provide stability. A probe is shown in the physician's right hand. Gentle pressure and a rolling motion are used to dilate the orifice of the vessel. The lower portion of the illustration shows a method of taping that fixes the catheter's position, preventing it from penetrating deeper or becoming dislodged. A light dressing can be placed over the umbilicus to guard against local infection.

umbilical vein and stump for signs of local infection should follow removal of the catheter.

Umbilical Artery Catheterization

Catheterization of the umbilical artery is accomplished in a manner similar to catheterization of the umbilical vein, and the equipment used is the same. Its purpose is to provide access to the arterial circulation for monitoring blood pressure and blood gases and for infusion of selected solutions. Even in skilled hands, the procedure carries risks of embolization, sepsis, extravasation of blood, and distal arterial insufficiency. These complications must be considered in any determination of the risk/benefit ratio before performance of the procedure. Samples from the radial and temporal arteries are of preductal arterial blood and for single-measurement purposes are safer and more precise than is umbilical artery catheterization. Catheter placement at the point of bifurcation of the aorta is desirable to avoid damage to the renal arteries. The shoulder-umbilical length is measured, and the distance to the bifurcation of the aorta is determined by the conversion method shown in Figure B-16.

Attention to aseptic techniques is essential. The heavy-walled artery may be dilated gently. A rim of vessel wall is picked up gently with fine-toothed forceps. The catheter, filled with heparinized saline and attached to a closed three-way stopcock, then is introduced into the artery. Advancement of the catheter may be hindered by vasospasm; this can be overcome by applying slow, gentle pressure. Forceful probing should be avoided. If the catheter cannot be advanced, the other umbilical artery should be used. If resistance again is encountered and gentle pressure fails to advance the catheter, 0.1 to 0.2 ml of 1% or 2% lidocaine, without epinephrine, is instilled into the lumen of the artery. After 2 or 3 minutes the catheter can be advanced more easily.

The position of the catheter at the bifurcation of the aorta should be verified by roentgenogram. The catheter must be fixed carefully to the cord stump with a purse-string suture and to the abdomen with adhesive tape. An antibiotic ointment and a sterile dressing should be applied lightly, so as not to obscure blood loss, and the dressing should be changed daily.

The danger of iatrogenic accidents must be emphasized. Dislodgment of the catheters, stopcock leakage, and inadequate tamponade on removal of the catheter may result in significant blood loss. Failure to record and replace blood removed from the catheter may result in anemia and a deficit of fluid. Catheter removal is indicated when signs of ischemia of the lower extremities are present.

Exchange Transfusion

Prepackaged exchange transfusion sets with appropriate four-way stopcocks are available commercially. The operator must take time to become familiar with the function of the stopcock. If two standard stopcocks are used rather than the four way, extra care must be taken to prevent accidents.[5,17]

The equipment needed includes material for an umbilical catheterization, a source of heat (preferably an overhead radiant warmer), surgical drapes, gown, cap, mask, monitors for pulse and respiration, blood matched to infant and mother, resuscitation equipment, and 5 to 10 ml of 10% calcium gluconate solution.

The blood should be warmed with a blood warmer. Contrived hot water baths may cause lysis of red cells and are potentially dangerous.

Acid-citrate-dextrose blood, citrate-phosphate-dextrose blood, or heparinized preserved blood may be used. The first is adequate and usually available. A two-volume exchange should be performed. The amount of blood required is 170 ml/kg body weight, up to 500 ml. If possible, the blood bank should adjust the hematocrit of the donor blood to 55%. The hydropic infant, however, may require a very slow, careful exchange with packed red blood cells, while the assistant monitors central venous pressure and observes the patient for signs of congestive heart failure.

The infant should be restrained and the stomach emptied. The umbilicus should be prepared and draped and the venous catheter inserted. Plastic tubing connects the stopcock to the waste bag, the donor blood, and the umbilical vein catheter. The central venous pressure, blood pressure, pulse, and respirations are recorded throughout the procedure.

Blood initially is withdrawn from the baby and sent to the laboratory for determination of the values for central hematocrit, bilirubin, glucose, total protein, and serum electrolytes (sodium, chloride, carbon dioxide, calcium, potassium, and blood urea nitrogen).

Aliquots of 5 to 20 ml may be withdrawn and replaced, depending on the infant's age and cardiovascular stability. A rate of 3 to 5 ml/kg/min, or 1 to 1½ minutes per aliquot withdrawn and replaced, is desirable.

An assistant is required to record the vital signs, each volume exchanged, and a running exchange total. A person skilled at resuscitation and appropriate equipment also should be available.

If acid-citrate-dextrose blood is used, 1 ml of 10% calcium gluconate should be given for every 100 ml replaced. Irritability, tachycardia, and prolongation of the QT interval on the ECG are signs of hypocalcemia. If heparinized blood is used, 0.5 mg of protamine is given intramuscularly after the procedure.

The box on the right lists the potential complications of exchange transfusions.

The final aliquot of blood removed is sent to the laboratory for typing and cross-matching and for hematocrit and electrolyte determinations. The catheter then is withdrawn, and a sterile dressing is applied to the umbilicus. The infant is monitored intensively over the next 4 hours for cardiovascular stability, pulse, and blood pressure. During this time the infant should receive nothing by mouth and have intravenous hydration. From 4 to 6 hours after the procedure, determinations of hematocrit, bilirubin, and calcium should be repeated.

COMPLICATIONS OF EXCHANGE TRANSFUSIONS

- Vascular
  - Embolization with air or clots
  - Thrombosis
- Cardiac
  - Arrhythmias
  - Volume overload
  - Arrest
- Electrolyte
  - Hyperkalemia
  - Hypernatremia
  - Hypocalcemia
  - Acidosis
- Hematological
  - Overheparinization
  - Thrombocytopenia
- Infectious
  - Bacteremia
  - Serum hepatitis
- Miscellaneous
  - Mechanical injury to donor cells
  - Hypothermia
  - Hypoglycemia

Tube Thoracostomy

Pneumothorax is a common complication in the emergency care of infants, children, and adolescents. Placement of a thoracostomy tube (for drainage of air and fluid that has accumulated in the pleural cavity) by blunt dissection of a tract in the intercostal space with a hemostat is more tedious but safer than using a trocar unless the operator is experienced in the latter technique. A 12 Fr catheter should be used for infants and children up to age 3, a 16 Fr catheter for children up to age 10, and a 20 Fr catheter for older children and adolescents.

The fourth or fifth intercostal space in the anterior axillary line is the appropriate site. The pectoralis muscle, the nipple, and the intercostal arteries (at the inferior aspect of each rib) are to be avoided. The infant or child is placed in the supine position with the arm restrained above the head with appropriate assistance. The site is prepared and draped aseptically. Local anesthetic is infiltrated into the skin overlying the fifth or sixth rib by using a 22-gauge, 1½-inch needle. While the needle is advanced subcutaneously within the fourth or fifth intercostal space, the anesthetic is infiltrated within the soft tissues down to the level of and including the pleura.

A 2 cm skin incision over the intercostal space is made, and with blunt dissection a hemostat is introduced through the previously anesthetized tissues into the pleural cavity, as illustrated in Figure B-18. The chest tube then is clamped in the curved jaws of the hemostat and advanced through the dissected intercostal space tract to the pleural cavity. The tube ideally should lie anterior to the lung at its apex. The lateral orifices of the catheter must be well within the pleural cavity. The tube is secured with skin sutures, one on either side of the incision, wrapped around the tube, and tied tightly enough to crimp the tube slightly. A minimal dressing is applied so that malpositioning may be detected. Bulky dressings are not warranted. The dissected tract heals rapidly.

Common errors in the placement of thoracostomy tubes are subcutaneous placement, resulting from incomplete blunt dissection, and dislodgment caused by inadequate securement. Bleeding and infection rarely are encountered.

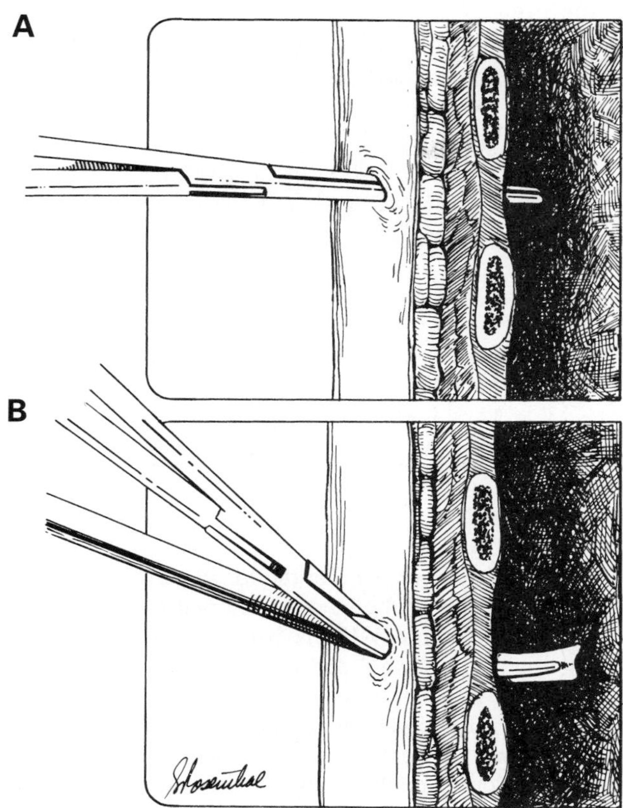

FIG. B-18 Placement of an intercostal chest tube. **A,** Formation of tract with hemostat. **B,** Insertion of tube with hemostat.

(From Wilkins EW Jr: *MGH textbook of emergency medicine*, ed 2, Baltimore, 1983, Williams & Wilkins.)

HAZARDS OF INTUBATION

Hyperextension or hyperflexion of the neck
Failure to clear the oropharynx of secretions
Failure to ventilate the patient manually with mask oxygen before and after unsuccessful attempts
Prolonged attempts, lasting longer than 30 seconds
Intubation of the esophagus
Intubation of the right main stem bronchus
Faulty or unavailable equipment
Haste

EQUIPMENT REQUIRED FOR INTUBATION

Laryngoscope handle: extra bulbs, batteries
Blades: Miller, sizes 00, 0, 1, and 2
Suction catheters: 5, 8, 10, 12, and 14 Fr
Source of suction
Endotracheal tubes: one size larger than deemed appropriate by age, one of adequate size, and one size smaller than deemed appropriate by age
Sterile lubricant
Oxygen supply
Ventilator bag with 15 mm universal female adapter (Hope, Ambu, Ohio)
Mask for ventilator bag: infant, child, and adult sizes
Tape
Tincture of benzoin
Nasogastric tubes

An alternative technique for immediate placement of a catheter in the chest for drainage involves using a guide wire and a pigtail catheter and is useful in emergencies and transport.

Endotracheal Intubation

It is essential for every physician who cares for children to master endotracheal intubation. Several hazards commonly accompany this process[5,8,17]; they are listed in the box above.

The key to success in intubation is approaching the procedure in a calm, deliberate way with a much-practiced technique and with equipment that is readily available and properly prepared. The equipment required for intubation is listed in the box above. A well-organized emergency tray, which is checked daily, is one of the most important items needed to perform this emergency procedure.

Preparation of the Patient. Protection of the airway and adequate oxygenation guarantee safe and successful intubation. Intubation always should be accompanied by administration of atropine (0.01 to 0.02 mg/kg, with a maximum dose of 1 mg). Use of a muscle relaxant to reduce respiratory effort may be indicated. When used, it should be accompanied by sedation. Succinylcholine (1 mg/kg given intravenously) is preferred as a muscle relaxant because it is metabolized rapidly.

Methohexital (Brevital) may be given as a light anesthetic during intubation (1 to 2 mg/kg intravenously), but it should be used with caution in a patient whose cardiovascular system is compromised secondary to shock or cyanotic congenital heart disease.

Midazolam is a useful, quick-acting induction agent. Atropine (0.01 mg/kg) should be administered because it blocks vagally induced bradycardia.

Emesis and subsequent aspiration are hazards encountered in emergency intubation. When the urgency of the situation does not allow for an anesthetist to be called, reasonable precautions can prevent complications.

Before any airway manipulation, a source of suction and a supply of suction catheters should be readily available. Downward pressure exerted on the cricoid cartilage effectively closes the esophagus and can prevent aspiration of oral or gastric material.

When possible, preoxygenation of the patient (3 minutes of breathing 100% oxygen) reduces complications. A pulse oximeter, ECG, and blood pressure monitor should be placed if time allows.

Technique of Intubation. During intubation, care must be taken to avoid damaging the teeth with the laryngoscope blade. A straight laryngoscope blade should be used; Portex or Murphy tubes are recommended because they are uniform in diameter and biologically nonreactive. A slight air leak is to be expected with a tube of appropriate size. The recommended sizes, according to the patient's weight and age, are shown in Table B-1.

Table B-1 Recommended Sizes of Endotracheal Tubes*

Patient's age	No. (Fr)	Internal diameter (mm)	Length (cm)	Adapter, internal diameter (mm)
Newborn				
<1 kg	11-12	2.5	10	3
>1 kg	13-14	3.0	11	3
1-6 mo	15-16	3.5	11	4
7-12 mo	17-18	4.0	12	4
13-18 mo	19-20	4.5	13	5
19-36 mo	21-22	5.0	14	5
3-4 yr	23-24	5.5	16	6
5 yr	25	6.0	18	6
6-7 yr	26	6.5	18	7
8-9 yr	27-28	7.0	20	7
10-11 yr	29-30	7.5	22	8
12-14 yr	32-34	8.0	24	8

*Tube should be of material labeled "I.T.-Z79" to satisfy standard tissue implant tests.

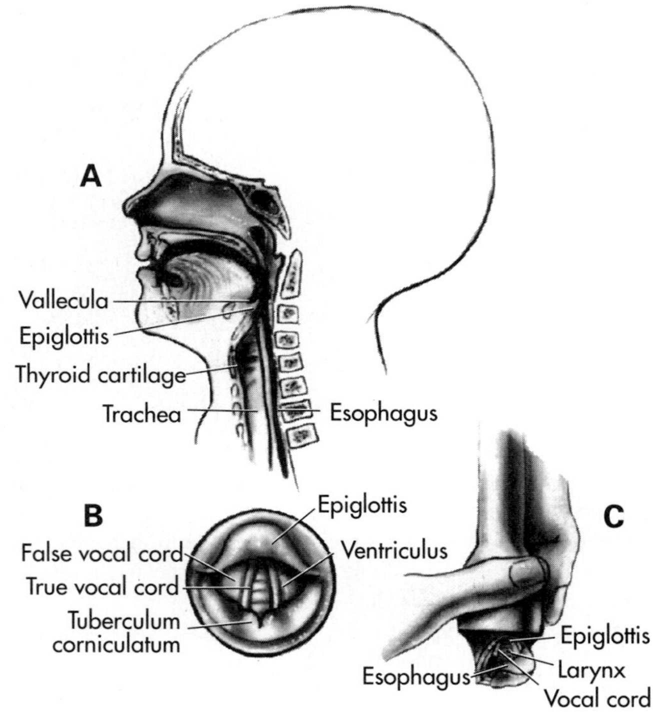

FIG. B-19 Endotracheal intubation. Relationship of the vallecula, the epiglottis, and the base of the tongue; note the cephalad position of the larynx in the infant **(A)**; an older child's larynx is positioned more caudally. **B,** The laryngeal structures as viewed from above. **C,** The small size and relative position of the vocal cords, the epiglottis, and the larynx as viewed through the laryngoscope.

Figure B-19 illustrates the relationship of the laryngoscope blade to the epiglottis and vocal cords. The endotracheal tube ideally should be positioned midway between the vocal cords and the carina. The patient should be placed on a firm surface with the head and neck in the so-called flower-sniffing position. The neck is extended only slightly and the jaw pulled forward only slightly. The nose and mouth are suctioned gently, and the patient is given oxygen by bag and mask for no more than 1 minute. The laryngoscope is held in the left hand. The blade is introduced into the mouth to the right of the tongue, so that the tongue will be deflected to the left. The tip of the blade is inserted to the vallecula. As illustrated in Figure B-19, the handle of the laryngoscope is tilted slightly backward and upward toward the operator. Care must be taken not to use the teeth or alveolar ridge as a fulcrum. The vocal cords should be in view. The tube can be advanced along the right side of the patient's mouth, inserted between the cords into the trachea, and advanced further to a position below the level of the vocal cords. Immediate auscultation of the lungs for symmetry of air movement is essential. If the right main stem bronchus is cannulated accidentally, the tube can be withdrawn to a safe position above the carina and checked again by auscultation. A chest roentgenogram should be obtained to ensure appropriate placement. The size, position of the tip of the tube in the trachea, and distance inserted from the patient's lip must be documented in the patient's record.[31]

Stabilizing the Tube. Stabilizing the tube is primarily a nursing care task and is subject to many variations. Figure B-20 illustrates one method. Some common problems encountered include the following:

1. Increased extension or flexion of the neck causes the tube to move up and down the trachea; therefore, care must be taken to stabilize the position of the neck when handling the patient. The rule of thumb is that the tip of the endotracheal tube follows the chin up or down.
2. Using too much tape may prevent adequate nasal and oral suctioning, and inspection for leaks and kinks in the tube may be hampered.
3. Tincture of benzoin may spill into the eyes.

Postintubation Care. The intubated infant or child requires exacting nursing care. The patient needs monitoring of vital signs and frequent physical examinations to ascertain the adequacy of ventilation. Pneumothorax, tube obstruction, and dislodgment of the tube must be anticipated in the care of these children.

Suctioning reduces tidal volume and available oxygen. It predisposes the patient to apnea and bradycardia. The physician and nurse should decide jointly how often suctioning should be done. Once an hour is a reasonable initial schedule. The need for this type of care is justification enough for referral to an intensive care unit. Suctioning of the tube is a

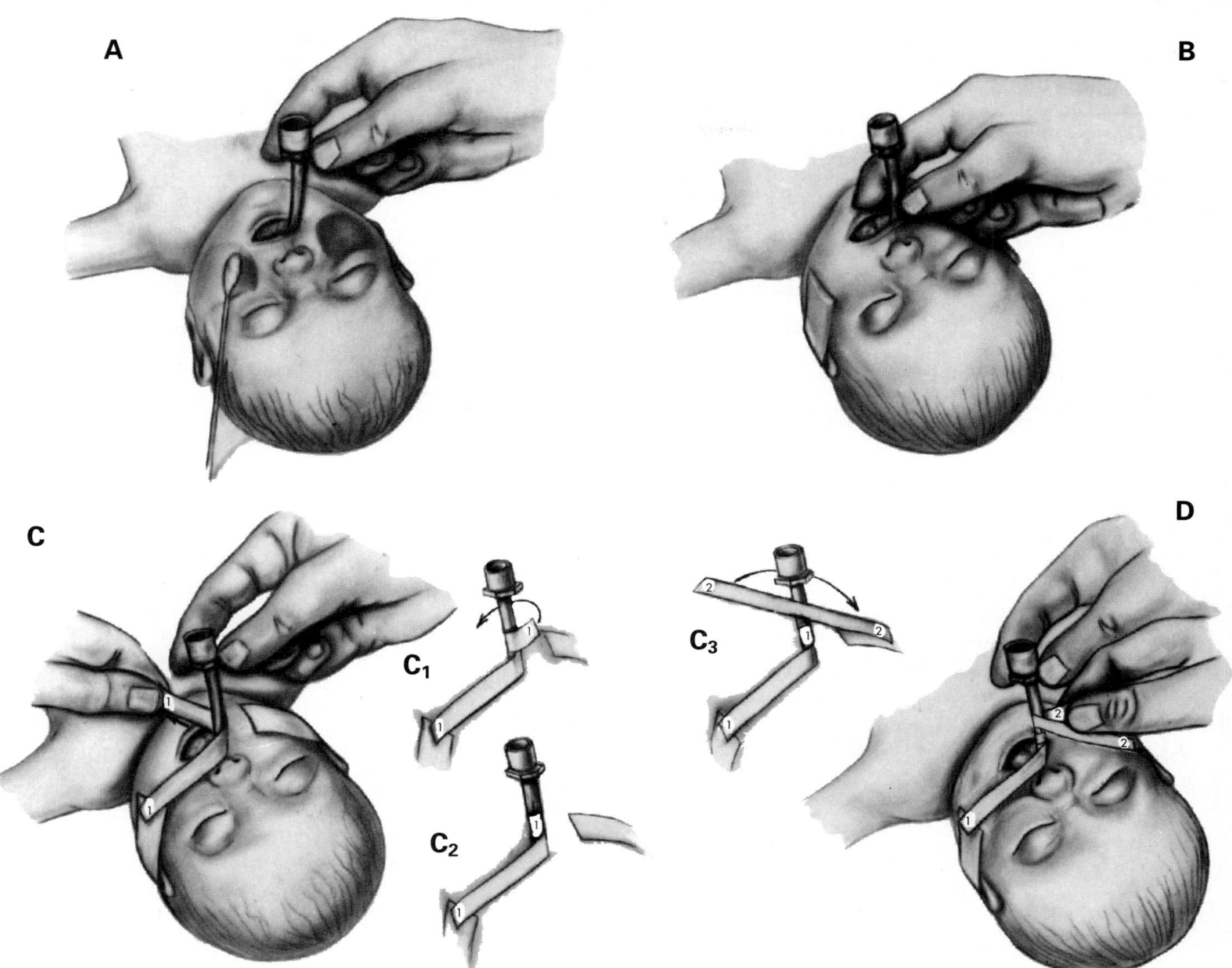

FIG. B-20 Securing an endotracheal tube. **A,** The cheeks and sides of the face are painted with tincture of benzoin (some neonatal intensive care units do not use benzoin because of its absorption and potential toxic effects). **B,** Wide pieces of elastic tape (Elastikon, Johnson & Johnson, New Brunswick, NJ) are placed over the sides of the face and pinnae. **C_1** to **C_2,** With the tube pulled to the right side of the mouth, a thin piece of tape *(1)* secures the tube on the left side of the face. **C_3** and **D,** Another piece of tape *(2)* then secures the tube on the right side of the face in a similar fashion.

nursing task primarily, but the physician should be aware of certain potential problems. The following is a safe method:

1. The endotracheal tube is disconnected from the ventilator.
2. Normal saline (0.25 to 0.5 ml) is instilled into the tube.
3. The infant receives ventilation for 60 seconds.
4. The head is turned to one side.
5. A sterile, end-hole catheter is passed a premeasured 1 to 2 cm beyond the tracheal tube's distal orifice.
6. Suction is applied after the catheter has been pulled back 1 cm.
7. Suction is applied as the catheter is withdrawn, over a 5-second interval.
8. The endotracheal tube is reconnected to the ventilator.
9. The head is turned to the opposite side, and the procedure is repeated.

REFERENCES

1. Anand KDJ, Hickey PR: Pain and its effects in the human neonate and fetus, *N Engl J Med* 317;1321, 1987.
2. Bauchner H: Procedures, pain, and parents: commentaries, *Pediatrics* 87:563, 1991.
3. Berde DB et al: Comparison of morphine and methadone for prevention of postoperative pain in 3- to 7-year-old children, *J Pediatr* 119:136, 1991.

4. Berg RA: Emergency infusion of catecholamines into bone marrow, *Am J Dis Child* 138:810, 1984.
5. Blumer JL, editor: *A practical guide to pediatric intensive care,* ed 3, St Louis, 1990, Mosby.
6. Butt W et al: Complications resulting from use of arterial catheters: retrograde flow and rapid elevation in blood pressure, *Pediatrics* 76:250, 1985.
7. Committee on Drugs, Section on Anesthesiology 1983-84: Guidelines for the elective use of conscious sedation, deep sedation, and general anesthesia in pediatric patients, *Pediatrics* 76:317, 1985.
8. Firestone L, Lebowitz P, Cook C: *Clinical anesthesia procedures of the Massachusetts General Hospital,* Boston, 1988, Little, Brown.
9. Fuhrman BP et al: Pleural drainage using modified pigtail catheters, *Crit Care Med* 15:575, 1986.
10. Halperin DL et al: Topical skin anesthesia for venous subcutaneous drug reservoir and lumbar punctures in children, *Pediatrics* 84:281, 1981.
11. Iserson KV, Criss EA: Pediatric venous cutdowns: utility in emergency situations, *Pediatr Emerg Care* 2:231, 1986.
12. Joyce TH III: Topical anesthesia and pain management before venipuncture, *J Pediatr* 122:S24, 1993.
13. Kanter RK et al: Central venous catheter insertion by femoral vein: safety and effectiveness for the pediatric patient, *Pediatrics* 77:842, 1986.
14. Kanter RK et al: Pediatric emergency intravenous access: evaluation of a protocol, *Am J Dis Child* 140:132, 1986.
15. Kanter RK et al: Anatomy of femoral vessels in infants and guidelines for venous catheterization, *Pediatrics* 83:1020, 1989.
16. Koren G: Use of the eutectic mixture of local anesthetics in young children for procedure-related pain, *J Pediatr* 122:S30, 1993.
17. Johnson KB, editor: *The Harriet Lane handbook: a manual for pediatric house officers,* ed 13, St Louis, 1993, Mosby.
18. Lawless S et al: New pigtail catheter for pleural drainage in pediatric patients, *Crit Care Med* 17:173, 1989.
19. Levy L, Pandit SK: Is midazolam a dangerous drug? *J Postanesth Nurs* 4:40, 1989.
20. McGrath PJ, McAlpine L: Psychologic perspectives on pediatric pain, *J Pediatr* 122:S2, 1993.
21. Neish SR et al: Intraosseous infusion of hypertonic glucose and dopamine, *Am J Dis Child* 142:878, 1988.
22. Orlowski JP: My kingdom for an intravenous line, *Am J Dis Child* 138:803, 1984.
23. Orlowski JP et al: Comparison study of intraosseous, central intravenous, and peripheral intravenous infusions of emergency drugs, *Am J Dis Child* 144:112, 1990.
24. Rosetti V et al: Difficulty and delay in intravenous access in pediatric arrest, *Ann Emerg Med* 13:406, 1984.
25. Shapiro JM et al: Midazolam infusion for sedation in the intensive care unit: effect on adrenal function, *Anesthesiology* 64:394, 1986.
26. Sievers TD et al: Midazolam for conscious sedation during pediatric oncology procedures: safety and recovery procedures, *Pediatrics* 88:1172, 1991.
27. Smith-Wright DL et al: Complications of vascular catheterization in critically ill children, *Crit Care Med* 12:1015, 1984.
28. Spivey WH: Intraosseous infusions, *J Pediatr* 111:639, 1987.
29. Stenzel JP et al: Percutaneous femoral venous catheterizations: a prospective study of complications, *J Pediatr* 114:411, 1989.
30. Swanson RS et al: Emergency intravenous access through the femoral vein, *Ann Emerg Med* 13:244, 1984.
31. Todres ID et al: Endotracheal tube displacement in the newborn infant, *J Pediatr* 89:126, 1976.
32. Tribett D, Brenner M: Peripheral and femoral vein cannulation. In Venus B, Mallory D, editors: *Problems in critical care,* ed 2, vol 2, Philadelphia, 1988, JB Lippincott.
33. Venkataraman ST, Orr RA, Thompson AE: Percutaneous infraclavicular subclavian vein catheterization in critically ill infants and children, *J Pediatr* 113:480, 1988.
34. Yaster M: The management of acute pain in children with a local anesthetic: a primer for the nonanesthesiologist, *Compr Ther* 15:14, 1989.
35. Yaster M et al: Pain sedation and postoperative anesthetic management in the pediatric intensive care unit. In Rogers MC, editor, *Textbook of pediatric intensive care,* Baltimore 1987, Williams & Wilkins.
36. Yaster M et al: Midazolam-fentanyl intravenous sedation in children: case report of respiratory arrest, *Pediatrics* 86:463, 1990.

C Miscellaneous Values

Kathleen A. Woodin

BONE AGE

Sontag Method

The Sontag method is used to evaluate the skeletal development of children from 1 to 60 months of age:

1. Roentgenograms are taken of all epiphyseal centers on the left side of the body: shoulder, elbow, wrist and hand, hip, knee (anteroposterior [AP] views before 24 months of age, lateral views after 24 months), and ankle and foot (AP views before 48 months of age, lateral views after 48 months).
2. All ossification centers in the left half of the body are counted. A center is counted as soon as it casts any shadow on the roentgenogram.
3. The number of ossification centers is compared with normal values for the patient's age (Table C-1).

Gruelich and Pyle Method

The Gruelich and Pyle method is used to evaluate the skeletal development of girls from 5 to 18 years of age and for boys from 5 to 19 years:

1. A roentgenogram is taken of the left hand and wrist.
2. Calculation of the skeletal development is based on the order of appearance and maturation of the epiphyseal centers. (For normal values, see Gruelich and Pyle's *Radiographic Atlas of Skeletal Development of the Hand and Wrist.*[1])

Table C-1 Mean Total Number of Centers on the Left Side of Body Ossified at Given Age Levels

	Boys		Girls	
Age (mo)	Mean	SD*	Mean	SD
1	4.11	1.41	4.58	1.76
3	6.63	1.86	7.78	2.16
6	9.61	1.95	11.44	2.53
9	11.88	2.66	15.36	4.92
12	13.96	3.96	22.40	6.93
18	19.27	6.61	34.10	8.44
24	29.21	8.10	43.44	6.65
30	37.59	7.40	48.91	6.50
36	43.42	5.34	52.73	5.48
42	47.06	5.26	56.61	3.98
48	51.24	4.59	57.94	3.91
54	53.94	4.35	59.89	3.36
60	56.24	4.07	61.52	2.69

From Sontag LW, Snell D, Anderson M: *Am J Dis Child* 58:949, 1939.
**SD,* Standard deviation.

DETERMINATION OF BODY SURFACE AREA

On the basis of the nomogram shown in Figure C-1, a straight line joining the patient's height and weight will intersect the center column at the calculated body surface area (BSA).

CONVERSION FORMULAS

Height (Length)

1 millimeter (mm) = 0.04 inch
1 centimeter = 0.4 inch
2.54 centimeters = 1 inch
1 meter (m) = 39.37 inches

Weight

60 milligrams (mg) = 1 grain
28.35 grams (g) = 1 ounce
454 grams = 1 pound
1000 grams (1 kilogram [kg]) = 2.2 pounds

Milligram-Milliequivalent Conversions

$$\text{mEq/L} = \text{mg/L} \times \frac{\text{Valence}}{\text{Atomic weight}}$$

$$\text{mg/L} = \text{mEq/L} \times \frac{\text{Atomic weight}}{\text{Valence}}$$

$$\text{Equivalent weight} = \frac{\text{Atomic weight}}{\text{Valence}}$$

Milliosmols

The milliequivalent (mEq) is roughly equivalent to the milliosmol (mOsm), the unit of measure of osmolarity or tonicity.

Prefixes for Decimal Factors

Prefix	Symbol	Factor
mega	m	10^{6}
kilo	k	10^{3}
hecto	h	10^{2}
deka	da	10^{1}
deci	d	10^{-1}
centi	c	10^{-2}
milli	m	10^{-3}
micro	μ	10^{-6}
nano	n	10^{-9}
pico	p	10^{-12}
femto	f	10^{-15}

ACID-BASE RESPONSE IN RESPIRATORY ACIDOSIS AND ALKALOSIS

The nomogram in Figure C-2 shows confidence bands for the normal adjustment in carbon dioxide content and pH

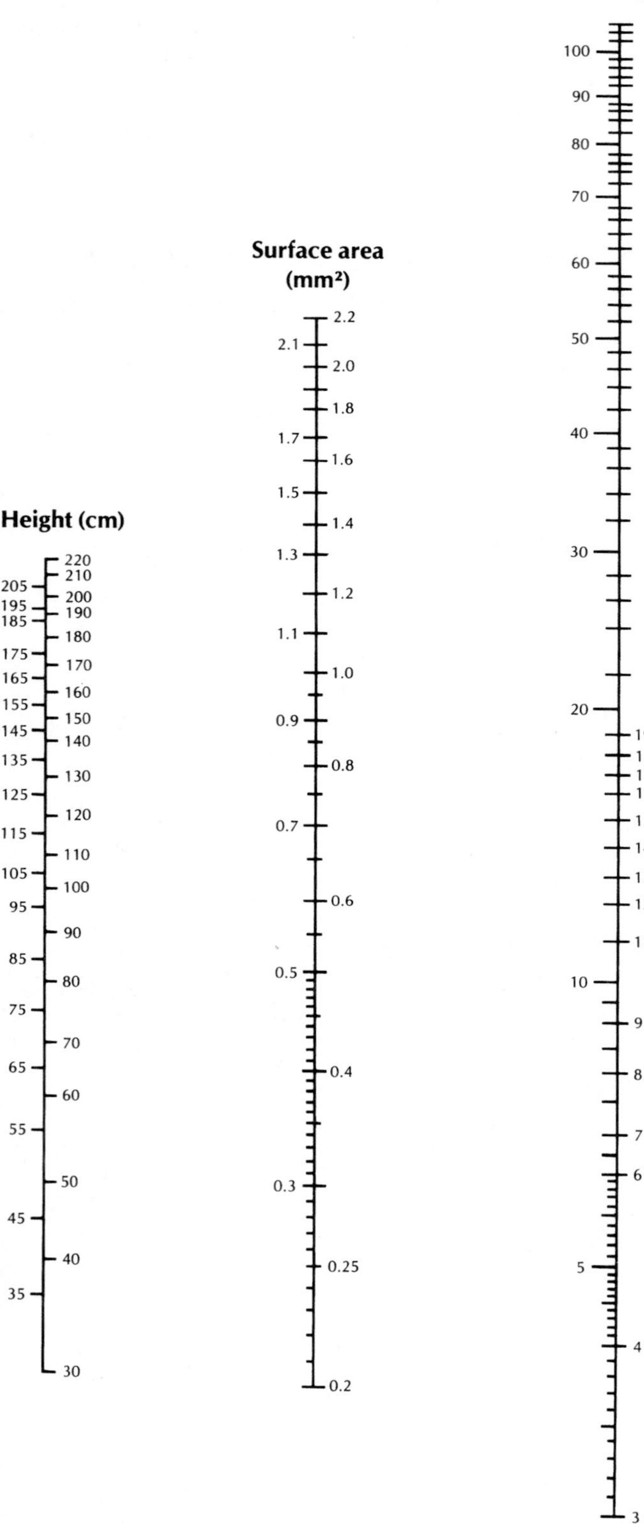

FIG. C-1 Nomogram to determine body surface area.

(Redrawn from Cole CH, editor: ***The Harriet Lane handbook,*** Chicago, 1984, Mosby. Based on data from Gelian EA, George SL: ***Cancer Chemother Rep*** 54:225, 1970.)

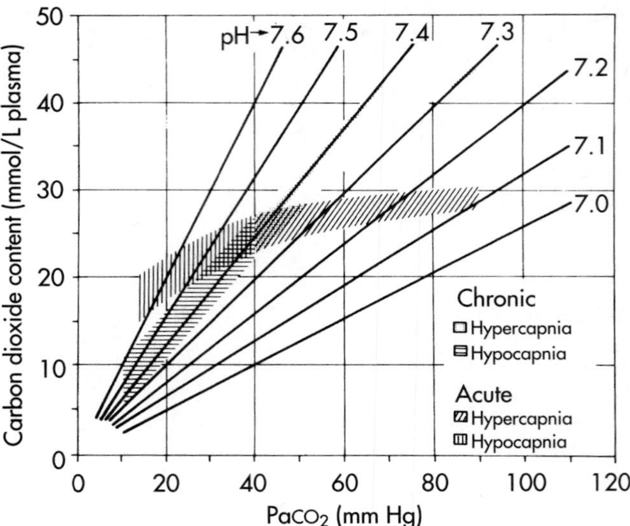

FIG. C-2 Acid-base response in respiratory acidosis and alkalosis.

(Modified from Arbus GS: ***Can Med Assoc J*** 109:291, 1973.)

made to accommodate acute and chronic changes in arterial P_{CO_2}.

1. The pH is determined on the nomogram from the plotted Pa_{CO_2} and carbon dioxide content obtained from blood gas measurements.
2. If the pH value is not within confidence bands, the change in carbon dioxide content and pH is different from that expected from a pure respiratory condition; thus a metabolic abnormality also is present.
3. To estimate the effect of acute and chronic changes in P_{CO_2} on pH, the following formulas are used:

Acute change in P_{CO_2}:

$$(\Delta\ P_{CO_2})\ (0.008) = \Delta\ pH$$

Chronic change in P_{CO_2}:

$$(\Delta\ P_{CO_2})\ (0.003) = \Delta\ pH$$

REFERENCE

1. Gruelich WW, Pyle SI: *Radiographic atlas of skeletal development of the hand and wrist,* San Francisco, 1974, Stanford University Press.

SUGGESTED READINGS

Normal laboratory values (case records of the Massachusetts General Hospital), *N Engl J Med* 314:39, 1986.

Queen PM, Wilson SE: Growth and nutrient requirements of infants. In Grand RJ, Sutphen JL, Dietz WH, editors: *Pediatric nutrition: theory and practice,* Boston, 1987, Butterworth.

Tietz NW, editor: *Clinical guide to laboratory tests,* Philadelphia, 1983, WB Saunders.

Young SD: Normal laboratory values in SI units, *N Engl J Med* 292:795, 1975.

Table C-2 Cerebrospinal Fluid

	Mean	Range	Polymorphonuclear cells
Cell count*			
Preterm newborn	9.0	0-29	57%
Term newborn	8.2	0-32	61%
Child (>1 mo)		0-6	
Glucose			
Preterm newborn	50 mg/dl	24-63 mg/dl	
Term newborn	52 mg/dl	34-119 mg/dl	
Child		40-80 mg/dl	
Pressure, opening			
Newborn	<110 mm H_2O		
Child	<200 mm H_2O		
Protein			
Preterm newborn	115 mg/dl	65-150 mg/dl	
Term newborn	90 mg/dl	20-170 mg/dl	
Child		5-40 mg/dl	
Volume			
Child	60-100 ml		
Adult	100-160 ml		

Data from Klein JO, Feigin RD, McCracken GH: *Pediatrics* 78(suppl):959, 1986; Portnoy JM, Olson LC: *Pediatrics* 75:484, 1985; Sarff LD, Platt LH, McCracken GH: *J Pediatr* 88:473, 1976.

*Traumatic lumbar punctures (>1000 red blood cells/mm^3) are uninterpretable because correction formulas may underestimate the true white blood cell count.

Table C-3 Synovial Fluid Analysis

	Cells per microliter (μl)	Polymorphonuclear leukocytes (PMNL)	Glucose (mg/dl)	Mucin clot	Protein (mg/dl)
Normal	50-200	<5%	>80	Good	1.8
Inflammatory*					
Bacterial	>10,000	>90%	<50	Poor	>4
Nonseptic	<10,000	<90%	50-80	Poor	2-4

Modified from Rudy P, DuPont HL: Infectious arthritis. In Pickering LK, DuPont HL, editors: *Infectious diseases of children and adults,* Menlo Park, Calif, 1986, Addison-Wesley.

*Fluid should be evaluated for the presence of urate crystals that occur in gout and pseudogout.

Table C-4 Clinical Chemistry

Determination	Standard units	Factor	SI units
Alanine aminotransferase (ALT or SGPT)			
Infant	5-54 U/L	NA	NA
Child	3-37 U/L	NA	NA
Adult	8-45 U/L	NA	NA
Alkaline phosphatase			
Newborn	35-213 U/L	1.00	35-213 U/L
Child	71-142 U/L	1.00	71-142 U/L
Adolescent	106-213 U/L	1.00	106-213 U/L
Adult	32-92 U/L	1.00	32-92 U/L
Aldolase			
Newborn	5.2-32.8 U/L	1.00	5.2-32.8 U/L
Child	2.6-16.4 U/L	1.00	2.6-16.4 U/L
Adult	1.3-8.2 U/L	1.00	1.3-8.2 U/L
Ammonia	15-49 μg/dl	0.7333	11-35 μmol/L
Amylase			
Serum	60-160 U/dl	NA*	NA
Urine	17-200 U/dl	NA	NA
Aspartate aminotransferase (AST or SGOT)			
Newborn	25-75 U/L	NA	NA
Infant	15-60 U/L	NA	NA
Child	20-50 U/L	NA	NA
Adult	8-40 U/L	NA	NA
Bicarbonate	18-25 mEq/L	1.00	8-25 mmol/L
Bilirubin (>1 mo)			
Total	<0.2-1.0 mg/dl	17.10	<3.4 μmol/L
Direct	<0.2 mg/dl	17.10	<3.4-17.1 μmol/L
Calcium			
Total	8.8-10.8 mg/dl	0.2495	2.20-2.70 mmol/L
Ionized	4.48-4.92 mg/dl	0.2495	1.12-1.23 mmol/L
Carotene			
Infant	20-70 μg/dl	0.0186	0.37-1.30 μmol/L
Adult	40-130 μg/dl	0.0186	0.74-2.42 μmol/L
Child	60-200 μg/dl	0.0186	1.12-3.72 μmol/L
Chloride	98-106 mEq/L	1.00	98-106 mmol/L
Cholesterol, fasting			
Newborn	53-135 mg/dl	0.0259	1.37-3.50 mmol/L
Infant	70-175 mg/dl	0.0259	1.81-4.53 mmol/L
Child	120-200 mg/dl	0.0259	3.11-5.18 mmol/L
Adolescent	120-210 mg/dl	0.0259	3.11-5.44 mmol/L
Adult	140-250 mg/dl	0.0259	3.63-6.48 mmol/L
Copper			
Infant	20-70 μg/dl	0.1574	3.14-10.99 μmol/L
Child	90-190 μg/dl	0.1574	14.13-29.83 μmol/L
Adolescent	80-160 μg/dl	0.1574	12.56-25.12 μmol/L
Adult	70-155 μg/dl	0.1574	10.99-24.34 μmol/L
Creatinine			
Newborn	0.8-1.4 mg/dl	88.4	70.7-123.8 μmol/L
Infant	0.7-1.7 mg/dl	88.4	61.9-150.3 μmol/L
Adult	0.6-1.5 mg/dl	88.4	53.133 μmol/L
Creatinine kinase			
Female	10-55 U/L	1.00	10-55 U/L
Male	12-80 U/L	1.00	12-80 U/L
Glucose	55-100 mg/dl	0.05551	3.055-5.55 mmol/L
Haptoglobin	40-336 mg/dl	0.01	0.4-3.36 g/L
Iron, serum			
Newborn	100-250 μg/dl	0.1791	17.90-44.75 μmol/L
Infant	40-100 μg/dl	0.1791	7.16-17.90 μmol/L
Child	50-120 μg/dl	0.1791	8.95-21.48 μmol/L
Adult	40-160 μg/dl	0.1791	7.16-28.64 μmol/L

**NA*, Not available or not applicable.

Table C-4 Clinical Chemistry—cont'd

Determination	Standard units	Factor	SI units
Iron-binding capacity, total (TIBC)			
Infant	100-400 μg/dl	0.1791	17.90-71.60 μmol/L
Child	250-400 μg/dl	0.1791	44.75-71.60 μmol/L
Adult	250-400 μg/dl	0.1791	44.75-71.60 μmol/L
Lactate	0.6-1.8 mEq/L	1.00	0.6-1.8 mmol/L
Lactic dehydrogenase			
Newborn	160-450 U/L	NA	NA
Infant	100-250 U/L	NA	NA
Child	60-170 U/L	NA	NA
Adult	45-90 U/L	NA	NA
Lead (child)	<10 μg/dl	0.0483	<0.48 μmol/L
Lipids			
Phospholipids	180-295 mg/dl	0.01	1.8-2.95 g/L
Triglycerides	40-150 mg/dl	0.01	0.4-1.5 g/L
Lipoprotein, HDL	150-330 mg/dl	0.01	1.5-3.3 g/L
Lipoprotein, LDL	28%-53% total		
Magnesium			
Newborn	1.0-1.8 mEq/L	0.5	0.5-0.9 mmol/L
Child	1.5-2.0 mEq/L	0.5	0.8-1.0 mmol/L
Osmolarity	275-295 mOsm/kg	1.00	275-295 mmol/kg
pH (arterial)	7.35-7.45	1.00	7.35-7.45
Pco_2	35-45 mm Hg	0.1333	4.7-6.0 kPa
Po_2	83-108 mm Hg	0.1333	11.04-14.36 kPa
Phosphorus, inorganic			
Newborn	5.5-9.5 mg/dl	0.3229	1.78-3.07 mmol/L
Infant	4.5-6.5 mg/dl	0.3229	1.45-2.10 mmol/L
Child	4.5-5.5 mg/dl	0.3229	1.45-1.78 mmol/L
Adult	2.7-4.5 mg/dl	0.3229	0.87-1.45 mmol/L
Potassium	3.5-5.1 mEq/L	1.00	3.5-5.1 mmol/L
Proteins (NOTE: Globulin = Total protein − Albumin)			
Albumin/total protein			
Newborn	2.4-4.8/4.6-7.0 g/dl	10.0	24-48/46-70 g/L
Infant	3.0-4.5/5.1-7.3 g/dl	10.0	30-45/51-73 g/L
Child	3.8-5.6/6.0-8.0 g/dl	10.0	38-56/60-80 g/L
Adult	3.5-5.5/6.4-8.3 g/dl	10.0	35-55/64-83 g/L
Sodium	136-145 mEq/L	1.00	136-145 mmol/L
Urea nitrogen			
Newborn	4-12 mg/dl	0.3569	1.4-4.3 mmol/L
Child/adult	5-18 mg/dl	0.3569	1.8-6.4 mmol/L
Uric acid	3.0-7.0 mg/dl	0.0595	0.18-0.42 mmol/L
Vitamin A	30-80 μg/dl	0.0349	1.05-2.79 μmol/L
Vitamin E (tocopherol)	0.5-2.0 mg/dl	23.22	11.6-46.4 μmol/L

Table C-5 Newborn Clinical Chemistry

Determination*	Cord sample†	Capillary samples†			
		1-12 hr	12-24 hr	24-48 hr	48-72 hr
Sodium (mmol/L)	147 (126-166)	143 (124-156)	145 (132-159)	148 (134-160)	149 (139-162)
Potassium (mmol/L)	7.8 (5.6-12)	6.4 (5.3-7.3)	6.3 (5.3-8.9)	6.0 (5.2-7.3)	5.9 (5.0-7.7)
Chloride (mmol/L)	103 (98-110)	100.7 (90-111)	103 (87-114)	102 (92-114)	103 (93-112)
Calcium (mg/dl)	9.3 (8.2-11.1)	8.4 (7.3-9.2)	7.8 (6.9-9.4)	8.0 (6.1-9.9)	7.9 (5.9-9.7)
Phosphorus (mg/dl)	5.6 (3.7-8.1)	6.1 (3.5-8.6)	5.7 (2.9-8.1)	5.9 (3.0-8.7)	5.8 (2.8-7.6)
Blood urea (mg/dl)	29 (21-40)	27 (8-34)	33 (9-63)	32 (13-77)	31 (13-68)
Total protein (g/dl)	6.1 (4.8-7.3)	6.6 (5.6-8.5)	6.6 (5.8-8.2)	6.9 (5.9-8.2)	7.2 (6.0-8.5)
Glucose (mg/dl)	73 (45-96)	63 (40-97)	63 (42-104)	56 (30-91)	59 (40-90)
Lactic acid (mg/dl)	19.5 (11-30)	14.6 (11-24)	14 (10-23)	14.3 (9-22)	13.5 (7-21)
Lactate (mmol/L)‡	2.0-3.0	2.0			

Modified from Avery GB: *Neonatology, pathophysiology and management in the newborn,* ed 3, Philadelphia, 1987, JB Lippincott.
*Acharya PT, Payne WW: *Arch Dis Child* 40:430, 1965.
†Numbers in parentheses indicate a normal range.
‡Daniel SS, Adamsons K Jr, James LS: *Pediatrics* 37:942, 1966.

Table C-6 Hematology

Age	Hemoglobin (grams %): mean (−2 SD)	Hematocrit (%) mean (−2 SD)	Mean cell volume (fluid) mean (−2 SD)	Mean corpuscular hemoglobin concentration (grams/%RBC) mean (−2 SD)	Reticulocytes (%)	WBC/mm^3 × 100 mean (−2 SD)	Platelets (10^3 mm^3) mean (±2 SD)
26-30 wk gestation*	13.4 (11)	41.5 (34.9)	118.2 (106.7)	37.9 (30.6)	—	4.4 (2.7)	254 (180-327)
28 wk	14.5	45	120	31	(5-10)	—	275
32 wk	15.0	47	118	32	(3-10)	—	290
Term† (cord)	16.5 (13.5)	51 (42)	108 (98)	33 (30)	(3-7)	18.1 (9-30)‡	290
1-3 days	18.5 (14.5)	56 (45)	108 (95)	33 (29)	(1.8-4.6)	18.9 (9.4-34)	192
2 wk	16.6 (13.4)	53 (41)	105 (88)	31.4 (28.1)		11.4 (5-20)	252
1 mo	13.9 (10.7)	44 (33)	101 (91)	31.8 (28.1)	(0.1-1.7)	10.8 (4-19.5)	
2 mo	11.2 (9.4)	35 (28)	95 (84)	31.8 (28.3)			
6 mo	12.6 (11.1)	36 (31)	76 (68)	35 (32.7)	(0.7-2.3)	11.9 (6-17.5)	
6 mo-2 yr	12 (10.5)	36 (33)	78 (70)	33 (30)		10.6 (6-17)	(150-350)
2-6 yr	12.5 (11.5)	37 (34)	81 (75)	34 (31)	(0.5-1.0)	8.5 (5-15.5)	(150-350)
6-12 yr	13.5 (11.5)	40 (35)	86 (77)	34 (31)	(0.5-1.0)	8.1 (4.5-13.5)	(150-350)
12-18 yr							
Male	14.5 (13)	43 (36)	88 (78)	34 (31)	(0.5-1.0)	7.8 (4.5-13.5)	(150-350)
Female	14 (12)	41 (37)	90 (78)	34 (31)	(0.5-1.0)	7.8 (4.5-13.5)	(150-350)
Adult							
Male	15.5 (13.5)	47 (41)	90 (80)	34 (31)	(0.8-2.5)	7.4 (4.5-11)	(150-350)
Female	14 (12)	41 (36)	90 (80)	34 (31)	(0.8-4.1)	7.4 (4.5-11)	(150-350)

Modified from Johnson KB, editor: *The Harriet Lane handbook,* ed 13, Chicago, 1993, Mosby.

*Values are from fetal samplings.

†Under 1 mo of age, capillary hemoglobin exceeds venous hemoglobin: age 1 hr—by 3.6 g; age 5 days—by 2.2 g; age 3 wk—by 1.1 g.

‡Mean (95% confidence limits).

Table C-7 Conversion of Centimeters to Inches

cm	in	cm	in	cm	in	cm	in
1	0.39	51	20.08	101	39.76	151	59.45
2	0.79	52	20.47	102	40.16	152	59.84
3	1.18	53	20.87	103	40.55	153	60.24
4	1.57	54	21.26	104	40.94	154	60.63
5	1.97	55	21.65	105	41.34	155	61.02
6	2.36	56	22.05	106	41.73	156	61.42
7	2.76	57	22.44	107	42.13	157	61.81
8	3.15	58	22.83	108	42.52	158	62.20
9	3.54	59	23.23	109	42.91	159	62.60
10	3.94	60	23.62	110	43.31	160	62.99
11	4.33	61	24.02	111	43.70	161	63.39
12	4.72	62	24.41	112	44.09	162	63.78
13	5.12	63	24.80	113	44.49	163	64.17
14	5.51	64	25.20	114	44.88	164	64.57
15	5.91	65	25.59	115	45.28	165	64.96
16	6.30	66	25.98	116	45.67	166	65.35
17	6.69	67	26.38	117	46.06	167	65.75
18	7.09	68	26.78	118	46.46	168	66.14
19	7.48	69	27.17	119	46.85	169	66.54
20	7.87	70	27.56	120	47.24	170	66.93
21	8.27	71	27.95	121	47.64	171	67.32
22	8.66	72	28.35	122	48.03	172	67.72
23	9.06	73	28.74	123	48.43	173	68.11
24	9.45	74	29.13	124	48.82	174	68.50
25	9.84	75	29.53	125	49.21	175	68.90
26	10.24	76	29.92	126	49.61	176	69.29
27	10.63	77	30.31	127	50.00	177	69.68
28	11.02	78	30.71	128	50.39	178	70.08
29	11.42	79	31.10	129	50.79	179	70.47
30	11.81	80	31.50	130	51.18	180	70.87
31	12.20	81	31.89	131	51.57	181	71.26
32	12.60	82	32.28	132	51.97	182	71.65
33	13.00	83	32.68	133	52.36	183	72.05
34	13.39	84	33.07	134	52.76	184	72.44
35	13.78	85	33.46	135	53.15	185	72.83
36	14.17	86	33.86	136	53.54	186	73.23
37	14.57	87	34.25	137	53.94	187	73.62
38	14.96	88	34.65	138	54.33	188	74.02
39	15.35	89	35.04	139	54.72	189	74.41
40	15.75	90	35.43	140	55.12	190	74.80
41	16.14	91	35.83	141	55.51	191	75.20
42	16.54	92	36.22	142	55.91	192	75.59
43	16.93	93	36.61	143	56.30	193	75.98
44	17.32	94	37.01	144	56.69	194	76.38
45	17.72	95	37.40	145	57.09	195	76.77
46	18.11	96	37.80	146	57.48	196	77.17
47	18.50	97	38.19	147	57.87	197	77.56
48	18.90	98	38.58	148	58.27	198	77.95
49	19.29	99	38.98	149	58.66	199	78.35
50	19.69	100	39.37	150	59.06	200	78.74

Table C-8 Conversion of Pounds to Grams

ounces	1 lb	2 lb	3 lb	4 lb	5 lb	6 lb	7 lb	8 lb
	Grams							
0	454	907	1361	1814	2268	2722	3175	3629
1	482	936	1389	1843	2296	2750	3204	3657
2	510	964	1418	1871	2325	2778	3232	3686
3	539	992	1446	1899	2353	2807	3260	3714
4	567	1021	1474	1928	2381	2835	3289	3742
5	595	1049	1503	1956	2410	2863	3317	3771
6	624	1077	1531	1985	2438	2892	3345	3799
7	652	1106	1559	2013	2466	2920	3374	3827
8	680	1134	1588	2041	2495	2948	3402	3856
9	709	1162	1616	2070	2523	2977	3430	3884
10	737	1191	1644	2098	2552	3005	3459	3912
11	765	1219	1673	2126	2580	3033	3487	3941
12	794	1247	1701	2155	2608	3062	3515	3969
13	822	1276	1729	2183	2637	3090	3544	3997
14	851	1304	1758	2211	2665	3119	3572	4026
15	879	1332	1786	2240	2693	3147	3600	4054

Table C-9 Temperature Equivalents

Celsius*	Fahrenheit†	Celsius*	Fahrenheit†
34.0	93.2	38.6	101.4
34.2	93.6	38.8	101.8
34.4	93.9	39.0	102.2
34.6	94.3	39.2	102.5
34.8	94.6	39.4	102.9
35.0	95.0	39.6	103.2
35.2	95.4	39.8	103.6
35.4	95.7	40.0	104.0
35.6	96.1	40.2	104.3
35.8	96.4	40.4	104.7
36.0	96.8	40.6	105.1
36.2	97.1	40.8	105.4
36.4	97.5	41.0	105.8
36.6	97.8	41.2	106.1
36.8	98.2	41.4	106.5
37.0	98.6	41.6	106.8
37.2	98.9	41.8	107.2
37.4	99.3	42.0	107.6
37.6	99.6	42.2	108.0
37.8	100.0	42.4	108.3
38.0	100.4	42.6	108.7
38.2	100.7	42.8	109.0
38.4	101.1	43.0	109.4

*To convert Celsius to Fahrenheit: 9/5 × (Temperature) + 32).
†To convert Fahrenheit to Celsius: 5/9 × (Temperature) − 32).

Table C-10 Laboratory Parameters of Acid-Base Disturbances*

	pH	Arterial carbon dioxide pressure (Pa_{CO_2})	Bicarbonate (HCO_3^-) (mEq/L)	Carbon dioxide (CO_2) content (mEq/L)
Normal values	7.35-7.45	35-45	24-26	25-28
Disturbances				
Metabolic acidosis	↓	↓	↓	↓
Acute respiratory acidosis	↓	↑	↔	Slight ↑
Compensated respiratory acidosis	↔ or slight↓	↑	↑	↑
Metabolic alkalosis	↑	Slight ↑	↑	↑
Acute respiratory alkalosis	↑	↓	↔	Slight ↓
Compensated respiratory alkalosis	↔ or slight ↑	↓	↓	↓

*Values obtained by arteriolized capillary blood or direct arterial puncture.

Table C-11 Components of Human Milk and Infant Formula

Product	Protein	Fat	Carbohydrate	Comments
Human milk	80% whey, 20% casein	Human milk fat	Lactose	
Alimentum	Hydrolized casein	50% MCT,* 40% safflower, 10% soy oils	Sucrose-modified tapioca starch	For malabsorption syndromes
Cow milk	80% casein, 20% whey	Butterfat	Lactose	
Enfamil and Enfamil with Iron	40% casein, 60% whey	55% coconut, 45% soy oils	Lactose	
Enfamil Premature	60% whey, 40% casein	40% MCT, 40% soy, 20% coconut oils	Corn syrup solids,† lactose	For premature infants
Evaporated milk base	80% casein, 20% whey	Butterfat	Lactose	Add 19 oz water and 2 tbsp. sugar to a 13 oz can of evaporated milk; supplement with multivitamins and iron
Isomil	Soy protein	60% soy, 40% coconut oils	Corn syrup solids, sucrose	For cow milk protein and/or lactose intolerance
Isomil SF	Soy protein	60% soy, 40% coconut oils	Corn syrup solids	For cow milk protein, lactose, and/or sucrose intolerance
Lofenalac	Casein hydrolysate processed to remove most of the phenylalanine	Corn oil	Corn syrup solids, modified tapioca starch	For phenylketonuria—low in phenylalanine
Nursoy‡	Soy protein	58% safflower, 27% coconut, 15% soy oils	Sucrose	For cow milk protein and/or lactose intolerance
Nutramigen	Casein hydrolysate	Corn oil	Corn syrup solids, corn starch	For sensitivity to intact milk protein or for lactose intolerance
Portagen	Sodium caseinate	85% MCT, 15% corn oil	Corn syrup solids, sucrose, lactose	For fat malabsorption disorders and lactose intolerance (liver disease)
Pregestimil	Casein hydrolysate with added L-cystine, L-tyrosine, and L-tryptophan	60% MCT, 20% corn, 20% safflower oils	Corn syrup solids, dextrose, corn starch	For many malabsorption syndromes
Prosobee	Soy protein isolate	55% coconut, 45% soy oils	Corn syrup solids	For lactose and cow milk protein intolerance, sucrose intolerance, and galactosemia
RCF (Ross Carbohydrate Free)	Soy protein isolate	Coconut, soy oils	None—selected by physician	
Similac and Similac with Iron	Nonfat cow milk	60% soy, 40% coconut oils	Lactose	
Similac PM 60/40	60% whey, 40% casein	60% coconut, 40% corn oils	Lactose	For infants predisposed to hypocalcemia (calcium/phosphorus ratio is 2:1); low salt content
Similac Special Care	60% whey, 40% casein	MCT, corn, coconut oils	Lactose, hydrolyzed corn starch	For premature infants
Similac Special Care 24	Nonfat cow milk, whey	50% MCT, coconut, soy oils	Lactose, hydrolyzed corn starch	Can be used for premature infants with fluid intolerance
SMA and SMA with Iron‡	Nonfat cow milk, demineralized whey	Oleo, oleic, coconut, soy oils	Lactose	Low salt content
SMA Preemie 24‡	60% whey, 40% casein	MCT, coconut, soy oils	Lactose, glucose	For premature infants

Modified from Johnson KB, editor: *The Harriet Lane handbook,* ed 13, Chicago, 1993, Mosby.

**MCT,* Medium-chain triglycerides.

†Corn syrup solids include dextrose, maltose, and other glucose polymers.

‡No longer available in the United States.

Table C-12 Composition of Human Milk and Infant Formulas

Formula	Calories per ounce (ml)*	Percentage of weight for volume (g/dl)*			
		Protein	Fat	Carbohydrate	Sodium (mEq/L)
Human milk	21 (0.70)	1.00 (6)	4.40 (55)	6.90 (39)	7
Alimentum	20 (0.67)	1.90 (11)	3.80 (48)	6.90 (41)	13
Cow milk	20 (0.67)	3.30 (21)	3.30 (49)	4.70 (30)	21
Enfamil 20†	20 (0.67)	1.50 (9)	3.80 (50)	6.98 (41)	8
Enfamil Premature†	20 (0.67)	2.00 (12)	3.40 (44)	7.40 (44)	11
Evaporated milk with sugar	20 (0.67)	2.80 (17)	3.20 (43)	6.80 (40)	22
Isomil	20 (0.67)	1.80 (11)	3.69 (49)	6.80 (40)	13
Isomil SF	20 (0.67)	2.00 (12)	3.60 (48)	6.80 (40)	13
Lofenalac	20 (0.67)	2.20 (13)	2.60 (35)	8.80 (52)	14
Nursoy	20 (0.67)	2.10 (12)	3.60 (48)	6.90 (40)	9
Nutramigen	20 (0.67)	1.90 (11)	2.64 (35)	9.09 (54)	14
Portagen	20 (0.67)	2.30 (14)	3.10 (40)	7.70 (46)	14
Pregestimil	20 (0.67)	1.90 (11)	3.80 (48)	6.90 (41)	12
Prosobee	20 (0.67)	2.00 (12)	3.60 (48)	6.80 (40)	11
RCF	Varies‡	2.00 (20)	3.60 (80)	0 (0)	13
Similac 20	20 (0.67)	1.50 (9)	3.63 (48)	7.23 (43)	8
Similac PM 60/40	20 (0.67)	1.58 (9)	3.76 (50)	6.88 (41)	7
Similac Special Care	20 (0.67)	1.83 (11)	3.67 (47)	7.17 (42)	13
Similac Special Care 24†	24 (0.80)	2.20 (11)	4.49 (47)	8.49 (42)	15
Similac whey	20 (0.67)	1.50 (9)	3.63 (48)	7.23 (43)	10
SMA 20†	20 (0.67)	1.50 (9)	3.60 (48)	7.20 (43)	6.5
SMA Preemie 24†	24 (0.80)	2.00 (10)	4.40 (48)	8.60 (42)	14

Modified from Johnson KB, editor: *The Harriet Lane handbook,* ed 13, Chicago, 1993, Mosby. also from manufacturers' information.
*Numbers in parentheses indicate percentage of calories supplied by this substance.
†Available with or without iron (≥12 mg/dl).
‡Varies with the amount of carbohydrate added.

Potassium (mEq/L)	Calcium (mg/L)	Phosphorus (mg/L)	Calcium/phosphorus ratio	Iron (mg/L)	Approximate solute load (mOsm/L) Renal	Gastrointestinal
13	320	140	2.3/1	0.3	75	273
20	710	510	1.39/1	12	122	370
39	1190	930	1.30/1	0.5-1	220	260
18	470	320	1.47/1	1.1/12.8	100	300
17	1120	510	2.1/1	1.7/12.8	124	244
35	1165	909	1.28/1	0.9	—	—
19	710	510	1.39/1	12	116	240
19	710	510	1.39/1	12	116	140
18	634	475	1.33/1	13	134	310
18	600	420	1.40/1	11.5	122	266
19	640	430	1.50/1	12.8	125	320
22	635	475	1.33/1	13	150	220
19	640	430	1.50/1	12.8	125	320
21	640	500	1.26/1	12.8	127	200
19	700	500	1.40/1	1.5	124	74
19	493	380	1.30/1	1.5/12	97	300
15	380	190	2.00/1	1.5	96	280
22	1220	610	2.00/1	2.5	124	300
27	1460	730	2.01/1	3/15	149	300
19	400	300	1.33/1	12	101	270
14	420	280	1.50/1	1.5/12	92	300
19	750	400	1.88/1	3	128	300

D Common Psychological and Educational Tests

Philip W. Davidson, Kyle D. Houser, Olle Jane Z. Sahler, and Jean M. Garrett

Over the past 15 years, the number of preschool and school-age children seeing allied health professionals for psychological and educational assessment has risen dramatically. At the same time, the assessment armamentarium of the psychoeducational specialist has expanded to the point that many of the materials commonly used are unfamiliar to the pediatrician. The physician frequently receives reports from psychologists and educational specialists, speech and language pathologists, and pediatric occupational therapists—reports that must be interpreted or explained to the parents. Because these materials must be described succinctly to simplify the physician's assignment, summaries are provided in the box on p. 1835 (which groups tests by the function they measure) and in Table D-1 (which lists tests alphabetically and gives some of the tests' characteristics).

The table provides a quick reference to a wide range of psychoeducational screening and diagnostic tools commonly used by school health teams, special-child educators, clinical and pediatric psychologists, and other allied health professionals. Included are only individually administered tests, inasmuch as they are less familiar to both parents and physicians than are the group-administered standardized tests used by schools.

The information provided for each procedure is useful in identifying the general nature of each, the usual professional training of the person administering the test, and whether it is "normed." For some procedures, special features or characteristics also are noted.

The list of tests is not all-inclusive. On the other hand, most procedures that are likely to be described in a typical consultant's report are included. Screening procedures are presented because more and more states are requiring preschool and kindergarten readiness screening for all children. These screening tools often trigger more extensive evaluations for children who do not pass, a decision in which the pediatrician should participate. The diagnostic procedures given include many standard methods, as well as a variety of nonstandard methods designed for children who have disabilities that may interfere with routine testing procedures. Finally, some "parent report" procedures also are included because many preschool assessments may depend on such tools.

Clearly, interpreting the results of a screening or complete diagnostic assessment cannot be accomplished fully by referring only to this table. Communicating directly with the evaluator is the only reliable means of clarifying results. Such contact often must be initiated by the pediatrician because personnel from many schools and mental health facilities may not communicate routinely with the primary health care provider.

REFERRAL BY THE PEDIATRICIAN FOR PSYCHOLOGICAL OR EDUCATIONAL TESTING

Under what circumstances should a pediatrician refer a patient for special testing? Often the primary care pediatrician is in the best position to identify a child's developmental or behavioral difficulties, such as developmental delay in the infant or preschool child, learning difficulty or school failure in the school-age child, or adjustment difficulty in the latency-age child or adolescent. In these and similar situations the pediatrician quite appropriately might consider initiating a referral for psychological or educational testing, or both.

Several types of resources are available to accept referrals. One resource is the local government or the school district, both of which are obliged by the Education for All Handicapped Children Act, as reauthorized in 1987 (PL-99-457), to provide evaluation and intervention plans for any child suspected of having an educational handicapping condition. This federal law is implemented differently for preschool children ages birth through 2 years 11 months, and for school-age children ages 3 to 21 years, but services must be provided at public expense and without cost to the family. Preschoolers may be evaluated by any community resource certified as qualified by the state agency administering Part H of the law (pertaining to preschoolers). Such resources must be interdisciplinary and must include a medical and a developmental examination and a family assessment. The results are incorporated in an Individualized Family Service Plan to be carried out by the school district or other local entity as designated by the state. For school-age children, the evaluations must be provided by the local school district and usually are performed by school psychologists, who typically specialize in standard educational testing and are less intensively trained in dealing with complex psychoeducational and emotional problems. Unfortunately, the referral may not be acted upon promptly because of the large caseloads carried by school psychologists, who usually serve many schools within a district. However, the benefit of this type of referral is that results, once available, may be acted on more expeditiously (because the psychologist is a member of the committee on special education, the school district–based, decision making mechanism required by law to address the needs of children who have educational handicaps).

Another resource is a private practicing psychologist or educational specialist. The reasons for selecting this option might include a need for an independent opinion after a school district evaluation, a limitation on the resources available in the school system for competent studies of children who have complex problems, or parental preference.

To determine both cognitive and emotional status by means

Text continued on p. 1844.

CLASSIFICATION OF COMMON PSYCHOLOGICAL AND EDUCATIONAL TESTS BY FUNCTION

Developmental scales

Battelle Developmental Inventory (BDI)
Bayley Scales of Infant Development-II (BSID-II)
Callier-Azusa Scale
Cattell Infant Intelligence Scale
Clinical Adaptive Test/Clinical Linguistic Auditory Milestone Scale (CAT/CLAMS)
Denver Developmental Screening Test (DDST)
Gesell Developmental Schedules
Infant Mullen Scales of Early Learning (Infant-MSEL)
Infant Psychological Development Scale
Kaufman Developmental Scale (KDS)
Kaufman Infant and Preschool Scale (KIPS)
Minnesota Child Development Inventory
Neonatal Behavioral Assessment Scale (Brazelton)
Ordinal Scales of Psychological Development
Prescreening Developmental Questionnaire (PDQ)
School Readiness Survey

Temperament measures

Infant Temperament Questionnaire (ITQ) (Carey-McDevitt)
Temperament Assessment Battery for Children (TABC)
Temperament Scales

Sensory/perceptual/motor/auditory/visual scales

Auditory Discrimination Test
Bender Visual Motor Gestalt Test
Bruininks-Oseretsky Test of Motor Proficiency
Developmental Test of Visual Motor Integration (DTVMI)
Frostig Developmental Test of Visual Perception
Goldman-Fristoe-Woodcock Auditory Skills Test Battery
Motor Free Test of Visual Perception (MFTVP)
Peabody Developmental Motor Scales and Activity Cards
Sequenced Inventory of Communication Development–Revised Edition
Southern California Sensory Integration Test

Intelligence/cognitive/neuropsychological tests

Columbia Mental Maturity Scale
Draw-A-Man
Goodenough-Harris Drawing Test
Halstead Reitan Neuropsychological Test Battery for Older Children
Kaufman Assessment Battery for Children (K-ABC)
Luria-Nebraska Neuropsychological Battery: Children's Revision (LNNB-C)
McCarthy Scales of Children's Abilities
Merrill-Palmer Scale
Raven's Progressive Matrices (RPM)
Reitan-Indiana Neuropsychological Test Battery for Children
Slosson Intelligence Test–Revised (SIT-R)
Stanford-Binet Intelligence Test–Fourth Edition (SBFE)
Wechsler Intelligence Scale for Children-III (WISC-III)
Wechsler Memory Scale-Revised (WMS-R)
Wechsler Preschool and Primary Scales of Intelligence–Revised (WPPSI-R)
Wisconsin Card Sorting Test (WCST)

Nonverbal/blind/deaf

Blind Learning Aptitude Test (BLAT)
French Pictorial Intelligence Test
Hiskey-Nebraska Test of Learning Aptitude
Leiter International Performance Scale (LIPS)
Perkins-Binet Test of Intelligence for the Blind
Test of Nonverbal Intelligence–Revised (TONI-2)

Adaptive behavior scales

AAMR Adaptive Behavior Scale (ABS)
Adaptive Behavior Inventory for Children (ABIC)
California Adaptive Behavior Scale
Vineland Adaptive Behavior Scale (VABS)

Behavior/personality/problem scales and checklists

Childhood Autism Rating Scale (CARS)
Child Behavior Checklist (CBC) and Revised Child Behavior Profile
Children's Apperception Test (CAT)
Connors Parent and Teacher Rating Scales
Devereux Child Behavior Rating Scale (DCB)
House-Tree-Person (H-T-P) Projective Technique
Kinetic Drawing System for Family and Schools (KFD and KSD)
Personality Inventory for Children–Revised Format (PIC-R)
Preschool Behavior Questionnaire
Rorschach Psychodiagnostic Test
Sentence Completion Test
Thematic Apperception Test (TAT)
Wisconsin Behavior Rating Scale (WBRS)

Achievement/aptitude/other educational tests

ADD-H Comprehensive Teacher's Rating Scale (ACTeRS)
Assessing Prelinguistic and Early Linguistic Behaviors
Attention Deficit Disorders Behavior Rating Scales (ADDBRS)
Autism Screening Instrument for Educational Planning (ASIEP)
Detroit Test of Learning Aptitude–3 (DTLA-3)
Illinois Test of Psycholinguistic Abilities–2 (ITPA-2)
Kaufman Test of Educational Achievement (K-TEA)
KeyMath Revised: A Diagnostic Inventory of Essential Mathematics
Peabody Individual Achievement Test–Revised (PIAT-R)
Peabody Picture Vocabulary Test–Revised (PPVT-R)
Physician Developmental Quick Screen for Speech Disorders
Piers-Harris Children's Self Concept Scale (PHCSCS)
Preschool Language Scale (PLS)
Receptive-Expressive Emergent Language Scale (REEL)
Silvaroli Reading Inventory
Stanford Measurement Series
Sucher-Allred Reading Placement Inventory
Test of Language Development–2 (TOLD-2)
Test of Written Language–2 (TOWL-2)
Test of Written Spelling–2 (TWS-2)
Wide Range Achievement Test–3 (WRAT-3)
Woodcock Reading Mastery Test–Revised (WRMT-R)
Woodcock-Johnson Psychoeducational Battery–Revised (WJ-R)

Table D-1 Common Psychological and Educational Tests

Test name	Age range	Purpose and description
AAMR Adaptive Behavior Scales (ABS) Residential and Community (ABS-RC:2) School (ABS-S:2)	3 yr–adult	The third and latest revision (1992) of this widely used scale; assesses social, daily living, domestic and other skills of children whose behavior indicates possible mental retardation, emotional disturbance, or other handicaps; used for screening and instructional planning as well as for documenting progress; generally administered by a psychologist or educational specialist.
Adaptive Behavior Inventory for Children (ABIC)	5-11 yr	Interview inventory to assess child's social role performance in family, peer group, and community; section two includes age-graded questions.
ADD-H Comprehensive Teacher's Rating Scale (ACTeRS)	Grade K–5	Also widely known as the ACTeRS; aids in assessing behavior in the classroom that may be relevant to a diagnosis of attention deficit disorder; four subscales include hyperactivity, social skills, oppositional, and attention; ACTeRS Profile for either boys or girls is generated; psychologist administers and interprets.
Assessing Prelinguistic and Early Linguistic Behaviors	9-24 mo	A "normed" measure containing five scales assessing prelinguistic and linguistic development, including cognitive antecedents to word meaning, play, communicative interaction, language comprehension, and language production; speech pathologist administers.
Attention Deficit Disorder Behavior Rating Scales (ADDBRS)	6-16 yr	A screening device used by a teacher or parent and evaluated by an examiner; results aid in the differential diagnosis of attention deficit with and without hyperactivity.
Auditory Discrimination Test (ADT)	4-8 yr 11 mo	Gross screening measure of auditory discrimination for preschool and early elementary school-age children; designed to measure a child's ability to hear spoken language accurately; administered by an educational specialist, psychologist, or speech pathologist.
Autism Screening Instrument for Educational Planning (ASIEP)	18 mo–adult	Battery of five tests useful in assessing children, adolescents, and adults who have autism; assesses interactional, vocal, and functional skills and provides a prognosis for learning rate; includes Autism Behavior Checklist (ABC); used to establish IEPs; administered by a psychologist or educational specialist.
Battelle Developmental Inventory (BDI)	Birth–8 yr	Developmental inventory encompassing five domains: personal-social, adaptive, motor, communication, and cognitive; uses a mixture of test item, interview, and observational data: results heavily dependent on an informant's ability to provide accurate information; administered by a psychologist or educational specialist.
Bayley Scales of Infant Development–II	1-42 mo	One of the most widely used tools for assessing developmental status; newly revised second edition has an extended age range that measures cognitive, perceptual, and motor behavior; scale yields normed developmental indices useful in comparing a child with age peers; generally administered by a psychologist.
Bender Visual Motor Gestalt Test	3 yr–adult	Widely known and used screening test of visual-motor integration, usually administered by a psychologist; two normed scoring forms: Koppitz for children ages 4-12 yr; Hutt for adolescents and adults; test also yields indicators of neurological and emotional status.
Blind Learning Aptitude Test (BLAT)	6-16 yr	Nonverbal cognitive test for use with blind children that assesses general reasoning and abstraction; test seems to work best with children ages 6-12 yr; should be used in conjunction with a verbal test; usually administered by a psychologist or other trained professional.

Table D-1 Common Psychological and Educational Tests—cont'd

Test name	Age range	Purpose and description
The Neonatal Behavioral Assessment Scale	Birth–1 mo	Diagnostic test of developmental status in infancy that evaluates early social behaviors; results give a profile of infant behavior rather than an overall score; subscale ratings for different item types (e.g., neurological development) can be obtained; administered by an examiner who must be certified in its administration and interpretation.
Callier-Azusa Scale–H	Severely and profoundly mentally retarded individuals	Developmental scale designed to assess communicative abilities of the deaf-blind and severely and profoundly handicapped; scale should be administered by individuals who are familiar with the child's behavior.
Bruininks-Oseretsky Test of Motor Proficiency	4½-14½ yr	A normed performance scale that assesses motor proficiency and neurological development; yields a gross and fine motor composite as well as a battery composite; age equivalents available; generally administered by an occupational or physical therapist.
California Adaptive Behavior Scale	Birth–18 yr	Measures overall adaptive behavior in the areas of self-help, socialization, language and gross motor, perceptual motor, vocational, independent living, and academic skills; also assesses school and vocational readiness; psychologist or educational specialist administers and interprets.
Cattell Infant Intelligence Scale	3-30 mo	Diagnostic test of developmental status in infancy that measures cognitive and perceptual adaptive behaviors; a well-established tool, but the norms are dated; has been displaced by the Bayley Scales; usually administered by a qualified developmental specialist (e.g., a pediatric psychologist).
Child Behavior Checklist and Revised Child Behavior Profile	2-16 yr	Commonly known as the CBC and CBCL and developed by Achenbach; assesses behavioral problems and competencies of children and adolescents; four versions available, including Parent, Teacher, Youth Self-Report, and Direct Observation; a version for evaluating the mentally retarded is available from the author.
Childhood Autism Rating Scale (CARS)	Child, adolescent	Useful in the diagnosis of children functioning on the autistic spectrum and for distinguishing them from developmentally delayed children and others who are not autistic; used in psychological, medical, and educational assessment.
Children's Apperception Test (CAT)	2-10 yr	Diagnostic test of personality and social development in children and adolescents that usually is administered by a psychologist; used to help characterize the child's interpersonal relationships; test has three forms: one based on picture stories of humans (CAT-H), another on picture stories of animals, (CAT-A) and a supplemental form based on animal figures in family situations (CAT-S).
Clinical Adaptive Test/Clinical Linguistic Auditory Milestone Scale (CAT/CLAMS)	1-36 mo	A parental report (CLAMS) and direct assessment (CAT) measure developed for pediatricians to assess early development; normed developmental quotients (DQ) provided for nonlanguage, visual, motor, and language abilities as well as a composite score; brief and easy to administer; reported to discriminate children who have mental retardation from those who have communication disorders; preliminary data suggest that individual and composite DQs correlate with Bayley Scales of Infant Development (BSID).
Columbia Mental Maturity Scale	3½-10 yr	Diagnostic test of cognitive ability used to evaluate children who have sensory or motor defects or difficulty speaking or writing; developmental index is derived from norms; usually administered by a psychologist.
Connors Parent and Teacher Rating Scale	School age	Screening test of personality and social development completed by teachers to evaluate possible hyperactivity and other patterns of behavior in students; used widely in research settings.

Continued.

Table D-1 Common Psychological and Educational Tests—cont'd

Test name	Age range	Purpose and description
Denver Developmental Screening Test (DDST)	Birth–6 yr	Office screening test of developmental status that evaluates performance in four developmental areas: gross motor, fine motor, language, and personal and social skills; can be administered by a physician, nurse, or other trained worker; requires multiple data points, and up to 10% of all results are either abnormal, questionable, or unobtainable; shorter form (DDST-R) available for preliminary screening (see Chapter 20, Eleven).
Detroit Test of Learning Aptitude–3	6-18 yr	Diagnostic test of learning potential that was revised in 1988; useful as a test of general intellectual ability; standard scores used for each of 11 subtests; usually administered by a trained psychologist or special educator.
Developmental Test of Visual Motor Integration (DTVMI or VMI)	4-13 yr	Sometimes known as the Beery, Beery-Buktenica, or simply the VMI; perceptual motor ability test that aids in identifying children who have visual perception, hand control, and eye-hand coordination problems; also used with developmentally delayed adults; usually administered by a psychologist, educational specialist, or occupational or physical therapist.
Devereux Child Behavior Rating Scale (DBC)	6-12 yr	Diagnostic and screening procedure used to assess overt behavior patterns in children; examiner evaluates ratings made by parent or caregiver on 17 subscales; also used with mentally retarded and emotionally disturbed children.
Draw-a-Man	3-16 yr	See Goodenough-Harris Drawing Test.
French Pictorial Intelligence Test	3-8 yr	Diagnostic test of cognitive development independent of verbal expression—requires "pointing" responses to visual stimuli; most often used with speech-, language-, or hearing-impaired children; yields a developmental quotient based on norms; administered by a trained psychologist.
Frostig Developmental Test of Visual Perception	Infancy–8 yr	Drawing and copying test of perceptual motor ability that measures five areas of visual perception, including eye-hand coordination, figure-ground perception, form constancy, position in space, and spatial relationships; usually administered by a psychologist or specially trained teacher.
Gesell Developmental Schedules	4 wk–5 yr	Assesses physical and mental abilities in the adaptive, gross motor, fine motor, language, and personal-social areas; infant performance usually observed by a psychologist; norms yield an age-equivalent score.
Goldman-Fristoe-Woodcock Auditory Skills Test Battery	3 yr–adult	A normed scale that assesses ability to hear clearly under difficult conditions; subtests measure auditory attention, discrimination, memory, and sound symbol skills; administered by an educational specialist or other qualified professional.
Goodenough-Harris Drawing Test	3-16 yr	Also informally known as Draw-A-Man Test; brief, nonverbal test of intelligence and mental maturity that requires child to draw a person; points are given for various body parts; Harris revision includes an extensive objective scoring system as well as Draw-A-Woman and Self-Drawing tests; assesses perception, abstraction, generalization, and concept formation; male and female norms; administered by a psychologist or skilled examiner.
Halstead-Reitan Neuropsychological Test Battery for Older Children	9-14 yr	Neuropsychological test battery that falls between the Reitan-Indiana Battery and the adult version of the Halstead-Reitan in age applicability; multihour battery of cognitive and perceptual measures that includes a version of the Wechsler Intelligence Scale for Children (WISC) and various sensory-perceptual, academic, and achievement measures; as with other neuropsychological batteries, it is administered by a psychologist or specialist trained in neuropsychological assessment; used to evaluate children suspected of brain damage and cognitive dysfunction; short screening battery available.

Table D-1 Common Psychological and Educational Tests—cont'd

Test name	Age range	Purpose and description
House-Tree-Person (H-T-P) Projective Technique	3 yr–adult	Diagnostic test of personality and cognitive status usually administered by a trained psychologist as a projective device to evaluate self-image and other ego functions.
Hiskey-Nebraska Test of Learning Aptitude	3-18 yr	Nonverbal diagnostic test of cognitive ability usually used for deaf and hearing-impaired children; separate norms available for deaf and for hearing children; usually administered by a trained psychologist.
Illinois Test of Psycholinguistic Abilities–Revised (ITPA-R)	2-10 yr	Normed diagnostic test of cognitive ability designed specifically to evaluate verbal abilities and auditory-verbal and visual-motor processing; can be administered by a psychologist, speech pathologist, or educator; the norms and the test's usefulness in a psychoeducational battery both have been questioned.
Infant Mullen Scales of Early Learning (Infant MSEL)	Birth–36 mo	Comprehensive scale of mental and motor ability; measures specific learning abilities and patterns in gross motor, visual, and language areas; yields strengths and weaknesses and generates an IEP predicated on child's receptive/expressive learning style; administered by a psychologist or educational specialist.
Infant Psychological Development Scale	2 wk–2 yr	Developed by Uzgiris and Hunt on the basis of Piagetian theory; measures cognitive processes associated with natural stages of development; subscales measure development of a specific ability and consist of a number of ordinal steps; can be useful in planning sequenced curriculum; has both clinical and educational use; administered by a psychologist or educational specialist.
Infant Temperament Questionnaire (ITQ)	4-8 mo	Helps to determine infant temperament; questions relate to the nine categories of behavior described by Thomas, Chess, and Birch (see Temperament Scales described later in this table); takes approximately 30 minutes; this questionnaire, which is completed by parents, can be used to supplement information about parent-child interaction derived from the clinical interview.
Kaufman Assessment Battery for Children (K-ABC)	2½-12½ yr	Diagnostic test that should be administered by a qualified professional; intended for use in schools and clinical settings to provide a measure of intelligence and achievement; does not include measures of verbal cognitive processes in the composite score.
Kaufman Developmental Scale (KDS)	Up to 9 yr	Evaluates school readiness and developmental deficiencies among children through age 9; yields a developmental age and developmental quotient, as well as individual age scores in several areas; also useful in evaluating mental retardation; administered by a psychologist.
Kaufman Infant and Preschool Scale (KIPS)	1 mo–4 yr	Screening test for early cognitive processes; indicates possible need for intervention in normal children and in mentally retarded individuals who have mental ages of 4 years or less; administered by a psychologist, physician, or special education teacher.
Kaufman Test of Educational Achievement (K-TEA)	6-18 yr	Screening measure of achievement in the areas of reading, mathematics, spelling, decoding, and comprehension; used for educational planning by a psychologist or educational specialist.
Key Math Test	Kindergarten–grade 8	Normed diagnostic test of arithmetic achievement that can be administered by a teacher or psychologist; evaluates 14 areas of mathematics content, including operations and applications; weak in the area of computation.
Kinetic Family Drawing	5 yr–adolescence	Diagnostic test of personality and social development that measures, in particular, family interactions; special features include identification of trends or characteristics commonly seen in various subgroups (e.g., learning disabled, developmentally disabled, or perceptual-motor-handicapped children); usually administered by a psychologist or trained clinician.

Continued.

Table D-1 Common Psychological and Educational Tests—cont'd

Test name	Age range	Purpose and description
Leiter International Performance Scale	2 yr–adult	Normed diagnostic test of cognitive development usually administered by a psychologist and particularly appropriate for evaluating speech- and hearing-impaired individuals.
Luria-Nebraska Neuropsychological Battery: Children's Revision (LNNB-C)	8-12 yr	Considered the downward extension of the Adolescent-Adult Luria-Nebraska Battery; a verbal observational adaption designed to assess cognitive strengths and weaknesses and aid in selection and assessment of rehabilitation programs; administered by a psychologist or specialist trained in neuropsychological evaluation.
McCarthy Scales of Children's Abilities	2½-8½ yr	Relatively new diagnostic test of cognitive and perceptual ability that yields IQ-like indices of verbal, memory, perceptual, quantitative, and motor function; the General Cognitive Index (GCI), an overall estimate of cognitive function, is derived also; must be administered by a trained professional; particularly useful for diagnosing learning disabilities.
Merrill-Palmer Intelligence Test	18 mo–4 yr	Diagnostic test of cognitive and adaptive skills usually performed by a psychologist; because the test contains many "timed" items, it is highly demanding of the child being examined; yields a normal cognitive level score; extended version also available.
Minnesota Child Development Inventory	12 mo–6 yr	Parent questionnaire inventory that assesses general development and fine motor, gross motor, expressive language, comprehension-cognition, self-help, and personal-social skills.
Motor Free Test of Visual Perception (MFTVP)	4-9 yr	Diagnostic test of cognitive ability that measures the same five areas of visual perception evaluated by the Frostig Test, except that the child is not required to give motor responses requiring eye-hand coordination; useful in differentiating perceptual-motor problems from purely visual-perceptual difficulties; can be administered by a psychologist or teacher.
Peabody Developmental Motor Scales and Activity Cards	Birth–7 yr	A normed task performance test consisting of a sequence of gross and fine motor skills; identifies children whose gross or fine motor skills are delayed; activity cards include 170 gross motor and 112 fine motor items; activities referenced to items on the test can be used to set developmental/instructional objectives; administered by an educational specialist, physical therapist, or occupational therapist.
Peabody Individual Achievement Test–Revised (PIAT-R)	5-18 yr	Achievement test usually administered by an educational specialist or psychologist; provides wide-range screening in six areas—general information, reading recognition, reading comprehension, mathematics, spelling, and written expression; useful in diagnosing an individual's general level of achievement, but does not provide in-depth assessment of specific areas of skill.
Peabody Picture Vocabulary Test–Revised (PPVT-R)	2½ yr–adult	Screening test of receptive vocabulary administered by a speech and language specialist, teacher, or psychologist; correlates highly with IQ tests but cannot be used in place of a more intensive test of cognitive ability.
Perkins-Binet Tests of Intelligence for the Blind	3 yr–adult	Test of general intelligence with two forms—one for children who have usable vision and one for children who have no usable vision; yields IQ score based on the same method as that used in the Stanford-Binet intelligence tests.
Personality Inventory for Children–Revised (PIC-R)	3-16 yr	Screening test of personality and social development completed by parents; areas evaluated are achievement, intellectual screening, somatic concerns, depression, family dysfunction, withdrawal, anxiety, psychosis, hyperactivity, and social skills.
Physician Developmental Quick Screen for Speech Disorders (PDQ)	6 mo–6 yr	Office screening test performed by a physician, nurse, or other trained individual; measures various aspects of language, rhythm of speech, articulation, speaking mechanisms, and voice.

Table D-1 Common Psychological and Educational Tests—cont'd

Test name	Age range	Purpose and description
Piers-Harris Children's Self-Concept Scale	4-12 yr	Screening test for personality and social development that evaluates six facets of self-concept, including physical, social, family, and school precepts; the face validity of this test appears to be quite good; usually administered by a psychologist or teacher.
Preschool Behavior Questionnaire	3-6 yr	Observational screening scale for behavior problems in preschool children; measures hostile-aggressive, anxious, and distractible behaviors; administered by a teacher or psychologist.
Preschool Language Scale (PLS)	1-7 yr	Diagnostic test measuring expressive and receptive language skills that yields normed age-equivalent score for each skill; usually administered by a teacher, psychologist, or speech and language pathologist; revised in 1993.
Prescreening Developmental Questionnaire (PDQ)	3 mo–6 yr	Parent questionnaire used to determine whether DDST screening is necessary; addresses motor, language, social, and cognitive items; either office staff members or parents can complete items.
Raven Progressive Matrices	5½ yr–adult	Normal diagnostic test of cognitive ability that relies heavily on visual-spatial abstract reasoning; claimed to be culture free; usually administered by a psychologist; Coloured Progressive Metrics (CPM) used for younger children and special populations.
Receptive-Expressive Emergent Language Scale (REEL)	Birth–36 mo	Sometimes prefaced by authors' names (Bzoch and League); 132-item scale assesses emerging factors of receptive and expressive language as being present or absent; identifies those needing further evaluation; items are answered by a parent or reliable correspondent and evaluated by an educational specialist or speech pathologist.
Reitan-Indiana Neuropsychological Test Battery for Children	5-8 yr	Related to the Halstead-Reitan Neuropsychological Test Battery, which is used with older children and adults; a 4- to 6-hour battery of cognitive and perceptual tests that includes a version of the Wechsler Intelligence Scale for Children (WISC), a modified Reitan, an Aphasia Screening Test, and other sensory-perceptual measures; used to evaluate children suspected of brain damage and cognitive dysfunction; administered by a psychologist or specialist trained in neuropsychological assessment.
Rorschach Psychodiagnostic Test	3 yr–adult	Projective test of personality and social development specifically designed to evaluate personality structure; administered by a trained psychologist; extensive scoring criteria required to interpret results.
School Readiness Survey	4-6 yr	Screening test of learning ability in children that can be administered by a teacher, psychologist, or parent; identifies areas in which a child may be ready for school or deficient with regard to entrance into kindergarten.
Sentence Completion Tests	All ages	Projective tests of personality and social development usually administered by a psychologist; responses differentiating between adjustment and maladjustment can be identified; a number of different versions of the technique are in use, some of which have been validated and others in which scoring usually is achieved by clinical interpretation.
Sequenced Inventory of Communication Development–Revised Edition	4 mo–4 yr	A normed 210-item inventory assessing language disorders in young children; behaviorally based receptive and expressive sections result in an overall Communication Profile; used in developing remedial programs for language disordered, mentally retarded, hearing-impaired, and visually impaired children; can also be used with autistic and other difficult to test children; administered by a psychologist, educational specialist, or speech pathologist.

Continued.

Table D-1 Common Psychological and Educational Tests—cont'd

Test name	Age range	Purpose and description
Silvaroli Reading Inventory	Preschool–grade 8	Screening test of achievement usually administered by an educational specialist; assesses word recognition, passage comprehension, and spelling; scores for children in kindergarten to grade 6 appear to be somewhat inflated; reliability appears to be better at higher grade levels.
Slosson Intelligence Test–Revised (SIT-R)	Birth–27 yr	Diagnostic test of cognitive ability usually administered by a teacher or psychologist; designed to be a quick assessment, is widely used in schools, and is less well normed than the more intensive individual intelligence tests.
Southern California Sensory Integration Test	4-8 yr	Test usually administered by a certified occupational therapist; 18 subtests evaluate sensory integration; findings are not widely accepted by many psychologists or educators, although a sizable literature suggests substantial construct validity.
Stanford-Binet Intelligence Test, fourth edition	2 yr–adult	Well-known diagnostic test of cognitive ability administered by a psychologist; yields 15 subtest scores organized into four areas, including verbal reasoning, quantitative reasoning, and short-term memory; full battery requires more than 2 hours to administer, making it perhaps the longest standardized test of general intelligence; an option to shorten the scales for briefer administration is available, but validity has not yet been established for shortened version; may not be as effective as the WISC-R for diagnosing educational difficulties and for language handicaps; because of uneven range of standard scores, profile analysis should be used with caution.
Stanford Measurement Series	School age	Not to be confused with the Stanford-Binet Intelligence Test; a series of tests that measures mathematics, reading, and overall achievement; may be used for diagnosing specific student needs; administered by an educational specialist.
Sucher-Allred Reading Placement Inventory	Kindergarten–grade 9	Diagnostic test of reading ability containing a word recognition test and an oral reading test; provides an informal measure of a child's reading ability, not an in-depth assessment of reading difficulties; usually administered by an educational specialist or a classroom teacher to screen students for placement in reading.
Temperament Assessment Battery for Children (TABC)	3-7 yr	Multiple-item measure assessing six temperamental variables: activity, adaptability, approach/withdrawal, intensity, distractibility, and persistence; each is rated on a 7-point scale; parent, teacher, and clinical forms available; administered by a psychologist or educational specialist.
Temperament Scales	Infancy	Uses nine scales (activity level, rhythmicity, response to new stimuli, adaptability, intensity, threshold of responsiveness, mood, distractibility, attention span) to assess infant temperament; evaluation usually performed by a trained clinician.
Test of Language Development–Primary (TOLD)	4 yr 8 mo–11 yr	Diagnostic test of language development in children usually administered by a speech and language pathologist but also can be administered by a teacher, psychologist, or other professional; measures spoken language, listening, semantics, and syntax; age scores and language quotients result from norms. Intermediate version available.
Test of Non-Verbal Intelligence (TONI-2)	5-86 yr	Language-free measure of intelligence that may be used for hearing-impaired, language-impaired, and motor-impaired persons; has been suggested that the TONI should be used only as a supplemental test (as part of a battery) and that it should not be used with children under age 7.
Test of Written Language (TOWL-2)	7-17 yr	Diagnostic test usually administered by an educational specialist; helps to determine a student's general writing proficiency and to recognize a student's strengths and weaknesses.

Table D-1 Common Psychological and Educational Tests—cont'd

Test name	Age range	Purpose and description
Test of Written Spelling–2 (TWS-2)	6½-18½ yr	Uses a dictated work format to measure student's ability to spell words with readily predictable and with less predictable sound-letter patterns; can provide diagnostic information relative to specific spelling strategies; an excellent instrument for assessing written spelling ability; can be administered by a teacher, psychologist, or other professional.
Thematic Apperception Test (TAT)	School age–adult	Projective test of personality and social development measuring interpersonal relationships and usually administered by a trained psychologist; useful in identifying emotional disorders; extensive scoring criteria are applied to interpret results.
Vineland Adaptive Behavior Scale (VABS)	Birth–19 yr	Assesses social competence of handicapped and nonhandicapped individuals; usually administered by a trained interviewer; has three versions: survey form, expanded form, and classroom edition; each version measures adaptive behavior in four domains: communication, daily living skills, socialization, and motor skills; survey and expanded forms include a maladaptive behavior domain; respondent is a caregiver, parent, or teacher; also used with mentally retarded and low-function adults.
Wechsler Intelligence Scale for Children–III	6-16 yr 11 mo	Intelligence test used most commonly for school-age child and adolescent; third edition published in 1991; gives separate verbal and performance quotients, as well as Full Scale IQ scores. Subscale profiles can be used to evaluate learning ability and special learning disabilities; also used as part of Halstead-Reitan and Reitan-Indiana neuropsychological test batteries; usually administered by a psychologist or school psychologist.
Wechsler Memory Scale–Revised (WMS-R)	16-74 yr	Used primarily in neuropsychological testing to assess memory functioning; also used to evaluate aphasic, brain-impaired, and elderly individuals; has subtests for verbal and nonverbal memory functioning; three new subtests and more explicit scoring guidelines are improvements over Wechsler's original memory scale; administered by a psychologist or skilled examiner.
Wechsler Preschool and Primary Scales of Intelligence–Revised (WPPSI-R)	3-7 yr	Wechsler test designed to be used with preschool children and designed similarly to the WISC–III.
Wide Range Achievement Test–3	5-74 yr	A commonly used and recently revised brief screening test of achievement; evaluates reading, spelling, and arithmetic; usually administered by an educational specialist.
Wisconsin Behavior Rating Scale (WBRS)	Birth–3 yr	An adaptive behavior rating scale designed for persons who function developmentally at or below the 3-year-old level; assesses basic survival skills, using items that are developmentally arranged and sequenced under several subcategories of adaptive behavior: gross motor, fine motor, expressive communication, play skills, socialization, domestic activities, eating, toileting, dressing, and grooming; usually administered by a trained interviewer.
Wisconsin Card Sorting Test (WCST)	16 yr–adult	Used primarily in neuropsychological testing to assess abstract thinking and perseveration; a nonverbal test that has an individual match card in two response decks to one of four stimulus cards based on color, form, or number; helps identify frontal lobe dysfunction; administered by a psychologist or skilled examiner.
Woodcock Reading Mastery Test–Revised (WRMT-R)	5 yr or older	Tests specifically for reading skills; usually administered by an educational specialist; measures word and letter identification, word attack, and passage and word comprehension; norms available.
Woodcock-Johnson Psychoeducational Battery–Revised (WJ-R)	All ages	Diagnostic test of achievement usually administered by an educational specialist; measures cognitive ability, achievement, and interest; more reliable at the elementary than the secondary educational level.

of psychological evaluations, the best resources are licensed psychologists. In most states, psychologists who are eligible for third-party reimbursement must be licensed. In general, licensed psychologists must hold a doctoral degree in psychology and have postdoctoral training. The postdoctoral subspecialization areas of most interest to pediatricians include clinical child psychology, pediatric psychology, counseling psychology, neuropsychology, and educational psychology. In some instances, referral to specialists would be appropriate. For example, a child who has a closed head injury or other trauma associated with neurological impairment routinely should be evaluated by a clinical neuropsychologist.

A child's age may determine which specialist should be consulted. For instance, almost all child neuropsychological tests are not suitable for children under age 6 or 7. Despite the new requirement for evaluation and intervention for preschoolers, relatively few school psychologists have extensive training in preschool evaluation. Although this situation is being corrected by school psychology graduate curriculum reform, it will be some time before local districts develop sufficient expertise. Thus, preschool children might better be referred to a clinical child psychologist or pediatric psychologist.

Some psychologists may perform psychoeducational assessments—evaluations of the child's learning styles and determination of the best teaching approaches. Alternative resources for these services include special educators and educational consultants. No licensure is required to practice in this specialty, nor are many of the services provided by educational consultants eligible for third-party reimbursement. Nevertheless, the pediatrician may decide that children who have certain complex problems require special education studies to clarify appropriate interventions and consider referral to such consultants as the most appropriate option.

Characteristics of a Good Psychoeducational or Psychological Report

A good evaluation should include a written report to the pediatrician. Because there is no single test that provides a comprehensive assessment, an evaluation of high quality will report the results of a number of measures, including intellectual ability, emotional status, visual-motor and linguistic functioning, and social-adaptive behaviors. Also, a complete report will include suggestions for intervention, including recommendations for placement, curriculum, therapies, and other referrals. Should any of these elements be missing from the report, the pediatrician should request this information from the consultant.

Usually, the psychologist will share the report with the child's parents. In cases in which this practice has not been followed, the pediatrician should ask the psychologist the reasons for withholding the data. It may be that the child refused to allow release of some part of the report to parents, or the psychologist may believe that release of some parts of the report are not in the child's or the family's best interest. Knowing this, the pediatrician is in a better position to preserve requested confidentiality and thus can be discrete in developing an effective management strategy that will be accepted by the child and the family.

SUGGESTED READINGS

Fewell RR: Trends in the assessment of infants and toddlers with disabilities, *Except Child* 58:166, 1991.

Gilbride KE: Developmental testing, *Pediatr Rev* 16:338, 1995.

Goldstein G, Hersen M: *Handbook of psychological assessment,* ed 2, New York, 1990, Pergamon Press.

Hebbeler KM, Smith BJ, Black TL: Federal early childhood special education policy: a model for the improvement of services for children with disabilities, *Except Child* 58:104, 1991.

Hoon AH Jr et al: Clinical Adaptive Test/Clinical Linguistic Auditory Milestone Scale in early cognitive assessment, *J Pediatr* 123:S1, 1993.

Keyser DJ, Sweetland RC: *Test critiques,* vol 1-9, Kansas City, Kan, 1984, Test Corp. of America.

Kramer JJ, Conoley JC: *The eleventh mental measure yearbook,* Lincoln, Neb, 1992, University of Nebraska Press.

Mitchell JV Jr: *Tests in print III,* Lincoln, Neb, 1983, University of Nebraska Press.

Sattler JM: *Assessment of children,* ed 3, San Diego, Calif, 1988, Jerome M Sattler.

Sweetland RC, Keyser DJ: *Tests: a comprehensive reference for assessments in psychology, education, and business,* ed 3, Austin, 1991, PRO-ED.

Index

W